2008

**INGENIX**®

# ICD-9-CM
# Expert

*for Hospitals*
*Volumes 1, 2 & 3*

*International Classification of Diseases*
*9th Revision*
*Clinical Modification*

*Sixth Edition*

*Edited by:*
*Anita C. Hart, RHIA, CCS, CCS-P*
*Melinda S. Stegman, MBA, CCS*

Ingenix is committed to providing you with the ICD-9-CM code update information you need to code accurately and to be in compliance with HIPAA regulations. In the case of adoption of additional ICD-9-CM code changes effective April 1, 2008, Ingenix will provide these code changes to you at no additional cost! Just check back at www.shopingenix.com/productalerts to review the latest information concerning any new code changes.

**Codes Valid October 1, 2007, through September 30, 2008**

Additional copies may be ordered from:

Your local bookstore

or

1-800-INGENIX (464-3649)

IHES ISBN 978-1-60151-037-2

## PUBLISHER'S NOTICE

All the codes, indexes and other material in the ICD-9-CM are compiled from official ICD-9-CM codes and instructions as well as the Medicare regulations and manuals issued or authorized by the Centers for Medicare and Medicaid Services. The code book is designed to provide accurate and authoritative information in regard to the subject covered, and every reasonable effort has been made to ensure the accuracy of the information within these pages. However, the ultimate responsibility for correct coding lies with the provider of services.

Ingenix, its employees, agents and staff make no representation, warranty or guarantee that this compilation of codes and narratives is error-free or that the use of this code book will prevent differences of opinion or disputes with Medicare or other third-party payers as to the codes that are accepted or the amounts that will be paid to providers of services, and will bear no responsibility or liability for the results or consequences of the use of this code book.

## CONTINUING EDUCATION UNITS FOR CERTIFIED MEMBERS OF THE AMERICAN ACADEMY OF PROFESSIONAL CODERS

This publication has prior approval by the American Academy of Professional Coders for continuing education units (CEUs). Granting of prior approval in no way constitutes endorsement by the Academy of the publication content nor the publisher. Instructions to submit CEUs are available within the "Preapproved CEU Vendor List" file at www.aapc.com/education/CEUs/ceus.html.

## OUR COMMITMENT TO ACCURACY

Ingenix is committed to producing accurate and reliable materials. To report corrections, please visit www.ingenixonline.com/accuracy or email accuracy@ingenix.com. You can also reach customer service by calling 1.800.INGENIX (464.3649), option 1.

## SPECIAL REPORTS AND ANNOUNCEMENTS

**Purchase of this publication entitles you to Special Reports and announcements via email. Please call customer service at 800 INGENIX (464-3649) or contact your bookstore to take advantage of this exciting free service that will keep you abreast of important code changes and regulatory developments.**

**Review, download, and print the Special Reports in .pdf format. Log on to www.shopingenix.com/productalerts**

# Preface

Since the federal government implemented diagnosis-related groups (DRGs) on October 1, 1983, medical record profes-sionals and others have had to refer to many sources for ICD-9-CM codes and coding and reimbursement principles.

*ICD-9-CM for Hospitals, Volumes 1, 2 & 3,* has been designed with the health information professional in mind. All three volumes of the most recent official government version of ICD-9-CM have been combined into one book.

Our technical experts have drawn upon their extensive hands-on experience to enhance the government's book with valuable features essential to correct coding and reimbursement. Without these enhancements, health information management departments would spend hours locating the information required to code each record accurately. Because of the thoroughness, accuracy, timeliness and ease of use of *ICD-9-CM for Hospitals,* health information departments nationwide have turned to them for their coding needs.

*ICD-9-CM for Hospitals* includes many of the enhancements described below in direct response to requests from our subscribers. As you review the content, you'll find the following:

- The complete ICD-9-CM official guidelines for coding and reporting, published by the U.S. Department of Health and Human Services and approved by the cooperating parties (American Hospital Association, American Health Information Management Association, Health Care Financing Administration and National Center for Health Statistics)
- All the official ICD-9-CM codes, indexes, notes, footnotes and symbols
- color-highlighted illustrations and clearly worded definitions integrated in the tabular, provide important clinical information
- Exclusive color coding, symbols, and footnotes that alert coders to coding and reimbursement issues, including the majority of the Medicare code edits and identification of conditions that significantly affect DRG assignment of cardiovascular and HIV cases.
- The complication and comorbidity (CC) exclusion list, integrated beneath the applicable codes makes it easier to determine complications and comorbidities excluded with a particular principal diagnosis
- The American Hospital Association (AHA's) *Coding Clinic for ICD-9-CM* references, integrated beneath the applicable codes to provide easy reference to official coding advice as designated by the four cooperating parties (AHA, AHIMA, CMS, and NCHS)
- Compliance symbol identifying diagnosis codes associated with DRGs targeted by the government for audit
- Check fourth- and fifth-digit symbols identify codes that require the addition of a fourth or fifth digit for code specificity and validity
- Symbols identify new codes and text revisions and pages are dated to indicate when the changes were made
- Synopsis of the code changes for the current year
- Color coding and symbol legend at the bottom of each page
- Exclusive QuickFlip Color Tabs for quick, easy location of terms and codes in the index and Tabular List

Please review "How to Use *ICD-9-CM for Hospitals (Volumes 1, 2 & 3)*" in this section to learn about the features that will help you assign and report correct codes, ensuring appropriate reimbursement.

## USE OF OFFICIAL SOURCES

The *ICD-9-CM for Hospitals* contains the official U.S. Department of Health and Human Services, Ninth Revision, Sixth Edition ICD-9-CM codes, effective for the current year.

The color-coding, footnotes and symbols, which identify coding and reimbursement issues, are derived from official federal government sources, including the Medicare Code Edits (MCE), Version 25.0.

The American Hospital Association's (AHA) *Coding Clinic for ICD-9-CM* references are used with permission of the AHA.

## IMPORTANT INFORMATION ABOUT YOUR SUBSCRIPTION SERVICE

If you have purchased the updateable *ICD-9-CM Expert for Hospitals,* your subscription includes an updating service throughout the year to keep the code book current and accurate. The February update includes new illustrations and definitions, *AHA Coding Clinic* references for third and fourth quarter, the latest MCEs, and official errata changes. In July you will receive a list of all new, revised, and invalid codes for the upcoming year.

## TECHNICAL EDITORS

**Anita C. Hart, RHIA, CCS, CCS-P**
*Product Manager, Ingenix*
Ms. Hart's experience includes conducting and publishing research in clinical medicine and human genetics for Yale University, Massachusetts General Hospital, and Massachusetts Institute of Technology. In addition, Ms. Hart has supervised medical records management, health information management, coding and reimbursement, and worker's compensation issues as the office manager for a physical therapy rehabilitation clinic. Ms. Hart is an expert in physician and facility coding, reimbursement systems, and compliance issues. Ms. Hart has developed and has served as technical consultant for numerous other publications for hospital and physician practices. Currrently, Ms. Hart is the Product Manager and Technical Editor for the ICD-9-CM and ICD-10-CM/PCS product lines.

**Melinda S. Stegman, MBA, CCS**
*Clinical/Technical Editor, Ingenix*
Ms. Stegman has 25 years of experience in the HIM profession and has been responsible for managing the clinical aspects of the HSS/Ingenix HIM Consulting practice in the Washington, DC area office. Her areas of specialization include training on inpatient and DRG coding, outpatient coding, and Ambulatory Payment Classifications (APCs) for HIM professionals, software developers, and other clients; developing an outpatient billing/coding compliance tool for a major accounting firm; and managing HIM consulting practices. Ms. Stegman is a regular contributing author for *Advance for Health Information Management Professionals* and for the *Journal of Health Care Compliance.* She has performed coding assessments and educational sessions throughout the country.

In addition to the editors, the following people have contributed to this book:

Michael E. Desposito, *Vice President, Coding and Referential*
Lynn Speirs, *Senior Director, Editorial/Desktop Publishing*
Stacy Perry, *Manager, Desktop Publishing*
Tracy Betzler, *Desktop Publishing Specialist*
Hope Dunn, *Desktop Publishing Specialist*
Kate Holden, *Editor*

## WHAT TO DO IF YOU HAVE QUESTIONS

If you have any questions call our customer service department toll-free at 800-INGENIX (464-3649), option 1.

If you have comments on the content of this book, please email them to customerservice@ingenix.com or fax to 801-982-4033.

## ADDITIONAL COPIES

Contact the customer service order department toll-free at 800-INGENIX (464-3649), option 1.

# Introduction

## HISTORY AND FUTURE OF ICD-9

The International Classification of Diseases, Ninth Revision, Clinical Modification (ICD-9-CM) is based on the official version of the World Health Organization's Ninth Revision, International Classification of Diseases (ICD-9). ICD-9 classifies morbidity and mortality information for statistical purposes, and for the indexing of hospital records by disease and operations, for data storage and retrieval.

This modification of ICD-9 supplants the Eighth Revision International Classification of Diseases, Adapted for Use in the United States (ICDA-8) and the Hospital Adaptation of ICDA (H-ICDA).

The concept of extending the International Classification of Diseases for use in hospital indexing was originally developed in response to a need for a more efficient basis for storage and retrieval of diagnostic data. In 1950, the U.S. Public Health Service and the Veterans Administration began independent tests of the International Classification of Diseases for hospital indexing purposes. The following year, the Columbia Presbyterian Medical Center in New York City adopted the International Classification of Diseases, Sixth Revision, with some modifications for use in its medical record department. A few years later, the Commission on Professional and Hospital Activities (CPHA) in Ann Arbor, Mich., adopted the International Classification of Diseases with similar modifications for use in hospitals participating in the Professional Activity Study.

The problem of adapting ICD for indexing hospital records was taken up by the U.S. National Committee on Vital and Health Statistics through its subcommittee on hospital statistics. The subcommittee reviewed the modifications made by the various users of ICD and proposed that uniform changes be made. This was done by a small working party.

In view of the growing interest in the use of the International Classification of Diseases for hospital indexing, a study was undertaken in 1956 by the American Hospital Association and the American Medical Record Association (then the American Association of Medical Record Librarians) of the relative efficiencies of coding systems for diagnostic indexing. This study indicated the International Classification of Diseases provided a suitable and efficient framework for indexing hospital records. The major users of the International Classification of Diseases for hospital indexing purposes then consolidated their experiences, and an adaptation was first published in December 1959. A revision was issued in 1962 and the first "Classification of Operations and Treatments" was included.

In 1966, the international conference for revising the International Classification of Diseases noted the eighth revision of ICD had been constructed with hospital indexing in mind and considered the revised classification suitable, in itself, for hospital use in some countries. However, it was recognized that the basic classification might provide inadequate detail for diagnostic indexing in other countries. A group of consultants was asked to study the eighth revision of ICD (ICD-8) for applicability to various users in the United States. This group recommended that further detail be provided for coding of hospital and morbidity data. The American Hospital Association was requested to develop the needed adaptation proposals. This was done by an advisory committee (the Advisory Committee to the Central Office on ICDA). In 1968 the United States Public Health Service published the product, Eighth Revision International Classification of Diseases, Adapted for Use in the United States. This became commonly known as ICDA-8, and beginning in 1968 it served as the basis for coding diagnostic data for both official morbidity and mortality statistics in the United States.

In 1968, the CPHA published the Hospital Adaptation of ICDA (H-ICDA) based on both the original ICD-8 and ICDA-8. In 1973, CPHA published a revision of H-ICDA, referred to as H-ICDA-2. Hospitals throughout the United States were divided in their use of these classifications until January 1979, when ICD-9-CM was made the single classification intended primarily for use in the United States, replacing these earlier related, but somewhat dissimilar, classifications.

Physicians have been required by law to submit diagnosis codes for Medicare reimbursement since the passage of the Medicare Catastrophic Coverage Act of 1988. This act requires physician offices to include the appropriate diagnosis codes when billing for services provided to Medicare beneficiaries on or after April 1, 1989. The Centers for Medicare and Medicaid Services (formerly known as Health Care Financing Administration) designated ICD-9-CM as the coding system physicians must use.

In 1993 the World Health Organization published the newest version of International Classification of Diseases, Tenth Revision, ICD-10. This version contains the greatest number of changes in the history of ICD. There are more codes (5,500 more than ICD-9) to allow more specific reporting of diseases and newly recognized conditions. ICD-10 consists of three volumes; Tabular List (volume I), instructions (volume 2) and the Alphabetic Index (volume 3). It contains 21 chapters including two supplementary ones. The codes are alphanumeric (A00–T98, V01–Y98 and Z00–Z99). Currently ICD-10 is being used in some European countries with implementation expected after the year 2011 in the United States.

## ICD-9-CM BACKGROUND

In February 1977, a steering committee was convened by the National Center for Health Statistics to provide advice and counsel in developing a clinical modification of ICD-9. The organizations represented on the steering committee included the following:

- American Association of Health Data Systems
- American Hospital Association
- American Medical Record Association
- Association for Health Records
- Council on Clinical Classifications
- Centers for Medicare and Medicaid Services, Department of Health and Human Services
- WHO Center for Classification of Diseases for North America, sponsored by the National Center for Health Statistics, Department of Health and Human Services

The Council on Clinical Classifications was sponsored by the following:

- American Academy of Pediatrics
- American College of Obstetricians and Gynecologists
- American College of Physicians
- American College of Surgeons
- American Psychiatric Association
- Commission on Professional and Hospital Activities

The steering committee met periodically in 1977. Clinical guidance and technical input were provided by task forces on classification from the Council on Clinical Classification's sponsoring organizations.

ICD-9-CM is a clinical modification of the World Health Organization's ICD-9. The term "clinical" is used to emphasize the modification's intent: to serve as a useful tool to classify morbidity data for indexing medical records, medical care review, and ambulatory and other medical care programs, as well as for basic health statistics. To describe the clinical picture of the patient, the codes must be more precise than those needed only for statistical groupings and trend analysis.

## CHARACTERISTICS OF ICD-9-CM

ICD-9-CM far exceeds its predecessors in the number of codes provided. The disease classification has been expanded to include health-related conditions and to provide greater specificity at the fifth-digit level of detail. These fifth digits are not optional; they are intended for use in recording the information substantiated in the clinical record.

Volume I (Tabular List) of ICD-9-CM contains four appendices:

| | |
|---|---|
| Appendix A: | Morphology of Neoplasms |
| Appendix B: | Deleted Effective October 1, 2004 |
| Appendix C: | Classification of Drugs by American Hospital Formulary Service List Number and Their ICD-9-CM Equivalents |

These appendices are included as a reference to provide further information about the patient's clinical picture, to further define a diagnostic statement, to aid in classifying new drugs or to reference three-digit categories.

Volume 2 (Alphabetic Index) of ICD-9-CM contains many diagnostic terms that do not appear in Volume I since the index includes most diagnostic terms currently in use.

Volume 3 (Procedure Index and Procedure Tabular) of ICD-9-CM contains codes for operations and procedures. The format for the tabular is the same as Volume 1 disease tabular, except the codes consist of two digits with one or two digits following the decimal point. Conventions in the index follow Volume 2 conventions except some subterms appear immediately below the main term rather than following alphabetizing rules.

# THE DISEASE CLASSIFICATION

ICD-9-CM is totally compatible with its parent system, ICD-9, thus meeting the need for comparability of morbidity and mortality statistics at the international level. A few fourth-digit codes were created in existing three-digit rubrics only when the necessary detail could not be accommodated by the use of a fifth-digit subclassification. To ensure that each rubric of ICD-9-CM collapses back to its ICD-9 counterpart the following specifications governed the ICD-9-CM disease classification:

Specifications for the Tabular List:

1.  Three-digit rubrics and their contents are unchanged from ICD-9.

2.  The sequence of three-digit rubrics is unchanged from ICD-9.

3.  Three-digit rubrics are not added to the main body of the classification.

4.  Unsubdivided three-digit rubrics are subdivided where necessary to
    *   add clinical detail
    *   isolate terms for clinical accuracy

5.  The modification in ICD-9-CM is accomplished by adding a fifth digit to existing ICD-9 rubrics, except as noted under #7 below.

6.  The optional dual classification in ICD-9 is modified.
    *   Duplicate rubrics are deleted:
        –   four-digit manifestation categories duplicating etiology entries
        –   manifestation inclusion terms duplicating etiology entries
    *   Manifestations of disease are identified, to the extent possible, by creating five-digit codes in the etiology rubrics.
    *   When the manifestation of a disease cannot be included in the etiology rubrics, provision for its identification is made by retaining the ICD-9 rubrics used for classifying manifestations of disease.

7.  The format of ICD-9-CM is revised from that used in ICD-9.
    *   American spelling of medical terms is used.
    *   Inclusion terms are indented beneath the titles of codes.
    *   Codes not to be used for primary tabulation of disease are printed in italics with the notation, "code first underlying disease."

Specifications for the Alphabetic Index:

1.  The format of the Alphabetic Index follows that of ICD-9.

2.  When two codes are required to indicate etiology and manifestation, the manifestation code appears in brackets (e.g., diabetic cataract 250.5 [366.41]).

# THE ICD-9-CM COORDINATION AND MAINTENANCE COMMITTEE

The four cooperating parties involved in maintaining the ICD-9-CM classification system include representatives of the American Hospital Association (AHA), the Centers for Medicare and Medicaid Services (CMS), the National Center for Health Statistics (NCHS), and the American Health Information Management Association (AHIMA).

Proposals for changes to the ICD-9-CM classification system are submitted and discussed in two open forum meetings held in April and October of each year at the Headquarters of the Centers for Medicare and Medicaid Services, Baltimore, Maryland. Comments received during and after the meetings are then discussed by the Committee. A notice of the new codes and code revisions approved by the Committee are published in the *Federal Register* as part of the proposed and final rule for the changes to the inpatient prospective payment system. The complete official document of changes to the classification system is released as the Addenda for the *International Classification of Diseases, Ninth Revision, Clinical Modification, Sixth Edition, Volumes 1, 2 and 3.*

# How to Use the ICD-9-CM for Hospitals (Volumes 1, 2 & 3)

This *ICD-9-CM for Hospitals* is based on the official version of the International Classification of Diseases, Ninth Revision, Clinical Modification, Sixth Edition, issued by the U.S. Department of Health and Human Services. Annual code changes are implemented by the government and are effective Oct. 1 and valid through Sept. 30 of the following year.

The code book is totally compatible with its parent system, ICD-9, thus meeting the need for comparability of morbidity and mortality statistics at the international level.

This book is consistent with the content of the government's version of ICD-9-CM. However, to accommodate the coder's approach to coding, the Alphabetic Index has been placed before the Tabular List in both the disease and procedure classifications. This allows the user to locate the correct codes in a logical, natural manner by locating the term in the index, then confirming the accuracy of the code in the Tabular List.

## STEPS TO CORRECT CODING

1.  Look up the main term in the Alphabetic Index and scan the subterm entries as appropriate. Follow any cross-references such as "*see*" and "*see also.*" Do not code from the Alphabetic Index without verifying the accuracy of the code in the Tabular List.

2.  Locate the code in the numerically arranged Tabular List.

3.  Observe the punctuation, footnotes, cross-references, color-coded prompts and other conventions described in the 'Conventions' section.

4.  To determine the appropriateness of the code selection, read all instructional material:

    *   "includes" and "*excludes*" notes
    *   "*see*," "*see also*" and "*see category*" cross-references
    *   "use additional code" and "*code first underlying disease*" instructions
    *   "code also" and "*omit code*" notes
    *   fourth- and fifth-digit requirements
    *   CC exclusions

5.  Consult definitions, relevant illustrations, CC exclusions, color coding and reimbursement prompts, the check fourth- and fifth-digit, age and sex symbols. Refer to the color/symbol legend at the bottom of each page for symbols. Refer to the list of footnotes that is included in the "Additional Conventions" section of this book for a full explanation of a footnote associated with a code.

6.  Consult the official ICD-9-CM guidelines for coding and reporting, and refer to the AHA's *Coding Clinic for ICD-9-CM* for coding guidelines governing the use of specific codes.

7.  Confirm and transcribe the correct code.

## ORGANIZATION

### Introduction
The introductory material in this book includes the history and future of ICD-9-CM as well as an overview of the classification system.

### Official ICD-9-CM Conventions
This section provides a full explanation of all the official footnotes, symbols, instructional notes, and conventions found in the official government version.

### Additional Conventions
Exclusive color-coding, symbols, and notations have been included in the *ICD-9-CM for Hospitals, Volumes 1, 2 & 3* to alert coders to important coding and reimbursement issues. This section provides a full explanation of the additional conventions used throughout this book.

### Coding Guidelines
Included in this book are the official ICD-9-CM coding guidelines as approved by the four cooperating parties of the ICD-9-CM Coordination and Maintenance Committee. Failure to comply with the official coding guidelines may result in denied or delayed claims.

### Summary of Code Changes
This section includes a complete listing of all new code changes for the current year.

### Summary of AHA's Coding Clinic for ICD-9-CM Topics
This is a brief summary of the official advice concerning coding topics covered in the latest issues of AHA's *Coding Clinic for ICD-9-CM* and is found only in the *ICD-9-CM Expert for Hospitals* updateable edition.

### Disease Classification: Alphabetic Index to Diseases
The Alphabetic Index to Diseases is separated by tabs labeled with the letters of the alphabet, contains diagnostic terms for illnesses, injuries and reasons for encounters with health care professionals. The Table of Drugs and Chemicals is easily located with the tab in this section.

The warning statement at the bottom of every page of the index, ▼ Subterms under main terms may continue to next column or page, is a reminder to always check for additional subterms before making final selection.

### Disease Classification: Tabular List of Diseases
The Tabular List of Diseases arranges the ICD-9-CM codes and descriptors numerically. QuickFlip color tabs divide this section into chapters, identified by the code range on the tab.

The Tabular List includes two supplementary classifications:

*   V Codes—Supplementary Classification of Factors Influencing Health Status and Contact with Health Services (V01–V86)
*   E Codes—Supplementary Classification of External Causes of Injury and Poisoning (E800–E999)

ICD-9-CM includes four official appendixes.

*   Appendix A          Morphology of Neoplasms
*   Appendix B:         Deleted Effective October 1, 2004
*   Appendix C          Classification of Drugs by AHFS List
*   Appendix D          Classification of Industrial Accidents According to Agency
*   Appendix E          List of Three-digit Categories

These appendices are included as a reference to provide further information about the patient's circumstances, help further define a diagnostic statement, maintain a tumor registry and aid in classifying new drugs.

### Procedure Classification: Alphabetic Index to Procedures
The Alphabetic Index to Procedures lists common surgical and procedural terminology.

The warning statement at the bottom of every page of the index, ▼ Subterms under main terms may continue to next column or page, is a reminder to always check for additional subterms before making final selection.

### Procedure Classification: Tabular List of Procedures
The Tabular List of Procedures numerically arranges the procedure codes and their descriptors.

## Resources

Listed below are the exclusive resources found ONLY in the *ICD-9-CM Expert for Hospitals, Volumes 1, 2 & 3* books.

### Mapping of CMS-DRG Version 24.0 to MS-DRG Version 25.0

This resource lists the official mapping of CMS-DRG Version 24.0 to the new MS-DRG Version 25.0 released by the Centers for Medicare and Medicaid Services (CMS).

### Dx/MDC/DRG List

Provides the complete list of principal diagnosis codes and the MDC and MS-DRG to which they group, with the exception of a combination of principal and secondary diagnosis affecting DRG assignment.

### MCC Condition List

A complete list of all codes considered MCC (Major Complications and Comorbidities) that will affect DRG assignment. This is an essential auditing tool for assigning the most appropriate DRG.

### CC Condition List

A complete list of all codes considered CC (Complications and Comorbidities) that will affect DRG assignment. This an essential auditing tool for assigning the most appropriate DRG.

### Pharmacological Listings

The most common generic and brand names of drugs are linked with the disease processes to assist in the identification of CC, thereby improving DRG assignment practices.

### Valid Three-digit Code Table

ICD-9-CM is composed of codes with either 3, 4, or 5 digits. A code is invalid if it has not been coded to the full number of digits required for that code. There are a certain number codes that are valid for reporting as three digit codes. A list of the valid three-digit code is included as a convenient reference when auditing claims.

### Present On Admission (POA) Indicator Tutorial

This resource presents an in-depth explanation of guidelines for assigning the present on admission (POA) indicators with case scenarios and exemptions. A table of official guidelines is included for quick reference regarding the use of information documented in the medical record.

# ICD-9-CM Official Conventions

## ICD-9-CM FOOTNOTES, SYMBOLS, INSTRUCTIONAL NOTES AND CONVENTIONS

This *ICD-9-CM for Hospitals* preserves all the footnotes, symbols, instructional notes and conventions found in the government's official version. Accurate coding depends upon understanding the meaning of these elements.

The following appear in the disease Tabular List, unless otherwise noted.

## OFFICIAL GOVERNMENT SYMBOLS

§    The section mark preceding a code denotes a footnote on the page. This symbol is used in the Tabular List of Diseases and in the Tabular List of Procedures.

## ICD-9-CM CONVENTIONS USED IN THE TABULAR LIST

In addition to the symbols and footnotes above, the ICD-9-CM disease tabular has certain abbreviations, punctuation, symbols and other conventions. Our *ICD-9-CM for Hospitals* preserves these conventions. Proper use of the conventions will lead to efficient and accurate coding.

### Abbreviations

**NEC**    Not elsewhere classifiable

This abbreviation is used when the ICD-9-CM system does not provide a code specific for the patient's condition.

**NOS**    Not otherwise specified

This abbreviation is the equivalent of 'unspecified' and is used only when the coder lacks the information necessary to code to a more specific four-digit subcategory.

[ ]    Brackets enclose synonyms, alternative terminology or explanatory phrases:

**482.2    Pneumonia due to Hemophilus influenzae [H. influenzae]**

Brackets that appear beneath a code indicate the fifth digits that are considered valid fifth digits for the code. This convention is applied for those instances in ICD-9-CM where not all common fifth digits are considered valid for each subcategory within a category.

**715.0    Osteoarthrosis, generalized**
[0,4,9]

Generalized arthrosis can only be assigned in cases for which the degenerative joint disease involves multiple joints. Therefore, this code is considered for arthrosis in the sites described as unspecified, hand (which consists of multiple joints), or multiple sites. Therefore, only fifth digits 0, 4, and 9 are valid with subcategory 715.0.

*[ ]*    Slanted brackets that appear in the Alphabetic Indexes indicate mandatory multiple coding. Both codes must be assigned to fully describe the condition and are sequenced in the order listed.

**Tachycardia**
    ventricular (paroxysmal)
      psychogenic 316 *[427.1]*

Psychogenic paroxysmal tachycardia is reported using both 316, Psychogenic factors associated with diseases classified elsewhere, and 427.1, Paroxysmal ventricular tachydcardia.

**Diversion**
    biliopancratic (BPD) 43.7 *[45.51] [45.91]*

Code assignment of biliopancratic diversion is reported using all three codes 43.7, Partial gastrectomy with anastomosis to jejunum, 45.51, Isolation of segment of small intestine, and 45.91, Small-to-small intestinal anastomosis.

( )    Parentheses enclose supplementary words, called nonessential modifiers, that may be present in the narrative description of a disease without affecting the code assignment:

**198.4    Other parts of nervous system**
    Meninges (cerebral) (spinal)

:    Colons are used in the Tabular List after an incomplete term that needs one or more of the modifiers that follow in order to make it assignable to a given category:

**021.1    Enteric tularemia**
    Tularemia:
      cryptogenic
      intestinal
      typhoidal

}    Braces enclose a series of terms, each of which is modified by the statement appearing to the right of the brace:

**560.2    Volvulus**
    Knotting
    Strangulation
    Torsion     } of intestine, bowel, or colon
    Twist

## OTHER CONVENTIONS

**Boldface**    Boldface type is used for all codes and titles in the Tabular List.

*Italicized*    Italicized type is used for all exclusion notes and to identify codes that should not be used for describing the primary diagnosis.

## INSTRUCTIONAL NOTES

These notes appear only in the Tabular List of Diseases:

**Includes:**    An includes note further defines or clarifies the content of the chapter, subchapter, category, sub-category or subclassification. The includes note in the example below applies only to category 461.

***Excludes:***    Terms following the word "*Excludes*" are not classified to the chapter, subchapter, category, subcategory or specific subclassification code under which it is found. The note also may provide the location of the excluded diagnosis. Excludes notes are italicized.

**461    Acute sinusitis**

    INCLUDES    abscess
                empyema        acute, of sinus
                infection        (accessory)
                inflammation   (nasal)
                suppuration

    EXCLUDES    *chronic or unspecified sinusitis (473.0-473.9)*

**Use additional code:**

This instruction signals the coder that an additional code should be used if the information is available to provide a more complete picture of that diagnosis.

**362.13    Changes in vascular appearance**
    Vascular sheathing of retina
    Use additional code for any associated atherosclerosis (440.8)

There are coding circumstances outside of the etiology/manifestation convention when multiple coding for a single condition is required. The 'Use additional code' note will be found under the associated condition code in the tabular. In the index, the multiple coding requirement is indicated by the use of the slanted bracket. The two codes are to be sequenced as listed in the index. For example, retinal arterisosclerosis must be coded using two codes sequenced as listed in the index.

**Arteriosclerosis, arteriosclerotic**
  retinal (vascular) 440.8 *[362.13]*

## Code first underlying disease:

The *Code first underlying disease* instructional note found under certain codes is a sequencing rule. Most often this sequencing rule applies to the etiology/manifestation convention and is found under at the manifestation code. The manifestation code may never be used alone or as a primary diagnosis (i.e., sequenced first). The instructional note, the code and its descriptor appear in italics in the Tabular List.

**590.81 *Pyelitis or pyelonephritis in diseases classified elsewhere***

  *Code first underlying disease as:*
    tuberculosis (016.0)

Not all codes with a 'Code first underlying disease' instructional note are part of the etiology/manifestation convention. The 'Code first' note will appear, but the title of the code and the instructional note are not in italics. These codes may be reported alone or as the secondary diagnosis. For example, disseminated chorioretinitis may be reported as a principal diagnosis. However, if the underlying condition that caused disseminated chorioretinitis is known, such as tuberculous disseminated chorioretinitis, two codes are required and sequenced as listed in the index.

**363.13 Disseminated choroiditis and chorioretinitis, generalized**

  Code first underlying disease as:
    tuberculosis (017.3)

## Code, if applicable, any causal condition first:

A code with this note indicates that this code may be assigned as a principal diagnosis when the causal condition is unknown or not applicable. If a causal condition is known, then the code for that condition should be sequenced as the principal or first-listed diagnosis.

**590.0 Chronic pyelonephritis**

  Chronic pyelitis
  Chronic pyonephrosis
  Code, if applicable, any causal condition first

## Omit code:

"*Omit code*" is used to instruct the coder that no code is to be assigned. When this instruction is found in the Alphabetic Index to Diseases the medical term should not be coded as a diagnosis.

**Metaplasia**

  cervix — *omit code*

When used in Volume 3, 'omit code' is meant to indicate procedures that do not merit separate code assignments, such as minor procedures preformed in conjunction with more extensive procedures or procedures that represent an operative approach.

**Arthrotomy 80.10**

  as operative approach — *omit code*

## *See* Condition:

The "*see* condition" note found in the Alphabetic Index to Disease instructs the coder to refer to a main term for the condition. This note will follow index terms that are nouns for anatomical sites or adjectival forms of disease term. In the example below, the index terms 'Cervix' and 'Diffuse' are followed by the — *see* condition. Coders should search the index using a condition term such as atrophy or prolapse.

**Cervix** — *see* condition
**Diffuse** — *see* condition

## Morphology Codes

For each neoplastic disease listed in the index, a morphology code is provided that identifies histological type and behavior.

*Example:*

**Myelolipoma** (M8870/0) — *see* Neoplasm, by site, benign

The histology is identified by the first four digits and the behavior is identified by the digit following the slash. Appendix A of Volume 1 contains a listing of morphology codes. This appendix is helpful when the pathology report identifies the neoplasm by using an M code. The coder may refer to Appendix A to determine the nomenclature of the neoplasm that will be the main term to search in the Index. The behavior classification is as follows:

  0    Benign
  1    Uncertain behavior
  2    Carcinoma in situ
  3    Malignant, primary site
  6    Malignant, secondary site.

# Additional Conventions

## NEW AND REVISED TEXT SYMBOLS

●   A bullet at a code or line of text indicates that that the entry is new.

▲   A triangle in the Tabular List indicates that the code title is revised. In the Alphabetic Index the triangle indicates that a code has changed.

►◄   These symbols appear at the beginning and at the end of a section of new or revised text.

When these symbols appear on a page there will be a date on the lower outside corner of the page indicating the date of the change, (e.g., October 2007).

## ADDITIONAL DIGITS REQUIRED

√3ʳᵈ   This symbol indicates that the code requires a third digit.

√4ᵗʰ   This symbol indicates that the code requires a fourth digit.

√5ᵗʰ   This symbol indicates that a code requires a fifth digit.

☑   This symbol found only in the Alphabetic Index sections and the Table of Drugs and Chemicals indicates that an additional digit is required. Referring to the tabular section is essential to locate the appropriate additional digit.

## DEFINITIONS

**DEF:**   This symbol indicates a definition of disease or procedure term. The definition will appear in blue type in the Disease and Procedure Tabular Lists.

## AHA's *CODING CLINIC FOR ICD-9-CM* REFERENCES

The four cooperating parties have designated the AHA's *Coding Clinic for ICD-9-CM* as the official publication for coding guidelines. The references are identified by the notation **AHA:** followed by the issue, year and page number.

In the example below, AHA's *Coding Clinic for ICD-9-CM*, third quarter 1991, page 15, contains a discussion on code assignment for vitreous hemorrhage:

> **379.23**   **Vitreous hemorrhage**
> **AHA:** 3Q, '91, 15

The table below explains the abbreviations in the *Coding Clinic* references:

| | |
|---|---|
| J-F | January/February |
| M-A | March/April |
| M-J | May/June |
| J-A | July/August |
| S-O | September/October |
| N-D | November/December |
| 1Q | First quarter |
| 2Q | Second quarter |
| 3Q | Third quarter |
| 4Q | Fourth quarter |

## MEDICARE CODE EDITS

Fiscal intermediaries use Medicare code edits (MCE) to check the coding accuracy on claims. The Medicare code edits are listed below:

- Invalid diagnosis or procedure code
- E-code as principal diagnosis
- Duplicate of principal diagnosis (PDx) (as applied to a secondary diagnosis)
- *Age conflict
- *Sex conflict
- *Manifestation code as principal diagnosis
- *Questionable admission
- *Unacceptable principal diagnosis

- *Noncovered procedure
- Open biopsy check
- *Bilateral procedure
- Invalid age
- Invalid sex
- Invalid discharge status
- *Limited coverage procedure

Starred edits are identified by colors, symbols or footnotes as described on the next page.

## Age and Sex Edit Symbols

The age edits below address MCE edit 4 and are used to detect inconsistencies between the patient's age and diagnosis. They appear in the Tabular List of Diseases to the right of the code description.

**Newborn Age: 0**

These diagnoses are intended for newborns and neonates and the patient's age must be 0 years

**Pediatric Age: 0-17**

These diagnoses are intended for children and the patient's age must between 0 and 17 years

**Maternity Age: 12-55**

These diagnoses are intended for the patients between the age of 12 and 55 years

**Adult Age: 15-124**

These diagnoses are intended for the patients between the age of 15 and 124 years.

The sex symbols below address MCE edit 5 and are used to detect inconsistencies between the patient's sex and diagnosis or procedure. They appear in the Tabular Lists to the right of the code description:

♂   **Male diagnosis or procedure only**

This symbol appears to the right of the code description. This reference appears in the disease and procedure Tabular List.

♀   **Female diagnosis or procedure only**

This symbol appears to the right of the code description. This reference appears in the disease and procedure Tabular List.

## Color Coding

For a quick reference to the color codes and their meaning, refer to the color/symbol legend located at the bottom of each page.

To alert the coder to important reimbursement issues affected by the code assignment, color bars have been added. The colors represent Medicare code edits as well as other reimbursement issues.

Color coding appears in both Tabular Lists. Some codes carry more than one color. Please note that the same color may appear in the disease and procedure Tabular Lists, but with different meanings.

### *Disease Tabular List*
**Manifestation Code**

These codes will appear in italic type as well as with a blue color bar over the code title. A manifestation code is not allowed to be reported as a primary diagnosis because each describes a manifestation of some other underlying disease, not the disease itself. This is referred to as mandatory multiple coding of etiology and manifestation. Code the underlying disease first. A 'Code first underlying disease' instructional note will appear with underlying disease codes identified. In the Alphabetic Index these codes are listed as the secondary code in slanted bracket with the code for the underlying disease listed first. Medicare code edit (MCE) 6

**Unacceptable PDx**

These codes will appear with a gray color bar over the code title. These codes do not describe a current illness or injury, but a circumstance which influences a patient's health status. These are considered an unacceptable principal diagnosis for inpatient admission.

### Questionable Admission

These codes will also appear with a gray color bar over the code title. These codes identify a condition that usually is insufficient justification for hospital admission. Since these codes are considered an unacceptable principal diagnoses for inpatient admission, they are color coded in the same manner as the "unacceptable PDx codes".

### Nonspecific PDx

Effective October 1, 2007 the Medicare code edit for Non-Specific Diagnoses was deactivated. Therefore, these codes will no longer be identified by a yellow color bar over the code title.

## Procedure Tabular List

### Nonspecific OR Procedure

Effective October 1, 2007 the Medicare code edit for Non-Specific OR was deactivated. Therefore, these codes will no longer be identified by a yellow color bar over the code title.

### Valid OR

A procedure that triggers a change in DRG assignment.

### Non-OR Procedure

A non-operating room procedure that affects DRG assignment.

### Adjunct Codes

These codes are not to be reported alone and are indicated by the red color bar over the code title. Adjunct codes are assigned only in addition to a primary procedure. Their purpose is to provide supplemental information about the primary procedure performed. Adjunct codes are not procedure codes, but serve to provide additional detail about the primary procedure.

*Example:*

PTCA balloon inflation of two vessels, with insertion of one intravascular coronary stent.

Code assignment:

**00.66 Percutaneous transluminal coronary angioplasty [PTCA] or athrectomy**

**00.41 Procedure on two vessels**

**00.45 Insertion of one vascular stent**

In the above example, codes 00.41 and 00.45 are adjunct codes that provide specific detail about the PTCA procedure performed.

## Footnotes

All footnotes are identified by a numerical superscript that appears to the upper left of the code:

**[1]427.41 Ventricular fibrillation**

The footnote 1 indicates "MCC = Only if patient is discharged alive'. This means that ventricular fibrillation is considered a major complication or comorbidity that may affect DRG assignment only if the patient is discharged alive. Otherwise ventricular fibrillation is assigned as a non CC condition.

The following list identifies the meaning of each footnote number and the classification in which the footnote appears:

### Disease Tabular

1. Major complication or comorbidity (MCC) that may affect DRG assignment only if the patient is discharged alive.

2. These V codes may be used as principal diagnosis on Medicare patients.

3. This V code, with the fourth digit of 1 or 2, is unacceptable as a principal diagnosis.

4. These codes, with the fourth digit of 0, may be used as a principal diagnosis for Medicare patients.

5. Rehabilitation codes acceptable as a principal diagnosis when accompanied by a secondary diagnosis reflecting the condition treated.

6. These V codes are acceptable as principal diagnosis when accompanied by a diagnosis of personal history of malignancy. These codes group to MS-DRG 949-950.

7. Diagnosis code with fifth digit of 0 is considered a "Questionable Admission" diagnosis when used as à principal diagnosis.

### Procedure Tabular

1. Valid OR procedure code if accompanied by one of the following codes: 37.80, 37.81, 37.82, 37.85, 37.86, 37.87.

2. Valid OR procedure code if accompanied by one of the following codes: 37.80, 37.83.

3. Valid OR procedure code if accompanied by one of the following codes: 37.80, 37.85, 37.86, 37.87.

4. Valid OR procedure code if accompanied by any one of the following codes: 37.80, 37.81, 37.82, 37.83, 37.85, 37.86, 37.87.

5. Valid OR procedure code if accompanied by any other pacemaker procedure except 37.72, 37.76.

6. Valid OR procedure code if accompanied by any other pacemaker procedure except 37.70, 37.71, 37.73, 37.76.

7. Non-covered except when reported with procedure code 00.65, Percutaneous insertion of intracranial vascular stent(s).

8. Non-covered procedure only when the following diagnoses are present as either a principal or secondary diagnosis: 204.00, 205.00, 205.10, 205.11, 206.00, 207.00, 208.00.

9. Non-covered procedure only when the following diagnoses are present as either a principal or secondary diagnosis: 203.00, 203.01.

10. Non-covered procedure unless reported with code 55.69 and a diagnosis code from 250.x0 or 250.x2 with 403.x1, 404.x2, 404.x3, 585.x, V42.0 or V42.89; or reported with a diagnosis code 250.x1 or 250.x3.

11. Non-covered except when the patient is 60 years old or less.

## Other Notations

### Alphabetic Indexes

**Subterms under main terms may continue to next column or page.**

This warning statement is a reminder to always check for additional subterms and information that may continue onto the next page or column before making a final selection.

### Disease Tabular

#### CC Condition

This symbol designates a complication or comorbidity diagnosis that may affect DRG assignment. A complication or comorbidity diagnosis, CC condition, is defined as a significant acute disease, a significant acute manifestation of a chronic disease, an advanced or end stage chronic disease, or a chronic disease associated with systemic physiological decompensation and debility that have consistently greater impact on hospital resources.

A CC listed with a digit or range of digits indicates that only the fifth-digit assignments stated for that code are to be considered CC conditions. For example, code 642.1 has a CC 3-4 which means that only codes 642.13 and 642.14 are considered CC conditions. Codes 642.11 and 642.12 are considered major complications or comorbidity (MCC) conditions. Code 642.10 is not designated as CC or MCC.

#### MCC Condition

This symbol designates a complication or comorbidity diagnosis that meets the criteria established for the revised CC list and was an AP-DRG major CC and was an APR-DRG default severity level 3 (major) or level 4 (extensive) with the exception of the newborn, maternity, and congenital anomalies which are APR-DRG default severity level 3 (major) or level 4 (extensive) only.

An MCC listed with a digit or range of digits indicates that only the fifth-digit assignments stated for that code are to be considered MCC conditions. For example; code 642.1 has a CC 3-4 which means that only codes 642.13 and 642.14 are considered CC conditions. Codes 642.11 and 642.12 are considered major complications or comorbidity (MCC) conditions and code 642.1 also has an MCC 1-2 designation. Code 642.10 is not designated as CC or MCC.

## CC Exclusion List

A exclusive feature of *ICD-9-CM for Hospitals* is the integration of the government's CC exclusion list with each affected code.

The CC exclusion list indicates secondary diagnosis codes that are excluded as CC conditions with certain principal diagnoses. This exclusion occurs because the cited conditions are inherent to the disease process of the principal diagnosis.

Listed below each code that is considered a complication or comorbidity (CC) diagnosis, are the codes or code ranges of principal diagnosis with which the CC code cannot be used.

In the example below, code 254.1 is considered a CC condition. However, the CC exclusion (CC Excl:) notation indicates that if a code from the listed code ranges is assigned as the principal diagnosis, the secondary diagnosis of 254.1 will not be recognized as a CC condition in DRG assignment.

**254.1   Abscess of thymus**   `CC`
   **CC Excl:** 254.0-254.9, 259.8-259.9

Please note that the same notation, CC Exclusion (**CC Excl:**), is used for both the MCC and CC conditions. Both MCC and CC are considered complication and comorbidity conditions. And for both, the same criteria are applied in determining which principal diagnosis for which the designated CC or MCC will not affect DRG assignment.

## HIV

This symbol indicates that the condition is considered a major HIV related diagnosis. When the condition is coded in combination with a diagnosis of human immunodeficiency virus (HIV), code 042, the case will move from MS-DRG 977 to MS-DRGs 974–976.

## Medicare as Secondary Payer (MSP)

**Note:** This edit is no longer included in the official Medicare Code Editor (MCE) for the inpatient prospective payment system (IPPS). The Medicare as Secondary Payer (MSP) alert identified trauma diagnoses that may be covered under automobile insurance, no-fault insurance, workmen's compensation or other types of liability insurance for which Medicare should be a secondary payer Providers must verify MSP information prior to submitting the claim to Medicare.

## V Code table

**Note:** Please note that while the official guidelines [Section 1. C.18.e.] include the V Code Table the reporting designations indicated by the Table are often in conflict with the Medicare code edits (MCE) for the inpatient prospective payment system (IPPS). Therefore, only the inpatient prospective payment system code edits are represented in this edition.

## *Procedure Tabular*
### Noncovered Procedure

A procedure not covered by Medicare. In some instances this procedure may also be identified as a valid operating room (OR) procedure that may trigger a DRG assignment. Even if a DRG assignment is made, Medicare may not reimburse for the noncovered procedure.

### Limited Coverage Procedure

A procedure whose medical complexity and serious nature incur associated costs that are deemed extraordinary and Medicare limits coverage to a portion of the cost.

### Bilateral Edit

Due to the lack of laterality in ICD-9-CM, there are certain lower extremity joint procedure codes that do not accurately reflect procedures that are performed in one admission on two or more different bilateral joints. To group to MS-DRG 461 or 462, Bilateral or Multiple Joint Procedures of Lower Extremity with or without MCC, a case must be coded with a combination of two or more different major lower extremity joint procedures. The bilateral procedure symbol identifies those procedure codes that when coded twice represent the same procedure performed on both of the same bilateral joints of the lower extremity. Otherwise, a code edit will instruct the fiscal intermediary to verify that the two different procedures were performed on two different bilateral joints.

# Summary of Code Changes

## DISEASE TABULAR LIST (VOLUME 1)

001-139 Chapter Excludes term revised
▲ 005.1 Botulism ▶food poisoning◀
  Includes note added
  Excludes note added
● 040.4 Other specified botulism
  Includes note added
  Excludes note added
● 040.41 Infant botulism
● 040.42 Wound botulism
  Includes note added
  Use additional code note added
041 Excludes term revised
049.8 Excludes note added
054.3 Excludes note added
057.8 Includes terms deleted
  Excludes note added
● OTHER HUMAN HERPESVIRUSES (058)
● 058 Other human herpesvirus
  Excludes note added
● 058.1 Roseola infantum
  Includes note added
● 058.10 Roseola infantum, unspecified
  Includes note added
● 058.11 Roseola infantum due to human
  herpesvirus 6
  Includes note added
● 058.12 Roseola infantum due to human
  herpesvirus 7
  Includes note added
● 058.2 Other human herpesvirus encephalitis
  Excludes note added
● 058.21 Human herpesvirus 6 encephalitis
● 058.29 Other human herpesvirus encephalitis
  Includes note added
● 058.8 Other human herpesvirus infections
● 058.81 Human herpesvirus 6 infection
● 058.82 Human herpesvirus 7 infection
● 058.89 Other human herpesvirus infection
  Includes note added
● 079.83 Parvovirus B19
  Includes note added
  Excludes note added
184 Excludes term revised
193 Includes term deleted
▲ 200 Lymphosarcoma and reticulosarcoma
  ▶and other specified malignant tumors of
  lymphatic tissue◀
● 200.3 Marginal zone lymphoma
  Includes note added
● 200.30 Marginal zone lymphoma, unspecified site,
  extranodal and solid organ sites
● 200.31 Marginal zone lymphoma, lymph nodes of
  head, face, and neck
● 200.32 Marginal zone lymphoma, intrathoracic
  lymph nodes
● 200.33 Marginal zone lymphoma, intra-abdominal
  lymph nodes
● 200.34 Marginal zone lymphoma, lymph nodes of
  axilla and upper limb
● 200.35 Marginal zone lymphoma, lymph nodes of
  inguinal region and lower limb
● 200.36 Marginal zone lymphoma, intrapelvic
  lymph nodes
● 200.37 Marginal zone lymphoma, spleen
● 200.38 Marginal zone lymphoma, lymph nodes of
  multiple sites
● 200.4 Mantle cell lymphoma
● 200.40 Mantle cell lymphoma, unspecified site,
  extranodal and solid organ sites
● 200.41 Mantle cell lymphoma, lymph nodes of
  head, face, and neck
● 200.42 Mantle cell lymphoma, intrathoracic lymph
  nodes
● 200.43 Mantle cell lymphoma, intra-abdominal
  lymph nodes
● 200.44 Mantle cell lymphoma, lymph nodes of
  axilla and upper limb
● 200.45 Mantle cell lymphoma, lymph nodes of
  inguinal region and lower limb
● 200.46 Mantle cell lymphoma, intrapelvic lymph
  nodes

● 200.47 Mantle cell lymphoma, spleen
● 200.48 Mantle cell lymphoma, lymph nodes of
  multiple sites
● 200.5 Primary central nervous system lymphoma
● 200.50 Primary central nervous system
  lymphoma, unspecified site, extranodal
  and solid organ sites
● 200.51 Primary central nervous system
  lymphoma, lymph nodes of head, face, and
  neck
● 200.52 Primary central nervous system
  lymphoma, intrathoracic lymph nodes
● 200.53 Primary central nervous system
  lymphoma, intra-abdominal lymph nodes
● 200.54 Primary central nervous system
  lymphoma, lymph nodes of axilla and
  upper limb
● 200.55 Primary central nervous system
  lymphoma, lymph nodes of inguinal region
  and lower limb
● 200.56 Primary central nervous system
  lymphoma, intrapelvic lymph nodes
● 200.57 Primary central nervous system
  lymphoma, spleen
● 200.58 Primary central nervous system
  lymphoma, lymph nodes of multiple sites
● 200.6 Anaplastic large cell lymphoma
● 200.60 Anaplastic large cell lymphoma,
  unspecified site, extranodal and solid
  organ sites
● 200.61 Anaplastic large cell lymphoma, lymph
  nodes of head, face, and neck
● 200.62 Anaplastic large cell lymphoma,
  intrathoracic lymph nodes
● 200.63 Anaplastic large cell lymphoma, intra-
  abdominal lymph nodes
● 200.64 Anaplastic large cell lymphoma, lymph
  nodes of axilla and upper limb
● 200.65 Anaplastic large cell lymphoma, lymph
  nodes of inguinal region and lower limb
● 200.66 Anaplastic large cell lymphoma, intrapelvic
  lymph nodes
● 200.67 Anaplastic large cell lymphoma, spleen
● 200.68 Anaplastic large cell lymphoma, lymph
  nodes of multiple sites
● 200.7 Large cell lymphoma
● 200.70 Large cell lymphoma, unspecified site,
  extranodal and solid organ sites
● 200.71 Large cell lymphoma, lymph nodes of head,
  face, and neck
● 200.72 Large cell lymphoma, intrathoracic lymph
  nodes
● 200.73 Large cell lymphoma, intra-abdominal
  lymph nodes
● 200.74 Large cell lymphoma, lymph nodes of axilla
  and upper limb
● 200.75 Large cell lymphoma, lymph nodes of
  inguinal region and lower limb
● 200.76 Large cell lymphoma, intrapelvic lymph
  nodes
● 200.77 Large cell lymphoma, spleen
● 200.78 Large cell lymphoma, lymph nodes of
  multiple sites
● 202.7 Peripheral T-cell lymphoma
● 202.70 Peripheral T-cell lymphoma, unspecified
  site, extranodal and solid organ sites
● 202.71 Peripheral T-cell lymphoma, lymph nodes
  of head, face, and neck
● 202.72 Peripheral T-cell lymphoma, intrathoracic
  lymph nodes
● 202.73 Peripheral T-cell lymphoma, intra-
  abdominal lymph nodes
● 202.74 Peripheral T-cell lymphoma, lymph nodes
  of axilla and upper limb
● 202.75 Peripheral T-cell lymphoma, lymph nodes
  of inguinal region and lower limb
● 202.76 Peripheral T-cell lymphoma, intrapelvic
  lymph nodes
● 202.77 Peripheral T-cell lymphoma, spleen
● 202.78 Peripheral T-cell lymphoma, lymph nodes
  of multiple sites
232.5 Excludes term revised
233.1 Includes term added

● 233.30 Unspecified female genital organ
  [Carcinoma in situ]
● 233.31 Vagina [Carcinoma in situ]
  Includes note added
● 233.32 Vulva [Carcinoma in situ]
  Includes note added
● 233.39 Other female genital organ
250 Excludes term revised
250.6 Use additional code note revised
255.4 Includes note deleted
● 255.41 Glucocorticoid deficiency
  Includes note added
● 255.42 Mineralocorticoid deficiency
  Includes note added
  Excludes note added
258.0 Includes term deleted
  Includes note added
  Use additional code note added
● 258.01 Multiple endocrine neoplasia [MEN] type I
  Includes note added
● 258.02 Multiple endocrine neoplasia [MEN]
  type IIA
  Includes note added
● 258.03 Multiple endocrine neoplasia [MEN]
  type IIB
268.1 Use additional code note deleted
  Code first note added
276.6 Excludes term revised
284.1 Excludes term revised
284.8 Includes note deleted
  Use additional code note deleted
● 284.81 Red cell aplasia (acquired) (adult) (with
  thymoma)
  Includes note added
● 284.89 Other specified aplastic anemias
  Includes note added
  Use additional code note revised
288.0 Use additional code note revised
● 288.66 Bandemia
  Includes note added
  Excludes note added
302.5 Includes note added
302.85 Use additional code note added
315.32 Includes term added
  Excludes term added
● 315.34 Speech and language developmental delay
  due to hearing loss
  Use additional code note added
331 Use additional code note added
331.1 Use additional code note deleted
331.3 Includes note added
  Excludes terms added
  Excludes term revised
331.4 Excludes terms added
  Excludes term revised
● 331.5 Idiopathic normal pressure hydrocephalus
  [INPH]
  Includes note added
  Excludes note added
331.82 Use additional code note deleted
353.1 Code first note added
358.1 Includes term deleted
  Code first note revised
359.2 Includes note deleted
  Excludes note added
● 359.21 Myotonic muscular dystrophy
  Includes note added
● 359.22 Myotonia congenita
  Includes note added
● 359.23 Myotonic chondrodystrophy
  Includes note added
● 359.24 Drug-induced myotonia
  Use additional code note added
● 359.29 Other specified myotonic disorder
  Includes note added
▲ 359.3 Familial pPeriodic paralysis
  Includes terms added
  Excludes note added
359.5 Code first note revised
364.8 Includes note deleted
  Excludes note deleted

---

▶◀ Revised Text    ● New Code    ▲ Revised Code Title

● 364.81 Floppy iris syndrome
　　Includes note added
　　Use additional code note added
● 364.89 Other disorders of iris and ciliary body
　　Includes note added
　　Excludes note added
　366.43 Code first note revised
● 388.45 Acquired auditory processing disorder
　　Includes note added
　　Excludes note added
　389.0 Excludes note added
● 389.05 Conductive hearing loss, unilateral
● 389.06 Conductive hearing loss, bilateral
　389.1 Excludes term added
● 389.13 Neural hearing loss, unilateral
▲ 389.14 Central hearing loss, bilateral
● 389.17 Sensory hearing loss, unilateral
● 389.17 Sensory hearing loss, unilateral
▲ 389.18 Sensorineural hearing loss of combined types, bilateral
　389.2 Includes note revised
● 389.20 Mixed hearing loss, unspecified
● 389.21 Mixed hearing loss, unilateral
● 389.22 Mixed hearing loss, bilateral
▲ 389.7 Deaf mutism, ▶nonspeaking,◀ not elsewhere classifiable
　　Includes note deleted
　414.0 Use additional code note added
● 414.2 Chronic total occlusion of coronary artery
　　Includes note added
　　Code first note added
　　Excludes note added
● 415.12 Septic pulmonary embolism
　　Includes note added
　　Code first note added
　　Excludes note added
● 423.3 Cardiac tamponade
　　Code first note added
　425.8 Code first note revised
　438 Excludes note added
　438.82 Use additional code note added
　440-449 Section title revised
　440.2 Use additional code note added
● 440.4 Chronic total occlusion of artery of the extremities
　　Includes note added
　　Code first note added
　　Excludes note added
　444 Excludes term added
● 449 Septic arterial embolism
　　Code first note added
　　Use additional coed note added
　　Excludes note added
　460-466 Section Excludes note revised
　480-488 Section title revised
　487 Excludes term added
● 488 Influenza due to identified avian influenza virus
　　Instructional note added
　　Excludes note added
● 525.71 Osseointegration failure of dental implant
　　Includes note added
● 525.72 Post-osseointegration biological failure of dental implant
　　Includes note added
● 525.73 Post-osseointegration mechanical failure of dental implant
　　Includes note added
　　Excludes note added
● 525.79 Other endosseous dental implant failure
　　Includes note added
　526.4 Excludes term added
　528.7 Excludes term revised
　536.3 Code first note added
　565.0 Includes note deleted
　　Excludes term added
　568.82 Excludes note revised
● 569.43 Anal sphincter tear (healed) (old)
　　Use additional code note added
　　Excludes note added
　572.2 Excludes note added
　585 Code first note revised
　608.22 Includes note added
　623.0 Includes note added
　　Excludes term revised
　　Excludes terms added
　624.0 Includes note deleted
　　Excludes term revised
　　Excludes terms added

● 624.01 Vulvar intraepithelial neoplasia I [VIN I]
　　Includes note added
● 624.02 Vulvar intraepithelial neoplasia II [VIN II]
　　Includes note added
● 624.09 Other dystrophy of vulva
　　Includes note added
　646.3 Excludes term revised
　654 Excludes note added
　654.8 Includes term added
　　Excludes term added
　661.2 Includes term added
　　Excludes note added
　664.2 Excludes term added
● 664.6 Anal sphincter tear complicating delivery, not associated with third-degree perineal laceration
　　Excludes note added
● 664.60 Anal sphincter tear complicating delivery, not associated with third-degree perineal laceration, unspecified as to episode of care or not applicable
● 664.61 Anal sphincter tear complicating delivery, not associated with third-degree perineal laceration, delivered, with or without mention of antepartum condition
● 664.64 Anal sphincter tear complicating delivery, not associated with third-degree perineal laceration, postpartum condition or complication
　666.1 Includes term added
　　Excludes term revised
　　Excludes term added
● 733.45 Jaw [Aseptic necrosis of bone]
　　Use additional code note added
　　Excludes note added
　756.4 Excludes term added
　771 Excludes term added
　780.39 Includes term added
　782.3 Excludes term revised
　784.1 Excludes term revised
　784.99 Includes term added
　　Excludes note added
　787.2 Includes note deleted
　　Code first note added
● 787.20 Dysphagia, unspecified
　　Includes note added
● 787.21 Dysphagia, oral phase
● 787.22 Dysphagia, oropharyngeal phase
● 787.23 Dysphagia, pharyngeal phase
● 787.24 Dysphagia, pharyngoesophageal phase
● 787.29 Other dysphagia
　　Includes note added
　789.3 Excludes term revised
● 789.51 Malignant ascites
　　Code first note added
● 789.59 Other ascites
　996 Excludes terms added
　996.62 Includes term revised
　　Excludes term added
　996.77 Use additional code note added
　998.5 Excludes term revised
　999 Use additional code note added
　999.3 Use additional code note added
● 999.31 Infection due to central venous catheter
　　Includes note added
　　Excludes note added
● 999.39 Infection following other infusion, injection, transfusion, or vaccination
● V12.53 Sudden cardiac arrest [Personal history of disease of circulatory system]
　　Includes note added
● V12.54 Transient ischemic attack [TIA], and cerebral infarction without residual deficits [Personal history of disease of circulatory system]
　　Includes note added
　　Excludes note added
　V13.2 Excludes term revised
● V13.22 Personal history of cervical dysplasia
　　Includes note added
　　Excludes note added
　V16.5 Includes note revised
● V16.52 Bladder [Family history of malignant neoplasm]
● V17.41 Family history of sudden cardiac death [SCD]
　　Excludes note added
● V17.49 Family history of other cardiovascular diseases

　　Includes note added
● V18.11 Multiple endocrine neoplasia [MEN] syndrome
● V18.19 Other endocrine and metabolic diseases
　V23.2 Excludes term revised
● V25.04 Counseling and instruction in natural family planning to avoid pregnancy
● V26.41 Procreative counseling and advice using natural family planning
● V26.49 Other procreative management, counseling and advice
● V26.81 Encounter for assisted reproductive fertility procedure cycle
　　Includes note added
　　Use additional code note added
　　Excludes note added
● V26.89 Other specified procreative management
● V49.85 Dual sensory impairment
　　Includes note added
　　Code first note added
　V58.69 Includes note revised
　V58.78 Excludes note added
　V64.05 Includes note added
　V65.4 Excludes term revised
　V68.0 Includes note deleted
● V68.01 Disability examination
　　Use additional code note added
● V68.09 Other issue of medical certificates
● V72.12 Encounter for hearing conservation and treatment
　V72.31 Use additional code note added
● V73.81 Human papillomavirus [HPV] [Special screening examination]
　V74.5 Includes note added
　　Excludes note added
　V76.2 Excludes term added
　V80.3 Excludes note revised
　V82.7 Excludes note revised
● V84.81 Genetic susceptibility to multiple endocrine neoplasia [MEN]
● V84.89 Genetic susceptibility to other disease
● E928.6 Environmental exposure to harmful algae and toxins
　　Includes note added
● E933.6 Oral bisphophonates
● E933.7 Intravenous bisphophonates

## PROCEDURE TABULAR (VOLUME 3)
▲ 00.18 Infusion of immunosuppressive antibody therapy during induction phase of solid organ transplantation
　　Includes term added
● 00.19 Disruption of blood brain barrier via infusion [BBBD]
　　Includes note added
　　Code also note added
　　Excludes note added
▲ 00.74 Hip replacement bearing surface, metal-on-polyethylene
▲ 00.75 Hip replacement bearing surface, metal-on-metal
▲ 00.76 Hip replacement bearing surface, ceramic-on-ceramic
▲ 00.77 Hip replacement bearing surface, ceramic-on-polyethylene
● 00.94 Intra-operative neurophysiologic monitoring
　　Includes note added
　　Excludes note added
● 01.10 Intracranial pressure monitoring
　　Includes note added
● 01.16 Intracranial oxygen monitoring
　　Includes note added
● 01.17 Brain temperature monitoring
　　Includes note added
　01.18 Excludes terms added
　03.09 Code also note added
▲ 07.81 ▶Other◀ partial excision of thymus
　　Includes term added
　　Excludes term added
▲ 07.82 ▶Other◀ total excision of thymus
　　Includes term added
　　Excludes term added
● 07.83 Thoracoscopic partial excision of thymus
　　Excludes note added
● 07.84 Thoracoscopic total excision of thymus
　　Excludes note added
▲ 07.92 ▶Other◀ incision of thymus
　　Includes term added
　　Excludes term added

▶◀ Revised Text　　● New Code　　▲ Revised Code Title

| ● 07.95 | Thoracoscopic incision of thymus |
| | Excludes note added |
| ● 07.98 | Other and unspecified thoracoscopic operations on thymus |
| ▲ 07.99 | Other ▶and unspecified operations on thymus◀ |
| | Includes term added |
| | Includes term deleted |
| | Excludes term added |
| 20.99 | Includes term added |
| ● 32.20 | Thoracoscopic excision of lesion or tissue of lung |
| | Includes note added |
| 32.25 | Excludes term added |
| 32.29 | Excludes term added |
| ● 32.30 | Thoracoscopic segmental resection of lung |
| ● 32.39 | Other and unspecified segmental resection of lung |
| | Excludes note added |
| ● 32.41 | Thoracoscopic lobectomy of lung |
| ● 32.49 | Other lobectomy of lung |
| | Excludes note added |
| ▲ 32.5 | ~~Complete P~~pneumonectomy |
| ● 32.50 | Thoracoscopic pneumonectomy |
| ● 32.59 | Other and unspecified pneumonectomy |
| | Excludes note added |
| ● 33.20 | Thoracoscopic lung biopsy |
| | Excludes note added |
| 33.26 | Includes terms added |
| | Excludes term added |
| 33.27 | Excludes term added |
| 34.04 | Excludes term added |
| ● 34.06 | Thoracoscopic drainage of pleural cavity |
| | Includes note added |
| ● 34.20 | Thoracoscopic pleural biopsy |
| ▲ 34.24 | ▶Other◀ pleural biopsy |
| | Excludes term added |
| 34.51 | Excludes term added |
| ● 34.52 | Thoracoscopic decortication of lung |
| ▲ 39.8 | Operations on carotid body▶, carotid sinus◀ and other vascular bodies |
| | Includes terms deleted |
| | Includes terms revised |
| | Includes term added |
| | Excludes term added |
| 48.74 | Includes term added |
| ● 50.13 | Transjugular liver biopsy |
| | Includes term added |
| | Excludes terms added |
| ● 50.14 | Laparoscopic liver biopsy |
| | Excludes terms added |
| 50.19 | Includes term deleted |
| | Excludes terms added |

| ▲ 53.41 | Repair of umbilical hernia with ▶graft or◀ prosthesis |
| ▲ 53.61 | Incisional hernia repair with ▶graft or◀ prosthesis |
| ▲ 53.69 | Repair of other hernia of anterior abdominal wall with ▶graft or◀ prosthesis |
| 54 | Includes term revised |
| | Excludes term deleted |
| 70.52 | Excludes terms added |
| ● 70.53 | Repair of cystocele and rectocele with graft or prosthesis |
| | Use additional code note added |
| ● 70.54 | Repair of cystocele with graft or prosthesis |
| | Includes note added |
| | Use additional code note added |
| ● 70.55 | Repair of rectocele with graft or prosthesis |
| | Includes note added |
| | Use additional code note added |
| ● 70.63 | Vaginal construction with graft or prosthesis |
| | Use additional code note added |
| | Excludes note added |
| ● 70.64 | Vaginal reconstruction with graft or prosthesis |
| | Use additional code note added |
| ● 70.78 | Vaginal suspension and fixation with graft or prosthesis |
| | Use additional code note added |
| ● 70.93 | Other operations on cul-de-sac with graft or prosthesis |
| | Includes note added |
| | Use additional code note added |
| ● 70.94 | Insertion of biological graft |
| | Includes note added |
| | Code first note added |
| ● 70.95 | Insertion of synthetic graft or prosthesis |
| | Includes note added |
| | Code first note added |
| 78.6 | Includes term added |
| | Excludes terms added |
| 80.0 | Includes term added |
| | Code also any note revised |
| | Excludes term added |
| 81.0 | Code also any note added |
| 81.3 | Code also any note added |
| 81.5 | Includes terms deleted |
| 81.51 | Code also any note revised |
| 81.52 | Code also any note revised |
| 81.53 | Code also any note revised |
| 84.56 | Includes term revised |
| 84.57 | Includes term revised |

| 84.58 | ~~Implantation of interspinous process decompression device~~ |
| 84.59 | Includes term deleted |
| | Excludes terms added |
| ● 84.8 | Insertion, replacement and revision of posterior spinal motion preservation device(s) |
| | Includes note added |
| | Code also note added |
| | Excludes note added |
| ● 84.80 | Insertion or replacement of interspinous process device(s) |
| | Includes note added |
| | Excludes note added |
| ● 84.81 | Revision of interspinous process device(s) |
| | Includes note added |
| | Excludes note added |
| ● 84.82 | Insertion or replacement of pedicle-based dynamic stabilization device(s) |
| | Excludes note added |
| ● 84.83 | Revision of pedicle-based dynamic stabilization device(s) |
| | Includes note added |
| | Excludes note added |
| ● 84.84 | Insertion or replacement of facet replacement device(s) |
| | Includes note added |
| | Excludes note added |
| ● 84.85 | Revision of facet replacement device(s) |
| | Includes note added |
| | Excludes note added |
| 86.05 | Includes term revised |
| 86.6 | Excludes term revised |
| 86.7 | Excludes term revised |
| 88.52 | Excludes term added |
| 88.53 | Excludes term added |
| 88.54 | Excludes term added |
| 88.55 | Excludes term added |
| 88.56 | Excludes term added |
| 88.57 | Excludes term added |
| ● 88.59 | Intra-operative fluorescence vascular angiography |
| | Includes note added |
| 92.25 | Excludes term added |
| ● 92.4 | Intra-operative radiation procedures |
| ● 92.41 | Intra-operative electron radiation therapy |
| | Includes terms added |
| 96.7 | Excludes term revised |
| 97.49 | Excludes term added |
| 98.15 | Excludes note added |
| ▲ 99.14 | Injection ▶or infusion◀ of gamma globulin |
| 99.25 | Use additional code note added |
| 99.29 | Excludes term added |

▶◀ Revised Text    ● New Code    ▲ Revised Code Title

# Coding Guidelines

## NEW GUIDELINES
Effective November 15, 2006

Narrative changes appear in bold text. Items underlined have been moved within the guidelines since December 2005. The guidelines include the updated V Code Table

The Centers for Medicare and Medicaid Services (CMS) and the National Center for Health Statistics (NCHS), two departments within the U. S. Federal Government's Department of Health and Human Services (DHHS) provide the following guidelines for coding and reporting using the International Classification of Diseases, 9th Revision, Clinical Modification (ICD-9-CM). These guidelines should be used as a companion document to the official version of the ICD-9-CM as published on CD-ROM by the U.S. Government Printing Office (GPO).

These guidelines have been approved by the four organizations that make up the Cooperating Parties for the ICD-9-CM: the American Hospital Association (AHA), the American Health Information Management Association (AHIMA), CMS, and NCHS. These guidelines are included on the official government version of the ICD-9-CM, and also appear in "Coding Clinic for ICD-9-CM" published by the AHA.

These guidelines are a set of rules that have been developed to accompany and complement the official conventions and instructions provided within the ICD-9-CM itself. These guidelines are based on the coding and sequencing instructions in Volumes I, II and III of ICD-9-CM, but provide additional instruction. Adherence to these guidelines when assigning ICD-9-CM diagnosis and procedure codes is required under the Health Insurance Portability and Accountability Act (HIPAA). The diagnosis codes (Volumes 1-2) have been adopted under HIPAA for all healthcare settings. Volume 3 procedure codes have been adopted for inpatient procedures reported by hospitals. A joint effort between the healthcare provider and the coder is essential to achieve complete and accurate documentation, code assignment, and reporting of diagnoses and procedures. These guidelines have been developed to assist both the healthcare provider and the coder in identifying those diagnoses and procedures that are to be reported. The importance of consistent, complete documentation in the medical record cannot be overemphasized. Without such documentation accurate coding cannot be achieved. The entire record should be reviewed to determine the specific reason for the encounter and the conditions treated.

The term encounter is used for all settings, including hospital admissions. In the context of these guidelines, the term provider is used throughout the guidelines to mean physician or any qualified health care practitioner who is legally accountable for establishing the patient's diagnosis. Only this set of guidelines, approved by the Cooperating Parties, is official.

The guidelines are organized into sections. Section I includes the structure and conventions of the classification and general guidelines that apply to the entire classification, and chapter-specific guidelines that correspond to the chapters as they are arranged in the classification. Section II includes guidelines for selection of principal diagnosis for non-outpatient settings. Section III includes guidelines for reporting additional diagnoses in non-outpatient settings. Section IV is for outpatient coding and reporting.

## Section I. Conventions, general coding guidelines and chapter-specific guidelines
A. Conventions for the ICD-9-CM
  1. Format
  2. Abbreviations
    a. Index abbreviations
    b. Tabular abbreviations
  3. Punctuation
  4. Includes and excludes notes and inclusion terms
  5. Other and Unspecified codes
    a. "Other" codes
    b. "Unspecified" codes
  6. Etiology/manifestation convention ("code first," "use additional code," and "in diseases classified elsewhere" notes)
  7. "And"
  8. "With"
  9. "See" and "see also"
B. General coding guidelines
  1. Use of both Alphabetic Index and Tabular List

  2. Locate each term in the Alphabetic Index
  3. Level of detail in coding
  4. Code or codes from 001.0 through V86.1
  5. Selection of codes 001.0 through 999.9
  6. Signs and symptoms
  7. Conditions that are an integral part of a disease process
  8. Conditions that are not an integral part of a disease process
  9. Multiple coding for a single condition
  10. Acute and chronic conditions
  11. Combination code
  12. Late effects
  13. Impending or threatened condition
C. Chapter-specific coding guidelines
  1. Chapter 1: Infectious and Parasitic Diseases (001–139)
    a. Human immunodeficiency virus (HIV) infections
    b. Septicemia, systemic inflammatory response syndrome (SIRS), sepsis, severe sepsis, and septic shock
  2. Chapter 2: Neoplasms (140–239)
    a. Treatment directed at the malignancy
    b. Treatment of secondary site
    c. Coding and sequencing of complications
    d. Primary malignancy previously excised
    e. Admissions/encounters involving chemotherapy and radiation therapy
    f. Admission/encounter to determine extent of malignancy
    g. Symptoms, signs, and ill-defined conditions listed in chapter 16
    **h. Admission/encounter for pain control/management**
  3. Chapter 3: Endocrine, Nutritional, and Metabolic Diseases and Immunity Disorders (240–279)
    a. Diabetes mellitus
  4. Chapter 4: Diseases of Blood and Blood-Forming Organs (280–289)
    a. Anemia of chronic disease
  5. Chapter 5: Mental Disorders (290–319)
    Reserved for future guideline expansion
  6. Chapter 6: Diseases of Nervous System and Sense Organs (320–389)
    **a. Pain—Category 338**
  7. Chapter 7: Diseases of Circulatory System (390–459)
    a. Hypertension
    b. Cerebral infarction/stroke/cerebrovascular accident (CVA)
    c. Postoperative cerebrovascular accident
    d. Late effects of cerebrovascular disease
    e. Acute myocardial infarction (AMI)
  8. Chapter 8: Diseases of Respiratory System (460–519)
    a. Chronic obstructive pulmonary disease [COPD] and asthma
    b. Chronic obstructive pulmonary disease [COPD] and bronchitis
    **c. Acute Respiratory Failure**
  9. Chapter 9: Diseases of Digestive System (520–579)
    Reserved for future guideline expansion
  10. Chapter 10: Diseases of Genitourinary System (580–629)
    **a. Chronic kidney disease**
  11. Chapter 11: Complications of Pregnancy, Childbirth, and the Puerperium (630–677)
    a. General rules for obstetric cases
    b. Selection of OB principal or first-listed diagnosis
    c. Fetal conditions affecting the management of the mother
    d. HIV infection in pregnancy, childbirth and the puerperium
    e. Current conditions complicating pregnancy
    f. Diabetes mellitus in pregnancy
    g. Gestational diabetes
    h. Normal delivery, code 650
    i. The postpartum and peripartum eriods
    j. Code 677 Late effect of complication of pregnancy
    k. Abortions
  12. Chapter 12: Diseases Skin and Subcutaneous Tissue (680–709)
    Reserved for future guideline expansion
  13. Chapter 13: Diseases of Musculoskeletal and Connective Tissue (710–739)
    **a. Coding of Pathologic Fractures**

## Section I. Conventions, general coding guidelines and chapter specific guidelines
The conventions, general guidelines and chapter-specific guidelines are applicable to all health care settings unless otherwise indicated.

**A. Conventions for the ICD-9-CM**—The conventions for the ICD-9-CM are the general rules for use of the classification independent of the guidelines. These conventions are incorporated within the index and tabular of the ICD-9-CM as instructional notes. The conventions are as follows:

1. **Format:**
   The ICD-9-CM uses an indented format for ease in reference

2. **Abbreviations**
   a. **Index abbreviations**
      NEC "Not elsewhere classifiable"
         This abbreviation in the index represents "other specified" when a specific code is not available for a condition the index directs the coder to the "other specified" code in the tabular.
   b. **Tabular abbreviations**
      NEC "Not elsewhere classifiable"
         This abbreviation in the tabular represents "other specified." When a specific code is not available for a condition the tabular includes an NEC entry under a code to identify the code as the "other specified" code.
         *(See Section I.A.5.a. "Other" codes)*
      NOS "Not otherwise specified"
         This abbreviation is the equivalent of unspecified.
         *(See Section I.A.5.b., "Unspecified" codes)*

3. **Punctuation**
   [ ] Brackets are used in the tabular list to enclose synonyms, alternative wording or explanatory phrases. Brackets are used in the index to identify manifestation codes.
      *(See Section I.A.6. "Etiology/manifestations")*
   ( ) Parentheses are used in both the index and tabular to enclose supplementary words that may be present or absent in the statement of a disease or procedure without affecting the code number to which it is assigned. The terms within the parentheses are referred to as nonessential modifiers.
   : Colons are used in the Tabular list after an incomplete term which needs one or more of the modifiers following the colon to make it assignable to a given category.

4. **Includes and Excludes notes and Inclusion terms**
   Includes: This note appears immediately under a three-digit code title to further define, or give examples of, the content of the category.
   Excludes: An excludes note under a code indicates that the terms excluded from the code are to be coded elsewhere. In some cases the codes for the excluded terms should not be used in conjunction with the code from which it is excluded. An example of this is a congenital condition excluded from an acquired form of the same condition. The congenital and acquired codes should not be used together. In other cases, the excluded terms may be used together with an excluded code. An example of this is when fractures of different bones are coded to different codes. Both codes may be used together if both types of fractures are present.

Inclusion terms: List of terms is included under certain four and five digit codes. These terms are the conditions for which that code number is to be used. The terms may be synonyms of the code title, or, in the case of "other specified" codes, the terms are a list of the various conditions assigned to that code. The inclusion terms are not necessarily exhaustive. Additional terms found only in the index may also be assigned to a code.

5. **Other and Unspecified codes**

    a. **"Other" codes**

    Codes titled "other" or "other specified" (usually a code with a 4th digit 8 or fifth-digit 9 for diagnosis codes) are for use when the information in the medical record provides detail for which a specific code does not exist. Index entries with NEC in the line designate "other" codes in the tabular. These index entries represent specific disease entities for which no specific code exists so the term is included within an "other" code.

    b. **"Unspecified" codes**

    Codes (usually a code with a 4th digit 9 or 5th digit 0 for diagnosis codes) titled "unspecified" are for use when the information in the medical record is insufficient to assign a more specific code.

6. **Etiology/manifestation convention ("code first," "use additional code" and "in diseases classified elsewhere" notes)**—Certain conditions have both an underlying etiology and multiple body system manifestations due to the underlying etiology. For such conditions, the ICD-9-CM has a coding convention that requires the underlying condition be sequenced first followed by the manifestation. Wherever such a combination exists, there is a "use additional code" note at the etiology code, and a "code first" note at the manifestation code. These instructional notes indicate the proper sequencing order of the codes, etiology followed by manifestation.

    In most cases the manifestation codes will have in the code title, "in diseases classified elsewhere." Codes with this title are a component of the etiology/ manifestation convention. The code title indicates that it is a manifestation code. "In diseases classified elsewhere" codes are never permitted to be used as first listed or principal diagnosis codes. They must be used in conjunction with an underlying condition code and they must be listed following the underlying condition.

    There are manifestation codes that do not have "in diseases classified elsewhere" in the title. For such codes a "use additional code" note will still be present and the rules for sequencing apply.

    In addition to the notes in the tabular, these conditions also have a specific index entry structure. In the index both conditions are listed together with the etiology code first followed by the manifestation codes in brackets. The code in brackets is always to be sequenced second.

    The most commonly used etiology/manifestation combinations are the codes for Diabetes mellitus, category 250. For each code under category 250 there is a use additional code note for the manifestation that is specific for that particular diabetic manifestation. Should a patient have more than one manifestation of diabetes, more than one code from category 250 may be used with as many manifestation codes as are needed to fully describe the patient's complete diabetic condition. The category 250 diabetes codes should be sequenced first, followed by the manifestation codes.

    "Code first" and "Use additional code" notes are also used as sequencing rules in the classification for certain codes that are not part of an etiology/ manifestation combination. *See Section I.B.9. "Multiple coding for a single conditon"*

7. **"And"**—The word "and" should be interpreted to mean either "and" or "or" when it appears in a title.

8. **"With"**—The word "with" in the alphabetic index is sequenced immediately following the main term, not in alphabetical order.

9. **"See" and "See Also"**—The "see" instruction following a main term in the index indicates that another term should be referenced. It is necessary to go to the main term referenced with the "see" note to locate the correct code.

    A "see also" instruction following a main term in the index instructs that there is another main term that may also be referenced that may provide additional index entries that may be

useful. It is not necessary to follow the "see also" note when the original main term provides the necessary code.

B. **General Coding Guidelines**

1. **Use of both Alphabetic Index and Tabular List**—Use both the Alphabetic Index and the Tabular List when locating and assigning a code. Reliance on only the Alphabetic Index or the Tabular List leads to errors in code assignments and less specificity in code selection.

2. **Locate each term in the Alphabetic Index**—Locate each term in the Alphabetic Index and verify the code selected in the Tabular List. Read and be guided by instructional notations that appear in both the Alphabetic Index and the Tabular List.

3. **Level of detail in coding**—Diagnosis and procedure codes are to be used at their highest number of digits available.

    ICD-9-CM diagnosis codes are composed of codes with either 3, 4, or 5 digits. Codes with three digits are included in ICD-9-CM as the heading of a category of codes that may be further subdivided by the use of fourth and/or fifth digits, which provide greater detail.

    A three-digit code is to be used only if it is not further subdivided. Where fourth-digit subcategories and/or fifth-digit subclassifications are provided, they must be assigned. A code is invalid if it has not been coded to the full number of digits required for that code. For example, Acute myocardial infarction, code 410, has fourth digits that describe the location of the infarction (e.g., 410.2, Of inferolateral wall), and fifth digits that identify the episode of care. It would be incorrect to report a code in category 410 without a fourth and fifth digit.

    ICD-9-CM Volume 3 procedure codes are composed of codes with either 3 or 4 digits. Codes with two digits are included in ICD-9-CM as the heading of a category of codes that may be further subdivided by the use of third and/or fourth digits, which provide greater detail.

4. **Code or codes from 001.0 through V86.1**—The appropriate code or codes from 001.0 through V86.1 must be used to identify diagnoses, symptoms, conditions, problems, complaints or other reason(s) for the encounter/visit.

5. **Selection of codes 001.0 through 999.9**—The selection of codes 001.0 through 999.9 will frequently be used to describe the reason for the admission/encounter. These codes are from the section of ICD-9-CM for the classification of diseases and injuries (e.g., infectious and parasitic diseases; neoplasms; symptoms, signs, and ill-defined conditions, etc.).

6. **Signs and symptoms**—Codes that describe symptoms and signs, as opposed to diagnoses, are acceptable for reporting purposes when a related definitive diagnosis has not been established (confirmed) by the provider. Chapter 16 of ICD-9-CM, Symptoms, Signs, and Ill-defined Conditions (codes 780.0–799.9) contain many, but not all codes for symptoms.

7. **Conditions that are an integral part of a disease process**—Signs and symptoms that are integral to the disease process should not be assigned as additional codes, **unless otherwise instructed by the classification.**

8. **Conditions that are not an integral part of a disease process**—Additional signs and symptoms that may not be associated routinely with a disease process should be coded when present.

9. **Multiple coding for a single condition**—In addition to the etiology/manifestation convention that requires two codes to fully describe a single condition that affects multiple body systems, there are other single conditions that also require more than one code. "Use additional code" notes are found in the tabular at codes that are not part of an etiology/manifestation pair where a secondary code is useful to fully describe a condition. The sequencing rule is the same as the etiology/manifestation pair, "use additional code" indicates that a secondary code should be added.

    For example, for infections that are not included in chapter 1, a secondary code from category 041 Bacterial infection in conditions classified elsewhere and of unspecified site, may be required to identify the bacterial organism causing the infection. A "use additional code" note will normally be found at the infectious disease code, indicating a need for the organism code to be added as a secondary code.

    "Code first" notes are also under certain codes that are not specifically manifestation codes but may be due to an underlying cause. When a "code first" note is present and an underlying condition is present the underlying condition should be sequenced first.

"Code, if applicable, any causal condition first," notes indicate that this code may be assigned as a principal diagnosis when the causal condition is unknown or not applicable. If a causal condition is known, then the code for that condition should be sequenced as the principal or first-listed diagnosis.

Multiple codes may be needed for late effects, complication codes and obstetric codes to more fully describe a condition. See the specific guidelines for these conditions for further instruction.

10. **Acute and Chronic Conditions**—If the same condition is described as both acute (subacute) and chronic, and separate subentries exist in the Alphabetic Index at the same indentation level, code both and sequence the acute (subacute) code first.

11. **Combination Code**—A combination code is a single code used to classify:
    - Two diagnoses, or
    - A diagnosis with an associated secondary process (manifestation)
    - A diagnosis with an associated complication

Combination codes are identified by referring to subterm entries in the Alphabetic Index and by reading the inclusion and exclusion notes in the Tabular List.

Assign only the combination code when that code fully identifies the diagnostic conditions involved or when the Alphabetic Index so directs. Multiple coding should not be used when the classification provides a combination code that clearly identifies all of the elements documented in the diagnosis. When the combination code lacks necessary specificity in describing the manifestation or complication, an additional code should be used as a secondary code.

12. **Late Effects**—A late effect is the residual effect (condition produced) after the acute phase of an illness or injury has terminated. There is no time limit on when a late effect code can be used. The residual may be apparent early, such as in cerebrovascular accident cases, or it may occur months or years later, such as that due to a previous injury. Coding of late effects generally requires two codes sequenced in the following order: The condition or nature of the late effect is sequenced first. The late effect code is sequenced second.

An exception to the above guidelines are those instances where the code for late effect is followed by a manifestation code identified in the Tabular List and title, or the late effect code has been expanded (at the fourth and fifth-digit levels) to include the manifestation(s). The code for the acute phase of an illness or injury that led to the late effect is never used with a code for the late effect.

13. **Impending or threatened condition**—Code any condition described at the time of discharge as "impending" or "threatened" as follows:
    - If it did occur, code as confirmed diagnosis.
    - If it did not occur, reference the Alphabetic Index to determine if the condition has a subentry term for "impending" or "threatened" and also reference main term entries for "Impending" and for "Threatened."
    - If the subterms are listed, assign the given code.
    - If the subterms are not listed, code the existing underlying condition(s) and not the condition described as impending or threatened.

**C. Chapter-Specific Coding Guidelines**—In addition to general coding guidelines, there are guidelines for specific diagnoses and/or conditions in the classification. Unless otherwise indicated, these guidelines apply to all health care settings. Please refer to Section II for guidelines on the selection of principal diagnosis.

1. **Chapter 1: Infectious and Parasitic Diseases (001-139)**
    a. **Human immunodeficiency virus (HIV) infections**
        1) **Code only confirmed cases**—Code only confirmed cases of HIV infection/illness. This is an exception to the hospital inpatient guideline Section II, H.

        In this context, "confirmation" does not require documentation of positive serology or culture for HIV; the provider's diagnostic statement that the patient is HIV positive, or has an HIV-related illness is sufficient.

    2) Selection and sequencing of HIV codes
        (a) **Patient admitted for HIV-related condition**—If a patient is admitted for an HIV-related condition, the principal diagnosis should be 042, followed by additional diagnosis codes for all reported HIV-related conditions.
        (b) **Patient with HIV didsase admitted for unrelated condition**—If a patient with HIV disease is admitted for an unrelated condition (such as a traumatic injury), the code for the unrelated condition (e.g., the nature of injury code) should be the principal diagnosis. Other diagnoses would be 042 followed by additional diagnosis codes for all reported HIV-related conditions.
        (c) **Whether the patient is newly diagnosed**—Whether the patient is newly diagnosed or has had previous admissions/encounters for HIV conditions is irrelevant to the sequencing decision.
        (d) **Asymptomatic human immunodefiency virus**—V08 Asymptomatic human immunodeficiency virus [HIV] infection, is to be applied when the patient without any documentation of symptoms is listed as being "HIV positive," "known HIV," "HIV test positive," or similar terminology. Do not use this code if the term "AIDS" is used or if the patient is treated for any HIV-related illness or is described as having any condition(s) resulting from his/her HIV positive status; use 042 in these cases.
        (e) **Patients with inconclusive HIV serology**—Patients with inconclusive HIV serology, but no definitive diagnosis or manifestations of the illness, may be assigned code 795.71, Inconclusive serologic test for human immunodeficiency virus [HIV].
        (f) **Previously diagnosed HIV-related illness**—Patients with any known prior diagnosis of an HIV-related illness should be coded to 042. Once a patient has developed an HIV-related illness, the patient should always be assigned code 042 on every subsequent admission/encounter. Patients previously diagnosed with any HIV illness (042) should never be assigned to 795.71 or V08.
        (g) **HIV infection in pregnancy, childbirth and the peuerperium**—During pregnancy, childbirth or the puerperium, a patient admitted (or presenting for a health care encounter) because of an HIV-related illness should receive a principal diagnosis code of 647.6X Other specified infectious and parasitic diseases in the mother classifiable elsewhere, but complicating the pregnancy, childbirth or the puerperium, followed by 042 and the code(s) for the HIV-related illness(es). Codes from Chapter 15 always take sequencing priority.

        Patients with asymptomatic HIV infection status admitted (or presenting for a health care encounter) during pregnancy, childbirth, or the puerperium should receive codes of 647.6X and V08.
        (h) **Encounters for testing HIV**—If a patient is being seen to determine his/her HIV status, use code V73.89, Screening for other specified viral disease. Use code V69.8, Other problems related to lifestyle, as a secondary code if an asymptomatic patient is in a known high risk group for HIV. Should a patient with signs or symptoms or illness, or a confirmed HIV related diagnosis be tested for HIV, code the signs and symptoms or the diagnosis. An additional counseling code V65.44 may be used if counseling is provided during the encounter for the test.

        When a patient returns to be informed of his/her HIV test results use code V65.44, HIV counseling, if the results of the test are negative.

        If the results are positive but the patient is asymptomatic use code V08, Asymptomatic HIV infection. If the results are positive and the patient is symptomatic use code 042, HIV infection, with codes for the HIV related symptoms or diagnosis. The HIV counseling code may also be used if counseling is provided for patients with positive test results.

b. **Septicemia, Systemic Inflammatory Response Syndrome (SIRS), Sepsis, Severe Sepsis, and Septic Shock**

   1) **SIRS, Septicemia, and Sepsis**

      (a) The terms *septicemia* and *sepsis* are often used interchangeably by providers, however they are not considered synonymous terms. The following descriptions are provided for reference but do not preclude querying the provider for clarification about terms used in the documentation:

         (i) Septicemia generally refers to a systemic disease associated with the presence of pathological microorganisms or toxins in the blood, which can include bacteria, viruses, fungi or other organisms.

         (ii) Systemic inflammatory response syndrome (SIRS) generally refers to the systemic response to infection, trauma/burns, or other insult (such as cancer) with symptoms including fever, tachycardia, tachypnea, and leukocytosis.

         (iii) Sepsis generally refers to SIRS due to infection.

         (iv) Severe sepsis generally refers to sepsis with associated acute organ dysfunction.

      (b) The coding of SIRS, sepsis and severe sepsis requires a minimum of 2 codes: a code for the underlying cause (such as infection or trauma) and a code from subcategory 995.9 Systemic inflammatory response syndrome (SIRS).

         (i) The code for the underlying cause (such as infection or trauma) must be sequenced before the code from subcategory 995.9 Systemic inflammatory response syndrome (SIRS).

         (ii) Sepsis and severe sepsis require a code for the systemic infection (038.xx, 112.5, etc.) and either code 995.91, Sepsis, or 995.92, Severe sepsis. If the causal organism is not documented, assign code 038.9, Unspecified septicemia.

         (iii) Severe sepsis requires additional code(s) for the associated acute organ dysfunction(s).

         (iv) If a patient has sepsis with multiple organ dysfunctions, follow the instructions for coding severe sepsis.

         (v) Either the term sepsis or SIRS must be documented to assign a code from subcategory 995.9.

         (vi) *See Section I.C.17.g, Injury and poisoning, for information regarding systematic inflammatory response syndrome (SIRS) due to trauma/burns and other noninfectious processes.*

      (c) Due to the complex nature of sepsis and severe sepsis, some cases may require querying the provider prior to assignment of the codes.

   2) **Sequencing sepsis and severe sepsis**

      (a) **Sepsis and severe sepsis as principal diagnosis—** If sepsis **or severe sepsis** is present on admission, and meets the definition of principal diagnosis, the **systemic infection code** (e.g., 038.xx, 112.5, etc.) should be assigned as the principal diagnosis, followed by code **995.91 Sepsis** or **995.92 Severe Sepsis**, as required by the sequencing rules in the Tabular List. Codes from subcategory 995.9 can never be assigned as a principal diagnosis. **A code should also be assigned for any localized infection, if present.**

      (b) **Sepsis and severe sepsis as secondary diagnoses—** When sepsis **or severe sepsis** develops during the encounter (it was not present on admission), the **systematic infection code and code 995.91 or 995.92 should be assigned** as secondary diagnoses.

      (c) **Documentation unclear as to whether sepsis or severe sepsis is present on admission—**Sepsis or severe sepsis may be present on admission but the

diagnosis may not be confirmed until sometime after admission. **If the documentation is not clear whether the sepsis or severe sepsis was present on admission, the provider should be queried.**

   3) **Sepsis/SIRS with localized infection**—If the reason for admission is both sepsis, severe sepsis, or SIRS and a localized infection, such as pneumonia or cellulitis, a code for the systemic infection (038.xx, 112.5, etc) should be assigned first, then code 995.91 or 995.92, followed by the code for the localized infection. If the patient is admitted with a localized infection, such as pneumonia, and sepsis/SIRS doesn't develop until after admission, see guideline 2b.

      Note: The term urosepsis is a nonspecific term. If that is the only term documented then only code 599.0 should be assigned based on the default for the term in the ICD-9-CM index, in addition to the code for the causal organism if known.

   4) **Bacterial sepsis and septicemia**—In most cases, it will be a code from category 038 Septicemia, that will be used in conjunction with a code from subcategory 995.9 such as the following:

      (a) Streptococcal sepsis—If the documentation in the record states streptococcal sepsis, codes 038.0 Streptococcal septicemia, and code 995.91 should be used, in that sequence.

      (b) Streptococcal septicemia—If the documentation states streptococcal septicemia, only code 038.0 should be assigned however, the provider should be queried whether the patient has sepsis, an infection with SIRS.

   5) **Acute organ dysfunction that is not clearly associated with the sepsis**—If a patient has sepsis and an acute organ dysfunction, but the medical record documentation indicates that the acute organ dysfunction is related to a medical condition other than the sepsis, do not assign code 995.92 Severe sepsis. An acute organ dysfunction must be associated with the sepsis in order to assign the severe sepsis code. If the documentation is not clear as to whether an acute organ dysfunction is related to the sepsis or another medical condition, query the provider.

   6) **Septic shock**

      (a) **Sequencing of septic shock**—Septic shock **generally refers to circulatory failure** associated with severe sepsis, **and, therefore, it represents a type of acute organ dysfunction. For all cases of septic shock, the code for the systemic infection should be sequenced first, followed by codes 995.92 and 785.52. Any additional codes for other acute organ dysfunctions should also be assigned.** As noted in the sequencing instructions in the Tabular List, the code for septic shock cannot be assigned as a principal diagnosis.

      (b) **Septic shock without documentation of severe sepsis**—Septic shock **indicates the presence of severe sepsis. Code 995.92 Severe sepsis, must be assigned with code 785.52 Septic shock, even if the term severe sepsis is not documented in the record.** The "use additional code" note and the "code first" note **in the tabular support this guideline.**

   7) **Sepsis and septic shock complicating abortion and pregnancy**—Sepsis and septic shock complicating abortion, ectopic pregnancy, and molar pregnancy are classified to category codes in Chapter 11 (630-639). *See section I.C.11.*

   8) **Negative or inconclusive blood cultures**—Negative or inconclusive blood cultures do not preclude a diagnosis of septicemia or sepsis in patients with clinical evidence of the condition, however, the provider should be queried.

9) **Newborn sepsis**—*See Section I.C.15.j for information on the coding of newborn sepsis.*

10) **Sepsis due to a postprocedural infection**—Sepsis resulting from a postprocedural infection is a complication of care. For such cases, **the postprocedural infection, such as code 998.59, Other postoperative infection, or 674.3x, Other complications of obstetrical surgical wounds**, should be coded first followed by the appropriate sepsis **codes (systemic infection code and either code 995.91or 995.92). An additional code(s) for any acute organ dysfunction should also be assigned for cases of severe sepsis.**

11) **External cause of injury codes with SIRS**—*Refer to Section I.C.19.a.7 for instruction on the use of external cause of injury codes with codes for SIRS resulting from trauma.*

12) <u>**Sepsis and severe sepsis associated with noninfectious process**</u>—**In some cases, a non-infectious process, such as trauma, may lead to an infection which can result in sepsis or severe sepsis. If sepsis or severe sepsis is documented as associated with a non-infectious condition, such as a burn or serious injury, and this condition meets the definition for principal diagnosis, the code for the non-infectious condition should be sequenced first, followed by the code for the systemic infection and either code 995.91, Sepsis, or 995.92, Severe sepsis. Additional codes for any associated acute organ dysfunction(s) should also be assigned for cases of severe sepsis. If the sepsis or severe sepsis meets the definition of principal diagnosis, the systemic infection and sepsis codes should be sequenced before the non-infectious condition.** *See Section I.C.1.b.2)(a) for guidelines pertaining to sepsis or severe sepsis as the principal diagnosis.* **When both the associated non-infectious condition and the sepsis or severe sepsis meet the definition of principal diagnosis, either may be assigned as principal diagnosis.**

**Only one SIRS code, representing the sepsis or severe sepsis, should be assigned for patients with sepsis or severe sepsis associated with trauma or other non-infectious condition. Do not assign codes 995.93, Systemic inflammatory response syndrome due to non-infectious process without acute organ dysfunction, or 995.94, Systemic inflammatory response syndrome due to noninfectious process with acute organ dysfunction, in addition to 995.91, Sepsis, or 995.92, Severe sepsis, if the patient has sepsis or severe sepsis associated with a non-infectious condition.**

*See Section I.C.17.g for information on the coding of SIRS due to trauma/burns or other non-infectious disease processes.*

2. **Chapter 2: Neoplasms (140-239)**

**General guidelines**

Chapter 2 of the ICD-9-CM contains the codes for most benign and all malignant neoplasms. Certain benign neoplasms, such as prostatic adenomas, may be found in the specific body system chapters. To properly code a neoplasm it is necessary to determine from the record if the neoplasm is benign, in-situ, malignant, or of uncertain histologic behavior. If malignant, any secondary (metastatic) sites should also be determined.

The neoplasm table in the Alphabetic Index should be referenced first. However, if the histological term is documented, that term should be referenced first, rather than going immediately to the Neoplasm Table, in order to determine which column in the Neoplasm Table is appropriate. For example, if the documentation indicates "adenoma," refer to the term in the Alphabetic Index to review the entries under this term and the instructional note to "see also neoplasm, by site, benign." The table provides the proper code based on the type of neoplasm and the site. It is important to select the proper column in the table that corresponds to the type of neoplasm. The tabular should then be referenced to verify that the correct code has been selected from the table and that a more specific site code does not exist.

*See Section I. C. 18.d.4. for information regarding V codes for genetic susceptibility to cancer.*

a. **Treatment directed at the malignancy**—If the treatment is directed at the malignancy, designate the malignancy as the principal diagnosis.

b. **Treatment of secondary site**—When a patient is admitted because of a primary neoplasm with metastasis and treatment is directed toward the secondary site only, the secondary neoplasm is designated as the principal diagnosis even though the primary malignancy is still present.

c. **Coding and sequencing of complications**—Coding and sequencing of complications associated with the malignancies or with the therapy thereof are subject to the following guidelines:

1) **Anemia associated with malignancy**—When admission/encounter is for management of an anemia associated with the malignancy, and the treatment is only for anemia, the appropriate anemia code (such as code 285.22, Anemia in neoplastic disease) is designated as the principal diagnosis and is followed by the appropriate code(s) for the malignancy.
Code 285.22 may also be used as a secondary code if the patient suffers from anemia and is being treated for the malignancy.

2) **Anemia associated with chemotherapy, immunotherapy and radiation therapy**—When the admission/encounter is for management of an anemia associated with chemotherapy, immunotherapy or radiotherapy and the only treatment is for the anemia, the anemia is sequenced first followed by code E933.1. The appropriate neoplasm code should be assigned as an additional code.

3) **Management of dehydration due to the malignancy**—When the admission/encounter is for management of dehydration due to the malignancy or the therapy, or a combination of both, and only the dehydration is being treated (intravenous rehydration), the dehydration is sequenced first, followed by the code(s) for the malignancy.

4) **Treatment of a complication resulting from a surgical procedure**—When the admission/encounter is for treatment of a complication resulting from a surgical procedure, designate the complication as the principal or first-listed diagnosis if treatment is directed at resolving the complication.

d. **Primary malignancy previously excised**—When a primary malignancy has been previously excised or eradicated from its site and there is no further treatment directed to that site and there is no evidence of any existing primary malignancy, a code from category V10, Personal history of malignant neoplasm, should be used to indicate the former site of the malignancy. Any mention of extension, invasion, or metastasis to another site is coded as a secondary malignant neoplasm to that site. The secondary site may be the principal or first-listed with the V10 code used as a secondary code.

e. **Admissions/encounters involving chemotherapy, immunotherapy and radiation therapy**

1) **Episode of care involves surgical removal of neoplasm**—When an episode of care involves the surgical removal of a neoplasm, primary or secondary site, followed by adjunct chemotherapy or radiation treatment during the same episode of care, the neoplasm code should be assigned as principal or first-listed diagnosis, using codes in the 140-198 series or where appropriate in the 200-203 series.

2) **Patient admission/encounter solely for administration of chemotherapy, immunotherapy and radiation therapy**—If a patient admission/encounter is solely for the administration of chemotherapy, immunotherapy or radiation therapy assign code V58.0, Encounter for radiation therapy, or V58.11, Encounter for antineoplastic chemotherapy, or V58.12, Encounter for antineoplastic immunotherapy as the first-listed or principal diagnosis. If a patient receives more than one of these therapies during the

same admission more than one of these codes may be assigned, in any sequence.

**3) Patient admitted for radiotherapy/chemotherapy and immunotherapy and develops complications—**When a patient is admitted for the purpose of radiotherapy, immunotherapy or chemotherapy and develops complications such as uncontrolled nausea and vomiting or dehydration, the principal or first-listed diagnosis is V58.0, Encounter for radiotherapy, or V58.11, Encounter for antineoplastic chemotherapy, or V58.12, Encounter for antineoplastic immunotherapy followed by any codes for the complications. *See Section I.C.18.d.7. for additional information regarding aftercare V codes.*

**f. Admission/encounter to determine extent of malignancy—**When the reason for admission/encounter is to determine the extent of the malignancy, or for a procedure such as paracentesis or thoracentesis, the primary malignancy or appropriate metastatic site is designated as the principal or first-listed diagnosis, even though chemotherapy or radiotherapy is administered.

**g. Symptoms, signs, and ill-defined conditions listed in Chapter 16—**Symptoms, signs, and ill-defined conditions listed in Chapter 16 characteristic of, or associated with, an existing primary or secondary site malignancy cannot be used to replace the malignancy as principal or first-listed diagnosis, regardless of the number of admissions or encounters for treatment and care of the neoplasm.
*See Section I.C.18.d.14, Encounter for prophylactic organ removal.*

**h. Admission/encounter for pain control/management—***See Section I.C.6.a.5 for information on coding admission/encounter for pain control/management.*

**3. Chapter 3: Endocrine, Nutritional, and Metabolic Diseases and Immunity Disorders (240-279)**

**a. Diabetes mellitus—**Codes under category 250, Diabetes mellitus, identify complications/manifestations associated with diabetes mellitus. A fifth-digit is required for all category 250 codes to identify the type of diabetes mellitus and whether the diabetes is controlled or uncontrolled.

**1) Fifth-digits for category 250:**
The following are the fifth-digits for the codes under category 250:

0 type II or unspecified type, not stated as uncontrolled
1 type I, [juvenile type], not stated as uncontrolled
2 type II or unspecified type, uncontrolled
3 type I, [juvenile type], uncontrolled

The age of a patient is not the sole determining factor, though most type I diabetics develop the condition before reaching puberty. For this reason type I diabetes mellitus is also referred to as juvenile diabetes.

**2) Type of diabetes mellitus not documented—**If the type of diabetes mellitus is not documented in the medical record the default is type II.

**3) Diabetes mellitus and the use of insulin—**All type I diabetics must use insulin to replace what their bodies do not produce. However, the use of insulin does not mean that a patient is a type I diabetic. Some patients with type II diabetes mellitus are unable to control their blood sugar through diet and oral medication alone and do require insulin. If the documentation in a medical record does not indicate the type of diabetes but does indicate that the patient uses insulin, the appropriate fifth-digit for type II must be used. For type II patients who routinely use insulin, code V58.67, Long-term (current) use of insulin, should also be assigned to indicate that the patient uses insulin. Code V58.67 should not be assigned if insulin is given temporarily to bring a type II patient's blood sugar under control during an encounter.

**4) Assigning and sequencing diabetes codes and associated conditions—**When assigning codes for diabetes and its associated conditions, the code(s) from category 250 must be sequenced before the codes for the associated conditions. The diabetes codes and the secondary codes that correspond to them are paired codes that follow the etiology/manifestation convention

of the classification (*See Section I.A.6., Etiology/manifestation convention*). Assign as many codes from category 250 as needed to identify all of the associated conditions that the patient has. The corresponding secondary codes are listed under each of the diabetes codes.

**(a) Diabetic retinopathy/diabetic macular edema—**Diabetic macular edema, code 362.07, is only present with diabetic retinopathy. Another code from subcategory 362.0, Diabetic retinopathy, must be used with code 362.07. Codes under subcategory 362.0 are diabetes manifestation codes, so they must be used following the appropriate diabetes code.

**5) Diabetes mellitus in pregnancy and gestational diabetes**

**(a)** For diabetes mellitus complicating pregnancy, see Section I.C.11.f., Diabetes mellitus in pregnancy.

**(b)** For gestational diabetes, see Section I.C.11, g., Gestational diabetes.

**6) Insulin pump malfunction**

**(a) Underdose of insulin due insulin pump failure—**An underdose of insulin due to an insulin pump failure should be assigned 996.57, Mechanical complication due to insulin pump, as the principal or first listed code, followed by the appropriate diabetes mellitus code based on documentation.

**(b) Overdose of insulin due to insulin pump failure—**The principal or first listed code for an encounter due to an insulin pump malfunction resulting in an overdose of insulin, should also be 996.57, Mechanical complication due to insulin pump, followed by code 962.3, Poisoning by insulins and antidiabetic agents, and the appropriate diabetes mellitus code based on documentation.

**4. Chapter 4: Diseases of Blood and Blood Forming Organs (280-289)**

**a. Anemia of chronic disease—**Subcategory 285.2, Anemia in chronic illness, has codes for anemia in chronic kidney disease, code 285.21; anemia in neoplastic disease, code 285.22; and anemia in other chronic illness, code 285.29. These codes can be used as the principal/first listed code if the reason for the encounter is to treat the anemia. They may also be used as secondary codes if treatment of the anemia is a component of an encounter, but not the primary reason for the encounter. When using a code from subcategory 285 it is also necessary to use the code for the chronic condition causing the anemia.

**1) Anemia in chronic kidney disease—**When assigning code 285.21, Anemia in chronic kidney disease, it is also necessary to assign a code from category 585, Chronic kidney disease, to indicate the stage of chronic kidney disease.
*See I.C.10.a. Chronic kidney disease (CKD).*

**2) Anemia in neoplastic disease—**When assigning code 285.22, Anemia in neoplastic disease, it is also necessary to assign the neoplasm code that is responsible for the anemia. Code 285.22 is for use for anemia that is due to the malignancy, not for anemia due to antineoplastic chemotherapy drugs, which is an adverse effect.
*See I.C.2.c.1 Anemia associated with malignancy.*
*See I.C.2.c.2 Anemia associated with chemotherapy, immunotherapy and radiation therapy.*
*See I.C.17.e.1. Adverse effects.*

**5. Chapter 5: Mental Disorders (290-319)**
Reserved for future guideline expansion

**6. Chapter 6: Diseases of Nervous System and Sense Organs (320-389)**

**a. Pain — Category 338**

**1) General coding information—Codes in category 338 may be used in conjunction with codes from other categories and chapters to provide more detail about acute or chronic pain and neoplasm-related pain. If the pain is not specified as acute or chronic, do not assign codes from**

category 338, except for post-thoracotomy pain, postoperative pain or neoplasm related pain.

A code from subcategories 338.1 and 338.2 should not be assigned if the underlying (definitive) diagnosis is known, unless the reason for the encounter is pain control/management and not management of the underlying condition.

(a) Category 338 codes as principal or first-listed diagnosis
Category 338 codes are acceptable as principal diagnosis or the first-listed code for reporting purposes:

- When the related definitive diagnosis has not been established (confirmed) by the provider, or
- When pain control or pain management is the reason for the admission/encounter (e.g., a patient with displaced intervertebral disc, nerve impingement and severe back pain presents for injection of steroid into the spinal canal). The underlying cause of the pain should be reported as an additional diagnosis, if known.

(b) Use of category 338 codes in conjunction with site specific pain codes

(i) Assigning category 338 codes and site-specific Pain Codes—Codes from category 338 may be used in conjunction with codes that identify the site of pain (including codes from chapter 16) if the category 338 code provides additional information. For example, if the code describes the site of the pain, but does not fully describe whether the pain is acute or chronic, then both codes should be assigned.

(ii) Sequencing of category 338 codes with site-specific pain codes—The sequencing of category 338 codes with site-specific pain codes (including chapter 16 codes), is dependent on the circumstances of the encounter/admission as follows:

- If the encounter is for pain control or pain management, assign the code from category 338 followed by the code identifying the specific site of pain (e.g., encounter for pain management for acute neck pain from trauma is assigned code 338.11, Acute pain due to trauma, followed by code 723.1, Cervicalgia, to identify the site of pain).
- If the encounter is for any other reason except pain control or pain management, and a related definitive diagnosis has not been established (confirmed) by the provider, assign the code for the specific site of pain first, followed by the appropriate code from category 338.

2) **Pain due to devices**—Pain associated with devices or foreign bodies left in a surgical site is assigned to the appropriate code(s) found in Chapter 17, Injury and Poisoning (for example painful retained suture).

3) **Postoperative pain**—Post-thoracotomy pain and other postoperative pain are classified to subcategories 338.1 and 338.2, depending on whether the pain is acute or chronic.

**The default for post-thoracotomy and other postoperative pain not specified as acute or chronic is the code for the acute form.**

**Postoperative pain not associated with a specific postoperative complication is assigned to the appropriate postoperative pain code in category 338.**

**Postoperative pain associated with a specific postoperative complication (such as a device left in the body) is assigned to the appropriate code(s) found in Chapter 17, Injury and Poisoning. Since the complication represents the underlying (definitive) diagnosis associated with the pain, no additional code should be assigned from category 338. If pain control/management is the reason for the encounter, a code from category 338 should be assigned as the principal or first-listed diagnosis in accordance with *Section I.C.6.a.1.a above*.**

Postoperative pain may be reported as the principal or first-listed diagnosis when the stated reason for the admission/encounter is documented as postoperative pain control/management.

Postoperative pain may be reported as a secondary diagnosis code when a patient presents for outpatient surgery and develops an unusual or inordinate amount of postoperative pain.

Routine or expected postoperative pain immediately after surgery should not be coded.

The provider's documentation should be used to guide the coding of postoperative pain, as well as Section III. Reporting Additional Diagnoses and Section IV. Diagnostic Coding and Reporting in the Outpatient Setting.

*See Section II.I.2 for information on sequencing of diagnoses for patients admitted to hospital inpatient care following post-operative observation.*

*See Section II.J for information on sequencing of diagnoses for patients admitted to hospital inpatient care from outpatient surgery.*

*See Section IV.A.2 for information on sequencing of diagnoses for patients admitted for observation.*

4) **Chronic pain**—Chronic pain is classified to subcategory 338.2. There is no time frame defining when pain becomes chronic pain. The provider's documentation should be used to guide use of these codes.

5) **Neoplasm related pain**—Code 338.3 is assigned to pain documented as being related, associated or due to cancer, primary or secondary malignancy, or tumor. This code is assigned regardless of whether the pain is acute or chronic.

This code may be assigned as the principal or first-listed code when the stated reason for the admission/encounter is documented as pain control/pain management. The underlying neoplasm should be reported as an additional diagnosis.

When the reason for the admission/encounter is management of the neoplasm and the pain associated with the neoplasm is also documented, code 338.3 may be assigned as an additional diagnosis.

*See Section I.C.2 for instructions on the sequencing of neoplasms for all other stated reasons for the admission/encounter (except for pain control/pain management).*

6) **Chronic pain syndrome**—This condition is different than the term "chronic pain," and therefore this code should only be used when the provider has specifically documented this condition.

7. Chapter 7: Diseases of Circulatory System (390-459)

a. Hypertension

**Hypertension Table**—The Hypertension Table, found under the main term, "Hypertension," in the Alphabetic Index, contains a complete listing of all conditions due to or associated with hypertension and classifies them according to malignant, benign, and unspecified.

1) **Hypertension, essential, or NOS**—Assign hypertension (arterial) (essential) (primary) (systemic) (NOS) to category code 401 with the appropriate fourth digit to indicate malignant (.0), benign (.1), or unspecified (.9). Do not use either .0 malignant or .1 benign unless medical record documentation supports such a designation.

2) **Hypertension with heart disease**—Heart conditions (425.8, 429.0-429.3, 429.8, 429.9) are assigned to a code from category 402 when a causal relationship is stated (due to hypertension) or implied (hypertensive). Use an additional code from category 428 to identify the type of heart failure in those patients with heart failure. More than one code from category 428 may be assigned if the patient has systolic or diastolic failure and congestive heart failure. The same heart conditions (425.8, 429.0-429.3, 429.8, 429.9) with hypertension, but without a stated causal relationship, are coded separately. Sequence according to the circumstances of the admission/encounter.

**3) Hypertensive <u>chronic</u> kidney disease**—Assign codes from category 403, Hypertensive **chronic** kidney disease, when conditions classified to categories 585-587 are present. Unlike hypertension with heart disease, ICD-9-CM presumes a cause-and-effect relationship and classifies **chronic kidney disease (CKD)** with hypertension as hypertensive **chronic** kidney disease.

**Fifth digits for category 403 should be assigned as follows:**

- **0 with CKD stage I through stage IV, or unspecified.**
- **1 with CKD stage V or end stage renal disease.**

**The appropriate code from category 585, Chronic kidney disease, should be used as a secondary code with a code from category 403 to identify the stage of chronic kidney disease.**

*See Section I.C.10.a for information on the coding of chronic kidney disease.*

**4) Hypertensive heart and <u>chronic</u> kidney disease**—Assign codes from combination category 404, Hypertensive heart and **chronic** kidney disease, when both hypertensive kidney disease and hypertensive heart disease are stated in the diagnosis. Assume a relationship between the hypertension and the **chronic** kidney disease, whether or not the condition is so designated. Assign an additional code from category 428, to identify the type of heart failure. More than one code from category 428 may be assigned if the patient has systolic or diastolic failure and congestive heart failure.

**Fifth digits for category 404 should be assigned as follows:**

- **0 without heart failure and with chronic kidney disease (CKD) stage I through stage IV, or unspecified**
- **1 with heart failure and with CKD stage I through stage IV, or unspecified**
- **2 without heart failure and with CKD stage V or end stage renal disease**
- **3 with heart failure and with CKD stage V or end stage renal disease**

**The appropriate code from category 585, Chronic kidney disease, should be used as a secondary code with a code from category 404 to identify the stage of kidney disease.**

*See Section I.C.10.a for information on the coding of chronic kidney disease.*

**5) Hypertensive cerebrovascular disease**—First assign codes from 430-438, Cerebrovascular disease, then the appropriate hypertension code from categories 401-405.

**6) Hypertensive retinopathy**—Two codes are necessary to identify the condition. First assign the code from subcategory 362.11, Hypertensive retinopathy, then the appropriate code from categories 401-405 to indicate the type of hypertension.

**7) Hypertension, secondary**—Two codes are required: one to identify the underlying etiology and one from category 405 to identify the hypertension. Sequencing of codes is determined by the reason for admission/encounter.

**8) Hypertension, transient**—Assign code 796.2, Elevated blood pressure reading without diagnosis of hypertension, unless patient has an established diagnosis of hypertension. Assign code 642.3x for transient hypertension of pregnancy.

**9) Hypertension, controlled**—Assign appropriate code from categories 401-405. This diagnostic statement usually refers to an existing state of hypertension under control by therapy.

**10) Hypertension, uncontrolled**—Uncontrolled hypertension may refer to untreated hypertension or hypertension not responding to current therapeutic regimen. In either case, assign the appropriate code from categories 401-405 to designate the stage and type of hypertension. Code to the type of hypertension.

**11) Elevated blood pressure**—For a statement of elevated blood pressure without further specificity, assign code 796.2, Elevated blood pressure reading without diagnosis of hypertension, rather than a code from category 401.

**b. Cerebral infarction/stroke/cerebrovascular accident (CVA)**—The terms stroke and CVA are often used interchangeably to refer to a cerebral infarction. The terms stroke, CVA, and cerebral infarction NOS are all indexed to the default code 434.91, Cerebral artery occlusion, unspecified, with infarction. Code 436, Acute, but ill-defined, cerebrovascular disease, should not be used when the documentation states stroke or CVA.

**c. Postoperative cerebrovascular accident**—A cerebrovascular hemorrhage or infarction that occurs as a result of medical intervention is coded to 997.02, Iatrogenic cerebrovascular infarction or hemorrhage. Medical record documentation should clearly specify the cause- and-effect relationship between the medical intervention and the cerebrovascular accident in order to assign this code. A secondary code from the code range 430-432 or from a code from subcategories 433 or 434 with a fifth digit of "1" should also be used to identify the type of hemorrhage or infarct.

This guideline conforms to the use additional code note instruction at category 997. Code 436, Acute, but ill-defined, cerebrovascular disease, should not be used as a secondary code with code 997.02.

**d. Late Effects of Cerebrovascular Disease**

**1) Category 438, Late Effects of Cerebrovascular disease**—Category 438 is used to indicate conditions classifiable to categories 430-437 as the causes of late effects (neurologic deficits), themselves classified elsewhere. These "late effects" include neurologic deficits that persist after initial onset of conditions classifiable to 430-437. The neurologic deficits caused by cerebrovascular disease may be present from the onset or may arise at any time after the onset of the condition classifiable to 430-437.

**2) Codes from category 438 with codes from 430-437**—Codes from category 438 may be assigned on a health care record with codes from 430-437, if the patient has a current cerebrovascular accident (CVA) and deficits from an old CVA.

**3) Code V12.59**—Assign code V12.59 (and not a code from category 438) as an additional code for history of cerebrovascular disease when no neurologic deficits are present.

**e. Acute myocardial infarction (AMI)**

**1) ST elevation myocardial infarction (STEMI) and non ST elevation myocardial infarction (NSTEMI)**—The ICD-9-CM codes for acute myocardial infarction (AMI) identify the site, such as anterolateral wall or true posterior wall. Subcategories 410.0-410.6 and 410.8 are used for ST elevation myocardial infarction (STEMI). Subcategory 410.7, Subendocardial infarction, is used for non ST elevation myocardial infarction (NSTEMI) and nontransmural MIs.

**2) Acute myocardial infarction, unspecified**—Subcategory 410.9 is the default for the unspecified term acute myocardial infarction. If only STEMI or transmural MI without the site is documented, query the provider as to the site, or assign a code from subcategory 410.9.

**3) AMI documented as nontransmural or subendocardial but site provided**—If an AMI is documented as nontransmural or subendocardial, but the site is provided, it is still coded as a subendocardial AMI. If NSTEMI evolves to STEMI, assign the STEMI code. If STEMI converts to NSTEMI due to thrombolytic therapy, it is still coded as STEMI.

**8. Chapter 8: Diseases of Respiratory System (460-519)**

**a. Chronic obstructive pulmonary disease [COPD] and asthma**

**1) Conditions that comprise COPD and asthma**—The conditions that comprise COPD are obstructive chronic bronchitis, subcategory 491.2, and emphysema, category 492. All asthma codes are under category 493, Asthma. Code 496, Chronic airway obstruction, not elsewhere classified, is a nonspecific code that should only be used when the documentation in a medical record does not specify the type of COPD being treated.

**2) Acute exacerbation of chronic obstructive bronchitis and asthma**—The codes for chronic obstructive bronchitis and asthma distinguish between uncomplicated cases and those in acute exacerbation. An acute exacerbation is a worsening or a decompensation of a chronic condition. An acute exacerbation is not equivalent to an infection superimposed on a chronic condition, though an exacerbation may be triggered by an infection.

**3) Overlapping nature of the conditions that comprise COPD and asthma**—Due to the overlapping nature of the conditions that make up COPD and asthma, there are many variations in the way these conditions are documented. Code selection must be based on the terms as documented. When selecting the correct code for the documented type of COPD and asthma, it is essential to first review the index, and then verify the code in the tabular list. There are many instructional notes under the different COPD subcategories and codes. It is important that all such notes be reviewed to assure correct code assignment.

**4) Acute exacerbation of asthma and status asthmaticus**—An acute exacerbation of asthma is an increased severity of the asthma symptoms, such as wheezing and shortness of breath. Status asthmaticus refers to a patient's failure to respond to therapy administered during an asthmatic episode and is a life threatening complication that requires emergency care. If status asthmaticus is documented by the provider with any type of COPD or with acute bronchitis, the status asthmaticus should be sequenced first. It supersedes any type of COPD including that with acute exacerbation or acute bronchitis. It is inappropriate to assign an asthma code with 5th digit 2, with acute exacerbation, together with an asthma code with 5th digit 1, with status asthmatics. Only the 5th digit 1 should be assigned.

**b. Chronic obstructive pulmonary disease [COPD] and bronchitis**

**1) Acute bronchitis with COPD**—Acute bronchitis, code 466.0, is due to an infectious organism. When acute bronchitis is documented with COPD, code 491.22, Obstructive chronic bronchitis with acute bronchitis, should be assigned. It is not necessary to also assign code 466.0. If a medical record documents acute bronchitis with COPD with acute exacerbation, only code 491.22 should be assigned. The acute bronchitis included in code 491.22 supersedes the acute exacerbation. If a medical record documents COPD with acute exacerbation without mention of acute bronchitis, only code 491.21 should be assigned.

**c. Acute Respiratory Failure**

**1) Acute respiratory failure as principal diagnosis**—**Code 518.81, Acute respiratory failure, may be assigned as a principal diagnosis when it is the condition established after study to be chiefly responsible for occasioning the admission to the hospital, and the selection is supported by the Alphabetic Index and Tabular List. However, chapter-specific coding guidelines (such as obstetrics, poisoning, HIV, newborn) that provide sequencing direction take precedence.**

**2) Acute respiratory failure as secondary diagnosis**—**Respiratory failure may be listed as a secondary diagnosis if it occurs after admission, or if it is present on admission, but does not meet the definition of principal diagnosis.**

**3) Sequencing of acute respiratory failure and another acute condition**—**When a patient is admitted with respiratory failure and another acute condition, (e.g., myocardial infarction, cerebrovascular accident), the principal diagnosis will not be the same in every situation. Selection of the principal diagnosis will be dependent on the circumstances of admission. If both the respiratory failure and the other acute condition are equally responsible for occasioning the admission to the hospital, and there are no chapter-specific sequencing rules, the guideline regarding two or more diagnoses that equally meet the definition for principal diagnosis (Section II, C.) may be applied in these situations. If the documentation is not clear as to whether acute respiratory failure and another condition are equally responsible for occasioning the admission, query the provider for clarification.**

**9. Chapter 9: Diseases of Digestive System (520-579)**
Reserved for future guideline expansion

**10. Chapter 10: Diseases of Genitourinary System (580-629)**

**a. Chronic kidney disease**

**1) Stages of chronic kidney disease (CKD)**—The ICD-9-CM classifies CKD based on severity. The severity of CKD is designated by stages I-V. Stage II, code 585.2, equates to mild CKD; stage III, code 585.3, equates to moderate CKD; and stage IV, code 585.4, equates to severe CKD. Code 585.6, End stage renal disease (ESRD), is assigned when the provider has documented end-stage-renal disease (ESRD).

If both a stage of CKD and ESRD are documented, assign code 585.6 only.

**2) Chronic kidney disease and kidney transplant status—Patients who have undergone kidney transplant may still have some form of CKD, because the kidney transplant may not fully restore kidney function. Therefore, the presence of CKD alone does not constitute a transplant complication. Assign the appropriate 585 code for the patient's stage of CKD and code V42.0. If a transplant complication such as failure or rejection is documented, *see section I.C.17.f.1.b for information on coding complications of a kidney transplant*. If the documentation is unclear as to whether the patient has a complication of the transplant, query the provider.**

**3) Chronic kidney disease with other conditions**—Patients with CKD may also suffer from other serious conditions, most commonly diabetes mellitus and hypertension. The sequencing of the CKD code in relationship to codes for other contributing conditions is based on the conventions in the tabular list.

*See I.C.3.a.4 for sequencing instructions for diabetes.*

*See I.C.4.a.1 for anemia in CKD.*

*See I.C.7.a.3 for hypertensive **chronic** kidney disease.*

*See I.C.17.f.1.b, Kidney transplant complications, for instructions on coding of documented rejection or failure.*

**11. Chapter 11: Complications of Pregnancy, Childbirth, and the Puerperium (630-677)**

**a. General rules for obstetric cases**

**1) Codes from chapter 11 and sequencing priority**—Obstetric cases require codes from chapter 11, codes in the range 630-677, Complications of Pregnancy, Childbirth, and the Puerperium. Chapter 11 codes have sequencing priority over codes from other chapters. Additional codes from other chapters may be used in conjunction with Chapter 11 codes to further specify conditions. Should the provider document that the pregnancy is incidental to the encounter, then code V22.2 should be used in place of any Chapter 11 codes. It is the provider's responsibility to state that the condition being treated is not affecting the pregnancy.

**2) Chapter 11 codes used only on the maternal record**—Chapter 11 codes are to be used only on the maternal record, never on the record of the newborn.

**3) Chapter 11 fifth-digits**—Categories 640-648, 651-676 have required fifth-digits, which indicate whether the encounter is antepartum, postpartum and whether a delivery has also occurred.

**4) Fifth-digits, appropriate for each code**—The fifth-digits, which are appropriate for each code number, are listed in brackets under each code. The fifth-digits on each code should all be consistent with each other. That is, should a delivery occur all of the fifth-digits should indicate the delivery.

**b. Selection of OB principal or first-listed diagnosis**

**1) Routine outpatient prenatal visits**—For routine outpatient prenatal visits when no complications are present codes V22.0, Supervision of normal first pregnancy, and V22.1, Supervision of other normal pregnancy, should be used as the first-listed diagnoses. These codes should not be used in conjunction with chapter 11 codes.

**2) Prenatal outpatient visits for high-risk patients**—For prenatal outpatient visits for patients with high-risk pregnancies, a code from category V23, Supervision of high-risk pregnancy, should be used as the principal or first-listed diagnosis. Secondary chapter 11 codes may be used in conjunction with these codes if appropriate.

**3) Episodes when no delivery occurs**—In episodes when no delivery occurs, the principal diagnosis should correspond to the principal complication of the pregnancy, which necessitated the encounter. Should more than one complication exist, all of which are treated or monitored, any of the complications codes may be sequenced first.

**4) When a delivery occurs**—When a delivery occurs, the principal diagnosis should correspond to the main circumstances or complication of the delivery. In cases of cesarean delivery, the selection of the principal diagnosis should correspond to the reason the cesarean delivery was performed unless the reason for admission/encounter was unrelated to the condition resulting in the cesarean delivery.

**5) Outcome of delivery**—An outcome of delivery code, V27.0-V27.9, should be included on every maternal record when a delivery has occurred. These codes are not to be used on subsequent records or on the newborn record.

**c. Fetal conditions affecting the management of the mother**

**1) Codes from category 655**—Known or suspected fetal abnormality affecting management of the mother, and category 656, Other fetal and placental problems affecting the management of the mother, are assigned only when the fetal condition is actually responsible for modifying the management of the mother, i.e., by requiring diagnostic studies, additional observation, special care, or termination of pregnancy. The fact that the fetal condition exists does not justify assigning a code from this series to the mother's record.

**2) In utero surgery**—In cases when surgery is performed on the fetus, a diagnosis code from category 655, Known or suspected fetal abnormalities affecting management of the mother, should be assigned identifying the fetal condition. Procedure code 75.36, Correction of fetal defect, should be assigned on the hospital inpatient record. No code from Chapter 15, the perinatal codes, should be used on the mother's record to identify fetal conditions. Surgery performed in utero on a fetus is still to be coded as an obstetric encounter.

**d. HIV infection in pregnancy, childbirth and the puerperium**—During pregnancy, childbirth or the puerperium, a patient admitted because of an HIV-related illness should receive a principal diagnosis of 647.6X, Other specified infectious and parasitic diseases in the mother classifiable elsewhere, but complicating the pregnancy, childbirth or the puerperium, followed by 042 and the code(s) for the HIV-related illness(es). Patients with asymptomatic HIV infection status admitted during pregnancy, childbirth, or the puerperium should receive codes of 647.6X and V08.

**e. Current conditions complicating pregnancy**—Assign a code from subcategory 648.x for patients that have current conditions when the condition affects the management of the pregnancy, childbirth, or the puerperium. Use additional secondary codes from other chapters to identify the conditions, as appropriate.

**f. Diabetes mellitus in pregnancy**—Diabetes mellitus is a significant complicating factor in pregnancy. Pregnant women who are diabetic should be assigned code 648.0x, Diabetes mellitus complicating pregnancy, and a secondary code from category 250, Diabetes mellitus, to identify the type of diabetes. Code V58.67, Long-term (current) use of insulin, should also be assigned if the diabetes mellitus is being treated with insulin.

**g. Gestational diabetes**—Gestational diabetes can occur during the second and third trimester of pregnancy in women who were not diabetic prior to pregnancy. Gestational diabetes can cause complications in the pregnancy similar to those of pre-existing diabetes mellitus. It also puts the woman at greater risk of developing diabetes after the pregnancy. Gestational diabetes is coded to 648.8x, Abnormal glucose tolerance. Codes 648.0x and 648.8x should never be used together on the same record. Code V58.67, Long-term (current) use of insulin, should also be assigned if the gestational diabetes is being treated with insulin.

**h. Normal delivery, code 650**

**1) Normal delivery**—Code 650 is for use in cases when a woman is admitted for a full-term normal delivery and delivers a single, healthy infant without any complications antepartum, during the delivery, or postpartum during the delivery episode. Code 650 is always a principal diagnosis. It is not to be used if any other code from chapter 11 is needed to describe a current complication of the antenatal, delivery, or perinatal period. Additional codes from other chapters may be used with code 650 if they are not related to or are in any way complicating the pregnancy.

**2) Normal delivery with resolved antepartum complication**—Code 650 may be used if the patient had a complication at some point during her pregnancy, but the complication is not present at the time of the admission for delivery.

**3) V27.0, Single liveborn, outcome of delivery**—V27.0, Single liveborn, is the only outcome of delivery code appropriate for use with 650.

**i. The postpartum and peripartum periods**

**1) Postpartum and peripartum periods**—The postpartum period begins immediately after delivery and continues for six weeks following delivery. The peripartum period is defined as the last month of pregnancy to five months postpartum.

**2) Postpartum complication**—A postpartum complication is any complication occurring within the six-week period.

**3) Pregnancy-related complications after 6 week period**—Chapter 11 codes may also be used to describe pregnancy-related complications after the six-week period should the provider document that a condition is pregnancy related.

**4) Postpartum complications occurring during the same admission as delivery**—Postpartum complications that occur during the same admission as the delivery are identified with a fifth digit of "2." Subsequent admissions/encounters for postpartum complications should be identified with a fifth digit of "4."

**5) Admission for routine postpartum care following delivery outside hospital**—When the mother delivers outside the hospital prior to admission and is admitted for routine postpartum care and no complications are noted, code V24.0, Postpartum care and examination immediately after delivery, should be assigned as the principal diagnosis.

**6) Admission following delivery outside hospital with postpartum conditions**—A delivery diagnosis code should not be used for a woman who has delivered prior to admission to the hospital. Any postpartum conditions and/or postpartum procedures should be coded.

**j. Code 677 Late effect of complication of pregnancy**

**1) Code 677**—Code 677, Late effect of complication of pregnancy, childbirth, and the puerperium is for use in those cases when an initial complication of a pregnancy develops a sequelae requiring care or treatment at a future date.

**2) After the initial postpartum period**—This code may be used at any time after the initial postpartum period.

**3) Sequencing of code 677**—This code, like all late effect codes, is to be sequenced following the code describing the sequelae of the complication.

**k. Abortions**

**1) Fifth-digits required for abortion categories**—Fifth-digits are required for abortion categories 634-637. Fifth-digit 1, incomplete, indicates that all of the products of conception have not been expelled from the uterus. Fifth-digit 2, complete, indicates that all products of conception have been expelled from the uterus prior to the episode of care.

**2) Code from categories 640-648 and 651-659**—A code from categories 640-648 and 651-659 may be used as additional codes with an abortion code to indicate the complication leading to the abortion. Fifth digit 3 is assigned with codes from these categories when used with an abortion code because the other fifth digits will not apply. Codes from the 660-669 series are not to be used for complications of abortion.

**3) Code 639 for complications**—Code 639 is to be used for all complications following abortion. Code 639 cannot be assigned with codes from categories 634-638.

**4) Abortion with liveborn fetus**—When an attempted termination of pregnancy results in a liveborn fetus assign code 644.21, Early onset of delivery, with an appropriate code from category V27, Outcome of Delivery. The procedure code for the attempted termination of pregnancy should also be assigned.

**5) Retained products of conception following an abortion**—Subsequent admissions for retained products of conception following a spontaneous or legally induced abortion are assigned the appropriate code from category 634, Spontaneous abortion, or 635 Legally induced abortion, with a fifth digit of "1" (incomplete). This advice is appropriate even when the patient was discharged previously with a discharge diagnosis of complete abortion.

12. **Chapter 12: Diseases Skin and Subcutaneous Tissue (680-709)**
Reserved for future guideline expansion

13. **Chapter 13: Diseases of Musculoskeletal and Connective Tissue (710-739)**

a. <u>Coding of pathologic fractures</u>

1) <u>Acute fractures vs. aftercare</u>—**Pathologic fractures are reported using subcategory 733.1, when the fracture is newly diagnosed. Subcategory 733.1 may be used while the patient is receiving active treatment for the fracture. Examples of active treatment are: surgical treatment, emergency department encounter, evaluation and treatment by a new physician.**

**Fractures are coded using the aftercare codes (subcategories V54.0, V54.2, V54.8 or V54.9) for encounters after the patient has completed active treatment of the fracture and is receiving routine care for the fracture during the healing or recovery phase. Examples of fracture aftercare are: cast change or removal, removal of external or internal fixation device, medication adjustment, and follow up visits following fracture treatment.**

**Care for complications of surgical treatment for fracture repairs during the healing or recovery phase should be coded with the appropriate complication codes.**

**Care of complications of fractures, such as malunion and nonunion, should be reported with the appropriate codes.**

*See Section I. C. 17.b for information on the coding of traumatic fractures.*

14. **Chapter 14: Congenital Anomalies (740-759)**

a. **Codes in categories 740-759, Congenital Anomalies**—Assign an appropriate code(s) from categories 740-759, Congenital Anomalies, when an anomaly is documented. A congenital anomaly may be the principal/first listed diagnosis on a record or a secondary diagnosis.

When a congenital anomaly does not have a unique code assignment, assign additional code(s) for any manifestations that may be present.

When the code assignment specifically identifies the congenital anomaly, manifestations that are an inherent component of the anomaly should not be coded separately. Additional codes should be assigned for manifestations that are not an inherent component.

Codes from Chapter 14 may be used throughout the life of the patient. If a congenital anomaly has been corrected, a personal history code should be used to identify the history of the anomaly. Although present at birth, a congenital anomaly may not be identified until later in life. Whenever the condition is diagnosed by the physician, it is appropriate to assign a code from codes 740-759.

For the birth admission, the appropriate code from category V30, Liveborn infants, according to type of birth should be sequenced as the principal diagnosis, followed by any congenital anomaly codes, 740-759.

15. **Chapter 15: Newborn (Perinatal) Guidelines (760-779)**—For coding and reporting purposes the perinatal period is defined as **before** birth through the 28th day following birth. The following guidelines are provided for reporting purposes. Hospitals may record other diagnoses as needed for internal data use.

a. **General perinatal rules**

1) **Chapter 15 codes**—They are never for use on the maternal record. Codes from Chapter 11, the obstetric chapter, are never permitted on the newborn record. Chapter 15 code may be used throughout the life of the patient if the condition is still present.

2) **Sequencing of perinatal codes**—Generally, codes from Chapter 15 should be sequenced as the principal/first-listed diagnosis on the newborn record, with the exception of the appropriate V30 code for the birth episode, followed by codes from any other chapter that provide additional detail. The "use additional code" note at the beginning of the chapter supports this guideline. If the index does not provide a specific code for a perinatal condition, assign code 779.89, Other specified conditions originating in the perinatal period, followed by the code from another chapter that specifies the condition. Codes for signs and symptoms may be assigned when a definitive diagnosis has not been established.

3) **Birth process or community acquired conditions**—If a newborn has a condition that may be either due to the birth process or community acquired and the documentation does not indicate which it is, the default is due to the birth process and the code from Chapter 15 should be used. If the condition is community-acquired, a code from Chapter 15 should not be assigned.

4) **Code all clinically significant conditions**—All clinically significant conditions noted on routine newborn examination should be coded. A condition is clinically significant if it requires:

- clinical evaluation; or
- therapeutic treatment; or
- diagnostic procedures; or
- extended length of hospital stay; or
- increased nursing care and/or monitoring; or
- has implications for future health care needs

Note: The perinatal guidelines listed above are the same as the general coding guidelines for "additional diagnoses", except for the final point regarding implications for future health care needs. Codes should be assigned for conditions that have been specified by the provider as having implications for future health care needs. Codes from the perinatal chapter should not be assigned unless the provider has established a definitive diagnosis.

b. **Use of codes V30-V39**—When coding the birth of an infant, assign a code from categories V30-V39, according to the type of birth. A code from this series is assigned as a principal diagnosis, and assigned only once to a newborn at the time of birth.

c. **Newborn transfers**—If the newborn is transferred to another institution, the V30 series is not used at the receiving hospital.

d. **Use of category V29**

1) **Assigning a code from category V29**—Assign a code from category V29, Observation and evaluation of newborns and infants for suspected conditions not found, to identify those instances when a healthy newborn is evaluated for a suspected condition that is determined after study not to be present. Do not use a code from category V29 when the patient has identified signs or symptoms of a suspected problem; in such cases, code the sign or symptom.

A code from category V29 may also be assigned as a principal code for readmissions or encounters when the V30 code no longer applies. Codes from category V29 are for use only for healthy newborns and infants for which no condition after study is found to be present.

2) **V29 code on a birth record**—A V29 code is to be used as a secondary code after the V30, Outcome of delivery, code.

**Revised text in bold font**

e.  **Use of other V codes on perinatal records**—V codes other than V30 and V29 may be assigned on a perinatal or newborn record code. The codes may be used as a principal or first-listed diagnosis for specific types of encounters or for readmissions or encounters when the V30 code no longer applies.

*See Section I.C.18 for information regarding the assignment of V codes.*

f.  **Maternal Causes of Perinatal Morbidity**—Codes from categories 760-763, Maternal causes of perinatal morbidity and mortality, are assigned only when the maternal condition has actually affected the fetus or newborn. The fact that the mother has an associated medical condition or experiences some complication of pregnancy, labor or delivery does not justify the routine assignment of codes from these categories to the newborn record.

g.  **Congenital Anomalies in Newborns**—For the birth admission, the appropriate code from category V30, Liveborn infants according to type of birth, should be used, followed by any congenital anomaly codes, categories 740-759. Use additional secondary codes from other chapters to specify conditions associated with the anomaly, if applicable.

*Also, see Section I.C.14 for information on the coding of congenital anomalies.*

h.  **Coding Additional Perinatal Diagnoses**

1)  **Assigning codes for conditions that require treatment**—Assign codes for conditions that require treatment or further investigation, prolong the length of stay, or require resource utilization.

2)  **Codes for conditions specified as having implications for future health care needs**—Assign codes for conditions that have been specified by the provider as having implications for future health care needs. Note: This guideline should not be used for adult patients.

3)  **Codes for newborn conditions originating in the perinatal period**—Assign a code for newborn conditions originating in the perinatal period (categories 760-779), as well as complications arising during the current episode of care classified in other chapters, only if the diagnoses have been documented by the responsible provider at the time of transfer or discharge as having affected the fetus or newborn.

i.  **Prematurity and Fetal Growth Retardation**—Providers utilize different criteria in determining prematurity. A code for prematurity should not be assigned unless it is documented. The 5th digit assignment for codes from category 764 and subcategories 765.0 and 765.1 should be based on the recorded birth weight and estimated gestational age.

A code from subcategory 765.2, Weeks of gestation, should be assigned as an additional code with category 764 and codes from 765.0 and 765.1 to specify weeks of gestation as documented by the provider in the record.

j.  **Newborn sepsis**—Code 771.81, Septicemia [sepsis] of newborn, should be assigned with a secondary code from category 041, Bacterial infections in conditions classified elsewhere and of unspecified site, to identify the organism. It is not necessary to use a code from subcategory 995.9, Systemic inflammatory response syndrome (SIRS), on a newborn record. A code from category 038, Septicemia, should not be used on a newborn record. Code 771.81 describes the sepsis.

16. **Chapter 16: Signs, Symptoms and Ill-Defined Conditions (780-799)**—Reserved for future guideline expansion

17. **Chapter 17: Injury and Poisoning (800-999)**

a.  **Coding of Injuries**—When coding injuries, assign separate codes for each injury unless a combination code is provided, in which case the combination code is assigned. Multiple injury codes are provided in ICD-9-CM, but should not be assigned unless information for a more specific code is not available. These codes are not to be used for normal, healing surgical wounds or to identify complications of surgical wounds.

The code for the most serious injury, as determined by the provider and the focus of treatment, is sequenced first.

1)  **Superficial injuries**—Superficial injuries such as abrasions or contusions are not coded when associated with more severe injuries of the same site.

2)  **Primary injury with damage to nerves/blood vessels**—When a primary injury results in minor damage to peripheral nerves or blood vessels, the primary injury is sequenced first with additional code(s) from categories 950-957, Injury to nerves and spinal cord, and/or 900-904, Injury to blood vessels. When the primary injury is to the blood vessels or nerves, that injury should be sequenced first.

b.  **Coding of Traumatic Fractures**—The principles of multiple coding of injuries should be followed in coding fractures. Fractures of specified sites are coded individually by site in accordance with both the provisions within categories 800-829 and the level of detail furnished by medical record content. Combination categories for multiple fractures are provided for use when there is insufficient detail in the medical record (such as trauma cases transferred to another hospital), when the reporting form limits the number of codes that can be used in reporting pertinent clinical data, or when there is insufficient specificity at the fourth-digit or fifth-digit level. More specific guidelines are as follows:

1)  **Acute Fractures vs. Aftercare**—Traumatic fractures are coded using the acute fracture codes (800-829) while the patient is receiving active treatment for the fracture. Examples of active treatment are: surgical treatment, emergency department encounter, and evaluation and treatment by a new physician. Fractures are coded using the aftercare codes (subcategories V54.0, V54.1, V54.8, or V54.9) for encounters after the patient has completed active treatment of the fracture and is receiving routine care for the fracture during the healing or recovery phase. Examples of fracture aftercare are: cast change or removal, removal of external or internal fixation device, medication adjustment, and follow up visits following fracture treatment.
Care for complications of surgical treatment for fracture repairs during the healing or recovery phase should be coded with the appropriate complication codes. Care of complications of fractures, such as malunion and nonunion, should be reported with the appropriate codes. Pathologic fractures are not coded in the 800-829 range, but instead are assigned to subcategory 733.1.
*See Section I.C.13.a for additional information.*

2)  **Multiple fractures of same limb**—Multiple fractures of same limb classifiable to the same three-digit or four-digit category are coded to that category.

3)  **Multiple unilateral or bilateral fractures of same bone**—Multiple unilateral or bilateral fractures of same bone(s) but classified to different fourth-digit subdivisions (bone part) within the same three-digit category are coded individually by site.

4)  **Multiple fracture categories 819 and 828**—Multiple fracture categories 819 and 828 classify bilateral fractures of both upper limbs (819) and both lower limbs (828), but without any detail at the fourth-digit level other than open and closed type of fractures.

5)  **Multiple fractures sequencing**—Multiple fractures are sequenced in accordance with the severity of the fracture. The provider should be asked to list the fracture diagnoses in the order of severity.

c.  **Coding of Burns**—Current burns (940-948) are classified by depth, extent and by agent (E code). Burns are classified by depth as first degree (erythema), second degree (blistering), and third degree (full-thickness involvement).

1)  **Sequencing of burn and related condition codes**—Sequence first the code that reflects the highest degree of burn when more than one burn is present.

a) When the reason for the admission or encounter is for treatment of external multiple burns, sequence first the code that reflects the burn of the highest degree.

b) When a patient has both internal and external burns, the circumstances of admission govern the selection of the principal diagnosis or first-listed diagnosis.

c) When a patient is admitted for burn injuries and other related conditions such as smoke inhalation and/or respiratory failure, the circumstances of admission govern the selection of the principal or first-listed diagnosis.

**2) Burns of the same local site**—Classify burns of the same local site (three-digit category level, 940-947) but of different degrees to the subcategory identifying the highest degree recorded in the diagnosis.

**3) Non-healing burns**—Non-healing burns are coded as acute burns. Necrosis of burned skin should be coded as a non-healed burn.

**4) Code 958.3, Posttraumatic wound infection**—Assign code 958.3, Posttraumatic wound infection, not elsewhere classified, as an additional code for any documented infected burn site.

**5) Assign separate codes for each burn site**—When coding burns, assign separate codes for each burn site. Category 946 Burns of Multiple specified sites, should only be used if the location of the burns are not documented. Category 949, Burn, unspecified, is extremely vague and should rarely be used.

**6) Assign codes from category 948, Burns**—Burns classified according to extent of body surface involved, when the site of the burn is not specified or when there is a need for additional data. It is advisable to use category 948 as additional coding when needed to provide data for evaluating burn mortality, such as that needed by burn units. It is also advisable to use category 948 as an additional code for reporting purposes when there is mention of a third-degree burn involving 20 percent or more of the body surface.

In assigning a code from category 948:

Fourth-digit codes are used to identify the percentage of total body surface involved in a burn (all degree).

Fifth-digits are assigned to identify the percentage of body surface involved in third-degree burn.

Fifth-digit zero (0) is assigned when less than 10 percent or when no body surface is involved in a third-degree burn.

Category 948 is based on the classic "rule of nines" in estimating body surface involved: head and neck are assigned nine percent, each arm nine percent, each leg 18 percent, the anterior trunk 18 percent, posterior trunk 18 percent, and genitalia one percent. Providers may change these percentage assignments where necessary to accommodate infants and children who have proportionately larger heads than adults and patients who have large buttocks, thighs, or abdomen that involve burns.

**7) Encounters for treatment of late effects of burns**—Encounters for the treatment of the late effects of burns (i.e., scars or joint contractures) should be coded to the residual condition (sequelae) followed by the appropriate late effect code (906.5-906.9). A late effect E code may also be used, if desired.

**8) Sequelae with a late effect code and current burn**—When appropriate, both a sequelae with a late effect code, and a current burn code may be assigned on the same record (when both a current burn and sequelae of an old burn exist).

**d. Coding of Debridement of Wound, Infection, or Burn**—Excisional debridement involves surgical removal or cutting away, as opposed to a mechanical (brushing, scrubbing, washing) debridement. For coding purposes, excisional debridement is assigned to code 86.22. Nonexcisional debridement is assigned to code 86.28.

**e. Adverse Effects, Poisoning and Toxic Effects**—The properties of certain drugs, medicinal and biological substances or combinations of such substances, may cause toxic reactions. The occurrence of drug toxicity is classified in ICD-9-CM as follows:

**1) Adverse Effect**—When the drug was correctly prescribed and properly administered, code the reaction plus the appropriate code from the E930-E949 series. Codes from the E930-E949 series must be used to identify the causative substance for an adverse effect of drug, medicinal and biological substances, correctly prescribed and properly administered. The effect, such as tachycardia, delirium, gastrointestinal hemorrhaging, vomiting, hypokalemia, hepatitis, renal failure, or respiratory failure, is coded and followed by the appropriate code from the E930-E949 series. Adverse effects of therapeutic substances correctly prescribed and properly administered (toxicity, synergistic reaction, side effect, and idiosyncratic reaction) may be due to (1) differences among patients, such as age, sex, disease, and genetic factors, and (2) drug-related factors, such as type of drug, route of administration, duration of therapy, dosage, and bioavailability.

**2) Poisoning**

**(a) Error was made in drug prescription**—Errors made in drug prescription or in the administration of the drug by provider, nurse, patient, or other person, use the appropriate poisoning code from the 960-979 series.

**(b) Overdose of a drug intentionally taken**—If an overdose of a drug was intentionally taken or administered and resulted in drug toxicity, it would be coded as a poisoning (960-979 series).

**(c) Nonprescribed drug taken with correctly prescribed and properly administered drug**—If a nonprescribed drug or medicinal agent was taken in combination with a correctly prescribed and properly administered drug, any drug toxicity or other reaction resulting from the interaction of the two drugs would be classified as a poisoning.

**(d) Sequencing of poisoning**—When coding a poisoning or reaction to the improper use of a medication (e.g., wrong dose, wrong substance, wrong route of administration) the poisoning code is sequenced first, followed by a code for the manifestation. If there is also a diagnosis of drug abuse or dependence to the substance, the abuse or dependence is coded as an additional code. *See Section I.C.3.a.6.b. if poisoning is the result of insulin pump malfunctions and Section I.C.19 for general use of E-codes.*

**3) Toxic Effects**

**(a) Toxic effect codes** —When a harmful substance is ingested or comes in contact with a person, this is classified as a toxic effect. The toxic effect codes are in categories 980-989.

**(b) Sequencing toxic effect codes** —A toxic effect code should be sequenced first, followed by the code(s) that identify the result of the toxic effect.

**(c) External cause codes for toxic effects**—An external cause code from categories E860-E869 for accidental exposure, codes E950.6 or E950.7 for intentional self-harm, category E962 for assault, or categories E980-E982, for undetermined, should also be assigned to indicate intent.

**f. Complications of care**

**1) Transplant complications**

**(a) Transplant complications other than kidney**—Codes under subcategory 996.8, Complications of transplanted organ, are for use for both complications and rejection of transplanted organs. A transplant complication code is only assigned if the complication affects the function of the transplanted organ. Two codes are required to fully describe a transplant complication, the appropriate code from subcategory 996.8 and a secondary code that identifies the complication.

Pre-existing conditions or conditions that develop after the transplant are not coded as complications unless they affect the function of the transplanted organs.

**(b) Kidney transplant complications—Code 996.81 should be assigned for documented complications of a kidney transplant, such as transplant failure**

or rejection. Code 996.81 should not be assigned for post kidney transplant patients who have chronic kidney (CKD) unless a transplant complication such as transplant failure or rejection is documented. If the documentation is unclear as to whether the patient has a complication of the transplant, query the provider.

For patients with CKD following a kidney transplant, but who do not have a complication such as failure or rejection, *see section I.C.10.a.2, Chronic kidney disease and kidney transplant status.*

g. SIRS due to non-infectious Process—The systemic inflammatory response syndrome (SIRS) can develop as a result of certain non-infectious disease processes, such as trauma, malignant neoplasm, or pancreatitis. When SIRS is documented with a noninfectious condition, and no subsequent infection is documented, the code for the underlying condition, such as an injury, should be assigned, followed by code 995.93, Systemic inflammatory response syndrome due to noninfectious process without acute organ dysfunction, or 995.94, Systemic inflammatory response syndrome due to non-infectious process with acute organ dysfunction. If an acute organ dysfunction is documented, the appropriate code(s) for the associated acute organ dysfunction(s) should be assigned in addition to code 995.94. If acute organ dysfunction is documented, but it cannot be determined if the acute organ dysfunction is associated with SIRS or due to another condition (e.g., directly due to the trauma), the provider should be queried. When the non-infectious condition has led to an infection that results in SIRS, *see Section I.C.1.b.11 for the guideline for sepsis and severe sepsis associated with a non-infectious process.*

18. **Classification of Factors Influencing Health Status and Contact with Health Service (Supplemental V01-V86)**

**Note:** The chapter specific guidelines provide additional information about the use of V codes for specified encounters.

a. **Introduction**—ICD-9-CM provides codes to deal with encounters for circumstances other than a disease or injury. The Supplementary Classification of Factors Influencing Health Status and Contact with Health Services (V01.0–V86.1) is provided to deal with occasions when circumstances other than a disease or injury (codes 001-999) are recorded as a diagnosis or problem.
There are four primary circumstances for the use of V codes:

1) A person who is not currently sick encounters the health services for some specific reason, such as to act as an organ donor, to receive prophylactic care, such as inoculations or health screenings, or to receive counseling on health related issues.

2) A person with a resolving disease or injury, or a chronic, long-term condition requiring continuous care, encounters the health care system for specific aftercare of that disease or injury (e.g., dialysis for renal disease; chemotherapy for malignancy; cast change). A diagnosis/symptom code should be used whenever a current, acute, diagnosis is being treated or a sign or symptom is being studied.

3) Circumstances or problems influence a person's health status but are not in themselves a current illness or injury.

4) Newborns, to indicate birth status

b. **V codes use in any healthcare setting**—V codes are for use in any healthcare setting. V codes may be used as either a first listed (principal diagnosis code in the inpatient setting) or secondary code, depending on the circumstances of the encounter. Certain V codes may only be used as first listed, others only as secondary codes. *See Section I.C.18.e, V Code Table*

c. **V Codes indicate a reason for an encounter**—They are not procedure codes. A corresponding procedure code must accompany a V code to describe the procedure performed.

d. **Categories of V Codes**

1) **Contact/Exposure**—Category V01 indicates contact with or exposure to communicable diseases. These codes are for patients who do not show any sign or symptom of a disease but have been exposed to it by close personal contact with an infected individual or are in an area where a disease is epidemic. These codes may be used as a first listed code to explain an encounter for testing, or, more commonly, as a secondary code to identify a potential risk.

2) **Inoculations and vaccinations**—Categories V03-V06 are for encounters for inoculations and vaccinations. They indicate that a patient is being seen to receive a prophylactic inoculation against a disease. The injection itself must be represented by the appropriate procedure code. A code from V03-V06 may be used as a secondary code if the inoculation is given as a routine part of preventive health care, such as a well-baby visit.

3) **Status**—Status codes indicate that a patient is either a carrier of a disease or has the sequelae or residual of a past disease or condition. This includes such things as the presence of prosthetic or mechanical devices resulting from past treatment. A status code is informative, because the status may affect the course of treatment and its outcome. A status code is distinct from a history code. The history code indicates that the patient no longer has the condition. A status code should not be used with a diagnosis code from one of the body system chapters, if the diagnosis code includes the information provided by the status code. For example, code V42.1, Heart transplant status, should not be used with code 996.83, Complications of transplanted heart. The status code does not provide additional information. The complication code indicates that the patient is a heart transplant patient.
The status V codes/categories are:

| | |
|---|---|
| V02 | Carrier or suspected carrier of infectious diseases<br>Carrier status indicates that a person harbors the specific organisms of a disease without manifest symptoms and is capable of transmitting the infection. |
| V08 | Asymptomatic HIV infection status: This code indicates that a patient has tested positive for HIV but has manifested no signs or symptoms of the disease. |
| V09 | Infection with drug-resistant microorganisms<br>This category indicates that a patient has an infection that is resistant to drug treatment.<br>Sequence the infection code first. |
| V21 | Constitutional states in development |
| V22.2 | Pregnant state, incidental<br>This code is a secondary code only for use when the pregnancy is in no way complicating the reason for visit. Otherwise, a code from the obstetric chapter is required. |
| V26.5x | Sterilization status |
| V42 | Organ or tissue replaced by transplant |
| V43 | Organ or tissue replaced by other means |
| V44 | Artificial opening status |
| V45 | Other postsurgical states |
| V46 | Other dependence on machines |
| V49.6 | Upper limb amputation status |
| V49.7 | Lower limb amputation status |
| V49.81 | Postmenopausal status |
| V49.82 | Dental sealant status |
| V49.83 | Awaiting organ transplant status |
| V58.6 | Long-term (current) drug use<br>This subcategory indicates a patient's continuous use of a prescribed drug |

(including such things as aspirin therapy) for the long-term treatment of a condition or for prophylactic use. It is not for use for patients who have addictions to drugs. Assign a code from subcategory V58.6, Long-term (current) drug use, if the patient is receiving a medication for an extended period as a prophylactic measure (such as for the prevention of deep vein thrombosis) or as treatment of a chronic condition (such as arthritis) or a disease requiring a lengthy course of treatment (such as cancer). Do not assign a code from subcategory V58.6 for medication being administered for a brief period of time to treat an acute illness or injury (such as a course of antibiotics to treat acute bronchitis).

V83    Genetic carrier status

Genetic carrier status indicates that a person carries a gene, associated with a particular disease, which may be passed to offspring who may develop that disease. The person does not have the disease and is not at risk of developing the disease.

V84    Genetic susceptibility status

Genetic susceptibility indicates that a person has a gene that increases the risk of that person developing the disease. Codes from category V84, Genetic susceptibility to disease, should not be used as principal or first-listed codes. If the patient has the condition to which he/she is susceptible, and that condition is the reason for the encounter, the code for the current condition should be sequenced first. If the patient is being seen for follow-up after completed treatment for this condition, and the condition no longer exists, a follow-up code should be sequenced first, followed by the appropriate personal history and genetic susceptibility codes. If the purpose of the encounter is genetic counseling associated with procreative management, a code from subcategory V26.3, Genetic counseling and testing, should be assigned as the first-listed code, followed by a code from category V84. Additional codes should be assigned for any applicable family or personal history.

*See Section I.C. 18.d.14 for information on prophylactic organ removal due to a genetic susceptibility.*

**V86**    **Estrogen receptor status**

**Note**: Categories V42-V46, and subcategories V49.6, V49.7 are for use only if there are no complications or malfunctions of the organ or tissue replaced, the amputation site or the equipment on which the patient is dependent.

4)   **History (of)**—There are two types of history V codes, personal and family. Personal history codes explain a patient's past medical condition that no longer exists and is not receiving any treatment, but that has the potential for recurrence, and therefore may require continued monitoring. The exceptions to this general rule are category V14, Personal history of allergy to medicinal agents, and subcategory V15.0, Allergy, other than to medicinal agents. A person who has had an allergic episode to a substance or food in the past should always be considered allergic to the substance.

Family history codes are for use when a patient has a family member(s) who has had a particular disease that causes the patient to be at higher risk of also contracting the disease.

Personal history codes may be used in conjunction with follow-up codes and family history codes may be used in conjunction with screening codes to explain the need for a test or procedure. History codes are also acceptable on any medical record regardless of the reason for visit. A history of an illness, even if no longer present, is important information that may alter the type of treatment ordered.

The history V code categories are:

| | |
|---|---|
| V10 | Personal history of malignant neoplasm |
| V12 | Personal history of certain other diseases |
| V13 | Personal history of other diseases Except: V13.4, Personal history of arthritis, and |
| V13.6 | Personal history of congenital malformations. These conditions are life-long so are not true history codes. |
| V14 | Personal history of allergy to medicinal agents |
| V15 | Other personal history presenting hazards to health Except: V15.7, Personal history of contraception. |
| V16 | Family history of malignant neoplasm |
| V17 | Family history of certain chronic disabling diseases |
| V18 | Family history of certain other specific diseases |
| V19 | Family history of other conditions |

5)   **Screening**—Screening is the testing for disease or disease precursors in seemingly well individuals so that early detection and treatment can be provided for those who test positive for the disease. Screenings that are recommended for many subgroups in a population include: routine mammograms for women over 40, a fecal occult blood test for everyone over 50, an amniocentesis to rule out a fetal anomaly for pregnant women over 35, because the incidence of breast cancer and colon cancer in these subgroups is higher than in the general population, as is the incidence of Down's syndrome in older mothers.

The testing of a person to rule out or confirm a suspected diagnosis because the patient has some sign or symptom is a diagnostic examination, not a screening. In these cases, the sign or symptom is used to explain the reason for the test.

A screening code may be a first listed code if the reason for the visit is specifically the screening exam. It may also be used as an additional code if the screening is done during an office visit for other health problems. A screening code is not necessary if the screening is inherent to a routine examination, such as a pap smear done during a routine pelvic examination.

Should a condition be discovered during the screening then the code for the condition may be assigned as an additional diagnosis.

The V code indicates that a screening exam is planned. A procedure code is required to confirm that the screening was performed.

The screening V code categories:

| | |
|---|---|
| V28 | Antenatal screening |
| V73-V82 | Special screening examinations |

6)   **Observation**—There are two observation V code categories. They are for use in very limited circumstances when a person is being observed for a suspected condition that is ruled out. The observation codes are not for use if an injury or illness or any signs or symptoms related to the suspected condition are present. In such cases the diagnosis/symptom code is used with the corresponding E code to identify any external cause.

The observation codes are to be used as principal diagnosis only. The only exception to this is when the principal diagnosis is required to be a code from the V30, Live born infant, category. Then the V29 observation code is sequenced after the V30 code.

Additional codes may be used in addition to the observation code but only if they are unrelated to the suspected condition being observed.

The observation V code categories:

V29     Observation and evaluation of newborns for suspected condition not found
For the birth encounter, a code from category V30 should be sequenced before the V29 code.

V71     Observation and evaluation for suspected condition not found

7) **Aftercare**—Aftercare visit codes cover situations when the initial treatment of a disease or injury has been performed and the patient requires continued care during the healing or recovery phase, or for the long-term consequences of the disease. The aftercare V code should not be used if treatment is directed at a current, acute disease or injury. The diagnosis code is to be used in these cases. Exceptions to this rule are codes V58.0, Radiotherapy, and codes from subcategory V58.1, Encounter for chemotherapy and immunotherapy for neoplastic conditions. These codes are to be first listed, followed by the diagnosis code when a patient's encounter is solely to receive radiation therapy or chemotherapy for the treatment of a neoplasm. Should a patient receive both chemotherapy and radiation therapy during the same encounter code V58.0 and V58.1 may be used together on a record with either one being sequenced first.

The aftercare codes are generally first listed to explain the specific reason for the encounter. An aftercare code may be used as an additional code when some type of aftercare is provided in addition to the reason for admission and no diagnosis code is applicable. An example of this would be the closure of a colostomy during an encounter for treatment of another condition.

Certain aftercare V code categories need a secondary diagnosis code to describe the resolving condition or sequelae, for others, the condition is inherent in the code title.

Additional V code aftercare category terms include, fitting and adjustment, and attention to artificial openings.

Status V codes may be used with aftercare V codes to indicate the nature of the aftercare. For example code V45.81, Aortocoronary bypass status, may be used with code V58.73, Aftercare following surgery of the circulatory system, NEC, to indicate the surgery for which the aftercare is being performed. Also, a transplant status code may be used following code V58.44, Aftercare following organ transplant, to identify the organ transplanted. A status code should not be used when the aftercare code indicates the type of status, such as using V55.0, Attention to tracheostomy with V44.0, Tracheostomy status.

The aftercare V category/codes:

V52     Fitting and adjustment of prosthetic device and implant

V53     Fitting and adjustment of other device

V54     Other orthopedic aftercare

V55     Attention to artificial openings

V56     Encounter for dialysis and dialysis catheter care

V57     Care involving the use of rehabilitation procedures

V58.0     Radiotherapy

V58.11     Encounter for antineoplastic chemotherapy

V58.12     Encounter for antineoplastic immunotherapy

**V58.3x**     **Attention to dressings and sutures**

V58.41     Encounter for planned post-operative wound closure

V58.42     Aftercare, surgery, neoplasm

V58.43     Aftercare, surgery, trauma

V58.44     Aftercare involving organ transplant

V58.49     Other specified aftercare following surgery

V58.7x     Aftercare following surgery

V58.81     Fitting and adjustment of vascular catheter

V58.82     Fitting and adjustment of non-vascular catheter

V58.83     Monitoring therapeutic drug

V58.89     Other specified aftercare

8) **Follow-up**—The follow-up codes are used to explain continuing surveillance following completed treatment of a disease, condition, or injury. They imply that the condition has been fully treated and no longer exists. They should not be confused with aftercare codes that explain current treatment for a healing condition or its sequelae. Follow-up codes may be used in conjunction with history codes to provide the full picture of the healed condition and its treatment. The follow-up code is sequenced first, followed by the history code.

A follow-up code may be used to explain repeated visits. Should a condition be found to have recurred on the follow-up visit, then the diagnosis code should be used in place of the follow-up code.

The follow-up V code categories:

V24     Postpartum care and evaluation

V67     Follow-up examination

9) **Donor**—Category V59 is the donor codes. They are used for living individuals who are donating blood or other body tissue. These codes are only for individuals donating for others, not for self donations. They are not for use to identify cadaveric donations.

10) **Counseling**—Counseling V codes are used when a patient or family member receives assistance in the aftermath of an illness or injury, or when support is required in coping with family or social problems. They are not necessary for use in conjunction with a diagnosis code when the counseling component of care is considered integral to standard treatment.

The counseling V categories/codes:

V25.0     General counseling and advice for contraceptive management

V26.3     Genetic counseling

V26.4     General counseling and advice for procreative management

V61     Other family circumstances

V65.1     Person consulted on behalf of another person

V65.3     Dietary surveillance and counseling

V65.4     Other counseling, not elsewhere classified

11) **Obstetrics and related conditions**—*See Section I.C.11., the Obstetrics guidelines for further instruction on the use of these codes.*

V codes for pregnancy are for use in those circumstances when none of the problems or complications included in the codes from the Obstetrics chapter exist (a routine prenatal visit or postpartum care). Codes V22.0, Supervision of normal first pregnancy, and V22.1, Supervision of other normal pregnancy, are always first listed and are not to be used with any other code from the OB chapter.

The outcome of delivery, category V27, should be included on all maternal delivery records. It is always a secondary code.

V codes for family planning (contraceptive) or procreative management and counseling should be included on an obstetric record either during the pregnancy or the postpartum stage, if applicable.

Obstetrics and related conditions V code categories:

V22     Normal pregnancy

V23     Supervision of high-risk pregnancy
Except: V23.2, Pregnancy with history of abortion. Code 646.3, Habitual aborter,

from the OB chapter is required to indicate a history of abortion during a pregnancy.

| | |
|---|---|
| V24 | Postpartum care and evaluation |
| V25 | Encounter for contraceptive management Except V25.0x (*See Section I.C.18.d.11, Counseling*) |
| V26 | Procreative management Except V26.5x, Sterilization status, V26.3 and V26.4 (*See Section I.C.18.d.11., Counseling*) |
| V27 | Outcome of delivery |
| V28 | Antenatal screening (*See Section I.C.18.d.6., Screening*) |

12) **Newborn, infant and child—***See Section I.C.15, the Newborn guidelines for further instruction on the use of these codes.*

Newborn V code categories:

| | |
|---|---|
| V20 | Health supervision of infant or child |
| V29 | Observation and evaluation of newborns for suspected condition not found (*See Section I.C.18.d.7, Observation*) |
| V30-V39 | Liveborn infant according to type of birth |

13) **Routine and administrative examinations—**The V codes allow for the description of encounters for routine examinations, such as, a general check-up, or, examinations for administrative purposes, such as, a pre-employment physical. The codes are not to be used if the examination is for diagnosis of a suspected condition or for treatment purposes. In such cases the diagnosis code is used. During a routine exam, should a diagnosis or condition be discovered, it should be coded as an additional code. Pre-existing and chronic conditions and history codes may also be included as additional codes as long as the examination is for administrative purposes and not focused on any particular condition.

Pre-operative examination V codes are for use only in those situations when a patient is being cleared for surgery and no treatment is given.

The V codes categories/code for routine and administrative examinations:

| | |
|---|---|
| V20.2 | Routine infant or child health check Any injections given should have a corresponding procedure code. |
| V70 | General medical examination |
| V72 | Special investigations and examinations |

**Codes V72.5 and V72.6 may be used if the reason for the patient encounter is for routine laboratory/radiology testing in the absence of any signs, symptoms, or associated diagnosis. If routine testing is performed during the same encounter as a test to evaluate a sign, symptom, or diagnosis, it is appropriate to assign both the V code and the code describing the reason for the non-routine test.**

14) **Miscellaneous V codes—**The miscellaneous V codes capture a number of other health care encounters that do not fall into one of the other categories. Certain of these codes identify the reason for the encounter, others are for use as additional codes that provide useful information on circumstances that may affect a patient's care and treatment.

**Prophylactic Organ Removal—**For encounters specifically for prophylactic removal of breasts, ovaries, or another organ due to a genetic susceptibility to cancer or a family history of cancer, the principal or first listed code should be a code from subcategory V50.4, Prophylactic organ removal, followed by the appropriate genetic susceptibility code and the appropriate family history code.

If the patient has a malignancy of one site and is having prophylactic removal at another site to prevent either a new primary malignancy or metastatic disease, a code for the malignancy should also be assigned in addition to a code from subcategory V50.4. A V50.4 code should not be assigned if the patient is having organ removal for treatment of a malignancy, such as the removal of the testes for the treatment of prostate cancer.

Miscellaneous V code categories/codes:

| | |
|---|---|
| V07 | Need for isolation and other prophylactic measures |
| V50 | Elective surgery for purposes other than remedying health states |
| V58.5 | Orthodontics |
| V60 | Housing, household, and economic circumstances |
| V62 | Other psychosocial circumstances |
| V63 | Unavailability of other medical facilities for care |
| V64 | Persons encountering health services for specific procedures, not carried out |
| V66 | Convalescence and Palliative Care |
| V68 | Encounters for administrative purposes |
| V69 | Problems related to lifestyle |
| **V85** | **Body Mass Index** |

15) **Nonspecific V codes—**Certain V codes are so non-specific, or potentially redundant with other codes in the classification, that there can be little justification for their use in the inpatient setting. Their use in the outpatient setting should be limited to those instances when there is no further documentation to permit more precise coding. Otherwise, any sign or symptom or any other reason for visit that is captured in another code should be used.

Nonspecific V code categories/codes:

| | |
|---|---|
| V11 | Personal history of mental disorder A code from the mental disorders chapter, with an in remission fifth-digit, should be used. |
| V13.4 | Personal history of arthritis |
| V13.69 | Personal history of congenital malformations |
| V13.9 | Personal history of unspecified disease |
| V15.7 | Personal history of contraception |
| V40 | Mental and behavioral problems |
| V41 | Problems with special senses and other special functions |
| V46.9 | Unspecified machine dependence |
| V47 | Other problems with internal organs |
| V48 | Problems with head, neck, and trunk |
| V49 | Problems with limbs and other problems Exceptions: |
| V49.6 | Upper limb amputation status |
| V49.7 | Lower limb amputation status |
| V49.81 | Postmenopausal status |
| V49.82 | Dental sealant status |
| V49.83 | Awaiting organ transplant status |
| V49.84 | Bed confinement status |
| V49.89 | Other specified conditions influencing health status |
| V51 | Aftercare involving the use of plastic surgery |
| V58.2 | Blood transfusion, without reported diagnosis |
| V58.5 | Other specified procedures or aftercare |
| V58.9 | Unspecified aftercare *See Section IV.K. and Section IV.L. of the Outpatient guidelines.* |
| V72.9 | Unspecified examination |

## V CODE TABLE
### October 1, 2006 (FY2007)

Items in bold indicate a new entry or change from the December 2005 table. Items underlined have been moved within the table since December 2005.

**This year's update includes a new V code table format that will make utilizing the table easier and more efficient to use and update. The table contains columns for 1st listed, 1st or additional, additional only, and non-specific. Each code or category is listed on the left hand column and the allowable sequencing of the code or codes within the category is noted under the appropriate column.**

| Code(s) | Description | 1st Dx Only[1] | 1st or Add'l Dx[2] | Add'l Dx Only[3] | Non-Specific Diagnosis[4] |
|---|---|---|---|---|---|
| V01.X | Contact with or exposure to communicable diseases | | X | | |
| V02.X | Carrier or suspected carrier of infectious diseases | | X | | |
| V03.X | Need for prophylactic vaccination and inoculation against bacterial diseases | | X | | |
| V04.X | Need for prophylactic vaccination and inoculation against certain diseases | | X | | |
| V05.X | Need for prophylactic vaccination and inoculation against single diseases | | X | | |
| V06.X | Need for prophylactic vaccination and inoculation against combinations of diseases | | X | | |
| V07.X | Need for isolation and other prophylactic measures | | X | | |
| V08 | Asymptomatic HIV infection status | | X | | |
| V09.X | Infection with drug resistant organisms | | | X | |
| V10.X | Personal history of malignant neoplasm | | X | | |
| V11.X | Personal history of mental disorder | | | | X |
| V12.X | Personal history of certain other diseases | | X | | |
| V13.0X | Personal history of other disorders of urinary system | | X | | |
| V13.1 | Personal history of trophoblastic disease | | X | | |
| V13.2X | Personal history of other genital system and obstetric disorders | | X | | |
| V13.3 | Personal history of diseases of skin and subcutaneous tissue | | X | | |
| V13.4 | Personal history of arthritis | | | | X |
| V13.5 | Personal history of other musculoskeletal disorders | | X | | |
| V13.61 | Personal history of hypospadias | | | X | |
| V13.69 | Personal history of congenital malformations | | | | X |
| V13.7 | Personal history of perinatal problems | | X | | |
| V13.8 | Personal history of other specified diseases | | X | | |
| V13.9 | Personal history of unspecified disease | | | | **X** |
| V14.X | Personal history of allergy to medicinal agents | | | X | |
| V15.0X | Personal history of allergy, other than to medicinal agents | | | X | |
| V15.1 | Personal history of surgery to heart and great vessels | | | X | |
| V15.2 | Personal history of surgery to other major organs | | | X | |
| V15.3 | Personal history of irradiation | | | X | |
| V15.4X | Personal history of psychological trauma | | | X | |
| V15.5 | Personal history of injury | | | X | |
| V15.6 | Personal history of poisoning | | | X | |
| V15.7 | Personal history of contraception | | | | X |
| V15.81 | Personal history of noncompliance with medical treatment | | | X | |
| V15.82 | Personal history of tobacco use | | | X | |
| V15.84 | Personal history of exposure to asbestos | | | X | |
| V15.85 | Personal history of exposure to potentially hazardous body fluids | | | X | |
| V15.86 | Personal history of exposure to lead | | | X | |
| V15.87 | Personal history of extracorporeal membrane oxygenation [ECMO] | | | X | |
| V15.88 | History of fall | | X | | |
| V15.89 | Other specified personal history presenting hazards to health | | | X | |
| V16.X | Family history of malignant neoplasm | | X | | |
| V17.X | Family history of certain chronic disabling diseases | | X | | |
| V18.X | Family history of certain other specific conditions | | X | | |
| V19.X | Family history of other conditions | | X | | |
| V20.X | Health supervision of infant or child | X | | | |
| V21.X | Constitutional states in development | | | X | |
| V22.0 | Supervision of normal first pregnancy | X | | | |
| V22.1 | Supervision of other normal pregnancy | X | | | |
| V22.2 | Pregnancy state, incidental | | | X | |
| V23.X | Supervision of high-risk pregnancy | | X | | |
| V24.X | Postpartum care and examination | X | | | |

[1] Generally for use as first listed only but may be used as additional if patient has more than one encounter on one day

[2] These codes may be used as first listed or additional codes

[3] These codes are only for use as additional codes

[4] These codes are primarily for use in the nonacute setting and should be limited to encounters for which no sign or symptom or reason for visit is documented in the record. Their use may be as either a first listed or additional code.

| Code(s) | Description | 1st Dx Only[1] | 1st or Add'l Dx[2] | Add'l Dx Only[3] | Non-Specific Diagnosis[4] |
|---------|-------------|----------------|--------------------|-------------------|---------------------------|
| V25.X | Encounter for contraceptive management | | X | | |
| V26.0 | Tuboplasty or vasoplasty after previous sterilization | | X | | |
| V26.1 | Artificial insemination | | X | | |
| V26.2X | Procreative management investigation and testing | | X | | |
| V26.3X | Procreative management, genetic counseling and testing | | X | | |
| V26.4 | Procreative management, genetic counseling and advice | | X | | |
| V26.5X | Procreative management, sterilization status | | | X | |
| V26.8 | Other specified procreative management | | X | | |
| V26.9 | Unspecified procreative management | | X | | |
| V27.X | Outcome of delivery | | | X | |
| **V28.X** | **Encounter for antenatal screening of mother** | | X | | |
| V29.X | Observation and evaluation of newborns for suspected condition not found | X | | | |
| V30.X | Single liveborn | X | | | |
| V31.X | Twin, mate liveborn | X | | | |
| V32.X | Twin, mate stillborn | X | | | |
| V33.X | Twin, unspecified | X | | | |
| V34.X | Other multiple, mates all liveborn | X | | | |
| V35.X | Other multiple, mates all stillborn | X | | | |
| V36.X | Other multiple, mates live- and stillborn | X | | | |
| V37.X | Other multiple, unspecified | X | | | |
| V39.X | Unspecified | X | | | |
| V40.X | Mental and behavioral problems | | | | X |
| V41.X | Problems with special senses and other special functions | | | | X |
| V42.X | Organ or tissue replaced by transplant | | | X | |
| V43.0 | Organ or tissue replaced by other means, eye globe | | | X | |
| V43.1 | Organ or tissue replaced by other means, lens | | | X | |
| V43.21 | Organ or tissue replaced by other means, heart assist device | | | X | |
| V43.22 | Fully implantable artificial heart status | | X | | |
| V43.3 | Organ or tissue replaced by other means, heart valve | | | X | |
| V43.4 | Organ or tissue replaced by other means, blood vessel | | | X | |
| V43.5 | Organ or tissue replaced by other means, bladder | | | X | |
| V43.6X | Organ or tissue replaced by other means, joint | | | X | |
| V43.7 | Organ or tissue replaced by other means, limb | | | X | |
| V43.8X | Other organ or tissue replaced by other means | | | X | |
| V44.X | Artificial opening status | | | X | |
| V45.0X | Cardiac device in situ | | | X | |
| V45.1 | Renal dialysis status | | | X | |
| V45.2 | Presence of cerebrospinal fluid drainage device | | | X | |
| V45.3 | Intestinal bypass or anastomosis status | | | X | |
| V45.4 | Arthrodesis status | | | X | |
| V45.5X | Presence of contraceptive device | | | X | |
| V45.6X | States following surgery of eye and adnexa | | | X | |
| V45.7X | Acquired absence of organ | | X | | |
| V45.8X | Other postprocedural status | | | X | |
| V46.0 | Other dependence on machines, aspirator | | | X | |
| V46.11 | Dependence on respiratory, status | | | X | |
| V46.12 | Encounter for respirator dependence during power failure | X | | | |
| V46.13 | Encounter for weaning from respirator [ventilator] | X | | | |
| V46.14 | Mechanical complication of respirator [ventilator] | | X | | |
| V46.2 | Other dependence on machines, supplemental oxygen | | | X | |
| V46.8 | Other dependence on other enabling machines | | | X | |

[1] Generally for use as first listed only but may be used as additional if patient has more than one encounter on one day
[2] These codes may be used as first listed or additional codes
[3] These codes are only for use as additional codes
[4] These codes are primarily for use in the nonacute setting and should be limited to encounters for which no sign or symptom or reason for visit is documented in the record. Their use may be as either a first listed or additional code.

| Code(s) | Description | 1st Dx Only[1] | 1st or Add'l Dx[2] | Add'l Dx Only[3] | Non-Specific Diagnosis[4] |
|---|---|---|---|---|---|
| V46.9 | Unspecified machine dependence | | | | **X** |
| V47.X | Other problems with internal organs | | | | X |
| V48.X | Problems with head, neck and trunk | | | | X |
| V49.0 | Deficiencies of limbs | | | | X |
| V49.1 | Mechanical problems with limbs | | | | X |
| V49.2 | Motor problems with limbs | | | | X |
| V49.3 | Sensory problems with limbs | | | | X |
| V49.4 | Disfigurements of limbs | | | | X |
| V49.5 | Other problems with limbs | | | | X |
| V49.6X | Upper limb amputation status | | X | | |
| V49.7X | Lower limb amputation status | | X | | |
| V49.81 | Asymptomatic postmenopausal status (age-related) (natural) | | X | | |
| V49.82 | Dental sealant status | | | X | |
| V49.83 | Awaiting organ transplant status | | | X | |
| V49.84 | Bed confinement status | | X | | |
| V49.89 | Other specified conditions influencing health status | | X | | |
| V49.9 | Unspecified condition influencing health status | | | | X |
| V50.X | Elective surgery for purposes other than remedying health states | | X | | |
| V51 | Aftercare involving the use of plastic surgery | | | | X |
| V52.X | Fitting and adjustment of prosthetic device and implant | | X | | |
| V53.X | Fitting and adjustment of other device | | X | | |
| V54.X | Other orthopedic aftercare | | X | | |
| V55.X | Attention to artificial openings | | X | | |
| V56.0 | Extracorporeal dialysis | X | | | |
| V56.1 | Encounter for fitting and adjustment of extracorporeal dialysis catheter | | X | | |
| V56.2 | Encounter for fitting and adjustment of peritoneal dialysis catheter | | X | | |
| V56.3X | Encounter for adequacy testing for dialysis | | X | | |
| V56.8 | Encounter for other dialysis and dialysis catheter care | | X | | |
| V57.X | Care involving use of rehabilitation procedures | X | | | |
| V58.0 | Radiotherapy | X | | | |
| V58.11 | Encounter for antineoplastic chemotherapy | X | | | |
| V58.12 | Encounter for antineoplastic immunotherapy | X | | | |
| V58.2 | Blood transfusion without reported diagnosis | | | | X |
| **V58.3X** | **Attention to dressings and sutures** | | X | | |
| V58.4X | Other aftercare following surgery | | X | | |
| V58.5 | Encounter for orthodontics | | | | X |
| V58.6X | Long term (current) drug use | | | X | |
| V58.7X | Aftercare following surgery to specified body systems, not elsewhere classified | | X | | |
| V58.8X | Other specified procedures and aftercare | | X | | |
| V58.9 | Unspecified aftercare | | | | X |
| V59.X | Donors | X | | | |
| V60.X | Housing, household, and economic circumstances | | | X | |
| V61.X | Other family circumstances | | X | | |
| V62.X | Other psychosocial circumstances | | | X | |
| V63.X | Unavailability of other medical facilities for care | | X | | |
| V64.X | Persons encountering health services for specified procedure, not carried out | | | X | |
| V65.X | Other persons seeking consultation without complaint or sickness | | X | | |
| V66.0 | Convalescence and palliative care following surgery | X | | | |
| V66.1 | Convalescence and palliative care following radiotherapy | X | | | |
| V66.2 | Convalescence and palliative care following chemotherapy | X | | | |
| V66.3 | Convalescence and palliative care following psychotherapy and other treatment for mental disorder | X | | | |

[1]  Generally for use as first listed only but may be used as additional if patient has more than one encounter on one day
[2]  These codes may be used as first listed or additional codes
[3]  These codes are only for use as additional codes
[4]  These codes are primarily for use in the nonacute setting and should be limited to encounters for which no sign or symptom or reason for visit is documented in the record.  Their use may be as either a first listed or additional code.

| Code(s) | Description | 1st Dx Only[1] | 1st or Add'l Dx[2] | Add'l Dx Only[3] | Non-Specific Diagnosis[4] |
|---------|-------------|----------------|--------------------|-------------------|---------------------------|
| V66.4 | Convalescence and palliative care following treatment of fracture | X | | | |
| V66.5 | Convalescence and palliative care following other treatment | X | | | |
| V66.6 | Convalescence and palliative care following combined treatment | X | | | |
| V66.7 | Encounter for palliative care | | | X | |
| V66.9 | Unspecified convalescence | X | | | |
| V67.X | Follow-up examination | | X | | |
| V68.X | Encounters for administrative purposes | X | | | |
| V69.X | Problems related to lifestyle | | X | | |
| V70.0 | Routine general medical examination at a health care facility | X | | | |
| V70.1 | General psychiatric examination, requested by the authority | X | | | |
| V70.2 | General psychiatric examination, other and unspecified | X | | | |
| V70.3 | Other medical examination for administrative purposes | X | | | |
| V70.4 | Examination for medicolegal reasons | X | | | |
| V70.5 | Health examination of defined subpopulations | X | | | |
| V70.6 | Health examination in population surveys | X | | | |
| V70.7 | Examination of participant in clinical trial | | X | | |
| V70.8 | Other specified general medical examinations | X | | | |
| V70.9 | Unspecified general medical examination | X | | | |
| V71.X | Observation and evaluation for suspected conditions not found | X | | | |
| V72.0 | Examination of eyes and vision | | **X** | | |
| **V72.1X** | Examination of ears and hearing | | **X** | | |
| V72.2 | Dental examination | | **X** | | |
| V72.3X | Gynecological examination | | **X** | | |
| V72.4X | Pregnancy examination or test | | X | | |
| V72.5 | Radiological examination, NEC | | X | | |
| V72.6 | Laboratory examination | | X | | |
| V72.7 | Diagnostic skin and sensitization tests | | **X** | | |
| V72.81 | Preoperative cardiovascular examination | | **X** | | |
| V72.82 | Preoperative respiratory examination | | **X** | | |
| V72.83 | Other specified preoperative examination | | **X** | | |
| V72.84 | Preoperative examination, unspecified | | **X** | | |
| V72.85 | Other specified examination | | X | | |
| V72.86 | Encounter for blood typing | | X | | |
| V72.9 | Unspecified examination | | | | **X** |
| V73.X | Special screening examination for viral and chlamydial diseases | | X | | |
| V74.X | Special screening examination for bacterial and spirochetal diseases | | X | | |
| V75.X | Special screening examination for other infectious diseases | | X | | |
| V76.X | Special screening examination for malignant neoplasms | | X | | |
| V77.X | Special screening examination for endocrine, nutritional, metabolic and immunity disorders | | X | | |
| V78.X | Special screening examination for disorders of blood and blood-forming organs | | X | | |
| V79.X | Special screening examination for mental disorders and developmental handicaps | | X | | |
| V80.X | Special screening examination for neurological, eye, and ear diseases | | X | | |
| V81.X | Special screening examination for cardiovascular, respiratory, and genitourinary diseases | | X | | |
| V82.X | Special screening examination for other conditions | | X | | |
| V83.X | Genetic carrier status | | X | | |
| V84 | Genetic susceptibility to disease | | | X | |
| V85 | Body mass index | | | X | |
| **V86** | **Estrogen receptor status** | | | **X** | |

[1]  Generally for use as first listed only but may be used as additional if patient has more than one encounter on one day
[2]  These codes may be used as first listed or additional codes
[3]  These codes are only for use as additional codes
[4]  These codes are primarily for use in the nonacute setting and should be limited to encounters for which no sign or symptom or reason for visit is documented in the record.  Their use may be as either a first listed or additional code.

19. **Supplemental Classification of External Causes of Injury and Poisoning (E-codes, E800- E999)**—Introduction: These guidelines are provided for those who are currently collecting E codes in order that there will be standardization in the process. If your institution plans to begin collecting E codes, these guidelines are to be applied. The use of E codes is supplemental to the application of ICD-9-CM diagnosis codes. E codes are never to be recorded as principal diagnoses (first-listed in non-inpatient setting) and are not required for reporting to CMS.

External causes of injury and poisoning codes (E codes) are intended to provide data for injury research and evaluation of injury prevention strategies. E codes capture how the injury or poisoning happened (cause), the intent (unintentional or accidental; or intentional, such as suicide or assault), and the place where the event occurred.

Some major categories of E codes include:

transport accidents

poisoning and adverse effects of drugs, medicinal substances and biologicals

accidental falls

accidents caused by fire and flames

accidents due to natural and environmental factors

late effects of accidents, assaults or self injury

assaults or purposely inflicted injury

suicide or self inflicted injury

These guidelines apply for the coding and collection of E codes from records in hospitals, outpatient clinics, emergency departments, other ambulatory care settings and provider offices, and nonacute care settings, except when other specific guidelines apply.

### a. General E code coding guidelines

1) **Used with any code in the range of 001-V86.1**—An E code may be used with any code in the range of 001-V86.1, which indicates an injury, poisoning, or adverse effect due to an external cause.

2) **Assign the appropriate E code for all initial treatments**—Assign the appropriate E code for the initial encounter of an injury, poisoning, or adverse effect of drugs, not for subsequent treatment.

   **External cause of injury codes (E codes) may be assigned while the acute fracture codes are still applicable.**

   *See Section I.C.17.b.1 for coding of acute fractures.*

3) **Use the full range of E codes**—Use the full range of E codes to completely describe the cause, the intent and the place of occurrence, if applicable, for all injuries, poisonings, and adverse effects of drugs.

4) **Assign as many E codes as necessary**—Assign as many E codes as necessary to fully explain each cause. If only one E code can be recorded, assign the E code most related to the principal diagnosis.

5) **The selection of the appropriate E code**—The selection of the appropriate E code is guided by the Index to External Causes, which is located after the alphabetical index to diseases and by Inclusion and Exclusion notes in the Tabular List.

6) **E code can never be a principal diagnosis**—An E code can never be a principal (first listed) diagnosis.

7) **External cause code(s) with systemic inflammatory response syndrome (SIRS)**—**An external cause code is not appropriate with a code from subcategory 995.9, unless the patient also has an injury, poisoning, or adverse effect of drugs.**

### b. Place of Occurrence Guideline

**Place of Occurrence Guideline**—Use an additional code from category E849 to indicate the Place of Occurrence for injuries and poisonings. The Place of Occurrence describes the place where the event occurred and not the patient's activity at the time of the event. Do not use E849.9 if the place of occurrence is not stated.

### c. Adverse Effects of Drugs, Medicinal and Biological Substances Guidelines

1) **Do not code directly from the Table of Drugs**—Do not code directly from the Table of Drugs and Chemicals. Always refer back to the Tabular List.

2) **Use as many codes as necessary to describe**—Use as many codes as necessary to describe completely all drugs, medicinal or biological substances.

3) **If the same E code would describe the causative agent**—If the same E code would describe the causative agent for more than one adverse reaction, assign the code only once.

4) **If two or more drugs, medicinal or biological substances**—If two or more drugs, medicinal or biological substances are reported, code each individually unless the combination code is listed in the Table of Drugs and Chemicals. In that case, assign the E code for the combination.

5) **When a reaction results from the interaction of a drug(s)**—When a reaction results from the interaction of a drug(s) and alcohol, use poisoning codes and E codes for both.

6) **If the reporting format limits the number of E codes**—If the reporting format limits the number of E codes that can be used in reporting clinical data, code the one most related to the principal diagnosis. Include at least one from each category (cause, intent, place) if possible.

   If there are different fourth digit codes in the same three digit category, use the code for "Other specified" of that category. If there is no "Other specified" code in that category, use the appropriate "Unspecified" code in that category.

   If the codes are in different three digit categories, assign the appropriate E code for other multiple drugs and medicinal substances.

7) **Codes from the E930-E949 series**—Codes from the E930-E949 series must be used to identify the causative substance for an adverse effect of drug, medicinal and biological substances, correctly prescribed and properly administered. The effect, such as tachycardia, delirium, gastrointestinal hemorrhaging, vomiting, hypokalemia, hepatitis, renal failure, or respiratory failure, is coded and followed by the appropriate code from the E930-E949 series.

### d. Multiple cause E code coding guidelines

**Multiple cause E code coding guidelines**—If two or more events cause separate injuries, an E code should be assigned for each cause. The first listed E code will be selected in the following order:

E codes for child and adult abuse take priority over all other E codes.

*See Section I.C.19.e., Child and Adult abuse guidelines.*

E codes for terrorism events take priority over all other E codes except child and adult abuse.

E codes for cataclysmic events take priority over all other E codes except child and adult abuse and terrorism.

E codes for transport accidents take priority over all other E codes except cataclysmic events and child and adult abuse and terrorism.

The first-listed E code should correspond to the cause of the most serious diagnosis due to an assault, accident, or self-harm, following the order of hierarchy listed above.

### e. Child and Adult Abuse Guideline

1) **Intentional injury**—When the cause of an injury or neglect is intentional child or adult abuse, the first listed E code should be assigned from categories E960-E968, Homicide and injury purposely inflicted by other persons, (except category E967). An E code from category E967, Child and adult battering and other maltreatment, should be added as an additional code to identify the perpetrator, if known.

2) **Accidental intent**—In cases of neglect when the intent is determined to be accidental E code E904.0, Abandonment or neglect of infant and helpless person, should be the first listed E code.

f.  **Unknown or Suspected Intent Guideline**

1) **If the intent (accident, self-harm, assault) of the cause of an injury or poisoning is unknown**

If the intent (accident, self-harm, assault) of the cause of an injury or poisoning is unknown or unspecified, code the intent as undetermined E980-E989.

2) **If the intent (accident, self-harm, assault) of the cause of an injury or poisoning is questionable**

If the intent (accident, self-harm, assault) of the cause of an injury or poisoning is questionable, probable or suspected, code the intent as undetermined E980-E989.

g.  **Undetermined Cause**—When the intent of an injury or poisoning is known, but the cause is unknown, use codes: E928.9, Unspecified accident, E958.9, Suicide and self-inflicted injury by unspecified means, and E968.9, Assault by unspecified means.

These E codes should rarely be used, as the documentation in the medical record, in both the inpatient outpatient and other settings, should normally provide sufficient detail to determine the cause of the injury.

h.  **Late Effects of External Cause Guidelines**

1) **Late effect E codes**—Late effect E codes exist for injuries and poisonings but not for adverse effects of drugs, misadventures and surgical complications.

2) **Late effect E codes (E929, E959, E969, E977, E989, or E999.1)**—A late effect E code (E929, E959, E969, E977, E989, or E999.1) should be used with any report of a late effect or sequela resulting from a previous injury or poisoning (905-909).

3) **Late effect E code with a related current injury**—A late effect E code should never be used with a related current nature of injury code.

4) **Use of late effect E codes for subsequent visits**—Use a late effect E code for subsequent visits when a late effect of the initial injury or poisoning is being treated. There is no late effect E code for adverse effects of drugs. Do not use a late effect E code for subsequent visits for follow-up care (e.g., to assess healing, to receive rehabilitative therapy) of the injury or poisoning when no late effect of the injury has been documented.

i.  **Misadventures and Complications of Care Guidelines**

1) **Code range E870-E876**—Assign a code in the range of E870-E876 if misadventures are stated by the provider.

2) **Code range E878-E879**—Assign a code in the range of E878-E879 if the provider attributes an abnormal reaction or later complication to a surgical or medical procedure, but does not mention misadventure at the time of the procedure as the cause of the reaction.

j.  **Terrorism Guidelines**

1) **Cause of injury identified by the Federal Government (FBI) as terrorism**—When the cause of an injury is identified by the Federal Government (FBI) as terrorism, the first-listed E-code should be a code from category E979, Terrorism. The definition of terrorism employed by the FBI is found at the inclusion note at E979. The terrorism E-code is the only E-code that should be assigned. Additional E codes from the assault categories should not be assigned.

2) **Cause of an injury is suspected to be the result of terrorism**—When the cause of an injury is suspected to be the result of terrorism a code from category E979 should not be assigned. Assign a code in the range of E codes based circumstances on the documentation of intent and mechanism.

3) **Code E979.9, Terrorism, secondary effects**—Assign code E979.9, Terrorism, secondary effects, for conditions occurring subsequent to the terrorist event. This code should not be assigned for conditions that are due to the initial terrorist act.

4) **Statistical tabulation of terrorism codes**—For statistical purposes these codes will be tabulated within the category for assault, expanding the current category from E960-E969 to include E979 and E999.1.

## Section II. Selection of Principal Diagnosis

The circumstances of inpatient admission always govern the selection of principal diagnosis. The principal diagnosis is defined in the Uniform Hospital Discharge Data Set (UHDDS) as "that condition established after study to be chiefly responsible for occasioning the admission of the patient to the hospital for care."

The UHDDS definitions are used by hospitals to report inpatient data elements in a standardized manner. These data elements and their definitions can be found in the July 31, 1985, Federal Register (Vol. 50, No, 147), pp. 31038-40.

Since that time the application of the UHDDS definitions has been expanded to include all non-outpatient settings (acute care, short term, long term care and psychiatric hospitals; home health agencies; rehab facilities; nursing homes, etc).

In determining principal diagnosis the coding conventions in the ICD-9-CM, Volumes I and II take precedence over these official coding guidelines.

*(See Section I.A., Conventions for the ICD-9-CM)*

The importance of consistent, complete documentation in the medical record cannot be overemphasized. Without such documentation the application of all coding guidelines is a difficult, if not impossible, task.

**A. Codes for symptoms, signs, and ill-defined conditions**—Codes for symptoms, signs, and ill-defined conditions from Chapter 16 are not to be used as principal diagnosis when a related definitive diagnosis has been established.

**B. Two or more interrelated conditions, each potentially meeting the definition for principal diagnosis**—When there are two or more interrelated conditions (such as diseases in the same ICD-9-CM chapter or manifestations characteristically associated with a certain disease) potentially meeting the definition of principal diagnosis, either condition may be sequenced first, unless the circumstances of the admission, the therapy provided, the Tabular List, or the Alphabetic Index indicate otherwise.

**C. Two or more diagnoses that equally meet the definition for principal diagnosis**—In the unusual instance when two or more diagnoses equally meet the criteria for principal diagnosis as determined by the circumstances of admission, diagnostic workup and/or therapy provided, and the Alphabetic Index, Tabular List, or another coding guidelines does not provide sequencing direction, any one of the diagnoses may be sequenced first.

**D. Two or more comparative or contrasting conditions**—In those rare instances when two or more contrasting or comparative diagnoses are documented as "either/or" (or similar terminology), they are coded as if the diagnoses were confirmed and the diagnoses are sequenced according to the circumstances of the admission. If no further determination can be made as to which diagnosis should be principal, either diagnosis may be sequenced first.

**E. A symptom(s) followed by contrasting/comparative diagnoses**—When a symptom(s) is followed by contrasting/comparative diagnoses, the symptom code is sequenced first. All the contrasting/comparative diagnoses should be coded as additional diagnoses.

**F. Original treatment plan not carried out**—Sequence as the principal diagnosis the condition, which after study occasioned the admission to the hospital, even though treatment may not have been carried out due to unforeseen circumstances.

**G. Complications of surgery and other medical care**—When the admission is for treatment of a complication resulting from surgery or other medical care, the complication code is sequenced as the principal diagnosis. If the complication is classified to the 996-999 series and the code lacks the necessary specificity in describing the complication, an additional code for the specific complication should be assigned.

**H. Uncertain Diagnosis**—If the diagnosis documented at the time of discharge is qualified as "probable," "suspected," "likely," "questionable," "possible," or "still to be ruled out," **or other similar terms indicating uncertainty**, code the condition as if it existed or was established. The bases for these guidelines are the diagnostic workup, arrangements for further workup or observation, and initial therapeutic approach that correspond most closely with the established diagnosis.

Note: This guideline is applicable only to short-term, acute, long-term care and psychiatric hospitals.

## I. Admission from Observation Unit

1. **Admission following medical observation**—When a patient is admitted to an observation unit for a medical condition, which either worsens or does not improve, and is subsequently admitted as an inpatient of the same hospital for this same medical condition, the principal diagnosis would be the medical condition which led to the hospital admission.

2. **Admission following post-operative observation**—When a patient is admitted to an observation unit to monitor a condition (or complication) that develops following outpatient surgery, and then is subsequently admitted as an inpatient of the same hospital, hospitals should apply the Uniform Hospital Discharge Data Set (UHDDS) definition of principal diagnosis as "that condition established after study to be chiefly responsible for occasioning the admission of the patient to the hospital for care."

**J. Admission from outpatient surgery**—When a patient receives surgery in the hospital's outpatient surgery department and is subsequently admitted for continuing inpatient care at the same hospital, the following guidelines should be followed in selecting the principal diagnosis for the inpatient admission:

- If the reason for the inpatient admission is a complication, assign the complication as the principal diagnosis.

- If no complication, or other condition, is documented as the reason for the inpatient admission, assign the reason for the outpatient surgery as the principal diagnosis.

- If the reason for the inpatient admission is another condition unrelated to the surgery, assign the unrelated condition as the principal diagnosis.

## Section III. Reporting Additional Diagnoses

### GENERAL RULES FOR OTHER (ADDITIONAL) DIAGNOSES

For reporting purposes the definition for "other diagnoses" is interpreted as additional conditions that affect patient care in terms of requiring:

clinical evaluation; or

therapeutic treatment; or

diagnostic procedures; or

extended length of hospital stay; or

increased nursing care and/or monitoring.

The UHDDS item #11-b defines Other Diagnoses as "all conditions that coexist at the time of admission, that develop subsequently, or that affect the treatment received and/or the length of stay. Diagnoses that relate to an earlier episode which have no bearing on the current hospital stay are to be excluded." UHDDS definitions apply to inpatients in acute care, short-term, long term care and psychiatric hospital setting. The UHDDS definitions are used by acute care short-term hospitals to report inpatient data elements in a standardized manner. These data elements and their definitions can be found in the July 31, 1985, Federal Register (Vol. 50, No, 147), pp. 31038-40.

Since that time the application of the UHDDS definitions has been expanded to include all non-outpatient settings (acute care, short term, long term care and psychiatric hospitals; home health agencies; rehab facilities; nursing homes, etc.).

The following guidelines are to be applied in designating "other diagnoses" when neither the Alphabetic Index nor the Tabular List in ICD-9-CM provide direction. The listing of the diagnoses in the patient record is the responsibility of the attending provider.

**A. Previous conditions**—If the provider has included a diagnosis in the final diagnostic statement, such as the discharge summary or the face sheet, it should ordinarily be coded. Some providers include in the diagnostic statement resolved conditions or diagnoses and status-post procedures from previous admission that have no bearing on the current stay. Such conditions are not to be reported and are coded only if required by hospital policy.

However, history codes (V10-V19) may be used as secondary codes if the historical condition or family history has an impact on current care or influences treatment.

**B. Abnormal findings**—Abnormal findings (laboratory, x-ray, pathologic, and other diagnostic results) are not coded and reported unless the provider indicates their clinical significance. If the findings are outside the normal range and the attending provider has ordered other tests to evaluate the condition or prescribed treatment, it is appropriate to ask the provider whether the abnormal finding should be added.

**Please note:** This differs from the coding practices in the outpatient setting for coding encounters for diagnostic tests that have been interpreted by a provider.

**C. Uncertain Diagnosis**—If the diagnosis documented at the time of discharge is qualified as "probable," "suspected," "likely," "questionable," "possible," or "still to be ruled out" **or other similar terms indicating uncertainty**, code the condition as if it existed or was established. The bases for these guidelines are the diagnostic workup, arrangements for further workup or observation, and initial therapeutic approach that correspond most closely with the established diagnosis.

**Note:** This guideline is applicable only to short-term, acute, long-term care and psychiatric hospitals.

## Section IV. Diagnostic Coding and Reporting Guidelines for Outpatient Services

These coding guidelines for outpatient diagnoses have been approved for use by hospitals/ providers in coding and reporting hospital-based outpatient services and provider-based office visits.

Information about the use of certain abbreviations, punctuation, symbols, and other conventions used in the ICD-9-CM Tabular List (code numbers and titles), can be found in Section IA of these guidelines, under "Conventions Used in the Tabular List." Information about the correct sequence to use in finding a code is also described in Section I.

The terms encounter and visit are often used interchangeably in describing outpatient service contacts and, therefore, appear together in these guidelines without distinguishing one from the other.

Though the conventions and general guidelines apply to all settings, coding guidelines for outpatient and provider reporting of diagnoses will vary in a number of instances from those for inpatient diagnoses, recognizing that:

> The Uniform Hospital Discharge Data Set (UHDDS) definition of principal diagnosis applies only to inpatients in acute, short-term, long-term care and psychiatric hospitals.
>
> Coding guidelines for inconclusive diagnoses (probable, suspected, rule out, etc.) were developed for inpatient reporting and do not apply to outpatients.

**A. Selection of first-listed condition**—In the outpatient setting, the term first-listed diagnosis is used in lieu of principal diagnosis.

In determining the first-listed diagnosis the coding conventions of ICD-9-CM, as well as the general and disease specific guidelines take precedence over the outpatient guidelines.

Diagnoses often are not established at the time of the initial encounter/visit. It may take two or more visits before the diagnosis is confirmed.

The most critical rule involves beginning the search for the correct code assignment through the Alphabetic Index. Never begin searching initially in the Tabular List as this will lead to coding errors.

1. **Outpatient surgery**—When a patient presents for outpatient surgery, code the reason for the surgery as the first-listed diagnosis (reason for the encounter), even if the surgery is not performed due to a contraindication.

2. **Observation stay**—When a patient is admitted for observation for a medical condition, assign a code for the medical condition as the first-listed diagnosis. When a patient presents for outpatient surgery and develops complications requiring admission to observation, code the reason for the surgery as the first reported diagnosis (reason for the encounter), followed by codes for the complications as secondary diagnoses.

**B. Codes from 001.0 through V86.1**—The appropriate code or codes from 001.0 through V86.1 must be used to identify diagnoses, symptoms, conditions, problems, complaints, or other reason(s) for the encounter/visit.

**C. Accurate reporting of ICD-9-CM diagnosis codes**—For accurate reporting of ICD-9-CM diagnosis codes, the documentation should describe the patient's condition, using terminology which includes specific diagnoses as well as symptoms, problems, or reasons for the encounter. There are ICD-9-CM codes to describe all of these.

**D. Selection of codes 001.0 through 999.9**—The selection of codes 001.0 through 999.9 will frequently be used to describe the reason for the encounter. These codes are from the section of ICD-9-CM for the classification of diseases and injuries (e.g. infectious and parasitic diseases; neoplasms; symptoms, signs, and ill-defined conditions, etc.).

**E. Codes that describe symptoms and signs**—Codes that describe symptoms and signs, as opposed to diagnoses, are acceptable for reporting purposes when a diagnosis has not been established (confirmed) by the provider. Chapter 16 of ICD-9-CM, Symptoms, Signs, and Ill-defined Conditions (codes 780.0 - 799.9) contain many, but not all codes for symptoms.

**F. Encounters for circumstances other than a disease or injury**—ICD-9-CM provides codes to deal with encounters for circumstances other than a disease or injury. The Supplementary Classification of factors Influencing Health Status and Contact with Health Services (V01.0- V84.8) is provided to deal with occasions when circumstances other than a disease or injury are recorded as diagnosis or problems. *See Section I.C. 18 for information on V codes.*

**G. Level of Detail in Coding**

1. **ICD-9-CM codes with 3, 4, or 5 digits**

   ICD-9-CM is composed of codes with either 3, 4, or 5 digits. Codes with three digits are included in ICD-9-CM as the heading of a category of codes that may be further subdivided by the use of fourth and/or fifth digits, which provide greater specificity.

2. **Use of full number of digits required for a code**

   A three-digit code is to be used only if it is not further subdivided. Where fourth-digit subcategories and/or fifth-digit subclassifications are provided, they must be assigned. A code is invalid if it has not been coded to the full number of digits required for that code. *See also discussion under Section I.b.3., General Coding Guidelines, Level of Detail in Coding.*

**H. ICD-9-CM code for the diagnosis, condition, problem, or other reason for encounter/visit**—List first the ICD-9-CM code for the diagnosis, condition, problem, or other reason for encounter/visit shown in the medical record to be chiefly responsible for the services provided. List additional codes that describe any coexisting conditions. In some cases the first-listed diagnosis may be a symptom when a diagnosis has not been established (confirmed) by the physician.

**I. Uncertain diagnosis**—Do not code diagnoses documented as "probable," "suspected," "questionable," "rule out," or "working diagnosis" **or other similar terms indicating uncertainty**. Rather, code the condition(s) to the highest degree of certainty for that encounter/visit, such as symptoms, signs, abnormal test results, or other reason for the visit.

**Please note**: This differs from the coding practices used by short-term, acute care, long-term care and psychiatric hospitals.

**J. Chronic diseases**—Chronic diseases treated on an ongoing basis may be coded and reported as many times as the patient receives treatment and care for the condition(s).

**K. Code all documented conditions that coexist**—Code all documented conditions that coexist at the time of the encounter/visit, and require or affect patient care treatment or management. Do not code conditions that were previously treated and no longer exist. However, history codes (V10-V19) may be used as secondary codes if the historical condition or family history has an impact on current care or influences treatment.

**L. Patients receiving diagnostic services only**—For patients receiving diagnostic services only during an encounter/visit, sequence first the diagnosis, condition, problem, or other reason for encounter/visit shown in the medical record to be chiefly responsible for the outpatient services provided during the encounter/visit. Codes for other diagnoses (e.g., chronic conditions) may be sequenced as additional diagnoses.

**For encounters for routine laboratory/radiology testing in the absence of any signs, symptoms, or associated diagnosis, assign V72.5 and V72.6. If routine testing is performed during the same encounter as a test to evaluate a sign, symptom, or diagnosis, it is appropriate to assign both the V code and the code describing the reason for the non-routine test.**

For outpatient encounters for diagnostic tests that have been interpreted by a physician, and the final report is available at the time of coding, code any confirmed or definitive diagnosis(es) documented in the interpretation. Do not code related signs and symptoms as additional diagnoses.

**Please note**: This differs from the coding practice in the hospital inpatient setting regarding abnormal findings on test results.

**M. Patients receiving therapeutic services only**—For patients receiving therapeutic services only during an encounter/visit, sequence first the diagnosis, condition, problem, or other reason for encounter/visit shown in the medical record to be chiefly responsible for the outpatient services provided during the encounter/visit. Codes for other diagnoses (e.g., chronic conditions) may be sequenced as additional diagnoses.

The only exception to this rule is that when the primary reason for the admission/encounter is chemotherapy, radiation therapy, or rehabilitation, the appropriate V code for the service is listed first, and the diagnosis or problem for which the service is being performed listed second.

**N. Patients receiving preoperative evaluations only**—For patients receiving preoperative evaluations only, sequence first a code from category V72.8, Other specified examinations, to describe the pre-op consultations. Assign a code for the condition to describe the reason for the surgery as an additional diagnosis. Code also any findings related to the pre-op evaluation.

**O. Ambulatory surgery**—For ambulatory surgery, code the diagnosis for which the surgery was performed. If the postoperative diagnosis is known to be different from the preoperative diagnosis at the time the diagnosis is confirmed, select the postoperative diagnosis for coding, since it is the most definitive.

**P. Routine outpatient prenatal visits**—For routine outpatient prenatal visits when no complications are present, codes V22.0, Supervision of normal first pregnancy, or V22.1 Supervision of other normal pregnancy, should be used as the principal diagnosis. These codes should not be used in conjunction with Chapter 11 codes.

## Appendix I Present on Admission Reporting Guidelines [Added to the Official Coding Guidelines October 1, 2006]

### Introduction

These guidelines are to be used as a supplement to the *ICD-9-CM Official Guidelines for Coding and Reporting* to facilitate the assignment of the Present on Admission (POA) indicator for each diagnosis and external cause of injury code reported on claim forms (UB-04 and 837 Institutional).

These guidelines are not intended to replace any guidelines in the main body of the *ICD-9-CM Official Guidelines for Coding and Reporting*. The POA guidelines are not intended to provide guidance on when a condition should be coded, but rather, how to apply the POA indicator to the final set of diagnosis codes that have been assigned in accordance with Sections I, II, and III of the official coding guidelines. Subsequent to the assignment of the ICD-9-CM codes, the POA indicator should then be assigned to those conditions that have been coded.

As stated in the Introduction to the ICD-9-CM Official Guidelines for Coding and Reporting, a joint effort between the healthcare provider and the coder is essential to achieve complete and accurate documentation, code assignment, and reporting of diagnoses and procedures. The importance of consistent, complete documentation in the medical record cannot be overemphasized. Medical record documentation from any provider involved in the care and treatment of the patient may be used to support the determination of whether a condition was present on admission or not. In the context of the official coding guidelines, the term "provider" means a physician or any qualified healthcare practitioner who is legally accountable for establishing the patient's diagnosis.

### General Reporting Requirements

All claims involving inpatient admissions to general acute care hospitals or other facilities that are subject to a law or regulation mandating collection of present on admission information.

Present on admission is defined as present at the time the order for inpatient admission occurs—conditions that develop during an outpatient encounter, including emergency department, observation, or outpatient surgery, are considered as present on admission.

POA indicator is assigned to principal and secondary diagnoses (as defined in Section II of the Official Guidelines for Coding and Reporting) and the external cause of injury codes.

Issues related to inconsistent, missing, conflicting or unclear documentation must still be resolved by the provider.

If a condition would not be coded and reported based on UHDDS definitions and current official coding guidelines, then the POA indicator would not be reported.

### Reporting Options

Y - Yes

N - No

U - Unknown

W – Clinically undetermined

Unreported/Not used – (Exempt from POA reporting)

### Reporting Definitions

Y = present at the time of inpatient admission

N = not present at the time of inpatient admission

U = documentation is insufficient to determine if condition is present on admission

W = provider is unable to clinically determine whether condition was present on admission or not

## Assigning the POA Indicator

### Condition is on the "Exempt from Reporting" list

Leave the "present on admission" field blank if the condition is on the list of ICD-9-CM codes for which this field is not applicable. This is the only circumstance in which the field may be left blank.

### POA Explicitly Documented

Assign Y for any condition the provider explicitly documents as being present on admission.

Assign N for any condition the provider explicitly documents as not present at the time of admission.

### Conditions diagnosed prior to inpatient admission

Assign "Y" for conditions that were diagnosed prior to admission (example: hypertension, diabetes mellitus, asthma)

### Conditions diagnosed during the admission but clearly present before admission

Assign "Y" for conditions diagnosed during the admission that were clearly present but not diagnosed until after admission occurred.

Diagnoses subsequently confirmed after admission are considered present on admission if at the time of admission they are documented as suspected, possible, rule out, differential diagnosis, or constitute an underlying cause of a symptom that is present at the time of admission.

### Condition develops during outpatient encounter prior to inpatient admission

Assign Y for any condition that develops during an outpatient encounter prior to a written order for inpatient admission.

### Documentation does not indicate whether condition was present on admission

Assign "U" when the medical record documentation is unclear as to whether the condition was present on admission. "U" should not be routinely assigned and used only in very limited circumstances. Coders are encouraged to query the providers when the documentation is unclear.

### Documentation states that it cannot be determined whether the condition was or was not present on admission

Assign "W" when the medical record documentation indicates that it cannot be clinically determined whether or not the condition was present on admission.

### Chronic condition with acute exacerbation during the admission

If the code is a combination code that identifies both the chronic condition and the acute exacerbation, see POA guidelines pertaining to combination codes.

If the combination code only identifies the chronic condition and not the acute exacerbation (e.g., acute exacerbation of CHF), assign "Y."

### Conditions documented as possible, probable, suspected, or rule out at the time of discharge

If the final diagnosis contains a possible, probable, suspected, or rule out diagnosis, and this diagnosis was suspected at the time of inpatient admission, assign "Y."

If the final diagnosis contains a possible, probable, suspected, or rule out diagnosis, and this diagnosis was based on symptoms or clinical findings that were not present on admission, assign "N".

### Conditions documented as impending or threatened at the time of discharge

If the final diagnosis contains an impending or threatened diagnosis, and this diagnosis is based on symptoms or clinical findings that were present on admission, assign "Y."

If the final diagnosis contains an impending or threatened diagnosis, and this diagnosis is based on symptoms or clinical findings that were not present on admission, assign "N."

### Acute and chronic conditions

Assign "Y" for acute conditions that are present at time of admission and N for acute conditions that are not present at time of admission.

Assign "Y" for chronic conditions, even though the condition may not be diagnosed until after admission.

If a single code identifies both an acute and chronic condition, see the POA guidelines for combination codes.

### Combination codes

Assign "N" if any part of the combination code was not present on admission (e.g., obstructive chronic bronchitis with acute exacerbation and the exacerbation was not present on admission; gastric ulcer that does not start bleeding until after admission; asthma patient develops status asthmaticus after admission).

Assign "Y" if all parts of the combination code were present on admission (e.g., patient with diabetic nephropathy is admitted with uncontrolled diabetes).

If the final diagnosis includes comparative or contrasting diagnoses, and both were present, or suspected, at the time of admission, assign "Y".

For infection codes that include the causal organism, assign "Y" if the infection (or signs of the infection) was present on admission, even though the culture results may not be known until after admission (e.g., patient is admitted with pneumonia and the provider documents pseudomonas as the causal organism a few days later).

### Obstetrical conditions

Whether or not the patient delivers during the current hospitalization does not affect assignment of the POA indicator. The determining factor for POA assignment is whether the pregnancy complication or obstetrical condition described by the code was present at the time of admission or not.

If the pregnancy complication or obstetrical condition was present on admission (e.g., patient admitted in preterm labor), assign "Y."

If the pregnancy complication or obstetrical condition was not present on admission (e.g., 2nd degree laceration during delivery, postpartum hemorrhage that occurred during current hospitalization, fetal distress develops after admission), assign "N."

If the obstetrical code includes more than one diagnosis and any of the diagnoses identified by the code were not present on admission assign "N."

(e.g., Code 642.7 Pre-eclampsia or eclampsia superimposed on preexisting hypertension).

If the obstetrical code includes information that is not a diagnosis, do not consider that information in the POA determination.

(e.g. Code 652.1x Breech or other malpresentation successfully converted to cephalic presentation should be reported as present on admission if the fetus was breech on admission but was converted to cephalic presentation after admission (since the conversion to cephalic presentation does not represent a diagnosis, the fact that the conversion occurred after admission has no bearing on the POA determination).

### Perinatal conditions

Newborns are not considered to be admitted until after birth. Therefore, any condition present at birth or that developed in utero is considered present at admission and should be assigned "Y." This includes conditions that occur during delivery (e.g., injury during delivery, meconium aspiration, exposure to streptococcus B in the vaginal canal).

### Congenital conditions and anomalies

Assign "Y" for congenital conditions and anomalies. Congenital conditions are always considered present on admission.

## External cause of injury codes

Assign "Y" for any E code representing an external cause of injury or poisoning that occurred prior to inpatient admission (e.g., patient fell out of bed at home, patient fell out of bed in emergency room prior to admission).

*Assign "N" for any E code representing an external cause of injury or poisoning that occurred during inpatient hospitalization (e.g., patient fell out of hospital bed during hospital stay, patient experienced an adverse reaction to a medication administered after inpatient admission).*

## Categories and Codes Exempt from Diagnosis Present on Admission Requirement

Note: "Diagnosis present on admission" for these code categories are exempt because they represent circumstances regarding the healthcare encounter or factors influencing health status that do not represent a current disease or injury or are always present on admission.

| | |
|---|---|
| 137-139 | Late effects of infectious and parasitic diseases |
| 268.1 | Rickets, late effect |
| 326 | Late effects of intracranial abscess or pyogenic infection |
| 438 | Late effects of cerebrovascular disease |
| 650 | Normal delivery |
| 660.7 | Failed forceps or vacuum extractor, unspecified |
| 677 | Late effect of complication of pregnancy, childbirth, and the puerperium |
| 905-909 | Late effects of injuries, poisonings, toxic effects, and other external causes |
| V02 | Carrier or suspected carrier of infectious diseases |
| V03 | Need for prophylactic vaccination and inoculation against bacterial diseases |
| V04 | Need for prophylactic vaccination and inoculation against certain viral diseases |
| V05 | Need for other prophylactic vaccination and inoculation against single diseases |
| V06 | Need for prophylactic vaccination and inoculation against combinations of diseases |
| V07 | Need for isolation and other prophylactic measures |
| V10 | Personal history of malignant neoplasm |
| V11 | Personal history of mental disorder |
| V12 | Personal history of certain other diseases |
| V13 | Personal history of other diseases |
| V14 | Personal history of allergy to medicinal agents |
| V15 | Other personal history presenting hazards to health |
| V16 | Family history of malignant neoplasm |
| V17 | Family history of certain chronic disabling diseases |
| V18 | Family history of certain other specific conditions |
| V19 | Family history of other conditions |
| V20 | Health supervision of infant or child |
| V21 | Constitutional states in development |
| V22 | Normal pregnancy |
| V23 | Supervision of high-risk pregnancy |
| V24 | Postpartum care and examination |
| V25 | Encounter for contraceptive management |
| V26 | Procreative management |
| V27 | Outcome of delivery |
| V28 | Antenatal screening |
| V29 | Observation and evaluation of newborns for suspected condition not found |
| V30-V39 | Liveborn infants according to type of birth |
| V42 | Organ or tissue replaced by transplant |
| V43 | Organ or tissue replaced by other means |
| V44 | Artificial opening status |
| V45 | Other postprocedural states |
| V46 | Other dependence on machines |
| V49.60-V49.77 | Upper and lower limb amputation status |
| V49.81-V49.84 | Other specified conditions influencing health status |
| V50 | Elective surgery for purposes other than remedying health states |
| V51 | Aftercare involving the use of plastic surgery |
| V52 | Fitting and adjustment of prosthetic device and implant |
| V53 | Fitting and adjustment of other device |
| V54 | Other orthopedic aftercare |
| V55 | Attention to artificial openings |
| V56 | Encounter for dialysis and dialysis catheter care |
| V57 | Care involving use of rehabilitation procedures |
| V58 | Encounter for other and unspecified procedures and aftercare |
| V59 | Donors |
| V60 | Housing, household, and economic circumstances |
| V61 | Other family circumstances |
| V62 | Other psychosocial circumstances |
| V64 | Persons encountering health services for specific procedures, not carried out |
| V65 | Other persons seeking consultation |
| V66 | Convalescence and palliative care |
| V67 | Follow-up examination |
| V68 | Encounters for administrative purposes |
| V69 | Problems related to lifestyle |
| V70 | General medical examination |
| V71 | Observation and evaluation for suspected condition not found |
| V72 | Special investigations and examinations |
| V73 | Special screening examination for viral and chlamydial diseases |
| V74 | Special screening examination for bacterial and spirochetal diseases |
| V75 | Special screening examination for other infectious diseases |
| V76 | Special screening for malignant neoplasms |
| V77 | Special screening for endocrine, nutritional, metabolic, and immunity disorders |
| V78 | Special screening for disorders of blood and blood-forming organs |
| V79 | Special screening for mental disorders and developmental handicaps |
| V80 | Special screening for neurological, eye, and ear diseases |
| V81 | Special screening for cardiovascular, respiratory, and genitourinary diseases |
| V82 | Special screening for other conditions |
| V83 | Genetic carrier status |
| V84 | Genetic susceptibility to disease |
| V85 | Body Mass Index |
| V86 | Estrogen receptor status |
| E800-E807 | Railway accidents |
| E810-E819 | Motor vehicle traffic accidents |
| E820-E825 | Motor vehicle nontraffic accidents |
| E826-E829 | Other road vehicle accidents |
| E830-E838 | Water transport accidents |
| E840-E845 | Air and space transport accidents |
| E846-E848 | Vehicle accidents not elsewhere classifiable |
| E849.0-E849.6 | Place of occurrence |
| E849.8-E849.9 | Place of occurrence |
| E883.1 | Accidental fall into well |
| E883.2 | Accidental fall into storm drain or manhole |
| E884.0 | Fall from playground equipment |
| E884.1 | Fall from cliff |
| E885.0 | Fall from (nonmotorized) scooter |
| E885.1 | Fall from roller skates |
| E885.2 | Fall from skateboard |
| E885.3 | Fall from skis |
| E885.4 | Fall from snowboard |
| E886.0 | Fall on same level from collision, pushing, or shoving, by or with other person, In sports |
| E890.0-E89.9 | Conflagration in private dwelling |
| E893.0 | Accident caused by ignition of clothing, from controlled fire in private dwelling |
| E893.2 | Accident caused by ignition of clothing, from controlled fire not in building or structure |
| E894 | Ignition of highly inflammable material |
| E895 | Accident caused by controlled fire in private dwelling |
| E897 | Accident caused by controlled fire not in building or structure |
| E898.0-E898.1 | Accident caused by other specified fire and flames |
| E917.0 | Striking against or struck accidentally by objects or persons, in sports without subsequent fall |
| E917.1 | Striking against or struck accidentally by objects or persons, caused by a crowd, by collective fear or panic without subsequent fall |
| E917.2 | Striking against or struck accidentally by objects or persons, in running water without subsequent fall |
| E917.5 | Striking against or struck accidentally by objects or persons, object in sports with subsequent fall |
| E917.6 | Striking against or struck accidentally by objects or persons, caused by a crowd, by collective fear or panic with subsequent fall |
| E919 | Accidents caused by machinery |
| E921.0-E921.9 | Accident caused by explosion of pressure vessel |

| | |
|---|---|
| E922.0-E922.9 | Accident caused by firearm and air gun missile |
| E924.1 | Caustic and corrosive substances |
| E926.2 | Visible and ultraviolet light sources |
| E927 | Overexertion and strenuous movements |
| E928.0-E928.8 | Other and unspecified environmental and accidental causes |
| E929.0-E929.9 | Late effects of accidental injury |
| E959 | Late effects of self-inflicted injury |
| E970-E978 | Legal intervention |
| E979 | Terrorism |
| E981.0-E980.9 | Poisoning by gases in domestic use, undetermined whether accidentally or purposely inflicted |
| E982.0-E982.9 | Poisoning by other gases, undetermined whether accidentally or purposely inflicted |
| E985.0-E985.7 | Injury by firearms, air guns and explosives, undetermined whether accidentally or purposely inflicted |
| E987.0 | Falling from high place, undetermined whether accidentally or purposely inflicted, residential premises |
| E987.2 | Falling from high place, undetermined whether accidentally or purposely inflicted, natural sites |
| E989 | Late effects of injury, undetermined whether accidentally or purposely inflicted |
| E990-E999 | Injury resulting from operations of war |

## POA Examples

### General Medical Surgical

1. Patient is admitted for diagnostic work-up for cachexia. The final diagnosis is malignant neoplasm of lung with metastasis.

   *Assign "Y" on the POA field for the malignant neoplasm. The malignant neoplasm was clearly present on admission, although it was not diagnosed until after the admission occurred.*

2. A patient undergoes outpatient surgery. During the recovery period, the patient develops atrial fibrillation and the patient is subsequently admitted to the hospital as an inpatient.

   *Assign "Y" on the POA field for the atrial fibrillation since it developed prior to a written order for inpatient admission.*

3. A patient is treated in observation and while in Observation, the patient falls out of bed and breaks a hip. The patient is subsequently admitted as an inpatient to treat the hip fracture.

   *Assign "Y" on the POA field for the hip fracture since it developed prior to a written order for inpatient admission.*

4. A patient with known congestive heart failure is admitted to the hospital after he develops decompensated congestive heart failure.

   *Assign "Y" on the POA field for the congestive heart failure. The ICD-9-CM code identifies the chronic condition and does not specify the acute exacerbation.*

5. A patient undergoes inpatient surgery. After surgery, the patient develops fever and is treated aggressively. The physician's final diagnosis documents "possible postoperative infection following surgery."

   *Assign "N" on the POA field for the postoperative infection since final diagnoses that contain the terms "possible," "probable," "suspected" or "rule out" and that are based on symptoms or clinical findings that were not present on admission should be reported as "N."*

6. A patient with severe cough and difficulty breathing was diagnosed during his hospitalization to have lung cancer.

   *Assign "Y" on the POA field for the lung cancer. Even though the cancer was not diagnosed until after admission, it is a chronic before the patient's admission.*

7. A patient is admitted to the hospital for a coronary artery bypass surgery. Postoperatively he developed a pulmonary embolism.

   *Assign "N" on the POA field for the pulmonary embolism. This is an acute condition that was not present on admission.*

8. A patient is admitted with a known history of coronary atherosclerosis, status post myocardial infarction five years ago is now admitted for treatment of impending myocardial infarction. The final diagnosis is documented as "impending myocardial infarction."

   *Assign "Y" to the impending myocardial infarction because the condition is present on admission.*

9. A patient with diabetes mellitus developed uncontrolled diabetes on day 3 of the hospitalization.

   *Assign "N" to the diabetes code because the "uncontrolled" component of the code was not present on admission.*

10. A patient is admitted with high fever and pneumonia. The patient rapidly deteriorates and becomes septic. The discharge diagnosis lists sepsis and pneumonia. The documentation is unclear as to whether the sepsis was present on admission or developed shortly after admission.

    *Query the physician as to whether the sepsis was present on admission, developed shortly after admission, or it cannot be clinically determined as to whether it was present on admission or not.*

11. A patient is admitted for repair of an abdominal aneurysm. However, the aneurysm ruptures after hospital admission.

    *Assign "N" for the ruptured abdominal aneurysm. Although the aneurysm was present on admission, the "ruptured" component of the code description did not occur until after admission.*

12. A patient with viral hepatitis B progresses to hepatic coma after admission.

    *Assign "N" for the viral hepatitis B with hepatic coma because part of the code description did not develop until after admission.*

13. A patient with a history of varicose veins and ulceration of the left lower extremity strikes the area against the side of his hospital bed during an inpatient hospitalization. It bleeds profusely. The final diagnosis lists varicose veins with ulcer and hemorrhage.

    *Assign "Y" for the varicose veins with ulcer. Although the hemorrhage occurred after admission, the code description for varicose veins with ulcer does not mention hemorrhage.*

### Obstetrics

1. A female patient was admitted to the hospital and underwent a normal delivery.

   *Leave the "present on admission" (POA) field blank. Code 650 Normal delivery, is on the "exempt from reporting" list.*

2. Patient admitted in late pregnancy due to excessive vomiting and dehydration. During admission patient goes into premature labor.

   *Assign "Y" for the excessive vomiting and the dehydration. Assign "N" for the premature labor.*

3. Patient admitted in active labor. During the stay, a breast abscess is noted when mother attempted to breast feed. Provider is unable to determine whether the abscess was present on admission.

   *Assign "W" for the breast abscess.*

4. Patient admitted in active labor. After 12 hours of labor it is noted that the infant is in fetal distress and a Cesarean section is performed.

   *Assign "N" for the fetal distress.*

### Newborn

1. A single liveborn infant was delivered in the hospital via Cesarean section. The physician documented fetal bradycardia during labor in the final diagnosis in the newborn record.

   *Assign " Y" because the bradycardia developed prior to the newborn admission (birth).*

2. A newborn developed diarrhea which was believed to be due to the hospital baby formula.

   *Assign " N" because the diarrhea developed after admission.*

## A

**AAT** (alpha-1 antitrypsin) deficiency 273.4
**AAV (disease) (illness) (infection)** — see Human immunodeficiency virus (disease) (illness) (infection)
**Abactio** — see Abortion, induced
**Abactus venter** — see Abortion, induced
**Abarognosis** 781.99
**Abasia** (-astasia) 307.9
  atactica 781.3
  choreic 781.3
  hysterical 300.11
  paroxysmal trepidant 781.3
  spastic 781.3
  trembling 781.3
  trepidans 781.3
**Abderhalden-Kaufmann-Lignac syndrome** (cystinosis) 270.0
**Abdomen, abdominal** — see also condition
  accordion 306.4
  acute 789.0 ☑
  angina 557.1
  burst 868.00
  convulsive equivalent (see also Epilepsy) 345.5 ☑
  heart 746.87
  muscle deficiency syndrome 756.79
  obstipum 756.79
**Abdominalgia** 789.0 ☑
  periodic 277.31
**Abduction contracture, hip or other joint** — see Contraction, joint
**Abercrombie's syndrome** (amyloid degeneration) 277.39
**Aberrant** (congenital) — see also Malposition, congenital
  adrenal gland 759.1
  blood vessel NEC 747.60
    arteriovenous NEC 747.60
    cerebrovascular 747.81
    gastrointestinal 747.61
    lower limb 747.64
    renal 747.62
    spinal 747.82
    upper limb 747.63
  breast 757.6
  endocrine gland NEC 759.2
  gastrointestinal vessel (peripheral) 747.61
  hepatic duct 751.69
  lower limb vessel (peripheral) 747.64
  pancreas 751.7
  parathyroid gland 759.2
  peripheral vascular vessel NEC 747.60
  pituitary gland (pharyngeal) 759.2
  renal blood vessel 747.62
  sebaceous glands, mucous membrane, mouth 750.26
  spinal vessel 747.82
  spleen 759.0
  testis (descent) 752.51
  thymus gland 759.2
  thyroid gland 759.2
  upper limb vessel (peripheral) 747.63
**Aberratio**
  lactis 757.6
  testis 752.51
**Aberration** — see also Anomaly
  chromosome — see Anomaly, chromosome(s)
  distantial 368.9
  mental (see also Disorder, mental, nonpsychotic) 300.9
**Abetalipoproteinemia** 272.5
**Abionarce** 780.79
**Abiotrophy** 799.89
**Ablatio**
  placentae — see Placenta, ablatio
  retinae (see also Detachment, retina) 361.9
**Ablation**
  pituitary (gland) (with hypofunction) 253.7
  placenta — see Placenta, ablatio

**Ablation** — continued
  uterus 621.8
**Ablepharia, ablepharon, ablephary** 743.62
**Ablepsia** — see Blindness
**Ablepsy** — see Blindness
**Ablutomania** 300.3
**Abnormal, abnormality, abnormalities** — see also Anomaly
  acid-base balance 276.4
    fetus or newborn — see Distress, fetal
  adaptation curve, dark 368.63
  alveolar ridge 525.9
  amnion 658.9 ☑
    affecting fetus or newborn 762.9
  anatomical relationship NEC 759.9
  apertures, congenital, diaphragm 756.6
  auditory perception NEC 388.40
  autosomes NEC 758.5
    13 758.1
    18 758.2
    21 or 22 758.0
    $D_1$ 758.1
    $E_3$ 758.2
    G 758.0
  ballistocardiogram 794.39
  basal metabolic rate (BMR) 794.7
  biosynthesis, testicular androgen 257.2
  blood level (of)
    cobalt 790.6
    copper 790.6
    iron 790.6
    lead 790.6
    lithium 790.6
    magnesium 790.6
    mineral 790.6
    zinc 790.6
  blood pressure
    elevated (without diagnosis of hypertension) 796.2
    low (see also Hypotension) 458.9
    reading (incidental) (isolated) (nonspecific) 796.3
  blood sugar 790.29 ●
  bowel sounds 787.5
  breathing behavior — see Respiration
  caloric test 794.19
  cervix (acquired) NEC 622.9
    congenital 752.40
    in pregnancy or childbirth 654.6 ☑
      causing obstructed labor 660.2 ☑
        affecting fetus or newborn 763.1
  chemistry, blood NEC 790.6
  chest sounds 786.7
  chorion 658.9 ☑
    affecting fetus or newborn 762.9
  chromosomal NEC 758.89
    analysis, nonspecific result 795.2
    autosomes (see also Abnormal, autosomes NEC) 758.5
    fetal, (suspected) affecting management of pregnancy 655.1 ☑
    sex 758.81
  clinical findings NEC 796.4
  communication — see Fistula
  configuration of pupils 379.49
  coronary
    artery 746.85
    vein 746.9
  cortisol-binding globulin 255.8
  course, Eustachian tube 744.24
  dentofacial NEC 524.9
    functional 524.50
    specified type NEC 524.89
  development, developmental NEC 759.9
    bone 756.9
    central nervous system 742.9
  direction, teeth 524.30
  Dynia (see also Defect, coagulation) 286.9

**Abnormal, abnormality, abnormalities**
  — see also Anomaly — continued
  Ebstein 746.2
  echocardiogram 793.2
  echoencephalogram 794.01
  echogram NEC — see Findings, abnormal, structure
  electrocardiogram (ECG) (EKG) 794.31
  electroencephalogram (EEG) 794.02
  electromyogram (EMG) 794.17
    ocular 794.14
  electro-oculogram (EOG) 794.12
  electroretinogram (ERG) 794.11
  erythrocytes 289.9
    congenital, with perinatal jaundice 282.9 [774.0]
  Eustachian valve 746.9
  excitability under minor stress 301.9
  fat distribution 782.9
  feces 787.7
  fetal heart rate — see Distress, fetal
  fetus NEC
    affecting management of pregnancy — see Pregnancy, management affected by, fetal
    causing disproportion 653.7 ☑
      affecting fetus or newborn 763.1
      causing obstructed labor 660.1 ☑
        affecting fetus or newborn 763.1
  findings without manifest disease — see Findings, abnormal
  fluid
    amniotic 792.3
    cerebrospinal 792.0
    peritoneal 792.9
    pleural 792.9
    synovial 792.9
    vaginal 792.9
  forces of labor NEC 661.9 ☑
    affecting fetus or newborn 763.7
  form, teeth 520.2
  function studies
    auditory 794.15
    bladder 794.9
    brain 794.00
    cardiovascular 794.30
    endocrine NEC 794.6
    kidney 794.4
    liver 794.8
    nervous system
      central 794.00
      peripheral 794.19
    oculomotor 794.14
    pancreas 794.9
    placenta 794.9
    pulmonary 794.2
    retina 794.11
    special senses 794.19
    spleen 794.9
    thyroid 794.5
    vestibular 794.16
  gait 781.2
    hysterical 300.11
  gastrin secretion 251.5
  globulin
    cortisol-binding 255.8
    thyroid-binding 246.8
  glucagon secretion 251.4
  glucose 790.29
    in pregnancy, childbirth, or puerperium 648.8 ☑
      fetus or newborn 775.0
    non-fasting 790.29
  gravitational (G) forces or states 994.9
  hair NEC 704.2
  hard tissue formation in pulp 522.3
  head movement 781.0
  heart
    rate
      fetus, affecting liveborn infant
        before the onset of labor 763.81
        during labor 763.82

**Abnormal, abnormality, abnormalities**
  — see also Anomaly — continued
  heart — continued
    rate — continued
      fetus, affecting liveborn infant — continued
        unspecified as to time of onset 763.83
      intrauterine
        before the onset of labor 763.81
        during labor 763.82
        unspecified as to time of onset 763.83
      newborn
        before the onset of labor 763.81
        during labor 763.82
        unspecified as to time of onset 763.83
    shadow 793.2
    sounds NEC 785.3
  hemoglobin (see also Disease, hemoglobin) 282.7
    trait — see Trait, hemoglobin, abnormal
  hemorrhage, uterus — see Hemorrhage, uterus
  histology NEC 795.4
  increase
    in
      appetite 783.6
      development 783.9
  involuntary movement 781.0
  jaw closure 524.51
  karyotype 795.2
  knee jerk 796.1
  labor NEC 661.9 ☑
    affecting fetus or newborn 763.7
  laboratory findings — see Findings, abnormal
  length, organ or site, congenital — see Distortion
  loss of height 781.91
  loss of weight 783.21
  lung shadow 793.1
  mammogram 793.80
    calcification 793.89
    calculus 793.89
    microcalcification 793.81
  Mantoux test 795.5
  membranes (fetal)
    affecting fetus or newborn 762.9
    complicating pregnancy 658.8 ☑
  menstruation — see Menstruation
  metabolism (see also condition) 783.9
  movement 781.0
    disorder NEC 333.90
      sleep related, unspecified 780.58
      specified NEC 333.99
    head 781.0
    involuntary 781.0
    specified type NEC 333.99
  muscle contraction, localized 728.85
  myoglobin (Aberdeen) (Annapolis) 289.9
  narrowness, eyelid 743.62
  optokinetic response 379.57
  organs or tissues of pelvis NEC
    in pregnancy or childbirth 654.9 ☑
      affecting fetus or newborn 763.89
      causing obstructed labor 660.2 ☑
        affecting fetus or newborn 763.1
  origin — see Malposition, congenital
  palmar creases 757.2
  Papanicolaou (smear)
    cervix 795.00

☑ Additional Digit Required — Refer to the Tabular List for Digit Selection        ▽ Subterms under main terms may continue to next column or page

**2008 ICD-9-CM**      ▶◀ Revised Text      ● New Line      ▲ Revised Code      **October 2007 • Volume 2 — 1**

**Abnormal, abnormality, abnormalities**
— see also Anomaly —
*continued*
Papanicolaou — *continued*
cervix — *continued*
with
atypical squamous cells
cannot exclude high grade
squamous intraep-
ithelial lesion (ASC-
H) 795.02
of undetermined signifi-
cance (ASC-US)
795.01
cytologic evidence of malignancy 795.06
high grade squamous intraepithelial lesion (HGSIL)
795.04
low grade squamous intraepithelial lesion (LGSIL)
795.03
nonspecific finding NEC 795.09
other site 795.1
parturition
affecting fetus or newborn 763.9
mother — see Delivery, complicated
pelvis (bony) — see Deformity, pelvis
percussion, chest 786.7
periods (grossly) (see also Menstruation) 626.9
phonocardiogram 794.39
placenta — see Placenta, abnormal
plantar reflex 796.1
plasma protein — see Deficiency,
plasma, protein
pleural folds 748.8
position (see also Malposition)
gravid uterus 654.4 ✔
causing obstructed labor
660.2 ✔
affecting fetus or newborn
763.1
posture NEC 781.92
presentation (fetus) — see Presentation, fetus, abnormal
product of conception NEC 631
puberty — see Puberty
pulmonary
artery 747.3
function, newborn 770.89
test results 794.2
ventilation, newborn 770.89
hyperventilation 786.01
pulsations in neck 785.1
pupil reflexes 379.40
quality of milk 676.8 ✔
radiological examination 793.99
abdomen NEC 793.6
biliary tract 793.3
breast 793.89
mammogram NOS 793.80
mammographic
calcification 793.89
calculus 793.89
microcalcification 793.81
gastrointestinal tract 793.4
genitourinary organs 793.5
head 793.0
image test inconclusive due to excess body fat 793.91
intrathoracic organ NEC 793.2
lung (field) 793.1
musculoskeletal system 793.7
retroperitoneum 793.6
skin and subcutaneous tissue
793.99
skull 793.0
red blood cells 790.09
morphology 790.09
volume 790.09
reflex NEC 796.1
renal function test 794.4
respiration signs — see Respiration
response to nerve stimulation 794.10

**Abnormal, abnormality, abnormalities**
— see also Anomaly —
*continued*
retinal correspondence 368.34
rhythm, heart (see also Arrhythmia)
fetus — see Distress, fetal
saliva 792.4
scan
brain 794.09
kidney 794.4
liver 794.8
lung 794.2
thyroid 794.5
secretion
gastrin 251.5
glucagon 251.4
semen 792.2
serum level (of)
acid phosphatase 790.5
alkaline phosphatase 790.5
amylase 790.5
enzymes NEC 790.5
lipase 790.5
shape
cornea 743.41
gallbladder 751.69
gravid uterus 654.4 ✔
affecting fetus or newborn
763.89
causing obstructed labor
660.2 ✔
affecting fetus or newborn
763.1
head (see also Anomaly, skull)
756.0
organ or site, congenital NEC —
see Distortion
sinus venosus 747.40
size
fetus, complicating delivery
653.5 ✔
causing obstructed labor
660.1 ✔
gallbladder 751.69
head (see also Anomaly, skull)
756.0
organ or site, congenital NEC —
see Distortion
teeth 520.2
skin and appendages, congenital NEC
757.9
soft parts of pelvis — see Abnormal,
organs or tissues of pelvis
spermatozoa 792.2
sputum (amount) (color) (excessive)
(odor) (purulent) 786.4
stool NEC 787.7
bloody 578.1
occult 792.1
bulky 787.7
color (dark) (light) 792.1
content (fat) (mucus) (pus) 792.1
occult blood 792.1
synchondrosis 756.9
test results without manifest disease
— see Findings, abnormal
thebesian valve 746.9
thermography — see Findings, abnormal, structure
threshold, cones or rods (eye) 368.63
thyroid-binding globulin 246.8
thyroid product 246.8
toxicology (findings) NEC 796.0
tracheal cartilage (congenital) 748.3
transport protein 273.8
ultrasound results — see Findings,
abnormal, structure
umbilical cord
affecting fetus or newborn 762.6
complicating delivery 663.9 ✔
specified NEC 663.8 ✔
union
cricoid cartilage and thyroid cartilage 748.3
larynx and trachea 748.3

**Abnormal, abnormality, abnormalities**
— see also Anomaly —
*continued*
union — *continued*
thyroid cartilage and hyoid bone
748.3
urination NEC 788.69
psychogenic 306.53
stream
intermittent 788.61
slowing 788.62
splitting 788.61
weak 788.62
urgency 788.63
urine (constituents) NEC 791.9
uterine hemorrhage (see also Hemorrhage, uterus) 626.9
climacteric 627.0
postmenopausal 627.1
vagina (acquired) (congenital)
in pregnancy or childbirth 654.7 ✔
affecting fetus or newborn
763.89
causing obstructed labor
660.2 ✔
affecting fetus or newborn
763.1
vascular sounds 785.9
vectorcardiogram 794.39
visually evoked potential (VEP) 794.13
vulva (acquired) (congenital)
in pregnancy or childbirth 654.8 ✔
affecting fetus or newborn
763.89
causing obstructed labor
660.2 ✔
affecting fetus or newborn
763.1
weight
gain 783.1
of pregnancy 646.1 ✔
with hypertension — see
Toxemia, of pregnancy
loss 783.21
x-ray examination — see Abnormal,
radiological examination
**Abnormally formed uterus** — see
Anomaly, uterus
**Abnormity** (any organ or part) — see
Anomaly
**ABO**
hemolytic disease 773.1
incompatibility reaction 999.6
**Abocclusion** 524.20
**Abolition, language** 784.69
**Aborter, habitual or recurrent** NEC
without current pregnancy 629.81
current abortion (see also Abortion,
spontaneous) 634.9 ✔
affecting fetus or newborn 761.8
observation in current pregnancy
646.3 ✔
**Abortion** (complete) (incomplete) (in-
evitable) (with retained products of
conception) 637.9 ✔

Note — Use the following fifth-digit
subclassification with categories
634–637:

0   unspecified

1   incomplete

2   complete

with
complication(s) (any) following previous abortion — see category 639 ✔
damage to pelvic organ (laceration)
(rupture) (tear) 637.2 ✔
embolism (air) (amniotic fluid)
(blood clot) (pulmonary)
(pyemic) (septic) (soap)
637.6 ✔
genital tract and pelvic infection
637.0 ✔

**Abortion** — *continued*
with — *continued*
hemorrhage, delayed or excessive
637.1 ✔
metabolic disorder 637.4 ✔
renal failure (acute) 637.3 ✔
sepsis (genital tract) (pelvic organ)
637.0 ✔
urinary tract 637.7 ✔
shock (postoperative) (septic)
637.5 ✔
specified complication NEC
637.7 ✔
toxemia 637.3 ✔
unspecified complication(s)
637.8 ✔
urinary tract infection 637.7 ✔
accidental — see Abortion, spontaneous
artificial — see Abortion, induced
attempted (failed) — see Abortion,
failed
criminal — see Abortion, illegal
early — see Abortion, spontaneous
elective — see Abortion, legal
failed (legal) 638.9
with
damage to pelvic organ (laceration) (rupture) (tear) 638.2
embolism (air) (amniotic fluid)
(blood clot) (pulmonary)
(pyemic) (septic) (soap)
638.6
genital tract and pelvic infection
638.0
hemorrhage, delayed or excessive 638.1
metabolic disorder 638.4
renal failure (acute) 638.3
sepsis (genital tract) (pelvic organ) 638.0
urinary tract 638.7
shock (postoperative) (septic)
638.5
specified complication NEC
638.7
toxemia 638.3
unspecified complication(s)
638.8
urinary tract infection 638.7
fetal indication — see Abortion, legal
fetus 779.6
following threatened abortion — see
Abortion, by type
habitual or recurrent (care during
pregnancy) 646.3 ✔
with current abortion (see also
Abortion, spontaneous)
634.9 ✔
affecting fetus or newborn 761.8
without current pregnancy 629.81
homicidal — see Abortion, illegal
illegal 636.9 ✔
with
damage to pelvic organ (laceration) (rupture) (tear)
636.2 ✔
embolism (air) (amniotic fluid)
(blood clot) (pulmonary)
(pyemic) (septic) (soap)
636.6 ✔
genital tract and pelvic infection
636.0 ✔
hemorrhage, delayed or excessive 636.1 ✔
metabolic disorder 636.4 ✔
renal failure 636.3 ✔
sepsis (genital tract) (pelvic organ) 636.0 ✔
urinary tract 636.7 ✔
shock (postoperative) (septic)
636.5 ✔
specified complication NEC
636.7 ✔
toxemia 636.3 ✔

---

**Abortion** — *continued*
illegal — *continued*
with — *continued*
unspecified complication(s) 636.8 ☑
urinary tract infection 636.7 ☑
fetus 779.6
induced 637.9 ☑
illegal — *see* Abortion, illegal
legal indications — *see* Abortion, legal
medical indications — *see* Abortion, legal
therapeutic — *see* Abortion, legal
late — *see* Abortion, spontaneous
legal (legal indication) (medical indication) (under medical supervision) 635.9 ☑
with
damage to pelvic organ (laceration) (rupture) (tear) 635.2 ☑
embolism (air) (amniotic fluid) (blood clot) (pulmonary) (pyemic) (septic) (soap) 635.6 ☑
genital tract and pelvic infection 635.0 ☑
hemorrhage, delayed or excessive 635.1 ☑
metabolic disorder 635.4 ☑
renal failure (acute) 635.3 ☑
sepsis (genital tract) (pelvic organ) 635.0 ☑
urinary tract 635.7 ☑
shock (postoperative) (septic) 635.5 ☑
specified complication NEC 635.7 ☑
toxemia 635.3 ☑
unspecified complication(s) 635.8 ☑
urinary tract infection 635.7 ☑
fetus 779.6
medical indication — *see* Abortion, legal
mental hygiene problem — *see* Abortion, legal
missed 632
operative — *see* Abortion, legal
psychiatric indication — *see* Abortion, legal
recurrent — *see* Abortion, spontaneous
self-induced — *see* Abortion, illegal
septic — *see* Abortion, by type, with sepsis
spontaneous 634.9 ☑
with
damage to pelvic organ (laceration) (rupture) (tear) 634.2 ☑
embolism (air) (amniotic fluid) (blood clot) (pulmonary) (pyemic) (septic) (soap) 634.6 ☑
genital tract and pelvic infection 634.0 ☑
hemorrhage, delayed or excessive 634.1 ☑
metabolic disorder 634.4 ☑
renal failure 634.3 ☑
sepsis (genital tract) (pelvic organ) 634.0 ☑
urinary tract 634.7 ☑
shock (postoperative) (septic) 634.5 ☑
specified complication NEC 634.7 ☑
toxemia 634.3 ☑
unspecified complication(s) 634.8 ☑
urinary tract infection 634.7 ☑
fetus 761.8
threatened 640.0 ☑

**Abortion** — *continued*
spontaneous — *continued*
threatened — *continued*
affecting fetus or newborn 762.1
surgical — *see* Abortion, legal
therapeutic — *see* Abortion, legal
threatened 640.0 ☑
affecting fetus or newborn 762.1
tubal — *see* Pregnancy, tubal
voluntary — *see* Abortion, legal
**Abortus fever** 023.9
**Aboulomania** 301.6
**Abrachia** 755.20
**Abrachiatism** 755.20
**Abrachiocephalia** 759.89
**Abrachiocephalus** 759.89
**Abrami's disease** (acquired hemolytic jaundice) 283.9
**Abramov-Fiedler myocarditis** (acute isolated myocarditis) 422.91
**Abrasion** — *see also* Injury, superficial, by site
cornea 918.1
dental 521.20
extending into
dentine 521.22
pulp 521.23
generalized 521.25
limited to enamel 521.21
localized 521.24
teeth, tooth (dentifrice) (habitual) (hard tissues) (occupational) (ritual) (traditional) (wedge defect) — *see also* Abrasion, dental 521.20
**Abrikossov's tumor** (M9580/0) — *see also* Neoplasm, connective tissue, benign
malignant (M9580/3) — *see* Neoplasm, connective tissue, malignant
**Abrism** 988.8
**Abruption, placenta** — *see* Placenta, abruptio
**Abruptio placentae** — *see* Placenta, abruptio
**Abscess** (acute) (chronic) (infectional) (lymphangitic) (metastatic) (multiple) (pyogenic) (septic) (with lymphangitis) — *see also* Cellulitis 682.9
abdomen, abdominal
cavity 567.22
wall 682.2
abdominopelvic 567.22
accessory sinus (chronic) (*see also* Sinusitis) 473.9
adrenal (capsule) (gland) 255.8
alveolar 522.5
with sinus 522.7
amebic 006.3
bladder 006.8
brain (with liver or lung abscess) 006.5
liver (without mention of brain or lung abscess) 006.3
with
brain abscess (and lung abscess) 006.5
lung abscess 006.4
lung (with liver abscess) 006.4
with brain abscess 006.5
seminal vesicle 006.8
specified site NEC 006.8
spleen 006.8
anaerobic 040.0
ankle 682.6
anorectal 566
antecubital space 682.3
antrum (chronic) (Highmore) (*see also* Sinusitis, maxillary) 473.0
anus 566
apical (tooth) 522.5
with sinus (alveolar) 522.7
appendix 540.1

**Abscess** — *see also* Cellulitis — *continued*
areola (acute) (chronic) (nonpuerperal) 611.0
puerperal, postpartum 675.1 ☑
arm (any part, above wrist) 682.3
artery (wall) 447.2
atheromatous 447.2
auditory canal (external) 380.10
auricle (ear) (staphylococcal) (streptococcal) 380.10
axilla, axillary (region) 682.3
lymph gland or node 683
back (any part) 682.2
Bartholin's gland 616.3
with
abortion — *see* Abortion, by type, with sepsis
ectopic pregnancy (*see also* categories 633.0–633.9) 639.0
molar pregnancy (*see also* categories 630–632) 639.0
complicating pregnancy or puerperium 646.6 ☑
following
abortion 639.0
ectopic or molar pregnancy 639.0
bartholinian 616.3
Bezold's 383.01
bile, biliary, duct or tract (*see also* Cholecystitis) 576.8
bilharziasis 120.1
bladder (wall) 595.89
amebic 006.8
bone (subperiosteal) (*see also* Osteomyelitis) 730.0 ☑
accessory sinus (chronic) (*see also* Sinusitis) 473.9
acute 730.0 ☑
chronic or old 730.1 ☑
jaw (lower) (upper) 526.4
mastoid — *see* Mastoiditis, acute
petrous (*see also* Petrositis) 383.20
spinal (tuberculous) (*see also* Tuberculosis) 015.0 ☑ [730.88]
nontuberculous 730.08
bowel 569.5
brain (any part) 324.0
amebic (with liver or lung abscess) 006.5
cystic 324.0
late effect — *see* category 326
otogenic 324.0
tuberculous (*see also* Tuberculosis) 013.3 ☑
breast (acute) (chronic) (nonpuerperal) 611.0
newborn 771.5
puerperal, postpartum 675.1 ☑
tuberculous (*see also* Tuberculosis) 017.9 ☑
broad ligament (chronic) (*see also* Disease, pelvis, inflammatory) 614.4
acute 614.3
Brodie's (chronic) (localized) (*see also* Osteomyelitis) 730.1 ☑
bronchus 519.19
buccal cavity 528.3
bulbourethral gland 597.0
bursa 727.89
pharyngeal 478.29
buttock 682.5
canaliculus, breast 611.0
canthus 372.20
cartilage 733.99
cecum 569.5
with appendicitis 540.1
cerebellum, cerebellar 324.0
late effect — *see* category 326
cerebral (embolic) 324.0
late effect — *see* category 326
cervical (neck region) 682.1
lymph gland or node 683

**Abscess** — *see also* Cellulitis — *continued*
cervical — *continued*
stump (*see also* Cervicitis) 616.0
cervix (stump) (uteri) (*see also* Cervicitis) 616.0
cheek, external 682.0
inner 528.3
chest 510.9
with fistula 510.0
wall 682.2
chin 682.0
choroid 363.00
ciliary body 364.3
circumtonsillar 475
cold (tuberculous) (*see also* Tuberculosis, abscess)
articular — *see also* Tuberculosis, joint
colon (wall) 569.5
colostomy or enterostomy 569.61
conjunctiva 372.00
connective tissue NEC 682.9
cornea 370.55
with ulcer 370.00
corpus
cavernosum 607.2
luteum (*see also* Salpingo-oophoritis) 614.2
Cowper's gland 597.0
cranium 324.0
cul-de-sac (Douglas') (posterior) (*see also* Disease, pelvis, inflammatory) 614.4
acute 614.3
dental 522.5
with sinus (alveolar) 522.7
dentoalveolar 522.5
with sinus (alveolar) 522.7
diaphragm, diaphragmatic 567.22
digit NEC 681.9
Douglas' cul-de-sac or pouch (*see also* Disease, pelvis, inflammatory) 614.4
acute 614.3
Dubois' 090.5
ductless gland 259.8
ear
acute 382.00
external 380.10
inner 386.30
middle — *see* Otitis media
elbow 682.3
endamebic — *see* Abscess, amebic
entamebic — *see* Abscess, amebic
enterostomy 569.61
epididymis 604.0
epidural 324.9
brain 324.0
late effect — *see* category 326
spinal cord 324.1
epiglottis 478.79
epiploon, epiploic 567.22
erysipelatous (*see also* Erysipelas) 035
esophagostomy 530.86
esophagus 530.19
ethmoid (bone) (chronic) (sinus) (*see also* Sinusitis, ethmoidal) 473.2
external auditory canal 380.10
extradural 324.9
brain 324.0
late effect — *see* category 326
spinal cord 324.1
extraperitoneal — *see* Abscess, peritoneum
eye 360.00
eyelid 373.13
face (any part, except eye) 682.0
fallopian tube (*see also* Salpingo-oophoritis) 614.2
fascia 728.89
fauces 478.29
fecal 569.5
femoral (region) 682.6
filaria, filarial (*see also* Infestation, filarial) 125.9

Abscess — *see also* Cellulitis — *continued*
finger (any) (intrathecal) (periosteal) (subcutaneous) (subcuticular) 681.00
fistulous NEC 682.9
flank 682.2
foot (except toe) 682.7
forearm 682.3
forehead 682.0
frontal (sinus) (chronic) (*see also* Sinusitis, frontal) 473.1
gallbladder (*see also* Cholecystitis, acute) 575.0
gastric 535.0 ☑
genital organ or tract NEC
　female 616.9
　　with
　　　abortion — *see* Abortion, by type, with sepsis
　　　ectopic pregnancy (*see also* categories 633.0–633.9) 639.0
　　　molar pregnancy (*see also* categories 630–632) 639.0
　　following
　　　abortion 639.0
　　　ectopic or molar pregnancy 639.0
　　puerperal, postpartum, childbirth 670.0 ☑
　male 608.4
genitourinary system, tuberculous (*see also* Tuberculosis) 016.9 ☑
gingival 523.30
gland, glandular (lymph) (acute) NEC 683
glottis 478.79
gluteal (region) 682.5
gonorrheal NEC (*see also* Gonococcus) 098.0
groin 682.2
gum 523.30
hand (except finger or thumb) 682.4
head (except face) 682.8
heart 429.89
heel 682.7
helminthic (*see also* Infestation, by specific parasite) 128.9
hepatic 572.0
　amebic (*see also* Abscess, liver, amebic) 006.3
　duct 576.8
hip 682.6
　tuberculous (active) (*see also* Tuberculosis) 015.1 ☑
ileocecal 540.1
ileostomy (bud) 569.61
iliac (region) 682.2
　fossa 540.1
iliopsoas 567.31
　nontuberculous 728.89
　tuberculous (*see also* Tuberculosis) 015.0 ☑ *[730.88]*
infraclavicular (fossa) 682.3
inguinal (region) 682.2
　lymph gland or node 683
intersphincteric (anus) 566
intestine, intestinal 569.5
　rectal 566
intra-abdominal (*see also* Abscess, peritoneum) 567.22
　postoperative 998.59
intracranial 324.0
　late effect — *see* category 326
intramammary — *see* Abscess, breast
intramastoid (*see also* Mastoiditis, acute) 383.00
intraorbital 376.01
intraperitoneal 567.22
intraspinal 324.1
　late effect — *see* category 326
intratonsillar 475
iris 364.3
ischiorectal 566

Abscess — *see also* Cellulitis — *continued*
jaw (bone) (lower) (upper) 526.4
　skin 682.0
joint (*see also* Arthritis, pyogenic) 711.0 ☑
　vertebral (tuberculous) (*see also* Tuberculosis)
　　015.0 ☑ *[730.88]*
　　nontuberculous 724.8
kidney 590.2
　with
　　abortion — *see* Abortion, by type, with urinary tract infection
　　calculus 592.0
　　ectopic pregnancy (*see also* categories 633.0–633.9) 639.8
　　molar pregnancy (*see also* categories 630–632) 639.8
　　complicating pregnancy or puerperium 646.6 ☑
　　　affecting fetus or newborn 760.1
　　following
　　　abortion 639.8
　　　ectopic or molar pregnancy 639.8
knee 682.6
　joint 711.06
　tuberculous (active) (*see also* Tuberculosis) 015.2 ☑
labium (majus) (minus) 616.4
　complicating pregnancy, childbirth, or puerperium 646.6 ☑
lacrimal (passages) (sac) (*see also* Dacryocystitis) 375.30
　caruncle 375.30
　gland (*see also* Dacryoadenitis) 375.00
lacunar 597.0
larynx 478.79
lateral (alveolar) 522.5
　with sinus 522.7
leg, except foot 682.6
lens 360.00
lid 373.13
lingual 529.0
　tonsil 475
lip 528.5
Littre's gland 597.0
liver 572.0
　amebic 006.3
　　with
　　　brain abscess (and lung abscess) 006.5
　　　lung abscess 006.4
　　due to Entamoeba histolytica 006.3
　　dysenteric (*see also* Abscess, liver, amebic) 006.3
　　pyogenic 572.0
　　tropical (*see also* Abscess, liver, amebic) 006.3
loin (region) 682.2
lumbar (tuberculous) (*see also* Tuberculosis) 015.0 ☑ *[730.88]*
　nontuberculous 682.2
lung (miliary) (putrid) 513.0
　amebic (with liver abscess) 006.4
　　with brain abscess 006.5
lymphangitic, acute — *see* Cellulitis
lymph, lymphatic, gland or node (acute) 683
　any site, except mesenteric 683
　mesentery 289.2
malar 526.4
mammary gland — *see* Abscess, breast
marginal (anus) 566
mastoid (process) (*see also* Mastoiditis, acute) 383.00
　subperiosteal 383.01
maxilla, maxillary 526.4
　molar (tooth) 522.5
　　with sinus 522.7
　premolar 522.5

Abscess — *see also* Cellulitis — *continued*
maxilla, maxillary — *continued*
　sinus (chronic) (*see also* Sinusitis, maxillary) 473.0
mediastinum 513.1
meibomian gland 373.12
meninges (*see also* Meningitis) 320.9
mesentery, mesenteric 567.22
mesosalpinx (*see also* Salpingo-oophoritis) 614.2
milk 675.1 ☑
Monro's (psoriasis) 696.1
mons pubis 682.2
mouth (floor) 528.3
multiple sites NEC 682.9
mural 682.2
muscle 728.89
　psoas 567.31
myocardium 422.92
nabothian (follicle) (*see also* Cervicitis) 616.0
nail (chronic) (with lymphangitis) 681.9
　finger 681.02
　toe 681.11
nasal (fossa) (septum) 478.19
　sinus (chronic) (*see also* Sinusitis) 473.9
nasopharyngeal 478.29
nates 682.5
navel 682.2
　newborn NEC 771.4
neck (region) 682.1
　lymph gland or node 683
nephritic (*see also* Abscess, kidney) 590.2
nipple 611.0
　puerperal, postpartum 675.0 ☑
nose (septum) 478.19
　external 682.0
omentum 567.22
operative wound 998.59
orbit, orbital 376.01
ossifluent — *see* Abscess, bone
ovary, ovarian (corpus luteum) (*see also* Salpingo-oophoritis) 614.2
oviduct (*see also* Salpingo-oophoritis) 614.2
palate (soft) 528.3
　hard 526.4
palmar (space) 682.4
pancreas (duct) 577.0
paradontal 523.30
parafrenal 607.2
parametric, parametrium (chronic) (*see also* Disease, pelvis, inflammatory) 614.4
　acute 614.3
paranephric 590.2
parapancreatic 577.0
parapharyngeal 478.22
pararectal 566
parasinus (*see also* Sinusitis) 473.9
parauterine (*see also* Disease, pelvis, inflammatory) 614.4
　acute 614.3
paravaginal (*see also* Vaginitis) 616.10
parietal region 682.8
parodontal 523.30
parotid (duct) (gland) 527.3
　region 528.3
parumbilical 682.2
　newborn 771.4
pectoral (region) 682.2
pelvirectal 567.22
pelvis, pelvic
　female (chronic) (*see also* Disease, pelvis, inflammatory) 614.4
　　acute 614.3
　male, peritoneal (cellular tissue) — *see* Abscess, peritoneum
　tuberculous (*see also* Tuberculosis) 016.9 ☑
penis 607.2
　gonococcal (acute) 098.0

Abscess — *see also* Cellulitis — *continued*
penis — *continued*
　gonococcal — *continued*
　　chronic or duration of 2 months or over 098.2
perianal 566
periapical 522.5
　with sinus (alveolar) 522.7
periappendiceal 540.1
pericardial 420.99
pericecal 540.1
pericemental 523.30
pericholecystic (*see also* Cholecystitis, acute) 575.0
pericoronal 523.30
peridental 523.30
perigastric 535.0 ☑
perimetric (*see also* Disease, pelvis, inflammatory) 614.4
　acute 614.3
perinephric, perinephritic (*see also* Abscess, kidney) 590.2
perineum, perineal (superficial) 682.2
　deep (with urethral involvement) 597.0
　urethra 597.0
periodontal (parietal) 523.31
　apical 522.5
periosteum, periosteal (*see also* Periostitis) 730.3 ☑
　with osteomyelitis (*see also* Osteomyelitis) 730.2 ☑
　　acute or subacute 730.0 ☑
　　chronic or old 730.1 ☑
peripleuritic 510.9
　with fistula 510.0
periproctic 566
periprostatic 601.2
perirectal (staphylococcal) 566
perirenal (tissue) (*see also* Abscess, kidney) 590.2
perisinuous (nose) (*see also* Sinusitis) 473.9
peritoneum, peritoneal (perforated) (ruptured) 567.22
　with
　　abortion — *see* Abortion, by type, with sepsis
　　appendicitis 540.1
　　ectopic pregnancy (*see also* categories 633.0–633.9) 639.0
　　molar pregnancy (*see also* categories 630–632) 639.0
　　following
　　　abortion 639.0
　　　ectopic or molar pregnancy 639.0
　　pelvic, female (*see also* Disease, pelvis, inflammatory) 614.4
　　　acute 614.3
　　postoperative 998.59
　　puerperal, postpartum, childbirth 670.0 ☑
　　tuberculous (*see also* Tuberculosis) 014.0 ☑
peritonsillar 475
perityphlic 540.1
periureteral 593.89
periurethral 597.0
　gonococcal (acute) 098.0
　　chronic or duration of 2 months or over 098.2
periuterine (*see also* Disease, pelvis, inflammatory) 614.4
　acute 614.3
perivesical 595.89
pernicious NEC 682.9
petrous bone — *see* Petrositis
phagedenic NEC 682.9
　chancroid 099.0
pharynx, pharyngeal (lateral) 478.29
phlegmonous NEC 682.9
pilonidal 685.0
pituitary (gland) 253.8

☑ Additional Digit Required — Refer to the Tabular List for Digit Selection　　　　　⬙ Subterms under main terms may continue to next column or page

4 — Volume 2　　　　▶◀ Revised Text　　　● New Line　　　▲ Revised Code　　　*2008 ICD-9-CM*

**Abscess** — *see also* Cellulitis — *continued*
  pleura 510.9
    with fistula 510.0
  popliteal 682.6
  postanal 566
  postcecal 540.1
  postlaryngeal 478.79
  postnasal 478.19
  postpharyngeal 478.24
  posttonsillar 475
  posttyphoid 002.0
  Pott's (*see also* Tuberculosis)
    015.0 ☑ *[730.88]*
  pouch of Douglas (chronic) (*see also* Disease, pelvis, inflammatory) 614.4
  premammary — *see* Abscess, breast
  prepatellar 682.6
  prostate (*see also* Prostatitis) 601.2
    gonococcal (acute) 098.12
      chronic or duration of 2 months or over 098.32
  psoas 567.31
    nontuberculous 728.89
    tuberculous (*see also* Tuberculosis) 015.0 ☑ *[730.88]*
  pterygopalatine fossa 682.8
  pubis 682.2
  puerperal — *see* Puerperal, abscess, by site
  pulmonary — *see* Abscess, lung
  pulp, pulpal (dental) 522.0
    finger 681.01
    toe 681.10
  pyemic — *see* Septicemia
  pyloric valve 535.0 ☑
  rectovaginal septum 569.5
  rectovesical 595.89
  rectum 566
  regional NEC 682.9
  renal (*see also* Abscess, kidney) 590.2
  retina 363.00
  retrobulbar 376.01
  retrocecal 567.22
  retrolaryngeal 478.79
  retromammary — *see* Abscess, breast
  retroperineal 682.2
  retroperitoneal 567.38
    postprocedural 998.59
  retropharyngeal 478.24
    tuberculous (*see also* Tuberculosis) 012.8 ☑
  retrorectal 566
  retrouterine (*see also* Disease, pelvis, inflammatory) 614.4
    acute 614.3
  retrovesical 595.89
  root, tooth 522.5
    with sinus (alveolar) 522.7
  round ligament (*see also* Disease, pelvis, inflammatory) 614.4
    acute 614.3
  rupture (spontaneous) NEC 682.9
  sacrum (tuberculous) (*see also* Tuberculosis) 015.0 ☑ *[730.88]*
    nontuberculous 730.08
  salivary duct or gland 527.3
  scalp (any part) 682.8
  scapular 730.01
  sclera 379.09
  scrofulous (*see also* Tuberculosis) 017.2 ☑
  scrotum 608.4
  seminal vesicle 608.0
    amebic 006.8
  septal, dental 522.5
    with sinus (alveolar) 522.7
  septum (nasal) 478.19
  serous (*see also* Periostitis) 730.3 ☑
  shoulder 682.3
  side 682.2
  sigmoid 569.5
  sinus (accessory) (chronic) (nasal) (*see also* Sinusitis) 473.9
    intracranial venous (any) 324.0

**Abscess** — *see also* Cellulitis — *continued*
  sinus (*see also* Sinusitis) — *continued*
    intracranial venous — *continued*
      late effect — *see* category 326
  Skene's duct or gland 597.0
  skin NEC 682.9
    tuberculous (primary) (*see also* Tuberculosis) 017.0 ☑
  sloughing NEC 682.9
  specified site NEC 682.8
    amebic 006.8
  spermatic cord 608.4
  sphenoidal (sinus) (*see also* Sinusitis, sphenoidal) 473.3
  spinal
    cord (any part) (staphylococcal) 324.1
      tuberculous (*see also* Tuberculosis) 013.5 ☑
    epidural 324.1
  spine (column) (tuberculous) (*see also* Tuberculosis) 015.0 ☑ *[730.88]*
    nontuberculous 730.08
  spleen 289.59
    amebic 006.8
  staphylococcal NEC 682.9
  stitch 998.59
  stomach (wall) 535.0 ☑
  strumous (tuberculous) (*see also* Tuberculosis) 017.2 ☑
  subarachnoid 324.9
    brain 324.0
    cerebral 324.0
    late effect — *see* category 326
    spinal cord 324.1
  subareolar (*see also* Abscess, breast)
    puerperal, postpartum 675.1 ☑
  subcecal 540.1
  subcutaneous NEC 682.9
  subdiaphragmatic 567.22
  subdorsal 682.2
  subdural 324.9
    brain 324.0
    late effect — *see* category 326
    spinal cord 324.1
  subgaleal 682.8
  subhepatic 567.22
  sublingual 528.3
    gland 527.3
  submammary — *see* Abscess, breast
  submandibular (region) (space) (triangle) 682.0
    gland 527.3
  submaxillary (region) 682.0
    gland 527.3
  submental (pyogenic) 682.0
    gland 527.3
  subpectoral 682.2
  subperiosteal — *see* Abscess, bone
  subperitoneal 567.22
  subphrenic (*see also* Abscess, peritoneum) 567.22
    postoperative 998.59
  subscapular 682.2
  subungual 681.9
  suburethral 597.0
  sudoriparous 705.89
  suppurative NEC 682.9
  supraclavicular (fossa) 682.3
  suprahepatic 567.22
  suprapelvic (*see also* Disease, pelvis, inflammatory) 614.4
    acute 614.3
  suprapubic 682.2
  suprarenal (capsule) (gland) 255.8
  sweat gland 705.89
  syphilitic 095.8
  teeth, tooth (root) 522.5
    with sinus (alveolar) 522.7
    supporting structures NEC 523.30
  temple 682.0
  temporal region 682.0
  temporosphenoidal 324.0

**Abscess** — *see also* Cellulitis — *continued*
  temporosphenoidal — *continued*
    late effect — *see* category 326
  tendon (sheath) 727.89
  testicle — *see* Orchitis
  thecal 728.89
  thigh (acquired) 682.6
  thorax 510.9
    with fistula 510.0
  throat 478.29
  thumb (intrathecal) (periosteal) (subcutaneous) (subcuticular) 681.00
  thymus (gland) 254.1
  thyroid (gland) 245.0
  toe (any) (intrathecal) (periosteal) (subcutaneous) (subcuticular) 681.10
  tongue (staphylococcal) 529.0
  tonsil(s) (lingual) 475
  tonsillopharyngeal 475
  tooth, teeth (root) 522.5
    with sinus (alveolar) 522.7
    supporting structure NEC 523.30
  trachea 478.9
  trunk 682.2
  tubal (*see also* Salpingo-oophoritis) 614.2
  tuberculous — *see* Tuberculosis, abscess
  tubo-ovarian (*see also* Salpingo-oophoritis) 614.2
  tunica vaginalis 608.4
  umbilicus NEC 682.2
    newborn 771.4
  upper arm 682.3
  upper respiratory 478.9
  urachus 682.2
  urethra (gland) 597.0
  urinary 597.0
  uterus, uterine (wall) (*see also* Endometritis) 615.9
    ligament (*see also* Disease, pelvis, inflammatory) 614.4
      acute 614.3
    neck (*see also* Cervicitis) 616.0
  uvula 528.3
  vagina (wall) (*see also* Vaginitis) 616.10
  vaginorectal (*see also* Vaginitis) 616.10
  vas deferens 608.4
  vermiform appendix 540.1
  vertebra (column) (tuberculous) (*see also* Tuberculosis) 015.0 ☑ *[730.88]*
    nontuberculous 730.0 ☑
  vesical 595.89
  vesicouterine pouch (*see also* Disease, pelvis, inflammatory) 614.4
  vitreous (humor) (pneumococcal) 360.04
  vocal cord 478.5
  von Bezold's 383.01
  vulva 616.4
    complicating pregnancy, childbirth, or puerperium 646.6 ☑
  vulvovaginal gland (*see also* Vaginitis) 616.3
  web-space 682.4
  wrist 682.4
**Absence** (organ or part) (complete or partial)
  acoustic nerve 742.8
  adrenal (gland) (congenital) 759.1
    acquired V45.79
  albumin (blood) 273.8
  alimentary tract (complete) (congenital) (partial) 751.8
    lower 751.5
    upper 750.8
  alpha-fucosidase 271.8
  alveolar process (acquired) 525.8
    congenital 750.26
  anus, anal (canal) (congenital) 751.2

**Absence** — *continued*
  aorta (congenital) 747.22
  aortic valve (congenital) 746.89
  appendix, congenital 751.2
  arm (acquired) V49.60
    above elbow V49.66
    below elbow V49.65
    congenital (*see also* Deformity, reduction, upper limb) 755.20
    lower — *see* Absence, forearm, congenital
    upper (complete) (partial) (with absence of distal elements, incomplete) 755.24
      with
        complete absence of distal elements 755.21
        forearm (incomplete) 755.23
  artery (congenital) (peripheral) NEC (*see also* Anomaly, peripheral vascular system) 747.60
    brain 747.81
    cerebral 747.81
    coronary 746.85
    pulmonary 747.3
    umbilical 747.5
  atrial septum 745.69
  auditory canal (congenital) (external) 744.01
  auricle (ear) (with stenosis or atresia of auditory canal), congenital 744.01
  bile, biliary duct (common) or passage (congenital) 751.61
  bladder (acquired) V45.74
    congenital 753.8
  bone (congenital) NEC 756.9
    marrow 284.9
      acquired (secondary) 284.89   ▲
      congenital 284.09
      hereditary 284.09
      idiopathic 284.9
    skull 756.0
  bowel sounds 787.5
  brain 740.0
    specified part 742.2
  breast(s) (acquired) V45.71
    congenital 757.6
  broad ligament (congenital) 752.19
  bronchus (congenital) 748.3
  calvarium, calvaria (skull) 756.0
  canaliculus lacrimalis, congenital 743.65
  carpal(s) (congenital) (complete) (partial) (with absence of distal elements, incomplete) (*see also* Deformity, reduction, upper limb) 755.28
    with complete absence of distal elements 755.21
  cartilage 756.9
  caudal spine 756.13
  cecum (acquired) (postoperative) (posttraumatic) V45.72
    congenital 751.2
  cementum 520.4
  cerebellum (congenital) (vermis) 742.2
  cervix (acquired) (uteri) V45.77
    congenital 752.49
  chin, congenital 744.89
  cilia (congenital) 743.63
    acquired 374.89
  circulatory system, part NEC 747.89
  clavicle 755.51
  clitoris (congenital) 752.49
  coccyx, congenital 756.13
  cold sense (*see also* Disturbance, sensation) 782.0
  colon (acquired) (postoperative) V45.72
    congenital 751.2
  congenital
    lumen — *see* Atresia

☑ Additional Digit Required — Refer to the Tabular List for Digit Selection      ▽ Subterms under main terms may continue to next column or page

*2008 ICD-9-CM*      ▶◀ Revised Text      ● New Line      ▲ Revised Code      October 2007 · Volume 2 — 5

**Absence** — *continued*
 congenital — *continued*
  organ or site NEC — *see* Agenesis
  septum — *see* Imperfect, closure
 corpus callosum (congenital) 742.2
 cricoid cartilage 748.3
 diaphragm (congenital) (with hernia) 756.6
  with obstruction 756.6
 digestive organ(s) or tract, congenital (complete) (partial) 751.8
  acquired V45.79
  lower 751.5
  upper 750.8
 ductus arteriosus 747.89
 duodenum (acquired) (postoperative) V45.72
  congenital 751.1
 ear, congenital 744.09
  acquired V45.79
  auricle 744.01
  external 744.01
  inner 744.05
  lobe, lobule 744.21
  middle, except ossicles 744.03
   ossicles 744.04
  ossicles 744.04
 ejaculatory duct (congenital) 752.89
 endocrine gland NEC (congenital) 759.2
 epididymis (congenital) 752.89
  acquired V45.77
 epiglottis, congenital 748.3
 epileptic (atonic) (typical) (*see also* Epilepsy) 345.0 ☑
 erythrocyte 284.9
 erythropoiesis 284.9
  congenital 284.01
 esophagus (congenital) 750.3
 Eustachian tube (congenital) 744.24
 extremity (acquired)
  congenital (*see also* Deformity, reduction) 755.4
  lower V49.70
  upper V49.60
 extrinsic muscle, eye 743.69
 eye (acquired) V45.78
  adnexa (congenital) 743.69
  congenital 743.00
  muscle (congenital) 743.69
 eyelid (fold), congenital 743.62
  acquired 374.89
 face
  bones NEC 756.0
  specified part NEC 744.89
 fallopian tube(s) (acquired) V45.77
  congenital 752.19
 femur, congenital (complete) (partial) (with absence of distal elements, incomplete) (*see also* Deformity, reduction, lower limb) 755.34
  with
   complete absence of distal elements 755.31
   tibia and fibula (incomplete) 755.33
 fibrin 790.92
 fibrinogen (congenital) 286.3
  acquired 286.6
 fibula, congenital (complete) (partial) (with absence of distal elements, incomplete) (*see also* Deformity, reduction, lower limb) 755.37
  with
   complete absence of distal elements 755.31
   tibia 755.35
    with
     complete absence of distal elements 755.31
     femur (incomplete) 755.33
      with complete absence of distal elements 755.31
 finger (acquired) V49.62

**Absence** — *continued*
 finger — *continued*
  congenital (complete) (partial) (*see also* Deformity, reduction, upper limb) 755.29
   meaning all fingers (complete) (partial) 755.21
   transverse 755.21
 fissures of lungs (congenital) 748.5
 foot (acquired) V49.73
  congenital (complete) 755.31
 forearm (acquired) V49.65
  congenital (complete) (partial) (with absence of distal elements, incomplete) (*see also* Deformity, reduction, upper limb) 755.25
   with
    complete absence of distal elements (hand and fingers) 755.21
    humerus (incomplete) 755.23
 fovea centralis 743.55
 fucosidase 271.8
 gallbladder (acquired) V45.79
  congenital 751.69
 gamma globulin (blood) 279.00
 genital organs
  acquired V45.77
  congenital
   female 752.89
    external 752.49
    internal NEC 752.89
   male 752.89
    penis 752.69
 genitourinary organs, congenital NEC 752.89
 glottis 748.3
 gonadal, congenital NEC 758.6
 hair (congenital) 757.4
  acquired — *see* Alopecia
 hand (acquired) V49.63
  congenital (complete) (*see also* Deformity, reduction, upper limb) 755.21
 heart (congenital) 759.89
  acquired — *see* Status, organ replacement
 heat sense (*see also* Disturbance, sensation) 782.0
 humerus, congenital (complete) (partial) (with absence of distal elements, incomplete) (*see also* Deformity, reduction, upper limb) 755.24
  with
   complete absence of distal elements 755.21
   radius and ulna (incomplete) 755.23
 hymen (congenital) 752.49
 ileum (acquired) (postoperative) (posttraumatic) V45.72
  congenital 751.1
 immunoglobulin, isolated NEC 279.03
  IgA 279.01
  IgG 279.03
  IgM 279.02
 incus (acquired) 385.24
  congenital 744.04
 internal ear (congenital) 744.05
 intestine (acquired) (small) V45.72
  congenital 751.1
   large 751.2
  large V45.72
   congenital 751.2
 iris (congenital) 743.45
 jaw — *see* Absence, mandible
 jejunum (acquired) V45.72
  congenital 751.1
 joint, congenital NEC 755.8
 kidney(s) (acquired) V45.73
  congenital 753.0
 labium (congenital) (majus) (minus) 752.49
 labyrinth, membranous 744.05

**Absence** — *continued*
 lacrimal apparatus (congenital) 743.65
 larynx (congenital) 748.3
 leg (acquired) V49.70
  above knee V49.76
  below knee V49.75
  congenital (partial) (unilateral) (*see also* Deformity, reduction, lower limb) 755.31
   lower (complete) (partial) (with absence of distal elements, incomplete) 755.35
    with
     complete absence of distal elements (foot and toes) 755.31
     thigh (incomplete) 755.33
      with complete absence of distal elements 755.31
   upper — *see* Absence, femur
 lens (congenital) 743.35
  acquired 379.31
 ligament, broad (congenital) 752.19
 limb (acquired)
  congenital (complete) (partial) (*see also* Deformity, reduction) 755.4
   lower 755.30
    complete 755.31
    incomplete 755.32
    longitudinal — *see* Deficiency, lower limb, longitudinal
    transverse 755.31
   upper 755.20
    complete 755.21
    incomplete 755.22
    longitudinal — *see* Deficiency, upper limb, longitudinal
    transverse 755.21
  lower NEC V49.70
  upper NEC V49.60
 lip 750.26
 liver (congenital) (lobe) 751.69
 lumbar (congenital) (vertebra) 756.13
  isthmus 756.11
  pars articularis 756.11
 lumen — *see* Atresia
 lung (bilateral) (congenital) (fissure) (lobe) (unilateral) 748.5
  acquired (any part) V45.76
 mandible (congenital) 524.09
 maxilla (congenital) 524.09
 menstruation 626.0
 metacarpal(s), congenital (complete) (partial) (with absence of distal elements, incomplete) (*see also* Deformity, reduction, upper limb) 755.28
  with all fingers, complete 755.21
 metatarsal(s), congenital (complete) (partial) (with absence of distal elements, incomplete) (*see also* Deformity, reduction, lower limb) 755.38
  with complete absence of distal elements 755.31
 muscle (congenital) (pectoral) 756.81
  ocular 743.69
 musculoskeletal system (congenital) NEC 756.9
 nail(s) (congenital) 757.5
 neck, part 744.89
 nerve 742.8
 nervous system, part NEC 742.8
 neutrophil 288.00
 nipple (congenital) 757.6
 nose (congenital) 748.1
  acquired 738.0
 nuclear 742.8
 ocular muscle (congenital) 743.69
 organ
  of Corti (congenital) 744.05

**Absence** — *continued*
 organ — *continued*
  or site
   acquired V45.79
   congenital NEC 759.89
 osseous meatus (ear) 744.03
 ovary (acquired) V45.77
  congenital 752.0
 oviduct (acquired) V45.77
  congenital 752.19
 pancreas (congenital) 751.7
  acquired (postoperative) (posttraumatic) V45.79
 parathyroid gland (congenital) 759.2
 parotid gland(s) (congenital) 750.21
 patella, congenital 755.64
 pelvic girdle (congenital) 755.69
 penis (congenital) 752.69
  acquired V45.77
 pericardium (congenital) 746.89
 perineal body (congenital) 756.81
 phalange(s), congenital 755.4
  lower limb (complete) (intercalary) (partial) (terminal) (*see also* Deformity, reduction, lower limb) 755.39
   meaning all toes (complete) (partial) 755.31
   transverse 755.31
  upper limb (complete) (intercalary) (partial) (terminal) (*see also* Deformity, reduction, upper limb) 755.29
   meaning all digits (complete) (partial) 755.21
   transverse 755.21
 pituitary gland (congenital) 759.2
 postoperative — *see* Absence, by site, acquired
 prostate (congenital) 752.89
  acquired V45.77
 pulmonary
  artery 747.3
  trunk 747.3
  valve (congenital) 746.01
  vein 747.49
 punctum lacrimale (congenital) 743.65
 radius, congenital (complete) (partial) (with absence of distal elements, incomplete) 755.26
  with
   complete absence of distal elements 755.21
   ulna 755.25
    with
     complete absence of distal elements 755.21
     humerus (incomplete) 755.23
 ray, congenital 755.4
  lower limb (complete) (partial) (*see also* Deformity, reduction, lower limb) 755.38
   meaning all rays 755.31
   transverse 755.31
  upper limb (complete) (partial) (*see also* Deformity, reduction, upper limb) 755.28
   meaning all rays 755.21
   transverse 755.21
 rectum (congenital) 751.2
  acquired V45.79
 red cell 284.9
  acquired (secondary) 284.81　▲
  congenital 284.01
  hereditary 284.01
  idiopathic 284.9
 respiratory organ (congenital) NEC 748.9
 rib (acquired) 738.3
  congenital 756.3
 roof of orbit (congenital) 742.0
 round ligament (congenital) 752.89
 sacrum, congenital 756.13
 salivary gland(s) (congenital) 750.21
 scapula 755.59

☑ Additional Digit Required — Refer to the Tabular List for Digit Selection　　　　　　　　🔻 Subterms under main terms may continue to next column or page

6 — Volume 2 · October 2007　　　　▶◀ Revised Text　　　　● New Line　　　　▲ Revised Code　　　　*2008 ICD-9-CM*

**Absence** — *continued*
  scrotum, congenital 752.89
  seminal tract or duct (congenital)
      752.89
    acquired V45.77
  septum (congenital) (*see also* Imper-
      fect, closure, septum)
    atrial 745.69
      and ventricular 745.7
    between aorta and pulmonary
        artery 745.0
    ventricular 745.3
      and atrial 745.7
  sex chromosomes 758.81
  shoulder girdle, congenital (complete)
      (partial) 755.59
  skin (congenital) 757.39
  skull bone 756.0
    with
      anencephalus 740.0
      encephalocele 742.0
      hydrocephalus 742.3
        with spina bifida (*see also*
            Spina bifida) 741.0 ☑
      microcephalus 742.1
  spermatic cord (congenital) 752.89
  spinal cord 742.59
  spine, congenital 756.13
  spleen (congenital) 759.0
    acquired V45.79
  sternum, congenital 756.3
  stomach (acquired) (partial) (postoper-
      ative) V45.75
    with postgastric surgery syndrome
        564.2
    congenital 750.7
  submaxillary gland(s) (congenital)
      750.21
  superior vena cava (congenital) 747.49
  tarsal(s), congenital (complete) (partial)
      (with absence of distal elements,
      incomplete) (*see also* Deformity,
      reduction, lower limb) 755.38
  teeth, tooth (congenital) 520.0
    with abnormal spacing 524.30
    acquired 525.10
      with malocclusion 524.30
      due to
        caries 525.13
        extraction 525.10
        periodontal disease 525.12
        trauma 525.11
  tendon (congenital) 756.81
  testis (congenital) 752.89
    acquired V45.77
  thigh (acquired) 736.89
  thumb (acquired) V49.61
    congenital 755.29
  thymus gland (congenital) 759.2
  thyroid (gland) (surgical) 246.8
    with hypothyroidism 244.0
    cartilage, congenital 748.3
    congenital 243
  tibia, congenital (complete) (partial)
      (with absence of distal elements,
      incomplete) (*see also* Deformity,
      reduction, lower limb) 755.36
    with
      complete absence of distal ele-
          ments 755.31
      fibula 755.35
        with
          complete absence of distal
              elements 755.31
          femur (incomplete) 755.33
            with complete absence
                of distal ele-
                ments 755.31
  toe (acquired) V49.72
    congenital (complete) (partial)
        755.39
      meaning all toes 755.31
      transverse 755.31
    great V49.71
  tongue (congenital) 750.11
  tooth, teeth (congenital) 520.0

**Absence** — *continued*
  tooth, teeth — *continued*
    with abnormal spacing 524.30
    acquired 525.10
      with malocclusion 524.30
      due to
        caries 525.13
        extraction 525.10
        periodontal disease 525.12
        trauma 525.11
  trachea (cartilage) (congenital) (rings)
      748.3
  transverse aortic arch (congenital)
      747.21
  tricuspid valve 746.1
  ulna, congenital (complete) (partial)
      (with absence of distal elements,
      incomplete) (*see also* Deformity,
      reduction, upper limb) 755.27
    with
      complete absence of distal ele-
          ments 755.21
      radius 755.25
        with
          complete absence of distal
              elements 755.21
          humerus (incomplete)
              755.23
  umbilical artery (congenital) 747.5
  ureter (congenital) 753.4
    acquired V45.74
  urethra, congenital 753.8
    acquired V45.74
  urinary system, part NEC, congenital
      753.8
    acquired V45.74
  uterus (acquired) V45.77
    congenital 752.3
  uvula (congenital) 750.26
  vagina, congenital 752.49
    acquired V45.77
  vas deferens (congenital) 752.89
    acquired V45.77
  vein (congenital) (peripheral) NEC (*see
      also* Anomaly, peripheral vascu-
      lar system) 747.60
    brain 747.81
    great 747.49
    portal 747.49
    pulmonary 747.49
  vena cava (congenital) (inferior) (supe-
      rior) 747.49
  ventral horn cell 742.59
  ventricular septum 745.3
  vermis of cerebellum 742.2
  vertebra, congenital 756.13
  vulva, congenital 752.49
**Absentia epileptica** — *see also* Epilepsy
    345.0 ☑
**Absinthemia** — *see also* Dependence
    304.6 ☑
**Absinthism** — *see also* Dependence
    304.6 ☑
**Absorbent system disease** 459.89
**Absorption**
  alcohol, through placenta or breast
      milk 760.71
  antibiotics, through placenta or breast
      milk 760.74
  anticonvulsants, through placenta or
      breast milk 760.77
  antifungals, through placenta or
      breast milk 760.74
  anti-infective, through placenta or
      breast milk 760.74
  antimetabolics, through placenta or
      breast milk 760.78
  chemical NEC 989.9
    specified chemical or substance —
        *see* Table of Drugs and
        Chemicals
    through placenta or breast milk
        (fetus or newborn) 760.70
      alcohol 760.71
      anticonvulsants 760.77
      antifungals 760.74

**Absorption** — *continued*
  chemical — *continued*
    through placenta or breast milk —
        *continued*
      anti-infective agents 760.74
      antimetabolics 760.78
      cocaine 760.75
      "crack" 760.75
      diethylstilbestrol [DES] 760.76
      hallucinogenic agents 760.73
      medicinal agents NEC 760.79
      narcotics 760.72
      obstetric anesthetic or analgesic
          drug 763.5
      specified agent NEC 760.79
      suspected, affecting manage-
          ment of pregnancy
          655.5 ☑
  cocaine, through placenta or breast
      milk 760.75
  drug NEC (*see also* Reaction, drug)
    through placenta or breast milk
        (fetus or newborn) 760.70
      alcohol 760.71
      anticonvulsants 760.77
      antifungals 760.74
      anti-infective agents 760.74
      antimetabolics 760.78
      cocaine 760.75
      "crack" 760.75
      diethylstilbestrol [DES] 760.76
      hallucinogenic agents 760.73
      medicinal agents NEC 760.79
      narcotics 760.72
      obstetric anesthetic or analgesic
          drug 763.5
      specified agent NEC 760.79
      suspected, affecting manage-
          ment of pregnancy
          655.5 ☑
  fat, disturbance 579.8
  hallucinogenic agents, through placen-
      ta or breast milk 760.73
  immune sera, through placenta or
      breast milk 760.79
  lactose defect 271.3
  medicinal agents NEC, through placen-
      ta or breast milk 760.79
  narcotics, through placenta or breast
      milk 760.72
  noxious substance — *see* Absorption,
      chemical
  protein, disturbance 579.8
  pus or septic, general — *see* Sep-
      ticemia
  quinine, through placenta or breast
      milk 760.74
  toxic substance — *see* Absorption,
      chemical
  uremic — *see* Uremia
**Abstinence symptoms or syndrome**
  alcohol 291.81
  drug 292.0
**Abt-Letterer-Siwe syndrome** (acute
    histiocytosis X) (M9722/3) 202.5 ☑
**Abulia** 799.89
**Abulomania** 301.6
**Abuse**
  adult 995.80
    emotional 995.82
    multiple forms 995.85
    neglect (nutritional) 995.84
    physical 995.81
    psychological 995.82
    sexual 995.83
  alcohol — *see also* Alcoholism
      305.0 ☑
    dependent 303.9 ☑
    non-dependent 305.0 ☑
  child 995.50
    counseling
      perpetrator
        non-parent V62.83
        parent V61.22
      victim V61.21
    emotional 995.51

**Abuse** — *continued*
  child — *continued*
    multiple forms 995.59
    neglect (nutritional) 995.52
    physical 995.54
      shaken infant syndrome 995.55
    psychological 995.51
    sexual 995.53
  drugs, nondependent 305.9 ☑

*Note — Use the following fifth-digit
subclassification with the following
codes: 305.0, 305.2–305.9:*

  *0   unspecified*
  *1   continuous*
  *2   episodic*
  *3   in remission*

    amphetamine type 305.7 ☑
    antidepressants 305.8 ☑
    anxiolytic 305.4 ☑
    barbiturates 305.4 ☑
    caffeine 305.9 ☑
    cannabis 305.2 ☑
    cocaine type 305.6 ☑
    hallucinogens 305.3 ☑
    hashish 305.2 ☑
    hypnotic 305.4 ☑
    inhalant 305.9 ☑
    LSD 305.3 ☑
    marijuana 305.2 ☑
    mixed 305.9 ☑
    morphine type 305.5 ☑
    opioid type 305.5 ☑
    phencyclidine (PCP) 305.9 ☑
    sedative 305.4 ☑
    specified NEC 305.9 ☑
    tranquilizers 305.4 ☑
  spouse 995.80
  tobacco 305.1
**Acalcerosis** 275.40
**Acalcicosis** 275.40
**Acalculia** 784.69
  developmental 315.1
**Acanthocheilonemiasis** 125.4
**Acanthocytosis** 272.5
**Acanthokeratodermia** 701.1
**Acantholysis** 701.8
  bullosa 757.39
**Acanthoma** (benign) (M8070/0) — *see
    also* Neoplasm, by site, benign
    malignant (M8070/3) — *see* Neo-
    plasm, by site, malignant
**Acanthosis** (acquired) (nigricans) 701.2
  adult 701.2
  benign (congenital) 757.39
  congenital 757.39
  glycogenic
    esophagus 530.89
  juvenile 701.2
  tongue 529.8
**Acanthrocytosis** 272.5
**Acapnia** 276.3
**Acarbia** 276.2
**Acardia** 759.89
**Acardiacus amorphus** 759.89
**Acardiotrophia** 429.1
**Acardius** 759.89
**Acariasis** 133.9
  sarcoptic 133.0
**Acaridiasis** 133.9
**Acarinosis** 133.9
**Acariosis** 133.9
**Acarodermatitis** 133.9
  urticarioides 133.9
**Acarophobia** 300.29
**Acatalasemia** 277.89
**Acatalasia** 277.89
**Acatamathesia** 784.69
**Acataphasia** 784.5
**Acathisia** 781.0
  due to drugs 333.99
**Acceleration, accelerated**
  atrioventricular conduction 426.7
  idioventricular rhythm 427.89

☑ Additional Digit Required — Refer to the Tabular List for Digit Selection          ▽ Subterms under main terms may continue to next column or page

*2008 ICD-9-CM*          ▶◀ Revised Text          ● New Line          ▲ Revised Code          Volume 2 — 7

**Accessory** (congenital)
adrenal gland 759.1
anus 751.5
appendix 751.5
atrioventricular conduction 426.7
auditory ossicles 744.04
auricle (ear) 744.1
autosome(s) NEC 758.5
  21 or 22 758.0
biliary duct or passage 751.69
bladder 753.8
blood vessels (peripheral) (congenital) NEC (*see also* Anomaly, peripheral vascular system) 747.60
  cerebral 747.81
  coronary 746.85
bone NEC 756.9
  foot 755.67
breast tissue, axilla 757.6
carpal bones 755.56
cecum 751.5
cervix 752.49
chromosome(s) NEC 758.5
  13-15 758.1
  16-18 758.2
  21 or 22 758.0
  autosome(s) NEC 758.5
  $D_1$ 758.1
  $E_3$ 758.2
  G 758.0
  sex 758.81
coronary artery 746.85
cusp(s), heart valve NEC 746.89
  pulmonary 746.09
cystic duct 751.69
digits 755.00
ear (auricle) (lobe) 744.1
endocrine gland NEC 759.2
external os 752.49
eyelid 743.62
eye muscle 743.69
face bone(s) 756.0
fallopian tube (fimbria) (ostium) 752.19
fingers 755.01
foreskin 605
frontonasal process 756.0
gallbladder 751.69
genital organ(s)
  female 752.89
    external 752.49
    internal NEC 752.89
  male NEC 752.89
    penis 752.69
genitourinary organs NEC 752.89
heart 746.89
  valve NEC 746.89
    pulmonary 746.09
hepatic ducts 751.69
hymen 752.49
intestine (large) (small) 751.5
kidney 753.3
lacrimal canal 743.65
leaflet, heart valve NEC 746.89
  pulmonary 746.09
ligament, broad 752.19
liver (duct) 751.69
lobule (ear) 744.1
lung (lobe) 748.69
muscle 756.82
navicular of carpus 755.56
nervous system, part NEC 742.8
nipple 757.6
nose 748.1
organ or site NEC — *see* Anomaly, specified type NEC
ovary 752.0
oviduct 752.19
pancreas 751.7
parathyroid gland 759.2
parotid gland (and duct) 750.22
pituitary gland 759.2
placental lobe — *see* Placenta, abnormal
preauricular appendage 744.1
prepuce 605

**Accessory** — *continued*
renal arteries (multiple) 747.62
rib 756.3
  cervical 756.2
roots (teeth) 520.2
salivary gland 750.22
sesamoids 755.8
sinus — *see* condition
skin tags 757.39
spleen 759.0
sternum 756.3
submaxillary gland 750.22
tarsal bones 755.67
teeth, tooth 520.1
  causing crowding 524.31
tendon 756.89
thumb 755.01
thymus gland 759.2
thyroid gland 759.2
toes 755.02
tongue 750.13
tragus 744.1
ureter 753.4
urethra 753.8
urinary organ or tract NEC 753.8
uterus 752.2
vagina 752.49
valve, heart NEC 746.89
  pulmonary 746.09
vertebra 756.19
vocal cords 748.3
vulva 752.49
**Accident, accidental** — *see also* condition
birth NEC 767.9
cardiovascular (*see also* Disease, cardiovascular) 429.2
cerebral (*see also* Disease, cerebrovascular, acute) 434.91
cerebrovascular (current) (CVA) (*see also* Disease, cerebrovascular, acute) 434.91
  aborted 434.91
  embolic 434.11
  healed or old V12.54
  hemorrhagic — *see* Hemorrhage, brain
  impending 435.9
  ischemic 434.91
  late effect — *see* Late effect(s) (of) cerebrovascular disease
  postoperative 997.02
  thrombotic 434.01
coronary (*see also* Infarct, myocardium) 410.9 ☑
craniovascular (*see also* Disease, cerebrovascular, acute) 436
during pregnancy, to mother, affecting fetus or newborn 760.5
heart, cardiac (*see also* Infarct, myocardium) 410.9 ☑
intrauterine 779.89
vascular — *see* Disease, cerebrovascular, acute
**Accommodation**
disorder of 367.51
  drug-induced 367.89
  toxic 367.89
insufficiency of 367.4
paralysis of 367.51
  hysterical 300.11
spasm of 367.53
**Accouchement** — *see* Delivery
**Accreta placenta** (without hemorrhage) 667.0 ☑
  with hemorrhage 666.0 ☑
**Accretio cordis** (nonrheumatic) 423.1
**Accretions on teeth** 523.6
**Accumulation secretion, prostate** 602.8
**Acephalia, acephalism, acephaly** 740.0
**Acephalic** 740.0
**Acephalobrachia** 759.89
**Acephalocardia** 759.89
**Acephalocardius** 759.89
**Acephalochiria** 759.89
**Acephalochirus** 759.89

**Acephalogaster** 759.89
**Acephalostomus** 759.89
**Acephalothorax** 759.89
**Acephalus** 740.0
**Acetonemia** 790.6
  diabetic 250.1 ☑
**Acetonglycosuria** 982.8
**Acetonuria** 791.6
**Achalasia** 530.0
  cardia 530.0
  digestive organs congenital NEC 751.8
  esophagus 530.0
  pelvirectal 751.3
  psychogenic 306.4
  pylorus 750.5
  sphincteral NEC 564.89
**Achard-Thiers syndrome** (adrenogenital) 255.2
**Ache(s)** — *see* Pain
**Acheilia** 750.26
**Acheiria** 755.21
**Achillobursitis** 726.71
**Achillodynia** 726.71
**Achlorhydria, achlorhydric** 536.0
  anemia 280.9
  diarrhea 536.0
  neurogenic 536.0
  postvagotomy 564.2
  psychogenic 306.4
  secondary to vagotomy 564.2
**Achloroblepsia** 368.52
**Achloropsia** 368.52
**Acholia** 575.8
**Acholuric jaundice** (familial) (splenomegalic) — *see also* Spherocytosis 282.0
  acquired 283.9
**Achondroplasia** 756.4
**Achrestic anemia** 281.8
**Achroacytosis, lacrimal gland** 375.00
  tuberculous (*see also* Tuberculosis) 017.3 ☑
**Achroma, cutis** 709.00
**Achromate** (congenital) 368.54
**Achromatopia** 368.54
**Achromatopsia** (congenital) 368.54
**Achromia**
  congenital 270.2
  parasitica 111.0
  unguium 703.8
**Achylia**
  gastrica 536.8
    neurogenic 536.3
    psychogenic 306.4
  pancreatica 577.1
**Achylosis** 536.8
**Acid**
burn (*see also* Burn, by site)
  from swallowing acid — *see* Burn, internal organs
deficiency
  amide nicotinic 265.2
  amino 270.9
  ascorbic 267
  folic 266.2
  nicotinic (amide) 265.2
  pantothenic 266.2
intoxication 276.2
peptic disease 536.8
stomach 536.8
  psychogenic 306.4
**Acidemia** 276.2
arginosuccinic 270.6
fetal
  affecting management of pregnancy 656.3 ☑
  before onset of labor, in liveborn infant 768.2
  during labor and delivery in liveborn infant 768.3
  intrauterine 656.3 ☑
  unspecified as to time of onset, in liveborn infant 768.4
newborn 775.81
pipecolic 270.7
**Acidity, gastric** (high) (low) 536.8

**Acidity, gastric** — *continued*
psychogenic 306.4
**Acidocytopenia** 288.59
**Acidocytosis** 288.3
**Acidopenia** 288.59
**Acidosis** 276.2
diabetic 250.1 ☑
fetal, affecting management of pregnancy 656.8 ☑
fetal, affecting newborn 775.81
kidney tubular 588.89
  newborn 775.81
lactic 276.2
metabolic NEC 276.2
  with respiratory acidosis 276.4
    of newborn 775.81
  late, of newborn 775.7
newborn 775.81
renal
  hyperchloremic 588.89
  tubular (distal) (proximal) 588.89
respiratory 276.2
  complicated by
    metabolic acidosis 276.4
      of newborn 775.81
    metabolic alkalosis 276.4
**Aciduria** 791.9
arginosuccinic 270.6
beta-aminoisobutyric (BAIB) 277.2
glutaric
  type I 270.7
  type II (type IIA, IIB, IIC) 277.85
  type III 277.86
glycolic 271.8
methylmalonic 270.3
  with glycinemia 270.7
organic 270.9
orotic (congenital) (hereditary) (pyrimidine deficiency) 281.4
**Acladiosis** 111.8
skin 111.8
**Aclasis**
diaphyseal 756.4
tarsoepiphyseal 756.59
**Acleistocardia** 745.5
**Aclusion** 524.4
**Acmesthesia** 782.0
**Acne** (pustular) (vulgaris) 706.1
agminata (*see also* Tuberculosis) 017.0 ☑
artificialis 706.1
atrophica 706.0
cachecticorum (Hebra) 706.1
conglobata 706.1
conjunctiva 706.1
cystic 706.1
decalvans 704.09
erythematosa 695.3
eyelid 706.1
frontalis 706.0
indurata 706.1
keloid 706.1
lupoid 706.0
necrotic, necrotica 706.0
  miliaris 704.8
neonatal 706.1
nodular 706.1
occupational 706.1
papulosa 706.1
rodens 706.0
rosacea 695.3
scorbutica 267
scrofulosorum (Bazin) (*see also* Tuberculosis) 017.0 ☑
summer 692.72
tropical 706.1
varioliformis 706.0
**Acneiform drug eruptions** 692.3
**Acnitis** (primary) — *see also* Tuberculosis 017.0 ☑
**Acomia** 704.00
**Acontractile bladder** 344.61
**Aconuresis** — *see also* Incontinence 788.30
**Acosta's disease** 993.2
**Acousma** 780.1

---

☑ Additional Digit Required — Refer to the Tabular List for Digit Selection      Subterms under main terms may continue to next column or page

8 — Volume 2 · October 2007      ▶◀ Revised Text      ● New Line      ▲ Revised Code      *2008 ICD-9-CM*

**Acoustic** — see condition
**Acousticophobia** 300.29
**Acquired** — see condition
**Acquired immune deficiency syndrome** — see Human immunodeficiency virus (disease) (illness) (infection)
**Acquired immunodeficiency syndrome** — see Human immunodeficiency virus (disease) (illness) (infection)
**Acragnosis** 781.99
**Acrania** 740.0
**Acroagnosis** 781.99
**Acroasphyxia, chronic** 443.89
**Acrobrachycephaly** 756.0
**Acrobystiolith** 608.89
**Acrobystitis** 607.2
**Acrocephalopolysyndactyly** 755.55
**Acrocephalosyndactyly** 755.55
**Acrocephaly** 756.0
**Acrochondrohyperplasia** 759.82
**Acrocyanosis** 443.89
  newborn 770.83
    meaning transient blue hands and feet — omit code
**Acrodermatitis** 686.8
  atrophicans (chronica) 701.8
  continua (Hallopeau) 696.1
  enteropathica 686.8
  Hallopeau's 696.1
  perstans 696.1
  pustulosa continua 696.1
  recalcitrant pustular 696.1
**Acrodynia** 985.0
**Acrodysplasia** 755.55
**Acrohyperhidrosis** — see also Hyperhidrosis 780.8
**Acrokeratosis verruciformis** 757.39
**Acromastitis** 611.0
**Acromegaly, acromegalia** (skin) 253.0
**Acromelalgia** 443.82
**Acromicria, acromikria** 756.59
**Acronyx** 703.0
**Acropachyderma** 757.39
**Acropachy, thyroid** — see also Thyrotoxicosis 242.9 ☑
**Acroparesthesia** 443.89
  simple (Schultz's type) 443.89
  vasomotor (Nothnagel's type) 443.89
**Acropathy thyroid** — see also Thyrotoxicosis 242.9 ☑
**Acrophobia** 300.29
**Acroposthitis** 607.2
**Acroscleriasis** — see also Scleroderma 710.1
**Acroscleroderma** — see also Scleroderma 710.1
**Acrosclerosis** — see also Scleroderma 710.1
**Acrophacelus** 785.4
**Acrosphenosyndactylia** 755.55
**Acrospiroma, eccrine** (M8402/0) — see Neoplasm, skin, benign
**Acrostealgia** 732.9
**Acrosyndactyly** — see also Syndactylism 755.10
**Acrotrophodynia** 991.4
**Actinic** — see also condition
  cheilitis (due to sun) 692.72
    chronic NEC 692.74
    due to radiation, except from sun 692.82
  conjunctivitis 370.24
  dermatitis (due to sun) (see also Dermatitis, actinic) 692.70
    due to
      roentgen rays or radioactive substance 692.82
      ultraviolet radiation, except from sun 692.82
      sun NEC 692.70
  elastosis solare 692.74
  granuloma 692.73
  keratitis 370.24
  ophthalmia 370.24
  reticuloid 692.73
**Actinobacillosis, general** 027.8

**Actinobacillus**
  lignieresii 027.8
  mallei 024
  muris 026.1
**Actinocutitis** NEC — see also Dermatitis, actinic 692.70
**Actinodermatitis** NEC — see also Dermatitis, actinic 692.70
**Actinomyces**
  israelii (infection) — see Actinomycosis
  muris-ratti (infection) 026.1
**Actinomycosis, actinomycotic** 039.9
  with
    pneumonia 039.1
  abdominal 039.2
  cervicofacial 039.3
  cutaneous 039.0
  pulmonary 039.1
  specified site NEC 039.8
  thoracic 039.1
**Actinoneuritis** 357.89
**Action, heart**
  disorder 427.9
    postoperative 997.1
  irregular 427.9
    postoperative 997.1
    psychogenic 306.2
**Active** — see condition
**Activity decrease, functional** 780.99
**Acute** — see also condition
  abdomen NEC 789.0 ☑
  gallbladder (see also Cholecystitis, acute) 575.0
**Acyanoblepsia** 368.53
**Acyanopsia** 368.53
**Acystia** 753.8
**Acystinervia** — see Neurogenic, bladder
**Acystineuria** — see Neurogenic, bladder
**Adactylia, adactyly** (congenital) 755.4
  lower limb (complete) (intercalary) (partial) (terminal) (see also Deformity, reduction, lower limb) 755.39
    meaning all digits (complete) (partial) 755.31
    transverse (complete) (partial) 755.31
  upper limb (complete) (intercalary) (partial) (terminal) (see also Deformity, reduction, upper limb) 755.29
    meaning all digits (complete) (partial) 755.21
    transverse (complete) (partial) 755.21
**Adair-Dighton syndrome** (brittle bones and blue sclera, deafness) 756.51
**Adamantinoblastoma** (M9310/0) — see Ameloblastoma
**Adamantinoma** (M9310/0) — see Ameloblastoma
**Adamantoblastoma** (M9310/0) — see Ameloblastoma
**Adams-Stokes (-Morgagni) disease or syndrome** (syncope with heart block) 426.9
**Adaptation reaction** — see also Reaction, adjustment 309.9
**Addiction** — see also Dependence
  absinthe 304.6 ☑
  alcoholic (ethyl) (methyl) (wood) 303.9 ☑
    complicating pregnancy, childbirth, or puerperium 648.4 ☑
      affecting fetus or newborn 760.71
      suspected damage to fetus affecting management of pregnancy 655.4 ☑
  drug (see also Dependence) 304.9 ☑
  ethyl alcohol 303.9 ☑
  heroin 304.0 ☑
  hospital 301.51
  methyl alcohol 303.9 ☑
  methylated spirit 303.9 ☑
  morphine (-like substances) 304.0 ☑

**Addiction** — see also Dependence — continued
  nicotine 305.1
  opium 304.0 ☑
  tobacco 305.1
  wine 303.9 ☑
**Addison's**
  anemia (pernicious) 281.0
  disease (bronze) (primary adrenal insufficiency) 255.41 ▲
    tuberculous (see also Tuberculosis) 017.6 ☑
  keloid (morphea) 701.0
  melanoderma (adrenal cortical hypofunction) 255.41 ▲
**Addison-Biermer anemia** (pernicious) 281.0
**Addison-Gull disease** — see Xanthoma
**Addisonian crisis or melanosis** (acute adrenocortical insufficiency) 255.41 ▲
**Additional** — see also Accessory
  chromosome(s) 758.5
    13-15 758.1
    16-18 758.2
    21 758.0
    autosome(s) NEC 758.5
    sex 758.81
**Adduction contracture, hip or other joint** — see Contraction, joint
**ADEM** (acute disseminated encephalomyelitis) (postinfectious) 136.9 [323.61]
  infectious 136.9 [323.61]
  noninfectious 323.81
**Adenasthenia gastrica** 536.0
**Aden fever** 061
**Adenitis** — see also Lymphadenitis 289.3
  acute, unspecified site 683
    epidemic infectious 075
  axillary 289.3
    acute 683
    chronic or subacute 289.1
  Bartholin's gland 616.89
  bulbourethral gland (see also Urethritis) 597.89
  cervical 289.3
    acute 683
    chronic or subacute 289.1
  chancroid (Ducrey's bacillus) 099.0
  chronic (any lymph node, except mesenteric) 289.1
    mesenteric 289.2
  Cowper's gland (see also Urethritis) 597.89
  epidemic, acute 075
  gangrenous 683
  gonorrheal NEC 098.89
  groin 289.3
    acute 683
    chronic or subacute 289.1
  infectious 075
  inguinal (region) 289.3
    acute 683
    chronic or subacute 289.1
  lymph gland or node, except mesenteric 289.3
    acute 683
    chronic or subacute 289.1
    mesenteric (acute) (chronic) (nonspecific) (subacute) 289.2
  mesenteric (acute) (chronic) (nonspecific) (subacute) 289.2
    due to Pasteurella multocida (P. septica) 027.2
  parotid gland (suppurative) 527.2
  phlegmonous 683
  salivary duct or gland (any) (recurring) (suppurative) 527.2
  scrofulous (see also Tuberculosis) 017.2 ☑
  septic 289.3
  Skene's duct or gland (see also Urethritis) 597.89

**Adenitis** — see also Lymphadenitis — continued
  strumous, tuberculous (see also Tuberculosis) 017.2 ☑
  subacute, unspecified site 289.1
  sublingual gland (suppurative) 527.2
  submandibular gland (suppurative) 527.2
  submaxillary gland (suppurative) 527.2
  suppurative 683
  tuberculous — see Tuberculosis, lymph gland
  urethral gland (see also Urethritis) 597.89
  venereal NEC 099.8
  Wharton's duct (suppurative) 527.2
**Adenoacanthoma** (M8570/3) — see Neoplasm, by site, malignant
**Adenoameloblastoma** (M9300/0) 213.1
  upper jaw (bone) 213.0
**Adenocarcinoma** (M8140/3) — see also Neoplasm, by site, malignant

> Note — The list of adjectival modifiers below is not exhaustive. A description of adenocarcinoma that does not appear in this list should be coded in the same manner as carcinoma with that description. Thus, "mixed acidophil-basophil adenocarcinoma," should be coded in the same manner as "mixed acidophil-basophil carcinoma," which appears in the list under "Carcinoma."
>
> Except where otherwise indicated, the morphological varieties of adenocarcinoma in the list below should be coded by site as for "Neoplasm, malignant."

  with
    apocrine metaplasia (M8573/3)
    cartilaginous (and osseous) metaplasia (M8571/3)
    osseous (and cartilaginous) metaplasia (M8571/3)
    spindle cell metaplasia (M8572/3)
    squamous metaplasia (M8570/3)
  acidophil (M8280/3)
    specified site — see Neoplasm, by site, malignant
    unspecified site 194.3
  acinar (M8550/3)
  acinic cell (M8550/3)
  adrenal cortical (M8370/3) 194.0
  alveolar (M8251/3)
    and
      epidermoid carcinoma, mixed (M8560/3)
      squamous cell carcinoma, mixed (M8560/3)
  apocrine (M8401/3)
    breast — see Neoplasm, breast, malignant
    specified site NEC — see Neoplasm, skin, malignant
    unspecified site 173.9
  basophil (M8300/3)
    specified site — see Neoplasm, by site, malignant
    unspecified site 194.3
  bile duct type (M8160/3)
    liver 155.1
    specified site NEC — see Neoplasm, by site, malignant
    unspecified site 155.1
  bronchiolar (M8250/3) — see Neoplasm, lung, malignant
  ceruminous (M8420/3) 173.2
  chromophobe (M8270/3)
    specified site — see Neoplasm, by site, malignant
    unspecified site 194.3

☑ Additional Digit Required — Refer to the Tabular List for Digit Selection        ▼ Subterms under main terms may continue to next column or page

**2008 ICD-9-CM**      ▶◀ Revised Text      ● New Line      ▲ Revised Code      **October 2007 · Volume 2 — 9**

Index

Adenocarcinoma — Adenoma

**Adenocarcinoma** — see also Neoplasm, by site, malignant — continued
clear cell (mesonephroid type) (M8310/3)
colloid (M8480/3)
cylindroid type (M8200/3)
diffuse type (M8145/3)
  specified site — see Neoplasm, by site, malignant
  unspecified site 151.9
duct (infiltrating) (M8500/3)
  with Paget's disease (M8541/3) — see Neoplasm, breast, malignant
  specified site — see Neoplasm, by site, malignant
  unspecified site 174.9
embryonal (M9070/3)
endometrioid (M8380/3) — see Neoplasm, by site, malignant
eosinophil (M8280/3)
  specified site — see Neoplasm, by site, malignant
  unspecified site 194.3
follicular (M8330/3)
  and papillary (M8340/3) 193
  moderately differentiated type (M8332/3) 193
  pure follicle type (M8331/3) 193
  specified site — see Neoplasm, by site, malignant
  trabecular type (M8332/3) 193
  unspecified type 193
  well differentiated type (M8331/3) 193
gelatinous (M8480/3)
granular cell (M8320/3)
Hürthle cell (M8290/3) 193
in
  adenomatous
    polyp (M8210/3)
    polyposis coli (M8220/3) 153.9
  polypoid adenoma (M8210/3)
  tubular adenoma (M8210/3)
  villous adenoma (M8261/3)
infiltrating duct (M8500/3)
  with Paget's disease (M8541/3) — see Neoplasm, breast, malignant
  specified site — see Neoplasm, by site, malignant
  unspecified site 174.9
inflammatory (M8530/3)
  specified site — see Neoplasm, by site, malignant
  unspecified site 174.9
in situ (M8140/2) — see Neoplasm, by site, in situ
intestinal type (M8144/3)
  specified site — see Neoplasm, by site, malignant
  unspecified site 151.9
intraductal (noninfiltrating) (M8500/2)
  papillary (M8503/2)
    specified site — see Neoplasm, by site, in situ
    unspecified site 233.0
  specified site — see Neoplasm, by site, in situ
  unspecified site 233.0
islet cell (M8150/3)
  and exocrine, mixed (M8154/3)
    specified site — see Neoplasm, by site, malignant
    unspecified site 157.9
  pancreas 157.4
  specified site NEC — see Neoplasm, by site, malignant
  unspecified site 157.4
lobular (M8520/3)
  specified site — see Neoplasm, by site, malignant
  unspecified site 174.9

**Adenocarcinoma** — see also Neoplasm, by site, malignant — continued
medullary (M8510/3)
mesonephric (M9110/3)
mixed cell (M8323/3)
mucinous (M8480/3)
mucin-producing (M8481/3)
mucoid (M8480/3) (see also Neoplasm, by site, malignant)
  cell (M8300/3)
    specified site — see Neoplasm, by site, malignant
    unspecified site 194.3
nonencapsulated sclerosing (M8350/3) 193
oncocytic (M8290/3)
oxyphilic (M8290/3)
papillary (M8260/3)
  and follicular (M8340/3) 193
  intraductal (noninfiltrating) (M8503/2)
    specified site — see Neoplasm, by site, in situ
    unspecified site 233.0
  serous (M8460/3)
    specified site — see Neoplasm, by site, malignant
    unspecified site 183.0
papillocystic (M8450/3)
  specified site — see Neoplasm, by site, malignant
  unspecified site 183.0
pseudomucinous (M8470/3)
  specified site — see Neoplasm, by site, malignant
  unspecified site 183.0
renal cell (M8312/3) 189.0
sebaceous (M8410/3)
serous (M8441/3) (see also Neoplasm, by site, malignant)
  papillary
    specified site — see Neoplasm, by site, malignant
    unspecified site 183.0
signet ring cell (M8490/3)
superficial spreading (M8143/3)
sweat gland (M8400/3) — see Neoplasm, skin, malignant
trabecular (M8190/3)
tubular (M8211/3)
villous (M8262/3)
water-clear cell (M8322/3) 194.1
**Adenofibroma** (M9013/0)
clear cell (M8313/0) — see Neoplasm, by site, benign
endometrioid (M8381/0) 220
  borderline malignancy (M8381/1) 236.2
  malignant (M8381/3) 183.0
mucinous (M9015/0)
  specified site — see Neoplasm, by site, benign
  unspecified site 220
prostate 600.20
  with
    other lower urinary tract symptoms (LUTS) 600.21
    urinary
      obstruction 600.21
      retention 600.21
serous (M9014/0)
  specified site — see Neoplasm, by site, benign
  unspecified site 220
specified site — see Neoplasm, by site, benign
unspecified site 220
**Adenofibrosis**
breast 610.2
endometrioid 617.0
**Adenoiditis** 474.01
acute 463
chronic 474.01
  with chronic tonsillitis 474.02
**Adenoids** (congenital) (of nasal fossa) 474.9

**Adenoids** — continued
hypertrophy 474.12
vegetations 474.2
**Adenolipomatosis** (symmetrical) 272.8
**Adenolymphoma** (M8561/0)
specified site — see Neoplasm, by site, benign
unspecified 210.2
**Adenomatosis** (M8220/0)
endocrine (multiple) (M8360/1)
  single specified site — see Neoplasm, by site, uncertain behavior
  two or more specified sites 237.4
  unspecified site 237.4
erosive of nipple (M8506/0) 217
pluriendocrine — see Adenomatosis, endocrine
pulmonary (M8250/1) 235.7
  malignant (M8250/3) — see Neoplasm, lung, malignant
specified site — see Neoplasm, by site, benign
unspecified site 211.3
**Adenomatous**
cyst, thyroid (gland) — see Goiter, nodular
goiter (nontoxic) (see also Goiter, nodular) 241.9
  toxic or with hyperthyroidism 242.3 ☑
**Adenoma** (sessile) (M8140/0) — see also Neoplasm, by site, benign

Note — Except where otherwise indicated, the morphological varieties of adenoma in the list below should be coded by site as for "Neoplasm, benign."

acidophil (M8280/0)
  specified site — see Neoplasm, by site, benign
  unspecified site 227.3
acinar (cell) (M8550/0)
acinic cell (M8550/0)
adrenal (cortex) (cortical) (functioning) (M8370/0) 227.0
  clear cell type (M8373/0) 227.0
  compact cell type (M8371/0) 227.0
  glomerulosa cell type (M8374/0) 227.0
  heavily pigmented variant (M8372/0) 227.0
  mixed cell type (M8375/0) 227.0
alpha cell (M8152/0)
  pancreas 211.7
  specified site NEC — see Neoplasm, by site, benign
  unspecified site 211.7
alveolar (M8251/0)
apocrine (M8401/0)
  breast 217
  specified site NEC — see Neoplasm, skin, benign
  unspecified site 216.9
basal cell (M8147/0)
basophil (M8300/0)
  specified site — see Neoplasm, by site, benign
  unspecified site 227.3
beta cell (M8151/0)
  pancreas 211.7
  specified site NEC — see Neoplasm, by site, benign
  unspecified site 211.7
bile duct (M8160/0) 211.5
black (M8372/0) 227.0
bronchial (M8140/1) 235.7
  carcinoid type (M8240/3) — see Neoplasm, lung, malignant
  cylindroid type (M8200/3) — see Neoplasm, lung, malignant
ceruminous (M8420/0) 216.2
chief cell (M8321/0) 227.1
chromophobe (M8270/0)
  specified site — see Neoplasm, by site, benign
  unspecified site 227.3

**Adenoma** — see also Neoplasm, by site, benign — continued
clear cell (M8310/0)
colloid (M8334/0)
  specified site — see Neoplasm, by site, benign
  unspecified site 226
cylindroid type, bronchus (M8200/3) — see Neoplasm, lung, malignant
duct (M8503/0)
embryonal (M8191/0)
endocrine, multiple (M8360/1)
  single specified site — see Neoplasm, by site, uncertain behavior
  two or more specified sites 237.4
  unspecified site 237.4
endometrioid (M8380/0) (see also Neoplasm, by site, benign)
  borderline malignancy (M8380/1) — see Neoplasm, by site, uncertain behavior
eosinophil (M8280/0)
  specified site — see Neoplasm, by site, benign
  unspecified site 227.3
fetal (M8333/0)
  specified site — see Neoplasm, by site, benign
  unspecified site 226
follicular (M8330/0)
  specified site — see Neoplasm, by site, benign
  unspecified site 226
hepatocellular (M8170/0) 211.5
Hürthle cell (M8290/0) 226
intracystic papillary (M8504/0)
islet cell (functioning) (M8150/0)
  pancreas 211.7
  specified site NEC — see Neoplasm, by site, benign
  unspecified site 211.7
liver cell (M8170/0) 211.5
macrofollicular (M8334/0)
  specified site NEC — see Neoplasm, by site, benign
  unspecified site 226
malignant, malignum (M8140/3) — see Neoplasm, by site, malignant
mesonephric (M9110/0)
microfollicular (M8333/0)
  specified site — see Neoplasm, by site, benign
  unspecified site 226
mixed cell (M8323/0)
monomorphic (M8146/0)
mucinous (M8480/0)
mucoid cell (M8300/0)
  specified site — see Neoplasm, by site, benign
  unspecified site 227.3
multiple endocrine (M8360/1)
  single specified site — see Neoplasm, by site, uncertain behavior
  two or more specified sites 237.4
  unspecified site 237.4
nipple (M8506/0) 217
oncocytic (M8290/0)
oxyphilic (M8290/0)
papillary (M8260/0) (see also Neoplasm, by site, benign)
  intracystic (M8504/0)
papillotubular (M8263/0)
Pick's tubular (M8640/0)
  specified site — see Neoplasm, by site, benign
  unspecified site
    female 220
    male 222.0
pleomorphic (M8940/0)
polypoid (M8210/0)
prostate (benign) 600.20

**Adenoma** — see also Neoplasm, by site, benign — continued
  prostate — continued
    with
      other lower urinary tract symptoms (LUTS) 600.21
      urinary
        obstruction 600.21
        retention 600.21
  rete cell 222.0
  sebaceous, sebaceum (gland) (senile) (M8410/0) (see also Neoplasm, skin, benign)
    disseminata 759.5
  Sertoli cell (M8640/0)
    specified site — see Neoplasm, by site, benign
    unspecified site
      female 220
      male 222.0
  skin appendage (M8390/0) — see Neoplasm, skin, benign
  sudoriferous gland (M8400/0) — see Neoplasm, skin, benign
  sweat gland or duct (M8400/0) — see Neoplasm, skin, benign
  testicular (M8640/0)
    specified site — see Neoplasm, by site, benign
    unspecified site
      female 220
      male 222.0
  thyroid 226
  trabecular (M8190/0)
  tubular (M8211/0) (see also Neoplasm, by site, benign)
    papillary (M8460/3)
    Pick's (M8640/0)
      specified site — see Neoplasm, by site, benign
      unspecified site
        female 220
        male 222.0
  tubulovillous (M8263/0)
  villoglandular (M8263/0)
  villous (M8261/1) — see Neoplasm, by site, uncertain behavior
  water-clear cell (M8322/0) 227.1
  wolffian duct (M9110/0)

**Adenomyoma** (M8932/0) — see also Neoplasm, by site, benign
  prostate 600.20
    with
      other lower urinary tract symptoms (LUTS) 600.21
      urinary
        obstruction 600.21
        retention 600.21

**Adenomyometritis** 617.0
**Adenomyosis** (uterus) (internal) 617.0
**Adenopathy** (lymph gland) 785.6
  inguinal 785.6
  mediastinal 785.6
  mesentery 785.6
  syphilitic (secondary) 091.4
  tracheobronchial 785.6
    tuberculous (see also Tuberculosis) 012.1 ☑
      primary, progressive 010.8 ☑
  tuberculous (see also Tuberculosis, lymph gland) 017.2 ☑
    tracheobronchial 012.1 ☑
      primary, progressive 010.8 ☑

**Adenopharyngitis** 462
**Adenophlegmon** 683
**Adenosalpingitis** 614.1
**Adenosarcoma** (M8960/3) 189.0
**Adenosclerosis** 289.3
**Adenosis**
  breast (sclerosing) 610.2
  vagina, congenital 752.49
**Adentia** (complete) (partial) — see also Absence, teeth 520.0
**Adherent**
  labium (minus) 624.4
  pericardium (nonrheumatic) 423.1

**Adherent** — continued
  pericardium — continued
    rheumatic 393
  placenta 667.0 ☑
    with hemorrhage 666.0 ☑
  prepuce 605
  scar (skin) NEC 709.2
  tendon in scar 709.2
**Adhesion(s), adhesive** (postinfectional) (postoperative)
  abdominal (wall) (see also Adhesions, peritoneum) 568.0
  amnion to fetus 658.8 ☑
    affecting fetus or newborn 762.8
  appendix 543.9
  arachnoiditis — see Meningitis
  auditory tube (Eustachian) 381.89
  bands (see also Adhesions, peritoneum)
    cervix 622.3
    uterus 621.5
  bile duct (any) 576.8
  bladder (sphincter) 596.8
  bowel (see also Adhesions, peritoneum) 568.0
  cardiac 423.1
    rheumatic 398.99
  cecum (see also Adhesions, peritoneum) 568.0
  cervicovaginal 622.3
    congenital 752.49
    postpartal 674.8 ☑
    old 622.3
  cervix 622.3
  clitoris 624.4
  colon (see also Adhesions, peritoneum) 568.0
  common duct 576.8
  congenital (see also Anomaly, specified type NEC)
    fingers (see also Syndactylism, fingers) 755.11
    labium (majus) (minus) 752.49
    omental, anomalous 751.4
    ovary 752.0
    peritoneal 751.4
    toes (see also Syndactylism, toes) 755.13
    tongue (to gum or roof of mouth) 750.12
  conjunctiva (acquired) (localized) 372.62
    congenital 743.63
    extensive 372.63
  cornea — see Opacity, cornea
  cystic duct 575.8
  diaphragm (see also Adhesions, peritoneum) 568.0
  due to foreign body — see Foreign body
  duodenum (see also Adhesions, peritoneum) 568.0
    with obstruction 537.3
  ear, middle — see Adhesions, middle ear
  epididymis 608.89
  epidural — see Adhesions, meninges
  epiglottis 478.79
  Eustachian tube 381.89
  eyelid 374.46
    postoperative 997.99
      surgically created V45.69
  gallbladder (see also Disease, gallbladder) 575.8
  globe 360.89
  heart 423.1
    rheumatic 398.99
  ileocecal (coil) (see also Adhesions, peritoneum) 568.0
  ileum (see also Adhesions, peritoneum) 568.0
  intestine (postoperative) (see also Adhesions, peritoneum) 568.0
    with obstruction 560.81
      with hernia (see also Hernia, by site, with obstruction)

**Adhesion(s), adhesive** — continued
  intestine (see also Adhesions, peritoneum) — continued
    with obstruction — continued
      with hernia (see also Hernia, by site, with obstruction) — continued
        gangrenous — see Hernia, by site, with gangrene
    intra-abdominal (see also Adhesions, peritoneum) 568.0
  iris 364.70
    to corneal graft 996.79
  joint (see also Ankylosis) 718.5 ☑
  kidney 593.89
  labium (majus) (minus), congenital 752.49
  liver 572.8
  lung 511.0
  mediastinum 519.3
  meninges 349.2
    cerebral (any) 349.2
      congenital 742.4
    congenital 742.8
    spinal (any) 349.2
      congenital 742.59
    tuberculous (cerebral) (spinal) (see also Tuberculosis, meninges) 013.0 ☑
  mesenteric (see also Adhesions, peritoneum) 568.0
  middle ear (fibrous) 385.10
    drum head 385.19
    to
      incus 385.11
      promontorium 385.13
      stapes 385.12
    specified NEC 385.19
  nasal (septum) (to turbinates) 478.19
  nerve NEC 355.9
    spinal 355.9
      root 724.9
        cervical NEC 723.4
        lumbar NEC 724.4
        lumbosacral 724.4
        thoracic 724.4
  ocular muscle 378.60
  omentum (see also Adhesions, peritoneum) 568.0
  organ or site, congenital NEC — see Anomaly, specified type NEC
  ovary 614.6
    congenital (to cecum, kidney, or omentum) 752.0
  parauterine 614.6
  parovarian 614.6
  pelvic (peritoneal)
    female (postoperative) (postinfection) 614.6
    male (postoperative) (postinfection) (see also Adhesions, peritoneum) 568.0
    postpartal (old) 614.6
    tuberculous (see also Tuberculosis) 016.9 ☑
  penis to scrotum (congenital) 752.69
  periappendiceal (see also Adhesions, peritoneum) 568.0
  pericardium (nonrheumatic) 423.1
    rheumatic 393
    tuberculous (see also Tuberculosis) 017.9 ☑ [420.0]
  pericholecystic 575.8
  perigastric (see also Adhesions, peritoneum) 568.0
  periovarian 614.6
  periprostatic 602.8
  perirectal (see also Adhesions, peritoneum) 568.0
  perirenal 593.89
  peritoneum, peritoneal (fibrous) (postoperative)
    with obstruction (intestinal) 560.81
      with hernia (see also Hernia, by site, with obstruction)

**Adhesion(s), adhesive** — continued
  peritoneum, peritoneal — continued
    with obstruction — continued
      with hernia (see also Hernia, by site, with obstruction) — continued
        gangrenous — see Hernia, by site, with gangrene
    duodenum 537.3
    congenital 751.4
    female (postoperative) (postinfective) 614.6
    pelvic, female 614.6
    pelvic, male 568.0
    postpartal, pelvic 614.6
    to uterus 614.6
  peritubal 614.6
  periureteral 593.89
  periuterine 621.5
  perivesical 596.8
  perivesicular (seminal vesicle) 608.89
  pleura, pleuritic 511.0
    tuberculous (see also Tuberculosis, pleura) 012.0 ☑
  pleuropericardial 511.0
  postoperative (gastrointestinal tract) (see also Adhesions, peritoneum) 568.0
    eyelid 997.99
      surgically created V45.69
    pelvic female 614.9
    pelvic male 568.0
    urethra 598.2
  postpartal, old 624.4
  preputial, prepuce 605
  pulmonary 511.0
  pylorus (see also Adhesions, peritoneum) 568.0
  Rosenmüller's fossa 478.29
  sciatic nerve 355.0
  seminal vesicle 608.89
  shoulder (joint) 726.0
  sigmoid flexure (see also Adhesions, peritoneum) 568.0
  spermatic cord (acquired) 608.89
    congenital 752.89
  spinal canal 349.2
    nerve 355.9
      root 724.9
        cervical NEC 723.4
        lumbar NEC 724.4
        lumbosacral 724.4
        thoracic 724.4
  stomach (see also Adhesions, peritoneum) 568.0
  subscapular 726.2
  tendonitis 726.90
    shoulder 726.0
  testicle 608.89
  tongue (congenital) (to gum or roof of mouth) 750.12
    acquired 529.8
  trachea 519.19
  tubo-ovarian 614.6
  tunica vaginalis 608.89
  ureter 593.89
  uterus 621.5
    to abdominal wall 614.6
    in pregnancy or childbirth 654.4 ☑
      affecting fetus or newborn 763.89
  vagina (chronic) (postoperative) (postradiation) 623.2
  vaginitis (congenital) 752.49
  vesical 596.8
  vitreous 379.29
**Adie (-Holmes) syndrome** (tonic pupillary reaction) 379.46
**Adiponecrosis neonatorum** 778.1
**Adiposa dolorosa** 272.8
**Adiposalgia** 272.8
**Adiposis**
  cerebralis 253.8
  dolorosa 272.8

☑ Additional Digit Required — Refer to the Tabular List for Digit Selection      ▽ Subterms under main terms may continue to next column or page

**2008 ICD-9-CM**    ▶◀ Revised Text    ● New Line    ▲ Revised Code    **Volume 2 — 11**

**Adiposis** — *continued*
  tuberosa simplex 272.8
**Adiposity** 278.02
  heart (*see also* Degeneration, myocardial) 429.1
  localized 278.1
**Adiposogenital dystrophy** 253.8
**Adjustment**
  prosthesis or other device — *see* Fitting of
  reaction — *see* Reaction, adjustment
**Administration, prophylactic**
  antibiotics V07.39
  antitoxin, any V07.2
  antivenin V07.2
  chemotherapeutic agent NEC V07.39
  chemotherapy NEC V07.39
  diphtheria antitoxin V07.2
  fluoride V07.31
  gamma globulin V07.2
  immune sera (gamma globulin) V07.2
  passive immunization agent V07.2
  RhoGAM V07.2
**Admission** (encounter)
  as organ donor — *see* Donor
  by mistake V68.9
  for
    adequacy testing (for)
      hemodialysis V56.31
      peritoneal dialysis V56.32
    adjustment (of)
      artificial
        arm (complete) (partial) V52.0
        eye V52.2
        leg (complete) (partial) V52.1
      brain neuropacemaker V53.02
      breast
        implant V52.4
        prosthesis V52.4
      cardiac device V53.39
        defibrillator, automatic implantable V53.32
        pacemaker V53.31
          carotid sinus V53.39
      catheter
        non-vascular V58.82
        vascular V58.81
      cerebral ventricle (communicating) shunt V53.01
      colostomy belt V55.3
      contact lenses V53.1
      cystostomy device V53.6
      dental prosthesis V52.3
      device, unspecified type V53.90
        abdominal V53.5
        cardiac V53.39
          defibrillator, automatic implantable V53.32
          pacemaker V53.31
        carotid sinus V53.39
        cerebral ventricle (communicating) shunt V53.01
        insulin pump V53.91
        intrauterine contraceptive V25.1
        nervous system V53.09
        orthodontic V53.4
        other device V53.99
        prosthetic V52.9
          breast V52.4
          dental V52.3
          eye V52.2
          specified type NEC V52.8
        special senses V53.09
        substitution
          auditory V53.09
          nervous system V53.09
          visual V53.09
        urinary V53.6
      dialysis catheter
        extracorporeal V56.1
        peritoneal V56.2
      diaphragm (contraceptive) V25.02
      growth rod V54.02

**Admission** — *continued*
  for — *continued*
    adjustment — *continued*
      hearing aid V53.2
      ileostomy device V55.2
      intestinal appliance or device NEC V53.5
      intrauterine contraceptive device V25.1
      neuropacemaker (brain) (peripheral nerve) (spinal cord) V53.02
      orthodontic device V53.4
      orthopedic (device) V53.7
        brace V53.7
        cast V53.7
        shoes V53.7
      pacemaker
        brain V53.02
        cardiac V53.31
          carotid sinus V53.39
        peripheral nerve V53.02
        spinal cord V53.02
      prosthesis V52.9
        arm (complete) (partial) V52.0
        breast V52.4
        dental V52.3
        eye V52.2
        leg (complete) (partial) V52.1
        specified type NEC V52.8
      spectacles V53.1
      wheelchair V53.8
    adoption referral or proceedings V68.89
    aftercare (*see also* Aftercare) V58.9
      cardiac pacemaker V53.31
      chemotherapy V58.11
      dialysis
        extracorporeal (renal) V56.0
        peritoneal V56.8
        renal V56.0
      fracture (*see also* Aftercare, fracture) V54.9
      medical NEC V58.89
      organ transplant V58.44
      orthopedic V54.9
        specified care NEC V54.89
      pacemaker device
        brain V53.02
        cardiac V53.31
        carotid sinus V53.39
        nervous system V53.02
        spinal cord V53.02
      postoperative NEC V58.49
        wound closure, planned V58.41
      postpartum
        immediately after delivery V24.0
        routine follow-up V24.2
      postradiation V58.0
      radiation therapy V58.0
      removal of
        non-vascular catheter V58.82
        vascular catheter V58.81
        specified NEC V58.89
        surgical NEC V58.49
          wound closure, planned V58.41
    antineoplastic
      chemotherapy V58.11
      immunotherapy V58.12
    artificial insemination V26.1
    assisted reproductive fertility ●
      procedure cycle V26.81 ●
    attention to artificial opening (of) V55.9
      artificial vagina V55.7
      colostomy V55.3
      cystostomy V55.5
      enterostomy V55.4
      gastrostomy V55.1
      ileostomy V55.2
      jejunostomy V55.4

**Admission** — *continued*
  for — *continued*
    attention to artificial opening — *continued*
      nephrostomy V55.6
      specified site NEC V55.8
        intestinal tract V55.4
        urinary tract V55.6
      tracheostomy V55.0
      ureterostomy V55.6
      urethrostomy V55.6
    battery replacement
      cardiac pacemaker V53.31
    blood typing V72.86
      Rh typing V72.86
    boarding V65.0
    breast
      augmentation or reduction V50.1
      removal, prophylactic V50.41
    change of
      cardiac pacemaker (battery) V53.31
      carotid sinus pacemaker V53.39
      catheter in artificial opening — *see* Attention to, artificial, opening
      drains V58.49
      dressing
        wound V58.30
          nonsurgical V58.30
          surgical V58.31
      fixation device
        external V54.89
        internal V54.01
      Kirschner wire V54.89
      neuropacemaker device (brain) (peripheral nerve) (spinal cord) V53.02
      nonsurgical wound dressing V58.30
      pacemaker device
        brain V53.02
        cardiac V53.31
        carotid sinus V53.39
        nervous system V53.02
      plaster cast V54.89
      splint, external V54.89
      Steinmann pin V54.89
      surgical wound dressing V58.31
      traction device V54.89
      wound packing V58.30
        nonsurgical V58.30
        surgical V58.31
    checkup only V70.0
    chemotherapy, antineoplastic V58.11
    circumcision, ritual or routine (in absence of medical indication) V50.2
    clinical research investigation (control) (normal comparison) (participant) V70.7
    closure of artificial opening — *see* Attention to, artificial, opening
    contraceptive
      counseling V25.09
        emergency V25.03
        postcoital V25.03
      management V25.9
        specified type NEC V25.8
    convalescence following V66.9
      chemotherapy V66.2
      psychotherapy V66.3
      radiotherapy V66.1
      surgery V66.0
      treatment (for) V66.5
        combined V66.6
        fracture V66.4
        mental disorder NEC V66.3
        specified condition NEC V66.5
    cosmetic surgery NEC V50.1
      following healed injury or operation V51

**Admission** — *continued*
  for — *continued*
    counseling (*see also* Counseling) V65.40
      without complaint or sickness V65.49
      contraceptive management V25.09
        emergency V25.03
        postcoital V25.03
      dietary V65.3 ·
      exercise V65.41
      for
        nonattending third party V65.19
        pediatric pre-birth visit for expectant mother V65.11
        victim of abuse
          child V61.21
          partner or spouse V61.11
      genetic V26.33
      gonorrhea V65.45
      HIV V65.44
      human immunodeficiency virus V65.44
      injury prevention V65.43
      insulin pump training V65.46
      natural family planning ●
        procreative V26.41 ●
        to avoid pregnancy V25.04 ●
      procreative management V26.49 ▲
        using natural family planning V26.41 ●
      sexually transmitted disease NEC V65.45
        HIV V65.44
      specified reason NEC V65.49
      substance use and abuse V65.42
      syphilis V65.45
      victim of abuse
        child V61.21
        partner or spouse V61.11
    desensitization to allergens V07.1
    dialysis V56.0
      catheter
        fitting and adjustment
          extracorporeal V56.1
          peritoneal V56.2
        removal or replacement
          extracorporeal V56.1
          peritoneal V56.2
      extracorporeal (renal) V56.0
      peritoneal V56.8
      renal V56.0
    dietary surveillance and counseling V65.3
    drug monitoring, therapeutic V58.83
    ear piercing V50.3
    elective surgery V50.9
      breast
        augmentation or reduction V50.1
        removal, prophylactic V50.41
      circumcision, ritual or routine (in absence of medical indication) V50.2
      cosmetic NEC V50.1
        following healed injury or operation V51
      ear piercing V50.3
      face-lift V50.1
      hair transplant V50.0
      plastic
        cosmetic NEC V50.1
        following healed injury or operation V51
      prophylactic organ removal V50.49
        breast V50.41
        ovary V50.42

---

**Admission** — *continued*
  for — *continued*
    elective surgery — *continued*
      repair of scarred tissue (follow-
        ing healed injury or opera-
        tion) V51
      specified type NEC V50.8
    end-of-life care V66.7
    examination (*see also* Examination)
      V70.9
      administrative purpose NEC
        V70.3
      adoption V70.3
      allergy V72.7
      at health care facility V70.0
      athletic team V70.3
      camp V70.3
      cardiovascular, preoperative
        V72.81
      clinical research investigation
        (control) (participant)
        V70.7
      dental V72.2
      developmental testing (child)
        (infant) V20.2
      donor (potential) V70.8
      driver's license V70.3
      ear V72.19
      employment V70.5
      eye V72.0
      follow-up (routine) — *see* Exam-
        ination, follow-up
      for admission to
        old age home V70.3
        school V70.3
      general V70.9
        specified reason NEC V70.8
      gynecological V72.31
      health supervision (child) (in-
        fant) V20.2
      hearing V72.19
        following failed hearing
          screening V72.11
      immigration V70.3
      infant, routine V20.2
      insurance certification V70.3
      laboratory V72.6
      marriage license V70.3
      medical (general) (*see also* Exam-
        ination, medical) V70.9
      medicolegal reasons V70.4
      naturalization V70.3
      pelvic (annual) (periodic) V72.31
      postpartum checkup V24.2
      pregnancy (possible) (uncon-
        firmed) V72.40
        negative result V72.41
        positive result V72.42
      preoperative V72.84
        cardiovascular V72.81
        respiratory V72.82
        specified NEC V72.83
      preprocedural V72.84
        cardiovascular V72.81
        general physical V72.83
        respiratory V72.82
        specified NEC V72.83
      prison V70.3
      psychiatric (general) V70.2
        requested by authority V70.1
      radiological NEC V72.5
      respiratory, preoperative V72.82
      school V70.3
      screening — *see* Screening
      skin hypersensitivity V72.7
      specified type NEC V72.85
      sport competition V70.3
      vision V72.0
      well baby and child care V20.2
    exercise therapy V57.1
    face-lift, cosmetic reason V50.1
    fitting (of)
      artificial
        arm (complete) (partial)
          V52.0
        eye V52.2

**Admission** — *continued*
  for — *continued*
    fitting — *continued*
      artificial — *continued*
        leg (complete) (partial) V52.1
      biliary drainage tube V58.82
      brain neuropacemaker V53.02
      breast V52.4
        implant V52.4
        prosthesis V52.4
      cardiac pacemaker V53.31
      catheter
        non-vascular V58.82
        vascular V58.81
      cerebral ventricle (communicat-
        ing) shunt V53.01
      chest tube V58.82
      colostomy belt V55.2
      contact lenses V53.1
      cystostomy device V53.6
      dental prosthesis V52.3
      device, unspecified type V53.90
        abdominal V53.5
        cerebral ventricle (communi-
          cating) shunt V53.01
        insulin pump V53.91
        intrauterine contraceptive
          V25.1
        nervous system V53.09
        orthodontic V53.4
        other device V53.99
        prosthetic V53.9
          breast V52.4
          dental V52.3
          eye V52.2
        special senses V53.09
        substitution
          auditory V53.09
          nervous system V53.09
          visual V53.09
      diaphragm (contraceptive)
        V25.02
      fistula (sinus tract) drainage
        tube V58.82
      growth rod V54.02
      hearing aid V53.2
      ileostomy device V55.2
      intestinal appliance or device
        NEC V53.5
      intrauterine contraceptive de-
        vice V25.1
      neuropacemaker (brain) (periph-
        eral nerve) (spinal cord)
        V53.02
      orthodontic device V53.4
      orthopedic (device) V53.7
        brace V53.7
        cast V53.7
        shoes V53.7
      pacemaker
        brain V53.02
        cardiac V53.31
        carotid sinus V53.39
        spinal cord V53.02
      pleural drainage tube V58.82
      prosthesis V52.9
        arm (complete) (partial)
          V52.0
        breast V52.4
        dental V52.3
        eye V52.2
        leg (complete) (partial) V52.1
        specified type NEC V52.8
      spectacles V53.1
      wheelchair V53.8
    follow-up examination (routine)
      (following) V67.9
      cancer chemotherapy V67.2
      chemotherapy V67.2
      high-risk medication NEC
        V67.51
      injury NEC V67.59
      psychiatric V67.3
      psychotherapy V67.3
      radiotherapy V67.1
      specified surgery NEC V67.09

**Admission** — *continued*
  for — *continued*
    follow-up examination — *contin-
      ued*
      surgery V67.00
        vaginal pap smear V67.01
      treatment (for) V67.9
        combined V67.6
        fracture V67.4
        involving high-risk medica-
          tion NEC V67.51
        mental disorder V67.3
        specified NEC V67.59
    hair transplant, for cosmetic rea-
      son V50.0
    health advice, education, or instruc-
      tion V65.4 ☑
    hearing conservation and treat- ●
      ment V72.12 ●
    hormone replacement therapy
      (postmenopausal) V07.4
    hospice care V66.7
    immunotherapy, antineoplastic
      V58.12
    insertion (of)
      subdermal implantable contra-
        ceptive V25.5
    insulin pump titration V53.91
    insulin pump training V65.46
    intrauterine device
      insertion V25.1
      management V25.42
    investigation to determine further
      disposition V63.8
    in vitro fertilization cycle V26.81 ●
    isolation V07.0
    issue of
      disability examination certifi- ●
        cate V68.01 ●
      medical certificate NEC
        V68.09 ▲
      repeat prescription NEC V68.1
        contraceptive device NEC
          V25.49
    kidney dialysis V56.0
    lengthening of growth rod V54.02
    mental health evaluation V70.2
      requested by authority V70.1
    natural family planning counsel- ●
      ing and advice ●
      procreative V26.41 ●
      to avoid pregnancy V25.04 ●
    nonmedical reason NEC V68.89
    nursing care evaluation V63.8
    observation (without need for fur-
      ther medical care) (*see also*
      Observation) V71.9
      accident V71.4
      alleged rape or seduction V71.5
      criminal assault V71.6
      following accident V71.4
        at work V71.3
      foreign body ingestion V71.89
      growth and development varia-
        tions, childhood V21.0
      inflicted injury NEC V71.6
      ingestion of deleterious agent or
        foreign body V71.89
      injury V71.6
      malignant neoplasm V71.1
      mental disorder V71.09
      newborn — *see* Observation,
        suspected, condition,
        newborn
      rape V71.5
      specified NEC V71.89
      suspected disorder V71.9
        abuse V71.81
        accident V71.4
          at work V71.3
        benign neoplasm V71.89
        cardiovascular V71.7
        exposure
          anthrax V71.82
          biological agent NEC
            V71.83

**Admission** — *continued*
  for — *continued*
    observation (*see also* Observation)
      — *continued*
      suspected disorder — *contin-
        ued*
        exposure — *continued*
          SARS V71.83
        heart V71.7
        inflicted injury NEC V71.6
        malignant neoplasm V71.1
        mental NEC V71.09
        neglect V71.81
        specified condition NEC
          V71.89
        tuberculosis V71.2
      tuberculosis V71.2
    occupational therapy V57.21
    organ transplant, donor — *see*
      Donor
    ovary, ovarian removal, prophylac-
      tic V50.42
    palliative care V66.7
    Papanicolaou smear
      cervix V76.2
        for suspected malignant
          neoplasm V76.2
        no disease found V71.1
        routine, as part of gynecolog-
          ical examination
          V72.31
        to confirm findings of recent
          normal smear following
          initial abnormal smear
          V72.32
      vaginal V76.47
        following hysterectomy for
          malignant condition
          V67.01
    passage of sounds or bougie in ar-
      tificial opening — *see* Atten-
      tion to, artificial, opening
    paternity testing V70.4
    peritoneal dialysis V56.32
    physical therapy NEC V57.1
    plastic surgery
      cosmetic NEC V50.1
      following healed injury or opera-
        tion V51
    postmenopausal hormone replace-
      ment therapy V07.4
    postpartum observation
      immediately after delivery V24.0
      routine follow-up V24.2
    poststerilization (for restoration)
      V26.0
    procreative management V26.9
      assisted reproductive fertility ●
        procedure cycle V26.81 ●
      in vitro fertilization cycle ●
        V26.81 ●
      specified type NEC V26.89 ▲
    prophylactic
      administration of
        antibiotics V07.39
        antitoxin, any V07.2
        antivenin V07.2
        chemotherapeutic agent NEC
          V07.39
        chemotherapy NEC V07.39
        diphtheria antitoxin V07.2
        fluoride V07.31
        gamma globulin V07.2
        immune sera (gamma globu-
          lin) V07.2
        RhoGAM V07.2
        tetanus antitoxin V07.2
      breathing exercises V57.0
      chemotherapy NEC V07.39
        fluoride V07.31
      measure V07.9
        specified type NEC V07.8
      organ removal V50.49
        breast V50.41
        ovary V50.42

**Admission** — *continued*
  for — *continued*
    psychiatric examination (general)
      V70.2
      requested by authority V70.1
    radiation management V58.0
    radiotherapy V58.0
    reforming of artificial opening —
      *see* Attention to, artificial,
      opening
    rehabilitation V57.9
      multiple types V57.89
      occupational V57.21
      orthoptic V57.4
      orthotic V57.81
      physical NEC V57.1
      specified type NEC V57.89
      speech V57.3
      vocational V57.22
    removal of
      cardiac pacemaker V53.31
      cast (plaster) V54.89
      catheter from artificial opening
        — *see* Attention to, artifi-
        cial, opening
      cerebral ventricle (communicat-
        ing) shunt V53.01
      cystostomy catheter V55.5
      device
        cerebral ventricle (communi-
          cating) shunt V53.01
        fixation
          external V54.89
          internal V54.01
        intrauterine contraceptive
          V25.42
        traction, external V54.89
      drains V58.49
      dressing
        wound V58.30
          nonsurgical V58.30
          surgical V58.31
      fixation device
        external V54.89
        internal V54.01
      intrauterine contraceptive de-
        vice V25.42
      Kirschner wire V54.89
      neuropacemaker (brain) (periph-
        eral nerve) (spinal cord)
        V53.02
      nonsurgical wound dressing
        V58.30
      orthopedic fixation device
        external V54.89
        internal V54.01
      pacemaker device
        brain V53.02
        cardiac V53.31
        carotid sinus V53.39
        nervous system V53.02
      plaster cast V54.89
      plate (fracture) V54.01
      rod V54.01
      screw (fracture) V54.01
      splint, traction V54.89
      staples V58.32
      Steinmann pin V54.89
      subdermal implantable contra-
        ceptive V25.43
      surgical wound dressing V58.31
      sutures V58.32
      traction device, external V54.89
      ureteral stent V53.6
      wound packing V58.30
        nonsurgical V58.30
        surgical V58.31
    repair of scarred tissue (following
      healed injury or operation)
      V51
    reprogramming of cardiac pacemak-
      er V53.31
    respirator [ventilator] dependence
      during
        mechanical failure V46.14
        power failure V46.12

**Admission** — *continued*
  for — *continued*
    respirator [ventilator] dependence
      — *continued*
      for weaning V46.13
    restoration of organ continuity
      (poststerilization) (tuboplasty)
      (vasoplasty) V26.0
    Rh typing V72.86
    sensitivity test (*see also* Test, skin)
      allergy NEC V72.7
      bacterial disease NEC V74.9
      Dick V74.8
      Kveim V82.89
      Mantoux V74.1
      mycotic infection NEC V75.4
      parasitic disease NEC V75.8
      Schick V74.3
      Schultz-Charlton V74.8
    social service (agency) referral or
      evaluation V63.8
    speech therapy V57.3
    sterilization V25.2
    suspected disorder (ruled out)
      (without need for further
      care) — *see* Observation
    terminal care V66.7
    tests only — *see* Test
    therapeutic drug monitoring
      V58.83
    therapy
      blood transfusion, without re-
        ported diagnosis V58.2
      breathing exercises V57.0
      chemotherapy, antineoplastic
        V58.11
        prophylactic NEC V07.39
        fluoride V07.31
      dialysis (intermittent) (treat-
        ment)
        extracorporeal V56.0
        peritoneal V56.8
        renal V56.0
        specified type NEC V56.8
      exercise (remedial) NEC V57.1
        breathing V57.0
      immunotherapy, antineoplastic
        V58.12
      long-term (current) drug use
        NEC V58.69
        antibiotics V58.62
        anticoagulants V58.61
        anti-inflammatories, non-
          steroidal (NSAID)
          V58.64
        antiplatelets V58.63
        antithrombotics V58.63
        aspirin V58.66
        high-risk medications NEC ●
          V58.69 ●
        insulin V58.67
        steroids V58.65
      occupational V57.21
      orthoptic V57.4
      physical NEC V57.1
      radiation V58.0
      speech V57.3
      vocational V57.22
    toilet or cleaning
      of artificial opening — *see* Atten-
        tion to, artificial, opening
      of non-vascular catheter V58.82
      of vascular catheter V58.81
    tubal ligation V25.2
    tuboplasty for previous sterilization
      V26.0
    vaccination, prophylactic (against)
      arthropod-borne virus, viral
        NEC V05.1
        disease NEC V05.1
        encephalitis V05.0
      Bacille Calmette Guérin (BCG)
        V03.2
      BCG V03.2
      chickenpox V05.4
      cholera alone V03.0

**Admission** — *continued*
  for — *continued*
    vaccination, prophylactic — *contin-*
      *ued*
      cholera alone — *continued*
        with typhoid-paratyphoid
          (cholera + TAB) V06.0
      common cold V04.7
      dengue V05.1
      diphtheria alone V03.5
      diphtheria-tetanus-pertussis
        (DTP) (DTaP) V06.1
        with
          poliomyelitis (DTP + polio)
            V06.3
          typhoid-paratyphoid (DTP
            + TAB) V06.2
      diphtheria-tetanus [Td] [DT]
        without pertussis V06.5
      disease (single) NEC V05.9
        bacterial NEC V03.9
          specified type NEC V03.89
        combinations NEC V06.9
          specified type NEC V06.8
        specified type NEC V05.8
        viral NEC V04.89
      encephalitis, viral, arthropod-
        borne V05.0
      Hemophilus influenzae, type B
        [Hib] V03.81
      hepatitis, viral V05.3
      human papillomavirus (HPV) ●
        V04.89 ●
      immune sera (gamma globulin)
        V07.2
      influenza V04.81
        with
          Streptococcus pneumoni-
            ae [pneumococcus]
            V06.6
      Leishmaniasis V05.2
      measles alone V04.2
      measles-mumps-rubella (MMR)
        V06.4
      mumps alone V04.6
        with measles and rubella
          (MMR) V06.4
      not done because of contraindi-
        cation V64.09
      pertussis alone V03.6
      plague V03.3
      pneumonia V03.82
      poliomyelitis V04.0
        with diphtheria-tetanus-per-
          tussis (DTP+ polio)
          V06.3
      rabies V04.5
      respiratory syncytial virus (RSV)
        V04.82
      rubella alone V04.3
        with measles and mumps
          (MMR) V06.4
      smallpox V04.1
      specified type NEC V05.8
      Streptococcus pneumoniae
        [pneumococcus] V03.82
        with
          influenza V06.6
      tetanus toxoid alone V03.7
        with diphtheria [Td] [DT]
          V06.5
          and pertussis (DTP)
            (DTaP) V06.1
      tuberculosis (BCG) V03.2
      tularemia V03.4
      typhoid alone V03.1
        with diphtheria-tetanus-per-
          tussis (TAB + DTP)
          V06.2
      typhoid-paratyphoid alone (TAB)
        V03.1
      typhus V05.8
      varicella (chicken pox) V05.4
      viral encephalitis, arthropod-
        borne V05.0
      viral hepatitis V05.3

**Admission** — *continued*
  for — *continued*
    vaccination, prophylactic — *contin-*
      *ued*
      yellow fever V04.4
    vasectomy V25.2
    vasoplasty for previous sterilization
      V26.0
    vision examination V72.0
    vocational therapy V57.22
    waiting period for admission to
      other facility V63.2
      undergoing social agency inves-
        tigation V63.8
    well baby and child care V20.2
    x-ray of chest
      for suspected tuberculosis
        V71.2
      routine V72.5
**Adnexitis** (suppurative) — *see also*
  Salpingo-oophoritis 614.2
**Adolescence** NEC V21.2
**Adoption**
  agency referral V68.89
  examination V70.3
  held for V68.89
**Adrenal gland** — *see* condition
**Adrenalism** 255.9
  tuberculous (*see also* Tuberculosis)
    017.6 ☑
**Adrenalitis, adrenitis** 255.8
  meningococcal hemorrhagic 036.3
**Adrenarche, precocious** 259.1
**Adrenocortical syndrome** 255.2
**Adrenogenital syndrome** (acquired)
  (congenital) 255.2
  iatrogenic, fetus or newborn 760.79
**Adrenoleukodystrophy** 277.86
  neonatal 277.86
  x-linked 277.86
**Adrenomyeloneuropathy** 277.86
**Adventitious bursa** — *see* Bursitis
**Adynamia** (episodica) (hereditary) (peri-
  odic) 359.3
**Adynamic**
  ileus or intestine (*see also* Ileus) 560.1
  ureter 753.22
**Aeration lung, imperfect, newborn**
  770.5
**Aerobullosis** 993.3
**Aerocele** — *see* Embolism, air
**Aerodermectasia**
  subcutaneous (traumatic) 958.7
    surgical 998.81
  surgical 998.81
**Aerodontalgia** 993.2
**Aeroembolism** 993.3
**Aerogenes capsulatus infection** — *see*
  *also* Gangrene, gas 040.0
**Aero-otitis media** 993.0
**Aerophagy, aerophagia** 306.4
  psychogenic 306.4
**Aerosinusitis** 993.1
**Aerotitis** 993.0
**Affection, affections** — *see also* Disease
  sacroiliac (joint), old 724.6
  shoulder region NEC 726.2
**Afibrinogenemia** 286.3
  acquired 286.6
  congenital 286.3
  postpartum 666.3 ☑
**African**
  sleeping sickness 086.5
  tick fever 087.1
  trypanosomiasis 086.5
    Gambian 086.3
    Rhodesian 086.4
**Aftercare** V58.9
  amputation stump V54.89
  artificial openings — *see* Attention to,
    artificial, opening
  blood transfusion without reported
    diagnosis V58.2
  breathing exercise V57.0
  cardiac device V53.39

**Aftercare** — *continued*
  cardiac device — *continued*
    defibrillator, automatic implantable V53.32
      pacemaker V53.31
        carotid sinus V53.39
    carotid sinus pacemaker V53.39
    cerebral ventricle (communicating) shunt V53.01
    chemotherapy session (adjunctive) (maintenance) V58.11
    defibrillator, automatic implantable cardiac V53.32
    exercise (remedial) (therapeutic) V57.1
      breathing V57.0
    extracorporeal dialysis (intermittent) (treatment) V56.0
    following surgery NEC V58.49
      for
        injury V58.43
        neoplasm V58.42
        organ transplant V58.44
        trauma V58.43
      joint replacement V54.81
      of
        circulatory system V58.73
        digestive system V58.75
        genital organs V58.76
        genitourinary system V58.76
        musculoskeletal system V58.78
        nervous system V58.72
        oral cavity V58.75
        respiratory system V58.74
        sense organs V58.71
        skin V58.77
        subcutaneous tissue V58.77
        teeth V58.75
        urinary system V58.76
      spinal — *see* Aftercare, following ●
        surgery, of, specified body ●
        system
      wound closure, planned V58.41
  fracture V54.9
    healing V54.89
      pathologic
        ankle V54.29
        arm V54.20
          lower V54.22
          upper V54.21
        finger V54.29
        foot V54.29
        hand V54.29
        hip V54.23
        leg V54.24
          lower V54.26
          upper V54.25
        pelvis V54.29
        specified site NEC V54.29
        toe(s) V54.29
        vertebrae V54.27
        wrist V54.29
      traumatic
        ankle V54.19
        arm V54.10
          lower V54.12
          upper V54.11
        finger V54.19
        foot V54.19
        hand V54.19
        hip V54.13
        leg V54.14
          lower V54.16
          upper V54.15
        pelvis V54.19
        specified site NEC V54.19
        toe(s) V54.19
        vertebrae V54.17
        wrist V54.19
    removal of
      external fixation device V54.89
      internal fixation device V54.01
    specified care NEC V54.89
  gait training V57.1
    for use of artificial limb(s) V57.81
  internal fixation device V54.09

**Aftercare** — *continued*
  involving
    dialysis (intermittent) (treatment)
      extracorporeal V56.0
      peritoneal V56.8
      renal V56.0
    gait training V57.1
      for use of artificial limb(s) V57.81
    growth rod
      adjustment V54.02
      lengthening V54.02
    internal fixation device V54.09
    orthoptic training V57.4
    orthotic training V57.81
    radiotherapy session V58.0
    removal of
      drains V58.49
      dressings
        wound V58.30
          nonsurgical V58.30
          surgical V58.31
      fixation device
        external V54.89
        internal V54.01
      fracture plate V54.01
      nonsurgical wound dressing V58.30
      pins V54.01
      plaster cast V54.89
      rods V54.01
      screws V58.32
      staples V58.32
      surgical wound dressings V58.31
      sutures V58.32
      traction device, external V54.89
      wound packing V58.30
        nonsurgical V58.30
        surgical V58.31
    neuropacemaker (brain) (peripheral nerve) (spinal cord) V53.02
    occupational therapy V57.21
    orthodontic V58.5
    orthopedic V54.9
      change of external fixation or traction device V54.89
      following joint replacement V54.81
      internal fixation device V54.09
      removal of fixation device
        external V54.89
        internal V54.01
      specified care NEC V54.89
    orthoptic training V57.4
    orthotic training V57.81
    pacemaker
      brain V53.02
      cardiac V53.31
      carotid sinus V53.39
      peripheral nerve V53.02
      spinal cord V53.02
    peritoneal dialysis (intermittent) (treatment) V56.8
    physical therapy NEC V57.1
      breathing exercises V57.0
    radiotherapy session V58.0
    rehabilitation procedure V57.9
      breathing exercises V57.0
      multiple types V57.89
      occupational V57.21
      orthoptic V57.4
      orthotic V57.81
      physical therapy NEC V57.1
      remedial exercises V57.1
      specified type NEC V57.89
      speech V57.3
      therapeutic exercises V57.1
      vocational V57.22
    renal dialysis (intermittent) (treatment) V56.0
    specified type NEC V58.89
      removal of non-vascular catheter V58.82
      removal of vascular catheter V58.81
    speech therapy V57.3

**Aftercare** — *continued*
    stump, amputation V54.89
    vocational rehabilitation V57.22
**After-cataract** 366.50
  obscuring vision 366.53
  specified type, not obscuring vision 366.52
**Agalactia** 676.4 ☑
**Agammaglobulinemia** 279.00
  with lymphopenia 279.2
  acquired (primary) (secondary) 279.06
  Bruton's X-linked 279.04
  infantile sex-linked (Bruton's) (congenital) 279.04
  Swiss-type 279.2
**Aganglionosis** (bowel) (colon) 751.3
**Age** (old) — *see also* Senile 797
**Agenesis** — *see also* Absence, by site, congenital
  acoustic nerve 742.8
  adrenal (gland) 759.1
  alimentary tract (complete) (partial) NEC 751.8
    lower 751.2
    upper 750.8
  anus, anal (canal) 751.2
  aorta 747.22
  appendix 751.2
  arm (complete) (partial) (*see also* Deformity, reduction, upper limb) 755.20
  artery (peripheral) NEC (*see also* Anomaly, peripheral vascular system) 747.60
    brain 747.81
    coronary 746.85
    pulmonary 747.3
    umbilical 747.5
  auditory (canal) (external) 744.01
  auricle (ear) 744.01
  bile, biliary duct or passage 751.61
  bone NEC 756.9
  brain 740.0
    specified part 742.2
  breast 757.6
  bronchus 748.3
  canaliculus lacrimalis 743.65
  carpus NEC (*see also* Deformity, reduction, upper limb) 755.28
  cartilage 756.9
  cecum 751.2
  cerebellum 742.2
  cervix 752.49
  chin 744.89
  cilia 743.63
  circulatory system, part NEC 747.89
  clavicle 755.51
  clitoris 752.49
  coccyx 756.13
  colon 751.2
  corpus callosum 742.2
  cricoid cartilage 748.3
  diaphragm (with hernia) 756.6
  digestive organ(s) or tract (complete) (partial) NEC 751.8
    lower 751.2
    upper 750.8
  ductus arteriosus 747.89
  duodenum 751.1
  ear NEC 744.09
    auricle 744.01
    lobe 744.21
  ejaculatory duct 752.89
  endocrine (gland) NEC 759.2
  epiglottis 748.3
  esophagus 750.3
  Eustachian tube 744.24
  extrinsic muscle, eye 743.69
  eye 743.00
    adnexa 743.69
  eyelid (fold) 743.62
  face
    bones NEC 756.0
    specified part NEC 744.89
  fallopian tube 752.19

**Agenesis** — *see also* Absence, by site, congenital — *continued*
  femur NEC (*see also* Absence, femur, congenital) 755.34
  fibula NEC (*see also* Absence, fibula, congenital) 755.37
  finger NEC (*see also* Absence, finger, congenital) 755.29
  foot (complete) (*see also* Deformity, reduction, lower limb) 755.31
  gallbladder 751.69
  gastric 750.8
  genitalia, genital (organ)
    female 752.89
      external 752.49
      internal NEC 752.89
    male 752.89
      penis 752.69
  glottis 748.3
  gonadal 758.6
  hair 757.4
  hand (complete) (*see also* Deformity, reduction, upper limb) 755.21
  heart 746.89
    valve NEC 746.89
      aortic 746.89
      mitral 746.89
      pulmonary 746.01
  hepatic 751.69
  humerus NEC (*see also* Absence, humerus, congenital) 755.24
  hymen 752.49
  ileum 751.1
  incus 744.04
  intestine (small) 751.1
    large 751.2
  iris (dilator fibers) 743.45
  jaw 524.09
  jejunum 751.1
  kidney(s) (partial) (unilateral) 753.0
  labium (majus) (minus) 752.49
  labyrinth, membranous 744.05
  lacrimal apparatus (congenital) 743.65
  larynx 748.3
  leg NEC (*see also* Deformity, reduction, lower limb) 755.30
  lens 743.35
  limb (complete) (partial) (*see also* Deformity, reduction) 755.4
    lower NEC 755.30
    upper 755.20
  lip 750.26
  liver 751.69
  lung (bilateral) (fissures) (lobe) (unilateral) 748.5
  mandible 524.09
  maxilla 524.09
  metacarpus NEC 755.28
  metatarsus NEC 755.38
  muscle (any) 756.81
  musculoskeletal system NEC 756.9
  nail(s) 757.5
  neck, part 744.89
  nerve 742.8
  nervous system, part NEC 742.8
  nipple 757.6
  nose 748.1
  nuclear 742.8
  organ
    of Corti 744.05
    or site not listed — *see* Anomaly, specified type NEC
  osseous meatus (ear) 744.03
  ovary 752.0
  oviduct 752.19
  pancreas 751.7
  parathyroid (gland) 759.2
  patella 755.64
  pelvic girdle (complete) (partial) 755.69
  penis 752.69
  pericardium 746.89
  perineal body 756.81
  pituitary (gland) 759.2
  prostate 752.89
  pulmonary
    artery 747.3

**Agenesis** — *see also* Absence, by site, congenital — *continued*
pulmonary — *continued*
  trunk 747.3
  vein 747.49
punctum lacrimale 743.65
radioulnar NEC (*see also* Absence, forearm, congenital) 755.25
radius NEC (*see also* Absence, radius, congenital) 755.26
rectum 751.2
renal 753.0
respiratory organ NEC 748.9
rib 756.3
roof of orbit 742.0
round ligament 752.89
sacrum 756.13
salivary gland 750.21
scapula 755.59
scrotum 752.89
seminal duct or tract 752.89
septum
  atrial 745.69
  between aorta and pulmonary artery 745.0
  ventricular 745.3
shoulder girdle (complete) (partial) 755.59
skull (bone) 756.0
  with
    anencephalus 740.0
    encephalocele 742.0
    hydrocephalus 742.3
      with spina bifida (*see also* Spina bifida) 741.0 ☑
    microcephalus 742.1
spermatic cord 752.89
spinal cord 742.59
spine 756.13
  lumbar 756.13
    isthmus 756.11
    pars articularis 756.11
spleen 759.0
sternum 756.3
stomach 750.7
tarsus NEC 755.38
tendon 756.81
testicular 752.89
testis 752.89
thymus (gland) 759.2
thyroid (gland) 243
  cartilage 748.3
tibia NEC (*see also* Absence, tibia, congenital) 755.36
tibiofibular NEC 755.35
toe (complete) (partial) (*see also* Absence, toe, congenital) 755.39
tongue 750.11
trachea (cartilage) 748.3
ulna NEC (*see also* Absence, ulna, congenital) 755.27
ureter 753.4
urethra 753.8
urinary tract NEC 753.8
uterus 752.3
uvula 750.26
vagina 752.49
vas deferens 752.89
vein(s) (peripheral) NEC (*see also* Anomaly, peripheral vascular system) 747.60
  brain 747.81
  great 747.49
  portal 747.49
  pulmonary 747.49
  vena cava (inferior) (superior) 747.49
vermis of cerebellum 742.2
vertebra 756.13
  lumbar 756.13
    isthmus 756.11
    pars articularis 756.11
vulva 752.49
**Ageusia** — *see also* Disturbance, sensation 781.1
**Aggressiveness** 301.3

**Aggressive outburst** — *see also* Disturbance, conduct 312.0 ☑
  in children or adolescents 313.9
**Aging skin** 701.8
**Agitated** — *see* condition
**Agitation** 307.9
  catatonic (*see also* Schizophrenia) 295.2 ☑
**Aglossia** (congenital) 750.11
**Aglycogenosis** 271.0
**Agnail** (finger) (with lymphangitis) 681.02
**Agnosia** (body image) (tactile) 784.69
  verbal 784.69
    auditory 784.69
      secondary to organic lesion 784.69
    developmental 315.8
      secondary to organic lesion 784.69
    visual 784.69
      developmental 315.8
      secondary to organic lesion 784.69
  visual 368.16
    developmental 315.31
**Agoraphobia** 300.22
  with panic disorder 300.21
**Agrammatism** 784.69
**Agranulocytopenia** — *see also* Agranulocytosis 288.09
**Agranulocytosis** (angina) 288.09
  chronic 288.09
  cyclical 288.02
  genetic 288.01
  infantile 288.01
  periodic 288.02
  pernicious 288.09
**Agraphia** (absolute) 784.69
  with alexia 784.61
  developmental 315.39
**Agrypnia** — *see also* Insomnia 780.52
**Ague** — *see also* Malaria 084.6
  brass-founders' 985.8
  dumb 084.6
  tertian 084.1
**Agyria** 742.2
**Ahumada-del Castillo syndrome** (nonpuerperal galactorrhea and amenorrhea) 253.1
**AIDS** 042
**AIDS-associated retrovirus** (disease) (illness) 042
  infection — *see* Human immunodeficiency virus, infection
**AIDS-associated virus** (disease) (illness) 042
  infection — *see* Human immunodeficiency virus, infection
**AIDS-like disease** (illness) (syndrome) 042
**AIDS-related complex** 042
**AIDS-related conditions** 042
**AIDS-related virus** (disease) (illness) 042
  infection — *see* Human immunodeficiency virus, infection
**AIDS virus** (disease) (illness) 042
  infection — *see* Human immunodeficiency virus, infection
**Ailment, heart** — *see* Disease, heart
**Ailurophobia** 300.29
**Ainhum** (disease) 136.0
**Air**
  anterior mediastinum 518.1
  compressed, disease 993.3
  embolism (any site) (artery) (cerebral) 958.0
    with
      abortion — *see* Abortion, by type, with embolism
      ectopic pregnancy (*see also* categories 633.0–633.9) 639.6
      molar pregnancy (*see also* categories 630–632) 639.6

**Air** — *continued*
  embolism — *continued*
    due to implanted device — *see* Complications, due to (presence of) any device, implant, or graft classified to 996.0–996.5 NEC
    following
      abortion 639.6
      ectopic or molar pregnancy 639.6
    infusion, perfusion, or transfusion 999.1
    in pregnancy, childbirth, or puerperium 673.0 ☑
    traumatic 958.0
  hunger 786.09
    psychogenic 306.1
  leak (lung) (pulmonary) (thorax) 512.8
    iatrogenic 512.1
    postoperative 512.1
  rarefied, effects of — *see* Effect, adverse, high altitude
  sickness 994.6
**Airplane sickness** 994.6
**Akathisia, acathisia** 781.0
  due to drugs 333.99
  neuroleptic-induced acute 333.99
**Akinesia algeria** 352.6
**Akiyami** 100.89
**Akureyri disease** (epidemic neuromyasthenia) 049.8
**Alacrima** (congenital) 743.65
**Alactasia** (hereditary) 271.3
**Alagille syndrome** 759.89
**Alalia** 784.3
  developmental 315.31
    receptive-expressive 315.32
  secondary to organic lesion 784.3
**Alaninemia** 270.8
**Alastrim** 050.1
**Albarrán's disease** (colibacilluria) 791.9
**Albers-Schönberg's disease** (marble bones) 756.52
**Albert's disease** 726.71
**Albinism, albino** (choroid) (cutaneous) (eye) (generalized) (isolated) (ocular) (oculocutaneous) (partial) 270.2
**Albinismus** 270.2
**Albright (-Martin) (-Bantam) disease** (pseudohypoparathyroidism) 275.49
**Albright (-McCune) (-Sternberg) syndrome** (osteitis fibrosa disseminata) 756.59
**Albuminous** — *see* condition
**Albuminuria, albuminuric** (acute) (chronic) (subacute) 791.0
  Bence-Jones 791.0
  cardiac 785.9
  complicating pregnancy, childbirth, or puerperium 646.2 ☑
    with hypertension — *see* Toxemia, of pregnancy
    affecting fetus or newborn 760.1
  cyclic 593.6
  gestational 646.2 ☑
  gravidarum 646.2 ☑
    with hypertension — *see* Toxemia, of pregnancy
    affecting fetus or newborn 760.1
  heart 785.9
  idiopathic 593.6
  orthostatic 593.6
  postural 593.6
  pre-eclamptic (mild) 642.4 ☑
    affecting fetus or newborn 760.0
    severe 642.5 ☑
      affecting fetus or newborn 760.0
  recurrent physiologic 593.6
  scarlatinal 034.1
**Albumosuria** 791.0
  Bence-Jones 791.0
  myelopathic (M9730/3) 203.0 ☑
**Alcaptonuria** 270.2

**Alcohol, alcoholic**
abstinence 291.81
acute intoxication 305.0 ☑
  with dependence 303.0 ☑
addiction (*see also* Alcoholism) 303.9 ☑
  maternal
    with suspected fetal damage affecting management of pregnancy 655.4 ☑
    affecting fetus or newborn 760.71
amnestic disorder, persisting 291.1
anxiety 291.89
brain syndrome, chronic 291.2
cardiopathy 425.5
chronic (*see also* Alcoholism) 303.9 ☑
cirrhosis (liver) 571.2
delirium 291.0
  acute 291.0
  chronic 291.1
  tremens 291.0
  withdrawal 291.0
dementia NEC 291.2
deterioration 291.2
drunkenness (simple) 305.0 ☑
hallucinosis (acute) 291.3
induced
  circadian rhythm sleep disorder 291.82
  hypersomnia 291.82
  insomnia 291.82
  mental disorder 291.9
    anxiety 291.89
    mood 291.89
    sexual 291.89
    sleep 291.82
    specified type 291.89
  parasomnia 291.82
  persisting
    amnestic disorder 291.1
    dementia 291.2
  psychotic disorder
    with
      delusions 291.5
      hallucinations 291.3
  sleep disorder 291.82
insanity 291.9
intoxication (acute) 305.0 ☑
  with dependence 303.0 ☑
  pathological 291.4
jealousy 291.5
Korsakoff's, Korsakov's, Korsakow's 291.1
liver NEC 571.3
  acute 571.1
  chronic 571.2
mania (acute) (chronic) 291.9
mood 291.89
paranoia 291.5
paranoid (type) psychosis 291.5
pellagra 265.2
poisoning, accidental (acute) NEC 980.9
  specified type of alcohol — *see* Table of Drugs and Chemicals
psychosis (*see also* Psychosis, alcoholic) 291.9
  Korsakoff's, Korsakov's, Korsakow's 291.1
  polyneuritic 291.1
  with
    delusions 291.5
    hallucinations 291.3
related disorder 291.9
withdrawal symptoms, syndrome NEC 291.81
  delirium 291.0
  hallucinosis 291.3

**Alcoholism** 303.9 ☑

Note — Use the following fifth-digit subclassification with category 303:

0    unspecified
1    continuous
2    episodic
3    in remission

with psychosis (see also Psychosis, alcoholic) 291.9
acute 303.0 ☑
chronic 303.9 ☑
   with psychosis 291.9
complicating pregnancy, childbirth, or puerperium 648.4 ☑
   affecting fetus or newborn 760.71
history V11.3
Korsakoff's, Korsakov's, Korsakow's 291.1
suspected damage to fetus affecting management of pregnancy 655.4 ☑
**Alder's anomaly or syndrome** (leukocyte granulation anomaly) 288.2
**Alder-Reilly anomaly** (leukocyte granulation) 288.2
**Aldosteronism** (primary) 255.10
congenital 255.10
familial type I 255.11
glucocorticoid-remediable 255.11
secondary 255.14
**Aldosteronoma** (M8370/1) 237.2
**Aldrich (-Wiskott) syndrome** (eczema-thrombocytopenia) 279.12
**Aleppo boil** 085.1
**Aleukemic** — see condition
**Aleukia**
congenital 288.09
hemorrhagica 284.9
   acquired (secondary) 284.89
   congenital 284.09
   idiopathic 284.9
splenica 289.4
**Alexia** (congenital) (developmental) 315.01
secondary to organic lesion 784.61
**Algoneurodystrophy** 733.7
**Algophobia** 300.29
**Alibert-Bazin disease** (M9700/3) 202.1 ☑
**Alibert's disease** (mycosis fungoides) (M9700/3) 202.1 ☑
**Alice in Wonderland syndrome** 293.89
**Alienation, mental** — see also Psychosis 298.9
**Alkalemia** 276.3
**Alkalosis** 276.3
metabolic 276.3
   with respiratory acidosis 276.4
respiratory 276.3
**Alkaptonuria** 270.2
**Allen-Masters syndrome** 620.6
**Allergic bronchopulmonary aspergillosis** 518.6
**Allergy, allergic** (reaction) 995.3
air-borne substance — see also Fever, hay 477.9
   specified allergen NEC 477.8
alveolitis (extrinsic) 495.9
   due to
     Aspergillus clavatus 495.4
     cryptostroma corticale 495.6
     organisms (fungal, thermophilic actinomyces, other) growing in ventilation (air conditioning systems) 495.7
     specified type NEC 495.8
anaphylactic shock 999.4
   due to food — see Anaphylactic shock, due to, food
angioneurotic edema 995.1
animal (cat) (dog) (epidermal) 477.8
   dander 477.2

**Allergy, allergic** — continued
animal — continued
   hair 477.2
arthritis (see also Arthritis, allergic) 716.2 ☑
asthma — see Asthma
bee sting (anaphylactic shock) 989.5
biological — see Allergy, drug
bronchial asthma — see Asthma
conjunctivitis (eczematous) 372.14
dander, animal (cat) (dog) 477.2
dandruff 477.8
dermatitis (venenata) — see Dermatitis
diathesis V15.09
drug, medicinal substance, and biological (any) (correct medicinal substance properly administered) (external) (internal) 995.27
   wrong substance given or taken NEC 977.9
     specified drug or substance — see Table of Drugs and Chemicals
dust (house) (stock) 477.8
eczema — see Eczema
endophthalmitis 360.19
epidermal (animal) 477.8
existing dental restorative material 525.66
feathers 477.8
food (any) (ingested) 693.1
   atopic 691.8
   in contact with skin 692.5
gastritis 535.4 ☑
gastroenteritis 558.3
gastrointestinal 558.3
grain 477.0
grass (pollen) 477.0
   asthma (see also Asthma) 493.0 ☑
   hay fever 477.0
hair, animal (cat) (dog) 477.2
hay fever (grass) (pollen) (ragweed) (tree) (see also Fever, hay) 477.9
history (of) V15.09
   to
     eggs V15.03
     food additives V15.05
     insect bite V15.06
     latex V15.07
     milk products V15.02
     nuts V15.05
       peanuts V15.01
     radiographic dye V15.08
     seafood V15.04
     specified food NEC V15.05
     spider bite V15.06
horse serum — see Allergy, serum
inhalant 477.9
   dust 477.8
   pollen 477.0
   specified allergen other than pollen 477.8
kapok 477.8
medicine — see Allergy, drug
migraine 346.2 ☑
milk protein 558.3
pannus 370.62
pneumonia 518.3
pollen (any) (hay fever) 477.0
   asthma (see also Asthma) 493.0 ☑
primrose 477.0
primula 477.0
purpura 287.0
ragweed (pollen) (Senecio jacobae) 477.0
   asthma (see also Asthma) 493.0 ☑
   hay fever 477.0
respiratory (see also Allergy, inhalant) 477.9
   due to
     drug — see Allergy, drug
     food — see Allergy, food
rhinitis (see also Fever, hay) 477.9
   due to food 477.1

**Allergy, allergic** — continued
rose 477.0
Senecio jacobae 477.0
serum (prophylactic) (therapeutic) 999.5
   anaphylactic shock 999.4
shock (anaphylactic) (due to adverse effect of correct medicinal substance properly administered) 995.0
   food — see Anaphylactic shock, due to, food
   from serum or immunization 999.5
     anaphylactic 999.4
sinusitis (see also Fever, hay) 477.9
skin reaction 692.9
   specified substance — see Dermatitis, due to
tree (any) (hay fever) (pollen) 477.0
   asthma (see also Asthma) 493.0 ☑
upper respiratory (see also Fever, hay) 477.9
urethritis 597.89
urticaria 708.0
vaccine — see Allergy, serum
**Allescheriosis** 117.6
**Alligator skin disease** (ichthyosis congenita) 757.1
acquired 701.1
**Allocheiria, allochiria** — see also Disturbance, sensation 782.0
**Almeida's disease** (Brazilian blastomycosis) 116.1
**Alopecia** (atrophicans) (pregnancy) (premature) (senile) 704.00
adnata 757.4
areata 704.01
celsi 704.01
cicatrisata 704.09
circumscripta 704.01
congenital, congenitalis 757.4
disseminata 704.01
effluvium (telogen) 704.02
febrile 704.09
generalisata 704.09
hereditaria 704.09
marginalis 704.01
mucinosa 704.09
postinfectional 704.09
seborrheica 704.09
specific 091.82
syphilitic (secondary) 091.82
telogen effluvium 704.02
totalis 704.09
toxica 704.09
universalis 704.09
x-ray 704.09
**Alpers' disease** 330.8
**Alpha-lipoproteinemia** 272.4
**Alpha thalassemia** 282.49
**Alphos** 696.1
**Alpine sickness** 993.2
**Alport's syndrome** (hereditary hematuria-nephropathy-deafness) 759.89
**Alteration** (of), altered
awareness 780.09
   transient 780.02
consciousness 780.09
   persistent vegetative state 780.03
   transient 780.02
mental status 780.97
   amnesia (retrograde) 780.93
   memory loss 780.93
**Alternaria** (infection) 118
**Alternating** — see condition
**Altitude, high** (effects) — see Effect, adverse, high altitude
**Aluminosis** (of lung) 503
**Alvarez syndrome** (transient cerebral ischemia) 435.9
**Alveolar capillary block syndrome** 516.3
**Alveolitis**
allergic (extrinsic) 495.9

**Alveolitis** — continued
allergic — continued
   due to organisms (fungal, thermophilic actinomycete, other) growing in ventilation (air conditioning systems) 495.7
   specified type NEC 495.8
due to
   Aspergillus clavatus 495.4
   Cryptostroma corticale 495.6
fibrosing (chronic) (cryptogenic) (lung) 516.3
   idiopathic 516.3
   rheumatoid 714.81
jaw 526.5
sicca dolorosa 526.5
**Alveolus, alveolar** — see condition
**Alymphocytosis** (pure) 279.2
**Alymphoplasia, thymic** 279.2
**Alzheimer's**
dementia (senile)
   with behavioral disturbance 331.0 [294.11]
   without behavioral disturbance 331.0 [294.10]
disease or sclerosis 331.0
   with dementia — see Alzheimer's, dementia
**Amastia** — see also Absence, breast 611.8
**Amaurosis** (acquired) (congenital) — see also Blindness 369.00
fugax 362.34
hysterical 300.11
Leber's (congenital) 362.76
tobacco 377.34
uremic — see Uremia
**Amaurotic familial idiocy** (infantile) (juvenile) (late) 330.1
**Ambisexual** 752.7
**Amblyopia** (acquired) (congenital) (partial) 368.00
color 368.59
   acquired 368.55
deprivation 368.02
ex anopsia 368.00
hysterical 300.11
nocturnal 368.60
   vitamin A deficiency 264.5
refractive 368.03
strabismic 368.01
suppression 368.01
tobacco 377.34
toxic NEC 377.34
uremic — see Uremia
**Ameba, amebic** (histolytica) — see also Amebiasis
abscess 006.3
   bladder 006.8
   brain (with liver and lung abscess) 006.5
   liver 006.3
     with
       brain abscess (and lung abscess) 006.5
       lung abscess 006.4
   lung (with liver abscess) 006.4
     with brain abscess 006.5
   seminal vesicle 006.8
   spleen 006.8
carrier (suspected of) V02.2
meningoencephalitis
   due to Naegleria (gruberi) 136.2
   primary 136.2
**Amebiasis** NEC 006.9
with
   brain abscess (with liver or lung abscess) 006.5
   liver abscess (without mention of brain or lung abscess) 006.3
   lung abscess (with liver abscess) 006.4
     with brain abscess 006.5
acute 006.0
bladder 006.8
chronic 006.1

☑ Additional Digit Required — Refer to the Tabular List for Digit Selection

☒ Subterms under main terms may continue to next column or page

*2008 ICD-9-CM*

▶◀ Revised Text     ● New Line     ▲ Revised Code

**October 2007 · Volume 2 — 17**

Alcoholism — Amebiasis

**Index**

**Amebiasis — Anemia**

**Amebiasis** — *continued*
cutaneous 006.6
cutis 006.6
due to organism other than Entamoeba histolytica 007.8
hepatic (*see also* Abscess, liver, amebic) 006.3
nondysenteric 006.2
seminal vesicle 006.8
specified
  organism NEC 007.8
  site NEC 006.8
**Ameboma** 006.8
**Amelia** 755.4
lower limb 755.31
upper limb 755.21
**Ameloblastoma** (M9310/0) 213.1
jaw (bone) (lower) 213.1
  upper 213.0
long bones (M9261/3) — *see* Neoplasm, bone, malignant
malignant (M9310/3) 170.1
  jaw (bone) (lower) 170.1
    upper 170.0
mandible 213.1
tibial (M9261/3) 170.7
**Amelogenesis imperfecta** 520.5
nonhereditaria (segmentalis) 520.4
**Amenorrhea** (primary) (secondary) 626.0
due to ovarian dysfunction 256.8
hyperhormonal 256.8
**Amentia** — *see also* Retardation, mental 319
Meynert's (nonalcoholic) 294.0
  alcoholic 291.1
nevoid 759.6
**American**
leishmaniasis 085.5
mountain tick fever 066.1
trypanosomiasis — *see* Trypanosomiasis, American
**Ametropia** — *see also* Disorder, accommodation 367.9
**Amianthosis** 501
**Amimia** 784.69
**Amino acid**
deficiency 270.9
  anemia 281.4
metabolic disorder (*see also* Disorder, amino acid) 270.9
**Aminoaciduria** 270.9
imidazole 270.5
**Amnesia** (retrograde) 780.93
auditory 784.69
  developmental 315.31
  secondary to organic lesion 784.69
dissociative 300.12
hysterical or dissociative type 300.12
psychogenic 300.12
transient global 437.7
**Amnestic** (confabulatory) **syndrome** 294.0
alcohol-induced persisting 291.1
drug-induced persisting 292.83
posttraumatic 294.0
**Amniocentesis screening** (for) V28.2
alphafetoprotein level, raised V28.1
chromosomal anomalies V28.0
**Amnion, amniotic** — *see also* condition
nodosum 658.8 ☑
**Amnionitis** (complicating pregnancy) 658.4 ☑
affecting fetus or newborn 762.7
**Amoral trends** 301.7
**Amotio retinae** — *see also* Detachment, retina 361.9
**Ampulla**
lower esophagus 530.89
phrenic 530.89
**Amputation**
any part of fetus, to facilitate delivery 763.89
cervix (supravaginal) (uteri) 622.8
  in pregnancy or childbirth 654.6 ☑
    affecting fetus or newborn 763.89

**Amputation** — *continued*
clitoris — *see* Wound, open, clitoris
congenital
  lower limb 755.31
  upper limb 755.21
neuroma (traumatic) (*see also* Injury, nerve, by site)
  surgical complication (late) 997.61
penis — *see* Amputation, traumatic, penis
status (without complication) — *see* Absence, by site, acquired
stump (surgical) (posttraumatic)
  abnormal, painful, or with complication (late) 997.60
  healed or old NEC (*see also* Absence, by site, acquired)
    lower V49.70
    upper V49.60
traumatic (complete) (partial)

> *Note* — "*Complicated*" *includes traumatic amputation with delayed healing, delayed treatment, foreign body, or infection.*

  arm 887.4
    at or above elbow 887.2
      complicated 887.3
    below elbow 887.0
      complicated 887.1
    both (bilateral) (any level(s)) 887.6
      complicated 887.7
    complicated 887.5
  finger(s) (one or both hands) 886.0
    with thumb(s) 885.0
      complicated 885.1
    complicated 886.1
  foot (except toe(s) only) 896.0
    and other leg 897.6
      complicated 897.7
    both (bilateral) 896.2
      complicated 896.3
    complicated 896.1
    toe(s) only (one or both feet) 895.0
      complicated 895.1
  genital organ(s) (external) NEC 878.8
    complicated 878.9
  hand (except finger(s) only) 887.0
    and other arm 887.6
      complicated 887.7
    both (bilateral) 887.6
      complicated 887.7
    complicated 887.1
    finger(s) (one or both hands) 886.0
      with thumb(s) 885.0
        complicated 885.1
      complicated 886.1
    thumb(s) (with fingers of either hand) 885.0
      complicated 885.1
  head 874.9
  late effect — *see* Late, effects (of), amputation
  leg 897.4
    and other foot 897.6
      complicated 897.7
    at or above knee 897.2
      complicated 897.3
    below knee 897.0
      complicated 897.1
    both (bilateral) 897.6
      complicated 897.7
    complicated 897.5
  lower limb(s) except toe(s) — *see* Amputation, traumatic, leg
  nose — *see* Wound, open, nose
  penis 878.0
    complicated 878.1
  sites other than limbs — *see* Wound, open, by site
  thumb(s) (with finger(s) of either hand) 885.0
    complicated 885.1

**Amputation** — *continued*
traumatic — *continued*
  toe(s) (one or both feet) 895.0
    complicated 895.1
  upper limb(s) — *see* Amputation, traumatic, arm
**Amputee** (bilateral) (old) — *see also* Absence, by site, acquired V49.70
**Amusia** 784.69
developmental 315.39
secondary to organic lesion 784.69
**Amyelencephalus** 740.0
**Amyelia** 742.59
**Amygdalitis** — *see* Tonsillitis
**Amygdalolith** 474.8
**Amyloid disease or degeneration** 277.30
heart 277.39 *[425.7]*
**Amyloidosis** (familial) (general) (generalized) (genetic) (primary) 277.39
with lung involvement 277.39 *[517.8]*
cardiac, hereditary 277.39
heart 277.39 *[425.7]*
nephropathic 277.39 *[583.81]*
neuropathic (Portuguese) (Swiss) 277.39 *[357.4]*
pulmonary 277.39 *[517.8]*
secondary 277.39
systemic, inherited 277.39
**Amylopectinosis** (brancher enzyme deficiency) 271.0
**Amylophagia** 307.52
**Amyoplasia, congenita** 756.89
**Amyotonia** 728.2
congenita 358.8
**Amyotrophia, amyotrophy, amyotrophic** 728.2
congenita 756.89
diabetic 250.6 ☑ *[353.1]* ▲
lateral sclerosis (syndrome) 335.20
neuralgic 353.5
sclerosis (lateral) 335.20
spinal progressive 335.21
**Anacidity, gastric** 536.0
psychogenic 306.4
**Anaerosis of newborn** 770.88
**Analbuminemia** 273.8
**Analgesia** — *see also* Anesthesia 782.0
**Analphalipoproteinemia** 272.5
**Anaphylactic shock or reaction** (correct substance properly administered) 995.0
due to
  food 995.60
    additives 995.66
    crustaceans 995.62
    eggs 995.68
    fish 995.65
    fruits 995.63
    milk products 995.67
    nuts (tree) 995.64
    peanuts 995.61
    seeds 995.64
    specified NEC 995.69
    tree nuts 995.64
    vegetables 995.63
  immunization 999.4
  overdose or wrong substance given or taken 977.9
    specified drug — *see* Table of Drugs and Chemicals
  serum 999.4
following sting(s) 989.5
purpura 287.0
serum 999.4
**Anaphylactoid shock or reaction** — *see* Anaphylactic shock
**Anaphylaxis** — *see* Anaphylactic shock
**Anaplasia, cervix** 622.10
**Anarthria** 784.5
**Anarthritic rheumatoid disease** 446.5
**Anasarca** 782.3
cardiac (*see also* Failure, heart) 428.0
fetus or newborn 778.0
lung 514
nutritional 262

**Anasarca** — *continued*
pulmonary 514
renal (*see also* Nephrosis) 581.9
**Anaspadias** 752.62
**Anastomosis**
aneurysmal — *see* Aneurysm
arteriovenous, congenital NEC (*see also* Anomaly, arteriovenous) 747.60
  ruptured, of brain (*see also* Hemorrhage, subarachnoid) 430
intestinal 569.89
  complicated NEC 997.4
    involving urinary tract 997.5
retinal and choroidal vessels 743.58
  acquired 362.17
**Anatomical narrow angle** (glaucoma) 365.02
**Ancylostoma** (infection) (infestation) 126.9
americanus 126.1
braziliense 126.2
caninum 126.8
ceylanicum 126.3
duodenale 126.0
Necator americanus 126.1
**Ancylostomiasis** (intestinal) 126.9
ancylostoma
  americanus 126.1
  caninum 126.8
  ceylanicum 126.3
  duodenale 126.0
braziliense 126.2
Necator americanus 126.1
**Anders' disease or syndrome** (adiposis tuberosa simplex) 272.8
**Andersen's glycogen storage disease** 271.0
**Anderson's disease** 272.7
**Andes disease** 993.2
**Andrews' disease** (bacterid) 686.8
**Androblastoma** (M8630/1)
benign (M8630/0)
  specified site — *see* Neoplasm, by site, benign
  unspecified site
    female 220
    male 222.0
malignant (M8630/3)
  specified site — *see* Neoplasm, by site, malignant
  unspecified site
    female 183.0
    male 186.9
specified site — *see* Neoplasm, by site, uncertain behavior
tubular (M8640/0)
  with lipid storage (M8641/0)
    specified site — *see* Neoplasm, by site, benign
    unspecified site
      female 220
      male 222.0
  specified site — *see* Neoplasm, by site, benign
  unspecified site
    female 220
    male 222.0
unspecified site
  female 236.2
  male 236.4
**Android pelvis** 755.69
with disproportion (fetopelvic) 653.3 ☑
  affecting fetus or newborn 763.1
  causing obstructed labor 660.1 ☑
    affecting fetus or newborn 763.1
**Anectasis, pulmonary** (newborn or fetus) 770.5
**Anemia** 285.9
with
  disorder of
    anaerobic glycolysis 282.3
    pentose phosphate pathway 282.2
  koilonychia 280.9

☑ Additional Digit Required — Refer to the Tabular List for Digit Selection          ⬚ Subterms under main terms may continue to next column or page

18 — Volume 2 • October 2007     ▶◀ Revised Text     ● New Line     ▲ Revised Code     **2008 ICD-9-CM**

**Anemia** — *continued*
  6-phosphogluconic dehydrogenase
    deficiency 282.2
  achlorhydric 280.9
  achrestic 281.8
  Addison's (pernicious) 281.0
  Addison-Biermer (pernicious) 281.0
  agranulocytic 288.09
  amino acid deficiency 281.4
  aplastic 284.9
    acquired (secondary) 284.81 ▲
    congenital 284.01
    constitutional 284.01
    due to
      chronic systemic disease
        284.89 ▲
      drugs 284.89 ▲
      infection 284.89 ▲
      radiation 284.89 ▲
    idiopathic 284.9
    myxedema 244.9
    of or complicating pregnancy
      648.2 ☑
    red cell (acquired) ▶(adult)◀ (with
      thymoma) 284.81 ▲
      congenital 284.01
      pure 284.01
    specified type NEC 284.89 ▲
    toxic (paralytic) 284.89 ▲
  aregenerative 284.9
    congenital 284.01
  asiderotic 280.9
  atypical (primary) 285.9
  autohemolysis of Selwyn and Dacie
    (type I) 282.2
  autoimmune hemolytic 283.0
  Baghdad Spring 282.2
  Balantidium coli 007.0
  Biermer's (pernicious) 281.0
  blood loss (chronic) 280.0
    acute 285.1
  bothriocephalus 123.4
  brickmakers' (*see also* Ancylostomia-
    sis) 126.9
  cerebral 437.8
  childhood 282.9
  chlorotic 280.9
  chronica congenita aregenerativa
    284.01
  chronic simple 281.9
  combined system disease NEC
    281.0 *[336.2]*
    due to dietary deficiency
      2⁵¹ *[336.2]*
  complic⟨ g pregnancy or childbirth
    64ᶜ ☑
  congenital (t⸱ wing fetal blood loss)
    776.5
    aplastic 284.01
    due to isoimmunization NEC 773.2
    Heinz-body 282.7
    hereditary hemolytic NEC 282.9
    nonspherocytic
      Type I 282.2
      Type II 282.3
    pernicious 281.0
    spherocytic (*see also* Spherocyto-
      sis) 282.0
  Cooley's (erythroblastic) 282.49
  crescent — *see* Disease, sickle-cell
  cytogenic 281.0
  Dacie's (nonspherocytic)
    type I 282.2
    type II 282.3
  Davidson's (refractory) 284.9
  deficiency 281.9
    2, 3 diphosphoglycurate mutase
      282.3
    2, 3 PG 282.3
    6-PGD 282.3
    6-phosphogluronic dehydrogenase
      282.2
    amino acid 281.4
    combined $B_{12}$ and folate 281.3
    enzyme, drug-induced (hemolytic)
      282.2

**Anemia** — *continued*
  deficiency — *continued*
    erythrocytic glutathione 282.2
    folate 281.2
      dietary 281.2
      drug-induced 281.2
    folic acid 281.2
      dietary 281.2
      drug-induced 281.2
    G-6-PD 282.2
    GGS-R 282.2
    glucose-6-phosphate dehydroge-
      nase (G-6-PD) 282.2
    glucose-phosphate isomerase 282.3
    glutathione peroxidase 282.2
    glutathione reductase 282.2
    glyceraldehyde phosphate dehydro-
      genase 282.3
    GPI 282.3
    G SH 282.2
    hexokinase 282.3
    iron (Fe) 280.9
      specified NEC 280.8
    nutritional 281.9
      with
        poor iron absorption 280.9
        specified deficiency NEC
          281.8
      due to inadequate dietary iron
        intake 280.1
      specified type NEC 281.8
    of or complicating pregnancy
      648.2 ☑
    pentose phosphate pathway 282.2
    PFK 282.3
    phosphofructo-aldolase 282.3
    phosphofructokinase 282.3
    phosphoglycerate kinase 282.3
    PK 282.3
    protein 281.4
    pyruvate kinase (PK) 282.3
    TPI 282.3
    triosephosphate isomerase 282.3
    vitamin $B_{12}$ NEC 281.1
      dietary 281.1
      pernicious 281.0
  Diamond-Blackfan (congenital hy-
    poplastic) 284.01
  dibothriocephalus 123.4
  dimorphic 281.9
  diphasic 281.8
  diphtheritic 032.89
  Diphyllobothrium 123.4
  drepanocytic (*see also* Disease, sickle-
    cell) 282.60
  due to
    blood loss (chronic) 280.0
      acute 285.1
    defect of Embden-Meyerhof path-
      way glycolysis 282.3
    disorder of glutathione metabolism
      282.2
    fetal blood loss 776.5
    fish tapeworm (D. latum) infesta-
      tion 123.4
    glutathione metabolism disorder
      282.2
    hemorrhage (chronic) 280.0
      acute 285.1
    hexose monophosphate (HMP)
      shunt deficiency 282.2
    impaired absorption 280.9
    loss of blood (chronic) 280.0
      acute 285.1
    myxedema 244.9
    Necator americanus 126.1
    prematurity 776.6
    selective vitamin $B_{12}$ malabsorp-
      tion with proteinuria 281.1
  Dyke-Young type (secondary)
    (symptomatic) 283.9
  dyserythropoietic (congenital) (types
    I, II, III) 285.8
  dyshemopoietic (congenital) 285.8
  Egypt (*see also* Ancylostomiasis) 126.9

**Anemia** — *continued*
  elliptocytosis (*see also* Elliptocytosis)
    282.1
  enzyme deficiency, drug-induced
    282.2
  epidemic (*see also* Ancylostomiasis)
    126.9
  EPO resistant 285.21
  erythroblastic
    familial 282.49
    fetus or newborn (*see also* Disease,
      hemolytic) 773.2
    late 773.5
  erythrocytic glutathione deficiency
    282.2
  erythropoietin-resistant (EPO resistant
    anemia) 285.21
  essential 285.9
  Faber's (achlorhydric anemia) 280.9
  factitious (self-induced blood letting)
    280.0
  familial erythroblastic (microcytic)
    282.49
  Fanconi's (congenital pancytopenia)
    284.09
  favism 282.2
  fetal, following blood loss 776.5
  fetus or newborn
    due to
      ABO
        antibodies 773.1
        incompatibility, maternal/fe-
          tal 773.1
        isoimmunization 773.1
      Rh
        antibodies 773.0
        incompatibility, maternal/fe-
          tal 773.0
        isoimmunization 773.0
    following fetal blood loss 776.5
  fish tapeworm (D. latum) infestation
    123.4
  folate (folic acid) deficiency 281.2
    dietary 281.2
    drug-induced 281.2
  folate malabsorption, congenital 281.2
  folic acid deficiency 281.2
    dietary 281.2
    drug-induced 281.2
  G-6-PD 282.2
  general 285.9
  glucose-6-phosphate dehydrogenase
    deficiency 282.2
  glutathione-reductase deficiency 282.2
  goat's milk 281.2
  granulocytic 288.09
  Heinz-body, congenital 282.7
  hemoglobin deficiency 285.9
  hemolytic 283.9
    acquired 283.9
      with hemoglobinuria NEC 283.2
      autoimmune (cold type) (idio-
        pathic) (primary) (sec-
        ondary) (symptomatic)
        (warm type) 283.0
      due to
        cold reactive antibodies
          283.0
        drug exposure 283.0
        warm reactive antibodies
          283.0
      fragmentation 283.19
      idiopathic (chronic) 283.9
      infectious 283.19
        autoimmune 283.0
      non-autoimmune 283.10
      toxic 283.19
      traumatic cardiac 283.19
    acute 283.9
      due to enzyme deficiency NEC
        282.3
      fetus or newborn (*see also* Dis-
        ease, hemolytic) 773.2
      late 773.5
    Lederer's (acquired infectious
      hemolytic anemia) 283.19

**Anemia** — *continued*
  hemolytic — *continued*
    autoimmune (acquired) 283.0
    chronic 282.9
      idiopathic 283.9
    cold type (secondary) (symptomatic)
      283.0
    congenital (spherocytic) (*see also*
      Spherocytosis) 282.0
      nonspherocytic — *see* Anemia,
        hemolytic, nonspherocyt-
        ic, congenital
    drug-induced 283.0
      enzyme deficiency 282.2
    due to
      cardiac conditions 283.19
      drugs 283.0
      enzyme deficiency NEC 282.3
        drug-induced 282.2
      presence of shunt or other inter-
        nal prosthetic device
        283.19
      thrombotic thrombocytopenic
        purpura 446.6
    elliptocytotic (*see also* Elliptocyto-
      sis) 282.1
    familial 282.9
    hereditary 282.9
      due to enzyme deficiency NEC
        282.3
      specified NEC 282.8
    idiopathic (chronic) 283.9
    infectious (acquired) 283.19
    mechanical 283.19
    microangiopathic 283.19
    non-autoimmune NEC 283.10
    nonspherocytic
      congenital or hereditary NEC
        282.3
        glucose-6-phosphate dehydro-
          genase deficiency
          282.2
        pyruvate kinase (PK) deficien-
          cy 282.3
        type I 282.2
        type II 282.3
      type I 282.2
      type II 282.3
    of or complicating pregnancy
      648.2 ☑
    resulting from presence of shunt
      or other internal prosthetic
      device 283.19
    secondary 283.19
      autoimmune 283.0
    sickle-cell — *see* Disease, sickle-
      cell
    Stransky-Regala type (Hb-E) (*see
      also* Disease, hemoglobin)
      282.7
    symptomatic 283.19
      autoimmune 283.0
    toxic (acquired) 283.19
    uremic (adult) (child) 283.11
    warm type (secondary) (symptomat-
      ic) 283.0
  hemorrhagic (chronic) 280.0
    acute 285.1
  HEMPAS 285.8
  hereditary erythroblast multinucleari-
    ty-positive acidified serum test
    285.8
  Herrick's (hemoglobin S disease)
    282.61
  hexokinase deficiency 282.3
  high $A_2$ 282.49
  hookworm (*see also* Ancylostomiasis)
    126.9
  hypochromic (idiopathic) (microcytic)
    (normoblastic) 280.9
    with iron loading 285.0
    due to blood loss (chronic) 280.0
      acute 285.1
    familial sex linked 285.0
    pyridoxine-responsive 285.0

---

☑ Additional Digit Required — Refer to the Tabular List for Digit Selection      ▽ Subterms under main terms may continue to next column or page

**Anemia** — *continued*
hypoplasia, red blood cells 284.81 ▲
congenital or familial 284.01
hypoplastic (idiopathic) 284.9
congenital 284.01
familial 284.01
of childhood 284.09
idiopathic 285.9
hemolytic, chronic 283.9
in
chronic illness NEC 285.29
chronic kidney disease 285.21
end-stage renal disease 285.21
neoplastic disease 285.22
infantile 285.9
infective, infectional 285.9
intertropical (*see also* Ancylostomiasis) 126.9
iron (Fe) deficiency 280.9
due to blood loss (chronic) 280.0
acute 285.1
of or complicating pregnancy 648.2 ☑
specified NEC 280.8
Jaksch's (pseudoleukemia infantum) 285.8
Joseph-Diamond-Blackfan (congenital hypoplastic) 284.01
labyrinth 386.50
Lederer's (acquired infectious hemolytic anemia) 283.19
leptocytosis (hereditary) 282.49
leukoerythroblastic 284.2
macrocytic 281.9
nutritional 281.2
of or complicating pregnancy 648.2 ☑
tropical 281.2
malabsorption (familial), selective B$_{12}$
with proteinuria 281.1
malarial (*see also* Malaria) 084.6
malignant (progressive) 281.0
malnutrition 281.9
marsh (*see also* Malaria) 084.6
Mediterranean (with hemoglobinopathy) 282.49
megaloblastic 281.9
combined B$_{12}$ and folate deficiency 281.3
nutritional (of infancy) 281.2
of infancy 281.2
of or complicating pregnancy 648.2 ☑
refractory 281.3
specified NEC 281.3
megalocytic 281.9
microangiopathic hemolytic 283.19
microcytic (hypochromic) 280.9
due to blood loss (chronic) 280.0
acute 285.1
familial 282.49
hypochromic 280.9
microdrepanocytosis 282.49
miners' (*see also* Ancylostomiasis) 126.9
myelopathic 285.8
myelophthisic (normocytic) 284.2
newborn (*see also* Disease, hemolytic) 773.2
due to isoimmunization (*see also* Disease, hemolytic) 773.2
late, due to isoimmunization 773.5
posthemorrhagic 776.5
nonregenerative 284.9
nonspherocytic hemolytic — *see* Anemia, hemolytic, nonspherocytic
normocytic (infectional) (not due to blood loss) 285.9
due to blood loss (chronic) 280.0
acute 285.1
myelophthisic 284.2
nutritional (deficiency) 281.9
with
poor iron absorption 280.9
specified deficiency NEC 281.8

**Anemia** — *continued*
nutritional — *continued*
due to inadequate dietary iron intake 280.1
megaloblastic (of infancy) 281.2
of childhood 282.9
of chronic
disease NEC 285.29
illness NEC 285.29
of or complicating pregnancy 648.2 ☑
affecting fetus or newborn 760.8
of prematurity 776.6
orotic aciduric (congenital) (hereditary) 281.4
osteosclerotic 289.89
ovalocytosis (hereditary) (*see also* Elliptocytosis) 282.1
paludal (*see also* Malaria) 084.6
pentose phosphate pathway deficiency 282.2
pernicious (combined system disease) (congenital) (dorsolateral spinal degeneration) (juvenile) (myelopathy) (neuropathy) (posterior sclerosis) (primary) (progressive) (spleen) 281.0
of or complicating pregnancy 648.2 ☑
pleochromic 285.9
of sprue 281.8
portal 285.8
posthemorrhagic (chronic) 280.0
acute 285.1
newborn 776.5
postoperative
due to ▶(acute)◀ blood loss 285.1
chronic blood loss 280.0 ●
other 285.9
postpartum 648.2 ☑
pressure 285.9
primary 285.9
profound 285.9
progressive 285.9
malignant 281.0
pernicious 281.0
protein-deficiency 281.4
pseudoleukemica infantum 285.8
puerperal 648.2 ☑
pure red cell 284.81 ▲
congenital 284.01
pyridoxine-responsive (hypochromic) 285.0
pyruvate kinase (PK) deficiency 282.3
refractoria sideroblastica 238.72
refractory (primary) 238.72
with
excess
blasts-1 (RAEB-1) 238.73
blasts-2 (RAEB-2) 238.73
hemochromatosis 238.72
ringed sideroblasts (RARS) 238.72
megaloblastic 281.3
sideroblastic 238.72
sideropenic 280.9
Rietti-Greppi-Micheli (thalassemia minor) 282.49
scorbutic 281.8
secondary (to) 285.9
blood loss (chronic) 280.0
acute 285.1
hemorrhage 280.0
acute 285.1
inadequate dietary iron intake 280.1
semiplastic 284.9
septic 285.9
sickle-cell (*see also* Disease, sickle-cell) 282.60
sideroachrestic 285.0
sideroblastic (acquired) (any type) (congenital) (drug-induced) (due to disease) (hereditary) (primary) (secondary) (sex-linked hypochromic) (vitamin B$_6$ responsive) 285.0

**Anemia** — *continued*
sideroblastic — *continued*
refractory 238.72
sideropenic (refractory) 280.9
due to blood loss (chronic) 280.0
acute 285.1
simple chronic 281.9
specified type NEC 285.8
spherocytic (hereditary) (*see also* Spherocytosis) 282.0
splenic 285.8
familial (Gaucher's) 272.7
splenomegalic 285.8
stomatocytosis 282.8
syphilitic 095.8
target cell (oval) 282.49
thalassemia 282.49
thrombocytopenic (*see also* Thrombocytopenia) 287.5
toxic 284.89 ▲
triosephosphate isomerase deficiency 282.3
tropical, macrocytic 281.2
tuberculous (*see also* Tuberculosis) 017.9 ☑
vegan's 281.1
vitamin
B$_6$-responsive 285.0
B$_{12}$ deficiency (dietary) 281.1
pernicious 281.0
von Jaksch's (pseudoleukemia infantum) 285.8
Witts' (achlorhydric anemia) 280.9
Zuelzer (-Ogden) (nutritional megaloblastic anemia) 281.2
**Anencephalus, anencephaly** 740.0
fetal, affecting management of pregnancy 655.0 ☑
**Anergasia** — *see also* Psychosis, organic 294.9
senile 290.0
**Anesthesia, anesthetic** 782.0
complication or reaction NEC 995.22
due to
correct substance properly administered 995.22
overdose or wrong substance given 968.4
specified anesthetic — *see* Table of Drugs and Chemicals
cornea 371.81
death from
correct substance properly administered 995.4
during delivery 668.9 ☑
overdose or wrong substance given 968.4
specified anesthetic — *see* Table of Drugs and Chemicals
eye 371.81
functional 300.11
hyperesthetic, thalamic 338.0
hysterical 300.11
local skin lesion 782.0
olfactory 781.1
sexual (psychogenic) 302.72
shock
due to
correct substance properly administered 995.4
overdose or wrong substance given 968.4
specified anesthetic — *see* Table of Drugs and Chemicals
skin 782.0
tactile 782.0
testicular 608.9
thermal 782.0
**Anetoderma** (maculosum) 701.3
**Aneuploidy** NEC 758.5
**Aneurin deficiency** 265.1
**Aneurysm** (anastomotic) (artery) (cirsoid) (diffuse) (false) (fusiform) (multiple) (ruptured) (saccular) (varicose) 442.9

**Aneurysm** — *continued*
abdominal (aorta) 441.4
ruptured 441.3
syphilitic 093.0
aorta, aortic (nonsyphilitic) 441.9
abdominal 441.4
dissecting 441.02
ruptured 441.3
syphilitic 093.0
arch 441.2
ruptured 441.1
arteriosclerotic NEC 441.9
ruptured 441.5
ascending 441.2
ruptured 441.1
congenital 747.29
descending 441.9
abdominal 441.4
ruptured 441.3
ruptured 441.5
thoracic 441.2
ruptured 441.1
dissecting 441.00
abdominal 441.02
thoracic 441.01
thoracoabdominal 441.03
due to coarctation (aorta) 747.10
ruptured 441.5
sinus, right 747.29
syphilitic 093.0
thoracoabdominal 441.7
ruptured 441.6
thorax, thoracic (arch) (nonsyphilitic) 441.2
dissecting 441.01
ruptured 441.1
syphilitic 093.0
transverse 441.2
ruptured 441.1
valve (heart) (*see also* Endocarditis, aortic) 424.1
arteriosclerotic NEC 442.9
cerebral 437.3
ruptured (*see also* Hemorrhage, subarachnoid) 430
arteriovenous (congenital) (peripheral) NEC (*see also* Anomaly, arteriovenous) 747.60
acquired NEC 447.0
brain 437.3
ruptured (*see also* Hemorrhage, subarachnoid) 430
coronary 414.11
pulmonary 417.0
brain (cerebral) 747.81
ruptured (*see also* Hemorrhage, subarachnoid) 430
coronary 746.85
pulmonary 747.3
retina 743.58
specified site NEC 747.89
acquired 447.0
traumatic (*see also* Injury, blood vessel, by site) 904.9
basal — *see* Aneurysm, brain
berry (congenital) (ruptured) (*see also* Hemorrhage, subarachnoid) 430
brain 437.3
arteriosclerotic 437.3
ruptured (*see also* Hemorrhage, subarachnoid) 430
arteriovenous 747.81
acquired 437.3
ruptured (*see also* Hemorrhage, subarachnoid) 430
ruptured (*see also* Hemorrhage, subarachnoid) 430
berry (congenital) (ruptured) (*see also* Hemorrhage, subarachnoid) 430
congenital 747.81
ruptured (*see also* Hemorrhage, subarachnoid) 430
meninges 437.3

☑ Additional Digit Required — Refer to the Tabular List for Digit Selection ⟨⟩ Subterms under main terms may continue to next column or page

20 — Volume 2 • October 2007 ▶◀ Revised Text ● New Line ▲ Revised Code **2008 ICD-9-CM**

**Aneurysm** — *continued*
  brain — *continued*
    meninges — *continued*
      ruptured (*see also* Hemorrhage, subarachnoid) 430
      miliary (congenital) (ruptured) (*see also* Hemorrhage, subarachnoid) 430
    mycotic 421.0
      ruptured (*see also* Hemorrhage, subarachnoid) 430
    nonruptured 437.3
    ruptured (*see also* Hemorrhage, subarachnoid) 430
    syphilitic 094.87
    syphilitic (hemorrhage) 094.87
    traumatic — *see* Injury, intracranial
  cardiac (false) (*see also* Aneurysm, heart) 414.10
  carotid artery (common) (external) 442.81
    internal (intracranial portion) 437.3
      extracranial portion 442.81
      ruptured into brain (*see also* Hemorrhage, subarachnoid) 430
    syphilitic 093.89
      intracranial 094.87
  cavernous sinus (*see also* Aneurysm, brain) 437.3
    arteriovenous 747.81
      ruptured (*see also* Hemorrhage, subarachnoid) 430
    congenital 747.81
      ruptured (*see also* Hemorrhage, subarachnoid) 430
  celiac 442.84
  central nervous system, syphilitic 094.89
  cerebral — *see* Aneurysm, brain
  chest — *see* Aneurysm, thorax
  circle of Willis (*see also* Aneurysm, brain) 437.3
    congenital 747.81
      ruptured (*see also* Hemorrhage, subarachnoid) 430
    ruptured (*see also* Hemorrhage, subarachnoid) 430
  common iliac artery 442.2
  congenital (peripheral) NEC 747.60
    brain 747.81
      ruptured (*see also* Hemorrhage, subarachnoid) 430
    cerebral — *see* Aneurysm, brain, congenital
    coronary 746.85
    gastrointestinal 747.61
    lower limb 747.64
    pulmonary 747.3
    renal 747.62
    retina 743.58
    specified site NEC 747.89
    spinal 747.82
    upper limb 747.63
  conjunctiva 372.74
  conus arteriosus (*see also* Aneurysm, heart) 414.10
  coronary (arteriosclerotic) (artery) (vein) (*see also* Aneurysm, heart) 414.11
    arteriovenous 746.85
    congenital 746.85
    syphilitic 093.89
  cylindrical 441.9
    ruptured 441.5
    syphilitic 093.9
  dissecting 442.9
    aorta 441.00
      abdominal 441.02
      thoracic 441.01
        thoracoabdominal 441.03
    syphilitic 093.9
  ductus arteriosus 747.0
  embolic — *see* Embolism, artery
  endocardial, infective (any valve) 421.0

**Aneurysm** — *continued*
  femoral 442.3
  gastroduodenal 442.84
  gastroepiploic 442.84
  heart (chronic or with a stated duration of over 8 weeks) (infectional) (wall) 414.10
    acute or with a stated duration of 8 weeks or less (*see also* Infarct, myocardium) 410.9 ☑
    congenital 746.89
    valve — *see* Endocarditis
  hepatic 442.84
  iliac (common) 442.2
  infective (any valve) 421.0
  innominate (nonsyphilitic) 442.89
    syphilitic 093.89
  interauricular septum (*see also* Aneurysm, heart) 414.10
  interventricular septum (*see also* Aneurysm, heart) 414.10
  intracranial — *see* Aneurysm, brain
  intrathoracic (nonsyphilitic) 441.2
    ruptured 441.1
    syphilitic 093.0
  jugular vein 453.8
  lower extremity 442.3
  lung (pulmonary artery) 417.1
  malignant 093.9
  mediastinal (nonsyphilitic) 442.89
    syphilitic 093.89
  miliary (congenital) (ruptured) (*see also* Hemorrhage, subarachnoid) 430
  mitral (heart) (valve) 424.0
  mural (arteriovenous) (heart) (*see also* Aneurysm, heart) 414.10
  mycotic, any site 421.0
    without endocarditis — *see* Aneurysm by site
    ruptured, brain (*see also* Hemorrhage, subarachnoid) 430
  myocardium (*see also* Aneurysm, heart) 414.10
  neck 442.81
  pancreaticoduodenal 442.84
  patent ductus arteriosus 747.0
  peripheral NEC 442.89
    congenital NEC (*see also* Aneurysm, congenital) 747.60
  popliteal 442.3
  pulmonary 417.1
    arteriovenous 747.3
      acquired 417.0
    syphilitic 093.89
    valve (heart) (*see also* Endocarditis, pulmonary) 424.3
  racemose 442.9
    congenital (peripheral) NEC 747.60
  radial 442.0
  Rasmussen's (*see also* Tuberculosis) 011.2 ☑
  renal 442.1
  retinal (acquired) 362.17
    congenital 743.58
    diabetic 250.5 ☑ *[362.01]*
  sinus, aortic (of Valsalva) 747.29
  specified site NEC 442.89
  spinal (cord) 442.89
    congenital 747.82
    syphilitic (hemorrhage) 094.89
  spleen, splenic 442.83
  subclavian 442.82
    syphilitic 093.89
  superior mesenteric 442.84
  syphilitic 093.9
    aorta 093.0
    central nervous system 094.89
    congenital 090.5
    spine, spinal 094.89
  thoracoabdominal 441.7
    ruptured 441.6
  thorax, thoracic (arch) (nonsyphilitic) 441.2
    dissecting 441.01

**Aneurysm** — *continued*
  thorax, thoracic — *continued*
    ruptured 441.1
    syphilitic 093.0
  traumatic (complication) (early) — *see* Injury, blood vessel, by site
  tricuspid (heart) (valve) — *see* Endocarditis, tricuspid
  ulnar 442.0
  upper extremity 442.0
  valve, valvular — *see* Endocarditis
  venous 456.8
    congenital NEC (*see also* Aneurysm, congenital) 747.60
  ventricle (arteriovenous) (*see also* Aneurysm, heart) 414.10
  visceral artery NEC 442.84
**Angiectasis** 459.89
**Angiectopia** 459.9
**Angiitis** 447.6
  allergic granulomatous 446.4
  hypersensitivity 446.20
    Goodpasture's syndrome 446.21
    specified NEC 446.29
  necrotizing 446.0
  Wegener's (necrotizing respiratory granulomatosis) 446.4
**Angina** (attack) (cardiac) (chest) (effort) (heart) (pectoris) (syndrome) (vasomotor) 413.9
  abdominal 557.1
  accelerated 411.1
  agranulocytic 288.03
  aphthous 074.0
  catarrhal 462
  crescendo 411.1
  croupous 464.4
  cruris 443.9
    due to atherosclerosis NEC (*see also* Arteriosclerosis, extremities) 440.20
  decubitus 413.0
  diphtheritic (membranous) 032.0
  erysipelatous 034.0
  erythematous 462
  exudative, chronic 476.0
  faucium 478.29
  gangrenous 462
    diphtheritic 032.0
  infectious 462
  initial 411.1
  intestinal 557.1
  ludovici 528.3
  Ludwig's 528.3
  malignant 462
    diphtheritic 032.0
  membranous 464.4
    diphtheritic 032.0
  mesenteric 557.1
  monocytic 075
  nocturnal 413.0
  phlegmonous 475
    diphtheritic 032.0
  preinfarctional 411.1
  Prinzmetal's 413.1
  progressive 411.1
  pseudomembranous 101
  psychogenic 306.2
  pultaceous, diphtheritic 032.0
  scarlatinal 034.1
  septic 034.0
  simple 462
  stable NEC 413.9
  staphylococcal 462
  streptococcal 034.0
  stridulous, diphtheritic 032.3
  syphilitic 093.9
    congenital 090.5
  tonsil 475
  trachealis 464.4
  unstable 411.1
  variant 413.1
  Vincent's 101

**Angioblastoma** (M9161/1) — *see* Neoplasm, connective tissue, uncertain behavior
**Angiocholecystitis** — *see also* Cholecystitis, acute 575.0
**Angiocholitis** — *see also* Cholecystitis, acute 576.1
**Angiodysgensis spinalis** 336.1
**Angiodysplasia** (intestinalis) (intestine) 569.84
  with hemorrhage 569.85
  duodenum 537.82
    with hemorrhage 537.83
  stomach 537.82
    with hemorrhage 537.83
**Angioedema** (allergic) (any site) (with urticaria) 995.1
  hereditary 277.6
**Angioendothelioma** (M9130/1) — *see also* Neoplasm, by site, uncertain behavior
  benign (M9130/0) (*see also* Hemangioma, by site) 228.00
  bone (M9260/3) — *see* Neoplasm, bone, malignant
  Ewing's (M9260/3) — *see* Neoplasm, bone, malignant
  nervous system (M9130/0) 228.09
**Angiofibroma** (M9160/0) — *see also* Neoplasm, by site, benign
  juvenile (M9160/0) 210.7
    specified site — *see* Neoplasm, by site, benign
    unspecified site 210.7
**Angiohemophilia** (A) (B) 286.4
**Angioid streaks** (choroid) (retina) 363.43
**Angiokeratoma** (M9141/0) — *see also* Neoplasm, skin, benign
  corporis diffusum 272.7
**Angiokeratosis**
  diffuse 272.7
**Angioleiomyoma** (M8894/0) — *see* Neoplasm, connective tissue, benign
**Angioleucitis** 683
**Angiolipoma** (M8861/0) — *see also* Lipoma, by site 214.9
  infiltrating (M8861/1) — *see* Neoplasm, connective tissue, uncertain behavior
**Angioma** (M9120/0) — *see also* Hemangioma, by site 228.00
  capillary 448.1
  hemorrhagicum hereditaria 448.0
  malignant (M9120/3) — *see* Neoplasm, connective tissue, malignant
  pigmentosum et atrophicum 757.33
  placenta — *see* Placenta, abnormal
  plexiform (M9131/0) — *see* Hemangioma, by site
  senile 448.1
  serpiginosum 709.1
  spider 448.1
  stellate 448.1
**Angiomatosis** 757.32
  bacillary 083.8
  corporis diffusum universale 272.7
  cutaneocerebral 759.6
  encephalocutaneous 759.6
  encephalofacial 759.6
  encephalotrigeminal 759.6
  hemorrhagic familial 448.0
  hereditary familial 448.0
  heredofamilial 448.0
  meningo-oculofacial 759.6
  multiple sites 228.09
  neuro-oculocutaneous 759.6
  retina (Hippel's disease) 759.6
  retinocerebellosa 759.6
  retinocerebral 759.6
  systemic 228.09
**Angiomyolipoma** (M8860/0)
  specified site — *see* Neoplasm, connective tissue, benign
  unspecified site 223.0

☑ Additional Digit Required — Refer to the Tabular List for Digit Selection      ▽ Subterms under main terms may continue to next column or page

*2008 ICD-9-CM*      ▶◀ Revised Text      ● New Line      ▲ Revised Code      **Volume 2 — 21**

**Angiomyoliposarcoma** (M8860/3) — *see* Neoplasm, connective tissue, malignant
**Angiomyoma** (M8894/0) — *see* Neoplasm, connective tissue, benign
**Angiomyosarcoma** (M8894/3) — *see* Neoplasm, connective tissue, malignant
**Angioneurosis** 306.2
**Angioneurotic edema** (allergic) (any site) (with urticaria) 995.1
  hereditary 277.6
**Angiopathia, angiopathy** 459.9
  diabetic (peripheral) 250.7 ☑ *[443.81]*
  peripheral 443.9
    diabetic 250.7 ☑ *[443.81]*
    specified type NEC 443.89
  retinae syphilitica 093.89
  retinalis (juvenilis) 362.18
    background 362.10
    diabetic 250.5 ☑ *[362.01]*
    proliferative 362.29
    tuberculous (*see also* Tuberculosis) 017.3 ☑ *[362.18]*
**Angiosarcoma** (M9120/3) — *see* Neoplasm, connective tissue, malignant
**Angiosclerosis** — *see* Arteriosclerosis
**Angioscotoma, enlarged** 368.42
**Angiospasm** 443.9
  brachial plexus 353.0
  cerebral 435.9
  cervical plexus 353.2
  nerve
    arm 354.9
      axillary 353.0
      median 354.1
      ulnar 354.2
    autonomic (*see also* Neuropathy, peripheral, autonomic) 337.9
    axillary 353.0
    leg 355.8
      plantar 355.6
    lower extremity — *see* Angiospasm, nerve, leg
    median 354.1
    peripheral NEC 355.9
    spinal NEC 355.9
    sympathetic (*see also* Neuropathy, peripheral, autonomic) 337.9
    ulnar 354.2
    upper extremity — *see* Angiospasm, nerve, arm
  peripheral NEC 443.9
  traumatic 443.9
    foot 443.9
    leg 443.9
  vessel 443.9
**Angiospastic disease or edema** 443.9
**Angle's**
  class I 524.21
  class II 524.22
  class III 524.23
**Anguillulosis** 127.2
**Angulation**
  cecum (*see also* Obstruction, intestine) 560.9
  coccyx (acquired) 738.6
    congenital 756.19
  femur (acquired) 736.39
    congenital 755.69
  intestine (large) (small) (*see also* Obstruction, intestine) 560.9
  sacrum (acquired) 738.5
    congenital 756.19
  sigmoid (flexure) (*see also* Obstruction, intestine) 560.9
  spine (*see also* Curvature, spine) 737.9
  tibia (acquired) 736.89
    congenital 755.69
  ureter 593.3
  wrist (acquired) 736.09
    congenital 755.59
**Angulus infectiosus** 686.8
**Anhedonia** 780.99 ▲

**Anhidrosis** (lid) (neurogenic) (thermogenic) 705.0
**Anhydration** 276.51
  with
    hypernatremia 276.0
    hyponatremia 276.1
**Anhydremia** 276.52
  with
    hypernatremia 276.0
    hyponatremia 276.1
**Anidrosis** 705.0
**Aniridia** (congenital) 743.45
**Anisakiasis** (infection) (infestation) 127.1
**Anisakis larva infestation** 127.1
**Aniseikonia** 367.32
**Anisocoria** (pupil) 379.41
  congenital 743.46
**Anisocytosis** 790.09
**Anisometropia** (congenital) 367.31
**Ankle** — *see* condition
**Ankyloblepharon** (acquired) (eyelid) 374.46
  filiforme (adnatum) (congenital) 743.62
  total 743.62
**Ankylodactly** — *see also* Syndactylism 755.10
**Ankyloglossia** 750.0
**Ankylosis** (fibrous) (osseous) 718.50
  ankle 718.57
  any joint, produced by surgical fusion V45.4
  cricoarytenoid (cartilage) (joint) (larynx) 478.79
  dental 521.6
  ear ossicle NEC 385.22
    malleus 385.21
  elbow 718.52
  finger 718.54
  hip 718.55
  incostapedial joint (infectional) 385.22
  joint, produced by surgical fusion NEC V45.4
  knee 718.56
  lumbosacral (joint) 724.6
  malleus 385.21
  multiple sites 718.59
  postoperative (status) V45.4
  sacroiliac (joint) 724.6
  shoulder 718.51
  specified site NEC 718.58
  spine NEC 724.9
  surgical V45.4
  teeth, tooth (hard tissues) 521.6
  temporomandibular joint 524.61
  wrist 718.53
**Ankylostoma** — *see* Ancylostoma
**Ankylostomiasis** (intestinal) — *see* Ancylostomiasis
**Ankylurethria** — *see also* Stricture, urethra 598.9
**Annular** — *see also* condition
  detachment, cervix 622.8
  organ or site, congenital NEC — *see* Distortion
  pancreas (congenital) 751.7
**Anodontia** (complete) (partial) (vera) 520.0
  with abnormal spacing 524.30
  acquired 525.10
    causing malocclusion 524.30
    due to
      caries 525.13
      extraction 525.10
      periodontal disease 525.12
      trauma 525.11
**Anomaly, anomalous** (congenital) (unspecified type) 759.9
  abdomen 759.9
  abdominal wall 756.70
  acoustic nerve 742.9
  adrenal (gland) 759.1
  Alder (-Reilly) (leukocyte granulation) 288.2
  alimentary tract 751.9
    lower 751.5

**Anomaly, anomalous** — *continued*
  alimentary tract — *continued*
    specified type NEC 751.8
    upper (any part, except tongue) 750.9
      tongue 750.10
        specified type NEC 750.19
  alveolar 524.70
    ridge (process) 525.8
    specified NEC 524.79
  ankle (joint) 755.69
  anus, anal (canal) 751.5
  aorta, aortic 747.20
    arch 747.21
    coarctation (postductal) (preductal) 747.10
    cusp or valve NEC 746.9
    septum 745.0
    specified type NEC 747.29
  aorticopulmonary septum 745.0
  apertures, diaphragm 756.6
  appendix 751.5
  aqueduct of Sylvius 742.3
    with spina bifida (*see also* Spina bifida) 741.0 ☑
  arm 755.50
    reduction (*see also* Deformity, reduction, upper limb) 755.20
  arteriovenous (congenital) (peripheral) NEC 747.60
    brain 747.81
    cerebral 747.81
    coronary 746.85
    gastrointestinal 747.61
      acquired — *see* Angiodysplasia
    lower limb 747.64
    renal 747.62
    specified site NEC 747.69
    spinal 747.82
    upper limb 747.63
  artery (*see also* Anomaly, peripheral vascular system) NEC 747.60
    brain 747.81
    cerebral 747.81
    coronary 746.85
    eye 743.9
    pulmonary 747.3
    renal 747.62
    retina 743.9
    umbilical 747.5
  arytenoepiglottic folds 748.3
  atrial
    bands 746.9
    folds 746.9
    septa 745.5
  atrioventricular
    canal 745.69
    common 745.69
    conduction 426.7
    excitation 426.7
    septum 745.4
  atrium — *see* Anomaly, atrial
  auditory canal 744.3
    specified type NEC 744.29
      with hearing impairment 744.02
  auricle
    ear 744.3
      causing impairment of hearing 744.02
    heart 746.9
      septum 745.5
  autosomes, autosomal NEC 758.5
  Axenfeld's 743.44
  back 759.9
  band
    atrial 746.9
    heart 746.9
    ventricular 746.9
  Bartholin's duct 750.9
  biliary duct or passage 751.60
    atresia 751.61
  bladder (neck) (sphincter) (trigone) 753.9
    specified type NEC 753.8
  blood vessel 747.9
    artery — *see* Anomaly, artery

**Anomaly, anomalous** — *continued*
  blood vessel — *continued*
    peripheral vascular — *see* Anomaly, peripheral vascular system
    vein — *see* Anomaly, vein
  bone NEC 756.9
    ankle 755.69
    arm 755.50
    chest 756.3
    cranium 756.0
    face 756.0
    finger 755.50
    foot 755.67
    forearm 755.50
    frontal 756.0
    head 756.0
    hip 755.63
    leg 755.60
    lumbosacral 756.10
    nose 748.1
    pelvic girdle 755.60
    rachitic 756.4
    rib 756.3
    shoulder girdle 755.50
    skull 756.0
      with
        anencephalus 740.0
        encephalocele 742.0
        hydrocephalus 742.3
          with spina bifida (*see also* Spina bifida) 741.0 ☑
        microcephalus 742.1
    toe 755.66
  brain 742.9
    multiple 742.4
    reduction 742.2
    specified type NEC 742.4
    vessel 747.81
  branchial cleft NEC 744.49
    cyst 744.42
    fistula 744.41
    persistent 744.41
    sinus (external) (internal) 744.41
  breast 757.9
  broad ligament 752.10
    specified type NEC 752.19
  bronchus 748.3
  bulbar septum 745.0
  bulbus cordis 745.9
    persistent (in left ventricle) 745.8
  bursa 756.9
  canal of Nuck 752.9
  canthus 743.9
  capillary NEC (*see also* Anomaly, peripheral vascular system) 747.60
  cardiac 746.9
    septal closure 745.9
      acquired 429.71
    valve NEC 746.9
      pulmonary 746.00
      specified type NEC 746.89
  cardiovascular system 746.9
    complicating pregnancy, childbirth, or puerperium 648.5 ☑
  carpus 755.50
  cartilage, trachea 748.3
  cartilaginous 756.9
  caruncle, lacrimal, lachrymal 743.9
  cascade stomach 750.7
  cauda equina 742.59
  cecum 751.5
  cerebral (*see also* Anomaly, brain vessels) 747.81
  cerebrovascular system 747.81
  cervix (uterus) 752.40
    with doubling of vagina and uterus 752.2
    in pregnancy or childbirth 654.6 ☑
      affecting fetus or newborn 763.89
      causing obstructed labor 660.2 ☑

☑ Additional Digit Required — Refer to the Tabular List for Digit Selection     Subterms under main terms may continue to next column or page

22 — Volume 2 · October 2007    ▶◀ Revised Text    ● New Line    ▲ Revised Code    **2008 ICD-9-CM**

Anomaly, anomalous — *continued*
cervix — *continued*
in pregnancy or childbirth — *continued*
causing obstructed labor — *continued*
affecting fetus or newborn 763.1
Chédiak-Higashi (-Steinbrinck) (congenital gigantism of peroxidase granules) 288.2
cheek 744.9
chest (wall) 756.3
chin 744.9
specified type NEC 744.89
chordae tendineae 746.9
choroid 743.9
plexus 742.9
chromosomes, chromosomal 758.9
13 (13-15) 758.1
18 (16-18) 758.2
21 or 22 758.0
autosomes NEC (*see also* Abnormal, autosomes) 758.5
deletion 758.39
Christchurch 758.39
D₁ 758.1
E₃ 758.2
G 758.0
mitochondrial 758.9
mosaics 758.89
sex 758.81
complement, XO 758.6
complement, XXX 758.81
complement, XXY 758.7
complement, XYY 758.81
gonadal dysgenesis 758.6
Klinefelter's 758.7
Turner's 758.6
trisomy 21 758.0
cilia 743.9
circulatory system 747.9
specified type NEC 747.89
clavicle 755.51
clitoris 752.40
coccyx 756.10
colon 751.5
common duct 751.60
communication
coronary artery 746.85
left ventricle with right atrium 745.4
concha (ear) 744.3
connection
renal vessels with kidney 747.62
total pulmonary venous 747.41
connective tissue 756.9
specified type NEC 756.89
cornea 743.9
shape 743.41
size 743.41
specified type NEC 743.49
coronary
artery 746.85
vein 746.89
cranium — *see* Anomaly, skull
cricoid cartilage 748.3
cushion, endocardial 745.60
specified type NEC 745.69
cystic duct 751.60
dental arch 524.20
specified NEC 524.29
dental arch relationship 524.20
angle's class I 524.21
angle's class II 524.22
angle's class III 524.23
articulation
anterior 524.27
posterior 524.27
reverse 524.27
disto-occlusion 524.22
division I 524.22
division II 524.22
excessive horizontal overlap 524.26
interarch distance (excessive) (inadequate) 524.28

Anomaly, anomalous — *continued*
dental arch relationship — *continued*
mesio-occlusion 524.23
neutro-occlusion 524.21
open
anterior occlusal relationship 524.24
posterior occlusal relationship 524.25
specified NEC 524.29
dentition 520.6
dentofacial NEC 524.9
functional 524.50
specified type NEC 524.89
dermatoglyphic 757.2
Descemet's membrane 743.9
specified type NEC 743.49
development
cervix 752.40
vagina 752.40
vulva 752.40
diaphragm, diaphragmatic (apertures) NEC 756.6
digestive organ(s) or system 751.9
lower 751.5
specified type NEC 751.8
upper 750.9
distribution, coronary artery 746.85
ductus
arteriosus 747.0
Botalli 747.0
duodenum 751.5
dura 742.9
brain 742.4
spinal cord 742.59
ear 744.3
causing impairment of hearing 744.00
specified type NEC 744.09
external 744.3
causing impairment of hearing 744.02
specified type NEC 744.29
inner (causing impairment of hearing) 744.05
middle, except ossicles (causing impairment of hearing) 744.03
ossicles 744.04
ossicles 744.04
prominent auricle 744.29
specified type NEC 744.29
with hearing impairment 744.09
Ebstein's (heart) 746.2
tricuspid valve 746.2
ectodermal 757.9
Eisenmenger's (ventricular septal defect) 745.4
ejaculatory duct 752.9
specified type NEC 752.89
elbow (joint) 755.50
endocardial cushion 745.60
specified type NEC 745.69
endocrine gland NEC 759.2
epididymis 752.9
epiglottis 748.3
esophagus 750.9
specified type NEC 750.4
Eustachian tube 744.3
specified type NEC 744.24
eye (any part) 743.9
adnexa 743.9
specified type NEC 743.69
anophthalmos 743.00
anterior
chamber and related structures 743.9
angle 743.9
specified type NEC 743.44
specified type NEC 743.44
segment 743.9
combined 743.48
multiple 743.48
specified type NEC 743.49
cataract (*see also* Cataract) 743.30

Anomaly, anomalous — *continued*
eye — *continued*
glaucoma (*see also* Buphthalmia) 743.20
lid 743.9
specified type NEC 743.63
microphthalmos (*see also* Microphthalmos) 743.10
posterior segment 743.9
specified type NEC 743.59
vascular 743.58
vitreous 743.9
specified type NEC 743.51
ptosis (eyelid) 743.61
retina 743.9
specified type NEC 743.59
sclera 743.9
specified type NEC 743.47
specified type NEC 743.8
eyebrow 744.89
eyelid 743.9
specified type NEC 743.63
face (any part) 744.9
bone(s) 756.0
specified type NEC 744.89
fallopian tube 752.10
specified type NEC 752.19
fascia 756.9
specified type NEC 756.89
femur 755.60
fibula 755.60
finger 755.50
supernumerary 755.01
webbed (*see also* Syndactylism, fingers) 755.11
fixation, intestine 751.4
flexion (joint) 755.9
hip or thigh (*see also* Dislocation, hip, congenital) 754.30
folds, heart 746.9
foot 755.67
foramen
Botalli 745.5
ovale 745.5
forearm 755.50
forehead (*see also* Anomaly, skull) 756.0
form, teeth 520.2
fovea centralis 743.9
frontal bone (*see also* Anomaly, skull) 756.0
gallbladder 751.60
Gartner's duct 752.41
gastrointestinal tract 751.9
specified type NEC 751.8
vessel 747.61
genitalia, genital organ(s) or system
female 752.9
external 752.40
specified type NEC 752.49
internal NEC 752.9
male (external and internal) 752.9
epispadias 752.62
hidden penis 752.65
hydrocele, congenital 778.6
hypospadias 752.61
micropenis 752.64
testis, undescended 752.51
retractile 752.52
specified type NEC 752.89
genitourinary NEC 752.9
Gerbode 745.4
globe (eye) 743.9
glottis 748.3
granulation or granulocyte, genetic 288.2
constitutional 288.2
leukocyte 288.2
gum 750.9
gyri 742.9
hair 757.9
specified type NEC 757.4
hand 755.50
hard tissue formation in pulp 522.3
head (*see also* Anomaly, skull) 756.0
heart 746.9

Anomaly, anomalous — *continued*
heart — *continued*
auricle 746.9
bands 746.9
fibroelastosis cordis 425.3
folds 746.9
malposition 746.87
maternal, affecting fetus or newborn 760.3
obstructive NEC 746.84
patent ductus arteriosus (Botalli) 747.0
septum 745.9
acquired 429.71
aortic 745.0
aorticopulmonary 745.0
atrial 745.5
auricular 745.5
between aorta and pulmonary artery 745.0
endocardial cushion type 745.60
specified type NEC 745.69
interatrial 745.5
interventricular 745.4
with pulmonary stenosis or atresia, dextraposition of aorta, and hypertrophy of right ventricle 745.2
acquired 429.71
specified type NEC 745.8
ventricular 745.4
with pulmonary stenosis or atresia, dextraposition of aorta, and hypertrophy of right ventricle 745.2
acquired 429.71
specified type NEC 746.89
tetralogy of Fallot 745.2
valve NEC 746.9
aortic 746.9
atresia 746.89
bicuspid valve 746.4
insufficiency 746.4
specified type NEC 746.89
stenosis 746.3
subaortic 746.81
supravalvular 747.22
mitral 746.9
atresia 746.89
insufficiency 746.6
specified type NEC 746.89
stenosis 746.5
pulmonary 746.00
atresia 746.01
insufficiency 746.09
stenosis 746.02
infundibular 746.83
subvalvular 746.83
tricuspid 746.9
atresia 746.1
stenosis 746.1
ventricle 746.9
heel 755.67
Hegglin's 288.2
hemianencephaly 740.0
hemicephaly 740.0
hemicrania 740.0
hepatic duct 751.60
hip (joint) 755.63
hourglass
bladder 753.8
gallbladder 751.69
stomach 750.7
humerus 755.50
hymen 752.40
hypersegmentation of neutrophils, hereditary 288.2
hypophyseal 759.2
ileocecal (coil) (valve) 751.5
ileum (intestine) 751.5
ilium 755.60
integument 757.9
specified type NEC 757.8

☑ Additional Digit Required — Refer to the Tabular List for Digit Selection ▽ Subterms under main terms may continue to next column or page

2008 ICD-9-CM ▶◀ Revised Text ● New Line ▲ Revised Code Volume 2 — 23

**Anomaly, anomalous** — *continued*
  interarch distance (excessive) (inadequate) 524.28
  intervertebral cartilage or disc 756.10
  intestine (large) (small) 751.5
    fixational type 751.4
  iris 743.9
    specified type NEC 743.46
  ischium 755.60
  jaw NEC 524.9
    closure 524.51
    size (major) NEC 524.00
    specified type NEC 524.89
  jaw-cranial base relationship 524.10
    specified NEC 524.19
  jejunum 751.5
  joint 755.9
    hip
      dislocation (*see also* Dislocation, hip, congenital) 754.30
      predislocation (*see also* Subluxation, congenital, hip) 754.32
      preluxation (*see also* Subluxation, congenital, hip) 754.32
      subluxation (*see also* Subluxation, congenital, hip) 754.32
    lumbosacral 756.10
      spondylolisthesis 756.12
      spondylosis 756.11
    multiple arthrogryposis 754.89
    sacroiliac 755.69
  Jordan's 288.2
  kidney(s) (calyx) (pelvis) 753.9
    vessel 747.62
  Klippel-Feil (brevicollis) 756.16
  knee (joint) 755.64
  labium (majus) (minus) 752.40
  labyrinth, membranous (causing impairment of hearing) 744.05
  lacrimal
    apparatus, duct or passage 743.9
      specified type NEC 743.65
    gland 743.9
      specified type NEC 743.64
  Langdon Down (mongolism) 758.0
  larynx, laryngeal (muscle) 748.3
    web, webbed 748.2
  leg (lower) (upper) 755.60
    reduction NEC (*see also* Deformity, reduction, lower limb) 755.30
  lens 743.9
    shape 743.36
    specified type NEC 743.39
  leukocytes, genetic 288.2
    granulation (constitutional) 288.2
  lid (fold) 743.9
  ligament 756.9
    broad 752.10
    round 752.9
  limb, except reduction deformity 755.9
    lower 755.60
      reduction deformity (*see also* Deformity, reduction, lower limb) 755.30
      specified type NEC 755.69
    upper 755.50
      reduction deformity (*see also* Deformity, reduction, upper limb) 755.20
      specified type NEC 755.59
  lip 750.9
    harelip (*see also* Cleft, lip) 749.10
    specified type NEC 750.26
  liver (duct) 751.60
    atresia 751.69
  lower extremity 755.60
    vessel 747.64
  lumbosacral (joint) (region) 756.10
  lung (fissure) (lobe) NEC 748.60
    agenesis 748.5
    specified type NEC 748.69
  lymphatic system 759.9
  Madelung's (radius) 755.54

**Anomaly, anomalous** — *continued*
  mandible 524.9
    size NEC 524.00
  maxilla 524.9
    size NEC 524.00
  May (-Hegglin) 288.2
  meatus urinarius 753.9
    specified type NEC 753.8
  meningeal bands or folds, constriction of 742.8
  meninges 742.9
    brain 742.4
    spinal 742.59
  meningocele (*see also* Spina bifida) 741.9 ☑
    acquired 349.2
  mesentery 751.9
  metacarpus 755.50
  metatarsus 755.67
  middle ear, except ossicles (causing impairment of hearing) 744.03
    ossicles 744.04
  mitral (leaflets) (valve) 746.9
    atresia 746.89
    insufficiency 746.6
    specified type NEC 746.89
    stenosis 746.5
  mouth 750.9
    specified type NEC 750.26
  multiple NEC 759.7
    specified type NEC 759.89
  muscle 756.9
    eye 743.9
      specified type NEC 743.69
    specified type NEC 756.89
  musculoskeletal system, except limbs 756.9
    specified type NEC 756.9
  nail 757.9
    specified type NEC 757.5
  narrowness, eyelid 743.62
  nasal sinus or septum 748.1
  neck (any part) 744.9
    specified type NEC 744.89
  nerve 742.9
    acoustic 742.9
      specified type NEC 742.8
    optic 742.9
      specified type NEC 742.8
    specified type NEC 742.8
  nervous system NEC 742.9
    brain 742.9
      specified type NEC 742.4
    specified type NEC 742.8
  neurological 742.9
  nipple 757.6
  nonteratogenic NEC 754.89
  nose, nasal (bone) (cartilage) (septum) (sinus) 748.1
  ocular muscle 743.9
  omphalomesenteric duct 751.0
  opening, pulmonary veins 747.49
  optic
    disc 743.9
      specified type NEC 743.57
    nerve 742.9
  opticociliary vessels 743.9
  orbit (eye) 743.9
    specified type NEC 743.66
  organ
    of Corti (causing impairment of hearing) 744.05
    or site 759.9
      specified type NEC 759.89
  origin
    both great arteries from same ventricle 745.11
    coronary artery 746.85
    innominate artery 747.69
    left coronary artery from pulmonary artery 746.85
    pulmonary artery 747.3
    renal vessels 747.62
    subclavian artery (left) (right) 747.21
  osseous meatus (ear) 744.03

**Anomaly, anomalous** — *continued*
  ovary 752.0
  oviduct 752.10
  palate (hard) (soft) 750.9
    cleft (*see also* Cleft, palate) 749.00
  pancreas (duct) 751.7
  papillary muscles 746.9
  parathyroid gland 759.2
  paraurethral ducts 753.9
  parotid (gland) 750.9
  patella 755.64
  Pelger-Huët (hereditary hyposegmentation) 288.2
  pelvic girdle 755.60
    specified type NEC 755.69
  pelvis (bony) 755.60
    complicating delivery 653.0 ☑
    rachitic 268.1
      fetal 756.4
  penis (glans) 752.69
  pericardium 746.89
  peripheral vascular system NEC 747.60
    gastrointestinal 747.61
    lower limb 747.64
    renal 747.62
    specified site NEC 747.69
    spinal 747.82
    upper limb 747.63
  Peter's 743.44
  pharynx 750.9
    branchial cleft 744.41
    specified type NEC 750.29
  Pierre Robin 756.0
  pigmentation 709.00
    congenital 757.33
    specified NEC 709.09
  pituitary (gland) 759.2
  pleural folds 748.8
  portal vein 747.40
  position tooth, teeth 524.30
    crowding 524.31
    displacement 524.30
      horizontal 524.33
      vertical 524.34
    distance
      interocclusal
        excessive 524.37
        insufficient 524.36
    excessive spacing 524.32
    rotation 524.35
    specified NEC 524.39
  preauricular sinus 744.46
  prepuce 752.9
  prostate 752.9
  pulmonary 748.60
    artery 747.3
    circulation 747.3
    specified type NEC 748.69
    valve 746.00
      atresia 746.01
      insufficiency 746.09
      specified type NEC 746.09
      stenosis 746.02
        infundibular 746.83
        subvalvular 746.83
    vein 747.40
    venous
      connection 747.49
        partial 747.42
        total 747.41
      return 747.49
        partial 747.42
        total (TAPVR) (complete) (subdiaphragmatic) (supradiaphragmatic) 747.41
  pupil 743.9
  pylorus 750.9
    hypertrophy 750.5
    stenosis 750.5
  rachitic, fetal 756.4
  radius 755.50
  rectovaginal (septum) 752.40
  rectum 751.5
  refraction 367.9

**Anomaly, anomalous** — *continued*
  renal 753.9
    vessel 747.62
  respiratory system 748.9
    specified type NEC 748.8
  rib 756.3
    cervical 756.2
  Rieger's 743.44
  rings, trachea 748.3
  rotation (*see also* Malrotation)
    hip or thigh (*see also* Subluxation, congenital, hip) 754.32
  round ligament 752.9
  sacroiliac (joint) 755.69
  sacrum 756.10
  saddle
    back 754.2
    nose 754.0
      syphilitic 090.5
  salivary gland or duct 750.9
    specified type NEC 750.26
  scapula 755.50
  sclera 743.9
    specified type NEC 743.47
  scrotum 752.9
  sebaceous gland 757.9
  seminal duct or tract 752.9
  sense organs 742.9
    specified type NEC 742.8
  septum
    heart — *see* Anomaly, heart, septum
    nasal 748.1
  sex chromosomes NEC (*see also* Anomaly, chromosomes) 758.81
  shoulder (girdle) (joint) 755.50
    specified type NEC 755.59
  sigmoid (flexure) 751.5
  sinus of Valsalva 747.29
  site NEC 759.9
  skeleton generalized NEC 756.50
  skin (appendage) 757.9
    specified type NEC 757.39
  skull (bone) 756.0
    with
      anencephalus 740.0
      encephalocele 742.0
      hydrocephalus 742.3
        with spina bifida (*see also* Spina bifida) 741.0 ☑
      microcephalus 742.1
  specified type NEC
    adrenal (gland) 759.1
    alimentary tract (complete) (partial) 751.8
      lower 751.5
      upper 750.8
    ankle 755.69
    anus, anal (canal) 751.5
    aorta, aortic 747.29
      arch 747.21
    appendix 751.5
    arm 755.59
    artery (peripheral) NEC (*see also* Anomaly, peripheral vascular system) 747.60
      brain 747.81
      coronary 746.85
      eye 743.58
      pulmonary 747.3
      retinal 743.58
      umbilical 747.5
    auditory canal 744.29
      causing impairment of hearing 744.02
    bile duct or passage 751.69
    bladder 753.8
      neck 753.8
    bone(s) 756.9
      arm 755.59
      face 756.0
      leg 755.69
      pelvic girdle 755.69
      shoulder girdle 755.59
      skull 756.0

☑ Additional Digit Required — Refer to the Tabular List for Digit Selection         Subterms under main terms may continue to next column or page

24 — Volume 2      ▶◀ Revised Text      ● New Line      ▲ Revised Code      *2008 ICD-9-CM*

**Anomaly, anomalous** — *continued*
  specified type — *continued*
    bone(s) — *continued*
      skull — *continued*
        with
          anencephalus 740.0
          encephalocele 742.0
          hydrocephalus 742.3
            with spina bifida (*see also* Spina bifida) 741.0 ☑
          microcephalus 742.1
    brain 742.4
    breast 757.6
    broad ligament 752.19
    bronchus 748.3
    canal of Nuck 752.89
    cardiac septal closure 745.8
    carpus 755.59
    cartilaginous 756.9
    cecum 751.5
    cervix 752.49
    chest (wall) 756.3
    chin 744.89
    ciliary body 743.46
    circulatory system 747.89
    clavicle 755.51
    clitoris 752.49
    coccyx 756.19
    colon 751.5
    common duct 751.69
    connective tissue 756.89
    cricoid cartilage 748.3
    cystic duct 751.69
    diaphragm 756.6
    digestive organ(s) or tract 751.8
      lower 751.5
      upper 750.8
    duodenum 751.5
    ear 744.29
      auricle 744.29
        causing impairment of hearing 744.02
      causing impairment of hearing 744.09
      inner (causing impairment of hearing) 744.05
      middle, except ossicles 744.03
        ossicles 744.04
    ejaculatory duct 752.89
    endocrine 759.2
    epiglottis 748.3
    esophagus 750.4
    Eustachian tube 744.24
    eye 743.8
      lid 743.63
      muscle 743.69
    face 744.89
      bone(s) 756.0
    fallopian tube 752.19
    fascia 756.89
    femur 755.69
    fibula 755.69
    finger 755.59
    foot 755.67
    fovea centralis 743.55
    gallbladder 751.69
    Gartner's duct 752.89
    gastrointestinal tract 751.8
    genitalia, genital organ(s)
      female 752.89
        external 752.49
        internal NEC 752.89
      male 752.89
        penis 752.69
        scrotal transposition 752.81
    genitourinary tract NEC 752.89
    glottis 748.3
    hair 757.4
    hand 755.59
    heart 746.89
      valve NEC 746.89
        pulmonary 746.09
    hepatic duct 751.69
    hydatid of Morgagni 752.89
    hymen 752.49

**Anomaly, anomalous** — *continued*
  specified type — *continued*
    integument 757.8
    intestine (large) (small) 751.5
      fixational type 751.4
    iris 743.46
    jejunum 751.5
    joint 755.8
    kidney 753.3
    knee 755.64
    labium (majus) (minus) 752.49
    labyrinth, membranous 744.05
    larynx 748.3
    leg 755.69
    lens 743.39
    limb, except reduction deformity 755.8
      lower 755.69
        reduction deformity (*see also* Deformity, reduction, lower limb) 755.30
      upper 755.59
        reduction deformity (*see also* Deformity, reduction, upper limb) 755.20
    lip 750.26
    liver 751.69
    lung (fissure) (lobe) 748.69
    meatus urinarius 753.8
    metacarpus 755.59
    mouth 750.26
    muscle 756.89
      eye 743.69
    musculoskeletal system, except limbs 756.9
    nail 757.5
    neck 744.89
    nerve 742.8
      acoustic 742.8
      optic 742.8
    nervous system 742.8
    nipple 757.6
    nose 748.1
    organ NEC 759.89
      of Corti 744.05
    osseous meatus (ear) 744.03
    ovary 752.0
    oviduct 752.19
    pancreas 751.7
    parathyroid 759.2
    patella 755.64
    pelvic girdle 755.69
    penis 752.69
    pericardium 746.89
    peripheral vascular system NEC (*see also* Anomaly, peripheral vascular system) 747.60
    pharynx 750.29
    pituitary 759.2
    prostate 752.89
    radius 755.59
    rectum 751.5
    respiratory system 748.8
    rib 756.3
    round ligament 752.89
    sacrum 756.19
    salivary duct or gland 750.26
    scapula 755.59
    sclera 743.47
    scrotum 752.89
      transposition 752.81
    seminal duct or tract 752.89
    shoulder girdle 755.59
    site NEC 759.89
    skin 757.39
    skull (bone(s)) 756.0
      with
        anencephalus 740.0
        encephalocele 742.0
        hydrocephalus 742.3
          with spina bifida (*see also* Spina bifida) 741.0 ☑
        microcephalus 742.1
    specified organ or site NEC 759.89
    spermatic cord 752.89

**Anomaly, anomalous** — *continued*
  specified type — *continued*
    spinal cord 742.59
    spine 756.19
    spleen 759.0
    sternum 756.3
    stomach 750.7
    tarsus 755.67
    tendon 756.89
    testis 752.89
    thorax (wall) 756.3
    thymus 759.2
    thyroid (gland) 759.2
      cartilage 748.3
    tibia 755.69
    toe 755.66
    tongue 750.19
    trachea (cartilage) 748.3
    ulna 755.59
    urachus 753.7
    ureter 753.4
      obstructive 753.29
    urethra 753.8
      obstructive 753.6
    urinary tract 753.8
    uterus 752.3
    uvula 750.26
    vagina 752.49
    vascular NEC (*see also* Anomaly, peripheral vascular system) 747.60
      brain 747.81
    vas deferens 752.89
    vein(s) (peripheral) NEC (*see also* Anomaly, peripheral vascular system) 747.60
      brain 747.81
      great 747.49
      portal 747.49
      pulmonary 747.49
    vena cava (inferior) (superior) 747.49
    vertebra 756.19
    vulva 752.49
  spermatic cord 752.9
  spine, spinal 756.10
    column 756.10
    cord 742.9
      meningocele (*see also* Spina bifida) 741.9 ☑
      specified type NEC 742.59
      spina bifida (*see also* Spina bifida) 741.9 ☑
      vessel 747.82
    meninges 742.59
    nerve root 742.9
  spleen 759.0
  Sprengel's 755.52
  sternum 756.3
  stomach 750.9
    specified type NEC 750.7
  submaxillary gland 750.9
  superior vena cava 747.40
  talipes — *see* Talipes
  tarsus 755.67
    with complete absence of distal elements 755.31
  teeth, tooth NEC 520.9
    position 524.30
      crowding 524.31
      displacement 524.30
        horizontal 524.33
        vertical 524.34
      distance
        interocclusal
          excessive 524.37
          insufficient 524.36
      excessive spacing 524.32
      rotation 524.35
      specified NEC 524.39
    spacing 524.30
  tendon 756.9
    specified type NEC 756.89
  termination
    coronary artery 746.85
  testis 752.9

**Anomaly, anomalous** — *continued*
  thebesian valve 746.9
  thigh 755.60
    flexion (*see also* Subluxation, congenital, hip) 754.32
  thorax (wall) 756.3
  throat 750.9
  thumb 755.50
    supernumerary 755.01
  thymus gland 759.2
  thyroid (gland) 759.2
    cartilage 748.3
  tibia 755.60
    saber 090.5
  toe 755.66
    supernumerary 755.02
    webbed (*see also* Syndactylism, toes) 755.13
  tongue 750.10
    specified type NEC 750.19
  trachea, tracheal 748.3
    cartilage 748.3
    rings 748.3
  tragus 744.3
  transverse aortic arch 747.21
  trichromata 368.59
  trichromatopsia 368.59
  tricuspid (leaflet) (valve) 746.9
    atresia 746.1
    Ebstein's 746.2
    specified type NEC 746.89
    stenosis 746.1
  trunk 759.9
  Uhl's (hypoplasia of myocardium, right ventricle) 746.84
  ulna 755.50
  umbilicus 759.9
    artery 747.5
  union, trachea with larynx 748.3
  unspecified site 759.9
  upper extremity 755.50
    vessel 747.63
  urachus 753.7
    specified type NEC 753.7
  ureter 753.9
    obstructive 753.20
    specified type NEC 753.4
      obstructive 753.29
  urethra (valve) 753.9
    obstructive 753.6
    specified type NEC 753.8
  urinary tract or system (any part, except urachus) 753.9
    specified type NEC 753.8
    urachus 753.7
  uterus 752.3
    with only one functioning horn 752.3
    in pregnancy or childbirth 654.0 ☑
      affecting fetus or newborn 763.89
      causing obstructed labor 660.2 ☑
        affecting fetus or newborn 763.1
  uvula 750.9
  vagina 752.40
  valleculae 748.3
  valve (heart) NEC 746.9
    formation, ureter 753.29
    pulmonary 746.00
    specified type NEC 746.89
  vascular NEC (*see also* Anomaly, peripheral vascular system) 747.60
    ring 747.21
  vas deferens 752.9
  vein(s) (peripheral) NEC (*see also* Anomaly, peripheral vascular system) 747.60
    brain 747.81
    cerebral 747.81
    coronary 746.89
    great 747.40
      specified type NEC 747.49
    portal 747.40

☑ Additional Digit Required — Refer to the Tabular List for Digit Selection      ▽ Subterms under main terms may continue to next column or page

*2008 ICD-9-CM*      ▶◀ Revised Text      ● New Line      ▲ Revised Code      **Volume 2 — 25**

**Anomaly, anomalous** — *continued*
vein(s) (*see also* Anomaly, peripheral vascular system) — *continued*
pulmonary 747.40
retina 743.9
vena cava (inferior) (superior) 747.40
venous return (pulmonary) 747.49
partial 747.42
total 747.41
ventricle, ventricular (heart) 746.9
bands 746.9
folds 746.9
septa 745.4
vertebra 756.10
vesicourethral orifice 753.9
vessels NEC (*see also* Anomaly, peripheral vascular system) 747.60
optic papilla 743.9
vitelline duct 751.0
vitreous humor 743.9
specified type NEC 743.51
vulva 752.40
wrist (joint) 755.50
**Anomia** 784.69
**Anonychia** 757.5
acquired 703.8
**Anophthalmos, anophthalmus** (clinical) (congenital) (globe) 743.00
acquired V45.78
**Anopsia** (altitudinal) (quadrant) 368.46
**Anorchia** 752.89
**Anorchism, anorchidism** 752.89
**Anorexia** 783.0
hysterical 300.11
nervosa 307.1
**Anosmia** — *see also* Disturbance, sensation 781.1
hysterical 300.11
postinfectional 478.9
psychogenic 306.7
traumatic 951.8
**Anosognosia** 780.99
**Anosphrasia** 781.1
**Anosteoplasia** 756.50
**Anotia** 744.09
**Anovulatory cycle** 628.0
**Anoxemia** 799.02
newborn 770.88
**Anoxia** 799.02
altitude 993.2
cerebral 348.1
with
abortion — *see* Abortion, by type, with specified complication NEC
ectopic pregnancy (*see also* categories 633.0–633.9) 639.8
molar pregnancy (*see also* categories 630–632) 639.8
complicating
delivery (cesarean) (instrumental) 669.4 ☑
ectopic or molar pregnancy 639.8
obstetric anesthesia or sedation 668.2 ☑
during or resulting from a procedure 997.01
following
abortion 639.8
ectopic or molar pregnancy 639.8
newborn (*see also* Distress, fetal, liveborn infant) 770.88
due to drowning 994.1
fetal, affecting newborn 770.88
heart — *see* Insufficiency, coronary
high altitude 993.2
intrauterine
fetal death (before onset of labor) 768.0
during labor 768.1
liveborn infant — *see* Distress, fetal, liveborn infant

**Anoxia** — *continued*
myocardial — *see* Insufficiency, coronary
newborn 768.9
mild or moderate 768.6
severe 768.5
pathological 799.02
**Anteflexion** — *see* Anteversion
**Antenatal**
care, normal pregnancy V22.1
first V22.0
screening of mother (for) V28.9
based on amniocentesis NEC V28.2
chromosomal anomalies V28.0
raised alphafetoprotein levels V28.1
chromosomal anomalies V28.0
fetal growth retardation using ulatrasonics V28.4
isoimmunization V28.5
malformations using ulatrasonics V28.3
raised alphafetoprotein levels in amniotic fluid V28.1
specified condition NEC V28.8
Streptococcus B V28.6
**Antepartum** — *see* condition
**Anterior** — *see also* condition
spinal artery compression syndrome 721.1
**Antero-occlusion** 524.24
**Anteversion**
cervix — *see* Anteversion, uterus
femur (neck), congenital 755.63
uterus, uterine (cervix) (postinfectional) (postpartal, old) 621.6
congenital 752.3
in pregnancy or childbirth 654.4 ☑
affecting fetus or newborn 763.89
causing obstructed labor 660.2 ☑
affecting fetus or newborn 763.1
**Anthracosilicosis** (occupational) 500
**Anthracosis** (lung) (occupational) 500
lingua 529.3
**Anthrax** 022.9
with pneumonia 022.1 *[484.5]*
colitis 022.2
cutaneous 022.0
gastrointestinal 022.2
intestinal 022.2
pulmonary 022.1
respiratory 022.1
septicemia 022.3
specified manifestation NEC 022.8
**Anthropoid pelvis** 755.69
with disproportion (fetopelvic) 653.2 ☑
affecting fetus or newborn 763.1
causing obstructed labor 660.1 ☑
affecting fetus or newborn 763.1
**Anthropophobia** 300.29
**Antibioma, breast** 611.0
**Antibodies**
maternal (blood group) (*see also* Incompatibility) 656.2 ☑
anti-D, cord blood 656.1 ☑
fetus or newborn 773.0
**Antibody deficiency syndrome**
agammaglobulinemic 279.00
congenital 279.04
hypogammaglobulinemic 279.00
**Anticoagulant, circulating** — *see also* Circulating anticoagulants 286.5
**Antimongolism syndrome** 758.39
**Antimonial cholera** 985.4
**Antisocial personality** 301.7
**Antithrombinemia** — *see also* Circulating anticoagulants 286.5
**Antithromboplastinemia** — *see also* Circulating anticoagulants 286.5
**Antithromboplastinogenemia** — *see also* Circulating anticoagulants 286.5

**Antitoxin complication or reaction** — *see* Complications, vaccination
**Anton (-Babinski) syndrome** (hemiasomatognosia) 307.9
**Antritis** (chronic) 473.0
maxilla 473.0
acute 461.0
stomach 535.4 ☑
**Antrum, antral** — *see* condition
**Anuria** 788.5
with
abortion — *see* Abortion, by type, with renal failure
ectopic pregnancy (*see also* categories 633.0–633.9) 639.3
molar pregnancy (*see also* categories 630–632) 639.3
calculus (impacted) (recurrent) 592.9
kidney 592.0
ureter 592.1
congenital 753.3
due to a procedure 997.5
following
abortion 639.3
ectopic or molar pregnancy 639.3
newborn 753.3
postrenal 593.4
puerperal, postpartum, childbirth 669.3 ☑
specified as due to a procedure 997.5
sulfonamide
correct substance properly administered 788.5
overdose or wrong substance given or taken 961.0
traumatic (following crushing) 958.5
**Anus, anal** — *see* condition
**Anusitis** 569.49
**Anxiety** (neurosis) (reaction) (state) 300.00
alcohol-induced 291.89
depression 300.4
drug-induced 292.89
due to or associated with physical condition 293.84
generalized 300.02
hysteria 300.20
in
acute stress reaction 308.0
transient adjustment reaction 309.24
panic type 300.01
separation, abnormal 309.21
syndrome (organic) (transient) 293.84
**Aorta, aortic** — *see* condition
**Aortectasia** 441.9
**Aortitis** (nonsyphilitic) 447.6
arteriosclerotic 440.0
calcific 447.6
Döhle-Heller 093.1
luetic 093.1
rheumatic (*see also* Endocarditis, acute, rheumatic) 391.1
rheumatoid — *see* Arthritis, rheumatoid
specific 093.1
syphilitic 093.1
congenital 090.5
**Apathetic thyroid storm** — *see also* Thyrotoxicosis 242.9 ☑
**Apepsia** 536.8
achlorhydric 536.0
psychogenic 306.4
**Aperistalsis, esophagus** 530.0
**Apert-Gallais syndrome** (adrenogenital) 255.2
**Apertognathia** 524.20
**Apert's syndrome** (acrocephalosyndactyly) 755.55
**Aphagia** 787.20 ▲
psychogenic 307.1
**Aphakia** (acquired) (bilateral) (postoperative) (unilateral) 379.31
congenital 743.35
**Aphalangia** (congenital) 755.4

**Aphalangia** — *continued*
lower limb (complete) (intercalary) (partial) (terminal) 755.39
meaning all digits (complete) (partial) 755.31
transverse 755.31
upper limb (complete) (intercalary) (partial) (terminal) 755.29
meaning all digits (complete) (partial) 755.21
transverse 755.21
**Aphasia** (amnestic) (ataxic) (auditory) (Broca's) (choreatic) (classic) (expressive) (global) (ideational) (ideokinetic) (ideomotor) (jargon) (motor) (nominal) (receptive) (semantic) (sensory) (syntactic) (verbal) (visual) (Wernicke's) 784.3
developmental 315.31
syphilis, tertiary 094.89
uremic — *see* Uremia
**Aphemia** 784.3
uremic — *see* Uremia
**Aphonia** 784.41
clericorum 784.49
hysterical 300.11
organic 784.41
psychogenic 306.1
**Aphthae, aphthous** — *see also* condition
Bednar's 528.2
cachectic 529.0
epizootic 078.4
fever 078.4
oral 528.2
stomatitis 528.2
thrush 112.0
ulcer (oral) (recurrent) 528.2
genital organ(s) NEC
female 616.50 ▲
male 608.89
larynx 478.79
**Apical** — *see* condition
**Apical ballooning syndrome** 429.83
**Aplasia** — *see also* Agenesis
alveolar process (acquired) 525.8
congenital 750.26
aorta (congenital) 747.22
aortic valve (congenital) 746.89
axialis extracorticalis (congenital) 330.0
bone marrow (myeloid) 284.9
acquired (secondary) 284.89 ▲
congenital 284.01
idiopathic 284.9
brain 740.0
specified part 742.2
breast 757.6
bronchus 748.3
cementum 520.4
cerebellar 742.2
congenital (pure) red cell 284.01
corpus callosum 742.2
erythrocyte 284.81 ▲
congenital 284.01
extracortical axial 330.0
eye (congenital) 743.00
fovea centralis (congenital) 743.55
germinal (cell) 606.0
iris 743.45
labyrinth, membranous 744.05
limb (congenital) 755.4
lower NEC 755.30
upper NEC 755.20
lung (bilateral) (congenital) (unilateral) 748.5
nervous system NEC 742.8
nuclear 742.8
ovary 752.0
Pelizaeus-Merzbacher 330.0
prostate (congenital) 752.89
red cell (with thymoma) ▶(adult)◀ 284.81 ▲
acquired (secondary) 284.81 ▲
congenital 284.01
hereditary 284.01
of infants 284.01

**Aplasia** — *see also* Agenesis — *continued*
  red cell — *continued*
    primary 284.01
    pure 284.01
  round ligament (congenital) 752.89
  salivary gland 750.21
  skin (congenital) 757.39
  spinal cord 742.59
  spleen 759.0
  testis (congenital) 752.89
  thymic, with immunodeficiency 279.2
  thyroid 243
  uterus 752.3
  ventral horn cell 742.59
**Apleuria** 756.3
**Apnea, apneic** (spells) 786.03
  newborn, neonatorum 770.81
    essential 770.81
    obstructive 770.82
    primary 770.81
    sleep 770.81
    specified NEC 770.82
  psychogenic 306.1
  sleep, unspecified 780.57
    with
      hypersomnia, unspecified 780.53
      hyposomnia, unspecified 780.51
      insomnia, unspecified 780.51
      sleep disturbance 780.57
    central, in conditions classified elsewhere 327.27
    obstructive (adult) (pediatric) 327.23
    organic 327.20
    other 327.29
    primary central 327.21
**Apneumatosis newborn** 770.4
**Apodia** 755.31
**Aponeurosis** 726.90
**Apophysitis** (bone) — *see also* Osteochondrosis 732.9
  calcaneus 732.5
  juvenile 732.6
**Apoplectiform convulsions** — *see also* Disease, cerebrovascular, acute 436
**Apoplexia, apoplexy, apoplectic** — *see also* Disease, cerebrovascular, acute 436
  abdominal 569.89
  adrenal 036.3
  attack 436
  basilar (*see also* Disease, cerebrovascular, acute) 436
  brain (*see also* Disease, cerebrovascular, acute) 436
  bulbar (*see also* Disease, cerebrovascular, acute) 436
  capillary (*see also* Disease, cerebrovascular, acute) 436
  cardiac (*see also* Infarct, myocardium) 410.9 ☑
  cerebral (*see also* Disease, cerebrovascular, acute) 436
  chorea (*see also* Disease, cerebrovascular, acute) 436
  congestive (*see also* Disease, cerebrovascular, acute) 436
    newborn 767.4
  embolic (*see also* Embolism, brain) 434.1 ☑
  fetus 767.0
  fit (*see also* Disease, cerebrovascular, acute) 436
  healed or old V12.54 ▲
  heart (auricle) (ventricle) (*see also* Infarct, myocardium) 410.9 ☑
  heat 992.0
  hemiplegia (*see also* Disease, cerebrovascular, acute) 436
  hemorrhagic (stroke) (*see also* Hemorrhage, brain) 432.9
  ingravescent (*see also* Disease, cerebrovascular, acute) 436

**Apoplexia, apoplexy, apoplectic** — *see also* Disease, cerebrovascular, acute — *continued*
  late effect — *see* Late effect(s) (of) cerebrovascular disease
  lung — *see* Embolism, pulmonary
  meninges, hemorrhagic (*see also* Hemorrhage, subarachnoid) 430
  neonatorum 767.0
  newborn 767.0
  pancreatitis 577.0
  placenta 641.2 ☑
  progressive (*see also* Disease, cerebrovascular, acute) 436
  pulmonary (artery) (vein) — *see* Embolism, pulmonary
  sanguineous (*see also* Disease, cerebrovascular, acute) 436
  seizure (*see also* Disease, cerebrovascular, acute) 436
  serous (*see also* Disease, cerebrovascular, acute) 436
  spleen 289.59
  stroke (*see also* Disease, cerebrovascular, acute) 436
  thrombotic (*see also* Thrombosis, brain) 434.0 ☑
  uremic — *see* Uremia
  uteroplacental 641.2 ☑
**Appendage**
  fallopian tube (cyst of Morgagni) 752.11
  intestine (epiploic) 751.5
  preauricular 744.1
  testicular (organ of Morgagni) 752.89
**Appendicitis** 541
  with
    perforation, peritonitis (generalized), or rupture 540.0
      with peritoneal abscess 540.1
    peritoneal abscess 540.1
  acute (catarrhal) (fulminating) (gangrenous) (inflammatory) (obstructive) (retrocecal) (suppurative) 540.9
    with
      perforation, peritonitis, or rupture 540.0
        with peritoneal abscess 540.1
      peritoneal abscess 540.1
  amebic 006.8
  chronic (recurrent) 542
  exacerbation — *see* Appendicitis, acute
  fulminating — *see* Appendicitis, acute
  gangrenous — *see* Appendicitis, acute
  healed (obliterative) 542
  interval 542
  neurogenic 542
  obstructive 542
  pneumococcal 541
  recurrent 542
  relapsing 542
  retrocecal 541
  subacute (adhesive) 542
  subsiding 542
  suppurative — *see* Appendicitis, acute
  tuberculous (*see also* Tuberculosis) 014.8 ☑
**Appendiclausis** 543.9
**Appendicolithiasis** 543.9
**Appendicopathia oxyurica** 127.4
**Appendix, appendicular** — *see also* condition
  Morgagni (male) 752.89
  fallopian tube 752.11
**Appetite**
  depraved 307.52
  excessive 783.6
    psychogenic 307.51
  lack or loss (*see also* Anorexia) 783.0
    nonorganic origin 307.59
  perverted 307.52
    hysterical 300.11

**Apprehension, apprehensiveness** (abnormal) (state) 300.00
  specified type NEC 300.09
**Approximal wear** 521.10
**Apraxia** (classic) (ideational) (ideokinetic) (ideomotor) (motor) 784.69
  oculomotor, congenital 379.51
  verbal 784.69
**Aptyalism** 527.7
**Aqueous misdirection** 365.83
**Arabicum elephantiasis** — *see also* Infestation, filarial 125.9
**Arachnidism** 989.5
**Arachnitis** — *see* Meningitis
**Arachnodactyly** 759.82
**Arachnoidism** 989.5
**Arachnoiditis** (acute) (adhesive) (basic) (brain) (cerebrospinal) (chiasmal) (chronic) (spinal) — *see also* Meningitis 322.9
  meningococcal (chronic) 036.0
  syphilitic 094.2
  tuberculous (*see also* Tuberculosis, meninges) 013.0 ☑
**Araneism** 989.5
**Arboencephalitis, Australian** 062.4
**Arborization block** (heart) 426.6
**Arbor virus, arbovirus** (infection) NEC 066.9
**ARC** 042
**Arches** — *see* condition
**Arcuatus uterus** 752.3
**Arcus** (cornea)
  juvenilis 743.43
    interfering with vision 743.42
  senilis 371.41
**Arc-welders' lung** 503
**Arc-welders' syndrome** (photokeratitis) 370.24
**Areflexia** 796.1
**Areola** — *see* condition
**Argentaffinoma** (M8241/1) — *see also* Neoplasm, by site, uncertain behavior
  benign (M8241/0) — *see* Neoplasm, by site, benign
  malignant (M8241/3) — *see* Neoplasm, by site, malignant
  syndrome 259.2
**Argentinian hemorrhagic fever** 078.7
**Arginosuccinicaciduria** 270.6
**Argonz-Del Castillo syndrome** (nonpuerperal galactorrhea and amenorrhea) 253.1
**Argyll-Robertson phenomenon, pupil, or syndrome** (syphilitic) 094.89
  atypical 379.45
  nonluetic 379.45
  nonsyphilitic 379.45
  reversed 379.45
**Argyria, argyriasis** NEC 985.8
  conjunctiva 372.55
  cornea 371.16
  from drug or medicinal agent
    correct substance properly administered 709.09
    overdose or wrong substance given or taken 961.2
**Arhinencephaly** 742.2
**Arias-Stella phenomenon** 621.30
**Ariboflavinosis** 266.0
**Arizona enteritis** 008.1
**Arm** — *see* condition
**Armenian disease** 277.31
**Arnold-Chiari obstruction or syndrome** — *see also* Spina bifida 741.0 ☑
  type I 348.4
  type II (*see also* Spina bifida) 741.0 ☑
  type III 742.0
  type IV 742.2
**Arousals**
  confusional 327.41
**Arrest, arrested**
  active phase of labor 661.1 ☑
    affecting fetus or newborn 763.7

**Arrest, arrested** — *continued*
  any plane in pelvis
    complicating delivery 660.1 ☑
      affecting fetus or newborn 763.1
  bone marrow (*see also* Anemia, aplastic) 284.9
  cardiac 427.5
    with
      abortion — *see* Abortion, by type, with specified complication NEC
      ectopic pregnancy (*see also* categories 633.0–633.9) 639.8
      molar pregnancy (*see also* categories 630–632) 639.8
    complicating
      anesthesia
        correct substance properly administered 427.5
        obstetric 668.1 ☑
        overdose or wrong substance given 968.4
        specified anesthetic — *see* Table of Drugs and Chemicals
      delivery (cesarean) (instrumental) 669.4 ☑
      ectopic or molar pregnancy 639.8
      surgery (nontherapeutic) (therapeutic) 997.1
    fetus or newborn 779.85
    following
      abortion 639.8
      ectopic or molar pregnancy 639.8
    personal history, successfully resuscitated V12.53 ●
    postoperative (immediate) 997.1
      long-term effect of cardiac surgery 429.4
  cardiorespiratory (*see also* Arrest, cardiac) 427.5
  deep transverse 660.3 ☑
    affecting fetus or newborn 763.1
  development or growth
    bone 733.91
    child 783.40
    fetus 764.9 ☑
      affecting management of pregnancy 656.5 ☑
    tracheal rings 748.3
  epiphyseal 733.91
  granulopoiesis 288.09
  heart — *see* Arrest, cardiac
  respiratory 799.1
    newborn 770.87
  sinus 426.6
  transverse (deep) 660.3 ☑
    affecting fetus or newborn 763.1
**Arrhenoblastoma** (M8630/1)
  benign (M8630/0)
    specified site — *see* Neoplasm, by site, benign
    unspecified site
      female 220
      male 222.0
  malignant (M8630/3)
    specified site — *see* Neoplasm, by site, malignant
    unspecified site
      female 183.0
      male 186.9
  specified site — *see* Neoplasm, by site, uncertain behavior
  unspecified site
    female 236.2
    male 236.4
**Arrhinencephaly** 742.2
  due to
    trisomy 13 (13-15) 758.1
    trisomy 18 (16-18) 758.2

---

☑ Additional Digit Required — Refer to the Tabular List for Digit Selection      ⬛ᵛ Subterms under main terms may continue to next column or page

**Arrhythmia** (auricle) (cardiac) (cordis) (gallop rhythm) (juvenile) (nodal) (reflex) (sinus) (supraventricular) (transitory) (ventricle) 427.9
  bigeminal rhythm 427.89
  block 426.9
  bradycardia 427.89
  contractions, premature 427.60
  coronary sinus 427.89
  ectopic 427.89
  extrasystolic 427.60
  postoperative 997.1
  psychogenic 306.2
  vagal 780.2
**Arrillaga-Ayerza syndrome** (pulmonary artery sclerosis with pulmonary hypertension) 416.0
**Arsenical**
  dermatitis 692.4
  keratosis 692.4
  pigmentation 985.1
    from drug or medicinal agent
      correct substance properly administered 709.09
      overdose or wrong substance given or taken 961.1
**Arsenism** 985.1
  from drug or medicinal agent
    correct substance properly administered 692.4
    overdose or wrong substance given or taken 961.1
**Arterial** — *see* condition
**Arteriectasis** 447.8
**Arteriofibrosis** — *see* Arteriosclerosis
**Arteriolar sclerosis** — *see* Arteriosclerosis
**Arteriolith** — *see* Arteriosclerosis
**Arteriolitis** 447.6
  necrotizing, kidney 447.5
  renal — *see* Hypertension, kidney
**Arteriolosclerosis** — *see* Arteriosclerosis
**Arterionephrosclerosis** — *see also* Hypertension, kidney 403.90
**Arteriopathy** 447.9
**Arteriosclerosis, arteriosclerotic** (artery) (deformans) (diffuse) (disease) (endarteritis) (general) (obliterans) (obliterative) (occlusive) (senile) (with calcification) 440.9
  with
    gangrene 440.24
    psychosis (*see also* Psychosis, arteriosclerotic) 290.40
    ulceration 440.23
  aorta 440.0
  arteries of extremities — *see* Arteriosclerosis, extremities
  basilar (artery) (*see also* Occlusion, artery, basilar) 433.0 ☑
  brain 437.0
  bypass graft
    coronary artery 414.05
      autologous artery (gastroepiploic) (internal mammary) 414.04
      autologous vein 414.02
      nonautologous biological 414.03
      of transplanted heart 414.07
    extremity 440.30
      autologous vein 440.31
      nonautologous biological 440.32
  cardiac — *see* Arteriosclerosis, coronary
  cardiopathy — *see* Arteriosclerosis, coronary
  cardiorenal (*see also* Hypertension, cardiorenal) 404.90
  cardiovascular (*see also* Disease, cardiovascular) 429.2
  carotid (artery) (common) (internal) (*see also* Occlusion, artery, carotid) 433.1 ☑
  central nervous system 437.0
  cerebral 437.0

**Arteriosclerosis, arteriosclerotic** — *continued*
  cerebral — *continued*
    late effect — *see* Late effect(s) (of) cerebrovascular disease
  cerebrospinal 437.0
  cerebrovascular 437.0
  coronary (artery) 414.00
    graft — *see* Arteriosclerosis, bypass graft
    native artery 414.01
      of transplanted heart 414.06
  extremities (native artery) NEC 440.20
    bypass graft 440.30
      autologous vein 440.31
      nonautologous biological 440.32
    claudication (intermittent) 440.21
    and
      gangrene 440.24
      rest pain 440.22
      and
        gangrene 440.24
        ulceration 440.23
        and gangrene 440.24
      ulceration 440.23
        and gangrene 440.24
    gangrene 440.24
    rest pain 440.22
      and
        gangrene 440.24
        ulceration 440.23
        and gangrene 440.24
    specified site NEC 440.29
    ulceration 440.23
      and gangrene 440.24
  heart (disease) (*see also* Arteriosclerosis, coronary)
    valve 424.99
      aortic 424.1
      mitral 424.0
      pulmonary 424.3
      tricuspid 424.2
  kidney (*see also* Hypertension, kidney) 403.90
  labyrinth, labyrinthine 388.00
  medial NEC (*see also* Arteriosclerosis, extremities) 440.20
  mesentery (artery) 557.1
  Mönckeberg's (*see also* Arteriosclerosis, extremities) 440.20
  myocarditis 429.0
  nephrosclerosis (*see also* Hypertension, kidney) 403.90
  peripheral (of extremities) — *see* Arteriosclerosis, extremities
  precerebral 433.9 ☑
    specified artery NEC 433.8 ☑
  pulmonary (idiopathic) 416.0
  renal (*see also* Hypertension, kidney) 403.90
    arterioles (*see also* Hypertension, kidney) 403.90
    artery 440.1
  retinal (vascular) 440.8 *[362.13]*
  specified artery NEC 440.8
    with gangrene 440.8 *[785.4]*
  spinal (cord) 437.0
  vertebral (artery) (*see also* Occlusion, artery, vertebral) 433.2 ☑
**Arteriospasm** 443.9
**Arteriovenous** — *see* condition
**Arteritis** 447.6
  allergic (*see also* Angiitis, hypersensitivity) 446.20
  aorta (nonsyphilitic) 447.6
    syphilitic 093.1
  aortic arch 446.7
  brachiocephalica 446.7
  brain 437.4
    syphilitic 094.89
  branchial 446.7
  cerebral 437.4
    late effect — *see* Late effect(s) (of) cerebrovascular disease
    syphilitic 094.89

**Arteritis** — *continued*
  coronary (artery) (*see also* Arteriosclerosis, coronary)
    rheumatic 391.9
      chronic 398.99
    syphilitic 093.89
  cranial (left) (right) 446.5
  deformans — *see* Arteriosclerosis
  giant cell 446.5
  necrosing or necrotizing 446.0
  nodosa 446.0
  obliterans (*see also* Arteriosclerosis)
    subclaviocarotica 446.7
  pulmonary 417.8
  retina 362.18
  rheumatic — *see* Fever, rheumatic
  senile — *see* Arteriosclerosis
  suppurative 447.2
  syphilitic (general) 093.89
    brain 094.89
    coronary 093.89
    spinal 094.89
  temporal 446.5
  young female, syndrome 446.7
**Artery, arterial** — *see* condition
**Arthralgia** — *see also* Pain, joint 719.4 ☑
  allergic (*see also* Pain, joint) 719.4 ☑
  in caisson disease 993.3
  psychogenic 307.89
  rubella 056.71
  Salmonella 003.23
  temporomandibular joint 524.62
**Arthritis, arthritic** (acute) (chronic) (subacute) 716.9 ☑
  meaning Osteoarthritis — *see* Osteoarthrosis

---

*Note — Use the following fifth-digit subclassification with categories 711–712, 715–716:*

| | |
|---|---|
| *0* | *site unspecified* |
| *1* | *shoulder region* |
| *2* | *upper arm* |
| *3* | *forearm* |
| *4* | *hand* |
| *5* | *pelvic region and thigh* |
| *6* | *lower leg* |
| *7* | *ankle and foot* |
| *8* | *other specified sites* |
| *9* | *multiple sites* |

---

  allergic 716.2 ☑
  ankylosing (crippling) (spine) 720.0
    sites other than spine 716.9 ☑
  atrophic 714.0
    spine 720.9
  back (*see also* Arthritis, spine) 721.90
  Bechterew's (ankylosing spondylitis) 720.0
  blennorrhagic 098.50
  cervical, cervicodorsal (*see also* Spondylosis, cervical) 721.0
  Charcôt's 094.0 *[713.5]*
    diabetic 250.6 ☑ *[713.5]*
    syringomyelic 336.0 *[713.5]*
    tabetic 094.0 *[713.5]*
  chylous (*see also* Filariasis) 125.9 *[711.7]*
  climacteric NEC 716.3 ☑
  coccyx 721.8
  cricoarytenoid 478.79
  crystal (-induced) — *see* Arthritis, due to crystals
  deformans (*see also* Osteoarthrosis) 715.9 ☑
    spine 721.90
      with myelopathy 721.91
  degenerative (*see also* Osteoarthrosis) 715.9 ☑
    idiopathic 715.09
    polyarticular 715.09
    spine 721.90
      with myelopathy 721.91

**Arthritis, arthritic** — *continued*
  dermatoarthritis, lipoid 272.8 *[713.0]*
  due to or associated with
    acromegaly 253.0 *[713.0]*
    actinomycosis 039.8 *[711.4]* ☑
    amyloidosis 277.39 *[713.7]*
    bacterial disease NEC 040.89 *[711.4]* ☑
    Behçet's syndrome 136.1 *[711.2]* ☑
    blastomycosis 116.0 *[711.6]* ☑
    brucellosis (*see also* Brucellosis) 023.9 *[711.4]* ☑
    caisson disease 993.3
    coccidioidomycosis 114.3 *[711.6]* ☑
    coliform (Escherichia coli) 711.0 ☑
    colitis, ulcerative (*see also* Colitis, ulcerative) 556.9 *[713.1]*
    cowpox 051.0 *[711.5]* ☑
    crystals (*see also* Gout)
      dicalcium phosphate 275.49 *[712.1]* ☑
      pyrophosphate 275.49 *[712.2]* ☑
      specified NEC 275.49 *[712.8]* ☑
    dermatoarthritis, lipoid 272.8 *[713.0]*
    dermatological disorder NEC 709.9 *[713.3]*
    diabetes 250.6 ☑ *[713.5]*
    diphtheria 032.89 *[711.4]* ☑
    dracontiasis 125.7 *[711.7]* ☑
    dysentery 009.0 *[711.3]* ☑
    endocrine disorder NEC 259.9 *[713.0]*
    enteritis NEC 009.1 *[711.3]* ☑
      infectious (*see also* Enteritis, infectious)
        009.0 *[711.3]* ☑
      specified organism NEC 008.8 *[711.3]* ☑
      regional (*see also* Enteritis, regional) 555.9 *[713.1]*
      specified organism NEC 008.8 *[711.3]* ☑
    epiphyseal slip, nontraumatic (old) 716.8 ☑
    erysipelas 035 *[711.4]* ☑
    erythema
      epidemic 026.1
      multiforme 695.1 *[713.3]*
      nodosum 695.2 *[713.3]*
    Escherichia coli 711.0 ☑
    filariasis NEC 125.9 *[711.7]* ☑
    gastrointestinal condition NEC 569.9 *[713.1]*
    glanders 024 *[711.4]* ☑
    Gonococcus 098.50
    gout 274.0
    helminthiasis NEC 128.9 *[711.7]* ☑
    hematological disorder NEC 289.9 *[713.2]*
    hemochromatosis 275.0 *[713.0]*
    hemoglobinopathy NEC (*see also* Disease, hemoglobin) 282.7 *[713.2]*
    hemophilia (*see also* Hemophilia) 286.0 *[713.2]*
    Hemophilus influenzae (H. influenzae) 711.0 ☑
    Henoch (-Schönlein) purpura 287.0 *[713.6]*
    H. influenzae 711.0 ☑
    histoplasmosis NEC (*see also* Histoplasmosis) 115.99 *[711.6]* ☑
    human parvovirus 079.83 *[711.5]* ☑ ●
    hyperparathyroidism 252.00 *[713.0]*
    hypersensitivity reaction NEC 995.3 *[713.6]*
    hypogammaglobulinemia (*see also* Hypogamma-globulinemia) 279.00 *[713.0]*
    hypothyroidism NEC 244.9 *[713.0]*

**Arthritis, arthritic** — *continued*
  due to or associated with — *continued*
    infection (*see also* Arthritis, infectious) 711.9 ☑
    infectious disease NEC 136.9 [711.8] ☑
    leprosy (*see also* Leprosy) 030.9 [711.4] ☑
    leukemia NEC (M9800/3) 208.9 [713.2]
    lipoid dermatoarthritis 272.8 [713.0]
    Lyme disease 088.81 [711.8] ☑
    Mediterranean fever, familial 277.31 [713.7]
    meningococcal infection 036.82
    metabolic disorder NEC 277.9 [713.0]
    multiple myelomatosis (M9730/3) 203.0 [713.2]
    mumps 072.79 [711.5] ☑
    mycobacteria 031.8 [711.4] ☑
    mycosis NEC 117.9 [711.6] ☑
    neurological disorder NEC 349.9 [713.5]
    ochronosis 270.2 [713.0]
    O'Nyong Nyong 066.3 [711.5] ☑
    parasitic disease NEC 136.9 [711.8] ☑
    paratyphoid fever (*see also* Fever, paratyphoid) 002.9 [711.3] ☑
    parvovirus B19 079.83 [711.5] ☑ ●
    Pneumococcus 711.0 ☑
    poliomyelitis (*see also* Poliomyelitis) 045.9 ☑ [711.5] ☑
    Pseudomonas 711.0 ☑
    psoriasis 696.0
    pyogenic organism (E. coli) (H. influenzae) (Pseudomonas) (Streptococcus) 711.0 ☑
    rat-bite fever 026.1 [711.4] ☑
    regional enteritis (*see also* Enteritis, regional) 555.9 [713.1]
    Reiter's disease 099.3 [711.1] ☑
    respiratory disorder NEC 519.9 [713.4]
    reticulosis, malignant (M9720/3) 202.3 [713.2]
    rubella 056.71
    salmonellosis 003.23
    sarcoidosis 135 [713.7]
    serum sickness 999.5 [713.6]
    Staphylococcus 711.0 ☑
    Streptococcus 711.0 ☑
    syphilis (*see also* Syphilis) 094.0 [711.4] ☑
    syringomyelia 336.0 [713.5]
    thalassemia 282.49 [713.2]
    tuberculosis (*see also* Tuberculosis, arthritis) 015.9 ☑ [711.4] ☑
    typhoid fever 002.0 [711.3] ☑
    ulcerative colitis (*see also* Colitis, ulcerative) 556.9 [713.1]
    urethritis
      nongonococcal (*see also* Urethritis, nongonococcal) 099.40 [711.1] ☑
      nonspecific (*see also* Urethritis, nongonococcal) 099.40 [711.1] ☑
      Reiter's 099.3
    viral disease NEC 079.99 [711.5] ☑
  erythema epidemic 026.1
  gonococcal 098.50
  gouty (acute) 274.0
  hypertrophic (*see also* Osteoarthrosis) 715.9 ☑
    spine 721.90
      with myelopathy 721.91
  idiopathic, blennorrheal 099.3
  in caisson disease 993.3 [713.8]
  infectious or infective (acute) (chronic) (subacute) NEC 711.9 ☑
    nonpyogenic 711.9 ☑
    spine 720.9

**Arthritis, arthritic** — *continued*
  inflammatory NEC 714.9
  juvenile rheumatoid (chronic) (polyarticular) 714.30
    acute 714.31
    monoarticular 714.33
    pauciarticular 714.32
  lumbar (*see also* Spondylosis, lumbar) 721.3
  meningococcal 036.82
  menopausal NEC 716.3 ☑
  migratory — *see* Fever, rheumatic
  neuropathic (Charcot's) 094.0 [713.5]
    diabetic 250.6 ☑ [713.5]
    nonsyphilitic NEC 349.9 [713.5]
    syringomyelic 336.0 [713.5]
    tabetic 094.0 [713.5]
  nodosa (*see also* Osteoarthrosis) 715.9 ☑
    spine 721.90
      with myelopathy 721.91
  nonpyogenic NEC 716.9 ☑
    spine 721.90
      with myelopathy 721.91
  ochronotic 270.2 [713.0]
  palindromic (see also Rheumatism, palindromic) 719.3 ☑
  pneumococcal 711.0 ☑
  postdysenteric 009.0 [711.3] ☑
  postrheumatic, chronic (Jaccoud's) 714.4
  primary progressive 714.0
    spine 720.9
  proliferative 714.0
    spine 720.0
  psoriatic 696.0
  purulent 711.0 ☑
  pyogenic or pyemic 711.0 ☑
  rheumatic 714.0
    acute or subacute — *see* Fever, rheumatic
    chronic 714.0
    spine 720.9
  rheumatoid (nodular) 714.0
    with
      splenoadenomegaly and leukopenia 714.1
      visceral or systemic involvement 714.2
    aortitis 714.89
    carditis 714.2
    heart disease 714.2
    juvenile (chronic) (polyarticular) 714.30
      acute 714.31
      monoarticular 714.33
      pauciarticular 714.32
      spine 720.0
  rubella 056.71
  sacral, sacroiliac, sacrococcygeal (*see also* Spondylosis, sacral) 721.3
  scorbutic 267
  senile or senescent (*see also* Osteoarthrosis) 715.9 ☑
    spine 721.90
      with myelopathy 721.91
  septic 711.0 ☑
  serum (nontherapeutic) (therapeutic) 999.5 [713.6]
  specified form NEC 716.8 ☑
  spine 721.90
    with myelopathy 721.91
    atrophic 720.9
    degenerative 721.90
      with myelopathy 721.91
    hypertrophic (with deformity) 721.90
      with myelopathy 721.91
    infectious or infective NEC 720.9
    Marie-Strümpell 720.0
    nonpyogenic 721.90
      with myelopathy 721.91
    pyogenic 720.9
    rheumatoid 720.0
    traumatic (old) 721.7

**Arthritis, arthritic** — *continued*
  spine — *continued*
    tuberculous (*see also* Tuberculosis) 015.0 ☑ [720.81]
  staphylococcal 711.0 ☑
  streptococcal 711.0 ☑
  suppurative 711.0 ☑
  syphilitic 094.0 [713.5]
    congenital 090.49 [713.5]
  syphilitica deformans (Charcôt) 094.0 [713.5]
  temporomandibular joint 524.69
  thoracic (*see also* Spondylosis, thoracic) 721.2
  toxic of menopause 716.3 ☑
  transient 716.4 ☑
  traumatic (chronic) (old) (post) 716.1 ☑
    current injury — *see* nature of injury
  tuberculous (*see also* Tuberculosis, arthritis) 015.9 ☑ [711.4] ☑
  urethritica 099.3 [711.1] ☑
  urica, uratic 274.0
  venereal 099.3 [711.1] ☑
  vertebral (*see also* Arthritis, spine) 721.90
  villous 716.8 ☑
  von Bechterew's 720.0

**Arthrocele** — *see also* Effusion, joint 719.0 ☑
**Arthrochondritis** — *see* Arthritis
**Arthrodesis status** V45.4
**Arthrodynia** — *see also* Pain, joint 719.4 ☑
  psychogenic 307.89
**Arthrodysplasia** 755.9
**Arthrofibrosis joint** — *see also* Ankylosis 718.5 ☑
**Arthrogryposis** 728.3
  multiplex, congenita 754.89
**Arthrokatadysis** 715.35
**Arthrolithiasis** 274.0
**Arthro-onychodysplasia** 756.89
**Arthro-osteo-onychodysplasia** 756.89
**Arthropathy** — *see also* Arthritis 716.9 ☑

*Note — Use the following fifth-digit subclassification with categories 711–712, 716:*

*0   site unspecified*
*1   shoulder region*
*2   upper arm*
*3   forearm*
*4   hand*
*5   pelvic region and thigh*
*6   lower leg*
*7   ankle and foot*
*8   other specified sites*
*9   multiple sites*

  Behçet's 136.1 [711.2] ☑
  Charcôt's 094.0 [713.5]
    diabetic 250.6 ☑ [713.5]
    syringomyelic 336.0 [713.5]
    tabetic 094.0 [713.5]
  crystal (-induced) — *see* Arthritis, due to crystals
  gouty 274.0
  neurogenic, neuropathic (Charcot's) (tabetic) 094.0 [713.5]
    diabetic 250.6 ☑ [713.5]
    nonsyphilitic NEC 349.9 [713.5]
    syringomyelic 336.0 [713.5]
  postdysenteric NEC 009.0 [711.3] ☑
  postrheumatic, chronic (Jaccoud's) 714.4
  psoriatic 696.0
  pulmonary 731.2
  specified NEC 716.8 ☑
  syringomyelia 336.0 [713.5]

**Arthropathy** — *see also* Arthritis — *continued*
  tabes dorsalis 094.0 [713.5]
  tabetic 094.0 [713.5]
  transient 716.4 ☑
  traumatic 716.1 ☑
  uric acid 274.0
**Arthrophyte** — *see also* Loose, body, joint 718.1 ☑
**Arthrophytis** 719.80
  ankle 719.87
  elbow 719.82
  foot 719.87
  hand 719.84
  hip 719.85
  knee 719.86
  multiple sites 719.89
  pelvic region 719.85
  shoulder (region) 719.81
  specified site NEC 719.88
  wrist 719.83
**Arthropyosis** — *see also* Arthritis, pyogenic 711.0 ☑
**Arthroscopic surgical procedure converted to open procedure** V64.43
**Arthrosis** (deformans) (degenerative) — *see also* Osteoarthrosis 715.9 ☑
  Charcôt's 094.0 [713.5]
  polyarticular 715.09
  spine (*see also* Spondylosis) 721.90
**Arthus phenomenon** 995.21
  due to
    correct substance properly administered 995.21
    overdose or wrong substance given or taken 977.9
      specified drug — *see* Table of Drugs and Chemicals
    serum 999.5
**Articular** — *see also* condition
  disc disorder (reducing or non-reducing) 524.63
  spondylolisthesis 756.12
**Articulation**
  anterior 524.27
  posterior 524.27
  reverse 524.27
**Artificial**
  device (prosthetic) — *see* Fitting, device
  insemination V26.1
  menopause (states) (symptoms) (syndrome) 627.4
  opening status (functioning) (without complication) V44.9
    anus (colostomy) V44.3
    colostomy V44.3
    cystostomy V44.50
      appendico-vesicostomy V44.52
      cutaneous-vesicostomy V44.51
      specified type NEC V44.59
    enterostomy V44.4
    gastrostomy V44.1
    ileostomy V44.2
    intestinal tract NEC V44.4
    jejunostomy V44.4
    nephrostomy V44.6
    specified site NEC V44.8
    tracheostomy V44.0
    ureterostomy V44.6
    urethrostomy V44.6
    urinary tract NEC V44.6
    vagina V44.7
    vagina status V44.7
**ARV** (disease) (illness) (infection) — *see* Human immunodeficiency virus (disease) (illness) (infection)
**Arytenoid** — *see* condition
**Asbestosis** (occupational) 501
**Asboe-Hansen's disease** (incontinentia pigmenti) 757.33
**Ascariasis** (intestinal) (lung) 127.0
**Ascaridiasis** 127.0
**Ascaridosis** 127.0
**Ascaris** 127.0
  lumbricoides (infestation) 127.0

☑ Additional Digit Required — Refer to the Tabular List for Digit Selection      ▽ Subterms under main terms may continue to next column or page

*2008 ICD-9-CM*     ▶◀ Revised Text     ● New Line     ▲ Revised Code     October 2007 · Volume 2 — 29

Ascaris — Astrocytoma

**Ascaris** — *continued*
pneumonia 127.0
**Ascending** — *see* condition
**ASC-H** (atypical squamous cells cannot exclude high grade squamous intraepithelial lesion) 795.02
**Aschoff's bodies** — *see also* Myocarditis, rheumatic 398.0
**Ascites** 789.59 ▲
abdominal NEC 789.59 ▲
cancerous (M8000/6) 789.51 ▲
cardiac 428.0
chylous (nonfilarial) 457.8
filarial (*see also* Infestation, filarial) 125.9
congenital 778.0
due to S. japonicum 120.2
fetal, causing fetopelvic disproportion 653.7 ☑
heart 428.0
joint (*see also* Effusion, joint) 719.0 ☑
malignant (M8000/6) 789.51 ▲
pseudochylous 789.59 ▲
syphilitic 095.2
tuberculous (*see also* Tuberculosis) 014.0 ☑
**Ascorbic acid** (vitamin C) **deficiency** (scurvy) 267
**ASC-US** (atypical squamous cells of undetermined significance) 795.01
**ASCVD** (arteriosclerotic cardiovascular disease) 429.2
**Aseptic** — *see* condition
**Asherman's syndrome** 621.5
**Asialia** 527.7
**Asiatic cholera** — *see also* Cholera 001.9
**Asocial personality or trends** 301.7
**Asomatognosia** 781.8
**Aspergillosis** 117.3
with pneumonia 117.3 [484.6]
allergic bronchopulmonary 518.6
nonsyphilitic NEC 117.3
**Aspergillus** (flavus) (fumigatus) (infection) (terreus) 117.3
**Aspermatogenesis** 606.0
**Aspermia** (testis) 606.0
**Asphyxia, asphyxiation** (by) 799.01
antenatal — *see* Distress, fetal
bedclothes 994.7
birth (*see also* Asphyxia, newborn) 768.9
bunny bag 994.7
carbon monoxide 986
caul (*see also* Asphyxia, newborn) 768.9
cave-in 994.7
crushing — *see* Injury, internal, intrathoracic organs
constriction 994.7
crushing — *see* Injury, internal, intrathoracic organs
drowning 994.1
fetal, affecting newborn 768.9
food or foreign body (in larynx) 933.1
bronchioles 934.8
bronchus (main) 934.1
lung 934.8
nasopharynx 933.0
nose, nasal passages 932
pharynx 933.0
respiratory tract 934.9
specified part NEC 934.8
throat 933.0
trachea 934.0
gas, fumes, or vapor NEC 987.9
specified — *see* Table of Drugs and Chemicals
gravitational changes 994.7
hanging 994.7
inhalation — *see* Inhalation
intrauterine
fetal death (before onset of labor) 768.0
during labor 768.1
liveborn infant — *see* Distress, fetal, liveborn infant

**Asphyxia, asphyxiation** — *continued*
local 443.0
mechanical 994.7
during birth (*see also* Distress, fetal) 768.9
mucus 933.1
bronchus (main) 934.1
larynx 933.1
lung 934.8
nasal passages 932
newborn 770.18
pharynx 933.0
respiratory tract 934.9
specified part NEC 934.8
throat 933.0
trachea 934.0
vaginal (fetus or newborn) 770.18
newborn 768.9
with neurologic involvement 768.5
blue 768.6
livida 768.6
mild or moderate 768.6
pallida 768.5
severe 768.5
white 768.5
pathological 799.01
plastic bag 994.7
postnatal (*see also* Asphyxia, newborn) 768.9
mechanical 994.7
pressure 994.7
reticularis 782.61
strangulation 994.7
submersion 994.1
traumatic NEC — *see* Injury, internal, intrathoracic organs
vomiting, vomitus — *see* Asphyxia, food or foreign body
**Aspiration**
acid pulmonary (syndrome) 997.3
obstetric 668.0 ☑
amniotic fluid 770.13
with respiratory symptoms 770.14
bronchitis 507.0
clear amniotic fluid 770.13
with
pneumonia 770.14
pneumonitis 770.14
respiratory symptoms 770.14
contents of birth canal 770.17
with respiratory symptoms 770.18
fetal 770.10
blood 770.15
with
pneumonia 770.16
pneumonitis 770.16
pneumonitis 770.18
food, foreign body, or gasoline (with asphyxiation) — *see* Asphyxia, food or foreign body
meconium 770.11
with
pneumonia 770.12
pneumonitis 770.12
respiratory symptoms 770.12
below vocal cords 770.11
with respiratory symptoms 770.12
mucus 933.1
into
bronchus (main) 934.1
lung 934.8
respiratory tract 934.9
specified part NEC 934.8
trachea 934.0
newborn 770.17
vaginal (fetus or newborn) 770.17
newborn 770.10
with respiratory symptoms 770.18
blood 770.15
with
pneumonia 770.16
pneumonitis 770.16
respiratory symptoms 770.16
pneumonia 507.0
fetus or newborn 770.18

**Aspiration** — *continued*
pneumonia — *continued*
fetus or newborn — *continued*
meconium 770.12
pneumonitis 507.0
fetus or newborn 770.18
meconium 770.12
obstetric 668.0 ☑
postnatal stomach contents 770.85
with
pneumonia 770.86
pneumonitis 770.86
respiratory symptoms 770.86
syndrome of newborn (massive) 770.18
meconium 770.12
vernix caseosa 770.12
**Asplenia** 759.0
with mesocardia 746.87
**Assam fever** 085.0
**Assimilation, pelvis**
with disproportion 653.2 ☑
affecting fetus or newborn 763.1
causing obstructed labor 660.1 ☑
affecting fetus or newborn 763.1
**Assmann's focus** — *see also* Tuberculosis 011.0 ☑
**Astasia** (-abasia) 307.9
hysterical 300.11
**Asteatosis** 706.8
cutis 706.8
**Astereognosis** 780.99
**Asterixis** 781.3
in liver disease 572.8
**Asteroid hyalitis** 379.22
**Asthenia, asthenic** 780.79
cardiac (*see also* Failure, heart) 428.9
psychogenic 306.2
cardiovascular (*see also* Failure, heart) 428.9
psychogenic 306.2
heart (*see also* Failure, heart) 428.9
psychogenic 306.2
hysterical 300.11
myocardial (*see also* Failure, heart) 428.9
psychogenic 306.2
nervous 300.5
neurocirculatory 306.2
neurotic 300.5
psychogenic 300.5
psychoneurotic 300.5
psychophysiologic 300.5
reaction, psychoneurotic 300.5
senile 797
Stiller's 780.79
tropical anhidrotic 705.1
**Asthenopia** 368.13
accommodative 367.4
hysterical (muscular) 300.11
psychogenic 306.7
**Asthenospermia** 792.2
**Asthma, asthmatic** (bronchial) (catarrh) (spasmodic) 493.9 ☑

*Note — Use the following fifth-digit subclassification with category 493:*

0  *without mention of status asthmaticus or acute exacerbation or unspecified*

1  *with status asthmaticus*

2  *with acute exacerbation*

with
chronic obstructive pulmonary disease (COPD) 493.2 ☑
hay fever 493.0 ☑
rhinitis, allergic 493.0 ☑
allergic 493.9 ☑
stated cause (external allergen) 493.0 ☑
atopic 493.0 ☑
cardiac (*see also* Failure, ventricular, left) 428.1
cardiobronchial (*see also* Failure, ventricular, left) 428.1

**Asthma, asthmatic** — *continued*
cardiorenal (*see also* Hypertension, cardiorenal) 404.90
childhood 493.0 ☑
Colliers' 500
cough variant 493.82
croup 493.9 ☑
detergent 507.8
due to
detergent 507.8
inhalation of fumes 506.3
internal immunological process 493.0 ☑
endogenous (intrinsic) 493.1 ☑
eosinophilic 518.3
exercise induced bronchospasm 493.81
exogenous (cosmetics) (dander or dust) (drugs) (dust) (feathers) (food) (hay) (platinum) (pollen) 493.0 ☑
extrinsic 493.0 ☑
grinders' 502
hay 493.0 ☑
heart (*see also* Failure, ventricular, left) 428.1
IgE 493.0 ☑
infective 493.1 ☑
intrinsic 493.1 ☑
Kopp's 254.8
late-onset 493.1 ☑
meat-wrappers' 506.9
Millar's (laryngismus stridulus) 478.75
millstone makers' 502
miners' 500
Monday morning 504
New Orleans (epidemic) 493.0 ☑
platinum 493.0 ☑
pneumoconiotic (occupational) NEC 505
potters' 502
psychogenic 316 [493.9] ☑
pulmonary eosinophilic 518.3
red cedar 495.8
Rostan's (*see also* Failure, ventricular, left) 428.1
sandblasters' 502
sequoiosis 495.8
stonemasons' 502
thymic 254.8
tuberculous (*see also* Tuberculosis, pulmonary) 011.9 ☑
Wichmann's (laryngismus stridulus) 478.75
wood 495.8
**Astigmatism** (compound) (congenital) 367.20
irregular 367.22
regular 367.21
**Astroblastoma** (M9430/3)
nose 748.1
specified site — *see* Neoplasm, by site, malignant
unspecified site 191.9
**Astrocytoma** (cystic) (M9400/3)
anaplastic type (M9401/3)
specified site — *see* Neoplasm, by site, malignant
unspecified site 191.9
fibrillary (M9420/3)
specified site — *see* Neoplasm, by site, malignant
unspecified site 191.9
fibrous (M9420/3)
specified site — *see* Neoplasm, by site, malignant
unspecified site 191.9
gemistocytic (M9411/3)
specified site — *see* Neoplasm, by site, malignant
unspecified site 191.9
juvenile (M9421/3)
specified site — *see* Neoplasm, by site, malignant
unspecified site 191.9

**Astrocytoma** — *continued*
　nose 748.1
　pilocytic (M9421/3)
　　specified site — *see* Neoplasm, by
　　　site, malignant
　　unspecified site 191.9
　piloid (M9421/3)
　　specified site — *see* Neoplasm, by
　　　site, malignant
　　unspecified site 191.9
　protoplasmic (M9410/3)
　　specified site — *see* Neoplasm, by
　　　site, malignant
　　unspecified site 191.9
　specified site — *see* Neoplasm, by site,
　　malignant
　subependymal (M9383/1) 237.5
　　giant cell (M9384/1) 237.5
　unspecified site 191.9
**Astroglioma** (M9400/3)
　nose 748.1
　specified site — *see* Neoplasm, by site,
　　malignant
　unspecified site 191.9
**Asymbolia** 784.60
**Asymmetrical breathing** 786.09
**Asymmetry** — *see also* Distortion
　chest 786.9
　face 754.0
　jaw NEC 524.12
　　maxillary 524.11
　pelvis with disproportion 653.0 ☑
　　affecting fetus or newborn 763.1
　　causing obstructed labor 660.1 ☑
　　　affecting fetus or newborn 763.1
**Asynergia** 781.3
**Asynergy** 781.3
　ventricular 429.89
**Asystole** (heart) — *see also* Arrest, car-
　diac 427.5
**Ataxia, ataxy, ataxic** 781.3
　acute 781.3
　brain 331.89
　cerebellar 334.3
　　hereditary (Marie's) 334.2
　　in
　　　alcoholism 303.9 ☑ *[334.4]*
　　　myxedema (*see also* Myxedema)
　　　　244.9 *[334.4]*
　　　neoplastic disease NEC
　　　　239.9 *[334.4]*
　cerebral 331.89
　family, familial 334.2
　　cerebral (Marie's) 334.2
　　spinal (Friedreich's) 334.0
　Friedreich's (heredofamilial) (spinal)
　　334.0
　frontal lobe 781.3
　gait 781.2
　　hysterical 300.11
　general 781.3
　hereditary NEC 334.2
　　cerebellar 334.2
　　spastic 334.1
　　spinal 334.0
　heredofamilial (Marie's) 334.2
　hysterical 300.11
　locomotor (progressive) 094.0
　　diabetic 250.6 ☑ *[337.1]*
　Marie's (cerebellar) (heredofamilial)
　　334.2
　nonorganic origin 307.9
　partial 094.0
　postchickenpox 052.7
　progressive locomotor 094.0
　psychogenic 307.9
　Sanger-Brown's 334.2
　spastic 094.0
　　hereditary 334.1
　　syphilitic 094.0
　spinal
　　hereditary 334.0
　　progressive locomotor 094.0
　telangiectasia 334.8
**Ataxia-telangiectasia** 334.8

**Atelectasis** (absorption collapse) (com-
　plete) (compression) (massive)
　(partial) (postinfective) (pressure
　collapse) (pulmonary) (relaxation)
　518.0
　newborn (congenital) (partial) 770.5
　　primary 770.4
　primary 770.4
　tuberculous (*see also* Tuberculosis,
　　pulmonary) 011.9 ☑
**Ateleiosis, ateliosis** 253.3
**Atelia** — *see* Distortion
**Ateliosis** 253.3
**Atelocardia** 746.9
**Atelomyelia** 742.59
**Athelia** 757.6
**Atheroembolism**
　extremity
　　lower 445.02
　　upper 445.01
　kidney 445.81
　specified site NEC 445.89
**Atheroma, atheromatous** — *see also*
　Arteriosclerosis 440.9
　aorta, aortic 440.0
　　valve (*see also* Endocarditis, aortic)
　　　424.1
　artery — *see* Arteriosclerosis
　basilar (artery) (*see also* Occlusion,
　　artery, basilar) 433.0 ☑
　carotid (artery) (common) (internal)
　　(*see also* Occlusion, artery,
　　carotid) 433.1 ☑
　cerebral (arteries) 437.0
　coronary (artery) — *see* Arterioscle-
　　rosis, coronary
　degeneration — *see* Arteriosclerosis
　heart, cardiac — *see* Arteriosclerosis,
　　coronary
　mitral valve 424.0
　myocardium, myocardial — *see* Arte-
　　riosclerosis, coronary
　pulmonary valve (heart) (*see also* En-
　　docarditis, pulmonary) 424.3
　skin 706.2
　tricuspid (heart) (valve) 424.2
　valve, valvular — *see* Endocarditis
　vertebral (artery) (*see also* Occlusion,
　　artery, vertebral) 433.2 ☑
**Atheromatosis** — *see also* Arteriosclero-
　sis
　arterial, congenital 272.8
**Atherosclerosis** — *see* Arteriosclerosis
**Athetosis** (acquired) 781.0
　bilateral 333.79
　congenital (bilateral) 333.6
　double 333.71
　unilateral 781.0
**Athlete's**
　foot 110.4
　heart 429.3
**Athletic team examination** V70.3
**Athrepsia** 261
**Athyrea** (acquired) — *see also* Hypothy-
　roidism 244.9
　congenital 243
**Athyreosis** (congenital) 243
　acquired — *see* Hypothyroidism
**Athyroidism** (acquired) — *see also* Hy-
　pothyroidism 244.9
　congenital 243
**Atmospheric pyrexia** 992.0
**Atonia, atony, atonic**
　abdominal wall 728.2
　bladder (sphincter) 596.4
　　neurogenic NEC 596.54
　　　with cauda equina syndrome
　　　　344.61
　capillary 448.9
　cecum 564.89
　　psychogenic 306.4
　colon 564.89
　　psychogenic 306.4
　congenital 779.89
　dyspepsia 536.3
　　psychogenic 306.4

**Atonia, atony, atonic** — *continued*
　intestine 564.89
　　psychogenic 306.4
　stomach 536.3
　　neurotic or psychogenic 306.4
　　psychogenic 306.4
　uterus 661.2 ☑　　　　　　　　　▲
　　with hemorrhage ▶(postpartum)◀
　　　666.1 ☑
　　without hemorrhage
　　　intrapartum 661.2 ☑　　　　●
　　　postpartum 669.8 ☑　　　　●
　vesical 596.4
**Atopy** NEC V15.09
**Atransferrinemia, congenital** 273.8
**Atresia, atretic** (congenital) 759.89
　alimentary organ or tract NEC 751.8
　　lower 751.2
　　upper 750.8
　ani, anus, anal (canal) 751.2
　aorta 747.22
　　with hypoplasia of ascending aorta
　　　and defective development of
　　　left ventricle (with mitral
　　　valve atresia) 746.7
　　arch 747.11
　　ring 747.21
　aortic (orifice) (valve) 746.89
　　arch 747.11
　aqueduct of Sylvius 742.3
　　with spina bifida (*see also* Spina
　　　bifida) 741.0 ☑
　artery NEC (*see also* Atresia, blood
　　vessel) 747.60
　　cerebral 747.81
　　coronary 746.85
　　eye 743.58
　　pulmonary 747.3
　　umbilical 747.5
　auditory canal (external) 744.02
　bile, biliary duct (common) or passage
　　751.61
　　acquired (*see also* Obstruction,
　　　biliary) 576.2
　bladder (neck) 753.6
　blood vessel (peripheral) NEC 747.60
　　cerebral 747.81
　　gastrointestinal 747.61
　　lower limb 747.64
　　pulmonary artery 747.3
　　renal 747.62
　　spinal 747.82
　　upper limb 747.63
　bronchus 748.3
　canal, ear 744.02
　cardiac
　　valve 746.89
　　　aortic 746.89
　　　mitral 746.89
　　　pulmonary 746.01
　　　tricuspid 746.1
　cecum 751.2
　cervix (acquired) 622.4
　　congenital 752.49
　　in pregnancy or childbirth 654.6 ☑
　　　affecting fetus or newborn
　　　　763.89
　　　causing obstructed labor
　　　　660.2 ☑
　　　　affecting fetus or newborn
　　　　　763.1
　choana 748.0
　colon 751.2
　cystic duct 751.61
　　acquired 575.8
　　　with obstruction (*see also* Ob-
　　　　struction, gallbladder)
　　　　575.2
　digestive organs NEC 751.8
　duodenum 751.1
　ear canal 744.02
　ejaculatory duct 752.89
　epiglottis 748.3
　esophagus 750.3
　Eustachian tube 744.24
　fallopian tube (acquired) 628.2

**Atresia, atretic** — *continued*
　fallopian tube — *continued*
　　congenital 752.19
　follicular cyst 620.0
　foramen of
　　Luschka 742.3
　　　with spina bifida (*see also* Spina
　　　　bifida) 741.0 ☑
　　Magendie 742.3
　　　with spina bifida (*see also* Spina
　　　　bifida) 741.0 ☑
　gallbladder 751.69
　genital organ
　　external
　　　female 752.49
　　　male NEC 752.89
　　　　penis 752.69
　　internal
　　　female 752.89
　　　male 752.89
　glottis 748.3
　gullet 750.3
　heart
　　valve NEC 746.89
　　　aortic 746.89
　　　mitral 746.89
　　　pulmonary 746.01
　　　tricuspid 746.1
　hymen 752.42
　　acquired 623.3
　　postinfective 623.3
　ileum 751.1
　intestine (small) 751.1
　　large 751.2
　iris, filtration angle (*see also* Buph-
　　thalmia) 743.20
　jejunum 751.1
　kidney 753.3
　lacrimal, apparatus 743.65
　　acquired — *see* Stenosis, lacrimal
　larynx 748.3
　ligament, broad 752.19
　lung 748.5
　meatus urinarius 753.6
　mitral valve 746.89
　　with atresia or hypoplasia of aortic
　　　orifice or valve, with hypopla-
　　　sia of ascending aorta and
　　　defective development of left
　　　ventricle 746.7
　nares (anterior) (posterior) 748.0
　nasolacrimal duct 743.65
　nasopharynx 748.8
　nose, nostril 748.0
　　acquired 738.0
　organ or site NEC — *see* Anomaly,
　　specified type NEC
　osseous meatus (ear) 744.03
　oviduct (acquired) 628.2
　　congenital 752.19
　parotid duct 750.23
　　acquired 527.8
　pulmonary (artery) 747.3
　　valve 746.01
　　vein 747.49
　pulmonic 746.01
　pupil 743.46
　rectum 751.2
　salivary duct or gland 750.23
　　acquired 527.8
　sublingual duct 750.23
　　acquired 527.8
　submaxillary duct or gland 750.23
　　acquired 527.8
　trachea 748.3
　tricuspid valve 746.1
　ureter 753.29
　ureteropelvic junction 753.21
　ureterovesical orifice 753.22
　urethra (valvular) 753.6
　urinary tract NEC 753.29
　uterus 752.3
　　acquired 621.8
　vagina (acquired) 623.2
　　congenital 752.49
　　postgonococcal (old) 098.2

---

☑ Additional Digit Required — Refer to the Tabular List for Digit Selection　　　　　　　▽ Subterms under main terms may continue to next column or page

**Atresia, atretic** — *continued*
vagina — *continued*
  postinfectional 623.2
  senile 623.2
vascular NEC (*see also* Atresia, blood
  vessel) 747.60
  cerebral 747.81
vas deferens 752.89
vein NEC (*see also* Atresia, blood vessel) 747.60
  cardiac 746.89
  great 747.49
  portal 747.49
  pulmonary 747.49
vena cava (inferior) (superior) 747.49
vesicourethral orifice 753.6
vulva 752.49
  acquired 624.8
**Atrichia, atrichosis** 704.00
congenital (universal) 757.4
**Atrioventricularis commune** 745.69
**At risk for falling** V15.88
**Atrophia** — *see also* Atrophy
alba 709.09
cutis 701.8
  idiopathica progressiva 701.8
  senilis 701.8
dermatological, diffuse (idiopathic)
  701.8
flava hepatis (acuta) (subacuta) (*see
  also* Necrosis, liver) 570
gyrata of choroid and retina (central)
  363.54
  generalized 363.57
senilis 797
  dermatological 701.8
unguium 703.8
  congenita 757.5
**Atrophoderma, atrophodermia** 701.9
diffusum (idiopathic) 701.8
maculatum 701.3
  et striatum 701.3
    due to syphilis 095.8
  syphilitic 091.3
neuriticum 701.8
pigmentosum 757.33
reticulatum symmetricum faciei 701.8
senile 701.8
symmetrical 701.8
vermiculata 701.8
**Atrophy, atrophic**
adrenal (autoimmune) (capsule) (cortex) (gland) 255.41 ▲
  with hypofunction 255.41 ▲
alveolar process or ridge (edentulous)
  525.20
  mandible 525.20
    minimal 525.21
    moderate 525.22
    severe 525.23
  maxilla 525.20
    minimal 525.24
    moderate 525.25
    severe 525.26
appendix 543.9
Aran-Duchenne muscular 335.21
arm 728.2
arteriosclerotic — *see* Arteriosclerosis
arthritis 714.0
  spine 720.9
bile duct (any) 576.8
bladder 596.8
blanche (of Milian) 701.3
bone (senile) 733.99
  due to
    disuse 733.7
    infection 733.99
    tabes dorsalis (neurogenic)
      094.0
  posttraumatic 733.99
brain (cortex) (progressive) 331.9
  with dementia 290.10
    Alzheimer's 331.0
      with dementia — *see*
        Alzheimer's, dementia
  circumscribed (Pick's) 331.11

**Atrophy, atrophic** — *continued*
brain — *continued*
  circumscribed — *continued*
    with dementia
      with behavioral disturbance
        331.11 *[294.11]*
      without behavioral distur-
        bance 331.11 *[294.10]*
  congenital 742.4
  hereditary 331.9
  senile 331.2
breast 611.4
  puerperal, postpartum 676.3 ☑
buccal cavity 528.9
cardiac (brown) (senile) (*see also* Degeneration, myocardial) 429.1
cartilage (infectional) (joint) 733.99
cast, plaster of Paris 728.2
cerebellar — *see* Atrophy, brain
cerebral — *see* Atrophy, brain
cervix (endometrium) (mucosa) (myometrium) (senile) (uteri) 622.8
  menopausal 627.8
Charcôt-Marie-Tooth 356.1
choroid 363.40
  diffuse secondary 363.42
  hereditary (*see also* Dystrophy,
    choroid) 363.50
    gyrate
      central 363.54
      diffuse 363.57
      generalized 363.57
  senile 363.41
ciliary body 364.57
colloid, degenerative 701.3
conjunctiva (senile) 372.89
corpus cavernosum 607.89
cortical (*see also* Atrophy, brain) 331.9
Cruveilhier's 335.21
cystic duct 576.8
dacryosialadenopathy 710.2
degenerative
  colloid 701.3
  senile 701.3
Déjérine-Thomas 333.0
diffuse idiopathic, dermatological
  701.8
disuse
  bone 733.7
  muscle 728.2
  pelvic muscles and anal sphincter
    618.83
Duchenne-Aran 335.21
ear 388.9
edentulous alveolar ridge 525.20
  mandible 525.20
    minimal 525.21
    moderate 525.22
    severe 525.23
  maxilla 525.20
    minimal 525.24
    moderate 525.25
    severe 525.26
emphysema, lung 492.8
endometrium (senile) 621.8
  cervix 622.8
enteric 569.89
epididymis 608.3
eyeball, cause unknown 360.41
eyelid (senile) 374.50
facial (skin) 701.9
facioscapulohumeral (Landouzy-
  Déjérine) 359.1
fallopian tube (senile), acquired 620.3
fatty, thymus (gland) 254.8
gallbladder 575.8
gastric 537.89
gastritis (chronic) 535.1 ☑
gastrointestinal 569.89
genital organ, male 608.89
glandular 289.3
globe (phthisis bulbi) 360.41
gum (*see also* Recession, gingival)
  523.20
hair 704.2

**Atrophy, atrophic** — *continued*
heart (brown) (senile) (*see also* Degeneration, myocardial) 429.1
hemifacial 754.0
  Romberg 349.89
hydronephrosis 591
infantile 261
  paralysis, acute (*see also* Poliomyeli-
    tis, with paralysis) 045.1 ☑
intestine 569.89
iris (generalized) (postinfectional)
  (sector shaped) 364.59
  essential 364.51
  progressive 364.51
  sphincter 364.54
kidney (senile) (*see also* Sclerosis, renal) 587
  with hypertension (*see also* Hyper-
    tension, kidney) 403.90
  congenital 753.0
  hydronephrotic 591
  infantile 753.0
lacrimal apparatus (primary) 375.13
  secondary 375.14
Landouzy-Déjérine 359.1
laryngitis, infection 476.0
larynx 478.79
Leber's optic 377.16
lip 528.5
liver (acute) (subacute) (*see also*
  Necrosis, liver) 570
  chronic (yellow) 571.8
  yellow (congenital) 570
    with
      abortion — *see* Abortion, by
        type, with specified
        complication NEC
      ectopic pregnancy (*see also*
        categories
        633.0–633.9) 639.8
      molar pregnancy (*see also*
        categories 630–632)
        639.8
    chronic 571.8
    complicating pregnancy
      646.7 ☑
    following
      abortion 639.8
      ectopic or molar pregnancy
        639.8
    from injection, inoculation or
      transfusion (onset within
      8 months after administra-
      tion) — *see* Hepatitis, viral
    healed 571.5
    obstetric 646.7 ☑
    postabortal 639.8
    postimmunization — *see* Hepati-
      tis, viral
    posttransfusion — *see* Hepatitis,
      viral
    puerperal, postpartum 674.8 ☑
lung (senile) 518.89
  congenital 748.69
macular (dermatological) 701.3
  syphilitic, skin 091.3
    striated 095.8
muscle, muscular 728.2
  disuse 728.2
  Duchenne-Aran 335.21
  extremity (lower) (upper) 728.2
  familial spinal 335.11
  general 728.2
  idiopathic 728.2
  infantile spinal 335.0
  myelopathic (progressive) 335.10
  myotonic 359.21 ▲
  neuritic 356.1
  neuropathic (peroneal) (progressive)
    356.1
  peroneal 356.1
  primary (idiopathic) 728.2
  progressive (familial) (hereditary)
    (pure) 335.21
    adult (spinal) 335.19
    infantile (spinal) 335.0

**Atrophy, atrophic** — *continued*
muscle, muscular — *continued*
  progressive — *continued*
    juvenile (spinal) 335.11
    spinal 335.10
      adult 335.19
      hereditary or familial 335.11
      infantile 335.0
  pseudohypertrophic 359.1
  spinal (progressive) 335.10
    adult 335.19
    Aran-Duchenne 335.21
    familial 335.11
    hereditary 335.11
    infantile 335.0
    juvenile 335.11
  syphilitic 095.6
myocardium (*see also* Degeneration,
  myocardial) 429.1
myometrium (senile) 621.8
  cervix 622.8
myotatic 728.2
myotonia 359.21 ▲
nail 703.8
  congenital 757.5
nasopharynx 472.2
nerve (*see also* Disorder, nerve)
  abducens 378.54
  accessory 352.4
  acoustic or auditory 388.5
  cranial 352.9
    first (olfactory) 352.0
    second (optic) (*see also* Atrophy,
      optic nerve) 377.10
    third (oculomotor) (partial)
      378.51
      total 378.52
    fourth (trochlear) 378.53
    fifth (trigeminal) 350.8
    sixth (abducens) 378.54
    seventh (facial) 351.8
    eighth (auditory) 388.5
    ninth (glossopharyngeal) 352.2
    tenth (pneumogastric) (vagus)
      352.3
    eleventh (accessory) 352.4
    twelfth (hypoglossal) 352.5
  facial 351.8
  glossopharyngeal 352.2
  hypoglossal 352.5
  oculomotor (partial) 378.51
    total 378.52
  olfactory 352.0
  peripheral 355.9
  pneumogastric 352.3
  trigeminal 350.8
  trochlear 378.53
  vagus (pneumogastric) 352.3
nervous system, congenital 742.8
neuritic (*see also* Disorder, nerve)
  355.9
neurogenic NEC 355.9
  bone
    tabetic 094.0
nutritional 261
old age 797
olivopontocerebellar 333.0
optic nerve (ascending) (descending)
  (infectional) (nonfamilial) (papil-
  lomacular bundle) (postretinal)
  (secondary NEC) (simple) 377.10
  associated with retinal dystrophy
    377.13
  dominant hereditary 377.16
  glaucomatous 377.14
  hereditary (dominant) (Leber's)
    377.16
  Leber's (hereditary) 377.16
  partial 377.15
  postinflammatory 377.12
  primary 377.11
  syphilitic 094.84
    congenital 090.49
    tabes dorsalis 094.0
orbit 376.45
ovary (senile), acquired 620.3

---

☑ Additional Digit Required — Refer to the Tabular List for Digit Selection          ⩫ Subterms under main terms may continue to next column or page

32 — Volume 2 • October 2007      ▶◀ Revised Text      ● New Line      ▲ Revised Code      *2008 ICD-9-CM*

**Atrophy, atrophic** — *continued*
  oviduct (senile), acquired 620.3
  palsy, diffuse 335.20
  pancreas (duct) (senile) 577.8
  papillary muscle 429.81
  paralysis 355.9
  parotid gland 527.0
  patches skin 701.3
    senile 701.8
  penis 607.89
  pharyngitis 472.1
  pharynx 478.29
  pluriglandular 258.8
  polyarthritis 714.0
  prostate 602.2
  pseudohypertrophic 359.1
  renal (*see also* Sclerosis, renal) 587
  reticulata 701.8
  retina (*see also* Degeneration, retina)
    362.60
    hereditary (*see also* Dystrophy,
      retina) 362.70
  rhinitis 472.0
  salivary duct or gland 527.0
  scar NEC 709.2
  sclerosis, lobar (of brain) 331.0
    with dementia
      with behavioral disturbance
        331.0 [294.11]
      without behavioral disturbance
        331.0 [294.10]
  scrotum 608.89
  seminal vesicle 608.89
  senile 797
    degenerative, of skin 701.3
  skin (patches) (senile) 701.8
  spermatic cord 608.89
  spinal (cord) 336.8
    acute 336.8
    muscular (chronic) 335.10
      adult 335.19
      familial 335.11
      juvenile 335.10
    paralysis 335.10
      acute (*see also* Poliomyelitis,
        with paralysis) 045.1 ☑
  spine (column) 733.99
  spleen (senile) 289.59
  spots (skin) 701.3
    senile 701.8
  stomach 537.89
  striate and macular 701.3
    syphilitic 095.8
  subcutaneous 701.9
    due to injection 999.9
  sublingual gland 527.0
  submaxillary gland 527.0
  Sudeck's 733.7
  suprarenal (autoimmune) (capsule)
    (gland) 255.41 ▲
    with hypofunction 255.41 ▲
  tarso-orbital fascia, congenital 743.66
  testis 608.3
  thenar, partial 354.0
  throat 478.29
  thymus (fat) 254.8
  thyroid (gland) 246.8
    with
      cretinism 243
      myxedema 244.9
    congenital 243
  tongue (senile) 529.8
    papillae 529.4
    smooth 529.4
  trachea 519.19
  tunica vaginalis 608.89
  turbinate 733.99
  tympanic membrane (nonflaccid)
    384.82
    flaccid 384.81
  ulcer (*see also* Ulcer, skin) 707.9
  upper respiratory tract 478.9
  uterus, uterine (acquired) (senile)
    621.8
    cervix 622.8

**Atrophy, atrophic** — *continued*
  uterus, uterine — *continued*
    due to radiation (intended effect)
      621.8
  vagina (senile) 627.3
  vascular 459.89
  vas deferens 608.89
  vertebra (senile) 733.99
  vulva (primary) (senile) 624.1
  Werdnig-Hoffmann 335.0
  yellow (acute) (congenital) (liver) (sub-
    acute) (*see also* Necrosis, liver)
    570
    chronic 571.8
    resulting from administration of
      blood, plasma, serum, or
      other biological substance
      (within 8 months of adminis-
      tration) — *see* Hepatitis, viral

**Attack**
  akinetic (*see also* Epilepsy) 345.0 ☑
  angina — *see* Angina
  apoplectic (*see also* Disease, cere-
    brovascular, acute) 436
  benign shuddering 333.93
  bilious — *see* Vomiting
  cataleptic 300.11
  cerebral (*see also* Disease, cerebrovas-
    cular, acute) 436
  coronary (*see also* Infarct, myocardi-
    um) 410.9 ☑
  cyanotic, newborn 770.83
  epileptic (*see also* Epilepsy) 345.9 ☑
  epileptiform 780.39
  heart (*see also* Infarct, myocardium)
    410.9 ☑
  hemiplegia (*see also* Disease, cere-
    brovascular, acute) 436
  hysterical 300.11
  jacksonian (*see also* Epilepsy) 345.5 ☑
  myocardium, myocardial (*see also* In-
    farct, myocardium) 410.9 ☑
  myoclonic (*see also* Epilepsy) 345.1 ☑
  panic 300.01
  paralysis (*see also* Disease, cerebrovas-
    cular, acute) 436
  paroxysmal 780.39
  psychomotor (*see also* Epilepsy)
    345.4 ☑
  salaam (*see also* Epilepsy) 345.6 ☑
  schizophreniform (*see also*
    Schizophrenia) 295.4 ☑
  sensory and motor 780.39
  syncope 780.2
  toxic, cerebral 780.39
  transient ischemic (TIA) 435.9
  unconsciousness 780.2
    hysterical 300.11
  vasomotor 780.2
  vasovagal (idiopathic) (paroxysmal)
    780.2

**Attention to**
  artificial opening (of) V55.9
    digestive tract NEC V55.4
    specified site NEC V55.8
    urinary tract NEC V55.6
    vagina V55.7
  colostomy V55.3
  cystostomy V55.5
  dressing
    wound V58.30
      nonsurgical V58.30
      surgical V58.31
  gastrostomy V55.1
  ileostomy V55.2
  jejunostomy V55.4
  nephrostomy V55.6
  surgical dressings V58.31
  sutures V58.32
  tracheostomy V55.0
  ureterostomy V55.6
  urethrostomy V55.6

**Attrition**
  gum (*see also* Recession, gingival)
    523.20
  teeth (hard tissues) 521.10

**Attrition** — *continued*
  teeth — *continued*
    excessive 521.10
    extending into
      dentine 521.12
      pulp 521.13
    generalized 521.15
    limited to enamel 521.11
    localized 521.14
**Atypical** — *see also* condition
  cells
    endocervical 795.00
    endometrial 795.00
    glandular 795.00
  distribution, vessel (congenital) (pe-
    ripheral) NEC 747.60
  endometrium 621.9
  kidney 593.89
**Atypism, cervix** 622.10
**Audible tinnitus** — *see also* Tinnitus
  388.30
**Auditory** — *see* condition
**Audry's syndrome** (acropachyderma)
  757.39
**Aujeszky's disease** 078.89
**Aura, jacksonian** — *see also* Epilepsy
  345.5 ☑
**Aurantiasis, cutis** 278.3
**Auricle, auricular** — *see* condition
**Auriculotemporal syndrome** 350.8
**Australian**
  Q fever 083.0
  X disease 062.4
**Autism, autistic** (child) (infantile)
  299.0 ☑
**Autodigestion** 799.89
**Autoerythrocyte sensitization** 287.2
**Autographism** 708.3
**Autoimmune**
  cold sensitivity 283.0
  disease NEC 279.4
  hemolytic anemia 283.0
  thyroiditis 245.2
**Autoinfection, septic** — *see* Septicemia
**Autointoxication** 799.89
**Automatism** 348.8
  epileptic (*see also* Epilepsy) 345.4 ☑
  paroxysmal, idiopathic (*see also*
    Epilepsy) 345.4 ☑
**Autonomic, autonomous**
  bladder 596.54
    neurogenic 596.54
      with cauda equina 344.61
  dysreflexia 337.3
  faciocephalalgia (*see also* Neuropathy,
    peripheral, autonomic) 337.9
  hysterical seizure 300.11
  imbalance (*see also* Neuropathy, pe-
    ripheral, autonomic) 337.9
**Autophony** 388.40
**Autopsy** 780.99
**Autosensitivity, erythrocyte** 287.2
**Autotopagnosia** 780.99
**Autotoxemia** 799.89
**Autumn** — *see* condition
**Avellis' syndrome** 344.89
**Aviators**
  disease or sickness (*see also* Effect,
    adverse, high altitude) 993.2
  ear 993.0
  effort syndrome 306.2
**Avitaminosis** (multiple NEC) — *see also*
  Deficiency, vitamin 269.2
  A 264.9
  B 266.9
    with
      beriberi 265.0
      pellagra 265.2
  B$_1$ 265.1
  B$_2$ 266.0
  B$_6$ 266.1
  B$_{12}$ 266.2
  C (with scurvy) 267
  D 268.9
    with
      osteomalacia 268.2

**Avitaminosis** — *see also* Deficiency,
  vitamin — *continued*
  D — *continued*
    with — *continued*
      rickets 268.0
  E 269.1
  G 266.0
  H 269.1
  K 269.0
  multiple 269.2
  nicotinic acid 265.2
  P 269.1
**Avulsion** (traumatic) 879.8
  blood vessel — *see* Injury, blood ves-
    sel, by site
  cartilage (*see also* Dislocation, by site)
    knee, current (*see also* Tear,
      meniscus) 836.2
    symphyseal (inner), complicating
      delivery 665.6 ☑
  complicated 879.9
  diaphragm — *see* Injury, internal, di-
    aphragm
  ear — *see* Wound, open, ear
  epiphysis of bone — *see* Fracture, by
    site
  external site other than limb — *see*
    Wound, open, by site
  eye 871.3
  fingernail — *see* Wound, open, finger
  fracture — *see* Fracture, by site
  genital organs, external — *see* Wound,
    open, genital organs
  head (intracranial) NEC (*see also* In-
    jury, intracranial, with open in-
    tracranial wound)
    complete 874.9
    external site NEC 873.8
      complicated 873.9
  internal organ or site — *see* Injury,
    internal, by site
  joint (*see also* Dislocation, by site)
    capsule — *see* Sprain, by site
  ligament — *see* Sprain, by site
  limb (*see also* Amputation, traumatic,
    by site)
    skin and subcutaneous tissue —
      *see* Wound, open, by site
  muscle — *see* Sprain, by site
  nerve (root) — *see* Injury, nerve, by
    site
  scalp — *see* Wound, open, scalp
  skin and subcutaneous tissue — *see*
    Wound, open, by site
  symphyseal cartilage (inner), compli-
    cating delivery 665.6 ☑
  tendon (*see also* Sprain, by site)
    with open wound — *see* Wound,
      open, by site
  toenail — *see* Wound, open, toe(s)
  tooth 873.63
    complicated 873.73
**Awaiting organ transplant status**
  V49.83
**Awareness of heart beat** 785.1
**Axe grinders' disease** 502
**Axenfeld's anomaly or syndrome**
  743.44
**Axilla, axillary** — *see also* condition
  breast 757.6
**Axonotmesis** — *see* Injury, nerve, by site
**Ayala's disease** 756.89
**Ayerza's disease or syndrome** (pul-
  monary artery sclerosis with pul-
  monary hypertension) 416.0
**Azoospermia** 606.0
**Azorean disease** (of the nervous system)
  334.8
**Azotemia** 790.6
  meaning uremia (*see also* Uremia) 586
**Aztec ear** 744.29
**Azygos lobe, lung** (fissure) 748.69

**B**

**Baader's syndrome** (erythema multiforme exudativum) 695.1

---

☑ Additional Digit Required — Refer to the Tabular List for Digit Selection      ⩒ Subterms under main terms may continue to next column or page

**2008 ICD-9-CM**      ▶◀ Revised Text      ● New Line      ▲ Revised Code      **October 2007 • Volume 2 — 33**

**Baastrup's syndrome** 721.5
**Babesiasis** 088.82
**Babesiosis** 088.82
**Babington's disease** (familial hemorrhagic telangiectasia) 448.0
**Babinski-Fröhlich syndrome** (adiposogenital dystrophy) 253.8
**Babinski-Nageotte syndrome** 344.89
**Babinski's syndrome** (cardiovascular syphilis) 093.89
**Bacillary** — see condition
**Bacilluria** 791.9
asymptomatic, in pregnancy or puerperium 646.5 ☑
tuberculous (see also Tuberculosis) 016.9 ☑
**Bacillus** — see also Infection, bacillus
abortus infection 023.1
anthracis infection 022.9
coli
infection 041.4
generalized 038.42
intestinal 008.00
pyemia 038.42
septicemia 038.42
Flexner's 004.1
fusiformis infestation 101
mallei infection 024
Shiga's 004.0
suipestifer infection (see also Infection, Salmonella) 003.9
**Back** — see condition
**Backache** (postural) 724.5
psychogenic 307.89
sacroiliac 724.6
**Backflow** (pyelovenous) — see also Disease, renal 593.9
**Backknee** — see also Genu, recurvatum 736.5
**Bacteremia** 790.7
newborn 771.83
**Bacteria**
in blood (see also Bacteremia) 790.7
in urine (see also Bacteriuria) 599.0
**Bacterial** — see condition
**Bactericholia** — see also Cholecystitis, acute 575.0
**Bacterid, bacteride** (Andrews' pustular) 686.8
**Bacteriuria, bacteruria** 791.9
with
urinary tract infection 599.0
asymptomatic 791.9
in pregnancy or puerperium 646.5 ☑
affecting fetus or newborn 760.1
**Bad**
breath 784.99
heart — see Disease, heart
trip (see also Abuse, drugs, nondependent) 305.3 ☑
**Baehr-Schiffrin disease** (thrombotic thrombocytopenic purpura) 446.6
**Baelz's disease** (cheilitis glandularis apostematosa) 528.5
**Baerensprung's disease** (eczema marginatum) 110.3
**Bagassosis** (occupational) 495.1
**Baghdad boil** 085.1
**Bagratuni's syndrome** (temporal arteritis) 446.5
**Baker's**
cyst (knee) 727.51
tuberculous (see also Tuberculosis) 015.2 ☑
itch 692.89
**Bakwin-Krida syndrome** (craniometaphyseal dysplasia) 756.89
**Balanitis** (circinata) (gangraenosa) (infectious) (vulgaris) 607.1
amebic 006.8
candidal 112.2
chlamydial 099.53
due to Ducrey's bacillus 099.0
erosiva circinata et gangraenosa 607.1
gangrenous 607.1

**Balanitis** — continued
gonococcal (acute) 098.0
chronic or duration of 2 months or over 098.2
nongonococcal 607.1
phagedenic 607.1
venereal NEC 099.8
xerotica obliterans 607.81
**Balanoposthitis** 607.1
chlamydial 099.53
gonococcal (acute) 098.0
chronic or duration of 2 months or over 098.2
ulcerative NEC 099.8
**Balanorrhagia** — see Balanitis
**Balantidiasis** 007.0
**Balantidiosis** 007.0
**Balbuties, balbutio** 307.0
**Bald**
patches on scalp 704.00
tongue 529.4
**Baldness** — see also Alopecia 704.00
**Balfour's disease** (chloroma) 205.3 ☑
**Balint's syndrome** (psychic paralysis of visual fixation) 368.16
**Balkan grippe** 083.0
**Ball**
food 938
hair 938
**Ballantyne (-Runge) syndrome** (postmaturity) 766.22
**Balloon disease** — see also Effect, adverse, high altitude 993.2
**Ballooning posterior leaflet syndrome** 424.0
**Baló's disease or concentric sclerosis** 341.1
**Bamberger's disease** (hypertrophic pulmonary osteoarthropathy) 731.2
**Bamberger-Marie disease** (hypertrophic pulmonary osteoarthropathy) 731.2
**Bamboo spine** 720.0
**Bancroft's filariasis** 125.0
**Band(s)**
adhesive (see also Adhesions, peritoneum) 568.0
amniotic 658.8 ☑
affecting fetus or newborn 762.8
anomalous or congenital (see also Anomaly, specified type NEC)
atrial 746.9
heart 746.9
intestine 751.4
omentum 751.4
ventricular 746.9
cervix 622.3
gallbladder (congenital) 751.69
intestinal (adhesive) (see also Adhesions, peritoneum) 568.0
congenital 751.4
obstructive (see also Obstruction, intestine) 560.81
periappendiceal (congenital) 751.4
peritoneal (adhesive) (see also Adhesions, peritoneum) 568.0
with intestinal obstruction 560.81
congenital 751.4
uterus 621.5
vagina 623.2
**Bandemia** (without diagnosis of specific ● infection) 288.66
**Bandl's ring** (contraction)
complicating delivery 661.4 ☑
affecting fetus or newborn 763.7
**Bang's disease** (Brucella abortus) 023.1
**Bangkok hemorrhagic fever** 065.4
**Bannister's disease** 995.1
**Bantam-Albright-Martin disease** (pseudohypoparathyroidism) 275.49
**Banti's disease or syndrome** (with cirrhosis) (with portal hypertension) — see Cirrhosis, liver
**Bar**
calcaneocuboid 755.67
calcaneonavicular 755.67
cubonavicular 755.67

**Bar** — continued
prostate 600.90
with
other lower urinary tract symptoms (LUTS) 600.91
urinary
obstruction 600.91
retention 600.91
talocalcaneal 755.67
**Baragnosis** 780.99
**Barasheh, barashek** 266.2
**Barcoo disease or rot** — see also Ulcer, skin 707.9
**Bard-Pic syndrome** (carcinoma, head of pancreas) 157.0
**Bärensprung's disease** (eczema marginatum) 110.3
**Baritosis** 503
**Barium lung disease** 503
**Barlow (-Möller) disease or syndrome** (meaning infantile scurvy) 267
**Barlow's syndrome** (meaning mitral valve prolapse) 424.0
**Barodontalgia** 993.2
**Baron Münchausen syndrome** 301.51
**Barosinusitis** 993.1
**Barotitis** 993.0
**Barotrauma** 993.2
odontalgia 993.2
otitic 993.0
sinus 993.1
**Barraquer's disease or syndrome** (progressive lipodystrophy) 272.6
**Barré-Guillain syndrome** 357.0
**Barrel chest** 738.3
**Barré-Liéou syndrome** (posterior cervical sympathetic) 723.2
**Barrett's esophagus** 530.85
**Barrett's syndrome or ulcer** (chronic peptic ulcer of esophagus) 530.85
**Bársony-Polgár syndrome** (corkscrew esophagus) 530.5
**Bársony-Teschendorf syndrome** (corkscrew esophagus) 530.5
**Bartholin's**
adenitis (see also Bartholinitis) 616.89
gland — see condition
**Bartholinitis** (suppurating) 616.89
gonococcal (acute) 098.0
chronic or duration of 2 months or over 098.2
**Barth syndrome** 759.89
**Bartonellosis** 088.0
**Bartter's syndrome** (secondary hyperaldosteronism with juxtaglomerular hyperplasia) 255.13
**Basal** — see condition
**Basan's** (hidrotic) **ectodermal dysplasia** 757.31
**Baseball finger** 842.13
**Basedow's disease or syndrome** (exophthalmic goiter) 242.0 ☑
**Basic** — see condition
**Basilar** — see condition
**Bason's** (hidrotic) **ectodermal dysplasia** 757.31
**Basopenia** 288.59
**Basophilia** 288.65
**Basophilism** (corticoadrenal) (Cushing's) (pituitary) (thymic) 255.0
**Bassen-Kornzweig syndrome** (abetalipoproteinemia) 272.5
**Bat ear** 744.29
**Bateman's**
disease 078.0
purpura (senile) 287.2
**Bathing cramp** 994.1
**Bathophobia** 300.23
**Batten's disease, retina** 330.1 [362.71]
**Batten-Mayou disease** 330.1 [362.71]
**Batten-Steinert syndrome** 359.21 ▲
**Battered**
adult (syndrome) 995.81
baby or child (syndrome) 995.54
spouse (syndrome) 995.81
**Battey mycobacterium infection** 031.0

**Battledore placenta** — see Placenta, abnormal
**Battle exhaustion** — see also Reaction, stress, acute 308.9
**Baumgarten-Cruveilhier** (cirrhosis) **disease, or syndrome** 571.5
**Bauxite**
fibrosis (of lung) 503
workers' disease 503
**Bayle's disease** (dementia paralytica) 094.1
**Bazin's disease** (primary) — see also Tuberculosis 017.1 ☑
**Beach ear** 380.12
**Beaded hair** (congenital) 757.4
**Beals syndrome** 759.82
**Beard's disease** (neurasthenia) 300.5
**Bearn-Kunkel (-Slater) syndrome** (lupoid hepatitis) 571.49
**Beat**
elbow 727.2
hand 727.2
knee 727.2
**Beats**
ectopic 427.60
escaped, heart 427.60
postoperative 997.1
premature (nodal) 427.60
atrial 427.61
auricular 427.61
postoperative 997.1
specified type NEC 427.69
supraventricular 427.61
ventricular 427.69
**Beau's**
disease or syndrome (see also Degeneration, myocardial) 429.1
lines (transverse furrows on fingernails) 703.8
**Bechterew's disease** (ankylosing spondylitis) 720.0
**Bechterew-Strümpell-Marie syndrome** (ankylosing spondylitis) 720.0
**Becker's**
disease
idiopathic mural endomyocardial ●
disease 425.2 ●
myotonia congenita, recessive ●
form 359.22 ●
dystrophy 359.22 ▲
**Beck's syndrome** (anterior spinal artery occlusion) 433.8 ☑
**Beckwith (-Wiedemann) syndrome** 759.89
**Bedclothes, asphyxiation or suffocation by** 994.7
**Bed confinement status** V49.84
**Bednar's aphthae** 528.2
**Bedsore** 707.00
with gangrene 707.00 [785.4]
**Bedwetting** — see also Enuresis 788.36
**Beer-drinkers' heart** (disease) 425.5
**Bee sting** (with allergic or anaphylactic shock) 989.5
**Begbie's disease** (exophthalmic goiter) 242.0 ☑
**Behavior disorder, disturbance** — see also Disturbance, conduct
antisocial, without manifest psychiatric disorder
adolescent V71.02
adult V71.01
child V71.02
dyssocial, without manifest psychiatric disorder
adolescent V71.02
adult V71.01
child V71.02
high risk — see Problem
**Behçet's syndrome** 136.1
**Behr's disease** 362.50
**Beigel's disease or morbus** (white piedra) 111.2
**Bejel** 104.0
**Bekhterev's disease** (ankylosing spondylitis) 720.0

**Bekhterev-Strümpell-Marie syndrome** (ankylosing spondylitis) 720.0
**Belching** — see also Eructation 787.3
**Bell's**
  disease (see also Psychosis, affective) 296.0 ☑
  mania (see also Psychosis, affective) 296.0 ☑
  palsy, paralysis 351.0
    infant 767.5
    newborn 767.5
    syphilitic 094.89
  spasm 351.0
**Bence-Jones albuminuria, albuminosuria, or proteinuria** 791.0
**Bends** 993.3
**Benedikt's syndrome** (paralysis) 344.89
**Benign** — see also condition
  cellular changes, cervix 795.09
  prostate
    with
      other lower urinary tract symptoms (LUTS) 600.21
      urinary
        obstruction 600.21
        retention 600.21
    hyperplasia 600.20
    neoplasm 222.2
**Bennett's**
  disease (leukemia) 208.9 ☑
  fracture (closed) 815.01
    open 815.11
**Benson's disease** 379.22
**Bent**
  back (hysterical) 300.11
  nose 738.0
    congenital 754.0
**Bereavement** V62.82
  as adjustment reaction 309.0
**Bergeron's disease** (hysteroepilepsy) 300.11
**Berger's paresthesia** (lower limb) 782.0
**Beriberi** (acute) (atrophic) (chronic) (dry) (subacute) (wet) 265.0
  with polyneuropathy 265.0 [357.4]
  heart (disease) 265.0 [425.7]
  leprosy 030.1
  neuritis 265.0 [357.4]
**Berlin's disease or edema** (traumatic) 921.3
**Berloque dermatitis** 692.72
**Bernard-Horner syndrome** — see also Neuropathy, peripheral, autonomic 337.9
**Bernard-Sergent syndrome** (acute adrenocortical insufficiency) 255.41 ▲
**Bernard-Soulier disease or thrombopathy** 287.1
**Bernhardt's disease or paresthesia** 355.1
**Bernhardt-Roth disease or syndrome** (paresthesia) 355.1
**Bernheim's syndrome** — see also Failure, heart 428.0
**Bertielliasis** 123.8
**Bertolotti's syndrome** (sacralization of fifth lumbar vertebra) 756.15
**Berylliosis** (acute) (chronic) (lung) (occupational) 503
**Besnier's**
  lupus pernio 135
  prurigo (atopic dermatitis) (infantile eczema) 691.8
**Besnier-Boeck disease or sarcoid** 135
**Besnier-Boeck-Schaumann disease** (sarcoidosis) 135
**Best's disease** 362.76
**Bestiality** 302.1
**Beta-adrenergic hyperdynamic circulatory state** 429.82
**Beta-aminoisobutyric aciduria** 277.2
**Beta-mercaptolactate-cysteine disulfiduria** 270.0
**Beta thalassemia** (major) (minor) (mixed) 282.49

**Beurmann's disease** (sporotrichosis) 117.1
**Bezoar** 938
  intestine 936
  stomach 935.2
**Bezold's abscess** — see also Mastoiditis 383.01
**Bianchi's syndrome** (aphasia-apraxia-alexia) 784.69
**Bicornuate or bicornis uterus** 752.3
  in pregnancy or childbirth 654.0 ☑
    with obstructed labor 660.2 ☑
      affecting fetus or newborn 763.1
    affecting fetus or newborn 763.89
**Bicuspid aortic valve** 746.4
**Biedl-Bardet syndrome** 759.89
**Bielschowsky's disease** 330.1
**Bielschowsky-Jansky**
  amaurotic familial idiocy 330.1
  disease 330.1
**Biemond's syndrome** (obesity, polydactyly, and mental retardation) 759.89
**Biermer's anemia or disease** (pernicious anemia) 281.0
**Biett's disease** 695.4
**Bifid** (congenital) — see also Imperfect, closure
  apex, heart 746.89
  clitoris 752.49
  epiglottis 748.3
  kidney 753.3
  nose 748.1
  patella 755.64
  scrotum 752.89
  toe 755.66
  tongue 750.13
  ureter 753.4
  uterus 752.3
  uvula 749.02
    with cleft lip (see also Cleft, palate, with cleft lip) 749.20
**Biforis uterus** (suprasimplex) 752.3
**Bifurcation** (congenital) — see also Imperfect, closure
  gallbladder 751.69
  kidney pelvis 753.3
  renal pelvis 753.3
  rib 756.3
  tongue 750.13
  trachea 748.3
  ureter 753.4
  urethra 753.8
  uvula 749.02
    with cleft lip (see also Cleft, palate, with cleft lip) 749.20
  vertebra 756.19
**Bigeminal pulse** 427.89
**Bigeminy** 427.89
**Big spleen syndrome** 289.4
**Bilateral** — see condition
**Bile duct** — see condition
**Bile pigments in urine** 791.4
**Bilharziasis** — see also Schistosomiasis 120.9
  chyluria 120.0
  cutaneous 120.3
  galacturia 120.0
  hematochyluria 120.0
  intestinal 120.1
  lipemia 120.9
  lipuria 120.0
  Oriental 120.2
  piarhemia 120.9
  pulmonary 120.2
  tropical hematuria 120.0
  vesical 120.0
**Biliary** — see condition
**Bilious** (attack) — see also Vomiting
  fever, hemoglobinuric 084.8
**Bilirubinuria** 791.4
**Biliuria** 791.4
**Billroth's disease**
  meningocele (see also Spina bifida) 741.9 ☑
**Bilobate placenta** — see Placenta, abnormal

**Bilocular**
  heart 745.7
  stomach 536.8
**Bing-Horton syndrome** (histamine cephalgia) 346.2 ☑
**Binswanger's disease or dementia** 290.12
**Biörck (-Thorson) syndrome** (malignant carcinoid) 259.2
**Biparta, bipartite** — see also Imperfect, closure
  carpal scaphoid 755.59
  patella 755.64
  placenta — see Placenta, abnormal
  vagina 752.49
**Bird**
  face 756.0
  fanciers' lung or disease 495.2
**Bird's disease** (oxaluria) 271.8
**Birth**
  abnormal fetus or newborn 763.9
  accident, fetus or newborn — see Birth, injury
  complications in mother — see Delivery, complicated
  compression during NEC 767.9
  defect — see Anomaly
  delayed, fetus 763.9
  difficult NEC, affecting fetus or newborn 763.9
  dry, affecting fetus or newborn 761.1
  forced, NEC, affecting fetus or newborn 763.89
  forceps, affecting fetus or newborn 763.2
  hematoma of sternomastoid 767.8
  immature 765.1 ☑
    extremely 765.0 ☑
  inattention, after or at 995.52
  induced, affecting fetus or newborn 763.89
  infant — see Newborn
  injury NEC 767.9
    adrenal gland 767.8
    basal ganglia 767.0
    brachial plexus (paralysis) 767.6
    brain (compression) (pressure) 767.0
    cerebellum 767.0
    cerebral hemorrhage 767.0
    conjunctiva 767.8
    eye 767.8
    fracture
      bone, any except clavicle or spine 767.3
      clavicle 767.2
      femur 767.3
      humerus 767.3
      long bone 767.3
      radius and ulna 767.3
      skeleton NEC 767.3
      skull 767.3
      spine 767.4
      tibia and fibula 767.3
    hematoma 767.8
      liver (subcapsular) 767.8
      mastoid 767.8
      skull 767.19
      sternomastoid 767.8
      testes 767.8
      vulva 767.8
    intracranial (edema) 767.0
    laceration
      brain 767.0
      by scalpel 767.8
      peripheral nerve 767.7
    liver 767.8
    meninges
      brain 767.0
      spinal cord 767.4
    nerves (cranial, peripheral) 767.7
      brachial plexus 767.6
      facial 767.5
    paralysis 767.7
      brachial plexus 767.6
      Erb (-Duchenne) 767.6

**Birth** — continued
  injury — continued
    paralysis — continued
      facial nerve 767.5
      Klumpke (-Déjérine) 767.6
      radial nerve 767.6
      spinal (cord) (hemorrhage) (laceration) (rupture) 767.4
    rupture
      intracranial 767.0
      liver 767.8
      spinal cord 767.4
      spleen 767.8
      viscera 767.8
    scalp 767.19
    scalpel wound 767.8
    skeleton NEC 767.3
    specified NEC 767.8
    spinal cord 767.4
    spleen 767.8
    subdural hemorrhage 767.0
    tentorial, tear 767.0
    testes 767.8
    vulva 767.8
  instrumental, NEC, affecting fetus or newborn 763.2
  lack of care, after or at 995.52
  multiple
    affected by maternal complications of pregnancy 761.5
    healthy liveborn — see Newborn, multiple
  neglect, after or at 995.52
  newborn — see Newborn
  palsy or paralysis NEC 767.7
  precipitate, fetus or newborn 763.6
  premature (infant) 765.1 ☑
  prolonged, affecting fetus or newborn 763.9
  retarded, fetus or newborn 763.9
  shock, newborn 779.89
  strangulation or suffocation
    due to aspiration of clear amniotic fluid 770.13
      with respiratory symptoms 770.14
    mechanical 767.8
  trauma NEC 767.9
  triplet
    affected by maternal complications of pregnancy 761.5
    healthy liveborn — see Newborn, multiple
  twin
    affected by maternal complications of pregnancy 761.5
    healthy liveborn — see Newborn, twin
  ventouse, affecting fetus or newborn 763.3
**Birthmark** 757.32
**Bisalbuminemia** 273.8
**Biskra button** 085.1
**Bite(s)**
  with intact skin surface — see Contusion
  animal — see Wound, open, by site
    intact skin surface — see Contusion
  centipede 989.5
  chigger 133.8
  fire ant 989.5
  flea — see Injury, superficial, by site
  human (open wound) (see also Wound, open, by site)
    intact skin surface — see Contusion
  insect
    nonvenomous — see Injury, superficial, by site
    venomous 989.5
  mad dog (death from) 071
  open
    anterior 524.24
    posterior 524.25
  poisonous 989.5

---

☑ Additional Digit Required — Refer to the Tabular List for Digit Selection      ▽ Subterms under main terms may continue to next column or page

**2008 ICD-9-CM**     ▶◀ Revised Text     ● New Line     ▲ Revised Code     **October 2007 · Volume 2 — 35**

**Bite(s)** — *continued*
  red bug 133.8
  reptile 989.5
    nonvenomous — *see* Wound, open,
      by site
  snake 989.5
    nonvenomous — *see* Wound, open,
      by site
  spider (venomous) 989.5
    nonvenomous — *see* Injury, super-
      ficial, by site
  venomous 989.5
**Biting**
  cheek or lip 528.9
  nail 307.9
**Black**
  death 020.9
  eye NEC 921.0
  hairy tongue 529.3
  heel 924.20
  lung disease 500
  palm 923.20
**Blackfan-Diamond anemia or syndrome**
  (congenital hypoplastic anemia)
  284.01
**Blackhead** 706.1
**Blackout** 780.2
**Blackwater fever** 084.8
**Bladder** — *see* condition
**Blast**
  blindness 921.3
  concussion — *see* Blast, injury
  injury 869.0
    with open wound into cavity 869.1
    abdomen or thorax — *see* Injury,
      internal, by site
    brain (*see also* Concussion, brain)
      850.9
      with skull fracture — *see* Frac-
        ture, skull
    ear (acoustic nerve trauma) 951.5
      with perforation, tympanic
        membrane — *see* Wound,
        open, ear, drum
    lung (*see also* Injury, internal,
      lung) 861.20
    otitic (explosive) 388.11
**Blastomycosis, blastomycotic** (chronic)
  (cutaneous) (disseminated) (lung)
  (pulmonary) (systemic) 116.0
  Brazilian 116.1
  European 117.5
  keloidal 116.2
  North American 116.0
  primary pulmonary 116.0
  South American 116.1
**Bleb(s)** 709.8
  emphysematous (bullous) (diffuse)
    (lung) (ruptured) (solitary) 492.0
  filtering, eye (postglaucoma) (status)
    V45.69
    with complication 997.99
      postcataract extraction (complica-
        tion) 997.99
  lung (ruptured) 492.0
    congenital 770.5
  subpleural (emphysematous) 492.0
**Bleeder** (familial) (hereditary) — *see also*
  Defect, coagulation 286.9
  nonfamilial 286.9
**Bleeding** — *see also* Hemorrhage 459.0
  anal 569.3
  anovulatory 628.0
  atonic, following delivery 666.1 ☑
  capillary 448.9
  due to subinvolution 621.1
    puerperal 666.2 ☑
  ear 388.69
  excessive, associated with menopausal
    onset 627.0
  familial (*see also* Defect, coagulation)
    286.9
  following intercourse 626.7
  gastrointestinal 578.9
  gums 523.8

**Bleeding** — *see also* Hemorrhage —
  *continued*
  hemorrhoids — *see* Hemorrhoids,
    bleeding
  intermenstrual
    irregular 626.6
    regular 626.5
  intraoperative 998.11
  irregular NEC 626.4
  menopausal 627.0
  mouth 528.9
  nipple 611.79
  nose 784.7
  ovulation 626.5
  postclimacteric 627.1
  postcoital 626.7
  postmenopausal 627.1
    following induced menopause
      627.4
  postoperative 998.11
  preclimacteric 627.0
  puberty 626.3
    excessive, with onset of menstrual
      periods 626.3
  rectum, rectal 569.3
  tendencies (*see also* Defect, coagula-
    tion) 286.9
  throat 784.8
  umbilical stump 772.3
  umbilicus 789.9
  unrelated to menstrual cycle 626.6
  uterus, uterine 626.9
    climacteric 627.0
    dysfunctional 626.8
    functional 626.8
    unrelated to menstrual cycle 626.6
  vagina, vaginal 623.8
    functional 626.8
  vicarious 625.8
**Blennorrhagia, blennorrhagic** — *see*
  Blennorrhea
**Blennorrhea** (acute) 098.0
  adultorum 098.40
  alveolaris 523.40
  chronic or duration of 2 months or
    over 098.2
  gonococcal (neonatorum) 098.40
  inclusion (neonatal) (newborn) 771.6
  neonatorum 098.40
**Blepharelosis** — *see also* Entropion
  374.00
**Blepharitis** (eyelid) 373.00
  angularis 373.01
  ciliaris 373.00
    with ulcer 373.01
  marginal 373.00
    with ulcer 373.01
  scrofulous (*see also* Tuberculosis)
    017.3 ☑ [373.00]
  squamous 373.02
  ulcerative 373.01
**Blepharochalasis** 374.34
  congenital 743.62
**Blepharoclonus** 333.81
**Blepharoconjunctivitis** — *see also*
  Conjunctivitis 372.20
  angular 372.21
  contact 372.22
**Blepharophimosis** (eyelid) 374.46
  congenital 743.62
**Blepharoplegia** 374.89
**Blepharoptosis** 374.30
  congenital 743.61
**Blepharopyorrhea** 098.49
**Blepharospasm** 333.81
  due to drugs 333.85
**Blessig's cyst** 362.62
**Blighted ovum** 631
**Blind**
  bronchus (congenital) 748.3
  eye (*see also* Blindness)
    hypertensive 360.42
    hypotensive 360.41
  loop syndrome (postoperative) 579.2
  sac, fallopian tube (congenital) 752.19
  spot, enlarged 368.42

**Blind** — *continued*
  tract or tube (congenital) NEC — *see*
    Atresia
**Blindness** (acquired) (congenital) (both
  eyes) 369.00
  with deafness V49.85     ●
  blast 921.3
    with nerve injury — *see* Injury,
      nerve, optic
  Bright's — *see* Uremia
  color (congenital) 368.59
    acquired 368.55
    blue 368.53
    green 368.52
    red 368.51
    total 368.54
  concussion 950.9
  cortical 377.75
  day 368.10
    acquired 368.10
    congenital 368.10
    hereditary 368.10
    specified type NEC 368.10
  due to
    injury NEC 950.9
    refractive error — *see* Error, refrac-
      tive
  eclipse (total) 363.31
  emotional 300.11
  hysterical 300.11
  legal (both eyes) (USA definition) 369.4
    with impairment of better (less im-
      paired) eye
      near-total 369.02
        with
          lesser eye impairment
            369.02
            near-total 369.04
            total 369.03
      profound 369.05
        with
          lesser eye impairment
            369.05
            near-total 369.07
            profound 369.08
            total 369.06
      severe 369.21
        with
          lesser eye impairment
            369.21
            blind 369.11
            near-total 369.13
            profound 369.14
            severe 369.22
            total 369.12
      total
        with lesser eye impairment
          total 369.01
  mind 784.69
  moderate
    both eyes 369.25
      with impairment of lesser eye
        (specified as)
        blind, not further specified
          369.15
        low vision, not further speci-
          fied 369.23
        near-total 369.17
        profound 369.18
        severe 369.24
        total 369.16
    one eye 369.74
      with vision of other eye (speci-
        fied as)
        near-normal 369.75
        normal 369.76
  near-total
    both eyes 369.04
      with impairment of lesser eye
        (specified as)
        blind, not further specified
          369.02
        total 369.03
    one eye 369.64

**Blindness** — *continued*
  near-total — *continued*
    one eye — *continued*
      with vision of other eye (speci-
        fied as)
        near-normal 369.65
        normal 369.66
  night 368.60
    acquired 368.62
    congenital (Japanese) 368.61
    hereditary 368.61
    specified type NEC 368.69
    vitamin A deficiency 264.5
  nocturnal — *see* Blindness, night
  one eye 369.60
    with low vision of other eye 369.10
  profound
    both eyes 369.08
      with impairment of lesser eye
        (specified as)
        blind, not further specified
          369.05
        near-total 369.07
        total 369.06
    one eye 369.67
      with vision of other eye (speci-
        fied as)
        near-normal 369.68
        normal 369.69
  psychic 784.69
  severe
    both eyes 369.22
      with impairment of lesser eye
        (specified as)
        blind, not further specified
          369.11
        low vision, not further speci-
          fied 369.21
        near-total 369.13
        profound 369.14
        total 369.12
    one eye 369.71
      with vision of other eye (speci-
        fied as)
        near-normal 369.72
        normal 369.73
  snow 370.24
  sun 363.31
  temporary 368.12
  total
    both eyes 369.01
    one eye 369.61
      with vision of other eye (speci-
        fied as)
        near-normal 369.62
        normal 369.63
  transient 368.12
  traumatic NEC 950.9
  word (developmental) 315.01
    acquired 784.61
    secondary to organic lesion 784.61
**Blister** — *see also* Injury, superficial, by
  site
  beetle dermatitis 692.89
  due to burn — *see* Burn, by site, sec-
    ond degree
  fever 054.9
  multiple, skin, nontraumatic 709.8
**Bloating** 787.3
**Bloch-Siemens syndrome** (incontinentia
  pigmenti) 757.33
**Bloch-Stauffer dyshormonal dermato-
  sis** 757.33
**Bloch-Sulzberger disease or syndrome**
  (incontinentia pigmenti)
  (melanoblastosis) 757.33
**Block**
  alveolar capillary 516.3
  arborization (heart) 426.6
  arrhythmic 426.9
  atrioventricular (AV) (incomplete)
    (partial) 426.10
    with
      2:1 atrioventricular response
        block 426.13

☑ Additional Digit Required — Refer to the Tabular List for Digit Selection          ▽ Subterms under main terms may continue to next column or page

36 — Volume 2 · October 2007      ►◄ Revised Text      ● New Line      ▲ Revised Code      *2008 ICD-9-CM*

**Block** — *continued*
  atrioventricular — *continued*
    with — *continued*
      atrioventricular dissociation
        426.0
      first degree (incomplete) 426.11
      second dcgree (Mobitz type I)
        426.13
        Mobitz (type) II 426.12
      third degree 426.0
      complete 426.0
        congenital 746.86
      congenital 746.86
      Mobitz (incomplete)
        type I (Wenckebach's) 426.13
        type II 426.12
      partial 426.13
  auriculoventricular (*see also* Block,
      atrioventricular) 426.10
    complete 426.0
      congenital 746.86
    congenital 746.86
  bifascicular (cardiac) 426.53
  bundle branch (complete) (false) (in-
      complete) 426.50
    bilateral 426.53
    left (complete) (main stem) 426.3
      with right bundle branch block
        426.53
      anterior fascicular 426.2
        with
          posterior fascicular block
            426.3
          right bundle branch block
            426.52
      hemiblock 426.2
      incomplete 426.2
        with right bundle branch
          block 426.53
      posterior fascicular 426.2
        with
          anterior fascicular block
            426.3
          right bundle branch block
            426.51
    right 426.4
      with
        left bundle branch block (in-
          complete) (main stem)
          426.53
        left fascicular block 426.53
          anterior 426.52
          posterior 426.51
    Wilson's type 426.4
  cardiac 426.9
  conduction 426.9
    complete 426.0
  Eustachian tube (*see also* Obstruc-
      tion, Eustachian tube) 381.60
  fascicular (left anterior) (left posterior)
      426.2
  foramen Magendie (acquired) 331.3
    congenital 742.3
      with spina bifida (*see also* Spina
        bifida) 741.0 ☑
  heart 426.9
    first degree (atrioventricular)
      426.11
    second degree (atrioventricular)
      426.13
    third degree (atrioventricular)
      426.0
    bundle branch (complete) (false)
      (incomplete) 426.50
      bilateral 426.53
      left (*see also* Block, bundle
        branch, left) 426.3
      right (*see also* Block, bundle
        branch, right) 426.4
    complete (atrioventricular) 426.0
      congenital 746.86
    incomplete 426.13
    intra-atrial 426.6
    intraventricular NEC 426.6
    sinoatrial 426.6
    specified type NEC 426.6

**Block** — *continued*
  hepatic vein 453.0
  intraventricular (diffuse) (myofibrillar)
    426.6
    bundle branch (complete) (false)
      (incomplete) 426.50
      bilateral 426.53
      left (*see also* Block, bundle
        branch, left) 426.3
      right (*see also* Block, bundle
        branch, right) 426.4
  kidney (*see also* Disease, renal) 593.9
    postcystoscopic 997.5
  myocardial (*see also* Block, heart)
    426.9
  nodal 426.10
  optic nerve 377.49
  organ or site (congenital) NEC — *see*
      Atresia
  parietal 426.6
  peri-infarction 426.6
  portal (vein) 452
  sinoatrial 426.6
  sinoauricular 426.6
  spinal cord 336.9
  trifascicular 426.54
  tubal 628.2
  vein NEC 453.9
**Blocq's disease or syndrome** (astasia-
    abasia) 307.9
**Blood**
  constituents, abnormal NEC 790.6
  disease 289.9
    specified NEC 289.89
  donor V59.01
    other blood components V59.09
    stem cells V59.02
    whole blood V59.01
  dyscrasia 289.9
    with
      abortion — *see* Abortion, by
        type, with hemorrhage,
        delayed or excessive
      ectopic pregnancy (*see also* cat-
        egories 633.0–633.9)
        639.1
      molar pregnancy (*see also* cate-
        gories 630–632) 639.1
    fetus or newborn NEC 776.9
    following
      abortion 639.1
      ectopic or molar pregnancy
        639.1
    puerperal, postpartum 666.3 ☑
  flukes NEC (*see also* Infestation,
      Schistosoma) 120.9
  in
    feces (*see also* Melena) 578.1
      occult 792.1
    urine (*see also* Hematuria) 599.7
  mole 631
  occult 792.1
  poisoning (*see also* Septicemia) 038.9
  pressure
    decreased, due to shock following
      injury 958.4
    fluctuating 796.4
    high (*see also* Hypertension) 401.9
      incidental reading (isolated)
        (nonspecific), without diag-
        nosis of hypertension
        796.2
    low (*see also* Hypotension) 458.9
      incidental reading (isolated)
        (nonspecific), without diag-
        nosis of hypotension
        796.3
  spitting (*see also* Hemoptysis) 786.3
  staining cornea 371.12
  transfusion
    without reported diagnosis V58.2
    donor V59.01
      stem cells V59.02
    reaction or complication — *see*
      Complications, transfusion
  tumor — *see* Hematoma

**Blood** — *continued*
  vessel rupture — *see* Hemorrhage
  vomiting (*see also* Hematemesis) 578.0
**Blood-forming organ disease** 289.9
**Bloodgood's disease** 610.1
**Bloodshot eye** 379.93
**Bloom (-Machacek) (-Torre) syndrome**
    757.39
**Blotch, palpebral** 372.55
**Blotch's disease** (tibia vara) 732.4
**Blount-Barber syndrome** (tibia vara)
    732.4
**Blount's disease** (tibia vara) 732.4
**Blue**
  baby 746.9
  bloater 491.20
    with
      acute bronchitis 491.22
      exacerbation (acute) 491.21
  diaper syndrome 270.0
  disease 746.9
  dome cyst 610.0
  drum syndrome 381.02
  sclera 743.47
    with fragility of bone and deafness
      756.51
  toe syndrome 445.02
**Blueness** — *see also* Cyanosis 782.5
**Blurring, visual** 368.8
**Blushing** (abnormal) (excessive) 782.62
**BMI** (body mass index)
  adult
    25.0-25.9 V85.21
    26.0-26.9 V85.22
    27.0-27.9 V85.23
    28.0-28.9 V85.24
    29.0-29.9 V85.25
    30.0-30.9 V85.30
    31.0-31.9 V85.31
    32.0-32.9 V85.32
    33.0-33.9 V85.33
    34.0-34.9 V85.34
    35.0-35.9 V85.35
    36.0-36.9 V85.36
    37.0-37.9 V85.37
    38.0-38.9 V85.38
    39.0-39.9 V85.39
    40 and over V85.4
    between 19-24 V85.1
    less than 19 V85.0
  pediatric
    5th percentile to less than 85th
      percentile for age V85.52
    85th percentile to less than 95th
      percentile for age V85.53
    greater than or equal to 95th per-
      centile for age V85.54
    less than 5th percentile for age
      V85.51
**Boarder, hospital** V65.0
  infant V65.0
**Bockhart's impetigo** (superficial folliculi-
    tis) 704.8
**Bodechtel-Guttmann disease** (subacute
    sclerosing panencephalitis) 046.2
**Boder-Sedgwick syndrome** (ataxia-
    telangiectasia) 334.8
**Body, bodies**
  Aschoff (*see also* Myocarditis,
      rheumatic) 398.0
  asteroid, vitreous 379.22
  choroid, colloid (degenerative) 362.57
    hereditary 362.77
  cytoid (retina) 362.82
  drusen (retina) (*see also* Drusen)
    362.57
    optic disc 377.21
  fibrin, pleura 511.0
  foreign — *see* Foreign body
  Hassall-Henle 371.41
  loose
    joint (*see also* Loose, body, joint)
      718.1 ☑
      knee 717.6
    knee 717.6
    sheath, tendon 727.82
  Mallory's 034.1

**Body, bodies** — *continued*
  mass index (BMI)
    adult
      25.0-25.9 V85.21
      26.0-26.9 V85.22
      27.0-27.9 V85.23
      28.0-28.9 V85.24
      29.0-29.9 V85.25
      30.0-30.9 V85.30
      31.0-31.9 V85.31
      32.0-32.9 V85.32
      33.0-33.9 V85.33
      34.0-34.9 V85.34
      36.0-36.9 V85.36
      37.0-37.9 V85.37
      38.0-38.9 V85.38
      39.0-39.9 V85.39
      40 and over V85.4
      between 19-24 V85.1
      less than 19 V85.0
    pediatric
      5th percentile to less than 85th
        percentile for age V85.52
      85th percentile to less than
        95th percentile for age
        V85.53
      greater than or equal to 95th
        percentile for age V85.54
      less than 5th percentile for age
        V85.51
  Mooser 081.0
  Negri 071
  rice (joint) (*see also* Loose, body, joint)
    718.1 ☑
    knee 717.6
  rocking 307.3
**Boeck's**
  disease (sarcoidosis) 135
  lupoid (miliary) 135
  sarcoid 135
**Boerhaave's syndrome** (spontaneous
    esophageal rupture) 530.4
**Boggy**
  cervix 622.8
  uterus 621.8
**Boil** — *see also* Carbuncle 680.9
  abdominal wall 680.2
  Aleppo 085.1
  ankle 680.6
  anus 680.5
  arm (any part, above wrist) 680.3
  auditory canal, external 680.0
  axilla 680.3
  back (any part) 680.2
  Baghdad 085.1
  breast 680.2
  buttock 680.5
  chest wall 680.2
  corpus cavernosum 607.2
  Delhi 085.1
  ear (any part) 680.0
  eyelid 373.13
  face (any part, except eye) 680.0
  finger (any) 680.4
  flank 680.2
  foot (any part) 680.7
  forearm 680.3
  Gafsa 085.1
  genital organ, male 608.4
  gluteal (region) 680.5
  groin 680.2
  hand (any part) 680.4
  head (any part, except face) 680.8
  heel 680.7
  hip 680.6
  knee 680.6
  labia 616.4
  lacrimal (*see also* Dacryocystitis)
    375.30
    gland (*see also* Dacryoadenitis)
      375.00
    passages (duct) (sac) (*see also*
      Dacryocystitis) 375.30
  leg, any part, except foot 680.6
  multiple sites 680.9
  natal 085.1

Block — Boil

☑ Additional Digit Required — Refer to the Tabular List for Digit Selection                                    Ⓦ Subterms under main terms may continue to next column or page

*2008 ICD-9-CM*          ▶◀ Revised Text          ● New Line          ▲ Revised Code                                **Volume 2 — 37**

**Boil** — see also Carbuncle —
    continued
  neck 680.1
  nose (external) (septum) 680.0
  orbit, orbital 376.01
  partes posteriores 680.5
  pectoral region 680.2
  penis 607.2
  perineum 680.2
  pinna 680.0
  scalp (any part) 680.8
  scrotum 608.4
  seminal vesicle 608.0
  shoulder 680.3
  skin NEC 680.9
  specified site NEC 680.8
  spermatic cord 608.4
  temple (region) 680.0
  testis 608.4
  thigh 680.6
  thumb 680.4
  toe (any) 680.7
  tropical 085.1
  trunk 680.2
  tunica vaginalis 608.4
  umbilicus 680.2
  upper arm 680.3
  vas deferens 608.4
  vulva 616.4
  wrist 680.4
**Bold hives** — see also Urticaria 708.9
**Bolivian hemorrhagic fever** 078.7
**Bombé, iris** 364.74
**Bomford-Rhoads anemia** (refractory)
    238.72
**Bone** — see condition
**Bonnevie-Ullrich syndrome** 758.6
**Bonnier's syndrome** 386.19
**Bonvale Dam fever** 780.79
**Bony block of joint** 718.80
  ankle 718.87
  elbow 718.82
  foot 718.87
  hand 718.84
  hip 718.85
  knee 718.86
  multiple sites 718.89
  pelvic region 718.85
  shoulder (region) 718.81
  specified site NEC 718.88
  wrist 718.83
**Borderline**
  intellectual functioning V62.89
  pelvis 653.1 ☑
    with obstruction during labor
      660.1 ☑
        affecting fetus or newborn 763.1
  psychosis (see also Schizophrenia)
    295.5 ☑
  of childhood (see also Psychosis,
    childhood) 299.8 ☑
  schizophrenia (see also Schizophrenia)
    295.5 ☑
**Borna disease** 062.9
**Bornholm disease** (epidemic pleurody-
    nia) 074.1
**Borrelia vincentii** (mouth) (pharynx)
    (tonsils) 101
**Bostock's catarrh** — see also Fever, hay
    477.9
**Boston exanthem** 048
**Botalli, ductus** (patent) (persistent)
    747.0
**Bothriocephalus latus infestation** 123.4
**Botulism** 005.1
  food poisoning 005.1                ●
  infant 040.41                       ●
  non-foodborne 040.42                ●
  wound 040.42                        ▲
**Bouba** — see also Yaws 102.9
**Bouffée délirante** 298.3
**Bouillaud's disease or syndrome**
    (rheumatic heart disease) 391.9
**Bourneville's disease** (tuberous sclero-
    sis) 759.5
**Boutonneuse fever** 082.1

**Boutonniere**
  deformity (finger) 736.21
  hand (intrinsic) 736.21
**Bouveret (-Hoffmann) disease or syn-
    drome** (paroxysmal tachycardia)
    427.2
**Bovine heart** — see Hypertrophy, car-
    diac
**Bowel** — see condition
**Bowen's**
  dermatosis (precancerous) (M8081/2)
    — see Neoplasm, skin, in situ
  disease (M8081/2) — see Neoplasm,
    skin, in situ
  epithelioma (M8081/2) — see Neo-
    plasm, skin, in situ
  type
    epidermoid carcinoma in situ
      (M8081/2) — see Neoplasm,
      skin, in situ
    intraepidermal squamous cell car-
      cinoma (M8081/2) — see
      Neoplasm, skin, in situ
**Bowing**
  femur 736.89
    congenital 754.42
  fibula 736.89
    congenital 754.43
  forearm 736.09
    away from midline (cubitus valgus)
      736.01
    toward midline (cubitus varus)
      736.02
  leg(s), long bones, congenital 754.44
  radius 736.09
    away from midline (cubitus valgus)
      736.01
    toward midline (cubitus varus)
      736.02
  tibia 736.89
    congenital 754.43
**Bowleg(s)** 736.42
  congenital 754.44
  rachitic 268.1
**Boyd's dysentery** 004.2
**Brachial** — see condition
**Brachman-de Lange syndrome** (Amster-
    dam dwarf, mental retardation, and
    brachycephaly) 759.89
**Brachycardia** 427.89
**Brachycephaly** 756.0
**Brachymorphism and ectopia lentis**
    759.89
**Bradley's disease** (epidemic vomiting)
    078.82
**Bradycardia** 427.89
  chronic (sinus) 427.81
  newborn 779.81
  nodal 427.89
  postoperative 997.1
  reflex 337.0
  sinoatrial 427.89
    with paroxysmal tachyarrhythmia
      or tachycardia 427.81
    chronic 427.81
  sinus 427.89
    with paroxysmal tachyarrhythmia
      or tachycardia 427.81
    chronic 427.81
    persistent 427.81
    severe 427.81
  tachycardia syndrome 427.81
  vagal 427.89
**Bradypnea** 786.09
**Brailsford's disease** 732.3
  radial head 732.3
  tarsal scaphoid 732.5
**Brailsford-Morquio disease or syn-
    drome** (mucopolysaccharidosis IV)
    277.5
**Brain** — see also condition
  death 348.8

**Brain** — see also condition —
    continued
  syndrome (acute) (chronic) (nonpsy-
    chotic) (organic) (with neurotic
    reaction) (with behavioral reac-
    tion) (see also Syndrome, brain)
    310.9
    with
      presenile brain disease 290.10
      psychosis, psychotic reaction
        (see also Psychosis, organ-
        ic) 294.9
  congenital (see also Retardation,
    mental) 319
**Branched-chain amino-acid disease**
    270.3
**Branchial** — see condition
**Brandt's syndrome** (acrodermatitis en-
    teropathica) 686.8
**Brash** (water) 787.1
**Brass-founders' ague** 985.8
**Bravais-Jacksonian epilepsy** — see also
    Epilepsy 345.5 ☑
**Braxton Hicks contractions** 644.1 ☑
**Braziers' disease** 985.8
**Brazilian**
  blastomycosis 116.1
  leishmaniasis 085.5
**BRBPR** (bright red blood per rectum)
    569.3
**Break**
  cardiorenal — see Hypertension, car-
    diorenal
  retina (see also Defect, retina) 361.30
**Breakbone fever** 061
**Breakdown**
  device, implant, or graft — see Compli-
    cations, mechanical
  nervous (see also Disorder, mental,
    nonpsychotic) 300.9
  perineum 674.2 ☑
**Breast** — see condition
**Breast feeding difficulties** 676.8 ☑
**Breath**
  foul 784.99
  holder, child 312.81
  holding spells 786.9
  shortness 786.05
**Breathing**
  asymmetrical 786.09
  bronchial 786.09
  exercises V57.0
  labored 786.09
  mouth 784.99
    causing malocclusion 524.59
  periodic 786.09
    high altitude 327.22
  tic 307.20
**Breathlessness** 786.09
**Breda's disease** — see also Yaws 102.9
**Breech**
  delivery, affecting fetus or newborn
    763.0
  extraction, affecting fetus or newborn
    763.0
  presentation (buttocks) (complete)
    (frank) 652.2 ☑
    with successful version 652.1 ☑
    before labor, affecting fetus or
      newborn 761.7
    during labor, affecting fetus or
      newborn 763.0
**Breisky's disease** (kraurosis vulvae)
    624.09                              ▲
**Brennemann's syndrome** (acute
    mesenteric lymphadenitis) 289.2
**Brenner's**
  tumor (benign) (M9000/0) 220
    borderline malignancy (M9000/1)
      236.2
    malignant (M9000/3) 183.0
    proliferating (M9000/1) 236.2
**Bretonneau's disease** (diphtheritic ma-
    lignant angina) 032.0
**Breus' mole** 631
**Brevicollis** 756.16

**Bricklayers' itch** 692.89
**Brickmakers' anemia** 126.9
**Bridge**
  myocardial 746.85
**Bright's**
  blindness — see Uremia
  disease (see also Nephritis) 583.9
    arteriosclerotic (see also Hyperten-
      sion, kidney) 403.90
**Bright red blood per rectum** (BRBPR)
    569.3
**Brill's disease** (recrudescent typhus)
    081.1
  flea-borne 081.0
  louse-borne 081.1
**Brill-Symmers disease** (follicular lym-
    phoma) (M9690/3) 202.0 ☑
**Brill-Zinsser disease** (recrudescent ty-
    phus) 081.1
**Brinton's disease** (linitis plastica)
    (M8142/3) 151.9
**Brion-Kayser disease** — see also Fever,
    paratyphoid 002.9
**Briquet's disorder or syndrome** 300.81
**Brissaud's**
  infantilism (infantile myxedema) 244.9
  motor-verbal tic 307.23
**Brissaud-Meige syndrome** (infantile
    myxedema) 244.9
**Brittle**
  bones (congenital) 756.51
  nails 703.8
    congenital 757.5
**Broad** — see also condition
  beta disease 272.2
  ligament laceration syndrome 620.6
**Brock's syndrome** (atelectasis due to
    enlarged lymph nodes) 518.0
**Brocq's disease** 691.8
  atopic (diffuse) neurodermatitis 691.8
  lichen simplex chronicus 698.3
  parakeratosis psoriasiformis 696.2
  parapsoriasis 696.2
**Brocq-Duhring disease** (dermatitis her-
    petiformis) 694.0
**Brodie's**
  abscess (localized) (chronic) (see also
    Osteomyelitis) 730.1 ☑
  disease (joint) (see also Osteomyelitis)
    730.1 ☑
**Broken**
  arches 734
    congenital 755.67
  back — see Fracture, vertebra, by site
  bone — see Fracture, by site
  compensation — see Disease, heart
  heart syndrome 429.83
  implant or internal device — see list-
    ing under Complications, me-
    chanical
  neck — see Fracture, vertebra, cervi-
    cal
  nose 802.0
    open 802.1
  tooth, teeth 873.63
    complicated 873.73
**Bromhidrosis** 705.89
**Bromidism, bromism**
  acute 967.3
    correct substance properly admin-
      istered 349.82
    overdose or wrong substance given
      or taken 967.3
  chronic (see also Dependence)
    304.1 ☑
**Bromidrosiphobia** 300.23
**Bromidrosis** 705.89
**Bronchi, bronchial** — see condition
**Bronchiectasis** (cylindrical) (diffuse)
    (fusiform) (localized) (moniliform)
    (postinfectious) (recurrent) (saccu-
    lar) 494.0
  with acute exacerbation 494.1
  congenital 748.61
  tuberculosis (see also Tuberculosis)
    011.5 ☑

☑ Additional Digit Required — Refer to the Tabular List for Digit Selection          ⓦ Subterms under main terms may continue to next column or page

38 — Volume 2 · October 2007          ▶◀ Revised Text          ● New Line          ▲ Revised Code          *2008 ICD-9-CM*

**Bronchiolectasis** — *see* Bronchiectasis
**Bronchiolitis** (acute) (infectious) (subacute) 466.19
with
  bronchospasm or obstruction 466.19
  influenza, flu, or grippe 487.1
catarrhal (acute) (subacute) 466.19
chemical 506.0
  chronic 506.4
chronic (obliterative) 491.8
due to external agent — *see* Bronchitis, acute, due to
fibrosa obliterans 491.8
influenzal 487.1
obliterans 491.8
  with organizing pneumonia (B.O.O.P.) 516.8
  status post lung transplant 996.84
obliterative (chronic) (diffuse) (subacute) 491.8
  due to fumes or vapors 506.4
respiratory syncytial virus 466.11
vesicular — *see* Pneumonia, broncho-
**Bronchitis** (diffuse) (hypostatic) (infectious) (inflammatory) (simple) 490
with
  emphysema — *see* Emphysema
  influenza, flu, or grippe 487.1
  obstruction airway, chronic 491.20
    with
      acute bronchitis 491.22
      exacerbation (acute) 491.21
  tracheitis 490
    acute or subacute 466.0
      with bronchospasm or obstruction 466.0
    chronic 491.8
acute or subacute 466.0
  with
    bronchospasm 466.0
    obstruction 466.0
    tracheitis 466.0
  chemical (due to fumes or vapors) 506.0
  due to
    fumes or vapors 506.0
    radiation 508.8
allergic (acute) (*see also* Asthma) 493.9 ☑
arachidic 934.1
aspiration 507.0
  due to fumes or vapors 506.0
asthmatic (acute) 493.90
  with
    acute exacerbation 493.92
    status asthmaticus 493.91
  chronic 493.2 ☑
capillary 466.19
  with bronchospasm or obstruction 466.19
  chronic 491.8
caseous (*see also* Tuberculosis) 011.3 ☑
Castellani's 104.8
catarrhal 490
  acute — *see* Bronchitis, acute
  chronic 491.0
chemical (acute) (subacute) 506.0
  chronic 506.4
  due to fumes or vapors (acute) (subacute) 506.0
    chronic 506.4
chronic 491.9
  with
    tracheitis (chronic) 491.8
  asthmatic 493.2 ☑
  catarrhal 491.0
  chemical (due to fumes and vapors) 506.4
  due to
    fumes or vapors (chemical) (inhalation) 506.4
    radiation 508.8
    tobacco smoking 491.0
  mucopurulent 491.1

**Bronchitis** — *continued*
chronic — *continued*
  obstructive 491.20
    with
      acute bronchitis 491.22
      exacerbation (acute) 491.21
  purulent 491.1
  simple 491.0
  specified type NEC 491.8
croupous 466.0
  with bronchospasm or obstruction 466.0
  due to fumes or vapors 506.0
emphysematous 491.20
  with
    acute bronchitis 491.22
    exacerbation (acute) 491.21
exudative 466.0
fetid (chronic) (recurrent) 491.1
fibrinous, acute or subacute 466.0
  with bronchospasm or obstruction 466.0
grippal 487.1
influenzal 487.1
membranous, acute or subacute 466.0
  with bronchospasm or obstruction 466.0
moulders' 502
mucopurulent (chronic) (recurrent) 491.1
  acute or subacute 466.0
obliterans 491.8
obstructive (chronic) 491.20
  with
    acute bronchitis 491.22
    exacerbation (acute) 491.21
pituitous 491.1
plastic (inflammatory) 466.0
pneumococcal, acute or subacute 466.0
  with bronchospasm or obstruction 466.0
pseudomembranous 466.0
purulent (chronic) (recurrent) 491.1
  acute or subacute 466.0
    with bronchospasm or obstruction 466.0
putrid 491.1
scrofulous (*see also* Tuberculosis) 011.3 ☑
senile 491.9
septic, acute or subacute 466.0
  with bronchospasm or obstruction 466.0
smokers' 491.0
spirochetal 104.8
suffocative, acute or subacute 466.0
summer (*see also* Asthma) 493.9 ☑
suppurative (chronic) 491.1
  acute or subacute 466.0
tuberculous (*see also* Tuberculosis) 011.3 ☑
ulcerative 491.8
Vincent's 101
viral, acute or subacute 466.0
**Bronchoalveolitis** 485
**Bronchoaspergillosis** 117.3
**Bronchocele**
meaning
  dilatation of bronchus 519.19
  goiter 240.9
**Bronchogenic carcinoma** 162.9
**Bronchohemisporosis** 117.9
**Broncholithiasis** 518.89
  tuberculous (*see also* Tuberculosis) 011.3 ☑
**Bronchomalacia** 748.3
**Bronchomoniliasis** 112.89
**Bronchomycosis** 112.89
**Bronchonocardiosis** 039.1
**Bronchopleuropneumonia** — *see* Pneumonia, broncho-
**Bronchopneumonia** — *see* Pneumonia, broncho-

**Bronchopneumonitis** — *see* Pneumonia, broncho-
**Bronchopulmonary** — *see* condition
**Bronchopulmonitis** — *see* Pneumonia, broncho-
**Bronchorrhagia** 786.3
newborn 770.3
tuberculous (*see also* Tuberculosis) 011.3 ☑
**Bronchorrhea** (chronic) (purulent) 491.0
acute 466.0
**Bronchospasm** 519.11
with
  asthma — *see* Asthma
  bronchiolitis, acute 466.19
    due to respiratory syncytial virus 466.11
  bronchitis — *see* Bronchitis
  chronic obstructive pulmonary disease (COPD) 496
  emphysema — *see* Emphysema
  due to external agent — *see* Condition, respiratory, acute, due to
acute 519.11
exercise induced 493.81
**Bronchospirochetosis** 104.8
**Bronchostenosis** 519.19
**Bronchus** — *see* condition
**Bronze, bronzed**
diabetes 275.0
disease (Addison's) (skin) 255.41 ▲
  tuberculous (*see also* Tuberculosis) 017.6 ☑
**Brooke's disease or tumor** (M8100/0) — *see* Neoplasm, skin, benign
**Brown enamel of teeth** (hereditary) 520.5
**Brown-Séquard's paralysis** (syndrome) 344.89
**Brown's tendon sheath syndrome** 378.61
**Brow presentation complicating delivery** 652.4 ☑
**Brucella, brucellosis** (infection) 023.9
abortus 023.1
canis 023.3
dermatitis, skin 023.9
melitensis 023.0
mixed 023.8
suis 023.2
**Bruck-de Lange disease or syndrome** (Amsterdam dwarf, mental retardation, and brachycephaly) 759.89
**Bruck's disease** 733.99
**Brugada syndrome** 746.89
**Brug's filariasis** 125.1
**Brugsch's syndrome** (acropachyderma) 757.39
**Bruhl's disease** (splenic anemia with fever) 285.8
**Bruise** (skin surface intact) — *see also* Contusion
with
  fracture — *see* Fracture, by site
  open wound — *see* Wound, open, by site
  internal organ (abdomen, chest, or pelvis) — *see* Injury, internal, by site
  umbilical cord 663.6 ☑
    affecting fetus or newborn 762.6
**Bruit** 785.9
arterial (abdominal) (carotid) 785.9
supraclavicular 785.9
**Brushburn** — *see* Injury, superficial, by site
**Bruton's X-linked agammaglobulinemia** 279.04
**Bruxism** 306.8
sleep related 327.53
**Bubbly lung syndrome** 770.7
**Bubo** 289.3
blennorrhagic 098.89
chancroidal 099.0
climatic 099.1

**Bubo** — *continued*
due to Hemophilus ducreyi 099.0
gonococcal 098.89
indolent NEC 099.8
inguinal NEC 099.8
  chancroidal 099.0
  climatic 099.1
  due to H. ducreyi 099.0
scrofulous (*see also* Tuberculosis) 017.2 ☑
soft chancre 099.0
suppurating 683
syphilitic 091.0
  congenital 090.0
tropical 099.1
venereal NEC 099.8
virulent 099.0
**Bubonic plague** 020.0
**Bubonocele** — *see* Hernia, inguinal
**Buccal** — *see* condition
**Buchanan's disease** (juvenile osteochondrosis of iliac crest) 732.1
**Buchem's syndrome** (hyperostosis corticalis) 733.3
**Buchman's disease** (osteochondrosis, juvenile) 732.1
**Bucket handle fracture** (semilunar cartilage) — *see also* Tear, meniscus 836.2
**Budd-Chiari syndrome** (hepatic vein thrombosis) 453.0
**Budgerigar-fanciers' disease or lung** 495.2
**Büdinger-Ludloff-Läwen disease** 717.89
**Buerger's disease** (thromboangiitis obliterans) 443.1
**Bulbar** — *see* condition
**Bulbus cordis** 745.9
persistent (in left ventricle) 745.8
**Bulging fontanels** (congenital) 756.0
**Bulimia** 783.6
nervosa 307.51
nonorganic origin 307.51
**Bulky uterus** 621.2
**Bulla(e)** 709.8
lung (emphysematous) (solitary) 492.0
**Bullet wound** — *see also* Wound, open, by site
fracture — *see* Fracture, by site, open
internal organ (abdomen, chest, or pelvis) — *see* Injury, internal, by site, with open wound
intracranial — *see* Laceration, brain, with open wound
**Bullis fever** 082.8
**Bullying** — *see also* Disturbance, conduct 312.0 ☑
**Bundle**
branch block (complete) (false) (incomplete) 426.50
  bilateral 426.53
  left (*see also* Block, bundle branch, left) 426.3
    hemiblock 426.2
  right (*see also* Block, bundle branch, right) 426.4
of His — *see* condition
of Kent syndrome (anomalous atrioventricular excitation) 426.7
**Bungpagga** 040.81
**Bunion** 727.1
**Bunionette** 727.1
**Bunyamwera fever** 066.3
**Buphthalmia, buphthalmos** (congenital) 743.20
associated with
  keratoglobus, congenital 743.22
  megalocornea 743.22
  ocular anomalies NEC 743.22
isolated 743.21
simple 743.21
**Bürger-Grütz disease or syndrome** (essential familial hyperlipemia) 272.3
**Buried roots** 525.3
**Burke's syndrome** 577.8

---

☑ Additional Digit Required — Refer to the Tabular List for Digit Selection                               ▽ Subterms under main terms may continue to next column or page

**Burkitt's**

tumor (M9750/3) 200.2 ☑
type malignant, lymphoma, lymphoblastic, or undifferentiated (M9750/3) 200.2 ☑

**Burn** (acid) (cathode ray) (caustic) (chemical) (electric heating appliance) (electricity) (fire) (flame) (hot liquid or object) (irradiation) (lime) (radiation) (steam) (thermal) (x-ray) 949.0

*Note — Use the following fifth-digit subclassification with category 948 to indicate the percent of body surface with third degree burn:*

*0　Less than 10% or unspecified*
*1　10–19%*
*2　20–29%*
*3　30–39%*
*4　40–49%*
*5　50–59%*
*6　60–69%*
*7　70–79%*
*8　80–89%*
*9　90% or more of body surface*

with
　blisters — *see* Burn, by site, second degree
　erythema — *see* Burn, by site, first degree
　skin loss (epidermal) (*see also* Burn, by site, second degree)
　full thickness (*see also* Burn, by site, third degree)
　　with necrosis of underlying tissues — *see* Burn, by site, third degree, deep
　first degree — *see* Burn, by site, first degree
　second degree — *see* Burn, by site, second degree
　third degree — *see* Burn, by site, third degree
　　deep — *see* Burn, by site, third degree, deep
abdomen, abdominal (muscle) (wall) 942.03
　with
　　trunk — *see* Burn, trunk, multiple sites
　first degree 942.13
　second degree 942.23
　third degree 942.33
　　deep 942.43
　　　with loss of body part 942.53
ankle 945.03
　with
　　lower limb(s) — *see* Burn, leg, multiple sites
　first degree 945.13
　second degree 945.23
　third degree 945.33
　　deep 945.43
　　　with loss of body part 945.53
anus — *see* Burn, trunk, specified site NEC
arm(s) 943.00
　first degree 943.10
　second degree 943.20
　third degree 943.30
　　deep 943.40
　　　with loss of body part 943.50
　lower — *see* Burn, forearm(s)
　multiple sites, except hand(s) or wrist(s) 943.09
　　first degree 943.19
　　second degree 943.29
　　third degree 943.39
　　　deep 943.49
　　　　with loss of body part 943.59

**Burn** — *continued*
arm(s) — *continued*
　upper 943.03
　　first degree 943.13
　　second degree 943.23
　　third degree 943.33
　　　deep 943.43
　　　　with loss of body part 943.53
auditory canal (external) — *see* Burn, ear
auricle (ear) — *see* Burn, ear
axilla 943.04
　with
　　upper limb(s), except hand(s) or wrist(s) — *see* Burn, arm(s), multiple sites
　first degree 943.14
　second degree 943.24
　third degree 943.34
　　deep 943.44
　　　with loss of body part 943.54
back 942.04
　with
　　trunk — *see* Burn, trunk, multiple sites
　first degree 942.14
　second degree 942.24
　third degree 942.34
　　deep 942.44
　　　with loss of body part 942.54
biceps
　brachii — *see* Burn, arm(s), upper
　femoris — *see* Burn, thigh
breast(s) 942.01
　with
　　trunk — *see* Burn, trunk, multiple sites
　first degree 942.11
　second degree 942.21
　third degree 942.31
　　deep 942.41
　　　with loss of body part 942.51
brow — *see* Burn, forehead
buttock(s) — *see* Burn, back
canthus (eye) 940.1
　chemical 940.0
cervix (uteri) 947.4
cheek (cutaneous) 941.07
　with
　　face or head — *see* Burn, head, multiple sites
　first degree 941.17
　second degree 941.27
　third degree 941.37
　　deep 941.47
　　　with loss of body part 941.57
chest wall (anterior) 942.02
　with
　　trunk — *see* Burn, trunk, multiple sites
　first degree 942.12
　second degree 942.22
　third degree 942.32
　　deep 942.42
　　　with loss of body part 942.52
chin 941.04
　with
　　face or head — *see* Burn, head, multiple sites
　first degree 941.14
　second degree 941.24
　third degree 941.34
　　deep 941.44
　　　with loss of body part 941.54
clitoris — *see* Burn, genitourinary organs, external
colon 947.3
conjunctiva (and cornea) 940.4
　chemical
　　acid 940.3
　　alkaline 940.2
cornea (and conjunctiva) 940.4
　chemical
　　acid 940.3
　　alkaline 940.2

**Burn** — *continued*
costal region — *see* Burn, chest wall
due to ingested chemical agent — *see* Burn, internal organs
ear (auricle) (canal) (drum) (external) 941.01
　with
　　face or head — *see* Burn, head, multiple sites
　first degree 941.11
　second degree 941.21
　third degree 941.31
　　deep 941.41
　　　with loss of a body part 941.51
elbow 943.02
　with
　　hand(s) and wrist(s) — *see* Burn, multiple specified sites
　　upper limb(s), except hand(s) or wrist(s) (*see also* Burn, arm(s), multiple sites)
　first degree 943.12
　second degree 943.22
　third degree 943.32
　　deep 943.42
　　　with loss of body part 943.52
electricity, electric current — *see* Burn, by site
entire body — *see* Burn, multiple, specified sites
epididymis — *see* Burn, genitourinary organs, external
epigastric region — *see* Burn, abdomen
epiglottis 947.1
esophagus 947.2
extent (percent of body surface)
　less than 10 percent 948.0 ☑
　10-19 percent 948.1 ☑
　20-29 percent 948.2 ☑
　30-39 percent 948.3 ☑
　40-49 percent 948.4 ☑
　50-59 percent 948.5 ☑
　60-69 percent 948.6 ☑
　70-79 percent 948.7 ☑
　80-89 percent 948.8 ☑
　90 percent or more 948.9 ☑
extremity
　lower — *see* Burn, leg
　upper — *see* Burn, arm(s)
eye(s) (and adnexa) (only) 940.9
　with
　　face, head, or neck 941.02
　　　first degree 941.12
　　　second degree 941.22
　　　third degree 941.32
　　　　deep 941.42
　　　　　with loss of body part 941.52
　　other sites (classifiable to more than one category in 940–945) — *see* Burn, multiple, specified sites
　　resulting rupture and destruction of eyeball 940.5
　specified part — *see* Burn, by site
eyeball (*see also* Burn, eye )
　with resulting rupture and destruction of eyeball 940.5
eyelid(s) 940.1
　chemical 940.0
face — *see* Burn, head
finger (nail) (subungual) 944.01
　with
　　hand(s) — *see* Burn, hand(s), multiple sites
　　other sites — *see* Burn, multiple, specified sites
　　thumb 944.04
　　　first degree 944.14
　　　second degree 944.24
　　　third degree 944.34
　　　　deep 944.44

**Burn** — *continued*
finger — *continued*
　with — *continued*
　　thumb — *continued*
　　　third degree — *continued*
　　　　deep — *continued*
　　　　　with loss of body part 944.54
　first degree 944.11
　second degree 944.21
　third degree 944.31
　　deep 944.41
　　　with loss of body part 944.51
　multiple (digits) 944.03
　　with thumb — *see* Burn, finger, with thumb
　　first degree 944.13
　　second degree 944.23
　　third degree 944.33
　　　deep 944.43
　　　　with loss of body part 944.53
flank — *see* Burn, abdomen
foot 945.02
　with
　　lower limb(s) — *see* Burn, leg, multiple sites
　first degree 945.12
　second degree 945.22
　third degree 945.32
　　deep 945.42
　　　with loss of body part 945.52
forearm(s) 943.01
　with
　　upper limb(s), except hand(s) or wrist(s) — *see* Burn, arm(s), multiple sites
　first degree 943.11
　second degree 943.21
　third degree 943.31
　　deep 943.41
　　　with loss of body part 943.51
forehead 941.07
　with
　　face or head — *see* Burn, head, multiple sites
　first degree 941.17
　second degree 941.27
　third degree 941.37
　　deep 941.47
　　　with loss of body part 941.57
fourth degree — *see* Burn, by site, third degree, deep
friction — *see* Injury, superficial, by site
from swallowing caustic or corrosive substance NEC — *see* Burn, internal organs
full thickness — *see* Burn, by site, third degree
gastrointestinal tract 947.3
genitourinary organs
　external 942.05
　　with
　　　trunk — *see* Burn, trunk, multiple sites
　　first degree 942.15
　　second degree 942.25
　　third degree 942.35
　　　deep 942.45
　　　　with loss of body part 942.55
　internal 947.8
globe (eye) — *see* Burn, eyeball
groin — *see* Burn, abdomen
gum 947.0
hand(s) (phalanges) (and wrist) 944.00
　first degree 944.10
　second degree 944.20
　third degree 944.30
　　deep 944.40
　　　with loss of body part 944.50
　back (dorsal surface) 944.06
　　first degree 944.16
　　second degree 944.26
　　third degree 944.36

☑ Additional Digit Required — Refer to the Tabular List for Digit Selection　　　　　　　　　Subterms under main terms may continue to next column or page

40 — Volume 2　　　　　▶◀ Revised Text　　　● New Line　　　▲ Revised Code　　　**2008 ICD-9-CM**

**Burn** — *continued*
  hand(s) — *continued*
    back — *continued*
      third degree — *continued*
        deep 944.46
          with loss of body part 944.56
        multiple sites 944.08
          first degree 944.18
          second degree 944.28
          third degree 944.38
            deep 944.48
              with loss of body part 944.58
    head (and face) 941.00
      first degree 941.10
      second degree 941.20
      third degree 941.30
        deep 941.40
          with loss of body part 941.50
      eye(s) only 940.9
        specified part — *see* Burn, by site
      multiple sites 941.09
        with eyes — *see* Burn, eyes, with face, head, or neck
        first degree 941.19
        second degree 941.29
        third degree 941.39
          deep 941.49
            with loss of body part 941.59
    heel — *see* Burn, foot
    hip — *see* Burn, trunk, specified site NEC
    iliac region — *see* Burn, trunk, specified site NEC
    infected 958.3
    inhalation (*see also* Burn, internal organs) 947.9
    internal organs 947.9
      from caustic or corrosive substance (swallowing) NEC 947.9
      specified NEC (*see also* Burn, by site) 947.8
    interscapular region — *see* Burn, back
    intestine (large) (small) 947.3
    iris — *see* Burn, eyeball
    knee 945.05
      with
        lower limb(s) — *see* Burn, leg, multiple sites
      first degree 945.15
      second degree 945.25
      third degree 945.35
        deep 945.45
          with loss of body part 945.55
    labium (majus) (minus) — *see* Burn, genitourinary organs, external
    lacrimal apparatus, duct, gland, or sac 940.1
      chemical 940.0
    larynx 947.1
    late effect — *see* Late, effects (of), burn
    leg 945.00
      first degree 945.10
      second degree 945.20
      third degree 945.30
        deep 945.40
          with loss of body part 945.50
      lower 945.04
        with other part(s) of lower limb(s) — *see* Burn, leg, multiple sites
        first degree 945.14
        second degree 945.24
        third degree 945.34
          deep 945.44
            with loss of body part 945.54
      multiple sites 945.09
        first degree 945.19
        second degree 945.29
        third degree 945.39
          deep 945.49

**Burn** — *continued*
  leg — *continued*
    multiple sites — *continued*
      third degree — *continued*
        deep — *continued*
          with loss of body part 945.59
      upper — *see* Burn, thigh
    lightning — *see* Burn, by site
    limb(s)
      lower (including foot or toe(s)) — *see* Burn, leg
      upper (except wrist and hand) — *see* Burn, arm(s)
    lip(s) 941.03
      with
        face or head — *see* Burn, head, multiple sites
      first degree 941.13
      second degree 941.23
      third degree 941.33
        deep 941.43
          with loss of body part 941.53
    lumbar region — *see* Burn, back
    lung 947.1
    malar region — *see* Burn, cheek
    mastoid region — *see* Burn, scalp
    membrane, tympanic — *see* Burn, ear
    midthoracic region — *see* Burn, chest wall
    mouth 947.0
    multiple (*see also* Burn, unspecified) 949.0
      specified sites classifiable to more than one category in 940-945 ☑, 946.0
        first degree 946.1
        second degree 946.2
        third degree 946.3
          deep 946.4
            with loss of body part 946.5
    muscle, abdominal — *see* Burn, abdomen
    nasal (septum) — *see* Burn, nose
    neck 941.08
      with
        face or head — *see* Burn, head, multiple sites
      first degree 941.18
      second degree 941.28
      third degree 941.38
        deep 941.48
          with loss of body part 941.58
    nose (septum) 941.05
      with
        face or head — *see* Burn, head, multiple sites
      first degree 941.15
      second degree 941.25
      third degree 941.35
        deep 941.45
          with loss of body part 941.55
    occipital region — *see* Burn, scalp
    orbit region 940.1
      chemical 940.0
    oronasopharynx 947.0
    palate 947.0
    palm(s) 944.05
      with
        hand(s) and wrist(s) — *see* Burn, hand(s), multiple sites
      first degree 944.15
      second degree 944.25
      third degree 944.35
        deep 944.45
          with loss of a body part 944.55
    parietal region — *see* Burn, scalp
    penis — *see* Burn, genitourinary organs, external
    perineum — *see* Burn, genitourinary organs, external
    periocular area 940.1
      chemical 940.0

**Burn** — *continued*
  pharynx 947.0
  pleura 947.1
  popliteal space — *see* Burn, knee
  prepuce — *see* Burn, genitourinary organs, external
  pubic region — *see* Burn, genitourinary organs, external
  pudenda — *see* Burn, genitourinary organs, external
  rectum 947.3
  sac, lacrimal 940.1
    chemical 940.0
  sacral region — *see* Burn, back
  salivary (ducts) (glands) 947.0
  scalp 941.06
    with
      face or neck — *see* Burn, head, multiple sites
    first degree 941.16
    second degree 941.26
    third degree 941.36
      deep 941.46
        with loss of body part 941.56
  scapular region 943.06
    with
      upper limb(s), except hand(s) or wrist(s) — *see* Burn, arm(s), multiple sites
    first degree 943.16
    second degree 943.26
    third degree 943.36
      deep 943.46
        with loss of body part 943.56
  sclera — *see* Burn, eyeball
  scrotum — *see* Burn, genitourinary organs, external
  septum, nasal — *see* Burn, nose
  shoulder(s) 943.05
    with
      hand(s) and wrist(s) — *see* Burn, multiple, specified sites
      upper limb(s), except hand(s) or wrist(s) — *see* Burn, arm(s), multiple sites
    first degree 943.15
    second degree 943.25
    third degree 943.35
      deep 943.45
        with loss of body part 943.55
  skin NEC (*see also* Burn, unspecified) 949.0
  skull — *see* Burn, head
  small intestine 947.3
  sternal region — *see* Burn, chest wall
  stomach 947.3
  subconjunctival — *see* Burn, conjunctiva
  subcutaneous — *see* Burn, by site, third degree
  submaxillary region — *see* Burn, head
  submental region — *see* Burn, chin
  sun — *see* Sunburn
  supraclavicular fossa — *see* Burn, neck
  supraorbital — *see* Burn, forehead
  temple — *see* Burn, scalp
  temporal region — *see* Burn, scalp
  testicle — *see* Burn, genitourinary organs, external
  testis — *see* Burn, genitourinary organs, external
  thigh 945.06
    with
      lower limb(s) — *see* Burn, leg, multiple sites
    first degree 945.16
    second degree 945.26
    third degree 945.36
      deep 945.46
        with loss of body part 945.56
  thorax (external) — *see* Burn, chest wall
  throat 947.0
  thumb(s) (nail) (subungual) 944.02

**Burn** — *continued*
  thumb(s) — *continued*
    with
      finger(s) — *see* Burn, finger, with other sites, thumb
      hand(s) and wrist(s) — *see* Burn, hand(s), multiple sites
    first degree 944.12
    second degree 944.22
    third degree 944.32
      deep 944.42
        with loss of body part 944.52
  toe (nail) (subungual) 945.01
    with
      lower limb(s) — *see* Burn, leg, multiple sites
    first degree 945.11
    second degree 945.21
    third degree 945.31
      deep 945.41
        with loss of body part 945.51
  tongue 947.0
  tonsil 947.0
  trachea 947.1
  trunk 942.00
    first degree 942.10
    second degree 942.20
    third degree 942.30
      deep 942.40
        with loss of body part 942.50
    multiple sites 942.09
      first degree 942.19
      second degree 942.29
      third degree 942.39
        deep 942.49
          with loss of body part 942.59
    specified site NEC 942.09
      first degree 942.19
      second degree 942.29
      third degree 942.39
        deep 942.49
          with loss of body part 942.59
  tunica vaginalis — *see* Burn, genitourinary organs, external
  tympanic membrane — *see* Burn, ear
  tympanum — *see* Burn, ear
  ultraviolet 692.82
  unspecified site (multiple) 949.0
    with extent of body surface involved specified
      less than 10 percent 948.0 ☑
      10-19 percent 948.1 ☑
      20-29 percent 948.2 ☑
      30-39 percent 948.3 ☑
      40-49 percent 948.4 ☑
      50-59 percent 948.5 ☑
      60-69 percent 948.6 ☑
      70-79 percent 948.7 ☑
      80-89 percent 948.8 ☑
      90 percent or more 948.9 ☑
    first degree 949.1
    second degree 949.2
    third degree 949.3
      deep 949.4
        with loss of body part 949.5
  uterus 947.4
  uvula 947.0
  vagina 947.4
  vulva — *see* Burn, genitourinary organs, external
  wrist(s) 944.07
    with
      hand(s) — *see* Burn, hand(s), multiple sites
    first degree 944.17
    second degree 944.27
    third degree 944.37
      deep 944.47
        with loss of body part 944.57
**Burnett's syndrome** (milk-alkali) 275.42
**Burnier's syndrome** (hypophyseal dwarfism) 253.3

☑ Additional Digit Required — Refer to the Tabular List for Digit Selection

�稜 Subterms under main terms may continue to next column or page

*2008 ICD-9-CM*

▶◀ Revised Text

● New Line

▲ Revised Code

Volume 2 — 41

**Burning**
feet syndrome 266.2
sensation (*see also* Disturbance, sensation) 782.0
tongue 529.6
**Burns' disease** (osteochondrosis, lower ulna) 732.3
**Bursa** — *see also* condition
pharynx 478.29
**Bursitis** NEC 727.3
Achilles tendon 726.71
adhesive 726.90
shoulder 726.0
ankle 726.79
buttock 726.5
calcaneal 726.79
collateral ligament
fibular 726.63
tibial 726.62
Duplay's 726.2
elbow 726.33
finger 726.8
foot 726.79
gonococcal 098.52
hand 726.4
hip 726.5
infrapatellar 726.69
ischiogluteal 726.5
knee 726.60
occupational NEC 727.2
olecranon 726.33
pes anserinus 726.61
pharyngeal 478.29
popliteal 727.51
prepatellar 726.65
radiohumeral 727.3
scapulohumeral 726.19
adhesive 726.0
shoulder 726.10
adhesive 726.0
subacromial 726.19
adhesive 726.0
subcoracoid 726.19
subdeltoid 726.19
adhesive 726.0
subpatellar 726.69
syphilitic 095.7
Thornwaldt's, Tornwaldt's (pharyngeal) 478.29
toe 726.79
trochanteric area 726.5
wrist 726.4
**Burst stitches or sutures** (complication of surgery) (external) 998.32
internal 998.31
**Buruli ulcer** 031.1
**Bury's disease** (erythema elevatum diutinum) 695.89
**Buschke's disease or scleredema** (adultorum) 710.1
**Busquet's disease** (osteoperiostitis) — *see also* Osteomyelitis 730.1 ☑
**Busse-Buschke disease** (cryptococcosis) 117.5
**Buttock** — *see* condition
**Button**
Biskra 085.1
Delhi 085.1
oriental 085.1
**Buttonhole hand** (intrinsic) 736.21
**Bwamba fever** (encephalitis) 066.3
**Byssinosis** (occupational) 504
**Bywaters' syndrome** 958.5

---

**C**

**Cacergasia** 300.9
**Cachexia** 799.4
cancerous (*see also* Neoplasm, by site, malignant) 799.4
cardiac — *see* Disease, heart
dehydration 276.51
with
hypernatremia 276.0
hyponatremia 276.1
due to malnutrition 799.4
exophthalmic 242.0 ☑

**Cachexia** — *continued*
heart — *see* Disease, heart
hypophyseal 253.2
hypopituitary 253.2
lead 984.9
specified type of lead — *see* Table of Drugs and Chemicals
malaria 084.9
malignant (*see also* Neoplasm, by site, malignant) 799.4
marsh 084.9
nervous 300.5
old age 797
pachydermic — *see* Hypothyroidism
paludal 084.9
pituitary (postpartum) 253.2
renal (*see also* Disease, renal) 593.9
saturnine 984.9
specified type of lead — *see* Table of Drugs and Chemicals
senile 797
Simmonds' (pituitary cachexia) 253.2
splenica 289.59
strumipriva (*see also* Hypothyroidism) 244.9
tuberculous NEC (*see also* Tuberculosis) 011.9 ☑
**Café au lait spots** 709.09
**Caffey's disease or syndrome** (infantile cortical hyperostosis) 756.59
**Caisson disease** 993.3
**Caked breast** (puerperal, postpartum) 676.2 ☑
**Cake kidney** 753.3
**Calabar swelling** 125.2
**Calcaneal spur** 726.73
**Calcaneoapophysitis** 732.5
**Calcaneonavicular bar** 755.67
**Calcareous** — *see* condition
**Calcicosis** (occupational) 502
**Calciferol** (vitamin D) **deficiency** 268.9
with
osteomalacia 268.2
rickets (*see also* Rickets) 268.0
**Calcification**
adrenal (capsule) (gland) 255.41 ▲
tuberculous (*see also* Tuberculosis) 017.6 ☑
aorta 440.0
artery (annular) — *see* Arteriosclerosis
auricle (ear) 380.89
bladder 596.8
due to S. hematobium 120.0
brain (cortex) — *see* Calcification, cerebral
bronchus 519.19
bursa 727.82
cardiac (*see also* Degeneration, myocardial) 429.1
cartilage (postinfectional) 733.99
cerebral (cortex) 348.8
artery 437.0
cervix (uteri) 622.8
choroid plexus 349.2
conjunctiva 372.54
corpora cavernosa (penis) 607.89
cortex (brain) — *see* Calcification, cerebral
dental pulp (nodular) 522.2
dentinal papilla 520.4
disc, intervertebral 722.90
cervical, cervicothoracic 722.91
lumbar, lumbosacral 722.93
thoracic, thoracolumbar 722.92
fallopian tube 620.8
falx cerebri — *see* Calcification, cerebral
fascia 728.89
gallbladder 575.8
general 275.40
heart (*see also* Degeneration, myocardial) 429.1
valve — *see* Endocarditis
intervertebral cartilage or disc (postinfectional) 722.90
cervical, cervicothoracic 722.91

**Calcification** — *continued*
intervertebral cartilage or disc — *continued*
lumbar, lumbosacral 722.93
thoracic, thoracolumbar 722.92
intracranial — *see* Calcification, cerebral
intraspinal ligament 728.89
joint 719.80
ankle 719.87
elbow 719.82
foot 719.87
hand 719.84
hip 719.85
knee 719.86
multiple sites 719.89
pelvic region 719.85
shoulder (region) 719.81
specified site NEC 719.88
wrist 719.83
kidney 593.89
tuberculous (*see also* Tuberculosis) 016.0 ☑
larynx (senile) 478.79
lens 366.8
ligament 728.89
intraspinal 728.89
knee (medial collateral) 717.89
lung 518.89
active 518.89
postinfectional 518.89
tuberculous (*see also* Tuberculosis, pulmonary) 011.9 ☑
lymph gland or node (postinfectional) 289.3
tuberculous (*see also* Tuberculosis, lymph gland) 017.2 ☑
mammographic 793.89
massive (paraplegic) 728.10
medial NEC (*see also* Arteriosclerosis, extremities) 440.20
meninges (cerebral) 349.2
metastatic 275.40
Mönckeberg's — *see* Arteriosclerosis
muscle 728.10
heterotopic, postoperative 728.13
myocardium, myocardial (*see also* Degeneration, myocardial) 429.1
ovary 620.8
pancreas 577.8
penis 607.89
periarticular 728.89
pericardium (*see also* Pericarditis) 423.8
pineal gland 259.8
pleura 511.0
postinfectional 518.89
tuberculous (*see also* Tuberculosis, pleura) 012.0 ☑
pulp (dental) (nodular) 522.2
renal 593.89
Rider's bone 733.99
sclera 379.16
semilunar cartilage 717.89
spleen 289.59
subcutaneous 709.3
suprarenal (capsule) (gland) 255.41 ▲
tendon (sheath) 727.82
with bursitis, synovitis or tenosynovitis 727.82
trachea 519.19
ureter 593.89
uterus 621.8
vitreous 379.29
**Calcified** — *see also* Calcification
hematoma NEC 959.9
**Calcinosis** (generalized) (interstitial) (tumoral) (universalis) 275.49
circumscripta 709.3
cutis 709.3
intervertebralis 275.49 [722.90]
Raynaud's phenomenonsclerodactylytelangiectasis (CRST) 710.1
**Calciphylaxis** — *see also* Calcification, by site 275.49

**Calcium**
blood
high (*see also* Hypercalcemia) 275.42
low (*see also* Hypocalcemia) 275.41
deposits (*see also* Calcification, by site)
in bursa 727.82
in tendon (sheath) 727.82
with bursitis, synovitis or tenosynovitis 727.82
salts or soaps in vitreous 379.22
**Calciuria** 791.9
**Calculi** — *see* Calculus
**Calculosis, intrahepatic** — *see* Choledocholithiasis
**Calculus, calculi, calculous** 592.9
ampulla of Vater — *see* Choledocholithiasis
anuria (impacted) (recurrent) 592.0
appendix 543.9
bile duct (any) — *see* Choledocholithiasis
biliary — *see* Cholelithiasis
bilirubin, multiple — *see* Cholelithiasis
bladder (encysted) (impacted) (urinary) 594.1
diverticulum 594.0
bronchus 518.89
calyx (kidney) (renal) 592.0
congenital 753.3
cholesterol (pure) (solitary) — *see* Cholelithiasis
common duct (bile) — *see* Choledocholithiasis
conjunctiva 372.54
cystic 594.1
duct — *see* Cholelithiasis
dental 523.6
subgingival 523.6
supragingival 523.6
epididymis 608.89
gallbladder (*see also* Cholelithiasis)
congenital 751.69
hepatic (duct) — *see* Choledocholithiasis
intestine (impaction) (obstruction) 560.39
kidney (impacted) (multiple) (pelvis) (recurrent) (staghorn) 592.0
congenital 753.3
lacrimal (passages) 375.57
liver (impacted) — *see* Choledocholithiasis
lung 518.89
mammographic 793.89
nephritic (impacted) (recurrent) 592.0
nose 478.19
pancreas (duct) 577.8
parotid duct 527.5
pelvis, encysted 592.0
prostate 602.0
pulmonary 518.89
renal (impacted) (recurrent) 592.0
congenital 753.3
salivary (duct) (gland) 527.5
seminal vesicle 608.89
staghorn 592.0
Stensen's duct 527.5
sublingual duct or gland 527.5
congenital 750.26
submaxillary duct, gland, or region 527.5
suburethral 594.8
tonsil 474.8
tooth, teeth 523.6
tunica vaginalis 608.89
ureter (impacted) (recurrent) 592.1
urethra (impacted) 594.2
urinary (duct) (impacted) (passage) (tract) 592.9
lower tract NEC 594.9
specified site 594.8
vagina 623.8
vesical (impacted) 594.1

**Calculus, calculi, calculous** —
*continued*
Wharton's duct 527.5
**Caliectasis** 593.89
**California**
disease 114.0
encephalitis 062.5
**Caligo cornea** 371.03
**Callositas, callosity** (infected) 700
**Callus** (infected) 700
bone 726.91
excessive, following fracture (*see also*
Late, effect (of), fracture)
**Calvé (-Perthes) disease** (osteochondrosis, femoral capital) 732.1
**Calvities** — *see also* Alopecia 704.00
**Cameroon fever** — *see also* Malaria
084.6
**Camptocormia** 300.11
**Camptodactyly** (congenital) 755.59
**Camurati-Engelmann disease** (diaphyseal sclerosis) 756.59
**Canal** — *see* condition
**Canaliculitis** (lacrimal) (acute) 375.31
Actinomyces 039.8
chronic 375.41
**Canavan's disease** 330.0
**Cancer** (M8000/3) — *see also* Neoplasm,
by site, malignant

*Note — The term "cancer" when modified by an adjective or adjectival phrase indicating a morphological type should be coded in the same manner as "carcinoma" with that adjective or phrase. Thus, "squamous-cell cancer" should be coded in the same manner as "squamous-cell carcinoma," which appears in the list under "Carcinoma."*

bile duct type (M8160/3), liver 155.1
hepatocellular (M8170/3) 155.0
**Cancerous** (M8000/3) — *see also* Neoplasm,
by site, malignant
**Cancerphobia** 300.29
**Cancrum oris** 528.1
**Candidiasis, candidal** 112.9
with pneumonia 112.4
balanitis 112.2
congenital 771.7
disseminated 112.5
endocarditis 112.81
esophagus 112.84
intertrigo 112.3
intestine 112.85
lung 112.4
meningitis 112.83
mouth 112.0
nails 112.3
neonatal 771.7
onychia 112.3
otitis externa 112.82
otomycosis 112.82
paronychia 112.3
perionyxis 112.3
pneumonia 112.4
pneumonitis 112.4
skin 112.3
specified site NEC 112.89
systemic 112.5
urogenital site NEC 112.2
vagina 112.1
vulva 112.1
vulvovaginitis 112.1
**Candidiosis** — *see* Candidiasis
**Candiru infection or infestation** 136.8
**Canities** (premature) 704.3
congenital 757.4
**Canker** (mouth) (sore) 528.2
rash 034.1
**Cannabinosis** 504
**Canton fever** 081.9
**Cap**
cradle 690.11
**Capillariasis** 127.5
**Capillary** — *see* condition
**Caplan-Colinet syndrome** 714.81
**Caplan's syndrome** 714.81

**Capsule** — *see* condition
**Capsulitis** (joint) 726.90
adhesive (shoulder) 726.0
hip 726.5
knee 726.60
labyrinthine 387.8
thyroid 245.9
wrist 726.4
**Caput**
crepitus 756.0
medusae 456.8
succedaneum 767.19
**Carapata disease** 087.1
**Carate** — *see* Pinta
**Carbohydrate-deficient glycoprotein
syndrome** (CGDS) 271.8
**Carboxyhemoglobinemia** 986
**Carbuncle** 680.9
abdominal wall 680.2
ankle 680.6
anus 680.5
arm (any part, above wrist) 680.3
auditory canal, external 680.0
axilla 680.3
back (any part) 680.2
breast 680.2
buttock 680.5
chest wall 680.2
corpus cavernosum 607.2
ear (any part) (external) 680.0
eyelid 373.13
face (any part, except eye) 680.0
finger (any) 680.4
flank 680.2
foot (any part) 680.7
forearm 680.3
genital organ (male) 608.4
gluteal (region) 680.5
groin 680.2
hand (any part) 680.4
head (any part, except face) 680.8
heel 680.7
hip 680.6
kidney (*see also* Abscess, kidney)
590.2
knee 680.6
labia 616.4
lacrimal
gland (*see also* Dacryoadenitis)
375.00
passages (duct) (sac) (*see also*
Dacryocystitis) 375.30
leg, any part except foot 680.6
lower extremity, any part except foot
680.6
malignant 022.0
multiple sites 680.9
neck 680.1
nose (external) (septum) 680.0
orbit, orbital 376.01
partes posteriores 680.5
pectoral region 680.2
penis 607.2
perineum 680.2
pinna 680.0
scalp (any part) 680.8
scrotum 608.4
seminal vesicle 608.0
shoulder 680.3
skin NEC 680.9
specified site NEC 680.8
spermatic cord 608.4
temple (region) 680.0
testis 608.4
thigh 680.6
thumb 680.4
toe (any) 680.7
trunk 680.2
tunica vaginalis 608.4
umbilicus 680.2
upper arm 680.3
urethra 597.0
vas deferens 608.4
vulva 616.4
wrist 680.4
**Carbunculus** — *see also* Carbuncle 680.9

**Carcinoid** (tumor) (M8240/1) — *see also*
Neoplasm, by site, uncertain behavior
and struma ovarii (M9091/1) 236.2
argentaffin (M8241/1) — *see* Neoplasm, by site, uncertain behavior
malignant (M8241/3) — *see* Neoplasm, by site, malignant
benign (M9091/0) 220
composite (M8244/3) — *see* Neoplasm, by site, malignant
goblet cell (M8243/3) — *see* Neoplasm, by site, malignant
malignant (M8240/3) — *see* Neoplasm, by site, malignant
nonargentaffin (M8242/1) (*see also*
Neoplasm, by site, uncertain
behavior)
malignant (M8242/3) — *see* Neoplasm, by site, malignant
strumal (M9091/1) 236.2
syndrome (intestinal) (metastatic)
259.2
type bronchial adenoma (M8240/3)
— *see* Neoplasm, lung, malignant
**Carcinoidosis** 259.2
**Carcinomaphobia** 300.29
**Carcinomatosis**
peritonei (M8010/6) 197.6
specified site NEC (M8010/3) — *see*
Neoplasm, by site, malignant
unspecified site (M8010/6) 199.0
**Carcinoma** (M8010/3) — *see also* Neoplasm, by site, malignant

*Note — Except where otherwise indicated, the morphological varieties of carcinoma in the list below should be coded by site as for "Neoplasm, malignant."*

with
apocrine metaplasia (M8573/3)
cartilaginous (and osseous) metaplasia (M8571/3)
osseous (and cartilaginous) metaplasia (M8571/3)
productive fibrosis (M8141/3)
spindle cell metaplasia (M8572/3)
squamous metaplasia (M8570/3)
acidophil (M8280/3)
specified site — *see* Neoplasm, by site, malignant
unspecified site 194.3
acidophil-basophil, mixed (M8281/3)
specified site — *see* Neoplasm, by site, malignant
unspecified site 194.3
acinar (cell) (M8550/3)
acinic cell (M8550/3)
adenocystic (M8200/3)
adenoid
cystic (M8200/3)
squamous cell (M8075/3)
adenosquamous (M8560/3)
adnexal (skin) (M8390/3) — *see* Neoplasm, skin, malignant
adrenal cortical (M8370/3) 194.0
alveolar (M8251/3)
cell (M8250/3) — *see* Neoplasm, lung, malignant
anaplastic type (M8021/3)
apocrine (M8401/3)
breast — *see* Neoplasm, breast, malignant
specified site NEC — *see* Neoplasm, skin, malignant
unspecified site 173.9
basal cell (pigmented) (M8090/3) (*see also* Neoplasm, skin, malignant)
fibro-epithelial type (M8093/3) — *see* Neoplasm, skin, malignant
morphea type (M8092/3) — *see* Neoplasm, skin, malignant
multicentric (M8091/3) — *see* Neoplasm, skin, malignant

**Carcinoma** — *see also* Neoplasm, by site,
malignant — *continued*
basaloid (M8123/3)
basal-squamous cell, mixed
(M8094/3) — *see* Neoplasm,
skin, malignant
basophil (M8300/3)
specified site — *see* Neoplasm, by site, malignant
unspecified site 194.3
basophil-acidophil, mixed (M8281/3)
specified site — *see* Neoplasm, by site, malignant
unspecified site 194.3
basosquamous (M8094/3) — *see*
Neoplasm, skin, malignant
bile duct type (M8160/3)
and hepatocellular, mixed
(M8180/3) 155.0
liver 155.1
specified site NEC — *see* Neoplasm, by site, malignant
unspecified site 155.1
branchial or branchiogenic 146.8
bronchial or bronchogenic — *see*
Neoplasm, lung, malignant
bronchiolar (terminal) (M8250/3) —
*see* Neoplasm, lung, malignant
bronchiolo-alveolar (M8250/3) — *see*
Neoplasm, lung, malignant
bronchogenic (epidermoid) 162.9
C cell (M8510/3)
specified site — *see* Neoplasm, by site, malignant
unspecified site 193
ceruminous (M8420/3) 173.2
chorionic (M9100/3)
specified site — *see* Neoplasm, by site, malignant
unspecified site
female 181
male 186.9
chromophobe (M8270/3)
specified site — *see* Neoplasm, by site, malignant
unspecified site 194.3
clear cell (mesonephroid type)
(M8310/3)
cloacogenic (M8124/3)
specified site — *see* Neoplasm, by site, malignant
unspecified site 154.8
colloid (M8480/3)
cribriform (M8201/3)
cylindroid type (M8200/3)
diffuse type (M8145/3)
specified site — *see* Neoplasm, by site, malignant
unspecified site 151.9
duct (cell) (M8500/3)
with Paget's disease (M8541/3) —
*see* Neoplasm, breast, malignant
infiltrating (M8500/3)
specified site — *see* Neoplasm, by site, malignant
unspecified site 174.9
ductal (M8500/3)
ductular, infiltrating (M8521/3)
embryonal (M9070/3)
and teratoma, mixed (M9081/3)
combined with choriocarcinoma
(M9101/3) — *see* Neoplasm,
by site, malignant
infantile type (M9071/3)
liver 155.0
polyembryonal type (M9072/3)
endometrioid (M8380/3)
eosinophil (M8280/3)
specified site — *see* Neoplasm, by site, malignant
unspecified site 194.3
epidermoid (M8070/3) (*see also* Carcinoma, squamous cell)

☑ Additional Digit Required — Refer to the Tabular List for Digit Selection          Ⓦ Subterms under main terms may continue to next column or page

*2008 ICD-9-CM*          ▶◀ Revised Text          ● New Line          ▲ Revised Code          **Volume 2 — 43**

**Carcinoma** — *see also* Neoplasm, by site, malignant — *continued*
epidermoid (*see also* Carcinoma, squamous cell) — *continued*
  and adenocarcinoma, mixed (M8560/3)
  in situ, Bowen's type (M8081/2) — *see* Neoplasm, skin, in situ
  intradermal — *see* Neoplasm, skin, in situ
fibroepithelial type basal cell (M8093/3) — *see* Neoplasm, skin, malignant
follicular (M8330/3)
  and papillary (mixed) (M8340/3) 193
  moderately differentiated type (M8332/3) 193
  pure follicle type (M8331/3) 193
  specified site — *see* Neoplasm, by site, malignant
  trabecular type (M8332/3) 193
  unspecified site 193
  well differentiated type (M8331/3) 193
gelatinous (M8480/3)
giant cell (M8031/3)
  and spindle cell (M8030/3)
granular cell (M8320/3)
granulosa cell (M8620/3) 183.0
hepatic cell (M8170/3) 155.0
hepatocellular (M8170/3) 155.0
  and bile duct, mixed (M8180/3) 155.0
hepatocholangiolitic (M8180/3) 155.0
Hürthle cell (thyroid) 193
hypernephroid (M8311/3)
in
  adenomatous
    polyp (M8210/3)
    polyposis coli (M8220/3) 153.9
  pleomorphic adenoma (M8940/3)
  polypoid adenoma (M8210/3)
  situ (M8010/3) — *see* Carcinoma, in situ
  tubular adenoma (M8210/3)
  villous adenoma (M8261/3)
infiltrating duct (M8500/3)
  with Paget's disease (M8541/3) — *see* Neoplasm, breast, malignant
  specified site — *see* Neoplasm, by site, malignant
  unspecified site 174.9
inflammatory (M8530/3)
  specified site — *see* Neoplasm, by site, malignant
  unspecified site 174.9
in situ (M8010/2) (*see also* Neoplasm, by site, in situ)
  epidermoid (M8070/2) (*see also* Neoplasm, by site, in situ)
    with questionable stromal invasion (M8076/2)
      specified site — *see* Neoplasm, by site, in situ
      unspecified site 233.1
    Bowen's type (M8081/2) — *see* Neoplasm, skin, in situ
  intraductal (M8500/2)
    specified site — *see* Neoplasm, by site, in situ
    unspecified site 233.0
  lobular (M8520/2)
    specified site — *see* Neoplasm, by site, in situ
    unspecified site 233.0
  papillary (M8050/2) — *see* Neoplasm, by site, in situ
  squamous cell (M8070/2) (*see also* Neoplasm, by site, in situ)
    with questionable stromal invasion (M8076/2)
    specified site — *see* Neoplasm, by site, in situ
    unspecified site 233.1

**Carcinoma** — *see also* Neoplasm, by site, malignant — *continued*
in situ (*see also* Neoplasm, by site, in situ) — *continued*
  transitional cell (M8120/2) — *see* Neoplasm, by site, in situ
intestinal type (M8144/3)
  specified site — *see* Neoplasm, by site, malignant
  unspecified site 151.9
intraductal (noninfiltrating) (M8500/2)
  papillary (M8503/2)
    specified site — *see* Neoplasm, by site, in situ
    unspecified site 233.0
  specified site — *see* Neoplasm, by site, in situ
  unspecified site 233.0
intraepidermal (M8070/2) (*see also* Neoplasm, skin, in situ)
  squamous cell, Bowen's type (M8081/2) — *see* Neoplasm, skin, in situ
intraepithelial (M8010/2) (*see also* Neoplasm, by site, in situ)
  squamous cell (M8072/2) — *see* Neoplasm, by site, in situ
intraosseous (M8170/3) 170.1
  upper jaw (bone) 170.0
islet cell (M8150/3)
  and exocrine, mixed (M8154/3)
    specified site — *see* Neoplasm, by site, malignant
    unspecified site 157.9
  pancreas 157.4
  specified site NEC — *see* Neoplasm, by site, malignant
  unspecified site 157.4
juvenile, breast (M8502/3) — *see* Neoplasm, breast, malignant
Kulchitsky's cell (carcinoid tumor of intestine) 259.2
large cell (M8012/3)
  squamous cell, non-keratinizing type (M8072/3)
Leydig cell (testis) (M8650/3)
  specified site — *see* Neoplasm, by site, malignant
  unspecified site 186.9
    female 183.0
    male 186.9
liver cell (M8170/3) 155.0
lobular (infiltrating) (M8520/3)
  non-infiltrating (M8520/2)
    specified site — *see* Neoplasm, by site, in situ
    unspecified site 233.0
  specified site — *see* Neoplasm, by site, malignant
  unspecified site 174.9
lymphoepithelial (M8082/3)
medullary (M8510/3)
  with
    amyloid stroma (M8511/3)
      specified site — *see* Neoplasm, by site, malignant
      unspecified site 193
    lymphoid stroma (M8512/3)
      specified site — *see* Neoplasm, by site, malignant
      unspecified site 174.9
mesometanephric (M9110/3)
mesonephric (M9110/3)
metastatic (M8010/6) — *see* Metastasis, cancer
metatypical (M8095/3) — *see* Neoplasm, skin, malignant
morphea type basal cell (M8092/3) — *see* Neoplasm, skin, malignant

**Carcinoma** — *see also* Neoplasm, by site, malignant — *continued*
mucinous (M8480/3)
mucin-producing (M8481/3)
mucin-secreting (M8481/3)
mucoepidermoid (M8430/3)
mucoid (M8480/3)
  cell (M8300/3)
    specified site — *see* Neoplasm, by site, malignant
    unspecified site 194.3
mucous (M8480/3)
nonencapsulated sclerosing (M8350/3) 193
noninfiltrating
  intracystic (M8504/2) — *see* Neoplasm, by site, in situ
  intraductal (M8500/2)
    papillary (M8503/2)
      specified site — *see* Neoplasm, by site, in situ
      unspecified site 233.0
    specified site — *see* Neoplasm, by site, in situ
    unspecified site 233.0
  lobular (M8520/2)
    specified site — *see* Neoplasm, by site, in situ
    unspecified site 233.0
oat cell (M8042/3)
  specified site — *see* Neoplasm, by site, malignant
  unspecified site 162.9
odontogenic (M9270/3) 170.1
  upper jaw (bone) 170.0
onocytic (M8290/3)
oxyphilic (M8290/3)
papillary (M8050/3)
  and follicular (mixed) (M8340/3) 193
  epidermoid (M8052/3)
  intraductal (noninfiltrating) (M8503/2)
    specified site — *see* Neoplasm, by site, in situ
    unspecified site 233.0
  serous (M8460/3)
    specified site — *see* Neoplasm, by site, malignant
    surface (M8461/3)
      specified site — *see* Neoplasm, by site, malignant
      unspecified site 183.0
    unspecified site 183.0
  squamous cell (M8052/3)
  transitional cell (M8130/3)
papillocystic (M8450/3)
  specified site — *see* Neoplasm, by site, malignant
  unspecified site 183.0
parafollicular cell (M8510/3)
  specified site — *see* Neoplasm, by site, malignant
  unspecified site 193
pleomorphic (M8022/3)
polygonal cell (M8034/3)
prickle cell (M8070/3)
pseudoglandular, squamous cell (M8075/3)
pseudomucinous (M8470/3)
  specified site — *see* Neoplasm, by site, malignant
  unspecified site 183.0
pseudosarcomatous (M8033/3)
regaud type (M8082/3) — *see* Neoplasm, nasopharynx, malignant
renal cell (M8312/3) 189.0
reserve cell (M8041/3)
round cell (M8041/3)
Schmincke (M8082/3) — *see* Neoplasm, nasopharynx, malignant
Schneiderian (M8121/3)
  specified site — *see* Neoplasm, by site, malignant
  unspecified site 160.0

**Carcinoma** — *see also* Neoplasm, by site, malignant — *continued*
scirrhous (M8141/3)
sebaceous (M8410/3) — *see* Neoplasm, skin, malignant
secondary (M8010/6) — *see* Neoplasm, by site, malignant, secondary
secretory, breast (M8502/3) — *see* Neoplasm, breast, malignant
serous (M8441/3)
  papillary (M8460/3)
    specified site — *see* Neoplasm, by site, malignant
    unspecified site 183.0
  surface, papillary (M8461/3)
    specified site — *see* Neoplasm, by site, malignant
    unspecified site 183.0
Sertoli cell (M8640/3)
  specified site — *see* Neoplasm, by site, malignant
  unspecified site 186.9
signet ring cell (M8490/3)
  metastatic (M8490/6) — *see* Neoplasm, by site, secondary
simplex (M8231/3)
skin appendage (M8390/3) — *see* Neoplasm, skin, malignant
small cell (M8041/3)
  fusiform cell type (M8043/3)
  squamous cell, non-keratinizing type (M8073/3)
solid (M8230/3)
  with amyloid stroma (M8511/3)
    specified site — *see* Neoplasm, by site, malignant
    unspecified site 193
spheroidal cell (M8035/3)
spindle cell (M8032/3)
  and giant cell (M8030/3)
spinous cell (M8070/3)
squamous (cell) (M8070/3)
  adenoid type (M8075/3)
  and adenocarcinoma, mixed (M8560/3)
  intraepidermal, Bowen's type — *see* Neoplasm, skin, in situ
  keratinizing type (large cell) (M8071/3)
  large cell, non-keratinizing type (M8072/3)
  microinvasive (M8076/3)
    specified site — *see* Neoplasm, by site, malignant
    unspecified site 180.9
  non-keratinizing type (M8072/3)
  papillary (M8052/3)
  pseudoglandular (M8075/3)
  small cell, non-keratinizing type (M8073/3)
  spindle cell type (M8074/3)
  verrucous (M8051/3)
superficial spreading (M8143/3)
sweat gland (M8400/3) — *see* Neoplasm, skin, malignant
theca cell (M8600/3) 183.0
thymic (M8580/3) 164.0
trabecular (M8190/3)
transitional (cell) (M8120/3)
  papillary (M8130/3)
  spindle cell type (M8122/3)
tubular (M8211/3)
undifferentiated type (M8020/3)
urothelial (M8120/3)
ventriculi 151.9
verrucous (epidermoid) (squamous cell) (M8051/3)
villous (M8262/3)
water-clear cell (M8322/3) 194.1
wolffian duct (M9110/3)
**Carcinosarcoma** (M8980/3) — *see also* Neoplasm, by site, malignant
embryonal type (M8981/3) — *see* Neoplasm, by site, malignant
**Cardiac** — *see also* condition

☑ Additional Digit Required — Refer to the Tabular List for Digit Selection     ⁽ᵗᵉᵇ⁾ Subterms under main terms may continue to next column or page

44 — Volume 2     ►◄ Revised Text     ● New Line     ▲ Revised Code     *2008 ICD-9-CM*

**Cardiac** — see also condition — continued
  death — see Disease, heart
  device
    defibrillator, automatic implantable V45.02
    in situ NEC V45.00
    pacemaker
      cardiac
        fitting or adjustment V53.31
        in situ V45.01
      carotid sinus
        fitting or adjustment V53.39
        in situ V45.09
  pacemaker — see Cardiac, device, pacemaker
  tamponade 423.3
**Cardia, cardial** — see condition
**Cardialgia** — see also Pain, precordial 786.51
**Cardiectasis** — see Hypertrophy, cardiac
**Cardiochalasia** 530.81
**Cardiomalacia** — see also Degeneration, myocardial 429.1
**Cardiomegalia glycogenica diffusa** 271.0
**Cardiomegaly** — see also Hypertrophy, cardiac 429.3
  congenital 746.89
  glycogen 271.0
  hypertensive (see also Hypertension, heart) 402.90
  idiopathic 429.3
**Cardiomyoliposis** — see also Degeneration, myocardial 429.1
**Cardiomyopathy** (congestive) (constrictive) (familial) (infiltrative) (obstructive) (restrictive) (sporadic) 425.4
  alcoholic 425.5
  amyloid 277.39 [425.7]
  beriberi 265.0 [425.7]
  cobalt-beer 425.5
  congenital 425.3
  due to
    amyloidosis 277.39 [425.7]
    beriberi 265.0 [425.7]
    cardiac glycogenosis 271.0 [425.7]
    Chagas' disease 086.0
    Friedreich's ataxia 334.0 [425.8]
    hypertension — see Hypertension, with, heart involvement
    mucopolysaccharidosis 277.5 [425.7]
    myotonia atrophica 359.21 [425.8]
    progressive muscular dystrophy 359.1 [425.8]
    sarcoidosis 135 [425.8]
  glycogen storage 271.0 [425.7]
  hypertensive — see Hypertension, with, heart involvement
  hypertrophic
    nonobstructive 425.4
    obstructive 425.1
      congenital 746.84
  idiopathic (concentric) 425.4
  in
    Chagas' disease 086.0
    sarcoidosis 135 [425.8]
  ischemic 414.8
  metabolic NEC 277.9 [425.7]
    amyloid 277.39 [425.7]
    thyrotoxic (see also Thyrotoxicosis) 242.9 ☑ [425.7]
    thyrotoxicosis (see also Thyrotoxicosis) 242.9 ☑ [425.7]
  newborn 425.4
    congenital 425.3
  nutritional 269.9 [425.7]
    beriberi 265.0 [425.7]
  obscure of Africa 425.2
  peripartum 674.5 ☑
  postpartum 674.5 ☑
  primary 425.4
  secondary 425.9
  stress inuced 429.83

**Cardiomyopathy** — continued
  takotsubo 429.83
  thyrotoxic (see also Thyrotoxicosis) 242.9 ☑ [425.7]
  toxic NEC 425.9
  tuberculous (see also Tuberculosis) 017.9 ☑ [425.8]
**Cardionephritis** — see Hypertension, cardiorenal
**Cardionephropathy** — see Hypertension, cardiorenal
**Cardionephrosis** — see Hypertension, cardiorenal
**Cardioneurosis** 306.2
**Cardiopathia nigra** 416.0
**Cardiopathy** — see also Disease, heart 429.9
  hypertensive (see also Hypertension, heart) 402.90
  idiopathic 425.4
  mucopolysaccharidosis 277.5 [425.7]
**Cardiopericarditis** — see also Pericarditis 423.9
**Cardiophobia** 300.29
**Cardioptosis** 746.87
**Cardiorenal** — see condition
**Cardiorrhexis** — see also Infarct, myocardium 410.9 ☑
**Cardiosclerosis** — see Arteriosclerosis, coronary
**Cardiosis** — see Disease, heart
**Cardiospasm** (esophagus) (reflex) (stomach) 530.0
  congenital 750.7
**Cardiostenosis** — see Disease, heart
**Cardiosymphysis** 423.1
**Cardiothyrotoxicosis** — see Hyperthyroidism
**Cardiovascular** — see condition
**Carditis** (acute) (bacterial) (chronic) (subacute) 429.89
  Coxsackie 074.20
  hypertensive (see also Hypertension, heart) 402.90
  meningococcal 036.40
  rheumatic — see Disease, heart, rheumatic
  rheumatoid 714.2
**Care** (of)
  child (routine) V20.1
  convalescent following V66.9
    chemotherapy V66.2
    medical NEC V66.5
    psychotherapy V66.3
    radiotherapy V66.1
    surgery V66.0
    surgical NEC V66.0
    treatment (for) V66.5
      combined V66.6
      fracture V66.4
      mental disorder NEC V66.3
      specified type NEC V66.5
  end-of-life V66.7
  family member (handicapped) (sick)
    creating problem for family V61.49
    provided away from home for holiday relief V60.5
    unavailable, due to
      absence (person rendering care) (sufferer) V60.4
      inability (any reason) of person rendering care V60.4
  holiday relief V60.5
  hospice V66.7
  lack of (at or after birth) (infant) (child) 995.52
    adult 995.84
  lactation of mother V24.1
  palliative V66.7
  postpartum
    immediately after delivery V24.0
    routine follow-up V24.2
  prenatal V22.1
    first pregnancy V22.0
    high-risk pregnancy V23.9
      specified problem NEC V23.89

**Care** — continued
  terminal V66.7
  unavailable, due to
    absence of person rendering care V60.4
    inability (any reason) of person rendering care V60.4
  well baby V20.1
**Caries** (bone) — see also Tuberculosis, bone 015.9 ☑ [730.8] ☑
  arrested 521.04
  cementum 521.03
  cerebrospinal (tuberculous) 015.0 ☑ [730.88]
  dental (acute) (chronic) (incipient) (infected) 521.00
    with pulp exposure 521.03
    extending to
      dentine 521.02
      pulp 521.03
    other specified NEC 521.09
    pit and fissure 521.06
    primary
      pit and fissure origin 521.06
      root surface 521.08
      smooth surface origin 521.07
    root surface 521.08
    smooth surface 521.07
  dentin (acute) (chronic) 521.02
  enamel (acute) (chronic) (incipient) 521.01
  external meatus 380.89
  hip (see also Tuberculosis) 015.1 ☑ [730.85]
  initial 521.01
  knee 015.2 ☑ [730.86]
  labyrinth 386.8
  limb NEC 015.7 ☑ [730.88]
  mastoid (chronic) (process) 383.1
  middle ear 385.89
  nose 015.7 ☑ [730.88]
  orbit 015.7 ☑ [730.88]
  ossicle 385.24
  petrous bone 383.20
  sacrum (tuberculous) 015.0 ☑ [730.88]
  spine, spinal (column) (tuberculous) 015.0 ☑ [730.88]
  syphilitic 095.5
    congenital 090.0 [730.8] ☑
  teeth (internal) 521.00
    initial 521.01
  vertebra (column) (tuberculous) 015.0 ☑ [730.88]
**Carini's syndrome** (ichthyosis congenita) 757.1
**Carious teeth** 521.00
**Carneous mole** 631
**Carnosinemia** 270.5
**Carotid body or sinus syndrome** 337.0
**Carotidynia** 337.0
**Carotinemia** (dietary) 278.3
**Carotinosis** (cutis) (skin) 278.3
**Carpal tunnel syndrome** 354.0
**Carpenter's syndrome** 759.89
**Carpopedal spasm** — see also Tetany 781.7
**Carpoptosis** 736.05
**Carrier** (suspected) of
  amebiasis V02.2
  bacterial disease (meningococcal, staphylococcal) NEC V02.59
  cholera V02.0
  cystic fibrosis gene V83.81
  defective gene V83.89
  diphtheria V02.4
  dysentery (bacillary) V02.3
    amebic V02.2
  Endamoeba histolytica V02.2
  gastrointestinal pathogens NEC V02.3
  genetic defect V83.89
  gonorrhea V02.7
  group B streptococcus V02.51
  HAA (hepatitis Australian-antigen) V02.61
  hemophilia A (asymptomatic) V83.01

**Carrier** (suspected) of — continued
  hemophilia A — continued
    symptomatic V83.02
  hepatitis V02.60
    Australian-antigen (HAA) V02.61
    B V02.61
    C V02.62
    serum V02.61
    specified type NEC V02.69
    viral V02.60
  infective organism NEC V02.9
  malaria V02.9
  paratyphoid V02.3
  Salmonella V02.3
    typhosa V02.1
  serum hepatitis V02.61
  Shigella V02.3
  Staphylococcus NEC V02.59
  Streptococcus NEC V02.52
    group B V02.51
  typhoid V02.1
  venereal disease NEC V02.8
**Carrión's disease** (Bartonellosis) 088.0
**Car sickness** 994.6
**Carter's**
  relapsing fever (Asiatic) 087.0
**Cartilage** — see condition
**Caruncle** (inflamed)
  abscess, lacrimal (see also Dacryocystitis) 375.30
  conjunctiva 372.00
    acute 372.00
  eyelid 373.00
  labium (majus) (minus) 616.89
  lacrimal 375.30
  urethra (benign) 599.3
  vagina (wall) 616.89
**Cascade stomach** 537.6
**Caseation lymphatic gland** — see also Tuberculosis 017.2 ☑
**Caseous**
  bronchitis — see Tuberculosis, pulmonary
  meningitis 013.0 ☑
  pneumonia — see Tuberculosis, pulmonary
**Cassidy (-Scholte) syndrome** (malignant carcinoid) 259.2
**Castellani's bronchitis** 104.8
**Castleman's tumor or lymphoma** (mediastinal lymph node hyperplasia) 785.6
**Castration, traumatic** 878.2
  complicated 878.3
**Casts in urine** 791.7
**Catalepsy** 300.11
  catatonic (acute) (see also Schizophrenia) 295.2 ☑
  hysterical 300.11
  schizophrenic (see also Schizophrenia) 295.2 ☑
**Cataphasia** 307.0
**Cataplexy** (idiopathic) — see Narcolepsy
**Cataract** (anterior cortical) (anterior polar) (black) (capsular) (central) (cortical) (hypermature) (immature) (incipient) (mature) 366.9
  anterior
    and posterior axial embryonal 743.33
    pyramidal 743.31
    subcapsular polar
      infantile, juvenile, or presenile 366.01
      senile 366.13
  associated with
    calcinosis 275.40 [366.42]
    craniofacial dysostosis 756.0 [366.44]
    galactosemia 271.1 [366.44]
    hypoparathyroidism 252.1 [366.42]
    myotonic disorders 359.21 [366.43]
    neovascularization 366.33
  blue dot 743.39
  cerulean 743.39

☑ Additional Digit Required — Refer to the Tabular List for Digit Selection      ▽ Subterms under main terms may continue to next column or page

2008 ICD-9-CM      ▶◀ Revised Text      ● New Line      ▲ Revised Code      October 2007 · Volume 2 — 45

**Cataract** — *continued*
  complicated NEC 366.30
  congenital 743.30
    capsular or subcapsular 743.31
    cortical 743.32
    nuclear 743.33
    specified type NEC 743.39
    total or subtotal 743.34
    zonular 743.32
  coronary (congenital) 743.39
    acquired 366.12
  cupuliform 366.14
  diabetic 250.5 ☑ *[366.41]*
  drug-induced 366.45
  due to
    chalcosis 360.24 *[366.34]*
    chronic choroiditis (*see also*
      Choroiditis) 363.20 *[366.32]*
    degenerative myopia
      360.21 *[366.34]*
    glaucoma (*see also* Glaucoma)
      365.9 *[366.31]*
    infection, intraocular NEC 366.32
    inflammatory ocular disorder NEC
      366.32
    iridocyclitis, chronic
      364.10 *[366.33]*
    pigmentary retinal dystrophy
      362.74 *[366.34]*
    radiation 366.46
  electric 366.46
  glassblowers' 366.46
  heat ray 366.46
  heterochromic 366.33
  in eye disease NEC 366.30
  infantile (*see also* Cataract, juvenile)
    366.00
  intumescent 366.12
  irradiational 366.46
  juvenile 366.00
    anterior subcapsular polar 366.01
    combined forms 366.09
    cortical 366.03
    lamellar 366.03
    nuclear 366.04
    posterior subcapsular polar 366.02
    specified NEC 366.09
    zonular 366.03
  lamellar 743.32
    infantile, juvenile, or presenile
      366.03
  morgagnian 366.18
  myotonic 359.21 *[366.43]*    ▲
  myxedema 244.9 *[366.44]*
  nuclear 366.16
  posterior, polar (capsular) 743.31
    infantile, juvenile, or presenile
      366.02
    senile 366.14
  presenile (*see also* Cataract, juvenile)
    366.00
  punctate
    acquired 366.12
    congenital 743.39
  secondary (membrane) 366.50
    obscuring vision 366.53
    specified type, not obscuring vision
      366.52
  senile 366.10
    anterior subcapsular polar 366.13
    combined forms 366.19
    cortical 366.15
    hypermature 366.18
    immature 366.12
    incipient 366.12
    mature 366.17
    nuclear 366.16
    posterior subcapsular polar 366.14
    specified NEC 366.19
    total or subtotal 366.17
  snowflake 250.5 ☑ *[366.41]*
  specified NEC 366.8
  subtotal (senile) 366.17
    congenital 743.34
  sunflower 360.24 *[366.34]*
  tetanic NEC 252.1 *[366.42]*

**Cataract** — *continued*
  total (mature) (senile) 366.17
    congenital 743.34
    localized 366.21
    traumatic 366.22
  toxic 366.45
  traumatic 366.20
    partially resolved 366.23
    total 366.22
  zonular (perinuclear) 743.32
    infantile, juvenile, or presenile
      366.03
**Cataracta** 366.10
  brunescens 366.16
  cerulea 743.39
  complicata 366.30
  congenita 743.30
  coralliformis 743.39
  coronaria (congenital) 743.39
    acquired 366.12
  diabetic 250.5 ☑ *[366.41]*
  floriformis 360.24 *[366.34]*
  membranacea
    accreta 366.50
    congenita 743.39
  nigra 366.16
**Catarrh, catarrhal** (inflammation) — *see*
    *also* condition 460
  acute 460
  asthma, asthmatic (*see also* Asthma)
    493.9 ☑
  Bostock's (*see also* Fever, hay) 477.9
  bowel — *see* Enteritis
  bronchial 490
    acute 466.0
    chronic 491.0
    subacute 466.0
  cervix, cervical (canal) (uteri) — *see*
    Cervicitis
  chest (*see also* Bronchitis) 490
  chronic 472.0
  congestion 472.0
  conjunctivitis 372.03
  due to syphilis 095.9
    congenital 090.0
  enteric — *see* Enteritis
  epidemic 487.1
  Eustachian 381.50
  eye (acute) (vernal) 372.03
  fauces (*see also* Pharyngitis) 462
  febrile 460
  fibrinous acute 466.0
  gastroenteric — *see* Enteritis
  gastrointestinal — *see* Enteritis
  gingivitis 523.00
  hay (*see also* Fever, hay) 477.9
  infectious 460
  intestinal — *see* Enteritis
  larynx (*see also* Laryngitis, chronic)
    476.0
  liver 070.1
    with hepatic coma 070.0
  lung (*see also* Bronchitis) 490
    acute 466.0
    chronic 491.0
  middle ear (chronic) — *see* Otitis me-
    dia, chronic
  mouth 528.00
  nasal (chronic) (*see also* Rhinitis)
    472.0
    acute 460
  nasobronchial 472.2
  nasopharyngeal (chronic) 472.2
    acute 460
  nose — *see* Catarrh, nasal
  ophthalmia 372.03
  pneumococcal, acute 466.0
  pulmonary (*see also* Bronchitis) 490
    acute 466.0
    chronic 491.0
  spring (eye) 372.13
  suffocating (*see also* Asthma) 493.9 ☑
  summer (hay) (*see also* Fever, hay)
    477.9
  throat 472.1
  tracheitis 464.10

**Catarrh, catarrhal** — *see also* condition
    — *continued*
  tracheitis — *continued*
    with obstruction 464.11
  tubotympanal 381.4
    acute (*see also* Otitis media, acute,
      nonsuppurative) 381.00
    chronic 381.10
  vasomotor (*see also* Fever, hay) 477.9
  vesical (bladder) — *see* Cystitis
**Catarrhus aestivus** — *see also* Fever,
    hay 477.9
**Catastrophe, cerebral** — *see also* Dis-
    ease, cerebrovascular, acute 436
**Catatonia, catatonic** (acute) 781.99
  with
    affective psychosis — *see* Psy-
      chosis, affective
  agitation 295.2 ☑
  dementia (praecox) 295.2 ☑
  due to or associated with physical
    condition 293.89
  excitation 295.2 ☑
  excited type 295.2 ☑
  in conditions classified elsewhere
    293.89
  schizophrenia 295.2 ☑
  stupor 295.2 ☑
**Cat's ear** 744.29
**Cat-scratch** — *see also* Injury, superfi-
    cial
  disease or fever 078.3
**Cauda equina** — *see also* condition
  syndrome 344.60
**Cauliflower ear** 738.7
**Caul over face** 768.9
**Causalgia** 355.9
  lower limb 355.71
  upper limb 354.4
**Cause**
  external, general effects NEC 994.9
  not stated 799.9
  unknown 799.9
**Caustic burn** — *see also* Burn, by site
  from swallowing caustic or corrosive
    substance — *see* Burn, internal
    organs
**Cavare's disease** (familial periodic
    paralysis) 359.3
**Cave-in, injury**
  crushing (severe) (*see also* Crush, by
    site) 869.1
  suffocation 994.7
**Cavernitis** (penis) 607.2
  lymph vessel — *see* Lymphangioma
**Cavernositis** 607.2
**Cavernous** — *see* condition
**Cavitation of lung** — *see also* Tubercu-
    losis 011.2 ☑
  nontuberculous 518.89
  primary, progressive 010.8 ☑
**Cavity**
  lung — *see* Cavitation of lung
  optic papilla 743.57
  pulmonary — *see* Cavitation of lung
  teeth 521.00
  vitreous (humor) 379.21
**Cavovarus foot, congenital** 754.59
**Cavus foot** (congenital) 754.71
  acquired 736.73
**Cazenave's**
  disease (pemphigus) NEC 694.4
  lupus (erythematosus) 695.4
**CDGS** (carbohydrate-deficient glycopro-
    tein syndrome) 271.8
**Cecitis** — *see* Appendicitis
**Cecocele** — *see* Hernia
**Cecum** — *see* condition
**Celiac**
  artery compression syndrome 447.4
  disease 579.0
  infantilism 579.0
**Cell, cellular** — *see also* condition
  anterior chamber (eye) (positive aque-
    ous ray) 364.04

**Cellulitis** (diffuse) (with lymphangitis) —
    *see also* Abscess 682.9
  abdominal wall 682.2
  anaerobic (*see also* Gas gangrene)
    040.0
  ankle 682.6
  anus 566
  areola 611.0
  arm (any part, above wrist) 682.3
  auditory canal (external) 380.10
  axilla 682.3
  back (any part) 682.2
  breast 611.0
    postpartum 675.1 ☑
  broad ligament (*see also* Disease,
    pelvis, inflammatory) 614.4
    acute 614.3
  buttock 682.5
  cervical (neck region) 682.1
  cervix (uteri) (*see also* Cervicitis) 616.0
  cheek, external 682.0
    internal 528.3
  chest wall 682.2
  chronic NEC 682.9
  colostomy 569.61
  corpus cavernosum 607.2
  digit 681.9
  Douglas' cul-de-sac or pouch (chronic)
    (*see also* Disease, pelvis, inflam-
    matory) 614.4
    acute 614.3
  drainage site (following operation)
    998.59
  ear, external 380.10
  enterostomy 569.61
  erysipelar (*see also* Erysipelas) 035
  esophagostomy 530.86
  eyelid 373.13
  face (any part, except eye) 682.0
  finger (intrathecal) (periosteal) (subcu-
    taneous) (subcuticular) 681.00
  flank 682.2
  foot (except toe) 682.7
  forearm 682.3
  gangrenous (*see also* Gangrene) 785.4
  genital organ NEC
    female — *see* Abscess, genital or-
      gan, female
    male 608.4
  glottis 478.71
  gluteal (region) 682.5
  gonococcal NEC 098.0
  groin 682.2
  hand (except finger or thumb) 682.4
  head (except face) NEC 682.8
  heel 682.7
  hip 682.6
  jaw (region) 682.0
  knee 682.6
  labium (majus) (minus) (*see also* Vul-
    vitis) 616.10
  larynx 478.71
  leg, except foot 682.6
  lip 528.5
  mammary gland 611.0
  mouth (floor) 528.3
  multiple sites NEC 682.9
  nasopharynx 478.21
  navel 682.2
    newborn NEC 771.4
  neck (region) 682.1
  nipple 611.0
  nose 478.19
    external 682.0
  orbit, orbital 376.01
  palate (soft) 528.3
  pectoral (region) 682.2
  pelvis, pelvic
    with
      abortion — *see* Abortion, by
        type, with sepsis
      ectopic pregnancy (*see also* cat-
        egories 633.0–633.9)
        639.0
      molar pregnancy (*see also* cate-
        gories 630–632) 639.0

☑ Additional Digit Required — Refer to the Tabular List for Digit Selection         Subterms under main terms may continue to next column or page

46 — Volume 2 • October 2007      ►◄ Revised Text      ● New Line      ▲ Revised Code      **2008 ICD-9-CM**

**Cellulitis** — *see also* Abscess — *continued*
  pelvis, pelvic — *continued*
    female (*see also* Disease, pelvis, inflammatory) 614.4
      acute 614.3
      following
        abortion 639.0
        ectopic or molar pregnancy 639.0
    male 567.21
    puerperal, postpartum, childbirth 670.0 ☑
  penis 607.2
  perineal, perineum 682.2
  perirectal 566
  peritonsillar 475
  periurethral 597.0
  periuterine (*see also* Disease, pelvis, inflammatory) 614.4
    acute 614.3
  pharynx 478.21
  phlegmonous NEC 682.9
  rectum 566
  retromammary 611.0
  retroperitoneal (*see also* Peritonitis) 567.2 ☑, 567.38
  round ligament (*see also* Disease, pelvis, inflammatory) 614.4
    acute 614.3
  scalp (any part) 682.8
    dissecting 704.8
  scrotum 608.4
  seminal vesicle 608.0
  septic NEC 682.9
  shoulder 682.3
  specified sites NEC 682.8
  spermatic cord 608.4
  submandibular (region) (space) (triangle) 682.0
    gland 527.3
  submaxillary 528.3
    gland 527.3
  submental (pyogenic) 682.0
    gland 527.3
  suppurative NEC 682.9
  testis 608.4
  thigh 682.6
  thumb (intrathecal) (periosteal) (subcutaneous) (subcuticular) 681.00
  toe (intrathecal) (periosteal) (subcutaneous) (subcuticular) 681.10
  tonsil 475
  trunk 682.2
  tuberculous (primary) (*see also* Tuberculosis) 017.0 ☑
  tunica vaginalis 608.4
  umbilical 682.2
    newborn NEC 771.4
  vaccinal 999.39 ▲
  vagina — *see* Vaginitis
  vas deferens 608.4
  vocal cords 478.5
  vulva (*see also* Vulvitis) 616.10
  wrist 682.4
**Cementoblastoma, benign** (M9273/0) 213.1
  upper jaw (bone) 213.0
**Cementoma** (M9273/0) 213.1
  gigantiform (M9276/0) 213.1
    upper jaw (bone) 213.0
  upper jaw (bone) 213.0
**Cementoperiostitis** 523.40
**Cephalgia, cephalagia** — *see also* Headache 784.0
  histamine 346.2 ☑
  nonorganic origin 307.81
  psychogenic 307.81
  tension 307.81
**Cephalhematocele, cephalematocele**
  due to birth injury 767.19
  fetus or newborn 767.19
  traumatic (*see also* Contusion, head) 920

**Cephalhematoma, cephalematoma** (calcified)
  due to birth injury 767.19
  fetus or newborn 767.19
  traumatic (*see also* Contusion, head) 920
**Cephalic** — *see* condition
**Cephalitis** — *see* Encephalitis
**Cephalocele** 742.0
**Cephaloma** — *see* Neoplasm, by site, malignant
**Cephalomenia** 625.8
**Cephalopelvic** — *see* condition
**Cercomoniasis** 007.3
**Cerebellitis** — *see* Encephalitis
**Cerebellum** (cerebellar) — *see* condition
**Cerebral** — *see* condition
**Cerebritis** — *see* Encephalitis
**Cerebrohepatorenal syndrome** 759.89
**Cerebromacular degeneration** 330.1
**Cerebromalacia** — *see also* Softening, brain 434.9 ☑
**Cerebrosidosis** 272.7
**Cerebrospasticity** — *see* Palsy, cerebral
**Cerebrospinal** — *see* condition
**Cerebrum** — *see* condition
**Ceroid storage disease** 272.7
**Cerumen** (accumulation) (impacted) 380.4
**Cervical** — *see also* condition
  auricle 744.43
  high risk human papillomavirus (HPV) DNA test positive 795.05
  intraepithelial glandular neoplasia 233.1
  low risk human papillomavirus (HPV) DNA test positive 795.09
  rib 756.2
**Cervicalgia** 723.1
**Cervicitis** (acute) (chronic) (nonvenereal) (subacute) (with erosion or ectropion) 616.0
  with
    abortion — *see* Abortion, by type, with sepsis
    ectopic pregnancy (*see also* categories 633.0–633.9) 639.0
    molar pregnancy (*see also* categories 630–632) 639.0
    ulceration 616.0
  chlamydial 099.53
  complicating pregnancy or puerperium 646.6 ☑
    affecting fetus or newborn 760.8
  following
    abortion 639.0
    ectopic or molar pregnancy 639.0
  gonococcal (acute) 098.15
    chronic or duration of 2 months or more 098.35
  senile (atrophic) 616.0
  syphilitic 095.8
  trichomonal 131.09
  tuberculous (*see also* Tuberculosis) 016.7 ☑
**Cervicoaural fistula** 744.49
**Cervicocolpitis** (emphysematosa) — *see also* Cervicitis 616.0
**Cervix** — *see* condition
**Cesarean delivery, operation or section** NEC 669.7 ☑
  affecting fetus or newborn 763.4
  post mortem, affecting fetus or newborn 761.6
  previous, affecting management of pregnancy 654.2 ☑
**Céstan-Chenais paralysis** 344.89
**Céstan-Raymond syndrome** 433.8 ☑
**Céstan's syndrome** 344.89
**Cestode infestation** NEC 123.9
  specified type NEC 123.8
**Cestodiasis** 123.9
**CGF** (congenital generalized fibromatosis) 759.89
**Chabert's disease** 022.9
**Chacaleh** 266.2

**Chafing** 709.8
**Chagas' disease** — *see also* Trypanosomiasis, American 086.2
  with heart involvement 086.0
**Chagres fever** 084.0
**Chalasia** (cardiac sphincter) 530.81
**Chalazion** 373.2
**Chalazoderma** 757.39
**Chalcosis** 360.24
  cornea 371.15
  crystalline lens 360.24 [366.34]
  retina 360.24
**Chalicosis** (occupational) (pulmonum) 502
**Chancre** (any genital site) (hard) (indurated) (infecting) (primary) (recurrent) 091.0
  congenital 090.0
  conjunctiva 091.2
  Ducrey's 099.0
  extragenital 091.2
  eyelid 091.2
  Hunterian 091.0
  lip (syphilis) 091.2
  mixed 099.8
  nipple 091.2
  Nisbet's 099.0
  of
    carate 103.0
    pinta 103.0
    yaws 102.0
  palate, soft 091.2
  phagedenic 099.0
  Ricord's 091.0
  Rollet's (syphilitic) 091.0
  seronegative 091.0
  seropositive 091.0
  simple 099.0
  soft 099.0
    bubo 099.0
  urethra 091.0
  yaws 102.0
**Chancriform syndrome** 114.1
**Chancroid** 099.0
  anus 099.0
  penis (Ducrey's bacillus) 099.0
  perineum 099.0
  rectum 099.0
  scrotum 099.0
  urethra 099.0
  vulva 099.0
**Chandipura fever** 066.8
**Chandler's disease** (osteochondritis dissecans, hip) 732.7
**Change(s)** (of) — *see also* Removal of
  arteriosclerotic — *see* Arteriosclerosis
  battery
    cardiac pacemaker V53.31
  bone 733.90
    diabetic 250.8 ☑ [731.8]
    in disease, unknown cause 733.90
  bowel habits 787.99
  cardiorenal (vascular) (*see also* Hypertension, cardiorenal) 404.90
  cardiovascular — *see* Disease, cardiovascular
  circulatory 459.9
  cognitive or personality change of other type, nonpsychotic 310.1
  color, teeth, tooth
    during formation 520.8
    extrinsic 523.6
    intrinsic posteruptive 521.7
  contraceptive device V25.42
  cornea, corneal
    degenerative NEC 371.40
    membrane NEC 371.30
    senile 371.41
  coronary (*see also* Ischemia, heart) 414.9
  degenerative
    chamber angle (anterior) (iris) 364.56
    ciliary body 364.57
    spine or vertebra (*see also* Spondylosis) 721.90

**Change(s)** — *see also* Removal of — *continued*
  dental pulp, regressive 522.2
  drains V58.49
  dressing
    wound V58.30
      nonsurgical V58.30
      surgical V58.31
  fixation device V54.89
    external V54.89
    internal V54.01
  heart (*see also* Disease, heart)
  hip joint 718.95
  hyperplastic larynx 478.79
  hypertrophic
    nasal sinus (*see also* Sinusitis) 473.9
    turbinate, nasal 478.0
    upper respiratory tract 478.9
  inflammatory — *see* Inflammation
  joint (*see also* Derangement, joint) 718.90
    sacroiliac 724.6
  Kirschner wire V54.89
  knee 717.9
  macular, congenital 743.55
  malignant (M— — /3) (*see also* Neoplasm, by site, malignant)

> *Note — for malignant change occurring in a neoplasm, use the appropriate M code with behavior digit /3 e.g., malignant change in uterine fibroid — M8890/3. For malignant change occurring in a nonneoplastic condition (e.g., gastric ulcer) use the M code M8000/3.*

  mental (status) NEC 780.97
    due to or associated with physical condition — *see* Syndrome, brain
  myocardium, myocardial — *see* Degeneration, myocardial
  of life (*see also* Menopause) 627.2
  pacemaker battery (cardiac) V53.31
  peripheral nerve 355.9
  personality (nonpsychotic) NEC 310.1
  plaster cast V54.89
  refractive, transient 367.81
  regressive, dental pulp 522.2
  retina 362.9
    myopic (degenerative) (malignant) 360.21
    vascular appearance 362.13
  sacroiliac joint 724.6
  scleral 379.19
    degenerative 379.16
  senile (*see also* Senility) 797
  sensory (*see also* Disturbance, sensation) 782.0
  skin texture 782.8
  spinal cord 336.9
  splint, external V54.89
  subdermal implantable contraceptive V25.5
  suture V58.32
  traction device V54.89
  trophic 355.9
    arm NEC 354.9
    leg NEC 355.8
    lower extremity NEC 355.8
    upper extremity NEC 354.9
  vascular 459.9
  vasomotor 443.9
  voice 784.49
    psychogenic 306.1
  wound packing V58.30
    nonsurgical V58.30
    surgical V58.31
**Changing sleep-work schedule, affecting sleep** 327.36
**Changuinola fever** 066.0
**Chapping skin** 709.8
**Character**
  depressive 301.12
**Charcôt's**
  arthropathy 094.0 [713.5]
  cirrhosis — *see* Cirrhosis, biliary

☑ Additional Digit Required — Refer to the Tabular List for Digit Selection     ⩘ Subterms under main terms may continue to next column or page

*2008 ICD-9-CM*    ▶◀ Revised Text    ● New Line    ▲ Revised Code    October 2007 • Volume 2 — 47

☑ Additional Digit Required — Refer to the Tabular List for Digit Selection          ᴺᴱᶜ Subterms under main terms may continue to next column or page

48 — Volume 2 · October 2007          ▶◀ Revised Text          ● New Line          ▲ Revised Code          **2008 ICD-9-CM**

**Cholesterolemia** — *continued*
  familial 272.0
  hereditary 272.0
**Cholesterosis, cholesterolosis** (gallbladder) 575.6
  with
    cholecystitis — *see* Cholecystitis
    cholelithiasis — *see* Cholelithiasis
    middle ear (*see also* Cholesteatoma) 385.30
**Cholocolic fistula** — *see also* Fistula, gallbladder 575.5
**Choluria** 791.4
**Chondritis** (purulent) 733.99
  auricle 380.03
  costal 733.6
    Tietze's 733.6
  patella, posttraumatic 717.7
  pinna 380.03
  posttraumatica patellae 717.7
  tuberculous (active) (*see also* Tuberculosis) 015.9 ☑
    intervertebral 015.0 ☑ *[730.88]*
**Chondroangiopathia calcarea seu punctate** 756.59
**Chondroblastoma** (M9230/0) — *see also* Neoplasm, bone, benign
  malignant (M9230/3) — *see* Neoplasm, bone, malignant
**Chondrocalcinosis** (articular) (crystal deposition) (dihydrate) — *see also* Arthritis, due to, crystals 275.49 *[712.3]* ☑
  due to
    calcium pyrophosphate 275.49 *[712.2]* ☑
    dicalcium phosphate crystals 275.49 *[712.1]* ☑
    pyrophosphate crystals 275.49 *[712.2]* ☑
**Chondrodermatitis nodularis helicis** 380.00
**Chondrodysplasia** 756.4
  angiomatose 756.4
  calcificans congenita 756.59
  epiphysialis punctata 756.59
  hereditary deforming 756.4
  rhizomelic punctata 277.86
**Chondrodystrophia** (fetalis) 756.4
  calcarea 756.4
  calcificans congenita 756.59
  fetalis hypoplastica 756.59
  hypoplastica calcinosa 756.59
  punctata 756.59
  tarda 277.5
**Chondrodystrophy** (familial) (hypoplastic) 756.4
  myotonic (congenital) 359.23 ●
**Chondroectodermal dysplasia** 756.55
**Chondrolysis** 733.99
**Chondroma** (M9220/0) — *see also* Neoplasm cartilage, benign
  juxtacortical (M9221/1) — *see* Neoplasm, bone, benign
  periosteal (M9221/0) — *see* Neoplasm, bone, benign
**Chondromalacia** 733.92
  epiglottis (congenital) 748.3
  generalized 733.92
  knee 717.7
  larynx (congenital) 748.3
  localized, except patella 733.92
  patella, patellae 717.7
  systemic 733.92
  tibial plateau 733.92
  trachea (congenital) 748.3
**Chondromatosis** (M9220/1) — *see* Neoplasm, cartilage, uncertain behavior
**Chondromyxosarcoma** (M9220/3) — *see* Neoplasm, cartilage, malignant
**Chondro-osteodysplasia** (Morquio-Brailsford type) 277.5
**Chondro-osteodystrophy** 277.5
**Chondro-osteoma** (M9210/0) — *see* Neoplasm, bone, benign

**Chondropathia tuberosa** 733.6
**Chondrosarcoma** (M9220/3) — *see also* Neoplasm, cartilage, malignant
  juxtacortical (M9221/3) — *see* Neoplasm, bone, malignant
  mesenchymal (M9240/3) — *see* Neoplasm, connective tissue, malignant
**Chordae tendineae rupture** (chronic) 429.5
**Chordee** (nonvenereal) 607.89
  congenital 752.63
  gonococcal 098.2
**Chorditis** (fibrinous) (nodosa) (tuberosa) 478.5
**Chordoma** (M9370/3) — *see* Neoplasm, by site, malignant
**Chorea** (gravis) (minor) (spasmodic) 333.5
  with
    heart involvement — *see* Chorea with rheumatic heart disease
    rheumatic heart disease (chronic, inactive, or quiescent) (conditions classifiable to 393–398) (*see also* rheumatic heart condition involved)
      active or acute (conditions classifiable to 391) 392.0
  acute — *see* Chorea, Sydenham's
  apoplectic (*see also* Disease, cerebrovascular, acute) 436
  chronic 333.4
  electric 049.8
  gravidarum — *see* Eclampsia, pregnancy
  habit 307.22
  hereditary 333.4
  Huntington's 333.4
  posthemiplegic 344.89
  pregnancy — *see* Eclampsia, pregnancy
  progressive 333.4
    chronic 333.4
    hereditary 333.4
  rheumatic (chronic) 392.9
    with heart disease or involvement — *see* Chorea, with rheumatic heart disease
  senile 333.5
  Sydenham's 392.9
    with heart involvement — *see* Chorea, with rheumatic heart disease
    nonrheumatic 333.5
  variabilis 307.23
**Choreoathetosis** (paroxysmal) 333.5
**Chorioadenoma** (destruens) (M9100/1) 236.1
**Chorioamnionitis** 658.4 ☑
  affecting fetus or newborn 762.7
**Chorioangioma** (M9120/0) 219.8
**Choriocarcinoma** (M9100/3)
  combined with
    embryonal carcinoma (M9101/3) — *see* Neoplasm, by site, malignant
    teratoma (M9101/3) — *see* Neoplasm, by site, malignant
  specified site — *see* Neoplasm, by site, malignant
  unspecified site
    female 181
    male 186.9
**Chorioencephalitis, lymphocytic** (acute) (serous) 049.0
**Chorioepithelioma** (M9100/3) — *see* Choriocarcinoma
**Choriomeningitis** (acute) (benign) (lymphocytic) (serous) 049.0
**Chorionepithelioma** (M9100/3) — *see* Choriocarcinoma
**Chorionitis** — *see also* Scleroderma 710.1
**Chorioretinitis** 363.20
  disseminated 363.10
    generalized 363.13

**Chorioretinitis** — *continued*
  disseminated — *continued*
    in
      neurosyphilis 094.83
      secondary syphilis 091.51
    peripheral 363.12
    posterior pole 363.11
    tuberculous (*see also* Tuberculosis) 017.3 ☑ *[363.13]*
  due to
    histoplasmosis (*see also* Histoplasmosis) 115.92
    toxoplasmosis (acquired) 130.2
      congenital (active) 771.2
  focal 363.00
    juxtapapillary 363.01
    peripheral 363.04
    posterior pole NEC 363.03
  juxtapapillaris, juxtapapillary 363.01
  progressive myopia (degeneration) 360.21
  syphilitic (secondary) 091.51
    congenital (early) 090.0 *[363.13]*
      late 090.5 *[363.13]*
    late 095.8 *[363.13]*
  tuberculous (*see also* Tuberculosis) 017.3 ☑ *[363.13]*
**Choristoma** — *see* Neoplasm, by site, benign
**Choroid** — *see* condition
**Choroideremia, choroidermia** (initial stage) (late stage) (partial or total atrophy) 363.55
**Choroiditis** — *see also* Chorioretinitis 363.20
  leprous 030.9 *[363.13]*
  senile guttate 363.41
  sympathetic 360.11
  syphilitic (secondary) 091.51
    congenital (early) 090.0 *[363.13]*
      late 090.5 *[363.13]*
    late 095.8 *[363.13]*
  Tay's 363.41
  tuberculous (*see also* Tuberculosis) 017.3 ☑ *[363.13]*
**Choroidopathy** NEC 363.9
  degenerative (*see also* Degeneration, choroid) 363.40
  hereditary (*see also* Dystrophy, choroid) 363.50
  specified type NEC 363.8
**Choroidoretinitis** — *see* Chorioretinitis
**Choroidosis, central serous** 362.41
**Choroidretinopathy, serous** 362.41
**Christian's syndrome** (chronic histiocytosis X) 277.89
**Christian-Weber disease** (nodular nonsuppurative panniculitis) 729.30
**Christmas disease** 286.1
**Chromaffinoma** (M8700/0) — *see also* Neoplasm, by site, benign
  malignant (M8700/3) — *see* Neoplasm, by site, malignant
**Chromatopsia** 368.59
**Chromhidrosis, chromidrosis** 705.89
**Chromoblastomycosis** 117.2
**Chromomycosis** 117.2
**Chromophytosis** 111.0
**Chromotrichomycosis** 111.8
**Chronic** — *see* condition
**Churg-Strauss syndrome** 446.4
**Chyle cyst, mesentery** 457.8
**Chylocele** (nonfilarial) 457.8
  filarial (*see also* Infestation, filarial) 125.9
  tunica vaginalis (nonfilarial) 608.84
    filarial (*see also* Infestation, filarial) 125.9
**Chylomicronemia** (fasting) (with hyperprebetalipoproteinemia) 272.3
**Chylopericardium** (acute) 420.90
**Chylothorax** (nonfilarial) 457.8
  filarial (*see also* Infestation, filarial) 125.9
**Chylous**
  ascites 457.8

**Chylous** — *continued*
  cyst of peritoneum 457.8
  hydrocele 603.9
  hydrothorax (nonfilarial) 457.8
    filarial (*see also* Infestation, filarial) 125.9
**Chyluria** 791.1
  bilharziasis 120.0
  due to
    Brugia (malayi) 125.1
    Wuchereria (bancrofti) 125.0
      malayi 125.1
  filarial (*see also* Infestation, filarial) 125.9
  filariasis (*see also* Infestation, filarial) 125.9
  nonfilarial 791.1
**Cicatricial** (deformity) — *see* Cicatrix
**Cicatrix** (adherent) (contracted) (painful) (vicious) 709.2
  adenoid 474.8
  alveolar process 525.8
  anus 569.49
  auricle 380.89
  bile duct (*see also* Disease, biliary) 576.8
  bladder 596.8
  bone 733.99
  brain 348.8
  cervix (postoperative) (postpartal) 622.3
    in pregnancy or childbirth 654.6 ☑
      causing obstructed labor 660.2 ☑
  chorioretinal 363.30
    disseminated 363.35
    macular 363.32
    peripheral 363.34
    posterior pole NEC 363.33
  choroid — *see* Cicatrix, chorioretinal
  common duct (*see also* Disease, biliary) 576.8
  congenital 757.39
  conjunctiva 372.64
  cornea 371.00
    tuberculous (*see also* Tuberculosis) 017.3 ☑ *[371.05]*
  duodenum (bulb) 537.3
  esophagus 530.3
  eyelid 374.46
    with
      ectropion — *see* Ectropion
      entropion — *see* Entropion
  hypopharynx 478.29
  knee, semilunar cartilage 717.5
  lacrimal
    canaliculi 375.53
    duct
      acquired 375.56
      neonatal 375.55
      punctum 375.52
      sac 375.54
  larynx 478.79
  limbus (cystoid) 372.64
  lung 518.89
  macular 363.32
    disseminated 363.35
    peripheral 363.34
  middle ear 385.89
  mouth 528.9
  muscle 728.89
  nasolacrimal duct
    acquired 375.56
    neonatal 375.55
  nasopharynx 478.29
  palate (soft) 528.9
  penis 607.89
  prostate 602.8
  rectum 569.49
  retina 363.30
    disseminated 363.35
    macular 363.32
    peripheral 363.34
    posterior pole NEC 363.33
  semilunar cartilage — *see* Derangement, meniscus

☑ Additional Digit Required — Refer to the Tabular List for Digit Selection          ▽ Subterms under main terms may continue to next column or page

*2008 ICD-9-CM*          ▶◀ Revised Text          ● New Line          ▲ Revised Code          October 2007 · Volume 2 — 49

**Cicatrix** — *continued*
seminal vesicle 608.89
skin 709.2
   infected 686.8
   postinfectional 709.2
   tuberculous (*see also* Tuberculosis)
      017.0 ☑
specified site NEC 709.2
throat 478.29
tongue 529.8
tonsil (and adenoid) 474.8
trachea 478.9
tuberculous NEC (*see also* Tuberculosis) 011.9 ☑
ureter 593.89
urethra 599.84
uterus 621.8
vagina 623.4
   in pregnancy or childbirth 654.7 ☑
      causing obstructed labor
         660.2 ☑
vocal cord 478.5
wrist, constricting (annular) 709.2
**CIDP** (chronic inflammatory demyelinat- ●
   ing polyneuropathy) 357.81        ●
**CIN I** [cervical intraepithelial neoplasia
   I] 622.11
**CIN II** [cervical intraepithelial neoplasia
   II] 622.12
**CIN III** [**cervical intraepithelial neoplasia III**] 233.1
**Cinchonism**
   correct substance properly adminis-
      tered 386.9
   overdose or wrong substance given or
      taken 961.4
**Circine herpes** 110.5
**Circle of Willis** — *see* condition
**Circular** — *see also* condition
   hymen 752.49
**Circulating anticoagulants** 286.5
   following childbirth 666.3 ☑
   postpartum 666.3 ☑
**Circulation**
   collateral (venous), any site 459.89
   defective 459.9
      congenital 747.9
      lower extremity 459.89
   embryonic 747.9
   failure 799.89
      fetus or newborn 779.89
      peripheral 785.59
   fetal, persistent 747.83
   heart, incomplete 747.9
**Circulatory system** — *see* condition
**Circulus senilis** 371.41
**Circumcision**
   in absence of medical indication V50.2
   ritual V50.2
   routine V50.2
   status (post), female 629.20
**Circumscribed** — *see* condition
**Circumvallata placenta** — *see* Placenta,
   abnormal
**Cirrhosis, cirrhotic** 571.5
   with alcoholism 571.2
   alcoholic (liver) 571.2
   atrophic (of liver) — *see* Cirrhosis,
      portal
   Baumgarten-Cruveilhier 571.5
   biliary (cholangiolitic) (cholangitic)
      (cholestatic) (extrahepatic) (hy-
      pertrophic) (intrahepatic)
      (nonobstructive) (obstructive)
      (pericholangiolitic) (posthepatic)
      (primary) (secondary) (xanthoma-
      tous) 571.6
      due to
         clonorchiasis 121.1
         flukes 121.3
   brain 331.9
   capsular — *see* Cirrhosis, portal
   cardiac 571.5
      alcoholic 571.2
   central (liver) — *see* Cirrhosis, liver
   Charcôt's 571.6

**Cirrhosis, cirrhotic** — *continued*
   cholangiolitic — *see* Cirrhosis, biliary
   cholangitic — *see* Cirrhosis, biliary
   cholestatic — *see* Cirrhosis, biliary
   clitoris (hypertrophic) 624.2
   coarsely nodular 571.5
   congestive (liver) — *see* Cirrhosis,
      cardiac
   Cruveilhier-Baumgarten 571.5
   cryptogenic (of liver) 571.5
      alcoholic 571.2
   dietary (*see also* Cirrhosis, portal)
      571.5
   due to
      bronzed diabetes 275.0
      congestive hepatomegaly — *see*
         Cirrhosis, cardiac
      cystic fibrosis 277.00
      hemochromatosis 275.0
      hepatolenticular degeneration
         275.1
      passive congestion (chronic) — *see*
         Cirrhosis, cardiac
      Wilson's disease 275.1
      xanthomatosis 272.2
   extrahepatic (obstructive) — *see* Cir-
      rhosis, biliary
   fatty 571.8
      alcoholic 571.0
   florid 571.2
   Glisson's — *see* Cirrhosis, portal
   Hanot's (hypertrophic) — *see* Cirrho-
      sis, biliary
   hepatic — *see* Cirrhosis, liver
   hepatolienal — *see* Cirrhosis, liver
   hobnail — *see* Cirrhosis, portal
   hypertrophic (*see also* Cirrhosis, liver)
      biliary — *see* Cirrhosis, biliary
      Hanot's — *see* Cirrhosis, biliary
   infectious NEC — *see* Cirrhosis, portal
   insular — *see* Cirrhosis, portal
   intrahepatic (obstructive) (primary)
      (secondary) — *see* Cirrhosis,
      biliary
   juvenile (*see also* Cirrhosis, portal)
      571.5
   kidney (*see also* Sclerosis, renal) 587
   Laennec's (of liver) 571.2
      nonalcoholic 571.5
   liver (chronic) (hepatolienal) (hyper-
      trophic) (nodular) (splenomegal-
      ic) (unilobar) 571.5
      with alcoholism 571.2
      alcoholic 571.2
      congenital (due to failure of obliter-
         ation of umbilical vein) 777.8
      cryptogenic 571.5
         alcoholic 571.2
      fatty 571.8
         alcoholic 571.0
      macronodular 571.5
         alcoholic 571.2
      micronodular 571.5
         alcoholic 571.2
      nodular, diffuse 571.5
         alcoholic 571.2
      pigmentary 275.0
      portal 571.5
         alcoholic 571.2
      postnecrotic 571.5
         alcoholic 571.2
      syphilitic 095.3
   lung (chronic) (*see also* Fibrosis, lung)
      515
   macronodular (of liver) 571.5
      alcoholic 571.2
   malarial 084.9
   metabolic NEC 571.5
   micronodular (of liver) 571.5
      alcoholic 571.2
   monolobular — *see* Cirrhosis, portal
   multilobular — *see* Cirrhosis, portal
   nephritis (*see also* Sclerosis, renal)
      587
   nodular — *see* Cirrhosis, liver
   nutritional (fatty) 571.5

**Cirrhosis, cirrhotic** — *continued*
   obstructive (biliary) (extrahepatic) (in-
      trahepatic) — *see* Cirrhosis, bil-
      iary
   ovarian 620.8
   paludal 084.9
   pancreas (duct) 577.8
   pericholangiolitic — *see* Cirrhosis,
      biliary
   periportal — *see* Cirrhosis, portal
   pigment, pigmentary (of liver) 275.0
   portal (of liver) 571.5
      alcoholic 571.2
   posthepatitic (*see also* Cirrhosis,
      postnecrotic) 571.5
   postnecrotic (of liver) 571.5
      alcoholic 571.2
   primary (intrahepatic) — *see* Cirrho-
      sis, biliary
   pulmonary (*see also* Fibrosis, lung)
      515
   renal (*see also* Sclerosis, renal) 587
   septal (*see also* Cirrhosis, postnecrot-
      ic) 571.5
   spleen 289.51
   splenomegalic (of liver) — *see* Cirrho-
      sis, liver
   stasis (liver) — *see* Cirrhosis, liver
   stomach 535.4 ☑
   Todd's (*see also* Cirrhosis, biliary)
      571.6
   toxic (nodular) — *see* Cirrhosis, post-
      necrotic
   trabecular — *see* Cirrhosis, postnecrot-
      ic
   unilobar — *see* Cirrhosis, liver
   vascular (of liver) — *see* Cirrhosis,
      liver
   xanthomatous (biliary) (*see also* Cir-
      rhosis, biliary) 571.6
      due to xanthomatosis (familial)
         (metabolic) (primary) 272.2
**Cistern, subarachnoid** 793.0
**Citrullinemia** 270.6
**Citrullinuria** 270.6
**Ciuffini-Pancoast tumor** (M8010/3)
   (carcinoma, pulmonary apex) 162.3
**Civatte's disease or poikiloderma**
   709.09
**Clam diggers' itch** 120.3
**Clap** — *see* Gonorrhea
**Clarke-Hadfield syndrome** (pancreatic
   infantilism) 577.8
**Clark's paralysis** 343.9
**Clastothrix** 704.2
**Claude Bernard-Horner syndrome** —
   *see also* Neuropathy, peripheral,
   autonomic 337.9
**Claude's syndrome** 352.6
**Claudication, intermittent** 443.9
   cerebral (artery) (*see also* Ischemia,
      cerebral, transient) 435.9
      due to atherosclerosis 440.21
   spinal cord (arteriosclerotic) 435.1
      syphilitic 094.89
   spinalis 435.1
   venous (axillary) 453.8
**Claudicatio venosa intermittens** 453.8
**Claustrophobia** 300.29
**Clavus** (infected) 700
**Clawfoot** (congenital) 754.71
   acquired 736.74
**Clawhand** (acquired) 736.06
   congenital 755.59
**Clawtoe** (congenital) 754.71
   acquired 735.5
**Clay eating** 307.52
**Clay shovelers' fracture** — *see* Fracture,
   vertebra, cervical
**Cleansing of artificial opening** — *see
   also* Attention to artificial opening
   V55.9
**Cleft** (congenital) — *see also* Imperfect,
   closure
   alveolar process 525.8
   branchial (persistent) 744.41

**Cleft** — *see also* Imperfect, closure —
   *continued*
   branchial — *continued*
      cyst 744.42
   clitoris 752.49
   cricoid cartilage, posterior 748.3
   facial (*see also* Cleft, lip) 749.10
   lip 749.10
      with cleft palate 749.20
         bilateral (lip and palate) 749.24
            with unilateral lip or palate
               749.25
            complete 749.23
            incomplete 749.24
         unilateral (lip and palate)
            749.22
            with bilateral lip or palate
               749.25
            complete 749.21
            incomplete 749.22
      bilateral 749.14
         with cleft palate, unilateral
            749.25
         complete 749.13
         incomplete 749.14
      unilateral 749.12
         with cleft palate, bilateral
            749.25
         complete 749.11
         incomplete 749.12
   nose 748.1
   palate 749.00
      with cleft lip 749.20
         bilateral (lip and palate) 749.24
            with unilateral lip or palate
               749.25
            complete 749.23
            incomplete 749.24
         unilateral (lip and palate)
            749.22
            with bilateral lip or palate
               749.25
            complete 749.21
            incomplete 749.22
      bilateral 749.04
         with cleft lip, unilateral 749.25
         complete 749.03
         incomplete 749.04
      unilateral 749.02
         with cleft lip, bilateral 749.25
         complete 749.01
         incomplete 749.02
   penis 752.69
   posterior, cricoid cartilage 748.3
   scrotum 752.89
   sternum (congenital) 756.3
   thyroid cartilage (congenital) 748.3
   tongue 750.13
   uvula 749.02
      with cleft lip (*see also* Cleft, lip,
         with cleft palate) 749.20
   water 366.12
**Cleft hand** (congenital) 755.58
**Cleidocranial dysostosis** 755.59
**Cleidotomy, fetal** 763.89
**Cleptomania** 312.32
**Clérambault's syndrome** 297.8
   erotomania 302.89
**Clergyman's sore throat** 784.49
**Click, clicking**
   systolic syndrome 785.2
**Clifford's syndrome** (postmaturity)
   766.22
**Climacteric** — *see also* Menopause
   627.2
   arthritis NEC (*see also* Arthritis, cli-
      macteric) 716.3 ☑
   depression (*see also* Psychosis, affec-
      tive) 296.2 ☑
   disease 627.2
      recurrent episode 296.3 ☑
      single episode 296.2 ☑
   female (symptoms) 627.2
   male (symptoms) (syndrome) 608.89
   melancholia (*see also* Psychosis, affec-
      tive) 296.2 ☑

**Climacteric** — see also Menopause — continued
  melancholia (see also Psychosis, affective) — continued
    recurrent episode 296.3 ☑
    single episode 296.2 ☑
  paranoid state 297.2
  paraphrenia 297.2
  polyarthritis NEC 716.39
    male 608.89
  symptoms (female) 627.2
**Clinical research investigation** (control) (participant) V70.7
**Clinodactyly** 755.59
**Clitoris** — see condition
**Cloaca, persistent** 751.5
**Clonorchiasis** 121.1
**Clonorchiosis** 121.1
**Clonorchis infection, liver** 121.1
**Clonus** 781.0
**Closed bite** 524.20
**Closed surgical procedure converted to open procedure**
  arthroscopic V64.43
  laparoscopic V64.41
  thoracoscopic V64.42
**Closure**
  artificial opening (see also Attention to artificial opening) V55.9
  congenital, nose 748.0
  cranial sutures, premature 756.0
  defective or imperfect NEC — see Imperfect, closure
  fistula, delayed — see Fistula
  fontanelle, delayed 756.0
  foramen ovale, imperfect 745.5
  hymen 623.3
  interauricular septum, defective 745.5
  interventricular septum, defective 745.4
  lacrimal duct 375.56
    congenital 743.65
    neonatal 375.55
  nose (congenital) 748.0
    acquired 738.0
  vagina 623.2
  valve — see Endocarditis
  vulva 624.8
**Clot** (blood)
  artery (obstruction) (occlusion) (see also Embolism) 444.9
  atrial appendage 429.89
  bladder 596.7
  brain (extradural or intradural) (see also Thrombosis, brain) 434.0 ☑
    late effect — see Late effect(s) (of) cerebrovascular disease
  circulation 444.9
  heart (see also Infarct, myocardium) 410.9 ☑
    without myocardial infarction 429.89
  vein (see also Thrombosis) 453.9
**Clotting defect** NEC — see also Defect, coagulation 286.9
**Clouded state** 780.09
  epileptic (see also Epilepsy) 345.9 ☑
  paroxysmal (idiopathic) (see also Epilepsy) 345.9 ☑
**Clouding**
  corneal graft 996.51
**Cloudy**
  antrum, antra 473.0
  dialysis effluent 792.5
**Clouston's (hidrotic) ectodermal dysplasia** 757.31
**Clubbing of fingers** 781.5
**Clubfinger** 736.29
  acquired 736.29
  congenital 754.89
**Clubfoot** (congenital) 754.70
  acquired 736.71
  equinovarus 754.51
  paralytic 736.71
**Club hand** (congenital) 754.89
  acquired 736.07

**Clubnail** (acquired) 703.8
  congenital 757.5
**Clump kidney** 753.3
**Clumsiness** 781.3
  syndrome 315.4
**Cluttering** 307.0
**Clutton's joints** 090.5
**Coagulation, intravascular** (diffuse) (disseminated) — see also Fibrinolysis 286.6
  newborn 776.2
**Coagulopathy** — see also Defect, coagulation 286.9
  consumption 286.6
  intravascular (disseminated) NEC 286.6
  newborn 776.2
**Coalition**
  calcaneoscaphoid 755.67
  calcaneus 755.67
  tarsal 755.67
**Coal miners'**
  elbow 727.2
  lung 500
**Coal workers' lung or pneumoconiosis** 500
**Coarctation**
  aorta (postductal) (preductal) 747.10
  pulmonary artery 747.3
**Coated tongue** 529.3
**Coats' disease** 362.12
**Cocainism** — see also Dependence 304.2 ☑
**Coccidioidal granuloma** 114.3
**Coccidioidomycosis** 114.9
  with pneumonia 114.0
  cutaneous (primary) 114.1
  disseminated 114.3
  extrapulmonary (primary) 114.1
  lung 114.5
    acute 114.0
    chronic 114.4
    primary 114.0
  meninges 114.2
  primary (pulmonary) 114.0
    acute 114.0
  prostate 114.3
  pulmonary 114.5
    acute 114.0
    chronic 114.4
    primary 114.0
  specified site NEC 114.3
**Coccidioidosis** 114.9
  lung 114.5
    acute 114.0
    chronic 114.4
    primary 114.0
  meninges 114.2
**Coccidiosis** (colitis) (diarrhea) (dysentery) 007.2
**Cocciuria** 791.9
**Coccus in urine** 791.9
**Coccydynia** 724.79
**Coccygodynia** 724.79
**Coccyx** — see condition
**Cochin-China**
  diarrhea 579.1
    anguilluliasis 127.2
  ulcer 085.1
**Cockayne's disease or syndrome** (microcephaly and dwarfism) 759.89
**Cockayne-Weber syndrome** (epidermolysis bullosa) 757.39
**Cocked-up toe** 735.2
**Cock's peculiar tumor** 706.2
**Codman's tumor** (benign chondroblastoma) (M9230/0) — see Neoplasm, bone, benign
**Coenurosis** 123.8
**Coffee workers' lung** 495.8
**Cogan's syndrome** 370.52
  congenital oculomotor apraxia 379.51
  nonsyphilitic interstitial keratitis 370.52
**Coiling, umbilical cord** — see Complications, umbilical cord

**Coitus, painful** (female) 625.0
  male 608.89
  psychogenic 302.76
**Cold** 460
  with influenza, flu, or grippe 487.1
  abscess (see also Tuberculosis, abscess)
    articular — see Tuberculosis, joint
  agglutinin
    disease (chronic) or syndrome 283.0
    hemoglobinuria 283.0
      paroxysmal (cold) (nocturnal) 283.2
  allergic (see also Fever, hay) 477.9
  bronchus or chest — see Bronchitis
    with grippe or influenza 487.1
  common (head) 460
    vaccination, prophylactic (against) V04.7
  deep 464.10
  effects of 991.9
    specified effect NEC 991.8
  excessive 991.9
    specified effect NEC 991.8
  exhaustion from 991.8
  exposure to 991.9
    specified effect NEC 991.8
  grippy 487.1
  head 460
  injury syndrome (newborn) 778.2
  intolerance 780.99
  on lung — see Bronchitis
  rose 477.0
  sensitivity, autoimmune 283.0
  virus 460
**Coldsore** — see also Herpes, simplex 054.9
**Colibacillosis** 041.4
  generalized 038.42
**Colibacilluria** 791.9
**Colic** (recurrent) 789.0 ☑
  abdomen 789.0 ☑
    psychogenic 307.89
  appendicular 543.9
  appendix 543.9
  bile duct — see Choledocholithiasis
  biliary — see Cholelithiasis
  bilious — see Cholelithiasis
  common duct — see Choledocholithiasis
  Devonshire NEC 984.9
    specified type of lead — see Table of Drugs and Chemicals
  flatulent 787.3
  gallbladder or gallstone — see Cholelithiasis
  gastric 536.8
  hepatic (duct) — see Choledocholithiasis
  hysterical 300.11
  infantile 789.0 ☑
  intestinal 789.0 ☑
  kidney 788.0
  lead NEC 984.9
    specified type of lead — see Table of Drugs and Chemicals
  liver (duct) — see Choledocholithiasis
  mucous 564.9
    psychogenic 316 [564.9]
  nephritic 788.0
  painter's NEC 984.9
  pancreas 577.8
  psychogenic 306.4
  renal 788.0
  saturnine NEC 984.9
    specified type of lead — see Table of Drugs and Chemicals
  spasmodic 789.0 ☑
  ureter 788.0
  urethral 599.84
    due to calculus 594.2
  uterus 625.8
    menstrual 625.3
  vermicular 543.9
  virus 460

**Colic** — continued
  worm NEC 128.9
**Colicystitis** — see also Cystitis 595.9
**Colitis** (acute) (catarrhal) (croupous) (cystica superficialis) (exudative) (hemorrhagic) (noninfectious) (phlegmonous) (presumed noninfectious) 558.9
  adaptive 564.9
  allergic 558.3
  amebic (see also Amebiasis) 006.9
    nondysenteric 006.2
  anthrax 022.2
  bacillary (see also Infection, Shigella) 004.9
  balantidial 007.0
  chronic 558.9
    ulcerative (see also Colitis, ulcerative) 556.9
  coccidial 007.2
  dietetic 558.9
  due to radiation 558.1
  functional 558.9
  gangrenous 009.0
  giardial 007.1
  granulomatous 555.1
  gravis (see also Colitis, ulcerative) 556.9
  infectious (see also Enteritis, due to, specific organism) 009.0
    presumed 009.1
  ischemic 557.9
    acute 557.0
    chronic 557.1
    due to mesenteric artery insufficiency 557.1
  membranous 564.9
    psychogenic 316 [564.9]
  mucous 564.9
    psychogenic 316 [564.9]
  necrotic 009.0
  polyposa (see also Colitis, ulcerative) 556.9
  protozoal NEC 007.9
  pseudomembranous 008.45
  pseudomucinous 564.9
  regional 555.1
  segmental 555.1
  septic (see also Enteritis, due to, specific organism) 009.0
  spastic 564.9
    psychogenic 316 [564.9]
  Staphylococcus 008.41
    food 005.0
  thromboulcerative 557.0
  toxic 558.2
  transmural 555.1
  trichomonal 007.3
  tuberculous (ulcerative) 014.8 ☑
  ulcerative (chronic) (idiopathic) (nonspecific) 556.9
    entero- 556.0
    fulminant 557.0
    ileo- 556.1
    left-sided 556.5
    procto- 556.2
    proctosigmoid 556.3
    psychogenic 316 [556] ☑
    specified NEC 556.8
    universal 556.6
**Collagen disease** NEC 710.9
  nonvascular 710.9
  vascular (allergic) (see also Angiitis, hypersensitivity) 446.20
**Collagenosis** — see also Collagen disease 710.9
  cardiovascular 425.4
  mediastinal 519.3
**Collapse** 780.2
  adrenal 255.8
  cardiorenal (see also Hypertension, cardiorenal) 404.90
  cardiorespiratory 785.51
    fetus or newborn 779.85
  cardiovascular (see also Disease, heart) 785.51

---

☑ Additional Digit Required — Refer to the Tabular List for Digit Selection

▼ Subterms under main terms may continue to next column or page

**Collapse** — *continued*
cardiovascular (*see also* Disease, heart) — *continued*
fetus or newborn 779.85
circulatory (peripheral) 785.59
with
abortion — *see* Abortion, by type, with shock
ectopic pregnancy (*see also* categories 633.0–633.9) 639.5
molar pregnancy (*see also* categories 630–632) 639.5
during or after labor and delivery 669.1 ☑
fetus or newborn 779.85
following
abortion 639.5
ectopic or molar pregnancy 639.5
during or after labor and delivery 669.1 ☑
fetus or newborn 779.89
external ear canal 380.50
secondary to
inflammation 380.53
surgery 380.52
trauma 380.51
general 780.2
heart — *see* Disease, heart
heat 992.1
hysterical 300.11
labyrinth, membranous (congenital) 744.05
lung (massive) (*see also* Atelectasis) 518.0
pressure, during labor 668.0 ☑
myocardial — *see* Disease, heart
nervous (*see also* Disorder, mental, nonpsychotic) 300.9
neurocirculatory 306.2
nose 738.0
postoperative (cardiovascular) 998.0
pulmonary (*see also* Atelectasis) 518.0
fetus or newborn 770.5
partial 770.5
primary 770.4
thorax 512.8
iatrogenic 512.1
postoperative 512.1
trachea 519.19
valvular — *see* Endocarditis
vascular (peripheral) 785.59
with
abortion — *see* Abortion, by type, with shock
ectopic pregnancy (*see also* categories 633.0–633.9) 639.5
molar pregnancy (*see also* categories 630–632) 639.5
cerebral (*see also* Disease, cerebrovascular, acute) 436
during or after labor and delivery 669.1 ☑
fetus or newborn 779.89
following
abortion 639.5
ectopic or molar pregnancy 639.5
vasomotor 785.59
vertebra 733.13
**Collateral** — *see also* condition
circulation (venous) 459.89
dilation, veins 459.89
**Colles' fracture** (closed) (reversed) (separation) 813.41
open 813.51
**Collet-Sicard syndrome** 352.6
**Collet's syndrome** 352.6
**Colliculitis urethralis** — *see also* Urethritis 597.89
**Colliers'**
asthma 500
lung 500

**Colliers'** — *continued*
phthisis (*see also* Tuberculosis) 011.4 ☑
**Collodion baby** (ichthyosis congenita) 757.1
**Colloid milium** 709.3
**Coloboma** NEC 743.49
choroid 743.59
fundus 743.52
iris 743.46
lens 743.36
lids 743.62
optic disc (congenital) 743.57
acquired 377.23
retina 743.56
sclera 743.47
**Coloenteritis** — *see* Enteritis
**Colon** — *see* condition
**Coloptosis** 569.89
**Color**
amblyopia NEC 368.59
acquired 368.55
blindness NEC (congenital) 368.59
acquired 368.55
**Colostomy**
attention to V55.3
fitting or adjustment V55.3
malfunctioning 569.62
status V44.3
**Colpitis** — *see also* Vaginitis 616.10
**Colpocele** 618.6
**Colpocystitis** — *see also* Vaginitis 616.10
**Colporrhexis** 665.4 ☑
**Colpospasm** 625.1
**Column, spinal, vertebral** — *see* condition
**Coma** 780.01
apoplectic (*see also* Disease, cerebrovascular, acute) 436
diabetic (with ketoacidosis) 250.3 ☑
hyperosmolar 250.2 ☑
eclamptic (*see also* Eclampsia) 780.39
epileptic 345.3
hepatic 572.2
hyperglycemic 250.2 ☑
hyperosmolar (diabetic) (nonketotic) 250.2 ☑
hypoglycemic 251.0
diabetic 250.3 ☑
insulin 250.3 ☑
hyperosmolar 250.2 ☑
non-diabetic 251.0
organic hyperinsulinism 251.0
Kussmaul's (diabetic) 250.3 ☑
liver 572.2
newborn 779.2
prediabetic 250.2 ☑
uremic — *see* Uremia
**Combat fatigue** — *see also* Reaction, stress, acute 308.9
**Combined** — *see* condition
**Comedo** 706.1
**Comedocarcinoma** (M8501/3) — *see also* Neoplasm, breast, malignant
noninfiltrating (M8501/2)
specified site — *see* Neoplasm, by site, in situ
unspecified site 233.0
**Comedomastitis** 610.4
**Comedones** 706.1
lanugo 757.4
**Comma bacillus, carrier** (suspected) of V02.3
**Comminuted fracture** — *see* Fracture, by site
**Common**
aortopulmonary trunk 745.0
atrioventricular canal (defect) 745.69
atrium 745.69
cold (head) 460
vaccination, prophylactic (against) V04.7
truncus (arteriosus) 745.0
ventricle 745.3

**Commotio** (current)
cerebri (*see also* Concussion, brain) 850.9
with skull fracture — *see* Fracture, skull, by site
retinae 921.3
spinalis — *see* Injury, spinal, by site
**Commotion** (current)
brain (without skull fracture) (*see also* Concussion, brain) 850.9
with skull fracture — *see* Fracture, skull, by site
spinal cord — *see* Injury, spinal, by site
**Communication**
abnormal (*see also* Fistula)
between
base of aorta and pulmonary artery 745.0
left ventricle and right atrium 745.4
pericardial sac and pleural sac 748.8
pulmonary artery and pulmonary vein 747.3
congenital, between uterus and anterior abdominal wall 752.3
bladder 752.3
intestine 752.3
rectum 752.3
left ventricular — right atrial 745.4
pulmonary artery — pulmonary vein 747.3
**Compartment syndrome** — *see* Syndrome, compartment
**Compensation**
broken — *see* Failure, heart
failure — *see* Failure, heart
neurosis, psychoneurosis 300.11
**Complaint** — *see also* Disease
bowel, functional 564.9
psychogenic 306.4
intestine, functional 564.9
psychogenic 306.4
kidney (*see also* Disease, renal) 593.9
liver 573.9
miners' 500
**Complete** — *see* condition
**Complex**
cardiorenal (*see also* Hypertension, cardiorenal) 404.90
castration 300.9
Costen's 524.60
ego-dystonic homosexuality 302.0
Eisenmenger's (ventricular septal defect) 745.4
homosexual, ego-dystonic 302.0
hypersexual 302.89
inferiority 301.9
jumped process
spine — *see* Dislocation, vertebra
primary, tuberculosis (*see also* Tuberculosis) 010.0 ☑
Taussig-Bing (transposition, aorta and overriding pulmonary artery) 745.11
**Complications**
abortion NEC — *see* categories 634-639 ☑
accidental puncture or laceration during a procedure 998.2
amputation stump (late) (surgical) 997.60
traumatic — *see* Amputation, traumatic
anastomosis (and bypass) (*see also* Complications, due to (presence of) any device, implant, or graft classified to 996.0–996.5 NEC)
hemorrhage NEC 998.11
intestinal (internal) NEC 997.4
involving urinary tract 997.5
mechanical — *see* Complications, mechanical, graft

**Complications** — *continued*
anastomosis (*see also* Complications, due to any device, implant, or graft classified to 996.0–996.5) — *continued*
urinary tract (involving intestinal tract) 997.5
anesthesia, anesthetic NEC (*see also* Anesthesia, complication) 995.22
in labor and delivery 668.9 ☑
affecting fetus or newborn 763.5
cardiac 668.1 ☑
central nervous system 668.2 ☑
pulmonary 668.0 ☑
specified type NEC 668.8 ☑
aortocoronary (bypass) graft 996.03
atherosclerosis — *see* Arteriosclerosis, coronary
embolism 996.72
occlusion NEC 996.72
thrombus 996.72
arthroplasty (*see also* Complications, prosthetic joint) 996.49
artificial opening
cecostomy 569.60
colostomy 569.60
cystostomy 997.5
enterostomy 569.60
esophagostomy 530.87
infection 530.86
mechanical 530.87
gastrostomy 536.40
ileostomy 569.60
jejunostomy 569.60
nephrostomy 997.5
tracheostomy 519.00
ureterostomy 997.5
urethrostomy 997.5
bariatric surgery 997.4
bile duct implant (prosthetic) NEC 996.79
infection or inflammation 996.69
mechanical 996.59
bleeding (intraoperative) (postoperative) 998.11
blood vessel graft 996.1
aortocoronary 996.03
atherosclerosis — *see* Arteriosclerosis, coronary
embolism 996.72
occlusion NEC 996.72
thrombus 996.72
atherosclerosis — *see* Arteriosclerosis, extremities
embolism 996.74
occlusion NEC 996.74
thrombus 996.74
bone growth stimulator NEC 996.78
infection or inflammation 996.67
bone marrow transplant 996.85
breast implant (prosthetic) NEC 996.79
infection or inflammation 996.69
mechanical 996.54
bypass (*see also* Complications, anastomosis)
aortocoronary 996.03
atherosclerosis — *see* Arteriosclerosis, coronary
embolism 996.72
occlusion NEC 996.72
thrombus 996.72
carotid artery 996.1
atherosclerosis — *see* Arteriosclerosis, extremities
embolism 996.74
occlusion NEC 996.74
thrombus 996.74
cardiac (*see also* Disease, heart) 429.9
device, implant, or graft NEC 996.72
infection or inflammation 996.61
long-term effect 429.4

**Complications** — *continued*
cardiac (*see also* Disease, heart) — *continued*
  device, implant, or graft — *continued*
    mechanical (*see also* Complications, mechanical, by type) 996.00
    valve prosthesis 996.71
      infection or inflammation 996.61
    postoperative NEC 997.1
    long-term effect 429.4
cardiorenal (*see also* Hypertension, cardiorenal) 404.90
carotid artery bypass graft 996.1
  atherosclerosis — *see* Arteriosclerosis, extremities
  embolism 996.74
  occlusion NEC 996.74
  thrombus 996.74
cataract fragments in eye 998.82
catheter device NEC (*see also* Complications, due to (presence of) any device, implant, or graft classified to 996.0–996.5 NEC)
  mechanical — *see* Complications, mechanical, catheter
cecostomy 569.60
cesarean section wound 674.3 ☑
chemotherapy (antineoplastic) ● 995.29
chin implant (prosthetic) NEC 996.79
  infection or inflammation 996.69
  mechanical 996.59
colostomy (enterostomy) 569.60
  specified type NEC 569.69
contraceptive device, intrauterine NEC 996.76
  infection 996.65
  inflammation 996.65
  mechanical 996.32
cord (umbilical) — *see* Complications, umbilical cord
cornea
  due to
    contact lens 371.82
coronary (artery) bypass (graft) NEC 996.03
  atherosclerosis — *see* Arteriosclerosis, coronary
  embolism 996.72
  infection or inflammation 996.61
  mechanical 996.03
  occlusion NEC 996.72
  specified type NEC 996.72
  thrombus 996.72
cystostomy 997.5
delivery 669.9 ☑
  procedure (instrumental) (manual) (surgical) 669.4 ☑
  specified type NEC 669.8 ☑
dialysis (hemodialysis) (peritoneal) (renal) NEC 999.9
  catheter NEC (*see also* Complications, due to (presence of) any device, implant, or graft classified to 996.0–996.5 NEC)
    infection or inflammation 996.62
      peritoneal 996.68
    mechanical 996.1
      peritoneal 996.56
drug NEC 995.29 ●
due to (presence of) any device, implant, or graft classified to 996.0–996.5 NEC 996.70
  with infection or inflammation — *see* Complications, infection or inflammation, due to (presence of) any device, implant, or graft classified to 996.0–996.5 NEC
  arterial NEC 996.74
    coronary NEC 996.03

**Complications** — *continued*
due to any device, implant, or graft classified to 996.0–996.5 — *continued*
  arterial — *continued*
    coronary — *continued*
      atherosclerosis — *see* Arteriosclerosis, coronary
      embolism 996.72
      occlusion NEC 996.72
      specified type NEC 996.72
      thrombus 996.72
    renal dialysis 996.73
  arteriovenous fistula or shunt NEC 996.74
  bone growth stimulator 996.78
  breast NEC 996.79
  cardiac NEC 996.72
    defibrillator 996.72
    pacemaker 996.72
    valve prosthesis 996.71
  catheter NEC 996.79
    spinal 996.75
    urinary, indwelling 996.76
    vascular NEC 996.74
      renal dialysis 996.73
    ventricular shunt 996.75
  coronary (artery) bypass (graft) NEC 996.03
    atherosclerosis — *see* Arteriosclerosis, coronary
    embolism 996.72
    occlusion NEC 996.72
    thrombus 996.72
  electrodes
    brain 996.75
    heart 996.72
  esophagostomy 530.87
  gastrointestinal NEC 996.79
  genitourinary NEC 996.76
  heart valve prosthesis NEC 996.71
  infusion pump 996.74
  insulin pump 996.57
  internal
    joint prosthesis 996.77
    orthopedic NEC 996.78
    specified type NEC 996.79
  intrauterine contraceptive device NEC 996.76
  joint prosthesis, internal NEC 996.77
  mechanical — *see* Complications, mechanical
  nervous system NEC 996.75
  ocular lens NEC 996.79
  orbital NEC 996.79
  orthopedic NEC 996.78
    joint, internal 996.77
  renal dialysis 996.73
  specified type NEC 996.79
  urinary catheter, indwelling 996.76
  vascular NEC 996.74
  ventricular shunt 996.75
during dialysis NEC 999.9
ectopic or molar pregnancy NEC 639.9
electroshock therapy NEC 999.9
enterostomy 569.60
  specified type NEC 569.69
esophagostomy 530.87
  infection 530.86
  mechanical 530.87
external (fixation) device with internal component(s) NEC 996.78
  infection or inflammation 996.67
  mechanical 996.49
extracorporeal circulation NEC 999.9
eye implant (prosthetic) NEC 996.79
  infection or inflammation 996.69
  mechanical
    ocular lens 996.53
    orbital globe 996.59
gastrointestinal, postoperative NEC (*see also* Complications, surgical procedures) 997.4
gastrostomy 536.40
  specified type NEC 536.49

**Complications** — *continued*
genitourinary device, implant or graft NEC 996.76
  infection or inflammation 996.65
    urinary catheter, indwelling 996.64
  mechanical (*see also* Complications, mechanical, by type) 996.30
    specified NEC 996.39
graft (bypass) (patch) (*see also* Complications, due to (presence of) any device, implant, or graft classified to 996.0–996.5 NEC)
  bone marrow 996.85
  corneal NEC 996.79
    infection or inflammation 996.69
    rejection or reaction 996.51
  mechanical — *see* Complications, mechanical, graft
  organ (immune or nonimmune cause) (partial) (total) 996.80
    bone marrow 996.85
    heart 996.83
    intestines 996.87
    kidney 996.81
    liver 996.82
    lung 996.84
    pancreas 996.86
    specified NEC 996.89
  skin NEC 996.79
    infection or inflammation 996.69
    rejection 996.52
      artificial 996.55
      decellularized allodermis 996.55
heart (*see also* Disease, heart transplant (immune or nonimmune cause)) 996.83
hematoma (intraoperative) (postoperative) 998.12
hemorrhage (intraoperative) (postoperative) 998.11
hyperalimentation therapy NEC 999.9
immunization (procedure) — *see* Complications, vaccination
implant (*see also* Complications, due to (presence of) any device, implant, or graft classified to 996.0–996.5 NEC)
  dental placement, hemorrhagic ● 525.71 ●
  mechanical — *see* Complications, mechanical, implant
infection and inflammation
  due to (presence of) any device, implant or graft classified to 996.0–996.5 NEC 996.60
    arterial NEC 996.62
      coronary 996.61
      renal dialysis 996.62
    arteriovenous fistula or shunt 996.62
    artificial heart 996.61
    bone growth stimulator 996.67
    breast 996.69
    cardiac 996.61
    catheter NEC 996.69
      central venous 999.31 ●
      Hickman 999.31 ●
      peripherally inserted central (PICC) 999.31 ●
      peritoneal 996.68
      spinal 996.63
      triple lumen 999.31 ●
      urinary, indwelling 996.64
      vascular ▶(arterial) (dialysis) (peripheral venous)◀ NEC 996.62
      ventricular shunt 996.63
    central venous catheter ● 999.31 ●
    coronary artery bypass 996.61

**Complications** — *continued*
infection and inflammation — *continued*
  due to any device, implant or graft classified to 996.0–996.5 — *continued*
    electrodes
      brain 996.63
      heart 996.61
    gastrointestinal NEC 996.69
    genitourinary NEC 996.65
      indwelling urinary catheter 996.64
    heart assist device 996.61
    heart valve 996.61
    Hickman catheter 999.31 ●
    infusion pump 996.62
    insulin pump 996.69
    intrauterine contraceptive device 996.65
    joint prosthesis, internal 996.66
    ocular lens 996.69
    orbital (implant) 996.69
    orthopedic NEC 996.67
      joint, internal 996.66
    peripherally inserted central ● catheter (PICC) 999.31 ●
    specified type NEC 996.69 ●
    triple lumen catheter 999.31 ●
    urinary catheter, indwelling 996.64
    ventricular shunt 996.63
infusion (procedure) 999.9
  blood — *see* Complications, transfusion
  infection NEC 999.39 ▲
  sepsis NEC 999.39 ▲
inhalation therapy NEC 999.9
injection (procedure) 999.9
  drug reaction (*see also* Reaction, drug) 995.27
  infection NEC 999.39 ▲
  sepsis NEC 999.39 ▲
  serum (prophylactic) (therapeutic) — *see* Complications, vaccination
  vaccine (any) — *see* Complications, vaccination
inoculation (any) — *see* Complications, vaccination
insulin pump 996.57
internal device (catheter) (electronic) (fixation) (prosthetic) (*see also* Complications, due to (presence of) any device, implant, or graft classified to 996.0–996.5 NEC)
  mechanical — *see* Complications, mechanical
intestinal transplant (immune or nonimmune cause) 996.87
intraoperative bleeding or hemorrhage 998.11
intrauterine contraceptive device (*see also* Complications, contraceptive device) 996.76
  with fetal damage affecting management of pregnancy 655.8 ☑
  infection or inflammation 996.65
jejunostomy 569.60
kidney transplant (immune or nonimmune cause) 996.81
labor 669.9 ☑
  specified condition NEC 669.8 ☑
liver transplant (immune or nonimmune cause) 996.82
lumbar puncture 349.0
mechanical
  anastomosis — *see* Complications, mechanical, graft
  artificial heart 996.09
  bypass — *see* Complications, mechanical, graft
  catheter NEC 996.59
    cardiac 996.09
    cystostomy 996.39
    dialysis (hemodialysis) 996.1

☑ Additional Digit Required — Refer to the Tabular List for Digit Selection
▽ Subterms under main terms may continue to next column or page
*2008 ICD-9-CM*
▶◀ Revised Text
● New Line
▲ Revised Code
October 2007 · Volume 2 — 53

**Complications** — *continued*
mechanical — *continued*
catheter — *continued*
dialysis — *continued*
peritoneal 996.56
during a procedure 998.2
urethral, indwelling 996.31
colostomy 569.62
device NEC 996.59
balloon (counterpulsation), intra-aortic 996.1
cardiac 996.00
automatic implantable defibrillator 996.04
long-term effect 429.4
specified NEC 996.09
contraceptive, intrauterine 996.32
counterpulsation, intra-aortic 996.1
fixation, external, with internal components 996.49
fixation, internal (nail, rod, plate) 996.40
genitourinary 996.30
specified NEC 996.39
insulin pump 996.57
nervous system 996.2
orthopedic, internal 996.40
prosthetic joint (*see also* Complications, mechanical, device, orthopedic, prosthetic, joint) 996.47
prosthetic NEC 996.59
joint (*see also* Complications, prosthetic joint) 996.47
articular bearing surface wear 996.46
aseptic loosening 996.41
breakage 996.43
dislocation 996.42
failure 996.43
fracture 996.43
around prosthetic 996.44
peri-prosthetic 996.44
instability 996.42
loosening 996.41
peri-prosthetic osteolysis 996.45
subluxation 996.42
wear 996.46
umbrella, vena cava 996.1
vascular 996.1
dorsal column stimulator 996.2
electrode NEC 996.59
brain 996.2
cardiac 996.01
spinal column 996.2
enterostomy 569.62
esophagostomy 530.87
fistula, arteriovenous, surgically created 996.1
gastrostomy 536.42
graft NEC 996.52
aortic (bifurcation) 996.1
aortocoronary bypass 996.03
blood vessel NEC 996.1
bone 996.49
cardiac 996.00
carotid artery bypass 996.1
cartilage 996.49
corneal 996.51
coronary bypass 996.03
decellularized allodermis 996.55
genitourinary 996.30
specified NEC 996.39
muscle 996.49
nervous system 996.2
organ (immune or nonimmune cause) 996.80
heart 996.83
intestines 996.87
kidney 996.81
liver 996.82

**Complications** — *continued*
mechanical — *continued*
graft — *continued*
organ — *continued*
lung 996.84
pancreas 996.86
specified NEC 996.89
orthopedic, internal 996.49
peripheral nerve 996.2
prosthetic NEC 996.59
skin 996.52
artificial 996.55
specified NEC 996.59
tendon 996.49
tissue NEC 996.52
tooth 996.59
ureter, without mention of resection 996.39
vascular 996.1
heart valve prosthesis 996.02
long-term effect 429.4
implant NEC 996.59
cardiac 996.00
automatic implantable defibrillator 996.04
long-term effect 429.4
specified NEC 996.09
electrode NEC 996.59
brain 996.2
cardiac 996.01
spinal column 996.2
genitourinary 996.30
nervous system 996.2
orthopedic, internal 996.49
prosthetic NEC 996.59
in
bile duct 996.59
breast 996.54
chin 996.59
eye
ocular lens 996.53
orbital globe 996.59
vascular 996.1
insulin pump 996.57
nonabsorbable surgical material 996.59
pacemaker NEC 996.59
brain 996.2
cardiac 996.01
nerve (phrenic) 996.2
patch — *see* Complications, mechanical, graft
prosthesis NEC 996.59
bile duct 996.59
breast 996.54
chin 996.59
ocular lens 996.53
reconstruction, vas deferens 996.39
reimplant NEC 996.59
extremity (*see also* Complications, reattached, extremity) 996.90
organ (*see also* Complications, transplant, organ, by site) 996.80
repair — *see* Complications, mechanical, graft
respirator [ventilator] V46.14
shunt NEC 996.59
arteriovenous, surgically created 996.1
ventricular (communicating) 996.2
stent NEC 996.59
tracheostomy 519.02
vas deferens reconstruction 996.39
ventilator [respirator] V46.14
medical care NEC 999.9
cardiac NEC 997.1
gastrointestinal NEC 997.4
nervous system NEC 997.00
peripheral vascular NEC 997.2
respiratory NEC 997.3
urinary NEC 997.5

**Complications** — *continued*
medical care — *continued*
vascular
mesenteric artery 997.71
other vessels 997.79
peripheral vessels 997.2
renal artery 997.72
nephrostomy 997.5
nervous system
device, implant, or graft NEC 349.1
mechanical 996.2
postoperative NEC 997.00
obstetric 669.9 ☑
procedure (instrumental) (manual) (surgical) 669.4 ☑
specified NEC 669.8 ☑
surgical wound 674.3 ☑
ocular lens implant NEC 996.79
infection or inflammation 996.69
mechanical 996.53
organ transplant — *see* Complications, transplant, organ, by site
orthopedic device, implant, or graft
internal (fixation) (nail) (plate) (rod) NEC 996.78
infection or inflammation 996.67
joint prosthesis 996.77
infection or inflammation 996.66
mechanical 996.40
pacemaker (cardiac) 996.72
infection or inflammation 996.61
mechanical 996.01
pancreas transplant (immune or non-immune cause) 996.86
perfusion NEC 999.9
perineal repair (obstetrical) 674.3 ☑
disruption 674.2 ☑
pessary (uterus) (vagina) — *see* Complications, contraceptive device
phototherapy 990
postcystoscopic 997.5
postmastoidectomy NEC 383.30
postoperative — *see* Complications, surgical procedures
pregnancy NEC 646.9 ☑
affecting fetus or newborn 761.9
prosthetic device, internal (*see also* Complications, due to (presence of) any device, implant or graft classified to 996.0–996.5 NEC)
mechanical NEC (*see also* Complications, mechanical) 996.59
puerperium NEC (*see also* Puerperal) 674.9 ☑
puncture, spinal 349.0
pyelogram 997.5
radiation 990
radiotherapy 990
reattached
body part, except extremity 996.99
extremity (infection) (rejection) 996.90
arm(s) 996.94
digit(s) (hand) 996.93
foot 996.95
finger(s) 996.93
foot 996.95
forearm 996.91
hand 996.92
leg 996.96
lower NEC 996.96
toe(s) 996.95
upper NEC 996.94
reimplant NEC (*see also* Complications, due to (presence of) any device, implant, or graft classified to 996.0–996.5 NEC)
bone marrow 996.85
extremity (*see also* Complications, reattached, extremity) 996.90
due to infection 996.90
mechanical — *see* Complications, mechanical, reimplant

**Complications** — *continued*
reimplant (*see also* Complications, due to any device, implant, or graft classified to 996.0–996.5) — *continued*
organ (immune or nonimmune cause) (partial) (total) (*see also* Complications, transplant, organ, by site) 996.80
renal allograft 996.81
renal dialysis — *see* Complications, dialysis
respirator [ventilator], mechanical V46.14
respiratory 519.9
device, implant or graft NEC 996.79
infection or inflammation 996.69
mechanical 996.59
distress syndrome, adult, following trauma or surgery 518.5
insufficiency, acute, postoperative 518.5
postoperative NEC 997.3
therapy NEC 999.9
sedation during labor and delivery 668.9 ☑
affecting fetus or newborn 763.5
cardiac 668.1 ☑
central nervous system 668.2 ☑
pulmonary 668.0 ☑
specified type NEC 668.8 ☑
seroma (intraoperative) (postoperative) (noninfected) 998.13
infected 998.51
shunt (*see also* Complications, due to (presence of) any device, implant, or graft classified to 996.0–996.5 NEC)
mechanical — *see* Complications, mechanical, shunt
specified body system NEC
device, implant, or graft — *see* Complications, due to (presence of) any device, implant, or graft classified to 996.0–996.5 NEC
postoperative NEC 997.99
spinal puncture or tap 349.0
stomach banding 997.4
stomach stapling 997.4
stoma, external
gastrointestinal tract
colostomy 569.60
enterostomy 569.60
esophagostomy 530.87
infection 530.86
mechanical 530.87
gastrostomy 536.40
urinary tract 997.5
surgical procedures 998.9
accidental puncture or laceration 998.2
amputation stump (late) 997.60
anastomosis — *see* Complications, anastomosis
burst stitches or sutures (external) 998.32
internal 998.31
cardiac 997.1
long-term effect following cardiac surgery 429.4
cataract fragments in eye 998.82
catheter device — *see* Complications, catheter device
cecostomy malfunction 569.62
colostomy malfunction 569.62
cystostomy malfunction 997.5
dehiscence (of incision) (external) 998.32
internal 998.31
dialysis NEC (*see also* Complications, dialysis) 999.9

**Complications** — *continued*
surgical procedures — *continued*
disruption
anastomosis (internal) — *see*
Complications, mechanical, graft
internal suture (line) 998.31
wound (external) 998.32
internal 998.31
dumping syndrome (postgastrectomy) 564.2
elephantiasis or lymphedema 997.99
postmastectomy 457.0
emphysema (surgical) 998.81
enterostomy malfunction 569.62
esophagostomy malfunction 530.87
evisceration 998.32
fistula (persistent postoperative) 998.6
foreign body inadvertently left in wound (sponge) (suture) (swab) 998.4
from nonabsorbable surgical material (Dacron) (mesh) (permanent suture) (reinforcing) (Teflon) — *see* Complications, due to (presence of) any device, implant, or graft classified to 996.0–996.5 NEC
gastrointestinal NEC 997.4
gastrostomy malfunction 536.42
hematoma 998.12
hemorrhage 998.11
ileostomy malfunction 569.62
internal prosthetic device NEC (*see also* Complications, internal device) 996.70
hemolytic anemia 283.19
infection or inflammation 996.60
malfunction — *see* Complications, mechanical
mechanical complication — *see* Complications, mechanical
thrombus 996.70
jejunostomy malfunction 569.62
nervous system NEC 997.00
obstruction, internal anastomosis — *see* Complications, mechanical, graft
other body system NEC 997.99
peripheral vascular NEC 997.2
postcardiotomy syndrome 429.4
postcholecystectomy syndrome 576.0
postcommissurotomy syndrome 429.4
postgastrectomy dumping syndrome 564.2
postmastectomy lymphedema syndrome 457.0
postmastoidectomy 383.30
cholesteatoma, recurrent 383.32
cyst, mucosal 383.31
granulation 383.33
inflammation, chronic 383.33
postvagotomy syndrome 564.2
postvalvulotomy syndrome 429.4
reattached extremity (infection) (rejection) (*see also* Complications, reattached, extremity) 996.90
respiratory NEC 997.3
seroma 998.13
shock (endotoxic) (hypovolemic) (septic) 998.0
shunt, prosthetic (thrombus) (*see also* Complications, due to (presence of) any device, implant, or graft classified to 996.0–996.5 NEC)
hemolytic anemia 283.19
specified complication NEC 998.89
stitch abscess 998.59

**Complications** — *continued*
surgical procedures — *continued*
transplant — *see* Complications, graft
ureterostomy malfunction 997.5
urethrostomy malfunction 997.5
urinary NEC 997.5
vascular
mesenteric artery 997.71
other vessels 997.79
peripheral vessels 997.2
renal artery 997.72
wound infection 998.59
therapeutic misadventure NEC 999.9
surgical treatment 998.9
tracheostomy 519.00
transfusion (blood) (lymphocytes) (plasma) NEC 999.8
acute lung injury (TRALI) 518.7
atrophy, liver, yellow, subacute (within 8 months of administration) — *see* Hepatitis, viral
bone marrow 996.85
embolism
air 999.1
thrombus 999.2
hemolysis NEC 999.8
bone marrow 996.85
hepatitis (serum) (type B) (within 8 months after administration) — *see* Hepatitis, viral
incompatibility reaction (ABO) (blood group) 999.6
Rh (factor) 999.7
infection 999.39 ▲
jaundice (serum) (within 8 months after administration) — *see* Hepatitis, viral
sepsis 999.39 ▲
shock or reaction NEC 999.8
bone marrow 996.85
subacute yellow atrophy of liver (within 8 months after administration) — *see* Hepatitis, viral
thromboembolism 999.2
transplant NEC (*see also* Complications, due to (presence of) any device, implant, or graft classified to 996.0–996.5 NEC)
bone marrow 996.85
organ (immune or nonimmune cause) (partial) (total) 996.80
bone marrow 996.85
heart 996.83
intestines 996.87
kidney 996.81
liver 996.82
lung 996.84
pancreas 996.86
specified NEC 996.89
trauma NEC (early) 958.8
ultrasound therapy NEC 999.9
umbilical cord
affecting fetus or newborn 762.6
complicating delivery 663.9 ☑
affecting fetus or newborn 762.6
specified type NEC 663.8 ☑
urethral catheter NEC 996.76
infection or inflammation 996.64
mechanical 996.31
urinary, postoperative NEC 997.5
vaccination 999.9
anaphylaxis NEC 999.4
cellulitis 999.39 ▲
encephalitis or encephalomyelitis 323.51
hepatitis (serum) (type B) (within 8 months after administration) — *see* Hepatitis, viral
infection (general) (local) NEC 999.39 ▲
jaundice (serum) (within 8 months after administration) — *see* Hepatitis, viral
meningitis 997.09 [321.8]

**Complications** — *continued*
vaccination — *continued*
myelitis 323.52
protein sickness 999.5
reaction (allergic) 999.5
Herxheimer's 995.0
serum 999.5
sepsis 999.39 ▲
serum intoxication, sickness, rash, or other serum reaction NEC 999.5
shock (allergic) (anaphylactic) 999.4
subacute yellow atrophy of liver (within 8 months after administration) — *see* Hepatitis, viral
vaccinia (generalized) 999.0
localized 999.39 ▲
vascular
device, implant, or graft NEC 996.74
infection or inflammation 996.62
mechanical NEC 996.1
cardiac (*see also* Complications, mechanical, by type) 996.00
following infusion, perfusion, or transfusion 999.2
postoperative NEC 997.2
mesenteric artery 997.71
other vessels 997.79
peripheral vessels 997.2
renal artery 997.72
ventilation therapy NEC 999.9
ventilator [respirator], mechanical V46.14
**Compound presentation, complicating delivery** 652.8 ☑
causing obstructed labor 660.0 ☑
**Compressed air disease** 993.3
**Compression**
with injury — *see* specific injury
arm NEC 354.9
artery 447.1
celiac, syndrome 447.4
brachial plexus 353.0
brain (stem) 348.4
due to
contusion, brain — *see* Contusion, brain
injury NEC (*see also* Hemorrhage, brain, traumatic)
birth — *see* Birth, injury, brain
laceration, brain — *see* Laceration, brain
osteopathic 739.0
bronchus 519.19
by cicatrix — *see* Cicatrix
cardiac 423.9
cauda equina 344.60
with neurogenic bladder 344.61
celiac (artery) (axis) 447.4
cerebral — *see* Compression, brain
cervical plexus 353.2
cord (umbilical) — *see* Compression, umbilical cord
cranial nerve 352.9
second 377.49
third (partial) 378.51
total 378.52
fourth 378.53
fifth 350.8
sixth 378.54
seventh 351.8
divers' squeeze 993.3
duodenum (external) (*see also* Obstruction, duodenum) 537.3
during birth 767.9
esophagus 530.3
congenital, external 750.3
Eustachian tube 381.63
facies (congenital) 754.0
fracture — *see* Fracture, by site

**Compression** — *continued*
heart — *see* Disease, heart
intestine (*see also* Obstruction, intestine) 560.9
with hernia — *see* Hernia, by site, with obstruction
laryngeal nerve, recurrent 478.79
leg NEC 355.8
lower extremity NEC 355.8
lumbosacral plexus 353.1
lung 518.89
lymphatic vessel 457.1
medulla — *see* Compression, brain
nerve NEC (*see also* Disorder, nerve)
arm NEC 354.9
autonomic nervous system (*see also* Neuropathy, peripheral, autonomic) 337.9
axillary 353.0
cranial NEC 352.9
due to displacement of intervertebral disc 722.2
with myelopathy 722.70
cervical 722.0
with myelopathy 722.71
lumbar, lumbosacral 722.10
with myelopathy 722.73
thoracic, thoracolumbar 722.11
with myelopathy 722.72
iliohypogastric 355.79
ilioinguinal 355.79
leg NEC 355.8
lower extremity NEC 355.8
median (in carpal tunnel) 354.0
obturator 355.79
optic 377.49
plantar 355.6
posterior tibial (in tarsal tunnel) 355.5
root (by scar tissue) NEC 724.9
cervical NEC 723.4
lumbar NEC 724.4
lumbosacral 724.4
thoracic 724.4
saphenous 355.79
sciatic (acute) 355.0
sympathetic 337.9
traumatic — *see* Injury, nerve
ulnar 354.2
upper extremity NEC 354.9
peripheral — *see* Compression, nerve
spinal (cord) (old or nontraumatic) 336.9
by displacement of intervertebral disc — *see* Displacement, intervertebral disc
nerve
root NEC 724.9
postoperative 722.80
cervical region 722.81
lumbar region 722.83
thoracic region 722.82
traumatic — *see* Injury, nerve, spinal
traumatic — *see* Injury, nerve, spinal
spondylogenic 721.91
cervical 721.1
lumbar, lumbosacral 721.42
thoracic 721.41
traumatic (*see also* Injury, spinal, by site)
with fracture, vertebra — *see* Fracture, vertebra, by site, with spinal cord injury
spondylogenic — *see* Compression, spinal cord, spondylogenic
subcostal nerve (syndrome) 354.8
sympathetic nerve NEC 337.9
syndrome 958.5
thorax 512.8
iatrogenic 512.1
postoperative 512.1
trachea 519.19
congenital 748.3

**Index**

**Compression** — *continued*
  ulnar nerve (by scar tissue) 354.2
  umbilical cord
    affecting fetus or newborn 762.5
      cord prolapsed 762.4
    complicating delivery 663.2 ☑
      cord around neck 663.1 ☑
      cord prolapsed 663.0 ☑
  upper extremity NEC 354.9
  ureter 593.3
  urethra — *see* Stricture, urethra
  vein 459.2
  vena cava (inferior) (superior) 459.2
  vertebral NEC — *see* Compression, spinal (cord)
**Compulsion, compulsive**
  eating 307.51
  neurosis (obsessive) 300.3
  personality 301.4
  states (mixed) 300.3
  swearing 300.3
    in Gilles de la Tourette's syndrome 307.23
  tics and spasms 307.22
  water drinking NEC (syndrome) 307.9
**Concato's disease** (pericardial polyserositis) 423.2
  peritoneal 568.82
  pleural — *see* Pleurisy
**Concavity, chest wall** 738.3
**Concealed**
  hemorrhage NEC 459.0
  penis 752.65
**Concentric fading** 368.12
**Concern** (normal) **about sick person in family** V61.49
**Concrescence** (teeth) 520.2
**Concretio cordis** 423.1
  rheumatic 393
**Concretion** — *see also* Calculus
  appendicular 543.9
  canaliculus 375.57
  clitoris 624.8
  conjunctiva 372.54
  eyelid 374.56
  intestine (impaction) (obstruction) 560.39
  lacrimal (passages) 375.57
  prepuce (male) 605
    female (clitoris) 624.8
  salivary gland (any) 527.5
  seminal vesicle 608.89
  stomach 537.89
  tonsil 474.8
**Concussion** (current) 850.9
  with
    loss of consciousness 850.5
      brief (less than one hour)
        30 minutes or less 850.11
        31-59 minutes 850.12
      moderate (1-24 hours) 850.2
      prolonged (more than 24 hours) (with complete recovery) (with return to pre-existing conscious level) 850.3
      without return to pre-existing conscious level 850.4
    mental confusion or disorientation (without loss of consciousness) 850.0
      with loss of consciousness — *see* Concussion, with, loss of consciousness
  without loss of consciousness 850.0
  blast (air) (hydraulic) (immersion) (underwater) 869.0
    with open wound into cavity 869.1
    abdomen or thorax — *see* Injury, internal, by site
    brain — *see* Concussion, brain
    ear (acoustic nerve trauma) 951.5
      with perforation, tympanic membrane — *see* Wound, open, ear drum

**Concussion** — *continued*
  blast — *continued*
    thorax — *see* Injury, internal, intrathoracic organs NEC
  brain or cerebral (without skull fracture) 850.9
    with
      loss of consciousness 850.5
        brief (less than one hour)
          30 minutes or less 850.11
          31-59 minutes 850.12
        moderate (1-24 hours) 850.2
        prolonged (more than 24 hours) (with complete recovery) (with return to pre-existing conscious level) 850.3
        without return to pre-existing conscious level 850.4
      mental confusion or disorientation (without loss of consciousness) 850.0
        with loss of consciousness — *see* Concussion, brain, with, loss of consciousness
      skull fracture — *see* Fracture, skull, by site
      without loss of consciousness 850.0
  cauda equina 952.4
  cerebral — *see* Concussion, brain
  conus medullaris (spine) 952.4
  hydraulic — *see* Concussion, blast
  internal organs — *see* Injury, internal, by site
  labyrinth — *see* Injury, intracranial
  ocular 921.3
  osseous labyrinth — *see* Injury, intracranial
  spinal (cord) (*see also* Injury, spinal, by site)
    due to
      broken
        back — *see* Fracture, vertebra, by site, with spinal cord injury
        neck — *see* Fracture, vertebra, cervical, with spinal cord injury
      fracture, fracture dislocation, or compression fracture of spine or vertebra — *see* Fracture, vertebra, by site, with spinal cord injury
  syndrome 310.2
  underwater blast — *see* Concussion, blast
**Condition** — *see also* Disease
  psychiatric 298.9
  respiratory NEC 519.9
    acute or subacute NEC 519.9
      due to
        external agent 508.9
          specified type NEC 508.8
        fumes or vapors (chemical) (inhalation) 506.3
        radiation 508.0
    chronic NEC 519.9
      due to
        external agent 508.9
          specified type NEC 508.8
        fumes or vapors (chemical) (inhalation) 506.4
        radiation 508.1
    due to
      external agent 508.9
        specified type NEC 508.8
      fumes or vapors (chemical) (inhalation) 506.9
**Conduct disturbance** — *see also* Disturbance, conduct 312.9
  adjustment reaction 309.3
  hyperkinetic 314.2

**Condyloma** NEC 078.10
  acuminatum 078.11
  gonorrheal 098.0
  latum 091.3
  syphilitic 091.3
    congenital 090.0
  venereal, syphilitic 091.3
**Confinement** — *see* Delivery
**Conflagration** — *see also* Burn, by site
  asphyxia (by inhalation of smoke, gases, fumes, or vapors) 987.9
    specified agent — *see* Table of Drugs and Chemicals
**Conflict**
  family V61.9
    specified circumstance NEC V61.8
  interpersonal NEC V62.81
  marital V61.10
    involving divorce or estrangement V61.0
  parent-child V61.20
  partner V61.10
**Confluent** — *see* condition
**Confusional arousals** 327.41
**Confusion, confused** (mental) (state) — *see also* State, confusional 298.9
  acute 293.0
  epileptic 293.0
  postoperative 293.9
  psychogenic 298.2
  reactive (from emotional stress, psychological trauma) 298.2
  subacute 293.1
**Congelation** 991.9
**Congenital** — *see also* condition
  aortic septum 747.29
  generalized fibromatosis (CGF) 759.89
  intrinsic factor deficiency 281.0
  malformation — *see* Anomaly
**Congestion, congestive**
  asphyxia, newborn 768.9
  bladder 596.8
  bowel 569.89
  brain (*see also* Disease, cerebrovascular NEC) 437.8
    malarial 084.9
  breast 611.79
  bronchi 519.19
  bronchial tube 519.19
  catarrhal 472.0
  cerebral — *see* Congestion, brain
  cerebrospinal — *see* Congestion, brain
  chest 786.9 ▲
  chill 780.99
    malarial (*see also* Malaria) 084.6
  circulatory NEC 459.9
  conjunctiva 372.71
  due to disturbance of circulation 459.9
  duodenum 537.3
  enteritis — *see* Enteritis
  eye 372.71
  fibrosis syndrome (pelvic) 625.5
  gastroenteritis — *see* Enteritis
  general 799.89
  glottis 476.0
  heart (*see also* Failure, heart) 428.0
  hepatic 573.0
  hypostatic (lung) 514
  intestine 569.89
  intracranial — *see* Congestion, brain
  kidney 593.89
  labyrinth 386.50
  larynx 476.0
  liver 573.0
  lung 786.9 ▲
    active or acute (*see also* Pneumonia) 486
    congenital 770.0
    chronic 514
    hypostatic 514
    idiopathic, acute 518.5
    passive 514
  malaria, malarial (brain) (fever) (*see also* Malaria) 084.6
  medulla — *see* Congestion, brain

**Congestion, congestive** — *continued*
  nasal 478.19
  nose 478.19 ●
  orbit, orbital 376.33
    inflammatory (chronic) 376.10
      acute 376.00
  ovary 620.8
  pancreas 577.8
  pelvic, female 625.5
  pleural 511.0
  prostate (active) 602.1
  pulmonary — *see* Congestion, lung
  renal 593.89
  retina 362.89
  seminal vesicle 608.89
  spinal cord 336.1
  spleen 289.51
    chronic 289.51
  stomach 537.89
  trachea 464.11
  urethra 599.84
  uterus 625.5
    with subinvolution 621.1
  viscera 799.89
**Congestive** — *see* Congestion
**Conical**
  cervix 622.6
  cornea 371.60
  teeth 520.2
**Conjoined twins** 759.4
  causing disproportion (fetopelvic) 653.7 ☑
**Conjugal maladjustment** V61.10
  involving divorce or estrangement V61.0
**Conjunctiva** — *see* condition
**Conjunctivitis** (exposure) (infectious) (nondiphtheritic) (pneumococcal) (pustular) (staphylococcal) (streptococcal) NEC 372.30
  actinic 370.24
  acute 372.00
    atopic 372.05
    contagious 372.03
    follicular 372.02
    hemorrhagic (viral) 077.4
  adenoviral (acute) 077.3
  allergic (chronic) 372.14
    with hay fever 372.05
  anaphylactic 372.05
  angular 372.03
  Apollo (viral) 077.4
  atopic 372.05
  blennorrhagic (neonatorum) 098.40
  catarrhal 372.03
  chemical 372.01
    allergic 372.05
    meaning corrosion — *see* Burn, conjunctiva
  chlamydial 077.98
    due to
      Chlamydia trachomatis — *see* Trachoma
    paratrachoma 077.0
  chronic 372.10
    allergic 372.14
    follicular 372.12
    simple 372.11
    specified type NEC 372.14
    vernal 372.13
  diphtheritic 032.81
  due to
    dust 372.05
    enterovirus type 70 077.4
    erythema multiforme 695.1 [372.33]
    filariasis (*see also* Filariasis) 125.9 [372.15]
    mucocutaneous
      disease NEC 372.33
      leishmaniasis 085.5 [372.15]
    Reiter's disease 099.3 [372.33]
    syphilis 095.8 [372.10]
    toxoplasmosis (acquired) 130.1
      congenital (active) 771.2
    trachoma — *see* Trachoma

☑ Additional Digit Required — Refer to the Tabular List for Digit Selection
🆕 Subterms under main terms may continue to next column or page
56 — Volume 2 • October 2007    ►◄ Revised Text    ● New Line    ▲ Revised Code    *2008 ICD-9-CM*

**Conjunctivitis** — *continued*
    dust 372.05
    eczematous 370.31
    epidemic 077.1
        hemorrhagic 077.4
    follicular (acute) 372.02
        adenoviral (acute) 077.3
        chronic 372.12
    glare 370.24
    gonococcal (neonatorum) 098.40
    granular (trachomatous) 076.1
        late effect 139.1
    hemorrhagic (acute) (epidemic) 077.4
    herpetic (simplex) 054.43
        zoster 053.21
    inclusion 077.0
    infantile 771.6
    influenzal 372.03
    Koch-Weeks 372.03
    light 372.05
    medicamentosa 372.05
    membranous 372.04
    meningococcic 036.89
    Morax-Axenfeld 372.02
    mucopurulent NEC 372.03
    neonatal 771.6
        gonococcal 098.40
    Newcastle's 077.8
    nodosa 360.14
    of Beal 077.3
    parasitic 372.15
        filariasis (*see also* Filariasis)
            125.9 *[372.15]*
        mucocutaneous leishmaniasis
            085.5 *[372.15]*
    Parinaud's 372.02
    petrificans 372.39
    phlyctenular 370.31
    pseudomembranous 372.04
        diphtheritic 032.81
    purulent 372.03
    Reiter's 099.3 *[372.33]*
    rosacea 695.3 *[372.31]*
    serous 372.01
        viral 077.99
    simple chronic 372.11
    specified NEC 372.39
    sunlamp 372.04
    swimming pool 077.0
    trachomatous (follicular) 076.1
        acute 076.0
        late effect 139.1
    traumatic NEC 372.39
    tuberculous (*see also* Tuberculosis)
        017.3 ✓ *[370.31]*
    tularemic 021.3
    tularensis 021.3
    vernal 372.13
        limbar 372.13 *[370.32]*
    viral 077.99
        acute hemorrhagic 077.4
        specified NEC 077.8
**Conjunctivochalasis** 372.81
**Conjunctoblepharitis** — *see* Conjunctivitis
**Connective tissue** — *see* condition
**Conn (-Louis) syndrome** (primary aldosteronism) 255.12
**Conradi (-Hünermann) syndrome or disease** (chondrodysplasia calcificans congenita) 756.59
**Consanguinity** V19.7
**Consecutive** — *see* condition
**Consolidated lung** (base) — *see* Pneumonia, lobar
**Constipation** 564.00
    atonic 564.09
    drug induced
        correct substance properly administered 564.09
        overdose or wrong substance given or taken 977.9
        specified drug — *see* Table of Drugs and Chemicals
    neurogenic 564.09
    other specified NEC 564.09

**Constipation** — *continued*
    outlet dysfunction 564.02
    psychogenic 306.4
    simple 564.00
    slow transit 564.01
    spastic 564.09
**Constitutional** — *see also* condition
    arterial hypotension (*see also* Hypotension) 458.9
    obesity 278.00
        morbid 278.01
    psychopathic state 301.9
    short stature in childhood 783.43
    state, developmental V21.9
        specified development NEC V21.8
    substandard 301.6
**Constitutionally substandard** 301.6
**Constriction**
    anomalous, meningeal bands or folds 742.8
    aortic arch (congenital) 747.10
    asphyxiation or suffocation by 994.7
    bronchus 519.19
    canal, ear (*see also* Stricture, ear canal, acquired) 380.50
    duodenum 537.3
    gallbladder (*see also* Obstruction, gallbladder) 575.2
        congenital 751.69
    intestine (*see also* Obstruction, intestine) 560.9
    larynx 478.74
        congenital 748.3
    meningeal bands or folds, anomalous 742.8
    organ or site, congenital NEC — *see* Atresia
    prepuce (congenital) 605
    pylorus 537.0
        adult hypertrophic 537.0
        congenital or infantile 750.5
        newborn 750.5
    ring (uterus) 661.4 ✓
        affecting fetus or newborn 763.7
    spastic (*see also* Spasm)
        ureter 593.3
        urethra — *see* Stricture, urethra
    stomach 537.89
    ureter 593.3
    urethra — *see* Stricture, urethra
    visual field (functional) (peripheral) 368.45
**Constrictive** — *see* condition
**Consultation**
    without complaint or sickness V65.9
        feared complaint unfounded V65.5
        specified reason NEC V65.8
    medical (*see also* Counseling, medical)
    specified reason NEC V65.8
**Consumption** — *see* Tuberculosis
**Contact**
    with
        AIDS virus V01.79
        anthrax V01.81
        cholera V01.0
        communicable disease V01.9
            specified type NEC V01.89
            viral NEC V01.79
        Escherichia coli (E. coli) V01.83
        German measles V01.4
        gonorrhea V01.6
        HIV V01.79
        human immunodeficiency virus V01.79
        meningococcus V01.84
        parasitic disease NEC V01.89
        poliomyelitis V01.2
        rabies V01.5
        rubella V01.4
        SARS-associated coronavirus V01.82
        smallpox V01.3
        syphilis V01.6
        tuberculosis V01.1
        varicella V01.71
        venereal disease V01.6

**Contact** — *continued*
    with — *continued*
        viral disease NEC V01.79
    dermatitis — *see* Dermatitis
**Contamination, food** — *see also* Poisoning, food 005.9
**Contraception, contraceptive**
    advice NEC V25.09
        family planning V25.09
        fitting of diaphragm V25.02
        prescribing or use of
            oral contraceptive agent V25.01
            specified agent NEC V25.02
    counseling NEC V25.09
        emergency V25.03
        family planning V25.09
        fitting of diaphragm V25.02
        prescribing or use of
            oral contraceptive agent V25.01
                emergency V25.03
                postcoital V25.03
            specified agent NEC V25.02
    device (in situ) V45.59
        causing menorrhagia 996.76
        checking V25.42
        complications 996.32
        insertion V25.1
        intrauterine V45.51
        reinsertion V25.42
        removal V25.42
        subdermal V45.52
    fitting of diaphragm V25.02
    insertion
        intrauterine contraceptive device V25.1
        subdermal implantable V25.5
    maintenance V25.40
        examination V25.40
            oral contraceptive V25.41
            specified method NEC V25.49
            subdermal implantable V25.43
                intrauterine device V25.42
        intrauterine device V25.42
        oral contraceptive V25.41
        specified method NEC V25.49
        subdermal implantable V25.43
    management NEC V25.49
    prescription
        oral contraceptive agent V25.01
            emergency V25.03
            postcoital V25.03
            repeat V25.41
        specified agent NEC V25.02
            repeat V25.49
    sterilization V25.2
    surveillance V25.40
        intrauterine device V25.42
        oral contraceptive agent V25.41
            subdermal implantable V25.43
        specified method NEC V25.49
**Contraction, contracture, contracted**
    Achilles tendon (*see also* Short, tendon, Achilles) 727.81
    anus 564.89
    axilla 729.9
    bile duct (*see also* Disease, biliary) 576.8
    bladder 596.8
        neck or sphincter 596.0
    bowel (*see also* Obstruction, intestine) 560.9
    Braxton Hicks 644.1 ✓
    bronchus 519.19
    burn (old) — *see* Cicatrix
    cecum (*see also* Obstruction, intestine) 560.9
    cervix (*see also* Stricture, cervix) 622.4
        congenital 752.49
    cicatricial — *see* Cicatrix
    colon (*see also* Obstruction, intestine) 560.9
    conjunctiva trachomatous, active 076.1
        late effect 139.1
    Dupuytren's 728.6
    eyelid 374.41

**Contraction, contracture, contracted** — *continued*
    eye socket (after enucleation) 372.64
    face 729.9
    fascia (lata) (postural) 728.89
        Dupuytren's 728.6
        palmar 728.6
        plantar 728.71
    finger NEC 736.29
        congenital 755.59
        joint (*see also* Contraction, joint) 718.44
    flaccid, paralytic
        joint (*see also* Contraction, joint) 718.4 ✓
        muscle 728.85
            ocular 378.50
    gallbladder (*see also* Obstruction, gallbladder) 575.2
    hamstring 728.89
        tendon 727.81
    heart valve — *see* Endocarditis
    Hicks' 644.1 ✓
    hip (*see also* Contraction, joint) 718.4 ✓
    hourglass
        bladder 596.8
            congenital 753.8
        gallbladder (*see also* Obstruction, gallbladder) 575.2
            congenital 751.69
        stomach 536.8
            congenital 750.7
            psychogenic 306.4
        uterus 661.4 ✓
            affecting fetus or newborn 763.7
    hysterical 300.11
    infantile (*see also* Epilepsy) 345.6 ✓
    internal os (*see also* Stricture, cervix) 622.4
    intestine (*see also* Obstruction, intestine) 560.9
    joint (abduction) (acquired) (adduction) (flexion) (rotation) 718.40
        ankle 718.47
        congenital NEC 755.8
            generalized or multiple 754.89
                lower limb joints 754.89
            hip (*see also* Subluxation, congenital, hip) 754.32
            lower limb (including pelvic girdle) not involving hip 754.89
            upper limb (including shoulder girdle) 755.59
        elbow 718.42
        foot 718.47
        hand 718.44
        hip 718.45
        hysterical 300.11
        knee 718.46
        multiple sites 718.49
        pelvic region 718.45
        shoulder (region) 718.41
        specified site NEC 718.48
        wrist 718.43
    kidney (granular) (secondary) (*see also* Sclerosis, renal) 587
        congenital 753.3
        hydronephritic 591
        pyelonephritic (*see also* Pyelitis, chronic) 590.00
        tuberculous (*see also* Tuberculosis) 016.0 ✓
    ligament 728.89
        congenital 756.89
    liver — *see* Cirrhosis, liver
    muscle (postinfectional) (postural) NEC 728.85
        congenital 756.89
            sternocleidomastoid 754.1
        extraocular 378.60
        eye (extrinsic) (*see also* Strabismus) 378.9
            paralytic (*see also* Strabismus, paralytic) 378.50

**Contraction, contracture, contracted**

**Contraction, contracture, contracted**
*— continued*
muscle *— continued*
  flaccid 728.85
  hysterical 300.11
  ischemic (Volkmann's) 958.6
  paralytic 728.85
  posttraumatic 958.6
  psychogenic 306.0
    specified as conversion reaction
      300.11
myotonic 728.85
neck (*see also* Torticollis) 723.5
  congenital 754.1
  psychogenic 306.0
ocular muscle (*see also* Strabismus)
  378.9
  paralytic (*see also* Strabismus,
    paralytic) 378.50
organ or site, congenital NEC *— see*
  Atresia
outlet (pelvis) *— see* Contraction,
  pelvis
palmar fascia 728.6
paralytic
  joint (*see also* Contraction, joint)
    718.4 ☑
  muscle 728.85
    ocular (*see also* Strabismus,
      paralytic) 378.50
pelvis (acquired) (general) 738.6
  affecting fetus or newborn 763.1
  complicating delivery 653.1 ☑
    causing obstructed labor
      660.1 ☑
    generally contracted 653.1 ☑
      causing obstructed labor
        660.1 ☑
    inlet 653.2 ☑
      causing obstructed labor
        660.1 ☑
    midpelvic 653.8 ☑
      causing obstructed labor
        660.1 ☑
    midplane 653.8 ☑
      causing obstructed labor
        660.1 ☑
    outlet 653.3 ☑
      causing obstructed labor
        660.1 ☑
plantar fascia 728.71
premature
  atrial 427.61
  auricular 427.61
  auriculoventricular 427.61
  heart (junctional) (nodal) 427.60
  supraventricular 427.61
  ventricular 427.69
prostate 602.8
pylorus (*see also* Pylorospasm) 537.81
rectosigmoid (*see also* Obstruction,
  intestine) 560.9
rectum, rectal (sphincter) 564.89
  psychogenic 306.4
ring (Bandl's) 661.4 ☑
  affecting fetus or newborn 763.7
scar *— see* Cicatrix
sigmoid (*see also* Obstruction, intestine) 560.9
socket, eye 372.64
spine (*see also* Curvature, spine)
  737.9
stomach 536.8
  hourglass 536.8
    congenital 750.7
  psychogenic 306.4
tendon (sheath) (*see also* Short, tendon) 727.81
toe 735.8
ureterovesical orifice (postinfectional)
  593.3
urethra 599.84
uterus 621.8
  abnormal 661.9 ☑
    affecting fetus or newborn 763.7

**Contraction, contracture, contracted**
*— continued*
uterus *— continued*
  clonic, hourglass or tetanic
    661.4 ☑
    affecting fetus or newborn 763.7
  dyscoordinate 661.4 ☑
    affecting fetus or newborn 763.7
  hourglass 661.4 ☑
    affecting fetus or newborn 763.7
  hypotonic NEC 661.2 ☑
    affecting fetus or newborn 763.7
  incoordinate 661.4 ☑
    affecting fetus or newborn 763.7
  inefficient or poor 661.2 ☑
    affecting fetus or newborn 763.7
  irregular 661.2 ☑
    affecting fetus or newborn 763.7
  tetanic 661.4 ☑
    affecting fetus or newborn 763.7
vagina (outlet) 623.2
vesical 596.8
  neck or urethral orifice 596.0
visual field, generalized 368.45
Volkmann's (ischemic) 958.6
**Contusion** (skin surface intact) 924.9
with
  crush injury *— see* Crush
  dislocation *— see* Dislocation, by
    site
  fracture *— see* Fracture, by site
  internal injury (*see also* Injury, in-
    ternal, by site)
    heart *— see* Contusion, cardiac
    kidney *— see* Contusion, kidney
    liver *— see* Contusion, liver
    lung *— see* Contusion, lung
    spleen *— see* Contusion, spleen
  intracranial injury *— see* Injury,
    intracranial
  nerve injury *— see* Injury, nerve
  open wound *— see* Wound, open,
    by site
abdomen, abdominal (muscle) (wall)
  922.2
  organ(s) NEC 868.00
adnexa, eye NEC 921.9
ankle 924.21
  with other parts of foot 924.20
arm 923.9
  lower (with elbow) 923.10
  upper 923.03
    with shoulder or axillary region
      923.09
auditory canal (external) (meatus) (and
  other part(s) of neck, scalp, or
  face, except eye) 920
auricle, ear (and other part(s) of neck,
  scalp, or face except eye) 920
axilla 923.02
  with shoulder or upper arm 923.09
back 922.31
bone NEC 924.9

**Contusion** *— continued*
brain (cerebral) (membrane) (with
  hemorrhage) 851.8 ☑

*Note — Use the following fifth–digit*
*subclassification with categories*
*851–854:*

| 0 | unspecified state of conscious-ness |
| 1 | with no loss of consciousness |
| 2 | with brief [less than one hour] loss of consciousness |
| 3 | with moderate [1–24 hours] loss of consciousness |
| 4 | with prolonged [more than 24 hours] loss of consciousness and return to pre–existing conscious level |
| 5 | with prolonged [more than 24 hours] loss of consciousness, without return to pre–existing conscious level |

*Use fifth–digit 5 to designate when a*
*patient is unconscious and dies before*
*regaining consciousness, regardless of*
*the duration of the loss of consciousness*

| 6 | with loss of consciousness of un-specified duration |
| 9 | with concussion, unspecified |

  with
    open intracranial wound
      851.9 ☑
    skull fracture *— see* Fracture,
      skull, by site
  cerebellum 851.4 ☑
    with open intracranial wound
      851.5 ☑
  cortex 851.0 ☑
    with open intracranial wound
      851.1 ☑
  occipital lobe 851.4 ☑
    with open intracranial wound
      851.5 ☑
  stem 851.4 ☑
    with open intracranial wound
      851.5 ☑
breast 922.0
brow (and other part(s) of neck, scalp,
  or face, except eye) 920
buttock 922.32
canthus 921.1
cardiac 861.01
  with open wound into thorax
    861.11
cauda equina (spine) 952.4
cerebellum *— see* Contusion, brain,
  cerebellum
cerebral *— see* Contusion, brain
cheek(s) (and other part(s) of neck,
  scalp, or face, except eye) 920
chest (wall) 922.1
chin (and other part(s) of neck, scalp,
  or face, except eye) 920
clitoris 922.4
conjunctiva 921.1
conus medullaris (spine) 952.4
cornea 921.3
corpus cavernosum 922.4
cortex (brain) (cerebral) *— see* Contusion, brain, cortex
costal region 922.1
ear (and other part(s) of neck, scalp,
  or face except eye) 920
elbow 923.11
  with forearm 923.10
epididymis 922.4
epigastric region 922.2
eye NEC 921.9
eyeball 921.3
eyelid(s) (and periocular area) 921.1
face (and neck, or scalp, any part, except eye) 920

**Contusion** *— continued*
femoral triangle 922.2
fetus or newborn 772.6
finger(s) (nail) (subungual) 923.3
flank 922.2
foot (with ankle) (excluding toe(s))
  924.20
forearm (and elbow) 923.10
forehead (and other part(s) of neck,
  scalp, or face, except eye) 920
genital organs, external 922.4
globe (eye) 921.3
groin 922.2
gum(s) (and other part(s) of neck,
  scalp, or face, except eye) 920
hand(s) (except fingers alone) 923.20
head (any part, except eye) (and face)
  (and neck) 920
heart *— see* Contusion, cardiac
heel 924.20
hip 924.01
  with thigh 924.00
iliac region 922.2
inguinal region 922.2
internal organs (abdomen, chest, or
  pelvis) NEC *— see* Injury, internal, by site
interscapular region 922.33
iris (eye) 921.3
kidney 866.01
  with open wound into cavity
    866.11
knee 924.11
  with lower leg 924.10
labium (majus) (minus) 922.4
lacrimal apparatus, gland, or sac
  921.1
larynx (and other part(s) of neck,
  scalp, or face, except eye) 920
late effect *— see* Late, effects (of),
  contusion
leg 924.5
  lower (with knee) 924.10
lens 921.3
lingual (and other part(s) of neck,
  scalp, or face, except eye) 920
lip(s) (and other part(s) of neck, scalp,
  or face, except eye) 920
liver 864.01
  with
    laceration *— see* Laceration,
      liver
    open wound into cavity 864.11
lower extremity 924.5
  multiple sites 924.4
lumbar region 922.31
lung 861.21
  with open wound into thorax
    861.31
malar region (and other part(s) of
  neck, scalp, or face, except eye)
  920
mandibular joint (and other part(s) of
  neck, scalp, or face, except eye)
  920
mastoid region (and other part(s) of
  neck, scalp, or face, except eye)
  920
membrane, brain *— see* Contusion,
  brain
midthoracic region 922.1
mouth (and other part(s) of neck,
  scalp, or face, except eye) 920
multiple sites (not classifiable to same
  three-digit category) 924.8
  lower limb 924.4
  trunk 922.8
  upper limb 923.8
muscle NEC 924.9
myocardium *— see* Contusion, cardiac
nasal (septum) (and other part(s) of
  neck, scalp, or face, except eye)
  920
neck (and scalp or face, any part, except eye) 920
nerve *— see* Injury, nerve, by site

**Contusion** — *continued*
nose (and other part(s) of neck, scalp, or face, except eye) 920
occipital region (scalp) (and neck or face, except eye) 920
lobe — *see* Contusion, brain, occipital lobe
orbit (region) (tissues) 921.2
palate (soft) (and other part(s) of neck, scalp, or face, except eye) 920
parietal region (scalp) (and neck, or face, except eye) 920
lobe — *see* Contusion, brain
penis 922.4
pericardium — *see* Contusion, cardiac
perineum 922.4
periocular area 921.1
pharynx (and other part(s) of neck, scalp, or face, except eye) 920
popliteal space (*see also* Contusion, knee) 924.11
prepuce 922.4
pubic region 922.4
pudenda 922.4
pulmonary — *see* Contusion, lung
quadriceps femoralis 924.00
rib cage 922.1
sacral region 922.32
salivary ducts or glands (and other part(s) of neck, scalp, or face, except eye) 920
scalp (and neck, or face any part, except eye) 920
scapular region 923.01
with shoulder or upper arm 923.09
sclera (eye) 921.3
scrotum 922.4
shoulder 923.00
with upper arm or axillar regions 923.09
skin NEC 924.9
skull 920
spermatic cord 922.4
spinal cord (*see also* Injury, spinal, by site)
cauda equina 952.4
conus medullaris 952.4
spleen 865.01
with open wound into cavity 865.11
sternal region 922.1
stomach — *see* Injury, internal, stomach
subconjunctival 921.1
subcutaneous NEC 924.9
submaxillary region (and other part(s) of neck, scalp, or face, except eye) 920
submental region (and other part(s) of neck, scalp, or face, except eye) 920
subperiosteal NEC 924.9
supraclavicular fossa (and other part(s) of neck, scalp, or face, except eye) 920
supraorbital (and other part(s) of neck, scalp, or face, except eye) 920
temple (region) (and other part(s) of neck, scalp, or face, except eye) 920
testis 922.4
thigh (and hip) 924.00
thorax 922.1
organ — *see* Injury, internal, intrathoracic
throat (and other part(s) of neck, scalp, or face, except eye) 920
thumb(s) (nail) (subungual) 923.3
toe(s) (nail) (subungual) 924.3
tongue (and other part(s) of neck, scalp, or face, except eye) 920
trunk 922.9
multiple sites 922.8
specified site — *see* Contusion, by site
tunica vaginalis 922.4

**Contusion** — *continued*
tympanum (membrane) (and other part(s) of neck, scalp, or face, except eye) 920
upper extremity 923.9
multiple sites 923.8
uvula (and other part(s) of neck, scalp, or face, except eye) 920
vagina 922.4
vocal cord(s) (and other part(s) of neck, scalp, or face, except eye) 920
vulva 922.4
wrist 923.21
with hand(s), except finger(s) alone 923.20
**Conus** (any type) (congenital) 743.57
acquired 371.60
medullaris syndrome 336.8
**Convalescence** (following) V66.9
chemotherapy V66.2
medical NEC V66.5
psychotherapy V66.3
radiotherapy V66.1
surgery NEC V66.0
treatment (for) NEC V66.5
combined V66.6
fracture V66.4
mental disorder NEC V66.3
specified disorder NEC V66.5
**Conversion**
closed surgical procedure to open procedure
arthroscopic V64.43
laparoscopic V64.41
thoracoscopic V64.42
hysteria, hysterical, any type 300.11
neurosis, any 300.11
reaction, any 300.11
**Converter, tuberculosis** (test reaction) 795.5
**Convulsions** (idiopathic) 780.39
apoplectiform (*see also* Disease, cerebrovascular, acute) 436
brain 780.39
cerebral 780.39
cerebrospinal 780.39
due to trauma NEC — *see* Injury, intracranial
eclamptic (*see also* Eclampsia) 780.39
epileptic (*see also* Epilepsy) 345.9 ☑
epileptiform (*see also* Seizure, epileptiform) 780.39
epileptoid (*see also* Seizure, epileptiform) 780.39
ether
anesthetic
correct substance properly administered 780.39
overdose or wrong substance given 968.2
other specified type — *see* Table of Drugs and Chemicals
febrile (simple) 780.31
complex 780.32
generalized 780.39
hysterical 300.11
infantile 780.39
epilepsy — *see* Epilepsy
internal 780.39
jacksonian (*see also* Epilepsy) 345.5 ☑
myoclonic 333.2
newborn 779.0
paretic 094.1
pregnancy (nephritic) (uremic) — *see* Eclampsia, pregnancy
psychomotor (*see also* Epilepsy) 345.4 ☑
puerperal, postpartum — *see* Eclampsia, pregnancy
recurrent 780.39
epileptic — *see* Epilepsy
reflex 781.0
repetitive 780.39
epileptic — *see* Epilepsy
salaam (*see also* Epilepsy) 345.6 ☑

**Convulsions** — *continued*
scarlatinal 034.1
spasmodic 780.39
tetanus, tetanic (*see also* Tetanus) 037
thymic 254.8
uncinate 780.39
uremic 586
**Convulsive** — *see also* Convulsions
disorder or state 780.39
epileptic — *see* Epilepsy
equivalent, abdominal (*see also* Epilepsy) 345.5 ☑
**Cooke-Apert-Gallais syndrome** (adrenogenital) 255.2
**Cooley's anemia** (erythroblastic) 282.49
**Coolie itch** 126.9
**Cooper's**
disease 610.1
hernia — *see* Hernia, Cooper's
**Coordination disturbance** 781.3
**Copper wire arteries, retina** 362.13
**Copra itch** 133.8
**Coprolith** 560.39
**Coprophilia** 302.89
**Coproporphyria, hereditary** 277.1
**Coprostasis** 560.39
with hernia (*see also* Hernia, by site, with obstruction)
gangrenous — *see* Hernia, by site, with gangrene
**Cor**
biloculare 745.7
bovinum — *see* Hypertrophy, cardiac
bovis (*see also* Hypertrophy, cardiac)
pulmonale (chronic) 416.9
acute 415.0
triatriatum, triatrium 746.82
triloculare 745.8
biatriatum 745.3
biventriculare 745.69
**Corbus' disease** 607.1
**Cord** — *see also* condition
around neck (tightly) (with compression)
affecting fetus or newborn 762.5
complicating delivery 663.1 ☑
without compression 663.3 ☑
affecting fetus or newborn 762.6
bladder NEC 344.61
tabetic 094.0
prolapse
affecting fetus or newborn 762.4
complicating delivery 663.0 ☑
**Cord's angiopathy** — *see also* Tuberculosis 017.3 ☑ *[362.18]*
**Cordis ectopia** 746.87
**Corditis** (spermatic) 608.4
**Corectopia** 743.46
**Cori type glycogen storage disease** — *see* Disease, glycogen storage
**Cork-handlers' disease or lung** 495.3
**Corkscrew esophagus** 530.5
**Corlett's pyosis** (impetigo) 684
**Corn** (infected) 700
**Cornea** — *see also* condition
donor V59.5
guttata (dystrophy) 371.57
plana 743.41
**Cornelia de Lange's syndrome** (Amsterdam dwarf, mental retardation, and brachycephaly) 759.89
**Cornual gestation or pregnancy** — *see* Pregnancy, cornual
**Cornu cutaneum** 702.8
**Coronary** (artery) — *see also* condition
arising from aorta or pulmonary trunk 746.85
**Corpora** — *see also* condition
amylacea (prostate) 602.8
cavernosa — *see* condition
**Corpulence** — *see* Obesity
**Corpus** — *see* condition
**Corrigan's disease** — *see* Insufficiency, aortic
**Corrosive burn** — *see* Burn, by site

**Corsican fever** — *see also* Malaria 084.6
**Cortical** — *see also* condition
blindness 377.75
necrosis, kidney (bilateral) 583.6
**Corticoadrenal** — *see* condition
**Corticosexual syndrome** 255.2
**Coryza** (acute) 460
with grippe or influenza 487.1
syphilitic 095.8
congenital (chronic) 090.0
**Costen's syndrome or complex** 524.60
**Costiveness** — *see also* Constipation 564.00
**Costochondritis** 733.6
**Cotard's syndrome** (paranoia) 297.1
**Cot death** 798.0
**Cotungo's disease** 724.3
**Cough** 786.2
with hemorrhage (*see also* Hemoptysis) 786.3
affected 786.2
bronchial 786.2
with grippe or influenza 487.1
chronic 786.2
epidemic 786.2
functional 306.1
hemorrhagic 786.3
hysterical 300.11
laryngeal, spasmodic 786.2
nervous 786.2
psychogenic 306.1
smokers' 491.0
tea tasters' 112.89
**Counseling** NEC V65.40
without complaint or sickness V65.49
abuse victim NEC V62.89
child V61.21
partner V61.11
spouse V61.11
child abuse, maltreatment, or neglect V61.21
contraceptive NEC V25.09
device (intrauterine) V25.02
maintenance V25.40
intrauterine contraceptive device V25.42
oral contraceptive (pill) V25.41
specified type NEC V25.49
subdermal implantable V25.43
management NEC V25.9
oral contraceptive (pill) V25.01
emergency V25.03
postcoital V25.03
prescription NEC V25.02
oral contraceptive (pill) V25.01
emergency V25.03
postcoital V25.03
repeat prescription V25.41
repeat prescription V25.40
subdermal implantable V25.43
surveillance NEC V25.40
dietary V65.3
exercise V65.41
expectant mother, pediatric pre-birth visit V65.11
explanation of
investigation finding NEC V65.49
medication NEC V65.49
family planning V25.09
natural ●
procreative V26.41 ●
to avoid pregnancy V25.04 ●
for nonattending third party V65.19
genetic V26.33
gonorrhea V65.45
health (advice) (education) (instruction) NEC V65.49
HIV V65.44
human immunodeficiency virus V65.44
injury prevention V65.43
insulin pump training V65.46
marital V61.10
medical (for) V65.9
boarding school resident V60.6
condition not demonstrated V65.5

☑ Additional Digit Required — Refer to the Tabular List for Digit Selection
▽ Subterms under main terms may continue to next column or page
*2008 ICD-9-CM*
▶◀ Revised Text
● New Line
▲ Revised Code
**October 2007 • Volume 2 — 59**

Contusion — Counseling

**Index**

**Counseling — Crush, crushed, crushing**

**Counseling** — *continued*
medical — *continued*
feared complaint and no disease found V65.5
institutional resident V60.6
on behalf of another V65.19
person living alone V60.3
natural family planning ●
procreative V26.41 ●
to avoid pregnancy V25.04 ●
parent-child conflict V61.20
specified problem NEC V61.29
partner abuse
perpetrator V61.12
victim V61.11
pediatric pre-birth visit for expectant mother V65.11
perpetrator of
child abuse V62.83
parental V61.22
partner abuse V61.12
spouse abuse V61.12
procreative V65.49
sex NEC V65.49
transmitted disease NEC V65.45
HIV V65.44
specified reason NEC V65.49
spousal abuse
perpetrator V61.12
victim V61.11
substance use and abuse V65.42
syphilis V65.45
victim (of)
abuse NEC V62.89
child abuse V61.21
partner abuse V61.11
spousal abuse V61.11
**Coupled rhythm** 427.89
**Couvelaire uterus** (complicating delivery) — *see* Placenta, separation
**Cowper's gland** — *see* condition
**Cowperitis** — *see also* Urethritis 597.89
gonorrheal (acute) 098.0
chronic or duration of 2 months or over 098.2
**Cowpox** (abortive) 051.0
due to vaccination 999.0
eyelid 051.0 [373.5]
postvaccination 999.0 [373.5]
**Coxa**
plana 732.1
valga (acquired) 736.31
congenital 755.61
late effect of rickets 268.1
vara (acquired) 736.32
congenital 755.61
late effect of rickets 268.1
**Coxae malum senilis** 715.25
**Coxalgia** (nontuberculous) 719.45
tuberculous (*see also* Tuberculosis) 015.1 ☑ [730.85]
**Coxalgic pelvis** 736.30
**Coxitis** 716.65
**Coxsackie** (infection) (virus) 079.2
central nervous system NEC 048
endocarditis 074.22
enteritis 008.67
meningitis (aseptic) 047.0
myocarditis 074.23
pericarditis 074.21
pharyngitis 074.0
pleurodynia 074.1
specific disease NEC 074.8
**Crabs, meaning pubic lice** 132.2
**Crack baby** 760.75
**Cracked**
nipple 611.2
puerperal, postpartum 676.1 ☑
tooth 521.81
**Cradle cap** 690.11
**Craft neurosis** 300.89
**Craigiasis** 007.8
**Cramp(s)** 729.82
abdominal 789.0 ☑
bathing 994.1
colic 789.0 ☑

**Cramp(s)** — *continued*
colic — *continued*
psychogenic 306.4
due to immersion 994.1
extremity (lower) (upper) NEC 729.82
fireman 992.2
heat 992.2
hysterical 300.11
immersion 994.1
intestinal 789.0 ☑
psychogenic 306.4
linotypist's 300.89
organic 333.84
muscle (extremity) (general) 729.82
due to immersion 994.1
hysterical 300.11
occupational (hand) 300.89
organic 333.84
psychogenic 307.89
salt depletion 276.1
sleep related leg 327.52
stoker 992.2
stomach 789.0 ☑
telegraphers' 300.89
organic 333.84
typists' 300.89
organic 333.84
uterus 625.8
menstrual 625.3
writers' 333.84
organic 333.84
psychogenic 300.89
**Cranial** — *see* condition
**Cranioclasis, fetal** 763.89
**Craniocleidodysostosis** 755.59
**Craniofenestria** (skull) 756.0
**Craniolacunia** (skull) 756.0
**Craniopagus** 759.4
**Craniopathy, metabolic** 733.3
**Craniopharyngeal** — *see* condition
**Craniopharyngioma** (M9350/1) 237.0
**Craniorachischisis** (totalis) 740.1
**Cranioschisis** 756.0
**Craniostenosis** 756.0
**Craniosynostosis** 756.0
**Craniotabes** (cause unknown) 733.3
rachitic 268.1
syphilitic 090.5
**Craniotomy, fetal** 763.89
**Cranium** — *see* condition
**Craw-craw** 125.3
**CRBSI** (catheter-related bloodstream ● infection) 999.31 ●
**Creaking joint** 719.60
ankle 719.67
elbow 719.62
foot 719.67
hand 719.64
hip 719.65
knee 719.66
multiple sites 719.69
pelvic region 719.65
shoulder (region) 719.61
specified site NEC 719.68
wrist 719.63
**Creeping**
eruption 126.9
palsy 335.21
paralysis 335.21
**Crenated tongue** 529.8
**Creotoxism** 005.9
**Crepitus**
caput 756.0
joint 719.60
ankle 719.67
elbow 719.62
foot 719.67
hand 719.64
hip 719.65
knee 719.66
multiple sites 719.69
pelvic region 719.65
shoulder (region) 719.61
specified site NEC 719.68
wrist 719.63

**Crescent or conus choroid, congenital** 743.57
**Cretin, cretinism** (athyrotic) (congenital) (endemic) (metabolic) (nongoitrous) (sporadic) 243
goitrous (sporadic) 246.1
pelvis (dwarf type) (male type) 243
with disproportion (fetopelvic) 653.1 ☑
affecting fetus or newborn 763.1
causing obstructed labor 660.1 ☑
affecting fetus or newborn 763.1
pituitary 253.3
**Cretinoid degeneration** 243
**Creutzfeldt-Jakob disease** (syndrome) (new variant) 046.1
with dementia
with behavioral disturbance 046.1 [294.11]
without behavioral disturbance 046.1 [294.10]
**Crib death** 798.0
**Cribriform hymen** 752.49
**Cri-du-chat syndrome** 758.31
**Crigler-Najjar disease or syndrome** (congenital hyperbilirubinemia) 277.4
**Crimean hemorrhagic fever** 065.0
**Criminalism** 301.7
**Crisis**
abdomen 789.0 ☑
addisonian (acute adrenocortical insufficiency) 255.41 ▲
adrenal (cortical) 255.41 ▲
asthmatic — *see* Asthma
brain, cerebral (*see also* Disease, cerebrovascular, acute) 436
celiac 579.0
Dietl's 593.4
emotional NEC 309.29
acute reaction to stress 308.0
adjustment reaction 309.9
specific to childhood or adolescence 313.9
gastric (tabetic) 094.0
glaucomatocyclitic 364.22
heart (*see also* Failure, heart) 428.9
hypertensive — *see* Hypertension
nitritoid
correct substance properly administered 458.29
overdose or wrong substance given or taken 961.1
oculogyric 378.87
psychogenic 306.7
Pel's 094.0
psychosexual identity 302.6
rectum 094.0
renal 593.81
sickle cell 282.62
stomach (tabetic) 094.0
tabetic 094.0
thyroid (*see also* Thyrotoxicosis) 242.9 ☑
thyrotoxic (*see also* Thyrotoxicosis) 242.9 ☑
vascular — *see* Disease, cerebrovascular, acute
**Crocq's disease** (acrocyanosis) 443.89
**Crohn's disease** — *see also* Enteritis, regional 555.9
**Cronkhite-Canada syndrome** 211.3
**Crooked septum, nasal** 470
**Cross**
birth (of fetus) complicating delivery 652.3 ☑
with successful version 652.1 ☑
causing obstructed labor 660.0 ☑
bite, anterior or posterior 524.27
eye (*see also* Esotropia) 378.00
**Crossed ectopia of kidney** 753.3
**Crossfoot** 754.50

**Croup, croupous** (acute) (angina) (catarrhal) (infective) (inflammatory) (laryngeal) (membranous) (nondiphtheritic) (pseudomembranous) 464.4
asthmatic (*see also* Asthma) 493.9 ☑
bronchial 466.0
diphtheritic (membranous) 032.3
false 478.75
spasmodic 478.75
diphtheritic 032.3
stridulous 478.75
diphtheritic 032.3
**Crouzon's disease** (craniofacial dysostosis) 756.0
**Crowding, teeth** 524.31
**CRST syndrome** (cutaneous systemic sclerosis) 710.1
**Cruchet's disease** (encephalitis lethargica) 049.8
**Cruelty in children** — *see also* Disturbance, conduct 312.9
**Crural ulcer** — *see also* Ulcer, lower extremity 707.10
**Crush, crushed, crushing** (injury) 929.9
abdomen 926.19
internal — *see* Injury, internal, abdomen
ankle 928.21
with other parts of foot 928.20
arm 927.9
lower (and elbow) 927.10
upper 927.03
with shoulder or axillary region 927.09
axilla 927.02
with shoulder or upper arm 927.09
back 926.11
breast 926.19
buttock 926.12
cheek 925.1
chest — *see* Injury, internal, chest
ear 925.1
elbow 927.11
with forearm 927.10
face 925.1
finger(s) 927.3
with hand(s) 927.20
and wrist(s) 927.21
flank 926.19
foot, excluding toe(s) alone (with ankle) 928.20
forearm (and elbow) 927.10
genitalia, external (female) (male) 926.0
internal — *see* Injury, internal, genital organ NEC
hand, except finger(s) alone (and wrist) 927.20
head — *see* Fracture, skull, by site
heel 928.20
hip 928.01
with thigh 928.00
internal organ (abdomen, chest, or pelvis) — *see* Injury, internal, by site
knee 928.11
with leg, lower 928.10
labium (majus) (minus) 926.0
larynx 925.2
late effect — *see* Late, effects (of), crushing
leg 928.9
lower 928.10
and knee 928.11
upper 928.00
limb
lower 928.9
multiple sites 928.8
upper 927.9
multiple sites 927.8
multiple sites NEC 929.0
neck 925.2
nerve — *see* Injury, nerve, by site
nose 802.0
open 802.1

**Crush, crushed, crushing —**
*continued*
penis 926.0
pharynx 925.2
scalp 925.1
scapular region 927.01
with shoulder or upper arm 927.09
scrotum 926.0
shoulder 927.00
with upper arm or axillary region 927.09
skull or cranium — *see* Fracture, skull, by site
spinal cord — *see* Injury, spinal, by site
syndrome (complication of trauma) 958.5
testis 926.0
thigh (with hip) 928.00
throat 925.2
thumb(s) (and fingers) 927.3
toe(s) 928.3
with foot 928.20
and ankle 928.21
tonsil 925.2
trunk 926.9
chest — *see* Injury, internal, intrathoracic organs NEC
internal organ — *see* Injury, internal, by site
multiple sites 926.8
specified site NEC 926.19
vulva 926.0
wrist 927.21
with hand(s), except fingers alone 927.20
**Crusta lactea** 690.11
**Crusts** 782.8
**Crutch paralysis** 953.4
**Cruveilhier-Baumgarten cirrhosis, disease, or syndrome** 571.5
**Cruveilhier's disease** 335.21
**Cruz-Chagas disease** — *see also* Trypanosomiasis 086.2
**Crying**
constant, continuous
adolescent 780.95
adult 780.95
baby 780.92
child 780.95
infant 780.92
newborn 780.92
excessive
adolescent 780.95
adult 780.95
baby 780.92
child 780.95
infant 780.92
newborn 780.92
**Cryoglobulinemia** (mixed) 273.2
**Crypt** (anal) (rectal) 569.49
**Cryptitis** (anal) (rectal) 569.49
**Cryptococcosis** (European) (pulmonary) (systemic) 117.5
**Cryptococcus** 117.5
epidermicus 117.5
neoformans, infection by 117.5
**Cryptopapillitis** (anus) 569.49
**Cryptophthalmos** (eyelid) 743.06
**Cryptorchid, cryptorchism, cryptorchidism** 752.51
**Cryptosporidiosis** 007.4
**Cryptotia** 744.29
**Crystallopathy**
calcium pyrophosphate (*see also* Arthritis) 275.49 *[712.2]* ☑
dicalcium phosphate (*see also* Arthritis) 275.49 *[712.1]* ☑
gouty 274.0
pyrophosphate NEC (*see also* Arthritis) 275.49 *[712.2]* ☑
uric acid 274.0
**Crystalluria** 791.9
**Csillag's disease** (lichen sclerosis et atrophicus) 701.0
**Cuban itch** 050.1

**Cubitus**
valgus (acquired) 736.01
congenital 755.59
late effect of rickets 268.1
varus (acquired) 736.02
congenital 755.59
late effect of rickets 268.1
**Cultural deprivation** V62.4
**Cupping of optic disc** 377.14
**Curling esophagus** 530.5
**Curling's ulcer** — *see* Ulcer, duodenum
**Curschmann (-Batten) (-Steinert) disease or syndrome** 359.21 ▲
**Curvature**
organ or site, congenital NEC — *see* Distortion
penis (lateral) 752.69
Pott's (spinal) (*see also* Tuberculosis) 015.0 ☑ *[737.43]*
radius, idiopathic, progressive (congenital) 755.54
spine (acquired) (angular) (idiopathic) (incorrect) (postural) 737.9
congenital 754.2
due to or associated with
Charcôt-Marie-Tooth disease 356.1 *[737.40]*
mucopolysaccharidosis 277.5 *[737.40]*
neurofibromatosis 237.71 *[737.40]*
osteitis
deformans 731.0 *[737.40]*
fibrosa cystica 252.01 *[737.40]*
osteoporosis (*see also* Osteoporosis) 733.00 *[737.40]*
poliomyelitis (*see also* Poliomyelitis) 138 *[737.40]*
tuberculosis (Pott's curvature) (*see also* Tuberculosis) 015.0 ☑ *[737.43]*
kyphoscoliotic (*see also* Kyphoscoliosis) 737.30
kyphotic (*see also* Kyphosis) 737.10
late effect of rickets 268.1 *[737.40]*
Pott's 015.0 ☑ *[737.40]*
scoliotic (*see also* Scoliosis) 737.30
specified NEC 737.8
tuberculous 015.0 ☑ *[737.40]*
**Cushing's**
basophilism, disease, or syndrome (iatrogenic) (idiopathic) (pituitary basophilism) (pituitary dependent) 255.0
ulcer — *see* Ulcer, peptic
**Cushingoid due to steroid therapy**
correct substance properly administered 255.0
overdose or wrong substance given or taken 962.0
**Cut** (external) — *see* Wound, open, by site
**Cutaneous** — *see also* condition
hemorrhage 782.7
horn (cheek) (eyelid) (mouth) 702.8
larva migrans 126.9
**Cutis** — *see also* condition
hyperelastic 756.83
acquired 701.8
laxa 756.83
senilis 701.8
marmorata 782.61
osteosis 709.3
pendula 756.83
acquired 701.8
rhomboidalis nuchae 701.8
verticis gyrata 757.39
acquired 701.8
**Cyanopathy, newborn** 770.83
**Cyanosis** 782.5
autotoxic 289.7
common atrioventricular canal 745.69
congenital 770.83
conjunctiva 372.71

**Cyanosis** — *continued*
due to
endocardial cushion defect 745.60
nonclosure, foramen botalli 745.5
patent foramen botalli 745.5
persistent foramen ovale 745.5
enterogenous 289.7
fetus or newborn 770.83
ostium primum defect 745.61
paroxysmal digital 443.0
retina, retinal 362.10
**Cycle**
anovulatory 628.0
menstrual, irregular 626.4
**Cyclencephaly** 759.89
**Cyclical vomiting** 536.2
psychogenic 306.4
**Cyclitic membrane** 364.74
**Cyclitis** — *see also* Iridocyclitis 364.3
acute 364.00
primary 364.01
recurrent 364.02
chronic 364.10
in
sarcoidosis 135 *[364.11]*
tuberculosis (*see also* Tuberculosis) 017.3 ☑ *[364.11]*
Fuchs' heterochromic 364.21
granulomatous 364.10
lens induced 364.23
nongranulomatous 364.00
posterior 363.21
primary 364.01
recurrent 364.02
secondary (noninfectious) 364.04
infectious 364.03
subacute 364.00
primary 364.01
recurrent 364.02
**Cyclokeratitis** — *see* Keratitis
**Cyclophoria** 378.44
**Cyclopia, cyclops** 759.89
**Cycloplegia** 367.51
**Cyclospasm** 367.53
**Cyclosporiasis** 007.5
**Cyclothymia** 301.13
**Cyclothymic personality** 301.13
**Cyclotropia** 378.33
**Cyesis** — *see* Pregnancy
**Cylindroma** (M8200/3) — *see also* Neoplasm, by site, malignant
eccrine dermal (M8200/0) — *see* Neoplasm, skin, benign
skin (M8200/0) — *see* Neoplasm, skin, benign
**Cylindruria** 791.7
**Cyllosoma** 759.89
**Cynanche**
diphtheritic 032.3
tonsillaris 475
**Cynorexia** 783.6
**Cyphosis** — *see* Kyphosis
**Cyprus fever** — *see also* Brucellosis 023.9
**Cyriax's syndrome** (slipping rib) 733.99

**Cyst** (mucus) (retention) (serous) (simple)

> *Note* — In general, cysts are not neoplastic and are classified to the appropriate category for disease of the specified anatomical site. This generalization does not apply to certain types of cysts which are neoplastic in nature, for example, dermoid, nor does it apply to cysts of certain structures, for example, branchial cleft, which are classified as developmental anomalies.
>
> The following listing includes some of the most frequently reported sites of cysts as well as qualifiers which indicate the type of cyst. The latter qualifiers usually are not repeated under the anatomical sites. Since the code assignment for a given site may vary depending upon the type of cyst, the coder should refer to the listings under the specified type of cyst before consideration is given to the site.

accessory, fallopian tube 752.11
adenoid (infected) 474.8
adrenal gland 255.8
congenital 759.1
air, lung 518.89
allantoic 753.7
alveolar process (jaw bone) 526.2
amnion, amniotic 658.8 ☑
anterior chamber (eye) 364.60
exudative 364.62
implantation (surgical) (traumatic) 364.61
parasitic 360.13
anterior nasopalatine 526.1
antrum 478.19
anus 569.49
apical (periodontal) (tooth) 522.8
appendix 543.9
arachnoid, brain 348.0
arytenoid 478.79
auricle 706.2
Baker's (knee) 727.51
tuberculous (*see also* Tuberculosis) 015.2 ☑
Bartholin's gland or duct 616.2
bile duct (*see also* Disease, biliary) 576.8
bladder (multiple) (trigone) 596.8
Blessig's 362.62
blood, endocardial (*see also* Endocarditis) 424.90
blue dome 610.0
bone (local) 733.20
aneurysmal 733.22
jaw 526.2
developmental (odontogenic) 526.0
fissural 526.1
latent 526.89
solitary 733.21
unicameral 733.21
brain 348.0
congenital 742.4
hydatid (*see also* Echinococcus) 122.9
third ventricle (colloid) 742.4
branchial (cleft) 744.42
branchiogenic 744.42
breast (benign) (blue dome) (pedunculated) (solitary) (traumatic) 610.0
involution 610.4
sebaceous 610.8
broad ligament (benign) 620.8
embryonic 752.11
bronchogenic (mediastinal) (sequestration) 518.89
congenital 748.4
buccal 528.4
bulbourethral gland (Cowper's) 599.89
bursa, bursal 727.49
pharyngeal 478.26

# Cyst

**Cyst** — *continued*
calcifying odontogenic (M9301/0) 213.1
    upper jaw (bone) 213.0
canal of Nuck (acquired) (serous) 629.1
    congenital 752.41
canthus 372.75
carcinomatous (M8010/3) — *see* Neoplasm, by site, malignant
cartilage (joint) — *see* Derangement, joint
cauda equina 336.8
cavum septi pellucidi NEC 348.0
celomic (pericardium) 746.89
cerebellopontine (angle) — *see* Cyst, brain
cerebellum — *see* Cyst, brain
cerebral — *see* Cyst, brain
cervical lateral 744.42
cervix 622.8
    embryonal 752.41
    nabothian (gland) 616.0
chamber, anterior (eye) 364.60
    exudative 364.62
    implantation (surgical) (traumatic) 364.61
    parasitic 360.13
chiasmal, optic NEC (*see also* Lesion, chiasmal) 377.54
chocolate (ovary) 617.1
choledochal (congenital) 751.69
    acquired 576.8
choledochus 751.69
chorion 658.8 ☑
choroid plexus 348.0
chyle, mesentery 457.8
ciliary body 364.60
    exudative 364.64
    implantation 364.61
    primary 364.63
clitoris 624.8
coccyx (*see also* Cyst, bone) 733.20
colloid
    third ventricle (brain) 742.4
    thyroid gland — *see* Goiter
colon 569.89
common (bile) duct (*see also* Disease, biliary) 576.8
congenital NEC 759.89
    adrenal glands 759.1
    epiglottis 748.3
    esophagus 750.4
    fallopian tube 752.11
    kidney 753.10
        multiple 753.19
        single 753.11
    larynx 748.3
    liver 751.62
    lung 748.4
    mediastinum 748.8
    ovary 752.0
    oviduct 752.11
    pancreas 751.7
    periurethral (tissue) 753.8
    prepuce NEC 752.69
        penis 752.69
    sublingual 750.26
    submaxillary gland 750.26
    thymus (gland) 759.2
    tongue 750.19
    ureterovesical orifice 753.4
    vulva 752.41
conjunctiva 372.75
cornea 371.23
corpora quadrigemina 348.0
corpus
    albicans (ovary) 620.2
    luteum (ruptured) 620.1
Cowper's gland (benign) (infected) 599.89
cranial meninges 348.0
craniobuccal pouch 253.8
craniopharyngeal pouch 253.8
cystic duct (*see also* Disease, gallbladder) 575.8

**Cyst** — *continued*
Cysticercus (any site) 123.1
Dandy-Walker 742.3
    with spina bifida (*see also* Spina bifida) 741.0 ☑
dental 522.8
    developmental 526.0
    eruption 526.0
    lateral periodontal 526.0
    primordial (keratocyst) 526.0
    root 522.8
dentigerous 526.0
    mandible 526.0
    maxilla 526.0
dermoid (M9084/0) (*see also* Neoplasm, by site, benign)
    with malignant transformation (M9084/3) 183.0
    implantation
        external area or site (skin) NEC 709.8
        iris 364.61
        skin 709.8
        vagina 623.8
        vulva 624.8
    mouth 528.4
    oral soft tissue 528.4
    sacrococcygeal 685.1
        with abscess 685.0
developmental of ovary, ovarian 752.0
dura (cerebral) 348.0
    spinal 349.2
ear (external) 706.2
echinococcal (*see also* Echinococcus) 122.9
embryonal
    cervix uteri 752.41
    genitalia, female external 752.41
    uterus 752.3
    vagina 752.41
endometrial 621.8
    ectopic 617.9
endometrium (uterus) 621.8
    ectopic — *see* Endometriosis
enteric 751.5
enterogenous 751.5
epidermal (inclusion) (*see also* Cyst, skin) 706.2
epidermoid (inclusion) (*see also* Cyst, skin) 706.2
    mouth 528.4
    not of skin — *see* Cyst, by site
    oral soft tissue 528.4
epididymis 608.89
epiglottis 478.79
epiphysis cerebri 259.8
epithelial (inclusion) (*see also* Cyst, skin) 706.2
epoophoron 752.11
eruption 526.0
esophagus 530.89
ethmoid sinus 478.19
eye (retention) 379.8
    congenital 743.03
    posterior segment, congenital 743.54
eyebrow 706.2
eyelid (sebaceous) 374.84
    infected 373.13
    sweat glands or ducts 374.84
falciform ligament (inflammatory) 573.8
fallopian tube 620.8
female genital organs NEC 629.89
fimbrial (congenital) 752.11
fissural (oral region) 526.1
follicle (atretic) (graafian) (ovarian) 620.0
    nabothian (gland) 616.0
follicular (atretic) (ovarian) 620.0
    dentigerous 526.0
frontal sinus 478.19
gallbladder or duct 575.8
ganglion 727.43
Gartner's duct 752.41
gas, of mesentery 568.89

**Cyst** — *continued*
gingiva 523.8
gland of moll 374.84
globulomaxillary 526.1
graafian follicle 620.0
granulosal lutein 620.2
hemangiomatous (M9121/0) (*see also* Hemangioma) 228.00
hydatid (*see also* Echinococcus) 122.9
    fallopian tube (Morgagni) 752.11
    liver NEC 122.8
    lung NEC 122.9
    Morgagni 752.89
        fallopian tube 752.11
    specified site NEC 122.9
hymen 623.8
    embryonal 752.41
hypopharynx 478.26
hypophysis, hypophyseal (duct) (recurrent) 253.8
    cerebri 253.8
implantation (dermoid)
    anterior chamber (eye) 364.61
    external area or site (skin) NEC 709.8
    iris 364.61
    vagina 623.8
    vulva 624.8
incisor, incisive canal 526.1
inclusion (epidermal) (epithelial) (epidermoid) (mucous) (squamous) (*see also* Cyst, skin) 706.2
    not of skin — *see* Neoplasm, by site, benign
intestine (large) (small) 569.89
intracranial — *see* Cyst, brain
intraligamentous 728.89
    knee 717.89
intrasellar 253.8
iris (idiopathic) 364.60
    exudative 364.62
    implantation (surgical) (traumatic) 364.61
    miotic pupillary 364.55
    parasitic 360.13
Iwanoff's 362.62
jaw (bone) (aneurysmal) (extravasation) (hemorrhagic) (traumatic) 526.2
    developmental (odontogenic) 526.0
    fissural 526.1
keratin 706.2
kidney (congenital) 753.10
    acquired 593.2
    calyceal (*see also* Hydronephrosis) 591
    multiple 753.19
    pyelogenic (*see also* Hydronephrosis) 591
    simple 593.2
    single 753.11
    solitary (not congenital) 593.2
labium (majus) (minus) 624.8
    sebaceous 624.8
lacrimal
    apparatus 375.43
    gland or sac 375.12
larynx 478.79
lens 379.39
    congenital 743.39
lip (gland) 528.5
liver 573.8
    congenital 751.62
    hydatid (*see also* Echinococcus) 122.8
        granulosis 122.0
        multilocularis 122.5
lung 518.89
    congenital 748.4
    giant bullous 492.0
lutein 620.1
lymphangiomatous (M9173/0) 228.1
lymphoepithelial
    mouth 528.4
    oral soft tissue 528.4
macula 362.54

**Cyst** — *continued*
malignant (M8000/3) — *see* Neoplasm, by site, malignant
mammary gland (sweat gland) (*see also* Cyst, breast) 610.0
mandible 526.2
    dentigerous 526.0
    radicular 522.8
maxilla 526.2
    dentigerous 526.0
    radicular 522.8
median
    anterior maxillary 526.1
    palatal 526.1
mediastinum (congenital) 748.8
meibomian (gland) (retention) 373.2
    infected 373.12
membrane, brain 348.0
meninges (cerebral) 348.0
    spinal 349.2
meniscus knee 717.5
mesentery, mesenteric (gas) 568.89
    chyle 457.8
    gas 568.89
mesonephric duct 752.89
mesothelial
    peritoneum 568.89
    pleura (peritoneal) 568.89
milk 611.5
miotic pupillary (iris) 364.55
Morgagni (hydatid) 752.89
    fallopian tube 752.11
mouth 528.4
mullerian duct 752.89
multilocular (ovary) (M8000/1) 239.5
myometrium 621.8
nabothian (follicle) (ruptured) 616.0
nasal sinus 478.19
nasoalveolar 528.4
nasolabial 528.4
nasopalatine (duct) 526.1
    anterior 526.1
nasopharynx 478.26
neoplastic (M8000/1) (*see also* Neoplasm, by site, unspecified nature)
    benign (M8000/0) — *see* Neoplasm, by site, benign
    uterus 621.8
nervous system — *see* Cyst, brain
neuroenteric 742.59
neuroepithelial ventricle 348.0
nipple 610.0
nose 478.19
    skin of 706.2
odontogenic, developmental 526.0
omentum (lesser) 568.89
    congenital 751.8
oral soft tissue (dermoid) (epidermoid) (lymphoepithelial) 528.4
ora serrata 361.19
orbit 376.81
ovary, ovarian (twisted) 620.2
    adherent 620.2
    chocolate 617.1
    corpus
        albicans 620.2
        luteum 620.1
    dermoid (M9084/0) 220
    developmental 752.0
    due to failure of involution NEC 620.2
    endometrial 617.1
    follicular (atretic) (graafian) (hemorrhagic) 620.0
    hemorrhagic 620.2
    in pregnancy or childbirth 654.4 ☑
        affecting fetus or newborn 763.89
        causing obstructed labor 660.2 ☑
            affecting fetus or newborn 763.1
    multilocular (M8000/1) 239.5
    pseudomucinous (M8470/0) 220
    retention 620.2

---

▶◀ Revised Text     ● New Line     ▲ Revised Code

Subterms under main terms may continue to next column or page

**Cyst** — *continued*
  ovary, ovarian — *continued*
    serous 620.2
    theca lutein 620.2
    tuberculous (*see also* Tuberculosis)
      016.6 ☑
    unspecified 620.2
  oviduct 620.8
  palatal papilla (jaw) 526.1
  palate 526.1
    fissural 526.1
    median (fissural) 526.1
  palatine, of papilla 526.1
  pancreas, pancreatic 577.2
    congenital 751.7
    false 577.2
    hemorrhagic 577.2
    true 577.2
  paranephric 593.2
  para ovarian 752.11
  paraphysis, cerebri 742.4
  parasitic NEC 136.9
  parathyroid (gland) 252.8
  paratubal (fallopian) 620.8
  paraurethral duct 599.89
  paroophoron 752.11
  parotid gland 527.6
    mucous extravasation or retention
      527.6
  parovarian 752.11
  pars planus 364.60
    exudative 364.64
    primary 364.63
  pelvis, female
    in pregnancy or childbirth 654.4 ☑
      affecting fetus or newborn
        763.89
      causing obstructed labor
        660.2 ☑
        affecting fetus or newborn
          763.1
  penis (sebaceous) 607.89
  periapical 522.8
  pericardial (congenital) 746.89
    acquired (secondary) 423.8
  pericoronal 526.0
  perineural (Tarlov's) 355.9
  periodontal 522.8
    lateral 526.0
  peripancreatic 577.2
  peripelvic (lymphatic) 593.2
  peritoneum 568.89
    chylous 457.8
  pharynx (wall) 478.26
  pilonidal (infected) (rectum) 685.1
    with abscess 685.0
    malignant (M9084/3) 173.5
  pituitary (duct) (gland) 253.8
  placenta (amniotic) — *see* Placenta,
    abnormal
  pleura 519.8
  popliteal 727.51
  porencephalic 742.4
    acquired 348.0
  postanal (infected) 685.1
    with abscess 685.0
  posterior segment of eye, congenital
    743.54
  postmastoidectomy cavity 383.31
  preauricular 744.47
  prepuce 607.89
    congenital 752.69
  primordial (jaw) 526.0
  prostate 600.3
  pseudomucinous (ovary) (M8470/0)
    220
  pudenda (sweat glands) 624.8
  pupillary, miotic 364.55
    sebaceous 624.8
  radicular (residual) 522.8
  radiculodental 522.8
  ranular 527.6
  Rathke's pouch 253.8
  rectum (epithelium) (mucous) 569.49
  renal — *see* Cyst, kidney
  residual (radicular) 522.8

**Cyst** — *continued*
  retention (ovary) 620.2
  retina 361.19
    macular 362.54
    parasitic 360.13
    primary 361.13
    secondary 361.14
  retroperitoneal 568.89
  sacrococcygeal (dermoid) 685.1
    with abscess 685.0
  salivary gland or duct 527.6
    mucous extravasation or retention
      527.6
  Sampson's 617.1
  sclera 379.19
  scrotum (sebaceous) 706.2
    sweat glands 706.2
  sebaceous (duct) (gland) 706.2
    breast 610.8
    eyelid 374.84
    genital organ NEC
      female 629.89
      male 608.89
    scrotum 706.2
  semilunar cartilage (knee) (multiple)
    717.5
  seminal vesicle 608.89
  serous (ovary) 620.2
  sinus (antral) (ethmoidal) (frontal)
    (maxillary) (nasal) (sphenoidal)
    478.19
  Skene's gland 599.89
  skin (epidermal) (epidermoid, inclu-
    sion) (epithelial) (inclusion) (re-
    tention) (sebaceous) 706.2
    breast 610.8
    eyelid 374.84
    genital organ NEC
      female 629.89
      male 608.89
    neoplastic 216.3
    scrotum 706.2
    sweat gland or duct 705.89
  solitary
    bone 733.21
    kidney 593.2
  spermatic cord 608.89
  sphenoid sinus 478.19
  spinal meninges 349.2
  spine (*see also* Cyst, bone) 733.20
  spleen NEC 289.59
    congenital 759.0
    hydatid (*see also* Echinococcus)
      122.9
  spring water (pericardium) 746.89
  subarachnoid 348.0
    intrasellar 793.0
  subdural (cerebral) 348.0
    spinal cord 349.2
  sublingual gland 527.6
    mucous extravasation or retention
      527.6
  submaxillary gland 527.6
    mucous extravasation or retention
      527.6
  suburethral 599.89
  suprarenal gland 255.8
  suprasellar — *see* Cyst, brain
  sweat gland or duct 705.89
  sympathetic nervous system 337.9
  synovial 727.40
    popliteal space 727.51
  Tarlov's 355.9
  tarsal 373.2
  tendon (sheath) 727.42
  testis 608.89
  theca-lutein (ovary) 620.2
  Thornwaldt's, Tornwaldt's 478.26
  thymus (gland) 254.8
  thyroglossal (duct) (infected) (persis-
    tent) 759.2
  thyroid (gland) 246.2
    adenomatous — *see* Goiter, nodu-
      lar
    colloid (*see also* Goiter) 240.9

**Cyst** — *continued*
  thyrolingual duct (infected) (persistent)
    759.2
  tongue (mucous) 529.8
  tonsil 474.8
  tooth (dental root) 522.8
  tubo-ovarian 620.8
    inflammatory 614.1
  tunica vaginalis 608.89
  turbinate (nose) (*see also* Cyst, bone)
    733.20
  Tyson's gland (benign) (infected)
    607.89
  umbilicus 759.89
  urachus 753.7
  ureter 593.89
  ureterovesical orifice 593.89
    congenital 753.4
  urethra 599.84
  urethral gland (Cowper's) 599.89
  uterine
    ligament 620.8
      embryonic 752.11
    tube 620.8
  uterus (body) (corpus) (recurrent)
    621.8
    embryonal 752.3
  utricle (ear) 386.8
    prostatic 599.89
  utriculus masculinus 599.89
  vagina, vaginal (squamous cell) (wall)
    623.8
    embryonal 752.41
    implantation 623.8
    inclusion 623.8
  vallecula, vallecular 478.79
  ventricle, neuroepithelial 348.0
  verumontanum 599.89
  vesical (orifice) 596.8
  vitreous humor 379.29
  vulva (sweat glands) 624.8
    congenital 752.41
    implantation 624.8
    inclusion 624.8
    sebaceous gland 624.8
  vulvovaginal gland 624.8
  wolffian 752.89
**Cystadenocarcinoma** (M8440/3) — *see
  also* Neoplasm, by site, malignant
  bile duct type (M8161/3) 155.1
  endometrioid (M8380/3) — *see* Neo-
    plasm, by site, malignant
  mucinous (M8470/3)
    papillary (M8471/3)
      specified site — *see* Neoplasm,
        by site, malignant
      unspecified site 183.0
    specified site — *see* Neoplasm, by
      site, malignant
    unspecified site 183.0
  papillary (M8450/3)
    mucinous (M8471/3)
      specified site — *see* Neoplasm,
        by site, malignant
      unspecified site 183.0
    pseudomucinous (M8471/3)
      specified site — *see* Neoplasm,
        by site, malignant
      unspecified site 183.0
    serous (M8460/3)
      specified site — *see* Neoplasm,
        by site, malignant
      unspecified site 183.0
    specified site — *see* Neoplasm, by
      site, malignant
    unspecified site 183.0
  pseudomucinous (M8470/3)
    papillary (M8471/3)
      specified site — *see* Neoplasm,
        by site, malignant
      unspecified site 183.0
    specified site — *see* Neoplasm, by
      site, malignant
    unspecified site 183.0

**Cystadenocarcinoma** — *see also*
  Neoplasm, by site, malignant —
  *continued*
  serous (M8441/3)
    papillary (M8460/3)
      specified site — *see* Neoplasm,
        by site, malignant
      unspecified site 183.0
    specified site — *see* Neoplasm, by
      site, malignant
    unspecified site 183.0
**Cystadenofibroma** (M9013/0)
  clear cell (M8313/0) — *see* Neoplasm,
    by site, benign
  endometrioid (M8381/0) 220
    borderline malignancy (M8381/1)
      236.2
    malignant (M8381/3) 183.0
  mucinous (M9015/0)
    specified site — *see* Neoplasm, by
      site, benign
    unspecified site 220
  serous (M9014/0)
    specified site — *see* Neoplasm, by
      site, benign
    unspecified site 220
  specified site — *see* Neoplasm, by site,
    benign
  unspecified site 220
**Cystadenoma** (M8440/0) — *see also*
  Neoplasm, by site, benign
  bile duct (M8161/0) 211.5
  endometrioid (M8380/0) (*see also*
    Neoplasm, by site, benign)
    borderline malignancy (M8380/1)
      — *see* Neoplasm, by site,
      uncertain behavior
    malignant (M8440/3) — *see* Neo-
      plasm, by site, malignant
  mucinous (M8470/0)
    borderline malignancy (M8470/1)
      specified site — *see* Neoplasm,
        uncertain behavior
      unspecified site 236.2
    papillary (M8471/0)
      borderline malignancy
        (M8471/1)
        specified site — *see* Neo-
          plasm, by site, uncer-
          tain behavior
        unspecified site 236.2
      specified site — *see* Neoplasm,
        by site, benign
      unspecified site 220
    specified site — *see* Neoplasm, by
      site, benign
    unspecified site 220
  papillary (M8450/0)
    borderline malignancy (M8450/1)
      specified site — *see* Neoplasm,
        by site, uncertain behav-
        ior
      unspecified site 236.2
    lymphomatosum (M8561/0) 210.2
    mucinous (M8471/0)
      borderline malignancy
        (M8471/1)
        specified site — *see* Neo-
          plasm, by site, uncer-
          tain behavior
        unspecified site 236.2
      specified site — *see* Neoplasm,
        by site, benign
      unspecified site 220
    pseudomucinous (M8471/0)
      borderline malignancy
        (M8471/1)
        specified site — *see* Neo-
          plasm, by site, uncer-
          tain behavior
        unspecified site 236.2
      specified site — *see* Neoplasm,
        by site, benign
      unspecified site 220

☑ Additional Digit Required — Refer to the Tabular List for Digit Selection
*2008 ICD-9-CM*
▶◀ Revised Text
● New Line
▲ Revised Code
〰 Subterms under main terms may continue to next column or page
Volume 2 — 63

## Cystadenoma

Cystadenoma — *see also* Neoplasm, by site, benign — *continued*
   papillary — *continued*
      serous (M8460/0)
         borderline malignancy (M8460/1)
            specified site — *see* Neoplasm, by site, uncertain behavior
            unspecified site 236.2
         specified site — *see* Neoplasm, by site, benign
         unspecified site 220
      specified site — *see* Neoplasm, by site, benign
      unspecified site 220
   pseudomucinous (M8470/0)
      borderline malignancy (M8470/1)
         specified site — *see* Neoplasm, by site, uncertain behavior
         unspecified site 236.2
      papillary (M8471/0)
         borderline malignancy (M8471/1)
            specified site — *see* Neoplasm, by site, uncertain behavior
            unspecified site 236.2
         specified site — *see* Neoplasm, by site, benign
         unspecified site 220
      specified site — *see* Neoplasm, by site, benign
      unspecified site 220
   serous (M8441/0)
      borderline malignancy (M8441/1)
         specified site — *see* Neoplasm, by site, uncertain behavior
         unspecified site 236.2
      papillary (M8460/0)
         borderline malignancy (M8460/1)
            specified site — *see* Neoplasm, by site, uncertain behavior
            unspecified site 236.2
         specified site — *see* Neoplasm, by site, benign
         unspecified site 220
      specified site — *see* Neoplasm, by site, benign
      unspecified site 220
   thyroid 226
Cystathioninemia 270.4
Cystathioninuria 270.4
Cystic — *see also* condition
   breast, chronic 610.1
   corpora lutea 620.1
   degeneration, congenital
      brain 742.4
      kidney (*see also* Cystic, disease, kidney) 753.10

Cystic — *see also* condition — *continued*
   disease
      breast, chronic 610.1
      kidney, congenital 753.10
         medullary 753.16
         multiple 753.19
         polycystic — *see* Polycystic, kidney
         single 753.11
         specified NEC 753.19
      liver, congenital 751.62
      lung 518.89
         congenital 748.4
      pancreas, congenital 751.7
      semilunar cartilage 717.5
   duct — *see* condition
   eyeball, congenital 743.03
   fibrosis (pancreas) 277.00
      with
         manifestations
            gastrointestinal 277.03
            pulmonary 277.02
            specified NEC 277.09
         meconium ileus 277.01
         pulmonary exacerbation 277.02
   hygroma (M9173/0) 228.1
   kidney, congenital 753.10
      medullary 753.16
      multiple 753.19
      polycystic — *see* Polycystic, kidney
      single 753.11
      specified NEC 753.19
   liver, congenital 751.62
   lung 518.89
      congenital 748.4
   mass — *see* Cyst
   mastitis, chronic 610.1
   ovary 620.2
   pancreas, congenital 751.7
Cysticerciasis 123.1
Cysticercosis (mammary) (subretinal) 123.1
Cysticercus 123.1
   cellulosae infestation 123.1
Cystinosis (malignant) 270.0
Cystinuria 270.0
Cystitis (bacillary) (colli) (diffuse) (exudative) (hemorrhagic) (purulent) (recurrent) (septic) (suppurative) (ulcerative) 595.9
   with
      abortion — *see* Abortion, by type, with urinary tract infection
      ectopic pregnancy (*see also* categories 633.0–633.9) 639.8
      fibrosis 595.1
      leukoplakia 595.1
      malakoplakia 595.1
      metaplasia 595.1
      molar pregnancy (*see also* categories 630–632) 639.8
   actinomycotic 039.8 *[595.4]*
   acute 595.0

Cystitis — *continued*
   acute — *continued*
      of trigone 595.3
   allergic 595.89
   amebic 006.8 *[595.4]*
   bilharzial 120.9 *[595.4]*
   blennorrhagic (acute) 098.11
      chronic or duration of 2 months or more 098.31
   bullous 595.89
   calculous 594.1
      chlamydial 099.53
   chronic 595.2
      interstitial 595.1
      of trigone 595.3
   complicating pregnancy, childbirth, or puerperium 646.6 ☑
      affecting fetus or newborn 760.1
   cystic(a) 595.81
   diphtheritic 032.84
   echinococcal
      granulosus 122.3 *[595.4]*
      multilocularis 122.6 *[595.4]*
   emphysematous 595.89
   encysted 595.81
   follicular 595.3
   following
      abortion 639.8
      ectopic or molar pregnancy 639.8
   gangrenous 595.89
   glandularis 595.89
   gonococcal (acute) 098.11
      chronic or duration of 2 months or more 098.31
   incrusted 595.89
   interstitial 595.1
   irradiation 595.82
   irritation 595.89
   malignant 595.89
   monilial 112.2
   of trigone 595.3
   panmural 595.1
   polyposa 595.89
   prostatic 601.3
   radiation 595.82
   Reiter's (abacterial) 099.3
   specified NEC 595.89
   subacute 595.2
   submucous 595.1
   syphilitic 095.8
   trichomoniasis 131.09
   tuberculous (*see also* Tuberculosis) 016.1 ☑
   ulcerative 595.1
Cystocele
   female (without uterine prolapse) 618.01
      with uterine prolapse 618.4
         complete 618.3
         incomplete 618.2
      lateral 618.02
      midline 618.01
      paravaginal 618.02
   in pregnancy or childbirth 654.4 ☑

Cystocele — *continued*
   in pregnancy or childbirth — *continued*
      affecting fetus or newborn 763.89
      causing obstructed labor 660.2 ☑
         affecting fetus or newborn 763.1
   male 596.8
Cystoid
   cicatrix limbus 372.64
   degeneration macula 362.53
Cystolithiasis 594.1
Cystoma (M8440/0) — *see also* Neoplasm, by site, benign
   endometrial, ovary 617.1
   mucinous (M8470/0)
      specified site — *see* Neoplasm, by site, benign
      unspecified site 220
   serous (M8470/0)
      specified site — *see* Neoplasm, by site, benign
      unspecified site 220
   simple (ovary) 620.2
Cystoplegia 596.53
Cystoptosis 596.8
Cystopyelitis — *see also* Pyelitis 590.80
Cystorrhagia 596.8
Cystosarcoma phyllodes (M9020/1) 238.3
   benign (M9020/0) 217
   malignant (M9020/3) — *see* Neoplasm, breast, malignant
Cystostomy status V44.50
   with complication 997.5
   appendico-vesicostomy V44.52
   cutaneous-vesicostomy V44.51
   specified type NEC V44.59
Cystourethritis — *see also* Urethritis 597.89
Cystourethrocele — *see also* Cystocele
   female (without uterine prolapse) 618.09
      with uterine prolapse 618.4
         complete 618.3
         incomplete 618.2
   male 596.8
Cytomegalic inclusion disease 078.5
   congenital 771.1
Cytomycosis, reticuloendothelial — *see also* Histoplasmosis, American 115.00
Cytopenia 289.9
   refractory
      with
         multilineage dysplasia (RCMD) 238.72
         and ringed sideroblasts (RCMD-RS) 238.72

Cystadenoma — Cytopenia

**D**

**Daae (-Finsen) disease** (epidemic pleurodynia) 074.1
**Dabney's grip** 074.1
**Da Costa's syndrome** (neurocirculatory asthenia) 306.2
**Dacryoadenitis, dacryadenitis** 375.00
  acute 375.01
  chronic 375.02
**Dacryocystitis** 375.30
  acute 375.32
  chronic 375.42
  neonatal 771.6
  phlegmonous 375.33
  syphilitic 095.8
    congenital 090.0
  trachomatous, active 076.1
    late effect 139.1
  tuberculous (see also Tuberculosis) 017.3 ☑
**Dacryocystoblenorrhea** 375.42
**Dacryocystocele** 375.43
**Dacryolith, dacryolithiasis** 375.57
**Dacryoma** 375.43
**Dacryopericystitis** (acute) (subacute) 375.32
  chronic 375.42
**Dacryops** 375.11
**Dacryosialadenopathy, atrophic** 710.2
**Dacryostenosis** 375.56
  congenital 743.65
**Dactylitis**
  bone (see also Osteomyelitis) 730.2 ☑
  sickle-cell 282.62
    Hb-C 282.64
    Hb-SS 282.62
    specified NEC 282.69
  syphilitic 095.5
  tuberculous (see also Tuberculosis) 015.5 ☑
**Dactylolysis spontanea** 136.0
**Dactylosymphysis** — see also Syndactylism 755.10
**Damage**
  arteriosclerotic — see Arteriosclerosis
  brain 348.9
    anoxic, hypoxic 348.1
      during or resulting from a procedure 997.01
      ischemic, in newborn 768.7
    child NEC 343.9
    due to birth injury 767.0
    minimal (child) (see also Hyperkinesia) 314.9
    newborn 767.0
  cardiac (see also Disease, heart)
  cardiorenal (vascular) (see also Hypertension, cardiorenal) 404.90
  central nervous system — see Damage, brain
  cerebral NEC — see Damage, brain
  coccyx, complicating delivery 665.6 ☑
  coronary (see also Ischemia, heart) 414.9
  eye, birth injury 767.8
  heart (see also Disease, heart)
    valve — see Endocarditis
  hypothalamus NEC 348.9
  liver 571.9
    alcoholic 571.3
  medication 995.20
  myocardium (see also Degeneration, myocardial) 429.1
  pelvic
    joint or ligament, during delivery 665.6 ☑
    organ NEC
      with
        abortion — see Abortion, by type, with damage to pelvic organs
        ectopic pregnancy (see also categories 633.0–633.9) 639.2

**Damage** — continued
  pelvic — continued
    organ — continued
      with — continued
        molar pregnancy (see also categories 630–632) 639.2
      during delivery 665.5 ☑
      following
        abortion 639.2
        ectopic or molar pregnancy 639.2
  renal (see also Disease, renal) 593.9
  skin, solar 692.79
    acute 692.72
    chronic 692.74
  subendocardium, subendocardial (see also Degeneration, myocardial) 429.1
  vascular 459.9
**Dameshek's syndrome** (erythroblastic anemia) 282.49
**Dana-Putnam syndrome** (subacute combined sclerosis with pernicious anemia) 281.0 [336.2]
**Danbolt (-Closs) syndrome** (acrodermatitis enteropathica) 686.8
**Dandruff** 690.18
**Dandy fever** 061
**Dandy-Walker deformity or syndrome** (atresia, foramen of Magendie) 742.3
  with spina bifida (see also Spina bifida) 741.0 ☑
**Dangle foot** 736.79
**Danielssen's disease** (anesthetic leprosy) 030.1
**Danlos' syndrome** 756.83
**Darier's disease** (congenital) (keratosis follicularis) 757.39
  due to vitamin A deficiency 264.8
  meaning erythema annulare centrifugum 695.0
**Darier-Roussy sarcoid** 135
**Darling's**
  disease (see also Histoplasmosis, American) 115.00
  histoplasmosis (see also Histoplasmosis, American) 115.00
**Dartre** 054.9
**Darwin's tubercle** 744.29
**Davidson's anemia** (refractory) 284.9
**Davies-Colley syndrome** (slipping rib) 733.99
**Davies' disease** 425.0
**Dawson's encephalitis** 046.2
**Day blindness** — see also Blindness, day 368.60
**Dead**
  fetus
    retained (in utero) 656.4 ☑
      early pregnancy (death before 22 completed weeks gestation) 632
      late (death after 22 completed weeks gestation) 656.4 ☑
    syndrome 641.3 ☑
  labyrinth 386.50
  ovum, retained 631
**Deaf and dumb** NEC 389.7
**Deaf mutism** (acquired) (congenital) NEC 389.7
  endemic 243
  hysterical 300.11
  syphilitic, congenital 090.0
**Deafness** (acquired) (complete) (congenital) (hereditary) (middle ear) (partial) 389.9
  with
    blindness V49.85
    blue sclera and fragility of bone 756.51
  auditory fatigue 389.9
  aviation 993.0
    nerve injury 951.5
  boilermakers' 951.5

**Deafness** — continued
  central 389.14
    with conductive hearing loss 389.20 ▲
      bilateral 389.22 ●
      unilateral 389.21 ●
  conductive (air) 389.00
    with sensorineural hearing loss 389.20 ▲
      bilateral 389.22 ●
      unilateral 389.21 ●
    bilateral 389.06 ●
    combined types 389.08
    external ear 389.01
    inner ear 389.04
    middle ear 389.03
    multiple types 389.08
    tympanic membrane 389.02
    unilateral 389.05 ●
  emotional (complete) 300.11
  functional (complete) 300.11
  high frequency 389.8
  hysterical (complete) 300.11
  injury 951.5
  low frequency 389.8
  mental 784.69
  mixed conductive and sensorineural 389.20 ▲
    bilateral 389.22 ●
    unilateral 389.21 ●
  nerve
    with conductive hearing loss 389.20 ▲
      bilateral 389.22 ●
      unilateral 389.21 ●
    bilateral 389.12 ●
    unilateral 389.13 ●
  neural
    with conductive hearing loss 389.20 ▲
      bilateral 389.22 ●
      unilateral 389.21 ●
    bilateral 389.12 ●
    unilateral 389.13 ●
  noise-induced 388.12
    nerve injury 951.5
  nonspeaking 389.7
  perceptive 389.10
    with conductive hearing loss 389.20 ▲
      bilateral 389.22 ●
      unilateral 389.21 ●
    central 389.14
    neural
      bilateral 389.12 ●
      unilateral 389.13 ●
    sensorineural 389.10
      asymmetrical 389.16
      bilateral 389.18
      unilateral 389.15
    sensory
      bilateral 389.11
      unilateral 389.17 ●
  psychogenic (complete) 306.7
  sensorineural (see also Deafness, perceptive) 389.10
    asymmetrical 389.16
    bilateral 389.18
    unilateral 389.15
  sensory
    with conductive hearing loss 389.20 ▲
      bilateral 389.22 ●
      unilateral 389.21 ●
    bilateral 389.11 ●
    unilateral 389.17 ●
  specified type NEC 389.8
  sudden NEC 388.2
  syphilitic 094.89
  transient ischemic 388.02
  transmission — see Deafness, conductive
  traumatic 951.5
  word (secondary to organic lesion) 784.69
    developmental 315.31

**Death**
  after delivery (cause not stated) (sudden) 674.9 ☑
  anesthetic
    due to
      correct substance properly administered 995.4
      overdose or wrong substance given 968.4
      specified anesthetic — see Table of Drugs and Chemicals
    during delivery 668.9 ☑
  brain 348.8
  cardiac ▶(sudden) (SCD)◀ — code to underlying condition◀
    family history of V17.41 ●
    personal history of, successfully ● resuscitated V12.53
  cause unknown 798.2
  cot (infant) 798.0
  crib (infant) 798.0
  fetus, fetal (cause not stated) (intrauterine) 779.9
    early, with retention (before 22 completed weeks gestation) 632
    from asphyxia or anoxia (before labor) 768.0
      during labor 768.1
    late, affecting management of pregnancy (after 22 completed weeks gestation) 656.4 ☑
  from pregnancy NEC 646.9 ☑
  instantaneous 798.1
  intrauterine (see also Death, fetus) 779.9
    complicating pregnancy 656.4 ☑
  maternal, affecting fetus or newborn 761.6
  neonatal NEC 779.9
  sudden (cause unknown) 798.1
    cardiac (SCD) ●
      family history of V17.41 ●
      personal history of, successfully resuscitated V12.53 ●
    during delivery 669.9 ☑
      under anesthesia NEC 668.9 ☑
    infant, syndrome (SIDS) 798.0
    puerperal, during puerperium 674.9 ☑
  unattended (cause unknown) 798.9
  under anesthesia NEC
    due to
      correct substance properly administered 995.4
      overdose or wrong substance given 968.4
      specified anesthetic — see Table of Drugs and Chemicals
    during delivery 668.9 ☑
  violent 798.1
**de Beurmann-Gougerot disease** (sporotrichosis) 117.1
**Debility** (general) (infantile) (postinfectional) 799.3
  with nutritional difficulty 269.9
  congenital or neonatal NEC 779.9
  nervous 300.5
  old age 797
  senile 797
**Débove's disease** (splenomegaly) 789.2
**Decalcification**
  bone (see also Osteoporosis) 733.00
  teeth 521.89
**Decapitation** 874.9
  fetal (to facilitate delivery) 763.89
**Decapsulation, kidney** 593.89
**Decay**
  dental 521.00
  senile 797
  tooth, teeth 521.00
**Decensus, uterus** — see Prolapse, uterus

**Deciduitis** (acute)
with
  abortion — *see* Abortion, by type, with sepsis
  ectopic pregnancy (*see also* categories 633.0–633.9) 639.0
  molar pregnancy (*see also* categories 630–632) 639.0
  affecting fetus or newborn 760.8
  following
    abortion 639.0
    ectopic or molar pregnancy 639.0
  in pregnancy 646.6 ☑
  puerperal, postpartum 670.0 ☑
**Deciduoma malignum** (M9100/3) 181
**Deciduous tooth** (retained) 520.6
**Decline** (general) — *see also* Debility 799.3
**Decompensation**
  cardiac (acute) (chronic) (*see also* Disease, heart) 429.9
    failure — *see* Failure, heart
  cardiorenal (*see also* Hypertension, cardiorenal) 404.90
  cardiovascular (*see also* Disease, cardiovascular) 429.2
  heart (*see also* Disease, heart) 429.9
    failure — *see* Failure, heart
  hepatic 572.2
  myocardial (acute) (chronic) (*see also* Disease, heart) 429.9
    failure — *see* Failure, heart
  respiratory 519.9
**Decompression sickness** 993.3
**Decrease, decreased**
  blood
    platelets (*see also* Thrombocytopenia) 287.5
    pressure 796.3
      due to shock following
        injury 958.4
        operation 998.0
    white cell count 288.50
      specified NEC 288.59
  cardiac reserve — *see* Disease, heart
  estrogen 256.39
    postablative 256.2
  fetal movements 655.7 ☑
  fragility of erythrocytes 289.89
  function
    adrenal (cortex) 255.41
      medulla 255.5
    ovary in hypopituitarism 253.4
    parenchyma of pancreas 577.8
    pituitary (gland) (lobe) (anterior) 253.2
      posterior (lobe) 253.8
  functional activity 780.99
  glucose 790.29
  haptoglobin (serum) NEC 273.8
  leukocytes 288.50
  libido 799.81
  lymphocytes 288.51
  platelets (*see also* Thrombocytopenia) 287.5
  pulse pressure 785.9
  respiration due to shock following injury 958.4
  sexual desire 799.81
  tear secretion NEC 375.15
  tolerance
    fat 579.8
    salt and water 276.9
  vision NEC 369.9
  white blood cell count 288.50
**Decubital gangrene** 707.00 [785.4]
**Decubiti** — *see also* Decubitus 707.00
**Decubitus** (ulcer) 707.00
  with gangrene 707.00 [785.4]
  ankle 707.06
  back
    lower 707.03
    upper 707.02
  buttock 707.05
  elbow 707.01
  head 707.09

**Decubitus** — *continued*
  heel 707.07
  hip 707.04
  other site 707.09
  sacrum 707.03
  shoulder blades 707.02
**Deepening acetabulum** 718.85
**Defect, defective** 759.9
  3-beta-hydroxysteroid dehydrogenase 255.2
  11-hydroxylase 255.2
  21-hydroxylase 255.2
  abdominal wall, congenital 756.70
  aorticopulmonary septum 745.0
  aortic septal 745.0
  atrial septal (ostium secundum type) 745.5
    acquired 429.71
    ostium primum type 745.61
    sinus venosus 745.8
  atrioventricular
    canal 745.69
    septum 745.4
      acquired 429.71
  atrium secundum 745.5
    acquired 429.71
  auricular septal 745.5
    acquired 429.71
  bilirubin excretion 277.4
  biosynthesis, testicular androgen 257.2
  bridge 525.60
  bulbar septum 745.0
  butanol-insoluble iodide 246.1
  chromosome — *see* Anomaly, chromosome
  circulation (acquired) 459.9
    congenital 747.9
    newborn 747.9
  clotting NEC (*see also* Defect, coagulation) 286.9
  coagulation (factor) (*see also* Deficiency, coagulation factor) 286.9
    with
      abortion — *see* Abortion, by type, with hemorrhage
      ectopic pregnancy (*see also* categories 634–638) 639.1
      molar pregnancy (*see also* categories 630–632) 639.1
    acquired (any) 286.7
    antepartum or intrapartum 641.3 ☑
      affecting fetus or newborn 762.1
    causing hemorrhage of pregnancy or delivery 641.3 ☑
    complicating pregnancy, childbirth, or puerperium 649.3 ☑
    due to
      liver disease 286.7
      vitamin K deficiency 286.7
    newborn, transient 776.3
    postpartum 666.3 ☑
    specified type NEC 286.9 ▲
  conduction (heart) 426.9
    bone (*see also* Deafness, conductive) 389.00
  congenital, organ or site NEC (*see also* Anomaly)
    circulation 747.9
    Descemet's membrane 743.9
      specified type NEC 743.49
    diaphragm 756.6
    ectodermal 757.9
    esophagus 750.9
    pulmonic cusps — *see* Anomaly, heart valve
    respiratory system 748.9
      specified type NEC 748.8
  crown 525.60
  cushion endocardial 745.60
  dental restoration 525.60
  dentin (hereditary) 520.5
  Descemet's membrane (congenital) 743.9
    acquired 371.30

**Defect, defective** — *continued*
  Descemet's membrane — *continued*
    specific type NEC 743.49
  deutan 368.52
  developmental (*see also* Anomaly, by site)
    cauda equina 742.59
    left ventricle 746.9
      with atresia or hypoplasia of aortic orifice or valve, with hypoplasia of ascending aorta 746.7
      in hypoplastic left heart syndrome 746.7
    testis 752.9
    vessel 747.9
  diaphragm
    with elevation, eventration, or hernia — *see* Hernia, diaphragm
    congenital 756.6
      with elevation, eventration, or hernia 756.6
      gross (with elevation, eventration, or hernia) 756.6
  ectodermal, congenital 757.9
  Eisenmenger's (ventricular septal defect) 745.4
  endocardial cushion 745.60
    specified type NEC 745.69
  esophagus, congenital 750.9
  extensor retinaculum 728.9
  fibrin polymerization (*see also* Defect, coagulation) 286.3
  filling
    biliary tract 793.3
    bladder 793.5
    dental 525.60
    gallbladder 793.3
    kidney 793.5
    stomach 793.4
    ureter 793.5
  fossa ovalis 745.5
  gene, carrier (suspected) of V83.89
  Gerbode 745.4
  glaucomatous, without elevated tension 365.89
  Hageman (factor) (*see also* Defect, coagulation) 286.3
  hearing (*see also* Deafness) 389.9
  high grade 317
  homogentisic acid 270.2
  interatrial septal 745.5
    acquired 429.71
  interauricular septal 745.5
    acquired 429.71
  interventricular septal 745.4
    with pulmonary stenosis or atresia, dextraposition of aorta, and hypertrophy of right ventricle 745.2
    acquired 429.71
    in tetralogy of Fallot 745.2
  iodide trapping 246.1
  iodotyrosine dehalogenase 246.1
  kynureninase 270.2
  learning, specific 315.2
  major osseous 731.3
  mental (*see also* Retardation, mental) 319
  osseous, major 731.3
  osteochondral NEC 738.8
  ostium
    primum 745.61
    secundum 745.5
  pericardium 746.89
  peroxidase-binding 246.1
  placental blood supply — *see* Placenta, insufficiency
  platelet (qualitative) 287.1
    constitutional 286.4
  postural, spine 737.9
  protan 368.51
  pulmonic cusps, congenital 746.00
  renal pelvis 753.9
    obstructive 753.29

**Defect, defective** — *continued*
  renal pelvis — *continued*
    specified type NEC 753.3
  respiratory system, congenital 748.9
    specified type NEC 748.8
  retina, retinal 361.30
    with detachment (*see also* Detachment, retina, with retinal defect) 361.00
    multiple 361.33
      with detachment 361.02
    nerve fiber bundle 362.85
    single 361.30
      with detachment 361.01
  septal (closure) (heart) NEC 745.9
    acquired 429.71
    atrial 745.5
    specified type NEC 745.8
  speech NEC 784.5
    developmental 315.39
    secondary to organic lesion 784.5
  Taussig-Bing (transposition, aorta and overriding pulmonary artery) 745.11
  teeth, wedge 521.20
  thyroid hormone synthesis 246.1
  tritan 368.53
  ureter 753.9
    obstructive 753.29
  vascular (acquired) (local) 459.9
    congenital (peripheral) NEC 747.60
      gastrointestinal 747.61
      lower limb 747.64
      renal 747.62
      specified NEC 747.69
      spinal 747.82
      upper limb 747.63
  ventricular septal 745.4
    with pulmonary stenosis or atresia, dextraposition of aorta, and hypertrophy of right ventricle 745.2
    acquired 429.71
    atrioventricular canal type 745.69
    between infundibulum and anterior portion 745.4
    in tetralogy of Fallot 745.2
    isolated anterior 745.4
  vision NEC 369.9
  visual field 368.40
    arcuate 368.43
    heteronymous, bilateral 368.47
    homonymous, bilateral 368.46
    localized NEC 368.44
    nasal step 368.44
    peripheral 368.44
    sector 368.43
  voice 784.40
  wedge, teeth (abrasion) 521.20
**Defeminization syndrome** 255.2
**Deferentitis** 608.4
  gonorrheal (acute) 098.14
    chronic or duration of 2 months or over 098.34
**Defibrination syndrome** — *see also* Fibrinolysis 286.6
**Deficiency, deficient**
  3-beta-hydroxysteroid dehydrogenase 255.2
  6-phosphogluconic dehydrogenase (anemia) 282.2
  11-beta-hydroxylase 255.2
  17-alpha-hydroxylase 255.2
  18-hydroxysteroid dehydrogenase 255.2
  20-alpha-hydroxylase 255.2
  21-hydroxylase 255.2
  AAT (alpha-1 antitrypsin) 273.4
  abdominal muscle syndrome 756.79
  accelerator globulin (Ac G) (blood) (*see also* Defect, coagulation) 286.3
  AC globulin (congenital) (*see also* Defect, coagulation) 286.3
    acquired 286.7
  activating factor (blood) (*see also* Defect, coagulation) 286.3

**Deficiency, deficient** — *continued*
  adenohypophyseal 253.2
  adenosine deaminase 277.2
  aldolase (hereditary) 271.2
  alpha-1-antitrypsin 273.4
  alpha-1-trypsin inhibitor 273.4
  alpha-fucosidase 271.8
  alpha-lipoprotein 272.5
  alpha-mannosidase 271.8
  amino acid 270.9
  anemia — *see* Anemia, deficiency
  aneurin 265.1
      with beriberi 265.0
  antibody NEC 279.00
  antidiuretic hormone 253.5
  antihemophilic
      factor (A) 286.0
        B 286.1
        C 286.2
      globulin (AHG) NEC 286.0
  antithrombin III 289.81
  antitrypsin 273.4
  argininosuccinate synthetase or lyase
      270.6
  ascorbic acid (with scurvy) 267
  autoprothrombin
      I (*see also* Defect, coagulation)
          286.3
      II 286.1
      C (*see also* Defect, coagulation)
          286.3
  bile salt 579.8
  biotin 266.2
  biotinidase 277.6
  bradykinase-1 277.6
  brancher enzyme (amylopectinosis)
      271.0
  calciferol 268.9
      with
          osteomalacia 268.2
          rickets (*see also* Rickets) 268.0
  calcium 275.40
      dietary 269.3
  calorie, severe 261
  carbamyl phosphate synthetase 270.6
  cardiac (*see also* Insufficiency, myocar-
      dial) 428.0
  carnitine 277.81
      due to
          hemodialysis 277.83
          inborn errors of metabolism
              277.82
          valproic acid therapy 277.83
      iatrogenic 277.83
      palmitoyltransferase (CPT1, CPT2)
          277.85
      palmityl transferase (CPT1, CPT2)
          277.85
      primary 277.81
      secondary 277.84
  carotene 264.9
  Carr factor (*see also* Defect, coagula-
      tion) 286.9
  central nervous system 349.9
  ceruloplasmin 275.1
  cevitamic acid (with scurvy) 267
  choline 266.2
  Christmas factor 286.1
  chromium 269.3
  citrin 269.1
  clotting (blood) (*see also* Defect, coag-
      ulation) 286.9
  coagulation factor NEC 286.9
      with
          abortion — *see* Abortion, by
              type, with hemorrhage
          ectopic pregnancy (*see also* cat-
              egories 634–638) 639.1
          molar pregnancy (*see also* cate-
              gories 630–632) 639.1
      acquired (any) 286.7
      antepartum or intrapartum
          641.3 ☑
          affecting fetus or newborn 762.1
      complicating pregnancy, childbirth,
          or puerperium 649.3 ☑

**Deficiency, deficient** — *continued*
  coagulation factor — *continued*
      due to
          liver disease 286.7
          vitamin K deficiency 286.7
      newborn, transient 776.3
      postpartum 666.3 ☑
      specified type NEC 286.3
  color vision (congenital) 368.59
      acquired 368.55
  combined glucocorticoid and miner-●
      alocorticoid 255.41 ●
  combined, two or more coagulation
      factors (*see also* Defect, coagula-
      tion) 286.9
  complement factor NEC 279.8
  contact factor (*see also* Defect, coagu-
      lation) 286.3
  copper NEC 275.1
  corticoadrenal 255.41                    ▲
  craniofacial axis 756.0
  cyanocobalamin (vitamin B₁₂) 266.2
  debrancher enzyme (limit dextrinosis)
      271.0
  desmolase 255.2
  diet 269.9
  dihydrofolate reductase 281.2
  dihydropteridine reductase 270.1
  disaccharidase (intestinal) 271.3
  disease NEC 269.9
  ear(s) V48.8
  edema 262
  endocrine 259.9
  enzymes, circulating NEC (*see also*
      Deficiency, by specific enzyme)
      277.6
  ergosterol 268.9
      with
          osteomalacia 268.2
          rickets (*see also* Rickets) 268.0
  erythrocytic glutathione (anemia)
      282.2
  eyelid(s) V48.8
  factor (*see also* Defect, coagulation)
      286.9
      I (congenital) (fibrinogen) 286.3
          antepartum or intrapartum
              641.3 ☑
              affecting fetus or newborn
                  762.1
          newborn, transient 776.3
          postpartum 666.3 ☑
      II (congenital) (prothrombin) 286.3
      V (congenital) (labile) 286.3
      VII (congenital) (stable) 286.3
      VIII (congenital) (functional) 286.0
          with
              functional defect 286.0
              vascular defect 286.4
      IX (Christmas) (congenital) (func-
          tional) 286.1
      X (congenital) (Stuart-Prower)
          286.3
      XI (congenital) (plasma thrombo-
          plastin antecedent) 286.2
      XII (congenital) (Hageman) 286.3
      XIII (congenital) (fibrin stabilizing)
          286.3
      Hageman 286.3
      multiple (congenital) 286.9
          acquired 286.7
  fibrinase (*see also* Defect, coagulation)
      286.3
  fibrinogen (congenital) (*see also* De-
      fect, coagulation) 286.3
      acquired 286.6
  fibrin-stabilizing factor (congenital)
      (*see also* Defect, coagulation)
      286.3
  finger — *see* Absence, finger
  fletcher factor (*see also* Defect, coagu-
      lation) 286.9
  fluorine 269.3
  folate, anemia 281.2
  folic acid (vitamin B꜀) 266.2
      anemia 281.2

**Deficiency, deficient** — *continued*
  follicle-stimulating hormone (FSH)
      253.4
  fructokinase 271.2
  fructose-1, 6-diphosphate 271.2
  fructose-1-phosphate aldolase 271.2
  FSH (follicle-stimulating hormone)
      253.4
  fucosidase 271.8
  galactokinase 271.1
  galactose-1-phosphate uridyl trans-
      ferase 271.1
  gamma globulin in blood 279.00
  glass factor (*see also* Defect, coagula-
      tion) 286.3
  glucocorticoid 255.41                    ▲
  glucose-6-phosphatase 271.0
  glucose-6-phosphate dehydrogenase
      anemia 282.2
  glucuronyl transferase 277.4
  glutathione-reductase (anemia) 282.2
  glycogen synthetase 271.0
  growth hormone 253.3
  Hageman factor (congenital) (*see also*
      Defect, coagulation) 286.3
  head V48.0
  hemoglobin (*see also* Anemia) 285.9
  hepatophosphorylase 271.0
  hexose monophosphate (HMP) shunt
      282.2
  HGH (human growth hormone) 253.3
  HG-PRT 277.2
  homogentisic acid oxidase 270.2
  hormone (*see also* Deficiency, by spe-
      cific hormone)
      anterior pituitary (isolated) (partial)
          NEC 253.4
          growth (human) 253.3
      follicle-stimulating 253.4
      growth (human) (isolated) 253.3
      human growth 253.3
      interstitial cell-stimulating 253.4
      luteinizing 253.4
      melanocyte-stimulating 253.4
      testicular 257.2
  human growth hormone 253.3
  humoral 279.00
      with
          hyper-IgM 279.05
              autosomal recessive 279.05
              X-linked 279.05
          increased IgM 279.05
      congenital hypogammaglobuline-
          mia 279.04
      non-sex-linked 279.06
      selective immunoglobulin NEC
          279.03
          IgA 279.01
          IgG 279.03
          IgM 279.02
              increased 279.05
      specified NEC 279.09
  hydroxylase 255.2
  hypoxanthine-guanine phosphoribo-
      syltransferase (HG-PRT) 277.2
  ICSH (interstitial cell-stimulating
      hormone) 253.4
  immunity NEC 279.3
      cell-mediated 279.10
          with
              hyperimmunoglobulinemia
                  279.2
              thrombocytopenia and
                  eczema 279.12
          specified NEC 279.19
      combined (severe) 279.2
          syndrome 279.2
      common variable 279.06
      humoral NEC 279.00
      IgA (secretory) 279.01
      IgG 279.03
      IgM 279.02
  immunoglobulin, selective NEC
      279.03
      IgA 279.01
      IgG 279.03

**Deficiency, deficient** — *continued*
  immunoglobulin, selective — *contin-*
      *ued*
      IgM 279.02
  inositol (B complex) 266.2
  interferon 279.4
  internal organ V47.0
  interstitial cell-stimulating hormone
      (ICSH) 253.4
  intrinsic factor (Castle's) (congenital)
      281.0
  intrinsic (urethral) sphincter (ISD)
      599.82
  invertase 271.3
  iodine 269.3
  iron, anemia 280.9
  labile factor (congenital) (*see also* De-
      fect, coagulation) 286.3
      acquired 286.7
  lacrimal fluid (acquired) 375.15
      congenital 743.64
  lactase 271.3
  Laki-Lorand factor (*see also* Defect,
      coagulation) 286.3
  lecithin-cholesterol acyltranferase
      272.5
  LH (luteinizing hormone) 253.4
  limb V49.0
      lower V49.0
          congenital (*see also* Deficiency,
              lower limb, congenital)
              755.30
      upper V49.0
          congenital (*see also* Deficiency,
              upper limb, congenital)
              755.20
  lipocaic 577.8
  lipoid (high-density) 272.5
  lipoprotein (familial) (high density)
      272.5
  liver phosphorylase 271.0
  long chain 3-hydroxyacyl CoA dehydro-
      genase (LCHAD) 277.85
  long chain/very long chain acyl CoA
      dehydrogenase (LCAD, VLCAD)
      277.85
  lower limb V49.0
      congenital 755.30
          with complete absence of distal
              elements 755.31
          longitudinal (complete) (partial)
              (with distal deficiencies,
              incomplete) 755.32
              with complete absence of
                  distal elements 755.31
              combined femoral, tibial,
                  fibular (incomplete)
                  755.33
              femoral 755.34
              fibular 755.37
              metatarsal(s) 755.38
              phalange(s) 755.39
                  meaning all digits 755.31
              tarsal(s) 755.38
              tibia 755.36
              tibiofibular 755.35
          transverse 755.31
  luteinizing hormone (LH) 253.4
  lysosomal alpha-1, 4 glucosidase
      271.0
  magnesium 275.2
  mannosidase 271.8
  medium chain acyl CoA dehydroge-
      nase (MCAD) 277.85
  melanocyte-stimulating hormone
      (MSH) 253.4
  menadione (vitamin K) 269.0
      newborn 776.0
  mental (familial) (hereditary) (*see also*
      Retardation, mental) 319
  methylenetetrahydrofolate reductase●
      (MTHFR) 270.4                        ●
  mineral NEC 269.3
  mineralocorticoid 255.42                ●
  molybdenum 269.3
  moral 301.7

☑ Additional Digit Required — Refer to the Tabular List for Digit Selection          ▽ Subterms under main terms may continue to next column or page

*2008 ICD-9-CM*          ▶◀ Revised Text          ● New Line          ▲ Revised Code          October 2007 · Volume 2 — 67

**Deficiency, deficient** — *continued*
　multiple, syndrome 260
　myocardial (*see also* Insufficiency, myocardial) 428.0
　myophosphorylase 271.0
　NADH-diaphorase or reductase (congenital) 289.7
　NADH (DPNH)-methemoglobin-reductase (congenital) 289.7
　neck V48.1
　niacin (amide) (-tryptophan) 265.2
　nicotinamide 265.2
　nicotinic acid (amide) 265.2
　nose V48.8
　number of teeth (*see also* Anodontia) 520.0
　nutrition, nutritional 269.9
　　specified NEC 269.8
　ornithine transcarbamylase 270.6
　ovarian 256.39
　oxygen (*see also* Anoxia) 799.02
　pantothenic acid 266.2
　parathyroid (gland) 252.1
　phenylalanine hydroxylase 270.1
　phosphoenolpyruvate carboxykinase 271.8
　phosphofructokinase 271.2
　phosphoglucomutase 271.0
　phosphohexosisomerase 271.0
　phosphomannomutase 271.8
　phosphomannose isomerase 271.8
　phosphomannosyl mutase 271.8
　phosphorylase kinase, liver 271.0
　pituitary (anterior) 253.2
　　posterior 253.5
　placenta — *see* Placenta, insufficiency
　plasma
　　cell 279.00
　　protein (paraproteinemia) (pyroglobulinemia) 273.8
　　　gamma globulin 279.00
　　thromboplastin
　　　antecedent (PTA) 286.2
　　　component (PTC) 286.1
　platelet NEC 287.1
　　constitutional 286.4
　polyglandular 258.9
　potassium (K) 276.8
　proaccelerin (congenital) (*see also* Defect, congenital) 286.3
　　acquired 286.7
　proconvertin factor (congenital) (*see also* Defect, coagulation) 286.3
　　acquired 286.7
　prolactin 253.4
　protein 260
　　anemia 281.4
　　C 289.81
　　plasma — *see* Deficiency, plasma, protein
　　S 289.81
　prothrombin (congenital) (*see also* Defect, coagulation) 286.3
　　acquired 286.7
　Prower factor (*see also* Defect, coagulation) 286.3
　PRT 277.2
　pseudocholinesterase 289.89
　psychobiological 301.6
　PTA 286.2
　PTC 286.1
　purine nucleoside phosphorylase 277.2
　pyracin (alpha) (beta) 266.1
　pyridoxal 266.1
　pyridoxamine 266.1
　pyridoxine (derivatives) 266.1
　pyruvate carboxylase 271.8
　pyruvate dehydrogenase 271.8
　pyruvate kinase (PK) 282.3
　riboflavin (vitamin B$_2$) 266.0
　saccadic eye movements 379.57
　salivation 527.7
　salt 276.1
　secretion
　　ovary 256.39

**Deficiency, deficient** — *continued*
　secretion — *continued*
　　salivary gland (any) 527.7
　　urine 788.5
　selenium 269.3
　serum
　　antitrypsin, familial 273.4
　　protein (congenital) 273.8
　short chain acyl CoA dehydrogenase (SCAD) 277.85
　short stature homeobox gene (SHOX)●
　　with
　　　dyschondrosteosis 756.89　●
　　　short stature (idiopathic) 783.43　●
　　　Turner's syndrome 758.6　●
　smooth pursuit movements (eye) 379.58
　sodium (Na) 276.1
　SPCA (*see also* Defect, coagulation) 286.3
　specified NEC 269.8
　stable factor (congenital) (*see also* Defect, coagulation) 286.3
　　acquired 286.7
　Stuart (-Prower) factor (*see also* Defect, coagulation) 286.3
　sucrase 271.3
　sucrase-isomaltase 271.3
　sulfite oxidase 270.0
　syndrome, multiple 260
　thiamine, thiaminic (chloride) 265.1
　thrombokinase (*see also* Defect, coagulation) 286.3
　　newborn 776.0
　thrombopoieten 287.39
　thymolymphatic 279.2
　thyroid (gland) 244.9
　tocopherol 269.1
　toe — *see* Absence, toe
　tooth bud (*see also* Anodontia) 520.0
　trunk V48.1
　UDPG-glycogen transferase 271.0
　upper limb V49.0
　vascular 459.9
　vasopressin 253.5
　viosterol (*see also* Deficiency, calciferol) 268.9
　vitamin (multiple) NEC 269.2
　　A 264.9
　　　with
　　　　Bitôt's spot 264.1
　　　　corneal 264.2
　　　　　with corneal ulceration 264.3
　　　　keratomalacia 264.4
　　　　keratosis, follicular 264.8
　　　　night blindness 264.5
　　　　scar of cornea, xerophthalmic 264.6
　　　　specified manifestation NEC 264.8
　　　　　ocular 264.7
　　　　xeroderma 264.8
　　　　xerophthalmia 264.7
　　　　xerosis
　　　　　conjunctival 264.0

**Deficiency, deficient** — *continued*
　vitamin — *continued*
　　A — *continued*
　　　with — *continued*
　　　　xerosis — *continued*
　　　　　conjunctival — *continued*
　　　　　　with Bitôt's spot 264.1
　　　　　corneal 264.2
　　　　　　with corneal ulceration 264.3
　　B (complex) NEC 266.9
　　　with
　　　　beriberi 265.0
　　　　pellagra 265.2
　　　specified type NEC 266.2
　　B$_1$ NEC 265.1
　　　beriberi 265.0
　　B$_2$ 266.0
　　B$_6$ 266.1
　　B$_{12}$ 266.2
　　B$_c$ (folic acid) 266.2
　　C (ascorbic acid) (with scurvy) 267
　　D (calciferol) (ergosterol) 268.9
　　　with
　　　　osteomalacia 268.2
　　　　rickets (*see also* Rickets) 268.0
　　E 269.1
　　folic acid 266.2
　　G 266.0
　　H 266.2
　　K 269.0
　　　of newborn 776.0
　　nicotinic acid 265.2
　　P 269.1
　　PP 265.2
　　specified NEC 269.1
　zinc 269.3
**Deficient** — *see also* Deficiency
　blink reflex 374.45
　craniofacial axis 756.0
　number of teeth (*see also* Anodontia) 520.0
　secretion of urine 788.5
**Deficit**
　neurologic NEC 781.99
　　due to
　　　cerebrovascular lesion (*see also* Disease, cerebrovascular, acute) 436
　　　late effect — *see* Late effect(s) (of) cerebrovascular disease
　　　transient ischemic attack 435.9
　　ischemic
　　　reversible (RIND) 434.91　●
　　　　history of (personal) V12.54●
　　　prolonged (PRIND) 434.91　●
　　　　history of (personal) V12.54　●
　oxygen 799.02
**Deflection**
　radius 736.09
　septum (acquired) (nasal) (nose) 470
　spine — *see* Curvature, spine
　turbinate (nose) 470
**Defluvium**
　capillorum (*see also* Alopecia) 704.00
　ciliorum 374.55
　unguium 703.8
**Deformity** 738.9
　abdomen, congenital 759.9
　abdominal wall
　　acquired 738.8
　　congenital 756.70
　　muscle deficiency syndrome 756.79
　acquired (unspecified site) 738.9
　　specified site NEC 738.8
　adrenal gland (congenital) 759.1
　alimentary tract, congenital 751.9
　　lower 751.5
　　　specified type NEC 751.8
　　upper (any part, except tongue) 750.9

**Deformity** — *continued*
　alimentary tract, congenital — *continued*
　　upper — *continued*
　　　specified type NEC 750.8
　　　tongue 750.10
　　　　specified type NEC 750.19
　ankle (joint) (acquired) 736.70
　　abduction 718.47
　　congenital 755.69
　　contraction 718.47
　　specified NEC 736.79
　anus (congenital) 751.5
　　acquired 569.49
　aorta (congenital) 747.20
　　acquired 447.8
　　arch 747.21
　　　acquired 447.8
　　coarctation 747.10
　aortic
　　arch 747.21
　　　acquired 447.8
　　cusp or valve (congenital) 746.9
　　　acquired (*see also* Endocarditis, aortic) 424.1
　　ring 747.21
　appendix 751.5
　arm (acquired) 736.89
　　congenital 755.50
　arteriovenous (congenital) (peripheral) NEC 747.60
　　gastrointestinal 747.61
　　lower limb 747.64
　　renal 747.62
　　specified NEC 747.69
　　spinal 747.82
　　upper limb 747.63
　artery (congenital) (peripheral) NEC (*see also* Deformity, vascular) 747.60
　　acquired 447.8
　　cerebral 747.81
　　coronary (congenital) 746.85
　　　acquired (*see also* Ischemia, heart) 414.9
　　retinal 743.9
　　umbilical 747.5
　atrial septal (congenital) (heart) 745.5
　auditory canal (congenital) (external) (*see also* Deformity, ear) 744.3
　　acquired 380.50
　auricle
　　ear (congenital) (*see also* Deformity, ear) 744.3
　　　acquired 380.32
　　heart (congenital) 746.9
　back (acquired) — *see* Deformity, spine
　Bartholin's duct (congenital) 750.9●
　bile duct (congenital) 751.60
　　acquired 576.8
　　　with calculus, choledocholithiasis, or stones — *see* Choledocholithiasis
　biliary duct or passage (congenital) 751.60
　　acquired 576.8
　　　with calculus, choledocholithiasis, or stones — *see* Choledocholithiasis
　bladder (neck) (sphincter) (trigone) (acquired) 596.8
　　congenital 753.9
　bone (acquired) NEC 738.9
　　congenital 756.9
　　turbinate 738.0
　boutonniere (finger) 736.21
　brain (congenital) 742.9
　　acquired 348.8
　　multiple 742.4
　　reduction 742.2
　　vessel (congenital) 747.81
　breast (acquired) 611.8
　　congenital 757.9
　bronchus (congenital) 748.3
　　acquired 519.19

☑ Additional Digit Required — Refer to the Tabular List for Digit Selection
　　　　　　　　　　　　　　　　　　　　　　 Subterms under main terms may continue to next column or page
68 — Volume 2 · October 2007
▶◀ Revised Text　　●  New Line　　▲ Revised Code
2008 ICD-9-CM

**Deformity** — *continued*
  bursa, congenital 756.9
  canal of Nuck 752.9
  canthus (congenital) 743.9
    acquired 374.89
  capillary (acquired) 448.9
    congenital NEC (*see also* Deformity, vascular) 747.60
  cardiac — *see* Deformity, heart
  cardiovascular system (congenital) 746.9
  caruncle, lacrimal (congenital) 743.9
    acquired 375.69
  cascade, stomach 537.6
  cecum (congenital) 751.5
    acquired 569.89
  cerebral (congenital) 742.9
    acquired 348.8
  cervix (acquired) (uterus) 622.8
    congenital 752.40
  cheek (acquired) 738.19
    congenital 744.9
  chest (wall) (acquired) 738.3
    congenital 754.89
    late effect of rickets 268.1
  chin (acquired) 738.19
    congenital 744.9
  choroid (congenital) 743.9
    acquired 363.8
    plexus (congenital) 742.9
      acquired 349.2
  cicatricial — *see* Cicatrix
  cilia (congenital) 743.9
    acquired 374.89
  circulatory system (congenital) 747.9
  clavicle (acquired) 738.8
    congenital 755.51
  clitoris (congenital) 752.40
    acquired 624.8
  clubfoot — *see* Clubfoot
  coccyx (acquired) 738.6
    congenital 756.10
  colon (congenital) 751.5
    acquired 569.89
  concha (ear) (congenital) (*see also* Deformity, ear) 744.3
    acquired 380.32
  congenital, organ or site not listed (*see also* Anomaly) 759.9
  cornea (congenital) 743.9
    acquired 371.70
  coronary artery (congenital) 746.85
    acquired (*see also* Ischemia, heart) 414.9
  cranium (acquired) 738.19
    congenital (*see also* Deformity, skull, congenital) 756.0
  cricoid cartilage (congenital) 748.3
    acquired 478.79
  cystic duct (congenital) 751.60
    acquired 575.8
  Dandy-Walker 742.3
    with spina bifida (*see also* Spina bifida) 741.0 ☑
  diaphragm (congenital) 756.6
    acquired 738.8
  digestive organ(s) or system (congenital) NEC 751.9
    specified type NEC 751.8
  ductus arteriosus 747.0
  duodenal bulb 537.89
  duodenum (congenital) 751.5
    acquired 537.89
  dura (congenital) 742.9
    brain 742.4
      acquired 349.2
    spinal 742.59
      acquired 349.2
  ear (congenital) 744.3
    acquired 380.32
    auricle 744.3
      causing impairment of hearing 744.02
    causing impairment of hearing 744.00
    external 744.3

**Deformity** — *continued*
  ear — *continued*
    external — *continued*
      causing impairment of hearing 744.02
    internal 744.05
    lobule 744.3
    middle 744.03
      ossicles 744.04
    ossicles 744.04
  ectodermal (congenital) NEC 757.9
    specified type NEC 757.8
  ejaculatory duct (congenital) 752.9
    acquired 608.89
  elbow (joint) (acquired) 736.00
    congenital 755.50
    contraction 718.42
  endocrine gland NEC 759.2
  epididymis (congenital) 752.9
    acquired 608.89
    torsion 608.24
  epiglottis (congenital) 748.3
    acquired 478.79
  esophagus (congenital) 750.9
    acquired 530.89
  Eustachian tube (congenital) NEC 744.3
    specified type NEC 744.24
  extremity (acquired) 736.9
    congenital, except reduction deformity 755.9
      lower 755.60
      upper 755.50
    reduction — *see* Deformity, reduction
  eye (congenital) 743.9
    acquired 379.8
    muscle 743.9
  eyebrow (congenital) 744.89
  eyelid (congenital) 743.9
    acquired 374.89
    specified type NEC 743.62
  face (acquired) 738.19
    congenital (any part) 744.9
      due to intrauterine malposition and pressure 754.0
  fallopian tube (congenital) 752.10
    acquired 620.8
  femur (acquired) 736.89
    congenital 755.60
  fetal
    with fetopelvic disproportion 653.7 ☑
      affecting fetus or newborn 763.1
    causing obstructed labor 660.1 ☑
      affecting fetus or newborn 763.1
    known or suspected, affecting management of pregnancy 655.9 ☑
  finger (acquired) 736.20
    boutonniere type 736.21
    congenital 755.50
    flexion contracture 718.44
    swan neck 736.22
  flexion (joint) (acquired) 736.9
    congenital NEC 755.9
    hip or thigh (acquired) 736.39
      congenital (*see also* Subluxation, congenital, hip) 754.32
  foot (acquired) 736.70
    cavovarus 736.75
    congenital 754.59
    congenital NEC 754.70
      specified type NEC 754.79
    valgus (acquired) 736.79
      congenital 754.60
        specified type NEC 754.69
    varus (acquired) 736.79
      congenital 754.50
        specified type NEC 754.59
  forearm (acquired) 736.00
    congenital 755.50
  forehead (acquired) 738.19
    congenital (*see also* Deformity, skull, congenital) 756.0

**Deformity** — *continued*
  frontal bone (acquired) 738.19
    congenital (*see also* Deformity, skull, congenital) 756.0
  gallbladder (congenital) 751.60
    acquired 575.8
  gastrointestinal tract (congenital) NEC 751.9
    acquired 569.89
    specified type NEC 751.8
  genitalia, genital organ(s) or system NEC
    congenital 752.9
    female (congenital) 752.9
      acquired 629.89
      external 752.40
      internal 752.9
    male (congenital) 752.9
      acquired 608.89
  globe (eye) (congenital) 743.9
    acquired 360.89
  gum (congenital) 750.9
    acquired 523.9
  gunstock 736.02
  hand (acquired) 736.00
    claw 736.06
    congenital 755.50
    minus (and plus) (intrinsic) 736.09
    pill roller (intrinsic) 736.09
    plus (and minus) (intrinsic) 736.09
    swan neck (intrinsic) 736.09
  head (acquired) 738.10
    congenital (*see also* Deformity, skull congenital) 756.0
    specified NEC 738.19
  heart (congenital) 746.9
    auricle (congenital) 746.9
    septum 745.9
      auricular 745.5
        specified type NEC 745.8
      ventricular 745.4
    valve (congenital) NEC 746.9
      acquired — *see* Endocarditis
      pulmonary (congenital) 746.00
        specified type NEC 746.89
    ventricle (congenital) 746.9
  heel (acquired) 736.76
    congenital 755.67
  hepatic duct (congenital) 751.60
    acquired 576.8
      with calculus, choledocholithiasis, or stones — *see* Choledocholithiasis
  hip (joint) (acquired) 736.30
    congenital NEC 755.63
    flexion 718.45
      congenital (*see also* Subluxation, congenital, hip) 754.32
  hourglass — *see* Contraction, hourglass
  humerus (acquired) 736.89
    congenital 755.50
  hymen (congenital) 752.40
  hypophyseal (congenital) 759.2
  ileocecal (coil) (valve) (congenital) 751.5
    acquired 569.89
  ileum (intestine) (congenital) 751.5
    acquired 569.89
  ilium (acquired) 738.6
    congenital 755.60
  integument (congenital) 757.9
  intervertebral cartilage or disc (acquired) (*see also* Displacement, intervertebral disc)
    congenital 756.10
  intestine (large) (small) (congenital) 751.5
    acquired 569.89
  iris (acquired) 364.75
    congenital 743.9
    prolapse 364.89 ▲
  ischium (acquired) 738.6
    congenital 755.60
  jaw (acquired) (congenital) NEC 524.9

**Deformity** — *continued*
  jaw — *continued*
    due to intrauterine malposition and pressure 754.0
  joint (acquired) NEC 738.8
    congenital 755.9
    contraction (abduction) (adduction) (extension) (flexion) — *see* Contraction, joint
  kidney(s) (calyx) (pelvis) (congenital) 753.9
    acquired 593.89
    vessel 747.62
      acquired 459.9
  Klippel-Feil (brevicollis) 756.16
  knee (acquired) NEC 736.6
    congenital 755.64
  labium (majus) (minus) (congenital) 752.40
    acquired 624.8
  lacrimal apparatus or duct (congenital) 743.9
    acquired 375.69
  larynx (muscle) (congenital) 748.3
    acquired 478.79
    web (glottic) (subglottic) 748.2
  leg (lower) (upper) (acquired) NEC 736.89
    congenital 755.60
    reduction — *see* Deformity, reduction, lower limb
  lens (congenital) 743.9
    acquired 379.39
  lid (fold) (congenital) 743.9
    acquired 374.89
  ligament (acquired) 728.9
    congenital 756.9
  limb (acquired) 736.9
    congenital, except reduction deformity 755.9
      lower 755.60
        reduction (*see also* Deformity, reduction, lower limb) 755.30
      upper 755.50
        reduction (*see also* Deformity, reduction, upper limb) 755.20
    specified NEC 736.89
  lip (congenital) NEC 750.9
    acquired 528.5
    specified type NEC 750.26
  liver (congenital) 751.60
    acquired 573.8
    duct (congenital) 751.60
      acquired 576.8
        with calculus, choledocholithiasis, or stones — *see* Choledocholithiasis
  lower extremity — *see* Deformity, leg
  lumbosacral (joint) (region) (congenital) 756.10
    acquired 738.5
  lung (congenital) 748.60
    acquired 518.89
    specified type NEC 748.69
  lymphatic system, congenital 759.9
  Madelung's (radius) 755.54
  maxilla (acquired) (congenital) 524.9
  meninges or membrane (congenital) 742.9
    brain 742.4
      acquired 349.2
    spinal (cord) 742.59
      acquired 349.2
  mesentery (congenital) 751.9
    acquired 568.89
  metacarpus (acquired) 736.00
    congenital 755.50
  metatarsus (acquired) 736.70
    congenital 754.70
  middle ear, except ossicles (congenital) 744.03
    ossicles 744.04

☑ Additional Digit Required — Refer to the Tabular List for Digit Selection
▽ Subterms under main terms may continue to next column or page

**2008 ICD-9-CM**
▶◀ Revised Text
● New Line
▲ Revised Code
October 2007 · Volume 2 — **69**

**Deformity** — *continued*
 mitral (leaflets) (valve) (congenital)
  746.9
  acquired — *see* Endocarditis, mitral
  Ebstein's 746.89
  parachute 746.5
  specified type NEC 746.89
  stenosis, congenital 746.5
 mouth (acquired) 528.9
  congenital NEC 750.9
   specified type NEC 750.26
 multiple, congenital NEC 759.7
  specified type NEC 759.89
 muscle (acquired) 728.9
  congenital 756.9
   specified type NEC 756.89
   sternocleidomastoid (due to in-
    trauterine malposition
    and pressure) 754.1
 musculoskeletal system, congenital
  NEC 756.9
  specified type NEC 756.9
 nail (acquired) 703.9
  congenital 757.9
 nasal — *see* Deformity, nose
 neck (acquired) NEC 738.2
  congenital (any part) 744.9
   sternocleidomastoid 754.1
 nervous system (congenital) 742.9
 nipple (congenital) 757.9
  acquired 611.8
 nose, nasal (cartilage) (acquired) 738.0
  bone (turbinate) 738.0
  congenital 748.1
   bent 754.0
   squashed 754.0
  saddle 738.0
   syphilitic 090.5
  septum 470
   congenital 748.1
  sinus (wall) (congenital) 748.1
   acquired 738.0
  syphilitic (congenital) 090.5
   late 095.8
 ocular muscle (congenital) 743.9
  acquired 378.60
 opticociliary vessels (congenital) 743.9
 orbit (congenital) (eye) 743.9
  acquired NEC 376.40
   associated with craniofacial de-
    formities 376.44
   due to
    bone disease 376.43
    surgery 376.47
    trauma 376.47
 organ of Corti (congenital) 744.05
 ovary (congenital) 752.0
  acquired 620.8
 oviduct (congenital) 752.10
  acquired 620.8
 palate (congenital) 750.9
  acquired 526.89
  cleft (congenital) (*see also* Cleft,
   palate) 749.00
  hard, acquired 526.89
  soft, acquired 528.9
 pancreas (congenital) 751.7
  acquired 577.8
 parachute, mitral valve 746.5
 parathyroid (gland) 759.2
 parotid (gland) (congenital) 750.9
  acquired 527.8
 patella (acquired) 736.6
  congenital 755.64
 pelvis, pelvic (acquired) (bony) 738.6
  with disproportion (fetopelvic)
   653.0 ☑
   affecting fetus or newborn 763.1
   causing obstructed labor
    660.1 ☑
    affecting fetus or newborn
     763.1
  congenital 755.60
  rachitic (late effect) 268.1
 penis (glans) (congenital) 752.9

**Deformity** — *continued*
 penis — *continued*
  acquired 607.89
 pericardium (congenital) 746.9
  acquired — *see* Pericarditis
 pharynx (congenital) 750.9
  acquired 478.29
 Pierre Robin (congenital) 756.0
 pinna (acquired) 380.32
  congenital 744.3
 pituitary (congenital) 759.2
 pleural folds (congenital) 748.8
 portal vein (congenital) 747.40
 posture — *see* Curvature, spine
 prepuce (congenital) 752.9
  acquired 607.89
 prostate (congenital) 752.9
  acquired 602.8
 pulmonary valve — *see* Endocarditis,
  pulmonary
 pupil (congenital) 743.9
  acquired 364.75
 pylorus (congenital) 750.9
  acquired 537.89
 rachitic (acquired), healed or old 268.1
 radius (acquired) 736.00
  congenital 755.50
   reduction — *see* Deformity, re-
    duction, upper limb
 rectovaginal septum (congenital)
  752.40
  acquired 623.8
 rectum (congenital) 751.5
  acquired 569.49
 reduction (extremity) (limb) 755.4
  brain 742.2
  lower limb 755.30
   with complete absence of distal
    elements 755.31
   longitudinal (complete) (partial)
    (with distal deficiencies,
    incomplete) 755.32
    with complete absence of
     distal elements 755.31
   combined femoral, tibial,
    fibular (incomplete)
    755.33
   femoral 755.34
   fibular 755.37
   metatarsal(s) 755.38
   phalange(s) 755.39
    meaning all digits 755.31
   tarsal(s) 755.38
   tibia 755.36
   tibiofibular 755.35
   transverse 755.31
  upper limb 755.20
   with complete absence of distal
    elements 755.21
   longitudinal (complete) (partial)
    (with distal deficiencies,
    incomplete) 755.22
    with complete absence of
     distal elements 755.21
   carpal(s) 755.28
   combined humeral, radial,
    ulnar (incomplete)
    755.23
   humeral 755.24
   metacarpal(s) 755.28
   phalange(s) 755.29
    meaning all digits 755.21
   radial 755.26
   radioulnar 755.25
   ulnar 755.27
   transverse (complete) (partial)
    755.21
 renal — *see* Deformity, kidney
 respiratory system (congenital) 748.9
  specified type NEC 748.8
 rib (acquired) 738.3
  congenital 756.3
   cervical 756.2
 rotation (joint) (acquired) 736.9
  congenital 755.9
  hip or thigh 736.39

**Deformity** — *continued*
 rotation — *continued*
  hip or thigh — *continued*
   congenital (*see also* Subluxa-
    tion, congenital, hip)
    754.32
 sacroiliac joint (congenital) 755.69
  acquired 738.5
 sacrum (acquired) 738.5
  congenital 756.10
 saddle
  back 737.8
  nose 738.0
   syphilitic 090.5
 salivary gland or duct (congenital)
  750.9
  acquired 527.8
 scapula (acquired) 736.89
  congenital 755.50
 scrotum (congenital) 752.9
  acquired 608.89
 sebaceous gland, acquired 706.8
 seminal tract or duct (congenital)
  752.9
  acquired 608.89
 septum (nasal) (acquired) 470
  congenital 748.1
 shoulder (joint) (acquired) 736.89
  congenital 755.50
   specified type NEC 755.59
  contraction 718.41
 sigmoid (flexure) (congenital) 751.5
  acquired 569.89
 sinus of Valsalva 747.29
 skin (congenital) 757.9
  acquired NEC 709.8
 skull (acquired) 738.19
  congenital 756.0
   with
    anencephalus 740.0
    encephalocele 742.0
    hydrocephalus 742.3
     with spina bifida (*see also*
      Spina bifida)
      741.0 ☑
    microcephalus 742.1
   due to intrauterine malposition
    and pressure 754.0
 soft parts, organs or tissues (of pelvis)
  in pregnancy or childbirth NEC
   654.9 ☑
   affecting fetus or newborn
    763.89
   causing obstructed labor
    660.2 ☑
    affecting fetus or newborn
     763.1
 spermatic cord (congenital) 752.9
  acquired 608.89
   torsion 608.22
    extravaginal 608.21
    intravaginal 608.22
 spinal
  column — *see* Deformity, spine
  cord (congenital) 742.9
   acquired 336.8
   vessel (congenital) 747.82
  nerve root (congenital) 742.9
   acquired 724.9
 spine (acquired) NEC 738.5
  congenital 756.10
   due to intrauterine malposition
    and pressure 754.2
  kyphoscoliotic (*see also* Kyphoscoliosis) 737.30
  kyphotic (*see also* Kyphosis)
   737.10
  lordotic (*see also* Lordosis) 737.20
  rachitic 268.1
  scoliotic (*see also* Scoliosis) 737.30
 spleen
  acquired 289.59
  congenital 759.0
 Sprengel's (congenital) 755.52
 sternum (acquired) 738.3
  congenital 756.3

**Deformity** — *continued*
 stomach (congenital) 750.9
  acquired 537.89
 submaxillary gland (congenital) 750.9
  acquired 527.8
 swan neck (acquired)
  finger 736.22
  hand 736.09
 talipes — *see* Talipes
 teeth, tooth NEC 520.9
 testis (congenital) 752.9
  acquired 608.89
   torsion 608.20
 thigh (acquired) 736.89
  congenital 755.60
 thorax (acquired) (wall) 738.3
  congenital 754.89
  late effect of rickets 268.1
 thumb (acquired) 736.20
  congenital 755.50
 thymus (tissue) (congenital) 759.2
 thyroid (gland) (congenital) 759.2
  cartilage 748.3
   acquired 478.79
 tibia (acquired) 736.89
  congenital 755.60
  saber 090.5
 toe (acquired) 735.9
  congenital 755.66
  specified NEC 735.8
 tongue (congenital) 750.10
  acquired 529.8
 tooth, teeth NEC 520.9
 trachea (rings) (congenital) 748.3
  acquired 519.19
 transverse aortic arch (congenital)
  747.21
 tricuspid (leaflets) (valve) (congenital)
  746.9
  acquired — *see* Endocarditis, tricuspid
  atresia or stenosis 746.1
  specified type NEC 746.89
 trunk (acquired) 738.3
  congenital 759.9
 ulna (acquired) 736.00
  congenital 755.50
 upper extremity — *see* Deformity, arm
 urachus (congenital) 753.7
 ureter (opening) (congenital) 753.9
  acquired 593.89
 urethra (valve) (congenital) 753.9
  acquired 599.84
 urinary tract or system (congenital)
  753.9
  urachus 753.7
 uterus (congenital) 752.3
  acquired 621.8
 uvula (congenital) 750.9
  acquired 528.9
 vagina (congenital) 752.40
  acquired 623.8
 valve, valvular (heart) (congenital)
  746.9
  acquired — *see* Endocarditis
  pulmonary 746.00
  specified type NEC 746.89
 vascular (congenital) (peripheral) NEC
  747.60
  acquired 459.9
  gastrointestinal 747.61
  lower limb 747.64
  renal 747.62
  specified site NEC 747.69
  spinal 747.82
  upper limb 747.63
 vas deferens (congenital) 752.9
  acquired 608.89
 vein (congenital) NEC (*see also* Deformity, vascular) 747.60
  brain 747.81
  coronary 746.9
  great 747.40
 vena cava (inferior) (superior) (congenital) 747.40
 vertebra — *see* Deformity, spine

☑ Additional Digit Required — Refer to the Tabular List for Digit Selection      ▽ Subterms under main terms may continue to next column or page

**70** — Volume 2      ▶◀ Revised Text      ● New Line      ▲ Revised Code      *2008 ICD-9-CM*

**Deformity** — *continued*
vesicourethral orifice (acquired) 596.8
  congenital NEC 753.9
    specified type NEC 753.8
vessels of optic papilla (congenital)
  743.9
visual field (contraction) 368.45
vitreous humor (congenital) 743.9
  acquired 379.29
vulva (congenital) 752.40
  acquired 624.8
wrist (joint) (acquired) 736.00
  congenital 755.50
  contraction 718.43
  valgus 736.03
    congenital 755.59
  varus 736.04
    congenital 755.59

**Degeneration, degenerative**
adrenal (capsule) (gland) 255.8
  with hypofunction 255.41                       ▲
  fatty 255.8
  hyaline 255.8
  infectional 255.8
  lardaceous 277.39
amyloid (any site) (general) 277.39
anterior cornua, spinal cord 336.8
aorta, aortic 440.0
  fatty 447.8
  valve (heart) (see also Endocarditis,
    aortic) 424.1
arteriovascular — see Arteriosclerosis
artery, arterial (atheromatous) (calcare-
    ous) (see also Arteriosclerosis)
  amyloid 277.39
  lardaceous 277.39
  medial NEC (see also Arteriosclero-
    sis, extremities) 440.20
articular cartilage NEC (see also Dis-
    order, cartilage, articular)
    718.0 ☑
  elbow 718.02
  knee 717.5
  patella 717.7
  shoulder 718.01
  spine (see also Spondylosis) 721.90
atheromatous — see Arteriosclerosis
bacony (any site) 277.39
basal nuclei or ganglia NEC 333.0
bone 733.90
brachial plexus 353.0
brain (cortical) (progressive) 331.9
  arteriosclerotic 437.0
  childhood 330.9
    specified type NEC 330.8
  congenital 742.4
  cystic 348.0
    congenital 742.4
  familial NEC 331.89
  grey matter 330.8
  heredofamilial NEC 331.89
  in
    alcoholism 303.9 ☑ [331.7]
    beriberi 265.0 [331.7]
    cerebrovascular disease
      437.9 [331.7]
    congenital hydrocephalus
      742.3 [331.7]
      with spina bifida (see also
        Spina bifida)
        741.0 ☑ [331.7]
    Fabry's disease 272.7 [330.2]
    Gaucher's disease 272.7 [330.2]
    Hunter's disease or syndrome
      277.5 [330.3]
    lipidosis
      cerebral 330.1
      generalized 272.7 [330.2]
    mucopolysaccharidosis
      277.5 [330.3]
    myxedema (see also Myxedema)
      244.9 [331.7]
    neoplastic disease NEC
      (M8000/1) 239.9 [331.7]
    Niemann-Pick disease
      272.7 [330.2]

**Degeneration, degenerative** —
  *continued*
brain — *continued*
  in — *continued*
    sphingolipidosis 272.7 [330.2]
    vitamin B$_{12}$ deficiency
      266.2 [331.7]
  motor centers 331.89
  senile 331.2
  specified type NEC 331.89
breast — see Disease, breast
Bruch's membrane 363.40
bundle of His 426.50
  left 426.3
  right 426.4
calcareous NEC 275.49
capillaries 448.9
  amyloid 277.39
  fatty 448.9
  lardaceous 277.39
cardiac (brown) (calcareous) (fatty) (fi-
    brous) (hyaline) (mural) (muscu-
    lar) (pigmentary) (senile) (with
    arteriosclerosis) (see also Degen-
    eration, myocardial) 429.1
  valve, valvular — see Endocarditis
cardiorenal (see also Hypertension,
    cardiorenal) 404.90
cardiovascular (see also Disease, car-
    diovascular) 429.2
  renal (see also Hypertension, car-
    diorenal) 404.90
cartilage (joint) — see Derangement,
    joint
cerebellar NEC 334.9
  primary (hereditary) (sporadic)
    334.2
cerebral — see Degeneration, brain
cerebromacular 330.1
cerebrovascular 437.1
  due to hypertension 437.2
  late effect — see Late effect(s) (of)
    cerebrovascular disease
cervical plexus 353.2
cervix 622.8
  due to radiation (intended effect)
    622.8
    adverse effect or misadventure
      622.8
changes, spine or vertebra (see also
    Spondylosis) 721.90
chitinous 277.39
chorioretinal 363.40
  congenital 743.53
  hereditary 363.50
choroid (colloid) (drusen) 363.40
  hereditary 363.50
  senile 363.41
    diffuse secondary 363.42
cochlear 386.8
collateral ligament (knee) (medial)
    717.82
  lateral 717.81
combined (spinal cord) (subacute)
    266.2 [336.2]
  with anemia (pernicious)
    281.0 [336.2]
  due to dietary deficiency
    281.1 [336.2]
  due to vitamin B$_{12}$ deficiency ane-
    mia (dietary) 281.1 [336.2]
conjunctiva 372.50
  amyloid 277.39 [372.50]
cornea 371.40
  calcerous 371.44
  familial (hereditary) (see also Dys-
    trophy, cornea) 371.50
    macular 371.55
    reticular 371.54
  hyaline (of old scars) 371.41
  marginal (Terrien's) 371.48
  mosaic (shagreen) 371.41
  nodular 371.46
  peripheral 371.48
  senile 371.41

**Degeneration, degenerative** —
  *continued*
cortical (cerebellar) (parenchymatous)
    334.2
  alcoholic 303.9 ☑ [334.4]
  diffuse, due to arteriopathy 437.0
corticostriatal-spinal 334.8
cretinoid 243
cruciate ligament (knee) (posterior)
    717.84
  anterior 717.83
cutis 709.3
  amyloid 277.39
dental pulp 522.2
disc disease — see Degeneration, in-
    tervertebral disc
dorsolateral (spinal cord) — see Degen-
    eration, combined
endocardial 424.90
extrapyramidal NEC 333.90
eye NEC 360.40
  macular (see also Degeneration,
    macula) 362.50
    congenital 362.75
    hereditary 362.76
fatty (diffuse) (general) 272.8
  liver 571.8
    alcoholic 571.0
  localized site — see Degeneration,
    by site, fatty
  placenta — see Placenta, abnormal
globe (eye) NEC 360.40
  macular — see Degeneration,
    macula
grey matter 330.8
heart (brown) (calcareous) (fatty) (fi-
    brous) (hyaline) (mural) (muscu-
    lar) (pigmentary) (senile) (with
    arteriosclerosis) (see also Degen-
    eration, myocardial) 429.1
  amyloid 277.39 [425.7]
  atheromatous — see Arteriosclero-
    sis, coronary
  gouty 274.82
  hypertensive (see also Hyperten-
    sion, heart) 402.90
  ischemic 414.9
  valve, valvular — see Endocarditis
hepatolenticular (Wilson's) 275.1
hepatorenal 572.4
heredofamilial
  brain NEC 331.89
  spinal cord NEC 336.8
hyaline (diffuse) (generalized) 728.9
  localized (see also Degeneration,
    by site)
    cornea 371.41
    keratitis 371.41
hypertensive vascular — see Hyperten-
    sion
infrapatellar fat pad 729.31
internal semilunar cartilage 717.3
intervertebral disc 722.6
  with myelopathy 722.70
  cervical, cervicothoracic 722.4
    with myelopathy 722.71
  lumbar, lumbosacral 722.52
    with myelopathy 722.73
  thoracic, thoracolumbar 722.51
    with myelopathy 722.72
intestine 569.89
  amyloid 277.39
  lardaceous 277.39
iris (generalized) (see also Atrophy,
    iris) 364.59
  pigmentary 364.53
  pupillary margin 364.54
ischemic — see Ischemia
joint disease (see also Osteoarthrosis)
    715.9 ☑
  multiple sites 715.09
  spine (see also Spondylosis) 721.90
kidney (see also Sclerosis, renal) 587
  amyloid 277.39 [583.81]
  cyst, cystic (multiple) (solitary)
    593.2

**Degeneration, degenerative** —
  *continued*
kidney (see also Sclerosis, renal) —
    *continued*
  cyst, cystic — *continued*
    congenital (see also Cystic, dis-
      ease, kidney) 753.10
    fatty 593.89
    fibrocystic (congenital) 753.19
    lardaceous 277.39 [583.81]
    polycystic (congenital) 753.12
      adult type (APKD) 753.13
      autosomal dominant 753.13
      autosomal recessive 753.14
      childhood type (CPKD) 753.14
      infantile 753.14
    waxy 277.39 [583.81]
Kuhnt-Junius (retina) 362.52
labyrinth, osseous 386.8
lacrimal passages, cystic 375.12
lardaceous (any site) 277.39
lateral column (posterior), spinal cord
    (see also Degeneration, com-
    bined) 266.2 [336.2]
lattice 362.63
lens 366.9
  infantile, juvenile, or presenile
    366.00
  senile 366.10
lenticular (familial) (progressive) (Wil-
    son's) (with cirrhosis of liver)
    275.1
  striate artery 437.0
lethal ball, prosthetic heart valve
    996.02
ligament
  collateral (knee) (medial) 717.82
    lateral 717.81
  cruciate (knee) (posterior) 717.84
    anterior 717.83
liver (diffuse) 572.8
  amyloid 277.39
  congenital (cystic) 751.62
  cystic 572.8
    congenital 751.62
  fatty 571.8
    alcoholic 571.0
  hypertrophic 572.8
  lardaceous 277.39
  parenchymatous, acute or suba-
    cute (see also Necrosis, liver)
    570
  pigmentary 572.8
  toxic (acute) 573.8
  waxy 277.39
lung 518.89
lymph gland 289.3
  hyaline 289.3
  lardaceous 277.39
macula (acquired) (senile) 362.50
  atrophic 362.51
  Best's 362.76
  congenital 362.75
  cystic 362.54
  cystoid 362.53
  disciform 362.52
  dry 362.51
  exudative 362.52
  familial pseudoinflammatory
    362.77
  hereditary 362.76
  hole 362.54
  juvenile (Stargardt's) 362.75
  nonexudative 362.51
  pseudohole 362.54
  wet 362.52
medullary — see Degeneration, brain
membranous labyrinth, congenital
    (causing impairment of hearing)
    744.05
meniscus — see Derangement, joint
microcystoid 362.62
mitral — see Insufficiency, mitral
Mönckeberg's (see also Arteriosclero-
    sis, extremities) 440.20
moral 301.7

**Degeneration, degenerative** — *continued*

motor centers, senile 331.2
mural (*see also* Degeneration, myocardial) 429.1
heart, cardiac (*see also* Degeneration, myocardial) 429.1
myocardium, myocardial (*see also* Degeneration, myocardial) 429.1
muscle 728.9
fatty 728.9
fibrous 728.9
heart (*see also* Degeneration, myocardial) 429.1
hyaline 728.9
muscular progressive 728.2
myelin, central nervous system NEC 341.9
myocardium, myocardial (brown) (calcareous) (fatty) (fibrous) (hyaline) (mural) (muscular) (pigmentary) (senile) (with arteriosclerosis) 429.1
with rheumatic fever (conditions classifiable to 390) 398.0
active, acute, or subacute 391.2
with chorea 392.0
inactive or quiescent (with chorea) 398.0
amyloid 277.39 [425.7]
congenital 746.89
fetus or newborn 779.89
gouty 274.82
hypertensive (*see also* Hypertension, heart) 402.90
ischemic 414.8
rheumatic (*see also* Degeneration, myocardium, with rheumatic fever) 398.0
syphilitic 093.82
nasal sinus (mucosa) (*see also* Sinusitis) 473.9
frontal 473.1
maxillary 473.0
nerve — *see* Disorder, nerve
nervous system 349.89
amyloid 277.39 [357.4]
autonomic (*see also* Neuropathy, peripheral, autonomic) 337.9
fatty 349.89
peripheral autonomic NEC (*see also* Neuropathy, peripheral, autonomic) 337.9
nipple 611.9
nose 478.19
oculoacousticocerebral, congenital (progressive) 743.8
olivopontocerebellar (familial) (hereditary) 333.0
osseous labyrinth 386.8
ovary 620.8
cystic 620.2
microcystic 620.2
pallidal, pigmentary (progressive) 333.0
pancreas 577.8
tuberculous (*see also* Tuberculosis) 017.9 ☑
papillary muscle 429.81
paving stone 362.61
penis 607.89
peritoneum 568.89
pigmentary (diffuse) (general)
localized — *see* Degeneration, by site
pallidal (progressive) 333.0
secondary 362.65
pineal gland 259.8
pituitary (gland) 253.8
placenta (fatty) (fibrinoid) (fibroid) — *see* Placenta, abnormal
popliteal fat pad 729.31
posterolateral (spinal cord) (*see also* Degeneration, combined) 266.2 [336.2]

**Degeneration, degenerative** — *continued*

pulmonary valve (heart) (*see also* Endocarditis, pulmonary) 424.3
pulp (tooth) 522.2
pupillary margin 364.54
renal (*see also* Sclerosis, renal) 587
fibrocystic 753.19
polycystic 753.12
adult type (APKD) 753.13
autosomal dominant 753.13
autosomal recessive 753.14
childhood type (CPKD) 753.14
infantile type 753.14
reticuloendothelial system 289.89
retina (peripheral) 362.60
with retinal defect (*see also* Detachment, retina, with retinal defect) 361.00
cystic (senile) 362.50
cystoid 362.53
hereditary (*see also* Dystrophy, retina) 362.70
cerebroretinal 362.71
congenital 362.75
juvenile (Stargardt's) 362.75
macula 362.76
Kuhnt-Junius 362.52
lattice 362.63
macular (*see also* Degeneration, macula) 362.50
microcystoid 362.62
palisade 362.63
paving stone 362.61
pigmentary (primary) 362.74
secondary 362.65
posterior pole (*see also* Degeneration, macula) 362.50
secondary 362.66
senile 362.60
cystic 362.53
reticular 362.64
saccule, congenital (causing impairment of hearing) 744.05
sacculocochlear 386.8
senile 797
brain 331.2
cardiac, heart, or myocardium (*see also* Degeneration, myocardial) 429.1
motor centers 331.2
reticule 362.64
retina, cystic 362.50
vascular — *see* Arteriosclerosis
silicone rubber poppet (prosthetic valve) 996.02
sinus (cystic) (*see also* Sinusitis) 473.9
polypoid 471.1
skin 709.3
amyloid 277.39
colloid 709.3
spinal (cord) 336.8
amyloid 277.39
column 733.90
combined (subacute) (*see also* Degeneration, combined) 266.2 [336.2]
with anemia (pernicious) 281.0 [336.2]
dorsolateral (*see also* Degeneration, combined) 266.2 [336.2]
familial NEC 336.8
fatty 336.8
funicular (*see also* Degeneration, combined) 266.2 [336.2]
heredofamilial NEC 336.8
posterolateral (*see also* Degeneration, combined) 266.2 [336.2]
subacute combined — *see* Degeneration, combined
tuberculous (*see also* Tuberculosis) 013.8 ☑
spine 733.90
spleen 289.59
amyloid 277.39
lardaceous 277.39

**Degeneration, degenerative** — *continued*

stomach 537.89
lardaceous 277.39
strionigral 333.0
sudoriparous (cystic) 705.89
suprarenal (capsule) (gland) 255.8 ▲
with hypofunction 255.41
sweat gland 705.89
synovial membrane (pulpy) 727.9
tapetoretinal 362.74
adult or presenile form 362.50
testis (postinfectional) 608.89
thymus (gland) 254.8
fatty 254.8
lardaceous 277.39
thyroid (gland) 246.8
tricuspid (heart) (valve) — *see* Endocarditis, tricuspid
tuberculous NEC (*see also* Tuberculosis) 011.9 ☑
turbinate 733.90
uterus 621.8
cystic 621.8
vascular (senile) (*see also* Arteriosclerosis)
hypertensive — *see* Hypertension
vitreoretinal (primary) 362.73
secondary 362.66
vitreous humor (with infiltration) 379.21
wallerian NEC — *see* Disorder, nerve
waxy (any site) 277.39
Wilson's hepatolenticular 275.1
**Deglutition**
paralysis 784.99
hysterical 300.11
pneumonia 507.0
**Degos' disease or syndrome** 447.8
**Degradation disorder, branched-chain amino acid** 270.3
**Dehiscence**
anastomosis — *see* Complications, anastomosis
cesarean wound 674.1 ☑
episiotomy 674.2 ☑
operation wound 998.32
internal 998.31
perineal wound (postpartum) 674.2 ☑
postoperative 998.32
abdomen 998.32
internal 998.31
internal 998.31
uterine wound 674.1 ☑
**Dehydration** (cachexia) 276.51
with
hypernatremia 276.0
hyponatremia 276.1
newborn 775.5
**Deiters' nucleus syndrome** 386.19
**Déjérine's disease** 356.0
**Déjérine-Klumpke paralysis** 767.6
**Déjérine-Roussy syndrome** 338.0
**Déjérine-Sottas disease or neuropathy** (hypertrophic) 356.0
**Déjérine-Thomas atrophy or syndrome** 333.0
**de Lange's syndrome** (Amsterdam dwarf, mental retardation, and brachycephaly) 759.89
**Delay, delayed**
adaptation, cones or rods 368.63
any plane in pelvis
affecting fetus or newborn 763.1
complicating delivery 660.1 ☑
birth or delivery NEC 662.1 ☑
affecting fetus or newborn 763.89
second twin, triplet, or multiple mate 662.3 ☑
closure (*see also* Fistula)
cranial suture 756.0
fontanel 756.0
coagulation NEC 790.92
conduction (cardiac) (ventricular) 426.9
delivery NEC 662.1 ☑

**Delay, delayed** — *continued*
delivery — *continued*
second twin, triplet, etc. 662.3 ☑
affecting fetus or newborn 763.89
development
in childhood 783.40
physiological 783.40
intellectual NEC 315.9
learning NEC 315.2
reading 315.00
sexual 259.0
speech 315.39
and language due to hearing ●
loss 315.34 ●
associated with hyperkinesis 314.1
spelling 315.09
gastric emptying 536.8
menarche 256.39
due to pituitary hypofunction 253.4
menstruation (cause unknown) 626.8
milestone in childhood 783.42
motility — *see* Hypomotility
passage of meconium (newborn) 777.1
primary respiration 768.9
puberty 259.0
separation of umbilical cord 779.83
sexual maturation, female 259.0
**Del Castillo's syndrome** (germinal aplasia) 606.0
**Déleage's disease** 359.89
**Deletion syndrome**
5p 758.31
22q11.2 758.32
autosomal NEC 758.39
constitutional 5q deletion 758.39
**Delhi** (boil) (button) (sore) 085.1
**Delinquency** (juvenile) 312.9
group (*see also* Disturbance, conduct) 312.2 ☑
neurotic 312.4
**Delirium, delirious** 780.09
acute (psychotic) 293.0
alcoholic 291.0
acute 291.0
chronic 291.1
alcoholicum 291.0
chronic (*see also* Psychosis) 293.89
due to or associated with physical condition — *see* Psychosis, organic
drug-induced 292.81
due to conditions classified elsewhere 293.0
eclamptic (*see also* Eclampsia) 780.39
exhaustion (*see also* Reaction, stress, acute) 308.9
hysterical 300.11
in
presenile dementia 290.11
senile dementia 290.3
induced by drug 292.81
manic, maniacal (acute) (*see also* Psychosis, affective) 296.0 ☑
recurrent episode 296.1 ☑
single episode 296.0 ☑
puerperal 293.9
senile 290.3
subacute (psychotic) 293.1
thyroid (*see also* Thyrotoxicosis) 242.9 ☑
traumatic (*see also* Injury, intracranial)
with
lesion, spinal cord — *see* Injury, spinal, by site
shock, spinal — *see* Injury, spinal, by site
tremens (impending) 291.0
uremic — *see* Uremia
withdrawal
alcoholic (acute) 291.0
chronic 291.1
drug 292.0

☑ Additional Digit Required — Refer to the Tabular List for Digit Selection        Subterms under main terms may continue to next column or page

72 — Volume 2 • October 2007        ▶◀ Revised Text        ● New Line        ▲ Revised Code        **2008 ICD-9-CM**

**Delivery**

Note — Use the following fifth-digit
subclassification with categories
640–648, 651–676:

0   unspecified as to episode of care

1   delivered, with or without mention
    of antepartum condition

2   delivered, with mention of postpar-
    tum complication

3   antepartum condition or complica-
    tion

4   postpartum condition or complica-
    tion

breech (assisted) (buttocks) (complete)
      (frank) (spontaneous) 652.2 ☑
   affecting fetus or newborn 763.0 ☑
   extraction NEC 669.6 ☑
cesarean (for) 669.7 ☑
   abnormal
      cervix 654.6 ☑
      pelvic organs or tissues 654.9 ☑
      pelvis (bony) (major) NEC
         653.0 ☑
      presentation or position
         652.9 ☑
         in multiple gestation 652.6 ☑
      size, fetus 653.5 ☑
      soft parts (of pelvis) 654.9 ☑
      uterus, congenital 654.0 ☑
      vagina 654.7 ☑
      vulva 654.8 ☑
   abruptio placentae 641.2 ☑
   acromion presentation 652.8 ☑
   affecting fetus or newborn 763.4 ☑
   anteversion, cervix or uterus
      654.4 ☑
   atony, uterus 661.2 ☑                     ▲
      with hemorrhage 666.1 ☑               ●
   bicornis or bicornuate uterus
      654.0 ☑
   breech presentation (buttocks)
      (complete) (frank) 652.2 ☑
   brow presentation 652.4 ☑
   cephalopelvic disproportion (nor-
      mally formed fetus) 653.4 ☑
   chin presentation 652.4 ☑
   cicatrix of cervix 654.6 ☑
   contracted pelvis (general) 653.1 ☑
      inlet 653.2 ☑
      outlet 653.3 ☑
   cord presentation or prolapse
      663.0 ☑
   cystocele 654.4 ☑
   deformity (acquired) (congenital)
      pelvic organs or tissues NEC
         654.9 ☑
      pelvis (bony) NEC 653.0 ☑
   displacement, uterus NEC 654.4 ☑
   disproportion NEC 653.9 ☑
   distress
      fetal 656.8 ☑
      maternal 669.0 ☑
   eclampsia 642.6 ☑
   face presentation 652.4 ☑
   failed
      forceps 660.7 ☑
      trial of labor NEC 660.6 ☑
      vacuum extraction 660.7 ☑
      ventouse 660.7 ☑
   fetal deformity 653.7 ☑
   fetal-maternal hemorrhage 656.0 ☑
   fetus, fetal
      distress 656.8 ☑
      prematurity 656.8 ☑
   fibroid (tumor) (uterus) 654.1 ☑
   footling 652.8 ☑
      with successful version 652.1 ☑
   hemorrhage (antepartum) (intra-
      partum) NEC 641.9 ☑
   hydrocephalic fetus 653.6 ☑
   incarceration of uterus 654.3 ☑

**Delivery** — continued
cesarean — continued
   incoordinate uterine action
      661.4 ☑
   inertia, uterus 661.2 ☑
      primary 661.0 ☑
      secondary 661.1 ☑
   lateroversion, uterus or cervix
      654.4 ☑
   mal lie 652.9 ☑
   malposition
      fetus 652.9 ☑
         in multiple gestation 652.6 ☑
      pelvic organs or tissues NEC
         654.9 ☑
      uterus NEC or cervix 654.4 ☑
   malpresentation NEC 652.9 ☑
      in multiple gestation 652.6 ☑
   maternal
      diabetes mellitus 648.0 ☑
      heart disease NEC 648.6 ☑
   meconium in liquor 656.8 ☑
      staining only 792.3
   oblique presentation 652.3 ☑
   oversize fetus 653.5 ☑
   pelvic tumor NEC 654.9 ☑
   placental insufficiency 656.5 ☑
   placenta previa 641.0 ☑
      with hemorrhage 641.1 ☑
   poor dilation, cervix 661.0 ☑
   pre-eclampsia 642.4 ☑
      severe 642.5 ☑
   previous
      cesarean delivery, section
         654.2 ☑
      surgery (to)
         cervix 654.6 ☑
         gynecological NEC 654.9 ☑
         rectum 654.8 ☑
         uterus NEC 654.9 ☑
            previous cesarean deliv-
               ery, section
               654.2 ☑
         vagina 654.7 ☑
   prolapse
      arm or hand 652.7 ☑
      uterus 654.4 ☑
   prolonged labor 662.1 ☑
   rectocele 654.4 ☑
   retroversion, uterus or cervix
      654.3 ☑
   rigid
      cervix 654.6 ☑
      pelvic floor 654.4 ☑
      perineum 654.8 ☑
      vagina 654.7 ☑
      vulva 654.8 ☑
   sacculation, pregnant uterus
      654.4 ☑
   scar(s)
      cervix 654.6 ☑
      cesarean delivery, section
         654.2 ☑
      uterus NEC 654.9 ☑
         due to previous cesarean de-
            livery, section 654.2 ☑
   Shirodkar suture in situ 654.5 ☑
   shoulder presentation 652.8 ☑
   stenosis or stricture, cervix
      654.6 ☑
   transverse presentation or lie
      652.3 ☑
   tumor, pelvic organs or tissues
      NEC 654.4 ☑
   umbilical cord presentation or
      prolapse 663.0 ☑
completely normal case — see category 650
complicated (by) NEC 669.9 ☑
   abdominal tumor, fetal 653.7 ☑
      causing obstructed labor
         660.1 ☑
   abnormal, abnormality of
      cervix 654.6 ☑

**Delivery** — continued
complicated — continued
   abnormal, abnormality of — contin-
      ued
      cervix — continued
         causing obstructed labor
            660.2 ☑
      forces of labor 661.9 ☑
      formation of uterus 654.0 ☑
      pelvic organs or tissues 654.9 ☑
         causing obstructed labor
            660.2 ☑
      pelvis (bony) (major) NEC
         653.0 ☑
         causing obstructed labor
            660.1 ☑
      presentation or position NEC
         652.9 ☑
         causing obstructed labor
            660.0 ☑
      size, fetus 653.5 ☑
         causing obstructed labor
            660.1 ☑
      soft parts (of pelvis) 654.9 ☑
         causing obstructed labor
            660.2 ☑
      uterine contractions NEC
         661.9 ☑
      uterus (formation) 654.0 ☑
         causing obstructed labor
            660.2 ☑
      vagina 654.7 ☑
         causing obstructed labor
            660.2 ☑
   abnormally formed uterus (any
      type) (congenital) 654.0 ☑
      causing obstructed labor
         660.2 ☑
   acromion presentation 652.8 ☑
      causing obstructed labor
         660.0 ☑
   adherent placenta 667.0 ☑
      with hemorrhage 666.0 ☑
   adhesions, uterus (to abdominal
      wall) 654.4 ☑
   advanced maternal age NEC
      659.6 ☑
      multigravida 659.6 ☑
      primigravida 659.5 ☑
   air embolism 673.0 ☑
   amnionitis 658.4 ☑
   amniotic fluid embolism 673.1 ☑
   anesthetic death 668.9 ☑
   annular detachment, cervix
      665.3 ☑
   antepartum hemorrhage — see
      Delivery, complicated, hemor-
      rhage
   anteversion, cervix or uterus
      654.4 ☑
      causing obstructed labor
         660.2 ☑
   apoplexy 674.0 ☑
      placenta 641.2 ☑
   arrested active phase 661.1 ☑
   asymmetrical pelvis bone 653.0 ☑
      causing obstructed labor
         660.1 ☑
   atony, uterus with hemorrhage
      (hypotonic) (inertia) 666.1 ☑
      hypertonic 661.4 ☑
   Bandl's ring 661.4 ☑
   battledore placenta — see Placenta,
      abnormal
   bicornis or bicornuate uterus
      654.0 ☑
      causing obstructed labor
         660.2 ☑
   birth injury to mother NEC
      665.9 ☑
   bleeding (see also Delivery, compli-
      cated, hemorrhage) 641.9 ☑
   breech presentation (assisted)
      (buttocks) (complete) (frank)
      (spontaneous) 652.2 ☑

**Delivery** — continued
complicated — continued
   breech presentation — contin-
      ued
      with successful version 652.1 ☑
   brow presentation 652.4 ☑
   cephalopelvic disproportion (nor-
      mally formed fetus) 653.4 ☑
      causing obstructed labor
         660.1 ☑
   cerebral hemorrhage 674.0 ☑      ▲
   cervical dystocia 661.2 ☑         ▲
   chin presentation 652.4 ☑
      causing obstructed labor
         660.0 ☑
   cicatrix
      cervix 654.6 ☑
         causing obstructed labor
            660.2 ☑
      vagina 654.7 ☑
         causing obstructed labor
            660.2 ☑
   coagulation defect 649.3 ☑
   colporrhexis 665.4 ☑
      with perineal laceration 664.0 ☑
   compound presentation 652.8 ☑
      causing obstructed labor
         660.0 ☑
   compression of cord (umbilical)
      663.2 ☑
      around neck 663.1 ☑
      cord prolapsed 663.0 ☑
   contraction, contracted pelvis
      653.1 ☑
      causing obstructed labor
         660.1 ☑
      general 653.1 ☑
         causing obstructed labor
            660.1 ☑
      inlet 653.2 ☑
         causing obstructed labor
            660.1 ☑
      midpelvic 653.8 ☑
         causing obstructed labor
            660.1 ☑
      midplane 653.8 ☑
         causing obstructed labor
            660.1 ☑
      outlet 653.3 ☑
         causing obstructed labor
            660.1 ☑
   contraction ring 661.4 ☑
   cord (umbilical) 663.9 ☑
      around neck, tightly or with
         compression 663.1 ☑
         without compression
            663.3 ☑
      bruising 663.6 ☑
      complication NEC 663.9 ☑
         specified type NEC 663.8 ☑
      compression NEC 663.2 ☑
      entanglement NEC 663.3 ☑
         with compression 663.2 ☑
      forelying 663.0 ☑
      hematoma 663.6 ☑
      marginal attachment 663.8 ☑
      presentation 663.0 ☑
      prolapse (complete) (occult)
         (partial) 663.0 ☑
      short 663.4 ☑
      specified complication NEC
         663.8 ☑
      thrombosis (vessels) 663.6 ☑
      vascular lesion 663.6 ☑
      velamentous insertion 663.8 ☑
   Couvelaire uterus 641.2 ☑
   cretin pelvis (dwarf type) (male
      type) 653.1 ☑
      causing obstructed labor
         660.1 ☑
   crossbirth 652.3 ☑
      with successful version 652.1 ☑
      causing obstructed labor
         660.0 ☑

☑ Additional Digit Required — Refer to the Tabular List for Digit Selection             ▽ Subterms under main terms may continue to next column or page

Delivery — Delivery

**Delivery** — *continued*
complicated — *continued*
cyst (Gartner's duct) 654.7 ☑
cystocele 654.4 ☑
causing obstructed labor
660.2 ☑
death of fetus (near term) 656.4 ☑
early (before 22 completed
weeks gestation) 632
deformity (acquired) (congenital)
fetus 653.7 ☑
causing obstructed labor
660.1 ☑
pelvic organs or tissues NEC
654.9 ☑
causing obstructed labor
660.2 ☑
pelvis (bony) NEC 653.0 ☑
causing obstructed labor
660.1 ☑
delay, delayed
delivery in multiple pregnancy
662.3 ☑
due to locked mates 660.5 ☑
following rupture of membranes
(spontaneous) 658.2 ☑
artificial 658.3 ☑
depressed fetal heart tones
659.7 ☑
diastasis recti 665.8 ☑
dilatation
bladder 654.4 ☑
causing obstructed labor
660.2 ☑
cervix, incomplete, poor or slow
661.0 ☑
diseased placenta 656.7 ☑
displacement uterus NEC 654.4 ☑
causing obstructed labor
660.2 ☑
disproportion NEC 653.9 ☑
causing obstructed labor
660.1 ☑
disruptio uteri — *see* Delivery,
complicated, rupture, uterus
distress
fetal 656.8 ☑
maternal 669.0 ☑
double uterus (congenital) 654.0 ☑
causing obstructed labor
660.2 ☑
dropsy amnion 657.0 ☑
dysfunction, uterus 661.9 ☑
hypertonic 661.4 ☑
hypotonic 661.2 ☑
primary 661.0 ☑
secondary 661.1 ☑
incoordinate 661.4 ☑
dystocia
cervical 661.2 ☑                      ▲
fetal — *see* Delivery, complicated, abnormal, presenta-
tion
maternal — *see* Delivery, complicated, prolonged labor
pelvic — *see* Delivery, complicated, contraction pelvis
positional 652.8 ☑
shoulder girdle 660.4 ☑
eclampsia 642.6 ☑
ectopic kidney 654.4 ☑
causing obstructed labor
660.2 ☑
edema, cervix 654.6 ☑
causing obstructed labor
660.2 ☑
effusion, amniotic fluid 658.1 ☑
elderly multigravida 659.6 ☑
elderly primigravida 659.5 ☑
embolism (pulmonary) 673.2 ☑
air 673.0 ☑
amniotic fluid 673.1 ☑
blood clot 673.2 ☑
cerebral 674.0 ☑
fat 673.8 ☑

**Delivery** — *continued*
complicated — *continued*
embolism — *continued*
pyemic 673.3 ☑
septic 673.3 ☑
entanglement, umbilical cord
663.3 ☑
with compression 663.2 ☑
around neck (with compression)
663.1 ☑
eversion, cervix or uterus 665.2 ☑
excessive
fetal growth 653.5 ☑
causing obstructed labor
660.1 ☑
size of fetus 653.5 ☑
causing obstructed labor
660.1 ☑
face presentation 652.4 ☑
causing obstructed labor
660.0 ☑
to pubes 660.3 ☑
failure, fetal head to enter pelvic
brim 652.5 ☑
causing obstructed labor
660.0 ☑
female genital mutilation 660.8 ☑
fetal
acid-base balance 656.8 ☑
death (near term) NEC 656.4 ☑
early (before 22 completed
weeks gestation) 632
deformity 653.7 ☑
causing obstructed labor
660.1 ☑
distress 656.8 ☑
heart rate or rhythm 659.7 ☑
reduction of multiple fetuses
reduced to single fetus
651.7 ☑
fetopelvic disproportion 653.4 ☑
causing obstructed labor
660.1 ☑
fever during labor 659.2 ☑
fibroid (tumor) (uterus) 654.1 ☑
causing obstructed labor
660.2 ☑
fibromyomata 654.1 ☑
causing obstructed labor
660.2 ☑
forelying umbilical cord 663.0 ☑
fracture of coccyx 665.6 ☑
hematoma 664.5 ☑
broad ligament 665.7 ☑
ischial spine 665.7 ☑
pelvic 665.7 ☑
perineum 664.5 ☑
soft tissues 665.7 ☑
subdural 674.0 ☑
umbilical cord 663.6 ☑
vagina 665.7 ☑
vulva or perineum 664.5 ☑
hemorrhage (uterine) (antepartum)
(intrapartum) (pregnancy)
641.9 ☑
accidental 641.2 ☑
associated with
afibrinogenemia 641.3 ☑
coagulation defect 641.3 ☑
hyperfibrinolysis 641.3 ☑
hypofibrinogenemia
641.3 ☑
cerebral 674.0 ☑
due to
low-lying placenta 641.1 ☑
placenta previa 641.1 ☑
premature separation of placenta (normally im-
planted) 641.2 ☑
retained placenta 666.0 ☑
trauma 641.8 ☑
uterine leiomyoma 641.8 ☑
marginal sinus rupture 641.2 ☑
placenta NEC 641.9 ☑

**Delivery** — *continued*
complicated — *continued*
hemorrhage — *continued*
postpartum (atonic) (immediate)
(within 24 hours) 666.1 ☑
with retained or trapped placenta 666.0 ☑
delayed 666.2 ☑
secondary 666.2 ☑
third stage 666.0 ☑
hourglass contraction, uterus
661.4 ☑
hydramnios 657.0 ☑
hydrocephalic fetus 653.6 ☑
causing obstructed labor
660.1 ☑
hydrops fetalis 653.7 ☑
causing obstructed labor
660.1 ☑
hypertension — *see* Hypertension,
complicating pregnancy
hypertonic uterine dysfunction
661.4 ☑
hypotonic uterine dysfunction
661.2 ☑
impacted shoulders 660.4 ☑
incarceration, uterus 654.3 ☑
causing obstructed labor
660.2 ☑
incomplete dilation (cervix)
661.0 ☑
incoordinate uterus 661.4 ☑
indication NEC 659.9 ☑
specified type NEC 659.8 ☑
inertia, uterus 661.2 ☑
hypertonic 661.4 ☑
hypotonic 661.2 ☑
primary 661.0 ☑
secondary 661.1 ☑
infantile
genitalia 654.4 ☑
causing obstructed labor
660.2 ☑
uterus (os) 654.4 ☑
causing obstructed labor
660.2 ☑
injury (to mother) NEC 665.9 ☑
intrauterine fetal death (near term)
NEC 656.4 ☑
early (before 22 completed
weeks gestation) 632
inversion, uterus 665.2 ☑
kidney, ectopic 654.4 ☑
causing obstructed labor
660.2 ☑
knot (true), umbilical cord 663.2 ☑
labor, premature (before 37 completed weeks gestation)
644.2 ☑
laceration 664.9 ☑
anus (sphincter) ▶(healed)
(old)◀ 654.8 ☑                ▲
with mucosa 664.3 ☑
not associated with third-  ●
degree perineal lacer-  ●
ation 664.6 ☑              ●
bladder (urinary) 665.5 ☑
bowel 665.5 ☑
central 664.4 ☑
cervix (uteri) 665.3 ☑
fourchette 664.0 ☑
hymen 664.0 ☑
labia (majora) (minora) 664.0 ☑
pelvic
floor 664.1 ☑
organ NEC 665.5 ☑
perineum, perineal 664.4 ☑
first degree 664.0 ☑
second degree 664.1 ☑
third degree 664.2 ☑
fourth degree 664.3 ☑
central 664.4 ☑
extensive NEC 664.4 ☑
muscles 664.1 ☑

**Delivery** — *continued*
complicated — *continued*
laceration — *continued*
perineum, perineal — *continued*
skin 664.0 ☑
slight 664.0 ☑
peritoneum 665.5 ☑
periurethral tissue
664.8 ☑                      ▲
rectovaginal (septum) (without
perineal laceration)
665.4 ☑
with perineum 664.2 ☑
with anal or rectal mu-
cosa 664.3 ☑
skin (perineum) 664.0 ☑
specified site or type NEC
664.8 ☑
sphincter ani ▶(healed) (old)◀
654.8 ☑                      ▲
with mucosa 664.3 ☑
not associated with third-  ●
degree perineal lacer-  ●
ation 664.6 ☑              ●
urethra 665.5 ☑
uterus 665.1 ☑
before labor 665.0 ☑
vagina, vaginal (deep) (high)
(sulcus) (wall) (without
perineal laceration)
665.4 ☑
with perineum 664.0 ☑
muscles, with perineum
664.1 ☑
vulva 664.0 ☑
lateroversion, uterus or cervix
654.4 ☑
causing obstructed labor
660.2 ☑
locked mates 660.5 ☑
low implantation of placenta — *see*
Delivery, complicated, placenta, previa
mal lie 652.9 ☑
malposition
fetus NEC 652.9 ☑
causing obstructed labor
660.0 ☑
pelvic organs or tissues NEC
654.9 ☑
causing obstructed labor
660.2 ☑
placenta 641.1 ☑
without hemorrhage 641.0 ☑
uterus NEC or cervix 654.4 ☑
causing obstructed labor
660.2 ☑
malpresentation 652.9 ☑
causing obstructed labor
660.0 ☑
marginal sinus (bleeding) (rupture)
641.2 ☑
maternal hypotension syndrome
669.2 ☑
meconium in liquor 656.8 ☑
membranes, retained — *see* Delivery, complicated, placenta,
retained
mentum presentation 652.4 ☑
causing obstructed labor
660.0 ☑
metrorrhagia (myopathia) — *see*
Delivery, complicated, hemorrhage
metrorrhexis — *see* Delivery, complicated, rupture, uterus
multiparity (grand) 659.4 ☑
myelomeningocele, fetus 653.7 ☑
causing obstructed labor
660.1 ☑
Nägele's pelvis 653.0 ☑
causing obstructed labor
660.1 ☑

---

☑ Additional Digit Required — Refer to the Tabular List for Digit Selection          🖑 Subterms under main terms may continue to next column or page

**Delivery** — *continued*
  complicated — *continued*
    nonengagement, fetal head
      652.5 ☑
      causing obstructed labor
        660.0 ☑
    oblique presentation 652.3 ☑
      causing obstructed labor
        660.0 ☑
    obstetric
      shock 669.1 ☑
      trauma NEC 665.9 ☑
    obstructed labor 660.9 ☑
      due to
        abnormality of pelvic organs
          or tissues (conditions
          classifiable to
          654.0–654.9) 660.2 ☑
        deep transverse arrest
          660.3 ☑
        impacted shoulders 660.4 ☑
        locked twins 660.5 ☑
        malposition and malpresenta-
          tion of fetus (condi-
          tions classifiable to
          652.0–652.9) 660.0 ☑
        persistent occipitoposterior
          660.3 ☑
        shoulder dystocia 660.4 ☑
    occult prolapse of umbilical cord
      663.0 ☑
    oversize fetus 653.5 ☑
      causing obstructed labor
        660.1 ☑
    pathological retraction ring, uterus
      661.4 ☑
    pelvic
      arrest (deep) (high) (of fetal
        head) (transverse)
        660.3 ☑
      deformity (bone) (*see also* Defor-
        mity, pelvis, with dispro-
        portion)
        soft tissue 654.9 ☑
          causing obstructed labor
            660.2 ☑
      tumor NEC 654.9 ☑
        causing obstructed labor
          660.2 ☑
    penetration, pregnant uterus by
      instrument 665.1 ☑
    perforation — *see* Delivery, compli-
      cated, laceration
    persistent
      hymen 654.8 ☑
        causing obstructed labor
          660.2 ☑
      occipitoposterior 660.3 ☑
    placenta, placental
      ablatio 641.2 ☑
      abnormality 656.7 ☑
        with hemorrhage 641.2 ☑
      abruptio 641.2 ☑
      accreta 667.0 ☑
        with hemorrhage 666.0 ☑
      adherent (without hemorrhage)
        667.0 ☑
        with hemorrhage 666.0 ☑
      apoplexy 641.2 ☑
      battledore placenta — *see* Pla-
        centa, abnormal
      detachment (premature)
        641.2 ☑
      disease 656.7 ☑
      hemorrhage NEC 641.9 ☑
      increta (without hemorrhage)
        667.0 ☑
        with hemorrhage 666.0 ☑
      low (implantation) 641.1 ☑
        without hemorrhage 641.0 ☑
      malformation 656.7 ☑
        with hemorrhage 641.2 ☑
      malposition 641.1 ☑
        without hemorrhage 641.0 ☑
      marginal sinus rupture 641.2 ☑

**Delivery** — *continued*
  complicated — *continued*
    placenta, placental — *continued*
      percreta 667.0 ☑
        with hemorrhage 666.0 ☑
      premature separation 641.2 ☑
      previa (central) (lateral)
        (marginal) (partial)
        641.1 ☑
        without hemorrhage 641.0 ☑
      retained (with hemorrhage)
        666.0 ☑
        without hemorrhage 667.0 ☑
      rupture of marginal sinus
        641.2 ☑
      separation (premature) 641.2 ☑
      trapped 666.0 ☑
        without hemorrhage 667.0 ☑
      vicious insertion 641.1 ☑
    polyhydramnios 657.0 ☑
    polyp, cervix 654.6 ☑
      causing obstructed labor
        660.2 ☑
    precipitate labor 661.3 ☑
    premature
      labor (before 37 completed
        weeks gestation) 644.2 ☑
      rupture, membranes 658.1 ☑
        delayed delivery following
          658.2 ☑
    presenting umbilical cord 663.0 ☑
    previous
      cesarean delivery, section
        654.2 ☑
      surgery
        cervix 654.6 ☑
          causing obstructed labor
            660.2 ☑
        gynecological NEC 654.9 ☑
          causing obstructed labor
            660.2 ☑
        perineum 654.8 ☑
        rectum 654.8 ☑
        uterus NEC 654.9 ☑
          due to previous cesarean
            delivery, section
            654.2 ☑
        vagina 654.7 ☑
          causing obstructed labor
            660.2 ☑
        vulva 654.8 ☑
    primary uterine inertia 661.0 ☑
    primipara, elderly or old 659.5 ☑
    prolapse
      arm or hand 652.7 ☑
        causing obstructed labor
          660.0 ☑
      cord (umbilical) 663.0 ☑
      fetal extremity 652.8 ☑
      foot or leg 652.8 ☑
        causing obstructed labor
          660.0 ☑
      umbilical cord (complete) (oc-
        cult) (partial) 663.0 ☑
      uterus 654.4 ☑
        causing obstructed labor
          660.2 ☑
    prolonged labor 662.1 ☑
      first stage 662.0 ☑
      second stage 662.2 ☑
      active phase 661.2 ☑
      due to
        cervical dystocia
          661.2 ☑ ▲
        contraction ring 661.4 ☑
        tetanic uterus 661.4 ☑
        uterine inertia 661.2 ☑
          primary 661.0 ☑
          secondary 661.1 ☑
        latent phase 661.0 ☑
    pyrexia during labor 659.2 ☑
    rachitic pelvis 653.2 ☑
      causing obstructed labor
        660.1 ☑

**Delivery** — *continued*
  complicated — *continued*
    rectocele 654.4 ☑
      causing obstructed labor
        660.2 ☑
    retained membranes or portions of
      placenta 666.2 ☑
      without hemorrhage 667.1 ☑
    retarded (prolonged) birth 662.1 ☑
    retention secundines (with hemor-
      rhage) 666.2 ☑
      without hemorrhage 667.1 ☑
    retroversion, uterus or cervix
      654.3 ☑
      causing obstructed labor
        660.2 ☑
    rigid
      cervix 654.6 ☑
        causing obstructed labor
          660.2 ☑
      pelvic floor 654.4 ☑
        causing obstructed labor
          660.2 ☑
      perineum or vulva 654.8 ☑
        causing obstructed labor
          660.2 ☑
      vagina 654.7 ☑
        causing obstructed labor
          660.2 ☑
    Robert's pelvis 653.0 ☑
      causing obstructed labor
        660.1 ☑
    rupture (*see also* Delivery, compli-
      cated, laceration)
      bladder (urinary) 665.5 ☑
      cervix 665.3 ☑
      marginal sinus 641.2 ☑
      membranes, premature 658.1 ☑
      pelvic organ NEC 665.5 ☑
      perineum (without mention of
        other laceration) — *see*
        Delivery, complicated,
        laceration, perineum
      peritoneum 665.5 ☑
      urethra 665.5 ☑
      uterus (during labor) 665.1 ☑
        before labor 665.0 ☑
    sacculation, pregnant uterus
      654.4 ☑
    sacral teratomas, fetal 653.7 ☑
      causing obstructed labor
        660.1 ☑
    scar(s)
      cervix 654.6 ☑
        causing obstructed labor
          660.2 ☑
      cesarean delivery, section
        654.2 ☑
        causing obstructed labor
          660.2 ☑
      perineum 654.8 ☑
        causing obstructed labor
          660.2 ☑
      uterus NEC 654.9 ☑
        causing obstructed labor
          660.2 ☑
        due to previous cesarean de-
          livery, section 654.2 ☑
      vagina 654.7 ☑
        causing obstructed labor
          660.2 ☑
      vulva 654.8 ☑
        causing obstructed labor
          660.2 ☑
    scoliotic pelvis 653.0 ☑
      causing obstructed labor
        660.1 ☑
    secondary uterine inertia 661.1 ☑
    secundines, retained — *see* Deliv-
      ery, complicated, placenta,
      retained
    separation
      placenta (premature) 641.2 ☑
      pubic bone 665.6 ☑
      symphysis pubis 665.6 ☑

**Delivery** — *continued*
  complicated — *continued*
    septate vagina 654.7 ☑
      causing obstructed labor
        660.2 ☑
    shock (birth) (obstetric) (puerperal)
      669.1 ☑
    short cord syndrome 663.4 ☑
    shoulder
      girdle dystocia 660.4 ☑
      presentation 652.8 ☑
        causing obstructed labor
          660.0 ☑
    Siamese twins 653.7 ☑
      causing obstructed labor
        660.1 ☑
    slow slope active phase 661.2 ☑
    spasm
      cervix 661.4 ☑
      uterus 661.4 ☑
    spondylolisthesis, pelvis 653.3 ☑
      causing obstructed labor
        660.1 ☑
    spondylolysis (lumbosacral)
      653.3 ☑
      causing obstructed labor
        660.1 ☑
    spondylosis 653.0 ☑
      causing obstructed labor
        660.1 ☑
    stenosis or stricture
      cervix 654.6 ☑
        causing obstructed labor
          660.2 ☑
      vagina 654.7 ☑
        causing obstructed labor
          660.2 ☑
    sudden death, unknown cause
      669.9 ☑
    tear (pelvic organ) (*see also* Deliv-
      ery, complicated, laceration)
      664.9 ☑
      anal sphincter (healed) (old) ●
        654.8 ☑ ●
        not associated with third- ●
          degree perineal lacer- ●
          ation 664.6 ☑ ●
    teratomas, sacral, fetal 653.7 ☑
      causing obstructed labor
        660.1 ☑
    tetanic uterus 661.4 ☑
    tipping pelvis 653.0 ☑
      causing obstructed labor
        660.1 ☑
    transverse
      arrest (deep) 660.3 ☑
      presentation or lie 652.3 ☑
        with successful version
          652.1 ☑
        causing obstructed labor
          660.0 ☑
    trauma (obstetrical) NEC 665.9 ☑
    tumor
      abdominal, fetal 653.7 ☑
        causing obstructed labor
          660.1 ☑
      pelvic organs or tissues NEC
        654.9 ☑
        causing obstructed labor
          660.2 ☑
    umbilical cord (*see also* Delivery,
      complicated, cord) 663.9 ☑
      around neck tightly, or with
        compression 663.1 ☑
      entanglement NEC 663.3 ☑
        with compression 663.2 ☑
      prolapse (complete) (occult)
        (partial) 663.0 ☑
    unstable lie 652.0 ☑
      causing obstructed labor
        660.0 ☑
    uterine
      inertia (*see also* Delivery, compli-
        cated, inertia, uterus)
        661.2 ☑

☑ Additional Digit Required — Refer to the Tabular List for Digit Selection                  ▽ Subterms under main terms may continue to next column or page

*2008 ICD-9-CM*            ▶◀ Revised Text            ● New Line            ▲ Revised Code            **October 2007 · Volume 2 — 75**

**Delivery** — *continued*
  complicated — *continued*
    uterine — *continued*
      spasm 661.4 ☑
      vasa previa 663.5 ☑
      velamentous insertion of cord
        663.8 ☑
      young maternal age 659.8 ☑
  delayed NEC 662.1 ☑
    following rupture of membranes
      (spontaneous) 658.2 ☑
      artificial 658.3 ☑
    second twin, triplet, etc. 662.3 ☑
  difficult NEC 669.9 ☑
    previous, affecting management of
      pregnancy or childbirth
      V23.49
    specified type NEC 669.8 ☑
  early onset (spontaneous) 644.2 ☑
  footling 652.8 ☑
    with successful version 652.1 ☑
  forceps NEC 669.5 ☑
    affecting fetus or newborn 763.2
  missed (at or near term) 656.4 ☑
  multiple gestation NEC 651.9 ☑
    with fetal loss and retention of one
      or more fetus(es) 651.6 ☑
    following (elective) fetal reduction
      651.7 ☑
    specified type NEC 651.8 ☑
      with fetal loss and retention of
        one or more fetus(es)
        651.6 ☑
      following (elective) fetal reduc-
        tion 651.7 ☑
  nonviable infant 656.4 ☑
  normal — *see* category 650
  precipitate 661.3 ☑
    affecting fetus or newborn 763.6
  premature NEC (before 37 completed
    weeks gestation) 644.2 ☑
    previous, affecting management of
      pregnancy V23.41
  quadruplet NEC 651.2 ☑
    with fetal loss and retention of one
      or more fetus(es) 651.5 ☑
    following (elective) fetal reduction
      651.7 ☑
  quintuplet NEC 651.8 ☑
    with fetal loss and retention of one
      or more fetus(es) 651.6 ☑
    following (elective) fetal reduction
      651.7 ☑
  sextuplet NEC 651.8 ☑
    with fetal loss and retention of one
      or more fetus(es) 651.6 ☑
    following (elective) fetal reduction
      651.7 ☑
  specified complication NEC 669.8 ☑
  stillbirth (near term) NEC 656.4 ☑
    early (before 22 completed weeks
      gestation) 632
  term pregnancy (live birth) NEC — *see*
    category 650
    stillbirth NEC 656.4 ☑
  threatened premature 644.2 ☑
  triplets NEC 651.1 ☑
    with fetal loss and retention of one
      or more fetus(es) 651.4 ☑
    delayed delivery (one or more
      mates) 662.3 ☑
    following (elective) fetal reduction
      651.7 ☑
    locked mates 660.5 ☑
  twins NEC 651.0 ☑
    with fetal loss and retention of one
      fetus 651.3 ☑
    delayed delivery (one or more
      mates) 662.3 ☑
    following (elective) fetal reduction
      651.7 ☑
    locked mates 660.5 ☑
  uncomplicated — *see* category 650
  vacuum extractor NEC 669.5 ☑
    affecting fetus or newborn 763.3

**Delivery** — *continued*
  ventouse NEC 669.5 ☑
    affecting fetus or newborn 763.3
**Dellen, cornea** 371.41
**Delusions** (paranoid) 297.9
  grandiose 297.1
  parasitosis 300.29
  systematized 297.1
**Dementia** 294.8
  alcohol-induced persisting (*see also*
    Psychosis, alcoholic) 291.2
  Alzheimer's — *see* Alzheimer's, demen-
    tia
  arteriosclerotic (simple type) (uncom-
    plicated) 290.40
    with
      acute confusional state 290.41
      delirium 290.41
      delusions 290.42
      depressed mood 290.43
    depressed type 290.43
    paranoid type 290.42
  Binswanger's 290.12
  catatonic (acute) (*see also*
    Schizophrenia) 295.2 ☑
  congenital (*see also* Retardation,
    mental) 319
  degenerative 290.9
    presenile-onset — *see* Dementia,
      presenile
    senile-onset — *see* Dementia, se-
      nile
  developmental (*see also* Schizophre-
    nia) 295.9 ☑
  dialysis 294.8
    transient 293.9
  drug-induced persisting (*see also*
    Psychosis, drug) 292.82
  due to or associated with condition(s)
    classified elsewhere
    Alzheimer's
      with behavioral disturbance
        331.0 *[294.11]*
      without behavioral disturbance
        331.0 *[294.10]*
    cerebral lipidoses
      with behavioral disturbance
        330.1 *[294.11]*
      without behavioral disturbance
        330.1 *[294.10]*
    epilepsy
      with behavioral disturbance
        345.9 ☑ *[294.11]*
      without behavioral disturbance
        345.9 ☑ *[294.10]*
    hepatolenticular degeneration
      with behavioral disturbance
        275.1 *[294.11]*
      without behavioral disturbance
        275.1 *[294.10]*
    HIV
      with behavioral disturbance
        042 *[294.11]*
      without behavioral disturbance
        042 *[294.10]*
    Huntington's chorea
      with behavioral disturbance
        333.4 *[294.11]*
      without behavioral disturbance
        333.4 *[294.10]*
    Jakob-Creutzfeldt disease (new
      variant)
      with behavioral disturbance
        046.1 *[294.11]*
      without behavioral disturbance
        046.1 *[294.10]*
    Lewy bodies
      with behavioral disturbance
        331.82 *[294.11]*
      without behavioral disturbance
        331.82 *[294.10]*
    multiple sclerosis
      with behavioral disturbance
        340 *[294.11]*
      without behavioral disturbance
        340 *[294.10]*

**Dementia** — *continued*
  due to or associated with condition(s)
    classified elsewhere — *contin-
    ued*
    neurosyphilis
      with behavioral disturbance
        094.9 *[294.11]*
      without behavioral disturbance
        094.9 *[294.10]*
    Parkinsonism
      with behavioral disturbance
        331.82 *[294.11]*
      without behavioral disturbance
        331.82 *[294.10]*
    Pelizaeus-Merzbacher disease
      with behavioral disturbance
        333.0 *[294.11]*
      without behavioral disturbance
        333.0 *[294.10]*
    Pick's disease
      with behavioral disturbance
        331.11 *[294.11]*
      without behavioral disturbance
        331.11 *[294.10]*
    polyarteritis nodosa
      with behavioral disturbance
        446.0 *[294.11]*
      without behavioral disturbance
        446.0 *[294.10]*
    syphilis
      with behavioral disturbance
        094.1 *[294.11]*
      without behavioral disturbance
        094.1 *[294.10]*
    Wilson's disease
      with behavioral disturbance
        275.1 *[294.11]*
      without behavioral disturbance
        275.1 *[294.10]*
  frontal 331.19
    with behavioral disturbance
      331.19 *[294.11]*
    without behavioral disturbance
      331.19 *[294.10]*
  frontotemporal 331.19
    with behavioral disturbance
      331.19 *[294.11]*
    without behavioral disturbance
      331.19 *[294.10]*
  hebephrenic (acute) 295.1 ☑
  Heller's (infantile psychosis) (*see also*
    Psychosis, childhood) 299.1 ☑
  idiopathic 290.9
    presenile-onset — *see* Dementia,
      presenile
    senile-onset — *see* Dementia, se-
      nile
  in
    arteriosclerotic brain disease
      290.40
    senility 290.0
  induced by drug 292.82
  infantile, infantilia (*see also* Psychosis,
    childhood) 299.0 ☑
  Lewy body 331.82
    with behavioral disturbance
      331.82 *[294.11]*
    without behavioral disturbance
      331.82 *[294.10]*
  multi-infarct (cerebrovascular) (*see
    also* Dementia, arteriosclerotic)
    290.40
  old age 290.0
  paralytica, paralytic 094.1
    juvenilis 090.40
    syphilitic 094.1
      congenital 090.40
    tabetic form 094.1
  paranoid (*see also* Schizophrenia)
    295.3 ☑
  paraphrenic (*see also* Schizophrenia)
    295.3 ☑
  paretic 094.1
  praecox (*see also* Schizophrenia)
    295.9 ☑
  presenile 290.10

**Dementia** — *continued*
  presenile — *continued*
    with
      acute confusional state 290.11
      delirium 290.11
      delusional features 290.12
      depressive features 290.13
    depressed type 290.13
    paranoid type 290.12
    simple type 290.10
    uncomplicated 290.10
  primary (acute) (*see also* Schizophre-
    nia) 295.0 ☑
  progressive, syphilitic 094.1
  puerperal — *see* Psychosis, puerperal
  schizophrenic (*see also* Schizophrenia)
    295.9 ☑
  senile 290.0
    with
      acute confusional state 290.3
      delirium 290.3
      delusional features 290.20
      depressive features 290.21
    depressed type 290.21
    exhaustion 290.0
    paranoid type 290.20
  simple type (acute) (*see also*
    Schizophrenia) 295.0 ☑
  simplex (acute) (*see also* Schizophre-
    nia) 295.0 ☑
  syphilitic 094.1
  uremic — *see* Uremia
  vascular 290.40
    with
      delirium 290.41
      delusions 290.42
      depressed mood 290.43
**Demerol dependence** — *see also* Dependence 304.0 ☑
**Demineralization, ankle** — *see also*
  Osteoporosis 733.00
**Demodex folliculorum** (infestation)
  133.8
**de Morgan's spots** (senile angiomas)
  448.1
**Demyelinating**
  polyneuritis, chronic inflammatory
    357.81
**Demyelination, demyelinization**
  central nervous system 341.9
    specified NEC 341.8
  corpus callosum (central) 341.8
  global 340
**Dengue** (fever) 061
  sandfly 061
  vaccination, prophylactic (against)
    V05.1
  virus hemorrhagic fever 065.4
**Dens**
  evaginatus 520.2
  in dente 520.2
  invaginatus 520.2
**Density**
  increased, bone (disseminated) (gener-
    alized) (spotted) 733.99
  lung (nodular) 518.89
**Dental** — *see also* condition
  examination only V72.2
**Dentia praecox** 520.6
**Denticles** (in pulp) 522.2
**Dentigerous cyst** 526.0
**Dentin**
  irregular (in pulp) 522.3
  opalescent 520.5
  secondary (in pulp) 522.3
  sensitive 521.89
**Dentinogenesis imperfecta** 520.5
**Dentinoma** (M9271/0) 213.1
  upper jaw (bone) 213.0
**Dentition** 520.7
  abnormal 520.6
  anomaly 520.6
  delayed 520.6
  difficult 520.7
  disorder of 520.6
  precocious 520.6

☑ Additional Digit Required — Refer to the Tabular List for Digit Selection ⮟ Subterms under main terms may continue to next column or page

76 — Volume 2      ▶◀ Revised Text      ● New Line      ▲ Revised Code      *2008 ICD-9-CM*

**Dentition** — *continued*
retarded 520.6
**Denture sore** (mouth) 528.9
**Dependence**

---

Note — Use the following fifth-digit subclassification with category 304:

0   unspecified

1   continuous

2   episodic

3   in remission

---

with
withdrawal symptoms
alcohol 291.81
drug 292.0
14-hydroxy-dihydromorphinone 304.0 ☑
absinthe 304.6 ☑
acemorphan 304.0 ☑
acetanilid(e) 304.6 ☑
acetophenetidin 304.6 ☑
acetorphine 304.0 ☑
acetyldihydrocodeine 304.0 ☑
acetyldihydrocodeinone 304.0 ☑
Adalin 304.1 ☑
Afghanistan black 304.3 ☑
agrypnal 304.1 ☑
alcohol, alcoholic (ethyl) (methyl) (wood) 303.9 ☑
maternal, with suspected fetal damage affecting management of pregnancy 655.4 ☑
allobarbitone 304.1 ☑
allonal 304.1 ☑
allylisopropylacetylurea 304.1 ☑
alphaprodine (hydrochloride) 304.0 ☑
Alurate 304.1 ☑
Alvodine 304.0 ☑
amethocaine 304.6 ☑
amidone 304.0 ☑
amidopyrine 304.6 ☑
aminopyrine 304.6 ☑
amobarbital 304.1 ☑
amphetamine(s) (type) (drugs classifiable to 969.7) 304.4 ☑
amylene hydrate 304.6 ☑
amylobarbitone 304.1 ☑
amylocaine 304.6 ☑
Amytal (sodium) 304.1 ☑
analgesic (drug) NEC 304.6 ☑
synthetic with morphine-like effect 304.0 ☑
anesthetic (agent) (drug) (gas) (general) (local) NEC 304.6 ☑
Angel dust 304.6 ☑
anileridine 304.0 ☑
antipyrine 304.6 ☑
anxiolytic 304.1 ☑
aprobarbital 304.1 ☑
aprobarbitone 304.1 ☑
atropine 304.6 ☑
Avertin (bromide) 304.6 ☑
barbenyl 304.1 ☑
barbital(s) 304.1 ☑
barbitone 304.1 ☑
barbiturate(s) (compounds) (drugs classifiable to 967.0) 304.1 ☑
barbituric acid (and compounds) 304.1 ☑
benzedrine 304.4 ☑
benzylmorphine 304.0 ☑
Beta-chlor 304.1 ☑
bhang 304.3 ☑
blue velvet 304.0 ☑
Brevital 304.1 ☑
bromal (hydrate) 304.1 ☑
bromide(s) NEC 304.1 ☑
bromine compounds NEC 304.1 ☑
bromisovalum 304.1 ☑
bromoform 304.1 ☑
Bromo-seltzer 304.1 ☑
bromural 304.1 ☑
butabarbital (sodium) 304.1 ☑

**Dependence** — *continued*
butabarpal 304.1 ☑
butallylonal 304.1 ☑
butethal 304.1 ☑
buthalitone (sodium) 304.1 ☑
Butisol 304.1 ☑
butobarbitone 304.1 ☑
butyl chloral (hydrate) 304.1 ☑
caffeine 304.4 ☑
cannabis (indica) (sativa) (resin) (derivatives) (type) 304.3 ☑
carbamazepine 304.6 ☑
Carbrital 304.1 ☑
carbromal 304.1 ☑
carisoprodol 304.6 ☑
Catha (edulis) 304.4 ☑
chloral (betaine) (hydrate) 304.1 ☑
chloralamide 304.1 ☑
chloralformamide 304.1 ☑
chloralose 304.1 ☑
chlordiazepoxide 304.1 ☑
Chloretone 304.1 ☑
chlorobutanol 304.1 ☑
chlorodyne 304.1 ☑
chloroform 304.6 ☑
Cliradon 304.0 ☑
coca (leaf) and derivatives 304.2 ☑
cocaine 304.2 ☑
hydrochloride 304.2 ☑
salt (any) 304.2 ☑
codeine 304.0 ☑
combination of drugs (excluding morphine or opioid type drug) NEC 304.8 ☑
morphine or opioid type drug with any other drug 304.7 ☑
croton-chloral 304.1 ☑
cyclobarbital 304.1 ☑
cyclobarbitone 304.1 ☑
dagga 304.3 ☑
Delvinal 304.1 ☑
Demerol 304.0 ☑
desocodeine 304.0 ☑
desomorphine 304.0 ☑
desoxyephedrine 304.4 ☑
DET 304.5 ☑
dexamphetamine 304.4 ☑
dexedrine 304.4 ☑
dextromethorphan 304.0 ☑
dextromoramide 304.0 ☑
dextronorpseudoephedrine 304.4 ☑
dextrorphan 304.0 ☑
diacetylmorphine 304.0 ☑
Dial 304.1 ☑
diallylbarbituric acid 304.1 ☑
diamorphine 304.0 ☑
diazepam 304.1 ☑
dibucaine 304.6 ☑
dichloroethane 304.6 ☑
diethyl barbituric acid 304.1 ☑
diethylsulfone-diethylmethane 304.1 ☑
difencloxazine 304.0 ☑
dihydrocodeine 304.0 ☑
dihydrocodeinone 304.0 ☑
dihydrohydroxycodeinone 304.0 ☑
dihydroisocodeine 304.0 ☑
dihydromorphine 304.0 ☑
dihydromorphinone 304.0 ☑
dihydroxcodeinone 304.0 ☑
Dilaudid 304.0 ☑
dimenhydrinate 304.6 ☑
dimethylmeperidine 304.0 ☑
dimethyltriptamine 304.5 ☑
Dionin 304.0 ☑
diphenoxylate 304.6 ☑
dipipanone 304.0 ☑
d-lysergic acid diethylamide 304.5 ☑
DMT 304.5 ☑
Dolophine 304.0 ☑
DOM 304.2 ☑
Doriden 304.1 ☑
dormiral 304.1 ☑
Dormison 304.1 ☑

**Dependence** — *continued*
Dromoran 304.0 ☑
drug NEC 304.9 ☑
analgesic NEC 304.6 ☑
combination (excluding morphine or opioid type drug) NEC 304.8 ☑
morphine or opioid type drug with any other drug 304.7 ☑
complicating pregnancy, childbirth, or puerperium 648.3 ☑
affecting fetus or newborn 779.5
hallucinogenic 304.5 ☑
hypnotic NEC 304.1 ☑
narcotic NEC 304.9 ☑
psychostimulant NEC 304.4 ☑
sedative 304.1 ☑
soporific NEC 304.1 ☑
specified type NEC 304.6 ☑
suspected damage to fetus affecting management of pregnancy 655.5 ☑
synthetic, with morphine-like effect 304.0 ☑
tranquilizing 304.1 ☑
duboisine 304.6 ☑
ectylurea 304.1 ☑
Endocaine 304.6 ☑
Equanil 304.1 ☑
Eskabarb 304.1 ☑
ethchlorvynol 304.1 ☑
ether (ethyl) (liquid) (vapor) (vinyl) 304.6 ☑
ethidene 304.6 ☑
ethinamate 304.1 ☑
ethoheptazine 304.6 ☑
ethyl
alcohol 303.9 ☑
bromide 304.6 ☑
carbamate 304.6 ☑
chloride 304.6 ☑
morphine 304.0 ☑
ethylene (gas) 304.6 ☑
dichloride 304.6 ☑
ethylidene chloride 304.6 ☑
etilfen 304.1 ☑
etorphine 304.0 ☑
etoval 304.1 ☑
eucodal 304.0 ☑
euneryl 304.1 ☑
Evipal 304.1 ☑
Evipan 304.1 ☑
fentanyl 304.0 ☑
ganja 304.3 ☑
gardenal 304.1 ☑
gardenpanyl 304.1 ☑
gelsemine 304.6 ☑
Gelsemium 304.6 ☑
Gemonil 304.1 ☑
glucochloral 304.1 ☑
glue (airplane) (sniffing) 304.6 ☑
glutethimide 304.1 ☑
hallucinogenics 304.5 ☑
hashish 304.3 ☑
headache powder NEC 304.6 ☑
Heavenly Blue 304.5 ☑
hedonal 304.1 ☑
hemp 304.3 ☑
heptabarbital 304.1 ☑
Heptalgin 304.0 ☑
heptobarbitone 304.1 ☑
heroin 304.0 ☑
salt (any) 304.0 ☑
hexethal (sodium) 304.1 ☑
hexobarbital 304.1 ☑
Hycodan 304.0 ☑
hydrocodone 304.0 ☑
hydromorphinol 304.0 ☑
hydromorphinone 304.0 ☑
hydromorphone 304.0 ☑
hydroxycodeine 304.0 ☑
hypnotic NEC 304.1 ☑
Indian hemp 304.3 ☑

**Dependence** — *continued*
inhalant 304.6 ☑
intranarcon 304.1 ☑
Kemithal 304.1 ☑
ketobemidone 304.0 ☑
khat 304.4 ☑
kif 304.3 ☑
Lactuca (virosa) extract 304.1 ☑
lactucarium 304.1 ☑
laudanum 304.0 ☑
Lebanese red 304.3 ☑
Leritine 304.0 ☑
lettuce opium 304.1 ☑
Levanil 304.1 ☑
Levo-Dromoran 304.0 ☑
levo-iso-methadone 304.0 ☑
levorphanol 304.0 ☑
Librium 304.1 ☑
Lomotil 304.6 ☑
Lotusate 304.1 ☑
LSD (-25) (and derivatives) 304.5 ☑
Luminal 304.1 ☑
lysergic acid 304.5 ☑
amide 304.5 ☑
maconha 304.3 ☑
magic mushroom 304.5 ☑
marihuana 304.3 ☑
MDA (methylene dioxyamphetamine) 304.4 ☑
Mebaral 304.1 ☑
Medinal 304.1 ☑
Medomin 304.1 ☑
megahallucinogenics 304.5 ☑
meperidine 304.0 ☑
mephobarbital 304.1 ☑
meprobamate 304.1 ☑
mescaline 304.5 ☑
methadone 304.0 ☑
methamphetamine(s) 304.4 ☑
methaqualone 304.1 ☑
metharbital 304.1 ☑
methitural 304.1 ☑
methobarbitone 304.1 ☑
methohexital 304.1 ☑
methopholine 304.6 ☑
methyl
alcohol 303.9 ☑
bromide 304.6 ☑
morphine 304.0 ☑
sulfonal 304.1 ☑
methylaparafynol 304.1 ☑
methylated spirit 303.9 ☑
methylbutinol 304.6 ☑
methyldihydromorphinone 304.0 ☑
methylene
chloride 304.6 ☑
dichloride 304.6 ☑
dioxyamphetamine (MDA) 304.4 ☑
methylphenidate 304.4 ☑
methyprylone 304.1 ☑
metopon 304.0 ☑
Miltown 304.1 ☑
morning glory seeds 304.5 ☑
morphinan(s) 304.0 ☑
morphine (sulfate) (sulfite) (type) (drugs classifiable to 965.00–965.09) 304.0 ☑
morphine or opioid type drug (drugs classifiable to 965.00–965.09) with any other drug 304.7 ☑
morphinol(s) 304.0 ☑
morphinon 304.0 ☑
morpholinylethylmorphine 304.0 ☑
mylomide 304.1 ☑
myristicin 304.5 ☑
narcotic (drug) NEC 304.9 ☑
nealbarbital 304.1 ☑
nealbarbitone 304.1 ☑
Nembutal 304.1 ☑
Neonal 304.1 ☑
Neraval 304.1 ☑
Neravan 304.1 ☑
neurobarb 304.1 ☑
nicotine 305.1

---

☑ Additional Digit Required — Refer to the Tabular List for Digit Selection    ▽ Subterms under main terms may continue to next column or page

**Dependence** — *continued*
Nisentil 304.0 ☑
nitrous oxide 304.6 ☑
Noctec 304.1 ☑
Noludar 304.1 ☑
nonbarbiturate sedatives and tranquilizers with similar effect 304.1 ☑
noptil 304.1 ☑
normorphine 304.0 ☑
noscapine 304.0 ☑
Novocaine 304.6 ☑
Numorphan 304.0 ☑
nunol 304.1 ☑
Nupercaine 304.6 ☑
Oblivon 304.1 ☑
on
    aspirator V46.0
    hemodialysis V45.1
    hyperbaric chamber V46.8
    iron lung V46.11
    machine (enabling) V46.9
      specified type NEC V46.8
    peritoneal dialysis V45.1
    Possum (Patient-Operated-Selector-Mechanism) V46.8
    renal dialysis machine V45.1
    respirator [ventilator] V46.11
      encounter
        during
          mechanical failure V46.14
          power failure V46.12
        for weaning V46.13
    supplemental oxygen V46.2
opiate 304.0 ☑
opioids 304.0 ☑
opioid type drug 304.0 ☑
    with any other drug 304.7 ☑
opium (alkaloids) (derivatives) (tincture) 304.0 ☑
ortal 304.1 ☑
Oxazepam 304.1 ☑
oxycodone 304.0 ☑
oxymorphone 304.0 ☑
Palfium 304.0 ☑
Panadol 304.6 ☑
pantopium 304.0 ☑
pantopon 304.0 ☑
papaverine 304.0 ☑
paracetamol 304.6 ☑
paracodin 304.0 ☑
paraldehyde 304.1 ☑
paregoric 304.0 ☑
Parzone 304.0 ☑
PCP (phencyclidine) 304.6 ☑
Pearly Gates 304.5 ☑
pentazocine 304.0 ☑
pentobarbital 304.1 ☑
pentobarbitone (sodium) 304.1 ☑
Pentothal 304.1 ☑
Percaine 304.6 ☑
Percodan 304.0 ☑
Perichlor 304.1 ☑
Pernocton 304.1 ☑
Pernoston 304.1 ☑
peronine 304.0 ☑
pethidine (hydrochloride) 304.0 ☑
petrichloral 304.1 ☑
peyote 304.5 ☑
Phanodron 304.1 ☑
phenacetin 304.6 ☑
phenadoxone 304.0 ☑
phenaglycodol 304.1 ☑
phenazocine 304.0 ☑
phencyclidine 304.6 ☑
phenmetrazine 304.4 ☑
phenobal 304.1 ☑
phenobarbital 304.1 ☑
phenobarbitone 304.1 ☑
phenomorphan 304.0 ☑
phenonyl 304.1 ☑
phenoperidine 304.0 ☑
pholcodine 304.0 ☑
piminodine 304.0 ☑
Pipadone 304.0 ☑

**Dependence** — *continued*
Pitkin's solution 304.6 ☑
Placidyl 304.1 ☑
polysubstance 304.8 ☑
Pontocaine 304.6 ☑
pot 304.3 ☑
potassium bromide 304.1 ☑
Preludin 304.4 ☑
Prinadol 304.0 ☑
probarbital 304.1 ☑
procaine 304.6 ☑
propanal 304.1 ☑
propoxyphene 304.6 ☑
psilocibin 304.5 ☑
psilocin 304.5 ☑
psilocybin 304.5 ☑
psilocyline 304.5 ☑
psilocyn 304.5 ☑
psychedelic agents 304.5 ☑
psychostimulant NEC 304.4 ☑
psychotomimetic agents 304.5 ☑
pyrahexyl 304.3 ☑
Pyramidon 304.6 ☑
quinalbarbitone 304.1 ☑
racemoramide 304.0 ☑
racemorphan 304.0 ☑
Rela 304.6 ☑
scopolamine 304.6 ☑
secobarbital 304.1 ☑
Seconal 304.1 ☑
sedative NEC 304.1 ☑
    nonbarbiturate with barbiturate effect 304.1 ☑
Sedormid 304.1 ☑
sernyl 304.1 ☑
sodium bromide 304.1 ☑
Soma 304.6 ☑
Somnal 304.1 ☑
Somnos 304.1 ☑
Soneryl 304.1 ☑
soporific (drug) NEC 304.1 ☑
specified drug NEC 304.6 ☑
speed 304.4 ☑
spinocaine 304.6 ☑
Stovaine 304.6 ☑
STP 304.5 ☑
stramonium 304.6 ☑
Sulfonal 304.1 ☑
sulfonethylmethane 304.1 ☑
sulfonmethane 304.1 ☑
Surital 304.1 ☑
synthetic drug with morphine-like effect 304.0 ☑
talbutal 304.1 ☑
tetracaine 304.6 ☑
tetrahydrocannabinol 304.3 ☑
tetronal 304.1 ☑
THC 304.3 ☑
thebacon 304.0 ☑
thebaine 304.0 ☑
thiamil 304.1 ☑
thiamylal 304.1 ☑
thiopental 304.1 ☑
tobacco 305.1
toluene, toluol 304.6 ☑
tranquilizer NEC 304.1 ☑
    nonbarbiturate with barbiturate effect 304.1 ☑
tribromacetaldehyde 304.6 ☑
tribromethanol 304.6 ☑
tribromomethane 304.6 ☑
trichloroethanol 304.6 ☑
trichoroethyl phosphate 304.1 ☑
triclofos 304.1 ☑
Trional 304.1 ☑
Tuinal 304.1 ☑
Turkish Green 304.3 ☑
urethan(e) 304.6 ☑
Valium 304.1 ☑
Valmid 304.1 ☑
veganin 304.0 ☑
veramon 304.1 ☑
Veronal 304.1 ☑
versidyne 304.6 ☑

**Dependence** — *continued*
vinbarbital 304.1 ☑
vinbarbitone 304.1 ☑
vinyl bitone 304.1 ☑
vitamin $B_6$ 266.1
wine 303.9 ☑
Zactane 304.6 ☑
**Dependency**
passive 301.6
reactions 301.6
**Depersonalization** (episode, in neurotic state) (neurotic) (syndrome) 300.6
**Depletion**
carbohydrates 271.9
complement factor 279.8
extracellular fluid 276.52
plasma 276.52
potassium 276.8
    nephropathy 588.89
salt or sodium 276.1
    causing heat exhaustion or prostration 992.4
    nephropathy 593.9
volume 276.50
    extracellular fluid 276.52
    plasma 276.52
**Deposit**
argentous, cornea 371.16
bone, in Boeck's sarcoid 135
calcareous, calcium — *see* Calcification
cholesterol
    retina 362.82
    skin 709.3
    vitreous (humor) 379.22
conjunctival 372.56
cornea, corneal NEC 371.10
    argentous 371.16
    in
      cystinosis 270.0 *[371.15]*
      mucopolysaccharidosis 277.5 *[371.15]*
crystalline, vitreous (humor) 379.22
hemosiderin, in old scars of cornea 371.11
metallic, in lens 366.45
skin 709.3
teeth, tooth (betel) (black) (green) (materia alba) (orange) (soft) (tobacco) 523.6
urate, in kidney (*see also* Disease, renal) 593.9
**Depraved appetite** 307.52
**Depression** 311
acute (*see also* Psychosis, affective) 296.2 ☑
    recurrent episode 296.3 ☑
    single episode 296.2 ☑
agitated (*see also* Psychosis, affective) 296.2 ☑
    recurrent episode 296.3 ☑
    single episode 296.2 ☑
anaclitic 309.21
anxiety 300.4
arches 734
    congenital 754.61
autogenous (*see also* Psychosis, affective) 296.2 ☑
    recurrent episode 296.3 ☑
    single episode 296.2 ☑
basal metabolic rate (BMR) 794.7
bone marrow 289.9
central nervous system 799.1
    newborn 779.2
cerebral 331.9
    newborn 779.2
cerebrovascular 437.8
    newborn 779.2
chest wall 738.3
endogenous (*see also* Psychosis, affective) 296.2 ☑
    recurrent episode 296.3 ☑
    single episode 296.2 ☑
functional activity 780.99
hysterical 300.11

**Depression** — *continued*
involutional, climacteric, or menopausal (*see also* Psychosis, affective) 296.2 ☑
    recurrent episode 296.3 ☑
    single episode 296.2 ☑
manic (*see also* Psychosis, affective) 296.80
medullary 348.8
    newborn 779.2
mental 300.4
metatarsal heads — *see* Depression, arches
metatarsus — *see* Depression, arches
monopolar (*see also* Psychosis, affective) 296.2 ☑
    recurrent episode 296.3 ☑
    single episode 296.2 ☑
nervous 300.4
neurotic 300.4
nose 738.0
postpartum 648.4 ☑
psychogenic 300.4
    reactive 298.0
psychoneurotic 300.4
psychotic (*see also* Psychosis, affective) 296.2 ☑
    reactive 298.0
    recurrent episode 296.3 ☑
    single episode 296.2 ☑
reactive 300.4
    neurotic 300.4
    psychogenic 298.0
    psychoneurotic 300.4
    psychotic 298.0
recurrent 296.3 ☑
respiratory center 348.8
    newborn 770.89
scapula 736.89
senile 290.21
situational (acute) (brief) 309.0
    prolonged 309.1
skull 754.0
sternum 738.3
visual field 368.40
**Depressive reaction** — *see also* Reaction, depressive
acute (transient) 309.0
    with anxiety 309.28
    prolonged 309.1
situational (acute) 309.0
    prolonged 309.1
**Deprivation**
cultural V62.4
emotional V62.89
    affecting
      adult 995.82
      infant or child 995.51
food 994.2
    specific substance NEC 269.8
protein (familial) (kwashiorkor) 260
sleep V69.4
social V62.4
    affecting
      adult 995.82
      infant or child 995.51
symptoms, syndrome
    alcohol 291.81
    drug 292.0
vitamins (*see also* Deficiency, vitamin) 269.2
water 994.3
**de Quervain's**
disease (tendon sheath) 727.04
thyroiditis (subacute granulomatous thyroiditis) 245.1
**Derangement**
ankle (internal) 718.97
    current injury (*see also* Dislocation, ankle) 837.0
    recurrent 718.37
cartilage (articular) NEC (*see also* Disorder, cartilage, articular) 718.0 ☑
    knee 717.9
      recurrent 718.36

---

☑ Additional Digit Required — Refer to the Tabular List for Digit Selection        ⊽ Subterms under main terms may continue to next column or page

**Derangement** — *continued*
  cartilage (*see also* Disorder, cartilage, articular) — *continued*
    recurrent 718.3 ☑
  collateral ligament (knee) (medial) (tibial) 717.82
    current injury 844.1
      lateral (fibular) 844.0
    lateral (fibular) 717.81
      current injury 844.0
  cruciate ligament (knee) (posterior) 717.84
    anterior 717.83
      current injury 844.2
    current injury 844.2
  elbow (internal) 718.92
    current injury (*see also* Dislocation, elbow) 832.00
    recurrent 718.32
  gastrointestinal 536.9
  heart — *see* Disease, heart
  hip (joint) (internal) (old) 718.95
    current injury (*see also* Dislocation, hip) 835.00
    recurrent 718.35
  intervertebral disc — *see* Displacement, intervertebral disc
  joint (internal) 718.90
    ankle 718.97
    current injury (*see also* Dislocation, by site)
      knee, meniscus or cartilage (*see also* Tear, meniscus) 836.2
    elbow 718.92
    foot 718.97
    hand 718.94
    hip 718.95
    knee 717.9
    multiple sites 718.99
    pelvic region 718.95
    recurrent 718.30
      ankle 718.37
      elbow 718.32
      foot 718.37
      hand 718.34
      hip 718.35
      knee 718.36
      multiple sites 718.39
      pelvic region 718.35
      shoulder (region) 718.31
      specified site NEC 718.38
      temporomandibular (old) 524.69
      wrist 718.33
    shoulder (region) 718.91
    specified site NEC 718.98
    spine NEC 724.9
    temporomandibular 524.69
    wrist 718.93
  knee (cartilage) (internal) 717.9
    current injury (*see also* Tear, meniscus) 836.2
    ligament 717.89
      capsular 717.85
      collateral — *see* Derangement, collateral ligament
      cruciate — *see* Derangement, cruciate ligament
      specified NEC 717.85
    recurrent 718.36
  low back NEC 724.9
  meniscus NEC (knee) 717.5
    current injury (*see also* Tear, meniscus) 836.2
    lateral 717.40
      anterior horn 717.42
      posterior horn 717.43
      specified NEC 717.49
    medial 717.3
      anterior horn 717.1
      posterior horn 717.2
    recurrent 718.3 ☑
    site other than knee — *see* Disorder, cartilage, articular
  mental (*see also* Psychosis) 298.9
  rotator cuff (recurrent) (tear) 726.10

**Derangement** — *continued*
  rotator cuff — *continued*
    current 840.4
  sacroiliac (old) 724.6
    current — *see* Dislocation, sacroiliac
  semilunar cartilage (knee) 717.5
    current injury 836.2
      lateral 836.1
      medial 836.0
    recurrent 718.3 ☑
  shoulder (internal) 718.91
    current injury (*see also* Dislocation, shoulder) 831.00
    recurrent 718.31
  spine (recurrent) NEC 724.9
    current — *see* Dislocation, spine
  temporomandibular (internal) (joint) (old) 524.69
    current — *see* Dislocation, jaw
**Dercum's disease or syndrome** (adiposis dolorosa) 272.8
**Derealization** (neurotic) 300.6
**Dermal** — *see* condition
**Dermaphytid** — *see* Dermatophytosis
**Dermatergosis** — *see* Dermatitis
**Dermatitis** (allergic) (contact) (occupational) (venenata) 692.9
  ab igne 692.82
  acneiform 692.9
  actinic (due to sun) 692.70
    acute 692.72
    chronic NEC 692.74
    other than from sun NEC 692.82
  ambustionis
    due to
      burn or scald — *see* Burn, by site
      sunburn (*see also* Sunburn) 692.71
  amebic 006.6
  ammonia 691.0
  anaphylactoid NEC 692.9
  arsenical 692.4
  artefacta 698.4
    psychogenic 316 [698.4]
  asthmatic 691.8
  atopic (allergic) (intrinsic) 691.8
    psychogenic 316 [691.8]
  atrophicans 701.8
    diffusa 701.8
    maculosa 701.3
  berlock, berloque 692.72
  blastomycetic 116.0
  blister beetle 692.89
  Brucella NEC 023.9
  bullosa 694.9
    striata pratensis 692.6
  bullous 694.9
    mucosynechial, atrophic 694.60
      with ocular involvement 694.61
    seasonal 694.8
  calorica
    due to
      burn or scald — *see* Burn, by site
      cold 692.89
      sunburn (*see also* Sunburn) 692.71
  caterpillar 692.89
  cercarial 120.3
  combustionis
    due to
      burn or scald — *see* Burn, by site
      sunburn (*see also* Sunburn) 692.71
  congelationis 991.5
  contusiformis 695.2
  diabetic 250.8 ☑
  diaper 691.0
  diphtheritica 032.85
  due to
    acetone 692.2
    acids 692.4
    adhesive plaster 692.4

**Dermatitis** — *continued*
  due to — *continued*
    alcohol (skin contact) (substances classifiable to 980.0–980.9) 692.4
      taken internally 693.8
    alkalis 692.4
    allergy NEC 692.9
    ammonia (household) (liquid) 692.4
    animal
      dander (cat) (dog) 692.84
      hair (cat) (dog) 692.84
    arnica 692.3
    arsenic 692.4
      taken internally 693.8
    blister beetle 692.89
    cantharides 692.3
    carbon disulphide 692.2
    caterpillar 692.89
    caustics 692.4
    cereal (ingested) 693.1
      contact with skin 692.5
    chemical(s) NEC 692.4
      internal 693.8
      irritant NEC 692.4
      taken internally 693.8
    chlorocompounds 692.2
    coffee (ingested) 693.1
      contact with skin 692.5
    cold weather 692.89
    cosmetics 692.81
    cyclohexanes 692.2
    dander, animal (cat) (dog) 692.84
    deodorant 692.81
    detergents 692.0
    dichromate 692.4
    drugs and medicinals (correct substance properly administered) (internal use) 693.0
      external (in contact with skin) 692.3
        wrong substance given or taken 976.9
          specified substance — *see* Table of Drugs and Chemicals
      wrong substance given or taken 977.9
        specified substance — *see* Table of Drugs and Chemicals
    dyes 692.89
      hair 692.89
    epidermophytosis — *see* Dermatophytosis
    esters 692.2
    external irritant NEC 692.9
      specified agent NEC 692.89
    eye shadow 692.81
    fish (ingested) 693.1
      contact with skin 692.5
    flour (ingested) 693.1
      contact with skin 692.5
    food (ingested) 693.1
      in contact with skin 692.5
    fruit (ingested) 693.1
      contact with skin 692.5
    fungicides 692.3
    furs 692.84
    glycols 692.2
    greases NEC 692.1
    hair, animal (cat) (dog) 692.84
    hair dyes 692.89
    hot
      objects and materials — *see* Burn, by site
      weather or places 692.89
    hydrocarbons 692.2
    infrared rays, except from sun 692.82
      solar NEC (*see also* Dermatitis, due to, sun) 692.70
    ingested substance 693.9
      drugs and medicinals (*see also* Dermatitis, due to, drugs and medicinals) 693.0

**Dermatitis** — *continued*
  due to — *continued*
    ingested substance — *continued*
      food 693.1
        specified substance NEC 693.8
    ingestion or injection of chemical 693.8
      drug (correct substance properly administered) 693.0
        wrong substance given or taken 977.9
          specified substance — *see* Table of Drugs and Chemicals
    insecticides 692.4
    internal agent 693.9
      drugs and medicinals (*see also* Dermatitis, due to, drugs and medicinals) 693.0
      food (ingested) 693.1
        in contact with skin 692.5
      specified agent NEC 693.8
    iodine 692.3
    iodoform 692.3
    irradiation 692.82
    jewelry 692.83
    keratolytics 692.3
    ketones 692.2
    lacquer tree (Rhus verniciflua) 692.6
    light (sun) NEC (*see also* Dermatitis, due to, sun) 692.70
      other 692.82
    low temperature 692.89
    mascara 692.81
    meat (ingested) 693.1
      contact with skin 692.5
    mercury, mercurials 692.3
    metals 692.83
    milk (ingested) 693.1
      contact with skin 692.5
    Neomycin 692.3
    nylon 692.4
    oils NEC 692.1
    paint solvent 692.2
    pediculocides 692.3
    petroleum products (substances classifiable to 981) 692.4
    phenol 692.3
    photosensitiveness, photosensitivity (sun) 692.72
      other light 692.82
    plants NEC 692.6
    plasters, medicated (any) 692.3
    plastic 692.4
    poison
      ivy (Rhus toxicodendron) 692.6
      oak (Rhus diversiloba) 692.6
      plant or vine 692.6
      sumac (Rhus venenata) 692.6
      vine (Rhus radicans) 692.6
    preservatives 692.89
    primrose (primula) 692.6
    primula 692.6
    radiation 692.82
      sun NEC (*see also* Dermatitis, due to, sun) 692.70
      tanning bed 692.82
    radioactive substance 692.82
    radium 692.82
    ragweed (Senecio jacobae) 692.6
    Rhus (diversiloba) (radicans) (toxicodendron) (venenata) (verniciflua) 692.6
    rubber 692.4
    scabicides 692.3
    Senecio jacobae 692.6
    solar radiation — *see* Dermatitis, due to, sun
    solvents (any) (substances classifiable to 982.0–982.8) 692.4
      chlorocompound group 692.2
      cyclohexane group 692.2
      ester group 692.2
      glycol group 692.2
      hydrocarbon group 692.2

Dermatitis — Detachment

**Dermatitis** — continued
due to — continued
solvents — continued
ketone group 692.2
paint 692.2
specified agent NEC 692.89
sun 692.70
acute 692.72
chronic NEC 692.74
specified NEC 692.79
sunburn (see also Sunburn)
692.71
sunshine NEC (see also Dermatitis,
due to, sun) 692.70
tanning bed 692.82
tetrachlorethylene 692.2
toluene 692.2
topical medications 692.3
turpentine 692.2
ultraviolet rays, except from sun
692.82
sun NEC (see also Dermatitis,
due to, sun) 692.70
vaccine or vaccination (correct
substance properly administered) 693.0
wrong substance given or taken
bacterial vaccine 978.8
specified — see Table of
Drugs and Chemi-
cals
other vaccines NEC 979.9
specified — see Table of
Drugs and Chemi-
cals
varicose veins (see also Varicose,
vein, inflamed or infected)
454.1
x-rays 692.82
dyshydrotic 705.81
dysmenorrheica 625.8
eczematoid NEC 692.9
infectious 690.8
eczematous NEC 692.9
epidemica 695.89
erysipelatosa 695.81
escharotica — see Burn, by site
exfoliativa, exfoliative 695.89
generalized 695.89
infantum 695.81
neonatorum 695.81
eyelid 373.31
allergic 373.32
contact 373.32
eczematous 373.31
herpes (zoster) 053.20
simplex 054.41
infective 373.5
due to
actinomycosis 039.3 [373.5]
herpes
simplex 054.41
zoster 053.20
impetigo 684 [373.5]
leprosy (see also Leprosy)
030.0 [373.4]
lupus vulgaris (tuberculous)
(see also Tuberculosis)
017.0 ☑ [373.4]
mycotic dermatitis (see also
Dermatomycosis)
111.9 [373.5]
vaccinia 051.0 [373.5]
postvaccination
999.0 [373.5]
yaws (see also Yaws)
102.9 [373.4]
facta, factitia 698.4
psychogenic 316 [698.4]
ficta 698.4
psychogenic 316 [698.4]
flexural 691.8
follicularis 704.8
friction 709.8
fungus 111.9
specified type NEC 111.8

**Dermatitis** — continued
gangrenosa, gangrenous (infantum)
(see also Gangrene) 785.4
gestationis 646.8 ☑
gonococcal 098.89
gouty 274.89
harvest mite 133.8
heat 692.89
herpetiformis (bullous) (erythematous)
(pustular) (vesicular) 694.0
juvenile 694.2
senile 694.5
hiemalis 692.89
hypostatic, hypostatica 454.1
with ulcer 454.2
impetiginous 684
infantile (acute) (chronic) (intertriginous) (intrinsic) (seborrheic)
690.12
infectiosa eczematoides 690.8
infectious (staphylococcal) (streptococcal) 686.9
eczematoid 690.8
infective eczematoid 690.8
Jacquet's (diaper dermatitis) 691.0
leptus 133.8
lichenified NEC 692.9
lichenoid, chronic 701.0
lichenoides purpurica pigmentosa
709.1
meadow 692.6
medicamentosa (correct substance
properly administered) (internal
use) (see also Dermatitis, due
to, drugs or medicinals) 693.0
due to contact with skin 692.3
mite 133.8
multiformis 694.0
juvenile 694.2
senile 694.5
napkin 691.0
neuro 698.3
neurotica 694.0
nummular NEC 692.9
osteatosis, osteatotic 706.8
papillaris capillitii 706.1
pellagrous 265.2
perioral 695.3
perstans 696.1
photosensitivity (sun) 692.72
other light 692.82
pigmented purpuric lichenoid 709.1
polymorpha dolorosa 694.0
primary irritant 692.9
pruriginosa 694.0
pruritic NEC 692.9
psoriasiform nodularis 696.2
psychogenic 316
purulent 686.00
pustular contagious 051.2
pyococcal 686.00
pyocyaneus 686.09
pyogenica 686.00
radiation 692.82
repens 696.1
Ritter's (exfoliativa) 695.81
Schamberg's (progressive pigmentary
dermatosis) 709.09
schistosome 120.3
seasonal bullous 694.8
seborrheic 690.10
infantile 690.12
sensitization NEC 692.9
septic (see also Septicemia) 686.00
gonococcal 098.89
solar, solare NEC (see also Dermatitis,
due to, sun) 692.70
stasis 459.81
due to
postphlebitic syndrome 459.12
with ulcer 459.13
varicose veins — see Varicose
ulcerated or with ulcer (varicose)
454.2
sunburn (see also Sunburn) 692.71
suppurative 686.00

**Dermatitis** — continued
traumatic NEC 709.8
trophoneurotica 694.0
ultraviolet, except from sun 692.82
due to sun NEC (see also Dermatitis, due to, sun) 692.82
varicose 454.1
with ulcer 454.2
vegetans 686.8
verrucosa 117.2
xerotic 706.8
**Dermatoarthritis, lipoid** 272.8 [713.0]
**Dermatochalasia, dermatochalasis**
374.87
**Dermatofibroma** (lenticulare) (M8832/0)
— see also Neoplasm, skin, benign
protuberans (M8832/1) — see Neoplasm, skin, uncertain behavior
**Dermatofibrosarcoma** (protuberans)
(M8832/3) — see Neoplasm, skin,
malignant
**Dermatographia** 708.3
**Dermatolysis** (congenital) (exfoliativa)
757.39
acquired 701.8
eyelids 374.34
palpebrarum 374.34
senile 701.8
**Dermatomegaly** NEC 701.8
**Dermatomucomyositis** 710.3
**Dermatomycosis** 111.9
furfuracea 111.0
specified type NEC 111.8
**Dermatomyositis** (acute) (chronic) 710.3
**Dermatoneuritis of children** 985.0
**Dermatophiliasis** 134.1
**Dermatophytide** — see Dermatophytosis
**Dermatophytosis** (Epidermophyton) (infection) (microsporum) (tinea) (Trichophyton) 110.9
beard 110.0
body 110.5
deep seated 110.6
fingernails 110.1
foot 110.4
groin 110.3
hand 110.2
nail 110.1
perianal (area) 110.3
scalp 110.0
scrotal 110.8
specified site NEC 110.8
toenails 110.1
vulva 110.8
**Dermatopolyneuritis** 985.0
**Dermatorrhexis** 756.83
acquired 701.8
**Dermatosclerosis** — see also Scleroderma 710.1
localized 701.0
**Dermatosis** 709.9
Andrews' 686.8
atopic 691.8
Bowen's (M8081/2) — see Neoplasm,
skin, in situ
bullous 694.9
specified type NEC 694.8
erythematosquamous 690.8
exfoliativa 695.89
factitial 698.4
gonococcal 098.89
herpetiformis 694.0
juvenile 694.2
senile 694.5
hysterical 300.11
linear IgA 694.8
menstrual NEC 709.8
neutrophilic, acute febrile 695.89
occupational (see also Dermatitis)
692.9
papulosa nigra 709.8
pigmentary NEC 709.00
progressive 709.09
Schamberg's 709.09
Siemens-Bloch 757.33
progressive pigmentary 709.09

**Dermatosis** — continued
psychogenic 316
pustular subcorneal 694.1
Schamberg's (progressive pigmentary)
709.09
senile NEC 709.3
specified NEC 702.8
Unna's (seborrheic dermatitis) 690.10
**Dermographia** 708.3
**Dermographism** 708.3
**Dermoid** (cyst) (M9084/0) — see also
Neoplasm, by site, benign
with malignant transformation
(M9084/3) 183.0
**Dermopathy**
infiltrative, with thyrotoxicosis
242.0 ☑
senile NEC 709.3
**Dermophytosis** — see Dermatophytosis
**Descemet's membrane** — see condition
**Descemetocele** 371.72
**Descending** — see condition
**Descensus uteri** (complete) (incomplete)
(partial) (without vaginal wall pro-
lapse) 618.1
with mention of vaginal wall prolapse
— see Prolapse, uterovaginal
**Desensitization to allergens** V07.1
**Desert**
rheumatism 114.0
sore (see also Ulcer, skin) 707.9
**Desertion** (child) (newborn) 995.52
adult 995.84
**Desmoid** (extra-abdominal) (tumor)
(M8821/1) — see also Neoplasm,
connective tissue, uncertain behavior
abdominal (M8822/1) — see Neoplasm, connective tissue, uncertain behavior
**Despondency** 300.4
**Desquamative dermatitis** NEC 695.89
**Destruction**
articular facet (see also Derangement,
joint) 718.9 ☑
vertebra 724.9
bone 733.90
syphilitic 095.5
joint (see also Derangement, joint)
718.9 ☑
sacroiliac 724.6
kidney 593.89
live fetus to facilitate birth NEC
763.89
ossicles (ear) 385.24
rectal sphincter 569.49
septum (nasal) 478.19
tuberculous NEC (see also Tuberculosis) 011.9 ☑
tympanic membrane 384.82
tympanum 385.89
vertebral disc — see Degeneration,
intervertebral disc
**Destructiveness** — see also Disturbance,
conduct 312.9
adjustment reaction 309.3
**Detachment**
cartilage (see also Sprain, by site)
knee — see Tear, meniscus
cervix, annular 622.8
complicating delivery 665.3 ☑
choroid (old) (postinfectional) (simple)
(spontaneous) 363.70
hemorrhagic 363.72
serous 363.71
knee, medial meniscus (old) 717.3
current injury 836.0
ligament — see Sprain, by site
placenta (premature) — see Placenta,
separation
retina (recent) 361.9
with retinal defect (rhegmatogenous) 361.00
giant tear 361.03
multiple 361.02

☑ Additional Digit Required — Refer to the Tabular List for Digit Selection          ᴺᴱᶜ Subterms under main terms may continue to next column or page

80 — Volume 2          ▶◀ Revised Text          ● New Line          ▲ Revised Code          *2008 ICD-9-CM*

**Detachment** — *continued*
retina — *continued*
with retinal defect — *continued*
partial
with
giant tear 361.03
multiple defects 361.02
retinal dialysis (juvenile) 361.04
single defect 361.01
retinal dialysis (juvenile) 361.04
single 361.01
subtotal 361.05
total 361.05
delimited (old) (partial) 361.06
old
delimited 361.06
partial 361.06
total or subtotal 361.07
pigment epithelium (RPE) (serous) 362.42
exudative 362.42
hemorrhagic 362.43
rhegmatogenous (*see also* Detachment, retina, with retinal defect) 361.00
serous (without retinal defect) 361.2
specified type NEC 361.89
traction (with vitreoretinal organization) 361.81
vitreous humor 379.21
**Detergent asthma** 507.8
**Deterioration**
epileptic
with behavioral disturbance 345.9 ☑ *[294.11]*
without behavioral disturbance 345.9 ☑ *[294.10]*
heart, cardiac (*see also* Degeneration, myocardial) 429.1
mental (*see also* Psychosis) 298.9
myocardial, myocardium (*see also* Degeneration, myocardial) 429.1
senile (simple) 797
transplanted organ — *see* Complications, transplant, organ, by site
**de Toni-Fanconi syndrome** (cystinosis) 270.0
**Deuteranomaly** 368.52
**Deuteranopia** (anomalous trichromat) (complete) (incomplete) 368.52
**Deutschländer's disease** — *see* Fracture, foot
**Development**
abnormal, bone 756.9
arrested 783.40
bone 733.91
child 783.40
due to malnutrition (protein-calorie) 263.2
fetus or newborn 764.9 ☑
tracheal rings (congenital) 748.3
defective, congenital (*see also* Anomaly)
cauda equina 742.59
left ventricle 746.9
with atresia or hypoplasia of aortic orifice or valve with hypoplasia of ascending aorta 746.7
in hypoplastic left heart syndrome 746.7
delayed (*see also* Delay, development) 783.40
arithmetical skills 315.1
language (skills) 315.31
and speech due to hearing ●
loss 315.34 ●
expressive 315.31
mixed receptive-expressive 315.32
learning skill, specified NEC 315.2
mixed skills 315.5
motor coordination 315.4
reading 315.00

**Development** — *continued*
delayed (*see also* Delay, development) — *continued*
specified
learning skill NEC 315.2
type NEC, except learning 315.8
speech 315.39
and language due to hearing ●
loss 315.34 ●
associated with hyperkinesia 314.1
phonological 315.39
spelling 315.09
written expression 315.2
imperfect, congenital (*see also* Anomaly)
heart 746.9
lungs 748.60
improper (fetus or newborn) 764.9 ☑
incomplete (fetus or newborn) 764.9 ☑
affecting management of pregnancy 656.5 ☑
bronchial tree 748.3
organ or site not listed — *see* Hypoplasia
respiratory system 748.9
sexual, precocious NEC 259.1
tardy, mental (*see also* Retardation, mental) 319
**Developmental** — *see* condition
**Devergie's disease** (pityriasis rubra pilaris) 696.4
**Deviation**
conjugate (eye) 378.87
palsy 378.81
spasm, spastic 378.82
esophagus 530.89
eye, skew 378.87
mandible, opening and closing 524.53
midline (jaw) (teeth) 524.29
specified site NEC — *see* Malposition
occlusal plane 524.76
organ or site, congenital NEC — *see* Malposition, congenital
septum (acquired) (nasal) 470
congenital 754.0
sexual 302.9
bestiality 302.1
coprophilia 302.89
ego-dystonic
homosexuality 302.0
lesbianism 302.0
erotomania 302.89
Clérambault's 297.8
exhibitionism (sexual) 302.4
fetishism 302.81
transvestic 302.3
frotteurism 302.89
homosexuality, ego-dystonic 302.0
pedophilic 302.2
lesbianism, ego-dystonic 302.0
masochism 302.83
narcissism 302.89
necrophilia 302.89
nymphomania 302.89
pederosis 302.2
pedophilia 302.2
sadism 302.84
sadomasochism 302.84
satyriasis 302.89
specified type NEC 302.89
transvestic fetishism 302.3
transvestism 302.3
voyeurism 302.82
zoophilia (erotica) 302.1
teeth, midline 524.29
trachea 519.19
ureter (congenital) 753.4
**Devic's disease** 341.0
**Device**
cerebral ventricle (communicating) in situ V45.2
contraceptive — *see* Contraceptive, device
drainage, cerebrospinal fluid V45.2

**Devil's**
grip 074.1
pinches (purpura simplex) 287.2
**Devitalized tooth** 522.9
**Devonshire colic** 984.9
specified type of lead — *see* Table of Drugs and Chemicals
**Dextraposition, aorta** 747.21
with ventricular septal defect, pulmonary stenosis or atresia, and hypertrophy of right ventricle 745.2
in tetralogy of Fallot 745.2
**Dextratransposition, aorta** 745.11
**Dextrinosis, limit** (debrancher enzyme deficiency) 271.0
**Dextrocardia** (corrected) (false) (isolated) (secondary) (true) 746.87
with
complete transposition of viscera 759.3
situs inversus 759.3
**Dextroversion, kidney** (left) 753.3
**Dhobie itch** 110.3
**Diabetes, diabetic** (brittle) (congenital) (familial) (mellitus) (poorly controlled) (severe) (slight) (without complication) 250.0 ☑

---

*Note* — Use the following fifth-digit subclassification with category 250:

0　type II or unspecified type, not stated as uncontrolled

*Fifth-digit 0 is for use for type II patients, even if the patient requires insulin*

1　type I [juvenile type], not stated as uncontrolled

2　type II or unspecified type, uncontrolled

*Fifth-digit 2 is for use for type II patients, even if the patient requires insulin*

3　type I [juvenile type], uncontrolled

---

with
coma (with ketoacidosis) 250.3 ☑
hyperosmolar (nonketotic) 250.2 ☑
complication NEC 250.9 ☑
specified NEC 250.8 ☑
gangrene 250.7 ☑ *[785.4]*
hyperosmolarity 250.2 ☑
ketosis, ketoacidosis 250.1 ☑
osteomyelitis 250.8 ☑ *[731.8]*
specified manisfestations NEC 250.8 ☑
acetonemia 250.1 ☑
acidosis 250.1 ☑
amyotrophy 250.6 ☑ *[353.1]*　　▲
angiopathy, peripheral 250.7 ☑ *[443.81]*
asymptomatic 790.29
autonomic neuropathy (peripheral) 250.6 ☑ *[337.1]*
bone change 250.8 ☑ *[731.8]*
bronze, bronzed 275.0
cataract 250.5 ☑ *[366.41]*
chemical 790.29
complicating pregnancy, childbirth, or puerperium 648.8 ☑
coma (with ketoacidosis) 250.3 ☑
hyperglycemic 250.3 ☑
hyperosmolar (nonketotic) 250.2 ☑
hypoglycemic 250.3 ☑
insulin 250.3 ☑
complicating pregnancy, childbirth, or puerperium (maternal) 648.0 ☑
affecting fetus or newborn 775.0
complication NEC 250.9 ☑
specified NEC 250.8 ☑
dorsal sclerosis 250.6 ☑ *[340]*

**Diabetes, diabetic** — *continued*
dwarfism-obesity syndrome 258.1
gangrene 250.7 ☑ *[785.4]*
gastroparesis 250.6 ☑ *[536.3]*
gestational 648.8 ☑
complicating pregnancy, childbirth, or puerperium 648.8 ☑
glaucoma 250.5 ☑ *[365.44]*
glomerulosclerosis (intercapillary) 250.4 ☑ *[581.81]*
glycogenosis, secondary 250.8 ☑ *[259.8]*
hemochromatosis 275.0
hyperosmolar coma 250.2 ☑
hyperosmolarity 250.2 ☑
hypertension-nephrosis syndrome 250.4 ☑ *[581.81]*
hypoglycemia 250.8 ☑
hypoglycemic shock 250.8 ☑
insipidus 253.5
nephrogenic 588.1
pituitary 253.5
vasopressin-resistant 588.1
intercapillary glomerulosclerosis 250.4 ☑ *[581.81]*
iritis 250.5 ☑ *[364.42]*
ketosis, ketoacidosis 250.1 ☑
Kimmelstiel (-Wilson) disease or syndrome (intercapillary glomerulosclerosis) 250.4 ☑ *[581.81]*
Lancereaux's (diabetes mellitus with marked emaciation) 250.8 ☑ *[261]*
latent (chemical) 790.29
complicating pregnancy, childbirth, or puerperium 648.8 ☑
lipoidosis 250.8 ☑ *[272.7]*
macular edema 250.5 ☑ *[362.07]*
maternal
with manifest disease in the infant 775.1
affecting fetus or newborn 775.0
microaneurysms, retinal 250.5 ☑ *[362.01]*
mononeuropathy 250.6 ☑ *[355.9]*
neonatal, transient 775.1
nephropathy 250.4 ☑ *[583.81]*
nephrosis (syndrome) 250.4 ☑ *[581.81]*
neuralgia 250.6 ☑ *[357.2]*
neuritis 250.6 ☑ *[357.2]*
neurogenic arthropathy 250.6 ☑ *[713.5]*
neuropathy 250.6 ☑ *[357.2]*
nonclinical 790.29
osteomyelitis 250.8 ☑ *[731.8]*
peripheral autonomic neuropathy 250.6 ☑ *[337.1]*
phosphate 275.3
polyneuropathy 250.6 ☑ *[357.2]*
renal (true) 271.4
retinal
edema 250.5 ☑ *[362.07]*
hemorrhage 250.5 ☑ *[362.01]*
microaneurysms 250.5 ☑ *[362.01]*
retinitis 250.5 ☑ *[362.01]*
retinopathy 250.5 ☑ *[362.01]*
background 250.5 ☑ *[362.01]*
nonproliverative 250.5 ☑ *[362.03]*
mild 250.5 ☑ *[362.04]*
moderate 250.5 ☑ *[362.05]*
severe 250.5 ☑ *[362.06]*
proliferative 250.5 ☑ *[362.02]*
steroid induced
correct substance properly administered 251.8
overdose or wrong substance given or taken 962.0
stress 790.29
subclinical 790.29
subliminal 790.29
sugar 250.0 ☑
ulcer (skin) 250.8 ☑ *[707.9]*
lower extremity 250.8 ☑ *[707.10]*
ankle 250.8 ☑ *[707.13]*

**Diabetes, diabetic** — *continued*
  ulcer — *continued*
    lower extremity — *continued*
      calf 250.8 ☑ *[707.12]*
      foot 250.8 ☑ *[707.15]*
      heel 250.8 ☑ *[707.14]*
      knee 250.8 ☑ *[707.19]*
      specified site NEC
        250.8 ☑ *[707.19]*
      thigh 250.8 ☑ *[707.11]*
      toes 250.8 ☑ *[707.15]*
    specified site NEC 250.8 ☑ *[707.8]*
    xanthoma 250.8 ☑ *[272.2]*
**Diacyclothrombopathia** 287.1
**Diagnosis deferred** 799.9
**Dialysis** (intermittent) (treatment)
  anterior retinal (juvenile) (with detachment) 361.04
  extracorporeal V56.0
  hemodialysis V56.0
    status only V45.1
  peritoneal V56.8
    status only V45.1
  renal V56.0
    status only V45.1
  specified type NEC V56.8
**Diamond-Blackfan anemia or syndrome** (congenital hypoplastic anemia) 284.01
**Diamond-Gardener syndrome** (autoerythrocyte sensitization) 287.2
**Diaper rash** 691.0
**Diaphoresis** (excessive) NEC — *see also* Hyperhidrosis) 780.8
**Diaphragm** — *see* condition
**Diaphragmalgia** 786.52
**Diaphragmitis** 519.4
**Diaphyseal aclasis** 756.4
**Diaphysitis** 733.99
**Diarrhea, diarrheal** (acute) (autumn) (bilious) (bloody) (catarrhal) (choleraic) (chronic) (gravis) (green) (infantile) (lienteric) (noninfectious) (presumed noninfectious) (putrefactive) (secondary) (sporadic) (summer) (symptomatic) (thermic) 787.91
  achlorhydric 536.0
  allergic 558.3
  amebic (*see also* Amebiasis) 006.9
    with abscess — *see* Abscess, amebic
    acute 006.0
    chronic 006.1
    nondysenteric 006.2
  bacillary — *see* Dysentery, bacillary
  bacterial NEC 008.5
  balantidial 007.0
  bile salt-induced 579.8
  cachectic NEC 787.91
  chilomastix 007.8
  choleriformis 001.1
  coccidial 007.2
  Cochin-China 579.1
    anguilluliasis 127.2
    psilosis 579.1
  Dientamoeba 007.8
  dietetic 787.91
  due to
    achylia gastrica 536.8
    Aerobacter aerogenes 008.2
    Bacillus coli — *see* Enteritis, E. coli
    bacteria NEC 008.5
    bile salts 579.8
    Capillaria
      hepatica 128.8
      philippinensis 127.5
    Clostridium perfringens (C) (F) 008.46
    Enterobacter aerogenes 008.2
    enterococci 008.49
    Escherichia coli — *see* Enteritis, E. coli
    Giardia lamblia 007.1
    Heterophyes heterophyes 121.6
    irritating foods 787.91

**Diarrhea, diarrheal** — *continued*
  due to — *continued*
    Metagonimus yokogawai 121.5
    Necator americanus 126.1
    Paracolobactrum arizonae 008.1
    Paracolon bacillus NEC 008.47
      Arizona 008.1
    Proteus (bacillus) (mirabilis) (Morganii) 008.3
    Pseudomonas aeruginosa 008.42
    S. japonicum 120.2
    specified organism NEC 008.8
      bacterial 008.49
      viral NEC 008.69
    Staphylococcus 008.41
    Streptococcus 008.49
      anaerobic 008.46
    Strongyloides stercoralis 127.2
    Trichuris trichiuria 127.3
    virus NEC (*see also* Enteritis, viral) 008.69
  dysenteric 009.2
    due to specified organism NEC 008.8
  dyspeptic 787.91
  endemic 009.3
    due to specified organism NEC 008.8
  epidemic 009.2
    due to specified organism NEC 008.8
  fermentative 787.91
  flagellate 007.9
  Flexner's (ulcerative) 004.1
  functional 564.5
    following gastrointestinal surgery 564.4
    psychogenic 306.4
  giardial 007.1
  Giardia lamblia 007.1
  hill 579.1
  hyperperistalsis (nervous) 306.4
  infectious 009.2
    due to specified organism NEC 008.8
    presumed 009.3
  inflammatory 787.91
    due to specified organism NEC 008.8
  malarial (*see also* Malaria) 084.6
  mite 133.8
  mycotic 117.9
  nervous 306.4
  neurogenic 564.5
  parenteral NEC 009.2
  postgastrectomy 564.4
  postvagotomy 564.4
  prostaglandin induced 579.8
  protozoal NEC 007.9
  psychogenic 306.4
  septic 009.2
    due to specified organism NEC 008.8
  specified organism NEC 008.8
    bacterial 008.49
    viral NEC 008.69
  Staphylococcus 008.41
  Streptococcus 008.49
    anaerobic 008.46
  toxic 558.2
  travelers' 009.2
    due to specified organism NEC 008.8
  trichomonal 007.3
  tropical 579.1
  tuberculous 014.8 ☑
  ulcerative (chronic) (*see also* Colitis, ulcerative) 556.9
  viral (*see also* Enteritis, viral) 008.8
  zymotic NEC 009.2
**Diastasis**
  cranial bones 733.99
    congenital 756.0
  joint (traumatic) — *see* Dislocation, by site
  muscle 728.84

**Diastasis** — *continued*
  muscle — *continued*
    congenital 756.89
  recti (abdomen) 728.84
    complicating delivery 665.8 ☑
    congenital 756.79
**Diastema, teeth, tooth** 524.30
**Diastematomyelia** 742.51
**Diataxia, cerebral, infantile** 343.0
**Diathesis**
  allergic V15.09
  bleeding (familial) 287.9
  cystine (familial) 270.0
  gouty 274.9
  hemorrhagic (familial) 287.9
    newborn NEC 776.0
  oxalic 271.8
  scrofulous (*see also* Tuberculosis) 017.2 ☑
  spasmophilic (*see also* Tetany) 781.7
  ulcer 536.9
  uric acid 274.9
**Diaz's disease or osteochondrosis** 732.5
**Dibothriocephaliasis** 123.4
  larval 123.5
**Dibothriocephalus** (infection) (infestation) (latus) 123.4
  larval 123.5
**Dicephalus** 759.4
**Dichotomy, teeth** 520.2
**Dichromat, dichromata** (congenital) 368.59
**Dichromatopsia** (congenital) 368.59
**Dichuchwa** 104.0
**Dicroceliasis** 121.8
**Didelphys, didelphic** — *see also* Double uterus 752.2
**Didymitis** — *see also* Epididymitis 604.90
**Died** — *see also* Death
  without
    medical attention (cause unknown) 798.9
    sign of disease 798.2
**Dientamoeba diarrhea** 007.8
**Dietary**
  inadequacy or deficiency 269.9
  surveillance and counseling V65.3
**Dietl's crisis** 593.4
**Dieulafoy lesion** (hemorrhagic)
  of
    duodenum 537.84
    esophagus 530.82
    intestine 569.86
    stomach 537.84
**Difficult**
  birth, affecting fetus or newborn 763.9
  delivery NEC 669.9 ☑
**Difficulty**
  feeding 783.3
    adult 783.3
    breast 676.8 ☑
    child 783.3
    elderly 783.3
    infant 783.3
    newborn 779.3
    nonorganic (infant) NEC 307.59
  mechanical, gastroduodenal stoma 537.89
  reading 315.00
  specific, spelling 315.09
  swallowing (*see also* Dysphagia) 787.20 ▲
  walking 719.7
**Diffuse** — *see* condition
**Diffused ganglion** 727.42
**Di George's syndrome** (thymic hypoplasia) 279.11
**Digestive** — *see* condition
**Di Guglielmo's disease or syndrome** (M9841/3) 207.0
**Diktyoma** (M9051/3) — *see* Neoplasm, by site, malignant
**Dilaceration, tooth** 520.4

**Dilatation**
  anus 564.89
    venule — *see* Hemorrhoids
  aorta (focal) (general) (*see also* Aneurysm, aorta) 441.9
    congenital 747.29
    infectional 093.0
    ruptured 441.5
    syphilitic 093.0
  appendix (cystic) 543.9
  artery 447.8
  bile duct (common) (cystic) (congenital) 751.69
    acquired 576.8
  bladder (sphincter) 596.8
    congenital 753.8
    in pregnancy or childbirth 654.4 ☑
      causing obstructed labor 660.2 ☑
        affecting fetus or newborn 763.1
  blood vessel 459.89
  bronchus, bronchi 494.0
    with acute exacerbation 494.1
  calyx (due to obstruction) 593.89
  capillaries 448.9
  cardiac (acute) (chronic) (*see also* Hypertrophy, cardiac) 429.3
    congenital 746.89
    valve NEC 746.89
      pulmonary 746.09
    hypertensive (*see also* Hypertension, heart) 402.90
  cavum septi pellucidi 742.4
  cecum 564.89
    psychogenic 306.4
  cervix (uteri) (*see also* Incompetency, cervix)
    incomplete, poor, slow
      affecting fetus or newborn 763.7
      complicating delivery 661.0 ☑
        affecting fetus or newborn 763.7
  colon 564.7
    congenital 751.3
    due to mechanical obstruction 560.89
    psychogenic 306.4
  common bile duct (congenital) 751.69
    acquired 576.8
      with calculus, choledocholithiasis, or stones — *see* Choledocholithiasis
  cystic duct 751.69
    acquired (any bile duct) 575.8
  duct, mammary 610.4
  duodenum 564.89
  esophagus 530.89
    congenital 750.4
    due to
      achalasia 530.0
      cardiospasm 530.0
  Eustachian tube, congenital 744.24
  fontanel 756.0
  gallbladder 575.8
    congenital 751.69
  gastric 536.8
    acute 536.1
    psychogenic 306.4
  heart (acute) (chronic) (*see also* Hypertrophy, cardiac) 429.3
    congenital 746.89
    hypertensive (*see also* Hypertension, heart) 402.90
    valve (*see also* Endocarditis)
      congenital 746.89
  ileum 564.89
    psychogenic 306.4
  inguinal rings — *see* Hernia, inguinal
  jejunum 564.89
    psychogenic 306.4
  kidney (calyx) (collecting structures) (cystic) (parenchyma) (pelvis) 593.89
  lacrimal passages 375.69
  lymphatic vessel 457.1

☑ Additional Digit Required — Refer to the Tabular List for Digit Selection      ᴺᴱᶜ Subterms under main terms may continue to next column or page

82 — Volume 2 • October 2007    ▶◀ Revised Text    ● New Line    ▲ Revised Code    *2008 ICD-9-CM*

**Dilatation** — *continued*
  mammary duct 610.4
  Meckel's diverticulum (congenital) 751.0
  meningeal vessels, congenital 742.8
  myocardium (acute) (chronic) (*see also* Hypertrophy, cardiac) 429.3
  organ or site, congenital NEC — *see* Distortion
  pancreatic duct 577.8
  pelvis, kidney 593.89
  pericardium — *see* Pericarditis
  pharynx 478.29
  prostate 602.8
  pulmonary
    artery (idiopathic) 417.8
      congenital 747.3
    valve, congenital 746.09
  pupil 379.43
  rectum 564.89
  renal 593.89
  saccule vestibularis, congenital 744.05
  salivary gland (duct) 527.8
  sphincter ani 564.89
  stomach 536.8
    acute 536.1
    psychogenic 306.4
  submaxillary duct 527.8
  trachea, congenital 748.3
  ureter (idiopathic) 593.89
    congenital 753.20
    due to obstruction 593.5
  urethra (acquired) 599.84
  vasomotor 443.9
  vein 459.89
  ventricular, ventricle (acute) (chronic) (*see also* Hypertrophy, cardiac) 429.3
    cerebral, congenital 742.4
    hypertensive (*see also* Hypertension, heart) 402.90
  venule 459.89
    anus — *see* Hemorrhoids
  vesical orifice 596.8
**Dilated, dilation** — *see* Dilatation
**Diminished**
  hearing (acuity) (*see also* Deafness) 389.9
  pulse pressure 785.9
  vision NEC 369.9
  vital capacity 794.2
**Diminuta taenia** 123.6
**Diminution, sense or sensation** (cold) (heat) (tactile) (vibratory) — *see also* Disturbance, sensation 782.0
**Dimitri-Sturge-Weber disease** (encephalocutaneous angiomatosis) 759.6
**Dimple**
  parasacral 685.1
    with abscess 685.0
  pilonidal 685.1
    with abscess 685.0
  postanal 685.1
    with abscess 685.0
**Dioctophyma renale** (infection) (infestation) 128.8
**Dipetalonemiasis** 125.4
**Diphallus** 752.69
**Diphtheria, diphtheritic** (gangrenous) (hemorrhagic) 032.9
  carrier (suspected) of V02.4
  cutaneous 032.85
  cystitis 032.84
  faucial 032.0
  infection of wound 032.85
  inoculation (anti) (not sick) V03.5
  laryngeal 032.3
  myocarditis 032.82
  nasal anterior 032.2
  nasopharyngeal 032.1
  neurological complication 032.89
  peritonitis 032.83
  specified site NEC 032.89
**Diphyllobothriasis** (intestine) 123.4

**Diphyllobothriasis** — *continued*
  larval 123.5
**Diplacusis** 388.41
**Diplegia** (upper limbs) 344.2
  brain or cerebral 437.8
  congenital 343.0
  facial 351.0
    congenital 352.6
  infantile or congenital (cerebral) (spastic) (spinal) 343.0
  lower limbs 344.1
  syphilitic, congenital 090.49
**Diplococcus, diplococcal** — *see* condition
**Diplomyelia** 742.59
**Diplopia** 368.2
  refractive 368.15
**Dipsomania** — *see also* Alcoholism 303.9 ☑
  with psychosis (*see also* Psychosis, alcoholic) 291.9
**Dipylidiasis** 123.8
  intestine 123.8
**Direction, teeth, abnormal** 524.30
**Dirt-eating child** 307.52
**Disability**
  heart — *see* Disease, heart
  learning NEC 315.2
  special spelling 315.09
**Disarticulation** — *see also* Derangement, joint 718.9 ☑
  meaning
    amputation
      status — *see* Absence, by site
      traumatic — *see* Amputation, traumatic
    dislocation, traumatic or congenital — *see* Dislocation
**Disaster, cerebrovascular** — *see also* Disease, cerebrovascular, acute 436
**Discharge**
  anal NEC 787.99
  breast (female) (male) 611.79
  conjunctiva 372.89
  continued locomotor idiopathic (*see also* Epilepsy) 345.5 ☑
  diencephalic autonomic idiopathic (*see also* Epilepsy) 345.5 ☑
  ear 388.60
    blood 388.69
    cerebrospinal fluid 388.61
  excessive urine 788.42
  eye 379.93
  nasal 478.19
  nipple 611.79
  patterned motor idiopathic (*see also* Epilepsy) 345.5 ☑
  penile 788.7
  postnasal — *see* Sinusitis
  sinus, from mediastinum 510.0
  umbilicus 789.9
  urethral 788.7
    bloody 599.84
  vaginal 623.5
**Discitis** 722.90
  cervical, cervicothoracic 722.91
  lumbar, lumbosacral 722.93
  thoracic, thoracolumbar 722.92
**Discogenic syndrome** — *see* Displacement, intervertebral disc
**Discoid**
  kidney 753.3
  meniscus, congenital 717.5
  semilunar cartilage 717.5
**Discoloration**
  mouth 528.9
  nails 703.8
  teeth 521.7
    due to
      drugs 521.7
      metals (copper) (silver) 521.7
      pulpal bleeding 521.7
    during formation 520.8
    extrinsic 523.6
    intrinsic posteruptive 521.7

**Discomfort**
  chest 786.59
  visual 368.13
**Discomycosis** — *see* Actinomycosis
**Discontinuity, ossicles, ossicular chain** 385.23
**Discrepancy**
  centric occlusion
    maximum intercuspation 524.55
    of teeth 524.55
  leg length (acquired) 736.81
  uterine size-date 649.6 ☑
**Discrimination**
  political V62.4
  racial V62.4
  religious V62.4
  sex V62.4
**Disease, diseased** — *see also* Syndrome
  Abrami's (acquired hemolytic jaundice) 283.9
  absorbent system 459.89
  accumulation — *see* Thesaurismosis
  acid-peptic 536.8
  Acosta's 993.2
  Adams-Stokes (-Morgagni) (syncope with heart block) 426.9
  Addison's (bronze) (primary adrenal insufficiency) 255.41 ▲
    anemia (pernicious) 281.0
    tuberculous (*see also* Tuberculosis) 017.6 ☑
  Addison-Gull — *see* Xanthoma
  adenoids (and tonsils) (chronic) 474.9
  adrenal (gland) (capsule) (cortex) 255.9
    hyperfunction 255.3
    hypofunction 255.41 ▲
    specified type NEC 255.8
  ainhum (dactylolysis spontanea) 136.0
  akamushi (scrub typhus) 081.2
  Akureyri (epidemic neuromyasthenia) 049.8
  Albarrán's (colibacilluria) 791.9
  Albers-Schönberg's (marble bones) 756.52
  Albert's 726.71
  Albright (-Martin) (-Bantam) 275.49
  Alibert's (mycosis fungoides) (M9700/3) 202.1 ☑
  Alibert-Bazin (M9700/3) 202.1 ☑
  alimentary canal 569.9
  alligator skin (ichthyosis congenita) 757.1
    acquired 701.1
  Almeida's (Brazilian blastomycosis) 116.1
  Alpers' 330.8
  alpine 993.2
  altitude 993.2
  alveoli, teeth 525.9
  Alzheimer's — *see* Alzheimer's
  amyloid (any site) 277.30
  anarthritic rheumatoid 446.5
  Anders' (adiposis tuberosa simplex) 272.8
  Andersen's (glycogenosis IV) 271.0
  Anderson's (angiokeratoma corporis diffusum) 272.7
  Andes 993.2
  Andrews' (bacterid) 686.8
  angiospastic, angiospasmodic 443.9
    cerebral 435.9
      with transient neurologic deficit 435.9
    vein 459.89
  anterior
    chamber 364.9
    horn cell 335.9
      specified type NEC 335.8
  antral (chronic) 473.0
    acute 461.0
  anus NEC 569.49
  aorta (nonsyphilitic) 447.9
    syphilitic NEC 093.89
  aortic (heart) (valve) (*see also* Endocarditis, aortic) 424.1

**Disease, diseased** — *see also* Syndrome — *continued*
  apollo 077.4
  aponeurosis 726.90
  appendix 543.9
  aqueous (chamber) 364.9
  arc-welders' lung 503
  Armenian 277.31
  Arnold-Chiari (*see also* Spina bifida) 741.0 ☑
  arterial 447.9
    occlusive (*see also* Occlusion, by site) 444.22
      with embolus or thrombus — *see* Occlusion, by site
      due to stricture or stenosis 447.1
    specified type NEC 447.8
  arteriocardiorenal (*see also* Hypertension, cardiorenal) 404.90
  arteriolar (generalized) (obliterative) 447.9
    specified type NEC 447.8
  arteriorenal — *see* Hypertension, kidney
  arteriosclerotic (*see also* Arteriosclerosis)
    cardiovascular 429.2
    coronary — *see* Arteriosclerosis, coronary
    heart — *see* Arteriosclerosis, coronary
    vascular — *see* Arteriosclerosis
  artery 447.9
    cerebral 437.9
    coronary — *see* Arteriosclerosis, coronary
    specified type NEC 447.8
  arthropod-borne NEC 088.9
    specified type NEC 088.89
  Asboe-Hansen's (incontinentia pigmenti) 757.33
  atticoantral, chronic (with posterior or superior marginal perforation of ear drum) 382.2
  auditory canal, ear 380.9
  Aujeszky's 078.89
  auricle, ear NEC 380.30
  Australian X 062.4
  autoimmune NEC 279.4
    hemolytic (cold type) (warm type) 283.0
    parathyroid 252.1
    thyroid 245.2
  aviators' (*see also* Effect, adverse, high altitude) 993.2
  ax(e)-grinders' 502
  Ayala's 756.89
  Ayerza's (pulmonary artery sclerosis with pulmonary hypertension) 416.0
  Azorean (of the nervous system) 334.8
  Babington's (familial hemorrhagic telangiectasia) 448.0
  back bone NEC 733.90
  bacterial NEC 040.89
    zoonotic NEC 027.9
      specified type NEC 027.8
  Baehr-Schiffrin (thrombotic thrombocytopenic purpura) 446.6
  Baelz's (cheilitis glandularis apostematosa) 528.5
  Baerensprung's (eczema marginatum) 110.3
  Balfour's (chloroma) 205.3 ☑
  balloon (*see also* Effect, adverse, high altitude) 993.2
  Baló's 341.1
  Bamberger (-Marie) (hypertrophic pulmonary osteoarthropathy) 731.2
  Bang's (Brucella abortus) 023.1
  Bannister's 995.1
  Banti's (with cirrhosis) (with portal hypertension) — *see* Cirrhosis, liver

☑ Additional Digit Required — Refer to the Tabular List for Digit Selection      ▽ Subterms under main terms may continue to next column or page

**2008 ICD-9-CM**      ►◄ Revised Text      ● New Line      ▲ Revised Code      **October 2007 · Volume 2 — 83**

**Disease, diseased** — *see also* Syndrome — *continued*

Barcoo (*see also* Ulcer, skin) 707.9
barium lung 503
Barlow (-Möller) (infantile scurvy) 267
barometer makers' 985.0
Barraquer (-Simons) (progressive lipodystrophy) 272.6
basal ganglia 333.90
    degenerative NEC 333.0
    specified NEC 333.89
Basedow's (exophthalmic goiter) 242.0 ☑
basement membrane NEC 583.89
    with
        pulmonary hemorrhage (Goodpasture's syndrome) 446.21 [583.81]
Bateman's 078.0
    purpura (senile) 287.2
Batten's 330.1 [362.71]
Batten-Mayou (retina) 330.1 [362.71]
Batten-Steinert 359.21 ▲
Battey 031.0
Baumgarten-Cruveilhier (cirrhosis of liver) 571.5
bauxite-workers' 503
Bayle's (dementia paralytica) 094.1
Bazin's (primary) (*see also* Tuberculosis) 017.1 ☑
Beard's (neurasthenia) 300.5
Beau's (*see also* Degeneration, myocardial) 429.1
Bechterew's (ankylosing spondylitis) 720.0
Becker's
    idiopathic mural endomyocardial disease 425.2 ●
    myotonia congenita, recessive form 359.22 ●
Begbie's (exophthalmic goiter) 242.0 ☑
Behr's 362.50
Beigel's (white piedra) 111.2
Bekhterev's (ankylosing spondylitis) 720.0
Bell's (*see also* Psychosis, affective) 296.0 ☑
Bennett's (leukemia) 208.9 ☑
Benson's 379.22
Bergeron's (hysteroepilepsy) 300.11
Berlin's 921.3
Bernard-Soulier (thrombopathy) 287.1
Bernhardt (-Roth) 355.1
beryllium 503
Besnier-Boeck (-Schaumann) (sarcoidosis) 135
Best's 362.76
Beurmann's (sporotrichosis) 117.1
Bielschowsky (-Jansky) 330.1
Biermer's (pernicious anemia) 281.0
Biett's (discoid lupus erythematosus) 695.4
bile duct (*see also* Disease, biliary) 576.9
biliary (duct) (tract) 576.9
    with calculus, choledocholithiasis, or stones — *see* Choledocholithiasis
Billroth's (meningocele) (*see also* Spina bifida) 741.9 ☑
Binswanger's 290.12
Bird's (oxaluria) 271.8
bird fanciers' 495.2
black lung 500
bladder 596.9
    specified NEC 596.8
bleeder's 286.0
Bloch-Sulzberger (incontinentia pigmenti) 757.33
Blocq's (astasia-abasia) 307.9
blood (-forming organs) 289.9
    specified NEC 289.89
    vessel 459.9
Bloodgood's 610.1
Blount's (tibia vara) 732.4
blue 746.9

**Disease, diseased** — *see also* Syndrome — *continued*

Bodechtel-Guttmann (subacute sclerosing panencephalitis) 046.2
Boeck's (sarcoidosis) 135
bone 733.90
    fibrocystic NEC 733.29
        jaw 526.2
    marrow 289.9
    Paget's (osteitis deformans) 731.0
    specified type NEC 733.99
    von Recklinghausen's (osteitis fibrosa cystica) 252.01
Bonfils' — *see* Disease, Hodgkin's
Borna 062.9
Bornholm (epidemic pleurodynia) 074.1
Bostock's (*see also* Fever, hay) 477.9
Bouchard's (myopathic dilatation of the stomach) 536.1
Bouillaud's (rheumatic heart disease) 391.9
Bourneville (-Brissaud) (tuberous sclerosis) 759.5
Bouveret (-Hoffmann) (paroxysmal tachycardia) 427.2
bowel 569.9
    functional 564.9
        psychogenic 306.4
Bowen's (M8081/2) — *see* Neoplasm, skin, in situ
Bozzolo's (multiple myeloma) (M9730/3) 203.0 ☑
Bradley's (epidemic vomiting) 078.82
Brailsford's 732.3
    radius, head 732.3
    tarsal, scaphoid 732.5
Brailsford-Morquio (mucopolysaccharidosis IV) 277.5
brain 348.9
    Alzheimer's 331.0
        with dementia — *see* Alzheimer's, dementia
    arterial, artery 437.9
    arteriosclerotic 437.0
    congenital 742.9
    degenerative — *see* Degeneration, brain
    inflammatory (*see also* Encephalitis)
        late effect — *see* category 326
    organic 348.9
        arteriosclerotic 437.0
    parasitic NEC 123.9
    Pick's 331.11
        with dementia
            with behavioral disturbance 331.11 [294.11]
            without behavioral disturbance 331.11 [294.10]
    senile 331.2
braziers' 985.8
breast 611.9
    cystic (chronic) 610.1
    fibrocystic 610.1
    inflammatory 611.0
    Paget's (M8540/3) 174.0
    puerperal, postpartum NEC 676.3 ☑
    specified NEC 611.8
Breda's (*see also* Yaws) 102.9
Breisky's (kraurosis vulvae) 624.09 ▲
Bretonneau's (diphtheritic malignant angina) 032.0
Bright's (*see also* Nephritis) 583.9
    arteriosclerotic (*see also* Hypertension, kidney) 403.90
Brill's (recrudescent typhus) 081.1
    flea-borne 081.0
    louse-borne 081.1
Brill-Symmers (follicular lymphoma) (M9690/3) 202.0 ☑
Brill-Zinsser (recrudescent typhus) 081.1

**Disease, diseased** — *see also* Syndrome — *continued*

Brinton's (leather bottle stomach) (M8142/3) 151.9
Brion-Kayser (*see also* Fever, paratyphoid) 002.9
broad
    beta 272.2
    ligament, noninflammatory 620.9
        specified NEC 620.8
Brocq's 691.8
    meaning
        atopic (diffuse) neurodermatitis 691.8
        dermatitis herpetiformis 694.0
        lichen simplex chronicus 698.3
        parapsoriasis 696.2
        prurigo 698.2
Brocq-Duhring (dermatitis herpetiformis) 694.0
Brodie's (joint) (*see also* Osteomyelitis) 730.1 ☑
bronchi 519.19
bronchopulmonary 519.19
bronze (Addison's) 255.41 ▲
    tuberculous (*see also* Tuberculosis) 017.6 ☑
Brown-Séquard 344.89
Bruck's 733.99
Bruck-de Lange (Amsterdam dwarf, mental retardation and brachycephaly) 759.89
Bruhl's (splenic anemia with fever) 285.8
Bruton's (X-linked agammaglobulinemia) 279.04
buccal cavity 528.9
Buchanan's (juvenile osteochondrosis, iliac crest) 732.1
Buchman's (osteochondrosis juvenile) 732.1
Budgerigar-Fanciers' 495.2
Büdinger-Ludloff-Läwen 717.89
Buerger's (thromboangiitis obliterans) 443.1
Bürger-Grütz (essential familial hyperlipemia) 272.3
Burns' (lower ulna) 732.3
bursa 727.9
Bury's (erythema elevatum diutinum) 695.89
Buschke's 710.1
Busquet's (*see also* Osteomyelitis) 730.1 ☑
Busse-Buschke (cryptococcosis) 117.5
C$_2$ (*see also* Alcoholism) 303.9 ☑
Caffey's (infantile cortical hyperostosis) 756.59
caisson 993.3
calculous 592.9
California 114.0
Calvé (-Perthes) (osteochondrosis, femoral capital) 732.1
Camurati-Engelmann (diaphyseal sclerosis) 756.59
Canavan's 330.0
capillaries 448.9
Carapata 087.1
cardiac — *see* Disease, heart
cardiopulmonary, chronic 416.9
cardiorenal (arteriosclerotic) (hepatic) (hypertensive) (vascular) (*see also* Hypertension, cardiorenal) 404.90
cardiovascular (arteriosclerotic) 429.2
    congenital 746.9
    hypertensive (*see also* Hypertension, heart) 402.90
        benign 402.10
        malignant 402.00
    renal (*see also* Hypertension, cardiorenal) 404.90
    syphilitic (asymptomatic) 093.9
carotid gland 259.8
Carrión's (Bartonellosis) 088.0
cartilage NEC 733.90

**Disease, diseased** — *see also* Syndrome — *continued*

cartilage — *continued*
    specified NEC 733.99
Castellani's 104.8
cat-scratch 078.3
Cavare's (familial periodic paralysis) 359.3
Cazenave's (pemphigus) 694.4
cecum 569.9
celiac (adult) 579.0
    infantile 579.0
cellular tissue NEC 709.9
central core 359.0
cerebellar, cerebellum — *see* Disease, brain
cerebral (*see also* Disease, brain) 348.9
    arterial, artery 437.9
    degenerative — *see* Degeneration, brain
cerebrospinal 349.9
cerebrovascular NEC 437.9
    acute 436
        embolic — *see* Embolism, brain
        late effect — *see* Late effect(s) (of) cerebrovascular disease
        puerperal, postpartum, childbirth 674.0 ☑
        thrombotic — *see* Thrombosis, brain
    arteriosclerotic 437.0
        embolic — *see* Embolism, brain
    ischemic, generalized NEC 437.1
        late effect — *see* Late effect(s) (of) cerebrovascular disease
    occlusive 437.1
    puerperal, postpartum, childbirth 674.0 ☑
    specified type NEC 437.8
    thrombotic — *see* Thrombosis, brain
ceroid storage 272.7
cervix (uteri)
    inflammatory 616.0 ▲
    noninflammatory 622.9
        specified NEC 622.8
Chabert's 022.9
Chagas' (*see also* Trypanosomiasis, American) 086.2
Chandler's (osteochondritis dissecans, hip) 732.7
Charcôt-Marie-Tooth 356.1
Charcôt's (joint) 094.0 [713.5]
    spinal cord 094.0
Charlouis' (*see also* Yaws) 102.9
Cheadle (-Möller) (-Barlow) (infantile scurvy) 267
Chédiak-Steinbrinck (-Higashi) (congenital gigantism of peroxidase granules) 288.2
cheek, inner 528.9
chest 519.9
Chiari's (hepatic vein thrombosis) 453.0
Chicago (North American blastomycosis) 116.0
chignon (white piedra) 111.2
chigoe, chigo (jigger) 134.1
childhood granulomatous 288.1
Chinese liver fluke 121.1
chlamydial NEC 078.88
cholecystic (*see also* Disease, gallbladder) 575.9
choroid 363.9
    degenerative (*see also* Degeneration, choroid) 363.40
    hereditary (*see also* Dystrophy, choroid) 363.50
    specified type NEC 363.8
Christian's (chronic histiocytosis X) 277.89
Christian-Weber (nodular nonsuppurative panniculitis) 729.30
Christmas 286.1

---

☑ Additional Digit Required — Refer to the Tabular List for Digit Selection

🔺 Subterms under main terms may continue to next column or page

▶◀ Revised Text     ● New Line     ▲ Revised Code

Disease, diseased — *Disease, diseased*

**Disease, diseased** — *see also* Syndrome
— *continued*
ciliary body 364.9
specified NEC 364.89 •
circulatory (system) NEC 459.9
chronic, maternal, affecting fetus
or newborn 760.3
specified NEC 459.89
syphilitic 093.9
congenital 090.5
Civatte's (poikiloderma) 709.09
climacteric 627.2
male 608.89
coagulation factor deficiency (congenital) (*see also* Defect, coagulation) 286.9
Coats' 362.12
coccidioidal pulmonary 114.5
acute 114.0
chronic 114.4
primary 114.0
residual 114.4
Cockayne's (microcephaly and
dwarfism) 759.89
Cogan's 370.52
cold
agglutinin 283.0
or hemoglobinuria 283.0
paroxysmal (cold) (nocturnal)
283.2
hemagglutinin (chronic) 283.0
collagen NEC 710.9
nonvascular 710.9
specified NEC 710.8
vascular (allergic) (*see also* Angiitis,
hypersensitivity) 446.20
colon 569.9
functional 564.9
congenital 751.3
ischemic 557.0
combined system (of spinal cord)
266.2 *[336.2]*
with anemia (pernicious)
281.0 *[336.2]*
compressed air 993.3
Concato's (pericardial polyserositis)
423.2
peritoneal 568.82
pleural — *see* Pleurisy
congenital NEC 799.89
conjunctiva 372.9
chlamydial 077.98
specified NEC 077.8
specified type NEC 372.89
viral 077.99
specified NEC 077.8
connective tissue, diffuse (*see also*
Disease, collagen) 710.9
Conor and Bruch's (boutonneuse
fever) 082.1
Conradi (-Hünermann) 756.59
Cooley's (erythroblastic anemia)
282.49
Cooper's 610.1
Corbus' 607.1
cork-handlers' 495.3
cornea (*see also* Keratopathy) 371.9
coronary (*see also* Ischemia, heart)
414.9
congenital 746.85
ostial, syphilitic 093.20
aortic 093.22
mitral 093.21
pulmonary 093.24
tricuspid 093.23
Corrigan's — *see* Insufficiency, aortic
Cotugno's 724.3
Coxsackie (virus) NEC 074.8
cranial nerve NEC 352.9
Creutzfeldt-Jakob (new variant) 046.1
with dementia
with behavioral disturbance
046.1 *[294.11]*
without behavioral disturbance
046.1 *[294.10]*

**Disease, diseased** — *see also* Syndrome
— *continued*
Crigler-Najjar (congenital hyperbilirubinemia) 277.4
Crocq's (acrocyanosis) 443.89
Crohn's (intestine) (*see also* Enteritis,
regional) 555.9
Crouzon's (craniofacial dysostosis)
756.0
Cruchet's (encephalitis lethargica)
049.8
Cruveilhier's 335.21
Cruz-Chagas (*see also* Trypanosomiasis, American) 086.2
crystal deposition (*see also* Arthritis,
due to, crystals) 712.9 ☑
Csillag's (lichen sclerosus et atrophicus) 701.0
Curschmann's 359.21 ▲
Cushing's (pituitary basophilism)
255.0
cystic
breast (chronic) 610.1
kidney, congenital (*see also* Cystic,
disease, kidney) 753.10
liver, congenital 751.62
lung 518.89
congenital 748.4
pancreas 577.2
congenital 751.7
renal, congenital (*see also* Cystic,
disease, kidney) 753.10
semilunar cartilage 717.5
cysticercus 123.1
cystine storage (with renal sclerosis)
270.0
cytomegalic inclusion (generalized)
078.5
with
pneumonia 078.5 *[484.1]*
congenital 771.1
Daae (-Finsen) (epidemic pleurodynia)
074.1
dancing 297.8
Danielssen's (anesthetic leprosy)
030.1
Darier's (congenital) (keratosis follicularis) 757.39
erythema annulare centrifugum
695.0
vitamin A deficiency 264.8
Darling's (histoplasmosis) (*see also*
Histoplasmosis, American)
115.00
Davies' 425.0
de Beurmann-Gougerot (sporotrichosis) 117.1
Débove's (splenomegaly) 789.2
deer fly (*see also* Tularemia) 021.9
deficiency 269.9
degenerative (*see also* Degeneration)
disc — *see* Degeneration, intervertebral disc
Degos' 447.8
Déjérine (-Sottas) 356.0
Déléage's 359.89
demyelinating, demyelinizating (brain
stem) (central nervous system)
341.9
multiple sclerosis 340
specified NEC 341.8
de Quervain's (tendon sheath) 727.04
thyroid (subacute granulomatous
thyroiditis) 245.1
Dercum's (adiposis dolorosa) 272.8
Deutschländer's — *see* Fracture, foot
Devergie's (pityriasis rubra pilaris)
696.4
Devic's 341.0
diaphorase deficiency 289.7
diaphragm 519.4
diarrheal, infectious 009.2
diatomaceous earth 502
Diaz's (osteochondrosis astragalus)
732.5
digestive system 569.9

**Disease, diseased** — *see also* Syndrome
— *continued*
Di Guglielmo's (erythemic myelosis)
(M9841/3) 207.0 ☑
Dimitri-Sturge-Weber (encephalocutaneous angiomatosis) 759.6
disc, degenerative — *see* Degeneration, intervertebral disc
discogenic (*see also* Disease, intervertebral disc) 722.90
diverticular — *see* Diverticula
Down's (mongolism) 758.0
Dubini's (electric chorea) 049.8
Dubois' (thymus gland) 090.5
Duchenne's 094.0
locomotor ataxia 094.0
muscular dystrophy 359.1
paralysis 335.22
pseudohypertrophy, muscles 359.1
Duchenne-Griesinger 359.1
ductless glands 259.9
Duhring's (dermatitis herpetiformis)
694.0
Dukes (-Filatov) 057.8
duodenum NEC 537.9
specified NEC 537.89
Duplay's 726.2
Dupré's (meningism) 781.6
Dupuytren's (muscle contracture)
728.6
Durand-Nicolas-Favre (climatic bubo)
099.1
Duroziez's (congenital mitral stenosis)
746.5
Dutton's (trypanosomiasis) 086.9
Eales' 362.18
ear (chronic) (inner) NEC 388.9
middle 385.9
adhesive (*see also* Adhesions,
middle ear) 385.10
specified NEC 385.89
Eberth's (typhoid fever) 002.0
Ebstein's
heart 746.2
meaning diabetes 250.4 ☑ *[581.81]*
Echinococcus (*see also* Echinococcus)
122.9
ECHO virus NEC 078.89
Economo's (encephalitis lethargica)
049.8
Eddowes' (brittle bones and blue
sclera) 756.51
Edsall's 992.2
Eichstedt's (pityriasis versicolor) 111.0
Ellis-van Creveld (chondroectodermal
dysplasia) 756.55
endocardium — *see* Endocarditis
endocrine glands or system NEC
259.9
specified NEC 259.8
endomyocardial, idiopathic mural
425.2
Engelmann's (diaphyseal sclerosis)
756.59
Engel-von Recklinghausen (osteitis fibrosa cystica) 252.01
English (rickets) 268.0
Engman's (infectious eczematoid dermatitis) 690.8
enteroviral, enterovirus NEC 078.89
central nervous system NEC 048
epidemic NEC 136.9
epididymis 608.9
epigastric, functional 536.9
psychogenic 306.4
Erb (-Landouzy) 359.1
Erb-Goldflam 358.00
Erichsen's (railway spine) 300.16
esophagus 530.9
functional 530.5
psychogenic 306.4
Eulenburg's (congenital paramyotonia)
359.29 ▲
Eustachian tube 381.9
Evans' (thrombocytopenic purpura)
287.32

**Disease, diseased** — *see also* Syndrome
— *continued*
external auditory canal 380.9
extrapyramidal NEC 333.90
eye 379.90
anterior chamber 364.9
inflammatory NEC 364.3
muscle 378.9
eyeball 360.9
eyelid 374.9
eyeworm of Africa 125.2
Fabry's (angiokeratoma corporis diffusum) 272.7
facial nerve (seventh) 351.9
newborn 767.5
Fahr-Volhard (malignant nephrosclerosis) 403.00
fallopian tube, noninflammatory 620.9
specified NEC 620.8
familial periodic 277.31
paralysis 359.3
Fanconi's (congenital pancytopenia)
284.09
Farber's (disseminated lipogranulomatosis) 272.8
fascia 728.9
inflammatory 728.9
Fauchard's (periodontitis) 523.40
Favre-Durand-Nicolas (climatic bubo)
099.1
Favre-Racouchot (elastoidosis cutanea
nodularis) 701.8
Fede's 529.0
Feer's 985.0
Felix's (juvenile osteochondrosis, hip)
732.1
Fenwick's (gastric atrophy) 537.89
Fernels' (aortic aneurysm) 441.9
fibrocaseous, of lung (*see also* Tuberculosis, pulmonary) 011.9 ☑
fibrocystic (*see also* Fibrocystic, disease)
newborn 277.01
Fiedler's (leptospiral jaundice) 100.0
fifth 057.0
Filatoff's (infectious mononucleosis)
075
Filatov's (infectious mononucleosis)
075
file-cutters' 984.9
specified type of lead — *see* Table
of Drugs and Chemicals
filterable virus NEC 078.89
fish skin 757.1
acquired 701.1
Flajani (-Basedow) (exophthalmic goiter) 242.0 ☑
Flatau-Schilder 341.1
flax-dressers' 504
Fleischner's 732.3
flint 502
fluke — *see* Infestation, fluke
Følling's (phenylketonuria) 270.1
foot and mouth 078.4
foot process 581.3
Forbes' (glycogenosis III) 271.0
Fordyce's (ectopic sebaceous glands)
(mouth) 750.26
Fordyce-Fox (apocrine miliaria) 705.82
Fothergill's
meaning scarlatina anginosa 034.1
neuralgia (*see also* Neuralgia,
trigeminal) 350.1
Fournier's 608.83
fourth 057.8
Fox (-Fordyce) (apocrine miliaria)
705.82
Francis' (*see also* Tularemia) 021.9
Franklin's (heavy chain) 273.2
Frei's (climatic bubo) 099.1
Freiberg's (flattening metatarsal) 732.5
Friedländer's (endarteritis obliterans)
— *see* Arteriosclerosis
Friedreich's
combined systemic or ataxia 334.0
facial hemihypertrophy 756.0

☑ Additional Digit Required — Refer to the Tabular List for Digit Selection
▽ Subterms under main terms may continue to next column or page
**2008 ICD-9-CM**
▶◀ Revised Text
● New Line
▲ Revised Code
**October 2007 • Volume 2 — 85**

Disease, diseased — *see also* Syndrome
— *continued*
Friedreich's — *continued*
myoclonia 333.2
Fröhlich's (adiposogenital dystrophy)
253.8
Frommel's 676.6 ☑
frontal sinus (chronic) 473.1
acute 461.1
Fuller's earth 502
fungus, fungous NEC 117.9
Gaisböck's (polycythemia hypertonica)
289.0
gallbladder 575.9
congenital 751.60
Gamna's (siderotic splenomegaly)
289.51
Gamstorp's (adynamia episodica
hereditaria) 359.3
Gandy-Nanta (siderotic splenomegaly)
289.51
Gannister (occupational) 502
Garré's (*see also* Osteomyelitis)
730.1 ☑
gastric (*see also* Disease, stomach)
537.9
gastrointestinal (tract) 569.9
amyloid 277.39
functional 536.9
psychogenic 306.4
Gaucher's (adult) (cerebroside lipidosis) (infantile) 272.7
Gayet's (superior hemorrhagic polioencephalitis) 265.1
Gee (-Herter) (-Heubner) (-Thaysen)
(nontropical sprue) 579.0
generalized neoplastic (M8000/6)
199.0
genital organs NEC
female 629.9
specified NEC 629.89
male 608.9
Gerhardt's (erythromelalgia) 443.82
Gerlier's (epidemic vertigo) 078.81
Gibert's (pityriasis rosea) 696.3
Gibney's (perispondylitis) 720.9
Gierke's (glycogenosis I) 271.0
Gilbert's (familial nonhemolytic jaundice) 277.4
Gilchrist's (North American blastomycosis) 116.0
Gilford (-Hutchinson) (progeria) 259.8
Gilles de la Tourette's (motor-verbal
tic) 307.23
Giovannini's 117.9
gland (lymph) 289.9
Glanzmann's (hereditary hemorrhagic
thrombasthenia) 287.1
glassblowers' 527.1
Glénard's (enteroptosis) 569.89
Glisson's (*see also* Rickets) 268.0
glomerular
membranous, idiopathic 581.1
minimal change 581.3
glycogen storage (Andersen's) (Cori
types 1-7) (Forbes') (McArdle-
Schmid-Pearson) (Pompe's)
(types I-VII) 271.0
cardiac 271.0 *[425.7]*
generalized 271.0
glucose–6–phosphatase deficiency
271.0
heart 271.0 *[425.7]*
hepatorenal 271.0
liver and kidneys 271.0
myocardium 271.0 *[425.7]*
von Gierke's (glycogenosis I) 271.0
Goldflam-Erb 358.00
Goldscheider's (epidermolysis bullosa)
757.39
Goldstein's (familial hemorrhagic
telangiectasia) 448.0
gonococcal NEC 098.0
Goodall's (epidemic vomiting) 078.82
Gordon's (exudative enteropathy)
579.8

Disease, diseased — *see also* Syndrome
— *continued*
Gougerot's (trisymptomatic) 709.1
Gougerot-Carteaud (confluent reticulate papillomatosis) 701.8
Gougerot-Hailey-Hailey (benign familial chronic pemphigus) 757.39
graft-versus-host (bone marrow)
996.85
due to organ transplant NEC — *see*
Complications, transplant,
organ
grain-handlers' 495.8
Grancher's (splenopneumonia) — *see*
Pneumonia
granulomatous (childhood) (chronic)
288.1
graphite lung 503
Graves' (exophthalmic goiter) 242.0 ☑
Greenfield's 330.0
green monkey 078.89
Griesinger's (*see also* Ancylostomiasis)
126.9
grinders' 502
Grisel's 723.5
Gruby's (tinea tonsurans) 110.0
Guertin's (electric chorea) 049.8
Guillain-Barré 357.0
Guinon's (motor-verbal tic) 307.23
Gull's (thyroid atrophy with myxede-
ma) 244.8
Gull and Sutton's — *see* Hypertension, kidney
gum NEC 523.9
Günther's (congenital erythropoietic
porphyria) 277.1
gynecological 629.9
specified NEC 629.89
H 270.0
Haas' 732.3
Habermann's (acute parapsoriasis
varioliformis) 696.2
Haff 985.1
Hageman (congenital factor XII defi-
ciency) (*see also* Defect, congen-
ital) 286.3
Haglund's (osteochondrosis os tibiale
externum) 732.5
Hagner's (hypertrophic pulmonary
osteoarthropathy) 731.2
Hailey-Hailey (benign familial chronic
pemphigus) 757.39
hair (follicles) NEC 704.9
specified type NEC 704.8
Hallervorden-Spatz 333.0
Hallopeau's (lichen sclerosus et atrophicus) 701.0
Hamman's (spontaneous mediastinal
emphysema) 518.1
hand, foot, and mouth 074.3
Hand-Schüller-Christian (chronic
histiocytosis X) 277.89
Hanot's — *see* Cirrhosis, biliary
Hansen's (leprosy) 030.9
benign form 030.1
malignant form 030.0
Harada's 363.22
Harley's (intermittent hemoglobinuria)
283.2
Hartnup (pellagra-cerebellar ataxia-
renal aminoaciduria) 270.0
Hart's (pellagra-cerebellar ataxia-renal
aminoaciduria) 270.0
Hashimoto's (struma lymphomatosa)
245.2
Hb — *see* Disease, hemoglobin
heart (organic) 429.9
with
acute pulmonary edema (*see
also* Failure, ventricular,
left) 428.1
hypertensive 402.91
with renal failure 404.93
benign 402.11
with renal failure
404.13

Disease, diseased — *see also* Syndrome
— *continued*
heart — *continued*
with — *continued*
acute pulmonary edema (*see also* Failure, ventricular,
left) — *continued*
hypertensive — *continued*
malignant 402.01
with renal failure
404.03
kidney disease — *see* Hypertension, cardiorenal
rheumatic fever (conditions
classifiable to 390)
active 391.9
with chorea 392.0
inactive or quiescent (with
chorea) 398.90
amyloid 277.39 *[425.7]*
aortic (valve) (*see also* Endocarditis, aortic) 424.1
arteriosclerotic or sclerotic (minimal) (senile) — *see* Arteriosclerosis, coronary
artery, arterial — *see* Arteriosclerosis, coronary
atherosclerotic — *see* Arteriosclerosis, coronary
beer drinkers' 425.5
beriberi 265.0 *[425.7]*
black 416.0
congenital NEC 746.9
cyanotic 746.9
maternal, affecting fetus or
newborn 760.3
specified type NEC 746.89
congestive (*see also* Failure, heart)
428.0
coronary 414.9
cryptogenic 429.9
due to
amyloidosis 277.39 *[425.7]*
beriberi 265.0 *[425.7]*
cardiac glycogenosis
271.0 *[425.7]*
Friedreich's ataxia 334.0 *[425.8]*
gout 274.82
mucopolysaccharidosis
277.5 *[425.7]*
myotonia atrophica
359.21 *[425.8]* ▲
progressive muscular dystrophy
359.1 *[425.8]*
sarcoidosis 135 *[425.8]*
fetal 746.9
inflammatory 746.89
fibroid (*see also* Myocarditis) 429.0
functional 427.9
postoperative 997.1
psychogenic 306.2
glycogen storage 271.0 *[425.7]*
gonococcal NEC 098.85
gouty 274.82
hypertensive (*see also* Hypertension, heart) 402.90
benign 402.10
malignant 402.00
hyperthyroid (*see also* Hyperthyroidism) 242.9 ☑ *[425.7]*
incompletely diagnosed — *see* Disease, heart
ischemic (chronic) (*see also* Ischemia, heart) 414.9
acute (*see also* Infarct, myocardium) 410.9 ☑
without myocardial infarction
411.89
with coronary (artery) occlusion 411.81
asymptomatic 412
diagnosed on ECG or other special investigation but currently presenting no
symptoms 412
kyphoscoliotic 416.1

Disease, diseased — *see also* Syndrome
— *continued*
heart — *continued*
mitral (*see also* Endocarditis, mitral) 394.9
muscular (*see also* Degeneration,
myocardial) 429.1
postpartum 674.8 ☑
psychogenic (functional) 306.2
pulmonary (chronic) 416.9
acute 415.0
specified NEC 416.8
rheumatic (chronic) (inactive) (old)
(quiescent) (with chorea)
398.90
active or acute 391.9
with chorea (active)
(rheumatic) (Syden-
ham's) 392.0
specified type NEC 391.8
maternal, affecting fetus or
newborn 760.3
rheumatoid — *see* Arthritis,
rheumatoid
sclerotic — *see* Arteriosclerosis,
coronary
senile (*see also* Myocarditis) 429.0
specified type NEC 429.89
syphilitic 093.89
aortic 093.1
aneurysm 093.0
asymptomatic 093.89
congenital 090.5
thyroid (gland) (*see also* Hyperthyroidism) 242.9 ☑ *[425.7]*
thyrotoxic (*see also* Thyrotoxicosis)
242.9 ☑ *[425.7]*
tuberculous (*see also* Tuberculosis)
017.9 ☑ *[425.8]*
valve, valvular (obstructive) (regurgitant) (*see also* Endocarditis)
congenital NEC (*see also*
Anomaly, heart, valve)
746.9
pulmonary 746.00
specified type NEC 746.89
vascular — *see* Disease, cardiovascular
heavy-chain (gamma G) 273.2
Heberden's 715.04
Hebra's
dermatitis exfoliativa 695.89
erythema multiforme exudativum
695.1
pityriasis
maculata et circinata 696.3
rubra 695.89
pilaris 696.4
prurigo 698.2
Heerfordt's (uveoparotitis) 135
Heidenhain's 290.10
with dementia 290.10
Heilmeyer-Schöner (M9842/3)
207.1 ☑
Heine-Medin (*see also* Poliomyelitis)
045.9 ☑
Heller's (*see also* Psychosis, childhood)
299.1 ☑
Heller-Döhle (syphilitic aortitis) 093.1
hematopoietic organs 289.9
hemoglobin (Hb) 282.7
with thalassemia 282.49
abnormal (mixed) NEC 282.7
with thalassemia 282.49
AS genotype 282.5
Bart's 282.49
C (Hb-C) 282.7
with other abnormal hemoglobin
NEC 282.7
elliptocytosis 282.7
Hb-S (without crisis) 282.63
with
crisis 282.64
vaso-occlusive pain
282.64

Disease, diseased — *see also* Syndrome
— *continued*
hemoglobin — *continued*
C — *continued*
sickle-cell (without crisis)
282.63
with
crisis 282.64
vaso-occlusive pain
282.64
thalassemia 282.49
constant spring 282.7
D (Hb-D) 282.7
with other abnormal hemoglobin
NEC 282.7
Hb-S (without crisis) 282.68
with crisis 282.69
sickle-cell (without crisis)
282.68
with crisis 282.69
thalassemia 282.49
E (Hb-E) 282.7
with other abnormal hemoglobin
NEC 282.7
Hb-S (without crisis) 282.68
with crisis 282.69
sickle-cell (without crisis)
282.68
with crisis 282.69
thalassemia 282.49
elliptocytosis 282.7
F (Hb-F) 282.7
G (Hb-G) 282.7
H (Hb-H) 282.49
hereditary persistence, fetal (HPFH)
("Swiss variety") 282.7
high fetal gene 282.7
I thalassemia 282.49
M 289.7
S (*see also* Disease, sickle-cell, Hb-
S)
thalassemia (without crisis)
282.41
with
crisis 282.42
vaso-occlusive pain
282.42
spherocytosis 282.7
unstable, hemolytic 282.7
Zurich (Hb-Zurich) 282.7
hemolytic (fetus) (newborn) 773.2
autoimmune (cold type) (warm
type) 283.0
due to or with
incompatibility
ABO (blood group) 773.1
blood (group) (Duffy) (Kell)
(Kidd) (Lewis) (M) (S)
NEC 773.2
Rh (blood group) (factor)
773.0
Rh negative mother 773.0
unstable hemoglobin 282.7
hemorrhagic 287.9
newborn 776.0
Henoch (-Schönlein) (purpura nervosa)
287.0
hepatic — *see* Disease, liver
hepatolenticular 275.1
heredodegenerative NEC
brain 331.89
spinal cord 336.8
Hers' (glycogenosis VI) 271.0
Herter (-Gee) (-Heubner) (nontropical
sprue) 579.0
Herxheimer's (diffuse idiopathic cutaneous atrophy) 701.8
Heubner's 094.89
Heubner-Herter (nontropical sprue)
579.0
high fetal gene or hemoglobin thalassemia 282.49
Hildenbrand's (typhus) 081.9
hip (joint) NEC 719.95
congenital 755.63
suppurative 711.05

Disease, diseased — *see also* Syndrome
— *continued*
hip — *continued*
tuberculous (*see also* Tuberculosis)
015.1 ☑ *[730.85]*
Hippel's (retinocerebral angiomatosis)
759.6
Hirschfeld's (acute diabetes mellitus)
(*see also* Diabetes) 250.0 ☑
Hirschsprung's (congenital megacolon)
751.3
His (-Werner) (trench fever) 083.1
HIV 042
Hodgkin's (M9650/3) 201.9 ☑

Note — *Use the following fifth-digit
subclassification with category 201:*

0   *unspecified site*
1   *lymph nodes of head, face, and
neck*
2   *intrathoracic lymph nodes*
3   *intra-abdominal lymph nodes*
4   *lymph nodes of axilla and upper
limb*
5   *lymph nodes of inguinal region
and lower limb*
6   *intrapelvic lymph nodes*
7   *spleen*
8   *lymph nodes of multiple sites*

lymphocytic
depletion (M9653/3) 201.7 ☑
diffuse fibrosis (M9654/3)
201.7 ☑
reticular type (M9655/3)
201.7 ☑
predominance (M9651/3)
201.4 ☑
lymphocytic-histiocytic predominance (M9651/3) 201.4 ☑
mixed cellularity (M9652/3)
201.6 ☑
nodular sclerosis (M9656/3)
201.5 ☑
cellular phase (M9657/3)
201.5 ☑
Hodgson's 441.9
ruptured 441.5
Hoffa (-Kastert) (liposynovitis
prepatellaris) 272.8
Holla (*see also* Spherocytosis) 282.0
homozygous-Hb-S 282.61
hoof and mouth 078.4
hookworm (*see also* Ancylostomiasis)
126.9
Horton's (temporal arteritis) 446.5
host-versus-graft (immune or nonimmune cause) 996.80
bone marrow 996.85
heart 996.83
intestines 996.87
kidney 996.81
liver 996.82
lung 996.84
pancreas 996.86
specified NEC 996.89
HPFH (hereditary persistence of fetal
hemoglobin) ("Swiss variety")
282.7
Huchard's disease (continued arterial
hypertension) 401.9
Huguier's (uterine fibroma) 218.9
human immunodeficiency (virus) 042
hunger 251.1
Hunt's
dyssynergia cerebellaris myoclonica
334.2
herpetic geniculate ganglionitis
053.11
Huntington's 333.4
Huppert's (multiple myeloma)
(M9730/3) 203.0 ☑

Disease, diseased — *see also* Syndrome
— *continued*
Hurler's (mucopolysaccharidosis I)
277.5
Hutchinson-Boeck (sarcoidosis) 135
Hutchinson-Gilford (progeria) 259.8
Hutchinson's, meaning
angioma serpiginosum 709.1
cheiropompholyx 705.81
prurigo estivalis 692.72
hyaline (diffuse) (generalized) 728.9
membrane (lung) (newborn) 769
hydatid (*see also* Echinococcus) 122.9
Hyde's (prurigo nodularis) 698.3
hyperkinetic (*see also* Hyperkinesia)
314.9
heart 429.82
hypertensive (*see also* Hypertension)
401.9
hypophysis 253.9
hyperfunction 253.1
hypofunction 253.2
Iceland (epidemic neuromyasthenia)
049.8
I cell 272.7
ill-defined 799.89
immunologic NEC 279.9
immunoproliferative 203.8 ☑
inclusion 078.5
salivary gland 078.5
infancy, early NEC 779.9
infective NEC 136.9
inguinal gland 289.9
internal semilunar cartilage, cystic
717.5
intervertebral disc 722.90
with myelopathy 722.70
cervical, cervicothoracic 722.91
with myelopathy 722.71
lumbar, lumbosacral 722.93
with myelopathy 722.73
thoracic, thoracolumbar 722.92
with myelopathy 722.72
intestine 569.9
functional 564.9
congenital 751.3
psychogenic 306.4
lardaceous 277.39
organic 569.9
protozoal NEC 007.9
iris 364.9
specified NEC 364.89            ●
iron
metabolism 275.0
storage 275.0
Isambert's (*see also* Tuberculosis,
larynx) 012.3 ☑
Iselin's (osteochondrosis, fifth
metatarsal) 732.5
island (scrub typhus) 081.2
itai-itai 985.5
Jadassohn's (maculopapular erythroderma) 696.2
Jadassohn-Pellizari's (anetoderma)
701.3
Jakob-Creutzfeldt (new variant) 046.1
with dementia
with behavioral disturbance
046.1 *[294.11]*
without behavioral disturbance
046.1 *[294.10]*
Jaksch (-Luzet) (pseudoleukemia infantum) 285.8
Janet's 300.89
Jansky-Bielschowsky 330.1
jaw NEC 526.9
fibrocystic 526.2
Jensen's 363.05
Jeune's (asphyxiating thoracic dystrophy) 756.4
jigger 134.1
Johnson-Stevens (erythema multiforme exudativum) 695.1
joint NEC 719.9 ☑
ankle 719.97
Charcôt 094.0 *[713.5]*

Disease, diseased — *see also* Syndrome
— *continued*
joint — *continued*
degenerative (*see also* Osteoarthrosis) 715.9 ☑
multiple 715.09
spine (*see also* Spondylosis)
721.90
elbow 719.92
foot 719.97
hand 719.94
hip 719.95
hypertrophic (chronic) (degenerative) (*see also* Osteoarthrosis)
715.9 ☑
spine (*see also* Spondylosis)
721.90
knee 719.96
Luschka 721.90
multiple sites 719.99
pelvic region 719.95
sacroiliac 724.6
shoulder (region) 719.91
specified site NEC 719.98
spine NEC 724.9
pseudarthrosis following fusion
733.82
sacroiliac 724.6
wrist 719.93
Jourdain's (acute gingivitis) 523.00
Jüngling's (sarcoidosis) 135
Kahler (-Bozzolo) (multiple myeloma)
(M9730/3) 203.0 ☑
Kalischer's 759.6
Kaposi's 757.33
lichen ruber 697.8
acuminatus 696.4
moniliformis 697.8
xeroderma pigmentosum 757.33
Kaschin-Beck (endemic polyarthritis)
716.00
ankle 716.07
arm 716.02
lower (and wrist) 716.03
upper (and elbow) 716.02
foot (and ankle) 716.07
forearm (and wrist) 716.03
hand 716.04
leg 716.06
lower 716.06
upper 716.05
multiple sites 716.09
pelvic region (hip) (thigh) 716.05
shoulder region 716.01
specified site NEC 716.08
Katayama 120.2
Kawasaki 446.1
Kedani (scrub typhus) 081.2
kidney (functional) (pelvis) (*see also*
Disease, renal) 593.9
chronic 585.9
requiring chronic dialysis 585.6
stage
I 585.1
II (mild) 585.2
III (moderate) 585.3
IV (severe) 585.4
V 585.5
cystic (congenital) 753.10
multiple 753.19
single 753.11
specified NEC 753.19
fibrocystic (congenital) 753.19
in gout 274.10
polycystic (congenital) 753.12
adult type (APKD) 753.13
autosomal dominant 753.13
autosomal recessive 753.14
childhood type (CPKD) 753.14
infantile type 753.14
Kienböck's (carpal lunate) (wrist)
732.3
Kimmelstiel (-Wilson) (intercapillary
glomerulosclerosis)
250.4 ☑ *[581.81]*

☑ Additional Digit Required — Refer to the Tabular List for Digit Selection       Ⓥ Subterms under main terms may continue to next column or page

*2008 ICD-9-CM*       ▶◀ Revised Text       ● New Line       ▲ Revised Code       October 2007 · Volume 2 — 87

**Disease, diseased** — *see also* Syndrome
— *continued*

Kinnier Wilson's (hepatolenticular degeneration) 275.1
kissing 075
Kleb's (*see also* Nephritis) 583.9
Klinger's 446.4
Klippel's 723.8
Klippel-Feil (brevicollis) 756.16
knight's 911.1
Köbner's (epidermolysis bullosa) 757.39
Koenig-Wichmann (pemphigus) 694.4
Köhler's
　first (osteoarthrosis juvenilis) 732.5
　second (Freiberg's infraction, metatarsal head) 732.5
　patellar 732.4
　tarsal navicular (bone) (osteoarthrosis juvenilis) 732.5
Köhler-Freiberg (infraction, metatarsal head) 732.5
Köhler-Mouchet (osteoarthrosis juvenilis) 732.5
Köhler-Pellegrini-Stieda (calcification, knee joint) 726.62
Kok 759.89
König's (osteochondritis dissecans) 732.7
Korsakoff's (nonalcoholic) 294.0
　alcoholic 291.1
Kostmann's (infantile genetic agranulocytosis) 288.01
Krabbe's 330.0
Kraepelin-Morel (*see also* Schizophrenia) 295.9 ✓
Kraft-Weber-Dimitri 759.6
Kufs' 330.1
Kugelberg-Welander 335.11
Kuhnt-Junius 362.52
Kümmell's (-Verneuil) (spondylitis) 721.7
Kundrat's (lymphosarcoma) 200.1 ✓
kuru 046.0
Kussmaul (-Meier) (polyarteritis nodosa) 446.0
Kyasanur Forest 065.2
Kyrle's (hyperkeratosis follicularis in cutem penetrans) 701.1
labia
　inflammatory 616.10　　　　　　　▲
　noninflammatory 624.9
　　specified NEC 624.8
labyrinth, ear 386.8
lacrimal system (apparatus) (passages) 375.9
　gland 375.00
　specified NEC 375.89
Lafora's 333.2
Lagleyze-von Hippel (retinocerebral angiomatosis) 759.6
Lancereaux-Mathieu (leptospiral jaundice) 100.0
Landry's 357.0
Lane's 569.89
lardaceous (any site) 277.39
Larrey-Weil (leptospiral jaundice) 100.0
Larsen (-Johansson) (juvenile osteopathia patellae) 732.4
larynx 478.70
Lasègue's (persecution mania) 297.9
Leber's 377.16
Lederer's (acquired infectious hemolytic anemia) 283.19
Legg's (capital femoral osteochondrosis) 732.1
Legg-Calvé-Perthes (capital femoral osteochondrosis) 732.1
Legg-Calvé-Waldenström (femoral capital osteochondrosis) 732.1
Legg-Perthes (femoral capital osteochondrosis) 732.1
Legionnaires' 482.84
Leigh's 330.8
Leiner's (exfoliative dermatitis) 695.89

**Disease, diseased** — *see also* Syndrome
— *continued*

Leloir's (lupus erythematosus) 695.4
Lenegre's 426.0
lens (eye) 379.39
Leriche's (osteoporosis, posttraumatic) 733.7
Letterer-Siwe (acute histiocytosis X) (M9722/3) 202.5 ✓
Lev's (acquired complete heart block) 426.0
Lewandowski's (*see also* Tuberculosis) 017.0 ✓
Lewandowski-Lutz (epidermodysplasia verruciformis) 078.19
Lewy body 331.82
　with dementia
　　with behavioral disturbance 331.82 [294.11]
　　without behavioral disturbance 331.82 [294.10]
Leyden's (periodic vomiting) 536.2
Libman-Sacks (verrucous endocarditis) 710.0 [424.91]
Lichtheim's (subacute combined sclerosis with pernicious anemia) 281.0 [336.2]
ligament 728.9
light chain 203.0 ✓
Lightwood's (renal tubular acidosis) 588.89
Lignac's (cystinosis) 270.0
Lindau's (retinocerebral angiomatosis) 759.6
Lindau-von Hippel (angiomatosis retinocerebellosa) 759.6
lip NEC 528.5
lipidosis 272.7
lipoid storage NEC 272.7
Lipschütz's 616.50
Little's — *see* Palsy, cerebral
liver 573.9
　alcoholic 571.3
　　acute 571.1
　　chronic 571.3
　chronic 571.9
　　alcoholic 571.3
　cystic, congenital 751.62
　drug-induced 573.3
　due to
　　chemicals 573.3
　　fluorinated agents 573.3
　　hypersensitivity drugs 573.3
　　isoniazids 573.3
　end stage NEC 572.8　　　　　　　●
　　due to hepatitis — *see* Hepati-●
　　　tis　　　　　　　　　　　　　●
　fibrocystic (congenital) 751.62
　glycogen storage 271.0
　organic 573.9
　polycystic (congenital) 751.62
Lobo's (keloid blastomycosis) 116.2
Lobstein's (brittle bones and blue sclera) 756.51
locomotor system 334.9
Lorain's (pituitary dwarfism) 253.3
Lou Gehrig's 335.20
Lucas-Championnière (fibrinous bronchitis) 466.0
Ludwig's (submaxillary cellulitis) 528.3
luetic — *see* Syphilis
lumbosacral region 724.6
lung NEC 518.89
　black 500
　congenital 748.60
　cystic 518.89
　　congenital 748.4
　fibroid (chronic) (*see also* Fibrosis, lung) 515
　fluke 121.2
　　oriental 121.2
　in
　　amyloidosis 277.39 [517.8]
　　polymyositis 710.4 [517.8]
　　sarcoidosis 135 [517.8]

**Disease, diseased** — *see also* Syndrome
— *continued*

lung — *continued*
　in — *continued*
　　Sjögren's syndrome 710.2 [517.8]
　　syphilis 095.1
　　systemic lupus erythematosus 710.0 [517.8]
　　systemic sclerosis 710.1 [517.2]
　interstitial (chronic) 515
　　acute 136.3
　nonspecific, chronic 496
　obstructive (chronic) (COPD) 496
　　with
　　　acute
　　　　bronchitis 491.22
　　　　exacerbation NEC 491.21
　　　alveolitis, allergic (*see also* Alveolitis, allergic) 495.9
　　　asthma (chronic) (obstructive) 493.2 ✓
　　　bronchiectasis 494.0
　　　　with acute exacerbation 494.1
　　　bronchitis (chronic) 491.20
　　　　with
　　　　　acute bronchitis 491.22
　　　　　exacerbation (acute) 491.21
　　　decompensated 491.21
　　　　with exacerbation 491.21
　　　emphysema NEC 492.8
　diffuse (with fibrosis) 496
　polycystic 518.89
　　asthma (chronic) (obstructive) 493.2 ✓
　　congenital 748.4
　purulent (cavitary) 513.0
　restrictive 518.89
　rheumatoid 714.81
　　diffuse interstitial 714.81
　specified NEC 518.89
Lutembacher's (atrial septal defect with mitral stenosis) 745.5
Lutz-Miescher (elastosis perforans serpiginosa) 701.1
Lutz-Splendore-de Almeida (Brazilian blastomycosis) 116.1
Lyell's (toxic epidermal necrolysis) 695.1
　due to drug
　　correct substance properly administered 695.1
　　overdose or wrong substance given or taken 977.9
　　specific drug — *see* Table of Drugs and Chemicals
Lyme 088.81
lymphatic (gland) (system) 289.9
　channel (noninfective) 457.9
　vessel (noninfective) 457.9
　　specified NEC 457.8
lymphoproliferative (chronic) (M9970/1) 238.79
Machado-Joseph 334.8
Madelung's (lipomatosis) 272.8
Madura (actinomycotic) 039.9
　mycotic 117.4
Magitot's 526.4
Majocchi's (purpura annularis telangiectodes) 709.1
malarial (*see also* Malaria) 084.6
Malassez's (cystic) 608.89
Malibu 919.8
　infected 919.9
malignant (M8000/3) (*see also* Neoplasm, by site, malignant)
　previous, affecting management of pregnancy V23.89
Manson's 120.1
maple bark 495.6
maple syrup (urine) 270.3
Marburg (virus) 078.89

**Disease, diseased** — *see also* Syndrome
— *continued*

Marchiafava (-Bignami) 341.8
Marfan's 090.49
　congenital syphilis 090.49
　meaning Marfan's syndrome 759.82
Marie-Bamberger (hypertrophic pulmonary osteoarthropathy) (secondary) 731.2
　primary or idiopathic (acropachyderma) 757.39
　pulmonary (hypertrophic osteoarthropathy) 731.2
Marie-Strümpell (ankylosing spondylitis) 720.0
Marion's (bladder neck obstruction) 596.0
Marsh's (exophthalmic goiter) 242.0 ✓
Martin's 715.27
mast cell 757.33
　systemic (M9741/3) 202.6 ✓
mastoid (*see also* Mastoiditis) 383.9
　process 385.9
maternal, unrelated to pregnancy NEC, affecting fetus or newborn 760.9
Mathieu's (leptospiral jaundice) 100.0
Mauclaire's 732.3
Mauriac's (erythema nodosum syphiliticum) 091.3
Maxcy's 081.0
McArdle (-Schmid-Pearson) (glycogenosis V) 271.0
mediastinum NEC 519.3
Medin's (*see also* Poliomyelitis) 045.9 ✓
Mediterranean (with hemoglobinopathy) 282.49
medullary center (idiopathic) (respiratory) 348.8
Meige's (chronic hereditary edema) 757.0
Meleda 757.39
Ménétrier's (hypertrophic gastritis) 535.2 ✓
Ménière's (active) 386.00
　cochlear 386.02
　cochleovestibular 386.01
　inactive 386.04
　in remission 386.04
　vestibular 386.03
meningeal — *see* Meningitis
mental (*see also* Psychosis) 298.9
Merzbacher-Pelizaeus 330.0
mesenchymal 710.9
mesenteric embolic 557.0
metabolic NEC 277.9
metal polishers' 502
metastatic — *see* Metastasis
Mibelli's 757.39
microdrepanocytic 282.49
microvascular — code to condition
Miescher's 709.3
Mikulicz's (dryness of mouth, absent or decreased lacrimation) 527.1
Milkman (-Looser) (osteomalacia with pseudofractures) 268.2
Miller's (osteomalacia) 268.2
Mills' 335.29
Milroy's (chronic hereditary edema) 757.0
Minamata 985.0
Minor's 336.1
Minot's (hemorrhagic disease, newborn) 776.0
Minot-von Willebrand-Jürgens (angiohemophilia) 286.4
Mitchell's (erythromelalgia) 443.82
mitral — *see* Endocarditis, mitral
Mljet (mal de Meleda) 757.39
Möbius', Moebius' 346.8 ✓
Moeller's 267
Möller (-Barlow) (infantile scurvy) 267
Mönckeberg's (*see also* Arteriosclerosis, extremities) 440.20

✓ Additional Digit Required — Refer to the Tabular List for Digit Selection　　　　　　　　　　　　　　　Subterms under main terms may continue to next column or page

88 — Volume 2 · October 2007　　　▶◀ Revised Text　　　● New Line　　　▲ Revised Code　　　**2008 ICD-9-CM**

Disease, diseased — *see also* Syndrome — *continued*

Mondor's (thrombophlebitis of breast) 451.89

Monge's 993.2

Morel-Kraepelin (*see also* Schizophrenia) 295.9 ☑

Morgagni's (syndrome) (hyperostosis frontalis interna) 733.3

Morgagni-Adams-Stokes (syncope with heart block) 426.9

Morquio (-Brailsford) (-Ullrich) (mucopolysaccharidosis IV) 277.5

Morton's (with metatarsalgia) 355.6

Morvan's 336.0

motor neuron (bulbar) (mixed type) 335.20

Mouchet's (juvenile osteochondrosis, foot) 732.5

mouth 528.9

Moyamoya 437.5

Mucha's (acute parapsoriasis varioliformis) 696.2

mu-chain 273.2

mucolipidosis (I) (II) (III) 272.7

Münchmeyer's (exostosis luxurians) 728.11

Murri's (intermittent hemoglobinuria) 283.2

muscle 359.9
  inflammatory 728.9
  ocular 378.9

musculoskeletal system 729.9

mushroom workers' 495.5

Myà's (congenital dilation, colon) 751.3

mycotic 117.9

myeloproliferative (chronic) (M9960/1) 238.79

myocardium, myocardial (*see also* Degeneration, myocardial) 429.1
  hypertensive (*see also* Hypertension, heart 402.90
  primary (idiopathic) 425.4

myoneural 358.9

Naegeli's 287.1

nail 703.9
  specified type NEC 703.8

Nairobi sheep 066.1

nasal 478.19
  cavity NEC 478.19
  sinus (chronic) — *see* Sinusitis

navel (newborn) NEC 779.89
  delayed separation of umbilical cord 779.83

nemaline body 359.0

neoplastic, generalized (M8000/6) 199.0

nerve — *see* Disorder, nerve

nervous system (central) 349.9
  autonomic, peripheral (*see also* Neuropathy, peripheral, autonomic) 337.9
  congenital 742.9
  inflammatory — *see* Encephalitis
  parasympathetic (*see also* Neuropathy, peripheral, autonomic) 337.9
  peripheral NEC 355.9
  specified NEC 349.89
  sympathetic (*see also* Neuropathy, peripheral, autonomic) 337.9
  vegetative (*see also* Neuropathy, peripheral, autonomic) 337.9

Nettleship's (urticaria pigmentosa) 757.33

Neumann's (pemphigus vegetans) 694.4

neurologic (central) NEC (*see also* Disease, nervous system) 349.9
  peripheral NEC 355.9

neuromuscular system NEC 358.9

Newcastle 077.8

Nicolas (-Durand) — Favre (climatic bubo) 099.1

Disease, diseased — *see also* Syndrome — *continued*

Niemann-Pick (lipid histiocytosis) 272.7

nipple 611.9
  Paget's (M8540/3) 174.0

Nishimoto (-Takeuchi) 437.5

nonarthropod-borne NEC 078.89
  central nervous system NEC 049.9
  enterovirus NEC 078.89

nonautoimmune hemolytic NEC 283.10

Nonne-Milroy-Meige (chronic hereditary edema) 757.0

Norrie's (congenital progressive oculoacousticocerebral degeneration) 743.8

nose 478.19

nucleus pulposus — *see* Disease, intervertebral disc

nutritional 269.9
  maternal, affecting fetus or newborn 760.4

oasthouse, urine 270.2

obliterative vascular 447.1

Odelberg's (juvenile osteochondrosis) 732.1

Oguchi's (retina) 368.61

Ohara's (*see also* Tularemia) 021.9

Ollier's (chondrodysplasia) 756.4

Opitz's (congestive splenomegaly) 289.51

Oppenheim's 358.8

Oppenheim-Urbach (necrobiosis lipoidica diabeticorum) 250.8 ☑ *[709.3]*

optic nerve NEC 377.49

orbit 376.9
  specified NEC 376.89

Oriental liver fluke 121.1

Oriental lung fluke 121.2

Ormond's 593.4

Osgood-Schlatter 732.4

Osgood's tibia (tubercle) 732.4

Osler (-Vaquez) (polycythemia vera) (M9950/1) 238.4

Osler-Rendu (familial hemorrhagic telangiectasia) 448.0

osteofibrocystic 252.01

Otto's 715.35

outer ear 380.9

ovary (noninflammatory) NEC 620.9
  cystic 620.2
  polycystic 256.4
  specified NEC 620.8

Owren's (congenital) (*see also* Defect, coagulation) 286.3

Paas' 756.59

Paget's (osteitis deformans) 731.0
  with infiltrating duct carcinoma of the breast (M8541/3) — *see* Neoplasm, breast, malignant
  bone 731.0
    osteosarcoma in (M9184/3) — *see* Neoplasm, bone, malignant
  breast (M8540/3) 174.0
  extramammary (M8542/3) (*see also* Neoplasm, skin, malignant)
    anus 154.3
    skin 173.5
  malignant (M8540/3)
    breast 174.0
    specified site NEC (M8542/3) — *see* Neoplasm, skin, malignant
    unspecified site 174.0
  mammary (M8540/3) 174.0
  nipple (M8540/3) 174.0

palate (soft) 528.9

Paltauf-Sternberg 201.9 ☑

pancreas 577.9
  cystic 577.2
    congenital 751.7
  fibrocystic 277.00

Panner's 732.3

Disease, diseased — *see also* Syndrome — *continued*

Panner's — *continued*
  capitellum humeri 732.3
  head of humerus 732.3
  tarsal navicular (bone) (osteochondrosis) 732.5

panvalvular — *see* Endocarditis, mitral

parametrium 629.9

parasitic NEC 136.9
  cerebral NEC 123.9
  intestinal NEC 129
  mouth 112.0
  skin NEC 134.9
  specified type — *see* Infestation
  tongue 112.0

parathyroid (gland) 252.9
  specified NEC 252.8

Parkinson's 332.0

parodontal 523.9

Parrot's (syphilitic osteochondritis) 090.0

Parry's (exophthalmic goiter) 242.0 ☑

Parson's (exophthalmic goiter) 242.0 ☑

Pavy's 593.6

Paxton's (white piedra) 111.2

Payr's (splenic flexure syndrome) 569.89

pearl-workers' (chronic osteomyelitis) (*see also* Osteomyelitis) 730.1 ☑

Pel-Ebstein — *see* Disease, Hodgkin's

Pelizaeus-Merzbacher 330.0
  with dementia
    with behavioral disturbance 330.0 *[294.11]*
    without behavioral disturbance 330.0 *[294.10]*

Pellegrini-Stieda (calcification, knee joint) 726.62

pelvis, pelvic
  female NEC 629.9
    specified NEC 629.89
  gonococcal (acute) 098.19
    chronic or duration of 2 months or over 098.39
  infection (*see also* Disease, pelvis, inflammatory) 614.9
  inflammatory (female) (PID) 614.9
    with
      abortion — *see* Abortion, by type, with sepsis
      ectopic pregnancy (*see also* categories 633.0–633.9) 639.0
      molar pregnancy (*see also* categories 630–632) 639.0
    acute 614.3
    chronic 614.4
    complicating pregnancy 646.6 ☑
      affecting fetus or newborn 760.8
    following
      abortion 639.0
      ectopic or molar pregnancy 639.0
    peritonitis (acute) 614.5
      chronic NEC 614.7
    puerperal, postpartum, childbirth 670.0 ☑
    specified NEC 614.8
  organ, female NEC 629.9
    specified NEC 629.89
  peritoneum, female NEC 629.9
    specified NEC 629.89

penis 607.9
  inflammatory 607.2

peptic NEC 536.9
  acid 536.8

periapical tissues NEC 522.9

pericardium 423.9
  specified type NEC 423.8

Disease, diseased — *see also* Syndrome — *continued*

perineum
  female
    inflammatory 616.9
      specified NEC 616.89
    noninflammatory 624.9
      specified NEC 624.8
  male (inflammatory) 682.2

periodic (familial) (Reimann's) NEC 277.31

paralysis 359.3

periodontal NEC 523.9
  specified NEC 523.8

periosteum 733.90

peripheral
  arterial 443.9
  autonomic nervous system (*see also* Neuropathy, autonomic) 337.9
  nerve NEC (*see also* Neuropathy) 356.9
    multiple — *see* Polyneuropathy
  vascular 443.9
    specified type NEC 443.89

peritoneum 568.9
  pelvic, female 629.9
    specified NEC 629.89

Perrin-Ferraton (snapping hip) 719.65

persistent mucosal (middle ear) (with posterior or superior marginal perforation of ear drum) 382.2

Perthes' (capital femoral osteochondrosis) 732.1

Petit's (*see also* Hernia, lumbar) 553.8

Peutz-Jeghers 759.6

Peyronie's 607.85

Pfeiffer's (infectious mononucleosis) 075

pharynx 478.20

Phocas' 610.1

photochromogenic (acid-fast bacilli) (pulmonary) 031.0
  nonpulmonary 031.9

Pick's
  brain 331.11
    with dementia
      with behavioral disturbance 331.11 *[294.11]*
      without behavioral disturbance 331.11 *[294.10]*
  cerebral atrophy 331.11
    with dementia
      with behavioral disturbance 331.11 *[294.11]*
      without behavioral disturbance 331.11 *[294.10]*
  lipid histiocytosis 272.7
  liver (pericardial pseudocirrhosis of liver) 423.2
  pericardium (pericardial pseudocirrhosis of liver) 423.2
  polyserositis (pericardial pseudocirrhosis of liver) 423.2

Pierson's (osteochondrosis) 732.1

pigeon fanciers' or breeders' 495.2

pineal gland 259.8

pink 985.0

Pinkus' (lichen nitidus) 697.1

pinworm 127.4

pituitary (gland) 253.9
  hyperfunction 253.1
  hypofunction 253.2

pituitary snuff-takers' 495.8

placenta
  affecting fetus or newborn 762.2
  complicating pregnancy or childbirth 656.7 ☑

pleura (cavity) (*see also* Pleurisy) 511.0

Plummer's (toxic nodular goiter) 242.3 ☑

pneumatic
  drill 994.9
  hammer 994.9

policeman's 729.2

☑ Additional Digit Required — Refer to the Tabular List for Digit Selection    ▽ Subterms under main terms may continue to next column or page

2008 ICD-9-CM    ▶◀ Revised Text    ● New Line    ▲ Revised Code    Volume 2 — 89

Disease, diseased — Disease, diseased

**Disease, diseased** — *see also* Syndrome — *continued*

Pollitzer's (hidradenitis suppurativa) 705.83
polycystic (congenital) 759.89
  congenital 748.4
    kidney or renal 753.12
      adult type (APKD) 753.13
      autosomal dominant 753.13
      autosomal recessive 753.14
      childhood type (CPKD) 753.14
      infantile type 753.14
    liver or hepatic 751.62
    lung or pulmonary 518.89
    ovary, ovaries 256.4
    spleen 759.0
Pompe's (glycogenosis II) 271.0
Poncet's (tuberculous rheumatism) (*see also* Tuberculosis) 015.9 ☑
Posada-Wernicke 114.9
Potain's (pulmonary edema) 514
Pott's (*see also* Tuberculosis) 015.0 ☑ *[730.88]*
  osteomyelitis 015.0 ☑ *[730.88]*
  paraplegia 015.0 ☑ *[730.88]*
  spinal curvature 015.0 ☑ *[737.43]*
  spondylitis 015.0 ☑ *[720.81]*
Potter's 753.0
Poulet's 714.2
pregnancy NEC (*see also* Pregnancy) 646.9 ☑
Preiser's (osteoporosis) 733.09
Pringle's (tuberous sclerosis) 759.5
Profichet's 729.9
prostate 602.9
  specified type NEC 602.8
protozoal NEC 136.8
  intestine, intestinal NEC 007.9
pseudo-Hurler's (mucolipidosis III) 272.7
psychiatric (*see also* Psychosis) 298.9
psychotic (*see also* Psychosis) 298.9
Puente's (simple glandular cheilitis) 528.5
puerperal NEC (*see also* Puerperal) 674.9 ☑
pulmonary (*see also* Disease, lung)
  amyloid 277.39 *[517.8]*
  artery 417.9
  circulation, circulatory 417.9
    specified NEC 417.8
  diffuse obstructive (chronic) 496
    with
      acute bronchitis 491.22
      asthma (chronic) (obstructive) 493.2 ☑
      exacerbation NEC (acute) 491.21
  heart (chronic) 416.9
    specified NEC 416.8
  hypertensive (vascular) 416.0
    cardiovascular 416.0
  obstructive diffuse (chronic) 496
    with
      acute bronchitis 491.22
      asthma (chronic) (obstructive) 493.2 ☑
      bronchitis (chronic) 491.20
        with
          exacerbation (acute) 491.21
        acute 491.22
        exacerbation NEC (acute) 491.21
      decompensated 491.21
        with exacerbation 491.21
  valve (*see also* Endocarditis, pulmonary) 424.3
  pulp (dental) NEC 522.9
pulseless 446.7
Putnam's (subacute combined sclerosis with pernicious anemia) 281.0 *[336.2]*
Pyle (-Cohn) (craniometaphyseal dysplasia) 756.89
pyramidal tract 333.90

**Disease, diseased** — *see also* Syndrome — *continued*

Quervain's
  tendon sheath 727.04
  thyroid (subacute granulomatous thyroiditis) 245.1
Quincke's — *see* Edema, angioneurotic
Quinquaud (acne decalvans) 704.09
rag sorters' 022.1
Raynaud's (paroxysmal digital cyanosis) 443.0
reactive airway — *see* Asthma
Recklinghausen's (M9540/1) 237.71
  bone (osteitis fibrosa cystica) 252.01
Recklinghausen-Applebaum (hemochromatosis) 275.0
Reclus' (cystic) 610.1
rectum NEC 569.49
Refsum's (heredopathia atactica polyneuritiformis) 356.3
Reichmann's (gastrosuccorrhea) 536.8
Reimann's (periodic) 277.31
Reiter's 099.3
renal (functional) (pelvis) (*see also* Disease, kidney) 593.9
  with
    edema (*see also* Nephrosis) 581.9
    exudative nephritis 583.89
    lesion of interstitial nephritis 583.89
    stated generalized cause — *see* Nephritis
  acute 593.9
  basement membrane NEC 583.89
    with
      pulmonary hemorrhage (Goodpasture's syndrome) 446.21 *[583.81]*
  chronic (*see also* Disease, kidney, chronic) 593.9
  complicating pregnancy or puerperium NEC 646.2 ☑
    with hypertension — *see* Toxemia, of pregnancy
    affecting fetus or newborn 760.1
  cystic, congenital (*see also* Cystic, disease, kidney) 753.10
  diabetic 250.4 ☑ *[583.81]*
  due to
    amyloidosis 277.39 *[583.81]*
    diabetes mellitus 250.4 ☑ *[583.81]*
    systemic lupus erythematosis 710.0 *[583.81]*
  end-stage 585.6
  exudative 583.89
  fibrocystic (congenital) 753.19
  gonococcal 098.19 *[583.81]*
  gouty 274.10
  hypertensive (*see also* Hypertension, kidney) 403.90
  immune complex NEC 583.89
  interstitial (diffuse) (focal) 583.89
  lupus 710.0 *[583.81]*
  maternal, affecting fetus or newborn 760.1
    hypertensive 760.0
  phosphate-losing (tubular) 588.0
  polycystic (congenital) 753.12
    adult type (APKD) 753.13
    autosomal dominant 753.13
    autosomal recessive 753.14
    childhood type (CPKD) 753.14
    infantile type 753.14
  specified lesion or cause NEC (*see also* Glomerulonephritis) 583.89
  subacute 581.9
  syphilitic 095.4
  tuberculous (*see also* Tuberculosis) 016.0 ☑ *[583.81]*
  tubular (*see also* Nephrosis, tubular) 584.5

**Disease, diseased** — *see also* Syndrome — *continued*

Rendu-Osler-Weber (familial hemorrhagic telangiectasia) 448.0
renovascular (arteriosclerotic) (*see also* Hypertension, kidney) 403.90
respiratory (tract) 519.9
  acute or subacute (upper) NEC 465.9
    due to fumes or vapors 506.3
    multiple sites NEC 465.8
    noninfectious 478.9
    streptococcal 034.0
  chronic 519.9
    arising in the perinatal period 770.7
    due to fumes or vapors 506.4
  due to
    aspiration of liquids or solids 508.9
    external agents NEC 508.9
      specified NEC 508.8
    fumes or vapors 506.9
      acute or subacute NEC 506.3
      chronic 506.4
  fetus or newborn NEC 770.9
  obstructive 496
  specified type NEC 519.8
  upper (acute) (infectious) NEC 465.9
    multiple sites NEC 465.8
    noninfectious NEC 478.9
    streptococcal 034.0
retina, retinal NEC 362.9
  Batten's or Batten-Mayou 330.1 *[362.71]*
  degeneration 362.89
  vascular lesion 362.17
rheumatic (*see also* Arthritis) 716.8 ☑
  heart — *see* Disease, heart, rheumatic
rheumatoid (heart) — *see* Arthritis, rheumatoid
rickettsial NEC 083.9
  specified type NEC 083.8
Riedel's (ligneous thyroiditis) 245.3
Riga (-Fede) (cachectic aphthae) 529.0
Riggs' (compound periodontitis) 523.40
Ritter's 695.81
Rivalta's (cervicofacial actinomycosis) 039.3
Robles' (onchocerciasis) 125.3 *[360.13]*
Roger's (congenital interventricular septal defect) 745.4
Rokitansky's (*see also* Necrosis, liver) 570
Romberg's 349.89
Rosenthal's (factor XI deficiency) 286.2
Rossbach's (hyperchlorhydria) 536.8
  psychogenic 306.4
Roth (-Bernhardt) 355.1
Runeberg's (progressive pernicious anemia) 281.0
Rust's (tuberculous spondylitis) (*see also* Tuberculosis) 015.0 ☑ *[720.81]*
Rustitskii's (multiple myeloma) (M9730/3) 203.0 ☑
Ruysch's (Hirschsprung's disease) 751.3
Sachs (-Tay) 330.1
sacroiliac NEC 724.6
salivary gland or duct NEC 527.9
  inclusion 078.5
    streptococcal 034.0
  virus 078.5
Sander's (paranoia) 297.1
Sandhoff's 330.1
sandworm 126.9
Savill's (epidemic exfoliative dermatitis) 695.89
Schamberg's (progressive pigmentary dermatosis) 709.09
Schaumann's (sarcoidosis) 135
Schenck's (sporotrichosis) 117.1

**Disease, diseased** — *see also* Syndrome — *continued*

Scheuermann's (osteochondrosis) 732.0
Schilder (-Flatau) 341.1
Schimmelbusch's 610.1
Schlatter-Osgood 732.4
Schlatter's tibia (tubercle) 732.4
Schmorl's 722.30
  cervical 722.39
  lumbar, lumbosacral 722.32
  specified region NEC 722.39
  thoracic, thoracolumbar 722.31
Scholz's 330.0
Schönlein (-Henoch) (purpura rheumatica) 287.0
Schottmüller's (*see also* Fever, paratyphoid) 002.9
Schüller-Christian (chronic histiocytosis X) 277.89
Schultz's (agranulocytosis) 288.09
Schwalbe-Ziehen-Oppenheimer 333.6
Schwartz-Jampel 359.23 ●
Schweninger-Buzzi (macular atrophy) 701.3
sclera 379.19
scrofulous (*see also* Tuberculosis) 017.2 ☑
scrotum 608.9
sebaceous glands NEC 706.9
Secretan's (posttraumatic edema) 782.3
semilunar cartilage, cystic 717.5
seminal vesicle 608.9
Senear-Usher (pemphigus erythematosus) 694.4
serum NEC 999.5
Sever's (osteochondrosis calcaneum) 732.5
sexually transmitted — *see* Disease, ●
  venereal ●
Sézary's (reticulosis) (M9701/3) 202.2 ☑
Shaver's (bauxite pneumoconiosis) 503
Sheehan's (postpartum pituitary necrosis) 253.2
shimamushi (scrub typhus) 081.2
shipyard 077.1
sickle cell 282.60
  with
    crisis 282.62
    Hb-S disease 282.61
    other abnormal hemoglobin (Hb-D) (Hb-E) (Hb-G) (Hb-J) (Hb-K) (Hb-O) (Hb-P) (high fetal gene) (without crisis) 282.68
      with crisis 282.69
  elliptocytosis 282.60
  Hb-C (without crisis) 282.63
    with
      crisis 282.64
      vaso-occlusive pain 282.64
  Hb-S 282.61
    with
      crisis 282.62
      Hb-C (without crisis) 282.63
        with
          crisis 282.64
          vaso-occlusive pain 282.64
      other abnormal hemoglobin (Hb-D) (Hb-E) (Hb-G) (Hb-J) (Hb-K) (Hb-O) (Hb-P) (high fetal gene) (without crisis) 282.68
      with crisis 282.69
  spherocytosis 282.60
  thalassemia (without crisis) 282.41
    with
      crisis 282.42
      vaso-occlusive pain 282.42
Siegal-Cattan-Mamou (periodic) 277.31
silo fillers' 506.9

☑ Additional Digit Required — Refer to the Tabular List for Digit Selection              Subterms under main terms may continue to next column or page

90 — Volume 2 • October 2007    ▶◀ Revised Text    ● New Line    ▲ Revised Code    *2008 ICD-9-CM*

Disease, diseased — *see also* Syndrome
— *continued*
  Simian B 054.3
  Simmonds' (pituitary cachexia) 253.2
  Simons' (progressive lipodystrophy)
    272.6
  Sinding-Larsen (juvenile osteopathia
    patellae) 732.4
  sinus (*see also* Sinusitis)
    brain 437.9
    specified NEC 478.19
  Sirkari's 085.0
  sixth ▶(*see also* Exanthem subitum)◀
    058.10                               ▲
  Sjögren (-Gougerot) 710.2
    with lung involvement
      710.2 [517.8]
  Skevas-Zerfus 989.5
  skin NEC 709.9
    due to metabolic disorder 277.9
    specified type NEC 709.8
  sleeping (*see also* Narcolepsy) 347.00
    meaning sleeping sickness (*see al-
      so* Trypanosomiasis) 086.5
  small vessel 443.9
  Smith-Strang (oasthouse urine) 270.2
  Sneddon-Wilkinson (subcorneal pus-
    tular dermatosis) 694.1
  South African creeping 133.8
  Spencer's (epidemic vomiting) 078.82
  Spielmeyer-Stock 330.1
  Spielmeyer-Vogt 330.1
  spine, spinal 733.90
    combined system (*see also* Degen-
      eration, combined)
        266.2 [336.2]
        with pernicious anemia
          281.0 [336.2]
    cord NEC 336.9
      congenital 742.9
    demyelinating NEC 341.8
    joint (*see also* Disease, joint, spine)
      724.9
    tuberculous 015.0 ☑ [730.8] ☑
  spinocerebellar 334.9
    specified NEC 334.8
  spleen (organic) (postinfectional)
    289.50
    amyloid 277.39
    lardaceous 277.39
    polycystic 759.0
    specified NEC 289.59
  sponge divers' 989.5
  Stanton's (melioidosis) 025
  Stargardt's 362.75
  Startle 759.89
  Steinert's 359.21                      ▲
  Sternberg's — *see* Disease, Hodgkin's
  Stevens-Johnson (erythema multi-
    forme exudativum) 695.1
  Sticker's (erythema infectiosum) 057.0
  Stieda's (calcification, knee joint)
    726.62
  Still's (juvenile rheumatoid arthritis)
    714.30
  Stiller's (asthenia) 780.79
  Stokes' (exophthalmic goiter) 242.0 ☑
  Stokes-Adams (syncope with heart
    block) 426.9
  Stokvis (-Talma) (enterogenous
    cyanosis) 289.7
  stomach NEC (organic) 537.9
    functional 536.9
      psychogenic 306.4
    lardaceous 277.39
  stonemasons' 502
  storage
    glycogen (*see also* Disease, glyco-
      gen storage) 271.0
    lipid 272.7
    mucopolysaccharide 277.5
  striatopallidal system 333.90
    specified NEC 333.89
  Strümpell-Marie (ankylosing
    spondylitis) 720.0

Disease, diseased — *see also* Syndrome
— *continued*
  Stuart's (congenital factor X deficien-
    cy) (*see also* Defect, coagulation)
      286.3
  Stuart-Prower (congenital factor X
    deficiency) (*see also* Defect, co-
      agulation) 286.3
  Sturge (-Weber) (-Dimitri) (encephalo-
    cutaneous angiomatosis) 759.6
  Stuttgart 100.89
  Sudeck's 733.7
  supporting structures of teeth NEC
    525.9
  suprarenal (gland) (capsule) 255.9
    hyperfunction 255.3
    hypofunction 255.41               ▲
  Sutton's 709.09
  Sutton and Gull's — *see* Hyperten-
    sion, kidney
  sweat glands NEC 705.9
    specified type NEC 705.89
  sweating 078.2
  Sweeley-Klionsky 272.4
  Swift (-Feer) 985.0
  swimming pool (bacillus) 031.1
  swineherd's 100.89
  Sylvest's (epidemic pleurodynia) 074.1
  Symmers (follicular lymphoma)
    (M9690/3) 202.0 ☑
  sympathetic nervous system (*see also*
    Neuropathy, peripheral, auto-
      nomic) 337.9
  synovium 727.9
  syphilitic — *see* Syphilis
  systemic tissue mast cell (M9741/3)
    202.6 ☑
  Taenzer's 757.4
  Takayasu's (pulseless) 446.7
  Talma's 728.85
  Tangier (familial high-density lipopro-
    tein deficiency) 272.5
  Tarral-Besnier (pityriasis rubra pilaris)
    696.4
  Taylor's 701.8
  Tay-Sachs 330.1
  tear duct 375.69
  teeth, tooth 525.9
    hard tissues 521.9
      specified NEC 521.89
    pulp NEC 522.9
  tendon 727.9
    inflammatory NEC 727.9
  terminal vessel 443.9
  testis 608.9
  Thaysen-Gee (nontropical sprue)
    579.0
  Thomsen's 359.22                     ▲
  Thomson's (congenital poikiloderma)
    757.33
  Thornwaldt's, Tornwaldt's (pharyngeal
    bursitis) 478.29
  throat 478.20
    septic 034.0
  thromboembolic (*see also* Embolism)
    444.9
  thymus (gland) 254.9
    specified NEC 254.8
  thyroid (gland) NEC 246.9
    heart (*see also* Hyperthyroidism)
      242.9 ☑ [425.7]
    lardaceous 277.39
    specified NEC 246.8
  Tietze's 733.6
  Tommaselli's
    correct substance properly admin-
      istered 599.7
    overdose or wrong substance given
      or taken 961.4
  tongue 529.9
  tonsils, tonsillar (and adenoids)
    (chronic) 474.9
    specified NEC 474.8
  tooth, teeth 525.9
    hard tissues 521.9
      specified NEC 521.89

Disease, diseased — *see also* Syndrome
— *continued*
  tooth, teeth — *continued*
    pulp NEC 522.9
  Tornwaldt's (pharyngeal bursitis)
    478.29
  Tourette's 307.23
  trachea 519.19
  tricuspid — *see* Endocarditis, tricus-
    pid
  triglyceride-storage, type I, II, III 272.7
  triple vessel (coronary arteries) — *see*
    Arteriosclerosis, coronary
  trisymptomatic, Gougerot's 709.1
  trophoblastic (*see also* Hydatidiform
    mole) 630
    previous, affecting management of
      pregnancy V23.1
  tsutsugamushi (scrub typhus) 081.2
  tube (fallopian), noninflammatory
    620.9
    specified NEC 620.8
  tuberculous NEC (*see also* Tuberculo-
    sis) 011.9 ☑
  tubo-ovarian
    inflammatory (*see also* Salpingo-
      oophoritis) 614.2
    noninflammatory 620.9
      specified NEC 620.8
  tubotympanic, chronic (with anterior
    perforation of ear drum) 382.1
  tympanum 385.9
  Uhl's 746.84
  umbilicus (newborn) NEC 779.89
    delayed separation 779.83
  Underwood's (sclerema neonatorum)
    778.1
  undiagnosed 799.9
  Unna's (seborrheic dermatitis) 690.18
  unstable hemoglobin hemolytic 282.7
  Unverricht (-Lundborg) 333.2
  Urbach-Oppenheim (necrobiosis
    lipoidica diabeticorum)
      250.8 ☑ [709.3]
  Urbach-Wiethe (lipoid proteinosis)
    272.8
  ureter 593.9
  urethra 599.9
    specified type NEC 599.84
  urinary (tract) 599.9
    bladder 596.9
      specified NEC 596.8
    maternal, affecting fetus or new-
      born 760.1
  Usher-Senear (pemphigus erythemato-
    sus) 694.4
  uterus (organic) 621.9
    infective (*see also* Endometritis)
      615.9
    inflammatory (*see also* Endometri-
      tis) 615.9
    noninflammatory 621.9
      specified type NEC 621.8
  uveal tract
    anterior 364.9
    posterior 363.9
  vagabonds' 132.1
  vagina, vaginal
    inflammatory 616.10            ▲
    noninflammatory 623.9
      specified NEC 623.8
  Valsuani's (progressive pernicious
    anemia, puerperal) 648.2 ☑
    complicating pregnancy or puerperi-
      um 648.2 ☑
  valve, valvular — *see* Endocarditis
  van Bogaert-Nijssen (-Peiffer) 330.0
  van Creveld-von Gierke (glycogenosis
    I) 271.0
  van den Bergh's (enterogenous
    cyanosis) 289.7
  van Neck's (juvenile osteochondrosis)
    732.1
  Vaquez (-Osler) (polycythemia vera)
    (M9950/1) 238.4
  vascular 459.9

Disease, diseased — *see also* Syndrome
— *continued*
  vascular — *continued*
    arteriosclerotic — *see* Arterioscle-ro-
      sis
    hypertensive — *see* Hypertension
    obliterative 447.1
      peripheral 443.9
    occlusive 459.9
    peripheral (occlusive) 443.9
      in diabetes mellitus
        250.7 ☑ [443.81]
      specified type NEC 443.89
  vas deferens 608.9
  vasomotor 443.9
  vasospastic 443.9
  vein 459.9
  venereal 099.9
    chlamydial NEC 099.50
      anus 099.52
      bladder 099.53
      cervix 099.53
      epididymis 099.54
      genitourinary NEC 099.55
        lower 099.53
        specified NEC 099.54
      pelvic inflammatory disease
        099.54
      perihepatic 099.56
      peritoneum 099.56
      pharynx 099.51
      rectum 099.52
      specified site NEC 099.59
      testis 099.54
      vagina 099.53
      vulva 099.53
    complicating pregnancy, childbirth,
      or puerperium 647.2 ☑
    fifth 099.1
    sixth 099.1
    specified nature or type NEC 099.8
      chlamydial — *see* Disease,
        venereal, chlamydial
  Verneuil's (syphilitic bursitis) 095.7
  Verse's (calcinosis intervertebralis)
    275.49 [722.90]
  vertebra, vertebral NEC 733.90
    disc — *see* Disease, Intervertebral
      disc
  vibration NEC 994.9
  Vidal's (lichen simplex chronicus)
    698.3
  Vincent's (trench mouth) 101
  Virchow's 733.99
  virus (filterable) NEC 078.89
    arbovirus NEC 066.9
    arthropod-borne NEC 066.9
    central nervous system NEC 049.9
      specified type NEC 049.8
    complicating pregnancy, childbirth,
      or puerperium 647.6 ☑
    contact (with) V01.79
      varicella V01.71
    exposure to V01.79
      varicella V01.71
    Marburg 078.89
    maternal
      with fetal damage affecting
        management of pregnancy
          655.3 ☑
    nonarthropod-borne NEC 078.89
      central nervous system NEC
        049.9
        specified NEC 049.8
    vaccination, prophylactic (against)
      V04.89
  vitreous 379.29
  vocal cords NEC 478.5
  Vogt's (Cecile) 333.71
  Vogt-Spielmeyer 330.1
  Volhard-Fahr (malignant nephroscle-
    rosis) 403.00
  Volkmann's
    acquired 958.6
  von Bechterew's (ankylosing
    spondylitis) 720.0

☑ Additional Digit Required — Refer to the Tabular List for Digit Selection          ⒉ Subterms under main terms may continue to next column or page

**2008 ICD-9-CM**          ▶◀ Revised Text          ● New Line          ▲ Revised Code          **October 2007 · Volume 2 — 91**

**Index**

**Disease, diseased — Dislocation**

**Disease, diseased** — *see also* Syndrome
— *continued*
von Economo's (encephalitis lethargica) 049.8
von Eulenburg's (congenital paramyotonia) 359.29 ▲
von Gierke's (glycogenosis I) 271.0
von Graefe's 378.72
von Hippel's (retinocerebral angiomatosis) 759.6
von Hippel-Lindau (angiomatosis
retinocerebellosa) 759.6
von Jaksch's (pseudoleukemia infantum) 285.8
von Recklinghausen's (M9540/1)
237.71
bone (osteitis fibrosa cystica)
252.01
von Recklinghausen-Applebaum
(hemochromatosis) 275.0
von Willebrand (-Jürgens) (angiohemophilia) 286.4
von Zambusch's (lichen sclerosus et
atrophicus) 701.0
Voorhoeve's (dyschondroplasia) 756.4
Vrolik's (osteogenesis imperfecta)
756.51
vulva
inflammatory 616.10 ▲
noninflammatory 624.9
specified NEC 624.8
Wagner's (colloid milium) 709.3
Waldenström's (osteochondrosis capital femoral) 732.1
Wallgren's (obstruction of splenic vein
with collateral circulation)
459.89
Wardrop's (with lymphangitis) 681.9
finger 681.02
toe 681.11
Wassilieff's (leptospiral jaundice)
100.0
wasting NEC 799.4
due to malnutrition 261
paralysis 335.21
Waterhouse-Friderichsen 036.3
waxy (any site) 277.39
Weber-Christian (nodular nonsuppurative panniculitis) 729.30
Wegner's (syphilitic osteochondritis)
090.0
Weil's (leptospiral jaundice) 100.0
of lung 100.0
Weir Mitchell's (erythromelalgia)
443.82
Werdnig-Hoffmann 335.0
Werlhof's (*see also* Purpura, thrombocytopenic) 287.39
Wermer's 258.01 ▲
Werner's (progeria adultorum) 259.8
Werner-His (trench fever) 083.1
Werner-Schultz (agranulocytosis)
288.09
Wernicke's (superior hemorrhagic po-
lioencephalitis) 265.1
Wernicke-Posadas 114.9
Whipple's (intestinal lipodystrophy)
040.2
whipworm 127.3
White's (congenital) (keratosis follicu-
laris) 757.39
white
blood cell 288.9
specified NEC 288.8
spot 701.0
Whitmore's (melioidosis) 025
Widal-Abrami (acquired hemolytic
jaundice) 283.9
Wilkie's 557.1
Wilkinson-Sneddon (subcorneal pustular dermatosis) 694.1
Willis' (diabetes mellitus) (*see also* Diabetes) 250.0 ☑
Wilson's (hepatolenticular degeneration) 275.1

**Disease, diseased** — *see also* Syndrome
— *continued*
Wilson-Brocq (dermatitis exfoliativa)
695.89
winter vomiting 078.82
Wise's 696.2
Wohlfart-Kugelberg-Welander 335.11
Woillez's (acute idiopathic pulmonary
congestion) 518.5
Wolman's (primary familial xanthomatosis) 272.7
wool-sorters' 022.1
Zagari's (xerostomia) 527.7
Zahorsky's (exanthem subitum)
058.10 ▲
Ziehen-Oppenheim 333.6
zoonotic, bacterial NEC 027.9
specified type NEC 027.8
**Disfigurement** (due to scar) 709.2
head V48.6
limb V49.4
neck V48.7
trunk V48.7
**Disgerminoma** — *see* Dysgerminoma
**Disinsertion, retina** 361.04
**Disintegration, complete, of the body**
799.89
traumatic 869.1
**Disk kidney** 753.3
**Dislocatable hip, congenital** — *see also*
Dislocation, hip, congenital 754.30
**Dislocation** (articulation) (closed) (displacement) (simple) (subluxation)
839.8

---

*Note — "Closed" includes simple, com-
plete, partial, uncomplicated, and unspecified dislocation.*

*"Open" includes dislocation specified
as infected or compound and dislocation
with foreign body.*

*"Chronic," "habitual," "old," or "recur-
rent" dislocations should be coded as
indicated under the entry "Dislocation,
recurrent," and "pathological" as indicated under the entry "Dislocation, pathological."*

*For late effect of dislocation see Late,
effect, dislocation.*

---

with fracture — *see* Fracture, by site
acromioclavicular (joint) (closed)
831.04
open 831.14
anatomical site (closed)
specified NEC 839.69
open 839.79
unspecified or ill-defined 839.8
open 839.9
ankle (scaphoid bone) (closed) 837.0
open 837.1
arm (closed) 839.8
open 839.9
astragalus (closed) 837.0
open 837.1
atlanto-axial (closed) 839.01
open 839.11
atlas (closed) 839.01
open 839.11
axis (closed) 839.02
open 839.12
back (closed) 839.8
open 839.9
Bell-Daly 723.8
breast bone (closed) 839.61
open 839.71
capsule, joint — *see* Dislocation, by
site
carpal (bone) — *see* Dislocation, wrist
carpometacarpal (joint) (closed) 833.04
open 833.14
cartilage (joint) (*see also* Dislocation,
by site)
knee — *see* Tear, meniscus

**Dislocation** — *continued*
cervical, cervicodorsal, or cervicothoracic (spine) (vertebra) — *see*
Dislocation, vertebra, cervical
chiropractic (*see also* Lesion, nonallopathic) 739.9
chondrocostal — *see* Dislocation,
costochondral
chondrosternal — *see* Dislocation,
costochondral
chronic — *see* Dislocation, recurrent
clavicle (closed) 831.04
open 831.14
coccyx (closed) 839.41
open 839.51
collar bone (closed) 831.04
open 831.14
compound (open) NEC 839.9
congenital NEC 755.8
hip (*see also* Dislocation, hip, congenital) 754.30
lens 743.37
rib 756.3
sacroiliac 755.69
spine NEC 756.19
vertebra 756.19
coracoid (closed) 831.09
open 831.19
costal cartilage (closed) 839.69
open 839.79
costochondral (closed) 839.69
open 839.79
cricoarytenoid articulation (closed)
839.69
open 839.79
cricothyroid (cartilage) articulation
(closed) 839.69
open 839.79
dorsal vertebrae (closed) 839.21
open 839.31
ear ossicle 385.23
elbow (closed) 832.00
anterior (closed) 832.01
open 832.11
congenital 754.89
divergent (closed) 832.09
open 832.19
lateral (closed) 832.04
open 832.14
medial (closed) 832.03
open 832.13
open 832.10
posterior (closed) 832.02
open 832.12
recurrent 718.32
specified type NEC 832.09
open 832.19
eye 360.81
lateral 376.36
eyeball 360.81
lateral 376.36
femur
distal end (closed) 836.50
anterior 836.52
open 836.62
lateral 836.53
open 836.63
medial 836.54
open 836.64
open 836.60
posterior 836.51
open 836.61
proximal end (closed) 835.00
anterior (pubic) 835.03
open 835.13
obturator 835.02
open 835.12
open 835.10
posterior 835.01
open 835.11
fibula
distal end (closed) 837.0
open 837.1
proximal end (closed) 836.59
open 836.69
finger(s) (phalanx) (thumb) (closed)
834.00
interphalangeal (joint) 834.02

**Dislocation** — *continued*
finger(s) — *continued*
interphalangeal — *continued*
open 834.12
metacarpal (bone), distal end
834.01
open 834.11
metacarpophalangeal (joint) 834.01
open 834.11
open 834.10
recurrent 718.34
foot (closed) 838.00
open 838.10
recurrent 718.37
forearm (closed) 839.8
open 839.9
fracture — *see* Fracture, by site
glenoid (closed) 831.09
open 831.19
habitual — *see* Dislocation, recurrent
hand (closed) 839.8
open 839.9
hip (closed) 835.00
anterior 835.03
obturator 835.02
open 835.12
open 835.13
congenital (unilateral) 754.30
with subluxation of other hip
754.35
bilateral 754.31
developmental 718.75
open 835.10
posterior 835.01
open 835.11
recurrent 718.35
humerus (closed) 831.00
distal end (*see also* Dislocation, elbow) 832.00
open 831.10
proximal end (closed) 831.00
anterior (subclavicular) (subcoracoid) (subglenoid)
(closed) 831.01
open 831.11
inferior (closed) 831.03
open 831.13
open 831.10
posterior (closed) 831.02
open 831.12
implant — *see* Complications, mechanical
incus 385.23
infracoracoid (closed) 831.01
open 831.11
innominate (pubic junction) (sacral
junction) (closed) 839.69
acetabulum (*see also* Dislocation,
hip) 835.00
open 839.79
interphalangeal (joint)
finger or hand (closed) 834.02
open 834.12
foot or toe (closed) 838.06
open 838.16
jaw (cartilage) (meniscus) (closed)
830.0
open 830.1
recurrent 524.69
joint NEC (closed) 839.8
developmental 718.7 ☑
open 839.9
pathological — *see* Dislocation,
pathological
recurrent — *see* Dislocation, recurrent
knee (closed) 836.50
anterior 836.51
open 836.61
congenital (with genu recurvatum)
754.41
habitual 718.36
lateral 836.54
open 836.64
medial 836.53
open 836.63

**Dislocation** — *continued*
　knee — *continued*
　　old 718.36
　　open 836.60
　　posterior 836.52
　　　open 836.62
　　recurrent 718.36
　　rotatory 836.59
　　　open 836.69
　lacrimal gland 375.16
　leg (closed) 839.8
　　open 839.9
　lens (crystalline) (complete) (partial)
　　　379.32
　　anterior 379.33
　　congenital 743.37
　　ocular implant 996.53
　　posterior 379.34
　　traumatic 921.3
　ligament — *see* Dislocation, by site
　lumbar (vertebrae) (closed) 839.20
　　open 839.30
　lumbosacral (vertebrae) (closed)
　　　839.20
　　congenital 756.19
　　open 839.30
　mandible (closed) 830.0
　　open 830.1
　maxilla (inferior) (closed) 830.0
　　open 830.1
　meniscus (knee) (*see also* Tear,
　　　meniscus)
　　other sites — *see* Dislocation, by
　　　site
　metacarpal (bone)
　　distal end (closed) 834.01
　　　open 834.11
　　proximal end (closed) 833.05
　　　open 833.15
　metacarpophalangeal (joint) (closed)
　　　834.01
　　open 834.11
　metatarsal (bone) (closed) 838.04
　　open 838.14
　metatarsophalangeal (joint) (closed)
　　　838.05
　　open 838.15
　midcarpal (joint) (closed) 833.03
　　open 833.13
　midtarsal (joint) (closed) 838.02
　　open 838.12
　Monteggia's — *see* Dislocation, hip
　multiple locations (except fingers only
　　　or toes only) (closed) 839.8
　　open 839.9
　navicular (bone) foot (closed) 837.0
　　open 837.1
　neck (*see also* Dislocation, vertebra,
　　　cervical) 839.00
　Nélaton's — *see* Dislocation, ankle
　nontraumatic (joint) — *see* Disloca-
　　　tion, pathological
　nose (closed) 839.69
　　open 839.79
　not recurrent, not current injury —
　　　*see* Dislocation, pathological
　occiput from atlas (closed) 839.01
　　open 839.11
　old — *see* Dislocation, recurrent
　open (compound) NEC 839.9
　ossicle, ear 385.23
　paralytic (flaccid) (spastic) — *see* Dis-
　　　location, pathological
　patella (closed) 836.3
　　congenital 755.64
　　open 836.4
　pathological NEC 718.20
　　ankle 718.27
　　elbow 718.22
　　foot 718.27
　　hand 718.24
　　hip 718.25
　　knee 718.26
　　lumbosacral joint 724.6
　　multiple sites 718.29
　　pelvic region 718.25

**Dislocation** — *continued*
　pathological — *continued*
　　sacroiliac 724.6
　　shoulder (region) 718.21
　　specified site NEC 718.28
　　spine 724.8
　　　sacroiliac 724.6
　　wrist 718.23
　pelvis (closed) 839.69
　　acetabulum (*see also* Dislocation,
　　　hip) 835.00
　　open 839.79
　phalanx
　　foot or toe (closed) 838.09
　　　open 838.19
　　hand or finger (*see also* Disloca-
　　　tion, finger) 834.00
　postpoliomyelitic — *see* Dislocation,
　　　pathological
　prosthesis, internal — *see* Complica-
　　　tions, mechanical
　radiocarpal (joint) (closed) 833.02
　　open 833.12
　radioulnar (joint)
　　distal end (closed) 833.01
　　　open 833.11
　　proximal end (*see also* Dislocation,
　　　elbow) 832.00
　radius
　　distal end (closed) 833.00
　　　open 833.10
　　proximal end (closed) 832.01
　　　open 832.11
　recurrent (*see also* Derangement,
　　　joint, recurrent) 718.3 ☑
　　elbow 718.32
　　hip 718.35
　　joint NEC 718.38
　　knee 718.36
　　lumbosacral (joint) 724.6
　　patella 718.36
　　sacroiliac 724.6
　　shoulder 718.31
　　temporomandibular 524.69
　rib (cartilage) (closed) 839.69
　　congenital 756.3
　　open 839.79
　sacrococcygeal (closed) 839.42
　　open 839.52
　sacroiliac (joint) (ligament) (closed)
　　　839.42
　　congenital 755.69
　　open 839.52
　　recurrent 724.6
　sacrum (closed) 839.42
　　open 839.52
　scaphoid (bone)
　　ankle or foot (closed) 837.0
　　　open 837.1
　　wrist (closed) (*see also* Dislocation,
　　　wrist) 833.00
　　　open 833.10
　scapula (closed) 831.09
　　open 831.19
　semilunar cartilage, knee — *see* Tear,
　　　meniscus
　septal cartilage (nose) (closed) 839.69
　　open 839.79
　septum (nasal) (old) 470
　sesamoid bone — *see* Dislocation, by
　　　site
　shoulder (blade) (ligament) (closed)
　　　831.00
　　anterior (subclavicular) (subcora-
　　　coid) (subglenoid) (closed)
　　　831.01
　　　open 831.11
　　chronic 718.31
　　inferior 831.03
　　　open 831.13
　　　open 831.10
　　posterior (closed) 831.02
　　　open 831.12
　　recurrent 718.31
　skull — *see* Injury, intracranial
　Smith's — *see* Dislocation, foot

**Dislocation** — *continued*
　spine (articular process) (*see also*
　　　Dislocation, vertebra) (closed)
　　　839.40
　　atlanto-axial (closed) 839.01
　　　open 839.11
　　　recurrent 723.8
　　cervical, cervicodorsal, cervicotho-
　　　racic (closed) (*see also* Dislo-
　　　cation, vertebrae, cervical)
　　　839.00
　　　open 839.10
　　　recurrent 723.8
　　coccyx 839.41
　　　open 839.51
　　congenital 756.19
　　due to birth trauma 767.4
　　open 839.50
　　recurrent 724.9
　　sacroiliac 839.42
　　　recurrent 724.6
　　sacrum (sacrococcygeal) (sacroiliac)
　　　839.42
　　　open 839.52
　spontaneous — *see* Dislocation,
　　　pathological
　sternoclavicular (joint) (closed) 839.61
　　open 839.71
　sternum (closed) 839.61
　　open 839.71
　subastragalar — *see* Dislocation, foot
　subglenoid (closed) 831.01
　　open 831.11
　symphysis
　　jaw (closed) 830.0
　　　open 830.1
　　mandibular (closed) 830.0
　　　open 830.1
　　pubis (closed) 839.69
　　　open 839.79
　tarsal (bone) (joint) 838.01
　　open 838.11
　tarsometatarsal (joint) 838.03
　　open 838.13
　temporomandibular (joint) (closed)
　　　830.0
　　open 830.1
　　recurrent 524.69
　thigh
　　distal end (*see also* Dislocation, fe-
　　　mur, distal end) 836.50
　　proximal end (*see also* Dislocation,
　　　hip) 835.00
　thoracic (vertebrae) (closed) 839.21
　　open 839.31
　thumb(s) (*see also* Dislocation, finger)
　　　834.00
　thyroid cartilage (closed) 839.69
　　open 839.79
　tibia
　　distal end (closed) 837.0
　　　open 837.1
　　proximal end (closed) 836.50
　　　anterior 836.51
　　　　open 836.61
　　　lateral 836.54
　　　　open 836.64
　　　medial 836.53
　　　　open 836.63
　　　open 836.60
　　　posterior 836.52
　　　　open 836.62
　　　rotatory 836.59
　　　　open 836.69
　tibiofibular
　　distal (closed) 837.0
　　　open 837.1
　　superior (closed) 836.59
　　　open 836.69
　toe(s) (closed) 838.09
　　open 838.19
　trachea (closed) 839.69
　　open 839.79
　ulna
　　distal end (closed) 833.09
　　　open 833.19

**Dislocation** — *continued*
　ulna — *continued*
　　proximal end — *see* Dislocation,
　　　elbow
　vertebra (articular process) (body)
　　　(closed) (traumatic) 839.40
　　cervical, cervicodorsal or cervicotho-
　　　racic (closed) 839.00
　　　first (atlas) 839.01
　　　　open 839.11
　　　second (axis) 839.02
　　　　open 839.12
　　　third 839.03
　　　　open 839.13
　　　fourth 839.04
　　　　open 839.14
　　　fifth 839.05
　　　　open 839.15
　　　sixth 839.06
　　　　open 839.16
　　　seventh 839.07
　　　　open 839.17
　　　congential 756.19
　　　multiple sites 839.08
　　　　open 839.18
　　　open 839.10
　　congenital 756.19
　　dorsal 839.21
　　　open 839.31
　　　recurrent 724.9
　　lumbar, lumbosacral 839.20
　　　open 839.30
　　non-traumatic — *see* Displace-
　　　ment, intervertebral disc
　　open NEC 839.50
　　recurrent 724.9
　　specified region NEC 839.49
　　　open 839.59
　　thoracic 839.21
　　　open 839.31
　wrist (carpal bone) (scaphoid)
　　　(semilunar) (closed) 833.00
　　carpometacarpal (joint) 833.04
　　　open 833.14
　　metacarpal bone, proximal end
　　　833.05
　　　open 833.15
　　midcarpal (joint) 833.03
　　　open 833.13
　　open 833.10
　　radiocarpal (joint) 833.02
　　　open 833.12
　　radioulnar (joint) 833.01
　　　open 833.11
　　recurrent 718.33
　　specified site NEC 833.09
　　　open 833.19
　xiphoid cartilage (closed) 839.61
　　open 839.71
**Dislodgement**
　artificial skin graft 996.55
　decellularized allodermis graft 996.55
**Disobedience, hostile** (covert) (overt) —
　　*see also* Disturbance, conduct
　　312.0 ☑
**Disorder** — *see also* Disease
　academic underachievement, child-
　　　hood and adolescence 313.83
　accommodation 367.51
　　drug-induced 367.89
　　toxic 367.89
　adjustment (*see also* Reaction, adjust-
　　　ment) 309.9
　　with
　　　anxiety 309.24
　　　anxiety and depressed mood
　　　　309.28
　　　depressed mood 309.0
　　　disturbance of conduct 309.3
　　　disturbance of emotions and
　　　　conduct 309.4
　adrenal (capsule) (cortex) (gland) 255.9
　　specified type NEC 255.8
　adrenogenital 255.2
　affective (*see also* Psychosis, affective)
　　　296.90

☑ Additional Digit Required — Refer to the Tabular List for Digit Selection　　　　　　▽ Subterms under main terms may continue to next column or page

*2008 ICD-9-CM*　　　　▶◀ Revised Text　　　　● New Line　　　　▲ Revised Code　　　　**Volume 2 — 93**

**Disorder** — *see also* Disease — *continued*
affective (*see also* Psychosis, affective) — *continued*
  atypical 296.81
aggressive, unsocialized (*see also* Disturbance, conduct) 312.0 ☑
alcohol, alcoholic (*see also* Alcohol) 291.9
allergic — *see* Allergy
amino acid (metabolic) (*see also* Disturbance, metabolism, amino acid) 270.9
  albinism 270.2
  alkaptonuria 270.2
  argininosuccinicaciduria 270.6
  beta-amino-isobutyricaciduria 277.2
  cystathioninuria 270.4
  cystinosis 270.0
  cystinuria 270.0
  glycinuria 270.0
  homocystinuria 270.4
  imidazole 270.5
  maple syrup (urine) disease 270.3
  neonatal, transitory 775.89
  oasthouse urine disease 270.2
  ochronosis 270.2
  phenylketonuria 270.1
  phenylpyruvic oligophrenia 270.1
  purine NEC 277.2
  pyrimidine NEC 277.2
  renal transport NEC 270.0
  specified type NEC 270.8
  transport NEC 270.0
    renal 270.0
  xanthinuria 277.2
amnestic (*see also* Amnestic syndrome) 294.8
  alcohol-induced persisting 291.1
  drug-induced persisting 292.83
  in conditions classified elsewhere 294.0
anaerobic glycolysis with anemia 282.3
anxiety (*see also* Anxiety) 300.00
  due to or associated with physical condition 293.84
arteriole 447.9
  specified type NEC 447.8
artery 447.9
  specified type NEC 447.8
articulation — *see* Disorder, joint
Asperger's 299.8 ☑
attachment of infancy or early childhood 313.89
attention deficit 314.00
  with hyperactivity 314.01
  predominantly
    combined hyperactive/inattentive 314.01
    hyperactive/impulsive 314.01
    inattentive 314.00
  residual type 314.8
auditory processing disorder 388.45 ●
  acquired 388.45 ●
  developmental 315.32 ●
autistic 299.0 ☑
autoimmune NEC 279.4
  hemolytic (cold type) (warm type) 283.0
  parathyroid 252.1
  thyroid 245.2
avoidant, childhood or adolescence 313.21
balance
  acid-base 276.9
    mixed (with hypercapnia) 276.4
  electrolyte 276.9
  fluid 276.9
behavior NEC (*see also* Disturbance, conduct) 312.9
  disruptive 312.9
bilirubin excretion 277.4

**Disorder** — *see also* Disease — *continued*
bipolar (affective) (alternating) 296.80

> *Note* — Use the following fifth-digit subclassification with categories 296.0–296.6:
>
> 0  *unspecified*
> 1  *mild*
> 2  *moderate*
> 3  *severe, without mention of psychotic behavior*
> 4  *severe, specified as with psychotic behavior*
> 5  *in partial or unspecified remission*
> 6  *in full remission*

  atypical 296.7
  currently
    depressed 296.5 ☑
    hypomanic 296.4 ☑
    manic 296.4 ☑
  mixed 296.6 ☑
  specified type NEC 296.89
  type I 296.7
    most recent episode (or current)
      depressed 296.5 ☑
      hypomanic 296.4 ☑
      manic 296.4 ☑
      mixed 296.6 ☑
      unspecified 296.7
    single manic episode 296.0 ☑
  type II (recurrent major depressive episodes with hypomania) 296.89
bladder 596.9
  functional NEC 596.59
  specified NEC 596.8
bleeding 286.9 ●
bone NEC 733.90
  specified NEC 733.99
brachial plexus 353.0
branched-chain amino-acid degradation 270.3
breast 611.9
  puerperal, postpartum 676.3 ☑
  specified NEC 611.8
Briquet's 300.81
bursa 727.9
  shoulder region 726.10
carbohydrate metabolism, congenital 271.9
cardiac, functional 427.9
  postoperative 997.1
  psychogenic 306.2
cardiovascular, psychogenic 306.2
cartilage NEC 733.90
  articular 718.00
    ankle 718.07
    elbow 718.02
    foot 718.07
    hand 718.04
    hip 718.05
    knee 717.9
    multiple sites 718.09
    pelvic region 718.05
    shoulder region 718.01
    specified
      site NEC 718.08
      type NEC 733.99
    wrist 718.03
catatonic — *see* Catatonia
central auditory processing 315.32
  acquired 388.45 ●
  developmental 315.32 ●
cervical region NEC 723.9
cervical root (nerve) NEC 353.2
character NEC (*see also* Disorder, personality) 301.9
ciliary body 364.9 ●
  specified NEC 364.89 ●
coagulation (factor) (*see also* Defect, coagulation) 286.9

**Disorder** — *see also* Disease — *continued*
coagulation (*see also* Defect, coagulation) — *continued*
  factor VIII (congenital) (functional) 286.0
  factor IX (congenital) (functional) 286.1
  neonatal, transitory 776.3
coccyx 724.70
  specified NEC 724.79
cognitive 294.9
colon 569.9
  functional 564.9
    congenital 751.3
communication 307.9
conduct (*see also* Disturbance, conduct) 312.9
  adjustment reaction 309.3
  adolescent onset type 312.82
  childhood onset type 312.81
  compulsive 312.30
    specified type NEC 312.39
  hyperkinetic 314.2
  onset unspecified 312.89
  socialized (type) 312.20
    aggressive 312.23
    unaggressive 312.21
  specified NEC 312.89
conduction, heart 426.9
  specified NEC 426.89
conflict
  sexual orientation 302.0
congenital
  glycosylation (CDG) 271.8
convulsive (secondary) (*see also* Convulsions) 780.39
  due to injury at birth 767.0
  idiopathic 780.39
coordination 781.3
cornea NEC 371.89
  due to contact lens 371.82
corticosteroid metabolism NEC 255.2
cranial nerve — *see* Disorder, nerve, cranial
cyclothymic 301.13
degradation, branched-chain amino acid 270.3
delusional 297.1
dentition 520.6
depersonalization 300.6
depressive NEC 311
  atypical 296.82
  major (*see also* Psychosis, affective) 296.2 ☑
    recurrent episode 296.3 ☑
    single episode 296.2 ☑
development, specific 315.9
  associated with hyperkinesia 314.1
  coordination 315.4
  language 315.31
    and speech due to hearing loss 315.34 ●
  learning 315.2
    arithmetical 315.1
    reading 315.00
  mixed 315.5
  motor coordination 315.4
  specified type NEC 315.8
  speech 315.39
    and language due to hearing loss 315.34 ●
diaphragm 519.4
digestive 536.9
  fetus or newborn 777.9
    specified NEC 777.8
  psychogenic 306.4
disintegrative, childhood 299.1 ☑
dissociative 300.15
  identity 300.14
  nocturnal 307.47
drug-related 292.9
dysmorphic body 300.7
dysthymic 300.4
ear 388.9
  degenerative NEC 388.00

**Disorder** — *see also* Disease — *continued*
ear — *continued*
  external 380.9
    specified 380.89
  pinna 380.30
  specified type NEC 388.8
  vascular NEC 388.00
eating NEC 307.50
electrolyte NEC 276.9
  with
    abortion — *see* Abortion, by type, with metabolic disorder
    ectopic pregnancy (*see also* categories 633.0–633.9) 639.4
    molar pregnancy (*see also* categories 630–632) 639.4
  acidosis 276.2
    metabolic 276.2
    respiratory 276.2
  alkalosis 276.3
    metabolic 276.3
    respiratory 276.3
  following
    abortion 639.4
    ectopic or molar pregnancy 639.4
  neonatal, transitory NEC 775.5
emancipation as adjustment reaction 309.22
emotional (*see also* Disorder, mental, nonpsychotic) V40.9
endocrine 259.9
  specified type NEC 259.8
esophagus 530.9
  functional 530.5
  psychogenic 306.4
explosive
  intermittent 312.34
  isolated 312.35
expressive language 315.31
eye 379.90
  globe — *see* Disorder, globe
  ill-defined NEC 379.99
  limited duction NEC 378.63
  specified NEC 379.8
eyelid 374.9
  degenerative 374.50
  sensory 374.44
  specified type NEC 374.89
  vascular 374.85
factitious (with combined psychological and physical signs and symptoms) (with predominantly physical signs and symptoms) 300.19
  with predominantly psychological signs and symptoms 300.16
factor, coagulation (*see also* Defect, coagulation) 286.9
  IX (congenital) (funcitonal) 286.1
  VIII (congenital) (functional) 286.0
fascia 728.9
fatty acid oxidation 277.85
feeding — *see* Feeding
female sexual arousal 302.72
fluid NEC 276.9
gastric (functional) 536.9
  motility 536.8
  psychogenic 306.4
  secretion 536.8
gastrointestinal (functional) NEC 536.9
  newborn (neonatal) 777.9
    specified NEC 777.8
  psychogenic 306.4
gender (child) 302.6
  adult 302.85
gender identity (childhood) 302.6
  adolescents 302.85
  adults (-life) 302.85
genitourinary system, psychogenic 306.50
globe 360.9

**Disorder** — *see also* Disease — *continued*
globe — *continued*
  degenerative 360.20
    specified NEC 360.29
    specified type NEC 360.89
hearing (*see also* Deafness)
  conductive type (air) (*see also* Deafness, conductive) 389.00
  mixed conductive and sensorineural 389.20 ▲
    bilateral 389.22 ●
    unilateral 389.21 ●
  nerve
    bilateral 389.12 ●
    unilateral 389.13 ●
  perceptive (*see also* Deafness, perceptive) 389.10
  sensorineural type NEC (*see also* Deafness, sensorineural) 389.10
heart action 427.9
  postoperative 997.1
hematological, transient neonatal 776.9
  specified type NEC 776.8
hematopoietic organs 289.9
hemorrhagic NEC 287.9
  due to intrinsic circulating anticoagulants 286.5
  specified type NEC 287.8
hemostasis (*see also* Defect, coagulation) 286.9
homosexual conflict 302.0
hypomanic (chronic) 301.11
identity
  childhood and adolescence 313.82
  gender 302.6
immune mechanism (immunity) 279.9
  single complement (C1-C9) 279.8
  specified type NEC 279.8
impulse control (*see also* Disturbance, conduct, compulsive) 312.30
infant sialic acid storage 271.8
integument, fetus or newborn 778.9
  specified type NEC 778.8
interactional psychotic (childhood) (*see also* Psychosis, childhood) 299.1 ☑
intermittent explosive 312.34
intervertebral disc 722.90
  cervical, cervicothoracic 722.91
  lumbar, lumbosacral 722.93
  thoracic, thoracolumbar 722.92
intestinal 569.9
  functional NEC 564.9
    congenital 751.3
    postoperative 564.4
  psychogenic 306.4
introverted, of childhood and adolescence 313.22
involuntary emotional expression (IEED) 310.8 ●
iris 364.9 ●
  specified NEC 364.89 ●
iron, metabolism 275.0
isolated explosive 312.35
joint NEC 719.90
  ankle 719.97
  elbow 719.92
  foot 719.97
  hand 719.94
  hip 719.95
  knee 719.96
  multiple sites 719.99
  pelvic region 719.95
  psychogenic 306.0
  shoulder (region) 719.91
  specified site NEC 719.98
  temporomandibular 524.60
    sounds on opening or closing 524.64
    specified NEC 524.69
  wrist 719.93
kidney 593.9
  functional 588.9

**Disorder** — *see also* Disease — *continued*
kidney — *continued*
  functional — *continued*
    specified NEC 588.89
labyrinth, labyrinthine 386.9
  specified type NEC 386.8
lactation 676.9 ☑
language (developmental) (expressive) 315.31
  mixed receptive-expressive 315.32
learning 315.9
ligament 728.9
ligamentous attachments, peripheral (*see also* Enthesopathy)
  spine 720.1
limb NEC 729.9
  psychogenic 306.0
lipid
  metabolism, congenital 272.9
  storage 272.7
lipoprotein deficiency (familial) 272.5
low back NEC 724.9
  psychogenic 306.0
lumbosacral
  plexus 353.1
  root (nerve) NEC 353.4
lymphoproliferative (chronic) NEC (M9970/1) 238.79
major depressive (*see also* Psychosis, affective) 296.2 ☑
  recurrent episode 296.3 ☑
  single episode 296.2 ☑
male erectile 607.84
  nonorganic origin 302.72
manic (*see also* Psychosis, affective) 296.0 ☑
  atypical 296.81
mathematics 315.1
meniscus NEC (*see also* Disorder, cartilage, articular) 718.0 ☑
menopausal 627.9
  specified NEC 627.8
menstrual 626.9
  psychogenic 306.52
  specified NEC 626.8
mental (nonpsychotic) 300.9
  affecting management of pregnancy, childbirth, or puerperium 648.4 ☑
  drug-induced 292.9
    hallucinogen persisting perception 292.89
    specified type NEC 292.89
  due to or associated with
    alcoholism 291.9
    drug consumption NEC 292.9
      specified type NEC 292.89
    physical condition NEC 293.9
  induced by drug 292.9
    specified type NEC 292.89
  neurotic (*see also* Neurosis) 300.9
  of infancy, childhood or adolescence 313.9
  persistent
    other
      due to conditions classified elsewhere 294.8
    unspecified
      due to conditions classified elsewhere 294.9
  presenile 310.1
    psychotic NEC 290.10
  previous, affecting management of pregnancy V23.89
  psychoneurotic (*see also* Neurosis) 300.9
  psychotic (*see also* Psychosis) 298.9
    brief 298.8
    senile 290.20
  specific, following organic brain damage 310.9
    cognitive or personality change of other type 310.1
    frontal lobe syndrome 310.0

**Disorder** — *see also* Disease — *continued*
mental — *continued*
  specific, following organic brain damage — *continued*
    postconcussional syndrome 310.2
    specified type NEC 310.8
  transient
    in conditions classified elsewhere 293.9
metabolism NEC 277.9
  with
    abortion — *see* Abortion, by type, with metabolic disorder
    ectopic pregnancy (*see also* categories 633.0–633.9) 639.4
    molar pregnancy (*see also* categories 630–632) 639.4
  alkaptonuria 270.2
  amino acid (*see also* Disorder, amino acid) 270.9
    specified type NEC 270.8
  ammonia 270.6
  arginine 270.6
  argininosuccinic acid 270.6
  basal 794.7
  bilirubin 277.4
  calcium 275.40
  carbohydrate 271.9
    specified type NEC 271.8
  cholesterol 272.9
  citrulline 270.6
  copper 275.1
  corticosteroid 255.2
  cystine storage 270.0
  cystinuria 270.0
  fat 272.9
  fatty acid oxidation 277.85
  following
    abortion 639.4
    ectopic or molar pregnancy 639.4
  fructosemia 271.2
  fructosuria 271.2
  fucosidosis 271.8
  galactose-1-phosphate uridyl transferase 271.1
  glutamine 270.7
  glycine 270.7
  glycogen storage NEC 271.0
    hepatorenal 271.0
  hemochromatosis 275.0
  in labor and delivery 669.0 ☑
  iron 275.0
  lactose 271.3
  lipid 272.9
    specified type NEC 272.8
    storage 272.7
  lipoprotein (*see also* Hyperlipemia deficiency (familial)) 272.5
  lysine 270.7
  magnesium 275.2
  mannosidosis 271.8
  mineral 275.9
    specified type NEC 275.8
  mitochondrial 277.87
  mucopolysaccharide 277.5
  nitrogen 270.9
  ornithine 270.6
  oxalosis 271.8
  pentosuria 271.8
  phenylketonuria 270.1
  phosphate 275.3
  phosphorous 275.3
  plasma protein 273.9
    specified type NEC 273.8
  porphyrin 277.1
  purine 277.2
  pyrimidine 277.2
  serine 270.7
  sodium 276.9
  specified type NEC 277.89
  steroid 255.2

**Disorder** — *see also* Disease — *continued*
metabolism — *continued*
  threonine 270.7
  urea cycle 270.6
  xylose 271.8
micturition NEC 788.69
  psychogenic 306.53
misery and unhappiness, of childhood and adolescence 313.1
mitochondrial metabolism 277.87
mitral valve 424.0
mood (*see also* Disorder, bipolar) 296.90
  episodic 296.90
    specified NEC 296.99
  in conditions classified elsewhere 293.83
motor tic 307.20
  chronic 307.22
  transient (childhood) 307.21
movement NEC 333.90
  hysterical 300.11
  medication-induced 333.90
  periodic limb 327.51
  sleep related, unspecified 780.58
    other organic 327.59
  specified type NEC 333.99
  stereotypic 307.3
mucopolysaccharide 277.5
muscle 728.9
  psychogenic 306.0
  specified type NEC 728.3
muscular attachments, peripheral (*see also* Enthesopathy)
  spine 720.1
musculoskeletal system NEC 729.9
  psychogenic 306.0
myeloproliferative (chronic) NEC (M9960/1) 238.79
myoneural 358.9
  due to lead 358.2
  specified type NEC 358.8
  toxic 358.2
myotonic 359.29 ▲
neck region NEC 723.9
nerve 349.9
  abducens NEC 378.54
  accessory 352.4
  acoustic 388.5
  auditory 388.5
  auriculotemporal 350.8
  axillary 353.0
  cerebral — *see* Disorder, nerve, cranial
  cranial 352.9
    first 352.0
    second 377.49
    third
      partial 378.51
      total 378.52
    fourth 378.53
    fifth 350.9
    sixth 378.54
    seventh NEC 351.9
    eighth 388.5
    ninth 352.2
    tenth 352.3
    eleventh 352.4
    twelfth 352.5
    multiple 352.6
  entrapment — *see* Neuropathy, entrapment
  facial 351.9
    specified NEC 351.8
  femoral 355.2
  glossopharyngeal NEC 352.2
  hypoglossal 352.5
  iliohypogastric 355.79
  ilioinguinal 355.79
  intercostal 353.8
  lateral
    cutaneous of thigh 355.1
    popliteal 355.3
  lower limb NEC 355.8
  medial, popliteal 355.4

☑ Additional Digit Required — Refer to the Tabular List for Digit Selection     ▲ Subterms under main terms may continue to next column or page

*2008 ICD-9-CM*    ▶◀ Revised Text    ● New Line    ▲ Revised Code    October 2007 · Volume 2 — 95

Disorder — Disorder

**Disorder** — *see also* Disease — *continued*

nerve — *continued*
median NEC 354.1
obturator 355.79
oculomotor
  partial 378.51
  total 378.52
olfactory 352.0
optic 377.49
  hypoplasia 377.43
  ischemic 377.41
  nutritional 377.33
  toxic 377.34
peroneal 355.3
phrenic 354.8
plantar 355.6
pneumogastric 352.3
posterior tibial 355.5
radial 354.3
recurrent laryngeal 352.3
root 353.9
  specified NEC 353.8
saphenous 355.79
sciatic NEC 355.0
specified NEC 355.9
  lower limb 355.79
  upper limb 354.8
spinal 355.9
sympathetic NEC 337.9
trigeminal 350.9
  specified NEC 350.8
trochlear 378.53
ulnar 354.2
upper limb NEC 354.9
vagus 352.3
nervous system NEC 349.9
autonomic (peripheral) (*see also*
  Neuropathy, peripheral, autonomic) 337.9
cranial 352.9
parasympathetic (*see also* Neuropathy, peripheral, autonomic)
  337.9
specified type NEC 349.89
sympathetic (*see also* Neuropathy,
  peripheral, autonomic) 337.9
vegetative (*see also* Neuropathy,
  peripheral, autonomic) 337.9
neurohypophysis NEC 253.6
neurological NEC 781.99
  peripheral NEC 355.9
neuromuscular NEC 358.9
  hereditary NEC 359.1
  specified NEC 358.8
  toxic 358.2
neurotic 300.9
  specified type NEC 300.89
neutrophil, polymorphonuclear (functional) 288.1
nightmare 307.47
night terror 307.46
obsessive-compulsive 300.3
oppositional defiant, childhood and
  adolescence 313.81
optic
chiasm 377.54
  associated with
    inflammatory disorders
      377.54
    neoplasm NEC 377.52
      pituitary 377.51
    pituitary disorders 377.51
    vascular disorders 377.53
nerve 377.49
radiations 377.63
tracts 377.63
orbit 376.9
  specified NEC 376.89
orgasmic
female 302.73
male 302.74
overanxious, of childhood and adolescence 313.0
oxidation, fatty acid 277.85

**Disorder** — *see also* Disease — *continued*

pancreas, internal secretion (other
  than diabetes mellitus) 251.9
  specified type NEC 251.8
panic 300.01
  with agoraphobia 300.21
papillary muscle NEC 429.81
paranoid 297.9
  induced 297.3
  shared 297.3
parathyroid 252.9
  specified type NEC 252.8
paroxysmal, mixed 780.39
pentose phosphate pathway with
  anemia 282.2
periodic limb movement 327.51
peroxisomal 277.86
personality 301.9
affective 301.10
aggressive 301.3
amoral 301.7
anancastic, anankastic 301.4
antisocial 301.7
asocial 301.7
asthenic 301.6
avoidant 301.82
borderline 301.83
compulsive 301.4
cyclothymic 301.13
dependent-passive 301.6
dyssocial 301.7
emotional instability 301.59
epileptoid 301.3
explosive 301.3
following organic brain damage
  310.1
histrionic 301.50
hyperthymic 301.11
hypomanic (chronic) 301.11
hypothymic 301.12
hysterical 301.50
immature 301.89
inadequate 301.6
introverted 301.21
labile 301.59
moral deficiency 301.7
narcissistic 301.81
obsessional 301.4
obsessive-compulsive 301.4
overconscientious 301.4
paranoid 301.0
passive (-dependent) 301.6
passive-aggressive 301.84
pathological NEC 301.9
pseudosocial 301.7
psychopathic 301.9
schizoid 301.20
  introverted 301.21
  schizotypal 301.22
schizotypal 301.22
seductive 301.59
type A 301.4
unstable 301.59
pervasive developmental 299.9 ☑
  childhood-onset 299.8 ☑
  specified NEC 299.8 ☑
phonological 315.39
pigmentation, choroid (congenital)
  743.53
pinna 380.30
  specified type NEC 380.39
pituitary, thalamic 253.9
  anterior NEC 253.4
  iatrogenic 253.7
  postablative 253.7
  specified NEC 253.8
pityriasis-like NEC 696.8
platelets (blood) 287.1
polymorphonuclear neutrophils
  (functional) 288.1
porphyrin metabolism 277.1
postmenopausal 627.9
  specified type NEC 627.8
posttraumatic stress 309.81
post-traumatic stress (PTSD) 309.81

**Disorder** — *see also* Disease — *continued*

post-traumatic stress — *continued*
acute 309.81
brief 309.81
chronic 309.81
premenstrual dysphoric (PMDD) 625.4
psoriatic-like NEC 696.8
psychic, with diseases classified elsewhere 316
psychogenic NEC (*see also* condition)
  300.9
allergic NEC
  respiratory 306.1
anxiety 300.00
  atypical 300.00
  generalized 300.02
appetite 307.59
articulation, joint 306.0
asthenic 300.5
blood 306.8
cardiovascular (system) 306.2
compulsive 300.3
cutaneous 306.3
depressive 300.4
digestive (system) 306.4
dysmenorrheic 306.52
dyspneic 306.1
eczematous 306.3
endocrine (system) 306.6
eye 306.7
feeding 307.59
functional NEC 306.9
gastric 306.4
gastrointestinal (system) 306.4
genitourinary (system) 306.50
heart (function) (rhythm) 306.2
hemic 306.8
hyperventilatory 306.1
hypochondriacal 300.7
hysterical 300.10
intestinal 306.4
joint 306.0
learning 315.2
limb 306.0
lymphatic (system) 306.8
menstrual 306.52
micturition 306.53
monoplegic NEC 306.0
motor 307.9
muscle 306.0
musculoskeletal 306.0
neurocirculatory 306.2
obsessive 300.3
occupational 300.89
organ or part of body NEC 306.9
organs of special sense 306.7
paralytic NEC 306.0
phobic 300.20
physical NEC 306.9
pruritic 306.3
rectal 306.4
respiratory (system) 306.1
rheumatic 306.0
sexual (function) 302.70
  specified type NEC 302.79
sexual orientation conflict 302.0
skin (allergic) (eczematous) (pruritic) 306.3
sleep 307.40
  initiation or maintenance
    307.41
    persistent 307.42
    transient 307.41
  movement 780.58
  sleep terror 307.46
  specified type NEC 307.49
specified part of body NEC 306.8
stomach 306.4
psychomotor NEC 307.9
  hysterical 300.11
psychoneurotic (*see also* Neurosis)
  300.9
  mixed NEC 300.89
psychophysiologic (*see also* Disorder,
  psychosomatic) 306.9

**Disorder** — *see also* Disease — *continued*

psychosexual identity (childhood)
  302.6
  adult-life 302.85
psychosomatic NEC 306.9
allergic NEC
  respiratory 306.1
articulation, joint 306.0
cardiovascular (system) 306.2
cutaneous 306.3
digestive (system) 306.4
dysmenorrheic 306.52
dyspneic 306.1
endocrine (system) 306.6
eye 306.7
gastric 306.4
gastrointestinal (system) 306.4
genitourinary (system) 306.50
heart (functional) (rhythm) 306.2
hyperventilatory 306.1
intestinal 306.4
joint 306.0
limb 306.0
lymphatic (system) 306.8
menstrual 306.52
micturition 306.53
monoplegic NEC 306.0
muscle 306.0
musculoskeletal 306.0
neurocirculatory 306.2
organs of special sense 306.7
paralytic NEC 306.0
pruritic 306.3
rectal 306.4
respiratory (system) 306.1
rheumatic 306.0
sexual (function) 302.70
skin 306.3
specified part of body NEC 306.8
specified type NEC 302.79
stomach 306.4
psychotic (*see also* Psychosis) 298.9
  brief 298.8
purine metabolism NEC 277.2
pyrimidine metabolism NEC 277.2
reactive attachment of infancy or early
  childhood 313.89
reading, developmental 315.00
reflex 796.1
REM sleep behavior 327.42
renal function, impaired 588.9
  specified type NEC 588.89
renal transport NEC 588.89
respiration, respiratory NEC 519.9
  due to
    aspiration of liquids or solids
      508.9
    inhalation of fumes or vapors
      506.9
  psychogenic 306.1
retina 362.9
  specified type NEC 362.89
rumination 307.53
sacroiliac joint NEC 724.6
sacrum 724.6
schizo-affective (*see also* Schizophrenia) 295.7 ☑
schizoid, childhood or adolescence
  313.22
schizophreniform 295.4 ☑
schizotypal personality 301.22
secretion, thyrocalcitonin 246.0
seizure 345.9 ☑
  recurrent 345.9 ☑
    epileptic — *see* Epilepsy
sense of smell 781.1
  psychogenic 306.7
separation anxiety 309.21
sexual (*see also* Deviation, sexual)
  302.9
  aversion 302.79
  desire, hypoactive 302.71
  function, psychogenic 302.70
shyness, of childhood and adolescence
  313.21

☑ Additional Digit Required — Refer to the Tabular List for Digit Selection          ⁽ᵃᵇᶜ⁾ Subterms under main terms may continue to next column or page

96 — Volume 2          ▶◀ Revised Text          ● New Line          ▲ Revised Code          *2008 ICD-9-CM*

**Disorder** — see also Disease —
continued
single complement (C1-C9) 279.8
skin NEC 709.9
　fetus or newborn 778.9
　　specified type 778.8
　psychogenic (allergic) (eczematous)
　　(pruritic) 306.3
　specified type NEC 709.8
　vascular 709.1
sleep 780.50
　with apnea — see Apnea, sleep
　alcohol induced 291.82
　arousal 307.46
　　confusional 327.41
　circadian rhythm 327.30
　　advanced sleep phase type
　　　327.32
　　alcohol induced 291.82
　　delayed sleep phase type 327.31
　　drug induced 292.85
　　free running type 327.34
　　in conditions classified else-
　　　where 327.37
　　irregular sleep-wake type
　　　327.33
　　jet lag type 327.35
　　other 327.39
　　shift work type 327.36
　drug induced 292.85
　initiation or maintenance (see also
　　Insomnia) 780.52
　nonorganic origin (transient)
　　307.41
　　persistent 307.42
　nonorganic origin 307.40
　　specified type NEC 307.49
　organic specified type NEC 327.8
　periodic limb movement 327.51
　specified NEC 780.59
　wake
　　cycle — see Disorder, sleep, cir-
　　　cadian rhythm
　　schedule — see Disorer, sleep,
　　　circadian rhythm
social, of childhood and adolescence
　313.22
soft tissue 729.9
somatization 300.81
somatoform (atypical) (undifferentiat-
　ed) 300.82
　severe 300.81
　specified type NEC 300.89
speech NEC 784.5
　nonorganic origin 307.9
spine NEC 724.9
　ligamentous or muscular attach-
　　ments, peripheral 720.1
steroid metabolism NEC 255.2
stomach (functional) (see also Disor-
　der, gastric) 536.9
　psychogenic 306.4
storage, iron 275.0
stress (see also Reaction, stress,
　acute) 308.3
　posttraumatic
　　acute 309.81
　　brief 309.81
　　chronic 309.81
substitution 300.11
suspected — see Observation
synovium 727.9
temperature regulation, fetus or new-
　born 778.4
temporomandibular joint NEC 524.60
　sounds on opening or closing
　　524.64
　specified NEC 524.69
tendon 727.9
　shoulder region 726.10
thoracic root (nerve) NEC 353.3
thyrocalcitonin secretion 246.0
thyroid (gland) NEC 246.9
　specified type NEC 246.8
tic 307.20
　chronic (motor or vocal) 307.22

**Disorder** — see also Disease —
continued
tic — continued
　motor-verbal 307.23
　organic origin 333.1
　transient (of childhood) 307.21
tooth NEC 525.9
　development NEC 520.9
　　specified type NEC 520.8
　eruption 520.6
　specified type NEC 525.8
Tourette's 307.23
transport, carbohydrate 271.9
　specified type NEC 271.8
tubular, phosphate-losing 588.0
tympanic membrane 384.9
unaggressive, unsocialized (see also
　Disturbance, conduct) 312.1 ☑
undersocialized, unsocialized (see also
　Disturbance, conduct)
　aggressive (type) 312.0 ☑
　unaggressive (type) 312.1 ☑
vision, visual NEC 368.9
　binocular NEC 368.30
　cortex 377.73
　　associated with
　　　inflammatory disorders
　　　　377.73
　　　neoplasms 377.71
　　　vascular disorders 377.72
　pathway NEC 377.63
　　associated with
　　　inflammatory disorders
　　　　377.63
　　　neoplasms 377.61
　　　vascular disorders 377.62
vocal tic
　chronic 307.22
wakefulness (see also Hypersomnia)
　780.54
　nonorganic origin (transient)
　　307.43
　　persistent 307.44
written expression 315.2
**Disorganized globe** 360.29
**Displacement, displaced**

Note — For acquired displacement of
bones, cartilage, joints, tendons, due to
injury, see also Dislocation.

Displacements at ages under one year
should be considered congenital, provided there is no indication the condition
was acquired after birth.

　acquired traumatic of bone, cartilage,
　　joint, tendon NEC (without
　　fracture) (see also Dislocation)
　　839.8
　　with fracture — see Fracture, by
　　　site
　adrenal gland (congenital) 759.1
　alveolus and teeth, vertical 524.75
　appendix, retrocecal (congenital) 751.5
　auricle (congenital) 744.29
　bladder (acquired) 596.8
　　congenital 753.8
　brachial plexus (congenital) 742.8
　brain stem, caudal 742.4
　canaliculus lacrimalis 743.65
　cardia, through esophageal hiatus
　　750.6
　cerebellum, caudal 742.4
　cervix — see Displacement, uterus
　colon (congenital) 751.4
　device, implant, or graft — see Compli-
　　cations, mechanical
　epithelium
　　columnar of cervix 622.10
　　cuboidal, beyond limits of external
　　　os (uterus) 752.49
　esophageal mucosa into cardia of
　　stomach, congenital 750.4
　esophagus (acquired) 530.89
　　congenital 750.4
　eyeball (acquired) (old) 376.36
　　congenital 743.8

**Displacement, displaced** —
continued
eyeball — continued
　current injury 871.3
　lateral 376.36
fallopian tube (acquired) 620.4
　congenital 752.19
　opening (congenital) 752.19
gallbladder (congenital) 751.69
gastric mucosa 750.7
　into
　　duodenum 750.7
　　esophagus 750.7
　　Meckel's diverticulum, congeni-
　　　tal 750.7
globe (acquired) (lateral) (old) 376.36
　current injury 871.3
graft
　artificial skin graft 996.55
　decellularized allodermis graft
　　996.55
heart (congenital) 746.87
　acquired 429.89
hymen (congenital) (upward) 752.49
internal prosthesis NEC — see Com-
　plications, mechanical
intervertebral disc (with neuritis,
　radiculitis, sciatica, or other
　pain) 722.2
　with myelopathy 722.70
　cervical, cervicodorsal, cervicotho-
　　racic 722.0
　　with myelopathy 722.71
　　due to major trauma — see
　　　Dislocation, vertebra, cer-
　　　vical
　due to trauma — see Dislocation,
　　vertebra
　lumbar, lumbosacral 722.10
　　with myelopathy 722.73
　　due to major trauma — see
　　　Dislocation, vertebra,
　　　lumbar
　thoracic, thoracolumbar 722.11
　　with myelopathy 722.72
　　due to major trauma — see
　　　Dislocation, vertebra, tho-
　　　racic
intrauterine device 996.32
kidney (acquired) 593.0
　congenital 753.3
lacrimal apparatus or duct (congeni-
　tal) 743.65
macula (congenital) 743.55
Meckel's diverticulum (congenital)
　751.0
nail (congenital) 757.5
　acquired 703.8
opening of Wharton's duct in mouth
　750.26
organ or site, congenital NEC — see
　Malposition, congenital
ovary (acquired) 620.4
　congenital 752.0
　free in peritoneal cavity (congenital)
　　752.0
　into hernial sac 620.4
oviduct (acquired) 620.4
　congenital 752.19
parathyroid (gland) 252.8
parotid gland (congenital) 750.26
punctum lacrimale (congenital) 743.65
sacroiliac (congenital) (joint) 755.69
　current injury — see Dislocation,
　　sacroiliac
　old 724.6
spine (congenital) 756.19
spleen, congenital 759.0
stomach (congenital) 750.7
　acquired 537.89
subglenoid (closed) 831.01
sublingual duct (congenital) 750.26
teeth, tooth 524.30
　horizontal 524.33
　vertical 524.34
tongue (congenital) (downward) 750.19

**Displacement, displaced** —
continued
trachea (congenital) 748.3
ureter or ureteric opening or orifice
　(congenital) 753.4
uterine opening of oviducts or fallopi-
　an tubes 752.19
uterus, uterine (see also Malposition,
　uterus) 621.6
　congenital 752.3
ventricular septum 746.89
　with rudimentary ventricle 746.89
xyphoid bone (process) 738.3
**Disproportion** 653.9 ☑
affecting fetus or newborn 763.1
caused by
　conjoined twins 653.7 ☑
　contraction, pelvis (general)
　　653.1 ☑
　　inlet 653.2 ☑
　　midpelvic 653.8 ☑
　　midplane 653.8 ☑
　　outlet 653.3 ☑
　fetal
　　ascites 653.7 ☑
　　hydrocephalus 653.6 ☑
　　hydrops 653.7 ☑
　　meningomyelocele 653.7 ☑
　　sacral teratoma 653.7 ☑
　　tumor 653.7 ☑
　hydrocephalic fetus 653.6 ☑
　pelvis, pelvic, abnormality (bony)
　　NEC 653.0 ☑
　unusually large fetus 653.5 ☑
causing obstructed labor 660.1 ☑
cephalopelvic, normally formed fetus
　653.4 ☑
　causing obstructed labor 660.1 ☑
fetal NEC 653.5 ☑
　causing obstructed labor 660.1 ☑
fetopelvic, normally formed fetus
　653.4 ☑
　causing obstructed labor 660.1 ☑
mixed maternal and fetal origin, nor-
　mally formed fetus 653.4 ☑
pelvis, pelvic (bony) NEC 653.1 ☑
　causing obstructed labor 660.1 ☑
specified type NEC 653.8 ☑
**Disruption**
cesarean wound 674.1 ☑
family V61.0
gastrointestinal anastomosis 997.4
ligament(s) (see also Sprain)
　knee
　　current injury — see Disloca-
　　　tion, knee
　　old 717.89
　　　capsular 717.85
　　　collateral (medial) 717.82
　　　　lateral 717.81
　　　cruciate (posterior) 717.84
　　　　anterior 717.83
　　　specified site NEC 717.85
marital V61.10
　involving divorce or estrangement
　　V61.0
operation wound (external) 998.32
　internal 998.31
organ transplant, anastomosis site —
　see Complications, transplant,
　organ, by site
ossicles, ossicular chain 385.23
　traumatic — see Fracture, skull,
　　base
parenchyma
　liver (hepatic) — see Laceration,
　　liver, major
　spleen — see Laceration, spleen,
　　parenchyma, massive
phase-shift, of 24-hour sleep-wake
　cycle, unspecified 780.55
　nonorganic origin 307.45
sleep-wake cycle (24-hour), unspeci-
　fied 780.55
　circadian rhythm 327.33
　nonorganic origin 307.45

☑ Additional Digit Required — Refer to the Tabular List for Digit Selection　　　　　　　⬇ Subterms under main terms may continue to next column or page

**2008 ICD-9-CM**　　　▶◀ Revised Text　　　● New Line　　　▲ Revised Code　　　**Volume 2 — 97**

Disorder — Disruption

**Disruption** — continued
    suture line (external) 998.32
        internal 998.31
    wound
        cesarean operation 674.1 ☑
        episiotomy 674.2 ☑
        operation 998.32
            cesarean 674.1 ☑
            internal 998.31
        perineal (obstetric) 674.2 ☑
        uterine 674.1 ☑
**Disruptio uteri** — see also Rupture, uterus
    complicating delivery — see Delivery, complicated, rupture, uterus
**Dissatisfaction with**
    employment V62.2
    school environment V62.3
**Dissecting** — see condition
**Dissection**
    aorta 441.00
        abdominal 441.02
        thoracic 441.01
        thoracoabdominal 441.03
    artery, arterial
        carotid 443.21
        coronary 414.12
        iliac 443.22
        renal 443.23
        specified NEC 443.29
        vertebral 443.24
    vascular 459.9
    wound — see Wound, open, by site
**Disseminated** — see condition
**Dissociated personality** NEC 300.15
**Dissociation**
    auriculoventricular or atrioventricular (any degree) (AV) 426.89
        with heart block 426.0
    interference 426.89
    isorhythmic 426.89
    rhythm
        atrioventricular (AV) 426.89
        interference 426.89
**Dissociative**
    identity disorder 300.14
    reaction NEC 300.15
**Dissolution, vertebra** — see also Osteoporosis 733.00
**Distention**
    abdomen (gaseous) 787.3
    bladder 596.8
    cecum 569.89
    colon 569.89
    gallbladder 575.8
    gaseous (abdomen) 787.3
    intestine 569.89
    kidney 593.89
    liver 573.9
    seminal vesicle 608.89
    stomach 536.8
        acute 536.1
        psychogenic 306.4
    ureter 593.5
    uterus 621.8
**Distichia, distichiasis** (eyelid) 743.63
**Distoma hepaticum infestation** 121.3
**Distomiasis** 121.9
    bile passages 121.3
        due to Clonorchis sinensis 121.1
    hemic 120.9
    hepatic (liver) 121.3
        due to Clonorchis sinensis (clonorchiasis) 121.1
    intestinal 121.4
    liver 121.3
        due to Clonorchis sinensis 121.1
    lung 121.2
    pulmonary 121.2
**Distomolar** (fourth molar) 520.1
    causing crowding 524.31
**Disto-occlusion** (division I) (division II) 524.22
**Distortion** (congenital)
    adrenal (gland) 759.1
    ankle (joint) 755.69

**Distortion** — continued
    anus 751.5
    aorta 747.29
    appendix 751.5
    arm 755.59
    artery (peripheral) NEC (see also Distortion, peripheral vascular system) 747.60
        cerebral 747.81
        coronary 746.85
        pulmonary 747.3
        retinal 743.58
        umbilical 747.5
    auditory canal 744.29
        causing impairment of hearing 744.02
    bile duct or passage 751.69
    bladder 753.8
    brain 742.4
    bronchus 748.3
    cecum 751.5
    cervix (uteri) 752.49
    chest (wall) 756.3
    clavicle 755.51
    clitoris 752.49
    coccyx 756.19
    colon 751.5
    common duct 751.69
    cornea 743.41
    cricoid cartilage 748.3
    cystic duct 751.69
    duodenum 751.5
    ear 744.29
        auricle 744.29
            causing impairment of hearing 744.02
        causing impairment of hearing 744.09
        external 744.29
            causing impairment of hearing 744.02
        inner 744.05
        middle, except ossicles 744.03
            ossicles 744.04
        ossicles 744.04
    endocrine (gland) NEC 759.2
    epiglottis 748.3
    Eustachian tube 744.24
    eye 743.8
        adnexa 743.69
    face bone(s) 756.0
    fallopian tube 752.19
    femur 755.69
    fibula 755.69
    finger(s) 755.59
    foot 755.67
    gallbladder 751.69
    genitalia, genital organ(s)
        female 752.89
            external 752.49
            internal NEC 752.89
        male 752.89
            penis 752.69
    glottis 748.3
    gyri 742.4
    hand bone(s) 755.59
    heart (auricle) (ventricle) 746.89
        valve (cusp) 746.89
    hepatic duct 751.69
    humerus 755.59
    hymen 752.49
    ileum 751.5
    intestine (large) (small) 751.5
        with anomalous adhesions, fixation or malrotation 751.4
    jaw NEC 524.89
    jejunum 751.5
    kidney 753.3
    knee (joint) 755.64
    labium (majus) (minus) 752.49
    larynx 748.3
    leg 755.69
    lens 743.36
    liver 751.69
    lumbar spine 756.19

**Distortion** — continued
    lumbar spine — continued
        with disproportion (fetopelvic) 653.0 ☑
            affecting fetus or newborn 763.1
            causing obstructed labor 660.1 ☑
    lumbosacral (joint) (region) 756.19
    lung (fissures) (lobe) 748.69
    nerve 742.8
    nose 748.1
    organ
        of Corti 744.05
        of site not listed — see Anomaly, specified type NEC
    ossicles, ear 744.04
    ovary 752.0
    oviduct 752.19
    pancreas 751.7
    parathyroid (gland) 759.2
    patella 755.64
    peripheral vascular system NEC 747.60
        gastrointestinal 747.61
        lower limb 747.64
        renal 747.62
        spinal 747.82
        upper limb 747.63
    pituitary (gland) 759.2
    radius 755.59
    rectum 751.5
    rib 756.3
    sacroiliac joint 755.69
    sacrum 756.19
    scapula 755.59
    shoulder girdle 755.59
    site not listed — see Anomaly, specified type NEC
    skull bone(s) 756.0
        with
            anencephalus 740.0
            encephalocele 742.0
            hydrocephalus 742.3
                with spina bifida (see also Spina bifida) 741.0 ☑
            microcephalus 742.1
    spinal cord 742.59
    spine 756.19
    spleen 759.0
    sternum 756.3
    thorax (wall) 756.3
    thymus (gland) 759.2
    thyroid (gland) 759.2
        cartilage 748.3
    tibia 755.69
    toe(s) 755.66
    tongue 750.19
    trachea (cartilage) 748.3
    ulna 755.59
    ureter 753.4
        causing obstruction 753.20
    urethra 753.8
        causing obstruction 753.6
    uterus 752.3
    vagina 752.49
    vein (peripheral) NEC (see also Distortion, peripheral vascular system) 747.60
        great 747.49
        portal 747.49
        pulmonary 747.49
    vena cava (inferior) (superior) 747.49
    vertebra 756.19
    visual NEC 368.15
        shape or size 368.14
    vulva 752.49
    wrist (bones) (joint) 755.59
**Distress**
    abdomen 789.0 ☑
    colon 564.9
    emotional V40.9
    epigastric 789.0 ☑
    fetal (syndrome) 768.4
        affecting management of pregnancy or childbirth 656.8 ☑
        liveborn infant 768.4

**Distress** — continued
    fetal — continued
        liveborn infant — continued
            first noted
                before onset of labor 768.2
                during labor and delivery 768.3
            stillborn infant (death before onset of labor) 768.0
                death during labor 768.1
    gastrointestinal (functional) 536.9
        psychogenic 306.4
    intestinal (functional) NEC 564.9
        psychogenic 306.4
    intrauterine — see Distress, fetal
    leg 729.5
    maternal 669.0 ☑
    mental V40.9
    respiratory 786.09
        acute (adult) 518.82
        adult syndrome (following shock, surgery, or trauma) 518.5
            specified NEC 518.82
        fetus or newborn 770.89
        syndrome (idiopathic) (newborn) 769
    stomach 536.9
        psychogenic 306.4
**Distribution vessel, atypical** NEC 747.60
    coronary artery 746.85
    spinal 747.82
**Districhiasis** 704.2
**Disturbance** — see also Disease
    absorption NEC 579.9
        calcium 269.3
        carbohydrate 579.8
        fat 579.8
        protein 579.8
        specified type NEC 579.8
        vitamin (see also Deficiency, vitamin) 269.2
    acid-base equilibrium 276.9
    activity and attention, simple, with hyperkinesis 314.01
    amino acid (metabolic) (see also Disorder, amino acid) 270.9
        imidazole 270.5
        maple syrup (urine) disease 270.3
        transport 270.0
    assimilation, food 579.9
    attention, simple 314.00
        with hyperactivity 314.01
    auditory, nerve, except deafness 388.5
    behavior (see also Disturbance, conduct) 312.9
    blood clotting (hypoproteinemia) (mechanism) (see also Defect, coagulation) 286.9
    central nervous system NEC 349.9
    cerebral nerve NEC 352.9
    circulatory 459.9
    conduct 312.9

Note — Use the following fifth-digit subclassification with categories 312.0–312.2:

    0    unspecified

    1    mild

    2    moderate

    3    severe

        adjustment reaction 309.3
        adolescent onset type 312.82
        childhood onset type 312.81
        compulsive 312.30
            intermittent explosive disorder 312.34
            isolated explosive disorder 312.35
            kleptomania 312.32
            pathological gambling 312.31
            pyromania 312.33
        hyperkinetic 314.2
        intermittent explosive 312.34
        isolated explosive 312.35

☑ Additional Digit Required — Refer to the Tabular List for Digit Selection          Subterms under main terms may continue to next column or page

98 — Volume 2          ▶◀ Revised Text          ● New Line          ▲ Revised Code          **2008 ICD-9-CM**

**Disturbance** — *see also* Disease — *continued*
  conduct — *continued*
    mixed with emotions 312.4
    socialized (type) 312.20
      aggressive 312.23
      unaggressive 312.21
    specified type NEC 312.89
    undersocialized, unsocialized
      aggressive (type) 312.0 ☑
      unaggressive (type) 312.1 ☑
  coordination 781.3
  cranial nerve NEC 352.9
  deep sensibility — *see* Disturbance, sensation
  digestive 536.9
    psychogenic 306.4
  electrolyte — *see* Imbalance, electrolyte
  emotions specific to childhood or adolescence 313.9
    with
      academic underachievement 313.83
      anxiety and fearfulness 313.0
      elective mutism 313.23
      identity disorder 313.82
      jealousy 313.3
      misery and unhappiness 313.1
      oppositional defiant disorder 313.81
      overanxiousness 313.0
      sensitivity 313.21
      shyness 313.21
      social withdrawal 313.22
      withdrawal reaction 313.22
    involving relationship problems 313.3
    mixed 313.89
    specified type NEC 313.89
  endocrine (gland) 259.9
    neonatal, transitory 775.9
      specified NEC 775.89
  equilibrium 780.4
  feeding (elderly) (infant) 783.3
    newborn 779.3
    nonorganic origin NEC 307.59
    psychogenic NEC 307.59
  fructose metabolism 271.2
  gait 781.2
    hysterical 300.11
  gastric (functional) 536.9
    motility 536.8
    psychogenic 306.4
    secretion 536.8
  gastrointestinal (functional) 536.9
    psychogenic 306.4
  habit, child 307.9
  hearing, except deafness 388.40
  heart, functional (conditions classifiable to 426, 427, 428)
    due to presence of (cardiac) prosthesis 429.4
    postoperative (immediate) 997.1
      long-term effect of cardiac surgery 429.4
    psychogenic 306.2
  hormone 259.9
  innervation uterus, sympathetic, parasympathetic 621.8
  keratinization NEC
    gingiva 523.10
    lip 528.5
    oral (mucosa) (soft tissue) 528.79
      residual ridge mucosa
        excessive 528.72
        minimal 528.71
    tongue 528.79
  labyrinth, labyrinthine (vestibule) 386.9
  learning, specific NEC 315.2
  memory (*see also* Amnesia) 780.93
    mild, following organic brain damage 310.8
  mental (*see also* Disorder, mental) 300.9

**Disturbance** — *see also* Disease — *continued*
  mental (*see also* Disorder, mental) — *continued*
    associated with diseases classified elsewhere 316
  metabolism (acquired) (congenital) (*see also* Disorder, metabolism) 277.9
    with
      abortion — *see* Abortion, by type, with metabolic disorder
      ectopic pregnancy (*see also* categories 633.0–633.9) 639.4
      molar pregnancy (*see also* categories 630–632) 639.4
    amino acid (*see also* Disorder, amino acid) 270.9
      aromatic NEC 270.2
      branched-chain 270.3
      specified type NEC 270.8
      straight-chain NEC 270.7
      sulfur-bearing 270.4
      transport 270.0
    ammonia 270.6
    arginine 270.6
    argininosuccinic acid 270.6
    carbohydrate NEC 271.9
    cholesterol 272.9
    citrulline 270.6
    cystathionine 270.4
    fat 272.9
    following
      abortion 639.4
      ectopic or molar pregnancy 639.4
    general 277.9
      carbohydrate 271.9
      iron 275.0
      phosphate 275.3
      sodium 276.9
    glutamine 270.7
    glycine 270.7
    histidine 270.5
    homocystine 270.4
    in labor or delivery 669.0 ☑
    iron 275.0
    isoleucine 270.3
    leucine 270.3
    lipid 272.9
      specified type NEC 272.8
    lysine 270.7
    methionine 270.4
    neonatal, transitory 775.9
      specified type NEC 775.89
    nitrogen 788.9
    ornithine 270.6
    phosphate 275.3
    phosphatides 272.7
    serine 270.7
    sodium NEC 276.9
    threonine 270.7
    tryptophan 270.2
    tyrosine 270.2
    urea cycle 270.6
    valine 270.3
  motor 796.1
  nervous functional 799.2
  neuromuscular mechanism (eye) due to syphilis 094.84
  nutritional 269.9
    nail 703.8
  ocular motion 378.87
    psychogenic 306.7
  oculogyric 378.87
    psychogenic 306.7
  oculomotor NEC 378.87
    psychogenic 306.7
  olfactory nerve 781.1
  optic nerve NEC 377.49
  oral epithelium, including tongue 528.79
    residual ridge mucosa
      excessive 528.72

**Disturbance** — *see also* Disease — *continued*
  oral epithelium, including tongue — *continued*
    residual ridge mucosa — *continued*
      minimal 528.71
  personality (pattern) (trait) (*see also* Disorder, personality) 301.9
    following organic brain damage 310.1
  polyglandular 258.9
  psychomotor 307.9
  pupillary 379.49
  reflex 796.1
  rhythm, heart 427.9
    postoperative (immediate) 997.1
      long-term effect of cardiac surgery 429.4
    psychogenic 306.2
  salivary secretion 527.7
  sensation (cold) (heat) (localization) (tactile discrimination localization) (texture) (vibratory) NEC 782.0
    hysterical 300.11
    skin 782.0
    smell 781.1
    taste 781.1
  sensory (*see also* Disturbance, sensation) 782.0
    innervation 782.0
  situational (transient) (*see also* Reaction, adjustment) 309.9
    acute 308.3
  sleep 780.50
    with apnea — *see* Apnea, sleep
    initiation or maintenance (*see also* Insomnia) 780.52
      nonorganic origin 307.41
    nonorganic origin 307.40
      specified type NEC 307.49
    specified NEC 780.59
      nonorganic origin 307.49
    wakefulness (*see also* Hypersomnia) 780.54
      nonorganic origin 307.43
  sociopathic 301.7
  speech NEC 784.5
    developmental 315.39
      associated with hyperkinesis 314.1
    secondary to organic lesion 784.5
  stomach (functional) (*see also* Disturbance, gastric) 536.9
  sympathetic (nerve) (*see also* Neuropathy, peripheral, autonomic) 337.9
  temperature sense 782.0
    hysterical 300.11
  tooth
    eruption 520.6
    formation 520.4
    structure, hereditary NEC 520.5
  touch (*see also* Disturbance, sensation) 782.0
  vascular 459.9
    arteriosclerotic — *see* Arteriosclerosis
  vasomotor 443.9
  vasospastic 443.9
  vestibular labyrinth 386.9
  vision, visual NEC 368.9
    psychophysical 368.16
    specified NEC 368.8
    subjective 368.10
  voice 784.40
  wakefulness (initiation or maintenance) (*see also* Hypersomnia) 780.54
    nonorganic origin 307.43
**Disulfiduria, beta-mercaptolactate-cysteine** 270.0
**Disuse atrophy, bone** 733.7
**Ditthomska syndrome** 307.81
**Diuresis** 788.42

**Divers'**
  palsy or paralysis 993.3
  squeeze 993.3
**Diverticula, diverticulosis, diverticulum** (acute) (multiple) (perforated) (ruptured) 562.10
  with diverticulitis 562.11
  aorta (Kommerell's) 747.21
  appendix (noninflammatory) 543.9
  bladder (acquired) (sphincter) 596.3
    congenital 753.8
  broad ligament 620.8
  bronchus (congenital) 748.3
    acquired 494.0
      with acute exacerbation 494.1
  calyx, calyceal (kidney) 593.89
  cardia (stomach) 537.1
  cecum 562.10
    with
      diverticulitis 562.11
        with hemorrhage 562.13
      hemorrhage 562.12
    congenital 751.5
  colon (acquired) 562.10
    with
      diverticulitis 562.11
        with hemorrhage 562.13
      hemorrhage 562.12
    congenital 751.5
  duodenum 562.00
    with
      diverticulitis 562.01
        with hemorrhage 562.03
      hemorrhage 562.02
    congenital 751.5
  epiphrenic (esophagus) 530.6
  esophagus (congenital) 750.4
    acquired 530.6
    epiphrenic 530.6
    pulsion 530.6
    traction 530.6
    Zenker's 530.6
  Eustachian tube 381.89
  fallopian tube 620.8
  gallbladder (congenital) 751.69
  gastric 537.1
  heart (congenital) 746.89
  ileum 562.00
    with
      diverticulitis 562.01
        with hemorrhage 562.03
      hemorrhage 562.02
  intestine (large) 562.10
    with
      diverticulitis 562.11
        with hemorrhage 562.13
      hemorrhage 562.12
    congenital 751.5
    small 562.00
      with
        diverticulitis 562.01
          with hemorrhage 562.03
        hemorrhage 562.02
      congenital 751.5
  jejunum 562.00
    with
      diverticulitis 562.01
        with hemorrhage 562.03
      hemorrhage 562.02
  kidney (calyx) (pelvis) 593.89
    with calculus 592.0
  Kommerell's 747.21
  laryngeal ventricle (congenital) 748.3
  Meckel's (displaced) (hypertrophic) 751.0
  midthoracic 530.6
  organ or site, congenital NEC — *see* Distortion
  pericardium (congenital) (cyst) 746.89
    acquired (true) 423.8
  pharyngoesophageal (pulsion) 530.6
  pharynx (congenital) 750.27
  pulsion (esophagus) 530.6
  rectosigmoid 562.10
    with
      diverticulitis 562.11

☑ Additional Digit Required — Refer to the Tabular List for Digit Selection ⬛ Subterms under main terms may continue to next column or page

**2008 ICD-9-CM**    ►◄ Revised Text    ● New Line    ▲ Revised Code    **Volume 2 — 99**

Disturbance — Diverticula, diverticulosis

**Diverticula, diverticulosis, diverticulum** — continued
  rectosigmoid — continued
    with — continued
      diverticulitis — continued
        with hemorrhage 562.13
      hemorrhage 562.12
      congenital 751.5
  rectum 562.10
    with
      diverticulitis 562.11
        with hemorrhage 562.13
      hemorrhage 562.12
  renal (calyces) (pelvis) 593.89
    with calculus 592.0
  Rokitansky's 530.6
  seminal vesicle 608.0
  sigmoid 562.10
    with
      diverticulitis 562.11
        with hemorrhage 562.13
      hemorrhage 562.12
    congenital 751.5
  small intestine 562.00
    with
      diverticulitis 562.01
        with hemorrhage 562.03
      hemorrhage 562.02
  stomach (cardia) (juxtacardia) (juxtapyloric) (acquired) 537.1
    congenital 750.7
  subdiaphragmatic 530.6
  trachea (congenital) 748.3
    acquired 519.19
  traction (esophagus) 530.6
  ureter (acquired) 593.89
    congenital 753.4
  ureterovesical orifice 593.89
  urethra (acquired) 599.2
    congenital 753.8
  ventricle, left (congenital) 746.89
  vesical (urinary) 596.3
    congenital 753.8
  Zenker's (esophagus) 530.6
**Diverticulitis** (acute) — see also Diverticula 562.11
  with hemorrhage 562.13
  bladder (urinary) 596.3
  cecum (perforated) 562.11
    with hemorrhage 562.13
  colon (perforated) 562.11
    with hemorrhage 562.13
  duodenum 562.01
    with hemorrhage 562.03
  esophagus 530.6
  ileum (perforated) 562.01
    with hemorrhage 562.03
  intestine (large) (perforated) 562.11
    with hemorrhage 562.13
    small 562.01
      with hemorrhage 562.03
  jejunum (perforated) 562.01
    with hemorrhage 562.03
  Meckel's (perforated) 751.0
  pharyngoesophageal 530.6
  rectosigmoid (perforated) 562.11
    with hemorrhage 562.13
  rectum 562.11
    with hemorrhage 562.13
  sigmoid (old) (perforated) 562.11
    with hemorrhage 562.13
  small intestine (perforated) 562.01
    with hemorrhage 562.03
  vesical (urinary) 596.3
**Diverticulosis** — see Diverticula
**Division**
  cervix uteri 622.8
    external os into two openings by frenum 752.49
  external (cervical) into two openings by frenum 752.49
  glans penis 752.69
  hymen 752.49
  labia minora (congenital) 752.49
  ligament (partial or complete) (current) (see also Sprain, by site)

**Division** — continued
  ligament (see also Sprain, by site) — continued
    with open wound — see Wound, open, by site
  muscle (partial or complete) (current) (see also Sprain, by site)
    with open wound — see Wound, open, by site
  nerve — see Injury, nerve, by site
  penis glans 752.69
  spinal cord — see Injury, spinal, by site
  vein 459.9
    traumatic — see Injury, vascular, by site
**Divorce** V61.0
**Dix-Hallpike neurolabyrinthitis** 386.12
**Dizziness** 780.4
  hysterical 300.11
  psychogenic 306.9
**Doan-Wiseman syndrome** (primary splenic neutropenia) 289.53
**Dog bite** — see Wound, open, by site
**Döhle body-panmyelopathic syndrome** 288.2
**Döhle-Heller aortitis** 093.1
**Dolichocephaly, dolichocephalus** 754.0
**Dolichocolon** 751.5
**Dolichostenomelia** 759.82
**Donohue's syndrome** (leprechaunism) 259.8
**Donor**
  blood V59.01
    other blood components V59.09
    stem cells V59.02
    whole blood V59.01
  bone V59.2
    marrow V59.3
  cornea V59.5
  egg (oocyte) (ovum) V59.70
    over age 35 V59.73
      anonymous recipient V59.73
      designated recipient V59.74
    under age 35 V59.71
      anonymous recipient V59.71
      designated recipient V59.72
  heart V59.8
  kidney V59.4
  liver V59.6
  lung V59.8
  lymphocyte V59.8
  organ V59.9
    specified NEC V59.8
  potential, examination of V70.8
  skin V59.1
  specified organ or tissue NEC V59.8
  sperm V59.8
  stem cells V59.02
  tissue V59.9
    specified type NEC V59.8
**Donovanosis** (granuloma venereum) 099.2
**DOPS** (diffuse obstructive pulmonary syndrome) 496
**Double**
  albumin 273.8
  aortic arch 747.21
  auditory canal 744.29
  auricle (heart) 746.82
  bladder 753.8
  external (cervical) os 752.49
  kidney with double pelvis (renal) 753.3
  larynx 748.3
  meatus urinarius 753.8
  organ or site NEC — see Accessory orifice
    heart valve NEC 746.89
      pulmonary 746.09
  outlet, right ventricle 745.11
  pelvis (renal) with double ureter 753.4
  penis 752.69
  tongue 750.13
  ureter (one or both sides) 753.4
    with double pelvis (renal) 753.4
  urethra 753.8

**Double** — continued
  urinary meatus 753.8
  uterus (any degree) 752.2
    with doubling of cervix and vagina 752.2
    in pregnancy or childbirth 654.0 ☑
      affecting fetus or newborn 763.89
  vagina 752.49
    with doubling of cervix and uterus 752.2
  vision 368.2
  vocal cords 748.3
  vulva 752.49
  whammy (syndrome) 360.81
**Douglas' pouch, cul-de-sac** — see condition
**Down's disease or syndrome** (mongolism) 758.0
**Down-growth, epithelial** (anterior chamber) 364.61
**Dracontiasis** 125.7
**Dracunculiasis** 125.7
**Dracunculosis** 125.7
**Drainage**
  abscess (spontaneous) — see Abscess
  anomalous pulmonary veins to hepatic veins or right atrium 747.41
  stump (amputation) (surgical) 997.62
  suprapubic, bladder 596.8
**Dream state, hysterical** 300.13
**Drepanocytic anemia** — see also Disease, sickle cell 282.60
**Dresbach's syndrome** (elliptocytosis) 282.1
**Dreschlera** (infection) 118
  hawaiiensis 117.8
**Dressler's syndrome** (postmyocardial infarction) 411.0
**Dribbling** (post-void) 788.35
**Drift, ulnar** 736.09
**Drinking (alcohol)** — see also Alcoholism
  excessive, to excess NEC (see also Abuse, drugs, nondependent) 305.0 ☑
    bouts, periodic 305.0 ☑
    continual 303.9 ☑
    episodic 305.0 ☑
    habitual 303.9 ☑
    periodic 305.0 ☑
**Drip, postnasal** (chronic) 784.91
  due to
    allergic rhinitis — see Rhinitis, allergic
    common cold 460
    gastroesophageal reflux — see Reflux, gastroesophageal
    nasopharyngitis — see Nasopharyngitis
    other known condition — code to condition
    sinusitis — see Sinusitis
**Drivers' license examination** V70.3
**Droop**
  Cooper's 611.8
  facial 781.94
**Drop**
  finger 736.29
  foot 736.79
  hematocrit (precipitous) 790.01
  toe 735.8
  wrist 736.05
**Dropped**
  dead 798.1
  heart beats 426.6
**Dropsy, dropsical** — see also Edema 782.3
  abdomen 789.59 ▲
  amnion (see also Hydramnios) 657.0 ☑
  brain — see Hydrocephalus
  cardiac (see also Failure, heart) 428.0
  cardiorenal (see also Hypertension, cardiorenal) 404.90
  chest 511.9

**Dropsy, dropsical** — see also Edema — continued
  fetus or newborn 778.0
    due to isoimmunization 773.3
  gangrenous (see also Gangrene) 785.4
  heart (see also Failure, heart) 428.0
  hepatic — see Cirrhosis, liver
  infantile — see Hydrops, fetalis
  kidney (see also Nephrosis) 581.9
  liver — see Cirrhosis, liver
  lung 514
  malarial (see also Malaria) 084.9
  neonatorum — see Hydrops, fetalis
  nephritic 581.9
  newborn — see Hydrops, fetalis
  nutritional 269.9
  ovary 620.8
  pericardium (see also Pericarditis) 423.9
  renal (see also Nephrosis) 581.9
  uremic — see Uremia
**Drowned, drowning** 994.1
  lung 518.5
**Drowsiness** 780.09
**Drug** — see also condition
  addiction (see also listing under Dependence) 304.9 ☑
  adverse effect NEC, correct substance properly administered 995.20
  allergy 995.27
  dependence (see also listing under Dependence) 304.9 ☑
  habit (see also listing under Dependence) 304.9 ☑
  hypersensitivity 995.27
  induced
    circadian rhythm sleep disorder 292.85
    hypersomnia 292.85
    insomnia 292.85
    mental disorder 292.9
      anxiety 292.89
      mood 292.84
      sexual 292.89
      sleep 292.85
      specified type 292.89
    parasomnia 292.85
    persisting
      amnestic disorder 292.83
      dementia 292.82
    psychotic disorder
      with
        delusions 292.11
        hallucinations 292.12
    sleep disorder 292.85
  intoxication 292.89
  overdose — see Table of Drugs and Chemicals
  poisoning — see Table of Drugs and Chemicals
  therapy (maintenance) status NEC
    chemotherapy, antineoplastic V58.11
    immunotherapy, antineoplastic V58.12
    long-term (current) use V58.69
      antibiotics V58.62
      anticoagulants V58.61
      anti-inflammatories, non-steroidal (NSAID) V58.64
      antiplatelets V58.63
      antithrombotics V58.63
      aspirin V58.66
      high-risk medications NEC ●
      V58.69 ●
      insulin V58.67
      steroids V58.65
  wrong substance given or taken in error — see Table of Drugs and Chemicals
**Drunkenness** — see also Abuse, drugs, nondependent 305.0 ☑
  acute in alcoholism (see also Alcoholism) 303.0 ☑
  chronic (see also Alcoholism) 303.9 ☑
  pathologic 291.4

☑ Additional Digit Required — Refer to the Tabular List for Digit Selection      ▧ Subterms under main terms may continue to next column or page

100 — Volume 2 · October 2007      ►◄ Revised Text    ● New Line    ▲ Revised Code      2008 ICD-9-CM

**Drunkenness** — *see also* Abuse, drugs,
   nondependent — *continued*
   simple (acute) 305.0 ☑
      in alcoholism 303.0 ☑
   sleep 307.47
**Drusen**
   optic disc or papilla 377.21
   retina (colloid) (hyaloid degeneration)
      362.57
      hereditary 362.77
**Drusenfieber** 075
**Dry, dryness** — *see also* condition
   eye 375.15
      syndrome 375.15
   larynx 478.79
   mouth 527.7
   nose 478.19
   skin syndrome 701.1
   socket (teeth) 526.5
   throat 478.29
**DSAP** (disseminated superficial actinic
   porokeratosis) 692.75
**Duane's retraction syndrome** 378.71
**Duane-Stilling-Türk syndrome** (ocular
   retraction syndrome) 378.71
**Dubini's disease** (electric chorea) 049.8
**Dubin-Johnson disease or syndrome**
   277.4
**Dubois' abscess or disease** 090.5
**Duchenne's**
   disease 094.0
      locomotor ataxia 094.0
      muscular dystrophy 359.1
      pseudohypertrophy, muscles 359.1
   paralysis 335.22
   syndrome 335.22
**Duchenne-Aran myelopathic, muscular
   atrophy** (nonprogressive) (progres-
   sive) 335.21
**Duchenne-Griesinger disease** 359.1
**Ducrey's**
   bacillus 099.0
   chancre 099.0
   disease (chancroid) 099.0
**Duct, ductus** — *see* condition
**Duengero** 061
**Duhring's disease** (dermatitis herpeti-
   formis) 694.0
**Dukes (-Filatov) disease** 057.8
**Dullness**
   cardiac (decreased) (increased) 785.3
**Dumb ague** — *see also* Malaria 084.6
**Dumbness** — *see also* Aphasia 784.3
**Dumdum fever** 085.0
**Dumping syndrome** (postgastrectomy)
   564.2
   nonsurgical 536.8
**Duodenitis** (nonspecific) (peptic) 535.60
   with hemorrhage 535.61
   due to
      Strongyloides stercoralis 127.2
**Duodenocholangitis** 575.8
**Duodenum, duodenal** — *see* condition
**Duplay's disease, periarthritis, or syn-
   drome** 726.2
**Duplex** — *see also* Accessory
   kidney 753.3
   placenta — *see* Placenta, abnormal
   uterus 752.2
**Duplication** — *see also* Accessory
   anus 751.5
   aortic arch 747.21
   appendix 751.5
   biliary duct (any) 751.69
   bladder 753.8
   cecum 751.5
      and appendix 751.5
   clitoris 752.49
   cystic duct 751.69
   digestive organs 751.8
   duodenum 751.5
   esophagus 750.4
   fallopian tube 752.19
   frontonasal process 756.0
   gallbladder 751.69
   ileum 751.5

**Duplication** — *see also* Accessory —
   *continued*
   intestine (large) (small) 751.5
   jejunum 751.5
   kidney 753.3
   liver 751.69
   nose 748.1
   pancreas 751.7
   penis 752.69
   respiratory organs NEC 748.9
   salivary duct 750.22
   spinal cord (incomplete) 742.51
   stomach 750.7
   ureter 753.4
   vagina 752.49
   vas deferens 752.89
   vocal cords 748.3
**Dupré's disease or syndrome**
   (meningism) 781.6
**Dupuytren's**
   contraction 728.6
   disease (muscle contracture) 728.6
   fracture (closed) 824.4
      ankle (closed) 824.4
         open 824.5
      fibula (closed) 824.4
         open 824.5
         open 824.5
      radius (closed) 813.42
         open 813.52
   muscle contracture 728.6
**Durand-Nicolas-Favre disease** (climatic
   bubo) 099.1
**Duroziez's disease** (congenital mitral
   stenosis) 746.5
**Dust**
   conjunctivitis 372.05
   reticulation (occupational) 504
**Dutton's**
   disease (trypanosomiasis) 086.9
   relapsing fever (West African) 087.1
**Dwarf, dwarfism** 259.4
   with infantilism (hypophyseal) 253.3
   achondroplastic 756.4
   Amsterdam 759.89
   bird-headed 759.89
   congenital 259.4
   constitutional 259.4
   hypophyseal 253.3
   infantile 259.4
   Levi type 253.3
   Lorain-Levi (pituitary) 253.3
   Lorain type (pituitary) 253.3
   metatropic 756.4
   nephrotic-glycosuric, with hypophos-
      phatemic rickets 270.0
   nutritional 263.2
   ovarian 758.6
   pancreatic 577.8
   pituitary 253.3
   polydystrophic 277.5
   primordial 253.3
   psychosocial 259.4
   renal 588.0
      with hypertension — *see* Hyperten-
         sion, kidney
   Russell's (uterine dwarfism and cran-
      iofacial dysostosis) 759.89
**Dyke-Young anemia or syndrome** (acquired macrocytic hemolytic anemia) (secondary) (symptomatic)
   283.9
**Dynia abnormality** — *see also* Defect,
   coagulation 286.9
**Dysacousis** 388.40
**Dysadrenocortism** 255.9
   hyperfunction 255.3
   hypofunction 255.41       ▲
**Dysarthria** 784.5
**Dysautonomia** — *see also* Neuropathy,
   peripheral, autonomic 337.9
   familial 742.8
**Dysbarism** 993.3
**Dysbasia** 719.7
   angiosclerotica intermittens 443.9
      due to atherosclerosis 440.21

**Dysbasia** — *continued*
   hysterical 300.11
   lordotica (progressiva) 333.6
   nonorganic origin 307.9
   psychogenic 307.9
**Dysbetalipoproteinemia** (familial) 272.2
**Dyscalculia** 315.1
**Dyschezia** — *see also* Constipation
   564.00
**Dyschondroplasia** (with hemangiomata)
   756.4
   Voorhoeve's 756.4
**Dyschondrosteosis** 756.59
**Dyschromia** 709.00
**Dyscollagenosis** 710.9
**Dyscoria** 743.41
**Dyscraniopyophalangy** 759.89
**Dyscrasia**
   blood 289.9
      with antepartum hemorrhage
         641.3 ☑
      fetus or newborn NEC 776.9
      hemorrhage, subungual 287.8
      puerperal, postpartum 666.3 ☑
   ovary 256.8
   plasma cell 273.9
   pluriglandular 258.9
   polyglandular 258.9
**Dysdiadochokinesia** 781.3
**Dysectasia, vesical neck** 596.8
**Dysendocrinism** 259.9
**Dysentery, dysenteric** (bilious)
   (catarrhal) (diarrhea) (epidemic)
   (gangrenous) (hemorrhagic) (infectious) (sporadic) (tropical) (ulcerative) 009.0
   abscess, liver (*see also* Abscess, ame-
      bic) 006.3
   amebic (*see also* Amebiasis) 006.9
      with abscess — *see* Abscess, ame-
         bic
      acute 006.0
      carrier (suspected) of V02.2
      chronic 006.1
   arthritis, due to (*see also* Arthritis, due to,
      dysentery) 009.0 *[711.3]* ☑
      bacillary 004.9 *[711.3]* ☑
   asylum 004.9
   bacillary 004.9
      arthritis 004.9 *[711.3]* ☑
      Boyd 004.2
      Flexner 004.1
      Schmitz (-Stutzer) 004.0
      Shiga 004.0
      Shigella 004.9
         group A 004.0
         group B 004.1
         group C 004.2
         group D 004.3
         specified type NEC 004.8
      Sonne 004.3
      specified type NEC 004.8
   bacterium 004.9
   balantidial 007.0
   Balantidium coli 007.0
   Boyd's 004.2
   Chilomastix 007.8
   Chinese 004.9
   choleriform 001.1
   coccidial 007.2
   Dientamoeba fragilis 007.8
   due to specified organism NEC — *see*
      Enteritis, due to, by organism
   Embadomonas 007.8
   Endolimax nana — *see* Dysentery,
      amebic
   Entamoba, entamebic — *see* Dysen-
      tery, amebic
   Flexner's 004.1
   Flexner-Boyd 004.2
   giardial 007.1
   Giardia lamblia 007.1
   Hiss-Russell 004.1
   lamblia 007.1
   leishmanial 085.0
   malarial (*see also* Malaria) 084.6

**Dysentery, dysenteric** — *continued*
   metazoal 127.9
   Monilia 112.89
   protozoal NEC 007.9
   Russell's 004.8
   salmonella 003.0
   schistosomal 120.1
   Schmitz (-Stutzer) 004.0
   Shiga 004.0
   Shigella NEC (*see also* Dysentery,
      bacillary) 004.9
      boydii 004.2
      dysenteriae 004.0
         Schmitz 004.0
         Shiga 004.0
      flexneri 004.1
      group A 004.0
      group B 004.1
      group C 004.2
      group D 004.3
      Schmitz 004.0
      Shiga 004.0
      Sonnei 004.3
   Sonne 004.3
   strongyloidiasis 127.2
   trichomonal 007.3
   tuberculous (*see also* Tuberculosis)
      014.8 ☑
   viral (*see also* Enteritis, viral) 008.8
**Dysequilibrium** 780.4
**Dysesthesia** 782.0
   hysterical 300.11
**Dysfibrinogenemia** (congenital) — *see
   also* Defect, coagulation 286.3
**Dysfunction**
   adrenal (cortical) 255.9
      hyperfunction 255.3
      hypofunction 255.41      ▲
   associated with sleep stages or
      arousal from sleep 780.56
      nonorganic origin 307.47
   bladder NEC 596.59
   bleeding, uterus 626.8
   brain, minimal (*see also* Hyperkinesia)
      314.9
   cerebral 348.30
   colon 564.9
      psychogenic 306.4
   colostomy or enterostomy 569.62
   cystic duct 575.8
   diastolic 429.9
      with heart failure — *see* Failure,
         heart
      due to
         cardiomyopathy — *see* Car-
            diomyopathy
         hypertension — *see* Hyperten-
            sion, heart
   endocrine NEC 259.9
   endometrium 621.8
   enteric stoma 569.62
   enterostomy 569.62
   erectile 607.84
      nonorganic origin 302.72
   esophagostomy 530.87
   Eustachian tube 381.81
   gallbladder 575.8
   gastrointestinal 536.9
   gland, glandular NEC 259.9
   heart 427.9
      postoperative (immediate) 997.1
         long-term effect of cardiac
            surgery 429.4
   hemoglobin 289.89
   hepatic 573.9
   hepatocellular NEC 573.9
   hypophysis 253.9
      hyperfunction 253.1
      hypofunction 253.2
      posterior lobe 253.6
         hypofunction 253.5
   kidney (*see also* Disease, renal) 593.9
   labyrinthine 386.50
      specified NEC 386.58
   liver 573.9
      constitutional 277.4

☑ Additional Digit Required — Refer to the Tabular List for Digit Selection           ▽ Subterms under main terms may continue to next column or page

*2008 ICD-9-CM*          ▶◀ Revised Text       ● New Line       ▲ Revised Code        October 2007 • Volume 2 — 101

Drunkenness — Dysfunction

**Dysfunction** — *continued*
minimal brain (child) (*see also* Hyperkinesis) 314.9
ovary, ovarian 256.9
  hyperfunction 256.1
    estrogen 256.0
  hypofunction 256.39
    postablative 256.2
  postablative 256.2
  specified NEC 256.8
papillary muscle 429.81
  with myocardial infarction 410.8 ☑
parathyroid 252.8
  hyperfunction 252.00
  hypofunction 252.1
pineal gland 259.8
pituitary (gland) 253.9
  hyperfunction 253.1
  hypofunction 253.2
  posterior 253.6
    hypofunction 253.5
placental — *see* Placenta, insufficiency
platelets (blood) 287.1
polyglandular 258.9
  specified NEC 258.8
psychosexual 302.70
  with
    dyspareunia (functional) (psychogenic) 302.76
    frigidity 302.72
    impotence 302.72
    inhibition
      orgasm
        female 302.73
        male 302.74
      sexual
        desire 302.71
        excitement 302.72
    premature ejaculation 302.75
    sexual aversion 302.79
    specified disorder NEC 302.79
    vaginismus 306.51
pylorus 537.9
rectum 564.9
  psychogenic 306.4
segmental (*see also* Dysfunction, somatic) 739.9
senile 797
sexual 302.70
sinoatrial node 427.81
somatic 739.9
  abdomen 739.9
  acromioclavicular 739.7
  cervical 739.1
  cervicothoracic 739.1
  costochondral 739.8
  costovertebral 739.8
  extremities
    lower 739.6
    upper 739.7
  head 739.0
  hip 739.5
  lumbar, lumbosacral 739.3
  occipitocervical 739.0
  pelvic 739.5
  pubic 739.5
  rib cage 739.8
  sacral 739.4
  sacrococcygeal 739.4
  sacroiliac 739.4
  specified site NEC 739.9
  sternochondral 739.8
  sternoclavicular 739.7
  temporomandibular 739.0
  thoracic, thoracolumbar 739.2
stomach 536.9
  psychogenic 306.4
suprarenal 255.9
  hyperfunction 255.3
  hypofunction 255.41 ▲
symbolic NEC 784.60
  specified type NEC 784.69
systolic 429.9
  with heart failure — *see* Failure, heart

**Dysfunction** — *continued*
temporomandibular (joint) (joint-pain-syndrome) NEC 524.60
  sounds on opening or closing 524.64
  specified NEC 524.69
testicular 257.9
  hyperfunction 257.0
  hypofunction 257.2
  specified type NEC 257.8
thymus 254.9
thyroid 246.9
  complicating pregnancy, childbirth, or puerperium 648.1 ☑
  hyperfunction — *see* Hyperthyroidism
  hypofunction — *see* Hypothyroidism
uterus, complicating delivery 661.9 ☑
  affecting fetus or newborn 763.7
  hypertonic 661.4 ☑
  hypotonic 661.2 ☑
    primary 661.0 ☑
    secondary 661.1 ☑
velopharyngeal (acquired) 528.9
  congenital 750.29
ventricular 429.9
  with congestive heart failure (*see also* Failure, heart) 428.0
  due to
    cardiomyopathy — *see* Cardiomyopathy
    hypertension — *see* Hypertension, heart
  left, reversible following sudden emotional stress 429.83
vesicourethral NEC 596.59
vestibular 386.50
  specified type NEC 386.58
**Dysgammaglobulinemia** 279.06
**Dysgenesis**
  gonadal (due to chromosomal anomaly) 758.6
    pure 752.7
  kidney(s) 753.0
  ovarian 758.6
  renal 753.0
  reticular 279.2
  seminiferous tubules 758.6
  tidal platelet 287.31
**Dysgerminoma** (M9060/3)
  specified site — *see* Neoplasm, by site, malignant
  unspecified site
    female 183.0
    male 186.9
**Dysgeusia** 781.1
**Dysgraphia** 781.3
**Dyshidrosis** 705.81
**Dysidrosis** 705.81
**Dysinsulinism** 251.8
**Dyskaryotic cervical smear** 795.09
**Dyskeratosis** — *see also* Keratosis 701.1
  bullosa hereditaria 757.39
  cervix 622.10
  congenital 757.39
  follicularis 757.39
    vitamin A deficiency 264.8
  gingiva 523.8
  oral soft tissue NEC 528.79
  tongue 528.79
  uterus NEC 621.8
**Dyskinesia** 781.3
  biliary 575.8
  esophagus 530.5
  hysterical 300.11
  intestinal 564.89
  neuroleptic-induced tardive 333.85
  nonorganic origin 307.9
  orofacial 333.82
    due to drugs 333.85
  psychogenic 307.9
  subacute, due to drugs 333.85
  tardive (oral) 333.85
**Dyslalia** 784.5
  developmental 315.39

**Dyslexia** 784.61
  developmental 315.02
  secondary to organic lesion 784.61
**Dyslipidemia** 272.4
**Dysmaturity** — *see also* Immaturity 765.1 ☑
  lung 770.4
  pulmonary 770.4
**Dysmenorrhea** (essential) (exfoliative) (functional) (intrinsic) (membranous) (primary) (secondary) 625.3
  psychogenic 306.52
**Dysmetabolic syndrome X** 277.7
**Dysmetria** 781.3
**Dysmorodystrophia mesodermalis congenita** 759.82
**Dysnomia** 784.3
**Dysorexia** 783.0
  hysterical 300.11
**Dysostosis**
  cleidocranial, cleidocranialis 755.59
  craniofacial 756.0
  Fairbank's (idiopathic familial generalized osteophytosis) 756.50
  mandibularis 756.0
  mandibulofacial, incomplete 756.0
  multiplex 277.5
  orodigitofacial 759.89
**Dyspareunia** (female) 625.0
  male 608.89
  psychogenic 302.76
**Dyspepsia** (allergic) (congenital) (fermentative) (flatulent) (functional) (gastric) (gastrointestinal) (neurogenic) (occupational) (reflex) 536.8
  acid 536.8
  atonic 536.3
    psychogenic 306.4
  diarrhea 787.91
    psychogenic 306.4
  intestinal 564.89
    psychogenic 306.4
  nervous 306.4
  neurotic 306.4
  psychogenic 306.4
**Dysphagia** 787.20                          ▲
  cervical 787.29                              ●
  functional 300.11
  hysterical 300.11
  nervous 300.11
  neurogenic 787.29                            ●
  oral phase 787.21                            ●
  oropharyngeal phase 787.22                   ●
  pharyngeal phase 787.23                      ●
  pharyngoesophageal phase 787.24 ●
  psychogenic 306.4
  sideropenic 280.8
  spastica 530.5
  specified NEC 787.29                         ●
**Dysphagocytosis, congenital** 288.1
**Dysphasia** 784.5
**Dysphonia** 784.49
  clericorum 784.49
  functional 300.11
  hysterical 300.11
  psychogenic 306.1
  spastica 478.79
**Dyspigmentation** — *see also* Pigmentation
  eyelid (acquired) 374.52
**Dyspituitarism** 253.9
  hyperfunction 253.1
  hypofunction 253.2
  posterior lobe 253.6
**Dysplasia** — *see also* Anomaly
  artery
    fibromuscular NEC 447.8
      carotid 447.8
      renal 447.3
  bladder 596.8
  bone (fibrous) NEC 733.29
    diaphyseal, progressive 756.59
    jaw 526.89
    monostotic 733.29
    polyostotic 756.54
    solitary 733.29

**Dysplasia** — *see also* Anomaly — *continued*
brain 742.9
bronchopulmonary, fetus or newborn 770.7
cervix (uteri) 622.10
  cervical intraepithelial neoplasia I [CIN I] 622.11
  cervical intraepithelial neoplasia II [CIN II] 622.12
  cervical intraepithelial neoplasia III [CIN III] 233.1
  CIN I 622.11
  CIN II 622.12
  CIN III 233.1
  mild 622.11
  moderate 622.12
  severe 233.1
chondroectodermal 756.55
chondromatose 756.4
colon 211.3
craniocarpotarsal 759.89
craniometaphyseal 756.89
dentinal 520.5
diaphyseal, progressive 756.59
ectodermal (anhidrotic) (Bason) (Clouston's) (congenital) (Feinmesser) (hereditary) (hidrotic) (Marshall) (Robinson's) 757.31
epiphysealis 756.9
  multiplex 756.56
  punctata 756.59
epiphysis 756.9
  multiple 756.56
epithelial
  epiglottis 478.79
  uterine cervix 622.10
erythroid NEC 289.89
eye (*see also* Microphthalmos) 743.10
familial metaphyseal 756.89
fibromuscular, artery NEC 447.8
  carotid 447.8
  renal 447.3
fibrous
  bone NEC 733.29
    diaphyseal, progressive 756.59
    jaw 526.89
    monostotic 733.29
    polyostotic 756.54
    solitary 733.29
high-grade, focal — *see* Neoplasm, by site, benign
hip (congenital) 755.63
  with dislocation (*see also* Dislocation, hip, congenital) 754.30
hypohidrotic ectodermal 757.31
joint 755.8
kidney 753.15
leg 755.69
linguofacialis 759.89
lung 748.5
macular 743.55
mammary (benign) (gland) 610.9
  cystic 610.1
  specified type NEC 610.8
metaphyseal 756.9
  familial 756.89
monostotic fibrous 733.29
muscle 756.89
myeloid NEC 289.89
nervous system (general) 742.9
neuroectodermal 759.6
oculoauriculovertebral 756.0
oculodentodigital 759.89
olfactogenital 253.4
osteo-onycho-arthro (hereditary) 756.89
periosteum 733.99
polyostotic fibrous 756.54
progressive diaphyseal 756.59
prostate 602.3
  intraepithelial neoplasia I [PIN I] 602.3
  intraepithelial neoplasia II [PIN II] 602.3

Index

Dysfunction — Dysplasia

**Dysplasia** — *see also* Anomaly — *continued*
  prostate — *continued*
    intraepithelial neoplasia III [PIN III] 233.4
  renal 753.15
  renofacialis 753.0
  retinal NEC 743.56
  retrolental 362.21
  spinal cord 742.9
  thymic, with immunodeficiency 279.2
  vagina 623.0
    severe 233.31 ●
  vocal cord 478.5
  vulva 624.8
    intraepithelial neoplasia I [VIN I] 624.01 ▲
    intraepithelial neoplasia II [VIN II] 624.02 ▲
    intraepithelial neoplasia III [VIN III] 233.32 ▲
    mild 624.01 ●
    moderate 624.02 ●
    severe 233.32 ●
    VIN I 624.01 ▲
    VIN II 624.02 ▲
    VIN III 233.32 ▲
**Dyspnea** (nocturnal) (paroxysmal) 786.09
  asthmatic (bronchial) (*see also* Asthma) 493.9 ☑
    with bronchitis (*see also* Asthma) 493.9 ☑
      chronic 493.2 ☑
  cardiac (*see also* Failure, ventricular, left) 428.1
  cardiac (*see also* Failure, ventricular, left) 428.1
  functional 300.11
  hyperventilation 786.01
  hysterical 300.11
  Monday morning 504
  newborn 770.89
  psychogenic 306.1
  uremic — *see* Uremia
**Dyspraxia** 781.3
  syndrome 315.4
**Dysproteinemia** 273.8
  transient with copper deficiency 281.4
**Dysprothrombinemia** (constitutional) — *see also* Defect, coagulation 286.3
**Dysreflexia, autonomic** 337.3
**Dysrhythmia**
  cardiac 427.9
    postoperative (immediate) 997.1
      long-term effect of cardiac surgery 429.4
    specified type NEC 427.89
  cerebral or cortical 348.30
**Dyssecretosis, mucoserous** 710.2
**Dyssocial reaction, without manifest psychiatric disorder**
  adolescent V71.02
  adult V71.01
  child V71.02
**Dyssomnia** NEC 780.56
  nonorganic origin 307.47
**Dyssplenism** 289.4
**Dyssynergia**
  biliary (*see also* Disease, biliary) 576.8
  cerebellaris myoclonica 334.2
  detrusor sphincter (bladder) 596.55
  ventricular 429.89
**Dystasia, hereditary areflexic** 334.3
**Dysthymia** 300.4
**Dysthymic disorder** 300.4
**Dysthyroidism** 246.9
**Dystocia** 660.9 ☑
  affecting fetus or newborn 763.1
  cervical 661.2 ☑ ▲
    affecting fetus or newborn 763.7
  contraction ring 661.4 ☑
    affecting fetus or newborn 763.7
  fetal 660.9 ☑
    abnormal size 653.5 ☑
    affecting fetus or newborn 763.1
    deformity 653.7 ☑

**Dystocia** — *continued*
  maternal 660.9 ☑
    affecting fetus or newborn 763.1
  positional 660.0 ☑
    affecting fetus or newborn 763.1
  shoulder (girdle) 660.4 ☑
    affecting fetus or newborn 763.1
  uterine NEC 661.4 ☑
    affecting fetus or newborn 763.7
**Dystonia**
  acute
    due to drugs 333.72
    neuroleptic-induced acute 333.72
  deformans progressiva 333.6
  lenticularis 333.6
  musculorum deformans 333.6
  torsion (idiopathic) 333.6
    acquired 333.79
    fragments (of) 333.89
    genetic 333.6
    symptomatic 333.79
**Dystonic**
  movements 781.0
**Dystopia kidney** 753.3
**Dystrophia myotonica** 359.2 ☑
**Dystrophy, dystrophia** 783.9
  adiposogenital 253.8
  asphyxiating thoracic 756.4
  Becker's type 359.22
  brevicollis 756.16
  Bruch's membrane 362.77
  cervical (sympathetic) NEC 337.0
  chondro-osseus with punctate epiphyseal dysplasia 756.59
  choroid (hereditary) 363.50
    central (areolar) (partial) 363.53
      total (gyrate) 363.54
    circinate 363.53
    circumpapillary (partial) 363.51
      total 363.52
    diffuse
      partial 363.56
      total 363.57
    generalized
      partial 363.56
      total 363.57
    gyrate
      central 363.54
      generalized 363.57
    helicoid 363.52
    peripapillary — *see* Dystrophy, choroid, circumpapillary
    serpiginous 363.54
  cornea (hereditary) 371.50
    anterior NEC 371.52
    Cogan's 371.52
    combined 371.57
    crystalline 371.56
    endothelial (Fuchs') 371.57
    epithelial 371.50
      juvenile 371.51
      microscopic cystic 371.52
    granular 371.53
    lattice 371.54
    macular 371.55
    marginal (Terrien's) 371.48
    Meesman's 371.51
    microscopic cystic (epithelial) 371.52
    nodular, Salzmann's 371.46
    polymorphous 371.58
    posterior NEC 371.58
    ring-like 371.52
    Salzmann's nodular 371.46
    stromal NEC 371.56
  dermatochondrocorneal 371.50
  Duchenne's 359.1
  due to malnutrition 263.9
  Erb's 359.1
  familial
    hyperplastic periosteal 756.59
    osseous 277.5
  foveal 362.77
  Fuchs', cornea 371.57
  Gowers' muscular 359.1
  hair 704.2

**Dystrophy, dystrophia** — *continued*
  hereditary, progressive muscular 359.1
  hypogenital, with diabetic tendency 759.81
  Landouzy-Déjérine 359.1
  Leyden-Möbius 359.1
  mesodermalis congenita 759.82
  muscular 359.1
    congenital (hereditary) 359.0
      myotonic 359.22 ▲
    distal 359.1
    Duchenne's 359.1
    Erb's 359.1
    fascioscapulohumeral 359.1
    Gowers' 359.1
    hereditary (progressive) 359.1
    Landouzy-Déjérine 359.1
    limb-girdle 359.1
    myotonic 359.21 ▲
    progressive (hereditary) 359.1
      Charcôt-Marie-Tooth 356.1
    pseudohypertrophic (infantile) 359.1
  myocardium, myocardial (*see also* Degeneration, myocardial) 429.1
  myotonic 359.21 ▲
  myotonica 359.21 ▲
  nail 703.8
    congenital 757.5
  neurovascular (traumatic) (*see also* Neuropathy, peripheral, autonomic) 337.9
  nutritional 263.9
  ocular 359.1
  oculocerebrorenal 270.8
  oculopharyngeal 359.1
  ovarian 620.8
  papillary (and pigmentary) 701.1
  pelvicrural atrophic 359.1
  pigmentary (*see also* Acanthosis) 701.2
  pituitary (gland) 253.8
  polyglandular 258.8
  posttraumatic sympathetic — *see* Dystrophy, sympathetic
  progressive ophthalmoplegic 359.1
  retina, retinal (hereditary) 362.70
    albipunctate 362.74
    Bruch's membrane 362.77
    cone, progressive 362.75
    hyaline 362.77
    in
      Bassen-Kornzweig syndrome 272.5 [362.72]
      cerebroretinal lipidosis 330.1 [362.71]
      Refsum's disease 356.3 [362.72]
      systemic lipidosis 272.7 [362.71]
    juvenile (Stargardt's) 362.75
    pigmentary 362.74
    pigment epithelium 362.76
    progressive cone (-rod) 362.75
    pseudoinflammatory foveal 362.77
    rod, progressive 362.75
    sensory 362.75
    vitelliform 362.76
  Salzmann's nodular 371.46
  scapuloperoneal 359.1
  skin NEC 709.9
  sympathetic (posttraumatic) (reflex) 337.20
    lower limb 337.22
    specified site NEC 337.29
    upper limb 337.21
  tapetoretinal NEC 362.74
  thoracic asphyxiating 756.4
  unguium 703.8
    congenital 757.5
  vitreoretinal (primary) 362.73
    secondary 362.66
  vulva 624.09 ▲
**Dysuria** 788.1
  psychogenic 306.53

### E

**Eagle-Barrett syndrome** 756.71
**Eales' disease** (syndrome) 362.18
**Ear** — *see also* condition
  ache 388.70
    otogenic 388.71
    referred 388.72
  lop 744.29
  piercing V50.3
  swimmers' acute 380.12
  tank 380.12
  tropical 111.8 [380.15]
  wax 380.4
**Earache** 388.70
  otogenic 388.71
  referred 388.72
**Early satiety** 780.94
**Eaton-Lambert syndrome** — *see also* Neoplasm, by site, malignant 199.1 [358.1]
**Eberth's disease** (typhoid fever) 002.0
**Ebstein's**
  anomaly or syndrome (downward displacement, tricuspid valve into right ventricle) 746.2
  disease (diabetes) 250.4 ☑ [581.81]
**Eccentro-osteochondrodysplasia** 277.5
**Ecchondroma** (M9210/0) — *see* Neoplasm, bone, benign
**Ecchondrosis** (M9210/1) 238.0
**Ecchordosis physaliphora** 756.0
**Ecchymosis** (multiple) 459.89
  conjunctiva 372.72
  eye (traumatic) 921.0
  eyelids (traumatic) 921.1
  newborn 772.6
  spontaneous 782.7
  traumatic — *see* Contusion
**Echinococciasis** — *see* Echinococcus
**Echinococcosis** — *see* Echinococcus
**Echinococcus** (infection) 122.9
  granulosus 122.4
    liver 122.0
    lung 122.1
    orbit 122.3 [376.13]
    specified site NEC 122.3
    thyroid 122.2
  liver NEC 122.8
    granulosus 122.0
    multilocularis 122.5
  lung NEC 122.9
    granulosus 122.1
    multilocularis 122.6
  multilocularis 122.7
    liver 122.5
    specified site NEC 122.6
  orbit 122.9 [376.13]
    granulosus 122.3 [376.13]
    multilocularis 122.6 [376.13]
  specified site NEC 122.9
    granulosus 122.3
    multilocularis 122.6 [376.13]
  thyroid NEC 122.9
    granulosus 122.2
    multilocularis 122.6
**Echinorhynchiasis** 127.7
**Echinostomiasis** 121.8
**Echolalia** 784.69
**ECHO virus infection** NEC 079.1
**Eclampsia, eclamptic** (coma) (convulsions) (delirium) 780.39
  female, child-bearing age NEC — *see* Eclampsia, pregnancy
  gravidarum — *see* Eclampsia, pregnancy
  male 780.39
  not associated with pregnancy or childbirth 780.39
  pregnancy, childbirth, or puerperium 642.6 ☑
    with pre-existing hypertension 642.7 ☑
    affecting fetus or newborn 760.0
  uremic 586
**Eclipse blindness** (total) 363.31

**Economic circumstance affecting care**
V60.9
specified type NEC V60.8
**Economo's disease** (encephalitis lethargica) 049.8
**Ectasia, ectasis**
aorta (see also Aneurysm, aorta) 441.9
ruptured 441.5
breast 610.4
capillary 448.9
cornea (marginal) (postinfectional) 371.71
duct (mammary) 610.4
gastric antral vascular (GAVE) 537.82 ●
with hemorrhage 537.83 ●
without hemorrhage 537.82 ●
kidney 593.89
mammary duct (gland) 610.4
papillary 448.9
renal 593.89
salivary gland (duct) 527.8
scar, cornea 371.71
sclera 379.11
**Ecthyma** 686.8
contagiosum 051.2
gangrenosum 686.09
infectiosum 051.2
**Ectocardia** 746.87
**Ectodermal dysplasia, congenital** 757.31
**Ectodermosis erosiva pluriorificialis** 695.1
**Ectopic, ectopia** (congenital) 759.89
abdominal viscera 751.8
due to defect in anterior abdominal wall 756.79
ACTH syndrome 255.0
adrenal gland 759.1
anus 751.5
auricular beats 427.61
beats 427.60
bladder 753.5
bone and cartilage in lung 748.69
brain 742.4
breast tissue 757.6
cardiac 746.87
cerebral 742.4
cordis 746.87
endometrium 617.9
gallbladder 751.69
gastric mucosa 750.7
gestation — see Pregnancy, ectopic
heart 746.87
hormone secretion NEC 259.3
hyperparathyroidism 259.3
kidney (crossed) (intrathoracic) (pelvis) 753.3
in pregnancy or childbirth 654.4 ☑
causing obstructed labor 660.2 ☑
lens 743.37
lentis 743.37
mole — see Pregnancy, ectopic
organ or site NEC — see Malposition, congenital
ovary 752.0
pancreas, pancreatic tissue 751.7
pregnancy — see Pregnancy, ectopic
pupil 364.75
renal 753.3
sebaceous glands of mouth 750.26
secretion
ACTH 255.0
adrenal hormone 259.3
adrenalin 259.3
adrenocorticotropin 255.0
antidiuretic hormone (ADH) 259.3
epinephrine 259.3
hormone NEC 259.3
norepinephrine 259.3
pituitary (posterior) 259.3
spleen 759.0
testis 752.51
thyroid 759.2
ureter 753.4

**Ectopic, ectopia** — continued
ventricular beats 427.69
vesicae 753.5
**Ectrodactyly** 755.4
finger (see also Absence, finger, congenital) 755.29
toe (see also Absence, toe, congenital) 755.39
**Ectromelia** 755.4
lower limb 755.30
upper limb 755.20
**Ectropion** 374.10
anus 569.49
cervix 622.0
with mention of cervicitis 616.0
cicatricial 374.14
congenital 743.62
eyelid 374.10
cicatricial 374.14
congenital 743.62
mechanical 374.12
paralytic 374.12
senile 374.11
spastic 374.13
iris (pigment epithelium) 364.54
lip (congenital) 750.26
acquired 528.5
mechanical 374.12
paralytic 374.12
rectum 569.49
senile 374.11
spastic 374.13
urethra 599.84
uvea 364.54
**Eczema** (acute) (allergic) (chronic) (erythematous) (fissum) (occupational) (rubrum) (squamous) 692.9
asteatotic 706.8
atopic 691.8
contact NEC 692.9
dermatitis NEC 692.9
due to specified cause — see Dermatitis, due to
dyshidrotic 705.81
external ear 380.22
flexural 691.8
gouty 274.89
herpeticum 054.0
hypertrophicum 701.8
hypostatic — see Varicose, vein
impetiginous 684
infantile (acute) (chronic) (due to any substance) (intertriginous) (seborrheic) 690.12
intertriginous NEC 692.9
infantile 690.12
intrinsic 691.8
lichenified NEC 692.9
marginatum 110.3
nummular 692.9
pustular 686.8
seborrheic 690.18
infantile 690.12
solare 692.72
stasis (lower extremity) 454.1
ulcerated 454.2
vaccination, vaccinatum 999.0
varicose (lower extremity) — see Varicose, vein
verrucosum callosum 698.3
**Eczematoid, exudative** 691.8
**Eddowes' syndrome** (brittle bones and blue sclera) 756.51
**Edema, edematous** 782.3
with nephritis (see also Nephrosis) 581.9
allergic 995.1
angioneurotic (allergic) (any site) (with urticaria) 995.1
hereditary 277.6
angiospastic 443.9
Berlin's (traumatic) 921.3
brain 348.5
due to birth injury 767.8
fetus or newborn 767.8
cardiac (see also Failure, heart) 428.0

**Edema, edematous** — continued
cardiovascular (see also Failure, heart) 428.0
cerebral — see Edema, brain
cerebrospinal vessel — see Edema, brain
cervix (acute) (uteri) 622.8
puerperal, postpartum 674.8 ☑
chronic hereditary 757.0
circumscribed, acute 995.1
hereditary 277.6
complicating pregnancy (gestational) 646.1 ☑
with hypertension — see Toxemia, of pregnancy
conjunctiva 372.73
connective tissue 782.3
cornea 371.20
due to contact lenses 371.24
idiopathic 371.21
secondary 371.22
cystoid macular 362.53
due to
lymphatic obstruction — see Edema, lymphatic
salt retention 276.0
epiglottis — see Edema, glottis
essential, acute 995.1
hereditary 277.6
extremities, lower — see Edema, legs
eyelid NEC 374.82
familial, hereditary (legs) 757.0
famine 262
fetus or newborn 778.5
genital organs
female 629.89
male 608.86
gestational 646.1 ☑
with hypertension — see Toxemia, of pregnancy
glottis, glottic, glottides (obstructive) (passive) 478.6
allergic 995.1
hereditary 277.6
due to external agent — see Condition, respiratory, acute, due to specified agent
heart (see also Failure, heart) 428.0
newborn 779.89
heat 992.7
hereditary (legs) 757.0
inanition 262
infectious 782.3
intracranial 348.5
due to injury at birth 767.8
iris 364.89
joint (see also Effusion, joint) 719.0 ☑
larynx (see also Edema, glottis) 478.6
legs 782.3
due to venous obstruction 459.2
hereditary 757.0
localized 782.3
due to venous obstruction 459.2
lower extremity 459.2
lower extremities — see Edema, legs
lung 514
acute 518.4
with heart disease or failure (see also Failure, ventricular, left) 428.1
congestive 428.0
chemical (due to fumes or vapors) 506.1
due to
external agent(s) NEC 508.9
specified NEC 508.8
fumes and vapors (chemical) (inhalation) 506.1
radiation 508.0
chemical (acute) 506.1
chronic 506.4
chronic 514
chemical (due to fumes or vapors) 506.4
due to
external agent(s) NEC 508.9

**Edema, edematous** — continued
lung — continued
chronic — continued
due to — continued
external agent(s) — continued
specified NEC 508.8
fumes or vapors (chemical) (inhalation) 506.4
radiation 508.1
due to
external agent 508.9
specified NEC 508.8
high altitude 993.2
near drowning 994.1
postoperative 518.4
terminal 514
lymphatic 457.1
due to mastectomy operation 457.0
macula 362.83
cystoid 362.53
diabetic 250.5 ☑ [362.07]
malignant (see also Gangrene, gas) 040.0
Milroy's 757.0
nasopharynx 478.25
neonatorum 778.5
nutritional (newborn) 262
with dyspigmentation, skin and hair 260
optic disc or nerve — see Papilledema
orbit 376.33
circulatory 459.89
palate (soft) (hard) 528.9
pancreas 577.8
penis 607.83
periodic 995.1
hereditary 277.6
pharynx 478.25
pitting 782.3
pulmonary — see Edema, lung
Quincke's 995.1
hereditary 277.6
renal (see also Nephrosis) 581.9
retina (localized) (macular) (peripheral) 362.83
cystoid 362.53
diabetic 250.5 ☑ [362.07]
salt 276.0
scrotum 608.86
seminal vesicle 608.86
spermatic cord 608.86
spinal cord 336.1
starvation 262
stasis (see also Hypertension, venous) 459.30
subconjunctival 372.73
subglottic (see also Edema, glottis) 478.6
supraglottic (see also Edema, glottis) 478.6
testis 608.86
toxic NEC 782.3
traumatic NEC 782.3
tunica vaginalis 608.86
vas deferens 608.86
vocal cord — see Edema, glottis
vulva (acute) 624.8
**Edentia** (complete) (partial) — see also Absence, tooth 520.0
acquired (see also Edentulism) 525.40
due to
caries 525.13
extraction 525.10
periodontal disease 525.12
specified NEC 525.19
trauma 525.11
causing malocclusion 524.30
congenital (deficiency of tooth buds) 520.0
**Edentulism** 525.40
complete 525.40
class I 525.41
class II 525.42
class III 525.43
class IV 525.44

**Edentulism** — *continued*
  partial 525.50
    class I 525.51
    class II 525.52
    class III 525.53
    class IV 525.54
**Edsall's disease** 992.2
**Educational handicap** V62.3
**Edwards' syndrome** 758.2
**Effect, adverse** NEC
  abnormal gravitational (G) forces or
    states 994.9
  air pressure — *see* Effect, adverse,
    atmospheric pressure
  altitude (high) — *see* Effect, adverse,
    high altitude
  anesthetic
    in labor and delivery NEC 668.9 ☑
      affecting fetus or newborn 763.5
  antitoxin — *see* Complications, vacci-
    nation
  atmospheric pressure 993.9
    due to explosion 993.4
    high 993.3
    low — *see* Effect, adverse, high al-
      titude
    specified effect NEC 993.8
  biological, correct substance properly
    administered (*see also* Effect,
    adverse, drug) 995.20
  blood (derivatives) (serum) (transfu-
    sion) — *see* Complications,
    transfusion
  chemical substance NEC 989.9
    specified — *see* Table of Drugs and
      Chemicals
  cobalt, radioactive (*see also* Effect,
    adverse, radioactive substance)
    990
  cold (temperature) (weather) 991.9
    chilblains 991.5
    frostbite — *see* Frostbite
    specified effect NEC 991.8
  drugs and medicinals 995.20
    correct substance properly admin-
      istered 995.20
    overdose or wrong substance given
      or taken 977.9
      specified drug — *see* Table of
        Drugs and Chemicals
  electric current (shock) 994.8
    burn — *see* Burn, by site
  electricity (electrocution) (shock) 994.8
    burn — *see* Burn, by site
  exertion (excessive) 994.5
  exposure 994.9
    exhaustion 994.4
  external cause NEC 994.9
  fallout (radioactive) NEC 990
  fluoroscopy NEC 990
  foodstuffs
    allergic reaction (*see also* Allergy,
      food) 693.1
    anaphylactic shock due to food
      NEC 995.60
    noxious 988.9
      specified type NEC (*see also*
        Poisoning, by name of
        noxious foodstuff) 988.8
  gases, fumes, or vapors — *see* Table
    of Drugs and Chemicals
  glue (airplane) sniffing 304.6 ☑
  heat — *see* Heat
  high altitude NEC 993.2
    anoxia 993.2
    on
      ears 993.0
      sinuses 993.1
    polycythemia 289.0
  hot weather — *see* Heat
  hunger 994.2
  immersion, foot 991.4
  immunization — *see* Complications,
    vaccination
  immunological agents — *see* Compli-
    cations, vaccination

**Effect, adverse** — *continued*
  implantation (removable) of isotope or
    radium NEC 990
  infrared (radiation) (rays) NEC 990
    burn — *see* Burn, by site
    dermatitis or eczema 692.82
  infusion — *see* Complications, infu-
    sion
  ingestion or injection of isotope (ther-
    apeutic) NEC 990
  irradiation NEC (*see also* Effect, ad-
    verse, radiation) 990
  isotope (radioactive) NEC 990
  lack of care (child) (infant) (newborn)
    995.52
    adult 995.84
  lightning 994.0
    burn — *see* Burn, by site
  Lirugin — *see* Complications, vaccina-
    tion
  medicinal substance, correct, properly
    administered (*see also* Effect,
    adverse, drugs) 995.20
  mesothorium NEC 990
  motion 994.6
  noise, inner ear 388.10
  other drug, medicinal and biological
    substance 995.29
  overheated places — *see* Heat
  polonium NEC 990
  psychosocial, of work environment
    V62.1
  radiation (diagnostic) (fallout) (in-
    frared) (natural source) (thera-
    peutic) (tracer) (ultraviolet) (x-
    ray) NEC 990
    with pulmonary manifestations
      acute 508.0
      chronic 508.1
    dermatitis or eczema 692.82
      due to sun NEC (*see also* Der-
        matitis, due to, sun)
        692.70
    fibrosis of lungs 508.1
    maternal with suspected damage
      to fetus affecting manage-
      ment of pregnancy 655.6 ☑
    pneumonitis 508.0
  radioactive substance NEC 990
    dermatitis or eczema 692.82
  radioactivity NEC 990
  radiotherapy NEC 990
    dermatitis or eczema 692.82
  radium NEC 990
  reduced temperature 991.9
    frostbite — *see* Frostbite
    immersion, foot (hand) 991.4
    specified effect NEC 991.8
  roentgenography NEC 990
  roentgenoscopy NEC 990
  roentgen rays NEC 990
  serum (prophylactic) (therapeutic)
    NEC 999.5
  specified NEC 995.89
    external cause NEC 994.9
  strangulation 994.7
  submersion 994.1
  teletherapy NEC 990
  thirst 994.3
  transfusion — *see* Complications,
    transfusion
  ultraviolet (radiation) (rays) NEC 990
    burn (*see also* Burn, by site)
      from sun (*see also* Sunburn)
        692.71
    dermatitis or eczema 692.82
      due to sun NEC (*see also* Der-
        matitis, due to, sun)
        692.70
  uranium NEC 990
  vaccine (any) — *see* Complications,
    vaccination
  weightlessness 994.9
  whole blood (*see also* Complications,
    transfusion)

**Effect, adverse** — *continued*
  whole blood (*see also* Complications,
    transfusion) — *continued*
    overdose or wrong substance given
      (*see also* Table of Drugs and
      Chemicals) 964.7
  working environment V62.1
  x-rays NEC 990
    dermatitis or eczema 692.82
**Effect, remote**
  of cancer — *see* condition
**Effects, late** — *see* Late, effect (of)
**Effluvium, telogen** 704.02
**Effort**
  intolerance 306.2
  syndrome (aviators) (psychogenic)
    306.2
**Effusion**
  amniotic fluid (*see also* Rupture,
    membranes, premature)
    658.1 ☑
  brain (serous) 348.5
  bronchial (*see also* Bronchitis) 490
  cerebral 348.5
  cerebrospinal (*see also* Meningitis)
    322.9
    vessel 348.5
  chest — *see* Effusion, pleura
  intracranial 348.5
  joint 719.00
    ankle 719.07
    elbow 719.02
    foot 719.07
    hand 719.04
    hip 719.05
    knee 719.06
    multiple sites 719.09
    pelvic region 719.05
    shoulder (region) 719.01
    specified site NEC 719.08
    wrist 719.03
  meninges (*see also* Meningitis) 322.9
  pericardium, pericardial (*see also*
    Pericarditis) 423.9
    acute 420.90
  peritoneal (chronic) 568.82
  pleura, pleurisy, pleuritic, pleuroperi-
    cardial 511.9
    bacterial, nontuberculous 511.1
    fetus or newborn 511.9
    malignant 197.2
    nontuberculous 511.9
      bacterial 511.1
    pneumococcal 511.1
    staphylococcal 511.1
    streptococcal 511.1
    traumatic 862.29
      with open wound 862.39
    tuberculous (*see also* Tuberculosis,
      pleura) 012.0 ☑
      primary progressive 010.1 ☑
  pulmonary — *see* Effusion, pleura
  spinal (*see also* Meningitis) 322.9
  thorax, thoracic — *see* Effusion,
    pleura
**Egg** (oocyte) (ovum)
  donor V59.70
    over age 35 V59.73
      anonymous recipient V59.73
      designated recipient V59.74
    under age 35 V59.71
      anonymous recipient V59.71
      designated recipient V59.72
**Eggshell nails** 703.8
  congenital 757.5
**Ego-dystonic**
  homosexuality 302.0
  lesbianism 302.0
  sexual orientation 302.0
**Egyptian splenomegaly** 120.1
**Ehlers-Danlos syndrome** 756.83
**Ehrlichiosis** 082.40
  chaffeensis 082.41
  specified type NEC 082.49
**Eichstedt's disease** (pityriasis versicolor)
  111.0

**Eisenmenger's complex or syndrome**
  (ventricular septal defect) 745.4
**Ejaculation, semen**
  painful 608.89
    psychogenic 306.59
  premature 302.75
  retrograde 608.87
**Ekbom syndrome** (restless legs) 333.94
**Ekman's syndrome** (brittle bones and
  blue sclera) 756.51
**Elastic skin** 756.83
  acquired 701.8
**Elastofibroma** (M8820/0) — *see* Neoplasm, connective tissue, benign
**Elastoidosis**
  cutanea nodularis 701.8
  cutis cystica et comedonica 701.8
**Elastoma** 757.39
  juvenile 757.39
  Miescher's (elastosis perforans serpig-
    inosa) 701.1
**Elastomyofibrosis** 425.3
**Elastosis** 701.8
  atrophicans 701.8
  perforans serpiginosa 701.1
  reactive perforating 701.1
  senilis 701.8
  solar (actinic) 692.74
**Elbow** — *see* condition
**Electric**
  current, electricity, effects (concus-
    sion) (fatal) (nonfatal) (shock)
    994.8
    burn — *see* Burn, by site
  feet (foot) syndrome 266.2
**Electrocution** 994.8
**Electrolyte imbalance** 276.9
  with
    abortion — *see* Abortion, by type,
      with metabolic disorder
    ectopic pregnancy (*see also* cate-
      gories 633.0–633.9) 639.4
    hyperemesis gravidarum (before 22
      completed weeks gestation)
      643.1 ☑
    molar pregnancy (*see also* cate-
      gories 630–632) 639.4
  following
    abortion 639.4
    ectopic or molar pregnancy 639.4
**Elephantiasis** (nonfilarial) 457.1
  arabicum (*see also* Infestation, filarial)
    125.9
  congenita hereditaria 757.0
  congenital (any site) 757.0
  due to
    Brugia (malayi) 125.1
    mastectomy operation 457.0
    Wuchereria (bancrofti) 125.0
      malayi 125.1
  eyelid 374.83
  filarial (*see also* Infestation, filarial)
    125.9
  filariensis (*see also* Infestation, filarial)
    125.9
  gingival 523.8
  glandular 457.1
  graecorum 030.9
  lymphangiectatic 457.1
  lymphatic vessel 457.1
    due to mastectomy operation 457.0
  neuromatosa 237.71
  postmastectomy 457.0
  scrotum 457.1
  streptococcal 457.1
  surgical 997.99
    postmastectomy 457.0
  telangiectodes 457.1
  vulva (nonfilarial) 624.8
**Elephant man syndrome** 237.71
**Elevated** — *see* Elevation
**Elevation**
  17-ketosteroids 791.9
  acid phosphatase 790.5
  alkaline phosphatase 790.5
  amylase 790.5

**Elevation** — continued
  antibody titers 795.79
  basal metabolic rate (BMR) 794.7
  blood pressure (see also Hypertension) 401.9
    reading (incidental) (isolated) (nonspecific), no diagnosis of hypertension 796.2
  blood sugar 790.29
  body temperature (of unknown origin) (see also Pyrexia) 780.6
  cancer antigen 125 [CA 125] 795.82
  carcinoembryonic antigen [CEA] 795.81
  cholesterol 272.0
    with triglycerides 272.2
  conjugate, eye 378.81
  C-reactive protein (CRP) 790.95
  CRP (C-reactive protein) 790.95
  diaphragm, congenital 756.6
  glucose
    fasting 790.21
    tolerance test 790.22
  immunoglobulin level 795.79
  indolacetic acid 791.9
  lactic acid dehydrogenase (LDH) level 790.4
  leukocytes 288.60
  lipase 790.5
  lipoprotein a level 272.8
  liver function test (LFT) 790.6
    alkaline phosphatase 790.5
    aminotransferase 790.4
    bilirubin 782.4
    hepatic enzyme NEC 790.5
    lactate dehydrogenase 790.4
  lymphocytes 288.61
  prostate specific antigen (PSA) 790.93
  renin 790.99
    in hypertension (see also Hypertension, renovascular) 405.91
  Rh titer 999.7
  scapula, congenital 755.52
  sedimentation rate 790.1
  SGOT 790.4
  SGPT 790.4
  transaminase 790.4
  triglycerides 272.1
    with cholesterol 272.2
  vanillylmandelic acid 791.9
  venous pressure 459.89
  VMA 791.9
  white blood cell count 288.60
    specified NEC 288.69
**Elliptocytosis** (congenital) (hereditary) 282.1
  Hb-C (disease) 282.7
  hemoglobin disease 282.7
  sickle-cell (disease) 282.60
    trait 282.5
**Ellison-Zollinger syndrome** (gastric hypersecretion with pancreatic islet cell tumor) 251.5
**Ellis-van Creveld disease or syndrome** (chondroectodermal dysplasia) 756.55
**Elongation, elongated** (congenital) — see also Distortion
  bone 756.9
  cervix (uteri) 752.49
    acquired 622.6
    hypertrophic 622.6
  colon 751.5
  common bile duct 751.69
  cystic duct 751.69
  frenulum, penis 752.69
  labia minora, acquired 624.8
  ligamentum patellae 756.89
  petiolus (epiglottidis) 748.3
  styloid bone (process) 733.99
  tooth, teeth 520.2
  uvula 750.26
    acquired 528.9
**Elschnig bodies or pearls** 366.51
**El Tor cholera** 001.1
**Emaciation** (due to malnutrition) 261

**Emancipation disorder** 309.22
**Embadomoniasis** 007.8
**Embarrassment heart, cardiac** — see Disease, heart
**Embedded tooth, teeth** 520.6
  root only 525.3
**Embolic** — see condition
**Embolism** 444.9
  with
    abortion — see Abortion, by type, with embolism
    ectopic pregnancy (see also categories 633.0–633.9) 639.6
    molar pregnancy (see also categories 630–632) 639.6
  air (any site) 958.0
    with
      abortion — see Abortion, by type, with embolism
      ectopic pregnancy (see also categories 633.0–633.9) 639.6
      molar pregnancy (see also categories 630–632) 639.6
    due to implanted device — see Complications, due to (presence of) any device, implant, or graft classified to 996.0–996.5 NEC
    following
      abortion 639.6
      ectopic or molar pregnancy 639.6
      infusion, perfusion, or transfusion 999.1
    in pregnancy, childbirth, or puerperium 673.0 ✓
    traumatic 958.0
  amniotic fluid (pulmonary) 673.1 ✓
    with
      abortion — see Abortion, by type, with embolism
      ectopic pregnancy (see also categories 633.0–633.9) 639.6
      molar pregnancy (see also categories 630–632) 639.6
    following
      abortion 639.6
      ectopic or molar pregnancy 639.6
  aorta, aortic 444.1
    abdominal 444.0
    bifurcation 444.0
    saddle 444.0
    thoracic 444.1
  artery 444.9
    auditory, internal 433.8 ✓
    basilar (see also Occlusion, artery, basilar) 433.0 ✓
    bladder 444.89
    carotid (common) (internal) (see also Occlusion, artery, carotid) 433.1 ✓
    cerebellar (anterior inferior) (posterior inferior) (superior) 433.8 ✓
    cerebral (see also Embolism, brain) 434.1 ✓
    choroidal (anterior) 433.8 ✓
    communicating posterior 433.8 ✓
    coronary (see also Infarct, myocardium) 410.9 ✓
      without myocardial infarction 411.81
    extremity 444.22
      lower 444.22
      upper 444.21
    hypophyseal 433.8 ✓
    mesenteric (with gangrene) 557.0
    ophthalmic (see also Occlusion, retina) 362.30
    peripheral 444.22
    pontine 433.8 ✓
    precerebral NEC — see Occlusion, artery, precerebral

**Embolism** — continued
  artery — continued
    pulmonary — see Embolism, pulmonary
    pyemic 449 ●
      pulmonary 415.12 ●
    renal 593.81
    retinal (see also Occlusion, retina) 362.30
    septic 449 ●
      pulmonary 415.12 ●
    specified site NEC 444.89
    vertebral (see also Occlusion, artery, vertebral) 433.2 ✓
  auditory, internal 433.8 ✓
  basilar (artery) (see also Occlusion, artery, basilar) 433.0 ✓
  birth, mother — see Embolism, obstetrical
  blood-clot
    with
      abortion — see Abortion, by type, with embolism
      ectopic pregnancy (see also categories 633.0–633.9) 639.6
      molar pregnancy (see also categories 630–632) 639.6
    following
      abortion 639.6
      ectopic or molar pregnancy 639.6
    in pregnancy, childbirth, or puerperium 673.2 ✓
  brain 434.1 ✓
    with
      abortion — see Abortion, by type, with embolism
      ectopic pregnancy (see also categories 633.0–633.9) 639.6
      molar pregnancy (see also categories 630–632) 639.6
    following
      abortion 639.6
      ectopic or molar pregnancy 639.6
    late effect — see Late effect(s) (of) cerebrovascular disease
    puerperal, postpartum, childbirth 674.0 ✓
  capillary 448.9
  cardiac (see also Infarct, myocardium) 410.9 ✓
  carotid (artery) (common) (internal) (see also Occlusion, artery, carotid) 433.1 ✓
  cavernous sinus (venous) — see Embolism, intracranial venous sinus
  cerebral (see also Embolism, brain) 434.1 ✓
  cholesterol — see Atheroembolism
  choroidal (anterior) (artery) 433.8 ✓
  coronary (artery or vein) (systemic) (see also Infarct, myocardium) 410.9 ✓
    without myocardial infarction 411.81
  due to (presence of) any device, implant, or graft classifiable to 996.0–996.5 — see Complications, due to (presence of) any device, implant, or graft classified to 996.0–996.5 NEC
  encephalomalacia (see also Embolism, brain) 434.1 ✓
  extremities 444.22
    lower 444.22
    upper 444.21
  eye 362.30
  fat (cerebral) (pulmonary) (systemic) 958.1
    with
      abortion — see Abortion, by type, with embolism

**Embolism** — continued
  fat — continued
    with — continued
      ectopic pregnancy (see also categories 633.0–633.9) 639.6
      molar pregnancy (see also categories 630–632) 639.6
      complicating delivery or puerperium 673.8 ✓
    following
      abortion 639.6
      ectopic or molar pregnancy 639.6
    in pregnancy, childbirth, or the puerperium 673.8 ✓
  femoral (artery) 444.22
    vein 453.8
      deep 453.41
  following
    abortion 639.6
    ectopic or molar pregnancy 639.6
    infusion, perfusion, or transfusion
      air 999.1
      thrombus 999.2
  heart (fatty) (see also Infarct, myocardium) 410.9 ✓
  hepatic (vein) 453.0
  iliac (artery) 444.81
  iliofemoral 444.81
  in pregnancy, childbirth, or puerperium (pulmonary) — see Embolism, obstetrical
  intestine (artery) (vein) (with gangrene) 557.0
  intracranial (see also Embolism, brain) 434.1 ✓
    venous sinus (any) 325
      late effect — see category 326
      nonpyogenic 437.6
        in pregnancy or puerperium 671.5 ✓
  kidney (artery) 593.81
  lateral sinus (venous) — see Embolism, intracranial venous sinus
  longitudinal sinus (venous) — see Embolism, intracranial venous sinus
  lower extremity 444.22
  lung (massive) — see Embolism, pulmonary
  meninges (see also Embolism, brain) 434.1 ✓
  mesenteric (artery) (with gangrene) 557.0
  multiple NEC 444.9
  obstetrical (pulmonary) 673.2 ✓
    air 673.0 ✓
    amniotic fluid (pulmonary) 673.1 ✓
    blood-clot 673.2 ✓
    cardiac 674.8 ✓
    fat 673.8 ✓
    heart 674.8 ✓
    pyemic 673.3 ✓
    septic 673.3 ✓
    specified NEC 674.8 ✓
  ophthalmic (see also Occlusion, retina) 362.30
  paradoxical NEC 444.9
  penis 607.82
  peripheral arteries NEC 444.22
    lower 444.22
    upper 444.21
  pituitary 253.8
  popliteal (artery) 444.22
  portal (vein) 452
  postoperative NEC 997.2
    cerebral 997.02
    mesenteric artery 997.71
    other vessels 997.79
    peripheral vascular 997.2
    pulmonary 415.11
      septic 415.12
    renal artery 997.72

**Embolism** — *continued*
  precerebral artery (*see also* Occlusion, artery, precerebral) 433.9 ☑
  puerperal — *see* Embolism, obstetrical
  pulmonary (artery) (vein) 415.19
    with
      abortion — *see* Abortion, by type, with embolism
      ectopic pregnancy (*see also* categories 633.0–633.9) 639.6
      molar pregnancy (*see also* categories 630–632) 639.6
    following
      abortion 639.6
      ectopic or molar pregnancy 639.6
    iatrogenic 415.11
    in pregnancy, childbirth, or puerperium — *see* Embolism, obstetrical
    postoperative 415.11
    septic 415.12 ●
  pyemic (multiple) ►(*see also* Septicemia)◄ 415.12 ▲
    with
      abortion — *see* Abortion, by type, with embolism
      ectopic pregnancy (*see also* categories 633.0–633.9) 639.6
      molar pregnancy (*see also* categories 630–632) 639.6
    Aerobacter aerogenes 415.12 ▲
    enteric gram-negative bacilli 415.12 ▲
    Enterobacter aerogenes 415.12 ▲
    Escherichia coli 415.12 ▲
    following
      abortion 639.6
      ectopic or molar pregnancy 639.6
    Hemophilus influenzae 415.12
    pneumococcal 415.12 ▲
    Proteus vulgaris 415.12 ▲
    Pseudomonas (aeruginosa) 415.12 ▲
    puerperal, postpartum, childbirth (any organism) 673.3 ☑
    Serratia 415.12 ▲
    specified organism NEC 415.12 ▲
    staphylococcal 415.12 ▲
      aureus 415.12 ▲
      specified organism NEC 415.12 ▲
    streptococcal 415.12 ▲
  renal (artery) 593.81
    vein 453.3
  retina, retinal (*see also* Occlusion, retina) 362.30
  saddle (aorta) 444.0
  septic 415.12 ●
    arterial 449
  septicemic — *see* Embolism, pyemic
  sinus — *see* Embolism, intracranial venous sinus
  soap
    with
      abortion — *see* Abortion, by type, with embolism
      ectopic pregnancy (*see also* categories 633.0–633.9) 639.6
      molar pregnancy (*see also* categories 630–632) 639.6
    following
      abortion 639.6
      ectopic or molar pregnancy 639.6
  spinal cord (nonpyogenic) 336.1
    in pregnancy or puerperium 671.5 ☑
    pyogenic origin 324.1

**Embolism** — *continued*
  spinal cord — *continued*
    pyogenic origin — *continued*
      late effect — *see* category 326
  spleen, splenic (artery) 444.89
  thrombus (thromboembolism) following infusion, perfusion, or transfusion 999.2
  upper extremity 444.21
  vein 453.9
    with inflammation or phlebitis — *see* Thrombophlebitis
    cerebral (*see also* Embolism, brain) 434.1 ☑
    coronary (*see also* Infarct, myocardium) 410.9 ☑
      without myocardial infarction 411.81
    hepatic 453.0
    lower extremity 453.8
      deep 453.40
        calf 453.42
        distal (lower leg) 453.42
        femoral 453.41
        iliac 453.41
        lower leg 453.42
        peroneal 453.42
        popliteal 453.41
        proximal (upper leg) 453.41
        thigh 453.41
        tibial 453.42
    mesenteric (with gangrene) 557.0
    portal 452
    pulmonary — *see* Embolism, pulmonary
    renal 453.3
    specified NEC 453.8
      with inflammation or phlebitis — *see* Thrombophlebitis
    vena cava (inferior) (superior) 453.2
    vessels of brain (*see also* Embolism, brain) 434.1 ☑
**Embolization** — *see* Embolism
**Embolus** — *see* Embolism
**Embryoma (M9080/1)** — *see also* Neoplasm, by site, uncertain behavior
  benign (M9080/0) — *see* Neoplasm, by site, benign
  kidney (M8960/3) 189.0
  liver (M8970/3) 155.0
  malignant (M9080/3) (*see also* Neoplasm, by site, malignant)
    kidney (M8960/3) 189.0
    liver (M8970/3) 155.0
    testis (M9070/3) 186.9
      undescended 186.0
  testis (M9070/3) 186.9
    undescended 186.0
**Embryonic**
  circulation 747.9
  heart 747.9
  vas deferens 752.89
**Embryopathia NEC** 759.9
**Embryotomy, fetal** 763.89
**Embryotoxon** 743.43
  interfering with vision 743.42
**Emesis** — *see also* Vomiting
  gravidarum — *see* Hyperemesis, gravidarum
**Emissions, nocturnal** (semen) 608.89
**Emotional**
  crisis — *see* Crisis, emotional
  disorder (*see also* Disorder, mental) 300.9
  instability (excessive) 301.3
  overlay — *see* Reaction, adjustment
  upset 300.9
**Emotionality, pathological** 301.3
**Emotogenic disease** — *see also* Disorder, psychogenic 306.9

**Emphysema** (atrophic) (centriacinar) (centrilobular) (chronic) (diffuse) (essential) (hypertrophic) (interlobular) (lung) (obstructive) (panlobular) (paracicatricial) (paracinar) (postural) (pulmonary) (senile) (subpleural) (traction) (unilateral) (unilobular) (vesicular) 492.8
  with bronchitis
    chronic 491.20
      with
        acute bronchitis 491.22
        exacerbation (acute) 491.21
  bullous (giant) 492.0
  cellular tissue 958.7
    surgical 998.81
  compensatory 518.2
  congenital 770.2
  conjunctiva 372.89
  connective tissue 958.7
    surgical 998.81
  due to fumes or vapors 506.4
  eye 376.89
  eyelid 374.85
    surgical 998.81
    traumatic 958.7
  fetus or newborn (interstitial) (mediastinal) (unilobular) 770.2
  heart 416.9
  interstitial 518.1
    congenital 770.2
    fetus or newborn 770.2
  laminated tissue 958.7
    surgical 998.81
  mediastinal 518.1
    fetus or newborn 770.2
  newborn (interstitial) (mediastinal) (unilobular) 770.2
  obstructive diffuse with fibrosis 492.8
  orbit 376.89
  subcutaneous 958.7
    due to trauma 958.7
    nontraumatic 518.1
    surgical 998.81
  surgical 998.81
  thymus (gland) (congenital) 254.8
  traumatic 958.7
  tuberculous (*see also* Tuberculosis, pulmonary) 011.9 ☑
**Employment examination** (certification) V70.5
**Empty sella (turcica) syndrome** 253.8
**Empyema** (chest) (diaphragmatic) (double) (encapsulated) (general) (interlobar) (lung) (medial) (necessitatis) (perforating chest wall) (pleura) (pneumococcal) (residual) (sacculated) (streptococcal) (supradiaphragmatic) 510.9
  with fistula 510.0
  accessory sinus (chronic) (*see also* Sinusitis) 473.9
  acute 510.9
    with fistula 510.0
  antrum (chronic) (*see also* Sinusitis, maxillary) 473.0
  brain (any part) (*see also* Abscess, brain) 324.0
  ethmoidal (sinus) (chronic) (*see also* Sinusitis, ethmoidal) 473.2
  extradural (*see also* Abscess, extradural) 324.9
  frontal (sinus) (chronic) (*see also* Sinusitis, frontal) 473.1
  gallbladder (*see also* Cholecystitis, acute) 575.0
  mastoid (process) (acute) (*see also* Mastoiditis, acute) 383.00
  maxilla, maxillary 526.4
    sinus (chronic) (*see also* Sinusitis, maxillary) 473.0
  nasal sinus (chronic) (*see also* Sinusitis) 473.9
  sinus (accessory) (nasal) (*see also* Sinusitis) 473.9

**Empyema** — *continued*
  sphenoidal (chronic) (sinus) (*see also* Sinusitis, sphenoidal) 473.3
  subarachnoid (*see also* Abscess, extradural) 324.9
  subdural (*see also* Abscess, extradural) 324.9
  tuberculous (*see also* Tuberculosis, pleura) 012.0 ☑
  ureter (*see also* Ureteritis) 593.89
  ventricular (*see also* Abscess, brain) 324.0
**Enameloma** 520.2
**Encephalitis** (bacterial) (chronic) (hemorrhagic) (idiopathic) (nonepidemic) (spurious) (subacute) 323.9
  acute (*see also* Encephalitis, viral)
    disseminated (postinfectious) NEC 136.9 *[323.61]*
      postimmunization or postvaccination 323.51
    inclusional 049.8
    inclusion body 049.8
    necrotizing 049.8
  arboviral, arbovirus NEC 064
  arthropod-borne (*see also* Encephalitis, viral, arthropod-borne) 064
  Australian X 062.4
  Bwamba fever 066.3
  California (virus) 062.5
  Central European 063.2
  Czechoslovakian 063.2
  Dawson's (inclusion body) 046.2
  diffuse sclerosing 046.2
  due to
    actinomycosis 039.8 *[323.41]*
    cat-scratch disease 078.3 *[323.01]*
    human herpesvirus NEC 058.29 ●
    human herpesvirus 6 058.21 ●
    human herpesvirus 7 058.29 ●
    infection classified elsewhere 136.9 *[323.41]*
    infectious mononucleosis 075 *[323.01]*
    malaria (*see also* Malaria) 084.6 *[323.2]*
    Negishi virus 064
    ornithosis 073.7 *[323.01]*
    prophylactic inoculation against smallpox 323.51
    rickettsiosis (*see also* Rickettsiosis) 083.9 *[323.1]*
    rubella 056.01
    toxoplasmosis (acquired) 130.0
      congenital (active) 771.2 *[323.41]*
    typhus (fever) (*see also* Typhus) 081.9 *[323.1]*
    vaccination (smallpox) 323.51
  Eastern equine 062.2
  endemic 049.8
  epidemic 049.8
  equine (acute) (infectious) (viral) 062.9
    Eastern 062.2
    Venezuelan 066.2
    Western 062.1
  Far Eastern 063.0
  following vaccination or other immunization procedure 323.51
  herpes 054.3
  human herpesvirus NEC 058.29 ●
  human herpesvirus 6 058.21 ●
  human herpesvirus 7 058.29 ●
  Ilheus (virus) 062.8
  inclusion body 046.2
  infectious (acute) (virus) NEC 049.8
  influenzal 487.8 *[323.41]*
    lethargic 049.8
  Japanese (B type) 062.0
  La Crosse 062.5
  Langat 063.8
  late effect — *see* Late, effect, encephalitis
  lead 984.9 *[323.71]*
  lethargic (acute) (infectious) (influenzal) 049.8

---

☑ Additional Digit Required — Refer to the Tabular List for Digit Selection        ⏷ Subterms under main terms may continue to next column or page

**Encephalitis** — *continued*
  lethargica 049.8
  louping ill 063.1
  lupus 710.0 *[323.81]*
  lymphatica 049.0
  Mengo 049.8
  meningococcal 036.1
  mumps 072.2
  Murray Valley 062.4
  myoclonic 049.8
  Negishi virus 064
  otitic NEC 382.4 *[323.41]*
  parasitic NEC 123.9 *[323.41]*
  periaxialis (concentrica) (diffusa) 341.1
  postchickenpox 052.0
  postexanthematous NEC
    057.9 *[323.62]*
  postimmunization 323.51
  postinfectious NEC 136.9 *[323.62]*
  postmeasles 055.0
  posttraumatic 323.81
  postvaccinal (smallpox) 323.51
  postvaricella 052.0
  postviral NEC 079.99 *[323.62]*
    postexanthematous 057.9 *[323.62]*
    specified NEC 057.8 *[323.62]*
  Powassan 063.8
  progressive subcortical (Binswanger's)
    290.12
  Rasmussen 323.81
  Rio Bravo 049.8
  rubella 056.01
  Russian
    autumnal 062.0
    spring-summer type (taiga) 063.0
  saturnine 984.9 *[323.71]*
  Semliki Forest 062.8
  serous 048
  slow-acting virus NEC 046.8
  specified cause NEC 323.81
  St. Louis type 062.3
  subacute sclerosing 046.2
  subcorticalis chronica 290.12
  summer 062.0
  suppurative 324.0
  syphilitic 094.81
    congenital 090.41
  tick-borne 063.9
  torula, torular 117.5 *[323.41]*
  toxic NEC 989.9 *[323.71]*
  toxoplasmic (acquired) 130.0
    congenital (active) 771.2 *[323.41]*
  trichinosis 124 *[323.41]*
  Trypanosomiasis (*see also* Trypanosomiasis) 086.9 *[323.2]*
  tuberculous (*see also* Tuberculosis)
    013.6 ☑
  type B (Japanese) 062.0
  type C 062.3
  van Bogaert's 046.2
  Venezuelan 066.2
  Vienna type 049.8
  viral, virus 049.9
    arthropod-borne NEC 064
      mosquito-borne 062.9
        Australian X disease 062.4
        California virus 062.5
        Eastern equine 062.2
        Ilheus virus 062.8
        Japanese (B type) 062.0
        Murray Valley 062.4
        specified type NEC 062.8
        St. Louis 062.3
        type B 062.0
        type C 062.3
        Western equine 062.1
      tick-borne 063.9
        biundulant 063.2
        Central European 063.2
        Czechoslovakian 063.2
        diphasic meningoencephalitis
          063.2
        Far Eastern 063.0
        Langat 063.8
        louping ill 063.1
        Powassan 063.8

**Encephalitis** — *continued*
  viral, virus — *continued*
    arthropod-borne — *continued*
      tick-borne — *continued*
        Russian spring-summer
          (taiga) 063.0
        specified type NEC 063.8
      vector unknown 064
      Western equine 062.1
    slow acting NEC 046.8
    specified type NEC 049.8
    vaccination, prophylactic (against)
      V05.0
  von Economo's 049.8
  Western equine 062.1
  West Nile type 066.41
**Encephalocele** 742.0
  orbit 376.81
**Encephalocystocele** 742.0
**Encephalomalacia** (brain) (cerebellar)
    (cerebral) (cerebrospinal) — *see also* Softening, brain 434.9 ☑
  due to
    hemorrhage (*see also* Hemorrhage,
      brain) 431
    recurrent spasm of artery 435.9
  embolic (cerebral) (*see also* Embolism,
    brain) 434.1 ☑
  subcorticalis chronicus arteriosclerotica 290.12
  thrombotic (*see also* Thrombosis,
    brain) 434.0 ☑
**Encephalomeningitis** — *see* Meningoencephalitis
**Encephalomeningocele** 742.0
**Encephalomeningomyelitis** — *see*
    Meningoencephalitis
**Encephalomeningopathy** — *see also*
    Meningoencephalitis 349.9
**Encephalomyelitis** (chronic) (granulomatous) (hemorrhagic necrotizing,
    acute) (myalgic, benign) — *see also*
    Encephalitis 323.9
  abortive disseminated 049.8
  acute disseminated (ADEM) (postinfectious) 136.9 *[323.61]*
    infectious 136.9 *[323.61]*
    noninfectious 323.81
    postimmunization 323.51
  due to
    cat-scratch disease 078.3 *[323.01]*
    infectious mononucleosis
      075 *[323.01]*
    ornithosis 073.7 *[323.01]*
    vaccination (any) 323.51
  equine (acute) (infectious) 062.9
    Eastern 062.2
    Venezuelan 066.2
    Western 062.1
  funicularis infectiosa 049.8
  late effect — *see* Late, effect, encephalitis
  Munch-Peterson's 049.8
  postchickenpox 052.0
  postimmunization 323.51
  postmeasles 055.0
  postvaccinal (smallpox) 323.51
  rubella 056.01
  specified cause NEC 323.81
  syphilitic 094.81
  West Nile 066.41
**Encephalomyelocele** 742.0
**Encephalomyelomeningitis** — *see*
    Meningoencephalitis
**Encephalomyeloneuropathy** 349.9
**Encephalomyelopathy** 349.9
  subacute necrotizing (infantile) 330.8
**Encephalomyeloradiculitis** (acute)
    357.0
**Encephalomyeloradiculoneuritis** (acute)
    357.0
**Encephalomyeloradiculopathy** 349.9
**Encephalomyocarditis** 074.23
**Encephalopathia hyperbilirubinemica,
    newborn** 774.7

**Encephalopathia hyperbilirubinemica,
    newborn** — *continued*
  due to isoimmunization (conditions
    classifiable to 773.0–773.2)
    773.4
**Encephalopathy** (acute) 348.30
  alcoholic 291.2
  anoxic — *see* Damage, brain, anoxic
  arteriosclerotic 437.0
    late effect — *see* Late effect(s) (of)
      cerebrovascular disease
  bilirubin, newborn 774.7
    due to isoimmunization 773.4
  congenital 742.9
  demyelinating (callosal) 341.8
  due to
    birth injury (intracranial) 767.8
    dialysis 294.8
      transient 293.9
    hyperinsulinism — *see* Hyperinsulinism
    influenza (virus) 487.8
    lack of vitamin (*see also* Deficiency,
      vitamin) 269.2
    nicotinic acid deficiency 291.2
    serum (nontherapeutic) (therapeutic) 999.5
    syphilis 094.81
    trauma (postconcussional) 310.2
      current (*see also* Concussion,
        brain) 850.9
        with skull fracture — *see*
          Fracture, skull, by site,
          with intracranial injury
    vaccination 323.51
  hepatic 572.2
  hyperbilirubinemic, newborn 774.7
    due to isoimmunization (conditions
      classifiable to 773.0–773.2)
      773.4
  hypertensive 437.2
  hypoglycemic 251.2
  hypoxic (*see also* Damage, brain,
    anoxic)
    ischemic (HIE) 768.7
  infantile cystic necrotizing (congenital)
    341.8
  lead 984.9 *[323.71]*
  leukopolio 330.0
  metabolic (*see also* Delirium) 348.31
    toxic 349.82
  necrotizing
    hemorrhagic 323.61
    subacute 330.8
  other specified type NEC 348.39
  pellagrous 265.2
  portal-systemic 572.2
  postcontusional 310.2
  posttraumatic 310.2
  saturnine 984.9 *[323.71]*
  septic 348.31
  spongioform, subacute (viral) 046.1
  subacute
    necrotizing 330.8
    spongioform 046.1
    viral, spongioform 046.1
  subcortical progressive (Schilder)
    341.1
    chronic (Binswanger's) 290.12
  toxic 349.82
    metabolic 349.82
  traumatic (postconcussional) 310.2
    current (*see also* Concussion,
      brain) 850.9
      with skull fracture — *see* Fracture, skull, by site, with
        intracranial injury
  vitamin B deficiency NEC 266.9
  Wernicke's (superior hemorrhagic polioencephalitis) 265.1
**Encephalorrhagia** — *see also* Hemorrhage, brain 432.9
  healed or old V12.54
  late effect — *see* Late effect(s) (of)
    cerebrovascular disease
**Encephalosis, posttraumatic** 310.2

**Enchondroma** (M9220/0) — *see also*
    Neoplasm, bone, benign
  multiple, congenital 756.4
**Enchondromatosis** (cartilaginous) (congenital) (multiple) 756.4
**Enchondroses, multiple** (cartilaginous)
    (congenital) 756.4
**Encopresis** — *see also* Incontinence, feces 787.6
  nonorganic origin 307.7
**Encounter for** — *see also* Admission for
    administrative purpose only V68.9
  referral of patient without examination or treatment V68.81
    specified purpose NEC V68.89
  chemotherapy, antineoplastic V58.11
  dialysis
    extracorporeal (renal) V56.0
    peritoneal V56.8
  disability examination V68.01          ●
  end-of-life care V66.7
  hospice care V66.7
  immunotherapy, antineoplastic
    V58.12
  palliative care V66.7
  paternity testing V70.4
  radiotherapy V58.0
  respirator [ventilator] dependence
    during
      mechanical failure V46.14
      power failure V46.12
    for weaning V46.13
  screening mammogram NEC V76.12
    for high-risk patient V76.11
  terminal care V66.7
  weaning from respirator [ventilator]
    V46.13
**Encystment** — *see* Cyst
**Endamebiasis** — *see* Amebiasis
**Endamoeba** — *see* Amebiasis
**Endarteritis** (bacterial, subacute) (infective) (septic) 447.6
  brain, cerebral or cerebrospinal 437.4
    late effect — *see* Late effect(s) (of)
      cerebrovascular disease
  coronary (artery) — *see* Arteriosclerosis, coronary
  deformans — *see* Arteriosclerosis
  embolic (*see also* Embolism) 444.9
  obliterans (*see also* Arteriosclerosis)
    pulmonary 417.8
  pulmonary 417.8
  retina 362.18
  senile — *see* Arteriosclerosis
  syphilitic 093.89
    brain or cerebral 094.89
    congenital 090.5
    spinal 094.89
  tuberculous (*see also* Tuberculosis)
    017.9 ☑
**Endemic** — *see* condition
**Endocarditis** (chronic) (indeterminate)
    (interstitial) (marantis) (nonbacterial thrombotic) (residual) (sclerotic)
    (sclerous) (senile) (valvular) 424.90
  with
    rheumatic fever (conditions classifiable to 390)
      active — *see* Endocarditis,
        acute, rheumatic
      inactive or quiescent (with
        chorea) 397.9
  acute or subacute 421.9
    rheumatic (aortic) (mitral) (pulmonary) (tricuspid) 391.1
      with chorea (acute) (rheumatic)
        (Sydenham's) 392.0
  aortic (heart) (nonrheumatic) (valve)
    424.1
    with
      mitral (valve) disease 396.9
        active or acute 391.1
          with chorea (acute)
            (rheumatic) (Sydenham's) 392.0
  bacterial 421.0

Endocarditis — *continued*
  aortic — *continued*
    with — *continued*
      rheumatic fever (conditions
          classifiable to 390)
        active — *see* Endocarditis,
            acute, rheumatic
        inactive or quiescent (with
            chorea) 395.9
          with mitral disease 396.9
      acute or subacute 421.9
      arteriosclerotic 424.1
      congenital 746.89
      hypertensive 424.1
      rheumatic (chronic) (inactive) 395.9
        with mitral (valve) disease 396.9
          active or acute 391.1
            with chorea (acute)
                (rheumatic) (Syden-
                ham's) 392.0
        active or acute 391.1
          with chorea (acute)
              (rheumatic) (Syden-
              ham's) 392.0
        specified cause, except rheumatic
            424.1
      syphilitic 093.22
    arteriosclerotic or due to arterioscle-
        sis 424.99
    atypical verrucous (Libman-Sacks)
        710.0 *[424.91]*
    bacterial (acute) (any valve) (chronic)
        (subacute) 421.0
    blastomycotic 116.0 *[421.1]*
    candidal 112.81
    congenital 425.3
    constrictive 421.0
    Coxsackie 074.22
    due to
      blastomycosis 116.0 *[421.1]*
      candidiasis 112.81
      Coxsackie (virus) 074.22
      disseminated lupus erythematosus
          710.0 *[424.91]*
      histoplasmosis (*see also* Histoplas-
          mosis) 115.94
      hypertension (benign) 424.99
      moniliasis 112.81
      prosthetic cardiac valve 996.61
      Q fever 083.0 *[421.1]*
      serratia marcescens 421.0
      typhoid (fever) 002.0 *[421.1]*
    fetal 425.3
    gonococcal 098.84
    hypertensive 424.99
    infectious or infective (acute) (any
        valve) (chronic) (subacute) 421.0
    lenta (acute) (any valve) (chronic)
        (subacute) 421.0
    Libman-Sacks 710.0 *[424.91]*
    Loeffler's (parietal fibroplastic) 421.0
    malignant (acute) (any valve) (chronic)
        (subacute) 421.0
    meningococcal 036.42
    mitral (chronic) (double) (fibroid)
        (heart) (inactive) (valve) (with
        chorea) 394.9
      with
        aortic (valve) disease 396.9
          active or acute 391.1
            with chorea (acute)
                (rheumatic) (Syden-
                ham's) 392.0
          rheumatic fever (conditions
              classifiable to 390)
            active — *see* Endocarditis,
                acute, rheumatic
            inactive or quiescent (with
                chorea) 394.9
              with aortic valve disease
                  396.9
        active or acute 391.1
          with chorea (acute) (rheumatic)
              (Sydenham's) 392.0
        bacterial 421.0
        arteriosclerotic 424.0

Endocarditis — *continued*
  mitral — *continued*
    congenital 746.89
    hypertensive 424.0
    nonrheumatic 424.0
      acute or subacute 421.9
    syphilitic 093.21
    monilial 112.81
    mycotic (acute) (any valve) (chronic)
        (subacute) 421.0
    pneumococcic (acute) (any valve)
        (chronic) (subacute) 421.0
    pulmonary (chronic) (heart) (valve)
        424.3
      with
        rheumatic fever (conditions
            classifiable to 390)
          active — *see* Endocarditis,
              acute, rheumatic
          inactive or quiescent (with
              chorea) 397.1
      acute or subacute 421.9
        rheumatic 391.1
          with chorea (acute)
              (rheumatic) (Syden-
              ham's) 392.0
    arteriosclerotic or due to arterioscle-
        rosis 424.3
    congenital 746.09
    hypertensive or due to hyperten-
        sion (benign) 424.3
    rheumatic (chronic) (inactive) (with
        chorea) 397.1
      active or acute 391.1
        with chorea (acute)
            (rheumatic) (Syden-
            ham's) 392.0
    syphilitic 093.24
    purulent (acute) (any valve) (chronic)
        (subacute) 421.0
    rheumatic (chronic) (inactive) (with
        chorea) 397.9
      active or acute (aortic) (mitral)
          (pulmonary) (tricuspid) 391.1
        with chorea (acute) (rheumatic)
            (Sydenham's) 392.0
    septic (acute) (any valve) (acute)
        (subacute) 421.0
    specified cause, except rheumatic
        424.99
    streptococcal (acute) (any valve)
        (chronic) (subacute) 421.0
    subacute — *see* Endocarditis, acute
    suppurative (any valve) (acute)
        (chronic) (subacute) 421.0
    syphilitic NEC 093.20
    toxic (*see also* Endocarditis, acute)
        421.9
    tricuspid (chronic) (heart) (inactive)
        (rheumatic) (valve) (with chorea)
        397.0
      with
        rheumatic fever (conditions
            classifiable to 390)
          active — *see* Endocarditis,
              acute, rheumatic
          inactive or quiescent (with
              chorea) 397.0
      active or acute 391.1
        with chorea (acute) (rheumatic)
            (Sydenham's) 392.0
    arteriosclerotic 424.2
    congenital 746.89
    hypertensive 424.2
    nonrheumatic 424.2
      acute or subacute 421.9
    specified cause, except rheumatic
        424.2
    syphilitic 093.23
    tuberculous (*see also* Tuberculosis)
        017.9 ☑ *[424.91]*
    typhoid 002.0 *[421.1]*
    ulcerative (acute) (any valve) (chronic)
        (subacute) 421.0
    vegetative (acute) (any valve) (chronic)
        (subacute) 421.0

Endocarditis — *continued*
  verrucous (acute) (any valve) (chronic)
      (subacute) NEC 710.0 *[424.91]*
    nonbacterial 710.0 *[424.91]*
    nonrheumatic 710.0 *[424.91]*
Endocardium, endocardial — *see also*
    condition
  cushion defect 745.60
    specified type NEC 745.69
Endocervicitis — *see also* Cervicitis
    616.0
  due to
    intrauterine (contraceptive) device
        996.65
  gonorrheal (acute) 098.15
    chronic or duration of 2 months or
        over 098.35
  hyperplastic 616.0
  syphilitic 095.8
  trichomonal 131.09
  tuberculous (*see also* Tuberculosis)
      016.7 ☑
Endocrine — *see* condition
Endocrinopathy, pluriglandular 258.9
Endodontitis 522.0
End-of-life care V66.7
Endomastoiditis — *see also* Mastoiditis
    383.9
Endometrioma 617.9
Endometriosis 617.9
  appendix 617.5
  bladder 617.8
  bowel 617.5
  broad ligament 617.3
  cervix 617.0
  colon 617.5
  cul-de-sac (Douglas') 617.3
  exocervix 617.0
  fallopian tube 617.2
  female genital organ NEC 617.8
  gallbladder 617.8
  in scar of skin 617.6
  internal 617.0
  intestine 617.5
  lung 617.8
  myometrium 617.0
  ovary 617.1
  parametrium 617.3
  pelvic peritoneum 617.3
  peritoneal (pelvic) 617.3
  rectovaginal septum 617.4
  rectum 617.5
  round ligament 617.3
  skin 617.6
  specified site NEC 617.8
  stromal (M8931/1) 236.0
  umbilicus 617.8
  uterus 617.0
    internal 617.0
  vagina 617.4
  vulva 617.8
Endometritis (nonspecific) (purulent)
    (septic) (suppurative) 615.9
  with
    abortion — *see* Abortion, by type,
        with sepsis
    ectopic pregnancy (*see also* cate-
        gories 633.0–633.9) 639.0
    molar pregnancy (*see also* cate-
        gories 630–632) 639.0
  acute 615.0
  blennorrhagic 098.16
    acute 098.16
    chronic or duration of 2 months or
        over 098.36
  cervix, cervical (*see also* Cervicitis)
      616.0
    hyperplastic 616.0
  chronic 615.1
  complicating pregnancy 646.6 ☑
    affecting fetus or newborn 760.8
  decidual 615.9
  following
    abortion 639.0
    ectopic or molar pregnancy 639.0
  gonorrheal (acute) 098.16

Endometritis — *continued*
  gonorrheal — *continued*
    chronic or duration of 2 months or
        over 098.36
  hyperplastic (*see also* Hyperplasia,
      endometrium) 621.30
    cervix 616.0
  polypoid — *see* Endometritis, hyper-
      plastic
  puerperal, postpartum, childbirth
      670.0 ☑
  senile (atrophic) 615.9
  subacute 615.0
  tuberculous (*see also* Tuberculosis)
      016.7 ☑
Endometrium — *see* condition
Endomyocardiopathy, South African
    425.2
Endomyocarditis — *see* Endocarditis
Endomyofibrosis 425.0
Endomyometritis — *see also* Endometri-
    tis 615.9
Endopericarditis — *see* Endocarditis
Endoperineuritis — *see* Disorder, nerve
Endophlebitis — *see also* Phlebitis 451.9
  leg 451.2
    deep (vessels) 451.19
    superficial (vessels) 451.0
  portal (vein) 572.1
  retina 362.18
  specified site NEC 451.89
  syphilitic 093.89
Endophthalmia — *see also* Endoph-
    thalmitis 360.00
  gonorrheal 098.42
Endophthalmitis (globe) (infective)
    (metastatic) (purulent) (subacute)
    360.00
  acute 360.01
  bleb associated 379.63
  chronic 360.03
  parasitic 360.13
  phacoanaphylactic 360.19
  specified type NEC 360.19
  sympathetic 360.11
Endosalpingioma (M9111/1) 236.2
Endosalpingiosis 629.89
Endosteitis — *see* Osteomyelitis
Endothelioma, bone (M9260/3) — *see*
    Neoplasm, bone, malignant
Endotheliosis 287.8
  hemorrhagic infectional 287.8
Endotoxemia — code to condition
Endotoxic shock 785.52
Endotrachelitis — *see also* Cervicitis
    616.0
Enema rash 692.89
Engelmann's disease (diaphyseal sclero-
    sis) 756.9
Engel-von Recklinghausen disease or
    syndrome (osteitis fibrosa cystica)
    252.01
English disease — *see also* Rickets
    268.0
Engman's disease (infectious eczematoid
    dermatitis) 690.8
Engorgement
  breast 611.79
    newborn 778.7
    puerperal, postpartum 676.2 ☑
  liver 573.9
  lung 514
  pulmonary 514
  retina, venous 362.37
  stomach 536.8
  venous, retina 362.37
Enlargement, enlarged — *see also* Hy-
    pertrophy
  abdomen 789.3 ☑
  adenoids 474.12
    and tonsils 474.10
  alveolar process or ridge 525.8
  apertures of diaphragm (congenital)
      756.6
  blind spot, visual field 368.42
  gingival 523.8

●

**Enlargement, enlarged** — see also
Hypertrophy — continued
heart, cardiac (see also Hypertrophy,
cardiac) 429.3
lacrimal gland, chronic 375.03
liver (see also Hypertrophy, liver)
789.1
lymph gland or node 785.6
orbit 376.46
organ or site, congenital NEC — see
Anomaly, specified type NEC
parathyroid (gland) 252.01
pituitary fossa 793.0
prostate (simple) (soft) 600.00
with
other lower urinary tract symptoms (LUTS) 600.01
urinary
obstruction 600.01
retention 600.01
sella turcica 793.0
spleen (see also Splenomegaly) 789.2
congenital 759.0
thymus (congenital) (gland) 254.0
thyroid (gland) (see also Goiter) 240.9
tongue 529.8
tonsils 474.11
and adenoids 474.10
uterus 621.2
**Enophthalmos** 376.50
due to
atrophy of orbital tissue 376.51
surgery 376.52
trauma 376.52
**Enostosis** 526.89
**Entamebiasis** — see Amebiasis
**Entamebic** — see Amebiasis
**Entanglement, umbilical cord(s)**
663.3 ☑
with compression 663.2 ☑
affecting fetus or newborn 762.5
around neck with compression
663.1 ☑
twins in monoamniotic sac 663.2 ☑
**Enteralgia** 789.0 ☑
**Enteric** — see condition
**Enteritis** (acute) (catarrhal) (choleraic)
(chronic) (congestive) (diarrheal)
(exudative) (follicular) (hemorrhagic) (infantile) (lienteric) (noninfectious) (perforative) (phlegmonous)
(presumed noninfectious) (pseudomembranous) 558.9
adaptive 564.9
aertrycke infection 003.0
allergic 558.3
amebic (see also Amebiasis) 006.9
with abscess — see Abscess, amebic
acute 006.0
with abscess — see Abscess,
amebic
nondysenteric 006.2
chronic 006.1
with abscess — see Abscess,
amebic
nondysenteric 006.2
nondysenteric 006.2
anaerobic (cocci) (gram-negative)
(gram-positive) (mixed) NEC
008.46
bacillary NEC 004.9
bacterial NEC 008.5
specified NEC 008.49
Bacteroides (fragilis) (melaninogenis-
cus) (oralis) 008.46
Butyrivibrio (fibriosolvens) 008.46
Campylobacter 008.43
Candida 112.85
Chilomastix 007.8
choleriformis 001.1
chronic 558.9
ulcerative (see also Colitis, ulcerative) 556.9
cicatrizing (chronic) 555.0

**Enteritis** — continued
Clostridium
botulinum 005.1
difficile 008.45
haemolyticum 008.46
novyi 008.46
perfringens (C) (F) 008.46
specified type NEC 008.46
coccidial 007.2
dietetic 558.9
due to
achylia gastrica 536.8
adenovirus 008.62
Aerobacter aerogenes 008.2
anaerobes (see also Enteritis,
anaerobic) 008.46
Arizona (bacillus) 008.1
astrovirus 008.66
Bacillus coli — see Enteritis, E. coli
bacteria NEC 008.5
specified NEC 008.49
Bacteroides (see also Enteritis,
Bacteroides) 008.46
Butyrivibrio (fibriosolvens) 008.46
Calcivirus 008.65
Camplyobacter 008.43
Clostridium — see Enteritis,
Clostridium
Cockle agent 008.64
Coxsackie (virus) 008.67
Ditchling agent 008.64
ECHO virus 008.67
Enterobacter aerogenes 008.2
enterococci 008.49
enterovirus NEC 008.67
Escherichia coli — see Enteritis,
E. coli
Eubacterium 008.46
Fusobacterium (nucleatum) 008.46
gram-negative bacteria NEC 008.47
anaerobic NEC 008.46
Hawaii agent 008.63
irritating foods 558.9
Klebsiella aerogenes 008.47
Marin County agent 008.66
Montgomery County agent 008.63
Norwalk-like agent 008.63
Norwalk virus 008.63
Otofuke agent 008.63
Paracolobactrum arizonae 008.1
paracolon bacillus NEC 008.47
Arizona 008.1
Paramatta agent 008.64
Peptococcus 008.46
Peptostreptococcus 008.46
Proprionibacterium 008.46
Proteus (bacillus) (mirabilis) (mor-
ganii) 008.3
Pseudomonas aeruginosa 008.42
Rotavirus 008.61
Sapporo agent 008.63
small round virus (SRV) NEC
008.64
featureless NEC 008.63
structured NEC 008.63
Snow Mountain (SM) agent 008.63
specified
bacteria NEC 008.49
organism, nonbacterial NEC
008.8
virus NEC 008.69
Staphylococcus 008.41
Streptococcus 008.49
anaerobic 008.46
Taunton agent 008.63
Torovirus 008.69
Treponema 008.46
Veillonella 008.46
virus 008.8
specified type NEC 008.69
Wollan (W) agent 008.64
Yersinia enterocolitica 008.44
dysentery — see Dysentery
E. coli 008.00
enterohemorrhagic 008.04
enteroinvasive 008.03

**Enteritis** — continued
E. coli — continued
enteropathogenic 008.01
enterotoxigenic 008.02
specified type NEC 008.09
el tor 001.1
embadomonial 007.8
epidemic 009.0
Eubacterium 008.46
fermentative 558.9
fulminant 557.0
Fusobacterium (nucleatum) 008.46
gangrenous (see also Enteritis, due
to, by organism) 009.0
giardial 007.1
gram-negative bacteria NEC 008.47
anaerobic NEC 008.46
infectious NEC (see also Enteritis, due
to, by organism) 009.0
presumed 009.1
influenzal 487.8
ischemic 557.9
acute 557.0
chronic 557.1
due to mesenteric artery insufficiency 557.1
membranous 564.9
mucous 564.9
myxomembranous 564.9
necrotic (see also Enteritis, due to, by
organism) 009.0
necroticans 005.2
necrotizing of fetus or newborn 777.5
neurogenic 564.9
newborn 777.8
necrotizing 777.5
parasitic NEC 129
paratyphoid (fever) (see also Fever,
paratyphoid) 002.9
Peptococcus 008.46
Peptostreptococcus 008.46
Proprionibacterium 008.46
protozoal NEC 007.9
radiation 558.1
regional (of) 555.9
intestine
large (bowel, colon, or rectum)
555.1
with small intestine 555.2
small (duodenum, ileum, or jejunum) 555.0
with large intestine 555.2
Salmonella infection 003.0
salmonellosis 003.0
segmental (see also Enteritis, regional)
555.9
septic (see also Enteritis, due to, by
organism) 009.0
Shigella 004.9
simple 558.9
spasmodic 564.9
spastic 564.9
staphylococcal 008.41
due to food 005.0
streptococcal 008.49
anaerobic 008.46
toxic 558.2
Treponema (denticola) (macrodentium)
008.46
trichomonal 007.3
tuberculous (see also Tuberculosis)
014.8 ☑
typhosa 002.0
ulcerative (chronic) (see also Colitis,
ulcerative) 556.9
Veillonella 008.46
viral 008.8
adenovirus 008.62
enterovirus 008.67
specified virus NEC 008.69
Yersinia enterocolitica 008.44
zymotic 009.0
**Enteroarticular syndrome** 099.3
**Enterobiasis** 127.4
**Enterobius vermicularis** 127.4
**Enterocele** — see also Hernia 553.9

**Enterocele** — see also Hernia —
continued
pelvis, pelvic (acquired) (congenital)
618.6
vagina, vaginal (acquired) (congenital)
618.6
**Enterocolitis** — see also Enteritis
fetus or newborn 777.8
necrotizing 777.5
fulminant 557.0
granulomatous 555.2
hemorrhagic (acute) 557.0
chronic 557.1
necrotizing (acute) (membranous)
557.0
primary necrotizing 777.5
pseudomembranous 008.45
radiation 558.1
newborn 777.5
ulcerative 556.0
**Enterocystoma** 751.5
**Enterogastritis** — see Enteritis
**Enterogenous cyanosis** 289.7
**Enterolith, enterolithiasis** (impaction)
560.39
with hernia (see also Hernia, by site,
with obstruction)
gangrenous — see Hernia, by site,
with gangrene
**Enteropathy** 569.9
exudative (of Gordon) 579.8
gluten 579.0
hemorrhagic, terminal 557.0
protein-losing 579.8
**Enteroperitonitis** — see also Peritonitis
567.9
**Enteroptosis** 569.89
**Enterorrhagia** 578.9
**Enterospasm** 564.9
psychogenic 306.4
**Enterostenosis** — see also Obstruction,
intestine 560.9
**Enterostomy status** V44.4
with complication 569.60
**Enthesopathy** 726.90
ankle and tarsus 726.70
elbow region 726.30
specified NEC 726.39
hip 726.5
knee 726.60
peripheral NEC 726.8
shoulder region 726.10
adhesive 726.0
spinal 720.1
wrist and carpus 726.4
**Entrance, air into vein** — see Embolism, air
**Entrapment, nerve** — see Neuropathy,
entrapment
**Entropion** (eyelid) 374.00
cicatricial 374.04
congenital 743.62
late effect of trachoma (healed) 139.1
mechanical 374.02
paralytic 374.02
senile 374.01
spastic 374.03
**Enucleation of eye** (current) (traumatic)
871.3
**Enuresis** 788.30
habit disturbance 307.6
nocturnal 788.36
psychogenic 307.6
nonorganic origin 307.6
psychogenic 307.6
**Enzymopathy** 277.9
**Eosinopenia** 288.59
**Eosinophilia** 288.3
allergic 288.3
hereditary 288.3
idiopathic 288.3
infiltrative 518.3
Loeffler's 518.3
myalgia syndrome 710.5
pulmonary (tropical) 518.3
secondary 288.3

**Eosinophilia** — *continued*
  tropical 518.3
**Eosinophilic** — *see also* condition
  fasciitis 728.89
  granuloma (bone) 277.89
  infiltration lung 518.3
**Ependymitis** (acute) (cerebral) (chronic)
    (granular) — *see also* Meningitis
    322.9
**Ependymoblastoma** (M9392/3)
  specified site — *see* Neoplasm, by site,
    malignant
  unspecified site 191.9
**Ependymoma** (epithelial) (malignant)
    (M9391/3)
  anaplastic type (M9392/3)
    specified site — *see* Neoplasm, by
      site, malignant
    unspecified site 191.9
  benign (M9391/0)
    specified site — *see* Neoplasm, by
      site, benign
    unspecified site 225.0
  myxopapillary (M9394/1) 237.5
  papillary (M9393/1) 237.5
  specified site — *see* Neoplasm, by site,
    malignant
  unspecified site 191.9
**Ependymopathy** 349.2
  spinal cord 349.2
**Ephelides, ephelis** 709.09
**Ephemeral fever** — *see also* Pyrexia
  780.6
**Epiblepharon** (congenital) 743.62
**Epicanthus, epicanthic fold** (congenital)
  (eyelid) 743.63
**Epicondylitis** (elbow) (lateral) 726.32
  medial 726.31
**Epicystitis** — *see also* Cystitis 595.9
**Epidemic** — *see* condition
**Epidermidalization, cervix** — *see* con-
  dition
**Epidermidization, cervix** — *see* condi-
  tion
**Epidermis, epidermal** — *see* condition
**Epidermization, cervix** — *see* condition
**Epidermodysplasia verruciformis**
  078.19
**Epidermoid**
  cholesteatoma — *see* Cholesteatoma
  inclusion (*see also* Cyst, skin) 706.2
**Epidermolysis**
  acuta (combustiformis) (toxica) 695.1
  bullosa 757.39
  necroticans combustiformis 695.1
    due to drug
      correct substance properly ad-
        ministered 695.1
      overdose or wrong substance
        given or taken 977.9
      specified drug — *see* Table
        of Drugs and Chemi-
        cals
**Epidermophytid** — *see* Dermatophytosis
**Epidermophytosis** (infected) — *see* Dermatophytosis
**Epidermosis, ear** (middle) — *see also*
  Cholesteatoma 385.30
**Epididymis** — *see* condition
**Epididymitis** (nonvenereal) 604.90
  with abscess 604.0
  acute 604.99
  blennorrhagic (acute) 098.0
    chronic or duration of 2 months or
      over 098.2
  caseous (*see also* Tuberculosis)
    016.4 ☑
  chlamydial 099.54
  diphtheritic 032.89 [604.91]
  filarial 125.9 [604.91]
  gonococcal (acute) 098.0
    chronic or duration of 2 months or
      over 098.2
  recurrent 604.99
  residual 604.99
  syphilitic 095.8 [604.91]

**Epididymitis** — *continued*
  tuberculous (*see also* Tuberculosis)
    016.4 ☑
**Epididymo-orchitis** — *see also* Epididymitis 604.90
  with abscess 604.0
  chlamydial 099.54
  gonococcal (acute) 098.13
    chronic or duration of 2 months or
      over 098.33
**Epidural** — *see* condition
**Epigastritis** — *see also* Gastritis 535.5 ☑
**Epigastrium, epigastric** — *see* condition
**Epigastrocele** — *see also* Hernia, epigastric 553.29
**Epiglottiditis** (acute) 464.30
  with obstruction 464.31
  chronic 476.1
  viral 464.30
    with obstruction 464.31
**Epiglottis** — *see* condition
**Epiglottitis** (acute) 464.30
  with obstruction 464.31
  chronic 476.1
  viral 464.30
    with obstruction 464.31
**Epignathus** 759.4
**Epilepsia**
  partialis continua (*see also* Epilepsy)
    345.7 ☑
  procursiva (*see also* Epilepsy) 345.8 ☑
**Epilepsy, epileptic** (idiopathic) 345.9 ☑

> *Note* — use the following fifth-digit sub-
> classification with categories 345.0,
> 345.1, 345.4–345.9:
>
> 0   *without mention of intractable*
>      *epilepsy*
>
> 1   *with intractable epilepsy*

  abdominal 345.5 ☑
  absence (attack) 345.0 ☑
  akinetic 345.0 ☑
    psychomotor 345.4 ☑
  automatism 345.4 ☑
  autonomic diencephalic 345.5 ☑
  brain 345.9 ☑
  Bravais-Jacksonian 345.5 ☑
  cerebral 345.9 ☑
  climacteric 345.9 ☑
  clonic 345.1 ☑
  clouded state 345.9 ☑
  coma 345.3
  communicating 345.4 ☑
  complicating pregnancy, childbirth,
    or the puerperium 649.4 ☑
  congenital 345.9 ☑
  convulsions 345.9 ☑
  cortical (focal) (motor) 345.5 ☑
  cursive (running) 345.8 ☑
  cysticercosis 123.1
  deterioration
    with behavioral disturbance
      345.9 [294.11]
    without behavioral disturbance
      345.9 [294.10]
  due to syphilis 094.89
  equivalent 345.5 ☑
  fit 345.9 ☑
  focal (motor) 345.5 ☑
  gelastic 345.8 ☑
  generalized 345.9 ☑
    convulsive 345.1 ☑
    flexion 345.1 ☑
    nonconvulsive 345.0 ☑
  grand mal (idiopathic) 345.1 ☑
  Jacksonian (motor) (sensory) 345.5 ☑
  Kojevnikoff's, Kojevnikov's, Kojew-
    nikoff's 345.7 ☑
  laryngeal 786.2
  limbic system 345.4 ☑

**Epilepsy, epileptic** — *continued*
  localization related (focal) (partial) and
    epileptic syndromes
    with
      complex partial seizures
        345.4 ☑
      simple partial seizures 345.5 ☑
  major (motor) 345.1 ☑
  minor 345.0 ☑
  mixed (type) 345.9 ☑
  motor partial 345.5 ☑
  musicogenic 345.1 ☑
  myoclonus, myoclonic 345.1 ☑
    progressive (familial) 333.2
  nonconvulsive, generalized 345.0 ☑
  parasitic NEC 123.9
  partial (focalized) 345.5 ☑
    with
      impairment of consciousness
        345.4 ☑
      memory and ideational distur-
        bances 345.4 ☑
    without impairment of conscious-
      ness 345.5 ☑
    abdominal type 345.5 ☑
    motor type 345.5 ☑
    psychomotor type 345.4 ☑
    psychosensory type 345.4 ☑
    secondarily generalized 345.4 ☑
    sensory type 345.5 ☑
    somatomotor type 345.5 ☑
    somatosensory type 345.5 ☑
    temporal lobe type 345.4 ☑
    visceral type 345.5 ☑
    visual type 345.5 ☑
  peripheral 345.9 ☑
  petit mal 345.0 ☑
  photokinetic 345.8 ☑
  progressive myoclonic (familial) 333.2
  psychic equivalent 345.5 ☑
  psychomotor 345.4 ☑
  psychosensory 345.4 ☑
  reflex 345.1 ☑
  seizure 345.9 ☑
  senile 345.9 ☑
  sensory-induced 345.5 ☑
  sleep (*see also* Narcolepsy) 347.00
  somatomotor type 345.5 ☑
  somatosensory 345.5 ☑
  specified type NEC 345.8 ☑
  status (grand mal) 345.3
    focal motor 345.7 ☑
    petit mal 345.2
    psychomotor 345.7 ☑
    temporal lobe 345.7 ☑
  symptomatic 345.9 ☑
  temporal lobe 345.4 ☑
  tonic (-clonic) 345.1 ☑
  traumatic (injury unspecified) 907.0
    injury specified — *see* Late, effect
      (of) specified injury
  twilight 293.0
  uncinate (gyrus) 345.4 ☑
  Unverricht (-Lundborg) (familial my-
    oclonic) 333.2
  visceral 345.5 ☑
  visual 345.5 ☑
**Epileptiform**
  convulsions 780.39
  seizure 780.39
**Epiloia** 759.5
**Epimenorrhea** 626.2
**Epipharyngitis** — *see also* Nasopharyngitis 460
**Epiphora** 375.20
  due to
    excess lacrimation 375.21
    insufficient drainage 375.22
**Epiphyseal arrest** 733.91
  femoral head 732.2
**Epiphyseolysis, epiphysiolysis** — *see*
  *also* Osteochondrosis 732.9
**Epiphysitis** — *see also* Osteochondrosis
  732.9
  juvenile 732.6

**Epiphysitis** — *see also* Osteochondrosis
  — *continued*
  marginal (Scheuermann's) 732.0
  os calcis 732.5
  syphilitic (congenital) 090.0
  vertebral (Scheuermann's) 732.0
**Epiplocele** — *see also* Hernia 553.9
**Epiploitis** — *see also* Peritonitis 567.9
**Epiplosarcomphalocele** — *see also*
  Hernia, umbilicus 553.1
**Episcleritis** 379.00
  gouty 274.89 [379.09]
  nodular 379.02
  periodica fugax 379.01
    angioneurotic — *see* Edema, an-
      gioneurotic
  specified NEC 379.09
  staphylococcal 379.00
  suppurative 379.00
  syphilitic 095.0
  tuberculous (*see also* Tuberculosis)
    017.3 ☑ [379.09]
**Episode**
  brain (*see also* Disease, cerebrovascu-
    lar, acute) 436
  cerebral (*see also* Disease, cerebrovas-
    cular, acute) 436
  depersonalization (in neurotic state)
    300.6
  hyporesponsive 780.09
  psychotic (*see also* Psychosis) 298.9
    organic, transient 293.9
  schizophrenic (acute) NEC (*see also*
    Schizophrenia) 295.4 ☑
**Epispadias**
  female 753.8
  male 752.62
**Episplenitis** 289.59
**Epistaxis** (multiple) 784.7
  hereditary 448.0
  vicarious menstruation 625.8
**Epithelioma** (malignant) (M8011/3) —
    *see also* Neoplasm, by site, malig-
    nant
  adenoides cysticum (M8100/0) — *see*
    Neoplasm, skin, benign
  basal cell (M8090/3) — *see* Neoplasm,
    skin, malignant
  benign (M8011/0) — *see* Neoplasm,
    by site, benign
  Bowen's (M8081/2) — *see* Neoplasm,
    skin, in situ
  calcifying (benign) (Malherbe's)
    (M8110/0) — *see* Neoplasm,
    skin, benign
  external site — *see* Neoplasm, skin,
    malignant
  intraepidermal, Jadassohn (M8096/0)
    — *see* Neoplasm, skin, benign
  squamous cell (M8070/3) — *see* Neo-
    plasm, by site, malignant
**Epitheliopathy**
  pigment, retina 363.15
  posterior multifocal placoid (acute)
    363.15
**Epithelium, epithelial** — *see* condition
**Epituberculosis** (allergic) (with atelectasis) — *see also* Tuberculosis
  010.8 ☑
**Eponychia** 757.5
**Epstein's**
  nephrosis or syndrome (*see also*
    Nephrosis) 581.9
  pearl (mouth) 528.4
**Epstein-Barr infection** (viral) 075
  chronic 780.79 [139.8]
**Epulis** (giant cell) (gingiva) 523.8
**Equinia** 024
**Equinovarus** (congenital) 754.51
  acquired 736.71
**Equivalent**
  convulsive (abdominal) (*see also*
    Epilepsy) 345.5 ☑
  epileptic (psychic) (*see also* Epilepsy)
    345.5 ☑

☑ Additional Digit Required — Refer to the Tabular List for Digit Selection           ▽ Subterms under main terms may continue to next column or page

**2008 ICD-9-CM**          ▶◀ Revised Text       ● New Line       ▲ Revised Code          **Volume 2 — 111**

**Erb's**
disease 359.1
palsy, paralysis (birth) (brachial) (newborn) 767.6
spinal (spastic) syphilitic 094.89
pseudohypertrophic muscular dystrophy 359.1
**Erb-Goldflam disease or syndrome** 358.00
**Erb (-Duchenne) paralysis** (birth injury) (newborn) 767.6
**Erdheim's syndrome** (acromegalic macrospondylitis) 253.0
**Erection, painful** (persistent) 607.3
**Ergosterol deficiency** (vitamin D) 268.9
with
osteomalacia 268.2
rickets (see also Rickets) 268.0
**Ergotism** (ergotized grain) 988.2
from ergot used as drug (migraine therapy)
correct substance properly administered 349.82
overdose or wrong substance given or taken 975.0
**Erichsen's disease** (railway spine) 300.16
**Erlacher-Blount syndrome** (tibia vara) 732.4
**Erosio interdigitalis blastomycetica** 112.3
**Erosion**
arteriosclerotic plaque — see Arteriosclerosis, by site
artery NEC 447.2
without rupture 447.8
bone 733.99
bronchus 519.19
cartilage (joint) 733.99
cervix (uteri) (acquired) (chronic) (congenital) 622.0
with mention of cervicitis 616.0
cornea (recurrent) (see also Keratitis) 371.42
traumatic 918.1
dental (idiopathic) (occupational) 521.30
extending into
dentine 521.32
pulp 521.33
generalized 521.35
limited to enamel 521.31
localized 521.34
duodenum, postpyloric — see Ulcer, duodenum
esophagus 530.89
gastric 535.4 ☑
intestine 569.89
lymphatic vessel 457.8
pylorus, pyloric (ulcer) 535.4 ☑
sclera 379.16
spine, aneurysmal 094.89
spleen 289.59
stomach 535.4 ☑
teeth (idiopathic) (occupational) (see also Erosion, dental) 521.30
due to
medicine 521.30
persistent vomiting 521.30
urethra 599.84
uterus 621.8
vertebra 733.99
**Erotomania** 302.89
Clérambault's 297.8
**Error**
in diet 269.9
refractive 367.9
astigmatism (see also Astigmatism) 367.20
drug-induced 367.89
hypermetropia 367.0
hyperopia 367.0
myopia 367.1
presbyopia 367.4
toxic 367.89
**Eructation** 787.3

**Eructation** — continued
nervous 306.4
psychogenic 306.4
**Eruption**
creeping 126.9
drug — see Dermatitis, due to, drug
Hutchinson, summer 692.72
Kaposi's varicelliform 054.0
napkin (psoriasiform) 691.0
polymorphous
light (sun) 692.72
other source 692.82
psoriasiform, napkin 691.0
recalcitrant pustular 694.8
ringed 695.89
skin (see also Dermatitis) 782.1
creeping (meaning hookworm) 126.9
due to
chemical(s) NEC 692.4
internal use 693.8
drug — see Dermatitis, due to, drug
prophylactic inoculation or vaccination against disease — see Dermatitis, due to, vaccine
smallpox vaccination NEC — see Dermatitis, due to, vaccine
erysipeloid 027.1
feigned 698.4
Hutchinson, summer 692.72
Kaposi's, varicelliform 054.0
vaccinia 999.0
lichenoid, axilla 698.3
polymorphous, due to light 692.72
toxic NEC 695.0
vesicular 709.8
teeth, tooth
accelerated 520.6
delayed 520.6
difficult 520.6
disturbance of 520.6
in abnormal sequence 520.6
incomplete 520.6
late 520.6
natal 520.6
neonatal 520.6
obstructed 520.6
partial 520.6
persistent primary 520.6
premature 520.6
prenatal 520.6
vesicular 709.8
**Erysipelas** (gangrenous) (infantile) (newborn) (phlegmonous) (suppurative) 035
external ear 035 [380.13]
puerperal, postpartum, childbirth 670.0 ☑
**Erysipelatoid** (Rosenbach's) 027.1
**Erysipeloid** (Rosenbach's) 027.1
**Erythema, erythematous** (generalized) 695.9
ab igne — see Burn, by site, first degree
annulare (centrifugum) (rheumaticum) 695.0
arthriticum epidemicum 026.1
brucellum (see also Brucellosis) 023.9
bullosum 695.1
caloricum — see Burn, by site, first degree
chronicum migrans 088.81
circinatum 695.1
diaper 691.0
due to
chemical (contact) NEC 692.4
internal 693.8
drug (internal use) 693.0
contact 692.3
elevatum diutinum 695.89
endemic 265.2
epidemic, arthritic 026.1
figuratum perstans 695.0

**Erythema, erythematous** — continued
gluteal 691.0
gyratum (perstans) (repens) 695.1
heat — see Burn, by site, first degree
ichthyosiforme congenitum 757.1
induratum (primary) (scrofulosorum) (see also Tuberculosis) 017.1 ☑
nontuberculous 695.2
infantum febrile 057.8
infectional NEC 695.9
infectiosum 057.0
inflammation NEC 695.9
intertrigo 695.89
iris 695.1
lupus (discoid) (localized) (see also Lupus, erythematosus) 695.4
marginatum 695.0
rheumaticum — see Fever, rheumatic
medicamentosum — see Dermatitis, due to, drug
migrans 529.1
chronicum 088.81
multiforme 695.1
bullosum 695.1
conjunctiva 695.1
exudativum (Hebra) 695.1
pemphigoides 694.5
napkin 691.0
neonatorum 778.8
nodosum 695.2
tuberculous (see also Tuberculosis) 017.1 ☑
nummular, nummulare 695.1
palmar 695.0
palmaris hereditarium 695.0
pernio 991.5
perstans solare 692.72
rash, newborn 778.8
scarlatiniform (exfoliative) (recurrent) 695.0
simplex marginatum 057.8
solare (see also Sunburn) 692.71
streptogenes 696.5
toxic, toxicum NEC 695.0
newborn 778.8
tuberculous (primary) (see also Tuberculosis) 017.0 ☑
venenatum 695.0
**Erythematosus** — see condition
**Erythematous** — see condition
**Erythermalgia** (primary) 443.82
**Erythralgia** 443.82
**Erythrasma** 039.0
**Erythredema** 985.0
polyneuritica 985.0
polyneuropathy 985.0
**Erythremia** (acute) (M9841/3) 207.0 ☑
chronic (M9842/3) 207.1 ☑
secondary 289.0
**Erythroblastopenia** (acquired) 284.89 ▲
congenital 284.01
**Erythroblastophthisis** 284.01
**Erythroblastosis** (fetalis) (newborn) 773.2
due to
ABO
antibodies 773.1
incompatibility, maternal/fetal 773.1
isoimmunization 773.1
Rh
antibodies 773.0
incompatibility, maternal/fetal 773.0
isoimmunization 773.0
**Erythrocyanosis** (crurum) 443.89
**Erythrocythemia** — see Erythremia
**Erythrocytopenia** 285.9
**Erythrocytosis** (megalosplenic)
familial 289.6
oval, hereditary (see also Elliptocytosis) 282.1
secondary 289.0

**Erythrocytosis** — continued
stress 289.0
**Erythroderma** — see also Erythema 695.9
desquamativa (in infants) 695.89
exfoliative 695.89
ichthyosiform, congenital 757.1
infantum 695.89
maculopapular 696.2
neonatorum 778.8
psoriaticum 696.1
secondary 695.9
**Erythrodysesthesia, palmar plantar ● (PPE)** 693.0 ●
**Erythrogenesis imperfecta** 284.09
**Erythroleukemia** (M9840/3) 207.0 ☑
**Erythromelalgia** 443.82
**Erythromelia** 701.8
**Erythropenia** 285.9
**Erythrophagocytosis** 289.9
**Erythrophobia** 300.23
**Erythroplakia**
oral mucosa 528.79
tongue 528.79
**Erythroplasia** (Queyrat) (M8080/2)
specified site — see Neoplasm, skin, in situ
unspecified site 233.5
**Erythropoiesis, idiopathic ineffective** 285.0
**Escaped beats, heart** 427.60
postoperative 997.1
**Esoenteritis** — see Enteritis
**Esophagalgia** 530.89
**Esophagectasis** 530.89
due to cardiospasm 530.0
**Esophagismus** 530.5
**Esophagitis** (alkaline) (chemical) (chronic) (infectional) (necrotic) (peptic) (postoperative) (regurgitant) 530.10
acute 530.12
candidal 112.84
reflux 530.11
specified NEC 530.19
tuberculous (see also Tuberculosis) 017.8 ☑
ulcerative 530.19
**Esophagocele** 530.6
**Esophagodynia** 530.89
**Esophagomalacia** 530.89
**Esophagoptosis** 530.89
**Esophagospasm** 530.5
**Esophagostenosis** 530.3
**Esophagostomiasis** 127.7
**Esophagostomy**
complication 530.87
infection 530.86
malfunctioning 530.87
mechanical 530.87
**Esophagotracheal** — see condition
**Esophagus** — see condition
**Esophoria** 378.41
convergence, excess 378.84
divergence, insufficiency 378.85
**Esotropia** (nonaccommodative) 378.00
accommodative 378.35
alternating 378.05
with
A pattern 378.06
specified noncomitancy NEC 378.08
V pattern 378.07
X pattern 378.08
Y pattern 378.08
intermittent 378.22
intermittent 378.22
alternating 378.22
monocular 378.21
monocular 378.01
with
A pattern 378.02
specified noncomitancy NEC 378.04
V pattern 378.03
X pattern 378.04
Y pattern 378.04

☑ Additional Digit Required — Refer to the Tabular List for Digit Selection ⏀ Subterms under main terms may continue to next column or page

112 — Volume 2 · October 2007    ▶◀ Revised Text    ● New Line    ▲ Revised Code    **2008 ICD-9-CM**

**Esotropia** — *continued*
  monocular — *continued*
    intermittent 378.21
**Espundia** 085.5
**Essential** — *see* condition
**Esterapenia** 289.89
**Esthesioneuroblastoma** (M9522/3)
  160.0
**Esthesioneurocytoma** (M9521/3) 160.0
**Esthesioneuroepithelioma** (M9523/3)
  160.0
**Esthiomene** 099.1
**Estivo-autumnal**
  fever 084.0
  malaria 084.0
**Estrangement** V61.0
**Estriasis** 134.0
**Ethanolaminuria** 270.8
**Ethanolism** — *see also* Alcoholism
  303.9 ☑
**Ether dependence, dependency** — *see
  also* Dependence 304.6 ☑
**Etherism** — *see also* Dependence
  304.6 ☑
**Ethmoid, ethmoidal** — *see* condition
**Ethmoiditis** (chronic) (nonpurulent)
  (purulent) — *see also* Sinusitis,
  ethmoidal 473.2
  influenzal 487.1
  Woakes' 471.1
**Ethylism** — *see also* Alcoholism 303.9 ☑
**Eulenburg's disease** (congenital
  paramyotonia) 359.29 ▲
**Eunuchism** 257.2
**Eunuchoidism** 257.2
  hypogonadotropic 257.2
**European blastomycosis** 117.5
**Eustachian** — *see* condition
**Euthyroidism** 244.9
**Euthyroid sick syndrome** 790.94
**Evaluation**
  fetal lung maturity 659.8 ☑
  for suspected condition (*see also* Ob-
    servation) V71.9
    abuse V71.81
    exposure
      anthrax V71.82
      biologic agent NEC V71.83
      SARS V71.83
    neglect V71.81
    newborn — *see* Observation, sus-
      pected, condition, newborn
    specified condition NEC V71.89
  mental health V70.2
    requested by authority V70.1
  nursing care V63.8
  social service V63.8
**Evans' syndrome** (thrombocytopenic
  purpura) 287.32
**Eventration**
  colon into chest — *see* Hernia, di-
    aphragm
  diaphragm (congenital) 756.6
**Eversion**
  bladder 596.8
  cervix (uteri) 622.0
    with mention of cervicitis 616.0
  foot NEC 736.79
    congenital 755.67
  lacrimal punctum 375.51
  punctum lacrimale (postinfectional)
    (senile) 375.51
  ureter (meatus) 593.89
  urethra (meatus) 599.84
  uterus 618.1
    complicating delivery 665.2 ☑
      affecting fetus or newborn
        763.89
    puerperal, postpartum 674.8 ☑
**Evidence**
  of malignancy
    cytologic
      without histologic confirmation
        795.06
**Evisceration**
  birth injury 767.8

**Evisceration** — *continued*
  bowel (congenital) — *see* Hernia, ven-
    tral
  congenital (*see also* Hernia, ventral)
    553.29
  operative wound 998.32
  traumatic NEC 869.1
    eye 871.3
**Evulsion** — *see* Avulsion
**Ewing's**
  angioendothelioma (M9260/3) — *see*
    Neoplasm, bone, malignant
  sarcoma (M9260/3) — *see* Neoplasm,
    bone, malignant
  tumor (M9260/3) — *see* Neoplasm,
    bone, malignant
**Exaggerated lumbosacral angle** (with
  impinging spine) 756.12
**Examination** (general) (routine) (of) (for)
  V70.9
  allergy V72.7
  annual V70.0
  cardiovascular preoperative V72.81
  cervical Papanicolaou smear V76.2
    as a part of routine gynecological
      examination V72.31
    to confirm findings of recent nor-
      mal smear following initial
      abnormal smear V72.32
  child care (routine) V20.2
  clinical research investigation (normal
    control patient) (participant)
    V70.7
  dental V72.2
  developmental testing (child) (infant)
    V20.2
  donor (potential) V70.8
  ear V72.19
  eye V72.0
  following
    accident (motor vehicle) V71.4
    alleged rape or seduction (victim or
      culprit) V71.5
    inflicted injury (victim or culprit)
      NEC V71.6
    rape or seduction, alleged (victim
      or culprit) V71.5
    treatment (for) V67.9
      combined V67.6
      fracture V67.4
      involving high-risk medication
        NEC V67.51
      mental disorder V67.3
      specified condition NEC V67.59
  follow-up (routine) (following) V67.9
    cancer chemotherapy V67.2
    chemotherapy V67.2
    disease NEC V67.59
    high-risk medication NEC V67.51
    injury NEC V67.59
    population survey V70.6
    postpartum V24.2
    psychiatric V67.3
    psychotherapy V67.3
    radiotherapy V67.1
    specified surgery NEC V67.09
    surgery V67.00
    vaginal pap smear V67.01
  gynecological V72.31
    for contraceptive maintenance
      V25.40
      intrauterine device V25.42
      pill V25.41
      specified method NEC V25.49
  health (of)
    armed forces personnel V70.5
    checkup V70.0
    child, routine V20.2
    defined subpopulation NEC V70.5
    inhabitants of institutions V70.5
    occupational V70.5
    pre-employment screening V70.5
    preschool children V70.5
      for admission to school V70.3
    prisoners V70.5
      for entrance into prison V70.3

**Examination** — *continued*
  health — *continued*
    prostitutes V70.5
    refugees V70.5
    school children V70.5
    students V70.5
  hearing V72.19
    following failed hearing screening
      V72.11
  infant V20.2
  laboratory V72.6
  lactating mother V24.1
  medical (for) (of) V70.9
    administrative purpose NEC V70.3
    admission to
      old age home V70.3
      prison V70.3
      school V70.3
    adoption V70.3
    armed forces personnel V70.5
    at health care facility V70.0
    camp V70.3
    child, routine V20.2
    clinical research (control) (normal
      comparison) (participant)
      V70.7
    defined subpopulation NEC V70.5
    donor (potential) V70.8
    driving license V70.3
    general V70.9
      routine V70.0
      specified reason NEC V70.8
    immigration V70.3
    inhabitants of institutions V70.5
    insurance certification V70.3
    marriage V70.3
    medicolegal reasons V70.4
    naturalization V70.3
    occupational V70.5
    population survey V70.6
    pre-employment V70.5
    preschool children V70.5
      for admission to school V70.3
    prison V70.3
    prisoners V70.5
      for entrance into prison V70.3
    prostitutes V70.5
    refugees V70.5
    school children V70.5
    specified reason NEC V70.8
    sport competition V70.3
    students V70.5
  medicolegal reason V70.4
  pelvic (annual) (periodic) V72.31
  periodic (annual) (routine) V70.0
  postpartum
    immediately after delivery V24.0
    routine follow-up V24.2
  pregnancy (unconfirmed) (possible)
    V72.40
    negative result V72.41
    positive result V72.42
  prenatal V22.1
    first pregnancy V22.0
    high-risk pregnancy V23.9
      specified problem NEC V23.89
  preoperative V72.84
    cardiovascular V72.81
    respiratory V72.82
    specified NEC V72.83
  preprocedural V72.84
    cardiovascular V72.81
    general physical V72.83
    respiratory V72.82
    specified NEC V72.83
  psychiatric V70.2
    follow-up not needing further care
      V67.3
    requested by authority V70.1
  radiological NEC V72.5
  respiratory preoperative V72.82
  screening — *see* Screening
  sensitization V72.7
  skin V72.7
    hypersensitivity V72.7
  special V72.9

**Examination** — *continued*
  specified type or reason NEC V72.85
    preoperative V72.83
      specified NEC V72.83
  teeth V72.2
  vaginal Papanicolaou smear V76.47
    following hysterectomy for malig-
      nant condition V67.01
  victim or culprit following
    alleged rape or seduction V71.5
    inflicted injury NEC V71.6
  vision V72.0
  well baby V20.2
**Exanthem, exanthema** — *see also* Rash
  782.1
  Boston 048
  epidemic, with meningitis 048
  lichenoid psoriasiform 696.2
  subitum 058.10 ▲
    due to ●
      human herpesvirus 6 058.11 ●
      human herpesvirus 7 058.12 ●
  viral, virus NEC 057.9
    specified type NEC 057.8
**Excess, excessive, excessively**
  alcohol level in blood 790.3
  carbohydrate tissue, localized 278.1
  carotene (dietary) 278.3
  cold 991.9
    specified effect NEC 991.8
  convergence 378.84
  crying 780.95
    of
      adolescent 780.95
      adult 780.95
      baby 780.92
      child 780.95
      infant (baby) 780.92
      newborn 780.92
  development, breast 611.1
  diaphoresis (*see also* Hyperhidrosis)
    780.8
  distance, interarch 524.28
  divergence 378.85
  drinking (alcohol) NEC (*see also*
    Abuse, drugs, nondependent)
    305.0 ☑
    continual (*see also* Alcoholism)
      303.9 ☑
    habitual (*see also* Alcoholism)
      303.9 ☑
  eating 783.6
  eyelid fold (congenital) 743.62
  fat 278.02
    in heart (*see also* Degeneration,
      myocardial) 429.1
    tissue, localized 278.1
  foreskin 605
  gas 787.3
  gastrin 251.5
  glucagon 251.4
  heat (*see also* Heat) 992.9
  horizontal
    overjet 524.26
    overlap 524.26
  interarch distance 524.28
  intermaxillary vertical dimension
    524.37
  interocclusal distance of teeth 524.37
  large
    colon 564.7
      congenital 751.3
    fetus or infant 766.0
      with obstructed labor 660.1 ☑
        affecting management of preg-
          nancy 656.6 ☑
      causing disproportion 653.5 ☑
      newborn (weight of 4500 grams or
        more) 766.0
    organ or site, congenital NEC —
      *see* Anomaly, specified type
      NEC
  lid fold (congenital) 743.62
  long
    colon 751.5

**Excess, excessive, excessively** — *continued*
  long — *continued*
    organ or site, congenital NEC — *see* Anomaly, specified type NEC
    umbilical cord (entangled)
      affecting fetus or newborn 762.5
      in pregnancy or childbirth 663.3 ☑
        with compression 663.2 ☑
  menstruation 626.2
  number of teeth 520.1
    causing crowding 524.31
  nutrients (dietary) NEC 783.6
  potassium (K) 276.7
  salivation (*see also* Ptyalism) 527.7
  secretion (*see also* Hypersecretion)
    milk 676.6 ☑
    sputum 786.4
    sweat (*see also* Hyperhidrosis) 780.8
  short
    organ or site, congenital NEC — *see* Anomaly, specified type NEC
    umbilical cord
      affecting fetus or newborn 762.6
      in pregnancy or childbirth 663.4 ☑
  skin NEC 701.9
    eyelid 743.62
      acquired 374.30
  sodium (Na) 276.0
  spacing of teeth 524.32
  sputum 786.4
  sweating (*see also* Hyperhidrosis) 780.8
  tearing (ducts) (eye) (*see also* Epiphora) 375.20
  thirst 783.5
    due to deprivation of water 994.3
  tuberosity 524.07
  vitamin
    A (dietary) 278.2
      administered as drug (chronic) (prolonged excessive intake) 278.2
        reaction to sudden overdose 963.5
    D (dietary) 278.4
      administered as drug (chronic) (prolonged excessive intake) 278.4
        reaction to sudden overdose 963.5
  weight 278.02
    gain 783.1
      of pregnancy 646.1 ☑
    loss 783.21
**Excitability, abnormal, under minor stress** 309.29
**Excitation**
  catatonic (*see also* Schizophrenia) 295.2 ☑
  psychogenic 298.1
  reactive (from emotional stress, psychological trauma) 298.1
**Excitement**
  manic (*see also* Psychosis, affective) 296.0 ☑
    recurrent episode 296.1 ☑
    single episode 296.0 ☑
  mental, reactive (from emotional stress, psychological trauma) 298.1
  state, reactive (from emotional stress, psychological trauma) 298.1
**Excluded pupils** 364.76
**Excoriation** (traumatic) — *see also* Injury, superficial, by site 919.8
  neurotic 698.4
**Excyclophoria** 378.44
**Excyclotropia** 378.33
**Exencephalus, exencephaly** 742.0

**Exercise**
  breathing V57.0
  remedial NEC V57.1
  therapeutic NEC V57.1
**Exfoliation, teeth due to systemic causes** 525.0
**Exfoliative** — *see also* condition
  dermatitis 695.89
**Exhaustion, exhaustive** (physical NEC) 780.79
  battle (*see also* Reaction, stress, acute) 308.9
  cardiac (*see also* Failure, heart) 428.9
  delirium (*see also* Reaction, stress, acute) 308.9
  due to
    cold 991.8
    excessive exertion 994.5
    exposure 994.4
  fetus or newborn 779.89
  heart (*see also* Failure, heart) 428.9
  heat 992.5
    due to
      salt depletion 992.4
      water depletion 992.3
  manic (*see also* Psychosis, affective) 296.0 ☑
    recurrent episode 296.1 ☑
    single episode 296.0 ☑
  maternal, complicating delivery 669.8 ☑
    affecting fetus or newborn 763.89
  mental 300.5
  myocardium, myocardial (*see also* Failure, heart) 428.9
  nervous 300.5
  old age 797
  postinfectional NEC 780.79
  psychogenic 300.5
  psychosis (*see also* Reaction, stress, acute) 308.9
  senile 797
    dementia 290.0
**Exhibitionism** (sexual) 302.4
**Exomphalos** 756.79
**Exophoria** 378.42
  convergence, insufficiency 378.83
  divergence, excess 378.85
**Exophthalmic**
  cachexia 242.0 ☑
  goiter 242.0 ☑
  ophthalmoplegia 242.0 ☑ [376.22]
**Exophthalmos** 376.30
  congenital 743.66
  constant 376.31
  endocrine NEC 259.9 [376.22]
  hyperthyroidism 242.0 ☑ [376.21]
  intermittent NEC 376.34
  malignant 242.0 ☑ [376.21]
  pulsating 376.35
    endocrine NEC 259.9 [376.22]
  thyrotoxic 242.0 ☑ [376.21]
**Exostosis** 726.91
  cartilaginous (M9210/0) — *see* Neoplasm, bone, benign
  congenital 756.4
  ear canal, external 380.81
  gonococcal 098.89
  hip 726.5
  intracranial 733.3
  jaw (bone) 526.81
  luxurians 728.11
  multiple (cancellous) (congenital) (hereditary) 756.4
  nasal bones 726.91
  orbit, orbital 376.42
  osteocartilaginous (M9210/0) — *see* Neoplasm, bone, benign
  spine 721.8
    with spondylosis — *see* Spondylosis
  syphilitic 095.5
  wrist 726.4
**Exotropia** 378.10
  alternating 378.15

**Exotropia** — *continued*
  alternating — *continued*
    with
      A pattern 378.16
      specified noncomitancy NEC 378.18
      V pattern 378.17
      X pattern 378.18
      Y pattern 378.18
    intermittent 378.24
  intermittent 378.20
    alternating 378.24
    monocular 378.23
  monocular 378.11
    with
      A pattern 378.12
      specified noncomitancy NEC 378.14
      V pattern 378.13
      X pattern 378.14
      Y pattern 378.14
    intermittent 378.23
**Explanation of**
  investigation finding V65.4 ☑
  medication V65.4 ☑
**Exposure** 994.9
  cold 991.9
    specified effect NEC 991.8
  effects of 994.9
  exhaustion due to 994.4
  to
    AIDS virus V01.79
    anthrax V01.81
    asbestos V15.84
    body fluids (hazardous) V15.85
    cholera V01.0
    communicable disease V01.9
      specified type NEC V01.89
    Escherichia coli (E. coli) V01.83
    German measles V01.4
    gonorrhea V01.6
    hazardous body fluids V15.85
    HIV V01.79
    human immunodeficiency virus V01.79
    lead V15.86
    meningococcus V01.84
    parasitic disease V01.89
    poliomyelitis V01.2
    potentially hazardous body fluids V15.85
    rabies V01.5
    rubella V01.4
    SARS-associated coronavirus V01.82
    smallpox V01.3
    syphilis V01.6
    tuberculosis V01.1
    varicella V01.71
    venereal disease V01.6
    viral disease NEC V01.79
    varicella V01.71
**Exsanguination, fetal** 772.0
**Exstrophy**
  abdominal content 751.8
  bladder (urinary) 753.5
**Extensive** — *see* condition
**Extra** — *see also* Accessory
  rib 756.3
    cervical 756.2
**Extraction**
  with hook 763.89
  breech NEC 669.6 ☑
    affecting fetus or newborn 763.0
  cataract postsurgical V45.61
  manual NEC 669.8 ☑
    affecting fetus or newborn 763.89
**Extrasystole** 427.60
  atrial 427.61
  postoperative 997.1
  ventricular 427.69
**Extrauterine gestation or pregnancy** — *see* Pregnancy, ectopic
**Extravasation**
  blood 459.0
    lower extremity 459.0

**Extravasation** — *continued*
  chyle into mesentery 457.8
  pelvicalyceal 593.4
  pyelosinus 593.4
  urine 788.8
    from ureter 788.8
**Extremity** — *see* condition
**Extrophy** — *see* Exstrophy
**Extroversion**
  bladder 753.5
  uterus 618.1
    complicating delivery 665.2 ☑
      affecting fetus or newborn 763.89
    postpartal (old) 618.1
**Extruded tooth** 524.34
**Extrusion**
  alveolus and teeth 524.75
  breast implant (prosthetic) 996.54
  device, implant, or graft — *see* Complications, mechanical
  eye implant (ball) (globe) 996.59
  intervertebral disc — *see* Displacement, intervertebral disc
  lacrimal gland 375.43
  mesh (reinforcing) 996.59
  ocular lens implant 996.53
  prosthetic device NEC — *see* Complications, mechanical
  vitreous 379.26
**Exudate, pleura** — *see* Effusion, pleura
**Exudates, retina** 362.82
**Exudative** — *see* condition
**Eye, eyeball, eyelid** — *see* condition
**Eyestrain** 368.13
**Eyeworm disease of Africa** 125.2

## F

**Faber's anemia or syndrome** (achlorhydric anemia) 280.9
**Fabry's disease** (angiokeratoma corporis diffusum) 272.7
**Face, facial** — *see* condition
**Facet of cornea** 371.44
**Faciocephalalgia, autonomic** — *see also* Neuropathy, peripheral, autonomic 337.9
**Facioscapulohumeral myopathy** 359.1
**Factitious disorder, illness** — *see* Illness, factitious
**Factor**
  deficiency — *see* Deficiency, factor
  psychic, associated with diseases classified elsewhere 316
  risk — *see* Problem
**Fahr-Volhard disease** (malignant nephrosclerosis) 403.00
**Failure, failed**
  adenohypophyseal 253.2
  attempted abortion (legal) (*see also* Abortion, failed) 638.9
  bone marrow (anemia) 284.9
    acquired (secondary) 284.89 ▲
    congenital 284.09
    idiopathic 284.9
  cardiac (*see also* Failure, heart) 428.9
    newborn 779.89
  cardiorenal (chronic) 428.9
    hypertensive (*see also* Hypertension, cardiorenal) 404.93
  cardiorespiratory 799.1
    specified during or due to a procedure 997.1
    long-term effect of cardiac surgery 429.4
  cardiovascular (chronic) 428.9
  cerebrovascular 437.8
  cervical dilatation in labor 661.0 ☑
    affecting fetus or newborn 763.7
  circulation, circulatory 799.89
    fetus or newborn 779.89
    peripheral 785.50
  compensation — *see* Disease, heart
  congestive (*see also* Failure, heart) 428.0

☑ Additional Digit Required — Refer to the Tabular List for Digit Selection
▽ Subterms under main terms may continue to next column or page
114 — Volume 2 · October 2007
▶◀ Revised Text   ● New Line   ▲ Revised Code
2008 ICD-9-CM

☑ Additional Digit Required — Refer to the Tabular List for Digit Selection    �📖 Subterms under main terms may continue to next column or page

**2008 ICD-9-CM**    ▶◀ Revised Text    ● New Line    ▲ Revised Code    **October 2007 · Volume 2 — 115**

**Fallopian**
  insufflation
    fertility testing V26.21
    following sterilization reversal
      V26.22
  tube — see condition
**Fallot's**
  pentalogy 745.2
  tetrad or tetralogy 745.2
  triad or trilogy 746.09
**Fallout, radioactive** (adverse effect) NEC
    990
**False** — see also condition
  bundle branch block 426.50
  bursa 727.89
  croup 478.75
  joint 733.82
  labor (pains) 644.1 ☑
  opening, urinary, male 752.69
  passage, urethra (prostatic) 599.4
  positive
    serological test for syphilis 795.6
    Wassermann reaction 795.6
  pregnancy 300.11
**Family, familial** — see also condition
  disruption V61.0
  hemophagocytic
    lymphohistiocytosis 288.4
    reticulosis 288.4
  Li-Fraumeni (syndrome) V84.01
  planning advice V25.09
    natural ●
      procreative V26.41 ●
      to avoid pregnancy V25.04 ●
  problem V61.9
    specified circumstance NEC V61.8
  retinoblastoma (syndrome) 190.5
**Famine** 994.2
  edema 262
**Fanconi's anemia** (congenital pancytope-
    nia) 284.09
**Fanconi (-de Toni) (-Debré) syndrome**
    (cystinosis) 270.0
**Farber (-Uzman) syndrome or disease**
    (disseminated lipogranulomatosis)
    272.8
**Farcin** 024
**Farcy** 024
**Farmers'**
  lung 495.0
  skin 692.74
**Farsightedness** 367.0
**Fascia** — see condition
**Fasciculation** 781.0
**Fasciculitis optica** 377.32
**Fasciitis** 729.4
  eosinophilic 728.89
  necrotizing 728.86
  nodular 728.79
  perirenal 593.4
  plantar 728.71
  pseudosarcomatous 728.79
  traumatic (old) NEC 728.79
    current — see Sprain, by site
**Fasciola hepatica infestation** 121.3
**Fascioliasis** 121.3
**Fasciolopsiasis** (small intestine) 121.4
**Fasciolopsis** (small intestine) 121.4
**Fast pulse** 785.0
**Fat**
  embolism (cerebral) (pulmonary) (sys-
    temic) 958.1
    with
      abortion — see Abortion, by
        type, with embolism
      ectopic pregnancy (see also cat-
        egories 633.0–633.9)
        639.6
      molar pregnancy (see also cate-
        gories 630–632) 639.6
    complicating delivery or puerperi-
      um 673.8 ☑
    following
      abortion 639.6
      ectopic or molar pregnancy
        639.6

**Fat** — continued
  embolism — continued
    in pregnancy, childbirth, or the
      puerperium 673.8 ☑
    excessive 278.02
      in heart (see also Degeneration,
        myocardial) 429.1
    general 278.02
    hernia, herniation 729.30
      eyelid 374.34
      knee 729.31
      orbit 374.34
      retro-orbital 374.34
      retropatellar 729.31
      specified site NEC 729.39
    indigestion 579.8
    in stool 792.1
    localized (pad) 278.1
      heart (see also Degeneration, my-
        ocardial) 429.1
      knee 729.31
      retropatellar 729.31
    necrosis (see also Fatty, degeneration)
      breast (aseptic) (segmental) 611.3
      mesentery 567.82
      omentum 567.82
      peritoneum 567.82
    pad 278.1
**Fatal syncope** 798.1
**Fatigue** 780.79
  auditory deafness (see also Deafness)
    389.9
  chronic, syndrome 780.71
  combat (see also Reaction, stress,
    acute) 308.9
  during pregnancy 646.8 ☑
  general 780.79
    psychogenic 300.5
  heat (transient) 992.6
  muscle 729.89
  myocardium (see also Failure, heart)
    428.9
  nervous 300.5
  neurosis 300.5
  operational 300.89
  postural 729.89
  posture 729.89
  psychogenic (general) 300.5
  senile 797
  syndrome NEC 300.5
    chronic 780.71
  undue 780.79
  voice 784.49
**Fatness** 278.02
**Fatty** — see also condition
  apron 278.1
  degeneration (diffuse) (general) NEC
    272.8
    localized — see Degeneration, by
      site, fatty
    placenta — see Placenta, abnormal
  heart (enlarged) (see also Degenera-
    tion, myocardial) 429.1
  infiltration (diffuse) (general) (see also
    Degeneration, by site, fatty)
    272.8
    heart (enlarged) (see also Degener-
      ation, myocardial) 429.1
  liver 571.8
    alcoholic 571.0
  necrosis — see Degeneration, fatty
  phanerosis 272.8
**Fauces** — see condition
**Fauchard's disease** (periodontitis)
    523.40
**Faucitis** 478.29
**Faulty** — see also condition
  position of teeth 524.30
**Favism** (anemia) 282.2
**Favre-Racouchot disease** (elastoidosis
    cutanea nodularis) 701.8
**Favus** 110.9
  beard 110.0
  capitis 110.0
  corporis 110.5
  eyelid 110.8

**Favus** — continued
  foot 110.4
  hand 110.2
  scalp 110.0
  specified site NEC 110.8
**Feared complaint unfounded** V65.5
**Fear, fearfulness** (complex) (reaction)
    300.20
  child 313.0
  of
    animals 300.29
    closed spaces 300.29
    crowds 300.29
    eating in public 300.23
    heights 300.29
    open spaces 300.22
      with panic attacks 300.21
    public speaking 300.23
    streets 300.22
      with panic attacks 300.21
    travel 300.22
      with panic attacks 300.21
    washing in public 300.23
  transient 308.0
**Febricula** (continued) (simple) — see also
    Pyrexia 780.6
**Febrile** — see also Pyrexia 780.6
  convulsion (simple) 780.31
    complex 780.32
  seizure (simple) 780.31
    atypical 780.32
    complex 780.32
    complicated 780.32
**Febris** — see also Fever 780.6
  aestiva (see also Fever, hay) 477.9
  flava (see also Fever, yellow) 060.9
  melitensis 023.9
  pestis (see also Plague) 020.9
  puerperalis 672.0 ☑
  recurrens (see also Fever, relapsing)
    087.9
    pediculo vestimenti 087.0
  rubra 034.1
  typhoidea 002.0
  typhosa 002.0
**Fecal** — see condition
**Fecalith** (impaction) 560.39
  with hernia (see also Hernia, by site,
    with obstruction)
    gangrenous — see Hernia, by site,
      with gangrene
  appendix 543.9
  congenital 777.1
**Fede's disease** 529.0
**Feeble-minded** 317
**Feeble rapid pulse due to shock follow-
    ing injury** 958.4
**Feeding**
  faulty (elderly) (infant) 783.3
    newborn 779.3
  formula check V20.2
  improper (elderly) (infant) 783.3
    newborn 779.3
  problem (elderly) (infant) 783.3
    newborn 779.3
    nonorganic origin 307.59
**Feeling of foreign body in throat** ●
    784.99 ●
**Feer's disease** 985.0
**Feet** — see condition
**Feigned illness** V65.2
**Feil-Klippel syndrome** (brevicollis)
    756.16
**Feinmesser's** (hidrotic) **ectodermal
    dysplasia** 757.31
**Felix's disease** (juvenile osteochondrosis,
    hip) 732.1
**Felon** (any digit) (with lymphangitis)
    681.01
  herpetic 054.6
**Felty's syndrome** (rheumatoid arthritis
    with splenomegaly and leukopenia)
    714.1
**Feminism in boys** 302.6
**Feminization, testicular** 259.5

**Feminization, testicular** —
    continued
  with pseudohermaphroditism, male
    259.5
**Femoral hernia** — see Hernia, femoral
**Femora vara** 736.32
**Femur, femoral** — see condition
**Fenestrata placenta** — see Placenta,
    abnormal
**Fenestration, fenestrated** — see also
    Imperfect, closure
  aorta-pulmonary 745.0
  aorticopulmonary 745.0
  aortopulmonary 745.0
  cusps, heart valve NEC 746.89
    pulmonary 746.09
  hymen 752.49
  pulmonic cusps 746.09
**Fenwick's disease** 537.89
**Fermentation** (gastric) (gastrointestinal)
    (stomach) 536.8
  intestine 564.89
    psychogenic 306.4
  psychogenic 306.4
**Fernell's disease** (aortic aneurysm)
    441.9
**Fertile eunuch syndrome** 257.2
**Fertility, meaning multiparity** — see
    Multiparity
**Fetal alcohol syndrome** 760.71
**Fetalis uterus** 752.3
**Fetid**
  breath 784.99
  sweat 705.89
**Fetishism** 302.81
  transvestic 302.3
**Fetomaternal hemorrhage**
  affecting management of pregnancy
    656.0 ☑
  fetus or newborn 772.0
**Fetus, fetal** — see also condition
  papyraceous 779.89
  type lung tissue 770.4
**Fever** 780.6
  with chills 780.6
    in malarial regions (see also
      Malaria) 084.6
  abortus NEC 023.9
  aden 061
  African tick-borne 087.1
  American
    mountain tick 066.1
    spotted 082.0
  and ague (see also Malaria) 084.6
  aphthous 078.4
  arbovirus hemorrhagic 065.9
  Assam 085.0
  Australian A or Q 083.0
  Bangkok hemorrhagic 065.4
  biliary, Charcôt's intermittent — see
    Choledocholithiasis
  bilious, hemoglobinuric 084.8
  blackwater 084.8
  blister 054.9
  Bonvale Dam 780.79
  boutonneuse 082.1
  brain 323.9
    late effect — see category 326
  breakbone 061
  Bullis 082.8
  Bunyamwera 066.3
  Burdwan 085.0
  Bwamba (encephalitis) 066.3
  Cameroon (see also Malaria) 084.6
  Canton 081.9
  catarrhal (acute) 460
    chronic 472.0
  cat-scratch 078.3
  cerebral 323.9
    late effect — see category 326
  cerebrospinal (meningococcal) (see
    also Meningitis, cerebrospinal)
    036.0
  Chagres 084.0
  Chandipura 066.8
  changuinola 066.0

**Fever** — *continued*
   Charcôt's (biliary) (hepatic) (intermit-
     tent) — *see* Choledocholithiasis
   Chikungunya (viral) 066.3
     hemorrhagic 065.4
   childbed 670.0 ☑
   Chitral 066.0
   Colombo (*see also* Fever, paratyphoid)
     002.9
   Colorado tick (virus) 066.1
   congestive
     malarial (*see also* Malaria) 084.6
     remittent (*see also* Malaria) 084.6
   Congo virus 065.0
   continued 780.6
     malarial 084.0
   Corsican (*see also* Malaria) 084.6
   Crimean hemorrhagic 065.0
   Cyprus (*see also* Brucellosis) 023.9
   dandy 061
   deer fly (*see also* Tularemia) 021.9
   dehydration, newborn 778.4
   dengue (virus) 061
     hemorrhagic 065.4
   desert 114.0
   due to heat 992.0
   Dumdum 085.0
   enteric 002.0
   ephemeral (of unknown origin) (*see*
     *also* Pyrexia) 780.6
   epidemic, hemorrhagic of the Far East
     065.0
   erysipelatous (*see also* Erysipelas) 035
   estivo-autumnal (malarial) 084.0
   etiocholanolone 277.31
   famine (*see also* Fever, relapsing)
     meaning typhus — *see* Typhus
   Far Eastern hemorrhagic 065.0
   five day 083.1
   Fort Bragg 100.89
   gastroenteric 002.0
   gastromalarial (*see also* Malaria) 084.6
   Gibraltar (*see also* Brucellosis) 023.9
   glandular 075
   Guama (viral) 066.3
   Haverhill 026.1
   hay (allergic) (with rhinitis) 477.9
     with
       asthma (bronchial) (*see also*
        Asthma) 493.0 ☑
     due to
       dander, animal (cat) (dog) 477.2
       dust 477.8
       fowl 477.8
       hair, animal (cat) (dog) 477.2
       pollen, any plant or tree 477.0
       specified allergen other than
        pollen 477.8
   heat (effects) 992.0
   hematuric, bilious 084.8
   hemoglobinuric (malarial) 084.8
     bilious 084.8
   hemorrhagic (arthropod-borne) NEC
     065.9
     with renal syndrome 078.6
     arenaviral 078.7
     Argentine 078.7
     Bangkok 065.4
     Bolivian 078.7
     Central Asian 065.0
     chikungunya 065.4
     Crimean 065.0
     dengue (virus) 065.4
     Ebola 065.8
     epidemic 078.6
       of Far East 065.0
     Far Eastern 065.0
     Junin virus 078.7
     Korean 078.6
     Kyasanur forest 065.2
     Machupo virus 078.7
     mite-borne NEC 065.8
     mosquito-borne 065.4
     Omsk 065.1
     Philippine 065.4
     Russian (Yaroslav) 078.6

**Fever** — *continued*
   hemorrhagic — *continued*
     Singapore 065.4
     Southeast Asia 065.4
     Thailand 065.4
     tick-borne NEC 065.3
   hepatic (*see also* Cholecystitis) 575.8
     intermittent (Charcôt's) — *see*
       Choledocholithiasis
   herpetic (*see also* Herpes) 054.9
   Hyalomma tick 065.0
   icterohemorrhagic 100.0
   inanition 780.6
     newborn 778.4
   infective NEC 136.9
   intermittent (bilious) (*see also* Malaria)
     084.6
     hepatic (Charcôt) — *see* Choledo-
       cholithiasis
     of unknown origin (*see also* Pyrex-
       ia) 780.6
     pernicious 084.0
   iodide
     correct substance properly admin-
       istered 780.6
     overdose or wrong substance given
       or taken 975.5
   Japanese river 081.2
   jungle yellow 060.0
   Junin virus, hemorrhagic 078.7
   Katayama 120.2
   Kedani 081.2
   Kenya 082.1
   Korean hemorrhagic 078.6
   Lassa 078.89
   Lone Star 082.8
   lung — *see* Pneumonia
   Machupo virus, hemorrhagic 078.7
   malaria, malarial (*see also* Malaria)
     084.6
   Malta (*see also* Brucellosis) 023.9
   Marseilles 082.1
   marsh (*see also* Malaria) 084.6
   Mayaro (viral) 066.3
   Mediterranean (*see also* Brucellosis)
     023.9
     familial 277.31
     tick 082.1
   meningeal — *see* Meningitis
   metal fumes NEC 985.8
   Meuse 083.1
   Mexican — *see* Typhus, Mexican
   Mianeh 087.1
   miasmatic (*see also* Malaria) 084.6
   miliary 078.2
   milk, female 672.0 ☑
   mill 504
   mite-borne hemorrhagic 065.8
   Monday 504
   mosquito-borne NEC 066.3
     hemorrhagic NEC 065.4
   mountain 066.1
     meaning
       Rocky Mountain spotted 082.0
       undulant fever (*see also* Brucel-
        losis) 023.9
     tick (American) 066.1
   Mucambo (viral) 066.3
   mud 100.89
   Neapolitan (*see also* Brucellosis) 023.9
   neutropenic 288.00
   nine-mile 083.0
   nonexanthematous tick 066.1
   North Asian tick-borne typhus 082.2
   Omsk hemorrhagic 065.1
   O'nyong-nyong (viral) 066.3
   Oropouche (viral) 066.3
   Oroya 088.0
   paludal (*see also* Malaria) 084.6
   Panama 084.0
   pappataci 066.0
   paratyphoid 002.9
     A 002.1
     B (Schottmüller's) 002.2
     C (Hirschfeld) 002.3
   parrot 073.9

**Fever** — *continued*
   periodic 277.31
   pernicious, acute 084.0
   persistent (of unknown origin) (*see*
     *also* Pyrexia) 780.6
   petechial 036.0
   pharyngoconjunctival 077.2
     adenoviral type 3 077.2
   Philippine hemorrhagic 065.4
   phlebotomus 066.0
   Piry 066.8
   Pixuna (viral) 066.3
   Plasmodium ovale 084.3
   pleural (*see also* Pleurisy) 511.0
   pneumonic — *see* Pneumonia
   polymer fume 987.8
   postoperative 998.89
     due to infection 998.59
   pretibial 100.89
   puerperal, postpartum 672.0 ☑
   putrid — *see* Septicemia
   pyemic — *see* Septicemia
   Q 083.0
     with pneumonia 083.0 *[484.8]*
   quadrilateral 083.0
   quartan (malaria) 084.2
   Queensland (coastal) 083.0
     seven-day 100.89
   Quintan (A) 083.1
   quotidian 084.0
   rabbit (*see also* Tularemia) 021.9
   rat-bite 026.9
     due to
       Spirillum minor or minus 026.0
       Spirochaeta morsus muris
        026.0
       Streptobacillus moniliformis
        026.1
   recurrent — *see* Fever, relapsing
   relapsing 087.9
     Carter's (Asiatic) 087.0
     Dutton's (West African) 087.1
     Koch's 087.9
     louse-borne (epidemic) 087.0
     Novy's (American) 087.1
     Obermeyer's (European) 087.0
     spirillum NEC 087.9
     tick-borne (endemic) 087.1
   remittent (bilious) (congestive) (gastric)
     (*see also* Malaria) 084.6
   rheumatic (active) (acute) (chronic)
     (subacute) 390
     with heart involvement 391.9
       carditis 391.9
       endocarditis (aortic) (mitral)
        (pulmonary) (tricuspid)
        391.1
       multiple sites 391.8
       myocarditis 391.2
       pancarditis, acute 391.8
       pericarditis 391.0
       specified type NEC 391.8
       valvulitis 391.1
     cardiac hypertrophy 398.99
     inactive or quiescent
       with cardiac hypertrophy
        398.99
       carditis 398.90
       endocarditis 397.9
        aortic (valve) 395.9
         with mitral (valve) disease
         396.9
        mitral (valve) 394.9
         with aortic (valve) disease
         396.9
        pulmonary (valve) 397.1
        tricuspid (valve) 397.0
       heart conditions (classifiable to
        429.3, 429.6, 429.9)
        398.99
       failure (congestive) (condi-
        tions classifiable to
        428.0, 428.9) 398.91
       left ventricular failure (condi-
        tions classifiable to 428.1)
        398.91

**Fever** — *continued*
   rheumatic — *continued*
     inactive or quiescent — *contin-*
       *ued*
       myocardial degeneration (condi-
        tions classifiable to 429.1)
        398.0
       myocarditis (conditions classifi-
        able to 429.0) 398.0
       pancarditis 398.99
       pericarditis 393
   Rift Valley (viral) 066.3
   Rocky Mountain spotted 082.0
   rose 477.0
   Ross river (viral) 066.3
   Russian hemorrhagic 078.6
   sandfly 066.0
   San Joaquin (valley) 114.0
   São Paulo 082.0
   scarlet 034.1
   septic — *see* Septicemia
   seven-day 061
     Japan 100.89
     Queensland 100.89
   shin bone 083.1
   Singapore hemorrhagic 065.4
   solar 061
   sore 054.9
   South African tick-bite 087.1
   Southeast Asia hemorrhagic 065.4
   spinal — *see* Meningitis
   spirillary 026.0
   splenic (*see also* Anthrax) 022.9
   spotted (Rocky Mountain) 082.0
     American 082.0
     Brazilian 082.0
     Colombian 082.0
     meaning
       cerebrospinal meningitis 036.0
       typhus 082.9
   spring 309.23
   steroid
     correct substance properly admin-
       istered 780.6
     overdose or wrong substance given
       or taken 962.0
   streptobacillary 026.1
   subtertian 084.0
   Sumatran mite 081.2
   sun 061
   swamp 100.89
   sweating 078.2
   swine 003.8
   sylvatic yellow 060.0
   Tahyna 062.5
   tertian — *see* Malaria, tertian
   Thailand hemorrhagic 065.4
   thermic 992.0
   three day 066.0
     with Coxsackie exanthem 074.8
   tick
     American mountain 066.1
     Colorado 066.1
     Kemerovo 066.1
     Mediterranean 082.1
     mountain 066.1
     nonexanthematous 066.1
     Quaranfil 066.1
   tick-bite NEC 066.1
   tick-borne NEC 066.1
     hemorrhagic NEC 065.3
   transitory of newborn 778.4
   trench 083.1
   tsutsugamushi 081.2
   typhogastric 002.0
   typhoid (abortive) (ambulant) (any site)
     (hemorrhagic) (infection) (inter-
     mittent) (malignant) (rheumatic)
     002.0
   typhomalarial (*see also* Malaria) 084.6
   typhus — *see* Typhus
   undulant (*see also* Brucellosis) 023.9
   unknown origin (*see also* Pyrexia)
     780.6
   uremic — *see* Uremia
   uveoparotid 135

---

☑ Additional Digit Required — Refer to the Tabular List for Digit Selection     ᵂᵇ Subterms under main terms may continue to next column or page

**2008 ICD-9-CM**     ▶◀ Revised Text     ● New Line     ▲ Revised Code     **Volume 2 — 117**

Fever — Fibrosis, fibrotic

**Fever** — *continued*
valley (Coccidioidomycosis) 114.0
Venezuelan equine 066.2
Volhynian 083.1
Wesselsbron (viral) 066.3
West
  African 084.8
  Nile (viral) 066.40
    with
      cranial nerve disorders 066.42
      encephalitis 066.41
      optic neuritis 066.42
      other complications 066.49
      other neurologic manifestations 066.42
      polyradiculitis 066.42
Whitmore's 025
Wolhynian 083.1
worm 128.9
Yaroslav hemorrhagic 078.6
yellow 060.9
  jungle 060.0
  sylvatic 060.0
  urban 060.1
  vaccination, prophylactic (against) V04.4
Zika (viral) 066.3
**Fibrillation**
atrial (established) (paroxysmal) 427.31
auricular (atrial) (established) 427.31
cardiac (ventricular) 427.41
coronary (*see also* Infarct, myocardium) 410.9 ☑
heart (ventricular) 427.41
muscular 728.9
postoperative 997.1
ventricular 427.41
**Fibrin**
ball or bodies, pleural (sac) 511.0
chamber, anterior (eye) (gelatinous exudate) 364.04
**Fibrinogenolysis** (hemorrhagic) — *see* Fibrinolysis
**Fibrinogenopenia** (congenital) (hereditary) — *see also* Defect, coagulation 286.3
acquired 286.6
**Fibrinolysis** (acquired) (hemorrhagic) (pathologic) 286.6
with
  abortion — *see* Abortion, by type, with hemorrhage, delayed or excessive
  ectopic pregnancy (*see also* categories 633.0–633.9) 639.1
  molar pregnancy (*see also* categories 630–632) 639.1
antepartum or intrapartum 641.3 ☑
  affecting fetus or newborn 762.1
following
  abortion 639.1
  ectopic or molar pregnancy 639.1
newborn, transient 776.2
postpartum 666.3 ☑
**Fibrinopenia** (hereditary) — *see also* Defect, coagulation 286.3
acquired 286.6
**Fibrinopurulent** — *see* condition
**Fibrinous** — *see* condition
**Fibroadenoma** (M9010/0)
cellular intracanalicular (M9020/0) 217
giant (intracanalicular) (M9020/0) 217
intracanalicular (M9011/0)
  cellular (M9020/0) 217
  giant (M9020/0) 217
  specified site — *see* Neoplasm, by site, benign
  unspecified site 217
juvenile (M9030/0) 217
pericanicular (M9012/0)
  specified site — *see* Neoplasm, by site, benign
  unspecified site 217

**Fibroadenoma** — *continued*
phyllodes (M9020/0) 217
prostate 600.20
  with
    other lower urinary tract symptoms (LUTS) 600.21
    urinary
      obstruction 600.21
      retention 600.21
specified site — *see* Neoplasm, by site, benign
unspecified site 217
**Fibroadenosis, breast** (chronic) (cystic) (diffuse) (periodic) (segmental) 610.2
**Fibroangioma** (M9160/0) — *see also* Neoplasm, by site, benign
juvenile (M9160/0)
  specified site — *see* Neoplasm, by site, benign
  unspecified site 210.7
**Fibrocellulitis progressiva ossificans** 728.11
**Fibrochondrosarcoma** (M9220/3) — *see* Neoplasm, cartilage, malignant
**Fibrocystic**
disease 277.00
  bone NEC 733.29
  breast 610.1
  jaw 526.2
  kidney (congenital) 753.19
  liver 751.62
  lung 518.89
    congenital 748.4
  pancreas 277.00
kidney (congenital) 753.19
**Fibrodysplasia ossificans multiplex** (progressiva) 728.11
**Fibroelastosis** (cordis) (endocardial) (endomyocardial) 425.3
**Fibroid** (tumor) (M8890/0) — *see also* Neoplasm, connective tissue, benign
disease, lung (chronic) (*see also* Fibrosis, lung) 515
heart (disease) (*see also* Myocarditis) 429.0
induration, lung (chronic) (*see also* Fibrosis, lung) 515
in pregnancy or childbirth 654.1 ☑
  affecting fetus or newborn 763.89
  causing obstructed labor 660.2 ☑
    affecting fetus or newborn 763.1
liver — *see* Cirrhosis, liver
lung (*see also* Fibrosis, lung) 515
pneumonia (chronic) (*see also* Fibrosis, lung) 515
uterus (M8890/0) (*see also* Leiomyoma, uterus) 218.9
**Fibrolipoma** (M8851/0) — *see also* Lipoma, by site 214.9
**Fibroliposarcoma** (M8850/3) — *see* Neoplasm, connective tissue, malignant
**Fibroma** (M8810/0) — *see also* Neoplasm, connective tissue, benign
ameloblastic (M9330/0) 213.1
  upper jaw (bone) 213.0
bone (nonossifying) 733.99
  ossifying (M9262/0) — *see* Neoplasm, bone, benign
cementifying (M9274/0) — *see* Neoplasm, bone, benign
chondromyxoid (M9241/0) — *see* Neoplasm, bone, benign
desmoplastic (M8823/1) — *see* Neoplasm, connective tissue, uncertain behavior
facial (M8813/0) — *see* Neoplasm, connective tissue, benign
invasive (M8821/1) — *see* Neoplasm, connective tissue, uncertain behavior
molle (M8851/0) (*see also* Lipoma, by site) 214.9

**Fibroma** — *see also* Neoplasm, connective tissue, benign — *continued*
myxoid (M8811/0) — *see* Neoplasm, connective tissue, benign
nasopharynx, nasopharyngeal (juvenile) (M9160/0) 210.7
nonosteogenic (nonossifying) — *see* Dysplasia, fibrous
odontogenic (M9321/0) 213.1
  upper jaw (bone) 213.0
ossifying (M9262/0) — *see* Neoplasm, bone, benign
periosteal (M8812/0) — *see* Neoplasm, bone, benign
prostate 600.20
  with
    other lower urinary tract symptoms (LUTS) 600.21
    urinary
      obstruction 600.21
      retention 600.21
soft (M8851/0) (*see also* Lipoma, by site) 214.9
**Fibromatosis** 728.79
abdominal (M8822/1) — *see* Neoplasm, connective tissue, uncertain behavior
aggressive (M8821/1) — *see* Neoplasm, connective tissue, uncertain behavior
congenital generalized (CGF) 759.89
Dupuytren's 728.6
gingival 523.8
plantar fascia 728.71
proliferative 728.79
pseudosarcomatous (proliferative) (subcutaneous) 728.79
subcutaneous pseudosarcomatous (proliferative) 728.79
**Fibromyalgia** 729.1
**Fibromyoma** (M8890/0) — *see also* Neoplasm, connective tissue, benign
uterus (corpus) (*see also* Leiomyoma, uterus) 218.9
  in pregnancy or childbirth 654.1 ☑
    affecting fetus or newborn 763.89
    causing obstructed labor 660.2 ☑
      affecting fetus or newborn 763.1
**Fibromyositis** — *see also* Myositis 729.1
scapulohumeral 726.2
**Fibromyxolipoma** (M8852/0) — *see also* Lipoma, by site 214.9
**Fibromyxoma** (M8811/0) — *see* Neoplasm, connective tissue, benign
**Fibromyxosarcoma** (M8811/3) — *see* Neoplasm, connective tissue, malignant
**Fibro-odontoma, ameloblastic** (M9290/0) 213.1
upper jaw (bone) 213.0
**Fibro-osteoma** (M9262/0) — *see* Neoplasm, bone, benign
**Fibroplasia, retrolental** 362.21
**Fibropurulent** — *see* condition
**Fibrosarcoma** (M8810/3) — *see also* Neoplasm, connective tissue, malignant
ameloblastic (M9330/3) 170.1
  upper jaw (bone) 170.0
congenital (M8814/3) — *see* Neoplasm, connective tissue, malignant
fascial (M8813/3) — *see* Neoplasm, connective tissue, malignant
infantile (M8814/3) — *see* Neoplasm, connective tissue, malignant
odontogenic (M9330/3) 170.1
  upper jaw (bone) 170.0
periosteal (M8812/3) — *see* Neoplasm, bone, malignant

**Fibrosclerosis**
breast 610.3
corpora cavernosa (penis) 607.89
familial multifocal NEC 710.8
multifocal (idiopathic) NEC 710.8
penis (corpora cavernosa) 607.89
**Fibrosis, fibrotic**
adrenal (gland) 255.8
alveolar (diffuse) 516.3
amnion 658.8 ☑
anal papillae 569.49
anus 569.49
appendix, appendiceal, noninflammatory 543.9
arteriocapillary — *see* Arteriosclerosis
bauxite (of lung) 503
biliary 576.8
  due to Clonorchis sinensis 121.1
bladder 596.8
  interstitial 595.1
  localized submucosal 595.1
  panmural 595.1
bone, diffuse 756.59
breast 610.3
capillary (*see also* Arteriosclerosis)
  lung (chronic) (*see also* Fibrosis, lung) 515
cardiac (*see also* Myocarditis) 429.0
cervix 622.8
chorion 658.8 ☑
corpus cavernosum 607.89
cystic (of pancreas) 277.00
  with
    manifestations
      gastrointestinal 277.03
      pulmonary 277.02
      specified NEC 277.09
    meconium ileus 277.01
    pulmonary exacerbation 277.02
due to (presence of) any device, implant, or graft — *see* Complications, due to (presence of) any device, implant, or graft classified to 996.0–996.5 NEC
ejaculatory duct 608.89
endocardium (*see also* Endocarditis) 424.90
endomyocardial (African) 425.0
epididymis 608.89
eye muscle 378.62
graphite (of lung) 503
heart (*see also* Myocarditis) 429.0
hepatic (*see also* Cirrhosis, liver)
  due to Clonorchis sinensis 121.1
hepatolienal — *see* Cirrhosis, liver
hepatosplenic — *see* Cirrhosis, liver
infrapatellar fat pad 729.31
interstitial pulmonary, newborn 770.7
intrascrotal 608.89
kidney (*see also* Sclerosis, renal) 587
liver — *see* Cirrhosis, liver
lung (atrophic) (capillary) (chronic) (confluent) (massive) (perialveolar) (peribronchial) 515
  with
    anthracosilicosis (occupational) 500
    anthracosis (occupational) 500
    asbestosis (occupational) 501
    bagassosis (occupational) 495.1
    bauxite 503
    berylliosis (occupational) 503
    byssinosis (occupational) 504
    calcicosis (occupational) 502
    chalicosis (occupational) 502
    dust reticulation (occupational) 504
    farmers' lung 495.0
    gannister disease (occupational) 502
    graphite 503
    pneumoconiosis (occupational) 505
    pneumosiderosis (occupational) 503
    siderosis (occupational) 503

**Fibrosis, fibrotic** — *continued*
  lung — *continued*
    with — *continued*
      silicosis (occupational) 502
      tuberculosis (*see also* Tuberculosis) 011.4 ☑
    diffuse (idiopathic) (interstitial) 516.3
    due to
      bauxite 503
      fumes or vapors (chemical) (inhalation) 506.4
      graphite 503
    following radiation 508.1
    postinflammatory 515
    silicotic (massive) (occupational) 502
    tuberculous (*see also* Tuberculosis) 011.4 ☑
  lymphatic gland 289.3
  median bar 600.90
    with
      other lower urinary tract symptoms (LUTS) 600.91
      urinary
        obstruction 600.91
        retention 600.91
  mediastinum (idiopathic) 519.3
  meninges 349.2
  muscle NEC 728.2
    iatrogenic (from injection) 999.9
  myocardium, myocardial (*see also* Myocarditis) 429.0
  oral submucous 528.8
  ovary 620.8
  oviduct 620.8
  pancreas 577.8
    cystic 277.00
      with
        manifestations
          gastrointestinal 277.03
          pulmonary 277.02
          specified NEC 277.09
        meconium ileus 277.01
        pulmonary exacerbation 277.02
  penis 607.89
  periappendiceal 543.9
  periarticular (*see also* Ankylosis) 718.5 ☑
  pericardium 423.1
  perineum, in pregnancy or childbirth 654.8 ☑
    affecting fetus or newborn 763.89
    causing obstructed labor 660.2 ☑
      affecting fetus or newborn 763.1
  perineural NEC 355.9
    foot 355.6
  periureteral 593.89
  placenta — *see* Placenta, abnormal
  pleura 511.0
  popliteal fat pad 729.31
  preretinal 362.56
  prostate (chronic) 600.90
    with
      other lower urinary tract symptoms (LUTS) 600.91
      urinary
        obstruction 600.91
        retention 600.91
  pulmonary (chronic) (*see also* Fibrosis, lung) 515
    alveolar capillary block 516.3
    interstitial
      diffuse (idiopathic) 516.3
      newborn 770.7
    radiation — *see* Effect, adverse, radiation
  rectal sphincter 569.49
  retroperitoneal, idiopathic 593.4
  sclerosing mesenteric (idiopathic) 567.82
  scrotum 608.89
  seminal vesicle 608.89
  senile 797
  skin NEC 709.2

**Fibrosis, fibrotic** — *continued*
  spermatic cord 608.89
  spleen 289.59
    bilharzial (*see also* Schistosomiasis) 120.9
  subepidermal nodular (M8832/0) — *see* Neoplasm, skin, benign
  submucous NEC 709.2
    oral 528.8
    tongue 528.8
  syncytium — *see* Placenta, abnormal
  testis 608.89
    chronic, due to syphilis 095.8
  thymus (gland) 254.8
  tunica vaginalis 608.89
  ureter 593.89
  urethra 599.84
  uterus (nonneoplastic) 621.8
    bilharzial (*see also* Schistosomiasis) 120.9
    neoplastic (*see also* Leiomyoma, uterus) 218.9
  vagina 623.8
  valve, heart (*see also* Endocarditis) 424.90
  vas deferens 608.89
  vein 459.89
    lower extremities 459.89
  vesical 595.1
**Fibrositis** (periarticular) (rheumatoid) 729.0
  humeroscapular region 726.2
  nodular, chronic
    Jaccoud's 714.4
    rheumatoid 714.4
  ossificans 728.11
  scapulohumeral 726.2
**Fibrothorax** 511.0
**Fibrotic** — *see* Fibrosis
**Fibrous** — *see* condition
**Fibroxanthoma** (M8831/0) — *see also* Neoplasm, connective tissue, benign
  atypical (M8831/1) — *see* Neoplasm, connective tissue, uncertain behavior
  malignant (M8831/3) — *see* Neoplasm, connective tissue, malignant
**Fibroxanthosarcoma** (M8831/3) — *see* Neoplasm, connective tissue, malignant
**Fiedler's**
  disease (leptospiral jaundice) 100.0
  myocarditis or syndrome (acute isolated myocarditis) 422.91
**Fiessinger-Leroy (-Reiter) syndrome** 099.3
**Fiessinger-Rendu syndrome** (erythema muliforme exudativum) 695.1
**Fifth disease** (eruptive) 057.0
  venereal 099.1
**Filaria, filarial** — *see* Infestation, filarial
**Filariasis** — *see also* Infestation, filarial 125.9
  bancroftian 125.0
  Brug's 125.1
  due to
    bancrofti 125.0
    Brugia (Wuchereria) (malayi) 125.1
    Loa loa 125.2
    malayi 125.1
    organism NEC 125.6
    Wuchereria (bancrofti) 125.0
      malayi 125.1
  Malayan 125.1
  ozzardi 125.5
  specified type NEC 125.6
**Filatoff's, Filatov's, Filatow's disease** (infectious mononucleosis) 075
**File-cutters' disease** 984.9
  specified type of lead — *see* Table of Drugs and Chemicals
**Filling defect**
  biliary tract 793.3
  bladder 793.5

**Filling defect** — *continued*
  duodenum 793.4
  gallbladder 793.3
  gastrointestinal tract 793.4
  intestine 793.4
  kidney 793.5
  stomach 793.4
  ureter 793.5
**Filtering bleb, eye** (postglaucoma) (status) V45.69
  with complication or rupture 997.99
  postcataract extraction (complication) 997.99
**Fimbrial cyst** (congenital) 752.11
**Fimbriated hymen** 752.49
**Financial problem affecting care** V60.2
**Findings, abnormal, without diagnosis** (examination) (laboratory test) 796.4
  17-ketosteroids, elevated 791.9
  acetonuria 791.6
  acid phosphatase 790.5
  albumin-globulin ratio 790.99
  albuminuria 791.0
  alcohol in blood 790.3
  alkaline phosphatase 790.5
  amniotic fluid 792.3
  amylase 790.5
  anisocytosis 790.09
  antenatal screening 796.5
  anthrax, positive 795.31
  antibody titers, elevated 795.79
  anticardiolipin antibody 795.79
  antigen-antibody reaction 795.79
  antiphospholipid antibody 795.79
  bacteriuria 791.9
  ballistocardiogram 794.39
  bicarbonate 276.9
  bile in urine 791.4
  bilirubin 277.4
  bleeding time (prolonged) 790.92
  blood culture, positive 790.7
  blood gas level (arterial) 790.91
  blood sugar level 790.29
    high 790.29
      fasting glucose 790.21
      glucose tolerance test 790.22
    low 251.2
  calcium 275.40
  cancer antigen 125 [CA 125] 795.82
  carbonate 276.9
  carcinoembryonic antigen [CEA] 795.81
  casts, urine 791.7
  catecholamines 791.9
  cells, urine 791.7
  cerebrospinal fluid (color) (content) (pressure) 792.0
  cervical
    high risk human papillomavirus (HPV) DNA test positive 795.05
    low risk human papillomavirus (HPV) DNA test positive 795.09
  chloride 276.9
  cholesterol 272.9
    high 272.0 ●
      with high triglycerides 272.2 ●
  chromosome analysis 795.2
  chyluria 791.1
  circulation time 794.39
  cloudy dialysis effluent 792.5
  cloudy urine 791.9
  coagulation study 790.92
  cobalt, blood 790.6
  color of urine (unusual) NEC 791.9
  copper, blood 790.6
  C-reactive protein (CRP) 790.95
  crystals, urine 791.9
  culture, positive NEC 795.39
    blood 790.7
    HIV V08
    human immunodeficiency virus V08
    nose 795.39

**Findings, abnormal, without diagnosis** — *continued*
  culture, positive — *continued*
    skin lesion NEC 795.39
    spinal fluid 792.0
    sputum 795.39
    stool 792.1
    throat 795.39
    urine 791.9
    viral
      human immunodeficiency V08
    wound 795.39
  echocardiogram 793.2
  echoencephalogram 794.01
  echogram NEC — *see* Findings, abnormal, structure
  electrocardiogram (ECG) (EKG) 794.31
  electroencephalogram (EEG) 794.02
  electrolyte level, urinary 791.9
  electromyogram (EMG) 794.17
    ocular 794.14
  electro-oculogram (EOG) 794.12
  electroretinogram (ERG) 794.11
  enzymes, serum NEC 790.5
  fibrinogen titer coagulation study 790.92
  filling defect — *see* Filling defect
  function study NEC 794.9
    auditory 794.15
    bladder 794.9
    brain 794.00
    cardiac 794.30
    endocrine NEC 794.6
      thyroid 794.5
    kidney 794.4
    liver 794.8
    nervous system
      central 794.00
      peripheral 794.19
    oculomotor 794.14
    pancreas 794.9
    placenta 794.9
    pulmonary 794.2
    retina 794.11
    special senses 794.19
    spleen 794.9
    vestibular 794.16
  gallbladder, nonvisualization 793.3
  glucose 790.29
    elevated
      fasting 790.21
      tolerance test 790.22
  glycosuria 791.5
  heart
    shadow 793.2
    sounds 785.3
  hematinuria 791.2
  hematocrit
    drop (precipitous) 790.01
    elevated 282.7
    low 285.9
  hematologic NEC 790.99
  hematuria 599.7
  hemoglobin
    elevated 282.7
    low 285.9
  hemoglobinuria 791.2
  histological NEC 795.4
  hormones 259.9
  immunoglobulins, elevated 795.79
  indolacetic acid, elevated 791.9
  iron 790.6
  karyotype 795.2
  ketonuria 791.6
  lactic acid dehydrogenase (LDH) 790.4
  lead 790.6
  lipase 790.5
  lipids NEC 272.9
  lithium, blood 790.6
  liver function test 790.6
  lung field (coin lesion) (shadow) 793.1
  magnesium, blood 790.6
  mammogram 793.80
    calcification 793.89
    calculus 793.89
    microcalcification 793.81

**Findings, abnormal, without diagnosis — continued**
mediastinal shift 793.2
melanin, urine 791.9
microbiologic NEC 795.39
mineral, blood NEC 790.6
myoglobinuria 791.3
nasal swab, anthrax 795.31
neonatal screening 796.6
nitrogen derivatives, blood 790.6
nonvisualization of gallbladder 793.3
nose culture, positive 795.39
odor of urine (unusual) NEC 791.9
oxygen saturation 790.91
Papanicolaou (smear) 795.1
  cervix 795.00
    with
      atypical squamous cells
        cannot exclude high grade
          squamous intraep-
          ithelial lesion (ASC-
          H) 795.02
        of undetermined signifi-
          cance (ASC-US)
          795.01
      cytologic evidence of malig-
        nancy 795.06
      high grade squamous intraep-
        ithelial lesion (HGSIL)
        795.04
      low grade squamous intraep-
        ithelial lesion (LGSIL)
        795.03
    dyskaryotic 795.09
    nonspecific finding NEC 795.09
  other site 795.1
peritoneal fluid 792.9
phonocardiogram 794.39
phosphorus 275.3
pleural fluid 792.9
pneumoencephalogram 793.0
PO2-oxygen ratio 790.91
poikilocytosis 790.09
potassium
  deficiency 276.8
  excess 276.7
PPD 795.5
prostate specific antigen (PSA) 790.93
protein, serum NEC 790.99
proteinuria 791.0
prothrombin time (partial) (prolonged) (PT) (PTT) 790.92
pyuria 791.9
radiologic (x-ray) 793.99
  abdomen 793.6
  biliary tract 793.3
  breast 793.89
    abnormal mammogram NOS
      793.80
    mammographic
      calcification 793.89
      calculus 793.89
      microcalcification 793.81
  gastrointestinal tract 793.4
  genitourinary organs 793.5
  head 793.0
  image test inconclusive due to ex-
    cess body fat 793.91
  intrathoracic organs NEC 793.2
  lung 793.1
  musculoskeletal 793.7
  placenta 793.99
  retroperitoneum 793.6
  skin 793.99
  skull 793.0
  subcutaneous tissue 793.99
red blood cell 790.09
  count 790.09
  morphology 790.09
  sickling 790.09
  volume 790.09
saliva 792.4
scan NEC 794.9
  bladder 794.9
  bone 794.9
  brain 794.09

**Findings, abnormal, without diagnosis — continued**
scan — continued
  kidney 794.4
  liver 794.8
  lung 794.2
  pancreas 794.9
  placental 794.9
  spleen 794.9
  thyroid 794.5
sedimentation rate, elevated 790.1
semen 792.2
serological (for)
  human immunodeficiency virus (HIV)
    inconclusive 795.71
    positive V08
  syphilis — see Findings, serology for syphilis
serology for syphilis
  false positive 795.6
  positive 097.1
    false 795.6
    follow-up of latent syphilis — see Syphilis, latent
    only finding — see Syphilis, latent
serum 790.99
  blood NEC 790.99
  enzymes NEC 790.5
  proteins 790.99
SGOT 790.4
SGPT 790.4
sickling of red blood cells 790.09
skin test, positive 795.79
  tuberculin (without active tubercu-losis) 795.5
sodium 790.6
  deficiency 276.1
  excess 276.0
spermatozoa 792.2
spinal fluid 792.0
  culture, positive 792.0
sputum culture, positive 795.39
  for acid-fast bacilli 795.39
stool NEC 792.1
  bloody 578.1
    occult 792.1
  color 792.1
  culture, positive 792.1
  occult blood 792.1
stress test 794.39
structure, body (echogram) (thermo-gram) (ultrasound) (x-ray) NEC 793.99
  abdomen 793.6
  breast 793.89
    abnormal mammogram 793.80
    mammographic
      calcification 793.89
      calculus 793.89
      microcalcification 793.81
  gastrointestinal tract 793.4
  genitourinary organs 793.5
  head 793.0
    echogram (ultrasound) 794.01
  intrathoracic organs NEC 793.2
  lung 793.1
  musculoskeletal 793.7
  placenta 793.99
  retroperitoneum 793.6
  skin 793.99
  subcutaneous tissue NEC 793.99
synovial fluid 792.9
thermogram — see Findings, abnor-mal, structure
throat culture, positive 795.39
thyroid (function) 794.5
  metabolism (rate) 794.5
  scan 794.5
  uptake 794.5
total proteins 790.99
toxicology (drugs) (heavy metals) 796.0
transaminase (level) 790.4
triglycerides 272.9
  high 272.1 ●

**Findings, abnormal, without diagnosis — continued**
triglycerides — continued
  high — continued
    with high cholesterol 272.2 ●
tuberculin skin test (without active tuberculosis) 795.5
tumor markers NEC 795.89
ultrasound (see also Findings, abnor-mal, structure)
  cardiogram 793.2
uric acid, blood 790.6
urine, urinary constituents 791.9
  acetone 791.6
  albumin 791.0
  bacteria 791.9
  bile 791.4
  blood 599.7
  casts or cells 791.7
  chyle 791.1
  culture, positive 791.9
  glucose 791.5
  hemoglobin 791.2
  ketone 791.6
  protein 791.0
  pus 791.9
  sugar 791.5
vaginal fluid 792.9
vanillylmandelic acid, elevated 791.9
vectorcardiogram (VCG) 794.39
ventriculogram (cerebral) 793.0
VMA, elevated 791.9
Wassermann reaction
  false positive 795.6
  positive 097.1
    follow-up of latent syphilis — see Syphilis, latent
    only finding — see Syphilis, latent
white blood cell 288.9
  count 288.9
    elevated 288.60
    low 288.50
  differential 288.9
  morphology 288.9
wound culture 795.39
xerography 793.89
zinc, blood 790.6
**Finger** — see condition
**Finnish type nephrosis** (congenital) ● 759.89 ●
**Fire, St. Anthony's** — see also Erysipelas 035
**Fish**
  hook stomach 537.89
  meal workers' lung 495.8
**Fisher's syndrome** 357.0
**Fissure, fissured**
  abdominal wall (congenital) 756.79
  anus, anal 565.0
    congenital 751.5
  buccal cavity 528.9
  clitoris (congenital) 752.49
  ear, lobule (congenital) 744.29
  epiglottis (congenital) 748.3
  larynx 478.79
    congenital 748.3
  lip 528.5
    congenital (see also Cleft, lip) 749.10
  nipple 611.2
    puerperal, postpartum 676.1 ☑
  palate (congenital) (see also Cleft, palate) 749.00
  postanal 565.0
  rectum 565.0
  skin 709.8
    streptococcal 686.9
  spine (congenital) (see also Spina bifi-da) 741.9 ☑
  sternum (congenital) 756.3
  tongue (acquired) 529.5
    congenital 750.13
**Fistula** (sinus) 686.9
  abdomen (wall) 569.81
    bladder 596.2

**Fistula** — continued
abdomen — continued
  intestine 569.81
  ureter 593.82
  uterus 619.2
abdominorectal 569.81
abdominosigmoidal 569.81
abdominothoracic 510.0
abdominouterine 619.2
  congenital 752.3
abdominovesical 596.2
accessory sinuses (see also Sinusitis) 473.9
actinomycotic — see Actinomycosis
alveolar
  antrum (see also Sinusitis, maxil-lary) 473.0
  process 522.7
anorectal 565.1
antrobuccal (see also Sinusitis, maxil-lary) 473.0
antrum (see also Sinusitis, maxillary) 473.0
anus, anal (infectional) (recurrent) 565.1
  congenital 751.5
  tuberculous (see also Tuberculosis) 014.8 ☑
aortic sinus 747.29
aortoduodenal 447.2
appendix, appendicular 543.9
arteriovenous (acquired) 447.0
  brain 437.3
    congenital 747.81
      ruptured (see also Hemor-rhage, subarachnoid) 430
    ruptured (see also Hemorrhage, subarachnoid) 430
  cerebral 437.3
    congenital 747.81
  congenital (peripheral) 747.60
    brain — see Fistula, arteriove-nous, brain, congenital
    coronary 746.85
    gastrointestinal 747.61
    lower limb 747.64
    pulmonary 747.3
    renal 747.62
    specified site NEC 747.69
    upper limb 747.63
  coronary 414.19
    congenital 746.85
  heart 414.19
  pulmonary (vessels) 417.0
    congenital 747.3
  surgically created (for dialysis) V45.1
    complication NEC 996.73
      atherosclerosis — see Arte-riosclerosis, extremi-ties
      embolism 996.74
      infection or inflammation 996.62
      mechanical 996.1
      occlusion NEC 996.74
      thrombus 996.74
    traumatic — see Injury, blood ves-sel, by site
artery 447.2
aural 383.81
  congenital 744.49
auricle 383.81
  congenital 744.49
Bartholin's gland 619.8
bile duct (see also Fistula, biliary) 576.4
biliary (duct) (tract) 576.4
  congenital 751.69
bladder (neck) (sphincter) 596.2
  into seminal vesicle 596.2
bone 733.99
brain 348.8
  arteriovenous — see Fistula, arteri-ovenous, brain

☑ Additional Digit Required — Refer to the Tabular List for Digit Selection ▽ Subterms under main terms may continue to next column or page

120 — Volume 2 · October 2007 ▶◀ Revised Text ● New Line ▲ Revised Code 2008 ICD-9-CM

Fistula — Fistula

**Fistula** — *continued*
branchial (cleft) 744.41
branchiogenous 744.41
breast 611.0
   puerperal, postpartum 675.1 ☑
bronchial 510.0
bronchocutaneous, bronchomediastinal, bronchopleural, bronchopleuromediastinal (infective)
   510.0
   tuberculous (*see also* Tuberculosis)
     011.3 ☑
bronchoesophageal 530.89
   congenital 750.3
buccal cavity (infective) 528.3
canal, ear 380.89
carotid-cavernous
   congenital 747.81
     with hemorrhage 430
   traumatic 900.82
     with hemorrhage (*see also*
       Hemorrhage, brain, trau-
       matic) 853.0 ☑
       late effect 908.3
cecosigmoidal 569.81
cecum 569.81
cerebrospinal (fluid) 349.81
cervical, lateral (congenital) 744.41
cervicoaural (congenital) 744.49
cervicosigmoidal 619.1
cervicovesical 619.0
cervix 619.8
chest (wall) 510.0
cholecystocolic (*see also* Fistula, gallbladder) 575.5
cholecystocolonic (*see also* Fistula,
   gallbladder) 575.5
cholecystoduodenal (*see also* Fistula,
   gallbladder) 575.5
cholecystoenteric (*see also* Fistula,
   gallbladder) 575.5
cholecystogastric (*see also* Fistula,
   gallbladder) 575.5
cholecystointestinal (*see also* Fistula,
   gallbladder) 575.5
choledochoduodenal 576.4
cholocolic (*see also* Fistula, gallbladder) 575.5
coccyx 685.1
   with abscess 685.0
colon 569.81
colostomy 569.69
colovaginal (acquired) 619.1
common duct (bile duct) 576.4
congenital, NEC — *see* Anomaly,
   specified type NEC
cornea, causing hypotony 360.32
coronary, arteriovenous 414.19
   congenital 746.85
costal region 510.0
cul-de-sac, Douglas' 619.8
cutaneous 686.9
cystic duct (*see also* Fistula, gallbladder) 575.5
   congenital 751.69
dental 522.7
diaphragm 510.0
   bronchovisceral 510.0
   pleuroperitoneal 510.0
   pulmonoperitoneal 510.0
duodenum 537.4
ear (canal) (external) 380.89
enterocolic 569.81
enterocutaneous 569.81
enteroenteric 569.81
entero-uterine 619.1
   congenital 752.3
enterovaginal 619.1
   congenital 752.49
enterovesical 596.1
epididymis 608.89
   tuberculous (*see also* Tuberculosis)
     016.4 ☑
esophagobronchial 530.89
   congenital 750.3
esophagocutaneous 530.89

**Fistula** — *continued*
esophagopleurocutaneous 530.89
esophagotracheal 530.84
   congenital 750.3
esophagus 530.89
   congenital 750.4
ethmoid (*see also* Sinusitis, ethmoidal)
   473.2
eyeball (cornea) (sclera) 360.32
eyelid 373.11
fallopian tube (external) 619.2
fecal 569.81
   congenital 751.5
from periapical lesion 522.7
frontal sinus (*see also* Sinusitis,
   frontal) 473.1
gallbladder 575.5
   with calculus, cholelithiasis, stones
     (*see also* Cholelithiasis)
     574.2 ☑
   congenital 751.69
gastric 537.4
gastrocolic 537.4
   congenital 750.7
   tuberculous (*see also* Tuberculosis)
     014.8 ☑
gastroenterocolic 537.4
gastroesophageal 537.4
gastrojejunal 537.4
gastrojejunocolic 537.4
genital
   organs
     female 619.9
       specified site NEC 619.8
     male 608.89
   tract-skin (female) 619.2
hepatopleural 510.0
hepatopulmonary 510.0
horseshoe 565.1
ileorectal 569.81
ileosigmoidal 569.81
ileostomy 569.69
ileovesical 596.1
ileum 569.81
in ano 565.1
   tuberculous (*see also* Tuberculosis)
     014.8 ☑
inner ear (*see also* Fistula, labyrinth)
   386.40
intestine 569.81
intestinocolonic (abdominal) 569.81
intestinoureteral 593.82
intestinouterine 619.1
intestinovaginal 619.1
   congenital 752.49
intestinovesical 596.1
involving female genital tract 619.9
   digestive-genital 619.1
   genital tract-skin 619.2
   specified site NEC 619.8
   urinary-genital 619.0
ischiorectal (fossa) 566
jejunostomy 569.69
jejunum 569.81
joint 719.80
   ankle 719.87
   elbow 719.82
   foot 719.87
   hand 719.84
   hip 719.85
   knee 719.86
   multiple sites 719.89
   pelvic region 719.85
   shoulder (region) 719.81
   specified site NEC 719.88
   tuberculous — *see* Tuberculosis,
     joint
   wrist 719.83
kidney 593.89
labium (majus) (minus) 619.8
labyrinth, labyrinthine NEC 386.40
   combined sites 386.48
   multiple sites 386.48
   oval window 386.42
   round window 386.41
   semicircular canal 386.43

**Fistula** — *continued*
lacrimal, lachrymal (duct) (gland) (sac)
   375.61
lacrimonasal duct 375.61
laryngotracheal 748.3
larynx 478.79
lip 528.5
   congenital 750.25
lumbar, tuberculous (*see also* Tuberculosis) 015.0 ☑ [730.8] ☑
lung 510.0
lymphatic (node) (vessel) 457.8
mamillary 611.0
mammary (gland) 611.0
   puerperal, postpartum 675.1 ☑
mastoid (process) (region) 383.1
maxillary (*see also* Sinusitis, maxillary) 473.0
mediastinal 510.0
mediastinobronchial 510.0
mediastinocutaneous 510.0
middle ear 385.89
mouth 528.3
nasal 478.19
   sinus (*see also* Sinusitis) 473.9
nasopharynx 478.29
nipple — *see* Fistula, breast
nose 478.19
oral (cutaneous) 528.3
   maxillary (*see also* Sinusitis, max-
     illary) 473.0
   nasal (with cleft palate) (*see also*
     Cleft, palate) 749.00
orbit, orbital 376.10
oro-antral (*see also* Sinusitis, maxillary) 473.0
oval window (internal ear) 386.42
oviduct (external) 619.2
palate (hard) 526.89
   soft 528.9
pancreatic 577.8
pancreaticoduodenal 577.8
parotid (gland) 527.4
   region 528.3
pelvoabdominointestinal 569.81
penis 607.89
perianal 565.1
pericardium (pleura) (sac) (*see also*
   Pericarditis) 423.8
pericecal 569.81
perineal — *see* Fistula, perineum
perineorectal 569.81
perineosigmoidal 569.81
perineo-urethroscrotal 608.89
perineum, perineal (with urethral involvement) NEC 599.1
   tuberculous (*see also* Tuberculosis)
     017.9 ☑
   ureter 593.82
perirectal 565.1
   tuberculous (*see also* Tuberculosis)
     014.8 ☑
peritoneum (*see also* Peritonitis)
   567.22
periurethral 599.1
pharyngo-esophageal 478.29
pharynx 478.29
   branchial cleft (congenital) 744.41
pilonidal (infected) (rectum) 685.1
   with abscess 685.0
pleura, pleural, pleurocutaneous,
   pleuroperitoneal 510.0
   stomach 510.0
   tuberculous (*see also* Tuberculosis)
     012.0 ☑
pleuropericardial 423.8
postauricular 383.81
postoperative, persistent 998.6
preauricular (congenital) 744.46
prostate 602.8
pulmonary 510.0
   arteriovenous 417.0
     congenital 747.3
   tuberculous (*see also* Tuberculosis,
     pulmonary) 011.9 ☑
pulmonoperitoneal 510.0

**Fistula** — *continued*
rectolabial 619.1
rectosigmoid (intercommunicating)
   569.81
rectoureteral 593.82
rectourethral 599.1
   congenital 753.8
rectouterine 619.1
   congenital 752.3
rectovaginal 619.1
   congenital 752.49
   old, postpartal 619.1
   tuberculous (*see also* Tuberculosis)
     014.8 ☑
rectovesical 596.1
   congenital 753.8
rectovesicovaginal 619.1
rectovulvar 619.1
   congenital 752.49
rectum (to skin) 565.1
   tuberculous (*see also* Tuberculosis)
     014.8 ☑
renal 593.89
retroauricular 383.81
round window (internal ear) 386.41
salivary duct or gland 527.4
   congenital 750.24
sclera 360.32
scrotum (urinary) 608.89
   tuberculous (*see also* Tuberculosis)
     016.5 ☑
semicircular canals (internal ear)
   386.43
sigmoid 569.81
   vesicoabdominal 596.1
sigmoidovaginal 619.1
   congenital 752.49
skin 686.9
   ureter 593.82
   vagina 619.2
sphenoidal sinus (*see also* Sinusitis,
   sphenoidal) 473.3
splenocolic 289.59
stercoral 569.81
stomach 537.4
sublingual gland 527.4
   congenital 750.24
submaxillary
   gland 527.4
     congenital 750.24
   region 528.3
thoracic 510.0
   duct 457.8
thoracicoabdominal 510.0
thoracicogastric 510.0
thoracicointestinal 510.0
thoracoabdominal 510.0
thoracogastric 510.0
thorax 510.0
thyroglossal duct 759.2
thyroid 246.8
trachea (congenital) (external) (internal) 748.3
tracheoesophageal 530.84
   congenital 750.3
   following tracheostomy 519.09
traumatic
   arteriovenous (*see also* Injury,
     blood vessel, by site) 904.9
   brain — *see* Injury, intracranial
tuberculous — *see* Tuberculosis, by
   site
typhoid 002.0
umbilical 759.89
umbilico-urinary 753.8
urachal, urachus 753.7
ureter (persistent) 593.82
ureteroabdominal 593.82
ureterocervical 593.82
ureterorectal 593.82
ureterosigmoido-abdominal 593.82
ureterovaginal 619.0
ureterovesical 596.2
urethra 599.1
   congenital 753.8

☑ Additional Digit Required — Refer to the Tabular List for Digit Selection       ☸ Subterms under main terms may continue to next column or page

**2008 ICD-9-CM**       ▶◀ Revised Text       ● New Line       ▲ Revised Code       **Volume 2 — 121**

**Fistula** — *continued*
urethra — *continued*
tuberculous (*see also* Tuberculosis) 016.3 ✓
urethroperineal 599.1
urethroperineovesical 596.2
urethrorectal 599.1
congenital 753.8
urethroscrotal 608.89
urethrovaginal 619.0
urethrovesical 596.2
urethrovesicovaginal 619.0
urinary (persistent) (recurrent) 599.1
uteroabdominal (anterior wall) 619.2
congenital 752.3
uteroenteric 619.1
uterofecal 619.1
uterointestinal 619.1
congenital 752.3
uterorectal 619.1
congenital 752.3
uteroureteric 619.0
uterovaginal 619.8
uterovesical 619.0
congenital 752.3
uterus 619.8
vagina (wall) 619.8
postpartal, old 619.8
vaginocutaneous (postpartal) 619.2
vaginoileal (acquired) 619.1
vaginoperineal 619.2
vesical NEC 596.2
vesicoabdominal 596.2
vesicocervicovaginal 619.0
vesicocolic 596.1
vesicocutaneous 596.2
vesicoenteric 596.1
vesicointestinal 596.1
vesicometrorectal 619.1
vesicoperineal 596.2
vesicorectal 596.1
congenital 753.8
vesicosigmoidal 596.1
vesicosigmoidovaginal 619.1
vesicoureteral 596.2
vesicoureterovaginal 619.0
vesicourethral 596.2
vesicourethrorectal 596.1
vesicouterine 619.0
congenital 752.3
vesicovaginal 619.0
vulvorectal 619.1
congenital 752.49
**Fit** 780.39
apoplectic (*see also* Disease, cerebrovascular, acute) 436
late effect — *see* Late effect(s) (of) cerebrovascular disease
epileptic (*see also* Epilepsy) 345.9 ✓
fainting 780.2
hysterical 300.11
newborn 779.0
**Fitting** (of)
artificial
arm (complete) (partial) V52.0
breast V52.4
eye(s) V52.2
leg(s) (complete) (partial) V52.1
brain neuropacemaker V53.02
cardiac pacemaker V53.31
carotid sinus pacemaker V53.39
cerebral ventricle (communicating) shunt V53.01
colostomy belt V53.5
contact lenses V53.1
cystostomy device V53.6
defibrillator, automatic implantable cardiac V53.32
dentures V52.3
device, unspecified type V53.90
abdominal V53.5
cardiac
defibrillator, automatic implantable V53.32
pacemaker V53.31
specified NEC V53.39

**Fitting** — *continued*
device, unspecified type — *continued*
cerebral ventricle (communicating) shunt V53.01
insulin pump V53.91
intrauterine contraceptive V25.1
nervous system V53.09
orthodontic V53.4
other device V53.99
prosthetic V52.9
breast V52.4
dental V52.3
eye V52.2
specified type NEC V52.8
special senses V53.09
substitution
auditory V53.09
nervous system V53.09
visual V53.09
urinary V53.6
diaphragm (contraceptive) V25.02
glasses (reading) V53.1
growth rod V54.02
hearing aid V53.2
ileostomy device V53.5
intestinal appliance or device NEC V53.5
intrauterine contraceptive device V25.1
neuropacemaker (brain) (peripheral nerve) (spinal cord) V53.02
orthodontic device V53.4
orthopedic (device) V53.7
brace V53.7
cast V53.7
corset V53.7
shoes V53.7
pacemaker (cardiac) V53.31
brain V53.02
carotid sinus V53.39
peripheral nerve V53.02
spinal cord V53.02
prosthesis V52.9
arm (complete) (partial) V52.0
breast V52.4
dental V52.3
eye V52.2
leg (complete) (partial) V52.1
specified type NEC V52.8
spectacles V53.1
wheelchair V53.8
**Fitz-Hugh and Curtis syndrome** 098.86
due to
Chlamydia trachomatis 099.56
Neisseria gonorrhoeae (gonococcal peritonitis) 098.86
**Fitz's syndrome** (acute hemorrhagic pancreatitis) 577.0
**Fixation**
joint — *see* Ankylosis
larynx 478.79
pupil 364.76
stapes 385.22
deafness (*see also* Deafness, conductive) 389.04
uterus (acquired) — *see* Malposition, uterus
vocal cord 478.5
**Flaccid** — *see also* condition
foot 736.79
forearm 736.09
palate, congenital 750.26
**Flail**
chest 807.4
newborn 767.3
joint (paralytic) 718.80
ankle 718.87
elbow 718.82
foot 718.87
hand 718.84
hip 718.85
knee 718.86
multiple sites 718.89
pelvic region 718.85

**Flail** — *continued*
joint — *continued*
shoulder (region) 718.81
specified site NEC 718.88
wrist 718.83
**Flajani (-Basedow) syndrome or disease** (exophthalmic goiter) 242.0 ✓
**Flap, liver** 572.8
**Flare, anterior chamber** (aqueous) (eye) 364.04
**Flashback phenomena** (drug) (hallucinogenic) 292.89
**Flat**
chamber (anterior) (eye) 360.34
chest, congenital 754.89
electroencephalogram (EEG) 348.8
foot (acquired) (fixed type) (painful) (postural) (spastic) 734
congenital 754.61
rocker bottom 754.61
vertical talus 754.61
rachitic 268.1
rocker bottom (congenital) 754.61
vertical talus, congenital 754.61
organ or site, congenital NEC — *see* Anomaly, specified type NEC
pelvis 738.6
with disproportion (fetopelvic) 653.2 ✓
affecting fetus or newborn 763.1
causing obstructed labor 660.1 ✓
affecting fetus or newborn 763.1
congenital 755.69
**Flatau-Schilder disease** 341.1
**Flattening**
head, femur 736.39
hip 736.39
lip (congenital) 744.89
nose (congenital) 754.0
acquired 738.0
**Flatulence** 787.3
**Flatus** 787.3
vaginalis 629.89
**Flax dressers' disease** 504
**Flea bite** — *see* Injury, superficial, by site
**Fleischer (-Kayser) ring** (corneal pigmentation) 275.1 *[371.14]*
**Fleischner's disease** 732.3
**Fleshy mole** 631
**Flexibilitas cerea** — *see also* Catalepsy 300.11
**Flexion**
cervix — *see* Flexion, uterus
contracture, joint (*see also* Contraction, joint) 718.4 ✓
deformity, joint (*see also* Contraction, joint) 736.9
hip, congenital (*see also* Subluxation, congenital, hip) 754.32
uterus (*see also* Malposition, uterus) 621.6
**Flexner's**
bacillus 004.1
diarrhea (ulcerative) 004.1
dysentery 004.1
**Flexner-Boyd dysentery** 004.2
**Flexure** — *see* condition
**Floater, vitreous** 379.24
**Floating**
cartilage (joint) (*see also* Disorder, cartilage, articular) 718.0 ✓
knee 717.6
gallbladder (congenital) 751.69
kidney 593.0
congenital 753.3
liver (congenital) 751.69
rib 756.3
spleen 289.59
**Flooding** 626.2
**Floor** — *see* condition
**Floppy**
infant NEC 781.99
iris syndrome 364.81

**Floppy** — *continued*
valve syndrome (mitral) 424.0
**Flu** — *see also* Influenza
gastric NEC 008.8
**Fluctuating blood pressure** 796.4
**Fluid**
abdomen 789.59 ▲
chest (*see also* Pleurisy, with effusion) 511.9
heart (*see also* Failure, heart) 428.0
joint (*see also* Effusion, joint) 719.0 ✓
loss (acute) 276.50
with
hypernatremia 276.0
hyponatremia 276.1
lung (*see also* Edema, lung)
encysted 511.8
peritoneal cavity 789.59 ▲
malignant 789.51 ●
pleural cavity (*see also* Pleurisy, with effusion) 511.9
retention 276.6
**Flukes** NEC — *see also* Infestation, fluke 121.9
blood NEC (*see also* Infestation, Schistosoma) 120.9
liver 121.3
**Fluor** (albus) (vaginalis) 623.5
trichomonal (Trichomonas vaginalis) 131.00
**Fluorosis** (dental) (chronic) 520.3
**Flushing** 782.62
menopausal 627.2
**Flush syndrome** 259.2
**Flutter**
atrial or auricular 427.32
heart (ventricular) 427.42
atrial 427.32
impure 427.32
postoperative 997.1
ventricular 427.42
**Flux** (bloody) (serosanguineous) 009.0
**Focal** — *see* condition
**Fochier's abscess** — *see* Abscess, by site
**Focus, Assmann's** — *see also* Tuberculosis 011.0 ✓
**Fogo selvagem** 694.4
**Foix-Alajouanine syndrome** 336.1
**Folds, anomalous** — *see also* Anomaly, specified type NEC
Bowman's membrane 371.31
Descemet's membrane 371.32
epicanthic 743.63
heart 746.89
posterior segment of eye, congenital 743.54
**Folie à deux** 297.3
**Follicle**
cervix (nabothian) (ruptured) 616.0
graafian, ruptured, with hemorrhage 620.0
nabothian 616.0
**Folliclis** (primary) — *see also* Tuberculosis 017.0 ✓
**Follicular** — *see also* condition
cyst (atretic) 620.0
**Folliculitis** 704.8
abscedens et suffodiens 704.8
decalvans 704.09
gonorrheal (acute) 098.0
chronic or duration of 2 months or more 098.2
keloid, keloidalis 706.1
pustular 704.8
ulerythematosa reticulata 701.8
**Folliculosis, conjunctival** 372.02
**Følling's disease** (phenylketonuria) 270.1
**Follow-up** (examination) (routine) (following) V67.9
cancer chemotherapy V67.2
chemotherapy V67.2
fracture V67.4
high-risk medication V67.51
injury NEC V67.59

**Follow-up** — *continued*
  postpartum
    immediately after delivery V24.0
    routine V24.2
  psychiatric V67.3
  psychotherapy V67.3
  radiotherapy V67.1
  specified condition NEC V67.59
  specified surgery NEC V67.09
  surgery V67.00
    vaginal pap smear V67.01
  treatment V67.9
    combined NEC V67.6
    fracture V67.4
    involving high-risk medication NEC
      V67.51
    mental disorder V67.3
    specified NEC V67.59
**Fong's syndrome** (hereditary osteoony-
    chodysplasia) 756.89
**Food**
  allergy 693.1
  anaphylactic shock — *see* Anaphylac-
    tic shock, due to, food
  asphyxia (from aspiration or inhala-
    tion) (*see also* Asphyxia, food)
    933.1
  choked on (*see also* Asphyxia, food)
    933.1
  deprivation 994.2
    specified kind of food NEC 269.8
  intoxication (*see also* Poisoning, food)
    005.9
  lack of 994.2
  poisoning (*see also* Poisoning, food)
    005.9
  refusal or rejection NEC 307.59
  strangulation or suffocation (*see also*
    Asphyxia, food) 933.1
  toxemia (*see also* Poisoning, food)
    005.9
**Foot** — *see also* condition
  and mouth disease 078.4
  process disease 581.3
**Foramen ovale** (nonclosure) (patent)
    (persistent) 745.5
**Forbes-Albright syndrome** (nonpuerper-
    al amenorrhea and lactation asso-
    ciated with pituitary tumor) 253.1
**Forbes'(glycogen storage) disease**
    271.0
**Forced birth or delivery** NEC 669.8 ☑
  affecting fetus or newborn NEC
    763.89
**Forceps**
  delivery NEC 669.5 ☑
    affecting fetus or newborn 763.2
**Fordyce's disease** (ectopic sebaceous
    glands) (mouth) 750.26
**Fordyce-Fox disease** (apocrine miliaria)
    705.82
**Forearm** — *see* condition
**Foreign body**

> *Note — For foreign body with open*
> *wound, or other injury, see Wound,*
> *open, or the type of injury specified.*

  accidentally left during a procedure
    998.4
  anterior chamber (eye) 871.6
    magnetic 871.5
      retained or old 360.51
    retained or old 360.61
  ciliary body (eye) 871.6
    magnetic 871.5
      retained or old 360.52
    retained or old 360.62
  entering through orifice (current) (old)
    accessory sinus 932
    air passage (upper) 933.0
      lower 934.8
    alimentary canal 938
    alveolar process 935.0
    antrum (Highmore) 932
    anus 937
    appendix 936

**Foreign body** — *continued*
  entering through orifice — *contin-
    ued*
    asphyxia due to (*see also* Asphyxia,
      food) 933.1
    auditory canal 931
    auricle 931
    bladder 939.0
    bronchioles 934.8
    bronchus (main) 934.1
    buccal cavity 935.0
    canthus (inner) 930.1
    cecum 936
    cervix (canal) uterine 939.1
    coil, ileocecal 936
    colon 936
    conjunctiva 930.1
    conjunctival sac 930.1
    cornea 930.0
    digestive organ or tract NEC 938
    duodenum 936
    ear (external) 931
    esophagus 935.1
    eye (external) 930.9
      combined sites 930.8
      intraocular — *see* Foreign body,
        by site
      specified site NEC 930.8
    eyeball 930.8
      intraocular — *see* Foreign body,
        intraocular
    eyelid 930.1
      retained or old 374.86
    frontal sinus 932
    gastrointestinal tract 938
    genitourinary tract 939.9
    globe 930.8
      penetrating 871.6
        magnetic 871.5
          retained or old 360.50
        retained or old 360.60
    gum 935.0
    Highmore's antrum 932
    hypopharynx 933.0
    ileocecal coil 936
    ileum 936
    inspiration (of) 933.1
    intestine (large) (small) 936
    lacrimal apparatus, duct, gland, or
      sac 930.2
    larynx 933.1
    lung 934.8
    maxillary sinus 932
    mouth 935.0
    nasal sinus 932
    nasopharynx 933.0
    nose (passage) 932
    nostril 932
    oral cavity 935.0
    palate 935.0
    penis 939.3
    pharynx 933.0
    pyriform sinus 933.0
    rectosigmoid 937
      junction 937
    rectum 937
    respiratory tract 934.9
      specified part NEC 934.8
    sclera 930.1
    sinus 932
      accessory 932
      frontal 932
      maxillary 932
      nasal 932
      pyriform 933.0
    small intestine 936
    stomach (hairball) 935.2
    suffocation by (*see also* Asphyxia,
      food) 933.1
    swallowed 938
      tongue 933.0
    tear ducts or glands 930.2
    throat 933.0
    tongue 935.0
      swallowed 933.0
    tonsil, tonsillar 933.0

**Foreign body** — *continued*
  entering through orifice — *contin-
    ued*
    tonsil, tonsillar — *continued*
      fossa 933.0
    trachea 934.0
    ureter 939.0
    urethra 939.0
    uterus (any part) 939.1
    vagina 939.2
    vulva 939.2
    wind pipe 934.0
  feeling of, in throat 784.99          ●
  granuloma (old) 728.82
    bone 733.99
    in operative wound (inadvertently
      left) 998.4
      due to surgical material inten-
        tionally left — *see* Compli-
        cations, due to (presence
        of) any device, implant, or
        graft classified to
        996.0–996.5 NEC
    muscle 728.82
    skin 709.4
    soft tissue 709.4
    subcutaneous tissue 709.4
  in
    bone (residual) 733.99
    open wound — *see* Wound, open,
      by site complicated
    soft tissue (residual) 729.6
  inadvertently left in operation wound
    (causing adhesions, obstruction,
    or perforation) 998.4
  ingestion, ingested NEC 938
  inhalation or inspiration (*see also* As-
    phyxia, food) 933.1
  internal organ, not entering through
    an orifice — *see* Injury, internal,
    by site, with open wound
  intraocular (nonmagnetic) 871.6
    combined sites 871.6
      magnetic 871.5
        retained or old 360.59
      retained or old 360.69
    magnetic 871.5
      retained or old 360.50
    retained or old 360.60
    specified site NEC 871.6
      magnetic 871.5
        retained or old 360.59
      retained or old 360.69
  iris (nonmagnetic) 871.6
    magnetic 871.5
      retained or old 360.52
    retained or old 360.62
  lens (nonmagnetic) 871.6
    magnetic 871.5
      retained or old 360.53
    retained or old 360.63
  lid, eye 930.1
  ocular muscle 870.4
    retained or old 376.6
  old or residual
    bone 733.99
    eyelid 374.86
    middle ear 385.83
    muscle 729.6
      ocular 376.6
    retrobulbar 376.6
    skin 729.6
      with granuloma 709.4
    soft tissue 729.6
      with granuloma 709.4
    subcutaneous tissue 729.6
      with granuloma 709.4
  operation wound, left accidentally
    998.4
  orbit 870.4
    retained or old 376.6
  posterior wall, eye 871.6
    magnetic 871.5
      retained or old 360.55
    retained or old 360.65
  respiratory tree 934.9

**Foreign body** — *continued*
  respiratory tree — *continued*
    specified site NEC 934.8
  retained (old) (nonmagnetic) (in)
    anterior chamber (eye) 360.61
      magnetic 360.51
    ciliary body 360.62
      magnetic 360.52
    eyelid 374.86
    globe 360.60
      magnetic 360.50
    intraocular 360.60
      magnetic 360.50
      specified site NEC 360.69
        magnetic 360.59
    iris 360.62
      magnetic 360.52
    lens 360.63
      magnetic 360.53
    muscle 729.6
    orbit 376.6
    posterior wall of globe 360.65
      magnetic 360.55
    retina 360.65
      magnetic 360.55
    retrobulbar 376.6
    skin 729.6
      with granuloma 709.4
    soft tissue 729.6
      with granuloma 709.4
    subcutaneous tissue 729.6
      with granuloma 709.4
    vitreous 360.64
      magnetic 360.54
  retina 871.6
    magnetic 871.5
      retained or old 360.55
    retained or old 360.65
  superficial, without major open wound
    (*see also* Injury, superficial, by
    site) 919.6
  swallowed NEC 938
  throat, feeling of 784.99          ●
  vitreous (humor) 871.6
    magnetic 871.5
      retained or old 360.54
    retained or old 360.64
**Forking, aqueduct of Sylvius** 742.3
  with spina bifida (*see also* Spina bifi-
    da) 741.0 ☑
**Formation**
  bone in scar tissue (skin) 709.3
  connective tissue in vitreous 379.25
  Elschnig pearls (postcataract extrac-
    tion) 366.51
  hyaline in cornea 371.49
  sequestrum in bone (due to infection)
    (*see also* Osteomyelitis) 730.1 ☑
  valve
    colon, congenital 751.5
    ureter (congenital) 753.29
**Formication** 782.0
**Fort Bragg fever** 100.89
**Fossa** — *see also* condition
  pyriform — *see* condition
**Foster-Kennedy syndrome** 377.04
**Fothergill's**
  disease, meaning scarlatina anginosa
    034.1
  neuralgia (*see also* Neuralgia, trigemi-
    nal) 350.1
**Foul breath** 784.99
**Found dead** (cause unknown) 798.9
**Foundling** V20.0
**Fournier's disease** (idiopathic gangrene)
    608.83
**Fourth**
  cranial nerve — *see* condition
  disease 057.8
  molar 520.1
**Foville's syndrome** 344.89
**Fox's**
  disease (apocrine miliaria) 705.82
  impetigo (contagiosa) 684
**Fox-Fordyce disease** (apocrine miliaria)
    705.82

**Fracture** (abduction) (adduction) (avulsion) (compression) (crush) (dislocation) (oblique) (separation) (closed) 829.0

> *Note* — *For fracture of any of the following sites with fracture of other bones — see Fracture, multiple.*
>
> *"Closed" includes the following descriptions of fractures, with or without delayed healing, unless they are specified as open or compound:*
>
> | | |
> |---|---|
> | comminuted | linear |
> | depressed | simple |
> | elevated | slipped epiphysis |
> | fissured | spiral |
> | greenstick | unspecified |
> | impacted | |
>
> *"Open" includes the following descriptions of fractures, with or without delayed healing:*
>
> | | |
> |---|---|
> | compound | puncture |
> | infected | with foreign body |
> | missile | |
>
> *For late effect of fracture, see Late, effect, fracture, by site.*

with
    internal injuries in same region (conditions classifiable to 860–869) (*see also* Injury, internal, by site)
    pelvic region — *see* Fracture, pelvis
acetabulum (with visceral injury) (closed) 808.0
    open 808.1
acromion (process) (closed) 811.01
    open 811.11
alveolus (closed) 802.8
    open 802.9
ankle (malleolus) (closed) 824.8
    bimalleolar (Dupuytren's) (Pott's) 824.4
      open 824.5
    bone 825.21
      open 825.31
    lateral malleolus only (fibular) 824.2
      open 824.3
    medial malleolus only (tibial) 824.0
      open 824.1
    open 824.9
    pathologic 733.16
    talus 825.21
      open 825.31
    trimalleolar 824.6
      open 824.7
antrum — *see* Fracture, skull, base
arm (closed) 818.0
    and leg(s) (any bones) 828.0
      open 828.1
    both (any bones) (with rib(s)) (with sternum) 819.0
      open 819.1
    lower 813.80
      open 813.90
    open 818.1
    upper — *see* Fracture, humerus
astragalus (closed) 825.21
    open 825.31
atlas — *see* Fracture, vertebra, cervical, first
axis — *see* Fracture, vertebra, cervical, second
back — *see* Fracture, vertebra, by site
Barton's — *see* Fracture, radius, lower end
basal (skull) — *see* Fracture, skull, base
Bennett's (closed) 815.01

Fracture — *continued*
Bennett's — *continued*
    open 815.11
bimalleolar (closed) 824.4
    open 824.5
bone (closed) NEC 829.0
    birth injury NEC 767.3
    open 829.1
    pathologic NEC (*see also* Fracture, pathologic) 733.10
    stress NEC (*see also* Fracture, stress) 733.95
boot top — *see* Fracture, fibula
boxers' — *see* Fracture, metacarpal bone(s)
breast bone — *see* Fracture, sternum
bucket handle (semilunar cartilage) — *see* Tear, meniscus
burst — *see* Fracture, traumatic, by site ●
bursting — *see* Fracture, phalanx, hand, distal
calcaneus (closed) 825.0
    open 825.1
capitate (bone) (closed) 814.07
    open 814.17
capitellum (humerus) (closed) 812.49
    open 812.59
carpal bone(s) (wrist NEC) (closed) 814.00
    open 814.10
    specified site NEC 814.09
      open 814.19
cartilage, knee (semilunar) — *see* Tear, meniscus
cervical — *see* Fracture, vertebra, cervical
chauffeur's — *see* Fracture, ulna, lower end
chisel — *see* Fracture, radius, upper end
clavicle (interligamentous part) (closed) 810.00
    acromial end 810.03
      open 810.13
    due to birth trauma 767.2
    open 810.10
    shaft (middle third) 810.02
      open 810.12
    sternal end 810.01
      open 810.11
clayshovelers' — *see* Fracture, vertebra, cervical
coccyx (*see also* Fracture, vertebra, coccyx)
    complicating delivery 665.6 ☑
collar bone — *see* Fracture, clavicle
Colles' (reversed) (closed) 813.41
    open 813.51
comminuted — *see* Fracture, by site
compression (*see also* Fracture, by site)
    nontraumatic — *see* Fracture, pathologic
congenital 756.9
coracoid process (closed) 811.02
    open 811.12
coronoid process (ulna) (closed) 813.02
    mandible (closed) 802.23
      open 802.33
    open 813.12
corpus cavernosum penis 959.13
costochondral junction — *see* Fracture, rib
costosternal junction — *see* Fracture, rib
cranium — *see* Fracture, skull, by site
cricoid cartilage (closed) 807.5
    open 807.6
cuboid (ankle) (closed) 825.23
    open 825.33
cuneiform
    foot (closed) 825.24
      open 825.34
    wrist (closed) 814.03

Fracture — *continued*
cuneiform — *continued*
    wrist — *continued*
      open 814.13
dental implant 525.73 ●
dental restorative material
    with loss of material 525.64
    without loss of material 525.63
due to
    birth injury — *see* Birth injury, fracture
    gunshot — *see* Fracture, by site, open
    neoplasm — *see* Fracture, pathologic
    osteoporosis — *see* Fracture, pathologic
Dupuytren's (ankle) (fibula) (closed) 824.4
    open 824.5
    radius 813.42
      open 813.52
Duverney's — *see* Fracture, ilium
elbow (*see also* Fracture, humerus, lower end)
    olecranon (process) (closed) 813.01
      open 813.11
    supracondylar (closed) 812.41
      open 812.51
ethmoid (bone) (sinus) — *see* Fracture, skull, base
face bone(s) (closed) NEC 802.8
    with
      other bone(s) — *see* Fracture, multiple, skull
      skull (*see also* Fracture, skull)
        involving other bones — *see* Fracture, multiple, skull
    open 802.9
fatigue — *see* Fracture, march
femur, femoral (closed) 821.00
    cervicotrochanteric 820.03
      open 820.13
    condyles, epicondyles 821.21
      open 821.31
    distal end — *see* Fracture, femur, lower end
    epiphysis (separation)
      capital 820.01
        open 820.11
      head 820.01
        open 820.11
      lower 821.22
        open 821.32
      trochanteric 820.01
        open 820.11
      upper 820.01
        open 820.11
    head 820.09
      open 820.19
    lower end or extremity (distal end) (closed) 821.20
      condyles, epicondyles 821.21
        open 821.31
      epiphysis (separation) 821.22
        open 821.32
      multiple sites 821.29
        open 821.39
      open 821.30
      specified site NEC 821.29
        open 821.39
      supracondylar 821.23
        open 821.33
      T-shaped 821.21
        open 821.31
    neck (closed) 820.8
      base (cervicotrochanteric) 820.03
        open 820.13
      extracapsular 820.20
        open 820.30
      intertrochanteric (section) 820.21
        open 820.31
      intracapsular 820.00

Fracture — *continued*
femur, femoral — *continued*
    neck — *continued*
      intracapsular — *continued*
        open 820.10
      intratrochanteric 820.21
        open 820.31
      midcervical 820.02
        open 820.12
      open 820.9
      pathologic 733.14
        specified part NEC 733.15
      specified site NEC 820.09
        open 820.19
      transcervical 820.02
        open 820.12
      transtrochanteric 820.20
        open 820.30
    open 821.10
    pathologic 733.14
      specified part NEC 733.15
    peritrochanteric (section) 820.20
      open 820.30
    shaft (lower third) (middle third) (upper third) 821.01
      open 821.11
    subcapital 820.09
      open 820.19
    subtrochanteric (region) (section) 820.22
      open 820.32
    supracondylar 821.23
      open 821.33
    transepiphyseal 820.01
      open 820.11
    trochanter (greater) (lesser) (*see also* Fracture, femur, neck, by site) 820.20
      open 820.30
    T-shaped, into knee joint 821.21
      open 821.31
    upper end 820.8
      open 820.9
fibula (closed) 823.81
    with tibia 823.82
      open 823.92
    distal end 824.8
      open 824.9
    epiphysis
      lower 824.8
        open 824.9
      upper — *see* Fracture, fibula, upper end
    head — *see* Fracture, fibula, upper end
    involving ankle 824.2
      open 824.3
    lower end or extremity 824.8
      open 824.9
    malleolus (external) (lateral) 824.2
      open 824.3
    open NEC 823.91
    pathologic 733.16
    proximal end — *see* Fracture, fibula, upper end
    shaft 823.21
      with tibia 823.22
        open 823.32
      open 823.31
    stress 733.93
    torus 823.41
      with tibia 823.42
    upper end or extremity (epiphysis) (head) (proximal end) (styloid) 823.01
      with tibia 823.02
        open 823.12
      open 823.11
finger(s), of one hand (closed) (*see also* Fracture, phalanx, hand) 816.00
    with
      metacarpal bone(s), of same hand 817.0
        open 817.1
      thumb of same hand 816.03
        open 816.13

☑ Additional Digit Required — Refer to the Tabular List for Digit Selection            🔳 Subterms under main terms may continue to next column or page

124 — Volume 2 · October 2007      ▶◀ Revised Text      ● New Line      ▲ Revised Code      *2008 ICD-9-CM*

**Fracture** — *continued*
finger(s), of one hand (*see also* Fracture, phalanx, hand) — *continued*
open 816.10
foot, except toe(s) alone (closed) 825.20
open 825.30
forearm (closed) NEC 813.80
lower end (distal end) (lower epiphysis) 813.40
open 813.50
open 813.90
shaft 813.20
open 813.30
upper end (proximal end) (upper epiphysis) 813.00
open 813.10
fossa, anterior, middle, or posterior — *see* Fracture, skull, base
Fracture (abduction) (adduction) (avulsion) (compression) (crush) (dislocation) (oblique) (separation) (closed) 829.0
frontal (bone) (*see also* Fracture, skull, vault)
sinus — *see* Fracture, skull, base
Galeazzi's — *see* Fracture, radius, lower end
glenoid (cavity) (fossa) (scapula) (closed) 811.03
open 811.13
Gosselin's — *see* Fracture, ankle
greenstick — *see* Fracture, by site
grenade-throwers' — *see* Fracture, humerus, shaft
gutter — *see* Fracture, skull, vault
hamate (closed) 814.08
open 814.18
hand, one (closed) 815.00
carpals 814.00
open 814.10
specified site NEC 814.09
open 814.19
metacarpals 815.00
open 815.10
multiple, bones of one hand 817.0
open 817.1
open 815.10
phalanges (*see also* Fracture, phalanx, hand) 816.00
open 816.10
healing
aftercare (*see also* Aftercare, fracture) V54.89
change of cast V54.89
complications — *see* condition
convalescence V66.4
removal of
cast V54.89
fixation device
external V54.89
internal V54.01
heel bone (closed) 825.0
open 825.1
hip (closed) (*see also* Fracture, femur, neck) 820.8
open 820.9
pathologic 733.14
humerus (closed) 812.20
anatomical neck 812.02
open 812.12
articular process (*see also* Fracture humerus, condyle(s)) 812.44
open 812.54
capitellum 812.49
open 812.59
condyle(s) 812.44
lateral (external) 812.42
open 812.52
medial (internal epicondyle) 812.43
open 812.53
open 812.54
distal end — *see* Fracture, humerus, lower end

**Fracture** — *continued*
humerus — *continued*
epiphysis
lower (*see also* Fracture, humerus, condyle(s)) 812.44
open 812.54
upper 812.09
open 812.19
external condyle 812.42
open 812.52
great tuberosity 812.03
open 812.13
head 812.09
open 812.19
internal epicondyle 812.43
open 812.53
lesser tuberosity 812.09
open 812.19
lower end or extremity (distal end) (*see also* Fracture, humerus, by site) 812.40
multiple sites NEC 812.49
open 812.59
open 812.50
specified site NEC 812.49
open 812.59
neck 812.01
open 812.11
open 812.30
pathologic 733.11
proximal end — *see* Fracture, humerus, upper end
shaft 812.21
open 812.31
supracondylar 812.41
open 812.51
surgical neck 812.01
open 812.11
trochlea 812.49
open 812.59
T-shaped 812.44
open 812.54
tuberosity — *see* Fracture, humerus, upper end
upper end or extremity (proximal end) (*see also* Fracture, humerus, by site) 812.00
open 812.10
specified site NEC 812.09
open 812.19
hyoid bone (closed) 807.5
open 807.6
hyperextension — *see* Fracture, radius, lower end
ilium (with visceral injury) (closed) 808.41
open 808.51
impaction, impacted — *see* Fracture, by site
incus — *see* Fracture, skull, base
innominate bone (with visceral injury) (closed) 808.49
open 808.59
instep, of one foot (closed) 825.20
with toe(s) of same foot 827.0
open 827.1
open 825.30
● insufficiency — *see* Fracture, pathologic, by site ●
internal
ear — *see* Fracture, skull, base
semilunar cartilage, knee — *see* Tear, meniscus, medial
intertrochanteric — *see* Fracture, femur, neck, intertrochanteric
ischium (with visceral injury) (closed) 808.42
open 808.52
jaw (bone) (lower) (closed) (*see also* Fracture, mandible) 802.20
angle 802.25
open 802.35
open 802.30
upper — *see* Fracture, maxilla

**Fracture** — *continued*
knee
cap (closed) 822.0
open 822.1
cartilage (semilunar) — *see* Tear, meniscus
labyrinth (osseous) — *see* Fracture, skull, base
larynx (closed) 807.5
open 807.6
late effect — *see* Late, effects (of), fracture
Le Fort's — *see* Fracture, maxilla
leg (closed) 827.0
with rib(s) or sternum 828.0
open 828.1
both (any bones) 828.0
open 828.1
lower — *see* Fracture, tibia
open 827.1
upper — *see* Fracture, femur
limb
lower (multiple) (closed) NEC 827.0
open 827.1
upper (multiple) (closed) NEC 818.0
open 818.1
long bones, due to birth trauma — *see* Birth injury, fracture
lower end or extremity (anterior lip) (posterior) 824.8
open 824.9
lumbar — *see* Fracture, vertebra, lumbar
lunate bone (closed) 814.02
open 814.12
malar bone (closed) 802.4
open 802.5
Malgaigne's (closed) 808.43
open 808.53
malleolus (closed) 824.8
bimalleolar 824.4
open 824.5
lateral 824.2
and medial (*see also* Fracture, malleolus, bimalleolar)
with lip of tibia — *see* Fracture, malleolus, trimalleolar
open 824.3
medial (closed) 824.0
and lateral (*see also* Fracture, malleolus, bimalleolar)
with lip of tibia — *see* Fracture, malleolus, trimalleolar
open 824.1
open 824.9
trimalleolar (closed) 824.6
open 824.7
malleus — *see* Fracture, skull, base
malunion 733.81
mandible (closed) 802.20
angle 802.25
open 802.35
body 802.28
alveolar border 802.27
open 802.37
open 802.38
symphysis 802.26
open 802.36
condylar process 802.21
open 802.31
coronoid process 802.23
open 802.33
multiple sites 802.29
open 802.39
open 802.30
ramus NEC 802.24
open 802.34
subcondylar 802.22
open 802.32
manubrium — *see* Fracture, sternum
march 733.95
fibula 733.93
metatarsals 733.94
tibia 733.93

**Fracture** — *continued*
maxilla, maxillary (superior) (upper jaw) (closed) 802.4
inferior — *see* Fracture, mandible
open 802.5
meniscus, knee — *see* Tear, meniscus
metacarpus, metacarpal (bone(s)), of one hand (closed) 815.00
with phalanx, phalanges, hand (finger(s)) (thumb) of same hand 817.0
open 817.1
base 815.02
first metacarpal 815.01
open 815.11
open 815.12
thumb 815.01
open 815.11
multiple sites 815.09
open 815.19
neck 815.04
open 815.14
open 815.10
shaft 815.03
open 815.13
metatarsus, metatarsal (bone(s)), of one foot (closed) 825.25
with tarsal bone(s) 825.29
open 825.39
open 825.35
Monteggia's (closed) 813.03
open 813.13
Moore's — *see* Fracture, radius, lower end
multangular bone (closed)
larger 814.05
open 814.15
smaller 814.06
open 814.16
multiple (closed) 829.0

*Note — Multiple fractures of sites classifiable to the same three- or four-digit category are coded to that category, except for sites classifiable to 810–818 or 820–827 in different limbs.*

*Multiple fractures of sites classifiable to different fourth-digit subdivisions within the same three–digit category should be dealt with according to coding rules.*

*Multiple fractures of sites classifiable to different three–digit categories (identifiable from the listing under "Fracture"), and of sites classifiable to 810–818 or 820–827 in different limbs should be coded according to the following list, which should be referred to in the following priority order: skull or face bones, pelvis or vertebral column, legs, arms.*

arm (multiple bones in same arm except in hand alone) (sites classifiable to 810–817 with sites classifiable to a different three–digit category in 810–817 in same arm) (closed) 818.0
open 818.1
arms, both or arm(s) with rib(s) or sternum (sites classifiable to 810–818 with sites classifiable to same range of categories in other limb or to 807) (closed) 819.0
open 819.1
bones of trunk NEC (closed) 809.0
open 809.1
hand, metacarpal bone(s) with phalanx or phalanges of same hand (sites classifiable to 815 with sites classifiable to 816 in same hand) (closed) 817.0
open 817.1

☑ Additional Digit Required — Refer to the Tabular List for Digit Selection
*2008 ICD-9-CM*
▶◀ Revised Text   ● New Line   ▲ Revised Code
▽ Subterms under main terms may continue to next column or page
**October 2007 • Volume 2 — 125**

**Fracture** — *continued*
  multiple — *continued*
    leg (multiple bones in same leg)
      (sites classifiable to 820–826
      with sites classifiable to a
      different three–digit category
      in that range in same leg)
      (closed) 827.0
        open 827.1
    legs, both or leg(s) with arm(s),
      rib(s), or sternum (sites clas-
      sifiable to 820–827 with sites
      classifiable to same range of
      categories in other leg or to
      807 or 810–819) (closed)
      828.0
        open 828.1
      open 829.1
    pelvis with other bones except skull
      or face bones (sites classifi-
      able to 808 with sites classi-
      fiable to 805–807 or
      810–829) (closed) 809.0
        open 809.1
    skull, specified or unspecified
      bones, or face bone(s) with
      any other bone(s) (sites clas-
      sifiable to 800–803 with sites
      classifiable to 805–829)
      (closed) 804.0 ☑

> *Note — Use the following fifth-digit*
> *subclassification with categories 800,*
> *801, 803, and 804:*
>
> 0   *unspecified state of conscious-*
>     *ness*
>
> 1   *with no loss of consciousness*
>
> 2   *with brief [less than one hour]*
>     *loss of consciousness*
>
> 3   *with moderate [1–24 hours] loss*
>     *of consciousness*
>
> 4   *with prolonged [more than 24*
>     *hours] loss of consciousness and*
>     *return to pre–existing conscious*
>     *level*
>
> 5   *with prolonged [more than 24*
>     *hours] loss of consciousness,*
>     *without return to pre–existing*
>     *conscious level*
>
> *Use fifth-digit 5 to designate when a*
> *patient is unconscious and dies before*
> *regaining consciousness, regardless of*
> *the duration of the loss of consciousness*
>
> 6   *with loss of consciousness of un-*
>     *specified duration*
>
> 9   *with concussion, unspecified*

      with
        contusion, cerebral 804.1 ☑
        epidural hemorrhage
          804.2 ☑
        extradural hemorrhage
          804.2 ☑
        hemorrhage (intracranial)
          NEC 804.3 ☑
        intracranial injury NEC
          804.4 ☑
        laceration, cerebral 804.1 ☑
        subarachnoid hemorrhage
          804.2 ☑
        subdural hemorrhage
          804.2 ☑
      open 804.5 ☑
        with
          contusion, cerebral
            804.6 ☑
          epidural hemorrhage
            804.7 ☑
          extradural hemorrhage
            804.7 ☑
          hemorrhage (intracranial)
            NEC 804.8 ☑

**Fracture** — *continued*
  multiple — *continued*
    skull, specified or unspecified
      bones, or face bone(s) with
      any other bone(s) — *contin-*
      *ued*
        open — *continued*
          with — *continued*
            intracranial injury NEC
              804.9 ☑
            laceration, cerebral
              804.6 ☑
            subarachnoid hemorrhage
              804.7 ☑
            subdural hemorrhage
              804.7 ☑
    vertebral column with other bones,
      except skull or face bones
      (sites classifiable to 805 or
      806 with sites classifiable to
      807–808 or 810–829) (closed)
      809.0
        open 809.1
  nasal (bone(s)) (closed) 802.0
    open 802.1
    sinus — *see* Fracture, skull, base
  navicular
    carpal (wrist) (closed) 814.01
      open 814.11
    tarsal (ankle) (closed) 825.22
      open 825.32
  neck — *see* Fracture, vertebra, cervi-
    cal
  neural arch — *see* Fracture, vertebra,
    by site
  nonunion 733.82
  nose, nasal, (bone) (septum) (closed)
    802.0
    open 802.1
  occiput — *see* Fracture, skull, base
  odontoid process — *see* Fracture,
    vertebra, cervical
  olecranon (process) (ulna) (closed)
    813.01
    open 813.11
  open 829.1
  orbit, orbital (bone) (region) (closed)
    802.8
    floor (blow-out) 802.6
      open 802.7
    open 802.9
    roof — *see* Fracture, skull, base
    specified part NEC 802.8
      open 802.9
  os
    calcis (closed) 825.0
      open 825.1
    magnum (closed) 814.07
      open 814.17
    pubis (with visceral injury) (closed)
      808.2
      open 808.3
    triquetrum (closed) 814.03
      open 814.13
  osseous
    auditory meatus — *see* Fracture,
      skull, base
    labyrinth — *see* Fracture, skull,
      base
    ossicles, auditory (incus) (malleus)
      (stapes) — *see* Fracture, skull,
      base
  osteoporotic — *see* Fracture, patholog-
    ic
  palate (closed) 802.8
    open 802.9
  paratrooper — *see* Fracture, tibia,
    lower end
  parietal bone — *see* Fracture, skull,
    vault
  parry — *see* Fracture, Monteggia's
  patella (closed) 822.0
    open 822.1
  pathologic (cause unknown) 733.10
    ankle 733.16
    femur (neck) 733.14

**Fracture** — *continued*
  pathologic — *continued*
    femur — *continued*
      specified NEC 733.15
    fibula 733.16
    hip 733.14
    humerus 733.11
    radius (distal) 733.12
    specified site NEC 733.19
    tibia 733.16
    ulna 733.12
    vertebrae (collapse) 733.13
    wrist 733.12
  pedicle (of vertebral arch) — *see*
    Fracture, vertebra, by site
  pelvis, pelvic (bone(s)) (with visceral
    injury) (closed) 808.8
    multiple (with disruption of pelvic
      circle) 808.43
      open 808.53
    open 808.9
    rim (closed) 808.49
      open 808.59
  peritrochanteric (closed) 820.20
    open 820.30
  phalanx, phalanges, of one
    foot (closed) 826.0
      with bone(s) of same lower limb
        827.0
        open 827.1
      open 826.1
    hand (closed) 816.00
      with metacarpal bone(s) of same
        hand 817.0
        open 817.1
      distal 816.02
        open 816.12
      middle 816.01
        open 816.11
      multiple sites NEC 816.03
        open 816.13
      open 816.10
      proximal 816.01
        open 816.11
  pisiform (closed) 814.04
    open 814.14
  pond — *see* Fracture, skull, vault
  Pott's (closed) 824.4
    open 824.5
  prosthetic device, internal — *see*
    Complications, mechanical
  pubis (with visceral injury) (closed)
    808.2
    open 808.3
  Quervain's (closed) 814.01
    open 814.11
  radius (alone) (closed) 813.81
    with ulna NEC 813.83
      open 813.93
    distal end — *see* Fracture, radius,
      lower end
    epiphysis
      lower — *see* Fracture, radius,
        lower end
      upper — *see* Fracture, radius,
        upper end
    head — *see* Fracture, radius, upper
      end
    lower end or extremity (distal end)
      (lower epiphysis) 813.42
      with ulna (lower end) 813.44
        open 813.54
      open 813.52
      torus 813.45
    neck — *see* Fracture, radius, upper
      end
    open NEC 813.91
    pathologic 733.12
    proximal end — *see* Fracture, ra-
      dius, upper end
    shaft (closed) 813.21
      with ulna (shaft) 813.23
        open 813.33
      open 813.31
    upper end 813.07
      with ulna (upper end) 813.08

**Fracture** — *continued*
  radius — *continued*
    upper end — *continued*
      with ulna — *continued*
        open 813.18
      epiphysis 813.05
        open 813.15
      head 813.05
        open 813.15
      multiple sites 813.07
        open 813.17
      neck 813.06
        open 813.16
      open 813.17
      specified site NEC 813.07
        open 813.17
  ramus
    inferior or superior (with visceral
      injury) (closed) 808.2
      open 808.3
    ischium — *see* Fracture, ischium
    mandible 802.24
      open 802.34
  rib(s) (closed) 807.0 ☑

> *Note — Use the following fifth-digit*
> *subclassification with categories*
> *807.0–807.1:*
>
> 0   *rib(s), unspecified*
>
> 1   *one rib*
>
> 2   *two ribs*
>
> 3   *three ribs*
>
> 4   *four ribs*
>
> 5   *five ribs*
>
> 6   *six ribs*
>
> 7   *seven ribs*
>
> 8   *eight or more ribs*
>
> 9   *multiple ribs, unspecified*

    with flail chest (open) 807.4
    open 807.1 ☑
  root, tooth 873.63
    complicated 873.73
  sacrum — *see* Fracture, vertebra,
    sacrum
  scaphoid
    ankle (closed) 825.22
      open 825.32
    wrist (closed) 814.01
      open 814.11
  scapula (closed) 811.00
    acromial, acromion (process)
      811.01
      open 811.11
    body 811.09
      open 811.19
    coracoid process 811.02
      open 811.12
    glenoid (cavity) (fossa) 811.03
      open 811.13
    neck 811.03
      open 811.13
    open 811.10
  semilunar
    bone, wrist (closed) 814.02
      open 814.12
    cartilage (interior) (knee) — *see*
      Tear, meniscus
  sesamoid bone — *see* Fracture, by site
  Shepherd's (closed) 825.21
    open 825.31
  shoulder (*see also* Fracture, humerus,
    upper end)
    blade — *see* Fracture, scapula
  silverfork — *see* Fracture, radius,
    lower end
  sinus (ethmoid) (frontal) (maxillary)
    (nasal) (sphenoidal) — *see*
    Fracture, skull, base
  Skillern's — *see* Fracture, radius,
    shaft

**Fracture** — *continued*
  skull (multiple NEC) (with face bones)
      (closed) 803.0 ☑

---

*Note* — *Use the following fifth-digit subclassification with categories 800, 801, 803, and 804:*

0    *unspecified state of consciousness*

1    *with no loss of consciousness*

2    *with brief [less than one hour] loss of consciousness*

3    *with moderate [1-24 hours] loss of consciousness*

4    *with prolonged [more than 24 hours] loss of consciousness and return to pre-existing conscious level*

5    *with prolonged [more than 24 hours] loss of consciousness, without return to pre-existing conscious level*

*Use fifth-digit 5 to designate when a patient is unconscious and dies before regaining consciousness, regardless of the duration of the loss of consciousness*

6    *with loss of consciousness of unspecified duration*

9    *with concussion, unspecified*

---

      with
          contusion, cerebral 803.1 ☑
          epidural hemorrhage
              803.2 ☑
          extradural hemorrhage
              803.2 ☑
          hemorrhage (intracranial)
              NEC 803.3 ☑
          intracranial injury NEC
              803.4 ☑
          laceration, cerebral 803.1 ☑
          other bones — *see* Fracture,
              multiple, skull
          subarachnoid hemorrhage
              803.2 ☑
          subdural hemorrhage
              803.2 ☑
      base (antrum) (ethmoid bone) (fossa) (internal ear) (nasal sinus) (occiput) (sphenoid)
          (temporal bone) (closed)
          801.0 ☑
          with
              contusion, cerebral
                  801.1 ☑
              epidural hemorrhage
                  801.2 ☑
              extradural hemorrhage
                  801.2 ☑
              hemorrhage (intracranial)
                  NEC 801.3 ☑
              intracranial injury NEC
                  801.4 ☑
              laceration, cerebral
                  801.1 ☑
              subarachnoid hemorrhage
                  801.2 ☑
              subdural hemorrhage
                  801.2 ☑
          open 801.5 ☑
              with
                  contusion, cerebral
                      801.6 ☑
                  epidural hemorrhage
                      801.7 ☑
                  extradural hemorrhage
                      801.7 ☑
                  hemorrhage (intracranial) NEC
                      801.8 ☑
                  intracranial injury NEC
                      801.9 ☑

**Fracture** — *continued*
  skull — *continued*
      base — *continued*
          open — *continued*
              with — *continued*
                  laceration, cerebral
                      801.6 ☑
                  subarachnoid hemorrhage 801.7 ☑
                  subdural hemorrhage
                      801.7 ☑
      birth injury 767.3
      face bones — *see* Fracture, face
          bones
      open 803.5 ☑
          with
              contusion, cerebral
                  803.6 ☑
              epidural hemorrhage
                  803.7 ☑
              extradural hemorrhage
                  803.7 ☑
              hemorrhage (intracranial)
                  NEC 803.8 ☑
              intracranial injury NEC
                  803.9 ☑
              laceration, cerebral
                  803.6 ☑
              subarachnoid hemorrhage
                  803.7 ☑
              subdural hemorrhage
                  803.7 ☑
      vault (frontal bone) (parietal bone)
          (vertex) (closed) 800.0 ☑
          with
              contusion, cerebral
                  800.1 ☑
              epidural hemorrhage
                  800.2 ☑
              extradural hemorrhage
                  800.2 ☑
              hemorrhage (intracranial)
                  NEC 800.3 ☑
              intracranial injury NEC
                  800.4 ☑
              laceration, cerebral
                  800.1 ☑
              subarachnoid hemorrhage
                  800.2 ☑
              subdural hemorrhage
                  800.2 ☑
          open 800.5 ☑
              with
                  contusion, cerebral
                      800.6 ☑
                  epidural hemorrhage
                      800.7 ☑
                  extradural hemorrhage
                      800.7 ☑
                  hemorrhage (intracranial) NEC
                      800.8 ☑
                  intracranial injury NEC
                      800.9 ☑
                  laceration, cerebral
                      800.6 ☑
                  subarachnoid hemorrhage 800.7 ☑
                  subdural hemorrhage
                      800.7 ☑
      Smith's 813.41
          open 813.51
      sphenoid (bone) (sinus) — *see* Fracture, skull, base
      spine (*see also* Fracture, vertebra, by site due to birth trauma) 767.4
      spinous process — *see* Fracture, vertebra, by site
      spontaneous — *see* Fracture, pathologic
      sprinters' — *see* Fracture, ilium
      stapes — *see* Fracture, skull, base
      stave (*see also* Fracture, metacarpus, metacarpal bone(s))

**Fracture** — *continued*
  stave (*see also* Fracture, metacarpus, metacarpal bone(s) — *continued*
      spine — *see* Fracture, tibia, upper
          end
  sternum (closed) 807.2
      with flail chest (open) 807.4
      open 807.3
  Stieda's — *see* Fracture, femur, lower
      end
  stress 733.95
      fibula 733.93
      metatarsals 733.94
      specified site NEC 733.95
      tibia 733.93
  styloid process
      metacarpal (closed) 815.02
          open 815.12
      radius — *see* Fracture, radius,
          lower end
      temporal bone — *see* Fracture,
          skull, base
      ulna — *see* Fracture, ulna, lower
          end
  supracondylar, elbow 812.41
      open 812.51
  symphysis pubis (with visceral injury)
      (closed) 808.2
      open 808.3
  talus (ankle bone) (closed) 825.21
      open 825.31
  tarsus, tarsal bone(s) (with metatarsus) of one foot (closed) NEC
      825.29
      open 825.39
  temporal bone (styloid) — *see* Fracture, skull, base
  tendon — *see* Sprain, by site
  thigh — *see* Fracture, femur, shaft
  thumb (and finger(s)) of one hand
      (closed) (*see also* Fracture, phalanx, hand) 816.00
      with metacarpal bone(s) of same
          hand 817.0
          open 817.1
      metacarpal(s) — *see* Fracture,
          metacarpus
      open 816.10
  thyroid cartilage (closed) 807.5
      open 807.6
  tibia (closed) 823.80
      with fibula 823.82
          open 823.92
      condyles — *see* Fracture, tibia,
          upper end
      distal end 824.8
          open 824.9
      epiphysis
          lower 824.8
              open 824.9
          upper — *see* Fracture, tibia,
              upper end
      head (involving knee joint) — *see*
          Fracture, tibia, upper end
      intercondyloid eminence — *see*
          Fracture, tibia, upper end
      involving ankle 824.0
          open 824.9
      lower end or extremity (anterior lip)
          (posterior lip) 824.8
          open 824.9
      malleolus (internal) (medial) 824.0
          open 824.1
      open NEC 823.90
      pathologic 733.16
      proximal end — *see* Fracture, tibia,
          upper end
      shaft 823.20
          with fibula 823.22
              open 823.32
          open 823.30
      spine — *see* Fracture, tibia, upper
          end
      stress 733.93
      torus 823.40

**Fracture** — *continued*
  tibia — *continued*
      torus — *continued*
          with fibula 823.42
      tuberosity — *see* Fracture, tibia,
          upper end
      upper end or extremity (condyle)
          (epiphysis) (head) (spine)
          (proximal end) (tuberosity)
          823.00
          with fibula 823.02
              open 823.12
          open 823.10
  toe(s), of one foot (closed) 826.0
      with bone(s) of same lower limb
          827.0
          open 827.1
      open 826.1
  tooth (root) 873.63
      complicated 873.73
  torus
      fibula 823.41
          with tibia 823.42
      radius 813.45
      tibia 823.40
          with fibula 823.42
  trachea (closed) 807.5
      open 807.6
  transverse process — *see* Fracture,
      vertebra, by site
  trapezium (closed) 814.05
      open 814.15
  trapezoid bone (closed) 814.06
      open 814.16
  trimalleolar (closed) 824.6
      open 824.7
  triquetral (bone) (closed) 814.03
      open 814.13
  trochanter (greater) (lesser) (closed)
      (*see also* Fracture, femur, neck,
      by site) 820.20
      open 820.30
  trunk (bones) (closed) 809.0
      open 809.1
  tuberosity (external) — *see* Fracture,
      by site
  ulna (alone) (closed) 813.82
      with radius NEC 813.83
          open 813.93
      coronoid process (closed) 813.02
          open 813.12
      distal end — *see* Fracture, ulna,
          lower end
      epiphysis
          lower — *see* Fracture, ulna,
              lower end
          upper — *see* Fracture, ulna,
              upper end
      head — *see* Fracture, ulna, lower
          end
      lower end (distal end) (head) (lower
          epiphysis) (styloid process)
          813.43
          with radius (lower end) 813.44
              open 813.54
          open 813.53
      olecranon process (closed) 813.01
          open 813.11
      open NEC 813.92
      pathologic 733.12
      proximal end — *see* Fracture, ulna,
          upper end
      shaft 813.22
          with radius (shaft) 813.23
              open 813.33
          open 813.32
      styloid process — *see* Fracture, ulna, lower end
      transverse — *see* Fracture, ulna,
          by site
      upper end (epiphysis) 813.04
          with radius (upper end) 813.08
              open 813.18
          multiple sites 813.04
              open 813.14
          open 813.14

---

☑ Additional Digit Required — Refer to the Tabular List for Digit Selection        🔺 Subterms under main terms may continue to next column or page

**2008 ICD-9-CM**        ▶◀ Revised Text        ● New Line        ▲ Revised Code        **Volume 2 — 127**

Index

Fracture — Furuncle

**Fracture** — *continued*
  ulna — *continued*
    upper end — *continued*
      specified site NEC 813.04
        open 813.14
  unciform (closed) 814.08
    open 814.18
  vertebra, vertebral (back) (body) (column) (neural arch) (pedicle) (spine) (spinous process) (transverse process) (closed) 805.8
    with
      hematomyelia — *see* Fracture, vertebra, by site, with spinal cord injury
      injury to
        cauda equina — *see* Fracture, vertebra, sacrum, with spinal cord injury
        nerve — *see* Fracture, vertebra, by site, with spinal cord injury
      paralysis — *see* Fracture, vertebra, by site, with spinal cord injury
      paraplegia — *see* Fracture, vertebra, by site, with spinal cord injury
      quadriplegia — *see* Fracture, vertebra, by site, with spinal cord injury
      spinal concussion — *see* Fracture, vertebra, by site, with spinal cord injury
      spinal cord injury (closed) NEC 806.8

*Note — Use the following fifth-digit subclassification with categories 806.0–806.3:*

$C_1$–$C_4$ *or unspecified level and* $D_1$–$D_6$ ($T_1$–$T_6$) *or unspecified level with*

0  *unspecified spinal cord injury*
1  *complete lesion of cord*
2  *anterior cord syndrome*
3  *central cord syndrome*
4  *specified injury NEC*

$C_5$–$C_7$ *level and* $D_7$–$D_{12}$ *level with:*

5  *unspecified spinal cord injury*
6  *complete lesion of cord*
7  *anterior cord syndrome*
8  *central cord syndrome*
9  *specified injury NEC*

        cervical 806.0 ☑
          open 806.1 ☑
        dorsal, dorsolumbar 806.2 ☑
          open 806.3 ☑
        open 806.9
        thoracic, thoracolumbar 806.2 ☑
          open 806.3 ☑
    atlanto-axial — *see* Fracture, vertebra, cervical
    cervical (hangman) (teardrop) (closed) 805.00
      with spinal cord injury — *see* Fracture, vertebra, with spinal cord injury, cervical
      first (atlas) 805.01
        open 805.11
      second (axis) 805.02
        open 805.12
      third 805.03
        open 805.13
      fourth 805.04
        open 805.14
      fifth 805.05
        open 805.15
      sixth 805.06

**Fracture** — *continued*
  vertebra, vertebral — *continued*
    cervical — *continued*
      sixth — *continued*
        open 805.16
      seventh 805.07
        open 805.17
      multiple sites 805.08
        open 805.18
      open 805.10
    chronic 733.13 ●
    coccyx (closed) 805.6
      with spinal cord injury (closed) 806.60
        cauda equina injury 806.62
          complete lesion 806.61
            open 806.71
          open 806.72
        open 806.70
        specified type NEC 806.69
          open 806.79
      open 805.7
    collapsed 733.13
    compression, not due to trauma 733.13
    dorsal (closed) 805.2
      with spinal cord injury — *see* Fracture, vertebra, with spinal cord injury, dorsal
      open 805.3
    dorsolumbar (closed) 805.2
      with spinal cord injury — *see* Fracture, vertebra, with spinal cord injury, dorsal
      open 805.3
    due to osteoporosis 733.13
    fetus or newborn 767.4
    lumbar (closed) 805.4
      with spinal cord injury (closed) 806.4
        open 806.5
      open 805.5
    nontraumatic 733.13
    open NEC 805.9
    pathologic (any site) 733.13
    sacrum (closed) 805.6
      with spinal cord injury 806.60
        cauda equina injury 806.62
          complete lesion 806.61
            open 806.71
          open 806.72
        open 806.70
        specified type NEC 806.69
          open 806.79
      open 805.7
    site unspecified (closed) 805.8
      with spinal cord injury (closed) 806.8
        open 806.9
      open 805.9
    stress (any site) 733.95
    thoracic (closed) 805.2
      with spinal cord injury — *see* Fracture, vertebra, with spinal cord injury, thoracic
      open 805.3
  vertex — *see* Fracture, skull, vault
  vomer (bone) 802.0
    open 802.1
  Wagstaffe's — *see* Fracture, ankle
  wrist (closed) 814.00
    open 814.10
    pathologic 733.12
  xiphoid (process) — *see* Fracture, sternum
  zygoma (zygomatic arch) (closed) 802.4
    open 802.5
**Fragile X syndrome** 759.83
**Fragilitas**
  crinium 704.2
  hair 704.2
  ossium 756.51
    with blue sclera 756.51
  unguium 703.8
    congenital 757.5

**Fragility**
  bone 756.51
    with deafness and blue sclera 756.51
  capillary (hereditary) 287.8
  hair 704.2
  nails 703.8
**Fragmentation** — *see* Fracture, by site
**Frambesia, frambesial** (tropica) — *see also* Yaws 102.9
  initial lesion or ulcer 102.0
  primary 102.0
**Frambeside**
  gummatous 102.4
  of early yaws 102.2
**Frambesioma** 102.1
**Franceschetti's syndrome** (mandibulofacial dysostosis) 756.0
**Francis' disease** — *see also* Tularemia 021.9
**Franklin's disease** (heavy chain) 273.2
**Frank's essential thrombocytopenia** — *see also* Purpura, thrombocytopenic 287.39
**Fraser's syndrome** 759.89
**Freckle** 709.09
  malignant melanoma in (M8742/3) — *see* Melanoma
  melanotic (of Hutchinson) (M8742/2) — *see* Neoplasm, skin, in situ
**Freeman-Sheldon syndrome** 759.89
**Freezing** 991.9
  specified effect NEC 991.8
**Freiberg's**
  disease (osteochondrosis, second metatarsal) 732.5
  infraction of metatarsal head 732.5
  osteochondrosis 732.5
**Frei's disease** (climatic bubo) 099.1
**Fremitus, friction, cardiac** 785.3
**Frenulum linguae** 750.0
**Frenum**
  external os 752.49
  tongue 750.0
**Frequency** (urinary) NEC 788.41
  micturition 788.41
  nocturnal 788.43
  polyuria 788.42
  psychogenic 306.53
**Frey's syndrome** (auriculotemporal syndrome) 705.22
**Friction**
  burn (*see also* Injury, superficial, by site) 919.0
  fremitus, cardiac 785.3
  precordial 785.3
  sounds, chest 786.7
**Friderichsen-Waterhouse syndrome or disease** 036.3
**Friedländer's**
  B (bacillus) NEC (*see also* condition) 041.3
  sepsis or septicemia 038.49
  disease (endarteritis obliterans) — *see* Arteriosclerosis
**Friedreich's**
  ataxia 334.0
  combined systemic disease 334.0
  disease 333.2
    combined systemic 334.0
  myoclonia 333.2
  sclerosis (spinal cord) 334.0
**Friedrich-Erb-Arnold syndrome** (acropachyderma) 757.39
**Frigidity** 302.72
  psychic or psychogenic 302.72
**Fröhlich's disease or syndrome** (adiposogenital dystrophy) 253.8
**Froin's syndrome** 336.8
**Frommel-Chiari syndrome** 676.6 ☑
**Frommel's disease** 676.6 ☑
**Frontal** — *see also* condition
  lobe syndrome 310.0
**Frostbite** 991.3
  face 991.0
  foot 991.2

**Frostbite** — *continued*
  hand 991.1
  specified site NEC 991.3
**Frotteurism** 302.89
**Frozen** 991.9
  pelvis 620.8
  shoulder 726.0
**Fructosemia** 271.2
**Fructosuria** (benign) (essential) 271.2
**Fuchs'**
  black spot (myopic) 360.21
  corneal dystrophy (endothelial) 371.57
  heterochromic cyclitis 364.21
**Fucosidosis** 271.8
**Fugue** 780.99
  dissociative 300.13
  hysterical (dissociative) 300.13
  reaction to exceptional stress (transient) 308.1
**Fukuhara syndrome** 277.87
**Fuller Albright's syndrome** (osteitis fibrosa disseminata) 756.59
**Fuller's earth disease** 502
**Fulminant, fulminating** — *see* condition
**Functional** — *see* condition
**Functioning**
  borderline intellectual V62.89
**Fundus** — *see also* condition
  flavimaculatus 362.76
**Fungemia** 117.9
**Fungus, fungous**
  cerebral 348.8
  disease NEC 117.9
  infection — *see* Infection, fungus
  testis (*see also* Tuberculosis) 016.5 ☑ *[608.81]*
**Funiculitis** (acute) 608.4
  chronic 608.4
  endemic 608.4
  gonococcal (acute) 098.14
    chronic or duration of 2 months or over 098.34
  tuberculous (*see also* Tuberculosis) 016.5 ☑
**Funnel**
  breast (acquired) 738.3
    congenital 754.81
    late effect of rickets 268.1
  chest (acquired) 738.3
    congenital 754.81
    late effect of rickets 268.1
  pelvis (acquired) 738.6
    with disproportion (fetopelvic) 653.3 ☑
      affecting fetus or newborn 763.1
      causing obstructed labor 660.1 ☑
        affecting fetus or newborn 763.1
    congenital 755.69
    tuberculous (*see also* Tuberculosis) 016.9 ☑
**FUO** — *see also* Pyrexia 780.6
**Furfur** 690.18
  microsporon 111.0
**Furor, paroxysmal** (idiopathic) — *see also* Epilepsy 345.8 ☑
**Furriers' lung** 495.8
**Furrowed tongue** 529.5
  congenital 750.13
**Furrowing nail(s)** (transverse) 703.8
  congenital 757.5
**Furuncle** 680.9
  abdominal wall 680.2
  ankle 680.6
  anus 680.5
  arm (any part, above wrist) 680.3
  auditory canal, external 680.0
  axilla 680.3
  back (any part) 680.2
  breast 680.2
  buttock 680.5
  chest wall 680.2
  corpus cavernosum 607.2
  ear (any part) 680.0
  eyelid 373.13

**Furuncle** — *continued*
face (any part, except eye) 680.0
finger (any) 680.4
flank 680.2
foot (any part) 680.7
forearm 680.3
gluteal (region) 680.5
groin 680.2
hand (any part) 680.4
head (any part, except face) 680.8
heel 680.7
hip 680.6
kidney (*see also* Abscess, kidney)
590.2
knee 680.6
labium (majus) (minus) 616.4
lacrimal
gland (*see also* Dacryoadenitis)
375.00
passages (duct) (sac) (*see also*
Dacryocystitis) 375.30
leg, any part except foot 680.6
malignant 022.0
multiple sites 680.9
neck 680.1
nose (external) (septum) 680.0
orbit 376.01
partes posteriores 680.5
pectoral region 680.2
penis 607.2
perineum 680.2
pinna 680.0
scalp (any part) 680.8
scrotum 608.4

**Furuncle** — *continued*
seminal vesicle 608.0
shoulder 680.3
skin NEC 680.9
specified site NEC 680.8
spermatic cord 608.4
temple (region) 680.0
testis 604.90
thigh 680.6
thumb 680.4
toe (any) 680.7
trunk 680.2
tunica vaginalis 608.4
umbilicus 680.2
upper arm 680.3
vas deferens 608.4
vulva 616.4
wrist 680.4
**Furunculosis** — *see also* Furuncle 680.9
external auditory meatus
680.0 [*380.13*]
**Fusarium** (infection) 118
**Fusion, fused** (congenital)
anal (with urogenital canal) 751.5
aorta and pulmonary artery 745.0
astragaloscaphoid 755.67
atria 745.5
atrium and ventricle 745.69
auditory canal 744.02
auricles, heart 745.5
binocular, with defective stereopsis
368.33
bone 756.9
cervical spine — *see* Fusion, spine

**Fusion, fused** — *continued*
choanal 748.0
commissure, mitral valve 746.5
cranial sutures, premature 756.0
cusps, heart valve NEC 746.89
mitral 746.5
tricuspid 746.89
ear ossicles 744.04
fingers (*see also* Syndactylism, fingers)
755.11
hymen 752.42
hymeno-urethral 599.89
causing obstructed labor 660.1 ☑
affecting fetus or newborn 763.1
joint (acquired) (*see also* Ankylosis)
congenital 755.8
kidneys (incomplete) 753.3
labium (majus) (minus) 752.49
larynx and trachea 748.3
limb 755.8
lower 755.69
upper 755.59
lobe, lung 748.5
lumbosacral (acquired) 724.6
congenital 756.15
surgical V45.4
nares (anterior) (posterior) 748.0
nose, nasal 748.0
nostril(s) 748.0
organ or site NEC — *see* Anomaly,
specified type NEC
ossicles 756.9
auditory 744.04

**Fusion, fused** — *continued*
pulmonary valve segment 746.02
pulmonic cusps 746.02
ribs 756.3
sacroiliac (acquired) (joint) 724.6
congenital 755.69
surgical V45.4
skull, imperfect 756.0
spine (acquired) 724.9
arthrodesis status V45.4
congenital (vertebra) 756.15
postoperative status V45.4
sublingual duct with submaxillary
duct at opening in mouth
750.26
talonavicular (bar) 755.67
teeth, tooth 520.2
testes 752.89
toes (*see also* Syndactylism, toes)
755.13
trachea and esophagus 750.3
twins 759.4
urethral-hymenal 599.89
vagina 752.49
valve cusps — *see* Fusion, cusps,
heart valve
ventricles, heart 745.4
vertebra (arch) — *see* Fusion, spine
vulva 752.49
**Fusospirillosis** (mouth) (tongue) (tonsil)
101
**Fussy infant** (baby) 780.91

☑ Additional Digit Required — Refer to the Tabular List for Digit Selection
**2008 ICD-9-CM**
▶◀ Revised Text
● New Line
▲ Revised Code

▽ Subterms under main terms may continue to next column or page

**Volume 2 — 129**

### G

**Gafsa boil** 085.1
**Gain, weight** (abnormal) (excessive) — *see also* Weight, gain 783.1
**Gaisböck's disease or syndrome** (polycythemia hypertonica) 289.0
**Gait**
abnormality 781.2
hysterical 300.11
ataxic 781.2
hysterical 300.11
disturbance 781.2
hysterical 300.11
paralytic 781.2
scissor 781.2
spastic 781.2
staggering 781.2
hysterical 300.11
**Galactocele** (breast) (infected) 611.5
puerperal, postpartum 676.8 ☑
**Galactophoritis** 611.0
puerperal, postpartum 675.2 ☑
**Galactorrhea** 676.6 ☑
not associated with childbirth 611.6
**Galactosemia** (classic) (congenital) 271.1
**Galactosuria** 271.1
**Galacturia** 791.1
bilharziasis 120.0
**Galen's vein** — *see* condition
**Gallbladder** — *see also* condition
acute (*see also* Disease, gallbladder) 575.0
**Gall duct** — *see* condition
**Gallop rhythm** 427.89
**Gallstone** (cholemic) (colic) (impacted) — *see also* Cholelithiasis
causing intestinal obstruction 560.31
**Gambling, pathological** 312.31
**Gammaloidosis** 277.39
**Gammopathy** 273.9
macroglobulinemia 273.3
monoclonal (benign) (essential) (idiopathic) (with lymphoplasmacytic dyscrasia) 273.1
**Gamna's disease** (siderotic splenomegaly) 289.51
**Gampsodactylia** (congenital) 754.71
**Gamstorp's disease** (adynamia episodica hereditaria) 359.3
**Gandy-Nanta disease** (siderotic splenomegaly) 289.51
**Gang activity, without manifest psychiatric disorder** V71.09
adolescent V71.02
adult V71.01
child V71.02
**Gangliocytoma** (M9490/0) — *see* Neoplasm, connective tissue, benign
**Ganglioglioma** (M9505/1) — *see* Neoplasm, by site, uncertain behavior
**Ganglion** 727.43
joint 727.41
of yaws (early) (late) 102.6
periosteal (*see also* Periostitis) 730.3 ☑
tendon sheath (compound) (diffuse) 727.42
tuberculous (*see also* Tuberculosis) 015.9 ☑
**Ganglioneuroblastoma** (M9490/3) — *see* Neoplasm, connective tissue, malignant
**Ganglioneuroma** (M9490/0) — *see also* Neoplasm, connective tissue, benign
malignant (M9490/3) — *see* Neoplasm, connective tissue, malignant
**Ganglioneuromatosis** (M9491/0) — *see* Neoplasm, connective tissue, benign
**Ganglionitis**
fifth nerve (*see also* Neuralgia, trigeminal) 350.1
gasserian 350.1

**Ganglionitis** — *continued*
geniculate 351.1
herpetic 053.11
newborn 767.5
herpes zoster 053.11
herpetic geniculate (Hunt's syndrome) 053.11
**Gangliosidosis** 330.1
**Gangosa** 102.5
**Gangrene, gangrenous** (anemia) (artery) (cellulitis) (dermatitis) (dry) (infective) (moist) (pemphigus) (septic) (skin) (stasis) (ulcer) 785.4
with
arteriosclerosis (native artery) 440.24
bypass graft 440.30
autologous vein 440.31
nonautologous biological 440.32
diabetes (mellitus) 250.7 ☑ [785.4]
abdomen (wall) 785.4
adenitis 683
alveolar 526.5
angina 462
diphtheritic 032.0
anus 569.49
appendices epiploicae — *see* Gangrene, mesentery
appendix — *see* Appendicitis, acute
arteriosclerotic — *see* Arteriosclerosis, with, gangrene
auricle 785.4
Bacillus welchii (*see also* Gangrene, gas) 040.0
bile duct (*see also* Cholangitis) 576.8
bladder 595.89
bowel — *see* Gangrene, intestine
cecum — *see* Gangrene, intestine
Clostridium perfringens or welchii (*see also* Gangrene, gas) 040.0
colon — *see* Gangrene, intestine
connective tissue 785.4
cornea 371.40
corpora cavernosa (infective) 607.2
noninfective 607.89
cutaneous, spreading 785.4
decubital (*see also* Decubitus) 707.00 [785.4]
diabetic (any site) 250.7 ☑ [785.4]
dropsical 785.4
emphysematous (*see also* Gangrene, gas) 040.0
epidemic (ergotized grain) 988.2
epididymis (infectional) (*see also* Epididymitis) 604.99
erysipelas (*see also* Erysipelas) 035
extremity (lower) (upper) 785.4
gallbladder or duct (*see also* Cholecystitis, acute) 575.0
gas (bacillus) 040.0
with
abortion — *see* Abortion, by type, with sepsis
ectopic pregnancy (*see also* categories 633.0–633.9) 639.0
molar pregnancy (*see also* categories 630–632) 639.0
following
abortion 639.0
ectopic or molar pregnancy 639.0
puerperal, postpartum, childbirth 670.0 ☑
glossitis 529.0
gum 523.8
hernia — *see* Hernia, by site, with gangrene
hospital noma 528.1
intestine, intestinal (acute) (hemorrhagic) (massive) 557.0
with
hernia — *see* Hernia, by site, with gangrene

**Gangrene, gangrenous** — *continued*
intestine, intestinal — *continued*
with — *continued*
mesenteric embolism or infarction 557.0
obstruction (*see also* Obstruction, intestine) 560.9
laryngitis 464.00
with obstruction 464.01
liver 573.8
lung 513.0
spirochetal 104.8
lymphangitis 457.2
Meleney's (cutaneous) 686.09
mesentery 557.0
with
embolism or infarction 557.0
intestinal obstruction (*see also* Obstruction, intestine) 560.9
mouth 528.1
noma 528.1
orchitis 604.90
ovary (*see also* Salpingo-oophoritis) 614.2
pancreas 577.0
penis (infectional) 607.2
noninfective 607.89
perineum 785.4
pharynx 462
pneumonia 513.0
Pott's 440.24
presenile 443.1
pulmonary 513.0
pulp, tooth 522.1
quinsy 475
Raynaud's (symmetric gangrene) 443.0 [785.4]
rectum 569.49
retropharyngeal 478.24
rupture — *see* Hernia, by site, with gangrene
scrotum 608.4
noninfective 608.83
senile 440.24
septic 034.0
septic 034.0
sore throat 462
spermatic cord 608.4
noninfective 608.89
spine 785.4
spirochetal NEC 104.8
spreading cutaneous 785.4
stomach 537.89
stomatitis 528.1
symmetrical 443.0 [785.4]
testis (infectional) (*see also* Orchitis) 604.99
noninfective 608.89
throat 462
diphtheritic 032.0
thyroid (gland) 246.8
tonsillitis (acute) 463
tooth (pulp) 522.1
tuberculous NEC (*see also* Tuberculosis) 011.9 ☑
tunica vaginalis 608.4
noninfective 608.89
umbilicus 785.4
uterus (*see also* Endometritis) 615.9
uvulitis 528.3
vas deferens 608.4
noninfective 608.89
vulva (*see also* Vulvitis) 616.10
**Gannister disease** (occupational) 502
with tuberculosis — *see* Tuberculosis, pulmonary
**Ganser's syndrome, hysterical** 300.16
**Gardner-Diamond syndrome** (autoerythrocyte sensitization) 287.2
**Gargoylism** 277.5
**Garré's**
disease (*see also* Osteomyelitis) 730.1 ☑
osteitis (sclerosing) (*see also* Osteomyelitis) 730.1 ☑

**Garré's** — *continued*
osteomyelitis (*see also* Osteomyelitis) 730.1 ☑
**Garrod's pads, knuckle** 728.79
**Gartner's duct**
cyst 752.41
persistent 752.41
**Gas** 787.3 ▲
asphyxia, asphyxiation, inhalation, poisoning, suffocation NEC 987.9
specified gas — *see* Table of Drugs and Chemicals
bacillus gangrene or infection — *see* Gas, gangrene
cyst, mesentery 568.89
excessive 787.3
gangrene 040.0
with
abortion — *see* Abortion, by type, with sepsis
ectopic pregnancy (*see also* categories 633.0–633.9) 639.0
molar pregnancy (*see also* categories 630–632) 639.0
following
abortion 639.0
ectopic or molar pregnancy 639.0
puerperal, postpartum, childbirth 670.0 ☑
on stomach 787.3
pains 787.3
**Gastradenitis** 535.0 ☑
**Gastralgia** 536.8
psychogenic 307.89
**Gastrectasis, gastrectasia** 536.1
psychogenic 306.4
**Gastric** — *see* condition
**Gastrinoma** (M8153/1)
malignant (M8153/3)
pancreas 157.4
specified site NEC — *see* Neoplasm, by site, malignant
unspecified site 157.4
specified site — *see* Neoplasm, by site, uncertain behavior
unspecified site 235.5
**Gastritis** 535.5 ☑

Note — *Use the following fifth-digit subclassification for category 535:*

0   *without mention of hemorrhage*

1   *with hemorrhage*

acute 535.0 ☑
alcoholic 535.3 ☑
allergic 535.4 ☑
antral 535.4 ☑
atrophic 535.1 ☑
atrophic-hyperplastic 535.1 ☑
bile-induced 535.4 ☑
catarrhal 535.0 ☑
chronic (atrophic) 535.1 ☑
cirrhotic 535.4 ☑
corrosive (acute) 535.4 ☑
dietetic 535.4 ☑
due to diet deficiency 269.9 [535.4] ☑
eosinophilic 535.4 ☑
erosive 535.4 ☑
follicular 535.4 ☑
chronic 535.1 ☑
giant hypertrophic 535.2 ☑
glandular 535.4 ☑
chronic 535.1 ☑
hypertrophic (mucosa) 535.2 ☑
chronic giant 211.1
irritant 535.4 ☑
nervous 306.4
phlegmonous 535.0 ☑
psychogenic 306.4
sclerotic 535.4 ☑
spastic 536.8
subacute 535.0 ☑
superficial 535.4 ☑

**Gastritis** — *continued*
  suppurative 535.0 ☑
  toxic 535.4 ☑
  tuberculous (*see also* Tuberculosis)
    017.9 ☑
**Gastrocarcinoma** (M8010/3) 151.9
**Gastrocolic** — *see* condition
**Gastrocolitis** — *see* Enteritis
**Gastrodisciasis** 121.8
**Gastroduodenitis** — *see also* Gastritis
  535.5 ☑
  catarrhal 535.0 ☑
  infectional 535.0 ☑
  virus, viral 008.8
    specified type NEC 008.69
**Gastrodynia** 536.8
**Gastroenteritis** (acute) (catarrhal) (congestive) (hemorrhagic) (noninfectious) — *see also* Enteritis 558.9
  aertrycke infection 003.0
  allergic 558.3
  chronic 558.9
    ulcerative (*see also* Colitis, ulcerative) 556.9
  dietetic 558.9
  due to
    food poisoning (*see also* Poisoning, food) 005.9
    radiation 558.1
  epidemic 009.0
  functional 558.9
  infectious (*see also* Enteritis, due to, by organism) 009.0
    presumed 009.1
  salmonella 003.0
  septic (*see also* Enteritis, due to, by organism) 009.0
  toxic 558.2
  tuberculous (*see also* Tuberculosis) 014.8 ☑
  ulcerative (*see also* Colitis, ulcerative) 556.9
  viral NEC 008.8
    specified type NEC 008.69
  zymotic 009.0
**Gastroenterocolitis** — *see* Enteritis
**Gastroenteropathy, protein-losing** 579.8
**Gastroenteroptosis** 569.89
**Gastroesophageal laceration-hemorrhage syndrome** 530.7
**Gastroesophagitis** 530.19
**Gastrohepatitis** — *see also* Gastritis 535.5 ☑
**Gastrointestinal** — *see* condition
**Gastrojejunal** — *see* condition
**Gastrojejunitis** — *see also* Gastritis 535.5 ☑
**Gastrojejunocolic** — *see* condition
**Gastroliths** 537.89
**Gastromalacia** 537.89
**Gastroparalysis** 536.3
  diabetic 250.6 ☑ *[536.3]*
**Gastroparesis** 536.3
  diabetic 250.6 ☑ *[536.3]*
**Gastropathy** 537.9
  congestive portal 537.89 ●
  erythematous 535.5 ☑
  exudative 579.8
  portal hypertensive 537.89 ●
**Gastroptosis** 537.5
**Gastrorrhagia** 578.0
**Gastrorrhea** 536.8
  psychogenic 306.4
**Gastroschisis** (congenital) 756.79
  acquired 569.89
**Gastrospasm** (neurogenic) (reflex) 536.8
  neurotic 306.4
  psychogenic 306.4
**Gastrostaxis** 578.0
**Gastrostenosis** 537.89
**Gastrostomy**
  attention to V55.1
  complication 536.40
    specified type 536.49
  infection 536.41

**Gastrostomy** — *continued*
  malfunctioning 536.42
  status V44.1
**Gastrosuccorrhea** (continuous) (intermittent) 536.8
  neurotic 306.4
  psychogenic 306.4
**Gaucher's**
  disease (adult) (cerebroside lipidosis) (infantile) 272.7
  hepatomegaly 272.7
  splenomegaly (cerebroside lipidosis) 272.7
**GAVE** (gastric antral vascular ectasia) ●
  537.82
  with hemorrhage 537.83 ●
  without hemorrhage 537.82 ●
**Gayet's disease** (superior hemorrhagic polioencephalitis) 265.1
**Gayet-Wernicke's syndrome** (superior hemorrhagic polioencephalitis) 265.1
**Gee (-Herter) (-Heubner) (-Thaysen) disease or syndrome** (nontropical sprue) 579.0
**Gélineau's syndrome** — *see also* Narcolepsy 347.00
**Gemination, teeth** 520.2
**Gemistocytoma** (M9411/3)
  specified site — *see* Neoplasm, by site, malignant
  unspecified site 191.9
**General, generalized** — *see* condtion
**Genetic**
  susceptibility to
    MEN (multiple endocrine neoplasia) V84.81 ●
    neoplasia ●
      multiple endocrine [MEN] ●
      V84.81 ●
    neoplasm
      malignant, of
        breast V84.01
        endometrium V84.04
        other V84.09
        ovary V84.02
        prostate V84.03
      ▶specified disease NEC◀
      V84.89 ▲
**Genital** — *see* condition
  warts 078.19
**Genito-anorectal syndrome** 099.1
**Genitourinary system** — *see* condition
**Genu**
  congenital 755.64
  extrorsum (acquired) 736.42
    congenital 755.64
    late effects of rickets 268.1
  introrsum (acquired) 736.41
    congenital 755.64
    late effects of rickets 268.1
  rachitic (old) 268.1
  recurvatum (acquired) 736.5
    congenital 754.40
      with dislocation of knee 754.41
    late effects of rickets 268.1
  valgum (acquired) (knock-knee) 736.41
    congenital 755.64
    late effects of rickets 268.1
  varum (acquired) (bowleg) 736.42
    congenital 755.64
    late effect of rickets 268.1
**Geographic tongue** 529.1
**Geophagia** 307.52
**Geotrichosis** 117.9
  intestine 117.9
  lung 117.9
  mouth 117.9
**Gephyrophobia** 300.29
**Gerbode defect** 745.4
**Gerhardt's**
  disease (erythromelalgia) 443.82
  syndrome (vocal cord paralysis) 478.30

**Gerlier's disease** (epidemic vertigo) 078.81
**German measles** 056.9
  exposure to V01.4
**Germinoblastoma** (diffuse) (M9614/3) 202.8 ☑
  follicular (M9692/3) 202.0 ☑
**Germinoma** (M9064/3) — *see* Neoplasm, by site, malignant
**Gerontoxon** 371.41
**Gerstmann's syndrome** (finger agnosia) 784.69
**Gestation** (period) — *see also* Pregnancy
  ectopic NEC (*see also* Pregnancy, ectopic) 633.90
    with intrauterine pregnancy 633.91
**Gestational proteinuria** 646.2 ☑
  with hypertension — *see* Toxemia, of pregnancy
**Ghon tubercle primary infection** — *see also* Tuberculosis 010.0 ☑
**Ghost**
  teeth 520.4
  vessels, cornea 370.64
**Ghoul hand** 102.3
**Gianotti Crosti syndrome** 057.8
  due to known virus — *see* Infection, virus
  due to unknown virus 057.8
**Giant**
  cell
    epulis 523.8
    peripheral (gingiva) 523.8
    tumor, tendon sheath 727.02
  colon (congenital) 751.3
  esophagus (congenital) 750.4
  kidney 753.3
  urticaria 995.1
    hereditary 277.6
**Giardia lamblia infestation** 007.1
**Giardiasis** 007.1
**Gibert's disease** (pityriasis rosea) 696.3
**Gibraltar fever** — *see* Brucellosis
**Giddiness** 780.4
  hysterical 300.11
  psychogenic 306.9
**Gierke's disease** (glycogenosis I) 271.0
**Gigantism** (cerebral) (hypophyseal) (pituitary) 253.0
**Gilbert's disease or cholemia** (familial nonhemolytic jaundice) 277.4
**Gilchrist's disease** (North American blastomycosis) 116.0
**Gilford (-Hutchinson) disease or syndrome** (progeria) 259.8
**Gilles de la Tourette's disease** (motorverbal tic) 307.23
**Gillespie's syndrome** (dysplasia oculo-dentodigitalis) 759.89
**Gingivitis** 523.10
  acute 523.00
    necrotizing 101
      non-plaque induced 523.01
      plaque induced 523.00
  catarrhal 523.00
  chronic 523.10
    non-plaque induced 523.11
  desquamative 523.10
  expulsiva 523.40
  hyperplastic 523.10
  marginal, simple 523.10
  necrotizing, acute 101
  non-plaque induced 523.11
  pellagrous 265.2
  plaque induced 523.10
  ulcerative 523.10
    acute necrotizing 101
  Vincent's 101
**Gingivoglossitis** 529.0
**Gingivopericementitis** 523.40
**Gingivosis** 523.10
**Gingivostomatitis** 523.10
  herpetic 054.2
**Giovannini's disease** 117.9
**GISA** (glycopeptide intermediate staphylococcus aureus) V09.8 ☑

**Glanders** 024
**Gland, glandular** — *see* condition
**Glanzmann (-Naegeli) disease or thrombasthenia** 287.1
**Glassblowers' disease** 527.1
**Glaucoma** (capsular) (inflammatory) (noninflammatory) (primary) 365.9
  with increased episcleral venous pressure 365.82
  absolute 360.42
  acute 365.22
    narrow angle 365.22
    secondary 365.60
  angle closure 365.20
    acute 365.22
    chronic 365.23
    intermittent 365.21
    interval 365.21
    residual stage 365.24
    subacute 365.21
  borderline 365.00
  chronic 365.11
    noncongestive 365.11
    open angle 365.11
    simple 365.11
  closed angle — *see* Glaucoma, angle closure
  congenital 743.20
    associated with other eye anomalies 743.22
    simple 743.21
  congestive — *see* Glaucoma, narrow angle
  corticosteroid-induced (glaucomatous stage) 365.31
    residual stage 365.32
  hemorrhagic 365.60
  hypersecretion 365.81
  infantile 365.14
    congenital 743.20
      associated with other eye anomalies 743.22
      simple 743.21
  in or with
    aniridia 743.45 *[365.42]*
    Axenfeld's anomaly 743.44 *[365.41]*
    concussion of globe 921.3 *[365.65]*
    congenital syndromes NEC 759.89 *[365.44]*
    dislocation of lens
      anterior 379.33 *[365.59]*
      posterior 379.34 *[365.59]*
    disorder of lens NEC 365.59
    epithelial down-growth 364.61 *[365.64]*
    glaucomatocyclitic crisis 364.22 *[365.62]*
    hypermature cataract 366.18 *[365.51]*
    hyphema 364.41 *[365.63]*
    inflammation, ocular 365.62
    iridocyclitis 364.3 *[365.62]*
    iris
      anomalies NEC 743.46 *[365.42]*
      atrophy, essential 364.51 *[365.42]*
      bombé 364.74 *[365.61]*
      rubeosis 364.42 *[365.63]*
    microcornea 743.41 *[365.43]*
    neurofibromatosis 237.71 *[365.44]*
    ocular
      cysts NEC 365.64
      disorders NEC 365.60
      trauma 365.65
      tumors NEC 365.64
    postdislocation of lens
      anterior 379.33 *[365.59]*
      posterior 379.34 *[365.59]*
    pseudoexfoliation of capsule 366.11 *[365.52]*
    pupillary block or seclusion 364.74 *[365.61]*
    recession of chamber angle 364.77 *[365.65]*
    retinal vein occlusion 362.35 *[365.63]*

☑ Additional Digit Required — Refer to the Tabular List for Digit Selection      ▽ Subterms under main terms may continue to next column or page

132 — Volume 2 • October 2007      ▶◀ Revised Text      ● New Line      ▲ Revised Code      **2008 ICD-9-CM**

**Glaucoma** — *continued*
 in or with — *continued*
  Rieger's anomaly or syndrome
   743.44 *[365.41]*
  rubeosis of iris 364.42 *[365.63]*
  seclusion of pupil 364.74 *[365.61]*
  spherophakia 743.36 *[365.59]*
  Sturge-Weber (-Dimitri) syndrome
   759.6 *[365.44]*
  systemic syndrome NEC 365.44
  tumor of globe 365.64
  vascular disorders NEC 365.63
 juvenile 365.14
 low tension 365.12
 malignant 365.83
 narrow angle (primary) 365.20
  acute 365.22
  chronic 365.23
  intermittent 365.21
  interval 365.21
  residual stage 365.24
  subacute 365.21
 newborn 743.20
  associated with other eye anomalies 743.22
  simple 743.21
 noncongestive (chronic) 365.11
 nonobstructive (chronic) 365.11
 obstructive 365.60
  due to lens changes 365.59
 open angle 365.10
  with
   borderline intraocular pressure
    365.01
   cupping of optic discs 365.01
   primary 365.11
   residual stage 365.15
 phacolytic 365.51
  with hypermature cataract
   366.18 *[365.51]*
 pigmentary 365.13
 postinfectious 365.60
 pseudoexfoliation 365.52
  with pseudoexfoliation of capsule
   366.11 *[365.52]*
 secondary NEC 365.60
 simple (chronic) 365.11
 simplex 365.11
 steroid responders 365.03
 suspect 365.00
 syphilitic 095.8
 traumatic NEC 365.65
  newborn 767.8
 tuberculous (*see also* Tuberculosis)
  017.3 ☑ *[365.62]*
 wide angle (*see also* Glaucoma, open
  angle) 365.10
**Glaucomatous flecks** (subcapsular)
 366.31
**Glazed tongue** 529.4
**Gleet** 098.2
**Glénard's disease or syndrome** (enteroptosis) 569.89
**Glinski-Simmonds syndrome** (pituitary
 cachexia) 253.2
**Glioblastoma** (multiforme) (M9440/3)
 with sarcomatous component
  (M9442/3)
   specified site — *see* Neoplasm, by
    site, malignant
   unspecified site 191.9
 giant cell (M9441/3)
  specified site — *see* Neoplasm, by
   site, malignant
  unspecified site 191.9
 specified site — *see* Neoplasm, by site,
  malignant
 unspecified site 191.9
**Glioma** (malignant) (M9380/3)
 astrocytic (M9400/3)
  specified site — *see* Neoplasm, by
   site, malignant
  unspecified site 191.9
 mixed (M9382/3)
  specified site — *see* Neoplasm, by
   site, malignant

**Glioma** — *continued*
 mixed — *continued*
  unspecified site 191.9
 nose 748.1
 specified site NEC — *see* Neoplasm,
  by site, malignant
 subependymal (M9383/1) 237.5
 unspecified site 191.9
**Gliomatosis cerebri** (M9381/3) 191.0
**Glioneuroma** (M9505/1) — *see* Neoplasm, by site, uncertain behavior
**Gliosarcoma** (M9380/3)
 specified site — *see* Neoplasm, by site,
  malignant
 unspecified site 191.9
**Gliosis** (cerebral) 349.89
 spinal 336.0
**Glisson's**
 cirrhosis — *see* Cirrhosis, portal
 disease (*see also* Rickets) 268.0
**Glissonitis** 573.3
**Globinuria** 791.2
**Globus** 306.4
 hystericus 300.11
**Glomangioma** (M8712/0) — *see also*
 Hemangioma 228.00
**Glomangiosarcoma** (M8710/3) — *see*
 Neoplasm, connective tissue, malignant
**Glomerular nephritis** — *see also*
 Nephritis 583.9
**Glomerulitis** — *see also* Nephritis 583.9
**Glomerulonephritis** — *see also* Nephritis
 583.9
 with
  edema (*see also* Nephrosis) 581.9
  lesion of
   exudative nephritis 583.89
   interstitial nephritis (diffuse)
    (focal) 583.89
   necrotizing glomerulitis 583.4
    acute 580.4
    chronic 582.4
   renal necrosis 583.9
    cortical 583.6
    medullary 583.7
   specified pathology NEC 583.89
    acute 580.89
    chronic 582.89
  necrosis, renal 583.9
   cortical 583.6
   medullary (papillary) 583.7
  specified pathology or lesion NEC
   583.89
 acute 580.9
  with
   exudative nephritis 580.89
   interstitial nephritis (diffuse)
    (focal) 580.89
   necrotizing glomerulitis 580.4
   extracapillary with epithelial cres-
    cents 580.4
   poststreptococcal 580.0
   proliferative (diffuse) 580.0
   rapidly progressive 580.4
   specified pathology NEC 580.89
  arteriolar (*see also* Hypertension, kidney) 403.90
  arteriosclerotic (*see also* Hypertension,
   kidney) 403.90
  ascending (*see also* Pyelitis) 590.80
  basement membrane NEC 583.89
   with
    pulmonary hemorrhage (Good-
     pasture's syndrome)
     446.21 *[583.81]*
  chronic 582.9
   with
    exudative nephritis 582.89
    interstitial nephritis (diffuse)
     (focal) 582.89
    necrotizing glomerulitis 582.4
    specified pathology or lesion
     NEC 582.89
   endothelial 582.2

**Glomerulonephritis** — *see also* Nephritis
 — *continued*
 chronic — *continued*
  extracapillary with epithelial crescents 582.4
  hypocomplementemic persistent
   582.2
  lobular 582.2
  membranoproliferative 582.2
  membranous 582.1
   and proliferative (mixed) 582.2
   sclerosing 582.1
  mesangiocapillary 582.2
  mixed membranous and proliferative 582.2
  proliferative (diffuse) 582.0
  rapidly progressive 582.4
  sclerosing 582.1
 cirrhotic — *see* Sclerosis, renal
 desquamative — *see* Nephrosis
 due to or associated with
  amyloidosis 277.39 *[583.81]*
   with nephrotic syndrome
    277.39 *[581.81]*
   chronic 277.39 *[582.81]*
  diabetes mellitus 250.4 ☑ *[583.81]*
   with nephrotic syndrome
    250.4 ☑ *[581.81]*
  diphtheria 032.89 *[580.81]*
  gonococcal infection (acute)
   098.19 *[583.81]*
   chronic or duration of 2 months
    or over 098.39 *[583.81]*
  infectious hepatitis 070.9 *[580.81]*
  malaria (with nephrotic syndrome)
   084.9 *[581.81]*
  mumps 072.79 *[580.81]*
  polyarteritis (nodosa) (with
   nephrotic syndrome)
   446.0 *[581.81]*
  specified pathology NEC 583.89
   acute 580.89
   chronic 582.89
  streptotrichosis 039.8 *[583.81]*
  subacute bacterial endocarditis
   421.0 *[580.81]*
  syphilis (late) 095.4
   congenital 090.5 *[583.81]*
   early 091.69 *[583.81]*
  systemic lupus erythematosus
   710.0 *[583.81]*
   with nephrotic syndrome
    710.0 *[581.81]*
   chronic 710.0 *[582.81]*
  tuberculosis (*see also* Tuberculosis)
   016.0 ☑ *[583.81]*
  typhoid fever 002.0 *[580.81]*
 extracapillary with epithelial crescents
  583.4
  acute 580.4
  chronic 582.4
 exudative 583.89
  acute 580.89
  chronic 582.89
 focal (*see also* Nephritis) 583.9
  embolic 580.4
 granular 582.89
 granulomatous 582.89
 hydremic (*see also* Nephrosis) 581.9
 hypocomplementemic persistent 583.2
  with nephrotic syndrome 581.2
  chronic 582.2
 immune complex NEC 583.89
 infective (*see also* Pyelitis) 590.80
 interstitial (diffuse) (focal) 583.89
  with nephrotic syndrome 581.89
  acute 580.89
  chronic 582.89
 latent or quiescent 582.9
 lobular 583.2
  with nephrotic syndrome 581.2
  chronic 582.2
 membranoproliferative 583.2
  with nephrotic syndrome 581.2
  chronic 582.2
 membranous 583.1

**Glomerulonephritis** — *see also* Nephritis
 — *continued*
 membranous — *continued*
  with nephrotic syndrome 581.1
  and proliferative (mixed) 583.2
   with nephrotic syndrome 581.2
   chronic 582.2
  chronic 582.1
  sclerosing 582.1
   with nephrotic syndrome 581.1
 mesangiocapillary 583.2
  with nephrotic syndrome 581.2
  chronic 582.2
 minimal change 581.3
 mixed membranous and proliferative
  583.2
  with nephrotic syndrome 581.2
  chronic 582.2
 necrotizing 583.4
  acute 580.4
  chronic 582.4
 nephrotic (*see also* Nephrosis) 581.9
 old — *see* Glomerulonephritis, chronic
 parenchymatous 581.89
 poststreptococcal 580.0
 proliferative (diffuse) 583.0
  with nephrotic syndrome 581.0
  acute 580.0
  chronic 582.0
 purulent (*see also* Pyelitis) 590.80
 quiescent — *see* Nephritis, chronic
 rapidly progressive 583.4
  acute 580.4
  chronic 582.4
 sclerosing membranous (chronic)
  582.1
  with nephrotic syndrome 581.1
 septic (*see also* Pyelitis) 590.80
 specified pathology or lesion NEC
  583.89
  with nephrotic syndrome 581.89
  acute 580.89
  chronic 582.89
 suppurative (acute) (disseminated)
  (*see also* Pyelitis) 590.80
 toxic — *see* Nephritis, acute
 tubal, tubular — *see* Nephrosis,
  tubular
 type II (Ellis) — *see* Nephrosis
 vascular — *see* Hypertension, kidney
**Glomerulosclerosis** — *see also* Sclerosis,
 renal 587
 focal 582.1
  with nephrotic syndrome 581.1
 intercapillary (nodular) (with diabetes)
  250.4 ☑ *[581.81]*
**Glossagra** 529.6
**Glossalgia** 529.6
**Glossitis** 529.0
 areata exfoliativa 529.1
 atrophic 529.4
 benign migratory 529.1
 gangrenous 529.0
 Hunter's 529.4
 median rhomboid 529.2
 Moeller's 529.4
 pellagrous 265.2
**Glossocele** 529.8
**Glossodynia** 529.6
 exfoliativa 529.4
**Glossoncus** 529.8
**Glossophytia** 529.3
**Glossoplegia** 529.8
**Glossoptosis** 529.8
**Glossopyrosis** 529.6
**Glossotrichia** 529.3
**Glossy skin** 701.9
**Glottis** — *see* condition
**Glottitis** — *see* Glossitis
**Glucagonoma** (M8152/0)
 malignant (M8152/3)
  pancreas 157.4
  specified site NEC — *see* Neoplasm,
   by site, malignant
  unspecified site 157.4
 pancreas 211.7

☑ Additional Digit Required — Refer to the Tabular List for Digit Selection

▽ Subterms under main terms may continue to next column or page

**Glucagonoma** — *continued*
  specified site NEC — *see* Neoplasm,
    by site, benign
  unspecified site 211.7
**Glucoglycinuria** 270.7
**Glue ear syndrome** 381.20
**Glue sniffing** (airplane glue) — *see also*
  Dependence 304.6 ☑
**Glycinemia** (with methylmalonic
  acidemia) 270.7
**Glycinuria** (renal) (with ketosis) 270.0
**Glycogen**
  infiltration (*see also* Disease, glycogen
    storage) 271.0
  storage disease (*see also* Disease,
    glycogen storage) 271.0
**Glycogenosis** — *see also* Disease, glycogen storage 271.0
  cardiac 271.0 *[425.7]*
  Cori, types I-VII 271.0
  diabetic, secondary 250.8 ☑ *[259.8]*
  diffuse (with hepatic cirrhosis) 271.0
  generalized 271.0
  glucose-6-phosphatase deficiency
    271.0
  hepatophosphorylase deficiency 271.0
  hepatorenal 271.0
  myophosphorylase deficiency 271.0
**Glycopenia** 251.2
**Glycopeptide**
  intermediate staphylococcus aureus
    (GISA) V09.8 ☑
  resistant
    enterococcus V09.8 ☑
    staphylococcus aureus (GRSA)
      V09.8 ☑
**Glycoprolinuria** 270.8
**Glycosuria** 791.5
  renal 271.4
**Gnathostoma** (spinigerum) (infection)
  (infestation) 128.1
  wandering swellings from 128.1
**Gnathostomiasis** 128.1
**Goiter** (adolescent) (colloid) (diffuse)
  (dipping) (due to iodine deficiency)
  (endemic) (euthyroid) (heart) (hyperplastic) (internal) (intrathoracic)
  (juvenile) (mixed type) (nonendemic)
  (parenchymatous) (plunging) (sporadic) (subclavicular) (substernal)
  240.9
  with
    hyperthyroidism (recurrent) (*see*
      *also* Goiter, toxic) 242.0 ☑
    thyrotoxicosis (*see also* Goiter,
      toxic) 242.0 ☑
  adenomatous (*see also* Goiter, nodu-
    lar) 241.9
  cancerous (M8000/3) 193
  complicating pregnancy, childbirth,
    or puerperium 648.1 ☑
  congenital 246.1
  cystic (*see also* Goiter, nodular) 241.9
  due to enzyme defect in synthesis of
    thyroid hormone (butane-insol-
    uble iodine) (coupling) (deiodi-
    nase) (iodide trapping or organi-
    fication) (iodotyrosine dehaloge-
    nase) (peroxidase) 246.1
  dyshormonogenic 246.1
  exophthalmic (*see also* Goiter, toxic)
    242.0 ☑
  familial (with deaf-mutism) 243
  fibrous 245.3
  lingual 759.2
  lymphadenoid 245.2
  malignant (M8000/3) 193
  multinodular (nontoxic) 241.1
    toxic or with hyperthyroidism (*see*
      *also* Goiter, toxic) 242.2 ☑
  nodular (nontoxic) 241.9
    with
      hyperthyroidism (*see also* Goi-
        ter, toxic) 242.3 ☑
      thyrotoxicosis (*see also* Goiter,
        toxic) 242.3 ☑

**Goiter** — *continued*
  nodular — *continued*
    endemic 241.9
    exophthalmic (diffuse) (*see also*
      Goiter, toxic) 242.0 ☑
    multinodular (nontoxic) 241.1
    sporadic 241.9
    toxic (*see also* Goiter, toxic)
      242.3 ☑
    uninodular (nontoxic) 241.0
  nontoxic (nodular) 241.9
    multinodular 241.1
    uninodular 241.0
  pulsating (*see also* Goiter, toxic)
    242.0 ☑
  simple 240.0
  toxic 242.0 ☑

> *Note — Use the following fifth-digit
> subclassification with category 242:*
>
> 0  *without mention of thyrotoxic cri-
>    sis or storm*
>
> 1  *with mention of thyrotoxic crisis
>    or storm*

    adenomatous 242.3 ☑
      multinodular 242.2 ☑
      uninodular 242.1 ☑
    multinodular 242.2 ☑
    nodular 242.3 ☑
      multinodular 242.2 ☑
      uninodular 242.1 ☑
    uninodular 242.1 ☑
  uninodular (nontoxic) 241.0
    toxic or with hyperthyroidism (*see
      also* Goiter, toxic) 242.1 ☑
**Goldberg (-Maxwell) (-Morris) syndrome**
  (testicular feminization) 259.5
**Goldblatt's**
  hypertension 440.1
  kidney 440.1
**Goldenhar's syndrome** (oculoauriculovertebral dysplasia) 756.0
**Goldflam-Erb disease or syndrome**
  358.00
**Goldscheider's disease** (epidermolysis
  bullosa) 757.39
**Goldstein's disease** (familial hemorrhagic telangiectasia) 448.0
**Golfer's elbow** 726.32
**Goltz-Gorlin syndrome** (dermal hypoplasia) 757.39
**Gonadoblastoma** (M9073/1)
  specified site — *see* Neoplasm, by site
    uncertain behavior
  unspecified site
    female 236.2
    male 236.4
**Gonecystitis** — *see also* Vesiculitis
  608.0
**Gongylonemiasis** 125.6
  mouth 125.6
**Goniosynechiae** 364.73
**Gonococcemia** 098.89
**Gonococcus, gonococcal** (disease) (infection) — *see also* condition 098.0
  anus 098.7
  bursa 098.52
  chronic NEC 098.2
  complicating pregnancy, childbirth,
    or puerperium 647.1 ☑
    affecting fetus or newborn 760.2
  conjunctiva, conjunctivitis (neonato-
    rum) 098.40
  dermatosis 098.89
  endocardium 098.84
  epididymo-orchitis 098.13
    chronic or duration of 2 months or
      over 098.33
  eye (newborn) 098.40
  fallopian tube (chronic) 098.37
    acute 098.17
  genitourinary (acute) (organ) (system)
    (tract) (*see also* Gonorrhea)
    098.0
    lower 098.0

**Gonococcus, gonococcal** — *see also*
  condition — *continued*
  genitourinary (*see also* Gonorrhea) —
    *continued*
    lower — *continued*
      chronic 098.2
    upper 098.10
      chronic 098.30
  heart NEC 098.85
  joint 098.50
  keratoderma 098.81
  keratosis (blennorrhagica) 098.81
  lymphatic (gland) (node) 098.89
  meninges 098.82
  orchitis (acute) 098.13
    chronic or duration of 2 months or
      over 098.33
  pelvis (acute) 098.19
    chronic or duration of 2 months or
      over 098.39
  pericarditis 098.83
  peritonitis 098.86
  pharyngitis 098.6
  pharynx 098.6
  proctitis 098.7
  pyosalpinx (chronic) 098.37
    acute 098.17
  rectum 098.7
  septicemia 098.89
  skin 098.89
  specified site NEC 098.89
  synovitis 098.51
  tendon sheath 098.51
  throat 098.6
  urethra (acute) 098.0
    chronic or duration of 2 months or
      over 098.2
  vulva (acute) 098.0
    chronic or duration of 2 months or
      over 098.2
**Gonocytoma** (M9073/1)
  specified site — *see* Neoplasm, by site,
    uncertain behavior
  unspecified site
    female 236.2
    male 236.4
**Gonorrhea** 098.0
  acute 098.0
  Bartholin's gland (acute) 098.0
    chronic or duration of 2 months or
      over 098.2
  bladder (acute) 098.11
    chronic or duration of 2 months or
      over 098.31
  carrier (suspected of) V02.7
  cervix (acute) 098.15
    chronic or duration of 2 months or
      over 098.35
  chronic 098.2
  complicating pregnancy, childbirth,
    or puerperium 647.1 ☑
    affecting fetus or newborn 760.2
  conjunctiva, conjunctivitis (neonato-
    rum) 098.40
  contact V01.6
  Cowper's gland (acute) 098.0
    chronic or duration of 2 months or
      over 098.2
  duration of two months or over 098.2
  exposure to V01.6
  fallopian tube (chronic) 098.37
    acute 098.17
  genitourinary (acute) (organ) (system)
    (tract) 098.0
    chronic 098.2
    duration of two months or over
      098.2
  kidney (acute) 098.19
    chronic or duration of 2 months or
      over 098.39
  ovary (acute) 098.19
    chronic or duration of 2 months or
      over 098.39
  pelvis (acute) 098.19
    chronic or duration of 2 months or
      over 098.39

**Gonorrhea** — *continued*
  penis (acute) 098.0
    chronic or duration of 2 months or
      over 098.2
  prostate (acute) 098.12
    chronic or duration of 2 months or
      over 098.32
  seminal vesicle (acute) 098.14
    chronic or duration of 2 months or
      over 098.34
  specified site NEC — *see* Gonococcus
  spermatic cord (acute) 098.14
    chronic or duration of 2 months or
      over 098.34
  urethra (acute) 098.0
    chronic or duration of 2 months or
      over 098.2
  vagina (acute) 098.0
    chronic or duration of 2 months or
      over 098.2
  vas deferens (acute) 098.14
    chronic or duration of 2 months or
      over 098.34
  vulva (acute) 098.0
    chronic or duration of 2 months or
      over 098.2
**Goodpasture's syndrome** (pneumorenal)
  446.21
**Good's syndrome** 279.06
**Gopalan's syndrome** (burning feet) 266.2
**Gordon's disease** (exudative enteropathy)
  579.8
**Gorlin-Chaudhry-Moss syndrome**
  759.89
**Gougerot-Blum syndrome** (pigmented
  purpuric lichenoid dermatitis)
  709.1
**Gougerot-Carteaud disease or syn-
  drome** (confluent reticulate papillomatosis) 701.8
**Gougerot-Hailey-Hailey disease** (benign
  familial chronic pemphigus) 757.39
**Gougerot (-Houwer) -Sjögren syndrome**
  (keratoconjunctivitis sicca) 710.2
**Gougerot's syndrome** (trisymptomatic)
  709.1
**Gouley's syndrome** (constrictive pericarditis) 423.2
**Goundou** 102.6
**Gout, gouty** 274.9
  with specified manifestations NEC
    274.89
  arthritis (acute) 274.0
  arthropathy 274.0
  degeneration, heart 274.82
  diathesis 274.9
  eczema 274.89
  episcleritis 274.89 *[379.09]*
  external ear (tophus) 274.81
  glomerulonephritis 274.10
  iritis 274.89 *[364.11]*
  joint 274.0
  kidney 274.10
  lead 984.9
    specified type of lead — *see* Table
      of Drugs and Chemicals
  nephritis 274.10
  neuritis 274.89 *[357.4]*
  phlebitis 274.89 *[451.9]*
  rheumatic 714.0
  saturnine 984.9
    specified type of lead — *see* Table
      of Drugs and Chemicals
  spondylitis 274.0
  synovitis 274.0
  syphilitic 095.8
  tophi 274.0
    ear 274.81
    heart 274.82
    specified site NEC 274.82
**Gowers'**
  muscular dystrophy 359.1
  syndrome (vasovagal attack) 780.2
**Gowers-Paton-Kennedy syndrome**
  377.04
**Gradenigo's syndrome** 383.02

---

☑ Additional Digit Required — Refer to the Tabular List for Digit Selection          ▽ Subterms under main terms may continue to next column or page

**Graft-versus-host disease** (bone marrow) 996.85
   due to organ transplant NEC — *see* Complications, transplant, organ
**Graham Steell's murmur** (pulmonic regurgitation) — *see also* Endocarditis, pulmonary 424.3
**Grain-handlers' disease or lung** 495.8
**Grain mite** (itch) 133.8
**Grand**
   mal (idiopathic) (*see also* Epilepsy) 345.1 ☑
     hysteria of Charcôt 300.11
     nonrecurrent or isolated 780.39
   multipara
     affecting management of labor and delivery 659.4 ☑
     status only (not pregnant) V61.5
**Granite workers' lung** 502
**Granular** — *see also* condition
   inflammation, pharynx 472.1
   kidney (contracting) (*see also* Sclerosis, renal) 587
   liver — *see* Cirrhosis, liver
   nephritis — *see* Nephritis
**Granulation tissue, abnormal** — *see also* Granuloma
   abnormal or excessive 701.5
   postmastoidectomy cavity 383.33
   postoperative 701.5
   skin 701.5
**Granulocytopenia, granulocytopenic** (primary) 288.00
   malignant 288.09
**Granuloma** NEC 686.1
   abdomen (wall) 568.89
     skin (pyogenicum) 686.1
       from residual foreign body 709.4
   annulare 695.89
   anus 569.49
   apical 522.6
   appendix 543.9
   aural 380.23
   beryllium (skin) 709.4
     lung 503
   bone (*see also* Osteomyelitis) 730.1 ☑
     eosinophilic 277.89
     from residual foreign body 733.99
   canaliculus lacrimalis 375.81
   cerebral 348.8
   cholesterin, middle ear 385.82
   coccidioidal (progressive) 114.3
     lung 114.4
     meninges 114.2
     primary (lung) 114.0
   colon 569.89
   conjunctiva 372.61
   dental 522.6
   ear, middle (cholesterin) 385.82
     with otitis media — *see* Otitis media
   eosinophilic 277.89
     bone 277.89
     lung 277.89
     oral mucosa 528.9
   exuberant 701.5
   eyelid 374.89
   facial
     lethal midline 446.3
     malignant 446.3
   faciale 701.8
   fissuratum (gum) 523.8
   foot NEC 686.1
   foreign body (in soft tissue) NEC 728.82
     bone 733.99
     in operative wound 998.4
     muscle 728.82
     skin 709.4
     subcutaneous tissue 709.4
   fungoides 202.1 ☑
   gangraenescens 446.3
   giant cell (central) (jaw) (reparative) 526.3
     gingiva 523.8

**Granuloma** — *continued*
   giant cell — *continued*
     peripheral (gingiva) 523.8
   gland (lymph) 289.3
   Hodgkin's (M9661/3) 201.1 ☑
   ileum 569.89
   infectious NEC 136.9
   inguinale (Donovan) 099.2
     venereal 099.2
   intestine 569.89
   iridocyclitis 364.10
   jaw (bone) 526.3
     reparative giant cell 526.3
   kidney (*see also* Infection, kidney) 590.9
   lacrimal sac 375.81
   larynx 478.79
   lethal midline 446.3
   lipid 277.89
   lipoid 277.89
   liver 572.8
   lung (infectious) (*see also* Fibrosis, lung) 515
     coccidioidal 114.4
     eosinophilic 277.89
   lymph gland 289.3
   Majocchi's 110.6
   malignant, face 446.3
   mandible 526.3
   mediastinum 519.3
   midline 446.3
   monilial 112.3
   muscle 728.82
     from residual foreign body 728.82
   nasal sinus (*see also* Sinusitis) 473.9
   operation wound 998.59
     foreign body 998.4
     stitch (external) 998.89
       internal wound 998.89
     talc 998.7
   oral mucosa, eosinophilic or pyogenic 528.9
   orbit, orbital 376.11
   paracoccidioidal 116.1
   penis, venereal 099.2
   periapical 522.6
   peritoneum 568.89
     due to ova of helminths NEC (*see also* Helminthiasis) 128.9
   postmastoidectomy cavity 383.33
   postoperative — *see* Granuloma, operation wound
   prostate 601.8
   pudendi (ulcerating) 099.2
   pudendorum (ulcerative) 099.2
   pulp, internal (tooth) 521.49
   pyogenic, pyogenicum (skin) 686.1
     maxillary alveolar ridge 522.6
     oral mucosa 528.9
   rectum 569.49
   reticulohistiocytic 277.89
   rubrum nasi 705.89
   sarcoid 135
   Schistosoma 120.9
   septic (skin) 686.1
   silica (skin) 709.4
   sinus (accessory) (infectional) (nasal) (*see also* Sinusitis) 473.9
   skin (pyogenicum) 686.1
     from foreign body or material 709.4
   sperm 608.89
   spine
     syphilitic (epidural) 094.89
     tuberculous (*see also* Tuberculosis) 015.0 ☑ [730.88]
   stitch (postoperative) 998.89
     internal wound 998.89
   suppurative (skin) 686.1
   suture (postoperative) 998.89
     internal wound 998.89
   swimming pool 031.1
   talc 728.82
     in operation wound 998.7
   telangiectaticum (skin) 686.1
   tracheostomy 519.09
   trichophyticum 110.6

**Granuloma** — *continued*
   tropicum 102.4
   umbilicus 686.1
     newborn 771.4
   urethra 599.84
   uveitis 364.10
   vagina 099.2
   venereum 099.2
   vocal cords 478.5
   Wegener's (necrotizing respiratory granulomatosis) 446.4
**Granulomatosis** NEC 686.1
   disciformis chronica et progressiva 709.3
   infantiseptica 771.2
   lipoid 277.89
   lipophagic, intestinal 040.2
   miliary 027.0
   necrotizing, respiratory 446.4
   progressive, septic 288.1
   Wegener's (necrotizing respiratory) 446.4
**Granulomatous tissue** — *see* Granuloma
**Granulosis rubra nasi** 705.89
**Graphite fibrosis** (of lung) 503
**Graphospasm** 300.89
   organic 333.84
**Grating scapula** 733.99
**Gravel** (urinary) — *see also* Calculus 592.9
**Graves' disease** (exophthalmic goiter) — *see also* Goiter, toxic 242.0 ☑
**Gravis** — *see* condition
**Grawitz's tumor** (hypernephroma) (M8312/3) 189.0
**Grayness, hair** (premature) 704.3
   congenital 757.4
**Gray or grey syndrome** (chloramphenicol) (newborn) 779.4
**Greenfield's disease** 330.0
**Green sickness** 280.9
**Greenstick fracture** — *see* Fracture, by site
**Greig's syndrome** (hypertelorism) 756.0
**Grief** 309.0 ●
**Griesinger's disease** — *see also* Ancylostomiasis 126.9
**Grinders'**
   asthma 502
   lung 502
   phthisis (*see also* Tuberculosis) 011.4 ☑
**Grinding, teeth** 306.8
**Grip**
   Dabney's 074.1
   devil's 074.1
**Grippe, grippal** — *see also* Influenza
   Balkan 083.0
   intestinal 487.8
   summer 074.8
**Grippy cold** 487.1
**Grisel's disease** 723.5
**Groin** — *see* condition
**Grooved**
   nails (transverse) 703.8
   tongue 529.5
     congenital 750.13
**Ground itch** 126.9
**Growing pains, children** 781.99
**Growth** (fungoid) (neoplastic) (new) (M8000/1) — *see also* Neoplasm, by site, unspecified nature
   adenoid (vegetative) 474.12
   benign (M8000/0) — *see* Neoplasm, by site, benign
   fetal, poor 764.9 ☑
     affecting management of pregnancy 656.5 ☑
   malignant (M8000/3) — *see* Neoplasm, by site, malignant
   rapid, childhood V21.0
   secondary (M8000/6) — *see* Neoplasm, by site, malignant, secondary
**GRSA** (glycopeptide resistant staphylococcus aureus) V09.8 ☑

**Gruber's hernia** — *see* Hernia, Gruber's
**Gruby's disease** (tinea tonsurans) 110.0
**G-trisomy** 758.0
**Guama fever** 066.3
**Gubler (-Millard) paralysis or syndrome** 344.89
**Guérin-Stern syndrome** (arthrogryposis multiplex congenita) 754.89
**Guertin's disease** (electric chorea) 049.8
**Guillain-Barré disease or syndrome** 357.0
**Guinea worms** (infection) (infestation) 125.7
**Guinon's disease** (motor-verbal tic) 307.23
**Gull and Sutton's disease** — *see* Hypertension, kidney
**Gull's disease** (thyroid atrophy with myxedema) 244.8
**Gum** — *see* condition
**Gumboil** 522.7
**Gumma** (syphilitic) 095.9
   artery 093.89
     cerebral or spinal 094.89
   bone 095.5
     of yaws (late) 102.6
   brain 094.89
   cauda equina 094.89
   central nervous system NEC 094.9
   ciliary body 095.8 [364.11]
   congenital 090.5
     testis 090.5
   eyelid 095.8 [373.5]
   heart 093.89
   intracranial 094.89
   iris 095.8 [364.11]
   kidney 095.4
   larynx 095.8
   leptomeninges 094.2
   liver 095.3
   meninges 094.2
   myocardium 093.82
   nasopharynx 095.8
   neurosyphilitic 094.9
   nose 095.8
   orbit 095.8
   palate (soft) 095.8
   penis 095.8
   pericardium 093.81
   pharynx 095.8
   pituitary 095.8
   scrofulous (*see also* Tuberculosis) 017.0 ☑
   skin 095.8
   specified site NEC 095.8
   spinal cord 094.89
   tongue 095.8
   tonsil 095.8
   trachea 095.8
   tuberculous (*see also* Tuberculosis) 017.0 ☑
   ulcerative due to yaws 102.4
   ureter 095.8
   yaws 102.4
     bone 102.6
**Gunn's syndrome** (jaw-winking syndrome) 742.8
**Gunshot wound** — *see also* Wound, open, by site
   fracture — *see* Fracture, by site, open
   internal organs (abdomen, chest, or pelvis) — *see* Injury, internal, by site, with open wound
   intracranial — *see* Laceration, brain, with open intracranial wound
**Günther's disease or syndrome** (congenital erythropoietic porphyria) 277.1
**Gustatory hallucination** 780.1
**Gynandrism** 752.7
**Gynandroblastoma** (M8632/1)
   specified site — *see* Neoplasm, by site, uncertain behavior
   unspecified site
     female 236.2
     male 236.4
**Gynandromorphism** 752.7

☑ Additional Digit Required — Refer to the Tabular List for Digit Selection
▽ Subterms under main terms may continue to next column or page

**2008 ICD-9-CM**
▶◀ Revised Text
● New Line
▲ Revised Code
**October 2007 • Volume 2 — 135**

**Gynatresia** (congenital) 752.49
**Gynecoid pelvis, male** 738.6
**Gynecological examination** V72.31
  for contraceptive maintenance V25.40
**Gynecomastia** 611.1
**Gynephobia** 300.29
**Gyrate scalp** 757.39

## H

**Haas' disease** (osteochondrosis head of
  humerus) 732.3
**Habermann's disease** (acute parapsoriasis varioliformis) 696.2
**Habit, habituation**
  chorea 307.22
  disturbance, child 307.9
  drug (see also Dependence) 304.9 ☑
  laxative (see also Abuse, drugs, non-
    dependent) 305.9 ☑
  spasm 307.20
    chronic 307.22
    transient (of childhood) 307.21
  tic 307.20
    chronic 307.22
    transient (of childhood) 307.21
  use of
    nonprescribed drugs (see also
      Abuse, drugs, nondependent)
      305.9 ☑
    patent medicines (see also Abuse,
      drugs, nondependent)
      305.9 ☑
  vomiting 536.2
**Hadfield-Clarke syndrome** (pancreatic
  infantilism) 577.8
**Haff disease** 985.1
**Hageman factor defect, deficiency, or
  disease** — see also Defect, coagula-
  tion 286.3
**Haglund's disease** (osteochondrosis os
  tibiale externum) 732.5
**Haglund-Läwen-Fründ syndrome**
  717.89
**Hagner's disease** (hypertrophic pul-
  monary osteoarthropathy) 731.2
**Hag teeth, tooth** 524.39
**Hailey-Hailey disease** (benign familial
  chronic pemphigus) 757.39
**Hair** — see also condition
  plucking 307.9
**Hairball in stomach** 935.2
**Hairy black tongue** 529.3
**Half vertebra** 756.14
**Halitosis** 784.99
**Hallermann-Streiff syndrome** 756.0
**Hallervorden-Spatz disease or syn-
  drome** 333.0
**Hallopeau's**
  acrodermatitis (continua) 696.1
  disease (lichen sclerosis et atrophicus)
    701.0
**Hallucination** (auditory) (gustatory) (olfactory) (tactile) 780.1
  alcohol-induced 291.3
  drug-induced 292.12
  visual 368.16
**Hallucinosis** 298.9
  alcohol-induced (acute) 291.3
  drug-induced 292.12
**Hallus** — see Hallux
**Hallux** 735.9
  limitus 735.8
  malleus (acquired) 735.3
  rigidus (acquired) 735.2
    congenital 755.66
    late effects of rickets 268.1
  valgus (acquired) 735.0
    congenital 755.66
  varus (acquired) 735.1
    congenital 755.66
**Halo, visual** 368.15
**Hamartoblastoma** 759.6
**Hamartoma** 759.6
  epithelial (gingival), odontogenic, cen-
    tral, or peripheral (M9321/0)
    213.1

**Hamartoma** — continued
  epithelial, odontogenic, central, or pe-
    ripheral — continued
    upper jaw (bone) 213.0
  vascular 757.32
**Hamartosis, hamartoses** NEC 759.6
**Hamman's disease or syndrome** (spontaneous mediastinal emphysema)
  518.1
**Hamman-Rich syndrome** (diffuse interstitial pulmonary fibrosis) 516.3
**Hammer toe** (acquired) 735.4
  congenital 755.66
  late effects of rickets 268.1
**Hand** — see condition
**Hand-foot syndrome** 693.0 ▲
**Hand-Schüller-Christian disease or
  syndrome** (chronic histiocytosis x)
  277.89
**Hanging** (asphyxia) (strangulation) (suffocation) 994.7
**Hangnail** (finger) (with lymphangitis)
  681.02
**Hangover** (alcohol) — see also Abuse,
  drugs, nondependent 305.0 ☑
**Hanot-Chauffard (-Troisier) syndrome**
  (bronze diabetes) 275.0
**Hanot's cirrhosis or disease** — see Cirrhosis, biliary
**Hansen's disease** (leprosy) 030.9
  benign form 030.1
  malignant form 030.0
**Harada's disease or syndrome** 363.22
**Hard chancre** 091.0
**Hardening**
  artery — see Arteriosclerosis
  brain 348.8
  liver 571.8
**Hard firm prostate** 600.10
  with
    urinary
      obstruction 600.11
      retention 600.11
**Harelip** — see also Cleft, lip 749.10
**Hare's syndrome** (M8010/3) (carcinoma,
  pulmonary apex) 162.3
**Harkavy's syndrome** 446.0
**Harlequin** (fetus) 757.1
  color change syndrome 779.89
**Harley's disease** (intermittent
  hemoglobinuria) 283.2
**Harris'**
  lines 733.91
  syndrome (organic hyperinsulinism)
    251.1
**Hart's disease or syndrome** (pellagra-
  cerebellar ataxia-renal
  aminoaciduria) 270.0
**Hartmann's pouch** (abnormal saccula-
  tion of gallbladder neck) 575.8
  of intestine V44.3
    attention to V55.3
**Hartnup disease** (pellagra-cerebellar
  ataxia-renal aminoaciduria) 270.0
**Harvester lung** 495.0
**Hashimoto's disease or struma** (struma
  lymphomatosa) 245.2
**Hassall-Henle bodies** (corneal warts)
  371.41
**Haut mal** — see also Epilepsy 345.1 ☑
**Haverhill fever** 026.1
**Hawaiian wood rose dependence**
  304.5 ☑
**Hawkins' keloid** 701.4
**Hay**
  asthma (see also Asthma) 493.0 ☑
  fever (allergic) (with rhinitis) 477.9
    with asthma (bronchial) (see also
      Asthma) 493.0 ☑
    allergic, due to grass, pollen, rag-
      weed, or tree 477.0
    conjunctivitis 372.05
    due to
      dander, animal (cat) (dog) 477.2
      dust 477.8
      fowl 477.8

**Hay** — continued
  fever — continued
    due to — continued
      hair, animal (cat) (dog) 477.2
      pollen 477.0
      specified allergen other than
        pollen 477.8
**Hayem-Faber syndrome** (achlorhydric
  anemia) 280.9
**Hayem-Widal syndrome** (acquired
  hemolytic jaundice) 283.9
**Haygarth's nodosities** 715.04
**Hazard-Crile tumor** (M8350/3) 193
**Hb** (abnormal)
  disease — see Disease, hemoglobin
  trait — see Trait
**H disease** 270.0
**Head** — see also condition
  banging 307.3
**Headache** 784.0
  allergic 346.2 ☑
  cluster 346.2 ☑
  due to
    loss, spinal fluid 349.0
    lumbar puncture 349.0
    saddle block 349.0
  emotional 307.81
  histamine 346.2 ☑
  lumbar puncture 349.0
  menopausal 627.2
  migraine 346.9 ☑
  nonorganic origin 307.81
  postspinal 349.0
  psychogenic 307.81
  psychophysiologic 307.81
  sick 346.1 ☑
  spinal 349.0
    complicating labor and delivery
      668.8 ☑
    postpartum 668.8 ☑
  spinal fluid loss 349.0
  tension 307.81
  vascular 784.0
    migraine type 346.9 ☑
  vasomotor 346.9 ☑
**Health**
  advice V65.4 ☑
  audit V70.0
  checkup V70.0
  education V65.4 ☑
  hazard (see also History of) V15.9
    falling V15.88
    specified cause NEC V15.89
  instruction V65.4 ☑
  services provided because (of)
    boarding school residence V60.6
    holiday relief for person providing
      home care V60.5
    inadequate
      housing V60.1
      resources V60.2
    lack of housing V60.0
    no care available in home V60.4
    person living alone V60.3
    poverty V60.3
    residence in institution V60.6
    specified cause NEC V60.8
    vacation relief for person providing
      home care V60.5
**Healthy**
  donor (see also Donor) V59.9
  infant or child
    accompanying sick mother V65.0
    receiving care V20.1
  person
    accompanying sick relative V65.0
    admitted for sterilization V25.2
    receiving prophylactic inoculation
      or vaccination (see also Vac-
      cination, prophylactic) V05.9
**Hearing**
  conservation and treatment V72.12 ●
  examination V72.19        ●
    following failed hearing screening ●
      V72.11
**Heart** — see condition

**Heartburn** 787.1
  psychogenic 306.4
**Heat** (effects) 992.9
  apoplexy 992.0
  burn (see also Burn, by site)
    from sun (see also Sunburn)
      692.71
  collapse 992.1
  cramps 992.2
  dermatitis or eczema 692.89
  edema 992.7
  erythema — see Burn, by site
  excessive 992.9
    specified effect NEC 992.8
  exhaustion 992.5
    anhydrotic 992.3
    due to
      salt (and water) depletion 992.4
      water depletion 992.3
  fatigue (transient) 992.6
  fever 992.0
  hyperpyrexia 992.0
  prickly 705.1
  prostration — see Heat, exhaustion
  pyrexia 992.0
  rash 705.1
  specified effect NEC 992.8
  stroke 992.0
  sunburn (see also Sunburn) 692.71
  syncope 992.1
**Heavy-chain disease** 273.2
**Heavy-for-dates** (fetus or infant) 766.1
  4500 grams or more 766.0
  exceptionally 766.0
**Hebephrenia, hebephrenic** (acute) —
  see also Schizophrenia 295.1 ☑
  dementia (praecox) (see also
    Schizophrenia) 295.1 ☑
  schizophrenia (see also Schizophrenia)
    295.1 ☑
**Heberden's**
  disease or nodes 715.04
  syndrome (angina pectoris) 413.9
**Hebra's disease**
  dermatitis exfoliativa 695.89
  erythema multiforme exudativum
    695.1
  pityriasis 695.89
    maculata et circinata 696.3
    rubra 695.89
    pilaris 696.4
  prurigo 698.2
**Hebra, nose** 040.1
**Hedinger's syndrome** (malignant carcinoid) 259.2
**Heel** — see condition
**Heerfordt's disease or syndrome**
  (uveoparotitis) 135
**Hegglin's anomaly or syndrome** 288.2
**Heidenhain's disease** 290.10
  with dementia 290.10
**Heilmeyer-Schöner disease** (M9842/3)
  207.1 ☑
**Heine-Medin disease** — see also Poliomyelitis 045.9 ☑
**Heinz-body anemia, congenital** 282.7
**Heller's disease or syndrome** (infantile
  psychosis) — see also Psychosis,
  childhood 299.1 ☑
**H.E.L.L.P** 642.5 ☑
**Helminthiasis** — see also Infestation, by
  specific parasite 128.9
  Ancylostoma (see also Ancylostoma)
    126.9
  intestinal 127.9
    mixed types (types classifiable to
      more than one of the cate-
      gories 120.0–127.7) 127.8
    specified type 127.7
  mixed types (intestinal) (types classifi-
    able to more than one of the
    categories 120.0–127.7) 127.8
  Necator americanus 126.1
  specified type NEC 128.8
  Trichinella 124
**Heloma** 700

☑ Additional Digit Required — Refer to the Tabular List for Digit Selection            🆕 Subterms under main terms may continue to next column or page

**Hemangioblastoma** (M9161/1) — *see also* Neoplasm, connective tissue, uncertain behavior
  malignant (M9161/3) — *see* Neoplasm, connective tissue, malignant
**Hemangioblastomatosis, cerebelloretinal** 759.6
**Hemangioendothelioma** (M9130/1) — *see also* Neoplasm, by site, uncertain behavior
  benign (M9130/0) 228.00
  bone (diffuse) (M9130/3) — *see* Neoplasm, bone, malignant
  malignant (M9130/3) — *see* Neoplasm, connective tissue, malignant
  nervous system (M9130/0) 228.09
**Hemangioendotheliosarcoma** (M9130/3) — *see* Neoplasm, connective tissue, malignant
**Hemangiofibroma** (M9160/0) — *see* Neoplasm, by site, benign
**Hemangiolipoma** (M8861/0) — *see* Lipoma
**Hemangioma** (M9120/0) 228.00
  arteriovenous (M9123/0) — *see* Hemangioma, by site
  brain 228.02
  capillary (M9131/0) — *see* Hemangioma, by site
  cavernous (M9121/0) — *see* Hemangioma, by site
  central nervous system NEC 228.09
  choroid 228.09
  heart 228.09
  infantile (M9131/0) — *see* Hemangioma, by site
  intra-abdominal structures 228.04
  intracranial structures 228.02
  intramuscular (M9132/0) — *see* Hemangioma, by site
  iris 228.09
  juvenile (M9131/0) — *see* Hemangioma, by site
  malignant (M9120/3) — *see* Neoplasm, connective tissue, malignant
  meninges 228.09
    brain 228.02
    spinal cord 228.09
  peritoneum 228.04
  placenta — *see* Placenta, abnormal
  plexiform (M9131/0) — *see* Hemangioma, by site
  racemose (M9123/0) — *see* Hemangioma, by site
  retina 228.03
  retroperitoneal tissue 228.04
  sclerosing (M8832/0) — *see* Neoplasm, skin, benign
  simplex (M9131/0) — *see* Hemangioma, by site
  skin and subcutaneous tissue 228.01
  specified site NEC 228.09
  spinal cord 228.09
  venous (M9122/0) — *see* Hemangioma, by site
  verrucous keratotic (M9142/0) — *see* Hemangioma, by site
**Hemangiomatosis** (systemic) 757.32
  involving single site — *see* Hemangioma
**Hemangiopericytoma** (M9150/1) — *see also* Neoplasm, connective tissue, uncertain behavior
  benign (M9150/0) — *see* Neoplasm, connective tissue, benign
  malignant (M9150/3) — *see* Neoplasm, connective tissue, malignant
**Hemangiosarcoma** (M9120/3) — *see* Neoplasm, connective tissue, malignant
**Hemarthrosis** (nontraumatic) 719.10
  ankle 719.17

**Hemarthrosis** — *continued*
  elbow 719.12
  foot 719.17
  hand 719.14
  hip 719.15
  knee 719.16
  multiple sites 719.19
  pelvic region 719.15
  shoulder (region) 719.11
  specified site NEC 719.18
  traumatic — *see* Sprain, by site
  wrist 719.13
**Hematemesis** 578.0
  with ulcer — *see* Ulcer, by site, with hemorrhage
  due to S. japonicum 120.2
  Goldstein's (familial hemorrhagic telangiectasia) 448.0
  newborn 772.4
    due to swallowed maternal blood 777.3
**Hematidrosis** 705.89
**Hematinuria** — *see also* Hemoglobinuria 791.2
  malarial 084.8
  paroxysmal 283.2
**Hematite miners' lung** 503
**Hematobilia** 576.8
**Hematocele** (congenital) (diffuse) (idiopathic) 608.83
  broad ligament 620.7
  canal of Nuck 629.0
  cord, male 608.83
  fallopian tube 620.8
  female NEC 629.0
  ischiorectal 569.89
  male NEC 608.83
  ovary 629.0
  pelvis, pelvic
    female 629.0
      with ectopic pregnancy (*see also* Pregnancy, ectopic) 633.90
        with intrauterine pregnancy 633.91
    male 608.83
  periuterine 629.0
  retrouterine 629.0
  scrotum 608.83
  spermatic cord (diffuse) 608.83
  testis 608.84
  traumatic — *see* Injury, internal, pelvis
  tunica vaginalis 608.83
  uterine ligament 629.0
  uterus 621.4
  vagina 623.6
  vulva 624.5
**Hematocephalus** 742.4
**Hematochezia** — *see also* Melena 578.1
**Hematochyluria** — *see also* Infestation, filarial 125.9
**Hematocolpos** 626.8
**Hematocornea** 371.12
**Hematogenous** — *see* condition
**Hematoma** (skin surface intact) (traumatic) — *see also* Contusion

*Note* — *Hematomas are coded according to origin and the nature and site of the hematoma or the accompanying injury. Hematomas of unspecified origin are coded as injuries of the sites involved, except:*

  (a) *hematomas of genital organs which are coded as diseases of the organ involved unless they complicate pregnancy or delivery*

  (b) *hematomas of the eye which are coded as diseases of the eye.*

*For late effect of hematoma classifiable to 920–924 see Late, effect, contusion*

  with
    crush injury — *see* Crush
    fracture — *see* Fracture, by site

**Hematoma** — *see also* Contusion — *continued*
  with — *continued*
    injury of internal organs (*see also* Injury, internal, by site)
      kidney — *see* Hematoma, kidney traumatic
      liver — *see* Hematoma, liver, traumatic
      spleen — *see* Hematoma, spleen
    nerve injury — *see* Injury, nerve
    open wound — *see* Wound, open, by site
    skin surface intact — *see* Contusion
  abdomen (wall) — *see* Contusion, abdomen
  amnion 658.8 ☑
  aorta, dissecting 441.00
    abdominal 441.02
    thoracic 441.01
    thoracoabdominal 441.03
  arterial (complicating trauma) 904.9
    specified site — *see* Injury, blood vessel, by site
  auricle (ear) 380.31
  birth injury 767.8
    skull 767.19
  brain (traumatic) 853.0 ☑

*Note* — *Use the following fifth-digit subclassification with categories 851–854:*

  0    *unspecified state of consciousness*

  1    *with no loss of consciousness*

  2    *with brief [less than one hour] loss of consciousness*

  3    *with moderate [1–24 hours] loss of consciousness*

  4    *with prolonged [more than 24 hours] loss of consciousness and return to pre–existing conscious level*

  5    *with prolonged [more than 24 hours] loss of consciousness, without return to pre–existing conscious level*

*Use fifth-digit 5 to designate when a patient is unconscious and dies before regaining consciousness, regardless of the duration of the loss of consciousness*

  6    *with loss of consciousness of unspecified duration*

  9    *with concussion, unspecified*

  with
    cerebral
      contusion — *see* Contusion, brain
      laceration — *see* Laceration, brain
    open intracranial wound 853.1 ☑
    skull fracture — *see* Fracture, skull, by site
  extradural or epidural 852.4 ☑
    with open intracranial wound 852.5 ☑
    fetus or newborn 767.0
    nontraumatic 432.0
  fetus or newborn NEC 767.0
  nontraumatic (*see also* Hemorrhage, brain) 431
    epidural or extradural 432.0
    newborn NEC 772.8
    subarachnoid, arachnoid, or meningeal (*see also* Hemorrhage, subarachnoid) 430
    subdural (*see also* Hemorrhage, subdural) 432.1

**Hematoma** — *see also* Contusion — *continued*
  brain — *continued*
    subarachnoid, arachnoid, or meningeal 852.0 ☑
      with open intracranial wound 852.1 ☑
      fetus or newborn 772.2
      nontraumatic (*see also* Hemorrhage, subarachnoid) 430
    subdural 852.2 ☑
      with open intracranial wound 852.3 ☑
      fetus or newborn (localized) 767.0
      nontraumatic (*see also* Hemorrhage, subdural) 432.1
  breast (nontraumatic) 611.8
  broad ligament (nontraumatic) 620.7
    complicating delivery 665.7 ☑
    traumatic — *see* Injury, internal, broad ligament
  calcified NEC 959.9
  capitis 920
    due to birth injury 767.19
    newborn 767.19
  cerebral — *see* Hematoma, brain
  cesarean section wound 674.3 ☑
  chorion — *see* Placenta, abnormal
  complicating delivery (perineum) (vulva) 664.5 ☑
    pelvic 665.7 ☑
    vagina 665.7 ☑
  corpus
    cavernosum (nontraumatic) 607.82
    luteum (nontraumatic) (ruptured) 620.1
  dura (mater) — *see* Hematoma, brain, subdural
  epididymis (nontraumatic) 608.83
  epidural (traumatic) (*see also* Hematoma, brain, extradural)
    spinal — *see* Injury, spinal, by site
  episiotomy 674.3 ☑
  external ear 380.31
  extradural (*see also* Hematoma, brain, extradural)
    fetus or newborn 767.0
    nontraumatic 432.0
      fetus or newborn 767.0
  fallopian tube 620.8
  genital organ (nontraumatic)
    female NEC 629.89
    male NEC 608.83
    traumatic (external site) 922.4
      internal — *see* Injury, internal, genital organ
  graafian follicle (ruptured) 620.0
  internal organs (abdomen, chest, or pelvis) (*see also* Injury, internal, by site)
    kidney — *see* Hematoma, kidney, traumatic
    liver — *see* Hematoma, liver, traumatic
    spleen — *see* Hematoma, spleen
  intracranial — *see* Hematoma, brain
  kidney, cystic 593.81
    traumatic 866.01
      with open wound into cavity 866.11
  labia (nontraumatic) 624.5
  lingual (and other parts of neck, scalp, or face, except eye) 920
  liver (subcapsular) 573.8
    birth injury 767.8
    fetus or newborn 767.8
    traumatic NEC 864.01
      with
        laceration — *see* Laceration, liver
        open wound into cavity 864.11
  mediastinum — *see* Injury, internal, mediastinum

☑ Additional Digit Required — Refer to the Tabular List for Digit Selection          ▼ Subterms under main terms may continue to next column or page

*2008 ICD-9-CM*          ▶◀ Revised Text          ● New Line          ▲ Revised Code          **Volume 2 — 137**

Hemangioblastoma — Hematoma

**Hematoma** — *see also* Contusion — *continued*
  meninges, meningeal (brain) (*see also* Hematoma, brain, subarachnoid)
    spinal — *see* Injury, spinal, by site
  mesosalpinx (nontraumatic) 620.8
    traumatic — *see* Injury, internal, pelvis
  muscle (traumatic) — *see* Contusion, by site
  nasal (septum) (and other part(s) of neck, scalp, or face, except eye) 920
  obstetrical surgical wound 674.3 ☑
  orbit, orbital (nontraumatic) 376.32
    traumatic 921.2
  ovary (corpus luteum) (nontraumatic) 620.1
    traumatic — *see* Injury, internal, ovary
  pelvis (female) (nontraumatic) 629.89
    complicating delivery 665.7 ☑
    male 608.83
    traumatic (*see also* Injury, internal, pelvis)
      specified organ NEC (*see also* Injury, internal, pelvis) 867.6
  penis (nontraumatic) 607.82
  pericranial (and neck, or face any part, except eye) 920
    due to injury at birth 767.19
  perineal wound (obstetrical) 674.3 ☑
    complicating delivery 664.5 ☑
  perirenal, cystic 593.81
  pinna 380.31
  placenta — *see* Placenta, abnormal
  postoperative 998.12
  retroperitoneal (nontraumatic) 568.81
    traumatic — *see* Injury, internal, retroperitoneum
  retropubic, male 568.81
  scalp (and neck, or face any part, except eye) 920
    fetus or newborn 767.19
  scrotum (nontraumatic) 608.83
    traumatic 922.4
  seminal vesicle (nontraumatic) 608.83
    traumatic — *see* Injury, internal, seminal, vesicle
  spermatic cord (*see also* Injury, internal, spermatic cord)
    nontraumatic 608.83
  spinal (cord) (meninges) (*see also* Injury, spinal, by site)
    fetus or newborn 767.4
    nontraumatic 336.1
  spleen 865.01
    with
      laceration — *see* Laceration, spleen
      open wound into cavity 865.11
  sternocleidomastoid, birth injury 767.8
  sternomastoid, birth injury 767.8
  subarachnoid (*see also* Hematoma, brain, subarachnoid)
    fetus or newborn 772.2
    nontraumatic (*see also* Hemorrhage, subarachnoid) 430
    newborn 772.2
  subdural (*see also* Hematoma, brain, subdural)
    fetus or newborn (localized) 767.0
    nontraumatic (*see also* Hemorrhage, subdural) 432.1
  subperiosteal (syndrome) 267
    traumatic — *see* Hematoma, by site
  superficial, fetus or newborn 772.6
  syncytium — *see* Placenta, abnormal
  testis (nontraumatic) 608.83
    birth injury 767.8
    traumatic 922.4

**Hematoma** — *see also* Contusion — *continued*
  tunica vaginalis (nontraumatic) 608.83
  umbilical cord 663.6 ☑
    affecting fetus or newborn 762.6
  uterine ligament (nontraumatic) 620.7
    traumatic — *see* Injury, internal, pelvis
  uterus 621.4
    traumatic — *see* Injury, internal, pelvis
  vagina (nontraumatic) (ruptured) 623.6
    complicating delivery 665.7 ☑
    traumatic 922.4
  vas deferens (nontraumatic) 608.83
    traumatic — *see* Injury, internal, vas deferens
  vitreous 379.23
  vocal cord 920
  vulva (nontraumatic) 624.5
    complicating delivery 664.5 ☑
    fetus or newborn 767.8
    traumatic 922.4
**Hematometra** 621.4
**Hematomyelia** 336.1
  with fracture of vertebra (*see also* Fracture, vertebra, by site, with spinal cord injury) 806.8
  fetus or newborn 767.4
**Hematomyelitis** 323.9
  late effect — *see* category 326
**Hematoperitoneum** — *see also* Hemoperitoneum 568.81
**Hematopneumothorax** — *see also* Hemothorax 511.8
**Hematopoiesis, cyclic** 288.02
**Hematoporphyria** (acquired) (congenital) 277.1
**Hematoporphyrinuria** (acquired) (congenital) 277.1
**Hematorachis, hematorrhachis** 336.1
  fetus or newborn 767.4
**Hematosalpinx** 620.8
  with
    ectopic pregnancy (*see also* categories 633.0–633.9) 639.2
    infectional (*see also* Salpingo-oophoritis) 614.2
    molar pregnancy (*see also* categories 630–632) 639.2
**Hematospermia** 608.82
**Hematothorax** — *see also* Hemothorax 511.8
**Hematotympanum** 381.03
**Hematuria** (benign) (essential) (idiopathic) 599.7
  due to S. hematobium 120.0
  endemic 120.0
  intermittent 599.7
  malarial 084.8
  paroxysmal 599.7
  sulfonamide
    correct substance properly administered 599.7
    overdose or wrong substance given or taken 961.0
  tropical (bilharziasis) 120.0
  tuberculous (*see also* Tuberculosis) 016.9 ☑
**Hematuric bilious fever** 084.8
**Hemeralopia** 368.10
**Hemiabiotrophy** 799.89
**Hemi-akinesia** 781.8
**Hemianalgesia** — *see also* Disturbance, sensation 782.0
**Hemianencephaly** 740.0
**Hemianesthesia** — *see also* Disturbance, sensation 782.0
**Hemianopia, hemianopsia** (altitudinal) (homonymous) 368.46
  binasal 368.47
  bitemporal 368.47
  heteronymous 368.47
  syphilitic 095.8

**Hemiasomatognosia** 307.9
**Hemiathetosis** 781.0
**Hemiatrophy** 799.89
  cerebellar 334.8
  face 349.89
    progressive 349.89
  fascia 728.9
  leg 728.2
  tongue 529.8
**Hemiballism** (us) 333.5
**Hemiblock** (cardiac) (heart) (left) 426.2
**Hemicardia** 746.89
**Hemicephalus, hemicephaly** 740.0
**Hemichorea** 333.5
**Hemicrania** 346.9 ☑
  congenital malformation 740.0
**Hemidystrophy** — *see* Hemiatrophy
**Hemiectromelia** 755.4
**Hemihypalgesia** — *see also* Disturbance, sensation 782.0
**Hemihypertrophy** (congenital) 759.89
  cranial 756.0
**Hemihypesthesia** — *see also* Disturbance, sensation 782.0
**Hemi-inattention** 781.8
**Hemimelia** 755.4
  lower limb 755.30
    paraxial (complete) (incomplete) (intercalary) (terminal) 755.32
      fibula 755.37
      tibia 755.36
    transverse (complete) (partial) 755.31
  upper limb 755.20
    paraxial (complete) (incomplete) (intercalary) (terminal) 755.22
      radial 755.26
      ulnar 755.27
    transverse (complete) (partial) 755.21
**Hemiparalysis** — *see also* Hemiplegia 342.9 ☑
**Hemiparesis** — *see also* Hemiplegia 342.9 ☑
**Hemiparesthesia** — *see also* Disturbance, sensation 782.0
**Hemiplegia** 342.9 ☑
  acute (*see also* Disease, cerebrovascular, acute) 436
  alternans facialis 344.89
  apoplectic (*see also* Disease, cerebrovascular, acute) 436
    late effect or residual
      affecting
        dominant side 438.21
        nondominant side 438.22
        unspecified side 438.20
  arteriosclerotic 437.0
    late effect or residual
      affecting
        dominant side 438.21
        nondominant side 438.22
        unspecified side 438.20
  ascending (spinal) NEC 344.89
  attack (*see also* Disease, cerebrovascular, acute) 436
  brain, cerebral (current episode) 437.8
    congenital 343.1
  cerebral — *see* Hemiplegia, brain
  congenital (cerebral) (spastic) (spinal) 343.1
  conversion neurosis (hysterical) 300.11
  cortical — *see* Hemiplegia, brain
  due to
    arteriosclerosis 437.0
      late effect or residual
        affecting
          dominant side 438.21
          nondominant side 438.22
          unspecified side 438.20
    cerebrovascular lesion (*see also* Disease, cerebrovascular, acute) 436

**Hemiplegia** — *continued*
  due to — *continued*
    cerebrovascular lesion (*see also* Disease, cerebrovascular, acute) — *continued*
      late effect
        affecting
          dominant side 438.21
          nondominant side 438.22
          unspecified side 438.20
    embolic (current) (*see also* Embolism, brain) 434.1 ☑
      late effect
        affecting
          dominant side 438.21
          nondominant side 438.22
          unspecified side 438.20
    flaccid 342.0 ☑
    hypertensive (current episode) 437.8
    infantile (postnatal) 343.4
    late effect
      birth injury, intracranial or spinal 343.4
      cerebrovascular lesion — *see* Late effect(s) (of) cerebrovascular disease
      viral encephalitis 139.0
    middle alternating NEC 344.89
    newborn NEC 767.0
    seizure (current episode) (*see also* Disease, cerebrovascular, acute) 436
    spastic 342.1 ☑
      congenital or infantile 343.1
    specified NEC 342.8 ☑
    thrombotic (current) (*see also* Thrombosis, brain) 434.0 ☑
      late effect — *see* Late effect(s) (of) cerebrovascular disease
**Hemisection, spinal cord** — *see* Fracture, vertebra, by site, with spinal cord injury
**Hemispasm** 781.0
  facial 781.0
**Hemispatial neglect** 781.8
**Hemisporosis** 117.9
**Hemitremor** 781.0
**Hemivertebra** 756.14
**Hemobilia** 576.8
**Hemocholecyst** 575.8
**Hemochromatosis** (acquired) (diabetic) (hereditary) (liver) (myocardium) (primary idiopathic) (secondary) 275.0
  with refractory anemia 238.72
**Hemodialysis** V56.0
**Hemoglobin** — *see also* condition
  abnormal (disease) — *see* Disease, hemoglobin
  AS genotype 282.5
  fetal, hereditary persistence 282.7
  high-oxygen-affinity 289.0
  low NEC 285.9
  S (Hb-S), heterozygous 282.5
**Hemoglobinemia** 283.2
  due to blood transfusion NEC 999.8
    bone marrow 996.85
  paroxysmal 283.2
**Hemoglobinopathy** (mixed) — *see also* Disease, hemoglobin 282.7
  with thalassemia 282.49
  sickle-cell 282.60
    with thalassemia (without crisis) 282.41
      with
        crisis 282.42
        vaso-occlusive pain 282.42
**Hemoglobinuria, hemoglobinuric** 791.2
  with anemia, hemolytic, acquired (chronic) NEC 283.2
  cold (agglutinin) (paroxysmal) (with Raynaud's syndrome) 283.2
  due to
    exertion 283.2
    hemolysis (from external causes) NEC 283.2

**Hemoglobinuria, hemoglobinuric** — *continued*
  exercise 283.2
  fever (malaria) 084.8
  infantile 791.2
  intermittent 283.2
  malarial 084.8
  march 283.2
  nocturnal (paroxysmal) 283.2
  paroxysmal (cold) (nocturnal) 283.2
**Hemolymphangioma** (M9175/0) 228.1
**Hemolysis**
  fetal — *see* Jaundice, fetus or newborn
  intravascular (disseminated) NEC 286.6
    with
      abortion — *see* Abortion, by type, with hemorrhage, delayed or excessive
      ectopic pregnancy (*see also* categories 633.0–633.9) 639.1
      hemorrhage of pregnancy 641.3 ☑
        affecting fetus or newborn 762.1
      molar pregnancy (*see also* categories 630–632) 639.1
    acute 283.2
    following
      abortion 639.1
      ectopic or molar pregnancy 639.1
  neonatal — *see* Jaundice, fetus or newborn
  transfusion NEC 999.8
    bone marrow 996.85
**Hemolytic** — *see also* condition
  anemia — *see* Anemia, hemolytic
  uremic syndrome 283.11
**Hemometra** 621.4
**Hemopericardium** (with effusion) 423.0
  newborn 772.8
  traumatic (*see also* Hemothorax, traumatic) 860.2
    with open wound into thorax 860.3
**Hemoperitoneum** 568.81
  infectional (*see also* Peritonitis) 567.29
  traumatic — *see* Injury, internal, peritoneum
**Hemophagocytic syndrome** 288.4
  infection-associated 288.4
**Hemophilia** (familial) (hereditary) 286.0
  A 286.0
    carrier (asymptomatic) V83.01
      symptomatic V83.02
  acquired 286.5
  B (Leyden) 286.1
  C 286.2
  calcipriva (*see also* Fibrinolysis) 286.7
  classical 286.0
  nonfamilial 286.7
  secondary 286.5
  vascular 286.4
**Hemophilus influenzae** NEC 041.5
  arachnoiditis (basic) (brain) (spinal) 320.0
    late effect — *see* category 326
  bronchopneumonia 482.2
  cerebral ventriculitis 320.0
    late effect — *see* category 326
  cerebrospinal inflammation 320.0
    late effect — *see* category 326
  infection NEC 041.5
  leptomeningitis 320.0
    late effect — *see* category 326
  meningitis (cerebral) (cerebrospinal) (spinal) 320.0
    late effect — *see* category 326
  meningomyelitis 320.0
    late effect — *see* category 326
  pachymeningitis (adhesive) (fibrous) (hemorrhagic) (hypertrophic) (spinal) 320.0
    late effect — *see* category 326

**Hemophilus influenzae** — *continued*
  pneumonia (broncho-) 482.2
**Hemophthalmos** 360.43
**Hemopneumothorax** — *see also* Hemothorax 511.8
  traumatic 860.4
    with open wound into thorax 860.5
**Hemoptysis** 786.3
  due to Paragonimus (westermani) 121.2
  newborn 770.3
  tuberculous (*see also* Tuberculosis, pulmonary) 011.9 ☑
**Hemorrhage, hemorrhagic** (nontraumatic) 459.0
  abdomen 459.0
  accidental (antepartum) 641.2 ☑
    affecting fetus or newborn 762.1
  adenoid 474.8
  adrenal (capsule) (gland) (medulla) 255.41 ▲
    newborn 772.5
  after labor — *see* Hemorrhage, postpartum
  alveolar
    lung, newborn 770.3
    process 525.8
  alveolus 525.8
  amputation stump (surgical) 998.11
    secondary, delayed 997.69
  anemia (chronic) 280.0
    acute 285.1
  antepartum — *see* Hemorrhage, pregnancy
  anus (sphincter) 569.3
  apoplexy (stroke) 432.9
  arachnoid — *see* Hemorrhage, subarachnoid
  artery NEC 459.0
    brain (*see also* Hemorrhage, brain) 431
    middle meningeal — *see* Hemorrhage, subarachnoid
  basilar (ganglion) (*see also* Hemorrhage, brain) 431
  bladder 596.8
  blood dyscrasia 289.9
  bowel 578.9
    newborn 772.4
  brain (miliary) (nontraumatic) 431
    with
      birth injury 767.0
      arachnoid — *see* Hemorrhage, subarachnoid
    due to
      birth injury 767.0
      rupture of aneurysm (congenital) (*see also* Hemorrhage, subarachnoid) 430
        mycotic 431
      syphilis 094.89
    epidural or extradural — *see* Hemorrhage, extradural
    fetus or newborn (anoxic) (hypoxic) (due to birth trauma) (nontraumatic) 767.0
    intraventricular 772.10
      grade I 772.11
      grade II 772.12
      grade III 772.13
      grade IV 772.14
    iatrogenic 997.02
    postoperative 997.02
    puerperal, postpartum, childbirth 674.0 ☑
    stem 431
    subarachnoid, arachnoid, or meningeal — *see* Hemorrhage, subarachnoid
    subdural — *see* Hemorrhage, subdural

**Hemorrhage, hemorrhagic** — *continued*
  brain — *continued*
    traumatic NEC 853.0 ☑

> *Note* — *Use the following fifth-digit subclassification with categories 851–854:*
>
> 0   *unspecified state of consciousness*
>
> 1   *with no loss of consciousness*
>
> 2   *with brief [less than one hour] loss of consciousness*
>
> 3   *with moderate [1–24 hours] loss of consciousness*
>
> 4   *with prolonged [more than 24 hours] loss of consciousness and return to pre-existing conscious level*
>
> 5   *with prolonged [more than 24 hours] loss of consciousness, without return to pre-existing conscious level*
>
> *Use fifth-digit 5 to designate when a patient is unconscious and dies before regaining consciousness, regardless of the duration of the loss of consciousness*
>
> 6   *with loss of consciousness of unspecified duration*
>
> 9   *with concussion, unspecified*

    with
      cerebral
        contusion — *see* Contusion, brain
        laceration — *see* Laceration, brain
      open intracranial wound 853.1 ☑
      skull fracture — *see* Fracture, skull, by site
    extradural or epidural 852.4 ☑
      with open intracranial wound 852.5 ☑
    subarachnoid 852.0 ☑
      with open intracranial wound 852.1 ☑
    subdural 852.2 ☑
      with open intracranial wound 852.3 ☑
  breast 611.79
  bronchial tube — *see* Hemorrhage, lung
  bronchopulmonary — *see* Hemorrhage, lung
  bronchus (cause unknown) (*see also* Hemorrhage, lung) 786.3
  bulbar (*see also* Hemorrhage, brain) 431
  bursa 727.89
  capillary 448.9
    primary 287.8
  capsular — *see* Hemorrhage, brain
  cardiovascular 429.89
  cecum 578.9
  cephalic (*see also* Hemorrhage, brain) 431
  cerebellar (*see also* Hemorrhage, brain) 431
  cerebellum (*see also* Hemorrhage, brain) 431
  cerebral (*see also* Hemorrhage, brain) 431
    fetus or newborn (anoxic) (traumatic) 767.0
  cerebromeningeal (*see also* Hemorrhage, brain) 431
  cerebrospinal (*see also* Hemorrhage, brain) 431
  cerebrovascular accident — *see* Hemorrhage, brain
  cerebrum (*see also* Hemorrhage, brain) 431

**Hemorrhage, hemorrhagic** — *continued*
  cervix (stump) (uteri) 622.8
  cesarean section wound 674.3 ☑
  chamber, anterior (eye) 364.41
  childbirth — *see* Hemorrhage, complicating, delivery
  choroid 363.61
    expulsive 363.62
  ciliary body 364.41
  cochlea 386.8
  colon — *see* Hemorrhage, intestine
  complicating
    delivery 641.9 ☑
      affecting fetus or newborn 762.1
      associated with
        afibrinogenemia 641.3 ☑
          affecting fetus or newborn 763.89
        coagulation defect 641.3 ☑
          affecting fetus or newborn 763.89
        hyperfibrinolysis 641.3 ☑
          affecting fetus or newborn 763.89
        hypofibrinogenemia 641.3 ☑
          affecting fetus or newborn 763.89
      due to
        low-lying placenta 641.1 ☑
          affecting fetus or newborn 762.0
        placenta previa 641.1 ☑
          affecting fetus or newborn 762.0
        premature separation of placenta 641.2 ☑
          affecting fetus or newborn 762.1
      retained
        placenta 666.0 ☑
        secundines 666.2 ☑
      trauma 641.8 ☑
        affecting fetus or newborn 763.89
      uterine leiomyoma 641.8 ☑
        affecting fetus or newborn 763.89
    surgical procedure 998.11
  complication(s)     ●
    of dental implant placement   ●
      525.71     ●
  concealed NEC 459.0
  congenital 772.9
  conjunctiva 372.72
    newborn 772.8
  cord, newborn 772.0
    slipped ligature 772.3
    stump 772.3
  corpus luteum (ruptured) 620.1
  cortical (*see also* Hemorrhage, brain) 431
  cranial 432.9
  cutaneous 782.7
    newborn 772.6
  cystitis — *see* Cystitis
  cyst, pancreas 577.2
  delayed
    with
      abortion — *see* Abortion, by type, with hemorrhage, delayed or excessive
      ectopic pregnancy (*see also* categories 633.0–633.9) 639.1
      molar pregnancy (*see also* categories 630–632) 639.1
    following
      abortion 639.1
      ectopic or molar pregnancy 639.1
    postpartum 666.2 ☑
  diathesis (familial) 287.9
    newborn 776.0
  disease 287.9
    newborn 776.0

☑ Additional Digit Required — Refer to the Tabular List for Digit Selection      ▽ Subterms under main terms may continue to next column or page

*2008 ICD-9-CM*      ▶◀ Revised Text      ● New Line      ▲ Revised Code      **October 2007 • Volume 2 — 139**

**Hemorrhage, hemorrhagic —**
*continued*
disease — *continued*
　　specified type NEC 287.8
disorder 287.9
　　due to intrinsic circulating antico-
　　　agulants 286.5
　　specified type NEC 287.8
due to
　　any device, implant or graft (pres-
　　　ence of) classifiable to
　　　996.0–996.5 — *see* Complica-
　　　tions, due to (presence of)
　　　any device, implant, or graft
　　　classified to 996.0–996.5NEC
　　intrinsic circulating anticoagulant
　　　286.5
duodenum, duodenal 537.89
　　ulcer — *see* Ulcer, duodenum, with
　　　hemorrhage
dura mater — *see* Hemorrhage, sub-
　　dural
endotracheal — *see* Hemorrhage, lung
epicranial subaponeurotic (massive)
　　767.11
epidural — *see* Hemorrhage, extradu-
　　ral
episiotomy 674.3 ☑
esophagus 530.82
　　varix (*see also* Varix, esophagus,
　　　bleeding) 456.0
excessive
　　with
　　　abortion — *see* Abortion, by
　　　　type, with hemorrhage,
　　　　delayed or excessive
　　　ectopic pregnancy (*see also* cat-
　　　　egories 633.0–633.9)
　　　　639.1
　　　molar pregnancy (*see also* cate-
　　　　gories 630–632) 639.1
　　　following
　　　　abortion 639.1
　　　　ectopic or molar pregnancy
　　　　　639.1
external 459.0
extradural (traumatic) (*see also* Hem-
　　orrhage, brain, traumatic, ex-
　　tradural)
　　birth injury 767.0
　　fetus or newborn (anoxic) (traumat-
　　　ic) 767.0
　　nontraumatic 432.0
eye 360.43
　　chamber (anterior) (aqueous)
　　　364.41
　　fundus 362.81
eyelid 374.81
fallopian tube 620.8
fetomaternal 772.0
　　affecting management of pregnancy
　　　or puerperium 656.0 ☑
fetus, fetal 772.0
　　from
　　　cut end of co-twin's cord 772.0
　　　placenta 772.0
　　　ruptured cord 772.0
　　　vasa previa 772.0
　　into
　　　co-twin 772.0
　　　mother's circulation 772.0
　　　　affecting management of
　　　　　pregnancy or puerperi-
　　　　　um 656.0 ☑
fever (*see also* Fever, hemorrhagic)
　　065.9
　　with renal syndrome 078.6
　　arthropod-borne NEC 065.9
　　Bangkok 065.4
　　Crimean 065.0
　　dengue virus 065.4
　　epidemic 078.6
　　Junin virus 078.7
　　Korean 078.6
　　Machupo virus 078.7
　　mite-borne 065.8

**Hemorrhage, hemorrhagic —**
*continued*
fever (*see also* Fever, hemorrhagic) —
　　*continued*
　　mosquito-borne 065.4
　　Philippine 065.4
　　Russian (Yaroslav) 078.6
　　Singapore 065.4
　　southeast Asia 065.4
　　Thailand 065.4
　　tick-borne NEC 065.3
fibrinogenolysis (*see also* Fibrinolysis)
　　286.6
fibrinolytic (acquired) (*see also* Fibri-
　　nolysis) 286.6
fontanel 767.19
from tracheostomy stoma 519.09
fundus, eye 362.81
funis
　　affecting fetus or newborn 772.0
　　complicating delivery 663.8 ☑
gastric (*see also* Hemorrhage, stom-
　　ach) 578.9
gastroenteric 578.9
　　newborn 772.4
gastrointestinal (tract) 578.9
　　newborn 772.4
genitourinary (tract) NEC 599.89
gingiva 523.8
globe 360.43
gravidarum — *see* Hemorrhage, preg-
　　nancy
gum 523.8
heart 429.89
hypopharyngeal (throat) 784.8
intermenstrual 626.6
　　irregular 626.6
　　regular 626.5
internal (organs) 459.0
　　capsule (*see also* Hemorrhage,
　　　brain) 431
　　ear 386.8
　　newborn 772.8
intestine 578.9
　　congenital 772.4
　　newborn 772.4
into
　　bladder wall 596.7
　　bursa 727.89
　　corpus luysii (*see also* Hemorrhage,
　　　brain) 431
intra-abdominal 459.0
　　during or following surgery 998.11
intra-alveolar, newborn (lung) 770.3
intracerebral (*see also* Hemorrhage,
　　brain) 431
intracranial NEC 432.9
　　puerperal, postpartum, childbirth
　　　674.0 ☑
　　traumatic — *see* Hemorrhage,
　　　brain, traumatic
intramedullary NEC 336.1
intraocular 360.43
intraoperative 998.11
intrapartum — *see* Hemorrhage,
　　complicating, delivery
intrapelvic
　　female 629.89
　　male 459.0
intraperitoneal 459.0
intrapontine (*see also* Hemorrhage,
　　brain) 431
intrauterine 621.4
　　complicating delivery — *see* Hemor-
　　　rhage, complicating, delivery
　　in pregnancy or childbirth — *see*
　　　Hemorrhage, pregnancy
　　postpartum (*see also* Hemorrhage,
　　　postpartum) 666.1 ☑
intraventricular (*see also* Hemorrhage,
　　brain) 431
　　fetus or newborn (anoxic) (traumat-
　　　ic) 772.10
　　　grade I 772.11
　　　grade II 772.12
　　　grade III 772.13

**Hemorrhage, hemorrhagic —**
*continued*
intraventricular (*see also* Hemorrhage,
　　brain) — *continued*
　　fetus or newborn — *continued*
　　　grade IV 772.14
intravesical 596.7
iris (postinfectional) (postinflammato-
　　ry) (toxic) 364.41
joint (nontraumatic) 719.10
　　ankle 719.17
　　elbow 719.12
　　foot 719.17
　　forearm 719.13
　　hand 719.14
　　hip 719.15
　　knee 719.16
　　lower leg 719.16
　　multiple sites 719.19
　　pelvic region 719.15
　　shoulder (region) 719.11
　　specified site NEC 719.18
　　thigh 719.15
　　upper arm 719.12
　　wrist 719.13
kidney 593.81
knee (joint) 719.16
labyrinth 386.8
leg NEC 459.0
lenticular striate artery (*see also*
　　Hemorrhage, brain) 431
ligature, vessel 998.11
liver 573.8
lower extremity NEC 459.0
lung 786.3
　　newborn 770.3
　　tuberculous (*see also* Tuberculosis,
　　　pulmonary) 011.9 ☑
malaria 084.8
marginal sinus 641.2 ☑
massive subaponeurotic, birth injury
　　767.11
maternal, affecting fetus or newborn
　　762.1
mediastinum 786.3
medulla (*see also* Hemorrhage, brain)
　　431
membrane (brain) (*see also* Hemor-
　　rhage, subarachnoid) 430
　　spinal cord — *see* Hemorrhage,
　　　spinal cord
meninges, meningeal (brain) (middle)
　　(*see also* Hemorrhage, subarach-
　　noid) 430
　　spinal cord — *see* Hemorrhage,
　　　spinal cord
mesentery 568.81
metritis 626.8
midbrain (*see also* Hemorrhage, brain)
　　431
mole 631
mouth 528.9
mucous membrane NEC 459.0
　　newborn 772.8
muscle 728.89
nail (subungual) 703.8
nasal turbinate 784.7
　　newborn 772.8
nasopharynx 478.29
navel, newborn 772.3
newborn 772.9
　　adrenal 772.5
　　alveolar (lung) 770.3
　　brain (anoxic) (hypoxic) (due to
　　　birth trauma) 767.0
　　cerebral (anoxic) (hypoxic) (due to
　　　birth trauma) 767.0
　　conjunctiva 772.8
　　cutaneous 772.6
　　diathesis 776.0
　　due to vitamin K deficiency 776.0
　　epicranial subaponeurotic (mas-
　　　sive) 767.11
　　gastrointestinal 772.4
　　internal (organs) 772.8
　　intestines 772.4

**Hemorrhage, hemorrhagic —**
*continued*
newborn — *continued*
　　intra-alveolar (lung) 770.3
　　intracranial (from any perinatal
　　　cause) 767.0
　　intraventricular (from any perinatal
　　　cause) 772.10
　　　grade I 772.11
　　　grade II 772.12
　　　grade III 772.13
　　　grade IV 772.14
　　lung 770.3
　　pulmonary (massive) 770.3
　　spinal cord, traumatic 767.4
　　stomach 772.4
　　subaponeurotic (massive) 767.11
　　subarachnoid (from any perinatal
　　　cause) 772.2
　　subconjunctival 772.8
　　subgaleal 767.11
　　umbilicus 772.0
　　　slipped ligature 772.3
　　　vasa previa 772.0
nipple 611.79
nose 784.7
　　newborn 772.8
obstetrical surgical wound 674.3 ☑
omentum 568.89
　　newborn 772.4
optic nerve (sheath) 377.42
orbit 376.32
ovary 620.1
oviduct 620.8
pancreas 577.8
parathyroid (gland) (spontaneous)
　　252.8
parturition — *see* Hemorrhage, com-
　　plicating, delivery
penis 607.82
pericardium, pericarditis 423.0
perineal wound (obstetrical) 674.3 ☑
peritoneum, peritoneal 459.0
peritonsillar tissue 474.8
　　after operation on tonsils 998.11
　　due to infection 475
petechial 782.7
pituitary (gland) 253.8
placenta NEC 641.9 ☑
　　affecting fetus or newborn 762.1
　　from surgical or instrumental
　　　damage 641.8 ☑
　　　affecting fetus or newborn 762.1
　　previa 641.1 ☑
　　　affecting fetus or newborn 762.0
pleura — *see* Hemorrhage, lung
polioencephalitis, superior 265.1
polymyositis — *see* Polymyositis
pons (*see also* Hemorrhage, brain) 431
pontine (*see also* Hemorrhage, brain)
　　431
popliteal 459.0
postcoital 626.7
postextraction (dental) 998.11
postmenopausal 627.1
postnasal 784.7
postoperative 998.11
postpartum (atonic) (following delivery
　　of placenta) 666.1 ☑
　　delayed or secondary (after 24
　　　hours) 666.2 ☑
　　retained placenta 666.0 ☑
　　third stage 666.0 ☑
pregnancy (concealed) 641.9 ☑
　　accidental 641.2 ☑
　　　affecting fetus or newborn 762.1
　　affecting fetus or newborn 762.1
　　before 22 completed weeks gesta-
　　　tion 640.9 ☑
　　　affecting fetus or newborn 762.1
　　due to
　　　abruptio placenta 641.2 ☑
　　　　affecting fetus or newborn
　　　　　762.1

☑ Additional Digit Required — Refer to the Tabular List for Digit Selection　　　　　　　　　　　　　▽ Subterms under main terms may continue to next column or page

140 — Volume 2　　　　　　　　　　　　▶◀ Revised Text　　　　　　● New Line　　　　　▲ Revised Code　　　　　　　**2008 ICD-9-CM**

**Hemorrhage, hemorrhagic —** *continued*
pregnancy — *continued*
due to — *continued*
afibrinogenemia or other coagulation or other coagulation defect (conditions classifiable to 286.0–286.9) 641.3 ☑
affecting fetus or newborn 762.1
coagulation defect 641.3 ☑
affecting fetus or newborn 762.1
hyperfibrinolysis 641.3 ☑
affecting fetus or newborn 762.1
hypofibrinogenemia 641.3 ☑
affecting fetus or newborn 762.1
leiomyoma, uterus 641.8 ☑
affecting fetus or newborn 762.1
low-lying placenta 641.1 ☑
affecting fetus or newborn 762.1
marginal sinus (rupture) 641.2 ☑
affecting fetus or newborn 762.1
placenta previa 641.1 ☑
affecting fetus or newborn 762.0
premature separation of placenta (normally implanted) 641.2 ☑
affecting fetus or newborn 762.1
threatened abortion 640.0 ☑
affecting fetus or newborn 762.1
trauma 641.8 ☑
affecting fetus or newborn 762.1
early (before 22 completed weeks gestation) 640.9 ☑
affecting fetus or newborn 762.1
previous, affecting management of pregnancy or childbirth V23.49
unavoidable — *see* Hemorrhage, pregnancy, due to placenta previa
prepartum (mother) — *see* Hemorrhage, pregnancy
preretinal, cause unspecified 362.81
prostate 602.1
puerperal (*see also* Hemorrhage, postpartum) 666.1 ☑
pulmonary (*see also* Hemorrhage, lung)
newborn (massive) 770.3
renal syndrome 446.21
purpura (primary) (*see also* Purpura, thrombocytopenic) 287.39
rectum (sphincter) 569.3
recurring, following initial hemorrhage at time of injury 958.2
renal 593.81
pulmonary syndrome 446.21
respiratory tract (*see also* Hemorrhage, lung) 786.3
retina, retinal (deep) (superficial) (vessels) 362.81
diabetic 250.5 ☑ *[362.01]*
due to birth injury 772.8
retrobulbar 376.89
retroperitoneal 459.0
retroplacental (*see also* Placenta, separation) 641.2 ☑
scalp 459.0
due to injury at birth 767.19
scrotum 608.83
secondary (nontraumatic) 459.0
following initial hemorrhage at time of injury 958.2
seminal vesicle 608.83

**Hemorrhage, hemorrhagic —** *continued*
skin 782.7
newborn 772.6
spermatic cord 608.83
spinal (cord) 336.1
aneurysm (ruptured) 336.1
syphilitic 094.89
due to birth injury 767.4
fetus or newborn 767.4
spleen 289.59
spontaneous NEC 459.0
petechial 782.7
stomach 578.9
newborn 772.4
ulcer — *see* Ulcer, stomach, with hemorrhage
subaponeurotic, newborn 767.11
massive (birth injury) 767.11
subarachnoid (nontraumatic) 430
fetus or newborn (anoxic) (traumatic) 772.2
puerperal, postpartum, childbirth 674.0 ☑
traumatic — *see* Hemorrhage, brain, traumatic, subarachnoid
subconjunctival 372.72
due to birth injury 772.8
newborn 772.8
subcortical (*see also* Hemorrhage, brain) 431
subcutaneous 782.7
subdiaphragmatic 459.0
subdural (nontraumatic) 432.1
due to birth injury 767.0
fetus or newborn (anoxic) (hypoxic) (due to birth trauma) 767.0
puerperal, postpartum, childbirth 674.0 ☑
spinal 336.1
traumatic — *see* Hemorrhage, brain, traumatic, subdural
subgaleal 767.11
subhyaloid 362.81
subperiosteal 733.99
subretinal 362.81
subtentorial (*see also* Hemorrhage, subdural) 432.1
subungual 703.8
due to blood dyscrasia 287.8
suprarenal (capsule) (gland) 255.41 ▲
fetus or newborn 772.5
tentorium (traumatic) (*see also* Hemorrhage, brain, traumatic)
fetus or newborn 767.0
nontraumatic — *see* Hemorrhage, subdural
testis 608.83
thigh 459.0
third stage 666.0 ☑
thorax — *see* Hemorrhage, lung
throat 784.8
thrombocythemia 238.71
thymus (gland) 254.8
thyroid (gland) 246.3
cyst 246.3
tongue 529.8
tonsil 474.8
postoperative 998.11
tooth socket (postextraction) 998.11
trachea — *see* Hemorrhage, lung
traumatic (*see also* nature of injury)
brain — *see* Hemorrhage, brain, traumatic
recurring or secondary (following initial hemorrhage at time of injury) 958.2
tuberculous NEC (*see also* Tuberculosis, pulmonary) 011.9 ☑
tunica vaginalis 608.83
ulcer — *see* Ulcer, by site, with hemorrhage
umbilicus, umbilical cord 772.0
after birth, newborn 772.3

**Hemorrhage, hemorrhagic —** *continued*
umbilicus, umbilical cord — *continued*
complicating delivery 663.8 ☑
affecting fetus or newborn 772.0
slipped ligature 772.3
stump 772.3
unavoidable (due to placenta previa) 641.1 ☑
affecting fetus or newborn 762.0
upper extremity 459.0
urethra (idiopathic) 599.84
uterus, uterine (abnormal) 626.9
climacteric 627.0
complicating delivery — *see* Hemorrhage, complicating, delivery
due to
intrauterine contraceptive device 996.76
perforating uterus 996.32
functional or dysfunctional 626.8
in pregnancy — *see* Hemorrhage, pregnancy
intermenstrual 626.6
irregular 626.6
regular 626.5
postmenopausal 627.1
postpartum (*see also* Hemorrhage, postpartum) 666.1 ☑
prepubertal 626.8
pubertal 626.3
puerperal (immediate) 666.1 ☑
vagina 623.8
vasa previa 663.5 ☑
affecting fetus or newborn 772.0
vas deferens 608.83
ventricular (*see also* Hemorrhage, brain) 431
vesical 596.8
viscera 459.0
newborn 772.8
vitreous (humor) (intraocular) 379.23
vocal cord 478.5
vulva 624.8
**Hemorrhoids** (anus) (rectum) (without complication) 455.6
bleeding, prolapsed, strangulated, or ulcerated NEC 455.8
external 455.5
internal 455.2
complicated NEC 455.8
complicating pregnancy and puerperium 671.8 ☑
external 455.3
with complication NEC 455.5
bleeding, prolapsed, strangulated, or ulcerated 455.5
thrombosed 455.4
internal 455.0
with complication NEC 455.2
bleeding, prolapsed, strangulated, or ulcerated 455.2
thrombosed 455.1
residual skin tag 455.9
sentinel pile 455.9
thrombosed NEC 455.7
external 455.4
internal 455.1
**Hemosalpinx** 620.8
**Hemosiderosis** 275.0
dietary 275.0
pulmonary (idiopathic) 275.0 *[516.1]*
transfusion NEC 999.8
bone marrow 996.85
**Hemospermia** 608.82
**Hemothorax** 511.8
bacterial, nontuberculous 511.1
newborn 772.8
nontuberculous 511.8
bacterial 511.1
pneumococcal 511.1
postoperative 998.11
staphylococcal 511.1
streptococcal 511.1
traumatic 860.2

**Hemothorax —** *continued*
traumatic — *continued*
with
open wound into thorax 860.3
pneumothorax 860.4
with open wound into thorax 860.5
tuberculous (*see also* Tuberculosis, pleura) 012.0 ☑
**Hemotympanum** 385.89
**Hench-Rosenberg syndrome** (palindromic arthritis) — *see also* Rheumatism, palindromic 719.3 ☑
**Henle's warts** 371.41
**Henoch (-Schönlein)**
disease or syndrome (allergic purpura) 287.0
purpura (allergic) 287.0
**Henpue, henpuye** 102.6
**Heparitinuria** 277.5
**Hepar lobatum** 095.3
**Hepatalgia** 573.8
**Hepatic** — *see also* condition
flexure syndrome 569.89
**Hepatitis** 573.3
acute (*see also* Necrosis, liver) 570
alcoholic 571.1
infective (HAA) 070.0
with hepatic coma 070.0
alcoholic 571.1
amebic — *see* Abscess, liver, amebic
anicteric (acute) — *see* Hepatitis, viral
antigen-associated (HAA) — *see* Hepatitis, viral, type B
Australian antigen (positive) — *see* Hepatitis, viral, type B
autoimmune 571.49
catarrhal (acute) 070.1
with hepatic coma 070.0
chronic 571.40
newborn 070.1
with hepatic coma 070.0
chemical 573.3
cholangiolitic 573.8
cholestatic 573.8
chronic 571.40
active 571.49
viral — *see* Hepatitis, viral
aggressive 571.49
persistent 571.41
viral — *see* Hepatitis, viral
cytomegalic inclusion virus 078.5 *[573.1]*
diffuse 573.3
"dirty needle" — *see* Hepatitis, viral
drug-induced 573.3
due to
Coxsackie 074.8 *[573.1]*
cytomegalic inclusion virus 078.5 *[573.1]*
infectious mononucleosis 075 *[573.1]*
malaria 084.9 *[573.2]*
mumps 072.71
secondary syphilis 091.62
toxoplasmosis (acquired) 130.5
congenital (active) 771.2
epidemic — *see* Hepatitis, viral, type A
fetus or newborn 774.4
fibrous (chronic) 571.49
acute 570
from injection, inoculation, or transfusion (blood) (other substance) (plasma) (serum) (onset within 8 months after administration) — *see* Hepatitis, viral
fulminant (viral) (*see also* Hepatitis, viral) 070.9
with hepatic coma 070.6
type A 070.1
with hepatic coma 070.0
type B — *see* Hepatitis, viral, type B
giant cell (neonatal) 774.4
hemorrhagic 573.8

**Hepatitis** — *continued*
  history of
    B V12.09
    C V12.09
  homologous serum — *see* Hepatitis, viral
  hypertrophic (chronic) 571.49
    acute 570
  infectious, infective (acute) (chronic) (subacute) 070.1
    with hepatic coma 070.0
  inoculation — *see* Hepatitis, viral
  interstitial (chronic) 571.49
    acute 570
  lupoid 571.49
  malarial 084.9 *[573.2]*
  malignant (*see also* Necrosis, liver) 570
  neonatal (toxic) 774.4
  newborn 774.4
  parenchymatous (acute) (*see also* Necrosis, liver) 570
  peliosis 573.3
  persistent, chronic 571.41
  plasma cell 571.49
  postimmunization — *see* Hepatitis, viral
  postnecrotic 571.49
  posttransfusion — *see* Hepatitis, viral
  recurrent 571.49
  septic 573.3
  serum — *see* Hepatitis, viral
    carrier (suspected of) V02.61
  subacute (*see also* Necrosis, liver) 570
  suppurative (diffuse) 572.0
  syphilitic (late) 095.3
    congenital (early) 090.0 *[573.2]*
      late 090.5 *[573.2]*
    secondary 091.62
  toxic (noninfectious) 573.3
    fetus or newborn 774.4
  tuberculous (*see also* Tuberculosis) 017.9 ☑
  viral (acute) (anicteric) (cholangiolitic) (cholestatic) (chronic) (subacute) 070.9
    with hepatic coma 070.6
    AU-SH type virus — *see* Hepatitis, viral, type B
    Australian antigen — *see* Hepatitis, viral, type B
    B-antigen — *see* Hepatitis, viral, type B
    Coxsackie 074.8 *[573.1]*
    cytomegalic inclusion 078.5 *[573.1]*
    IH (virus) — *see* Hepatitis, viral, type A
    infectious hepatitis virus — *see* Hepatitis, viral, type A
    serum hepatitis virus — *see* Hepatitis, viral, type B
    SH — *see* Hepatitis, viral, type B
    specified type NEC 070.59
      with hepatic coma 070.49
    type A 070.1
      with hepatic coma 070.0
    type B (acute) 070.30
      with
        hepatic coma 070.20
          with hepatitis delta 070.21
        hepatitis delta 070.31
          with hepatic coma 070.21
      carrier status V02.61
      chronic 070.32
        with
          hepatic coma 070.22
            with hepatitis delta 070.23
          hepatitis delta 070.33
            with hepatic coma 070.23
    type C
      acute 070.51
        with hepatic coma 070.41
      carrier status V02.62

**Hepatitis** — *continued*
  viral — *continued*
    type C — *continued*
      chronic 070.54
        with hepatic coma 070.44
      in remission 070.54
      unspecified 070.70
        with hepatic coma 070.71
    type delta (with hepatitis B carrier state) 070.52
      with
        active hepatitis B disease — *see* Hepatitis, viral, type B
        hepatic coma 070.42
    type E 070.53
      with hepatic coma 070.43
    vaccination and inoculation (prophylactic) V05.3
  Waldenström's (lupoid hepatitis) 571.49
**Hepatization, lung** (acute) — *see also* Pneumonia, lobar
  chronic (*see also* Fibrosis, lung) 515
**Hepatoblastoma** (M8970/3) 155.0
**Hepatocarcinoma** (M8170/3) 155.0
**Hepatocholangiocarcinoma** (M8180/3) 155.0
**Hepatocholangioma, benign** (M8180/0) 211.5
**Hepatocholangitis** 573.8
**Hepatocystitis** — *see also* Cholecystitis 575.10
**Hepatodystrophy** 570
**Hepatolenticular degeneration** 275.1
**Hepatolithiasis** — *see* Choledocholithiasis
**Hepatoma** (malignant) (M8170/3) 155.0
  benign (M8170/0) 211.5
  congenital (M8970/3) 155.0
  embryonal (M8970/3) 155.0
**Hepatomegalia glycogenica diffusa** 271.0
**Hepatomegaly** — *see also* Hypertrophy, liver 789.1
  congenital 751.69
    syphilitic 090.0
  due to Clonorchis sinensis 121.1
  Gaucher's 272.7
  syphilitic (congenital) 090.0
**Hepatoptosis** 573.8
**Hepatorrhexis** 573.8
**Hepatosis, toxic** 573.8
**Hepatosplenomegaly** 571.8
  due to S. japonicum 120.2
  hyperlipemic (Bürger-Grutz type) 272.3
**Herald patch** 696.3
**Hereditary** — *see* condition
**Heredodegeneration** 330.9
  macular 362.70
**Heredopathia atactica polyneuritiformis** 356.3
**Heredosyphilis** — *see also* Syphilis, congenital 090.9
**Hermaphroditism** (true) 752.7
  with specified chromosomal anomaly — *see* Anomaly, chromosomes, sex
**Hernia, hernial** (acquired) (recurrent) 553.9
  with
    gangrene (obstructed) NEC 551.9
    obstruction NEC 552.9
      and gangrene 551.9
  abdomen (wall) — *see* Hernia, ventral
  abdominal, specified site NEC 553.8
    with
      gangrene (obstructed) 551.8
      obstruction 552.8
        and gangrene 551.8
  appendix 553.8
    with
      gangrene (obstructed) 551.8
      obstruction 552.8
        and gangrene 551.8

**Hernia, hernial** — *continued*
  bilateral (inguinal) — *see* Hernia, inguinal
  bladder (sphincter)
    congenital (female) (male) 756.71
    female (*see also* Cystocele, female) 618.01
    male 596.8
  brain 348.4
    congenital 742.0
  broad ligament 553.8
  cartilage, vertebral — *see* Displacement, intervertebral disc
  cerebral 348.4
    congenital 742.0
    endaural 742.0
  ciliary body 364.89                                      ▲
    traumatic 871.1
  colic 553.9
    with
      gangrene (obstructed) 551.9
      obstruction 552.9
        and gangrene 551.9
  colon 553.9
    with
      gangrene (obstructed) 551.9
      obstruction 552.9
        and gangrene 551.9
  colostomy (stoma) 569.69
  Cooper's (retroperitoneal) 553.8
    with
      gangrene (obstructed) 551.8
      obstruction 552.8
        and gangrene 551.8
  crural — *see* Hernia, femoral
  diaphragm, diaphragmatic 553.3
    with
      gangrene (obstructed) 551.3
      obstruction 552.3
        and gangrene 551.3
    congenital 756.6
    due to gross defect of diaphragm 756.6
    traumatic 862.0
      with open wound into cavity 862.1
  direct (inguinal) — *see* Hernia, inguinal
  disc, intervertebral — *see* Displacement, intervertebral disc
  diverticulum, intestine 553.9
    with
      gangrene (obstructed) 551.9
      obstruction 552.9
        and gangrene 551.9
  double (inguinal) — *see* Hernia, inguinal
  due to adhesion with obstruction 560.81
  duodenojejunal 553.8
    with
      gangrene (obstructed) 551.8
      obstruction 552.8
        and gangrene 551.8
  en glissade — *see* Hernia, inguinal
  enterostomy (stoma) 569.69
  epigastric 553.29
    with
      gangrene (obstruction) 551.29
      obstruction 552.29
        and gangrene 551.29
    recurrent 553.21
      with
        gangrene (obstructed) 551.21
        obstruction 552.21
          and gangrene 551.21
  esophageal hiatus (sliding) 553.3
    with
      gangrene (obstructed) 551.3
      obstruction 552.3
        and gangrene 551.3
    congenital 750.6
  external (inguinal) — *see* Hernia, inguinal
  fallopian tube 620.4
  fascia 728.89

**Hernia, hernial** — *continued*
  fat 729.30
    eyelid 374.34
    orbital 374.34
    pad 729.30
      eye, eyelid 374.34
      knee 729.31
      orbit 374.34
      popliteal (space) 729.31
      specified site NEC 729.39
  femoral (unilateral) 553.00
    with
      gangrene (obstructed) 551.00
      obstruction 552.00
        with gangrene 551.00
    bilateral 553.02
      gangrenous (obstructed) 551.02
      obstructed 552.02
        with gangrene 551.02
      recurrent 553.03
        gangrenous (obstructed) 551.03
        obstructed 552.03
          with gangrene 551.03
    recurrent (unilateral) 553.01
      bilateral 553.03
        gangrenous (obstructed) 551.03
        obstructed 552.03
          with gangrene 551.01
      gangrenous (obstructed) 551.01
      obstructed 552.01
        with gangrene 551.01
  foramen
    Bochdalek 553.3
      with
        gangrene (obstructed) 551.3
        obstruction 552.3
          and gangrene 551.3
      congenital 756.6
    magnum 348.4
    Morgagni, Morgagnian 553.3
      with
        gangrene 551.3
        obstruction 552.3
          and gangrene 551.3
      congenital 756.6
  funicular (umbilical) 553.1
    with
      gangrene (obstructed) 551.1
      obstruction 552.1
        and gangrene 551.1
    spermatic cord — *see* Hernia, inguinal
  gangrenous — *see* Hernia, by site, with gangrene
  gastrointestinal tract 553.9
    with
      gangrene (obstructed) 551.9
      obstruction 552.9
        and gangrene 551.9
  gluteal — *see* Hernia, femoral
  Gruber's (internal mesogastric) 553.8
    with
      gangrene (obstructed) 551.8
      obstruction 552.8
        and gangrene 551.8
  Hesselbach's 553.8
    with
      gangrene (obstructed) 551.8
      obstruction 552.8
        and gangrene 551.8
  hiatal (esophageal) (sliding) 553.3
    with
      gangrene (obstructed) 551.3
      obstruction 552.3
        and gangrene 551.3
    congenital 750.6
  incarcerated (*see also* Hernia, by site, with obstruction) 552.9
    gangrenous (*see also* Hernia, by site, with gangrene) 551.9
  incisional 553.21
    with
      gangrene (obstructed) 551.21
      obstruction 552.21

**Hernia, hernial** — *continued*
  incisional — *continued*
    with — *continued*
      obstruction — *continued*
        and gangrene 551.21
    lumbar — *see* Hernia, lumbar
    recurrent 553.21
      with
        gangrene (obstructed) 551.21
        obstruction 552.21
          and gangrene 551.21
  indirect (inguinal) — *see* Hernia, in-guinal
  infantile — *see* Hernia, inguinal
  infrapatellar fat pad 729.31
  inguinal (direct) (double) (encysted) (external) (funicular) (indirect) (infantile) (internal) (interstitial) (oblique) (scrotal) (sliding) 550.9 ☑

Note — Use the following fifth-digit subclassification with category 550:

0  unilateral or unspecified (not specified as recurrent)

1  unilateral or unspecified, recurrent

2  bilateral (not specified as recurrent)

3  bilateral, recurrent

    with
      gangrene (obstructed) 550.0 ☑
      obstruction 550.1 ☑
        and gangrene 550.0 ☑
  internal 553.8
    with
      gangrene (obstructed) 551.8
      obstruction 552.8
        and gangrene 551.8
    inguinal — *see* Hernia, inguinal
  interstitial 553.9
    with
      gangrene (obstructed) 551.9
      obstruction 552.9
        and gangrene 551.9
    inguinal — *see* Hernia, inguinal
  intervertebral cartilage or disc — *see* Displacement, intervertebral disc
  intestine, intestinal 553.9
    with
      gangrene (obstructed) 551.9
      obstruction 552.9
        and gangrene 551.9
  intra-abdominal 553.9
    with
      gangrene (obstructed) 551.9
      obstruction 552.9
        and gangrene 551.9
  intraparietal 553.9
    with
      gangrene (obstructed) 551.9
      obstruction 552.9
        and gangrene 551.9
  iris 364.89  ▲
    traumatic 871.1
  irreducible (*see also* Hernia, by site, with obstruction) 552.9
    gangrenous (with obstruction) (*see also* Hernia, by site, with gangrene) 551.9
  ischiatic 553.8
    with
      gangrene (obstructed) 551.8
      obstruction 552.8
        and gangrene 551.8
  ischiorectal 553.8
    with
      gangrene (obstructed) 551.8
      obstruction 552.8
        and gangrene 551.8
  lens 379.32
    traumatic 871.1
  linea
    alba — *see* Hernia, epigastric

**Hernia, hernial** — *continued*
  linea — *continued*
    semilunaris — *see* Hernia, spigelian
  Littre's (diverticular) 553.9
    with
      gangrene (obstructed) 551.9
      obstruction 552.9
        and gangrene 551.9
  lumbar 553.8
    with
      gangrene (obstructed) 551.8
      obstruction 552.8
        and gangrene 551.8
    intervertebral disc 722.10
  lung (subcutaneous) 518.89
    congenital 748.69
  mediastinum 519.3
  mesenteric (internal) 553.8
    with
      gangrene (obstructed) 551.8
      obstruction 552.8
        and gangrene 551.8
  mesocolon 553.8
    with
      gangrene (obstructed) 551.8
      obstruction 552.8
        and gangrene 551.8
  muscle (sheath) 728.89
  nucleus pulposus — *see* Displacement, intervertebral disc
  oblique (inguinal) — *see* Hernia, inguinal
  obstructive (*see also* Hernia, by site, with obstruction) 552.9
    gangrenous (with obstruction) (*see also* Hernia, by site, with gangrene) 551.9
  obturator 553.8
    with
      gangrene (obstructed) 551.8
      obstruction 552.8
        and gangrene 551.8
  omental 553.8
    with
      gangrene (obstructed) 551.8
      obstruction 552.8
        and gangrene 551.8
  orbital fat (pad) 374.34
  ovary 620.4
  oviduct 620.4
  paracolostomy (stoma) 569.69
  paraduodenal 553.8
    with
      gangrene (obstructed) 551.8
      obstruction 552.8
        and gangrene 551.8
  paraesophageal 553.3
    with
      gangrene (obstructed) 551.3
      obstruction 552.3
        and gangrene 551.3
    congenital 750.6
  parahiatal 553.3
    with
      gangrene (obstructed) 551.3
      obstruction 552.3
        and gangrene 551.3
  paraumbilical 553.1
    with
      gangrene (obstructed) 551.1
      obstruction 552.1
        and gangrene 551.1
  parietal 553.9
    with
      gangrene (obstructed) 551.9
      obstruction 552.9
        and gangrene 551.9
  perineal 553.8
    with
      gangrene (obstructed) 551.8
      obstruction 552.8
        and gangrene 551.8
  peritoneal sac, lesser 553.8
    with
      gangrene (obstructed) 551.8

**Hernia, hernial** — *continued*
  peritoneal sac, lesser — *continued*
    with — *continued*
      obstruction 552.8
        and gangrene 551.8
  popliteal fat pad 729.31
  postoperative 553.21
    with
      gangrene (obstructed) 551.21
      obstruction 552.21
        and gangrene 551.21
  pregnant uterus 654.4 ☑
  prevesical 596.8
  properitoneal 553.8
    with
      gangrene (obstructed) 551.8
      obstruction 552.8
        and gangrene 551.8
  pudendal 553.8
    with
      gangrene (obstructed) 551.8
      obstruction 552.8
        and gangrene 551.8
  rectovaginal 618.6
  retroperitoneal 553.8
    with
      gangrene (obstructed) 551.8
      obstruction 552.8
        and gangrene 551.8
  Richter's (parietal) 553.9
    with
      gangrene (obstructed) 551.9
      obstruction 552.9
        and gangrene 551.9
  Rieux's, Riex's (retrocecal) 553.8
    with
      gangrene (obstructed) 551.8
      obstruction 552.8
        and gangrene 551.8
  sciatic 553.8
    with
      gangrene (obstructed) 551.8
      obstruction 552.8
        and gangrene 551.8
  scrotum, scrotal — *see* Hernia, inguinal
  sliding (inguinal) (*see also* Hernia, inguinal)
    hiatus — *see* Hernia, hiatal
  spigelian 553.29
    with
      gangrene (obstructed) 551.29
      obstruction 552.29
        and gangrene 551.29
  spinal (*see also* Spina bifida) 741.9 ☑
    with hydrocephalus 741.0 ☑
  strangulated (*see also* Hernia, by site, with obstruction) 552.9
    gangrenous (with obstruction) (*see also* Hernia, by site, with gangrene) 551.9
  supraumbilicus (linea alba) — *see* Hernia, epigastric
  tendon 727.9
  testis (nontraumatic) 550.9 ☑
    meaning
      scrotal hernia 550.9 ☑
      symptomatic late syphilis 095.8
  Treitz's (fossa) 553.8
    with
      gangrene (obstructed) 551.8
      obstruction 552.8
        and gangrene 551.8
  tunica
    albuginea 608.89
    vaginalis 752.89
  umbilicus, umbilical 553.1
    with
      gangrene (obstructed) 551.1
      obstruction 552.1
        and gangrene 551.1
  ureter 593.89
    with obstruction 593.4
  uterus 621.8
    pregnant 654.4 ☑
  vaginal (posterior) 618.6

**Hernia, hernial** — *continued*
  Velpeau's (femoral) (*see also* Hernia, femoral) 553.00
  ventral 553.20
    with
      gangrene (obstructed) 551.20
      obstruction 552.20
        and gangrene 551.20
    incisional 553.21
    recurrent 553.21
      with
        gangrene (obstructed) 551.21
        obstruction 552.21
          and gangrene 551.21
  vesical
    congenital (female) (male) 756.71
    female (*see also* Cystocele, female) 618.01
    male 596.8
  vitreous (into anterior chamber) 379.21
    traumatic 871.1
**Herniation** — *see also* Hernia
  brain (stem) 348.4
  cerebral 348.4
  gastric mucosa (into duodenal bulb) 537.89
  mediastinum 519.3
  nucleus pulposus — *see* Displacement, intervertebral disc
**Herpangina** 074.0
**Herpes, herpetic** 054.9
  auricularis (zoster) 053.71
    simplex 054.73
  blepharitis (zoster) 053.20
    simplex 054.41
  circinate 110.5
  circinatus 110.5
    bullous 694.5
  conjunctiva (simplex) 054.43
    zoster 053.21
  cornea (simplex) 054.43
    disciform (simplex) 054.43
    zoster 053.21
  encephalitis 054.3
  eye (zoster) 053.29
    simplex 054.40
  eyelid (zoster) 053.20
    simplex 054.41
  febrilis 054.9
  fever 054.9
  geniculate ganglionitis 053.11
  genital, genitalis 054.10
    specified site NEC 054.19
  gestationis 646.8 ☑
  gingivostomatitis 054.2
  iridocyclitis (simplex) 054.44
    zoster 053.22
  iris (any site) 695.1
  iritis (simplex) 054.44
  keratitis (simplex) 054.43
    dendritic 054.42
    disciform 054.43
    interstitial 054.43
    zoster 053.21
  keratoconjunctivitis (simplex) 054.43
    zoster 053.21
  labialis 054.9
    meningococcal 036.89
  lip 054.9
  meningitis (simplex) 054.72
    zoster 053.0
  ophthalmicus (zoster) 053.20
    simplex 054.40
  otitis externa (zoster) 053.71
    simplex 054.73
  penis 054.13
  perianal 054.10
  pharyngitis 054.79
  progenitalis 054.10
  scrotum 054.19
  septicemia 054.5
  simplex 054.9
    complicated 054.8
      ophthalmic 054.40
        specified NEC 054.49

**Herpes, herpetic** — *continued*
  simplex — *continued*
    complicated — *continued*
      specified NEC 054.79
    congenital 771.2
    external ear 054.73
    keratitis 054.43
      dendritic 054.42
    meningitis 054.72
    myelitis 054.74
    neuritis 054.79
    specified complication NEC 054.79
      ophthalmic 054.49
    visceral 054.71
  stomatitis 054.2
  tonsurans 110.0
    maculosus (of Hebra) 696.3
  visceral 054.71
  vulva 054.12
  vulvovaginitis 054.11
  whitlow 054.6
  zoster 053.9
    auricularis 053.71
    complicated 053.8
      specified NEC 053.79
    conjunctiva 053.21
    cornea 053.21
    ear 053.71
    eye 053.29
    geniculate 053.11
    keratitis 053.21
      interstitial 053.21
    myelitis 053.14
    neuritis 053.10
    ophthalmicus(a) 053.20
    oticus 053.71
    otitis externa 053.71
    specified complication NEC 053.79
    specified site NEC 053.9
  zosteriform, intermediate type 053.9
**Herrick's**
  anemia (hemoglobin S disease) 282.61
  syndrome (hemoglobin S disease) 282.61
**Hers' disease** (glycogenosis VI) 271.0
**Herter (-Gee) disease or syndrome** (nontropical sprue) 579.0
**Herter's infantilism** (nontropical sprue) 579.0
**Herxheimer's disease** (diffuse idiopathic cutaneous atrophy) 701.8
**Herxheimer's reaction** 995.0
**Hesitancy, urinary** 788.64
**Hesselbach's hernia** — *see* Hernia, Hesselbach's
**Heterochromia** (congenital) 743.46
  acquired 364.53
  cataract 366.33
  cyclitis 364.21
  hair 704.3
  iritis 364.21
  retained metallic foreign body 360.62
    magnetic 360.52
  uveitis 364.21
**Heterophoria** 378.40
  alternating 378.45
  vertical 378.43
**Heterophyes, small intestine** 121.6
**Heterophyiasis** 121.6
**Heteropsia** 368.8
**Heterotopia, heterotopic** — *see also* Malposition, congenital
  cerebralis 742.4
  pancreas, pancreatic 751.7
  spinalis 742.59
**Heterotropia** 378.30
  intermittent 378.20
    vertical 378.31
  vertical (constant) (intermittent) 378.31
**Heubner's disease** 094.89
**Heubner-Herter disease or syndrome** (nontropical sprue) 579.0
**Hexadactylism** 755.0 ☑
**Heyd's syndrome** (hepatorenal) 572.4

**HGSIL** (high grade squamous intraepithelial lesion) ▶(cytologic finding) (Pap smear finding)◀ 795.04
  biopsy finding — code to CIN II or ● CIN III
**Hibernoma (M8880/0)** — *see* Lipoma
**Hiccough** 786.8
  epidemic 078.89
  psychogenic 306.1
**Hiccup** — *see also* Hiccough 786.8
**Hicks (-Braxton) contractures** 644.1 ☑
**Hidden penis** 752.65
**Hidradenitis** (axillaris) (suppurative) 705.83
**Hidradenoma** (nodular) (M8400/0) — *see also* Neoplasm, skin, benign
  clear cell (M8402/0) — *see* Neoplasm, skin, benign
  papillary (M8405/0) — *see* Neoplasm, skin, benign
**Hidrocystoma** (M8404/0) — *see* Neoplasm, skin, benign
**HIE** (hypoxic-ischemic encephalopathy) 768.7
**High**
  A$_2$ anemia 282.49
  altitude effects 993.2
    anoxia 993.2
    on
      ears 993.0
      sinuses 993.1
    polycythemia 289.0
  arch
    foot 755.67
    palate 750.26
  artery (arterial) tension (*see also* Hypertension) 401.9
    without diagnosis of hypertension 796.2
  basal metabolic rate (BMR) 794.7
  blood pressure (*see also* Hypertension) 401.9
    incidental reading (isolated) (nonspecific), no diagnosis of hypertension 796.2
  cholesterol 272.0 ●
    with high triglycerides 272.2 ●
  compliance bladder 596.4
  diaphragm (congenital) 756.6
  frequency deafness (congenital) (regional) 389.8
  head at term 652.5 ☑
    affecting fetus or newborn 763.1
  output failure (cardiac) (*see also* Failure, heart) 428.9
  oxygen-affinity hemoglobin 289.0
  palate 750.26
  risk
    behavior — *see* Problem
    cervical, human papillomavirus (HPV) DNA test positive 795.05
    family situation V61.9
      specified circumstance NEC V61.8
    individual NEC V62.89
    infant NEC V20.1
    patient taking drugs (prescribed) V67.51
      nonprescribed (*see also* Abuse, drugs, nondependent) 305.9 ☑
    pregnancy V23.9
      inadequate prenatal care V23.7
      specified problem NEC V23.89
  temperature (of unknown origin) (*see also* Pyrexia) 780.6
  thoracic rib 756.3
  triglycerides 272.1 ●
    with high cholesterol 272.2 ●
**Hildenbrand's disease** (typhus) 081.9
**Hilger's syndrome** 337.0
**Hill diarrhea** 579.1
**Hilliard's lupus** — *see also* Tuberculosis 017.0 ☑
**Hilum** — *see* condition

**Hip** — *see* condition
**Hippel's disease** (retinocerebral angiomatosis) 759.6
**Hippus** 379.49
**Hirschfeld's disease** (acute diabetes mellitus) — *see also* Diabetes 250.0 ☑
**Hirschsprung's disease or megacolon** (congenital) 751.3
**Hirsuties** — *see also* Hypertrichosis 704.1
**Hirsutism** — *see also* Hypertrichosis 704.1
**Hirudiniasis** (external) (internal) 134.2
**Hiss-Russell dysentery** 004.1
**Histamine cephalgia** 346.2 ☑
**Histidinemia** 270.5
**Histidinuria** 270.5
**Histiocytic syndromes** 288.4
**Histiocytoma (M8832/0)** — *see also* Neoplasm, skin, benign
  fibrous (M8830/0) (*see also* Neoplasm, skin, benign)
    atypical (M8830/1) — *see* Neoplasm, connective tissue, uncertain behavior
    malignant (M8830/3) — *see* Neoplasm, connective tissue, malignant
**Histiocytosis** (acute) (chronic) (subacute) 277.89
  acute differentiated progressive (M9722/3) 202.5 ☑
  cholesterol 277.89
  essential 277.89
  lipid, lipoid (essential) 272.7
  lipochrome (familial) 288.1
  malignant (M9720/3) 202.3 ☑
  X (chronic) 277.89
    acute (progressive) (M9722/3) 202.5 ☑
**Histoplasmosis** 115.90
  with
    endocarditis 115.94
    meningitis 115.91
    pericarditis 115.93
    pneumonia 115.95
    retinitis 115.92
    specified manifestation NEC 115.99
  African (due to Histoplasma duboisii) 115.10
    with
      endocarditis 115.14
      meningitis 115.11
      pericarditis 115.13
      pneumonia 115.15
      retinitis 115.12
      specified manifestation NEC 115.19
  American (due to Histoplasma capsulatum) 115.00
    with
      endocarditis 115.04
      meningitis 115.01
      pericarditis 115.03
      pneumonia 115.05
      retinitis 115.02
      specified manifestation NEC 115.09
  Darling's — *see* Histoplasmosis, American
  large form (*see also* Histoplasmosis, African) 115.10
  lung 115.05
  small form (*see also* Histoplasmosis, American) 115.00
**History** (personal) of
  abuse
    emotional V15.42
    neglect V15.42
    physical V15.41
    sexual V15.41
  affective psychosis V11.1
  alcoholism V11.3

**History** of — *continued*
  alcoholism — *continued*
    specified as drinking problem (*see also* Abuse, drugs, nondependent) 305.0 ☑
  allergy to
    analgesic agent NEC V14.6
    anesthetic NEC V14.4
    antibiotic agent NEC V14.1
      penicillin V14.0
    anti-infective agent NEC V14.3
    diathesis V15.09
    drug V14.9
      specified type NEC V14.8
    eggs V15.03
    food additives V15.05
    insect bite V15.06
    latex V15.07
    medicinal agents V14.9
      specified type NEC V14.8
    milk products V15.02
    narcotic agent NEC V14.5
    nuts V15.05
      peanuts V15.01
    penicillin V14.0
    radiographic dye V15.08
    seafood V15.04
    serum V14.7
    specified food NEC V15.05
    specified nonmedicinal agents NEC V15.09
    spider bite V15.06
    sulfa V14.2
    sulfonamides V14.2
    therapeutic agent NEC V15.09
    vaccine V14.7
  anemia V12.3
  arrest, sudden cardiac V12.53 ●
  arthritis V13.4
  attack, transient ischemic (TIA) ● V12.54 ●
  benign neoplasm of brain V12.41
  blood disease V12.3
  calculi, urinary V13.01
  cardiovascular disease V12.50
    myocardial infarction 412
  child abuse V15.41
  cigarette smoking V15.82
  circulatory system disease V12.50
    myocardial infarction 412
  congenital malformation V13.69
  contraception V15.7
  death, sudden, successfully resusci- ● tated V12.53 ●
  deficit ●
    prolonged reversible ischemic ● neurologic (PRIND) V12.54 ●
    reversible ischemic neurologic ● (RIND) V12.54 ●
  diathesis, allergic V15.09
  digestive system disease V12.70
    peptic ulcer V12.71
    polyps, colonic V12.72
    specified NEC V12.79
  disease (of) V13.9
    blood V12.3
    blood-forming organs V12.3
    cardiovascular system V12.50
    circulatory system V12.50
      specified NEC V12.59 ●
    digestive system V12.70
      peptic ulcer V12.71
      polyps, colonic V12.72
      specified NEC V12.79
    infectious V12.00
      malaria V12.03
      poliomyelitis V12.02
      specified NEC V12.09
      tuberculosis V12.01
    parasitic V12.00
      specified NEC V12.09
    respiratory system V12.60
      pneumonia V12.61
      specified NEC V12.69
    skin V13.3
    specified site NEC V13.8

☑ Additional Digit Required — Refer to the Tabular List for Digit Selection

⬛ Subterms under main terms may continue to next column or page

Index

History — History

**History** of — *continued*
  myocardial infarction 412
  neglect (emotional) V15.42
  nephrotic syndrome V13.03
  nervous system disorder V12.40
    specified type NEC V12.49
  neurosis V11.2
  noncompliance with medical treatment V15.81
  nutritional deficiency V12.1
  obstetric disorder V13.29
    affecting management of current pregnancy V23.49
      pre-term labor V23.41
    pre-term labor V13.21
  parasitic disease V12.00
    specified NEC V12.09
  perinatal problems V13.7
    low birth weight (*see also* Status, low birth weight) V21.30
  physical abuse V15.41
  poisoning V15.6
  poliomyelitis V12.02
  polyps, colonic V12.72
  poor obstetric V13.29
    affecting management of current pregnancy V23.49
      pre-term labor V23.41
    pre-term labor V13.21
  prolonged reversible ischemic neuro- ●
    logic deficit (PRIND) V12.54      ●
  psychiatric disorder V11.9
    affective type V11.1
    manic-depressive V11.1
    neurosis V11.2
    schizophrenia V11.0
    specified type NEC V11.8
  psychological trauma V15.49
    emotional abuse V15.42
    neglect V15.42
    physical abuse V15.41
    rape V15.41
  psychoneurosis V11.2
  radiation therapy V15.3
  rape V15.41
  respiratory system disease V12.60
    pneumonia V12.61
    specified NEC V12.69
  reticulosarcoma V10.71
  reversible ischemic neurologic deficit ●
    (RIND) V12.54                     ●
  schizophrenia V11.0
  skin disease V13.3
  smoking (tobacco) V15.82
  stroke without residual deficits    ●
    V12.54                            ●
  subcutaneous tissue disease V13.3
  sudden                              ●
    cardiac                           ●
      arrest V12.53                   ●
      death (successfully resuscitat- ●
        ed) V12.53                    ●
  surgery (major) to
    great vessels V15.1
    heart V15.1
    major organs NEC V15.2
  syndrome, nephrotic V13.03
  thrombophlebitis V12.52
  thrombosis V12.51
  tobacco use V15.82
  trophoblastic disease V13.1
    affecting management of pregnancy V23.1
  tuberculosis V12.01
  ulcer, peptic V12.71
  urinary system disorder V13.00
    calculi V13.01
    infection V13.02
    nephrotic syndrome V13.03
    specified NEC V13.09
**His-Werner disease** (trench fever) 083.1
**Hives** (bold) — *see also* Urticaria 708.9
**HIV infection** (disease) (illness) — *see* Human immunodeficiency virus (disease) (illness) (infection)
**Hoarseness** 784.49

**Hobnail liver** — *see* Cirrhosis, portal
**Hobo, hoboism** V60.0
**Hodgkin's**
  disease (M9650/3) 201.9 ☑
    lymphocytic
      depletion (M9653/3) 201.7 ☑
        diffuse fibrosis (M9654/3) 201.7 ☑
        reticular type (M9655/3) 201.7 ☑
      predominance (M9651/3) 201.4 ☑
    lymphocytic-histiocytic predominance (M9651/3) 201.4 ☑
    mixed cellularity (M9652/3) 201.6 ☑
    nodular sclerosis (M9656/3) 201.5 ☑
      cellular phase (M9657/3) 201.5 ☑
  granuloma (M9661/3) 201.1 ☑
  lymphogranulomatosis (M9650/3) 201.9 ☑
  lymphoma (M9650/3) 201.9 ☑
  lymphosarcoma (M9650/3) 201.9 ☑
  paragranuloma (M9660/3) 201.0 ☑
  sarcoma (M9662/3) 201.2 ☑
**Hodgson's disease** (aneurysmal dilatation of aorta) 441.9
  ruptured 441.5
**Hodi-potsy** 111.0
**Hoffa (-Kastert) disease or syndrome** (liposynovitis prepatellaris) 272.8
**Hoffmann-Bouveret syndrome** (paroxysmal tachycardia) 427.2
**Hoffman's syndrome** 244.9 *[359.5]*
**Hole**
  macula 362.54
  optic disc, crater-like 377.22
  retina (macula) 362.54
    round 361.31
      with detachment 361.01
**Holla disease** — *see also* Spherocytosis 282.0
**Holländer-Simons syndrome** (progressive lipodystrophy) 272.6
**Hollow foot** (congenital) 754.71
  acquired 736.73
**Holmes' syndrome** (visual disorientation) 368.16
**Holoprosencephaly** 742.2
  due to
    trisomy 13 758.1
    trisomy 18 758.2
**Holthouse's hernia** — *see* Hernia, inguinal
**Homesickness** 309.89
**Homocystinemia** 270.4
**Homocystinuria** 270.4
**Homologous serum jaundice** (prophylactic) (therapeutic) — *see* Hepatitis, viral
**Homosexuality** — omit code
  ego-dystonic 302.0
  pedophilic 302.2
  problems with 302.0
**Homozygous Hb-S disease** 282.61
**Honeycomb lung** 518.89
  congenital 748.4
**Hong Kong ear** 117.3
**HOOD** (hereditary osteo-onychodysplasia) 756.89
**Hooded**
  clitoris 752.49
  penis 752.69
**Hookworm** (anemia) (disease) (infestation) — *see* Ancylostomiasis
**Hoppe-Goldflam syndrome** 358.00
**Hordeolum** (external) (eyelid) 373.11
  internal 373.12
**Horn**
  cutaneous 702.8
    cheek 702.8
    eyelid 702.8
    penis 702.8
    iliac 756.89

**Horn** — *continued*
  nail 703.8
    congenital 757.5
  papillary 700
**Horner's**
  syndrome (*see also* Neuropathy, peripheral, autonomic) 337.9
    traumatic 954.0
  teeth 520.4
**Horseshoe kidney** (congenital) 753.3
**Horton's**
  disease (temporal arteritis) 446.5
  headache or neuralgia 346.2 ☑
**Hospice care** V66.7
**Hospitalism (in children) NEC** 309.83
**Hourglass contraction, contracture**
  bladder 596.8
  gallbladder 575.2
    congenital 751.69
  stomach 536.8
    congenital 750.7
    psychogenic 306.4
  uterus 661.4 ☑
    affecting fetus or newborn 763.7
**Household circumstance affecting care** V60.9
  specified type NEC V60.8
**Housemaid's knee** 727.2
**Housing circumstance affecting care** V60.9
  specified type NEC V60.8
**HTLV-I infection** 079.51
**HTLV-II infection** 079.52
**HTLV-III/LAV** (disease) (illness) (infection) — *see* Human immunodeficiency virus (disease) (illness) (infection)
**HTLV-III** (disease) (illness) (infection) — *see* Human immunodeficiency virus (disease) (illness) (infection)
**Huchard's disease** (continued arterial hypertension) 401.9
**Hudson-Stähli lines** 371.11
**Huguier's disease** (uterine fibroma) 218.9
**Human bite** (open wound) — see also Wound, open, by site
  intact skin surface — *see* Contusion
**Human immunodeficiency virus** (disease) (illness) 042
  infection V08
    with symptoms, symptomatic 042
**Human immunodeficiency virus-2 infection** 079.53
**Human immunovirus** (disease) (illness) (infection) — *see* Human immunodeficiency virus (disease) (illness) (infection)
**Human papillomavirus** 079.4
  cervical
    high risk, DNA test positive 795.05
    low risk, DNA test positive 795.09
**Human parvovirus** 079.83           ●
**Human T-cell lymphotrophic virus-I infection** 079.51
**Human T-cell lymphotrophic virus-II infection** 079.52
**Human T-cell lymphotrophic virus-III** (disease) (illness) (infection) — *see* Human immunodeficiency virus (disease) (illness) (infection)
**Humpback** (acquired) 737.9
  congenital 756.19
**Hum, venous** — omit code
**Hunchback** (acquired) 737.9
  congenital 756.19
**Hunger** 994.2
  air, psychogenic 306.1
  disease 251.1
**Hunner's ulcer** — *see also* Cystitis 595.1
**Hunt's**
  neuralgia 053.11
  syndrome (herpetic geniculate ganglionitis) 053.11
    dyssynergia cerebellaris myoclonica 334.2

**Hunter's glossitis** 529.4
**Hunterian chancre** 091.0
**Hunter (-Hurler) syndrome** (mucopolysaccharidosis II) 277.5
**Huntington's**
  chorea 333.4
  disease 333.4
**Huppert's disease** (multiple myeloma) (M9730/3) 203.0 ☑
**Hurler (-Hunter) disease or syndrome** (mucopolysaccharidosis II) 277.5
**Hürthle cell**
  adenocarcinoma (M8290/3) 193
  adenoma (M8290/0) 226
  carcinoma (M8290/3) 193
  tumor (M8290/0) 226
**Hutchinson's**
  disease meaning
    angioma serpiginosum 709.1
    cheiropompholyx 705.81
    prurigo estivalis 692.72
    summer eruption, or summer prurigo 692.72
  incisors 090.5
  melanotic freckle (M8742/2) (*see also* Neoplasm, skin, in situ)
    malignant melanoma in (M8742/3) — *see* Melanoma
  teeth or incisors (congenital syphilis) 090.5
**Hutchinson-Boeck disease or syndrome** (sarcoidosis) 135
**Hutchinson-Gilford disease or syndrome** (progeria) 259.8
**Hyaline**
  degeneration (diffuse) (generalized) 728.9
    localized — *see* Degeneration, by site
  membrane (disease) (lung) (newborn) 769
**Hyalinosis cutis et mucosae** 272.8
**Hyalin plaque, sclera, senile** 379.16
**Hyalitis** (asteroid) 379.22
  syphilitic 095.8
**Hydatid**
  cyst or tumor (*see also* Echinococcus)
    fallopian tube 752.11
    mole — *see* Hydatidiform mole
    Morgagni (congenital) 752.89
      fallopian tube 752.11
**Hydatidiform mole** (benign) (complicating pregnancy) (delivered) (undelivered) 630
  invasive (M9100/1) 236.1
  malignant (M9100/1) 236.1
  previous, affecting management of pregnancy V23.1
**Hydatidosis** — *see* Echinococcus
**Hyde's disease** (prurigo nodularis) 698.3
**Hydradenitis** 705.83
**Hydradenoma** (M8400/0) — *see* Hidradenoma
**Hydralazine lupus or syndrome**
  correct substance properly administered 695.4
  overdose or wrong substance given or taken 972.6
**Hydramnios** 657.0 ☑
  affecting fetus or newborn 761.3
**Hydrancephaly** 742.3
  with spina bifida (*see also* Spina bifida) 741.0 ☑
**Hydranencephaly** 742.3
  with spina bifida (*see also* Spina bifida) 741.0 ☑
**Hydrargyrism NEC** 985.0
**Hydrarthrosis** — *see also* Effusion, joint 719.0 ☑
  gonococcal 098.50
  intermittent (*see also* Rheumatism, palindromic) 719.3 ☑
  of yaws (early) (late) 102.6
  syphilitic 095.8
    congenital 090.5
**Hydremia** 285.9

**Hydrencephalocele** (congenital) 742.0
**Hydrencephalomeningocele** (congenital) 742.0
**Hydroa** 694.0
  aestivale 692.72
  gestationis 646.8 ☑
  herpetiformis 694.0
  pruriginosa 694.0
  vacciniforme 692.72
**Hydroadenitis** 705.83
**Hydrocalycosis** — see also Hydronephrosis 591
  congenital 753.29
**Hydrocalyx** — see also Hydronephrosis 591
**Hydrocele** (calcified) (chylous) (idiopathic) (infantile) (inguinal canal) (recurrent) (senile) (spermatic cord) (testis) (tunica vaginalis) 603.9
  canal of Nuck (female) 629.1
    male 603.9
  congenital 778.6
  encysted 603.0
    congenital 778.6
  female NEC 629.89
  infected 603.1
  round ligament 629.89
  specified type NEC 603.8
    congenital 778.6
  spinalis (see also Spina bifida) 741.9 ☑
  vulva 624.8
**Hydrocephalic fetus**
  affecting management or pregnancy 655.0 ☑
  causing disproportion 653.6 ☑
    with obstructed labor 660.1 ☑
      affecting fetus or newborn 763.1
**Hydrocephalus** (acquired) (external) (internal) (malignant) (noncommunicating) (obstructive) (recurrent) 331.4
  aqueduct of Sylvius stricture 742.3
    with spina bifida (see also Spina bifida) 741.0 ☑
  chronic 742.3
    with spina bifida (see also Spina bifida) 741.0 ☑
  communicating 331.3
  congenital (external) (internal) 742.3
    with spina bifida (see also Spina bifida) 741.0 ☑
  due to
    stricture of aqueduct of Sylvius 742.3
      with spina bifida (see also Spina bifida) 741.0 ☑
    toxoplasmosis (congenital) 771.2
  fetal affecting management of pregnancy 655.0 ☑
  foramen Magendie block (acquired) 331.3
    congenital 742.3
      with spina bifida (see also Spina bifida) 741.0 ☑
  newborn 742.3
    with spina bifida (see also Spina bifida) 741.0 ☑
  normal pressure 331.5 ●
    idiopathic (INPH) 331.5 ●
    secondary 331.3 ●
  otitic 348.2
  syphilitic, congenital 090.49
  tuberculous (see also Tuberculosis) 013.8 ☑
**Hydrocolpos** (congenital) 623.8
**Hydrocystoma** (M8404/0) — see Neoplasm, skin, benign
**Hydroencephalocele** (congenital) 742.0
**Hydroencephalomeningocele** (congenital) 742.0
**Hydrohematopneumothorax** — see also Hemothorax 511.8
**Hydromeningitis** — see Meningitis
**Hydromeningocele** (spinal) — see also Spina bifida 741.9 ☑

**Hydromeningocele** — see also Spina bifida — continued
  cranial 742.0
**Hydrometra** 621.8
**Hydrometrocolpos** 623.8
**Hydromicrocephaly** 742.1
**Hydromphalus** (congenital) (since birth) 757.39
**Hydromyelia** 742.53
**Hydromyelocele** — see also Spina bifida 741.9 ☑
**Hydronephrosis** 591
  atrophic 591
  congenital 753.29
  due to S. hematobium 120.0
  early 591
  functionless (infected) 591
  infected 591
  intermittent 591
  primary 591
  secondary 591
  tuberculous (see also Tuberculosis) 016.0 ☑
**Hydropericarditis** — see also Pericarditis 423.9
**Hydropericardium** — see also Pericarditis 423.9
**Hydroperitoneum** 789.59 ▲
**Hydrophobia** 071
**Hydrophthalmos** — see also Buphthalmia 743.20
**Hydropneumohemothorax** — see also Hemothorax 511.8
**Hydropneumopericarditis** — see also Pericarditis 423.9
**Hydropneumopericardium** — see also Pericarditis 423.9
**Hydropneumothorax** 511.8
  nontuberculous 511.8
    bacterial 511.1
    pneumococcal 511.1
    staphylococcal 511.1
    streptococcal 511.1
  traumatic 860.0
    with open wound into thorax 860.1
  tuberculous (see also Tuberculosis, pleura) 012.0 ☑
**Hydrops** 782.3
  abdominis 789.59 ▲
  amnii (complicating pregnancy) (see also Hydramnios) 657.0 ☑
  articulorum intermittens (see also Rheumatism, palindromic) 719.3 ☑
  cardiac (see also Failure, heart) 428.0
  congenital — see Hydrops, fetalis
  endolymphatic (see also Disease, Ménière's) 386.00
  fetal(is) or newborn 778.0
    due to isoimmunization 773.3
    not due to isoimmunization 778.0
  gallbladder 575.3
  idiopathic (fetus or newborn) 778.0
  joint (see also Effusion, joint) 719.0 ☑
  labyrinth (see also Disease, Ménière's) 386.00
  meningeal NEC 331.4
  nutritional 262
  pericardium — see Pericarditis
  pleura (see also Hydrothorax) 511.8
  renal (see also Nephrosis) 581.9
  spermatic cord (see also Hydrocele) 603.9
**Hydropyonephrosis** — see also Pyelitis 590.80
  chronic 590.00
**Hydrorachis** 742.53
**Hydrorrhea** (nasal) 478.19
  gravidarum 658.1 ☑
  pregnancy 658.1 ☑
**Hydrosadenitis** 705.83
**Hydrosalpinx** (fallopian tube) (follicularis) 614.1
**Hydrothorax** (double) (pleural) 511.8
  chylous (nonfilarial) 457.8

**Hydrothorax** — continued
  chylous — continued
    filaria (see also Infestation, filarial) 125.9
  nontuberculous 511.8
    bacterial 511.1
    pneumococcal 511.1
    staphylococcal 511.1
    streptococcal 511.1
  traumatic 862.29
    with open wound into thorax 862.39
  tuberculous (see also Tuberculosis, pleura) 012.0 ☑
**Hydroureter** 593.5
  congenital 753.22
**Hydroureteronephrosis** — see also Hydronephrosis 591
**Hydrourethra** 599.84
**Hydroxykynureninuria** 270.2
**Hydroxyprolinemia** 270.8
**Hydroxyprolinuria** 270.8
**Hygroma** (congenital) (cystic) (M9173/0) 228.1
  prepatellar 727.3
  subdural — see Hematoma, subdural
**Hymen** — see condition
**Hymenolepiasis** (diminuta) (infection) (infestation) (nana) 123.6
**Hymenolepis** (diminuta) (infection) (infestation) (nana) 123.6
**Hypalgesia** — see also Disturbance, sensation 782.0
**Hyperabduction syndrome** 447.8
**Hyperacidity, gastric** 536.8
  psychogenic 306.4
**Hyperactive, hyperactivity** 314.01 ▲
  basal cell, uterine cervix 622.10
  bladder 596.51
  bowel (syndrome) 564.9
    sounds 787.5
  cervix epithelial (basal) 622.10
  child 314.01
  colon 564.9
  gastrointestinal 536.8
    psychogenic 306.4
  intestine 564.9
  labyrinth (unilateral) 386.51
    with loss of labyrinthine reactivity 386.58
    bilateral 386.52
  nasal mucous membrane 478.19
  stomach 536.8
  thyroid (gland) (see also Thyrotoxicosis) 242.9 ☑
**Hyperacusis** 388.42
**Hyperadrenalism** (cortical) 255.3
  medullary 255.6
**Hyperadrenocorticism** 255.3
  congenital 255.2
  iatrogenic
    correct substance properly administered 255.3
    overdose or wrong substance given or taken 962.0
**Hyperaffectivity** 301.11
**Hyperaldosteronism** (atypical) (hyperplastic) (normoaldosteronal) (normotensive) (primary) 255.10
  secondary 255.14
**Hyperalgesia** — see also Disturbance, sensation 782.0
**Hyperalimentation** 783.6
  carotene 278.3
  specified NEC 278.8
  vitamin A 278.2
  vitamin D 278.4
**Hyperaminoaciduria** 270.9
  arginine 270.6
  citrulline 270.6
  cystine 270.0
  glycine 270.0
  lysine 270.7
  ornithine 270.6
  renal (types I, II, III) 270.0
**Hyperammonemia** (congenital) 270.6

**Hyperamnesia** 780.99
**Hyperamylasemia** 790.5
**Hyperaphia** 782.0
**Hyperazotemia** 791.9
**Hyperbetalipoproteinemia** (acquired) (essential) (familial) (hereditary) (primary) (secondary) 272.0
  with prebetalipoproteinemia 272.2
**Hyperbilirubinemia** 782.4
  congenital 277.4
  constitutional 277.4
  neonatal (transient) (see also Jaundice, fetus or newborn) 774.6
  of prematurity 774.2
**Hyperbilirubinemica encephalopathia, newborn** 774.7
  due to isoimmunization 773.4
**Hypercalcemia, hypercalcemic** (idiopathic) 275.42
  nephropathy 588.89
**Hypercalcinuria** 275.40
**Hypercapnia** 786.09
  with mixed acid-based disorder 276.4
  fetal, affecting newborn 770.89
**Hypercarotinemia** 278.3
**Hypercementosis** 521.5
**Hyperchloremia** 276.9
**Hyperchlorhydria** 536.8
  neurotic 306.4
  psychogenic 306.4
**Hypercholesterinemia** — see Hypercholesterolemia
**Hypercholesterolemia** 272.0
  with hyperglyceridemia, endogenous 272.2
  essential 272.0
  familial 272.0
  hereditary 272.0
  primary 272.0
  pure 272.0
**Hypercholesterolosis** 272.0
**Hyperchylia gastrica** 536.8
  psychogenic 306.4
**Hyperchylomicronemia** (familial) (with hyperbetalipoproteinemia) 272.3
**Hypercoagulation syndrome** (primary) 289.81
  secondary 289.82
**Hypercorticosteronism**
  correct substance properly administered 255.3
  overdose or wrong substance given or taken 962.0
**Hypercortisonism**
  correct substance properly administered 255.3
  overdose or wrong substance given or taken 962.0
**Hyperdynamic beta-adrenergic state or syndrome** (circulatory) 429.82
**Hyperekplexia** 759.89
**Hyperelectrolytemia** 276.9
**Hyperemesis** 536.2
  arising during pregnancy — see Hyperemesis, gravidarum
  gravidarum (mild) (before 22 completed weeks gestation) 643.0 ☑
    with
      carbohydrate depletion 643.1 ☑
      dehydration 643.1 ☑
      electrolyte imbalance 643.1 ☑
      metabolic disturbance 643.1 ☑
    affecting fetus or newborn 761.8
    severe (with metabolic disturbance) 643.1 ☑
  psychogenic 306.4
**Hyperemia** (acute) 780.99
  anal mucosa 569.49
  bladder 596.7
  cerebral 437.8
  conjunctiva 372.71
  ear, internal, acute 386.30
  enteric 564.89
  eye 372.71
  eyelid (active) (passive) 374.82
  intestine 564.89

**Hyperemia** — *continued*
- iris 364.41
- kidney 593.81
- labyrinth 386.30
- liver (active) (passive) 573.8
- lung 514
- ovary 620.8
- passive 780.99
- pulmonary 514
- renal 593.81
- retina 362.89
- spleen 289.59
- stomach 537.89

**Hyperesthesia** (body surface) — *see also* Disturbance, sensation 782.0
- larynx (reflex) 478.79
    - hysterical 300.11
- pharynx (reflex) 478.29

**Hyperestrinism** 256.0
**Hyperestrogenism** 256.0
**Hyperestrogenosis** 256.0
**Hyperexplexia** 759.89
**Hyperextension, joint** 718.80
- ankle 718.87
- elbow 718.82
- foot 718.87
- hand 718.84
- hip 718.85
- knee 718.86
- multiple sites 718.89
- pelvic region 718.85
- shoulder (region) 718.81
- specified site NEC 718.88
- wrist 718.83

**Hyperfibrinolysis** — *see* Fibrinolysis
**Hyperfolliculinism** 256.0
**Hyperfructosemia** 271.2
**Hyperfunction**
- adrenal (cortex) 255.3
    - androgenic, acquired benign 255.3
    - medulla 255.6
    - virilism 255.2
- corticoadrenal NEC 255.3
- labyrinth — *see* Hyperactive, labyrinth
- medulloadrenal 255.6
- ovary 256.1
    - estrogen 256.0
- pancreas 577.8
- parathyroid (gland) 252.00
- pituitary (anterior) (gland) (lobe) 253.1
- testicular 257.0

**Hypergammaglobulinemia** 289.89
- monoclonal, benign (BMH) 273.1
- polyclonal 273.0
- Waldenström's 273.0

**Hyperglobulinemia** 273.8
**Hyperglycemia** 790.29
- maternal
    - affecting fetus or newborn 775.0
    - manifest diabetes in infant 775.1
- postpancreatectomy (complete) (partial) 251.3

**Hyperglyceridemia** 272.1
- endogenous 272.1
- essential 272.1
- familial 272.1
- mixed 272.3
- pure 272.1

**Hyperglycinemia** 270.7
**Hypergonadism**
- ovarian 256.1
- testicular (infantile) (primary) 257.0

**Hyperheparinemia** — *see also* Circulating anticoagulants 286.5
**Hyperhidrosis, hyperidrosis** 705.21
- axilla 705.21
- face 705.21
- focal (localized) 705.21
    - primary 705.21
        - axilla 705.21
        - face 705.21
        - palms 705.21
        - soles 705.21
    - secondary 705.22
        - axilla 705.22

**Hyperhidrosis, hyperidrosis** — *continued*
- focal — *continued*
    - secondary — *continued*
        - face 705.22
        - palms 705.22
        - soles 705.22
- generalized 780.8
- palms 705.21
- psychogenic 306.3
- secondary 780.8
- soles 705.21

**Hyperhistidinemia** 270.5
**Hyperinsulinism** (ectopic) (functional) (organic) NEC 251.1
- iatrogenic 251.0
- reactive 251.2
- spontaneous 251.2
- therapeutic misadventure (from administration of insulin) 962.3

**Hyperiodemia** 276.9
**Hyperirritability** (cerebral), in newborn 779.1
**Hyperkalemia** 276.7
**Hyperkeratosis** — *see also* Keratosis 701.1
- cervix 622.2
- congenital 757.39
- cornea 371.89
- due to yaws (early) (late) (palmar or plantar) 102.3
- eccentrica 757.39
- figurata centrifuga atrophica 757.39
- follicularis 757.39
    - in cutem penetrans 701.1
- limbic 371.89
- palmoplantaris climacterica 701.1
- pinta (carate) 103.1
- senile (with pruritus) 702.0
- tongue 528.79
- universalis congenita 757.1
- vagina 623.1
- vocal cord 478.5
- vulva 624.09

**Hyperkinesia, hyperkinetic** (disease) (reaction) (syndrome) 314.9
- with
    - attention deficit — *see* Disorder, attention deficit
    - conduct disorder 314.2
    - developmental delay 314.1
    - simple disturbance of activity and attention 314.01
    - specified manifestation NEC 314.8
- heart (disease) 429.82
- of childhood or adolescence NEC 314.9

**Hyperlacrimation** — *see also* Epiphora 375.21
**Hyperlipemia** — *see also* Hyperlipidemia 272.4
**Hyperlipidemia** 272.4
- carbohydrate-induced 272.1
- combined 272.4
- endogenous 272.1
- exogenous 272.3
- fat-induced 272.3
- group
    - A 272.0
    - B 272.1
    - C 272.2
    - D 272.3
- mixed 272.2
- specified type NEC 272.4

**Hyperlipidosis** 272.7
- hereditary 272.7

**Hyperlipoproteinemia** (acquired) (essential) (familial) (hereditary) (primary) (secondary) 272.4
- Fredrickson type
    - I 272.3
    - IIa 272.0
    - IIb 272.2
    - III 272.2
    - IV 272.1
    - V 272.3

**Hyperlipoproteinemia** — *continued*
- low-density-lipoid-type (LDL) 272.0
- very-low-density-lipoid-type (VLDL) 272.1

**Hyperlucent lung, unilateral** 492.8
**Hyperluteinization** 256.1
**Hyperlysinemia** 270.7
**Hypermagnesemia** 275.2
- neonatal 775.5

**Hypermaturity** (fetus or newborn)
- post-term infant 766.21
- prolonged gestation infant 766.22

**Hypermenorrhea** 626.2
**Hypermetabolism** 794.7
**Hypermethioninemia** 270.4
**Hypermetropia** (congenital) 367.0
**Hypermobility**
- cecum 564.9
- coccyx 724.71
- colon 564.9
    - psychogenic 306.4
- ileum 564.89
- joint (acquired) 718.80
    - ankle 718.87
    - elbow 718.82
    - foot 718.87
    - hand 718.84
    - hip 718.85
    - knee 718.86
    - multiple sites 718.89
    - pelvic region 718.85
    - shoulder (region) 718.81
    - specified site NEC 718.88
    - wrist 718.83
- kidney, congenital 753.3
- meniscus (knee) 717.5
- scapula 718.81
- stomach 536.8
    - psychogenic 306.4
- syndrome 728.5
- testis, congenital 752.52
- urethral 599.81

**Hypermotility**
- gastrointestinal 536.8
- intestine 564.9
    - psychogenic 306.4
- stomach 536.8

**Hypernasality** 784.49
**Hypernatremia** 276.0
- with water depletion 276.0

**Hypernephroma** (M8312/3) 189.0
**Hyperopia** 367.0
**Hyperorexia** 783.6
**Hyperornithinemia** 270.6
**Hyperosmia** — *see also* Disturbance, sensation 781.1
**Hyperosmolality** 276.0
**Hyperosteogenesis** 733.99
**Hyperostosis** 733.99
- calvarial 733.3
- cortical 733.3
    - infantile 756.59
- frontal, internal of skull 733.3
- interna frontalis 733.3
- monomelic 733.99
- skull 733.3
    - congenital 756.0
- vertebral 721.8
    - with spondylosis — *see* Spondylosis
    - ankylosing 721.6

**Hyperovarianism** 256.1
**Hyperovarism, hyperovaria** 256.1
**Hyperoxaluria** (primary) 271.8
**Hyperoxia** 987.8
**Hyperparathyroidism** 252.00
- ectopic 259.3
- other 252.08
- primary 252.01
- secondary (of renal origin) 588.81
    - non-renal 252.02
- tertiary 252.08

**Hyperpathia** — *see also* Disturbance, sensation 782.0
- psychogenic 307.80

**Hyperperistalsis** 787.4

**Hyperperistalsis** — *continued*
- psychogenic 306.4

**Hyperpermeability, capillary** 448.9
**Hyperphagia** 783.6
**Hyperphenylalaninemia** 270.1
**Hyperphoria** 378.40
- alternating 378.45

**Hyperphosphatemia** 275.3
**Hyperpiesia** — *see also* Hypertension 401.9
**Hyperpiesis** — *see also* Hypertension 401.9
**Hyperpigmentation** — *see* Pigmentation
**Hyperpinealism** 259.8
**Hyperpipecolatemia** 270.7
**Hyperpituitarism** 253.1
**Hyperplasia, hyperplastic**
- adenoids (lymphoid tissue) 474.12
    - and tonsils 474.10
- adrenal (capsule) (cortex) (gland) 255.8
    - with
        - sexual precocity (male) 255.2
        - virilism, adrenal 255.2
        - virilization (female) 255.2
    - congenital 255.2
    - due to excess ACTH (ectopic) (pituitary) 255.0
    - medulla 255.8
- alpha cells (pancreatic)
    - with
        - gastrin excess 251.5
        - glucagon excess 251.4
- appendix (lymphoid) 543.0
- artery, fibromuscular NEC 447.8
    - carotid 447.8
    - renal 447.3
- bone 733.99
    - marrow 289.9
- breast (*see also* Hypertrophy, breast) 611.1
- carotid artery 447.8
- cementation, cementum (teeth) (tooth) 521.5
- cervical gland 785.6
- cervix (uteri) 622.10
    - basal cell 622.10
    - congenital 752.49
    - endometrium 622.10
    - polypoid 622.10
- chin 524.05
- clitoris, congenital 752.49
- dentin 521.5
- endocervicitis 616.0
- endometrium, endometrial (adenomatous) (atypical) (cystic) (glandular) (polypoid) (uterus) 621.30
    - with atypia 621.33
    - without atypia
        - complex 621.32
        - simple 621.31
    - cervix 622.10
- epithelial 709.8
    - focal, oral, including tongue 528.79
        - mouth (focal) 528.79
    - nipple 611.8
    - skin 709.8
    - tongue (focal) 528.79
    - vaginal wall 623.0
- erythroid 289.9
- fascialis ossificans (progressiva) 728.11
- fibromuscular, artery NEC 447.8
    - carotid 447.8
    - renal 447.3
- genital
    - female 629.89
    - male 608.89
- gingiva 523.8
- glandularis
    - cystica uteri 621.30
    - endometrium (uterus) 621.30
    - interstitialis uteri 621.30
- granulocytic 288.69
- gum 523.8
- hymen, congenital 752.49
- islands of Langerhans 251.1

☑ Additional Digit Required — Refer to the Tabular List for Digit Selection

148 — Volume 2 · October 2007     ▶◀ Revised Text     ● New Line     ▲ Revised Code     Subterms under main terms may continue to next column or page     *2008 ICD-9-CM*

**Hyperplasia, hyperplastic —** *continued*
  islet cell (pancreatic) 251.9
    alpha cells
      with excess
        gastrin 251.5
        glucagon 251.4
    beta cells 251.1
  juxtaglomerular (complex) (kidney) 593.89
  kidney (congenital) 753.3
  liver (congenital) 751.69
  lymph node (gland) 785.6
  lymphoid (diffuse) (nodular) 785.6
    appendix 543.0
    intestine 569.89
  mandibular 524.02
    alveolar 524.72
    unilateral condylar 526.89
  Marchand multiple nodular (liver) — *see* Cirrhosis, postnecrotic
  maxillary 524.01
    alveolar 524.71
  medulla, adrenal 255.8
  myometrium, myometrial 621.2
  nose (lymphoid) (polypoid) 478.19
  oral soft tissue (inflammatory) (irritative) (mucosa) NEC 528.9
    gingiva 523.8
    tongue 529.8
  organ or site, congenital NEC — *see* Anomaly, specified type NEC
  ovary 620.8
  palate, papillary 528.9
  pancreatic islet cells 251.9
    alpha
      with excess
        gastrin 251.5
        glucagon 251.4
    beta 251.1
  parathyroid (gland) 252.01
  persistent, vitreous (primary) 743.51
  pharynx (lymphoid) 478.29
  prostate 600.90
    with
      other lower urinary tract symptoms (LUTS) 600.91
      urinary
        obstruction 600.91
        retention 600.91

**Hyperplasia, hyperplastic —** *continued*
  prostate — *continued*
    adenofibromatous 600.20
      with
        other lower urinary tract symptoms (LUTS) 600.21
        urinary
          obstruction 600.21
          retention 600.21
    nodular 600.10
      with
        urinary
          obstruction 600.11
          retention 600.11
  renal artery (fibromuscular) 447.3
  reticuloendothelial (cell) 289.9
  salivary gland (any) 527.1
  Schimmelbusch's 610.1
  suprarenal (capsule) (gland) 255.8
  thymus (gland) (persistent) 254.0
  thyroid (*see also* Goiter) 240.9
    primary 242.0 ☑
    secondary 242.2 ☑
  tonsil (lymphoid tissue) 474.11
    and adenoids 474.10
  urethrovaginal 599.89
  uterus, uterine (myometrium) 621.2
    endometrium (*see also* Hyperplasia, endometrium) 621.30
  vitreous (humor), primary persistent 743.51
  vulva 624.3
  zygoma 738.11
**Hyperpnea** — *see also* Hyperventilation 786.01
**Hyperpotassemia** 276.7
**Hyperprebetalipoproteinemia** 272.1
  with chylomicronemia 272.3
  familial 272.1
**Hyperprolactinemia** 253.1
**Hyperprolinemia** 270.8
**Hyperproteinemia** 273.8
**Hyperprothrombinemia** 289.89
**Hyperpselaphesia** 782.0
**Hyperpyrexia** 780.6
  heat (effects of) 992.0
  malarial (*see also* Malaria) 084.6
  malignant, due to anesthetic 995.86

**Hyperpyrexia** — *continued*
  rheumatic — *see* Fever, rheumatic
  unknown origin (*see also* Pyrexia) 780.6
**Hyperreactor, vascular** 780.2
**Hyperreflexia** 796.1
  bladder, autonomic 596.54
    with cauda equina 344.61
  detrusor 344.61
**Hypersalivation** — *see also* Ptyalism 527.7
**Hypersarcosinemia** 270.8
**Hypersecretion**
  ACTH 255.3
  androgens (ovarian) 256.1
  calcitonin 246.0
  corticoadrenal 255.3
  cortisol 255.0
  estrogen 256.0
  gastric 536.8
    psychogenic 306.4
  gastrin 251.5
  glucagon 251.4
  hormone
    ACTH 255.3
    anterior pituitary 253.1
    growth NEC 253.0
    ovarian androgen 256.1
    testicular 257.0
    thyroid stimulating 242.8 ☑
  insulin — *see* Hyperinsulinism
  lacrimal glands (*see also* Epiphora) 375.20
  medulloadrenal 255.6
  milk 676.6 ☑
  ovarian androgens 256.1
  pituitary (anterior) 253.1
  salivary gland (any) 527.7
  testicular hormones 257.0
  thyrocalcitonin 246.0
  upper respiratory 478.9
**Hypersegmentation, hereditary** 288.2
  eosinophils 288.2
  neutrophil nuclei 288.2
**Hypersensitive, hypersensitiveness, hypersensitivity** — *see also* Allergy
  angiitis 446.20
    specified NEC 446.29
  carotid sinus 337.0

**Hypersensitive, hypersensitiveness, hypersensitivity** — *see also* Allergy — *continued*
  colon 564.9
    psychogenic 306.4
  DNA (deoxyribonucleic acid) NEC 287.2
  drug (*see also* Allergy, drug) 995.27
  esophagus 530.89
  insect bites — *see* Injury, superficial, by site
  labyrinth 386.58
  pain (*see also* Disturbance, sensation) 782.0
  pneumonitis NEC 495.9
  reaction (*see also* Allergy) 995.3
    upper respiratory tract NEC 478.8
  stomach (allergic) (nonallergic) 536.8
    psychogenic 306.4
**Hypersomatotropism** (classic) 253.0
**Hypersomnia, unspecified** 780.54
  with sleep apnea, unspecified 780.53
  alcohol induced 291.82
  drug induced 292.85
  due to
    medical condition classified elsewhere 327.14
    mental disorder 327.15
  idiopathic
    with long sleep time 327.11
    without long sleep time 327.12
  menstrual related 327.13
  nonorganic origin 307.43
    persistent (primary) 307.44
    transient 307.43
  organic 327.10
    other 327.19
  primary 307.44
  recurrent 327.13
**Hypersplenia** 289.4
**Hypersplenism** 289.4
**Hypersteatosis** 706.3
**Hyperstimulation, ovarian** 256.1
**Hypersuprarenalism** 255.3
**Hypersusceptibility** — *see* Allergy
**Hyper-TBG-nemia** 246.8
**Hypertelorism** 756.0
  orbit, orbital 376.41

| | Malignant | Benign | Unspecified |
|---|---|---|---|
| **Hypertension, hypertensive** (arterial) (arteriolar) (crisis) (degeneration) (disease) (essential) (fluctuating) (idiopathic) (intermittent) (labile) (low renin) (orthostatic) (paroxysmal) (primary) (systemic) (uncontrolled) (vascular) | 401.0 | 401.1 | 401.9 |
| with | | | |
| chronic kidney disease | | | |
| stage I through stage IV, or unspecified | 403.00 | 403.10 | 403.90 |
| stage V or end stage renal disese | 403.01 | 403.11 | 403.91 |
| heart involvement (conditions classifiable to 429.0–429.3, 429.8, 429.9 due to hypertension) (see also Hypertension, heart) | 402.00 | 402.10 | 402.90 |
| with kidney involvement — see Hypertension, cardiorenal | | | |
| renal involvement (only conditions classifiable to 585, 586, 587) (excludes conditions classifiable to 584) (see also Hypertension, kidney) | 403.00 | 403.10 | 403.90 |
| with heart involvement — see Hypertension, cardiorenal | | | |
| failure (and sclerosis) (see also Hypertension, kidney) | 403.01 | 403.11 | 403.91 |
| sclerosis without failure (see also Hypertension, kidney) | 403.00 | 403.10 | 403.90 |
| accelerated (see also Hypertension, by type, malignant)) | 401.0 | — | |
| antepartum — see Hypertension, complicating pregnancy, childbirth, or the puerperium | | | |
| cardiorenal (disease) | 404.00 | 404.10 | 404.90 |
| with | | | |
| chronic kidney disease | | | |
| stage I through stage IV, or unspecified | 404.00 | 404.10 | 404.90 |
| and heart failure | 404.01 | 404.11 | 404.91 |
| stage V or end stage renal disease | 404.02 | 404.12 | 404.92 |
| and heart failure | 404.03 | 404.13 | 404.93 |
| heart failure | 404.01 | 404.11 | 404.91 |
| and chronic kidney disease | 404.01 ▲ | 404.11 ▲ | 404.91 ▲ |
| stage I through stage IV or unspecified | 404.01 ▲ | 404.11 ▲ | 404.91 ▲ |
| stave V or end stage renal disease | 404.03 | 404.13 | 404.93 |
| cardiovascular disease (arteriosclerotic) (sclerotic) | 402.00 | 402.10 | 402.90 |
| with | | | |
| heart failure | 402.01 | 402.11 | 402.91 |
| renal involvement (conditions classifiable to 403) (see also Hypertension, cardiorenal) | 404.00 | 404.10 | 404.90 |
| cardiovascular renal (disease) (sclerosis) (see also Hypertension, cardiorenal) | 404.00 | 404.10 | 404.90 |
| cerebrovascular disease NEC | 437.2 | 437.2 | 437.2 |
| complicating pregnancy, childbirth, or the puerperium | 642.2 ☑ | 642.0 ☑ | 642.9 ☑ |
| with | | | |
| albuminuria (and edema) (mild) | — | — | 642.4 ☑ |
| severe | — | — | 642.5 ☑ |
| chronic kidney disesae | 642.2 ☑ | 642.2 ☑ | 642.2 ☑ |
| and heart disease | 642.2 ☑ | 642.2 ☑ | 642.2 ☑ |
| edema (mild) | — | — | 642.4 ☑ |
| severe | — | — | 642.5 ☑ |
| heart disease | 642.2 ☑ | 642.2 ☑ | 642.2 ☑ |
| and chronic kidney disease | 642.2 ☑ | 642.2 ☑ | 642.2 ☑ |
| renal disease | 642.2 ☑ | 642.2 ☑ | 642.2 ☑ |
| and heart disease | 642.2 ☑ | 642.2 ☑ | 642.2 ☑ |
| chronic | 642.2 ☑ | 642.0 ☑ | 642.0 ☑ |
| with pre-eclampsia or eclampsia | 642.7 ☑ | 642.7 ☑ | 642.7 ☑ |
| fetus or newborn | 760.0 | 760.0 | 760.0 |
| essential | — | 642.0 ☑ | 642.0 ☑ |
| with pre-eclampsia or eclampsia | — | 642.7 ☑ | 642.7 ☑ |
| fetus or newborn | 760.0 | 760.0 | 760.0 |
| fetus or newborn | 760.0 | 760.0 | 760.0 |
| gestational | — | — | 642.3 ☑ |
| pre-existing | 642.2 ☑ | 642.0 ☑ | 642.0 ☑ |
| with pre-eclampsia or eclampsia | 642.7 ☑ | 642.7 ☑ | 642.7 ☑ |
| fetus or newborn | 760.0 | 760.0 | 760.0 |
| secondary to renal disease | 642.1 ☑ | 642.1 ☑ | 642.1 ☑ |
| with pre-eclampsia or eclampsia | 642.7 ☑ | 642.7 ☑ | 642.7 ☑ |
| fetus or newborn | 760.0 | 760.0 | 760.0 |
| transient | — | — | 642.3 ☑ |
| due to | | | |
| aldosteronism, primary | 405.09 | 405.19 | 405.99 |
| brain tumor | 405.09 | 405.19 | 405.99 |
| bulbar poliomyelitis | 405.09 | 405.19 | 405.99 |
| calculus | | | |
| kidney | 405.09 | 405.19 | 405.99 |
| ureter | 405.09 | 405.19 | 405.99 |
| coarctation, aorta | 405.09 | 405.19 | 405.99 |
| Cushing's disease | 405.09 | 405.19 | 405.99 |
| glomerulosclerosis (see also Hypertension, kidney) | 403.00 | 403.10 | 403.90 |
| periarteritis nodosa | 405.09 | 405.19 | 405.99 |
| pheochromocytoma | 405.09 | 405.19 | 405.99 |
| polycystic kidney(s) | 405.09 | 405.19 | 405.99 |
| polycythemia | 405.09 | 405.19 | 405.99 |
| porphyria | 405.09 | 405.19 | 405.99 |
| pyelonephritis | 405.09 | 405.19 | 405.99 |
| renal (artery) | | | |

| | Malignant | Benign | Unspecified |
|---|---|---|---|
| **Hypertension, hypertensive** — continued | | | |
| due to — continued | | | |
| renal — continued | | | |
| aneurysm | 405.01 | 405.11 | 405.91 |
| anomaly | 405.01 | 405.11 | 405.91 |
| embolism | 405.01 | 405.11 | 405.91 |
| fibromuscular hyperplasia | 405.01 | 405.11 | 405.91 |
| occlusion | 405.01 | 405.11 | 405.91 |
| stenosis | 405.01 | 405.11 | 405.91 |
| thrombosis | 405.01 | 405.11 | 405.91 |
| encephalopathy | 437.2 | 437.2 | 437.2 |
| gestational (transient) NEC | — | — | 642.3 ☑ |
| Goldblatt's | 440.1 | 440.1 | 440.1 |
| heart (disease) (conditions classifiable to 429.0–429.3, 429.8, 429.9 | | | |
| due to hypertension) | 402.00 | 402.10 | 402.90 |
| with heart failure | 402.01 | 402.11 | 402.91 |
| hypertensive kidney disease (conditions classifiable to 403) (see also Hypertension, cardiorenal) | 404.00 | 404.10 | 404.90 |
| renal sclerosis (see also Hypertension, cardiorenal) | 404.00 | 404.10 | 404.90 |
| intracranial, benign | — | 348.2 | — |
| intraocular | — | — | 365.04 |
| kidney | 403.00 | 403.10 | 403.90 |
| with | | | |
| chronic kidney disease | | | |
| stage I through stage IV, or unspecified | 403.00 | 403.10 | 403.90 |
| stage V or end stage renal disese | 403.01 | 403.11 | 403.91 |
| heart involvement (conditions classifiable to 429.0–429.3, 429.8, 429.9 due to hypertension) (see also Hypertension, cardiorenal) | 404.00 | 404.10 | 404.90 |
| hypertensive heart (disease) (conditions classifiable to 402) (see also Hypertension, cardiorenal) | 404.00 | 404.10 | 404.90 |
| lesser circulation | — | — | 416.0 |
| necrotizing | 401.0 | — | — |
| ocular | — | — | 365.04 |
| portal (due to chronic liver disease) | — | — | 572.3 |
| postoperative | — | — | 997.91 |
| psychogenic | — | — | 306.2 |
| puerperal, postpartum — see Hypertension, complicating pregnancy, childbirth, or the puerperium | | | |
| pulmonary (artery) | — | — | 416.8 |
| with cor pulmonale (chronic) | — | — | 416.8 |
| acute | — | — | 415.0 |
| idiopathic | — | — | 416.0 |
| primary | — | — | 416.0 |
| of newborn | — | — | 747.83 |
| secondary | — | — | 416.8 |
| renal (disease) (see also Hypertension, kidney) | 403.00 | 403.10 | 403.90 |
| renovascular NEC | 405.01 | 405.11 | 405.91 |
| secondary NEC | 405.09 | 405.19 | 405.99 |
| due to | | | |
| aldosteronism, primary | 405.09 | 405.19 | 405.99 |
| brain tumor | 405.09 | 405.19 | 405.99 |
| bulbar poliomyelitis | 405.09 | 405.19 | 405.99 |
| calculus | | | |
| kidney | 405.09 | 405.19 | 405.99 |
| ureter | 405.09 | 405.19 | 405.99 |
| coarctation, aorta | 405.09 | 405.19 | 405.99 |
| Cushing's disease | 405.09 | 405.19 | 405.99 |
| glomerulosclerosis (see also Hypertension, kidney) | 403.00 | 403.10 | 403.90 |
| periarteritis nodosa | 405.09 | 405.19 | 405.99 |
| pheochromocytoma | 405.09 | 405.19 | 405.99 |
| polycystic kidney(s) | 405.09 | 405.19 | 405.99 |
| polycythemia | 405.09 | 405.19 | 405.99 |
| porphyria | 405.09 | 405.19 | 405.99 |
| pyelonephritis | 405.09 | 405.19 | 405.99 |
| renal (artery) | | | |
| aneurysm | 405.01 | 405.11 | 405.91 |
| anomaly | 405.01 | 405.11 | 405.91 |
| embolism | 405.01 | 405.11 | 405.91 |
| fibromuscular hyperplasia | 405.01 | 405.11 | 405.91 |
| occlusion | 405.01 | 405.11 | 405.91 |
| stenosis | 405.01 | 405.11 | 405.91 |
| thrombosis | 405.01 | 405.11 | 405.91 |
| transient | — | — | 796.2 |
| of pregnancy | — | — | 642.3 ☑ |
| vascular degeneration | 401.0 | 401.1 | 401.9 |
| venous, chronic (asymptomatic) (idiopathic) | — | — | 459.30 |
| with | | | |
| complication, NEC | — | — | 459.39 |
| inflammation | — | — | 459.32 |
| with ulcer | — | — | 459.33 |
| ulcer | — | — | 459.31 |
| with inflammation | — | — | 459.33 |
| due to | | | |
| deep vein thrombosis (see also Syndrome, postphlebetic) | — | — | 459.10 |

☑ Additional Digit Required — Refer to the Tabular List for Digit Selection

⬙ Subterms under main terms may continue to next column or page

▶◀ Revised Text    ● New Line    ▲ Revised Code

**Hyperthecosis, ovary** 256.8
**Hyperthermia** (of unknown origin) — *see also* Pyrexia 780.6
  malignant (due to anesthesia) 995.86
  newborn 778.4
**Hyperthymergasia** — *see also* Psychosis, affective 296.0 ☑
  reactive (from emotional stress, psychological trauma) 298.1
  recurrent episode 296.1 ☑
  single episode 296.0 ☑
**Hyperthymism** 254.8
**Hyperthyroid** (recurrent) — *see* Hyperthyroidism
**Hyperthyroidism** (latent) (preadult) (recurrent) (without goiter) 242.9 ☑

> *Note — Use the following fifth-digit subclassification with category 242:*
> 0  *without mention of thyrotoxic crisis or storm*
> 1  *with mention of thyrotoxic crisis or storm*

  with
    goiter (diffuse) 242.0 ☑
      adenomatous 242.3 ☑
        multinodular 242.2 ☑
        uninodular 242.1 ☑
      nodular 242.3 ☑
        multinodular 242.2 ☑
        uninodular 242.1 ☑
    thyroid nodule 242.1 ☑
  complicating pregnancy, childbirth, or puerperium 648.1 ☑
  neonatal (transient) 775.3
**Hypertonia** — *see* Hypertonicity
**Hypertonicity**
  bladder 596.51
  fetus or newborn 779.89
  gastrointestinal (tract) 536.8
  infancy 779.89
    due to electrolyte imbalance 779.89
  muscle 728.85
  stomach 536.8
    psychogenic 306.4
  uterus, uterine (contractions) 661.4 ☑
    affecting fetus or newborn 763.7
**Hypertony** — *see* Hypertonicity
**Hypertransaminemia** 790.4
**Hypertrichosis** 704.1
  congenital 757.4
  eyelid 374.54
  lanuginosa 757.4
    acquired 704.1
**Hypertriglyceridemia, essential** 272.1
**Hypertrophy, hypertrophic**
  adenoids (infectional) 474.12
    and tonsils (faucial) (infective) (lingual) (lymphoid) 474.10
  adrenal 255.8
  alveolar process or ridge 525.8
  anal papillae 569.49
  apocrine gland 705.82
  artery NEC 447.8
    carotid 447.8
    congenital (peripheral) NEC 747.60
      gastrointestinal 747.61
      lower limb 747.64
      renal 747.62
      specified NEC 747.69
      spinal 747.82
      upper limb 747.63
    renal 447.3
  arthritis (chronic) (*see also* Osteoarthrosis) 715.9 ☑
    spine (*see also* Spondylosis) 721.90
  arytenoid 478.79
  asymmetrical (heart) 429.9
  auricular — *see* Hypertrophy, cardiac
  Bartholin's gland 624.8
  bile duct 576.8
  bladder (sphincter) (trigone) 596.8
  blind spot, visual field 368.42
  bone 733.99
  brain 348.8

**Hypertrophy, hypertrophic —** *continued*
  breast 611.1
    cystic 610.1
    fetus or newborn 778.7
    fibrocystic 610.1
    massive pubertal 611.1
    puerperal, postpartum 676.3 ☑
    senile (parenchymatous) 611.1
  cardiac (chronic) (idiopathic) 429.3
    with
      rheumatic fever (conditions classifiable to 390)
        active 391.8
          with chorea 392.0
        inactive or quiescent (with chorea) 398.99
    congenital NEC 746.89
    fatty (*see also* Degeneration, myocardial) 429.1
    hypertensive (*see also* Hypertension, heart) 402.90
    rheumatic (with chorea) 398.99
      active or acute 391.8
        with chorea 392.0
    valve (*see also* Endocarditis) 424.90
      congenital NEC 746.89
  cartilage 733.99
  cecum 569.89
  cervix (uteri) 622.6
    congenital 752.49
    elongation 622.6
  clitoris (cirrhotic) 624.2
    congenital 752.49
  colon 569.89
    congenital 751.3
  conjunctiva, lymphoid 372.73
  cornea 371.89
  corpora cavernosa 607.89
  duodenum 537.89
  endometrium (uterus) (*see also* Hyperplasia, endometrium) 621.30
    cervix 622.6
  epididymis 608.89
  esophageal hiatus (congenital) 756.6
    with hernia — *see* Hernia, diaphragm
  eyelid 374.30
  falx, skull 733.99
  fat pad 729.30
    infrapatellar 729.31
    knee 729.31
    orbital 374.34
    popliteal 729.31
    prepatellar 729.31
    retropatellar 729.31
    specified site NEC 729.39
  foot (congenital) 755.67
  frenum, frenulum (tongue) 529.8
    linguae 529.8
    lip 528.5
  gallbladder or cystic duct 575.8
  gastric mucosa 535.2 ☑
  gingiva 523.8
  gland, glandular (general) NEC 785.6
  gum (mucous membrane) 523.8
  heart (idiopathic) (*see also* Hypertrophy, cardiac)
    valve (*see also* Endocarditis)
      congenital NEC 746.89
  hemifacial 754.0
  hepatic — *see* Hypertrophy, liver
  hiatus (esophageal) 756.6
  hilus gland 785.6
  hymen, congenital 752.49
  ileum 569.89
  infrapatellar fat pad 729.31
  intestine 569.89
  jejunum 569.89
  kidney (compensatory) 593.1
    congenital 753.3
  labial frenulum 528.5
  labium (majus) (minus) 624.3
  lacrimal gland, chronic 375.03
  ligament 728.9

**Hypertrophy, hypertrophic —** *continued*
  ligament — *continued*
    spinal 724.8
  linguae frenulum 529.8
  lingual tonsil (infectional) 474.11
  lip (frenum) 528.5
    congenital 744.81
  liver 789.1
    acute 573.8
    cirrhotic — *see* Cirrhosis, liver
    congenital 751.69
    fatty — *see* Fatty, liver
  lymph gland 785.6
    tuberculous — *see* Tuberculosis, lymph gland
  mammary gland — *see* Hypertrophy, breast
  maxillary frenulum 528.5
  Meckel's diverticulum (congenital) 751.0
  medial meniscus, acquired 717.3
  median bar 600.90
    with
      other lower urinary tract symptoms (LUTS) 600.91
      urinary
        obstruction 600.91
        retention 600.91
  mediastinum 519.3
  meibomian gland 373.2
  meniscus, knee, congenital 755.64
  metatarsal head 733.99
  metatarsus 733.99
  mouth 528.9
  mucous membrane
    alveolar process 523.8
    nose 478.19
    turbinate (nasal) 478.0
  muscle 728.9
  muscular coat, artery NEC 447.8
    carotid 447.8
    renal 447.3
  myocardium (*see also* Hypertrophy, cardiac) 429.3
    idiopathic 425.4
  myometrium 621.2
  nail 703.8
    congenital 757.5
  nasal 478.19
    alae 478.19
    bone 738.0
    cartilage 478.19
    mucous membrane (septum) 478.19
    sinus (*see also* Sinusitis) 473.9
    turbinate 478.0
  nasopharynx, lymphoid (infectional) (tissue) (wall) 478.29
  neck, uterus 622.6
  nipple 611.1
  normal aperture diaphragm (congenital) 756.6
  nose (*see also* Hypertrophy, nasal) 478.19
  orbit 376.46
  organ or site, congenital NEC — *see* Anomaly, specified type NEC
  osteoarthropathy (pulmonary) 731.2
  ovary 620.8
  palate (hard) 526.89
    soft 528.9
  pancreas (congenital) 751.7
  papillae
    anal 569.49
    tongue 529.3
  parathyroid (gland) 252.01
  parotid gland 527.1
  penis 607.89
  phallus 607.89
    female (clitoris) 624.2
  pharyngeal tonsil 474.12
  pharyngitis 472.1
  pharynx 478.29
    lymphoid (infectional) (tissue) (wall) 478.29

**Hypertrophy, hypertrophic —** *continued*
  pituitary (fossa) (gland) 253.8
  popliteal fat pad 729.31
  preauricular (lymph) gland (Hampstead) 785.6
  prepuce (congenital) 605
    female 624.2
  prostate (asymptomatic) (early) (recurrent) 600.90
    with
      other lower urinary tract symptlms (LUTS) 600.91
      urinary
        obstruction 600.91
        retention 600.91
    adenofibromatous 600.20
      with
        other lower urinary tract symptoms (LUTS) 600.21
        urinary
          obstruction 600.21
          retention 600.21
    benign 600.00
      with
        other lower urinary tract symptoms (LUTS) 600.01
        urinary
          obstruction 600.01
          retention 600.01
    congenital 752.89
  pseudoedematous hypodermal 757.0
  pseudomuscular 359.1
  pylorus (muscle) (sphincter) 537.0
    congenital 750.5
    infantile 750.5
  rectal sphincter 569.49
  rectum 569.49
  renal 593.1
  rhinitis (turbinate) 472.0
  salivary duct or gland 527.1
    congenital 750.26
  scaphoid (tarsal) 733.99
  scar 701.4
  scrotum 608.89
  sella turcica 253.8
  seminal vesicle 608.89
  sigmoid 569.89
  skin condition NEC 701.9
  spermatic cord 608.89
  spinal ligament 724.8
  spleen — *see* Splenomegaly
  spondylitis (spine) (*see also* Spondylosis) 721.90
  stomach 537.89
  subaortic stenosis (idiopathic) 425.1
  sublingual gland 527.1
    congenital 750.26
  submaxillary gland 527.1
  suprarenal (gland) 255.8
  tendon 727.9
  testis 608.89
    congenital 752.89
  thymic, thymus (congenital) (gland) 254.0
  thyroid (gland) (*see also* Goiter) 240.9
    primary 242.0 ☑
    secondary 242.2 ☑
  toe (congenital) 755.65
    acquired 735.8
  tongue 529.8
    congenital 750.15
    frenum 529.8
    papillae (foliate) 529.3
  tonsil (faucial) (infective) (lingual) (lymphoid) 474.11
    with
      adenoiditis 474.01
      tonsillitis 474.00
        and adenoiditis 474.02
    and adenoids 474.10
  tunica vaginalis 608.89
  turbinate (mucous membrane) 478.0
  ureter 593.89

☑ Additional Digit Required — Refer to the Tabular List for Digit Selection    ▽ Subterms under main terms may continue to next column or page

**2008 ICD-9-CM**    ▶◀ Revised Text    ● New Line    ▲ Revised Code    **Volume 2 — 151**

**Hypoplasia, hypoplasis** — *continued*
erythropoietic, chronic acquired 284.81 ▲
esophagus 750.3
Eustachian tube 744.24
eye (*see also* Microphthalmos) 743.10
lid 743.62
face 744.89
bone(s) 756.0
fallopian tube 752.19
femur (*see also* Absence, femur, congenital) 755.34
fibula (*see also* Absence, fibula, congenital) 755.37
finger (*see also* Absence, finger, congenital) 755.29
focal dermal 757.39
foot 755.31
gallbladder 751.69
genitalia, genital organ(s)
female 752.89
external 752.49
internal NEC 752.89
in adiposogenital dystrophy 253.8
male 752.89
penis 752.69
glottis 748.3
hair 757.4
hand 755.21
heart 746.89
left (complex) (syndrome) 746.7
valve NEC 746.89
pulmonary 746.01
humerus (*see also* Absence, humerus, congenital) 755.24
hymen 752.49
intestine (small) 751.1
large 751.2
iris 743.46
jaw 524.09
kidney(s) 753.0
labium (majus) (minus) 752.49
labyrinth, membranous 744.05
lacrimal duct (apparatus) 743.65
larynx 748.3
leg (*see also* Absence, limb, congenital, lower) 755.30
limb 755.4
lower (*see also* Absence, limb, congenital, lower) 755.30
upper (*see also* Absence, limb, congenital, upper) 755.20
liver 751.69
lung (lobe) 748.5
mammary (areolar) 757.6
mandibular 524.04
alveolar 524.74
unilateral condylar 526.89
maxillary 524.03
alveolar 524.73
medullary 284.9
megakaryocytic 287.30
metacarpus (*see also* Absence, metacarpal, congenital) 755.28
metatarsus (*see also* Absence, metatarsal, congenital) 755.38
muscle 756.89
eye 743.69
myocardium (congenital) (Uhl's anomaly) 746.84
nail(s) 757.5
nasolacrimal duct 743.65
nervous system NEC 742.8
neural 742.8
nose, nasal 748.1
ophthalmic (*see also* Microphthalmos) 743.10
optic nerve 377.43
organ
of Corti 744.05
or site NEC — *see* Anomaly, by site
osseous meatus (ear) 744.03
ovary 752.0

**Hypoplasia, hypoplasis** — *continued*
oviduct 752.19
pancreas 751.7
parathyroid (gland) 759.2
parotid gland 750.26
patella 755.64
pelvis, pelvic girdle 755.69
penis 752.69
peripheral vascular system (congenital) NEC 747.60
gastrointestinal 747.61
lower limb 747.64
renal 747.62
specified NEC 747.69
spinal 747.82
upper limb 747.63
pituitary (gland) 759.2
pulmonary 748.5
arteriovenous 747.3
artery 747.3
valve 746.01
punctum lacrimale 743.65
radioulnar (*see also* Absence, radius, congenital, with ulna) 755.25
radius (*see also* Absence, radius, congenital) 755.26
rectum 751.2
respiratory system NEC 748.9
rib 756.3
sacrum 756.19
scapula 755.59
shoulder girdle 755.59
skin 757.39
skull (bone) 756.0
with
anencephalus 740.0
encephalocele 742.0
hydrocephalus 742.3
with spina bifida (*see also* Spina bifida) 741.0 ☑
microcephalus 742.1
spinal (cord) (ventral horn cell) 742.59
vessel 747.82
spine 756.19
spleen 759.0
sternum 756.3
tarsus (*see also* Absence, tarsal, congenital) 755.38
testis, testicle 752.89
thymus (gland) 279.11
thyroid (gland) 243
cartilage 748.3
tibiofibular (*see also* Absence, tibia, congenital, with fibula) 755.35
toe (*see also* Absence, toe, congenital) 755.39
tongue 750.16
trachea (cartilage) (rings) 748.3
Turner's (tooth) 520.4
ulna (*see also* Absence, ulna, congenital) 755.27
umbilical artery 747.5
ureter 753.29
uterus 752.3
vagina 752.49
vascular (peripheral) NEC (*see also* Hypoplasia, peripheral vascular system) 747.60
brain 747.81
vein(s) (peripheral) NEC (*see also* Hypoplasia, peripheral vascular system) 747.60
brain 747.81
cardiac 746.89
great 747.49
portal 747.49
pulmonary 747.49
vena cava (inferior) (superior) 747.49
vertebra 756.19
vulva 752.49
zonule (ciliary) 743.39
zygoma 738.12
**Hypopotassemia** 276.8

**Hypoproaccelerinemia** — *see also* Defect, coagulation 286.3
**Hypoproconvertinemia** (congenital) — *see also* Defect, coagulation 286.3
**Hypoproteinemia** (essential) (hypermetabolic) (idiopathic) 273.8
**Hypoproteinosis** 260
**Hypoprothrombinemia** (congenital) (hereditary) (idiopathic) — *see also* Defect, coagulation 286.3
acquired 286.7
newborn 776.3
**Hypopselaphesia** 782.0
**Hypopyon** (anterior chamber) (eye) 364.05
iritis 364.05
ulcer (cornea) 370.04
**Hypopyrexia** 780.99
**Hyporeflex** 796.1
**Hyporeninemia, extreme** 790.99
in primary aldosteronism 255.10
**Hyporesponsive episode** 780.09
**Hyposecretion**
ACTH 253.4
ovary 256.39
postablative 256.2
salivary gland (any) 527.7
**Hyposegmentation of neutrophils, hereditary** 288.2
**Hyposiderinemia** 280.9
**Hyposmolality** 276.1
syndrome 276.1
**Hyposomatotropism** 253.3
**Hyposomnia, unspecified** — *see also* Insomnia 780.52
with sleep apnea, unspecified 780.51
**Hypospadias** (male) 752.61
female 753.8
**Hypospermatogenesis** 606.1
**Hyposphagma** 372.72
**Hyposplenism** 289.59
**Hypostasis, pulmonary** 514
**Hypostatic** — *see* condition
**Hyposthenuria** 593.89
**Hyposuprarenalism** 255.41 ▲
**Hypo-TBG-nemia** 246.8
**Hypotension** (arterial) (constitutional) 458.9
chronic 458.1
iatrogenic 458.29
maternal, syndrome (following labor and delivery) 669.2 ☑
of hemodialysis 458.21
orthostatic (chronic) 458.0
dysautonomic-dyskinetic syndrome 333.0
permanent idiopathic 458.1
postoperative 458.29
postural 458.0
specified type NEC 458.8
transient 796.3
**Hypothermia** (accidental) 991.6
anesthetic 995.89
newborn NEC 778.3
not associated with low environmental temperature 780.99
**Hypothymergasia** — *see also* Psychosis, affective 296.2 ☑
recurrent episode 296.3 ☑
single episode 296.2 ☑
**Hypothyroidism** (acquired) 244.9
complicating pregnancy, childbirth, or puerperium 648.1 ☑
congenital 243
due to
ablation 244.1
radioactive iodine 244.1
surgical 244.0
iodine (administration) (ingestion) 244.2
radioactive 244.1
irradiation therapy 244.1
p-aminosalicylic acid (PAS) 244.3

**Hypothyroidism** — *continued*
due to — *continued*
phenylbutazone 244.3
resorcinol 244.3
specified cause NEC 244.8
surgery 244.0
goitrous (sporadic) 246.1
iatrogenic NEC 244.3
iodine 244.2
pituitary 244.8
postablative NEC 244.1
postsurgical 244.0
primary 244.9
secondary NEC 244.8
specified cause NEC 244.8
sporadic goitrous 246.1
**Hypotonia, hypotonicity, hypotony** 781.3
benign congenital 358.8
bladder 596.4
congenital 779.89
benign 358.8
eye 360.30
due to
fistula 360.32
ocular disorder NEC 360.33
following loss of aqueous or vitreous 360.33
primary 360.31
infantile muscular (benign) 359.0
muscle 728.9
uterus, uterine (contractions) — *see* Inertia, uterus
**Hypotrichosis** 704.09
congenital 757.4
lid (congenital) 757.4
acquired 374.55
postinfectional NEC 704.09
**Hypotropia** 378.32
**Hypoventilation** 786.09
congenital central alveolar syndrome 327.25
idiopathic sleep related nonobstructive alveolar 327.24
sleep related, in conditions classifiable elsewhere 327.26
**Hypovitaminosis** — *see also* Deficiency, vitamin 269.2
**Hypovolemia** 276.52
surgical shock 998.0
traumatic (shock) 958.4
**Hypoxemia** — *see also* Anoxia 799.02
sleep related, in conditions classifiable elsewhere 327.26
**Hypoxia** — *see also* Anoxia 799.02
cerebral 348.1
during or resulting from a procedure 997.01
newborn 770.88
mild or moderate 768.6
severe 768.5
fetal, affecting newborn 770.88
intrauterine — *see* Distress, fetal
myocardial (*see also* Insufficiency, coronary) 411.89
arteriosclerotic — *see* Arteriosclerosis, coronary
newborn 770.88
sleep related 327.24
**Hypoxic-ischemic encephalopathy** (HIE) 768.7
**Hypsarrhythmia** — *see also* Epilepsy 345.6 ☑
**Hysteralgia, pregnant uterus** 646.8 ☑
**Hysteria, hysterical** 300.10
anxiety 300.20
Charcôt's gland 300.11
conversion (any manifestation) 300.11
dissociative type NEC 300.15
psychosis, acute 298.1
**Hysteroepilepsy** 300.11
**Hysterotomy, affecting fetus or newborn** 763.89

## I

**Iatrogenic syndrome of excess cortisol** 255.0

**Iceland disease** (epidemic neuromyasthenia) 049.8

**Ichthyosis** (congenita) 757.1
- acquired 701.1
- fetalis gravior 757.1
- follicularis 757.1
- hystrix 757.39
- lamellar 757.1
- lingual 528.6
- palmaris and plantaris 757.39
- simplex 757.1
- vera 757.1
- vulgaris 757.1

**Ichthyotoxism** 988.0
- bacterial (see also Poisoning, food) 005.9

**Icteroanemia, hemolytic** (acquired) 283.9
- congenital (see also Spherocytosis) 282.0

**Icterus** — see also Jaundice 782.4
- catarrhal — see Icterus, infectious
- conjunctiva 782.4
  - newborn 774.6
- epidemic — see Icterus, infectious
- febrilis — see Icterus, infectious
- fetus or newborn — see Jaundice, fetus or newborn
- gravis (see also Necrosis, liver) 570
  - complicating pregnancy 646.7 ☑
    - affecting fetus or newborn 760.8
  - fetus or newborn NEC 773.0
  - obstetrical 646.7 ☑
    - affecting fetus or newborn 760.8
- hematogenous (acquired) 283.9
- hemolytic (acquired) 283.9
  - congenital (see also Spherocytosis) 282.0
- hemorrhagic (acute) 100.0
  - leptospiral 100.0
  - newborn 776.0
  - spirochetal 100.0
- infectious 070.1
  - with hepatic coma 070.0
  - leptospiral 100.0
  - spirochetal 100.0
- intermittens juvenilis 277.4
- malignant (see also Necrosis, liver) 570
- neonatorum (see also Jaundice, fetus or newborn) 774.6
- pernicious (see also Necrosis, liver) 570
- spirochetal 100.0

**Ictus solaris, solis** 992.0

**Ideation**
- suicidal V62.84

**Identity disorder** 313.82
- dissociative 300.14
- gender role (child) 302.6
  - adult 302.85
- psychosexual (child) 302.6
  - adult 302.85

**Idioglossia** 307.9

**Idiopathic** — see condition

**Idiosyncrasy** — see also Allergy 995.3
- drug, medicinal substance, and biological — see Allergy, drug

**Idiot, idiocy** (congenital) 318.2
- amaurotic (Bielschowsky) (-Jansky) (family) (infantile (late)) (juvenile (late)) (Vogt-Spielmeyer) 330.1
- microcephalic 742.1
- Mongolian 758.0
- oxycephalic 756.0

**Id reaction** (due to bacteria) 692.89

**IEED** (involuntary emotional expression disorder) 310.8 ●

**IFIS** (intraoperative floppy iris syndrome) 364.81 ●

**IgE asthma** 493.0 ☑ ●

**Ileitis** (chronic) — see also Enteritis 558.9

**Ileitis** — see also Enteritis — continued
- infectious 009.0
- noninfectious 558.9
- regional (ulcerative) 555.0
  - with large intestine 555.2
- segmental 555.0
  - with large intestine 555.2
- terminal (ulcerative) 555.0
  - with large intestine 555.2

**Ileocolitis** — see also Enteritis 558.9
- infectious 009.0
- regional 555.2
- ulcerative 556.1

**Ileostomy status** V44.2
- with complication 569.60

**Ileotyphus** 002.0

**Ileum** — see condition

**Ileus** (adynamic) (bowel) (colon) (inhibitory) (intestine) (neurogenic) (paralytic) 560.1
- arteriomesenteric duodenal 537.2
- due to gallstone (in intestine) 560.31
- duodenal, chronic 537.2
- following gastrointestinal surgery 997.4
- gallstone 560.31
- mechanical (see also Obstruction, intestine) 560.9
- meconium 777.1
  - due to cystic fibrosis 277.01
- myxedema 564.89
- postoperative 997.4
- transitory, newborn 777.4

**Iliac** — see condition

**Iliotibial band friction syndrome** 728.89

**Illegitimacy** V61.6

**Ill, louping** 063.1

**Illness** — see also Disease
- factitious 300.19
  - with
    - combined psychological and physical signs and symptoms 300.19
  - predominantly
    - physical signs and symptoms 300.19
    - psychological symptoms 300.16
  - chronic (with physical symptoms) 301.51
- heart — see Disease, heart
- manic-depressive (see also Psychosis, affective) 296.80
- mental (see also Disorder, mental) 300.9

**Imbalance** 781.2
- autonomic (see also Neuropathy, peripheral, autonomic) 337.9
- electrolyte 276.9
  - with
    - abortion — see Abortion, by type, with metabolic disorder
    - ectopic pregnancy (see also categories 633.0–633.9) 639.4
    - hyperemesis gravidarum (before 22 completed weeks gestation) 643.1 ☑
    - molar pregnancy (see also categories 630–632) 639.4
  - following
    - abortion 639.4
    - ectopic or molar pregnancy 639.4
  - neonatal, transitory NEC 775.5
- endocrine 259.9
- eye muscle NEC 378.9
  - heterophoria — see Heterophoria
- glomerulotubular NEC 593.89
- hormone 259.9
- hysterical (see also Hysteria) 300.10
- labyrinth NEC 386.50
- posture 729.9

**Imbalance** — continued
- sympathetic (see also Neuropathy, peripheral, autonomic) 337.9

**Imbecile, imbecility** 318.0
- moral 301.7
- old age 290.9
- senile 290.9
- specified IQ — see IQ
- unspecified IQ 318.0

**Imbedding, intrauterine device** 996.32

**Imbibition, cholesterol** (gallbladder) 575.6

**Imerslund (-Gräsbeck) syndrome** (anemia due to familial selective vitamin $B_{12}$ malabsorption) 281.1

**Iminoacidopathy** 270.8

**Iminoglycinuria, familial** 270.8

**Immature** — see also Immaturity
- personality 301.89

**Immaturity** 765.1 ☑
- extreme 765.0 ☑
- fetus or infant light-for-dates — see Light-for-dates
- lung, fetus or newborn 770.4
- organ or site NEC — see Hypoplasia
- pulmonary, fetus or newborn 770.4
- reaction 301.89
- sexual (female) (male) 259.0

**Immersion** 994.1
- foot 991.4
- hand 991.4

**Immobile, immobility**
- intestine 564.89
- joint — see Ankylosis
- syndrome (paraplegic) 728.3

**Immunization**
- ABO
  - affecting management of pregnancy 656.2 ☑
  - fetus or newborn 773.1
- complication — see Complications, vaccination
- Rh factor
  - affecting management of pregnancy 656.1 ☑
  - fetus or newborn 773.0
  - from transfusion 999.7

**Immunodeficiency** 279.3
- with
  - adenosine-deaminase deficiency 279.2
  - defect, predominant
    - B-cell 279.00
    - T-cell 279.10
  - hyperimmunoglobulinemia 279.2
  - lymphopenia, hereditary 279.2
  - thrombocytopenia and eczema 279.12
  - thymic
    - aplasia 279.2
    - dysplasia 279.2
- autosomal recessive, Swiss-type 279.2
- common variable 279.06
- severe combined (SCID) 279.2
- to Rh factor
  - affecting management of pregnancy 656.1 ☑
  - fetus or newborn 773.0
- X-linked, with increased IgM 279.05

**Immunotherapy, prophylactic** V07.2
- antineoplastic V58.12

**Impaction, impacted**
- bowel, colon, rectum 560.30
  - with hernia (see also Hernia, by site, with obstruction)
    - gangrenous — see Hernia, by site, with gangrene
  - by
    - calculus 560.39
    - gallstone 560.31
    - fecal 560.39
    - specified type NEC 560.39
- calculus — see Calculus
- cerumen (ear) (external) 380.4
- cuspid 520.6
- dental 520.6

**Impaction, impacted** — continued
- fecal, feces 560.39
  - with hernia (see also Hernia, by site, with obstruction)
    - gangrenous — see Hernia, by site, with gangrene
  - fracture — see Fracture, by site
  - gallbladder — see Cholelithiasis
  - gallstone(s) — see Cholelithiasis
  - in intestine (any part) 560.31
- intestine(s) 560.30
  - with hernia (see also Hernia, by site, with obstruction)
    - gangrenous — see Hernia, by site, with gangrene
  - by
    - calculus 560.39
    - gallstone 560.31
  - fecal 560.39
  - specified type NEC 560.39
- intrauterine device (IUD) 996.32
- molar 520.6
- shoulder 660.4 ☑
  - affecting fetus or newborn 763.1
- tooth, teeth 520.6
- turbinate 733.99

**Impaired, impairment** (function)
- arm V49.1
  - movement, involving
    - musculoskeletal system V49.1
    - nervous system V49.2
- auditory discrimination 388.43
- back V48.3
- body (entire) V49.89
- cognitive, mild, so stated 331.83
- combined visual hearing V49.85 ●
- dual sensory V49.85 ●
- glucose
  - fasting 790.21
  - tolerance test (oral) 790.22
- hearing (see also Deafness) 389.9
  - combined with visual impairment V49.85 ●
- heart — see Disease, heart
- kidney (see also Disease, renal) 593.9
  - disorder resulting from 588.9
    - specified NEC 588.89
- leg V49.1
  - movement, involving
    - musculoskeletal system V49.1
    - nervous system V49.2
- limb V49.1
  - movement, involving
    - musculoskeletal system V49.1
    - nervous system V49.2
- liver 573.8
- mastication 524.9
- mild cognitive, so stated 331.83
- mobility
  - ear ossicles NEC 385.22
  - incostapedial joint 385.22
  - malleus 385.21
- myocardium, myocardial (see also Insufficiency, myocardial) 428.0
- neuromusculoskeletal NEC V49.89
  - back V48.3
  - head V48.2
  - limb V49.2
  - neck V48.3
  - spine V48.3
  - trunk V48.3
- rectal sphincter 787.99
- renal (see also Disease, renal) 593.9
  - disorder resulting from 588.9
    - specified NEC 588.89
- spine V48.3
- vision NEC 369.9
  - both eyes NEC 369.3
  - combined with hearing impairment V49.85 ●
  - moderate 369.74
    - both eyes 369.25
      - with impairment of lesser eye (specified as)
        - blind, not further specified 369.15

**Impaired, impairment** — *continued*
　vision — *continued*
　　moderate — *continued*
　　　both eyes — *continued*
　　　　with impairment of lesser eye
　　　　　— *continued*
　　　　　low vision, not further
　　　　　　specified 369.23
　　　　　near-total 369.17
　　　　　profound 369.18
　　　　　severe 369.24
　　　　　total 369.16
　　　　one eye 369.74
　　　　　with vision of other eye
　　　　　　(specified as)
　　　　　　near-normal 369.75
　　　　　　normal 369.76
　　　near-total 369.64
　　　　both eyes 369.04
　　　　　with impairment of lesser eye
　　　　　　(specified as)
　　　　　　blind, not further speci-
　　　　　　　fied 369.02
　　　　　　total 369.03
　　　　one eye 369.64
　　　　　with vision of other eye
　　　　　　(specified as)
　　　　　　near normal 369.65
　　　　　　normal 369.66
　　　one eye 369.60
　　　　with low vision of other eye
　　　　　369.10
　　　profound 369.67
　　　　both eyes 369.08
　　　　　with impairment of lesser eye
　　　　　　(specified as)
　　　　　　blind, not further speci-
　　　　　　　fied 369.05
　　　　　　near-total 369.07
　　　　　　total 369.06
　　　　one eye 369.67
　　　　　with vision of other eye
　　　　　　(specified as)
　　　　　　near-normal 369.68
　　　　　　normal 369.69
　　　severe 369.71
　　　　both eyes 369.22
　　　　　with impairment of lesser eye
　　　　　　(specified as)
　　　　　　blind, not further speci-
　　　　　　　fied 369.11
　　　　　　low vision, not further
　　　　　　　specified 369.21
　　　　　　near-total 369.13
　　　　　　profound 369.14
　　　　　　total 369.12
　　　　one eye 369.71
　　　　　with vision of other eye
　　　　　　(specified as)
　　　　　　near-normal 369.72
　　　　　　normal 369.73
　　　total
　　　　both eyes 369.01
　　　　one eye 369.61
　　　　　with vision of other eye
　　　　　　(specified as)
　　　　　　near-normal 369.62
　　　　　　normal 369.63
**Impaludism** — *see* Malaria
**Impediment, speech** NEC 784.5
　psychogenic 307.9
　secondary to organic lesion 784.5
**Impending**
　cerebrovascular accident or attack
　　435.9
　coronary syndrome 411.1
　delirium tremens 291.0
　myocardial infarction 411.1
**Imperception, auditory** (acquired)
　(congenital) 389.9
**Imperfect**
　aeration, lung (newborn) 770.5
　closure (congenital)
　　alimentary tract NEC 751.8
　　　lower 751.5
　　　upper 750.8

**Imperfect** — *continued*
　closure — *continued*
　　atrioventricular ostium 745.69
　　atrium (secundum) 745.5
　　　primum 745.61
　　branchial cleft or sinus 744.41
　　choroid 743.59
　　cricoid cartilage 748.3
　　cusps, heart valve NEC 746.89
　　　pulmonary 746.09
　　ductus
　　　arteriosus 747.0
　　　Botalli 747.0
　　ear drum 744.29
　　　causing impairment of hearing
　　　　744.03
　　endocardial cushion 745.60
　　epiglottis 748.3
　　esophagus with communication to
　　　bronchus or trachea 750.3
　　Eustachian valve 746.89
　　eyelid 743.62
　　face, facial (*see also* Cleft, lip)
　　　749.10
　　foramen
　　　Botalli 745.5
　　　ovale 745.5
　　genitalia, genital organ(s) or system
　　　female 752.89
　　　　external 752.49
　　　　internal NEC 752.89
　　　　uterus 752.3
　　　male 752.89
　　　　penis 752.69
　　glottis 748.3
　　heart valve (cusps) NEC 746.89
　　interatrial ostium or septum 745.5
　　interauricular ostium or septum
　　　745.5
　　interventricular ostium or septum
　　　745.4
　　iris 743.46
　　kidney 753.3
　　larynx 748.3
　　lens 743.36
　　lip (*see also* Cleft, lip) 749.10
　　nasal septum or sinus 748.1
　　nose 748.1
　　omphalomesenteric duct 751.0
　　optic nerve entry 743.57
　　organ or site NEC — *see* Anomaly,
　　　specified type, by site
　　ostium
　　　interatrial 745.5
　　　interauricular 745.5
　　　interventricular 745.4
　　palate (*see also* Cleft, palate)
　　　749.00
　　preauricular sinus 744.46
　　retina 743.56
　　roof of orbit 742.0
　　sclera 743.47
　　septum
　　　aortic 745.0
　　　aorticopulmonary 745.0
　　　atrial (secundum) 745.5
　　　　primum 745.61
　　　between aorta and pulmonary
　　　　artery 745.0
　　　heart 745.9
　　　interatrial (secundum) 745.5
　　　　primum 745.61
　　　interauricular (secundum) 745.5
　　　　primum 745.61
　　　interventricular 745.4
　　　　with pulmonary stenosis or
　　　　　atresia, dextraposition
　　　　　of aorta, and hypertro-
　　　　　phy of right ventricle
　　　　　745.2
　　　　　in tetralogy of Fallot 745.2
　　　nasal 748.1
　　　ventricular 745.4

**Imperfect** — *continued*
　closure — *continued*
　　septum — *continued*
　　　ventricular — *continued*
　　　　with pulmonary stenosis or
　　　　　atresia, dextraposition
　　　　　of aorta, and hypertro-
　　　　　phy of right ventricle
　　　　　745.2
　　　　　in tetralogy of Fallot 745.2
　　skull 756.0
　　　with
　　　　anencephalus 740.0
　　　　encephalocele 742.0
　　　　hydrocephalus 742.3
　　　　　with spina bifida (*see also*
　　　　　　Spina bifida)
　　　　　　741.0 ☑
　　　　microcephalus 742.1
　　spine (with meningocele) (*see also*
　　　Spina bifida) 741.90
　　thyroid cartilage 748.3
　　trachea 748.3
　　tympanic membrane 744.29
　　　causing impairment of hearing
　　　　744.03
　　uterus (with communication to
　　　bladder, intestine, or rectum)
　　　752.3
　　uvula 749.02
　　　with cleft lip (*see also* Cleft,
　　　　palate, with cleft lip)
　　　　749.20
　　vitelline duct 751.0
　development — *see* Anomaly, by site
　erection 607.84
　fusion — *see* Imperfect, closure
　inflation lung (newborn) 770.5
　intestinal canal 751.5
　poise 729.9
　rotation — *see* Malrotation
　septum, ventricular 745.4
**Imperfectly descended testis** 752.51
**Imperforate** (congenital) — *see also*
　Atresia
　anus 751.2
　bile duct 751.61
　cervix (uteri) 752.49
　esophagus 750.3
　hymen 752.42
　intestine (small) 751.1
　　large 751.2
　jejunum 751.1
　pharynx 750.29
　rectum 751.2
　salivary duct 750.23
　urethra 753.6
　urinary meatus 753.6
　vagina 752.49
**Impervious** (congenital) — *see also*
　Atresia
　anus 751.2
　bile duct 751.61
　esophagus 750.3
　intestine (small) 751.1
　　large 751.5
　rectum 751.2
　urethra 753.6
**Impetiginization of other dermatoses**
　684
**Impetigo** (any organism) (any site) (bul-
　lous) (circinate) (contagiosa)
　(neonatorum) (simplex) 684
　Bockhart's (superficial folliculitis)
　　704.8
　external ear 684 *[380.13]*
　eyelid 684 *[373.5]*
　Fox's (contagiosa) 684
　furfuracea 696.5
　herpetiformis 694.3
　　nonobstetrical 694.3
　staphylococcal infection 684
　ulcerative 686.8
　vulgaris 684
**Impingement, soft tissue between**
　**teeth** 524.89

**Impingement, soft tissue between**
　**teeth** — *continued*
　anterior 524.81
　posterior 524.82
**Implantation**
　anomalous (*see also* Anomaly, speci-
　　fied type, by site)
　　ureter 753.4
　cyst
　　external area or site (skin) NEC
　　　709.8
　　iris 364.61
　　vagina 623.8
　　vulva 624.8
　dermoid (cyst)
　　external area or site (skin) NEC
　　　709.8
　　iris 364.61
　　vagina 623.8
　　vulva 624.8
　placenta, low or marginal — *see* Pla-
　　centa previa
**Implant, endometrial** 617.9
**Impotence** (sexual) 607.84
　organic origin NEC 607.84
　psychogenic 302.72
**Impoverished blood** 285.9
**Impression, basilar** 756.0
**Imprisonment** V62.5
**Improper**
　development, infant 764.9 ☑
**Improperly tied umbilical cord** (causing
　hemorrhage) 772.3
**Impulses, obsessional** 300.3
**Impulsive neurosis** 300.3
**Inaction, kidney** — *see also* Disease,
　renal 593.9
**Inactive** — *see* condition
**Inadequate, inadequacy**
　aesthetics of dental ►restoration◄
　　525.67
　biologic 301.6
　cardiac and renal — *see* Hypertension,
　　cardiorenal
　constitutional 301.6
　development
　　child 783.40
　　fetus 764.9 ☑
　　　affecting management of preg-
　　　　nancy 656.5 ☑
　　genitalia
　　　after puberty NEC 259.0
　　　congenital — *see* Hypoplasia,
　　　　genitalia
　　lungs 748.5
　　organ or site NEC — *see* Hypopla-
　　　sia, by site
　dietary 269.9
　distance, interarch 524.28
　education V62.3
　environment
　　economic problem V60.2
　　household condition NEC V60.1
　　poverty V60.2
　　unemployment V62.0
　functional 301.6
　household care, due to
　　family member
　　　handicapped or ill V60.4
　　　temporarily away from home
　　　　V60.4
　　　on vacation V60.5
　　technical defects in home V60.1
　　temporary absence from home of
　　　person rendering care V60.4
　housing (heating) (space) V60.1
　interarch distance 524.28
　material resources V60.2
　mental (*see also* Retardation, mental)
　　319
　nervous system 799.2
　personality 301.6
　prenatal care in current pregnancy
　　V23.7
　pulmonary
　　function 786.09

**Inadequate, inadequacy** — *continued*
  pulmonary — *continued*
    function — *continued*
      newborn 770.89
    ventilation, newborn 770.89
  respiration 786.09
    newborn 770.89
  sample, Papanicolaou smear 795.08
  social 301.6
**Inanition** 263.9
  with edema 262
  due to
    deprivation of food 994.2
    malnutrition 263.9
  fever 780.6
**Inappropriate secretion**
  ACTH 255.0
  antidiuretic hormone (ADH) (excessive) 253.6
    deficiency 253.5
  ectopic hormone NEC 259.3
  pituitary (posterior) 253.6
**Inattention after or at birth** 995.52
**Inborn errors of metabolism** — *see*
  Disorder, metabolism
**Incarceration, incarcerated**
  bubonocele (*see also* Hernia, inguinal, with obstruction)
    gangrenous — *see* Hernia, inguinal, with gangrene
  colon (by hernia) (*see also* Hernia, by site with obstruction)
    gangrenous — *see* Hernia, by site, with gangrene
  enterocele 552.9
    gangrenous 551.9
  epigastrocele 552.29
    gangrenous 551.29
  epiplocele 552.9
    gangrenous 551.9
  exomphalos 552.1
    gangrenous 551.1
  fallopian tube 620.8
  hernia (*see also* Hernia, by site, with obstruction)
    gangrenous — *see* Hernia, by site, with gangrene
  iris, in wound 871.1
  lens, in wound 871.1
  merocele (*see also* Hernia, femoral, with obstruction) 552.00
  omentum (by hernia) (*see also* Hernia, by site, with obstruction)
    gangrenous — *see* Hernia, by site, with gangrene
  omphalocele 756.79
  rupture (meaning hernia) (*see also* Hernia, by site, with obstruction) 552.9
    gangrenous (*see also* Hernia, by site, with gangrene) 551.9
  sarcoepiplocele 552.9
    gangrenous 551.9
  sarcoepiplomphalocele 552.1
    with gangrene 551.1
  uterus 621.8
    gravid 654.3 ☑
      causing obstructed labor 660.2 ☑
      affecting fetus or newborn 763.1
**Incident, cerebrovascular** — *see also* Disease, cerebrovascular, acute 436
**Incineration** (entire body) (from fire, conflagration, electricity, or lightning) — *see* Burn, multiple, specified sites
**Incised wound**
  external — *see* Wound, open, by site
  internal organs (abdomen, chest, or pelvis) — *see* Injury, internal, by site, with open wound
**Incision, incisional**
  hernia — *see* Hernia, incisional

**Incision, incisional** — *continued*
  surgical, complication — *see* Complications, surgical procedures
  traumatic
    external — *see* Wound, open, by site
    internal organs (abdomen, chest, or pelvis) — *see* Injury, internal, by site, with open wound
**Inclusion**
  azurophilic leukocytic 288.2
  blennorrhea (neonatal) (newborn) 771.6
  cyst — *see* Cyst, skin
  gallbladder in liver (congenital) 751.69
**Incompatibility**
  ABO
    affecting management of pregnancy 656.2 ☑
    fetus or newborn 773.1
    infusion or transfusion reaction 999.6
  blood (group) (Duffy) (E) (K(ell)) (Kidd) (Lewis) (M) (N) (P) (S) NEC
    affecting management of pregnancy 656.2 ☑
    fetus or newborn 773.2
    infusion or transfusion reaction 999.6
  contour of existing restoration of tooth with oral health 525.65
  marital V61.10
    involving divorce or estrangement V61.0
  Rh (blood group) (factor)
    affecting management of pregnancy 656.1 ☑
    fetus or newborn 773.0
    infusion or transfusion reaction 999.7
  Rhesus — *see* Incompatibility, Rh
**Incompetency, incompetence, incompetent**
  annular
    aortic (valve) (*see also* Insufficiency, aortic) 424.1
    mitral (valve) (*see also* Insufficiency, mitral) 424.0
    pulmonary valve (heart) (*see also* Endocarditis, pulmonary) 424.3
  aortic (valve) (*see also* Insufficiency, aortic) 424.1
    syphilitic 093.22
  cardiac (orifice) 530.0
    valve — *see* Endocarditis
  cervix, cervical (os) 622.5
    in pregnancy 654.5 ☑
      affecting fetus or newborn 761.0
  esophagogastric (junction) (sphincter) 530.0
  heart valve, congenital 746.89
  mitral (valve) — *see* Insufficiency, mitral
  papillary muscle (heart) 429.81
  pelvic fundus
    pubocervical tissue 618.81
    rectovaginal tissue 618.82
  pulmonary valve (heart) (*see also* Endocarditis, pulmonary) 424.3
    congenital 746.09
  tricuspid (annular) (rheumatic) (valve) (*see also* Endocarditis, tricuspid) 397.0
  valvular — *see* Endocarditis
  vein, venous (saphenous) (varicose) (*see also* Varicose, vein) 454.9
  velopharyngeal (closure)
    acquired 528.9
    congenital 750.29
**Incomplete** — *see also* condition
  bladder emptying 788.21
  expansion lungs (newborn) 770.5
  gestation (liveborn) — *see* Immaturity
  rotation — *see* Malrotation
**Incontinence** 788.30

**Incontinence** — *continued*
  without sensory awareness 788.34
  anal sphincter 787.6
  continuous leakage 788.37
  feces 787.6
    due to hysteria 300.11
    nonorganic origin 307.7
  hysterical 300.11
  mixed (male) (female) (urge and stress) 788.33
  overflow 788.38
  paradoxical 788.39
  rectal 787.6
  specified NEC 788.39
  stress (female) 625.6
    male NEC 788.32
  urethral sphincter 599.84
  urge 788.31
    and stress (male) (female) 788.33
  urine 788.30
    active 788.30
    male 788.30
      stress 788.32
      and urge 788.33
    neurogenic 788.39
    nonorganic origin 307.6
    stress (female) 625.6
      male NEC 788.32
    urge 788.31
      and stress 788.33
**Incontinentia pigmenti** 757.33
**Incoordinate**
  uterus (action) (contractions) 661.4 ☑
    affecting fetus or newborn 763.7
**Incoordination**
  esophageal-pharyngeal (newborn) 787.24 ▲
  muscular 781.3
  papillary muscle 429.81
**Increase, increased**
  abnormal, in development 783.9
  androgens (ovarian) 256.1
  anticoagulants (antithrombin) (anti-VIIIa) (anti-IXa) (anti-Xa) (anti-XIa) 286.5
    postpartum 666.3 ☑
  cold sense (*see also* Disturbance, sensation) 782.0
  estrogen 256.0
  function
    adrenal (cortex) 255.3
      medulla 255.6
    pituitary (anterior) (gland) (lobe) 253.1
      posterior 253.6
  heat sense (*see also* Disturbance, sensation) 782.0
  intracranial pressure 781.99
    injury at birth 767.8
  light reflex of retina 362.13
  permeability, capillary 448.9
  pressure
    intracranial 781.99
      injury at birth 767.8
    intraocular 365.00
  pulsations 785.9
  pulse pressure 785.9
  sphericity, lens 743.36
  splenic activity 289.4
  venous pressure 459.89
    portal 572.3
**Incrustation, cornea, lead or zinc** 930.0
**Incyclophoria** 378.44
**Incyclotropia** 378.33
**Indeterminate sex** 752.7
**India rubber skin** 756.83
**Indicanuria** 270.2
**Indigestion** (bilious) (functional) 536.8
  acid 536.8
  catarrhal 536.8
  due to decomposed food NEC 005.9
  fat 579.8
  nervous 306.4
  psychogenic 306.4
**Indirect** — *see* condition
**Indolent bubo** NEC 099.8

**Induced**
  abortion — *see* Abortion, induced
  birth, affecting fetus or newborn 763.89
  delivery — *see* Delivery
  labor — *see* Delivery
**Induration, indurated**
  brain 348.8
  breast (fibrous) 611.79
    puerperal, postpartum 676.3 ☑
  broad ligament 620.8
  chancre 091.0
    anus 091.1
    congenital 090.0
    extragenital NEC 091.2
  corpora cavernosa (penis) (plastic) 607.89
  liver (chronic) 573.8
    acute 573.8
  lung (black) (brown) (chronic) (fibroid) (*see also* Fibrosis, lung) 515
    essential brown 275.0 *[516.1]*
  penile 607.89
  phlebitic — *see* Phlebitis
  skin 782.8
  stomach 537.89
**Induratio penis plastica** 607.89
**Industrial** — *see* condition
**Inebriety** — *see also* Abuse, drugs, nondependent 305.0 ☑
**Inefficiency**
  kidney (*see also* Disease, renal) 593.9
  thyroid (acquired) (gland) 244.9
**Inelasticity, skin** 782.8
**Inequality, leg** (acquired) (length) 736.81
  congenital 755.30
**Inertia**
  bladder 596.4
    neurogenic 596.54
      with cauda equina syndrome 344.61
  stomach 536.8
    psychogenic 306.4
  uterus, uterine 661.2 ☑
    affecting fetus or newborn 763.7
    primary 661.0 ☑
    secondary 661.1 ☑
  vesical 596.4
    neurogenic 596.54
      with cauda equina 344.61
**Infant** — *see also* condition
  excessive crying of 780.92
  fussy (baby) 780.91
  held for adoption V68.89
  newborn — *see* Newborn
  post-term (gestation period over 40 completed weeks to 42 completed weeks) 766.21
  prolonged gestation of (period over 42 completed weeks) 766.22
  syndrome of diabetic mother 775.0
**"Infant Hercules" syndrome** 255.2
**Infantile** — *see also* condition
  genitalia, genitals 259.0
    in pregnancy or childbirth NEC 654.4 ☑
      affecting fetus or newborn 763.89
      causing obstructed labor 660.2 ☑
        affecting fetus or newborn 763.1
  heart 746.9
  kidney 753.3
  lack of care 995.52
  macula degeneration 362.75
  melanodontia 521.05
  os, uterus (*see also* Infantile, genitalia) 259.0
  pelvis 738.6
    with disproportion (fetopelvic) 653.1 ☑
      affecting fetus or newborn 763.1
      causing obstructed labor 660.1 ☑

**Infantile** — see also condition — continued
  pelvis — continued
    with disproportion — continued
      causing obstructed labor — continued
        affecting fetus or newborn 763.1
  penis 259.0
  testis 257.2
  uterus (see also Infantile, genitalia) 259.0
  vulva 752.49
**Infantilism** 259.9
  with dwarfism (hypophyseal) 253.3
  Brissaud's (infantile myxedema) 244.9
  celiac 579.0
  Herter's (nontropical sprue) 579.0
  hypophyseal 253.3
  hypothalamic (with obesity) 253.8
  idiopathic 259.9
  intestinal 579.0
  pancreatic 577.8
  pituitary 253.3
  renal 588.0
  sexual (with obesity) 259.0
**Infants, healthy liveborn** — see Newborn
**Infarct, infarction**
  adrenal (capsule) (gland) 255.41 ▲
  amnion 658.8 ☑
  anterior (with contiguous portion of intraventricular septum) NEC (see also Infarct, myocardium) 410.1 ☑
  appendices epiploicae 557.0
  bowel 557.0
  brain (stem) 434.91
    embolic (see also Embolism, brain) 434.11
    healed or old without residuals V12.54 ▲
    iatrogenic 997.02
    lacunar 434.91
    late effect — see Late effect(s) (of) cerebrovascular disease
    postoperative 997.02
    puerperal, postpartum, childbirth 674.0 ☑
    thrombotic (see also Thrombosis, brain) 434.01
  breast 611.8
  Brewer's (kidney) 593.81
  cardiac (see also Infarct, myocardium) 410.9 ☑
  cerebellar (see also Infarct, brain) 434.91
    embolic (see also Embolism, brain) 434.11
  cerebral (see also Infarct, brain) 434.91
    aborted 434.91 ●
    embolic (see also Embolism, brain) 434.11
    thrombotic (see also Infarct, brain) 434.01
  chorion 658.8 ☑
  colon (acute) (agnogenic) (embolic) (hemorrhagic) (nonocclusive) (nonthrombotic) (occlusive) (segmental) (thrombotic) (with gangrene) 557.0
  coronary artery (see also Infarct, myocardium) 410.9 ☑
  cortical 434.91
  embolic (see also Embolism) 444.9
  fallopian tube 620.8
  gallbladder 575.8
  heart (see also Infarct, myocardium) 410.9 ☑
  hepatic 573.4
  hypophysis (anterior lobe) 253.8
  impending (myocardium) 411.1

**Infarct, infarction** — continued
  intestine (acute) (agnogenic) (embolic) (hemorrhagic) (nonocclusive) (nonthrombotic) (occlusive) (thrombotic) (with gangrene) 557.0
  kidney 593.81
  lacunar 434.91
  liver 573.4
  lung (embolic) (thrombotic) 415.19
    with
      abortion — see Abortion, by type, with, embolism
      ectopic pregnancy (see also categories 633.0–633.9) 639.6
      molar pregnancy (see also categories 630–632) 639.6
    following
      abortion 639.6
      ectopic or molar pregnancy 639.6
    iatrogenic 415.11
    in pregnancy, childbirth, or puerperium — see Embolism, obstetrical
    postoperative 415.11
    septic 415.12 ●
  lymph node or vessel 457.8
  medullary (brain) — see Infarct, brain
  meibomian gland (eyelid) 374.85
  mesentery, mesenteric (embolic) (thrombotic) (with gangrene) 557.0
  midbrain — see Infarct, brain
  myocardium, myocardial (acute or with a stated duration of 8 weeks or less) (with hypertension) 410.9 ☑

---
Note — Use the following fifth-digit subclassification with category 410:

0   episode unspecified

1   initial episode

2   subsequent episode without recurrence
---

    with symptoms after 8 weeks from date of infarction 414.8
    anterior (wall) (with contiguous portion of intraventricular septum) NEC 410.1 ☑
    anteroapical (with contiguous portion of intraventricular septum) 410.1 ☑
    anterolateral (wall) 410.0 ☑
    anteroseptal (with contiguous portion of intraventricular septum) 410.1 ☑
    apical-lateral 410.5 ☑
    atrial 410.8 ☑
    basal-lateral 410.5 ☑
    chronic (with symptoms after 8 weeks from date of infarction) 414.8
    diagnosed on ECG, but presenting no symptoms 412
    diaphragmatic wall (with contiguous portion of intraventricular septum) 410.4 ☑
    healed or old, currently presenting no symptoms 412
    high lateral 410.5 ☑
    impending 411.1
    inferior (wall) (with contiguous portion of intraventricular septum) 410.4 ☑
    inferolateral (wall) 410.2 ☑
    inferoposterior wall 410.3 ☑
    intraoperative 997.1 ●
    lateral wall 410.5 ☑
    non-Q wave 410.7 ☑
    non-ST elevation (NSTEMI) 410.7 ☑
    nontransmural 410.7 ☑
    papillary muscle 410.8 ☑

**Infarct, infarction** — continued
  myocardium, myocardial — continued
    past (diagnosed on ECG or other special investigation, but currently presenting no symptoms) 412
      with symptoms NEC 414.8
    posterior (strictly) (true) (wall) 410.6 ☑
    posterobasal 410.6 ☑
    posteroinferior 410.3 ☑
    posterolateral 410.5 ☑
    postprocedural 997.1 ●
    previous, currently presenting no symptoms 412
    Q wave (see also Infarct, myocardium, by site) 410.9 ☑ ●
    septal 410.8 ☑
    specified site NEC 410.8 ☑
    ST elevation (STEMI) 410.9 ☑
      anterior (wall) 410.1 ☑
      anterolateral (wall) 410.0 ☑
      inferior (wall) 410.4 ☑
      inferolateral (wall) 410.2 ☑
      inferoposterior wall 410.3 ☑
      lateral wall 410.5 ☑
      posterior (strictly) (true) (wall) 410.6 ☑
      specified site NEC 410.8 ☑
    subendocardial 410.7 ☑
    syphilitic 093.82
  non-ST elevation myocardial infarction (NSTEMI) 410.7 ☑
  nontransmural 410.7 ☑
  omentum 557.0
  ovary 620.8
  pancreas 577.8
  papillary muscle (see also Infarct, myocardium) 410.8 ☑
  parathyroid gland 252.8
  pituitary (gland) 253.8
  placenta (complicating pregnancy) 656.7 ☑
    affecting fetus or newborn 762.2
  pontine — see Infarct, brain
  posterior NEC (see also Infarct, myocardium) 410.6 ☑
  prostate 602.8
  pulmonary (artery) (hemorrhagic) (vein) 415.19
    with
      abortion — see Abortion, by type, with embolism
      ectopic pregnancy (see also categories 633.0–633.9) 639.6
      molar pregnancy (see also categories 630–632) 639.6
    following
      abortion 639.6
      ectopic or molar pregnancy 639.6
    iatrogenic 415.11
    in pregnancy, childbirth, or puerperium — see Embolism, obstetrical
    postoperative 415.11
    septic 415.12 ●
  renal 593.81
    embolic or thrombotic 593.81
  retina, retinal 362.84
    with occlusion — see Occlusion, retina
  spinal (acute) (cord) (embolic) (nonembolic) 336.1
  spleen 289.59
    embolic or thrombotic 444.89
  subchorionic — see Infarct, placenta
  subendocardial (see also Infarct, myocardium) 410.7 ☑
  suprarenal (capsule) (gland) 255.41 ▲
  syncytium — see Infarct, placenta
  testis 608.83

**Infarct, infarction** — continued
  thrombotic (see also Thrombosis) 453.9
    artery, arterial — see Embolism
  thyroid (gland) 246.3
  ventricle (heart) (see also Infarct, myocardium) 410.9 ☑
**Infecting** — see condition
**Infection, infected, infective** (opportunistic) 136.9
  with lymphangitis — see Lymphangitis
  abortion — see Abortion, by type, with, sepsis
  abscess (skin) — see Abscess, by site
  Absidia 117.7
  Acanthocheilonema (perstans) 125.4
    streptocerca 125.6
  accessory sinus (chronic) (see also Sinusitis) 473.9
  Achorion — see Dermatophytosis
  Acremonium falciforme 117.4
  acromioclavicular (joint) 711.91
  actinobacillus
    lignieresii 027.8
    mallei 024
    muris 026.1
  actinomadura — see Actinomycosis
  Actinomyces (israelii) (see also Actinomycosis)
    muris-ratti 026.1
  Actinomycetales (actinomadura) (Actinomyces) (Nocardia) (Streptomyces) — see Actinomycosis
  actinomycotic NEC (see also Actinomycosis) 039.9
  adenoid (chronic) 474.01
    acute 463
    and tonsil (chronic) 474.02
      acute or subacute 463
  adenovirus NEC 079.0
    in diseases classified elsewhere — see category 079 ☑
    unspecified nature or site 079.0
  Aerobacter aerogenes NEC 041.85
    enteritis 008.2
  aerogenes capsulatus (see also Gangrene, gas) 040.0
  aertrycke (see also Infection, Salmonella) 003.9
  ajellomyces dermatitidis 116.0
  alimentary canal NEC (see also Enteritis, due to, by organism) 009.0
  Allescheria boydii 117.6
  Alternaria 118
  alveolus, alveolar (process) (pulpal origin) 522.4
  ameba, amebic (histolytica) (see also Amebiasis) 006.9
    acute 006.0
    chronic 006.1
    free-living 136.2
    hartmanni 007.8
    specified
      site NEC 006.8
      type NEC 007.8
  amniotic fluid or cavity 658.4 ☑
    affecting fetus or newborn 762.7
  anaerobes (cocci) (gram-negative) (gram-positive) (mixed) NEC 041.84
  anal canal 569.49
  Ancylostoma braziliense 126.2
  Angiostrongylus cantonensis 128.8
  anisakiasis 127.1
  Anisakis larva 127.1
  anthrax (see also Anthrax) 022.9
  antrum (chronic) (see also Sinusitis, maxillary) 473.0
  anus (papillae) (sphincter) 569.49
  arbor virus NEC 066.9
  arbovirus NEC 066.9
  argentophil-rod 027.0
  Ascaris lumbricoides 127.0
  ascomycetes 117.4
  Aspergillus (flavus) (fumigatus) (terreus) 117.3

☑ Additional Digit Required — Refer to the Tabular List for Digit Selection
**2008 ICD-9-CM**
▶◀ Revised Text    ● New Line    ▲ Revised Code
▽ Subterms under main terms may continue to next column or page
October 2007 · Volume 2 — 157

**Infection, infected, infective** — *continued*
atypical
  acid-fast (bacilli) (*see also* Mycobacterium, atypical) 031.9
  mycobacteria (*see also* Mycobacterium, atypical) 031.9
auditory meatus (circumscribed) (diffuse) (external) (*see also* Otitis, externa) 380.10
auricle (ear) (*see also* Otitis, externa) 380.10
axillary gland 683
Babesiasis 088.82
Babesiosis 088.82
Bacillus NEC 041.89
  abortus 023.1
  anthracis (*see also* Anthrax) 022.9
  cereus (food poisoning) 005.89
  coli — *see* Infection, Escherichia coli
  coliform NEC 041.85
  Ducrey's (any location) 099.0
  Flexner's 004.1
  Friedländer's NEC 041.3
  fusiformis 101
  gas (gangrene) (*see also* Gangrene, gas) 040.0
  mallei 024
  melitensis 023.0
  paratyphoid, paratyphosus 002.9
    A 002.1
    B 002.2
    C 002.3
  Schmorl's 040.3
  Shiga 004.0
  suipestifer (*see also* Infection, Salmonella) 003.9
  swimming pool 031.1
  typhosa 002.0
  welchii (*see also* Gangrene, gas) 040.0
  Whitmore's 025
bacterial NEC 041.9
  specified NEC 041.89
    anaerobic NEC 041.84
    gram-negative NEC 041.85
      anaerobic NEC 041.84
Bacterium
  paratyphosum 002.9
    A 002.1
    B 002.2
    C 002.3
  typhosum 002.0
Bacteroides (fragilis) (melaninogenicus) (oralis) NEC 041.82
balantidium coli 007.0
Bartholin's gland 616.89
Basidiobolus 117.7
Bedsonia 079.98
  specified NEC 079.88
bile duct 576.1
bladder (*see also* Cystitis) 595.9
Blastomyces, blastomycotic 116.0
  brasiliensis 116.1
  dermatitidis 116.0
  European 117.5
  loboi 116.2
  North American 116.0
  South American 116.1
bleb
  postprocedural 379.60
    stage 1 379.61
    stage 2 379.62
    stage 3 379.63
blood stream — *see* ▶*also*◀ Septicemia
  catheter-related (CRBSI) 999.31 ●
bone 730.9 ☑
  specified — *see* Osteomyelitis
Bordetella 033.9
  bronchiseptica 033.8
  parapertussis 033.1
  pertussis 033.0
Borrelia
  bergdorfi 088.81

**Infection, infected, infective** — *continued*
Borrelia — *continued*
  vincentii (mouth) (pharynx) (tonsil) 101
brain (*see also* Encephalitis) 323.9
  late effect — *see* category 326
  membranes (*see also* Meningitis) 322.9
  septic 324.0
    late effect — *see* category 326
    meninges (*see also* Meningitis) 320.9
branchial cyst 744.42
breast 611.0
  puerperal, postpartum 675.2 ☑
    with nipple 675.9 ☑
      specified type NEC 675.8 ☑
    nonpurulent 675.2 ☑
    purulent 675.1 ☑
bronchus (*see also* Bronchitis) 490
  fungus NEC 117.9
Brucella 023.9
  abortus 023.1
  canis 023.3
  melitensis 023.0
  mixed 023.8
  suis 023.2
Brugia (Wuchereria) malayi 125.1
bursa — *see* Bursitis
buttocks (skin) 686.9
Candida (albicans) (tropicalis) (*see also* Candidiasis) 112.9
  congenital 771.7
Candiru 136.8
Capillaria
  hepatica 128.8
  philippinensis 127.5
cartilage 733.99
catheter-related bloodstream (CRB-● SI) 999.31 ●
cat liver fluke 121.0
cellulitis — *see* Cellulitis, by site
Cephalosporum falciforme 117.4
Cercomonas hominis (intestinal) 007.3
cerebrospinal (*see also* Meningitis) 322.9
  late effect — *see* category 326
cervical gland 683
cervix (*see also* Cervicitis) 616.0
cesarean section wound 674.3 ☑
Chilomastix (intestinal) 007.8
Chlamydia 079.98
  specified NEC 079.88
cholera (*see also* Cholera) 001.9
chorionic plate 658.8 ☑
Cladosporium
  bantianum 117.8
  carrionii 117.2
  mansoni 111.1
  trichoides 117.8
  wernecki 111.1
Clonorchis (sinensis) (liver) 121.1
Clostridium (haemolyticum) (novyi) NEC 041.84
  botulinum 005.1
  histolyticum (*see also* Gangrene, gas) 040.0
  oedematiens (*see also* Gangrene, gas) 040.0
  perfringens 041.83
    due to food 005.2
  septicum (*see also* Gangrene, gas) 040.0
  sordellii (*see also* Gangrene, gas) 040.0
  welchii (*see also* Gangrene, gas) 040.0
    due to food 005.2
Coccidioides (immitis) (*see also* Coccidioidomycosis) 114.9
coccus NEC 041.89
colon (*see also* Enteritis, due to, by organism) 009.0
  bacillus — *see* Infection, Escherichia coli

**Infection, infected, infective** — *continued*
colostomy or enterostomy 569.61
common duct 576.1
complicating pregnancy, childbirth, or puerperium NEC 647.9 ☑
  affecting fetus or newborn 760.2
Condiobolus 117.7
congenital NEC 771.89
  Candida albicans 771.7
  chronic 771.2
  cytomegalovirus 771.1
  hepatitis, viral 771.2
  herpes simplex 771.2
  listeriosis 771.2
  malaria 771.2
  poliomyelitis 771.2
  rubella 771.0
  toxoplasmosis 771.2
  tuberculosis 771.2
  urinary (tract) 771.82
  vaccinia 771.2
coronavirus 079.89
  SARS-associated 079.82
corpus luteum (*see also* Salpingo-oophoritis) 614.2
Corynebacterium diphtheriae — *see* Diphtheria
Coxsackie (*see also* Coxsackie) 079.2
  endocardium 074.22
  heart NEC 074.20
  in diseases classified elsewhere — *see* category 079 ☑
  meninges 047.0
  myocardium 074.23
  pericardium 074.21
  pharynx 074.0
  specified disease NEC 074.8
  unspecified nature or site 079.2
Cryptococcus neoformans 117.5
Cryptosporidia 007.4
Cunninghamella 117.7
cyst — *see* Cyst
Cysticercus cellulosae 123.1
cytomegalovirus 078.5
  congenital 771.1
dental (pulpal origin) 522.4
deuteromycetes 117.4
Dicrocoelium dendriticum 121.8
Dipetalonema (perstans) 125.4
  streptocerca 125.6
diphtherial — *see* Diphtheria
Diphyllobothrium (adult) (latum) (pacificum) 123.4
  larval 123.5
Diplogonoporus (grandis) 123.8
Dipylidium (caninum) 123.8
Dirofilaria 125.6
dog tapeworm 123.8
Dracunculus medinensis 125.7
Dreschlera 118
  hawaiiensis 117.8
Ducrey's bacillus (any site) 099.0
due to or resulting from
  central venous catheter 999.31 ●
  device, implant, or graft (any) (presence of) — *see* Complications, infection and inflammation, due to (presence of) any device, implant, or graft classified to 996.0–996.5 NEC
  injection, inoculation, infusion, transfusion, or vaccination (prophylactic) (therapeutic) 999.39 ▲
  injury NEC — *see* Wound, open, by site, complicated
  surgery 998.59
duodenum 535.6 ☑
ear (*see also* Otitis)
  external (*see also* Otitis, externa) 380.10
  inner (*see also* Labyrinthitis) 386.30
  middle — *see* Otitis, media

**Infection, infected, infective** — *continued*
Eaton's agent NEC 041.81
Eberthella typhosa 002.0
Ebola 078.89
echinococcosis 122.9
Echinococcus (*see also* Echinococcus) 122.9
Echinostoma 121.8
ECHO virus 079.1
  in diseases classified elsewhere — *see* category 079 ☑
  unspecified nature or site 079.1
Ehrlichiosis 082.40
  chaffeensis 082.41
  specified type NEC 082.49
Endamoeba — *see* Infection, ameba
endocardium (*see also* Endocarditis) 421.9
endocervix (*see also* Cervicitis) 616.0
Entamoeba — *see* Infection, ameba
enteric (*see also* Enteritis, due to, by organism) 009.0
Enterobacter aerogenes NEC 041.85
Enterobacter sakazakii 041.85
Enterobius vermicularis 127.4
enterococcus NEC 041.04
enterovirus NEC 079.89
  central nervous system NEC 048
  enteritis 008.67
  meningitis 047.9
Entomophthora 117.7
Epidermophyton — *see* Dermatophytosis
epidermophytosis — *see* Dermatophytosis
episiotomy 674.3 ☑
Epstein-Barr virus 075
  chronic 780.79 [139.8]
erysipeloid 027.1
Erysipelothrix (insidiosa) (rhusiopathiae) 027.1
erythema infectiosum 057.0
Escherichia coli NEC 041.4
  enteritis — *see* Enteritis, E. coli
  generalized 038.42
  intestinal — *see* Enteritis, E. coli
esophagostomy 530.86
ethmoidal (chronic) (sinus) (*see also* Sinusitis, ethmoidal) 473.2
Eubacterium 041.84
Eustachian tube (ear) 381.50
  acute 381.51
  chronic 381.52
exanthema subitum ▶(*see also* Exanthem subitum)◀ 058.10 ▲
external auditory canal (meatus) (*see also* Otitis, externa) 380.10
eye NEC 360.00
eyelid 373.9
  specified NEC 373.8
fallopian tube (*see also* Salpingo-oophoritis) 614.2
fascia 728.89
Fasciola
  gigantica 121.3
  hepatica 121.3
Fasciolopsis (buski) 121.4
fetus (intra-amniotic) — *see* Infection, congenital
filarial — *see* Infestation, filarial
finger (skin) 686.9
  abscess (with lymphangitis) 681.00
    pulp 681.01
  cellulitis (with lymphangitis) 681.00
  distal closed space (with lymphangitis) 681.00
  nail 681.02
    fungus 110.1
fish tapeworm 123.4
  larval 123.5
flagellate, intestinal 007.9
fluke — *see* Infestation, fluke
focal
  teeth (pulpal origin) 522.4

**Infection, infected, infective —**
*continued*
  focal — *continued*
    tonsils 474.00
      and adenoids 474.02
  Fonsecaea
    compactum 117.2
    pedrosoi 117.2
  food (*see also* Poisoning, food) 005.9
  foot (skin) 686.9
    fungus 110.4
  Francisella tularensis (*see also* Tularemia) 021.9
  frontal sinus (chronic) (*see also* Sinusitis, frontal) 473.1
  fungus NEC 117.9
    beard 110.0
    body 110.5
    dermatiacious NEC 117.8
    foot 110.4
    groin 110.3
    hand 110.2
    nail 110.1
    pathogenic to compromised host only 118
    perianal (area) 110.3
    scalp 110.0
    scrotum 110.8
    skin 111.9
      foot 110.4
      hand 110.2
    toenails 110.1
    trachea 117.9
  Fusarium 118
  Fusobacterium 041.84
  gallbladder (*see also* Cholecystitis, acute) 575.0
  Gardnerella vaginalis 041.89
  gas bacillus (*see also* Gas, gangrene) 040.0
  gastric (*see also* Gastritis) 535.5 ☑
  Gastrodiscoides hominis 121.8
  gastroenteric (*see also* Enteritis, due to, by organism) 009.0
  gastrointestinal (*see also* Enteritis, due to, by organism) 009.0
  gastrostomy 536.41
  generalized NEC (*see also* Septicemia) 038.9
  genital organ or tract NEC
    female 614.9
      with
        abortion — *see* Abortion, by type, with sepsis
        ectopic pregnancy (*see also* categories 633.0–633.9) 639.0
        molar pregnancy (*see also* categories 630–632) 639.0
      complicating pregnancy 646.6 ☑
        affecting fetus or newborn 760.8
      following
        abortion 639.0
        ectopic or molar pregnancy 639.0
      puerperal, postpartum, childbirth 670.0 ☑
      minor or localized 646.6 ☑
        affecting fetus or newborn 760.8
    male 608.4
  genitourinary tract NEC 599.0
  Ghon tubercle, primary (*see also* Tuberculosis) 010.0 ☑
  Giardia lamblia 007.1
  gingival (chronic) 523.10
    acute 523.00
    Vincent's 101
  glanders 024
  Glenosporopsis amazonica 116.2
  Gnathostoma spinigerum 128.1
  Gongylonema 125.6

**Infection, infected, infective —**
*continued*
  gonococcal NEC (*see also* Gonococcus) 098.0
  gram-negative bacilli NEC 041.85
    anaerobic 041.84
  guinea worm 125.7
  gum (*see also* Infection, gingival) 523.10
  Hantavirus 079.81
  heart 429.89
  Helicobacter pylori (H. pylori) 041.86
  helminths NEC 128.9
    intestinal 127.9
      mixed (types classifiable to more than one category in 120.0–127.7) 127.8
      specified type NEC 127.7
    specified type NEC 128.8
  Hemophilus influenzae NEC 041.5
    generalized 038.41
  herpes (simplex) (*see also* Herpes, simplex) 054.9
    congenital 771.2
    zoster (*see also* Herpes, zoster) 053.9
      eye NEC 053.29
  Heterophyes heterophyes 121.6
  Histoplasma (*see also* Histoplasmosis) 115.90
    capsulatum (*see also* Histoplasmosis, American) 115.00
    duboisii (*see also* Histoplasmosis, African) 115.10
  HIV V08
    with symptoms, symptomatic 042
  hookworm (*see also* Ancylostomiasis) 126.9
  human herpesvirus NEC 058.89 ●
  human herpesvirus 6 058.81 ●
  human herpesvirus 7 058.82 ●
  human herpesvirus 8 058.89 ●
  human immunodeficiency virus V08
    with symptoms, symptomatic 042
  human papillomavirus 079.4
  hydrocele 603.1
  hydronephrosis 591
  Hymenolepis 123.6
  hypopharynx 478.29
  inguinal glands 683
    due to soft chancre 099.0
  intestine, intestinal (*see also* Enteritis, due to, by organism) 009.0
  intrauterine (*see also* Endometritis) 615.9
    complicating delivery 646.6 ☑
  isospora belli or hominis 007.2
  Japanese B encephalitis 062.0
  jaw (bone) (acute) (chronic) (lower) (subacute) (upper) 526.4
  joint — *see* Arthritis, infectious or infective
  Kaposi's sarcoma-associated herpesvirus 058.89 ●  ●
  kidney (cortex) (hematogenous) 590.9
    with
      abortion — *see* Abortion, by type, with urinary tract infection
      calculus 592.0
      ectopic pregnancy (*see also* categories 633.0–633.9) 639.8
      molar pregnancy (*see also* categories 630–632) 639.8
    complicating pregnancy or puerperium 646.6 ☑
      affecting fetus or newborn 760.1
    following
      abortion 639.8
      ectopic or molar pregnancy 639.8
    pelvis and ureter 590.3
  Klebsiella pneumoniae NEC 041.3
  knee (skin) NEC 686.9
    joint — *see* Arthritis, infectious

**Infection, infected, infective —**
*continued*
  Koch's (*see also* Tuberculosis, pulmonary) 011.9 ☑
  labia (majora) (minora) (*see also* Vulvitis) 616.10
  lacrimal
    gland (*see also* Dacryoadenitis) 375.00
    passages (duct) (sac) (*see also* Dacryocystitis) 375.30
  larynx NEC 478.79
  leg (skin) NEC 686.9
  Leishmania (*see also* Leishmaniasis) 085.9
    braziliensis 085.5
    donovani 085.0
    ethiopica 085.3
    furunculosa 085.1
    infantum 085.0
    mexicana 085.4
    tropica (minor) 085.1
      major 085.2
  Leptosphaeria senegalensis 117.4
  leptospira (*see also* Leptospirosis) 100.9
    Australis 100.89
    Bataviae 100.89
    pyrogenes 100.89
    specified type NEC 100.89
  leptospirochetal NEC (*see also* Leptospirosis) 100.9
  Leptothrix — *see* Actinomycosis
  Listeria monocytogenes (listeriosis) 027.0
    congenital 771.2
  liver fluke — *see* Infestation, fluke, liver
  Loa loa 125.2
    eyelid 125.2 [373.6]
  Loboa loboi 116.2
  local, skin (staphylococcal) (streptococcal) NEC 686.9
    abscess — *see* Abscess, by site
    cellulitis — *see* Cellulitis, by site
    ulcer (*see also* Ulcer, skin) 707.9
  Loefflerella
    mallei 024
    whitmori 025
  lung 518.89
    atypical Mycobacterium 031.0
      tuberculous (*see also* Tuberculosis, pulmonary) 011.9 ☑
    basilar 518.89
    chronic 518.89
    fungus NEC 117.9
    spirochetal 104.8
    virus — *see* Pneumonia, virus
  lymph gland (axillary) (cervical) (inguinal) 683
    mesenteric 289.2
  lymphoid tissue, base of tongue or posterior pharynx, NEC 474.00
  madurella
    grisea 117.4
    mycetomii 117.4
  major
    with
      abortion — *see* Abortion, by type, with sepsis
      ectopic pregnancy (*see also* categories 633.0–633.9) 639.0
      molar pregnancy (*see also* categories 630–632) 639.0
    following
      abortion 639.0
      ectopic or molar pregnancy 639.0
    puerperal, postpartum, childbirth 670.0 ☑
  Malassezia furfur 111.0
  Malleomyces
    mallei 024
    pseudomallei 025
  mammary gland 611.0

**Infection, infected, infective —**
*continued*
  mammary gland — *continued*
    puerperal, postpartum 675.2 ☑
  Mansonella (ozzardi) 125.5
  mastoid (suppurative) — *see* Mastoiditis
  maxilla, maxillary 526.4
    sinus (chronic) (*see also* Sinusitis, maxillary) 473.0
  mediastinum 519.2
  medina 125.7
  meibomian
    cyst 373.12
    gland 373.12
  melioidosis 025
  meninges (*see also* Meningitis) 320.9
  meningococcal (*see also* condition) 036.9
    brain 036.1
    cerebrospinal 036.0
    endocardium 036.42
    generalized 036.2
    meninges 036.0
    meningococcemia 036.2
    specified site NEC 036.89
  mesenteric lymph nodes or glands NEC 289.2
  Metagonimus 121.5
  metatarsophalangeal 711.97
  microorganism resistant to drugs — *see* Resistance (to), drugs by microorganisms
  Microsporidia 136.8
  microsporum, microsporic — *see* Dermatophytosis
  Mima polymorpha NEC 041.85
  mixed flora NEC 041.89
  Monilia (*see also* Candidiasis) 112.9
    neonatal 771.7
  monkeypox 057.8
  Monosporium apiospermum 117.6
  mouth (focus) NEC 528.9
    parasitic 136.9
  Mucor 117.7
  muscle NEC 728.89
  mycelium NEC 117.9
  mycetoma
    actinomycotic NEC (*see also* Actinomycosis) 039.9
    mycotic NEC 117.4
  Mycobacterium, mycobacterial (*see also* Mycobacterium) 031.9
  Mycoplasma NEC 041.81
  mycotic NEC 117.9
    pathogenic to compromised host only 118
    skin NEC 111.9
    systemic 117.9
  myocardium NEC 422.90
  nail (chronic) (with lymphangitis) 681.9
    finger 681.02
      fungus 110.1
    ingrowing 703.0
    toe 681.11
      fungus 110.1
  nasal sinus (chronic) (*see also* Sinusitis) 473.9
  nasopharynx (chronic) 478.29
    acute 460
  navel 686.9
    newborn 771.4
  Neisserian — *see* Gonococcus
  Neotestudina rosatii 117.4
  newborn, generalized 771.89
  nipple 611.0
    puerperal, postpartum 675.0 ☑
      with breast 675.9 ☑
        specified type NEC 675.8 ☑
  Nocardia — *see* Actinomycosis
  nose 478.19
  nostril 478.19
  obstetrical surgical wound 674.3 ☑
  Oesophagostomum (apiostomum) 127.7

**Infection, infected, infective —** *continued*

Oestrus ovis 134.0
Oidium albicans (see also Candidiasis) 112.9
Onchocerca (volvulus) 125.3
  eye 125.3 [360.13]
  eyelid 125.3 [373.6]
operation wound 998.59
Opisthorchis (felineus) (tenuicollis) (viverrini) 121.0
orbit 376.00
  chronic 376.10
ovary (see also Salpingo-oophoritis) 614.2
Oxyuris vermicularis 127.4
pancreas 577.0
Paracoccidioides brasiliensis 116.1
Paragonimus (westermani) 121.2
parainfluenza virus 079.89
parameningococcus NEC 036.9
  with meningitis 036.0
parasitic NEC 136.9
paratyphoid 002.9
  type A 002.1
  type B 002.2
  type C 002.3
paraurethral ducts 597.89
parotid gland 527.2
Pasteurella NEC 027.2
  multocida (cat-bite) (dog-bite) 027.2
  pestis (see also Plague) 020.9
  pseudotuberculosis 027.2
  septica (cat-bite) (dog-bite) 027.2
  tularensis (see also Tularemia) 021.9
pelvic, female (see also Disease, pelvis, inflammatory) 614.9
penis (glans) (retention) NEC 607.2
  herpetic 054.13
Peptococcus 041.84
Peptostreptococcus 041.84
periapical (pulpal origin) 522.4
peridental 523.30
perineal wound (obstetrical) 674.3 ☑
periodontal 523.31
periorbital 376.00
  chronic 376.10
perirectal 569.49
perirenal (see also Infection, kidney) 590.9
peritoneal (see also Peritonitis) 567.9
periureteral 593.89
periurethral 597.89
Petriellidium boydii 117.6
pharynx 478.29
  Coxsackie virus 074.0
  phlegmonous 462
  posterior, lymphoid 474.00
Phialophora
  gougerotii 117.8
  jeanselmei 117.8
  verrucosa 117.2
Piedraia hortai 111.3
pinna, acute 380.11
pinta 103.9
  intermediate 103.1
  late 103.2
  mixed 103.3
  primary 103.0
pinworm 127.4
pityrosporum furfur 111.0
pleuropneumonia-like organisms NEC (PPLO) 041.81
pneumococcal NEC 041.2
  generalized (purulent) 038.2
Pneumococcus NEC 041.2
postoperative wound 998.59
posttraumatic NEC 958.3
postvaccinal 999.39 ▲
prepuce NEC 607.1
Proprionibacterium 041.84
prostate (capsule) (see also Prostatitis) 601.9
Proteus (mirabilis) (morganii) (vulgaris) NEC 041.6

**Infection, infected, infective —** *continued*

Proteus — *continued*
  enteritis 008.3
protozoal NEC 136.8
  intestinal NEC 007.9
Pseudomonas NEC 041.7
  mallei 024
  pneumonia 482.1
  pseudomallei 025
psittacosis 073.9
puerperal, postpartum (major) 670.0 ☑
  minor 646.6 ☑
pulmonary — see Infection, lung
purulent — see Abscess
putrid, generalized — see Septicemia
pyemic — see Septicemia
Pyrenochaeta romeroi 117.4
Q fever 083.0
rabies 071
rectum (sphincter) 569.49
renal (see also Infection, kidney) 590.9
  pelvis and ureter 590.3
resistant to drugs — see Resistance (to), drugs by microorganisms
respiratory 519.8
  chronic 519.8
  influenzal (acute) (upper) 487.1
  lung 518.89
  rhinovirus 460
  syncytial virus 079.6
  upper (acute) (infectious) NEC 465.9
    with flu, grippe, or influenza 487.1
    influenzal 487.1
    multiple sites NEC 465.8
    streptococcal 034.0
    viral NEC 465.9
respiratory syncytial virus (RSV) 079.6
resulting from presence of shunt or other internal prosthetic device — see Complications, infection and inflammation, due to (presence of) any device, implant, or graft classified to 996.0–996.5 NEC
retroperitoneal 567.39
retrovirus 079.50
  human immunodeficiency virus type 2 [HIV2] 079.53
  human T-cell lymphotrophic virus type I [HTLV-I] 079.51
  human T-cell lymphotrophic virus type II [HTLV-II] 079.52
  specified NEC 079.59
Rhinocladium 117.1
Rhinosporidium — see beri 117.0
rhinovirus
  in diseases classified elsewhere — see category 079 ☑
  unspecified nature or site 079.3
Rhizopus 117.7
rickettsial 083.9
rickettsialpox 083.2
rubella (see also Rubella) 056.9
  congenital 771.0
Saccharomyces (see also Candidiasis) 112.9
Saksenaea 117.7
salivary duct or gland (any) 527.2
Salmonella (aertrycke) (callinarum) (choleraesuis) (enteritidis) (suipestifer) (typhimurium) 003.9
  with
    arthritis 003.23
    gastroenteritis 003.0
    localized infection 003.20
      specified type NEC 003.29
    meningitis 003.21
    osteomyelitis 003.24
    pneumonia 003.22
    septicemia 003.1

**Infection, infected, infective —** *continued*

Salmonella — *continued*
  with — *continued*
    specified manifestation NEC 003.8
  due to food (poisoning) (any serotype) (see also Poisoning, food, due to, Salmonella)
  hirschfeldii 002.3
  localized 003.20
    specified type NEC 003.29
  paratyphi 002.9
    A 002.1
    B 002.2
    C 002.3
  schottmuelleri 002.2
  specified type NEC 003.8
  typhi 002.0
  typhosa 002.0
saprophytic 136.8
Sarcocystis, lindemanni 136.5
SARS-associated coronavirus 079.82
scabies 133.0
Schistosoma — see Infestation, Schistosoma
Schmorl's bacillus 040.3
scratch or other superficial injury — see Injury, superficial, by site
scrotum (acute) NEC 608.4
secondary, burn or open wound (dislocation) (fracture) 958.3
seminal vesicle (see also Vesiculitis) 608.0
septic
  generalized — see Septicemia
  localized, skin (see also Abscess) 682.9
septicemic — see Septicemia
seroma 998.51
Serratia (marcescens) 041.85
  generalized 038.44
sheep liver fluke 121.3
Shigella 004.9
  boydii 004.2
  dysenteriae 004.0
  flexneri 004.1
  group
    A 004.0
    B 004.1
    C 004.2
    D 004.3
  Schmitz (-Stutzer) 004.0
  schmitzii 004.0
  Shiga 004.0
  sonnei 004.3
  specified type NEC 004.8
Sin Nombre virus 079.81
sinus (see also Sinusitis) 473.9
  pilonidal 685.1
    with abscess 685.0
  skin NEC 686.9
Skene's duct or gland (see also Urethritis) 597.89
skin (local) (staphylococcal) (streptococcal) NEC 686.9
  abscess — see Abscess, by site
  cellulitis — see Cellulitis, by site
  due to fungus 111.9
    specified type NEC 111.8
  mycotic 111.9
    specified type NEC 111.8
  ulcer (see also Ulcer, skin) 707.9
slow virus 046.9
  specified condition NEC 046.8
Sparganum (mansoni) (proliferum) 123.5
spermatic cord NEC 608.4
sphenoidal (chronic) (sinus) (see also Sinusitis, sphenoidal) 473.3
Spherophorus necrophorus 040.3
spinal cord NEC (see also Encephalitis) 323.9
  abscess 324.1
    late effect — see category 326
  late effect — see category 326

**Infection, infected, infective —** *continued*

spinal cord (see also Encephalitis) — *continued*
  meninges — see Meningitis
  streptococcal 320.2
Spirillum
  minus or minor 026.0
  morsus muris 026.0
  obermeieri 087.0
spirochetal NEC 104.9
  lung 104.8
  specified nature or site NEC 104.8
spleen 289.59
Sporothrix schenckii 117.1
Sporotrichum (schenckii) 117.1
Sporozoa 136.8
staphylococcal NEC 041.10
  aureus 041.11
  food poisoning 005.0
  generalized (purulent) 038.10
    aureus 038.11
    specified organism NEC 038.19
  pneumonia 482.40
    aureus 482.41
    specified type NEC 482.49
  septicemia 038.10
    aureus 038.11
    specified organism NEC 038.19
  specified NEC 041.19
steatoma 706.2
Stellantchasmus falcatus 121.6
Streptobacillus moniliformis 026.1
streptococcal NEC 041.00
  generalized (purulent) 038.0
  Group
    A 041.01
    B 041.02
    C 041.03
    D [enterococcus] 041.04
    G 041.05
  pneumonia — see Pneumonia, streptococcal
  septicemia 038.0
  sore throat 034.0
  specified NEC 041.09
Streptomyces — see Actinomycosis
streptotrichosis — see Actinomycosis
Strongyloides (stercoralis) 127.2
stump (amputation) (posttraumatic) (surgical) 997.62
  traumatic — see Amputation, traumatic, by site, complicated
subcutaneous tissue, local NEC 686.9
submaxillary region 528.9
suipestifer (see also Infection, Salmonella) 003.9
swimming pool bacillus 031.1
syphilitic — see Syphilis
systemic — see Septicemia
Taenia — see Infestation, Taenia
Taeniarhynchus saginatus 123.2
tapeworm — see Infestation, tapeworm
tendon (sheath) 727.89
Ternidens diminutus 127.7
testis (see also Orchitis) 604.90
thigh (skin) 686.9
threadworm 127.4
throat 478.29
  pneumococcal 462
  staphylococcal 462
  streptococcal 034.0
  viral NEC (see also Pharyngitis) 462
thumb (skin) 686.9
  abscess (with lymphangitis) 681.00
    pulp 681.01
  cellulitis (with lymphangitis) 681.00
  nail 681.02
thyroglossal duct 529.8
toe (skin) 686.9
  abscess (with lymphangitis) 681.10

**Infection, infected, infective** — *continued*
toe — *continued*
cellulitis (with lymphangitis) 681.10
nail 681.11
fungus 110.1
tongue NEC 529.0
parasitic 112.0
tonsil (faucial) (lingual) (pharyngeal) 474.00
acute or subacute 463
and adenoid 474.02
tag 474.00
tooth, teeth 522.4
periapical (pulpal origin) 522.4
peridental 523.30
periodontal 523.31
pulp 522.0
socket 526.5
Torula histolytica 117.5
Toxocara (cani) (cati) (felis) 128.0
Toxoplasma gondii (*see also* Toxoplasmosis) 130.9
trachea, chronic 491.8
fungus 117.9
traumatic NEC 958.3
trematode NEC 121.9
trench fever 083.1
Treponema
denticola 041.84
macrodenticum 041.84
pallidum (*see also* Syphilis) 097.9
Trichinella (spiralis) 124
Trichomonas 131.9
bladder 131.09
cervix 131.09
hominis 007.3
intestine 007.3
prostate 131.03
specified site NEC 131.8
urethra 131.02
urogenitalis 131.00
vagina 131.01
vulva 131.01
Trichophyton, trichophytid — *see* Dermatophytosis
Trichosporon (beigelii) cutaneum 111.2
Trichostrongylus 127.6
Trichuris (trichiuria) 127.3
Trombicula (irritans) 133.8
Trypanosoma (*see also* Trypanosomiasis) 086.9
cruzi 086.2
tubal (*see also* Salpingo-oophoritis) 614.2
tuberculous NEC (*see also* Tuberculosis) 011.9 ☑
tubo-ovarian (*see also* Salpingo-oophoritis) 614.2
tunica vaginalis 608.4
tympanic membrane — *see* Myringitis
typhoid (abortive) (ambulant) (bacillus) 002.0
typhus 081.9
flea-borne (endemic) 081.0
louse-borne (epidemic) 080
mite-borne 081.2
recrudescent 081.1
tick-borne 082.9
African 082.1
North Asian 082.2
umbilicus (septic) 686.9
newborn NEC 771.4
ureter 593.89
urethra (*see also* Urethritis) 597.80
urinary (tract) NEC 599.0
with
abortion — *see* Abortion, by type, with urinary tract infection
ectopic pregnancy (*see also* categories 633.0–633.9) 639.8

**Infection, infected, infective** — *continued*
urinary — *continued*
with — *continued*
molar pregnancy (*see also* categories 630–632) 639.8
candidal 112.2
complicating pregnancy, childbirth, or puerperium 646.6 ☑
affecting fetus or newborn 760.1
asymptomatic 646.5 ☑
affecting fetus or newborn 760.1
diplococcal (acute) 098.0
chronic 098.2
due to Trichomonas (vaginalis) 131.00
following
abortion 639.8
ectopic or molar pregnancy 639.8
gonococcal (acute) 098.0
chronic or duration of 2 months or over 098.2
newborn 771.82
trichomonal 131.00
tuberculous (*see also* Tuberculosis) 016.3 ☑
uterus, uterine (*see also* Endometritis) 615.9
utriculus masculinus NEC 597.89
vaccination 999.39 ▲
vagina (granulation tissue) (wall) (*see also* Vaginitis) 616.10
varicella 052.9
varicose veins — *see* Varicose, veins
variola 050.9
major 050.0
minor 050.1
vas deferens NEC 608.4
Veillonella 041.84
verumontanum 597.89
vesical (*see also* Cystitis) 595.9
Vibrio
cholerae 001.0
El Tor 001.1
parahaemolyticus (food poisoning) 005.4
vulnificus 041.85
Vincent's (gums) (mouth) (tonsil) 101
vaccination 999.39 ▲
virus, viral 079.99
adenovirus
in diseases classified elsewhere — *see* category 079 ☑
unspecified nature or site 079.0
central nervous system NEC 049.9
enterovirus 048
meningitis 047.9
specified type NEC 047.8
slow virus 046.9
specified condition NEC 046.8
chest 519.8
conjunctivitis 077.99
specified type NEC 077.8
coronavirus 079.89
SARS-associated 079.82
Coxsackie (*see also* Infection, Coxsackie) 079.2
Ebola 065.8
ECHO
in diseases classified elsewhere — *see* category 079 ☑
unspecified nature or site 079.1
encephalitis 049.9
arthropod-borne NEC 064
tick-borne 063.9
specified type NEC 063.8
enteritis NEC (*see also* Enteritis, viral) 008.8
exanthem NEC 057.9
Hantavirus 079.81
human papilloma 079.4

**Infection, infected, infective** — *continued*
virus, viral — *continued*
in diseases classified elsewhere — *see* category 079 ☑
intestine (*see also* Enteritis, viral) 008.8
lung — *see* Pneumonia, viral
respiratory syncytial (RSV) 079.6
retrovirus 079.50
rhinovirus
in diseases classified elsewhere — *see* category 079 ☑
unspecified nature or site 079.3
salivary gland disease 078.5
slow 046.9
specified condition NEC 046.8
specified type NEC 079.89
in diseases classified elsewhere — *see* category 079 ☑
unspecified nature or site 079.99
warts NEC 078.10
vulva (*see also* Vulvitis) 616.10
whipworm 127.3
Whitmore's bacillus 025
wound (local) (posttraumatic) NEC 958.3
with
dislocation — *see* Dislocation, by site, open
fracture — *see* Fracture, by site, open
open wound — *see* Wound, open, by site, complicated
postoperative 998.59
surgical 998.59
Wuchereria 125.0
bancrofti 125.0
malayi 125.1
yaws — *see* Yaws
yeast (*see also* Candidiasis) 112.9
yellow fever (*see also* Fever, yellow) 060.9
Yersinia pestis (*see also* Plague) 020.9
Zeis' gland 373.12
zoonotic bacterial NEC 027.9
Zopfia senegalensis 117.4
**Infective, infectious** — *see* condition
**Inferiority complex** 301.9
constitutional psychopathic 301.9
**Infertility**
female 628.9
age related 628.8
associated with
adhesions, peritubal 614.6 *[628.2]*
anomaly
cervical mucus 628.4
congenital
cervix 628.4
fallopian tube 628.2
uterus 628.3
vagina 628.4
anovulation 628.0
dysmucorrhea 628.4
endometritis, tuberculous (*see also* Tuberculosis) 016.7 ☑ *[628.3]*
Stein-Leventhal syndrome 256.4 *[628.0]*
due to
adiposogenital dystrophy 253.8 *[628.1]*
anterior pituitary disorder NEC 253.4 *[628.1]*
hyperfunction 253.1 *[628.1]*
cervical anomaly 628.4
fallopian tube anomaly 628.2
ovarian failure 256.39 *[628.0]*
Stein-Leventhal syndrome 256.4 *[628.0]*
uterine anomaly 628.3
vaginal anomaly 628.4
nonimplantation 628.3
origin
cervical 628.4

**Infertility** — *continued*
female — *continued*
origin — *continued*
pituitary-hypothalamus NEC 253.8 *[628.1]*
anterior pituitary NEC 253.4 *[628.1]*
hyperfunction NEC 253.1 *[628.1]*
dwarfism 253.3 *[628.1]*
panhypopituitarism 253.2 *[628.1]*
specified NEC 628.8
tubal (block) (occlusion) (stenosis) 628.2
adhesions 614.6 *[628.2]*
uterine 628.3
vaginal 628.4
previous, requiring supervision of pregnancy V23.0
male 606.9
absolute 606.0
due to
azoospermia 606.0
drug therapy 606.8
extratesticular cause NEC 606.8
germinal cell
aplasia 606.0
desquamation 606.1
hypospermatogenesis 606.1
infection 606.8
obstruction, afferent ducts 606.8
oligospermia 606.1
radiation 606.8
spermatogenic arrest (complete) 606.0
incomplete 606.1
systemic disease 606.8
**Infestation** 134.9
Acanthocheilonema (perstans) 125.4
streptocerca 125.6
Acariasis 133.9
demodex folliculorum 133.8
Sarcoptes scabiei 133.0
trombiculae 133.8
Agamofilaria streptocerca 125.6
Ancylostoma, Ankylostoma 126.9
americanum 126.1
braziliense 126.2
canium 126.8
ceylanicum 126.3
duodenale 126.0
new world 126.1
old world 126.0
Angiostrongylus cantonensis 128.8
anisakiasis 127.1
Anisakis larva 127.1
arthropod NEC 134.1
Ascaris lumbricoides 127.0
Bacillus fusiformis 101
Balantidium coli 007.0
beef tapeworm 123.2
Bothriocephalus (latus) 123.4
larval 123.5
broad tapeworm 123.4
larval 123.5
Brugia malayi 125.1
Candiru 136.8
Capillaria
hepatica 128.8
philippinensis 127.5
cat liver fluke 121.0
Cercomonas hominis (intestinal) 007.3
cestodes 123.9
specified type NEC 123.8
chigger 133.8
chigoe 134.1
Chilomastix 007.8
Clonorchis (sinensis) (liver) 121.1
coccidia 007.2
complicating pregnancy, childbirth, or puerperium 647.9 ☑
affecting fetus or newborn 760.8
Cysticercus cellulosae 123.1
Demodex folliculorum 133.8

☑ Additional Digit Required — Refer to the Tabular List for Digit Selection      ▽ Subterms under main terms may continue to next column or page

*2008 ICD-9-CM*     ►◄ Revised Text     ● New Line     ▲ Revised Code     October 2007 · Volume 2 — 161

**Infestation** — *continued*
Dermatobia (hominis) 134.0
Dibothriocephalus (latus) 123.4
  larval 123.5
Dicrocoelium dendriticum 121.8
Diphyllobothrium (adult) (intestinal)
  (latum) (pacificum) 123.4
  larval 123.5
Diplogonoporus (grandis) 123.8
Dipylidium (caninum) 123.8
Distoma hepaticum 121.3
dog tapeworm 123.8
Dracunculus medinensis 125.7
dragon worm 125.7
dwarf tapeworm 123.6
Echinococcus (*see also* Echinococcus)
  122.9
Echinostoma ilocanum 121.8
Embadomonas 007.8
Endamoeba (histolytica) — *see* Infection, ameba
Entamoeba (histolytica) — *see* Infection, ameba
Enterobius vermicularis 127.4
Epidermophyton — *see* Dermatophytosis
eyeworm 125.2
Fasciola
  gigantica 121.3
  hepatica 121.3
Fasciolopsis (buski) (small intestine)
  121.4
blood NEC (*see also* Schistosomiasis) 120.9
cat liver 121.0
filarial 125.9
  due to
    Acanthocheilonema (per-
     stans) 125.4
      streptocerca 125.6
    Brugia (Wuchereria) malayi
     125.1
    Dracunculus medinensis
     125.7
    guinea worms 125.7
    Mansonella (ozzardi) 125.5
    Onchocerca volvulus 125.3
     eye 125.3 *[360.13]*
     eyelid 125.3 *[373.6]*
    Wuchereria (bancrofti) 125.0
     malayi 125.1
  specified type NEC 125.6
fish tapeworm 123.4
  larval 123.5
fluke 121.9
intestinal (giant) 121.4
liver (sheep) 121.3
  cat 121.0
  Chinese 121.1
  clonorchiasis 121.1
  fascioliasis 121.3
  Oriental 121.1
lung (oriental) 121.2
sheep liver 121.3
fly larva 134.0
Gasterophilus (intestinalis) 134.0
Gastrodiscoides hominis 121.8
Giardia lamblia 007.1
Gnathostoma (spinigerum) 128.1
Gongylonema 125.6
guinea worm 125.7
helminth NEC 128.9
  intestinal 127.9
    mixed (types classifiable to more
     than one category in
     120.0–127.7) 127.8
    specified type NEC 127.7
  specified type NEC 128.8
Heterophyes heterophyes (small intestine) 121.6
hookworm (*see also* Infestation, ancylostoma) 126.9
Hymenolepis (diminuta) (nana) 123.6
intestinal NEC 129
leeches (aquatic) (land) 134.2
Leishmania — *see* Leishmaniasis

**Infestation** — *continued*
lice (*see also* Infestation, pediculus)
  132.9
Linguatulidae, linguatula (pentas-
  toma) (serrata) 134.1
Loa loa 125.2
  eyelid 125.2 *[373.6]*
louse (*see also* Infestation, pediculus)
  132.9
  body 132.1
  head 132.0
  pubic 132.2
maggots 134.0
Mansonella (ozzardi) 125.5
medina 125.7
Metagonimus yokogawai (small intestine) 121.5
Microfilaria streptocerca 125.3
  eye 125.3 *[360.13]*
  eyelid 125.3 *[373.6]*
Microsporon furfur 111.0
microsporum — *see* Dermatophytosis
mites 133.9
  scabic 133.0
  specified type NEC 133.8
monilia (albicans) (*see also* Candidiasis) 112.9
  vagina 112.1
  vulva 112.1
mouth 112.0
Necator americanus 126.1
nematode (intestinal) 127.9
  Ancylostoma (*see also* Ancy-
    lostoma) 126.9
  Ascaris lumbricoides 127.0
  conjunctiva NEC 128.9
  Dioctophyma 128.8
  Enterobius vermicularis 127.4
  Gnathostoma spinigerum 128.1
  Oesophagostomum (apiostomum)
    127.7
  Physaloptera 127.4
  specified type NEC 127.7
  Strongyloides stercoralis 127.2
  Ternidens diminutus 127.7
  Trichinella spiralis 124
  Trichostrongylus 127.6
  Trichuris (trichiuria) 127.3
Oesophagostomum (apiostomum)
  127.7
Oestrus ovis 134.0
Onchocerca (volvulus) 125.3
  eye 125.3 *[360.13]*
  eyelid 125.3 *[373.6]*
Opisthorchis (felineus) (tenuicollis)
  (viverrini) 121.0
Oxyuris vermicularis 127.4
Paragonimus (westermani) 121.2
parasite, parasitic NEC 136.9
  eyelid 134.9 *[373.6]*
  intestinal 129
  mouth 112.0
  orbit 376.13
  skin 134.9
  tongue 112.0
pediculus 132.9
  capitis (humanus) (any site) 132.0
  corporis (humanus) (any site) 132.1
  eyelid 132.0 *[373.6]*
  mixed (classifiable to more than
    one category in 132.0–132.2)
    132.3
  pubis (any site) 132.2
phthirus (pubis) (any site) 132.2
  with any infestation classifiable to
    132.0, 132.1 and 132.3
pinworm 127.4
pork tapeworm (adult) 123.0
protozoal NEC 136.8
pubic louse 132.2
rat tapeworm 123.6
red bug 133.8
roundworm (large) NEC 127.0
sand flea 134.1
saprophytic NEC 136.8
Sarcoptes scabiei 133.0

**Infestation** — *continued*
scabies 133.0
Schistosoma 120.9
  bovis 120.8
  cercariae 120.3
  hematobium 120.0
  intercalatum 120.8
  japonicum 120.2
  mansoni 120.1
  mattheii 120.8
  specified
    site — *see* Schistosomiasis
    type NEC 120.8
  spindale 120.8
screw worms 134.0
skin NEC 134.9
Sparganum (mansoni) (proliferum)
  123.5
  larval 123.5
specified type NEC 134.8
Spirometra larvae 123.5
Sporozoa NEC 136.8
Stellantchasmus falcatus 121.6
Strongyloides 127.2
Strongylus (gibsoni) 127.7
Taenia 123.3
  diminuta 123.6
  Echinococcus (*see also* Echinococ-
    cus) 122.9
  mediocanellata 123.2
  nana 123.6
  saginata (mediocanellata) 123.2
  solium (intestinal form) 123.0
    larval form 123.1
Taeniarhynchus saginatus 123.2
tapeworm 123.9
  beef 123.2
  broad 123.4
    larval 123.5
  dog 123.8
  dwarf 123.6
  fish 123.4
    larval 123.5
  pork 123.0
  rat 123.6
Ternidens diminutus 127.7
Tetranychus molestissimus 133.8
threadworm 127.4
tongue 112.0
Toxocara (cani) (cati) (felis) 128.0
trematode(s) NEC 121.9
Trichina spiralis 124
Trichinella spiralis 124
Trichocephalus 127.3
Trichomonas 131.9
  bladder 131.09
  cervix 131.09
  intestine 007.3
  prostate 131.03
  specified site NEC 131.8
  urethra (female) (male) 131.02
  urogenital 131.00
  vagina 131.01
  vulva 131.01
Trichophyton — *see* Dermatophytosis
Trichostrongylus instabilis 127.6
Trichuris (trichiuria) 127.3
Trombicula (irritans) 133.8
Trypanosoma — *see* Trypanosomiasis
Tunga penetrans 134.1
Uncinaria americana 126.1
whipworm 127.3
worms NEC 128.9
  intestinal 127.9
Wuchereria 125.0
  bancrofti 125.0
  malayi 125.1

**Infiltrate, infiltration**
with an iron compound 275.0
amyloid (any site) (generalized) 277.39
calcareous (muscle) NEC 275.49
  localized — *see* Degeneration, by
    site
calcium salt (muscle) 275.49
corneal (*see also* Edema, cornea)
  371.20

**Infiltrate, infiltration** — *continued*
eyelid 373.9
fatty (diffuse) (generalized) 272.8
  localized — *see* Degeneration, by
    site, fatty
glycogen, glycogenic (*see also* Disease,
  glycogen storage) 271.0
heart, cardiac
  fatty (*see also* Degeneration, my-
    ocardial) 429.1
  glycogenic 271.0 *[425.7]*
inflammatory in vitreous 379.29
kidney (*see also* Disease, renal) 593.9
leukemic (M9800/3) — *see* Leukemia
liver 573.8
  fatty — *see* Fatty, liver
  glycogen (*see also* Disease, glyco-
    gen storage) 271.0
lung (*see also* Infiltrate, pulmonary)
  518.3
  eosinophilic 518.3
  x-ray finding only 793.1
lymphatic (*see also* Leukemia, lymphatic) 204.9 ☑
  gland, pigmentary 289.3
muscle, fatty 728.9
myelogenous (*see also* Leukemia,
  myeloid) 205.9 ☑
myocardium, myocardial
  fatty (*see also* Degeneration, my-
    ocardial) 429.1
  glycogenic 271.0 *[425.7]*
pulmonary 518.3
  with
    eosinophilia 518.3
    pneumonia — *see* Pneumonia,
     by type
  x-ray finding only 793.1
  Ranke's primary (*see also* Tuberculo-
    sis) 010.0 ☑
skin, lymphocytic (benign) 709.8
thymus (gland) (fatty) 254.8
urine 788.8
vitreous humor 379.29
**Infirmity** 799.89
senile 797
**Inflammation, inflamed, inflammatory**
(with exudation)
abducens (nerve) 378.54
accessory sinus (chronic) (*see also* Sinusitis) 473.9
adrenal (gland) 255.8
alimentary canal — *see* Enteritis
alveoli (teeth) 526.5
  scorbutic 267
amnion — *see* Amnionitis
anal canal 569.49
antrum (chronic) (*see also* Sinusitis,
  maxillary) 473.0
anus 569.49
appendix (*see also* Appendicitis) 541
arachnoid — *see* Meningitis
areola 611.0
  puerperal, postpartum 675.0 ☑
areolar tissue NEC 686.9
artery — *see* Arteritis
auditory meatus (external) (*see also*
  Otitis, externa) 380.10
Bartholin's gland 616.89
bile duct or passage 576.1
bladder (*see also* Cystitis) 595.9
bleb
  postprocedural 379.60
    stage 1 379.61
    stage 2 379.62
    stage 3 379.63
bone — *see* Osteomyelitis
bowel (*see also* Enteritis) 558.9
brain (*see also* Encephalitis) 323.9
  late effect — *see* category 326
  membrane — *see* Meningitis
breast 611.0
  puerperal, postpartum 675.2 ☑
broad ligament (*see also* Disease,
  pelvis, inflammatory) 614.4
  acute 614.3

**Inflammation, inflamed, inflammatory**
— *continued*
bronchus — *see* Bronchitis
bursa — *see* Bursitis
capsule
   liver 573.3
   spleen 289.59
catarrhal (*see also* Catarrh) 460
   vagina 616.10
cecum (*see also* Appendicitis) 541
cerebral (*see also* Encephalitis) 323.9
   late effect — *see* category 326
   membrane — *see* Meningitis
cerebrospinal (*see also* Meningitis)
   322.9
   late effect — *see* category 326
   meningococcal 036.0
   tuberculous (*see also* Tuberculosis)
    013.6 ☑
cervix (uteri) (*see also* Cervicitis) 616.0
chest 519.9
choroid NEC (*see also* Choroiditis)
   363.20
cicatrix (tissue) — *see* Cicatrix
colon (*see also* Enteritis) 558.9
   granulomatous 555.1
   newborn 558.9
connective tissue (diffuse) NEC 728.9
cornea (*see also* Keratitis) 370.9
   with ulcer (*see also* Ulcer, cornea)
    370.00
corpora cavernosa (penis) 607.2
cranial nerve — *see* Disorder, nerve,
   cranial
diarrhea — *see* Diarrhea
disc (intervertebral) (space) 722.90
   cervical, cervicothoracic 722.91
   lumbar, lumbosacral 722.93
   thoracic, thoracolumbar 722.92
Douglas' cul-de-sac or pouch (chronic)
   (*see also* Disease, pelvis, inflammatory) 614.4
   acute 614.3
due to (presence of) any device, implant, or graft classifiable to
   996.0–996.5 — *see* Complications, infection and inflammation, due to (presence of) any
   device, implant, or graft classified to 996.0–996.5 NEC
duodenum 535.6 ☑
dura mater — *see* Meningitis
ear (*see also* Otitis)
   external (*see also* Otitis, externa)
    380.10
   inner (*see also* Labyrinthitis)
    386.30
   middle — *see* Otitis media
esophagus 530.10
ethmoidal (chronic) (sinus) (*see also*
   Sinusitis, ethmoidal) 473.2
Eustachian tube (catarrhal) 381.50
   acute 381.51
   chronic 381.52
extrarectal 569.49
eye 379.99
eyelid 373.9
   specified NEC 373.8
fallopian tube (*see also* Salpingo-
   oophoritis) 614.2
fascia 728.9
fetal membranes (acute) 658.4 ☑
   affecting fetus or newborn 762.7
follicular, pharynx 472.1
frontal (chronic) (sinus) (*see also* Sinusitis, frontal) 473.1
gallbladder (*see also* Cholecystitis,
   acute) 575.0
gall duct (*see also* Cholecystitis)
   575.10
gastrointestinal (*see also* Enteritis)
   558.9
genital organ (diffuse) (internal)
   female 614.9

**Inflammation, inflamed, inflammatory**
— *continued*
genital organ — *continued*
   female — *continued*
    with
     abortion — *see* Abortion, by
      type, with sepsis
     ectopic pregnancy (*see also*
      categories
      633.0–633.9) 639.0
     molar pregnancy (*see also*
      categories 630–632)
      639.0
     complicating pregnancy, child-
      birth, or puerperium
      646.6 ☑
     affecting fetus or newborn
      760.8
    following
     abortion 639.0
     ectopic or molar pregnancy
      639.0
   male 608.4
gland (lymph) (*see also* Lymphadenitis) 289.3
glottis (*see also* Laryngitis) 464.00
   with obstruction 464.01
granular, pharynx 472.1
gum 523.10
heart (*see also* Carditis) 429.89
hepatic duct 576.8
hernial sac — *see* Hernia, by site
ileum (*see also* Enteritis) 558.9
   terminal or regional 555.0
    with large intestine 555.2
intervertebral disc 722.90
   cervical, cervicothoracic 722.91
   lumbar, lumbosacral 722.93
   thoracic, thoracolumbar 722.92
intestine (*see also* Enteritis) 558.9
jaw (acute) (bone) (chronic) (lower)
   (suppurative) (upper) 526.4
jejunum — *see* Enteritis
joint NEC (*see also* Arthritis) 716.9 ☑
   sacroiliac 720.2
kidney (*see also* Nephritis) 583.9
knee (joint) 716.66
   tuberculous (active) (*see also* Tuber-
    culosis) 015.2 ☑
labium (majus) (minus) (*see also* Vulvitis) 616.10
lacrimal
   gland (*see also* Dacryoadenitis)
    375.00
   passages (duct) (sac) (*see also*
    Dacryocystitis) 375.30
larynx (*see also* Laryngitis) 464.00
   with obstruction 464.01
   diphtheritic 032.3
leg NEC 686.9
lip 528.5
liver (capsule) (*see also* Hepatitis)
   573.3
   acute 570
   chronic 571.40
   suppurative 572.0
lung (acute) (*see also* Pneumonia) 486
   chronic (interstitial) 518.89
lymphatic vessel (*see also* Lymphangitis) 457.2
lymph node or gland (*see also* Lymphadenitis) 289.3
mammary gland 611.0
   puerperal, postpartum 675.2 ☑
maxilla, maxillary 526.4
   sinus (chronic) (*see also* Sinusitis,
    maxillary) 473.0
membranes of brain or spinal cord —
   *see* Meningitis
meninges — *see* Meningitis
mouth 528.00
muscle 728.9
myocardium (*see also* Myocarditis)
   429.0
nasal sinus (chronic) (*see also* Sinusitis) 473.9

**Inflammation, inflamed, inflammatory**
— *continued*
nasopharynx — *see* Nasopharyngitis
navel 686.9
   newborn NEC 771.4
nerve NEC 729.2
nipple 611.0
   puerperal, postpartum 675.0 ☑
nose 478.19
   suppurative 472.0
oculomotor nerve 378.51
optic nerve 377.30
orbit (chronic) 376.10
   acute 376.00
   chronic 376.10
ovary (*see also* Salpingo-oophoritis)
   614.2
oviduct (*see also* Salpingo-oophoritis)
   614.2
pancreas — *see* Pancreatitis
parametrium (chronic) (*see also* Disease, pelvis, inflammatory)
   614.4
   acute 614.3
parotid region 686.9
   gland 527.2
pelvis, female (*see also* Disease, pelvis,
   inflammatory) 614.9
penis (corpora cavernosa) 607.2
perianal 569.49
pericardium (*see also* Pericarditis)
   423.9
perineum (female) (male) 686.9
perirectal 569.49
peritoneum (*see also* Peritonitis) 567.9
periuterine (*see also* Disease, pelvis,
   inflammatory) 614.9
perivesical (*see also* Cystitis) 595.9
petrous bone (*see also* Petrositis)
   383.20
pharynx (*see also* Pharyngitis) 462
   follicular 472.1
   granular 472.1
pia mater — *see* Meningitis
pleura — *see* Pleurisy
postmastoidectomy cavity 383.30
   chronic 383.33
prostate (*see also* Prostatitis) 601.9
rectosigmoid — *see* Rectosigmoiditis
rectum (*see also* Proctitis) 569.49
respiratory, upper (*see also* Infection,
   respiratory, upper) 465.9
   chronic, due to external agent —
    *see* Condition, respiratory,
    chronic, due to, external
    agent
   due to
    fumes or vapors (chemical) (in-
     halation) 506.2
    radiation 508.1
retina (*see also* Retinitis) 363.20
retrocecal (*see also* Appendicitis) 541
retroperitoneal (*see also* Peritonitis)
   567.9
salivary duct or gland (any) (suppurative) 527.2
scorbutic, alveoli, teeth 267
scrotum 608.4
sigmoid — *see* Enteritis
sinus (*see also* Sinusitis) 473.9
Skene's duct or gland (*see also* Urethritis) 597.89
skin 686.9
spermatic cord 608.4
sphenoidal (sinus) (*see also* Sinusitis,
   sphenoidal) 473.3
spinal
   cord (*see also* Encephalitis) 323.9
    late effect — *see* category 326
   membrane — *see* Meningitis
   nerve — *see* Disorder, nerve
spine (*see also* Spondylitis) 720.9
spleen (capsule) 289.59
stomach — *see* Gastritis
stricture, rectum 569.49
subcutaneous tissue NEC 686.9

**Inflammation, inflamed, inflammatory**
— *continued*
suprarenal (gland) 255.8
synovial (fringe) (membrane) — *see*
   Bursitis
tendon (sheath) NEC 726.90
testis (*see also* Orchitis) 604.90
thigh 686.9
throat (*see also* Sore throat) 462
thymus (gland) 254.8
thyroid (gland) (*see also* Thyroiditis)
   245.9
tongue 529.0
tonsil — *see* Tonsillitis
trachea — *see* Tracheitis
trochlear nerve 378.53
tubal (*see also* Salpingo-oophoritis)
   614.2
tuberculous NEC (*see also* Tuberculosis) 011.9 ☑
tubo-ovarian (*see also* Salpingo-
   oophoritis) 614.2
tunica vaginalis 608.4
tympanic membrane — *see* Myringitis
umbilicus, umbilical 686.9
   newborn NEC 771.4
uterine ligament (*see also* Disease,
   pelvis, inflammatory) 614.4
   acute 614.3
uterus (catarrhal) (*see also* Endometritis) 615.9
uveal tract (anterior) (*see also* Iridocyclitis) 364.3
   posterior — *see* Chorioretinitis
   sympathetic 360.11
vagina (*see also* Vaginitis) 616.10
vas deferens 608.4
vein (*see also* Phlebitis) 451.9
   thrombotic 451.9
    cerebral (*see also* Thrombosis,
     brain) 434.0 ☑
    leg 451.2
     deep (vessels) NEC 451.19
     superficial (vessels) 451.0
    lower extremity 451.2
     deep (vessels) NEC 451.19
     superficial (vessels) 451.0
vocal cord 478.5
vulva (*see also* Vulvitis) 616.10
**Inflation, lung imperfect** (newborn)
   770.5
**Influenza, influenzal** 487.1
   with
    bronchitis 487.1
    bronchopneumonia 487.0
    cold (any type) 487.1
    digestive manifestations 487.8
    hemoptysis 487.1
    involvement of
     gastrointestinal tract 487.8
     nervous system 487.8
    laryngitis 487.1
    manifestations NEC 487.8
     respiratory 487.1
      pneumonia 487.0
    pharyngitis 487.1
    pneumonia (any form classifiable
     to 480–483, 485–486) 487.0
    respiratory manifestations NEC
     487.1
    sinusitis 487.1
    sore throat 487.1
    tonsillitis 487.1
    tracheitis 487.1
    upper respiratory infection (acute)
     487.1
   abdominal 487.8
   Asian 487.1
   bronchial 487.1
   bronchopneumonia 487.0
   catarrhal 487.1
   due to identified avian influenza   ●
    virus 488   ●
   epidemic 487.1
   gastric 487.8
   intestinal 487.8

---

☑ Additional Digit Required — Refer to the Tabular List for Digit Selection          ▽ Subterms under main terms may continue to next column or page

**Influenza, influenzal** — *continued*
  laryngitis 487.1
  maternal affecting fetus or newborn
    760.2
    manifest influenza in infant 771.2
  pharyngitis 487.1
  pneumonia (any form) 487.0
  respiratory (upper) 487.1
  stomach 487.8
  vaccination, prophylactic (against)
    V04.81
**Influenza-like disease** 487.1
**Infraction, Freiberg's** (metatarsal head)
  732.5
**Infraeruption, teeth** 524.34
**Infusion complication, misadventure,
  or reaction** — *see* Complication,
    infusion
**Ingestion**
  chemical — *see* Table of Drugs and
    Chemicals
  drug or medicinal substance
    overdose or wrong substance given
      or taken 977.9
      specified drug — *see* Table of
        Drugs and Chemicals
  foreign body NEC (*see also* Foreign
    body) 938
**Ingrowing**
  hair 704.8
  nail (finger) (toe) (infected) 703.0
**Inguinal** — *see also* condition
  testis 752.51
**Inhalation**
  carbon monoxide 986
  flame
    lung 947.1
    mouth 947.0
  food or foreign body (*see also* Asphyx-
    ia, food or foreign body) 933.1
  gas, fumes, or vapor (noxious) 987.9
    specified agent — *see* Table of
      Drugs and Chemicals
  liquid or vomitus (*see also* Asphyxia,
    food or foreign body) 933.1
    lower respiratory tract NEC 934.9
  meconium (fetus or newborn) 770.11
    with respiratory symptoms 770.12
  mucus (*see also* Asphyxia, mucus)
    933.1
  oil (causing suffocation) (*see also* As-
    phyxia, food or foreign body)
    933.1
  pneumonia — *see* Pneumonia, aspira-
    tion
  smoke 987.9
  steam 987.9
  stomach contents or secretions (*see
    also* Asphyxia, food or foreign
    body) 933.1
    in labor and delivery 668.0 ☑
**Inhibition, inhibited**
  academic as adjustment reaction
    309.23
  orgasm
    female 302.73
    male 302.74
  sexual
    desire 302.71
    excitement 302.72
  work as adjustment reaction 309.23
**Inhibitor, systemic lupus erythemato-
  sus** (presence of) 286.5
**Iniencephalus, iniencephaly** 740.2
**Injected eye** 372.74

**Injury** 959.9

*Note — For abrasion, insect bite (nonven-
omous), blister, or scratch, see Injury,
superficial.*

*For laceration, traumatic rupture, tear,
or penetrating wound of internal organs,
such as heart, lung, liver, kidney, pelvic
organs, whether or not accompanied by
open wound in the same region, see Injury, internal.*

*For nerve injury, see Injury, nerve.*

*For late effect of injuries classifiable to
850–854, 860–869, 900–919, 950–959,
see Late, effect, injury, by type.*

  abdomen, abdominal (viscera) (*see al-
    so* Injury, internal, abdomen)
    muscle or wall 959.12
  acoustic, resulting in deafness 951.5
  adenoid 959.09
  adrenal (gland) — *see* Injury, internal,
    adrenal
  alveolar (process) 959.09
  ankle (and foot) (and knee) (and leg,
    except thigh) 959.7
  anterior chamber, eye 921.3
  anus 959.19
  aorta (thoracic) 901.0
    abdominal 902.0
  appendix — *see* Injury, internal, ap-
    pendix
  arm, upper (and shoulder) 959.2
  artery (complicating trauma) (*see also*
    Injury, blood vessel, by site)
    904.9
    cerebral or meningeal (*see also*
      Hemorrhage, brain, traumat-
      ic, subarachnoid) 852.0 ☑
  auditory canal (external) (meatus)
    959.09
  auricle, auris, ear 959.09
  axilla 959.2
  back 959.19
  bile duct — *see* Injury, internal, bile
    duct
  birth (*see also* Birth, injury)
    canal NEC, complicating delivery
      665.9 ☑
  bladder (sphincter) — *see* Injury, inter-
    nal, bladder
  blast (air) (hydraulic) (immersion)
    (underwater) NEC 869.0
    with open wound into cavity NEC
      869.1
    abdomen or thorax — *see* Injury,
      internal, by site
    brain — *see* Concussion, brain
    ear (acoustic nerve trauma) 951.5
      with perforation of tympanic
        membrane — *see* Wound,
        open, ear, drum
  blood vessel NEC 904.9
    abdomen 902.9
      multiple 902.87
      specified NEC 902.89
    aorta (thoracic) 901.0
      abdominal 902.0
    arm NEC 903.9
    axillary 903.00
      artery 903.01
      vein 903.02
    azygos vein 901.89
    basilic vein 903.1
    brachial (artery) (vein) 903.1
    bronchial 901.89
    carotid artery 900.00
      common 900.01
      external 900.02
      internal 900.03
    celiac artery 902.20
      specified branch NEC 902.24
    cephalic vein (arm) 903.1
    colica dextra 902.26
    cystic
      artery 902.24

**Injury** — *continued*
  blood vessel — *continued*
    cystic — *continued*
      vein 902.39
    deep plantar 904.6
    digital (artery) (vein) 903.5
    due to accidental puncture or lac-
      eration during procedure
      998.2
    extremity
      lower 904.8
        multiple 904.7
        specified NEC 904.7
      upper 903.9
        multiple 903.8
        specified NEC 903.8
    femoral
      artery (superficial) 904.1
        above profunda origin 904.0
        common 904.0
      vein 904.2
    gastric
      artery 902.21
      vein 902.39
    head 900.9
      intracranial — *see* Injury, in-
        tracranial
      multiple 900.82
      specified NEC 900.89
    hemiazygos vein 901.89
    hepatic
      artery 902.22
      vein 902.11
    hypogastric 902.59
      artery 902.51
      vein 902.52
    ileocolic
      artery 902.26
      vein 902.31
    iliac 902.50
      artery 902.53
      specified branch NEC 902.59
      vein 902.54
    innominate
      artery 901.1
      vein 901.3
    intercostal (artery) (vein) 901.81
    jugular vein (external) 900.81
      internal 900.1
    leg NEC 904.8
    mammary (artery) (vein) 901.82
    mesenteric
      artery 902.20
        inferior 902.27
        specified branch NEC 902.29
        superior (trunk) 902.25
          branches, primary 902.26
      vein 902.39
        inferior 902.32
        superior (and primary subdi-
          visions) 902.31
    neck 900.9
      multiple 900.82
      specified NEC 900.89
    ovarian 902.89
      artery 902.81
      vein 902.82
    palmar artery 903.4
    pelvis 902.9
      multiple 902.87
      specified NEC 902.89
    plantar (deep) (artery) (vein) 904.6
    popliteal 904.40
      artery 904.41
      vein 904.42
    portal 902.33
    pulmonary 901.40
      artery 901.41
      vein 901.42
    radial (artery) (vein) 903.2
    renal 902.40
      artery 902.41
      specified NEC 902.49
      vein 902.42
    saphenous
      artery 904.7

**Injury** — *continued*
  blood vessel — *continued*
    saphenous — *continued*
      vein (greater) (lesser) 904.3
    splenic
      artery 902.23
      vein 902.34
    subclavian
      artery 901.1
      vein 901.3
    suprarenal 902.49
    thoracic 901.9
      multiple 901.83
      specified NEC 901.89
    tibial 904.50
      artery 904.50
        anterior 904.51
        posterior 904.53
      vein 904.50
        anterior 904.52
        posterior 904.54
    ulnar (artery) (vein) 903.3
    uterine 902.59
      artery 902.55
      vein 902.56
    vena cava
      inferior 902.10
        specified branches NEC
          902.19
      superior 901.2
  brachial plexus 953.4
    newborn 767.6
  brain NEC (*see also* Injury, intracra-
    nial) 854.0 ☑
  breast 959.19
  broad ligament — *see* Injury, internal,
    broad ligament
  bronchus, bronchi — *see* Injury, inter-
    nal, bronchus
  brow 959.09
  buttock 959.19
  canthus, eye 921.1
  cathode ray 990
  cauda equina 952.4
    with fracture, vertebra — *see*
      Fracture, vertebra, sacrum
  cavernous sinus (*see also* Injury, in-
    tracranial) 854.0 ☑
  cecum — *see* Injury, internal, cecum
  celiac ganglion or plexus 954.1
  cerebellum (*see also* Injury, intracra-
    nial) 854.0 ☑
  cervix (uteri) — *see* Injury, internal,
    cervix
  cheek 959.09
  chest (*see also* Injury, internal, chest)
    wall 959.11
  childbirth (*see also* Birth, injury)
    maternal NEC 665.9 ☑
  chin 959.09
  choroid (eye) 921.3
  clitoris 959.14
  coccyx 959.19
    complicating delivery 665.6 ☑
  colon — *see* Injury, internal, colon
  common duct — *see* Injury, internal,
    common duct
  conjunctiva 921.1
    superficial 918.2
  cord
    spermatic — *see* Injury, internal,
      spermatic cord
    spinal — *see* Injury, spinal, by site
  cornea 921.3
    abrasion 918.1
    due to contact lens 371.82
    penetrating — *see* Injury, eyeball,
      penetrating
    superficial 918.1
      due to contact lens 371.82
  cortex (cerebral) (*see also* Injury, in-
    tracranial) 854.0 ☑
    visual 950.3
  costal region 959.11
  costochondral 959.11

☑ Additional Digit Required — Refer to the Tabular List for Digit Selection                    ᴴᴱˢ Subterms under main terms may continue to next column or page

164 — Volume 2          ▶◀ Revised Text          ● New Line          ▲ Revised Code          *2008 ICD-9-CM*

**Injury** — *continued*
  cranial
    bones — *see* Fracture, skull, by
      site
    cavity (*see also* Injury, intracranial)
      854.0 ☑
    nerve — *see* Injury, nerve, cranial
  crushing — *see* Crush
  cutaneous sensory nerve
    lower limb 956.4
    upper limb 955.5
  delivery (*see also* Birth, injury)
    maternal NEC 665.9 ☑
  Descemet's membrane — *see* Injury,
    eyeball, penetrating
  diaphragm — *see* Injury, internal, di-
    aphragm
  diffuse axonal — *see* Injury, intracra-
    nial
  duodenum — *see* Injury, internal,
    duodenum
  ear (auricle) (canal) (drum) (external)
    959.09
  elbow (and forearm) (and wrist) 959.3
  epididymis 959.14
  epigastric region 959.12
  epiglottis 959.09
  epiphyseal, current — *see* Fracture,
    by site
  esophagus — *see* Injury, internal,
    esophagus
  Eustachian tube 959.09
  extremity (lower) (upper) NEC 959.8
  eye 921.9
    penetrating eyeball — *see* Injury,
      eyeball, penetrating
    superficial 918.9
  eyeball 921.3
    penetrating 871.7
      with
        partial loss (of intraocular
          tissue) 871.2
        prolapse or exposure (of in-
          traocular tissue) 871.1
      without prolapse 871.0
      foreign body (nonmagnetic)
        871.6
        magnetic 871.5
    superficial 918.9
  eyebrow 959.09
  eyelid(s) 921.1
    laceration — *see* Laceration, eyelid
    superficial 918.0
  face (and neck) 959.09
  fallopian tube — *see* Injury, internal,
    fallopian tube
  finger(s) (nail) 959.5
  flank 959.19
  foot (and ankle) (and knee) (and leg,
    except thigh) 959.7
  forceps NEC 767.9
    scalp 767.19
  forearm (and elbow) (and wrist) 959.3
  forehead 959.09
  gallbladder — *see* Injury, internal,
    gallbladder
  gasserian ganglion 951.2
  gastrointestinal tract — *see* Injury,
    internal, gastrointestinal tract
  genital organ(s)
    with
      abortion — *see* Abortion, by
        type, with, damage to
        pelvic organs
      ectopic pregnancy (*see also* cat-
        egories 633.0–633.9)
        639.2
      molar pregnancy (*see also* cate-
        gories 630–632) 639.2
    external 959.14
      fracture of corpus cavernosum
        penis 959.13
    following
      abortion 639.2
      ectopic or molar pregnancy
        639.2

**Injury** — *continued*
  genital organ(s) — *continued*
    internal — *see* Injury, internal,
      genital organs
    obstetrical trauma NEC 665.9 ☑
      affecting fetus or newborn
        763.89
  gland
    lacrimal 921.1
      laceration 870.8
    parathyroid 959.09
    salivary 959.09
    thyroid 959.09
  globe (eye) (*see also* Injury, eyeball)
    921.3
  grease gun — *see* Wound, open, by
    site, complicated
  groin 959.19
  gum 959.09
  hand(s) (except fingers) 959.4
  head NEC 959.01
    with
      loss of consciousness 850.5
      skull fracture — *see* Fracture,
        skull, by site
  heart — *see* Injury, internal, heart
  heel 959.7
  hip (and thigh) 959.6
  hymen 959.14
  hyperextension (cervical) (vertebra)
    847.0
  ileum — *see* Injury, internal, ileum
  iliac region 959.19
  infrared rays NEC 990
  instrumental (during surgery) 998.2
    birth injury — *see* Birth, injury
    nonsurgical (*see also* Injury, by
      site) 959.9
    obstetrical 665.9 ☑
      affecting fetus or newborn
        763.89
      bladder 665.5 ☑
      cervix 665.3 ☑
      high vaginal 665.4 ☑
      perineal NEC 664.9 ☑
      urethra 665.5 ☑
      uterus 665.5 ☑
  internal 869.0

> *Note* — *For injury of internal organ(s)*
> *by foreign body entering through a nat-*
> *ural orifice (e.g., inhaled, ingested, or*
> *swallowed) — see Foreign body, enter-*
> *ing through orifice.*
>
> *For internal injury of any of the follow-*
> *ing sites with internal injury of any of*
> *other of the sites — see Injury, internal,*
> *multiple.*

    with
      fracture
        pelvis — *see* Fracture, pelvis
        specified site, except pelvis
          — *see* Injury, internal,
          by site
      open wound into cavity 869.1
    abdomen, abdominal (viscera) NEC
      868.00
      with
        fracture, pelvis — *see* Frac-
          ture, pelvis
        open wound into cavity
          868.10
      specified site NEC 868.09
        with open wound into
          cavity 868.19
    adrenal (gland) 868.01
      with open wound into cavity
        868.11
    aorta (thoracic) 901.0
      abdominal 902.0
    appendix 863.85
      with open wound into cavity
        863.95
    bile duct 868.02
      with open wound into cavity
        868.12

**Injury** — *continued*
  internal — *continued*
    bladder (sphincter) 867.0
      with
        abortion — *see* Abortion, by
          type, with damage to
          pelvic organs
        ectopic pregnancy (*see also*
          categories
          633.0–633.9) 639.2
        molar pregnancy (*see also*
          categories 630–632)
          639.2
        open wound into cavity 867.1
      following
        abortion 639.2
        ectopic or molar pregnancy
          639.2
      obstetrical trauma 665.5 ☑
        affecting fetus or newborn
          763.89
    blood vessel — *see* Injury, blood
      vessel, by site
    broad ligament 867.6
      with open wound into cavity
        867.7
    bronchus, bronchi 862.21
      with open wound into cavity
        862.31
    cecum 863.89
      with open wound into cavity
        863.99
    cervix (uteri) 867.4
      with
        abortion — *see* Abortion, by
          type, with damage to
          pelvic organs
        ectopic pregnancy (*see also*
          categories
          633.0–633.9) 639.2
        molar pregnancy (*see also*
          categories 630–632)
          639.2
        open wound into cavity 867.5
      following
        abortion 639.2
        ectopic or molar pregnancy
          639.2
      obstetrical trauma 665.3 ☑
        affecting fetus or newborn
          763.89
    chest (*see also* Injury, internal, in-
      trathoracic organs) 862.8
      with open wound into cavity
        862.9
    colon 863.40
      with
        open wound into cavity
          863.50
        rectum 863.46
          with open wound into
            cavity 863.56
      ascending (right) 863.41
        with open wound into cavity
          863.51
      descending (left) 863.43
        with open wound into cavity
          863.53
      multiple sites 863.46
        with open wound into cavity
          863.56
      sigmoid 863.44
        with open wound into cavity
          863.54
      specified site NEC 863.49
        with open wound into cavity
          863.59
      transverse 863.42
        with open wound into
          cavity 863.52
    common duct 868.02
      with open wound into cavity
        868.12
    complicating delivery 665.9 ☑
      affecting fetus or newborn
        763.89

**Injury** — *continued*
  internal — *continued*
    diaphragm 862.0
      with open wound into cavity
        862.1
    duodenum 863.21
      with open wound into cavity
        863.31
    esophagus (intrathoracic) 862.22
      with open wound into cavity
        862.32
      cervical region 874.4
        complicated 874.5
    fallopian tube 867.6
      with open wound into cavity
        867.7
    gallbladder 868.02
      with open wound into cavity
        868.12
    gastrointestinal tract NEC 863.80
      with open wound into cavity
        863.90
    genital organ NEC 867.6
      with open wound into cavity
        867.7
    heart 861.00
      with open wound into thorax
        861.10
    ileum 863.29
      with open wound into cavity
        863.39
    intestine NEC 863.89
      with open wound into cavity
        863.99
      large NEC 863.40
        with open wound into cavity
          863.50
      small NEC 863.20
        with open wound into cavity
          863.30
    intra-abdominal (organ) 868.00
      with open wound into cavity
        868.10
      multiple sites 868.09
        with open wound into cavity
          868.19
      specified site NEC 868.09
        with open wound into cavity
          868.19
    intrathoracic organs (multiple)
      862.8
      with open wound into cavity
        862.9
      diaphragm (only) — *see* Injury,
        internal, diaphragm
      heart (only) — *see* Injury, inter-
        nal, heart
      lung (only) — *see* Injury, inter-
        nal, lung
      specified site NEC 862.29
        with open wound into cavity
          862.39
    intrauterine (*see also* Injury, inter-
      nal, uterus) 867.4
      with open wound into cavity
        867.5
    jejunum 863.29
      with open wound into cavity
        863.39
    kidney (subcapsular) 866.00
      with
        disruption of parenchyma
          (complete) 866.03
          with open wound into
            cavity 866.13
        hematoma (without rupture
          of capsule) 866.01
          with open wound into
            cavity 866.11
        laceration 866.02
          with open wound into
            cavity 866.12
        open wound into cavity
          866.10
    liver 864.00

☑ Additional Digit Required — Refer to the Tabular List for Digit Selection      Ⓑ Subterms under main terms may continue to next column or page

*2008 ICD-9-CM*      ▶◀ Revised Text      ● New Line      ▲ Revised Code      **Volume 2 — 165**

**Injury** — *continued*
  internal — *continued*
    liver — *continued*
      with
        contusion 864.01
          with open wound into
            cavity 864.11
        hematoma 864.01
          with open wound into
            cavity 864.11
        laceration 864.05
          with open wound into
            cavity 864.15
          major (disruption of hepat-
            ic parenchyma)
            864.04
            with open wound into
              cavity 864.14
          minor (capsule only)
            864.02
            with open wound into
              cavity 864.12
          moderate (involving
            parenchyma)
            864.03
            with open wound into
              cavity 864.13
          multiple 864.04
          stellate 864.04
            with open wound into
              cavity 864.14
        open wound into cavity
          864.10
      lung 861.20
        with open wound into thorax
          861.30
        hemopneumothorax — *see*
          Hemopneumothorax,
          traumatic
        hemothorax — *see* Hemothorax,
          traumatic
        pneumohemothorax — *see*
          Pneumohemothorax,
          traumatic
        pneumothorax — *see* Pneumoth-
          orax, traumatic
        transfusion related, acute
          (TRALI) 518.7
      mediastinum 862.29
        with open wound into cavity
          862.39
      mesentery 863.89
        with open wound into cavity
          863.99
      mesosalpinx 867.6
        with open wound into cavity
          867.7
      multiple 869.0

> *Note — Multiple internal injuries of sites classifiable to the same three- or four-digit category should be classified to that category.*
>
> *Multiple injuries classifiable to different fourth-digit subdivisions of 861 (heart and lung injuries) should be dealt with according to coding rules.*

      internal
        with open wound into cavity
          869.1
        intra–abdominal organ (sites
          classifiable to 863–868)
          with
            intrathoracic organ(s)
              (sites classifiable to
              861–862) 869.0
              with open wound into
                cavity 869.1
            other intra–abdominal or-
              gan(s) (sites classifi-
              able to 863–868,
              except where classi-
              fiable to the same
              three–digit category)
              868.09

**Injury** — *continued*
  internal — *continued*
    multiple — *continued*
      intra–abdominal organ — *contin-*
        *ued*
        with — *continued*
          other intra–abdominal or-
            gan(s) — *contin-*
            *ued*
            with open wound into
              cavity 868.19
      intrathoracic organ (sites classi-
        fiable to 861–862)
        with
          intra–abdominal organ(s)
            (sites classifiable to
            863–868) 869.0
            with open wound into
              cavity 869.1
          other intrathoracic or-
            gan(s) (sites classifi-
            able to 861–862,
            except where classi-
            fiable to the same
            three–digit category)
            862.8
            with open wound into
              cavity 862.9
      myocardium — *see* Injury, internal,
        heart
      ovary 867.6
        with open wound into cavity
          867.7
      pancreas (multiple sites) 863.84
        with open wound into cavity
          863.94
        body 863.82
          with open wound into cavity
           863.92
        head 863.81
          with open wound into cavity
           863.91
        tail 863.83
          with open wound into cavity
           863.93
      pelvis, pelvic (organs) (viscera)
        867.8
        with
          fracture, pelvis — *see* Frac-
           ture, pelvis
          open wound into cavity 867.9
        specified site NEC 867.6
          with open wound into cavity
           867.7
      peritoneum 868.03
        with open wound into cavity
          868.13
      pleura 862.29
        with open wound into cavity
          862.39
      prostate 867.6
        with open wound into cavity
          867.7
      rectum 863.45
        with
          colon 863.46
            with open wound into
              cavity 863.56
          open wound into cavity
           863.55
      retroperitoneum 868.04
        with open wound into cavity
          868.14
      round ligament 867.6
        with open wound into cavity
          867.7
      seminal vesicle 867.6
        with open wound into cavity
          867.7
      spermatic cord 867.6
        with open wound into cavity
          867.7
        scrotal — *see* Wound, open,
          spermatic cord
      spleen 865.00

**Injury** — *continued*
  internal — *continued*
    spleen — *continued*
      with
        disruption of parenchyma
          (massive) 865.04
          with open wound into
           cavity 865.14
        hematoma (without rupture
          of capsule) 865.01
          with open wound into
           cavity 865.11
        open wound into cavity
          865.10
        tear, capsular 865.02
          with open wound into
           cavity 865.12
          extending into parenchy-
           ma 865.03
           with open wound into
            cavity 865.13
      stomach 863.0
        with open wound into cavity
          863.1
      suprarenal gland (multiple) 868.01
        with open wound into cavity
          868.11
      thorax, thoracic (cavity) (organs)
        (multiple) (*see also* Injury,
        internal, intrathoracic or-
        gans) 862.8
        with open wound into cavity
          862.9
      thymus (gland) 862.29
        with open wound into cavity
          862.39
      trachea (intrathoracic) 862.29
        with open wound into cavity
          862.39
        cervical region (*see also* Wound,
          open, trachea) 874.02
      ureter 867.2
        with open wound into cavity
          867.3
      urethra (sphincter) 867.0
        with
          abortion — *see* Abortion, by
           type, with damage to
           pelvic organs
          ectopic pregnancy (*see also*
           categories
           633.0–633.9) 639.2
          molar pregnancy (*see also*
           categories 630–632)
           639.2
          open wound into cavity 867.1
        following
          abortion 639.2
          ectopic or molar pregnancy
           639.2
        obstetrical trauma 665.5 ☑
          affecting fetus or newborn
           763.89
      uterus 867.4
        with
          abortion — *see* Abortion, by
           type, with damage to
           pelvic organs
          ectopic pregnancy (*see also*
           categories
           633.0–633.9) 639.2
          molar pregnancy (*see also*
           categories 630–632)
           639.2
          open wound into cavity 867.5
        following
          abortion 639.2
          ectopic or molar pregnancy
           639.2
        obstetrical trauma NEC 665.5 ☑
          affecting fetus or newborn
           763.89
      vas deferens 867.6
        with open wound into cavity
          867.7
      vesical (sphincter) 867.0

**Injury** — *continued*
  internal — *continued*
    vesical — *continued*
      with open wound into cavity
        867.1
    viscera (abdominal) (*see also* In-
      jury, internal, multiple)
      868.00
      with
        fracture, pelvis — *see* Frac-
          ture, pelvis
        open wound into cavity
          868.10
        thoracic NEC (*see also* Injury,
          internal, intrathoracic or-
          gans) 862.8
          with open wound into cavity
           862.9
  interscapular region 959.19
  intervertebral disc 959.19
  intestine — *see* Injury, internal, intes-
    tine
  intra–abdominal (organs) NEC — *see*
    Injury, internal, intra-abdominal
  intracranial 854.0 ☑

> *Note — Use the following fifth-digit subclassification with categories 851–854:*
>
> *0    unspecified state of conscious-ness*
>
> *1    with no loss of consciousness*
>
> *2    with brief [less than one hour] loss of consciousness*
>
> *3    with moderate [1–24 hours] loss of consciousness*
>
> *4    with prolonged [more than 24 hours] loss of consciousness and return to pre–existing conscious level*
>
> *5    with prolonged [more than 24 hours] loss of consciousness, without return to pre–existing conscious level*
>
> *Use fifth-digit 5 to designate when a patient is unconscious and dies before regaining consciousness, regardless of the duration of the loss of consciousness*
>
> *6    with loss of consciousness of un-specified duration*
>
> *9    with concussion, unspecified*

    with
      open intracranial wound
        854.1 ☑
      skull fracture — *see* Fracture,
        skull, by site
    contusion 851.8 ☑
      with open intracranial wound
        851.9 ☑
      brain stem 851.4 ☑
        with open intracranial wound
          851.5 ☑
      cerebellum 851.4 ☑
        with open intracranial wound
          851.5 ☑
      cortex (cerebral) 851.0 ☑
        with open intracranial wound
          851.2 ☑
    hematoma — *see* Injury, intracra-
      nial, hemorrhage
    hemorrhage 853.0 ☑
      with
        laceration — *see* Injury, in-
          tracranial, laceration
        open intracranial wound
          853.1 ☑
      extradural 852.4 ☑
        with open intracranial wound
          852.5 ☑
      subarachnoid 852.0 ☑
        with open intracranial wound
          852.1 ☑

☑ Additional Digit Required — Refer to the Tabular List for Digit Selection           Subterms under main terms may continue to next column or page

166 — Volume 2        ▶◀ Revised Text      ● New Line      ▲ Revised Code      *2008 ICD-9-CM*

**Injury** — *continued*
intracranial — *continued*
  hemorrhage — *continued*
    subdural 852.2 ☑
      with open intracranial wound
        852.3 ☑
    laceration 851.8 ☑
      with open intracranial wound
        851.9 ☑
      brain stem 851.6 ☑
        with open intracranial wound
          851.7 ☑
      cerebellum 851.6 ☑
        with open intracranial wound
          851.7 ☑
      cortex (cerebral) 851.2 ☑
        with open intracranial wound
          851.3 ☑
  intraocular — *see* Injury, eyeball, penetrating
  intrathoracic organs (multiple) — *see* Injury, internal, intrathoracic organs
  intrauterine — *see* Injury, internal, intrauterine
  iris 921.3
    penetrating — *see* Injury, eyeball, penetrating
  jaw 959.09
  jejunum — *see* Injury, internal, jejunum
  joint NEC 959.9
    old or residual 718.80
      ankle 718.87
      elbow 718.82
      foot 718.87
      hand 718.84
      hip 718.85
      knee 718.86
      multiple sites 718.89
      pelvic region 718.85
      shoulder (region) 718.81
      specified site NEC 718.88
      wrist 718.83
  kidney — *see* Injury, internal, kidney
  knee (and ankle) (and foot) (and leg, except thigh) 959.7
  labium (majus) (minus) 959.14
  labyrinth, ear 959.09
  lacrimal apparatus, gland, or sac 921.1
    laceration 870.8
  larynx 959.09
  late effect — *see* Late, effects (of), injury
  leg, except thigh (and ankle) (and foot) (and knee) 959.7
    upper or thigh 959.6
  lens, eye 921.3
    penetrating — *see* Injury, eyeball, penetrating
  lid, eye — *see* Injury, eyelid
  lip 959.09
  liver — *see* Injury, internal, liver
  lobe, parietal — *see* Injury, intracranial
  lumbar (region) 959.19
    plexus 953.5
  lumbosacral (region) 959.19
    plexus 953.5
  lung — *see* Injury, internal, lung
  malar region 959.09
  mastoid region 959.09
  maternal, during pregnancy, affecting fetus or newborn 760.5
  maxilla 959.09
  mediastinum — *see* Injury, internal, mediastinum
  membrane
    brain (*see also* Injury, intracranial) 854.0 ☑
    tympanic 959.09
  meningeal artery — *see* Hemorrhage, brain, traumatic, subarachnoid
  meninges (cerebral) — *see* Injury, intracranial

**Injury** — *continued*
mesenteric
  artery — *see* Injury, blood vessel, mesenteric, artery
  plexus, inferior 954.1
  vein — *see* Injury, blood vessel, mesenteric, vein
mesentery — *see* Injury, internal, mesentery
mesosalpinx — *see* Injury, internal, mesosalpinx
middle ear 959.09
midthoracic region 959.11
mouth 959.09
multiple (sites not classifiable to the same four–digit category in 959.0–959.7) 959.8
  internal 869.0
    with open wound into cavity 869.1
musculocutaneous nerve 955.4
nail
  finger 959.5
  toe 959.7
nasal (septum) (sinus) 959.09
nasopharynx 959.09
neck (and face) 959.09
nerve 957.9
  abducens 951.3
  abducent 951.3
  accessory 951.6
  acoustic 951.5
  ankle and foot 956.9
  anterior crural, femoral 956.1
  arm (*see also* Injury, nerve, upper limb) 955.9
  auditory 951.5
  axillary 955.0
  brachial plexus 953.4
  cervical sympathetic 954.0
  cranial 951.9
    first or olfactory 951.8
    second or optic 950.0
    third or oculomotor 951.0
    fourth or trochlear 951.1
    fifth or trigeminal 951.2
    sixth or abducens 951.3
    seventh or facial 951.4
    eighth, acoustic, or auditory 951.5
    ninth or glossopharyngeal 951.8
    tenth, pneumogastric, or vagus 951.8
    eleventh or accessory 951.6
    twelfth or hypoglossal 951.7
    newborn 767.7
  cutaneous sensory
    lower limb 956.4
    upper limb 955.5
  digital (finger) 955.6
    toe 956.5
  facial 951.4
    newborn 767.5
  femoral 956.1
  finger 955.9
  foot and ankle 956.9
  forearm 955.9
  glossopharyngeal 951.8
  hand and wrist 955.9
  head and neck, superficial 957.0
  hypoglossal 951.7
  involving several parts of body 957.8
  leg (*see also* Injury, nerve, lower limb) 956.9
  lower limb 956.9
    multiple 956.8
    specified site NEC 956.5
  lumbar plexus 953.5
  lumbosacral plexus 953.5
  median 955.1
    forearm 955.1
    wrist and hand 955.1

**Injury** — *continued*
nerve — *continued*
  multiple (in several parts of body) (sites not classifiable to the same three-digit category) 957.8
  musculocutaneous 955.4
  musculospiral 955.3
    upper arm 955.3
  oculomotor 951.0
  olfactory 951.8
  optic 950.0
  pelvic girdle 956.9
    multiple sites 956.8
    specified site NEC 956.5
  peripheral 957.9
    multiple (in several regions) (sites not classifiable to the same three-digit category) 957.8
    specified site NEC 957.1
  peroneal 956.3
    ankle and foot 956.3
    lower leg 956.3
  plantar 956.5
  plexus 957.9
    celiac 954.1
    mesenteric, inferior 954.1
    spinal 953.9
      brachial 953.4
      lumbosacral 953.5
      multiple sites 953.8
      sympathetic NEC 954.1
  pneumogastric 951.8
  radial 955.3
    wrist and hand 955.3
  sacral plexus 953.5
  sciatic 956.0
    thigh 956.0
  shoulder girdle 955.9
    multiple 955.8
    specified site NEC 955.7
  specified site NEC 957.1
  spinal 953.9
    plexus — *see* Injury, nerve, plexus, spinal
    root 953.9
      cervical 953.0
      dorsal 953.1
      lumbar 953.2
      multiple sites 953.8
      sacral 953.3
  splanchnic 954.1
  sympathetic NEC 954.1
    cervical 954.0
  thigh 956.9
  tibial 956.5
    ankle and foot 956.2
    lower leg 956.5
    posterior 956.2
  toe 956.9
  trigeminal 951.2
  trochlear 951.1
  trunk, excluding shoulder and pelvic girdles 954.9
    specified site NEC 954.8
    sympathetic NEC 954.1
  ulnar 955.2
    forearm 955.2
    wrist (and hand) 955.2
  upper limb 955.9
    multiple 955.8
    specified site NEC 955.7
  vagus 951.8
  wrist and hand 955.9
nervous system, diffuse 957.8
nose (septum) 959.09
obstetrical NEC 665.9 ☑
  affecting fetus or newborn 763.89
occipital (region) (scalp) 959.09
  lobe (*see also* Injury, intracranial) 854.0 ☑
optic 950.9
  chiasm 950.1
  cortex 950.3
  nerve 950.0

**Injury** — *continued*
optic — *continued*
  pathways 950.2
orbit, orbital (region) 921.2
  penetrating 870.3
    with foreign body 870.4
ovary — *see* Injury, internal, ovary
paint-gun — *see* Wound, open, by site, complicated
palate (soft) 959.09
pancreas — *see* Injury, internal, pancreas
parathyroid (gland) 959.09
parietal (region) (scalp) 959.09
  lobe — *see* Injury, intracranial
pelvic
  floor 959.19
    complicating delivery 664.1 ☑
      affecting fetus or newborn 763.89
  joint or ligament, complicating delivery 665.6 ☑
    affecting fetus or newborn 763.89
  organs (*see also* Injury, internal, pelvis)
    with
      abortion — *see* Abortion, by type, with damage to pelvic organs
      ectopic pregnancy (*see also* categories 633.0–633.9) 639.2
      molar pregnancy (*see also* categories 633.0–633.9) 639.2
    following
      abortion 639.2
      ectopic or molar pregnancy 639.2
    obstetrical trauma 665.5 ☑
      affecting fetus or newborn 763.89
pelvis 959.19
penis 959.14
  fracture of corpus cavernosum 959.13
perineum 959.14
peritoneum — *see* Injury, internal, peritoneum
periurethral tissue
  with
    abortion — *see* Abortion, by type, with damage to pelvic organs
    ectopic pregnancy (*see also* categories 633.0–633.9) 639.2
    molar pregnancy (*see also* categories 630–632) 639.2
  complicating delivery 665.5 ☑
    affecting fetus or newborn 763.89
  following
    abortion 639.2
    ectopic or molar pregnancy 639.2
phalanges
  foot 959.7
  hand 959.5
pharynx 959.09
pleura — *see* Injury, internal, pleura
popliteal space 959.7
post-cardiac surgery (syndrome) 429.4
prepuce 959.14
prostate — *see* Injury, internal, prostate
pubic region 959.19
pudenda 959.14
radiation NEC 990
radioactive substance or radium NEC 990
rectovaginal septum 959.14
rectum — *see* Injury, internal, rectum
retina 921.3

☑ Additional Digit Required — Refer to the Tabular List for Digit Selection     ⬇ Subterms under main terms may continue to next column or page

*2008 ICD-9-CM*     ▶◀ Revised Text     ● New Line     ▲ Revised Code     Volume 2 — 167

**Index**

**Injury — Injury**

**Injury** — *continued*
  retina — *continued*
    penetrating — *see* Injury, eyeball,
        penetrating
    retroperitoneal — *see* Injury, internal,
        retroperitoneum
  roentgen rays NEC 990
  round ligament — *see* Injury, internal,
      round ligament
  sacral (region) 959.19
    plexus 953.5
  sacroiliac ligament NEC 959.19
  sacrum 959.19
  salivary ducts or glands 959.09
  scalp 959.09
    due to birth trauma 767.19
    fetus or newborn 767.19
  scapular region 959.2
  sclera 921.3
    penetrating — *see* Injury, eyeball,
        penetrating
    superficial 918.2
  scrotum 959.14
  seminal vesicle — *see* Injury, internal,
      seminal vesicle
  shoulder (and upper arm) 959.2
  sinus
    cavernous (*see also* Injury, intracra-
        nial) 854.0 ☑
    nasal 959.09
  skeleton NEC, birth injury 767.3
  skin NEC 959.9
  skull — *see* Fracture, skull, by site
  soft tissue (of external sites) (severe)
      — *see* Wound, open, by site
  specified site NEC 959.8
  spermatic cord — *see* Injury, internal,
      spermatic cord
  spinal (cord) 952.9
    with fracture, vertebra — *see*
        Fracture, vertebra, by site,
        with spinal cord injury
    cervical (C₁-C₄) 952.00
      with
        anterior cord syndrome
            952.02
        central cord syndrome
            952.03
        complete lesion of cord
            952.01
        incomplete lesion NEC
            952.04
        posterior cord syndrome
            952.04
      C₅-C₇ level 952.05
      with
        anterior cord syndrome
            952.07
        central cord syndrome
            952.08
        complete lesion of cord
            952.06
        incomplete lesion NEC
            952.09
        posterior cord syndrome
            952.09
      specified type NEC 952.09
      specified type NEC 952.04
    dorsal (D₁-D₆) (T₁-T₆) (thoracic)
        952.10
      with
        anterior cord syndrome
            952.12
        central cord syndrome
            952.13
        complete lesion of cord
            952.11
        incomplete lesion NEC
            952.14
        posterior cord syndrome
            952.14
      D₇-D₁₂ level (T₇-T₁₂) 952.15
      with
        anterior cord syndrome
            952.17

**Injury** — *continued*
  spinal — *continued*
    dorsal — *continued*
      D₇-D₁₂ level — *continued*
        with — *continued*
          central cord syndrome
              952.18
          complete lesion of cord
              952.16
          incomplete lesion NEC
              952.19
          posterior cord syndrome
              952.19
        specified type NEC 952.19
      specified type NEC 952.14
    lumbar 952.2
    multiple sites 952.8
    nerve (root) NEC — *see* Injury,
        nerve, spinal, root
    plexus 953.9
      brachial 953.4
      lumbosacral 953.5
      multiple sites 953.8
    sacral 952.3
    thoracic (*see also* Injury, spinal,
        dorsal) 952.10
  spleen — *see* Injury, internal, spleen
  stellate ganglion 954.1
  sternal region 959.11
  stomach — *see* Injury, internal,
      stomach
  subconjunctival 921.1
  subcutaneous 959.9
  subdural — *see* Injury, intracranial
  submaxillary region 959.09
  submental region 959.09
  subungual
    fingers 959.5
    toes 959.7
  superficial 919 ☑

---

*Note — Use the following fourth-digit
subdivisions with categories 910–919:*

0   *Abrasion or friction burn without
    mention of infection*

1   *Abrasion or friction burn, infected*

2   *Blister without mention of infec-
    tion*

3   *Blister, infected*

4   *Insect bite, nonvenomous, without
    mention of infection*

5   *Insect bite, nonvenomous, infect-
    ed*

6   *Superficial foreign body (splinter)
    without major open wound and
    without mention of infection*

7   *Superficial foreign body (splinter)
    without major open wound, infect-
    ed*

8   *Other and unspecified superficial
    injury without mention of infection*

9   *Other and unspecified superficial
    injury, infected*

*For late effects of superficial injury, see
category 906.2.*

---

    abdomen, abdominal (muscle)
        (wall) (and other part(s) of
        trunk) 911 ☑
    ankle (and hip, knee, leg, or thigh)
        916 ☑
    anus (and other part(s) of trunk)
        911 ☑
    arm 913 ☑
      upper (and shoulder) 912 ☑
    auditory canal (external) (meatus)
        (and other part(s) of face,
        neck, or scalp, except eye)
        910 ☑
    axilla (and upper arm) 912 ☑
    back (and other part(s) of trunk)
        911 ☑

**Injury** — *continued*
  superficial — *continued*
    breast (and other part(s) of trunk)
        911 ☑
    brow (and other part(s) of face,
        neck, or scalp, except eye)
        910 ☑
    buttock (and other part(s) of trunk)
        911 ☑
    canthus, eye 918.0
    cheek(s) (and other part(s) of face,
        neck, or scalp, except eye)
        910 ☑
    chest wall (and other part(s) of
        trunk) 911 ☑
    chin (and other part(s) of face,
        neck, or scalp, except eye)
        910 ☑
    clitoris (and other part(s) of trunk)
        911 ☑
    conjunctiva 918.2
    cornea 918.1
      due to contact lens 371.82
    costal region (and other part(s) of
        trunk) 911 ☑
    ear(s) (auricle) (canal) (drum) (exter-
        nal) (and other part(s) of face,
        neck, or scalp, except eye)
        910 ☑
    elbow (and forearm) (and wrist)
        913 ☑
    epididymis (and other part(s) of
        trunk) 911 ☑
    epigastric region (and other part(s)
        of trunk) 911 ☑
    epiglottis (and other part(s) of face,
        neck, or scalp, except eye)
        910 ☑
    eye(s) (and adnexa) NEC 918.9
    eyelid(s) (and periocular area)
        918.0
    face (any part(s), except eye) (and
        neck or scalp) 910 ☑
    finger(s) (nail) (any) 915 ☑
    flank (and other part(s) of trunk)
        911 ☑
    foot (phalanges) (and toe(s)) 917 ☑
    forearm (and elbow) (and wrist)
        913 ☑
    forehead (and other part(s) of face,
        neck, or scalp, except eye)
        910 ☑
    globe (eye) 918.9
    groin (and other part(s) of trunk)
        911 ☑
    gum(s) (and other part(s) of face,
        neck, or scalp, except eye)
        910 ☑
    hand(s) (except fingers alone)
        914 ☑
    head (and other part(s) of face,
        neck, or scalp, except eye)
        910 ☑
    heel (and foot or toe) 917 ☑
    hip (and ankle, knee, leg, or thigh)
        916 ☑
    iliac region (and other part(s) of
        trunk) 911 ☑
    interscapular region (and other
        part(s) of trunk) 911 ☑
    iris 918.9
    knee (and ankle, hip, leg, or thigh)
        916 ☑
    labium (majus) (minus) (and other
        part(s) of trunk) 911 ☑
    lacrimal (apparatus) (gland) (sac)
        918.0
    leg (lower) (upper) (and ankle, hip,
        knee, or thigh) 916 ☑
    lip(s) (and other part(s) of face,
        neck, or scalp, except eye)
        910 ☑
    lower extremity (except foot) 916 ☑
    lumbar region (and other part(s) of
        trunk) 911 ☑

**Injury** — *continued*
  superficial — *continued*
    malar region (and other part(s) of
        face, neck, or scalp, except
        eye) 910 ☑
    mastoid region (and other part(s)
        of face, neck, or scalp, except
        eye) 910 ☑
    midthoracic region (and other
        part(s) of trunk) 911 ☑
    mouth (and other part(s) of face,
        neck, or scalp, except eye)
        910 ☑
    multiple sites (not classifiable to
        the same three-digit catego-
        ry) 919 ☑
    nasal (septum) (and other part(s)
        of face, neck, or scalp, except
        eye) 910 ☑
    neck (and face or scalp, any part(s),
        except eye) 910 ☑
    nose (septum) (and other part(s) of
        face, neck, or scalp, except
        eye) 910 ☑
    occipital region (and other part(s)
        of face, neck, or scalp, except
        eye) 910 ☑
    orbital region 918.0
    palate (soft) (and other part(s) of
        face, neck, or scalp, except
        eye) 910 ☑
    parietal region (and other part(s) of
        face, neck, or scalp, except
        eye) 910 ☑
    penis (and other part(s) of trunk)
        911 ☑
    perineum (and other part(s) of
        trunk) 911 ☑
    periocular area 918.0
    pharynx (and other part(s) of face,
        neck, or scalp, except eye)
        910 ☑
    popliteal space (and ankle, hip, leg,
        or thigh) 916 ☑
    prepuce (and other part(s) of trunk)
        911 ☑
    pubic region (and other part(s) of
        trunk) 911 ☑
    pudenda (and other part(s) of
        trunk) 911 ☑
    sacral region (and other part(s) of
        trunk) 911 ☑
    salivary (ducts) (glands) (and other
        part(s) of face, neck, or scalp,
        except eye) 910 ☑
    scalp (and other part(s) of face or
        neck, except eye) 910 ☑
    scapular region (and upper arm)
        912 ☑
    sclera 918.2
    scrotum (and other part(s) of trunk)
        911 ☑
    shoulder (and upper arm) 912 ☑
    skin NEC 919 ☑
    specified site(s) NEC 919 ☑
    sternal region (and other part(s) of
        trunk) 911 ☑
    subconjunctival 918.2
    subcutaneous NEC 919 ☑
    submaxillary region (and other
        part(s) of face, neck, or scalp,
        except eye) 910 ☑
    submental region (and other part(s)
        of face, neck, or scalp, except
        eye) 910 ☑
    supraclavicular fossa (and other
        part(s) of face, neck, or scalp,
        except eye) 910 ☑
    supraorbital 918.0
    temple (and other part(s) of face,
        neck, or scalp, except eye)
        910 ☑
    temporal region (and other part(s)
        of face, neck, or scalp, except
        eye) 910 ☑

---

☑ Additional Digit Required — Refer to the Tabular List for Digit Selection                    ᴺᴱᶜ̌ Subterms under main terms may continue to next column or page

**Injury** — *continued*
  superficial — *continued*
    testis (and other part(s) of trunk) 911 ☑
    thigh (and ankle, hip, knee, or leg) 916 ☑
    thorax, thoracic (external) (and other part(s) of trunk) 911 ☑
    throat (and other part(s) of face, neck, or scalp, except eye) 910 ☑
    thumb(s) (nail) 915 ☑
    toe(s) (nail) (subungual) (and foot) 917 ☑
    tongue (and other part(s) of face, neck, or scalp, except eye) 910 ☑
    tooth, teeth (*see also* Abrasion, dental) 521.20
    trunk (any part(s)) 911 ☑
    tunica vaginalis 959.14
    tympanum, tympanic membrane (and other part(s) of face, neck, or scalp, except eye) 910 ☑
    upper extremity NEC 913 ☑
    uvula (and other part(s) of face, neck, or scalp, except eye) 910 ☑
    vagina (and other part(s) of trunk) 911 ☑
    vulva (and other part(s) of trunk) 911 ☑
    wrist (and elbow) (and forearm) 913 ☑
  supraclavicular fossa 959.19
  supraorbital 959.09
  surgical complication (external or internal site) 998.2
  symphysis pubis 959.19
    complicating delivery 665.6 ☑
      affecting fetus or newborn 763.89
  temple 959.09
  temporal region 959.09
  testis 959.14
  thigh (and hip) 959.6
  thorax, thoracic (external) 959.11
    cavity — *see* Injury, internal, thorax
    internal — *see* Injury, internal, intrathoracic organs
  throat 959.09
  thumb(s) (nail) 959.5
  thymus — *see* Injury, internal, thymus
  thyroid (gland) 959.09
  toe (nail) (any) 959.7
  tongue 959.09
  tonsil 959.09
  tooth NEC 873.63
    complicated 873.73
  trachea — *see* Injury, internal, trachea
  trunk 959.19
  tunica vaginalis 959.14
  tympanum, tympanic membrane 959.09
  ultraviolet rays NEC 990
  ureter — *see* Injury, internal, ureter
  urethra (sphincter) — *see* Injury, internal, urethra
  uterus — *see* Injury, internal, uterus
  uvula 959.09
  vagina 959.14
  vascular — *see* Injury, blood vessel
  vas deferens — *see* Injury, internal, vas deferens
  vein (*see also* Injury, blood vessel, by site) 904.9
  vena cava
    inferior 902.10
    superior 901.2
  vesical (sphincter) — *see* Injury, internal, vesical

**Injury** — *continued*
  viscera (abdominal) — *see* Injury, internal, viscera
    with fracture, pelvis — *see* Fracture, pelvis
  visual 950.9
    cortex 950.3
  vitreous (humor) 871.2
  vulva 959.14
  whiplash (cervical spine) 847.0
  wringer — *see* Crush, by site
  wrist (and elbow) (and forearm) 959.3
  x-ray NEC 990
**Inoculation** — *see also* Vaccination
  complication or reaction — *see* Complication, vaccination
**INPH** (idiopathic normal pressure hydrocephalus) 331.5 ●
**Insanity, insane** — *see also* Psychosis 298.9
  adolescent (*see also* Schizophrenia) 295.9
  alternating (*see also* Psychosis, affective, circular) 296.7
  confusional 298.9
    acute 293.0
    subacute 293.1
  delusional 298.9
  paralysis, general 094.1
    progressive 094.1
  paresis, general 094.1
  senile 290.20
**Insect**
  bite — *see* Injury, superficial, by site
  venomous, poisoning by 989.5
**Insemination, artificial** V26.1
**Insensitivity**
  adrenocorticotropin hormone (ACTH) ● 255.41
  androgen 259.5
    partial 259.5
**Insertion**
  cord (umbilical) lateral or velamentous 663.8 ☑
    affecting fetus or newborn 762.6
  intrauterine contraceptive device V25.1
  placenta, vicious — *see* Placenta, previa
  subdermal implantable contraceptive V25.5
  velamentous, umbilical cord 663.8 ☑
    affecting fetus or newborn 762.6
**Insolation** 992.0
  meaning sunstroke 992.0
**Insomnia, unspecified** 780.52
  with sleep apnea, unspecified 780.51
  adjustment 307.41
  alcohol induced 291.82
  behavioral, of childhood V69.5
  drug induced 292.85
  due to
    medical condition classified elsewhere 327.01
    mental disorder 327.02
  idiopathic 307.42
  nonorganic origin 307.41
    persistent (primary) 307.42
    transient 307.41
  organic 327.00
    other 327.09
  paradoxical 307.42
  primary 307.42
  psychophysiological 307.42
  subjective complaint 307.49
**Inspiration**
  food or foreign body (*see also* Asphyxia, food or foreign body) 933.1
  mucus (*see also* Asphyxia, mucus) 933.1
**Inspissated bile syndrome, newborn** 774.4
**Instability**
  detrusor 596.59
  emotional (excessive) 301.3
  joint (posttraumatic) 718.80

**Instability** — *continued*
  joint — *continued*
    ankle 718.87
    elbow 718.82
    foot 718.87
    hand 718.84
    hip 718.85
    knee 718.86
    lumbosacral 724.6
    multiple sites 718.89
    pelvic region 718.85
    sacroiliac 724.6
    shoulder (region) 718.81
    specified site NEC 718.88
    wrist 718.83
  lumbosacral 724.6
  nervous 301.89
  personality (emotional) 301.59
  thyroid, paroxysmal 242.9 ☑
  urethral 599.83
  vasomotor 780.2
**Insufficiency, insufficient**
  accommodation 367.4
  adrenal (gland) (acute) (chronic) 255.41 ▲
    medulla 255.5
    primary 255.41 ▲
    specified site NEC 255.5
  adrenocortical 255.41 ▲
  anterior (occlusal) guidance 524.54
  anus 569.49
  aortic (valve) 424.1
    with
      mitral (valve) disease 396.1
        insufficiency, incompetence, or regurgitation 396.3
        stenosis or obstruction 396.1
      stenosis or obstruction 424.1
        with mitral (valve) disease 396.8
    congenital 746.4
    rheumatic 395.1
      with
        mitral (valve) disease 396.1
          insufficiency, incompetence, or regurgitation 396.3
          stenosis or obstruction 396.1
        stenosis or obstruction 395.2
          with mitral (valve) disease 396.8
    specified cause NEC 424.1
    syphilitic 093.22
  arterial 447.1
    basilar artery 435.0
    carotid artery 435.8
    cerebral 437.1
    coronary (acute or subacute) 411.89
    mesenteric 557.1
    peripheral 443.9
    precerebral 435.9
    vertebral artery 435.1
    vertebrobasilar 435.3
  arteriovenous 459.9
  basilar artery 435.0
  biliary 575.8
  cardiac (*see also* Insufficiency, myocardial) 428.0
    complicating surgery 997.1
    due to presence of (cardiac) prosthesis 429.4
    postoperative 997.1
      long-term effect of cardiac surgery 429.4
    specified during or due to a procedure 997.1
      long-term effect of cardiac surgery 429.4
  cardiorenal (*see also* Hypertension, cardiorenal) 404.90
  cardiovascular (*see also* Disease, cardiovascular) 429.2
    renal (*see also* Hypertension, cardiorenal) 404.90

**Insufficiency, insufficient** — *continued*
  carotid artery 435.8
  cerebral (vascular) 437.9
  cerebrovascular 437.9
    with transient focal neurological signs and symptoms 435.9
    acute 437.1
      with transient focal neurological signs and symptoms 435.9
  circulatory NEC 459.9
    fetus or newborn 779.89
  convergence 378.83
  coronary (acute or subacute) 411.89
    chronic or with a stated duration of over 8 weeks 414.8
  corticoadrenal 255.41 ▲
  dietary 269.9
  divergence 378.85
  food 994.2
  gastroesophageal 530.89
  gonadal
    ovary 256.39
    testis 257.2
  gonadotropic hormone secretion 253.4
  heart (*see also* Insufficiency, myocardial)
    fetus or newborn 779.89
    valve (*see also* Endocarditis) 424.90
      congenital NEC 746.89
  hepatic 573.8
  idiopathic autonomic 333.0
  interocclusal distance of teeth (ridge) 524.36
  kidney
    acute 593.9
    chronic 585.9
  labyrinth, labyrinthine (function) 386.53
    bilateral 386.54
    unilateral 386.53
  lacrimal 375.15
  liver 573.8
  lung (acute) (*see also* Insufficiency, pulmonary) 518.82
    following trauma, surgery, or shock 518.5
    newborn 770.89
  mental (congenital) (*see also* Retardation, mental) 319
  mesenteric 557.1
  mitral (valve) 424.0
    with
      aortic (valve) disease 396.3
        insufficiency, incompetence, or regurgitation 396.3
        stenosis or obstruction 396.2
      obstruction or stenosis 394.2
        with aortic valve disease 396.8
    congenital 746.6
    rheumatic 394.1
      with
        aortic (valve) disease 396.3
          insufficiency, incompetence, or regurgitation 396.3
          stenosis or obstruction 396.2
        obstruction or stenosis 394.2
          with aortic valve disease 396.8
      active or acute 391.1
        with chorea, rheumatic (Sydenham's) 392.0
    specified cause, except rheumatic 424.0
  muscle
    heart — *see* Insufficiency, myocardial
  ocular (*see also* Strabismus) 378.9
  myocardial, myocardium (with arteriosclerosis) 428.0

---

☑ Additional Digit Required — Refer to the Tabular List for Digit Selection　　　　　ᴺᴱᶜ Subterms under main terms may continue to next column or page

**Insufficiency, insufficient —** *continued*
  myocardial, myocardium — *continued*
    with rheumatic fever (conditions classifiable to 390)
      active, acute, or subacute 391.2
        with chorea 392.0
      inactive or quiescent (with chorea) 398.0
    congenital 746.89
    due to presence of (cardiac) prosthesis 429.4
    fetus or newborn 779.89
    following cardiac surgery 429.4
    hypertensive (*see also* Hypertension, heart) 402.91
      benign 402.11
      malignant 402.01
    postoperative 997.1
      long-term effect of cardiac surgery 429.4
    rheumatic 398.0
      active, acute, or subacute 391.2
        with chorea (Sydenham's) 392.0
    syphilitic 093.82
  nourishment 994.2
  organic 799.89
  ovary 256.39
    postablative 256.2
  pancreatic 577.8
  parathyroid (gland) 252.1
  peripheral vascular (arterial) 443.9
  pituitary (anterior) 253.2
    posterior 253.5
  placental — *see* Placenta, insufficiency
  platelets 287.5
  prenatal care in current pregnancy V23.7
  progressive pluriglandular 258.9
  pseudocholinesterase 289.89
  pulmonary (acute) 518.82
    following
      shock 518.5
      surgery 518.5
      trauma 518.5
    newborn 770.89
    valve (*see also* Endocarditis, pulmonary) 424.3
      congenital 746.09
  pyloric 537.0
  renal 593.9
    acute 593.9
    chronic 585.9
    due to a procedure 997.5
  respiratory 786.09
    acute 518.82
      following shock, surgery, or trauma 518.5
    newborn 770.89
  rotation — *see* Malrotation
  suprarenal 255.41 ▲
    medulla 255.5
  tarso-orbital fascia, congenital 743.66
  tear film 375.15
  testis 257.2
  thyroid (gland) (acquired) (*see also* Hypothyroidism)
    congenital 243
  tricuspid (*see also* Endocarditis, tricuspid) 397.0
    congenital 746.89
    syphilitic 093.23
  urethral sphincter 599.84
  valve, valvular (heart) (*see also* Endocarditis) 424.90
  vascular 459.9
    intestine NEC 557.9
    mesenteric 557.1
    peripheral 443.9
    renal (*see also* Hypertension, kidney) 403.90
  velopharyngeal
    acquired 528.9
    congenital 750.29

**Insufficiency, insufficient —** *continued*
  venous (peripheral) 459.81
  ventricular — *see* Insufficiency, myocardial
  vertebral artery 435.1
  vertebrobasilar artery 435.3
  weight gain during pregnancy 646.8 ☑
  zinc 269.3
**Insufflation**
  fallopian
    fertility testing V26.21
    following sterilization reversal V26.22
  meconium 770.11
    with respiratory symptoms 770.12
**Insular** — *see* condition
**Insulinoma** (M8151/0)
  malignant (M8151/3)
    pancreas 157.4
    specified site — *see* Neoplasm, by site, malignant
    unspecified site 157.4
  pancreas 211.7
  specified site — *see* Neoplasm, by site, benign
  unspecified site 211.7
**Insuloma** — *see* Insulinoma
**Insult**
  brain 437.9
    acute 436
  cerebral 437.9
    acute 436
  cerebrovascular 437.9
    acute 436
  vascular NEC 437.9
    acute 436
**Insurance examination** (certification) V70.3
**Intemperance** — *see also* Alcoholism 303.9 ☑
**Interception of pregnancy** (menstrual extraction) V25.3
**Interference**
  balancing side 524.56
  non-working side 524.56
**Intermenstrual**
  bleeding 626.6
    irregular 626.6
    regular 626.5
  hemorrhage 626.6
    irregular 626.6
    regular 626.5
  pain(s) 625.2
**Intermittent** — *see* condition
**Internal** — *see* condition
**Interproximal wear** 521.10
**Interruption**
  aortic arch 747.11
  bundle of His 426.50
  fallopian tube (for sterilization) V25.2
  phase-shift, sleep cycle 307.45
  repeated REM-sleep 307.48
  sleep
    due to perceived environmental disturbances 307.48
    phase-shift, of 24-hour sleep-wake cycle 307.45
    repeated REM-sleep type 307.48
  vas deferens (for sterilization) V25.2
**Intersexuality** 752.7
**Interstitial** — *see* condition
**Intertrigo** 695.89
  labialis 528.5
**Intervertebral disc** — *see* condition
**Intestine, intestinal** — *see also* condition
  flu 487.8
**Intolerance**
  carbohydrate NEC 579.8
  cardiovascular exercise, with pain (at rest) (with less than ordinary activity) (with ordinary activity) V47.2
  cold 780.99
  dissacharide (hereditary) 271.3

**Intolerance** — *continued*
  drug
    correct substance properly administered 995.27
    wrong substance given or taken in error 977.9
      specified drug — *see* Table of Drugs and Chemicals
  effort 306.2
  fat NEC 579.8
  foods NEC 579.8
  fructose (hereditary) 271.2
  glucose (-galactose) (congenital) 271.3
  gluten 579.0
  lactose (hereditary) (infantile) 271.3
  lysine (congenital) 270.7
  milk NEC 579.8
  protein (familial) 270.7
  starch NEC 579.8
  sucrose (-isomaltose) (congenital) 271.3
**Intoxicated** NEC — *see also* Alcoholism 305.0 ☑
**Intoxication**
  acid 276.2
  acute
    alcoholic 305.0 ☑
      with alcoholism 303.0 ☑
      hangover effects 305.0 ☑
    caffeine 305.9 ☑
    hallucinogenic (*see also* Abuse, drugs, nondependent) 305.3 ☑
  alcohol (acute) 305.0 ☑
    with alcoholism 303.0 ☑
    hangover effects 305.0 ☑
    idiosyncratic 291.4
    pathological 291.4
  alimentary canal 558.2
  ammonia (hepatic) 572.2
  caffeine 305.9 ☑
  chemical (*see also* Table of Drugs and Chemicals)
    via placenta or breast milk 760.70
      alcohol 760.71
      anticonvulsants
      antifungals
      anti-infective agents 760.74
      antimetabolics
      cocaine 760.75
      "crack" 760.75
      hallucinogenic agents NEC 760.73
      medicinal agents NEC 760.79
      narcotics 760.72
      obstetric anesthetic or analgesic drug 763.5
      specified agent NEC 760.79
      suspected, affecting management of pregnancy 655.5 ☑
  cocaine, through placenta or breast milk 760.75
  delirium
    alcohol 291.0
    drug 292.81
  drug 292.89
    with delirium 292.81
    correct substance properly administered (*see also* Allergy, drug) 995.27
    newborn 779.4
    obstetric anesthetic or sedation 668.9 ☑
      affecting fetus or newborn 763.5
    overdose or wrong substance given or taken — *see* Table of Drugs and Chemicals
  pathologic 292.2
  specific to newborn 779.4
  via placenta or breast milk 760.70
    alcohol 760.71
    anticonvulsants 760.77
    antifungals 760.74
    anti-infective agents 760.74
    antimetabolics 760.78

**Intoxication** — *continued*
  drug — *continued*
    via placenta or breast milk — *continued*
      cocaine 760.75
      "crack" 760.75
      hallucinogenic agents 760.73
      medicinal agents NEC 760.79
      narcotics 760.72
      obstetric anesthetic or analgesic drug 763.5
      specified agent NEC 760.79
      suspected, affecting management of pregnancy 655.5 ☑
  enteric — *see* Intoxication, intestinal
  fetus or newborn, via placenta or breast milk 760.70
    alcohol 760.71
    anticonvulsants 760.77
    antifungals 760.74
    anti-infective agents 760.74
    antimetabolics 760.78
    cocaine 760.75
    "crack" 760.75
    hallucinogenic agents 760.73
    medicinal agents NEC 760.79
    narcotics 760.72
    obstetric anesthetic or analgesic drug 763.5
    specified agent NEC 760.79
    suspected, affecting management of pregnancy 655.5 ☑
  food — *see* Poisoning, food
  gastrointestinal 558.2
  hallucinogenic (acute) 305.3 ☑
  hepatocerebral 572.2
  idiosyncratic alcohol 291.4
  intestinal 569.89
    due to putrefaction of food 005.9
  methyl alcohol (*see also* Alcoholism) 305.0 ☑
    with alcoholism 303.0 ☑
  non-foodborne due to toxins of ●
    Clostridium botulinum [C. bo-●
    tulinum] — *see* Botulism ●
  pathologic 291.4
    drug 292.2
  potassium (K) 276.7
  septic
    with
      abortion — *see* Abortion, by type, with sepsis
      ectopic pregnancy (*see also* categories 633.0–633.9) 639.0
      molar pregnancy (*see also* categories 630–632) 639.0
    during labor 659.3 ☑
    following
      abortion 639.0
      ectopic or molar pregnancy 639.0
    generalized — *see* Septicemia
    puerperal, postpartum, childbirth 670.0 ☑
  serum (prophylactic) (therapeutic) 999.5
  uremic — *see* Uremia
  water 276.6
**Intracranial** — *see* condition
**Intrahepatic gallbladder** 751.69
**Intraligamentous** — *see also* condition
  pregnancy — *see* Pregnancy, cornual
**Intraocular** — *see also* condition
  sepsis 360.00
**Intrathoracic** — *see also* condition
  kidney 753.3
  stomach — *see* Hernia, diaphragm
**Intrauterine contraceptive device**
  checking V25.42
  insertion V25.1
  in situ V45.51
  management V25.42
  prescription V25.02
  repeat V25.42

☑ Additional Digit Required — Refer to the Tabular List for Digit Selection    ᴺᴱᶜ Subterms under main terms may continue to next column or page

170 — Volume 2 • October 2007    ▶◀ Revised Text    ● New Line    ▲ Revised Code    *2008 ICD-9-CM*

**Intrauterine contraceptive device** — *continued*
reinsertion V25.42
removal V25.42
**Intraventricular** — *see condition*
**Intrinsic deformity** — *see* Deformity
**Intruded tooth** 524.34
**Intrusion, repetitive, of sleep** (due to environmental disturbances) (with atypical polysomnographic features) 307.48
**Intumescent, lens** (eye) NEC 366.9
senile 366.12
**Intussusception** (colon) (enteric) (intestine) (rectum) 560.0
appendix 543.9
congenital 751.5
fallopian tube 620.8
ileocecal 560.0
ileocolic 560.0
ureter (with obstruction) 593.4
**Invagination**
basilar 756.0
colon or intestine 560.0
**Invalid** (since birth) 799.89
**Invalidism** (chronic) 799.89
**Inversion**
albumin-globulin (A-G) ratio 273.8
bladder 596.8
cecum (*see also* Intussusception) 560.0
cervix 622.8
nipple 611.79
congenital 757.6
puerperal, postpartum 676.3 ☑
optic papilla 743.57
organ or site, congenital NEC — *see* Anomaly, specified type NEC
sleep rhythm 327.39
nonorganic origin 307.45
testis (congenital) 752.51
uterus (postinfectional) (postpartal, old) 621.7
chronic 621.7
complicating delivery 665.2 ☑
affecting fetus or newborn 763.89
vagina — *see* Prolapse, vagina
**Investigation**
allergens V72.7
clinical research (control) (normal comparison) (participant) V70.7
**Inviability** — *see* Immaturity
**Involuntary movement, abnormal** 781.0
**Involution, involutional** — *see also* condition
breast, cystic or fibrocystic 610.1
depression (*see also* Psychosis, affective) 296.2 ☑
recurrent episode 296.3 ☑
single episode 296.2 ☑
melancholia (*see also* Psychosis, affective) 296.2 ☑
recurrent episode 296.3 ☑
single episode 296.2 ☑
ovary, senile 620.3
paranoid state (reaction) 297.2
paraphrenia (climacteric) (menopause) 297.2
psychosis 298.8
thymus failure 254.8
**IQ**
under 20 318.2
20-34 318.1
35-49 318.0
50-70 317
**IRDS** 769
**Irideremia** 743.45
**Iridis rubeosis** 364.42
diabetic 250.5 ☑ *[364.42]*
**Iridochoroiditis** (panuveitis) 360.12
**Iridocyclitis** NEC 364.3
acute 364.00
primary 364.01
recurrent 364.02

**Iridocyclitis** — *continued*
chronic 364.10
in
lepromatous leprosy 030.0 *[364.11]*
sarcoidosis 135 *[364.11]*
tuberculosis (*see also* Tuberculosis) 017.3 ☑ *[364.11]*
due to allergy 364.04
endogenous 364.01
gonococcal 098.41
granulomatous 364.10
herpetic (simplex) 054.44
zoster 053.22
hypopyon 364.05
lens induced 364.23
nongranulomatous 364.00
primary 364.01
recurrent 364.02
rheumatic 364.10
secondary 364.04
infectious 364.03
noninfectious 364.04
subacute 364.00
primary 364.01
recurrent 364.02
sympathetic 360.11
syphilitic (secondary) 091.52
tuberculous (chronic) (*see also* Tuberculosis) 017.3 ☑ *[364.11]*
**Iridocyclochoroiditis** (panuveitis) 360.12
**Iridodialysis** 364.76
**Iridodonesis** 364.89 ▲
**Iridoplegia** (complete) (partial) (reflex) 379.49
**Iridoschisis** 364.52
**Iris** — *see* condition
**Iritis** 364.3
acute 364.00
primary 364.01
recurrent 364.02
chronic 364.10
in
sarcoidosis 135 *[364.11]*
tuberculosis (*see also* Tuberculosis) 017.3 ☑ *[364.11]*
diabetic 250.5 ☑ *[364.42]*
due to
allergy 364.04
herpes simplex 054.44
leprosy 030.0 *[364.11]*
endogenous 364.01
gonococcal 098.41
gouty 274.89 *[364.11]*
granulomatous 364.10
hypopyon 364.05
lens induced 364.23
nongranulomatous 364.00
papulosa 095.8 *[364.11]*
primary 364.01
recurrent 364.02
rheumatic 364.10
secondary 364.04
infectious 364.03
noninfectious 364.04
subacute 364.00
primary 364.01
recurrent 364.02
sympathetic 360.11
syphilitic (secondary) 091.52
congenital 090.0 *[364.11]*
late 095.8 *[364.11]*
tuberculous (*see also* Tuberculosis) 017.3 ☑ *[364.11]*
uratic 274.89 *[364.11]*
**Iron**
deficiency anemia 280.9
metabolism disease 275.0
storage disease 275.0
**Iron-miners' lung** 503
**Irradiated enamel** (tooth, teeth) 521.89
**Irradiation**
burn — *see* Burn, by site
effects, adverse 990

**Irreducible, irreducibility** — *see* condition
**Irregular, irregularity**
action, heart 427.9
alveolar process 525.8
bleeding NEC 626.4
breathing 786.09
colon 569.89
contour of cornea 743.41
acquired 371.70
dentin in pulp 522.3
eye movements NEC 379.59
menstruation (cause unknown) 626.4
periods 626.4
prostate 602.9
pupil 364.75
respiratory 786.09
septum (nasal) 470
shape, organ or site, congenital NEC — *see* Distortion
sleep-wake rhythm (non-24-hour) 327.39
nonorganic origin 307.45
vertebra 733.99
**Irritability** (nervous) 799.2
bladder 596.8
neurogenic 596.54
with cauda equina syndrome 344.61
bowel (syndrome) 564.1
bronchial (*see also* Bronchitis) 490
cerebral, newborn 779.1
colon 564.1
psychogenic 306.4
duodenum 564.89
heart (psychogenic) 306.2
ileum 564.89
jejunum 564.89
myocardium 306.2
rectum 564.89
stomach 536.9
psychogenic 306.4
sympathetic (nervous system) (*see also* Neuropathy, peripheral, autonomic) 337.9
urethra 599.84
ventricular (heart) (psychogenic) 306.2
**Irritable** — *see* Irritability
**Irritation**
anus 569.49
axillary nerve 353.0
bladder 596.8
brachial plexus 353.0
brain (traumatic) (*see also* Injury, intracranial) 854.0 ☑
nontraumatic — *see* Encephalitis
bronchial (*see also* Bronchitis) 490
cerebral (traumatic) (*see also* Injury, intracranial) 854.0 ☑
nontraumatic — *see* Encephalitis
cervical plexus 353.2
cervix (*see also* Cervicitis) 616.0
choroid, sympathetic 360.11
cranial nerve — *see* Disorder, nerve, cranial
digestive tract 536.9
psychogenic 306.4
gastric 536.9
psychogenic 306.4
gastrointestinal (tract) 536.9
functional 536.9
psychogenic 306.4
globe, sympathetic 360.11
intestinal (bowel) 564.9
labyrinth 386.50
lumbosacral plexus 353.1
meninges (traumatic) (*see also* Injury, intracranial) 854.0 ☑
nontraumatic — *see* Meningitis
myocardium 306.2
nerve — *see* Disorder, nerve
nervous 799.2
nose 478.19
penis 607.89
perineum 709.9

**Irritation** — *continued*
peripheral
autonomic nervous system (*see also* Neuropathy, peripheral, autonomic) 337.9
nerve — *see* Disorder, nerve
peritoneum (*see also* Peritonitis) 567.9
pharynx 478.29
plantar nerve 355.6
spinal (cord) (traumatic) (*see also* Injury, spinal, by site)
nerve (*see also* Disorder, nerve)
root NEC 724.9
traumatic — *see* Injury, nerve, spinal
nontraumatic — *see* Myelitis
stomach 536.9
psychogenic 306.4
sympathetic nerve NEC (*see also* Neuropathy, peripheral, autonomic) 337.9
ulnar nerve 354.2
vagina 623.9
**Isambert's disease** 012.3 ☑
**Ischemia, ischemic** 459.9
basilar artery (with transient neurologic deficit) 435.0
bone NEC 733.40
bowel (transient) 557.9
acute 557.0
chronic 557.1
due to mesenteric artery insufficiency 557.1
brain (*see also* Ischemia, cerebral)
recurrent focal 435.9
cardiac (*see also* Ischemia, heart) 414.9
cardiomyopathy 414.8
carotid artery (with transient neurologic deficit) 435.8
cerebral (chronic) (generalized) 437.1
arteriosclerotic 437.0
intermittent (with transient neurologic deficit) 435.9
newborn 779.2
puerperal, postpartum, childbirth 674.0 ☑
recurrent focal (with transient neurologic deficit) 435.9
transient (with transient neurologic deficit) 435.9
colon 557.9
acute 557.0
chronic 557.1
due to mesenteric artery insufficiency 557.1
coronary (chronic) (*see also* Ischemia, heart) 414.9
heart (chronic or with a stated duration of over 8 weeks) 414.9
acute or with a stated duration of 8 weeks or less (*see also* Infarct, myocardium) 410.9 ☑
without myocardial infarction 411.89
with coronary (artery) occlusion 411.81
subacute 411.89
intestine (transient) 557.9
acute 557.0
chronic 557.1
due to mesenteric artery insufficiency 557.1
kidney 593.81
labyrinth 386.50
muscles, leg 728.89
myocardium, myocardial (chronic or with a stated duration of over 8 weeks) 414.8
acute (*see also* Infarct, myocardium) 410.9 ☑
without myocardial infarction 411.89
with coronary (artery) occlusion 411.81
renal 593.81

☑ Additional Digit Required — Refer to the Tabular List for Digit Selection
**2008 ICD-9-CM**
▶◀ Revised Text
● New Line
▲ Revised Code
▽ Subterms under main terms may continue to next column or page
October 2007 • Volume 2 — 171

**Ischemia, ischemic** — *continued*
  retina, retinal 362.84
  small bowel 557.9
    acute 557.0
    chronic 557.1
    due to mesenteric artery insufficien-
      cy 557.1
  spinal cord 336.1
  subendocardial (*see also* Insufficiency,
    coronary) 411.89
  vertebral artery (with transient neuro-
    logic deficit) 435.1
**Ischialgia** — *see also* Sciatica 724.3
**Ischiopagus** 759.4
**Ischium, ischial** — *see* condition
**Ischomenia** 626.8
**Ischuria** 788.5
**Iselin's disease or osteochondrosis**
  732.5
**Islands of**
  parotid tissue in
    lymph nodes 750.26
    neck structures 750.26
  submaxillary glands in
    fascia 750.26
    lymph nodes 750.26

**Islands of** — *continued*
  submaxillary glands in — *contin-*
    *ued*
    neck muscles 750.26
**Islet cell tumor, pancreas** (M8150/0)
  211.7
**Isoimmunization** NEC — *see also* Incompatibility 656.2 ☑
  anti-E 656.2 ☑                                    ●
  fetus or newborn 773.2
    ABO blood groups 773.1
    Rhesus (Rh) factor 773.0
**Isolation** V07.0
  social V62.4
**Isosporosis** 007.2
**Issue**
  medical certificate NEC V68.09        ▲
    cause of death V68.09                ▲
    disability examination V68.01        ●
    fitness V68.09                       ▲
    incapacity V68.09                    ▲
  repeat prescription NEC V68.1
    appliance V68.1
    contraceptive V25.40
      device NEC V25.49
        intrauterine V25.42

**Issue** — *continued*
  repeat prescription — *continued*
    contraceptive — *continued*
      device — *continued*
        specified type NEC V25.49
      pill V25.41
    glasses V68.1
    medicinal substance V68.1
**Itch** — *see also* Pruritus 698.9
  bakers' 692.89
  barbers' 110.0
  bricklayers' 692.89
  cheese 133.8
  clam diggers' 120.3
  coolie 126.9
  copra 133.8
  Cuban 050.1
  dew 126.9
  dhobie 110.3
  eye 379.99
  filarial (*see also* Infestation, filarial)
    125.9
  grain 133.8
  grocers' 133.8
  ground 126.9
  harvest 133.8

**Itch** — *see also* Pruritus — *continued*
  jock 110.3
  Malabar 110.9
    beard 110.0
    foot 110.4
    scalp 110.0
  meaning scabies 133.0
  Norwegian 133.0
  perianal 698.0
  poultrymen's 133.8
  sarcoptic 133.0
  scrub 134.1
  seven year V61.10
    meaning scabies 133.0
  straw 133.8
  swimmers' 120.3
  washerwoman's 692.4
  water 120.3
  winter 698.8
**Itsenko-Cushing syndrome** (pituitary
  basophilism) 255.0
**Ivemark's syndrome** (asplenia with
  congenital heart disease) 759.0
**Ivory bones** 756.52
**Ixodes** 134.8
**Ixodiasis** 134.8

☑ Additional Digit Required — Refer to the Tabular List for Digit Selection
                                    Subterms under main terms may continue to next column or page
**172** — Volume 2 • October 2007    ►◄ Revised Text    ● New Line    ▲ Revised Code    ***2008 ICD-9-CM***

### J

**Jaccoud's nodular fibrositis, chronic** (Jaccoud's syndrome) 714.4
**Jackson's**
  membrane 751.4
  paralysis or syndrome 344.89
  veil 751.4
**Jacksonian**
  epilepsy (*see also* Epilepsy) 345.5 ☑
  seizures (focal) (*see also* Epilepsy) 345.5 ☑
**Jacob's ulcer** (M8090/3) — *see* Neoplasm, skin, malignant, by site
**Jacquet's dermatitis** (diaper dermatitis) 691.0
**Jadassohn's**
  blue nevus (M8780/0) — *see* Neoplasm, skin, benign
  disease (maculopapular erythroderma) 696.2
  intraepidermal epithelioma (M8096/0) — *see* Neoplasm, skin, benign
**Jadassohn-Lewandowski syndrome** (pachyonychia congenita) 757.5
**Jadassohn-Pellizari's disease** (anetoderma) 701.3
**Jadassohn-Tièche nevus** (M8780/0) — *see* Neoplasm, skin, benign
**Jaffe-Lichtenstein (-Uehlinger) syndrome** 252.01
**Jahnke's syndrome** (encephalocutaneous angiomatosis) 759.6
**Jakob-Creutzfeldt disease (syndrome) (new variant)** 046.1
  with dementia
    with behavioral disturbance 046.1 [294.11]
    without behavioral disturbance 046.1 [294.10]
**Jaksch (-Luzet) disease or syndrome** (pseudoleukemia infantum) 285.8
**Jamaican**
  neuropathy 349.82
  paraplegic tropical ataxic-spastic syndrome 349.82
**Janet's disease** (psychasthenia) 300.89
**Janiceps** 759.4
**Jansky-Bielschowsky amaurotic familial idiocy** 330.1
**Japanese**
  B type encephalitis 062.0
  river fever 081.2
  seven-day fever 100.89
**Jaundice** (yellow) 782.4
  acholuric (familial) (splenomegalic) (*see also* Spherocytosis) 282.0
    acquired 283.9
  breast milk 774.39
  catarrhal (acute) 070.1
    with hepatic coma 070.0
    chronic 571.9
    epidemic — *see* Jaundice, epidemic
  cholestatic (benign) 782.4
  chronic idiopathic 277.4
  epidemic (catarrhal) 070.1
    with hepatic coma 070.0
    leptospiral 100.0
    spirochetal 100.0
  febrile (acute) 070.1
    with hepatic coma 070.0
    leptospiral 100.0
    spirochetal 100.0
  fetus or newborn 774.6
    due to or associated with
      ABO
        absence or deficiency of enzyme system for bilirubin conjugation (congenital) 774.39
        antibodies 773.1
        blood group incompatibility NEC 773.2
        breast milk inhibitors to conjugation 774.39
          associated with preterm delivery 774.2
        bruising 774.1

**Jaundice** — *continued*
  fetus or newborn — *continued*
    due to or associated with — *continued*
      Crigler-Najjar syndrome 277.4 [774.31]
      delayed conjugation 774.30
        associated with preterm delivery 774.2
      development 774.39
      drugs or toxins transmitted from mother 774.1
      G-6-PD deficiency 282.2 [774.0]
      galactosemia 271.1 [774.5]
      Gilbert's syndrome 277.4 [774.31]
      hepatocellular damage 774.4
      hereditary hemolytic anemia (*see also* Anemia, hemolytic) 282.9 [774.0]
      hypothyroidism, congenital 243 [774.31]
      incompatibility, maternal/fetal NEC 773.2
      incompatibility, maternal/fetal 773.1
      infection 774.1
      inspissated bile syndrome 774.4
      isoimmunization NEC 773.2
      isoimmunization 773.1
      mucoviscidosis 277.01 [774.5]
      obliteration of bile duct, congenital 751.61 [774.5]
      polycythemia 774.1
      preterm delivery 774.2
      red cell defect 282.9 [774.0]
      Rh
        antibodies 773.0
        incompatibility, maternal/fetal 773.0
        isoimmunization 773.0
      spherocytosis (congenital) 282.0 [774.0]
      swallowed maternal blood 774.1
    physiological NEC 774.6
  from injection, inoculation, infusion, or transfusion (blood) (plasma) (serum) (other substance) (onset within 8 months after administration) — *see* Hepatitis, viral
  Gilbert's (familial nonhemolytic) 277.4
  hematogenous 283.9
  hemolytic (acquired) 283.9
    congenital (*see also* Spherocytosis) 282.0
  hemorrhagic (acute) 100.0
    leptospiral 100.0
    newborn 776.0
    spirochetal 100.0
  hepatocellular 573.8
  homologous (serum) — *see* Hepatitis, viral
  idiopathic, chronic 277.4
  infectious (acute) (subacute) 070.1
    with hepatic coma 070.0
    leptospiral 100.0
    spirochetal 100.0
  leptospiral 100.0
  malignant (*see also* Necrosis, liver) 570
  newborn (physiological) (*see also* Jaundice, fetus or newborn) 774.6
  nonhemolytic, congenital familial (Gilbert's) 277.4
  nuclear, newborn (*see also* Kernicterus of newborn) 774.7
  obstructive NEC (*see also* Obstruction, biliary) 576.8
  postimmunization — *see* Hepatitis, viral
  posttransfusion — *see* Hepatitis, viral
  regurgitation (*see also* Obstruction, biliary) 576.8

**Jaundice** — *continued*
  serum (homologous) (prophylactic) (therapeutic) — *see* Hepatitis, viral
  spirochetal (hemorrhagic) 100.0
  symptomatic 782.4
    newborn 774.6
**Jaw** — *see* condition
**Jaw-blinking** 374.43
  congenital 742.8
**Jaw-winking phenomenon or syndrome** 742.8
**Jealousy**
  alcoholic 291.5
  childhood 313.3
  sibling 313.3
**Jejunitis** — *see also* Enteritis 558.9
**Jejunostomy status** V44.4
**Jejunum, jejunal** — *see* condition
**Jensen's disease** 363.05
**Jericho boil** 085.1
**Jerks, myoclonic** 333.2
**Jervell-Lange-Nielsen syndrome** 426.82
**Jeune's disease or syndrome** (asphyxiating thoracic dystrophy) 756.4
**Jigger disease** 134.1
**Job's syndrome** (chronic granulomatous disease) 288.1
**Jod-Basedow phenomenon** 242.8 ☑
**Johnson-Stevens disease** (erythema multiforme exudativum) 695.1
**Joint** — *see also* condition
  Charcôt's 094.0 [713.5]
  false 733.82
  flail — *see* Flail, joint
  mice — *see* Loose, body, joint, by site
  sinus to bone 730.9 ☑
  von Gies' 095.8
**Jordan's anomaly or syndrome** 288.2
**Josephs-Diamond-Blackfan anemia** (congenital hypoplastic) 284.01
**Joubert syndrome** 759.89
**Jumpers' knee** 727.2
**Jungle yellow fever** 060.0
**Jüngling's disease** (sarcoidosis) 135
**Junin virus hemorrhagic fever** 078.7
**Juvenile** — *see* condition
  delinquent 312.9
    group (*see also* Disturbance, conduct) 312.2 ☑
    neurotic 312.4

### K

**Kabuki syndrome** 759.89
**Kahler (-Bozzolo) disease** (multiple myeloma) (M9730/3) 203.0 ☑
**Kakergasia** 300.9
**Kakke** 265.0
**Kala-azar** (Indian) (infantile) (Mediterranean) (Sudanese) 085.0
**Kalischer's syndrome** (encephalocutaneous angiomatosis) 759.6
**Kallmann's syndrome** (hypogonadotropic hypogonadism with anosmia) 253.4
**Kanner's syndrome** (autism) — *see also* Psychosis, childhood 299.0 ☑
**Kaolinosis** 502
**Kaposi's**
  disease 757.33
    lichen ruber 696.4
      acuminatus 696.4
      moniliformis 697.8
    xeroderma pigmentosum 757.33
  sarcoma (M9140/3) 176.9
    adipose tissue 176.1
    aponeurosis 176.1
    artery 176.1
    associated herpesvirus infection ● 058.89     ●
    blood vessel 176.1
    bursa 176.1
    connective tissue 176.1
    external genitalia 176.8
    fascia 176.1
    fatty tissue 176.1

**Kaposi's** — *continued*
  sarcoma — *continued*
    fibrous tissue 176.1
    gastrointestinal tract NEC 176.3
    ligament 176.1
    lung 176.4
    lymph
      gland(s) 176.5
      node(s) 176.5
    lymphatic(s) NEC 176.1
    muscle (skeletal) 176.1
    oral cavity NEC 176.8
    palate 176.2
    scrotum 176.8
    skin 176.0
    soft tissue 176.1
    specified site NEC 176.8
    subcutaneous tissue 176.1
    synovia 176.1
    tendon (sheath) 176.1
    vein 176.1
    vessel 176.1
    viscera NEC 176.9
    vulva 176.8
  varicelliform eruption 054.0
  vaccinia 999.0
**Kartagener's syndrome or triad** (sinusitis, bronchiectasis, situs inversus) 759.3
**Kasabach-Merritt syndrome** (capillary hemangioma associated with thrombocytopenic purpura) 287.39
**Kaschin-Beck disease** (endemic polyarthritis) — *see* Disease, Kaschin-Beck
**Kast's syndrome** (dyschondroplasia with hemangiomas) 756.4
**Katatonia** — *see* Catatonia
**Katayama disease or fever** 120.2
**Kathisophobia** 781.0
**Kawasaki disease** 446.1
**Kayser-Fleischer ring** (cornea) (pseudosclerosis) 275.1 [371.14]
**Kaznelson's syndrome** (congenital hypoplastic anemia) 284.01
**Kearns-Sayre syndrome** 277.87
**Kedani fever** 081.2
**Kelis** 701.4
**Kelly (-Patterson) syndrome** (sideropenic dysphagia) 280.8
**Keloid, cheloid** 701.4
  Addison's (morphea) 701.0
  cornea 371.00
  Hawkins' 701.4
  scar 701.4
**Keloma** 701.4
**Kenya fever** 082.1
**Keratectasia** 371.71
  congenital 743.41
**Keratinization NEC**
  alveolar ridge mucosa
    excessive 528.72
    minimal 528.71
**Keratitis** (nodular) (nonulcerative) (simple) (zonular) NEC 370.9
  with ulceration (*see also* Ulcer, cornea) 370.00
  actinic 370.24
  arborescens 054.42
  areolar 370.22
  bullosa 370.8
  deep — *see* Keratitis, interstitial
  dendritic(a) 054.42
  desiccation 370.34
  diffuse interstitial 370.52
  disciform(is) 054.43
    varicella 052.7 [370.44]
  epithelialis vernalis 372.13 [370.32]
  exposure 370.34
  filamentary 370.23
  gonococcal (congenital) (prenatal) 098.43
  herpes, herpetic (simplex) NEC 054.43
    zoster 053.21
  hypopyon 370.04

☑ Additional Digit Required — Refer to the Tabular List for Digit Selection            ⓦ Subterms under main terms may continue to next column or page

**2008 ICD-9-CM**      ▶◀ Revised Text      ● New Line      ▲ Revised Code      **October 2007 · Volume 2 — 173**

**Keratitis** — continued
  in
    chickenpox 052.7 [370.44]
    exanthema (see also Exanthem)
      057.9 [370.44]
    paravaccinia (see also Paravac-
      cinia) 051.9 [370.44]
    smallpox (see also Smallpox)
      050.9 [370.44]
    vernal conjunctivitis
      372.13 [370.32]
  interstitial (nonsyphilitic) 370.50
    with ulcer (see also Ulcer, cornea)
      370.00
    diffuse 370.52
    herpes, herpetic (simplex) 054.43
      zoster 053.21
    syphilitic (congenital) (hereditary)
      090.3
    tuberculous (see also Tuberculosis)
      017.3 ☑ [370.59]
  lagophthalmic 370.34
  macular 370.22
  neuroparalytic 370.35
  neurotrophic 370.35
  nummular 370.22
  oyster-shuckers' 370.8
  parenchymatous — see Keratitis, in-
    terstitial
  petrificans 370.8
  phlyctenular 370.31
  postmeasles 055.71
  punctata, punctate 370.21
    leprosa 030.0 [370.21]
    profunda 090.3
    superficial (Thygeson's) 370.21
  purulent 370.8
  pustuliformis profunda 090.3
  rosacea 695.3 [370.49]
  sclerosing 370.54
  specified type NEC 370.8
  stellate 370.22
  striate 370.22
  superficial 370.20
    with conjunctivitis (see also Kerato-
      conjunctivitis) 370.40
    punctate (Thygeson's) 370.21
  suppurative 370.8
  syphilitic (congenital) (prenatal) 090.3
  trachomatous 076.1
    late effect 139.1
  tuberculous (phlyctenular) (see also
    Tuberculosis) 017.3 ☑ [370.31]
  ulcerated (see also Ulcer, cornea)
    370.00
  vesicular 370.8
  welders' 370.24
  xerotic (see also Keratomalacia)
    371.45
    vitamin A deficiency 264.4
**Keratoacanthoma** 238.2
**Keratocele** 371.72
**Keratoconjunctivitis** — see also Keratitis 370.40
  adenovirus type 8 077.1
  epidemic 077.1
  exposure 370.34
  gonococcal 098.43
  herpetic (simplex) 054.43
    zoster 053.21
  in
    chickenpox 052.7 [370.44]
    exanthema (see also Exanthem)
      057.9 [370.44]
    paravaccinia (see also Paravac-
      cinia) 051.9 [370.44]
    smallpox (see also Smallpox)
      050.9 [370.44]
  infectious 077.1
  neurotrophic 370.35
  phlyctenular 370.31
  postmeasles 055.71
  shipyard 077.1
  sicca (Sjögren's syndrome) 710.2
    not in Sjögren's syndrome 370.33
  specified type NEC 370.49

**Keratoconjunctivitis** — see also
  Keratitis — continued
  tuberculous (phlyctenular) (see also
    Tuberculosis) 017.3 ☑ [370.31]
**Keratoconus** 371.60
  acute hydrops 371.62
  congenital 743.41
  stable 371.61
**Keratocyst** (dental) 526.0
**Keratoderma, keratodermia** (congenital)
  (palmaris et plantaris) (symmetrical) 757.39
  acquired 701.1
  blennorrhagica 701.1
    gonococcal 098.81
  climacterium 701.1
  eccentrica 757.39
  gonorrheal 098.81
  punctata 701.1
  tylodes, progressive 701.1
**Keratodermatocele** 371.72
**Keratoglobus** 371.70
  congenital 743.41
    associated with buphthalmos
      743.22
**Keratohemia** 371.12
**Keratoiritis** — see also Iridocyclitis
  364.3
  syphilitic 090.3
  tuberculous (see also Tuberculosis)
    017.3 ☑ [364.11]
**Keratolysis exfoliativa** (congenital)
  757.39
  acquired 695.89
  neonatorum 757.39
**Keratoma** 701.1
  congenital 757.39
  malignum congenitale 757.1
  palmaris et plantaris hereditarium
    757.39
  senile 702.0
**Keratomalacia** 371.45
  vitamin A deficiency 264.4
**Keratomegaly** 743.41
**Keratomycosis** 111.1
  nigricans (palmaris) 111.1
**Keratopathy** 371.40
  band (see also Keratitis) 371.43
  bullous (see also Keratitis) 371.23
  degenerative (see also Degeneration,
    cornea) 371.40
  hereditary (see also Dystrophy,
    cornea) 371.50
  discrete colliquative 371.49
**Keratoscleritis, tuberculous** — see also
  Tuberculosis 017.3 ☑ [370.31]
**Keratosis** 701.1
  actinic 702.0
  arsenical 692.4
  blennorrhagica 701.1
    gonococcal 098.81
  congenital (any type) 757.39
  ear (middle) (see also Cholesteatoma)
    385.30
  female genital (external) 629.89
  follicularis 757.39
    acquired 701.1
    congenital (acneiformis) (Siemens')
      757.39
    spinulosa (decalvans) 757.39
    vitamin A deficiency 264.8
  follicular, vitamin A deficiency 264.8
  gonococcal 098.81
  larynx, laryngeal 478.79
  male genital (external) 608.89
  middle ear (see also Cholesteatoma)
    385.30
  nigricans 701.2
    congenital 757.39
  obturans 380.21
  oral epithelium
    residual ridge mucosa
      excessive 528.72
      minimal 528.71
  palmaris et plantaris (symmetrical)
    757.39

**Keratosis** — continued
  penile 607.89
  pharyngeus 478.29
  pilaris 757.39
    acquired 701.1
  punctata (palmaris et plantaris) 701.1
  scrotal 608.89
  seborrheic 702.19
    inflamed 702.11
  senilis 702.0
  solar 702.0
  suprafollicularis 757.39
  tonsillaris 478.29
  vagina 623.1
  vegetans 757.39
  vitamin A deficiency 264.8
**Kerato-uveitis** — see also Iridocyclitis
  364.3
**Keraunoparalysis** 994.0
**Kerion** (celsi) 110.0
**Kernicterus of newborn** (not due to
  isoimmunization) 774.7
  due to isoimmunization (conditions
    classifiable to 773.0–773.2)
    773.4
**Ketoacidosis** 276.2
  diabetic 250.1 ☑
**Ketonuria** 791.6
  branched-chain, intermittent 270.3
**Ketosis** 276.2
  diabetic 250.1 ☑
**Kidney** — see condition
**Kienböck's**
  disease 732.3
    adult 732.8
  osteochondrosis 732.3
**Kimmelstiel (-Wilson) disease or syn-
  drome** (intercapillary glomerulosclerosis) 250.4 ☑ [581.81]
**Kink, kinking**
  appendix 543.9
  artery 447.1
  cystic duct, congenital 751.61
  hair (acquired) 704.2
  ileum or intestine (see also Obstruc-
    tion, intestine) 560.9
  Lane's (see also Obstruction, intestine)
    560.9
  organ or site, congenital NEC — see
    Anomaly, specified type NEC,
    by site
  ureter (pelvic junction) 593.3
    congenital 753.20
  vein(s) 459.2
    caval 459.2
    peripheral 459.2
**Kinnier Wilson's disease** (hepatolenticular degeneration) 275.1
**Kissing**
  osteophytes 721.5
  spine 721.5
  vertebra 721.5
**Klauder's syndrome** (erythema multi-
  forme, exudativum) 695.1
**Klebs' disease** — see also Nephritis
  583.9
**Kleine-Levin syndrome** 327.13
**Klein-Waardenburg syndrome** (ptosisepi-
  canthus) 270.2
**Kleptomania** 312.32
**Klinefelter's syndrome** 758.7
**Klinger's disease** 446.4
**Klippel's disease** 723.8
**Klippel-Feil disease or syndrome** (bre-
  vicollis) 756.16
**Klippel-Trenaunay syndrome** 759.89
**Klumpke (-Déjérine) palsy, paralysis**
  (birth) (newborn) 767.6
**Klüver-Bucy (-Terzian) syndrome** 310.0
**Knee** — see condition
**Knifegrinders' rot** — see also Tubercu-
  losis 011.4 ☑
**Knock-knee** (acquired) 736.41
  congenital 755.64
**Knot**
  intestinal, syndrome (volvulus) 560.2

**Knot** — continued
  umbilical cord (true) 663.2 ☑
    affecting fetus or newborn 762.5
**Knots, surfer** 919.8
  infected 919.9
**Knotting** (of)
  hair 704.2
  intestine 560.2
**Knuckle pads** (Garrod's) 728.79
**Köbner's disease** (epidermolysis bullosa)
  757.39
**Koch's**
  infection (see also Tuberculosis, pul-
    monary) 011.9 ☑
  relapsing fever 087.9
**Koch-Weeks conjunctivitis** 372.03
**Koenig-Wichman disease** (pemphigus)
  694.4
**Köhler's disease** (osteochondrosis) 732.5
  first (osteochondrosis juvenilis) 732.5
  second (Freiburg's infarction,
    metatarsal head) 732.5
  patellar 732.4
  tarsal navicular (bone) (osteoarthrosis
    juvenilis) 732.5
**Köhler-Mouchet disease** (osteoarthrosis
  juvenilis) 732.5
**Köhler-Pellegrini-Stieda disease or
  syndrome** (calcification, knee joint)
  726.62
**Koilonychia** 703.8
  congenital 757.5
**Kojevnikov's, Kojewnikoff's epilepsy**
  — see also Epilepsy 345.7 ☑
**König's**
  disease (osteochondritis dissecans)
    732.7
  syndrome 564.89
**Koniophthisis** — see also Tuberculosis
  011.4 ☑
**Koplik's spots** 055.9
**Kopp's asthma** 254.8
**Korean hemorrhagic fever** 078.6
**Korsakoff (-Wernicke) disease, psy-
  chosis, or syndrome** (nonalcoholic) 294.0
  alcoholic 291.1
**Korsakov's disease** — see Korsakoff's
  disease
**Korsakow's disease** — see Korsakoff's
  disease
**Kostmann's disease or syndrome** (infan-
  tile genetic agranulocytosis) 288.01
**Krabbe's**
  disease (leukodystrophy) 330.0
  syndrome
    congenital muscle hypoplasia
      756.89
    cutaneocerebral angioma 759.6
**Kraepelin-Morel disease** — see also
  Schizophrenia 295.9 ☑
**Kraft-Weber-Dimitri disease** 759.6
**Kraurosis**
  ani 569.49
  penis 607.0
  vagina 623.8
  vulva 624.09   ▲
**Kreotoxism** 005.9
**Krukenberg's**
  spindle 371.13
  tumor (M8490/6) 198.6
**Kufs' disease** 330.1
**Kugelberg-Welander disease** 335.11
**Kuhnt-Junius degeneration or disease**
  362.52
**Kulchitsky's cell carcinoma** (carcinoid
  tumor of intestine) 259.2
**Kümmell's disease or spondylitis** 721.7
**Kundrat's disease** (lymphosarcoma)
  200.1 ☑
**Kunekune** — see Dermatophytosis
**Kunkel syndrome** (lupoid hepatitis)
  571.49
**Kupffer cell sarcoma** (M9124/3) 155.0
**Kuru** 046.0

☑ Additional Digit Required — Refer to the Tabular List for Digit Selection     ▽ Subterms under main terms may continue to next column or page

174 — Volume 2 • October 2007    ▶◀ Revised Text    ● New Line    ▲ Revised Code    **2008 ICD-9-CM**

**Kussmaul's**
　coma (diabetic) 250.3 ☑
　disease (polyarteritis nodosa) 446.0
　respiration (air hunger) 786.09
**Kwashiorkor** (marasmus type) 260
**Kyasanur Forest disease** 065.2
**Kyphoscoliosis, kyphoscoliotic** (acquired) — see also Scoliosis 737.30
　congenital 756.19
　due to radiation 737.33
　heart (disease) 416.1
　idiopathic 737.30
　　infantile
　　　progressive 737.32
　　　resolving 737.31
　late effect of rickets 268.1 [737.43]
　specified NEC 737.39
　thoracogenic 737.34
　tuberculous (see also Tuberculosis)
　　015.0 ☑ [737.43]
**Kyphosis, kyphotic** (acquired) (postural) 737.10
　adolescent postural 737.0
　congenital 756.19
　dorsalis juvenilis 732.0
　due to or associated with
　　Charcôt-Marie-Tooth disease
　　　356.1 [737.41]
　　mucopolysaccharidosis
　　　277.5 [737.41]
　　neurofibromatosis 237.71 [737.41]
　　osteitis
　　　deformans 731.0 [737.41]
　　　fibrosa cystica 252.01 [737.41]
　　osteoporosis (see also Osteoporosis)
　　　733.0 ☑ [737.41]
　　poliomyelitis (see also Poliomyelitis)
　　　138 [737.41]
　　radiation 737.11
　　tuberculosis (see also Tuberculosis)
　　　015.0 ☑ [737.41]
　Kümmell's 721.7
　late effect of rickets 268.1 [737.41]
　Morquio-Brailsford type (spinal)
　　277.5 [737.41]
　pelvis 738.6
　postlaminectomy 737.12
　specified cause NEC 737.19
　syphilitic, congenital 090.5 [737.41]
　tuberculous (see also Tuberculosis)
　　015.0 ☑ [737.41]
**Kyrle's disease** (hyperkeratosis follicularis in cutem penetrans) 701.1

## L

**Labia, labium** — see condition
**Labiated hymen** 752.49
**Labile**
　blood pressure 796.2
　emotions, emotionality 301.3
　vasomotor system 443.9
**Labioglossal paralysis** 335.22
**Labium leporinum** — see also Cleft, lip
　749.10
**Labor** — see also Delivery
　with complications — see Delivery,
　　complicated
　abnormal NEC 661.9 ☑
　　affecting fetus or newborn 763.7
　arrested active phase 661.1 ☑
　　affecting fetus or newborn 763.7
　desultory 661.2 ☑
　　affecting fetus or newborn 763.7
　dyscoordinate 661.4 ☑
　　affecting fetus or newborn 763.7
　early onset (22-36 weeks gestation)
　　644.2 ☑
　failed
　　induction 659.1 ☑
　　　mechanical 659.0 ☑
　　　medical 659.1 ☑
　　　surgical 659.0 ☑
　　trial (vaginal delivery) 660.6 ☑
　false 644.1 ☑

**Labor** — see also Delivery — continued
　forced or induced, affecting fetus or
　　newborn 763.89
　hypertonic 661.4 ☑
　　affecting fetus or newborn 763.7
　hypotonic 661.2 ☑
　　primary 661.0 ☑
　　　affecting fetus or newborn 763.7
　　secondary 661.1 ☑
　　　affecting fetus or newborn 763.7
　incoordinate 661.4 ☑
　　affecting fetus or newborn 763.7
　irregular 661.2 ☑
　　affecting fetus or newborn 763.7
　long — see Labor, prolonged
　missed (at or near term) 656.4 ☑
　obstructed NEC 660.9 ☑
　　affecting fetus or newborn 763.1
　　due to female genital mutilation
　　　660.8 ☑
　　specified cause NEC 660.8 ☑
　　　affecting fetus or newborn 763.1
　pains, spurious 644.1 ☑
　precipitate 661.3 ☑
　　affecting fetus or newborn 763.6
　premature 644.2 ☑
　　threatened 644.0 ☑
　prolonged or protracted 662.1 ☑
　　first stage 662.0 ☑
　　　affecting fetus or newborn
　　　　763.89
　　second stage 662.2 ☑
　　　affecting fetus or newborn
　　　　763.89
　　affecting fetus or newborn 763.89
　threatened NEC 644.1 ☑
　undelivered 644.1 ☑
**Labored breathing** — see also Hyperventilation 786.09
**Labyrinthitis** (inner ear) (destructive)
　(latent) 386.30
　circumscribed 386.32
　diffuse 386.31
　focal 386.32
　purulent 386.33
　serous 386.31
　suppurative 386.33
　syphilitic 095.8
　toxic 386.34
　viral 386.35
**Laceration** — see also Wound, open, by
　site
　accidental, complicating surgery 998.2
　Achilles tendon 845.09
　　with open wound 892.2
　anus (sphincter) 879.6
　　with
　　　abortion — see Abortion, by
　　　　type, with damage to
　　　　pelvic organs
　　　ectopic pregnancy (see also categories 633.0–633.9)
　　　　639.2
　　　molar pregnancy (see also categories 630–632) 639.2
　　complicated 879.7
　　complicating delivery ▶(healed)
　　　(old)◀ 654.8 ☑　　　　　　▲
　　　with laceration of anal or rectal
　　　　mucosa 664.3 ☑
　　　not associated with third-de- ●
　　　　gree perineal laceration ●
　　　　664.6 ☑　　　　　　　　 ●
　　following
　　　abortion 639.2
　　　ectopic or molar pregnancy
　　　　639.2
　　nontraumatic, nonpuerperal
　　　▶(healed) (old)◀ 569.43
　bladder (urinary)
　　with
　　　abortion — see Abortion, by
　　　　type, with damage to
　　　　pelvic organs

**Laceration** — see also Wound, open, by
　site — continued
　bladder — continued
　　with — continued
　　　ectopic pregnancy (see also categories 633.0–633.9)
　　　　639.2
　　　molar pregnancy (see also categories 630–632) 639.2
　　following
　　　abortion 639.2
　　　ectopic or molar pregnancy
　　　　639.2
　　obstetrical trauma 665.5 ☑
　blood vessel — see Injury, blood vessel, by site
　bowel
　　with
　　　abortion — see Abortion, by
　　　　type, with damage to
　　　　pelvic organs
　　　ectopic pregnancy (see also categories 633.0–633.9)
　　　　639.2
　　　molar pregnancy (see also categories 630–632) 639.2
　　following
　　　abortion 639.2
　　　ectopic or molar pregnancy
　　　　639.2
　　obstetrical trauma 665.5 ☑
　brain (cerebral) (membrane) (with
　　hemorrhage) 851.8 ☑

Note — Use the following fifth-digit
subclassification with categories
851–854:

0　unspecified state of consciousness

1　with no loss of consciousness

2　with brief [less than one hour]
　loss of consciousness

3　with moderate [1–24 hours] loss
　of consciousness

4　with prolonged [more than 24
　hours] loss of consciousness and
　return to pre–existing conscious
　level

5　with prolonged [more than 24
　hours] loss of consciousness,
　without return to pre–existing
　conscious level

Use fifth-digit 5 to designate when a
patient is unconscious and dies before
regaining consciousness, regardless of
the duration of the loss of consciousness

6　with loss of consciousness of unspecified duration

9　with concussion, unspecified

　　with
　　　open intracranial wound
　　　　851.9 ☑
　　　skull fracture — see Fracture,
　　　　skull, by site
　　cerebellum 851.6 ☑
　　　with open intracranial wound
　　　　851.7 ☑
　　cortex 851.2 ☑
　　　with open intracranial wound
　　　　851.3 ☑
　　during birth 767.0
　　stem 851.6 ☑
　　　with open intracranial wound
　　　　851.7 ☑
　broad ligament
　　with
　　　abortion — see Abortion, by
　　　　type, with damage to
　　　　pelvic organs
　　　ectopic pregnancy (see also categories 633.0–633.9)
　　　　639.2

**Laceration** — see also Wound, open, by
　site — continued
　broad ligament — continued
　　with — continued
　　　molar pregnancy (see also categories 630–632) 639.2
　　following
　　　abortion 639.2
　　　ectopic or molar pregnancy
　　　　639.2
　　nontraumatic 620.6
　　obstetrical trauma 665.6 ☑
　　syndrome (nontraumatic) 620.6
　capsule, joint — see Sprain, by site
　cardiac — see Laceration, heart
　causing eversion of cervix uteri (old)
　　622.0
　central, complicating delivery 664.4 ☑
　cerebellum — see Laceration, brain,
　　cerebellum
　cerebral (see also Laceration, brain)
　　during birth 767.0
　cervix (uteri)
　　with
　　　abortion — see Abortion, by
　　　　type, with damage to
　　　　pelvic organs
　　　ectopic pregnancy (see also categories 633.0–633.9)
　　　　639.2
　　　molar pregnancy (see also categories 630–632) 639.2
　　following
　　　abortion 639.2
　　　ectopic or molar pregnancy
　　　　639.2
　　nonpuerperal/nontraumatic 622.3
　　obstetrical trauma (current)
　　　665.3 ☑
　　old (postpartal) 622.3
　　traumatic — see Injury, internal,
　　　cervix
　chordae heart 429.5
　complicated 879.9
　cornea — see Laceration, eyeball
　　superficial 918.1
　cortex (cerebral) — see Laceration,
　　brain, cortex
　esophagus 530.89
　eye(s) — see Laceration, ocular
　eyeball NEC 871.4
　　with prolapse or exposure of intraocular tissue 871.1
　　penetrating — see Penetrating
　　　wound, eyeball
　　specified as without prolapse of intraocular tissue 871.0
　eyelid NEC 870.8
　　full thickness 870.1
　　　involving lacrimal passages
　　　　870.2
　　skin (and periocular area) 870.0
　　　penetrating — see Penetrating
　　　　wound, orbit
　fourchette
　　with
　　　abortion — see Abortion, by
　　　　type, with damage to
　　　　pelvic organs
　　　ectopic pregnancy (see also categories 633.0–633.9)
　　　　639.2
　　　molar pregnancy (see also categories 630–632) 639.2
　　complicating delivery 664.0 ☑
　　following
　　　abortion 639.2
　　　ectopic or molar pregnancy
　　　　639.2
　heart (without penetration of heart
　　chambers) 861.02
　　with
　　　open wound into thorax 861.12
　　　penetration of heart chambers
　　　　861.03

Kussmaul's — Laceration

☑ Additional Digit Required — Refer to the Tabular List for Digit Selection　　　　　　　　　　　📖 Subterms under main terms may continue to next column or page

*2008 ICD-9-CM*　　　　　　　▶◀ Revised Text　　　　　● New Line　　　　▲ Revised Code　　　　　October 2007 • Volume 2 — 175

**Laceration** — *see also* Wound, open, by site — *continued*
heart — *continued*
with — *continued*
penetration of heart chambers — *continued*
with open wound into thorax 861.13
hernial sac — *see* Hernia, by site
internal organ (abdomen) (chest) (pelvis) NEC — *see* Injury, internal, by site
NEC — *see* Injury, internal, by site
kidney (parenchyma) 866.02
with
complete disruption of parenchyma (rupture) 866.03
with open wound into cavity 866.13
open wound into cavity 866.12
labia
complicating delivery 664.0 ☑
ligament (*see also* Sprain, by site)
with open wound — *see* Wound, open, by site
liver 864.05
with open wound into cavity 864.15
major (disruption of hepatic parenchyma) 864.04
with open wound into cavity 864.14
minor (capsule only) 864.02
with open wound into cavity 864.12
moderate (involving parenchyma without major disruption) 864.03
with open wound into cavity 864.13
multiple 864.04
with open wound into cavity 864.14
stellate 864.04
with open wound into cavity 864.14
lung 861.22
with open wound into thorax 861.32
meninges — *see* Laceration, brain
meniscus (knee) (*see also* Tear, meniscus) 836.2
old 717.5
site other than knee (*see also* Sprain, by site)
old NEC (*see also* Disorder, cartilage, articular) 718.0
muscle (*see also* Sprain, by site)
with open wound — *see* Wound, open, by site
myocardium — *see* Laceration, heart
nerve — *see* Injury, nerve, by site
ocular NEC (*see also* Laceration, eyeball) 871.4
adnexa NEC 870.8
penetrating 870.3
with foreign body 870.4
orbit (eye) 870.8
penetrating 870.3
with foreign body 870.4
pelvic
floor (muscles)
with
abortion — *see* Abortion, by type, with damage to pelvic organs
ectopic pregnancy (*see also* categories 633.0–633.9) 639.2
molar pregnancy (*see also* categories 630–632) 639.2
complicating delivery 664.1 ☑
following
abortion 639.2

**Laceration** — *see also* Wound, open, by site — *continued*
pelvic — *continued*
floor — *continued*
following — *continued*
ectopic or molar pregnancy 639.2
nonpuerperal 618.7
old (postpartal) 618.7
organ NEC
with
abortion — *see* Abortion, by type, with damage to pelvic organs
ectopic pregnancy (*see also* categories 633.0–633.9) 639.2
molar pregnancy (*see also* categories 630–632) 639.2
complicating delivery 665.5 ☑
affecting fetus or newborn 763.89
following
abortion 639.2
ectopic or molar pregnancy 639.2
obstetrical trauma 665.5 ☑
perineum, perineal (old) (postpartal) 618.7
with
abortion — *see* Abortion, by type, with damage to pelvic floor
ectopic pregnancy (*see also* categories 633.0–633.9) 639.2
molar pregnancy (*see also* categories 630–632) 639.2
complicating delivery 664.4 ☑
first degree 664.0 ☑
second degree 664.1 ☑
third degree 664.2 ☑
fourth degree 664.3 ☑
anal sphincter (healed) (old) 654.8 ☑
not associated with third-degree perineal laceration 664.6 ☑
sphincter (anal) (healed) (old) 654.8 ☑
not associated with third-degree perineal laceration 664.6 ☑
central 664.4 ☑
involving
anal sphincter 664.2 ☑
fourchette 664.0 ☑
hymen 664.0 ☑
labia 664.0 ☑
pelvic floor 664.1 ☑
perineal muscles 664.1 ☑
rectovaginal septum 664.2 ☑
with anal mucosa 664.3 ☑
skin 664.0 ☑
sphincter (anal) 664.2 ☑
with anal mucosa 664.3 ☑
vagina 664.0 ☑
vaginal muscles 664.1 ☑
vulva 664.0 ☑
secondary 674.2 ☑
following
abortion 639.2
ectopic or molar pregnancy 639.2
male 879.6
complicated 879.7
muscles, complicating delivery 664.1 ☑
nonpuerperal, current injury 879.6
complicated 879.7
secondary (postpartal) 674.2 ☑

**Laceration** — *see also* Wound, open, by site — *continued*
peritoneum
with
abortion — *see* Abortion, by type, with damage to pelvic organs
ectopic pregnancy (*see also* categories 633.0–633.9) 639.2
molar pregnancy (*see also* categories 630–632) 639.2
following
abortion 639.2
ectopic or molar pregnancy 639.2
obstetrical trauma 665.5 ☑
periurethral tissue
with
abortion — *see* Abortion, by type, with damage to pelvic organs
ectopic pregnancy (*see also* categories 633.0–633.9) 639.2
molar pregnancy (*see also* categories 630–632) 639.2
following
abortion 639.2
ectopic or molar pregnancy 639.2
obstetrical trauma 665.5 ☑
rectovaginal (septum)
with
abortion — *see* Abortion, by type, with damage to pelvic organs
ectopic pregnancy (*see also* categories 633.0–633.9) 639.2
molar pregnancy (*see also* categories 630–632) 639.2
complicating delivery 665.4 ☑
with perineum 664.2 ☑
involving anal or rectal mucosa 664.3 ☑
following
abortion 639.2
ectopic or molar pregnancy 639.2
nonpuerperal 623.4
old (postpartal) 623.4
spinal cord (meninges) (*see also* Injury, spinal, by site)
due to injury at birth 767.4
fetus or newborn 767.4
spleen 865.09
with
disruption of parenchyma (massive) 865.04
with open wound into cavity 865.14
open wound into cavity 865.19
capsule (without disruption of parenchyma) 865.02
with open wound into cavity 865.12
parenchyma 865.03
with open wound into cavity 865.13
massive disruption (rupture) 865.04
with open wound into cavity 865.14
tendon 848.9
with open wound — *see* Wound, open, by site
Achilles 845.09
with open wound 892.2
lower limb NEC 844.9
with open wound NEC 894.2
upper limb NEC 840.9
with open wound NEC 884.2
tentorium cerebelli — *see* Laceration, brain, cerebellum
tongue 873.64

**Laceration** — *see also* Wound, open, by site — *continued*
tongue — *continued*
complicated 873.74
urethra
with
abortion — *see* Abortion, by type, with damage to pelvic organs
ectopic pregnancy (*see also* categories 633.0–633.9) 639.2
molar pregnancy (*see also* categories 630–632) 639.2
following
abortion 639.2
ectopic or molar pregnancy 639.2
nonpuerperal, nontraumatic 599.84
obstetrical trauma 665.5 ☑
uterus
with
abortion — *see* Abortion, by type, with damage to pelvic organs
ectopic pregnancy (*see also* categories 633.0–633.9) 639.2
molar pregnancy (*see also* categories 630–632) 639.2
following
abortion 639.2
ectopic or molar pregnancy 639.2
nonpuerperal, nontraumatic 621.8
obstetrical trauma NEC 665.5 ☑
old (postpartal) 621.8
vagina
with
abortion — *see* Abortion, by type, with damage to pelvic organs
ectopic pregnancy (*see also* categories 633.0–633.9) 639.2
molar pregnancy (*see also* categories 630–632) 639.2
perineal involvement, complicating delivery 664.0 ☑
complicating delivery 665.4 ☑
first degree 664.0 ☑
second degree 664.1 ☑
third degree 664.2 ☑
fourth degree 664.3 ☑
high 665.4 ☑
muscles 664.1 ☑
sulcus 665.4 ☑
wall 665.4 ☑
following
abortion 639.2
ectopic or molar pregnancy 639.2
nonpuerperal, nontraumatic 623.4
old (postpartal) 623.4
valve, heart — *see* Endocarditis
vulva
with
abortion — *see* Abortion, by type, with damage to pelvic organs
ectopic pregnancy (*see also* categories 633.0–633.9) 639.2
molar pregnancy (*see also* categories 630–632) 639.2
complicating delivery 664.0 ☑
following
abortion 639.2
ectopic or molar pregnancy 639.2
nonpuerperal, nontraumatic 624.4
old (postpartal) 624.4
**Lachrymal** — *see* condition
**Lachrymonasal duct** — *see* condition

**Lack of**
adequate intermaxillary vertical dimension 524.36
appetite (see also Anorexia) 783.0
care
in home V60.4
of adult 995.84
of infant (at or after birth) 995.52
coordination 781.3
development (see also Hypoplasia)
physiological in childhood 783.40
education V62.3
energy 780.79
financial resources V60.2
food 994.2
in environment V60.8
growth in childhood 783.43
heating V60.1
housing (permanent) (temporary) V60.0
adequate V60.1
material resources V60.2
medical attention 799.89
memory (see also Amnesia) 780.93
mild, following organic brain damage 310.1
ovulation 628.0
person able to render necessary care V60.4
physical exercise V69.0
physiologic development in childhood 783.40
posterior occlusal support 524.57
prenatal care in current pregnancy V23.7
shelter V60.0
sleep V69.4
water 994.3
**Lacrimal** — see condition
**Lacrimation, abnormal** — see also Epiphora 375.20
**Lacrimonasal duct** — see condition
**Lactation, lactating** (breast) (puerperal) (postpartum)
defective 676.4 ☑
disorder 676.9 ☑
specified type NEC 676.8 ☑
excessive 676.6 ☑
failed 676.4 ☑
mastitis NEC 675.2 ☑
mother (care and/or examination) V24.1
nonpuerperal 611.6
suppressed 676.5 ☑
**Lacticemia** 271.3
excessive 276.2
**Lactosuria** 271.3
**Lacunar skull** 756.0
**Laennec's cirrhosis** (alcoholic) 571.2
nonalcoholic 571.5
**Lafora's disease** 333.2
**Lagleyze-von Hippel disease** (retinocerebral angiomatosis) 759.6
**Lag, lid** (nervous) 374.41
**Lagophthalmos** (eyelid) (nervous) 374.20
cicatricial 374.23
keratitis (see also Keratitis) 370.34
mechanical 374.22
paralytic 374.21
**La grippe** — see Influenza
**Lahore sore** 085.1
**Lakes, venous** (cerebral) 437.8
**Laki-Lorand factor deficiency** — see also Defect, coagulation 286.3
**Lalling** 307.9
**Lambliasis** 007.1
**Lame back** 724.5
**Lancereaux's diabetes** (diabetes mellitus with marked emaciation) 250.8 ☑ [261]
**Landouzy-Déjérine dystrophy** (fascioscapulohumeral atrophy) 359.1
**Landry's disease or paralysis** 357.0
**Landry-Guillain-Barré syndrome** 357.0
**Lane's**
band 751.4

**Lane's** — continued
disease 569.89
kink (see also Obstruction, intestine) 560.9
**Langdon Down's syndrome** (mongolism) 758.0
**Language abolition** 784.69
**Lanugo** (persistent) 757.4
**Laparoscopic surgical procedure converted to open procedure** V64.41
**Lardaceous**
degeneration (any site) 277.39
disease 277.39
kidney 277.39 [583.81]
liver 277.39
**Large**
baby (regardless of gestational age) 766.1
exceptionally (weight of 4500 grams or more) 766.0
of diabetic mother 775.0
ear 744.22
fetus (see also Oversize, fetus)
causing disproportion 653.5 ☑
with obstructed labor 660.1 ☑
for dates
fetus or newborn (regardless of gestational age) 766.1
affecting management of pregnancy 656.6 ☑
exceptionally (weight of 4500 grams or more) 766.0
physiological cup 743.57
stature 783.9
waxy liver 277.39
white kidney — see Nephrosis
**Larsen-Johansson disease** (juvenile osteopathia patellae) 732.4
**Larsen's syndrome** (flattened facies and multiple congenital dislocations) 755.8
**Larva migrans**
cutaneous NEC 126.9
ancylostoma 126.9
of Diptera in vitreous 128.0
visceral NEC 128.0
**Laryngeal** — see also condition 786.2
syncope 786.2
**Laryngismus** (acute) (infectious) (stridulous) 478.75
congenital 748.3
diphtheritic 032.3
**Laryngitis** (acute) (edematous) (fibrinous) (gangrenous) (infective) (infiltrative) (malignant) (membranous) (phlegmonous) (pneumococcal) (pseudomembranous) (septic) (subglottic) (suppurative) (ulcerative) (viral) 464.00
with
influenza, flu, or grippe 487.1
obstruction 464.01
tracheitis (see also Laryngotracheitis) 464.20
with obstruction 464.21
acute 464.20
with obstruction 464.21
chronic 476.1
atrophic 476.0
Borrelia vincentii 101
catarrhal 476.0
chronic 476.0
with tracheitis (chronic) 476.1
due to external agent — see Condition, respiratory, chronic, due to
diphtheritic (membranous) 032.3
due to external agent — see Inflammation, respiratory, upper, due to
Hemophilus influenzae 464.00
with obstruction 464.01
H. influenzae 464.00
with obstruction 464.01
hypertrophic 476.0
influenzal 487.1
pachydermic 478.79

**Laryngitis** — continued
sicca 476.0
spasmodic 478.75
acute 464.00
with obstruction 464.01
streptococcal 034.0
stridulous 478.75
syphilitic 095.8
congenital 090.5
tuberculous (see also Tuberculosis, larynx) 012.3 ☑
Vincent's 101
**Laryngocele** (congenital) (ventricular) 748.3
**Laryngofissure** 478.79
congenital 748.3
**Laryngomalacia** (congenital) 748.3
**Laryngopharyngitis** (acute) 465.0
chronic 478.9
due to external agent — see Condition, respiratory, chronic, due to
due to external agent — see Inflammation, respiratory, upper, due to
septic 034.0
**Laryngoplegia** — see also Paralysis, vocal cord 478.30
**Laryngoptosis** 478.79
**Laryngospasm** 478.75
due to external agent — see Condition, respiratory, acute, due to
**Laryngostenosis** 478.74
congenital 748.3
**Laryngotracheitis** (acute) (infectional) (viral) — see also Laryngitis 464.20
with obstruction 464.21
atrophic 476.1
Borrelia vincenti 101
catarrhal 476.1
chronic 476.1
due to external agent — see Condition, respiratory, chronic, due to
diphtheritic (membranous) 032.3
due to external agent — see Inflammation, respiratory, upper, due to
H. influenzae 464.20
with obstruction 464.21
hypertrophic 476.1
influenzal 487.1
pachydermic 478.75
sicca 476.1
spasmodic 478.75
acute 464.20
with obstruction 464.21
streptococcal 034.0
stridulous 478.75
syphilitic 095.8
congenital 090.5
tuberculous (see also Tuberculosis, larynx) 012.3 ☑
Vincent's 101
**Laryngotracheobronchitis** — see also Bronchitis 490
acute 466.0
chronic 491.8
viral 466.0
**Laryngotracheobronchopneumonitis** — see Pneumonia, broncho-
**Larynx, laryngeal** — see condition
**Lasègue's disease** (persecution mania) 297.9
**Lassa fever** 078.89
**Lassitude** — see also Weakness 780.79
**Late** — see also condition
effect(s) (of) (see also condition)
abscess
intracranial or intraspinal (conditions classifiable to 324) — see category 326
adverse effect of drug, medicinal or biological substance 909.5
allergic reaction 909.9
amputation
postoperative (late) 997.60

**Late** — see also condition — continued
effect(s) (see also condition) — continued
amputation — continued
traumatic (injury classifiable to 885–887 and 895–897) 905.9
burn (injury classifiable to 948–949) 906.9
extremities NEC (injury classifiable to 943 or 945) 906.7
hand or wrist (injury classifiable to 944) 906.6
eye (injury classifiable to 940) 906.5
face, head, and neck (injury classifiable to 941) 906.5
specified site NEC (injury classifiable to 942 and 946–947) 906.8
cerebrovascular disease (conditions classifiable to 430–437) 438.9
with
alterations of sensations 438.6
aphasia 438.11
apraxia 438.81
ataxia 438.84
cognitive deficits 438.0
disturbances of vision 438.7
dysphagia 438.82
dysphasia 438.12
facial droop 438.83
facial weakness 438.83
hemiplegia/hemiparesis affecting
dominant side 438.21
nondominant side 438.22
unspecified side 438.20
monoplegia of lower limb affecting
dominant side 438.41
nondominant side 438.42
unspecified side 438.40
monoplegia of upper limb affecting
dominant side 438.31
nondominant side 438.32
unspecified side 438.30
paralytic syndrome NEC affecting
bilateral 438.53
dominant side 438.51
nondominant side 438.52
unspecified side 438.50
specified type NEC 438.19
speech and language deficit 438.10
vertigo 438.85
specified type NEC 438.89
childbirth complication(s) 677
complication(s) of
childbirth 677
delivery 677
pregnancy 677
puerperium 677
surgical and medical care (conditions classifiable to 996–999) 909.3
trauma (conditions classifiable to 958) 908.6
contusion (injury classifiable to 920–924) 906.3
crushing (injury classifiable to 925–929) 906.4
delivery complication(s) 677

**Late** — *see also* condition — *continued*
effect(s) (*see also* condition) — *continued*
dislocation (injury classifiable to 830–839) 905.6
encephalitis or encephalomyelitis (conditions classifiable to 323) — *see* category 326
in infectious diseases 139.8
viral (conditions classifiable to 049.8, 049.9, 062–064) 139.0
external cause NEC (conditions classifiable to 995) 909.9
certain conditions classifiable to categories 991-994 909.4
foreign body in orifice (injury classifiable to 930–939) 908.5
fracture (multiple) (injury classifiable to 828–829) 905.5
extremity
lower (injury classifiable to 821–827) 905.4
neck of femur (injury classifiable to 820) 905.3
upper (injury classifiable to 810–819) 905.2
face and skull (injury classifiable to 800–804) 905.0
skull and face (injury classifiable to 800–804) 905.0
spine and trunk (injury classifiable to 805 and 807–809) 905.1
with spinal cord lesion (injury classifiable to 806) 907.2
infection
pyogenic, intracranial — *see* category 326
infectious diseases (conditions classifiable to 001–136) NEC 139.8
injury (injury classifiable to 959) 908.9
blood vessel 908.3
abdomen and pelvis (injury classifiable to 902) 908.4
extremity (injury classifiable to 903–904) 908.3
head and neck (injury classifiable to 900) 908.3
intracranial (injury classifiable to 850–854) 907.0
with skull fracture 905.0
thorax (injury classifiable to 901) 908.4
internal organ NEC (injury classifiable to 867 and 869) 908.2
abdomen (injury classifiable to 863–866 and 868) 908.1
thorax (injury classifiable to 860–862) 908.0
intracranial (injury classifiable to 850–854) 907.0
with skull fracture (injury classifiable to 800–801 and 803–804) 905.0
nerve NEC (injury classifiable to 957) 907.9
cranial (injury classifiable to 950–951) 907.1
peripheral NEC (injury classifiable to 957) 907.9
lower limb and pelvic girdle (injury classifiable to 956) 907.5

**Late** — *see also* condition — *continued*
effect(s) (*see also* condition) — *continued*
injury — *continued*
nerve — *continued*
peripheral — *continued*
upper limb and shoulder girdle (injury classifiable to 955) 907.4
roots and plexus(es), spinal (injury classifiable to 953) 907.3
trunk (injury classifiable to 954) 907.3
spinal
cord (injury classifiable to 806 and 952) 907.2
nerve root(s) and plexus(es) (injury classifiable to 953) 907.3
superficial (injury classifiable to 910–919) 906.2
tendon (tendon injury classifiable to 840–848, 880–884 with .2, and 890–894 with .2) 905.8
meningitis
bacterial (conditions classifiable to 320) — *see* category 326
unspecified cause (conditions classifiable to 322) — *see* category 326
myelitis (*see also* Late, effect(s) (of), encephalitis) — *see* category 326
parasitic diseases (conditions classifiable to 001–136 NEC) 139.8
phlebitis or thrombophlebitis of intracranial venous sinuses (conditions classifiable to 325) — *see* category 326
poisoning due to drug, medicinal or biological substance (conditions classifiable to 960–979) 909.0
poliomyelitis, acute (conditions classifiable to 045) 138
pregnancy complication(s) 677
puerperal complication(s) 677
radiation (conditions classifiable to 990) 909.2
rickets 268.1
sprain and strain without mention of tendon injury (injury classifiable to 840–848, except tendon injury) 905.7
tendon involvement 905.8
toxic effect of
drug, medicinal or biological substance (conditions classifiable to 960–979) 909.0
nonmedical substance (conditions classifiable to 980–989) 909.1
trachoma (conditions classifiable to 076) 139.1
tuberculosis 137.0
bones and joints (conditions classifiable to 015) 137.3
central nervous system (conditions classifiable to 013) 137.1
genitourinary (conditions classifiable to 016) 137.2
pulmonary (conditions classifiable to 010–012) 137.0
specified organs NEC (conditions classifiable to 014, 017–018) 137.4
viral encephalitis (conditions classifiable to 049.8, 049.9, 062–064) 139.0

**Late** — *see also* condition — *continued*
effect(s) (*see also* condition) — *continued*
wound, open
extremity (injury classifiable to 880–884 and 890–894, except .2) 906.1
tendon (injury classifiable to 880–884 with .2 and 890–894 with .2) 905.8
head, neck, and trunk (injury classifiable to 870–879) 906.0
infant
post-term (gestation period over 40 completed weeks to 42 completed weeks) 766.21
prolonged gestation (period over 42 completed weeks) 766.22
**Latent** — *see* condition
**Lateral** — *see* condition
**Laterocession** — *see* Lateroversion
**Lateroflexion** — *see* Lateroversion
**Lateroversion**
cervix — *see* Lateroversion, uterus
uterus, uterine (*see also* Lateroversion, uterus) (postinfectional) (postpartal, old) 621.6
congenital 752.3
in pregnancy or childbirth 654.4 ☑
affecting fetus or newborn 763.89
**Lathyrism** 988.2
**Launois-Bensaude's lipomatosis** 272.8
**Launois-Cléret syndrome** (adiposogenital dystrophy) 253.8
**Launois' syndrome** (pituitary gigantism) 253.0
**Laurence-Moon-Biedl syndrome** (obesity, polydactyly, and mental retardation) 759.89
**LAV** (disease) (illness) (infection) — *see* Human immunodeficiency virus (disease) (illness) (infection)
**LAV/HTLV-III** (disease) (illness) (infection) — *see* Human immunodeficiency virus (disease) (illness) (infection)
**Lawford's syndrome** (encephalocutaneous angiomatosis) 759.6
**Laxative habit** — *see also* Abuse, drugs, nondependent 305.9 ☑
**Lax, laxity** — *see also* Relaxation
ligament 728.4
skin (acquired) 701.8
congenital 756.83
**Lazy leukocyte syndrome** 288.09
**LCAD** (long chain/very long chain acyl CoA dehydrogenase deficiency, VLCAD) 277.85
**LCHAD** (long chain 3-hydroxyacyl CoA dehydrogenase deficiency) 277.85
**Lead** — *see also* condition
exposure to V15.86
incrustation of cornea 371.15
poisoning 984.9
specified type of lead — *see* Table of Drugs and Chemicals
**Lead miners' lung** 503
**Leakage**
amniotic fluid 658.1 ☑
with delayed delivery 658.2 ☑
affecting fetus or newborn 761.1
bile from drainage tube (T tube) 997.4
blood (microscopic), fetal, into maternal circulation 656.0 ☑
affecting management of pregnancy or puerperium 656.0 ☑
device, implant, or graft — *see* Complications, mechanical
spinal fluid at lumbar puncture site 997.09
urine, continuous 788.37
**Leaky heart** — *see* Endocarditis
**Learning defect, specific** NEC (strephosymbolia) 315.2

**Leather bottle stomach** (M8142/3) 151.9
**Leber's**
congenital amaurosis 362.76
optic atrophy (hereditary) 377.16
**Lederer's anemia or disease** (acquired infectious hemolytic anemia) 283.19
**Lederer-Brill syndrome** (acquired infectious hemolytic anemia) 283.19
**Leeches** (aquatic) (land) 134.2
**Left-sided neglect** 781.8
**Leg** — *see* condition
**Legal investigation** V62.5
**Legg (-Calvé) -Perthes disease or syndrome** (osteochondrosis, femoral capital) 732.1
**Legionnaires' disease** 482.84
**Leigh's disease** 330.8
**Leiner's disease** (exfoliative dermatitis) 695.89
**Leiofibromyoma** (M8890/0) — *see also* Leiomyoma
uterus (cervix) (corpus) (*see also* Leiomyoma, uterus) 218.9
**Leiomyoblastoma** (M8891/1) — *see* Neoplasm, connective tissue, uncertain behavior
**Leiomyofibroma** (M8890/0) — *see also* Neoplasm, connective tissue, benign
uterus (cervix) (corpus) (*see also* Leiomyoma, uterus) 218.9
**Leiomyoma** (M8890/0) — *see also* Neoplasm, connective tissue, benign
bizarre (M8893/0) — *see* Neoplasm, connective tissue, benign
cellular (M8892/1) — *see* Neoplasm, connective tissue, uncertain behavior
epithelioid (M8891/1) — *see* Neoplasm, connective tissue, uncertain behavior
prostate (polypoid) 600.20
with
other lower urinary tract symptoms (LUTS) 600.21
urinary
obstruction 600.21
retention 600.21
uterus (cervix) (corpus) 218.9
interstitial 218.1
intramural 218.1
submucous 218.0
subperitoneal 218.2
subserous 218.2
vascular (M8894/0) — *see* Neoplasm, connective tissue, benign
**Leiomyomatosis** (intravascular) (M8890/1) — *see* Neoplasm, connective tissue, uncertain behavior
**Leiomyosarcoma** (M8890/3) — *see also* Neoplasm, connective tissue, malignant
epithelioid (M8891/3) — *see* Neoplasm, connective tissue, malignant
**Leishmaniasis** 085.9
American 085.5
cutaneous 085.4
mucocutaneous 085.5
Asian desert 085.2
Brazilian 085.5
cutaneous 085.9
acute necrotizing 085.2
American 085.4
Asian desert 085.2
diffuse 085.3
dry form 085.1
Ethiopian 085.3
eyelid 085.5 [373.6]
late 085.1
lepromatous 085.3
recurrent 085.1
rural 085.2
ulcerating 085.1

**Leishmaniasis** — continued
  cutaneous — continued
    urban 085.1
    wet form 085.2
    zoonotic form 085.2
  dermal (see also Leishmaniasis, cutaneous)
    post kala-azar 085.0
  eyelid 085.5 [373.6]
  infantile 085.0
  Mediterranean 085.0
  mucocutaneous (American) 085.5
  naso-oral 085.5
  nasopharyngeal 085.5
  Old World 085.1
  tegumentaria diffusa 085.4
  vaccination, prophylactic (against) V05.2
  visceral (Indian) 085.0
**Leishmanoid, dermal** — see also Leishmaniasis, cutaneous
  post kala-azar 085.0
**Leloir's disease** 695.4
**Lemiere syndrome** 451.89
**Lenegre's disease** 426.0
**Lengthening, leg** 736.81
**Lennox-Gastaut syndrome** 345.0 ☑
  with tonic seizures 345.1 ☑
**Lennox's syndrome** — see also Epilepsy 345.0 ☑
**Lens** — see condition
**Lenticonus** (anterior) (posterior) (congenital) 743.36
**Lenticular degeneration, progressive** 275.1
**Lentiglobus** (posterior) (congenital) 743.36
**Lentigo** (congenital) 709.09
  juvenile 709.09
  Maligna (M8742/2) (see also Neoplasm, skin, in situ)
    melanoma (M8742/3) — see Melanoma
  senile 709.09
**Leonine leprosy** 030.0
**Leontiasis**
  ossium 733.3
  syphilitic 095.8
    congenital 090.5
**Léopold-Lévi's syndrome** (paroxysmal thyroid instability) 242.9 ☑
**Lepore hemoglobin syndrome** 282.49
**Lepothrix** 039.0
**Lepra** 030.9
  Willan's 696.1
**Leprechaunism** 259.8
**Lepromatous leprosy** 030.0
**Leprosy** 030.9
  anesthetic 030.1
  beriberi 030.1
  borderline (group B) (infiltrated) (neuritic) 030.3
  cornea (see also Leprosy, by type) 030.9 [371.89]
  dimorphous (group B) (infiltrated) (lepromatous) (neuritic) (tuberculoid) 030.3
  eyelid 030.0 [373.4]
  indeterminate (group I) (macular) (neuritic) (uncharacteristic) 030.2
  leonine 030.0
  lepromatous (diffuse) (infiltrated) (macular) (neuritic) (nodular) (type L) 030.0
  macular (early) (neuritic) (simple) 030.2
  maculoanesthetic 030.1
  mixed 030.0
  neuro 030.1
  nodular 030.0
  primary neuritic 030.3
  specified type or group NEC 030.8
  tubercular 030.1

**Leprosy** — continued
  tuberculoid (macular) (maculoanesthetic) (major) (minor) (neuritic) (type T) 030.1
**Leptocytosis, hereditary** 282.49
**Leptomeningitis** (chronic) (circumscribed) (hemorrhagic) (nonsuppurative) — see also Meningitis 322.9
  aseptic 047.9
    adenovirus 049.1
    Coxsackie virus 047.0
    ECHO virus 047.1
    enterovirus 047.9
    lymphocytic choriomeningitis 049.0
  epidemic 036.0
  late effect — see category 326
  meningococcal 036.0
  pneumococcal 320.1
  syphilitic 094.2
  tuberculous (see also Tuberculosis, meninges) 013.0 ☑
**Leptomeningopathy** — see also Meningitis 322.9
**Leptospiral** — see condition
**Leptospirochetal** — see condition
**Leptospirosis** 100.9
  autumnalis 100.89
  canicula 100.89
  grippotyphosa 100.89
  hebdomidis 100.89
  icterohemorrhagica 100.0
  nanukayami 100.89
  pomona 100.89
  Weil's disease 100.0
**Leptothricosis** — see Actinomycosis
**Leptothrix infestation** — see Actinomycosis
**Leptotricosis** — see Actinomycosis
**Leptus dermatitis** 133.8
**Leriche's syndrome** (aortic bifurcation occlusion) 444.0
**Léris pleonosteosis** 756.89
**Léri-Weill syndrome** 756.59
**Lermoyez's syndrome** — see also Disease, Ménière's 386.00
**Lesbianism** — omit code
  ego-dystonic 302.0
  problems with 302.0
**Lesch-Nyhan syndrome** (hypoxanthineguanine-phosphoribosyltransferase deficiency) 277.2
**Lesion(s)**
  abducens nerve 378.54
  alveolar process 525.8
  anorectal 569.49
  aortic (valve) — see Endocarditis, aortic
  auditory nerve 388.5
  basal ganglion 333.90
  bile duct (see also Disease, biliary) 576.8
  bladder 596.9
  bone 733.90
  brachial plexus 353.0
  brain 348.8
    congenital 742.9
    vascular (see also Lesion, cerebrovascular) 437.9
      degenerative 437.1
      healed or old without residuals V12.54 ▲
      hypertensive 437.2
      late effect — see Late effect(s) (of) cerebrovascular disease
  buccal 528.9
  calcified — see Calcification
  canthus 373.9
  carate — see Pinta, lesions
  cardia 537.89
  cardiac — see also Disease, heart
    congenital 746.9
    valvular — see Endocarditis
  cauda equina 344.60
    with neurogenic bladder 344.61
  cecum 569.89

**Lesion(s)** — continued
  cerebral — see Lesion, brain
  cerebrovascular (see also Disease, cerebrovascular NEC) 437.9
    degenerative 437.1
      healed or old without residuals V12.54 ▲
    hypertensive 437.2
    specified type NEC 437.8
  cervical root (nerve) NEC 353.2
  chiasmal 377.54
    associated with
      inflammatory disorders 377.54
      neoplasm NEC 377.52
        pituitary 377.51
      pituitary disorders 377.51
      vascular disorders 377.53
  chorda tympani 351.8
  coin, lung 793.1
  colon 569.89
  congenital — see Anomaly
  conjunctiva 372.9
  coronary artery (see also Ischemia, heart) 414.9
  cranial nerve 352.9
    first 352.0
    second 377.49
    third
      partial 378.51
      total 378.52
    fourth 378.53
    fifth 350.9
    sixth 378.54
    seventh 351.9
    eighth 388.5
    ninth 352.2
    tenth 352.3
    eleventh 352.4
    twelfth 352.5
  cystic — see Cyst
  degenerative — see Degeneration
  dermal (skin) 709.9
  Dieulafoy (hemorrhagic)
    of
      duodenum 537.84
      intestine 569.86
      stomach 537.84
  duodenum 537.89
    with obstruction 537.3
  eyelid 373.9
  gasserian ganglion 350.8
  gastric 537.89
  gastroduodenal 537.89
  gastrointestinal 569.89
  glossopharyngeal nerve 352.2
  heart (organic) (see also Disease, heart)
    vascular — see Disease, cardiovascular
  helix (ear) 709.9
  high grade myelodysplastic syndrome 238.73
  hyperchromic, due to pinta (carate) 103.1
  hyperkeratotic (see also Hyperkeratosis) 701.1
  hypoglossal nerve 352.5
  hypopharynx 478.29
  hypothalamic 253.9
  ileocecal coil 569.89
  ileum 569.89
  iliohypogastric nerve 355.79
  ilioinguinal nerve 355.79
  in continuity — see Injury, nerve, by site
  inflammatory — see Inflammation
  intestine 569.89
  intracerebral — see Lesion, brain
  intrachiasmal (optic) (see also Lesion, chiasmal) 377.54
  intracranial, space-occupying NEC 784.2
  joint 719.90
    ankle 719.97
    elbow 719.92
    foot 719.97

**Lesion(s)** — continued
  joint — continued
    hand 719.94
    hip 719.95
    knee 719.96
    multiple sites 719.99
    pelvic region 719.95
    sacroiliac (old) 724.6
    shoulder (region) 719.91
    specified site NEC 719.98
    wrist 719.93
  keratotic (see also Keratosis) 701.1
  kidney (see also Disease, renal) 593.9
  laryngeal nerve (recurrent) 352.3
  leonine 030.0
  lip 528.5
  liver 573.8
  low grade myelodysplastic syndrome 238.72
  lumbosacral
    plexus 353.1
    root (nerve) NEC 353.4
  lung 518.89
    coin 793.1
  maxillary sinus 473.0
  mitral — see Endocarditis, mitral
  motor cortex 348.4
  nerve (see also Disorder, nerve) 355.9
  nervous system 349.9
    congenital 742.9
  nonallopathic NEC 739.9
    in region (of)
      abdomen 739.9
      acromioclavicular 739.7
      cervical, cervicothoracic 739.1
      costochondral 739.8
      costovertebral 739.8
      extremity
        lower 739.6
        upper 739.7
      head 739.0
      hip 739.5
      lower extremity 739.6
      lumbar, lumbosacral 739.3
      occipitocervical 739.0
      pelvic 739.5
      pubic 739.5
      rib cage 739.8
      sacral, sacrococcygeal, sacroiliac 739.4
      sternochondral 739.8
      sternoclavicular 739.7
      thoracic, thoracolumbar 739.2
      upper extremity 739.7
  nose (internal) 478.19
  obstructive — see Obstruction
  obturator nerve 355.79
  occlusive
    artery — see Embolism, artery
  organ or site NEC — see Disease, by site
  osteolytic 733.90
  paramacular, of retina 363.32
  peptic 537.89
  periodontal, due to traumatic occlusion 523.8
  perirectal 569.49
  peritoneum (granulomatous) 568.89
  pigmented (skin) 709.00
  pinta — see Pinta, lesions
  polypoid — see Polyp
  prechiasmal (optic) (see also Lesion, chiasmal) 377.54
  primary (see also Syphilis, primary)
    carate 103.0
    pinta 103.0
    yaws 102.0
  pulmonary 518.89
    valve (see also Endocarditis, pulmonary) 424.3
  pylorus 537.89
  radiation NEC 990
  radium NEC 990
  rectosigmoid 569.89
  retina, retinal (see also Retinopathy)
    vascular 362.17

☑ Additional Digit Required — Refer to the Tabular List for Digit Selection      ᵂᴮ Subterms under main terms may continue to next column or page

**2008 ICD-9-CM**      ▶◀ Revised Text      ● New Line      ▲ Revised Code      **October 2007 · Volume 2 — 179**

**Lesion(s)** — continued
retroperitoneal 568.89
romanus 720.1
sacroiliac (joint) 724.6
salivary gland 527.8
benign lymphoepithelial 527.8
saphenous nerve 355.79
secondary — see Syphilis, secondary
sigmoid 569.89
sinus (accessory) (nasal) (see also Sinusitis) 473.9
skin 709.9
suppurative 686.00
SLAP (superior glenoid labrum) 840.7
space-occupying, intracranial NEC 784.2
spinal cord 336.9
congenital 742.9
traumatic (complete) (incomplete) (transverse) (see also Injury, spinal, by site)
with
broken
back — see Fracture, vertebra, by site, with spinal cord injury
neck — see Fracture, vertebra, cervical, with spinal cord injury
fracture, vertebra — see Fracture, vertebra, by site, with spinal cord injury
spleen 289.50
stomach 537.89
superior glenoid labrum (SLAP) 840.7
syphilitic — see Syphilis
tertiary — see Syphilis, tertiary
thoracic root (nerve) 353.3
tonsillar fossa 474.9
tooth, teeth 525.8
white spot 521.01
traumatic NEC (see also nature and site of injury) 959.9
tricuspid (valve) — see Endocarditis, tricuspid
trigeminal nerve 350.9
ulcerated or ulcerative — see Ulcer
uterus NEC 621.9
vagina 623.8
vagus nerve 352.3
valvular — see Endocarditis
vascular 459.9
affecting central nervous system (see also Lesion, cerebrovascular) 437.9
following trauma (see also Injury, blood vessel, by site) 904.9
retina 362.17
traumatic — see Injury, blood vessel, by site
umbilical cord 663.6 ☑
affecting fetus or newborn 762.6
visual
cortex NEC (see also Disorder, visual, cortex) 377.73
pathway NEC (see also Disorder, visual, pathway) 377.63
warty — see Verruca
white spot, on teeth 521.01
x-ray NEC 990
**Lethargic** — see condition
**Lethargy** 780.79
**Letterer-Siwe disease** (acute histiocytosis X) (M9722/3) 202.5 ☑
**Leucinosis** 270.3
**Leucocoria** 360.44
**Leucosarcoma** (M9850/3) 207.8 ☑
**Leukasmus** 270.2

**Leukemia, leukemic** (congenital) (M9800/3) 208.9 ☑

Note — Use the following fifth-digit subclassification for categories 203–208:
0    without mention of remission
1    with remission

acute NEC (M9801/3) 208.0 ☑
aleukemic NEC (M9804/3) 208.8 ☑
granulocytic (M9864/3) 205.8 ☑
basophilic (M9870/3) 205.1 ☑
blast (cell) (M9801/3) 208.0 ☑
blastic (M9801/3) 208.0 ☑
granulocytic (M9861/3) 205.0 ☑
chronic NEC (M9803/3) 208.1 ☑
compound (M9810/3) 207.8 ☑
eosinophilic (M9880/3) 205.1 ☑
giant cell (M9910/3) 207.2 ☑
granulocytic (M9860/3) 205.9 ☑
acute (M9861/3) 205.0 ☑
aleukemic (M9864/3) 205.8 ☑
blastic (M9861/3) 205.0 ☑
chronic (M9863/3) 205.1 ☑
subacute (M9862/3) 205.2 ☑
subleukemic (M9864/3) 205.8 ☑
hairy cell (M9940/3) 202.4 ☑
hemoblastic (M9801/3) 208.0 ☑
histiocytic (M9890/3) 206.9 ☑
lymphatic (M9820/3) 204.9 ☑
acute (M9821/3) 204.0 ☑
aleukemic (M9824/3) 204.8 ☑
chronic (M9823/3) 204.1 ☑
subacute (M9822/3) 204.2 ☑
subleukemic (M9824/3) 204.8 ☑
lymphoblastic (M9821/3) 204.0 ☑
lymphocytic (M9820/3) 204.9 ☑
acute (M9821/3) 204.0 ☑
aleukemic (M9824/3) 204.8 ☑
chronic (M9823/3) 204.1 ☑
subacute (M9822/3) 204.2 ☑
subleukemic (M9824/3) 204.8 ☑
lymphogenous (M9820/3) — see Leukemia, lymphoid
lymphoid (M9820/3) 204.9 ☑
acute (M9821/3) 204.0 ☑
aleukemic (M9824/3) 204.8 ☑
blastic (M9821/3) 204.0 ☑
chronic (M9823/3) 204.1 ☑
subacute (M9822/3) 204.2 ☑
subleukemic (M9824/3) 204.8 ☑
lymphosarcoma cell (M9850/3) 207.8 ☑
mast cell (M9900/3) 207.8 ☑
megakaryocytic (M9910/3) 207.2 ☑
megakaryocytoid (M9910/3) 207.2 ☑
mixed (cell) (M9810/3) 207.8 ☑
monoblastic (M9891/3) 206.0 ☑
monocytic (Schilling-type) (M9890/3) 206.9 ☑
acute (M9891/3) 206.0 ☑
aleukemic (M9894/3) 206.8 ☑
chronic (M9893/3) 206.1 ☑
Naegeli-type (M9863/3) 205.1 ☑
subacute (M9892/3) 206.2 ☑
subleukemic (M9894/3) 206.8 ☑
monocytoid (M9890/3) 206.9 ☑
acute (M9891/3) 206.0 ☑
aleukemic (M9894/3) 206.8 ☑
chronic (M9893/3) 206.1 ☑
myelogenous (M9863/3) 205.1 ☑
subacute (M9892/3) 206.2 ☑
subleukemic (M9894/3) 206.8 ☑
monomyelocytic (M9860/3) — see Leukemia, myelomonocytic
myeloblastic (M9861/3) 205.0 ☑
myelocytic (M9863/3) 205.1 ☑
acute (M9861/3) 205.0 ☑
myelogenous (M9860/3) 205.9 ☑
acute (M9861/3) 205.0 ☑
aleukemic (M9864/3) 205.8 ☑
chronic (M9863/3) 205.1 ☑
monocytoid (M9863/3) 205.1 ☑

**Leukemia, leukemic** — continued
myelogenous — continued
subacute (M9862/3) 205.2 ☑
subleukemic (M9864/3) 205.8 ☑
myeloid (M9860/3) 205.9 ☑
acute (M9861/3) 205.0 ☑
aleukemic (M9864/3) 205.8 ☑
chronic (M9863/3) 205.1 ☑
subacute (M9862/3) 205.2 ☑
subleukemic (M9864/3) 205.8 ☑
myelomonocytic (M9860/3) 205.9 ☑
acute (M9861/3) 205.0 ☑
chronic (M9863/3) 205.1 ☑
Naegeli-type monocytic (M9863/3) 205.1 ☑
neutrophilic (M9865/3) 205.1 ☑
plasma cell (M9830/3) 203.1 ☑
plasmacytic (M9830/3) 203.1 ☑
prolymphocytic (M9825/3) — see Leukemia, lymphoid
promyelocytic, acute (M9866/3) 205.0 ☑
Schilling-type monocytic (M9890/3) — see Leukemia, monocytic
stem cell (M9801/3) 208.0 ☑
subacute NEC (M9802/3) 208.2 ☑
subleukemic NEC (M9804/3) 208.8 ☑
thrombocytic (M9910/3) 207.2 ☑
undifferentiated (M9801/3) 208.0 ☑
**Leukemoid reaction** (basophilic) (lymphocytic) (monocytic) (myelocytic) (neutrophilic) 288.62
**Leukoclastic vasculitis** 446.29
**Leukocoria** 360.44
**Leukocythemia** — see Leukemia
**Leukocytopenia** 288.50
**Leukocytosis** 288.60
basophilic 288.8
eosinophilic 288.3
lymphocytic 288.8
monocytic 288.8
neutrophilic 288.8
**Leukoderma** 709.09
syphilitic 091.3
late 095.8
**Leukodermia** — see also Leukoderma 709.09
**Leukodystrophy** (cerebral) (globoid cell) (metachromatic) (progressive) (sudanophilic) 330.0
**Leukoedema, mouth or tongue** 528.79
**Leukoencephalitis**
acute hemorrhagic (postinfectious) NEC 136.9 [323.61]
postimmunization or postvaccinal 323.51
subacute sclerosing 046.2
van Bogaert's 046.2
van Bogaert's (sclerosing) 046.2
**Leukoencephalopathy** — see also Encephalitis 323.9
acute necrotizing hemorrhagic (postinfectious) 136.9 [323.61]
postimmunization or postvaccinal 323.51
metachromatic 330.0
multifocal (progressive) 046.3
progressive multifocal 046.3
**Leukoerythroblastosis** 289.9
**Leukoerythrosis** 289.0
**Leukokeratosis** — see also Leukoplakia 702.8
mouth 528.6
nicotina palati 528.79
tongue 528.6
**Leukokoria** 360.44
**Leukokraurosis vulva, vulvae** 624.09 ▲
**Leukolymphosarcoma** (M9850/3) 207.8 ☑
**Leukoma** (cornea) (interfering with central vision) 371.03
adherent 371.04
**Leukomalacia, periventricular** 779.7
**Leukomelanopathy, hereditary** 288.2
**Leukonychia** (punctata) (striata) 703.8

**Leukonychia** — continued
congenital 757.5
**Leukopathia** 703.8
unguium 703.8
congenital 757.5
**Leukopenia** 288.50
basophilic 288.59
cyclic 288.02
eosinophilic 288.59
familial 288.59
malignant (see also Agranulocytosis) 288.09
periodic 288.02
transitory neonatal 776.7
**Leukopenic** — see condition
**Leukoplakia** 702.8
anus 569.49
bladder (postinfectional) 596.8
buccal 528.6
cervix (uteri) 622.2
esophagus 530.83
gingiva 528.6
kidney (pelvis) 593.89
larynx 478.79
lip 528.6
mouth 528.6
oral soft tissue (including tongue) (mucosa) 528.6
palate 528.6
pelvis (kidney) 593.89
penis (infectional) 607.0
rectum 569.49
syphilitic 095.8
tongue 528.6
tonsil 478.29
ureter (postinfectional) 593.89
urethra (postinfectional) 599.84
uterus 621.8
vagina 623.1
vesical 596.8
vocal cords 478.5
vulva 624.09 ▲
**Leukopolioencephalopathy** 330.0
**Leukorrhea** (vagina) 623.5
due to trichomonas (vaginalis) 131.00
trichomonal (Trichomonas vaginalis) 131.00
**Leukosarcoma** (M9850/3) 207.8 ☑
**Leukosis** (M9800/3) — see Leukemia
**Lev's disease or syndrome** (acquired complete heart block) 426.0
**Levi's syndrome** (pituitary dwarfism) 253.3
**Levocardia** (isolated) 746.87
with situs inversus 759.3
**Levulosuria** 271.2
**Lewandowski's disease** (primary) — see also Tuberculosis 017.0 ☑
**Lewandowski-Lutz disease** (epidermodysplasia verruciformis) 078.19
**Lewy body dementia** 331.82
**Lewy body disease** 331.82
**Leyden's disease** (periodic vomiting) 536.2
**Leyden-Möbius dystrophy** 359.1
**Leydig cell**
carcinoma (M8650/3)
specified site — see Neoplasm, by site, malignant
unspecified site
female 183.0
male 186.9
tumor (M8650/1)
benign (M8650/0)
specified site — see Neoplasm, by site, benign
unspecified site
female 220
male 222.0
malignant (M8650/3)
specified site — see Neoplasm, by site, malignant
unspecified site
female 183.0
male 186.9

☑ Additional Digit Required — Refer to the Tabular List for Digit Selection
180 — Volume 2 · October 2007
▶◀ Revised Text    ● New Line    ▲ Revised Code
▽ Subterms under main terms may continue to next column or page
2008 ICD-9-CM

**Leydig cell** — *continued*
  tumor — *continued*
    specified site — *see* Neoplasm, by
      site, uncertain behavior
    unspecified site
      female 236.2
      male 236.4
**Leydig-Sertoli cell tumor** (M8631/0)
  specified site — *see* Neoplasm, by site,
    benign
  unspecified site
    female 220
    male 222.0
**LGSIL** (low grade squamous intraepithelial lesion) 795.03
**Liar, pathologic** 301.7
**Libman-Sacks disease or syndrome** 710.0 *[424.91]*
**Lice** (infestation) 132.9
  body (pediculus corporis) 132.1
  crab 132.2
  head (pediculus capitis) 132.0
  mixed (classifiable to more than one
    of the categories 132.0–132.2)
    132.3
  pubic (pediculus pubis) 132.2
**Lichen** 697.9
  albus 701.0
  annularis 695.89
  atrophicus 701.0
  corneus obtusus 698.3
  myxedematous 701.8
  nitidus 697.1
  pilaris 757.39
    acquired 701.1
  planopilaris 697.0
  planus (acute) (chronicus) (hypertrophic) (verrucous) 697.0
    morphoeicus 701.0
    sclerosus (et atrophicus) 701.0
  ruber 696.4
    acuminatus 696.4
    moniliformis 697.8
    obtusus corneus 698.3
    of Wilson 697.0
    planus 697.0
  sclerosus (et atrophicus) 701.0
  scrofulosus (primary) (*see also* Tuberculosis) 017.0 ☑
  simplex (Vidal's) 698.3
    chronicus 698.3
    circumscriptus 698.3
  spinulosus 757.39
    mycotic 117.9
  striata 697.8
  urticatus 698.2
**Lichenification** 698.3
  nodular 698.3
**Lichenoides tuberculosis** (primary) — *see also* Tuberculosis 017.0 ☑
**Lichtheim's disease or syndrome** (subacute combined sclerosis with pernicious anemia) 281.0 *[336.2]*
**Lien migrans** 289.59
**Lientery** — *see also* Diarrhea 787.91
  infectious 009.2
**Life circumstance problem** NEC V62.89
**Li-Fraumeni cancer syndrome** V84.01
**Ligament** — *see* condition
**Light-for-dates** (infant) 764.0 ☑
  with signs of fetal malnutrition 764.1 ☑
  affecting management of pregnancy 656.5 ☑
**Light-headedness** 780.4
**Lightning** (effects) (shock) (stroke) (struck by) 994.0
  burn — *see* Burn, by site
  foot 266.2
**Lightwood's disease or syndrome** (renal tubular acidosis) 588.89
**Lignac's disease** (cystinosis) 270.0
**Lignac (-Fanconi) syndrome** (cystinosis) 270.0
**Lignac (-de Toni) (-Fanconi) (-Debré) syndrome** (cystinosis) 270.0

**Ligneous thyroiditis** 245.3
**Likoff's syndrome** (angina in menopausal women) 413.9
**Limb** — *see* condition
**Limitation of joint motion** — *see also* Stiffness, joint 719.5 ☑
  sacroiliac 724.6
**Limit dextrinosis** 271.0
**Limited**
  cardiac reserve — *see* Disease, heart
  duction, eye NEC 378.63
  mandibular range of motion 524.52
**Lindau's disease** (retinocerebral angiomatosis) 759.6
**Lindau (-von Hippel) disease** (angiomatosis retinocerebellosa) 759.6
**Linea corneae senilis** 371.41
**Lines**
  Beau's (transverse furrows on fingernails) 703.8
  Harris' 733.91
  Hudson-Stähli 371.11
  Stähli's 371.11
**Lingua**
  geographical 529.1
  nigra (villosa) 529.3
  plicata 529.5
    congenital 750.13
  tylosis 528.6
**Lingual** (tongue) — *see also* condition
  thyroid 759.2
**Linitis** (gastric) 535.4 ☑
  plastica (M8142/3) 151.9
**Lioderma essentialis** (cum melanosis et telangiectasia) 757.33
**Lip** — *see also* condition
  biting 528.9
**Lipalgia** 272.8
**Lipedema** — *see* Edema
**Lipemia** — *see also* Hyperlipidemia 272.4
  retina, retinalis 272.3
**Lipidosis** 272.7
  cephalin 272.7
  cerebral (infantile) (juvenile) (late) 330.1
  cerebroretinal 330.1 *[362.71]*
  cerebroside 272.7
  cerebrospinal 272.7
  chemically-induced 272.7
  cholesterol 272.7
  diabetic 250.8 ☑ *[272.7]*
  dystopic (hereditary) 272.7
  glycolipid 272.7
  hepatosplenomegalic 272.3
  hereditary, dystopic 272.7
  sulfatide 330.0
**Lipoadenoma** (M8324/0) — *see* Neoplasm, by site, benign
**Lipoblastoma** (M8881/0) — *see* Lipoma, by site
**Lipoblastomatosis** (M8881/0) — *see* Lipoma, by site
**Lipochondrodystrophy** 277.5
**Lipochrome histiocytosis** (familial) 288.1
**Lipodystrophia progressiva** 272.6
**Lipodystrophy** (progressive) 272.6
  insulin 272.6
  intestinal 040.2
  mesenteric 567.82
**Lipofibroma** (M8851/0) — *see* Lipoma, by site
**Lipoglycoproteinosis** 272.8
**Lipogranuloma, sclerosing** 709.8
**Lipogranulomatosis** (disseminated) 272.8
  kidney 272.8
**Lipoid** — *see also* condition
  histiocytosis 272.7
    essential 272.7
  nephrosis (*see also* Nephrosis) 581.3
  proteinosis of Urbach 272.8
**Lipoidemia** — *see also* Hyperlipidemia 272.4
**Lipoidosis** — *see also* Lipidosis 272.7
**Lipoma** (M8850/0) 214.9

**Lipoma** — *continued*
  breast (skin) 214.1
  face 214.0
  fetal (M8881/0) (*see also* Lipoma, by site)
    fat cell (M8880/0) — *see* Lipoma, by site
  infiltrating (M8856/0) — *see* Lipoma, by site
  intra-abdominal 214.3
  intramuscular (M8856/0) — *see* Lipoma, by site
  intrathoracic 214.2
  kidney 214.3
  mediastinum 214.2
  muscle 214.8
  peritoneum 214.3
  retroperitoneum 214.3
  skin 214.1
    face 214.0
  spermatic cord 214.4
  spindle cell (M8857/0) — *see* Lipoma, by site
  stomach 214.3
  subcutaneous tissue 214.1
    face 214.0
  thymus 214.2
  thyroid gland 214.2
**Lipomatosis** (dolorosa) 272.8
  epidural 214.8
  fetal (M8881/0) — *see* Lipoma, by site
  Launois-Bensaude's 272.8
**Lipomyohemangioma** (M8860/0)
  specified site — *see* Neoplasm, connective tissue, benign
  unspecified site 223.0
**Lipomyoma** (M8860/0)
  specified site — *see* Neoplasm, connective tissue, benign
  unspecified site 223.0
**Lipomyxoma** (M8852/0) — *see* Lipoma, by site
**Lipomyxosarcoma** (M8852/3) — *see* Neoplasm, connective tissue, malignant
**Lipophagocytosis** 289.89
**Lipoproteinemia** (alpha) 272.4
  broad-beta 272.2
  floating-beta 272.2
  hyper-pre-beta 272.1
**Lipoproteinosis** (Rössle-Urbach-Wiethe) 272.8
**Liposarcoma** (M8850/3) — *see also* Neoplasm, connective tissue, malignant
  differentiated type (M8851/3) — *see* Neoplasm, connective tissue, malignant
  embryonal (M8852/3) — *see* Neoplasm, connective tissue, malignant
  mixed type (M8855/3) — *see* Neoplasm, connective tissue, malignant
  myxoid (M8852/3) — *see* Neoplasm, connective tissue, malignant
  pleomorphic (M8854/3) — *see* Neoplasm, connective tissue, malignant
  round cell (M8853/3) — *see* Neoplasm, connective tissue, malignant
  well differentiated type (M8851/3) — *see* Neoplasm, connective tissue, malignant
**Liposynovitis prepatellaris** 272.8
**Lipping**
  cervix 622.0
  spine (*see also* Spondylosis) 721.90
  vertebra (*see also* Spondylosis) 721.90
**Lip pits** (mucus), congenital 750.25
**Lipschütz disease or ulcer** 616.50
**Lipuria** 791.1
  bilharziasis 120.0
**Liquefaction, vitreous humor** 379.21
**Lisping** 307.9

**Lissauer's paralysis** 094.1
**Lissencephalia, lissencephaly** 742.2
**Listerellose** 027.0
**Listeriose** 027.0
**Listeriosis** 027.0
  congenital 771.2
  fetal 771.2
  suspected fetal damage affecting management of pregnancy 655.4 ☑
**Listlessness** 780.79
**Lithemia** 790.6
**Lithiasis** — *see also* Calculus
  hepatic (duct) — *see* Choledocholithiasis
  urinary 592.9
**Lithopedion** 779.9
  affecting management of pregnancy 656.8 ☑
**Lithosis** (occupational) 502
  with tuberculosis — *see* Tuberculosis, pulmonary
**Lithuria** 791.9
**Litigation** V62.5
**Little**
  league elbow 718.82
  stroke syndrome 435.9
**Little's disease** — *see* Palsy, cerebral
**Littre's**
  gland — *see* condition
  hernia — *see* Hernia, Littre's
**Littritis** — *see also* Urethritis 597.89
**Livedo** 782.61
  annularis 782.61
  racemose 782.61
  reticularis 782.61
**Live flesh** 781.0
**Liver** — *see also* condition
  donor V59.6
**Livida, asphyxia**
  newborn 768.6
**Living**
  alone V60.3
    with handicapped person V60.4
**Lloyd's syndrome** 258.1
**Loa loa** 125.2
**Lobe, lobar** — *see* condition
**Lobo's disease or blastomycosis** 116.2
**Lobomycosis** 116.2
**Lobotomy syndrome** 310.0
**Lobstein's disease** (brittle bones and blue sclera) 756.51
**Lobster-claw hand** 755.58
**Lobulation** (congenital) — *see also* Anomaly, specified type NEC, by site
  kidney, fetal 753.3
  liver, abnormal 751.69
  spleen 759.0
**Lobule, lobular** — *see* condition
**Local, localized** — *see* condition
**Locked bowel or intestine** — *see also* Obstruction, intestine 560.9
**Locked-in state** 344.81
**Locked twins** 660.5 ☑
  affecting fetus or newborn 763.1
**Locking**
  joint (*see also* Derangement, joint) 718.90
  knee 717.9
**Lockjaw** — *see also* Tetanus 037
**Locomotor ataxia** (progressive) 094.0
**Löffler's**
  endocarditis 421.0
  eosinophilia or syndrome 518.3
  pneumonia 518.3
  syndrome (eosinophilic pneumonitis) 518.3
**Löfgren's syndrome** (sarcoidosis) 135
**Loiasis** 125.2
  eyelid 125.2 *[373.6]*
**Loneliness** V62.89
**Lone star fever** 082.8
**Longitudinal stripes or grooves, nails** 703.8

☑ Additional Digit Required — Refer to the Tabular List for Digit Selection
**2008 ICD-9-CM**
▶◀ Revised Text    ● New Line    ▲ Revised Code

ᴺᴱᶜ Subterms under main terms may continue to next column or page
**Volume 2 — 181**

☑ Additional Digit Required — Refer to the Tabular List for Digit Selection
182 — Volume 2 · October 2007
▶◀ Revised Text
● New Line
▲ Revised Code
Subterms under main terms may continue to next column or page
2008 ICD-9-CM

Left margin: Index · Longitudinal stripes or grooves, nails — Lupus

**Lupus** — *continued*
nephritis 710.0 *[583.81]*
acute 710.0 *[580.81]*
chronic 710.0 *[582.81]*
nontuberculous, not disseminated 695.4
pernio (Besnier) 135
tuberculous (*see also* Tuberculosis) 017.0 ☑
eyelid (*see also* Tuberculosis) 017.0 ☑ *[373.4]*
vulgaris 017.0 ☑
**Luschka's joint disease** 721.90
**Luteinoma** (M8610/0) 220
**Lutembacher's disease or syndrome** (atrial septal defect with mitral stenosis) 745.5
**Luteoma** (M8610/0) 220
**Lutz-Miescher disease** (elastosis perforans serpiginosa) 701.1
**Lutz-Splendore-de Almeida disease** (Brazilian blastomycosis) 116.1
**Luxatio**
bulbi due to birth injury 767.8
coxae congenita (*see also* Dislocation, hip, congenital) 754.30
erecta — *see* Dislocation, shoulder
imperfecta — *see* Sprain, by site
perinealis — *see* Dislocation, hip
**Luxation** (*see also* Dislocation, by site)
eyeball 360.81
due to birth injury 767.8
lateral 376.36
genital organs (external) NEC — *see* Wound, open, genital organs
globe (eye) 360.81
lateral 376.36
lacrimal gland (postinfectional) 375.16
lens (old) (partial) 379.32
congenital 743.37
syphilitic 090.49 *[379.32]*
Marfan's disease 090.49
spontaneous 379.32
penis — *see* Wound, open, penis
scrotum — *see* Wound, open, scrotum
testis — *see* Wound, open, testis
**L-xyloketosuria** 271.8
**Lycanthropy** — *see also* Psychosis 298.9
**Lyell's disease or syndrome** (toxic epidermal necrolysis) 695.1
due to drug
correct substance properly administered 695.1
overdose or wrong substance given or taken 977.9
specified drug — *see* Table of Drugs and Chemicals
**Lyme disease** 088.81
**Lymph**
gland or node — *see* condition
scrotum (*see also* Infestation, filarial) 125.9
**Lymphadenitis** 289.3
with
abortion — *see* Abortion, by type, with sepsis
ectopic pregnancy (*see also* categories 633.0–633.9) 639.0
molar pregnancy (*see also* categories 630–632) 639.0
acute 683
mesenteric 289.2
any site, except mesenteric 289.3
acute 683
chronic 289.1
mesenteric (acute) (chronic) (nonspecific) (subacute) 289.2
subacute 289.1
mesenteric 289.2
breast, puerperal, postpartum 675.2 ☑
chancroidal (congenital) 099.0
chronic 289.1
mesenteric 289.2
dermatopathic 695.89

**Lymphadenitis** — *continued*
due to
anthracosis (occupational) 500
Brugia (Wuchereria) malayi 125.1
diphtheria (toxin) 032.89
lymphogranuloma venereum 099.1
Wuchereria bancrofti 125.0
following
abortion 639.0
ectopic or molar pregnancy 639.0
generalized 289.3
gonorrheal 098.89
granulomatous 289.1
infectional 683
mesenteric (acute) (chronic) (nonspecific) (subacute) 289.2
due to Bacillus typhi 002.0
tuberculous (*see also* Tuberculosis) 014.8 ☑
mycobacterial 031.8
purulent 683
pyogenic 683
regional 078.3
septic 683
streptococcal 683
subacute, unspecified site 289.1
suppurative 683
syphilitic (early) (secondary) 091.4
late 095.8
tuberculous — *see* Tuberculosis, lymph gland
venereal 099.1
**Lymphadenoid goiter** 245.2
**Lymphadenopathy** (general) 785.6
due to toxoplasmosis (acquired) 130.7
congenital (active) 771.2
**Lymphadenopathy-associated virus** (disease) (illness) (infection) — *see* Human immunodeficiency virus (disease) (illness) (infection)
**Lymphadenosis** 785.6
acute 075
**Lymphangiectasis** 457.1
conjunctiva 372.89
postinfectional 457.1
scrotum 457.1
**Lymphangiectatic elephantiasis, non-filarial** 457.1
**Lymphangioendothelioma** (M9170/0) 228.1
malignant (M9170/3) — *see* Neoplasm, connective tissue, malignant
**Lymphangioma** (M9170/0) 228.1
capillary (M9171/0) 228.1
cavernous (M9172/0) 228.1
cystic (M9173/0) 228.1
malignant (M9170/3) — *see* Neoplasm, connective tissue, malignant
**Lymphangiomyoma** (M9174/0) 228.1
**Lymphangiomyomatosis** (M9174/1) — *see* Neoplasm, connective tissue, uncertain behavior
**Lymphangiosarcoma** (M9170/3) — *see* Neoplasm, connective tissue, malignant
**Lymphangitis** 457.2
with
abortion — *see* Abortion, by type, with sepsis
abscess — *see* Abscess, by site
cellulitis — *see* Abscess, by site
ectopic pregnancy (*see also* categories 633.0–633.9) 639.0
molar pregnancy (*see also* categories 630–632) 639.0
acute (with abscess or cellulitis) 682.9
specified site — *see* Abscess, by site
breast, puerperal, postpartum 675.2 ☑
chancroidal 099.0
chronic (any site) 457.2
due to
Brugia (Wuchereria) malayi 125.1

**Lymphangitis** — *continued*
due to — *continued*
Wuchereria bancrofti 125.0
following
abortion 639.0
ectopic or molar pregnancy 639.0
gangrenous 457.2
penis
acute 607.2
gonococcal (acute) 098.0
chronic or duration of 2 months or more 098.2
puerperal, postpartum, childbirth 670.0 ☑
strumous, tuberculous (*see also* Tuberculosis) 017.2 ☑
subacute (any site) 457.2
tuberculous — *see* Tuberculosis, lymph gland
**Lymphatic** (vessel) — *see* condition
**Lymphatism** 254.8
scrofulous (*see also* Tuberculosis) 017.2 ☑
**Lymphectasia** 457.1
**Lymphedema** — *see also* Elephantiasis 457.1
acquired (chronic) 457.1
chronic hereditary 757.0
congenital 757.0
idiopathic hereditary 757.0
praecox 457.1
secondary 457.1
surgical NEC 997.99
postmastectomy (syndrome) 457.0
**Lymph-hemangioma** (M9120/0) — *see* Hemangioma, by site
**Lymphoblastic** — *see* condition
**Lymphoblastoma** (diffuse) (M9630/3) 200.1 ☑
giant follicular (M9690/3) 202.0 ☑
macrofollicular (M9690/3) 202.0 ☑
**Lymphoblastosis, acute benign** 075
**Lymphocele** 457.8
**Lymphocythemia** 288.51
**Lymphocytic** — *see also* condition
chorioencephalitis (acute) (serous) 049.0
choriomeningitis (acute) (serous) 049.0
**Lymphocytoma** (diffuse) (malignant) (M9620/3) 200.1 ☑
**Lymphocytomatosis** (M9620/3) 200.1 ☑
**Lymphocytopenia** 288.51
**Lymphocytosis** (symptomatic) 288.61
infectious (acute) 078.89
**Lymphoepithelioma** (M8082/3) — *see* Neoplasm, by site, malignant
**Lymphogranuloma** (malignant) (M9650/3) 201.9 ☑
inguinale 099.1
venereal (any site) 099.1
with stricture of rectum 099.1
venereum 099.1
**Lymphogranulomatosis** (malignant) (M9650/3) 201.9 ☑
benign (Boeck's sarcoid) (Schaumann's) 135
Hodgkin's (M9650/3) 201.9 ☑
**Lymphohistiocytosis, familial hemophagocytic** 288.4
**Lymphoid** — *see* condition
**Lympholeukoblastoma** (M9850/3) 207.8 ☑
**Lympholeukosarcoma** (M9850/3) 207.8 ☑

**Lymphoma** (malignant) (M9590/3) 202.8 ☑

*Note* — *Use the following fifth-digit subclassification with categories 200–202:*

| | |
|---|---|
| 0 | *unspecified site, extranodal and solid organ sites* |
| 1 | *lymph nodes of head, face, and neck* |
| 2 | *intrathoracic lymph nodes* |
| 3 | *intra–abdominal lymph nodes* |
| 4 | *lymph nodes of axilla and upper limb* |
| 5 | *lymph nodes of inguinal region and lower limb* |
| 6 | *intrapelvic lymph nodes* |
| 7 | *spleen* |
| 8 | *lymph nodes of multiple sites* |

benign (M9590/0) — *see* Neoplasm, by site, benign
Burkitt's type (lymphoblastic) (undifferentiated) (M9750/3) 200.2 ☑
Castleman's (mediastinal lymph node hyperplasia) 785.6
centroblastic-centrocytic
diffuse (M9614/3) 202.8 ☑
follicular (M9692/3) 202.0 ☑
centroblastic type (diffuse) (M9632/3) 202.8 ☑
follicular (M9697/3) 202.0 ☑
centrocytic (M9622/3) 202.8 ☑
compound (M9613/3) 200.8 ☑
convoluted cell type (lymphoblastic) (M9602/3) 202.8 ☑
diffuse NEC (M9590/3) 202.8 ☑
large B cell 202.8 ☑ ●
follicular (giant) (M9690/3) 202.0 ☑
center cell (diffuse) (M9615/3) 202.8 ☑
cleaved (diffuse) (M9623/3) 202.8 ☑
follicular (M9695/3) 202.0 ☑
non-cleaved (diffuse) (M9633/3) 202.8 ☑
follicular (M9698/3) 202.0 ☑
centroblastic-centrocytic (M9692/3) 202.0 ☑
centroblastic type (M9697/3) 202.0 ☑
lymphocytic
intermediate differentiation (M9694/3) 202.0 ☑
poorly differentiated (M9696/3) 202.0 ☑
mixed (cell type) (lymphocytic-histiocytic) (small cell and large cell) (M9691/3) 202.0 ☑
germinocytic (M9622/3) 202.8 ☑
giant, follicular or follicle (M9690/3) 202.0 ☑
histiocytic (diffuse) (M9640/3) 200.0 ☑
nodular (M9642/3) 200.0 ☑
pleomorphic cell type (M9641/3) 200.0 ☑
Hodgkin's (M9650/3) (*see also* Disease, Hodgkin's) 201.9 ☑
immunoblastic (type) (M9612/3) 200.8 ☑
large cell (M9640/3) 200.7 ☑ ▲
anaplastic 200.6 ☑ ●
nodular (M9642/3) 200.0 ☑
pleomorphic cell type (M9641/3) 200.0 ☑
lymphoblastic (diffuse) (M9630/3) 200.1 ☑
Burkitt's type (M9750/3) 200.2 ☑
convoluted cell type (M9602/3) 202.8 ☑

☑ Additional Digit Required — Refer to the Tabular List for Digit Selection

▽ Subterms under main terms may continue to next column or page

*2008 ICD-9-CM*

▶◀ Revised Text

● New Line

▲ Revised Code

October 2007 · Volume 2 — 183

Lupus — Lymphoma

**Lymphoma** — *continued*
  lymphocytic (cell type) (diffuse)
      (M9620/3) 200.1 ☑
    with plasmacytoid differentiation,
        diffuse (M9611/3) 200.8 ☑
    intermediate differentiation (dif-
        fuse) (M9621/3) 200.1 ☑
      follicular (M9694/3) 202.0 ☑
      nodular (M9694/3) 202.0 ☑
    nodular (M9690/3) 202.0 ☑
    poorly differentiated (diffuse)
        (M9630/3) 200.1 ☑
      follicular (M9696/3) 202.0 ☑
      nodular (M9696/3) 202.0 ☑
    well differentiated (diffuse)
        (M9620/3) 200.1 ☑
      follicular (M9693/3) 202.0 ☑
      nodular (M9693/3) 202.0 ☑
  lymphocytic-histiocytic, mixed (dif-
      fuse) (M9613/3) 200.8 ☑
    follicular (M9691/3) 202.0 ☑
    nodular (M9691/3) 202.0 ☑
  lymphoplasmacytoid type (M9611/3)
      200.8 ☑
  lymphosarcoma type (M9610/3)
      200.1 ☑
  macrofollicular (M9690/3) 202.0 ☑
  mantle cell 200.4 ☑                          ●
  marginal zone 200.3 ☑                        ●
    extranodal B-cell 200.3 ☑                  ●
    nodal B-cell 200.3 ☑                       ●
    splenic B-cell 200.3 ☑                     ●
  mixed cell type (diffuse) (M9613/3)
      200.8 ☑
    follicular (M9691/3) 202.0 ☑
    nodular (M9691/3) 202.0 ☑
  nodular (M9690/3) 202.0 ☑
    histiocytic (M9642/3) 200.0 ☑
    lymphocytic (M9690/3) 202.0 ☑
      intermediate differentiation
          (M9694/3) 202.0 ☑
      poorly differentiated (M9696/3)
          202.0 ☑
    mixed (cell type) (lymphocytic-histi-
        ocytic) (small cell and large
        cell) (M9691/3) 202.0 ☑
  non-Hodgkin's type NEC (M9591/3)
      202.8 ☑
  peripheral T-cell 202.7 ☑                    ●
  primary central nervous system
      200.5 ☑                                  ●
  reticulum cell (type) (M9640/3)
      200.0 ☑
  small cell and large cell, mixed (dif-
      fuse) (M9613/3) 200.8 ☑
    follicular (M9691/3) 202.0 ☑
    nodular (9691/3) 202.0 ☑
  stem cell (type) (M9601/3) 202.8 ☑
  T-cell 202.1 ☑
    peripheral 202.7 ☑                         ●
  undifferentiated (cell type) (non-
      Burkitt's) (M9600/3) 202.8 ☑
    Burkitt's type (M9750/3) 200.2 ☑
**Lymphomatosis** (M9590/3) — *see also*
      Lymphoma
  granulomatous 099.1
**Lymphopathia**
  venereum 099.1
  veneris 099.1
**Lymphopenia** 288.51
  familial 279.2
**Lymphoreticulosis, benign** (of inocula-
      tion) 078.3
**Lymphorrhea** 457.8
**Lymphosarcoma** (M9610/3) 200.1 ☑
  diffuse (M9610/3) 200.1 ☑
    with plasmacytoid differentiation
        (M9611/3) 200.8 ☑
    lymphoplasmacytic (M9611/3)
        200.8 ☑
  follicular (giant) (M9690/3) 202.0 ☑
    lymphoblastic (M9696/3) 202.0 ☑
    lymphocytic, intermediate differen-
        tiation (M9694/3) 202.0 ☑
    mixed cell type (M9691/3) 202.0 ☑

**Lymphosarcoma** — *continued*
  giant follicular (M9690/3) 202.0 ☑
  Hodgkin's (M9650/3) 201.9 ☑
  immunoblastic (M9612/3) 200.8 ☑
  lymphoblastic (diffuse) (M9630/3)
      200.1 ☑
    follicular (M9696/3) 202.0 ☑
    nodular (M9696/3) 202.0 ☑
  lymphocytic (diffuse) (M9620/3)
      200.1 ☑
    intermediate differentiation (dif-
        fuse) (M9621/3) 200.1 ☑
      follicular (M9694/3) 202.0 ☑
      nodular (M9694/3) 202.0 ☑
  mixed cell type (diffuse) (M9613/3)
      200.8 ☑
    follicular (M9691/3) 202.0 ☑
    nodular (M9691/3) 202.0 ☑
  nodular (M9690/3) 202.0 ☑
    lymphoblastic (M9696/3) 202.0 ☑
    lymphocytic, intermediate differen-
        tiation (M9694/3) 202.0 ☑
    mixed cell type (M9691/3) 202.0 ☑
  prolymphocytic (M9631/3) 200.1 ☑
  reticulum cell (M9640/3) 200.0 ☑
**Lymphostasis** 457.8
**Lypemania** — *see also* Melancholia
      296.2 ☑
**Lyssa** 071

## M

**Macacus ear** 744.29
**Maceration**
  fetus (cause not stated) 779.9
  wet feet, tropical (syndrome) 991.4
**Machado-Joseph disease** 334.8
**Machupo virus hemorrhagic fever**
      078.7
**Macleod's syndrome** (abnormal transra-
      diancy, one lung) 492.8
**Macrocephalia, macrocephaly** 756.0
**Macrocheilia** (congenital) 744.81
**Macrochilia** (congenital) 744.81
**Macrocolon** (congenital) 751.3
**Macrocornea** 743.41
  associated with buphthalmos 743.22
**Macrocytic** — *see* condition
**Macrocytosis** 289.89
**Macrodactylia, macrodactylism** (fin-
      gers) (thumbs) 755.57
  toes 755.65
**Macrodontia** 520.2
**Macroencephaly** 742.4
**Macrogenia** 524.05
**Macrogenitosomia** (female) (male)
      (praecox) 255.2
**Macrogingivae** 523.8
**Macroglobulinemia** (essential) (idiopath-
      ic) (monoclonal) (primary) (syn-
      drome) (Waldenström's) 273.3
**Macroglossia** (congenital) 750.15
  acquired 529.8
**Macrognathia, macrognathism** (congen-
      ital) 524.00
  mandibular 524.02
    alveolar 524.72
  maxillary 524.01
    alveolar 524.71
**Macrogyria** (congenital) 742.4
**Macrohydrocephalus** — *see also* Hydro-
      cephalus 331.4
**Macromastia** — *see also* Hypertrophy,
      breast 611.1
**Macrophage activation syndrome** 288.4
**Macropsia** 368.14
**Macrosigmoid** 564.7
  congenital 751.3
**Macrospondylitis, acromegalic** 253.0
**Macrostomia** (congenital) 744.83
**Macrotia** (external ear) (congenital)
      744.22
**Macula**
  cornea, corneal
    congenital 743.43
      interfering with vision 743.42

**Macula** — *continued*
  cornea, corneal — *continued*
    interfering with central vision
        371.03
    not interfering with central vision
        371.02
  degeneration (*see also* Degeneration,
      macula) 362.50
    hereditary (*see also* Dystrophy,
        retina) 362.70
  edema, cystoid 362.53
**Maculae ceruleae** 132.1
**Macules and papules** 709.8
**Maculopathy, toxic** 362.55
**Madarosis** 374.55
**Madelung's**
  deformity (radius) 755.54
  disease (lipomatosis) 272.8
  lipomatosis 272.8
**Madness** — *see also* Psychosis 298.9
  myxedema (acute) 293.0
    subacute 293.1
**Madura**
  disease (actinomycotic) 039.9
    mycotic 117.4
  foot (actinomycotic) 039.4
    mycotic 117.4
**Maduromycosis** (actinomycotic) 039.9
  mycotic 117.4
**Maffucci's syndrome** (dyschondroplasia
      with hemangiomas) 756.4
**Magenblase syndrome** 306.4
**Main en griffe** (acquired) 736.06
  congenital 755.59
**Maintenance**
  chemotherapy regimen or treatment
      V58.11
  dialysis regimen or treatment
    extracorporeal (renal) V56.0
    peritoneal V56.8
    renal V56.0
  drug therapy or regimen
    chemotherapy, antineoplastic
        V58.11
    immunotherapy, antineoplastic
        V58.12
  external fixation NEC V54.89
  radiotherapy V58.0
  traction NEC V54.89
**Majocchi's**
  disease (purpura annularis telangiec-
      todes) 709.1
  granuloma 110.6
**Major** — *see* condition
**Mal**
  cerebral (idiopathic) (*see also* Epilepsy)
      345.9 ☑
  comital (*see also* Epilepsy) 345.9 ☑
  de los pintos (*see also* Pinta) 103.9
  de Meleda 757.39
  de mer 994.6
  lie — *see* Presentation, fetal
  perforant (*see also* Ulcer, lower extrem-
      ity) 707.15
**Malabar itch** 110.9
  beard 110.0
  foot 110.4
  scalp 110.0
**Malabsorption** 579.9
  calcium 579.8
  carbohydrate 579.8
  disaccharide 271.3
  drug-induced 579.8
  due to bacterial overgrowth 579.8
  fat 579.8
  folate, congenital 281.2
  galactose 271.1
  glucose-galactose (congenital) 271.3
  intestinal 579.9
  isomaltose 271.3
  lactose (hereditary) 271.3
  methionine 270.4
  monosaccharide 271.8
  postgastrectomy 579.3
  postsurgical 579.3
  protein 579.8

**Malabsorption** — *continued*
  sucrose (-isomaltose) (congenital)
      271.3
  syndrome 579.9
    postgastrectomy 579.3
    postsurgical 579.3
**Malacia, bone** 268.2
  juvenile (*see also* Rickets) 268.0
  Kienböck's (juvenile) (lunate) (wrist)
      732.3
    adult 732.8
**Malacoplakia**
  bladder 596.8
  colon 569.89
  pelvis (kidney) 593.89
  ureter 593.89
  urethra 599.84
**Malacosteon** 268.2
  juvenile (*see also* Rickets) 268.0
**Maladaptation** — *see* Maladjustment
**Maladie de Roger** 745.4
**Maladjustment**
  conjugal V61.10
    involving divorce or estrangement
        V61.0
  educational V62.3
  family V61.9
    specified circumstance NEC V61.8
  marital V61.10
    involving divorce or estrangement
        V61.0
  occupational V62.2
  simple, adult (*see also* Reaction, ad-
      justment) 309.9
  situational acute (*see also* Reaction,
      adjustment) 309.9
  social V62.4
**Malaise** 780.79
**Malakoplakia** — *see* Malacoplakia
**Malaria, malarial** (fever) 084.6
  algid 084.9
  any type, with
    algid malaria 084.9
    blackwater fever 084.8
    fever
      blackwater 084.8
      hemoglobinuric (bilious) 084.8
    hemoglobinuria, malarial 084.8
    hepatitis 084.9 [573.2]
    nephrosis 084.9 [581.81]
    pernicious complication NEC 084.9
      cardiac 084.9
      cerebral 084.9
  cardiac 084.9
  carrier (suspected) of V02.9
  cerebral 084.9
  complicating pregnancy, childbirth,
      or puerperium 647.4 ☑
  congenital 771.2
  congestion, congestive 084.6
    brain 084.9
  continued 084.0
  estivo-autumnal 084.0
  falciparum (malignant tertian) 084.0
  hematinuria 084.8
  hematuria 084.8
  hemoglobinuria 084.8
  hemorrhagic 084.6
  induced (therapeutically) 084.7
    accidental — *see* Malaria, by type
  liver 084.9 [573.2]
  malariae (quartan) 084.2
  malignant (tertian) 084.0
  mixed infections 084.5
  monkey 084.4
  ovale 084.3
  pernicious, acute 084.0
  Plasmodium, P.
    falciparum 084.0
    malariae 084.2
    ovale 084.3
    vivax 084.1
  quartan 084.2
  quotidian 084.0
  recurrent 084.6
    induced (therapeutically) 084.7

☑ Additional Digit Required — Refer to the Tabular List for Digit Selection           ▽ Subterms under main terms may continue to next column or page

184 — Volume 2 • October 2007          ▶◀ Revised Text          ● New Line          ▲ Revised Code          *2008 ICD-9-CM*

**Malaria, malarial** — *continued*
  recurrent — *continued*
    induced — *continued*
      accidental — *see* Malaria, by
        type
  remittent 084.6
  specified types NEC 084.4
  spleen 084.6
  subtertian 084.0
  tertian (benign) 084.1
    malignant 084.0
  tropical 084.0
  typhoid 084.6
  vivax (benign tertian) 084.1
**Malassez's disease** (testicular cyst)
  608.89
**Malassimilation** 579.9
**Maldescent, testis** 752.51
**Maldevelopment** — *see also* Anomaly,
  by site
  brain 742.9
  colon 751.5
  hip (joint) 755.63
    congenital dislocation (*see also*
      Dislocation, hip, congenital)
      754.30
  mastoid process 756.0
  middle ear, except ossicles 744.03
    ossicles 744.04
  newborn (not malformation) 764.9 ☑
  ossicles, ear 744.04
  spine 756.10
  toe 755.66
**Male type pelvis** 755.69
  with disproportion (fetopelvic) 653.2 ☑
    affecting fetus or newborn 763.1
    causing obstructed labor 660.1 ☑
      affecting fetus or newborn 763.1
**Malformation** (congenital) — *see also*
  Anomaly
  bone 756.9
  bursa 756.9
  Chiari
    type I 348.4
    type II (*see also* Spina bifida)
      741.0 ☑
    type III 742.0
    type IV 742.2
  circulatory system NEC 747.9
    specified type NEC 747.89
  cochlea 744.05
  digestive system NEC 751.9
    lower 751.5
    specified type NEC 751.8
    upper 750.9
  eye 743.9
  gum 750.9
  heart NEC 746.9
    specified type NEC 746.89
    valve 746.9
  internal ear 744.05
  joint NEC 755.9
    specified type NEC 755.8
  Mondini's (congenital) (malformation,
    cochlea) 744.05
  muscle 756.9
  nervous system (central) 742.9
  pelvic organs or tissues
    in pregnancy or childbirth 654.9 ☑
      affecting fetus or newborn
        763.89
      causing obstructed labor
        660.2 ☑
        affecting fetus or newborn
          763.1
  placenta (*see also* Placenta, abnormal)
    656.7 ☑
  respiratory organs 748.9
    specified type NEC 748.8
  Rieger's 743.44
  sense organs NEC 742.9
    specified type NEC 742.8
  skin 757.9
    specified type NEC 757.8
  spinal cord 742.9
  teeth, tooth NEC 520.9

**Malformation** — *see also* Anomaly —
  *continued*
  tendon 756.9
  throat 750.9
  umbilical cord (complicating delivery)
    663.9 ☑
    affecting fetus or newborn 762.6
  umbilicus 759.9
  urinary system NEC 753.9
    specified type NEC 753.8
**Malfunction** — *see also* Dysfunction
  arterial graft 996.1
  cardiac pacemaker 996.01
  catheter device — *see* Complications,
    mechanical, catheter
  colostomy 569.62
    valve 569.62
  cystostomy 997.5
  device, implant, or graft NEC — *see*
    Complications, mechanical
  enteric stoma 569.62
  enterostomy 569.62
  esophagostomy 530.87
  gastroenteric 536.8
  gastrostomy 536.42
  ileostomy
    valve 569.62
  nephrostomy 997.5
  pacemaker — *see* Complications, me-
    chanical, pacemaker
  prosthetic device, internal — *see*
    Complications, mechanical
  tracheostomy 519.02
  valve
    colostomy 569.62
    ileostomy 569.62
  vascular graft or shunt 996.1
**Malgaigne's fracture** (closed) 808.43
  open 808.53
**Malherbe's**
  calcifying epithelioma (M8110/0) —
    *see* Neoplasm, skin, benign
  tumor (M8110/0) — *see* Neoplasm,
    skin, benign
**Malibu disease** 919.8
  infected 919.9
**Malignancy** (M8000/3) — *see* Neoplasm,
  by site, malignant
**Malignant** — *see* condition
**Malingerer, malingering** V65.2
**Mallet, finger** (acquired) 736.1
  congenital 755.59
  late effect of rickets 268.1
**Malleus** 024
**Mallory's bodies** 034.1
**Mallory-Weiss syndrome** 530.7
**Malnutrition** (calorie) 263.9
  complicating pregnancy 648.9 ☑
  degree
    first 263.1
    second 263.0
    third 262
    mild 263.1
    moderate 263.0
    severe 261
      protein-calorie 262
  fetus 764.2 ☑
    "light-for-dates" 764.1 ☑
  following gastrointestinal surgery
    579.3
  intrauterine or fetal 764.2 ☑
    fetus or infant "light-for-dates"
      764.1 ☑
  lack of care, or neglect (child) (infant)
    995.52
    adult 995.84
  malignant 260
  mild 263.1
  moderate 263.0
  protein 260
  protein-calorie 263.9
    severe 262
    specified type NEC 263.8
  severe 261
    protein-calorie NEC 262
**Malocclusion** (teeth) 524.4

**Malocclusion** — *continued*
  angle's class I 524.21
  angle's class II 524.22
  angle's class III 524.23
  due to
    abnormal swallowing 524.59
    accessory teeth (causing crowding)
      524.31
    dentofacial abnormality NEC
      524.89
    impacted teeth (causing crowding)
      520.6
    missing teeth 524.30
    mouth breathing 524.59
    sleep postures 524.59
    supernumerary teeth (causing
      crowding) 524.31
    thumb sucking 524.59
    tongue, lip, or finger habits 524.59
  temporomandibular (joint) 524.69
**Malposition**
  cardiac apex (congenital) 746.87
  cervix — *see* Malposition, uterus
  congenital
    adrenal (gland) 759.1
    alimentary tract 751.8
      lower 751.5
      upper 750.8
    aorta 747.21
    appendix 751.5
    arterial trunk 747.29
    artery (peripheral) NEC (*see also*
      Malposition, congenital, pe-
      ripheral vascular system)
      747.60
      coronary 746.85
      pulmonary 747.3
    auditory canal 744.29
      causing impairment of hearing
        744.02
    auricle (ear) 744.29
      causing impairment of hearing
        744.02
      cervical 744.43
    biliary duct or passage 751.69
    bladder (mucosa) 753.8
      exteriorized or extroverted 753.5
    brachial plexus 742.8
    brain tissue 742.4
    breast 757.6
    bronchus 748.3
    cardiac apex 746.87
    cecum 751.5
    clavicle 755.51
    colon 751.5
    digestive organ or tract NEC 751.8
      lower 751.5
      upper 750.8
    ear (auricle) (external) 744.29
      ossicles 744.04
    endocrine (gland) NEC 759.2
    epiglottis 748.3
    Eustachian tube 744.24
    eye 743.8
    facial features 744.89
    fallopian tube 752.19
    finger(s) 755.59
      supernumerary 755.01
    foot 755.67
    gallbladder 751.69
    gastrointestinal tract 751.8
    genitalia, genital organ(s) or tract
      female 752.89
        external 752.49
        internal NEC 752.89
      male 752.89
        penis 752.69
        scrotal transposition 752.81
    glottis 748.3
    hand 755.59
    heart 746.87
      dextrocardia 746.87
        with complete transposition
          of viscera 759.3
    hepatic duct 751.69

**Malposition** — *continued*
  congenital — *continued*
    hip (joint) (*see also* Dislocation,
      hip, congenital) 754.30
    intestine (large) (small) 751.5
      with anomalous adhesions, fixa-
        tion, or malrotation 751.4
    joint NEC 755.8
    kidney 753.3
    larynx 748.3
    limb 755.8
      lower 755.69
      upper 755.59
    liver 751.69
    lung (lobe) 748.69
    nail(s) 757.5
    nerve 742.8
    nervous system NEC 742.8
    nose, nasal (septum) 748.1
    organ or site NEC — *see* Anomaly,
      specified type NEC, by site
    ovary 752.0
    pancreas 751.7
    parathyroid (gland) 759.2
    patella 755.64
    peripheral vascular system 747.60
      gastrointestinal 747.61
      lower limb 747.64
      renal 747.62
      specified NEC 747.69
      spinal 747.82
      upper limb 747.63
    pituitary (gland) 759.2
    respiratory organ or system NEC
      748.9
    rib (cage) 756.3
      supernumerary in cervical re-
        gion 756.2
    scapula 755.59
    shoulder 755.59
    spinal cord 742.59
    spine 756.19
    spleen 759.0
    sternum 756.3
    stomach 750.7
    symphysis pubis 755.69
    testis (undescended) 752.51
    thymus (gland) 759.2
    thyroid (gland) (tissue) 759.2
      cartilage 748.3
    toe(s) 755.66
      supernumerary 755.02
    tongue 750.19
    trachea 748.3
    uterus 752.3
    vein(s) (peripheral) NEC (*see also*
      Malposition, congenital, pe-
      ripheral vascular system)
      747.60
      great 747.49
      portal 747.49
      pulmonary 747.49
      vena cava (inferior) (superior)
        747.49
  device, implant, or graft — *see* Compli-
    cations, mechanical
  fetus NEC (*see also* Presentation, fetal)
    652.9 ☑
    with successful version 652.1 ☑
    affecting fetus or newborn 763.1
    before labor, affecting fetus or
      newborn 761.7
    causing obstructed labor 660.0 ☑
    in multiple gestation (one fetus or
      more) 652.6 ☑
      with locking 660.5 ☑
      causing obstructed labor
        660.0 ☑
  gallbladder (*see also* Disease, gallblad-
    der) 575.8
  gastrointestinal tract 569.89
    congenital 751.8
  heart (*see also* Malposition, congeni-
    tal, heart) 746.87
  intestine 569.89
    congenital 751.5

☑ Additional Digit Required — Refer to the Tabular List for Digit Selection      ▼ Subterms under main terms may continue to next column or page

*2008 ICD-9-CM*      ►◄ Revised Text      ● New Line      ▲ Revised Code      **Volume 2 — 185**

**Malposition** — *continued*
  pelvic organs or tissues
    in pregnancy or childbirth 654.4 ☑
      affecting fetus or newborn
        763.89
      causing obstructed labor
        660.2 ☑
        affecting fetus or newborn
          763.1
  placenta — *see* Placenta, previa
  stomach 537.89
    congenital 750.7
  tooth, teeth 524.30
    with impaction 520.6
  uterus (acquired) (acute) (adherent)
    (any degree) (asymptomatic)
    (postinfectional) (postpartal, old)
    621.6
    anteflexion or anteversion (*see also*
      Anteversion, uterus) 621.6
    congenital 752.3
    flexion 621.6
      lateral (*see also* Lateroversion,
        uterus) 621.6
    in pregnancy or childbirth 654.4 ☑
      affecting fetus or newborn
        763.89
      causing obstructed labor
        660.2 ☑
        affecting fetus or newborn
          763.1
    inversion 621.6
    lateral (flexion) (version) (*see also*
      Lateroversion, uterus) 621.6
    lateroflexion (*see also* Laterover-
      sion, uterus) 621.6
    lateroversion (*see also* Laterover-
      sion, uterus) 621.6
    retroflexion or retroversion (*see al-
      so* Retroversion, uterus)
      621.6
**Malposture** 729.9
**Malpresentation, fetus** — *see also* Presentation, fetal 652.9 ☑
**Malrotation**
  cecum 751.4
  colon 751.4
  intestine 751.4
  kidney 753.3
**MALT** (mucosa associated lymphoid ●
  tissue) 200.3 ☑           ●
**Malta fever** — *see also* Brucellosis 023.9
**Maltosuria** 271.3
**Maltreatment** (of)
  adult 995.80
    emotional 995.82
    multiple forms 995.85
    neglect (nutritional) 995.84
    physical 995.81
    psychological 995.82
    sexual 995.83
  child 995.50
    emotional 995.51
    multiple forms 995.59
    neglect (nutritional) 995.52
    physical 995.54
      shaken infant syndrome 995.55
    psychological 995.51
    sexual 995.53
  spouse (*see also* Maltreatment, adult)
    995.80
**Malt workers' lung** 495.4
**Malum coxae senilis** 715.25
**Malunion, fracture** 733.81
**Mammillitis** — *see also* Mastitis 611.0
  puerperal, postpartum 675.2 ☑
**Mammitis** — *see also* Mastitis 611.0
  puerperal, postpartum 675.2 ☑
**Mammographic**
  calcification 793.89
  calculus 793.89
  microcalcification 793.81
**Mammoplasia** 611.1
**Management**
  contraceptive V25.9
    specified type NEC V25.8

**Management** — *continued*
  procreative V26.9
    specified type NEC V26.89   ▲
**Mangled** NEC — *see also* nature and site
  of injury 959.9
**Mania** (monopolar) — *see also* Psychosis,
  affective 296.0 ☑
  alcoholic (acute) (chronic) 291.9
  Bell's — *see* Mania, chronic
  chronic 296.0 ☑
    recurrent episode 296.1 ☑
    single episode 296.0 ☑
  compulsive 300.3
  delirious (acute) 296.0 ☑
    recurrent episode 296.1 ☑
    single episode 296.0 ☑
  epileptic (*see also* Epilepsy) 345.4 ☑
  hysterical 300.10
  inhibited 296.89
  puerperal (after delivery) 296.0 ☑
    recurrent episode 296.1 ☑
    single episode 296.0 ☑
  recurrent episode 296.1 ☑
  senile 290.8
  single episode 296.0 ☑
  stupor 296.89
  stuporous 296.89
  unproductive 296.89
**Manic-depressive insanity, psychosis,**
  **reaction, or syndrome** — *see also*
  Psychosis, affective 296.80
  circular (alternating) 296.7
    currently
      depressed 296.5 ☑
      episode unspecified 296.7
      hypomanic, previously de-
        pressed 296.4 ☑
      manic 296.4 ☑
      mixed 296.6 ☑
  depressed (type), depressive 296.2 ☑
    atypical 296.82
    recurrent episode 296.3 ☑
    single episode 296.2 ☑
  hypomanic 296.0 ☑
    recurrent episode 296.1 ☑
    single episode 296.0 ☑
  manic 296.0 ☑
    atypical 296.81
    recurrent episode 296.1 ☑
    single episode 296.0 ☑
  mixed NEC 296.89
  perplexed 296.89
  stuporous 296.89
**Manifestations, rheumatoid**
  lungs 714.81
  pannus — *see* Arthritis, rheumatoid
  subcutaneous nodules — *see* Arthri-
    tis, rheumatoid
**Mankowsky's syndrome** (familial dysplastic osteopathy) 731.2
**Mannoheptulosuria** 271.8
**Mannosidosis** 271.8
**Manson's**
  disease (schistosomiasis) 120.1
  pyosis (pemphigus contagiosus) 684
  schistosomiasis 120.1
**Mansonellosis** 125.5
**Manual** — *see* condition
**Maple bark disease** 495.6
**Maple bark-strippers' lung** 495.6
**Maple syrup (urine) disease or syn-**
  **drome** 270.3
**Marable's syndrome** (celiac artery compression) 447.4
**Marasmus** 261
  brain 331.9
  due to malnutrition 261
  intestinal 569.89
  nutritional 261
  senile 797
  tuberculous NEC (*see also* Tuberculo-
    sis) 011.9 ☑
**Marble**
  bones 756.52
  skin 782.61
**Marburg disease** (virus) 078.89

**March**
  foot 733.94
  hemoglobinuria 283.2
**Marchand multiple nodular hyperplasia**
  (liver) 571.5
**Marchesani (-Weill) syndrome** (brachymorphism and ectopia lentis)
  759.89
**Marchiafava (-Bignami) disease or**
  **syndrome** 341.8
**Marchiafava-Micheli syndrome** (paroxysmal nocturnal hemoglobinuria)
  283.2
**Marcus Gunn's syndrome** (jaw-winking
  syndrome) 742.8
**Marfan's**
  congenital syphilis 090.49
  disease 090.49
  syndrome (arachnodactyly) 759.82
    meaning congenital syphilis 090.49
    with luxation of lens
      090.49 *[379.32]*
**Marginal**
  implantation, placenta — *see* Placen-
    ta, previa
  placenta — *see* Placenta, previa
  sinus (hemorrhage) (rupture) 641.2 ☑
    affecting fetus or newborn 762.1
**Marie's**
  cerebellar ataxia 334.2
  syndrome (acromegaly) 253.0
**Marie-Bamberger disease or syndrome**
  (hypertrophic) (pulmonary) (secondary) 731.2
  idiopathic (acropachyderma) 757.39
  primary (acropachyderma) 757.39
**Marie-Charcôt-Tooth** neuropathic atrophy, muscle 356.1
**Marie-Strümpell arthritis or disease**
  (ankylosing spondylitis) 720.0
**Marihuana, marijuana**
  abuse (*see also* Abuse, drugs, nonde-
    pendent) 305.2 ☑
  dependence (*see also* Dependence)
    304.3 ☑
**Marion's disease** (bladder neck obstruction) 596.0
**Marital conflict** V61.10
**Mark**
  port wine 757.32
  raspberry 757.32
  strawberry 757.32
  stretch 701.3
  tattoo 709.09
**Maroteaux-Lamy syndrome** (mucopolysaccharidosis VI) 277.5
**Marriage license examination** V70.3
**Marrow** (bone)
  arrest 284.9
  megakaryocytic 287.30
  poor function 289.9
**Marseilles fever** 082.1
**Marshall's** (hidrotic) **ectodermal dyspla-**
  **sia** 757.31
**Marsh's disease** (exophthalmic goiter)
  242.0 ☑
**Marsh fever** — *see also* Malaria 084.6
**Martin-Albright syndrome** (pseudohypoparathyroidism) 275.49
**Martin's disease** 715.27
**Martorell-Fabre syndrome** (pulseless
  disease) 446.7
**Masculinization, female** , with adrenal
  hyperplasia 255.2
**Masculinovoblastoma** (M8670/0) 220
**Masochism** 302.83
**Masons' lung** 502
**Mass**
  abdominal 789.3 ☑
  anus 787.99
  bone 733.90
  breast 611.72
  cheek 784.2
  chest 786.6
  cystic — *see* Cyst
  ear 388.8

**Mass** — *continued*
  epigastric 789.3 ☑
  eye 379.92
  female genital organ 625.8
  gum 784.2
  head 784.2
  intracranial 784.2
  joint 719.60
    ankle 719.67
    elbow 719.62
    foot 719.67
    hand 719.64
    hip 719.65
    knee 719.66
    multiple sites 719.69
    pelvic region 719.65
    shoulder (region) 719.61
    specified site NEC 719.68
    wrist 719.63
  kidney (*see also* Disease, kidney)
    593.9
  lung 786.6
  lymph node 785.6
  malignant (M8000/3) — *see* Neo-
    plasm, by site, malignant
  mediastinal 786.6
  mouth 784.2
  muscle (limb) 729.89
  neck 784.2
  nose or sinus 784.2
  palate 784.2
  pelvis, pelvic 789.3 ☑
  penis 607.89
  perineum 625.8
  rectum 787.99
  scrotum 608.89
  skin 782.2
  specified organ NEC — *see* Disease of
    specified organ or site
  splenic 789.2
  substernal 786.6
    thyroid (*see also* Goiter) 240.9
  superficial (localized) 782.2
  testes 608.89
  throat 784.2
  tongue 784.2
  umbilicus 789.3 ☑
  uterus 625.8
  vagina 625.8
  vulva 625.8
**Massive** — *see* condition
**Mastalgia** 611.71
  psychogenic 307.89
**Mast cell**
  disease 757.33
    systemic (M9741/3) 202.6 ☑
  leukemia (M9900/3) 207.8 ☑
  sarcoma (M9742/3) 202.6 ☑
  tumor (M9740/1) 238.5
    malignant (M9740/3) 202.6 ☑
**Masters-Allen syndrome** 620.6
**Mastitis** (acute) (adolescent) (diffuse)
  (interstitial) (lobular) (nonpuerperal) (nonsuppurative) (parenchymatous) (phlegmonous) (simple) (subacute) (suppurative) 611.0
  chronic (cystic) (fibrocystic) 610.1
  cystic 610.1
    Schimmelbusch's type 610.1
  fibrocystic 610.1
  infective 611.0
  lactational 675.2 ☑
  lymphangitis 611.0
  neonatal (noninfective) 778.7
    infective 771.5
  periductal 610.4
  plasma cell 610.4
  puerperalis 675.2 ☑
  puerperal, postpartum, (interstitial)
    (nonpurulent) (parenchymatous)
    675.2 ☑
    purulent 675.1 ☑
    stagnation 676.2 ☑
  retromammary 611.0
    puerperal, postpartum 675.1 ☑
  submammary 611.0

☑ Additional Digit Required — Refer to the Tabular List for Digit Selection              ▽ Subterms under main terms may continue to next column or page

186 — Volume 2 · October 2007        ▶◀ Revised Text        ● New Line        ▲ Revised Code        *2008 ICD-9-CM*

**Mastitis** — *continued*
  submammary — *continued*
    puerperal, postpartum 675.1 ☑
**Mastocytoma** (M9740/1) 238.5
  malignant (M9740/3) 202.6 ☑
**Mastocytosis** 757.33
  malignant (M9741/3) 202.6 ☑
  systemic (M9741/3) 202.6 ☑
**Mastodynia** 611.71
  psychogenic 307.89
**Mastoid** — *see condition*
**Mastoidalgia** — *see also* Otalgia 388.70
**Mastoiditis** (coalescent) (hemorrhagic)
  (pneumococcal) (streptococcal)
  (suppurative) 383.9
  acute or subacute 383.00
    with
      Gradenigo's syndrome 383.02
      petrositis 383.02
      specified complication NEC
        383.02
      subperiosteal abscess 383.01
  chronic (necrotic) (recurrent) 383.1
  tuberculous (*see also* Tuberculosis)
    015.6 ☑
**Mastopathy, mastopathia** 611.9
  chronica cystica 610.1
  diffuse cystic 610.1
  estrogenic 611.8
  ovarian origin 611.8
**Mastoplasia** 611.1
**Masturbation** 307.9
**Maternal condition, affecting fetus or newborn**
  acute yellow atrophy of liver 760.8
  albuminuria 760.1
  anesthesia or analgesia 763.5
  blood loss 762.1
  chorioamnionitis 762.7
  circulatory disease, chronic (condi-
    tions classifiable to 390–459,
    745–747) 760.3
  congenital heart disease (conditions
    classifiable to 745–746) 760.3
  cortical necrosis of kidney 760.1
  death 761.6
  diabetes mellitus 775.0
    manifest diabetes in the infant
      775.1
  disease NEC 760.9
    circulatory system, chronic (condi-
      tions classifiable to 390–459,
      745–747) 760.3
    genitourinary system (conditions
      classifiable to 580–599)
      760.1
    respiratory (conditions classifiable
      to 490–519, 748) 760.3
  eclampsia 760.0
  hemorrhage NEC 762.1
  hepatitis acute, malignant, or suba-
    cute 760.8
  hyperemesis (gravidarum) 761.8
  hypertension (arising during pregnan-
    cy) (conditions classifiable to
    642) 760.0
  infection
    disease classifiable to
      001-136 ☑, 760.2
    genital tract NEC 760.8
    urinary tract 760.1
  influenza 760.2
    manifest influenza in the infant
      771.2
  injury (conditions classifiable to
    800–996) 760.5
  malaria 760.2
    manifest malaria in infant or fetus
      771.2
  malnutrition 760.4
  necrosis of liver 760.8
  nephritis (conditions classifiable to
    580–583) 760.1
  nephrosis (conditions classifiable to
    581) 760.1

**Maternal condition, affecting fetus or newborn** — *continued*
  noxious substance transmitted via
    breast milk or placenta 760.70
    alcohol 760.71
    anticonvulsants 760.77
    antifungals 760.74
    anti-infective agents 760.74
    antimetabolics 760.78
    cocaine 760.75
    "crack" 760.75
    diethylstilbestrol [DES] 760.76
    hallucinogenic agents 760.73
    medicinal agents NEC 760.79
    narcotics 760.72
    obstetric anesthetic or analgesic
      drug 760.72
    specified agent NEC 760.79
  nutritional disorder (conditions classi-
    fiable to 260–269) 760.4
  operation unrelated to current delivery
    760.6
  pre-eclampsia 760.0
  pyelitis or pyelonephritis, arising dur-
    ing pregnancy (conditions clas-
    sifiable to 590) 760.1
  renal disease or failure 760.1
  respiratory disease, chronic (condi-
    tions classifiable to 490–519,
    748) 760.3
  rheumatic heart disease (chronic)
    (conditions classifiable to
    393–398) 760.3
  rubella (conditions classifiable to 056)
    760.2
    manifest rubella in the infant or
      fetus 771.0
  surgery unrelated to current delivery
    760.6
    to uterus or pelvic organs 763.89
  syphilis (conditions classifiable to
    090–097) 760.2
    manifest syphilis in the infant or
      fetus 090.0
  thrombophlebitis 760.3
  toxemia (of pregnancy) 760.0
    pre-eclamptic 760.0
  toxoplasmosis (conditions classifiable
    to 130) 760.2
    manifest toxoplasmosis in the in-
      fant or fetus 771.2
  transmission of chemical substance
    through the placenta 760.70
    alcohol 760.71
    anticonvulsants 760.77
    antifungals 760.74
    anti-infective 760.74
    antimetabolics 760.78
    cocaine 760.75
    "crack" 760.75
    diethylstilbestrol [DES] 760.76
    hallucinogenic agents 760.73
    narcotics 760.72
    specified substance NEC 760.79
  uremia 760.1
  urinary tract conditions (conditions
    classifiable to 580–599) 760.1
  vomiting (pernicious) (persistent) (vi-
    cious) 761.8
**Maternity** — *see* Delivery
**Matheiu's disease** (leptospiral jaundice)
  100.0
**Mauclaire's disease or osteochondrosis**
  732.3
**Maxcy's disease** 081.0
**Maxilla, maxillary** — *see condition*
**May (-Hegglin) anomaly or syndrome**
  288.2
**Mayaro fever** 066.3
**Mazoplasia** 610.8
**MBD** (minimal brain dysfunction), child
  — *see also* Hyperkinesia 314.9
**MCAD** (medium chain acyl CoA dehydro-
  genase deficiency) 277.85
**McArdle (-Schmid-Pearson) disease or
  syndrome** (glycogenosis V) 271.0

**McCune-Albright syndrome** (osteitis fibrosa disseminata) 756.59
**MCLS** (mucocutaneous lymph node syndrome) 446.1
**McQuarrie's syndrome** (idiopathic familial hypoglycemia) 251.2
**Measles** (black) (hemorrhagic) (suppressed) 055.9
  with
    encephalitis 055.0
    keratitis 055.71
    keratoconjunctivitis 055.71
    otitis media 055.2
    pneumonia 055.1
  complication 055.8
    specified type NEC 055.79
  encephalitis 055.0
  French 056.9
  German 056.9
  keratitis 055.71
  keratoconjunctivitis 055.71
  liberty 056.9
  otitis media 055.2
  pneumonia 055.1
  specified complications NEC 055.79
  vaccination, prophylactic (against)
    V04.2
**Meatitis, urethral** — *see also* Urethritis
  597.89
**Meat poisoning** — *see* Poisoning, food
**Meatus, meatal** — *see condition*
**Meat-wrappers' asthma** 506.9
**Meckel's**
  diverticulitis 751.0
  diverticulum (displaced) (hypertrophic)
    751.0
**Meconium**
  aspiration 770.11
    with
      pneumonia 770.12
      pneumonitis 770.12
      respiratory symptoms 770.12
    below vocal cords 770.11
      with respiratory symptoms
        770.12
    syndrome 770.12
  delayed passage in newborn 777.1
  ileus 777.1
    due to cystic fibrosis 277.01
  in liquor 792.3
    noted during delivery 656.8 ☑
  insufflation 770.11
    with respiratory symptoms 770.12
  obstruction
    fetus or newborn 777.1
      in mucoviscidosis 277.01
  passage of 792.3
    noted during delivery 763.84
  peritonitis 777.6
  plug syndrome (newborn) NEC 777.1
  staining 779.84
**Median** — *see also* condition
  arcuate ligament syndrome 447.4
  bar (prostate) 600.90
    with
      other lower urinary tract symp-
        toms (LUTS) 600.91
      urinary
        obstruction 600.91
        retention 600.91
  rhomboid glossitis 529.2
  vesical orifice 600.90
    with
      other lower urinary tract symp-
        toms (LUTS) 600.91
      urinary
        obstruction 600.91
        retention 600.91
**Mediastinal shift** 793.2
**Mediastinitis** (acute) (chronic) 519.2
  actinomycotic 039.8
  syphilitic 095.8
  tuberculous (*see also* Tuberculosis)
    012.8 ☑
**Mediastinopericarditis** — *see also*
  Pericarditis 423.9

**Mediastinopericarditis** — *see also*
  Pericarditis — *continued*
  acute 420.90
  chronic 423.8
    rheumatic 393
  rheumatic, chronic 393
**Mediastinum, mediastinal** — *see* condition
**Medical services provided for** — *see*
  Health, services provided because
  (of)
**Medicine poisoning** (by overdose) (wrong
  substance given or taken in error)
  977.9
  specified drug or substance — *see*
    Table of Drugs and Chemicals
**Medin's disease** (poliomyelitis) 045.9 ☑
**Mediterranean**
  anemia (with other hemoglobinopathy)
    282.49
  disease or syndrome (hemipathic)
    282.49
  fever (*see also* Brucellosis) 023.9
    familial 277.31
  kala-azar 085.0
  leishmaniasis 085.0
  tick fever 082.1
**Medulla** — *see* condition
**Medullary**
  cystic kidney 753.16
  sponge kidney 753.17
**Medullated fibers**
  optic (nerve) 743.57
  retina 362.85
**Medulloblastoma** (M9470/3)
  desmoplastic (M9471/3) 191.6
  specified site — *see* Neoplasm, by site,
    malignant
  unspecified site 191.6
**Medulloepithelioma** (M9501/3) — *see
  also* Neoplasm, by site, malignant
  teratoid (M9502/3) — *see* Neoplasm,
    by site, malignant
**Medullomyoblastoma** (M9472/3)
  specified site — *see* Neoplasm, by site,
    malignant
  unspecified site 191.6
**Meekeren-Ehlers-Danlos syndrome**
  756.83
**Megacaryocytic** — *see* condition
**Megacolon** (acquired) (functional) (not
  Hirschsprung's disease) 564.7
  aganglionic 751.3
  congenital, congenitum 751.3
  Hirschsprung's (disease) 751.3
  psychogenic 306.4
  toxic (*see also* Colitis, ulcerative)
    556.9
**Megaduodenum** 537.3
**Megaesophagus** (functional) 530.0
  congenital 750.4
**Megakaryocytic** — *see* condition
**Megalencephaly** 742.4
**Megalerythema** (epidermicum) (infectio-
  sum) 057.0
**Megalia, cutis et ossium** 757.39
**Megaloappendix** 751.5
**Megalocephalus, megalocephaly** NEC
  756.0
**Megalocornea** 743.41
  associated with buphthalmos 743.22
**Megalocytic anemia** 281.9
**Megalodactylia** (fingers) (thumbs) 755.57
  toes 755.65
**Megaloduodenum** 751.5
**Megaloesophagus** (functional) 530.0
  congenital 750.4
**Megalogastria** (congenital) 750.7
**Megalomania** 307.9
**Megalophthalmos** 743.8
**Megalopsia** 368.14
**Megalosplenia** — *see also* Splenomegaly
  789.2
**Megaloureter** 593.89
  congenital 753.22
**Megarectum** 569.49

**Megasigmoid** 564.7
  congenital 751.3
**Megaureter** 593.89
  congenital 753.22
**Megrim** 346.9 ☑
**Meibomian**
  cyst 373.2
    infected 373.12
  gland — see condition
  infarct (eyelid) 374.85
  stye 373.11
**Meibomitis** 373.12
**Meige**
  -Milroy disease (chronic hereditary edema) 757.0
  syndrome (blepharospasm-oro-mandibular dystonia) 333.82
**Melalgia, nutritional** 266.2
**Melancholia** — see also Psychosis, affective 296.90
  climacteric 296.2 ☑
    recurrent episode 296.3 ☑
    single episode 296.2 ☑
  hypochondriac 300.7
  intermittent 296.2 ☑
    recurrent episode 296.3 ☑
    single episode 296.2 ☑
  involutional 296.2 ☑
    recurrent episode 296.3 ☑
    single episode 296.2 ☑
  menopausal 296.2 ☑
    recurrent episode 296.3 ☑
    single episode 296.2 ☑
  puerperal 296.2 ☑
  reactive (from emotional stress, psychological trauma) 298.0
  recurrent 296.3 ☑
  senile 290.21
  stuporous 296.2 ☑
    recurrent episode 296.3 ☑
    single episode 296.2 ☑
**Melanemia** 275.0
**Melanoameloblastoma** (M9363/0) — see Neoplasm, bone, benign
**Melanoblastoma** (M8720/3) — see Melanoma
**Melanoblastosis**
  Block-Sulzberger 757.33
  cutis linearis sive systematisata 757.33
**Melanocarcinoma** (M8720/3) — see Melanoma
**Melanocytoma, eyeball** (M8726/0) 224.0
**Melanoderma, melanodermia** 709.09
  Addison's (primary adrenal insufficiency) 255.41 ▲
**Melanodontia, infantile** 521.05
**Melanodontoclasia** 521.05
**Melanoepithelioma** (M8720/3) — see Melanoma
**Melanoma** (malignant) (M8720/3) 172.9

Note — Except where otherwise indicated, the morphological varieties of melanoma in the list below should be coded by site as for "Melanoma (malignant)". Internal sites should be coded to malignant neoplasm of those sites.

  abdominal wall 172.5
  ala nasi 172.3
  amelanotic (M8730/3) — see Melanoma, by site
  ankle 172.7
  anus, anal 154.3
    canal 154.2
  arm 172.6
  auditory canal (external) 172.2
  auricle (ear) 172.2
  auricular canal (external) 172.2
  axilla 172.5
  axillary fold 172.5
  back 172.5
  balloon cell (M8722/3) — see Melanoma, by site

**Melanoma** — continued
  benign (M8720/0) — see Neoplasm, skin, benign
  breast (female) (male) 172.5
  brow 172.3
  buttock 172.5
  canthus (eye) 172.1
  cheek (external) 172.3
  chest wall 172.5
  chin 172.3
  choroid 190.6
  conjunctiva 190.3
  ear (external) 172.2
  epithelioid cell (M8771/3) (see also Melanoma, by site)
    and spindle cell, mixed (M8775/3) — see Melanoma, by site
  external meatus (ear) 172.2
  eye 190.9
  eyebrow 172.3
  eyelid (lower) (upper) 172.1
  face NEC 172.3
  female genital organ (external) NEC 184.4
  finger 172.6
  flank 172.5
  foot 172.7
  forearm 172.6
  forehead 172.3
  foreskin 187.1
  gluteal region 172.5
  groin 172.5
  hand 172.6
  heel 172.7
  helix 172.2
  hip 172.7
  in
    giant pigmented nevus (M8761/3) — see Melanoma, by site
    Hutchinson's melanotic freckle (M8742/3) — see Melanoma, by site
    junctional nevus (M8740/3) — see Melanoma, by site
    precancerous melanosis (M8741/3) — see Melanoma, by site
  interscapular region 172.5
  iris 190.0
  jaw 172.3
  juvenile (M8770/0) — see Neoplasm, skin, benign
  knee 172.7
  labium
    majus 184.1
    minus 184.2
  lacrimal gland 190.2
  leg 172.7
  lip (lower) (upper) 172.0
  liver 197.7
  lower limb NEC 172.7
  male genital organ (external) NEC 187.9
  meatus, acoustic (external) 172.2
  meibomian gland 172.1
  metastatic
    of or from specified site — see Melanoma, by site
    site not of skin — see Neoplasm, by site, malignant, secondary
    to specified site — see Neoplasm, by site, malignant, secondary
    unspecified site 172.9
  nail 172.9
    finger 172.6
    toe 172.7
  neck 172.4
  nodular (M8721/3) — see Melanoma, by site
  nose, external 172.3
  orbit 190.1
  penis 187.4
  perianal skin 172.5
  perineum 172.5
  pinna 172.2
  popliteal (fossa) (space) 172.7
  prepuce 187.1

**Melanoma** — continued
  pubes 172.5
  pudendum 184.4
  retina 190.5
  scalp 172.4
  scrotum 187.7
  septum nasal (skin) 172.3
  shoulder 172.6
  skin NEC 172.8
  spindle cell (M8772/3) (see also Melanoma, by site)
    type A (M8773/3) 190.0
    type B (M8774/3) 190.0
  submammary fold 172.5
  superficial spreading (M8743/3) — see Melanoma, by site
  temple 172.3
  thigh 172.7
  toe 172.7
  trunk NEC 172.5
  umbilicus 172.5
  upper limb NEC 172.6
  vagina vault 184.0
  vulva 184.4
**Melanoplakia** 528.9
**Melanosarcoma** (M8720/3) — see also Melanoma
  epithelioid cell (M8771/3) — see Melanoma
**Melanosis** 709.09
  addisonian (primary adrenal insufficiency) 255.41 ▲
    tuberculous (see also Tuberculosis) 017.6 ☑
  adrenal 255.41 ▲
  colon 569.89
  conjunctiva 372.55
    congenital 743.49
  corii degenerativa 757.33
  cornea (presenile) (senile) 371.12
    congenital 743.43
      interfering with vision 743.42
  eye 372.55
    congenital 743.49
  jute spinners' 709.09
  lenticularis progressiva 757.33
  liver 573.8
  precancerous (M8741/2) (see also Neoplasm, skin, in situ)
    malignant melanoma in (M8741/3) — see Melanoma
  prenatal 743.43
    interfering with vision 743.42
  Riehl's 709.09
  sclera 379.19
    congenital 743.47
  suprarenal 255.41 ▲
  tar 709.09
  toxic 709.09
**Melanuria** 791.9
**Melasma** 709.09
  adrenal (gland) 255.41 ▲
  suprarenal (gland) 255.41 ▲
**MELAS syndrome** (mitochondrial encephalopathy, lactic acidosis and stroke-like episodes) 277.87
**Melena** 578.1
  due to
    swallowed maternal blood 777.3
    ulcer — see Ulcer, by site, with hemorrhage
  newborn 772.4
    due to swallowed maternal blood 777.3
**Meleney's**
  gangrene (cutaneous) 686.09
  ulcer (chronic undermining) 686.09
**Melioidosis** 025
**Melitensis, febris** 023.0
**Melitococcosis** 023.0
**Melkersson (-Rosenthal) syndrome** 351.8
**Mellitus, diabetes** — see Diabetes
**Melorheostosis** (bone) (leri) 733.99
**Meloschisis** 744.83
**Melotia** 744.29

**Membrana**
  capsularis lentis posterior 743.39
  epipapillaris 743.57
**Membranacea placenta** — see Placenta, abnormal
**Membranaceous uterus** 621.8
**Membrane, membranous** — see also condition
  folds, congenital — see Web
  Jackson's 751.4
  over face (causing asphyxia), fetus or newborn 768.9
  premature rupture — see Rupture, membranes, premature
  pupillary 364.74
    persistent 743.46
  retained (complicating delivery) (with hemorrhage) 666.2 ☑
    without hemorrhage 667.1 ☑
  secondary (eye) 366.50
  unruptured (causing asphyxia) 768.9
  vitreous humor 379.25
**Membranitis, fetal** 658.4 ☑
  affecting fetus or newborn 762.7
**Memory disturbance, loss or lack** — see also Amnesia 780.93
  mild, following organic brain damage 310.1
**MEN** (multiple endocrine neoplasia) ●
  **syndromes** ●
  type I 258.01 ●
  type IIA 258.02 ●
  type IIB 258.03 ●
**Menadione** (vitamin K) **deficiency** 269.0
**Menarche, precocious** 259.1
**Mendacity, pathologic** 301.7
**Mendelson's syndrome** (resulting from a procedure) 997.3
  obstetric 668.0 ☑
**Mende's syndrome** (ptosis-epicanthus) 270.2
**Ménétrier's disease or syndrome** (hypertrophic gastritis) 535.2 ☑
**Ménière's disease, syndrome, or vertigo** 386.00
  cochlear 386.02
  cochleovestibular 386.01
  inactive 386.04
  in remission 386.04
  vestibular 386.03
**Meninges, meningeal** — see condition
**Meningioma** (M9530/0) — see also Neoplasm, meninges, benign
  angioblastic (M9535/0) — see Neoplasm, meninges, benign
  angiomatous (M9534/0) — see Neoplasm, meninges, benign
  endotheliomatous (M9531/0) — see Neoplasm, meninges, benign
  fibroblastic (M9532/0) — see Neoplasm, meninges, benign
  fibrous (M9532/0) — see Neoplasm, meninges, benign
  hemangioblastic (M9535/0) — see Neoplasm, meninges, benign
  hemangiopericytic (M9536/0) — see Neoplasm, meninges, benign
  malignant (M9530/3) — see Neoplasm, meninges, malignant
  meningiothelial (M9531/0) — see Neoplasm, meninges, benign
  meningotheliomatous (M9531/0) — see Neoplasm, meninges, benign
  mixed (M9537/0) — see Neoplasm, meninges, benign
  multiple (M9530/1) 237.6
  papillary (M9538/1) 237.6
  psammomatous (M9533/0) — see Neoplasm, meninges, benign
  syncytial (M9531/0) — see Neoplasm, meninges, benign
  transitional (M9537/0) — see Neoplasm, meninges, benign
**Meningiomatosis** (diffuse) (M9530/1) 237.6

**Meningism** — *see also* Meningismus
781.6
**Meningismus** (infectional) (pneumococcal) 781.6
  due to serum or vaccine
    997.09 *[321.8]*
  influenzal NEC 487.8
**Meningitis** (basal) (basic) (basilar) (brain)
  (cerebral) (cervical) (congestive)
  (diffuse) (hemorrhagic) (infantile)
  (membranous) (metastatic) (nonspecific) (pontine) (progressive) (simple)
  (spinal) (subacute) (sympathetica)
  (toxic) 322.9
  abacterial NEC (*see also* Meningitis,
    aseptic) 047.9
  actinomycotic 039.8 *[320.7]*
  adenoviral 049.1
  Aerobacter aerogenes 320.82
    anaerobes (cocci) (gram-negative)
      (gram-positive) (mixed) (NEC)
      320.81
  arbovirus NEC 066.9 *[321.2]*
    specified type NEC 066.8 *[321.2]*
  aseptic (acute) NEC 047.9
    adenovirus 049.1
    Coxsackie virus 047.0
    due to
      adenovirus 049.1
      Coxsackie virus 047.0
      ECHO virus 047.1
      enterovirus 047.9
      mumps 072.1
      poliovirus (*see also* Poliomyeli-
        tis) 045.2 ☑ *[321.2]*
    ECHO virus 047.1
    herpes (simplex) virus 054.72
      zoster 053.0
    leptospiral 100.81
    lymphocytic choriomeningitis 049.0
    noninfective 322.0
  Bacillus pyocyaneus 320.89
  bacterial NEC 320.9
    anaerobic 320.81
    gram-negative 320.82
      anaerobic 320.81
  Bacteroides (fragilis) (oralis)
    (melaninogenicus) 320.81
  cancerous (M8000/6) 198.4
  candidal 112.83
  carcinomatous (M8010/6) 198.4
  caseous (*see also* Tuberculosis,
    meninges) 013.0 ☑
  cerebrospinal (acute) (chronic) (diplo-
    coccal) (endemic) (epidemic)
    (fulminant) (infectious) (malig-
    nant) (meningococcal) (sporadic)
    036.0
    carrier (suspected) of V02.59
  chronic NEC 322.2
  clear cerebrospinal fluid NEC 322.0
  Clostridium (haemolyticum) (novyi)
    NEC 320.81
  coccidioidomycosis 114.2
  Coxsackie virus 047.0
  cryptococcal 117.5 *[321.0]*
  diplococcal 036.0
    gram-negative 036.0
    gram-positive 320.1
  Diplococcus pneumoniae 320.1
  due to
    actinomycosis 039.8 *[320.7]*
    adenovirus 049.1
    coccidiomycosis 114.2
    enterovirus 047.9
      specified NEC 047.8
    histoplasmosis (*see also* Histoplas-
      mosis) 115.91
    Listerosis 027.0 *[320.7]*
    Lyme disease 088.81 *[320.7]*
    moniliasis 112.83
    mumps 072.1
    neurosyphilis 094.2
    nonbacterial organisms NEC 321.8
    oidiomycosis 112.83

**Meningitis** — *continued*
  due to — *continued*
    poliovirus (*see also* Poliomyelitis)
      045.2 ☑ *[321.2]*
    preventive immunization, inocula-
      tion, or vaccination
      997.09 *[321.8]*
    sarcoidosis 135 *[321.4]*
    sporotrichosis 117.1 *[321.1]*
    syphilis 094.2
      acute 091.81
      congenital 090.42
      secondary 091.81
    trypanosomiasis (*see also* Try-
      panosomiasis) 086.9 *[321.3]*
    whooping cough 033.9 *[321.7]*
  ECHO virus 047.1
  E. coli 320.82
  endothelial-leukocytic, benign, recur-
    rent 047.9
  Enterobacter aerogenes 320.82
  enteroviral 047.9
    specified type NEC 047.8
  enterovirus 047.9
    specified NEC 047.8
  eosinophilic 322.1
  epidemic NEC 036.0
  Escherichia coli (E. coli) 320.82
  Eubacterium 320.81
  fibrinopurulent NEC 320.9
    specified type NEC 320.89
  Friedländer (bacillus) 320.82
  fungal NEC 117.9 *[321.1]*
  Fusobacterium 320.81
  gonococcal 098.82
  gram-negative bacteria NEC 320.82
    anaerobic 320.81
    cocci 036.0
      specified NEC 320.82
  gram-negative cocci NEC 036.0
    specified NEC 320.82
  gram-positive cocci NEC 320.9
  herpes (simplex) virus 054.72
    zoster 053.0
  H. influenzae 320.0
  infectious NEC 320.9
  influenzal 320.0
  Klebsiella pneumoniae 320.82
  late effect — *see* Late, effect, meningi-
    tis
  leptospiral (aseptic) 100.81
  Listerella (monocytogenes)
    027.0 *[320.7]*
  Listeria monocytogenes 027.0 *[320.7]*
  lymphocytic (acute) (benign) (serous)
    049.0
    choriomeningitis virus 049.0
  meningococcal (chronic) 036.0
  Mima polymorpha 320.82
  Mollaret's 047.9
  monilial 112.83
  mumps (virus) 072.1
  mycotic NEC 117.9 *[321.1]*
  Neisseria 036.0
  neurosyphilis 094.2
  nonbacterial NEC (*see also* Meningitis,
    aseptic) 047.9
  nonpyogenic NEC 322.0
  oidiomycosis 112.83
  ossificans 349.2
  Peptococcus 320.81
  Peptostreptococcus 320.81
  pneumococcal 320.1
  poliovirus (*see also* Poliomyelitis)
    045.2 ☑ *[321.2]*
  Proprionibacterium 320.81
  Proteus morganii 320.82
  Pseudomonas (aeruginosa) (pyocya-
    neus) 320.82
  purulent NEC 320.9
    specified organism NEC 320.89
  pyogenic NEC 320.9
    specified organism NEC 320.89
  Salmonella 003.21
  septic NEC 320.9
    specified organism NEC 320.89

**Meningitis** — *continued*
  serosa circumscripta NEC 322.0
  serous NEC (*see also* Meningitis,
    aseptic) 047.9
    lymphocytic 049.0
    syndrome 348.2
  Serratia (marcescens) 320.82
  specified organism NEC 320.89
  sporadic cerebrospinal 036.0
  sporotrichosis 117.1 *[321.1]*
  staphylococcal 320.3
  sterile 997.09
  streptococcal (acute) 320.2
  suppurative 320.9
    specified organism NEC 320.89
  syphilitic 094.2
    acute 091.81
    congenital 090.42
    secondary 091.81
  torula 117.5 *[321.0]*
  traumatic (complication of injury)
    958.8
  Treponema (denticola) (macroden-
    ticum) 320.81
  trypanosomiasis 086.1 *[321.3]*
  tuberculous (*see also* Tuberculosis,
    meninges) 013.0 ☑
  typhoid 002.0 *[320.7]*
  Veillonella 320.81
  Vibrio vulnificus 320.82
  viral, virus NEC (*see also* Meningitis,
    aseptic) 047.9
  Wallgren's (*see also* Meningitis, asep-
    tic) 047.9
**Meningocele** (congenital) (spinal) — *see*
  *also* Spina bifida 741.9 ☑
  acquired (traumatic) 349.2
  cerebral 742.0
  cranial 742.0
**Meningocerebritis** — *see* Meningoencephalitis
**Meningococcemia** (acute) (chronic)
  036.2
**Meningococcus, meningococcal** — *see*
  *also* condition 036.9
  adrenalitis, hemorrhagic 036.3
  carditis 036.40
  carrier (suspected) of V02.59
  cerebrospinal fever 036.0
  encephalitis 036.1
  endocarditis 036.42
  exposure to V01.84
  infection NEC 036.9
  meningitis (cerebrospinal) 036.0
  myocarditis 036.43
  optic neuritis 036.81
  pericarditis 036.41
  septicemia (chronic) 036.2
**Meningoencephalitis** — *see also* Encephalitis 323.9
  acute NEC 048
  bacterial, purulent, pyogenic, or septic
    — *see* Meningitis
  chronic NEC 094.1
  diffuse NEC 094.1
  diphasic 063.2
  due to
    actinomycosis 039.8 *[320.7]*
    blastomycosis NEC (*see also* Blas-
      tomycosis) 116.0 *[323.41]*
    free-living amebae 136.2
    Listeria monocytogenes
      027.0 *[320.7]*
    Lyme disease 088.81 *[320.7]*
    mumps 072.2
    Naegleria (amebae) (gruberi) (organ-
      isms) 136.2
    rubella 056.01
    sporotrichosis 117.1 *[321.1]*
    toxoplasmosis (acquired) 130.0
      congenital (active)
        771.2 *[323.41]*
    Trypanosoma 086.1 *[323.2]*
  epidemic 036.0
  herpes 054.3
  herpetic 054.3

**Meningoencephalitis** — *see also*
  Encephalitis — *continued*
    H. influenzae 320.0
  infectious (acute) 048
  influenzal 320.0
  late effect — *see* category 326
  Listeria monocytogenes 027.0 *[320.7]*
  lymphocytic (serous) 049.0
  mumps 072.2
  parasitic NEC 123.9 *[323.41]*
  pneumococcal 320.1
  primary amebic 136.2
  rubella 056.01
  serous 048
    lymphocytic 049.0
  specific 094.2
  staphylococcal 320.3
  streptococcal 320.2
  syphilitic 094.2
  toxic NEC 989.9 *[323.71]*
    due to
      carbon tetrachloride
        987.8 *[323.71]*
      hydroxyquinoline derivatives
        poisoning 961.3 *[323.71]*
      lead 984.9 *[323.71]*
      mercury 985.0 *[323.71]*
      thallium 985.8 *[323.71]*
  toxoplasmosis (acquired) 130.0
  trypanosomic 086.1 *[323.2]*
  tuberculous (*see also* Tuberculosis,
    meninges) 013.0 ☑
  virus NEC 048
**Meningoencephalocele** 742.0
  syphilitic 094.89
  congenital 090.49
**Meningoencephalomyelitis** — *see also*
  Meningoencephalitis 323.9
  acute NEC 048
    disseminated (postinfectious)
      136.9 *[323.61]*
      postimmunization or postvacci-
        nation 323.51
  due to
    actinomycosis 039.8 *[320.7]*
    torula 117.5 *[323.41]*
    toxoplasma or toxoplasmosis (ac-
      quired) 130.0
      congenital (active)
        771.2 *[323.41]*
  late effect — *see* category 326
**Meningoencephalomyelopathy** — *see*
  *also* Meningoencephalomyelitis
  349.9
**Meningoencephalopathy** — *see also*
  Meningoencephalitis 348.39
**Meningoencephalopoliomyelitis** — *see*
  *also* Poliomyelitis, bulbar 045.0 ☑
  late effect 138
**Meningomyelitis** — *see also* Meningoencephalitis 323.9
  blastomycotic NEC (*see also* Blastomy-
    cosis) 116.0 *[323.41]*
  due to
    actinomycosis 039.8 *[320.7]*
    blastomycosis (*see also* Blastomy-
      cosis) 116.0 *[323.41]*
    Meningococcus 036.0
    sporotrichosis 117.1 *[323.41]*
    torula 117.5 *[323.41]*
  late effect — *see* category 326
  lethargic 049.8
  meningococcal 036.0
  syphilitic 094.2
  tuberculous (*see also* Tuberculosis,
    meninges) 013.0 ☑
**Meningomyelocele** — *see also* Spina
  bifida 741.9 ☑
  syphilitic 094.89
**Meningomyeloneuritis** — *see* Meningoencephalitis
**Meningoradiculitis** — *see* Meningitis
**Meningovascular** — *see* condition
**Meniscocytosis** 282.60
**Menkes' syndrome** — *see* Syndrome,
  Menkes'

☑ Additional Digit Required — Refer to the Tabular List for Digit Selection        ▿ Subterms under main terms may continue to next column or page

**2008 ICD-9-CM**      ▶◀ Revised Text      ● New Line      ▲ Revised Code      **Volume 2 — 189**

**Index**

**Menolipsis — Microdeletions NEC**

**Menolipsis** 626.0
**Menometrorrhagia** 626.2
**Menopause, menopausal** (symptoms) (syndrome) 627.2
  arthritis (any site) NEC 716.3 ☑
  artificial 627.4
  bleeding 627.0
  crisis 627.2
  depression (see also Psychosis, affective) 296.2 ☑
    agitated 296.2 ☑
      recurrent episode 296.3 ☑
      single episode 296.2 ☑
    psychotic 296.2 ☑
      recurrent episode 296.3 ☑
      single episode 296.2 ☑
    recurrent episode 296.3 ☑
    single episode 296.2 ☑
    melancholia (see also Psychosis, affective) 296.2 ☑
      recurrent episode 296.3 ☑
      single episode 296.2 ☑
  paranoid state 297.2
  paraphrenia 297.2
  postsurgical 627.4
  premature 256.31
    postirradiation 256.2
    postsurgical 256.2
  psychoneurosis 627.2
  psychosis NEC 298.8
  surgical 627.4
  toxic polyarthritis NEC 716.39
**Menorrhagia** (primary) 626.2
  climacteric 627.0
  menopausal 627.0
  postclimacteric 627.1
  postmenopausal 627.1
  preclimacteric 627.0
  premenopausal 627.0
  puberty (menses retained) 626.3
**Menorrhalgia** 625.3
**Menoschesis** 626.8
**Menostaxis** 626.2
**Menses, retention** 626.8
**Menstrual** — see also Menstruation
  cycle, irregular 626.4
  disorders NEC 626.9
  extraction V25.3
  fluid, retained 626.8
  molimen 625.4
  period, normal V65.5
  regulation V25.3
**Menstruation**
  absent 626.0
  anovulatory 628.0
  delayed 626.8
  difficult 625.3
  disorder 626.9
    psychogenic 306.52
    specified NEC 626.8
  during pregnancy 640.8 ☑
  excessive 626.2
  frequent 626.2
  infrequent 626.1
  irregular 626.4
  latent 626.8
  membranous 626.8
  painful (primary) (secondary) 625.3
    psychogenic 306.52
  passage of clots 626.2
  precocious 626.8
  protracted 626.8
  retained 626.8
  retrograde 626.8
  scanty 626.1
  suppression 626.8
  vicarious (nasal) 625.8
**Mentagra** — see also Sycosis 704.8
**Mental** — see also condition
  deficiency (see also Retardation, mental) 319
  deterioration (see also Psychosis) 298.9
  disorder (see also Disorder, mental) 300.9
  exhaustion 300.5

**Mental** — see also condition — continued
  insufficiency (congenital) (see also Retardation, mental) 319
  observation without need for further medical care NEC V71.09
  retardation (see also Retardation, mental) 319
  subnormality (see also Retardation, mental) 319
    mild 317
    moderate 318.0
    profound 318.2
    severe 318.1
  upset (see also Disorder, mental) 300.9
**Meralgia paresthetica** 355.1
**Mercurial** — see condition
**Mercurialism** NEC 985.0
**Merergasia** 300.9
**Merkel cell tumor** — see Neoplasm, by site, malignant
**Merocele** — see also Hernia, femoral 553.00
**Meromelia** 755.4
  lower limb 755.30
    intercalary 755.32
      femur 755.34
        tibiofibular (complete) (incomplete) 755.33
      fibula 755.37
      metatarsal(s) 755.38
      tarsal(s) 755.38
      tibia 755.36
      tibiofibular 755.35
    terminal (complete) (partial) (transverse) 755.31
    longitudinal 755.32
      metatarsal(s) 755.38
      phalange(s) 755.39
      tarsal(s) 755.38
    transverse 755.31
  upper limb 755.20
    intercalary 755.22
      carpal(s) 755.28
      humeral 755.24
        radioulnar (complete) (incomplete) 755.23
      metacarpal(s) 755.28
      phalange(s) 755.29
      radial 755.26
      radioulnar 755.25
      ulnar 755.27
    terminal (complete) (partial) (transverse) 755.21
    longitudinal 755.22
      carpal(s) 755.28
      metacarpal(s) 755.28
      phalange(s) 755.29
    transverse 755.21
**Merosmia** 781.1
**MERRF syndrome** (myoclonus with epilepsy and with ragged red fibers) 277.87
**Merycism** — see also Vomiting
  psychogenic 307.53
**Merzbacher-Pelizaeus disease** 330.0
**Mesaortitis** — see Aortitis
**Mesarteritis** — see Arteritis
**Mesencephalitis** — see also Encephalitis 323.9
  late effect — see category 326
**Mesenchymoma** (M8990/1) — see also Neoplasm, connective tissue, uncertain behavior
  benign (M8990/0) — see Neoplasm, connective tissue, benign
  malignant (M8990/3) — see Neoplasm, connective tissue, malignant
**Mesenteritis**
  retractile 567.82
  sclerosing 567.82
**Mesentery, mesenteric** — see condition
**Mesiodens, mesiodentes** 520.1
  causing crowding 524.31

**Mesio-occlusion** 524.23
**Mesocardia** (with asplenia) 746.87
**Mesocolon** — see condition
**Mesonephroma** (malignant) (M9110/3) — see also Neoplasm, by site, malignant
  benign (M9110/0) — see Neoplasm, by site, benign
**Mesophlebitis** — see Phlebitis
**Mesostromal dysgenesis** 743.51
**Mesothelioma** (malignant) (M9050/3) — see also Neoplasm, by site, malignant
  benign (M9050/0) — see Neoplasm, by site, benign
  biphasic type (M9053/3) (see also Neoplasm, by site, malignant)
    benign (M9053/0) — see Neoplasm, by site, benign
  epithelioid (M9052/3) (see also Neoplasm, by site, malignant)
    benign (M9052/0) — see Neoplasm, by site, benign
  fibrous (M9051/3) (see also Neoplasm, by site, malignant)
    benign (M9051/0) — see Neoplasm, by site, benign
**Metabolic syndrome** 277.7
**Metabolism disorder** 277.9
  specified type NEC 277.89
**Metagonimiasis** 121.5
**Metagonimus infestation** (small intestine) 121.5
**Metal**
  pigmentation (skin) 709.00
  polishers' disease 502
**Metalliferous miners' lung** 503
**Metamorphopsia** 368.14
**Metaplasia**
  bone, in skin 709.3
  breast 611.8
  cervix — omit code
  endometrium (squamous) 621.8
  esophagus 530.85
  intestinal, of gastric mucosa 537.89
  kidney (pelvis) (squamous) (see also Disease, renal) 593.89
  myelogenous 289.89
  myeloid 289.89
    agnogenic 238.76
    megakaryocytic 238.76
  spleen 289.59
  squamous cell
    amnion 658.8 ☑
    bladder 596.8
    cervix — see condition
    trachea 519.19
    tracheobronchial tree 519.19
    uterus 621.8
    cervix — see condition
**Metastasis, metastatic**
  abscess — see Abscess
  calcification 275.40
  cancer, neoplasm, or disease
    from specified site (M8000/3) — see Neoplasm, by site, malignant
    to specified site (M8000/6) — see Neoplasm, by site, malignant
  deposits (in) (M8000/6) — see Neoplasm, by site, secondary
  pneumonia 038.8 [484.8]
  spread (to) (M8000/6) — see Neoplasm, by site, secondary
**Metatarsalgia** 726.70
  anterior 355.6
  due to Freiberg's disease 732.5
  Morton's 355.6
**Metatarsus, metatarsal** — see also condition
  abductus valgus (congenital) 754.60
  adductus varus (congenital) 754.53
  primus varus 754.52
  valgus (adductus) (congenital) 754.60
  varus (abductus) (congenital) 754.53
    primus 754.52

**Methemoglobinemia** 289.7
  acquired (with sulfhemoglobinemia) 289.7
  congenital 289.7
  enzymatic 289.7
  Hb-M disease 289.7
  hereditary 289.7
  toxic 289.7
**Methemoglobinuria** — see also Hemoglobinuria 791.2
**Methicillin-resistant staphylococcus aureus** (MRSA) V09.0
**Methioninemia** 270.4
**Metritis** (catarrhal) (septic) (suppurative) — see also Endometritis 615.9
  blennorrhagic 098.16
    chronic or duration of 2 months or over 098.36
  cervical (see also Cervicitis) 616.0
  gonococcal 098.16
    chronic or duration of 2 months or over 098.36
  hemorrhagic 626.8
  puerperal, postpartum, childbirth 670.0 ☑
  tuberculous (see also Tuberculosis) 016.7 ☑
**Metropathia hemorrhagica** 626.8
**Metroperitonitis** — see also Peritonitis, pelvic, female 614.5
**Metrorrhagia** 626.6
  arising during pregnancy — see Hemorrhage, pregnancy
  postpartum NEC 666.2 ☑
  primary 626.6
  psychogenic 306.59
  puerperal 666.2 ☑
**Metrorrhexis** — see Rupture, uterus
**Metrosalpingitis** — see also Salpingo-oophoritis 614.2
**Metrostaxis** 626.6
**Metrovaginitis** — see also Endometritis 615.9
  gonococcal (acute) 098.16
    chronic or duration of 2 months or over 098.36
**Mexican fever** — see Typhus, Mexican
**Meyenburg-Altherr-Uehlinger syndrome** 733.99
**Meyer-Schwickerath and Weyers syndrome** (dysplasia oculodentodigitalis) 759.89
**Meynert's amentia** (nonalcoholic) 294.0
  alcoholic 291.1
**Mibelli's disease** 757.39
**Mice, joint** — see also Loose, body, joint 718.1 ☑
  knee 717.6
**Micheli-Rietti syndrome** (thalassemia minor) 282.49
**Michotte's syndrome** 721.5
**Micrencephalon, micrencephaly** 742.1
**Microalbuminuria** 791.0
**Microaneurysm, retina** 362.14
  diabetic 250.5 ☑ [362.01]
**Microangiopathy** 443.9
  diabetic (peripheral) 250.7 ☑ [443.81]
    retinal 250.5 ☑ [362.01]
  peripheral 443.9
    diabetic 250.7 ☑ [443.81]
  retinal 362.18
    diabetic 250.5 ☑ [362.01]
  thrombotic 446.6
    Moschcowitz's (thrombotic thrombocytopenic purpura) 446.6
**Microcalcification, mammographic** 793.81
**Microcephalus, microcephalic**, microcephaly 742.1
  due to toxoplasmosis (congenital) 771.2
**Microcheilia** 744.82
**Microcolon** (congenital) 751.5
**Microcornea** (congenital) 743.41
**Microcytic** — see condition
**Microdeletions NEC** 758.33

**Microdontia** 520.2
**Microdrepanocytosis** (thalassemia-Hb-S disease) 282.49
**Microembolism**
  atherothrombotic — *see* Atheroembolism
  retina 362.33
**Microencephalon** 742.1
**Microfilaria streptocerca infestation** 125.3
**Microgastria** (congenital) 750.7
**Microgenia** 524.06
**Microgenitalia** (congenital) 752.89
  penis 752.64
**Microglioma** (M9710/3)
  specified site — *see* Neoplasm, by site, malignant
  unspecified site 191.9
**Microglossia** (congenital) 750.16
**Micrognathia, micrognathism** (congenital) 524.00
  mandibular 524.04
    alveolar 524.74
  maxillary 524.03
    alveolar 524.73
**Microgyria** (congenital) 742.2
**Microinfarct, heart** — *see also* Insufficiency, coronary 411.89
**Microlithiasis, alveolar, pulmonary** 516.2
**Micromyelia** (congenital) 742.59
**Micropenis** 752.64
**Microphakia** (congenital) 743.36
**Microphthalmia** (congenital) — *see also* Microphthalmos 743.10
**Microphthalmos** (congenital) 743.10
  associated with eye and adnexal anomalies NEC 743.12
  due to toxoplasmosis (congenital) 771.2
  isolated 743.11
  simple 743.11
  syndrome 759.89
**Micropsia** 368.14
**Microsporidiosis** 136.8
**Microsporon furfur infestation** 111.0
**Microsporosis** — *see also* Dermatophytosis 110.9
  nigra 111.1
**Microstomia** (congenital) 744.84
**Microthelia** 757.6
**Microthromboembolism** — *see* Embolism
**Microtia** (congenital) (external ear) 744.23
**Microtropia** 378.34
**Micturition**
  disorder NEC 788.69
    psychogenic 306.53
  frequency 788.41
    psychogenic 306.53
  nocturnal 788.43
  painful 788.1
    psychogenic 306.53
**Middle**
  ear — *see* condition
  lobe (right) syndrome 518.0
**Midplane** — *see* condition
**Miescher's disease** 709.3
  cheilitis 351.8
  granulomatosis disciformis 709.3
**Miescher-Leder syndrome or granulomatosis** 709.3
**Mieten's syndrome** 759.89
**Migraine** (idiopathic) 346.9 ☑
  with aura 346.0 ☑
  abdominal (syndrome) 346.2 ☑
  allergic (histamine) 346.2 ☑
  atypical 346.1 ☑
  basilar 346.2 ☑
  classical 346.0 ☑
  common 346.1 ☑
  hemiplegic 346.8 ☑
  lower-half 346.2 ☑
  menstrual 625.4
  ophthalmic 346.8 ☑

**Migraine** — *continued*
  ophthalmoplegic 346.8 ☑
  retinal 346.2 ☑
  variant 346.2 ☑
**Migrant, social** V60.0
**Migratory, migrating** — *see also* condition
  person V60.0
  testis, congenital 752.52
**Mikulicz's disease or syndrome** (dryness of mouth, absent or decreased lacrimation) 527.1
**Milian atrophia blanche** 701.3
**Miliaria** (crystallina) (rubra) (tropicalis) 705.1
  apocrine 705.82
**Miliary** — *see* condition
**Milium** — *see also* Cyst, sebaceous 706.2
  colloid 709.3
  eyelid 374.84
**Milk**
  crust 690.11
  excess secretion 676.6 ☑
  fever, female 672.0 ☑
  poisoning 988.8
  retention 676.2 ☑
  sickness 988.8
  spots 423.1
**Milkers' nodes** 051.1
**Milk-leg** (deep vessels) 671.4 ☑
  complicating pregnancy 671.3 ☑
  nonpuerperal 451.19
  puerperal, postpartum, childbirth 671.4 ☑
**Milkman (-Looser) disease or syndrome** (osteomalacia with pseudofractures) 268.2
**Milky urine** — *see also* Chyluria 791.1
**Millar's asthma** (laryngismus stridulus) 478.75
**Millard-Gubler-Foville paralysis** 344.89
**Millard-Gubler paralysis or syndrome** 344.89
**Miller-Dieker syndrome** 758.33
**Miller's disease** (osteomalacia) 268.2
**Miller Fisher's syndrome** 357.0
**Milles' syndrome** (encephalocutaneous angiomatosis) 759.6
**Mills' disease** 335.29
**Millstone makers' asthma or lung** 502
**Milroy's disease** (chronic hereditary edema) 757.0
**Miners'** — *see also* condition
  asthma 500
  elbow 727.2
  knee 727.2
  lung 500
  nystagmus 300.89
  phthisis (*see also* Tuberculosis) 011.4 ☑
  tuberculosis (see also Tuberculosis) 011.4 ☑
**Minkowski-Chauffard syndrome** — *see also* Spherocytosis 282.0
**Minor** — *see* condition
**Minor's disease** 336.1
**Minot's disease** (hemorrhagic disease, newborn) 776.0
**Minot-von Willebrand (-Jürgens) disease or syndrome** (angiohemophilia) 286.4
**Minus (and plus) hand** (intrinsic) 736.09
**Miosis** (persistent) (pupil) 379.42
**Mirizzi's syndrome** (hepatic duct stenosis) — *see also* Obstruction, biliary 576.2
  with calculus, cholelithiasis, or stones — *see* Choledocholithiasis
**Mirror writing** 315.09
  secondary to organic lesion 784.69
**Misadventure** (prophylactic) (therapeutic) — *see also* Complications 999.9
  administration of insulin 962.3
  infusion — *see* Complications, infusion

**Misadventure** — *see also* Complications — *continued*
  local applications (of fomentations, plasters, etc.) 999.9
    burn or scald — *see* Burn, by site
  medical care (early) (late) NEC 999.9
    adverse effect of drugs or chemicals — *see* Table of Drugs and Chemicals
    burn or scald — *see* Burn, by site
  radiation NEC 990
  radiotherapy NEC 990
  surgical procedure (early) (late) — *see* Complications, surgical procedure
  transfusion — *see* Complications, transfusion
  vaccination or other immunological procedure — *see* Complications, vaccination
**Misanthropy** 301.7
**Miscarriage** — *see* Abortion, spontaneous
**Mischief, malicious, child** — *see also* Disturbance, conduct 312.0 ☑
**Misdirection**
  aqueous 365.83
**Mismanagement, feeding** 783.3
**Misplaced, misplacement**
  kidney (*see also* Disease, renal) 593.0
    congenital 753.3
  organ or site, congenital NEC — *see* Malposition, congenital
**Missed**
  abortion 632
  delivery (at or near term) 656.4 ☑
  labor (at or near term) 656.4 ☑
**Missing** — *see also* Absence
  teeth (acquired) 525.10
    congenital (see also Anodontia) 520.0
    due to
      caries 525.13
      extraction 525.10
      periodontal disease 525.12
      specified NEC 525.19
      trauma 525.11
  vertebrae (congenital) 756.13
**Misuse of drugs** NEC — *see also* Abuse, drug, nondependent 305.9 ☑
**Mitchell's disease** (erythromelalgia) 443.82
**Mite(s)**
  diarrhea 133.8
  grain (itch) 133.8
  hair follicle (itch) 133.8
  in sputum 133.8
**Mitochondrial encephalopathy, lactic** acidosis and stroke-like episodes (MELAS syndrome) 277.87
**Mitochondrial neurogastrointestinal** encephalopathy syndrome (MNGIE) 277.87
**Mitral** — *see* condition
**Mittelschmerz** 625.2
**Mixed** — *see* condition
**Mljet disease** (mal de Meleda) 757.39
**Mobile, mobility**
  cecum 751.4
  coccyx 733.99
  excessive — *see* Hypermobility
  gallbladder 751.69
  kidney 593.0
    congenital 753.3
  organ or site, congenital NEC — *see* Malposition, congenital
  spleen 289.59
**Mobitz heart block** (atrioventricular) 426.10
  type I (Wenckebach's) 426.13
  type II 426.12
**Möbius'**
  disease 346.8 ☑
  syndrome
    congenital oculofacial paralysis 352.6

**Möbius'** — *continued*
  syndrome — *continued*
    ophthalmoplegic migraine 346.8 ☑
**Moeller (-Barlow) disease** (infantile scurvy) 267
  glossitis 529.4
**Mohr's syndrome** (types I and II) 759.89
**Mola destruens** (M9100/1) 236.1
**Molarization, premolars** 520.2
**Molar pregnancy** 631
  hydatidiform (delivered) (undelivered) 630
**Molding, head** (during birth) — *omit code*
**Mold(s)** in vitreous 117.9
**Mole** (pigmented) (M8720/0) — *see also* Neoplasm, skin, benign
  blood 631
  Breus' 631
  cancerous (M8720/3) — *see* Melanoma
  carneous 631
  destructive (M9100/1) 236.1
  ectopic — *see* Pregnancy, ectopic
  fleshy 631
  hemorrhagic 631
  hydatid, hydatidiform (benign) (complicating pregnancy) (delivered) (undelivered) (*see also* Hydatidiform mole) 630
    invasive (M9100/1) 236.1
    malignant (M9100/1) 236.1
    previous, affecting management of pregnancy V23.1
  invasive (hydatidiform) (M9100/1) 236.1
  malignant
    meaning
      malignant hydatidiform mole (9100/1) 236.1
      melanoma (M8720/3) — *see* Melanoma
  nonpigmented (M8730/0) — *see* Neoplasm, skin, benign
  pregnancy NEC 631
  skin (M8720/0) — *see* Neoplasm, skin, benign
  tubal — *see* Pregnancy, tubal
  vesicular (*see also* Hydatidiform mole) 630
**Molimen, molimina** (menstrual) 625.4
**Mollaret's meningitis** 047.9
**Mollities** (cerebellar) (cerebral) 437.8
  ossium 268.2
**Molluscum**
  contagiosum 078.0
  epitheliale 078.0
  fibrosum (M8851/0) — *see* Lipoma, by site
  pendulum (M8851/0) — *see* Lipoma, by site
**Mönckeberg's arteriosclerosis, degeneration, disease, or sclerosis** — *see also* Arteriosclerosis, extremities 440.20
**Monday fever** 504
**Monday morning dyspnea or asthma** 504
**Mondini's malformation** (cochlea) 744.05
**Mondor's disease** (thrombophlebitis of breast) 451.89
**Mongolian, mongolianism, mongolism, mongoloid** 758.0
  spot 757.33
**Monilethrix** (congenital) 757.4
**Monilia infestation** — *see* Candidiasis
**Moniliasis** — *see also* Candidiasis
  neonatal 771.7
  vulvovaginitis 112.1
**Monkeypox** 057.8
**Monoarthritis** 716.60
  ankle 716.67
  arm 716.62
    lower (and wrist) 716.63
    upper (and elbow) 716.62
  foot (and ankle) 716.67

**Monoarthritis** — *continued*
forearm (and wrist) 716.63
hand 716.64
leg 716.66
lower 716.66
upper 716.65
pelvic region (hip) (thigh) 716.65
shoulder (region) 716.61
specified site NEC 716.68
**Monoblastic** — *see* condition
**Monochromatism** (cone) (rod) 368.54
**Monocytic** — *see* condition
**Monocytopenia** 288.59
**Monocytosis** (symptomatic) 288.63
**Monofixation syndrome** 378.34
**Monomania** — *see also* Psychosis 298.9
**Mononeuritis** 355.9
cranial nerve — *see* Disorder, nerve, cranial
femoral nerve 355.2
lateral
cutaneous nerve of thigh 355.1
popliteal nerve 355.3
lower limb 355.8
specified nerve NEC 355.79
medial popliteal nerve 355.4
median nerve 354.1
multiplex 354.5
plantar nerve 355.6
posterior tibial nerve 355.5
radial nerve 354.3
sciatic nerve 355.0
ulnar nerve 354.2
upper limb 354.9
specified nerve NEC 354.8
vestibular 388.5
**Mononeuropathy** — *see also* Mononeuritis 355.9
diabetic NEC 250.6 ✓ *[355.9]*
lower limb 250.6 ✓ *[355.8]*
upper limb 250.6 ✓ *[354.9]*
iliohypogastric nerve 355.79
ilioinguinal nerve 355.79
obturator nerve 355.79
saphenous nerve 355.79
**Mononucleosis, infectious** 075
with hepatitis 075 *[573.1]*
**Monoplegia** 344.5
brain (current episode) (*see also* Paralysis, brain) 437.8
fetus or newborn 767.8
cerebral (current episode) (*see also* Paralysis, brain) 437.8
congenital or infantile (cerebral) (spastic) (spinal) 343.3
embolic (current) (*see also* Embolism, brain) 434.1 ✓
late effect — *see* Late effect(s) (of) cerebrovascular disease
infantile (cerebral) (spastic) (spinal) 343.3
lower limb 344.30
affecting
dominant side 344.31
nondominant side 344.32
due to late effect of cerebrovascular accident — *see* Late effect(s) (of) cerebrovascular accident
newborn 767.8
psychogenic 306.0
specified as conversion reaction 300.11
thrombotic (current) (*see also* Thrombosis, brain) 434.0 ✓
late effect — *see* Late effect(s) (of) cerebrovascular disease
transient 781.4
upper limb 344.40
affecting
dominant side 344.41
nondominant side 344.42
due to late effect of cerebrovascular accident — *see* Late effect(s) (of) cerebrovascular accident
**Monorchism, monorchidism** 752.89
**Monteggia's fracture** (closed) 813.03

**Monteggia's fracture** — *continued*
open 813.13
**Mood swings**
brief compensatory 296.99
rebound 296.99
**Mooren's ulcer** (cornea) 370.07
**Moore's syndrome** — *see also* Epilepsy 345.5 ✓
**Mooser bodies** 081.0
**Mooser-Neill reaction** 081.0
**Moral**
deficiency 301.7
imbecility 301.7
**Morax-Axenfeld conjunctivitis** 372.03
**Morbilli** — *see also* Measles 055.9
**Morbus**
anglicus, anglorum 268.0
Beigel 111.2
caducus (*see also* Epilepsy) 345.9 ✓
caeruleus 746.89
celiacus 579.0
comitialis (see also Epilepsy) 345.9 ✓
cordis (*see also* Disease, heart)
valvulorum — *see* Endocarditis
coxae 719.95
tuberculous (*see also* Tuberculosis) 015.1 ✓
hemorrhagicus neonatorum 776.0
maculosus neonatorum 772.6
renum 593.0
senilis (*see also* Osteoarthrosis) 715.9 ✓
**Morel-Kraepelin disease** — *see also* Schizophrenia 295.9 ✓
**Morel-Moore syndrome** (hyperostosis frontalis interna) 733.3
**Morel-Morgagni syndrome** (hyperostosis frontalis interna) 733.3
**Morgagni**
cyst, organ, hydatid, or appendage 752.89
fallopian tube 752.11
disease or syndrome (hyperostosis frontalis interna) 733.3
**Morgagni-Adams-Stokes syndrome** (syncope with heart block) 426.9
**Morgagni-Stewart-Morel syndrome** (hyperostosis frontalis interna) 733.3
**Moria** — *see also* Psychosis 298.9
**Morning sickness** 643.0 ✓
**Moron** 317
**Morphea** (guttate) (linear) 701.0
**Morphine dependence** — *see also* Dependence 304.0 ✓
**Morphinism** — *see also* Dependence 304.0 ✓
**Morphinomania** — *see also* Dependence 304.0 ✓
**Morphoea** 701.0
**Morquio (-Brailsford) (-Ullrich) disease or syndrome** (mucopolysaccharidosis IV) 277.5
kyphosis 277.5
**Morris syndrome** (testicular feminization) 259.5
**Morsus humanus** (open wound) — *see also* Wound, open, by site
skin surface intact — *see* Contusion
**Mortification** (dry) (moist) — *see also* Gangrene 785.4
**Morton's**
disease 355.6
foot 355.6
metatarsalgia (syndrome) 355.6
neuralgia 355.6
neuroma 355.6
syndrome (metatarsalgia) (neuralgia) 355.6
toe 355.6
**Morvan's disease** 336.0
**Mosaicism, mosaic** (chromosomal) 758.9
autosomal 758.5
sex 758.81
**Moschcowitz's syndrome** (thrombotic thrombocytopenic purpura) 446.6

**Mother yaw** 102.0
**Motion sickness** (from travel, any vehicle) (from roundabouts or swings) 994.6
**Mottled teeth** (enamel) (endemic) (nonendemic) 520.3
**Mottling enamel** (endemic) (nonendemic) (teeth) 520.3
**Mouchet's disease** 732.5
**Mould(s)** (in vitreous) 117.9
**Moulders'**
bronchitis 502
tuberculosis (*see also* Tuberculosis) 011.4 ✓
**Mounier-Kuhn syndrome** 748.3
with
acute exacerbation 494.1
bronchiectasis 494.0
with (acute) exacerbation 494.1
acquired 519.19
with bronchiectasis 494.0
with (acute) exacerbation 494.1
**Mountain**
fever — *see* Fever, mountain
sickness 993.2
with polycythemia, acquired 289.0
acute 289.0
tick fever 066.1
**Mouse, joint** — *see also* Loose, body, joint 718.1 ✓
knee 717.6
**Mouth** — *see* condition
**Movable**
coccyx 724.71
kidney (*see also* Disease, renal) 593.0
congenital 753.3
organ or site, congenital NEC — *see* Malposition, congenital
spleen 289.59
**Movement**
abnormal (dystonic) (involuntary) 781.0
decreased fetal 655.7 ✓
paradoxical facial 374.43
**Moya Moya disease** 437.5
**Mozart's ear** 744.29
**MRSA** (methicillin-resistant staphylococcus aureus) V09.0
**Mucha's disease** (acute parapsoriasis varioliformis) 696.2
**Mucha-Haberman syndrome** (acute parapsoriasis varioliformis) 696.2
**Mu-chain disease** 273.2
**Mucinosis** (cutaneous) (papular) 701.8
**Mucocele**
appendix 543.9
buccal cavity 528.9
gallbladder (*see also* Disease, gallbladder) 575.3
lacrimal sac 375.43
orbit (eye) 376.81
salivary gland (any) 527.6
sinus (accessory) (nasal) 478.19
turbinate (bone) (middle) (nasal) 478.19
uterus 621.8
**Mucocutaneous lymph node syndrome** (acute) (febrile) (infantile) 446.1
**Mucoenteritis** 564.9
**Mucolipidosis I, II, III** 272.7
**Mucopolysaccharidosis** (types 1-6) 277.5
cardiopathy 277.5 *[425.7]*
**Mucormycosis** (lung) 117.7
**Mucosa associated lymphoid tissue** ● (MALT) 200.3 ✓ ●
**Mucositis** — *see also* Inflammation, by site 528.00
cervix (ulcerative) 616.81
due to
antineoplastic therapy (ulcerative) 528.01
other drugs (ulcerative) 528.02
specified NEC 528.09
gastrointestinal (ulcerative) 538
nasal (ulcerative) 478.11

**Mucositis** — *see also* Inflammation, by site — *continued*
necroticans agranulocytica (*see also* Agranulocytosis) 288.09
ulcerative 528.00
vagina (ulcerative) 616.81
vulva (ulcerative) 616.81
**Mucous** — *see also* condition
patches (syphilitic) 091.3
congenital 090.0
**Mucoviscidosis** 277.00
with meconium obstruction 277.01
**Mucus**
asphyxia or suffocation (*see also* Asphyxia, mucus) 933.1
newborn 770.18
in stool 792.1
plug (*see also* Asphyxia, mucus) 933.1
aspiration, of newborn 770.17
tracheobronchial 519.19
newborn 770.18
**Muguet** 112.0
**Mulberry molars** 090.5
**Mullerian mixed tumor** (M8950/3) — *see* Neoplasm, by site, malignant
**Multicystic kidney** 753.19
**Multilobed placenta** — *see* Placenta, abnormal
**Multinodular prostate** 600.10
with
urinary
obstruction 600.11
retention 600.11
**Multiparity** V61.5
affecting
fetus or newborn 763.89
management of
labor and delivery 659.4 ✓
pregnancy V23.3
requiring contraceptive management (*see also* Contraception) V25.9
**Multipartita placenta** — *see* Placenta, abnormal
**Multiple, multiplex** — *see also* condition
birth
affecting fetus or newborn 761.5
healthy liveborn — *see* Newborn, multiple
digits (congenital) 755.00
fingers 755.01
toes 755.02
organ or site NEC — *see* Accessory
personality 300.14
renal arteries 747.62
**Mumps** 072.9
with complication 072.8
specified type NEC 072.79
encephalitis 072.2
hepatitis 072.71
meningitis (aseptic) 072.1
meningoencephalitis 072.2
oophoritis 072.79
orchitis 072.0
pancreatitis 072.3
polyneuropathy 072.72
vaccination, prophylactic (against) V04.6
**Mumu** — *see also* Infestation, filarial 125.9
**Münchausen syndrome** 301.51
**Münchmeyer's disease or syndrome** (exostosis luxurians) 728.11
**Mural** — *see* condition
**Murmur** (cardiac) (heart) (nonorganic) (organic) 785.2
abdominal 787.5
aortic (valve) (*see also* Endocarditis, aortic) 424.1
benign — *omit code*
cardiorespiratory 785.2
diastolic — *see* condition
Flint (*see also* Endocarditis, aortic) 424.1

**Murmur** — *continued*
functional — *omit code*
Graham Steell (pulmonic regurgitation) (*see also* Endocarditis, pulmonary) 424.3
innocent — *omit code*
insignificant — *omit code*
midsystolic 785.2
mitral (valve) — *see* Stenosis, mitral
physiologic — *see* condition
presystolic, mitral — *see* Insufficiency, mitral
pulmonic (valve) (*see also* Endocarditis, pulmonary) 424.3
Still's (vibratory) — *omit code*
systolic (valvular) — *see* condition
tricuspid (valve) — *see* Endocarditis, tricuspid
undiagnosed 785.2
valvular — *see* condition
vibratory — *omit code*
**Murri's disease** (intermittent hemoglobinuria) 283.2
**Muscae volitantes** 379.24
**Muscle, muscular** — *see* condition
**Musculoneuralgia** 729.1
**Mushrooming hip** 718.95
**Mushroom workers' (pickers') lung** 495.5
**Mutation**
factor V leiden 289.81
prothrombin gene 289.81
**Mutism** — *see also* Aphasia 784.3
akinetic 784.3
deaf (acquired) (congenital) 389.7
hysterical 300.11
selective (elective) 313.23
adjustment reaction 309.83
**Myà's disease** (congenital dilation, colon) 751.3
**Myalgia** (intercostal) 729.1
eosinophilia syndrome 710.5
epidemic 074.1
cervical 078.89
psychogenic 307.89
traumatic NEC 959.9
**Myasthenia** 358.00
cordis — *see* Failure, heart
gravis 358.00
with exacerbation (acute) 358.01
in crisis 358.01
neonatal 775.2
pseudoparalytica 358.00
stomach 536.8
psychogenic 306.4
syndrome
in
botulism 005.1 *[358.1]*
diabetes mellitus 250.6 ☑ *[358.1]*
hypothyroidism (*see also* Hypothyroidism) 244.9 *[358.1]*
malignant neoplasm NEC 199.1 *[358.1]*
pernicious anemia 281.0 *[358.1]*
thyrotoxicosis (*see also* Thyrotoxicosis) 242.9 ☑ *[358.1]*
**Myasthenic** 728.87
**Mycelium infection** NEC 117.9
**Mycetismus** 988.1
**Mycetoma** (actinomycotic) 039.9
bone 039.8
mycotic 117.4
foot 039.4
mycotic 117.4
madurae 039.9
mycotic 117.4
maduromycotic 039.9
mycotic 117.4
mycotic 117.4
nocardial 039.9
**Mycobacteriosis** — *see* Mycobacterium
**Mycobacterium, mycobacterial** (infection) 031.9
acid-fast (bacilli) 031.9

**Mycobacterium, mycobacterial** — *continued*
anonymous (*see also* Mycobacterium, atypical) 031.9
atypical (acid-fast bacilli) 031.9
cutaneous 031.1
pulmonary 031.0
tuberculous (*see also* Tuberculosis, pulmonary) 011.9 ☑
specified site NEC 031.8
avium 031.0
intracellulare complex bacteremia (MAC) 031.2
balnei 031.1
Battey 031.0
cutaneous 031.1
disseminated 031.2
avium-intracellulare complex (DMAC) 031.2
fortuitum 031.0
intracellulare (battey bacillus) 031.0
kakerifu 031.8
kansasii 031.0
kasongo 031.8
leprae — *see* Leprosy
luciflavum 031.0
marinum 031.1
pulmonary 031.0
tuberculous (*see also* Tuberculosis, pulmonary) 011.9 ☑
scrofulaceum 031.1
tuberculosis (human, bovine) (*see also* Tuberculosis)
avian type 031.0
ulcerans 031.1
xenopi 031.0
**Mycosis, mycotic** 117.9
cutaneous NEC 111.9
ear 111.8 *[380.15]*
fungoides (M9700/3) 202.1 ☑
mouth 112.0
pharynx 117.9
skin NEC 111.9
stomatitis 112.0
systemic NEC 117.9
tonsil 117.9
vagina, vaginitis 112.1
**Mydriasis** (persistent) (pupil) 379.43
**Myelatelia** 742.59
**Myelinoclasis, perivascular**, acute (postinfectious) NEC 136.9 *[323.61]*
postimmunization or postvaccinal 323.51
**Myelinosis, central pontine** 341.8
**Myelitis** (ascending) (cerebellar) (childhood) (chronic) (descending) (diffuse) (disseminated) (pressure) (progressive) (spinal cord) (subacute) — *see also* Encephalitis 323.9
acute (transverse) 341.20
idiopathic 341.22
in conditions classified elsewhere 341.21
due to
infection classified elsewhere 136.9 *[323.42]*
specified cause NEC 323.82
vaccination (any) 323.52
viral diseases classified elsewhere 323.02
herpes simplex 054.74
herpes zoster 053.14
late effect — *see* category 326
optic neuritis in 341.0
postchickenpox 052.2
postimmunization 323.52
postinfectious 136.9 *[323.63]*
postvaccinal 323.52
postvaricella 052.2
syphilitic (transverse) 094.89
toxic 989.9 *[323.72]*
transverse 323.82
acute 341.20
idiopathic 341.22
in conditions classified elsewhere 341.21

**Myelitis** — *see also* Encephalitis — *continued*
transverse — *continued*
idiopathic 341.22
tuberculous (*see also* Tuberculosis) 013.6 ☑
virus 049.9
**Myeloblastic** — *see* condition
**Myelocele** — *see also* Spina bifida 741.9 ☑
with hydrocephalus 741.0 ☑
**Myelocystocele** — *see also* Spina bifida 741.9 ☑
**Myelocytic** — *see* condition
**Myelocytoma** 205.1 ☑
**Myelodysplasia** (spinal cord) 742.59
meaning myelodysplastic syndrome — *see* Syndrome, myelodysplastic
**Myeloencephalitis** — *see* Encephalitis
**Myelofibrosis** 289.83
with myeloid metaplasia 238.76
idiopathic (chronic) 238.76
megakaryocytic 238.79
primary 238.76
secondary 289.83
**Myelogenous** — *see* condition
**Myeloid** — *see* condition
**Myelokathexis** 288.09
**Myeloleukodystrophy** 330.0
**Myelolipoma** (M8870/0) — *see* Neoplasm, by site, benign
**Myeloma** (multiple) (plasma cell) (plasmacytic) (M9730/3) 203.0 ☑
monostotic (M9731/1) 238.6
solitary (M9731/1) 238.6
**Myelomalacia** 336.8
**Myelomata, multiple** (M9730/3) 203.0 ☑
**Myelomatosis** (M9730/3) 203.0 ☑
**Myelomeningitis** — *see* Meningoencephalitis
**Myelomeningocele** (spinal cord) — *see also* Spina bifida 741.9 ☑
fetal, causing fetopelvic disproportion 653.7 ☑
**Myelo-osteo-musculodysplasia** hereditaria 756.89
**Myelopathic** — *see* condition
**Myelopathy** (spinal cord) 336.9
cervical 721.1
diabetic 250.6 ☑ *[336.3]*
drug-induced 336.8
due to or with
carbon tetrachloride 987.8 *[323.72]*
degeneration or displacement, intervertebral disc 722.70
cervical, cervicothoracic 722.71
lumbar, lumbosacral 722.73
thoracic, thoracolumbar 722.72
hydroxyquinoline derivatives 961.3 *[323.72]*
infection — *see* Encephalitis
intervertebral disc disorder 722.70
cervical, cervicothoracic 722.71
lumbar, lumbosacral 722.73
thoracic, thoracolumbar 722.72
lead 984.9 *[323.72]*
mercury 985.0 *[323.72]*
neoplastic disease (*see also* Neoplasm, by site) 239.9 *[336.3]*
pernicious anemia 281.0 *[336.3]*
spondylosis 721.91
cervical 721.1
lumbar, lumbosacral 721.42
thoracic 721.41
thallium 985.8 *[323.72]*
lumbar, lumbosacral 721.42
necrotic (subacute) 336.1
radiation-induced 336.8
spondylogenic NEC 721.91
cervical 721.1
lumbar, lumbosacral 721.42
thoracic 721.41
thoracic 721.41
toxic NEC 989.9 *[323.72]*

**Myelopathy** — *continued*
transverse (*see also* Myelitis) 323.82
vascular 336.1
**Myelophthisis** 284.2
**Myeloproliferative disease** (M9960/1) 238.79
**Myeloradiculitis** — *see also* Polyneuropathy 357.0
**Myeloradiculodysplasia** (spinal) 742.59
**Myelosarcoma** (M9930/3) 205.3 ☑
**Myelosclerosis** 289.89
with myeloid metaplasia (M9961/1) 238.76
disseminated, of nervous system 340
megakaryocytic (M9961/1) 238.79
**Myelosis** (M9860/3) — *see also* Leukemia, myeloid 205.9 ☑
acute (M9861/3) 205.0 ☑
aleukemic (M9864/3) 205.8 ☑
chronic (M9863/3) 205.1 ☑
erythremic (M9840/3) 207.0 ☑
acute (M9841/3) 207.0 ☑
megakaryocytic (M9920/3) 207.2 ☑
nonleukemic (chronic) 288.8
subacute (M9862/3) 205.2 ☑
**Myesthenia** — *see* Myasthenia
**Myiasis** (cavernous) 134.0
orbit 134.0 *[376.13]*
**Myoadenoma, prostate** 600.20
with
other lower urinary tract symptoms (LUTS) 600.21
urinary
obstruction 600.21
retention 600.21
**Myoblastoma**
granular cell (M9580/0) (*see also* Neoplasm, connective tissue, benign)
malignant (M9580/3) — *see* Neoplasm, connective tissue, malignant
tongue (M9580/0) 210.1
**Myocardial** — *see* condition
**Myocardiopathy** (congestive) (constrictive) (familial) (hypertrophic nonobstructive) (idiopathic) (infiltrative) (obstructive) (primary) (restrictive) (sporadic) 425.4
alcoholic 425.5
amyloid 277.39 *[425.7]*
beriberi 265.0 *[425.7]*
cobalt-beer 425.5
due to
amyloidosis 277.39 *[425.7]*
beriberi 265.0 *[425.7]*
cardiac glycogenosis 271.0 *[425.7]*
Chagas' disease 086.0
Friedreich's ataxia 334.0 *[425.8]*
influenza 487.8 *[425.8]*
mucopolysaccharidosis 277.5 *[425.7]*
myotonia atrophica 359.21 *[425.8]* ▲
progressive muscular dystrophy 359.1 *[425.8]*
sarcoidosis 135 *[425.8]*
glycogen storage 271.0 *[425.7]*
hypertrophic obstructive 425.1
metabolic NEC 277.9 *[425.7]*
nutritional 269.9 *[425.7]*
obscure (African) 425.2
peripartum 674.5 ☑
postpartum 674.5 ☑
secondary 425.9
thyrotoxic (*see also* Thyrotoxicosis) 242.9 ☑ *[425.7]*
toxic NEC 425.9
**Myocarditis** (fibroid) (interstitial) (old) (progressive) (senile) (with arteriosclerosis) 429.0
with
rheumatic fever (conditions classifiable to 390) 398.0
active (*see also* Myocarditis, acute, rheumatic) 391.2

☑ Additional Digit Required — Refer to the Tabular List for Digit Selection
▽ Subterms under main terms may continue to next column or page
**2008 ICD-9-CM**
▶◀ Revised Text ● New Line ▲ Revised Code
**October 2007 · Volume 2 — 193**

**Myocarditis** — *continued*
  with — *continued*
    rheumatic fever — *continued*
      inactive or quiescent (with chorea) 398.0
  active (nonrheumatic) 422.90
    rheumatic 391.2
      with chorea (acute) (rheumatic) (Sydenham's) 392.0
  acute or subacute (interstitial) 422.90
    due to Streptococcus (beta-hemolytic) 391.2
    idiopathic 422.91
    rheumatic 391.2
      with chorea (acute) (rheumatic) (Sydenham's) 392.0
    specified type NEC 422.99
  aseptic of newborn 074.23
  bacterial (acute) 422.92
  chagasic 086.0
  chronic (interstitial) 429.0
  congenital 746.89
  constrictive 425.4
  Coxsackie (virus) 074.23
  diphtheritic 032.82
  due to or in
    Coxsackie (virus) 074.23
    diphtheria 032.82
    epidemic louse-borne typhus 080 [422.0]
    influenza 487.8 [422.0]
    Lyme disease 088.81 [422.0]
    scarlet fever 034.1 [422.0]
    toxoplasmosis (acquired) 130.3
    tuberculosis (*see also* Tuberculosis) 017.9 ☑ [422.0]
    typhoid 002.0 [422.0]
    typhus NEC 081.9 [422.0]
  eosinophilic 422.91
  epidemic of newborn 074.23
  Fiedler's (acute) (isolated) (subacute) 422.91
  giant cell (acute) (subacute) 422.91
  gonococcal 098.85
  granulomatous (idiopathic) (isolated) (nonspecific) 422.91
  hypertensive (*see also* Hypertension, heart) 402.90
  idiopathic 422.91
    granulomatous 422.91
  infective 422.92
  influenzal 487.8 [422.0]
  isolated (diffuse) (granulomatous) 422.91
  malignant 422.99
  meningococcal 036.43
  nonrheumatic, active 422.90
  parenchymatous 422.90
  pneumococcal (acute) (subacute) 422.92
  rheumatic (chronic) (inactive) (with chorea) 398.0
    active or acute 391.2
      with chorea (acute) (rheumatic) (Sydenham's) 392.0
  septic 422.92
  specific (giant cell) (productive) 422.91
  staphylococcal (acute) (subacute) 422.92
  suppurative 422.92
  syphilitic (chronic) 093.82
  toxic 422.93
    rheumatic (*see also* Myocarditis, acute rheumatic) 391.2
  tuberculous (*see also* Tuberculosis) 017.9 ☑ [422.0]
  typhoid 002.0 [422.0]
  valvular — *see* Endocarditis
  viral, except Coxsackie 422.91
    Coxsackie 074.23
    of newborn (Coxsackie) 074.23
**Myocardium, myocardial** — *see* condition
**Myocardosis** — *see also* Cardiomyopathy 425.4
**Myoclonia** (essential) 333.2

**Myoclonia** — *continued*
  epileptica 333.2
  Friedrich's 333.2
  massive 333.2
**Myoclonic**
  epilepsy, familial (progressive) 333.2
  jerks 333.2
**Myoclonus** (familial essential) (multifocal) (simplex) 333.2
  with epilepsy and with ragged red fibers (MERRF syndrome) 277.87
  facial 351.8
  massive (infantile) 333.2
  pharyngeal 478.29
**Myodiastasis** 728.84
**Myoendocarditis** — *see also* Endocarditis
  acute or subacute 421.9
**Myoepithelioma** (M8982/0) — *see* Neoplasm, by site, benign
**Myofascitis** (acute) 729.1
  low back 724.2
**Myofibroma** (M8890/0) — *see also* Neoplasm, connective tissue, benign
  uterus (cervix) (corpus) (*see also* Leiomyoma) 218.9
**Myofibromatosis**
  infantile 759.89
**Myofibrosis** 728.2
  heart (*see also* Myocarditis) 429.0
  humeroscapular region 726.2
  scapulohumeral 726.2
**Myofibrositis** — *see also* Myositis 729.1
  scapulohumeral 726.2
**Myogelosis** (occupational) 728.89
**Myoglobinuria** 791.3
**Myoglobulinuria, primary** 791.3
**Myokymia** — *see also* Myoclonus
  facial 351.8
**Myolipoma** (M8860/0)
  specified site — *see* Neoplasm, connective tissue, benign
  unspecified site 223.0
**Myoma** (M8895/0) — *see also* Neoplasm, connective tissue, benign
  cervix (stump) (uterus) (*see also* Leiomyoma) 218.9
  malignant (M8895/3) — *see* Neoplasm, connective tissue, malignant
  prostate 600.20
    with
      other lower urinary tract symptoms (LUTS) 600.21
      urinary
        obstruction 600.21
        retention 600.21
  uterus (cervix) (corpus) (*see also* Leiomyoma) 218.9
    in pregnancy or childbirth 654.1 ☑
      affecting fetus or newborn 763.89
      causing obstructed labor 660.2 ☑
        affecting fetus or newborn 763.1
**Myomalacia** 728.9
  cordis, heart (*see also* Degeneration, myocardial) 429.1
**Myometritis** — *see also* Endometritis 615.9
**Myometrium** — *see* condition
**Myonecrosis, clostridial** 040.0
**Myopathy** 359.9
  alcoholic 359.4
  amyloid 277.39 [359.6]
  benign, congenital 359.0
  central core 359.0
  centronuclear 359.0
  congenital (benign) 359.0
  critical illness 359.81
  distal 359.1
  due to drugs 359.4
  endocrine 259.9 [359.5]
    specified type NEC 259.8 [359.5]

**Myopathy** — *continued*
  extraocular muscles 376.82
  facioscapulohumeral 359.1
  in
    Addison's disease 255.41 [359.5] ▲
    amyloidosis 277.39 [359.6]
    cretinism 243 [359.5]
    Cushing's syndrome 255.0 [359.5]
    disseminated lupus erythematosus 710.0 [359.6]
    giant cell arteritis 446.5 [359.6]
    hyperadrenocorticism NEC 255.3 [359.5]
    hyperparathyroidism 252.01 [359.5]
    hypopituitarism 253.2 [359.5]
    hypothyroidism (*see also* Hypothyroidism) 244.9 [359.5]
    malignant neoplasm NEC (M8000/3) 199.1 [359.6]
    myxedema (*see also* Myxedema) 244.9 [359.5]
    polyarteritis nodosa 446.0 [359.6]
    rheumatoid arthritis 714.0 [359.6]
    sarcoidosis 135 [359.6]
    scleroderma 710.1 [359.6]
    Sjögren's disease 710.2 [359.6]
    thyrotoxicosis (*see also* Thyrotoxicosis) 242.9 ☑ [359.5]
  inflammatory 359.89
  intensive care (ICU) 359.81
  limb-girdle 359.1
  myotubular 359.0
  necrotizing, acute 359.81
  nemaline 359.0
  ocular 359.1
  oculopharyngeal 359.1
  of critical illness 359.81
  primary 359.89
  progressive NEC 359.89
  proximal myotonic (PROMM) 359.21 ●
  quadriplegic, acute 359.81
  rod body 359.0
  scapulohumeral 359.1
  specified type NEC 359.89
  toxic 359.4
**Myopericarditis** — *see also* Pericarditis 423.9
**Myopia** (axial) (congenital) (increased curvature or refraction, nucleus of lens) 367.1
  degenerative, malignant 360.21
  malignant 360.21
  progressive high (degenerative) 360.21
**Myosarcoma** (M8895/3) — *see* Neoplasm, connective tissue, malignant
**Myosis** (persistent) 379.42
  stromal (endolymphatic) (M8931/1) 236.0
**Myositis** 729.1
  clostridial 040.0
  due to posture 729.1
  epidemic 074.1
  fibrosa or fibrous (chronic) 728.2
    Volkmann's (complicating trauma) 958.6
  infective 728.0
  interstitial 728.81
  multiple — *see* Polymyositis
  occupational 729.1
  orbital, chronic 376.12
  ossificans 728.12
    circumscribed 728.12
    progressive 728.11
    traumatic 728.12
  progressive fibrosing 728.11
  purulent 728.0
  rheumatic 729.1
  rheumatoid 729.1
  suppurative 728.0
  syphilitic 095.6
  traumatic (old) 729.1
**Myospasia impulsiva** 307.23

**Myotonia** (acquisita) (intermittens) 728.85
  atrophica 359.21 ▲
  congenita 359.22 ▲
    acetazolamide responsive 359.22 ●
    dominant form 359.22 ●
    recessive form 359.22 ●
  drug-induced 359.24 ●
  dystrophica 359.21 ▲
  fluctuans 359.29 ●
  levior 359.29 ●
  permanens 359.29 ●
**Myotonic pupil** 379.46
**Myriapodiasis** 134.1
**Myringitis**
  with otitis media — *see* Otitis media
  acute 384.00
    specified type NEC 384.09
  bullosa hemorrhagica 384.01
  bullous 384.01
  chronic 384.1
**Mysophobia** 300.29
**Mytilotoxism** 988.0
**Myxadenitis labialis** 528.5
**Myxedema** (adult) (idiocy) (infantile) (juvenile) (thyroid gland) — *see also* Hypothyroidism 244.9
  circumscribed 242.9 ☑
  congenital 243
  cutis 701.8
  localized (pretibial) 242.9 ☑
  madness (acute) 293.0
    subacute 293.1
  papular 701.8
  pituitary 244.9
  postpartum 674.8 ☑
  pretibial 242.9 ☑
  primary 244.9
**Myxochondrosarcoma** (M9220/3) — *see* Neoplasm, cartilage, malignant
**Myxofibroma** (M8811/0) — *see also* Neoplasm, connective tissue, benign
  odontogenic (M9320/0) 213.1
  upper jaw (bone) 213.0
**Myxofibrosarcoma** (M8811/3) — *see* Neoplasm, connective tissue, malignant
**Myxolipoma** (M8852/0) — *see also* Lipoma, by site 214.9
**Myxoliposarcoma** (M8852/3) — *see* Neoplasm, connective tissue, malignant
**Myxoma** (M8840/0) — *see also* Neoplasm, connective tissue, benign
  odontogenic (M9320/0) 213.1
  upper jaw (bone) 213.0
**Myxosarcoma** (M8840/3) — *see* Neoplasm, connective tissue, malignant

## N

**Naegeli's**
  disease (hereditary hemorrhagic thrombasthenia) 287.1
  leukemia, monocytic (M9863/3) 205.1 ☑
  syndrome (incontinentia pigmenti) 757.33
**Naffziger's syndrome** 353.0
**Naga sore** — *see also* Ulcer, skin 707.9
**Nägele's pelvis** 738.6
  with disproportion (fetopelvic) 653.0 ☑
    affecting fetus or newborn 763.1
    causing obstructed labor 660.1 ☑
      affecting fetus or newborn 763.1
**Nager-de Reynier syndrome** (dysostosis mandibularis) 756.0
**Nail** — *see also* condition
  biting 307.9
  patella syndrome (hereditary osteoonychodysplasia) 756.89
**Nanism, nanosomia** — *see also* Dwarfism 259.4
  hypophyseal 253.3
  pituitary 253.3

☑ Additional Digit Required — Refer to the Tabular List for Digit Selection      ⤸ Subterms under main terms may continue to next column or page

194 — Volume 2 • October 2007      ►◄ Revised Text      ● New Line      ▲ Revised Code      *2008 ICD-9-CM*

**Nanism, nanosomia** — see also Dwarfism — continued
  renis, renalis 588.0
**Nanukayami** 100.89
**Napkin rash** 691.0
**Narcissism** 301.81
**Narcolepsy** 347.00
  with cataplexy 347.01
  in conditions classified elsewhere 347.10
    with cataplexy 347.11
**Narcosis**
  carbon dioxide (respiratory) 786.09
  due to drug
    correct substance properly administered 780.09
    overdose or wrong substance given or taken 977.9
    specified drug — see Table of Drugs and Chemicals
**Narcotism (chronic)** — see also Dependence 304.9 ☑
  acute
    correct substance properly administered 349.82
    overdose or wrong substance given or taken 967.8
    specified drug — see Table of Drugs and Chemicals
**NARP** (ataxia and retinitis pigmentosa) 277.87
**Narrow**
  anterior chamber angle 365.02
  pelvis (inlet) (outlet) — see Contraction, pelvis
**Narrowing**
  artery NEC 447.1
    auditory, internal 433.8 ☑
    basilar 433.0 ☑
      with other precerebral artery 433.3 ☑
      bilateral 433.3 ☑
    carotid 433.1 ☑
      with other precerebral artery 433.3 ☑
      bilateral 433.3 ☑
    cerebellar 433.8 ☑
    choroidal 433.8 ☑
    communicating posterior 433.8 ☑
    coronary (see also Arteriosclerosis, coronary)
      congenital 746.85
      due to syphilis 090.5
    hypophyseal 433.8 ☑
    pontine 433.8 ☑
    precerebral NEC 433.9 ☑
      multiple or bilateral 433.3 ☑
      specified NEC 433.8 ☑
    vertebral 433.2 ☑
      with other precerebral artery 433.3 ☑
      bilateral 433.3 ☑
  auditory canal (external) (see also Stricture, ear canal, acquired) 380.50
  cerebral arteries 437.0
  cicatricial — see Cicatrix
  congenital — see Anomaly, congenital
  coronary artery — see Narrowing, artery, coronary
  ear, middle 385.22
  Eustachian tube (see also Obstruction, Eustachian tube) 381.60
  eyelid 374.46
    congenital 743.62
  intervertebral disc or space NEC — see Degeneration, intervertebral disc
  joint space, hip 719.85
  larynx 478.74
  lids 374.46
    congenital 743.62
  mesenteric artery (with gangrene) 557.0
  palate 524.89
  palpebral fissure 374.46

**Narrowing** — continued
  retinal artery 362.13
  ureter 593.3
  urethra (see also Stricture, urethra) 598.9
**Narrowness, abnormal, eyelid** 743.62
**Nasal** — see condition
**Nasolacrimal** — see condition
**Nasopharyngeal** — see also condition
  bursa 478.29
  pituitary gland 759.2
  torticollis 723.5
**Nasopharyngitis** (acute) (infective) (subacute) 460
  chronic 472.2
    due to external agent — see Condition, respiratory, chronic, due to
  due to external agent — see Condition, respiratory, due to
  septic 034.0
  streptococcal 034.0
  suppurative (chronic) 472.2
  ulcerative (chronic) 472.2
**Nasopharynx, nasopharyngeal** — see condition
**Natal tooth, teeth** 520.6
**Nausea** — see also Vomiting 787.02
  with vomiting 787.01
  epidemic 078.82
  gravidarum — see Hyperemesis, gravidarum
  marina 994.6
**Navel** — see condition
**Neapolitan fever** — see also Brucellosis 023.9
**Nearsightedness** 367.1
**Near-syncope** 780.2
**Nebécourt's syndrome** 253.3
**Nebula, cornea** (eye) 371.01
  congenital 743.43
  interfering with vision 743.42
**Necator americanus infestation** 126.1
**Necatoriasis** 126.1
**Neck** — see condition
**Necrencephalus** — see also Softening, brain 437.8
**Necrobacillosis** 040.3
**Necrobiosis** 799.89
  brain or cerebral (see also Softening, brain) 437.8
  lipoidica 709.3
    diabeticorum 250.8 ☑ [709.3]
**Necrodermolysis** 695.1
**Necrolysis, toxic epidermal** 695.1
  due to drug
    correct substance properly administered 695.1
    overdose or wrong substance given or taken 977.9
    specified drug — see Table of Drugs and Chemicals
**Necrophilia** 302.89
**Necrosis, necrotic**
  adrenal (capsule) (gland) 255.8
  antrum, nasal sinus 478.19
  aorta (hyaline) (see also Aneurysm, aorta) 441.9
    cystic medial 441.00
      abdominal 441.02
      thoracic 441.01
      thoracoabdominal 441.03
    ruptured 441.5
  arteritis 446.0
  artery 447.5
  aseptic, bone 733.40
    femur (head) (neck) 733.42
      medial condyle 733.43
    humoral head 733.41
    jaw 733.45 ●
    medial femoral condyle 733.43
    specific site NEC 733.49
    talus 733.44
  avascular, bone NEC (see also Necrosis, aseptic, bone) 733.40
  bladder (aseptic) (sphincter) 596.8

**Necrosis, necrotic** — continued
  bone (see also Osteomyelitis) 730.1 ☑
    acute 730.0 ☑
    aseptic or avascular 733.40
      femur (head) (neck) 733.42
        medial condyle 733.43
      humoral head 733.41
      jaw 733.45 ●
      medial femoral condyle 733.43
      specified site NEC 733.49
      talus 733.44
    ethmoid 478.19
    ischemic 733.40
    jaw 526.4
      aseptic 733.45 ●
    marrow 289.89
    Paget's (osteitis deformans) 731.0
    tuberculous — see Tuberculosis, bone
  brain (softening) (see also Softening, brain) 437.8
  breast (aseptic) (fat) (segmental) 611.3
  bronchus, bronchi 519.19
  central nervous system NEC (see also Softening, brain) 437.8
  cerebellar (see also Softening, brain) 437.8
  cerebral (softening) (see also Softening, brain) 437.8
  cerebrospinal (softening) (see also Softening, brain) 437.8
  colon 557.0 ●
  cornea (see also Keratitis) 371.40
  cortical, kidney 583.6
  cystic medial (aorta) 441.00
    abdominal 441.02
    thoracic 441.01
    thoracoabdominal 441.03
  dental 521.09
    pulp 522.1
  due to swallowing corrosive substance — see Burn, by site
  ear (ossicle) 385.24
  esophagus 530.89
  ethmoid (bone) 478.19
  eyelid 374.50
  fat, fatty (generalized) (see also Degeneration, fatty) 272.8
    abdominal wall 567.82
    breast (aseptic) (segmental) 611.3
    intestine 569.89
    localized — see Degeneration, by site, fatty
    mesentery 567.82
    omentum 567.82
    pancreas 577.8
    peritoneum 567.82
    skin (subcutaneous) 709.3
      newborn 778.1
  femur (aseptic) (avascular) 733.42
    head 733.42
    medial condyle 733.43
    neck 733.42
  gallbladder (see also Cholecystitis, acute) 575.0
  gangrenous 785.4
  gastric 537.89
  glottis 478.79
  heart (myocardium) — see Infarct, myocardium
  hepatic (see also Necrosis, liver) 570
  hip (aseptic) (avascular) 733.42
  intestine (acute) (hemorrhagic) (massive) 557.0
  ischemic 785.4
  jaw 526.4
    aseptic 733.45 ●
  kidney (bilateral) 583.9
    acute 584.9
    cortical 583.6
      acute 584.6
        with
          abortion — see Abortion, by type, with renal failure

**Necrosis, necrotic** — continued
  kidney — continued
    cortical — continued
      acute — continued
        with — continued
          ectopic pregnancy (see also categories 633.0–633.9) 639.3
          molar pregnancy (see also categories 630–632) 639.3
        complicating pregnancy 646.2 ☑
          affecting fetus or newborn 760.1
        following labor and delivery 669.3 ☑
    medullary (papillary) (see also Pyelitis) 590.80
    in
      acute renal failure 584.7
      nephritis, nephropathy 583.7
    papillary (see also Pyelitis) 590.80
    in
      acute renal failure 584.7
      nephritis, nephropathy 583.7
    tubular 584.5
      with
        abortion — see Abortion, by type, with renal failure
        ectopic pregnancy (see also categories 633.0–633.9) 639.3
        molar pregnancy (see also categories 630–632) 639.3
      complicating
        abortion 639.3
        ectopic or molar pregnancy 639.3
        pregnancy 646.2 ☑
          affecting fetus or newborn 760.1
      following labor and delivery 669.3 ☑
      traumatic 958.5
  larynx 478.79
  liver (acute) (congenital) (diffuse) (massive) (subacute) 570
    with
      abortion — see Abortion, by type, with specified complication NEC
      ectopic pregnancy (see also categories 633.0–633.9) 639.8
      molar pregnancy (see also categories 630–632) 639.8
    complicating pregnancy 646.7 ☑
      affecting fetus or newborn 760.8
    following
      abortion 639.8
      ectopic or molar pregnancy 639.8
    obstetrical 646.7 ☑
    postabortal 639.8
    puerperal, postpartum 674.8 ☑
    toxic 573.3
  lung 513.0
  lymphatic gland 683
  mammary gland 611.3
  mastoid (chronic) 383.1
  mesentery 557.0
    fat 567.82
  mitral valve — see Insufficiency, mitral
  myocardium, myocardial — see Infarct, myocardium
  nose (septum) 478.19
  omentum 557.0
    with mesenteric infarction 557.0
    fat 567.82
  orbit, orbital 376.10
  ossicles, ear (aseptic) 385.24
  ovary (see also Salpingo-oophoritis) 614.2

---

☑ Additional Digit Required — Refer to the Tabular List for Digit Selection      ▽ Subterms under main terms may continue to next column or page

**2008 ICD-9-CM**    ▶◀ Revised Text    ● New Line    ▲ Revised Code    **October 2007 · Volume 2 — 195**

**Necrosis, necrotic** — *continued*
  pancreas (aseptic) (duct) (fat) 577.8
    acute 577.0
    infective 577.0
  papillary, kidney (*see also* Pyelitis) 590.80
  perineum 624.8
  peritoneum 557.0
    with mesenteric infarction 557.0
    fat 567.82
  pharynx 462
    in granulocytopenia 288.09
  phosphorus 983.9
  pituitary (gland) (postpartum) (Sheehan) 253.2
  placenta (*see also* Placenta, abnormal) 656.7 ☑
  pneumonia 513.0
  pulmonary 513.0
  pulp (dental) 522.1
  pylorus 537.89
  radiation — *see* Necrosis, by site
  radium — *see* Necrosis, by site
  renal — *see* Necrosis, kidney
  sclera 379.19
  scrotum 608.89
  skin or subcutaneous tissue 709.8

**Necrosis, necrotic** — *continued*
  skin or subcutaneous tissue — *continued*
    due to burn — *see* Burn, by site
    gangrenous 785.4
  spine, spinal (column) 730.18
    acute 730.18
    cord 336.1
  spleen 289.59
  stomach 537.89
  stomatitis 528.1
  subcutaneous fat 709.3
    fetus or newborn 778.1
  subendocardial — *see* Infarct, myocardium
  suprarenal (capsule) (gland) 255.8
  teeth, tooth 521.09
  testis 608.89
  thymus (gland) 254.8
  tonsil 474.8
  trachea 519.19
  tuberculous NEC — *see* Tuberculosis
  tubular (acute) (anoxic) (toxic) 584.5
    due to a procedure 997.5
  umbilical cord, affecting fetus or newborn 762.6
  vagina 623.8

**Necrosis, necrotic** — *continued*
  vertebra (lumbar) 730.18
    acute 730.18
    tuberculous (*see also* Tuberculosis) 015.0 ☑ [730.8] ☑
  vesical (aseptic) (bladder) 596.8
  vulva 624.8
  x-ray — *see* Necrosis, by site
**Necrospermia** 606.0
**Necrotizing angiitis** 446.0
**Negativism** 301.7
**Neglect** (child) (newborn) NEC 995.52
  adult 995.84
  after or at birth 995.52
  hemispatial 781.8
  left-sided 781.8
  sensory 781.8
  visuospatial 781.8
**Negri bodies** 071
**Neill-Dingwall syndrome** (microcephaly and dwarfism) 759.89
**Neisserian infection** NEC — *see* Gonococcus
**Nematodiasis** NEC — *see also* Infestation, Nematode 127.9
  ancylostoma (*see also* Ancylostomiasis) 126.9

**Neoformans cryptococcus infection** 117.5
**Neonatal** — *see also* condition
  adrenoleukodystrophy 277.86
  teeth, tooth 520.6
**Neonatorum** — *see* condition
**Neoplasia** ●
  multiple endocrine [MEN] ●
    type I 258.01 ●
    type IIA 258.02 ●
    type IIB 258.03 ●
  vaginal intraepithelial I [VAIN I] 623.0 ●
  vaginal intraepithelial II [VAIN II] 623.0 ●
  vaginal intraepithelial III [VAIN III] 233.31 ●
  vulvular intraepithelial I [VIN I] 624.01 ●
  vulvular intraepithelial II [VIN II] 624.02 ●
  vulvular intraepithelial III [VIN III] 233.32 ●

☑ Additional Digit Required — Refer to the Tabular List for Digit Selection      Subterms under main terms may continue to next column or page

196 — Volume 2 • October 2007      ►◄ Revised Text     ● New Line     ▲ Revised Code      *2008 ICD-9-CM*

| | Malignant | | | | | |
|---|---|---|---|---|---|---|
| | Primary | Secondary | Ca in situ | Benign | Uncertain Behavior | Unspecified |
| Neoplasm, neoplastic ........ | 199.1 | 199.1 | 234.9 | 229.9 | 238.9 | 239.9 |

Notes — 1. The list below gives the code numbers for neoplasms by anatomical site. For each site there are six possible code numbers according to whether the neoplasm in question is malignant, benign, in situ, of uncertain behavior, or of unspecified nature. The description of the neoplasm will often indicate which of the six columns is appropriate; e.g., malignant melanoma of skin, benign fibroadenoma of breast, carcinoma in situ of cervix uteri.

Where such descriptors are not present, the remainder of the Index should be consulted where guidance is given to the appropriate column for each morphological (histological) variety listed; e.g., Mesonephroma — see Neoplasm, malignant; Embryoma — see also Neoplasm, uncertain behavior; Disease, Bowen's — see Neoplasm, skin, in situ. However, the guidance in the Index can be overridden if one of the descriptors mentioned above is present; e.g., malignant adenoma of colon is coded to 153.9 and not to 211.3 as the adjective "malignant" overrides the Index entry "Adenoma — see also Neoplasm, benign."

2. Sites marked with the sign * (e.g., face NEC*) should be classified to malignant neoplasm of skin of these sites if the variety of neoplasm is a squamous cell carcinoma or an epidermoid carcinoma, and to benign neoplasm of skin of these sites if the variety of neoplasm is a papilloma (any type).

| | Primary | Secondary | Ca in situ | Benign | Uncertain Behavior | Unspecified |
|---|---|---|---|---|---|---|
| abdomen, abdominal ........ | 195.2 | 198.89 | 234.8 | 229.8 | 238.8 | 239.8 |
| cavity .............................. | 195.2 | 198.89 | 234.8 | 229.8 | 238.8 | 239.8 |
| organ ............................. | 195.2 | 198.89 | 234.8 | 229.8 | 238.8 | 239.8 |
| viscera ........................... | 195.2 | 198.89 | 234.8 | 229.8 | 238.8 | 239.8 |
| wall ............................... | 173.5 | 198.2 | 232.5 | 216.5 | 238.2 | 239.2 |
| connective tissue ...... | 171.5 | 198.89 | — | 215.5 | 238.1 | 239.2 |
| abdominopelvic ............... | 195.8 | 198.89 | 234.8 | 229.8 | 238.8 | 239.8 |
| accessory sinus — see Neoplasm, sinus | | | | | | |
| acoustic nerve ................ | 192.0 | 198.4 | — | 225.1 | 237.9 | 239.7 |
| acromion (process) ........... | 170.4 | 198.5 | — | 213.4 | 238.0 | 239.2 |
| adenoid (pharynx) (tissue) ........................ | 147.1 | 198.89 | 230.0 | 210.7 | 235.1 | 239.0 |
| adipose tissue (see also Neoplasm, connective tissue) ............................ | 171.9 | 198.89 | — | 215.9 | 238.1 | 239.2 |
| adnexa (uterine) ............. | 183.9 | 198.82 | 233.39 ▲ | 221.8 | 236.3 | 239.5 |
| adrenal (cortex) (gland) (medulla) .................. | 194.0 | 198.7 | 234.8 | 227.0 | 237.2 | 239.7 |
| ala nasi (external) ......... | 173.3 | 198.2 | 232.3 | 216.3 | 238.2 | 239.2 |
| alimentary canal or tract NEC ............................. | 159.9 | 197.8 | 230.9 | 211.9 | 235.5 | 239.0 |
| alveolar ......................... | 143.9 | 198.89 | 230.0 | 210.4 | 235.1 | 239.0 |
| mucosa ......................... | 143.9 | 198.89 | 230.0 | 210.4 | 235.1 | 239.0 |
| lower ......................... | 143.1 | 198.89 | 230.0 | 210.4 | 235.1 | 239.0 |
| upper ......................... | 143.0 | 198.89 | 230.0 | 210.4 | 235.1 | 239.0 |
| ridge or process ........... | 170.1 | 198.5 | — | 213.1 | 238.0 | 239.2 |
| carcinoma ................... | 143.9 | — | — | — | — | — |
| lower ...................... | 143.1 | — | — | — | — | — |
| upper ...................... | 143.0 | — | — | — | — | — |
| lower ......................... | 170.1 | 198.5 | — | 213.1 | 238.0 | 239.2 |
| mucosa .................... | 143.9 | 198.89 | 230.0 | 210.4 | 235.1 | 239.0 |
| lower ...................... | 143.1 | 198.89 | 230.0 | 210.4 | 235.1 | 239.0 |
| upper ...................... | 143.0 | 198.89 | 230.0 | 210.4 | 235.1 | 239.0 |
| upper ......................... | 170.0 | 198.5 | — | 213.0 | 238.0 | 239.2 |
| sulcus ........................... | 145.1 | 198.89 | 230.0 | 210.4 | 235.1 | 239.0 |
| alveolus ......................... | 143.9 | 198.89 | 230.0 | 210.4 | 235.1 | 239.0 |
| lower ............................. | 143.1 | 198.89 | 230.0 | 210.4 | 235.1 | 239.0 |
| upper ............................. | 143.0 | 198.89 | 230.0 | 210.4 | 235.1 | 239.0 |
| ampulla of Vater ............. | 156.2 | 197.8 | 230.8 | 211.5 | 235.3 | 239.0 |
| ankle NEC* ..................... | 195.5 | 198.89 | 232.7 | 229.8 | 238.8 | 239.8 |
| anorectum, anorectal (junction) ..................... | 154.8 | 197.5 | 230.7 | 211.4 | 235.2 | 239.0 |
| antecubital fossa or space* ......................... | 195.4 | 198.89 | 232.6 | 229.8 | 238.8 | 239.8 |
| antrum (Highmore) (maxillary) .................. | 160.2 | 197.3 | 231.8 | 212.0 | 235.9 | 239.1 |
| pyloric ........................... | 151.2 | 197.8 | 230.2 | 211.1 | 235.2 | 239.0 |
| tympanicum .................. | 160.1 | 197.3 | 231.8 | 212.0 | 235.9 | 239.1 |
| anus, anal ...................... | 154.3 | 197.5 | 230.6 | 211.4 | 235.5 | 239.0 |
| canal ............................. | 154.2 | 197.5 | 230.5 | 211.4 | 235.5 | 239.0 |
| contiguous sites with rectosigmoid junction or rectum ................. | 154.8 | — | — | — | — | — |
| margin .......................... | 173.5 | 198.2 | 232.5 | 216.5 | 238.2 | 239.2 |
| skin ............................... | 173.5 | 198.2 | 232.5 | 216.5 | 238.2 | 239.2 |
| sphincter ....................... | 154.2 | 197.5 | 230.5 | 211.4 | 235.5 | 239.0 |
| aorta (thoracic) .............. | 171.4 | 198.89 | — | 215.4 | 238.1 | 239.2 |

| | Primary | Secondary | Ca in situ | Benign | Uncertain Behavior | Unspecified |
|---|---|---|---|---|---|---|
| **Neoplasm, neoplastic —** *continued* | | | | | | |
| aorta — *continued* | | | | | | |
| abdominal ..................... | 171.5 | 198.89 | — | 215.5 | 238.1 | 239.2 |
| aortic body ..................... | 194.6 | 198.89 | — | 227.6 | 237.3 | 239.7 |
| aponeurosis ................... | 171.9 | 198.89 | — | 215.9 | 238.1 | 239.2 |
| palmar .......................... | 171.2 | 198.89 | — | 215.2 | 238.1 | 239.2 |
| plantar .......................... | 171.3 | 198.89 | — | 215.3 | 238.1 | 239.2 |
| appendix ........................ | 153.5 | 197.5 | 230.3 | 211.3 | 235.2 | 239.0 |
| arachnoid (cerebral) ......... | 192.1 | 198.4 | — | 225.2 | 237.6 | 239.7 |
| spinal ........................... | 192.3 | 198.4 | — | 225.4 | 237.6 | 239.7 |
| areola (female) ............... | 174.0 | 198.81 | 233.0 | 217 | 238.3 | 239.3 |
| male ............................. | 175.0 | 198.81 | 233.0 | 217 | 238.3 | 239.3 |
| arm NEC* ...................... | 195.4 | 198.89 | 232.6 | 229.8 | 238.8 | 239.8 |
| artery — *see* Neoplasm, connective tissue | | | | | | |
| aryepiglottic fold ............. | 148.2 | 198.89 | 230.0 | 210.8 | 235.1 | 239.0 |
| hypopharyngeal aspect ........................ | 148.2 | 198.89 | 230.0 | 210.8 | 235.1 | 239.0 |
| laryngeal aspect ........... | 161.1 | 197.3 | 231.0 | 212.1 | 235.6 | 239.1 |
| marginal zone ............... | 148.2 | 198.89 | 230.0 | 210.8 | 235.1 | 239.0 |
| arytenoid (cartilage) ........ | 161.3 | 197.3 | 231.0 | 212.1 | 235.6 | 239.1 |
| fold — *see* Neoplasm, aryepiglottic | | | | | | |
| atlas ............................... | 170.2 | 198.5 | — | 213.2 | 238.0 | 239.2 |
| atrium, cardiac ................ | 164.1 | 198.89 | — | 212.7 | 238.8 | 239.8 |
| auditory | | | | | | |
| canal (external) (skin) ........................ | 173.2 | 198.2 | 232.2 | 216.2 | 238.2 | 239.2 |
| internal ..................... | 160.1 | 197.3 | 231.8 | 212.0 | 235.9 | 239.1 |
| nerve ........................... | 192.0 | 198.4 | — | 225.1 | 237.9 | 239.7 |
| tube ............................. | 160.1 | 197.3 | 231.8 | 212.0 | 235.9 | 239.1 |
| Eustachian ............... | 160.1 | 197.3 | 231.8 | 212.0 | 235.9 | 239.1 |
| opening .................. | 147.2 | 198.89 | 230.0 | 210.7 | 235.1 | 239.0 |
| auricle, ear ..................... | 173.2 | 198.2 | 232.2 | 216.2 | 238.2 | 239.2 |
| cartilage ........................ | 171.0 | 198.89 | — | 215.0 | 238.1 | 239.2 |
| auricular canal (external) ..................... | 173.2 | 198.2 | 232.2 | 216.2 | 238.2 | 239.2 |
| internal ......................... | 160.1 | 197.3 | 231.8 | 212.0 | 235.9 | 239.1 |
| autonomic nerve or nervous system NEC ................... | 171.9 | 198.89 | — | 215.9 | 238.1 | 239.2 |
| axilla, axillary ................. | 195.1 | 198.89 | 234.8 | 229.8 | 238.8 | 239.8 |
| fold .............................. | 173.5 | 198.2 | 232.5 | 216.5 | 238.2 | 239.2 |
| back NEC* ..................... | 195.8 | 198.89 | 232.5 | 229.8 | 238.8 | 239.8 |
| Bartholin's gland ............. | 184.1 | 198.82 | 233.32 ▲ | 221.2 | 236.3 | 239.5 |
| basal ganglia .................. | 191.0 | 198.3 | — | 225.0 | 237.5 | 239.6 |
| basis pedunculi ............... | 191.7 | 198.3 | — | 225.0 | 237.5 | 239.6 |
| bile or biliary (tract) ........ | 156.9 | 197.8 | 230.8 | 211.5 | 235.3 | 239.0 |
| canaliculi (biliferi) (intrahepatic) ........... | 155.1 | 197.8 | 230.8 | 211.5 | 235.3 | 239.0 |
| canals, interlobular ....... | 155.1 | 197.8 | 230.8 | 211.5 | 235.3 | 239.0 |
| contiguous sites ......... | 156.8 | — | | | | |
| duct or passage (common) (cystic) (extrahepatic) ........... | 156.1 | 197.8 | 230.8 | 211.5 | 235.3 | 239.0 |
| contiguous sites with gallbladder .......... | 156.8 | — | — | — | — | — |
| interlobular ............... | 155.1 | 197.8 | 230.8 | 211.5 | 235.3 | 239.0 |
| intrahepatic .............. | 155.1 | 197.8 | 230.8 | 211.5 | 235.3 | 239.0 |
| and extrahepatic ..... | 156.9 | 197.8 | 230.8 | 211.5 | 235.3 | 239.0 |
| bladder (urinary) ............. | 188.9 | 198.1 | 233.7 | 223.3 | 236.7 | 239.4 |
| contiguous sites ........... | 188.8 | — | — | — | — | — |
| dome ............................ | 188.1 | 198.1 | 233.7 | 223.3 | 236.7 | 239.4 |
| neck ............................. | 188.5 | 198.1 | 233.7 | 223.3 | 236.7 | 239.4 |
| orifice ........................... | 188.9 | 198.1 | 233.7 | 223.3 | 236.7 | 239.4 |
| ureteric ...................... | 188.6 | 198.1 | 233.7 | 223.3 | 236.7 | 239.4 |
| urethral ...................... | 188.5 | 198.1 | 233.7 | 223.3 | 236.7 | 239.4 |
| sphincter ....................... | 188.8 | 198.1 | 233.7 | 223.3 | 236.7 | 239.4 |
| trigone .......................... | 188.0 | 198.1 | 233.7 | 223.3 | 236.7 | 239.4 |
| urachus ........................ | 188.7 | — | 233.7 | 223.3 | 236.7 | 239.4 |
| wall .............................. | 188.9 | 198.1 | 233.7 | 223.3 | 236.7 | 239.4 |
| anterior ...................... | 188.3 | 198.1 | 233.7 | 223.3 | 236.7 | 239.4 |
| lateral ........................ | 188.2 | 198.1 | 233.7 | 223.3 | 236.7 | 239.4 |
| posterior .................... | 188.4 | 198.1 | 233.7 | 223.3 | 236.7 | 239.4 |
| blood vessel — *see* Neoplasm, connective tissue | | | | | | |

☑ Additional Digit Required — Refer to the Tabular List for Digit Selection    ▽ Subterms under main terms may continue to next column or page

*2008 ICD-9-CM*    ▶◀ Revised Text    ● New Line    ▲ Revised Code    **October 2007 · Volume 2 — 197**

Neoplasm, neoplastic — *continued*

| | Malignant | | | Benign | Uncertain Behavior | Unspecified |
|---|---|---|---|---|---|---|
| | Primary | Secondary | Ca in situ | | | |
| bone (periosteum) | 170.9 | 198.5 | — | 213.9 | 238.0 | 239.2 |

*Note* — Carcinomas and adenocarcinomas, of any type other than intraosseous or odontogenic, of the sites listed under "Neoplasm, bone" should be considered as constituting metastatic spread from an unspecified primary site and coded to 198.5 for morbidity coding and to 199.1 for underlying cause of death coding.

| | Primary | Secondary | Ca in situ | Benign | Uncertain Behavior | Unspecified |
|---|---|---|---|---|---|---|
| acetabulum | 170.6 | 198.5 | — | 213.6 | 238.0 | 239.2 |
| acromion (process) | 170.4 | 198.5 | — | 213.4 | 238.0 | 239.2 |
| ankle | 170.8 | 198.5 | — | 213.8 | 238.0 | 239.2 |
| arm NEC | 170.4 | 198.5 | — | 213.4 | 238.0 | 239.2 |
| astragalus | 170.8 | 198.5 | — | 213.8 | 238.0 | 239.2 |
| atlas | 170.2 | 198.5 | — | 213.2 | 238.0 | 239.2 |
| axis | 170.2 | 198.5 | — | 213.2 | 238.0 | 239.2 |
| back NEC | 170.2 | 198.5 | — | 213.2 | 238.0 | 239.2 |
| calcaneus | 170.8 | 198.5 | — | 213.8 | 238.0 | 239.2 |
| calvarium | 170.0 | 198.5 | — | 213.0 | 238.0 | 239.2 |
| carpus (any) | 170.5 | 198.5 | — | 213.5 | 238.0 | 239.2 |
| cartilage NEC | 170.9 | 198.5 | — | 213.9 | 238.0 | 239.2 |
| clavicle | 170.3 | 198.5 | — | 213.3 | 238.0 | 239.2 |
| clivus | 170.0 | 198.5 | — | 213.0 | 238.0 | 239.2 |
| coccygeal vertebra | 170.6 | 198.5 | — | 213.6 | 238.0 | 239.2 |
| coccyx | 170.6 | 198.5 | — | 213.6 | 238.0 | 239.2 |
| costal cartilage | 170.3 | 198.5 | — | 213.3 | 238.0 | 239.2 |
| costovertebral joint | 170.3 | 198.5 | — | 213.3 | 238.0 | 239.2 |
| cranial | 170.0 | 198.5 | — | 213.0 | 238.0 | 239.2 |
| cuboid | 170.8 | 198.5 | — | 213.8 | 238.0 | 239.2 |
| cuneiform | 170.9 | 198.5 | — | 213.9 | 238.0 | 239.2 |
| ankle | 170.8 | 198.5 | — | 213.8 | 238.0 | 239.2 |
| wrist | 170.5 | 198.5 | — | 213.5 | 238.0 | 239.2 |
| digital | 170.9 | 198.5 | — | 213.9 | 238.0 | 239.2 |
| finger | 170.5 | 198.5 | — | 213.5 | 238.0 | 239.2 |
| toe | 170.8 | 198.5 | — | 213.8 | 238.0 | 239.2 |
| elbow | 170.4 | 198.5 | — | 213.4 | 238.0 | 239.2 |
| ethmoid (labyrinth) | 170.0 | 198.5 | — | 213.0 | 238.0 | 239.2 |
| face | 170.0 | 198.5 | — | 213.0 | 238.0 | 239.2 |
| lower jaw | 170.1 | 198.5 | — | 213.1 | 238.0 | 239.2 |
| femur (any part) | 170.7 | 198.5 | — | 213.7 | 238.0 | 239.2 |
| fibula (any part) | 170.7 | 198.5 | — | 213.7 | 238.0 | 239.2 |
| finger (any) | 170.5 | 198.5 | — | 213.5 | 238.0 | 239.2 |
| foot | 170.8 | 198.5 | — | 213.8 | 238.0 | 239.2 |
| forearm | 170.4 | 198.5 | — | 213.4 | 238.0 | 239.2 |
| frontal | 170.0 | 198.5 | — | 213.0 | 238.0 | 239.2 |
| hand | 170.5 | 198.5 | — | 213.5 | 238.0 | 239.2 |
| heel | 170.8 | 198.5 | — | 213.8 | 238.0 | 239.2 |
| hip | 170.6 | 198.5 | — | 213.6 | 238.0 | 239.2 |
| humerus (any part) | 170.4 | 198.5 | — | 213.4 | 238.0 | 239.2 |
| hyoid | 170.0 | 198.5 | — | 213.0 | 238.0 | 239.2 |
| ilium | 170.6 | 198.5 | — | 213.6 | 238.0 | 239.2 |
| innominate | 170.6 | 198.5 | — | 213.6 | 238.0 | 239.2 |
| intervertebral cartilage or disc | 170.2 | 198.5 | — | 213.2 | 238.0 | 239.2 |
| ischium | 170.6 | 198.5 | — | 213.6 | 238.0 | 239.2 |
| jaw (lower) | 170.1 | 198.5 | — | 213.1 | 238.0 | 239.2 |
| upper | 170.0 | 198.5 | — | 213.0 | 238.0 | 239.2 |
| knee | 170.7 | 198.5 | — | 213.7 | 238.0 | 239.2 |
| leg NEC | 170.7 | 198.5 | — | 213.7 | 238.0 | 239.2 |
| limb NEC | 170.9 | 198.5 | — | 213.9 | 238.0 | 239.2 |
| lower (long bones) | 170.7 | 198.5 | — | 213.7 | 238.0 | 239.2 |
| short bones | 170.8 | 198.5 | — | 213.8 | 238.0 | 239.2 |
| upper (long bones) | 170.4 | 198.5 | — | 213.4 | 238.0 | 239.2 |
| short bones | 170.5 | 198.5 | — | 213.5 | 238.0 | 239.2 |
| long | 170.9 | 198.5 | — | 213.9 | 238.0 | 239.2 |
| lower limbs NEC | 170.7 | 198.5 | — | 213.7 | 238.0 | 239.2 |
| upper limbs NEC | 170.4 | 198.5 | — | 213.4 | 238.0 | 239.2 |
| malar | 170.0 | 198.5 | — | 213.0 | 238.0 | 239.2 |
| mandible | 170.1 | 198.5 | — | 213.1 | 238.0 | 239.2 |
| marrow NEC | 202.9 ☑ | 198.5 | — | — | — | 238.79 |
| mastoid | 170.0 | 198.5 | — | 213.0 | 238.0 | 239.2 |
| maxilla, maxillary (superior) | 170.0 | 198.5 | — | 213.0 | 238.0 | 239.2 |
| inferior | 170.1 | 198.5 | — | 213.1 | 238.0 | 239.2 |
| metacarpus (any) | 170.5 | 198.5 | — | 213.5 | 238.0 | 239.2 |
| metatarsus (any) | 170.8 | 198.5 | — | 213.8 | 238.0 | 239.2 |
| navicular (ankle) | 170.8 | 198.5 | — | 213.8 | 238.0 | 239.2 |
| hand | 170.5 | 198.5 | — | 213.5 | 238.0 | 239.2 |

Neoplasm, neoplastic — *continued*

bone — *continued*

| | Primary | Secondary | Ca in situ | Benign | Uncertain Behavior | Unspecified |
|---|---|---|---|---|---|---|
| nose, nasal | 170.0 | 198.5 | — | 213.0 | 238.0 | 239.2 |
| occipital | 170.0 | 198.5 | — | 213.0 | 238.0 | 239.2 |
| orbit | 170.0 | 198.5 | — | 213.0 | 238.0 | 239.2 |
| parietal | 170.0 | 198.5 | — | 213.0 | 238.0 | 239.2 |
| patella | 170.8 | 198.5 | — | 213.8 | 238.0 | 239.2 |
| pelvic | 170.6 | 198.5 | — | 213.6 | 238.0 | 239.2 |
| phalanges | 170.9 | 198.5 | — | 213.9 | 238.0 | 239.2 |
| foot | 170.8 | 198.5 | — | 213.8 | 238.0 | 239.2 |
| hand | 170.5 | 198.5 | — | 213.5 | 238.0 | 239.2 |
| pubic | 170.6 | 198.5 | — | 213.6 | 238.0 | 239.2 |
| radius (any part) | 170.4 | 198.5 | — | 213.4 | 238.0 | 239.2 |
| rib | 170.3 | 198.5 | — | 213.3 | 238.0 | 239.2 |
| sacral vertebra | 170.6 | 198.5 | — | 213.6 | 238.0 | 239.2 |
| sacrum | 170.6 | 198.5 | — | 213.6 | 238.0 | 239.2 |
| scaphoid (of hand) | 170.5 | 198.5 | — | 213.5 | 238.0 | 239.2 |
| of ankle | 170.8 | 198.5 | — | 213.8 | 238.0 | 239.2 |
| scapula (any part) | 170.4 | 198.5 | — | 213.4 | 238.0 | 239.2 |
| sella turcica | 170.0 | 198.5 | — | 213.0 | 238.0 | 239.2 |
| short | 170.9 | 198.5 | — | 213.9 | 238.0 | 239.2 |
| lower limb | 170.8 | 198.5 | — | 213.8 | 238.0 | 239.2 |
| upper limb | 170.5 | 198.5 | — | 213.5 | 238.0 | 239.2 |
| shoulder | 170.4 | 198.5 | — | 213.4 | 238.0 | 239.2 |
| skeleton, skeletal NEC | 170.9 | 198.5 | — | 213.9 | 238.0 | 239.2 |
| skull | 170.0 | 198.5 | — | 213.0 | 238.0 | 239.2 |
| sphenoid | 170.0 | 198.5 | — | 213.0 | 238.0 | 239.2 |
| spine, spinal (column) | 170.2 | 198.5 | — | 213.2 | 238.0 | 239.2 |
| coccyx | 170.6 | 198.5 | — | 213.6 | 238.0 | 239.2 |
| sacrum | 170.6 | 198.5 | — | 213.6 | 238.0 | 239.2 |
| sternum | 170.3 | 198.5 | — | 213.3 | 238.0 | 239.2 |
| tarsus (any) | 170.8 | 198.5 | — | 213.8 | 238.0 | 239.2 |
| temporal | 170.0 | 198.5 | — | 213.0 | 238.0 | 239.2 |
| thumb | 170.5 | 198.5 | — | 213.5 | 238.0 | 239.2 |
| tibia (any part) | 170.7 | 198.5 | — | 213.7 | 238.0 | 239.2 |
| toe (any) | 170.8 | 198.5 | — | 213.8 | 238.0 | 239.2 |
| trapezium | 170.5 | 198.5 | — | 213.5 | 238.0 | 239.2 |
| trapezoid | 170.5 | 198.5 | — | 213.5 | 238.0 | 239.2 |
| turbinate | 170.0 | 198.5 | — | 213.0 | 238.0 | 239.2 |
| ulna (any part) | 170.4 | 198.5 | — | 213.4 | 238.0 | 239.2 |
| unciform | 170.5 | 198.5 | — | 213.5 | 238.0 | 239.2 |
| vertebra (column) | 170.2 | 198.5 | — | 213.2 | 238.0 | 239.2 |
| coccyx | 170.6 | 198.5 | — | 213.6 | 238.0 | 239.2 |
| sacrum | 170.6 | 198.5 | — | 213.6 | 238.0 | 239.2 |
| vomer | 170.0 | 198.5 | — | 213.0 | 238.0 | 239.2 |
| wrist | 170.5 | 198.5 | — | 213.5 | 238.0 | 239.2 |
| xiphoid process | 170.3 | 198.5 | — | 213.3 | 238.0 | 239.2 |
| zygomatic | 170.0 | 198.5 | — | 213.0 | 238.0 | 239.2 |
| book-leaf (mouth) | 145.8 | 198.89 | 230.0 | 210.4 | 235.1 | 239.0 |
| bowel — *see* Neoplasm, intestine | | | | | | |
| brachial plexus | 171.2 | 198.89 | — | 215.2 | 238.1 | 239.2 |
| brain NEC | 191.9 | 198.3 | — | 225.0 | 237.5 | 239.6 |
| basal ganglia | 191.0 | 198.3 | — | 225.0 | 237.5 | 239.6 |
| cerebellopontine angle | 191.6 | 198.3 | — | 225.0 | 237.5 | 239.6 |
| cerebellum NOS | 191.6 | 198.3 | — | 225.0 | 237.5 | 239.6 |
| cerebrum | 191.0 | 198.3 | — | 225.0 | 237.5 | 239.6 |
| choroid plexus | 191.5 | 198.3 | — | 225.0 | 237.5 | 239.6 |
| contiguous sites | 191.8 | — | — | — | — | — |
| corpus callosum | 191.8 | 198.3 | — | 225.0 | 237.5 | 239.6 |
| corpus striatum | 191.0 | 198.3 | — | 225.0 | 237.5 | 239.6 |
| cortex (cerebral) | 191.0 | 198.3 | — | 225.0 | 237.5 | 239.6 |
| frontal lobe | 191.1 | 198.3 | — | 225.0 | 237.5 | 239.6 |
| globus pallidus | 191.0 | 198.3 | — | 225.0 | 237.5 | 239.6 |
| hippocampus | 191.2 | 198.3 | — | 225.0 | 237.5 | 239.6 |
| hypothalamus | 191.0 | 198.3 | — | 225.0 | 237.5 | 239.6 |
| internal capsule | 191.0 | 198.3 | — | 225.0 | 237.5 | 239.6 |
| medulla oblongata | 191.7 | 198.3 | — | 225.0 | 237.5 | 239.6 |
| meninges | 192.1 | 198.4 | — | 225.2 | 237.6 | 239.7 |
| midbrain | 191.7 | 198.3 | — | 225.0 | 237.5 | 239.6 |
| occipital lobe | 191.4 | 198.3 | — | 225.0 | 237.5 | 239.6 |
| parietal lobe | 191.3 | 198.3 | — | 225.0 | 237.5 | 239.6 |
| peduncle | 191.7 | 198.3 | — | 225.0 | 237.5 | 239.6 |
| pons | 191.7 | 198.3 | — | 225.0 | 237.5 | 239.6 |
| stem | 191.7 | 198.3 | — | 225.0 | 237.5 | 239.6 |

☑ Additional Digit Required — Refer to the Tabular List for Digit Selection  ▽ Subterms under main terms may continue to next column or page

**198 — Volume 2**  ▶◀ Revised Text  ● New Line  ▲ Revised Code  *2008 ICD-9-CM*

Left margin: Index • Neoplasm, bone — Neoplasm, brain

| | Malignant | | | | | |
| --- | --- | --- | --- | --- | --- | --- |
| | Primary | Secondary | Ca in situ | Benign | Uncertain Behavior | Unspecified |
| **Neoplasm, neoplastic —** *continued* | | | | | | |
| brain — *continued* | | | | | | |
| tapetum | 191.8 | 198.3 | — | 225.0 | 237.5 | 239.6 |
| temporal lobe | 191.2 | 198.3 | — | 225.0 | 237.5 | 239.6 |
| thalamus | 191.0 | 198.3 | — | 225.0 | 237.5 | 239.6 |
| uncus | 191.2 | 198.3 | — | 225.0 | 237.5 | 239.6 |
| ventricle (floor) | 191.5 | 198.3 | — | 225.0 | 237.5 | 239.6 |
| branchial (cleft) (vestiges) | 146.8 | 198.89 | 230.0 | 210.6 | 235.1 | 239.0 |
| breast (connective tissue) (female) (glandular tissue) (soft parts) | 174.9 | 198.81 | 233.0 | 217 | 238.3 | 239.3 |
| areola | 174.0 | 198.81 | 233.0 | 217 | 238.3 | 239.3 |
| male | 175.0 | 198.81 | 233.0 | 217 | 238.3 | 239.3 |
| axillary tail | 174.6 | 198.81 | 233.0 | 217 | 238.3 | 239.3 |
| central portion | 174.1 | 198.81 | 233.0 | 217 | 238.3 | 239.3 |
| contiguous sites | 174.8 | — | — | — | — | — |
| ectopic sites | 174.8 | 198.81 | 233.0 | 217 | 238.3 | 239.3 |
| inner | 174.8 | 198.81 | 233.0 | 217 | 238.3 | 239.3 |
| lower | 174.8 | 198.81 | 233.0 | 217 | 238.3 | 239.3 |
| lower-inner quadrant | 174.3 | 198.81 | 233.0 | 217 | 238.3 | 239.3 |
| lower-outer quadrant | 174.5 | 198.81 | 233.0 | 217 | 238.3 | 239.3 |
| male | 175.9 | 198.81 | 233.0 | 217 | 238.3 | 239.3 |
| areola | 175.0 | 198.81 | 233.0 | 217 | 238.3 | 239.3 |
| ectopic tissue | 175.9 | 198.81 | 233.0 | 217 | 238.3 | 239.3 |
| nipple | 175.0 | 198.81 | 233.0 | 217 | 238.3 | 239.3 |
| mastectomy site (skin) | 173.5 | 198.2 | — | — | — | — |
| specified as breast tissue | 174.8 | 198.81 | — | — | — | — |
| midline | 174.8 | 198.81 | 233.0 | 217 | 238.3 | 239.3 |
| nipple | 174.0 | 198.81 | 233.0 | 217 | 238.3 | 239.3 |
| male | 175.0 | 198.81 | 233.0 | 217 | 238.3 | 239.3 |
| outer | 174.8 | 198.81 | 233.0 | 217 | 238.3 | 239.3 |
| skin | 173.5 | 198.2 | 232.5 | 216.5 | 238.2 | 239.2 |
| tail (axillary) | 174.6 | 198.81 | 233.0 | 217 | 238.3 | 239.3 |
| upper | 174.8 | 198.81 | 233.0 | 217 | 238.3 | 239.3 |
| upper-inner quadrant | 174.2 | 198.81 | 233.0 | 217 | 238.3 | 239.3 |
| upper-outer quadrant | 174.4 | 198.81 | 233.0 | 217 | 238.3 | 239.3 |
| broad ligament | 183.3 | 198.82 | 233.39▲ | 221.0 | 236.3 | 239.5 |
| bronchiogenic, bronchogenic (lung) | 162.9 | 197.0 | 231.2 | 212.3 | 235.7 | 239.1 |
| bronchiole | 162.9 | 197.0 | 231.2 | 212.3 | 235.7 | 239.1 |
| bronchus | 162.9 | 197.0 | 231.2 | 212.3 | 235.7 | 239.1 |
| carina | 162.2 | 197.0 | 231.2 | 212.3 | 235.7 | 239.1 |
| contiguous sites with lung or trachea | 162.8 | — | — | — | — | — |
| lower lobe of lung | 162.5 | 197.0 | 231.2 | 212.3 | 235.7 | 239.1 |
| main | 162.2 | 197.0 | 231.2 | 212.3 | 235.7 | 239.1 |
| middle lobe of lung | 162.4 | 197.0 | 231.2 | 212.3 | 235.7 | 239.1 |
| upper lobe of lung | 162.3 | 197.0 | 231.2 | 212.3 | 235.7 | 239.1 |
| brow | 173.3 | 198.2 | 232.3 | 216.3 | 238.2 | 239.2 |
| buccal (cavity) | 145.9 | 198.89 | 230.0 | 210.4 | 235.1 | 239.0 |
| commissure | 145.0 | 198.89 | 230.0 | 210.4 | 235.1 | 239.0 |
| groove (lower) (upper) | 145.1 | 198.89 | 230.0 | 210.4 | 235.1 | 239.0 |
| mucosa | 145.0 | 198.89 | 230.0 | 210.4 | 235.1 | 239.0 |
| sulcus (lower) (upper) | 145.1 | 198.89 | 230.0 | 210.4 | 235.1 | 239.0 |
| bulbourethral gland | 189.3 | 198.1 | 233.9 | 223.81 | 236.99 | 239.5 |
| bursa — *see* Neoplasm, connective tissue | | | | | | |
| buttock NEC* | 195.3 | 198.89 | 232.5 | 229.8 | 238.8 | 239.8 |
| calf* | 195.5 | 198.89 | 232.7 | 229.8 | 238.8 | 239.8 |
| calvarium | 170.0 | 198.5 | — | 213.0 | 238.0 | 239.2 |
| calyx, renal | 189.1 | 198.0 | 233.9 | 223.1 | 236.91 | 239.5 |
| canal | | | | | | |
| anal | 154.2 | 197.5 | 230.5 | 211.4 | 235.5 | 239.0 |
| auditory (external) | 173.2 | 198.2 | 232.2 | 216.2 | 238.2 | 239.2 |
| auricular (external) | 173.2 | 198.2 | 232.2 | 216.2 | 238.2 | 239.2 |
| canaliculi, biliary (biliferi) (intrahepatic) | 155.1 | 197.8 | 230.8 | 211.5 | 235.3 | 239.0 |
| **Neoplasm, neoplastic —** *continued* | | | | | | |
| canthus (eye) (inner) (outer) | 173.1 | 198.2 | 232.1 | 216.1 | 238.2 | 239.2 |
| capillary — *see* Neoplasm, connective tissue | | | | | | |
| caput coli | 153.4 | 197.5 | 230.3 | 211.3 | 235.2 | 239.0 |
| cardia (gastric) | 151.0 | 197.8 | 230.2 | 211.1 | 235.2 | 239.0 |
| cardiac orifice (stomach) | 151.0 | 197.8 | 230.2 | 211.1 | 235.2 | 239.0 |
| cardio-esophageal junction | 151.0 | 197.8 | 230.2 | 211.1 | 235.2 | 239.0 |
| cardio-esophagus | 151.0 | 197.8 | 230.2 | 211.1 | 235.2 | 239.0 |
| carina (bronchus) | 162.2 | 197.0 | 231.2 | 212.3 | 235.7 | 239.1 |
| carotid (artery) | 171.0 | 198.89 | — | 215.0 | 238.1 | 239.2 |
| body | 194.5 | 198.89 | — | 227.5 | 237.3 | 239.7 |
| carpus (any bone) | 170.5 | 198.5 | — | 213.5 | 238.0 | 239.2 |
| cartilage (articular) (joint) NEC (*see also* Neoplasm, bone) | 170.9 | 198.5 | — | 213.9 | 238.0 | 239.2 |
| arytenoid | 161.3 | 197.3 | 231.0 | 212.1 | 235.6 | 239.1 |
| auricular | 171.0 | 198.89 | — | 215.0 | 238.1 | 239.2 |
| bronchi | 162.2 | 197.3 | — | 212.3 | 235.7 | 239.1 |
| connective tissue — *see* Neoplasm, connective tissue | | | | | | |
| costal | 170.3 | 198.5 | — | 213.3 | 238.0 | 239.2 |
| cricoid | 161.3 | 197.3 | 231.0 | 212.1 | 235.6 | 239.1 |
| cuneiform | 161.3 | 197.3 | 231.0 | 212.1 | 235.6 | 239.1 |
| ear (external) | 171.0 | 198.89 | — | 215.0 | 238.1 | 239.2 |
| ensiform | 170.3 | 198.5 | — | 213.3 | 238.0 | 239.2 |
| epiglottis | 161.1 | 197.3 | 231.0 | 212.1 | 235.6 | 239.1 |
| anterior surface | 146.4 | 198.89 | 230.0 | 210.6 | 235.1 | 239.0 |
| eyelid | 171.0 | 198.89 | — | 215.0 | 238.1 | 239.2 |
| intervertebral | 170.2 | 198.5 | — | 213.2 | 238.0 | 239.2 |
| larynx, laryngeal | 161.3 | 197.3 | 231.0 | 212.1 | 235.6 | 239.1 |
| nose, nasal | 160.0 | 197.3 | 231.8 | 212.0 | 235.9 | 239.1 |
| pinna | 171.0 | 198.89 | — | 215.0 | 238.1 | 239.2 |
| rib | 170.3 | 198.5 | — | 213.3 | 238.0 | 239.2 |
| semilunar (knee) | 170.7 | 198.5 | — | 213.7 | 238.0 | 239.2 |
| thyroid | 161.3 | 197.3 | 231.0 | 212.1 | 235.6 | 239.1 |
| trachea | 162.0 | 197.3 | 231.1 | 212.2 | 235.7 | 239.1 |
| cauda equina | 192.2 | 198.3 | — | 225.3 | 237.5 | 239.7 |
| cavity | | | | | | |
| buccal | 145.9 | 198.89 | 230.0 | 210.4 | 235.1 | 239.0 |
| nasal | 160.0 | 197.3 | 231.8 | 212.0 | 235.9 | 239.1 |
| oral | 145.9 | 198.89 | 230.0 | 210.4 | 235.1 | 239.0 |
| peritoneal | 158.9 | 197.6 | — | 211.8 | 235.4 | 239.0 |
| tympanic | 160.1 | 197.3 | 231.8 | 212.0 | 235.9 | 239.1 |
| cecum | 153.4 | 197.5 | 230.3 | 211.3 | 235.2 | 239.0 |
| central | | | | | | |
| nervous system — *see* Neoplasm, nervous system | | | | | | |
| white matter | 191.0 | 198.3 | — | 225.0 | 237.5 | 239.6 |
| cerebellopontine (angle) | 191.6 | 198.3 | — | 225.0 | 237.5 | 239.6 |
| cerebellum, cerebellar | 191.6 | 198.3 | — | 225.0 | 237.5 | 239.6 |
| cerebrum, cerebral (cortex) (hemisphere) (white matter) | 191.0 | 198.3 | — | 225.0 | 237.5 | 239.6 |
| meninges | 192.1 | 198.4 | — | 225.2 | 237.6 | 239.7 |
| peduncle | 191.7 | 198.3 | — | 225.0 | 237.5 | 239.6 |
| ventricle (any) | 191.5 | 198.3 | — | 225.0 | 237.5 | 239.6 |
| cervical region | 195.0 | 198.89 | 234.8 | 229.8 | 238.8 | 239.8 |
| cervix (cervical) (uteri) (uterus) | 180.9 | 198.82 | 233.1 | 219.0 | 236.0 | 239.5 |
| canal | 180.0 | 198.82 | 233.1 | 219.0 | 236.0 | 239.5 |
| contiguous sites | 180.8 | — | — | — | — | — |
| endocervix (canal) (gland) | 180.0 | 198.82 | 233.1 | 219.0 | 236.0 | 239.5 |
| exocervix | 180.1 | 198.82 | 233.1 | 219.0 | 236.0 | 239.5 |
| external os | 180.1 | 198.82 | 233.1 | 219.0 | 236.0 | 239.5 |
| internal os | 180.0 | 198.82 | 233.1 | 219.0 | 236.0 | 239.5 |
| nabothian gland | 180.0 | 198.82 | 233.1 | 219.0 | 236.0 | 239.5 |
| squamocolumnar junction | 180.8 | 198.82 | 233.1 | 219.0 | 236.0 | 239.5 |
| stump | 180.8 | 198.82 | 233.1 | 219.0 | 236.0 | 239.5 |

Neoplasm, cheek — Neoplasm, cord

| Neoplasm, neoplastic — continued | Primary | Secondary | Ca in situ | Benign | Uncertain Behavior | Unspecified |
|---|---|---|---|---|---|---|
| cheek | 195.0 | 198.89 | 234.8 | 229.8 | 238.8 | 239.8 |
| external | 173.3 | 198.2 | 232.3 | 216.3 | 238.2 | 239.2 |
| inner aspect | 145.0 | 198.89 | 230.0 | 210.4 | 235.1 | 239.0 |
| internal | 145.0 | 198.89 | 230.0 | 210.4 | 235.1 | 239.0 |
| mucosa | 145.0 | 198.89 | 230.0 | 210.4 | 235.1 | 239.0 |
| chest (wall) NEC | 195.1 | 198.89 | 234.8 | 229.8 | 238.8 | 239.8 |
| chiasma opticum | 192.0 | 198.4 | — | 225.1 | 237.9 | 239.7 |
| chin | 173.3 | 198.2 | 232.3 | 216.3 | 238.2 | 239.2 |
| choana | 147.3 | 198.89 | 230.0 | 210.7 | 235.1 | 239.0 |
| cholangiole | 155.1 | 197.8 | 230.8 | 211.5 | 235.3 | 239.0 |
| choledochal duct | 156.1 | 197.8 | 230.8 | 211.5 | 235.3 | 239.0 |
| choroid | 190.6 | 198.4 | 234.0 | 224.6 | 238.8 | 239.8 |
| plexus | 191.5 | 198.3 | — | 225.0 | 237.5 | 239.6 |
| ciliary body | 190.0 | 198.4 | 234.0 | 224.0 | 238.8 | 239.8 |
| clavicle | 170.3 | 198.5 | — | 213.3 | 238.0 | 239.2 |
| clitoris | 184.3 | 198.82 | 233.32 ▲ | 221.2 | 236.3 | 239.5 |
| clivus | 170.0 | 198.5 | — | 213.0 | 238.0 | 239.2 |
| cloacogenic zone | 154.8 | 197.5 | 230.7 | 211.4 | 235.5 | 239.0 |
| coccygeal | | | | | | |
| body or glomus | 194.6 | 198.89 | — | 227.6 | 237.3 | 239.7 |
| vertebra | 170.6 | 198.5 | — | 213.6 | 238.0 | 239.2 |
| coccyx | 170.6 | 198.5 | — | 213.6 | 238.0 | 239.2 |
| colon (see also Neoplasm, intestine, large) | | | | | | |
| and rectum | 154.0 | 197.5 | 230.4 | 211.4 | 235.2 | 239.0 |
| columnella | 173.3 | 198.2 | 232.3 | 216.3 | 238.2 | 239.2 |
| column, spinal — see Neoplasm, spine | | | | | | |
| commissure | | | | | | |
| labial, lip | 140.6 | 198.89 | 230.0 | 210.4 | 235.1 | 239.0 |
| laryngeal | 161.0 | 197.3 | 231.0 | 212.1 | 235.6 | 239.1 |
| common (bile) duct | 156.1 | 197.8 | 230.8 | 211.5 | 235.3 | 239.0 |
| concha | 173.2 | 198.2 | 232.2 | 216.2 | 238.2 | 239.2 |
| nose | 160.0 | 197.3 | 231.8 | 212.0 | 235.9 | 239.1 |
| conjunctiva | 190.3 | 198.4 | 234.0 | 224.3 | 238.8 | 239.8 |
| connective tissue NEC | 171.9 | 198.89 | — | 215.9 | 238.1 | 239.2 |

*Note — For neoplasms of connective tissue (blood vessel, bursa, fascia, ligament, muscle, peripheral nerves, sympathetic and parasympathetic nerves and ganglia, synovia, tendon, etc.) or of morphological types that indicate connective tissue, code according to the list under "Neoplasm, connective tissue"; for sites that do not appear in this list, code to neoplasm of that site; e.g.,*

*liposarcoma, shoulder 171.2*

*leiomyosarcoma, stomach 151.9*

*neurofibroma, chest wall 215.4*

*Morphological types that indicate connective tissue appear in the proper place in the alphabetic index with the instruction "see Neoplasm, connective tissue..."*

| | Primary | Secondary | Ca in situ | Benign | Uncertain Behavior | Unspecified |
|---|---|---|---|---|---|---|
| abdomen | 171.5 | 198.89 | — | 215.5 | 238.1 | 239.2 |
| abdominal wall | 171.5 | 198.89 | — | 215.5 | 238.1 | 239.2 |
| ankle | 171.3 | 198.89 | — | 215.3 | 238.1 | 239.2 |
| antecubital fossa or space | 171.2 | 198.89 | — | 215.2 | 238.1 | 239.2 |
| arm | 171.2 | 198.89 | — | 215.2 | 238.1 | 239.2 |
| auricle (ear) | 171.0 | 198.89 | — | 215.0 | 238.1 | 239.2 |
| axilla | 171.4 | 198.89 | — | 215.4 | 238.1 | 239.2 |
| back | 171.7 | 198.89 | — | 215.7 | 238.1 | 239.2 |
| breast (female) (see also Neoplasm, breast) | 174.9 | 198.81 | 233.0 | 217 | 238.3 | 239.3 |
| male | 175.9 | 198.81 | 233.0 | 217 | 238.3 | 239.3 |
| buttock | 171.6 | 198.89 | — | 215.6 | 238.1 | 239.2 |
| calf | 171.3 | 198.89 | — | 215.3 | 238.1 | 239.2 |
| cervical region | 171.0 | 198.89 | — | 215.0 | 238.1 | 239.2 |
| cheek | 171.0 | 198.89 | — | 215.0 | 238.1 | 239.2 |
| chest (wall) | 171.4 | 198.89 | — | 215.4 | 238.1 | 239.2 |
| chin | 171.0 | 198.89 | — | 215.0 | 238.1 | 239.2 |
| contiguous sites | 171.8 | — | — | — | — | — |
| diaphragm | 171.4 | 198.89 | — | 215.4 | 238.1 | 239.2 |
| ear (external) | 171.0 | 198.89 | — | 215.0 | 238.1 | 239.2 |
| elbow | 171.2 | 198.89 | — | 215.2 | 238.1 | 239.2 |
| extrarectal | 171.6 | 198.89 | — | 215.6 | 238.1 | 239.2 |
| extremity | 171.8 | 198.89 | — | 215.8 | 238.1 | 239.2 |
| lower | 171.3 | 198.89 | — | 215.3 | 238.1 | 239.2 |
| upper | 171.2 | 198.89 | — | 215.2 | 238.1 | 239.2 |

| Neoplasm, neoplastic — continued connective tissue — continued | Primary | Secondary | Ca in situ | Benign | Uncertain Behavior | Unspecified |
|---|---|---|---|---|---|---|
| eyelid | 171.0 | 198.89 | — | 215.0 | 238.1 | 239.2 |
| face | 171.0 | 198.89 | — | 215.0 | 238.1 | 239.2 |
| finger | 171.2 | 198.89 | — | 215.2 | 238.1 | 239.2 |
| flank | 171.7 | 198.89 | — | 215.7 | 238.1 | 239.2 |
| foot | 171.3 | 198.89 | — | 215.3 | 238.1 | 239.2 |
| forearm | 171.2 | 198.89 | — | 215.2 | 238.1 | 239.2 |
| forehead | 171.0 | 198.89 | — | 215.0 | 238.1 | 239.2 |
| gastric | 171.5 | 198.89 | — | 215.5 | 238.1 | — |
| gastrointestinal | 171.5 | 198.89 | — | 215.5 | 238.1 | — |
| gluteal region | 171.6 | 198.89 | — | 215.6 | 238.1 | 239.2 |
| great vessels NEC | 171.4 | 198.89 | — | 215.4 | 238.1 | 239.2 |
| groin | 171.6 | 198.89 | — | 215.6 | 238.1 | 239.2 |
| hand | 171.2 | 198.89 | — | 215.2 | 238.1 | 239.2 |
| head | 171.0 | 198.89 | — | 215.0 | 238.1 | 239.2 |
| heel | 171.3 | 198.89 | — | 215.3 | 238.1 | 239.2 |
| hip | 171.3 | 198.89 | — | 215.3 | 238.1 | 239.2 |
| hypochondrium | 171.5 | 198.89 | — | 215.5 | 238.1 | 239.2 |
| iliopsoas muscle | 171.6 | 198.89 | — | 215.5 | 238.1 | 239.2 |
| infraclavicular region | 171.4 | 198.89 | — | 215.4 | 238.1 | 239.2 |
| inguinal (canal) (region) | 171.6 | 198.89 | — | 215.6 | 238.1 | 239.2 |
| intestine | 171.5 | 198.89 | — | 215.5 | 238.1 | — |
| intrathoracic | 171.4 | 198.89 | — | 215.4 | 238.1 | 239.2 |
| ischiorectal fossa | 171.6 | 198.89 | — | 215.6 | 238.1 | 239.2 |
| jaw | 143.9 | 198.89 | 230.0 | 210.4 | 235.1 | 239.0 |
| knee | 171.3 | 198.89 | — | 215.3 | 238.1 | 239.2 |
| leg | 171.3 | 198.89 | — | 215.3 | 238.1 | 239.2 |
| limb NEC | 171.9 | 198.89 | — | 215.8 | 238.1 | 239.2 |
| lower | 171.3 | 198.89 | — | 215.3 | 238.1 | 239.2 |
| upper | 171.2 | 198.89 | — | 215.2 | 238.1 | 239.2 |
| nates | 171.6 | 198.89 | — | 215.6 | 238.1 | 239.2 |
| neck | 171.0 | 198.89 | — | 215.0 | 238.1 | 239.2 |
| orbit | 190.1 | 198.4 | 234.0 | 224.1 | 238.8 | 239.8 |
| pararectal | 171.6 | 198.89 | — | 215.6 | 238.1 | 239.2 |
| para-urethral | 171.6 | 198.89 | — | 215.6 | 238.1 | 239.2 |
| paravaginal | 171.6 | 198.89 | — | 215.6 | 238.1 | 239.2 |
| pelvis (floor) | 171.6 | 198.89 | — | 215.6 | 238.1 | 239.2 |
| pelvo-abdominal | 171.8 | 198.89 | — | 215.8 | 238.1 | 239.2 |
| perineum | 171.6 | 198.89 | — | 215.6 | 238.1 | 239.2 |
| perirectal (tissue) | 171.6 | 198.89 | — | 215.6 | 238.1 | 239.2 |
| periurethral (tissue) | 171.6 | 198.89 | — | 215.6 | 238.1 | 239.2 |
| popliteal fossa or space | 171.3 | 198.89 | — | 215.3 | 238.1 | 239.2 |
| presacral | 171.6 | 198.89 | — | 215.6 | 238.1 | 239.2 |
| psoas muscle | 171.5 | 198.89 | — | 215.5 | 238.1 | 239.2 |
| pterygoid fossa | 171.0 | 198.89 | — | 215.0 | 238.1 | 239.2 |
| rectovaginal septum or wall | 171.6 | 198.89 | — | 215.6 | 238.1 | 239.2 |
| rectovesical | 171.6 | 198.89 | — | 215.6 | 238.1 | 239.2 |
| retroperitoneum | 158.0 | 197.6 | — | 211.8 | 235.4 | 239.0 |
| sacrococcygeal region | 171.6 | 198.89 | — | 215.6 | 238.1 | 239.2 |
| scalp | 171.0 | 198.89 | — | 215.0 | 238.1 | 239.2 |
| scapular region | 171.4 | 198.89 | — | 215.4 | 238.1 | 239.2 |
| shoulder | 171.2 | 198.89 | — | 215.2 | 238.1 | 239.2 |
| skin (dermis) NEC | 173.9 | 198.2 | 232.9 | 216.9 | 238.2 | 239.2 |
| stomach | 171.5 | 198.89 | — | 215.5 | 238.1 | — |
| submental | 171.0 | 198.89 | — | 215.0 | 238.1 | 239.2 |
| supraclavicular region | 171.0 | 198.89 | — | 215.0 | 238.1 | 239.2 |
| temple | 171.0 | 198.89 | — | 215.0 | 238.1 | 239.2 |
| temporal region | 171.0 | 198.89 | — | 215.0 | 238.1 | 239.2 |
| thigh | 171.3 | 198.89 | — | 215.3 | 238.1 | 239.2 |
| thoracic (duct) (wall) | 171.4 | 198.89 | — | 215.4 | 238.1 | 239.2 |
| thorax | 171.4 | 198.89 | — | 215.4 | 238.1 | 239.2 |
| thumb | 171.2 | 198.89 | — | 215.2 | 238.1 | 239.2 |
| toe | 171.3 | 198.89 | — | 215.3 | 238.1 | 239.2 |
| trunk | 171.7 | 198.89 | — | 215.7 | 238.1 | 239.2 |
| umbilicus | 171.5 | 198.89 | — | 215.5 | 238.1 | 239.2 |
| vesicorectal | 171.6 | 198.89 | — | 215.6 | 238.1 | 239.2 |
| wrist | 171.2 | 198.89 | — | 215.2 | 238.1 | 239.2 |
| conus medullaris | 192.2 | 198.3 | — | 225.3 | 237.5 | 239.7 |
| cord (true) (vocal) | 161.0 | 197.3 | 231.0 | 212.1 | 235.6 | 239.1 |

| | Malignant | | | | | |
|---|---|---|---|---|---|---|
| | Primary | Secondary | Ca in situ | Benign | Uncertain Behavior | Unspecified |
| **Neoplasm, neoplastic —** *continued* | | | | | | |
| cord — *continued* | | | | | | |
| false | 161.1 | 197.3 | 231.0 | 212.1 | 235.6 | 239.1 |
| spermatic | 187.6 | 198.82 | 233.6 | 222.8 | 236.6 | 239.5 |
| spinal (cervical) (lumbar) (thoracic) | 192.2 | 198.3 | — | 225.3 | 237.5 | 239.7 |
| cornea (limbus) | 190.4 | 198.4 | 234.0 | 224.4 | 238.8 | 239.8 |
| corpus | | | | | | |
| albicans | 183.0 | 198.6 | 233.39 ▲ | 220 | 236.2 | 239.5 |
| callosum, brain | 191.8 | 198.3 | — | 225.0 | 237.5 | 239.6 |
| cavernosum | 187.3 | 198.82 | 233.5 | 222.1 | 236.6 | 239.5 |
| gastric | 151.4 | 197.8 | 230.2 | 211.1 | 235.2 | 239.0 |
| penis | 187.3 | 198.82 | 233.5 | 222.1 | 236.6 | 239.5 |
| striatum, cerebrum | 191.0 | 198.3 | — | 225.0 | 237.5 | 239.6 |
| uteri | 182.0 | 198.82 | 233.2 | 219.1 | 236.0 | 239.5 |
| isthmus | 182.1 | 198.82 | 233.2 | 219.1 | 236.0 | 239.5 |
| cortex | | | | | | |
| adrenal | 194.0 | 198.7 | 234.8 | 227.0 | 237.2 | 239.7 |
| cerebral | 191.0 | 198.3 | — | 225.0 | 237.5 | 239.6 |
| costal cartilage | 170.3 | 198.5 | — | 213.3 | 238.0 | 239.2 |
| costovertebral joint | 170.3 | 198.5 | — | 213.3 | 238.0 | 239.2 |
| Cowper's gland | 189.3 | 198.1 | 233.9 | 223.81 | 236.99 | 239.5 |
| cranial (fossa, any) | 191.9 | 198.3 | — | 225.0 | 237.5 | 239.6 |
| meninges | 192.1 | 198.4 | — | 225.2 | 237.6 | 239.7 |
| nerve (any) | 192.0 | 198.4 | — | 225.1 | 237.9 | 239.7 |
| craniobuccal pouch | 194.3 | 198.89 | 234.8 | 227.3 | 237.0 | 239.7 |
| craniopharyngeal (duct) (pouch) | 194.3 | 198.89 | 234.8 | 227.3 | 237.0 | 239.7 |
| cricoid | 148.0 | 198.89 | 230.0 | 210.8 | 235.1 | 239.0 |
| cartilage | 161.3 | 197.3 | 231.0 | 212.1 | 235.6 | 239.1 |
| cricopharynx | 148.0 | 198.89 | 230.0 | 210.8 | 235.1 | 239.0 |
| crypt of Morgagni | 154.8 | 197.5 | 230.7 | 211.4 | 235.2 | 239.0 |
| crystalline lens | 190.0 | 198.4 | 234.0 | 224.0 | 238.8 | 239.8 |
| cul-de-sac (Douglas') | 158.8 | 197.6 | — | 211.8 | 235.4 | 239.0 |
| cuneiform cartilage | 161.3 | 197.3 | 231.0 | 212.1 | 235.6 | 239.1 |
| cutaneous — *see* Neoplasm, skin | | | | | | |
| cutis — *see* Neoplasm, skin | | | | | | |
| cystic (bile) duct (common) | 156.1 | 197.8 | 230.8 | 211.5 | 235.3 | 239.0 |
| dermis — *see* Neoplasm, skin | | | | | | |
| diaphragm | 171.4 | 198.89 | — | 215.4 | 238.1 | 239.2 |
| digestive organs, system, tube, or tract NEC | 159.9 | 197.8 | 230.9 | 211.9 | 235.5 | 239.0 |
| contiguous sites with peritoneum | 159.8 | — | — | — | — | — |
| disc, intervertebral | 170.2 | 198.5 | — | 213.2 | 238.0 | 239.2 |
| disease, generalized | 199.0 | 199.0 | 234.9 | 229.9 | 238.9 | 199.0 |
| disseminated | 199.0 | 199.0 | 234.9 | 229.9 | 238.9 | 199.0 |
| Douglas' cul-de-sac or pouch | 158.8 | 197.6 | — | 211.8 | 235.4 | 239.0 |
| duodenojejunal junction | 152.8 | 197.4 | 230.7 | 211.2 | 235.2 | 239.0 |
| duodenum | 152.0 | 197.4 | 230.7 | 211.2 | 235.2 | 239.0 |
| dura (cranial) (mater) | 192.1 | 198.4 | — | 225.2 | 237.6 | 239.7 |
| cerebral | 192.1 | 198.4 | — | 225.2 | 237.6 | 239.7 |
| spinal | 192.3 | 198.4 | — | 225.4 | 237.6 | 239.7 |
| ear (external) | 173.2 | 198.2 | 232.2 | 216.2 | 238.2 | 239.2 |
| auricle or auris | 173.2 | 198.2 | 232.2 | 216.2 | 238.2 | 239.2 |
| canal, external | 173.2 | 198.2 | 232.2 | 216.2 | 238.2 | 239.2 |
| cartilage | 171.0 | 198.89 | — | 215.0 | 238.1 | 239.2 |
| external meatus | 173.2 | 198.2 | 232.2 | 216.2 | 238.2 | 239.2 |
| inner | 160.1 | 197.3 | 231.8 | 212.0 | 235.9 | 239.8 |
| lobule | 173.2 | 198.2 | 232.2 | 216.2 | 238.2 | 239.2 |
| middle | 160.1 | 197.3 | 231.8 | 212.0 | 235.9 | 239.8 |
| contiguous sites with accessory sinuses or nasal cavities | 160.8 | — | — | — | — | — |
| skin | 173.2 | 198.2 | 232.2 | 216.2 | 238.2 | 239.2 |
| earlobe | 173.2 | 198.2 | 232.2 | 216.2 | 238.2 | 239.2 |
| ejaculatory duct | 187.8 | 198.82 | 233.6 | 222.8 | 236.6 | 239.5 |
| elbow NEC* | 195.4 | 198.89 | 232.6 | 229.8 | 238.8 | 239.8 |
| endocardium | 164.1 | 198.89 | — | 212.7 | 238.8 | 239.8 |
| **Neoplasm, neoplastic —** *continued* | | | | | | |
| endocervix (canal) (gland) | 180.0 | 198.82 | 233.1 | 219.0 | 236.0 | 239.5 |
| endocrine gland NEC | 194.9 | 198.89 | — | 227.9 | 237.4 | 239.7 |
| pluriglandular NEC | 194.8 | 198.89 | 234.8 | 227.8 | 237.4 | 239.7 |
| endometrium (gland) (stroma) | 182.0 | 198.82 | 233.2 | 219.1 | 236.0 | 239.5 |
| ensiform cartilage | 170.3 | 198.5 | — | 213.3 | 238.0 | 239.2 |
| enteric — *see* Neoplasm, intestine | | | | | | |
| ependyma (brain) | 191.5 | 198.3 | — | 225.0 | 237.5 | 239.6 |
| epicardium | 164.1 | 198.89 | — | 212.7 | 238.8 | 239.8 |
| epididymis | 187.5 | 198.82 | 233.6 | 222.3 | 236.6 | 239.5 |
| epidural | 192.9 | 198.4 | — | 225.9 | 237.9 | 239.7 |
| epiglottis | 161.1 | 197.3 | 231.0 | 212.1 | 235.6 | 239.1 |
| anterior aspect or surface | 146.4 | 198.89 | 230.0 | 210.6 | 235.1 | 239.0 |
| cartilage | 161.3 | 197.3 | 231.0 | 212.1 | 235.6 | 239.1 |
| free border (margin) | 146.4 | 198.89 | 230.0 | 210.6 | 235.1 | 239.0 |
| junctional region | 146.5 | 198.89 | 230.0 | 210.6 | 235.1 | 239.0 |
| posterior (laryngeal) surface | 161.1 | 197.3 | 231.0 | 212.1 | 235.6 | 239.1 |
| suprahyoid portion | 161.1 | 197.3 | 231.0 | 212.1 | 235.6 | 239.1 |
| esophagogastric junction | 151.0 | 197.8 | 230.2 | 211.1 | 235.2 | 239.0 |
| esophagus | 150.9 | 197.8 | 230.1 | 211.0 | 235.5 | 239.0 |
| abdominal | 150.2 | 197.8 | 230.1 | 211.0 | 235.5 | 239.0 |
| cervical | 150.0 | 197.8 | 230.1 | 211.0 | 235.5 | 239.0 |
| contiguous sites | 150.8 | — | — | — | — | — |
| distal (third) | 150.5 | 197.8 | 230.1 | 211.0 | 235.5 | 239.0 |
| lower (third) | 150.5 | 197.8 | 230.1 | 211.0 | 235.5 | 239.0 |
| middle (third) | 150.4 | 197.8 | 230.1 | 211.0 | 235.5 | 239.0 |
| proximal (third) | 150.3 | 197.8 | 230.1 | 211.0 | 235.5 | 239.0 |
| specified part NEC | 150.8 | 197.8 | 230.1 | 211.0 | 235.5 | 239.0 |
| thoracic | 150.1 | 197.8 | 230.1 | 211.0 | 235.5 | 239.0 |
| upper (third) | 150.3 | 197.8 | 230.1 | 211.0 | 235.5 | 239.0 |
| ethmoid (sinus) | 160.3 | 197.3 | 231.8 | 212.0 | 235.9 | 239.1 |
| bone or labyrinth | 170.0 | 198.5 | — | 213.0 | 238.0 | 239.2 |
| Eustachian tube | 160.1 | 197.3 | 231.8 | 212.0 | 235.9 | 239.1 |
| exocervix | 180.1 | 198.82 | 233.1 | 219.0 | 236.0 | 239.5 |
| external | | | | | | |
| meatus (ear) | 173.2 | 198.2 | 232.2 | 216.2 | 238.2 | 239.2 |
| os, cervix uteri | 180.1 | 198.82 | 233.1 | 219.0 | 236.0 | 239.5 |
| extradural | 192.9 | 198.4 | — | 225.9 | 237.9 | 239.7 |
| extrahepatic (bile) duct | 156.1 | 197.8 | 230.8 | 211.5 | 235.3 | 239.0 |
| contiguous sites with gallbladder | 156.8 | — | — | — | — | — |
| extraocular muscle | 190.1 | 198.4 | 234.0 | 224.1 | 238.8 | 239.8 |
| extrarectal | 195.3 | 198.89 | 234.8 | 229.8 | 238.8 | 239.8 |
| extremity* | 195.8 | 198.89 | 232.8 | 229.8 | 238.8 | 239.8 |
| lower* | 195.5 | 198.89 | 232.7 | 229.8 | 238.8 | 239.8 |
| upper* | 195.4 | 198.89 | 232.6 | 229.8 | 238.8 | 239.8 |
| eye NEC | 190.9 | 198.4 | 234.0 | 224.9 | 238.8 | 239.8 |
| contiguous sites | 190.8 | — | — | — | — | — |
| specified sites NEC | 190.8 | 198.4 | 234.0 | 224.8 | 238.8 | 239.8 |
| eyeball | 190.0 | 198.4 | 234.0 | 224.0 | 238.8 | 239.8 |
| eyebrow | 173.3 | 198.2 | 232.3 | 216.3 | 238.2 | 239.2 |
| eyelid (lower) (skin) (upper) | 173.1 | 198.2 | 232.1 | 216.1 | 238.2 | 239.2 |
| cartilage | 171.0 | 198.89 | — | 215.0 | 238.1 | 239.2 |
| face NEC* | 195.0 | 198.89 | 232.3 | 229.8 | 238.8 | 239.8 |
| fallopian tube (accessory) | 183.2 | 198.82 | 233.39 ▲ | 221.0 | 236.3 | 239.5 |
| falx (cerebelli) (cerebri) | 192.1 | 198.4 | — | 225.2 | 237.6 | 239.7 |
| fascia (*see also* Neoplasm, connective tissue) | | | | | | |
| palmar | 171.2 | 198.89 | — | 215.2 | 238.1 | 239.2 |
| plantar | 171.3 | 198.89 | — | 215.3 | 238.1 | 239.2 |
| fatty tissue — *see* Neoplasm, connective tissue | | | | | | |
| fauces, faucial NEC | 146.9 | 198.89 | 230.0 | 210.6 | 235.1 | 239.0 |
| pillars | 146.2 | 198.89 | 230.0 | 210.6 | 235.1 | 239.0 |
| tonsil | 146.0 | 198.89 | 230.0 | 210.5 | 235.1 | 239.0 |
| femur (any part) | 170.7 | 198.5 | — | 213.7 | 238.0 | 239.2 |
| fetal membrane | 181 | 198.82 | 233.2 | 219.8 | 236.1 | 239.5 |

---

☑ Additional Digit Required — Refer to the Tabular List for Digit Selection

▽ Subterms under main terms may continue to next column or page

| | Malignant | | | | | |
|---|---|---|---|---|---|---|
| | Primary | Secondary | Ca in situ | Benign | Uncertain Behavior | Unspecified |

**Neoplasm, neoplastic —** *continued*

| | Primary | Secondary | Ca in situ | Benign | Uncertain Behavior | Unspecified |
|---|---|---|---|---|---|---|
| fibrous tissue — *see* Neoplasm, connective tissue | | | | | | |
| fibula (any part) | 170.7 | 198.5 | — | 213.7 | 238.0 | 239.2 |
| filum terminale | 192.2 | 198.3 | — | 225.3 | 237.5 | 239.7 |
| finger NEC* | 195.4 | 198.89 | 232.6 | 229.8 | 238.8 | 239.8 |
| flank NEC* | 195.8 | 198.89 | 232.5 | 229.8 | 238.8 | 239.8 |
| follicle, nabothian | 180.0 | 198.82 | 233.1 | 219.0 | 236.0 | 239.5 |
| foot NEC* | 195.5 | 198.89 | 232.7 | 229.8 | 238.8 | 239.8 |
| forearm NEC* | 195.4 | 198.89 | 232.6 | 229.8 | 238.8 | 239.8 |
| forehead (skin) | 173.3 | 198.2 | 232.3 | 216.3 | 238.2 | 239.2 |
| foreskin | 187.1 | 198.82 | 233.5 | 222.1 | 236.6 | 239.5 |
| fornix | | | | | | |
| pharyngeal | 147.3 | 198.89 | 230.0 | 210.7 | 235.1 | 239.0 |
| vagina | 184.0 | 198.82 | 233.31 ▲ | 221.1 | 236.3 | 239.5 |
| fossa (of) | | | | | | |
| anterior (cranial) | 191.9 | 198.3 | — | 225.0 | 237.5 | 239.6 |
| cranial | 191.9 | 198.3 | — | 225.0 | 237.5 | 239.6 |
| ischiorectal | 195.3 | 198.89 | 234.8 | 229.8 | 238.8 | 239.8 |
| middle (cranial) | 191.9 | 198.3 | — | 225.0 | 237.5 | 239.6 |
| pituitary | 194.3 | 198.89 | 234.8 | 227.3 | 237.0 | 239.7 |
| posterior (cranial) | 191.9 | 198.3 | — | 225.0 | 237.5 | 239.6 |
| pterygoid | 171.0 | 198.89 | — | 215.0 | 238.1 | 239.2 |
| pyriform | 148.1 | 198.89 | 230.0 | 210.8 | 235.1 | 239.0 |
| Rosenmüller | 147.2 | 198.89 | 230.0 | 210.7 | 235.1 | 239.0 |
| tonsillar | 146.1 | 198.89 | 230.0 | 210.6 | 235.1 | 239.0 |
| fourchette | 184.4 | 198.82 | 233.32 ▲ | 221.2 | 236.3 | 239.5 |
| frenulum | | | | | | |
| labii — *see* Neoplasm, lip, internal | | | | | | |
| linguae | 141.3 | 198.89 | 230.0 | 210.1 | 235.1 | 239.0 |
| frontal | | | | | | |
| bone | 170.0 | 198.5 | — | 213.0 | 238.0 | 239.2 |
| lobe, brain | 191.1 | 198.3 | — | 225.0 | 237.5 | 239.6 |
| meninges | 192.1 | 198.4 | — | 225.2 | 237.6 | 239.7 |
| pole | 191.1 | 198.3 | — | 225.0 | 237.5 | 239.6 |
| sinus | 160.4 | 197.3 | 231.8 | 212.0 | 235.9 | 239.1 |
| fundus | | | | | | |
| stomach | 151.3 | 197.8 | 230.2 | 211.1 | 235.2 | 239.0 |
| uterus | 182.0 | 198.82 | 233.2 | 219.1 | 236.0 | 239.5 |
| gallbladder | 156.0 | 197.8 | 230.8 | 211.5 | 235.3 | 239.0 |
| contiguous sites with extrahepatic bile ducts | 156.8 | — | — | — | — | — |
| gall duct | | | | | | |
| (extrahepatic) | 156.1 | 197.8 | 230.8 | 211.5 | 235.3 | 239.0 |
| intrahepatic | 155.1 | 197.8 | 230.8 | 211.5 | 235.3 | 239.0 |
| ganglia (*see also* Neoplasm, connective tissue) | 171.9 | 198.89 | — | 215.9 | 238.1 | 239.2 |
| basal | 191.0 | 198.3 | — | 225.0 | 237.5 | 239.6 |
| ganglion (*see also* Neoplasm, connective tissue) | 171.9 | 198.89 | — | 215.9 | 238.1 | 239.2 |
| cranial nerve | 192.0 | 198.4 | — | 225.1 | 237.9 | 239.7 |
| Gartner's duct | 184.0 | 198.82 | 233.31 ▲ | 221.1 | 236.3 | 239.5 |
| gastric — *see* Neoplasm, stomach | | | | | | |
| gastrocolic | 159.8 | 197.8 | 230.9 | 211.9 | 235.5 | 239.0 |
| gastroesophageal junction | 151.0 | 197.8 | 230.2 | 211.1 | 235.2 | 239.0 |
| gastrointestinal (tract) NEC | 159.9 | 197.8 | 230.9 | 211.9 | 235.5 | 239.0 |
| generalized | 199.0 | 199.0 | 234.9 | 229.9 | 238.9 | 199.0 |
| genital organ or tract | | | | | | |
| female NEC | 184.9 | 198.82 | 233.39 ▲ | 221.9 | 236.3 | 239.5 |
| contiguous sites | 184.8 | — | — | — | — | — |
| specified site NEC | 184.8 | 198.82 | 233.39 ▲ | 221.8 | 236.3 | 239.5 |
| male NEC | 187.9 | 198.82 | 233.6 | 222.9 | 236.6 | 239.5 |
| contiguous sites | 187.8 | — | — | — | — | — |
| specified site NEC | 187.8 | 198.82 | 233.6 | 222.8 | 236.6 | 239.5 |
| genitourinary tract | | | | | | |
| female | 184.9 | 198.82 | 233.39 ▲ | 221.9 | 236.3 | 239.5 |
| male | 187.9 | 198.82 | 233.6 | 222.9 | 236.6 | 239.5 |

**Neoplasm, neoplastic —** *continued*

| | Primary | Secondary | Ca in situ | Benign | Uncertain Behavior | Unspecified |
|---|---|---|---|---|---|---|
| gingiva (alveolar) (marginal) | 143.9 | 198.89 | 230.0 | 210.4 | 235.1 | 239.0 |
| lower | 143.1 | 198.89 | 230.0 | 210.4 | 235.1 | 239.0 |
| mandibular | 143.1 | 198.89 | 230.0 | 210.4 | 235.1 | 239.0 |
| maxillary | 143.0 | 198.89 | 230.0 | 210.4 | 235.1 | 239.0 |
| upper | 143.0 | 198.89 | 230.0 | 210.4 | 235.1 | 239.0 |
| gland, glandular (lymphatic) (system) (*see also* Neoplasm, lymph gland) | | | | | | |
| endocrine NEC | 194.9 | 198.89 | — | 227.9 | 237.4 | 239.7 |
| salivary — *see* Neoplasm, salivary, gland | | | | | | |
| glans penis | 187.2 | 198.82 | 233.5 | 222.1 | 236.6 | 239.5 |
| globus pallidus | 191.0 | 198.3 | — | 225.0 | 237.5 | 239.6 |
| glomus | | | | | | |
| coccygeal | 194.6 | 198.89 | — | 227.6 | 237.3 | 239.7 |
| jugularis | 194.6 | 198.89 | — | 227.6 | 237.3 | 239.7 |
| glosso-epiglottic fold(s) | 146.4 | 198.89 | 230.0 | 210.6 | 235.1 | 239.0 |
| glossopalatine fold | 146.2 | 198.89 | 230.0 | 210.6 | 235.1 | 239.0 |
| glossopharyngeal sulcus | 146.1 | 198.89 | 230.0 | 210.6 | 235.1 | 239.0 |
| glottis | 161.0 | 197.3 | 231.0 | 212.1 | 235.6 | 239.1 |
| gluteal region* | 195.3 | 198.89 | 232.5 | 229.8 | 238.8 | 239.8 |
| great vessels NEC | 171.4 | 198.89 | — | 215.4 | 238.1 | 239.2 |
| groin NEC | 195.3 | 198.89 | 232.5 | 229.8 | 238.8 | 239.8 |
| gum | 143.9 | 198.89 | 230.0 | 210.4 | 235.1 | 239.0 |
| contiguous sites | 143.8 | — | — | — | — | — |
| lower | 143.1 | 198.89 | 230.0 | 210.4 | 235.1 | 239.0 |
| upper | 143.0 | 198.89 | 230.0 | 210.4 | 235.1 | 239.0 |
| hand NEC* | 195.4 | 198.89 | 232.6 | 229.8 | 238.8 | 239.8 |
| head NEC* | 195.0 | 198.89 | 232.4 | 229.8 | 238.8 | 239.8 |
| heart | 164.1 | 198.89 | — | 212.7 | 238.8 | 239.8 |
| contiguous sites with mediastinum or thymus | 164.8 | — | — | — | — | — |
| heel NEC* | 195.5 | 198.89 | 232.7 | 229.8 | 238.8 | 239.8 |
| helix | 173.2 | 198.2 | 232.2 | 216.2 | 238.2 | 239.2 |
| hematopoietic, hemopoietic tissue NEC | 202.8 ☑ | 198.89 | — | — | — | 238.79 |
| hemisphere, cerebral | 191.0 | 198.3 | — | 225.0 | 237.5 | 239.6 |
| hemorrhoidal zone | 154.2 | 197.5 | 230.5 | 211.4 | 235.5 | 239.0 |
| hepatic | 155.2 | 197.7 | 230.8 | 211.5 | 235.3 | 239.0 |
| duct (bile) | 156.1 | 197.8 | 230.8 | 211.5 | 235.3 | 239.0 |
| flexure (colon) | 153.0 | 197.5 | 230.3 | 211.3 | 235.2 | 239.0 |
| primary | 155.0 | — | — | — | — | — |
| hilus of lung | 162.2 | 197.0 | 231.2 | 212.3 | 235.7 | 239.1 |
| hip NEC* | 195.5 | 198.89 | 232.7 | 229.8 | 238.8 | 239.8 |
| hippocampus, brain | 191.2 | 198.3 | — | 225.0 | 237.5 | 239.6 |
| humerus (any part) | 170.4 | 198.5 | — | 213.4 | 238.0 | 239.2 |
| hymen | 184.0 | 198.82 | 233.31 ▲ | 221.1 | 236.3 | 239.5 |
| hypopharynx, hypopharyngeal NEC | 148.9 | 198.89 | 230.0 | 210.8 | 235.1 | 239.0 |
| contiguous sites | 148.8 | — | — | — | — | — |
| postcricoid region | 148.0 | 198.89 | 230.0 | 210.8 | 235.1 | 239.0 |
| posterior wall | 148.3 | 198.89 | 230.0 | 210.8 | 235.1 | 239.0 |
| pyriform fossa (sinus) | 148.1 | 198.89 | 230.0 | 210.8 | 235.1 | 239.0 |
| specified site NEC | 148.8 | 198.89 | 230.0 | 210.8 | 235.1 | 239.0 |
| wall | 148.9 | 198.89 | 230.0 | 210.8 | 235.1 | 239.0 |
| posterior | 148.3 | 198.89 | 230.0 | 210.8 | 235.1 | 239.0 |
| hypophysis | 194.3 | 198.89 | 234.8 | 227.3 | 237.0 | 239.7 |
| hypothalamus | 191.0 | 198.3 | — | 225.0 | 237.5 | 239.6 |
| ileocecum, ileocecal (coil) (junction) (valve) | 153.4 | 197.5 | 230.3 | 211.3 | 235.2 | 239.0 |
| ileum | 152.2 | 197.4 | 230.7 | 211.2 | 235.2 | 239.0 |
| ilium | 170.6 | 198.5 | — | 213.6 | 238.0 | 239.2 |
| immunoproliferative NEC | 203.8 ☑ | — | — | — | — | — |
| infraclavicular (region)* | 195.1 | 198.89 | 232.5 | 229.8 | 238.8 | 239.8 |
| inguinal (region)* | 195.3 | 198.89 | 232.5 | 229.8 | 238.8 | 239.8 |
| insula | 191.0 | 198.3 | — | 225.0 | 237.5 | 239.6 |

| | Malignant | | | | | |
| --- | Primary | Secondary | Ca in situ | Benign | Uncertain Behavior | Unspecified |
| --- | --- | --- | --- | --- | --- | --- |
| **Neoplasm, neoplastic —** continued | | | | | | |
| insular tissue | | | | | | |
| (pancreas) | 157.4 | 197.8 | 230.9 | 211.7 | 235.5 | 239.0 |
| brain | 191.0 | 198.3 | — | 225.0 | 237.5 | 239.6 |
| interarytenoid fold | 148.2 | 198.89 | 230.0 | 210.8 | 235.1 | 239.0 |
| hypopharyngeal aspect | 148.2 | 198.89 | 230.0 | 210.8 | 235.1 | 239.0 |
| laryngeal aspect | 161.1 | 197.3 | 231.0 | 212.1 | 235.6 | 239.1 |
| marginal zone | 148.2 | 198.89 | 230.0 | 210.8 | 235.1 | 239.0 |
| interdental papillae | 143.9 | 198.89 | 230.0 | 210.4 | 235.1 | 239.0 |
| lower | 143.1 | 198.89 | 230.0 | 210.4 | 235.1 | 239.0 |
| upper | 143.0 | 198.89 | 230.0 | 210.4 | 235.1 | 239.0 |
| internal | | | | | | |
| capsule | 191.0 | 198.3 | — | 225.0 | 237.5 | 239.6 |
| os (cervix) | 180.0 | 198.82 | 233.1 | 219.0 | 236.0 | 239.5 |
| intervertebral cartilage or disc | 170.2 | 198.5 | — | 213.2 | 238.0 | 239.2 |
| intestine, intestinal | 159.0 | 197.8 | 230.7 | 211.9 | 235.2 | 239.0 |
| large | 153.9 | 197.5 | 230.3 | 211.3 | 235.2 | 239.0 |
| appendix | 153.5 | 197.5 | 230.3 | 211.3 | 235.2 | 239.0 |
| caput coli | 153.4 | 197.5 | 230.3 | 211.3 | 235.2 | 239.0 |
| cecum | 153.4 | 197.5 | 230.3 | 211.3 | 235.2 | 239.0 |
| colon | 153.9 | 197.5 | 230.3 | 211.3 | 235.2 | 239.0 |
| and rectum | 154.0 | 197.5 | 230.4 | 211.4 | 235.2 | 239.0 |
| ascending | 153.6 | 197.5 | 230.3 | 211.3 | 235.2 | 239.0 |
| caput | 153.4 | 197.5 | 230.3 | 211.3 | 235.2 | 239.0 |
| contiguous sites | 153.8 | — | — | — | — | — |
| descending | 153.2 | 197.5 | 230.3 | 211.3 | 235.2 | 239.0 |
| distal | 153.2 | 197.5 | 230.3 | 211.3 | 235.2 | 239.0 |
| left | 153.2 | 197.5 | 230.3 | 211.3 | 235.2 | 239.0 |
| pelvic | 153.3 | 197.5 | 230.3 | 211.3 | 235.2 | 239.0 |
| right | 153.6 | 197.5 | 230.3 | 211.3 | 235.2 | 239.0 |
| sigmoid (flexure) | 153.3 | 197.5 | 230.3 | 211.3 | 235.2 | 239.0 |
| transverse | 153.1 | 197.5 | 230.3 | 211.3 | 235.2 | 239.0 |
| contiguous sites | 153.8 | — | — | — | — | — |
| hepatic flexure | 153.0 | 197.5 | 230.3 | 211.3 | 235.2 | 239.0 |
| ileocecum, ileocecal (coil) (valve) | 153.4 | 197.5 | 230.3 | 211.3 | 235.2 | 239.0 |
| sigmoid flexure (lower) (upper) | 153.3 | 197.5 | 230.3 | 211.3 | 235.2 | 239.0 |
| splenic flexure | 153.7 | 197.5 | 230.3 | 211.3 | 235.2 | 239.0 |
| small | 152.9 | 197.4 | 230.7 | 211.2 | 235.2 | 239.0 |
| contiguous sites | 152.8 | — | — | — | — | — |
| duodenum | 152.0 | 197.4 | 230.7 | 211.2 | 235.2 | 239.0 |
| ileum | 152.2 | 197.4 | 230.7 | 211.2 | 235.2 | 239.0 |
| jejunum | 152.1 | 197.4 | 230.7 | 211.2 | 235.2 | 239.0 |
| tract NEC | 159.0 | 197.8 | 230.7 | 211.9 | 235.2 | 239.0 |
| intra-abdominal | 195.2 | 198.89 | 234.8 | 229.8 | 238.8 | 239.8 |
| intracranial NEC | 191.9 | 198.3 | — | 225.0 | 237.5 | 239.6 |
| intrahepatic (bile) duct | 155.1 | 197.8 | 230.8 | 211.5 | 235.3 | 239.0 |
| intraocular | 190.0 | 198.4 | 234.0 | 224.0 | 238.8 | 239.8 |
| intraorbital | 190.1 | 198.4 | 234.0 | 224.1 | 238.8 | 239.8 |
| intrasellar | 194.3 | 198.89 | 234.8 | 227.3 | 237.0 | 239.7 |
| intrathoracic (cavity) (organs NEC) | 195.1 | 198.89 | 234.8 | 229.8 | 238.8 | 239.8 |
| contiguous sites with respiratory organs | 165.8 | — | — | — | — | — |
| iris | 190.0 | 198.4 | 234.0 | 224.0 | 238.8 | 239.8 |
| ischiorectal (fossa) | 195.3 | 198.89 | 234.8 | 229.8 | 238.8 | 239.8 |
| ischium | 170.6 | 198.5 | — | 213.6 | 238.0 | 239.2 |
| island of Reil | 191.0 | 198.3 | — | 225.0 | 237.5 | 239.6 |
| islands or islets of Langerhans | 157.4 | 197.8 | 230.9 | 211.7 | 235.5 | 239.0 |
| isthmus uteri | 182.1 | 198.82 | 233.2 | 219.1 | 236.0 | 239.5 |
| jaw | 195.0 | 198.89 | 234.8 | 229.8 | 238.8 | 239.8 |
| bone | 170.1 | 198.5 | — | 213.1 | 238.0 | 239.2 |
| carcinoma | 143.9 | — | — | — | — | — |
| lower | 143.1 | — | — | — | — | — |
| upper | 143.0 | — | — | — | — | — |
| lower | 170.1 | 198.5 | — | 213.1 | 238.0 | 239.2 |
| upper | 170.0 | 198.5 | — | 213.0 | 238.0 | 239.2 |
| carcinoma (any type) (lower)(upper) | 195.0 | — | — | — | — | — |
| skin | 173.3 | 198.2 | 232.3 | 216.3 | 238.2 | 239.2 |
| **Neoplasm, neoplastic —** continued | | | | | | |
| jaw — continued | | | | | | |
| soft tissues | 143.9 | 198.89 | 230.0 | 210.4 | 235.1 | 239.0 |
| lower | 143.1 | 198.89 | 230.0 | 210.4 | 235.1 | 239.0 |
| upper | 143.0 | 198.89 | 230.0 | 210.4 | 235.1 | 239.0 |
| jejunum | 152.1 | 197.4 | 230.7 | 211.2 | 235.2 | 239.0 |
| joint NEC (see also Neoplasm, bone) | 170.9 | 198.5 | — | 213.9 | 238.0 | 239.2 |
| acromioclavicular | 170.4 | 198.5 | — | 213.4 | 238.0 | 239.2 |
| bursa or synovial membrane — see Neoplasm, connective tissue | | | | | | |
| costovertebral | 170.3 | 198.5 | — | 213.3 | 238.0 | 239.2 |
| sternocostal | 170.3 | 198.5 | — | 213.3 | 238.0 | 239.2 |
| temporomandibular | 170.1 | 198.5 | — | 213.1 | 238.0 | 239.2 |
| junction | | | | | | |
| anorectal | 154.8 | 197.5 | 230.7 | 211.4 | 235.5 | 239.0 |
| cardioesophageal | 151.0 | 197.8 | 230.2 | 211.1 | 235.2 | 239.0 |
| esophagogastric | 151.0 | 197.8 | 230.2 | 211.1 | 235.2 | 239.0 |
| gastroesophageal | 151.0 | 197.8 | 230.2 | 211.1 | 235.2 | 239.0 |
| hard and soft palate | 145.5 | 198.89 | 230.0 | 210.4 | 235.1 | 239.0 |
| ileocecal | 153.4 | 197.5 | 230.3 | 211.3 | 235.2 | 239.0 |
| pelvirectal | 154.0 | 197.5 | 230.4 | 211.4 | 235.2 | 239.0 |
| pelviureteric | 189.1 | 198.0 | 233.9 | 223.1 | 236.91 | 239.5 |
| rectosigmoid | 154.0 | 197.5 | 230.4 | 211.4 | 235.2 | 239.0 |
| squamocolumnar, of cervix | 180.8 | 198.82 | 233.1 | 219.0 | 236.0 | 239.5 |
| kidney (parenchyma) | 189.0 | 198.0 | 233.9 | 223.0 | 236.91 | 239.5 |
| calyx | 189.1 | 198.0 | 233.9 | 223.1 | 236.91 | 239.5 |
| hilus | 189.1 | 198.0 | 233.9 | 223.1 | 236.91 | 239.5 |
| pelvis | 189.1 | 198.0 | 233.9 | 223.1 | 236.91 | 239.5 |
| knee NEC* | 195.5 | 198.89 | 232.7 | 229.8 | 238.8 | 239.8 |
| labia (skin) | 184.4 | 198.82 | 233.32 ▲ | 221.2 | 236.3 | 239.5 |
| majora | 184.1 | 198.82 | 233.32 ▲ | 221.2 | 236.3 | 239.5 |
| minora | 184.2 | 198.82 | 233.32 ▲ | 221.2 | 236.3 | 239.5 |
| labial (see also Neoplasm, lip) | | | | | | |
| sulcus (lower) (upper) | 145.1 | 198.89 | 230.0 | 210.4 | 235.1 | 239.0 |
| labium (skin) | 184.4 | 198.82 | 233.32 ▲ | 221.2 | 236.3 | 239.5 |
| majus | 184.1 | 198.82 | 233.32 ▲ | 221.2 | 236.3 | 239.5 |
| minus | 184.2 | 198.82 | 233.32 ▲ | 221.2 | 236.3 | 239.5 |
| lacrimal | | | | | | |
| canaliculi | 190.7 | 198.4 | 234.0 | 224.7 | 238.8 | 239.8 |
| duct (nasal) | 190.7 | 198.4 | 234.0 | 224.7 | 238.8 | 239.8 |
| gland | 190.2 | 198.4 | 234.0 | 224.2 | 238.8 | 239.8 |
| punctum | 190.7 | 198.4 | 234.0 | 224.7 | 238.8 | 239.8 |
| sac | 190.7 | 198.4 | 234.0 | 224.7 | 238.8 | 239.8 |
| Langerhans, islands or islets | 157.4 | 197.8 | 230.9 | 211.7 | 235.5 | 239.0 |
| laryngopharynx | 148.9 | 198.89 | 230.0 | 210.8 | 235.1 | 239.0 |
| larynx, laryngeal NEC | 161.9 | 197.3 | 231.0 | 212.1 | 235.6 | 239.1 |
| aryepiglottic fold | 161.1 | 197.3 | 231.0 | 212.1 | 235.6 | 239.1 |
| cartilage (arytenoid) (cricoid) (cuneiform) (thyroid) | 161.3 | 197.3 | 231.0 | 212.1 | 235.6 | 239.1 |
| commissure (anterior) (posterior) | 161.0 | 197.3 | 231.0 | 212.1 | 235.6 | 239.1 |
| contiguous sites | 161.8 | — | — | — | — | — |
| extrinsic NEC | 161.1 | 197.3 | 231.0 | 212.1 | 235.6 | 239.1 |
| meaning hypopharynx | 148.9 | 198.89 | 230.0 | 210.8 | 235.1 | 239.0 |
| interarytenoid fold | 161.1 | 197.3 | 231.0 | 212.1 | 235.6 | 239.1 |
| intrinsic | 161.0 | 197.3 | 231.0 | 212.1 | 235.6 | 239.1 |
| ventricular band | 161.1 | 197.3 | 231.0 | 212.1 | 235.6 | 239.1 |
| leg NEC* | 195.5 | 198.89 | 232.7 | 229.8 | 238.8 | 239.8 |
| lens, crystalline | 190.0 | 198.4 | 234.0 | 224.0 | 238.8 | 239.8 |
| lid (lower) (upper) | 173.1 | 198.2 | 232.1 | 216.1 | 238.2 | 239.2 |
| ligament (see also Neoplasm, connective tissue) | | | | | | |
| broad | 183.3 | 198.82 | 233.39 ▲ | 221.0 | 236.3 | 239.5 |
| Mackenrodt's | 183.8 | 198.82 | 233.39 ▲ | 221.8 | 236.3 | 239.5 |
| non-uterine — see Neoplasm, connective tissue | | | | | | |

☑ Additional Digit Required — Refer to the Tabular List for Digit Selection      ᴺᴱᶜ Subterms under main terms may continue to next column or page

**2008 ICD-9-CM**    ▶◀ Revised Text    ● New Line    ▲ Revised Code    **October 2007 • Volume 2 — 203**

| | Malignant | | | | | |
|---|---|---|---|---|---|---|
| Neoplasm, neoplastic — *continued* | Primary | Secondary | Ca in situ | Benign | Uncertain Behavior | Unspecified |
| ligament (*see also* Neoplasm, connective tissue) — *continued* | | | | | | |
| round | 183.5 | 198.82 | — | 221.0 | 236.3 | 239.5 |
| sacro-uterine | 183.4 | 198.82 | — | 221.0 | 236.3 | 239.5 |
| uterine | 183.4 | 198.82 | — | 221.0 | 236.3 | 239.5 |
| utero-ovarian | 183.8 | 198.82 | 233.39 ▲ | 221.8 | 236.3 | 239.5 |
| uterosacral | 183.4 | 198.82 | — | 221.0 | 236.3 | 239.5 |
| limb* | 195.8 | 198.89 | 232.8 | 229.8 | 238.8 | 239.8 |
| lower* | 195.5 | 198.89 | 232.7 | 229.8 | 238.8 | 239.8 |
| upper* | 195.4 | 198.89 | 232.6 | 229.8 | 238.8 | 239.8 |
| limbus of cornea | 190.4 | 198.4 | 234.0 | 224.4 | 238.8 | 239.8 |
| lingual NEC (*see also* Neoplasm, tongue) | 141.9 | 198.89 | 230.0 | 210.1 | 235.1 | 239.0 |
| lingula, lung | 162.3 | 197.0 | 231.2 | 212.3 | 235.7 | 239.1 |
| lip (external) (lipstick area) (vermillion border) | 140.9 | 198.89 | 230.0 | 210.0 | 235.1 | 239.0 |
| buccal aspect — *see* Neoplasm, lip, internal | | | | | | |
| commissure | 140.6 | 198.89 | 230.0 | 210.4 | 235.1 | 239.0 |
| contiguous sites | 140.8 | — | — | — | — | — |
| with oral cavity or pharynx | 149.8 | — | — | — | — | — |
| frenulum — *see* Neoplasm, lip, internal | | | | | | |
| inner aspect — *see* Neoplasm, lip, internal | | | | | | |
| internal (buccal) (frenulum) (mucosa) (oral) | 140.5 | 198.89 | 230.0 | 210.0 | 235.1 | 239.0 |
| lower | 140.4 | 198.89 | 230.0 | 210.0 | 235.1 | 239.0 |
| upper | 140.3 | 198.89 | 230.0 | 210.0 | 235.1 | 239.0 |
| lower | 140.1 | 198.89 | 230.0 | 210.0 | 235.1 | 239.0 |
| internal (buccal) (frenulum) (mucosa) (oral) | 140.4 | 198.89 | 230.0 | 210.0 | 235.1 | 239.0 |
| mucosa — *see* Neoplasm, lip, internal | | | | | | |
| oral aspect — *see* Neoplasm, lip, internal | | | | | | |
| skin (commissure) (lower) (upper) | 173.0 | 198.2 | 232.0 | 216.0 | 238.2 | 239.2 |
| upper | 140.0 | 198.89 | 230.0 | 210.0 | 235.1 | 239.0 |
| internal (buccal) (frenulum) (mucosa) (oral) | 140.3 | 198.89 | 230.0 | 210.0 | 235.1 | 239.0 |
| liver | 155.2 | 197.7 | 230.8 | 211.5 | 235.3 | 239.0 |
| primary | 155.0 | — | — | — | — | — |
| lobe | | | | | | |
| azygos | 162.3 | 197.0 | 231.2 | 212.3 | 235.7 | 239.1 |
| frontal | 191.1 | 198.3 | — | 225.0 | 237.5 | 239.6 |
| lower | 162.5 | 197.0 | 231.2 | 212.3 | 235.7 | 239.1 |
| middle | 162.4 | 197.0 | 231.2 | 212.3 | 235.7 | 239.1 |
| occipital | 191.4 | 198.3 | — | 225.0 | 237.5 | 239.6 |
| parietal | 191.3 | 198.3 | — | 225.0 | 237.5 | 239.6 |
| temporal | 191.2 | 198.3 | — | 225.0 | 237.5 | 239.6 |
| upper | 162.3 | 197.0 | 231.2 | 212.3 | 235.7 | 239.1 |
| lumbosacral plexus | 171.6 | 198.4 | — | 215.6 | 238.1 | 239.2 |
| lung | 162.9 | 197.0 | 231.2 | 212.3 | 235.7 | 239.1 |
| azygos lobe | 162.3 | 197.0 | 231.2 | 212.3 | 235.7 | 239.1 |
| carina | 162.2 | 197.0 | 231.2 | 212.3 | 235.7 | 239.1 |
| contiguous sites with bronchus or trachea | 162.8 | — | — | — | — | — |
| hilus | 162.2 | 197.0 | 231.2 | 212.3 | 235.7 | 239.1 |
| lingula | 162.3 | 197.0 | 231.2 | 212.3 | 235.7 | 239.1 |
| lobe NEC | 162.9 | 197.0 | 231.2 | 212.3 | 235.7 | 239.1 |
| lower lobe | 162.5 | 197.0 | 231.2 | 212.3 | 235.7 | 239.1 |

| | Malignant | | | | | |
|---|---|---|---|---|---|---|
| Neoplasm, neoplastic — *continued* | Primary | Secondary | Ca in situ | Benign | Uncertain Behavior | Unspecified |
| lung — *continued* | | | | | | |
| main bronchus | 162.2 | 197.0 | 231.2 | 212.3 | 235.7 | 239.1 |
| middle lobe | 162.4 | 197.0 | 231.2 | 212.3 | 235.7 | 239.1 |
| upper lobe | 162.3 | 197.0 | 231.2 | 212.3 | 235.7 | 239.1 |
| lymph, lymphatic | | | | | | |
| channel NEC (*see also* Neoplasm, connective tissue) | 171.9 | 198.89 | — | 215.9 | 238.1 | 239.2 |
| gland (secondary) | — | 196.9 | — | 229.0 | 238.8 | 239.8 |
| abdominal | — | 196.2 | — | 229.0 | 238.8 | 239.8 |
| aortic | — | 196.2 | — | 229.0 | 238.8 | 239.8 |
| arm | — | 196.3 | — | 229.0 | 238.8 | 239.8 |
| auricular (anterior) (posterior) | — | 196.0 | — | 229.0 | 238.8 | 239.8 |
| axilla, axillary | — | 196.3 | — | 229.0 | 238.8 | 239.8 |
| brachial | — | 196.3 | — | 229.0 | 238.8 | 239.8 |
| bronchial | — | 196.1 | — | 229.0 | 238.8 | 239.8 |
| bronchopulmonary | — | 196.1 | — | 229.0 | 238.8 | 239.8 |
| celiac | — | 196.2 | — | 229.0 | 238.8 | 239.8 |
| cervical | — | 196.0 | — | 229.0 | 238.8 | 239.8 |
| cervicofacial | — | 196.0 | — | 229.0 | 238.8 | 239.8 |
| Cloquet | — | 196.5 | — | 229.0 | 238.8 | 239.8 |
| colic | — | 196.2 | — | 229.0 | 238.8 | 239.8 |
| common duct | — | 196.2 | — | 229.0 | 238.8 | 239.8 |
| cubital | — | 196.3 | — | 229.0 | 238.8 | 239.8 |
| diaphragmatic | — | 196.1 | — | 229.0 | 238.8 | 239.8 |
| epigastric, inferior | — | 196.6 | — | 229.0 | 238.8 | 239.8 |
| epitrochlear | — | 196.3 | — | 229.0 | 238.8 | 239.8 |
| esophageal | — | 196.1 | — | 229.0 | 238.8 | 239.8 |
| face | — | 196.0 | — | 229.0 | 238.8 | 239.8 |
| femoral | — | 196.5 | — | 229.0 | 238.8 | 239.8 |
| gastric | — | 196.2 | — | 229.0 | 238.8 | 239.8 |
| groin | — | 196.5 | — | 229.0 | 238.8 | 239.8 |
| head | — | 196.0 | — | 229.0 | 238.8 | 239.8 |
| hepatic | — | 196.2 | — | 229.0 | 238.8 | 239.8 |
| hilar (pulmonary) | — | 196.1 | — | 229.0 | 238.8 | 239.8 |
| splenic | — | 196.2 | — | 229.0 | 238.8 | 239.8 |
| hypogastric | — | 196.6 | — | 229.0 | 238.8 | 239.8 |
| ileocolic | — | 196.2 | — | 229.0 | 238.8 | 239.8 |
| iliac | — | 196.6 | — | 229.0 | 238.8 | 239.8 |
| infraclavicular | — | 196.3 | — | 229.0 | 238.8 | 239.8 |
| inguina, inguinal | — | 196.5 | — | 229.0 | 238.8 | 239.8 |
| innominate | — | 196.1 | — | 229.0 | 238.8 | 239.8 |
| intercostal | — | 196.1 | — | 229.0 | 238.8 | 239.8 |
| intestinal | — | 196.2 | — | 229.0 | 238.8 | 239.8 |
| intra-abdominal | — | 196.2 | — | 229.0 | 238.8 | 239.8 |
| intrapelvic | — | 196.6 | — | 229.0 | 238.8 | 239.8 |
| intrathoracic | — | 196.1 | — | 229.0 | 238.8 | 239.9 |
| jugular | — | 196.0 | — | 229.0 | 238.8 | 239.8 |
| leg | — | 196.5 | — | 229.0 | 238.8 | 239.8 |
| limb | | | | | | |
| lower | — | 196.5 | — | 229.0 | 238.8 | 239.8 |
| upper | — | 196.3 | — | 229.0 | 238.8 | 239.8 |
| lower limb | — | 196.5 | — | 229.0 | 238.8 | 238.9 |
| lumbar | — | 196.2 | — | 229.0 | 238.8 | 239.8 |
| mandibular | — | 196.0 | — | 229.0 | 238.8 | 239.8 |
| mediastinal | — | 196.1 | — | 229.0 | 238.8 | 239.8 |
| mesenteric (inferior) (superior) | — | 196.2 | — | 229.0 | 238.8 | 239.8 |
| midcolic | — | 196.2 | — | 229.0 | 238.8 | 239.8 |
| multiple sites in categories 196.0–196.6 | — | 196.8 | — | 229.0 | 238.8 | 239.8 |
| neck | — | 196.0 | — | 229.0 | 238.8 | 239.8 |
| obturator | — | 196.6 | — | 229.0 | 238.8 | 239.8 |
| occipital | — | 196.0 | — | 229.0 | 238.8 | 239.8 |
| pancreatic | — | 196.2 | — | 229.0 | 238.8 | 239.8 |
| para-aortic | — | 196.2 | — | 229.0 | 238.8 | 239.8 |
| paracervical | — | 196.6 | — | 229.0 | 238.8 | 239.8 |
| parametrial | — | 196.6 | — | 229.0 | 238.8 | 239.8 |
| parasternal | — | 196.1 | — | 229.0 | 238.8 | 239.8 |
| parotid | — | 196.0 | — | 229.0 | 238.8 | 239.8 |
| pectoral | — | 196.3 | — | 229.0 | 238.8 | 239.8 |
| pelvic | — | 196.6 | — | 229.0 | 238.8 | 239.8 |
| peri-aortic | — | 196.2 | — | 229.0 | 238.8 | 239.8 |

☑ Additional Digit Required — Refer to the Tabular List for Digit Selection      ꜙꜙꜙ Subterms under main terms may continue to next column or page

204 — Volume 2 · October 2007     ▶◀ Revised Text     ● New Line     ▲ Revised Code     *2008 ICD-9-CM*

| Neoplasm, neoplastic — continued | Malignant | | | Benign | Uncertain Behavior | Unspecified |
|---|---|---|---|---|---|---|
| | Primary | Secondary | Ca in situ | | | |
| lymph, lymphatic — *continued* | | | | | | |
| gland — *continued* | | | | | | |
| peripancreatic | — | 196.2 | — | 229.0 | 238.8 | 239.8 |
| popliteal | — | 196.5 | — | 229.0 | 238.8 | 239.8 |
| porta hepatis | — | 196.2 | — | 229.0 | 238.8 | 239.8 |
| portal | — | 196.2 | — | 229.0 | 238.8 | 239.8 |
| preauricular | — | 196.0 | — | 229.0 | 238.8 | 239.8 |
| prelaryngeal | — | 196.0 | — | 229.0 | 238.8 | 239.8 |
| presymphysial | — | 196.6 | — | 229.0 | 238.8 | 239.8 |
| pretracheal | — | 196.0 | — | 229.0 | 238.8 | 239.8 |
| primary (any site) NEC | 202.9 ☑ | — | — | — | — | — |
| pulmonary (hiler) | — | 196.1 | — | 229.0 | 238.8 | 239.8 |
| pyloric | — | 196.2 | — | 229.0 | 238.8 | 239.8 |
| retroperitoneal | — | 196.2 | — | 229.0 | 238.8 | 239.8 |
| retropharyngeal | — | 196.0 | — | 229.0 | 238.8 | 239.8 |
| Rosenmüller's | — | 196.5 | — | 229.0 | 238.8 | 239.8 |
| sacral | — | 196.6 | — | 229.0 | 238.8 | 239.8 |
| scalene | — | 196.0 | — | 229.0 | 238.8 | 239.8 |
| site NEC | — | 196.9 | — | 229.0 | 238.8 | 239.8 |
| splenic (hilar) | — | 196.2 | — | 229.0 | 238.8 | 239.8 |
| subclavicular | — | 196.3 | — | 229.0 | 238.8 | 239.8 |
| subinguinal | — | 196.5 | — | 229.0 | 238.8 | 239.8 |
| sublingual | — | 196.0 | — | 229.0 | 238.8 | 239.8 |
| submandibular | — | 196.0 | — | 229.0 | 238.8 | 239.8 |
| submaxillary | — | 196.0 | — | 229.0 | 238.8 | 239.8 |
| submental | — | 196.0 | — | 229.0 | 238.8 | 239.8 |
| subscapular | — | 196.3 | — | 229.0 | 238.8 | 239.8 |
| supraclavicular | — | 196.0 | — | 229.0 | 238.8 | 239.8 |
| thoracic | — | 196.1 | — | 229.0 | 238.8 | 239.8 |
| tibial | — | 196.5 | — | 229.0 | 238.8 | 239.8 |
| tracheal | — | 196.1 | — | 229.0 | 238.8 | 239.8 |
| tracheobronchial | — | 196.1 | — | 229.0 | 238.8 | 239.8 |
| upper limb | — | 196.3 | — | 229.0 | 238.8 | 239.8 |
| Virchow's | — | 196.0 | — | 229.0 | 238.8 | 239.8 |
| node (*see also* Neoplasm, lymph gland) primary NEC | 202.9 ☑ | — | — | — | — | — |
| vessel (*see also* Neoplasm, connective tissue) | 171.9 | 198.89 | — | 215.9 | 238.1 | 239.2 |
| ►Mackenrodt's◄ ligament | 183.8 | 198.82 | 233.39 ▲ | 221.8 | 236.3 | 239.5 |
| malar | 170.0 | 198.5 | — | 213.0 | 238.0 | 239.2 |
| region — *see* Neoplasm, cheek | | | | | | |
| mammary gland — *see* Neoplasm, breast | | | | | | |
| mandible | 170.1 | 198.5 | — | 213.1 | 238.0 | 239.2 |
| alveolar | | | | | | |
| mucose | 143.1 | 198.89 | 230.0 | 210.4 | 235.1 | 239.0 |
| ridge or process | 170.1 | 198.5 | — | 213.1 | 238.0 | 239.2 |
| carcinoma | 143.1 | — | — | — | — | — |
| carcinoma | 143.1 | — | — | — | — | — |
| marrow (bone) NEC | 202.9 ☑ | 198.5 | — | — | — | 238.79 |
| mastectomy site (skin) | 173.5 | 198.2 | — | — | — | — |
| specified as breast tissue | 174.8 | 198.81 | — | — | — | — |
| mastoid (air cells) (antrum) (cavity) | 160.1 | 197.3 | 231.8 | 212.0 | 235.9 | 239.1 |
| bone or process | 170.0 | 198.5 | — | 213.0 | 238.0 | 239.2 |
| maxilla, maxillary (superior) | 170.0 | 198.5 | — | 213.0 | 238.0 | 239.2 |
| alveolar | | | | | | |
| mucosa | 143.0 | 198.89 | 230.0 | 210.4 | 235.1 | 239.0 |
| ridge or process | 170.0 | 198.5 | — | 213.0 | 238.0 | 239.2 |
| carcinoma | 143.0 | — | — | — | — | — |
| antrum | 160.2 | 197.3 | 231.8 | 212.0 | 235.9 | 239.1 |
| carcinoma | 143.0 | — | — | — | — | — |
| inferior — *see* Neoplasm, mandible | | | | | | |
| sinus | 160.2 | 197.3 | 231.8 | 212.0 | 235.9 | 239.1 |
| meatus | | | | | | |
| external (ear) | 173.2 | 198.2 | 232.2 | 216.2 | 238.2 | 239.2 |

| Neoplasm, neoplastic — continued | Malignant | | | Benign | Uncertain Behavior | Unspecified |
|---|---|---|---|---|---|---|
| | Primary | Secondary | Ca in situ | | | |
| Meckel's diverticulum | 152.3 | 197.4 | 230.7 | 211.2 | 235.2 | 239.0 |
| mediastinum, mediastinal | 164.9 | 197.1 | — | 212.5 | 235.8 | 239.8 |
| anterior | 164.2 | 197.1 | — | 212.5 | 235.8 | 239.8 |
| contiguous sites with heart and thymus | 164.8 | — | — | — | — | — |
| posterior | 164.3 | 197.1 | — | 212.5 | 235.8 | 239.8 |
| medulla | | | | | | |
| adrenal | 194.0 | 198.7 | 234.8 | 227.0 | 237.2 | 239.7 |
| oblongata | 191.7 | 198.3 | — | 225.0 | 237.5 | 239.6 |
| meibomian gland | 173.1 | 198.2 | 232.1 | 216.1 | 238.2 | 239.2 |
| meninges (brain) (cerebral) (cranial) (intracranial) | 192.1 | 198.4 | — | 225.2 | 237.6 | 239.7 |
| spinal (cord) | 192.3 | 198.4 | — | 225.4 | 237.6 | 239.7 |
| meniscus, knee joint (lateral) (medial) | 170.7 | 198.5 | — | 213.7 | 238.0 | 239.2 |
| mesentery, mesenteric | 158.8 | 197.6 | — | 211.8 | 235.4 | 239.0 |
| mesoappendix | 158.8 | 197.6 | — | 211.8 | 235.4 | 239.0 |
| mesocolon | 158.8 | 197.6 | — | 211.8 | 235.4 | 239.0 |
| mesopharynx — *see* Neoplasm, oropharynx | | | | | | |
| mesosalpinx | 183.3 | 198.82 | 233.39 ▲ | 221.0 | 236.3 | 239.5 |
| mesovarium | 183.3 | 198.82 | 233.39 ▲ | 221.0 | 236.3 | 239.5 |
| metacarpus (any bone) | 170.5 | 198.5 | — | 213.5 | 238.0 | 239.2 |
| metastatic NEC (*see also* Neoplasm, by site, secondary) | — | 199.1 | — | — | — | — |
| metatarsus (any bone) | 170.8 | 198.5 | — | 213.8 | 238.0 | 239.2 |
| midbrain | 191.7 | 198.3 | — | 225.0 | 237.5 | 239.6 |
| milk duct — *see* Neoplasm, breast | | | | | | |
| mons | | | | | | |
| pubis | 184.4 | 198.82 | 233.32 ▲ | 221.2 | 236.3 | 239.5 |
| veneris | 184.4 | 198.82 | 233.32 ▲ | 221.2 | 236.3 | 239.5 |
| motor tract | 192.9 | 198.4 | — | 225.9 | 237.9 | 239.7 |
| brain | 191.9 | 198.3 | — | 225.0 | 237.5 | 239.6 |
| spinal | 192.2 | 198.3 | — | 225.3 | 237.5 | 239.7 |
| mouth | 145.9 | 198.89 | 230.0 | 210.4 | 235.1 | 239.0 |
| contiguous sites | 145.8 | — | — | — | — | — |
| floor | 144.9 | 198.89 | 230.0 | 210.3 | 235.1 | 239.0 |
| anterior portion | 144.0 | 198.89 | 230.0 | 210.3 | 235.1 | 239.0 |
| contiguous sites | 144.8 | — | — | — | — | — |
| lateral portion | 144.1 | 198.89 | 230.0 | 210.3 | 235.1 | 239.0 |
| roof | 145.5 | 198.89 | 230.0 | 210.4 | 235.1 | 239.0 |
| specified part NEC | 145.8 | 198.89 | 230.0 | 210.4 | 235.1 | 239.0 |
| vestibule | 145.1 | 198.89 | 230.0 | 210.4 | 235.1 | 239.0 |
| mucosa | | | | | | |
| alveolar (ridge or process) | 143.9 | 198.89 | 230.0 | 210.4 | 235.1 | 239.0 |
| lower | 143.1 | 198.89 | 230.0 | 210.4 | 235.1 | 239.0 |
| upper | 143.0 | 198.89 | 230.0 | 210.4 | 235.1 | 239.0 |
| buccal | 145.0 | 198.89 | 230.0 | 210.4 | 235.1 | 239.0 |
| cheek | 145.0 | 198.89 | 230.0 | 210.4 | 235.1 | 239.0 |
| lip — *see* Neoplasm, lip, internal | | | | | | |
| nasal | 160.0 | 197.3 | 231.8 | 212.0 | 235.9 | 239.1 |
| oral | 145.0 | 198.89 | 230.0 | 210.4 | 235.1 | 239.0 |
| Müllerian duct | | | | | | |
| female | 184.8 | 198.82 | 233.39 ▲ | 221.8 | 236.3 | 239.5 |
| male | 187.8 | 198.82 | 233.6 | 222.8 | 236.6 | 239.5 |
| multiple sites NEC | 199.0 | 199.0 | 234.9 | 229.9 | 238.9 | 199.0 |
| muscle (*see also* Neoplasm, connective tissue) | | | | | | |
| extraocular | 190.1 | 198.4 | 234.0 | 224.1 | 238.8 | 239.8 |
| myocardium | 164.1 | 198.89 | — | 212.7 | 238.8 | 239.8 |
| myometrium | 182.0 | 198.82 | 233.2 | 219.1 | 236.0 | 239.5 |
| myopericardium | 164.1 | 198.89 | — | 212.7 | 238.8 | 239.8 |
| nabothian gland (follicle) | 180.0 | 198.82 | 233.1 | 219.0 | 236.0 | 239.5 |
| nail | 173.9 | 198.2 | 232.9 | 216.9 | 238.2 | 239.2 |
| finger | 173.6 | 198.2 | 232.6 | 216.6 | 238.2 | 239.2 |
| toe | 173.7 | 198.2 | 232.7 | 216.7 | 238.2 | 239.2 |

☑ Additional Digit Required — Refer to the Tabular List for Digit Selection     ⬆ Subterms under main terms may continue to next column or page

Index — Neoplasm, nares, naris — Neoplasm, paraganglion

| | Malignant | | | | | |
|---|---|---|---|---|---|---|
| | Primary | Secondary | Ca in situ | Benign | Uncertain Behavior | Unspecified |
| **Neoplasm, neoplastic —** *continued* | | | | | | |
| nares, naris (anterior) (posterior) | 160.0 | 197.3 | 231.8 | 212.0 | 235.9 | 239.1 |
| nasal — *see* Neoplasm, nose | | | | | | |
| nasolabial groove | 173.3 | 198.2 | 232.3 | 216.3 | 238.2 | 239.2 |
| nasolacrimal duct | 190.7 | 198.4 | 234.0 | 224.7 | 238.8 | 239.8 |
| nasopharynx, nasopharyngeal | 147.9 | 198.89 | 230.0 | 210.7 | 235.1 | 239.0 |
| contiguous sites | 147.8 | — | — | — | — | — |
| floor | 147.3 | 198.89 | 230.0 | 210.7 | 235.1 | 239.0 |
| roof | 147.0 | 198.89 | 230.0 | 210.7 | 235.1 | 239.0 |
| specified site NEC | 147.8 | 198.89 | 230.0 | 210.7 | 235.1 | 239.0 |
| wall | 147.9 | 198.89 | 230.0 | 210.7 | 235.1 | 239.0 |
| anterior | 147.3 | 198.89 | 230.0 | 210.7 | 235.1 | 239.0 |
| lateral | 147.2 | 198.89 | 230.0 | 210.7 | 235.1 | 239.0 |
| posterior | 147.1 | 198.89 | 230.0 | 210.7 | 235.1 | 239.0 |
| superior | 147.0 | 198.89 | 230.0 | 210.7 | 235.1 | 239.0 |
| nates | 173.5 | 198.2 | 232.5 | 216.5 | 238.2 | 239.2 |
| neck NEC* | 195.0 | 198.89 | 234.8 | 229.8 | 238.8 | 239.8 |
| nerve (autonomic) (ganglion) (parasympathetic) (peripheral) (sympathetic) (*see also* Neoplasm, connective tissue) | | | | | | |
| abducens | 192.0 | 198.4 | — | 225.1 | 237.9 | 239.7 |
| accessory (spinal) | 192.0 | 198.4 | — | 225.1 | 237.9 | 239.7 |
| acoustic | 192.0 | 198.4 | — | 225.1 | 237.9 | 239.7 |
| auditory | 192.0 | 198.4 | — | 225.1 | 237.9 | 239.7 |
| brachial | 171.2 | 198.89 | — | 215.2 | 238.1 | 239.2 |
| cranial (any) | 192.0 | 198.4 | — | 225.1 | 237.9 | 239.7 |
| facial | 192.0 | 198.4 | — | 225.1 | 237.9 | 239.7 |
| femoral | 171.3 | 198.89 | — | 215.3 | 238.1 | 239.2 |
| glossopharyngeal | 192.0 | 198.4 | — | 225.1 | 237.9 | 239.7 |
| hypoglossal | 192.0 | 198.4 | — | 225.1 | 237.9 | 239.7 |
| intercostal | 171.4 | 198.89 | — | 215.4 | 238.1 | 239.2 |
| lumbar | 171.7 | 198.89 | — | 215.7 | 238.1 | 239.2 |
| median | 171.2 | 198.89 | — | 215.2 | 238.1 | 239.2 |
| obturator | 171.3 | 198.89 | — | 215.3 | 238.1 | 239.2 |
| oculomotor | 192.0 | 198.4 | — | 225.1 | 237.9 | 239.7 |
| olfactory | 192.0 | 198.4 | — | 225.1 | 237.9 | 239.7 |
| optic | 192.0 | 198.4 | — | 225.1 | 237.9 | 239.7 |
| peripheral NEC | 171.9 | 198.89 | — | 215.9 | 238.1 | 239.2 |
| radial | 171.2 | 198.89 | — | 215.2 | 238.1 | 239.2 |
| sacral | 171.6 | 198.89 | — | 215.6 | 238.1 | 239.2 |
| sciatic | 171.3 | 198.89 | — | 215.3 | 238.1 | 239.2 |
| spinal NEC | 171.9 | 198.89 | — | 215.9 | 238.1 | 239.2 |
| trigeminal | 192.0 | 198.4 | — | 225.1 | 237.9 | 239.7 |
| trochlear | 192.0 | 198.4 | — | 225.1 | 237.9 | 239.7 |
| ulnar | 171.2 | 198.89 | — | 215.2 | 238.1 | 239.2 |
| vagus | 192.0 | 198.4 | — | 225.1 | 237.9 | 239.7 |
| nervous system (central) NEC | 192.9 | 198.4 | — | 225.9 | 237.9 | 239.7 |
| autonomic NEC | 171.9 | 198.89 | — | 215.9 | 238.1 | 239.2 |
| brain (*see also* Neoplasm, brain) | | | | | | |
| membrane or meninges | 192.1 | 198.4 | — | 225.2 | 237.6 | 239.7 |
| contiguous sites | 192.8 | — | — | — | — | — |
| parasympathetic NEC | 171.9 | 198.89 | — | 215.9 | 238.1 | 239.2 |
| sympathetic NEC | 171.9 | 198.89 | — | 215.9 | 238.1 | 239.2 |
| nipple (female) | 174.0 | 198.81 | 233.0 | 217 | 238.3 | 239.3 |
| male | 175.0 | 198.81 | 233.0 | 217 | 238.3 | 239.3 |
| nose, nasal | 195.0 | 198.89 | 234.8 | 229.8 | 238.8 | 239.8 |
| ala (external) | 173.3 | 198.2 | 232.3 | 216.3 | 238.2 | 239.2 |
| bone | 170.0 | 198.5 | — | 213.0 | 238.0 | 239.2 |
| cartilage | 160.0 | 197.3 | 231.8 | 212.0 | 235.9 | 239.1 |
| cavity | 160.0 | 197.3 | 231.8 | 212.0 | 235.9 | 239.1 |
| contiguous sites with accessory sinuses or middle ear | 160.8 | — | — | — | — | — |
| choana | 147.3 | 198.89 | 230.0 | 210.7 | 235.1 | 239.0 |
| external (skin) | 173.3 | 198.2 | 232.3 | 216.3 | 238.2 | 239.2 |
| fossa | 160.0 | 197.3 | 231.8 | 212.0 | 235.9 | 239.1 |
| internal | 160.0 | 197.3 | 231.8 | 212.0 | 235.9 | 239.1 |

| | Malignant | | | | | |
|---|---|---|---|---|---|---|
| | Primary | Secondary | Ca in situ | Benign | Uncertain Behavior | Unspecified |
| **Neoplasm, neoplastic —** *continued* | | | | | | |
| nose, nasal — *continued* | | | | | | |
| mucosa | 160.0 | 197.3 | 231.8 | 212.0 | 235.9 | 239.1 |
| septum | 160.0 | 197.3 | 231.8 | 212.0 | 235.9 | 239.1 |
| posterior margin | 147.3 | 198.89 | 230.0 | 210.7 | 235.1 | 239.0 |
| sinus — *see* Neoplasm, sinus | | | | | | |
| skin | 173.3 | 198.2 | 232.3 | 216.3 | 238.2 | 239.2 |
| turbinate (mucosa) | 160.0 | 197.3 | 231.8 | 212.0 | 235.9 | 239.1 |
| bone | 170.0 | 198.5 | — | 213.0 | 238.0 | 239.2 |
| vestibule | 160.0 | 197.3 | 231.8 | 212.0 | 235.9 | 239.1 |
| nostril | 160.0 | 197.3 | 231.8 | 212.0 | 235.9 | 239.1 |
| nucleus pulposus | 170.2 | 198.5 | — | 213.2 | 238.0 | 239.2 |
| occipital bone | 170.0 | 198.5 | — | 213.0 | 238.0 | 239.2 |
| lobe or pole, brain | 191.4 | 198.3 | — | 225.0 | 237.5 | 239.6 |
| odontogenic — *see* Neoplasm, jaw bone | | | | | | |
| oesophagus — *see* Neoplasm, esophagus | | | | | | |
| olfactory nerve or bulb | 192.0 | 198.4 | — | 225.1 | 237.9 | 239.7 |
| olive (brain) | 191.7 | 198.3 | — | 225.0 | 237.5 | 239.6 |
| omentum | 158.8 | 197.6 | — | 211.8 | 235.4 | 239.0 |
| operculum (brain) | 191.0 | 198.3 | — | 225.0 | 237.5 | 239.6 |
| optic nerve, chiasm, or tract | 192.0 | 198.4 | — | 225.1 | 237.9 | 239.7 |
| oral (cavity) | 145.9 | 198.89 | 230.0 | 210.4 | 235.1 | 239.0 |
| contiguous sites with lip or pharynx | 149.8 | — | — | — | — | — |
| ill-defined | 149.9 | 198.89 | 230.0 | 210.4 | 235.1 | 239.0 |
| mucosa | 145.9 | 198.89 | 230.0 | 210.4 | 235.1 | 239.0 |
| orbit | 190.1 | 198.4 | 234.0 | 224.1 | 238.8 | 239.8 |
| bone | 170.0 | 198.5 | — | 213.0 | 238.0 | 239.2 |
| eye | 190.1 | 198.4 | 234.0 | 224.1 | 238.8 | 239.8 |
| soft parts | 190.1 | 198.4 | 234.0 | 224.1 | 238.8 | 239.8 |
| organ of Zuckerkandl | 194.6 | 198.89 | — | 227.6 | 237.3 | 239.7 |
| oropharynx | 146.9 | 198.89 | 230.0 | 210.6 | 235.1 | 239.0 |
| branchial cleft (vestige) | 146.8 | 198.89 | 230.0 | 210.6 | 235.1 | 239.0 |
| contiguous sites | 146.8 | — | — | — | — | — |
| junctional region | 146.5 | 198.89 | 230.0 | 210.6 | 235.1 | 239.0 |
| lateral wall | 146.6 | 198.89 | 230.0 | 210.6 | 235.1 | 239.0 |
| pillars of fauces | 146.2 | 198.89 | 230.0 | 210.6 | 235.1 | 239.0 |
| posterior wall | 146.7 | 198.89 | 230.0 | 210.6 | 235.1 | 239.0 |
| specified part NEC | 146.8 | 198.89 | 230.0 | 210.6 | 235.1 | 239.0 |
| vallecula | 146.3 | 198.89 | 230.0 | 210.6 | 235.1 | 239.0 |
| os external | 180.1 | 198.82 | 233.1 | 219.0 | 236.0 | 239.5 |
| internal | 180.0 | 198.82 | 233.1 | 219.0 | 236.0 | 239.5 |
| ovary | 183.0 | 198.6 | 233.39 ▲ | 220 | 236.2 | 239.5 |
| oviduct | 183.2 | 198.82 | 233.39 ▲ | 221.0 | 236.3 | 239.5 |
| palate | 145.5 | 198.89 | 230.0 | 210.4 | 235.1 | 239.0 |
| hard | 145.2 | 198.89 | 230.0 | 210.4 | 235.1 | 239.0 |
| junction of hard and soft palate | 145.5 | 198.89 | 230.0 | 210.4 | 235.1 | 239.0 |
| soft | 145.3 | 198.89 | 230.0 | 210.4 | 235.1 | 239.0 |
| nasopharyngeal surface | 147.3 | 198.89 | 230.0 | 210.7 | 235.1 | 239.0 |
| posterior surface | 147.3 | 198.89 | 230.0 | 210.7 | 235.1 | 239.0 |
| superior surface | 147.3 | 198.89 | 230.0 | 210.7 | 235.1 | 239.0 |
| palatoglossal arch | 146.2 | 198.89 | 230.0 | 210.6 | 235.1 | 239.0 |
| palatopharyngeal arch | 146.2 | 198.89 | 230.0 | 210.6 | 235.1 | 239.0 |
| pallium | 191.0 | 198.3 | — | 225.0 | 237.5 | 239.6 |
| palpebra | 173.1 | 198.2 | 232.1 | 216.1 | 238.2 | 239.2 |
| pancreas | 157.9 | 197.8 | 230.9 | 211.6 | 235.5 | 239.0 |
| body | 157.1 | 197.8 | 230.9 | 211.6 | 235.5 | 239.0 |
| contiguous sites | 157.8 | — | — | — | — | — |
| duct (of Santorini) (of Wirsung) | 157.3 | 197.8 | 230.9 | 211.6 | 235.5 | 239.0 |
| ectopic tissue | 157.8 | 197.8 | 230.9 | 211.6 | 235.5 | 239.0 |
| head | 157.0 | 197.8 | 230.9 | 211.6 | 235.5 | 239.0 |
| islet cells | 157.4 | 197.8 | 230.9 | 211.7 | 235.5 | 239.0 |
| neck | 157.8 | 197.8 | 230.9 | 211.6 | 235.5 | 239.0 |
| tail | 157.2 | 197.8 | 230.9 | 211.6 | 235.5 | 239.0 |
| para-aortic body | 194.6 | 198.89 | — | 227.6 | 237.3 | 239.7 |
| paraganglion NEC | 194.6 | 198.89 | — | 227.6 | 237.3 | 239.7 |

☑ Additional Digit Required — Refer to the Tabular List for Digit Selection     ◔ Subterms under main terms may continue to next column or page

**Neoplasm, neoplastic — continued**

| | Malignant Primary | Secondary | Ca in situ | Benign | Uncertain Behavior | Unspecified |
|---|---|---|---|---|---|---|
| parametrium | 183.4 | 198.82 | — | 221.0 | 236.3 | 239.5 |
| paranephric | 158.0 | 197.6 | — | 211.8 | 235.4 | 239.0 |
| pararectal | 195.3 | 198.89 | — | 229.8 | 238.8 | 239.8 |
| parasagittal (region) | 195.0 | 198.89 | 234.8 | 229.8 | 238.8 | 239.8 |
| parasellar | 192.9 | 198.4 | — | 225.9 | 237.9 | 239.7 |
| parathyroid (gland) | 194.1 | 198.89 | 234.8 | 227.1 | 237.4 | 239.7 |
| paraurethral | 195.3 | 198.89 | — | 229.8 | 238.8 | 239.8 |
|   gland | 189.4 | 198.1 | 233.9 | 223.89 | 236.99 | 239.5 |
| paravaginal | 195.3 | 198.89 | — | 229.8 | 238.8 | 239.8 |
| parenchyma, kidney | 189.0 | 198.0 | 233.9 | 223.0 | 236.91 | 239.5 |
| parietal | | | | | | |
|   bone | 170.0 | 198.5 | — | 213.0 | 238.0 | 239.2 |
|   lobe, brain | 191.3 | 198.3 | — | 225.0 | 237.5 | 239.6 |
| paroophoron | 183.3 | 198.82 | 233.39 ▲ | 221.0 | 236.3 | 239.5 |
| parotid (duct) (gland) | 142.0 | 198.89 | 230.0 | 210.2 | 235.0 | 239.0 |
| parovarium | 183.3 | 198.82 | 233.39 ▲ | 221.0 | 236.3 | 239.5 |
| patella | 170.8 | 198.5 | — | 213.8 | 238.0 | 239.2 |
| peduncle, cerebral | 191.7 | 198.3 | — | 225.0 | 237.5 | 239.6 |
| pelvirectal junction | 154.0 | 197.5 | 230.4 | 211.4 | 235.2 | 239.0 |
| pelvis, pelvic | 195.3 | 198.89 | 234.8 | 229.8 | 238.8 | 239.8 |
|   bone | 170.6 | 198.5 | — | 213.6 | 238.0 | 239.2 |
|   floor | 195.3 | 198.89 | 234.8 | 229.8 | 238.8 | 239.8 |
|   renal | 189.1 | 198.0 | 233.9 | 223.1 | 236.91 | 239.5 |
|   viscera | 195.3 | 198.89 | 234.8 | 229.8 | 238.8 | 239.8 |
|   wall | 195.3 | 198.89 | 234.8 | 229.8 | 238.8 | 239.8 |
| pelvo-abdominal | 195.8 | 198.89 | 234.8 | 229.8 | 238.8 | 239.8 |
| penis | 187.4 | 198.82 | 233.5 | 222.1 | 236.6 | 239.5 |
|   body | 187.3 | 198.82 | 233.5 | 222.1 | 236.6 | 239.5 |
|   corpus | | | | | | |
|     (cavernosum) | 187.3 | 198.82 | 233.5 | 222.1 | 236.6 | 239.5 |
|   glans | 187.2 | 198.82 | 233.5 | 222.1 | 236.6 | 239.5 |
|   skin NEC | 187.4 | 198.82 | 233.5 | 222.1 | 236.6 | 239.5 |
| periadrenal (tissue) | 158.0 | 197.6 | — | 211.8 | 235.4 | 239.0 |
| perianal (skin) | 173.5 | 198.2 | 232.5 | 216.5 | 238.2 | 239.2 |
| pericardium | 164.1 | 198.89 | — | 212.7 | 238.8 | 239.8 |
| perinephric | 158.0 | 197.6 | — | 211.8 | 235.4 | 239.0 |
| perineum | 195.3 | 198.89 | 234.8 | 229.8 | 238.8 | 239.8 |
| periodontal tissue | | | | | | |
|   NEC | 143.9 | 198.89 | 230.0 | 210.4 | 235.1 | 239.0 |
| periosteum — see Neoplasm, bone | | | | | | |
| peripancreatic | 158.0 | 197.6 | — | 211.8 | 235.4 | 239.0 |
| peripheral nerve NEC | 171.9 | 198.89 | — | 215.9 | 238.1 | 239.2 |
| perirectal (tissue) | 195.3 | 198.89 | — | 229.8 | 238.8 | 239.8 |
| perirenal (tissue) | 158.0 | 197.6 | — | 211.8 | 235.4 | 239.0 |
| peritoneum, peritoneal | | | | | | |
|   (cavity) | 158.9 | 197.6 | — | 211.8 | 235.4 | 239.0 |
|   contiguous sites | 158.8 | — | — | — | — | — |
|     with digestive organs | 159.8 | — | — | — | — | — |
|   parietal | 158.8 | 197.6 | — | 211.8 | 235.4 | 239.0 |
|   pelvic | 158.8 | 197.6 | — | 211.8 | 235.4 | 239.0 |
|   specified part NEC | 158.8 | 197.6 | — | 211.8 | 235.4 | 239.0 |
| peritonsillar (tissue) | 195.0 | 198.89 | 234.8 | 229.8 | 238.8 | 239.8 |
| periurethral tissue | 195.3 | 198.89 | — | 229.8 | 238.8 | 239.8 |
| phalanges | 170.9 | 198.5 | — | 213.9 | 238.0 | 239.2 |
|   foot | 170.8 | 198.5 | — | 213.8 | 238.0 | 239.2 |
|   hand | 170.5 | 198.5 | — | 213.5 | 238.0 | 239.2 |
| pharynx, pharyngeal | 149.0 | 198.89 | 230.0 | 210.9 | 235.1 | 239.0 |
|   bursa | 147.1 | 198.89 | 230.0 | 210.7 | 235.1 | 239.0 |
|   fornix | 147.3 | 198.89 | 230.0 | 210.7 | 235.1 | 239.0 |
|   recess | 147.2 | 198.89 | 230.0 | 210.7 | 235.1 | 239.0 |
|   region | 149.0 | 198.89 | 230.0 | 210.9 | 235.1 | 239.0 |
|   tonsil | 147.1 | 198.89 | 230.0 | 210.7 | 235.1 | 239.0 |
|   wall (lateral) | | | | | | |
|     (posterior) | 149.0 | 198.89 | 230.0 | 210.9 | 235.1 | 239.0 |
| pia mater (cerebral) | | | | | | |
|   (cranial) | 192.1 | 198.4 | — | 225.2 | 237.6 | 239.7 |
|   spinal | 192.3 | 198.4 | — | 225.4 | 237.6 | 239.7 |
| pillars of fauces | 146.2 | 198.89 | 230.0 | 210.6 | 235.1 | 239.0 |
| pineal (body) (gland) | 194.4 | 198.89 | 234.8 | 227.4 | 237.1 | 239.7 |
| pinna (ear) NEC | 173.2 | 198.2 | 232.2 | 216.2 | 238.2 | 239.2 |
|   cartilage | 171.0 | 198.89 | — | 215.0 | 238.1 | 239.2 |
| piriform fossa or | | | | | | |
|   sinus | 148.1 | 198.89 | 230.0 | 210.8 | 235.1 | 239.0 |
| pituitary (body) (fossa) | | | | | | |
|   (gland) (lobe) | 194.3 | 198.89 | 234.8 | 227.3 | 237.0 | 239.7 |

**Neoplasm, neoplastic — continued**

| | Malignant Primary | Secondary | Ca in situ | Benign | Uncertain Behavior | Unspecified |
|---|---|---|---|---|---|---|
| placenta | 181 | 198.82 | 233.2 | 219.8 | 236.1 | 239.5 |
| pleura, pleural (cavity) | 163.9 | 197.2 | — | 212.4 | 235.8 | 239.1 |
|   contiguous sites | 163.8 | — | — | — | — | — |
|   parietal | 163.0 | 197.2 | — | 212.4 | 235.8 | 239.1 |
|   visceral | 163.1 | 197.2 | — | 212.4 | 235.8 | 239.1 |
| plexus | | | | | | |
|   brachial | 171.2 | 198.89 | — | 215.2 | 238.1 | 239.2 |
|   cervical | 171.0 | 198.89 | — | 215.0 | 238.1 | 239.2 |
|   choroid | 191.5 | 198.3 | — | 225.0 | 237.5 | 239.6 |
|   lumbosacral | 171.6 | 198.89 | — | 215.6 | 238.1 | 239.2 |
|   sacral | 171.6 | 198.89 | — | 215.6 | 238.1 | 239.2 |
| pluri-endocrine | 194.8 | 198.89 | 234.8 | 227.8 | 237.4 | 239.7 |
| pole | | | | | | |
|   frontal | 191.1 | 198.3 | — | 225.0 | 237.5 | 239.6 |
|   occipital | 191.4 | 198.3 | — | 225.0 | 237.5 | 239.6 |
| pons (varolii) | 191.7 | 198.3 | — | 225.0 | 237.5 | 239.6 |
| popliteal fossa or | | | | | | |
|   space* | 195.5 | 198.89 | 234.8 | 229.8 | 238.8 | 239.8 |
| postcricoid (region) | 148.0 | 198.89 | 230.0 | 210.8 | 235.1 | 239.0 |
| posterior fossa (cranial) | 191.9 | 198.3 | — | 225.0 | 237.5 | 239.6 |
| postnasal space | 147.9 | 198.89 | 230.0 | 210.7 | 235.1 | 239.0 |
| prepuce | 187.1 | 198.82 | 233.5 | 222.1 | 236.6 | 239.5 |
| prepylorus | 151.1 | 197.8 | 230.2 | 211.1 | 235.2 | 239.0 |
| presacral (region) | 195.3 | 198.89 | — | 229.8 | 238.8 | 239.8 |
| prostate (gland) | 185 | 198.82 | 233.4 | 222.2 | 236.5 | 239.5 |
|   utricle | 189.3 | 198.1 | 233.9 | 223.81 | 236.99 | 239.5 |
| pterygoid fossa | 171.0 | 198.89 | — | 215.0 | 238.1 | 239.2 |
| pubic bone | 170.6 | 198.5 | — | 213.6 | 238.0 | 239.2 |
| pudenda, pudendum | | | | | | |
|   (female) | 184.4 | 198.82 | 233.32 ▲ | 221.2 | 236.3 | 239.5 |
| pulmonary | 162.9 | 197.0 | 231.2 | 212.3 | 235.7 | 239.1 |
| putamen | 191.0 | 198.3 | — | 225.0 | 237.5 | 239.6 |
| pyloric | | | | | | |
|   antrum | 151.2 | 197.8 | 230.2 | 211.1 | 235.2 | 239.0 |
|   canal | 151.1 | 197.8 | 230.2 | 211.1 | 235.2 | 239.0 |
| pylorus | 151.1 | 197.8 | 230.2 | 211.1 | 235.2 | 239.0 |
| pyramid (brain) | 191.7 | 198.3 | — | 225.0 | 237.5 | 239.6 |
| pyriform fossa or | | | | | | |
|   sinus | 148.1 | 198.89 | 230.0 | 210.8 | 235.1 | 239.0 |
| radius (any part) | 170.4 | 198.5 | — | 213.4 | 238.0 | 239.2 |
| Rathke's pouch | 194.3 | 198.89 | 234.8 | 227.3 | 237.0 | 239.7 |
| rectosigmoid (colon) | | | | | | |
|   (junction) | 154.0 | 197.5 | 230.4 | 211.4 | 235.2 | 239.0 |
|   contiguous sites with anus or rectum | 154.8 | — | — | — | — | — |
| rectouterine pouch | 158.8 | 197.6 | — | 211.8 | 235.4 | 239.0 |
| rectovaginal septum or | | | | | | |
|   wall | 195.3 | 198.89 | 234.8 | 229.8 | 238.8 | 239.8 |
| rectovesical septum | 195.3 | 198.89 | 234.8 | 229.8 | 238.8 | 239.8 |
| rectum (ampulla) | 154.1 | 197.5 | 230.4 | 211.4 | 235.2 | 239.0 |
|   and colon | 154.0 | 197.5 | 230.4 | 211.4 | 235.2 | 239.0 |
|   contiguous sites with anus or rectosigmoid junction | 154.8 | — | — | — | — | — |
| renal | 189.0 | 198.0 | 233.9 | 223.0 | 236.91 | 239.5 |
|   calyx | 189.1 | 198.0 | 233.9 | 223.1 | 236.91 | 239.5 |
|   hilus | 189.1 | 198.0 | 233.9 | 223.1 | 236.91 | 239.5 |
|   parenchyma | 189.0 | 198.0 | 233.9 | 223.0 | 236.91 | 239.5 |
|   pelvis | 189.1 | 198.0 | 233.9 | 223.1 | 236.91 | 239.5 |
| respiratory | | | | | | |
|   organs or system | | | | | | |
|     NEC | 165.9 | 197.3 | 231.9 | 212.9 | 235.9 | 239.1 |
|     contiguous sites with intrathoracic organs | 165.8 | — | — | — | — | — |
|   specified sites | | | | | | |
|     NEC | 165.8 | 197.3 | 231.8 | 212.8 | 235.9 | 239.1 |
|   tract NEC | 165.9 | 197.3 | 231.9 | 212.9 | 235.9 | 239.1 |
|     upper | 165.0 | 197.3 | 231.9 | 212.9 | 235.9 | 239.1 |
| retina | 190.5 | 198.4 | 234.0 | 224.5 | 238.8 | 239.8 |
| retrobulbar | 190.1 | 198.4 | — | 224.1 | 238.8 | 239.8 |
| retrocecal | 158.0 | 197.6 | — | 211.8 | 235.4 | 239.0 |
| retromolar (area) (triangle) | | | | | | |
|   (trigone) | 145.6 | 198.89 | 230.0 | 210.4 | 235.1 | 239.0 |
| retro-orbital | 195.0 | 198.89 | 234.8 | 229.8 | 238.8 | 239.8 |

☑ Additional Digit Required — Refer to the Tabular List for Digit Selection       ⓥᴵᴵ Subterms under main terms may continue to next column or page

2008 ICD-9-CM    ▶◀ Revised Text    ● New Line    ▲ Revised Code    October 2007 • Volume 2 — 207

**Neoplasm, neoplastic — continued**

| | Malignant | | | | | |
|---|---|---|---|---|---|---|
| | Primary | Secondary | Ca in situ | Benign | Uncertain Behavior | Unspecified |
| retroperitoneal (space) (tissue) | 158.0 | 197.6 | — | 211.8 | 235.4 | 239.0 |
| contiguous sites | 158.8 | — | — | — | — | — |
| retroperitoneum | 158.0 | 197.6 | — | 211.8 | 235.4 | 239.0 |
| contiguous sites | 158.8 | — | — | — | — | — |
| retropharyngeal | 149.0 | 198.89 | 230.0 | 210.9 | 235.1 | 239.0 |
| retrovesical (septum) | 195.3 | 198.89 | 234.8 | 229.8 | 238.8 | 239.8 |
| rhinencephalon | 191.0 | 198.3 | — | 225.0 | 237.5 | 239.6 |
| rib | 170.3 | 198.5 | — | 213.3 | 238.0 | 239.2 |
| Rosenmüller's fossa | 147.2 | 198.89 | 230.0 | 210.7 | 235.1 | 239.0 |
| round ligament | 183.5 | 198.82 | — | 221.0 | 236.3 | 239.5 |
| sacrococcyx, sacrococcygeal | 170.6 | 198.5 | — | 213.6 | 238.0 | 239.2 |
| region | 195.3 | 198.89 | 234.8 | 229.8 | 238.8 | 239.8 |
| sacrouterine ligament | 183.4 | 198.82 | — | 221.0 | 236.3 | 239.5 |
| sacrum, sacral (vertebra) | 170.6 | 198.5 | — | 213.6 | 238.0 | 239.2 |
| salivary gland or duct (major) | 142.9 | 198.89 | 230.0 | 210.2 | 235.0 | 239.0 |
| contiguous sites | 142.8 | — | — | — | — | — |
| minor NEC | 145.9 | 198.89 | 230.0 | 210.4 | 235.1 | 239.0 |
| parotid | 142.0 | 198.89 | 230.0 | 210.2 | 235.0 | 239.0 |
| pluriglandular | 142.8 | 198.89 | — | 210.2 | 235.0 | 239.0 |
| sublingual | 142.2 | 198.89 | 230.0 | 210.2 | 235.0 | 239.0 |
| submandibular | 142.1 | 198.89 | 230.0 | 210.2 | 235.0 | 239.0 |
| submaxillary | 142.1 | 198.89 | 230.0 | 210.2 | 235.0 | 239.0 |
| salpinx (uterine) | 183.2 | 198.82 | 233.39▲ | 221.0 | 236.3 | 239.5 |
| Santorini's duct | 157.3 | 197.8 | 230.9 | 211.6 | 235.5 | 239.0 |
| scalp | 173.4 | 198.2 | 232.4 | 216.4 | 238.2 | 239.2 |
| scapula (any part) | 170.4 | 198.5 | — | 213.4 | 238.0 | 239.2 |
| scapular region | 195.1 | 198.89 | 234.8 | 229.8 | 238.8 | 239.8 |
| scar NEC (see also Neoplasm, skin) | 173.9 | 198.2 | 232.9 | 216.9 | 238.2 | 239.2 |
| sciatic nerve | 171.3 | 198.89 | — | 215.3 | 238.1 | 239.2 |
| sclera | 190.0 | 198.4 | 234.0 | 224.0 | 238.8 | 239.8 |
| scrotum (skin) | 187.7 | 198.82 | — | 222.4 | 236.6 | 239.5 |
| sebaceous gland — see Neoplasm, skin | | | | | | |
| sella turcica | 194.3 | 198.89 | 234.8 | 227.3 | 237.0 | 239.7 |
| bone | 170.0 | 198.5 | — | 213.0 | 238.0 | 239.2 |
| semilunar cartilage (knee) | 170.7 | 198.5 | — | 213.7 | 238.0 | 239.2 |
| seminal vesicle | 187.8 | 198.82 | 233.6 | 222.8 | 236.6 | 239.5 |
| septum nasal | 160.0 | 197.3 | 231.8 | 212.0 | 235.9 | 239.1 |
| posterior margin | 147.3 | 198.89 | 230.0 | 210.7 | 235.1 | 239.0 |
| rectovaginal | 195.3 | 198.89 | 234.8 | 229.8 | 238.8 | 239.8 |
| rectovesical | 195.3 | 198.89 | 234.8 | 229.8 | 238.8 | 239.8 |
| urethrovaginal | 184.9 | 198.82 | 233.39▲ | 221.9 | 236.3 | 239.5 |
| vesicovaginal | 184.9 | 198.82 | 233.39▲ | 221.9 | 236.3 | 239.5 |
| shoulder NEC* | 195.4 | 198.89 | 232.6 | 229.8 | 238.8 | 239.8 |
| sigmoid flexure (lower) (upper) | 153.3 | 197.5 | 230.3 | 211.3 | 235.2 | 239.0 |
| sinus (accessory) | 160.9 | 197.3 | 231.8 | 212.0 | 235.9 | 239.1 |
| bone (any) | 170.0 | 198.5 | — | 213.0 | 238.0 | 239.2 |
| contiguous sites with middle ear or nasal cavities | 160.8 | — | — | — | — | — |
| ethmoidal | 160.3 | 197.3 | 231.8 | 212.0 | 235.9 | 239.1 |
| frontal | 160.4 | 197.3 | 231.8 | 212.0 | 235.9 | 239.1 |
| maxillary | 160.2 | 197.3 | 231.8 | 212.0 | 235.9 | 239.1 |
| nasal, paranasal NEC | 160.9 | 197.3 | 231.8 | 212.0 | 235.9 | 239.1 |
| pyriform | 148.1 | 198.89 | 230.0 | 210.8 | 235.1 | 239.0 |
| sphenoidal | 160.5 | 197.3 | 231.8 | 212.0 | 235.9 | 239.1 |
| skeleton, skeletal NEC | 170.9 | 198.5 | — | 213.9 | 238.0 | 239.2 |
| Skene's gland | 189.4 | 198.1 | 233.9 | 223.89 | 236.99 | 239.5 |
| skin NEC | 173.9 | 198.2 | 232.9 | 216.9 | 238.2 | 239.2 |
| abdominal wall | 173.5 | 198.2 | 232.5 | 216.5 | 238.2 | 239.2 |
| ala nasi | 173.3 | 198.2 | 232.3 | 216.3 | 238.2 | 239.2 |
| ankle | 173.7 | 198.2 | 232.7 | 216.7 | 238.2 | 239.2 |
| antecubital space | 173.6 | 198.2 | 232.6 | 216.6 | 238.2 | 239.2 |
| anus | 173.5 | 198.2 | 232.5 | 216.5 | 238.2 | 239.2 |
| arm | 173.6 | 198.2 | 232.6 | 216.6 | 238.2 | 239.2 |
| auditory canal (external) | 173.2 | 198.2 | 232.2 | 216.2 | 238.2 | 239.2 |

**Neoplasm, neoplastic — continued / skin — continued**

| | Primary | Secondary | Ca in situ | Benign | Uncertain Behavior | Unspecified |
|---|---|---|---|---|---|---|
| auricle (ear) | 173.2 | 198.2 | 232.2 | 216.2 | 238.2 | 239.2 |
| auricular canal (external) | 173.2 | 198.2 | 232.2 | 216.2 | 238.2 | 239.2 |
| axilla, axillary fold | 173.5 | 198.2 | 232.5 | 216.5 | 238.2 | 239.2 |
| back | 173.5 | 198.2 | 232.5 | 216.5 | 238.2 | 239.2 |
| breast | 173.5 | 198.2 | 232.5 | 216.5 | 238.2 | 239.2 |
| brow | 173.3 | 198.2 | 232.3 | 216.3 | 238.2 | 239.2 |
| buttock | 173.5 | 198.2 | 232.5 | 216.5 | 238.2 | 239.2 |
| calf | 173.7 | 198.2 | 232.7 | 216.7 | 238.2 | 239.2 |
| canthus (eye) (inner) (outer) | 173.1 | 198.2 | 232.1 | 216.1 | 238.2 | 239.2 |
| cervical region | 173.4 | 198.2 | 232.4 | 216.4 | 238.2 | 239.2 |
| cheek (external) | 173.3 | 198.2 | 232.3 | 216.3 | 238.2 | 239.2 |
| chest (wall) | 173.5 | 198.2 | 232.5 | 216.5 | 238.2 | 239.2 |
| chin | 173.3 | 198.2 | 232.3 | 216.3 | 238.2 | 239.2 |
| clavicular area | 173.5 | 198.2 | 232.5 | 216.5 | 238.2 | 239.2 |
| clitoris | 184.3 | 198.82 | 233.32▲ | 221.2 | 236.3 | 239.5 |
| columnella | 173.3 | 198.2 | 232.3 | 216.3 | 238.2 | 239.2 |
| concha | 173.2 | 198.2 | 232.2 | 216.2 | 238.2 | 239.2 |
| contiguous sites | 173.8 | — | — | — | — | — |
| ear (external) | 173.2 | 198.2 | 232.2 | 216.2 | 238.2 | 239.2 |
| elbow | 173.6 | 198.2 | 232.6 | 216.6 | 238.2 | 239.2 |
| eyebrow | 173.3 | 198.2 | 232.3 | 216.3 | 238.2 | 239.2 |
| eyelid | 173.1 | 198.2 | 232.1 | — | 238.2 | 239.2 |
| face NEC | 173.3 | 198.2 | 232.3 | 216.3 | 238.2 | 239.2 |
| female genital organs (external) | 184.4 | 198.82 | 233.30▲ | 221.2 | 236.3 | 239.5 |
| clitoris | 184.3 | 198.82 | 233.32▲ | 221.2 | 236.3 | 239.5 |
| labium NEC | 184.4 | 198.82 | 233.32▲ | 221.2 | 236.3 | 239.5 |
| majus | 184.1 | 198.82 | 233.32▲ | 221.2 | 236.3 | 239.5 |
| minus | 184.2 | 198.82 | 233.32▲ | 221.2 | 236.3 | 239.5 |
| pudendum | 184.4 | 198.82 | 233.32▲ | 221.2 | 236.3 | 239.5 |
| vulva | 184.4 | 198.82 | 233.32▲ | 221.2 | 236.3 | 239.5 |
| finger | 173.6 | 198.2 | 232.6 | 216.6 | 238.2 | 239.2 |
| flank | 173.5 | 198.2 | 232.5 | 216.5 | 238.2 | 239.2 |
| foot | 173.7 | 198.2 | 232.7 | 216.7 | 238.2 | 239.2 |
| forearm | 173.6 | 198.2 | 232.6 | 216.6 | 238.2 | 239.2 |
| forehead | 173.3 | 198.2 | 232.3 | 216.3 | 238.2 | 239.2 |
| glabella | 173.3 | 198.2 | 232.3 | 216.3 | 238.2 | 239.2 |
| gluteal region | 173.5 | 198.2 | 232.5 | 216.5 | 238.2 | 239.2 |
| groin | 173.5 | 198.2 | 232.5 | 216.5 | 238.2 | 239.2 |
| hand | 173.6 | 198.2 | 232.6 | 216.6 | 238.2 | 239.2 |
| head NEC | 173.4 | 198.2 | 232.4 | 216.4 | 238.2 | 239.2 |
| heel | 173.7 | 198.2 | 232.7 | 216.7 | 238.2 | 239.2 |
| helix | 173.2 | 198.2 | — | 216.2 | 238.2 | 239.2 |
| hip | 173.7 | 198.2 | 232.7 | 216.7 | 238.2 | 239.2 |
| infraclavicular region | 173.5 | 198.2 | 232.5 | 216.5 | 238.2 | 239.2 |
| inguinal region | 173.5 | 198.2 | 232.5 | 216.5 | 238.2 | 239.2 |
| jaw | 173.3 | 198.2 | 232.3 | 216.3 | 238.2 | 239.2 |
| knee | 173.7 | 198.2 | 232.7 | 216.7 | 238.2 | 239.2 |
| labia majora | 184.1 | 198.82 | 233.32▲ | 221.2 | 236.3 | 239.5 |
| minora | 184.2 | 198.82 | 233.32▲ | 221.2 | 236.3 | 239.5 |
| leg | 173.7 | 198.2 | 232.7 | 216.7 | 238.2 | 239.2 |
| lid (lower) (upper) | — | 198.2 | 232.1 | 216.1 | 238.2 | 239.2 |
| limb NEC | 173.9 | 198.2 | 232.9 | 216.9 | 238.2 | 239.5 |
| lower | 173.7 | 198.2 | 232.7 | 216.7 | 238.2 | 239.2 |
| upper | 173.6 | 198.2 | 232.6 | 216.6 | 238.2 | 239.2 |
| lip (lower) (upper) | 173.0 | 198.2 | 232.0 | 216.0 | 238.2 | 239.2 |
| male genital organs | 187.9 | 198.82 | 233.6 | 222.9 | 236.6 | 239.5 |
| penis | 187.4 | 198.82 | 233.5 | 222.1 | 236.6 | 239.5 |
| prepuce | 187.1 | 198.82 | 233.5 | 222.1 | 236.6 | 239.5 |
| scrotum | 187.7 | 198.82 | 233.6 | 222.4 | 236.6 | 239.5 |
| mastectomy site | 173.5 | 198.2 | — | — | — | — |
| specified as breast tissue | 174.8 | 198.81 | — | — | — | — |
| meatus, acoustic (external) | 173.2 | 198.2 | 232.2 | 216.2 | 238.2 | 239.2 |
| nates | 173.5 | 198.2 | 232.5 | 216.5 | 238.2 | 239.0 |
| neck | 173.4 | 198.2 | 232.4 | 216.4 | 238.2 | 239.2 |
| nose (external) | 173.3 | 198.2 | 232.3 | 216.3 | 238.2 | 239.2 |
| palm | 173.6 | 198.2 | 232.6 | 216.6 | 238.2 | 239.2 |
| palpebra | 173.1 | 198.2 | 232.1 | 216.1 | 238.2 | 239.2 |
| penis NEC | 187.4 | 198.82 | 233.5 | 222.1 | 236.6 | 239.5 |
| perianal | 173.5 | 198.2 | 232.5 | 216.5 | 238.2 | 239.2 |

☑ Additional Digit Required — Refer to the Tabular List for Digit Selection       Subterms under main terms may continue to next column or page

208 — Volume 2 · October 2007     ▶◀ Revised Text     ● New Line     ▲ Revised Code     **2008 ICD-9-CM**

Neoplasm, neoplastic — continued
skin — continued

| | Malignant | | | | | |
| | Primary | Secondary | Ca in situ | Benign | Uncertain Behavior | Unspecified |
|---|---|---|---|---|---|---|
| perineum | 173.5 | 198.2 | 232.5 | 216.5 | 238.2 | 239.2 |
| pinna | 173.2 | 198.2 | 232.2 | 216.2 | 238.2 | 239.2 |
| plantar | 173.7 | 198.2 | 232.7 | 216.7 | 238.2 | 239.2 |
| popliteal fossa or space | 173.7 | 198.2 | 232.7 | 216.7 | 238.2 | 239.2 |
| prepuce | 187.1 | 198.82 | 233.5 | 222.1 | 236.6 | 239.5 |
| pubes | 173.5 | 198.2 | 232.5 | 216.5 | 238.2 | 239.2 |
| sacrococcygeal region | 173.5 | 198.2 | 232.5 | 216.5 | 238.2 | 239.2 |
| scalp | 173.4 | 198.2 | 232.4 | 216.4 | 238.2 | 239.2 |
| scapular region | 173.5 | 198.2 | 232.5 | 216.5 | 238.2 | 239.2 |
| scrotum | 187.7 | 198.82 | 233.6 | 222.4 | 236.6 | 239.5 |
| shoulder | 173.6 | 198.2 | 232.6 | 216.6 | 238.2 | 239.2 |
| sole (foot) | 173.7 | 198.2 | 232.7 | 216.7 | 238.2 | 239.2 |
| specified sites NEC | 173.8 | 198.2 | 232.8 | 216.8 | 232.8 | 239.2 |
| submammary fold | 173.5 | 198.2 | 232.5 | 216.5 | 238.2 | 239.2 |
| supraclavicular region | 173.4 | 198.2 | 232.4 | 216.4 | 238.2 | 239.2 |
| temple | 173.3 | 198.2 | 232.3 | 216.3 | 238.2 | 239.2 |
| thigh | 173.7 | 198.2 | 232.7 | 216.7 | 238.2 | 239.2 |
| thoracic wall | 173.5 | 198.2 | 232.5 | 216.5 | 238.2 | 239.2 |
| thumb | 173.6 | 198.2 | 232.6 | 216.6 | 238.2 | 239.2 |
| toe | 173.7 | 198.2 | 232.7 | 216.7 | 238.2 | 239.2 |
| tragus | 173.2 | 198.2 | 232.2 | 216.2 | 238.2 | 239.2 |
| trunk | 173.5 | 198.2 | 232.5 | 216.5 | 238.2 | 239.2 |
| umbilicus | 173.5 | 198.2 | 232.5 | 216.5 | 238.2 | 239.2 |
| vulva | 184.4 | 198.82 | 233.32 ▲ | 221.2 | 236.3 | 239.5 |
| wrist | 173.6 | 198.2 | 232.6 | 216.6 | 238.2 | 239.2 |
| skull | 170.0 | 198.5 | — | 213.0 | 238.0 | 239.2 |
| soft parts or tissues — see Neoplasm, connective tissue | | | | | | |
| specified site NEC | 195.8 | 198.89 | 234.8 | 229.8 | 238.8 | 239.8 |
| specified site — see Neoplasm, skin | | | | | | |
| spermatic cord | 187.6 | 198.82 | 233.6 | 222.8 | 236.6 | 239.5 |
| sphenoid | 160.5 | 197.3 | 231.8 | 212.0 | 235.9 | 239.1 |
|   bone | 170.0 | 198.5 | — | 213.0 | 238.0 | 239.2 |
|   sinus | 160.5 | 197.3 | 231.8 | 212.0 | 235.9 | 239.1 |
| sphincter | | | | | | |
|   anal | 154.2 | 197.5 | 230.5 | 211.4 | 235.5 | 239.0 |
|   of Oddi | 156.1 | 197.8 | 230.8 | 211.5 | 235.3 | 239.0 |
| spine, spinal (column) | 170.2 | 198.5 | — | 213.2 | 238.0 | 239.2 |
|   bulb | 191.7 | 198.3 | — | 225.0 | 237.5 | 239.6 |
|   coccyx | 170.6 | 198.5 | — | 213.6 | 238.0 | 239.2 |
|   cord (cervical) (lumbar) (sacral) (thoracic) | 192.2 | 198.3 | — | 225.3 | 237.5 | 239.7 |
|   dura mater | 192.3 | 198.4 | — | 225.4 | 237.6 | 239.7 |
|   lumbosacral | 170.2 | 198.5 | — | 213.2 | 238.0 | 239.2 |
|   membrane | 192.3 | 198.4 | — | 225.4 | 237.6 | 239.7 |
|   meninges | 192.3 | 198.4 | — | 225.4 | 237.6 | 239.7 |
|   nerve (root) | 171.9 | 198.89 | — | 215.9 | 238.1 | 239.2 |
|   pia mater | 192.3 | 198.4 | — | 225.4 | 237.6 | 239.7 |
|   root | 171.9 | 198.89 | — | 215.9 | 238.1 | 239.2 |
|   sacrum | 170.6 | 198.5 | — | 213.6 | 238.0 | 239.2 |
| spleen, splenic NEC | 159.1 | 197.8 | 230.9 | 211.9 | 235.5 | 239.0 |
|   flexure (colon) | 153.7 | 197.5 | 230.3 | 211.3 | 235.2 | 239.0 |
| stem, brain | 191.7 | 198.3 | — | 225.0 | 237.5 | 239.6 |
| Stensen's duct | 142.0 | 198.89 | 230.0 | 210.2 | 235.0 | 239.0 |
| sternum | 170.3 | 198.5 | — | 213.3 | 238.0 | 239.2 |
| stomach | 151.9 | 197.8 | 230.2 | 211.1 | 235.2 | 239.0 |
|   antrum (pyloric) | 151.2 | 197.8 | 230.2 | 211.1 | 235.2 | 239.0 |
|   body | 151.4 | 197.8 | 230.2 | 211.1 | 235.2 | 239.0 |
|   cardia | 151.0 | 197.8 | 230.2 | 211.1 | 235.2 | 239.0 |
|   cardiac orifice | 151.0 | 197.8 | 230.2 | 211.1 | 235.2 | 239.0 |
|   contiguous sites | 151.8 | — | — | — | — | — |
|   corpus | 151.4 | 197.8 | 230.2 | 211.1 | 235.2 | 239.0 |
|   fundus | 151.3 | 197.8 | 230.2 | 211.1 | 235.2 | 239.0 |
|   greater curvature NEC | 151.6 | 197.8 | 230.2 | 211.1 | 235.2 | 239.0 |
|   lesser curvature NEC | 151.5 | 197.8 | 230.2 | 211.1 | 235.2 | 239.0 |
|   prepylorus | 151.1 | 197.8 | 230.2 | 211.1 | 235.2 | 239.0 |
|   pylorus | 151.1 | 197.8 | 230.2 | 211.1 | 235.2 | 239.0 |
|   wall NEC | 151.9 | 197.8 | 230.2 | 211.1 | 235.2 | 239.0 |

Neoplasm, neoplastic — continued
stomach — continued
  wall — continued

| | Malignant | | | | | |
| | Primary | Secondary | Ca in situ | Benign | Uncertain Behavior | Unspecified |
|---|---|---|---|---|---|---|
|     anterior NEC | 151.8 | 197.8 | 230.2 | 211.1 | 235.2 | 239.0 |
|     posterior NEC | 151.8 | 197.8 | 230.2 | 211.1 | 235.2 | 239.0 |
| stroma, endometrial | 182.0 | 198.82 | 233.2 | 219.1 | 236.0 | 239.5 |
| stump, cervical | 180.8 | 198.82 | 233.1 | 219.0 | 236.0 | 239.5 |
| subcutaneous (nodule) (tissue) NEC — see Neoplasm, connective tissue | | | | | | |
| subdural | 192.1 | 198.4 | — | 225.2 | 237.6 | 239.7 |
| subglottis, subglottic | 161.2 | 197.3 | 231.0 | 212.1 | 235.6 | 239.1 |
| sublingual | 144.9 | 198.89 | 230.0 | 210.3 | 235.1 | 239.0 |
|   gland or duct | 142.2 | 198.89 | 230.0 | 210.2 | 235.0 | 239.0 |
| submandibular gland | 142.1 | 198.89 | 230.0 | 210.2 | 235.0 | 239.0 |
| submaxillary gland or duct | 142.1 | 198.89 | 230.0 | 210.2 | 235.0 | 239.0 |
| submental | 195.0 | 198.89 | 234.8 | 229.8 | 238.8 | 239.8 |
| subpleural | 162.9 | 197.0 | — | 212.3 | 235.7 | 239.1 |
| substernal | 164.2 | 197.1 | — | 212.5 | 235.8 | 239.8 |
| sudoriferous, sudoriparous gland, site | | | | | | |
|   unspecified | 173.9 | 198.2 | 232.9 | 216.9 | 238.2 | 239.2 |
|   specified site — see Neoplasm, skin | | | | | | |
| supraclavicular region | 195.0 | 198.89 | 234.8 | 229.8 | 238.8 | 239.8 |
| supraglottis | 161.1 | 197.3 | 231.0 | 212.1 | 235.6 | 239.1 |
| suprarenal (capsule) (cortex) (gland) (medulla) | 194.0 | 198.7 | 234.8 | 227.0 | 237.2 | 239.7 |
| suprasellar (region) | 191.9 | 198.3 | — | 225.0 | 237.5 | 239.6 |
| sweat gland (apocrine) (eccrine), site | | | | | | |
|   unspecified | 173.9 | 198.2 | 232.9 | 216.9 | 238.2 | 239.2 |
| sympathetic nerve or nervous system NEC | 171.9 | 198.89 | — | 215.9 | 238.1 | 239.2 |
| symphysis pubis | 170.6 | 198.5 | — | 213.6 | 238.0 | 239.2 |
| synovial membrane — see Neoplasm, connective tissue | | | | | | |
| tapetum, brain | 191.8 | 198.3 | — | 225.0 | 237.5 | 239.6 |
| tarsus (any bone) | 170.8 | 198.5 | — | 213.8 | 238.0 | 239.2 |
| temple (skin) | 173.3 | 198.2 | 232.3 | 216.3 | 238.2 | 239.2 |
| temporal | | | | | | |
|   bone | 170.0 | 198.5 | — | 213.0 | 238.0 | 239.2 |
|   lobe or pole | 191.2 | 198.3 | — | 225.0 | 237.5 | 239.6 |
|   region | 195.0 | 198.89 | 234.8 | 229.8 | 238.8 | 239.8 |
|   skin | 173.3 | 198.2 | 232.3 | 216.3 | 238.2 | 239.2 |
| tendon (sheath) — see Neoplasm, connective tissue | | | | | | |
| tentorium (cerebelli) | 192.1 | 198.4 | — | 225.2 | 237.6 | 239.7 |
| testis, testes (descended) (scrotal) | 186.9 | 198.82 | 233.6 | 222.0 | 236.4 | 239.5 |
|   ectopic | 186.0 | 198.82 | 233.6 | 222.0 | 236.4 | 239.5 |
|   retained | 186.0 | 198.82 | 233.6 | 222.0 | 236.4 | 239.5 |
|   undescended | 186.0 | 198.82 | 233.6 | 222.0 | 236.4 | 239.5 |
| thalamus | 191.0 | 198.3 | — | 225.0 | 237.5 | 239.6 |
| thigh NEC* | 195.5 | 198.89 | 234.8 | 229.8 | 238.8 | 239.8 |
| thorax, thoracic (cavity) (organs NEC) | 195.1 | 198.89 | 234.8 | 229.8 | 238.8 | 239.8 |
|   duct | 171.4 | 198.89 | — | 215.4 | 238.1 | 239.2 |
|   wall NEC | 195.1 | 198.89 | 234.8 | 229.8 | 238.8 | 239.8 |
| throat | 149.0 | 198.89 | 230.0 | 210.9 | 235.1 | 239.0 |
| thumb NEC* | 195.4 | 198.89 | 232.6 | 229.8 | 238.8 | 239.8 |
| thymus (gland) | 164.0 | 198.89 | — | 212.6 | 235.8 | 239.8 |
|   contiguous sites with heart and mediastinum | 164.8 | — | — | — | — | — |
| thyroglossal duct | 193 | 198.89 | 234.8 | 226 | 237.4 | 239.7 |
| thyroid (gland) | 193 | 198.89 | 234.8 | 226 | 237.4 | 239.7 |
|   cartilage | 161.3 | 197.3 | 231.0 | 212.1 | 235.6 | 239.1 |
| tibia (any part) | 170.7 | 198.5 | — | 213.7 | 238.0 | 239.2 |
| toe NEC* | 195.5 | 198.89 | 232.7 | 229.8 | 238.8 | 239.8 |
| tongue | 141.9 | 198.89 | 230.0 | 210.1 | 235.1 | 239.0 |
|   anterior (two-thirds) NEC | 141.4 | 198.89 | 230.0 | 210.1 | 235.1 | 239.0 |

| Neoplasm, neoplastic — continued | Malignant Primary | Malignant Secondary | Malignant Ca in situ | Benign | Uncertain Behavior | Unspecified |
|---|---|---|---|---|---|---|
| tongue — continued | | | | | | |
| anterior — continued | | | | | | |
| dorsal surface | 141.1 | 198.89 | 230.0 | 210.1 | 235.1 | 239.0 |
| ventral surface | 141.3 | 198.89 | 230.0 | 210.1 | 235.1 | 239.0 |
| base (dorsal surface) | 141.0 | 198.89 | 230.0 | 210.1 | 235.1 | 239.0 |
| border (lateral) | 141.2 | 198.89 | 230.0 | 210.1 | 235.1 | 239.0 |
| contiguous sites | 141.8 | — | — | — | — | — |
| dorsal surface NEC | 141.1 | 198.89 | 230.0 | 210.1 | 235.1 | 239.0 |
| fixed part NEC | 141.0 | 198.89 | 230.0 | 210.1 | 235.1 | 239.0 |
| foreamen cecum | 141.1 | 198.89 | 230.0 | 210.1 | 235.1 | 239.0 |
| frenulum linguae | 141.3 | 198.89 | 230.0 | 210.1 | 235.1 | 239.0 |
| junctional zone | 141.5 | 198.89 | 230.0 | 210.1 | 235.1 | 239.0 |
| margin (lateral) | 141.2 | 198.89 | 230.0 | 210.1 | 235.1 | 239.0 |
| midline NEC | 141.1 | 198.89 | 230.0 | 210.1 | 235.1 | 239.0 |
| mobile part NEC | 141.4 | 198.89 | 230.0 | 210.1 | 235.1 | 239.0 |
| posterior (third) | 141.0 | 198.89 | 230.0 | 210.1 | 235.1 | 239.0 |
| root | 141.0 | 198.89 | 230.0 | 210.1 | 235.1 | 239.0 |
| surface (dorsal) | 141.1 | 198.89 | 230.0 | 210.1 | 235.1 | 239.0 |
| base | 141.0 | 198.89 | 230.0 | 210.1 | 235.1 | 239.0 |
| ventral | 141.3 | 198.89 | 230.0 | 210.1 | 235.1 | 239.0 |
| tip | 141.2 | 198.89 | 230.0 | 210.1 | 235.1 | 239.0 |
| tonsil | 141.6 | 198.89 | 230.0 | 210.1 | 235.1 | 239.0 |
| tonsil | 146.0 | 198.89 | 230.0 | 210.5 | 235.1 | 239.0 |
| fauces, faucial | 146.0 | 198.89 | 230.0 | 210.5 | 235.1 | 239.0 |
| lingual | 141.6 | 198.89 | 230.0 | 210.1 | 235.1 | 239.0 |
| palatine | 146.0 | 198.89 | 230.0 | 210.5 | 235.1 | 239.0 |
| pharyngeal | 147.1 | 198.89 | 230.0 | 210.7 | 235.1 | 239.0 |
| pillar (anterior) (posterior) | 146.2 | 198.89 | 230.0 | 210.6 | 235.1 | 239.0 |
| tonsillar fossa | 146.1 | 198.89 | 230.0 | 210.6 | 235.1 | 239.0 |
| tooth socket NEC | 143.9 | 198.89 | 230.0 | 210.4 | 235.1 | 239.0 |
| trachea (cartilage) (mucosa) | 162.0 | 197.3 | 231.1 | 212.2 | 235.7 | 239.1 |
| contiguous sites with bronchus or lung | 162.8 | — | — | — | — | — |
| tracheobronchial | 162.8 | 197.3 | 231.1 | 212.2 | 235.7 | 239.1 |
| contiguous sites with lung | 162.8 | — | — | — | — | — |
| tragus | 173.2 | 198.2 | 232.2 | 216.2 | 238.2 | 239.2 |
| trunk NEC* | 195.8 | 198.89 | 232.5 | 229.8 | 238.8 | 239.8 |
| tubo-ovarian | 183.8 | 198.82 | 233.39 ▲ | 221.8 | 236.3 | 239.5 |
| tunica vaginalis | 187.8 | 198.82 | 233.6 | 222.8 | 236.6 | 239.5 |
| turbinate (bone) | 170.0 | 198.5 | — | 213.0 | 238.0 | 239.2 |
| nasal | 160.0 | 197.3 | 231.8 | 212.0 | 235.9 | 239.1 |
| tympanic cavity | 160.1 | 197.3 | 231.8 | 212.0 | 235.9 | 239.1 |
| ulna (any part) | 170.4 | 198.5 | — | 213.4 | 238.0 | 239.2 |
| umbilicus, umbilical | 173.5 | 198.2 | 232.5 | 216.5 | 238.2 | 239.2 |
| uncus, brain | 191.2 | 198.3 | — | 225.0 | 237.5 | 239.6 |
| unknown site or unspecified | 199.1 | 199.1 | 234.9 | 229.9 | 238.9 | 239.9 |
| urachus | 188.7 | 198.1 | 233.7 | 223.3 | 236.7 | 239.4 |
| ureter-bladder junction | 188.6 | 198.1 | 233.7 | 223.3 | 236.7 | 239.4 |
| ureter, ureteral | 189.2 | 198.1 | 233.9 | 223.2 | 236.91 | 239.5 |
| orifice (bladder) | 188.6 | 198.1 | 233.7 | 223.3 | 236.7 | 239.4 |
| urethra, urethral (gland) | 189.3 | 198.1 | 233.9 | 223.81 | 236.99 | 239.5 |
| orifice, internal | 188.5 | 198.1 | 233.7 | 223.3 | 236.7 | 239.4 |
| urethrovaginal (septum) | 184.9 | 198.82 | 233.39 ▲ | 221.9 | 236.3 | 239.5 |
| urinary organ or system NEC | 189.9 | 198.1 | 233.9 | 223.9 | 236.99 | 239.5 |
| bladder — see Neoplasm, bladder | | | | | | |
| contiguous sites | 189.8 | — | — | — | — | — |
| specified sites NEC | 189.8 | 198.1 | 233.9 | 223.89 | 236.99 | 239.5 |
| utero-ovarian | 183.8 | 198.82 | 233.39 ▲ | 221.8 | 236.3 | 239.5 |
| ligament | 183.3 | 198.82 | — | 221.0 | 236.3 | 239.5 |
| uterosacral ligament | 183.4 | 198.82 | — | 221.0 | 236.3 | 239.5 |
| uterus, uteri, uterine | 179 | 198.82 | 233.2 | 219.9 | 236.0 | 239.5 |
| adnexa NEC | 183.9 | 198.82 | 233.39 ▲ | 221.8 | 236.3 | 239.5 |
| contiguous sites | 183.8 | — | — | — | — | — |
| body | 182.0 | 198.82 | 233.2 | 219.1 | 236.0 | 239.5 |
| contiguous sites | 182.8 | — | — | — | — | — |
| cervix | 180.9 | 198.82 | 233.1 | 219.0 | 236.0 | 239.5 |

| Neoplasm, neoplastic — continued | Malignant Primary | Malignant Secondary | Malignant Ca in situ | Benign | Uncertain Behavior | Unspecified |
|---|---|---|---|---|---|---|
| uterus, uteri, uterine — continued | | | | | | |
| cornu | 182.0 | 198.82 | 233.2 | 219.1 | 236.0 | 239.5 |
| corpus | 182.0 | 198.82 | 233.2 | 219.1 | 236.0 | 239.5 |
| endocervix (canal) (gland) | 180.0 | 198.82 | 233.1 | 219.0 | 236.0 | 239.5 |
| endometrium | 182.0 | 198.82 | 233.2 | 219.1 | 236.0 | 239.5 |
| exocervix | 180.1 | 198.82 | 233.1 | 219.0 | 236.0 | 239.5 |
| external os | 180.1 | 198.82 | 233.1 | 219.0 | 236.0 | 239.5 |
| fundus | 182.0 | 198.82 | 233.2 | 219.1 | 236.0 | 239.5 |
| internal os | 180.0 | 198.82 | 233.1 | 219.0 | 236.0 | 239.5 |
| isthmus | 182.1 | 198.82 | 233.2 | 219.1 | 236.0 | 239.5 |
| ligament | 183.4 | 198.82 | — | 221.0 | 236.3 | 239.5 |
| broad | 183.3 | 198.82 | 233.39 ▲ | 221.0 | 236.3 | 239.5 |
| round | 183.5 | 198.82 | — | 221.0 | 236.3 | 239.5 |
| lower segment | 182.1 | 198.82 | 233.2 | 219.1 | 236.0 | 239.5 |
| myometrium | 182.0 | 198.82 | 233.2 | 219.1 | 236.0 | 239.5 |
| squamocolumnar junction | 180.8 | 198.82 | 233.1 | 219.0 | 236.0 | 239.5 |
| tube | 183.2 | 198.82 | 233.39 ▲ | 221.0 | 236.3 | 239.5 |
| utricle, prostatic | 189.3 | 198.1 | 233.9 | 223.81 | 236.99 | 239.5 |
| uveal tract | 190.0 | 198.4 | 234.0 | 224.0 | 238.8 | 239.8 |
| uvula | 145.4 | 198.89 | 230.0 | 210.4 | 235.1 | 239.0 |
| vagina, vaginal (fornix) (vault) (wall) | 184.0 | 198.82 | 233.31 ▲ | 221.1 | 236.3 | 239.5 |
| vaginovesical | 184.9 | 198.82 | 233.39 ▲ | 221.9 | 236.3 | 239.5 |
| septum | 194.9 | 198.82 | 233.39 ▲ | 221.9 | 236.3 | 239.5 |
| vallecula (epiglottis) | 146.3 | 198.89 | 230.0 | 210.6 | 235.1 | 239.0 |
| vascular — see Neoplasm, connective tissue | | | | | | |
| vas deferens | 187.6 | 198.82 | 233.6 | 222.8 | 236.6 | 239.5 |
| Vater's ampulla | 156.2 | 197.8 | 230.8 | 211.5 | 235.3 | 239.0 |
| vein, venous — see Neoplasm, connective tissue | | | | | | |
| vena cava (abdominal) (inferior) | 171.5 | 198.89 | — | 215.5 | 238.1 | 239.2 |
| superior | 171.4 | 198.89 | — | 215.4 | 238.1 | 239.2 |
| ventricle (cerebral) (floor) (fourth) (lateral) (third) | 191.5 | 198.3 | — | 225.0 | 237.5 | 239.6 |
| cardiac (left) (right) | 164.1 | 198.89 | — | 212.7 | 238.8 | 239.8 |
| ventricular band of larynx | 161.1 | 197.3 | 231.0 | 212.1 | 235.6 | 239.1 |
| ventriculus — see Neoplasm, stomach | | | | | | |
| vermillion border — see Neoplasm, lip | | | | | | |
| vermis, cerebellum | 191.6 | 198.3 | — | 225.0 | 237.5 | 239.6 |
| vertebra (column) | 170.2 | 198.5 | — | 213.2 | 238.0 | 239.2 |
| coccyx | 170.6 | 198.5 | — | 213.6 | 238.0 | 239.2 |
| sacrum | 170.6 | 198.5 | — | 213.6 | 238.0 | 239.2 |
| vesical — see Neoplasm, bladder | | | | | | |
| vesicle, seminal | 187.8 | 198.82 | 233.6 | 222.8 | 236.6 | 239.5 |
| vesicocervical tissue | 184.9 | 198.82 | 233.39 ▲ | 221.9 | 236.3 | 239.5 |
| vesicorectal | 195.3 | 198.89 | 234.8 | 229.8 | 238.8 | 239.8 |
| vesicovaginal | 184.9 | 198.82 | 233.39 ▲ | 221.9 | 236.3 | 239.5 |
| septum | 184.9 | 198.82 | 233.39 ▲ | 221.9 | 236.3 | 239.5 |
| vessel (blood) — see Neoplasm, connective tissue | | | | | | |
| vestibular gland, greater | 184.1 | 198.82 | 233.32 ▲ | 221.2 | 236.3 | 239.5 |
| vestibule | | | | | | |
| mouth | 145.1 | 198.89 | 230.0 | 210.4 | 235.1 | 239.0 |
| nose | 160.0 | 197.3 | 231.8 | 212.0 | 235.9 | 239.1 |
| Virchow's gland | — | 196.0 | — | 229.0 | 238.8 | 239.8 |
| viscera NEC | 195.8 | 198.89 | 234.8 | 229.8 | 238.8 | 239.8 |
| vocal cords (true) | 161.0 | 197.3 | 231.0 | 212.1 | 235.6 | 239.1 |
| false | 161.1 | 197.3 | 231.0 | 212.1 | 235.6 | 239.1 |
| vomer | 170.0 | 198.5 | — | 213.0 | 238.0 | 239.2 |
| vulva | 184.4 | 198.82 | 233.32 ▲ | 221.2 | 236.3 | 239.5 |
| vulvovaginal gland | 184.4 | 198.82 | 233.32 ▲ | 221.2 | 236.3 | 239.5 |
| Waldeyer's ring | 149.1 | 198.89 | 230.0 | 210.9 | 235.1 | 239.0 |
| Wharton's duct | 142.1 | 198.89 | 230.0 | 210.2 | 235.0 | 239.0 |

☑ Additional Digit Required — Refer to the Tabular List for Digit Selection

▽ Subterms under main terms may continue to next column or page

▶◀ Revised Text  ● New Line  ▲ Revised Code

| | Malignant | | | | | |
| | Primary | Secondary | Ca in situ | Benign | Uncertain Behavior | Unspecified |
|---|---|---|---|---|---|---|
| **Neoplasm, neoplastic** — *continued* | | | | | | |
| white matter (central) | | | | | | |
|   (cerebral) ..................... | 191.0 | 198.3 | — | 225.0 | 237.5 | 239.6 |
| windpipe .......................... | 162.0 | 197.3 | 231.1 | 212.2 | 235.7 | 239.1 |
| Wirsung's duct ................ | 157.3 | 197.8 | 230.9 | 211.6 | 235.5 | 239.0 |
| wolffian (body) (duct) | | | | | | |
|   female .......................... | 184.8 | 198.82 | 233.39 ▲ | 221.8 | 236.3 | 239.5 |
|   male ............................. | 187.8 | 198.82 | 233.6 | 222.8 | 236.6 | 239.5 |
| womb — *see* Neoplasm, uterus | | | | | | |
| wrist NEC* ...................... | 195.4 | 198.89 | 232.6 | 229.8 | 238.8 | 239.8 |
| xiphoid process ............... | 170.3 | 198.5 | — | 213.3 | 238.0 | 239.2 |
| Zuckerkandl's organ .......... | 194.6 | 198.89 | — | 227.6 | 237.3 | 239.7 |

☑ Additional Digit Required — Refer to the Tabular List for Digit Selection

*2008 ICD-9-CM*

►◄ Revised Text

● New Line    ▲ Revised Code

▽ Subterms under main terms may continue to next column or page

**October 2007 · Volume 2 — 211**

**Neovascularization**
- choroid 362.16
- ciliary body 364.42
- cornea 370.60
  - deep 370.63
  - localized 370.61
- iris 364.42
- retina 362.16
- subretinal 362.16

**Nephralgia** 788.0

**Nephritis, nephritic** (albuminuric) (azotemic) (congenital) (degenerative) (diffuse) (disseminated) (epithelial) (familial) (focal) (granulomatous) (hemorrhagic) (infantile) (nonsuppurative, excretory) (uremic) 583.9
- with
  - edema — see Nephrosis
  - lesion of
    - glomerulonephritis
      - hypocomplementemic persistent 583.2
        - with nephrotic syndrome 581.2
        - chronic 582.2
      - lobular 583.2
        - with nephrotic syndrome 581.2
        - chronic 582.2
      - membranoproliferative 583.2
        - with nephrotic syndrome 581.2
        - chronic 582.2
      - membranous 583.1
        - with nephrotic syndrome 581.1
        - chronic 582.1
      - mesangiocapillary 583.2
        - with nephrotic syndrome 581.2
        - chronic 582.2
      - mixed membranous and proliferative 583.2
        - with nephrotic syndrome 581.2
        - chronic 582.2
      - proliferative (diffuse) 583.0
        - with nephrotic syndrome 581.0
        - acute 580.0
        - chronic 582.0
        - rapidly progressive 583.4
          - acute 580.4
          - chronic 582.4
    - interstitial nephritis (diffuse) (focal) 583.89
      - with nephrotic syndrome 581.89
      - acute 580.89
      - chronic 582.89
    - necrotizing glomerulitis 583.4
      - acute 580.4
      - chronic 582.4
    - renal necrosis 583.9
      - cortical 583.6
      - medullary 583.7
    - specified pathology NEC 583.89
      - with nephrotic syndrome 581.89
      - acute 580.89
      - chronic 582.89
  - necrosis, renal 583.9
    - cortical 583.6
    - medullary (papillary) 583.7
  - nephrotic syndrome (see also Nephrosis) 581.9
  - papillary necrosis 583.7
  - specified pathology NEC 583.89
- acute 580.9
  - extracapillary with epithelial crescents 580.4
  - hypertensive (see also Hypertension, kidney) 403.90
  - necrotizing 580.4
  - poststreptococcal 580.0

**Nephritis, nephritic** — continued
- acute — continued
  - proliferative (diffuse) 580.0
  - rapidly progressive 580.4
  - specified pathology NEC 580.89
- amyloid 277.39 [583.81]
  - chronic 277.39 [582.81]
- arteriolar (see also Hypertension, kidney) 403.90
- arteriosclerotic (see also Hypertension, kidney) 403.90
- ascending (see also Pyelitis) 590.80
- atrophic 582.9
- basement membrane NEC 583.89
  - with
    - pulmonary hemorrhage (Goodpasture's syndrome) 446.21 [583.81]
- calculous, calculus 592.0
- cardiac (see also Hypertension, kidney) 403.90
- cardiovascular (see also Hypertension, kidney) 403.90
- chronic 582.9
  - arteriosclerotic (see also Hypertension, kidney) 403.90
  - hypertensive (see also Hypertension, kidney) 403.90
- cirrhotic (see also Sclerosis, renal) 587
- complicating pregnancy, childbirth, or puerperium 646.2 ☑
  - with hypertension 642.1 ☑
    - affecting fetus or newborn 760.0
  - affecting fetus or newborn 760.1
- croupous 580.9
- desquamative — see Nephrosis
- due to
  - amyloidosis 277.39 [583.81]
    - chronic 277.39 [582.81]
  - arteriosclerosis (see also Hypertension, kidney) 403.90
  - diabetes mellitus 250.4 ☑ [583.81]
    - with nephrotic syndrome 250.4 ☑ [581.81]
  - diphtheria 032.89 [580.81]
  - gonococcal infection (acute) 098.19 [583.81]
    - chronic or duration of 2 months or over 098.39 [583.81]
  - gout 274.10
  - infectious hepatitis 070.9 [580.81]
  - mumps 072.79 [580.81]
  - specified kidney pathology NEC 583.89
    - acute 580.89
    - chronic 582.89
  - streptotrichosis 039.8 [583.81]
  - subacute bacterial endocarditis 421.0 [580.81]
  - systemic lupus erythematosus 710.0 [583.81]
    - chronic 710.0 [582.81]
  - typhoid fever 002.0 [580.81]
- endothelial 582.2
- end stage (chronic) (terminal) NEC 585.6
- epimembranous 581.1
- exudative 583.89
  - with nephrotic syndrome 581.89
  - acute 580.89
  - chronic 582.89
- gonococcal (acute) 098.19 [583.81]
  - chronic or duration of 2 months or over 098.39 [583.81]
- gouty 274.10
- hereditary (Alport's syndrome) 759.89
- hydremic — see Nephrosis
- hypertensive (see also Hypertension, kidney) 403.90
- hypocomplementemic persistent 583.2
  - with nephrotic syndrome 581.2
  - chronic 582.2
- immune complex NEC 583.89
- infective (see also Pyelitis) 590.80
- interstitial (diffuse) (focal) 583.89
  - with nephrotic syndrome 581.89

**Nephritis, nephritic** — continued
- interstitial — continued
  - acute 580.89
  - chronic 582.89
- latent or quiescent — see Nephritis, chronic
- lead 984.9
  - specified type of lead — see Table of Drugs and Chemicals
- lobular 583.2
  - with nephrotic syndrome 581.2
  - chronic 582.2
- lupus 710.0 [583.81]
  - acute 710.0 [580.81]
  - chronic 710.0 [582.81]
- membranoproliferative 583.2
  - with nephrotic syndrome 581.2
  - chronic 582.2
- membranous 583.1
  - with nephrotic syndrome 581.1
  - chronic 582.1
- mesangiocapillary 583.2
  - with nephrotic syndrome 581.2
  - chronic 582.2
- minimal change 581.3
- mixed membranous and proliferative 583.2
  - with nephrotic syndrome 581.2
  - chronic 582.2
- necrotic, necrotizing 583.4
  - acute 580.4
  - chronic 582.4
- nephrotic — see Nephrosis
- old — see Nephritis, chronic
- parenchymatous 581.89
- polycystic 753.12
  - adult type (APKD) 753.13
  - autosomal dominant 753.13
  - autosomal recessive 753.14
  - childhood type (CPKD) 753.14
  - infantile type 753.14
- poststreptococcal 580.0
- pregnancy — see Nephritis, complicating pregnancy
- proliferative 583.0
  - with nephrotic syndrome 581.0
  - acute 580.0
  - chronic 582.0
- purulent (see also Pyelitis) 590.80
- rapidly progressive 583.4
  - acute 580.4
  - chronic 582.4
- salt-losing or salt-wasting (see also Disease, renal) 593.9
- saturnine 984.9
  - specified type of lead — see Table of Drugs and Chemicals
- septic (see also Pyelitis) 590.80
- specified pathology NEC 583.89
  - acute 580.89
  - chronic 582.89
- staphylococcal (see also Pyelitis) 590.80
- streptotrichosis 039.8 [583.81]
- subacute (see also Nephrosis) 581.9
- suppurative (see also Pyelitis) 590.80
- syphilitic (late) 095.4
  - congenital 090.5 [583.81]
  - early 091.69 [583.81]
- terminal (chronic) (end-stage) NEC 585.6
- toxic — see Nephritis, acute
- tubal, tubular — see Nephrosis, tubular
- tuberculous (see also Tuberculosis) 016.0 ☑ [583.81]
- type II (Ellis) — see Nephrosis
- vascular — see Hypertension, kidney
- war 580.9

**Nephroblastoma** (M8960/3) 189.0
- epithelial (M8961/3) 189.0
- mesenchymal (M8962/3) 189.0

**Nephrocalcinosis** 275.49

**Nephrocystitis, pustular** — see also Pyelitis 590.80

**Nephrolithiasis** (congenital) (pelvis) (recurrent) 592.0
- uric acid 274.11

**Nephroma** (M8960/3) 189.0
- mesoblastic (M8960/1) 236.9 ☑

**Nephronephritis** — see also Nephrosis 581.9

**Nephronopthisis** 753.16

**Nephropathy** — see also Nephritis 583.9
- with
  - exudative nephritis 583.89
  - interstitial nephritis (diffuse) (focal) 583.89
  - medullary necrosis 583.7
  - necrosis 583.9
    - cortical 583.6
    - medullary or papillary 583.7
  - papillary necrosis 583.7
  - specified lesion or cause NEC 583.89
- analgesic 583.89
  - with medullary necrosis, acute 584.7
- arteriolar (see also Hypertension, kidney) 403.90
- arteriosclerotic (see also Hypertension, kidney) 403.90
- complicating pregnancy 646.2 ☑
- diabetic 250.4 ☑ [583.81]
- gouty 274.10
  - specified type NEC 274.19
- hereditary amyloid 277.31
- hypercalcemic 588.89
- hypertensive (see also Hypertension, kidney) 403.90
- hypokalemic (vacuolar) 588.89
- IgA 583.9
- obstructive 593.89
  - congenital 753.20
- phenacetin 584.7
- phosphate-losing 588.0
- potassium depletion 588.89
- proliferative (see also Nephritis, proliferative) 583.0
- protein-losing 588.89
- salt-losing or salt-wasting (see also Disease, renal) 593.9
- sickle-cell (see also Disease, sickle-cell) 282.60 [583.81]
- toxic 584.5
- vasomotor 584.5
- water-losing 588.89

**Nephroptosis** — see also Disease, renal 593.0
- congenital (displaced) 753.3

**Nephropyosis** — see also Abscess, kidney 590.2

**Nephrorrhagia** 593.81

**Nephrosclerosis** (arteriolar) (arteriosclerotic) (chronic) (hyaline) — see also Hypertension, kidney 403.90
- gouty 274.10
- hyperplastic (arteriolar) (see also Hypertension, kidney) 403.90
- senile (see also Sclerosis, renal) 587

**Nephrosis, nephrotic** (Epstein's) (syndrome) 581.9
- with
  - lesion of
    - focal glomerulosclerosis 581.1
    - glomerulonephritis
      - endothelial 581.2
      - hypocomplementemic persistent 581.2
      - lobular 581.2
      - membranoproliferative 581.2
      - membranous 581.1
      - mesangiocapillary 581.2
      - minimal change 581.3
      - mixed membranous and proliferative 581.2
      - proliferative 581.2
      - segmental hyalinosis 581.1
      - specified pathology NEC 581.89
- acute — see Nephrosis, tubular
- anoxic — see Nephrosis, tubular

**Nephrosis, nephrotic** — *continued*
arteriosclerotic (*see also* Hypertension, kidney) 403.90
chemical — *see* Nephrosis, tubular
cholemic 572.4
complicating pregnancy, childbirth, or puerperium — *see* Nephritis, complicating pregnancy
diabetic 250.4 ☑ *[581.81]*
Finnish type (congenital) 759.89 ●
hemoglobinuric — *see* Nephrosis, tubular
in
amyloidosis 277.39 *[581.81]*
diabetes mellitus 250.4 ☑ *[581.81]*
epidemic hemorrhagic fever 078.6
malaria 084.9 *[581.81]*
polyarteritis 446.0 *[581.81]*
systemic lupus erythematosus 710.0 *[581.81]*
ischemic — *see* Nephrosis, tubular
lipoid 581.3
lower nephron — *see* Nephrosis, tubular
lupoid 710.0 *[581.81]*
lupus 710.0 *[581.81]*
malarial 084.9 *[581.81]*
minimal change 581.3
necrotizing — *see* Nephrosis, tubular
osmotic (sucrose) 588.89
polyarteritic 446.0 *[581.81]*
radiation 581.9
specified lesion or cause NEC 581.89
syphilitic 095.4
toxic — *see* Nephrosis, tubular
tubular (acute) 584.5
due to a procedure 997.5
radiation 581.9
**Nephrosonephritis hemorrhagic** (endemic) 078.6
**Nephrostomy status** V44.6
with complication 997.5
**Nerve** — *see* condition
**Nerves** 799.2
**Nervous** — *see also* condition 799.2
breakdown 300.9
heart 306.2
stomach 306.4
tension 799.2
**Nervousness** 799.2
**Nesidioblastoma** (M8150/0)
pancreas 211.7
specified site NEC — *see* Neoplasm, by site, benign
unspecified site 211.7
**Netherton's syndrome** (ichthyosiform erythroderma) 757.1
**Nettle rash** 708.8
**Nettleship's disease** (urticaria pigmentosa) 757.33
**Neumann's disease** (pemphigus vegetans) 694.4
**Neuralgia, neuralgic** (acute) — *see also* Neuritis 729.2
accessory (nerve) 352.4
acoustic (nerve) 388.5
ankle 355.8
anterior crural 355.8
anus 787.99
arm 723.4
auditory (nerve) 388.5
axilla 353.0
bladder 788.1
brachial 723.4
brain — *see* Disorder, nerve, cranial
broad ligament 625.9
cerebral — *see* Disorder, nerve, cranial
ciliary 346.2 ☑
cranial nerve (*see also* Disorder, nerve, cranial)
fifth or trigeminal (*see also* Neuralgia, trigeminal) 350.1
ear 388.71
middle 352.1
facial 351.8

**Neuralgia, neuralgic** — *see also* Neuritis — *continued*
finger 354.9
flank 355.8
foot 355.8
forearm 354.9
Fothergill's (*see also* Neuralgia, trigeminal) 350.1
postherpetic 053.12
glossopharyngeal (nerve) 352.1
groin 355.8
hand 354.9
heel 355.8
Horton's 346.2 ☑
Hunt's 053.11
hypoglossal (nerve) 352.5
iliac region 355.8
infraorbital (*see also* Neuralgia, trigeminal) 350.1
inguinal 355.8
intercostal (nerve) 353.8
postherpetic 053.19
jaw 352.1
kidney 788.0
knee 355.8
loin 355.8
malarial (*see also* Malaria) 084.6
mastoid 385.89
maxilla 352.1
median thenar 354.1
metatarsal 355.6
middle ear 352.1
migrainous 346.2 ☑
Morton's 355.6
nerve, cranial — *see* Disorder, nerve, cranial
nose 352.0
occipital 723.8
olfactory (nerve) 352.0
ophthalmic 377.30
postherpetic 053.19
optic (nerve) 377.30
penis 607.9
perineum 355.8
pleura 511.0
postherpetic NEC 053.19
geniculate ganglion 053.11
ophthalmic 053.19
trifacial 053.12
trigeminal 053.12
pubic region 355.8
radial (nerve) 723.4
rectum 787.99
sacroiliac joint 724.3
sciatic (nerve) 724.3
scrotum 608.9
seminal vesicle 608.9
shoulder 354.9
Sluder's 337.0
specified nerve NEC — *see* Disorder, nerve
spermatic cord 608.9
sphenopalatine (ganglion) 337.0
subscapular (nerve) 723.4
suprascapular (nerve) 723.4
testis 608.89
thenar (median) 354.1
thigh 355.8
tongue 352.5
trifacial (nerve) (*see also* Neuralgia, trigeminal) 350.1
trigeminal (nerve) 350.1
postherpetic 053.12
tympanic plexus 388.71
ulnar (nerve) 723.4
vagus (nerve) 352.3
wrist 354.9
writers' 300.89
organic 333.84
**Neurapraxia** — *see* Injury, nerve, by site
**Neurasthenia** 300.5
cardiac 306.2
gastric 306.4
heart 306.2
postfebrile 780.79
postviral 780.79

**Neurilemmoma** (M9560/0) — *see also* Neoplasm, connective tissue, benign
acoustic (nerve) 225.1
malignant (M9560/3) (*see also* Neoplasm, connective tissue, malignant)
acoustic (nerve) 192.0
**Neurilemmosarcoma** (M9560/3) — *see* Neoplasm, connective tissue, malignant
**Neurilemoma** — *see* Neurilemmoma
**Neurinoma** (M9560/0) — *see* Neurilemmoma
**Neurinomatosis** (M9560/1) — *see also* Neoplasm, connective tissue, uncertain behavior
centralis 759.5
**Neuritis** — *see also* Neuralgia 729.2
abducens (nerve) 378.54
accessory (nerve) 352.4
acoustic (nerve) 388.5
syphilitic 094.86
alcoholic 357.5
with psychosis 291.1
amyloid, any site 277.39 *[357.4]*
anterior crural 355.8
arising during pregnancy 646.4 ☑
arm 723.4
ascending 355.2
auditory (nerve) 388.5
brachial (nerve) NEC 723.4
due to displacement, intervertebral disc 722.0
cervical 723.4
chest (wall) 353.8
costal region 353.8
cranial nerve (*see also* Disorder, nerve, cranial)
first or olfactory 352.0
second or optic 377.30
third or oculomotor 378.52
fourth or trochlear 378.53
fifth or trigeminal (*see also* Neuralgia, trigeminal) 350.1
sixth or abducens 378.54
seventh or facial 351.8
newborn 767.5
eighth or acoustic 388.5
ninth or glossopharyngeal 352.1
tenth or vagus 352.3
eleventh or accessory 352.4
twelfth or hypoglossal 352.5
Déjérine-Sottas 356.0
diabetic 250.6 ☑ *[357.2]*
diphtheritic 032.89 *[357.4]*
due to
beriberi 265.0 *[357.4]*
displacement, prolapse, protrusion, or rupture of intervertebral disc 722.2
cervical 722.0
lumbar, lumbosacral 722.10
thoracic, thoracolumbar 722.11
herniation, nucleus pulposus 722.2
cervical 722.0
lumbar, lumbosacral 722.10
thoracic, thoracolumbar 722.11
endemic 265.0 *[357.4]*
facial (nerve) 351.8
newborn 767.5
general — *see* Polyneuropathy
geniculate ganglion 351.1
due to herpes 053.11
glossopharyngeal (nerve) 352.1
gouty 274.89 *[357.4]*
hypoglossal (nerve) 352.5
ilioinguinal (nerve) 355.8
in diseases classified elsewhere — *see* Polyneuropathy, in
infectious (multiple) 357.0
intercostal (nerve) 353.8
interstitial hypertrophic progressive NEC 356.9
leg 355.8

**Neuritis** — *see also* Neuralgia — *continued*
lumbosacral NEC 724.4
median (nerve) 354.1
thenar 354.1
multiple (acute) (infective) 356.9
endemic 265.0 *[357.4]*
multiplex endemica 265.0 *[357.4]*
nerve root (*see also* Radiculitis) 729.2
oculomotor (nerve) 378.52
olfactory (nerve) 352.0
optic (nerve) 377.30
in myelitis 341.0
meningococcal 036.81
pelvic 355.8
peripheral (nerve) (*see also* Neuropathy, peripheral)
complicating pregnancy or puerperium 646.4 ☑
specified nerve NEC — *see* Mononeuritis
pneumogastric (nerve) 352.3
postchickenpox 052.7
postherpetic 053.19
progressive hypertrophic interstitial NEC 356.9
puerperal, postpartum 646.4 ☑
radial (nerve) 723.4
retrobulbar 377.32
syphilitic 094.85
rheumatic (chronic) 729.2
sacral region 355.8
sciatic (nerve) 724.3
due to displacement of intervertebral disc 722.10
serum 999.5
specified nerve NEC — *see* Disorder, nerve
spinal (nerve) 355.9
root (*see also* Radiculitis) 729.2
subscapular (nerve) 723.4
suprascapular (nerve) 723.4
syphilitic 095.8
thenar (median) 354.1
thoracic NEC 724.4
toxic NEC 357.7
trochlear (nerve) 378.53
ulnar (nerve) 723.4
vagus (nerve) 352.3
**Neuroangiomatosis, encephalofacial** 759.6
**Neuroastrocytoma** (M9505/1) — *see* Neoplasm, by site, uncertain behavior
**Neuro-avitaminosis** 269.2
**Neuroblastoma** (M9500/3)
olfactory (M9522/3) 160.0
specified site — *see* Neoplasm, by site, malignant
unspecified site 194.0
**Neurochorioretinitis** — *see also* Chorioretinitis 363.20
**Neurocirculatory asthenia** 306.2
**Neurocytoma** (M9506/0) — *see* Neoplasm, by site, benign
**Neurodermatitis** (circumscribed) (circumscripta) (local) 698.3
atopic 691.8
diffuse (Brocq) 691.8
disseminated 691.8
nodulosa 698.3
**Neuroencephalomyelopathy, optic** 341.0
**Neuroepithelioma** (M9503/3) — *see also* Neoplasm, by site, malignant
olfactory (M9521/3) 160.0
**Neurofibroma** (M9540/0) — *see also* Neoplasm, connective tissue, benign
melanotic (M9541/0) — *see* Neoplasm, connective tissue, benign
multiple (M9540/1) 237.70
type 1 237.71
type 2 237.72
plexiform (M9550/0) — *see* Neoplasm, connective tissue, benign

☑ Additional Digit Required — Refer to the Tabular List for Digit Selection
2008 ICD-9-CM
►◄ Revised Text
● New Line
▲ Revised Code
🆆 Subterms under main terms may continue to next column or page
October 2007 · Volume 2 — 213

**Neurofibromatosis** (multiple) (M9540/1) 237.70
  acoustic 237.72
  malignant (M9540/3) — *see* Neoplasm, connective tissue, malignant
  type 1 237.71
  type 2 237.72
  von Recklinghausen's 237.71
**Neurofibrosarcoma** (M9540/3) — *see* Neoplasm, connective tissue, malignant
**Neurogenic** — *see also* condition
  bladder (atonic) (automatic) (autonomic) (flaccid) (hypertonic) (hypotonic) (inertia) (infranuclear) (irritable) (motor) (nonreflex) (nuclear) (paralysis) (reflex) (sensory) (spastic) (supranuclear) (uninhibited) 596.54
    with cauda equina syndrome 344.61
  bowel 564.81
  heart 306.2
**Neuroglioma (M9505/1)** — *see* Neoplasm, by site, uncertain behavior
**Neurolabyrinthitis** (of Dix and Hallpike) 386.12
**Neurolathyrism** 988.2
**Neuroleprosy** 030.1
**Neuroleptic malignant syndrome** 333.92
**Neurolipomatosis** 272.8
**Neuroma** (M9570/0) — *see also* Neoplasm, connective tissue, benign
  acoustic (nerve) (M9560/0) 225.1
  amputation (traumatic) (*see also* Injury, nerve, by site)
    surgical complication (late) 997.61
  appendix 211.3
  auditory nerve 225.1
  digital 355.6
    toe 355.6
  interdigital (toe) 355.6
  intermetatarsal 355.6
  Morton's 355.6
  multiple 237.70
    type 1 237.71
    type 2 237.72
  nonneoplastic 355.9
    arm NEC 354.9
    leg NEC 355.8
    lower extremity NEC 355.8
    specified site NEC — *see* Mononeuritis, by site
    upper extremity NEC 354.9
  optic (nerve) 225.1
  plantar 355.6
  plexiform (M9550/0) — *see* Neoplasm, connective tissue, benign
  surgical (nonneoplastic) 355.9
    arm NEC 354.9
    leg NEC 355.8
    lower extremity NEC 355.8
    upper extremity NEC 354.9
  traumatic (*see also* Injury, nerve, by site)
    old — *see* Neuroma, nonneoplastic
**Neuromyalgia** 729.1
**Neuromyasthenia** (epidemic) 049.8
**Neuromyelitis** 341.8
  ascending 357.0
  optica 341.0
**Neuromyopathy** NEC 358.9
**Neuromyositis** 729.1
**Neuronevus** (M8725/0) — *see* Neoplasm, skin, benign
**Neuronitis** 357.0
  ascending (acute) 355.2
  vestibular 386.12
**Neuroparalytic** — *see* condition
**Neuropathy, neuropathic** — *see also* Disorder, nerve 355.9
  acute motor 357.82
  alcoholic 357.5
    with psychosis 291.1

**Neuropathy, neuropathic** — *see also* Disorder, nerve — *continued*
  arm NEC 354.9
  ataxia and retinitis pigmentosa (NARP syndrome) 277.87
  autonomic (peripheral) — *see* Neuropathy, peripheral, autonomic
  axillary nerve 353.0
  brachial plexus 353.0
  cervical plexus 353.2
  chronic
    progressive segmentally demyelinating 357.89
    relapsing demyelinating 357.89
  congenital sensory 356.2
  Déjérine-Sottas 356.0
  diabetic 250.6 ✓ *[357.2]*
  entrapment 355.9
    iliohypogastric nerve 355.79
    ilioinguinal nerve 355.79
    lateral cutaneous nerve of thigh 355.1
    median nerve 354.0
    obturator nerve 355.79
    peroneal nerve 355.3
    posterior tibial nerve 355.5
    saphenous nerve 355.79
    ulnar nerve 354.2
  facial nerve 351.9
  hereditary 356.9
    peripheral 356.0
    sensory (radicular) 356.2
  hypertrophic
    Charcôt-Marie-Tooth 356.1
    Déjérine-Sottas 356.0
    interstitial 356.9
    Refsum 356.3
  intercostal nerve 354.8
  ischemic — *see* Disorder, nerve
  Jamaican (ginger) 357.7
  leg NEC 355.8
  lower extremity NEC 355.8
  lumbar plexus 353.1
  median nerve 354.1
  motor
    acute 357.82
  multiple (acute) (chronic) (*see also* Polyneuropathy) 356.9
  optic 377.39
    ischemic 377.41
    nutritional 377.33
    toxic 377.34
  peripheral (nerve) (*see also* Polyneuropathy) 356.9
    arm NEC 354.9
    autonomic 337.9
      amyloid 277.39 *[337.1]*
      idiopathic 337.0
      in
        amyloidosis 277.39 *[337.1]*
        diabetes (mellitus) 250.6 ✓ *[337.1]*
        diseases classified elsewhere 337.1
        gout 274.89 *[337.1]*
        hyperthyroidism 242.9 ✓ *[337.1]*
    due to
      antitetanus serum 357.6
      arsenic 357.7
      drugs 357.6
      lead 357.7
      organophosphate compounds 357.7
      toxic agent NEC 357.7
    hereditary 356.0
    idiopathic 356.9
      progressive 356.4
      specified type NEC 356.8
    in diseases classified elsewhere — *see* Polyneuropathy, in
    leg NEC 355.8
    lower extremity NEC 355.8
    upper extremity NEC 354.9
  plantar nerves 355.6

**Neuropathy, neuropathic** — *see also* Disorder, nerve — *continued*
  progressive hypertrophic interstitial 356.9
  radicular NEC 729.2
    brachial 723.4
    cervical NEC 723.4
    hereditary sensory 356.2
    lumbar 724.4
    lumbosacral 724.4
    thoracic NEC 724.4
  sacral plexus 353.1
  sciatic 355.0
  spinal nerve NEC 355.9
    root (*see also* Radiculitis) 729.2
  toxic 357.7
  trigeminal sensory 350.8
  ulnar nerve 354.2
  upper extremity NEC 354.9
  uremic 585.9 *[357.4]*
  vitamin $B_{12}$ 266.2 *[357.4]*
    with anemia (pernicious) 281.0 *[357.4]*
      due to dietary deficiency 281.1 *[357.4]*
**Neurophthisis** — *see also* Disorder, nerve
  diabetic 250.6 ✓ *[357.2]*
  peripheral 356.9
**Neuropraxia** — *see* Injury, nerve
**Neuroretinitis** 363.05
  syphilitic 094.85
**Neurosarcoma** (M9540/3) — *see* Neoplasm, connective tissue, malignant
**Neurosclerosis** — *see* Disorder, nerve
**Neurosis, neurotic** 300.9
  accident 300.16
  anancastic, anankastic 300.3
  anxiety (state) 300.00
    generalized 300.02
    panic type 300.01
  asthenic 300.5
  bladder 306.53
  cardiac (reflex) 306.2
  cardiovascular 306.2
  climacteric, unspecified type 627.2
  colon 306.4
  compensation 300.16
  compulsive, compulsion 300.3
  conversion 300.11
  craft 300.89
  cutaneous 306.3
  depersonalization 300.6
  depressive (reaction) (type) 300.4
  endocrine 306.6
  environmental 300.89
  fatigue 300.5
  functional (*see also* Disorder, psychosomatic) 306.9
  gastric 306.4
  gastrointestinal 306.4
  genitourinary 306.50
  heart 306.2
  hypochondriacal 300.7
  hysterical 300.10
    conversion type 300.11
    dissociative type 300.15
  impulsive 300.3
  incoordination 306.0
    larynx 306.1
    vocal cord 306.1
  intestine 306.4
  larynx 306.1
    hysterical 300.11
    sensory 306.1
  menopause, unspecified type 627.2
  mixed NEC 300.89
  musculoskeletal 306.0
  obsessional 300.3
    phobia 300.3
  obsessive-compulsive 300.3
  occupational 300.89
  ocular 306.7
  oral 307.0

**Neurosis, neurotic** — *continued*
  organ (*see also* Disorder, psychosomatic) 306.9
  pharynx 306.1
  phobic 300.20
  posttraumatic (acute) (situational) 309.81
    chronic 309.81
  psychasthenic (type) 300.89
  railroad 300.16
  rectum 306.4
  respiratory 306.1
  rumination 306.4
  senile 300.89
  sexual 302.70
  situational 300.89
  specified type NEC 300.89
  state 300.9
    with depersonalization episode 300.6
  stomach 306.4
  vasomotor 306.2
  visceral 306.4
  war 300.16
**Neurospongioblastosis diffusa** 759.5
**Neurosyphilis** (arrested) (early) (inactive) (late) (latent) (recurrent) 094.9
  with ataxia (cerebellar) (locomotor) (spastic) (spinal) 094.0
  acute meningitis 094.2
  aneurysm 094.89
  arachnoid (adhesive) 094.2
  arteritis (any artery) 094.89
  asymptomatic 094.3
  congenital 090.40
  dura (mater) 094.89
  general paresis 094.1
  gumma 094.9
  hemorrhagic 094.9
  juvenile (asymptomatic) (meningeal) 090.40
  leptomeninges (aseptic) 094.2
  meningeal 094.2
  meninges (adhesive) 094.2
  meningovascular (diffuse) 094.2
  optic atrophy 094.84
  parenchymatous (degenerative) 094.1
  paresis (*see also* Paresis, general) 094.1
  paretic (*see also* Paresis, general) 094.1
  relapse 094.9
  remission in (sustained) 094.9
  serological 094.3
  specified nature or site NEC 094.89
  tabes (dorsalis) 094.0
    juvenile 090.40
  tabetic 094.0
    juvenile 090.40
  taboparesis 094.1
    juvenile 090.40
  thrombosis 094.89
  vascular 094.89
**Neurotic** — *see also* Neurosis 300.9
  excoriation 698.4
  psychogenic 306.3
**Neurotmesis** — *see* Injury, nerve, by site
**Neurotoxemia** — *see* Toxemia
**Neuro-occlusion** 524.21
**Neutropenia, neutropenic** (idiopathic) (pernicious) (primary) 288.00
  chronic 288.09
    hypoplastic 288.09
  congenital (nontransient) 288.01
  cyclic 288.02
  drug induced 288.03
  due to infection 288.04
  fever 288.00
  genetic 288.01
  immune 288.09
  infantile 288.01
  malignant 288.09
  neonatal, transitory (isoimmune) (maternal transfer) 776.7
  periodic 288.02
  splenic 289.53

✓ Additional Digit Required — Refer to the Tabular List for Digit Selection      Subterms under main terms may continue to next column or page

**214 — Volume 2**      ▶◀ Revised Text    ● New Line    ▲ Revised Code      *2008 ICD-9-CM*

**Neutropenia, neutropenic** — *continued*
  splenomegaly 289.53
  toxic 288.09
**Neutrophilia, hereditary giant** 288.2
**Nevocarcinoma** (M8720/3) — *see* Melanoma
**Nevus** (M8720/0) — *see also* Neoplasm, skin, benign

Note — *Except where otherwise indicated, varieties of nevus in the list below that are followed by a morphology code number (M----/0) should be coded by site as for "Neoplasm, skin, benign."*

  acanthotic 702.8
  achromic (M8730/0)
  amelanotic (M8730/0)
  anemic, anemicus 709.09
  angiomatous (M9120/0) (*see also* Hemangioma) 228.00
  araneus 448.1
  avasculosus 709.09
  balloon cell (M8722/0)
  bathing trunk (M8761/1) 238.2
  blue (M8780/0)
    cellular (M8790/0)
    giant (M8790/0)
    Jadassohn's (M8780/0)
    malignant (M8780/3) — *see* Melanoma
  capillary (M9131/0) (*see also* Hemangioma) 228.00
  cavernous (M9121/0) (*see also* Hemangioma) 228.00
  cellular (M8720/0)
    blue (M8790/0)
  comedonicus 757.33
  compound (M8760/0)
  conjunctiva (M8720/0) 224.3
  dermal (M8750/0)
    and epidermal (M8760/0)
  epithelioid cell (and spindle cell) (M8770/0)
  flammeus 757.32
    osteohypertrophic 759.89
  hairy (M8720/0)
  halo (M8723/0)
  hemangiomatous (M9120/0) (*see also* Hemangioma) 228.00
  intradermal (M8750/0)
  intraepidermal (M8740/0)
  involuting (M8724/0)
  Jadassohn's (blue) (M8780/0)
  junction, junctional (M8740/0)
    malignant melanoma in (M8740/3) — *see* Melanoma
  juvenile (M8770/0)
  lymphatic (M9170/0) 228.1
  magnocellular (M8726/0)
    specified site — *see* Neoplasm, by site, benign
    unspecified site 224.0
  malignant (M8720/3) — *see* Melanoma
  meaning hemangioma (M9120/0) (*see also* Hemangioma) 228.00
  melanotic (pigmented) (M8720/0)
  multiplex 759.5
  nonneoplastic 448.1
  nonpigmented (M8730/0)
  nonvascular (M8720/0)
  oral mucosa, white sponge 750.26
  osteohypertrophic, flammeus 759.89
  papillaris (M8720/0)
  papillomatosus (M8720/0)
  pigmented (M8720/0)
    giant (M8761/1) (*see also* Neoplasm, skin, uncertain behavior)
      malignant melanoma in (M8761/3) — *see* Melanoma
    systematicus 757.33
  pilosus (M8720/0)
  port wine 757.32
  sanguineous 757.32

**Nevus** — *see also* Neoplasm, skin, benign — *continued*
  sebaceous (senile) 702.8
  senile 448.1
  spider 448.1
  spindle cell (and epithelioid cell) (M8770/0)
  stellar 448.1
  strawberry 757.32
  syringocystadenomatous papilliferous (M8406/0)
  unius lateris 757.33
  Unna's 757.32
  vascular 757.32
  verrucous 757.33
  white sponge (oral mucosa) 750.26
**Newborn** (infant) (liveborn)
  affected by maternal abuse of drugs (gestational) (via placenta) (via breast milk) (*see also* Noxious, substances transmitted through placenta or breast milk affecting fetus or newborn) 760.70
  apnea 770.81
    obstructive 770.82
    specified NEC 770.82
  cardiomyopathy 425.4
    congenital 425.3
  convulsion 779.0
  electrolyte imbalance NEC (transitory) 775.5
  gestation
    24 completed weeks 765.22
    25-26 completed weeks 765.23
    27-28 completed weeks 765.24
    29-30 completed weeks 765.25
    31-32 completed weeks 765.26
    33-34 completed weeks 765.27
    35-36 completed weeks 765.28
    37 or more completed weeks 765.29
    less than 24 completed weeks 765.21
    unspecified completed weeks 765.20
  infection 771.89
    candida 771.7
    mastitis 771.5
    specified NEC 771.89
    urinary tract 771.82
  mastitis 771.5
  multiple NEC
    born in hospital (without mention of cesarean delivery or section) V37.00
      with cesarean delivery or section V37.01
    born outside hospital
      hospitalized V37.1
      not hospitalized V37.2
    mates all liveborn
      born in hospital (without mention of cesarean delivery or section) V34.00
        with cesarean delivery or section V34.01
      born outside hospital
        hospitalized V34.1
        not hospitalized V34.2
    mates all stillborn
      born in hospital (without mention of cesarean delivery or section) V35.00
        with cesarean delivery or section V35.01
      born outside hospital
        hospitalized V35.1
        not hospitalized V35.2
    mates liveborn and stillborn
      born in hospital (without mention of cesarean delivery or section) V36.00
        with cesarean delivery or section V36.01
      born outside hospital
        hospitalized V36.1

**Newborn** — *continued*
  multiple — *continued*
    mates liveborn and stillborn — *continued*
      born outside hospital — *continued*
        not hospitalized V36.2
  omphalitis 771.4
  seizure 779.0
  sepsis 771.81
  single
    born in hospital (without mention of cesarean delivery or section) V30.00
      with cesarean delivery or section V30.01
    born outside hospital
      hospitalized V30.1
      not hospitalized V30.2
  specified condition NEC 779.89
  twin NEC
    born in hospital (without mention of cesarean delivery or section) V33.00
      with cesarean delivery or section V33.01
    born outside hospital
      hospitalized V33.1
      not hospitalized V33.2
    mate liveborn
      born in hospital V31.0 ☑
      born outside hospital
        hospitalized V31.1
        not hospitalized V31.2
    mate stillborn
      born in hospital V32.0 ☑
      born outside hospital
        hospitalized V32.1
        not hospitalized V32.2
  unspecified as to single or multiple birth
    born in hospital (without mention of cesarean delivery or section) V39.00
      with cesarean delivery or section V39.01
    born outside hospital
      hospitalized V39.1
      not hospitalized V39.2
**Newcastle's conjunctivitis or disease** 077.8
**Nezelof's syndrome** (pure alymphocytosis) 279.13
**Niacin** (amide) **deficiency** 265.2
**Nicolas-Durand-Favre disease** (climatic bubo) 099.1
**Nicolas-Favre disease** (climatic bubo) 099.1
**Nicotinic acid** (amide) **deficiency** 265.2
**Niemann-Pick disease** (lipid histiocytosis) (splenomegaly) 272.7
**Night**
  blindness (*see also* Blindness, night) 368.60
    congenital 368.61
    vitamin A deficiency 264.5
  cramps 729.82
  sweats 780.8
  terrors, child 307.46
**Nightmare** 307.47
  REM-sleep type 307.47
**Nipple** — *see* condition
**Nisbet's chancre** 099.0
**Nishimoto** (-Takeuchi) **disease** 437.5
**Nitritoid crisis or reaction** — *see* Crisis, nitritoid
**Nitrogen retention, extrarenal** 788.9
**Nitrosohemoglobinemia** 289.89
**Njovera** 104.0
**No**
  diagnosis 799.9
  disease (found) V71.9
  room at the inn V65.0
**Nocardiasis** — *see* Nocardiosis
**Nocardiosis** 039.9
  with pneumonia 039.1

**Nocardiosis** — *continued*
  lung 039.1
  specified type NEC 039.8
**Nocturia** 788.43
  psychogenic 306.53
**Nocturnal** — *see also* condition
  dyspnea (paroxysmal) 786.09
  emissions 608.89
  enuresis 788.36
    psychogenic 307.6
  frequency (micturition) 788.43
    psychogenic 306.53
**Nodal rhythm disorder** 427.89
**Nodding of head** 781.0
**Node(s)** — *see also* Nodule(s)
  Heberden's 715.04
  larynx 478.79
  lymph — *see* condition
  milkers' 051.1
  Osler's 421.0
  rheumatic 729.89
  Schmorl's 722.30
    lumbar, lumbosacral 722.32
    specified region NEC 722.39
    thoracic, thoracolumbar 722.31
  singers' 478.5
  skin NEC 782.2
  tuberculous — *see* Tuberculosis, lymph gland
  vocal cords 478.5
**Nodosities, Haygarth's** 715.04
**Nodule(s), nodular**
  actinomycotic (*see also* Actinomycosis) 039.9
  arthritic — *see* Arthritis, nodosa
  cutaneous 782.2
  Haygarth's 715.04
  inflammatory — *see* Inflammation
  juxta-articular 102.7
    syphilitic 095.7
    yaws 102.7
  larynx 478.79
  lung, solitary 518.89
    emphysematous 492.8
  milkers' 051.1
  prostate 600.10
    with
      urinary
        obstruction 600.11
        retention 600.11
  rheumatic 729.89
  rheumatoid — *see* Arthritis, rheumatoid
  scrotum (inflammatory) 608.4
  singers' 478.5
  skin NEC 782.2
  solitary, lung 518.89
    emphysematous 492.8
  subcutaneous 782.2
  thyroid (gland) (nontoxic) (uninodular) 241.0
    with
      hyperthyroidism 242.1 ☑
      thyrotoxicosis 242.1 ☑
    toxic or with hyperthyroidism 242.1 ☑
  vocal cords 478.5
**Noma** (gangrenous) (hospital) (infective) 528.1
  auricle (*see also* Gangrene) 785.4
  mouth 528.1
  pudendi (*see also* Vulvitis) 616.10
  vulvae (*see also* Vulvitis) 616.10
**Nomadism** V60.0
**Non-adherence**
  artificial skin graft 996.55
  decellularized allodermis graft 996.55
**Non-autoimmune hemolytic anemia** NEC 283.10
**Nonclosure** — *see also* Imperfect, closure
  ductus
    arteriosus 747.0
    Botalli 747.0
  Eustachian valve 746.89
  foramen
    Botalli 745.5

☑ Additional Digit Required — Refer to the Tabular List for Digit Selection      ▽ Subterms under main terms may continue to next column or page

**2008 ICD-9-CM**      ▶◀ Revised Text      ● New Line      ▲ Revised Code      **Volume 2 — 215**

**Nonclosure** — *see also* Imperfect, closure
— *continued*
  foramen — *continued*
    ovale 745.5
**Noncompliance with medical treatment** V15.81
**Nondescent (congenital)** — *see also*
  Malposition, congenital
  cecum 751.4
  colon 751.4
  testis 752.51
**Nondevelopment**
  brain 742.1
    specified part 742.2
  heart 746.89
  organ or site, congenital NEC — *see*
    Hypoplasia
**Nonengagement**
  head NEC 652.5 ☑
    in labor 660.1 ☑
      affecting fetus or newborn 763.1
**Nonexanthematous tick fever** 066.1
**Nonexpansion, lung** (newborn) NEC
  770.4
**Nonfunctioning**
  cystic duct (*see also* Disease, gallbladder) 575.8
  gallbladder (*see also* Disease, gallbladder) 575.8
  kidney (*see also* Disease, renal) 593.9
  labyrinth 386.58
**Nonhealing**
  stump (surgical) 997.69
  wound, surgical 998.83
**Nonimplantation of ovum, causing infertility** 628.3
**Noninsufflation, fallopian tube** 628.2
**Nonne-Milroy-Meige syndrome** (chronic hereditary edema) 757.0
**Nonovulation** 628.0
**Nonpatent fallopian tube** 628.2
**Nonpneumatization, lung** NEC 770.4
**Nonreflex bladder** 596.54
  with cauda equina 344.61
**Nonretention of food** — *see* Vomiting
**Nonrotation** — *see* Malrotation
**Nonsecretion, urine** — *see also* Anuria
  788.5

**Nonsecretion, urine** — *see also* Anuria
— *continued*
  newborn 753.3
**Nonunion**
  fracture 733.82
  organ or site, congenital NEC — *see*
    Imperfect, closure
  symphysis pubis, congenital 755.69
  top sacrum, congenital 756.19
**Nonviability** 765.0 ☑
**Nonvisualization, gallbladder** 793.3
**Nonvitalized tooth** 522.9
**Non-working side interference** 524.56
**Normal**
  delivery — *see* category 650
  menses V65.5
  state (feared complaint unfounded)
    V65.5
**Normoblastosis** 289.89
**Normocytic anemia** (infectional) 285.9
  due to blood loss (chronic) 280.0
    acute 285.1
**Norrie's disease** (congenital) (progressive oculoacousticocerebral degeneration) 743.8
**North American blastomycosis** 116.0
**Norwegian itch** 133.0
**Nosebleed** 784.7
**Nose, nasal** — *see* condition
**Nosomania** 298.9
**Nosophobia** 300.29
**Nostalgia** 309.89
**Notched lip, congenital** — *see also*
  Cleft, lip 749.10
**Notching nose, congenital** (tip) 748.1
**Notch of iris** 743.46
**Nothnagel's**
  syndrome 378.52
  vasomotor acroparesthesia 443.89
**Novy's relapsing fever** (American) 087.1
**Noxious**
  foodstuffs, poisoning by
    fish 988.0
    fungi 988.1
    mushrooms 988.1
    plants (food) 988.2
    shellfish 988.0
    specified type NEC 988.8

**Noxious** — *continued*
  foodstuffs, poisoning by — *continued*
    toadstool 988.1
  substances transmitted through placenta or breast milk (affecting fetus or newborn) 760.70
    acetretin 760.78
    alcohol 760.71
    aminopterin 760.78
    antiandrogens 760.79
    anticonvulsant 760.77
    antifungal 760.74
    anti-infective agents 760.74
    antimetabolic 760.78
    atorvastatin 760.78
    carbamazepine 760.77
    cocaine 760.75
    "crack" 760.75
    diethylstilbestrol (DES) 760.76
    divalproex sodium 760.77
    endocrine disrupting chemicals 760.79
    estrogens 760.79
    etretinate 760.78
    fluconazole 760.74
    fluvastatin 760.78
    hallucinogenic agents NEC 760.73
    hormones 760.79
    lithium 760.79
    lovastatin 760.78
    medicinal agents NEC 760.79
    methotrexate 760.78
    misoprostil 760.79
    narcotics 760.72
    obstetric anesthetic or analgesic 763.5
    phenobarbital 760.77
    phenytoin 760.77
    pravastatin 760.78
    progestins 760.79
    retinoic acid 760.78
    simvastatin 760.78
    solvents 760.79
    specified agent NEC 760.79
    statins 760.78
    suspected, affecting management of pregnancy 655.5 ☑

**Noxious** — *continued*
  substances transmitted through placenta or breast milk — *continued*
    tetracycline 760.74
    thalidomide 760.79
    trimethadione 760.77
    valproate 760.77
    valproic acid 760.77
    vitamin A 760.78
**Nuchal hitch** (arm) 652.8 ☑
**Nucleus pulposus** — *see* condition
**Numbness** 782.0
**Nuns' knee** 727.2
**Nursemaid's**
  elbow 832.0 ☑
  shoulder 831.0 ☑
**Nutmeg liver** 573.8
**Nutrition, deficient or insufficient** (particular kind of food) 269.9
  due to
    insufficient food 994.2
    lack of
      care (child) (infant) 995.52
        adult 995.84
      food 994.2
**Nyctalopia** — *see also* Blindness, night
  368.60
  vitamin A deficiency 264.5
**Nycturia** 788.43
  psychogenic 306.53
**Nymphomania** 302.89
**Nystagmus** 379.50
  associated with vestibular system disorders 379.54
  benign paroxysmal positional 386.11
  central positional 386.2
  congenital 379.51
  deprivation 379.53
  dissociated 379.55
  latent 379.52
  miners' 300.89
  positional
    benign paroxysmal 386.11
    central 386.2
  specified NEC 379.56
  vestibular 379.54
  visual deprivation 379.53

---

☑ Additional Digit Required — Refer to the Tabular List for Digit Selection          🖎 Subterms under main terms may continue to next column or page

## O

**Oasthouse urine disease** 270.2
**Obermeyer's relapsing fever** (European) 087.0
**Obesity** (constitutional) (exogenous) (familial) (nutritional) (simple) 278.00
  adrenal 255.8
  complicating pregnancy, childbirth, or puerperium 649.1 ☑
  due to hyperalimentation 278.00
  endocrine NEC 259.9
  endogenous 259.9
  Fröhlich's (adiposogenital dystrophy) 253.8
  glandular NEC 259.9
  hypothyroid (see also Hypothyroidism) 244.9
  morbid 278.01
  of pregnancy 649.1 ☑
  pituitary 253.8
  severe 278.01
  thyroid (see also Hypothyroidism) 244.9
**Oblique** — see also condition
  lie before labor, affecting fetus or newborn 761.7
**Obliquity, pelvis** 738.6
**Obliteration**
  abdominal aorta 446.7
  appendix (lumen) 543.9
  artery 447.1
  ascending aorta 446.7
  bile ducts 576.8
    with calculus, choledocholithiasis, or stones — see Choledocholithiasis
    congenital 751.61
      jaundice from 751.61 [774.5]
  common duct 576.8
    with calculus, choledocholithiasis, or stones — see Choledocholithiasis
    congenital 751.61
  cystic duct 575.8
    with calculus, choledocholithiasis, or stones — see Choledocholithiasis
  disease, arteriolar 447.1
  endometrium 621.8
  eye, anterior chamber 360.34
  fallopian tube 628.2
  lymphatic vessel 457.1
    postmastectomy 457.0
  organ or site, congenital NEC — see Atresia
  placental blood vessels — see Placenta, abnormal
  supra-aortic branches 446.7
  ureter 593.89
  urethra 599.84
  vein 459.9
  vestibule (oral) 525.8
**Observation** (for) V71.9
  without need for further medical care V71.9
  accident NEC V71.4
    at work V71.3
  criminal assault V71.6
  deleterious agent ingestion V71.89
  disease V71.9
    cardiovascular V71.7
    heart V71.7
    mental V71.09
    specified condition NEC V71.89
  foreign body ingestion V71.89
  growth and development variations V21.8
  injuries (accidental) V71.4
    inflicted NEC V71.6
      during alleged rape or seduction V71.5
  malignant neoplasm, suspected V71.1
  postpartum
    immediately after delivery V24.0
    routine follow-up V24.2

**Observation** — continued
  pregnancy
    high-risk V23.9
      specified problem NEC V23.89
    normal (without complication) V22.1
      with nonobstetric complication V22.2
    first V22.0
  rape or seduction, alleged V71.5
    injury during V71.5
  suicide attempt, alleged V71.89
  suspected (undiagnosed) (unproven)
    abuse V71.81
    cardiovascular disease V71.7
    child or wife battering victim V71.6
    concussion (cerebral) V71.6
    condition NEC V71.89
      infant — see Observation, suspected, condition, newborn
    newborn V29.9
      cardiovascular disease V29.8
      congenital anomaly V29.8
      genetic V29.3
      infectious V29.0
      ingestion foreign object V29.8
      injury V29.8
      metabolic V29.3
      neoplasm V29.8
      neurological V29.1
      poison, poisoning V29.8
      respiratory V29.2
      specified NEC V29.8
    exposure
      anthrax V71.82
      biologic agent NEC V71.83
      SARS V71.83
    infectious disease not requiring isolation V71.89
    malignant neoplasm V71.1
    mental disorder V71.09
    neglect V71.81
    neoplasm
      benign V71.89
      malignant V71.1
    specified condition NEC V71.89
    tuberculosis V71.2
  tuberculosis, suspected V71.2
**Obsession, obsessional** 300.3
  ideas and mental images 300.3
  impulses 300.3
  neurosis 300.3
  phobia 300.3
  psychasthenia 300.3
  ruminations 300.3
  state 300.3
  syndrome 300.3
**Obsessive-compulsive** 300.3
  neurosis 300.3
  personality 301.4
  reaction 300.3
**Obstetrical trauma** NEC (complicating delivery) 665.9 ☑
  with
    abortion — see Abortion, by type, with damage to pelvic organs
    ectopic pregnancy (see also categories 633.0–633.9) 639.2
    molar pregnancy (see also categories 630–632) 639.2
  affecting fetus or newborn 763.89
  following
    abortion 639.2
    ectopic or molar pregnancy 639.2
**Obstipation** — see also Constipation 564.00
  psychogenic 306.4
**Obstruction, obstructed, obstructive**
  airway NEC 519.8
    with
      allergic alveolitis NEC 495.9
      asthma NEC (see also Asthma) 493.9 ☑
      bronchiectasis 494.0

**Obstruction, obstructed, obstructive** — continued
  airway — continued
    with — continued
      bronchiectasis — continued
        with acute exacerbation 494.1
      bronchitis (chronic) (see also Bronchitis, with, obstruction) 491.20
      emphysema NEC 492.8
    chronic 496
      with
        allergic alveolitis NEC 495.5
        asthma NEC (see also Asthma) 493.2 ☑
        bronchiectasis 494.0
          with acute exacerbation 494.1
        bronchitis (chronic) (see also Bronchitis, with, obstruction) 491.20
        emphysema NEC 492.8
    due to
      bronchospasm 519.11
      foreign body 934.9
      inhalation of fumes or vapors 506.9
      laryngospasm 478.75
  alimentary canal (see also Obstruction, intestine) 560.9
  ampulla of Vater 576.2
    with calculus, cholelithiasis, or stones — see Choledocholithiasis
  aortic (heart) (valve) (see also Stenosis, aortic) 424.1
    rheumatic (see also Stenosis, aortic, rheumatic) 395.0
  aortoiliac 444.0
  aqueduct of Sylvius 331.4
    congenital 742.3
      with spina bifida (see also Spina bifida) 741.0 ☑
  Arnold-Chiari (see also Spina bifida) 741.0 ☑
  artery (see also Embolism, artery) 444.9
    basilar (complete) (partial) (see also Occlusion, artery, basilar) 433.0 ☑
    carotid (complete) (partial) (see also Occlusion, artery, carotid) 433.1 ☑
    precerebral — see Occlusion, artery, precerebral NEC
    retinal (central) (see also Occlusion, retina) 362.30
    vertebral (complete) (partial) (see also Occlusion, artery, vertebral) 433.2 ☑
  asthma (chronic) (with obstructive pulmonary disease) 493.2 ☑
  band (intestinal) 560.81
  bile duct or passage (see also Obstruction, biliary) 576.2
    congenital 751.61
      jaundice from 751.61 [774.5]
  biliary (duct) (tract) 576.2
    with calculus 574.51
      with cholecystitis (chronic) 574.41
        acute 574.31
    congenital 751.61
      jaundice from 751.61 [774.5]
    gallbladder 575.2
      with calculus 574.21
        with cholecystitis (chronic) 574.11
          acute 574.01
  bladder neck (acquired) 596.0
    congenital 753.6
  bowel (see also Obstruction, intestine) 560.9
  bronchus 519.19

**Obstruction, obstructed, obstructive** — continued
  canal, ear (see also Stricture, ear canal, acquired) 380.50
  cardia 537.89
  caval veins (inferior) (superior) 459.2
  cecum (see also Obstruction, intestine) 560.9
  circulatory 459.9
  colon (see also Obstruction, intestine) 560.9
    sympathicotonic 560.89
  common duct (see also Obstruction, biliary) 576.2
    congenital 751.61
  coronary (artery) (heart) (see also Arteriosclerosis, coronary)
    acute (see also Infarct, myocardium) 410.9 ☑
      without myocardial infarction 411.81
  cystic duct (see also Obstruction, gallbladder) 575.2
    congenital 751.61
  device, implant, or graft — see Complications, due to (presence of) any device, implant, or graft classified to 996.0–996.5 NEC
  due to foreign body accidentally left in operation wound 998.4
  duodenum 537.3
    congenital 751.1
    due to
      compression NEC 537.3
      cyst 537.3
      intrinsic lesion or disease NEC 537.3
      scarring 537.3
      torsion 537.3
      ulcer 532.91
      volvulus 537.3
  ejaculatory duct 608.89
  endocardium 424.90
    arteriosclerotic 424.99
    specified cause, except rheumatic 424.99
  esophagus 530.3
  eustachian tube (complete) (partial) 381.60
    cartilaginous
      extrinsic 381.63
      intrinsic 381.62
    due to
      cholesteatoma 381.61
      osseous lesion NEC 381.61
      polyp 381.61
    osseous 381.61
  fallopian tube (bilateral) 628.2
  fecal 560.39
    with hernia (see also Hernia, by site, with obstruction)
      gangrenous — see Hernia, by site, with gangrene
  foramen of Monro (congenital) 742.3
    with spina bifida (see also Spina bifida) 741.0 ☑
  foreign body — see Foreign body
  gallbladder 575.2
    with calculus, cholelithiasis, or stones 574.21
      with cholecystitis (chronic) 574.11
        acute 574.01
    congenital 751.69
      jaundice from 751.69 [774.5]
  gastric outlet 537.0
  gastrointestinal (see also Obstruction, intestine) 560.9
  glottis 478.79
  hepatic 573.8
    duct (see also Obstruction, biliary) 576.2
      congenital 751.61
  icterus (see also Obstruction, biliary) 576.8
    congenital 751.61

**Obstruction, obstructed, obstructive**
— *continued*
  ileocecal coil (*see also* Obstruction,
    intestine) 560.9
  ileum (*see also* Obstruction, intestine)
    560.9
  iliofemoral (artery) 444.81
  internal anastomosis — *see* Complica-
    tions, mechanical, graft
  intestine (mechanical) (neurogenic)
    (paroxysmal) (postinfectional)
    (reflex) 560.9
    with
        adhesions (intestinal) (peri-
          toneal) 560.81
        hernia (*see also* Hernia, by site,
          with obstruction)
            gangrenous — *see* Hernia, by
              site, with gangrene
    adynamic (*see also* Ileus) 560.1
    by gallstone 560.31
    congenital or infantile (small) 751.1
        large 751.2
    due to
        Ascaris lumbricoides 127.0
        mural thickening 560.89
        procedure 997.4
            involving urinary tract 997.5
    impaction 560.39
    infantile — *see* Obstruction, intes-
      tine, congenital
    newborn
        due to
            fecaliths 777.1
            inspissated milk 777.2
            meconium (plug) 777.1
                in mucoviscidosis 277.01
            transitory 777.4
        specified cause NEC 560.89
        transitory, newborn 777.4
        volvulus 560.2
  intracardiac ball valve prosthesis
    996.02
  jaundice (*see also* Obstruction, biliary)
    576.8
    congenital 751.61
  jejunum (*see also* Obstruction, intes-
    tine) 560.9
  kidney 593.89
  labor 660.9 ☑
    affecting fetus or newborn 763.1
    by
        bony pelvis (conditions classifi-
          able to 653.0–653.9)
          660.1 ☑
        deep transverse arrest 660.3 ☑
        impacted shoulder 660.4 ☑
        locked twins 660.5 ☑
        malposition (fetus) (conditions
          classifiable to
          652.0–652.9) 660.0 ☑
            head during labor 660.3 ☑
        persistent occipitoposterior posi-
          tion 660.3 ☑
        soft tissue, pelvic (conditions
          classifiable to
          654.0–654.9) 660.2 ☑
  lacrimal
    canaliculi 375.53
    congenital 743.65
    punctum 375.52
    sac 375.54
  lacrimonasal duct 375.56
    congenital 743.65
    neonatal 375.55
  lacteal, with steatorrhea 579.2
  laryngitis (*see also* Laryngitis) 464.01
  larynx 478.79
    congenital 748.3
  liver 573.8
    cirrhotic (*see also* Cirrhosis, liver)
      571.5
  lung 518.89
    with
        asthma — *see* Asthma
        bronchitis (chronic) 491.20

**Obstruction, obstructed, obstructive**
— *continued*
  lung — *continued*
    with — *continued*
        emphysema NEC 492.8
    airway, chronic 496
    chronic NEC 496
        with
            asthma (chronic) (obstruc-
              tive) 493.2 ☑
    disease, chronic 496
        with
            asthma (chronic) (obstruc-
              tive) 493.2 ☑
    emphysematous 492.8
  lymphatic 457.1
  meconium
    fetus or newborn 777.1
        in mucoviscidosis 277.01
    newborn due to fecaliths 777.1
  mediastinum 519.3
  mitral (rheumatic) — *see* Stenosis,
    mitral
  nasal 478.19
    duct 375.56
        neonatal 375.55
    sinus — *see* Sinusitis
  nasolacrimal duct 375.56
    congenital 743.65
    neonatal 375.55
  nasopharynx 478.29
  nose 478.19
  organ or site, congenital NEC — *see*
    Atresia
  pancreatic duct 577.8
  parotid gland 527.8
  pelviureteral junction (*see also* Ob-
    struction, ureter) 593.4
  pharynx 478.29
  portal (circulation) (vein) 452
  prostate 600.90
    with
        other lower urinary tract symp-
          toms (LUTS) 600.91
        urinary
            obstruction 600.91
            retention 600.91
    valve (urinary) 596.0
  pulmonary
    valve (heart) (*see also* Endocarditis,
      pulmonary) 424.3
    vein, isolated 747.49
  pyemic — *see* Septicemia
  pylorus (acquired) 537.0
    congenital 750.5
    infantile 750.5
  rectosigmoid (*see also* Obstruction,
    intestine) 560.9
  rectum 569.49
  renal 593.89
  respiratory 519.8
    chronic 496
  retinal (artery) (vein) (central) (*see also*
    Occlusion, retina) 362.30
  salivary duct (any) 527.8
    with calculus 527.5
  sigmoid (*see also* Obstruction, intes-
    tine) 560.9
  sinus (accessory) (nasal) (*see also* Si-
    nusitis) 473.9
  Stensen's duct 527.8
  stomach 537.89
    acute 536.1
    congenital 750.7
  submaxillary gland 527.8
    with calculus 527.5
  thoracic duct 457.1
  thrombotic — *see* Thrombosis
  tooth eruption 520.6
  trachea 519.19
  tracheostomy airway 519.09
  tricuspid — *see* Endocarditis, tricus-
    pid
  upper respiratory, congenital 748.8
  ureter (functional) 593.4
    congenital 753.20

**Obstruction, obstructed, obstructive**
— *continued*
  ureter — *continued*
    due to calculus 592.1
    ureteropelvic junction, congenital
      753.21
    ureterovesical junction, congenital
      753.22
  urethra 599.60
    congenital 753.6
  urinary (moderate) 599.60
    organ or tract (lower) 599.60
        due to
            benign prostatic hypertrophy
              (BPH) - see category
              600
        specified NEC 599.69
            due to
                benign prostatic hypertro-
                  phy (BPH) — see
                  category 600
    prostatic valve 596.0
  uropathy 599.60
  uterus 621.8
  vagina 623.2
  valvular — *see* Endocarditis
  vascular graft or shunt 996.1
    atherosclerosis — *see* Arteriosclero-
      sis, coronary
    embolism 996.74
    occlusion NEC 996.74
    thrombus 996.74
    vein, venous 459.2
        caval (inferior) (superior) 459.2
        thrombotic — *see* Thrombosis
    vena cava (inferior) (superior) 459.2
  ventricular shunt 996.2
  vesical 596.0
  vesicourethral orifice 596.0
  vessel NEC 459.9
**Obturator** — *see* condition
**Occlusal**
  plane deviation 524.76
  wear, teeth 521.10
**Occlusion**
  anus 569.49
    congenital 751.2
    infantile 751.2
  aortoiliac (chronic) 444.0
  aqueduct of Sylvius 331.4
    congenital 742.3
        with spina bifida (*see also* Spina
          bifida) 741.0 ☑
  arteries of extremities, lower 444.22
    without thrombus or embolus (*see
      also* Arteriosclerosis, extrem-
      ities) 440.20
    due to stricture or stenosis 447.1
    upper 444.21
        without thrombus or embolus
          (*see also* Arteriosclerosis,
          extremities) 440.20
        due to stricture or stenosis
          447.1
  artery NEC (*see also* Embolism, artery)
    444.9
    auditory, internal 433.8 ☑
    basilar 433.0 ☑
        with other precerebral artery
          433.3 ☑
        bilateral 433.3 ☑
    brain or cerebral (*see also* Infarct,
      brain) 434.9 ☑
    carotid 433.1 ☑
        with other precerebral artery
          433.3 ☑
        bilateral 433.3 ☑
    cerebellar (anterior inferior) (poste-
      rior inferior) (superior)
      433.8 ☑
    cerebral (*see also* Infarct, brain)
      434.9 ☑
    choroidal (anterior) 433.8 ☑
    chronic total                                      ●
        coronary 414.2                                 ●
        extremity(ies) 440.4                           ●

**Occlusion** — *continued*
  artery (*see also* Embolism, artery) —
    *continued*
        communicating posterior 433.8 ☑
        complete                                       ●
            coronary 414.2                             ●
            extremity(ies) 440.4                       ●
        coronary (thrombotic) (*see also* In-
          farct, myocardium) 410.9 ☑
            acute 410.9 ☑
                without myocardial infarction
                  411.81
            chronic total 414.2                        ●
            complete 414.2                             ●
            healed or old 412
            total 414.2                                ●
        extremity(ies)                                 ●
            chronic total 440.4                        ●
            complete 440.4                             ●
            total 440.4                                ●
        hypophyseal 433.8 ☑
        iliac (artery) 444.81
        mesenteric (embolic) (thrombotic)
          (with gangrene) 557.0
        pontine 433.8 ☑
        precerebral NEC 433.9 ☑
            late effect — *see* Late effect(s)
              (of) cerebrovascular dis-
              ease
            multiple or bilateral 433.3 ☑
            puerperal, postpartum, child-
              birth 674.0 ☑
            specified NEC 433.8 ☑
        renal 593.81
        retinal — *see* Occlusion, retina,
          artery
        spinal 433.8 ☑
        vertebral 433.2 ☑
            with other precerebral artery
              433.3 ☑
            bilateral 433.3 ☑
  basilar (artery) — *see* Occlusion,
    artery, basilar
  bile duct (any) (*see also* Obstruction,
    biliary) 576.2
  bowel (*see also* Obstruction, intestine)
    560.9
  brain (artery) (vascular) (*see also* In-
    farct, brain) 434.9 ☑
  breast (duct) 611.8
  carotid (artery) (common) (internal) —
    *see* Occlusion, artery, carotid
  cerebellar (anterior inferior) (artery)
    (posterior inferior) (superior)
    433.8 ☑
  cerebral (artery) (*see also* Infarct,
    brain) 434.9 ☑
  cerebrovascular (*see also* Infarct,
    brain) 434.9 ☑
    diffuse 437.0
  cervical canal (*see also* Stricture,
    cervix) 622.4
    by falciparum malaria 084.0
  cervix (uteri) (*see also* Stricture,
    cervix) 622.4
  choanal 748.0
  choroidal (artery) 433.8 ☑
  colon (*see also* Obstruction, intestine)
    560.9
  communicating posterior artery
    433.8 ☑
  coronary (artery) (thrombotic) (*see also*
    Infarct, myocardium) 410.9 ☑
    without myocardial infarction
      411.81
    acute 410.9 ☑
        without myocardial infarction
          411.81
    healed or old 412
  cystic duct (*see also* Obstruction,
    gallbladder) 575.2
    congenital 751.69
  disto
    division I 524.22
    division II 524.22
  embolic — *see* Embolism

---

☑ Additional Digit Required — Refer to the Tabular List for Digit Selection          ⱽᴱᴰ Subterms under main terms may continue to next column or page

**218 — Volume 2 · October 2007**        ►◄ Revised Text        ● New Line        ▲ Revised Code                    **2008 ICD-9-CM**

**Occlusion** — *continued*
  fallopian tube 628.2
    congenital 752.19
  gallbladder (*see also* Obstruction,
      gallbladder) 575.2
    congenital 751.69
      jaundice from 751.69 *[774.5]*
  gingiva, traumatic 523.8
  hymen 623.3
    congenital 752.42
  hypophyseal (artery) 433.8 ☑
  iliac artery 444.81
  intestine (*see also* Obstruction, intes-
      tine) 560.9
  kidney 593.89
  lacrimal apparatus — *see* Stenosis,
      lacrimal
  lung 518.89
  lymph or lymphatic channel 457.1
  mammary duct 611.8
  mesenteric artery (embolic) (thrombot-
      ic) (with gangrene) 557.0
  nose 478.1 ☑
    congenital 748.0
  organ or site, congenital NEC — *see*
      Atresia
  oviduct 628.2
    congenital 752.19
  periodontal, traumatic 523.8
  peripheral arteries (lower extremity)
      444.22
    without thrombus or embolus (*see
        also* Arteriosclerosis, extrem-
        ities) 440.20
    due to stricture or stenosis 447.1
    upper extremity 444.21
      without thrombus or embolus
          (*see also* Arteriosclerosis,
          extremities) 440.20
      due to stricture or stenosis
          447.1
  pontine (artery) 433.8 ☑
  posterior lingual, of mandibular teeth
      524.29
  precerebral artery — *see* Occlusion,
      artery, precerebral NEC
  puncta lacrimalia 375.52
  pupil 364.74
  pylorus (*see also* Stricture, pylorus)
      537.0
  renal artery 593.81
  retina, retinal (vascular) 362.30
    artery, arterial 362.30
      branch 362.32
      central (total) 362.31
      partial 362.33
      transient 362.34
      tributary 362.32
    vein 362.30
      branch 362.36
      central (total) 362.35
      incipient 362.37
      partial 362.37
      tributary 362.36
  spinal artery 433.8 ☑
  stent
    coronary 996.72
  teeth (mandibular) (posterior lingual)
      524.29
  thoracic duct 457.1
  tubal 628.2
  ureter (complete) (partial) 593.4
    congenital 753.29
  urethra (*see also* Stricture, urethra)
      598.9
    congenital 753.6
  uterus 621.8
  vagina 623.2
  vascular NEC 459.9
  vein — *see* Thrombosis
  vena cava (inferior) (superior) 453.2
  ventricle (brain) NEC 331.4
  vertebral (artery) — *see* Occlusion,
      artery, vertebral
  vessel (blood) NEC 459.9
  vulva 624.8

**Occlusio pupillae** 364.74
**Occupational**
  problems NEC V62.2
  therapy V57.21
**Ochlophobia** 300.29
**Ochronosis** (alkaptonuric) (congenital)
    (endogenous) 270.2
  with chloasma of eyelid 270.2
**Ocular muscle** — *see also* condition
  myopathy 359.1
  torticollis 781.93
**Oculoauriculovertebral dysplasia** 756.0
**Oculogyric**
  crisis or disturbance 378.87
    psychogenic 306.7
**Oculomotor syndrome** 378.81
**Oddi's sphincter spasm** 576.5
**Odelberg's disease** (juvenile osteochon-
    drosis) 732.1
**Odontalgia** 525.9
**Odontoameloblastoma** (M9311/0) 213.1
  upper jaw (bone) 213.0
**Odontoclasia** 521.05
**Odontoclasis** 873.63
  complicated 873.73
**Odontodysplasia, regional** 520.4
**Odontogenesis imperfecta** 520.5
**Odontoma** (M9280/0) 213.1
  ameloblastic (M9311/0) 213.1
    upper jaw (bone) 213.0
  calcified (M9280/0) 213.1
    upper jaw (bone) 213.0
  complex (M9282/0) 213.1
    upper jaw (bone) 213.0
  compound (M9281/0) 213.1
    upper jaw (bone) 213.0
  fibroameloblastic (M9290/0) 213.1
    upper jaw (bone) 213.0
  follicular 526.0
  upper jaw (bone) 213.0
**Odontomyelitis** (closed) (open) 522.0
**Odontonecrosis** 521.09
**Odontorrhagia** 525.8
**Odontosarcoma, ameloblastic**
    (M9290/3) 170.1
  upper jaw (bone) 170.0
**Odynophagia** 787.20                              ▲
**Oesophagostomiasis** 127.7
**Oesophagostomum infestation** 127.7
**Oestriasis** 134.0
**Ogilvie's syndrome** (sympathicotonic
    colon obstruction) 560.89
**Oguchi's disease** (retina) 368.61
**Ohara's disease** — *see also* Tularemia
    021.9
**Oidiomycosis** — *see also* Candidiasis
    112.9
**Oidiomycotic meningitis** 112.83
**Oidium albicans infection** — *see also*
    Candidiasis 112.9
**Old age** 797
  dementia (of) 290.0
**Olfactory** — *see* condition
**Oligemia** 285.9
**Oligergasia** — *see also* Retardation,
    mental 319
**Oligoamnios** 658.0 ☑
  affecting fetus or newborn 761.2
**Oligoastrocytoma, mixed** (M9382/3)
  specified site — *see* Neoplasm, by site,
      malignant
  unspecified site 191.9
**Oligocythemia** 285.9
**Oligodendroblastoma** (M9460/3)
  specified site — *see* Neoplasm, by site,
      malignant
  unspecified site 191.9
**Oligodendroglioma** (M9450/3)
  anaplastic type (M9451/3)
    specified site — *see* Neoplasm, by
        site, malignant
    unspecified site 191.9
  specified site — *see* Neoplasm, by
      site, malignant
  unspecified site 191.9

**Oligodendroma** — *see* Oligoden-
    droglioma
**Oligodontia** — *see also* Anodontia 520.0
**Oligoencephalon** 742.1
**Oligohydramnios** 658.0 ☑
  affecting fetus or newborn 761.2
  due to premature rupture of mem-
      branes 658.1 ☑
    affecting fetus or newborn 761.2
**Oligohydrosis** 705.0
**Oligomenorrhea** 626.1
**Oligophrenia** — *see also* Retardation,
    mental 319
  phenylpyruvic 270.1
**Oligospermia** 606.1
**Oligotrichia** 704.09
  congenita 757.4
**Oliguria** 788.5
  with
    abortion — *see* Abortion, by type,
        with renal failure
    ectopic pregnancy (*see also* cate-
        gories 633.0–633.9) 639.3
    molar pregnancy (*see also* cate-
        gories 630–632) 639.3
  complicating
    abortion 639.3
    ectopic or molar pregnancy 639.3
    pregnancy 646.2 ☑
      with hypertension — *see* Tox-
          emia, of pregnancy
  due to a procedure 997.5
  following labor and delivery 669.3 ☑
  heart or cardiac — *see* Failure, heart
  puerperal, postpartum 669.3 ☑
  specified due to a procedure 997.5
**Ollier's disease** (chondrodysplasia) 756.4
**Omentitis** — *see also* Peritonitis 567.9
**Omentocele** — *see also* Hernia, omental
    553.8
**Omentum, omental** — *see* condition
**Omphalitis** (congenital) (newborn) 771.4
  not of newborn 686.9
  tetanus 771.3
**Omphalocele** 756.79
**Omphalomesenteric duct, persistent**
    751.0
**Omphalorrhagia, newborn** 772.3
**Omsk hemorrhagic fever** 065.1
**Onanism** 307.9
**Onchocerciasis** 125.3
  eye 125.3 *[360.13]*
**Onchocercosis** 125.3
**Oncocytoma** (M8290/0) — *see* Neo-
    plasm, by site, benign
**Ondine's curse** 348.8
**Oneirophrenia** — *see also* Schizophrenia
    295.4 ☑
**Onychauxis** 703.8
  congenital 757.5
**Onychia** (with lymphangitis) 681.9
  dermatophytic 110.1
  finger 681.02
  toe 681.11
**Onychitis** (with lymphangitis) 681.9
  finger 681.02
  toe 681.11
**Onychocryptosis** 703.0
**Onychodystrophy** 703.8
  congenital 757.5
**Onychogryphosis** 703.8
**Onychogryposis** 703.8
**Onycholysis** 703.8
**Onychomadesis** 703.8
**Onychomalacia** 703.8
**Onychomycosis** 110.1
  finger 110.1
  toe 110.1
**Onycho-osteodysplasia** 756.89
**Onychophagy** 307.9
**Onychoptosis** 703.8
**Onychorrhexis** 703.8
  congenital 757.5
**Onychoschizia** 703.8
**Onychotrophia** — *see also* Atrophy, nail
    703.8

**O'nyong-nyong fever** 066.3
**Onyxis** (finger) (toe) 703.0
**Onyxitis** (with lymphangitis) 681.9
  finger 681.02
  toe 681.11
**Oocyte** (egg) (ovum)
  donor V59.70
    over age 35 V59.73
      anonymous recipient V59.73
      designated recipient V59.74
    under age 35 V59.71
      anonymous recipient V59.71
      designated recipient V59.72
**Oophoritis** (cystic) (infectional) (intersti-
    tial) — *see also* Salpingo-oophoritis
    614.2
  complicating pregnancy 646.6 ☑
  fetal (acute) 752.0
  gonococcal (acute) 098.19
    chronic or duration of 2 months or
        over 098.39
  tuberculous (*see also* Tuberculosis)
    016.6 ☑
**Opacity, opacities**
  cornea 371.00
    central 371.03
    congenital 743.43
      interfering with vision 743.42
    degenerative (*see also* Degenera-
        tion, cornea) 371.40
    hereditary (*see also* Dystrophy,
        cornea) 371.50
    inflammatory (*see also* Keratitis)
        370.9
    late effect of trachoma (healed)
        139.1
    minor 371.01
    peripheral 371.02
  enamel (fluoride) (nonfluoride) (teeth)
      520.3
  lens (*see also* Cataract) 366.9
  snowball 379.22
  vitreous (humor) 379.24
    congenital 743.51
**Opalescent dentin** (hereditary) 520.5
**Open, opening**
  abnormal, organ or site, congenital —
      *see* Imperfect, closure
  angle with
    borderline intraocular pressure
        365.01
    cupping of discs 365.01
  bite
    anterior 524.24                              ●
    posterior 524.25                             ●
  false — *see* Imperfect, closure
  margin on tooth restoration 525.61
  restoration margins 525.61
  wound — *see* Wound, open, by site
**Operation**
  causing mutilation of fetus 763.89
  destructive, on live fetus, to facilitate
      birth 763.89
  for delivery, fetus or newborn 763.89
  maternal, unrelated to current deliv-
      ery, affecting fetus or newborn
      760.6
**Operational fatigue** 300.89
**Operative** — *see* condition
**Operculitis** (chronic) 523.40
  acute 523.30
**Operculum, retina** 361.32
  with detachment 361.01
**Ophiasis** 704.01
**Ophthalmia** — *see also* Conjunctivitis
    372.30
  actinic rays 370.24
  allergic (acute) 372.05
    chronic 372.14
  blennorrhagic (neonatorum) 098.40
  catarrhal 372.03
  diphtheritic 032.81
  Egyptian 076.1
  electric, electrica 370.24
  gonococcal (neonatorum) 098.40
  metastatic 360.11

☑ Additional Digit Required — Refer to the Tabular List for Digit Selection        ꟿ Subterms under main terms may continue to next column or page

*2008 ICD-9-CM*        ▶◀ Revised Text        ● New Line        ▲ Revised Code        **October 2007 · Volume 2 — 219**

**Ophthalmia** — *see also* Conjunctivitis— *continued*
migraine 346.8 ☑
neonatorum, newborn 771.6
gonococcal 098.40
nodosa 360.14
phlyctenular 370.31
with ulcer (*see also* Ulcer, cornea) 370.00
sympathetic 360.11
**Ophthalmitis** — *see* Ophthalmia
**Ophthalmocele** (congenital) 743.66
**Ophthalmoneuromyelitis** 341.0
**Ophthalmopathy, infiltrative with thyrotoxicosis** 242.0 ☑
**Ophthalmoplegia** — *see also* Strabismus 378.9
anterior internuclear 378.86
ataxia-areflexia syndrome 357.0
bilateral 378.9
diabetic 250.5 ☑ *[378.86]*
exophthalmic 242.0 ☑ *[376.22]*
external 378.55
progressive 378.72
total 378.56
internal (complete) (total) 367.52
internuclear 378.86
migraine 346.8 ☑
painful 378.55
Parinaud's 378.81
progressive external 378.72
supranuclear, progressive 333.0
total (external) 378.56
internal 367.52
unilateral 378.9
**Opisthognathism** 524.00
**Opisthorchiasis** (felineus) (tenuicollis) (viverrini) 121.0
**Opisthotonos, opisthotonus** 781.0
**Opitz's disease** (congenital splenomegaly) 289.51
**Opiumism** — *see also* Dependence 304.0 ☑
**Oppenheim's disease** 358.8
**Oppenheim-Urbach disease or syndrome** (necrobiosis lipoidica diabeticorum) 250.8 ☑ *[709.3]*
**Opsoclonia** 379.59
**Optic nerve** — *see* condition
**Orbit** — *see* condition
**Orchioblastoma** (M9071/3) 186.9
**Orchitis** (nonspecific) (septic) 604.90
with abscess 604.0
blennorrhagic (acute) 098.13
chronic or duration of 2 months or over 098.33
diphtheritic 032.89 *[604.91]*
filarial 125.9 *[604.91]*
gangrenous 604.99
gonococcal (acute) 098.13
chronic or duration of 2 months or over 098.33
mumps 072.0
parotidea 072.0
suppurative 604.99
syphilitic 095.8 *[604.91]*
tuberculous (*see also* Tuberculosis) 016.5 ☑ *[608.81]*
**Orf** 051.2
**Organic** — *see also* condition
heart — *see* Disease, heart
insufficiency 799.89
**Oriental**
bilharziasis 120.2
schistosomiasis 120.2
sore 085.1
**Orientation**
ego-dystonic sexual 302.0
**Orifice** — *see* condition
**Origin, both great vessels from right ventricle** 745.11
**Ormond's disease or syndrome** 593.4
**Ornithosis** 073.9
with
complication 073.8
specified NEC 073.7

**Ornithosis** — *continued*
with — *continued*
pneumonia 073.0
pneumonitis (lobular) 073.0
**Orodigitofacial dysostosis** 759.89
**Oropouche fever** 066.3
**Orotaciduria, oroticaciduria** (congenital) (hereditary) (pyrimidine deficiency) 281.4
**Oroya fever** 088.0
**Orthodontics** V58.5
adjustment V53.4
aftercare V58.5
fitting V53.4
**Orthopnea** 786.02
**Orthoptic training** V57.4
**Osgood-Schlatter**
disease 732.4
osteochondrosis 732.4
**Osler's**
disease (M9950/1) (polycythemia vera) 238.4
nodes 421.0
**Osler-Rendu disease** (familial hemorrhagic telangiectasia) 448.0
**Osler-Vaquez disease** (M9950/1) (polycythemia vera) 238.4
**Osler-Weber-Rendu syndrome** (familial hemorrhagic telangiectasia) 448.0
**Osmidrosis** 705.89
**Osseous** — *see* condition
**Ossification**
artery — *see* Arteriosclerosis
auricle (ear) 380.39
bronchus 519.19
cardiac (*see also* Degeneration, myocardial) 429.1
cartilage (senile) 733.99
coronary (artery) — *see* Arteriosclerosis, coronary
diaphragm 728.10
ear 380.39
middle (*see also* Otosclerosis) 387.9
falx cerebri 349.2
fascia 728.10
fontanel
defective or delayed 756.0
premature 756.0
heart (*see also* Degeneration, myocardial) 429.1
valve — *see* Endocarditis
larynx 478.79
ligament
posterior longitudinal 724.8
cervical 723.7
meninges (cerebral) 349.2
spinal 336.8
multiple, eccentric centers 733.99
muscle 728.10
heterotopic, postoperative 728.13
myocardium, myocardial (*see also* Degeneration, myocardial) 429.1
penis 607.81
periarticular 728.89
sclera 379.16
tendon 727.82
trachea 519.19
tympanic membrane (*see also* Tympanosclerosis) 385.00
vitreous (humor) 360.44
**Osteitis** — *see also* Osteomyelitis 730.2 ☑
acute 730.0 ☑
alveolar 526.5
chronic 730.1 ☑
condensans (ilii) 733.5
deformans (Paget's) 731.0
due to or associated with malignant neoplasm (*see also* Neoplasm, bone, malignant) 170.9 *[731.1]*
due to yaws 102.6
fibrosa NEC 733.29
cystica (generalisata) 252.01
disseminata 756.59
osteoplastica 252.01

**Osteitis** — *see also* Osteomyelitis — *continued*
fragilitans 756.51
Garré's (sclerosing) 730.1 ☑
infectious (acute) (subacute) 730.0 ☑
chronic or old 730.1 ☑
jaw (acute) (chronic) (lower) (neonatal) (suppurative) (upper) 526.4
parathyroid 252.01
petrous bone (*see also* Petrositis) 383.20
pubis 733.5
sclerotic, nonsuppurative 730.1 ☑
syphilitic 095.5
tuberculosa
cystica (of Jüngling) 135
multiplex cystoides 135
**Osteoarthritica spondylitis** (spine) — *see also* Spondylosis 721.90
**Osteoarthritis** — *see also* Osteoarthrosis 715.9 ☑
distal interphalangeal 715.9 ☑
hyperplastic 731.2
interspinalis (*see also* Spondylosis) 721.90
spine, spinal NEC (*see also* Spondylosis) 721.90
**Osteoarthropathy** — *see also* Osteoarthrosis 715.9 ☑
chronic idiopathic hypertrophic 757.39
familial idiopathic 757.39
hypertrophic pulmonary 731.2
secondary 731.2
idiopathic hypertrophic 757.39
primary hypertrophic 731.2
pulmonary hypertrophic 731.2
secondary hypertrophic 731.2
**Osteoarthrosis** (degenerative) (hypertrophic) (rheumatoid) 715.9 ☑

*Note* — *Use the following fifth-digit subclassification with category 715:*

| | |
|---|---|
| 0 | site unspecified |
| 1 | shoulder region |
| 2 | upper arm |
| 3 | forearm |
| 4 | hand |
| 5 | pelvic region and thigh |
| 6 | lower leg |
| 7 | ankle and foot |
| 8 | other specified sites except spine |
| 9 | multiple sites |

Deformans alkaptonurica 270.2
generalized 715.09
juvenilis (Köhler's) 732.5
localized 715.3 ☑
idiopathic 715.1 ☑
primary 715.1 ☑
secondary 715.2 ☑
multiple sites, not specified as generalized 715.89
polyarticular 715.09
spine (*see also* Spondylosis) 721.90
temporomandibular joint 524.69
**Osteoblastoma** (M9200/0) — *see* Neoplasm, bone, benign
**Osteochondritis** — *see also* Osteochondrosis 732.9
dissecans 732.7
hip 732.7
ischiopubica 732.1
multiple 756.59
syphilitic (congenital) 090.0
**Osteochondrodermodysplasia** 756.59
**Osteochondrodystrophy** 277.5
deformans 277.5
familial 277.5
fetalis 756.4
**Osteochondrolysis** 732.7
**Osteochondroma** (M9210/0) — *see also* Neoplasm, bone, benign

**Osteochondroma** — *see also* Neoplasm, bone, benign — *continued*
multiple, congenital 756.4
**Osteochondromatosis** (M9210/1) 238.0
synovial 727.82
**Osteochondromyxosarcoma** (M9180/3) — *see* Neoplasm, bone, malignant
**Osteochondropathy** NEC 732.9
**Osteochondrosarcoma** (M9180/3) — *see* Neoplasm, bone, malignant
**Osteochondrosis** 732.9
acetabulum 732.1
adult spine 732.8
astragalus 732.5
Blount's 732.4
Buchanan's (juvenile osteochondrosis of iliac crest) 732.1
Buchman's (juvenile osteochondrosis) 732.1
Burns' 732.3
calcaneus 732.5
capitular epiphysis (femur) 732.1
carpal
lunate (wrist) 732.3
scaphoid 732.3
coxae juvenilis 732.1
deformans juvenilis (coxae) (hip) 732.1
Scheuermann's 732.0
spine 732.0
tibia 732.4
vertebra 732.0
Diaz's (astragalus) 732.5
dissecans (knee) (shoulder) 732.7
femoral capital epiphysis 732.1
femur (head) (juvenile) 732.1
foot (juvenile) 732.5
Freiberg's (disease) (second metatarsal) 732.5
Haas' 732.3
Haglund's (os tibiale externum) 732.5
hand (juvenile) 732.3
head of
femur 732.1
humerus (juvenile) 732.3
hip (juvenile) 732.1
humerus (juvenile) 732.3
iliac crest (juvenile) 732.1
ilium (juvenile) 732.1
ischiopubic synchondrosis 732.1
Iselin's (osteochondrosis fifth metatarsal) 732.5
juvenile, juvenilis 732.6
arm 732.3
capital femoral epiphysis 732.1
capitellum humeri 732.3
capitular epiphysis 732.1
carpal scaphoid 732.3
clavicle, sternal epiphysis 732.6
coxae 732.1
deformans 732.1
foot 732.5
hand 732.3
hip and pelvis 732.1
lower extremity, except foot 732.4
lunate, wrist 732.3
medial cuneiform bone 732.5
metatarsal (head) 732.5
metatarsophalangeal 732.5
navicular, ankle 732.5
patella 732.4
primary patellar center (of Köhler) 732.4
specified site NEC 732.6
spine 732.0
tarsal scaphoid 732.5
tibia (epiphysis) (tuberosity) 732.4
upper extremity 732.3
vertebra (body) (Calvé) 732.0
epiphyseal plates (of Scheuermann) 732.0
Kienböck's (disease) 732.3
Köhler's (disease) (navicular, ankle) 732.5
patellar 732.4
tarsal navicular 732.5
Legg-Calvé-Perthes (disease) 732.1

**Osteochondrosis** — *continued*
  lower extremity (juvenile) 732.4
  lunate bone 732.3
  Mauclaire's 732.3
  metacarpal heads (of Mauclaire) 732.3
  metatarsal (fifth) (head) (second) 732.5
  navicular, ankle 732.5
  os calcis 732.5
  Osgood-Schlatter 732.4
  os tibiale externum 732.5
  Panner's 732.3
  patella (juvenile) 732.4
  patellar center
    primary (of Köhler) 732.4
    secondary (of Sinding-Larsen) 732.4
  pelvis (juvenile) 732.1
  Pierson's 732.1
  radial head (juvenile) 732.3
  Scheuermann's 732.0
  Sever's (calcaneum) 732.5
  Sinding-Larsen (secondary patellar center) 732.4
  spine (juvenile) 732.0
    adult 732.8
  symphysis pubis (of Pierson) (juvenile) 732.1
  syphilitic (congenital) 090.0
  tarsal (navicular) (scaphoid) 732.5
  tibia (proximal) (tubercle) 732.4
  tuberculous — *see* Tuberculosis, bone 732.3
  ulna 732.3
  upper extremity (juvenile) 732.3
  van Neck's (juvenile osteochondrosis) 732.1
  vertebral (juvenile) 732.0
    adult 732.8
**Osteoclastoma** (M9250/1) 238.0
  malignant (M9250/3) — *see* Neoplasm, bone, malignant
**Osteocopic pain** 733.90
**Osteodynia** 733.90
**Osteodystrophy**
  azotemic 588.0
  chronica deformans hypertrophica 731.0
  congenital 756.50
    specified type NEC 756.59
  deformans 731.0
  fibrosa localisata 731.0
  parathyroid 252.01
  renal 588.0
**Osteofibroma** (M9262/0) — *see* Neoplasm, bone, benign
**Osteofibrosarcoma** (M9182/3) — *see* Neoplasm, bone, malignant
**Osteogenesis imperfecta** 756.51
**Osteogenic** — *see* condition
**Osteoma** (M9180/0) — *see also* Neoplasm, bone, benign
  osteoid (M9191/0) (*see also* Neoplasm, bone, benign)
    giant (M9200/0) — *see* Neoplasm, bone, benign
**Osteomalacia** 268.2
  chronica deformans hypertrophica 731.0
  due to vitamin D deficiency 268.2
  infantile (*see also* Rickets) 268.0
  juvenile (*see also* Rickets) 268.0
  pelvis 268.2
  vitamin D-resistant 275.3
**Osteomalacic bone** 268.2
**Osteomalacosis** 268.2

**Osteomyelitis** (general) (infective) (localized) (neonatal) (purulent) (pyogenic) (septic) (staphylococcal) (streptococcal) (suppurative) (with periostitis) 730.2 ☑

> *Note* — Use the following fifth-digit subclassification with category 730:
> 0   *site unspecified*
> 1   *shoulder region*
> 2   *upper arm*
> 3   *forearm*
> 4   *hand*
> 5   *pelvic region and thigh*
> 6   *lower leg*
> 7   *ankle and foot*
> 8   *other specified sites*
> 9   *multiple sites*

  acute or subacute 730.0 ☑
  chronic or old 730.1 ☑
  due to or associated with
    diabetes mellitus 250.8 ☑ *[731.8]* ☑
    tuberculosis (*see also* Tuberculosis, bone) 015.9 ☑ *[730.8]* ☑
      limb bones 015.5 ☑ *[730.8]* ☑
      specified bones NEC 015.7 ☑ *[730.8]* ☑
      spine 015.0 ☑ *[730.8]* ☑
    typhoid 002.0 *[730.8]* ☑
  Garré's 730.1 ☑
  jaw (acute) (chronic) (lower) (neonatal) (suppurative) (upper) 526.4
  nonsuppurating 730.1 ☑
  orbital 376.03
  petrous bone (*see also* Petrositis) 383.20
  Salmonella 003.24
  sclerosing, nonsuppurative 730.1 ☑
  sicca 730.1 ☑
  syphilitic 095.5
    congenital 090.0 *[730.8]* ☑
  tuberculous — *see* Tuberculosis, bone
  typhoid 002.0 *[730.8]* ☑
**Osteomyelofibrosis** 289.89
**Osteomyelosclerosis** 289.89
**Osteonecrosis** 733.40
  meaning osteomyelitis 730.1 ☑
**Osteo-onycho-arthro dysplasia** 756.89
**Osteo-onychodysplasia, hereditary** 756.89
**Osteopathia**
  condensans disseminata 756.53
  hyperostotica multiplex infantilis 756.59
  hypertrophica toxica 731.2
  striata 756.4
**Osteopathy resulting from poliomyelitis** — *see also* Poliomyelitis 045.9 ☑ *[730.7]* ☑
  familial dysplastic 731.2
**Osteopecilia** 756.53
**Osteopenia** 733.90
**Osteoperiostitis** — *see also* Osteomyelitis 730.2 ☑
  ossificans toxica 731.2
  toxica ossificans 731.2
**Osteopetrosis** (familial) 756.52
**Osteophyte** — *see* Exostosis
**Osteophytosis** — *see* Exostosis
**Osteopoikilosis** 756.53
**Osteoporosis** (generalized) 733.00
  circumscripta 731.0
  disuse 733.03
  drug-induced 733.09
  idiopathic 733.02
  postmenopausal 733.01
  posttraumatic 733.7
  screening V82.81
  senile 733.01
  specified type NEC 733.09

**Osteoporosis-osteomalacia syndrome** 268.2
**Osteopsathyrosis** 756.51
**Osteoradionecrosis, jaw** 526.89
**Osteosarcoma** (M9180/3) — *see also* Neoplasm, bone, malignant
  chondroblastic (M9181/3) — *see* Neoplasm, bone, malignant
  fibroblastic (M9182/3) — *see* Neoplasm, bone, malignant
  in Paget's disease of bone (M9184/3) — *see* Neoplasm, bone, malignant
  juxtacortical (M9190/3) — *see* Neoplasm, bone, malignant
  parosteal (M9190/3) — *see* Neoplasm, bone, malignant
  telangiectatic (M9183/3) — *see* Neoplasm, bone, malignant
**Osteosclerosis** 756.52
  fragilis (generalisata) 756.52
**Osteosclerotic anemia** 289.89
**Osteosis**
  acromegaloid 757.39
  cutis 709.3
  parathyroid 252.01
  renal fibrocystic 588.0
**Österreicher-Turner syndrome** 756.89
**Ostium**
  atrioventriculare commune 745.69
  primum (arteriosum) (defect) (persistent) 745.61
  secundum (arteriosum) (defect) (patent) (persistent) 745.5
**Ostrum-Furst syndrome** 756.59
**Os, uterus** — *see* condition
**Otalgia** 388.70
  otogenic 388.71
  referred 388.72
**Othematoma** 380.31
**Otitic hydrocephalus** 348.2
**Otitis** 382.9
  with effusion 381.4
    purulent 382.4
    secretory 381.4
    serous 381.4
    suppurative 382.4
  acute 382.9
  adhesive (*see also* Adhesions, middle ear) 385.10
  chronic 382.9
    with effusion 381.3
    mucoid, mucous (simple) 381.20
    purulent 382.3
    secretory 381.3
    serous 381.10
    suppurative 382.3
  diffuse parasitic 136.8
  externa (acute) (diffuse) (hemorrhagica) 380.10
    actinic 380.22
    candidal 112.82
    chemical 380.22
    chronic 380.23
      mycotic — *see* Otitis, externa, mycotic
      specified type NEC 380.23
    circumscribed 380.10
    contact 380.22
    due to
      erysipelas 035 *[380.13]*
      impetigo 684 *[380.13]*
      seborrheic dermatitis 690.10 *[380.13]*
    eczematoid 380.22
    furuncular 680.0 *[380.13]*
    infective 380.10
      chronic 380.16
    malignant 380.14
    mycotic (chronic) 380.15
      due to
        aspergillosis 117.3 *[380.15]*
        moniliasis 112.82
        otomycosis 111.8 *[380.15]*
    reactive 380.22
    specified type NEC 380.22

**Otitis** — *continued*
  externa — *continued*
    tropical 111.8 *[380.15]*
  insidiosa (*see also* Otosclerosis) 387.9
  interna (*see also* Labyrinthitis) 386.30
  media (hemorrhagic) (staphylococcal) (streptococcal) 382.9
    acute 382.9
      with effusion 381.00
      allergic 381.04
        mucoid 381.05
        sanguineous 381.06
        serous 381.04
      catarrhal 381.00
      exudative 381.00
      mucoid 381.02
        allergic 381.05
      necrotizing 382.00
        with spontaneous rupture of ear drum 382.01
        in
          influenza 487.8 *[382.02]*
          measles 055.2
          scarlet fever 034.1 *[382.02]*
      nonsuppurative 381.00
      purulent 382.00
        with spontaneous rupture of ear drum 382.01
      sanguineous 381.03
        allergic 381.06
      secretory 381.01
      seromucinous 381.02
      serous 381.01
        allergic 381.04
      suppurative 382.00
        with spontaneous rupture of ear drum 382.01
        due to
          influenza 487.8 *[382.02]*
          scarlet fever 034.1 *[382.02]*
      transudative 381.00
    adhesive (*see also* Adhesions, middle ear) 385.10
    allergic 381.4
      acute 381.04
        mucoid 381.05
        sanguineous 381.06
        serous 381.04
      chronic 381.3
    catarrhal 381.4
      acute 381.00
      chronic (simple) 381.10
    chronic 382.9
      with effusion 381.3
      adhesive (*see also* Adhesions, middle ear) 385.10
      allergic 381.3
      atticoantral, suppurative (with posterior or superior marginal perforation of ear drum) 382.2
      benign suppurative (with anterior or perforation of ear drum) 382.1
      catarrhal 381.10
      exudative 381.3
      mucinous 381.20
      mucoid, mucous (simple) 381.20
      mucosanguineous 381.29
      nonsuppurative 381.3
      purulent 382.3
      secretory 381.3
      seromucinous 381.3
      serosanguineous 381.19
      serous (simple) 381.10
      suppurative 382.3
        atticoantral (with posterior or superior marginal perforation of ear drum) 382.2
        benign (with anterior perforation of ear drum) 382.1

**Otitis** — *continued*
  media — *continued*
    chronic — *continued*
      suppurative — *continued*
        tuberculous (*see also* Tuberculosis) 017.4 ☑
        tubotympanic 382.1
        transudative 381.3
      exudative 381.4
        acute 381.00
        chronic 381.3
      fibrotic (*see also* Adhesions, middle ear) 385.10
      mucoid, mucous 381.4
        acute 381.02
        chronic (simple) 381.20
      mucosanguineous, chronic 381.29
      nonsuppurative 381.4
        acute 381.00
        chronic 381.3
      postmeasles 055.2
      purulent 382.4
        acute 382.00
          with spontaneous rupture of ear drum 382.01
        chronic 382.3
      sanguineous, acute 381.03
        allergic 381.06
      secretory 381.4
        acute or subacute 381.01
        chronic 381.3
      seromucinous 381.4
        acute or subacute 381.02
        chronic 381.3
      serosanguineous, chronic 381.19
      serous 381.4
        acute or subacute 381.01
        chronic (simple) 381.10
      subacute — *see* Otitis, media, acute
      suppurative 382.4
        acute 382.00
          with spontaneous rupture of ear drum 382.01
        chronic 382.3
          atticoantral 382.2
          benign 382.1
          tuberculous (*see also* Tuberculosis) 017.4 ☑
          tubotympanic 382.1
      transudative 381.4
        acute 381.00
        chronic 381.3
      tuberculous (*see also* Tuberculosis) 017.4 ☑
    postmeasles 055.2
**Otoconia** 386.8
**Otolith syndrome** 386.19
**Otomycosis** 111.8 *[380.15]*
  in
    aspergillosis 117.3 *[380.15]*
    moniliasis 112.82
**Otopathy** 388.9
**Otoporosis** — *see also* Otosclerosis 387.9
**Otorrhagia** 388.69
  traumatic — *see* nature of injury
**Otorrhea** 388.60
  blood 388.69
  cerebrospinal (fluid) 388.61
**Otosclerosis** (general) 387.9
  cochlear (endosteal) 387.2
  involving
    otic capsule 387.2
    oval window
      nonobliterative 387.0
      obliterative 387.1
    round window 387.2
  nonobliterative 387.0
  obliterative 387.1
  specified type NEC 387.8
**Otospongiosis** — *see also* Otosclerosis 387.9
**Otto's disease or pelvis** 715.35
**Outburst, aggressive** — *see also* Disturbance, conduct 312.0 ☑
  in children or adolescents 313.9

**Outcome of delivery**
  multiple birth NEC V27.9
    all liveborn V27.5
    all stillborn V27.7
    some liveborn V27.6
    unspecified V27.9
  single V27.9
    liveborn V27.0
    stillborn V27.1
  twins V27.9
    both liveborn V27.2
    both stillborn V27.4
    one liveborn, one stillborn V27.3
**Outlet** — *see also* condition
  syndrome (thoracic) 353.0
**Outstanding ears** (bilateral) 744.29
**Ovalocytosis** (congenital) (hereditary) — *see also* Elliptocytosis 282.1
**Ovarian** — *see also* condition
  pregnancy — *see* Pregnancy, ovarian
  remnant syndrome 620.8
  vein syndrome 593.4
**Ovaritis** (cystic) — *see also* Salpingo-oophoritis 614.2
**Ovary, ovarian** — *see* condition
**Overactive** — *see also* Hyperfunction
  bladder 596.51
  eye muscle (*see also* Strabismus) 378.9
  hypothalamus 253.8
  thyroid (*see also* Thyrotoxicosis) 242.9 ☑
**Overactivity, child** 314.01
**Overbite** (deep) (excessive) (horizontal) (vertical) 524.29
**Overbreathing** — *see also* Hyperventilation 786.01
**Overconscientious personality** 301.4
**Overdevelopment** — *see also* Hypertrophy
  breast (female) (male) 611.1
  nasal bones 738.0
  prostate, congenital 752.89
**Overdistention** — *see* Distention
**Overdose overdosage** (drug) 977.9
  specified drug or substance — *see* Table of Drugs and Chemicals
**Overeating** 783.6
  nonorganic origin 307.51
**Overexertion** (effects) (exhaustion) 994.5
**Overexposure** (effects) 994.9
  exhaustion 994.4
**Overfeeding** — *see also* Overeating 783.6
**Overfill, endodontic** 526.62
**Overgrowth, bone** NEC 733.99
**Overhanging**
  tooth restoration 525.62
  unrepairable, dental restorative materials 525.62
**Overheated** (effects) (places) — *see* Heat
**Overinhibited child** 313.0
**Overjet** 524.29
  excessive horizontal 524.26
**Overlaid, overlying** (suffocation) 994.7
**Overlap**
  excessive horizontal 524.26
**Overlapping toe** (acquired) 735.8
  congenital (fifth toe) 755.66
**Overload**
  fluid 276.6
  potassium (K) 276.7
  sodium (Na) 276.0
**Overnutrition** — *see also* Hyperalimentation 783.6
**Overproduction** — *see also* Hypersecretion
  ACTH 255.3
  cortisol 255.0
  growth hormone 253.0
  thyroid-stimulating hormone (TSH) 242.8 ☑
**Overriding**
  aorta 747.21
  finger (acquired) 736.29
    congenital 755.59
  toe (acquired) 735.8

**Overriding** — *continued*
  toe — *continued*
    congenital 755.66
**Oversize**
  fetus (weight of 4500 grams or more) 766.0
    affecting management of pregnancy 656.6 ☑
    causing disproportion 653.5 ☑
      with obstructed labor 660.1 ☑
    affecting fetus or newborn 763.1
**Overstimulation, ovarian** 256.1
**Overstrained** 780.79
  heart — *see* Hypertrophy, cardiac
**Overweight** — *see also* Obesity 278.00
**Overwork** 780.79
**Oviduct** — *see* condition
**Ovotestis** 752.7
**Ovulation** (cycle)
  failure or lack of 628.0
  pain 625.2
**Ovum**
  blighted 631
  donor V59.70
    over age 35 V59.73
      anonymous recipient V59.73
      designated recipient V59.74
    under age 35 V59.71
      anonymous recipient V59.71
      designated recipient V59.72
  dropsical 631
  pathologic 631
**Owren's disease or syndrome** (parahemophilia) — *see also* Defect, coagulation 286.3
**Oxalosis** 271.8
**Oxaluria** 271.8
**Ox heart** — *see* Hypertrophy, cardiac
**OX syndrome** 758.6
**Oxycephaly, oxycephalic** 756.0
  syphilitic, congenital 090.0
**Oxyuriasis** 127.4
**Oxyuris vermicularis** (infestation) 127.4
**Ozena** 472.0

**P**

**Pacemaker syndrome** 429.4
**Pachyderma, pachydermia** 701.8
  laryngis 478.5
  laryngitis 478.79
  larynx (verrucosa) 478.79
**Pachydermatitis** 701.8
**Pachydermatocele** (congenital) 757.39
  acquired 701.8
**Pachydermatosis** 701.8
**Pachydermoperiostitis**
  secondary 731.2
**Pachydermoperiostosis**
  primary idiopathic 757.39
  secondary 731.2
**Pachymeningitis** (adhesive) (basal) (brain) (cerebral) (cervical) (chronic) (circumscribed) (external) (fibrous) (hemorrhagic) (hypertrophic) (internal) (purulent) (spinal) (suppurative) — *see also* Meningitis 322.9
  gonococcal 098.82
**Pachyonychia** (congenital) 757.5
  acquired 703.8
**Pachyperiosteodermia**
  primary or idiopathic 757.39
  secondary 731.2
**Pachyperiostosis**
  primary or idiopathic 757.39
  secondary 731.2
**Pacinian tumor** (M9507/0) — *see* Neoplasm, skin, benign
**Pads, knuckle or Garrod's** 728.79
**Paget's disease** (osteitis deformans) 731.0
  with infiltrating duct carcinoma of the breast (M8541/3) — *see* Neoplasm, breast, malignant
  bone 731.0
    osteosarcoma in (M9184/3) — *see* Neoplasm, bone, malignant

**Paget's disease** — *continued*
  breast (M8540/3) 174.0
  extramammary (M8542/3) (*see also* Neoplasm, skin, malignant)
    anus 154.3
    skin 173.5
  malignant (M8540/3)
    breast 174.0
    specified site NEC (M8542/3) — *see* Neoplasm, skin, malignant
    unspecified site 174.0
  mammary (M8540/3) 174.0
  necrosis of bone 731.0
  nipple (M8540/3) 174.0
  osteitis deformans 731.0
**Paget-Schroetter syndrome** (intermittent venous claudication) 453.8
**Pain(s)** ▶(*see also* Painful)◀ 780.96
  abdominal 789.0 ☑
    acute 338.19
      due to trauma 338.11
      postoperative 338.18
        post-thoracotomy 338.12
  adnexa (uteri) 625.9
  alimentary, due to vascular insufficiency 557.9
  anginoid (*see also* Pain, precordial) 786.51
  anus 569.42
  arch 729.5
  arm 729.5
  axillary 729.5
  back (postural) 724.5
    low 724.2
    psychogenic 307.89
  bile duct 576.9
  bladder 788.9
  bone 733.90
  breast 611.71
    psychogenic 307.89
  broad ligament 625.9
  cancer associated 338.3
  cartilage NEC 733.90
  cecum 789.0 ☑
  cervicobrachial 723.3
  chest (central) 786.50
    atypical 786.59
    midsternal 786.51
    musculoskeletal 786.59
    noncardiac 786.59
    substernal 786.51
    wall (anterior) 786.52
  chronic 338.29
    associated with significant psychosocial dysfunction 338.4
    due to trauma 338.21
    postoperative 338.28
      post-thoracotomy 338.22
    syndrome 338.4
  coccyx 724.79
  colon 789.0 ☑
  common duct 576.9
  coronary — *see* Angina
  costochondral 786.52
  diaphragm 786.52
  due to (presence of) any device, implant, or graft classifiable to 996.0–996.5 — *see* Complications, due to (presence of) any device, implant, or graft classified to 996.0–996.5 NEC
  malignancy (primary) (secondary) 338.3
  ear (*see also* Otalgia) 388.70
  epigastric, epigastrium 789.06
  extremity (lower) (upper) 729.5
  eye 379.91
  face, facial 784.0
    atypical 350.2
    nerve 351.8
  false (labor) 644.1 ☑
  female genital organ NEC 625.9
    psychogenic 307.89
  finger 729.5
  flank 789.0 ☑

☑ Additional Digit Required — Refer to the Tabular List for Digit Selection

▶◀ Revised Text          ● New Line          ▲ Revised Code

⑭⑮⑯ Subterms under main terms may continue to next column or page

**Pain(s)** ▶(see also Painful)◀ —
   continued
  foot 729.5
  gallbladder 575.9
  gas (intestinal) 787.3
  gastric 536.8
  generalized 780.96
  genital organ
    female 625.9
    male 608.9
    psychogenic 307.89
  groin 789.0 ☑
  growing 781.99
  hand 729.5
  head (see also Headache) 784.0
  heart (see also Pain, precordial)
    786.51
  infraorbital (see also Neuralgia,
    trigeminal) 350.1
  intermenstrual 625.2
  jaw 526.9
  joint 719.40
    ankle 719.47
    elbow 719.42
    foot 719.47
    hand 719.44
    hip 719.45
    knee 719.46
    multiple sites 719.49
    pelvic region 719.45
    psychogenic 307.89
    shoulder (region) 719.41
    specified site NEC 719.48
    wrist 719.43
  kidney 788.0
  labor, false or spurious 644.1 ☑
  laryngeal 784.1
  leg 729.5
  limb 729.5
  low back 724.2
  lumbar region 724.2
  mastoid (see also Otalgia) 388.70
  maxilla 526.9
  menstrual 625.3 ●
  metacarpophalangeal (joint) 719.44
  metatarsophalangeal (joint) 719.47
  mouth 528.9
  muscle 729.1
    intercostal 786.59
  musculoskeletal (see also Pain, by
    site) 729.1
  nasal 478.19
  nasopharynx 478.29
  neck NEC 723.1
    psychogenic 307.89
  neoplasm related (acute) (chronic)
    338.3
  nerve NEC 729.2
  neuromuscular 729.1
  nose 478.19
  ocular 379.91
  ophthalmic 379.91
  orbital region 379.91
  osteocopic 733.90
  ovary 625.9
    psychogenic 307.89
  over heart (see also Pain, precordial)
    786.51
  ovulation 625.2
  pelvic (female) 625.9
    male NEC 789.0 ☑
      psychogenic 307.89
    psychogenic 307.89
  penis 607.9
    psychogenic 307.89
  pericardial (see also Pain, precordial)
    786.51
  perineum
    female 625.9
    male 608.9
  pharynx 478.29
  pleura, pleural, pleuritic 786.52
  postoperative 338.18
    acute 338.18
    chronic 338.28
  post-thoracotomy 338.12

**Pain(s)** ▶(see also Painful)◀ —
   continued
  post-thoracotomy — continued
    acute 338.12
    chronic 338.22
  preauricular 388.70
  precordial (region) 786.51
    psychogenic 307.89
  premenstrual 625.4
  psychogenic 307.80
    cardiovascular system 307.89
    gastrointestinal system 307.89
    genitourinary system 307.89
    heart 307.89
    musculoskeletal system 307.89
    respiratory system 307.89
    skin 306.3
  radicular (spinal) (see also Radiculitis)
    729.2
  rectum 569.42
  respiration 786.52
  retrosternal 786.51
  rheumatic NEC 729.0
    muscular 729.1
  rib 786.50
  root (spinal) (see also Radiculitis)
    729.2
  round ligament (stretch) 625.9
  sacroiliac 724.6
  sciatic 724.3
  scrotum 608.9
    psychogenic 307.89
  seminal vesicle 608.9
  sinus 478.19
  skin 782.0
  spermatic cord 608.9
  spinal root (see also Radiculitis) 729.2
  stomach 536.8
    psychogenic 307.89
  substernal 786.51
  temporomandibular (joint) 524.62
  temporomaxillary joint 524.62
  testis 608.9
    psychogenic 307.89
  thoracic spine 724.1
    with radicular and visceral pain
      724.4
  throat 784.1
  tibia 733.90
  toe 729.5
  tongue 529.6
  tooth 525.9
  total hip replacement 996.77 ●
  total knee replacement 996.77 ●
  trigeminal (see also Neuralgia,
    trigeminal) 350.1
  tumor associated 338.3
  umbilicus 789.05
  ureter 788.0
  urinary (organ) (system) 788.0
  uterus 625.9
    psychogenic 307.89
  vagina 625.9
  vertebrogenic (syndrome) 724.5
  vesical 788.9
  vulva 625.9
  xiphoid 733.90
**Painful** — see also Pain
  arc syndrome 726.19
  coitus
    female 625.0
    male 608.89
    psychogenic 302.76
  ejaculation (semen) 608.89
    psychogenic 302.79
  erection 607.3
  feet syndrome 266.2
  menstruation 625.3
    psychogenic 306.52
  micturition 788.1
  ophthalmoplegia 378.55
  respiration 786.52
  scar NEC 709.2
  urination 788.1
  wire sutures 998.89
**Painters' colic** 984.9

**Painters' colic** — continued
  specified type of lead — see Table of
    Drugs and Chemicals
**Palate** — see condition
**Palatoplegia** 528.9
**Palatoschisis** — see also Cleft, palate
  749.00
**Palilalia** 784.69
● **Palindromic arthritis** — see also
  Rheumatism, palindromic 719.3 ☑
**Palliative care** V66.7
**Pallor** 782.61
  temporal, optic disc 377.15
**Palmar** — see also condition
  fascia — see condition
**Palpable**
  cecum 569.89
  kidney 593.89
  liver 573.9
  lymph nodes 785.6
  ovary 620.8
  prostate 602.9
  spleen (see also Splenomegaly) 789.2
  uterus 625.8
**Palpitation** (heart) 785.1
  psychogenic 306.2
**Palsy** — see also Paralysis 344.9
  atrophic diffuse 335.20
  Bell's 351.0
    newborn 767.5
  birth 767.7
  brachial plexus 353.0
    fetus or newborn 767.6
  brain (see also Palsy, cerebral)
    noncongenital or noninfantile
      344.89
      late effect — see Late effect(s)
        (of) cerebrovascular dis-
        ease
    syphilitic 094.89
      congenital 090.49
  bulbar (chronic) (progressive) 335.22
    pseudo NEC 335.23
    supranuclear NEC 344.8 ☑
  cerebral (congenital) (infantile) (spas-
    tic) 343.9
    athetoid 333.71
    diplegic 343.0
      late effect — see Late effect(s)
        (of) cerebrovascular dis-
        ease
    hemiplegic 343.1
    monoplegic 343.3
    noncongenital or noninfantile
      437.8
      late effect — see Late effect(s)
        (of) cerebrovascular dis-
        ease
    paraplegic 343.0
    quadriplegic 343.2
    spastic, not congenital or infantile
      344.89
    syphilitic 094.89
      congenital 090.49
    tetraplegic 343.2
  cranial nerve (see also Disorder,
    nerve, cranial)
    multiple 352.6
  creeping 335.21
  divers' 993.3
  Erb's (birth injury) 767.6
  facial 351.0
    newborn 767.5
  glossopharyngeal 352.2
  Klumpke (-Déjérine) 767.6
  lead 984.9
    specified type of lead — see Table
      of Drugs and Chemicals
  median nerve (tardy) 354.0
  peroneal nerve (acute) (tardy) 355.3
  progressive supranuclear 333.0
  pseudobulbar NEC 335.23
  radial nerve (acute) 354.3
  seventh nerve 351.0
    newborn 767.5
  shaking (see also Parkinsonism) 332.0

**Palsy** — see also Paralysis —
   continued
  spastic (cerebral) (spinal) 343.9
    hemiplegic 343.1
  specified nerve NEC — see Disorder,
    nerve
  supranuclear NEC 356.8
    progressive 333.0
  ulnar nerve (tardy) 354.2
  wasting 335.21
**Paltauf-Sternberg disease** 201.9 ☑
**Paludism** — see Malaria
**Panama fever** 084.0
**Panaris** (with lymphangitis) 681.9
  finger 681.02
  toe 681.11
**Panaritium** (with lymphangitis) 681.9
  finger 681.02
  toe 681.11
**Panarteritis** (nodosa) 446.0
  brain or cerebral 437.4
**Pancake heart** 793.2
  with cor pulmonale (chronic) 416.9
**Pancarditis** (acute) (chronic) 429.89
  with
    rheumatic
      fever (active) (acute) (chronic)
        (subacute) 391.8
        inactive or quiescent 398.99
  rheumatic, acute 391.8
    chronic or inactive 398.99
**Pancoast's syndrome or tumor** (carcinoma, pulmonary apex) (M8010/3)
  162.3
**Pancoast-Tobias syndrome** (M8010/3)
  (carcinoma, pulmonary apex) 162.3
**Pancolitis** 556.6
**Pancreas, pancreatic** — see condition
**Pancreatitis** 577.0
  acute (edematous) (hemorrhagic) (re-
    current) 577.0
  annular 577.0
  apoplectic 577.0
  calcerceous 577.0
  chronic (infectious) 577.1
    recurrent 577.1
  cystic 577.2
  fibrous 577.8
  gangrenous 577.0
  hemorrhagic (acute) 577.0
  interstitial (chronic) 577.1
    acute 577.0
  malignant 577.0
  mumps 072.3
  painless 577.1
  recurrent 577.1
  relapsing 577.1
  subacute 577.1
  suppurative 577.0
  syphilitic 095.8
**Pancreatolithiasis** 577.8
**Pancytolysis** 289.9
**Pancytopenia** (acquired) 284.1
  with malformations 284.09
  congenital 284.09
**Panencephalitis** — see also Encephalitis
  subacute, sclerosing 046.2
**Panhematopenia** 284.81 ▲
  congenital 284.09
  constitutional 284.09
  splenic, primary 289.4
**Panhemocytopenia** 284.81 ▲
  congenital 284.09
  constitutional 284.09
**Panhypogonadism** 257.2
**Panhypopituitarism** 253.2
  prepubertal 253.3
**Panic** (attack) (state) 300.01
  reaction to exceptional stress (tran-
    sient) 308.0
**Panmyelopathy, familial constitutional**
  284.09
**Panmyelophthisis** 284.2
  acquired (secondary) 284.81 ▲
  congenital 284.2
  idiopathic 284.9

☑ Additional Digit Required — Refer to the Tabular List for Digit Selection               ▼ Subterms under main terms may continue to next column or page

**2008 ICD-9-CM**        ▶◀ Revised Text       ● New Line      ▲ Revised Code       **October 2007 · Volume 2 — 223**

**Panmyelosis** (acute) (M9951/1) 238.79
**Panner's disease** 732.3
  capitellum humeri 732.3
  head of humerus 732.3
  tarsal navicular (bone) (osteochondro-
    sis) 732.5
**Panneuritis endemica** 265.0 [357.4]
**Panniculitis** 729.30
  back 724.8
  knee 729.31
  mesenteric 567.82
  neck 723.6
  nodular, nonsuppurative 729.30
  sacral 724.8
  specified site NEC 729.39
**Panniculus adiposus** (abdominal) 278.1
**Pannus** (corneal) 370.62
  abdominal (symptomatic) 278.1
  allergic eczematous 370.62
  degenerativus 370.62
  keratic 370.62
  rheumatoid — see Arthritis, rheuma-
    toid
  trachomatosus, trachomatous (active)
    076.1 [370.62]
    late effect 139.1
**Panophthalmitis** 360.02
**Panotitis** — see Otitis media
**Pansinusitis** (chronic) (hyperplastic)
  (nonpurulent) (purulent) 473.8
  acute 461.8
  due to fungus NEC 117.9
  tuberculous (see also Tuberculosis)
    012.8 ☑
**Panuveitis** 360.12
  sympathetic 360.11
**Panvalvular disease** — see Endocarditis,
  mitral
**Papageienkrankheit** 073.9
**Papanicolaou smear**
  cervix (screening test) V76.2
    as part of gynecological examina-
      tion V72.31
    for suspected malignant neoplasm
      V76.2
      no disease found V71.1
    inadequate sample 795.08
    nonspecific abnormal finding
      795.00
      with
        atypical squamous cells
          cannot exclude high grade
            squamous intraep-
            ithelial lesion (ASC-
            H) 795.02
          of undetermined signifi-
            cance (ASC-US)
            795.01
        cytologic evidence of malig-
          nancy 795.06
        high grade squamous intraep-
          ithelial lesion (HGSIL)
          795.04
        low grade squamous intraep-
          ithelial lesion (LGSIL)
          795.03
        nonspecific finding NEC 795.09
    to confirm findings of recent
      normal smear following
      initial abnormal smear
      V72.32
    unsatisfactory 795.08
  other specified site (see also Screen-
    ing, malignant neoplasm)
    for suspected malignant neoplasm
      (see also Screening, malig-
      nant neoplasm)
      no disease found V71.1
    nonspecific abnormal finding 795.1
    vagina V76.47
    following hysterectomy for malig-
      nant condition V67.01
**Papilledema** 377.00
  associated with
    decreased ocular pressure 377.02

**Papilledema** — continued
  associated with — continued
    increased intracranial pressure
      377.01
    retinal disorder 377.03
  choked disc 377.00
  infectional 377.00
**Papillitis** 377.31
  anus 569.49
  chronic lingual 529.4
  necrotizing, kidney 584.7
  optic 377.31
  rectum 569.49
  renal, necrotizing 584.7
  tongue 529.0
**Papilloma** (M8050/0) — see also Neoplasm, by site, benign

> *Note — Except where otherwise indicat-
> ed, the morphological varieties of papil-
> loma in the list below should be coded
> by site as for "Neoplasm, benign."*

  acuminatum (female) (male) 078.11
  bladder (urinary) (transitional cell)
    (M8120/1) 236.7
    benign (M8120/0) 223.3
  choroid plexus (M9390/0) 225.0
    anaplastic type (M9390/3) 191.5
    malignant (M9390/3) 191.5
  ductal (M8503/0)
  dyskeratotic (M8052/0)
  epidermoid (M8052/0)
  hyperkeratotic (M8052/0)
  intracystic (M8504/0)
  intraductal (M8503/0)
  inverted (M8053/0)
  keratotic (M8052/0)
  parakeratotic (M8052/0)
  pinta (primary) 103.0
  renal pelvis (transitional cell)
    (M8120/1) 236.99
    benign (M8120/0) 223.1
  Schneiderian (M8121/0)
    specified site — see Neoplasm, by
      site, benign
    unspecified site 212.0
  serous surface (M8461/0)
    borderline malignancy (M8461/1)
      specified site — see Neoplasm,
        by site, uncertain behav-
        ior
      unspecified site 236.2
    specified site — see Neoplasm, by
      site, benign
    unspecified site 220
  squamous (cell) (M8052/0)
  transitional (cell) (M8120/0)
    bladder (urinary) (M8120/1) 236.7
    inverted type (M8121/1) — see
      Neoplasm, by site, uncertain
      behavior
    renal pelvis (M8120/1) 236.91
    ureter (M8120/1) 236.91
  ureter (transitional cell) (M8120/1)
    236.91
    benign (M8120/0) 223.2
  urothelial (M8120/1) — see Neoplasm,
    by site, uncertain behavior
  verrucous (M8051/0)
  villous (M8261/1) — see Neoplasm,
    by site, uncertain behavior
  yaws, plantar or palmar 102.1
**Papillomata, multiple, of yaws** 102.1
**Papillomatosis** (M8060/0) — see also
  Neoplasm, by site, benign
  confluent and reticulate 701.8
  cutaneous 701.8
  ductal, breast 610.1
  Gougerot-Carteaud (confluent reticu-
    late) 701.8
  intraductal (diffuse) (M8505/0) — see
    Neoplasm, by site, benign
  subareolar duct (M8506/0) 217
**Papillon-Léage and Psaume syndrome**
  (orodigitofacial dysostosis) 759.89
**Papule** 709.8
  carate (primary) 103.0

**Papule** — continued
  fibrous, of nose (M8724/0) 216.3
  pinta (primary) 103.0
**Papulosis, malignant** 447.8
**Papyraceous fetus** 779.89
  complicating pregnancy 646.0 ☑
**Paracephalus** 759.7
**Parachute mitral valve** 746.5
**Paracoccidioidomycosis** 116.1
  mucocutaneous-lymphangitic 116.1
  pulmonary 116.1
  visceral 116.1
**Paracoccidiomycosis** — see Paracoccidioidomycosis
**Paracusis** 388.40
**Paradentosis** 523.5
**Paradoxical facial movements** 374.43
**Paraffinoma** 999.9
**Paraganglioma** (M8680/1)
  adrenal (M8700/0) 227.0
    malignant (M8700/3) 194.0
  aortic body (M8691/1) 237.3
    malignant (M8691/3) 194.6
  carotid body (M8692/1) 237.3
    malignant (M8692/3) 194.5
  chromaffin (M8700/0) (see also Neo-
    plasm, by site, benign)
    malignant (M8700/3) — see Neo-
      plasm, by site, malignant
  extra-adrenal (M8693/1)
    malignant (M8693/3)
      specified site — see Neoplasm,
        by site, malignant
      unspecified site 194.6
    specified site — see Neoplasm, by
      site, uncertain behavior
    unspecified site 237.3
  glomus jugulare (M8690/1) 237.3
    malignant (M8690/3) 194.6
  jugular (M8690/1) 237.3
    malignant (M8680/3)
      specified site — see Neoplasm,
        by site, malignant
      unspecified site 194.6
  nonchromaffin (M8693/1)
    malignant (M8693/3)
      specified site — see Neoplasm,
        by site, malignant
      unspecified site 194.6
    specified site — see Neoplasm, by
      site, uncertain behavior
    unspecified site 237.3
  parasympathetic (M8682/1)
    specified site — see Neoplasm, by
      site, uncertain behavior
    unspecified site 237.3
  specified site — see Neoplasm, by site,
    uncertain behavior
  sympathetic (M8681/1)
    specified site — see Neoplasm, by
      site, uncertain behavior
    unspecified site 237.3
  unspecified site 237.3
**Parageusia** 781.1
  psychogenic 306.7
**Paragonimiasis** 121.2
**Paragranuloma, Hodgkin's** (M9660/3)
  201.0 ☑
**Parahemophilia** — see also Defect, coagulation 286.3
**Parakeratosis** 690.8
  psoriasiformis 696.2
  variegata 696.2
**Paralysis, paralytic** (complete) (incomplete) 344.9
  with
    broken
      back — see Fracture, vertebra,
        by site, with spinal cord
        injury
      neck — see Fracture, vertebra,
        cervical, with spinal cord
        injury
    fracture, vertebra — see Fracture,
      vertebra, by site, with spinal
      cord injury

**Paralysis, paralytic** — continued
  with — continued
    syphilis 094.89
  abdomen and back muscles 355.9
  abdominal muscles 355.9
  abducens (nerve) 378.54
  abductor 355.9
    lower extremity 355.8
    upper extremity 354.9
  accessory nerve 352.4
  accommodation 367.51
    hysterical 300.11
  acoustic nerve 388.5
  agitans 332.0
    arteriosclerotic 332.0
  alternating 344.89
    oculomotor 344.89
  amyotrophic 335.20
  ankle 355.8
  anterior serratus 355.9
  anus (sphincter) 569.49
  apoplectic (current episode) (see also
    Disease, cerebrovascular, acute)
    436
    late effect — see Late effect(s) (of)
      cerebrovascular disease
  arm 344.40
    affecting
      dominant side 344.41
      nondominant side 344.42
    both 344.2
    hysterical 300.11
    late effect — see Late effect(s) (of)
      cerebrovascular disease
    psychogenic 306.0
    transient 781.4
    traumatic NEC (see also Injury,
      nerve, upper limb) 955.9
  arteriosclerotic (current episode) 437.0
    late effect — see Late effect(s) (of)
      cerebrovascular disease
  ascending (spinal), acute 357.0
  associated, nuclear 344.89
  asthenic bulbar 358.00
  ataxic NEC 334.9
    general 094.1
  athetoid 333.71
  atrophic 356.9
    infantile, acute (see also Poliomyeli-
      tis, with paralysis) 045.1 ☑
    muscle NEC 355.9
    progressive 335.21
    spinal (acute) (see also Poliomyeli-
      tis, with paralysis) 045.1 ☑
  attack (see also Disease, cerebrovas-
    cular, acute) 436
  axillary 353.0
  Babinski-Nageotte's 344.89
  Bell's 351.0
    newborn 767.5
  Benedikt's 344.89
  birth (injury) 767.7
    brain 767.0
    intracranial 767.0
    spinal cord 767.4
  bladder (sphincter) 596.53
    neurogenic 596.54
      with cauda equina syndrome
        344.61
    puerperal, postpartum, childbirth
      665.5 ☑
    sensory 596.54
      with cauda equina 344.61
    spastic 596.54
      with cauda equina 344.61
  bowel, colon, or intestine (see also
    Ileus) 560.1
  brachial plexus 353.0
    due to birth injury 767.6
    newborn 767.6
  brain
    congenital — see Palsy, cerebral
    current episode 437.8
    diplegia 344.2
    hemiplegia 342.9 ☑

**Paralysis, paralytic** — *continued*
  brain — *continued*
    hemiplegia — *continued*
      late effect — *see* Late effect(s) (of) cerebrovascular disease
    infantile — *see* Palsy, cerebral
    late effect — *see* Late effect(s) (of) cerebrovascular disease
    monoplegia (*see also* Monoplegia)
      late effect — *see* Late effect(s) (of) cerebrovascular disease
    paraplegia 344.1
    quadriplegia — *see* Quadriplegia
    syphilitic, congenital 090.49
    triplegia 344.89
  bronchi 519.19
  Brown-Séquard's 344.89
  bulbar (chronic) (progressive) 335.22
    infantile (*see also* Poliomyelitis, bulbar) 045.0 ☑
    poliomyelitic (*see also* Poliomyelitis, bulbar) 045.0 ☑
    pseudo 335.23
    supranuclear 344.89
  bulbospinal 358.00
  cardiac (*see also* Failure, heart) 428.9
  cerebral
    current episode 437.8
    spastic, infantile — *see* Palsy, cerebral
  cerebrocerebellar 437.8
    diplegic infantile 343.0
  cervical
    plexus 353.2
    sympathetic NEC 337.0
  Céstan-Chenais 344.89
  Charcôt-Marie-Tooth type 356.1
  childhood — *see* Palsy, cerebral
  Clark's 343.9
  colon (*see also* Ileus) 560.1
  compressed air 993.3
  compression
    arm NEC 354.9
    cerebral — *see* Paralysis, brain
    leg NEC 355.8
    lower extremity NEC 355.8
    upper extremity NEC 354.9
  congenital (cerebral) (spastic) (spinal) — *see* Palsy, cerebral
  conjugate movement (of eye) 378.81
    cortical (nuclear) (supranuclear) 378.81
  convergence 378.83
  cordis (*see also* Failure, heart) 428.9
  cortical (*see also* Paralysis, brain) 437.8
  cranial or cerebral nerve (*see also* Disorder, nerve, cranial) 352.9
  creeping 335.21
  crossed leg 344.89
  crutch 953.4
  deglutition 784.99
    hysterical 300.11
  dementia 094.1
  descending (spinal) NEC 335.9
  diaphragm (flaccid) 519.4
    due to accidental section of phrenic nerve during procedure 998.2
  digestive organs NEC 564.89
  diplegic — *see* Diplegia
  divergence (nuclear) 378.85
  divers' 993.3
  Duchenne's 335.22
  due to intracranial or spinal birth injury — *see* Palsy, cerebral
  embolic (current episode) (*see also* Embolism, brain) 434.1 ☑
    late effect — *see* Late effect(s) (of) cerebrovascular disease
  enteric (*see also* Ileus) 560.1
    with hernia — *see* Hernia, by site, with obstruction

**Paralysis, paralytic** — *continued*
  Erb (-Duchenne) (birth) (newborn) 767.6
  Erb's syphilitic spastic spinal 094.89
  esophagus 530.89
  essential, infancy (*see also* Poliomyelitis) 045.9 ☑
  extremity
    lower — *see* Paralysis, leg
      spastic (hereditary) 343.3
        noncongenital or noninfantile 344.1
        transient (cause unknown) 781.4
    upper — *see* Paralysis, arm
  eye muscle (extrinsic) 378.55
    intrinsic 367.51
  facial (nerve) 351.0
    birth injury 767.5
    congenital 767.5
    following operation NEC 998.2
    newborn 767.5
  familial 359.3
    periodic 359.3
    spastic 334.1
  fauces 478.29
  finger NEC 354.9
  foot NEC 355.8
  gait 781.2
  gastric nerve 352.3
  gaze 378.81
  general 094.1
    ataxic 094.1
    insane 094.1
    juvenile 090.40
    progressive 094.1
    tabetic 094.1
  glossopharyngeal (nerve) 352.2
  glottis (*see also* Paralysis, vocal cord) 478.30
  gluteal 353.4
  Gubler (-Millard) 344.89
  hand 354.9
    hysterical 300.11
    psychogenic 306.0
  heart (*see also* Failure, heart) 428.9
  hemifacial, progressive 349.89
  hemiplegic — *see* Hemiplegia
  hyperkalemic periodic (familial) 359.3
  hypertensive (current episode) 437.8
  hypoglossal (nerve) 352.5
  hypokalemic periodic 359.3
  Hyrtl's sphincter (rectum) 569.49
  hysterical 300.11
  ileus (*see also* Ileus) 560.1
  infantile (*see also* Poliomyelitis) 045.9 ☑
    atrophic acute 045.1 ☑
    bulbar 045.0 ☑
    cerebral — *see* Palsy, cerebral
    paralytic 045.1 ☑
    progressive acute 045.9 ☑
    spastic — *see* Palsy, cerebral
    spinal 045.9 ☑
  infective (*see also* Poliomyelitis) 045.9 ☑
  inferior nuclear 344.9
  insane, general or progressive 094.1
  internuclear 378.86
  interosseous 355.9
  intestine (*see also* Ileus) 560.1
  intracranial (current episode) (*see also* Paralysis, brain) 437.8
    due to birth injury 767.0
  iris 379.49
    due to diphtheria (toxin) 032.81 [379.49]
  ischemic, Volkmann's (complicating trauma) 958.6
  isolated sleep, recurrent
  Jackson's 344.89
  jake 357.7
  Jamaica ginger (jake) 357.7
  juvenile general 090.40
  Klumpke (-Déjérine) (birth) (newborn) 767.6

**Paralysis, paralytic** — *continued*
  labioglossal (laryngeal) (pharyngeal) 335.22
  Landry's 357.0
  laryngeal nerve (recurrent) (superior) (*see also* Paralysis, vocal cord) 478.30
  larynx (*see also* Paralysis, vocal cord) 478.30
    due to diphtheria (toxin) 032.3
  late effect
    due to
      birth injury, brain or spinal (cord) — *see* Palsy, cerebral
      edema, brain or cerebral — *see* Paralysis, brain
    lesion
      late effect — *see* Late effect(s) (of) cerebrovascular disease
    spinal (cord) — *see* Paralysis, spinal
  lateral 335.24
  lead 984.9
    specified type of lead — *see* Table of Drugs and Chemicals
  left side — *see* Hemiplegia
  leg 344.30
    affecting
      dominant side 344.31
      nondominant side 344.32
    both (*see also* Paraplegia) 344.1
    crossed 344.89
    hysterical 300.11
    psychogenic 306.0
    transient or transitory 781.4
      traumatic NEC (*see also* Injury, nerve, lower limb) 956.9
  levator palpebrae superioris 374.31
  limb NEC 344.5
    all four — *see* Quadriplegia
    quadriplegia — *see* Quadriplegia
  lip 528.5
  Lissauer's 094.1
  local 355.9
  lower limb (*see also* Paralysis, leg)
    both (*see also* Paraplegia) 344.1
  lung 518.89
    newborn 770.89
  median nerve 354.1
  medullary (tegmental) 344.89
  mesencephalic NEC 344.89
    tegmental 344.89
  middle alternating 344.89
  Millard-Gubler-Foville 344.89
  monoplegic — *see* Monoplegia
  motor NEC 344.9
    cerebral — *see* Paralysis, brain
    spinal — *see* Paralysis, spinal
  multiple
    cerebral — *see* Paralysis, brain
    spinal — *see* Paralysis, spinal
  muscle (flaccid) 359.9
    due to nerve lesion NEC 355.9
    eye (extrinsic) 378.55
      intrinsic 367.51
      oblique 378.51
    iris sphincter 364.89                          ▲
    ischemic (complicating trauma) (Volkmann's) 958.6
    pseudohypertrophic 359.1
  muscular (atrophic) 359.9
    progressive 335.21
  musculocutaneous nerve 354.9
  musculospiral 354.9
  nerve (*see also* Disorder, nerve)
    third or oculomotor (partial) 378.51
      total 378.52
    fourth or trochlear 378.53
    sixth or abducens 378.54
    seventh or facial 351.0
      birth injury 767.5
      due to
        injection NEC 999.9
        operation NEC 997.09

**Paralysis, paralytic** — *continued*
  nerve (*see also* Disorder, nerve) — *continued*
    seventh or facial — *continued*
      newborn 767.5
    accessory 352.4
    auditory 388.5
    birth injury 767.7
    cranial or cerebral (*see also* Disorder, nerve, cranial) 352.9
    facial 351.0
      birth injury 767.5
      newborn 767.5
    laryngeal (*see also* Paralysis, vocal cord) 478.30
    newborn 767.7
    phrenic 354.8
      newborn 767.7
    radial 354.3
      birth injury 767.6
      newborn 767.6
    syphilitic 094.89
    traumatic NEC (*see also* Injury, nerve, by site) 957.9
    trigeminal 350.9
    ulnar 354.2
  newborn NEC 767.0
  normokalemic periodic 359.3
  obstetrical, newborn 767.7
  ocular 378.9
  oculofacial, congenital 352.6
  oculomotor (nerve) (partial) 378.51
    alternating 344.89
    external bilateral 378.55
    total 378.52
  olfactory nerve 352.0
  palate 528.9
  palatopharyngolaryngeal 352.6
  paratrigeminal 350.9
  periodic (familial) (hyperkalemic) (hypokalemic) (normokalemic) ▶(potassium sensitive)◄ (secondary) 359.3
  peripheral
    autonomic nervous system — *see* Neuropathy, peripheral, autonomic
    nerve NEC 355.9
  peroneal (nerve) 355.3
  pharynx 478.29
  phrenic nerve 354.8
  plantar nerves 355.6
  pneumogastric nerve 352.3
  poliomyelitis (current) (*see also* Poliomyelitis, with paralysis) 045.1 ☑
    bulbar 045.0 ☑
  popliteal nerve 355.3
  pressure (*see also* Neuropathy, entrapment) 355.9
  progressive 335.21
    atrophic 335.21
    bulbar 335.22
    general 094.1
    hemifacial 349.89
    infantile, acute (*see also* Poliomyelitis) 045.9 ☑
    multiple 335.20
  pseudobulbar 335.23
  pseudohypertrophic 359.1
    muscle 359.1
  psychogenic 306.0
  pupil, pupillary 379.49
  quadriceps 355.8
  quadriplegic (*see also* Quadriplegia) 344.0 ☑
  radial nerve 354.3
    birth injury 767.6
  rectum (sphincter) 569.49
  rectus muscle (eye) 378.55
  recurrent
    isolated sleep 327.43
    laryngeal nerve (*see also* Paralysis, vocal cord) 478.30
  respiratory (muscle) (system) (tract) 786.09

☑ Additional Digit Required — Refer to the Tabular List for Digit Selection
**2008 ICD-9-CM**                    ▶◄ Revised Text              ● New Line        ▲ Revised Code

▽ Subterms under main terms may continue to next column or page
**October 2007 · Volume 2 — 225**

**Paralysis, paralytic** — *continued*
  respiratory — *continued*
    center NEC 344.89
      fetus or newborn 770.87
    congenital 768.9
    newborn 768.9
  right side — *see* Hemiplegia
  Saturday night 354.3
  saturnine 984.9
    specified type of lead — *see* Table
      of Drugs and Chemicals
  sciatic nerve 355.0
  secondary — *see* Paralysis, late effect
  seizure (cerebral) (current episode)
    (*see also* Disease, cerebrovascu-
    lar, acute) 436
    late effect — *see* Late effect(s) (of)
      cerebrovascular disease
  senile NEC 344.9
  serratus magnus 355.9
  shaking (*see also* Parkinsonism) 332.0
  shock (*see also* Disease, cerebrovascu-
    lar, acute) 436
    late effect — *see* Late effect(s) (of)
      cerebrovascular disease
  shoulder 354.9
  soft palate 528.9
  spasmodic — *see* Paralysis, spastic
  spastic 344.9
    cerebral infantile — *see* Palsy,
      cerebral
    congenital (cerebral) — *see* Palsy,
      cerebral
    familial 334.1
    hereditary 334.1
    infantile 343.9
    noncongenital or noninfantile,
      cerebral 344.9
    syphilitic 094.0
      spinal 094.89
  sphincter, bladder (*see also* Paralysis,
    bladder) 596.53
  spinal (cord) NEC 344.1
    accessory nerve 352.4
    acute (*see also* Poliomyelitis)
      045.9 ☑
    ascending acute 357.0
    atrophic (acute) (*see also* Poliomyeli-
      tis, with paralysis) 045.1 ☑
      spastic, syphilitic 094.89
    congenital NEC 343.9
    hemiplegic — *see* Hemiplegia
    hereditary 336.8
    infantile (*see also* Poliomyelitis)
      045.9 ☑
    late effect NEC 344.89
    monoplegic — *see* Monoplegia
    nerve 355.9
    progressive 335.10
    quadriplegic — *see* Quadriplegia
    spastic NEC 343.9
    traumatic — *see* Injury, spinal, by
      site
  sternomastoid 352.4
  stomach 536.3
    diabetic 250.6 ☑ [536.3]
    nerve (nondiabetic) 352.3
  stroke (current episode) — *see* Infarct,
    brain
    late effect — *see* Late effect(s) (of)
      cerebrovascular disease
  subscapularis 354.8
  superior nuclear NEC 334.9
  supranuclear 356.8
  sympathetic
    cervical NEC 337.0
    nerve NEC (*see also* Neuropathy,
      peripheral, autonomic) 337.9
    nervous system — *see* Neuropathy,
      peripheral, autonomic
  syndrome 344.9
    specified NEC 344.89
  syphilitic spastic spinal (Erb's) 094.89
  tabetic general 094.1
  thigh 355.8
  throat 478.29

**Paralysis, paralytic** — *continued*
  throat — *continued*
    diphtheritic 032.0
    muscle 478.29
  thrombotic (current episode) (*see also*
    Thrombosis, brain) 434.0 ☑
    late effect — *see* Late effect(s) (of)
      cerebrovascular disease
  thumb NEC 354.9
  tick (-bite) 989.5
  Todd's (postepileptic transitory paral-
    ysis) 344.89
  toe 355.6
  tongue 529.8
  transient
    arm or leg NEC 781.4
    traumatic NEC (*see also* Injury,
      nerve, by site) 957.9
  trapezius 352.4
  traumatic, transient NEC (*see also*
    Injury, nerve, by site) 957.9
  trembling (*see also* Parkinsonism)
    332.0
  triceps brachii 354.9
  trigeminal nerve 350.9
  trochlear nerve 378.53
  ulnar nerve 354.2
  upper limb (*see also* Paralysis, arm)
    both (*see also* Diplegia) 344.2
  uremic — *see* Uremia
  uveoparotitic 135
  uvula 528.9
    hysterical 300.11
    postdiphtheritic 032.0
  vagus nerve 352.3
  vasomotor NEC 337.9
  velum palati 528.9
  vesical (*see also* Paralysis, bladder)
    596.53
  vestibular nerve 388.5
  visual field, psychic 368.16
  vocal cord 478.30
    bilateral (partial) 478.33
      complete 478.34
    complete (bilateral) 478.34
    unilateral (partial) 478.31
      complete 478.32
  Volkmann's (complicating trauma)
    958.6
  wasting 335.21
  Weber's 344.89
  wrist NEC 354.9
**Paramedial orifice, urethrovesical**
  753.8
**Paramenia** 626.9
**Parametritis** (chronic) — *see also* Disease, pelvis, inflammatory 614.4
  acute 614.3
  puerperal, postpartum, childbirth
    670.0 ☑
**Parametrium, parametric** — *see* condition
**Paramnesia** — *see also* Amnesia 780.93
**Paramolar** 520.1
  causing crowding 524.31
**Paramyloidosis** 277.30
**Paramyoclonus multiplex** 333.2
**Paramyotonia** 359.29 ▲
  congenita ▶(of von Eulenburg)◀
    359.29 ▲
**Paraneoplastic syndrome** — *see* condition
**Parangi** — *see also* Yaws 102.9
**Paranoia** 297.1
  alcoholic 291.5
  querulans 297.8
  senile 290.20
**Paranoid**
  dementia (*see also* Schizophrenia)
    295.3 ☑
    praecox (acute) 295.3 ☑
    senile 290.20
  personality 301.0
  psychosis 297.9
    alcoholic 291.5
    climacteric 297.2

**Paranoid** — *continued*
  psychosis — *continued*
    drug-induced 292.11
    involutional 297.2
    menopausal 297.2
    protracted reactive 298.4
    psychogenic 298.4
      acute 298.3
    senile 290.20
  reaction (chronic) 297.9
    acute 298.3
  schizophrenia (acute) (*see also*
    Schizophrenia) 295.3 ☑
  state 297.9
    alcohol-induced 291.5
    climacteric 297.2
    drug-induced 292.11
    due to or associated with
      arteriosclerosis (cerebrovascu-
      lar) 290.42
      presenile brain disease 290.12
      senile brain disease 290.20
    involutional 297.2
    menopausal 297.2
    senile 290.20
    simple 297.0
    specified type NEC 297.8
  tendencies 301.0
  traits 301.0
  trends 301.0
  type, psychopathic personality 301.0
**Paraparesis** — *see also* ▶Paraplegia◀
  344.1 ▲
**Paraphasia** 784.3
**Paraphilia** — *see also* Deviation, sexual
  302.9
**Paraphimosis** (congenital) 605
  chancroidal 099.0
**Paraphrenia, paraphrenic** (late) 297.2
  climacteric 297.2
  dementia (*see also* Schizophrenia)
    295.3 ☑
  involutional 297.2
  menopausal 297.2
  schizophrenia (acute) (*see also*
    Schizophrenia) 295.3 ☑
**Paraplegia** 344.1
  with
    broken back — *see* Fracture, verte-
      bra, by site, with spinal cord
      injury
    fracture, vertebra — *see* Fracture,
      vertebra, by site, with spinal
      cord injury
  ataxic — *see* Degeneration, combined,
    spinal cord
  brain (current episode) (*see also*
    Paralysis, brain) 437.8
  cerebral (current episode) (*see also*
    Paralysis, brain) 437.8
  congenital or infantile (cerebral)
    (spastic) (spinal) 343.0
  cortical — *see* Paralysis, brain
  familial spastic 334.1
  functional (hysterical) 300.11
  hysterical 300.11
  infantile 343.0
  late effect 344.1
  Pott's (*see also* Tuberculosis)
    015.0 ☑ [730.88]
  psychogenic 306.0
  spastic
    Erb's spinal 094.89
    hereditary 334.1
    not infantile or congenital 344.1
  spinal (cord)
    traumatic NEC — *see* Injury,
      spinal, by site
  syphilitic (spastic) 094.89
  traumatic NEC — *see* Injury, spinal,
    by site
**Paraproteinemia** 273.2
  benign (familial) 273.1
  monoclonal 273.1
  secondary to malignant or inflamma-
    tory disease 273.1

**Parapsoriasis** 696.2
  en plaques 696.2
  guttata 696.2
  lichenoides chronica 696.2
  retiformis 696.2
  varioliformis (acuta) 696.2
**Parascarlatina** 057.8
**Parasitic** — *see also* condition
  disease NEC (*see also* Infestation,
    parasitic) 136.9
    contact V01.89
    exposure to V01.89
    intestinal NEC 129
    skin NEC 134.9
  stomatitis 112.0
  sycosis 110.0
    beard 110.0
    scalp 110.0
  twin 759.4
**Parasitism** NEC 136.9
  intestinal NEC 129
  skin NEC 134.9
  specified — *see* Infestation
**Parasitophobia** 300.29
**Parasomnia** 307.47
  alcohol induced 291.82
  drug induced 292.85
  nonorganic origin 307.47
  organic 327.40
    in conditions classified elsewhere
      327.44
    other 327.49
**Paraspadias** 752.69
**Paraspasm facialis** 351.8
**Parathyroid gland** — *see* condition
**Parathyroiditis** (autoimmune) 252.1
**Parathyroprival tetany** 252.1
**Paratrachoma** 077.0
**Paratyphilitis** — *see also* Appendicitis
  541
**Paratyphoid** (fever) — *see* Fever, paraty-
  phoid
**Paratyphus** — *see* Fever, paratyphoid
**Paraurethral duct** 753.8
**Para-urethritis** 597.89
  gonococcal (acute) 098.0
    chronic or duration of 2 months or
      over 098.2
**Paravaccinia** NEC 051.9
  milkers' node 051.1
**Paravaginitis** — *see also* Vaginitis
  616.10
**Parencephalitis** — *see also* Encephalitis
  323.9
  late effect — *see* category 326
**Parergasia** 298.9
**Paresis** — *see also* Paralysis 344.9
  accommodation 367.51
  bladder (spastic) (sphincter) (*see also*
    Paralysis, bladder) 596.53
    tabetic 094.0
  bowel, colon, or intestine (*see also*
    Ileus) 560.1
  brain or cerebral — *see* Paralysis,
    brain
  extrinsic muscle, eye 378.55
  general 094.1
    arrested 094.1
    brain 094.1
    cerebral 094.1
    insane 094.1
    juvenile 090.40
      remission 090.49
    progressive 094.1
    remission (sustained) 094.1
    tabetic 094.1
  heart (*see also* Failure, heart) 428.9
  infantile (*see also* Poliomyelitis)
    045.9 ☑
  insane 094.1
  juvenile 090.40
  late effect — *see* Paralysis, late effect
  luetic (general) 094.1
  peripheral progressive 356.9
  pseudohypertrophic 359.1
  senile NEC 344.9

---

☑ Additional Digit Required — Refer to the Tabular List for Digit Selection
                                                  Subterms under main terms may continue to next column or page

**Paresis** — *see also* Paralysis —
  *continued*
  stomach 536.3
    diabetic 250.6 ☑ *[536.3]*
  syphilitic (general) 094.1
    congenital 090.40
  transient, limb 781.4
  vesical (sphincter) NEC 596.53
**Paresthesia** — *see also* Disturbance,
    sensation 782.0
  Berger's (paresthesia of lower limb)
    782.0
  Bernhardt 355.1
  Magnan's 782.0
**Paretic** — *see* condition
**Parinaud's**
  conjunctivitis 372.02
  oculoglandular syndrome 372.02
  ophthalmoplegia 378.81
  syndrome (paralysis of conjugate up-
    ward gaze) 378.81
**Parkes Weber and Dimitri syndrome**
    (encephalocutaneous angiomatosis)
    759.6
**Parkinson's disease, syndrome, or**
  **tremor** — *see* Parkinsonism
**Parkinsonism** (arteriosclerotic) (idiopath-
    ic) (primary) 332.0
  associated with orthostatic hypoten-
    sion (idiopathic) (symptomatic)
    333.0
  due to drugs 332.1
  neuroleptic-induced 332.1
  secondary 332.1
  syphilitic 094.82
**Parodontitis** 523.40
**Parodontosis** 523.5
**Paronychia** (with lymphangitis) 681.9
  candidal (chronic) 112.3
  chronic 681.9
    candidal 112.3
    finger 681.02
    toe 681.11
  finger 681.02
  toe 681.11
  tuberculous (primary) (*see also* Tuber-
    culosis) 017.0 ☑
**Parorexia** NEC 307.52
  hysterical 300.11
**Parosmia** 781.1
  psychogenic 306.7
**Parotid gland** — *see* condition
**Parotiditis** — *see also* Parotitis 527.2
  epidemic 072.9
  infectious 072.9
**Parotitis** 527.2
  allergic 527.2
  chronic 527.2
  epidemic (*see also* Mumps) 072.9
  infectious (*see also* Mumps) 072.9
  noninfectious 527.2
  nonspecific toxic 527.2
  not mumps 527.2
  postoperative 527.2
  purulent 527.2
  septic 527.2
  suppurative (acute) 527.2
  surgical 527.2
  toxic 527.2
**Paroxysmal** — *see also* condition
  dyspnea (nocturnal) 786.09
**Parrot's disease** (syphilitic osteochondri-
    tis) 090.0
**Parrot fever** 073.9
**Parry's disease or syndrome** (exoph-
    thalmic goiter) 242.0 ☑
**Parry-Romberg syndrome** 349.89
**Parsonage-Aldren-Turner syndrome**
    353.5
**Parsonage-Turner syndrome** 353.5
**Parson's disease** (exophthalmic goiter)
    242.0 ☑
**Pars planitis** 363.21
**Particolored infant** 757.39
**Parturition** — *see* Delivery
**Parvovirus** 079.83

**Parvovirus** — *continued*
● B19 079.83
● human 079.83
**Passage**
  false, urethra 599.4
  meconium noted during delivery
    763.84
  of sounds or bougies (*see also* Atten-
    tion to artificial opening) V55.9
**Passive** — *see* condition
**Pasteurella septica** 027.2
**Pasteurellosis** — *see also* Infection,
    Pasteurella 027.2
**PAT** (paroxysmal atrial tachycardia)
    427.0
**Patau's syndrome** (trisomy D1) 758.1
**Patch**
  herald 696.3
**Patches**
  mucous (syphilitic) 091.3
    congenital 090.0
  smokers' (mouth) 528.6
**Patellar** — *see* condition
**Patellofemoral syndrome** 719.46
**Patent** — *see also* Imperfect closure
  atrioventricular ostium 745.69
  canal of Nuck 752.41
  cervix 622.5
    complicating pregnancy 654.5 ☑
      affecting fetus or newborn 761.0
  ductus arteriosus or Botalli 747.0
  Eustachian
    tube 381.7
    valve 746.89
  foramen
    Botalli 745.5
    ovale 745.5
  interauricular septum 745.5
  interventricular septum 745.4
  omphalomesenteric duct 751.0
  os (uteri) — *see* Patent, cervix
  ostium secundum 745.5
  urachus 753.7
  vitelline duct 751.0
**Paternity testing** V70.4
**Paterson-Kelly syndrome or web**
    (sideropenic dysphagia) 280.8
**Paterson (-Brown) (-Kelly) syndrome**
    (sideropenic dysphagia) 280.8
**Paterson's syndrome** (sideropenic dys-
    phagia) 280.8
**Pathologic, pathological** — *see also*
    condition
  asphyxia 799.01
  drunkenness 291.4
  emotionality 301.3
  fracture — *see* Fracture, pathologic
  liar 301.7
  personality 301.9
  resorption, tooth 521.40
    external 521.42
    internal 521.41
    specified NEC 521.49
  sexuality (*see also* Deviation, sexual)
    302.9
**Pathology** (of) — *see also* Disease
  periradicular, associated with previous
    endodontic treatment 526.69
**Patterned motor discharge, idiopathic**
    — *see also* Epilepsy 345.5 ☑
**Patulous** — *see also* Patent
  anus 569.49
  Eustachian tube 381.7
**Pause, sinoatrial** 427.81
**Pavor nocturnus** 307.46
**Pavy's disease** 593.6
**Paxton's disease** (white piedra) 111.2
**Payr's disease or syndrome** (splenic
    flexure syndrome) 569.89
**PBA** (pseudobulbar affect) 310.8
**Pearls**
  Elschnig 366.51
  enamel 520.2
**Pearl-workers' disease** (chronic os-
    teomyelitis) — *see also* Osteomyeli-
    tis 730.1 ☑

**Pectenitis** 569.49
**Pectenosis** 569.49
**Pectoral** — *see* condition
**Pectus**
  carinatum (congenital) 754.82
    acquired 738.3
    rachitic (*see also* Rickets) 268.0
  excavatum (congenital) 754.81
    acquired 738.3
    rachitic (*see also* Rickets) 268.0
  recurvatum (congenital) 754.81
    acquired 738.3
**Pedatrophia** 261
**Pederosis** 302.2
**Pediculosis** (infestation) 132.9
  capitis (head louse) (any site) 132.0
  corporis (body louse) (any site) 132.1
  eyelid 132.0 *[373.6]*
  mixed (classifiable to more than one
    category in 132.0–132.2) 132.3
  pubis (pubic louse) (any site) 132.2
  vestimenti 132.1
  vulvae 132.2
**Pediculus** (infestation) — *see* Pediculosis
**Pedophilia** 302.2
**Peg-shaped teeth** 520.2
**Pelade** 704.01
**Pel's crisis** 094.0
**Pel-Ebstein disease** — *see* Disease,
    Hodgkin's
**Pelger-Huët anomaly or syndrome**
    (hereditary hyposegmentation)
    288.2
**Peliosis** (rheumatica) 287.0
**Pelizaeus-Merzbacher**
  disease 330.0
  sclerosis, diffuse cerebral 330.0
**Pellagra** (alcoholic or with alcoholism)
    265.2
  with polyneuropathy 265.2 *[357.4]*
**Pellagra-cerebellar-ataxia-renal**
  **aminoaciduria syndrome** 270.0
**Pellegrini's disease** (calcification, knee
    joint) 726.62
**Pellegrini (-Stieda) disease or syn-**
  **drome** (calcification, knee joint)
    726.62
**Pellizzi's syndrome** (pineal) 259.8
**Pelvic** — *see also* condition
  congestion-fibrosis syndrome 625.5
  kidney 753.3
**Pelvioectasis** 591
**Pelviolithiasis** 592.0
**Pelviperitonitis**
  female (*see also* Peritonitis, pelvic, fe-
    male) 614.5
  male (*see also* Peritonitis) 567.21
**Pelvis, pelvic** — *see also* condition or
    type
  infantile 738.6
  Nägele's 738.6
  obliquity 738.6
  Robert's 755.69
**Pemphigoid** 694.5
  benign, mucous membrane 694.60
    with ocular involvement 694.61
  bullous 694.5
  cicatricial 694.60
    with ocular involvement 694.61
  juvenile 694.2
**Pemphigus** 694.4
  benign 694.5
    chronic familial 757.39
  Brazilian 694.4
  circinatus 694.0
  congenital, traumatic 757.39
  conjunctiva 694.61
  contagiosus 684
  erythematodes 694.4
  erythematosus 694.4
  foliaceus 694.4
  frambesiodes 694.4
  gangrenous (*see also* Gangrene) 785.4
  malignant 694.4
  neonatorum, newborn 684
  ocular 694.61

**Pemphigus** — *continued*
  papillaris 694.4
  seborrheic 694.4
  South American 694.4
  syphilitic (congenital) 090.0
  vegetans 694.4
  vulgaris 694.4
  wildfire 694.4
**Pendred's syndrome** (familial goiter with
    deaf-mutism) 243
**Pendulous**
  abdomen 701.9
    in pregnancy or childbirth 654.4 ☑
      affecting fetus or newborn
        763.89
  breast 611.8
**Penetrating wound** — *see also* Wound,
    open, by site
  with internal injury — *see* Injury, in-
    ternal, by site, with open wound
  eyeball 871.7
    with foreign body (nonmagnetic)
      871.6
      magnetic 871.5
  ocular (*see also* Penetrating wound,
    eyeball) 871.7
    adnexa 870.3
      with foreign body 870.4
    orbit 870.3
      with foreign body 870.4
**Penetration, pregnant uterus by instru-**
  **ment**
  with
    abortion — *see* Abortion, by type,
      with damage to pelvic organs
    ectopic pregnancy (*see also* cate-
      gories 633.0–633.9) 639.2
    molar pregnancy (*see also* cate-
      gories 630–632) 639.2
  complication of delivery 665.1 ☑
    affecting fetus or newborn 763.89
  following
    abortion 639.2
    ectopic or molar pregnancy 639.2
**Penfield's syndrome** — *see also* Epilepsy
    345.5 ☑
**Penicilliosis of lung** 117.3
**Penis** — *see* condition
**Penitis** 607.2
**Pentalogy** (of Fallot) 745.2
**Penta X syndrome** 758.81
**Pentosuria** (benign) (essential) 271.8
**Peptic acid disease** 536.8
**Peregrinating patient** V65.2
**Perforated** — *see* Perforation
**Perforation, perforative** (nontraumatic)
  antrum (*see also* Sinusitis, maxillary)
    473.0
  appendix 540.0
    with peritoneal abscess 540.1
  atrial septum, multiple 745.5
  attic, ear 384.22
    healed 384.81
  bile duct, except cystic (*see also* Dis-
    ease, biliary) 576.3
    cystic 575.4
  bladder (urinary) 596.6
    with
      abortion — *see* Abortion, by
        type, with damage to
        pelvic organs
      ectopic pregnancy (*see also* cat-
        egories 633.0–633.9)
        639.2
      molar pregnancy (*see also* cate-
        gories 630–632) 639.2
    following
      abortion 639.2
      ectopic or molar pregnancy
        639.2
    obstetrical trauma 665.5 ☑
  bowel 569.83
    with
      abortion — *see* Abortion, by
        type, with damage to
        pelvic organs

☑ Additional Digit Required — Refer to the Tabular List for Digit Selection
*2008 ICD-9-CM*          ▶◀ Revised Text          ● New Line          ▲ Revised Code
     ▽ Subterms under main terms may continue to next column or page
                              **October 2007 · Volume 2 — 227**

Perforation, perforative — *continued*
bowel — *continued*
with — *continued*
ectopic pregnancy (*see also* categories 633.0–633.9) 639.2
molar pregnancy (*see also* categories 630–632) 639.2
fetus or newborn 777.6
following
abortion 639.2
ectopic or molar pregnancy 639.2
obstetrical trauma 665.5 ☑
broad ligament
with
abortion — *see* Abortion, by type, with damage to pelvic organs
ectopic pregnancy (*see also* categories 633.0–633.9) 639.2
molar pregnancy (*see also* categories 630–632) 639.2
following
abortion 639.2
ectopic or molar pregnancy 639.2
obstetrical trauma 665.6 ☑
by
device, implant, or graft — *see* Complications, mechanical
foreign body left accidentally in operation wound 998.4
instrument (any) during a procedure, accidental 998.2
cecum 540.0
with peritoneal abscess 540.1
cervix (uteri) (*see also* Injury, internal, cervix)
with
abortion — *see* Abortion, by type, with damage to pelvic organs
ectopic pregnancy (*see also* categories 633.0–633.9) 639.2
molar pregnancy (*see also* categories 630–632) 639.2
following
abortion 639.2
ectopic or molar pregnancy 639.2
obstetrical trauma 665.3 ☑
colon 569.83
common duct (bile) 576.3
cornea (*see also* Ulcer, cornea) 370.00
due to ulceration 370.06
cystic duct 575.4
diverticulum (*see also* Diverticula) 562.10
small intestine 562.00
duodenum, duodenal (ulcer) — *see* Ulcer, duodenum, with perforation
ear drum — *see* Perforation, tympanum
enteritis — *see* Enteritis
esophagus 530.4
ethmoidal sinus (*see also* Sinusitis, ethmoidal) 473.2
foreign body (external site) (*see also* Wound, open, by site, complicated)
internal site, by ingested object — *see* Foreign body
frontal sinus (*see also* Sinusitis, frontal) 473.1
gallbladder or duct (*see also* Disease, gallbladder) 575.4
gastric (ulcer) — *see* Ulcer, stomach, with perforation
heart valve — *see* Endocarditis
ileum (*see also* Perforation, intestine) 569.83

Perforation, perforative — *continued*
instrumental
external — *see* Wound, open, by site
pregnant uterus, complicating delivery 665.9 ☑
surgical (accidental) (blood vessel) (nerve) (organ) 998.2
intestine 569.83
with
abortion — *see* Abortion, by type, with damage to pelvic organs
ectopic pregnancy (*see also* categories 633.0–633.9) 639.2
molar pregnancy (*see also* categories 630–632) 639.2
fetus or newborn 777.6
obstetrical trauma 665.5 ☑
ulcerative NEC 569.83
jejunum, jejunal 569.83
ulcer — *see* Ulcer, gastrojejunal, with perforation
mastoid (antrum) (cell) 383.89
maxillary sinus (*see also* Sinusitis, maxillary) 473.0
membrana tympani — *see* Perforation, tympanum
nasal
septum 478.19
congenital 748.1
syphilitic 095.8
sinus (*see also* Sinusitis) 473.9
congenital 748.1
palate (hard) 526.89
soft 528.9
syphilitic 095.8
syphilitic 095.8
palatine vault 526.89
syphilitic 095.8
congenital 090.5
pelvic
floor
with
abortion — *see* Abortion, by type, with damage to pelvic organs
ectopic pregnancy (*see also* categories 633.0–633.9) 639.2
molar pregnancy (*see also* categories 630–632) 639.2
obstetrical trauma 664.1 ☑
organ
with
abortion — *see* Abortion, by type, with damage to pelvic organs
ectopic pregnancy (*see also* categories 633.0–633.9) 639.2
molar pregnancy (*see also* categories 630–632) 639.2
following
abortion 639.2
ectopic or molar pregnancy 639.2
obstetrical trauma 665.5 ☑
perineum — *see* Laceration, perineum
periurethral tissue
with
abortion — *see* Abortion, by type, with damage to pelvic organs
ectopic pregnancy (*see also* categories 630–632) 639.2
molar pregnancy (*see also* categories 630–632) 639.2
pharynx 478.29
pylorus, pyloric (ulcer) — *see* Ulcer, stomach, with perforation
rectum 569.49
root canal space 526.61

Perforation, perforative — *continued*
sigmoid 569.83
sinus (accessory) (chronic) (nasal) (*see also* Sinusitis) 473.9
sphenoidal sinus (*see also* Sinusitis, sphenoidal) 473.3
stomach (due to ulcer) — *see* Ulcer, stomach, with perforation
surgical (accidental) (by instrument) (blood vessel) (nerve) (organ) 998.2
traumatic
external — *see* Wound, open, by site
eye (*see also* Penetrating wound, ocular) 871.7
internal organ — *see* Injury, internal, by site
tympanum (membrane) (persistent posttraumatic) (postinflammatory) 384.20
with
otitis media — *see* Otitis media
attic 384.22
central 384.21
healed 384.81
marginal NEC 384.23
multiple 384.24
pars flaccida 384.22
total 384.25
traumatic — *see* Wound, open, ear, drum
typhoid, gastrointestinal 002.0
ulcer — *see* Ulcer, by site, with perforation
ureter 593.89
urethra
with
abortion — *see* Abortion, by type, with damage to pelvic organs
ectopic pregnancy (*see also* categories 633.0–633.9) 639.2
molar pregnancy (*see also* categories 630–632) 639.2
following
abortion 639.2
ectopic or molar pregnancy 639.2
obstetrical trauma 665.5 ☑
uterus (*see also* Injury, internal, uterus)
with
abortion — *see* Abortion, by type, with damage to pelvic organs
ectopic pregnancy (*see also* categories 633.0–633.9) 639.2
molar pregnancy (*see also* categories 630–632) 639.2
by intrauterine contraceptive device 996.32
following
abortion 639.2
ectopic or molar pregnancy 639.2
obstetrical trauma — *see* Injury, internal, uterus, obstetrical trauma
uvula 528.9
syphilitic 095.8
vagina — *see* Laceration, vagina
viscus NEC 799.89
traumatic 868.00
with open wound into cavity 868.10
**Periadenitis mucosa necrotica recurrens** 528.2
**Periangiitis** 446.0
**Periantritis** 535.4 ☑
**Periappendicitis** (acute) — *see also* Appendicitis 541
**Periarteritis** (disseminated) (infectious) (necrotizing) (nodosa) 446.0

**Periarthritis** (joint) 726.90
Duplay's 726.2
gonococcal 098.50
humeroscapularis 726.2
scapulohumeral 726.2
shoulder 726.2
wrist 726.4
**Periarthrosis** (angioneural) — *see* Periarthritis
**Peribronchitis** 491.9
tuberculous (*see also* Tuberculosis) 011.3 ☑
**Pericapsulitis, adhesive** (shoulder) 726.0
**Pericarditis** (granular) (with decompensation) (with effusion) 423.9
with
rheumatic fever (conditions classifiable to 390)
active (*see also* Pericarditis, rheumatic) 391.0
inactive or quiescent 393
actinomycotic 039.8 [420.0]
acute (nonrheumatic) 420.90
with chorea (acute) (rheumatic) (Sydenham's) 392.0
bacterial 420.99
benign 420.91
hemorrhagic 420.90
idiopathic 420.91
infective 420.90
nonspecific 420.91
rheumatic 391.0
with chorea (acute) (rheumatic) (Sydenham's) 392.0
sicca 420.90
viral 420.91
adhesive or adherent (external) (internal) 423.1
acute — *see* Pericarditis, acute
rheumatic (external) (internal) 393
amebic 006.8 [420.0]
bacterial (acute) (subacute) (with serous or seropurulent effusion) 420.99
calcareous 423.2
cholesterol (chronic) 423.8
acute 420.90
chronic (nonrheumatic) 423.8
rheumatic 393
constrictive 423.2
Coxsackie 074.21
due to
actinomycosis 039.8 [420.0]
amebiasis 006.8 [420.0]
Coxsackie (virus) 074.21
histoplasmosis (*see also* Histoplasmosis) 115.93
nocardiosis 039.8 [420.0]
tuberculosis (*see also* Tuberculosis) 017.9 ☑ [420.0]
fibrinocaseous 017.9 ☑ [420.0]
fibrinopurulent 420.99
fibrinous — *see* Pericarditis, rheumatic
fibropurulent 420.99
fibrous 423.1
gonococcal 098.83
hemorrhagic 423.0
idiopathic (acute) 420.91
infective (acute) 420.90
meningococcal 036.41
neoplastic (chronic) 423.8
acute 420.90
nonspecific 420.91
obliterans, obliterating 423.1
plastic 423.1
pneumococcal (acute) 420.99
postinfarction 411.0
purulent (acute) 420.99
rheumatic (active) (acute) (with effusion) (with pneumonia) 391.0
with chorea (acute) (rheumatic) (Sydenham's) 392.0

**Pericarditis** — *continued*
  rheumatic — *continued*
    chronic or inactive (with chorea) 393
  septic (acute) 420.99
  serofibrinous — *see* Pericarditis, rheumatic
  staphylococcal (acute) 420.99
  streptococcal (acute) 420.99
  suppurative (acute) 420.99
  syphilitic 093.81
  tuberculous (acute) (chronic) (*see also* Tuberculosis) 017.9 ☑ *[420.0]*
  uremic 585.9 *[420.0]*
  viral (acute) 420.91
**Pericardium, pericardial** — *see* condition
**Pericellulitis** — *see also* Cellulitis 682.9
**Pericementitis** 523.40
  acute 523.30
  chronic (suppurative) 523.40
**Pericholecystitis** — *see also* Cholecystitis 575.10
**Perichondritis**
  auricle 380.00
    acute 380.01
    chronic 380.02
  bronchus 491.9
  ear (external) 380.00
    acute 380.01
    chronic 380.02
  larynx 478.71
    syphilitic 095.8
    typhoid 002.0 *[478.71]*
  nose 478.19
  pinna 380.00
    acute 380.01
    chronic 380.02
  trachea 478.9
**Periclasia** 523.5
**Pericolitis** 569.89
**Pericoronitis** (chronic) 523.40
  acute 523.30
**Pericystitis** — *see also* Cystitis 595.9
**Pericytoma** (M9150/1) — *see also* Neoplasm, connective tissue, uncertain behavior
  benign (M9150/0) — *see* Neoplasm, connective tissue, benign
  malignant (M9150/3) — *see* Neoplasm, connective tissue, malignant
**Peridacryocystitis, acute** 375.32
**Peridiverticulitis** — *see also* Diverticulitis 562.11
**Periduodenitis** 535.6 ☑
**Periendocarditis** — *see also* Endocarditis 424.90
  acute or subacute 421.9
**Periepididymitis** — *see also* Epididymitis 604.90
**Perifolliculitis** (abscedens) 704.8
  capitis, abscedens et suffodiens 704.8
  dissecting, scalp 704.8
  scalp 704.8
  superficial pustular 704.8
**Perigastritis** (acute) 535.0 ☑
**Perigastrojejunitis** (acute) 535.0 ☑
**Perihepatitis** (acute) 573.3
  chlamydial 099.56
  gonococcal 098.86
**Peri-ileitis** (subacute) 569.89
**Perilabyrinthitis** (acute) — *see* Labyrinthitis
**Perimeningitis** — *see* Meningitis
**Perimetritis** — *see also* Endometritis 615.9
**Perimetrosalpingitis** — *see also* Salpingo-oophoritis 614.2
**Perineocele** 618.05
**Perinephric** — *see* condition
**Perinephritic** — *see* condition
**Perinephritis** — *see also* Infection, kidney 590.9
  purulent (*see also* Abscess, kidney) 590.2

**Perineum, perineal** — *see* condition
**Perineuritis** NEC 729.2
**Periodic** — *see also* condition
  disease (familial) 277.31
  edema 995.1
    hereditary 277.6
  fever 277.31
  limb movement disorder 327.51
  paralysis (familial) 359.3
  peritonitis 277.31
  polyserositis 277.31
  somnolence (*see also* Narcolepsy) 347.00
**Periodontal**
  cyst 522.8
  pocket 523.8
**Periodontitis** (chronic) (complex) (compound) (simplex) 523.40
  acute 523.33
  aggressive 523.30
    generalized 523.32
    localized 523.31
  apical 522.6
    acute (pulpal origin) 522.4
  generalized 523.42
  localized 523.41
**Periodontoclasia** 523.5
**Periodontosis** 523.5
**Periods** — *see also* Menstruation
  heavy 626.2
  irregular 626.4
**Perionychia** (with lymphangitis) 681.9
  finger 681.02
  toe 681.11
**Perioophoritis** — *see also* Salpingo-oophoritis 614.2
**Periorchitis** — *see also* Orchitis 604.90
**Periosteum, periosteal** — *see* condition
**Periostitis** (circumscribed) (diffuse) (infective) 730.3 ☑

> *Note* — *Use the following fifth-digit subclassification with category 730:*
> 0  *site unspecified*
> 1  *shoulder region*
> 2  *upper arm*
> 3  *forearm*
> 4  *hand*
> 5  *pelvic region and thigh*
> 6  *lower leg*
> 7  *ankle and foot*
> 8  *other specified sites*
> 9  *multiple sites*

  with osteomyelitis (*see also* Osteomyelitis) 730.2 ☑
    acute or subacute 730.0 ☑
    chronic or old 730.1 ☑
  albuminosa, albuminosus 730.3 ☑
  alveolar 526.5
  alveolodental 526.5
  dental 526.5
  gonorrheal 098.89
  hyperplastica, generalized 731.2
  jaw (lower) (upper) 526.4
  monomelic 733.99
  orbital 376.02
  syphilitic 095.5
    congenital 090.0 *[730.8]* ☑
    secondary 091.61
  tuberculous (*see also* Tuberculosis, bone) 015.9 ☑ *[730.8]* ☑
  yaws (early) (hypertrophic) (late) 102.6
**Periostosis** — *see also* Periostitis 730.3 ☑
  with osteomyelitis (*see also* Osteomyelitis) 730.2 ☑
    acute or subacute 730.0 ☑
    chronic or old 730.1 ☑
  hyperplastic 756.59
**Peripartum cardiomyopathy** 674.5 ☑
**Periphlebitis** — *see also* Phlebitis 451.9
  lower extremity 451.2

**Periphlebitis** — *see also* Phlebitis — *continued*
  lower extremity — *continued*
    deep (vessels) 451.19
    superficial (vessels) 451.0
  portal 572.1
  retina 362.18
  superficial (vessels) 451.0
  tuberculous (*see also* Tuberculosis) 017.9 ☑
    retina 017.3 ☑ *[362.18]*
**Peripneumonia** — *see* Pneumonia
**Periproctitis** 569.49
**Periprostatitis** — *see also* Prostatitis 601.9
**Perirectal** — *see* condition
**Perirenal** — *see* condition
**Perisalpingitis** — *see also* Salpingo-oophoritis 614.2
**Perisigmoiditis** 569.89
**Perisplenitis** (infectional) 289.59
**Perispondylitis** — *see* Spondylitis
**Peristalsis reversed or visible** 787.4
**Peritendinitis** — *see also* Tenosynovitis 726.90
  adhesive (shoulder) 726.0
**Perithelioma** (M9150/1) — *see* Pericytoma
**Peritoneum, peritoneal** — *see also* condition
  equilibration test V56.32
**Peritonitis** (acute) (adhesive) (fibrinous) (hemorrhagic) (idiopathic) (localized) (perforative) (primary) (with adhesions) (with effusion) 567.9
  with or following
    abortion — *see* Abortion, by type, with sepsis
    abscess 567.21
    appendicitis 540.0
      with peritoneal abscess 540.1
    ectopic pregnancy (*see also* categories 633.0–633.9) 639.0
    molar pregnancy (*see also* categories 630–632) 639.0
  aseptic 998.7
  bacterial 567.29
    spontaneous 567.23
  bile, biliary 567.81
  chemical 998.7
  chlamydial 099.56
  chronic proliferative 567.89
  congenital NEC 777.6
  diaphragmatic 567.22
  diffuse NEC 567.29
  diphtheritic 032.83
  disseminated NEC 567.29
  due to
    bile 567.81
    foreign
      body or object accidentally left during a procedure (instrument) (sponge) (swab) 998.4
      substance accidentally left during a procedure (chemical) (powder) (talc) 998.7
    talc 998.7
    urine 567.89
  fibrinopurulent 567.29
  fibrinous 567.29
  fibrocaseous (*see also* Tuberculosis) 014.0 ☑
  fibropurulent 567.29
  general, generalized (acute) 567.21
  gonococcal 098.86
  in infective disease NEC 136.9 *[567.0]*
  meconium (newborn) 777.6
  pancreatic 577.8
  paroxysmal, benign 277.31
  pelvic
    female (acute) 614.5
      chronic NEC 614.7
        with adhesions 614.6
      puerperal, postpartum, childbirth 670.0 ☑

**Peritonitis** — *continued*
  pelvic — *continued*
    male (acute) 567.21
  periodic (familial) 277.31
  phlegmonous 567.29
  pneumococcal 567.1
  postabortal 639.0
  proliferative, chronic 567.89
  puerperal, postpartum, childbirth 670.0 ☑
  purulent 567.29
  septic 567.29
  spontaneous bacterial 567.23
  staphylococcal 567.29
  streptococcal 567.29
  subdiaphragmatic 567.29
  subphrenic 567.29
  suppurative 567.29
  syphilitic 095.2
    congenital 090.0 *[567.0]*
  talc 998.7
  tuberculous (*see also* Tuberculosis) 014.0 ☑
  urine 567.89
**Peritonsillar** — *see* condition
**Peritonsillitis** 475
**Perityphlitis** — *see also* Appendicitis 541
**Periureteritis** 593.89
**Periurethral** — *see* condition
**Periurethritis** (gangrenous) 597.89
**Periuterine** — *see* condition
**Perivaginitis** — *see also* Vaginitis 616.10
**Perivasculitis, retinal** 362.18
**Perivasitis** (chronic) 608.4
**Periventricular leukomalacia** 779.7
**Perivesiculitis** (seminal) — *see also* Vesiculitis 608.0
**Perlèche** 686.8
  due to
    moniliasis 112.0
    riboflavin deficiency 266.0
**Pernicious** — *see* condition
**Pernio, perniosis** 991.5
**Persecution**
  delusion 297.9
  social V62.4
**Perseveration** (tonic) 784.69
**Persistence, persistent** (congenital) 759.89
  anal membrane 751.2
  arteria stapedia 744.04
  atrioventricular canal 745.69
  bloody ejaculate 792.2
  branchial cleft 744.41
  bulbus cordis in left ventricle 745.8
  canal of Cloquet 743.51
  capsule (opaque) 743.51
  cilioretinal artery or vein 743.51
  cloaca 751.5
  communication — *see* Fistula, congenital
  convolutions
    aortic arch 747.21
    fallopian tube 752.19
    oviduct 752.19
    uterine tube 752.19
  double aortic arch 747.21
  ductus
    arteriosus 747.0
    Botalli 747.0
  fetal
    circulation 747.83
    form of cervix (uteri) 752.49
    hemoglobin (hereditary) ("Swiss variety") 282.7
    pulmonary hypertension 747.83
  foramen
    Botalli 745.5
    ovale 745.5
  Gartner's duct 752.41
  hemoglobin, fetal (hereditary) (HPFH) 282.7
  hyaloid
    artery (generally incomplete) 743.51

☑ Additional Digit Required — Refer to the Tabular List for Digit Selection
Ⓦ Subterms under main terms may continue to next column or page
*2008 ICD-9-CM*
▶◀ Revised Text    ● New Line    ▲ Revised Code
**Volume 2 — 229**

**Persistence, persistent** — *continued*
 hyaloid — *continued*
  system 743.51
 hymen (tag)
  in pregnancy or childbirth 654.8 ☑
   causing obstructed labor 660.2 ☑
 lanugo 757.4
 left
  posterior cardinal vein 747.49
  root with right arch of aorta 747.21
  superior vena cava 747.49
 Meckel's diverticulum 751.0
 mesonephric duct 752.89
  fallopian tube 752.11
 mucosal disease (middle ear) (with posterior or superior marginal perforation of ear drum) 382.2
 nail(s), anomalous 757.5
 occiput, anterior or posterior 660.3 ☑
  fetus or newborn 763.1
 omphalomesenteric duct 751.0
 organ or site NEC — *see* Anomaly, specified type NEC
 ostium
  atrioventriculare commune 745.69
  primum 745.61
  secundum 745.5
 ovarian rests in fallopian tube 752.19
 pancreatic tissue in intestinal tract 751.5
 primary (deciduous)
  teeth 520.6
  vitreous hyperplasia 743.51
 pulmonary hypertension 747.83
 pupillary membrane 743.46
  iris 743.46
 Rhesus (Rh) titer 999.7
 right aortic arch 747.21
 sinus
  urogenitalis 752.89
  venosus with imperfect incorporation in right auricle 747.49
 thymus (gland) 254.8
  hyperplasia 254.0
 thyroglossal duct 759.2
 thyrolingual duct 759.2
 truncus arteriosus or communis 745.0
 tunica vasculosa lentis 743.39
 umbilical sinus 753.7
 urachus 753.7
 vegetative state 780.03
 vitelline duct 751.0
 wolffian duct 752.89
**Person** (with)
 admitted for clinical research, as participant or control subject V70.7
 awaiting admission to adequate facility elsewhere V63.2
  undergoing social agency investigation V63.8
 concern (normal) about sick person in family V61.49
 consulting on behalf of another V65.19
  pediatric pre-birth visit for expectant mother V65.11
 feared
  complaint in whom no diagnosis was made V65.5
  condition not demonstrated V65.5
 feigning illness V65.2
 healthy, accompanying sick person V65.0
 living (in)
  without
   adequate
    financial resources V60.2
    housing (heating) (space) V60.1
   housing (permanent) (temporary) V60.0
   material resources V60.2
   person able to render necessary care V60.4

**Person** — *continued*
 living — *continued*
  without — *continued*
   shelter V60.0
   alone V60.3
   boarding school V60.6
   residence remote from hospital or medical care facility V63.0
   residential institution V60.6
  medical services in home not available V63.1
  on waiting list V63.2
   undergoing social agency investigation V63.8
  sick or handicapped in family V61.49
  "worried well" V65.5
**Personality**
 affective 301.10
 aggressive 301.3
 amoral 301.7
 anancastic, anankastic 301.4
 antisocial 301.7
 asocial 301.7
 asthenic 301.6
 avoidant 301.82
 borderline 301.83
 change 310.1
 compulsive 301.4
 cycloid 301.13
 cyclothymic 301.13
 dependent 301.6
 depressive (chronic) 301.12
 disorder, disturbance NEC 301.9
  with
   antisocial disturbance 301.7
   pattern disturbance NEC 301.9
   sociopathic disturbance 301.7
   trait disturbance 301.9
 dual 300.14
 dyssocial 301.7
 eccentric 301.89
  "haltlose" type 301.89
 emotionally unstable 301.59
 epileptoid 301.3
 explosive 301.3
 fanatic 301.0
 histrionic 301.50
 hyperthymic 301.11
 hypomanic 301.11
 hypothymic 301.12
 hysterical 301.50
 immature 301.89
 inadequate 301.6
 labile 301.59
 masochistic 301.89
 morally defective 301.7
 multiple 300.14
 narcissistic 301.81
 obsessional 301.4
 obsessive-compulsive 301.4
 overconscientious 301.4
 paranoid 301.0
 passive (-dependent) 301.6
 passive-aggressive 301.84
 pathologic NEC 301.9
 pattern defect or disturbance 301.9
 pseudosocial 301.7
 psychoinfantile 301.59
 psychoneurotic NEC 301.89
 psychopathic 301.9
  with
   amoral trend 301.7
   antisocial trend 301.7
   asocial trend 301.7
   pathologic sexuality (*see also* Deviation, sexual) 302.9
  mixed types 301.9
 schizoid 301.20
 type A 301.4
 unstable (emotional) 301.59
**Perthes' disease** (capital femoral osteochondrosis) 732.1
**Pertussis** — *see also* Whooping cough 033.9
 vaccination, prophylactic (against) V03.6

**Peruvian wart** 088.0
**Perversion, perverted**
 appetite 307.52
  hysterical 300.11
 function
  pineal gland 259.8
  pituitary gland 253.9
   anterior lobe
    deficient 253.2
    excessive 253.1
   posterior lobe 253.6
  placenta — *see* Placenta, abnormal
 sense of smell or taste 781.1
  psychogenic 306.7
 sexual (*see also* Deviation, sexual) 302.9
**Pervious, congenital** — *see also* Imperfect, closure
 ductus arteriosus 747.0
**Pes** (congenital) — *see also* Talipes 754.70
 abductus (congenital) 754.60
  acquired 736.79
 acquired NEC 736.79
  planus 734
 adductus (congenital) 754.79
  acquired 736.79
 cavus 754.71
  acquired 736.73
 planovalgus (congenital) 754.69
  acquired 736.79
 planus (acquired) (any degree) 734
  congenital 754.61
  rachitic 268.1
 valgus (congenital) 754.61
  acquired 736.79
 varus (congenital) 754.50
  acquired 736.79
**Pest** — *see also* Plague 020.9
**Pestis** — *see also* Plague 020.9
 bubonica 020.0
 fulminans 020.0
 minor 020.8
 pneumonica — *see* Plague, pneumonic
**Petechial**
 fever 036.0
 typhus 081.9
**Petechia, petechiae** 782.7
 fetus or newborn 772.6
**Petges-Cléjat or Petges-Clégat syndrome** (poikilodermatomyositis) 710.3
**Petit's**
 disease (*see also* Hernia, lumbar) 553.8
**Petit mal** (idiopathic) — *see also* Epilepsy 345.0 ☑
 status 345.2
**Petrellidosis** 117.6
**Petrositis** 383.20
 acute 383.21
 chronic 383.22
**Peutz-Jeghers disease or syndrome** 759.6
**Peyronie's disease** 607.85
**Pfeiffer's disease** 075
**Phacentocele** 379.32
 traumatic 921.3
**Phacoanaphylaxis** 360.19
**Phacocele** (old) 379.32
 traumatic 921.3
**Phaehyphomycosis** 117.8
**Phagedena** (dry) (moist) — *see also* Gangrene 785.4
 arteriosclerotic 440.24
 geometric 686.09
 penis 607.89
 senile 440.2 ☑ [785.4]
 sloughing 785.4
 tropical (*see also* Ulcer, skin) 707.9
 vulva 616.50
**Phagedenic** — *see also* condition
 abscess (*see also* Abscess)
  chancroid 099.0
 bubo NEC 099.8
 chancre 099.0

**Phagedenic** — *see also* condition — *continued*
 ulcer (tropical) (*see also* Ulcer, skin) 707.9
**Phagomania** 307.52
**Phakoma** 362.89
**Phantom limb** (syndrome) 353.6
**Pharyngeal** — *see also* condition
 arch remnant 744.41
 pouch syndrome 279.11
**Pharyngitis** (acute) (catarrhal) (gangrenous) (infective) (malignant) (membranous) (phlegmonous) (pneumococcal) (pseudomembranous) (simple) (staphylococcal) (subacute) (suppurative) (ulcerative) (viral) 462
 with influenza, flu, or grippe 487.1
 aphthous 074.0
 atrophic 472.1
 chlamydial 099.51
 chronic 472.1
 Coxsackie virus 074.0
 diphtheritic (membranous) 032.0
 follicular 472.1
 fusospirochetal 101
 gonococcal 098.6
 granular (chronic) 472.1
 herpetic 054.79
 hypertrophic 472.1
 infectional, chronic 472.1
 influenzal 487.1
 lymphonodular, acute 074.8
 septic 034.0
 streptococcal 034.0
 tuberculous (*see also* Tuberculosis) 012.8 ☑
 vesicular 074.0
**Pharyngoconjunctival fever** 077.2
**Pharyngoconjunctivitis, viral** 077.2
**Pharyngolaryngitis** (acute) 465.0
 chronic 478.9
 septic 034.0
**Pharyngoplegia** 478.29
**Pharyngotonsillitis** 465.8
 tuberculous 012.8 ☑
**Pharyngotracheitis** (acute) 465.8
 chronic 478.9
**Pharynx, pharyngeal** — *see* condition
**Phase of life problem** NEC V62.89
**Phenomenon**
 Arthus' 995.21
 flashback (drug) 292.89
 jaw-winking 742.8
 Jod-Basedow 242.8 ☑
 L. E. cell 710.0
 lupus erythematosus cell 710.0
 Pelger-Huët (hereditary hyposegmentation) 288.2
 Raynaud's (paroxysmal digital cyanosis) (secondary) 443.0
 Reilly's (*see also* Neuropathy, peripheral, autonomic) 337.9
 vasomotor 780.2
 vasospastic 443.9
 vasovagal 780.2
 Wenckebach's, heart block (second degree) 426.13
**Phenylketonuria** (PKU) 270.1
**Phenylpyruvicaciduria** 270.1
**Pheochromoblastoma** (M8700/3)
 specified site — *see* Neoplasm, by site, malignant
 unspecified site 194.0
**Pheochromocytoma** (M8700/0)
 malignant (M8700/3)
  specified site — *see* Neoplasm, by site, malignant
  unspecified site 194.0
 specified site — *see* Neoplasm, by site, benign
 unspecified site 227.0
**Phimosis** (congenital) 605
 chancroidal 099.0
 due to infection 605

**Phlebectasia** — see also Varicose, vein 454.9
- congenital NEC 747.60
- esophagus (see also Varix, esophagus) 456.1
  - with hemorrhage (see also Varix, esophagus, bleeding) 456.0

**Phlebitis** (infective) (pyemic) (septic) (suppurative) 451.9
- antecubital vein 451.82
- arm NEC 451.84
  - axillary vein 451.89
  - basilic vein 451.82
  - deep 451.83
  - superficial 451.82
- axillary vein 451.89
- basilic vein 451.82
- blue 451.9
- brachial vein 451.83
- breast, superficial 451.89
- cavernous (venous) sinus — see Phlebitis, intracranial sinus
- cephalic vein 451.82
- cerebral (venous) sinus — see Phlebitis, intracranial sinus
- chest wall, superficial 451.89
- complicating pregnancy or puerperium 671.9 ☑
  - affecting fetus or newborn 760.3
- cranial (venous) sinus — see Phlebitis, intracranial sinus
- deep (vessels) 451.19
  - femoral vein 451.11
  - specified vessel NEC 451.19
- due to implanted device — see Complications, due to (presence of) any device, implant, or graft classified to 996.0–996.5 NEC
- during or resulting from a procedure 997.2
- femoral vein (deep) (superficial) 451.11
- femoropopliteal 451.19
- following infusion, perfusion, or transfusion 999.2
- gouty 274.89 [451.9]
- hepatic veins 451.89
- iliac vein 451.81
- iliofemoral 451.11
- intracranial sinus (any) (venous) 325
  - late effect — see category 326
  - nonpyogenic 437.6
    - in pregnancy or puerperium 671.5 ☑
- jugular vein 451.89
- lateral (venous) sinus — see Phlebitis, intracranial sinus
- leg 451.2
  - deep (vessels) 451.19
    - femoral vein 451.11
    - specified vessel NEC 451.19
  - superficial (vessels) 451.0
    - femoral vein 451.11
- longitudinal sinus — see Phlebitis, intracranial sinus
- lower extremity 451.2
  - deep (vessels) 451.19
    - femoral vein 451.11
    - specified vessel NEC 451.19
  - migrans, migrating (superficial) 453.1
  - superficial (vessels) 451.0
    - femoral vein 451.11
- pelvic
  - with
    - abortion — see Abortion, by type, with sepsis
    - ectopic pregnancy (see also categories 633.0–633.9) 639.0
    - molar pregnancy (see also categories 630–632) 639.0
  - following
    - abortion 639.0
    - ectopic or molar pregnancy 639.0
  - puerperal, postpartum 671.4 ☑

**Phlebitis** — continued
- popliteal vein 451.19
- portal (vein) 572.1
- postoperative 997.2
- pregnancy 671.9 ☑
  - deep 671.3 ☑
  - specified type NEC 671.5 ☑
  - superficial 671.2 ☑
- puerperal, postpartum, childbirth 671.9 ☑
  - deep 671.4 ☑
  - lower extremities 671.2 ☑
  - pelvis 671.4 ☑
  - specified site NEC 671.5 ☑
  - superficial 671.2 ☑
- radial vein 451.83
- retina 362.18
- saphenous (great) (long) 451.0
  - accessory or small 451.0
- sinus (meninges) — see Phlebitis, intracranial sinus
- specified site NEC 451.89
- subclavian vein 451.89
- syphilitic 093.89
- tibial vein 451.19
- ulcer, ulcerative 451.9
  - leg 451.2
    - deep (vessels) 451.19
      - femoral vein 451.11
      - specified vessel NEC 451.19
    - superficial (vessels) 451.0
      - femoral vein 451.11
    - lower extremity 451.2
      - deep (vessels) 451.19
        - femoral vein 451.11
        - specified vessel NEC 451.19
      - superficial (vessels) 451.0
- ulnar vein 451.83
- umbilicus 451.89
- upper extremity (see also Phlebitis, arm)
  - deep (veins) 451.83
    - brachial vein 451.83
    - radial vein 451.83
    - ulnar vein 451.83
  - superficial (veins) 451.82
    - antecubital vein 451.82
    - basilica vein 451.82
    - cephalic vein 451.82
- uterus (septic) (see also Endometritis) 615.9
- varicose (leg) (lower extremity) (see also Varicose, vein) 454.1

**Phlebofibrosis** 459.89
**Phleboliths** 459.89
**Phlebosclerosis** 459.89
**Phlebothrombosis** — see Thrombosis
**Phlebotomus fever** 066.0
**Phlegmasia**
- alba dolens (deep vessels) 451.19
  - complicating pregnancy 671.3 ☑
  - nonpuerperal 451.19
  - puerperal, postpartum, childbirth 671.4 ☑
- cerulea dolens 451.19

**Phlegm, choked on** 933.1
**Phlegmon** — see also Abscess 682.9
- erysipelatous (see also Erysipelas) 035
- iliac 682.2
  - fossa 540.1
- throat 478.29
**Phlegmonous** — see condition
**Phlyctenulosis** (allergic) (keratoconjunctivitis) (nontuberculous) 370.31
- cornea 370.31
  - with ulcer (see also Ulcer, cornea) 370.00
- tuberculous (see also Tuberculosis) 017.3 ☑ [370.31]
**Phobia, phobic** (reaction) 300.20
- animal 300.29
- isolated NEC 300.29
- obsessional 300.3
- simple NEC 300.29
- social 300.23
- specified NEC 300.29

**Phobia, phobic** — continued
- state 300.20
**Phocas' disease** 610.1
**Phocomelia** 755.4
- lower limb 755.32
  - complete 755.33
  - distal 755.35
  - proximal 755.34
- upper limb 755.22
  - complete 755.23
  - distal 755.25
  - proximal 755.24
**Phoria** — see also Heterophoria 378.40
**Phosphate-losing tubular disorder** 588.0
**Phosphatemia** 275.3
**Phosphaturia** 275.3
**Photoallergic response** 692.72
**Photocoproporphyria** 277.1
**Photodermatitis** (sun) 692.72
- light other than sun 692.82
**Photokeratitis** 370.24
**Photo-ophthalmia** 370.24
**Photophobia** 368.13
**Photopsia** 368.15
**Photoretinitis** 363.31
**Photoretinopathy** 363.31
**Photosensitiveness** (sun) 692.72
- light other than sun 692.82
**Photosensitization** (skin) (sun) 692.72
- light other than sun 692.82
**Phototoxic response** 692.72
**Phrenitis** 323.9
**Phrynoderma** 264.8
**Phthiriasis** (pubis) (any site) 132.2
- with any infestation classifiable to 132.0, 132.1, 132.3
**Phthirus infestation** — see Phthiriasis
**Phthisis** — see also Tuberculosis 011.9 ☑
- bulbi (infectional) 360.41
- colliers' 011.4 ☑
- cornea 371.05
- eyeball (due to infection) 360.41
- millstone makers' 011.4 ☑
- miners' 011.4 ☑
- potters' 011.4 ☑
- sandblasters' 011.4 ☑
- stonemasons' 011.4 ☑
**Phycomycosis** 117.7
**Physalopteriasis** 127.7
**Physical therapy** NEC V57.1
- breathing exercises V57.0
**Physiological cup, optic papilla**
- borderline, glaucoma suspect 365.00
- enlarged 377.14
- glaucomatous 377.14
**Phytobezoar** 938
- intestine 936
- stomach 935.2
**Pian** — see also Yaws 102.9
**Pianoma** 102.1
**Piarhemia, piarrhemia** — see also Hyperlipemia 272.4
- bilharziasis 120.9
**Pica** 307.52
- hysterical 300.11
**Pick's**
- cerebral atrophy 331.11
  - with dementia
    - with behavioral disturbance 331.11 [294.11]
    - without behavioral disturbance 331.11 [294.10]
- disease
  - brain 331.11
    - dementia in
      - with behavioral disturbance 331.11 [294.11]
      - without behavioral disturbance 331.11 [294.10]
  - lipid histiocytosis 272.7
  - liver (pericardial pseudocirrhosis of liver) 423.2
  - pericardium (pericardial pseudocirrhosis of liver) 423.2

**Pick's** — continued
- polyserositis (pericardial pseudocirrhosis of liver) 423.2
- syndrome
  - heart (pericardial pseudocirrhosis of liver) 423.2
  - liver (pericardial pseudocirrhosis of liver) 423.2
- tubular adenoma (M8640/0)
  - specified site — see Neoplasm, by site, benign
  - unspecified site
    - female 220
    - male 222.0
**Pick-Herxheimer syndrome** (diffuse idiopathic cutaneous atrophy) 701.8
**Pick-Niemann disease** (lipid histiocytosis) 272.7
**Pickwickian syndrome** (cardiopulmonary obesity) 278.8
**Piebaldism, classic** 709.09
**Piedra** 111.2
- beard 111.2
  - black 111.3
  - white 111.2
- black 111.3
- scalp 111.2
  - black 111.3
  - white 111.2
- white 111.2
**Pierre Marie-Bamberger syndrome** (hypertrophic pulmonary osteoarthropathy) 731.2
**Pierre Marie's syndrome** (pulmonary hypertrophic osteoarthropathy) 731.2
**Pierre Mauriac's syndrome** (diabetes-dwarfism-obesity) 258.1
**Pierre Robin deformity or syndrome** (congenital) 756.0
**Pierson's disease or osteochondrosis** 732.1
**Pigeon**
- breast or chest (acquired) 738.3
  - congenital 754.82
  - rachitic (see also Rickets) 268.0
- breeders' disease or lung 495.2
- fanciers' disease or lung 495.2
- toe 735.8
**Pigmentation** (abnormal) 709.00
- anomaly 709.00
  - congenital 757.33
  - specified NEC 709.09
- conjunctiva 372.55
- cornea 371.10
  - anterior 371.11
  - posterior 371.13
  - stromal 371.12
- lids (congenital) 757.33
  - acquired 374.52
- limbus corneae 371.10
- metals 709.00
- optic papilla, congenital 743.57
- retina (congenital) (grouped) (nevoid) 743.53
  - acquired 362.74
- scrotum, congenital 757.33
**Piles** — see Hemorrhoids
**Pili**
- annulati or torti (congenital) 757.4
- incarnati 704.8
**Pill roller hand** (intrinsic) 736.09
**Pilomatrixoma** (M8110/0) — see Neoplasm, skin, benign
**Pilonidal** — see condition
**Pimple** 709.8
**PIN I** (prostatic intraepithelial neoplasia I) 602.3
**PIN II** (prostatic intraepithelial neoplasia II) 602.3
**PIN III** (prostatic intraepithelial neoplasia III) 233.4
**Pinched nerve** — see Neuropathy, entrapment
**Pineal body or gland** — see condition
**Pinealoblastoma** (M9362/3) 194.4

☑ Additional Digit Required — Refer to the Tabular List for Digit Selection      ▽ Subterms under main terms may continue to next column or page

**2008 ICD-9-CM**    ▶◀ Revised Text    ● New Line    ▲ Revised Code    **Volume 2 — 231**

**Pinealoma** (M9360/1) 237.1
  malignant (M9360/3) 194.4
**Pineoblastoma** (M9362/3) 194.4
**Pineocytoma** (M9361/1) 237.1
**Pinguecula** 372.51
**Pinhole meatus** — *see also* Stricture,
  urethra 598.9
**Pink**
  disease 985.0
  eye 372.03
  puffer 492.8
**Pinkus' disease** (lichen nitidus) 697.1
**Pinpoint**
  meatus (*see also* Stricture, urethra)
    598.9
  os uteri (*see also* Stricture, cervix)
    622.4
**Pinselhaare** (congenital) 757.4
**Pinta** 103.9
  cardiovascular lesions 103.2
  chancre (primary) 103.0
  erythematous plaques 103.1
  hyperchromic lesions 103.1
  hyperkeratosis 103.1
  lesions 103.9
    cardiovascular 103.2
    hyperchromic 103.1
    intermediate 103.1
    late 103.2
    mixed 103.3
    primary 103.0
    skin (achromic) (cicatricial)
      (dyschromic) 103.2
      hyperchromic 103.1
      mixed (achromic and hyper-
        chromic) 103.3
  papule (primary) 103.0
  skin lesions (achromic) (cicatricial)
    (dyschromic) 103.2
    hyperchromic 103.1
    mixed (achromic and hyper-
      chromic) 103.3
  vitiligo 103.2
**Pintid** 103.0
**Pinworms** (disease) (infection) (infesta-
  tion) 127.4
**Piry fever** 066.8
**Pistol wound** — *see* Gunshot wound
**Pitchers' elbow** 718.82
**Pithecoid pelvis** 755.69
  with disproportion (fetopelvic) 653.2 ☑
    affecting fetus or newborn 763.1
    causing obstructed labor 660.1 ☑
**Pithiatism** 300.11
**Pit, lip** (mucus), **congenital** 750.25
**Pitted** — *see also* Pitting
  teeth 520.4
**Pitting** (edema) — *see also* Edema 782.3
  lip 782.3
  nail 703.8
    congenital 757.5
**Pituitary gland** — *see* condition
**Pituitary snuff-takers' disease** 495.8
**Pityriasis** 696.5
  alba 696.5
  capitis 690.11
  circinata (et maculata) 696.3
  Hebra's (exfoliative dermatitis) 695.89
  lichenoides et varioliformis 696.2
  maculata (et circinata) 696.3
  nigra 111.1
  pilaris 757.39
    acquired 701.1
    Hebra's 696.4
  rosea 696.3
  rotunda 696.3
  rubra (Hebra) 695.89
    pilaris 696.4
  sicca 690.18
  simplex 690.18
  specified type NEC 696.5
  streptogenes 696.5
  versicolor 111.0
    scrotal 111.0
**Placenta, placental**
  ablatio 641.2 ☑

**Placenta, placental** — *continued*
  ablatio — *continued*
    affecting fetus or newborn 762.1
  abnormal, abnormality 656.7 ☑
    with hemorrhage 641.8 ☑
      affecting fetus or newborn 762.1
    affecting fetus or newborn 762.2
  abruptio 641.2 ☑
    affecting fetus or newborn 762.1
  accessory lobe — *see* Placenta, abnor-
    mal
  accreta (without hemorrhage) 667.0 ☑
    with hemorrhage 666.0 ☑
  adherent (without hemorrhage)
    667.0 ☑
    with hemorrhage 666.0 ☑
  apoplexy — *see* Placenta, separation
  battledore — *see* Placenta, abnormal
  bilobate — *see* Placenta, abnormal
  bipartita — *see* Placenta, abnormal
  carneous mole 631
  centralis — *see* Placenta, previa
  circumvallata — *see* Placenta, abnor-
    mal
  cyst (amniotic) — *see* Placenta, abnor-
    mal
  deficiency — *see* Placenta, insufficien-
    cy
  degeneration — *see* Placenta, insuffi-
    ciency
  detachment (partial) (premature) (with
    hemorrhage) 641.2 ☑
    affecting fetus or newborn 762.1
  dimidiata — *see* Placenta, abnormal
  disease 656.7 ☑
    affecting fetus or newborn 762.2
  duplex — *see* Placenta, abnormal
  dysfunction — *see* Placenta, insuffi-
    ciency
  fenestrata — *see* Placenta, abnormal
  fibrosis — *see* Placenta, abnormal
  fleshy mole 631
  hematoma — *see* Placenta, abnormal
  hemorrhage NEC — *see* Placenta,
    separation
  hormone disturbance or malfunction
    — *see* Placenta, abnormal
  hyperplasia — *see* Placenta, abnormal
  increta (without hemorrhage) 667.0 ☑
    with hemorrhage 666.0 ☑
  infarction 656.7 ☑
    affecting fetus or newborn 762.2
  insertion, vicious — *see* Placenta,
    previa
  insufficiency
    affecting
      fetus or newborn 762.2
      management of pregnancy
        656.5 ☑
  lateral — *see* Placenta, previa
  low implantation or insertion — *see*
    Placenta, previa
  low-lying — *see* Placenta, previa
  malformation — *see* Placenta, abnor-
    mal
  malposition — *see* Placenta, previa
  marginalis, marginata — *see* Placenta,
    previa
  marginal sinus (hemorrhage) (rupture)
    641.2 ☑
    affecting fetus or newborn 762.1
  membranacea — *see* Placenta, abnor-
    mal
  multilobed — *see* Placenta, abnormal
  multipartita — *see* Placenta, abnormal
  necrosis — *see* Placenta, abnormal
  percreta (without hemorrhage)
    667.0 ☑
    with hemorrhage 666.0 ☑
  polyp 674.4 ☑
  previa (central) (centralis) (complete)
    (lateral) (marginal) (marginalis)
    (partial) (partialis) (total) (with
    hemorrhage) 641.1 ☑

**Placenta, placental** — *continued*
  previa — *continued*
    without hemorrhage (before labor
      and delivery) (during pregnan-
      cy) 641.0 ☑
    affecting fetus or newborn 762.0
    noted
      before labor, without hemor-
        rhage (with cesarean deliv-
        ery) 641.0 ☑
      during pregnancy (without
        hemorrhage) 641.0 ☑
    retention (with hemorrhage) 666.0 ☑
      without hemorrhage 667.0 ☑
    fragments, complicating puerperi-
      um (delayed hemorrhage)
      666.2 ☑
      without hemorrhage 667.1 ☑
    postpartum, puerperal 666.2 ☑
  separation (normally implanted) (par-
    tial) (premature) (with hemor-
    rhage) 641.2 ☑
    affecting fetus or newborn 762.1
  septuplex — *see* Placenta, abnormal
  small — *see* Placenta, insufficiency
  softening (premature) — *see* Placenta,
    abnormal
  spuria — *see* Placenta, abnormal
  succenturiata — *see* Placenta, abnor-
    mal
  syphilitic 095.8
  transfusion syndromes 762.3
  transmission of chemical substance
    — *see* Absorption, chemical,
    through placenta
  trapped (with hemorrhage) 666.0 ☑
    without hemorrhage 667.0 ☑
  trilobate — *see* Placenta, abnormal
  tripartita — *see* Placenta, abnormal
  triplex — *see* Placenta, abnormal
  varicose vessel — *see* Placenta, abnor-
    mal
  vicious insertion — *see* Placenta, pre-
    via
**Placentitis**
  affecting fetus or newborn 762.7
  complicating pregnancy 658.4 ☑
**Plagiocephaly** (skull) 754.0
**Plague** 020.9
  abortive 020.8
  ambulatory 020.8
  bubonic 020.0
  cellulocutaneous 020.1
  lymphatic gland 020.0
  pneumonic 020.5
    primary 020.3
    secondary 020.4
  pulmonary — *see* Plague, pneumonic
  pulmonic — *see* Plague, pneumonic
  septicemic 020.2
  tonsillar 020.9
    septicemic 020.2
  vaccination, prophylactic (against)
    V03.3
**Planning, family** V25.09
  contraception V25.9
  natural              ●
    procreative V26.41     ●
    to avoid pregnancy V25.04  ●
  procreation V26.49       ▲
    natural V26.41         ●
**Plaque**
  artery, arterial — *see* Arteriosclerosis
  calcareous — *see* Calcification
  Hollenhorst's (retinal) 362.33
  tongue 528.6
**Plasma cell myeloma** 203.0 ☑
**Plasmacytoma, plasmocytoma** (solitary)
  (M9731/1) 238.6
  benign (M9731/0) — *see* Neoplasm,
    by site, benign
  malignant (M9731/3) 203.8 ☑
**Plasmacytopenia** 288.59
**Plasmacytosis** 288.64
**Plaster ulcer** — *see also* Decubitus
  707.00

**Platybasia** 756.0
**Platyonychia** (congenital) 757.5
  acquired 703.8
**Platypelloid pelvis** 738.6
  with disproportion (fetopelvic) 653.2 ☑
    affecting fetus or newborn 763.1
    causing obstructed labor 660.1 ☑
      affecting fetus or newborn 763.1
  congenital 755.69
**Platyspondylia** 756.19
**Plethora** 782.62
  newborn 776.4
**Pleuralgia** 786.52
**Pleura, pleural** — *see* condition
**Pleurisy** (acute) (adhesive) (chronic)
  (costal) (diaphragmatic) (double)
  (dry) (fetid) (fibrinous) (fibrous) (interlobar) (latent) (lung) (old) (plastic)
  (primary) (residual) (sicca) (sterile)
  (subacute) (unresolved) (with adherent pleura) 511.0
  with
    effusion (without mention of cause)
      511.9
      bacterial, nontuberculous 511.1
      nontuberculous NEC 511.9
        bacterial 511.1
      pneumococcal 511.1
      specified type NEC 511.8
      staphylococcal 511.1
      streptococcal 511.1
      tuberculous (*see also* Tubercu-
        losis, pleura) 012.0 ☑
        primary, progressive 010.1 ☑
    influenza, flu, or grippe 487.1
    tuberculosis — *see* Pleurisy, tuber-
      culous
  encysted 511.8
  exudative (*see also* Pleurisy, with effu-
    sion) 511.9
    bacterial, nontuberculous 511.1
  fibrinopurulent 510.9
    with fistula 510.0
  fibropurulent 510.9
    with fistula 510.0
  hemorrhagic 511.8
  influenzal 487.1
  pneumococcal 511.0
    with effusion 511.1
  purulent 510.9
    with fistula 510.0
  septic 510.9
    with fistula 510.0
  serofibrinous (*see also* Pleurisy, with
    effusion) 511.9
    bacterial, nontuberculous 511.1
  seropurulent 510.9
    with fistula 510.0
  serous (*see also* Pleurisy, with effu-
    sion) 511.9
    bacterial, nontuberculous 511.1
  staphylococcal 511.0
    with effusion 511.1
  streptococcal 511.0
    with effusion 511.1
  suppurative 510.9
    with fistula 510.0
  traumatic (post) (current) 862.29
    with open wound into cavity
      862.39
  tuberculous (with effusion) (*see also*
    Tuberculosis, pleura) 012.0 ☑
    primary, progressive 010.1 ☑
**Pleuritis sicca** — *see* Pleurisy
**Pleurobronchopneumonia** — *see also*
  Pneumonia, broncho- 485
**Pleurodynia** 786.52
  epidemic 074.1
  viral 074.1
**Pleurohepatitis** 573.8
**Pleuropericarditis** — *see also* Pericarditis 423.9
  acute 420.90
**Pleuropneumonia** (acute) (bilateral)
  (double) (septic) — *see also* Pneumonia 486

---

☑ Additional Digit Required — Refer to the Tabular List for Digit Selection                    ▽ Subterms under main terms may continue to next column or page

**Pleuropneumonia** — *see also* Pneumonia
— *continued*
  chronic (*see also* Fibrosis, lung) 515
**Pleurorrhea** — *see also* Hydrothorax
  511.8
**Plexitis, brachial** 353.0
**Plica**
  knee 727.83
  polonica 132.0
  syndrome 727.83
  tonsil 474.8
**Plicae dysphonia ventricularis** 784.49
**Plicated tongue** 529.5
  congenital 750.13
**Plug**
  bronchus NEC 519.19
  meconium (newborn) NEC 777.1
  mucus — *see* Mucus, plug
**Plumbism** 984.9
  specified type of lead — *see* Table of
    Drugs and Chemicals
**Plummer's disease** (toxic nodular goiter)
  242.3 ☑
**Plummer-Vinson syndrome** (sideropenic
  dysphagia) 280.8
**Pluricarential syndrome of infancy** 260
**Plurideficiency syndrome of infancy**
  260
**Plus (and minus) hand** (intrinsic)
  736.09
**PMDD** (premenstrual dysphoric disorder)
  625.4
**PMS** 625.4
**Pneumathemia** — *see* Air, embolism,
  by type
**Pneumatic drill or hammer disease**
  994.9
**Pneumatocele** (lung) 518.89
  intracranial 348.8
  tension 492.0
**Pneumatosis**
  cystoides intestinalis 569.89
  peritonei 568.89
  pulmonum 492.8
**Pneumaturia** 599.84
**Pneumoblastoma** (M8981/3) — *see*
  Neoplasm, lung, malignant
**Pneumocephalus** 348.8
**Pneumococcemia** 038.2
**Pneumococcus, pneumococcal** — *see*
  condition
**Pneumoconiosis** (due to) (inhalation of)
  505
  aluminum 503
  asbestos 501
  bagasse 495.1
  bauxite 503
  beryllium 503
  carbon electrode makers' 503
  coal
    miners' (simple) 500
    workers' (simple) 500
  cotton dust 504
  diatomite fibrosis 502
  dust NEC 504
    inorganic 503
    lime 502
    marble 502
    organic NEC 504
  fumes or vapors (from silo) 506.9
  graphite 503
  hard metal 503
  mica 502
  moldy hay 495.0
  rheumatoid 714.81
  silica NEC 502
    and carbon 500
  silicate NEC 502
  talc 502
**Pneumocystis carinii pneumonia** 136.3
**Pneumocystis jiroveci pneumonia**
  136.3
**Pneumocystosis** 136.3
  with pneumonia 136.3
**Pneumoenteritis** 025

**Pneumohemopericardium** — *see also*
  Pericarditis 423.9
**Pneumohemothorax** — *see also*
  Hemothorax 511.8
  traumatic 860.4
    with open wound into thorax 860.5
**Pneumohydropericardium** — *see also*
  Pericarditis 423.9
**Pneumohydrothorax** — *see also* Hydrothorax 511.8
**Pneumomediastinum** 518.1
  congenital 770.2
  fetus or newborn 770.2
**Pneumomycosis** 117.9
**Pneumonia** (acute) (Alpenstich) (benign)
  (bilateral) (brain) (cerebral) (circumscribed) (congestive) (creeping) (delayed resolution) (double) (epidemic) (fever) (flash) (fulminant) (fungoid) (granulomatous) (hemorrhagic) (incipient) (infantile) (infectious)
  (infiltration) (insular) (intermittent)
  (latent) (lobe) (migratory) (newborn)
  (organized) (overwhelming) (primary) (progressive) (pseudolobar) (purulent) (resolved) (secondary) (senile) (septic) (suppurative) (terminal) (true) (unresolved) (vesicular)
  486
  with influenza, flu, or grippe 487.0
  adenoviral 480.0
  adynamic 514
  alba 090.0
  allergic 518.3
  alveolar — *see* Pneumonia, lobar
  anaerobes 482.81
  anthrax 022.1 *[484.5]*
  apex, apical — *see* Pneumonia, lobar
  ascaris 127.0 *[484.8]*
  aspiration 507.0
    due to
      aspiration of microorganisms
        bacterial 482.9
          specified type NEC 482.89
        specified organism NEC
          483.8
            bacterial NEC 482.89
        viral 480.9
          specified type NEC 480.8
      food (regurgitated) 507.0
      gastric secretions 507.0
      milk 507.0
      oils, essences 507.1
      solids, liquids NEC 507.8
      vomitus 507.0
    fetal 770.18
      due to
        blood 770.16
        clear amniotic fluid 770.14
        meconium 770.12
        postnatal stomach contents
          770.86
    newborn 770.18
      due to
        blood 770.16
        clear amniotic fluid 770.14
        meconium 770.12
        postnatal stomach contents
          770.86
  asthenic 514
  atypical (disseminated) (focal) (prima-
    ry) 486
    with influenza 487.0
  bacillus 482.9
    specified type NEC 482.89
  bacterial 482.9
    specified type NEC 482.89
  Bacteroides (fragilis) (oralis)
    (melaninogenicus) 482.81
  basal, basic, basilar — *see* Pneumo-
    nia, lobar
  broncho-, bronchial (confluent)
    (croupous) (diffuse) (disseminat-
    ed) (hemorrhagic) (involving
    lobes) (lobar) (terminal) 485
    with influenza 487.0

**Pneumonia** — *continued*
  broncho-, bronchial — *continued*
    allergic 518.3
    aspiration (*see also* Pneumonia,
      aspiration) 507.0
    bacterial 482.9
      specified type NEC 482.89
    capillary 466.19
      with bronchospasm or obstruc-
        tion 466.19
    chronic (*see also* Fibrosis, lung)
      515
    congenital (infective) 770.0
    diplococcal 481
    Eaton's agent 483.0
    Escherichia coli (E. coli) 482.82
    Friedländer's bacillus 482.0
    Hemophilus influenzae 482.2
    hiberno-vernal 083.0 *[484.8]*
    hypostatic 514
    influenzal 487.0
    inhalation (*see also* Pneumonia,
      aspiration) 507.0
      due to fumes or vapors (chemi-
        cal) 506.0
    Klebsiella 482.0
    lipid 507.1
      endogenous 516.8
    Mycoplasma (pneumoniae) 483.0
    ornithosis 073.0
    pleuropneumonia-like organisms
      (PPLO) 483.0
    pneumococcal 481
    Proteus 482.83
    Pseudomonas 482.1
    specified organism NEC 483.8
      bacterial NEC 482.89
    staphylococcal 482.40
      aureus 482.41
      specified type NEC 482.49
    streptococcal — *see* Pneumonia,
      streptococcal
    typhoid 002.0 *[484.8]*
    viral, virus (*see also* Pneumonia,
      viral) 480.9
  Butyrivibrio (fibriosolvens) 482.81
  Candida 112.4
  capillary 466.19
    with bronchospasm or obstruction
      466.19
  caseous (*see also* Tuberculosis)
    011.6 ☑
  catarrhal — *see* Pneumonia, broncho-
  central — *see* Pneumonia, lobar
  Chlamydia, chlamydial 483.1
    pneumoniae 483.1
    psittaci 073.0
    specified type NEC 483.1
    trachomatis 483.1
  cholesterol 516.8
  chronic (*see also* Fibrosis, lung) 515
  cirrhotic (chronic) (*see also* Fibrosis,
    lung) 515
  Clostridium (haemolyticum) (novyi)
    NEC 482.81
  confluent — *see* Pneumonia, broncho-
  congenital (infective) 770.0
    aspiration 770.18
  croupous — *see* Pneumonia, lobar
  cytomegalic inclusion 078.5 *[484.1]*
  deglutition (*see also* Pneumonia, aspi-
    ration) 507.0
  desquamative interstitial 516.8
  diffuse — *see* Pneumonia, broncho-
  diplococcal, diplococcus (broncho-)
    (lobar) 481
  disseminated (focal) — *see* Pneumo-
    nia, broncho-
  due to
    adenovirus 480.0
    anaerobes 482.81
    Bacterium anitratum 482.83
    Chlamydia, chlamydial 483.1
      pneumoniae 483.1
      psittaci 073.0
      specified type NEC 483.1

**Pneumonia** — *continued*
  due to — *continued*
    Chlamydia, chlamydial — *contin-
      ued*
      trachomatis 483.1
    coccidioidomycosis 114.0
    Diplococcus (pneumoniae) 481
    Eaton's agent 483.0
    Escherichia coli (E. coli) 482.82
    Friedländer's bacillus 482.0
    fumes or vapors (chemical) (inhala-
      tion) 506.0
    fungus NEC 117.9 *[484.7]*
      coccidioidomycosis 114.0
    Hemophilus influenzae (H. influen-
      zae) 482.2
    Herellea 482.83
    influenza 487.0
    Klebsiella pneumoniae 482.0
    Mycoplasma (pneumoniae) 483.0
    parainfluenza virus 480.2
    pleuropneumonia-like organism
      (PPLO) 483.0
    Pneumococcus 481
    Pneumocystis carinii 136.3
    Pneumocystis jiroveci 136.3
    Proteus 482.83
    Pseudomonas 482.1
    respiratory syncytial virus 480.1
    rickettsia 083.9 *[484.8]*
    SARS-associated coronavirus 480.3
    specified
      bacteria NEC 482.89
      organism NEC 483.8
      virus NEC 480.8
    Staphylococcus 482.40
      aureus 482.41
      specified type NEC 482.49
    Streptococcus (*see also* Pneumo-
      nia, streptococcal)
      pneumoniae 481
    virus (*see also* Pneumonia, viral)
      480.9
      SARS-associated coronavirus
        480.3
  Eaton's agent 483.0
  embolic, embolism — (*see* Embolism,
    pulmonary
  eosinophilic 518.3
  Escherichia coli (E. coli) 482.82
  Eubacterium 482.81
  fibrinous — *see* Pneumonia, lobar
  fibroid (chronic) (*see also* Fibrosis,
    lung) 515
  fibrous (*see also* Fibrosis, lung) 515
  Friedländer's bacillus 482.0
  Fusobacterium (nucleatum) 482.81
  gangrenous 513.0
  giant cell (*see also* Pneumonia, viral)
    480.9
  gram-negative bacteria NEC 482.83
    anaerobic 482.81
  grippal 487.0
  Hemophilus influenzae (bronchial)
    (lobar) 482.2
  hypostatic (broncho-) (lobar) 514
  in
    actinomycosis 039.1
    anthrax 022.1 *[484.5]*
    aspergillosis 117.3 *[484.6]*
    candidiasis 112.4
    coccidioidomycosis 114.0
    cytomegalic inclusion disease
      078.5 *[484.1]*
    histoplasmosis (*see also* Histoplas-
      mosis) 115.95
    infectious disease NEC
      136.9 *[484.8]*
    measles 055.1
    mycosis, systemic NEC
      117.9 *[484.7]*
    nocardiasis, nocardiosis 039.1
    ornithosis 073.0
    pneumocystosis 136.3
    psittacosis 073.0
    Q fever 083.0 *[484.8]*

---

☑ Additional Digit Required — Refer to the Tabular List for Digit Selection

▽ Subterms under main terms may continue to next column or page

**Pneumonia** — *continued*
  in — *continued*
    salmonellosis 003.22
    toxoplasmosis 130.4
    tularemia 021.2
    typhoid (fever) 002.0 *[484.8]*
    varicella 052.1
    whooping cough (*see also* Whooping cough) 033.9 *[484.3]*
  infective, acquired prenatally 770.0
  influenzal (broncho) (lobar) (virus) 487.0
  inhalation (*see also* Pneumonia, aspiration) 507.0
    fumes or vapors (chemical) 506.0
  interstitial 516.8
    with influenzal 487.0
    acute 136.3
    chronic (*see also* Fibrosis, lung) 515
    desquamative 516.8
    hypostatic 514
    lipoid 507.1
    lymphoid 516.8
    plasma cell 136.3
    Pseudomonas 482.1
  intrauterine (infective) 770.0
    aspiration 770.18
      blood 770.16
      clear amniotic fluid 770.14
      meconium 770.12
      postnatal stomach contents 770.86
  Klebsiella pneumoniae 482.0
  Legionnaires' 482.84
  lipid, lipoid (exogenous) (interstitial) 507.1
    endogenous 516.8
  lobar (diplococcal) (disseminated) (double) (interstitial) (pneumococcal, any type) 481
    with influenza 487.0
    bacterial 482.9
      specified type NEC 482.89
    chronic (*see also* Fibrosis, lung) 515
    Escherichia coli (E. coli) 482.82
    Friedländer's bacillus 482.0
    Hemophilus influenzae (H. influenzae) 482.2
    hypostatic 514
    influenzal 487.0
    Klebsiella 482.0
    ornithosis 073.0
    Proteus 482.83
    Pseudomonas 482.1
    psittacosis 073.0
    specified organism NEC 483.8
      bacterial NEC 482.89
    staphylococcal 482.40
      aureus 482.41
      specified type NEC 482.49
    streptococcal — *see* Pneumonia, streptococcal
    viral, virus (*see also* Pneumonia, viral) 480.9
  lobular (confluent) — *see* Pneumonia, broncho-
  Löffler's 518.3
  massive — *see* Pneumonia, lobar
  meconium aspiration 770.12
  metastatic NEC 038.8 *[484.8]*
  Mycoplasma (pneumoniae) 483.0
  necrotic 513.0
  nitrogen dioxide 506.9
  orthostatic 514
  parainfluenza virus 480.2
  parenchymatous (*see also* Fibrosis, lung) 515
  passive 514
  patchy — *see* Pneumonia, broncho-
  Peptococcus 482.81
  Peptostreptococcus 482.81
  plasma cell 136.3
  pleurolobar — *see* Pneumonia, lobar

**Pneumonia** — *continued*
  pleuropneumonia-like organism (PP-LO) 483.0
  pneumococcal (broncho) (lobar) 481
  Pneumocystis (carinii) (jiroveci) 136.3
  postinfectional NEC 136.9 *[484.8]*
  postmeasles 055.1
  postoperative 997.3
  primary atypical 486
  Proprionibacterium 482.81
  Proteus 482.83
  Pseudomonas 482.1
  psittacosis 073.0
  radiation 508.0
  respiratory syncytial virus 480.1
  resulting from a procedure 997.3
  rheumatic 390 *[517.1]*
  Salmonella 003.22
  SARS-associated coronavirus 480.3
  segmented, segmental — *see* Pneumonia, broncho-
  Serratia (marcescens) 482.83
  specified
    bacteria NEC 482.89
    organism NEC 483.8
    virus NEC 480.8
  spirochetal 104.8 *[484.8]*
  staphylococcal (broncho) (lobar) 482.40
    aureus 482.41
    specified type NEC 482.49
  static, stasis 514
  streptococcal (broncho) (lobar) NEC 482.30
    Group
      A 482.31
      B 482.32
      specified NEC 482.39
    pneumoniae 481
    specified type NEC 482.39
  Streptococcus pneumoniae 481
  traumatic (complication) (early) (secondary) 958.8
  tuberculous (any) (*see also* Tuberculosis) 011.6 ☑
  tularemic 021.2
  TWAR agent 483.1
  varicella 052.1
  Veillonella 482.81
  ventilator associated 999.9 ●
  viral, virus (broncho) (interstitial) (lobar) 480.9
    with influenza, flu, or grippe 487.0
    adenoviral 480.0
    parainfluenza 480.2
    respiratory syncytial 480.1
    SARS-associated coronavirus 480.3
    specified type NEC 480.8
  white (congenital) 090.0
**Pneumonic** — *see* condition
**Pneumonitis** (acute) (primary) — *see also* Pneumonia 486
  allergic 495.9
    specified type NEC 495.8
  aspiration 507.0
    due to fumes or gases 506.0
    fetal 770.18
      due to
        blood 770.16
        clear amniotic fluid 770.14
        meconium 770.12
        postnatal stomach contents 770.86
    newborn 770.18
      due to
        blood 770.16
        clear amniotic fluid 770.14
        meconium 770.12
        postnatal stomach contents 770.86
    obstetric 668.0 ☑
  chemical 506.0
    due to fumes or gases 506.0
  cholesterol 516.8
  chronic (*see also* Fibrosis, lung) 515
  congenital rubella 771.0

**Pneumonitis** — *see also* Pneumonia — *continued*
  crack 506.0
  due to
    crack (cocaine) 506.0
    fumes or vapors 506.0
    inhalation
      food (regurgitated), milk, vomitus 507.0
      oils, essences 507.1
      saliva 507.0
      solids, liquids NEC 507.8
    toxoplasmosis (acquired) 130.4
      congenital (active) 771.2 *[484.8]*
  eosinophilic 518.3
  fetal aspiration 770.18
    due to
      blood 770.16
      clear amniotic fluid 770.14
      meconium 770.12
      postnatal stomach contents 770.86
  hypersensitivity 495.9
  interstitial (chronic) (*see also* Fibrosis, lung) 515
    lymphoid 516.8
  lymphoid, interstitial 516.8
  meconium aspiration 770.12
  postanesthetic
    correct substance properly administered 507.0
    obstetric 668.0 ☑
    overdose or wrong substance given 968.4
      specified anesthetic — *see* Table of Drugs and Chemicals
  postoperative 997.3
    obstetric 668.0 ☑
  radiation 508.0
  rubella, congenital 771.0
  "ventilation" 495.7
  wood-dust 495.8
**Pneumoconiosis** — *see* Pneumoconiosis
**Pneumoparotid** 527.8
**Pneumopathy** NEC 518.89
  alveolar 516.9
    specified NEC 516.8
  due to dust NEC 504
  parietoalveolar 516.9
    specified condition NEC 516.8
**Pneumopericarditis** — *see also* Pericarditis 423.9
  acute 420.90
**Pneumopericardium** — *see also* Pericarditis
  congenital 770.2
  fetus or newborn 770.2
  traumatic (post) (*see also* Pneumothorax, traumatic) 860.0
    with open wound into thorax 860.1
**Pneumoperitoneum** 568.89
  fetus or newborn 770.2
**Pneumophagia** (psychogenic) 306.4
**Pneumopleurisy, pneumopleuritis** — *see also* Pneumonia 486
**Pneumopyopericardium** 420.99
**Pneumopyothorax** — *see also* Pyopneumothorax 510.9
  with fistula 510.0
**Pneumorrhagia** 786.3
  newborn 770.3
  tuberculous (*see also* Tuberculosis, pulmonary) 011.9 ☑
**Pneumosiderosis** (occupational) 503
**Pneumothorax** (acute) (chronic) 512.8
  congenital 770.2
  due to operative injury of chest wall or lung 512.1
    accidental puncture or laceration 512.1
  fetus or newborn 770.2
  iatrogenic 512.1
  postoperative 512.1
  spontaneous 512.8
    fetus or newborn 770.2

**Pneumothorax** — *continued*
  spontaneous — *continued*
    tension 512.0
  sucking 512.8
    iatrogenic 512.1
    postoperative 512.1
  tense valvular, infectional 512.0
  tension 512.0
    iatrogenic 512.1
    postoperative 512.1
    spontaneous 512.0
  traumatic 860.0
    with
      hemothorax 860.4
        with open wound into thorax 860.5
      open wound into thorax 860.1
  tuberculous (*see also* Tuberculosis) 011.7 ☑
**Pocket(s)**
  endocardial (*see also* Endocarditis) 424.90
  periodontal 523.8
**Podagra** 274.9
**Podencephalus** 759.89
**Poikilocytosis** 790.09
**Poikiloderma** 709.09
  Civatte's 709.09
  congenital 757.33
  vasculare atrophicans 696.2
**Poikilodermatomyositis** 710.3
**Pointed ear** 744.29
**Poise imperfect** 729.9
**Poisoned** — *see* Poisoning
**Poisoning** (acute) — *see also* Table of Drugs and Chemicals
  Bacillus, B.
    aertrycke (*see also* Infection, Salmonella) 003.9
    botulinus 005.1
    cholerae (suis) (*see also* Infection, Salmonella) 003.9
    paratyphosus (*see also* Infection, Salmonella) 003.9
    suipestifer (*see also* Infection, Salmonella) 003.9
  bacterial toxins NEC 005.9
  berries, noxious 988.2
  blood (general) — *see* Septicemia
  botulism 005.1
  bread, moldy, mouldy — *see* Poisoning, food
  Ciguatera 988.0 ●
  damaged meat — *see* Poisoning, food
  death-cap (Amanita phalloides) (Amanita verna) 988.1
  decomposed food — *see* Poisoning, food
  diseased food — *see* Poisoning, food
  drug — *see* Table of Drugs and Chemicals
  epidemic, fish, meat, or other food — *see* Poisoning, food
  fava bean 282.2
  fish (bacterial) (*see also* Poisoning, food)
    noxious 988.0
  food (acute) (bacterial) (diseased) (infected) NEC 005.9
    due to
      bacillus
        aertrycke (*see also* Poisoning, food, due to Salmonella) 003.9
        botulinus 005.1
        cereus 005.89
        choleraesuis (*see also* Poisoning, food, due to Salmonella) 003.9
        paratyphosus (*see also* Poisoning, food, due to Salmonella) 003.9
        suipestifer (*see also* Poisoning, food, due to Salmonella) 003.9
      Clostridium 005.3

**Poisoning** — *see also* Table of Drugs and Chemicals — *continued*
food — *continued*
  due to — *continued*
    Clostridium — *continued*
      botulinum 005.1
      perfringens 005.2
      welchii 005.2
      Salmonella (aertrycke) (callinarum) (choleraesuis) (enteritidis) (paratyphi) (suipestifer) 003.9
      with
        gastroenteritis 003.0
        localized infection(s) (*see also* Infection, Salmonella) 003.20
        septicemia 003.1
        specified manifestation NEC 003.8
     specified bacterium NEC 005.89
     Staphylococcus 005.0
     Streptococcus 005.89
     Vibrio parahaemolyticus 005.4
     Vibrio vulnificus 005.81
    noxious or naturally toxic 988.0
     berries 988.2
     fish 988.0
     mushroom 988.1
     plants NEC 988.2
  ice cream — *see* Poisoning, food
  ichthyotoxism (bacterial) 005.9
  kreotoxism, food 005.9
  malarial — *see* Malaria
  meat — *see* Poisoning, food
  mushroom (noxious) 988.1
  mussel (*see also* Poisoning, food) noxious 988.0
  noxious foodstuffs (*see also* Poisoning, food, noxious) 988.9
    specified type NEC 988.8
  plants, noxious 988.2
  pork (*see also* Poisoning, food) specified NEC 988.8
    Trichinosis 124
  ptomaine — *see* Poisoning, food
  putrefaction, food — *see* Poisoning, food
  radiation 508.0
  Salmonella (*see also* Infection, Salmonella) 003.9
  sausage (*see also* Poisoning, food) Trichinosis 124
  saxitoxin 988.0
  shellfish (*see also* Poisoning, food) noxious ▶(amnesic) (azaspiracid) (diarrheic) (neurotoxic) (paralytic)◀ 988.0
  Staphylococcus, food 005.0
  toxic, from disease NEC 799.89
  truffles — *see* Poisoning, food
  uremic — *see* Uremia
  uric acid 274.9
  water 276.6    ●
**Poison ivy, oak, sumac or other plant dermatitis** 692.6
**Poker spine** 720.0
**Policeman's disease** 729.2
**Polioencephalitis** (acute) (bulbar) — *see also* Poliomyelitis, bulbar 045.0 ☑
  inferior 335.22
  influenzal 487.8
  superior hemorrhagic (acute) (Wernicke's) 265.1
  Wernicke's (superior hemorrhagic) 265.1
**Polioencephalomyelitis** (acute) (anterior) (bulbar) — *see also* Polioencephalitis 045.0 ☑
**Polioencephalopathy, superior hemorrhagic** 265.1
  with
    beriberi 265.0
    pellagra 265.2
**Poliomeningoencephalitis** — *see* Meningoencephalitis

**Poliomyelitis** (acute) (anterior) (epidemic) 045.9 ☑

> **Note** — Use the following fifth-digit subclassification with category 045:
>
> 0  poliovirus, unspecified type
> 1  poliovirus, type I
> 2  poliovirus, type II
> 3  poliovirus, type III

  with
    paralysis 045.1 ☑
      bulbar 045.0 ☑
  abortive 045.2 ☑
  ascending 045.9 ☑
    progressive 045.9 ☑
  bulbar 045.0 ☑
  cerebral 045.0 ☑
  chronic 335.21
  congenital 771.2
  contact V01.2
  deformities 138
  exposure to V01.2
  late effect 138
  nonepidemic 045.9 ☑
  nonparalytic 045.2 ☑
  old with deformity 138
  posterior, acute 053.19
  residual 138
  sequelae 138
  spinal, acute 045.9 ☑
  syphilitic (chronic) 094.89
  vaccination, prophylactic (against) V04.0
**Poliosis** (eyebrow) (eyelashes) 704.3
  circumscripta (congenital) 757.4
    acquired 704.3
  congenital 757.4
**Pollakiuria** 788.41
  psychogenic 306.53
**Pollinosis** 477.0
**Pollitzer's disease** (hidradenitis suppurativa) 705.83
**Polyadenitis** — *see also* Adenitis 289.3
  malignant 020.0
**Polyalgia** 729.9
**Polyangiitis** (essential) 446.0
**Polyarteritis** (nodosa) (renal) 446.0
**Polyarthralgia** 719.49
  psychogenic 306.0
**Polyarthritis, polyarthropathy** NEC 716.59
  due to or associated with other specified conditions — *see* Arthritis, due to or associated with
  endemic (*see also* Disease, Kaschin-Beck) 716.0 ☑
  inflammatory 714.9
    specified type NEC 714.89
  juvenile (chronic) 714.30
    acute 714.31
  migratory — *see* Fever, rheumatic
  rheumatic 714.0
    fever (acute) — *see* Fever, rheumatic
**Polycarential syndrome of infancy** 260
**Polychondritis** (atrophic) (chronic) (relapsing) 733.99
**Polycoria** 743.46
**Polycystic** (congenital) (disease) 759.89
  degeneration, kidney — *see* Polycystic, kidney
  kidney (congenital) 753.12
    adult type (APKD) 753.13
    autosomal dominant 753.13
    autosomal recessive 753.14
    childhood type (CPKD) 753.14
    infantile type 753.14
  liver 751.62
  lung 518.89
    congenital 748.4
  ovary, ovaries 256.4
  spleen 759.0
**Polycythemia** (primary) (rubra) (vera) (M9950/1) 238.4

**Polycythemia** — *continued*
  acquired 289.0
  benign 289.0
    familial 289.6
  due to
    donor twin 776.4
    fall in plasma volume 289.0
    high altitude 289.0
    maternal-fetal transfusion 776.4
    stress 289.0
  emotional 289.0
  erythropoietin 289.0
  familial (benign) 289.6
  Gaisböck's (hypertonica) 289.0
  high altitude 289.0
  hypertonica 289.0
  hypoxemic 289.0
  neonatorum 776.4
  nephrogenous 289.0
  relative 289.0
  secondary 289.0
  spurious 289.0
  stress 289.0
**Polycytosis cryptogenica** 289.0
**Polydactylism, polydactyly** 755.00
  fingers 755.01
  toes 755.02
**Polydipsia** 783.5
**Polydystrophic oligophrenia** 277.5
**Polyembryoma** (M9072/3) — *see* Neoplasm, by site, malignant
**Polygalactia** 676.6 ☑
**Polyglandular**
  deficiency 258.9
  dyscrasia 258.9
  dysfunction 258.9
  syndrome 258.8
**Polyhydramnios** — *see also* Hydramnios 657.0 ☑
**Polymastia** 757.6
**Polymenorrhea** 626.2
**Polymicrogyria** 742.2
**Polymyalgia** 725
  arteritica 446.5
  rheumatica 725
**Polymyositis** (acute) (chronic) (hemorrhagic) 710.4
  with involvement of
    lung 710.4 [517.8]
    skin 710.3
  ossificans (generalisata) (progressiva) 728.19
  Wagner's (dermatomyositis) 710.3
**Polyneuritis, polyneuritic** — *see also* Polyneuropathy 356.9
  alcoholic 357.5
    with psychosis 291.1
  cranialis 352.6
  demyelinating, chronic inflammatory ▶(CIDP)◀ 357.81
  diabetic 250.6 ☑ *[357.2]*
  due to lack of vitamin NEC 269.2 *[357.4]*
  endemic 265.0 *[357.4]*
  erythredema 985.0
  febrile 357.0
  hereditary ataxic 356.3
  idiopathic, acute 357.0
  infective (acute) 357.0
  nutritional 269.9 *[357.4]*
  postinfectious 357.0
**Polyneuropathy** (peripheral) 356.9
  alcoholic 357.5
  amyloid 277.39 *[357.4]*
  arsenical 357.7
  critical illness 357.82
  demyelinating, chronic inflammatory● (CIDP) 357.81
  diabetic 250.6 ☑ *[357.2]*
  due to
    antitetanus serum 357.6
    arsenic 357.7
    drug or medicinal substance 357.6
      correct substance properly administered 357.6

**Polyneuropathy** — *continued*
  due to — *continued*
    drug or medicinal substance — *continued*
      overdose or wrong substance given or taken 977.9
      specified drug — *see* Table of Drugs and Chemicals
    lack of vitamin NEC 269.2 *[357.4]*
    lead 357.7
    organophosphate compounds 357.7
    pellagra 265.2 *[357.4]*
    porphyria 277.1 *[357.4]*
    serum 357.6
    toxic agent NEC 357.7
  hereditary 356.0
  idiopathic 356.9
    progressive 356.4
  in
    amyloidosis 277.39 *[357.4]*
    avitaminosis 269.2 *[357.4]*
      specified NEC 269.1 *[357.4]*
    beriberi 265.0 *[357.4]*
    collagen vascular disease NEC 710.9 *[357.1]*
    deficiency
      B-complex NEC 266.2 *[357.4]*
      vitamin B 266.1 *[357.4]*
      vitamin B6 266.9 *[357.4]*
    diabetes 250.6 ☑ *[357.2]*
    diphtheria (*see also* Diphtheria) 032.89 *[357.4]*
    disseminated lupus erythematosus 710.0 *[357.1]*
    herpes zoster 053.13
    hypoglycemia 251.2 *[357.4]*
    malignant neoplasm (M8000/3) NEC 199.1 *[357.3]*
    mumps 072.72
    pellagra 265.2 *[357.4]*
    polyarteritis nodosa 446.0 *[357.1]*
    porphyria 277.1 *[357.4]*
    rheumatoid arthritis 714.0 *[357.1]*
    sarcoidosis 135 *[357.4]*
    uremia 585.9 *[357.4]*
  lead 357.7
  nutritional 269.9 *[357.4]*
    specified NEC 269.8 *[357.4]*
  postherpetic 053.13
  progressive 356.4
  sensory (hereditary) 356.2
  specified NEC 356.8   ●
**Polyonychia** 757.5
**Polyopia** 368.2
  refractive 368.15
**Polyorchism, polyorchidism** (three testes) 752.89
**Polyorrhymenitis** (peritoneal) — *see also* Polyserositis 568.82
  pericardial 423.2
**Polyostotic fibrous dysplasia** 756.54
**Polyotia** 744.1
**Polyphagia** 783.6
**Polypoid** — *see* condition
**Polyposis** — *see also* Polyp
  coli (adenomatous) (M8220/0) 211.3
    adenocarcinoma in (M8220/3) 153.9
    carcinoma in (M8220/3) 153.9
  familial (M8220/0) 211.3
  intestinal (adenomatous) (M8220/0) 211.3
  multiple (M8221/0) — *see* Neoplasm, by site, benign

**Polyp, polypus**

> **Note** — Polyps of organs or sites that do not appear in the list below should be coded to the residual category for diseases of the organ or site concerned.

  accessory sinus 471.8
  adenoid tissue 471.0
  adenomatous (M8210/0) (*see also* Neoplasm, by site, benign)

☑ Additional Digit Required — Refer to the Tabular List for Digit Selection

2008 ICD-9-CM

▶◀ Revised Text

▽ Subterms under main terms may continue to next column or page

● New Line   ▲ Revised Code

October 2007 · Volume 2 — 235

**Polyp, polypus** — *continued*
adenomatous (*see also* Neoplasm, by
site, benign) — *continued*
adenocarcinoma in (M8210/3) —
*see* Neoplasm, by site, malignant
carcinoma in (M8210/3) — *see*
Neoplasm, by site, malignant
multiple (M8221/0) — *see* Neoplasm, by site, benign
antrum 471.8
anus, anal (canal) (nonadenomatous)
569.0
adenomatous 211.4
Bartholin's gland 624.6
bladder (M8120/1) 236.7
broad ligament 620.8
cervix (uteri) 622.7
adenomatous 219.0
in pregnancy or childbirth 654.6 ☑
affecting fetus or newborn
763.89
causing obstructed labor
660.2 ☑
mucous 622.7
nonneoplastic 622.7
choanal 471.0
cholesterol 575.6
clitoris 624.6
colon (M8210/0) (*see also* Polyp, adenomatous) 211.3
corpus uteri 621.0
dental 522.0
ear (middle) 385.30
endometrium 621.0
ethmoidal (sinus) 471.8
fallopian tube 620.8
female genital organs NEC 624.8
frontal (sinus) 471.8
gallbladder 575.6
gingiva 523.8
gum 523.8
labia 624.6
larynx (mucous) 478.4
malignant (M8000/3) — *see* Neoplasm, by site, malignant
maxillary (sinus) 471.8
middle ear 385.30
myometrium 621.0
nares
anterior 471.9
posterior 471.0
nasal (mucous) 471.9
cavity 471.0
septum 471.9
nasopharyngeal 471.0
neoplastic (M8210/0) — *see* Neoplasm, by site, benign
nose (mucous) 471.9
oviduct 620.8
paratubal 620.8
pharynx 478.29
congenital 750.29
placenta, placental 674.4 ☑
prostate 600.20
with
other lower urinary tract symptoms (LUTS) 600.21
urinary
obstruction 600.21
retention 600.21
pudenda 624.6
pulp (dental) 522.0
rectosigmoid 211.4
rectum (nonadenomatous) 569.0
adenomatous 211.4
septum (nasal) 471.9
sinus (accessory) (ethmoidal) (frontal)
(maxillary) (sphenoidal) 471.8
sphenoidal (sinus) 471.8
stomach (M8210/0) 211.1
tube, fallopian 620.8
turbinate, mucous membrane 471.8
ureter 593.89
urethra 599.3

**Polyp, polypus** — *continued*
uterine
ligament 620.8
tube 620.8
uterus (body) (corpus) (mucous) 621.0
in pregnancy or childbirth 654.1 ☑
affecting fetus or newborn
763.89
causing obstructed labor
660.2 ☑
vagina 623.7
vocal cord (mucous) 478.4
vulva 624.6
**Polyradiculitis** (acute) 357.0
**Polyradiculoneuropathy** (acute) (segmen-
tally demyelinating) 357.0
**Polysarcia** 278.00
**Polyserositis** (peritoneal) 568.82
due to pericarditis 423.2
paroxysmal (familial) 277.31
pericardial 423.2
periodic (familial) 277.31
pleural — *see* Pleurisy
recurrent 277.31
tuberculous (*see also* Tuberculosis,
polyserositis) 018.9 ☑
**Polysialia** 527.7
**Polysplenia syndrome** 759.0
**Polythelia** 757.6
**Polytrichia** — *see also* Hypertrichosis
704.1
**Polyunguia** (congenital) 757.5
acquired 703.8
**Polyuria** 788.42
**Pompe's disease** (glycogenosis II) 271.0
**Pompholyx** 705.81
**Poncet's disease** (tuberculous rheumatism) — *see also* Tuberculosis
015.9 ☑
**Pond fracture** — *see* Fracture, skull,
vault
**Ponos** 085.0
**Pons, pontine** — *see* condition
**Poor**
aesthetics of existing restoration of
tooth 525.67
contractions, labor 661.2 ☑
affecting fetus or newborn 763.7
fetal growth NEC 764.9 ☑
affecting management of pregnancy
656.5 ☑
incorporation
artificial skin graft 996.55
decellularized allodermis graft
996.55
obstetrical history V13.29
affecting management of current
pregnancy V23.49
pre-term labor V23.41
pre-term labor V13.21
sucking reflex (newborn) 796.1
vision NEC 369.9
**Poradenitis, nostras** 099.1
**Porencephaly** (congenital) (developmental) (true) 742.4
acquired 348.0
nondevelopmental 348.0
traumatic (post) 310.2
**Porocephaliasis** 134.1
**Porokeratosis** 757.39
disseminated superficial actinic
(DSAP) 692.75
**Poroma, eccrine** (M8402/0) — *see* Neoplasm, skin, benign
**Porphyria** (acute) (congenital) (constitutional) (erythropoietic) (familial)
(hepatica) (idiopathic) (idiosyncratic) (intermittent) (latent) (mixed
hepatic) (photosensitive) (South
African genetic) (Swedish) 277.1
acquired 277.1
cutaneatarda
hereditaria 277.1
symptomatica 277.1

**Porphyria** — *continued*
due to drugs
correct substance properly administered 277.1
overdose or wrong substance given
or taken 977.9
specified drug — *see* Table of
Drugs and Chemicals
secondary 277.1
toxic NEC 277.1
variegata 277.1
**Porphyrinuria** (acquired) (congenital)
(secondary) 277.1
**Porphyruria** (acquired) (congenital) 277.1
**Portal** — *see* condition
**Port wine nevus or mark** 757.32
**Posadas-Wernicke disease** 114.9
**Position**
fetus, abnormal (*see also* Presentation, fetal) 652.9 ☑
teeth, faulty (*see also* Anomaly, position tooth) 524.30
**Positive**
culture (nonspecific) 795.39
AIDS virus V08
blood 790.7
HIV V08
human immunodeficiency virus
V08
nose 795.39
skin lesion NEC 795.39
spinal fluid 792.0
sputum 795.39
stool 792.1
throat 795.39
urine 791.9
wound 795.39
findings, anthrax 795.31
HIV V08
human immunodeficiency virus (HIV)
V08
PPD 795.5
serology
AIDS virus V08
inconclusive 795.71
HIV V08
inconclusive 795.71
human immunodeficiency virus
(HIV) V08
inconclusive 795.71
syphilis 097.1
with signs or symptoms — *see*
Syphilis, by site and stage
false 795.6
skin test 795.7 ☑
tuberculin (without active tuberculosis) 795.5
VDRL 097.1
with signs or symptoms — *see*
Syphilis, by site and stage
false 795.6
Wassermann reaction 097.1
false 795.6
**Postcardiotomy syndrome** 429.4
**Postcaval ureter** 753.4
**Postcholecystectomy syndrome** 576.0
**Postclimacteric bleeding** 627.1
**Postcommissurotomy syndrome** 429.4
**Postconcussional syndrome** 310.2
**Postcontusional syndrome** 310.2
**Postcricoid region** — *see* condition
**Post-dates** (pregnancy) — *see* Pregnancy
**Postencephalitic** — *see also* condition
syndrome 310.8
**Posterior** — *see* condition
**Posterolateral sclerosis** (spinal cord) —
*see* Degeneration, combined
**Postexanthematous** — *see* condition
**Postfebrile** — *see* condition
**Postgastrectomy dumping syndrome**
564.2
**Posthemiplegic chorea** 344.89
**Posthemorrhagic anemia** (chronic)
280.0
acute 285.1
newborn 776.5

**Posthepatitis syndrome** 780.79
**Postherpetic neuralgia** (intercostal)
(syndrome) (zoster) 053.19
geniculate ganglion 053.11
ophthalmica 053.19
trigeminal 053.12
**Posthitis** 607.1
**Postimmunization complication or re-
action** — *see* Complications, vaccination
**Postinfectious** — *see* condition
**Postinfluenzal syndrome** 780.79
**Postlaminectomy syndrome** 722.80
cervical, cervicothoracic 722.81
kyphosis 737.12
lumbar, lumbosacral 722.83
thoracic, thoracolumbar 722.82
**Postleukotomy syndrome** 310.0
**Postlobectomy syndrome** 310.0
**Postmastectomy lymphedema** (syndrome) 457.0
**Postmaturity, postmature** (fetus or
newborn) (gestation period over 42
completed weeks) 766.22
affecting management of pregnancy
post-term pregnancy 645.1 ☑
prolonged pregnancy 645.2 ☑
syndrome 766.22
**Postmeasles** — *see also* condition
complication 055.8
specified NEC 055.79
**Postmenopausal**
endometrium (atrophic) 627.8
suppurative (*see also* Endometritis)
615.9
hormone replacement therapy V07.4
status (age related) (natural) V49.81
**Postnasal drip** 784.91
**Postnatal** — *see* condition
**Postoperative** — *see also* condition
confusion state 293.9
psychosis 293.9
status NEC (*see also* Status (post))
V45.89
**Postpancreatectomy hyperglycemia**
251.3
**Postpartum** — *see also* condition
anemia 648.2 ☑
cardiomyopathy 674.5 ☑
observation
immediately after delivery V24.0
routine follow-up V24.2
**Postperfusion syndrome** NEC 999.8
bone marrow 996.85
**Postpoliomyelitic** — *see* condition
**Postsurgery status** NEC — *see also*
Status (post V45.89
**Post-term** (pregnancy) 645.1 ☑
infant (gestation period over 40 com-
pleted weeks to 42 completed
weeks) 766.21
**Posttraumatic** — *see* condition
**Posttraumatic brain syndrome,
nonpsychotic** 310.2
**Post-traumatic stress disorder** (PTSD)
309.81
**Post-typhoid abscess** 002.0
**Postures, hysterical** 300.11
**Postvaccinal reaction or complication**
— *see* Complications, vaccination
**Postvagotomy syndrome** 564.2
**Postvalvulotomy syndrome** 429.4
**Postvasectomy sperm count** V25.8
**Potain's disease** (pulmonary edema) 514
**Potain's syndrome** (gastrectasis with
dyspepsia) 536.1
**Pott's**
curvature (spinal) (*see also* Tuberculosis) 015.0 ☑ *[737.43]*
disease or paraplegia (*see also* Tuberculosis) 015.0 ☑ *[730.88]*
fracture (closed) 824.4
open 824.5
gangrene 440.24
osteomyelitis (*see also* Tuberculosis)
015.0 ☑ *[730.88]*

**Pott's** — *continued*
spinal curvature (*see also* Tuberculosis) 015.0 ☑ *[737.43]*
tumor, puffy (*see also* Osteomyelitis) 730.2 ☑
**Potter's**
asthma 502
disease 753.0
facies 754.0
lung 502
syndrome (with renal agenesis) 753.0
**Pouch**
bronchus 748.3
Douglas' — *see* condition
esophagus, esophageal (congenital) 750.4
acquired 530.6
gastric 537.1
Hartmann's (abnormal sacculation of gallbladder neck) 575.8
of intestine V44.3
attention to V55.3
pharynx, pharyngeal (congenital) 750.27
**Poulet's disease** 714.2
**Poultrymen's itch** 133.8
**Poverty** V60.2
**PPE** (palmar plantar erythrodysesthesia) 693.0 ●
**Prader-Labhart-Willi-Fanconi syndrome** (hypogenital dystrophy with diabetic tendency) 759.81
**Prader-Willi syndrome** (hypogenital dystrophy with diabetic tendency) 759.81
**Preachers' voice** 784.49
**Pre-AIDS** — *see* Human immunodeficiency virus (disease) (illness) (infection)
**Preauricular appendage** 744.1
**Prebetalipoproteinemia** (acquired) (essential) (familial) (hereditary) (primary) (secondary) 272.1
with chylomicronemia 272.3
**Precipitate labor** 661.3 ☑
affecting fetus or newborn 763.6
**Preclimacteric bleeding** 627.0
menorrhagia 627.0
**Precocious**
adrenarche 259.1
menarche 259.1
menstruation 626.8
pubarche 259.1
puberty NEC 259.1
sexual development NEC 259.1
thelarche 259.1
**Precocity, sexual** (constitutional) (cryptogenic) (female) (idiopathic) (male) NEC 259.1
with adrenal hyperplasia 255.2
**Precordial pain** 786.51
psychogenic 307.89
**Predeciduous teeth** 520.2
**Prediabetes, prediabetic** 790.29
complicating pregnancy, childbirth, or puerperium 648.8 ☑
fetus or newborn 775.89
**Predislocation status of hip, at birth** — *see also* Subluxation, congenital, hip 754.32
**Preeclampsia** (mild) 642.4 ☑
with pre-existing hypertension 642.7 ☑
affecting fetus or newborn 760.0
severe 642.5 ☑
superimposed on pre-existing hypertensive disease 642.7 ☑
**Preeruptive color change, teeth, tooth** 520.8
**Preexcitation** 426.7
atrioventricular conduction 426.7
ventricular 426.7
**Preglaucoma** 365.00

**Pregnancy** (single) (uterine) (without sickness) V22.2

> Note — Use the following fifth-digit subclassification with categories 640–648, 651–676:
>
> 0　unspecified as to episode of care
> 1　delivered, with or without mention of antepartum condition
> 2　delivered, with mention of postpartum complication
> 3　antepartum condition or complication
> 4　postpartum condition or complication

abdominal (ectopic) 633.00
with intrauterine pregnancy 633.01
affecting fetus or newborn 761.4
abnormal NEC 646.9
ampullar — *see* Pregnancy, tubal
broad ligament — *see* Pregnancy, cornual
cervical — *see* Pregnancy, cornual
combined (extrauterine and intrauterine) — *see* Pregnancy, cornual
complicated (by)
abnormal, abnormality NEC 646.9 ☑
cervix 654.6 ☑
cord (umbilical) 663.9 ☑
glucose tolerance (conditions classifiable to 790.21–790.29) 648.8 ☑
pelvic organs or tissues NEC 654.9 ☑
pelvis (bony) 653.0 ☑
perineum or vulva 654.8 ☑
placenta, placental (vessel) 656.7 ☑
position
cervix 654.4 ☑
placenta 641.1 ☑
without hemorrhage 641.0 ☑
uterus 654.4 ☑
size, fetus 653.5 ☑
uterus (congenital) 654.0 ☑
abscess or cellulitis
bladder 646.6 ☑
genitourinary tract (conditions classifiable to 590, 595, 597, 599.0, 614.0–614.5, 614.7–614.9, 615) 646.6 ☑
kidney 646.6 ☑
urinary tract NEC 646.6 ☑
adhesion, pelvic peritoneal 648.9 ☑
air embolism 673.0 ☑
albuminuria 646.2 ☑
with hypertension — *see* Toxemia, of pregnancy
amnionitis 658.4 ☑
amniotic fluid embolism 673.1 ☑
anemia (conditions classifiable to 280–285) 648.2 ☑
appendicitis 648.9 ☑
atrophy, yellow (acute) (liver) (subacute) 646.7 ☑
bacilluria, asymptomatic 646.5 ☑
bacteriuria, asymptomatic 646.5 ☑
bariatric surgery status 649.2 ☑
bicornis or bicornuate uterus 654.0 ☑
biliary problems 646.8 ☑
bone and joint disorders (conditions classifiable to 720–724 or conditions affecting lower limbs classifiable to 711–719, 725–738) 648.7 ☑
breech presentation (buttocks) (complete) (frank) 652.2 ☑
with successful version 652.1 ☑

**Pregnancy** — *continued*
complicated — *continued*
cardiovascular disease (conditions classifiable to 390–398, 410–429) 648.6 ☑
congenital (conditions classifiable to 745–747) 648.5 ☑
cerebrovascular disorders (conditions classifiable to 430–434, 436–437) 674.0 ☑
cervicitis (conditions classifiable to 616.0) 646.6 ☑
chloasma (gravidarum) 646.8 ☑
cholelithiasis 646.8 ☑
chorea (gravidarum) — *see* Eclampsia, pregnancy
coagulation defect 649.3 ☑
contraction, pelvis (general) 653.1 ☑
inlet 653.2 ☑
outlet 653.3 ☑
convulsions (eclamptic) (uremic) 642.6 ☑
with pre-existing hypertension 642.7 ☑
current disease or condition (nonobstetric)
abnormal glucose tolerance 648.8 ☑
anemia 648.2 ☑
bone and joint (lower limb) 648.7 ☑
cardiovascular 648.6 ☑
congenital 648.5 ☑
cerebrovascular 674.0 ☑
diabetic 648.0 ☑
drug dependence 648.3 ☑
female genital mutilation 648.9 ☑
genital organ or tract 646.6 ☑
gonorrheal 647.1 ☑
hypertensive 642.2 ☑
chronic kidney 642.2 ☑
renal 642.1 ☑
infectious 647.9 ☑
specified type NEC 647.8 ☑
liver 646.7 ☑
malarial 647.4 ☑
nutritional deficiency 648.9 ☑
parasitic NEC 647.8 ☑
periodontal disease 648.9 ☑
renal 646.2 ☑
hypertensive 642.1 ☑
rubella 647.5 ☑
specified condition NEC 648.9 ☑
syphilitic 647.0 ☑
thyroid 648.1 ☑
tuberculous 647.3 ☑
urinary 646.6 ☑
venereal 647.2 ☑
viral NEC 647.6 ☑
cystitis 646.6 ☑
cystocele 654.4 ☑
death of fetus (near term) 656.4 ☑
early pregnancy (before 22 completed weeks gestation) 632
deciduitis 646.6 ☑
decreased fetal movements 655.7 ☑
diabetes (mellitus) (conditions classifiable to 250) 648.0 ☑
disorders of liver 646.7 ☑
displacement, uterus NEC 654.4 ☑
disproportion — *see* Disproportion
double uterus 654.0 ☑
drug dependence (conditions classifiable to 304) 648.3 ☑
dysplasia, cervix 654.6 ☑
early onset of delivery (spontaneous) 644.2 ☑
eclampsia, eclamptic (coma) (convulsions) (delirium) (nephritis) (uremia) 642.6 ☑

**Pregnancy** — *continued*
complicated — *continued*
eclampsia, eclamptic — *continued*
with pre-existing hypertension 642.7 ☑
edema 646.1 ☑
with hypertension — *see* Toxemia, of pregnancy
effusion, amniotic fluid 658.1 ☑
delayed delivery following 658.2 ☑
embolism
air 673.0 ☑
amniotic fluid 673.1 ☑
blood-clot 673.2 ☑
cerebral 674.0 ☑
pulmonary NEC 673.2 ☑
pyemic 673.3 ☑
septic 673.3 ☑
emesis (gravidarum) — *see* Pregnancy, complicated, vomiting
endometritis (conditions classifiable to 615.0–615.9) 670 ☑ ▲
decidual 646.6 ☑
epilepsy 649.4 ☑
excessive weight gain NEC 646.1 ☑
face presentation 652.4 ☑
failure, fetal head to enter pelvic brim 652.5 ☑
false labor (pains) 644.1 ☑
fatigue 646.8 ☑
fatty metamorphosis of liver 646.7 ☑
female genital mutilation 648.9 ☑
fetal
death (near term) 656.4 ☑
early (before 22 completed weeks gestation) 632
deformity 653.7 ☑
distress 656.8 ☑
reduction of multiple fetuses reduced to single fetus 651.7 ☑
fibroid (tumor) (uterus) 654.1 ☑
footling presentation 652.8 ☑
with successful version 652.1 ☑
gallbladder disease 646.8 ☑
gastric banding status 649.2 ☑
gastric bypass status for obesity 648.1 ☑
goiter 648.1 ☑
gonococcal infection (conditions classifiable to 098) 647.1 ☑
gonorrhea (conditions classifiable to 098) 647.1 ☑
hemorrhage 641.9 ☑
accidental 641.2 ☑
before 22 completed weeks gestation NEC 640.9 ☑
cerebrovascular 674.0 ☑
due to
afibrinogenemia or other coagulation defect (conditions classifiable to 286.0–286.9) 641.3 ☑
leiomyoma, uterine 641.8 ☑
marginal sinus (rupture) 641.2 ☑
premature separation, placenta 641.2 ☑
trauma 641.8 ☑
early (before 22 completed weeks gestation) 640.9 ☑
threatened abortion 640.0 ☑
unavoidable 641.1 ☑
hepatitis (acute) (malignant) (subacute) 646.7 ☑
viral 647.6 ☑
herniation of uterus 654.4 ☑
high head at term 652.5 ☑
hydatidiform mole (delivered) (undelivered) 630
hydramnios 657.0 ☑
hydrocephalic fetus 653.6 ☑

☑ Additional Digit Required — Refer to the Tabular List for Digit Selection
**2008 ICD-9-CM**
▶◀ Revised Text
● New Line
▲ Revised Code
⬇ Subterms under main terms may continue to next column or page
**October 2007 · Volume 2 — 237**

**Pregnancy** — *continued*
  complicated — *continued*
    hydrops amnii 657.0 ☑
    hydrorrhea 658.1 ☑
    hyperemesis (gravidarum) — *see*
      Hyperemesis, gravidarum
    hypertension — *see* Hypertension,
      complicating pregnancy
    hypertensive
      chronic kidney disease 642.2 ☑
      heart and chronic kidney dis-
        ease 642.2 ☑
      heart and renal disease 642.2 ☑
      heart disease 642.2 ☑
      renal disease 642.2 ☑
    hypertensive heart and chronic
      kidney disease 642.2 ☑
    hyperthyroidism 648.1 ☑
    hypothyroidism 648.1 ☑
    hysteralgia 646.8 ☑
    icterus gravis 646.7 ☑
    incarceration, uterus 654.3 ☑
    incompetent cervix (os) 654.5 ☑
    infection 647.9 ☑
      amniotic fluid 658.4 ☑
      bladder 646.6 ☑
      genital organ (conditions classi-
        fiable to 614.0–614.5,
        614.7–614.9, 615)
        646.6 ☑
      kidney (conditions classifiable
        to 590.0–590.9) 646.6 ☑
      urinary (tract) 646.6 ☑
        asymptomatic 646.5 ☑
    infective and parasitic diseases
      NEC 647.8 ☑
    inflammation
      bladder 646.6 ☑
      genital organ (conditions classi-
        fiable to 614.0–614.5,
        614.7–614.9, 615)
        646.6 ☑
      urinary tract NEC 646.6 ☑
    insufficient weight gain 646.8 ☑
    intrauterine fetal death (near term)
      NEC 656.4 ☑
      early (before 22 completed
        weeks' gestation) 632
    malaria (conditions classifiable to
      084) 647.4 ☑
    malformation, uterus (congenital)
      654.0 ☑
    malnutrition (conditions classifi-
      able to 260–269) 648.9 ☑
    malposition
      fetus — *see* Pregnancy, compli-
        cated, malpresentation
      uterus or cervix 654.4 ☑
    malpresentation 652.9 ☑
      with successful version 652.1 ☑
      in multiple gestation 652.6 ☑
      specified type NEC 652.8 ☑
    marginal sinus hemorrhage or
      rupture 641.2 ☑
    maternal obesity syndrome
      646.1 ☑
    menstruation 640.8 ☑
    mental disorders (conditions classi-
      fiable to 290–303, 305.0,
      305.2-305.9, 306–316,
      317–319) 648.4 ☑
    mentum presentation 652.4 ☑
    missed
      abortion 632
      delivery (at or near term)
        656.4 ☑
      labor (at or near term) 656.4 ☑
    necrosis
      genital organ or tract (condi-
        tions classifiable to
        614.0–614.5,
        614.7–614.9, 615)
        646.6 ☑
      liver (conditions classifiable to
        570) 646.7 ☑

**Pregnancy** — *continued*
  complicated — *continued*
    necrosis — *continued*
      renal, cortical 646.2 ☑
    nephritis or nephrosis (conditions
      classifiable to 580–589)
      646.2 ☑
      with hypertension 642.1 ☑
    nephropathy NEC 646.2 ☑
    neuritis (peripheral) 646.4 ☑
    nutritional deficiency (conditions
      classifiable to 260–269)
      648.9 ☑
    obesity 649.1 ☑
      surgery status 649.2 ☑
    oblique lie or presentation 652.3 ☑
      with successful version 652.1 ☑
    obstetrical trauma NEC 665.9 ☑
    oligohydramnios NEC 658.0 ☑
    onset of contractions before 37
      weeks 644.0 ☑
    oversize fetus 653.5 ☑
    papyraceous fetus 646.0 ☑
    patent cervix 654.5 ☑
    pelvic inflammatory disease (condi-
      tions classifiable to
      614.0–614.5, 614.7–614.9,
      615) 646.6 ☑
    pelvic peritoneal adhesion 648.9 ☑
    placenta, placental
      abnormality 656.7 ☑
      abruptio or ablatio 641.2 ☑
      detachment 641.2 ☑
      disease 656.7 ☑
      infarct 656.7 ☑
      low implantation 641.1 ☑
        without hemorrhage 641.0 ☑
      malformation 656.7 ☑
      malposition 641.1 ☑
        without hemorrhage 641.0 ☑
      marginal sinus hemorrhage
        641.2 ☑
      previa 641.1 ☑
        without hemorrhage 641.0 ☑
      separation (premature) (undeliv-
        ered) 641.2 ☑
    placentitis 658.4 ☑
    polyhydramnios 657.0 ☑
    postmaturity
      post-term 645.1 ☑
      prolonged 645.2 ☑
    prediabetes 648.8 ☑
    pre-eclampsia (mild) 642.4 ☑
      severe 642.5 ☑
      superimposed on pre-existing
        hypertensive disease
        642.7 ☑
    premature rupture of membranes
      658.1 ☑
      with delayed delivery 658.2 ☑
    previous
      infertility V23.0
      nonobstetric condition V23.89
      poor obstetrical history V23.49
      premature delivery V23.41
      trophoblastic disease (condi-
        tions classifiable to 630)
        V23.1
    prolapse, uterus 654.4 ☑
    proteinuria (gestational) 646.2 ☑
      with hypertension — *see* Tox-
        emia, of pregnancy
    pruritus (neurogenic) 646.8 ☑
    psychosis or psychoneurosis
      648.4 ☑
    ptyalism 646.8 ☑
    pyelitis (conditions classifiable to
      590.0–590.9) 646.6 ☑
    renal disease or failure NEC
      646.2 ☑
      with secondary hypertension
        642.1 ☑
      hypertensive 642.2 ☑
    retention, retained dead ovum 631
    retroversion, uterus 654.3 ☑

**Pregnancy** — *continued*
  complicated — *continued*
    Rh immunization, incompatibility,
      or sensitization 656.1 ☑
    rubella (conditions classifiable to
      056) 647.5 ☑
    rupture
      amnion (premature) 658.1 ☑
        with delayed delivery
          658.2 ☑
      marginal sinus (hemorrhage)
        641.2 ☑
      membranes (premature)
        658.1 ☑
        with delayed delivery
          658.2 ☑
      uterus (before onset of labor)
        665.0 ☑
    salivation (excessive) 646.8 ☑
    salpingo–oophoritis (conditions
      classifiable to 614.0–614.2)
      646.6 ☑
    septicemia (conditions classifiable
      to 038.0–038.9) 647.8 ☑
      postpartum 670.0 ☑
      puerperal 670.0 ☑
    smoking 649.0 ☑
    spasms, uterus (abnormal)
      646.8 ☑
    specified condition NEC 646.8 ☑
    spotting 649.5 ☑
    spurious labor pains 644.1 ☑
    status post
      bariatric surgery 649.2 ☑
      gastric banding 649.2 ☑
      gastric bypass for obesity
        649.2 ☑
      obesity surgery 649.2 ☑
    superfecundation 651.9 ☑
    superfetation 651.9 ☑
    syphilis (conditions classifiable to
      090–097) 647.0 ☑
    threatened
      abortion 640.0 ☑
      premature delivery 644.2 ☑
      premature labor 644.0 ☑
    thrombophlebitis (superficial)
      671.2 ☑
      deep 671.3 ☑
    thrombosis 671.9 ☑
      venous (superficial) 671.2 ☑
        deep 671.3 ☑
    thyroid dysfunction (conditions
      classifiable to 240–246)
      648.1 ☑
    thyroiditis 648.1 ☑
    thyrotoxicosis 648.1 ☑
    tobacco use disorder 649.0 ☑
    torsion of uterus 654.4 ☑
    toxemia — *see* Toxemia, of pregnan-
      cy
    transverse lie or presentation
      652.3 ☑
      with successful version 652.1 ☑
    trauma 648.9 ☑
      obstetrical 665.9 ☑
    tuberculosis (conditions classifiable
      to 010–018) 647.3 ☑
    tumor
      cervix 654.6 ☑
      ovary 654.4 ☑
      pelvic organs or tissue NEC
        654.4 ☑
      uterus (body) 654.1 ☑
        cervix 654.6 ☑
      vagina 654.7 ☑
      vulva 654.8 ☑
    unstable lie 652.0 ☑
    uremia — *see* Pregnancy, compli-
      cated, renal disease
    urethritis 646.6 ☑
    vaginitis or vulvitis (conditions
      classifiable to 616.1) 646.6 ☑
    varicose
      placental vessels 656.7 ☑

**Pregnancy** — *continued*
  complicated — *continued*
    varicose — *continued*
      veins (legs) 671.0 ☑
        perineum 671.1 ☑
        vulva 671.1 ☑
      varicosity, labia or vulva 671.1 ☑
    venereal disease NEC (conditions
      classifiable to 099) 647.2 ☑
    viral disease NEC (conditions clas-
      sifiable to 042, 050–055,
      057–079) 647.6 ☑
    vomiting (incoercible) (pernicious)
      (persistent) (uncontrollable)
      (vicious) 643.9 ☑
      due to organic disease or other
        cause 643.8 ☑
      early — *see* Hyperemesis, gravi-
        darum
      late (after 22 completed weeks
        gestation) 643.2 ☑
    young maternal age 659.8 ☑
  complications NEC 646.9 ☑
  cornual 633.80
    with intrauterine pregnancy 633.81
    affecting fetus or newborn 761.4
  death, maternal NEC 646.9 ☑
  delivered — *see* Delivery
  ectopic (ruptured) NEC 633.90
    with intrauterine pregnancy 633.91
    abdominal — *see* Pregnancy, ab-
      dominal
    affecting fetus or newborn 761.4
    combined (extrauterine and in-
      trauterine) — *see* Pregnancy,
      cornual
    ovarian — *see* Pregnancy, ovarian
    specified type NEC 633.80
      with intrauterine pregnancy
        633.81
      affecting fetus or newborn 761.4
    tubal — *see* Pregnancy, tubal
  examination, pregnancy
    negative result V72.41
    not confirmed V72.40
    positive result V72.42
  extrauterine — *see* Pregnancy, ectopic
  fallopian — *see* Pregnancy, tubal
  false 300.11
    labor (pains) 644.1 ☑
  fatigue 646.8 ☑
  illegitimate V61.6
  incidental finding V22.2
  in double uterus 654.0 ☑
  interstitial — *see* Pregnancy, cornual
  intraligamentous — *see* Pregnancy,
    cornual
  intramural — *see* Pregnancy, cornual
  intraperitoneal — *see* Pregnancy, ab-
    dominal
  isthmian — *see* Pregnancy, tubal
  management affected by
    abnormal, abnormality
      fetus (suspected) 655.9 ☑
        specified NEC 655.8 ☑
      placenta 656.7 ☑
    advanced maternal age NEC
      659.6 ☑
      multigravida 659.6 ☑
      primigravida 659.5 ☑
    antibodies (maternal)
      anti-c 656.1 ☑
      anti-d 656.1 ☑
      anti-e 656.1 ☑
      blood group (ABO) 656.2 ☑
        Rh(esus) 656.1 ☑
    appendicitis 648.9 ☑
    bariatric surgery status 649.2 ☑
    coagulation defect 649.3 ☑
    elderly multigravida 659.6 ☑
    elderly primigravida 659.5 ☑
    epilepsy 649.4 ☑
    fetal (suspected)
      abnormality 655.9 ☑
        acid-base balance 656.8 ☑

**Pregnancy** — *continued*
management affected by — *continued*
  fetal — *continued*
    abnormality — *continued*
      heart rate or rhythm 659.7 ☑
      specified NEC 655.8 ☑
    acidemia 656.3 ☑
    anencephaly 655.0 ☑
    bradycardia 659.7 ☑
    central nervous system malfor-
      mation 655.0 ☑
    chromosomal abnormalities
      (conditions classifiable to
      758.0–758.9) 655.1 ☑
    damage from
      drugs 655.5 ☑
        obstetric, anesthetic, or
          sedative 655.5 ☑
      environmental toxins
        655.8 ☑
      intrauterine contraceptive
        device 655.8 ☑
    maternal
      alcohol addiction 655.4 ☑
      disease NEC 655.4 ☑
      drug use 655.5 ☑
      listeriosis 655.4 ☑
      rubella 655.3 ☑
      toxoplasmosis 655.4 ☑
      viral infection 655.3 ☑
    radiation 655.6 ☑
    death (near term) 656.4 ☑
      early (before 22 completed
        weeks' gestation) 632
    distress 656.8 ☑
    excessive growth 656.6 ☑
    fetal-maternal hemorrhage
      656.0 ☑
    growth retardation 656.5 ☑
    hereditary disease 655.2 ☑
    hereditary disease in family
      (possibly) affecting fetus
      655.2 ☑
    hydrocephalus 655.0 ☑
    incompatibility, blood groups
      (ABO) 656.2 ☑
    intrauterine death 656.4 ☑
    poor growth 656.5 ☑
    Rh(esus) 656.1 ☑
    spina bifida (with
      myelomeningocele)
      655.0 ☑
  gastric banding status 649.2 ☑
  gastric bypass status for obesity
    649.2 ☑
  insufficient prenatal care V23.7
  intrauterine death 656.4 ☑
  isoimmunization (ABO) 656.2 ☑
    Rh(esus) 656.1 ☑
  large-for-dates fetus 656.6 ☑
  light-for-dates fetus 656.5 ☑
  meconium in liquor 656.8 ☑
  mental disorder (conditions classi-
    fiable to 290–303, 305.0,
    305.2–305.9, 306–316,
    317–319) 648.4 ☑
  multiparity (grand) 659.4 ☑
  obesity 649.1 ☑
    surgery status 649.2 ☑
  poor obstetric history V23.49
    pre-term labor V23.41
  postmaturity
    post-term 645.1 ☑
    prolonged 645.2 ☑
  post-term pregnancy 645.1 ☑
  previous
    abortion V23.2
      habitual 646.3 ☑
    cesarean delivery 654.2 ☑
    difficult delivery V23.49
    forceps delivery V23.49
    habitual abortions 646.3 ☑
    hemorrhage, antepartum or
      postpartum V23.49

**Pregnancy** — *continued*
management affected by — *continued*
  previous — *continued*
    hydatidiform mole V23.1
    infertility V23.0
    malignancy NEC V23.89
    nonobstetrical conditions
      V23.8
    premature delivery V23.41
    trophoblastic disease (condi-
      tions in 630) V23.1
    vesicular mole V23.1
  prolonged pregnancy 645.2 ☑
  small-for-dates fetus 656.5 ☑
  smoking 649.0 ☑
  spotting 649.5 ☑
  tobacco use disorder 649.0 ☑
  young maternal age 659.8 ☑
maternal death NEC 646.9 ☑
mesometric (mural) — *see* Pregnancy,
  cornual
molar 631
  hydatidiform (*see also* Hydatidiform
    mole) 630
    previous, affecting management
      of pregnancy V23.1
  previous, affecting management of
    pregnancy V23.49
multiple NEC 651.9 ☑
  with fetal loss and retention of one
    or more fetus(es) 651.6 ☑
  affecting fetus or newborn 761.5
  following (elective) fetal reduction
    651.7 ☑
  specified type NEC 651.8 ☑
    with fetal loss and retention of
      one or more fetus(es)
      651.6 ☑
    following (elective) fetal reduc-
      tion 651.7 ☑
mural — *see* Pregnancy, cornual
observation NEC V22.1
  first pregnancy V22.0
  high-risk V23.9
    specified problem NEC V23.89
ovarian 633.20
  with intrauterine pregnancy 633.21
  affecting fetus or newborn 761.4
possible, not (yet) confirmed V72.40
postmature
  post-term 645.1 ☑
  prolonged 645.2 ☑
post-term 645.1 ☑
prenatal care only V22.1
  first pregnancy V22.0
  high-risk V23.9
    specified problem NEC V23.89
prolonged 645.2 ☑
quadruplet NEC 651.2 ☑
  with fetal loss and retention of one
    or more fetus(es) 651.5 ☑
  affecting fetus or newborn 761.5
  following (elective) fetal reduction
    651.7 ☑
quintuplet NEC 651.8 ☑
  with fetal loss and retention of one
    or more fetus(es) 651.6 ☑
  affecting fetus or newborn 761.5
  following (elective) fetal reduction
    651.7 ☑
sextuplet NEC 651.8 ☑
  with fetal loss and retention of one
    or more fetus(es) 651.6 ☑
  affecting fetus or newborn 761.5
  following (elective) fetal reduction
    651.7 ☑
spurious 300.11
superfecundation NEC 651.9 ☑
  with fetal loss and retention of one
    or more fetus(es) 651.6 ☑
  following (elective) fetal reduction
    651.7 ☑
superfetation NEC 651.9 ☑

**Pregnancy** — *continued*
superfetation — *continued*
  with fetal loss and retention of one
    or more fetus(es) 651.6 ☑
  following (elective) fetal reduction
    651.7 ☑
supervision (of) (for) (*see also* Pregnancy, management affected by)
  elderly
    multigravida V23.82
    primigravida V23.81
  high-risk V23.9
    insufficient prenatal care V23.7
    specified problem NEC V23.89
  multiparity V23.3
  normal NEC V22.1
    first V22.0
  poor
    obstetric history V23.49
      pre-term labor V23.41
    reproductive history V23.5
  previous
    abortion V23.2
    hydatidiform mole V23.1
    infertility V23.0
    neonatal death V23.5
    stillbirth V23.5
    trophoblastic disease V23.1
    vesicular mole V23.1
  specified problem NEC V23.89
  young
    multigravida V23.84
    primigravida V23.83
triplet NEC 651.1 ☑
  with fetal loss and retention of one
    or more fetus(es) 651.4 ☑
  affecting fetus or newborn 761.5
  following (elective) fetal reduction
    651.7 ☑
tubal (with rupture) 633.10
  with intrauterine pregnancy 633.11
  affecting fetus or newborn 761.4
twin NEC 651.0 ☑
  with fetal loss and retention of one
    fetus 651.3 ☑
  affecting fetus or newborn 761.5
  following (elective) fetal reduction
    651.7 ☑
unconfirmed V72.40
undelivered (no other diagnosis) V22.2
  with false labor 644.1 ☑
  high-risk V23.9
    specified problem NEC V23.89
unwanted NEC V61.7
**Pregnant uterus** — *see* condition
**Preiser's disease** (osteoporosis) 733.09
**Prekwashiorkor** 260
**Preleukemia** 238.75
**Preluxation of hip, congenital** — *see
  also* Subluxation, congenital, hip
  754.32
**Premature** — *see also* condition
beats (nodal) 427.60
  atrial 427.61
  auricular 427.61
  postoperative 997.1
  specified type NEC 427.69
  supraventricular 427.61
  ventricular 427.69
birth NEC 765.1 ☑
closure
  cranial suture 756.0
  fontanel 756.0
  foramen ovale 745.8
contractions 427.60
  atrial 427.61
  auricular 427.61
  auriculoventricular 427.61
  heart (extrasystole) 427.60
  junctional 427.60
  nodal 427.60
  postoperative 997.1
  ventricular 427.69
ejaculation 302.75
infant NEC 765.1 ☑
  excessive 765.0 ☑

**Premature** — *see also* condition —
  *continued*
infant — *continued*
  light-for-dates — *see* Light-for-
    dates
labor 644.2 ☑
  threatened 644.0 ☑
lungs 770.4
menopause 256.31
puberty 259.1
rupture of membranes or amnion
  658.1 ☑
  affecting fetus or newborn 761.1
  delayed delivery following 658.2 ☑
senility (syndrome) 259.8
separation, placenta (partial) — *see*
  Placenta, separation
ventricular systole 427.69
**Prematurity** NEC 765.1 ☑
extreme 765.0 ☑
**Premenstrual syndrome** 625.4
**Premenstrual tension** 625.4
**Premolarization, cuspids** 520.2
**Premyeloma** 273.1
**Prenatal**
care, normal pregnancy V22.1
  first V22.0
death, cause unknown — *see* Death,
  fetus
screening — *see* Antenatal, screening
teeth 520.6
**Prepartum** — *see* condition
**Preponderance, left or right ventricu-
lar** 429.3
**Prepuce** — *see* condition
**PRES** (posterior reversible encephalopathy syndrome) 348.39
**Presbycardia** 797
hypertensive (*see also* Hypertension,
  heart) 402.90
**Presbycusis** 388.01
**Presbyesophagus** 530.89
**Presbyophrenia** 310.1
**Presbyopia** 367.4
**Prescription of contraceptives** NEC
  V25.02
diaphragm V25.02
oral (pill) V25.01
  emergency V25.03
  postcoital V25.03
  repeat V25.41
repeat V25.40
  oral (pill) V25.41
**Presenile** — *see also* condition
aging 259.8
dementia (*see also* Dementia, presenile) 290.10
**Presenility** 259.8
**Presentation, fetal**
abnormal 652.9 ☑
  with successful version 652.1 ☑
  before labor, affecting fetus or
    newborn 761.7
  causing obstructed labor 660.0 ☑
    affecting fetus or newborn, any,
      except breech 763.1
  in multiple gestation (one or more)
    652.6 ☑
  specified NEC 652.8 ☑
arm 652.7 ☑
  causing obstructed labor 660.0 ☑
breech (buttocks) (complete) (frank)
  652.2 ☑
  with successful version 652.1 ☑
  before labor, affecting fetus or
    newborn 761.7
  before labor, affecting fetus or
    newborn 761.7
brow 652.4 ☑
  causing obstructed labor 660.0 ☑
buttocks 652.2 ☑
chin 652.4 ☑
complete 652.2 ☑
compound 652.8 ☑
cord 663.0 ☑
extended head 652.4 ☑

**Presentation, fetal** — *continued*
　face 652.4 ☑
　　to pubes 652.8 ☑
　footling 652.8 ☑
　frank 652.2 ☑
　hand, leg, or foot NEC 652.8 ☑
　incomplete 652.8 ☑
　mentum 652.4 ☑
　multiple gestation (one fetus or more) 652.6 ☑
　oblique 652.3 ☑
　　with successful version 652.1 ☑
　shoulder 652.8 ☑
　　affecting fetus or newborn 763.1
　transverse 652.3 ☑
　　with successful version 652.1 ☑
　umbilical cord 663.0 ☑
　unstable 652.0 ☑
**Prespondylolisthesis** (congenital) (lumbosacral) 756.11
**Pressure**
　area, skin ulcer (*see also* Decubitus) 707.00
　atrophy, spine 733.99
　birth, fetus or newborn NEC 767.9
　brachial plexus 353.0
　brain 348.4
　　injury at birth 767.0
　cerebral — *see* Pressure, brain
　chest 786.59
　cone, tentorial 348.4
　　injury at birth 767.0
　funis — *see* Compression, umbilical cord
　hyposystolic (*see also* Hypotension) 458.9
　increased
　　intracranial 781.99
　　　due to
　　　　benign intracranial hypertension 348.2
　　　　hydrocephalus — *see* hydrocephalus
　　　　injury at birth 767.8
　　intraocular 365.00
　lumbosacral plexus 353.1
　mediastinum 519.3
　necrosis (chronic) (skin) (*see also* Decubitus) 707.00
　nerve — *see* Compression, nerve
　paralysis (*see also* Neuropathy, entrapment) 355.9
　sore (chronic) (*see also* Decubitus) 707.00
　spinal cord 336.9
　ulcer (chronic) (*see also* Decubitus) 707.00
　umbilical cord — *see* Compression, umbilical cord
　venous, increased 459.89
**Pre-syncope** 780.2
**Preterm infant NEC** 765.1 ☑
　extreme 765.0 ☑
**Priapism** (penis) 607.3
**Prickling sensation** — *see* Disturbance, sensation 782.0
**Prickly heat** 705.1
**Primary** — *see* condition
**Primigravida, elderly**
　affecting
　　fetus or newborn 763.89
　　management of pregnancy, labor, and delivery 659.5 ☑
**Primipara, old**
　affecting
　　fetus or newborn 763.89
　　management of pregnancy, labor, and delivery 659.5 ☑
**Primula dermatitis** 692.6
**Primus varus** (bilateral) (metatarsus) 754.52
**PRIND** ▶(prolonged reversible ischemic neurologic deficit)◀ 434.91 ▲
　history of (personal) V12.54 ●
**Pringle's disease** (tuberous sclerosis) 759.5

**Prinzmetal's angina** 413.1
**Prinzmetal-Massumi syndrome** (anterior chest wall) 786.52
**Prizefighter ear** 738.7
**Problem** (with) V49.9
　academic V62.3
　acculturation V62.4
　adopted child V61.29
　aged
　　in-law V61.3
　　parent V61.3
　　person NEC V61.8
　alcoholism in family V61.41
　anger reaction (*see also* Disturbance, conduct) 312.0 ☑
　behavioral V40.9
　　specified NEC V40.3
　behavior, child 312.9
　betting V69.3
　cardiorespiratory NEC V47.2
　career choice V62.2
　care of sick or handicapped person in family or household V61.49
　communication V40.1
　conscience regarding medical care V62.6
　delinquency (juvenile) 312.9
　diet, inappropriate V69.1
　digestive NEC V47.3
　ear NEC V41.3
　eating habits, inappropriate V69.1
　economic V60.2
　　affecting care V60.9
　　　specified type NEC V60.8
　educational V62.3
　enuresis, child 307.6
　exercise, lack of V69.0
　eye NEC V41.1
　family V61.9
　　specified circumstance NEC V61.8
　fear reaction, child 313.0
　feeding (elderly) (infant) 783.3
　　newborn 779.3
　　nonorganic 307.59
　fetal, affecting management of pregnancy 656.9 ☑
　　specified type NEC 656.8 ☑
　financial V60.2
　foster child V61.29
　　specified NEC V41.8
　functional V41.9
　　specified type NEC V41.8
　gambling V69.3
　genital NEC V47.5
　head V48.9
　　deficiency V48.0
　　disfigurement V48.6
　　mechanical V48.2
　　motor V48.2
　　movement of V48.2
　　sensory V48.4
　　specified condition NEC V48.8
　hearing V41.2
　high-risk sexual behavior V69.2
　identity 313.82
　influencing health status NEC V49.89
　internal organ NEC V47.9
　　deficiency V47.0
　　mechanical or motor V47.1
　interpersonal NEC V62.81
　jealousy, child 313.3
　learning V40.0
　legal V62.5
　life circumstance NEC V62.89
　lifestyle V69.9
　　specified NEC V69.8
　limb V49.9
　　deficiency V49.0
　　disfigurement V49.4
　　mechanical V49.1
　　motor V49.2
　　movement, involving
　　　musculoskeletal system V49.1
　　　nervous system V49.2
　　sensory V49.3
　　specified condition NEC V49.5

**Problem** — *continued*
　litigation V62.5
　living alone V60.3
　loneliness NEC V62.89
　marital V61.10
　　involving
　　　divorce V61.0
　　　estrangement V61.0
　　　psychosexual disorder 302.9
　　　sexual function V41.7
　　　relationship V61.10
　mastication V41.6
　medical care, within family V61.49
　mental V40.9
　　specified NEC V40.2
　mental hygiene, adult V40.9
　multiparity V61.5
　nail biting, child 307.9
　neck V48.9
　　deficiency V48.1
　　disfigurement V48.7
　　mechanical V48.3
　　motor V48.3
　　movement V48.3
　　sensory V48.5
　　specified condition NEC V48.8
　neurological NEC 781.99
　none (feared complaint unfounded) V65.5
　occupational V62.2
　parent-child V61.20
　　relationship V61.20
　partner V61.10
　　relationship V61.10
　personal NEC V62.89
　　interpersonal conflict NEC V62.81
　personality (*see also* Disorder, personality) 301.9
　phase of life V62.89
　placenta, affecting management of pregnancy 656.9 ☑
　　specified type NEC 656.8 ☑
　poverty V60.2
　presence of sick or handicapped person in family or household V61.49
　psychiatric 300.9
　psychosocial V62.9
　　specified type NEC V62.89
　relational NEC V62.81
　relationship, childhood 313.3
　religious or spiritual belief
　　other than medical care V62.89
　　regarding medical care V62.6
　self-damaging behavior V69.8
　sexual
　　behavior, high-risk V69.2
　　function NEC V41.7
　sibling
　　relational V61.8
　　relationship V61.8
　sight V41.0
　sleep disorder, child 307.40
　sleep, lack of V69.4
　smell V41.5
　speech V40.1
　spite reaction, child (*see also* Disturbance, conduct) 312.0 ☑
　spoiled child reaction (*see also* Disturbance, conduct) 312.1 ☑
　swallowing V41.6
　tantrum, child (*see also* Disturbance, conduct) 312.1 ☑
　taste V41.5
　thumb sucking, child 307.9
　tic (child) 307.21
　trunk V48.9
　　deficiency V48.1
　　disfigurement V48.7
　　mechanical V48.3
　　motor V48.3
　　movement V48.3
　　sensory V48.5
　　specified condition NEC V48.8
　unemployment V62.0
　urinary NEC V47.4

**Problem** — *continued*
　voice production V41.4
**Procedure** (surgical) **not done** NEC V64.3
　because of
　　contraindication V64.1
　　patient's decision V64.2
　　　for reasons of conscience or religion V62.6
　　specified reason NEC V64.3
**Procidentia**
　anus (sphincter) 569.1
　rectum (sphincter) 569.1
　stomach 537.89
　uteri 618.1
**Proctalgia** 569.42
　fugax 564.6
　spasmodic 564.6
　psychogenic 307.89
**Proctitis** 569.49
　amebic 006.8
　chlamydial 099.52
　gonococcal 098.7
　granulomatous 555.1
　idiopathic 556.2
　　with ulcerative sigmoiditis 556.3
　tuberculous (*see also* Tuberculosis) 014.8 ☑
　ulcerative (chronic) (nonspecific) 556.2
　　with ulcerative sigmoiditis 556.3
**Proctocele**
　female (without uterine prolapse) 618.04
　　with uterine prolapse 618.4
　　　complete 618.3
　　　incomplete 618.2
　male 569.49
**Proctocolitis, idiopathic** 556.2
　with ulcerative sigmoiditis 556.3
**Proctoptosis** 569.1
**Proctosigmoiditis** 569.89
　ulcerative (chronic) 556.3
**Proctospasm** 564.6
　psychogenic 306.4
**Prodromal-AIDS** — *see* Human immunodeficiency virus (disease) (illness) (infection)
**Profichet's disease or syndrome** 729.9
**Progeria** (adultorum) (syndrome) 259.8
**Prognathism** (mandibular) (maxillary) 524.00
**Progonoma** (melanotic) (M9363/0) — *see* Neoplasm, by site, benign
**Progressive** — *see* condition
**Prolapse, prolapsed**
　anus, anal (canal) (sphincter) 569.1
　arm or hand, complicating delivery 652.7 ☑
　　causing obstructed labor 660.0 ☑
　　　affecting fetus or newborn 763.1
　　fetus or newborn 763.1
　bladder (acquired) (mucosa) (sphincter)
　　congenital (female) (male) 756.71
　　female (*see also* Cystocele, female) 618.01
　　male 596.8
　breast implant (prosthetic) 996.54
　cecostomy 569.69
　cecum 569.89
　cervix, cervical (hypertrophied) 618.1
　　anterior lip, obstructing labor 660.2 ☑
　　　affecting fetus or newborn 763.1
　　congenital 752.49
　　postpartal (old) 618.1
　　stump 618.84
　ciliary body 871.1
　colon (pedunculated) 569.89
　colostomy 569.69
　conjunctiva 372.73
　cord — *see* Prolapse, umbilical cord
　disc (intervertebral) — *see* Displacement, intervertebral disc
　duodenum 537.89
　eye implant (orbital) 996.59

**Prolapse, prolapsed** — *continued*
eye implant — *continued*
lens (ocular) 996.53
fallopian tube 620.4
fetal extremity, complicating delivery 652.8 ☑
causing obstructed labor 660.0 ☑
fetus or newborn 763.1
funis — *see* Prolapse, umbilical cord
gastric (mucosa) 537.89
genital, female 618.9
specified NEC 618.89
globe 360.81
ileostomy bud 569.69
intervertebral disc — *see* Displacement, intervertebral disc
intestine (small) 569.89
iris 364.89 ▲
traumatic 871.1
kidney (*see also* Disease, renal) 593.0
congenital 753.3
laryngeal muscles or ventricle 478.79
leg, complicating delivery 652.8 ☑
causing obstructed labor 660.0 ☑
fetus or newborn 763.1
liver 573.8
meatus urinarius 599.5
mitral valve 424.0
ocular lens implant 996.53
organ or site, congenital NEC — *see* Malposition, congenital
ovary 620.4
pelvic (floor), female 618.89
perineum, female 618.89
pregnant uterus 654.4 ☑
rectum (mucosa) (sphincter) 569.1
due to Trichuris trichiuria 127.3
spleen 289.59
stomach 537.89
umbilical cord
affecting fetus or newborn 762.4
complicating delivery 663.0 ☑
ureter 593.89
with obstruction 593.4
ureterovesical orifice 593.89
urethra (acquired) (infected) (mucosa) 599.5
congenital 753.8
uterovaginal 618.4
complete 618.3
incomplete 618.2
specified NEC 618.89
uterus (first degree) (second degree) (third degree) (complete) (without vaginal wall prolapse) 618.1
with mention of vaginal wall prolapse — *see* Prolapse, uterovaginal
congenital 752.3
in pregnancy or childbirth 654.4 ☑
affecting fetus or newborn 763.1
causing obstructed labor 660.2 ☑
affecting fetus or newborn 763.1
postpartal (old) 618.1
uveal 871.1
vagina (anterior) (posterior) (vault) (wall) (without uterine prolapse) 618.00
with uterine prolapse 618.4
complete 618.3
incomplete 618.2
paravaginal 618.02
posthysterectomy 618.5
specified NEC 618.09
vitreous (humor) 379.26
traumatic 871.1
womb — *see* Prolapse, uterus
**Prolapsus, female** 618.9
**Proliferative** — *see* condition
**Prolinemia** 270.8
**Prolinuria** 270.8
**Prolonged, prolongation**
bleeding time (*see also* Defect, coagulation) 790.92

**Prolonged, prolongation** — *continued*
bleeding time (*see also* Defect, coagulation) — *continued*
"idiopathic" (in von Willebrand's disease) 286.4
coagulation time (*see also* Defect, coagulation) 790.92
gestation syndrome 766.22
labor 662.1 ☑
affecting fetus or newborn 763.89
first stage 662.0 ☑
second stage 662.2 ☑
pregnancy 645.2 ☑
PR interval 426.11
prothrombin time (*see also* Defect, coagulation) 790.92
QT interval 794.31
syndrome 426.82
rupture of membranes (24 hours or more prior to onset of labor) 658.2 ☑
uterine contractions in labor 661.4 ☑
affecting fetus or newborn 763.7
**Prominauris** 744.29
**Prominence**
auricle (ear) (congenital) 744.29
acquired 380.32
ischial spine or sacral promontory
with disproportion (fetopelvic) 653.3 ☑
affecting fetus or newborn 763.1
causing obstructed labor 660.1 ☑
affecting fetus or newborn 763.1
nose (congenital) 748.1
acquired 738.0
**PROMM** (proximal myotonic myotonia) ●
359.21 ●
**Pronation**
ankle 736.79
foot 736.79
congenital 755.67
**Prophylactic**
administration of
antibiotics V07.39
antitoxin, any V07.2
antivenin V07.2
chemotherapeutic agent NEC V07.39
fluoride V07.31
diphtheria antitoxin V07.2
drug V07.39 ●
gamma globulin V07.2
immune sera (gamma globulin) V07.2
RhoGAM V07.2
tetanus antitoxin V07.2
chemotherapy NEC V07.39
fluoride V07.31
hormone replacement (postmenopausal) V07.4
immunotherapy V07.2
measure V07.9
specified type NEC V07.8
medication V07.39 ●
postmenopausal hormone replacement V07.4
sterilization V25.2
**Proptosis** (ocular) — *see also* Exophthalmos 376.30
thyroid 242.0 ☑
**Propulsion**
eyeball 360.81
**Prosecution, anxiety concerning** V62.5
**Prostate, prostatic** — *see* condition
**Prostatism** 600.90
with
other lower urinary tract symptoms (LUTS) 600.91
urinary
obstruction 600.91
retention 600.91
**Prostatitis** (congestive) (suppurative) 601.9

**Prostatitis** — *continued*
acute 601.0
cavitary 601.8
chlamydial 099.54
chronic 601.1
diverticular 601.8
due to Trichomonas (vaginalis) 131.03
fibrous 600.90
with
other lower urinary tract symptoms (LUTS) 600.91
urinary
obstruction 600.91
retention 600.91
gonococcal (acute) 098.12
chronic or duration of 2 months or over 098.32
granulomatous 601.8
hypertrophic 600.00
with
other lower urinary tract symptoms (LUTS) 600.01
urinary
obstruction 600.01
retention 600.01
specified type NEC 601.8
subacute 601.1
trichomonal 131.03
tuberculous (*see also* Tuberculosis) 016.5 ☑ *[601.4]*
**Prostatocystitis** 601.3
**Prostatorrhea** 602.8
**Prostatoseminovesiculitis, trichomonal** 131.03
**Prostration** 780.79
heat 992.5
anhydrotic 992.3
due to
salt (and water) depletion 992.4
water depletion 992.3
nervous 300.5
newborn 779.89
senile 797
**Protanomaly** 368.51
**Protanopia** (anomalous trichromat) (complete) (incomplete) 368.51
**Protection** (against) (from) — *see* Pro- ●
phylactic ●
**Protein**
deficiency 260
malnutrition 260
sickness (prophylactic) (therapeutic) 999.5
**Proteinemia** 790.99
**Proteinosis**
alveolar, lung or pulmonary 516.0
lipid 272.8
lipoid (of Urbach) 272.8
**Proteinuria** — *see also* Albuminuria 791.0
Bence-Jones NEC 791.0
gestational 646.2 ☑
with hypertension — *see* Toxemia, of pregnancy
orthostatic 593.6
postural 593.6
**Proteolysis, pathologic** 286.6
**Protocoproporphyria** 277.1
**Protoporphyria** (erythrohepatic) (erythropoietic) 277.1
**Protrusio acetabuli** 718.65
**Protrusion**
acetabulum (into pelvis) 718.65
device, implant, or graft — *see* Complications, mechanical
ear, congenital 744.29
intervertebral disc — *see* Displacement, intervertebral disc
nucleus pulposus — *see* Displacement, intervertebral disc
**Proud flesh** 701.5
**Prune belly** (syndrome) 756.71
**Prurigo** (ferox) (gravis) (Hebra's) (hebrae) (mitis) (simplex) 698.2
agria 698.3
asthma syndrome 691.8

**Prurigo** — *continued*
Besnier's (atopic dermatitis) (infantile eczema) 691.8
eczematodes allergicum 691.8
estivalis (Hutchinson's) 692.72
Hutchinson's 692.72
nodularis 698.3
psychogenic 306.3
**Pruritus, pruritic** 698.9
ani 698.0
psychogenic 306.3
conditions NEC 698.9
psychogenic 306.3
due to Onchocerca volvulus 125.3
ear 698.9
essential 698.9
genital organ(s) 698.1
psychogenic 306.3
gravidarum 646.8 ☑
hiemalis 698.8
neurogenic (any site) 306.3
perianal 698.0
psychogenic (any site) 306.3
scrotum 698.1
psychogenic 306.3
senile, senilis 698.8
Trichomonas 131.9
vulva, vulvae 698.1
psychogenic 306.3
**Psammocarcinoma** (M8140/3) — *see* Neoplasm, by site, malignant
**Pseudarthrosis, pseudoarthrosis** (bone) 733.82
joint following fusion V45.4
**Pseudoacanthosis**
nigricans 701.8
**Pseudoaneurysm** — *see* Aneurysm
**Pseudoangina** (pectoris) — *see* Angina
**Pseudoangioma** 452
**Pseudo-Argyll-Robertson pupil** 379.45
**Pseudoarteriosus** 747.89
**Pseudoarthrosis** — *see* Pseudarthrosis
**Pseudoataxia** 799.89
**Pseudobulbar affect** (PBA) 310.8
**Pseudobursa** 727.89
**Pseudocholera** 025
**Pseudochromidrosis** 705.89
**Pseudocirrhosis, liver, pericardial** 423.2
**Pseudocoarctation** 747.21
**Pseudocowpox** 051.1
**Pseudocoxalgia** 732.1
**Pseudocroup** 478.75
**Pseudocyesis** 300.11
**Pseudocyst**
lung 518.89
pancreas 577.2
retina 361.19
**Pseudodementia** 300.16
**Pseudoelephantiasis neuroarthritica** 757.0
**Pseudoemphysema** 518.89
**Pseudoencephalitis**
superior (acute) hemorrhagic 265.1
**Pseudoerosion cervix, congenital** 752.49
**Pseudoexfoliation, lens capsule** 366.11
**Pseudofracture** (idiopathic) (multiple) (spontaneous) (symmetrical) 268.2
**Pseudoglanders** 025
**Pseudoglioma** 360.44
**Pseudogout** — *see* Chondrocalcinosis
**Pseudohallucination** 780.1
**Pseudohemianesthesia** 782.0
**Pseudohemophilia** (Bernuth's) (hereditary) (typeB) 286.4
type A 287.8
vascular 287.8
**Pseudohermaphroditism** 752.7
with chromosomal anomaly — *see* Anomaly, chromosomal
adrenal 255.2
female (without adrenocortical disorder) 752.7
with adrenocortical disorder 255.2
adrenal 255.2

☑ Additional Digit Required — Refer to the Tabular List for Digit Selection      ▽ Subterms under main terms may continue to next column or page

**2008 ICD-9-CM**      ▶◀ Revised Text      ● New Line      ▲ Revised Code      **October 2007 · Volume 2 — 241**

**Pseudohermaphroditism —** *continued*
  male (without gonadal disorder) 752.7
    with
      adrenocortical disorder 255.2
      cleft scrotum 752.7
      feminizing testis 259.5
      gonadal disorder 257.9
    adrenal 255.2
**Pseudohole, macula** 362.54
**Pseudo-Hurler's disease** (mucolipidosis III) 272.7
**Pseudohydrocephalus** 348.2
**Pseudohypertrophic muscular dystrophy** (Erb's) 359.1
**Pseudohypertrophy, muscle** 359.1
**Pseudohypoparathyroidism** 275.49
**Pseudoinfluenza** 487.1
**Pseudoinsomnia** 307.49
**Pseudoleukemia** 288.8
  infantile 285.8
**Pseudomembranous** — *see* condition
**Pseudomeningocele** (cerebral) (infective) 349.2
  postprocedural 997.01
  spinal 349.2
**Pseudomenstruation** 626.8
**Pseudomucinous**
  cyst (ovary) (M8470/0) 220
  peritoneum 568.89
**Pseudomyeloma** 273.1
**Pseudomyxoma peritonei** (M8480/6) 197.6
**Pseudoneuritis optic** (nerve) 377.24
  papilla 377.24
    congenital 743.57
**Pseudoneuroma** — *see* Injury, nerve, by site
**Pseudo-obstruction**
  intestine (chronic) (idiopathic) (intermittent secondary) (primary) 564.89
    acute 560.89
**Pseudopapilledema** 377.24
**Pseudoparalysis**
  arm or leg 781.4
  atonic, congenital 358.8
**Pseudopelade** 704.09
**Pseudophakia** V43.1
**Pseudopolycythemia** 289.0
**Pseudopolyposis, colon** 556.4
**Pseudoporencephaly** 348.0
**Pseudopseudohypoparathyroidism** 275.49
**Pseudopsychosis** 300.16
**Pseudopterygium** 372.52
**Pseudoptosis** (eyelid) 374.34
**Pseudorabies** 078.89
**Pseudoretinitis, pigmentosa** 362.65
**Pseudorickets** 588.0
  senile (Pozzi's) 731.0
**Pseudorubella** 057.8
**Pseudoscarlatina** 057.8
**Pseudoscarlatina** 778.1
**Pseudosclerema** 778.1
**Pseudosclerosis** (brain)
  Jakob's 046.1
  of Westphal (-Strümpell) (hepatolenticular degeneration) 275.1
  spastic 046.1
    with dementia
      with behavioral disturbance 046.1 *[294.11]*
      without behavioral disturbance 046.1 *[294.10]*
**Pseudoseizure** 780.39
  non-psychiatric 780.39
  psychiatric 300.11
**Pseudotabes** 799.89
  diabetic 250.6 ☑ *[337.1]*
**Pseudotetanus** — *see also* Convulsions 780.39
**Pseudotetany** 781.7
  hysterical 300.11
**Pseudothalassemia** 285.0
**Pseudotrichinosis** 710.3
**Pseudotruncus arteriosus** 747.29

**Pseudotuberculosis, pasteurella** (infection) 027.2
**Pseudotumor**
  cerebri 348.2
  orbit (inflammatory) 376.11
**Pseudo-Turner's syndrome** 759.89
**Pseudoxanthoma elasticum** 757.39
**Psilosis** (sprue) (tropical) 579.1
  Monilia 112.89
  nontropical 579.0
  not sprue 704.00
**Psittacosis** 073.9
**Psoitis** 728.89
**Psora** NEC 696.1
**Psoriasis** 696.1
  any type, except arthropathic 696.1
  arthritic, arthropathic 696.0
  buccal 528.6
  flexural 696.1
  follicularis 696.1
  guttate 696.1
  inverse 696.1
  mouth 528.6
  nummularis 696.1
  psychogenic 316 *[696.1]*
  punctata 696.1
  pustular 696.1
  rupioides 696.1
  vulgaris 696.1
**Psorospermiasis** 136.4
**Psorospermosis** 136.4
  follicularis (vegetans) 757.39
**Psychalgia** 307.80
**Psychasthenia** 300.89
  compulsive 300.3
  mixed compulsive states 300.3
  obsession 300.3
**Psychiatric disorder or problem** NEC 300.9
**Psychogenic** — *see also* condition
  factors associated with physical conditions 316
**Psychoneurosis, psychoneurotic** — *see also* Neurosis 300.9
  anxiety (state) 300.00
  climacteric 627.2
  compensation 300.16
  compulsion 300.3
  conversion hysteria 300.11
  depersonalization 300.6
  depressive type 300.4
  dissociative hysteria 300.15
  hypochondriacal 300.7
  hysteria 300.10
    conversion type 300.11
    dissociative type 300.15
  mixed NEC 300.89
  neurasthenic 300.5
  obsessional 300.3
  obsessive-compulsive 300.3
  occupational 300.89
  personality NEC 301.89
  phobia 300.20
  senile NEC 300.89
**Psychopathic** — *see also* condition
  constitution, posttraumatic 310.2
    with psychosis 293.9
  personality 301.9
    amoral trends 301.7
    antisocial trends 301.7
    asocial trends 301.7
    mixed types 301.7
  state 301.9
**Psychopathy, sexual** — *see also* Deviation, sexual 302.9
**Psychophysiologic, psychophysiological condition** — *see* Reaction, psychophysiologic
**Psychose passionelle** 297.8
**Psychosexual identity disorder** 302.6
  adult-life 302.85
  childhood 302.6
**Psychosis** 298.9
  acute hysterical 298.1

**Psychosis** — *continued*
  affecting management of pregnancy, childbirth, or puerperium 648.4 ☑
  affective (*see also* Disorder, mood) 296.90

> *Note* — Use the following fifth-digit subclassification with categories 296.0–296.6:
>
> 0   unspecified
>
> 1   mild
>
> 2   moderate
>
> 3   severe, without mention of psychotic behavior
>
> 4   severe, specified as with psychotic behavior
>
> 5   in partial or unspecified remission
>
> 6   in full remission

    drug-induced 292.84
    due to or associated with physical condition 293.83
    involutional 293.83
      recurrent episode 296.3 ☑
      single episode 296.2 ☑
    manic-depressive 296.80
      circular (alternating) 296.7
        currently depressed 296.5 ☑
        currently manic 296.4 ☑
      depressed type 296.2 ☑
        atypical 296.82
        recurrent episode 296.3 ☑
        single episode 296.2 ☑
      manic 296.0 ☑
        atypical 296.81
        recurrent episode 296.1 ☑
        single episode 296.0 ☑
      mixed type NEC 296.89
      specified type NEC 296.89
    senile 290.21
    specified type NEC 296.99
  alcoholic 291.9
    with
      anxiety 291.89
      delirium tremens 291.0
      delusions 291.5
      dementia 291.2
      hallucinosis 291.3
      jealousy 291.5
      mood disturbance 291.89
      paranoia 291.5
      persisting amnesia 291.1
      sexual dysfunction 291.89
      sleep disturbance 291.89
    amnestic confabulatory 291.1
    delirium tremens 291.0
    hallucinosis 291.3
    Korsakoff's, Korsakov's, Korsakow's 291.1
    paranoid type 291.5
    pathological intoxication 291.4
    polyneuritic 291.1
    specified type NEC 291.89
  alternating (*see also* Psychosis, manic-depressive, circular) 296.7
  anergastic (*see also* Psychosis, organic) 294.9
  arteriosclerotic 290.40
    with
      acute confusional state 290.41
      delirium 290.41
      delusions 290.42
      depressed mood 290.43
    depressed type 290.43
    paranoid type 290.42
    simple type 290.40
    uncomplicated 290.40
  atypical 298.9
    depressive 296.82
    manic 296.81
  borderline (schizophrenia) (*see also* Schizophrenia) 295.5 ☑

**Psychosis** — *continued*
  borderline (*see also* Schizophrenia) — *continued*
    of childhood (*see also* Psychosis, childhood) 299.8 ☑
    prepubertal 299.8 ☑
  brief reactive 298.8
  childhood, with origin specific to 299.9 ☑

> *Note* — Use the following fifth-digit subclassification with category 299:
>
> 0   current or active state
>
> 1   residual state

  atypical 299.8 ☑
    specified type NEC 299.8 ☑
  circular (*see also* Psychosis, manic-depressive, circular) 296.7
  climacteric (*see also* Psychosis, involutional) 298.8
  confusional 298.9
    acute 293.0
    reactive 298.2
    subacute 293.1
  depressive (*see also* Psychosis, affective) 296.2 ☑
    atypical 296.82
    involutional 296.2 ☑
      with hypomania (bipolar II) 296.89
      recurrent episode 296.3 ☑
      single episode 296.2 ☑
    psychogenic 298.0
    reactive (emotional stress) (psychological trauma) 298.0
    recurrent episode 296.3 ☑
      with hypomania (bipolar II) 296.89
    single episode 296.2 ☑
  disintegrative, childhood (*see also* Psychosis, childhood) 299.1 ☑
  drug 292.9
    with
      affective syndrome 292.84
      amnestic syndrome 292.83
      anxiety 292.89
      delirium 292.81
        withdrawal 292.0
      delusions 292.11
      dementia 292.82
      depressive state 292.84
      hallucinations 292.12
      hallucinosis 292.12
      mood disorder 292.84
      mood disturbance 292.84
      organic personality syndrome NEC 292.89
      sexual dysfunction 292.89
      sleep disturbance 292.89
      withdrawal syndrome (and delirium) 292.0
    affective syndrome 292.84
    delusions 292.11
    hallucinatory state 292.12
    hallucinosis 292.12
    paranoid state 292.11
    specified type NEC 292.89
    withdrawal syndrome (and delirium) 292.0
  due to or associated with physical condition (*see also* Psychosis, organic) 293.9
  epileptic NEC 294.8
  excitation (psychogenic) (reactive) 298.1
  exhaustive (*see also* Reaction, stress, acute) 308.9
  hypomanic (*see also* Psychosis, affective) 296.0 ☑
    recurrent episode 296.1 ☑
    single episode 296.0 ☑
  hysterical 298.8
    acute 298.1

**Psychosis** — *continued*
in
  conditions classified elsewhere
    with
      delusions 293.81
      hallucinations 293.82
  pregnancy, childbirth, or puerperi-
    um 648.4 ☑
incipient 298.8
  schizophrenic (*see also*
    Schizophrenia) 295.5 ☑
induced 297.3
infantile (*see also* Psychosis, childhood) 299.0 ☑
infective 293.9
  acute 293.0
  subacute 293.1
interactional (childhood) (*see also*
  Psychosis, childhood) 299.1 ☑
involutional 298.8
  depressive (*see also* Psychosis, af-
    fective) 296.2 ☑
    recurrent episode 296.3 ☑
    single episode 296.2 ☑
  melancholic 296.2 ☑
    recurrent episode 296.3 ☑
    single episode 296.2 ☑
  paranoid state 297.2
  paraphrenia 297.2
Korsakoff's, Korakov's, Korsakow's
  (nonalcoholic) 294.0
  alcoholic 291.1
mania (phase) (*see also* Psychosis, affective) 296.0 ☑
  recurrent episode 296.1 ☑
  single episode 296.0 ☑
manic (*see also* Psychosis, affective)
  296.0 ☑
  atypical 296.81
  recurrent episode 296.1 ☑
  single episode 296.0 ☑
manic-depressive 296.80
  circular 296.7
    currently
      depressed 296.5 ☑
      manic 296.4 ☑
      mixed 296.6 ☑
  depressive 296.2 ☑
    recurrent episode 296.3 ☑
      with hypomania (bipolar II)
      296.89
    single episode 296.2 ☑
  hypomanic 296.0 ☑
    recurrent episode 296.1 ☑
    single episode 296.0 ☑
  manic 296.0 ☑
    atypical 296.81
    recurrent episode 296.1 ☑
    single episode 296.0 ☑
  mixed NEC 296.89
  perplexed 296.89
  stuporous 296.89
menopausal (*see also* Psychosis, involutional) 298.8
mixed schizophrenic and affective (*see
  also* Schizophrenia) 295.7 ☑
multi-infarct (cerebrovascular) (*see
  also* Psychosis, arteriosclerotic)
  290.40
organic NEC 294.9
  due to or associated with
    addiction
      alcohol (*see also* Psychosis,
        alcoholic) 291.9
      drug (*see also* Psychosis,
        drug) 292.9
    alcohol intoxication, acute (*see
      also* Psychosis, alcoholic)
      291.9
    alcoholism (*see also* Psychosis,
      alcoholic) 291.9
    arteriosclerosis (cerebral) (*see
      also* Psychosis, arterioscle-
      rotic) 290.40

**Psychosis** — *continued*
organic — *continued*
  due to or associated with — *contin-
    ued*
    cerebrovascular disease
      acute (psychosis) 293.0
      arteriosclerotic (*see also* Psy-
        chosis, arteriosclerotic)
        290.40
    childbirth — *see* Psychosis,
      puerperal
    dependence
      alcohol (*see also* Psychosis,
        alcoholic) 291.9
      drug 292.9
    disease
      alcoholic liver (*see also* Psy-
        chosis, alcoholic) 291.9
      brain
        arteriosclerotic (*see also*
          Psychosis, arte-
          riosclerotic) 290.40
      cerebrovascular
        acute (psychosis) 293.0
        arteriosclerotic (*see also*
          Psychosis, arte-
          riosclerotic) 290.40
      endocrine or metabolic 293.9
        acute (psychosis) 293.0
        subacute (psychosis)
          293.1
      Jakob-Creutzfeldt (new vari-
        ant)
        with behavioral distur-
          bance
          046.1 *[294.11]*
        without behavioral distur-
          bance
          046.1 *[294.10]*
      liver, alcoholic (*see also* Psy-
        chosis, alcoholic) 291.9
    disorder
      cerebrovascular
        acute (psychosis) 293.0
      endocrine or metabolic 293.9
        acute (psychosis) 293.0
        subacute (psychosis)
          293.1
    epilepsy
      with behavioral disturbance
        345.9 *[294.11]*
      without behavioral distur-
        bance
        345.9 *[294.10]*
      transient (acute) 293.0
    Huntington's chorea
      with behavioral disturbance
        333.4 *[294.11]*
      without behavioral distur-
        bance 333.4 *[294.10]*
    infection
      brain 293.9
        acute (psychosis) 293.0
        chronic 294.8
        subacute (psychosis)
          293.1
      intracranial NEC 293.9
        acute (psychosis) 293.0
        chronic 294.8
        subacute (psychosis)
          293.1
    intoxication
      alcoholic (acute) (*see also*
        Psychosis, alcoholic)
        291.9
        pathological 291.4
      drug (*see also* Psychosis,
        drug) 292.2
    ischemia
      cerebrovascular (generalized)
        (*see also* Psychosis, ar-
        teriosclerotic) 290.40
    Jakob-Creutzfeldt disease (syn-
      drome) (new variant)
      with behavioral disturbance
        046.1 *[294.11]*

**Psychosis** — *continued*
organic — *continued*
  due to or associated with — *contin-
    ued*
    Jakob-Creutzfeldt disease —
      *continued*
      without behavioral distur-
        bance 046.1 *[294.10]*
    multiple sclerosis
      with behavioral disturbance
        340 *[294.11]*
      without behavioral distur-
        bance 340 *[294.10]*
    physical condition NEC 293.9
      with
        delusions 293.81
        hallucinations 293.82
    presenility 290.10
    puerperium — *see* Psychosis,
      puerperal
    sclerosis, multiple
      with behavioral disturbance
        340 *[294.11]*
      without behavioral distur-
        bance 340 *[294.10]*
    senility 290.20
    status epilepticus
      with behavioral disturbance
        345.3 *[294.11]*
      without behavioral distur-
        bance 345.3 *[294.10]*
    trauma
      brain (birth) (from electrical
        current) (surgical)
        293.9
        acute (psychosis) 293.0
        chronic 294.8
        subacute (psychosis)
          293.1
      unspecified physical con-
        dition 293.9
        with
          delusion 293.81
          hallucinations
            293.82
  infective 293.9
    acute (psychosis) 293.0
    subacute 293.1
  posttraumatic 293.9
    acute 293.0
    subacute 293.1
  specified type NEC 294.8
  transient 293.9
    with
      anxiety 293.84
      delusions 293.81
      depression 293.83
      hallucinations 293.82
    depressive type 293.83
    hallucinatory type 293.82
    paranoid type 293.81
    specified type NEC 293.89
paranoic 297.1
paranoid (chronic) 297.9
  alcoholic 291.5
  chronic 297.1
  climacteric 297.2
  involutional 297.2
  menopausal 297.2
  protracted reactive 298.4
  psychogenic 298.4
    acute 298.3
  schizophrenic (*see also*
    Schizophrenia) 295.3 ☑
  senile 290.20
paroxysmal 298.9
  senile 290.20
polyneuritic, alcoholic 291.1
postoperative 293.9
postpartum — *see* Psychosis, puerperal
prepsychotic (*see also* Schizophrenia)
  295.5 ☑
presbyophrenic (type) 290.8
presenile (*see also* Dementia, presenile) 290.10

**Psychosis** — *continued*
prison 300.16
psychogenic 298.8
  depressive 298.0
  paranoid 298.4
    acute 298.3
puerperal
  specified type — *see* categories
    295-298 ☑
  unspecified type 293.89
    acute 293.0
    chronic 293.89
    subacute 293.1
reactive (emotional stress) (psychological trauma) 298.8
  brief 298.8
  confusion 298.2
  depressive 298.0
  excitation 298.1
schizo-affective (depressed) (excited)
  (*see also* Schizophrenia)
  295.7 ☑
schizophrenia, schizophrenic (*see also*
  Schizophrenia) 295.9 ☑
  borderline type 295.5 ☑
    of childhood (*see also* Psychosis,
      childhood) 299.8 ☑
  catatonic (excited) (withdrawn)
    295.2 ☑
  childhood type (*see also* Psychosis,
    childhood) 299.9 ☑
  hebephrenic 295.1 ☑
  incipient 295.5 ☑
  latent 295.5 ☑
  paranoid 295.3 ☑
  prepsychotic 295.5 ☑
  prodromal 295.5 ☑
  pseudoneurotic 295.5 ☑
  pseudopsychopathic 295.5 ☑
  schizophreniform 295.4 ☑
  simple 295.0 ☑
  undifferentiated type 295.9 ☑
schizophreniform 295.4 ☑
senile NEC 290.20
  with
    delusional features 290.20
    depressive features 290.21
  depressed type 290.21
  paranoid type 290.20
  simple deterioration 290.20
  specified type — *see* categories
    295-298 ☑
shared 297.3
situational (reactive) 298.8
symbiotic (childhood) (*see also* Psychosis, childhood) 299.1 ☑
toxic (acute) 293.9
**Psychotic** — *see also* condition 298.9
episode 298.9
  due to or associated with physical
    conditions (*see also* Psy-
    chosis, organic) 293.9
**Pterygium** (eye) 372.40
central 372.43
colli 744.5
double 372.44
peripheral (stationary) 372.41
  progressive 372.42
recurrent 372.45
**Ptilosis** 374.55
**Ptomaine** (poisoning) — *see also* Poisoning, food 005.9
**Ptosis** (adiposa) 374.30
breast 611.8
cecum 569.89
colon 569.89
congenital (eyelid) 743.61
  specified site NEC — *see* Anomaly,
    specified type NEC
epicanthus syndrome 270.2
eyelid 374.30
  congenital 743.61
  mechanical 374.33
  myogenic 374.32
  paralytic 374.31
gastric 537.5

**Ptosis** — continued
  intestine 569.89
  kidney (see also Disease, renal) 593.0
    congenital 753.3
  liver 573.8
  renal (see also Disease, renal) 593.0
    congenital 753.3
  splanchnic 569.89
  spleen 289.59
  stomach 537.5
  viscera 569.89
**PTSD** (Post-traumatic stress disorder) 309.81
**Ptyalism** 527.7
  hysterical 300.11
  periodic 527.2
  pregnancy 646.8 ☑
  psychogenic 306.4
**Ptyalolithiasis** 527.5
**Pubalgia** 848.8
**Pubarche, precocious** 259.1
**Pubertas praecox** 259.1
**Puberty** V21.1
  abnormal 259.9
  bleeding 626.3
  delayed 259.0
  precocious (constitutional) (crypto-genic) (idiopathic) NEC 259.1
    due to
      adrenal
        cortical hyperfunction 255.2
        hyperplasia 255.2
      cortical hyperfunction 255.2
      ovarian hyperfunction 256.1
        estrogen 256.0
      pineal tumor 259.8
      testicular hyperfunction 257.0
  premature 259.1
    due to
      adrenal cortical hyperfunction 255.2
      pineal tumor 259.8
      pituitary (anterior) hyperfunction 253.1
**Puckering, macula** 362.56
**Pudenda, pudendum** — see condition
**Puente's disease** (simple glandular cheilitis) 528.5
**Puerperal**
  abscess
    areola 675.1 ☑
    Bartholin's gland 646.6 ☑
    breast 675.1 ☑
    cervix (uteri) 670.0 ☑
    fallopian tube 670.0 ☑
    genital organ 670.0 ☑
    kidney 646.6 ☑
    mammary 675.1 ☑
    mesosalpinx 670.0 ☑
    nabothian 646.6 ☑
    nipple 675.0 ☑
    ovary, ovarian 670.0 ☑
    oviduct 670.0 ☑
    parametric 670.0 ☑
    para-uterine 670.0 ☑
    pelvic 670.0 ☑
    perimetric 670.0 ☑
    periuterine 670.0 ☑
    retro-uterine 670.0 ☑
    subareolar 675.1 ☑
    suprapelvic 670.0 ☑
    tubal (ruptured) 670.0 ☑
    tubo-ovarian 670.0 ☑
    urinary tract NEC 646.6 ☑
    uterine, uterus 670.0 ☑
    vagina (wall) 646.6 ☑
    vaginorectal 646.6 ☑
    vulvovaginal gland 646.6 ☑
  accident 674.9 ☑
  adnexitis 670.0 ☑
  afibrinogenemia, or other coagulation defect 666.3 ☑
  albuminuria (acute) (subacute) 646.2 ☑
    pre-eclamptic 642.4 ☑

**Puerperal** — continued
  anemia (conditions classifiable to 280–285) 648.2 ☑
  anuria 669.3 ☑
  apoplexy 674.0 ☑
  asymptomatic bacteriuria 646.5 ☑
  atrophy, breast 676.3 ☑
  blood dyscrasia 666.3 ☑
  caked breast 676.2 ☑
  cardiomyopathy 674.5 ☑
  cellulitis — see Puerperal, abscess
  cerebrovascular disorder (conditions classifiable to 430–434, 436–437) 674.0 ☑
  cervicitis (conditions classifiable to 616.0) 646.6 ☑
  coagulopathy (any) 666.3 ☑
  complications 674.9 ☑
    specified type NEC 674.8 ☑
  convulsions (eclamptic) (uremic) 642.6 ☑
    with pre-existing hypertension 642.7 ☑
  cracked nipple 676.1 ☑
  cystitis 646.6 ☑
  cystopyelitis 646.6 ☑
  deciduitis (acute) 670.0 ☑
  delirium NEC 293.9
  diabetes (mellitus) (conditions classifiable to 250) 648.0 ☑
  disease 674.9 ☑
    breast NEC 676.3 ☑
    cerebrovascular (acute) 674.0 ☑
    nonobstetric NEC (see also Pregnancy, complicated, current disease or condition) 648.9 ☑
    pelvis inflammatory 670.0 ☑
    renal NEC 646.2 ☑
    tubo-ovarian 670.0 ☑
    Valsuani's (progressive pernicious anemia) 648.2 ☑
  disorder
    lactation 676.9 ☑
      specified type NEC 676.8 ☑
    nonobstetric NEC (see also Pregnancy, complicated, current disease or condition) 648.9 ☑
  disruption
    cesarean wound 674.1 ☑
    episiotomy wound 674.2 ☑
    perineal laceration wound 674.2 ☑
  drug dependence (conditions classifiable to 304) 648.3 ☑
  eclampsia 642.6 ☑
    with pre-existing hypertension 642.7 ☑
  embolism (pulmonary) 673.2 ☑
    air 673.0 ☑
    amniotic fluid 673.1 ☑
    blood-clot 673.2 ☑
    brain or cerebral 674.0 ☑
    cardiac 674.8 ☑
    fat 673.8 ☑
    intracranial sinus (venous) 671.5 ☑
    pyemic 673.3 ☑
    septic 673.3 ☑
    spinal cord 671.5 ☑
  endometritis (conditions classifiable to 615.0–615.9) 670.0 ☑
  endophlebitis — see Puerperal, phlebitis
  endotrachelitis 646.6 ☑
  engorgement, breasts 676.2 ☑
  erysipelas 670.0 ☑
  failure
    lactation 676.4 ☑
    renal, acute 669.3 ☑
  fever 670.0 ☑
    meaning pyrexia (of unknown origin) 672.0 ☑
    meaning sepsis 670.0 ☑
  fissure, nipple 676.1 ☑

**Puerperal** — continued
  fistula
    breast 675.1 ☑
    mammary gland 675.1 ☑
    nipple 675.0 ☑
  galactophoritis 675.2 ☑
  galactorrhea 676.6 ☑
  gangrene
    gas 670.0 ☑
    uterus 670.0 ☑
  gonorrhea (conditions classifiable to 098) 647.1 ☑
  hematoma, subdural 674.0 ☑
  hematosalpinx, infectional 670.0 ☑
  hemiplegia, cerebral 674.0 ☑
  hemorrhage 666.1 ☑
    brain 674.0 ☑
    bulbar 674.0 ☑
    cerebellar 674.0 ☑
    cerebral 674.0 ☑
    cortical 674.0 ☑
    delayed (after 24 hours) (uterine) 666.2 ☑
    extradural 674.0 ☑
    internal capsule 674.0 ☑
    intracranial 674.0 ☑
    intrapontine 674.0 ☑
    meningeal 674.0 ☑
    pontine 674.0 ☑
    subarachnoid 674.0 ☑
    subcortical 674.0 ☑
    subdural 674.0 ☑
    uterine, delayed 666.2 ☑
    ventricular 674.0 ☑
  hemorrhoids 671.8 ☑
  hepatorenal syndrome 674.8 ☑
  hypertrophy
    breast 676.3 ☑
    mammary gland 676.3 ☑
  induration breast (fibrous) 676.3 ☑
  infarction
    lung — see Puerperal, embolism
    pulmonary — see Puerperal, embolism
  infection
    Bartholin's gland 646.6 ☑
    breast 675.2 ☑
      with nipple 675.9 ☑
        specified type NEC 675.8 ☑
    cervix 646.6 ☑
    endocervix 646.6 ☑
    fallopian tube 670.0 ☑
    generalized 670.0 ☑
    genital tract (major) 670.0 ☑
      minor or localized 646.6 ☑
    kidney (bacillus coli) 646.6 ☑
    mammary gland 675.2 ☑
      with nipple 675.9 ☑
        specified type NEC 675.8 ☑
    nipple 675.0 ☑
      with breast 675.9 ☑
        specified type NEC 675.8 ☑
    ovary 670.0 ☑
    pelvic 670.0 ☑
    peritoneum 670.0 ☑
    renal 646.6 ☑
    tubo-ovarian 670.0 ☑
    urinary (tract) NEC 646.6 ☑
      asymptomatic 646.5 ☑
    uterus, uterine 670.0 ☑
    vagina 646.6 ☑
  inflammation (see also Puerperal, infection)
    areola 675.1 ☑
    Bartholin's gland 646.6 ☑
    breast 675.2 ☑
    broad ligament 670.0 ☑
    cervix (uteri) 646.6 ☑
    fallopian tube 670.0 ☑
    genital organs 670.0 ☑
      localized 646.6 ☑
    mammary gland 675.2 ☑
    nipple 675.0 ☑
    ovary 670.0 ☑

**Puerperal** — continued
  inflammation (see also Puerperal, infection) — continued
    oviduct 670.0 ☑
    pelvis 670.0 ☑
    periuterine 670.0 ☑
    tubal 670.0 ☑
    vagina 646.6 ☑
    vein — see Puerperal, phlebitis
  inversion, nipple 676.3 ☑
  ischemia, cerebral 674.0 ☑
  lymphangitis 670.0 ☑
    breast 675.2 ☑
  malaria (conditions classifiable to 084) 647.4 ☑
  malnutrition 648.9 ☑
  mammillitis 675.0 ☑
  mammitis 675.2 ☑
  mania 296.0 ☑
    recurrent episode 296.1 ☑
    single episode 296.0 ☑
  mastitis 675.2 ☑
    purulent 675.1 ☑
    retromammary 675.1 ☑
    submammary 675.1 ☑
  melancholia 296.2 ☑
    recurrent episode 296.3 ☑
    single episode 296.2 ☑
  mental disorder (conditions classifiable to 290–303, 305.0, 305.2–305.9, 306–316, 317–319) 648.4 ☑
  metritis (septic) (suppurative) 670.0 ☑
  metroperitonitis 670.0 ☑
  metrorrhagia 666.2 ☑
  metrosalpingitis 670.0 ☑
  metrovaginitis 670.0 ☑
  milk leg 671.4 ☑
  monoplegia, cerebral 674.0 ☑
  necrosis
    kidney, tubular 669.3 ☑
    liver (acute) (subacute) (conditions classifiable to 570) 674.8 ☑
    ovary 670.0 ☑
    renal cortex 669.3 ☑
  nephritis or nephrosis (conditions classifiable to 580–589) 646.2 ☑
    with hypertension 642.1 ☑
  nutritional deficiency (conditions classifiable to 260–269) 648.9 ☑
  occlusion, precerebral artery 674.0 ☑
  oliguria 669.3 ☑
  oophoritis 670.0 ☑
  ovaritis 670.0 ☑
  paralysis
    bladder (sphincter) 665.5 ☑
    cerebral 674.0 ☑
  paralytic stroke 674.0 ☑
  parametritis 670.0 ☑
  paravaginitis 646.6 ☑
  pelviperitonitis 670.0 ☑
  perimetritis 670.0 ☑
  perimetrosalpingitis 670.0 ☑
  perinephritis 646.6 ☑
  perioophoritis 670.0 ☑
  periphlebitis — see Puerperal, phlebitis
  perisalpingitis 670.0 ☑
  peritoneal infection 670.0 ☑
  peritonitis (pelvic) 670.0 ☑
  perivaginitis 646.6 ☑
  phlebitis 671.9 ☑
    deep 671.4 ☑
    intracranial sinus (venous) 671.5 ☑
    pelvic 671.4 ☑
    specified site NEC 671.5 ☑
    superficial 671.2 ☑
  phlegmasia alba dolens 671.4 ☑
  placental polyp 674.4 ☑
  pneumonia, embolic — see Puerperal, embolism
  prediabetes 648.8 ☑
  pre-eclampsia (mild) 642.4 ☑

---

☑ Additional Digit Required — Refer to the Tabular List for Digit Selection

⤷ Subterms under main terms may continue to next column or page

**Puerperal** — *continued*
  pre-eclampsia — *continued*
    with pre-existing hypertension 642.7 ☑
    severe 642.5 ☑
  psychosis, unspecified (*see also* Psychosis, puerperal) 293.89
  pyelitis 646.6 ☑
  pyelocystitis 646.6 ☑
  pyelohydronephrosis 646.6 ☑
  pyelonephritis 646.6 ☑
  pyelonephrosis 646.6 ☑
  pyemia 670.0 ☑
  pyocystitis 646.6 ☑
  pyohemia 670.0 ☑
  pyometra 670.0 ☑
  pyonephritis 646.6 ☑
  pyonephrosis 646.6 ☑
  pyo-oophoritis 670.0 ☑
  pyosalpingitis 670.0 ☑
  pyosalpinx 670.0 ☑
  pyrexia (of unknown origin) 672.0 ☑
  renal
    disease NEC 646.2 ☑
    failure, acute 669.3 ☑
  retention
    decidua (fragments) (with delayed hemorrhage) 666.2 ☑
     without hemorrhage 667.1 ☑
    placenta (fragments) (with delayed hemorrhage) 666.2 ☑
     without hemorrhage 667.1 ☑
    secundines (fragments) (with delayed hemorrhage) 666.2 ☑
     without hemorrhage 667.1 ☑
  retracted nipple 676.0 ☑
  rubella (conditions classifiable to 056) 647.5 ☑
  salpingitis 670.0 ☑
  salpingo-oophoritis 670.0 ☑
  salpingo-ovaritis 670.0 ☑
  salpingoperitonitis 670.0 ☑
  sapremia 670.0 ☑
  secondary perineal tear 674.2 ☑
  sepsis (pelvic) 670.0 ☑
  septicemia 670.0 ☑
  subinvolution (uterus) 674.8 ☑
  sudden death (cause unknown) 674.9 ☑
  suppuration — *see* Puerperal, abscess
  syphilis (conditions classifiable to 090–097) 647.0 ☑
  tetanus 670.0 ☑
  thelitis 675.0 ☑
  thrombocytopenia 666.3 ☑
  thrombophlebitis (superficial) 671.2 ☑
    deep 671.4 ☑
    pelvic 671.4 ☑
    specified site NEC 671.5 ☑
  thrombosis (venous) — *see* Thrombosis, puerperal
  thyroid dysfunction (conditions classifiable to 240–246) 648.1 ☑
  toxemia (*see also* Toxemia, of pregnancy) 642.4 ☑
    eclamptic 642.6 ☑
     with pre-existing hypertension 642.7 ☑
    pre-eclamptic (mild) 642.4 ☑
     with
      convulsions 642.6 ☑
      pre-existing hypertension 642.7 ☑
     severe 642.5 ☑
  tuberculosis (conditions classifiable to 010–018) 647.3 ☑
  uremia 669.3 ☑
  vaginitis (conditions classifiable to 616.1) 646.6 ☑
  varicose veins (legs) 671.0 ☑
    vulva or perineum 671.1 ☑
  vulvitis (conditions classifiable to 616.1) 646.6 ☑

**Puerperal** — *continued*
  vulvovaginitis (conditions classifiable to 616.1) 646.6 ☑
  white leg 671.4 ☑
**Pulled muscle** — *see* Sprain, by site
**Pulmolithiasis** 518.89
**Pulmonary** — *see* condition
**Pulmonitis** (unknown etiology) 486
**Pulpitis** (acute) (anachoretic) (chronic) (hyperplastic) (putrescent) (suppurative) (ulcerative) 522.0
**Pulpless tooth** 522.9
**Pulse**
  alternating 427.89
    psychogenic 306.2
  bigeminal 427.89
  fast 785.0
  feeble, rapid, due to shock following injury 958.4
  rapid 785.0
  slow 427.89
  strong 785.9
  trigeminal 427.89
  water-hammer (*see also* Insufficiency, aortic) 424.1
  weak 785.9
**Pulseless disease** 446.7
**Pulsus**
  alternans or trigeminy 427.89
    psychogenic 306.2
**Punch drunk** 310.2
**Puncta lacrimalia occlusion** 375.52
**Punctiform hymen** 752.49
**Puncture** (traumatic) — *see also* Wound, open, by site
  accidental, complicating surgery 998.2
  bladder, nontraumatic 596.6
  by
    device, implant, or graft — *see* Complications, mechanical
    foreign body
     internal organs (*see also* Injury, internal, by site)
      by ingested object — *see* Foreign body
     left accidentally in operation wound 998.4
    instrument (any) during a procedure, accidental 998.2
  internal organs, abdomen, chest, or pelvis — *see* Injury, internal, by site
  kidney, nontraumatic 593.89
**Pupil** — *see* condition
**Pupillary membrane** 364.74
  persistent 743.46
**Pupillotonia** 379.46
  pseudotabetic 379.46
**Purpura** 287.2
  abdominal 287.0
  allergic 287.0
  anaphylactoid 287.0
  annularis telangiectodes 709.1
  arthritic 287.0
  autoerythrocyte sensitization 287.2
  autoimmune 287.0
  bacterial 287.0
  Bateman's (senile) 287.2
  capillary fragility (hereditary) (idiopathic) 287.8
  cryoglobulinemic 273.2
  devil's pinches 287.2
  fibrinolytic (*see also* Fibrinolysis) 286.6
  fulminans, fulminous 286.6
  gangrenous 287.0
  hemorrhagic (*see also* Purpura, thrombocytopenic) 287.39
    nodular 272.7
    nonthrombocytopenic 287.0
    thrombocytopenic 287.39
  Henoch's (purpura nervosa) 287.0
  Henoch-Schönlein (allergic) 287.0
  hypergammaglobulinemic (benign primary) (Waldenström's) 273.0
  idiopathic 287.31

**Purpura** — *continued*
  idiopathic — *continued*
    nonthrombocytopenic 287.0
    thrombocytopenic 287.31
  immune thrombocytopenic 287.31
  infectious 287.0
  malignant 287.0
  neonatorum 772.6
  nervosa 287.0
  newborn NEC 772.6
  nonthrombocytopenic 287.2
    hemorrhagic 287.0
    idiopathic 287.0
  nonthrombopenic 287.2
  peliosis rheumatica 287.0
  pigmentaria, progressiva 709.09
  posttransfusion 287.4
  primary 287.0
  primitive 287.0
  red cell membrane sensitivity 287.2
  rheumatica 287.0
  Schönlein (-Henoch) (allergic) 287.0
  scorbutic 267
  senile 287.2
  simplex 287.2
  symptomatica 287.0
  telangiectasia annularis 709.1
  thrombocytopenic (*see also* Thrombocytopenia) 287.30
    congenital 287.33
    essential 287.30
    hereditary 287.31
    idiopathic 287.31
    immune 287.31
    neonatal, transitory (*see also* Thrombocytopenia, neonatal transitory) 776.1
    primary 287.30
    puerperal, postpartum 666.3 ☑
    thrombotic 446.6
  thrombohemolytic (*see also* Fibrinolysis) 286.6
  thrombopenic (*see also* Thrombocytopenia) 287.30
    congenital 287.33
    essential 287.30
    thrombotic 446.6
     thrombocytic 446.6
     thrombocytopenic 446.6
  toxic 287.0
  variolosa 050.0
  vascular 287.0
  visceral symptoms 287.0
  Werlhof's (*see also* Purpura, thrombocytopenic) 287.39
**Purpuric spots** 782.7
**Purulent** — *see* condition
**Pus**
  absorption, general — *see* Septicemia
  in
    stool 792.1
    urine 791.9
  tube (rupture) (*see also* Salpingo-oophoritis) 614.2
**Pustular rash** 782.1
**Pustule** 686.9
  malignant 022.0
  nonmalignant 686.9
**Putnam-Dana syndrome** (subacute combined sclerosis with pernicious anemia) 281.0 *[336.2]*
**Putnam's disease** (subacute combined sclerosis with pernicious anemia) 281.0 *[336.2]*
**Putrefaction, intestinal** 569.89
**Putrescent pulp** (dental) 522.1
**Pyarthritis** — *see* Pyarthrosis
**Pyarthrosis** — *see also* Arthritis, pyogenic 711.0 ☑
  tuberculous — *see* Tuberculosis, joint
**Pycnoepilepsy, pycnolepsy** (idiopathic) — *see also* Epilepsy 345.0 ☑
**Pyelectasia** 593.89
**Pyelectasis** 593.89
**Pyelitis** (congenital) (uremic) 590.80

**Pyelitis** — *continued*
  with
    abortion — *see* Abortion, by type, with specified complication NEC
    contracted kidney 590.00
    ectopic pregnancy (*see also* categories 633.0–633.9) 639.8
    molar pregnancy (*see also* categories 630–632) 639.8
  acute 590.10
    with renal medullary necrosis 590.11
  chronic 590.00
    with
     renal medullary necrosis 590.01
    complicating pregnancy, childbirth, or puerperium 646.6 ☑
     affecting fetus or newborn 760.1
  cystica 590.3
    following
     abortion 639.8
     ectopic or molar pregnancy 639.8
  gonococcal 098.19
    chronic or duration of 2 months or over 098.39
  tuberculous (*see also* Tuberculosis) 016.0 ☑ *[590.81]*
**Pyelocaliectasis** 593.89
**Pyelocystitis** — *see also* Pyelitis 590.80
**Pyelohydronephrosis** 591
**Pyelonephritis** — *see also* Pyelitis 590.80
  acute 590.10
    with renal medullary necrosis 590.11
  chronic 590.00
  syphilitic (late) 095.4
  tuberculous (*see also* Tuberculosis) 016.0 ☑ *[590.81]*
**Pyelonephrosis** — *see also* Pyelitis 590.80
  chronic 590.00
**Pyelophlebitis** 451.89
**Pyelo-ureteritis cystica** 590.3
**Pyemia, pyemic** (purulent) — *see also* Septicemia 038.9
  abscess — *see* Abscess
  arthritis (*see also* Arthritis, pyogenic) 711.0 ☑
  Bacillus coli 038.42
  embolism ►(*see also* Septicemia)◄ 415.12 ▲
  fever 038.9
  infection 038.9
  joint (*see also* Arthritis, pyogenic) 711.0 ☑
  liver 572.1
  meningococcal 036.2
  newborn 771.81
  phlebitis — *see* Phlebitis
  pneumococcal 038.2
  portal 572.1
  postvaccinal 999.39 ▲
  specified organism NEC 038.8
  staphylococcal 038.10
    aureus 038.11
    specified organism NEC 038.19
  streptococcal 038.0
  tuberculous — *see* Tuberculosis, miliary
**Pygopagus** 759.4
**Pykno-epilepsy, pyknolepsy** (idiopathic) — *see also* Epilepsy 345.0 ☑
**Pyle (-Cohn) disease** (craniometaphyseal dysplasia) 756.89
**Pylephlebitis** (suppurative) 572.1
**Pylethrombophlebitis** 572.1
**Pylethrombosis** 572.1
**Pyloritis** — *see also* Gastritis 535.5 ☑
**Pylorospasm** (reflex) 537.81
  congenital or infantile 750.5
  neurotic 306.4
  newborn 750.5
  psychogenic 306.4

**Pylorus, pyloric** — see condition
**Pyoarthrosis** — see Pyarthrosis
**Pyocele**
 mastoid 383.00
 sinus (accessory) (nasal) (see also Sinusitis) 473.9
 turbinate (bone) 473.9
 urethra (see also Urethritis) 597.0
**Pyococcal dermatitis** 686.00
**Pyococcide, skin** 686.00
**Pyocolpos** — see also Vaginitis 616.10
**Pyocyaneus dermatitis** 686.09
**Pyocystis** — see Cystitis 595.9
**Pyoderma, pyodermia** 686.00
 gangrenosum 686.01
 specified type NEC 686.09
 vegetans 686.8
**Pyodermatitis** 686.00
 vegetans 686.8
**Pyogenic** — see condition
**Pyohemia** — see Septicemia
**Pyohydronephrosis** — see also Pyelitis 590.80
**Pyometra** 615.9
**Pyometritis** — see also Endometritis 615.9
**Pyometrium** — see also Endometritis 615.9
**Pyomyositis** 728.0
 ossificans 728.19
 tropical (bungpagga) 040.81
**Pyonephritis** — see also Pyelitis 590.80
 chronic 590.00
**Pyonephrosis** (congenital) — see also Pyelitis 590.80
 acute 590.10
**Pyo-oophoritis** — see also Salpingooophoritis 614.2
**Pyo-ovarium** — see also Salpingooophoritis 614.2
**Pyopericarditis** 420.99
**Pyopericardium** 420.99
**Pyophlebitis** — see Phlebitis
**Pyopneumopericardium** 420.99
**Pyopneumothorax** (infectional) 510.9
 with fistula 510.0
 subdiaphragmatic (see also Peritonitis) 567.29
 subphrenic (see also Peritonitis) 567.29
 tuberculous (see also Tuberculosis, pleura) 012.0 ☑
**Pyorrhea** (alveolar) (alveolaris) 523.40
 degenerative 523.5
**Pyosalpingitis** — see also Salpingooophoritis 614.2
**Pyosalpinx** — see also Salpingooophoritis 614.2
**Pyosepticemia** — see Septicemia
**Pyosis**
 Corlett's (impetigo) 684
 Manson's (pemphigus contagiosus) 684
**Pyothorax** 510.9
 with fistula 510.0
 tuberculous (see also Tuberculosis, pleura) 012.0 ☑
**Pyoureter** 593.89
 tuberculous (see also Tuberculosis) 016.2 ☑
**Pyramidopallidonigral syndrome** 332.0
**Pyrexia** (of unknown origin) (P.U.O.) 780.6
 atmospheric 992.0
 during labor 659.2 ☑
 environmentally-induced newborn 778.4
 heat 992.0
 newborn, environmentally-induced 778.4
 puerperal 672.0 ☑
**Pyroglobulinemia** 273.8
**Pyromania** 312.33
**Pyrosis** 787.1
**Pyrroloporphyria** 277.1
**Pyuria** (bacterial) 791.9

## Q

**Q fever** 083.0
 with pneumonia 083.0 [484.8]
**Quadricuspid aortic valve** 746.89
**Quadrilateral fever** 083.0
**Quadriparesis** — see Quadriplegia
 meaning muscle weakness 728.87
**Quadriplegia** 344.00
 with fracture, vertebra (process) — see Fracture, vertebra, cervical, with spinal cord injury
 brain (current episode) 437.8
 C1-C4
  complete 344.01
  incomplete 344.02
 C5-C7
  complete 344.03
  incomplete 344.04
 cerebral (current episode) 437.8
 congenital or infantile (cerebral) (spastic) (spinal) 343.2
 cortical 437.8
 embolic (current episode) (see also Embolism, brain) 434.1 ☑
 infantile (cerebral) (spastic) (spinal) 343.2
 newborn NEC 767.0
 specified NEC 344.09
 thrombotic (current episode) (see also Thrombosis, brain) 434.0 ☑
 traumatic — see Injury, spinal, cervical
**Quadruplet**
 affected by maternal complications of pregnancy 761.5
 healthy liveborn — see Newborn, multiple
 pregnancy (complicating delivery) NEC 651.8 ☑
  with fetal loss and retention of one or more fetus(es) 651.5 ☑
  following (elective) fetal reduction 651.7 ☑
**Quarrelsomeness** 301.3
**Quartan**
 fever 084.2
 malaria (fever) 084.2
**Queensland fever** 083.0
 coastal 083.0
 seven-day 100.89
**Quervain's disease** 727.04
 thyroid (subacute granulomatous thyroiditis) 245.1
**Queyrat's erythroplasia** (M8080/2)
 specified site — see Neoplasm, skin, in situ
 unspecified site 233.5
**Quincke's disease or edema** — see Edema, angioneurotic
**Quinquaud's disease** (acne decalvans) 704.09
**Quinsy** (gangrenous) 475
**Quintan fever** 083.1
**Quintuplet**
 affected by maternal complications of pregnancy 761.5
 healthy liveborn — see Newborn, multiple
 pregnancy (complicating delivery) NEC 651.2 ☑
  with fetal loss and retention of one or more fetus(es) 651.6 ☑
  following (elective) fetal reduction 651.7 ☑
**Quotidian**
 fever 084.0
 malaria (fever) 084.0

## R

**Rabbia** 071
**Rabbit fever** — see also Tularemia 021.9
**Rabies** 071
 contact V01.5
 exposure to V01.5
 inoculation V04.5

**Rabies** — continued
 inoculation — continued
  reaction — see Complications, vaccination
 vaccination, prophylactic (against) V04.5
**Rachischisis** — see also Spina bifida 741.9 ☑
**Rachitic** — see also condition
 deformities of spine 268.1
 pelvis 268.1
  with disproportion (fetopelvic) 653.2 ☑
   affecting fetus or newborn 763.1
   causing obstructed labor 660.1 ☑
    affecting fetus or newborn 763.1
**Rachitis, rachitism** — see also Rickets
 acute 268.0
 fetalis 756.4
 renalis 588.0
 tarda 268.0
**Racket nail** 757.5
**Radial nerve** — see condition
**Radiation effects or sickness** — see also Effect, adverse, radiation
 cataract 366.46
 dermatitis 692.82
  sunburn (see also Sunburn) 692.71
**Radiculitis** (pressure) (vertebrogenic) 729.2
 accessory nerve 723.4
 anterior crural 724.4
 arm 723.4
 brachial 723.4
 cervical NEC 723.4
 due to displacement of intervertebral disc — see Neuritis, due to, displacement intervertebral disc
 leg 724.4
 lumbar NEC 724.4
 lumbosacral 724.4
 rheumatic 729.2
 syphilitic 094.89
 thoracic (with visceral pain) 724.4
**Radiculomyelitis** 357.0
 toxic, due to
  Clostridium tetani 037
  Corynebacterium diphtheriae 032.89
**Radiculopathy** — see also Radiculitis 729.2
**Radioactive substances, adverse effect** — see Effect, adverse, radioactive substance
**Radiodermal burns** (acute) (chronic) (occupational) — see Burn, by site
**Radiodermatitis** 692.82
**Radionecrosis** — see Effect, adverse, radiation
**Radiotherapy session** V58.0
**Radium, adverse effect** — see Effect, adverse, radioactive substance
**Raeder-Harbitz syndrome** (pulseless disease) 446.7
**Rage** — see also Disturbance, conduct 312.0 ☑
 meaning rabies 071
**Rag sorters' disease** 022.1
**Raillietiniasis** 123.8
**Railroad neurosis** 300.16
**Railway spine** 300.16
**Raised** — see Elevation
**Raiva** 071
**Rake teeth, tooth** 524.39
**Rales** 786.7
**Ramifying renal pelvis** 753.3
**Ramsay Hunt syndrome** (herpetic geniculate ganglionitis) 053.11
 meaning dyssynergia cerebellaris myoclonica 334.2
**Ranke's primary infiltration** — see also Tuberculosis 010.0 ☑
**Ranula** 527.6

**Ranula** — continued
 congenital 750.26
**Rape**
 adult 995.83
 alleged, observation or examination V71.5
 child 995.53
**Rapid**
 feeble pulse, due to shock, following injury 958.4
 heart (beat) 785.0
  psychogenic 306.2
 respiration 786.06
  psychogenic 306.1
 second stage (delivery) 661.3 ☑
  affecting fetus or newborn 763.6
 time-zone change syndrome 327.35
**Rarefaction, bone** 733.99
**Rash** 782.1
 canker 034.1
 diaper 691.0
 drug (internal use) 693.0
  contact 692.3
 ECHO 9 virus 078.89
 enema 692.89
 food (see also Allergy, food) 693.1
 heat 705.1
 napkin 691.0
 nettle 708.8
 pustular 782.1
 rose 782.1
  epidemic 056.9
  of infants 057.8
 scarlet 034.1
 serum (prophylactic) (therapeutic) 999.5
 toxic 782.1
 wandering tongue 529.1
**Rasmussen's aneurysm** — see also Tuberculosis 011.2 ☑
**Rat-bite fever** 026.9
 due to Streptobacillus moniliformis 026.1
 spirochetal (morsus muris) 026.0
**Rathke's pouch tumor** (M9350/1) 237.0
**Raymond (-Céstan) syndrome** 433.8 ☑
**Raynaud's**
 disease or syndrome (paroxysmal digital cyanosis) 443.0
 gangrene (symmetric) 443.0 [785.4]
 phenomenon (paroxysmal digital cyanosis) (secondary) 443.0
**RDS** 769
**Reaction**
 acute situational maladjustment (see also Reaction, adjustment) 309.9
 adaptation (see also Reaction, adjustment) 309.9
 adjustment 309.9
  with
   anxious mood 309.24
    with depressed mood 309.28
   conduct disturbance 309.3
    combined with disturbance of emotions 309.4
   depressed mood 309.0
    brief 309.0
     with anxious mood 309.28
    prolonged 309.1
   elective mutism 309.83
   mixed emotions and conduct 309.4
   mutism, elective 309.83
   physical symptoms 309.82
   predominant disturbance (of)
    conduct 309.3
    emotions NEC 309.29
     mixed 309.28
    mixed, emotions and conduct 309.4
   specified type NEC 309.89
   specific academic or work inhibition 309.23
   withdrawal 309.83

**Reaction** — *continued*
adjustment — *continued*
  depressive 309.0
    with conduct disturbance 309.4
    brief 309.0
    prolonged 309.1
    specified type NEC 309.89
  adverse food NEC 995.7
  affective (*see also* Psychosis, affective) 296.90
    specified type NEC 296.99
  aggressive 301.3
    unsocialized (*see also* Disturbance, conduct) 312.0 ☑
  allergic (*see also* Allergy) 995.3
    drug, medicinal substance, and biological — *see* Allergy, drug
    food — *see* Allergy, food
    serum 999.5
  anaphylactic — *see* Shock, anaphylactic
  anesthesia — *see* Anesthesia, complication
  anger 312.0 ☑
  antisocial 301.7
  antitoxin (prophylactic) (therapeutic) — *see* Complications, vaccination
  anxiety 300.00
  Arthus 995.21
  asthenic 300.5
  compulsive 300.3
  conversion (anesthetic) (autonomic) (hyperkinetic) (mixed paralytic) (paresthetic) 300.11
  deoxyribonuclease (DNA) (DNase) hypersensitivity NEC 287.2
  depressive 300.4
    acute 309.0
    affective (*see also* Psychosis, affective) 296.2 ☑
      recurrent episode 296.3 ☑
      single episode 296.2 ☑
    brief 309.0
    manic (*see also* Psychosis, affective) 296.80
    neurotic 300.4
    psychoneurotic 300.4
    psychotic 298.0
  dissociative 300.15
  drug NEC (*see also* Table of Drugs and Chemicals) 995.20
    allergic (*see also* Allergy, drug) 995.27
    correct substance properly administered 995.20
    obstetric anesthetic or analgesic NEC 668.9 ☑
      affecting fetus or newborn 763.5
    specified drug — *see* Table of Drugs and Chemicals
    overdose or poisoning 977.9
      specified drug — *see* Table of Drugs and Chemicals
    specific to newborn 779.4
    transmitted via placenta or breast milk — *see* Absorption, drug, through placenta
    withdrawal NEC 292.0
      infant of dependent mother 779.5
    wrong substance given or taken in error 977.9
      specified drug — *see* Table of Drugs and Chemicals
  dyssocial 301.7
  dystonic, acute, due to drugs 333.72
  erysipeloid 027.1
  fear 300.20
    child 313.0
  fluid loss, cerebrospinal 349.0
  food (*see also* Allergy, food)
    adverse NEC 995.7
    anaphylactic shock — *see* Anaphylactic shock, due to, food

**Reaction** — *continued*
foreign
  body NEC 728.82
    in operative wound (inadvertently left) 998.4
    due to surgical material intentionally left — *see* Complications, due to (presence of) any device, implant, or graft classified to 996.0–996.5 NEC
    substance accidentally left during a procedure (chemical) (powder) (talc) 998.7
    body or object (instrument) (sponge) (swab) 998.4
  graft-versus-host (GVH) 996.85
  grief (acute) (brief) 309.0
    prolonged 309.1
  gross stress (*see also* Reaction, stress, acute) 308.9
  group delinquent (*see also* Disturbance, conduct) 312.2 ☑
  Herxheimer's 995.0
  hyperkinetic (*see also* Hyperkinesia) 314.9
  hypochondriacal 300.7
  hypoglycemic, due to insulin 251.0
    therapeutic misadventure 962.3
  hypomanic (*see also* Psychosis, affective) 296.0 ☑
    recurrent episode 296.1 ☑
    single episode 296.0 ☑
  hysterical 300.10
    conversion type 300.11
    dissociative 300.15
  id (bacterial cause) 692.89
  immaturity NEC 301.89
    aggressive 301.3
    emotional instability 301.59
  immunization — *see* Complications, vaccination
  incompatibility
    blood group (ABO) (infusion) (transfusion) 999.6
    Rh (factor) (infusion) (transfusion) 999.7
  inflammatory — *see* Infection
  infusion — *see* Complications, infusion
  inoculation (immune serum) — *see* Complications, vaccination
  insulin 995.23
  involutional
    paranoid 297.2
    psychotic (*see also* Psychosis, affective, depressive) 296.2 ☑
  leukemoid (basophilic) (lymphocytic) (monocytic) (myelocytic) (neutrophilic) 288.62
  LSD (*see also* Abuse, drugs, nondependent) 305.3 ☑
  lumbar puncture 349.0
  manic-depressive (*see also* Psychosis, affective) 296.80
    depressed 296.2 ☑
      recurrent episode 296.3 ☑
      single episode 296.2 ☑
    hypomanic 296.0 ☑
  neurasthenic 300.5
  neurogenic (*see also* Neurosis) 300.9
  neurotic NEC 300.9
  neurotic-depressive 300.4
  nitritoid — *see* Crisis, nitritoid
  obsessive compulsive 300.3
  organic 293.9
    acute 293.0
    subacute 293.1
  overanxious, child or adolescent 313.0
  paranoid (chronic) 297.9
    acute 298.3
    climacteric 297.2
    involutional 297.2
    menopausal 297.2
    senile 290.20

**Reaction** — *continued*
paranoid — *continued*
  simple 297.0
  passive
    aggressive 301.84
    dependency 301.6
  personality (*see also* Disorder, personality) 301.9
  phobic 300.20
  postradiation — *see* Effect, adverse, radiation
  psychogenic NEC 300.9
  psychoneurotic (*see also* Neurosis) 300.9
    anxiety 300.00
    compulsive 300.3
    conversion 300.11
    depersonalization 300.6
    depressive 300.4
    dissociative 300.15
    hypochondriacal 300.7
    hysterical 300.10
      conversion type 300.11
      dissociative type 300.15
    neurasthenic 300.5
    obsessive 300.3
    obsessive-compulsive 300.3
    phobic 300.20
    tension state 300.9
  psychophysiologic NEC (*see also* Disorder, psychosomatic) 306.9
    cardiovascular 306.2
    digestive 306.4
    endocrine 306.6
    gastrointestinal 306.4
    genitourinary 306.50
    heart 306.2
    hemic 306.8
    intestinal (large) (small) 306.4
    laryngeal 306.1
    lymphatic 306.8
    musculoskeletal 306.0
    pharyngeal 306.1
    respiratory 306.1
    skin 306.3
    special sense organs 306.7
  psychosomatic (*see also* Disorder, psychosomatic) 306.9
  psychotic (*see also* Psychosis) 298.9
    depressive 298.0
    due to or associated with physical condition (*see also* Psychosis, organic) 293.9
    involutional (*see also* Psychosis, affective) 296.2 ☑
      recurrent episode 296.3 ☑
      single episode 296.2 ☑
  pupillary (myotonic) (tonic) 379.46
  radiation — *see* Effect, adverse, radiation
  runaway (*see also* Disturbance, conduct)
    socialized 312.2 ☑
    undersocialized, unsocialized 312.1 ☑
  scarlet fever toxin — *see* Complications, vaccination
  schizophrenic (*see also* Schizophrenia) 295.9 ☑
    latent 295.5 ☑
  serological for syphilis — *see* Serology for syphilis
  serum (prophylactic) (therapeutic) 999.5
    immediate 999.4
  situational (*see also* Reaction, adjustment) 309.9
    acute, to stress 308.3
    adjustment (*see also* Reaction, adjustment) 309.9
  somatization (*see also* Disorder, psychosomatic) 306.9
  spinal puncture 349.0
  spite, child (*see also* Disturbance, conduct) 312.0 ☑
  stress, acute 308.9

**Reaction** — *continued*
stress, acute — *continued*
  with predominant disturbance (of)
    consciousness 308.1
    emotions 308.0
    mixed 308.4
    psychomotor 308.2
    specified type NEC 308.3
  bone or cartilage — *see* Fracture, stress
  surgical procedure — *see* Complications, surgical procedure
  tetanus antitoxin — *see* Complications, vaccination
  toxin-antitoxin — *see* Complications, vaccination
  transfusion (blood) (bone marrow) (lymphocytes) (allergic) — *see* Complications, transfusion
  tuberculin skin test, nonspecific (without active tuberculosis) 795.5
    positive (without active tuberculosis) 795.5
  ultraviolet — *see* Effect, adverse, ultraviolet
  undersocialized, unsocialized (*see also* Disturbance, conduct)
    aggressive (type) 312.0 ☑
    unaggressive (type) 312.1 ☑
  vaccination (any) — *see* Complications, vaccination
  white graft (skin) 996.52
  withdrawing, child or adolescent 313.22
  x-ray — *see* Effect, adverse, x-rays
**Reactive depression** — *see also* Reaction, depressive 300.4
  neurotic 300.4
  psychoneurotic 300.4
  psychotic 298.0
**Rebound tenderness** 789.6 ☑
**Recalcitrant patient** V15.81
**Recanalization, thrombus** — *see* Thrombosis
**Recession, receding**
  chamber angle (eye) 364.77
  chin 524.06
  gingival (postinfective) (postoperative) 523.20
    generalized 523.25
    localized 523.24
    minimal 523.21
    moderate 523.22
    severe 523.23
**Recklinghausen-Applebaum disease** (hemochromatosis) 275.0
**Recklinghausen's disease** (M9540/1) 237.71
  bones (osteitis fibrosa cystica) 252.01
**Reclus' disease** (cystic) 610.1
**Recrudescent typhus** (fever) 081.1
**Recruitment, auditory** 388.44
**Rectalgia** 569.42
**Rectitis** 569.49
**Rectocele**
  female (without uterine prolapse) 618.04
    with uterine prolapse 618.4
      complete 618.3
      incomplete 618.2
  in pregnancy or childbirth 654.4 ☑
    causing obstructed labor 660.2 ☑
      affecting fetus or newborn 763.1
  male 569.49
  vagina, vaginal (outlet) 618.04
**Rectosigmoiditis** 569.89
  ulcerative (chronic) 556.3
**Rectosigmoid junction** — *see* condition
**Rectourethral** — *see* condition
**Rectovaginal** — *see* condition
**Rectovesical** — *see* condition
**Rectum, rectal** — *see* condition
**Recurrent** — *see* condition
**Red bugs** 133.8
**Red cedar asthma** 495.8

☑ Additional Digit Required — Refer to the Tabular List for Digit Selection      ▽ Subterms under main terms may continue to next column or page

**2008 ICD-9-CM**      ▶◀ Revised Text      ● New Line      ▲ Revised Code      **Volume 2 — 247**

Index     Reaction — Red cedar asthma

**Redness**
- conjunctiva 379.93
- eye 379.93
- nose 478.19

**Reduced ventilatory or vital capacity** 794.2

**Reduction**
- function
  - kidney (see also Disease, renal) 593.9
  - liver 573.8
- ventilatory capacity 794.2
- vital capacity 794.2

**Redundant, redundancy**
- abdomen 701.9
- anus 751.5
- cardia 537.89
- clitoris 624.2
- colon (congenital) 751.5
- foreskin (congenital) 605
- intestine 751.5
- labia 624.3
- organ or site, congenital NEC — see Accessory
- panniculus (abdominal) 278.1
- prepuce (congenital) 605
- pylorus 537.89
- rectum 751.5
- scrotum 608.89
- sigmoid 751.5
- skin (of face) 701.9
  - eyelids 374.30
- stomach 537.89
- uvula 528.9
- vagina 623.8

**Reduplication** — see Duplication

**Referral**
- adoption (agency) V68.89
- nursing care V63.8
- patient without examination or treatment V68.81
- social services V63.8

**Reflex** — see also condition
- blink, deficient 374.45
- hyperactive gag 478.29
- neurogenic bladder NEC 596.54
  - atonic 596.54
    - with cauda equina syndrome 344.61
- vasoconstriction 443.9
- vasovagal 780.2

**Reflux**
- esophageal 530.81
  - with esophagitis 530.11
- esophagitis 530.11
- gastroesophageal 530.81
- mitral — see Insufficiency, mitral
- ureteral — see Reflux, vesicoureteral
- vesicoureteral 593.70
  - with
    - reflux nephropathy 593.73
      - bilateral 593.72
      - unilateral 593.71

**Reformed gallbladder** 576.0

**Reforming, artificial openings** — see also Attention to, artificial, opening V55.9

**Refractive error** — see also Error, refractive 367.9

**Refsum's disease or syndrome** (heredopathia atactica polyneuritiformis) 356.3

**Refusal of**
- food 307.59
  - hysterical 300.11
- treatment because of, due to patient's decision NEC V64.2
  - reason of conscience or religion V62.6

**Regaud**
- tumor (M8082/3) — see Neoplasm, nasopharynx, malignant
- type carcinoma (M8082/3) — see Neoplasm, nasopharynx, malignant

**Regional** — see condition

**Regulation feeding** (elderly) (infant) 783.3
- newborn 779.3

**Regurgitated**
- food, choked on 933.1
- stomach contents, choked on 933.1

**Regurgitation** 787.03 ▲
- aortic (valve) (see also Insufficiency, aortic) 424.1
  - congenital 746.4
  - syphilitic 093.22
- food (see also Vomiting)
  - with reswallowing — see Rumination
  - newborn 779.3
- gastric contents — see Vomiting
- heart — see Endocarditis
- mitral (valve) (see also Insufficiency, mitral)
  - congenital 746.6
- myocardial — see Endocarditis
- pulmonary (heart) (valve) (see also Endocarditis, pulmonary) 424.3
- stomach — see Vomiting
- tricuspid — see Endocarditis, tricuspid
- valve, valvular — see Endocarditis
- vesicoureteral — see Reflux, vesicoureteral

**Rehabilitation** V57.9
- multiple types V57.89
- occupational V57.21
- specified type NEC V57.89
- speech V57.3
- vocational V57.22

**Reichmann's disease or syndrome** (gastrosuccorrhea) 536.8

**Reifenstein's syndrome** (hereditary familial hypogonadism, male) 259.5

**Reilly's syndrome or phenomenon** — see Neuropathy, peripheral, autonomic 337.9

**Reimann's periodic disease** 277.31

**Reinsertion, contraceptive device** V25.42

**Reiter's disease, syndrome, or urethritis** 099.3 [711.1] ☑

**Rejection**
- food, hysterical 300.11
- transplant 996.80
  - bone marrow 996.85
  - corneal 996.51
  - organ (immune or nonimmune cause) 996.80
    - bone marrow 996.85
    - heart 996.83
    - intestines 996.87
    - kidney 996.81
    - liver 996.82
    - lung 996.84
    - pancreas 996.86
    - specified NEC 996.89
  - skin 996.52
    - artificial 996.55
    - decellularized allodermis 996.55

**Relapsing fever** 087.9
- Carter's (Asiatic) 087.0
- Dutton's (West African) 087.1
- Koch's 087.9
- louse-borne (epidemic) 087.0
- Novy's (American) 087.1
- Obermeyer's (European) 087.0
- Spirillum 087.9
- tick-borne (endemic) 087.1

**Relaxation**
- anus (sphincter) 569.49
  - due to hysteria 300.11
- arch (foot) 734
  - congenital 754.61
- back ligaments 728.4
- bladder (sphincter) 596.59
- cardio-esophageal 530.89
- cervix (see also Incompetency, cervix) 622.5
- diaphragm 519.4
- inguinal rings — see Hernia, inguinal

**Relaxation** — continued
- joint (capsule) (ligament) (paralytic) (see also Derangement, joint) 718.90
  - congenital 755.8
- lumbosacral joint 724.6
- pelvic floor 618.89
- pelvis 618.89
- perineum 618.89
- posture 729.9
- rectum (sphincter) 569.49
- sacroiliac (joint) 724.6
- scrotum 608.89
- urethra (sphincter) 599.84
- uterus (outlet) 618.89
- vagina (outlet) 618.89
- vesical 596.59

**Remains**
- canal of Cloquet 743.51
- capsule (opaque) 743.51

**Remittent fever** (malarial) 084.6

**Remnant**
- canal of Cloquet 743.51
- capsule (opaque) 743.51
- cervix, cervical stump (acquired) (postoperative) 622.8
- cystic duct, postcholecystectomy 576.0
- fingernail 703.8
  - congenital 757.5
- meniscus, knee 717.5
- thyroglossal duct 759.2
- tonsil 474.8
  - infected 474.00
- urachus 753.7

**Remote effect of cancer** — see condition

**Removal** (of)
- catheter (urinary) (indwelling) V53.6
  - from artificial opening — see Attention to, artificial, opening
    - non-vascular V58.82
    - vascular V58.81
- cerebral ventricle (communicating) shunt V53.01
- device (see also Fitting (of))
  - contraceptive V25.42
  - fixation
    - external V54.89
    - internal V54.01
  - traction V54.89
- drains V58.49
- dressing
  - wound V58.30
    - nonsurgical V58.30
    - surgical V58.31
- ileostomy V55.2
- Kirschner wire V54.89
- nonvascular catheter V58.82
- pin V54.01
- plaster cast V54.89
- plate (fracture) V54.01
- rod V54.01
- screw V54.01
- splint, external V54.89
- staples V58.32
- subdermal implantable contraceptive V25.43
- sutures V58.32
- traction device, external V54.89
- vascular catheter V58.81
- wound packing V58.30
  - nonsurgical V58.30
  - surgical V58.31

**Ren**
- arcuatus 753.3
- mobile, mobilis (see also Disease, renal) 593.0
  - congenital 753.3
- unguliformis 753.3

**Renal** — see also condition
- glomerulohyalinosis-diabetic syndrome 250.4 ☑ [581.81]

**Rendu-Osler-Weber disease or syndrome** (familial hemorrhagic telangiectasia) 448.0

**Reninoma** (M8361/1) 236.91

**Rénon-Delille syndrome** 253.8

**Repair**
- pelvic floor, previous, in pregnancy or childbirth 654.4 ☑
  - affecting fetus or newborn 763.89
- scarred tissue V51

**Replacement by artificial or mechanical device or prosthesis of** — see also Fitting (of)
- artificial skin V43.83
- bladder V43.5
- blood vessel V43.4
- breast V43.82
- eye globe V43.0
- heart
  - with
    - assist device V43.21
    - fully implantable artificial heart V43.22
  - valve V43.3
- intestine V43.89
- joint V43.60
  - ankle V43.66
  - elbow V43.62
  - finger V43.69
  - hip (partial) (total) V43.64
  - knee V43.65
  - shoulder V43.61
  - specified NEC V43.69
  - wrist V43.63
- kidney V43.89
- larynx V43.81
- lens V43.1
- limb(s) V43.7
- liver V43.89
- lung V43.89
- organ NEC V43.89
- pancreas V43.89
- skin (artificial) V43.83
- tissue NEC V43.89

**Reprogramming**
- cardiac pacemaker V53.31

**Request for expert evidence** V68.2

**Reserve, decreased or low**
- cardiac — see Disease, heart
- kidney (see also Disease, renal) 593.9

**Residual** — see also condition
- bladder 596.8
- foreign body — see Retention, foreign body
- state, schizophrenic (see also Schizophrenia) 295.6 ☑
- urine 788.69

**Resistance, resistant** (to)
- activated protein C 289.81

Note — use the following subclassification for categories V09.5, V09.7, V09.8, V09.9:

| 0 | without mention of resistance to multiple drugs |
| 1 | with resistance to multiple drugs |

V09.5 quinolones and fluoroquinolones

V09.7 antimycobacterial agents

V09.8 specified drugs NEC

V09.9 unspecified drugs

- drugs by microorganisms V09.9 ☑
  - Amikacin V09.4
  - aminoglycosides V09.4
  - Amodiaquine V09.5 ☑
  - Amoxicillin V09.0
  - Ampicillin V09.0
  - antimycobacterial agents V09.7 ☑
  - Azithromycin V09.2
  - Azlocillin V09.0
  - Aztreonam V09.1
  - Bacampicillin V09.0
  - Bacitracin V09.8 ☑
  - Benznidazole V09.8 ☑
  - B-lactam antibiotics V09.1

**Resistance, resistant** — *continued*
drugs by microorganisms — *continued*
  Capreomycin V09.7 ☑
  Carbenicillin V09.0
  Cefaclor V09.1
  Cefadroxil V09.1
  Cefamandole V09.1
  Cefatetan V09.1
  Cefazolin V09.1
  Cefixime V09.1
  Cefonicid V09.1
  Cefoperazone V09.1
  Ceforanide V09.1
  Cefotaxime V09.1
  Cefoxitin V09.1
  Ceftazidime V09.1
  Ceftizoxime V09.1
  Ceftriaxone V09.1
  Cefuroxime V09.1
  Cephalexin V09.1
  Cephaloglycin V09.1
  Cephaloridine V09.1
  Cephalosporins V09.1
  Cephalothin V09.1
  Cephapirin V09.1
  Cephradine V09.1
  Chloramphenicol V09.8 ☑
  Chloroquine V09.5 ☑
  Chlorguanide V09.8 ☑
  Chlorproguanil V09.8 ☑
  Chlortetracyline V09.3
  Cinoxacin V09.5 ☑
  Ciprofloxacin V09.5 ☑
  Clarithromycin V09.2
  Clindamycin V09.8 ☑
  Clioquinol V09.5 ☑
  Clofazimine V09.7 ☑
  Cloxacillin V09.0
  Cyclacillin V09.0
  Cycloserine V09.7 ☑
  Dapsone [DZ] V09.7 ☑
  Demeclocycline V09.3
  Dicloxacillin V09.0
  Doxycycline V09.3
  Enoxacin V09.5 ☑
  Erythromycin V09.2
  Ethambutol [EMB] V09.7 ☑
  Ethionamide [ETA] V09.7 ☑
  fluoroquinolones V09.5 ☑
  Gentamicin V09.4
  Halofantrine V09.8 ☑
  Imipenem V09.1
  Iodoquinol V09.5 ☑
  Isoniazid [INH] V09.7 ☑
  Kanamycin V09.4
  macrolides V09.2
  Mafenide V09.6
  MDRO (multiple drug resistant organisms) NOS V09.91
  Mefloquine V09.8 ☑
  Melasoprol V09.8 ☑
  Methacycline V09.3
  Methenamine V09.8 ☑
  Methicillin V09.0
  Metronidazole V09.8 ☑
  Mezlocillin V09.0
  Minocycline V09.3
  multiple drug resistant organisms NOS V09.91
  Nafcillin V09.0
  Nalidixic acid V09.5 ☑
  Natamycin V09.2
  Neomycin V09.4
  Netilmicin V09.4
  Nimorazole V09.8 ☑
  Nitrofurantoin V09.8 ☑
  Nitrofurtimox V09.8 ☑
  Norfloxacin V09.5 ☑
  Nystatin V09.2
  Ofloxacin V09.5 ☑
  Oleandomycin V09.2
  Oxacillin V09.0
  Oxytetracycline V09.3

**Resistance, resistant** — *continued*
drugs by microorganisms — *continued*
  Para-amino salicylic acid [PAS] V09.7 ☑
  Paromomycin V09.4
  Penicillin (G) (V) (VK) V09.0
  penicillins V09.0
  Pentamidine V09.8 ☑
  Piperacillin V09.0
  Primaquine V09.5 ☑
  Proguanil V09.8 ☑
  Pyrazinamide [PZA] V09.7 ☑
  Pyrimethamine/Sulfalene V09.8 ☑
  Pyrimethamine/Sulfodoxine V09.8 ☑
  Quinacrine V09.5 ☑
  Quinidine V09.8 ☑
  Quinine V09.8 ☑
  quinolones V09.5 ☑
  Rifabutin V09.7 ☑
  Rifampin [RIF] V09.7 ☑
  Rifamycin V09.7 ☑
  Rolitetracycline V09.3
  specified drugs NEC V09.8 ☑
  Spectinomycin V09.8 ☑
  Spiramycin V09.2
  Streptomycin [SM] V09.4
  Sulfacetamide V09.6
  Sulfacytine V09.6
  Sulfadiazine V09.6
  Sulfadoxine V09.6
  Sulfamethoxazole V09.6
  Sulfapyridine V09.6
  Sulfasalizine V09.6
  Sulfasoxazole V09.6
  sulfonamides V09.6
  Sulfoxone V09.7 ☑
  tetracycline V09.3
  tetracyclines V09.3
  Thiamphenicol V09.8 ☑
  Ticarcillin V09.0
  Tinidazole V09.8 ☑
  Tobramycin V09.4
  Triamphenicol V09.8 ☑
  Trimethoprim V09.8 ☑
  Vancomycin V09.8 ☑
insulin 277.7
thyroid hormone 246.8
**Resorption**
biliary 576.8
  purulent or putrid (*see also* Cholecystitis) 576.8
dental (roots) 521.40
  alveoli 525.8
  pathological
    external 521.42
    internal 521.41
    specified NEC 521.49
septic — *see* Septicemia
teeth (roots) 521.40
  pathological
    external 521.42
    internal 521.41
    specified NEC 521.49
**Respiration**
asymmetrical 786.09
bronchial 786.09
Cheyne-Stokes (periodic respiration) 786.04
decreased, due to shock following injury 958.4
disorder of 786.00
  psychogenic 306.1
  specified NEC 786.09
failure 518.81
  acute 518.81
  acute and chronic 518.84
  chronic 518.83
  newborn 770.84
insufficiency 786.09
  acute 518.82
  newborn NEC 770.89
Kussmaul (air hunger) 786.09
painful 786.52
periodic 786.09

**Respiration** — *continued*
periodic — *continued*
  high altitude 327.22
poor 786.09
  newborn NEC 770.89
sighing 786.7
  psychogenic 306.1
wheezing 786.07
**Respiratory** — *see also* condition
distress 786.09
  acute 518.82
  fetus or newborn NEC 770.89
  syndrome (newborn) 769
    adult (following shock, surgery, or trauma) 518.5
    specified NEC 518.82
failure 518.81
  acute 518.81
  acute and chronic 518.84
  chronic 518.83
**Respiratory syncytial virus (RSV)** 079.6
bronchiolitis 466.11
pneumonia 480.1
vaccination, prophylactic (against) V04.82
**Response**
photoallergic 692.72
phototoxic 692.72
**Restless legs syndrome (RLS)** 333.94
**Restlessness** 799.2
**Restoration of organ continuity from previous sterilization** (tuboplasty) (vasoplasty) V26.0
**Rest, rests**
mesonephric duct 752.89
  fallopian tube 752.11
ovarian, in fallopian tubes 752.19
wolffian duct 752.89
**Restriction of housing space** V60.1
**Restzustand, schizophrenic** — *see also*
Schizophrenia 295.6 ☑
**Retained** — *see* Retention
**Retardation**
development, developmental, specific (*see also* Disorder, development, specific) 315.9
  learning, specific 315.2
    arithmetical 315.1
    language (skills) 315.31
      expressive 315.31
      mixed receptive-expressive 315.32
    mathematics 315.1
    reading 315.00
      phonological 315.39
    written expression 315.2
  motor 315.4
endochondral bone growth 733.91
growth (physical) in childhood 783.43
  due to malnutrition 263.2
  fetal (intrauterine) 764.9 ☑
    affecting management of pregnancy 656.5 ☑
intrauterine growth 764.9 ☑
  affecting management of pregnancy 656.5 ☑
mental 319
  borderline V62.89
  mild, IQ 50-70 317
  moderate, IQ 35-49 318.0
  profound, IQ under 20 318.2
  severe, IQ 20-34 318.1
motor, specific 315.4
physical 783.43
  child 783.43
  due to malnutrition 263.2
  fetus (intrauterine) 764.9 ☑
    affecting management of pregnancy 656.5 ☑
psychomotor NEC 307.9
reading 315.00
**Retching** — *see* Vomiting
**Retention, retained**
bladder (*see also* Retention, urine) 788.20
  psychogenic 306.53

**Retention, retained** — *continued*
carbon dioxide 276.2
cyst — *see* Cyst
dead
  fetus (after 22 completed weeks gestation) 656.4 ☑
    early fetal death (before 22 completed weeks gestation) 632
  ovum 631
decidua (following delivery) (fragments) (with hemorrhage) 666.2 ☑
  without hemorrhage 667.1 ☑
deciduous tooth 520.6
dental root 525.3
fecal (*see also* Constipation) 564.00
fluid 276.6
foreign body (*see also* Foreign body, retained)
  bone 733.99
  current trauma — *see* Foreign body, by site or type
  middle ear 385.83
  muscle 729.6
  soft tissue NEC 729.6
gastric 536.8
membranes (following delivery) (with hemorrhage) 666.2 ☑
  with abortion — *see* Abortion, by type
  without hemorrhage 667.1 ☑
menses 626.8
milk (puerperal) 676.2 ☑
nitrogen, extrarenal 788.9
placenta (total) (with hemorrhage) 666.0 ☑
  with abortion — *see* Abortion, by type
  without hemorrhage 667.0 ☑
  portions or fragments 666.2 ☑
    without hemorrhage 667.1 ☑
products of conception
  early pregnancy (fetal death before 22 completed weeks gestation) 632
  following
    abortion — *see* Abortion, by type
    delivery 666.2 ☑
      with hemorrhage 666.2 ☑
      without hemorrhage 667.1 ☑
secundines (following delivery) (with hemorrhage) 666.2 ☑
  with abortion — *see* Abortion, by type
  without hemorrhage 667.1 ☑
  complicating puerperium (delayed hemorrhage) 666.2 ☑
smegma, clitoris 624.8
urine NEC 788.20
  bladder, incomplete emptying 788.21
  due to
    benign prostatic hypertrophy (BPH) — *see* category 600
  due to
    benign prostatic hypertrophy (BPH) — *see* category 600
  psychogenic 306.53
  specified NEC 788.29
water (in tissue) (*see also* Edema) 782.3
**Reticulation, dust** (occupational) 504
**Reticulocytosis** NEC 790.99
**Reticuloendotheliosis**
acute infantile (M9722/3) 202.5 ☑
leukemic (M9940/3) 202.4 ☑
malignant (M9720/3) 202.3 ☑
nonlipid (M9722/3) 202.5 ☑
**Reticulohistiocytoma** (giant cell) 277.89
**Reticulohistiocytosis, multicentric** 272.8
**Reticulolymphosarcoma** (diffuse) (M9613/3) 200.8 ☑
follicular (M9691/3) 202.0 ☑

☑ Additional Digit Required — Refer to the Tabular List for Digit Selection      ▽ Subterms under main terms may continue to next column or page

**2008 ICD-9-CM**     ▶◀ Revised Text     ● New Line     ▲ Revised Code     **Volume 2 — 249**

**Reticulolymphosarcoma —**
*continued*
    nodular (M9691/3) 202.0 ☑
**Reticulosarcoma** (M9640/3) 200.0 ☑
    nodular (M9642/3) 200.0 ☑
    pleomorphic cell type (M9641/3)
        200.0 ☑
**Reticulosis** (skin)
    acute of infancy (M9722/3) 202.5 ☑
    familial hemophagocytic 288.4
    histiocytic medullary (M9721/3)
        202.3 ☑
    lipomelanotic 695.89
    malignant (M9720/3) 202.3 ☑
    Sézary's (M9701/3) 202.2 ☑
**Retina, retinal** — *see* condition
**Retinitis** — *see also* Chorioretinitis
        363.20
    albuminurica 585.9 *[363.10]*
    arteriosclerotic 440.8 *[362.13]*
    central angiospastic 362.41
    Coat's 362.12
    diabetic 250.5 ☑ *[362.01]*
    disciformis 362.52
    disseminated 363.10
        metastatic 363.14
        neurosyphilitic 094.83
        pigment epitheliopathy 363.15
    exudative 362.12
    focal 363.00
        in histoplasmosis 115.92
            capsulatum 115.02
            duboisii 115.12
        juxtapapillary 363.05
        macular 363.06
        paramacular 363.06
        peripheral 363.08
        posterior pole NEC 363.07
    gravidarum 646.8 ☑
    hemorrhagica externa 362.12
    juxtapapillary (Jensen's) 363.05
    luetic — *see* Retinitis, syphilitic
    metastatic 363.14
    pigmentosa 362.74
    proliferans 362.29
    proliferating 362.29
    punctata albescens 362.76
    renal 585.9 *[363.13]*
    syphilitic (secondary) 091.51
        congenital 090.0 *[363.13]*
        early 091.51
        late 095.8 *[363.13]*
    syphilitica, central, recurrent
        095.8 *[363.13]*
    tuberculous (*see also* Tuberculous)
        017.3 ☑ *[363.13]*
**Retinoblastoma** (M9510/3) 190.5
    differentiated type (M9511/3) 190.5
    undifferentiated type (M9512/3) 190.5
**Retinochoroiditis** — *see also* Chorioretinitis 363.20
    central angiospastic 362.41
    disseminated 363.10
        metastatic 363.14
        neurosyphilitic 094.83
        pigment epitheliopathy 363.15
        syphilitic 094.83
    due to toxoplasmosis (acquired) (focal)
        130.2
    focal 363.00
        in histoplasmosis 115.92
            capsulatum 115.02
            duboisii 115.12
        juxtapapillary (Jensen's) 363.05
        macular 363.06
        paramacular 363.06
        peripheral 363.08
        posterior pole NEC 363.07
    juxtapapillaris 363.05
    syphilitic (disseminated) 094.83
**Retinopathy** (background) 362.10
    arteriosclerotic 440.8 *[362.13]*
    atherosclerotic 440.8 *[362.13]*
    central serous 362.41
    circinate 362.10
    Coat's 362.12

**Retinopathy** — *continued*
    diabetic 250.5 ☑ *[362.01]*
        nonproliferative 250.5 ☑ *[362.03]*
            mild 250.5 ☑ *[362.04]*
            moderate 250.5 ☑ *[362.05]*
            severe 250.5 ☑ *[362.06]*
        proliferative 250.5 ☑ *[362.02]*
    exudative 362.12
    hypertensive 362.11
    nonproliferative
        diabetic 250.5 ☑ *[362.03]*
            mild 250.5 ☑ *[362.04]*
            moderate 250.5 ☑ *[362.05]*
            severe 250.5 ☑ *[362.06]*
    of prematurity 362.21
    pigmentary, congenital 362.74
    proliferative 362.29
        diabetic 250.5 ☑ *[362.02]*
        sickle-cell 282.60 *[362.29]*
    solar 363.31
**Retinoschisis** 361.10
    bullous 361.12
    congenital 743.56
    flat 361.11
    juvenile 362.73
**Retractile testis** 752.52
**Retraction**
    cervix — *see* Retraction, uterus
    drum (membrane) 384.82
    eyelid 374.41
    finger 736.29
    head 781.0
    lid 374.41
    lung 518.89
    mediastinum 519.3
    nipple 611.79
        congenital 757.6
        puerperal, postpartum 676.0 ☑
    palmar fascia 728.6
    pleura (*see also* Pleurisy) 511.0
    ring, uterus (Bandl's) (pathological)
        661.4 ☑
        affecting fetus or newborn 763.7
    sternum (congenital) 756.3
        acquired 738.3
        during respiration 786.9
    substernal 738.3
    supraclavicular 738.8
    syndrome (Duane's) 378.71
    uterus 621.6
    valve (heart) — *see* Endocarditis
**Retrobulbar** — *see* condition
**Retrocaval ureter** 753.4
**Retrocecal** — *see also* condition
    appendix (congenital) 751.5
**Retrocession** — *see* Retroversion
**Retrodisplacement** — *see* Retroversion
**Retroflection, retroflexion** — *see*
    Retroversion
**Retrognathia, retrognathism**
    (mandibular) (maxillary) 524.10
**Retrograde**
    ejaculation 608.87
    menstruation 626.8
**Retroiliac ureter** 753.4
**Retroperineal** — *see* condition
**Retroperitoneal** — *see* condition
**Retroperitonitis** 567.39
**Retropharyngeal** — *see* condition
**Retroplacental** — *see* condition
**Retroposition** — *see* Retroversion
**Retrosternal thyroid** (congenital) 759.2
**Retroversion, retroverted**
    cervix — *see* Retroversion, uterus
    female NEC (*see also* Retroversion,
        uterus) 621.6
    iris 364.70
    testis (congenital) 752.51
    uterus, uterine (acquired) (acute) (adherent) (any degree) (asymptomatic) (cervix) (postinfectional)
        (postpartal, old) 621.6
        congenital 752.3
        in pregnancy or childbirth 654.3 ☑
            affecting fetus or newborn
                763.89

**Retroversion, retroverted —**
*continued*
    uterus, uterine — *continued*
        in pregnancy or childbirth — *continued*
            causing obstructed labor
                660.2 ☑
                affecting fetus or newborn
                    763.1
**Retrusion, premaxilla** (developmental)
    524.04
**Rett's syndrome** 330.8
**Reverse, reversed**
    peristalsis 787.4
**Reye-Sheehan syndrome** (postpartum
    pituitary necrosis) 253.2
**Reye's syndrome** 331.81
**Rh** (factor)
    hemolytic disease 773.0
    incompatibility, immunization, or
        sensitization
        affecting management of pregnancy
            656.1 ☑
        fetus or newborn 773.0
        transfusion reaction 999.7
    negative mother, affecting fetus or
        newborn 773.0
    titer elevated 999.7
    transfusion reaction 999.7
**Rhabdomyolysis** (idiopathic) 728.88
**Rhabdomyoma** (M8900/0) — *see also*
    Neoplasm, connective tissue, benign
    adult (M8904/0) — *see* Neoplasm,
        connective tissue, benign
    fetal (M8903/0) — *see* Neoplasm,
        connective tissue, benign
    glycogenic (M8904/0) — *see* Neoplasm, connective tissue, benign
**Rhabdomyosarcoma** (M8900/3) — *see
    also* Neoplasm, connective tissue,
    malignant
    alveolar (M8920/3) — *see* Neoplasm,
        connective tissue, malignant
    embryonal (M8910/3) — *see* Neoplasm, connective tissue, malignant
    mixed type (M8902/3) — *see* Neoplasm, connective tissue, malignant
    pleomorphic (M8901/3) — *see* Neoplasm, connective tissue, malignant
**Rhabdosarcoma** (M8900/3) — *see*
    Rhabdomyosarcoma
**Rhesus** (factor) (Rh) incompatibility —
    *see* Rh, incompatibility
**Rheumaticosis** — *see* Rheumatism
**Rheumatism, rheumatic** (acute NEC)
    729.0
    adherent pericardium 393
    arthritis
        acute or subacute — *see* Fever,
            rheumatic
        chronic 714.0
            spine 720.0
        articular (chronic) NEC (*see also*
            Arthritis) 716.9 ☑
        acute or subacute — *see* Fever,
            rheumatic
    back 724.9
    blennorrhagic 098.59
    carditis — *see* Disease, heart,
        rheumatic
    cerebral — *see* Fever, rheumatic
    chorea (acute) — *see* Chorea,
        rheumatic
    chronic NEC 729.0
    coronary arteritis 391.9
        chronic 398.99
    degeneration, myocardium (*see also*
        Degeneration, myocardium, with
        rheumatic fever) 398.0
    desert 114.0
    febrile — *see* Fever, rheumatic
    fever — *see* Fever, rheumatic

**Rheumatism, rheumatic —**
*continued*
    gonococcal 098.59
    gout 274.0
    heart
        disease (*see also* Disease, heart,
            rheumatic) 398.90
        failure (chronic) (congestive) (inactive) 398.91
        hemopericardium — *see* Rheumatic,
            pericarditis
        hydropericardium — *see* Rheumatic,
            pericarditis
        inflammatory (acute) (chronic) (subacute) — *see* Fever, rheumatic
    intercostal 729.0
        meaning Tietze's disease 733.6
    joint (chronic) NEC (*see also* Arthritis)
        716.9 ☑
        acute — *see* Fever, rheumatic
    mediastinopericarditis — *see*
        Rheumatic, pericarditis
    muscular 729.0
    myocardial degeneration (*see also*
        Degeneration, myocardial, with
        rheumatic fever) 398.0
    myocarditis (chronic) (inactive) (with
        chorea) 398.0
        active or acute 391.2
            with chorea (acute) (rheumatic)
                (Sydenham's) 392.0
    myositis 729.1
    neck 724.9
    neuralgic 729.0
    neuritis (acute) (chronic) 729.2
    neuromuscular 729.0
    nodose — *see* Arthritis, nodosa
    nonarticular 729.0
    palindromic 719.30
        ankle 719.37
        elbow 719.32
        foot 719.37
        hand 719.34
        hip 719.35
        knee 719.36
        multiple sites 719.39
        pelvic region 719.35
        shoulder (region) 719.31
        specified site NEC 719.38
        wrist 719.33
    pancarditis, acute 391.8
        with chorea (acute) (rheumatic)
            (Sydenham's) 392.0
        chronic or inactive 398.99
    pericarditis (active) (acute) (with effusion) (with pneumonia) 391.0
        with chorea (acute) (rheumatic)
            (Sydenham's) 392.0
        chronic or inactive 393
    pericardium — *see* Rheumatic, pericarditis
    pleuropericarditis — *see* Rheumatic,
        pericarditis
    pneumonia 390 *[517.1]*
    pneumonitis 390 *[517.1]*
    pneumopericarditis — *see* Rheumatic,
        pericarditis
    polyarthritis
        acute or subacute — *see* Fever,
            rheumatic
        chronic 714.0
    polyarticular NEC (*see also* Arthritis)
        716.9 ☑
    psychogenic 306.0
    radiculitis 729.2
    sciatic 724.3
    septic — *see* Fever, rheumatic
    spine 724.9
    subacute NEC 729.0
    torticollis 723.5
    tuberculous NEC (*see also* Tuberculosis) 015.9 ☑
    typhoid fever 002.0
**Rheumatoid** — *see also* condition
    lungs 714.81

**Rhinitis** (atrophic) (catarrhal) (chronic) (croupous) (fibrinous) (hyperplastic) (hypertrophic) (membranous) (purulent) (suppurative) (ulcerative) 472.0
  with
    hay fever (see also Fever, hay) 477.9
      with asthma (bronchial) 493.0 ☑
    sore throat — see Nasopharyngitis
  acute 460
  allergic (nonseasonal) (seasonal) (see also Fever, hay) 477.9
    with asthma (see also Asthma) 493.0 ☑
    due to food 477.1
  granulomatous 472.0
  infective 460
  obstructive 472.0
  pneumococcal 460
  syphilitic 095.8
    congenital 090.0
  tuberculous (see also Tuberculosis) 012.8 ☑
  vasomotor (see also Fever, hay) 477.9
**Rhinoantritis** (chronic) 473.0
  acute 461.0
**Rhinodacryolith** 375.57
**Rhinolalia** (aperta) (clausa) (open) 784.49
**Rhinolith** 478.19
  nasal sinus (see also Sinusitis) 473.9
**Rhinomegaly** 478.19
**Rhinopharyngitis** (acute) (subacute) — see also Nasopharyngitis 460
  chronic 472.2
  destructive ulcerating 102.5
  mutilans 102.5
**Rhinophyma** 695.3
**Rhinorrhea** 478.19
  cerebrospinal (fluid) 349.81
  paroxysmal (see also Fever, hay) 477.9
  spasmodic (see also Fever, hay) 477.9
**Rhinosalpingitis** 381.50
  acute 381.51
  chronic 381.52
**Rhinoscleroma** 040.1
**Rhinosporidiosis** 117.0
**Rhinovirus infection** 079.3
**Rhizomelic chrondrodysplasia punctata** 277.86
**Rhizomelique, pseudopolyarthritic** 446.5
**Rhoads and Bomford anemia** (refractory) 238.72
**Rhus**
  diversiloba dermatitis 692.6
  radicans dermatitis 692.6
  toxicodendron dermatitis 692.6
  venenata dermatitis 692.6
  verniciflua dermatitis 692.6
**Rhythm**
  atrioventricular nodal 427.89
  disorder 427.9
    coronary sinus 427.89
    ectopic 427.89
    nodal 427.89
  escape 427.89
  heart, abnormal 427.9
    fetus or newborn — see Abnormal, heart rate
  idioventricular 426.89
    accelerated 427.89
  nodal 427.89
  sleep, inversion 327.39
    nonorganic origin 307.45
**Rhytidosis facialis** 701.8
**Rib** — see also condition
  cervical 756.2
**Riboflavin deficiency** 266.0
**Rice bodies** — see also Loose, body, joint 718.1 ☑
  knee 717.6
**Richter's hernia** — see Hernia, Richter's
**Ricinism** 988.2

**Rickets** (active) (acute) (adolescent) (adult) (chest wall) (congenital) (current) (infantile) (intestinal) 268.0
  celiac 579.0
  fetal 756.4
  hemorrhagic 267
  hypophosphatemic with nephroticglycosuric dwarfism 270.0
  kidney 588.0
  late effect 268.1
  renal 588.0
  scurvy 267
  vitamin D-resistant 275.3
**Rickettsial disease** 083.9
  specified type NEC 083.8
**Rickettsialpox** 083.2
**Rickettsiosis** NEC 083.9
  specified type NEC 083.8
  tick-borne 082.9
    specified type NEC 082.8
  vesicular 083.2
**Ricord's chancre** 091.0
**Riddoch's syndrome** (visual disorientation) 368.16
**Rider's**
  bone 733.99
  chancre 091.0
**Ridge, alveolus** — see also condition
  edentulous
    atrophy 525.20
      mandible 525.20
        minimal 525.21
        moderate 525.22
        severe 525.23
      maxilla 525.20
        minimal 525.24
        moderate 525.25
        severe 525.26
    flabby 525.20
**Ridged ear** 744.29
**Riedel's**
  disease (ligneous thyroiditis) 245.3
  lobe, liver 751.69
  struma (ligneous thyroiditis) 245.3
  thyroiditis (ligneous) 245.3
**Rieger's anomaly or syndrome** (mesodermal dysgenesis, anterior ocular segment) 743.44
**Riehl's melanosis** 709.09
**Rietti-Greppi-Micheli anemia or syndrome** 282.49
**Rieux's hernia** — see Hernia, Rieux's
**Rift Valley fever** 066.3
**Riga's disease** (cachectic aphthae) 529.0
**Riga-Fede disease** (cachectic aphthae) 529.0
**Riggs' disease** (compound periodontitis) 523.40
**Right middle lobe syndrome** 518.0
**Rigid, rigidity** — see also condition
  abdominal 789.4 ☑
  articular, multiple congenital 754.89
  back 724.8
  cervix uteri
    in pregnancy or childbirth 654.6 ☑
      affecting fetus or newborn 763.89
      causing obstructed labor 660.2 ☑
      affecting fetus or newborn 763.1
  hymen (acquired) (congenital) 623.3
  nuchal 781.6
  pelvic floor
    in pregnancy or childbirth 654.4 ☑
      affecting fetus or newborn 763.89
      causing obstructed labor 660.2 ☑
      affecting fetus or newborn 763.1
  perineum or vulva
    in pregnancy or childbirth 654.8 ☑
      affecting fetus or newborn 763.89

**Rigid, rigidity** — see also condition — continued
  perineum or vulva — continued
    in pregnancy or childbirth — continued
      causing obstructed labor 660.2 ☑
      affecting fetus or newborn 763.1
  spine 724.8
  vagina
    in pregnancy or childbirth 654.7 ☑
      affecting fetus or newborn 763.89
      causing obstructed labor 660.2 ☑
      affecting fetus or newborn 763.1
**Rigors** 780.99
**Riley-Day syndrome** (familial dysautonomia) 742.8
**RIND** (reversible ischemic neurological deficit) 434.91 ●
  history of (personal) V12.54 ●
**Ring(s)**
  aorta 747.21
  Bandl's, complicating delivery 661.4 ☑
    affecting fetus or newborn 763.7
  contraction, complicating delivery 661.4 ☑
    affecting fetus or newborn 763.7
  esophageal (congenital) 750.3
  Fleischer (-Kayser) (cornea) 275.1 [371.14]
  hymenal, tight (acquired) (congenital) 623.3
  Kayser-Fleischer (cornea) 275.1 [371.14]
  retraction, uterus, pathological 661.4 ☑
    affecting fetus or newborn 763.7
  Schatzki's (esophagus) (congenital) (lower) 750.3
    acquired 530.3
  Soemmering's 366.51
  trachea, abnormal 748.3
  vascular (congenital) 747.21
  Vossius' 921.3
    late effect 366.21
**Ringed hair** (congenital) 757.4
**Ringing in the ear** — see also Tinnitus 388.30
**Ringworm** 110.9
  beard 110.0
  body 110.5
  Burmese 110.9
  corporeal 110.5
  foot 110.4
  groin 110.3
  hand 110.2
  honeycomb 110.0
  nails 110.1
  perianal (area) 110.3
  scalp 110.0
  specified site NEC 110.8
  Tokelau 110.5
**Rise, venous pressure** 459.89
**Risk**
  factor — see Problem
  falling
    suicidal 300.9
**Ritter's disease** (dermatitis exfoliativa neonatorum) 695.81
**Rivalry, sibling** 313.3
**Rivalta's disease** (cervicofacial actinomycosis) 039.3
**River blindness** 125.3 [360.13]
**Robert's pelvis** 755.69
  with disproportion (fetopelvic) 653.0 ☑
    affecting fetus or newborn 763.1
    causing obstructed labor 660.1 ☑
      affecting fetus or newborn 763.1
**Robinson's** (hidrotic) **ectodermal dysplasia** 757.31
**Robin's syndrome** 756.0

**Robles' disease** (onchocerciasis) 125.3 [360.13]
**Rochalimea** — see Rickettsial disease
**Rocky Mountain fever** (spotted) 082.0
**Rodent ulcer** (M8090/3) — see also Neoplasm, skin, malignant
  cornea 370.07
**Roentgen ray, adverse effect** — see Effect, adverse, x-ray
**Roetheln** 056.9
**Roger's disease** (congenital interventricular septal defect) 745.4
**Rokitansky's**
  disease (see also Necrosis, liver) 570
  tumor 620.2
**Rokitansky-Aschoff sinuses** (mucosal outpouching of gallbladder) — see also Disease, gallbladder 575.8
**Rokitansky-Kuster-Hauser syndrome** (congenital absence vagina) 752.49
**Rollet's chancre** (syphilitic) 091.0
**Rolling of head** 781.0
**Romano-Ward syndrome** (prolonged QT interval syndrome) 426.82
**Romanus lesion** 720.1
**Romberg's disease or syndrome** 349.89
**Roof, mouth** — see condition
**Rosacea** 695.3
  acne 695.3
  keratitis 695.3 [370.49]
**Rosary, rachitic** 268.0
**Rose**
  cold 477.0
  fever 477.0
  rash 782.1
    epidemic 056.9
    of infants 057.8
**Rosenbach's erysipelatoid or erysipeloid** 027.1
**Rosen-Castleman-Liebow syndrome** (pulmonary proteinosis) 516.0
**Rosenthal's disease** (factor XI deficiency) 286.2
**Roseola** 057.8
  infantum, infantilis ▶(see also Exanthem subitum)◀ 058.10 ▲
**Rossbach's disease** (hyperchlorhydria) 536.8
  psychogenic 306.4
**Rössle-Urbach-Wiethe lipoproteinosis** 272.8
**Ross river fever** 066.3
**Rostan's asthma** (cardiac) — see also Failure, ventricular, left 428.1
**Rot**
  Barcoo (see also Ulcer, skin) 707.9
  knife-grinders' (see also Tuberculosis) 011.4 ☑
**Rotation**
  anomalous, incomplete or insufficient — see Malrotation
  cecum (congenital) 751.4
  colon (congenital) 751.4
  manual, affecting fetus or newborn 763.89
  spine, incomplete or insufficient 737.8
  tooth, teeth 524.35
  vertebra, incomplete or insufficient 737.8
**Rot-Bernhardt disease** 355.1
**Röteln** 056.9
**Roth-Bernhardt disease or syndrome** 355.1
**Roth's disease or meralgia** 355.1
**Rothmund (-Thomson) syndrome** 757.33
**Rotor's disease or syndrome** (idiopathic hyperbilirubinemia) 277.4
**Rotundum ulcus** — see Ulcer, stomach
**Round**
  back (with wedging of vertebrae) 737.10
    late effect of rickets 268.1
  hole, retina 361.31
    with detachment 361.01
  ulcer (stomach) — see Ulcer, stomach

---

☑ Additional Digit Required — Refer to the Tabular List for Digit Selection
           ▽ Subterms under main terms may continue to next column or page

**Round** — *continued*
   worms (infestation) (large) NEC 127.0
**Roussy-Lévy syndrome** 334.3
**Routine postpartum follow-up** V24.2
**Roy (-Jutras) syndrome** (acropachyderma) 757.39
**Rubella** (German measles) 056.9
   complicating pregnancy, childbirth, or puerperium 647.5 ☑
   complication 056.8
     neurological 056.00
      encephalomyelitis 056.01
       specified type NEC 056.09
      specified type NEC 056.79
   congenital 771.0
   contact V01.4
   exposure to V01.4
   maternal
     with suspected fetal damage affecting management of pregnancy 655.3 ☑
     affecting fetus or newborn 760.2
      manifest rubella in infant 771.0
   specified complications NEC 056.79
   vaccination, prophylactic (against) V04.3
**Rubeola** (measles) — *see also* Measles 055.9
   complicated 055.8
   meaning rubella (*see also* Rubella) 056.9
   scarlatinosis 057.8
**Rubeosis iridis** 364.42
   diabetica 250.5 ☑ *[364.42]*
**Rubinstein-Taybi's syndrome** (brachydactylia, short stature and mental retardation) 759.89
**Rudimentary** (congenital) — *see also* Agenesis
   arm 755.22
   bone 756.9
   cervix uteri 752.49
   eye (*see also* Microphthalmos) 743.10
   fallopian tube 752.19
   leg 755.32
   lobule of ear 744.21
   patella 755.64
   respiratory organs in thoracopagus 759.4
   tracheal bronchus 748.3
   uterine horn 752.3
   uterus 752.3
     in male 752.7
     solid or with cavity 752.3
   vagina 752.49
**Rud's syndrome** (mental deficiency, epilepsy, and infantilism) 759.89
**Ruiter-Pompen (-Wyers) syndrome** (angiokeratoma corporis diffusum) 272.7
**Ruled out condition** — *see also* Observation, suspected V71.9
**Rumination** — *see also* Vomiting
   disorder 307.53
   neurotic 300.3
   obsessional 300.3
   psychogenic 307.53
**Runaway reaction** — *see also* Disturbance, conduct
   socialized 312.2 ☑
   undersocialized, unsocialized 312.1 ☑
**Runeberg's disease** (progressive pernicious anemia) 281.0
**Runge's syndrome** (postmaturity) 766.22
**Runny nose** 784.99 ●
**Rupia** 091.3
   congenital 090.0
   tertiary 095.9
**Rupture, ruptured** 553.9
   abdominal viscera NEC 799.89
     obstetrical trauma 665.5 ☑
   abscess (spontaneous) — *see* Abscess, by site
   amnion — *see* Rupture, membranes
   aneurysm — *see* Aneurysm

**Rupture, ruptured** — *continued*
   anus (sphincter) — *see* Laceration, anus
   aorta, aortic 441.5
     abdominal 441.3
     arch 441.1
     ascending 441.1
     descending 441.5
      abdominal 441.3
      thoracic 441.1
     syphilitic 093.0
     thoracoabdominal 441.6
     thorax, thoracic 441.1
     transverse 441.1
     traumatic (thoracic) 901.0
      abdominal 902.0
     valve or cusp (*see also* Endocarditis, aortic) 424.1
   appendix (with peritonitis) 540.0
     with peritoneal abscess 540.1
     traumatic — *see* Injury, internal, gastrointestinal tract
   arteriovenous fistula, brain (congenital) 430
   artery 447.2
     brain (*see also* Hemorrhage, brain) 431
     coronary (*see also* Infarct, myocardium) 410.9 ☑
     heart (*see also* Infarct, myocardium) 410.9 ☑
     pulmonary 417.8
     traumatic (complication) (*see also* Injury, blood vessel, by site) 904.9
   bile duct, except cystic (*see also* Disease, biliary) 576.3
     cystic 575.4
     traumatic — *see* Injury, internal, intra-abdominal
   bladder (sphincter) 596.6
     with
      abortion — *see* Abortion, by type, with damage to pelvic organs
      ectopic pregnancy (*see also* categories 633.0–633.9) 639.2
      molar pregnancy (*see also* categories 630–632) 639.2
     following
      abortion 639.2
      ectopic or molar pregnancy 639.2
     nontraumatic 596.6
     obstetrical trauma 665.5 ☑
     spontaneous 596.6
     traumatic — *see* Injury, internal, bladder
   blood vessel (*see also* Hemorrhage) 459.0
     brain (*see also* Hemorrhage, brain) 431
     heart (*see also* Infarct, myocardium) 410.9 ☑
     traumatic (complication) (*see also* Injury, blood vessel, by site) 904.9
   bone — *see* Fracture, by site
   bowel 569.89
     traumatic — *see* Injury, internal, intestine
   Bowman's membrane 371.31
   brain
     aneurysm (congenital) (*see also* Hemorrhage, subarachnoid) 430
     late effect — *see* Late effect(s) (of) cerebrovascular disease
     syphilitic 094.87
     hemorrhagic (*see also* Hemorrhage, brain) 431
     injury at birth 767.0
     syphilitic 094.89
   capillaries 448.9

**Rupture, ruptured** — *continued*
   cardiac (*see also* Infarct, myocardium) 410.9 ☑
   cartilage (articular) (current) (*see also* Sprain, by site)
     knee — *see* Tear, meniscus
     semilunar — *see* Tear, meniscus
   cecum (with peritonitis) 540.0
     with peritoneal abscess 540.1
     traumatic 863.89
      with open wound into cavity 863.99
   cerebral aneurysm (congenital) (*see also* Hemorrhage, subarachnoid) 430
     late effect — *see* Late effect(s) (of) cerebrovascular disease
   cervix (uteri)
     with
      abortion — *see* Abortion, by type, with damage to pelvic organs
      ectopic pregnancy (*see also* categories 633.0–633.9) 639.2
      molar pregnancy (*see also* categories 630–632) 639.2
     following
      abortion 639.2
      ectopic or molar pregnancy 639.2
     obstetrical trauma 665.3 ☑
     traumatic — *see* Injury, internal, cervix
   chordae tendineae 429.5
   choroid (direct) (indirect) (traumatic) 363.63
   circle of Willis (*see also* Hemorrhage, subarachnoid) 430
     late effect — *see* Late effect(s) (of) cerebrovascular disease
   colon 569.89
     traumatic — *see* Injury, internal, colon
   cornea (traumatic) (*see also* Rupture, eye)
     due to ulcer 370.00
   coronary (artery) (thrombotic) (*see also* Infarct, myocardium) 410.9 ☑
   corpus luteum (infected) (ovary) 620.1
   cyst — *see* Cyst
   cystic duct (*see also* Disease, gallbladder) 575.4
   Descemet's membrane 371.33
     traumatic — *see* Rupture, eye
   diaphragm (*see also* Hernia, diaphragm)
     traumatic — *see* Injury, internal, diaphragm
   diverticulum
     bladder 596.3
     intestine (large) (*see also* Diverticula) 562.10
      small 562.00
   duodenal stump 537.89
   duodenum (ulcer) — *see* Ulcer, duodenum, with perforation
   ear drum (*see also* Perforation, tympanum) 384.20
     with otitis media — *see* Otitis media
     traumatic — *see* Wound, open, ear
   esophagus 530.4
     traumatic 862.22
      with open wound into cavity 862.32
      cervical region — *see* Wound, open, esophagus
   eye (without prolapse of intraocular tissue) 871.0
     with
      exposure of intraocular tissue 871.1
      partial loss of intraocular tissue 871.2

**Rupture, ruptured** — *continued*
   eye — *continued*
     with — *continued*
      prolapse of intraocular tissue 871.1
     due to burn 940.5
   fallopian tube 620.8
     due to pregnancy — *see* Pregnancy, tubal
     traumatic — *see* Injury, internal, fallopian tube
   fontanel 767.3
   free wall (ventricle) (*see also* Infarct, myocardium) 410.9 ☑
   gallbladder or duct (*see also* Disease, gallbladder) 575.4
     traumatic — *see* Injury, internal, gallbladder
   gastric (*see also* Rupture, stomach) 537.89
     vessel 459.0
   globe (eye) (traumatic) — *see* Rupture, eye
   graafian follicle (hematoma) 620.0
   heart (auricle) (ventricle) (*see also* Infarct, myocardium) 410.9 ☑
     infectional 422.90
     traumatic — *see* Rupture, myocardium, traumatic
   hymen 623.8
   internal
     organ, traumatic (*see also* Injury, internal, by site)
      heart — *see* Rupture, myocardium, traumatic
      kidney — *see* Rupture, kidney
      liver — *see* Rupture, liver
      spleen — *see* Rupture, spleen, traumatic
     semilunar cartilage — *see* Tear, meniscus
   intervertebral disc — *see* Displacement, intervertebral disc
     traumatic (current) — *see* Dislocation, vertebra
   intestine 569.89
     traumatic — *see* Injury, internal, intestine
   intracranial, birth injury 767.0
   iris 364.76
     traumatic — *see* Rupture, eye
   joint capsule — *see* Sprain, by site
   kidney (traumatic) 866.03
     with open wound into cavity 866.13
     due to birth injury 767.8
     nontraumatic 593.89
   lacrimal apparatus (traumatic) 870.2
   lens (traumatic) 366.20
   ligament (*see also* Sprain, by site)
     with open wound — *see* Wound, open, by site
     old (*see also* Disorder, cartilage, articular) 718.0 ☑
   liver (traumatic) 864.04
     with open wound into cavity 864.14
     due to birth injury 767.8
     nontraumatic 573.8
   lymphatic (node) (vessel) 457.8
   marginal sinus (placental) (with hemorrhage) 641.2 ☑
     affecting fetus or newborn 762.1
   meaning hernia — *see* Hernia
   membrana tympani (*see also* Perforation, tympanum) 384.20
     with otitis media — *see* Otitis media
     traumatic — *see* Wound, open, ear
   membranes (spontaneous)
     artificial
      delayed delivery following 658.3 ☑
       affecting fetus or newborn 761.1
     fetus or newborn 761.1

**Rupture, ruptured** — *continued*
  membranes — *continued*
    delayed delivery following 658.2 ☑
      affecting fetus or newborn 761.1
    premature (less than 24 hours prior to onset of labor) 658.1 ☑
      affecting fetus or newborn 761.1
      delayed delivery following 658.2 ☑
        affecting fetus or newborn 761.1
  meningeal artery (*see also* Hemorrhage, subarachnoid) 430
    late effect — *see* Late effect(s) (of) cerebrovascular disease
  meniscus (knee) (*see also* Tear, meniscus)
    old (*see also* Derangement, meniscus) 717.5
      site other than knee — *see* Disorder, cartilage, articular
    site other than knee — *see* Sprain, by site
  mesentery 568.89
    traumatic — *see* Injury, internal, mesentery
  mitral — *see* Insufficiency, mitral
  muscle (traumatic) NEC (*see also* Sprain, by site)
    with open wound — *see* Wound, open, by site
    nontraumatic 728.83
  musculotendinous cuff (nontraumatic) (shoulder) 840.4
  mycotic aneurysm, causing cerebral hemorrhage (*see also* Hemorrhage, subarachnoid) 430
    late effect — *see* Late effect(s) (of) cerebrovascular disease
  myocardium, myocardial (*see also* Infarct, myocardium) 410.9 ☑
    traumatic 861.03
      with open wound into thorax 861.13
  nontraumatic (meaning hernia) (*see also* Hernia, by site) 553.9
  obstructed (*see also* Hernia, by site, with obstruction) 552.9
    gangrenous (*see also* Hernia, by site, with gangrene) 551.9
  operation wound 998.32
    internal 998.31
  ovary, ovarian 620.8
    corpus luteum 620.1
    follicle (graafian) 620.0
  oviduct 620.8
    due to pregnancy — *see* Pregnancy, tubal
  pancreas 577.8
    traumatic — *see* Injury, internal, pancreas
  papillary muscle (ventricular) 429.6
  pelvic
    floor, complicating delivery 664.1 ☑
    organ NEC — *see* Injury, pelvic, organs
  penis (traumatic) — *see* Wound, open, penis
  perineum 624.8
    during delivery (*see also* Laceration, perineum, complicating delivery) 664.4 ☑
  pharynx (nontraumatic) (spontaneous) 478.29

**Rupture, ruptured** — *continued*
  pregnant uterus (before onset of labor) 665.0 ☑
  prostate (traumatic) — *see* Injury, internal, prostate
  pulmonary
    artery 417.8
    valve (heart) (*see also* Endocarditis, pulmonary) 424.3
    vein 417.8
    vessel 417.8
  pupil, sphincter 364.75
  pus tube (*see also* Salpingo-oophoritis) 614.2
  pyosalpinx (*see also* Salpingo-oophoritis) 614.2
  rectum 569.49
    traumatic — *see* Injury, internal, rectum
  retina, retinal (traumatic) (without detachment) 361.30
    with detachment (*see also* Detachment, retina, with retinal defect) 361.00
  rotator cuff (capsule) (traumatic) 840.4
    nontraumatic, complete 727.61
  sclera 871.0
  semilunar cartilage, knee (*see also* Tear, meniscus) 836.2
    old (*see also* Derangement, meniscus) 717.5
  septum (cardiac) 410.8 ☑
  sigmoid 569.89
    traumatic — *see* Injury, internal, colon, sigmoid
  sinus of Valsalva 747.29
  spinal cord (*see also* Injury, spinal, by site)
    due to injury at birth 767.4
    fetus or newborn 767.4
    syphilitic 094.89
    traumatic (*see also* Injury, spinal, by site)
      with fracture — *see* Fracture, vertebra, by site, with spinal cord injury
  spleen 289.59
    congenital 767.8
    due to injury at birth 767.8
    malarial 084.9
    nontraumatic 289.59
    spontaneous 289.59
    traumatic 865.04
      with open wound into cavity 865.14
  splenic vein 459.0
  stomach 537.89
    due to injury at birth 767.8
    traumatic — *see* Injury, internal, stomach
    ulcer — *see* Ulcer, stomach, with perforation
  synovium 727.50
    specified site NEC 727.59
  tendon (traumatic) (*see also* Sprain, by site)
    with open wound — *see* Wound, open, by site
    Achilles 845.09
      nontraumatic 727.67
    ankle 845.09
      nontraumatic 727.68
    biceps (long head) 840.8
      nontraumatic 727.62
    foot 845.10
      interphalangeal (joint) 845.13

**Rupture, ruptured** — *continued*
  tendon (*see also* Sprain, by site) — *continued*
    foot — *continued*
      metatarsophalangeal (joint) 845.12
      nontraumatic 727.68
      specified site NEC 845.19
      tarsometatarsal (joint) 845.11
    hand 842.10
      carpometacarpal (joint) 842.11
      interphalangeal (joint) 842.13
      metacarpophalangeal (joint) 842.12
      nontraumatic 727.63
        extensors 727.63
        flexors 727.64
      specified site NEC 842.19
    nontraumatic 727.60
      specified site NEC 727.69
    patellar 844.8
      nontraumatic 727.66
    quadriceps 844.8
      nontraumatic 727.65
    rotator cuff (capsule) 840.4
      nontraumatic, complete 727.61
    wrist 842.00
      carpal (joint) 842.01
      nontraumatic 727.63
        extensors 727.63
        flexors 727.64
      radiocarpal (joint) (ligament) 842.02
      radioulnar (joint), distal 842.09
      specified site NEC 842.09
  testis (traumatic) 878.2
    complicated 878.3
    due to syphilis 095.8
  thoracic duct 457.8
  tonsil 474.8
  traumatic
    with open wound — *see* Wound, open, by site
    aorta — *see* Rupture, aorta, traumatic
    ear drum — *see* Wound, open, ear, drum
    external site — *see* Wound, open, by site
    eye 871.2
    globe (eye) — *see* Wound, open, eyeball
    internal organ (abdomen, chest, or pelvis) (*see also* Injury, internal, by site)
      heart — *see* Rupture, myocardium, traumatic
      kidney — *see* Rupture, kidney
      liver — *see* Rupture, liver
      spleen — *see* Rupture, spleen, traumatic
    ligament, muscle, or tendon (*see also* Sprain, by site)
      with open wound — *see* Wound, open, by site
      meaning hernia — *see* Hernia
  tricuspid (heart) (valve) — *see* Endocarditis, tricuspid
  tube, tubal 620.8
    abscess (*see also* Salpingo-oophoritis) 614.2
    due to pregnancy — *see* Pregnancy, tubal
  tympanum, tympanic (membrane) (*see also* Perforation, tympanum) 384.20

**Rupture, ruptured** — *continued*
  tympanum, tympanic (*see also* Perforation, tympanum) — *continued*
    with otitis media — *see* Otitis media
    traumatic — *see* Wound, open, ear, drum
  umbilical cord 663.8 ☑
    fetus or newborn 772.0
  ureter (traumatic) (*see also* Injury, internal, ureter) 867.2
    nontraumatic 593.89
  urethra 599.84
    with
      abortion — *see* Abortion, by type, with damage to pelvic organs
      ectopic pregnancy (*see also* categories 633.0–633.9) 639.2
      molar pregnancy (*see also* categories 630–632) 639.2
    following
      abortion 639.2
      ectopic or molar pregnancy 639.2
    obstetrical trauma 665.5 ☑
    traumatic — *see* Injury, internal urethra
  uterosacral ligament 620.8
  uterus (traumatic) (*see also* Injury, internal uterus)
    affecting fetus or newborn 763.89
    during labor 665.1 ☑
    nonpuerperal, nontraumatic 621.8
    nontraumatic 621.8
    pregnant (during labor) 665.1 ☑
      before labor 665.0 ☑
  vagina 878.6
    complicated 878.7
    complicating delivery — *see* Laceration, vagina, complicating delivery
  valve, valvular (heart) — *see* Endocarditis
  varicose vein — *see* Varicose, vein
  varix — *see* Varix
  vena cava 459.0
  ventricle (free wall) (left) (*see also* Infarct, myocardium) 410.9 ☑
  vesical (urinary) 596.6
    traumatic — *see* Injury, internal, bladder
  vessel (blood) 459.0
    pulmonary 417.8
  viscus 799.89
  vulva 878.4
    complicated 878.5
    complicating delivery 664.0 ☑

**Russell's dwarf** (uterine dwarfism and craniofacial dysostosis) 759.89
**Russell's dysentery** 004.8
**Russell (-Silver) syndrome** (congenital hemihypertrophy and short stature) 759.89
**Russian spring-summer type encephalitis** 063.0
**Rust's disease** (tuberculous spondylitis) 015.0 *[720.81]*
**Rustitskii's disease** (multiple myeloma) (M9730/3) 203.0 ☑
**Ruysch's disease** (Hirschsprung's disease) 751.3
**Rytand-Lipsitch syndrome** (complete atrioventricular block) 426.0

☑ Additional Digit Required — Refer to the Tabular List for Digit Selection      ⬗ Subterms under main terms may continue to next column or page

**2008 ICD-9-CM**      ▶◀ Revised Text      ● New Line      ▲ Revised Code      **Volume 2 — 253**

## S

**Saber**
- shin 090.5
- tibia 090.5

**Saccharomyces infection** — see also Candidiasis 112.9

**Saccharopinuria** 270.7

**Saccular** — see condition

**Sacculation**
- aorta (nonsyphilitic) (see also Aneurysm, aorta) 441.9
  - ruptured 441.5
  - syphilitic 093.0
- bladder 596.3
- colon 569.89
- intralaryngeal (congenital) (ventricular) 748.3
- larynx (congenital) (ventricular) 748.3
- organ or site, congenital — see Distortion
- pregnant uterus, complicating delivery 654.4 ☑
  - affecting fetus or newborn 763.1
    - causing obstructed labor 660.2 ☑
      - affecting fetus or newborn 763.1
- rectosigmoid 569.89
- sigmoid 569.89
- ureter 593.89
- urethra 599.2
- vesical 596.3

**Sachs (-Tay) disease** (amaurotic familial idiocy) 330.1

**Sacks-Libman disease** 710.0 [424.91]

**Sac, lacrimal** — see condition

**Sacralgia** 724.6

**Sacralization**
- fifth lumbar vertebra 756.15
- incomplete (vertebra) 756.15

**Sacrodynia** 724.6

**Sacroiliac joint** — see condition

**Sacroiliitis** NEC 720.2

**Sacrum** — see condition

**Saddle**
- back 737.8
- embolus, aorta 444.0
- nose 738.0
  - congenital 754.0
  - due to syphilis 090.5

**Sadism** (sexual) 302.84

**Saemisch's ulcer** 370.04

**Saenger's syndrome** 379.46

**Sago spleen** 277.39

**Sailors' skin** 692.74

**Saint**
- Anthony's fire (see also Erysipelas) 035
- Guy's dance — see Chorea
- Louis-type encephalitis 062.3
- triad (see also Hernia, diaphragm) 553.3
- Vitus' dance — see Chorea

**Salicylism**
- correct substance properly administered 535.4 ☑
- overdose or wrong substance given or taken 965.1

**Salivary duct or gland** — see condition
- virus disease 078.5

**Salivation** (excessive) — see also Ptyalism 527.7

**Salmonella** (aertrycke) (choleraesuis) (enteritidis) (gallinarum) (suipestifer) (typhimurium) — see also Infection, Salmonella 003.9
- arthritis 003.23
- carrier (suspected) of V02.3
- meningitis 003.21
- osteomyelitis 003.24
- pneumonia 003.22
- septicemia 003.1
- typhosa 002.0
  - carrier (suspected) of V02.1

**Salmonellosis** 003.0

**Salmonellosis** — continued
- with pneumonia 003.22

**Salpingitis** (catarrhal) (fallopian tube) (nodular) (pseudofollicular) (purulent) (septic) — see also Salpingo-oophoritis 614.2
- ear 381.50
  - acute 381.51
  - chronic 381.52
- Eustachian (tube) 381.50
  - acute 381.51
  - chronic 381.52
- follicularis 614.1
- gonococcal (chronic) 098.37
  - acute 098.17
- interstitial, chronic 614.1
- isthmica nodosa 614.1
- old — see Salpingo-oophoritis, chronic
- puerperal, postpartum, childbirth 670.0 ☑
- specific (chronic) 098.37
  - acute 098.17
- tuberculous (acute) (chronic) (see also Tuberculosis) 016.6 ☑
- venereal (chronic) 098.37
  - acute 098.17

**Salpingocele** 620.4

**Salpingo-oophoritis** (catarrhal) (purulent) (ruptured) (septic) (suppurative) 614.2
- acute 614.0
  - with
    - abortion — see Abortion, by type, with sepsis
    - ectopic pregnancy (see also categories 633.0–633.9) 639.0
    - molar pregnancy (see also categories 630–632) 639.0
  - following
    - abortion 639.0
    - ectopic or molar pregnancy 639.0
  - gonococcal 098.17
  - puerperal, postpartum, childbirth 670.0 ☑
  - tuberculous (see also Tuberculosis) 016.6 ☑
- chronic 614.1
  - gonococcal 098.37
  - tuberculous (see also Tuberculosis) 016.6 ☑
- complicating pregnancy 646.6 ☑
  - affecting fetus or newborn 760.8
- gonococcal (chronic) 098.37
  - acute 098.17
- old — see Salpingo-oophoritis, chronic
- puerperal 670.0 ☑
- specific — see Salpingo-oophoritis, gonococcal
- subacute (see also Salpingo-oophoritis, acute) 614.0
- tuberculous (acute) (chronic) (see also Tuberculosis) 016.6 ☑
- venereal — see Salpingo-oophoritis, gonococcal

**Salpingo-ovaritis** — see also Salpingo-oophoritis 614.2

**Salpingoperitonitis** — see also Salpingo-oophoritis 614.2

**Salt-losing**
- nephritis (see also Disease, renal) 593.9
- syndrome (see also Disease, renal) 593.9

**Salt-rheum** — see also Eczema 692.9

**Salzmann's nodular dystrophy** 371.46

**Sampson's cyst or tumor** 617.1

**Sandblasters'**
- asthma 502
- lung 502

**Sander's disease** (paranoia) 297.1

**Sandfly fever** 066.0

**Sandhoff's disease** 330.1

**Sanfilippo's syndrome** (mucopolysaccharidosis III) 277.5

**Sanger-Brown's ataxia** 334.2

**San Joaquin Valley fever** 114.0

**Sao Paulo fever or typhus** 082.0

**Saponification, mesenteric** 567.89

**Sapremia** — see Septicemia

**Sarcocele** (benign)
- syphilitic 095.8
  - congenital 090.5

**Sarcoepiplocele** — see also Hernia 553.9

**Sarcoepiplomphalocele** — see also Hernia, umbilicus 553.1

**Sarcoid** (any site) 135
- with lung involvement 135 [517.8]
- Boeck's 135
- Darier-Roussy 135
- Spiegler-Fendt 686.8

**Sarcoidosis** 135
- cardiac 135 [425.8]
- lung 135 [517.8]

**Sarcoma** (M8800/3) — see also Neoplasm, connective tissue, malignant
- alveolar soft part (M9581/3) — see Neoplasm, connective tissue, malignant
- ameloblastic (M9330/3) 170.1
  - upper jaw (bone) 170.0
- botryoid (M8910/3) — see Neoplasm, connective tissue, malignant
- botryoides (M8910/3) — see Neoplasm, connective tissue, malignant
- cerebellar (M9480/3) 191.6
  - circumscribed (arachnoidal) (M9471/3) 191.6
- circumscribed (arachnoidal) cerebellar (M9471/3) 191.6
- clear cell, of tendons and aponeuroses (M9044/3) — see Neoplasm, connective tissue, malignant
- embryonal (M8991/3) — see Neoplasm, connective tissue, malignant
- endometrial (stromal) (M8930/3) 182.0
  - isthmus 182.1
- endothelial (M9130/3) (see also Neoplasm, connective tissue, malignant)
  - bone (M9260/3) — see Neoplasm, bone, malignant
- epithelioid cell (M8804/3) — see Neoplasm, connective tissue, malignant
- Ewing's (M9260/3) — see Neoplasm, bone, malignant
- follicular dendritic cell 202.9 ☑
- germinoblastic (diffuse) (M9632/3) 202.8 ☑
  - follicular (M9697/3) 202.0 ☑
- giant cell (M8802/3) (see also Neoplasm, connective tissue, malignant)
  - bone (M9250/3) — see Neoplasm, bone, malignant
- glomoid (M8710/3) — see Neoplasm, connective tissue, malignant
- granulocytic (M9930/3) 205.3 ☑
- hemangioendothelial (M9130/3) — see Neoplasm, connective tissue, malignant
- hemorrhagic, multiple (M9140/3) — see Kaposi's, sarcoma
- Hodgkin's (M9662/3) 201.2 ☑
- immunoblastic (M9612/3) 200.8 ☑
- interdigitating dendritic cell 202.9 ☑
- Kaposi's (M9140/3) — see Kaposi's, sarcoma
- Kupffer cell (M9124/3) 155.0
- Langerhans cell 202.9 ☑
- leptomeningeal (M9530/3) — see Neoplasm, meninges, malignant
- lymphangioendothelial (M9170/3) — see Neoplasm, connective tissue, malignant

**Sarcoma** — see also Neoplasm, connective tissue, malignant — continued
- lymphoblastic (M9630/3) 200.1 ☑
- lymphocytic (M9620/3) 200.1 ☑
- mast cell (M9740/3) 202.6 ☑
- melanotic (M8720/3) — see Melanoma
- meningeal (M9530/3) — see Neoplasm, meninges, malignant
- meningothelial (M9530/3) — see Neoplasm, meninges, malignant
- mesenchymal (M8800/3) (see also Neoplasm, connective tissue, malignant)
  - mixed (M8990/3) — see Neoplasm, connective tissue, malignant
- mesothelial (M9050/3) — see Neoplasm, by site, malignant
- monstrocellular (M9481/3)
  - specified site — see Neoplasm, by site, malignant
  - unspecified site 191.9
- myeloid (M9930/3) 205.3 ☑
- neurogenic (M9540/3) — see Neoplasm, connective tissue, malignant
- odontogenic (M9270/3) 170.1
  - upper jaw (bone) 170.0
- osteoblastic (M9180/3) — see Neoplasm, bone, malignant
- osteogenic (M9180/3) (see also Neoplasm, bone, malignant)
  - juxtacortical (M9190/3) — see Neoplasm, bone, malignant
  - periosteal (M9190/3) — see Neoplasm, bone, malignant
- periosteal (M8812/3) (see also Neoplasm, bone, malignant)
  - osteogenic (M9190/3) — see Neoplasm, bone, malignant
- plasma cell (M9731/3) 203.8 ☑
- pleomorphic cell (M8802/3) — see Neoplasm, connective tissue, malignant
- reticuloendothelial (M9720/3) 202.3 ☑
- reticulum cell (M9640/3) 200.0 ☑
  - nodular (M9642/3) 200.0 ☑
  - pleomorphic cell type (M9641/3) 200.0 ☑
- round cell (M8803/3) — see Neoplasm, connective tissue, malignant
- small cell (M8803/3) — see Neoplasm, connective tissue, malignant
- spindle cell (M8801/3) — see Neoplasm, connective tissue, malignant
- stromal (endometrial) (M8930/3) 182.0
  - isthmus 182.1
- synovial (M9040/3) (see also Neoplasm, connective tissue, malignant)
  - biphasic type (M9043/3) — see Neoplasm, connective tissue, malignant
  - epithelioid cell type (M9042/3) — see Neoplasm, connective tissue, malignant
  - spindle cell type (M9041/3) — see Neoplasm, connective tissue, malignant

**Sarcomatosis**
- meningeal (M9539/3) — see Neoplasm, meninges, malignant
- specified site NEC (M8800/3) — see Neoplasm, connective tissue, malignant
- unspecified site (M8800/6) 171.9

**Sarcosinemia** 270.8

**Sarcosporidiosis** 136.5

**Satiety, early** 780.94

**Saturnine** — see condition

**Saturnism** 984.9

☑ Additional Digit Required — Refer to the Tabular List for Digit Selection     ▽ Subterms under main terms may continue to next column or page

**2008 ICD-9-CM**     ▶◀ Revised Text     ● New Line     ▲ Revised Code     **Volume 2 — 255**

**Saturnism** — *continued*
  specified type of lead — *see* Table of Drugs and Chemicals
**Satyriasis** 302.89
**Sauriasis** — *see* Ichthyosis
**Sauriderma** 757.39
**Sauriosis** — *see* Ichthyosis
**Savill's disease** (epidemic exfoliative dermatitis) 695.89
**SBE** (subacute bacterial endocarditis) 421.0
**Scabies** (any site) 133.0
**Scabs** 782.8
**Scaglietti-Dagnini syndrome** (acromegalic macrospondylitis) 253.0
**Scald, scalded** — *see also* Burn, by site
  skin syndrome 695.1
**Scalenus anticus (anterior) syndrome** 353.0
**Scales** 782.8
**Scalp** — *see* condition
**Scaphocephaly** 756.0
**Scaphoiditis, tarsal** 732.5
**Scapulalgia** 733.90
**Scapulohumeral myopathy** 359.1
**Scarabiasis** 134.1
**Scarlatina** 034.1
  anginosa 034.1
  maligna 034.1
  myocarditis, acute 034.1 *[422.0]*
    old (*see also* Myocarditis) 429.0
  otitis media 034.1 *[382.02]*
  ulcerosa 034.1
**Scarlatinella** 057.8
**Scarlet fever** (albuminuria) (angina) (convulsions) (lesions of lid) (rash) 034.1
**Scar, scarring** — *see also* Cicatrix 709.2
  adherent 709.2
  atrophic 709.2
  cervix
    in pregnancy or childbirth 654.6 ☑
      affecting fetus or newborn 763.89
      causing obstructed labor 660.2 ☑
        affecting fetus or newborn 763.1
  cheloid 701.4
  chorioretinal 363.30
    disseminated 363.35
    macular 363.32
    peripheral 363.34
    posterior pole NEC 363.33
  choroid (*see also* Scar, chorioretinal) 363.30
  compression, pericardial 423.9
  congenital 757.39
  conjunctiva 372.64
  cornea 371.00
    xerophthalmic 264.6
  due to previous cesarean delivery, complicating pregnancy or childbirth 654.2 ☑
    affecting fetus or newborn 763.89
  duodenal (bulb) (cap) 537.3
  hypertrophic 701.4
  keloid 701.4
  labia 624.4
  lung (base) 518.89
  macula 363.32
    disseminated 363.35
    peripheral 363.34
  muscle 728.89
  myocardium, myocardial 412
  painful 709.2
  papillary muscle 429.81
  posterior pole NEC 363.33
    macular — *see* Scar, macula
  postnecrotic (hepatic) (liver) 571.9
  psychic V15.49
  retina (*see also* Scar, chorioretinal) 363.30
  trachea 478.9
  uterus 621.8

**Scar, scarring** — *see also* Cicatrix — *continued*
  uterus — *continued*
    in pregnancy or childbirth NEC 654.9 ☑
      affecting fetus or newborn 763.89
      due to previous cesarean delivery 654.2 ☑
  vulva 624.4
**Schamberg's disease, dermatitis, or dermatosis** (progressive pigmentary dermatosis) 709.09
**Schatzki's ring** (esophagus) (lower) (congenital) 750.3
  acquired 530.3
**Schaufenster krankheit** 413.9
**Schaumann's**
  benign lymphogranulomatosis 135
  disease (sarcoidosis) 135
  syndrome (sarcoidosis) 135
**Scheie's syndrome** (mucopolysaccharidosis IS) 277.5
**Schenck's disease** (sporotrichosis) 117.1
**Scheuermann's disease or osteochondrosis** 732.0
**Scheuthauer-Marie-Sainton syndrome** (cleidocranialis dysostosis) 755.59
**Schilder (-Flatau) disease** 341.1
**Schilling-type monocytic leukemia** (M9890/3) 206.9 ☑
**Schimmelbusch's disease, cystic mastitis, or hyperplasia** 610.1
**Schirmer's syndrome** (encephalocutaneous angiomatosis) 759.6
**Schistocelia** 756.79
**Schistoglossia** 750.13
**Schistosoma infestation** — *see* Infestation, Schistosoma
**Schistosomiasis** 120.9
  Asiatic 120.2
  bladder 120.0
  chestermani 120.8
  colon 120.1
  cutaneous 120.3
  due to
    S. hematobium 120.0
    S. japonicum 120.2
    S. mansoni 120.1
    S. mattheii 120.8
  eastern 120.2
  genitourinary tract 120.0
  intestinal 120.1
  lung 120.2
  Manson's (intestinal) 120.1
  Oriental 120.2
  pulmonary 120.2
  specified type NEC 120.8
  vesical 120.0
**Schizencephaly** 742.4
**Schizo-affective psychosis** — *see also* Schizophrenia 295.7 ☑
**Schizodontia** 520.2
**Schizoid personality** 301.20
  introverted 301.21
  schizotypal 301.22
**Schizophrenia, schizophrenic** (reaction) 295.9 ☑

*Note — Use the following fifth-digit subclassification with category 295:*

| 0 | *unspecified* |
|---|---|
| 1 | *subchronic* |
| 2 | *chronic* |
| 3 | *subchronic with acute exacerbation* |
| 4 | *chronic with acute exacerbation* |
| 5 | *in remission* |

  acute (attack) NEC 295.8 ☑
    episode 295.4 ☑
  atypical form 295.8 ☑
  borderline 295.5 ☑
  catalepsy 295.2 ☑

**Schizophrenia, schizophrenic** — *continued*
  catatonic (type) (acute) (excited) (withdrawn) 295.2 ☑
  childhood (type) (*see also* Psychosis, childhood) 299.9 ☑
  chronic NEC 295.6 ☑
  coenesthesiopathic 295.8 ☑
  cyclic (type) 295.7 ☑
  disorganized (type) 295.1 ☑
  flexibilitas cerea 295.2 ☑
  hebephrenic (type) (acute) 295.1 ☑
  incipient 295.5 ☑
  latent 295.5 ☑
  paranoid (type) (acute) 295.3 ☑
  paraphrenic (acute) 295.3 ☑
  prepsychotic 295.5 ☑
  primary (acute) 295.0 ☑
  prodromal 295.5 ☑
  pseudoneurotic 295.5 ☑
  pseudopsychopathic 295.5 ☑
  reaction 295.9 ☑
  residual type (state) 295.6 ☑
  restzustand 295.6 ☑
  schizo-affective (type) (depressed) (excited) 295.7 ☑
  schizophreniform type 295.4 ☑
  simple (type) (acute) 295.0 ☑
  simplex (acute) 295.0 ☑
  specified type NEC 295.8 ☑
  syndrome of childhood NEC (*see also* Psychosis, childhood) 299.9 ☑
  undifferentiated type 295.9 ☑
    acute 295.8 ☑
    chronic 295.6 ☑
**Schizothymia** 301.20
  introverted 301.21
  schizotypal 301.22
**Schlafkrankheit** 086.5
**Schlatter-Osgood disease** (osteochondrosis, tibial tubercle) 732.4
**Schlatter's tibia** (osteochondrosis) 732.4
**Schloffer's tumor** — *see also* Peritonitis 567.29
**Schmidt's syndrome**
  sphallo-pharyngo-laryngeal hemiplegia 352.6
  thyroid-adrenocortical insufficiency 258.1
  vagoaccessory 352.6
**Schmincke**
  carcinoma (M8082/3) — *see* Neoplasm, nasopharynx, malignant
  tumor (M8082/3) — *see* Neoplasm, nasopharynx, malignant
**Schmitz (-Stutzer) dysentery** 004.0
**Schmorl's disease or nodes** 722.30
  lumbar, lumbosacral 722.32
  specified region NEC 722.39
  thoracic, thoracolumbar 722.31
**Schneiderian**
  carcinoma (M8121/3)
    specified site — *see* Neoplasm, by site, malignant
    unspecified site 160.0
  papilloma (M8121/0)
    specified site — *see* Neoplasm, by site, benign
    unspecified site 212.0
**Schneider's syndrome** 047.9
**Schnitzler syndrome** 273.1
**Schoffer's tumor** — *see also* Peritonitis 567.29
**Scholte's syndrome** (malignant carcinoid) 259.2
**Scholz's disease** 330.0
**Scholz (-Bielschowsky-Henneberg) syndrome** 330.0
**Schönlein (-Henoch) disease** (primary) (purpura) (rheumatic) 287.0
**School examination** V70.3
**Schottmüller's disease** — *see also* Fever, paratyphoid 002.9
**Schroeder's syndrome** (endocrine-hypertensive) 255.3

**Schüller-Christian disease or syndrome** (chronic histiocytosis X) 277.89
**Schultz's disease or syndrome** (agranulocytosis) 288.09
**Schultze's acroparesthesia, simple** 443.89
**Schwalbe-Ziehen-Oppenheimer disease** 333.6
**Schwannoma** (M9560/0) — *see also* Neoplasm, connective tissue, benign
  malignant (M9560/3) — *see* Neoplasm, connective tissue, malignant
**Schwartz-Bartter syndrome** (inappropriate secretion of antidiuretic hormone) 253.6
**Schwartz (-Jampel) syndrome** 359.23 ▲
**Schweninger-Buzzi disease** (macular atrophy) 701.3
**Sciatic** — *see* condition
**Sciatica** (infectional) 724.3
  due to
    displacement of intervertebral disc 722.10
    herniation, nucleus pulposus 722.10
  wallet 724.3
**Scimitar syndrome** (anomalous venous drainage, right lung to inferior vena cava) 747.49
**Sclera** — *see* condition
**Sclerectasia** 379.11
**Scleredema**
  adultorum 710.1
  Buschke's 710.1
  newborn 778.1
**Sclerema**
  adiposum (newborn) 778.1
  adultorum 710.1
  edematosum (newborn) 778.1
  neonatorum 778.1
  newborn 778.1
**Scleriasis** — *see* Scleroderma
**Scleritis** 379.00
  with corneal involvement 379.05
  anterior (annular) (localized) 379.03
  brawny 379.06
  granulomatous 379.09
  posterior 379.07
  specified NEC 379.09
  suppurative 379.09
  syphilitic 095.0
  tuberculous (nodular) (*see also* Tuberculosis) 017.3 ☑ *[379.09]*
**Sclerochoroiditis** — *see also* Scleritis 379.00
**Scleroconjunctivitis** — *see also* Scleritis 379.00
**Sclerocystic ovary** (syndrome) 256.4
**Sclerodactylia** 701.0
**Scleroderma, sclerodermia** (acrosclerotic) (diffuse) (generalized) (progressive) (pulmonary) 710.1
  circumscribed 701.0
  linear 701.0
  localized (linear) 701.0
  newborn 778.1
**Sclerokeratitis** 379.05
  meaning sclerosing keratitis 370.54
  tuberculous (*see also* Tuberculosis) 017.3 ☑ *[379.09]*
**Scleromalacia**
  multiple 731.0
  perforans 379.04
**Scleroma, trachea** 040.1
**Scleromyxedema** 701.8
**Scleroperikeratitis** 379.05
**Sclerose en plaques** 340
**Sclerosis, sclerotic**
  adrenal (gland) 255.8
  Alzheimer's 331.0
    with dementia — *see* Alzheimer's, dementia
  amyotrophic (lateral) 335.20

**Sclerosis, sclerotic** — *continued*
  annularis fibrosi
    aortic 424.1
    mitral 424.0
  aorta, aortic 440.0
    valve (*see also* Endocarditis, aortic)
        424.1
  artery, arterial, arteriolar, arteriovas-
      cular — *see* Arteriosclerosis
  ascending multiple 340
  Baló's (concentric) 341.1
  basilar — *see* Sclerosis, brain
  bone (localized) NEC 733.99
  brain (general) (lobular) 341.9
    Alzheimer's — *see* Alzheimer's, de-
        mentia
    artery, arterial 437.0
    atrophic lobar 331.0
      with dementia
        with behavioral disturbance
            331.0 [294.11]
        without behavioral distur-
            bance 331.0 [294.10]
    diffuse 341.1
      familial (chronic) (infantile)
          330.0
      infantile (chronic) (familial)
          330.0
      Pelizaeus-Merzbacher type
          330.0
    disseminated 340
    hereditary 334.2
    infantile (degenerative) (diffuse)
        330.0
    insular 340
    Krabbe's 330.0
    miliary 340
    multiple 340
    Pelizaeus-Merzbacher 330.0
    progressive familial 330.0
    senile 437.0
    tuberous 759.5
  bulbar, progressive 340
  bundle of His 426.50
    left 426.3
    right 426.4
  cardiac — *see* Arteriosclerosis, coro-
      nary
  cardiorenal (*see also* Hypertension,
      cardiorenal) 404.90
  cardiovascular (*see also* Disease, car-
      diovascular) 429.2
    renal (*see also* Hypertension, car-
        diorenal) 404.90
  centrolobar, familial 330.0
  cerebellar — *see* Sclerosis, brain
  cerebral — *see* Sclerosis, brain
  cerebrospinal 340
    disseminated 340
    multiple 340
  cerebrovascular 437.0
  choroid 363.40
    diffuse 363.56
  combined (spinal cord) (*see also* De-
      generation, combined)
    multiple 340
  concentric, Baló's 341.1
  cornea 370.54
  coronary (artery) — *see* Arteriosclero-
      sis, coronary
  corpus cavernosum
    female 624.8
    male 607.89
  Dewitzky's
    aortic 424.1
    mitral 424.0
  diffuse NEC 341.1
  disease, heart — *see* Arteriosclerosis,
      coronary
  disseminated 340
  dorsal 340
  dorsolateral (spinal cord) — *see* Degen-
      eration, combined
  endometrium 621.8
  extrapyramidal 333.90
  eye, nuclear (senile) 366.16

**Sclerosis, sclerotic** — *continued*
  Friedreich's (spinal cord) 334.0
  funicular (spermatic cord) 608.89
  gastritis 535.4 ☑
  general (vascular) — *see* Arteriosclero-
      sis
  gland (lymphatic) 457.8
  hepatic 571.9
  hereditary
    cerebellar 334.2
    spinal 334.0
  idiopathic cortical (Garré's) (*see also*
      Osteomyelitis) 730.1 ☑
  ilium, piriform 733.5
  insular 340
    pancreas 251.8
  Islands of Langerhans 251.8
  kidney — *see* Sclerosis, renal
  larynx 478.79
  lateral 335.24
    amyotrophic 335.20
    descending 335.24
    primary 335.24
    spinal 335.24
  liver 571.9
  lobar, atrophic (of brain) 331.0
    with dementia
      with behavioral disturbance
          331.0 [294.11]
      without behavioral disturbance
          331.0 [294.10]
  lung (*see also* Fibrosis, lung) 515
  mastoid 383.1
  mitral — *see* Endocarditis, mitral
  Mönckeberg's (medial) (*see also* Arte-
      riosclerosis, extremities) 440.20
  multiple (brain stem) (cerebral) (gener-
      alized) (spinal cord) 340
  myocardium, myocardial — *see* Arte-
      riosclerosis, coronary
  nuclear (senile), eye 366.16
  ovary 620.8
  pancreas 577.8
  penis 607.89
  peripheral arteries (*see also* Arte-
      riosclerosis, extremities) 440.20
  plaques 340
  pluriglandular 258.8
  polyglandular 258.8
  posterior (spinal cord) (syphilitic)
      094.0
  posterolateral (spinal cord) — *see* De-
      generation, combined
  prepuce 607.89
  primary lateral 335.24
  progressive systemic 710.1
  pulmonary (*see also* Fibrosis, lung)
      515
    artery 416.0
    valve (heart) (*see also* Endocarditis,
        pulmonary) 424.3
  renal 587
    with
      cystine storage disease 270.0
      hypertension (*see also* Hyperten-
          sion, kidney) 403.90
      hypertensive heart disease
          (conditions classifiable to
          402) (*see also* Hyperten-
          sion, cardiorenal) 404.90
      arteriolar (hyaline) (*see also* Hyper-
          tension, kidney) 403.90
      hyperplastic (*see also* Hyperten-
          sion, kidney) 403.90
  retina (senile) (vascular) 362.17
  rheumatic
    aortic valve 395.9
    mitral valve 394.9
  Schilder's 341.1
  senile — *see* Arteriosclerosis
  spinal (cord) (general) (progressive)
      (transverse) 336.8
    ascending 357.0
    combined (*see also* Degeneration,
        combined)
      multiple 340

**Sclerosis, sclerotic** — *continued*
  spinal — *continued*
    combined (*see also* Degeneration,
        combined) — *continued*
      syphilitic 094.89
    disseminated 340
    dorsolateral — *see* Degeneration,
        combined
    hereditary (Friedreich's) (mixed
        form) 334.0
    lateral (amyotrophic) 335.24
    multiple 340
    posterior (syphilitic) 094.0
  stomach 537.89
  subendocardial, congenital 425.3
  systemic (progressive) 710.1
    with lung involvement
        710.1 [517.2]
  tricuspid (heart) (valve) — *see* Endo-
      carditis, tricuspid
  tuberous (brain) 759.5
  tympanic membrane (*see also* Tym-
      panosclerosis) 385.00
  valve, valvular (heart) — *see* Endo-
      carditis
  vascular — *see* Arteriosclerosis
  vein 459.89
**Sclerotenonitis** 379.07
**Sclerotitis** — *see also* Scleritis 379.00
  syphilitic 095.0
  tuberculous (*see also* Tuberculosis)
      017.3 ☑ [379.09]
**Scoliosis** (acquired) (postural) 737.30
  congenital 754.2
  due to or associated with
    Charcôt-Marie-Tooth disease
        356.1 [737.43]
    mucopolysaccharidosis
        277.5 [737.43]
    neurofibromatosis 237.71 [737.43]
    osteitis
      deformans 731.0 [737.43]
      fibrosa cystica 252.01 [737.43]
    osteoporosis (*see also* Osteoporosis)
        733.00 [737.43]
    poliomyelitis 138 [737.43]
    radiation 737.33
    tuberculosis (*see also* Tuberculosis)
        015.0 ☑ [737.43]
  idiopathic 737.30
    infantile
      progressive 737.32
      resolving 737.31
  paralytic 737.39
  rachitic 268.1
  sciatic 724.3
  specified NEC 737.39
  thoracogenic 737.34
  tuberculous (*see also* Tuberculosis)
      015.0 ☑ [737.43]
**Scoliotic pelvis** 738.6
  with disproportion (fetopelvic) 653.0 ☑
    affecting fetus or newborn 763.1
    causing obstructed labor 660.1 ☑
      affecting fetus or newborn 763.1
**Scorbutus, scorbutic** 267
  anemia 281.8
**Scotoma** (ring) 368.44
  arcuate 368.43
  Bjerrum 368.43
  blind spot area 368.42
  central 368.41
  centrocecal 368.41
  paracecal 368.42
  paracentral 368.41
  scintillating 368.12
  Seidel 368.43
**Scratch** — *see* Injury, superficial, by site
**Scratchy throat** 784.99　●
**Screening** (for) V82.9
  alcoholism V79.1
  anemia, deficiency NEC V78.1
    iron V78.0
  anomaly, congenital V82.89
  antenatal, of mother V28.9

**Screening** — *continued*
  antenatal, of mother — *continued*
    alphafetoprotein levels, raised
        V28.1
      based on amniocentesis V28.2
        chromosomal anomalies V28.0
        raised alphafetoprotein levels
            V28.1
    fetal growth retardation using ultra-
        sonics V28.4
      ultrasonics V28.4
    isoimmunization V28.5
    malformations using ultrasonics
        V28.3
    raised alphafetoprotein levels V28.1
    specified condition NEC V28.8
    Streptococcus B V28.6
  arterial hypertension V81.1
  arthropod-borne viral disease NEC
      V73.5
  asymptomatic bacteriuria V81.5
  bacterial
    and spirochetal sexually transmit- ●
        ted diseases V74.5　　　　　●
    conjunctivitis V74.4
    disease V74.9
      sexually transmitted V74.5　　●
      specified condition NEC V74.8
  bacteriuria, asymptomatic V81.5
  blood disorder NEC V78.9
    specified type NEC V78.8
  bronchitis, chronic V81.3
  brucellosis V74.8
  cancer — *see* Screening, malignant
      neoplasm
  cardiovascular disease NEC V81.2
  cataract V80.2
  Chagas' disease V75.3
  chemical poisoning V82.5
  cholera V74.0
  cholesterol level V77.91
  chromosomal
    anomalies
      by amniocentesis, antenatal
          V28.0
      maternal postnatal V82.4
    athletes V70.3
  condition
    cardiovascular NEC V81.2
    eye NEC V80.2
    genitourinary NEC V81.6
    neurological V80.0
    respiratory NEC V81.4
    skin V82.0
    specified NEC V82.89
  congenital
    anomaly V82.89
      eye V80.2
    dislocation of hip V82.3
    eye condition or disease V80.2
  conjunctivitis, bacterial V74.4
  contamination NEC (*see also* Poison-
      ing) V82.5
  coronary artery disease V81.0
  cystic fibrosis V77.6
  deficiency anemia NEC V78.1
    iron V78.0
  dengue fever V73.5
  depression V79.0
  developmental handicap V79.9
    in early childhood V79.3
    specified type NEC V79.8
  diabetes mellitus V77.1
  diphtheria V74.3
  disease or disorder V82.9
    bacterial V74.9
      specified NEC V74.8
    blood V78.9
      specified type NEC V78.8
    blood-forming organ V78.9
      specified type NEC V78.8
    cardiovascular NEC V81.2
      hypertensive V81.1
      ischemic V81.0
    Chagas' V75.3
    chlamydial V73.98

☑ Additional Digit Required — Refer to the Tabular List for Digit Selection　　　　　　　　　　　　　　▒ Subterms under main terms may continue to next column or page

**2008 ICD-9-CM**　　　　　　　▶◀ Revised Text　　　　　● New Line　　　　▲ Revised Code　　　　　　　**October 2007 · Volume 2 — 257**

**Screening** — *continued*
  disease or disorder — *continued*
    chlamydial — *continued*
      specified NEC V73.88
    ear NEC V80.3
    endocrine NEC V77.99
    eye NEC V80.2
    genitourinary NEC V81.6
    heart NEC V81.2
      hypertensive V81.1
      ischemic V81.0
    HPV (human papillomavirus) ●
      V73.81 ●
    human papillomavirus V73.81 ●
    immunity NEC V77.99
    infectious NEC V75.9
    lipoid NEC V77.91
    mental V79.9
      specified type NEC V79.8
    metabolic NEC V77.99
      inborn NEC V77.7
    neurological V80.0
    nutritional NEC V77.99
    rheumatic NEC V82.2
    rickettsial V75.0
    sexually transmitted V74.5 ●
      bacterial V74.5 ●
      spirochetal V74.5 ●
    sickle-cell V78.2
      trait V78.2
    specified type NEC V82.89
    thyroid V77.0
    vascular NEC V81.2
      ischemic V81.0
    venereal V74.5
    viral V73.99
      arthropod-borne NEC V73.5
      specified type NEC V73.89
  dislocation of hip, congenital V82.3
  drugs in athletes V70.3
  emphysema (chronic) V81.3
  encephalitis, viral (mosquito or tick
    borne) V73.5
  endocrine disorder NEC V77.99
  eye disorder NEC V80.2
    congenital V80.2
  fever
    dengue V73.5
    hemorrhagic V73.5
    yellow V73.4
  filariasis V75.6
  galactosemia V77.4
  genetic V82.79
    disease carrier status V82.71
  genitourinary condition NEC V81.6
  glaucoma V80.1
  gonorrhea V74.5
  gout V77.5
  Hansen's disease V74.2
  heart disease NEC V81.2
    hypertensive V81.1
    ischemic V81.0
  heavy metal poisoning V82.5
  helminthiasis, intestinal V75.7
  hematopoietic malignancy V76.89
  hemoglobinopathies NEC V78.3
  hemorrhagic fever V73.5
  Hodgkin's disease V76.89
  hormones in athletes V70.3
  HPV (human papillomavirus) V73.81●
  human papillomavirus (HPV) V73.81●
  hypercholesterolemia V77.91
  hyperlipidemia V77.91
  hypertension V81.1
  immunity disorder NEC V77.99
  inborn errors of metabolism NEC
    V77.7
  infection
    bacterial V74.9
      specified type NEC V74.8
    mycotic V75.4
    parasitic NEC V75.8
  infectious disease V75.9
    specified type NEC V75.8
  ingestion of radioactive substance
    V82.5

**Screening** — *continued*
  intestinal helminthiasis V75.7
  iron deficiency anemia V78.0
  ischemic heart disease V81.0
  lead poisoning V82.5
  leishmaniasis V75.2
  leprosy V74.2
  leptospirosis V74.8
  leukemia V76.89
  lipoid disorder NEC V77.91
  lymphoma V76.89
  malaria V75.1
  malignant neoplasm (of) V76.9
    bladder V76.3
    blood V76.89
    breast V76.10
      mammogram NEC V76.12
        for high-risk patient V76.11
      specified type NEC V76.19
    cervix V76.2
    colon V76.51
    colorectal V76.51
    hematopoietic system V76.89
    intestine V76.50
      colon V76.51
      small V76.52
    lung V76.0
    lymph (glands) V76.89
    nervous system V76.81
    oral cavity V76.42
    other specified neoplasm NEC
      V76.89
    ovary V76.46
    prostate V76.44
    rectum V76.41
    respiratory organs V76.0
    skin V76.43
    specified sites NEC V76.49
    testis V76.45
    vagina V76.47
      following hysterectomy for malig-
        nant condition V67.01
  malnutrition V77.2
  mammogram NEC V76.12
    for high-risk patient V76.11
  maternal postnatal chromosomal
    anomalies V82.4
  measles V73.2
  mental
    disorder V79.9
      specified type NEC V79.8
    retardation V79.2
  metabolic disorder NEC V77.99
  metabolic errors, inborn V77.7
  mucoviscidosis V77.6
  multiphasic V82.6
  mycosis V75.4
  mycotic infection V75.4
  nephropathy V81.5
  neurological condition V80.0
  nutritional disorder V77.99
  obesity V77.8
  osteoporosis V82.81
  parasitic infection NEC V75.8
  phenylketonuria V77.3
  plague V74.8
  poisoning
    chemical NEC V82.5
    contaminated water supply V82.5
      heavy metal V82.5
  poliomyelitis V73.0
  postnatal chromosomal anomalies,
    maternal V82.4
  prenatal — *see* Screening, antenatal
  pulmonary tuberculosis V74.1
  radiation exposure V82.5
  renal disease V81.5
  respiratory condition NEC V81.4
  rheumatic disorder NEC V82.2
  rheumatoid arthritis V82.1
  rickettsial disease V75.0
  rubella V73.3
  schistosomiasis V75.5
  senile macular lesions of eye V80.2
  sexually transmitted diseases V74.5●
    bacterial V74.5 ●

**Screening** — *continued*
  sexually transmitted diseases — *con-*
    *tinued*
    spirochetal V74.5 ●
  sickle-cell anemia, disease, or trait
    V78.2
  skin condition V82.0
  sleeping sickness V75.3
  smallpox V73.1
  special V82.9
    specified condition NEC V82.89
  specified type NEC V82.89
  spirochetal disease V74.9
    sexually transmitted V74.5 ●
    specified type NEC V74.8
  stimulants in athletes V70.3
  syphilis V74.5
  tetanus V74.8
  thyroid disorder V77.0
  trachoma V73.6
  trypanosomiasis V75.3
  tuberculosis, pulmonary V74.1
  venereal disease V74.5
  viral encephalitis
    mosquito-borne V73.5
    tick-borne V73.5
  whooping cough V74.8
  worms, intestinal V75.7
  yaws V74.6
  yellow fever V73.4
**Scrofula** — *see also* Tuberculosis
  017.2 ☑
**Scrofulide** (primary) — *see also* Tuberculosis 017.0 ☑
**Scrofuloderma, scrofulodermia** (any
  site) (primary) — *see also* Tuberculosis 017.0 ☑
**Scrofulosis** (universal) — *see also* Tuberculosis 017.2 ☑
**Scrofulosis lichen** (primary) — *see also*
  Tuberculosis 017.0 ☑
**Scrofulous** — *see* condition
**Scrotal tongue** 529.5
  congenital 750.13
**Scrotum** — *see* condition
**Scurvy** (gum) (infantile) (rickets) (scorbutic) 267
**Sea-blue histiocyte syndrome** 272.7
**Seabright-Bantam syndrome** (pseudohypoparathyroidism) 275.49
**Seasickness** 994.6
**Seatworm** 127.4
**Sebaceous**
  cyst (*see also* Cyst, sebaceous) 706.2
  gland disease NEC 706.9
**Sebocystomatosis** 706.2
**Seborrhea, seborrheic** 706.3
  adiposa 706.3
  capitis 690.11
  congestiva 695.4
  corporis 706.3
  dermatitis 690.10
    infantile 690.12
  diathesis in infants 695.89
  eczema 690.18
    infantile 690.12
  keratosis 702.19
    inflamed 702.11
  nigricans 705.89
  sicca 690.18
  wart 702.19
    inflamed 702.11
**Seckel's syndrome** 759.89
**Seclusion pupil** 364.74
**Seclusiveness, child** 313.22
**Secondary** — *see also* condition
  neoplasm — *see* Neoplasm, by site,
    malignant, secondary
**Secretan's disease or syndrome** (posttraumatic edema) 782.3
**Secretion**
  antidiuretic hormone, inappropriate
    (syndrome) 253.6
  catecholamine, by pheochromocytoma
    255.6

**Secretion** — *continued*
  hormone
    antidiuretic, inappropriate (syn-
      drome) 253.6
    by
      carcinoid tumor 259.2
      pheochromocytoma 255.6
    ectopic NEC 259.3
  urinary
    excessive 788.42
    suppression 788.5
**Section**
  cesarean
    affecting fetus or newborn 763.4
    post mortem, affecting fetus or
      newborn 761.6
    previous, in pregnancy or child-
      birth 654.2 ☑
      affecting fetus or newborn
        763.89
  nerve, traumatic — *see* Injury, nerve,
    by site
**Seeligmann's syndrome** (ichthyosis
  congenita) 757.1
**Segmentation, incomplete** (congenital)
  — *see also* Fusion
  bone NEC 756.9
  lumbosacral (joint) 756.15
  vertebra 756.15
    lumbosacral 756.15
**Seizure►(s)◄** 780.39
  akinetic (idiopathic) (*see also* Epilepsy)
    345.0 ☑
    psychomotor 345.4 ☑
  apoplexy, apoplectic (*see also* Disease,
    cerebrovascular, acute) 436
  atonic (*see also* Epilepsy) 345.0 ☑
  autonomic 300.11
  brain or cerebral (*see also* Disease,
    cerebrovascular, acute) 436
  convulsive (*see also* Convulsions)
    780.39
  cortical (focal) (motor) (*see also*
    Epilepsy) 345.5 ☑
  due to stroke 438.89 ●
  epilepsy, epileptic (cryptogenic) (*see*
    *also* Epilepsy) 345.9 ☑
  epileptiform, epileptoid 780.39
    focal (*see also* Epilepsy) 345.5 ☑
  febrile (simple) 780.31
    with status epilepticus 345.3
    atypical 780.32
    complex 780.32
    complicated 780.32
  heart — *see* Disease, heart
  hysterical 300.11
  Jacksonian (focal) (*see also* Epilepsy)
    345.5 ☑
    motor type 345.5 ☑
    sensory type 345.5 ☑
  newborn 779.0
  paralysis (*see also* Disease, cerebrovas-
    cular, acute) 436
  recurrent 345.9 ☑
    epileptic — *see* Epilepsy
  repetitive 780.39
    epileptic — *see* Epilepsy
  salaam (*see also* Epilepsy) 345.6 ☑
  uncinate (*see also* Epilepsy) 345.4 ☑
**Self-mutilation** 300.9
**Semicoma** 780.09
**Semiconsciousness** 780.09
**Seminal**
  vesicle — *see* condition
  vesiculitis (*see also* Vesiculitis) 608.0
**Seminoma** (M9061/3)
  anaplastic type (M9062/3)
    specified site — *see* Neoplasm, by
      site, malignant
    unspecified site 186.9
  specified site — *see* Neoplasm, by site,
    malignant
  spermatocytic (M9063/3)
    specified site — *see* Neoplasm, by
      site, malignant
    unspecified site 186.9

---

☑ Additional Digit Required — Refer to the Tabular List for Digit Selection      ▽ Subterms under main terms may continue to next column or page

**Seminoma** — *continued*
  unspecified site 186.9
**Semliki Forest encephalitis** 062.8
**Senear-Usher disease or syndrome**
  (pemphigus erythematosus) 694.4
**Senecio jacobae dermatitis** 692.6
**Senectus** 797
**Senescence** 797
**Senile** — *see also* condition 797
  cervix (atrophic) 622.8
  degenerative atrophy, skin 701.3
  endometrium (atrophic) 621.8
  fallopian tube (atrophic) 620.3
  heart (failure) 797
  lung 492.8
  ovary (atrophic) 620.3
  syndrome 259.8
  vagina, vaginitis (atrophic) 627.3
  wart 702.0
**Senility** 797
  with
    acute confusional state 290.3
    delirium 290.3
    mental changes 290.9
    psychosis NEC (*see also* Psychosis,
      senile) 290.20
  premature (syndrome) 259.8
**Sensation**
  burning (*see also* Disturbance, sensa-
    tion) 782.0
    tongue 529.6
  choking 784.99
  loss of (*see also* Disturbance, sensa-
    tion) 782.0
  prickling (*see also* Disturbance, sensa-
    tion) 782.0
  tingling (*see also* Disturbance, sensa-
    tion) 782.0
**Sense loss** (touch) — *see also* Disturbance, sensation 782.0
  smell 781.1
  taste 781.1
**Sensibility disturbance NEC** (cortical)
  (deep) (vibratory) — *see also* Disturbance, sensation 782.0
**Sensitive dentine** 521.89
**Sensitiver Beziehungswahn** 297.8
**Sensitivity, sensitization** — *see also*
  Allergy
  autoerythrocyte 287.2
  carotid sinus 337.0
  child (excessive) 313.21
  cold, autoimmune 283.0
  methemoglobin 289.7
  suxamethonium 289.89
  tuberculin, without clinical or radio-
    logical symptoms 795.5
**Sensory**
  extinction 781.8
  neglect 781.8
**Separation**
  acromioclavicular — *see* Dislocation,
    acromioclavicular
  anxiety, abnormal 309.21
  apophysis, traumatic — *see* Fracture,
    by site
  choroid 363.70
    hemorrhagic 363.72
    serous 363.71
  costochondral (simple) (traumatic) —
    *see* Dislocation, costochondral
  delayed
    umbilical cord 779.83
  epiphysis, epiphyseal
    nontraumatic 732.9
      upper femoral 732.2
    traumatic — *see* Fracture, by site
  fracture — *see* Fracture, by site
  infundibulum cardiac from right ven-
    tricle by a partition 746.83
  joint (current) (traumatic) — *see* Dislo-
    cation, by site
  placenta (normally implanted) — *see*
    Placenta, separation
  pubic bone, obstetrical trauma
    665.6 ☑

**Separation** — *continued*
  retina, retinal (*see also* Detachment,
    retina) 361.9
    layers 362.40
      sensory (*see also* Retinoschisis)
        361.10
      pigment epithelium (exudative)
        362.42
      hemorrhagic 362.43
  sternoclavicular (traumatic) — *see*
    Dislocation, sternoclavicular
  symphysis pubis, obstetrical trauma
    665.6 ☑
  tracheal ring, incomplete (congenital)
    748.3
**Sepsis** (generalized) 995.91
  with
    abortion — *see* Abortion, by type,
      with sepsis
    acute organ dysfunction 995.92
    ectopic pregnancy (*see also* cate-
      gories 633.0–633.9) 639.0
    molar pregnancy (*see also* cate-
      gories 630–632) 639.0
    multiple organ dysfunction (MOD)
      995.92
  buccal 528.3
  complicating labor 659.3 ☑
  dental (pulpal origin) 522.4
  female genital organ NEC 614.9
  fetus (intrauterine) 771.81
  following
    abortion 639.0
    ectopic or molar pregnancy 639.0
    infusion, perfusion, or transfusion
      999.39 ▲
  Friedländer's 038.49
  intraocular 360.00
  localized
    in operation wound 998.59
    skin (*see also* Abscess) 682.9
  malleus 024
  nadir 038.9
  newborn (organism unspecified) NEC
    771.81
  oral 528.3
  puerperal, postpartum, childbirth
    (pelvic) 670.0 ☑
  resulting from infusion, injection,
    transfusion, or vaccination
    999.39 ▲
  severe 995.92
  skin, localized (*see also* Abscess)
    682.9
  umbilical (newborn) (organism unspec-
    ified) 771.89
    tetanus 771.3
  urinary 599.0
    meaning sepsis 995.91
    meaning urinary tract infection
      599.0
**Septate** — *see also* Septum
**Septic** — *see also* condition
  adenoids 474.01
    and tonsils 474.02
  arm (with lymphangitis) 682.3
  embolus — *see* Embolism
  finger (with lymphangitis) 681.00
  foot (with lymphangitis) 682.7
  gallbladder (*see also* Cholecystitis)
    575.8
  hand (with lymphangitis) 682.4
  joint (*see also* Arthritis, septic)
    711.0 ☑
  kidney (*see also* Infection, kidney)
    590.9
  leg (with lymphangitis) 682.6
  mouth 528.3
  nail 681.9
    finger 681.02
    toe 681.11
  shock (endotoxic) 785.52
  sore (*see also* Abscess) 682.9
    throat 034.0
      milk-borne 034.0
      streptococcal 034.0

**Septic** — *see also* condition —
  *continued*
  spleen (acute) 289.59
  teeth (pulpal origin) 522.4
  throat 034.0
  thrombus — *see* Thrombosis
  toe (with lymphangitis) 681.10
  tonsils 474.00
    and adenoids 474.02
  umbilical cord (newborn) (organism
    unspecified) 771.89
  uterus (*see also* Endometritis) 615.9
**Septicemia, septicemic** (generalized)
  (suppurative) 038.9
  with
    abortion — *see* Abortion, by type,
      with sepsis
    ectopic pregnancy (*see also* cate-
      gories 633.0–633.9) 639.0
    molar pregnancy (*see also* cate-
      gories 630–632) 639.0
  Aerobacter aerogenes 038.49
  anaerobic 038.3
  anthrax 022.3
  Bacillus coli 038.42
  Bacteroides 038.3
  Clostridium 038.3
  complicating labor 659.3 ☑
  cryptogenic 038.9
  enteric gram-negative bacilli 038.40
  Enterobacter aerogenes 038.49
  Erysipelothrix (insidiosa) (rhusiopathi-
    ae) 027.1
  Escherichia coli 038.42
  following
    abortion 639.0
    ectopic or molar pregnancy 639.0
    infusion, injection, transfusion, or
      vaccination 999.39 ▲
  Friedländer's (bacillus) 038.49
  gangrenous 038.9
  gonococcal 098.89
  gram-negative (organism) 038.40
    anaerobic 038.3
  Hemophilus influenzae 038.41
  herpes (simplex) 054.5
  herpetic 054.5
  Listeria monocytogenes 027.0
  meningeal — *see* Meningitis
  meningococcal (chronic) (fulminating)
    036.2
  navel, newborn (organism unspecified)
    771.89
  newborn (organism unspecified)
    771.81
  plague 020.2
  pneumococcal 038.2
  postabortal 639.0
  postoperative 998.59
  Proteus vulgaris 038.49
  Pseudomonas (aeruginosa) 038.43
  puerperal, postpartum 670.0 ☑
  Salmonella (aertrycke) (callinarum)
    (choleraesuis) (enteritidis)
    (suipestifer) 003.1
  Serratia 038.44
  Shigella (*see also* Dysentery, bacillary)
    004.9
  specified organism NEC 038.8
  staphylococcal 038.10
    aureus 038.11
    specified organism NEC 038.19
  streptococcal (anaerobic) 038.0
  Streptococcus pneumoniae 038.2
  suipestifer 003.1
  umbilicus, newborn (organism unspec-
    ified) 771.89
  viral 079.99
  Yersinia enterocolitica 038.49
**Septum, septate** (congenital) — *see also*
  Anomaly, specified type NEC
  anal 751.2
  aqueduct of Sylvius 742.3
    with spina bifida (*see also* Spina
      bifida) 741.0 ☑
  hymen 752.49

**Septum, septate** — *see also* Anomaly,
  specified type — *continued*
  uterus (*see also* Double, uterus) 752.2
  vagina 752.49
    in pregnancy or childbirth 654.7 ☑
      affecting fetus or newborn
        763.89
      causing obstructed labor
        660.2 ☑
        affecting fetus or newborn
          763.1
**Sequestration**
  lung (congenital) (extralobar) (intralo-
    bar) 748.5
  orbit 376.10
  pulmonary artery (congenital) 747.3
  splenic 289.52
**Sequestrum**
  bone (*see also* Osteomyelitis) 730.1 ☑
    jaw 526.4
  dental 525.8
  jaw bone 526.4
  sinus (accessory) (nasal) (*see also* Si-
    nusitis) 473.9
    maxillary 473.0
**Sequoiosis asthma** 495.8
**Serology for syphilis**
  doubtful
    with signs or symptoms — *see*
      Syphilis, by site and stage
    follow-up of latent syphilis — *see*
      Syphilis, latent
  false positive 795.6
  negative, with signs or symptoms —
    *see* Syphilis, by site and stage
  positive 097.1
    with signs or symptoms — *see*
      Syphilis, by site and stage
    false 795.6
    follow-up of latent syphilis — *see*
      Syphilis, latent
    only finding — *see* Syphilis, latent
  reactivated 097.1
**Seroma** (postoperative) (non-infected)
  998.13
  infected 998.51
**Seropurulent** — *see* condition
**Serositis, multiple** 569.89
  pericardial 423.2
  peritoneal 568.82
  pleural — *see* Pleurisy
**Serotonin syndrome** 333.99
**Serous** — *see* condition
**Sertoli cell**
  adenoma (M8640/0)
    specified site — *see* Neoplasm, by
      site, benign
    unspecified site
      female 220
      male 222.0
  carcinoma (M8640/3)
    specified site — *see* Neoplasm, by
      site, malignant
    unspecified site 186.9
  syndrome (germinal aplasia) 606.0
  tumor (M8640/0)
    with lipid storage (M8641/0)
      specified site — *see* Neoplasm,
        by site, benign
      unspecified site
        female 220
        male 222.0
    specified site — *see* Neoplasm, by
      site, benign
    unspecified site
      female 220
      male 222.0
**Sertoli-Leydig cell tumor** (M8631/0)
  specified site — *see* Neoplasm, by site,
    benign
  unspecified site
    female 220
    male 222.0
**Serum**
  allergy, allergic reaction 999.5
    shock 999.4

☑ Additional Digit Required — Refer to the Tabular List for Digit Selection      ▼ Subterms under main terms may continue to next column or page

*2008 ICD-9-CM*     ▶◀ Revised Text     ● New Line     ▲ Revised Code     October 2007 • Volume 2 — 259

**Serum** — *continued*
  arthritis 999.5 *[713.6]*
  complication or reaction NEC 999.5
  disease NEC 999.5
    hepatitis 070.3 ☑
  intoxication 999.5
  jaundice (homologous) — *see* Hepatitis, viral, type B
  neuritis 999.5
  poisoning NEC 999.5
  rash NEC 999.5
  reaction NEC 999.5
  sickness NEC 999.5
**Sesamoiditis** 733.99
**Seven-day fever** 061
  of
    Japan 100.89
    Queensland 100.89
**Sever's disease or osteochondrosis** (calcaneum) 732.5
**Sex chromosome mosaics** 758.81
**Sex reassignment surgery status** (*see* ●
  *also* Trans-sexualism 302.50     ●
**Sextuplet**
  affected by maternal complications of pregnancy 761.5
  healthy liveborn — *see* Newborn, multiple
  pregnancy (complicating delivery) NEC 651.8 ☑
    with fetal loss and retention of one or more fetus(es) 651.6 ☑
    following (elective) fetal reduction 651.7 ☑
**Sexual**
  anesthesia 302.72
  deviation (*see also* Deviation, sexual) 302.9
  disorder (*see also* Deviation, sexual) 302.9
  frigidity (female) 302.72
  function, disorder of (psychogenic) 302.70
    specified type NEC 302.79
  immaturity (female) (male) 259.0
  impotence 607.84
    organic origin NEC 607.84
    psychogenic 302.72
  precocity (constitutional) (cryptogenic) (female) (idiopathic) (male) NEC 259.1
    with adrenal hyperplasia 255.2
  sadism 302.84
**Sexuality, pathological** — *see also* Deviation, sexual 302.9
**Sézary's disease, reticulosis, or syndrome** (M9701/3) 202.2 ☑
**Shadow, lung** 793.1
**Shaken infant syndrome** 995.55
**Shaking**
  head (tremor) 781.0
  palsy or paralysis (*see also* Parkinsonism) 332.0
**Shallowness, acetabulum** 736.39
**Shaver's disease or syndrome** (bauxite pneumoconiosis) 503
**Shearing**
  artificial skin graft 996.55
  decellularized allodermis graft 996.55
**Sheath** (tendon) — *see* condition
**Shedding**
  nail 703.8
  teeth, premature, primary (deciduous) 520.6
**Sheehan's disease or syndrome** (postpartum pituitary necrosis) 253.2
**Shelf, rectal** 569.49
**Shell**
  shock (current) (*see also* Reaction, stress, acute) 308.9
    lasting state 300.16
  teeth 520.5
**Shield kidney** 753.3
**Shifting**
  pacemaker 427.89

**Shifting** — *continued*
  sleep-work schedule (affecting sleep) 327.36
**Shift, mediastinal** 793.2
**Shiga's**
  bacillus 004.0
  dysentery 004.0
**Shigella** (dysentery) — *see also* Dysentery, bacillary 004.9
  carrier (suspected) of V02.3
**Shigellosis** — *see also* Dysentery, bacillary 004.9
**Shingles** — *see also* Herpes, zoster 053.9
  eye NEC 053.29
**Shin splints** 844.9
**Shipyard eye or disease** 077.1
**Shirodkar suture, in pregnancy** 654.5 ☑
**Shock** 785.50
  with
    abortion — *see* Abortion, by type, with shock
    ectopic pregnancy (*see also* categories 633.0–633.9) 639.5
    molar pregnancy (*see also* categories 630–632) 639.5
  allergic — *see* Shock, anaphylactic
  anaclitic 309.21
  anaphylactic 995.0
    chemical — *see* Table of Drugs and Chemicals
    correct medicinal substance properly administered 995.0
    drug or medicinal substance
      correct substance properly administered 995.0
      overdose or wrong substance given or taken 977.9
      specified drug — *see* Table of Drugs and Chemicals
    following sting(s) 989.5
    food — *see* Anaphylactic shock, due to, food
    immunization 999.4
    serum 999.4
  anaphylactoid — *see* Shock, anaphylactic
  anesthetic
    correct substance properly administered 995.4
    overdose or wrong substance given 968.4
    specified anesthetic — *see* Table of Drugs and Chemicals
  birth, fetus or newborn NEC 779.89
  cardiogenic 785.51
  chemical substance — *see* Table of Drugs and Chemicals
  circulatory 785.59
  complicating
    abortion — *see* Abortion, by type, with shock
    ectopic pregnancy (*see also* categories 633.0–633.9) 639.5
    labor and delivery 669.1 ☑
    molar pregnancy (*see also* categories 630–632) 639.5
  culture 309.29
  due to
    drug 995.0
      correct substance properly administered 995.0
      overdose or wrong substance given or taken 977.9
      specified drug — *see* Table of Drugs and Chemicals
    food — *see* Anaphylactic shock, due to, food
  during labor and delivery 669.1 ☑
  electric 994.8
  endotoxic 785.52
    due to surgical procedure 998.0
  following
    abortion 639.5

**Shock** — *continued*
  following — *continued*
    ectopic or molar pregnancy 639.5
    injury (immediate) (delayed) 958.4
    labor and delivery 669.1 ☑
  gram-negative 785.52
  hematogenic 785.59
  hemorrhagic
    due to
      disease 785.59
      surgery (intraoperative) (postoperative) 998.0
      trauma 958.4
  hypovolemic NEC 785.59
    surgical 998.0
    traumatic 958.4
  insulin 251.0
    therapeutic misadventure 962.3
  kidney 584.5
    traumatic (following crushing) 958.5
  lightning 994.0
  lung 518.5
  nervous (*see also* Reaction, stress, acute) 308.9
  obstetric 669.1 ☑
    with
      abortion — *see* Abortion, by type, with shock
      ectopic pregnancy (*see also* categories 633.0–633.9) 639.5
      molar pregnancy (*see also* categories 630–632) 639.5
    following
      abortion 639.5
      ectopic or molar pregnancy 639.5
  paralysis, paralytic (*see also* Disease, cerebrovascular, acute) 436
    late effect — *see* Late effect(s) (of) cerebrovascular disease
  pleural (surgical) 998.0
    due to trauma 958.4
  postoperative 998.0
    with
      abortion — *see* Abortion, by type, with shock
      ectopic pregnancy (*see also* categories 633.0–633.9) 639.5
      molar pregnancy (*see also* categories 630–632) 639.5
    following
      abortion 639.5
      ectopic or molar pregnancy 639.5
  psychic (*see also* Reaction, stress, acute) 308.9
    past history (of) V15.49
  psychogenic (*see also* Reaction, stress, acute) 308.9
  septic 785.52
    with
      abortion — *see* Abortion, by type, with shock
      ectopic pregnancy (*see also* categories 633.0–633.9) 639.5
      molar pregnancy (*see also* categories 630–632) 639.5
    due to
      surgical procedure 998.0
      transfusion NEC 999.8
        bone marrow 996.85
    following
      abortion 639.5
      ectopic or molar pregnancy 639.5
      surgical procedure 998.0
      transfusion NEC 999.8
        bone marrow 996.85
  spinal (*see also* Injury, spinal, by site)
    with spinal bone injury — *see* Fracture, vertebra, by site, with spinal cord injury

**Shock** — *continued*
  surgical 998.0
  therapeutic misadventure NEC (*see also* Complications) 998.89
  thyroxin 962.7
  toxic 040.82
  transfusion — *see* Complications, transfusion
  traumatic (immediate) (delayed) 958.4
**Shoemakers' chest** 738.3
**Short, shortening, shortness**
  Achilles tendon (acquired) 727.81
  arm 736.89
    congenital 755.20
  back 737.9
  bowel syndrome 579.3
  breath 786.05
  chain acyl CoA dehydrogenase deficiency (SCAD) 277.85
  common bile duct, congenital 751.69
  cord (umbilical) 663.4 ☑
    affecting fetus or newborn 762.6
  cystic duct, congenital 751.69
  esophagus (congenital) 750.4
  femur (acquired) 736.81
    congenital 755.34
  frenulum linguae 750.0
  frenum, lingual 750.0
  hamstrings 727.81
  hip (acquired) 736.39
    congenital 755.63
  leg (acquired) 736.81
    congenital 755.30
  metatarsus (congenital) 754.79
    acquired 736.79
  organ or site, congenital NEC — *see* Distortion
  palate (congenital) 750.26
  P-R interval syndrome 426.81
  radius (acquired) 736.09
    congenital 755.26
  round ligament 629.89
  sleeper 307.49
  stature, constitutional (hereditary) ▶(idiopathic)◄ 783.43
  tendon 727.81
    Achilles (acquired) 727.81
      congenital 754.79
  thigh (acquired) 736.81
    congenital 755.34
  tibialis anticus 727.81
  umbilical cord 663.4 ☑
    affecting fetus or newborn 762.6
  urethra 599.84
  uvula (congenital) 750.26
  vagina 623.8
**Shortsightedness** 367.1
**Shoshin** (acute fulminating beriberi) 265.0
**Shoulder** — *see* condition
**Shovel-shaped incisors** 520.2
**Shower, thromboembolic** — *see* Embolism
**Shunt** (status)
  aortocoronary bypass V45.81
  arterial-venous (dialysis) V45.1
  arteriovenous, pulmonary (acquired) 417.0
    congenital 747.3
    traumatic (complication) 901.40
  cerebral ventricle (communicating) in situ V45.2
  coronary artery bypass V45.81
  surgical, prosthetic, with complications — *see* Complications, shunt
  vascular NEC V45.89
**Shutdown**
  renal 586
    with
      abortion — *see* Abortion, by type, with renal failure
      ectopic pregnancy (*see also* categories 633.0–633.9) 639.3

---

**Shutdown** — *continued*
  renal — *continued*
    with — *continued*
      molar pregnancy (*see also* categories 630–632) 639.3
      complicating
        abortion 639.3
        ectopic or molar pregnancy 639.3
      following labor and delivery 669.3 ☑
**Shwachman's syndrome** 288.02
**Shy-Drager syndrome** (orthostatic hypotension with multisystem degeneration) 333.0
**Sialadenitis** (any gland) (chronic) (suppurative) 527.2
  epidemic — *see* Mumps
**Sialadenosis, periodic** 527.2
**Sialaporia** 527.7
**Sialectasia** 527.8
**Sialitis** 527.2
**Sialoadenitis** — *see also* Sialadenitis 527.2
**Sialoangitis** 527.2
**Sialodochitis** (fibrinosa) 527.2
**Sialodocholithiasis** 527.5
**Sialolithiasis** 527.5
**Sialorrhea** — *see also* Ptyalism 527.7
  periodic 527.2
**Sialosis** 527.8
  rheumatic 710.2
**Siamese twin** 759.4
**Sicard's syndrome** 352.6
**Sicca syndrome** (keratoconjunctivitis) 710.2
**Sick** 799.9
  cilia syndrome 759.89
  or handicapped person in family V61.49
**Sickle-cell**
  anemia (see also Disease, sickle-cell) 282.60
  disease (see also Disease, sickle-cell) 282.60
  hemoglobin
    C disease (without crisis) 282.63
      with
        crisis 282.64
          vaso-occlusive pain 282.64
    D disease (without crisis) 282.68
      with crisis 282.69
    E disease (without crisis) 282.68
      with crisis 282.69
  thalassemia (without crisis) 282.41
    with
      crisis 282.42
      vaso-occlusive pain 282.42
  trait 282.5
**Sicklemia** — *see also* Disease, sickle-cell 282.60
  trait 282.5
**Sickness**
  air (travel) 994.6
  airplane 994.6
  alpine 993.2
  altitude 993.2
  Andes 993.2
  aviators' 993.2
  balloon 993.2
  car 994.6
  compressed air 993.3
  decompression 993.3
  green 280.9
  harvest 100.89
  milk 988.8
  morning 643.0 ☑
  motion 994.6
  mountain 993.2
    acute 289.0
  protein (*see also* Complications, vaccination) 999.5
  radiation NEC 990
  roundabout (motion) 994.6
  sea 994.6
  serum NEC 999.5

**Sickness** — *continued*
  sleeping (African) 086.5
    by Trypanosoma 086.5
      gambiense 086.3
      rhodesiense 086.4
    Gambian 086.3
    late effect 139.8
    Rhodesian 086.4
  sweating 078.2
  swing (motion) 994.6
  train (railway) (travel) 994.6
  travel (any vehicle) 994.6
**Sick sinus syndrome** 427.81
**Sideropenia** — *see also* Anemia, iron deficiency 280.9
**Siderosis** (lung) (occupational) 503
  cornea 371.15
  eye (bulbi) (vitreous) 360.23
  lens 360.23
**Siegal-Cattan-Mamou disease** (periodic) 277.31
**Siemens' syndrome**
  ectodermal dysplasia 757.31
  keratosis follicularis spinulosa (decalvans) 757.39
**Sighing respiration** 786.7
**Sigmoid**
  flexure — *see* condition
  kidney 753.3
**Sigmoiditis** — *see* Enteritis
**Silfverskiöld's syndrome** 756.50
**Silicosis, silicotic** (complicated) (occupational) (simple) 502
  fibrosis, lung (confluent) (massive) (occupational) 502
  non-nodular 503
  pulmonum 502
**Silicotuberculosis** — *see also* Tuberculosis 011.4 ☑
**Silo fillers' disease** 506.9
**Silver's syndrome** (congenital hemihypertrophy and short stature) 759.89
**Silver wire arteries, retina** 362.13
**Silvestroni-Bianco syndrome** (thalassemia minima) 282.49
**Simian crease** 757.2
**Simmonds' cachexia or disease** (pituitary cachexia) 253.2
**Simons' disease or syndrome** (progressive lipodystrophy) 272.6
**Simple, simplex** — *see* condition
**Sinding-Larsen disease** (juvenile osteopathia patellae) 732.4
**Singapore hemorrhagic fever** 065.4
**Singers' node or nodule** 478.5
**Single**
  atrium 745.69
  coronary artery 746.85
  umbilical artery 747.5
  ventricle 745.3
**Singultus** 786.8
  epidemicus 078.89
**Sinus** — *see also* Fistula
  abdominal 569.81
  arrest 426.6
  arrhythmia 427.89
  bradycardia 427.89
    chronic 427.81
  branchial cleft (external) (internal) 744.41
  coccygeal (infected) 685.1
    with abscess 685.0
  dental 522.7
  dermal (congenital) 685.1
    with abscess 685.0
  draining — *see* Fistula
  infected, skin NEC 686.9
  marginal, ruptured or bleeding 641.2 ☑
    affecting fetus or newborn 762.1
  pause 426.6
  pericranii 742.0
  pilonidal (infected) (rectum) 685.1
    with abscess 685.0
  preauricular 744.46

**Sinus** — *see also* Fistula — *continued*
  rectovaginal 619.1
  sacrococcygeal (dermoid) (infected) 685.1
    with abscess 685.0
  skin
    infected NEC 686.9
    noninfected — *see* Ulcer, skin
  tachycardia 427.89
  tarsi syndrome 726.79
  testis 608.89
  tract (postinfectional) — *see* Fistula
  urachus 753.7
**Sinuses, Rokitansky-Aschoff** — *see also* Disease, gallbladder 575.8
**Sinusitis** (accessory) (nasal) (hyperplastic) (nonpurulent) (purulent) (chronic) 473.9
  with influenza, flu, or grippe 487.1
  acute 461.9
    ethmoidal 461.2
    frontal 461.1
    maxillary 461.0
    specified type NEC 461.8
    sphenoidal 461.3
  allergic (*see also* Fever, hay) 477.9
  antrum — *see* Sinusitis, maxillary
  due to
    fungus, any sinus 117.9
    high altitude 993.1
  ethmoidal 473.2
    acute 461.2
  frontal 473.1
    acute 461.1
  influenzal 478.19
  maxillary 473.0
    acute 461.0
  specified site NEC 473.8
  sphenoidal 473.3
    acute 461.3
  syphilitic, any sinus 095.8
  tuberculous, any sinus (*see also* Tuberculosis) 012.8 ☑
**Sinusitis-bronchiectasis-situs inversus** (syndrome) (triad) 759.3
**Sioloangitis** 527.2
**Sipple's syndrome** (medullary thyroid carcinoma-pheochromocytoma) 258.02 ▲
**Sirenomelia** 759.89
**Siriasis** 992.0
**Sirkari's disease** 085.0
**SIRS** (systemic inflammatory response syndrome) 995.90
  due to
    infectious process 995.91
      with acute organ dysfunction 995.92
    non-infectious process 995.93
      with acute organ dysfunction 995.94
**Siti** 104.0
**Sitophobia** 300.29
**Situational**
  disturbance (transient) (*see also* Reaction, adjustment) 309.9
    acute 308.3
  maladjustment, acute (*see also* Reaction, adjustment) 309.9
  reaction (*see also* Reaction, adjustment) 309.9
    acute 308.3
**Situation, psychiatric** 300.9
**Situs inversus or transversus** 759.3
  abdominalis 759.3
  thoracis 759.3
**Sixth disease**
  due to       ●
    human herpesvirus 6 058.11  ●
    human herpesvirus 7 058.12  ●
**Sjögren-Larsson syndrome** (ichthyosis congenita) 757.1
**Sjögren (-Gougerot) syndrome or disease** (keratoconjunctivitis sicca) 710.2
  with lung involvement 710.2 *[517.8]*

**Skeletal** — *see* condition
**Skene's gland** — *see* condition
**Skenitis** — *see also* Urethritis 597.89
  gonorrheal (acute) 098.0
    chronic or duration of 2 months or over 098.2
**Skerljevo** 104.0
**Skevas-Zerfus disease** 989.5
**Skin** — *see also* condition
  donor V59.1
  hidebound 710.9
**SLAP lesion** (superior glenoid labrum) 840.7
**Slate-dressers' lung** 502
**Slate-miners' lung** 502
**Sleep**
  deprivation V69.4
  disorder 780.50
    with apnea — *see* Apnea, sleep
    child 307.40
    movement, unspecified 780.58
    nonorganic origin 307.40
      specified type NEC 307.49
  disturbance 780.50
    with apnea — *see* Apnea, sleep
    nonorganic origin 307.40
      specified type NEC 307.49
  drunkenness 307.47
  movement disorder, unspecified 780.58
  paroxysmal (*see also* Narcolepsy) 347.00
  related movement disorder, unspecified 780.58
  rhythm inversion 327.39
    nonorganic origin 307.45
  walking 307.46
    hysterical 300.13
**Sleeping sickness** 086.5
  late effect 139.8
**Sleeplessness** — *see also* Insomnia 780.52
  menopausal 627.2
  nonorganic origin 307.41
**Slipped, slipping**
  epiphysis (postinfectional) 732.9
    traumatic (old) 732.9
      current — *see* Fracture, by site
      upper femoral (nontraumatic) 732.2
  intervertebral disc — *see* Displacement, intervertebral disc
  ligature, umbilical 772.3
  patella 717.89
  rib 733.99
  sacroiliac joint 724.6
  tendon 727.9
  ulnar nerve, nontraumatic 354.2
  vertebra NEC (*see also* Spondylolisthesis) 756.12
**Slocumb's syndrome** 255.3
**Sloughing** (multiple) (skin) 686.9
  abscess — *see* Abscess, by site
  appendix 543.9
  bladder 596.8
  fascia 728.9
  graft — *see* Complications, graft
  phagedena (*see also* Gangrene) 785.4
  reattached extremity (*see also* Complications, reattached extremity) 996.90
  rectum 569.49
  scrotum 608.89
  tendon 727.9
  transplanted organ (*see also* Rejection, transplant, organ, by site) 996.80
  ulcer (*see also* Ulcer, skin) 707.9
**Slow**
  feeding newborn 779.3
  fetal, growth NEC 764.9 ☑
    affecting management of pregnancy 656.5 ☑
**Slowing**
  heart 427.89
  urinary stream 788.62

☑ Additional Digit Required — Refer to the Tabular List for Digit Selection        ☝ Subterms under main terms may continue to next column or page

**2008 ICD-9-CM**          ▶◀ Revised Text       ● New Line    ▲ Revised Code       **October 2007 · Volume 2 — 261**

**Sluder's neuralgia or syndrome** 337.0
**Slurred, slurring, speech** 784.5
**Small-for-dates** — see also Light-for-
dates 764.0 ☑
affecting management of pregnancy
656.5 ☑
**Smallpox** 050.9
contact V01.3
exposure to V01.3
hemorrhagic (pustular) 050.0
malignant 050.0
modified 050.2
vaccination
complications — see Complications, vaccination
prophylactic (against) V04.1
**Small, smallness**
cardiac reserve — see Disease, heart
for dates
fetus or newborn 764.0 ☑
with malnutrition 764.1 ☑
affecting management of pregnancy 656.5 ☑
infant, term 764.0 ☑
with malnutrition 764.1 ☑
affecting management of pregnancy
656.5 ☑
introitus, vagina 623.3
kidney, unknown cause 589.9
bilateral 589.1
unilateral 589.0
ovary 620.8
pelvis
with disproportion (fetopelvic)
653.1 ☑
affecting fetus or newborn 763.1
causing obstructed labor 660.1 ☑
affecting fetus or newborn 763.1
placenta — see Placenta, insufficiency
uterus 621.8
white kidney 582.9
**Smith's fracture** (separation) (closed)
813.41
open 813.51
**Smith-Lemli Opitz syndrome** (cerebrohepatorenal syndrome) 759.89
**Smith-Magenis syndrome** 758.33
**Smith-Strang disease** (oasthouse urine)
270.2
**Smokers'**
bronchitis 491.0
cough 491.0
syndrome (see also Abuse, drugs,
nondependent) 305.1
throat 472.1
tongue 528.6
**Smoking complicating pregnancy,
childbirth, or the puerperium**
649.0 ☑
**Smothering spells** 786.09
**Snaggle teeth, tooth** 524.39
**Snapping**
finger 727.05
hip 719.65
jaw 524.69
temporomandibular joint sounds
on opening or closing 524.64
knee 717.9
thumb 727.05
**Sneddon-Wilkinson disease or syn-
drome** (subcorneal pustular dermatosis) 694.1
**Sneezing** 784.99
intractable 478.19
**Sniffing**
cocaine (see also Dependence)
304.2 ☑
ether (see also Dependence) 304.6 ☑
glue (airplane) (see also Dependence)
304.6 ☑
**Snoring** 786.09
**Snow blindness** 370.24
**Snuffles** (nonsyphilitic) 460
syphilitic (infant) 090.0
**Social migrant** V60.0
**Sodoku** 026.0

**Soemmering's ring** 366.51
**Soft** — see also condition
enlarged prostate 600.00
with
other lower urinary tract symptoms (LUTS) 600.01
urinary
obstruction 600.01
retention 600.01
nails 703.8
**Softening**
bone 268.2
brain (necrotic) (progressive) 434.9 ☑
arteriosclerotic 437.0
congenital 742.4
embolic (see also Embolism, brain)
434.1 ☑
hemorrhagic (see also Hemorrhage,
brain) 431
occlusive 434.9 ☑
thrombotic (see also Thrombosis,
brain) 434.0 ☑
cartilage 733.92
cerebellar — see Softening, brain
cerebral — see Softening, brain
cerebrospinal — see Softening, brain
myocardial, heart (see also Degeneration, myocardial) 429.1
nails 703.8
spinal cord 336.8
stomach 537.89
**Solar fever** 061
**Soldier's**
heart 306.2
patches 423.1
**Solitary**
cyst
bone 733.21
kidney 593.2
kidney (congenital) 753.0
tubercle, brain (see also Tuberculosis,
brain) 013.2 ☑
ulcer, bladder 596.8
**Somatization reaction, somatic reac-
tion** — see also Disorder, psychosomatic 306.9
disorder 300.81
**Somatoform disorder** 300.82
atypical 300.82
severe 300.81
undifferentiated 300.82
**Somnambulism** 307.46
hysterical 300.13
**Somnolence** 780.09
nonorganic origin 307.43
periodic 349.89
**Sonne dysentery** 004.3
**Soor** 112.0
**Sore**
Delhi 085.1
desert (see also Ulcer, skin) 707.9
eye 379.99
Lahore 085.1
mouth 528.9
canker 528.2
due to dentures 528.9
muscle 729.1
Naga (see also Ulcer, skin) 707.9
oriental 085.1
pressure (see also Decubitus) 707.00
with gangrene (see also Decubitus)
707.00 [785.4]
skin NEC 709.9
soft 099.0
throat 462
with influenza, flu, or grippe 487.1
acute 462
chronic 472.1
clergyman's 784.49
coxsackie (virus) 074.0
diphtheritic 032.0
epidemic 034.0
gangrenous 462
herpetic 054.79
influenzal 487.1
malignant 462

**Sore** — continued
throat — continued
purulent 462
putrid 462
septic 034.0
streptococcal (ulcerative) 034.0
ulcerated 462
viral NEC 462
Coxsackie 074.0
tropical (see also Ulcer, skin) 707.9
veldt (see also Ulcer, skin) 707.9
**Sotos' syndrome** (cerebral gigantism)
253.0
**Sounds**
friction, pleural 786.7
succussion, chest 786.7
temporomandibular joint
on opening or closing 524.64
**South African cardiomyopathy syn-
drome** 425.2
**South American**
blastomycosis 116.1
trypanosomiasis — see Trypanosomiasis
**Southeast Asian hemorrhagic fever**
065.4
**Spacing, teeth, abnormal** 524.30
excessive 524.32
**Spade-like hand** (congenital) 754.89
**Spading nail** 703.8
congenital 757.5
**Spanemia** 285.9
**Spanish collar** 605
**Sparganosis** 123.5
**Spasmodic** — see condition
**Spasmophilia** — see also Tetany 781.7
**Spasm, spastic, spasticity** — see also
condition 781.0
accommodation 367.53
ampulla of Vater (see also Disease,
gallbladder) 576.8
anus, ani (sphincter) (reflex) 564.6
psychogenic 306.4
artery NEC 443.9
basilar 435.0
carotid 435.8
cerebral 435.9
specified artery NEC 435.8
retinal (see also Occlusion, retinal,
artery) 362.30
vertebral 435.1
vertebrobasilar 435.3
Bell's 351.0
bladder (sphincter, external or internal) 596.8
bowel 564.9
psychogenic 306.4
bronchus, bronchiole 519.11
cardia 530.0
cardiac — see Angina
carpopedal (see also Tetany) 781.7
cecum 564.9
psychogenic 306.4
cerebral (arteries) (vascular) 435.9
specified artery NEC 435.8
cerebrovascular 435.9
cervix, complicating delivery 661.4 ☑
affecting fetus or newborn 763.7
ciliary body (of accommodation)
367.53
colon 564.1
psychogenic 306.4
common duct (see also Disease, biliary) 576.8
compulsive 307.22
conjugate 378.82
convergence 378.84
coronary (artery) — see Angina
diaphragm (reflex) 786.8
psychogenic 306.1
duodenum, duodenal (bulb) 564.89
esophagus (diffuse) 530.5
psychogenic 306.4
facial 351.8
fallopian tube 620.8
gait 781.2

**Spasm, spastic, spasticity** — see also
condition — continued
gastrointestinal (tract) 536.8
psychogenic 306.4
glottis 478.75
hysterical 300.11
psychogenic 306.1
specified as conversion reaction
300.11
reflex through recurrent laryngeal
nerve 478.75
habit 307.20
chronic 307.22
transient (of childhood) 307.21
heart — see Angina
hourglass — see Contraction, hourglass
hysterical 300.11
infantile (see also Epilepsy) 345.6 ☑
internal oblique, eye 378.51
intestinal 564.9
psychogenic 306.4
larynx, laryngeal 478.75
hysterical 300.11
psychogenic 306.1
specified as conversion reaction
300.11
levator palpebrae superioris 333.81
lightning (see also Epilepsy) 345.6 ☑
mobile 781.0
muscle 728.85
back 724.8
psychogenic 306.0
nerve, trigeminal 350.1
nervous 306.0
nodding 307.3
infantile (see also Epilepsy)
345.6 ☑
occupational 300.89
oculogyric 378.87
ophthalmic artery 362.30
orbicularis 781.0
perineal 625.8
peroneo-extensor (see also Flat, foot)
734
pharynx (reflex) 478.29
hysterical 300.11
psychogenic 306.1
specified as conversion reaction
300.11
pregnant uterus, complicating delivery
661.4 ☑
psychogenic 306.0
pylorus 537.81
adult hypertrophic 537.0
congenital or infantile 750.5
psychogenic 306.4
rectum (sphincter) 564.6
psychogenic 306.4
retinal artery NEC (see also Occlusion,
retina, artery) 362.30
sacroiliac 724.6
salaam (infantile) (see also Epilepsy)
345.6 ☑
saltatory 781.0
sigmoid 564.9
psychogenic 306.4
sphincter of Oddi (see also Disease,
gallbladder) 576.5
stomach 536.8
neurotic 306.4
throat 478.29
hysterical 300.11
psychogenic 306.1
specified as conversion reaction
300.11
tic 307.20
chronic 307.22
transient (of childhood) 307.21
tongue 529.8
torsion 333.6
trigeminal nerve 350.1
postherpetic 053.12
ureter 593.89
urethra (sphincter) 599.84
uterus 625.8

**Spasm, spastic, spasticity** — see also
condition — continued
uterus — continued
complicating labor 661.4 ☑
affecting fetus or newborn 763.7
vagina 625.1
psychogenic 306.51
vascular NEC 443.9
vasomotor NEC 443.9
vein NEC 459.89
vesical (sphincter, external or internal)
596.8
viscera 789.0 ☑
**Spasmus nutans** 307.3
**Spastic** — see also Spasm
child 343.9
**Spasticity** — see also Spasm
cerebral, child 343.9
**Speakers' throat** 784.49
**Specific, specified** — see condition
**Speech**
defect, disorder, disturbance, impediment NEC 784.5
psychogenic 307.9
therapy V57.3
**Spells** 780.39
breath-holding 786.9
**Spencer's disease** (epidemic vomiting)
078.82
**Spens' syndrome** (syncope with heart
block) 426.9
**Spermatic cord** — see condition
**Spermatocele** 608.1
congenital 752.89
**Spermatocystitis** 608.4
**Spermatocytoma** (M9063/3)
specified site — see Neoplasm, by site,
malignant
unspecified site 186.9
**Spermatorrhea** 608.89
**Sperm counts**
fertility testing V26.21
following sterilization reversal V26.22
postvasectomy V25.8
**Sphacelus** — see also Gangrene 785.4
**Sphenoidal** — see condition
**Sphenoiditis** (chronic) — see also Sinusitis, sphenoidal 473.3
**Sphenopalatine ganglion neuralgia**
337.0
**Sphericity, increased, lens** 743.36
**Spherocytosis** (congenital) (familial)
(hereditary) 282.0
hemoglobin disease 282.7
sickle-cell (disease) 282.60
**Spherophakia** 743.36
**Sphincter** — see condition
**Sphincteritis, sphincter of Oddi** — see
also Cholecystitis 576.8
**Sphingolipidosis** 272.7
**Sphingolipodystrophy** 272.7
**Sphingomyelinosis** 272.7
**Spicule tooth** 520.2
**Spider**
finger 755.59
nevus 448.1
vascular 448.1
**Spiegler-Fendt sarcoid** 686.8
**Spielmeyer-Stock disease** 330.1
**Spielmeyer-Vogt disease** 330.1
**Spina bifida** (aperta) 741.9 ☑

Note — Use the following fifth-digit
subclassification with category 741:

0   unspecified region

1   cervical region

2   dorsal [thoracic} region

3   lumbar region

with hydrocephalus 741.0 ☑
fetal (suspected), affecting management of pregnancy 655.0 ☑
occulta 756.17
**Spindle, Krukenberg's** 371.13
**Spine, spinal** — see condition

**Spiradenoma** (eccrine) (M8403/0) — see
Neoplasm, skin, benign
**Spirillosis** NEC — see also Fever, relapsing 087.9
**Spirillum minus** 026.0
**Spirillum obermeieri infection** 087.0
**Spirochetal** — see condition
**Spirochetosis** 104.9
arthritic, arthritica 104.9 [711.8]
bronchopulmonary 104.8
icterohemorrhagica 100.0
lung 104.8
**Spitting blood** — see also Hemoptysis
786.3
**Splanchnomegaly** 569.89
**Splanchnoptosis** 569.89
**Spleen, splenic** — see also condition
agenesis 759.0
flexure syndrome 569.89
neutropenia syndrome 289.53
sequestration syndrome 289.52
**Splenectasis** — see also Splenomegaly
789.2
**Splenitis** (interstitial) (malignant) (nonspecific) 289.59
malarial (see also Malaria) 084.6
tuberculous (see also Tuberculosis)
017.7 ☑
**Splenocele** 289.59
**Splenomegalia** — see Splenomegaly
**Splenomegalic** — see condition
**Splenomegaly** 789.2
Bengal 789.2
cirrhotic 289.51
congenital 759.0
congestive, chronic 289.51
cryptogenic 789.2
Egyptian 120.1
Gaucher's (cerebroside lipidosis) 272.7
idiopathic 789.2
malarial (see also Malaria) 084.6
neutropenic 289.53
Niemann-Pick (lipid histiocytosis)
272.7
siderotic 289.51
syphilitic 095.8
congenital 090.0
tropical (Bengal) (idiopathic) 789.2
**Splenopathy** 289.50
**Splenopneumonia** — see Pneumonia
**Splenoptosis** 289.59
**Splinter** — see Injury, superficial, by site
**Split, splitting**
heart sounds 427.89
lip, congenital (see also Cleft, lip)
749.10
nails 703.8
urinary stream 788.61
**Spoiled child reaction** — see also Disturbance, conduct 312.1 ☑
**Spondylarthritis** — see also Spondylosis
721.90
**Spondylarthrosis** — see also Spondylosis 721.90
**Spondylitis** 720.9
ankylopoietica 720.0
ankylosing (chronic) 720.0
atrophic 720.9
ligamentosa 720.9
chronic (traumatic) (see also Spondylosis) 721.90
deformans (chronic) (see also
Spondylosis) 721.90
gonococcal 098.53
gouty 274.0
hypertrophic (see also Spondylosis)
721.90
infectious NEC 720.9
juvenile (adolescent) 720.0
Kümmell's 721.7
Marie-Strümpell (ankylosing) 720.0
muscularis 720.9
ossificans ligamentosa 721.6
osteoarthritica (see also Spondylosis)
721.90
posttraumatic 721.7

**Spondylitis** — continued
proliferative 720.0
rheumatoid 720.0
rhizomelica 720.0
sacroiliac NEC 720.2
senescent (see also Spondylosis)
721.90
senile (see also Spondylosis) 721.90
static (see also Spondylosis) 721.90
traumatic (chronic) (see also Spondylosis) 721.90
tuberculous (see also Tuberculosis)
015.0 ☑ [720.81]
typhosa 002.0 [720.81]
**Spondyloarthrosis** — see also Spondylosis 721.90
**Spondylolisthesis** (congenital) (lumbosacral) 756.12
with disproportion (fetopelvic) 653.3 ☑
affecting fetus or newborn 763.1
causing obstructed labor 660.1 ☑
affecting fetus or newborn 763.1
acquired 738.4
degenerative 738.4
traumatic 738.4
acute (lumbar) — see Fracture,
vertebra, lumbar
site other than lumbosacral —
see Fracture, vertebra, by
site
**Spondylolysis** (congenital) 756.11
acquired 738.4
cervical 756.19
lumbosacral region 756.11
with disproportion (fetopelvic)
653.3 ☑
affecting fetus or newborn 763.1
causing obstructed labor
660.1 ☑
affecting fetus or newborn
763.1
**Spondylopathy**
inflammatory 720.9
specified type NEC 720.89
traumatic 721.7
**Spondylose rhizomelique** 720.0
**Spondylosis** 721.90
with
disproportion 653.3 ☑
affecting fetus or newborn 763.1
causing obstructed labor
660.1 ☑
affecting fetus or newborn
763.1
myelopathy NEC 721.91
cervical, cervicodorsal 721.0
with myelopathy 721.1
inflammatory 720.9
lumbar, lumbosacral 721.3
with myelopathy 721.42
sacral 721.3
with myelopathy 721.42
thoracic 721.2
with myelopathy 721.41
traumatic 721.7
**Sponge**
divers' disease 989.5
inadvertently left in operation wound
998.4
kidney (medullary) 753.17
**Spongioblastoma** (M9422/3)
multiforme (M9440/3)
specified site — see Neoplasm, by
site, malignant
unspecified site 191.9
polare (M9423/3)
specified site — see Neoplasm, by
site, malignant
unspecified site 191.9
primitive polar (M9443/3)
specified site — see Neoplasm, by
site, malignant
unspecified site 191.9
specified site — see Neoplasm, by site,
malignant
unspecified site 191.9

**Spongiocytoma** (M9400/3)
specified site — see Neoplasm, by site,
malignant
unspecified site 191.9
**Spongioneuroblastoma** (M9504/3) —
see Neoplasm, by site, malignant
**Spontaneous** — see also condition
fracture — see Fracture, pathologic
**Spoon nail** 703.8
congenital 757.5
**Sporadic** — see condition
**Sporotrichosis** (bones) (cutaneous) (disseminated) (epidermal) (lymphatic)
(lymphocutaneous) (mucous membranes) (pulmonary) (skeletal) (visceral) 117.1
**Sporotrichum schenckii infection**
117.1
**Spots, spotting**
atrophic (skin) 701.3
Bitôt's (in the young child) 264.1
café au lait 709.09
cayenne pepper 448.1
complicating pregnancy 649.5 ☑
cotton wool (retina) 362.83
de Morgan's (senile angiomas) 448.1
Fúchs' black (myopic) 360.21
intermenstrual
irregular 626.6
regular 626.5
interpalpebral 372.53
Koplik's 055.9
liver 709.09
Mongolian (pigmented) 757.33
of pregnancy 641.9 ☑
purpuric 782.7
ruby 448.1
**Spotted fever** — see Fever, spotted
**Sprain, strain** (joint) (ligament) (muscle)
(tendon) 848.9
abdominal wall (muscle) 848.8
Achilles tendon 845.09
acromioclavicular 840.0
ankle 845.00
and foot 845.00
anterior longitudinal, cervical 847.0
arm 840.9
upper 840.9
and shoulder 840.9
astragalus 845.00
atlanto-axial 847.0
atlanto-occipital 847.0
atlas 847.0
axis 847.0
back (see also Sprain, spine) 847.9
breast bone 848.40
broad ligament — see Injury, internal,
broad ligament
calcaneofibular 845.02
carpal 842.01
carpometacarpal 842.11
cartilage
costal, without mention of injury
to sternum 848.3
involving sternum 848.42
ear 848.8
knee 844.9
with current tear (see also Tear,
meniscus) 836.2
semilunar (knee) 844.8
with current tear (see also Tear,
meniscus) 836.2
septal, nose 848.0
thyroid region 848.2
xiphoid 848.49
cervical, cervicodorsal, cervicothoracic
847.0
chondrocostal, without mention of injury to sternum 848.3
involving sternum 848.42
chondrosternal 848.42
chronic (joint) — see Derangement,
joint
clavicle 840.9
coccyx 847.4
collar bone 840.9

☑ Additional Digit Required — Refer to the Tabular List for Digit Selection

**2008 ICD-9-CM**

▶◀ Revised Text

● New Line

▲ Revised Code

▽ Subterms under main terms may continue to next column or page

**Volume 2 — 263**

**Sprain, strain** — *continued*
  collateral, knee (medial) (tibial) 844.1
    lateral (fibular) 844.0
      recurrent or old 717.89
        lateral 717.81
        medial 717.82
  coracoacromial 840.8
  coracoclavicular 840.1
  coracohumeral 840.2
  coracoid (process) 840.9
  coronary, knee 844.8
  costal cartilage, without mention of
      injury to sternum 848.3
    involving sternum 848.42
  cricoarytenoid articulation 848.2
  cricothyroid articulation 848.2
  cruciate
    knee 844.2
    old 717.89
      anterior 717.83
      posterior 717.84
  deltoid
    ankle 845.01
    shoulder 840.8
  dorsal (spine) 847.1
  ear cartilage 848.8
  elbow 841.9
    and forearm 841.9
    specified site NEC 841.8
  femur (proximal end) 843.9
    distal end 844.9
  fibula (proximal end) 844.9
    distal end 845.00
  fibulocalcaneal 845.02
  finger(s) 842.10
  foot 845.10
    and ankle 845.00
  forearm 841.9
    and elbow 841.9
    specified site NEC 841.8
  glenoid (shoulder) (*see also* SLAP le-
      sion) 840.8
  hand 842.10
  hip 843.9
    and thigh 843.9
  humerus (proximal end) 840.9
    distal end 841.9
  iliofemoral 843.0
  infraspinatus 840.3
  innominate
    acetabulum 843.9
    pubic junction 848.5
    sacral junction 846.1
  internal
    collateral, ankle 845.01
    semilunar cartilage 844.8
      with current tear (*see also* Tear,
          meniscus) 836.2
      old 717.5
  interphalangeal
    finger 842.13
    toe 845.13
  ischiocapsular 843.1
  jaw (cartilage) (meniscus) 848.1
    old 524.69
  knee 844.9
    and leg 844.9
    old 717.5
      collateral
        lateral 717.81
        medial 717.82
      cruciate
        anterior 717.83
        posterior 717.84
  late effect — *see* Late, effects (of),
      sprain
  lateral collateral, knee 844.0
    old 717.81
  leg 844.9
    and knee 844.9
  ligamentum teres femoris 843.8
  low back 846.9
  lumbar (spine) 847.2
  lumbosacral 846.0
    chronic or old 724.6
  mandible 848.1

**Sprain, strain** — *continued*
  mandible — *continued*
    old 524.69
  maxilla 848.1
  medial collateral, knee 844.1
    old 717.82
  meniscus
    jaw 848.1
      old 524.69
    knee 844.8
      with current tear (*see also* Tear,
          meniscus) 836.2
      old 717.5
    mandible 848.1
      old 524.69
    specified site NEC 848.8
  metacarpal 842.10
    distal 842.12
    proximal 842.11
  metacarpophalangeal 842.12
  metatarsal 845.10
  metatarsophalangeal 845.12
  midcarpal 842.19
  midtarsal 845.19
  multiple sites, except fingers alone or
      toes alone 848.8
  neck 847.0
  nose (septal cartilage) 848.0
  occiput from atlas 847.0
  old — *see* Derangement, joint
  orbicular, hip 843.8
  patella(r) 844.8
    old 717.89
  pelvis 848.5
  phalanx
    finger 842.10
    toe 845.10
  radiocarpal 842.02
  radiohumeral 841.2
  radioulnar 841.9
    distal 842.09
  radius, radial (proximal end) 841.9
    and ulna 841.9
      distal 842.09
    collateral 841.0
    distal end 842.00
  recurrent — *see* Sprain, by site
  rib (cage), without mention of injury
      to sternum 848.3
    involving sternum 848.42
  rotator cuff (capsule) 840.4
  round ligament (*see also* Injury, inter-
      nal, round ligament)
    femur 843.8
  sacral (spine) 847.3
  sacrococcygeal 847.3
  sacroiliac (region) 846.9
    chronic or old 724.6
    ligament 846.1
    specified site NEC 846.8
  sacrospinatus 846.2
  sacrospinous 846.2
  sacrotuberous 846.3
  scaphoid bone, ankle 845.00
  scapula(r) 840.9
  semilunar cartilage (knee) 844.8
    with current tear (*see also* Tear,
        meniscus) 836.2
    old 717.5
  septal cartilage (nose) 848.0
  shoulder 840.9
    and arm, upper 840.9
    blade 840.9
  specified site NEC 848.8
  spine 847.9
    cervical 847.0
    coccyx 847.4
    dorsal 847.1
    lumbar 847.2
    lumbosacral 846.0
      chronic or old 724.6
    sacral 847.3
    sacroiliac (*see also* Sprain, sacroil-
        iac) 846.9
      chronic or old 724.6
    thoracic 847.1

**Sprain, strain** — *continued*
  sternoclavicular 848.41
  sternum 848.40
  subglenoid (*see also* SLAP lesion)
      840.8
  subscapularis 840.5
  supraspinatus 840.6
  symphysis
    jaw 848.1
      old 524.69
    mandibular 848.1
      old 524.69
    pubis 848.5
  talofibular 845.09
  tarsal 845.10
  tarsometatarsal 845.11
  temporomandibular 848.1
    old 524.69
  teres
    ligamentum femoris 843.8
    major or minor 840.8
  thigh (proximal end) 843.9
    and hip 843.9
    distal end 844.9
  thoracic (spine) 847.1
  thorax 848.8
  thumb 842.10
  thyroid cartilage or region 848.2
  tibia (proximal end) 844.9
    distal end 845.00
  tibiofibular
    distal 845.03
    superior 844.3
  toe(s) 845.10
  trachea 848.8
  trapezoid 840.8
  ulna, ulnar (proximal end) 841.9
    collateral 841.1
    distal end 842.00
  ulnohumeral 841.3
  vertebrae (*see also* Sprain, spine)
      847.9
    cervical, cervicodorsal, cervicotho-
        racic 847.0
  wrist (cuneiform) (scaphoid) (semilu-
      nar) 842.00
  xiphoid cartilage 848.49
**Sprengel's deformity** (congenital) 755.52
**Spring fever** 309.23
**Sprue** 579.1
  celiac 579.0
  idiopathic 579.0
  meaning thrush 112.0
  nontropical 579.0
  tropical 579.1
**Spur** — *see also* Exostosis
  bone 726.91
    calcaneal 726.73
  calcaneal 726.73
  iliac crest 726.5
  nose (septum) 478.19
    bone 726.91
  septal 478.19
**Spuria placenta** — *see* Placenta, abnor-
    mal
**Spurway's syndrome** (brittle bones and
    blue sclera) 756.51
**Sputum, abnormal** (amount) (color) (ex-
    cessive) (odor) (purulent) 786.4
  bloody 786.3
**Squamous** — *see also* condition
  cell metaplasia
    bladder 596.8
    cervix — *see* condition
  epithelium in
    cervical canal (congenital) 752.49
    uterine mucosa (congenital) 752.3
  metaplasia
    bladder 596.8
    cervix — *see* condition
**Squashed nose** 738.0
  congenital 754.0
**Squeeze, divers'** 993.3
**Squint** — *see also* Strabismus 378.9
  accommodative (*see also* Esotropia)
      378.00

**Squint** — *see also* Strabismus —
    *continued*
  concomitant (*see also* Heterotropia)
      378.30
**Stab** — *see also* Wound, open, by site
  internal organs — *see* Injury, internal,
      by site, with open wound
**Staggering gait** 781.2
  hysterical 300.11
**Staghorn calculus** 592.0
**Stain, staining**
  meconium 779.84
  port wine 757.32
  tooth, teeth (hard tissues) 521.7
    due to
      accretions 523.6
      deposits (betel) (black) (green)
          (materia alba) (orange)
          (tobacco) 523.6
      metals (copper) (silver) 521.7
      nicotine 523.6
      pulpal bleeding 521.7
      tobacco 523.6
**Stälh's**
  ear 744.29
  pigment line (cornea) 371.11
**Stälhi's pigment lines** (cornea) 371.11
**Stammering** 307.0
**Standstill**
  atrial 426.6
  auricular 426.6
  cardiac (*see also* Arrest, cardiac) 427.5
  sinoatrial 426.6
  sinus 426.6
  ventricular (*see also* Arrest, cardiac)
      427.5
**Stannosis** 503
**Stanton's disease** (melioidosis) 025
**Staphylitis** (acute) (catarrhal) (chronic)
    (gangrenous) (membranous) (sup-
    purative) (ulcerative) 528.3
**Staphylococcemia** 038.10
  aureus 038.11
  specified organism NEC 038.19
**Staphylococcus, staphylococcal** — *see*
    condition
**Staphyloderma** (skin) 686.00
**Staphyloma** 379.11
  anterior, localized 379.14
  ciliary 379.11
  cornea 371.73
  equatorial 379.13
  posterior 379.12
  posticum 379.12
  ring 379.15
  sclera NEC 379.11
**Starch eating** 307.52
**Stargardt's disease** 362.75
**Starvation** (inanition) (due to lack of
    food) 994.2
  edema 262
  voluntary NEC 307.1
**Stasis**
  bile (duct) (*see also* Disease, biliary)
      576.8
  bronchus (*see also* Bronchitis) 490
  cardiac (*see also* Failure, heart) 428.0
  cecum 564.89
  colon 564.89
  dermatitis (*see also* Varix, with stasis
      dermatitis) 454.1
  duodenal 536.8
  eczema (*see also* Varix, with stasis
      dermatitis) 454.1
  edema (*see also* Hypertension, venous)
      459.30
  foot 991.4
  gastric 536.3
  ileocecal coil 564.89
  ileum 564.89
  intestinal 564.89
  jejunum 564.89
  kidney 586
  liver 571.9
    cirrhotic — *see* Cirrhosis, liver
  lymphatic 457.8

☑ Additional Digit Required — Refer to the Tabular List for Digit Selection        ᵛ Subterms under main terms may continue to next column or page

**264 — Volume 2**        ▶◀ Revised Text        ● New Line        ▲ Revised Code        *2008 ICD-9-CM*

**Stasis** — *continued*
  pneumonia 514
  portal 571.9
  pulmonary 514
  rectal 564.89
  renal 586
    tubular 584.5
  stomach 536.3
  ulcer
    with varicose veins 454.0
    without varicose veins 459.81
  urine NEC (*see also* Retention, urine)
      788.20
  venous 459.81
**State**
  affective and paranoid, mixed, organic
      psychotic 294.8
  agitated 307.9
    acute reaction to stress 308.2
  anxiety (neurotic) (*see also* Anxiety)
      300.00
    specified type NEC 300.09
  apprehension (*see also* Anxiety)
      300.00
    specified type NEC 300.09
  climacteric, female 627.2
    following induced menopause
        627.4
  clouded
    epileptic (*see also* Epilepsy)
        345.9 ☑
    paroxysmal (idiopathic) (*see also*
        Epilepsy) 345.9 ☑
  compulsive (mixed) (with obsession)
      300.3
  confusional 298.9
    acute 293.0
      with
        arteriosclerotic dementia
            290.41
        presenile brain disease
            290.11
        senility 290.3
      alcoholic 291.0
      drug-induced 292.81
    epileptic 293.0
    postoperative 293.9
    reactive (emotional stress) (psycho-
        logical trauma) 298.2
    subacute 293.1
  constitutional psychopathic 301.9
  convulsive (*see also* Convulsions)
      780.39
  depressive NEC 311
    induced by drug 292.84
    neurotic 300.4
  dissociative 300.15
  hallucinatory 780.1
    induced by drug 292.12
  hypercoagulable (primary) 289.81
    secondary 289.82
  hyperdynamic beta-adrenergic circu-
      latory 429.82
  locked-in 344.81
  menopausal 627.2
    artificial 627.4
    following induced menopause
        627.4
  neurotic NEC 300.9
    with depersonalization episode
        300.6
  obsessional 300.3
  oneiroid (*see also* Schizophrenia)
      295.4 ☑
  panic 300.01
  paranoid 297.9
    alcohol-induced 291.5
    arteriosclerotic 290.42
    climacteric 297.2
    drug-induced 292.11
    in
      presenile brain disease 290.12
      senile brain disease 290.20
    involutional 297.2
    menopausal 297.2
    senile 290.20

**State** — *continued*
  paranoid — *continued*
    simple 297.0
  postleukotomy 310.0
  pregnant (*see also* Pregnancy) V22.2
  psychogenic, twilight 298.2
  psychotic, organic (*see also* Psychosis,
      organic) 294.9
    mixed paranoid and affective 294.8
    senile or presenile NEC 290.9
    transient NEC 293.9
      with
        anxiety 293.84
        delusions 293.81
        depression 293.83
        hallucinations 293.82
  residual schizophrenic (*see also*
      Schizophrenia) 295.6 ☑
  tension (*see also* Anxiety) 300.9
  transient organic psychotic 293.9
    anxiety type 293.84
    depressive type 293.83
    hallucinatory type 293.83
    paranoid type 293.81
    specified type NEC 293.89
  twilight
    epileptic 293.0
    psychogenic 298.2
  vegetative (persistent) 780.03
**Status** (post)
  absence
    epileptic (*see also* Epilepsy) 345.2
    of organ, acquired (postsurgical) —
        *see* Absence, by site, ac-
        quired
  anastomosis of intestine (for bypass)
      V45.3
  anginosus 413.9
  angioplasty, percutaneous translumi-
      nal coronary V45.82
  ankle prosthesis V43.66
  aortocoronary bypass or shunt V45.81
  arthrodesis V45.4
  artificially induced condition NEC
      V45.89
  artificial opening (of) V44.9
    gastrointestinal tract NEC V44.4
    specified site NEC V44.8
    urinary tract NEC V44.6
    vagina V44.7
  aspirator V46.0
  asthmaticus (*see also* Asthma)
      493.9 ☑
  awaiting organ transplant V49.83
  bariatric surgery V45.86
    complicating pregnancy, childbirth,
        or the puerperium 649.2 ☑
  bed confinement V49.84
  breast implant removal V45.83
  cardiac
    device (in situ) V45.00
      carotid sinus V45.09
        fitting or adjustment V53.39
      defibrillator, automatic im-
          plantable V45.02
      pacemaker V45.01
        fitting or adjustment V53.31
  carotid sinus stimulator V45.09
  cataract extraction V45.61
  chemotherapy V66.2
    current V58.69
  circumcision, female 629.20
  clitorectomy (female genital mutilation
      type I) 629.21
    with excision of labia minora (fe-
        male genital mutilation type
        II) 629.22
  colostomy V44.3
  contraceptive device V45.59
    intrauterine V45.51
    subdermal V45.52
  convulsivus idiopathicus (*see also*
      Epilepsy) 345.3
  coronary artery bypass or shunt
      V45.81

**Status** — *continued*
  cutting
    female genital 629.20
      specified NEC 629.29
      type I 629.21
      type II 629.22
      type III 629.23
      type IV 629.29
  cystostomy V44.50
    appendico-vesicostomy V44.52
    cutaneous-vesicostomy V44.51
    specified type NEC V44.59
  defibrillator, automatic implantable
      cardiac V45.02
  dental crowns V45.84
  dental fillings V45.84
  dental restoration V45.84
  dental sealant V49.82
  dialysis (hemo) (peritoneal) V45.1
  donor V59.9
  drug therapy or regimen V67.59
    high-risk medication NEC V67.51
  elbow prosthesis V43.62
  enterostomy V44.4
  epileptic, epilepticus (absence) (grand
      mal) (*see also* Epilepsy) 345.3
    focal motor 345.7 ☑
    partial 345.7 ☑
    petit mal 345.2
    psychomotor 345.7 ☑
    temporal lobe 345.7 ☑
  estrogen receptor
    negative [ER-] V86.1
    positive [ER+] V86.0
  eye (adnexa) surgery V45.69
  female genital
    cutting 629.20
      specified NEC 629.29
      type I 629.21
      type II 629.22
      type III 629.23
      type IV 629.29
    mutilation 629.20
      type I 629.21
      type II 629.22
      type III 629.23
      type IV 629.29
  filtering bleb (eye) (postglaucoma)
      V45.69
    with rupture or complication
        997.99
    postcataract extraction (complica-
        tion) 997.99
  finger joint prosthesis V43.69
  gastric
    banding V45.86
      complicating pregnancy, child-
          birth, or the puerperium
          649.2 ☑
    bypass for obesity V45.86
      complicating pregnancy, child-
          birth, or the puerperium
          649.2 ☑
  gastrostomy V44.1
  grand mal 345.3
  heart valve prosthesis V43.3
  hemodialysis V45.1
  hip prosthesis (joint) (partial) (total)
      V43.64
  ileostomy V44.2
  infibulation (female genital mutilation
      type III) 629.23
  insulin pump V45.85
  intestinal bypass V45.3
  intrauterine contraceptive device
      V45.51
  jejunostomy V44.4
  knee joint prosthesis V43.65
  lacunaris 437.8
  lacunosis 437.8
  low birth weight V21.30
    less than 500 grams V21.31
    1000–1499 grams V21.33
    1500–1999 grams V21.34
    2000–2500 grams V21.35
    500–999 grams V21.32

**Status** — *continued*
  lymphaticus 254.8
  malignant neoplasm, ablated or ex-
      cised — *see* History, malignant
      neoplasm
  marmoratus 333.79
  mutilation, female 629.20
    type I 629.21
    type II 629.22
    type III 629.23
    type IV 629.29
  nephrostomy V44.6
  neuropacemaker NEC V45.89
    brain V45.89
    carotid sinus V45.09
    neurologic NEC V45.89
  obesity surgery V45.86
    compliating pregnancy, childbirth,
        or the puerperium 649.2 ☑
  organ replacement
    by artificial or mechanical device
        or prosthesis of
      artery V43.4
      artificial skin V43.83
      bladder V43.5
      blood vessel V43.4
      breast V43.82
      eye globe V43.0
      heart
        assist device V43.21
        fully implantable artificial
            heart V43.22
        valve V43.3
      intestine V43.89
      joint V43.60
        ankle V43.66
        elbow V43.62
        finger V43.69
        hip (partial) (total) V43.64
        knee V43.65
        shoulder V43.61
        specified NEC V43.69
        wrist V43.63
      kidney V43.89
      larynx V43.81
      lens V43.1
      limb(s) V43.7
      liver V43.89
      lung V43.89
      organ NEC V43.89
      pancreas V43.89
      skin (artificial) V43.83
      tissue NEC V43.89
      vein V43.4
    by organ transplant (heterologous)
        (homologous) — *see* Status,
        transplant
  pacemaker
    brain V45.89
    cardiac V45.01
    carotid sinus V45.09
    neurologic NEC V45.89
    specified site NEC V45.89
  percutaneous transluminal coronary
      angioplasty V45.82
  peritoneal dialysis V45.1
  petit mal 345.2
  postcommotio cerebri 310.2
  postmenopausal (age related) (natural)
      V49.81
  postoperative NEC V45.89
  postpartum NEC V24.2
    care immediately following delivery
        V24.0
    routine follow-up V24.2
  postsurgical NEC V45.89
  renal dialysis V45.1
  respirator [ventilator] V46.11
    encounter
      during
        mechanical failure V46.14
        power failure V46.12
      for weaning V46.13
  reversed jejunal transposition (for by-
      pass) V45.3

---

☑ Additional Digit Required — Refer to the Tabular List for Digit Selection                        ⑥ Subterms under main terms may continue to next column or page

Status — Stenosis

**Status** — *continued*
  sex reassignment surgery (*see also* ●
     Trans-sexualism) 302.50    ●
  shoulder prosthesis V43.61
  shunt
    aortocoronary bypass V45.81
    arteriovenous (for dialysis) V45.1
    cerebrospinal fluid V45.2
    vascular NEC V45.89
      aortocoronary (bypass) V45.81
      ventricular (communicating) (for
        drainage) V45.2
  sterilization
    tubal ligation V26.51
    vasectomy V26.52
  subdermal contraceptive device
    V45.52
  thymicolymphaticus 254.8
  thymicus 254.8
  thymolymphaticus 254.8
  tooth extraction 525.10
  tracheostomy V44.0
  transplant
    blood vessel V42.89
    bone V42.4
      marrow V42.81
    cornea V42.5
    heart V42.1
      valve V42.2
    intestine V42.84
    kidney V42.0
    liver V42.7
    lung V42.6
    organ V42.9
      specified site NEC V42.89
    pancreas V42.83
    peripheral stem cells V42.82
    skin V42.3
    stem cells, peripheral V42.82
    tissue V42.9
      specified type NEC V42.89
    vessel, blood V42.89
  tubal ligation V26.51
  ureterostomy V44.6
  urethrostomy V44.6
  vagina, artificial V44.7
  vascular shunt NEC V45.89
    aortocoronary (bypass) V45.81
  vasectomy V26.52
  ventilator [respirator] V46.11
    encounter
      during
        mechanical failure V46.14
        power failure V46.12
      for weaning V46.13
  wrist prosthesis V43.63
**Stave fracture** — *see* Fracture,
  metacarpus, metacarpal bone(s)
**Steal**
  subclavian artery 435.2
  vertebral artery 435.1
**Stealing, solitary, child problem** — *see*
  *also* Disturbance, conduct 312.1 ☑
**Steam burn** — *see* Burn, by site
**Steatocystoma multiplex** 706.2
**Steatoma** (infected) 706.2
  eyelid (cystic) 374.84
    infected 373.13
**Steatorrhea** (chronic) 579.8
  with lacteal obstruction 579.2
  idiopathic 579.0
    adult 579.0
    infantile 579.0
  pancreatic 579.4
  primary 579.0
  secondary 579.8
  specified cause NEC 579.8
  tropical 579.1
**Steatosis** 272.8
  heart (*see also* Degeneration, myocar-
    dial) 429.1
  kidney 593.89
  liver 571.8
**Steele-Richardson (-Olszewski) Syn-
  drome** 333.0

**Steinbrocker's syndrome** — *see also*
  Neuropathy, peripheral, autonomic
  337.9
**Steinert's disease** 359.21   ▲
**Stein-Leventhal syndrome** (polycystic
  ovary) 256.4
**Stein's syndrome** (polycystic ovary)
  256.4
**STEMI** (ST elevation myocardial infarction — *see also* — Infarct, myocardium, ST elevation 410.9 ☑
**Stenocardia** — *see also* Angina 413.9
**Stenocephaly** 756.0
**Stenosis** (cicatricial) — *see also* Stricture
  ampulla of Vater 576.2
    with calculus, cholelithiasis, or
      stones — *see* Choledocholithi-
      asis
  anus, anal (canal) (sphincter) 569.2
    congenital 751.2
  aorta (ascending) 747.22
    arch 747.10
    arteriosclerotic 440.0
    calcified 440.0
  aortic (valve) 424.1
    with
      mitral (valve)
        insufficiency or incompe-
          tence 396.2
        stenosis or obstruction 396.0
    atypical 396.0
    congenital 746.3
    rheumatic 395.0
      with
        insufficiency, incompetency
          or regurgitation 395.2
          with mitral (valve) disease
            396.8
        mitral (valve)
          disease (stenosis) 396.0
          insufficiency or incompe-
            tence 396.2
          stenosis or obstruction
            396.0
    specified cause, except rheumatic
      424.1
    syphilitic 093.22
  aqueduct of Sylvius (congenital) 742.3
    with spina bifida (*see also* Spina
      bifida) 741.0 ☑
    acquired 331.4
  artery NEC ▶(*see also* Arteriosclero-
    sis)◀ 447.1
    basilar — *see* Narrowing, artery,
      basilar
    carotid (common) (internal) — *see*
      Narrowing, artery, carotid
    celiac 447.4
    cerebral 437.0
      due to
        embolism (*see also* Em-
          bolism, brain) 434.1 ☑
        thrombus (*see also* Thrombo-
          sis, brain) 434.0 ☑
    extremities 440.20    ●
    precerebral — *see* Narrowing,
      artery, precerebral
    pulmonary (congenital) 747.3
      acquired 417.8
    renal 440.1
    vertebral — *see* Narrowing, artery,
      vertebral
  bile duct or biliary passage (*see also*
    Obstruction, biliary) 576.2
    congenital 751.61
  bladder neck (acquired) 596.0
    congenital 753.6
  brain 348.8
  bronchus 519.19
    syphilitic 095.8
  cardia (stomach) 537.89
    congenital 750.7
  cardiovascular (*see also* Disease, car-
    diovascular) 429.2
  carotid artery — *see* Narrowing,
    artery, carotid

**Stenosis** — *see also* Stricture —
  *continued*
  cervix, cervical (canal) 622.4
    congenital 752.49
    in pregnancy or childbirth 654.6 ☑
      affecting fetus or newborn
        763.89
      causing obstructed labor
        660.2 ☑
        affecting fetus or newborn
          763.1
  colon (*see also* Obstruction, intestine)
    560.9
    congenital 751.2
  colostomy 569.62
  common bile duct (*see also* Obstruc-
    tion, biliary) 576.2
    congenital 751.61
  coronary (artery) — *see* Arterioscle-
    sis, coronary
  cystic duct (*see also* Obstruction,
    gallbladder) 575.2
    congenital 751.61
  due to (presence of) any device, im-
    plant, or graft classifiable to
    996.0–996.5 — *see* Complica-
    tions, due to (presence of) any
    device, implant, or graft classi-
    fied to 996.0–996.5 NEC
  duodenum 537.3
    congenital 751.1
  ejaculatory duct NEC 608.89
  endocervical os — *see* Stenosis, cervix
  enterostomy 569.62
  esophagostomy 530.87
  esophagus 530.3
    congenital 750.3
    syphilitic 095.8
      congenital 090.5
  external ear canal 380.50
    secondary to
      inflammation 380.53
      surgery 380.52
      trauma 380.51
  gallbladder (*see also* Obstruction,
    gallbladder) 575.2
  glottis 478.74
  heart valve (acquired) (*see also* Endo-
    carditis)
    congenital NEC 746.89
      aortic 746.3
      mitral 746.5
      pulmonary 746.02
      tricuspid 746.1
  hepatic duct (*see also* Obstruction,
    biliary) 576.2
  hymen 623.3
  hypertrophic subaortic (idiopathic)
    425.1
  infundibulum cardiac 746.83
  intestine (*see also* Obstruction, intes-
    tine) 560.9
    congenital (small) 751.1
      large 751.2
  lacrimal
    canaliculi 375.53
    duct 375.56
      congenital 743.65
    punctum 375.52
      congenital 743.65
    sac 375.54
      congenital 743.65
  lacrimonasal duct 375.56
    congenital 743.65
    neonatal 375.55
  larynx 478.74
    congenital 748.3
    syphilitic 095.8
      congenital 090.5
  mitral (valve) (chronic) (inactive) 394.0
    with
      aortic (valve)
        disease (insufficiency) 396.1
        insufficiency or incompe-
          tence 396.1
        stenosis or obstruction 396.0

**Stenosis** — *see also* Stricture —
  *continued*
  mitral — *continued*
    with — *continued*
      incompetency, insufficiency or
        regurgitation 394.2
        with aortic valve disease
          396.8
    active or acute 391.1
      with chorea (acute) (rheumatic)
        (Sydenham's) 392.0
    congenital 746.5
    specified cause, except rheumatic
      424.0
    syphilitic 093.21
  myocardium, myocardial (*see also*
    Degeneration, myocardial) 429.1
    hypertrophic subaortic (idiopathic)
      425.1
  nares (anterior) (posterior) 478.19
    congenital 748.0
  nasal duct 375.56
    congenital 743.65
  nasolacrimal duct 375.56
    congenital 743.65
    neonatal 375.55
  organ or site, congenital NEC — *see*
    Atresia
  papilla of Vater 576.2
    with calculus, cholelithiasis, or
      stones — *see* Choledocholithi-
      asis
  pulmonary (artery) (congenital) 747.3
    with ventricular septal defect, dex-
      traposition of aorta and hy-
      pertrophy of right ventricle
      745.2
    acquired 417.8
    infundibular 746.83
    in tetralogy of Fallot 745.2
    subvalvular 746.83
    valve (*see also* Endocarditis, pul-
      monary) 424.3
      congenital 746.02
    vein 747.49
      acquired 417.8
    vessel NEC 417.8
  pulmonic (congenital) 746.02
    infundibular 746.83
    subvalvular 746.83
  pylorus (hypertrophic) 537.0
    adult 537.0
    congenital 750.5
    infantile 750.5
  rectum (sphincter) (*see also* Stricture,
    rectum) 569.2
  renal artery 440.1
  salivary duct (any) 527.8
  sphincter of Oddi (*see also* Obstruc-
    tion, biliary) 576.2
  spinal 724.00
    cervical 723.0
    lumbar, lumbosacral 724.02
    nerve (root) NEC 724.9
    specified region NEC 724.09
    thoracic, thoracolumbar 724.01
  stomach, hourglass 537.6
  subaortic 746.81
    hypertrophic (idiopathic) 425.1
  supra (valvular)-aortic 747.22
  trachea 519.19
    congenital 748.3
    syphilitic 095.8
    tuberculous (*see also* Tuberculosis)
      012.8 ☑
  tracheostomy 519.02
  tricuspid (valve) (*see also* Endocardi-
    tis, tricuspid) 397.0
    congenital 746.1
    nonrheumatic 424.2
  tubal 628.2
  ureter (*see also* Stricture, ureter)
    593.3
    congenital 753.29
  urethra (*see also* Stricture, urethra)
    598.9

---

**Stenosis** — see also Stricture — continued
vagina 623.2
congenital 752.49
in pregnancy or childbirth 654.7 ☑
affecting fetus or newborn 763.89
causing obstructed labor 660.2 ☑
affecting fetus or newborn 763.1
valve (cardiac) (heart) (see also Endocarditis) 424.90
congenital NEC 746.89
aortic 746.3
mitral 746.5
pulmonary 746.02
tricuspid 746.1
urethra 753.6
valvular (see also Endocarditis) 424.90
congenital NEC 746.89
urethra 753.6
vascular graft or shunt 996.1
atherosclerosis — see Arteriosclerosis, extremities
embolism 996.74
occlusion NEC 996.74
thrombus 996.74
vena cava (inferior) (superior) 459.2
congenital 747.49
ventricular shunt 996.2
vulva 624.8
**Stercolith** — see also Fecalith 560.39
appendix 543.9
**Stercoraceous, stercoral ulcer** 569.82
anus or rectum 569.41
**Stereopsis, defective**
with fusion 368.33
without fusion 368.32
**Stereotypes** NEC 307.3
**Sterility**
female — see Infertility, female
male (see also Infertility, male) 606.9
**Sterilization, admission for** V25.2
status
tubal ligation V26.51
vasectomy V26.52
**Sternalgia** — see also Angina 413.9
**Sternopagus** 759.4
**Sternum bifidum** 756.3
**Sternutation** 784.99
**Steroid**
effects (adverse) (iatrogenic)
cushingoid
correct substance properly administered 255.0
overdose or wrong substance given or taken 962.0
diabetes
correct substance properly administered 251.8
overdose or wrong substance given or taken 962.0
due to
correct substance properly administered 255.8
overdose or wrong substance given or taken 962.0
fever
correct substance properly administered 780.6
overdose or wrong substance given or taken 962.0
withdrawal
correct substance properly administered 255.41 ▲
overdose or wrong substance given or taken 962.0
responder 365.03
**Stevens-Johnson disease or syndrome** (erythema multiforme exudativum) 695.1
**Stewart-Morel syndrome** (hyperostosis frontalis interna) 733.3

**Sticker's disease** (erythema infectiosum) 057.0
**Stickler syndrome** 759.89
**Sticky eye** 372.03
**Stieda's disease** (calcification, knee joint) 726.62
**Stiff**
back 724.8
neck (see also Torticollis) 723.5
**Stiff-baby** 759.89
**Stiff-man syndrome** 333.91
**Stiffness, joint** NEC 719.50
ankle 719.57
back 724.8
elbow 719.52
finger 719.54
hip 719.55
knee 719.56
multiple sites 719.59
sacroiliac 724.6
shoulder 719.51
specified site NEC 719.58
spine 724.9
surgical fusion V45.4
wrist 719.53
**Stigmata, congenital syphilis** 090.5
**Stillbirth, stillborn** NEC 779.9
**Still's disease or syndrome** 714.30
**Stiller's disease** (asthenia) 780.79
**Still-Felty syndrome** (rheumatoid arthritis with splenomegaly and leukopenia) 714.1
**Stilling-Türk-Duane syndrome** (ocular retraction syndrome) 378.71
**Stimulation, ovary** 256.1
**Sting** (animal) (bee) (fish) (insect) (jellyfish) (Portuguese man-o-war) (wasp) (venomous) 989.5
anaphylactic shock or reaction 989.5
plant 692.6
**Stippled epiphyses** 756.59
**Stitch**
abscess 998.59
burst (in external operation wound) 998.32
internal 998.31
in back 724.5
**Stojano's** (subcostal) **syndrome** 098.86
**Stokes-Adams syndrome** (syncope with heart block) 426.9
**Stokes' disease** (exophthalmic goiter) 242.0
**Stokvis' (-Talma) disease** (enterogenous cyanosis) 289.7
**Stomach** — see condition
**Stoma malfunction**
colostomy 569.62
cystostomy 997.5
enterostomy 569.62
esophagostomy 530.87
gastrostomy 536.42
ileostomy 569.62
nephrostomy 997.5
tracheostomy 519.02
ureterostomy 997.5
**Stomatitis** 528.00
angular 528.5
due to dietary or vitamin deficiency 266.0
aphthous 528.2
candidal 112.0
catarrhal 528.00
denture 528.9
diphtheritic (membranous) 032.0
due to
dietary deficiency 266.0
thrush 112.0
vitamin deficiency 266.0
epidemic 078.4
epizootic 078.4
follicular 528.00
gangrenous 528.1
herpetic 054.2
herpetiformis 528.2
malignant 528.00
membranous acute 528.00

**Stomatitis** — continued
monilial 112.0
mycotic 112.0
necrotic 528.1
ulcerative 101
necrotizing ulcerative 101
parasitic 112.0
septic 528.00
specified NEC 528.09
spirochetal 101
suppurative (acute) 528.00
ulcerative 528.00
necrotizing 101
ulceromembranous 101
vesicular 528.00
with exanthem 074.3
Vincent's 101
**Stomatocytosis** 282.8
**Stomatomycosis** 112.0
**Stomatorrhagia** 528.9
**Stone(s)** — see also Calculus
bladder 594.1
diverticulum 594.0
cystine 270.0
heart syndrome (see also Failure, ventricular, left) 428.1
kidney 592.0
prostate 602.0
pulp (dental) 522.2
renal 592.0
salivary duct or gland (any) 527.5
ureter 592.1
urethra (impacted) 594.2
urinary (duct) (impacted) (passage) 592.9
bladder 594.1
diverticulum 594.0
lower tract NEC 594.9
specified site 594.8
xanthine 277.2
**Stonecutters' lung** 502
tuberculous (see also Tuberculosis) 011.4 ☑
**Stonemasons'**
asthma, disease, or lung 502
tuberculous (see also Tuberculosis) 011.4 ☑
phthisis (see also Tuberculosis) 011.4 ☑
**Stoppage**
bowel (see also Obstruction, intestine) 560.9
heart (see also Arrest, cardiac) 427.5
intestine (see also Obstruction, intestine) 560.9
urine NEC (see also Retention, urine) 788.20
**Storm, thyroid** (apathetic) — see also Thyrotoxicosis 242.9 ☑
**Strabismus** (alternating) (congenital) (nonparalytic) 378.9
concomitant (see also Heterotropia) 378.30
convergent (see also Esotropia) 378.00
divergent (see also Exotropia) 378.10
convergent (see also Esotropia) 378.00
divergent (see also Exotropia) 378.10
due to adhesions, scars — see Strabismus, mechanical
in neuromuscular disorder NEC 378.73
intermittent 378.20
vertical 378.31
latent 378.40
convergent (esophoria) 378.41
divergent (exophoria) 378.42
vertical 378.43
mechanical 378.60
due to
Brown's tendon sheath syndrome 378.61
specified musculofascial disorder NEC 378.62
paralytic 378.50

**Strabismus** — continued
paralytic — continued
third or oculomotor nerve (partial) 378.51
total 378.52
fourth or trochlear nerve 378.53
sixth or abducens nerve 378.54
specified type NEC 378.73
vertical (hypertropia) 378.31
**Strain** — see also Sprain, by site
eye NEC 368.13
heart — see Disease, heart
meaning gonorrhea — see Gonorrhea
on urination 788.65
physical NEC V62.89
postural 729.9
psychological NEC V62.89
**Strands**
conjunctiva 372.62
vitreous humor 379.25
**Strangulation, strangulated** 994.7
appendix 543.9
asphyxiation or suffocation by 994.7
bladder neck 596.0
bowel — see Strangulation, intestine
colon — see Strangulation, intestine
cord (umbilical) — see Compression, umbilical cord
due to birth injury 767.8
food or foreign body (see also Asphyxia, food) 933.1
hemorrhoids 455.8
external 455.5
internal 455.2
hernia (see also Hernia, by site, with obstruction)
gangrenous — see Hernia, by site, with gangrene
intestine (large) (small) 560.2
with hernia (see also Hernia, by site, with obstruction)
gangrenous — see Hernia, by site, with gangrene
congenital (small) 751.1
large 751.2
mesentery 560.2
mucus (see also Asphyxia, mucus) 933.1
newborn 770.18
omentum 560.2
organ or site, congenital NEC — see Atresia
ovary 620.8
due to hernia 620.4
penis 607.89
foreign body 939.3
rupture (see also Hernia, by site, with obstruction) 552.9
gangrenous (see also Hernia, by site, with gangrene) 551.9
stomach, due to hernia (see also Hernia, by site, with obstruction) 552.9
with gangrene (see also Hernia, by site, with gangrene) 551.9
umbilical cord — see Compression, umbilical cord
vesicourethral orifice 596.0
**Strangury** 788.1
**Strawberry**
gallbladder (see also Disease, gallbladder) 575.6
mark 757.32
tongue (red) (white) 529.3
**Straw itch** 133.8
**Streak, ovarian** 752.0
**Strephosymbolia** 315.01
secondary to organic lesion 784.69
**Streptobacillary fever** 026.1
**Streptobacillus moniliformis** 026.1
**Streptococcemia** 038.0
**Streptococcicosis** — see Infection, streptococcal
**Streptococcus, streptococcal** — see condition
**Streptoderma** 686.00

---

**Streptomycosis** — *see* Actinomycosis
**Streptothricosis** — *see* Actinomycosis
**Streptothrix** — *see* Actinomycosis
**Streptotrichosis** — *see* Actinomycosis
**Stress** 308.9 ▲
  fracture — *see* Fracture, stress
  polycythemia 289.0
  reaction (gross) (*see also* Reaction, stress, acute) 308.9
**Stretching, nerve** — *see* Injury, nerve, by site
**Striae** (albicantes) (atrophicae) (cutis distensae) (distensae) 701.3
**Striations of nails** 703.8
**Stricture** — *see also* Stenosis 799.89
  ampulla of Vater 576.2
    with calculus, cholelithiasis, or stones — *see* Choledocholithiasis
  anus (sphincter) 569.2
    congenital 751.2
    infantile 751.2
  aorta (ascending) 747.22
    arch 747.10
    arteriosclerotic 440.0
    calcified 440.0
  aortic (valve) (*see also* Stenosis, aortic) 424.1
    congenital 746.3
  aqueduct of Sylvius (congenital) 742.3
    with spina bifida (*see also* Spina bifida) 741.0 ☑
    acquired 331.4
  artery 447.1
    basilar — *see* Narrowing, artery, basilar
    carotid (common) (internal) — *see* Narrowing, artery, carotid
    celiac 447.4
    cerebral 437.0
      congenital 747.81
      due to
        embolism (*see also* Embolism, brain) 434.1 ☑
        thrombus (*see also* Thrombosis, brain) 434.0 ☑
    congenital (peripheral) 747.60
      cerebral 747.81
      coronary 746.85
      gastrointestinal 747.61
      lower limb 747.64
      renal 747.62
      retinal 743.58
      specified NEC 747.69
      spinal 747.82
      umbilical 747.5
      upper limb 747.63
    coronary — *see* Arteriosclerosis, coronary
      congenital 746.85
    precerebral — *see* Narrowing, artery, precerebral NEC
    pulmonary (congenital) 747.3
      acquired 417.8
    renal 440.1
    vertebral — *see* Narrowing, artery, vertebral
  auditory canal (congenital) (external) 744.02
    acquired (*see also* Stricture, ear canal, acquired) 380.50
  bile duct or passage (any) (postoperative) (*see also* Obstruction, biliary) 576.2
    congenital 751.61
  bladder 596.8
    congenital 753.6
    neck 596.0
      congenital 753.6
  bowel (*see also* Obstruction, intestine) 560.9
  brain 348.8
  bronchus 519.19
    syphilitic 095.8
  cardia (stomach) 537.89
    congenital 750.7

**Stricture** — *see also* Stenosis — *continued*
  cardiac (*see also* Disease, heart)
    orifice (stomach) 537.89
  cardiovascular (*see also* Disease, cardiovascular) 429.2
  carotid artery — *see* Narrowing, artery, carotid
  cecum (*see also* Obstruction, intestine) 560.9
  cervix, cervical (canal) 622.4
    congenital 752.49
    in pregnancy or childbirth 654.6 ☑
      affecting fetus or newborn 763.89
      causing obstructed labor 660.2 ☑
        affecting fetus or newborn 763.1
  colon (*see also* Obstruction, intestine) 560.9
    congenital 751.2
  colostomy 569.62
  common bile duct (*see also* Obstruction, biliary) 576.2
    congenital 751.61
  coronary (artery) — *see* Arteriosclerosis, coronary
    congenital 746.85
  cystic duct (*see also* Obstruction, gallbladder) 575.2
    congenital 751.61
  cystostomy 997.5
  digestive organs NEC, congenital 751.8
  duodenum 537.3
    congenital 751.1
  ear canal (external) (congenital) 744.02
    acquired 380.50
      secondary to
        inflammation 380.53
        surgery 380.52
        trauma 380.51
  ejaculatory duct 608.85
  enterostomy 569.62
  esophagostomy 530.87
  esophagus (corrosive) (peptic) 530.3
    congenital 750.3
    syphilitic 095.8
      congenital 090.5
  eustachian tube (*see also* Obstruction, Eustachian tube) 381.60
    congenital 744.24
  fallopian tube 628.2
    gonococcal (chronic) 098.37
      acute 098.17
    tuberculous (*see also* Tuberculosis) 016.6 ☑
  gallbladder (*see also* Obstruction, gallbladder) 575.2
    congenital 751.69
  glottis 478.74
  heart (*see also* Disease, heart)
    congenital NEC 746.89
    valve (*see also* Endocarditis)
      congenital NEC 746.89
        aortic 746.3
        mitral 746.5
        pulmonary 746.02
        tricuspid 746.1
  hepatic duct (*see also* Obstruction, biliary) 576.2
  hourglass, of stomach 537.6
  hymen 623.3
  hypopharynx 478.29
  intestine (*see also* Obstruction, intestine) 560.9
    congenital (small) 751.1
      large 751.2
    ischemic 557.1
  lacrimal
    canaliculi 375.53
      congenital 743.65
    punctum 375.52
      congenital 743.65

**Stricture** — *see also* Stenosis — *continued*
  lacrimal — *continued*
    sac 375.54
      congenital 743.65
  lacrimonasal duct 375.56
    congenital 743.65
    neonatal 375.55
  larynx 478.79
    congenital 748.3
    syphilitic 095.8
      congenital 090.5
  lung 518.89
  meatus
    ear (congenital) 744.02
      acquired (*see also* Stricture, ear canal, acquired) 380.50
    osseous (congenital) (ear) 744.03
      acquired (*see also* Stricture, ear canal, acquired) 380.50
    urinarius (*see also* Stricture, urethra) 598.9
      congenital 753.6
  mitral (valve) (*see also* Stenosis, mitral) 394.0
    congenital 746.5
    specified cause, except rheumatic 424.0
  myocardium, myocardial (*see also* Degeneration, myocardial) 429.1
    hypertrophic subaortic (idiopathic) 425.1
  nares (anterior) (posterior) 478.19
    congenital 748.0
  nasal duct 375.56
    congenital 743.65
    neonatal 375.55
  nasolacrimal duct 375.56
    congenital 743.65
    neonatal 375.55
  nasopharynx 478.29
    syphilitic 095.8
  nephrostomy 997.5
  nose 478.19
    congenital 748.0
  nostril (anterior) (posterior) 478.19
    congenital 748.0
  organ or site, congenital NEC — *see* Atresia
  osseous meatus (congenital) (ear) 744.03
    acquired (*see also* Stricture, ear canal, acquired) 380.50
  os uteri (*see also* Stricture, cervix) 622.4
  oviduct — *see* Stricture, fallopian tube
  pelviureteric junction 593.3
  pharynx (dilation) 478.29
  prostate 602.8
  pulmonary, pulmonic
    artery (congenital) 747.3
      acquired 417.8
      noncongenital 417.8
    infundibulum (congenital) 746.83
    valve (*see also* Endocarditis, pulmonary) 424.3
      congenital 746.02
    vein (congenital) 747.49
      acquired 417.8
    vessel NEC 417.8
  punctum lacrimale 375.52
    congenital 743.65
  pylorus (hypertrophic) 537.0
    adult 537.0
    congenital 750.5
    infantile 750.5
  rectosigmoid 569.89
  rectum (sphincter) 569.2
    congenital 751.2
    due to
      chemical burn 947.3
      irradiation 569.2
      lymphogranuloma venereum 099.1
    gonococcal 098.7
    inflammatory 099.1

**Stricture** — *see also* Stenosis — *continued*
  rectum — *continued*
    syphilitic 095.8
    tuberculous (*see also* Tuberculosis) 014.8 ☑
  renal artery 440.1
  salivary duct or gland (any) 527.8
  sigmoid (flexure) (*see also* Obstruction, intestine) 560.9
  spermatic cord 608.85
  stoma (following) (of)
    colostomy 569.62
    cystostomy 997.5
    enterostomy 569.62
    esophagostomy 530.87
    gastrostomy 536.42
    ileostomy 569.62
    nephrostomy 997.5
    tracheostomy 519.02
    ureterostomy 997.5
  stomach 537.89
    congenital 750.7
    hourglass 537.6
  subaortic 746.81
    hypertrophic (acquired) (idiopathic) 425.1
  subglottic 478.74
  syphilitic NEC 095.8
  tendon (sheath) 727.81
  trachea 519.19
    congenital 748.3
    syphilitic 095.8
    tuberculous (*see also* Tuberculosis) 012.8 ☑
  tracheostomy 519.02
  tricuspid (valve) (*see also* Endocarditis, tricuspid) 397.0
    congenital 746.1
    nonrheumatic 424.2
  tunica vaginalis 608.85
  ureter (postoperative) 593.3
    congenital 753.29
    tuberculous (*see also* Tuberculosis) 016.2 ☑
  ureteropelvic junction 593.3
    congenital 753.21
  ureterovesical orifice 593.3
    congenital 753.22
  urethra (anterior) (meatal) (organic) (posterior) (spasmodic) 598.9
    associated with schistosomiasis (*see also* Schistosomiasis) 120.9 *[598.01]*
    congenital (valvular) 753.6
    due to
      infection 598.00
        syphilis 095.8 *[598.01]*
      trauma 598.1
    gonococcal 098.2 *[598.01]*
    gonorrheal 098.2 *[598.01]*
    infective 598.00
    late effect of injury 598.1
    postcatheterization 598.2
    postobstetric 598.1
    postoperative 598.2
    specified cause NEC 598.8
    syphilitic 095.8 *[598.01]*
    traumatic 598.1
    valvular, congenital 753.6
  urinary meatus (*see also* Stricture, urethra) 598.9
    congenital 753.6
  uterus, uterine 621.5
    os (external) (internal) — *see* Stricture, cervix
  vagina (outlet) 623.2
    congenital 752.49
  valve (cardiac) (heart) (*see also* Endocarditis) 424.90
    congenital (cardiac) (heart) NEC 746.89
      aortic 746.3
      mitral 746.5
      pulmonary 746.02
      tricuspid 746.1

☑ Additional Digit Required — Refer to the Tabular List for Digit Selection
▽ Subterms under main terms may continue to next column or page
268 — Volume 2 · October 2007
►◄ Revised Text    ● New Line    ▲ Revised Code
2008 ICD-9-CM

**Stricture** — *see also* Stenosis — *continued*
- valve (*see also* Endocarditis) — *continued*
  - congenital — *continued*
    - urethra 753.6
- valvular (*see also* Endocarditis) 424.90
- vascular graft or shunt 996.1
  - atherosclerosis — see Arteriosclerosis, extremities
  - embolism 996.74
  - occlusion NEC 996.74
  - thrombus 996.74
- vas deferens 608.85
  - congenital 752.89
- vein 459.2
- vena cava (inferior) (superior) NEC 459.2
  - congenital 747.49
- ventricular shunt 996.2
- vesicourethral orifice 596.0
  - congenital 753.6
- vulva (acquired) 624.8

**Stridor** 786.1
- congenital (larynx) 748.3

**Stridulous** — *see* condition

**Strippling of nails** 703.8

**Stroke** 434.91
- apoplectic (*see also* Disease, cerebrovascular, acute) 436
- brain — see Infarct, brain
- embolic 434.11
- epileptic — see Epilepsy
- healed or old V12.54 ▲
- heart — see Disease, heart
- heat 992.0
- hemorrhagic — see Hemorrhage, brain
- iatrogenic 997.02
- in evolution 434.91 ▲
- ischemic 434.91
- late effect — see Late effect(s) (of) cerebrovascular disease
- lightning 994.0
- paralytic — see Infarct, brain
- postoperative 997.02
- progressive 435.9
- thrombotic 434.01

**Stromatosis, endometrial** (M8931/1) 236.0

**Strong pulse** 785.9

**Strongyloides stercoralis infestation** 127.2

**Strongyloidiasis** 127.2

**Strongyloidosis** 127.2

**Strongylus** (gibsoni) infestation 127.7

**Strophulus** (newborn) 779.89
- pruriginosus 698.2

**Struck by lightning** 994.0

**Struma** — *see also* Goiter 240.9
- fibrosa 245.3
- Hashimoto (struma lymphomatosa) 245.2
- lymphomatosa 245.2
- nodosa (simplex) 241.9
  - endemic 241.9
  - multinodular 241.1
  - sporadic 241.9
  - toxic or with hyperthyroidism 242.3 ☑
    - multinodular 242.2 ☑
    - uninodular 242.1 ☑
  - toxicosa 242.3 ☑
    - multinodular 242.2 ☑
    - uninodular 242.1 ☑
  - uninodular 241.0
- ovarii (M9090/0) 220
  - and carcinoid (M9091/1) 236.2
  - malignant (M9090/3) 183.0
- Riedel's (ligneous thyroiditis) 245.3
- scrofulous (*see also* Tuberculosis) 017.2 ☑
- tuberculous (*see also* Tuberculosis) 017.2 ☑
  - abscess 017.2 ☑
  - adenitis 017.2 ☑

**Struma** — *see also* Goiter — *continued*
- tuberculous (*see also* Tuberculosis) — *continued*
  - lymphangitis 017.2 ☑
  - ulcer 017.2 ☑

**Strumipriva cachexia** — *see also* Hypothyroidism 244.9

**Strümpell-Marie disease or spine** (ankylosing spondylitis) 720.0

**Strümpell-Westphal pseudosclerosis** (hepatolenticular degeneration) 275.1

**Stuart's disease** (congenital factor X deficiency) — *see also* Defect, coagulation 286.3

**Stuart-Prower factor deficiency** (congenital factor X deficiency) — *see also* Defect, coagulation 286.3

**Students' elbow** 727.2

**Stuffy nose** 478.19

**Stump** — *see also* Amputation
- cervix, cervical (healed) 622.8

**Stupor** 780.09
- catatonic (*see also* Schizophrenia) 295.2 ☑
- circular (*see also* Psychosis, manic-depressive, circular) 296.7
- manic 296.89
- manic-depressive (*see also* Psychosis, affective) 296.89
- mental (anergic) (delusional) 298.9
- psychogenic 298.8
- reaction to exceptional stress (transient) 308.2
- traumatic NEC (*see also* Injury, intracranial)
  - with spinal (cord)
    - lesion — see Injury, spinal, by site
    - shock — see Injury, spinal, by site

**Sturge (-Weber) (-Dimitri) disease or syndrome** (encephalocutaneous angiomatosis) 759.6

**Sturge-Kalischer-Weber syndrome** (encephalocutaneous angiomatosis) 759.6

**Stuttering** 307.0

**Sty, stye** 373.11
- external 373.11
- internal 373.12
- meibomian 373.12

**Subacidity, gastric** 536.8
- psychogenic 306.4

**Subacute** — *see* condition

**Subarachnoid** — *see* condition

**Subclavian steal syndrome** 435.2

**Subcortical** — *see* condition

**Subcostal syndrome** 098.86
- nerve compression 354.8

**Subcutaneous, subcuticular** — *see* condition

**Subdelirium** 293.1

**Subdural** — *see* condition

**Subendocardium** — *see* condition

**Subependymoma** (M9383/1) 237.5

**Suberosis** 495.3

**Subglossitis** — *see* Glossitis

**Subhemophilia** 286.0

**Subinvolution** (uterus) 621.1
- breast (postlactational) (postpartum) 611.8
- chronic 621.1
- puerperal, postpartum 674.8 ☑

**Sublingual** — *see* condition

**Sublinguitis** 527.2

**Subluxation** — *see also* Dislocation, by site
- congenital NEC (*see also* Malposition, congenital)
  - hip (unilateral) 754.32
    - with dislocation of other hip 754.35
    - bilateral 754.33

**Subluxation** — *see also* Dislocation, by site — *continued*
- congenital (*see also* Malposition, congenital) — *continued*
  - joint
    - lower limb 755.69
    - shoulder 755.59
    - upper limb 755.59
  - lower limb (joint) 755.69
  - shoulder (joint) 755.59
  - upper limb (joint) 755.59
- lens 379.32
  - anterior 379.33
  - posterior 379.34
- rotary, cervical region of spine — *see* Fracture, vertebra, cervical

**Submaxillary** — *see* condition

**Submersion** (fatal) (nonfatal) 994.1

**Submissiveness** (undue), in child 313.0

**Submucous** — *see* condition

**Subnormal, subnormality**
- accommodation (*see also* Disorder, accommodation) 367.9
- mental (*see also* Retardation, mental) 319
  - mild 317
  - moderate 318.0
  - profound 318.2
  - severe 318.1
- temperature (accidental) 991.6
  - not associated with low environmental temperature 780.99

**Subphrenic** — *see* condition

**Subscapular nerve** — *see* condition

**Subseptus uterus** 752.3

**Subsiding appendicitis** 542

**Substernal thyroid** — *see also* Goiter 240.9
- congenital 759.2

**Substitution disorder** 300.11

**Subtentorial** — *see* condition

**Subtertian**
- fever 084.0
- malaria (fever) 084.0

**Subthyroidism** (acquired) — *see also* Hypothyroidism 244.9
- congenital 243

**Succenturiata placenta** — *see* Placenta, abnormal

**Succussion sounds, chest** 786.7

**Sucking thumb, child** 307.9

**Sudamen** 705.1

**Sudamina** 705.1

**Sudanese kala-azar** 085.0

**Sudden**
- death, cause unknown (less than 24 hours) 798.1
  - cardiac (SCD)     ●
    - family history of V17.41    ●
    - personal history of, successful-●
      - ly resuscitated V12.53   ●
  - during childbirth 669.9 ☑
  - infant 798.0
  - puerperal, postpartum 674.9 ☑
- hearing loss NEC 388.2
- heart failure (*see also* Failure, heart) 428.9
- infant death syndrome 798.0

**Sudeck's atrophy, disease, or syndrome** 733.7

**SUDS** (sudden unexplained death) 798.2

**Suffocation** — *see also* Asphyxia 799.01
- by
  - bed clothes 994.7
  - bunny bag 994.7
  - cave-in 994.7
  - constriction 994.7
  - drowning 994.1
  - inhalation
    - food or foreign body (*see also* Asphyxia, food or foreign body) 933.1
    - oil or gasoline (*see also* Asphyxia, food or foreign body) 933.1
  - overlying 994.7

**Suffocation** — *see also* Asphyxia — *continued*
- by — *continued*
  - plastic bag 994.7
  - pressure 994.7
  - strangulation 994.7
- during birth 768.1
- mechanical 994.7

**Sugar**
- blood
  - high 790.29
  - low 251.2
- in urine 791.5

**Suicide, suicidal** (attempted)
- by poisoning — see Table of Drugs and Chemicals
- ideation V62.84
- risk 300.9
- tendencies 300.9
- trauma NEC (*see also* nature and site of injury) 959.9

**Suipestifer infection** — *see also* Infection, Salmonella 003.9

**Sulfatidosis** 330.0

**Sulfhemoglobinemia, sulphemoglobinemia** (acquired) (congenital) 289.7

**Sumatran mite fever** 081.2

**Summer** — *see* condition

**Sunburn** 692.71
- first degree 692.71
- second degree 692.76
- third degree 692.77
- dermatitis 692.71
- due to
  - other ultraviolet radiation 692.82
  - tanning bed 692.82

**Sunken**
- acetabulum 718.85
- fontanels 756.0

**Sunstroke** 992.0

**Superfecundation** 651.9 ☑
- with fetal loss and retention of one or more fetus(es) 651.6 ☑
- following (elective) fetal reduction 651.7 ☑

**Superfetation** 651.9 ☑
- with fetal loss and retention of one or more fetus(es) 651.6 ☑
- following (elective) fetal reduction 651.7 ☑

**Superinvolution uterus** 621.8

**Supernumerary** (congenital)
- aortic cusps 746.89
- auditory ossicles 744.04
- bone 756.9
- breast 757.6
- carpal bones 755.56
- cusps, heart valve NEC 746.89
  - mitral 746.5
  - pulmonary 746.09
- digit(s) 755.00
  - finger 755.01
  - toe 755.02
- ear (lobule) 744.1
- fallopian tube 752.19
- finger 755.01
- hymen 752.49
- kidney 753.3
- lacrimal glands 743.64
- lacrimonasal duct 743.65
- lobule (ear) 744.1
- mitral cusps 746.5
- muscle 756.82
- nipples 757.6
- organ or site NEC — see Accessory
- ossicles, auditory 744.04
- ovary 752.0
- oviduct 752.19
- pulmonic cusps 746.09
- rib 756.3
  - cervical or first 756.2
  - syndrome 756.2
- roots (of teeth) 520.2
- spinal vertebra 756.19
- spleen 759.0
- tarsal bones 755.67

☑ Additional Digit Required — Refer to the Tabular List for Digit Selection            ▽ Subterms under main terms may continue to next column or page

*2008 ICD-9-CM*      ▶◀ Revised Text      ● New Line      ▲ Revised Code      **October 2007 · Volume 2 — 269**

**Supernumerary** — *continued*
  teeth 520.1
    causing crowding 524.31
  testis 752.89
  thumb 755.01
  toe 755.02
  uterus 752.2
  vagina 752.49
  vertebra 756.19
**Supervision** (of)
  contraceptive method previously prescribed V25.40
    intrauterine device V25.42
    oral contraceptive (pill) V25.41
    specified type NEC V25.49
    subdermal implantable contraceptive V25.43
  dietary (for) V65.3
    allergy (food) V65.3
    colitis V65.3
    diabetes mellitus V65.3
    food allergy intolerance V65.3
    gastritis V65.3
    hypercholesterolemia V65.3
    hypoglycemia V65.3
    intolerance (food) V65.3
    obesity V65.3
    specified NEC V65.3
  lactation V24.1
  pregnancy — *see* Pregnancy, supervision of
**Supplemental teeth** 520.1
  causing crowding 524.31
**Suppression**
  binocular vision 368.31
  lactation 676.5 ☑
  menstruation 626.8
  ovarian secretion 256.39
  renal 586
  urinary secretion 788.5
  urine 788.5
**Suppuration, suppurative** — *see also*
  condition
  accessory sinus (chronic) (*see also* Sinusitis) 473.9
  adrenal gland 255.8
  antrum (chronic) (*see also* Sinusitis, maxillary) 473.0
  bladder (*see also* Cystitis) 595.89
  bowel 569.89
  brain 324.0
    late effect 326
  breast 611.0
    puerperal, postpartum 675.1 ☑
  dental periosteum 526.5
  diffuse (skin) 686.00
  ear (middle) (*see also* Otitis media) 382.4
    external (*see also* Otitis, externa) 380.10
    internal 386.33
  ethmoidal (sinus) (chronic) (*see also* Sinusitis, ethmoidal) 473.2
  fallopian tube (*see also* Salpingo-oophoritis) 614.2
  frontal (sinus) (chronic) (*see also* Sinusitis, frontal) 473.1
  gallbladder (*see also* Cholecystitis, acute) 575.0
  gum 523.30
  hernial sac — *see* Hernia, by site
  intestine 569.89
  joint (*see also* Arthritis, suppurative) 711.0 ☑
  labyrinthine 386.33
  lung 513.0
  mammary gland 611.0
    puerperal, postpartum 675.1 ☑
  maxilla, maxillary 526.4
    sinus (chronic) (*see also* Sinusitis, maxillary) 473.0
  muscle 728.0
  nasal sinus (chronic) (*see also* Sinusitis) 473.9
  pancreas 577.0
  parotid gland 527.2

**Suppuration, suppurative** — *see also*
  condition — *continued*
  pelvis, pelvic
    female (*see also* Disease, pelvis, inflammatory) 614.4
      acute 614.3
    male (*see also* Peritonitis) 567.21
  pericranial (*see also* Osteomyelitis) 730.2 ☑
  salivary duct or gland (any) 527.2
  sinus (nasal) (*see also* Sinusitis) 473.9
  sphenoidal (sinus) (chronic) (*see also* Sinusitis, sphenoidal) 473.3
  thymus (gland) 254.1
  thyroid (gland) 245.0
  tonsil 474.8
  uterus (*see also* Endometritis) 615.9
  vagina 616.10
  wound (*see also* Wound, open, by site, complicated)
    dislocation — *see* Dislocation, by site, compound
    fracture — *see* Fracture, by site, open
    scratch or other superficial injury — *see* Injury, superficial, by site
**Supraeruption, teeth** 524.34
**Supraglottitis** 464.50
  with obstruction 464.51
**Suprapubic drainage** 596.8
**Suprarenal** (gland) — *see* condition
**Suprascapular nerve** — *see* condition
**Suprasellar** — *see* condition
**Supraspinatus syndrome** 726.10
**Surfer knots** 919.8
  infected 919.9
**Surgery**
  cosmetic NEC V50.1
    following healed injury or operation V51
    hair transplant V50.0
  elective V50.9
    breast augmentation or reduction V50.1
    circumcision, ritual or routine (in absence of medical indication) V50.2
    cosmetic NEC V50.1
    ear piercing V50.3
    face-lift V50.1
    following healed injury or operation V51
    hair transplant V50.0
  not done because of
    contraindication V64.1
    patient's decision V64.2
    specified reason NEC V64.3
  plastic
    breast augmentation or reduction V50.1
    cosmetic V50.1
    face-lift V50.1
    following healed injury or operation V51
    repair of scarred tissue (following healed injury or operation) V51
    specified type NEC V50.8
  previous, in pregnancy or childbirth
    cervix 654.6 ☑
      affecting fetus or newborn 763.89
      causing obstructed labor 660.2 ☑
        affecting fetus or newborn 763.1
    pelvic soft tissues NEC 654.9 ☑
      affecting fetus or newborn 763.89
      causing obstructed labor 660.2 ☑
        affecting fetus or newborn 763.1
    perineum or vulva 654.8 ☑
    uterus NEC 654.9 ☑

**Surgery** — *continued*
  previous, in pregnancy or childbirth — *continued*
    uterus — *continued*
      affecting fetus or newborn 763.89
      causing obstructed labor 660.2 ☑
        affecting fetus or newborn 763.1
      due to previous cesarean delivery 654.2 ☑
    vagina 654.7 ☑
**Surgical**
  abortion — *see* Abortion, legal
  emphysema 998.81
  kidney (*see also* Pyelitis) 590.80
  operation NEC 799.9
  procedures, complication or misadventure — *see* Complications, surgical procedure
  shock 998.0
**Susceptibility**
  genetic
    to
      MEN (multiple endocrine neoplasia) V84.81 ●
      neoplasia ●
        multiple endocrine [MEN] V84.81 ●
      neoplasm
        malignant, of
          breast V84.01
          endometrium V84.04
          other V84.09
          ovary V84.02
          prostate V84.03
        ▶specified◀ disease V84.89 ▲
**Suspected condition, ruled out** — *see also* Observation, suspected V71.9
  specified condition NEC V71.89
**Suspended uterus, in pregnancy or childbirth** 654.4 ☑
  affecting fetus or newborn 763.89
  causing obstructed labor 660.2 ☑
    affecting fetus or newborn 763.1
**Sutton and Gull's disease** (arteriolar nephrosclerosis) — *see also* Hypertension, kidney 403.90
**Sutton's disease** 709.09
**Suture**
  burst (in external operation wound) 998.32
    internal 998.31
  inadvertently left in operation wound 998.4
  removal V58.32
  Shirodkar, in pregnancy (with or without cervical incompetence) 654.5 ☑
**Swab inadvertently left in operation wound** 998.4
**Swallowed, swallowing**
  difficulty (*see also* Dysphagia) 787.20 ▲
  foreign body NEC (*see also* Foreign body) 938
**Swamp fever** 100.89
**Swan neck hand** (intrinsic) 736.09
**Sweat(s), sweating**
  disease or sickness 078.2
  excessive (*see also* Hyperhidrosis) 780.8
  fetid 705.89
  fever 078.2
  gland disease 705.9
    specified type NEC 705.89
  miliary 078.2
  night 780.8
**Sweeley-Klionsky disease** (angiokeratoma corporis diffusum) 272.7
**Sweet's syndrome** (acute febrile neutrophilic dermatosis) 695.89
**Swelling** 782.3 ▲
  abdominal (not referable to specific organ) 789.3 ☑

**Swelling** — *continued*
  adrenal gland, cloudy 255.8
  ankle 719.07
  anus 787.99
  arm 729.81
  breast 611.72
  Calabar 125.2
  cervical gland 785.6
  cheek 784.2
  chest 786.6
  ear 388.8
  epigastric 789.3 ☑
  extremity (lower) (upper) 729.81
  eye 379.92
  female genital organ 625.8
  finger 729.81
  foot 729.81
  glands 785.6
  gum 784.2
  hand 729.81
  head 784.2
  inflammatory — *see* Inflammation
  joint (*see also* Effusion, joint) 719.0 ☑
    tuberculous — *see* Tuberculosis, joint
  kidney, cloudy 593.89
  leg 729.81
  limb 729.81
  liver 573.8
  lung 786.6
  lymph nodes 785.6
  mediastinal 786.6
  mouth 784.2
  muscle (limb) 729.81
  neck 784.2
  nose or sinus 784.2
  palate 784.2
  pelvis 789.3 ☑
  penis 607.83
  perineum 625.8
  rectum 787.99
  scrotum 608.86
  skin 782.2
  splenic (*see also* Splenomegaly) 789.2
  substantial 786.6
  superficial, localized (skin) 782.2
  testicle 608.86
  throat 784.2
  toe 729.81
  tongue 784.2
  tubular (*see also* Disease, renal) 593.9
  umbilicus 789.3 ☑
  uterus 625.8
  vagina 625.8
  vulva 625.8
  wandering, due to Gnathostoma (spinigerum) 128.1
  white — *see* Tuberculosis, arthritis
**Swift's disease** 985.0
**Swimmers'**
  ear (acute) 380.12
  itch 120.3
**Swimming in the head** 780.4
**Swollen** — *see also* Swelling
  glands 785.6
**Swyer-James syndrome** (unilateral hyperlucent lung) 492.8
**Swyer's syndrome** (XY pure gonadal dysgenesis) 752.7
**Sycosis** 704.8
  barbae (not parasitic) 704.8
  contagiosa 110.0
  lupoid 704.8
  mycotic 110.0
  parasitic 110.0
  vulgaris 704.8
**Sydenham's chorea** — *see* Chorea, Sydenham's
**Sylvatic yellow fever** 060.0
**Sylvest's disease** (epidemic pleurodynia) 074.1
**Symblepharon** 372.63
  congenital 743.62
**Symonds' syndrome** 348.2
**Sympathetic** — *see* condition

---

☑ Additional Digit Required — Refer to the Tabular List for Digit Selection          ▽ Subterms under main terms may continue to next column or page

270 — Volume 2 · October 2007          ▶◀ Revised Text          ● New Line          ▲ Revised Code          *2008 ICD-9-CM*

Sympatheticotonia — see also Neuropathy, peripheral, autonomic 337.9
Sympathicoblastoma (M9500/3)
specified site — see Neoplasm, by site, malignant
unspecified site 194.0
Sympathicogonioma (M9500/3) — see Sympathicoblastoma
Sympathoblastoma (M9500/3) — see Sympathicoblastoma
Sympathogonioma (M9500/3) — see Sympathicoblastoma
Symphalangy — see also Syndactylism 755.10
Symptoms, specified (general) NEC 780.99
abdomen NEC 789.9
bone NEC 733.90
breast NEC 611.79
cardiac NEC 785.9
cardiovascular NEC 785.9
chest NEC 786.9
development NEC 783.9
digestive system NEC 787.99
eye NEC 379.99
gastrointestinal tract NEC 787.99
genital organs NEC
female 625.9
male 608.9
head and neck NEC 784.99
heart NEC 785.9
joint NEC 719.60
ankle 719.67
elbow 719.62
foot 719.67
hand 719.64
hip 719.65
knee 719.66
multiple sites 719.69
pelvic region 719.65
shoulder (region) 719.61
specified site NEC 719.68
wrist 719.63
larynx NEC 784.99
limbs NEC 729.89
lymphatic system NEC 785.9
menopausal 627.2
metabolism NEC 783.9
mouth NEC 528.9
muscle NEC 728.9
musculoskeletal NEC 781.99
limbs NEC 729.89
nervous system NEC 781.99
neurotic NEC 300.9
nutrition, metabolism, and development NEC 783.9
pelvis NEC 789.9
female 625.9
peritoneum NEC 789.9
respiratory system NEC 786.9
skin and integument NEC 782.9
subcutaneous tissue NEC 782.9
throat NEC 784.99
tonsil NEC 784.99
urinary system NEC 788.9
vascular NEC 785.9
Sympus 759.89
Synarthrosis 719.80
ankle 719.87
elbow 719.82
foot 719.87
hand 719.84
hip 719.85
knee 719.86
multiple sites 719.89
pelvic region 719.85
shoulder (region) 719.81
specified site NEC 719.88
wrist 719.83
Syncephalus 759.4
Synchondrosis 756.9
abnormal (congenital) 756.9
ischiopubic (van Neck's) 732.1
Synchysis (senile) (vitreous humor) 379.21
scintillans 379.22

Syncope (near) (pre-) 780.2
anginosa 413.9
bradycardia 427.89
cardiac 780.2
carotid sinus 337.0
complicating delivery 669.2 ☑
due to lumbar puncture 349.0
fatal 798.1
heart 780.2
heat 992.1
laryngeal 786.2
tussive 786.2
vasoconstriction 780.2
vasodepressor 780.2
vasomotor 780.2
vasovagal 780.2
Syncytial infarct — see Placenta, abnormal
Syndactylism, syndactyly (multiple sites) 755.10
fingers (without fusion of bone) 755.11
with fusion of bone 755.12
toes (without fusion of bone) 755.13
with fusion of bone 755.14
Syndrome — see also Disease
with 5q deletion 238.74
5q minus 238.74
abdominal
acute 789.0 ☑
migraine 346.2 ☑
muscle deficiency 756.79
Abercrombie's (amyloid degeneration) 277.39
abnormal innervation 374.43
abstinence
alcohol 291.81
drug 292.0
Abt-Letterer-Siwe (acute histiocytosis X) (M9722/3) 202.5 ☑
Achard-Thiers (adrenogenital) 255.2
acid pulmonary aspiration 997.3
obstetric (Mendelson's) 668.0 ☑
acquired immune deficiency 042
acquired immunodeficiency 042
acrocephalosyndactylism 755.55
acute abdominal 789.0 ☑
acute chest 517.3
acute coronary 411.1
Adair-Dighton (brittle bones and blue sclera, deafness) 756.51
Adams-Stokes (-Morgagni) (syncope with heart block) 426.9
Addisonian 255.41                          ▲
Adie (-Holmes) (pupil) 379.46
adiposogenital 253.8
adrenal
hemorrhage 036.3
meningococcic 036.3
adrenocortical 255.3
adrenogenital (acquired) (congenital) 255.2
feminizing 255.2
iatrogenic 760.79
virilism (acquired) (congenital) 255.2
affective organic NEC 293.89
drug-induced 292.84
afferent loop NEC 537.89
African macroglobulinemia 273.3
Ahumada-Del Castillo (nonpuerperal galactorrhea and amenorrhea) 253.1
air blast concussion — see Injury, internal, by site
Alagille 759.89
Albright (-Martin) (pseudohypoparathyroidism) 275.49
Albright-McCune-Sternberg (osteitis fibrosa disseminata) 756.59
alcohol withdrawal 291.81
Alder's (leukocyte granulation anomaly) 288.2
Aldrich (-Wiskott) (eczema-thrombocytopenia) 279.12
Alibert-Bazin (mycosis fungoides) (M9700/3) 202.1 ☑

Syndrome — see also Disease — continued
Alice in Wonderland 293.89
Allen-Masters 620.6
Alligator baby (ichthyosis congenita) 757.1
Alport's (hereditary hematuria-nephropathy-deafness) 759.89
Alvarez (transient cerebral ischemia) 435.9
alveolar capillary block 516.3
Alzheimer's 331.0
with dementia — see Alzheimer's, dementia
amnestic (confabulatory) 294.0
alcohol-induced persisting 291.1
drug-induced 292.83
posttraumatic 294.0
amotivational 292.89
amyostatic 275.1
amyotrophic lateral sclerosis 335.20
androgen insensitivity 259.5
Angelman 759.89
angina (see also Angina) 413.9
ankyloglossia superior 750.0
anterior
chest wall 786.52
compartment (tibial) 958.8
spinal artery 433.8 ☑
compression 721.1
tibial (compartment) 958.8
antibody deficiency 279.00
agammaglobulinemic 279.00
congenital 279.04
hypogammaglobulinemic 279.00
anticardiolipin antibody 795.79
antimongolism 758.39
antiphospholipid antibody 795.79
Anton (-Babinski) (hemiasomatognosia) 307.9
anxiety (see also Anxiety) 300.00
organic 293.84
aortic
arch 446.7
bifurcation (occlusion) 444.0
ring 747.21
Apert's (acrocephalosyndactyly) 755.55
Apert-Gallais (adrenogenital) 255.2
aphasia-apraxia-alexia 784.69
apical ballooning 429.83
"approximate answers" 300.16
arcuate ligament (-celiac axis) 447.4
arcus aortae 446.7
arc welders' 370.24
argentaffin, argintaffinoma 259.2
Argonz-Del Castillo (nonpuerperal galactorrhea and amenorrhea) 253.1
Argyll Robertson's (syphilitic) 094.89
nonsyphilitic 379.45
Armenian 277.31
arm-shoulder (see also Neuropathy, peripheral, autonomic) 337.9
Arnold-Chiari (see also Spina bifida) 741.0 ☑
type I 348.4
type II 741.0 ☑
type III 742.0
type IV 742.2
Arrillaga-Ayerza (pulmonary artery sclerosis with pulmonary hypertension) 416.0
arteriomesenteric duodenum occlusion 537.89
arteriovenous steal 996.73
arteritis, young female (obliterative brachiocephalic) 446.7
aseptic meningitis — see Meningitis, aseptic
Asherman's 621.5
Asperger's 299.8 ☑
asphyctic (see also Anxiety) 300.00
aspiration, of newborn (massive) 770.18
meconium 770.12

Syndrome — see also Disease — continued
ataxia-telangiectasia 334.8
Audry's (acropachyderma) 757.39
auriculotemporal 350.8
autosomal (see also Abnormal, autosomes NEC)
deletion 758.39
5p 758.31
22q11.2 758.32
Avellis' 344.89
Axenfeld's 743.44
Ayerza (-Arrillaga) (pulmonary artery sclerosis with pulmonary hypertension) 416.0
Baader's (erythema multiforme exudativum) 695.1
Baastrup's 721.5
Babinski (-Vaquez) (cardiovascular syphilis) 093.89
Babinski-Fröhlich (adiposogenital dystrophy) 253.8
Babinski-Nageotte 344.89
Bagratuni's (temporal arteritis) 446.5
Bakwin-Krida (craniometaphyseal dysplasia) 756.89
Balint's (psychic paralysis of visual disorientation) 368.16
Ballantyne (-Runge) (postmaturity) 766.22
ballooning posterior leaflet 424.0
Banti's — see Cirrhosis, liver
Bardet-Biedl (obesity, polydactyly, and mental retardation) 759.89
Bard-Pic's (carcinoma, head of pancreas) 157.0
Barlow's (mitral valve prolapse) 424.0
Barlow (-Möller) (infantile scurvy) 267
Baron Munchausen's 301.51
Barré-Guillain 357.0
Barré-Liéou (posterior cervical sympathetic) 723.2
Barrett's (chronic peptic ulcer of esophagus) 530.85
Bársony-Polgár (corkscrew esophagus) 530.5
Bársony-Teschendorf (corkscrew esophagus) 530.5
Barth 759.89
Bartter's (secondary hyperaldosteronism with juxtaglomerular hyperplasia) 255.13
Basedow's (exophthalmic goiter) 242.0 ☑
basilar artery 435.0
basofrontal 377.04
Bassen-Kornzweig (abetalipoproteinemia) 272.5
Batten-Steinert 359.21                     ▲
battered
adult 995.81
baby or child 995.54
spouse 995.81
Baumgarten-Cruveilhier (cirrhosis of liver) 571.5
Beals 759.82
Bearn-Kunkel (-Slater) (lupoid hepatitis) 571.49
Beau's (see also Degeneration, myocardial) 429.1
Bechterew-Strümpell-Marie (ankylosing spondylitis) 720.0
Beck's (anterior spinal artery occlusion) 433.8 ☑
Beckwith (-Wiedemann) 759.89
Behçet's 136.1
Bekhterev-Strümpell-Marie (ankylosing spondylitis) 720.0
Benedikt's 344.89
Béquez César (-Steinbrinck-Chédiak-Higashi) (congenital gigantism of peroxidase granules) 288.2
Bernard-Horner (see also Neuropathy, peripheral, autonomic) 337.9
Bernard-Sergent (acute adrenocortical insufficiency) 255.41         ▲

---

☑ Additional Digit Required — Refer to the Tabular List for Digit Selection          ⓥ Subterms under main terms may continue to next column or page

**Syndrome** — *see also* Disease —
*continued*
Bernhardt-Roth 355.1
Bernheim's (*see also* Failure, heart)
428.0
Bertolotti's (sacralization of fifth lumbar vertebra) 756.15
Besnier-Boeck-Schaumann (sarcoidosis) 135
Bianchi's (aphasia-apraxia-alexia
syndrome) 784.69
Biedl-Bardet (obesity, polydactyly, and
mental retardation) 759.89
Biemond's (obesity, polydactyly, and
mental retardation) 759.89
big spleen 289.4
bilateral polycystic ovarian 256.4
Bing-Horton's 346.2 ☑
Biörck (-Thorson) (malignant carcinoid) 259.2
Blackfan-Diamond (congenital hypoplastic anemia) 284.01
black lung 500
black widow spider bite 989.5
bladder neck (*see also* Incontinence,
urine) 788.30
blast (concussion) — *see* Blast, injury
blind loop (postoperative) 579.2
Bloch-Siemens (incontinentia pigmenti) 757.33
Bloch-Sulzberger (incontinentia pigmenti) 757.33
Bloom (-Machacek) (-Torre) 757.39
Blount-Barber (tibia vara) 732.4
blue
bloater 491.20
with
acute bronchitis 491.22
exacerbation (acute) 491.21
diaper 270.0
drum 381.02
sclera 756.51
toe 445.02
Boder-Sedgwick (ataxia-telangiectasia)
334.8
Boerhaave's (spontaneous esophageal
rupture) 530.4
Bonnevie-Ullrich 758.6
Bonnier's 386.19
Borjeson-Forssman-Lehmann 759.89
Bouillaud's (rheumatic heart disease)
391.9
Bourneville (-Pringle) (tuberous sclerosis) 759.5
Bouveret (-Hoffmann) (paroxysmal
tachycardia) 427.2
brachial plexus 353.0
Brachman-de Lange (Amsterdam
dwarf, mental retardation, and
brachycephaly) 759.89
bradycardia-tachycardia 427.81
Brailsford-Morquio (dystrophy) (mucopolysaccharidosis IV) 277.5
brain (acute) (chronic) (nonpsychotic)
(organic) (with behavioral reaction) (with neurotic reaction)
310.9
with
presenile brain disease (*see also*
Dementia, presenile)
290.10
psychosis, psychotic reaction
(*see also* Psychosis, organic) 294.9
chronic alcoholic 291.2
congenital (*see also* Retardation,
mental) 319
postcontusional 310.2
posttraumatic
nonpsychotic 310.2
psychotic 293.9
acute 293.0
chronic (*see also* Psychosis,
organic) 294.8
subacute 293.1

**Syndrome** — *see also* Disease —
*continued*
brain — *continued*
psycho-organic (*see also* Syndrome, psycho-organic)
310.9
psychotic (*see also* Psychosis, organic) 294.9
senile (*see also* Dementia, senile)
290.0
branchial arch 744.41
Brandt's (acrodermatitis enteropathica) 686.8
Brennemann's 289.2
Briquet's 300.81
Brissaud-Meige (infantile myxedema)
244.9
broad ligament laceration 620.6
Brock's (atelectasis due to enlarged
lymph nodes) 518.0
broken heart 429.83
Brown-Séquard 344.89
brown spot 756.59
Brown's tendon sheath 378.61
Brugada 746.89
Brugsch's (acropachyderma) 757.39
bubbly lung 770.7
Buchem's (hyperostosis corticalis)
733.3
Budd-Chiari (hepatic vein thrombosis)
453.0
Büdinger-Ludloff-Läwen 717.89
bulbar 335.22
lateral (*see also* Disease, cerebrovascular, acute) 436
Bullis fever 082.8
bundle of Kent (anomalous atrioventricular excitation) 426.7
Bürger-Grütz (essential familial hyperlipemia) 272.3
Burke's (pancreatic insufficiency and
chronic neutropenia) 577.8
Burnett's (milk-alkali) 275.42
Burnier's (hypophyseal dwarfism)
253.3
burning feet 266.2
Bywaters' 958.5
Caffey's (infantile cortical hyperostosis) 756.59
Calvé-Legg-Perthes (osteochondrosis,
femoral capital) 732.1
Caplan (-Colinet) syndrome 714.81
capsular thrombosis (*see also*
Thrombosis, brain) 434.0 ☑
carbohydrate-deficient glycoprotein
(CDGS) 271.8
carcinogenic thrombophlebitis 453.1
carcinoid 259.2
cardiac asthma (*see also* Failure,
ventricular, left) 428.1
cardiacos negros 416.0
cardiopulmonary obesity 278.8
cardiorenal (*see also* Hypertension,
cardiorenal) 404.90
cardiorespiratory distress (idiopathic),
newborn 769
cardiovascular renal (*see also* Hypertension, cardiorenal) 404.90
cardiovasorenal 272.7
Carini's (ichthyosis congenita) 757.1
carotid
artery (internal) 435.8
body or sinus 337.0
carpal tunnel 354.0
Carpenter's 759.89
Cassidy (-Scholte) (malignant carcinoid) 259.2
cat-cry 758.31
cauda equina 344.60
causalgia 355.9
lower limb 355.71
upper limb 354.4
cavernous sinus 437.6
celiac 579.0
artery compression 447.4
axis 447.4

**Syndrome** — *see also* Disease —
*continued*
central pain 338.0
cerebellomedullary malformation (*see
also* Spina bifida) 741.0 ☑
cerebral gigantism 253.0
cerebrohepatorenal 759.89
cervical (root) (spine) NEC 723.8
disc 722.71
posterior, sympathetic 723.2
rib 353.0
sympathetic paralysis 337.0
traumatic (acute) NEC 847.0
cervicobrachial (diffuse) 723.3
cervicocranial 723.2
cervicodorsal outlet 353.2
Céstan's 344.89
Céstan (-Raymond) 433.8 ☑
Céstan-Chenais 344.89
chancriform 114.1
Charcôt's (intermittent claudication)
443.9
angina cruris 443.9
due to atherosclerosis 440.21
Charcôt-Marie-Tooth 356.1
Charcôt-Weiss-Baker 337.0
CHARGE association 759.89
Cheadle (-Möller) (-Barlow) (infantile
scurvy) 267
Chédiak-Higashi (-Steinbrinck) (congenital gigantism of peroxidase
granules) 288.2
chest wall 786.52
Chiari's (hepatic vein thrombosis)
453.0
Chiari-Frommel 676.6 ☑
chiasmatic 368.41
Chilaiditi's (subphrenic displacement,
colon) 751.4
chondroectodermal dysplasia 756.55
chorea-athetosis-agitans 275.1
Christian's (chronic histiocytosis X)
277.89
chromosome 4 short arm deletion
758.39
chronic pain 338.4
Churg-Strauss 446.4
Clarke-Hadfield (pancreatic infantilism) 577.8
Claude's 352.6
Claude Bernard-Horner (*see also*
Neuropathy, peripheral, autonomic) 337.9
Clé rambault's
automatism 348.8
erotomania 297.8
Clifford's (postmaturity) 766.22
climacteric 627.2
Clouston's (hidrotic ectodermal dysplasia) 757.31
clumsiness 315.4
Cockayne's (microencephaly and
dwarfism) 759.89
Cockayne-Weber (epidermolysis bullosa) 757.39
Coffin-Lowry 759.89
Cogan's (nonsyphilitic interstitial keratitis) 370.52
cold injury (newborn) 778.2
Collet (-Sicard) 352.6
combined immunity deficiency 279.2
compartment(al) (anterior) (deep)
(posterior) 958.8
nontraumatic
abdomen 729.73
arm 729.71
buttock 729.72
fingers 729.71
foot 729.72
forearm 729.71
hand 729.71
hip 729.72
leg 729.72
lower extremity 729.72
shoulder 729.71
specified site NEC 729.79

**Syndrome** — *see also* Disease —
*continued*
compartment — *continued*
nontraumatic — *continued*
thigh 729.72
toes 729.72
upper extremity 729.71
wrist 729.71
traumatic 958.90
adomen 958.93
arm 958.91
buttock 958.92
fingers 958.91
foot 958.92
forearm 958.91
hand 958.91
hip 958.92
leg 958.92
lower extremity 958.92
shoulder 958.91
specified site NEC 958.99
thigh 958.92
tibial 958.92
toes 958.92
upper extremity 958.91
wrist 958.91
compression 958.5
cauda equina 344.60
with neurogenic bladder 344.61
concussion 310.2
congenital
affecting more than one system
759.7
specified type NEC 759.89
congenital central alveolar hypoventilation 327.25
facial diplegia 352.6
muscular hypertrophy-cerebral
759.89
congestion-fibrosis (pelvic) 625.5
conjunctivourethrosynovial 099.3
Conn (-Louis) (primary aldosteronism)
255.12
Conradi (-Hünermann) (chondrodysplasia calcificans congenita)
756.59
conus medullaris 336.8
Cooke-Apert-Gallais (adrenogenital)
255.2
Cornelia de Lange's (Amsterdam
dwarf, mental retardation, and
brachycephaly) 759.8 ☑
coronary insufficiency or intermediate
411.1
cor pulmonale 416.9
corticosexual 255.2
Costen's (complex) 524.60
costochondral junction 733.6
costoclavicular 353.0
costovertebral 253.0
Cotard's (paranoia) 297.1
Cowden 759.6
craniovertebral 723.2
Creutzfeldt-Jakob (new variant) 046.1
with dementia
with behavioral disturbance
046.1 [294.11]
without behavioral disturbance
046.1 [294.10]
crib death 798.0
cricopharyngeal 787.20 ▲
cri-du-chat 758.31
Crigler-Najjar (congenital hyperbilirubinemia) 277.4
crocodile tears 351.8
Cronkhite-Canada 211.3
croup 464.4
CRST (cutaneous systemic sclerosis)
710.1
crush 958.5
crushed lung (*see also* Injury, internal, lung) 861.20
Cruveilhier-Baumgarten (cirrhosis of
liver) 571.5
cubital tunnel 354.2

Syndrome — *see also* Disease — *continued*

Cuiffini-Pancoast (M8010/3) (carcinoma, pulmonary apex) 162.3
Curschmann (-Batten) (-Steinert) 359.21 ▲
Cushing's (iatrogenic) (idiopathic) (pituitary basophilism) (pituitary-dependent) 255.0
　overdose or wrong substance given or taken 962.0
Cyriax's (slipping rib) 733.99
cystic duct stump 576.0
Da Costa's (neurocirculatory asthenia) 306.2
Dameshek's (erythroblastic anemia) 282.49
Dana-Putnam (subacute combined sclerosis with pernicious anemia) 281.0 *[336.2]*
Danbolt (-Closs) (acrodermatitis enteropathica) 686.8
Dandy-Walker (atresia, foramen of Magendie) 742.3
　with spina bifida (*see also* Spina bifida) 741.0 ☑
Danlos' 756.83
Davies-Colley (slipping rib) 733.99
dead fetus 641.3 ☑
defeminization 255.2
defibrination (*see also* Fibrinolysis) 286.6
Degos' 447.8
Deiters' nucleus 386.19
Déjérine-Roussy 338.0
Déjérine-Thomas 333.0
de Lange's (Amsterdam dwarf, mental retardation, and brachycephaly) (Cornelia) 759.89
Del Castillo's (germinal aplasia) 606.0
deletion chromosomes 758.39
delusional
　induced by drug 292.11
dementia-aphonia, of childhood (*see also* Psychosis, childhood) 299.1 ☑
demyelinating NEC 341.9
denial visual hallucination 307.9
depersonalization 300.6
Dercum's (adiposis dolorosa) 272.8
de Toni-Fanconi (-Debré) (cystinosis) 270.0
diabetes-dwarfism-obesity (juvenile) 258.1
diabetes mellitus-hypertension-nephrosis 250.4 ☑ *[581.81]*
diabetes mellitus in newborn infant 775.1
diabetes-nephrosis 250.4 ☑ *[581.81]*
diabetic amyotrophy 250.6 ☑ *[353.1]* ▲
Diamond-Blackfan (congenital hypoplastic anemia) 284.01
Diamond-Gardener (autoerythrocyte sensitization) 287.2
DIC (diffuse or disseminated intravascular coagulopathy) (*see also* Fibrinolysis) 286.6
diencephalohypophyseal NEC 253.8
diffuse cervicobrachial 723.3
diffuse obstructive pulmonary 496
DiGeorge's (thymic hypoplasia) 279.11
Dighton's 756.51
Di Guglielmo's (erythremic myelosis) (M9841/3) 207.0 ☑
disequilibrium 276.9
disseminated platelet thrombosis 446.6
Ditthomska 307.81
Doan-Wisemann (primary splenic neutropenia) 289.53
Döhle body-panmyelopathic 288.2
Donohue's (leprechaunism) 259.8
dorsolateral medullary (*see also* Disease, cerebrovascular, acute) 436

Syndrome — *see also* Disease — *continued*

double athetosis 333.71
double whammy 360.81
Down's (mongolism) 758.0
Dresbach's (elliptocytosis) 282.1
Dressler's (postmyocardial infarction) 411.0
　hemoglobinuria 283.2
　postcardiotomy 429.4
drug withdrawal, infant, of dependent mother 779.5
dry skin 701.1
　eye 375.15
DSAP (disseminated superficial actinic porokeratosis) 692.75
Duane's (retraction) 378.71
Duane-Stilling-Türk (ocular retraction syndrome) 378.71
Dubin-Johnson (constitutional hyperbilirubinemia) 277.4
Dubin-Sprinz (constitutional hyperbilirubinemia) 277.4
Duchenne's 335.22
due to abnormality
　autosomal NEC (*see also* Abnormal, autosomes NEC) 758.5
　　13 758.1
　　18 758.2
　　21 or 22 758.0
　　D1 758.1
　　E3 758.2
　　G 758.0
　chromosomal 758.89
　　sex 758.81
dumping 564.2
　nonsurgical 536.8
Duplay's 726.2
Dupré's (meningism) 781.6
Dyke-Young (acquired macrocytic hemolytic anemia) 283.9
dyspraxia 315.4
dystocia, dystrophia 654.9 ☑
Eagle-Barret 756.71
Eales' 362.18
Eaton-Lambert (*see also* Neoplasm, by site, malignant) 199.1 *[358.1]*
Ebstein's (downward displacement, tricuspid valve into right ventricle) 746.2
ectopic ACTH secretion 255.0
eczema-thrombocytopenia 279.12
Eddowes' (brittle bones and blue sclera) 756.51
Edwards' 758.2
efferent loop 537.89
effort (aviators') (psychogenic) 306.2
Ehlers-Danlos 756.83
Eisenmenger's (ventricular septal defect) 745.4
Ekbom's (restless legs) 333.94
Ekman's (brittle bones and blue sclera) 756.51
electric feet 266.2
Elephant man 237.71
Ellison-Zollinger (gastric hypersecretion with pancreatic islet cell tumor) 251.5
Ellis-van Creveld (chondroectodermal dysplasia) 756.55
embryonic fixation 270.2
empty sella (turcica) 253.8
endocrine-hypertensive 255.3
Engel-von Recklinghausen (osteitis fibrosa cystica) 252.01
enteroarticular 099.3
entrapment — *see* Neuropathy, entrapment
eosinophilia myalgia 710.5
epidemic vomiting 078.82
Epstein's — *see* Nephrosis
Erb (-Oppenheim)-Goldflam 358.00
Erdheim's (acromegalic macrospondylitis) 253.0
Erlacher-Blount (tibia vara) 732.4
erythrocyte fragmentation 283.19

Syndrome — *see also* Disease — *continued*

euthyroid sick 790.94
Evans' (thrombocytopenic purpura) 287.32
excess cortisol, iatrogenic 255.0
exhaustion 300.5
extrapyramidal 333.90
eyelid-malar-mandible 756.0
eye retraction 378.71
Faber's (achlorhydric anemia) 280.9
Fabry (-Anderson) (angiokeratoma corporis diffusum) 272.7
facet 724.8
Fallot's 745.2
falx (*see also* Hemorrhage, brain) 431
familial eczema-thrombocytopenia 279.12
Fanconi (-de Toni) (-Debré) (cystinosis) 270.0
Fanconi's (anemia) (congenital pancytopenia) 284.09
Farber (-Uzman) (disseminated lipogranulomatosis) 272.8
fatigue NEC 300.5
　chronic 780.71
faulty bowel habit (idiopathic megacolon) 564.7
FDH (focal dermal hypoplasia) 757.39
fecal reservoir 560.39
Feil-Klippel (brevicollis) 756.16
Felty's (rheumatoid arthritis with splenomegaly and leukopenia) 714.1
fertile eunuch 257.2
fetal alcohol 760.71
　late effect 760.71
fibrillation-flutter 427.32
fibrositis (periarticular) 729.0
Fiedler's (acute isolated myocarditis) 422.91
Fiessinger-Leroy (-Reiter) 099.3
Fiessinger-Rendu (erythema multiforme exudativum) 695.1
first arch 756.0
Fisher's 357.0
fish odor 270.8
Fitz's (acute hemorrhagic pancreatitis) 577.0
Fitz-Hugh and Curtis 098.86
　due to
　　Chlamydia trachomatis 099.56
　　Neisseria gonorrhoeae (gonococcal peritonitis) 098.86
Flajani (-Basedow) (exophthalmic goiter) 242.0 ☑
floppy
　infant 781.99
　iris 364.81
　valve (mitral) 424.0
flush 259.2
Foix-Alajouanine 336.1
Fong's (hereditary osteo-onychodysplasia) 756.89
foramen magnum 348.4
Forbes-Albright (nonpuerperal amenorrhea and lactation associated with pituitary tumor) 253.1
Foster-Kennedy 377.04
Foville's (peduncular) 344.89
fragile X 759.83
Franceschetti's (mandibulofacial dysostosis) 756.0
Fraser's 759.89
Freeman-Sheldon 759.89
Frey's (auriculotemporal) 705.22
Friderichsen-Waterhouse 036.3
Friedrich-Erb-Arnold (acropachyderma) 757.39
Fröhlich's (adiposogenital dystrophy) 253.8
Froin's 336.8
Frommel-Chiari 676.6 ☑
frontal lobe 310.0
Fukuhara 277.87

Syndrome — *see also* Disease — *continued*

Fuller Albright's (osteitis fibrosa disseminata) 756.59
functional
　bowel 564.9
　prepubertal castrate 752.89
Gaisböck's (polycythemia hypertonica) 289.0
ganglion (basal, brain) 333.90
　geniculi 351.1
Ganser's, hysterical 300.16
Gardner-Diamond (autoerythrocyte sensitization) 287.2
gastroesophageal junction 530.0
gastroesophageal laceration-hemorrhage 530.7
gastrojejunal loop obstruction 537.89
Gayet-Wernicke's (superior hemorrhagic polioencephalitis) 265.1
Gee-Herter-Heubner (nontropical sprue) 579.0
Gélineau's (*see also* Narcolepsy) 347.00
genito-anorectal 099.1
Gerhardt's (vocal cord paralysis) 478.30
Gerstmann's (finger agnosia) 784.69
Gianotti Crosti 057.8
　due to known virus — *see* Infection, virus
　due to unknown virus 057.8
Gilbert's 277.4
Gilford (-Hutchinson) (progeria) 259.8
Gilles de la Tourette's 307.23
Gillespie's (dysplasia oculodentodigitalis) 759.89
Glénard's (enteroptosis) 569.89
Glinski-Simmonds (pituitary cachexia) 253.2
glucuronyl transferase 277.4
glue ear 381.20
Goldberg (-Maxwell) (-Morris) (testicular feminization) 259.5
Goldenhar's (oculoauriculovertebral dysplasia) 756.0
Goldflam-Erb 358.00
Goltz-Gorlin (dermal hypoplasia) 757.39
Good's 279.06
Goodpasture's (pneumorenal) 446.21
Gopalan's (burning feet) 266.2
Gorlin-Chaudhry-Moss 759.89
Gougerot-Blum (pigmented purpuric lichenoid dermatitis) 709.1
Gougerot-Carteaud (confluent reticulate papillomatosis) 701.8
Gougerot (-Houwer)-Sjögren (keratoconjunctivitis sicca) 710.2
Gouley's (constrictive pericarditis) 423.2
Gowers' (vasovagal attack) 780.2
Gowers-Paton-Kennedy 377.04
Gradenigo's 383.02
gray or grey (chloramphenicol) (newborn) 779.4
Greig's (hypertelorism) 756.0
Gubler-Millard 344.89
Guérin-Stern (arthrogryposis multiplex congenita) 754.89
Guillain-Barré (-Strohl) 357.0
Gunn's (jaw-winking syndrome) 742.8
Günther's (congenital erythropoietic porphyria) 277.1
gustatory sweating 350.8
H3O 759.81
Hadfield-Clarke (pancreatic infantilism) 577.8
Haglund-Läwen-Fründ 717.89
hairless women 257.8
hair tourniquet (*see also* Injury, superficial, by site)
　finger 915.8
　　infected 915.9
　penis 911.8
　　infected 911.9

☑ Additional Digit Required — Refer to the Tabular List for Digit Selection
**2008 ICD-9-CM**　　　　　▶◀ Revised Text　　　　●  New Line　　　　▲ Revised Code
▽ Subterms under main terms may continue to next column or page
**October 2007 • Volume 2 — 273**

**Syndrome** — *see also* Disease — *continued*

hair tourniquet (*see also* Injury, superficial, by site) — *continued*
  toe 917.8
    infected 917.9
Hallermann-Streiff 756.0
Hallervorden-Spatz 333.0
Hamman's (spontaneous mediastinal emphysema) 518.1
Hamman-Rich (diffuse interstitial pulmonary fibrosis) 516.3
hand-foot 693.0 ▲
Hand-Schüller-Christian (chronic histiocytosis X) 277.89
Hanot-Chauffard (-Troisier) (bronze diabetes) 275.0
Harada's 363.22
Hare's (M8010/3) (carcinoma, pulmonary apex) 162.3
Harkavy's 446.0
harlequin color change 779.89
Harris' (organic hyperinsulinism) 251.1
Hart's (pellagra-cerebellar ataxia-renal aminoaciduria) 270.0
Hayem-Faber (achlorhydric anemia) 280.9
Hayem-Widal (acquired hemolytic jaundice) 283.9
Heberden's (angina pectoris) 413.9
Hedinger's (malignant carcinoid) 259.2
Hegglin's 288.2
Heller's (infantile psychosis) (*see also* Psychosis, childhood) 299.1 ☑
H.E.L.L.P 642.5 ☑
hemolytic-uremic (adult) (child) 283.11
hemophagocytic 288.4
  infection-associated 288.4
Hench-Rosenberg (palindromic arthritis) (*see also* Rheumatism, palindromic) 719.3 ☑
Henoch-Schönlein (allergic purpura) 287.0
hepatic flexure 569.89
hepatorenal 572.4
  due to a procedure 997.4
  following delivery 674.8 ☑
hepatourologic 572.4
Herrick's (hemoglobin S disease) 282.61
Herter (-Gee) (nontropical sprue) 579.0
Heubner-Herter (nontropical sprue) 579.0
Heyd's (hepatorenal) 572.4
HHHO 759.81
high grade myelodysplastic 238.73
  with 5q deletion 238.73
Hilger's 337.0
histiocytic 288.4
Hoffa (-Kastert) (liposynovitis prepatellaris) 272.8
Hoffmann's 244.9 [359.5]
Hoffmann-Bouveret (paroxysmal tachycardia) 427.2
Hoffmann-Werdnig 335.0
Holländer-Simons (progressive lipodystrophy) 272.6
Holmes' (visual disorientation) 368.16
Holmes-Adie 379.46
Hoppe-Goldflam 358.00
Horner's (*see also* Neuropathy, peripheral, autonomic) 337.9
  traumatic — *see* Injury, nerve, cervical sympathetic
hospital addiction 301.51
Hunt's (herpetic geniculate ganglionitis) 053.11
  dyssynergia cerebellaris myoclonica 334.2
Hunter (-Hurler) (mucopolysaccharidosis II) 277.5
hunterian glossitis 529.4
Hurler (-Hunter) (mucopolysaccharidosis II) 277.5

**Syndrome** — *see also* Disease — *continued*

Hutchinson-Boeck (sarcoidosis) 135
Hutchinson-Gilford (progeria) 259.8
Hutchinson's incisors or teeth 090.5
hydralazine
  correct substance properly administered 695.4
  overdose or wrong substance given or taken 972.6
hydraulic concussion (abdomen) (*see also* Injury, internal, abdomen) 868.00
hyperabduction 447.8
hyperactive bowel 564.9
hyperaldosteronism with hypokalemic alkalosis (Bartter's) 255.13
hypercalcemic 275.42
hypercoagulation NEC 289.89
hypereosinophilic (idiopathic) 288.3
hyperkalemic 276.7
hyperkinetic (*see also* Hyperkinesia) heart 429.82
hyperlipemia-hemolytic anemia-icterus 571.1
hypermobility 728.5
hypernatremia 276.0
hyperosmolarity 276.0
hyperperfusion 997.01 ●
hypersomnia-bulimia 349.89
hypersplenic 289.4
hypersympathetic (*see also* Neuropathy, peripheral, autonomic) 337.9
hypertransfusion, newborn 776.4
hyperventilation, psychogenic 306.1
hyperviscosity (of serum) NEC 273.3
  polycythemic 289.0
  sclerothymic 282.8
hypoglycemic (familial) (neonatal) 251.2
  functional 251.1
hypokalemic 276.8
hypophyseal 253.8
hypophyseothalamic 253.8
hypopituitarism 253.2
hypoplastic left heart 746.7
hypopotassemia 276.8
hyposmolality 276.1
hypotension, maternal 669.2 ☑
hypothenar hammer 443.89 ●
hypotonia-hypomentia-hypogonadism-obesity 759.81
ICF (intravascular coagulation-fibrinolysis) (*see also* Fibrinolysis) 286.6
idiopathic cardiorespiratory distress, newborn 769
idiopathic nephrotic (infantile) 581.9
iliotibial band 728.89
Imerslund (-Gräsbeck) (anemia due to familial selective vitamin B$_{12}$ malabsorption) 281.1
immobility (paraplegic) 728.3
immunity deficiency, combined 279.2
impending coronary 411.1
impingement
  shoulder 726.2
  vertebral bodies 724.4
inappropriate secretion of antidiuretic hormone (ADH) 253.6
incomplete
  mandibulofacial 756.0
infant
  death, sudden (SIDS) 798.0
  Hercules 255.2
  of diabetic mother 775.0
  shaken 995.55
infantilism 253.3
inferior vena cava 459.2
influenza-like 487.1
inspissated bile, newborn 774.4
insufficient sleep 307.44
intermediate coronary (artery) 411.1
internal carotid artery (*see also* Occlusion, artery, carotid) 433.1 ☑

**Syndrome** — *see also* Disease — *continued*

interspinous ligament 724.8
intestinal
  carcinoid 259.2
  gas 787.3
  knot 560.2
intraoperative floppy iris (IFIS) 364.81 ●
intravascular
  coagulation-fibrinolysis (ICF) (*see also* Fibrinolysis) 286.6
  coagulopathy (*see also* Fibrinolysis) 286.6
inverted Marfan's 759.89
IRDS (idiopathic respiratory distress, newborn) 769
irritable
  bowel 564.1
  heart 306.2
  weakness 300.5
ischemic bowel (transient) 557.9
  chronic 557.1
  due to mesenteric artery insufficiency 557.1
Itsenko-Cushing (pituitary basophilism) 255.0
IVC (intravascular coagulopathy) (*see also* Fibrinolysis) 286.6
Ivemark's (asplenia with congenital heart disease) 759.0
Jaccoud's 714.4
Jackson's 344.89
Jadassohn-Lewandowski (pachyonchia congenita) 757.5
Jaffe-Lichtenstein (-Uehlinger) 252.01
Jahnke's (encephalocutaneous angiomatosis) 759.6
Jakob-Creutzfeldt (new variant) 046.1
  with dementia
    with behavioral disturbance 046.1 [294.11]
    without behavioral disturbance 046.1 [294.10]
Jaksch's (pseudoleukemia infantum) 285.8
Jaksch-Hayem (-Luzet) (pseudoleukemia infantum) 285.8
jaw-winking 742.8
jejunal 564.2
Jervell-Lange-Nielsen 426.82
jet lag 327.35
Jeune's (asphyxiating thoracic dystrophy of newborn) 756.4
Job's (chronic granulomatous disease) 288.1
Jordan's 288.2
Joseph-Diamond-Blackfan (congenital hypoplastic anemia) 284.01
Joubert 759.89
jugular foramen 352.6
Kabuki 759.89
Kahler's (multiple myeloma) (M9730/3) 203.0 ☑
Kalischer's (encephalocutaneous angiomatosis) 759.6
Kallmann's (hypogonadotropic hypogonadism with anosmia) 253.4
Kanner's (autism) (*see also* Psychosis, childhood) 299.0 ☑
Kartagener's (sinusitis, bronchiectasis, situs inversus) 759.3
Kasabach-Merritt (capillary hemangioma associated with thrombocytopenic purpura) 287.39
Kast's (dyschondroplasia with hemangiomas) 756.4
Kaznelson's (congenital hypoplastic anemia) 284.01
Kearns-Sayre 277.87
Kelly's (sideropenic dysphagia) 280.8
Kimmelstiel-Wilson (intercapillary glomerulosclerosis) 250.4 ☑ [581.81]
Klauder's (erythema multiforme exudativum) 695.1

**Syndrome** — *see also* Disease — *continued*

Kleine-Levin 327.13
Klein-Waardenburg (ptosis-epicanthus) 270.2
Klinefelter's 758.7
Klippel-Feil (brevicollis) 756.16
Klippel-Trenaunay 759.89
Klumpke (-Déjerine) (injury to brachial plexus at birth) 767.6
Klüver-Bucy (-Terzian) 310.0
Köhler-Pellegrini-Stieda (calcification, knee joint) 726.62
König's 564.89
Korsakoff's (nonalcoholic) 294.0
Korsakoff (-Wernicke) (nonalcoholic) 294.0
  alcoholic 291.1
  alcoholic 291.1
Kostmann's (infantile genetic agranulocytosis) 288.01
Krabbe's
  congenital muscle hypoplasia 756.89
  cutaneocerebral angioma 759.6
Kunkel (lupoid hepatitis) 571.49
labyrinthine 386.50
laceration, broad ligament 620.6
Langdon Down (mongolism) 758.0
Larsen's (flattened facies and multiple congenital dislocations) 755.8
lateral
  cutaneous nerve of thigh 355.1
  medullary (*see also* Disease, cerebrovascular acute) 436
Launois' (pituitary gigantism) 253.0
Launois-Cléret (adiposogenital dystrophy) 253.8
Laurence-Moon (-Bardet)-Biedl (obesity, polydactyly, and mental retardation) 759.89
Lawford's (encephalocutaneous angiomatosis) 759.6
lazy
  leukocyte 288.09
  posture 728.3
Lederer-Brill (acquired infectious hemolytic anemia) 283.19
Legg-Calvé-Perthes (osteochondrosis capital femoral) 732.1
Lemiere 451.89
Lennox's (*see also* Epilepsy) 345.0 ☑
Lennox-Gastaut syndrome 345.0 ☑
  with tonic seizures 345.1 ☑
lenticular 275.1
Léopold-Lévi's (paroxysmal thyroid instability) 242.9 ☑
Lepore hemoglobin 282.49
Leriche's (aortic bifurcation occlusion) 444.0
Léri-Weill 756.59
Lermoyez's (*see also* Disease, Ménière's) 386.00
Lesch-Nyhan (hypoxanthine-guanine-phosphoribosyltransferase deficiency) 277.2
Lev's (acquired complete heart block) 426.0
Levi's (pituitary dwarfism) 253.3
Lévy-Roussy 334.3
Lichtheim's (subacute combined sclerosis with pernicious anemia) 281.0 [336.2]
Li-Fraumeni V84.01
Lightwood's (renal tubular acidosis) 588.89
Lignac (-de Toni) (-Fanconi) (-Debré) (cystinosis) 270.0
Likoff's (angina in menopausal women) 413.9
liver-kidney 572.4
Lloyd's 258.1
lobotomy 310.0
Löffler's (eosinophilic pneumonitis) 518.3
Löfgren's (sarcoidosis) 135

☑ Additional Digit Required — Refer to the Tabular List for Digit Selection
**2008 ICD-9-CM**
▶◀ Revised Text
● New Line
▲ Revised Code
🦅 Subterms under main terms may continue to next column or page
**October 2007 · Volume 2 — 275**

**Syndrome** — *see also* Disease — *continued*

painful — *continued*
  arc 726.19
  bruising 287.2
  feet 266.2
Pancoast's (carcinoma, pulmonary apex) (M8010/3) 162.3
panhypopituitary (postpartum) 253.2
papillary muscle 429.81
  with myocardial infarction 410.8 ☑
Papillon-Léage and Psaume (orodigito-facial dysostosis) 759.89
parabiotic (transfusion)
  donor (twin) 772.0
  recipient (twin) 776.4
paralysis agitans 332.0
paralytic 344.9
  specified type NEC 344.89
paraneoplastic — *see* condition
Parinaud's (paralysis of conjugate upward gaze) 378.81
  oculoglandular 372.02
Parkes Weber and Dimitri (encephalo-cutaneous angiomatosis) 759.6
Parkinson's (*see also* Parkinsonism) 332.0
parkinsonian (*see also* Parkinsonism) 332.0
Parry's (exophthalmic goiter) 242.0 ☑
Parry-Romberg 349.89
Parsonage-Aldren-Turner 353.5
Parsonage-Turner 353.5
Patau's (trisomy D1) 758.1
patella clunk 719.66 ●
patellofemoral 719.46
Paterson (-Brown) (-Kelly) (sideropenic dysphagia) 280.8
Payr's (splenic flexure syndrome) 569.89
pectoral girdle 447.8
pectoralis minor 447.8
Pelger-Huët (hereditary hyposegmentation) 288.2
pellagra-cerebellar ataxia-renal aminoaciduria 270.0
pellagroid 265.2
Pellegrini-Stieda 726.62
Pellizzi's (pineal) 259.8
pelvic congestion (-fibrosis) 625.5
Pendred's (familial goiter with deaf-mutism) 243
Penfield's (*see also* Epilepsy) 345.5 ☑
Penta X 758.81
peptic ulcer — *see* Ulcer, peptic 533.9 ☑
perabduction 447.8
periodic 277.31
periurethral fibrosis 593.4
persistent fetal circulation 747.83
Petges-Cléjat (poikilodermatomyositis) 710.3
Peutz-Jeghers 759.6
Pfeiffer (acrocephalosyndactyly) 755.55
phantom limb 353.6
pharyngeal pouch 279.11
Pick's (pericardial pseudocirrhosis of liver) 423.2
  heart 423.2
  liver 423.2
Pick-Herxheimer (diffuse idiopathic cutaneous atrophy) 701.8
Pickwickian (cardiopulmonary obesity) 278.8
PIE (pulmonary infiltration with eosinophilia) 518.3
Pierre Marie-Bamberger (hypertrophic pulmonary osteoarthropathy) 731.2
Pierre Mauriac's (diabetes-dwarfism-obesity) 258.1
Pierre Robin 756.0
pigment dispersion, iris 364.53
pineal 259.8
pink puffer 492.8

**Syndrome** — *see also* Disease — *continued*

pituitary 253.0
placental
  dysfunction 762.2
  insufficiency 762.2
  transfusion 762.3
plantar fascia 728.71
plica knee 727.83
Plummer-Vinson (sideropenic dysphagia) 280.8
pluricarential of infancy 260
plurideficiency of infancy 260
pluriglandular (compensatory) 258.8
polycarential of infancy 260
polyglandular 258.8
polysplenia 759.0
pontine 433.8 ☑
popliteal
  artery entrapment 447.8
  web 756.89
postartificial menopause 627.4
postcardiac injury
  postcardiotomy 429.4
  postmyocardial infarction 411.0
postcardiotomy 429.4
postcholecystectomy 576.0
postcommissurotomy 429.4
postconcussional 310.2
postcontusional 310.2
postencephalitic 310.8
posterior
  cervical sympathetic 723.2
  fossa compression 348.4
  inferior cerebellar artery (*see also* Disease, cerebrovascular, acute) 436
  reversible encephalopathy (PRES) 348.39
postgastrectomy (dumping) 564.2
post-gastric surgery 564.2
posthepatitis 780.79
postherpetic (neuralgia) (zoster) 053.19
  geniculate ganglion 053.11
  ophthalmica 053.19
postimmunization — *see* Complications, vaccination
postinfarction 411.0
postinfluenza (asthenia) 780.79
postirradiation 990
postlaminectomy 722.80
  cervical, cervicothoracic 722.81
  lumbar, lumbosacral 722.83
  thoracic, thoracolumbar 722.82
postleukotomy 310.0
postlobotomy 310.0
postmastectomy lymphedema 457.0
postmature (of newborn) 766.22
postmyocardial infarction 411.0
postoperative NEC 998.9
  blind loop 579.2
postpartum panhypopituitary 253.2
postperfusion NEC 999.8
  bone marrow 996.85
postpericardiotomy 429.4
postphlebitic (asymptomatic) 459.10
  with
    complications NEC 459.19
    inflammation 459.12
      and ulcer 459.13
    stasis dermatitis 459.12
      with ulcer 459.13
    ulcer 459.11
      with inflammation 459.13
postpolio (myelitis) 138
postvagotomy 564.2
postvalvulotomy 429.4
postviral (asthenia) NEC 780.79
Potain's (gastrectasis with dyspepsia) 536.1
potassium intoxication 276.7
Potter's 753.0
Prader (-Labhart) -Willi (-Fanconi) 759.81
preinfarction 411.1

**Syndrome** — *see also* Disease — *continued*

preleukemic 238.75
premature senility 259.8
premenstrual 625.4
premenstrual tension 625.4
pre ulcer 536.9
Prinzmetal-Massumi (anterior chest wall syndrome) 786.52
Profichet's 729.9
progeria 259.8
progressive pallidal degeneration 333.0
prolonged gestation 766.22
Proteus (dermal hypoplasia) 757.39
prune belly 756.71
prurigo-asthma 691.8
pseudocarpal tunnel (sublimis) 354.0
pseudohermaphroditism-virilism-hirsutism 255.2
pseudoparalytica 358.00
pseudo-Turner's 759.89
psycho-organic 293.9
  acute 293.0
  anxiety type 293.84
  depressive type 293.83
  hallucinatory type 293.82
  nonpsychotic severity 310.1
    specified focal (partial) NEC 310.8
  paranoid type 293.81
  specified type NEC 293.89
  subacute 293.1
pterygolymphangiectasia 758.6
ptosis-epicanthus 270.2
pulmonary
  arteriosclerosis 416.0
  hypoperfusion (idiopathic) 769
  renal (hemorrhagic) 446.21
pulseless 446.7
Putnam-Dana (subacute combined sclerosis with pernicious anemia) 281.0 *[336.2]*
pyloroduodenal 537.89
pyramidopallidonigral 332.0
pyriformis 355.0
QT interval prolongation 426.82
radicular NEC 729.2
  lower limbs 724.4
  upper limbs 723.4
    newborn 767.4
Raeder-Harbitz (pulseless disease) 446.7
Ramsay Hunt's
  dyssynergia cerebellaris myoclonica 334.2
  herpetic geniculate ganglionitis 053.11
rapid time-zone change 327.35
Raymond (-Céstan) 433.8 ☑
Raynaud's (paroxysmal digital cyanosis) 443.0
RDS (respiratory distress syndrome, newborn) 769
Refsum's (heredopathia atactica polyneuritiformis) 356.3
Reichmann's (gastrosuccorrhea) 536.8
Reifenstein's (hereditary familial hypogonadism, male) 259.5
Reilly's (*see also* Neuropathy, peripheral, autonomic) 337.9
Reiter's 099.3
renal glomerulohyalinosis-diabetic 250.4 ☑ *[581.81]*
Rendu-Osler-Weber (familial hemorrhagic telangiectasia) 448.0
renofacial (congenital biliary fibroangiomatosis) 753.0
Rénon-Delille 253.8
respiratory distress (idiopathic) (newborn) 769
  adult (following shock, surgery, or trauma) 518.5
  specified NEC 518.82
  type II 770.6
restless legs (RLS) 333.94

**Syndrome** — *see also* Disease — *continued*

retinoblastoma (familial) 190.5
retraction (Duane's) 378.71
retroperitoneal fibrosis 593.4
retroviral seroconversion (acute) V08
Rett's 330.8
Reye's 331.81
Reye-Sheehan (postpartum pituitary necrosis) 253.2
Riddoch's (visual disorientation) 368.16
Ridley's (*see also* Failure, ventricular, left) 428.1
Rieger's (mesodermal dysgenesis, anterior ocular segment) 743.44
Rietti-Greppi-Micheli (thalassemia minor) 282.49
right ventricular obstruction — *see* Failure, heart
Riley-Day (familial dysautonomia) 742.8
Robin's 756.0
Rokitansky-Kuster-Hauser (congenital absence, vagina) 752.49
Romano-Ward (prolonged QT interval syndrome) 426.82
Romberg's 349.89
Rosen-Castleman-Liebow (pulmonary proteinosis) 516.0
rotator cuff, shoulder 726.10
Roth's 355.1
Rothmund's (congenital poikiloderma) 757.33
Rotor's (idiopathic hyperbilirubinemia) 277.4
Roussy-Lévy 334.3
Roy (-Jutras) (acropachyderma) 757.39
rubella (congenital) 771.0
Rubinstein-Taybi's (brachydactylia, short stature, and mental retardation) 759.89
Rud's (mental deficiency, epilepsy, and infantilism) 759.89
Ruiter-Pompen (-Wyers) (angiokeratoma corporis diffusum) 272.7
Runge's (postmaturity) 766.22
Russell (-Silver) (congenital hemihypertrophy and short stature) 759.89
Rytand-Lipsitch (complete atrioventricular block) 426.0
sacralization-scoliosis-sciatica 756.15
sacroiliac 724.6
Saenger's 379.46
salt
  depletion (*see also* Disease, renal) 593.9
    due to heat NEC 992.8
      causing heat exhaustion or prostration 992.4
  low (*see also* Disease, renal) 593.9
salt-losing (*see also* Disease, renal) 593.9
Sanfilippo's (mucopolysaccharidosis III) 277.5
Scaglietti-Dagnini (acromegalic macrospondylitis) 253.0
scalded skin 695.1
scalenus anticus (anterior) 353.0
scapulocostal 354.8
scapuloperoneal 359.1
scapulovertebral 723.4
Schaumann's (sarcoidosis) 135
Scheie's (mucopolysaccharidosis IS) 277.5
Scheuthauer-Marie-Sainton (cleidocranialis dysostosis) 755.59
Schirmer's (encephalocutaneous angiomatosis) 759.6
schizophrenic, of childhood NEC (*see also* Psychosis, childhood) 299.9 ☑

---

☑ Additional Digit Required — Refer to the Tabular List for Digit Selection

Subterms under main terms may continue to next column or page

**Syndrome** — *see also* Disease — *continued*

Schmidt's
  sphallo-pharyngo-laryngeal hemiplegia 352.6
  thyroid-adrenocortical insufficiency 258.1
  vagoaccessory 352.6
Schneider's 047.9
Schnitzler 273.1
Scholte's (malignant carcinoid) 259.2
Scholz (-Bielschowsky-Henneberg) 330.0
Schroeder's (endocrine-hypertensive) 255.3
Schüller-Christian (chronic histiocytosis X) 277.89
Schultz's (agranulocytosis) 288.09
Schwartz (-Jampel) 359.23 ▲
Schwartz-Bartter (inappropriate secretion of antidiuretic hormone) 253.6
Scimitar (anomalous venous drainage, right lung to inferior vena cava) 747.49
sclerocystic ovary 256.4
sea-blue histiocyte 272.7
Seabright-Bantam (pseudohypoparathyroidism) 275.49
Seckel's 759.89
Secretan's (posttraumatic edema) 782.3
secretoinhibitor (keratoconjunctivitis sicca) 710.2
Seeligmann's (ichthyosis congenita) 757.1
Senear-Usher (pemphigus erythematosus) 694.4
senilism 259.8
seroconversion, retroviral (acute) V08
serotonin 333.99
serous meningitis 348.2
Sertoli cell (germinal aplasia) 606.0
sex chromosome mosaic 758.81
Sézary's (reticulosis) (M9701/3) 202.2 ☑
shaken infant 995.55
Shaver's (bauxite pneumoconiosis) 503
Sheehan's (postpartum pituitary necrosis) 253.2
shock (traumatic) 958.4
  kidney 584.5
    following crush injury 958.5
  lung 518.5
  neurogenic 308.9
  psychic 308.9
short
  bowel 579.3
  P-R interval 426.81
shoulder-arm (*see also* Neuropathy, peripheral, autonomic) 337.9
shoulder-girdle 723.4
shoulder-hand (*see also* Neuropathy, peripheral, autonomic) 337.9
Shwachman's 288.02
Shy-Drager (orthostatic hypotension with multisystem degeneration) 333.0
Sicard's 352.6
sicca (keratoconjunctivitis) 710.2
sick
  cell 276.1
  cilia 759.89
  sinus 427.81
sideropenic 280.8
Siemens'
  ectodermal dysplasia 757.31
  keratosis follicularis spinulosa (decalvans) 757.39
Silfverskiöld's (osteochondrodystrophy, extremities) 756.50
Silver's (congenital hemihypertrophy and short stature) 759.89
Silvestroni-Bianco (thalassemia minima) 282.49

**Syndrome** — *see also* Disease — *continued*

Simons' (progressive lipodystrophy) 272.6
sinusitis-bronchiectasis-situs inversus 759.3
sinus tarsi 726.79
Sipple's (medullary thyroid carcinoma-pheochromocytoma) 258.02 ▲
Sjögren (-Gougerot) (keratoconjunctivitis sicca) 710.2
  with lung involvement 710.2 [517.8]
Sjögren-Larsson (ichthyosis congenita) 757.1
Slocumb's 255.3
Sluder's 337.0
Smith-Lemli-Opitz (cerebrohepatorenal syndrome) 759.89
Smith-Magenis 758.33
smokers' 305.1
Sneddon-Wilkinson (subcorneal pustular dermatosis) 694.1
Sotos' (cerebral gigantism) 253.0
South African cardiomyopathy 425.2
spasmodic
  upward movement, eye(s) 378.82
  winking 307.20
Spens' (syncope with heart block) 426.9
spherophakia-brachymorphia 759.89
spinal cord injury (*see also* Injury, spinal, by site)
  with fracture, vertebra — *see* Fracture, vertebra, by site, with spinal cord injury
  cervical — *see* Injury, spinal, cervical
  fluid malabsorption (acquired) 331.3
splenic
  agenesis 759.0
  flexure 569.89
  neutropenia 289.53
  sequestration 289.52
Spurway's (brittle bones and blue sclera) 756.51
staphylococcal scalded skin 695.1
Stein's (polycystic ovary) 256.4
Steinbrocker's (*see also* Neuropathy, peripheral, autonomic) 337.9
Stein-Leventhal (polycystic ovary) 256.4
Stevens-Johnson (erythema multiforme exudativum) 695.1
Stewart-Morel (hyperostosis frontalis interna) 733.3
Stickler 759.89
stiff-baby 759.89
stiff-man 333.91
Still's (juvenile rheumatoid arthritis) 714.30
Still-Felty (rheumatoid arthritis with splenomegaly and leukopenia) 714.1
Stilling-Türk-Duane (ocular retraction syndrome) 378.71
Stojano's (subcostal) 098.86
Stokes (-Adams) (syncope with heart block) 426.9
Stokvis-Talma (enterogenous cyanosis) 289.7
stone heart (*see also* Failure, ventricular, left) 428.1
straight-back 756.19
stroke (*see also* Disease, cerebrovascular, acute) 436
  little 435.9
Sturge-Kalischer-Weber (encephalotrigeminal angiomatosis) 759.6
Sturge-Weber (-Dimitri) (encephalocutaneous angiomatosis) 759.6
subclavian-carotid obstruction (chronic) 446.7

**Syndrome** — *see also* Disease — *continued*

subclavian steal 435.2
subcoracoid-pectoralis minor 447.8
subcostal 098.86
  nerve compression 354.8
subperiosteal hematoma 267
subphrenic interposition 751.4
sudden infant death (SIDS) 798.0
Sudeck's 733.7
Sudeck-Leriche 733.7
superior
  cerebellar artery (*see also* Disease, cerebrovascular, acute) 436
  mesenteric artery 557.1
  pulmonary sulcus (tumor) (M8010/3) 162.3
  vena cava 459.2
suprarenal cortical 255.3
supraspinatus 726.10
swallowed blood 777.3
sweat retention 705.1
Sweet's (acute febrile neutrophilic dermatosis) 695.89
Swyer's (XY pure gonadal dysgenesis) 752.7
Swyer-James (unilateral hyperlucent lung) 492.8
Symonds' 348.2
sympathetic
  cervical paralysis 337.0
  pelvic 625.5
syndactylic oxycephaly 755.55
syphilitic-cardiovascular 093.89
systemic
  fibrosclerosing 710.8
  inflammatory response (SIRS) 995.90
  due to
    infectious process 995.91
      with acute organ dysfunction 995.92
    non-infectious process 995.93
      with acute organ dysfunction 995.94
systolic click (-murmur) 785.2
Tabagism 305.1
tachycardia-bradycardia 427.81
Takayasu (-Onishi) (pulseless disease) 446.7
Takotsubo 429.83
Tapia's 352.6
tarsal tunnel 355.5
Taussig-Bing (transposition, aorta and overriding pulmonary artery) 745.11
Taybi's (otopalatodigital) 759.89
Taylor's 625.5
teething 520.7
tegmental 344.89
telangiectasis-pigmentation-cataract 757.33
temporal 383.02
  lobectomy behavior 310.0
temporomandibular joint-pain-dysfunction [TMJ] NEC 524.60
  specified NEC 524.69
Terry's 362.21
testicular feminization 259.5
testis, nonvirilizing 257.8
tethered (spinal) cord 742.59
thalamic 338.0
Thibierge-Weissenbach (cutaneous systemic sclerosis) 710.1
Thiele 724.6
thoracic outlet (compression) 353.0
thoracogenous rheumatic (hypertrophic pulmonary osteoarthropathy) 731.2
Thorn's (*see also* Disease, renal) 593.9
Thorson-Biörck (malignant carcinoid) 259.2
thrombopenia-hemangioma 287.39
thyroid-adrenocortical insufficiency 258.1

**Syndrome** — *see also* Disease — *continued*

Tietze's 733.6
time-zone (rapid) 327.35
Tobias' (carcinoma, pulmonary apex) (M8010/3) 162.3
toilet seat 926.0
Tolosa-Hunt 378.55
Toni-Fanconi (cystinosis) 270.0
Touraine's (hereditary osteo-onychodysplasia) 756.89
Touraine-Solente-Golé (acropachyderma) 757.39
toxic
  oil 710.5
  shock 040.82
transfusion
  fetal-maternal 772.0
  twin
    donor (infant) 772.0
    recipient (infant) 776.4
transient left ventricular apical ballooning 429.83
Treacher Collins' (incomplete mandibulofacial dysostosis) 756.0
trigeminal plate 259.8
triple X female 758.81
trisomy NEC 758.5
  13 or $D_1$ 758.1
  16-18 or E 758.2
  18 or $E_3$ 758.2
  20 758.5
  21 or G (mongolism) 758.0
  22 or G (mongolism) 758.0
  G 758.0
Troisier-Hanot-Chauffard (bronze diabetes) 275.0
tropical wet feet 991.4
Trousseau's (thrombophlebitis migrans visceral cancer) 453.1
Türk's (ocular retraction syndrome) 378.71
Turner's 758.6
Turner-Varny 758.6
twin-to-twin transfusion 762.3
  recipient twin 776.4
Uehlinger's (acropachyderma) 757.39
Ullrich (-Bonnevie) (-Turner) 758.6
Ullrich-Feichtiger 759.89
underwater blast injury (abdominal) (*see also* Injury, internal, abdomen) 868.00
universal joint, cervix 620.6
Unverricht (-Lundborg) 333.2
Unverricht-Wagner (dermatomyositis) 710.3
upward gaze 378.81
Urbach-Oppenheim (necrobiosis lipoidica diabeticorum) 250.8 ☑ [709.3]
Urbach-Wiethe (lipoid proteinosis) 272.8
uremia, chronic 585.9
urethral 597.81
urethro-oculoarticular 099.3
urethro-oculosynovial 099.3
urohepatic 572.4
uveocutaneous 364.24
uveomeningeal, uveomeningitis 363.22
vagohypoglossal 352.6
vagovagal 780.2
van Buchem's (hyperostosis corticalis) 733.3
van der Hoeve's (brittle bones and blue sclera, deafness) 756.51
van der Hoeve-Halbertsma-Waardenburg (ptosis-epicanthus) 270.2
van der Hoeve-Waardenburg-Gualdi (ptosis-epicanthus) 270.2
vanishing twin 651.33
van Neck-Odelberg (juvenile osteochondrosis) 732.1
vascular splanchnic 557.0
vasomotor 443.9

☑ Additional Digit Required — Refer to the Tabular List for Digit Selection      ▽ Subterms under main terms may continue to next column or page

**2008 ICD-9-CM**      ▶◀ Revised Text      ● New Line      ▲ Revised Code      **October 2007 · Volume 2 — 277**

**Syndrome** — *see also* Disease — *continued*
vasovagal 780.2
VATER 759.89
Velo-cardio-facial 758.32
vena cava (inferior) (superior) (obstruction) 459.2
Verbiest's (claudicatio intermittens spinalis) 435.1
Vernet's 352.6
vertebral
artery 435.1
compression 721.1
lumbar 724.4
steal 435.1
vertebrogenic (pain) 724.5
vertiginous NEC 386.9
video display tube 723.8
Villaret's 352.6
Vinson-Plummer (sideropenic dysphagia) 280.8
virilizing adrenocortical hyperplasia, congenital 255.2
virus, viral 079.99
visceral larval migrans 128.0
visual disorientation 368.16
vitamin B₆ deficiency 266.1
vitreous touch 997.99
Vogt's (corpus striatum) 333.71
Vogt-Koyanagi 364.24
Volkmann's 958.6
von Bechterew-Strümpell (ankylosing spondylitis) 720.0
von Graefe's 378.72
von Hippel-Lindau (angiomatosis retinocerebellosa) 759.6
von Schroetter's (intermittent venous claudication) 453.8
von Willebrand (-Jürgens) (angiohemophilia) 286.4
Waardenburg-Klein (ptosis epicanthus) 270.2
Wagner (-Unverricht) (dermatomyositis) 710.3
Waldenström's (macroglobulinemia) 273.3
Waldenström-Kjellberg (sideropenic dysphagia) 280.8
Wallenberg's (posterior inferior cerebellar artery) (*see also* Disease, cerebrovascular, acute) 436
Waterhouse (-Friderichsen) 036.3
water retention 276.6
Weber's 344.89
Weber-Christian (nodular nonsuppurative panniculitis) 729.30
Weber-Cockayne (epidermolysis bullosa) 757.39
Weber-Dimitri (encephalocutaneous angiomatosis) 759.6
Weber-Gubler 344.89
Weber-Leyden 344.89
Weber-Osler (familial hemorrhagic telangiectasia) 448.0
Wegener's (necrotizing respiratory granulomatosis) 446.4
Weill-Marchesani (brachymorphism and ectopia lentis) 759.89
Weingarten's (tropical eosinophilia) 518.3
Weiss-Baker (carotid sinus syncope) 337.0
Weissenbach-Thibierge (cutaneous systemic sclerosis) 710.1
Werdnig-Hoffmann 335.0
Werlhof-Wichmann (*see also* Purpura, thrombocytopenic) 287.39
Wermer's (polyendocrine adenomatosis) 258.01 ▲
Werner's (progeria adultorum) 259.8
Wernicke's (nonalcoholic) (superior hemorrhagic polioencephalitis) 265.1
Wernicke-Korsakoff (nonalcoholic) 294.0
alcoholic 291.1

**Syndrome** — *see also* Disease — *continued*
Westphal-Strümpell (hepatolenticular degeneration) 275.1
wet
brain (alcoholic) 303.9 ☑
feet (maceration) (tropical) 991.4
lung
adult 518.5
newborn 770.6
whiplash 847.0
Whipple's (intestinal lipodystrophy) 040.2
"whistling face" (craniocarpotarsal dystrophy) 759.89
Widal (-Abrami) (acquired hemolytic jaundice) 283.9
Wilkie's 557.1
Wilkinson-Sneddon (subcorneal pustular dermatosis) 694.1
Willan-Plumbe (psoriasis) 696.1
Willebrand (-Jürgens) (angiohemophilia) 286.4
Willi-Prader (hypogenital dystrophy with diabetic tendency) 759.81
Wilson's (hepatolenticular degeneration) 275.1
Wilson-Mikity 770.7
Wiskott-Aldrich (eczema-thrombocytopenia) 279.12
withdrawal
alcohol 291.81
drug 292.0
infant of dependent mother 779.5
Woakes' (ethmoiditis) 471.1
Wolff-Parkinson-White (anomalous atrioventricular excitation) 426.7
Wright's (hyperabduction) 447.8
X
cardiac 413.9
dysmetabolic 277.7
xiphoidalgia 733.99
XO 758.6
XXX 758.81
XXXXY 758.81
XXY 758.7
yellow vernix (placental dysfunction) 762.2
Zahorsky's 074.0
Zellweger 277.86
Zieve's (jaundice, hyperlipemia and hemolytic anemia) 571.1
Zollinger-Ellison (gastric hypersecretion with pancreatic islet cell tumor) 251.5
Zuelzer-Ogden (nutritional megaloblastic anemia) 281.2
**Synechia** (iris) (pupil) 364.70
anterior 364.72
peripheral 364.73
intrauterine (traumatic) 621.5
posterior 364.71
vulvae, congenital 752.49
**Synesthesia** — *see also* Disturbance, sensation 782.0
**Synodontia** 520.2
**Synophthalmus** 759.89
**Synorchidism** 752.89
**Synorchism** 752.89
**Synostosis** (congenital) 756.59
astragaloscaphoid 755.67
radioulnar 755.53
talonavicular (bar) 755.67
tarsal 755.67
**Synovial** — *see* condition
**Synovioma** (M9040/3) — *see also* Neoplasm, connective tissue, malignant
benign (M9040/0) — *see* Neoplasm, connective tissue, benign
**Synoviosarcoma** (M9040/3) — *see* Neoplasm, connective tissue, malignant
**Synovitis** 727.00

**Synovitis** — *continued*
chronic crepitant, wrist 727.2
due to crystals — *see* Arthritis, due to crystals
gonococcal 098.51
gouty 274.0
syphilitic 095.7
congenital 090.0
traumatic, current — *see* Sprain, by site
tuberculous — *see* Tuberculosis, synovitis
villonodular 719.20
ankle 719.27
elbow 719.22
foot 719.27
hand 719.24
hip 719.25
knee 719.26
multiple sites 719.29
pelvic region 719.25
shoulder (region) 719.21
specified site NEC 719.28
wrist 719.23
**Syphilide** 091.3
congenital 090.0
newborn 090.0
tubercular 095.8
congenital 090.0
**Syphilis, syphilitic** (acquired) 097.9
with lung involvement 095.1
abdomen (late) 095.2
acoustic nerve 094.86
adenopathy (secondary) 091.4
adrenal (gland) 095.8
with cortical hypofunction 095.8
age under 2 years NEC (*see also* Syphilis, congenital) 090.9
acquired 097.9
alopecia (secondary) 091.82
anemia 095.8
aneurysm (artery) (ruptured) 093.89
aorta 093.0
central nervous system 094.89
congenital 090.5
anus 095.8
primary 091.1
secondary 091.3
aorta, aortic (arch) (abdominal) (insufficiency) (pulmonary) (regurgitation) (stenosis) (thoracic) 093.89
aneurysm 093.0
arachnoid (adhesive) 094.2
artery 093.89
cerebral 094.89
spinal 094.89
arthropathy (neurogenic) (tabetic) 094.0 [713.5]
asymptomatic — *see* Syphilis, latent
ataxia, locomotor (progressive) 094.0
atrophoderma maculatum 091.3
auricular fibrillation 093.89
Bell's palsy 094.89
bladder 095.8
bone 095.5
secondary 091.61
brain 094.89
breast 095.8
bronchus 095.8
bubo 091.0
bulbar palsy 094.89
bursa (late) 095.7
cardiac decompensation 093.89
cardiovascular (early) (late) (primary) (secondary) (tertiary) 093.9
specified type and site NEC 093.89
causing death under 2 years of age (*see also* Syphilis, congenital) 090.9
stated to be acquired NEC 097.9
central nervous system (any site) (early) (late) (latent) (primary) (recurrent) (relapse) (secondary) (tertiary) 094.9
with
ataxia 094.0

**Syphilis, syphilitic** — *continued*
central nervous system — *continued*
with — *continued*
paralysis, general 094.1
juvenile 090.40
paresis (general) 094.1
juvenile 090.40
tabes (dorsalis) 094.0
juvenile 090.40
taboparesis 094.1
juvenile 090.40
aneurysm (ruptured) 094.87
congenital 090.40
juvenile 090.40
remission in (sustained) 094.9
serology doubtful, negative, or positive 094.9
specified nature or site NEC 094.89
vascular 094.89
cerebral 094.89
meningovascular 094.2
nerves 094.89
sclerosis 094.89
thrombosis 094.89
cerebrospinal 094.89
tabetic 094.0
cerebrovascular 094.89
cervix 095.8
chancre (multiple) 091.0
extragenital 091.2
Rollet's 091.2
Charcôt's joint 094.0 [713.5]
choked disc 094.89 [377.00]
chorioretinitis 091.51
congenital 090.0 [363.13]
late 094.83
choroiditis 091.51
congenital 090.0 [363.13]
late 094.83
prenatal 090.0 [363.13]
choroidoretinitis (secondary) 091.51
congenital 090.0 [363.13]
late 094.83
ciliary body (secondary) 091.52
late 095.8 [364.11]
colon (late) 095.8
combined sclerosis 094.89
complicating pregnancy, childbirth or puerperium 647.0 ☑
affecting fetus or newborn 760.2
condyloma (latum) 091.3
congenital 090.9
with
encephalitis 090.41
paresis (general) 090.40
tabes (dorsalis) 090.40
taboparesis 090.40
chorioretinitis, choroiditis 090.0 [363.13]
early or less than 2 years after birth NEC 090.2
with manifestations 090.0
latent (without manifestations) 090.1
negative spinal fluid test 090.1
serology, positive 090.1
symptomatic 090.0
interstitial keratitis 090.3
juvenile neurosyphilis 090.40
late or 2 years or more after birth NEC 090.7
chorioretinitis, choroiditis 090.5 [363.13]
interstitial keratitis 090.3
juvenile neurosyphilis NEC 090.40
latent (without manifestations) 090.6
negative spinal fluid test 090.6
serology, positive 090.6
symptomatic or with manifestations NEC 090.5
interstitial keratitis 090.3

**Syphilis, syphilitic** — continued
  conjugal 097.9
    tabes 094.0
  conjunctiva 095.8 [372.10]
  contact V01.6
  cord, bladder 094.0
  cornea, late 095.8 [370.59]
  coronary (artery) 093.89
    sclerosis 093.89
  coryza 095.8
    congenital 090.0
  cranial nerve 094.89
  cutaneous — see Syphilis, skin
  dacryocystitis 095.8
  degeneration, spinal cord 094.89
  d'emblée 095.8
  dementia 094.1
    paralytica 094.1
      juvenilis 090.40
  destruction of bone 095.5
  dilatation, aorta 093.0
  due to blood transfusion 097.9
  dura mater 094.89
  ear 095.8
    inner 095.8
      nerve (eighth) 094.86
      neurorecurrence 094.86
  early NEC 091.0
    cardiovascular 093.9
    central nervous system 094.9
      paresis 094.1
      tabes 094.0
    latent (without manifestations) (less
      than 2 years after infection)
      092.9
      negative spinal fluid test 092.9
      serological relapse following
        treatment 092.0
      serology positive 092.9
    paresis 094.1
    relapse (treated, untreated) 091.7
    skin 091.3
    symptomatic NEC 091.89
      extragenital chancre 091.2
      primary, except extragenital
        chancre 091.0
      secondary (see also Syphilis,
        secondary) 091.3
        relapse (treated, untreated)
          091.7
    tabes 094.0
    ulcer 091.3
  eighth nerve 094.86
  endemic, nonvenereal 104.0
  endocarditis 093.20
    aortic 093.22
    mitral 093.21
    pulmonary 093.24
    tricuspid 093.23
  epididymis (late) 095.8
  epiglottis 095.8
  epiphysitis (congenital) 090.0
  esophagus 095.8
  Eustachian tube 095.8
  exposure to V01.6
  eye 095.8 [363.13]
    neuromuscular mechanism 094.85
  eyelid 095.8 [373.5]
    with gumma 095.8 [373.5]
    ptosis 094.89
  fallopian tube 095.8
  fracture 095.5
  gallbladder (late) 095.8
  gastric 095.8
    crisis 094.0
    polyposis 095.8
  general 097.9
    paralysis 094.1
      juvenile 090.40
  genital (primary) 091.0
  glaucoma 095.8
  gumma (late) NEC 095.9
    cardiovascular system 093.9
    central nervous system 094.9
    congenital 090.5
    heart or artery 093.89

**Syphilis, syphilitic** — continued
  heart 093.89
    block 093.89
    decompensation 093.89
    disease 093.89
    failure 093.89
    valve (see also Syphilis, endocardi-
      tis) 093.20
  hemianesthesia 094.89
  hemianopsia 095.8
  hemiparesis 094.89
  hemiplegia 094.89
  hepatic artery 093.89
  hepatitis 095.3
  hepatomegaly 095.3
    congenital 090.0
  hereditaria tarda (see also Syphilis,
    congenital, late) 090.7
  hereditary (see also Syphilis, congeni-
    tal) 090.9
    interstitial keratitis 090.3
  Hutchinson's teeth 090.5
  hyalitis 095.8
  inactive — see Syphilis, latent
  infantum NEC (see also Syphilis,
    congenital) 090.9
  inherited — see Syphilis, congenital
  internal ear 095.8
  intestine (late) 095.8
  iris, iritis (secondary) 091.52
    late 095.8 [364.11]
  joint (late) 095.8
  keratitis (congenital) (early) (intersti-
    tial) (late) (parenchymatous)
    (punctata profunda) 090.3
  kidney 095.4
  lacrimal apparatus 095.8
  laryngeal paralysis 095.8
  larynx 095.8
  late 097.0
    cardiovascular 093.9
    central nervous system 094.9
    latent or 2 years or more after infec-
      tion (without manifestations)
      096
      negative spinal fluid test 096
      serology positive 096
    paresis 094.1
    specified site NEC 095.8
    symptomatic or with symptoms
      095.9
    tabes 094.0
  latent 097.1
    central nervous system 094.9
    date of infection unspecified 097.1
    early or less than 2 years after in-
      fection 092.9
    late or 2 years or more after infec-
      tion 096
    serology
      doubtful
        follow-up of latent syphilis
          097.1
          central nervous system
            094.9
          date of infection unspeci-
            fied 097.1
          early or less than 2 years
            after infection 092.9
          late or 2 years or more af-
            ter infection 096
      positive, only finding 097.1
        date of infection unspecified
          097.1
        early or less than 2 years af-
          ter infection 097.1
        late or 2 years or more after
          infection 097.1
  lens 095.8
  leukoderma 091.3
    late 095.8
  lienis 095.8
  lip 091.3
    chancre 091.2
    late 095.8
    primary 091.2

**Syphilis, syphilitic** — continued
  Lissauer's paralysis 094.1
  liver 095.3
    secondary 091.62
  locomotor ataxia 094.0
  lung 095.1
  lymphadenitis (secondary) 091.4
  lymph gland (early) (secondary) 091.4
    late 095.8
  macular atrophy of skin 091.3
    striated 095.8
  maternal, affecting fetus or newborn
    760.2
    manifest syphilis in newborn — see
      Syphilis, congenital
  mediastinum (late) 095.8
  meninges (adhesive) (basilar) (brain)
    (spinal cord) 094.2
  meningitis 094.2
    acute 091.81
    congenital 090.42
  meningoencephalitis 094.2
  meningovascular 094.2
    congenital 090.49
  mesarteritis 093.89
    brain 094.89
    spine 094.89
  middle ear 095.8
  mitral stenosis 093.21
  monoplegia 094.89
  mouth (secondary) 091.3
    late 095.8
  mucocutaneous 091.3
    late 095.8
  mucous
    membrane 091.3
      late 095.8
    patches 091.3
      congenital 090.0
  mulberry molars 090.5
  muscle 095.6
  myocardium 093.82
  myositis 095.6
  nasal sinus 095.8
  neonatorum NEC (see also Syphilis,
    congenital) 090.9
  nerve palsy (any cranial nerve) 094.89
  nervous system, central 094.9
  neuritis 095.8
    acoustic nerve 094.86
  neurorecidive of retina 094.83
  neuroretinitis 094.85
  newborn (see also Syphilis, congenital)
    090.9
  nodular superficial 095.8
  nonvenereal, endemic 104.0
  nose 095.8
    saddle back deformity 090.5
    septum 095.8
      perforated 095.8
  occlusive arterial disease 093.89
  ophthalmic 095.8 [363.13]
  ophthalmoplegia 094.89
  optic nerve (atrophy) (neuritis) (papilla)
    094.84
  orbit (late) 095.8
  orchitis 095.8
  organic 097.9
  osseous (late) 095.5
  osteochondritis (congenital) 090.0
  osteoporosis 095.5
  ovary 095.8
  oviduct 095.8
  palate 095.8
    gumma 095.8
    perforated 090.5
  pancreas (late) 095.8
  pancreatitis 095.8
  paralysis 094.89
    general 094.1
    juvenile 090.40
  paraplegia 094.89
  paresis (general) 094.1
    juvenile 090.40
  paresthesia 094.89

**Syphilis, syphilitic** — continued
  Parkinson's disease or syndrome
    094.82
  paroxysmal tachycardia 093.89
  pemphigus (congenital) 090.0
  penis 091.0
    chancre 091.0
    late 095.8
  pericardium 093.81
  perichondritis, larynx 095.8
  periosteum 095.5
    congenital 090.0
    early 091.61
    secondary 091.61
  peripheral nerve 095.8
  petrous bone (late) 095.5
  pharynx 095.8
    secondary 091.3
  pituitary (gland) 095.8
  placenta 095.8
  pleura (late) 095.8
  pneumonia, white 090.0
  pontine (lesion) 094.89
  portal vein 093.89
  primary NEC 091.2
    anal 091.1
    and secondary (see also Syphilis,
      secondary) 091.9
    cardiovascular 093.9
    central nervous system 094.9
    extragenital chancre NEC 091.2
    fingers 091.2
    genital 091.0
    lip 091.2
    specified site NEC 091.2
    tonsils 091.2
  prostate 095.8
  psychosis (intracranial gumma)
    094.89
  ptosis (eyelid) 094.89
  pulmonary (late) 095.1
    artery 093.89
  pulmonum 095.1
  pyelonephritis 095.4
  recently acquired, symptomatic NEC
    091.89
  rectum 095.8
  respiratory tract 095.8
  retina
    late 094.83
    neurorecidive 094.83
  retrobulbar neuritis 094.85
  salpingitis 095.8
  sclera (late) 095.0
  sclerosis
    cerebral 094.89
    coronary 093.89
    multiple 094.89
    subacute 094.89
  scotoma (central) 095.8
  scrotum 095.8
  secondary (and primary) 091.9
    adenopathy 091.4
    anus 091.3
    bone 091.61
    cardiovascular 093.9
    central nervous system 094.9
    chorioretinitis, choroiditis 091.51
    hepatitis 091.62
    liver 091.62
    lymphadenitis 091.4
    meningitis, acute 091.81
    mouth 091.3
    mucous membranes 091.3
    periosteum 091.61
    periostitis 091.61
    pharynx 091.3
    relapse (treated) (untreated) 091.7
    skin 091.3
    specified form NEC 091.89
    tonsil 091.3
    ulcer 091.3
    viscera 091.69
    vulva 091.3
  seminal vesicle (late) 095.8

☑ Additional Digit Required — Refer to the Tabular List for Digit Selection                    ▽ Subterms under main terms may continue to next column or page

**Syphilis, syphilitic** — *continued*
  seronegative
    with signs or symptoms — *see* Syphilis, by site or stage
  seropositive
    with signs or symptoms — *see* Syphilis, by site and stage
    follow-up of latent syphilis — *see* Syphilis, latent
    only finding — *see* Syphilis, latent
  seventh nerve (paralysis) 094.89
  sinus 095.8
  sinusitis 095.8
  skeletal system 095.5
  skin (early) (secondary) (with ulceration) 091.3
    late or tertiary 095.8
  small intestine 095.8
  spastic spinal paralysis 094.0
  spermatic cord (late) 095.8
  spinal (cord) 094.89
    with
      paresis 094.1
      tabes 094.0
  spleen 095.8
  splenomegaly 095.8
  spondylitis 095.5
  staphyloma 095.8
  stigmata (congenital) 090.5
  stomach 095.8
  synovium (late) 095.7
  tabes dorsalis (early) (late) 094.0
    juvenile 090.40
  tabetic type 094.0
    juvenile 090.40
  taboparesis 094.1
    juvenile 090.40
  tachycardia 093.89
  tendon (late) 095.7
  tertiary 097.0
    with symptoms 095.8
    cardiovascular 093.9
    central nervous system 094.9
    multiple NEC 095.8
    specified site NEC 095.8
  testis 095.8
  thorax 095.8
  throat 095.8
  thymus (gland) 095.8
  thyroid (late) 095.8
  tongue 095.8
  tonsil (lingual) 095.8
    primary 091.2
    secondary 091.3
  trachea 095.8
  tricuspid valve 093.23
  tumor, brain 094.89
  tunica vaginalis (late) 095.8
  ulcer (any site) (early) (secondary) 091.3
    late 095.9
    perforating 095.9
      foot 094.0
  urethra (stricture) 095.8
  urogenital 095.8
  uterus 095.8
  uveal tract (secondary) 091.50
    late 095.8 *[363.13]*
  uveitis (secondary) 091.50
    late 095.8 *[363.13]*
  uvula (late) 095.8
    perforated 095.8
  vagina 091.0
    late 095.8
  valvulitis NEC 093.20
  vascular 093.89
    brain or cerebral 094.89
  vein 093.89
    cerebral 094.89
  ventriculi 095.8
  vesicae urinariae 095.8
  viscera (abdominal) 095.2
    secondary 091.69
  vitreous (hemorrhage) (opacities) 095.8
  vulva 091.0

**Syphilis, syphilitic** — *continued*
  vulva — *continued*
    late 095.8
    secondary 091.3
**Syphiloma** 095.9
  cardiovascular system 093.9
  central nervous system 094.9
  circulatory system 093.9
  congenital 090.5
**Syphilophobia** 300.29
**Syringadenoma** (M8400/0) — *see also* Neoplasm, skin, benign
  papillary (M8406/0) — *see* Neoplasm, skin, benign
**Syringobulbia** 336.0
**Syringocarcinoma** (M8400/3) — *see* Neoplasm, skin, malignant
**Syringocystadenoma** (M8400/0) — *see also* Neoplasm, skin, benign
  papillary (M8406/0) — *see* Neoplasm, skin, benign
**Syringocystoma** (M8407/0) — *see* Neoplasm, skin, benign
**Syringoma** (M8407/0) — *see also* Neoplasm, skin, benign
  chondroid (M8940/0) — *see* Neoplasm, by site, benign
**Syringomyelia** 336.0
**Syringomyelitis** 323.9
  late effect — *see* category 326
**Syringomyelocele** — *see also* Spina bifida 741.9 ☑
**Syringopontia** 336.0
  disease, combined — *see* Degeneration, combined
  fibrosclerosing syndrome 710.8
  inflammatory response syndrome (SIRS) 995.90
    due to
      infectious process 995.91
        with organ dysfunction 995.92
      non-infectious process 995.93
        with organ dysfunction 995.94
  lupus erythematosus 710.0
    inhibitor 286.5
**System, systemic** — *see also* condition
  disease, combined — *see* Degeneration, combined
  fibrosclerosing syndrome 710.8
  inflammatory response syndrome (SIRS) 995.90
    due to
      infectious process 995.91
        with acute organ dysfunction 995.92
      non-infectious process 995.93
        with acute organ dysfunction 995.94
  lupus erythematosus 710.0
    inhibitor 286.5

**T**

**Tab** — *see* Tag
**Tabacism** 989.84
**Tabacosis** 989.84
**Tabardillo** 080
  flea-borne 081.0
  louse-borne 080
**Tabes, tabetic**
  with
    central nervous system syphilis 094.0
    Charcôt's joint 094.0 *[713.5]*
    cord bladder 094.0
    crisis, viscera (any) 094.0
    paralysis, general 094.1
    paresis (general) 094.1
    perforating ulcer 094.0
  arthropathy 094.0 *[713.5]*
  bladder 094.0
  bone 094.0
  cerebrospinal 094.0
  congenital 090.40
  conjugal 094.0

**Tabes, tabetic** — *continued*
  dorsalis 094.0
    neurosyphilis 094.0
  early 094.0
  juvenile 090.40
  latent 094.0
  mesenterica (*see also* Tuberculosis) 014.8 ☑
  paralysis insane, general 094.1
  peripheral (nonsyphilitic) 799.89
  spasmodic 094.0
    not dorsal or dorsalis 343.9
  syphilis (cerebrospinal) 094.0
**Taboparalysis** 094.1
**Taboparesis** (remission) 094.1
  with
    Charcôt's joint 094.1 *[713.5]*
    cord bladder 094.1
    perforating ulcer 094.1
  juvenile 090.40
**Tache noir** 923.20
**Tachyalimentation** 579.3
**Tachyarrhythmia, tachyrhythmia** — *see also* Tachycardia
  paroxysmal with sinus bradycardia 427.81
**Tachycardia** 785.0
  atrial 427.89
  auricular 427.89
  AV nodal re-entry (re-entrant) 427.89
  junctional ectopic 427.0            ●
  newborn 779.82
  nodal 427.89
    nonparoxysmal atrioventricular 426.89
    nonparoxysmal atrioventricular (nodal) 426.89
  paroxysmal 427.2
    with sinus bradycardia 427.81
    atrial (PAT) 427.0
      psychogenic 316 *[427.0]*
    atrioventricular (AV) 427.0
      psychogenic 316 *[427.0]*
    essential 427.2
    junctional 427.0
    nodal 427.0
    psychogenic 316 *[427.2]*
      atrial 316 *[427.0]*
      supraventricular 316 *[427.0]*
      ventricular 316 *[427.1]*
    supraventricular 427.0
      psychogenic 316 *[427.0]*
    ventricular 427.1
      psychogenic 316 *[427.1]*
  postoperative 997.1
  psychogenic 306.2
  sick sinus 427.81
  sinoauricular 427.89
  sinus 427.89
  supraventricular 427.89
  ventricular (paroxysmal) 427.1
    psychogenic 316 *[427.1]*
**Tachygastria** 536.8
**Tachypnea** 786.06
  hysterical 300.11
  newborn (idiopathic) (transitory) 770.6
  psychogenic 306.1
  transitory, of newborn 770.6
**Taenia** (infection) (infestation) — *see also* Infestation, taenia 123.3
  diminuta 123.6
  echinococcal infestation (*see also* Echinococcus) 122.9
  nana 123.6
  saginata infestation 123.2
  solium (intestinal form) 123.0
    larval form 123.1
**Taeniasis** (intestine) — *see also* Infestation, taenia 123.3
  saginata 123.2
  solium 123.0
**Taenzer's disease** 757.4
**Tag** (hypertrophied skin) (infected) 701.9
  adenoid 474.8
  anus 455.9

**Tag** — *continued*
  endocardial (*see also* Endocarditis) 424.90
  hemorrhoidal 455.9
  hymen 623.8
  perineal 624.8
  preauricular 744.1
  rectum 455.9
  sentinel 455.9
  skin 701.9
    accessory 757.39
    anus 455.9
    congenital 757.39
    preauricular 744.1
    rectum 455.9
  tonsil 474.8
  urethra, urethral 599.84
  vulva 624.8
**Tahyna fever** 062.5
**Takayasu (-Onishi) disease or syndrome** (pulseless disease) 446.7
**Takotsubo syndrome** 429.83
**Talc granuloma** 728.82
  in operation wound 998.7
**Talcosis** 502
**Talipes** (congenital) 754.70
  acquired NEC 736.79
    planus 734
  asymmetric 754.79
    acquired 736.79
  calcaneovalgus 754.62
    acquired 736.76
  calcaneovarus 754.59
    acquired 736.76
  calcaneus 754.79
    acquired 736.76
  cavovarus 754.59
    acquired 736.75
  cavus 754.71
    acquired 736.73
  equinovalgus 754.69
    acquired 736.72
  equinovarus 754.51
    acquired 736.71
  equinus 754.79
    acquired, NEC 736.72
  percavus 754.71
    acquired 736.73
  planovalgus 754.69
    acquired 736.79
  planus (acquired) (any degree) 734
    congenital 754.61
    due to rickets 268.1
  valgus 754.60
    acquired 736.79
  varus 754.50
    acquired 736.79
**Talma's disease** 728.85
**Talon noir** 924.20
  hand 923.20
  heel 924.20
  toe 924.3
**Tamponade heart** (Rose's) — *see also* Pericarditis 423.3            ▲
**Tanapox** 078.89
**Tangier disease** (familial high-density lipoprotein deficiency) 272.5
**Tank ear** 380.12
**Tantrum** (childhood) — *see also* Disturbance, conduct 312.1 ☑
**Tapeworm** (infection) (infestation) — *see also* Infestation, tapeworm 123.9
**Tapia's syndrome** 352.6
**Tarantism** 297.8
**Target-oval cell anemia** 282.49
**Tarlov's cyst** 355.9
**Tarral-Besnier disease** (pityriasis rubra pilaris) 696.4
**Tarsalgia** 729.2
**Tarsal tunnel syndrome** 355.5
**Tarsitis** (eyelid) 373.00
  syphilitic 095.8 *[373.00]*
  tuberculous (*see also* Tuberculosis) 017.0 ☑ *[373.4]*
**Tartar** (teeth) 523.6
**Tattoo** (mark) 709.09

☑ Additional Digit Required — Refer to the Tabular List for Digit Selection                                    ▽ Subterms under main terms may continue to next column or page

280 — Volume 2 • October 2007          ▶◀ Revised Text          ● New Line          ▲ Revised Code                    *2008 ICD-9-CM*

**Taurodontism** 520.2
**Taussig-Bing defect, heart, or syndrome** (transposition, aorta and overriding pulmonary artery) 745.11
**Taybi's syndrome** (otopalatodigital) 759.89
**Tay's choroiditis** 363.41
**Taylor's**
   disease (diffuse idiopathic cutaneous atrophy) 701.8
   syndrome 625.5
**Tay-Sachs**
   amaurotic familial idiocy 330.1
   disease 330.1
**Tear stone** 375.57
**Tear, torn** (traumatic) — *see also* Wound, open, by site
   anus, anal (sphincter) 863.89
      with open wound in cavity 863.99
      complicating delivery ▶(healed) (old)◀ 654.8 ☑ ▲
         with mucosa 664.3 ☑
         not associated with third-degree perineal laceration 664.6 ☑ ●
      nontraumatic, nonpuerperal ▶(healed) (old)◀ 569.43 ▲
   articular cartilage, old (*see also* Disorder, cartilage, articular) 718.0 ☑
   bladder
      with
         abortion — *see* Abortion, by type, with damage to pelvic organs
         ectopic pregnancy (*see also* categories 633.0–633.9) 639.2
         molar pregnancy (*see also* categories 630–632) 639.2
         following
            abortion 639.2
            ectopic or molar pregnancy 639.2
         obstetrical trauma 665.5 ☑
   bowel
      with
         abortion — *see* Abortion, by type, with damage to pelvic organs
         ectopic pregnancy (*see also* categories 633.0–633.9) 639.2
         molar pregnancy (*see also* categories 630–632) 639.2
         following
            abortion 639.2
            ectopic or molar pregnancy 639.2
         obstetrical trauma 665.5 ☑
   broad ligament
      with
         abortion — *see* Abortion, by type, with damage to pelvic organs
         ectopic pregnancy (*see also* categories 633.0–633.9) 639.2
         molar pregnancy (*see also* categories 630–632) 639.2
         following
            abortion 639.2
            ectopic or molar pregnancy 639.2
         obstetrical trauma 665.6 ☑
   bucket handle (knee) (meniscus) — *see* Tear, meniscus
   capsule
      joint — *see* Sprain, by site
      spleen — *see* Laceration, spleen, capsule
   cartilage (*see also* Sprain, by site)
      articular, old (*see also* Disorder, cartilage, articular) 718.0 ☑
      knee — *see* Tear, meniscus

**Tear, torn** — *see also* Wound, open, by site — *continued*
   cartilage (*see also* Sprain, by site) — *continued*
      semilunar (knee) (current injury) — *see* Tear, meniscus
   cervix
      with
         abortion — *see* Abortion, by type, with damage to pelvic organs
         ectopic pregnancy (*see also* categories 633.0–633.9) 639.2
         molar pregnancy (*see also* categories 630–632) 639.2
      following
         abortion 639.2
         ectopic or molar pregnancy 639.2
      obstetrical trauma (current) 665.3 ☑
      old 622.3
   dural 998.2 ●
   internal organ (abdomen, chest, or pelvis) — *see* Injury, internal, by site
   ligament (*see also* Sprain, by site)
      with open wound — *see* Wound, open by site
   meniscus (knee) (current injury) 836.2
      bucket handle 836.0
         old 717.0
      lateral 836.1
         anterior horn 836.1
            old 717.42
         bucket handle 836.1
            old 717.41
         old 717.40
         posterior horn 836.1
            old 717.43
         specified site NEC 836.1
            old 717.49
      medial 836.0
         anterior horn 836.0
            old 717.1
         bucket handle 836.0
            old 717.0
         old 717.3
         posterior horn 836.0
            old 717.2
      old NEC 717.5
      site other than knee — *see* Sprain, by site
   muscle (*see also* Sprain, by site)
      with open wound — *see* Wound, open by site
   pelvic
      floor, complicating delivery 664.1 ☑
      organ NEC
         with
            abortion — *see* Abortion, by type, with damage to pelvic organs
            ectopic pregnancy (*see also* categories 633.0–633.9) 639.2
            molar pregnancy (*see also* categories 630–632) 639.2
            following
               abortion 639.2
               ectopic or molar pregnancy 639.2
            obstetrical trauma 665.5 ☑
   perineum (*see also* Laceration, perineum)
      obstetrical trauma 665.5 ☑
   periurethral tissue
      with
         abortion — *see* Abortion, by type, with damage to pelvic organs

**Tear, torn** — *see also* Wound, open, by site — *continued*
   periurethral tissue — *continued*
      with — *continued*
         ectopic pregnancy (*see also* categories 633.0–633.9) 639.2
         molar pregnancy (*see also* categories 630–632) 639.2
      following
         abortion 639.2
         ectopic or molar pregnancy 639.2
      obstetrical trauma 665.5 ☑
   rectovaginal septum — *see* Laceration, rectovaginal septum
   retina, retinal (recent) (with detachment) 361.00
      without detachment 361.30
      dialysis (juvenile) (with detachment) 361.04
      giant (with detachment) 361.03
      horseshoe (without detachment) 361.32
      multiple (with detachment) 361.02
         without detachment 361.33
      old
         delimited (partial) 361.06
         partial 361.06
         total or subtotal 361.07
      partial (without detachment)
         giant 361.03
         multiple defects 361.02
         old (delimited) 361.06
         single defect 361.01
      round hole (without detachment) 361.31
      single defect (with detachment) 361.01
      total or subtotal (recent) 361.05
         old 361.07
   rotator cuff (traumatic) 840.4
      current injury 840.4
      degenerative 726.10
      nontraumatic 727.61
   semilunar cartilage, knee (*see also* Tear, meniscus) 836.2
      old 717.5
   tendon (*see also* Sprain, by site)
      with open wound — *see* Wound, open by site
   tentorial, at birth 767.0
   umbilical cord
      affecting fetus or newborn 772.0
      complicating delivery 663.8 ☑
   urethra
      with
         abortion — *see* Abortion, by type, with damage to pelvic organs
         ectopic pregnancy (*see also* categories 633.0–633.9) 639.2
         molar pregnancy (*see also* categories 630–632) 639.2
      following
         abortion 639.2
         ectopic or molar pregnancy 639.2
      obstetrical trauma 665.5 ☑
   uterus — *see* Injury, internal, uterus
   vagina — *see* Laceration, vagina
   vessel, from catheter 998.2
   vulva, complicating delivery 664.0 ☑
**Teething** 520.7
   syndrome 520.7
**Teeth, tooth** — *see also* condition
   grinding 306.8
   prenatal 520.6
**Tegmental syndrome** 344.89
**Telangiectasia, telangiectasis** (verrucous) 448.9
   ataxic (cerebellar) 334.8
   familial 448.0
   hemorrhagic, hereditary (congenital) (senile) 448.0

**Telangiectasia, telangiectasis** — *continued*
   hereditary hemorrhagic 448.0
   retina 362.15
   spider 448.1
**Telecanthus** (congenital) 743.63
**Telescoped bowel or intestine** — *see also* Intussusception 560.0
**Teletherapy, adverse effect** NEC 990
**Telogen effluvium** 704.02
**Temperature**
   body, high (of unknown origin) (*see also* Pyrexia) 780.6
   cold, trauma from 991.9
      newborn 778.2
      specified effect NEC 991.8
   high
      body (of unknown origin) (*see also* Pyrexia) 780.6
      trauma from — *see* Heat
**Temper tantrum** (childhood) — *see also* Disturbance, conduct 312.1 ☑
**Temple** — *see* condition
**Temporal** — *see also* condition
   lobe syndrome 310.0
**Temporomandibular joint-pain-dysfunction syndrome** 524.60
**Temporosphenoidal** — *see* condition
**Tendency**
   bleeding (*see also* Defect, coagulation) 286.9
   homosexual, ego-dystonic 302.0
   paranoid 301.0
   suicide 300.9
**Tenderness**
   abdominal (generalized) (localized) 789.6 ☑
   rebound 789.6 ☑
   skin 782.0
**Tendinitis, tendonitis** — *see also* Tenosynovitis 726.90
   Achilles 726.71
   adhesive 726.90
      shoulder 726.0
   calcific 727.82
      shoulder 726.11
   gluteal 726.5
   patellar 726.64
   peroneal 726.79
   pes anserinus 726.61
   psoas 726.5
   tibialis (anterior) (posterior) 726.72
   trochanteric 726.5
**Tendon** — *see* condition
**Tendosynovitis** — *see* Tenosynovitis
**Tendovaginitis** — *see* Tenosynovitis
**Tenesmus** 787.99
   rectal 787.99
   vesical 788.9
**Tenia** — *see* Taenia
**Teniasis** — *see* Taeniasis
**Tennis elbow** 726.32
**Tenonitis** — *see also* Tenosynovitis
   eye (capsule) 376.04
**Tenontosynovitis** — *see* Tenosynovitis
**Tenontothecitis** — *see* Tenosynovitis
**Tenophyte** 727.9
**Tenosynovitis** 727.00
   adhesive 726.90
      shoulder 726.0
   ankle 727.06
   bicipital (calcifying) 726.12
   buttock 727.09
   due to crystals — *see* Arthritis, due to crystals
   elbow 727.09
   finger 727.05
   foot 727.06
   gonococcal 098.51
   hand 727.05
   hip 727.09
   knee 727.09
   radial styloid 727.04
   shoulder 726.10
      adhesive 726.0
   spine 720.1

☑ Additional Digit Required — Refer to the Tabular List for Digit Selection
**2008 ICD-9-CM**
▶◀ Revised Text     ● New Line     ▲ Revised Code
Subterms under main terms may continue to next column or page
**October 2007 · Volume 2 — 281**

**Tenosynovitis** — *continued*
supraspinatus 726.10
toe 727.06
tuberculous — *see* Tuberculosis, tenosynovitis
wrist 727.05
**Tenovaginitis** — *see* Tenosynovitis
**Tension**
arterial, high (*see also* Hypertension) 401.9
without diagnosis of hypertension 796.2
headache 307.81
intraocular (elevated) 365.00
nervous 799.2
ocular (elevated) 365.00
pneumothorax 512.0
iatrogenic 512.1
postoperative 512.1
spontaneous 512.0
premenstrual 625.4
state 300.9
**Tentorium** — *see* condition
**Teratencephalus** 759.89
**Teratism** 759.7
**Teratoblastoma** (malignant) (M9080/3) — *see* Neoplasm, by site, malignant
**Teratocarcinoma** (M9081/3) — *see also* Neoplasm, by site, malignant
liver 155.0
**Teratoma** (solid) (M9080/1) — *see also* Neoplasm, by site, uncertain behavior
adult (cystic) (M9080/0) — *see* Neoplasm, by site, benign
and embryonal carcinoma, mixed (M9081/3) — *see* Neoplasm, by site, malignant
benign (M9080/0) — *see* Neoplasm, by site, benign
combined with choriocarcinoma (M9101/3) — *see* Neoplasm, by site, malignant
cystic (adult) (M9080/0) — *see* Neoplasm, by site, benign
differentiated type (M9080/0) — *see* Neoplasm, by site, benign
embryonal (M9080/3) (*see also* Neoplasm, by site, malignant)
liver 155.0
fetal
sacral, causing fetopelvic disproportion 653.7 ☑
immature (M9080/3) — *see* Neoplasm, by site, malignant
liver (M9080/3) 155.0
adult, benign, cystic, differentiated type or mature (M9080/0) 211.5
malignant (M9080/3) (*see also* Neoplasm, by site, malignant)
anaplastic type (M9082/3) — *see* Neoplasm, by site, malignant
intermediate type (M9083/3) — *see* Neoplasm, by site, malignant
liver (M9080/3) 155.0
trophoblastic (M9102/3)
specified site — *see* Neoplasm, by site, malignant
unspecified site 186.9
undifferentiated type (M9082/3) — *see* Neoplasm, by site, malignant
mature (M9080/0) — *see* Neoplasm, by site, benign
malignant (M9080/3) — *see* Neoplasm, by site, malignant ●
ovary (M9080/0) 220
embryonal, immature, or malignant (M9080/3) 183.0
suprasellar (M9080/3) — *see* Neoplasm, by site, malignant
testis (M9080/3) 186.9
adult, benign, cystic, differentiated type or mature (M9080/0) 222.0

**Teratoma** — *see also* Neoplasm, by site, uncertain behavior — *continued*
testis — *continued*
undescended 186.0
**Terminal care** V66.7
**Termination**
anomalous (*see also* Malposition, congenital)
portal vein 747.49
right pulmonary vein 747.42
pregnancy (legal) (therapeutic) — *see* Abortion, legal 635.9 ☑
fetus NEC 779.6
illegal (*see also* Abortion, illegal) 636.9 ☑
**Ternidens diminutus infestation** 127.7
**Terrors, night** (child) 307.46
**Terry's syndrome** 362.21
**Tertiary** — *see* condition
**Tessellated fundus, retina** (tigroid) 362.89
**Test(s)**
adequacy
hemodialysis V56.31
peritoneal dialysis V56.32
AIDS virus V72.6
allergen V72.7
bacterial disease NEC (*see also* Screening, by name of disease) V74.9
basal metabolic rate V72.6
blood-alcohol V70.4
blood-drug V70.4
for therapeutic drug monitoring V58.83
blood typing V72.86
Rh typing V72.86
developmental, infant or child V20.2
Dick V74.8
fertility V26.21
genetic
female V26.32
for genetic disease carrier status
female V26.31
male V26.34
male V26.39
hearing V72.19
following failed hearing screening V72.11
HIV V72.6
human immunodeficiency virus V72.6
Kveim V82.89
laboratory V72.6
for medicolegal reason V70.4
male partner of habitual aborter V26.35
Mantoux (for tuberculosis) V74.1
mycotic organism V75.4
parasitic agent NEC V75.8
paternity V70.4
peritoneal equilibration V56.32
pregnancy
negative result V72.41
positive result V72.42
first pregnancy V72.42
unconfirmed V72.40
preoperative V72.84
cardiovascular V72.81
respiratory V72.82
specified NEC V72.83
procreative management NEC V26.29
genetic disease carrier status
female V26.31
male V26.34
Rh typing V72.86
sarcoidosis V82.89
Schick V74.3
Schultz-Charlton V74.8
skin, diagnostic
allergy V72.7
bacterial agent NEC (*see also* Screening, by name of disease) V74.9
Dick V74.8
hypersensitivity V72.7
Kveim V82.89

**Test(s)** — *continued*
skin, diagnostic — *continued*
Mantoux V74.1
mycotic organism V75.4
parasitic agent NEC V75.8
sarcoidosis V82.89
Schick V74.3
Schultz-Charlton V74.8
tuberculin V74.1
specified type NEC V72.85
tuberculin V74.1
vision V72.0
Wassermann
positive (*see also* Serology for syphilis, positive) 097.1
false 795.6
**Testicle, testicular, testis** — *see also* condition
feminization (syndrome) 259.5
**Tetanus, tetanic** (cephalic) (convulsions) 037
with
abortion — *see* Abortion, by type, with sepsis
ectopic pregnancy (*see also* categories 633.0–633.9) 639.0
molar pregnancy — *see* categories 630–632 639.0
following
abortion 639.0
ectopic or molar pregnancy 639.0
inoculation V03.7
reaction (due to serum) — *see* Complications, vaccination
neonatorum 771.3
puerperal, postpartum, childbirth 670.0 ☑
**Tetany, tetanic** 781.7
alkalosis 276.3
associated with rickets 268.0
convulsions 781.7
hysterical 300.11
functional (hysterical) 300.11
hyperkinetic 781.7
hysterical 300.11
hyperpnea 786.01
hysterical 300.11
psychogenic 306.1
hyperventilation 786.01
hysterical 300.11
psychogenic 306.1
hypocalcemic, neonatal 775.4
hysterical 300.11
neonatal 775.4
parathyroid (gland) 252.1
parathyroprival 252.1
postoperative 252.1
postthyroidectomy 252.1
pseudotetany 781.7
hysterical 300.11
psychogenic 306.1
specified as conversion reaction 300.11
**Tetralogy of Fallot** 745.2
**Tetraplegia** — *see* Quadriplegia
**Thailand hemorrhagic fever** 065.4
**Thalassanemia** 282.49
**Thalassemia** (alpha) (beta) (disease) (Hb-C) (Hb-D) (Hb-E) (Hb-H) (Hb-I) (high fetal gene) (high fetal hemoglobin) (intermedia) (major) (minima) (minor) (mixed) (trait) (with other hemoglobinopathy) 282.49
Hb-S (without crisis) 282.41
with
crisis 282.42
vaso-occlusive pain 282.42
sickle-cell (without crisis) 282.41
with
crisis 282.42
vaso-occlusive pain 282.42
**Thalassemic variants** 282.49
**Thaysen-Gee disease** (nontropical sprue) 579.0
**Thecoma** (M8600/0) 220
malignant (M8600/3) 183.0

**Thelarche, precocious** 259.1
**Thelitis** 611.0
puerperal, postpartum 675.0 ☑
**Therapeutic** — *see* condition
**Therapy** V57.9
blood transfusion, without reported diagnosis V58.2
breathing V57.0
chemotherapy, antineoplastic V58.11
fluoride V07.31
prophylactic NEC V07.39
dialysis (intermittent) (treatment)
extracorporeal V56.0
peritoneal V56.8
renal V56.0
specified type NEC V56.8
exercise NEC V57.1
breathing V57.0
extracorporeal dialysis (renal) V56.0
fluoride prophylaxis V07.31
hemodialysis V56.0
hormone replacement (postmenopausal) V07.4
immunotherapy antineoplastic V58.12
long term oxygen therapy V46.2
occupational V57.21
orthoptic V57.4
orthotic V57.81
peritoneal dialysis V56.8
physical NEC V57.1
postmenopausal hormone replacement V07.4
radiation V58.0
speech V57.3
vocational V57.22
**Thermalgesia** 782.0
**Thermalgia** 782.0
**Thermanalgesia** 782.0
**Thermanesthesia** 782.0
**Thermic** — *see* condition
**Thermography** (abnormal) 793.99
breast 793.89
**Thermoplegia** 992.0
**Thesaurismosis**
amyloid 277.39
bilirubin 277.4
calcium 275.40
cystine 270.0
glycogen (*see also* Disease, glycogen storage) 271.0
kerasin 272.7
lipoid 272.7
melanin 255.41 ▲
phosphatide 272.7
urate 274.9
**Thiaminic deficiency** 265.1
with beriberi 265.0
**Thibierge-Weissenbach syndrome** (cutaneous systemic sclerosis) 710.1
**Thickened endometrium** 793.5
**Thickening**
bone 733.99
extremity 733.99
breast 611.79
hymen 623.3
larynx 478.79
nail 703.8
congenital 757.5
periosteal 733.99
pleura (*see also* Pleurisy) 511.0
skin 782.8
subepiglottic 478.79
tongue 529.8
valve, heart — *see* Endocarditis
**Thiele syndrome** 724.6
**Thigh** — *see* condition
**Thinning vertebra** — *see also* Osteoporosis 733.00
**Thirst, excessive** 783.5
due to deprivation of water 994.3
**Thomsen's disease** 359.22 ▲
**Thomson's disease** (congenital poikiloderma) 757.33
**Thoracic** — *see also* condition
kidney 753.3
outlet syndrome 353.0

**Thoracic** — see also condition —
  continued
    stomach — see Hernia, diaphragm
**Thoracogastroschisis** (congenital)
  759.89
**Thoracopagus** 759.4
**Thoracoschisis** 756.3
**Thoracoscopic surgical procedure**
  **converted to open procedure**
  V64.42
**Thorax** — see condition
**Thorn's syndrome** — see also Disease,
  renal 593.9
**Thornwaldt's, Tornwaldt's**
  bursitis (pharyngeal) 478.29
  cyst 478.26
  disease (pharyngeal bursitis) 478.29
**Thorson-Biörck syndrome** (malignant
  carcinoid) 259.2
**Threadworm** (infection) (infestation)
  127.4
**Threatened**
  abortion or miscarriage 640.0 ☑
    with subsequent abortion (see also
      Abortion, spontaneous)
      634.9 ☑
    affecting fetus 762.1
  labor 644.1 ☑
    affecting fetus or newborn 761.8
    premature 644.0 ☑
  miscarriage 640.0 ☑
    affecting fetus 762.1
  premature
    delivery 644.2 ☑
      affecting fetus or newborn 761.8
    labor 644.0 ☑
      before 22 completed weeks ges-
        tation 640.0 ☑
**Three-day fever** 066.0
**Threshers' lung** 495.0
**Thrix annulata** (congenital) 757.4
**Throat** — see condition
**Thrombasthenia** (Glanzmann's) (hemorrhagic) (hereditary) 287.1
**Thromboangiitis** 443.1
  obliterans (general) 443.1
    cerebral 437.1
    vessels
      brain 437.1
      spinal cord 437.1
**Thromboarteritis** — see Arteritis
**Thromboasthenia** (Glanzmann's) (hemorrhagic) (hereditary) 287.1
**Thrombocytasthenia** (Glanzmann's)
  287.1
**Thrombocythemia** (primary) (M9962/1)
  238.71
  essential 238.71
  hemorrhagic 238.71
  idiopathic (hemorrhagic) (M9962/1)
    238.71
**Thrombocytopathy** (dystrophic) (granu-
  lopenic) 287.1
**Thrombocytopenia, thrombocytopenic**
  287.5
  with
    absent radii (TAR) syndrome
    giant hemangioma
    amegakaryocytic, congenital 287.33
  congenital 287.33
  cyclic 287.39
  dilutional 287.4
  due to
    drugs 287.4
    extracorporeal circulation of blood
      287.4
    massive blood transfusion 287.4
    platelet alloimmunization 287.4
  essential 287.30
  hereditary 287.33
  Kasabach-Merritt 287.39
  neonatal, transitory 776.1
    due to
      exchange transfusion 776.1
      idiopathic maternal thrombocy-
        topenia 776.1

**Thrombocytopenia, thrombocytopenic**
  — continued
    neonatal, transitory — continued
      due to — continued
        isoimmunization 776.1
    primary 287.30
    puerperal, postpartum 666.3 ☑
    purpura (see also Purpura, thrombo-
      cytopenic) 287.30
      thrombotic 446.6
    secondary 287.4
    sex-linked 287.39
**Thrombocytosis** 238.71
  essential 238.71
  primary 238.71
**Thromboembolism** — see Embolism
**Thrombopathy** (Bernard-Soulier) 287.1
  constitutional 286.4
  Willebrand-Jürgens (angiohemophilia)
    286.4
**Thrombopenia** — see also Thrombocytopenia 287.5
**Thrombophlebitis** 451.9
  antecubital vein 451.82
  antepartum (superficial) 671.2 ☑
    affecting fetus or newborn 760.3
    deep 671.3 ☑
  arm 451.89
    deep 451.83
    superficial 451.82
  breast, superficial 451.89
  cavernous (venous) sinus — see
    Thrombophlebitis, intracranial
    venous sinus
  cephalic vein 451.82
  cerebral (sinus) (vein) 325
    late effect — see category 326
    nonpyogenic 437.6
      in pregnancy or puerperium
        671.5 ☑
      late effect — see Late effect(s)
        (of) cerebrovascular dis-
        ease
  due to implanted device — see Compli-
    cations, due to (presence of) any
    device, implant or graft classi-
    fied to 996.0–996.5 NEC
  during or resulting from a procedure
    NEC 997.2
  femoral 451.11
  femoropopliteal 451.19
  following infusion, perfusion, or
    transfusion 999.2
  hepatic (vein) 451.89
  idiopathic, recurrent 453.1
  iliac vein 451.81
  iliofemoral 451.11
  intracranial venous sinus (any) 325
    late effect — see category 326
    nonpyogenic 437.6
      in pregnancy or puerperium
        671.5 ☑
      late effect — see Late effect(s)
        (of) cerebrovascular dis-
        ease
  jugular vein 451.89
  lateral (venous) sinus — see Throm-
    bophlebitis, intracranial venous
    sinus
  leg 451.2
    deep (vessels) 451.19
      femoral vein 451.11
      specified vessel NEC 451.19
    superficial (vessels) 451.0
      femoral vein 451.11
  longitudinal (venous) sinus — see
    Thrombophlebitis, intracranial
    venous sinus
  lower extremity 451.2
    deep (vessels) 451.19
      femoral vein 451.11
      specified vessel NEC 451.19
    superficial (vessels) 451.0
  migrans, migrating 453.1

**Thrombophlebitis** — continued
  pelvic
    with
      abortion — see Abortion, by
        type, with sepsis
      ectopic pregnancy (see also cat-
        egories 633.0–633.9)
        639.0
      molar pregnancy (see also cate-
        gories 630–632) 639.0
    following
      abortion 639.0
      ectopic or molar pregnancy
        639.0
    puerperal 671.4 ☑
  popliteal vein 451.19
  portal (vein) 572.1
  postoperative 997.2
  pregnancy (superficial) 671.2 ☑
    affecting fetus or newborn 760.3
    deep 671.3 ☑
  puerperal, postpartum, childbirth
    (extremities) (superficial)
    671.2 ☑
    deep 671.4 ☑
    pelvic 671.4 ☑
    specified site NEC 671.5 ☑
  radial vein 451.83
  saphenous (greater) (lesser) 451.0
  sinus (intracranial) — see Throm-
    bophlebitis, intracranial venous
    sinus
  specified site NEC 451.89
  tibial vein 451.19
**Thrombosis, thrombotic** (marantic)
  (multiple) (progressive) (vein) (vessel) 453.9
  with childbirth or during the puerperi-
    um — see Thrombosis, puerper-
    al, postpartum
  antepartum — see Thrombosis, preg-
    nancy
  aorta, aortic 444.1
    abdominal 444.0
    bifurcation 444.0
    saddle 444.0
    terminal 444.0
    thoracic 444.1
    valve — see Endocarditis, aortic
  apoplexy (see also Thrombosis, brain)
    434.0 ☑
    late effect — see Late effect(s) (of)
      cerebrovascular disease
  appendix, septic — see Appendicitis,
    acute
  arteriolar-capillary platelet, dissemi-
    nated 446.6
  artery, arteries (postinfectional) 444.9
    auditory, internal 433.8 ☑
    basilar (see also Occlusion, artery,
      basilar) 433.0 ☑
    carotid (common) (internal) (see
      also Occlusion, artery,
      carotid) 433.1 ☑
      with other precerebral artery
        433.3 ☑
    cerebellar (anterior inferior) (poste-
      rior inferior) (superior)
      433.8 ☑
    cerebral (see also Thrombosis,
      brain) 434.0 ☑
    choroidal (anterior) 433.8 ☑
    communicating posterior 433.8 ☑
    coronary (see also Infarct, my-
      ocardium) 410.9 ☑
      without myocardial infarction
        411.81
      due to syphilis 093.89
      healed or specified as old 412
    extremities 444.22
      lower 444.22
      upper 444.21
    femoral 444.22
    hepatic 444.89
    hypophyseal 433.8 ☑

**Thrombosis, thrombotic** —
  continued
    artery, arteries — continued
      meningeal, anterior or posterior
        433.8 ☑
      mesenteric (with gangrene) 557.0
      ophthalmic (see also Occlusion,
        retina) 362.30
      pontine 433.8 ☑
      popliteal 444.22
      precerebral — see Occlusion,
        artery, precerebral NEC
      pulmonary 415.19
        iatrogenic 415.11
        postoperative 415.11
        septic 415.12                    ●
      renal 593.81
      retinal (see also Occlusion, retina)
        362.30
      specified site NEC 444.89
      spinal, anterior or posterior
        433.8 ☑
      traumatic (complication) (early) (see
        also Injury, blood vessel, by
        site) 904.9
      vertebral (see also Occlusion,
        artery, vertebral) 433.2 ☑
        with other precerebral artery
          433.3 ☑
  atrial (endocardial) 424.90
    without endocarditis 429.89
    due to syphilis 093.89
  auricular (see also Infarct, myocardi-
    um) 410.9 ☑
  axillary (vein) 453.8
  basilar (artery) (see also Occlusion,
    artery, basilar) 433.0 ☑
  bland NEC 453.9
  brain (artery) (stem) 434.0 ☑
    due to syphilis 094.89
    iatrogenic 997.02
    late effect — see Late effect(s) (of)
      cerebrovascular disease
    postoperative 997.02
    puerperal, postpartum, childbirth
      674.0 ☑
    sinus (see also Thrombosis, in-
      tracranial venous sinus) 325
  capillary 448.9
    arteriolar, generalized 446.6
  cardiac (see also Infarct, myocardium)
    410.9 ☑
    due to syphilis 093.89
    healed or specified as old 412
    valve — see Endocarditis
  carotid (artery) (common) (internal)
    (see also Occlusion, artery,
    carotid) 433.1 ☑
    with other precerebral artery
      433.3 ☑
  cavernous sinus (venous) — see
    Thrombosis, intracranial venous
    sinus
  cerebellar artery (anterior inferior)
    (posterior inferior) (superior)
    433.8 ☑
    late effect — see Late effect(s) (of)
      cerebrovascular disease
  cerebral (arteries) (see also Thrombo-
    sis, brain) 434.0 ☑
    late effect — see Late effect(s) (of)
      cerebrovascular disese
  coronary (artery) (see also Infarct,
    myocardium) 410.9 ☑
    without myocardial infarction
      411.81
    due to syphilis 093.89
    healed or specified as old 412
  corpus cavernosum 607.82
  cortical (see also Thrombosis, brain)
    434.0 ☑

**Thrombosis, thrombotic —**
*continued*
due to (presence of) any device, implant, or graft classifiable to 996.0–996.5 — *see* Complications, due to (presence of) any device, implant, or graft classified to 996.0–996.5 NEC
effort 453.8
endocardial — *see* Infarct, myocardium
eye (*see also* Occlusion, retina) 362.30
femoral (vein) 453.8
with inflammation or phlebitis 451.11
artery 444.22
deep 453.41
genital organ, male 608.83
heart (chamber) (*see also* Infarct, myocardium) 410.9 ☑
hepatic (vein) 453.0
artery 444.89
infectional or septic 572.1
iliac (vein) 453.8
with inflammation or phlebitis 451.81
artery (common) (external) (internal) 444.81
inflammation, vein — *see* Thrombophlebitis
internal carotid artery (*see also* Occlusion, artery, carotid) 433.1 ☑
with other precerebral artery 433.3 ☑
intestine (with gangrene) 557.0
intracranial (*see also* Thrombosis, brain) 434.0 ☑
venous sinus (any) 325
nonpyogenic origin 437.6
in pregnancy or puerperium 671.5 ☑
intramural (*see also* Infarct, myocardium) 410.9 ☑
without
cardiac condition 429.89
coronary artery disease 429.89
myocardial infarction 429.89
healed or specified as old 412
jugular (bulb) 453.8
kidney 593.81
artery 593.81
lateral sinus (venous) — *see* Thrombosis, intracranial venous sinus
leg 453.8
with inflammation or phlebitis — *see* Thrombophlebitis
deep (vessels) 453.40
lower (distal) 453.42
upper (proximal) 453.41
superficial (vessels) 453.8
liver (venous) 453.0
artery 444.89
infectional or septic 572.1
portal vein 452
longitudinal sinus (venous) — *see* Thrombosis, intracranial venous sinus
lower extremity 453.8
deep vessels 453.40
calf 453.42
distal (lower leg) 453.42
femoral 453.41
iliac 453.41
lower leg 453.42
peroneal 453.42
popliteal 453.41
proximal (upper leg) 453.41
thigh 453.41
tibial 453.42
lung 415.19
iatrogenic 415.11
postoperative 415.11
septic 415.12
marantic, dural sinus 437.6
meninges (brain) (*see also* Thrombosis, brain) 434.0 ☑

**Thrombosis, thrombotic —**
*continued*
mesenteric (artery) (with gangrene) 557.0
vein (inferior) (superior) 557.0
mitral — *see* Insufficiency, mitral
mural (heart chamber) (*see also* Infarct, myocardium) 410.9 ☑
without
cardiac condition 429.89
coronary artery disease 429.89
myocardial infarction 429.89
due to syphilis 093.89
following myocardial infarction 429.79
healed or specified as old 412
omentum (with gangrene) 557.0
ophthalmic (artery) (*see also* Occlusion, retina) 362.30
pampiniform plexus (male) 608.83
female 620.8
parietal (*see also* Infarct, myocardium) 410.9 ☑
penis, penile 607.82
peripheral arteries 444.22
lower 444.22
upper 444.21
platelet 446.6
portal 452
due to syphilis 093.89
infectional or septic 572.1
precerebral artery (*see also* Occlusion, artery, precerebral NEC)
pregnancy 671.9 ☑
deep (vein) 671.3 ☑
superficial (vein) 671.2 ☑
puerperal, postpartum, childbirth 671.9 ☑
brain (artery) 674.0 ☑
venous 671.5 ☑
cardiac 674.8 ☑
cerebral (artery) 674.0 ☑
venous 671.5 ☑
deep (vein) 671.4 ☑
intracranial sinus (nonpyogenic) (venous) 671.5 ☑
pelvic 671.4 ☑
pulmonary (artery) 673.2 ☑
specified site NEC 671.5 ☑
superficial 671.2 ☑
pulmonary (artery) (vein) 415.19
iatrogenic 415.11
postoperative 415.11
septic 415.12
renal (artery) 593.81
vein 453.3
resulting from presence of shunt or other internal prosthetic device — *see* Complications, due to (presence of) any device, implant, or graft classified to 996.0–996.5 NEC
retina, retinal (artery) 362.30
arterial branch 362.32
central 362.31
partial 362.33
vein
central 362.35
tributary (branch) 362.36
scrotum 608.83
seminal vesicle 608.83
sigmoid (venous) sinus — *see* Thrombosis, intracranial venous sinus 325
silent NEC 453.9
sinus, intracranial (venous) (any) (*see also* Thrombosis, intracranial venous sinus) 325
softening, brain (*see also* Thrombosis, brain) 434.0 ☑
specified site NEC 453.8
spermatic cord 608.83
spinal cord 336.1
due to syphilis 094.89
in pregnancy or puerperium 671.5 ☑

**Thrombosis, thrombotic —**
*continued*
spinal cord — *continued*
pyogenic origin 324.1
late effect — *see* category 326
spleen, splenic 289.59
artery 444.89
testis 608.83
traumatic (complication) (early) (*see also* Injury, blood vessel, by site) 904.9
tricuspid — *see* Endocarditis, tricuspid
tumor — *see* Neoplasm, by site
tunica vaginalis 608.83
umbilical cord (vessels) 663.6 ☑
affecting fetus or newborn 762.6
vas deferens 608.83
vein
deep 453.40
lower extremity — *see* Thrombosis, lower extremity
vena cava (inferior) (superior) 453.2
**Thrombus** — *see* Thrombosis
**Thrush** 112.0
newborn 771.7
**Thumb** — *see also* condition
gamekeeper's 842.12
sucking (child problem) 307.9
**Thygeson's superficial punctate keratitis** 370.21
**Thymergasia** — *see also* Psychosis, affective 296.80
**Thymitis** 254.8
**Thymoma** (benign) (M8580/0) 212.6
malignant (M8580/3) 164.0
**Thymus, thymic** (gland) — *see* condition
**Thyrocele** — *see also* Goiter 240.9
**Thyroglossal** — *see also* condition
cyst 759.2
duct, persistent 759.2
**Thyroid** (body) (gland) — *see also* condition
hormone resistance 246.8
lingual 759.2
**Thyroiditis** 245.9
acute (pyogenic) (suppurative) 245.0
nonsuppurative 245.0
autoimmune 245.2
chronic (nonspecific) (sclerosing) 245.8
fibrous 245.3
lymphadenoid 245.2
lymphocytic 245.2
lymphoid 245.2
complicating pregnancy, childbirth, or puerperium 648.1 ☑
de Quervain's (subacute granulomatous) 245.1
fibrous (chronic) 245.3
giant (cell) (follicular) 245.1
granulomatous (de Quervain's) (subacute) 245.1
Hashimoto's (struma lymphomatosa) 245.2
iatrogenic 245.4
invasive (fibrous) 245.3
ligneous 245.3
lymphocytic (chronic) 245.2
lymphoid 245.2
lymphomatous 245.2
pseudotuberculous 245.1
pyogenic 245.0
radiation 245.4
Riedel's (ligneous) 245.3
subacute 245.1
suppurative 245.0
tuberculous (*see also* Tuberculosis) 017.5 ☑
viral 245.1
woody 245.3
**Thyrolingual duct, persistent** 759.2
**Thyromegaly** 240.9
**Thyrotoxic**
crisis or storm (*see also* Thyrotoxicosis) 242.9 ☑

**Thyrotoxic** — *continued*
heart failure (*see also* Thyrotoxicosis) 242.9 ☑ *[425.7]*
**Thyrotoxicosis** 242.9 ☑

*Note — Use the following fifth-digit subclassification with category 242:*

| | |
|---|---|
| 0 | *without mention of thyrotoxic crisis or storm* |
| 1 | *with mention of thyrotoxic crisis or storm* |

with
goiter (diffuse) 242.0 ☑
adenomatous 242.3 ☑
multinodular 242.2 ☑
uninodular 242.1 ☑
nodular 242.3 ☑
multinodular 242.2 ☑
uninodular 242.1 ☑
infiltrative
dermopathy 242.0 ☑
ophthalmopathy 242.0 ☑
thyroid acropachy 242.0 ☑
complicating pregnancy, childbirth, or puerperium 648.1 ☑
due to
ectopic thyroid nodule 242.4 ☑
ingestion of (excessive) thyroid material 242.8 ☑
specified cause NEC 242.8 ☑
factitia 242.8 ☑
heart 242.9 ☑ *[425.7]*
neonatal (transient) 775.3
**TIA** (transient ischemic attack) 435.9
with transient neurologic deficit 435.9
late effect — *see* Late effect(s) (of) cerebrovascular disease
**Tibia vara** 732.4
**Tic** 307.20
breathing 307.20
child problem 307.21
compulsive 307.22
convulsive 307.20
degenerative (generalized) (localized) 333.3
facial 351.8
douloureux (*see also* Neuralgia, trigeminal) 350.1
atypical 350.2
habit 307.20
chronic (motor or vocal) 307.22
transient (of childhood) 307.21
lid 307.20
transient (of childhood) 307.21
motor-verbal 307.23
occupational 300.89
orbicularis 307.20
transient (of childhood) 307.21
organic origin 333.3
postchoreic — *see* Chorea
psychogenic 307.20
compulsive 307.22
salaam 781.0
spasm 307.20
chronic (motor or vocal) 307.22
transient (of childhood) 307.21
**Tick-bite fever** NEC 066.1
African 087.1
Colorado (virus) 066.1
Rocky Mountain 082.0
**Tick (-borne) fever** NEC 066.1
American mountain 066.1
Colorado 066.1
hemorrhagic NEC 065.3
Crimean 065.0
Kyasanur Forest 065.2
Omsk 065.1
mountain 066.1
nonexanthematous 066.1
**Tick paralysis** 989.5
**Tics and spasms, compulsive** 307.22
**Tietze's disease or syndrome** 733.6
**Tight, tightness**
anus 564.89
chest 786.59

---

☑ Additional Digit Required — Refer to the Tabular List for Digit Selection

☒ Subterms under main terms may continue to next column or page

**Tight, tightness** — *continued*
  fascia (lata) 728.9
  foreskin (congenital) 605
  hymen 623.3
  introitus (acquired) (congenital) 623.3
  rectal sphincter 564.89
  tendon 727.81
    Achilles (heel) 727.81
  urethral sphincter 598.9
**Tilting vertebra** 737.9
**Timidity, child** 313.21
**Tinea** (intersecta) (tarsi) 110.9
  amiantacea 110.0
  asbestina 110.0
  barbae 110.0
  beard 110.0
  black dot 110.0
  blanca 111.2
  capitis 110.0
  corporis 110.5
  cruris 110.3
  decalvans 704.09
  flava 111.0
  foot 110.4
  furfuracea 111.0
  imbricata (Tokelau) 110.5
  lepothrix 039.0
  manuum 110.2
  microsporic (*see also* Dermatophytosis) 110.9
  nigra 111.1
  nodosa 111.2
  pedis 110.4
  scalp 110.0
  specified site NEC 110.8
  sycosis 110.0
  tonsurans 110.0
  trichophytic (*see also* Dermatophytosis) 110.9
  unguium 110.1
  versicolor 111.0
**Tingling sensation** — *see also* Disturbance, sensation 782.0
**Tin-miners' lung** 503
**Tinnitus** (aurium) 388.30
  audible 388.32
  objective 388.32
  subjective 388.31
**Tipped, teeth** 524.33
**Tipping**
  pelvis 738.6
    with disproportion (fetopelvic) 653.0 ☑
      affecting fetus or newborn 763.1
      causing obstructed labor 660.1 ☑
        affecting fetus or newborn 763.1
  teeth 524.33
**Tiredness** 780.79
**Tissue** — *see* condition
**Tobacco**
  abuse (affecting health) NEC (*see also* Abuse, drugs, nondependent) 305.1
  heart 989.84
  use disorder complicating pregnancy, childbirth, or the puerperium 649.0 ☑
**Tobias' syndrome** (carcinoma, pulmonary apex) (M8010/3) 162.3
**Tocopherol deficiency** 269.1
**Todd's**
  cirrhosis — *see* Cirrhosis, biliary
  paralysis (postepileptic transitory paralysis) 344.89
**Toe** — *see* condition
**Toilet, artificial opening** — *see also* Attention to, artificial, opening V55.9
**Tokelau ringworm** 110.5
**Tollwut** 071
**Tolosa-Hunt syndrome** 378.55
**Tommaselli's disease**
  correct substance properly administered 599.7

**Tommaselli's disease** — *continued*
  overdose or wrong substance given or taken 961.4
**Tongue** — *see also* condition
  worms 134.1
**Tongue tie** 750.0
**Tonic pupil** 379.46
**Toni-Fanconi syndrome** (cystinosis) 270.0
**Tonsil** — *see* condition
**Tonsillitis** (acute) (catarrhal) (croupous) (follicular) (gangrenous) (infective) (lacunar) (lingual) (malignant) (membranous) (phlegmonous) (pneumococcal) (pseudomembranous) (purulent) (septic) (staphylococcal) (subacute) (suppurative) (toxic) (ulcerative) (vesicular) (viral) 463
  with influenza, flu, or grippe 487.1
  chronic 474.00
  diphtheritic (membranous) 032.0
  hypertrophic 474.00
  influenzal 487.1
  parenchymatous 475
  streptococcal 034.0
  tuberculous (*see also* Tuberculosis) 012.8 ☑
  Vincent's 101
**Tonsillopharyngitis** 465.8
**Toothache** 525.9
**Tooth, teeth** — *see* condition
**Topagnosis** 782.0
**Tophi** (gouty) 274.0
  ear 274.81
  heart 274.82
  specified site NEC 274.82
**Torn** — *see* Tear, torn
**Tornwaldt's bursitis** (disease) (pharyngeal bursitis) 478.29
  cyst 478.26
**Torpid liver** 573.9
**Torsion**
  accessory tube 620.5
  adnexa (female) 620.5
  aorta (congenital) 747.29
    acquired 447.1
  appendix
    epididymis 608.24
    testis 608.23
  bile duct 576.8
    with calculus, choledocholithiasis or stones — *see* Choledocholithiasis
    congenital 751.69
  bowel, colon, or intestine 560.2
  cervix — *see* Malposition, uterus
  duodenum 537.3
  dystonia — *see* Dystonia, torsion
  epididymis 608.24
    appendix 608.24
  fallopian tube 620.5
  gallbladder (*see also* Disease, gallbladder) 575.8
    congenital 751.69
  gastric 537.89
  hydatid of Morgagni (female) 620.5
  kidney (pedicle) 593.89
  Meckel's diverticulum (congenital) 751.0
  mesentery 560.2
  omentum 560.2
  organ or site, congenital NEC — *see* Anomaly, specified type NEC
  ovary (pedicle) 620.5
    congenital 752.0
  oviduct 620.5
  penis 607.89
    congenital 752.69
  renal 593.89
  spasm — *see* Dystonia, torsion
  spermatic cord 608.22
    extravaginal 608.21
    intravaginal 608.22
  spleen 289.59
  testicle, testis 608.20

**Torsion** — *continued*
  testicle, testis — *continued*
    appendix 608.23
  tibia 736.89
  umbilical cord — *see* Compression, umbilical cord
  uterus (*see also* Malposition, uterus) 621.6
**Torticollis** (intermittent) (spastic) 723.5
  congenital 754.1
    sternomastoid 754.1
  due to birth injury 767.8
  hysterical 300.11
  ocular 781.93
  psychogenic 306.0
    specified as conversion reaction 300.11
  rheumatic 723.5
  rheumatoid 714.0
  spasmodic 333.83
  traumatic, current NEC 847.0
**Tortuous**
  artery 447.1
  fallopian tube 752.19
  organ or site, congenital NEC — *see* Distortion
  renal vessel (congenital) 747.62
  retina vessel (congenital) 743.58
    acquired 362.17
  ureter 593.4
  urethra 599.84
  vein — *see* Varicose, vein
**Torula, torular** (infection) 117.5
  histolytica 117.5
  lung 117.5
**Torulosis** 117.5
**Torus**
  fracture
    fibula 823.41
      with tibia 823.42
    radius 813.45
    tibia 823.40
      with fibula 823.42
  mandibularis 526.81
  palatinus 526.81
**Touch, vitreous** 997.99
**Touraine-Solente-Golé syndrome** (acropachyderma) 757.39
**Touraine's syndrome** (hereditary osteoonychodysplasia) 756.89
**Tourette's disease** (motor-verbal tic) 307.23
**Tower skull** 756.0
  with exophthalmos 756.0
**Toxemia** 799.89
  with
    abortion — *see* Abortion, by type, with toxemia
  bacterial — *see* Septicemia
  biliary (*see also* Disease, biliary) 576.8
  burn — *see* Burn, by site
  congenital NEC 779.89
  eclamptic 642.6 ☑
    with pre-existing hypertension 642.7 ☑
  erysipelatous (*see also* Erysipelas) 035
  fatigue 799.89
  fetus or newborn NEC 779.89
  food (*see also* Poisoning, food) 005.9
  gastric 537.89
  gastrointestinal 558.2
  intestinal 558.2
  kidney (*see also* Disease, renal) 593.9
  lung 518.89
  malarial NEC (*see also* Malaria) 084.6
  maternal (of pregnancy), affecting fetus or newborn 760.0
  myocardial — *see* Myocarditis, toxic
  of pregnancy (mild) (pre-eclamptic) 642.4 ☑
    with
      convulsions 642.6 ☑
      pre-existing hypertension 642.7 ☑
    affecting fetus or newborn 760.0
    severe 642.5 ☑

**Toxemia** — *continued*
  pre-eclamptic — *see* Toxemia, of pregnancy
  puerperal, postpartum — *see* Toxemia, of pregnancy
  pulmonary 518.89
  renal (*see also* Disease, renal) 593.9
  septic (*see also* Septicemia) 038.9
  small intestine 558.2
  staphylococcal 038.10
    aureus 038.11
    due to food 005.0
    specified organism NEC 038.19
  stasis 799.89
  stomach 537.89
  uremic (*see also* Uremia) 586
  urinary 586
**Toxemica cerebropathia psychica** (nonalcoholic) 294.0
  alcoholic 291.1
**Toxic** (poisoning) — *see also* condition
  from drug or poison — *see* Table of Drugs and Chemicals
  oil syndrome 710.5
  shock syndrome 040.82
  thyroid (gland) (*see also* Thyrotoxicosis) 242.9 ☑
**Toxicemia** — *see* Toxemia
**Toxicity**
  dilantin
    asymptomatic 796.0
    symptomatic — *see* Table of Drugs and Chemicals
  drug
    asymptomatic 796.0
    symptomatic — *see* Table of Drugs and Chemicals
  fava bean 282.2
  from drug or poison
    asymptomatic 796.0
    symptomatic — *see* Table of Drugs and Chemicals
**Toxicosis** — *see also* Toxemia 799.89
  capillary, hemorrhagic 287.0
**Toxinfection** 799.89
  gastrointestinal 558.2
**Toxocariasis** 128.0
**Toxoplasma infection, generalized** 130.9
**Toxoplasmosis** (acquired) 130.9
  with pneumonia 130.4
  congenital, active 771.2
  disseminated (multisystemic) 130.8
  maternal
    with suspected damage to fetus affecting management of pregnancy 655.4 ☑
    affecting fetus or newborn 760.2
    manifest toxoplasmosis in fetus or newborn 771.2
  multiple sites 130.8
  multisystemic disseminated 130.8
  specified site NEC 130.7
**Trabeculation, bladder** 596.8
**Trachea** — *see* condition
**Tracheitis** (acute) (catarrhal) (infantile) (membranous) (plastic) (pneumococcal) (septic) (suppurative) (viral) 464.10
  with
    bronchitis 490
      acute or subacute 466.0
      chronic 491.8
      tuberculosis — *see* Tuberculosis, pulmonary
    laryngitis (acute) 464.20
      with obstruction 464.21
      chronic 476.1
      tuberculous (*see also* Tuberculosis, larynx) 012.3 ☑
    obstruction 464.11
  chronic 491.8
    with
      bronchitis (chronic) 491.8
      laryngitis (chronic) 476.1

☑ Additional Digit Required — Refer to the Tabular List for Digit Selection
▽ Subterms under main terms may continue to next column or page

**2008 ICD-9-CM**
▶◀ Revised Text
● New Line
▲ Revised Code
**Volume 2 — 285**

**Trichocephaliasis** 127.3
**Trichocephalosis** 127.3
**Trichocephalus infestation** 127.3
**Trichoclasis** 704.2
**Trichoepithelioma** (M8100/0) — *see also* Neoplasm, skin, benign
  breast 217
  genital organ NEC — *see* Neoplasm, by site, benign
  malignant (M8100/3) — *see* Neoplasm, skin, malignant
**Trichofolliculoma** (M8101/0) — *see* Neoplasm, skin, benign
**Tricholemmoma** (M8102/0) — *see* Neoplasm, skin, benign
**Trichomatosis** 704.2
**Trichomoniasis** 131.9
  bladder 131.09
  cervix 131.09
  intestinal 007.3
  prostate 131.03
  seminal vesicle 131.09
  specified site NEC 131.8
  urethra 131.02
  urogenitalis 131.00
  vagina 131.01
  vulva 131.01
  vulvovaginal 131.01
**Trichomycosis** 039.0
  axillaris 039.0
  nodosa 111.2
  nodularis 111.2
  rubra 039.0
**Trichonocardiosis** (axillaris) (palmellina) 039.0
**Trichonodosis** 704.2
**Trichophytide** — *see* Dermatophytosis
**Trichophytid, trichophyton infection** — *see also* Dermatophytosis 110.9
**Trichophytobezoar** 938
  intestine 936
  stomach 935.2
**Trichophytosis** — *see* Dermatophytosis
**Trichoptilosis** 704.2
**Trichorrhexis** (nodosa) 704.2
**Trichosporosis nodosa** 111.2
**Trichostasis spinulosa** (congenital) 757.4
**Trichostrongyliasis** (small intestine) 127.6
**Trichostrongylosis** 127.6
**Trichostrongylus** (instabilis) infection 127.6
**Trichotillomania** 312.39
**Trichromat, anomalous** (congenital) 368.59
**Trichromatopsia, anomalous** (congenital) 368.59
**Trichuriasis** 127.3
**Trichuris trichiuria** (any site) (infection) (infestation) 127.3
**Tricuspid** (valve) — *see* condition
**Trifid** — *see also* Accessory
  kidney (pelvis) 753.3
  tongue 750.13
**Trigeminal neuralgia** — *see also* Neuralgia, trigeminal 350.1
**Trigeminoencephaloangiomatosis** 759.6
**Trigeminy** 427.89
  postoperative 997.1
**Trigger finger** (acquired) 727.03
  congenital 756.89
**Trigonitis** (bladder) (chronic) (pseudomembranous) 595.3
  tuberculous (*see also* Tuberculosis) 016.1 ☑
**Trigonocephaly** 756.0
**Trihexosidosis** 272.7
**Trilobate placenta** — *see* Placenta, abnormal
**Trilocular heart** 745.8
**Trimethylaminuria** 270.8
**Tripartita placenta** — *see* Placenta, abnormal
**Triple** — *see also* Accessory

**Triple** — *see also* Accessory — continued
  kidneys 753.3
  uteri 752.2
  X female 758.81
**Triplegia** 344.89
  congenital or infantile 343.8
**Triplet**
  affected by maternal complications of pregnancy 761.5
  healthy liveborn — *see* Newborn, multiple
  pregnancy (complicating delivery) NEC 651.1 ☑
    with fetal loss and retention of one or more fetus(es) 651.4 ☑
    following (elective) fetal reduction 651.7 ☑
**Triplex placenta** — *see* Placenta, abnormal
**Triplication** — *see* Accessory
**Trismus** 781.0
  neonatorum 771.3
  newborn 771.3
**Trisomy** (syndrome) NEC 758.5
  13 (partial) 758.1
  16-18 758.2
  18 (partial) 758.2
  21 (partial) 758.0
  22 758.0
  autosomes NEC 758.5
  $D_1$ 758.1
  $E_3$ 758.2
  G (group) 758.0
  group $D_1$ 758.1
  group E 758.2
  group G 758.0
**Tritanomaly** 368.53
**Tritanopia** 368.53
**Troisier-Hanot-Chauffard syndrome** (bronze diabetes) 275.0
**Trombidiosis** 133.8
**Trophedema** (hereditary) 757.0
  congenital 757.0
**Trophoblastic disease** — *see also* Hydatidiform mole 630
  previous, affecting management of pregnancy V23.1
**Tropholymphedema** 757.0
**Trophoneurosis** NEC 356.9
  arm NEC 354.9
  disseminated 710.1
  facial 349.89
  leg NEC 355.8
  lower extremity NEC 355.8
  upper extremity NEC 354.9
**Tropical** — *see also* condition
  maceration feet (syndrome) 991.4
  wet foot (syndrome) 991.4
**Trouble** — *see also* Disease
  bowel 569.9
  heart — *see* Disease, heart
  intestine 569.9
  kidney (*see also* Disease, renal) 593.9
  nervous 799.2
  sinus (*see also* Sinusitis) 473.9
**Trousseau's syndrome** (thrombophlebitis migrans) 453.1
**Truancy, childhood** — *see also* Disturbance, conduct
  socialized 312.2 ☑
  undersocialized, unsocialized 312.1 ☑
**Truncus**
  arteriosus (persistent) 745.0
  common 745.0
  communis 745.0
**Trunk** — *see* condition
**Trychophytide** — *see* Dermatophytosis
**Trypanosoma infestation** — *see* Trypanosomiasis
**Trypanosomiasis** 086.9
  with meningoencephalitis 086.9 [323.2]
  African 086.5
    due to Trypanosoma 086.5
      gambiense 086.3

**Trypanosomiasis** — continued
  African — continued
    due to Trypanosoma — continued
      rhodesiense 086.4
  American 086.2
    with
      heart involvement 086.0
      other organ involvement 086.1
    without mention of organ involvement 086.2
  Brazilian — *see* Trypanosomiasis, American
  Chagas' — *see* Trypanosomiasis, American
  due to Trypanosoma
    cruzi — *see* Trypanosomiasis, American
    gambiense 086.3
    rhodesiense 086.4
  gambiensis, Gambian 086.3
  North American — *see* Trypanosomiasis, American
  rhodesiense, Rhodesian 086.4
  South American — *see* Trypanosomiasis, American
**T-shaped incisors** 520.2
**Tsutsugamushi fever** 081.2
**Tubercle** — *see also* Tuberculosis
  brain, solitary 013.2 ☑
  Darwin's 744.29
  epithelioid noncaseating 135
  Ghon, primary infection 010.0 ☑
**Tuberculid, tuberculide** (indurating) (lichenoid) (miliary) (papulonecrotic) (primary) (skin) (subcutaneous) — *see also* Tuberculosis 017.0 ☑
**Tuberculoma** — *see also* Tuberculosis
  brain (any part) 013.2 ☑
  meninges (cerebral) (spinal) 013.1 ☑
  spinal cord 013.4 ☑
**Tuberculosis, tubercular, tuberculous** (calcification) (calcified) (caseous) (chromogenic acid-fast bacilli) (congenital) (degeneration) (disease) (fibrocaseous) (fistula) (gangrene) (interstitial) (isolated circumscribed lesions) (necrosis) (parenchymatous) (ulcerative) 011.9 ☑

---

*Note* — *Use the following fifth-digit subclassification with categories 010–018:*

0   *unspecified*

1   *bacteriological or histological examination not done*

2   *bacteriological or histological examination unknown (at present)*

3   *tubercle bacilli found (in sputum) by microscopy*

4   *tubercle bacilli not found (in sputum) by microscopy, but found by bacterial culture*

5   *tubercle bacilli not found by bacteriological exam–ination, but tuberculosis confirmed histologically*

6   *tubercle bacilli not found by bacteriological or histological examination, but tuberculosis confirmed by other methods [inoculation of animals]*

*For tuberculous conditions specified as late effects or sequelae, see category 137.*

---

  abdomen 014.8 ☑
    lymph gland 014.8 ☑
  abscess 011.9 ☑
    arm 017.9 ☑
    bone (*see also* Osteomyelitis, due to, tuberculosis) 015.9 ☑ [730.8]
      hip 015.1 ☑ [730.85]

**Tuberculosis, tubercular, tuberculous** — continued
  abscess — continued
    bone (*see also* Osteomyelitis, due to, tuberculosis) — continued
      knee 015.2 ☑ [730.86]
      sacrum 015.0 ☑ [730.88]
      specified site NEC 015.7 ☑ [730.88]
      spinal 015.0 ☑ [730.88]
      vertebra 015.0 ☑ [730.88]
    brain 013.3 ☑
    breast 017.9 ☑
    Cowper's gland 016.5 ☑
    dura (mater) 013.8 ☑
      brain 013.3 ☑
      spinal cord 013.5 ☑
    epidural 013.8 ☑
      brain 013.3 ☑
      spinal cord 013.5 ☑
    frontal sinus — *see* Tuberculosis, sinus
    genital organs NEC 016.9 ☑
      female 016.7 ☑
      male 016.5 ☑
    genitourinary NEC 016.9 ☑
    gland (lymphatic) — *see* Tuberculosis, lymph gland
    hip 015.1 ☑
    iliopsoas 015.0 ☑ [730.88]
    intestine 014.8 ☑
    ischiorectal 014.8 ☑
    joint 015.9 ☑
      hip 015.1 ☑
      knee 015.2 ☑
      specified joint NEC 015.8 ☑
      vertebral 015.0 ☑ [730.88]
    kidney 016.0 ☑ [590.81]
    knee 015.2 ☑
    lumbar 015.0 ☑ [730.88]
    lung 011.2 ☑
      primary, progressive 010.8 ☑
    meninges (cerebral) (spinal) 013.0 ☑
    pelvic 016.9 ☑
      female 016.7 ☑
      male 016.5 ☑
    perianal 014.8 ☑
      fistula 014.8 ☑
    perinephritic 016.0 ☑ [590.81]
    perineum 017.9 ☑
    perirectal 014.8 ☑
    psoas 015.0 ☑ [730.88]
    rectum 014.8 ☑
    retropharyngeal 012.8 ☑
    sacrum 015.0 ☑ [730.88]
    scrofulous 017.2 ☑
    scrotum 016.5 ☑
    skin 017.0 ☑
      primary 017.0 ☑
    spinal cord 013.5 ☑
    spine or vertebra (column) 015.0 ☑ [730.88]
    strumous 017.2 ☑
    subdiaphragmatic 014.8 ☑
    testis 016.5 ☑
    thigh 017.9 ☑
    urinary 016.3 ☑
      kidney 016.0 ☑ [590.81]
    uterus 016.7 ☑
  accessory sinus — *see* Tuberculosis, sinus
  Addison's disease 017.6 ☑
  adenitis (*see also* Tuberculosis, lymph gland) 017.2 ☑
  adenoids 012.8 ☑
  adenopathy (*see also* Tuberculosis, lymph gland) 017.2 ☑
    tracheobronchial 012.1 ☑
      primary progressive 010.8 ☑
  adherent pericardium 017.9 ☑ [420.0]
  adnexa (uteri) 016.7 ☑
  adrenal (capsule) (gland) 017.6 ☑

☑ Additional Digit Required — Refer to the Tabular List for Digit Selection      ▽ Subterms under main terms may continue to next column or page

**2008 ICD-9-CM**      ▶◀ Revised Text      ● New Line      ▲ Revised Code      **Volume 2 — 287**

Tuberculosis, tubercular, tuberculous

**Tuberculosis, tubercular, tuberculous**
— *continued*
　miliary — *continued*
　　acute 018.0 ☑
　　chronic 018.8 ☑
　　specified type NEC 018.8 ☑
　millstone makers' 011.4 ☑
　miners' 011.4 ☑
　moulders' 011.4 ☑
　mouth 017.9 ☑
　multiple 018.9 ☑
　　acute 018.0 ☑
　　chronic 018.8 ☑
　muscle 017.9 ☑
　myelitis 013.6 ☑
　myocarditis 017.9 ☑ *[422.0]*
　myocardium 017.9 ☑ *[422.0]*
　nasal (passage) (sinus) 012.8 ☑
　nasopharynx 012.8 ☑
　neck gland 017.2 ☑
　nephritis 016.0 ☑ *[583.81]*
　nerve 017.9 ☑
　nose (septum) 012.8 ☑
　ocular 017.3 ☑
　old NEC 137.0
　　without residuals V12.01
　omentum 014.8 ☑
　oophoritis (acute) (chronic) 016.6 ☑
　optic 017.3 ☑ *[377.39]*
　　nerve trunk 017.3 ☑ *[377.39]*
　　papilla, papillae 017.3 ☑ *[377.39]*
　orbit 017.3 ☑
　orchitis 016.5 ☑ *[608.81]*
　organ, specified NEC 017.9 ☑
　orificialis (primary) 017.0 ☑
　osseous (*see also* Tuberculosis, bone)
　　015.9 ☑ *[730.8]* ☑
　osteitis (*see also* Tuberculosis, bone)
　　015.9 ☑ *[730.8]* ☑
　osteomyelitis (*see also* Tuberculosis,
　　bone) 015.9 ☑ *[730.8]* ☑
　otitis (media) 017.4 ☑
　ovaritis (acute) (chronic) 016.6 ☑
　ovary (acute) (chronic) 016.6 ☑
　oviducts (acute) (chronic) 016.6 ☑
　pachymeningitis 013.0 ☑
　palate (soft) 017.9 ☑
　pancreas 017.9 ☑
　papulonecrotic (primary) 017.0 ☑
　parathyroid glands 017.9 ☑
　paronychia (primary) 017.0 ☑
　parotid gland or region 017.9 ☑
　pelvic organ NEC 016.9 ☑
　　female 016.7 ☑
　　male 016.5 ☑
　pelvis (bony) 015.7 ☑ *[730.85]*
　penis 016.5 ☑
　peribronchitis 011.3 ☑
　pericarditis 017.9 ☑ *[420.0]*
　pericardium 017.9 ☑ *[420.0]*
　perichondritis, larynx 012.3 ☑
　perineum 017.9 ☑
　periostitis (*see also* Tuberculosis,
　　bone) 015.9 ☑ *[730.8]* ☑
　periphlebitis 017.9 ☑
　　eye vessel 017.3 ☑ *[362.18]*
　　retina 017.3 ☑ *[362.18]*
　perirectal fistula 014.8 ☑
　peritoneal gland 014.8 ☑
　peritoneum 014.0 ☑
　peritonitis 014.0 ☑
　pernicious NEC (*see also* Tuberculo-
　　sis, pulmonary) 011.9 ☑
　pharyngitis 012.8 ☑
　pharynx 012.8 ☑
　phlyctenulosis (conjunctiva)
　　017.3 ☑ *[370.31]*
　phthisis NEC (*see also* Tuberculosis,
　　pulmonary) 011.9 ☑
　pituitary gland 017.9 ☑
　placenta 016.7 ☑

**Tuberculosis, tubercular, tuberculous**
— *continued*
　pleura, pleural, pleurisy, pleuritis
　　(fibrinous) (obliterative) (puru-
　　lent) (simple plastic) (with effu-
　　sion) 012.0 ☑
　　primary, progressive 010.1 ☑
　pneumonia, pneumonic 011.6 ☑
　pneumothorax 011.7 ☑
　polyserositis 018.9 ☑
　　acute 018.0 ☑
　　chronic 018.8 ☑
　potters' 011.4 ☑
　prepuce 016.5 ☑
　primary 010.9 ☑
　　complex 010.0 ☑
　　complicated 010.8 ☑
　　　with pleurisy or effusion
　　　　010.1 ☑
　　progressive 010.8 ☑
　　　with pleurisy or effusion
　　　　010.1 ☑
　　skin 017.0 ☑
　proctitis 014.8 ☑
　prostate 016.5 ☑ *[601.4]*
　prostatitis 016.5 ☑ *[601.4]*
　pulmonaris (*see also* Tuberculosis,
　　pulmonary) 011.9 ☑
　pulmonary (artery) (incipient) (malig-
　　nant) (multiple round foci) (per-
　　nicious) (reinfection stage)
　　011.9 ☑
　　cavitated or with cavitation
　　　011.2 ☑
　　　primary, progressive 010.8 ☑
　　childhood type or first infection
　　　010.0 ☑
　　chromogenic acid-fast bacilli
　　　795.39
　　fibrosis or fibrotic 011.4 ☑
　　infiltrative 011.0 ☑
　　　primary, progressive 010.9 ☑
　　nodular 011.1 ☑
　　specified NEC 011.8 ☑
　　sputum positive only 795.39
　　status following surgical collapse
　　　of lung NEC 011.9 ☑
　pyelitis 016.0 ☑ *[590.81]*
　pyelonephritis 016.0 ☑ *[590.81]*
　pyemia — *see* Tuberculosis, miliary
　pyonephrosis 016.0 ☑
　pyopneumothorax 012.0 ☑
　pyothorax 012.0 ☑
　rectum (with abscess) 014.8 ☑
　　fistula 014.8 ☑
　reinfection stage (*see also* Tuberculo-
　　sis, pulmonary) 011.9 ☑
　renal 016.0 ☑
　renis 016.0 ☑
　reproductive organ 016.7 ☑
　respiratory NEC (*see also* Tuberculo-
　　sis, pulmonary) 011.9 ☑
　　specified site NEC 012.8 ☑
　retina 017.3 ☑ *[363.13]*
　retroperitoneal (lymph gland or node)
　　014.8 ☑
　　gland 014.8 ☑
　retropharyngeal abscess 012.8 ☑
　rheumatism 015.9 ☑
　rhinitis 012.8 ☑
　sacroiliac (joint) 015.8 ☑
　sacrum 015.0 ☑ *[730.88]*
　salivary gland 017.9 ☑
　salpingitis (acute) (chronic) 016.6 ☑
　sandblasters' 011.4 ☑
　sclera 017.3 ☑ *[379.09]*
　scoliosis 015.0 ☑ *[737.43]*
　scrofulous 017.2 ☑
　scrotum 016.5 ☑
　seminal tract or vesicle
　　016.5 ☑ *[608.81]*
　senile NEC (*see also* Tuberculosis,
　　pulmonary) 011.9 ☑

**Tuberculosis, tubercular, tuberculous**
— *continued*
　septic NEC (*see also* Tuberculosis,
　　miliary) 018.9 ☑
　shoulder 015.8 ☑
　　blade 015.7 ☑ *[730.8]* ☑
　sigmoid 014.8 ☑
　sinus (accessory) (nasal) 012.8 ☑
　　bone 015.7 ☑ *[730.88]*
　　epididymis 016.4 ☑
　skeletal NEC (*see also* Osteomyelitis,
　　due to tuberculosis)
　　015.9 ☑ *[730.8]* ☑
　skin (any site) (primary) 017.0 ☑
　small intestine 014.8 ☑
　soft palate 017.9 ☑
　spermatic cord 016.5 ☑
　spinal
　　column 015.0 ☑ *[730.88]*
　　cord 013.4 ☑
　　disease 015.0 ☑ *[730.88]*
　　medulla 013.4 ☑
　　membrane 013.0 ☑
　　meninges 013.0 ☑
　spine 015.0 ☑ *[730.88]*
　spleen 017.7 ☑
　splenitis 017.7 ☑
　spondylitis 015.0 ☑ *[720.81]*
　spontaneous pneumothorax — *see*
　　Tuberculosis, pulmonary
　sternoclavicular joint 015.8 ☑
　stomach 017.9 ☑
　stonemasons' 011.4 ☑
　struma 017.2 ☑
　subcutaneous tissue (cellular) (prima-
　　ry) 017.0 ☑
　subcutis (primary) 017.0 ☑
　subdeltoid bursa 017.9 ☑
　submaxillary 017.9 ☑
　　region 017.9 ☑
　supraclavicular gland 017.2 ☑
　suprarenal (capsule) (gland) 017.6 ☑
　swelling, joint (*see also* Tuberculosis,
　　joint) 015.9 ☑
　symphysis pubis 015.7 ☑ *[730.88]*
　synovitis 015.9 ☑ *[727.01]*
　　hip 015.1 ☑ *[727.01]*
　　knee 015.2 ☑ *[727.01]*
　　specified site NEC 015.8 ☑ *[727.01]*
　　spine or vertebra 015.0 ☑ *[727.01]*
　systemic — *see* Tuberculosis, miliary
　tarsitis (eyelid) 017.0 ☑ *[373.4]*
　　ankle (bone) 015.5 ☑ *[730.87]*
　tendon (sheath) — *see* Tuberculosis,
　　tenosynovitis
　tenosynovitis 015.9 ☑ *[727.01]*
　　hip 015.1 ☑ *[727.01]*
　　knee 015.2 ☑ *[727.01]*
　　specified site NEC 015.8 ☑ *[727.01]*
　　spine or vertebra 015.0 ☑ *[727.01]*
　testis 016.5 ☑ *[608.81]*
　throat 012.8 ☑
　thymus gland 017.9 ☑
　thyroid gland 017.5 ☑
　toe 017.9 ☑
　tongue 017.9 ☑
　tonsil (lingual) 012.8 ☑
　tonsillitis 012.8 ☑
　trachea, tracheal 012.8 ☑
　　gland 012.1 ☑
　　　primary, progressive 010.8 ☑
　　isolated 012.2 ☑
　tracheobronchial 011.3 ☑
　　glandular 012.1 ☑
　　　primary, progressive 010.8 ☑
　　isolated 012.2 ☑
　　lymph gland or node 012.1 ☑
　　　primary, progressive 010.8 ☑
　tubal 016.6 ☑
　tunica vaginalis 016.5 ☑
　typhlitis 014.8 ☑
　ulcer (primary) (skin) 017.0 ☑
　　bowel or intestine 014.8 ☑

**Tuberculosis, tubercular, tuberculous**
— *continued*
　ulcer — *continued*
　　specified site NEC — *see* Tubercu-
　　　losis, by site
　　unspecified site — *see* Tuberculosis,
　　　pulmonary
　ureter 016.2 ☑
　urethra, urethral 016.3 ☑
　urinary organ or tract 016.3 ☑
　　kidney 016.0 ☑
　uterus 016.7 ☑
　uveal tract 017.3 ☑ *[363.13]*
　uvula 017.9 ☑
　vaccination, prophylactic (against)
　　V03.2
　vagina 016.7 ☑
　vas deferens 016.5 ☑
　vein 017.9 ☑
　verruca (primary) 017.0 ☑
　verrucosa (cutis) (primary) 017.0 ☑
　vertebra (column) 015.0 ☑ *[730.88]*
　vesiculitis 016.5 ☑ *[608.81]*
　viscera NEC 014.8 ☑
　vulva 016.7 ☑ *[616.51]*
　wrist (joint) 015.8 ☑
　　bone 015.5 ☑ *[730.83]*

**Tuberculum**
　auriculae 744.29
　occlusal 520.2
　paramolare 520.2

**Tuberosity**
　jaw, excessive 524.07
　maxillary, entire 524.07

**Tuberous sclerosis** (brain) 759.5

**Tube, tubal, tubular** — *see also* condi-
　tion
　ligation, admission for V25.2

**Tubo-ovarian** — *see* condition

**Tuboplasty, after previous sterilization**
　V26.0

**Tubotympanitis** 381.10

**Tularemia** 021.9
　with
　　conjunctivitis 021.3
　　pneumonia 021.2
　bronchopneumonic 021.2
　conjunctivitis 021.3
　cryptogenic 021.1
　disseminated 021.8
　enteric 021.1
　generalized 021.8
　glandular 021.8
　intestinal 021.1
　oculoglandular 021.3
　ophthalmic 021.3
　pneumonia 021.2
　pulmonary 021.2
　specified NEC 021.8
　typhoidal 021.1
　ulceroglandular 021.0
　vaccination, prophylactic (against)
　　V03.4

**Tularensis conjunctivitis** 021.3

**Tumefaction** — *see also* Swelling
　liver (*see also* Hypertrophy, liver)
　　789.1

**Tumor** (M8000/1) — *see also* Neoplasm,
　　by site, unspecified nature
　Abrikossov's (M9580/0) (*see also*
　　Neoplasm, connective tissue,
　　benign)
　　malignant (M9580/3) — *see* Neo-
　　　plasm, connective tissue,
　　　malignant
　acinar cell (M8550/1) — *see* Neo-
　　plasm, by site, uncertain behav-
　　ior
　acinic cell (M8550/1) — *see* Neo-
　　plasm, by site, uncertain behav-
　　ior
　adenomatoid (M9054/0) (*see also*
　　Neoplasm, by site, benign)
　　odontogenic (M9300/0) 213.1
　　　upper jaw (bone) 213.0

---

☑ Additional Digit Required — Refer to the Tabular List for Digit Selection　　　　　　▽ Subterms under main terms may continue to next column or page

**2008 ICD-9-CM**　　　　▶◀ Revised Text　　　　● New Line　　　　▲ Revised Code　　　　**Volume 2 — 289**

**Tumor** — *see also* Neoplasm, by site, unspecified nature — *continued*
adnexal (skin) (M8390/0) — *see* Neoplasm, skin, benign
adrenal
  cortical (benign) (M8370/0) 227.0
    malignant (M8370/3) 194.0
  rest (M8671/0) — *see* Neoplasm, by site, benign
alpha cell (M8152/0)
  malignant (M8152/3)
    pancreas 157.4
    specified site NEC — *see* Neoplasm, by site, malignant
    unspecified site 157.4
  pancreas 211.7
  specified site NEC — *see* Neoplasm, by site, benign
  unspecified site 211.7
aneurysmal (*see also* Aneurysm) 442.9
aortic body (M8691/1) 237.3
  malignant (M8691/3) 194.6
argentaffin (M8241/1) — *see* Neoplasm, by site, uncertain behavior
basal cell (M8090/1) (*see also* Neoplasm, skin, uncertain behavior)
benign (M8000/0) — *see* Neoplasm, by site, benign
beta cell (M8151/0)
  malignant (M8151/3)
    pancreas 157.4
    specified site — *see* Neoplasm, by site, malignant
    unspecified site 157.4
  pancreas 211.7
  specified site NEC — *see* Neoplasm, by site, benign
  unspecified site 211.7
blood — *see* Hematoma
Brenner (M9000/0) 220
  borderline malignancy (M9000/1) 236.2
  malignant (M9000/3) 183.0
  proliferating (M9000/1) 236.2
Brooke's (M8100/0) — *see* Neoplasm, skin, benign
brown fat (M8880/0) — *see* Lipoma, by site
Burkitt's (M9750/3) 200.2 ☑
calcifying epithelial odontogenic (M9340/0) 213.1
  upper jaw (bone) 213.0
carcinoid (M8240/1) — *see* Carcinoid
carotid body (M8692/1) 237.3
  malignant (M8692/3) 194.5
Castleman's (mediastinal lymph node hyperplasia) 785.6
cells (M8001/1) (*see also* Neoplasm, by site, unspecified nature)
  benign (M8001/0) — *see* Neoplasm, by site, benign
  malignant (M8001/3) — *see* Neoplasm, by site, malignant
  uncertain whether benign or malignant (M8001/1) — *see* Neoplasm, by site, uncertain nature
cervix
  in pregnancy or childbirth 654.6 ☑
    affecting fetus or newborn 763.89
    causing obstructed labor 660.2 ☑
      affecting fetus or newborn 763.1
chondromatous giant cell (M9230/0) — *see* Neoplasm, bone, benign
chromaffin (M8700/0) (*see also* Neoplasm, by site, benign)
  malignant (M8700/3) — *see* Neoplasm, by site, malignant
Cock's peculiar 706.2
Codman's (benign chondroblastoma) (M9230/0) — *see* Neoplasm, bone, benign

**Tumor** — *see also* Neoplasm, by site, unspecified nature — *continued*
dentigerous, mixed (M9282/0) 213.1
  upper jaw (bone) 213.0
dermoid (M9084/0) — *see* Neoplasm, by site, benign
  with malignant transformation (M9084/3) 183.0
desmoid (extra-abdominal) (M8821/1) (*see also* Neoplasm, connective tissue, uncertain behavior)
  abdominal (M8822/1) — *see* Neoplasm, connective tissue, uncertain behavior
embryonal (mixed) (M9080/1) (*see also* Neoplasm, by site, uncertain behavior)
  liver (M9080/3) 155.0
endodermal sinus (M9071/3)
  specified site — *see* Neoplasm, by site, malignant
  unspecified site
    female 183.0
    male 186.9
epithelial
  benign (M8010/0) — *see* Neoplasm, by site, benign
  malignant (M8010/0) — *see* Neoplasm, by site, malignant
Ewing's (M9260/3) — *see* Neoplasm, bone, malignant
fatty — *see* Lipoma
fetal, causing disproportion 653.7 ☑
  causing obstructed labor 660.1 ☑
fibroid (M8890/0) — *see* Leiomyoma
G cell (M8153/1)
  malignant (M8153/3)
    pancreas 157.4
    specified site NEC — *see* Neoplasm, by site, malignant
    unspecified site 157.4
  specified site — *see* Neoplasm, by site, uncertain behavior
  unspecified site 235.5
giant cell (type) (M8003/1) (*see also* Neoplasm, by site, unspecified nature)
  bone (M9250/1) 238.0
    malignant (M9250/3) — *see* Neoplasm, bone, malignant
  chondromatous (M9230/0) — *see* Neoplasm, bone, benign
  malignant (M8003/3) — *see* Neoplasm, by site, malignant
  peripheral (gingiva) 523.8
  soft parts (M9251/1) (*see also* Neoplasm, connective tissue, uncertain behavior)
    malignant (M9251/3) — *see* Neoplasm, connective tissue, malignant
  tendon sheath 727.02
glomus (M8711/0) (*see also* Hemangioma, by site)
  jugulare (M8690/1) 237.3
    malignant (M8690/3) 194.6
gonadal stromal (M8590/1) — *see* Neoplasm, by site, uncertain behavior
granular cell (M9580/0) (*see also* Neoplasm, connective tissue, benign)
  malignant (M9580/3) — *see* Neoplasm, connective tissue, malignant
granulosa cell (M8620/1) 236.2
  malignant (M8620/3) 183.0
granulosa cell-theca cell (M8621/1) 236.2
  malignant (M8621/3) 183.0
Grawitz's (hypernephroma) (M8312/3) 189.0
hazard-crile (M8350/3) 193
hemorrhoidal — *see* Hemorrhoids
hilar cell (M8660/0) 220

**Tumor** — *see also* Neoplasm, by site, unspecified nature — *continued*
Hürthle cell (benign) (M8290/0) 226
  malignant (M8290/3) 193
hydatid (*see also* Echinococcus) 122.9
hypernephroid (M8311/1) (*see also* Neoplasm, by site, uncertain behavior)
interstitial cell (M8650/1) (*see also* Neoplasm, by site, uncertain behavior)
  benign (M8650/0) — *see* Neoplasm, by site, benign
  malignant (M8650/3) — *see* Neoplasm, by site, malignant
islet cell (M8150/0)
  malignant (M8150/3)
    pancreas 157.4
    specified site — *see* Neoplasm, by site, malignant
    unspecified site 157.4
  pancreas 211.7
  specified site NEC — *see* Neoplasm, by site, benign
  unspecified site 211.7
juxtaglomerular (M8361/1) 236.91
Krukenberg's (M8490/6) 198.6
Leydig cell (M8650/1)
  benign (M8650/0)
    specified site — *see* Neoplasm, by site, benign
    unspecified site
      female 220
      male 222.0
  malignant (M8650/3)
    specified site — *see* Neoplasm, by site, malignant
    unspecified site
      female 183.0
      male 186.9
  specified site — *see* Neoplasm, by site, uncertain behavior
  unspecified site
    female 236.2
    male 236.4
lipid cell, ovary (M8670/0) 220
lipoid cell, ovary (M8670/0) 220
lymphomatous, benign (M9590/0) (*see also* Neoplasm, by site, benign)
Malherbe's (M8110/0) — *see* Neoplasm, skin, benign
malignant (M8000/3) (*see also* Neoplasm, by site, malignant)
  fusiform cell (type) (M8004/3) — *see* Neoplasm, by site, malignant
  giant cell (type) (M8003/3) — *see* Neoplasm, by site, malignant
  mixed NEC (M8940/3) — *see* Neoplasm, by site, malignant
  small cell (type) (M8002/3) — *see* Neoplasm, by site, malignant
  spindle cell (type) (M8004/3) — *see* Neoplasm, by site, malignant
mast cell (M9740/1) 238.5
  malignant (M9740/3) 202.6 ☑
melanotic, neuroectodermal (M9363/0) — *see* Neoplasm, by site, benign
Merkel cell — *see* Neoplasm, by site, malignant
mesenchymal
  malignant (M8800/3) — *see* Neoplasm, connective tissue, malignant
  mixed (M8990/1) — *see* Neoplasm, connective tissue, uncertain behavior
mesodermal, mixed (M8951/3) (*see also* Neoplasm, by site, malignant)
  liver 155.0
mesonephric (M9110/1) (*see also* Neoplasm, by site, uncertain behavior)

**Tumor** — *see also* Neoplasm, by site, unspecified nature — *continued*
mesonephric (*see also* Neoplasm, by site, uncertain behavior) — *continued*
  malignant (M9110/3) — *see* Neoplasm, by site, malignant
metastatic
  from specified site (M8000/3) — *see* Neoplasm, by site, malignant
  to specified site (M8000/6) — *see* Neoplasm, by site, malignant, secondary
mixed NEC (M8940/0) (*see also* Neoplasm, by site, benign)
  malignant (M8940/3) — *see* Neoplasm, by site, malignant
mucocarcinoid, malignant (M8243/3) — *see* Neoplasm, by site, malignant
mucoepidermoid (M8430/1) — *see* Neoplasm, by site, uncertain behavior
Mullerian, mixed (M8950/3) — *see* Neoplasm, by site, malignant
myoepithelial (M8982/0) — *see* Neoplasm, by site, benign
neurogenic olfactory (M9520/3) 160.0
nonencapsulated sclerosing (M8350/3) 193
odontogenic (M9270/1) 238.0
  adenomatoid (M9300/0) 213.1
    upper jaw (bone) 213.0
  benign (M9270/0) 213.1
    upper jaw (bone) 213.0
  calcifying epithelial (M9340/0) 213.1
    upper jaw (bone) 213.0
  malignant (M9270/3) 170.1
    upper jaw (bone) 170.0
  squamous (M9312/0) 213.1
    upper jaw (bone) 213.0
ovarian stromal (M8590/1) 236.2
ovary
  in pregnancy or childbirth 654.4 ☑
    affecting fetus or newborn 763.89
    causing obstructed labor 660.2 ☑
      affecting fetus or newborn 763.1
pacinian (M9507/0) — *see* Neoplasm, skin, benign
Pancoast's (M8010/3) 162.3
papillary — *see* Papilloma
pelvic, in pregnancy or childbirth 654.9 ☑
  affecting fetus or newborn 763.89
  causing obstructed labor 660.2 ☑
  affecting fetus or newborn 763.1
phantom 300.11
plasma cell (M9731/1) 238.6
  benign (M9731/0) — *see* Neoplasm, by site, benign
  malignant (M9731/3) 203.8 ☑
polyvesicular vitelline (M9071/3)
  specified site — *see* Neoplasm, by site, malignant
  unspecified site
    female 183.0
    male 186.9
Pott's puffy (*see also* Osteomyelitis) 730.2 ☑
Rathke's pouch (M9350/1) 237.0
regaud's (M8082/3) — *see* Neoplasm, nasopharynx, malignant
rete cell (M8140/0) 222.0
retinal anlage (M9363/0) — *see* Neoplasm, by site, benign
Rokitansky's 620.2
salivary gland type, mixed (M8940/0) (*see also* Neoplasm, by site, benign)
  malignant (M8940/3) — *see* Neoplasm, by site, malignant

---

☑ Additional Digit Required — Refer to the Tabular List for Digit Selection      🖋 Subterms under main terms may continue to next column or page

290 — Volume 2      ▶◀ Revised Text      ● New Line      ▲ Revised Code      *2008 ICD-9-CM*

**Tumor** — see also Neoplasm, by site, unspecified nature — continued
Sampson's 617.1
Schloffer's (see also Peritonitis) 567.29
Schmincke (M8082/3) — see Neoplasm, nasopharynx, malignant
sebaceous (see also Cyst, sebaceous) 706.2
secondary (M8000/6) — see Neoplasm, by site, secondary
Sertoli cell (M8640/0)
  with lipid storage (M8641/0)
    specified site — see Neoplasm, by site, benign
    unspecified site
      female 220
      male 222.0
  specified site — see Neoplasm, by site, benign
  unspecified site
    female 220
    male 222.0
Sertoli-Leydig cell (M8631/0)
  specified site, — see Neoplasm, by site, benign
  unspecified site
    female 220
    male 222.0
sex cord (-stromal) (M8590/1) — see Neoplasm, by site, uncertain behavior
skin appendage (M8390/0) — see Neoplasm, skin, benign
soft tissue
  benign (M8800/0) — see Neoplasm, connective tissue, benign
  malignant (M8800/3) — see Neoplasm, connective tissue, malignant
sternomastoid 754.1
stromal
  abdomen
    benign 215.5
    malignant 171.5
    uncertain behavior 238.1
  digestive system 238.1
    benign 215.5
    malignant 171.5
    uncertain behavior 238.1
  gastric 238.1
    benign 215.5
    malignant 171.5
    uncertain behavior 238.1
  gastrointestinal 238.1
    benign 215.5
    malignant 171.5
    uncertain behavior 238.1
  intestine (small) (large) 238.1
    benign 215.5
    malignant 171.5
    uncertain behavior 238.1
  stomach 238.1
    benign 215.5
    malignant 171.5
    uncertain behavior 238.1
superior sulcus (lung) (pulmonary) (syndrome) (M8010/3) 162.3
suprasulcus (M8010/3) 162.3
sweat gland (M8400/1) (see also Neoplasm, skin, uncertain behavior)
  benign (M8400/0) — see Neoplasm, skin, benign
  malignant (M8400/3) — see Neoplasm, skin, malignant
syphilitic brain 094.89
  congenital 090.49
testicular stromal (M8590/1) 236.4
theca cell (M8600/0) 220
theca cell-granulosa cell (M8621/1) 236.2
theca-lutein (M8610/0) 220
turban (M8200/0) 216.4
uterus
  in pregnancy or childbirth 654.1 ☑

**Tumor** — see also Neoplasm, by site, unspecified nature — continued
uterus — continued
  in pregnancy or childbirth — continued
    affecting fetus or newborn 763.89
    causing obstructed labor 660.2 ☑
      affecting fetus or newborn 763.1
vagina
  in pregnancy or childbirth 654.7 ☑
    affecting fetus or newborn 763.89
    causing obstructed labor 660.2 ☑
      affecting fetus or newborn 763.1
varicose (see also Varicose, vein) 454.9
von Recklinghausen's (M9540/1) 237.71
vulva
  in pregnancy or childbirth 654.8 ☑
    affecting fetus or newborn 763.89
    causing obstructed labor 660.2 ☑
      affecting fetus or newborn 763.1
Warthin's (salivary gland) (M8561/0) 210.2
white (see also Tuberculosis, arthritis)
White-Darier 757.39
Wilms' (nephroblastoma) (M8960/3) 189.0
yolk sac (M9071/3)
  specified site — see Neoplasm, by site, malignant
  unspecified site
    female 183.0
    male 186.9
**Tumorlet (M8040/1)** — see Neoplasm, by site, uncertain behavior
**Tungiasis** 134.1
**Tunica vasculosa lentis** 743.39
**Tunnel vision** 368.45
**Turban tumor** (M8200/0) 216.4
**Türck's trachoma** (chronic catarrhal laryngitis) 476.0
**Türk's syndrome** (ocular retraction syndrome) 378.71
**Turner's**
hypoplasia (tooth) 520.4
syndrome 758.6
tooth 520.4
**Turner-Kieser syndrome** (hereditary osteo-onychodysplasia) 756.89
**Turner-Varny syndrome** 758.6
**Turricephaly** 756.0
**Tussis convulsiva** — see also Whooping cough 033.9
**Twin**
affected by maternal complications of pregnancy 761.5
conjoined 759.4
healthy liveborn — see Newborn, twin
pregnancy (complicating delivery) NEC 651.0 ☑
  with fetal loss and retention of one fetus 651.3 ☑
following (elective) fetal reduction
**Twinning, teeth** 520.2
**Twist, twisted**
bowel, colon, or intestine 560.2
hair (congenital) 757.4
mesentery 560.2
omentum 560.2
organ or site, congenital NEC — see Anomaly, specified type NEC
ovarian pedicle 620.5
  congenital 752.0
umbilical cord — see Compression, umbilical cord
**Twitch** 781.0
**Tylosis** 700

**Tylosis** — continued
buccalis 528.6
gingiva 523.8
linguae 528.6
palmaris et plantaris 757.39
**Tympanism** 787.3
**Tympanites** (abdominal) (intestine) 787.3
**Tympanitis** — see Myringitis
**Tympanosclerosis** 385.00
involving
  combined sites NEC 385.09
    with tympanic membrane 385.03
  tympanic membrane 385.01
    with ossicles 385.02
      and middle ear 385.03
**Tympanum** — see condition
**Tympany**
abdomen 787.3
chest 786.7
**Typhlitis** — see also Appendicitis 541
**Typhoenteritis** 002.0
**Typhogastric fever** 002.0
**Typhoid** (abortive) (ambulant) (any site) (fever) (hemorrhagic) (infection) (intermittent) (malignant) (rheumatic) 002.0
with pneumonia 002.0 [484.8]
abdominal 002.0
carrier (suspected) of V02.1
cholecystitis (current) 002.0
clinical (Widal and blood test negative) 002.0
endocarditis 002.0 [421.1]
inoculation reaction — see Complications, vaccination
meningitis 002.0 [320.7]
mesenteric lymph nodes 002.0
myocarditis 002.0 [422.0]
osteomyelitis (see also Osteomyelitis, due to, typhoid) 002.0 [730.8] ☑
perichondritis, larynx 002.0 [478.71]
pneumonia 002.0 [484.8]
spine 002.0 [720.81]
ulcer (perforating) 002.0
vaccination, prophylactic (against) V03.1
Widal negative 002.0
**Typhomalaria** (fever) — see also Malaria 084.6
**Typhomania** 002.0
**Typhoperitonitis** 002.0
**Typhus** (fever) 081.9
abdominal, abdominalis 002.0
African tick 082.1
amarillic (see also Fever, Yellow) 060.9
brain 081.9
cerebral 081.9
classical 080
endemic (flea-borne) 081.0
epidemic (louse-borne) 080
exanthematic NEC 080
exanthematicus SAI 080
  brillii SAI 081.1
  Mexicanus SAI 081.0
  pediculo vestimenti causa 080
  typhus murinus 081.0
flea-borne 081.0
Indian tick 082.1
Kenya tick 082.1
louse-borne 080
Mexican 081.0
  flea-borne 081.0
  louse-borne 080
  tabardillo 080
mite-borne 081.2
murine 081.0
North Asian tick-borne 082.2
petechial 081.9
Queensland tick 082.3
rat 081.0
recrudescent 081.1
recurrent (see also Fever, relapsing) 087.9
São Paulo 082.0

**Typhus** — continued
scrub (China) (India) (Malaya) (New Guinea) 081.2
shop (of Malaya) 081.0
Siberian tick 082.2
tick-borne NEC 082.9
tropical 081.2
vaccination, prophylactic (against) V05.8
**Tyrosinemia** 270.2
neonatal 775.89
**Tyrosinosis** (Medes) (Sakai) 270.2
**Tyrosinuria** 270.2
**Tyrosyluria** 270.2

## U

**Uehlinger's syndrome** (acropachyderma) 757.39
**Uhl's anomaly or disease** (hypoplasia of myocardium, right ventricle) 746.84
**Ulcerosa scarlatina** 034.1
**Ulcer, ulcerated, ulcerating, ulceration, ulcerative** 707.9
with gangrene 707.9 [785.4]
abdomen (wall) (see also Ulcer, skin) 707.8
ala, nose 478.19
alveolar process 526.5
amebic (intestine) 006.9
  skin 006.6
anastomotic — see Ulcer, gastrojejunal
anorectal 569.41
antral — see Ulcer, stomach
anus (sphincter) (solitary) 569.41
  varicose — see Varicose, ulcer, anus
aorta — see Aneuysm
aphthous (oral) (recurrent) 528.2
  genital organ(s)
    female 616.50 ▲
    male 608.89
  mouth 528.2
arm (see also Ulcer, skin) 707.8
arteriosclerotic plaque — see Arteriosclerosis, by site
artery NEC 447.2
  without rupture 447.8
atrophic NEC — see Ulcer, skin
Barrett's (chronic peptic ulcer of esophagus) 530.85
bile duct 576.8
bladder (solitary) (sphincter) 596.8
  bilharzial (see also Schistosomiasis) 120.9 [595.4]
  submucosal (see also Cystitis) 595.1
  tuberculous (see also Tuberculosis) 016.1 ☑
bleeding NEC — see Ulcer, peptic, with hemorrhage
bone 730.9 ☑
bowel (see also Ulcer, intestine) 569.82
breast 611.0
bronchitis 491.8
bronchus 519.19
buccal (cavity) (traumatic) 528.9
burn (acute) — see Ulcer, duodenum
Buruli 031.1
buttock (see also Ulcer, skin) 707.8
  decubitus (see also Ulcer, decubitus) 707.00
cancerous (M8000/3) — see Neoplasm, by site, malignant
cardia — see Ulcer, stomach
cardio-esophageal (peptic) 530.20
  with bleeding 530.21
cecum (see also Ulcer, intestine) 569.82
cervix (uteri) (trophic) 622.0
  with mention of cervicitis 616.0
chancroidal 099.0
chest (wall) (see also Ulcer, skin) 707.8

☑ Additional Digit Required — Refer to the Tabular List for Digit Selection
▲ Subterms under main terms may continue to next column or page
**2008 ICD-9-CM**
▶◀ Revised Text
● New Line
▲ Revised Code
**October 2007 • Volume 2 — 291**

Tumor — Ulcer, ulcerated, ulcerating

**Ulcer, ulcerated, ulcerating, ulceration, ulcerative** — *continued*
Chiclero 085.4
chin (pyogenic) (*see also* Ulcer, skin) 707.8
chronic (cause unknown) (*see also* Ulcer, skin)
  penis 607.89
Cochin-China 085.1
colitis — *see* Colitis, ulcerative
colon (*see also* Ulcer, intestine) 569.82
conjunctiva (acute) (postinfectional) 372.00
cornea (infectional) 370.00
  with perforation 370.06
  annular 370.02
  catarrhal 370.01
  central 370.03
  dendritic 054.42
  marginal 370.01
  mycotic 370.05
  phlyctenular, tuberculous (*see also* Tuberculosis) 017.3 ☑ [370.31]
  ring 370.02
  rodent 370.07
  serpent, serpiginous 370.04
  superficial marginal 370.01
  tuberculous (*see also* Tuberculosis) 017.3 ☑ [370.31]
corpus cavernosum (chronic) 607.89
crural — *see* Ulcer, lower extremity
Curling's — *see* Ulcer, duodenum
Cushing's — *see* Ulcer, peptic
cystitis (interstitial) 595.1
decubitus (unspecified site) 707.00
  with gangrene 707.00 [785.4]
  ankle 707.06
  back
    lower 707.03
    upper 707.02
  buttock 707.05
  elbow 707.01
  head 707.09
  heel 707.07
  hip 707.04
  other site 707.09
  sacrum 707.03
  shoulder blades 707.02
dendritic 054.42
diabetes, diabetic (mellitus) 250.8 ☑ [707.9]
  lower limb 250.8 ☑ [707.10]
    ankle 250.8 ☑ [707.13]
    calf 250.8 ☑ [707.12]
    foot 250.8 ☑ [707.15]
    heel 250.8 ☑ [707.14]
    knee 250.8 ☑ [707.19]
    specified site NEC 250.8 ☑ [707.19]
    thigh 250.8 ☑ [707.11]
    toes 250.8 ☑ [707.15]
  specified site NEC 250.8 ☑ [707.8]
Dieulafoy — *see* Lesion, Dieulafoy
due to
  infection NEC — *see* Ulcer, skin
  radiation, radium — *see* Ulcer, by site
  trophic disturbance (any region) — *see* Ulcer, skin
  x-ray — *see* Ulcer, by site
duodenum, duodenal (eroded) (peptic) 532.9 ☑

*Note — Use the following fifth-digit subclassification with categories 531–534:*
0  *without mention of obstruction*
1  *with obstruction*

  with
    hemorrhage (chronic) 532.4 ☑
      and perforation 532.6 ☑
    perforation (chronic) 532.5 ☑
      and hemorrhage 532.6 ☑
  acute 532.3 ☑

**Ulcer, ulcerated, ulcerating, ulceration, ulcerative** — *continued*
duodenum, duodenal — *continued*
  acute — *continued*
    with
      hemorrhage 532.0 ☑
        and perforation 532.2 ☑
      perforation 532.1 ☑
        and hemorrhage 532.2 ☑
    bleeding (recurrent) — *see* Ulcer, duodenum, with hemorrhage
  chronic 532.7 ☑
    with
      hemorrhage 532.4 ☑
        and perforation 532.6 ☑
      perforation 532.5 ☑
        and hemorrhage 532.6 ☑
  penetrating — *see* Ulcer, duodenum, with perforation
  perforating — *see* Ulcer, duodenum, with perforation
dysenteric NEC 009.0
elusive 595.1
endocarditis (any valve) (acute) (chronic) (subacute) 421.0
enteritis — *see* Colitis, ulcerative
enterocolitis 556.0
epiglottis 478.79
esophagus (peptic) 530.20
  with bleeding 530.21
  due to ingestion
    aspirin 530.20
    chemicals 530.20
    medicinal agents 530.20
  fungal 530.20
  infectional 530.20
  varicose (*see also* Varix, esophagus) 456.1
    bleeding (*see also* Varix, esophagus, bleeding) 456.0
eye NEC 360.00
  dendritic 054.42
eyelid (region) 373.01
face (*see also* Ulcer, skin) 707.8
fauces 478.29
Fenwick (-Hunner) (solitary) (*see also* Cystitis) 595.1
fistulous NEC — *see* Ulcer, skin
foot (indolent) (*see also* Ulcer, lower extremity) 707.15
  perforating 707.15
    leprous 030.1
    syphilitic 094.0
  trophic 707.15
  varicose 454.0
    inflamed or infected 454.2
frambesial, initial or primary 102.0
gallbladder or duct 575.8
gall duct 576.8
gangrenous (*see also* Gangrene) 785.4
gastric — *see* Ulcer, stomach
gastrocolic — *see* Ulcer, gastrojejunal
gastroduodenal — *see* Ulcer, peptic
gastroesophageal — *see* Ulcer, stomach
gastrohepatic — *see* Ulcer, stomach
gastrointestinal — *see* Ulcer, gastrojejunal
gastrojejunal (eroded) (peptic) 534.9 ☑

*Note — Use the following fifth-digit subclassification with categories 531–534:*
0  *without mention of obstruction*
1  *with obstruction*

  with
    hemorrhage (chronic) 534.4 ☑
      and perforation 534.6 ☑
    perforation 534.5 ☑
      and hemorrhage 534.6 ☑
  acute 534.3 ☑
    with
      hemorrhage 534.0 ☑
        and perforation 534.2 ☑
      perforation 534.1 ☑

**Ulcer, ulcerated, ulcerating, ulceration, ulcerative** — *continued*
gastrojejunal — *continued*
  acute — *continued*
    with — *continued*
      perforation — *continued*
        and hemorrhage 534.2 ☑
    bleeding (recurrent) — *see* Ulcer, gastrojejunal, with hemorrhage
  chronic 534.7 ☑
    with
      hemorrhage 534.4 ☑
        and perforation 534.6 ☑
      perforation 534.5 ☑
        and hemorrhage 534.6 ☑
  penetrating — *see* Ulcer, gastrojejunal, with perforation
  perforating — *see* Ulcer, gastrojejunal, with perforation
gastrojejunocolic — *see* Ulcer, gastrojejunal
genital organ
  female 629.89
  male 608.89
gingiva 523.8
gingivitis 523.10
glottis 478.79
granuloma of pudenda 099.2
groin (*see also* Ulcer, skin) 707.8
gum 523.8
gumma, due to yaws 102.4
hand (*see also* Ulcer, skin) 707.8
hard palate 528.9
heel (*see also* Ulcer, lower extremity) 707.14
  decubitus (*see also* Ulcer, decubitus) 707.07
hemorrhoids 455.8
  external 455.5
  internal 455.2
hip (*see also* Ulcer, skin) 707.8
  decubitus (*see also* Ulcer, decubitus) 707.04
Hunner's 595.1
hypopharynx 478.29
hypopyon (chronic) (subacute) 370.04
hypostaticum — *see* Ulcer, varicose
ileocolitis 556.1
ileum (*see also* Ulcer, intestine) 569.82
intestine, intestinal 569.82
  with perforation 569.83
  amebic 006.9
  duodenal — *see* Ulcer, duodenum
  granulocytopenic (with hemorrhage) 288.09
  marginal 569.82
  perforating 569.83
  small, primary 569.82
  stercoraceous 569.82
  stercoral 569.82
  tuberculous (*see also* Tuberculosis) 014.8 ☑
  typhoid (fever) 002.0
  varicose 456.8
ischemic 707.9
  lower extremity (*see also* Ulcer, lower extremity) 707.10
    ankle 707.13
    calf 707.12
    foot 707.15
    heel 707.14
    knee 707.19
    specified site NEC 707.19
    thigh 707.11
    toes 707.15
jejunum, jejunal — *see* Ulcer, gastrojejunal
keratitis (*see also* Ulcer, cornea) 370.00
knee — *see* Ulcer, lower extremity
labium (majus) (minus) 616.50
laryngitis (*see also* Laryngitis) 464.00
  with obstruction 464.01
larynx (aphthous) (contact) 478.79

**Ulcer, ulcerated, ulcerating, ulceration, ulcerative** — *continued*
larynx — *continued*
  diphtheritic 032.3
leg — *see* Ulcer, lower extremity
lip 528.5
Lipschütz's 616.50
lower extremity (atrophic) (chronic) (neurogenic) (perforating) (pyogenic) (trophic) (tropical) 707.10
  with gangrene (*see also* Ulcer, lower extremity) 707.10 [785.4]
    arteriosclerotic 440.24
  ankle 707.13
  arteriosclerotic 440.23
    with gangrene 440.24
  calf 707.12
  decubitus 707.00
    with gangrene 707.00 [785.4]
    ankle 707.06
    buttock 707.05
    heel 707.07
    hip 707.04
  foot 707.15
  heel 707.14
  knee 707.19
  specified site NEC 707.19
  thigh 707.11
  toes 707.15
  varicose 454.0
    inflamed or infected 454.2
luetic — *see* Ulcer, syphilitic
lung 518.89
  tuberculous (*see also* Tuberculosis) 011.2 ☑
malignant (M8000/3) — *see* Neoplasm, by site, malignant
marginal NEC — *see* Ulcer, gastrojejunal
meatus (urinarius) 597.89
Meckel's diverticulum 751.0
Meleney's (chronic undermining) 686.09
Mooren's (cornea) 370.07
mouth (traumatic) 528.9
mycobacterial (skin) 031.1
nasopharynx 478.29
navel cord (newborn) 771.4
neck (*see also* Ulcer, skin) 707.8
  uterus 622.0
neurogenic NEC — *see* Ulcer, skin
nose, nasal (infectional) (passage) 478.19
  septum 478.19
    varicose 456.8
  skin — *see* Ulcer, skin
  spirochetal NEC 104.8
oral mucosa (traumatic) 528.9
palate (soft) 528.9
penetrating NEC — *see* Ulcer, peptic, with perforation
penis (chronic) 607.89
peptic (site unspecified) 533.9 ☑

*Note — Use the following fifth-digit subclassification with categories 531–534:*
0  *without mention of obstruction*
1  *with obstruction*

  with
    hemorrhage 533.4 ☑
      and perforation 533.6 ☑
    perforation (chronic) 533.5 ☑
      and hemorrhage 533.6 ☑
  acute 533.3 ☑
    with
      hemorrhage 533.0 ☑
        and perforation 533.2 ☑
      perforation 533.1 ☑
        and hemorrhage 533.2 ☑
  bleeding (recurrent) — *see* Ulcer, peptic, with hemorrhage
  chronic 533.7 ☑
    with
      hemorrhage 533.4 ☑

☑ Additional Digit Required — Refer to the Tabular List for Digit Selection
Ⓥ Subterms under main terms may continue to next column or page
292 — Volume 2
►◄ Revised Text    ● New Line    ▲ Revised Code
2008 ICD-9-CM

**Ulcer, ulcerated, ulcerating, ulceration, ulcerative** — *continued*
peptic — *continued*
  chronic — *continued*
    with — *continued*
      hemorrhage — *continued*
        and perforation 533.6 ☑
      perforation 533.5 ☑
        and hemorrhage 533.6 ☑
  penetrating — *see* Ulcer, peptic, with perforation
  perforating NEC (*see also* Ulcer, peptic, with perforation) 533.5 ☑
skin 707.9
perineum (*see also* Ulcer, skin) 707.8
peritonsillar 474.8
phagedenic (tropical) NEC — *see* Ulcer, skin
pharynx 478.29
phlebitis — *see* Phlebitis
plaster (*see also* Ulcer, decubitus) 707.00
popliteal space — *see* Ulcer, lower extremity
postpyloric — *see* Ulcer, duodenum
prepuce 607.89
prepyloric — *see* Ulcer, stomach
pressure (*see also* Ulcer, decubitus) 707.00
primary of intestine 569.82
  with perforation 569.83
proctitis 556.2
  with ulcerative sigmoiditis 556.3
prostate 601.8
pseudopeptic — *see* Ulcer, peptic
pyloric — *see* Ulcer, stomach
rectosigmoid 569.82
  with perforation 569.83
rectum (sphincter) (solitary) 569.41
  stercoraceous, stercoral 569.41
  varicose — *see* Varicose, ulcer, anus
retina (*see also* Chorioretinitis) 363.20
rodent (M8090/3) (*see also* Neoplasm, skin, malignant)
  cornea 370.07
round — *see* Ulcer, stomach
sacrum (region) (*see also* Ulcer, skin) 707.8
Saemisch's 370.04
scalp (*see also* Ulcer, skin) 707.8
sclera 379.09
scrofulous (*see also* Tuberculosis) 017.2 ☑
scrotum 608.89
  tuberculous (*see also* Tuberculosis) 016.5 ☑
  varicose 456.4
seminal vesicle 608.89
sigmoid 569.82
  with perforation 569.83
skin (atrophic) (chronic) (neurogenic) (non-healing) (perforating) (pyogenic) (trophic) 707.9
  with gangrene 707.9 *[785.4]*
  amebic 006.6
  decubitus (*see also* Ulcer, decubitus) 707.00
    with gangrene 707.00 *[785.4]*
    in granulocytopenia 288.09
  lower extremity (*see also* Ulcer, lower extremity) 707.10
    with gangrene 707.10 *[785.4]*
      arteriosclerotic 440.24
    ankle 707.13
    arteriosclerotic 440.23
      with gangrene 440.24
    calf 707.12
    foot 707.15
    heel 707.14
    knee 707.19
    specified site NEC 707.19
    thigh 707.11
    toes 707.15
  mycobacterial 031.1
  syphilitic (early) (secondary) 091.3

**Ulcer, ulcerated, ulcerating, ulceration, ulcerative** — *continued*
skin — *continued*
  tuberculous (primary) (*see also* Tuberculosis) 017.0 ☑
  varicose — *see* Ulcer, varicose
  sloughing NEC — *see* Ulcer, skin
soft palate 528.9
solitary, anus or rectum (sphincter) 569.41
sore throat 462
  streptococcal 034.0
spermatic cord 608.89
spine (tuberculous) 015.0 ☑ *[730.88]*
stasis (leg) (venous) 454.0
  with varicose veins 454.0
  without varicose veins 459.81
  inflamed or infected 454.2
stercoral, stercoraceous 569.82
  with perforation 569.83
  anus or rectum 569.41
stomach (eroded) (peptic) (round) 531.9 ☑

*Note* — *Use the following fifth-digit subclassification with categories 531–534:*

*0*   *without mention of obstruction*

*1*   *with obstruction*

  with
    hemorrhage 531.4 ☑
      and perforation 531.6 ☑
    perforation (chronic) 531.5 ☑
      and hemorrhage 531.6 ☑
  acute 531.3 ☑
    with
      hemorrhage 531.0 ☑
        and perforation 531.2 ☑
      perforation 531.1 ☑
        and hemorrhage 531.2 ☑
  bleeding (recurrent) — *see* Ulcer, stomach, with hemorrhage
  chronic 531.7 ☑
    with
      hemorrhage 531.4 ☑
        and perforation 531.6 ☑
      perforation 531.5 ☑
        and hemorrhage 531.6 ☑
  penetrating — *see* Ulcer, stomach, with perforation
  perforating — *see* Ulcer, stomach, with perforation
stoma, stomal — *see* Ulcer, gastrojejunal
stomatitis 528.00
stress — *see* Ulcer, peptic
strumous (tuberculous) (*see also* Tuberculosis) 017.2 ☑
submental (*see also* Ulcer, skin) 707.8
submucosal, bladder 595.1
syphilitic (any site) (early) (secondary) 091.3
  late 095.9
  perforating 095.9
    foot 094.0
testis 608.89
thigh — *see* Ulcer, lower extremity
throat 478.29
  diphtheritic 032.0
toe — *see* Ulcer, lower extremity
tongue (traumatic) 529.0
tonsil 474.8
  diphtheritic 032.0
trachea 519.19
trophic — *see* Ulcer, skin
tropical NEC (*see also* Ulcer, skin) 707.9
tuberculous — *see* Tuberculosis, ulcer
tunica vaginalis 608.89
turbinate 730.9 ☑
typhoid (fever) 002.0
  perforating 002.0
umbilicus (newborn) 771.4
unspecified site NEC — *see* Ulcer, skin

**Ulcer, ulcerated, ulcerating, ulceration, ulcerative** — *continued*
urethra (meatus) (*see also* Urethritis) 597.89
uterus 621.8
  cervix 622.0
    with mention of cervicitis 616.0
  neck 622.0
    with mention of cervicitis 616.0
  vagina 616.89
valve, heart 421.0
varicose (lower extremity, any part) 454.0
  anus — *see* Varicose, ulcer, anus
  broad ligament 456.5
  esophagus (*see also* Varix, esophagus) 456.1
    bleeding (*see also* Varix, esophagus, bleeding) 456.0
    inflamed or infected 454.2
  nasal septum 456.8
  perineum 456.6
  rectum — *see* Varicose, ulcer, anus
  scrotum 456.4
  specified site NEC 456.8
  sublingual 456.3
  vulva 456.6
vas deferens 608.89
vesical (*see also* Ulcer, bladder) 596.8
vulva (acute) (infectional) 616.50
  Behçet's syndrome 136.1 *[616.51]*
  herpetic 054.12
  tuberculous 016.7 ☑ *[616.51]*
vulvobuccal, recurring 616.50
x-ray — *see* Ulcer, by site
yaws 102.4
**Ulcus** — *see also* Ulcer
cutis tuberculosum (*see also* Tuberculosis) 017.0 ☑
duodeni — *see* Ulcer, duodenum
durum 091.0
  extragenital 091.2
gastrojejunale — *see* Ulcer, gastrojejunal
hypostaticum — *see* Ulcer, varicose
molle (cutis) (skin) 099.0
serpens corneae (pneumococcal) 370.04
ventriculi — *see* Ulcer, stomach
**Ulegyria** 742.4
**Ulerythema**
acneiforma 701.8
centrifugum 695.4
ophryogenes 757.4
**Ullrich-Feichtiger syndrome** 759.89
**Ullrich (-Bonnevie) (-Turner) syndrome** 758.6
**Ulnar** — *see* condition
**Ulorrhagia** 523.8
**Ulorrhea** 523.8
**Umbilicus, umbilical** — *see also* condition
cord necrosis, affecting fetus or newborn 762.6
**Unacceptable**
existing dental restoration
  contours 525.65
  morphology 525.65
**Unavailability of medical facilities** (at) V63.9
due to
  investigation by social service agency V63.8
  lack of services at home V63.1
  remoteness from facility V63.0
  waiting list V63.2
home V63.1
outpatient clinic V63.0
specified reason NEC V63.8
**Uncinaria americana infestation** 126.1
**Uncinariasis** — *see also* Ancylostomiasis 126.9
**Unconscious, unconsciousness** 780.09
**Underdevelopment** — *see also* Undeveloped
sexual 259.0

**Underfill, endodontic** 526.63
**Undernourishment** 269.9
**Undernutrition** 269.9
**Under observation** — *see* Observation
**Underweight** 783.22
for gestational age — *see* Light-for-dates
**Underwood's disease** (sclerema neonatorum) 778.1
**Undescended** — *see also* Malposition, congenital
cecum 751.4
colon 751.4
testis 752.51
**Undetermined diagnosis or cause** 799.9
**Undeveloped, undevelopment** — *see also* Hypoplasia
brain (congenital) 742.1
cerebral (congenital) 742.1
fetus or newborn 764.9 ☑
heart 746.89
lung 748.5
testis 257.2
uterus 259.0
**Undiagnosed** (disease) 799.9
**Undulant fever** — *see also* Brucellosis 023.9
**Unemployment, anxiety concerning** V62.0
**Unequal leg** (acquired) (length) 736.81
congenital 755.30
**Unerupted teeth, tooth** 520.6
**Unextracted dental root** 525.3
**Unguis incarnatus** 703.0
**Unicornis uterus** 752.3
**Unicorporeus uterus** 752.3
**Uniformis uterus** 752.3
**Unilateral** — *see also* condition
development, breast 611.8
organ or site, congenital NEC — *see* Agenesis
vagina 752.49
**Unilateralis uterus** 752.3
**Unilocular heart** 745.8
**Uninhibited** bladder 596.54
with cauda equina syndrome 344.61
neurogenic — *see* Neurogenic, bladder 596.54
**Union, abnormal** — *see also* Fusion
divided tendon 727.89
larynx and trachea 748.3
**Universal**
joint, cervix 620.6
mesentery 751.4
**Unknown**
cause of death 799.9
diagnosis 799.9
**Unna's disease** (seborrheic dermatitis) 690.10
**Unresponsiveness, adrenocorticotropin** (ACTH) 255.41 ▲
**Unsatisfactory**
restoration, tooth (existing) 525.60
  specified NEC 525.69
smear 795.08
**Unsoundness of mind** — *see also* Psychosis 298.9
**Unspecified cause of death** 799.9
**Unstable**
back NEC 724.9
colon 569.89
joint — *see* Instability, joint
lie 652.0 ☑
  affecting fetus or newborn (before labor) 761.7
  causing obstructed labor 660.0 ☑
    affecting fetus or newborn 763.1
lumbosacral joint (congenital) 756.19
  acquired 724.6
sacroiliac 724.6
spine NEC 724.9
**Untruthfulness, child problem** — *see also* Disturbance, conduct 312.0 ☑
**Unverricht (-Lundborg) disease, syndrome, or epilepsy** 333.2

☑ Additional Digit Required — Refer to the Tabular List for Digit Selection      ▽ Subterms under main terms may continue to next column or page

**2008 ICD-9-CM**      ▶◀ Revised Text      ● New Line      ▲ Revised Code      **October 2007 · Volume 2 — 293**

**Unverricht-Wagner syndrome** (dermatomyositis) 710.3
**Upper respiratory** — see condition
**Upset**
    gastric 536.8
        psychogenic 306.4
    gastrointestinal 536.8
        psychogenic 306.4
        virus (see also Enteritis, viral) 008.8
    intestinal (large) (small) 564.9
        psychogenic 306.4
    menstruation 626.9
    mental 300.9
    stomach 536.8
        psychogenic 306.4
**Urachus** — see also condition
    patent 753.7
    persistent 753.7
**Uratic arthritis** 274.0
**Urbach's lipoid proteinosis** 272.8
**Urbach-Oppenheim disease or syndrome** (necrobiosis lipoidica diabeticorum) 250.8 ☑ [709.3]
**Urbach-Wiethe disease or syndrome** (lipoid proteinosis) 272.8
**Urban yellow fever** 060.1
**Urea, blood, high** — see Uremia
**Uremia, uremic** (absorption) (amaurosis) (amblyopia) (aphasia) (apoplexy) (coma) (delirium) (dementia) (dropsy) (dyspnea) (fever) (intoxication) (mania) (paralysis) (poisoning) (toxemia) (vomiting) 586
    with
        abortion — see Abortion, by type, with renal failure
        ectopic pregnancy (see also categories 633.0–633.9) 639.3
        hypertension (see also Hypertension, kidney) 403.91
        molar pregnancy (see also categories 630–632) 639.3
    chronic 585.9
    complicating
        abortion 639.3
        ectopic or molar pregnancy 639.3
        hypertension (see also Hypertension, kidney) 403.91
        labor and delivery 669.3 ☑
    congenital 779.89
    extrarenal 788.9
    hypertensive (chronic) (see also Hypertension, kidney) 403.91
    maternal NEC, affecting fetus or newborn 760.1
    neuropathy 585.9 [357.4]
    pericarditis 585.9 [420.0]
    prerenal 788.9
    pyelitic (see also Pyelitis) 590.80
**Ureteralgia** 788.0
**Ureterectasis** 593.89
**Ureteritis** 593.89
    cystica 590.3
    due to calculus 592.1
    gonococcal (acute) 098.19
        chronic or duration of 2 months or over 098.39
    nonspecific 593.89
**Ureterocele** (acquired) 593.89
    congenital 753.23
**Ureterolith** 592.1
**Ureterolithiasis** 592.1

**Ureterostomy status** V44.6
    with complication 997.5
**Ureter, ureteral** — see condition
**Urethralgia** 788.9
**Urethra, urethral** — see condition
**Urethritis** (abacterial) (acute) (allergic) (anterior) (chronic) (nonvenereal) (posterior) (recurrent) (simple) (subacute) (ulcerative) (undifferentiated) 597.80
    diplococcal (acute) 098.0
        chronic or duration of 2 months or over 098.2
    due to Trichomonas (vaginalis) 131.02
    gonococcal (acute) 098.0
        chronic or duration of 2 months or over 098.2
    nongonococcal (sexually transmitted) 099.40
        Chlamydia trachomatis 099.41
        Reiter's 099.3
        specified organism NEC 099.49
    nonspecific (sexually transmitted) (see also Urethritis, nongonococcal) 099.40
    not sexually transmitted 597.80
    Reiter's 099.3
    trichomonal or due to Trichomonas (vaginalis) 131.02
    tuberculous (see also Tuberculosis) 016.3 ☑
    venereal NEC (see also Urethritis, nongonococcal) 099.40
**Urethrocele**
    female 618.03
        with uterine prolapse 618.4
            complete 618.3
            incomplete 618.2
    male 599.5
**Urethrolithiasis** 594.2
**Urethro-oculoarticular syndrome** 099.3
**Urethro-oculosynovial syndrome** 099.3
**Urethrorectal** — see condition
**Urethrorrhagia** 599.84
**Urethrorrhea** 788.7
**Urethrostomy status** V44.6
    with complication 997.5
**Urethrotrigonitis** 595.3
**Urethrovaginal** — see condition
**Urhidrosis, uridrosis** 705.89
**Uric acid**
    diathesis 274.9
    in blood 790.6
**Uricacidemia** 790.6
**Uricemia** 790.6
**Uricosuria** 791.9
**Urination**
    frequent 788.41
    painful 788.1
    urgency 788.63
**Urinemia** — see Uremia
**Urine, urinary** — see also condition
    abnormality NEC 788.69
    blood in (see also Hematuria) 599.7
    discharge, excessive 788.42
    enuresis 788.30
        nonorganic origin 307.6
    extravasation 788.8
    frequency 788.41
    hesitancy 788.64
    incontinence 788.30
        active 788.30
        female 788.30

**Urine, urinary** — see also condition — continued
    incontinence — continued
        female — continued
            stress 625.6
                and urge 788.33
        male 788.30
            stress 788.32
                and urge 788.33
        mixed (stress and urge) 788.33
        neurogenic 788.39
        nonorganic origin 307.6
        overflow 788.38
        stress (female) 625.6
            male NEC 788.32
    intermittent stream 788.61
    pus in 791.9
    retention or stasis NEC 788.20
        bladder, incomplete emptying 788.21
        psychogenic 306.53
        specified NEC 788.29
    secretion
        deficient 788.5
        excessive 788.42
        frequency 788.41
    strain 788.65
    stream
        intermittent 788.61
        slowing 788.62
        splitting 788.61
        weak 788.62
    urgency 788.63
**Urinoma** NEC 599.9
    bladder 596.8
    kidney 593.89
    renal 593.89
    ureter 593.89
    urethra 599.84
**Uroarthritis, infectious** 099.3
**Urodialysis** 788.5
**Urodynia** 788.1
**Urolithiasis** 592.9
**Uronephrosis** 593.89
**Uropathy** 599.9
    obstructive 599.60
**Urosepsis** 599.0
    meaning sepsis 995.91
    meaning urinary tract infection 599.0
**Urticaria** 708.9
    with angioneurotic edema 995.1
        hereditary 277.6
    allergic 708.0
    cholinergic 708.5
    chronic 708.8
    cold, familial 708.2
    dermatographic 708.3
    due to
        cold or heat 708.2
        drugs 708.0
        food 708.0
        inhalants 708.0
        plants 708.8
        serum 999.5
    factitial 708.3
    giant 995.1
        hereditary 277.6
    gigantea 995.1
        hereditary 277.6
    idiopathic 708.1
    larynx 995.1
        hereditary 277.6
    neonatorum 778.8
    nonallergic 708.1

**Urticaria** — continued
    papulosa (Hebra) 698.2
    perstans hemorrhagica 757.39
    pigmentosa 757.33
    recurrent periodic 708.8
    serum 999.5
    solare 692.72
    specified type NEC 708.8
    thermal (cold) (heat) 708.2
    vibratory 708.4
**Urticarioides acarodermatitis** 133.9
**Use of**
    nonprescribed drugs (see also Abuse, drugs, nondependent) 305.9 ☑
    patent medicines (see also Abuse, drugs, nondependent) 305.9 ☑
**Usher-Senear disease** (pemphigus erythematosus) 694.4
**Uta** 085.5
**Uterine size-date discrepancy** 649.6 ☑
**Uteromegaly** 621.2
**Uterovaginal** — see condition
**Uterovesical** — see condition
**Uterus** — see condition
**Utriculitis** (utriculus prostaticus) 597.89
**Uveal** — see condition
**Uveitis** (anterior) — see also Iridocyclitis 364.3
    acute or subacute 364.00
        due to or associated with
            gonococcal infection 098.41
            herpes (simplex) 054.44
                zoster 053.22
        primary 364.01
        recurrent 364.02
        secondary (noninfectious) 364.04
            infectious 364.03
    allergic 360.11
    chronic 364.10
        due to or associated with
            sarcoidosis 135 [364.11]
            tuberculosis (see also Tuberculosis) 017.3 ☑ [364.11]
    due to
        operation 360.11
        toxoplasmosis (acquired) 130.2
            congenital (active) 771.2
    granulomatous 364.10
    heterochromic 364.21
    lens-induced 364.23
    nongranulomatous 364.00
    posterior 363.20
        disseminated — see Chorioretinitis, disseminated
        focal — see Chorioretinitis, focal
    recurrent 364.02
    sympathetic 360.11
    syphilitic (secondary) 091.50
        congenital 090.0 [363.13]
        late 095.8 [363.13]
    tuberculous (see also Tuberculosis) 017.3 ☑ [364.11]
**Uveoencephalitis** 363.22
**Uveokeratitis** — see also Iridocyclitis 364.3
**Uveoparotid fever** 135
**Uveoparotitis** 135
**Uvula** — see condition
**Uvulitis** (acute) (catarrhal) (chronic) (gangrenous) (membranous) (suppurative) (ulcerative) 528.3

## V

**Vaccination**
complication or reaction — *see* Complications, vaccination
not carried out V64.00
because of
acute illness V64.01
allergy to vaccine or component V64.04
caregiver refusal V64.05
chronic illness V64.02
guardian refusal V64.05 ●
immune compromised state V64.03
parent refusal V64.05 ●
patient had disease being vaccinated against V64.08
patient refusal V64.06
reason NEC V64.09
religious reasons V64.07
prophylactic (against) V05.9
arthropod-borne viral
disease NEC V05.1
encephalitis V05.0
chickenpox V05.4
cholera (alone) V03.0
with typhoid-paratyphoid (cholera + TAB) V06.0
common cold V04.7
diphtheria (alone) V03.5
with
poliomyelitis (DTP+ polio) V06.3
tetanus V06.5
pertussis combined (DTP) (DTaP) V06.1
typhoid-paratyphoid (DTP + TAB) V06.2
disease (single) NEC V05.9
bacterial NEC V03.9
specified type NEC V03.89
combination NEC V06.9
specified type NEC V06.8
specified type NEC V05.8
encephalitis, viral, arthropod-borne V05.0
Hemophilus influenzae, type B [Hib] V03.81
hepatitis, viral V05.3
influenza V04.81
with
Streptococcus pneumoniae [pneumococcus] V06.6
leishmaniasis V05.2
measles (alone) V04.2
with mumps-rubella (MMR) V06.4
mumps (alone) V04.6
with measles and rubella (MMR) V06.4
pertussis alone V03.6
plague V03.3
poliomyelitis V04.0
with diphtheria-tetanus-pertussis (DTP + polio) V06.3
rabies V04.5
respiratory syncytial virus (RSV) V04.82
rubella (alone) V04.3
with measles and mumps (MMR) V06.4
smallpox V04.1
Streptococcus pneumoniae [pneumococcus] V03.82
with
influenza V06.6
tetanus toxoid (alone) V03.7
with diphtheria [Td] [DT] V06.5
with
pertussis (DTP) (DTaP) V06.1
with poliomyelitis (DTP+polio) V06.3
tuberculosis (BCG) V03.2
tularemia V03.4

**Vaccination** — *continued*
prophylactic — *continued*
typhoid-paratyphoid (TAB) (alone) V03.1
with diphtheria-tetanus-pertussis (TAB + DTP) V06.2
varicella V05.4
viral
disease NEC V04.89
encephalitis, arthropod-borne V05.0
hepatitis V05.3
yellow fever V04.4
**Vaccinia** (generalized) 999.0
without vaccination 051.0
congenital 771.2
conjunctiva 999.39 ▲
eyelids 999.0 *[373.5]*
localized 999.39 ▲
nose 999.39 ▲
not from vaccination 051.0
eyelid 051.0 *[373.5]*
sine vaccinatione 051.0
**Vacuum**
extraction of fetus or newborn 763.3
in sinus (accessory) (nasal) (*see also* Sinusitis) 473.9
**Vagabond** V60.0
**Vagabondage** V60.0
**Vagabonds' disease** 132.1
**Vaginalitis** (tunica) 608.4
**Vagina, vaginal** — *see condition*
**Vaginismus** (reflex) 625.1
functional 306.51
hysterical 300.11
psychogenic 306.51
**Vaginitis** (acute) (chronic) (circumscribed) (diffuse) (emphysematous) (Hemophilus vaginalis) (nonspecific) (nonvenereal) (ulcerative) 616.10
with
abortion — *see* Abortion, by type, with sepsis
ectopic pregnancy (*see also* categories 633.0–633.9) 639.0
molar pregnancy (*see also* categories 630–632) 639.0
adhesive, congenital 752.49
atrophic, postmenopausal 627.3
bacterial 616.10
blennorrhagic (acute) 098.0
chronic or duration of 2 months or over 098.2
candidal 112.1
chlamydial 099.53
complicating pregnancy or puerperium 646.6 ☑
affecting fetus or newborn 760.8
congenital (adhesive) 752.49
due to
C. albicans 112.1
Trichomonas (vaginalis) 131.01
following
abortion 639.0
ectopic or molar pregnancy 639.0
gonococcal (acute) 098.0
chronic or duration of 2 months or over 098.2
granuloma 099.2
Monilia 112.1
mycotic 112.1
pinworm 127.4 *[616.11]*
postirradiation 616.10
postmenopausal atrophic 627.3
senile (atrophic) 627.3
syphilitic (early) 091.0
late 095.8
trichomonal 131.01
tuberculous (*see also* Tuberculosis) 016.7 ☑
venereal NEC 099.8
**Vaginosis** — *see* Vaginitis
**Vagotonia** 352.3
**Vagrancy** V60.0
**VAIN I** (vaginal intraepithelial neoplasia ●
I) 623.0 ●

**VAIN II** (vaginal intraepithelial neoplasia II) 623.0 ●
**VAIN III** (vaginal intraepithelial neoplasia III) 233.31 ●
**Vallecula** — *see* condition
**Valley fever** 114.0
**Valsuani's disease** (progressive pernicious anemia, puerperal) 648.2 ☑
**Valve, valvular** (formation) — *see also* condition
cerebral ventricle (communicating) in situ V45.2
cervix, internal os 752.49
colon 751.5
congenital NEC — *see* Atresia
formation, congenital NEC — *see* Atresia
heart defect — *see* Anomaly, heart, valve
ureter 753.29
pelvic junction 753.21
vesical orifice 753.22
urethra 753.6
**Valvulitis** (chronic) — *see also* Endocarditis 424.90
rheumatic (chronic) (inactive) (with chorea) 397.9
active or acute (aortic) (mitral) (pulmonary) (tricuspid) 391.1
syphilitic NEC 093.20
aortic 093.22
mitral 093.21
pulmonary 093.24
tricuspid 093.23
**Valvulopathy** — *see* Endocarditis
**van Bogaert-Nijssen (-Peiffer) disease** 330.0
**van Bogaert's leukoencephalitis** (sclerosing) (subacute) 046.2
**van Buchem's syndrome** (hyperostosis corticalis) 733.3
**Vancomycin** (glycopeptide)
intermediate staphylococcus aureus (VISA/GISA) V09.8 ☑
resistant
enterococcus (VRE) V09.8 ☑
staphylococcus aureus (VRSA/GRSA) V09.8 ☑
**van Creveld-von Gierke disease** (glycogenosis I) 271.0
**van den Bergh's disease** (enterogenous cyanosis) 289.7
**van der Hoeve-Halbertsma-Waardenburg syndrome** (ptosis-epicanthus) 270.2
**van der Hoeve-Waardenburg-Gualdi syndrome** (ptosis epicanthus) 270.2
**van der Hoeve's syndrome** (brittle bones and blue sclera, deafness) 756.51
**Vanillism** 692.89
**Vanishing lung** 492.0
**Vanishing twin** 651.33
**van Neck (-Odelberg) disease or syndrome** (juvenile osteochondrosis) 732.1
**Vapor asphyxia or suffocation NEC** 987.9
specified agent — *see* Table of Drugs and Chemicals
**Vaquez's disease** (M9950/1) 238.4
**Vaquez-Osler disease** (polycythemia vera) (M9950/1) 238.4
**Variance, lethal ball, prosthetic heart valve** 996.02
**Variants, thalassemic** 282.49
**Variations in hair color** 704.3
**Varicella** 052.9
with
complication 052.8
specified NEC 052.7
pneumonia 052.1
vaccination and inoculation (prophylactic) V05.4
exposure to V01.71

**Varicella** — *continued*
vaccination and inoculation (against) (prophylactic) V05.4
**Varices** — *see* Varix
**Varicocele** (scrotum) (thrombosed) 456.4
ovary 456.5
perineum 456.6
spermatic cord (ulcerated) 456.4
**Varicose**
aneurysm (ruptured) (*see also* Aneurysm) 442.9
dermatitis (lower extremity) — *see* Varicose, vein, inflamed or infected
eczema — *see* Varicose, vein
phlebitis — *see* Varicose, vein, inflamed or infected
placental vessel — *see* Placenta, abnormal
tumor — *see* Varicose, vein
ulcer (lower extremity, any part) 454.0
anus 455.8
external 455.5
internal 455.2
esophagus (*see also* Varix, esophagus) 456.1
bleeding (*see also* Varix, esophagus, bleeding) 456.0
inflamed or infected 454.2
nasal septum 456.8
perineum 456.6
rectum — *see* Varicose, ulcer, anus
scrotum 456.4
specified site NEC 456.8
vein (lower extremity) (ruptured) (*see also* Varix) 454.9
with
complications NEC 454.8
edema 454.8
inflammation or infection 454.1
ulcerated 454.2
pain 454.8
stasis dermatitis 454.1
with ulcer 454.2
swelling 454.8
ulcer 454.0
inflamed or infected 454.2
anus — *see* Hemorrhoids
broad ligament 456.5
congenital (peripheral) 747.60
gastrointestinal 747.61
lower limb 747.64
renal 747.62
specified NEC 747.69
upper limb 747.63
esophagus (ulcerated) (*see also* Varix, esophagus) 456.1
bleeding (*see also* Varix, esophagus, bleeding) 456.0
inflamed or infected 454.1
with ulcer 454.2
in pregnancy or puerperium 671.0 ☑
vulva or perineum 671.1 ☑
nasal septum (with ulcer) 456.8
pelvis 456.5
perineum 456.6
in pregnancy, childbirth, or puerperium 671.1 ☑
rectum — *see* Hemorrhoids
scrotum (ulcerated) 456.4
specified site NEC 456.8
sublingual 456.3
ulcerated 454.0
inflamed or infected 454.2
umbilical cord, affecting fetus or newborn 762.6
urethra 456.8
vulva 456.6
in pregnancy, childbirth, or puerperium 671.1 ☑
vessel (*see also* Varix)
placenta — *see* Placenta, abnormal
**Varicosis, varicosities, varicosity** — *see also* Varix 454.9
**Variola** 050.9

☑ Additional Digit Required — Refer to the Tabular List for Digit Selection     Subterms under main terms may continue to next column or page

**2008 ICD-9-CM**     ►◄ Revised Text     ● New Line     ▲ Revised Code     **October 2007 · Volume 2 — 295**

**Variola** — continued
  hemorrhagic (pustular) 050.0
  major 050.0
  minor 050.1
  modified 050.2
**Varioloid** 050.2
**Variolosa, purpura** 050.0
**Varix** (lower extremity) (ruptured) 454.9
  with
    complications NEC 454.8
    edema 454.8
    inflammation or infection 454.1
      with ulcer 454.2
    pain 454.8
    stasis dermatitis 454.1
      with ulcer 454.2
    swelling 454.8
    ulcer 454.0
      with inflammation or infection
        454.2
  aneurysmal (see also Aneurysm) 442.9
  anus — see Hemorrhoids
  arteriovenous (congenital) (peripheral)
    NEC 747.60
    gastrointestinal 747.61
    lower limb 747.64
    renal 747.62
    specified NEC 747.69
    spinal 747.82
    upper limb 747.63
  bladder 456.5
  broad ligament 456.5
  congenital (peripheral) 747.60
  esophagus (ulcerated) 456.1
    bleeding 456.0
    in
      cirrhosis of liver
        571.5 [456.20]
      portal hypertension
        572.3 [456.20]
    congenital 747.69
    in
      cirrhosis of liver
        571.5 [456.21]
        with bleeding
          571.5 [456.20]
      portal hypertension
        572.3 [456.21]
        with bleeding
          572.3 [456.20]
  gastric 456.8
  inflamed or infected 454.1
    ulcerated 454.2
  in pregnancy or puerperium 671.0 ☑
    perineum 671.1 ☑
    vulva 671.1 ☑
  labia (majora) 456.6
  orbit 456.8
    congenital 747.69
  ovary 456.5
  papillary 448.1
  pelvis 456.5
  perineum 456.6
    in pregnancy or puerperium
      671.1 ☑
  pharynx 456.8
  placenta — see Placenta, abnormal
  prostate 456.8
  rectum — see Hemorrhoids
  renal papilla 456.8
  retina 362.17
  scrotum (ulcerated) 456.4
  sigmoid colon 456.8
  specified site NEC 456.8
  spinal (cord) (vessels) 456.8
  spleen, splenic (vein) (with phlebolith)
    456.8
  sublingual 456.3
  ulcerated 456.8
    inflamed or infected 454.2
  umbilical cord, affecting fetus or new-
    born 762.6
  uterine ligament 456.5
  vocal cord 456.8
  vulva 456.6

**Varix** — continued
  vulva — continued
    in pregnancy, childbirth, or puer-
      perium 671.1 ☑
**Vasa previa** 663.5 ☑
  affecting fetus or newborn 762.6
  hemorrhage from, affecting fetus or
    newborn 772.0
**Vascular** — see also condition
  loop on papilla (optic) 743.57
  sheathing, retina 362.13
  spasm 443.9
  spider 448.1
**Vascularity, pulmonary, congenital**
  747.3
**Vascularization**
  choroid 362.16
  cornea 370.60
    deep 370.63
    localized 370.61
  retina 362.16
  subretinal 362.16
**Vasculitis** 447.6
  allergic 287.0
  cryoglobulinemic 273.2
  disseminated 447.6
  kidney 447.8
  leukocytoclastic 446.29
  nodular 695.2
  retinal 362.18
  rheumatic — see Fever, rheumatic
**Vasculopathy**
  cardiac allograft 996.83
**Vas deferens** — see condition
**Vas deferentitis** 608.4
**Vasectomy, admission for** V25.2
**Vasitis** 608.4
  nodosa 608.4
  scrotum 608.4
  spermatic cord 608.4
  testis 608.4
  tuberculous (see also Tuberculosis)
    016.5 ☑
  tunica vaginalis 608.4
  vas deferens 608.4
**Vasodilation** 443.9
**Vasomotor** — see condition
**Vasoplasty, after previous sterilization**
  V26.0
**Vasoplegia, splanchnic** — see also
  Neuropathy, peripheral, autonomic
  337.9
**Vasospasm** 443.9
  cerebral (artery) 435.9
    with transient neurologic deficit
      435.9
  coronary 413.1
  nerve
    arm NEC 354.9
    autonomic 337.9
    brachial plexus 353.0
    cervical plexus 353.2
    leg NEC 355.8
    lower extremity NEC 355.8
    peripheral NEC 355.9
    spinal NEC 355.9
    sympathetic 337.9
    upper extremity NEC 354.9
  peripheral NEC 443.9
  retina (artery) (see also Occlusion,
    retinal, artery) 362.30
**Vasospastic** — see condition
**Vasovagal attack** (paroxysmal) 780.2
  psychogenic 306.2
**Vater's ampulla** — see condition
**VATER syndrome** 759.89
**Vegetation, vegetative**
  adenoid (nasal fossa) 474.2
  consciousness (persistent) 780.03
  endocarditis (acute) (any valve)
    (chronic) (subacute) 421.0
  heart (mycotic) (valve) 421.0
  state (persistent) 780.03
**Veil**
  Jackson's 751.4
  over face (causing asphyxia) 768.9

**Vein, venous** — see condition
**Veldt sore** — see also Ulcer, skin 707.9
**Velo-cardio-facial syndrome** 758.32
**Velpeau's hernia** — see Hernia, femoral
**Venereal**
  balanitis NEC 099.8
  bubo 099.1
  disease 099.9
    specified nature or type NEC 099.8
  granuloma inguinale 099.2
  lymphogranuloma (Durand-Nicolas-
    Favre), any site 099.1
  salpingitis 098.37
  urethritis (see also Urethritis, non-
    gonococcal) 099.40
  vaginitis NEC 099.8
  warts 078.19
**Vengefulness, in child** — see also Disturbance, conduct 312.0 ☑
**Venofibrosis** 459.89
**Venom, venomous**
  bite or sting (animal or insect) 989.5
  poisoning 989.5
**Venous** — see condition
**Ventouse delivery** NEC 669.5 ☑
  affecting fetus or newborn 763.3
**Ventral** — see condition
**Ventricle, ventricular** — see also condition
  escape 427.69
  standstill (see also Arrest, cardiac)
    427.5
**Ventriculus, cerebral** — see also
  Meningitis 322.9
**Ventriculostomy status** V45.2
**Verbiest's syndrome** (claudicatio intermittens spinalis) 435.1
**Vernet's syndrome** 352.6
**Verneuil's disease** (syphilitic bursitis)
  095.7
**Verruca** (filiformis) 078.10
  acuminata (any site) 078.11
  necrogenica (primary) (see also Tuber-
    culosis) 017.0 ☑
  peruana 088.0
  peruviana 088.0
  plana (juvenilis) 078.19
  plantaris 078.19
  seborrheica 702.19
    inflamed 702.11
  senilis 702.0
  tuberculosa (primary) (see also Tuber-
    culosis) 017.0 ☑
  venereal 078.19
  viral NEC 078.10
**Verrucosities** — see also Verruca 078.10
**Verrucous endocarditis** (acute) (any
  valve) (chronic) (subacute)
  710.0 [424.91]
  nonbacterial 710.0 [424.91]
**Verruga**
  peruana 088.0
  peruviana 088.0
**Verse's disease** (calcinosis intervertebralis) 275.49 [722.90]
**Version**
  before labor, affecting fetus or new-
    born 761.7
  cephalic (correcting previous malposi-
    tion) 652.1 ☑
    affecting fetus or newborn 763.1
  cervix — see Version, uterus
  uterus (postinfectional) (postpartal,
    old) (see also Malposition,
    uterus) 621.6
    forward — see Anteversion, uterus
    lateral — see Lateroversion, uterus
**Vertebra, vertebral** — see condition
**Vertigo** 780.4
  auditory 386.19
  aural 386.19
  benign paroxysmal positional 386.11
  central origin 386.2
  cerebral 386.2
  Dix and Hallpike (epidemic) 386.12
  endemic paralytic 078.81

**Vertigo** — continued
  epidemic 078.81
    Dix and Hallpike 386.12
    Gerlier's 078.81
    Pedersen's 386.12
    vestibular neuronitis 386.12
  epileptic — see Epilepsy
  Gerlier's (epidemic) 078.81
  hysterical 300.11
  labyrinthine 386.10
  laryngeal 786.2
  malignant positional 386.2
  Ménière's (see also Disease, Ménière's)
    386.00
  menopausal 627.2
  otogenic 386.19
  paralytic 078.81
  paroxysmal positional, benign 386.11
  Pedersen's (epidemic) 386.12
  peripheral 386.10
    specified type NEC 386.19
  positional
    benign paroxysmal 386.11
    malignant 386.2
**Verumontanitis** (chronic) — see also
  Urethritis 597.89
**Vesania** — see also Psychosis 298.9
**Vesical** — see condition
**Vesicle**
  cutaneous 709.8
  seminal — see condition
  skin 709.8
**Vesicocolic** — see condition
**Vesicoperineal** — see condition
**Vesicorectal** — see condition
**Vesicourethrorectal** — see condition
**Vesicovaginal** — see condition
**Vesicular** — see condition
**Vesiculitis** (seminal) 608.0
  amebic 006.8
  gonorrheal (acute) 098.14
    chronic or duration of 2 months or
      over 098.34
  trichomonal 131.09
  tuberculous (see also Tuberculosis)
    016.5 ☑ [608.81]
**Vestibulitis** (ear) — see also Labyrinthitis
  386.30
  nose (external) 478.19
  vulvar 616.10
**Vestibulopathy, acute peripheral** (recur-
  rent) 386.12
**Vestige, vestigial** — see also Persistence
  branchial 744.41
  structures in vitreous 743.51
**Vibriosis NEC** 027.9
**Vidal's disease** (lichen simplex chronicus) 698.3
**Video display tube syndrome** 723.8
**Vienna-type encephalitis** 049.8
**Villaret's syndrome** 352.6
**Villous** — see condition
**VIN I** (vulvar intraepithelial neoplasia I)
  624.01                                  ▲
**VIN II** (vulvar intraepithelial neoplasia
  II) 624.02                              ▲
**VIN III** (vulvar intraepithelial neoplasia
  III) 233.32                             ▲
**Vincent's**
  angina 101
  bronchitis 101
  disease 101
  gingivitis 101
  infection (any site) 101
  laryngitis 101
  stomatitis 101
  tonsillitis 101
**Vinson-Plummer syndrome** (sideropenic
  dysphagia) 280.8
**Viosterol deficiency** — see also Deficiency, calciferol 268.9
**Virchow's disease** 733.99
**Viremia** 790.8
**Virilism** (adrenal) (female) NEC 255.2

**Virilism** — *continued*
  with
    3-beta-hydroxysteroid dehydrogenase defect 255.2
    11-hydroxylase defect 255.2
    21-hydroxylase defect 255.2
    adrenal
      hyperplasia 255.2
      insufficiency (congenital) 255.2
    cortical hyperfunction 255.2
**Virilization** (female) (suprarenal) — *see also* Virilism 255.2
  isosexual 256.4
**Virulent bubo** 099.0
**Virus, viral** — *see also* condition
  infection NEC (*see also* Infection, viral) 079.99
  septicemia 079.99
**VISA** (vancomycin intermediate staphylococcus aureus) V09.8 ☑
**Viscera, visceral** — *see* condition
**Visceroptosis** 569.89
**Visible peristalsis** 787.4
**Vision, visual**
  binocular, suppression 368.31
  blurred, blurring 368.8
    hysterical 300.11
  defect, defective (*see also* Impaired, vision) 369.9
  disorientation (syndrome) 368.16
  disturbance NEC (*see also* Disturbance, vision) 368.9
    hysterical 300.11
  examination V72.0
  field, limitation 368.40
  fusion, with defective steropsis 368.33
  hallucinations 368.16
  halos 368.16
  loss 369.9
    both eyes (*see also* Blindness, both eyes) 369.3
    complete (*see also* Blindness, both eyes) 369.00
    one eye 369.8
    sudden 368.16
  low (both eyes) 369.20
    one eye (other eye normal) (*see also* Impaired, vision) 369.70
      blindness, other eye 369.10
  perception, simultaneous without fusion 368.32
  tunnel 368.45
**Vitality, lack or want of** 780.79
  newborn 779.89
**Vitamin deficiency** NEC — *see also* Deficiency, vitamin 269.2
**Vitelline duct, persistent** 751.0
**Vitiligo** 709.01
  due to pinta (carate) 103.2
  eyelid 374.53
  vulva 624.8
**Vitium cordis** — *see* Disease, heart
**Vitreous** — *see also* condition
  touch syndrome 997.99
**VLCAD** (long chain/very long chain acyl CoA dehydrogenase deficiency, LCAD) 277.85
**Vocal cord** — *see* condition
**Vocational rehabilitation** V57.22
**Vogt's (Cecile) disease or syndrome** 333.7 ☑
**Vogt-Koyanagi syndrome** 364.24
**Vogt-Spielmeyer disease** (amaurotic familial idiocy) 330.1
**Voice**
  change (*see also* Dysphonia) 784.49
  loss (*see also* Aphonia) 784.41
**Volhard-Fahr disease** (malignant nephrosclerosis) 403.00
**Volhynian fever** 083.1
**Volkmann's ischemic contracture or paralysis** (complicating trauma) 958.6
**Voluntary starvation** 307.1
**Volvulus** (bowel) (colon) (intestine) 560.2

**Volvulus** — *continued*
  with
    hernia (*see also* Hernia, by site, with obstruction)
      gangrenous — *see* Hernia, by site, with gangrene
    perforation 560.2
  congenital 751.5
  duodenum 537.3
  fallopian tube 620.5
  oviduct 620.5
  stomach (due to absence of gastrocolic ligament) 537.89
**Vomiting** 787.03
  with nausea 787.01
  allergic 535.4 ☑
  asphyxia 933.1
  bilious (cause unknown) 787.0 ☑
    following gastrointestinal surgery 564.3
  blood (*see also* Hematemesis) 578.0
  causing asphyxia, choking, or suffocation (*see also* Asphyxia, food) 933.1
  cyclical 536.2
    psychogenic 306.4
  epidemic 078.82
  fecal matter 569.89
  following gastrointestinal surgery 564.3
  functional 536.8
    psychogenic 306.4
  habit 536.2
  hysterical 300.11
  nervous 306.4
  neurotic 306.4
  newborn 779.3
  of or complicating pregnancy 643.9 ☑
    due to
      organic disease 643.8 ☑
      specific cause NEC 643.8 ☑
    early — *see* Hyperemesis, gravidarum
    late (after 22 completed weeks of gestation) 643.2 ☑
  pernicious or persistent 536.2
    complicating pregnancy — *see* Hyperemesis, gravidarum
    psychogenic 306.4
  physiological 787.0 ☑
  psychic 306.4
  psychogenic 307.54
  stercoral 569.89
  uncontrollable 536.2
    psychogenic 306.4
  uremic — *see* Uremia
  winter 078.82
**von Bechterew (-Strumpell) disease or syndrome** (ankylosing spondylitis) 720.0
**von Bezold's abscess** 383.01
**von Economo's disease** (encephalitis lethargica) 049.8
**von Eulenburg's disease** (congenital paramyotonia) 359.29 ▲
**von Gierke's disease** (glycogenosis I) 271.0
**von Gies' joint** 095.8
**von Graefe's disease or syndrome** 378.72
**von Hippel (-Lindau) disease or syndrome** (retinocerebral angiomatosis) 759.6
**von Jaksch's anemia or disease** (pseudoleukemia infantum) 285.8
**von Recklinghausen-Applebaum disease** (hemochromatosis) 275.0
**von Recklinghausen's**
  disease or syndrome (nerves) (skin) (M9540/1) 237.71
    bones (osteitis fibrosa cystica) 252.01
  tumor (M9540/1) 237.71
**von Schroetter's syndrome** (intermittent venous claudication) 453.8

**von Willebrand (-Jürgens) (-Minot) disease or syndrome** (angiohemophilia) 286.4
**von Zambusch's disease** (lichen sclerosus et atrophicus) 701.0
**Voorhoeve's disease or dyschondroplasia** 756.4
**Vossius' ring** 921.3
  late effect 366.21
**Voyeurism** 302.82
**VRE** (vancomycin resistant enterococcus) V09.8 ☑
**Vrolik's disease** (osteogenesis imperfecta) 756.51
**VRSA** (vancomycin resistant staphylococcus aureus) V09.8 ☑
**Vulva** — *see* condition
**Vulvismus** 625.1
**Vulvitis** (acute) (allergic) (chronic) (gangrenous) (hypertrophic) (intertriginous) 616.10
  with
    abortion — *see* Abortion, by type, with sepsis
    ectopic pregnancy (*see also* categories 633.0–633.9) 639.0
    molar pregnancy (*see also* categories 630–632) 639.0
  adhesive, congenital 752.49
  blennorrhagic (acute) 098.0
    chronic or duration of 2 months or over 098.2
  chlamydial 099.53
  complicating pregnancy or puerperium 646.6 ☑
  due to Ducrey's bacillus 099.0
  following
    abortion 639.0
    ectopic or molar pregnancy 639.0
  gonococcal (acute) 098.0
    chronic or duration of 2 months or over 098.2
  herpetic 054.11
  leukoplakic 624.09 ▲
  monilial 112.1
  puerperal, postpartum, childbirth 646.6 ☑
  syphilitic (early) 091.0
    late 095.8
  trichomonal 131.01
**Vulvodynia** 625.8 ▲
**Vulvorectal** — *see* condition
**Vulvovaginitis** — *see also* Vulvitis 616.10
  amebic 006.8
  chlamydial 099.53
  gonococcal (acute) 098.0
    chronic or duration of 2 months or over 098.2
  herpetic 054.11
  monilial 112.1
  trichomonal (Trichomonas vaginalis) 131.01
**Watermelon stomach** 537.82 ●
  with hemorrhage 537.83 ●
  without hemorrhage 537.82 ●

## W

**Waardenburg-Klein syndrome** (ptosis-epicanthus) 270.2
**Waardenburg's syndrome** 756.89
  meaning ptosis-epicanthus 270.2
**Wagner's disease** (colloid milium) 709.3
**Wagner (-Unverricht) syndrome** (dermatomyositis) 710.3
**Waiting list, person on** V63.2
  undergoing social agency investigation V63.8
**Wakefulness disorder** — *see also* Hypersomnia 780.54
  nonorganic origin 307.43
**Waldenström's**
  disease (osteochondrosis, capital femoral) 732.1
  hepatitis (lupoid hepatitis) 571.49
  hypergammaglobulinemia 273.0

**Waldenström's** — *continued*
  macroglobulinemia 273.3
  purpura, hypergammaglobulinemic 273.0
  syndrome (macroglobulinemia) 273.3
**Waldenström-Kjellberg syndrome** (sideropenic dysphagia) 280.8
**Walking**
  difficulty 719.7
    psychogenic 307.9
  sleep 307.46
    hysterical 300.13
**Wall, abdominal** — *see* condition
**Wallenberg's syndrome** (posterior inferior cerebellar artery) — *see also* Disease, cerebrovascular, acute 436
**Wallgren's**
  disease (obstruction of splenic vein with collateral circulation) 459.89
  meningitis (*see also* Meningitis, aseptic) 047.9
**Wandering**
  acetabulum 736.39
  gallbladder 751.69
  kidney, congenital 753.3
  organ or site, congenital NEC — *see* Malposition, congenital
  pacemaker (atrial) (heart) 427.89
  spleen 289.59
**Wardrop's disease** (with lymphangitis) 681.9
  finger 681.02
  toe 681.11
**War neurosis** 300.16
**Wart** (common) (digitate) (filiform) (infectious) (viral) 078.10
  external genital organs (venereal) 078.19
  fig 078.19
  Hassall-Henle's (of cornea) 371.41
  Henle's (of cornea) 371.41
  juvenile 078.19
  moist 078.10
  Peruvian 088.0
  plantar 078.19
  prosector (*see also* Tuberculosis) 017.0 ☑
  seborrheic 702.19
    inflamed 702.11
  senile 702.0
  specified NEC 078.19
  syphilitic 091.3
  tuberculous (*see also* Tuberculosis) 017.0 ☑
  venereal (female) (male) 078.19
**Warthin's tumor** (salivary gland) (M8561/0) 210.2
**Washerwoman's itch** 692.4
**Wassilieff's disease** (leptospiral jaundice) 100.0
**Wasting**
  disease 799.4
    due to malnutrition 261
  extreme (due to malnutrition) 261
  muscular NEC 728.2
  palsy, paralysis 335.21
  pelvic muscle 618.83
**Water**
  clefts 366.12
  deprivation of 994.3
  in joint (*see also* Effusion, joint) 719.0 ☑
  intoxication 276.6
  itch 120.3
  lack of 994.3
  loading 276.6
  on
    brain — *see* Hydrocephalus
    chest 511.8
  poisoning 276.6
**Waterbrash** 787.1
**Water-hammer pulse** — *see also* Insufficiency, aortic 424.1

**Waterhouse (-Friderichsen) disease or syndrome** 036.3
**Water-losing nephritis** 588.89
**Wax in ear** 380.4
**Waxy**
  degeneration, any site 277.39
  disease 277.39
  kidney 277.39 *[583.81]*
  liver (large) 277.39
  spleen 277.39
**Weak, weakness** (generalized) 780.79
  arches (acquired) 734
    congenital 754.61
  bladder sphincter 596.59
  congenital 779.89
  eye muscle — *see* Strabismus
  facial 781.94
  foot (double) — *see* Weak, arches
  heart, cardiac (*see also* Failure, heart) 428.9
    congenital 746.9
  mind 317
  muscle (generalized) 728.87
  myocardium (*see also* Failure, heart) 428.9
  newborn 779.89
  pelvic fundus
    pubocervical tissue 618.81
    rectovaginal tissue 618.82
  pulse 785.9
  senile 797
  urinary stream 788.62
  valvular — *see* Endocarditis
**Wear, worn, tooth, teeth** (approximal) (hard tissues) (interproximal) (occlusal) — *see also* Attrition, teeth 521.10
**Weather, weathered**
  effects of
    cold NEC 991.9
      specified effect NEC 991.8
    hot (*see also* Heat) 992.9
  skin 692.74
**Weber-Christian disease or syndrome** (nodular nonsuppurative panniculitis) 729.30
**Weber-Cockayne syndrome** (epidermolysis bullosa) 757.39
**Weber-Dimitri syndrome** 759.6
**Weber-Gubler syndrome** 344.89
**Weber-Leyden syndrome** 344.89
**Weber-Osler syndrome** (familial hemorrhagic telangiectasia) 448.0
**Weber's paralysis or syndrome** 344.89
**Web, webbed** (congenital) — *see also* Anomaly, specified type NEC
  canthus 743.63
  digits (*see also* Syndactylism) 755.10
  duodenal 751.5
  esophagus 750.3
  fingers (*see also* Syndactylism, fingers) 755.11
  larynx (glottic) (subglottic) 748.2
  neck (pterygium colli) 744.5
  Paterson-Kelly (sideropenic dysphagia) 280.8
  popliteal syndrome 756.89
  toes (*see also* Syndactylism, toes) 755.13
**Wedge-shaped or wedging vertebra** — *see also* Osteoporosis 733.00
**Wegener's granulomatosis or syndrome** 446.4
**Wegner's disease** (syphilitic osteochondritis) 090.0
**Weight**
  gain (abnormal) (excessive) 783.1
    during pregnancy 646.1 ☑
      insufficient 646.8 ☑
  less than 1000 grams at birth 765.0 ☑
  loss (cause unknown) 783.21
**Weightlessness** 994.9
**Weil's disease** (leptospiral jaundice) 100.0
**Weill-Marchesani syndrome** (brachymorphism and ectopia lentis) 759.89

**Weingarten's syndrome** (tropical eosinophilia) 518.3
**Weir Mitchell's disease** (erythromelalgia) 443.82
**Weiss-Baker syndrome** (carotid sinus syncope) 337.0
**Weissenbach-Thibierge syndrome** (cutaneous systemic sclerosis) 710.1
**Wen** — *see also* Cyst, sebaceous 706.2
**Wenckebach's phenomenon, heart block** (second degree) 426.13
**Werdnig-Hoffmann syndrome** (muscular atrophy) 335.0
**Werlhof-Wichmann syndrome** — *see also* Purpura, thrombocytopenic 287.39
**Werlhof's disease** — *see also* Purpura, thrombocytopenic 287.39
**Wermer's syndrome or disease** (polyendocrine adenomatosis) 258.01 ▲
**Werner's disease or syndrome** (progeria adultorum) 259.8
**Werner-His disease** (trench fever) 083.1
**Werner-Schultz disease** (agranulocytosis) 288.09
**Wernicke's encephalopathy, disease, or syndrome** (superior hemorrhagic polioencephalitis) 265.1
**Wernicke-Korsakoff syndrome or psychosis** (nonalcoholic) 294.0
  alcoholic 291.1
**Wernicke-Posadas disease** — *see also* Coccidioidomycosis 114.9
**Wesselsbron fever** 066.3
**West African fever** 084.8
**West Nile**
  encephalitis 066.41
  encephalomyelitis 066.41
  fever 066.40
    with
      cranial nerve disorders 066.42
      encephalitis 066.41
      optic neuritis 066.42
      other complications 066.49
      other neurologic manifestations 066.42
      polyradiculitis 066.42
  virus 066.40
**Westphal-Strümpell syndrome** (hepatolenticular degeneration) 275.1
**Wet**
  brain (alcoholic) (*see also* Alcoholism) 303.9 ☑
  feet, tropical (syndrome) (maceration) 991.4
  lung (syndrome)
    adult 518.5
    newborn 770.6
**Wharton's duct** — *see* condition
**Wheal** 709.8
**Wheezing** 786.07
**Whiplash injury or syndrome** 847.0
**Whipple's disease or syndrome** (intestinal lipodystrophy) 040.2
**Whipworm** 127.3
**"Whistling face" syndrome** (craniocarpotarsal dystrophy) 759.89
**White** — *see also* condition
  kidney
    large — *see* Nephrosis
    small 582.9
  leg, puerperal, postpartum, childbirth 671.4 ☑
    nonpuerperal 451.19
  mouth 112.0
  patches of mouth 528.6
  sponge nevus of oral mucosa 750.26
  spot lesions, teeth 521.01
**White's disease** (congenital) (keratosis follicularis) 757.39
**Whitehead** 706.2
**Whitlow** (with lymphangitis) 681.01
  herpetic 054.6
**Whitmore's disease or fever** (melioidosis) 025

**Whooping cough** 033.9
  with pneumonia 033.9 *[484.3]*
  due to
    Bordetella
      bronchoseptica 033.8
        with pneumonia 033.8 *[484.3]*
      parapertussis 033.1
        with pneumonia 033.1 *[484.3]*
      pertussis 033.0
        with pneumonia 033.0 *[484.3]*
    specified organism NEC 033.8
      with pneumonia 033.8 *[484.3]*
  vaccination, prophylactic (against) V03.6
**Wichmann's asthma** (laryngismus stridulus) 478.75
**Widal (-Abrami) syndrome** (acquired hemolytic jaundice) 283.9
**Widening aorta** — *see also* Aneurysm, aorta 441.9
  ruptured 441.5
**Wilkie's disease or syndrome** 557.1
**Wilkinson-Sneddon disease or syndrome** (subcorneal pustular dermatosis) 694.1
**Willan's lepra** 696.1
**Willan-Plumbe syndrome** (psoriasis) 696.1
**Willebrand (-Jürgens) syndrome or thrombopathy** (angiohemophilia) 286.4
**Willi-Prader syndrome** (hypogenital dystrophy with diabetic tendency) 759.81
**Willis' disease** (diabetes mellitus) — *see also* Diabetes 250.0 ☑
**Wilms' tumor or neoplasm** (nephroblastoma) (M8960/3) 189.0
**Wilson's**
  disease or syndrome (hepatolenticular degeneration) 275.1
  hepatolenticular degeneration 275.1
  lichen ruber 697.0
**Wilson-Brocq disease** (dermatitis exfoliativa) 695.89
**Wilson-Mikity syndrome** 770.7
**Window** — *see also* Imperfect, closure
  aorticopulmonary 745.0
**Winged scapula** 736.89
**Winter** — *see also* condition
  vomiting disease 078.82
**Wise's disease** 696.2
**Wiskott-Aldrich syndrome** (eczema-thrombocytopenia) 279.12
**Withdrawal symptoms, syndrome**
  alcohol 291.81
    delirium (acute) 291.0
      chronic 291.1
    newborn 760.71
  drug or narcotic 292.0
    newborn, infant of dependent mother 779.5
  steroid NEC
    correct substance properly administered 255.41 ▲
    overdose or wrong substance given or taken 962.0
**Withdrawing reaction, child or adolescent** V313.22
**Witts' anemia** (achlorhydric anemia) 280.9
**Witzelsucht** 301.9
**Woakes' syndrome** (ethmoiditis) 471.1
**Wohlfart-Kugelberg-Welander disease** 335.11
**Woillez' disease** (acute idiopathic pulmonary congestion) 518.5
**Wolff-Parkinson-White syndrome** (anomalous atrioventricular excitation) 426.7
**Wolhynian fever** 083.1
**Wolman's disease** (primary familial xanthomatosis) 272.7

**Wood asthma** 495.8
**Woolly, wooly hair** (congenital) (nevus) 757.4
**Wool-sorters' disease** 022.1
**Word**
  blindness (congenital) (developmental) 315.01
    secondary to organic lesion 784.61
  deafness (secondary to organic lesion) 784.69
    developmental 315.31
**Worm(s)** (colic) (fever) (infection) (infestation) — *see also* Infestation 128.9
  guinea 125.7
  in intestine NEC 127.9
**Worm-eaten soles** 102.3
**Worn out** — *see also* Exhaustion 780.79
**"Worried well"** V65.5
**Wound, open** (by cutting or piercing instrument) (by firearms) (cut) (dissection) (incised) (laceration) (penetration) (perforating) (puncture) (with initial hemorrhage, not internal) 879.8

*Note — For fracture with open wound, see Fracture.*

*For laceration, traumatic rupture, tear or penetrating wound of internal organs, such as heart, lung, liver, kidney, pelvic organs, etc., whether or not accompanied by open wound or fracture in the same region, see Injury, internal.*

*For contused wound, see Contusion. For crush injury, see Crush. For abrasion, insect bite (nonvenomous), blister, or scratch, see Injury, superficial.*

*Complicated includes wounds with:*
  *delayed healing*
  *delayed treatment*
  *foreign body*
  *primary infection*

*For late effect of open wound, see Late, effect, wound, open, by site.*

  abdomen, abdominal (external) (muscle) 879.2
    complicated 879.3
    wall (anterior) 879.2
      complicated 879.3
      lateral 879.4
        complicated 879.5
  alveolar (process) 873.62
    complicated 873.72
  ankle 891.0
    with tendon involvement 891.2
    complicated 891.1
  anterior chamber, eye (*see also* Wound, open, intraocular) 871.9
  anus 879.6
    complicated 879.7
  arm 884.0
    with tendon involvement 884.2
    complicated 884.1
    forearm 881.00
      with tendon involvement 881.20
      complicated 881.10
    multiple sites — *see* Wound, open, multiple, upper limb
    upper 880.03
      with tendon involvement 880.23
      complicated 880.13
      multiple sites (with axillary or shoulder regions) 880.09
        with tendon involvement 880.29
        complicated 880.19
  artery — *see* Injury, blood vessel, by site
  auditory
    canal (external) (meatus) 872.02
      complicated 872.12
    ossicles (incus) (malleus) (stapes) 872.62

☑ Additional Digit Required — Refer to the Tabular List for Digit Selection   ▦ Subterms under main terms may continue to next column or page

298 — Volume 2 · October 2007   ▶◀ Revised Text   ● New Line   ▲ Revised Code   **2008 ICD-9-CM**

**Wound, open** — *continued*
auditory — *continued*
ossicles — *continued*
complicated 872.72
auricle, ear 872.01
complicated 872.11
axilla 880.02
with tendon involvement 880.22
complicated 880.12
with tendon involvement 880.29
involving other sites of upper arm 880.09
complicated 880.19
back 876.0
complicated 876.1
bladder — *see* Injury, internal, bladder
blood vessel — *see* Injury, blood vessel, by site
brain — *see* Injury, intracranial, with open intracranial wound
breast 879.0
complicated 879.1
brow 873.42
complicated 873.52
buccal mucosa 873.61
complicated 873.71
buttock 877.0
complicated 877.1
calf 891.0
with tendon involvement 891.2
complicated 891.1
canaliculus lacrimalis 870.8
with laceration of eyelid 870.2
canthus, eye 870.8
laceration — *see* Laceration, eyelid
cavernous sinus — *see* Injury, intracranial
cerebellum — *see* Injury, intracranial
cervical esophagus 874.4
complicated 874.5
cervix — *see* Injury, internal, cervix
cheek(s) (external) 873.41
complicated 873.51
internal 873.61
complicated 873.71
chest (wall) (external) 875.0
complicated 875.1
chin 873.44
complicated 873.54
choroid 363.63
ciliary body (eye) (*see also* Wound, open, intraocular) 871.9
clitoris 878.8
complicated 878.9
cochlea 872.64
complicated 872.74
complicated 879.9
conjunctiva — *see* Wound, open, intraocular
cornea (nonpenetrating) (*see also* Wound, open, intraocular) 871.9
costal region 875.0
complicated 875.1
Descemet's membrane (*see also* Wound, open, intraocular) 871.9
digit(s)
foot 893.0
with tendon involvement 893.2
complicated 893.1
hand 883.0
with tendon involvement 883.2
complicated 883.1
drumhead, ear 872.61
complicated 872.71
ear 872.8
canal 872.02
complicated 872.12
complicated 872.9
drum 872.61
complicated 872.71
external 872.00
complicated 872.10
multiple sites 872.69
complicated 872.79

ear — *continued*
ossicles (incus) (malleus) (stapes) 872.62
complicated 872.72
specified part NEC 872.69
complicated 872.79
elbow 881.01
with tendon involvement 881.21
complicated 881.11
epididymis 878.2
complicated 878.3
epigastric region 879.2
complicated 879.3
epiglottis 874.01
complicated 874.11
esophagus (cervical) 874.4
complicated 874.5
thoracic — *see* Injury, internal, esophagus
Eustachian tube 872.63
complicated 872.73
extremity
lower (multiple) NEC 894.0
with tendon involvement 894.2
complicated 894.1
upper (multiple) NEC 884.0
with tendon involvement 884.2
complicated 884.1
eye(s) (globe) — *see* Wound, open, intraocular
eyeball NEC 871.9
laceration (*see also* Laceration, eyeball) 871.4
penetrating (*see also* Penetrating wound, eyeball) 871.7
eyebrow 873.42
complicated 873.52
eyelid NEC 870.8
laceration — *see* Laceration, eyelid
face 873.40
complicated 873.50
multiple sites 873.49
complicated 873.59
specified part NEC 873.49
complicated 873.59
fallopian tube — *see* Injury, internal, fallopian tube
finger(s) (nail) (subungual) 883.0
with tendon involvement 883.2
complicated 883.1
flank 879.4
complicated 879.5
foot (any part except toe(s) alone) 892.0
with tendon involvement 892.2
complicated 892.1
forearm 881.00
with tendon involvement 881.20
complicated 881.10
forehead 873.42
complicated 873.52
genital organs (external) NEC 878.8
complicated 878.9
internal — *see* Injury, internal, by site
globe (eye) (*see also* Wound, open, eyeball) 871.9
groin 879.4
complicated 879.5
gum(s) 873.62
complicated 873.72
hand (except finger(s) alone) 882.0
with tendon involvement 882.2
complicated 882.1
head NEC 873.8
with intracranial injury — *see* Injury, intracranial
due to or associated with skull fracture — *see* Fracture, skull
complicated 873.9
scalp — *see* Wound, open, scalp
heel 892.0
with tendon involvement 892.2
complicated 892.1

high-velocity (grease gun) — *see* Wound, open, complicated, by site
hip 890.0
with tendon involvement 890.2
complicated 890.1
hymen 878.6
complicated 878.7
hypochondrium 879.4
complicated 879.5
hypogastric region 879.2
complicated 879.3
iliac (region) 879.4
complicated 879.5
incidental to
dislocation — *see* Dislocation, open, by site
fracture — *see* Fracture, open, by site
intracranial injury — *see* Injury, intracranial, with open intracranial wound
nerve injury — *see* Injury, nerve, by site
inguinal region 879.4
complicated 879.5
instep 892.0
with tendon involvement 892.2
complicated 892.1
interscapular region 876.0
complicated 876.1
intracranial — *see* Injury, intracranial, with open intracranial wound
intraocular 871.9
with
partial loss (of intraocular tissue) 871.2
prolapse or exposure (of intraocular tissue) 871.1
without prolapse (of intraocular tissue) 871.0
laceration (*see also* Laceration, eyeball) 871.4
penetrating 871.7
with foreign body (nonmagnetic) 871.6
magnetic 871.5
iris (*see also* Wound, open, eyeball) 871.9
jaw (fracture not involved) 873.44
with fracture — *see* Fracture, jaw
complicated 873.54
knee 891.0
with tendon involvement 891.2
complicated 891.1
labium (majus) (minus) 878.4
complicated 878.5
lacrimal apparatus, gland, or sac 870.8
with laceration of eyelid 870.2
larynx 874.01
with trachea 874.00
complicated 874.10
complicated 874.11
leg (multiple) 891.0
with tendon involvement 891.2
complicated 891.1
lower 891.0
with tendon involvement 891.2
complicated 891.1
thigh 890.0
with tendon involvement 890.2
complicated 890.1
upper 890.0
with tendon involvement 890.2
complicated 890.1
lens (eye) (alone) (*see also* Cataract, traumatic) 366.20
with involvement of other eye structures — *see* Wound, open, eyeball
limb
lower (multiple) NEC 894.0
with tendon involvement 894.2
complicated 894.1

limb — *continued*
upper (multiple) NEC 884.0
with tendon involvement 884.2
complicated 884.1
lip 873.43
complicated 873.53
loin 876.0
complicated 876.1
lumbar region 876.0
complicated 876.1
malar region 873.41
complicated 873.51
mastoid region 873.49
complicated 873.59
mediastinum — *see* Injury, internal, mediastinum
midthoracic region 875.0
complicated 875.1
mouth 873.60
complicated 873.70
floor 873.64
complicated 873.74
multiple sites 873.69
complicated 873.79
specified site NEC 873.69
complicated 873.79
multiple, unspecified site(s) 879.8

> *Note — Multiple open wounds of sites classifiable to the same four-digit category should be classified to that category unless they are in different limbs.*
>
> *Multiple open wounds of sites classifiable to different four-digit categories, or to different limbs, should be coded separately.*

complicated 879.9
lower limb(s) (one or both) (sites classifiable to more than one three-digit category in 890 to 893) 894.0
with tendon involvement 894.2
complicated 894.1
upper limb(s) (one or both) (sites classifiable to more than one three-digit category in 880 to 883) 884.0
with tendon involvement 884.2
complicated 884.1
muscle — *see* Sprain, by site
nail
finger(s) 883.0
complicated 883.1
thumb 883.0
complicated 883.1
toe(s) 893.0
complicated 893.1
nape (neck) 874.8
complicated 874.9
specified part NEC 874.8
complicated 874.9
nasal (*see also* Wound, open, nose)
cavity 873.22
complicated 873.32
septum 873.21
complicated 873.31
sinuses 873.23
complicated 873.33
nasopharynx 873.22
complicated 873.32
neck 874.8
complicated 874.9
nape 874.8
complicated 874.9
specified part NEC 874.8
complicated 874.9
nerve — *see* Injury, nerve, by site
non-healing surgical 998.83
nose 873.20
complicated 873.30
multiple sites 873.29
complicated 873.39
septum 873.21
complicated 873.31
sinuses 873.23

---

☑ Additional Digit Required — Refer to the Tabular List for Digit Selection       ▽ Subterms under main terms may continue to next column or page

**Index**

**Wound, open — Yersinia septica**

**Wound, open** — *continued*
  nose — *continued*
    sinuses — *continued*
      complicated 873.33
  occipital region — *see* Wound, open, scalp
  ocular NEC 871.9
    adnexa 870.9
      specified region NEC 870.8
    laceration (*see also* Laceration, ocular) 871.4
    muscle (extraocular) 870.3
      with foreign body 870.4
      eyelid 870.1
      intraocular — *see* Wound, open, eyeball
    penetrating (*see also* Penetrating wound, ocular) 871.7
  orbit 870.8
    penetrating 870.3
      with foreign body 870.4
  orbital region 870.9
  ovary — *see* Injury, internal, pelvic organs
  palate 873.65
    complicated 873.75
  palm 882.0
    with tendon involvement 882.2
    complicated 882.1
  parathyroid (gland) 874.2
    complicated 874.3
  parietal region — *see* Wound, open, scalp
  pelvic floor or region 879.6
    complicated 879.7
  penis 878.0
    complicated 878.1
  perineum 879.6
    complicated 879.7
  periocular area 870.8
    laceration of skin 870.0
  pharynx 874.4
    complicated 874.5
  pinna 872.01
    complicated 872.11
  popliteal space 891.0
    with tendon involvement 891.2
    complicated 891.1
  prepuce 878.0
    complicated 878.1
  pubic region 879.2
    complicated 879.3
  pudenda 878.8
    complicated 878.9
  rectovaginal septum 878.8
    complicated 878.9
  sacral region 877.0
    complicated 877.1
  sacroiliac region 877.0
    complicated 877.1
  salivary (ducts) (glands) 873.69
    complicated 873.79
  scalp 873.0
    complicated 873.1
  scalpel, fetus or newborn 767.8
  scapular region 880.01
    with tendon involvement 880.21
    complicated 880.11
    involving other sites of upper arm 880.09
      with tendon involvement 880.29
      complicated 880.19
  sclera (*see also* Wound, open, intraocular) 871.9
  scrotum 878.2
    complicated 878.3
  seminal vesicle — *see* Injury, internal, pelvic organs
  shin 891.0
    with tendon involvement 891.2
    complicated 891.1
  shoulder 880.00
    with tendon involvement 880.20
    complicated 880.10
    involving other sites of upper arm 880.09

**Wound, open** — *continued*
  shoulder — *continued*
    involving other sites of upper arm — *continued*
      with tendon involvement 880.29
      complicated 880.19
  skin NEC 879.8
    complicated 879.9
  skull (*see also* Injury, intracranial, with open intracranial wound)
    with skull fracture — *see* Fracture, skull
  spermatic cord (scrotal) 878.2
    complicated 878.3
    pelvic region — *see* Injury, internal, spermatic cord
  spinal cord — *see* Injury, spinal
  sternal region 875.0
    complicated 875.1
  subconjunctival — *see* Wound, open, intraocular
  subcutaneous NEC 879.8
    complicated 879.9
  submaxillary region 873.44
    complicated 873.54
  submental region 873.44
    complicated 873.54
  subungual
    finger(s) (thumb) — *see* Wound, open, finger
    toe(s) — *see* Wound, open, toe
  supraclavicular region 874.8
    complicated 874.9
  supraorbital 873.42
    complicated 873.52
  surgical, non-healing 998.83
  temple 873.49
    complicated 873.59
  temporal region 873.49
    complicated 873.59
  testis 878.2
    complicated 878.3
  thigh 890.0
    with tendon involvement 890.2
    complicated 890.1
  thorax, thoracic (external) 875.0
    complicated 875.1
  throat 874.8
    complicated 874.9
  thumb (nail) (subungual) 883.0
    with tendon involvement 883.2
    complicated 883.1
  thyroid (gland) 874.2
    complicated 874.3
  toe(s) (nail) (subungual) 893.0
    with tendon involvement 893.2
    complicated 893.1
  tongue 873.64
    complicated 873.74
  tonsil — *see* Wound, open, neck
  trachea (cervical region) 874.02
    with larynx 874.00
      complicated 874.10
    complicated 874.12
    intrathoracic — *see* Injury, internal, trachea
  trunk (multiple) NEC 879.6
    complicated 879.7
    specified site NEC 879.6
      complicated 879.7
  tunica vaginalis 878.2
    complicated 878.3
  tympanic membrane 872.61
    complicated 872.71
  tympanum 872.61
    complicated 872.71
  umbilical region 879.2
    complicated 879.3
  ureter — *see* Injury, internal, ureter
  urethra — *see* Injury, internal, urethra
  uterus — *see* Injury, internal, uterus
  uvula 873.69
    complicated 873.79
  vagina 878.6
    complicated 878.7

**Wound, open** — *continued*
  vas deferens — *see* Injury, internal, vas deferens
  vitreous (humor) 871.2
  vulva 878.4
    complicated 878.5
  wrist 881.02
    with tendon involvement 881.22
    complicated 881.12
**Wright's syndrome** (hyperabduction) 447.8
  pneumonia 390 [517.1]
**Wringer injury** — *see* Crush injury, by site
**Wrinkling of skin** 701.8
**Wrist** — *see also* condition
  drop (acquired) 736.05
**Wrong drug** (given in error) NEC 977.9
  specified drug or substance — *see* Table of Drugs and Chemicals
**Wry neck** — *see also* Torticollis
  congenital 754.1
**Wuchereria infestation** 125.0
  bancrofti 125.0
  Brugia malayi 125.1
  malayi 125.1
**Wuchereriasis** 125.0
**Wuchereriosis** 125.0
**Wuchernde struma langhans** (M8332/3) 193

## X

**Xanthelasma** 272.2
  eyelid 272.2 [374.51]
  palpebrarum 272.2 [374.51]
**Xanthelasmatosis** (essential) 272.2
**Xanthelasmoidea** 757.33
**Xanthine stones** 277.2
**Xanthinuria** 277.2
**Xanthofibroma** (M8831/0) — *see* Neoplasm, connective tissue, benign
**Xanthoma(s), xanthomatosis** 272.2
  with
    hyperlipoproteinemia
      type I 272.3
      type III 272.2
      type IV 272.1
      type V 272.3
  bone 272.7
  craniohypophyseal 277.89
  cutaneotendinous 272.7
  diabeticorum 250.8 ☑ [272.2]
  disseminatum 272.7
  eruptive 272.2
  eyelid 272.2 [374.51]
  familial 272.7
  hereditary 272.7
  hypercholesterinemic 272.0
  hypercholesterolemic 272.0
  hyperlipemic 272.4
  hyperlipidemic 272.4
  infantile 272.7
  joint 272.7
  juvenile 272.7
  multiple 272.7
  multiplex 272.7
  primary familial 272.7
  tendon (sheath) 272.7
  tuberosum 272.2
  tuberous 272.2
  tubo-eruptive 272.2
**Xanthosis** 709.09
  surgical 998.81
**Xenophobia** 300.29
**Xeroderma** (congenital) 757.39
  acquired 701.1
    eyelid 373.33
  eyelid 373.33
  pigmentosum 757.33
  vitamin A deficiency 264.8
**Xerophthalmia** 372.53
  vitamin A deficiency 264.7
**Xerosis**
  conjunctiva 372.53
    with Bitôt's spot 372.53
      vitamin A deficiency 264.1

**Xerosis** — *continued*
  conjunctiva — *continued*
    vitamin A deficiency 264.0
  cornea 371.40
    with corneal ulceration 370.00
      vitamin A deficiency 264.3
    vitamin A deficiency 264.2
  cutis 706.8
  skin 706.8
**Xerostomia** 527.7
**Xiphodynia** 733.90
**Xiphoidalgia** 733.90
**Xiphoiditis** 733.99
**Xiphopagus** 759.4
**XO syndrome** 758.6
**X-ray**
  effects, adverse, NEC 990
  of chest
    for suspected tuberculosis V71.2
    routine V72.5
**XXX syndrome** 758.81
**XXXXY syndrome** 758.81
**XXY syndrome** 758.7
**Xyloketosuria** 271.8
**Xylosuria** 271.8
**Xylulosuria** 271.8
**XYY syndrome** 758.81

## Y

**Yawning** 786.09
  psychogenic 306.1
**Yaws** 102.9
  bone or joint lesions 102.6
  butter 102.1
  chancre 102.0
  cutaneous, less than five years after infection 102.2
  early (cutaneous) (macular) (maculopapular) (micropapular) (papular) 102.2
    frambeside 102.2
    skin lesions NEC 102.2
  eyelid 102.9 [373.4]
  ganglion 102.6
  gangosis, gangosa 102.5
  gumma, gummata 102.4
    bone 102.6
  gummatous
    frambeside 102.4
    osteitis 102.6
    periostitis 102.6
  hydrarthrosis 102.6
  hyperkeratosis (early) (late) (palmar) (plantar) 102.3
  initial lesions 102.0
  joint lesions 102.6
  juxta-articular nodules 102.7
  late nodular (ulcerated) 102.4
  latent (without clinical manifestations) (with positive serology) 102.8
  mother 102.0
  mucosal 102.7
  multiple papillomata 102.1
  nodular, late (ulcerated) 102.4
  osteitis 102.6
  papilloma, papillomata (palmar) (plantar) 102.1
  periostitis (hypertrophic) 102.6
  ulcers 102.4
  wet crab 102.1
**Yeast infection** — *see also* Candidiasis 112.9
**Yellow**
  atrophy (liver) 570
    chronic 571.8
    resulting from administration of blood, plasma, serum, or other biological substance (within 8 months of administration) — *see* Hepatitis, viral
  fever — *see* Fever, yellow
  jack (*see also* Fever, yellow) 060.9
  jaundice (*see also* Jaundice) 782.4
  vernix syndrome 762.2
**Yersinia septica** 027.8

☑ Additional Digit Required — Refer to the Tabular List for Digit Selection      ⁿᵉʷ Subterms under main terms may continue to next column or page

**300 — Volume 2**      ▶◀ Revised Text      ● New Line      ▲ Revised Code      *2008 ICD-9-CM*

**Z**

**Zagari's disease** (xerostomia) 527.7
**Zahorsky's disease** (exanthema subitum)
▶(*see also* Exanthem subitum)◀
058.10 ▲
syndrome (herpangina) 074.0
**Zellweger syndrome** 277.86

**Zenker's diverticulum** (esophagus)
530.6
**Ziehen-Oppenheim disease** 333.6
**Zieve's syndrome** (jaundice, hyperlipemia, and hemolytic anemia)
571.1
**Zika fever** 066.3

**Zollinger-Ellison syndrome** (gastric hy-
persecretion with pancreatic islet
cell tumor) 251.5
**Zona** — *see also* Herpes, zoster 053.9
**Zoophilia** (erotica) 302.1
**Zoophobia** 300.29
**Zoster** (herpes) — *see also* Herpes, zoster
053.9

**Zuelzer (-Ogden) anemia or syndrome**
(nutritional megaloblastic anemia)
281.2
**Zygodactyly** — *see also* Syndactylism
755.10
**Zygomycosis** 117.7
**Zymotic** — *see* condition

# SECTION 2

## Alphabetic Index to Poisoning and External Causes of Adverse Effects of Drugs and Other Chemical Substances

### TABLE OF DRUGS AND CHEMICALS

This table contains a classification of drugs and other chemical substances to identify poisoning states and external causes of adverse effects.

Each of the listed substances in the table is assigned a code according to the poisoning classification (960-989). These codes are used when there is a statement of poisoning, overdose, wrong substance given or taken, or intoxication.

The table also contains a listing of external causes of adverse effects. An adverse effect is a pathologic manifestation due to ingestion or exposure to drugs or other chemical substances (e.g., dermatitis, hypersensitivity reaction, aspirin gastritis). The adverse effect is to be identified by the appropriate code found in Section 1, Index to Diseases and Injuries. An external cause code can then be used to identify the circumstances involved. The table headings pertaining to external causes are defined below:

**Accidental poisoning (E850-E869)** — accidental overdose of drug, wrong substance given or taken, drug taken inadvertently, accidents in the usage of drugs and biologicals in medical and surgical procedures, and to show external causes of poisonings classifiable to 980-989.

**Therapeutic use (E930-E949)** — a correct substance properly administered in therapeutic or prophylactic dosage as the external cause of adverse effects.

**Suicide attempt (E950-E952)** — instances in which self-inflicted injuries or poisonings are involved.

**Assault (E96I-E962)** — injury or poisoning inflicted by another person with the intent to injure or kill.

**Undetermined (E980-E982)** — to be used when the intent of the poisoning or injury cannot be determined whether it was intentional or accidental.

The American Hospital Formulary Service list numbers are included in the table to help classify new drugs not identified in the table by name. The AHFS list numbers are keyed to the continually revised American Hospital Formulary Service (AHFS).* These listings are found in the table under the main term **Drug**.

Excluded from the table are radium and other radioactive substances. The classification of adverse effects and complications pertaining to these substances will be found in Section 1, Index to Diseases and Injuries, and Section 3, Index to External Causes of Injuries.

Although certain substances are indexed with one or more subentries, the majority are listed according to one use or state. It is recognized that many substances may be used in various ways, in medicine and in industry, and may cause adverse effects whatever the state of the agent (solid, liquid, or fumes arising from a liquid). In cases in which the reported data indicates a use or state not in the table, or which is clearly different from the one listed, an attempt should be made to classify the substance in the form which most nearly expresses the reported facts.

*American Hospital Formulary Service, 2 vol. (Washington, D.C.: American Society of Hospital Pharmacists, 1959-)

☑ Additional Digit Required — Refer to the Tabular List for Digit Selection       ▽ Subterms under main terms may continue to next column or page

*2008 ICD-9-CM*          ▶◀ Revised Text          ● New Line          ▲ Revised Code          **Volume 2 — 303**

| | | External Cause (E-Code) | | | | |
|---|---|---|---|---|---|---|
| | Poisoning | Accident | Therapeutic Use | Suicide Attempt | Assault | Undetermined |
| **1-propanol** | 980.3 | E860.4 | — | E950.9 | E962.1 | E980.9 |
| **2-propanol** | 980.2 | E860.3 | — | E950.9 | E962.1 | E980.9 |
| **2, 4-D** (dichlorophenoxyacetic acid) | 989.4 | E863.5 | — | E950.6 | E962.1 | E980.7 |
| **2, 4-toluene diisocyanate** | 983.0 | E864.0 | — | E950.7 | E962.1 | E980.6 |
| **2, 4, 5-T** (trichlorophenoxyacetic acid) | 989.2 | E863.5 | — | E950.6 | E962.1 | E980.7 |
| **14-hydroxydihydromorphinone** | 965.09 | E850.2 | E935.2 | E950.0 | E962.0 | E980.0 |
| **ABOB** | 961.7 | E857 | E931.7 | E950.4 | E962.0 | E980.4 |
| **Abrus** (seed) | 988.2 | E865.3 | — | E950.9 | E962.1 | E980.9 |
| **Absinthe** | 980.0 | E860.1 | — | E950.9 | E962.1 | E980.9 |
| beverage | 980.0 | E860.0 | — | E950.9 | E962.1 | E980.9 |
| **Acenocoumarin, acenocoumarol** | 964.2 | E858.2 | E934.2 | E950.4 | E962.0 | E980.4 |
| **Acepromazine** | 969.1 | E853.0 | E939.1 | E950.3 | E962.0 | E980.3 |
| **Acetal** | 982.8 | E862.4 | — | E950.9 | E962.1 | E980.9 |
| **Acetaldehyde** (vapor) | 987.8 | E869.8 | — | E952.8 | E962.2 | E982.8 |
| liquid | 989.89 | E866.8 | — | E950.9 | E962.1 | E980.9 |
| **Acetaminophen** | 965.4 | E850.4 | E935.4 | E950.0 | E962.0 | E980.0 |
| **Acetaminosalol** | 965.1 | E850.3 | E935.3 | E950.0 | E962.0 | E980.0 |
| **Acetanilid(e)** | 965.4 | E850.4 | E935.4 | E950.0 | E962.0 | E980.0 |
| **Acetarsol, acetarsone** | 961.1 | E857 | E931.1 | E950.4 | E962.0 | E980.4 |
| **Acetazolamide** | 974.2 | E858.5 | E944.2 | E950.4 | E962.0 | E980.4 |
| **Acetic** | | | | | | |
| acid | 983.1 | E864.1 | — | E950.7 | E962.1 | E980.6 |
| with sodium acetate (ointment) | 976.3 | E858.7 | E946.3 | E950.4 | E962.0 | E980.4 |
| irrigating solution | 974.5 | E858.5 | E944.5 | E950.4 | E962.0 | E980.4 |
| lotion | 976.2 | E858.7 | E946.2 | E950.4 | E962.0 | E980.4 |
| anhydride | 983.1 | E864.1 | — | E950.7 | E962.1 | E980.6 |
| ether (vapor) | 982.8 | E862.4 | — | E950.9 | E962.1 | E980.9 |
| **Acetohexamide** | 962.3 | E858.0 | E932.3 | E950.4 | E962.0 | E980.4 |
| **Acetomenaphthone** | 964.3 | E858.2 | E934.3 | E950.4 | E962.0 | E980.4 |
| **Acetomorphine** | 965.01 | E850.0 | E935.0 | E950.0 | E962.0 | E980.0 |
| **Acetone** (oils) (vapor) | 982.8 | E862.4 | — | E950.9 | E962.1 | E980.9 |
| **Acetophenazine** (maleate) | 969.1 | E853.0 | E939.1 | E950.3 | E962.0 | E980.3 |
| **Acetophenetidin** | 965.4 | E850.4 | E935.4 | E950.0 | E962.0 | E980.0 |
| **Acetophenone** | 982.0 | E862.4 | — | E950.9 | E962.1 | E980.9 |
| **Acetorphine** | 965.09 | E850.2 | E935.2 | E950.0 | E962.0 | E980.0 |
| **Acetosulfone** (sodium) | 961.8 | E857 | E931.8 | E950.4 | E962.0 | E980.4 |
| **Acetrizoate** (sodium) | 977.8 | E858.8 | E947.8 | E950.4 | E962.0 | E980.4 |
| **Acetylcarbromal** | 967.3 | E852.2 | E937.3 | E950.2 | E962.0 | E980.2 |
| **Acetylcholine** (chloride) | 971.0 | E855.3 | E941.0 | E950.4 | E962.0 | E980.4 |
| **Acetylcysteine** | 975.5 | E858.6 | E945.5 | E950.4 | E962.0 | E980.4 |
| **Acetyldigitoxin** | 972.1 | E858.3 | E942.1 | E950.4 | E962.0 | E980.4 |
| **Acetyldihydrocodeine** | 965.09 | E850.2 | E935.2 | E950.0 | E962.0 | E980.0 |
| **Acetyldihydrocodeinone** | 965.09 | E850.2 | E935.2 | E950.0 | E962.0 | E980.0 |
| **Acetylene** (gas) (industrial) | 987.1 | E868.1 | — | E951.8 | E962.2 | E981.8 |
| incomplete combustion of — see Carbon monoxide, fuel, utility | | | | | | |
| tetrachloride (vapor) | 982.3 | E862.4 | — | E950.9 | E962.1 | E980.9 |
| **Acetyliodosalicylic acid** | 965.1 | E850.3 | E935.3 | E950.0 | E962.0 | E980.0 |
| **Acetylphenylhydrazine** | 965.8 | E850.8 | E935.8 | E950.0 | E962.0 | E980.0 |
| **Acetylsalicylic acid** | 965.1 | E850.3 | E935.3 | E950.0 | E962.0 | E980.0 |
| **Achromycin** | 960.4 | E856 | E930.4 | E950.4 | E962.0 | E980.4 |
| ophthalmic preparation | 976.5 | E858.7 | E946.5 | E950.4 | E962.0 | E980.4 |
| topical NEC | 976.0 | E858.7 | E946.0 | E950.4 | E962.0 | E980.4 |
| **Acidifying agents** | 963.2 | E858.1 | E933.2 | E950.4 | E962.0 | E980.4 |
| **Acids (corrosive) NEC** | 983.1 | E864.1 | — | E950.7 | E962.1 | E980.6 |
| **Aconite** (wild) | 988.2 | E865.4 | — | E950.9 | E962.1 | E980.9 |
| **Aconitine** (liniment) | 976.8 | E858.7 | E946.8 | E950.4 | E962.0 | E980.4 |
| **Aconitum ferox** | 988.2 | E865.4 | — | E950.9 | E962.1 | E980.9 |
| **Acridine** | 983.0 | E864.0 | — | E950.7 | E962.1 | E980.6 |
| vapor | 987.8 | E869.8 | — | E952.8 | E962.2 | E982.8 |
| **Acriflavine** | 961.9 | E857 | E931.9 | E950.4 | E962.0 | E980.4 |
| **Acrisorcin** | 976.0 | E858.7 | E946.0 | E950.4 | E962.0 | E980.4 |
| **Acrolein** (gas) | 987.8 | E869.8 | — | E952.8 | E962.2 | E982.8 |
| liquid | 989.89 | E866.8 | — | E950.9 | E962.1 | E980.9 |
| **Actaea spicata** | 988.2 | E865.4 | — | E950.9 | E962.1 | E980.9 |
| **Acterol** | 961.5 | E857 | E931.5 | E950.4 | E962.0 | E980.4 |
| **ACTH** | 962.4 | E858.0 | E932.4 | E950.4 | E962.0 | E980.4 |
| **Acthar** | 962.4 | E858.0 | E932.4 | E950.4 | E962.0 | E980.4 |
| **Actinomycin** (C) (D) | 960.7 | E856 | E930.7 | E950.4 | E962.0 | E980.4 |
| **Adalin** (acetyl) | 967.3 | E852.2 | E937.3 | E950.2 | E962.0 | E980.2 |
| **Adenosine** (phosphate) | 977.8 | E858.8 | E947.8 | E950.4 | E962.0 | E980.4 |
| **ADH** | 962.5 | E858.0 | E932.5 | E950.4 | E962.0 | E980.4 |
| **Adhesives** | 989.89 | E866.6 | — | E950.9 | E962.1 | E980.9 |
| **Adicillin** | 960.0 | E856 | E930.0 | E950.4 | E962.0 | E980.4 |
| **Adiphenine** | 975.1 | E855.6 | E945.1 | E950.4 | E962.0 | E980.4 |
| **Adjunct, pharmaceutical** | 977.4 | E858.8 | E947.4 | E950.4 | E962.0 | E980.4 |
| **Adrenal** (extract, cortex or medulla) (glucocorticoids) (hormones) (mineralocorticoids) | 962.0 | E858.0 | E932.0 | E950.4 | E962.0 | E980.4 |
| ENT agent | 976.6 | E858.7 | E946.6 | E950.4 | E962.0 | E980.4 |
| ophthalmic preparation | 976.5 | E858.7 | E946.5 | E950.4 | E962.0 | E980.4 |
| topical NEC | 976.0 | E858.7 | E946.0 | E950.4 | E962.0 | E980.4 |
| **Adrenalin** | 971.2 | E855.5 | E941.2 | E950.4 | E962.0 | E980.4 |
| **Adrenergic blocking agents** | 971.3 | E855.6 | E941.3 | E950.4 | E962.0 | E980.4 |
| **Adrenergics** | 971.2 | E855.5 | E941.2 | E950.4 | E962.0 | E980.4 |
| **Adrenochrome** (derivatives) | 972.8 | E858.3 | E942.8 | E950.4 | E962.0 | E980.4 |
| **Adrenocorticotropic hormone** | 962.4 | E858.0 | E932.4 | E950.4 | E962.0 | E980.4 |
| **Adrenocorticotropin** | 962.4 | E858.0 | E932.4 | E950.4 | E962.0 | E980.4 |
| **Adriamycin** | 960.7 | E856 | E930.7 | E950.4 | E962.0 | E980.4 |
| **Aerosol spray** — see Sprays | | | | | | |
| **Aerosporin** | 960.8 | E856 | E930.8 | E950.4 | E962.0 | E980.4 |
| ENT agent | 976.6 | E858.7 | E946.6 | E950.4 | E962.0 | E980.4 |
| ophthalmic preparation | 976.5 | E858.7 | E946.5 | E950.4 | E962.0 | E980.4 |
| topical NEC | 976.0 | E858.7 | E946.0 | E950.4 | E962.0 | E980.4 |
| **Aethusa cynapium** | 988.2 | E865.4 | — | E950.9 | E962.1 | E980.9 |
| **Afghanistan black** | 969.6 | E854.1 | E939.6 | E950.3 | E962.0 | E980.3 |
| **Aflatoxin** | 989.7 | E865.9 | — | E950.9 | E962.1 | E980.9 |
| **African boxwood** | 988.2 | E865.4 | — | E950.9 | E962.1 | E980.9 |
| **Agar (-agar)** | 973.3 | E858.4 | E943.3 | E950.4 | E962.0 | E980.4 |
| **Agricultural agent NEC** | 989.89 | E863.9 | — | E950.6 | E962.1 | E980.7 |
| **Agrypnal** | 967.0 | E851 | E937.0 | E950.1 | E962.0 | — |
| **Air contaminant(s),** source or type not specified | 987.9 | E869.9 | — | E952.9 | E962.2 | E982.9 |
| specified type — see specific substance | | | | | | |
| **Akee** | 988.2 | E865.4 | — | E950.9 | E962.1 | E980.9 |
| **Akrinol** | 976.0 | E858.7 | E946.0 | E950.4 | E962.0 | E980.4 |
| **Alantolactone** | 961.6 | E857 | E931.6 | E950.4 | E962.0 | E980.4 |
| **Albamycin** | 960.8 | E856 | E930.8 | E950.4 | E962.0 | E980.4 |
| **Albumin** (normal human serum) | 964.7 | E858.2 | E934.7 | E950.4 | E962.0 | E980.4 |
| **Albuterol** | 975.7 | E858.6 | E945.7 | E950.4 | E962.0 | E980.4 |
| **Alcohol** | 980.9 | E860.9 | — | E950.9 | E962.1 | E980.9 |
| absolute | 980.0 | E860.1 | — | E950.9 | E962.1 | E980.9 |
| beverage | 980.0 | E860.0 | E947.8 | E950.9 | E962.1 | E980.9 |
| amyl | 980.3 | E860.4 | — | E950.9 | E962.1 | E980.9 |
| antifreeze | 980.1 | E860.2 | — | E950.9 | E962.1 | E980.9 |
| butyl | 980.3 | E860.4 | — | E950.9 | E962.1 | E980.9 |
| dehydrated | 980.0 | E860.1 | — | E950.9 | E962.1 | E980.9 |
| beverage | 980.0 | E860.0 | E947.8 | E950.9 | E962.1 | E980.9 |
| denatured | 980.0 | E860.1 | — | E950.9 | E962.1 | E980.9 |
| deterrents | 977.3 | E858.8 | E947.3 | E950.4 | E962.0 | E980.4 |
| diagnostic (gastric function) | 977.8 | E858.8 | E947.8 | E950.4 | E962.0 | E980.4 |
| ethyl | 980.0 | E860.1 | — | E950.9 | E962.1 | E980.9 |
| beverage | 980.0 | E860.0 | E947.8 | E950.9 | E962.1 | E980.9 |
| grain | 980.0 | E860.1 | — | E950.9 | E962.1 | E980.9 |
| beverage | 980.0 | E860.0 | E947.8 | E950.9 | E962.1 | E980.9 |
| industrial | 980.9 | E860.9 | — | E950.9 | E962.1 | E980.9 |
| isopropyl | 980.2 | E860.3 | — | E950.9 | E962.1 | E980.9 |
| methyl | 980.1 | E860.2 | — | E950.9 | E962.1 | E980.9 |
| preparation for consumption | 980.0 | E860.0 | E947.8 | E950.9 | E962.1 | E980.9 |
| propyl | 980.3 | E860.4 | — | E950.9 | E962.1 | E980.9 |
| secondary | 980.2 | E860.3 | — | E950.9 | E962.1 | E980.9 |
| radiator | 980.1 | E860.2 | — | E950.9 | E962.1 | E980.9 |
| rubbing | 980.2 | E860.3 | — | E950.9 | E962.1 | E980.9 |
| specified type NEC | 980.8 | E860.8 | — | E950.9 | E962.1 | E980.9 |
| surgical | 980.9 | E860.9 | — | E950.9 | E962.1 | E980.9 |
| vapor (from any type of alcohol) | 987.8 | E869.8 | — | E952.8 | E962.2 | E982.8 |
| wood | 980.1 | E860.2 | — | E950.9 | E962.1 | E980.9 |
| **Alcuronium chloride** | 975.2 | E858.6 | E945.2 | E950.4 | E962.0 | E980.4 |
| **Aldactone** | 974.4 | E858.5 | E944.4 | E950.4 | E962.0 | E980.4 |
| **Aldicarb** | 989.3 | E863.2 | — | E950.6 | E962.1 | E980.7 |
| **Aldomet** | 972.6 | E858.3 | E942.6 | E950.4 | E962.0 | E980.4 |
| **Aldosterone** | 962.0 | E858.0 | E932.0 | E950.4 | E962.0 | E980.4 |
| **Aldrin** (dust) | 989.2 | E863.0 | — | E950.6 | E962.1 | E980.7 |
| **Algeldrate** | 973.0 | E858.4 | E943.0 | E950.4 | E962.0 | E980.4 |
| **Alidase** | 963.4 | E858.1 | E933.4 | E950.4 | E962.0 | E980.4 |
| **Aliphatic thiocyanates** | 989.0 | E866.8 | — | E950.9 | E962.1 | E980.9 |
| **Alkaline antiseptic solution** (aromatic) | 976.6 | E858.7 | E946.6 | E950.4 | E962.0 | E980.4 |

☑ Additional Digit Required — Refer to the Tabular List for Digit Selection     ⍟ Subterms under main terms may continue to next column or page

304 — Volume 2     ▶◀ Revised Text    ● New Line    ▲ Revised Code     **2008 ICD-9-CM**

| | Poisoning | Accident | Therapeutic Use | Suicide Attempt | Assault | Undetermined |
|---|---|---|---|---|---|---|
| **Alkalinizing agents** | | | | | | |
| (medicinal) | 963.3 | E858.1 | E933.3 | E950.4 | E962.0 | E980.4 |
| **Alkalis, caustic** | 983.2 | E864.2 | — | E950.7 | E962.1 | E980.6 |
| **Alkalizing agents** | | | | | | |
| (medicinal) | 963.3 | E858.1 | E933.3 | E950.4 | E962.0 | E980.4 |
| **Alka-seltzer** | 965.1 | E850.3 | E935.3 | E950.0 | E962.0 | E980.0 |
| **Alkavervir** | 972.6 | E858.3 | E942.6 | E950.4 | E962.0 | E980.4 |
| **Allegron** | 969.0 | E854.0 | E939.0 | E950.3 | E962.0 | E980.3 |
| **Alleve** — Naproxen | | | | | | |
| **Allobarbital, allobarbitone** | 967.0 | E851 | E937.0 | E950.1 | E962.0 | E980.1 |
| **Allopurinol** | 974.7 | E858.5 | E944.7 | E950.4 | E962.0 | E980.4 |
| **Allylestrenol** | 962.2 | E858.0 | E932.2 | E950.4 | E962.0 | E980.4 |
| **Allylisopropylacetylurea** | 967.8 | E852.8 | E937.8 | E950.2 | E962.0 | E980.2 |
| **Allylisopropylmalonylurea** | 967.0 | E851 | E937.0 | E950.1 | E962.0 | E980.1 |
| **Allyltribromide** | 967.3 | E852.2 | E937.3 | E950.2 | E962.0 | E980.2 |
| **Aloe, aloes, aloin** | 973.1 | E858.4 | E943.1 | E950.4 | E962.0 | E980.4 |
| **Alosetron** | 973.8 | E858.4 | E943.8 | E950.4 | E962.0 | E980.4 |
| **Aloxidone** | 966.0 | E855.0 | E936.0 | E950.4 | E962.0 | E980.4 |
| **Aloxiprin** | 965.1 | E850.3 | E935.3 | E950.0 | E962.0 | E980.0 |
| **Alpha-1 blockers** ● | 971.3 | E855.6 | E941.3 | E950.4 | E962.0 | E980.4 |
| **Alpha amylase** | 963.4 | E858.1 | E933.4 | E950.4 | E962.0 | E980.4 |
| **Alphaprodine** | | | | | | |
| (hydrochloride) | 965.09 | E850.2 | E935.2 | E950.0 | E962.0 | E980.0 |
| **Alpha tocopherol** | 963.5 | E858.1 | E933.5 | E950.4 | E962.0 | E980.4 |
| **Alseroxylon** | 972.6 | E858.3 | E942.6 | E950.4 | E962.0 | E980.4 |
| **Alum** (ammonium) | | | | | | |
| (potassium) | 983.2 | E864.2 | — | E950.7 | E962.1 | E980.6 |
| medicinal (astringent) NEC | 976.2 | E858.7 | E946.2 | E950.4 | E962.0 | E980.4 |
| **Aluminium, aluminum** (gel) | | | | | | |
| (hydroxide) | 973.0 | E858.4 | E943.0 | E950.4 | E962.0 | E980.4 |
| acetate solution | 976.2 | E858.7 | E946.2 | E950.4 | E962.0 | E980.4 |
| aspirin | 965.1 | E850.3 | E935.3 | E950.0 | E962.0 | E980.0 |
| carbonate | 973.0 | E858.4 | E943.0 | E950.4 | E962.0 | E980.4 |
| glycinate | 973.0 | E858.4 | E943.0 | E950.4 | E962.0 | E980.4 |
| nicotinate | 972.2 | E858.3 | E942.2 | E950.4 | E962.0 | E980.4 |
| ointment (surgical) (topical) | 976.3 | E858.7 | E946.3 | E950.4 | E962.0 | E980.4 |
| phosphate | 973.0 | E858.4 | E943.0 | E950.4 | E962.0 | E980.4 |
| subacetate | 976.2 | E858.7 | E946.2 | E950.4 | E962.0 | E980.4 |
| topical NEC | 976.3 | E858.7 | E946.3 | E950.4 | E962.0 | E980.4 |
| **Alurate** | 967.0 | E851 | E937.0 | E950.1 | E962.0 | E980.1 |
| **Alverine** (citrate) | 975.1 | E858.6 | E945.1 | E950.4 | E962.0 | E980.4 |
| **Alvodine** | 965.09 | E850.2 | E935.2 | E950.0 | E962.0 | E980.0 |
| **Amanita phalloides** | 988.1 | E865.5 | — | E950.9 | E962.1 | E980.9 |
| **Amantadine** (hydrochloride) | 966.4 | E855.0 | E936.4 | E950.4 | E962.0 | E980.4 |
| **Ambazone** | 961.9 | E857 | E931.9 | E950.4 | E962.0 | E980.4 |
| **Ambenonium** | 971.0 | E855.3 | E941.0 | E950.4 | E962.0 | E980.4 |
| **Ambutonium bromide** | 971.1 | E855.4 | E941.1 | E950.4 | E962.0 | E980.4 |
| **Ametazole** | 977.8 | E858.8 | E947.8 | E950.4 | E962.0 | E980.4 |
| **Amethocaine** (infiltration) | | | | | | |
| (topical) | 968.5 | E855.2 | E938.5 | E950.4 | E962.0 | E980.4 |
| nerve block (peripheral) | | | | | | |
| (plexus) | 968.6 | E855.2 | E938.6 | E950.4 | E962.0 | E980.4 |
| spinal | 968.7 | E855.2 | E938.7 | E950.4 | E962.0 | E980.4 |
| **Amethopterin** | 963.1 | E858.1 | E933.1 | E950.4 | E962.0 | E980.4 |
| **Amfepramone** | 977.0 | E858.8 | E947.0 | E950.4 | E962.0 | E980.4 |
| **Amidon** | 965.02 | E850.1 | E935.1 | E950.0 | E962.0 | E980.0 |
| **Amidopyrine** | 965.5 | E850.5 | E935.5 | E950.0 | E962.0 | E980.0 |
| **Aminacrine** | 976.0 | E858.7 | E946.0 | E950.4 | E962.0 | E980.4 |
| **Aminitrozole** | 961.5 | E857 | E931.5 | E950.4 | E962.0 | E980.4 |
| **Aminoacetic acid** | 974.5 | E858.5 | E944.5 | E950.4 | E962.0 | E980.4 |
| **Amino acids** | 974.5 | E858.5 | E944.5 | E950.4 | E962.0 | E980.4 |
| **Aminocaproic acid** | 964.4 | E858.2 | E934.4 | E950.4 | E962.0 | E980.4 |
| **Aminoethylisothiourium** | 963.8 | E858.1 | E933.8 | E950.4 | E962.0 | E980.4 |
| **Aminoglutethimide** | 966.3 | E855.0 | E936.3 | E950.4 | E962.0 | E980.4 |
| **Aminometradine** | 974.3 | E858.5 | E944.3 | E950.4 | E962.0 | E980.4 |
| **Aminopentamide** | 971.1 | E855.4 | E941.1 | E950.4 | E962.0 | E980.4 |
| **Aminophenazone** | 965.5 | E850.5 | E935.5 | E950.0 | E962.0 | E980.0 |
| **Aminophenol** | 983.0 | E864.0 | — | E950.7 | E962.1 | E980.6 |
| **Aminophenylpyridone** | 969.5 | E853.8 | E939.5 | E950.3 | E962.0 | E980.3 |
| **Aminophyllin** | 975.7 | E858.6 | E945.7 | E950.4 | E962.0 | E980.4 |
| **Aminopterin** | 963.1 | E858.1 | E933.1 | E950.4 | E962.0 | E980.4 |
| **Aminopyrine** | 965.5 | E850.5 | E935.5 | E950.0 | E962.0 | E980.0 |
| **Aminosalicylic acid** | 961.8 | E857 | E931.8 | E950.4 | E962.0 | E980.4 |
| **Amiphenazole** | 970.1 | E854.3 | E940.1 | E950.4 | E962.0 | E980.4 |
| **Amiquinsin** | 972.6 | E858.3 | E942.6 | E950.4 | E962.0 | E980.4 |
| **Amisometradine** | 974.3 | E858.5 | E944.3 | E950.4 | E962.0 | E980.4 |
| **Amitriptyline** | 969.0 | E854.0 | E939.0 | E950.3 | E962.0 | E980.3 |
| **Ammonia** (fumes) (gas) | | | | | | |
| (vapor) | 987.8 | E869.8 | — | E952.8 | E962.2 | E982.8 |
| liquid (household) NEC | 983.2 | E861.4 | — | E950.7 | E962.1 | E980.6 |

| | Poisoning | Accident | Therapeutic Use | Suicide Attempt | Assault | Undetermined |
|---|---|---|---|---|---|---|
| **Ammonia** — continued | | | | | | |
| spirit, aromatic | 970.8 | E854.3 | E940.8 | E950.4 | E962.0 | E980.4 |
| **Ammoniated mercury** | 976.0 | E858.7 | E946.0 | E950.4 | E962.0 | E980.4 |
| **Ammonium** | | | | | | |
| carbonate | 983.2 | E864.2 | — | E950.7 | E962.1 | E980.6 |
| chloride (acidifying agent) | 963.2 | E858.1 | E933.2 | E950.4 | E962.0 | E980.4 |
| expectorant | 975.5 | E858.6 | E945.5 | E950.4 | E962.0 | E980.4 |
| compounds (household) | | | | | | |
| NEC | 983.2 | E861.4 | — | E950.7 | E962.1 | E980.6 |
| fumes (any usage) | 987.8 | E869.8 | — | E952.8 | E962.2 | E982.8 |
| industrial | 983.2 | E864.2 | — | E950.7 | E962.1 | E980.6 |
| ichthyosulfonate | 976.4 | E858.7 | E946.4 | E950.4 | E962.0 | E980.4 |
| mandelate | 961.9 | E857 | E931.9 | E950.4 | E962.0 | E980.4 |
| **Amobarbital** | 967.0 | E851 | E937.0 | E950.1 | E962.0 | E980.1 |
| **Amodiaquin(e)** | 961.4 | E857 | E931.4 | E950.4 | E962.0 | E980.4 |
| **Amopyroquin(e)** | 961.4 | E857 | E931.4 | E950.4 | E962.0 | E980.4 |
| **Amphenidone** | 969.5 | E853.8 | E939.5 | E950.3 | E962.0 | E980.3 |
| **Amphetamine** | 969.7 | E854.2 | E939.7 | E950.3 | E962.0 | E980.3 |
| **Amphomycin** | 960.8 | E856 | E930.8 | E950.4 | E962.0 | E980.4 |
| **Amphotericin B** | 960.1 | E856 | E930.1 | E950.4 | E962.0 | E980.4 |
| topical | 976.0 | E858.7 | E946.0 | E950.4 | E962.0 | E980.4 |
| **Ampicillin** | 960.0 | E856 | E930.0 | E950.4 | E962.0 | E980.4 |
| **Amprotropine** | 971.1 | E855.4 | E941.1 | E950.4 | E962.0 | E980.4 |
| **Amygdalin** | 977.8 | E858.8 | E947.8 | E950.4 | E962.0 | E980.4 |
| **Amyl** | | | | | | |
| acetate (vapor) | 982.8 | E862.4 | — | E950.9 | E962.1 | E980.9 |
| alcohol | 980.3 | E860.4 | — | E950.9 | E962.1 | E980.9 |
| nitrite (medicinal) | 972.4 | E858.3 | E942.4 | E950.4 | E962.0 | E980.4 |
| **Amylase** (alpha) | 963.4 | E858.1 | E933.4 | E950.4 | E962.0 | E980.4 |
| **Amylene hydrate** | 980.8 | E860.8 | — | E950.9 | E962.1 | E980.9 |
| **Amylobarbitone** | 967.0 | E851 | E937.0 | E950.1 | E962.0 | E980.1 |
| **Amylocaine** | 968.9 | E855.2 | E938.9 | E950.4 | E962.0 | E980.4 |
| infiltration (subcutaneous) | 968.5 | E855.2 | E938.5 | E950.4 | E962.0 | E980.4 |
| nerve block (peripheral) | | | | | | |
| (plexus) | 968.6 | E855.2 | E938.6 | E950.4 | E962.0 | E980.4 |
| spinal | 968.7 | E855.2 | E938.7 | E950.4 | E962.0 | E980.4 |
| topical (surface) | 968.5 | E855.2 | E938.5 | E950.4 | E962.0 | E980.4 |
| **Amytal** (sodium) | 967.0 | E851 | E937.0 | E950.1 | E962.0 | E980.1 |
| **Analeptics** | 970.0 | E854.3 | E940.0 | E950.4 | E962.0 | E980.4 |
| **Analgesics** | 965.9 | E850.9 | E935.9 | E950.0 | E962.0 | E980.0 |
| aromatic NEC | 965.4 | E850.4 | E935.4 | E950.0 | E962.0 | E980.0 |
| non-narcotic NEC | 965.7 | E850.7 | E935.7 | E950.0 | E962.0 | E980.0 |
| specified NEC | 965.8 | E850.8 | E935.8 | E950.0 | E962.0 | E980.0 |
| **Anamirta cocculus** | 988.2 | E865.3 | — | E950.9 | E962.1 | E980.9 |
| **Ancillin** | 960.0 | E856 | E930.0 | E950.4 | E962.0 | E980.4 |
| **Androgens** (anabolic congeners) | 962.1 | E858.0 | E932.1 | E950.4 | E962.0 | E980.4 |
| **Androstalone** | 962.1 | E858.0 | E932.1 | E950.4 | E962.0 | E980.4 |
| **Androsterone** | 962.1 | E858.0 | E932.1 | E950.4 | E962.0 | E980.4 |
| **Anemone pulsatilla** | 988.2 | E865.4 | — | E950.9 | E962.1 | E980.9 |
| **Anesthesia, anesthetic** (general) | | | | | | |
| NEC | 968.4 | E855.1 | E938.4 | E950.4 | E962.0 | E980.4 |
| block (nerve) (plexus) | 968.6 | E855.2 | E938.6 | E950.4 | E962.0 | E980.4 |
| gaseous NEC | 968.2 | E855.1 | E938.2 | E950.4 | E962.0 | E980.4 |
| halogenated hydrocarbon derivatives NEC | 968.2 | E855.1 | E938.2 | E950.4 | E962.0 | E980.4 |
| infiltration (intradermal) (subcutaneous) (submucosal) | 968.5 | E855.2 | E938.5 | E950.4 | E962.0 | E980.4 |
| intravenous | 968.3 | E855.1 | E938.3 | E950.4 | E962.0 | E980.4 |
| local NEC | 968.9 | E855.2 | E938.9 | E950.4 | E962.0 | E980.4 |
| nerve blocking (peripheral) (plexus) | 968.6 | E855.2 | E938.6 | E950.4 | E962.0 | E980.4 |
| rectal NEC | 968.3 | E855.1 | E938.3 | E950.4 | E962.0 | E980.4 |
| spinal | 968.7 | E855.2 | E938.7 | E950.4 | E962.0 | E980.4 |
| surface | 968.5 | E855.2 | E938.5 | E950.4 | E962.0 | E980.4 |
| topical | 968.5 | E855.2 | E938.5 | E950.4 | E962.0 | E980.4 |
| **Aneurine** | 963.5 | E858.1 | E933.5 | E950.4 | E962.0 | E980.4 |
| **Anginine** — see Glyceryl trinitrate | | | | | | |
| **Angio-Conray** | 977.8 | E858.8 | E947.8 | E950.4 | E962.0 | E980.4 |
| **Angiotensin** | 971.2 | E855.5 | E941.2 | E950.4 | E962.0 | E980.4 |
| **Anhydrohydroxyprogesterone** | 962.2 | E858.0 | E932.2 | E950.4 | E962.0 | E980.4 |
| **Anhydron** | 974.3 | E858.5 | E944.3 | E950.4 | E962.0 | E980.4 |
| **Anileridine** | 965.09 | E850.2 | E935.2 | E950.0 | E962.0 | E980.0 |
| **Aniline** (dye) (liquid) | 983.0 | E864.0 | — | E950.7 | E962.1 | E980.6 |
| analgesic | 965.4 | E850.4 | E935.4 | E950.0 | E962.0 | E980.0 |
| derivatives, therapeutic NEC | 965.4 | E850.4 | E935.4 | E950.0 | E962.0 | E980.0 |
| vapor | 987.8 | E869.8 | — | E952.8 | E962.2 | E982.8 |
| **Aniscoropine** | 971.1 | E855.4 | E941.1 | E950.4 | E962.0 | E980.4 |

☑ Additional Digit Required — Refer to the Tabular List for Digit Selection

▽ Subterms under main terms may continue to next column or page

| Substance | Poisoning | Accident | Therapeutic Use | Suicide Attempt | Assault | Undetermined |
|---|---|---|---|---|---|---|
| Anisindione | 964.2 | E858.2 | E934.2 | E950.4 | E962.0 | E980.4 |
| Anorexic agents | 977.0 | E858.8 | E947.0 | E950.4 | E962.0 | E980.4 |
| Ant (bite) (sting) | — | E905.5 | — | E950.9 | E962.1 | E980.9 |
| Antabuse | 977.3 | E858.8 | E947.3 | E950.4 | E962.0 | E980.4 |
| Antacids | 973.0 | E858.4 | E943.0 | E950.4 | E962.0 | E980.4 |
| Antazoline | 963.0 | E858.1 | E933.0 | E950.4 | E962.0 | E980.4 |
| Anthralin | 976.4 | E858.7 | E946.4 | E950.4 | E962.0 | E980.4 |
| Anthramycin | 960.7 | E856 | E930.7 | E950.4 | E962.0 | E980.4 |
| Antiadrenergics | 971.3 | E855.6 | E941.3 | E950.4 | E962.0 | E980.4 |
| Antiallergic agents | 963.0 | E858.1 | E933.0 | E950.4 | E962.0 | E980.4 |
| Antianemic agents NEC | 964.1 | E858.2 | E934.1 | E950.4 | E962.0 | E980.4 |
| Antiaris toxicaria | 988.2 | E865.4 | — | E950.9 | E962.1 | E980.9 |
| Antiarteriosclerotic agents | 972.2 | E858.3 | E942.2 | E950.4 | E962.0 | E980.4 |
| Antiasthmatics | 975.7 | E858.6 | E945.7 | E950.4 | E962.0 | E980.4 |
| Antibiotics | 960.9 | E856 | E930.9 | E950.4 | E962.0 | E980.4 |
|   antifungal | 960.1 | E856 | E930.1 | E950.4 | E962.0 | E980.4 |
|   antimycobacterial | 960.6 | E856 | E930.6 | E950.4 | E962.0 | E980.4 |
|   antineoplastic | 960.7 | E856 | E930.7 | E950.4 | E962.0 | E980.4 |
|   cephalosporin (group) | 960.5 | E856 | E930.5 | E950.4 | E962.0 | E980.4 |
|   chloramphenicol (group) | 960.2 | E856 | E930.2 | E950.4 | E962.0 | E980.4 |
|   macrolides | 960.3 | E856 | E930.3 | E950.4 | E962.0 | E980.4 |
|   specified NEC | 960.8 | E856 | E930.8 | E950.4 | E962.0 | E980.4 |
|   tetracycline (group) | 960.4 | E856 | E930.4 | E950.4 | E962.0 | E980.4 |
| Anticancer agents NEC | 963.1 | E858.1 | E933.1 | E950.4 | E962.0 | E980.4 |
|   antibiotics | 960.7 | E856 | E930.7 | E950.4 | E962.0 | E980.4 |
| Anticholinergics | 971.1 | E855.4 | E941.1 | E950.4 | E962.0 | E980.4 |
| Anticholinesterase (organophosphorus) (reversible) | 971.0 | E855.3 | E941.0 | E950.4 | E962.0 | E980.4 |
| Anticoagulants | 964.2 | E858.2 | E934.2 | E950.4 | E962.0 | E980.4 |
|   antagonists | 964.5 | E858.2 | E934.5 | E950.4 | E962.0 | E980.4 |
| Anti-common cold agents NEC | 975.6 | E858.6 | E945.6 | E950.4 | E962.0 | E980.4 |
| Anticonvulsants NEC | 966.3 | E855.0 | E936.3 | E950.4 | E962.0 | E980.4 |
| Antidepressants | 969.0 | E854.0 | E939.0 | E950.3 | E962.0 | E980.3 |
| Antidiabetic agents | 962.3 | E858.0 | E932.3 | E950.4 | E962.0 | E980.4 |
| Antidiarrheal agents | 973.5 | E858.4 | E943.5 | E950.4 | E962.0 | E980.4 |
| Antidiuretic hormone | 962.5 | E858.0 | E932.5 | E950.4 | E962.0 | E980.4 |
| Antidotes NEC | 977.2 | E858.8 | E947.2 | E950.4 | E962.0 | E980.4 |
| Antiemetic agents | 963.0 | E858.1 | E933.0 | E950.4 | E962.0 | E980.4 |
| Antiepilepsy agent NEC | 966.3 | E855.0 | E936.3 | E950.4 | E962.0 | E980.4 |
| Antifertility pills | 962.2 | E858.0 | E932.2 | E950.4 | E962.0 | E980.4 |
| Antiflatulents | 973.8 | E858.4 | E943.8 | E950.4 | E962.0 | E980.4 |
| Antifreeze | 989.89 | E866.8 | — | E950.9 | E962.1 | E980.9 |
|   alcohol | 980.1 | E860.2 | — | E950.9 | E962.1 | E980.9 |
|   ethylene glycol | 982.8 | E862.4 | — | E950.9 | E962.1 | E980.9 |
| Antifungals (nonmedicinal) (sprays) | 989.4 | E863.6 | — | E950.6 | E962.1 | E980.7 |
|   medicinal NEC | 961.9 | E857 | E931.9 | E950.4 | E962.0 | E980.4 |
|   antibiotic | 960.1 | E856 | E930.1 | E950.4 | E962.0 | E980.4 |
|   topical | 976.0 | E858.7 | E946.0 | E950.4 | E962.0 | E980.4 |
| Antigastric secretion agents | 973.0 | E858.4 | E943.0 | E950.4 | E962.0 | E980.4 |
| Antihelmintics | 961.6 | E857 | E931.6 | E950.4 | E962.0 | E980.4 |
| Antihemophilic factor (human) | 964.7 | E858.2 | E934.7 | E950.4 | E962.0 | E980.4 |
| Antihistamine | 963.0 | E858.1 | E933.0 | E950.4 | E962.0 | E980.4 |
| Antihypertensive agents NEC | 972.6 | E858.3 | E942.6 | E950.4 | E962.0 | E980.4 |
| Anti-infectives NEC | 961.9 | E857 | E931.9 | E950.4 | E962.0 | E980.4 |
|   antibiotics | 960.9 | E856 | E930.9 | E950.4 | E962.0 | E980.4 |
|     specified NEC | 960.8 | E856 | E930.8 | E950.4 | E962.0 | E980.4 |
|   antihelmintic | 961.6 | E857 | E931.6 | E950.4 | E962.0 | E980.4 |
|   antimalarial | 961.4 | E857 | E931.4 | E950.4 | E962.0 | E980.4 |
|   antimycobacterial NEC | 961.8 | E857 | E931.8 | E950.4 | E962.0 | E980.4 |
|     antibiotics | 960.6 | E856 | E930.6 | E950.4 | E962.0 | E980.4 |
|   antiprotozoal NEC | 961.5 | E857 | E931.5 | E950.4 | E962.0 | — |
|     blood | 961.4 | E857 | E931.4 | E950.4 | E962.0 | E980.4 |
|   antiviral | 961.7 | E857 | E931.7 | E950.4 | E962.0 | E980.4 |
|   arsenical | 961.1 | E857 | E931.1 | E950.4 | E962.0 | E980.4 |
|   ENT agents | 976.6 | E858.7 | E946.6 | E950.4 | E962.0 | E980.4 |
|   heavy metals NEC | 961.2 | E857 | E931.2 | E950.4 | E962.0 | E980.4 |
|   local | 976.0 | E858.7 | E946.0 | E950.4 | E962.0 | E980.4 |
|   ophthalmic preparation | 976.5 | E858.7 | E946.5 | E950.4 | E962.0 | E980.4 |
|   topical NEC | 976.0 | E858.7 | E946.0 | E950.4 | E962.0 | E980.4 |
| Anti-inflammatory agents (topical) | 976.0 | E858.7 | E946.0 | E950.4 | E962.0 | E980.4 |
| Antiknock (tetraethyl lead) | 984.1 | E862.1 | — | E950.9 | — | E980.9 |
| Antilipemics | 972.2 | E858.3 | E942.2 | E950.4 | E962.0 | E980.4 |
| Antimalarials | 961.4 | E857 | E931.4 | E950.4 | E962.0 | E980.4 |

| Substance | Poisoning | Accident | Therapeutic Use | Suicide Attempt | Assault | Undetermined |
|---|---|---|---|---|---|---|
| Antimony (compounds) (vapor) NEC | 985.4 | E866.2 | — | E950.9 | E962.1 | E980.9 |
|   anti-infectives | 961.2 | E857 | E931.2 | E950.4 | E962.0 | E980.4 |
|   pesticides (vapor) | 985.4 | E863.4 | — | E950.6 | E962.2 | E980.7 |
|   potassium tartrate | 961.2 | E857 | E931.2 | E950.4 | E962.0 | E980.4 |
|   tartrated | 961.2 | E857 | E931.2 | E950.4 | E962.0 | E980.4 |
| Antimuscarinic agents | 971.1 | E855.4 | E941.1 | E950.4 | E962.0 | E980.4 |
| Antimycobacterials NEC | 961.8 | E857 | E931.8 | E950.4 | E962.0 | E980.4 |
|   antibiotics | 960.6 | E856 | E930.6 | E950.4 | E962.0 | E980.4 |
| Antineoplastic agents | 963.1 | E858.1 | E933.1 | E950.4 | E962.0 | E980.4 |
|   antibiotics | 960.7 | E856 | E930.7 | E950.4 | E962.0 | E980.4 |
| Anti-Parkinsonism agents | 966.4 | E855.0 | E936.4 | E950.4 | E962.0 | E980.4 |
| Antiphlogistics | 965.69 | E850.6 | E935.6 | E950.0 | E962.0 | E980.0 |
| Antiprotozoals NEC | 961.5 | E857 | E931.5 | E950.4 | E962.0 | E980.4 |
|   blood | 961.4 | E857 | E931.4 | E950.4 | E962.0 | E980.4 |
| Antipruritics (local) | 976.1 | E858.7 | E946.1 | E950.4 | E962.0 | E980.4 |
| Antipsychotic agents NEC | 969.3 | E853.8 | E939.3 | E950.3 | E962.0 | E980.3 |
| Antipyretics | 965.9 | E850.9 | E935.9 | E950.0 | E962.0 | E980.0 |
|   specified NEC | 965.8 | E850.8 | E935.8 | E950.0 | E962.0 | E980.0 |
| Antipyrine | 965.5 | E850.5 | E935.5 | E950.0 | E962.0 | E980.0 |
| Antirabies serum (equine) | 979.9 | E858.8 | E949.9 | E950.4 | E962.0 | E980.4 |
| Antirheumatics | 965.69 | E850.6 | E935.6 | E950.0 | E962.0 | E980.0 |
| Antiseborrheics | 976.4 | E858.7 | E946.4 | E950.4 | E962.0 | E980.4 |
| Antiseptics (external) (medicinal) | 976.0 | E858.7 | E946.0 | E950.4 | E962.0 | E980.4 |
| Antistine | 963.0 | E858.1 | E933.0 | E950.4 | E962.0 | E980.4 |
| Antithyroid agents | 962.8 | E858.0 | E932.8 | E950.4 | E962.0 | E980.4 |
| Antitoxin, any | 979.9 | E858.8 | E949.9 | E950.4 | E962.0 | E980.4 |
| Antituberculars | 961.8 | E857 | E931.8 | E950.4 | E962.0 | E980.4 |
|   antibiotics | 960.6 | E856 | E930.6 | E950.4 | E962.0 | E980.4 |
| Antitussives | 975.4 | E858.6 | E945.4 | E950.4 | E962.0 | E980.4 |
| Antivaricose agents (sclerosing) | 972.7 | E858.3 | E942.7 | E950.4 | E962.0 | E980.4 |
| Antivenin (crotaline) (spider-bite) | 979.9 | E858.8 | E949.9 | E950.4 | E962.0 | E980.4 |
| Antivert | 963.0 | E858.1 | E933.0 | E950.4 | E962.0 | E980.4 |
| Antivirals NEC | 961.7 | E857 | E931.7 | E950.4 | E962.0 | E980.4 |
| Ant poisons — *see* Pesticides | | | | | | |
| Antrol | 989.4 | E863.4 | — | E950.6 | E962.1 | E980.7 |
|   fungicide | 989.4 | E863.6 | — | E950.6 | E962.1 | E980.7 |
| Apomorphine hydrochloride (emetic) | 973.6 | E858.4 | E943.6 | E950.4 | E962.0 | E980.4 |
| Appetite depressants, central | 977.0 | E858.8 | E947.0 | E950.4 | E962.0 | E980.4 |
| Apresoline | 972.6 | E858.3 | E942.6 | E950.4 | E962.0 | E980.4 |
| Aprobarbital, aprobarbitone | 967.0 | E851 | E937.0 | E950.1 | E962.0 | E980.1 |
| Apronalide | 967.8 | E852.8 | E937.8 | E950.2 | E962.0 | E980.2 |
| Aqua fortis | 983.1 | E864.1 | — | E950.7 | E962.1 | E980.6 |
| Arachis oil (topical) | 976.3 | E858.7 | E946.3 | E950.4 | E962.0 | E980.4 |
|   cathartic | 973.2 | E858.4 | E943.2 | E950.4 | E962.0 | E980.4 |
| Aralen | 961.4 | E857 | E931.4 | E950.4 | E962.0 | E980.4 |
| Arginine salts | 974.5 | E858.5 | E944.5 | E950.4 | E962.0 | E980.4 |
| Argyrol | 976.0 | E858.7 | E946.0 | E950.4 | E962.0 | E980.4 |
|   ENT agent | 976.6 | E858.7 | E946.6 | E950.4 | E962.0 | E980.4 |
|   ophthalmic preparation | 976.5 | E858.7 | E946.5 | E950.4 | E962.0 | E980.4 |
| Aristocort | 962.0 | E858.0 | E932.0 | E950.4 | E962.0 | E980.4 |
|   ENT agent | 976.6 | E858.7 | E946.6 | E950.4 | E962.0 | E980.4 |
|   ophthalmic preparation | 976.5 | E858.7 | E946.5 | E950.4 | E962.0 | E980.4 |
|   topical NEC | 976.0 | E858.7 | E946.0 | E950.4 | E962.0 | E980.4 |
| Aromatics, corrosive | 983.0 | E864.0 | — | E950.7 | E962.1 | E980.6 |
|   disinfectants | 983.0 | E861.4 | — | E950.7 | E962.1 | E980.6 |
| Arsenate of lead (insecticide) | 985.1 | E863.4 | — | E950.8 | E962.1 | E980.8 |
|   herbicide | 985.1 | E863.5 | — | E950.8 | E962.1 | E980.8 |
| Arsenic, arsenicals (compounds) (dust) (fumes) (vapor) NEC | 985.1 | E866.3 | — | E950.8 | E962.1 | E980.8 |
|   anti-infectives | 961.1 | E857 | E931.1 | E950.4 | E962.0 | E980.4 |
|   pesticide (dust) (fumes) | 985.1 | E863.4 | — | E950.8 | E962.1 | E980.8 |
| Arsine (gas) | 985.1 | E866.3 | — | E950.8 | E962.1 | E980.8 |
| Arsphenamine (silver) | 961.1 | E857 | E931.1 | E950.4 | E962.0 | E980.4 |
| Arsthinol | 961.1 | E857 | E931.1 | E950.4 | E962.0 | E980.4 |
| Artane | 971.1 | E855.4 | E941.1 | E950.4 | E962.0 | E980.4 |
| Arthropod (venomous) NEC | 989.5 | E905.5 | — | E950.9 | E962.1 | E980.9 |
| Asbestos | 989.81 | E866.8 | — | E950.9 | E962.1 | E980.9 |
| Ascaridole | 961.6 | E857 | E931.6 | E950.4 | E962.0 | E980.4 |
| Ascorbic acid | 963.5 | E858.1 | E933.5 | E950.4 | E962.0 | E980.4 |
| Asiaticoside | 976.0 | E858.7 | E946.0 | E950.4 | E962.0 | E980.4 |
| Aspidium (oleoresin) | 961.6 | E857 | E931.6 | E950.4 | E962.0 | E980.4 |

☑ Additional Digit Required — Refer to the Tabular List for Digit Selection      ▽ Subterms under main terms may continue to next column or page

| | Poisoning | Accident | Therapeutic Use | Suicide Attempt | Assault | Undetermined |
|---|---|---|---|---|---|---|
| | | **External Cause (E-Code)** | | | | |
| Aspirin | 965.1 | E850.3 | E935.3 | E950.0 | E962.0 | E980.0 |
| Astringents (local) | 976.2 | E858.7 | E946.2 | E950.4 | E962.0 | E980.4 |
| Atabrine | 961.3 | E857 | E931.3 | E950.4 | E962.0 | E980.4 |
| Ataractics | 969.5 | E853.8 | E939.5 | E950.3 | E962.0 | E980.3 |
| Atonia drug, intestinal | 973.3 | E858.4 | E943.3 | E950.4 | E962.0 | E980.4 |
| Atophan | 974.7 | E858.5 | E944.7 | E950.4 | E962.0 | E980.4 |
| Atropine | 971.1 | E855.4 | E941.1 | E950.4 | E962.0 | E980.4 |
| Attapulgite | 973.5 | E858.4 | E943.5 | E950.4 | E962.0 | E980.4 |
| Attenuvax | 979.4 | E858.8 | E949.4 | E950.4 | E962.0 | E980.4 |
| Aureomycin | 960.4 | E856 | E930.4 | E950.4 | E962.0 | E980.4 |
|   ophthalmic preparation | 976.5 | E858.7 | E946.5 | E950.4 | E962.0 | E980.4 |
|   topical NEC | 976.0 | E858.7 | E946.0 | E950.4 | E962.0 | E980.4 |
| Aurothioglucose | 965.69 | E850.6 | E935.6 | E950.0 | E962.0 | E980.0 |
| Aurothioglycanide | 965.69 | E850.6 | E935.6 | E950.0 | E962.0 | E980.0 |
| Aurothiomalate | 965.69 | E850.6 | E935.6 | E950.0 | E962.0 | E980.0 |
| Automobile fuel | 981 | E862.1 | — | E950.9 | E962.1 | E980.9 |
| Autonomic nervous system agents NEC | 971.9 | E855.9 | E941.9 | E950.4 | E962.0 | E980.4 |
| Avlosulfon | 961.8 | E857 | E931.8 | E950.4 | E962.0 | E980.4 |
| Avomine | 967.8 | E852.8 | E937.8 | E950.2 | E962.0 | E980.2 |
| Azacyclonol | 969.5 | E853.8 | E939.5 | E950.3 | E962.0 | E980.3 |
| Azapetine | 971.3 | E855.6 | E941.3 | E950.4 | E962.0 | E980.4 |
| Azaribine | 963.1 | E858.1 | E933.1 | E950.4 | E962.0 | E980.4 |
| Azaserine | 960.7 | E856 | E930.7 | E950.4 | E962.0 | E980.4 |
| Azathioprine | 963.1 | E858.1 | E933.1 | E950.4 | E962.0 | E980.4 |
| Azosulfamide | 961.0 | E857 | E931.0 | E950.4 | E962.0 | E980.4 |
| Azulfidine | 961.0 | E857 | E931.0 | E950.4 | E962.0 | E980.4 |
| Azuresin | 977.8 | E858.8 | E947.8 | E950.4 | E962.0 | E980.4 |
| Bacimycin | 976.0 | E858.7 | E946.0 | E950.4 | E962.0 | E980.4 |
|   ophthalmic preparation | 976.5 | E858.7 | E946.5 | E950.4 | E962.0 | E980.4 |
| Bacitracin | 960.8 | E856 | E930.8 | E950.4 | E962.0 | E980.4 |
|   ENT agent | 976.6 | E858.7 | E946.6 | E950.4 | E962.0 | E980.4 |
|   ophthalmic preparation | 976.5 | E858.7 | E946.5 | E950.4 | E962.0 | E980.4 |
|   topical NEC | 976.0 | E858.7 | E946.0 | E950.4 | E962.0 | E980.4 |
| Baking soda | 963.3 | E858.1 | E933.3 | E950.4 | E962.0 | E980.4 |
| BAL | 963.8 | E858.1 | E933.8 | E950.4 | E962.0 | E980.4 |
| Bamethan (sulfate) | 972.5 | E858.3 | E942.5 | E950.4 | E962.0 | E980.4 |
| Bamipine | 963.0 | E858.1 | E933.0 | E950.4 | E962.0 | E980.4 |
| Baneberry | 988.2 | E865.4 | — | E950.9 | E962.1 | E980.9 |
| Banewort | 988.2 | E865.4 | — | E950.9 | E962.1 | E980.9 |
| Barbenyl | 967.0 | E851 | E937.0 | E950.1 | E962.0 | E980.1 |
| Barbital, barbitone | 967.0 | E851 | E937.0 | E950.1 | E962.0 | E980.1 |
| Barbiturates, barbituric acid | 967.0 | E851 | E937.0 | E950.1 | E962.0 | E980.1 |
|   anesthetic (intravenous) | 968.3 | E855.1 | E938.3 | E950.4 | E962.0 | E980.4 |
| Barium (carbonate) (chloride) (sulfate) | 985.8 | E866.4 | — | E950.9 | E962.1 | E980.9 |
|   diagnostic agent | 977.8 | E858.8 | E947.8 | E950.4 | E962.0 | E980.4 |
|   pesticide | 985.8 | E863.4 | — | E950.6 | E962.1 | E980.7 |
|   rodenticide | 985.8 | E863.7 | — | E950.6 | E962.1 | E980.7 |
| Barrier cream | 976.3 | E858.7 | E946.3 | E950.4 | E962.0 | E980.4 |
| Battery acid or fluid | 983.1 | E864.1 | — | E950.7 | E962.1 | E980.6 |
| Bay rum | 980.8 | E860.8 | — | E950.9 | E962.1 | E980.9 |
| BCG vaccine | 978.0 | E858.8 | E948.0 | E950.4 | E962.0 | E980.4 |
| Bearsfoot | 988.2 | E865.4 | — | E950.9 | E962.1 | E980.9 |
| Beclamide | 966.3 | E855.0 | E936.3 | E950.4 | E962.0 | E980.4 |
| Bee (sting) (venom) | 989.5 | E905.3 | — | E950.9 | E962.1 | E980.9 |
| Belladonna (alkaloids) | 971.1 | E855.4 | E941.1 | E950.4 | E962.0 | E980.4 |
| Bemegride | 970.0 | E854.3 | E940.0 | E950.4 | E962.0 | E980.4 |
| Benactyzine | 969.8 | E855.8 | E939.8 | E950.3 | E962.0 | E980.3 |
| Benadryl | 963.0 | E858.1 | E933.0 | E950.4 | E962.0 | E980.4 |
| Bendrofluazide | 974.3 | E858.5 | E944.3 | E950.4 | E962.0 | E980.4 |
| Bendroflumethiazide | 974.3 | E858.5 | E944.3 | E950.4 | E962.0 | E980.4 |
| Benemid | 974.7 | E858.5 | E944.7 | E950.4 | E962.0 | E980.4 |
| Benethamine penicillin G | 960.0 | E856 | E930.0 | E950.4 | E962.0 | E980.4 |
| Benisone | 976.0 | E858.7 | E946.0 | E950.4 | E962.0 | E980.4 |
| Benoquin | 976.8 | E858.7 | E946.8 | E950.4 | E962.0 | E980.4 |
| Benoxinate | 968.5 | E855.2 | E938.5 | E950.4 | E962.0 | E980.4 |
| Bentonite | 976.3 | E858.7 | E946.3 | E950.4 | E962.0 | E980.4 |
| Benzalkonium (chloride) | 976.0 | E858.7 | E946.0 | E950.4 | E962.0 | E980.4 |
|   ophthalmic preparation | 976.5 | E858.7 | E946.5 | E950.4 | E962.0 | E980.4 |
| Benzamidosalicylate (calcium) | 961.8 | E857 | E931.8 | E950.4 | E962.0 | E980.4 |
| Benzathine penicillin | 960.0 | E856 | E930.0 | E950.4 | E962.0 | E980.4 |
| Benzcarbimine | 963.1 | E858.1 | E933.1 | E950.4 | E962.0 | E980.4 |
| Benzedrex | 971.2 | E855.5 | E941.2 | E950.4 | E962.0 | E980.4 |
| Benzedrine (amphetamine) | 969.7 | E854.2 | E939.7 | E950.3 | E962.0 | E980.3 |
| Benzene (acetyl) (dimethyl) (methyl) (solvent) (vapor) | 982.0 | E862.4 | — | E950.9 | E962.1 | E980.9 |
|   hexachloride (gamma) (insecticide) (vapor) | 989.2 | E863.0 | — | E950.6 | E962.1 | E980.7 |
| Benzethonium | 976.0 | E858.7 | E946.0 | E950.4 | E962.0 | E980.4 |
| Benzhexol (chloride) | 966.4 | E855.0 | E936.4 | E950.4 | E962.0 | E980.4 |
| Benzilonium | 971.1 | E855.4 | E941.1 | E950.4 | E962.0 | E980.4 |
| Benzin(e) — *see* Ligroin | | | | | | |
| Benziodarone | 972.4 | E858.3 | E942.4 | E950.4 | E962.0 | E980.4 |
| Benzocaine | 968.5 | E855.2 | E938.5 | E950.4 | E962.0 | E980.4 |
| Benzodiapin | 969.4 | E853.2 | E939.4 | E950.3 | E962.0 | E980.3 |
| Benzodiazepines (tranquilizers) NEC | 969.4 | E853.2 | E939.4 | E950.3 | E962.0 | E980.3 |
| Benzoic acid (with salicylic acid) (anti-infective) | 976.0 | E858.7 | E946.0 | E950.4 | E962.0 | E980.4 |
| Benzoin | 976.3 | E858.7 | E946.3 | E950.4 | E962.0 | E980.4 |
| Benzol (vapor) | 982.0 | E862.4 | — | E950.9 | E962.1 | E980.9 |
| Benzomorphan | 965.09 | E850.2 | E935.2 | E950.0 | E962.0 | E980.0 |
| Benzonatate | 975.4 | E858.6 | E945.4 | E950.4 | E962.0 | E980.4 |
| Benzothiadiazides | 974.3 | E858.5 | E944.3 | E950.4 | E962.0 | E980.4 |
| Benzoylpas | 961.8 | E857 | E931.8 | E950.4 | E962.0 | E980.4 |
| Benzperidol | 969.5 | E853.8 | E939.5 | E950.3 | E962.0 | E980.3 |
| Benzphetamine | 977.0 | E858.8 | E947.0 | E950.4 | E962.0 | E980.4 |
| Benzpyrinium | 971.0 | E855.3 | E941.0 | E950.4 | E962.0 | E980.4 |
| Benzquinamide | 963.0 | E858.1 | E933.0 | E950.4 | E962.0 | E980.4 |
| Benzthiazide | 974.3 | E858.5 | E944.3 | E950.4 | E962.0 | E980.4 |
| Benztropine | 971.1 | E855.4 | E941.1 | E950.4 | E962.0 | E980.4 |
| Benzyl | | | | | | |
|   acetate | 982.8 | E862.4 | — | E950.9 | E962.1 | E980.9 |
|   benzoate (anti-infective) | 976.0 | E858.7 | E946.0 | E950.4 | E962.0 | E980.4 |
|   morphine | 965.09 | E850.2 | E935.2 | E950.0 | E962.0 | E980.0 |
|   penicillin | 960.0 | E856 | E930.0 | E950.4 | E962.0 | E980.4 |
| Bephenium hydroxynapthoate | 961.6 | E857 | E931.6 | E950.4 | E962.0 | E980.4 |
| Bergamot oil | 989.89 | E866.8 | — | E950.9 | E962.1 | E980.9 |
| Berries, poisonous | 988.2 | E865.3 | — | E950.9 | E962.1 | E980.9 |
| Beryllium (compounds) (fumes) | 985.3 | E866.4 | — | E950.9 | E962.1 | E980.9 |
| Beta-carotene | 976.3 | E858.7 | E946.3 | E950.4 | E962.0 | E980.4 |
| Beta-Chlor | 967.1 | E852.0 | E937.1 | E950.2 | E962.0 | E980.2 |
| Betamethasone | 962.0 | E858.0 | E932.0 | E950.4 | E962.0 | E980.4 |
|   topical | 976.0 | E858.7 | E946.0 | E950.4 | E962.0 | E980.4 |
| Betazole | 977.8 | E858.8 | E947.8 | E950.4 | E962.0 | E980.4 |
| Bethanechol | 971.0 | E855.3 | E941.0 | E950.4 | E962.0 | E980.4 |
| Bethanidine | 972.6 | E858.3 | E942.6 | E950.4 | E962.0 | E980.4 |
| Betula oil | 976.3 | E858.7 | E946.3 | E950.4 | E962.0 | E980.4 |
| Bhang | 969.6 | E854.1 | E939.6 | E950.3 | E962.0 | E980.3 |
| Bialamicol | 961.5 | E857 | E931.5 | E950.4 | E962.0 | E980.4 |
| Bichloride of mercury — *see* Mercury, chloride | | | | | | |
| Bichromates (calcium) (crystals) (potassium) (sodium) | 983.9 | E864.3 | — | E950.7 | E962.1 | E980.6 |
|   fumes | 987.8 | E869.8 | — | E952.8 | E962.2 | E982.8 |
| Biguanide derivatives, oral | 962.3 | E858.0 | E932.3 | E950.4 | E962.0 | E980.4 |
| Biligrafin | 977.8 | E858.8 | E947.8 | E950.4 | E962.0 | E980.4 |
| Bilopaque | 977.8 | E858.8 | E947.8 | E950.4 | E962.0 | E980.4 |
| Bioflavonoids | 972.8 | E858.3 | E942.8 | E950.4 | E962.0 | E980.4 |
| Biological substance NEC | 979.9 | E858.8 | E949.9 | E950.4 | E962.0 | E980.4 |
| Biperiden | 966.4 | E855.0 | E936.4 | E950.4 | E962.0 | E980.4 |
| Bisacodyl | 973.1 | E858.4 | E943.1 | E950.4 | E962.0 | E980.4 |
| Bishydroxycoumarin | 964.2 | E858.2 | E934.2 | E950.4 | E962.0 | E980.4 |
| Bismarsen | 961.1 | E857 | E931.1 | E950.4 | E962.0 | E980.4 |
| Bismuth (compounds) NEC | 985.8 | E866.4 | — | E950.9 | E962.1 | E980.9 |
|   anti-infectives | 961.2 | E857 | E931.2 | E950.4 | E962.0 | E980.4 |
|   subcarbonate | 973.5 | E858.4 | E943.5 | E950.4 | E962.0 | E980.4 |
|   sulfarsphenamine | 961.1 | E857 | E931.1 | E950.4 | E962.0 | E980.4 |
| Bisphosphonates ● | | | | | | |
|   intravenous ● | 963.1 | E858.1 | E933.7 | E950.4 | E962.0 | E980.4 |
|   oral ● | 963.1 | E858.1 | E933.6 | E950.4 | E962.0 | E980.4 |
| Bithionol | 961.6 | E857 | E931.6 | E950.4 | E962.0 | E980.4 |
| Bitter almond oil | 989.0 | E866.8 | — | E950.9 | E962.1 | E980.9 |
| Bittersweet | 988.2 | E865.4 | — | E950.9 | E962.1 | E930.9 |
| Black | | | | | | |
|   flag | 989.4 | E863.4 | — | E950.6 | E962.1 | E980.7 |
|   henbane | 988.2 | E865.4 | — | E950.9 | E962.1 | E980.9 |
|   leaf (40) | 989.4 | E863.4 | — | E950.6 | E962.1 | E980.7 |
|   widow spider (bite) | 989.5 | E905.1 | — | E950.9 | E962.1 | E980.9 |
|     antivenin | 979.9 | E858.8 | E949.9 | E950.4 | E962.0 | E980.4 |
| Blast furnace gas (carbon monoxide from) | 986 | E868.8 | — | E952.1 | E962.2 | E982.1 |
| Bleach NEC | 983.9 | E864.3 | — | E950.7 | E962.1 | E980.6 |
| Bleaching solutions | 983.9 | E864.3 | — | E950.7 | E962.1 | E980.6 |
| **Bleomycin** (sulfate) | 960.7 | E856 | E930.7 | E950.4 | E962.0 | E980.4 |

☑ Additional Digit Required — Refer to the Tabular List for Digit Selection　　　　　　　　　▽ Subterms under main terms may continue to next column or page

**2008 ICD-9-CM**　　　►◄ Revised Text　　　● New Line　　　▲ Revised Code　　　**October 2007 · Volume 2 — 307**

| | | External Cause (E-Code) | | | | |
|---|---|---|---|---|---|---|
| | Poisoning | Accident | Therapeutic Use | Suicide Attempt | Assault | Undetermined |
| **Blockain** | 968.9 | E855.2 | E938.9 | E950.4 | E962.0 | E980.4 |
| infiltration (subcutaneous) | 968.5 | E855.2 | E938.5 | E950.4 | E962.0 | E980.4 |
| nerve block (peripheral) | | | | | | |
| (plexus) | 968.6 | E855.2 | E938.6 | E950.4 | E962.0 | E980.4 |
| topical (surface) | 968.5 | E855.2 | E938.5 | E950.4 | E962.0 | E980.4 |
| **Blood** (derivatives) (natural) | | | | | | |
| (plasma) (whole) | 964.7 | E858.2 | E934.7 | E950.4 | E962.0 | E980.4 |
| affecting agent | 964.9 | E858.2 | E934.9 | E950.4 | E962.0 | E980.4 |
| specified NEC | 964.8 | E858.2 | E934.8 | E950.4 | E962.0 | E980.4 |
| substitute | | | | | | |
| (macromolecular) | 964.8 | E858.2 | E934.8 | E950.4 | E962.0 | E980.4 |
| **Blue velvet** | 965.09 | E850.2 | E935.2 | E950.0 | E962.0 | E980.0 |
| **Bone meal** | 989.89 | E866.5 | — | E950.9 | E962.1 | E980.9 |
| **Bonine** | 963.0 | E858.1 | E933.0 | E950.4 | E962.0 | E980.4 |
| **Boracic acid** | 976.0 | E858.7 | E946.0 | E950.4 | E962.0 | E980.4 |
| ENT agent | 976.6 | E858.7 | E946.6 | E950.4 | E962.0 | E980.4 |
| ophthalmic preparation | 976.5 | E858.7 | E946.5 | E950.4 | E962.0 | E980.4 |
| **Borate** (cleanser) (sodium) | 989.6 | E861.3 | — | E950.9 | E962.1 | E980.9 |
| **Borax** (cleanser) | 989.6 | E861.3 | — | E950.9 | E962.1 | E980.9 |
| **Boric acid** | 976.0 | E858.7 | E946.0 | E950.4 | E962.0 | E980.4 |
| ENT agent | 976.6 | E858.7 | E946.6 | E950.4 | E962.0 | E980.4 |
| ophthalmic preparation | 976.5 | E858.7 | E946.5 | E950.4 | E962.0 | E980.4 |
| **Boron hydride NEC** | 989.89 | E866.8 | — | E950.9 | E962.1 | E980.9 |
| fumes or gas | 987.8 | E869.8 | — | E952.8 | E962.2 | E982.8 |
| **Botox** | 975.3 | E858.6 | E945.3 | E950.4 | E962.0 | E980.4 |
| **Brake fluid vapor** | 987.8 | E869.8 | — | E952.8 | E962.2 | E982.8 |
| **Brass** (compounds) (fumes) | 985.8 | E866.4 | — | E950.9 | E962.1 | E980.9 |
| **Brasso** | 981 | E861.3 | — | E950.9 | E962.1 | E980.9 |
| **Bretylium** (tosylate) | 972.6 | E858.3 | E942.6 | E950.4 | E962.0 | E980.4 |
| **Brevital** (sodium) | 968.3 | E855.1 | E938.3 | E950.4 | E962.0 | E980.4 |
| **British antilewisite** | 963.8 | E858.1 | E933.8 | E950.4 | E962.0 | E980.4 |
| **Bromal** (hydrate) | 967.3 | E852.2 | E937.3 | E950.2 | E962.0 | E980.2 |
| **Bromelains** | 963.4 | E858.1 | E933.4 | E950.4 | E962.0 | E980.4 |
| **Bromides NEC** | 967.3 | E852.2 | E937.3 | E950.2 | E962.0 | E980.2 |
| **Bromine** (vapor) | 987.8 | E869.8 | — | E952.8 | E962.2 | E982.8 |
| compounds (medicinal) | 967.3 | E852.2 | E937.3 | E950.2 | E962.0 | E980.2 |
| **Bromisovalum** | 967.3 | E852.2 | E937.3 | E950.2 | E962.0 | E980.2 |
| **Bromobenzyl cyanide** | 987.5 | E869.3 | — | E952.8 | E962.2 | E982.8 |
| **Bromodiphenhydramine** | 963.0 | E858.1 | E933.0 | E950.4 | E962.0 | E980.4 |
| **Bromoform** | 967.3 | E852.2 | E937.3 | E950.2 | E962.0 | E980.2 |
| **Bromophenol blue** | | | | | | |
| reagent | 977.8 | E858.8 | E947.8 | E950.4 | E962.0 | E980.4 |
| **Bromosalicylhydroxamic** | | | | | | |
| acid | 961.8 | E857 | E931.8 | E950.4 | E962.0 | E980.4 |
| **Bromo-seltzer** | 965.4 | E850.4 | E935.4 | E950.0 | E962.0 | E980.0 |
| **Brompheniramine** | 963.0 | E858.1 | E933.0 | E950.4 | E962.0 | E980.4 |
| **Bromural** | 967.3 | E852.2 | E937.3 | E950.2 | E962.0 | E980.2 |
| **Brown spider** (bite) (venom) | 989.5 | E905.1 | — | E950.9 | E962.1 | E980.9 |
| **Brucia** | 988.2 | E865.3 | — | E950.9 | E962.1 | E980.9 |
| **Brucine** | 989.1 | E863.7 | — | E950.6 | E962.1 | E980.7 |
| **Brunswick green** — see Copper | | | | | | |
| **Bruten** — see Ibuprofen | | | | | | |
| **Bryonia** (alba) (dioica) | 988.2 | E865.4 | — | E950.9 | E962.1 | E980.9 |
| **Buclizine** | 969.5 | E853.8 | E939.5 | E950.3 | E962.0 | E980.3 |
| **Bufferin** | 965.1 | E850.3 | E935.3 | E950.0 | E962.0 | E980.0 |
| **Bufotenine** | 969.6 | E854.1 | E939.6 | E950.3 | E962.0 | E980.3 |
| **Buphenine** | 971.2 | E855.5 | E941.2 | E950.4 | E962.0 | E980.4 |
| **Bupivacaine** | 968.9 | E855.2 | E938.9 | E950.4 | E962.0 | E980.4 |
| infiltration (subcutaneous) | 968.5 | E855.2 | E938.5 | E950.4 | E962.0 | E980.4 |
| nerve block (peripheral) | | | | | | |
| (plexus) | 968.6 | E855.2 | E938.6 | E950.4 | E962.0 | E980.4 |
| **Busulfan** | 963.1 | E858.1 | E933.1 | E950.4 | E962.0 | E980.4 |
| **Butabarbital** (sodium) | 967.0 | E851 | E937.0 | E950.1 | E962.0 | E980.1 |
| **Butabarbitone** | 967.0 | E851 | E937.0 | E950.1 | E962.0 | E980.1 |
| **Butabarpal** | 967.0 | E851 | E937.0 | E950.1 | E962.0 | E980.1 |
| **Butacaine** | 968.5 | E855.2 | E938.5 | E950.4 | E962.0 | E980.4 |
| **Butallylonal** | 967.0 | E851 | E937.0 | E950.1 | E962.0 | E980.1 |
| **Butane** (distributed in mobile | | | | | | |
| container) | 987.0 | E868.0 | — | E951.1 | E962.2 | E981.1 |
| distributed through pipes | 987.0 | E867 | — | E951.0 | E962.2 | E981.0 |
| incomplete combustion of — see | | | | | | |
| Carbon monoxide, butane | | | | | | |
| **Butanol** | 980.3 | E860.4 | — | E950.9 | E962.1 | E980.9 |
| **Butanone** | 982.8 | E862.4 | — | E950.9 | E962.1 | E980.9 |
| **Butaperazine** | 969.1 | E853.0 | E939.1 | E950.3 | E962.0 | E980.3 |
| **Butazolidin** | 965.5 | E850.5 | E935.5 | E950.0 | E962.0 | E980.0 |
| **Butethal** | 967.0 | E851 | E937.0 | E950.1 | E962.0 | E980.1 |
| **Butethamate** | 971.1 | E855.4 | E941.1 | E950.4 | E962.0 | E980.4 |
| **Buthalitone** (sodium) | 968.3 | E855.1 | E938.3 | E950.4 | E962.0 | E980.4 |
| **Butisol** (sodium) | 967.0 | E851 | E937.0 | E950.1 | E962.0 | E980.1 |

| | | External Cause (E-Code) | | | | |
|---|---|---|---|---|---|---|
| | Poisoning | Accident | Therapeutic Use | Suicide Attempt | Assault | Undetermined |
| **Butobarbital,** | | | | | | |
| **butobarbitone** | 967.0 | E851 | E937.0 | E950.1 | E962.0 | E980.1 |
| **Butriptyline** | 969.0 | E854.0 | E939.0 | E950.3 | E962.0 | E980.3 |
| **Buttercups** | 988.2 | E865.4 | — | E950.9 | E962.1 | E980.9 |
| **Butter of antimony** — see | | | | | | |
| Antimony | | | | | | |
| **Butyl** | | | | | | |
| acetate (secondary) | 982.8 | E862.4 | — | E950.9 | E962.1 | E980.9 |
| alcohol | 980.3 | E860.4 | — | E950.9 | E962.1 | E980.9 |
| carbinol | 980.8 | E860.8 | — | E950.9 | E962.1 | E980.9 |
| carbitol | 982.8 | E862.4 | — | E950.9 | E962.1 | E980.9 |
| cellosolve | 982.8 | E862.4 | — | E950.9 | E962.1 | E980.9 |
| chloral (hydrate) | 967.1 | E852.0 | E937.1 | E950.2 | E962.0 | E980.2 |
| formate | 982.8 | E862.4 | — | E950.9 | E962.1 | E980.9 |
| scopolammonium bromide | 971.1 | E855.4 | E941.1 | E950.4 | E962.0 | E980.4 |
| **Butyn** | 968.5 | E855.2 | E938.5 | E950.4 | E962.0 | E980.4 |
| **Butyrophenone** (-based | | | | | | |
| tranquilizers) | 969.2 | E853.1 | E939.2 | E950.3 | E962.0 | E980.3 |
| **Cacodyl, cacodylic acid** — see | | | | | | |
| Arsenic | | | | | | |
| **Cactinomycin** | 960.7 | E856 | E930.7 | E950.4 | E962.0 | E980.4 |
| **Cade oil** | 976.4 | E858.7 | E946.4 | E950.4 | E962.0 | E980.4 |
| **Cadmium** (chloride) (compounds) | | | | | | |
| (dust) (fumes) (oxide) | 985.5 | E866.4 | — | E950.9 | E962.1 | E980.9 |
| sulfide (medicinal) NEC | 976.4 | E858.7 | E946.4 | E950.4 | E962.0 | E980.4 |
| **Caffeine** | 969.7 | E854.2 | E939.7 | E950.3 | E962.0 | E980.3 |
| **Calabar bean** | 988.2 | E865.4 | — | E950.9 | E962.1 | E980.9 |
| **Caladium seguinium** | 988.2 | E865.4 | — | E950.9 | E962.1 | E980.9 |
| **Calamine** (liniment) (lotion) | 976.3 | E858.7 | E946.3 | E950.4 | E962.0 | E980.4 |
| **Calciferol** | 963.5 | E858.1 | E933.5 | E950.4 | E962.0 | E980.4 |
| **Calcium** (salts) NEC | 974.5 | E858.5 | E944.5 | E950.4 | E962.0 | E980.4 |
| acetylsalicylate | 965.1 | E850.3 | E935.3 | E950.0 | E962.0 | E980.0 |
| benzamidosalicylate | 961.8 | E857 | E931.8 | E950.4 | E962.0 | E980.4 |
| carbaspirin | 965.1 | E850.3 | E935.3 | E950.0 | E962.0 | E980.0 |
| carbimide (citrated) | 977.3 | E858.8 | E947.3 | E950.4 | E962.0 | E980.4 |
| carbonate (antacid) | 973.0 | E858.4 | E943.0 | E950.4 | E962.0 | E980.4 |
| cyanide (citrated) | 977.3 | E858.8 | E947.3 | E950.4 | E962.0 | E980.4 |
| dioctyl sulfosuccinate | 973.2 | E858.4 | E943.2 | E950.4 | E962.0 | E980.4 |
| disodium edathamil | 963.8 | E858.1 | E933.8 | E950.4 | E962.0 | E980.4 |
| disodium edetate | 963.8 | E858.1 | E933.8 | E950.4 | E962.0 | E980.4 |
| EDTA | 963.8 | E858.1 | E933.8 | E950.4 | E962.0 | E980.4 |
| hydrate, hydroxide | 983.2 | E864.2 | — | E950.7 | E962.1 | E980.6 |
| mandelate | 961.9 | E857 | E931.9 | E950.4 | E962.0 | E980.4 |
| oxide | 983.2 | E864.2 | — | E950.7 | E962.1 | E980.6 |
| **Calomel** — see Mercury, chloride | | | | | | |
| **Caloric agents NEC** | 974.5 | E858.5 | E944.5 | E950.4 | E962.0 | E980.4 |
| **Calusterone** | 963.1 | E858.1 | E933.1 | E950.4 | E962.0 | E980.4 |
| **Camoquin** | 961.4 | E857 | E931.4 | E950.4 | E962.0 | E980.4 |
| **Camphor** (oil) | 976.1 | E858.7 | E946.1 | E950.4 | E962.0 | E980.4 |
| **Candeptin** | 976.0 | E858.7 | E946.0 | E950.4 | E962.0 | E980.4 |
| **Candicidin** | 976.0 | E858.7 | E946.0 | E950.4 | E962.0 | E980.4 |
| **Cannabinols** | 969.6 | E854.1 | E939.6 | E950.3 | E962.0 | E980.3 |
| **Cannabis** (derivatives) (indica) | | | | | | |
| (sativa) | 969.6 | E854.1 | E939.6 | E950.3 | E962.0 | E980.3 |
| **Canned heat** | 980.1 | E860.2 | — | E950.9 | E962.1 | E980.9 |
| **Cantharides, cantharidin,** | | | | | | |
| **cantharis** | 976.8 | E858.7 | E946.8 | E950.4 | E962.0 | E980.4 |
| **Capillary agents** | 972.8 | E858.3 | E942.8 | E950.4 | E962.0 | E980.4 |
| **Capreomycin** | 960.6 | E856 | E930.6 | E950.4 | E962.0 | E980.4 |
| **Captodiame,** | | | | | | |
| **captodiamine** | 969.5 | E853.8 | E939.5 | E950.3 | E962.0 | E980.3 |
| **Caramiphen** (hydrochloride) | 971.1 | E855.4 | E941.1 | E950.4 | E962.0 | E980.4 |
| **Carbachol** | 971.0 | E855.3 | E941.0 | E950.4 | E962.0 | E980.4 |
| **Carbacrylamine resins** | 974.5 | E858.5 | E944.5 | E950.4 | E962.0 | E980.4 |
| **Carbamate** (sedative) | 967.8 | E852.8 | E937.8 | E950.2 | E962.0 | E980.2 |
| herbicide | 989.3 | E863.5 | — | E950.6 | E962.1 | E980.7 |
| insecticide | 989.3 | E863.2 | — | E950.6 | E962.1 | E980.7 |
| **Carbamazepine** | 966.3 | E855.0 | E936.3 | E950.4 | E962.0 | E980.4 |
| **Carbamic esters** | 967.8 | E852.8 | E937.8 | E950.2 | E962.0 | E980.2 |
| **Carbamide** | 974.4 | E858.5 | E944.4 | E950.4 | E962.0 | E980.4 |
| topical | 976.8 | E858.7 | E946.8 | E950.4 | E962.0 | E980.4 |
| **Carbamylcholine chloride** | 971.0 | E855.3 | E941.0 | E950.4 | E962.0 | E980.4 |
| **Carbarsone** | 961.1 | E857 | E931.1 | E950.4 | E962.0 | E980.4 |
| **Carbaryl** | 989.3 | E863.2 | — | E950.6 | E962.1 | E980.7 |
| **Carbaspirin** | 965.1 | E850.3 | E935.3 | E950.0 | E962.0 | E980.0 |
| **Carbazochrome** | 972.8 | E858.3 | E942.8 | E950.4 | E962.0 | E980.4 |
| **Carbenicillin** | 960.0 | E856 | E930.0 | E950.4 | E962.0 | E980.4 |
| **Carbenoxolone** | 973.8 | E858.4 | E943.8 | E950.4 | E962.0 | E980.4 |
| **Carbetapentane** | 975.4 | E858.6 | E945.4 | E950.4 | E962.0 | E980.4 |
| **Carbimazole** | 962.8 | E858.0 | E932.8 | E950.4 | E962.0 | E980.4 |
| **Carbinol** | 980.1 | E860.2 | — | E950.9 | E962.1 | E980.9 |

☑ Additional Digit Required — Refer to the Tabular List for Digit Selection     ▽ Subterms under main terms may continue to next column or page

308 — Volume 2     ▶◀ Revised Text    ● New Line    ▲ Revised Code    *2008 ICD-9-CM*

| | Poisoning | Accident | Therapeutic Use | Suicide Attempt | Assault | Undetermined |
|---|---|---|---|---|---|---|
| Carbinoxamine | 963.0 | E858.1 | E933.0 | E950.4 | E962.0 | E980.4 |
| Carbitol | 982.8 | E862.4 | — | E950.9 | E962.1 | E980.9 |
| Carbocaine | 968.9 | E855.2 | E938.9 | E950.4 | E962.0 | E980.4 |
| infiltration (subcutaneous) | 968.5 | E855.2 | E938.5 | E950.4 | E962.0 | E980.4 |
| nerve block (peripheral) | | | | | | |
| (plexus) | 968.6 | E855.2 | E938.6 | E950.4 | E962.0 | E980.4 |
| topical (surface) | 968.5 | E855.2 | E938.5 | E950.4 | E962.0 | E980.4 |
| Carbol-fuchsin solution | 976.0 | E858.7 | E946.0 | E950.4 | E962.0 | E980.4 |
| Carbolic acid — see also Phenol | 963.0 | E864.0 | — | E950.7 | E962.1 | E980.6 |
| Carbomycin | 960.8 | E856 | E930.8 | E950.4 | E962.0 | E980.4 |
| Carbon | | | | | | |
| bisulfide (liquid)(vapor) | 982.2 | E862.4 | — | E950.9 | E962.1 | E980.9 |
| dioxide (gas) | 987.8 | E869.8 | — | E952.8 | E962.2 | E982.8 |
| disulfide (liquid)(vapor) | 982.2 | E862.4 | — | E950.9 | E962.1 | E980.9 |
| monoxide (from incomplete combustion of) (in) | | | | | | |
| NEC | 986 | E868.9 | — | E952.1 | E962.2 | E982.1 |
| blast furnace gas | 986 | E868.8 | — | E952.1 | E962.2 | E982.1 |
| butane (distributed in mobile container) | 986 | E868.0 | — | E951.1 | E962.2 | E981.1 |
| distributed through pipes | 986 | E867 | — | E951.0 | E962.2 | E981.0 |
| charcoal fumes | 986 | E868.3 | — | E952.1 | E962.2 | E982.1 |
| coal | | | | | | |
| gas (piped) | 986 | E867 | — | E951.0 | E962.2 | E981.0 |
| solid (in domestic stoves, fireplaces) | 986 | E868.3 | — | E952.1 | E962.2 | E982.1 |
| coke (in domestic stoves, fireplaces) | 986 | E868.3 | — | E952.1 | E962.2 | E982.1 |
| exhaust gas (motor) not in transit | 986 | E868.2 | — | E952.0 | E962.2 | E982.0 |
| combustion engine, any not in watercraft | 986 | E868.2 | — | E952.0 | E962.2 | E982.0 |
| farm tractor, not in transit | 986 | E868.2 | — | E952.0 | E962.2 | E982.0 |
| gas engine | 986 | E868.2 | — | E952.0 | E962.2 | E982.0 |
| motor pump | 986 | E868.2 | — | E952.0 | E962.2 | E982.0 |
| motor vehicle, not in transit | 986 | E868.2 | — | E952.0 | E962.2 | E982.0 |
| fuel (in domestic use) | 986 | E868.3 | — | E952.1 | E962.2 | E982.1 |
| gas (piped) | 986 | E867 | — | E951.0 | E962.2 | E981.0 |
| in mobile container | 986 | E868.0 | — | E951.1 | E962.2 | E981.1 |
| utility | 986 | E868.1 | — | E951.8 | E962.2 | E981.8 |
| in mobile container | 986 | E868.0 | — | E951.1 | E962.2 | E981.1 |
| piped (natural) | 986 | E867 | — | E951.0 | E962.2 | E981.0 |
| illuminating gas | 986 | E868.1 | — | E951.8 | E962.2 | E981.8 |
| industrial fuels or gases, any | 986 | E868.8 | — | E952.1 | E962.2 | E982.1 |
| kerosene (in domestic stoves, fireplaces) | 986 | E868.3 | — | E952.1 | E962.2 | E982.1 |
| kiln gas or vapor | 986 | E868.8 | — | E952.1 | E962.2 | E982.1 |
| motor exhaust gas, not in transit | 986 | E868.2 | — | E952.0 | E962.2 | E982.0 |
| piped gas (manufactured) (natural) | 986 | E867 | — | E951.0 | E962.2 | E981.0 |
| producer gas | 986 | E868.8 | — | E952.1 | E962.2 | E982.1 |
| propane (distributed in mobile container) | 986 | E868.0 | — | E951.1 | E962.2 | E981.1 |
| distributed through pipes | 986 | E867 | — | E951.0 | E962.2 | E981.0 |
| specified source NEC | 986 | E868.8 | — | E952.1 | E962.2 | E982.1 |
| stove gas | 986 | E868.1 | — | E951.8 | E962.2 | E981.8 |
| piped | 986 | E867 | — | E951.0 | E962.2 | E981.0 |
| utility gas | 986 | E868.1 | — | E951.8 | E962.2 | E981.8 |
| piped | 986 | E867 | — | E951.0 | E962.2 | E981.0 |
| water gas | 986 | E868.1 | — | E951.8 | E962.2 | E981.8 |
| wood (in domestic stoves, fireplaces) | 986 | E868.3 | — | E952.1 | E962.2 | E982.1 |
| tetrachloride (vapor) NEC | 987.8 | E869.8 | — | E952.8 | E962.2 | E982.8 |
| liquid (cleansing agent) NEC | 982.1 | E861.3 | — | E950.9 | E962.1 | E980.9 |
| solvent | 982.1 | E862.4 | — | E950.9 | E962.1 | E980.9 |
| Carbonic acid (gas) | 987.8 | E869.8 | — | E952.8 | E962.2 | E982.8 |
| anhydrase inhibitors | 974.2 | E858.5 | E944.2 | E950.4 | E962.0 | E980.4 |
| Carbowax | 976.3 | E858.7 | E946.3 | E950.4 | E962.0 | E980.4 |
| Carbrital | 967.0 | E851 | E937.0 | E950.1 | E962.0 | E980.1 |
| Carbromal (derivatives) | 967.3 | E852.2 | E937.3 | E950.2 | E962.0 | E980.2 |
| Cardiac | | | | | | |
| depressants | 972.0 | E858.3 | E942.0 | E950.4 | E962.0 | E980.4 |
| rhythm regulators | 972.0 | E858.3 | E942.0 | E950.4 | E962.0 | E980.4 |
| Cardiografin | 977.8 | E858.8 | E947.8 | E950.4 | E962.0 | E980.4 |
| Cardio-green | 977.8 | E858.8 | E947.8 | E950.4 | E962.0 | E980.4 |
| Cardiotonic glycosides | 972.1 | E858.3 | E942.1 | E950.4 | E962.0 | E980.4 |
| Cardiovascular agents NEC | 972.9 | E858.3 | E942.9 | E950.4 | E962.0 | E980.4 |
| Cardrase | 974.2 | E858.5 | E944.2 | E950.4 | E962.0 | E980.4 |
| Carfusin | 976.0 | E858.7 | E946.0 | E950.4 | E962.0 | E980.4 |
| Carisoprodol | 968.0 | E855.1 | E938.0 | E950.4 | E962.0 | E980.4 |
| Carmustine | 963.1 | E858.1 | E933.1 | E950.4 | E962.0 | E980.4 |
| Carotene | 963.5 | E858.1 | E933.5 | E950.4 | E962.0 | E980.4 |
| Carphenazine (maleate) | 969.1 | E853.0 | E939.1 | E950.3 | E962.0 | E980.3 |
| Carter's Little Pills | 973.1 | E858.4 | E943.1 | E950.4 | E962.0 | E980.4 |
| Cascara (sagrada) | 973.1 | E858.4 | E943.1 | E950.4 | E962.0 | E980.4 |
| Cassava | 988.2 | E865.4 | — | E950.9 | E962.1 | E980.9 |
| Castellani's paint | 976.0 | E858.7 | E946.0 | E950.4 | E962.0 | E980.4 |
| Castor | | | | | | |
| bean | 988.2 | E865.3 | — | E950.9 | E962.1 | E980.9 |
| oil | 973.1 | E858.4 | E943.1 | E950.4 | E962.0 | E980.4 |
| Caterpillar (sting) | 989.5 | E905.5 | — | E950.9 | E962.1 | E980.9 |
| Catha (edulis) | 970.8 | E854.3 | E940.8 | E950.4 | E962.0 | E980.4 |
| Cathartics NEC | 973.3 | E858.4 | E943.3 | E950.4 | E962.0 | E980.4 |
| contact | 973.1 | E858.4 | E943.1 | E950.4 | E962.0 | E980.4 |
| emollient | 973.2 | E858.4 | E943.2 | E950.4 | E962.0 | E980.4 |
| intestinal irritants | 973.1 | E858.4 | E943.1 | E950.4 | E962.0 | E980.4 |
| saline | 973.3 | E858.4 | E943.3 | E950.4 | E962.0 | E980.4 |
| Cathomycin | 960.8 | E856 | E930.8 | E950.4 | E962.0 | E980.4 |
| Caustic(s) | 983.9 | E864.4 | — | E950.7 | E962.1 | E980.6 |
| alkali | 983.2 | E864.2 | — | E950.7 | E962.1 | E980.6 |
| hydroxide | 983.2 | E864.2 | — | E950.7 | E962.1 | E980.6 |
| potash | 983.2 | E864.2 | — | E950.7 | E962.1 | E980.6 |
| soda | 983.2 | E864.2 | — | E950.7 | E962.1 | E980.6 |
| specified NEC | 983.9 | E864.3 | — | E950.7 | E962.1 | E980.6 |
| Ceepryn | 976.0 | E858.7 | E946.0 | E950.4 | E962.0 | E980.4 |
| ENT agent | 976.6 | E858.7 | E946.6 | E950.4 | E962.0 | E980.4 |
| lozenges | 976.6 | E858.7 | E946.6 | E950.4 | E962.0 | E980.4 |
| Celestone | 962.0 | E858.0 | E932.0 | E950.4 | E962.0 | E980.4 |
| topical | 976.0 | E858.7 | E946.0 | E950.4 | E962.0 | E980.4 |
| Cellosolve | 982.8 | E862.4 | — | E950.9 | E962.1 | E980.9 |
| Cell stimulants and proliferants | 976.8 | E858.7 | E946.8 | E950.4 | E962.0 | E980.4 |
| Cellulose derivatives, cathartic | 973.3 | E858.4 | E943.3 | E950.4 | E962.0 | E980.4 |
| nitrates (topical) | 976.3 | E858.7 | E946.3 | E950.4 | E962.0 | E980.4 |
| Centipede (bite) | 989.5 | E905.4 | — | E950.9 | E962.1 | E980.9 |
| Central nervous system | | | | | | |
| depressants | 968.4 | E855.1 | E938.4 | E950.4 | E962.0 | E980.4 |
| anesthetic (general) NEC | 968.4 | E855.1 | E938.4 | E950.4 | E962.0 | E980.4 |
| gases NEC | 968.2 | E855.1 | E938.2 | E950.4 | E962.0 | E980.4 |
| intravenous | 968.3 | E855.1 | E938.3 | E950.4 | E962.0 | E980.4 |
| barbiturates | 967.0 | E851 | E937.0 | E950.1 | E962.0 | E980.1 |
| bromides | 967.3 | E852.2 | E937.3 | E950.2 | E962.0 | E980.2 |
| cannabis sativa | 969.6 | E854.1 | E939.6 | E950.3 | E962.0 | E980.3 |
| chloral hydrate | 967.1 | E852.0 | E937.1 | E950.2 | E962.0 | E980.2 |
| hallucinogenics | 969.6 | E854.1 | E939.6 | E950.3 | E962.0 | E980.3 |
| hypnotics | 967.9 | E852.9 | E937.9 | E950.2 | E962.0 | E980.2 |
| specified NEC | 967.8 | E852.8 | E937.8 | E950.2 | E962.0 | E980.2 |
| muscle relaxants | 968.0 | E855.1 | E938.0 | E950.4 | E962.0 | E980.4 |
| paraldehyde | 967.2 | E852.1 | E937.2 | E950.2 | E962.0 | E980.2 |
| sedatives | 967.9 | E852.9 | E937.9 | E950.2 | E962.0 | E980.2 |
| mixed NEC | 967.6 | E852.5 | E937.6 | E950.2 | E962.0 | E980.2 |
| specified NEC | 967.8 | E852.8 | E937.8 | E950.2 | E962.0 | E980.2 |
| muscle-tone depressants | — | — | — | — | — | E980.4 |
| stimulants | 970.9 | E854.3 | E940.9 | E950.4 | E962.0 | E980.4 |
| amphetamines | 969.7 | E854.2 | E939.7 | E950.3 | E962.0 | E980.3 |
| analeptics | 970.0 | E854.3 | E940.0 | E950.4 | E962.0 | E980.4 |
| antidepressants | 969.0 | E854.0 | E939.0 | E950.3 | E962.0 | E980.3 |
| opiate antagonists | 970.1 | E854.3 | E940.0 | E950.4 | E962.0 | E980.4 |
| specified NEC | 970.8 | E854.3 | E940.8 | E950.4 | E962.0 | E980.4 |
| Cephalexin | 960.5 | E856 | E930.5 | E950.4 | E962.0 | E980.4 |
| Cephaloglycin | 960.5 | E856 | E930.5 | E950.4 | E962.0 | E980.4 |
| Cephaloridine | 960.5 | E856 | E930.5 | E950.4 | E962.0 | E980.4 |
| Cephalosporins NEC | 960.5 | E856 | E930.5 | E950.4 | E962.0 | E980.4 |
| N (adicillin) | 960.0 | E856 | E930.0 | E950.4 | E962.0 | E980.4 |
| Cephalothin (sodium) | 960.5 | E856 | E930.5 | E950.4 | E962.0 | E980.4 |
| Cerbera (odollam) | 988.2 | E865.4 | — | E950.9 | E962.1 | E980.9 |
| Cerberin | 972.1 | E858.3 | E942.1 | E950.4 | E962.0 | E980.4 |
| Cerebral stimulants | 970.9 | E854.3 | E940.9 | E950.4 | E962.0 | E980.4 |
| psychotherapeutic | 969.7 | E854.2 | E939.7 | E950.3 | E962.0 | E980.3 |
| specified NEC | 970.8 | E854.3 | E940.8 | E950.4 | E962.0 | E980.4 |
| Cetalkonium (chloride) | 976.0 | E858.7 | E946.0 | E950.4 | E962.0 | E980.4 |
| Cetoxime | 963.0 | E858.1 | E933.0 | E950.4 | E962.0 | E980.4 |
| Cetrimide | 976.2 | E858.7 | E946.2 | E950.4 | E962.0 | E980.4 |

☑ Additional Digit Required — Refer to the Tabular List for Digit Selection     ▽ Subterms under main terms may continue to next column or page

| | Poisoning | Accident | Therapeutic Use | Suicide Attempt | Assault | Undetermined |
|---|---|---|---|---|---|---|
| | | | **External Cause (E-Code)** | | | |
| **Cetylpyridinium** | 976.0 | E858.7 | E946.0 | E950.4 | E962.0 | E980.4 |
| ENT agent | 976.6 | E858.7 | E946.6 | E950.4 | E962.0 | E980.4 |
| lozenges | 976.6 | E858.7 | E946.6 | E950.4 | E962.0 | E980.4 |
| **Cevadilla** — see Sabadilla | | | | | | |
| **Cevitamic acid** | 963.5 | E858.1 | E933.5 | E950.4 | E962.0 | E980.4 |
| **Chalk, precipitated** | 973.0 | E858.4 | E943.0 | E950.4 | E962.0 | E980.4 |
| **Charcoal** | | | | | | |
| fumes (carbon monoxide) | 986 | E868.3 | — | E952.1 | E962.2 | E982.1 |
| industrial | 986 | E868.8 | — | E952.1 | E962.2 | E982.1 |
| medicinal (activated) | 973.0 | E858.4 | E943.0 | E950.4 | E962.0 | E980.4 |
| **Chelating agents NEC** | 977.2 | E858.8 | E947.2 | E950.4 | E962.0 | E980.4 |
| **Chelidonium majus** | 988.2 | E865.4 | — | E950.9 | E962.1 | E980.9 |
| **Chemical substance** | 989.9 | E866.9 | — | E950.9 | E962.1 | E980.9 |
| specified NEC | 989.89 | E866.8 | — | E950.9 | E962.1 | E980.9 |
| **Chemotherapy, antineoplastic** | 963.1 | E858.1 | E933.1 | E950.4 | E962.0 | E980.4 |
| **Chenopodium** (oil) | 961.6 | E857 | E931.6 | E950.4 | E962.0 | E980.4 |
| **Cherry laurel** | 988.2 | E865.4 | — | E950.9 | E962.1 | E980.9 |
| **Chiniofon** | 961.3 | E857 | E931.3 | E950.4 | E962.0 | E980.4 |
| **Chlophedianol** | 975.4 | E858.6 | E945.4 | E950.4 | E962.0 | E980.4 |
| **Chloral** (betaine) (formamide) (hydrate) | 967.1 | E852.0 | E937.1 | E950.2 | E962.0 | E980.2 |
| **Chloralamide** | 967.1 | E852.0 | E937.1 | E950.2 | E962.0 | E980.2 |
| **Chlorambucil** | 963.1 | E858.1 | E933.1 | E950.4 | E962.0 | E980.4 |
| **Chloramphenicol** | 960.2 | E856 | E930.2 | E950.4 | E962.0 | E980.4 |
| ENT agent | 976.6 | E858.7 | E946.6 | E950.4 | E962.0 | E980.4 |
| ophthalmic preparation | 976.5 | E858.7 | E946.5 | E950.4 | E962.0 | E980.4 |
| topical NEC | 976.0 | E858.7 | E946.0 | E950.4 | E962.0 | E980.4 |
| **Chlorate(s)** (potassium) (sodium) NEC | 983.9 | E864.3 | — | E950.7 | E962.1 | E980.6 |
| herbicides | 989.4 | E863.5 | — | E950.6 | E962.1 | E980.7 |
| **Chlorcylizine** | 963.0 | E858.1 | E933.0 | E950.4 | E962.0 | E980.4 |
| **Chlordan(e)** (dust) | 989.2 | E863.0 | — | E950.6 | E962.1 | E980.7 |
| **Chlordantoin** | 976.0 | E858.7 | E946.0 | E950.4 | E962.0 | E980.4 |
| **Chlordiazepoxide** | 969.4 | E853.2 | E939.4 | E950.3 | E962.0 | E980.3 |
| **Chloresium** | 976.8 | E858.7 | E946.8 | E950.4 | E962.0 | E980.4 |
| **Chlorethiazol** | 967.1 | E852.0 | E937.1 | E950.2 | E962.0 | E980.2 |
| **Chlorethyl** — see Ethyl, chloride | | | | | | |
| **Chloretone** | 967.1 | E852.0 | E937.1 | E950.2 | E962.0 | E980.2 |
| **Chlorex** | 982.3 | E862.4 | — | E950.9 | E962.1 | E980.9 |
| **Chlorhexadol** | 967.1 | E852.0 | E937.1 | E950.2 | E962.0 | E980.2 |
| **Chlorhexidine** (hydrochloride) | 976.0 | E858.7 | E946.0 | E950.4 | E962.0 | E980.4 |
| **Chlorhydroxyquinolin** | 976.0 | E858.7 | E946.0 | E950.4 | E962.0 | E980.4 |
| **Chloride of lime** (bleach) | 983.9 | E864.3 | — | E950.7 | E962.1 | E980.6 |
| **Chlorinated** | | | | | | |
| camphene | 989.2 | E863.0 | — | E950.6 | E962.1 | E980.7 |
| diphenyl | 989.89 | E866.8 | — | E950.9 | E962.1 | E980.9 |
| hydrocarbons NEC | 989.2 | E863.0 | — | E950.6 | E962.1 | E980.7 |
| solvent | 982.3 | E862.4 | — | E950.9 | E962.1 | E980.9 |
| lime (bleach) | 983.9 | E864.3 | — | E950.7 | E962.1 | E980.6 |
| naphthalene — see Naphthalene | | | | | | |
| pesticides NEC | 989.2 | E863.0 | — | E950.6 | E962.1 | E980.7 |
| soda — see Sodium, hypochlorite | | | | | | |
| **Chlorine** (fumes) (gas) | 987.6 | E869.8 | — | E952.8 | E962.2 | E982.8 |
| bleach | 983.9 | E864.3 | — | E950.7 | E962.1 | E980.6 |
| compounds NEC | 983.9 | E864.3 | — | E950.7 | E962.1 | E980.6 |
| disinfectant | 983.9 | E861.4 | — | E950.7 | E962.1 | E980.6 |
| releasing agents NEC | 983.9 | E864.3 | — | E950.7 | E962.1 | E980.6 |
| **Chlorisondamine** | 972.3 | E858.3 | E942.3 | E950.4 | E962.0 | E980.4 |
| **Chlormadinone** | 962.2 | E858.0 | E932.2 | E950.4 | E962.0 | E980.4 |
| **Chlormerodrin** | 974.0 | E858.5 | E944.0 | E950.4 | E962.0 | E980.4 |
| **Chlormethiazole** | 967.1 | E852.0 | E937.1 | E950.2 | E962.0 | E980.2 |
| **Chlormethylenecycline** | 960.4 | E856 | E930.4 | E950.4 | E962.0 | E980.4 |
| **Chlormezanone** | 969.5 | E853.8 | E939.5 | E950.3 | E962.0 | E980.3 |
| **Chloroacetophenone** | 987.5 | E869.3 | — | E952.8 | E962.2 | E982.8 |
| **Chloroaniline** | 983.0 | E864.0 | — | E950.7 | E962.1 | E980.6 |
| **Chlorobenzene, chlorobenzol** | 982.0 | E862.4 | — | E950.9 | E962.1 | E980.9 |
| **Chlorobutanol** | 967.1 | E852.0 | E937.1 | E950.2 | E962.0 | E980.2 |
| **Chlorodinitrobenzene** | 983.0 | E864.0 | — | E950.7 | E962.1 | E980.6 |
| dust or vapor | 987.8 | E869.8 | — | E952.8 | E962.2 | E982.8 |
| **Chloroethane** — see Ethyl, chloride | | | | | | |
| **Chloroform** (fumes) (vapor) | 987.8 | E869.8 | — | E952.8 | E962.2 | E982.8 |
| anesthetic (gas) | 968.2 | E855.1 | E938.2 | E950.4 | E962.0 | E980.4 |
| liquid NEC | 968.4 | E855.1 | E938.4 | E950.4 | E962.0 | E980.4 |
| solvent | 982.3 | E862.4 | — | E950.9 | E962.1 | E980.9 |
| **Chloroguanide** | 961.4 | E857 | E931.4 | E950.4 | E962.0 | E980.4 |

| | Poisoning | Accident | Therapeutic Use | Suicide Attempt | Assault | Undetermined |
|---|---|---|---|---|---|---|
| | | | **External Cause (E-Code)** | | | |
| **Chloromycetin** | 960.2 | E856 | E930.2 | E950.4 | E962.0 | E980.4 |
| ENT agent | 976.6 | E858.7 | E946.6 | E950.4 | E962.0 | E980.4 |
| ophthalmic preparation | 976.5 | E858.7 | E946.5 | E950.4 | E962.0 | E980.4 |
| otic solution | 976.6 | E858.7 | E946.6 | E950.4 | E962.0 | E980.4 |
| topical NEC | 976.0 | E858.7 | E946.0 | E950.4 | E962.0 | E980.4 |
| **Chloronitrobenzene** | 983.0 | E864.0 | — | E950.7 | E962.1 | E980.6 |
| dust or vapor | 987.8 | E869.8 | — | E952.8 | E962.2 | E982.8 |
| **Chlorophenol** | 983.0 | E864.0 | — | E950.7 | E962.1 | E980.6 |
| **Chlorophenothane** | 989.2 | E863.0 | — | E950.6 | E962.1 | E980.7 |
| **Chlorophyll** (derivatives) | 976.8 | E858.7 | E946.8 | E950.4 | E962.0 | E980.4 |
| **Chloropicrin** (fumes) | 987.8 | E869.8 | — | E952.8 | E962.2 | E982.8 |
| fumigant | 989.4 | E863.8 | — | E950.6 | E962.1 | E980.7 |
| fungicide | 989.4 | E863.6 | — | E950.6 | E962.1 | E980.7 |
| pesticide (fumes) | 989.4 | E863.4 | — | E950.6 | E962.1 | E980.7 |
| **Chloroprocaine** | 968.9 | E855.2 | E938.9 | E950.4 | E962.0 | E980.4 |
| infiltration (subcutaneous) | 968.5 | E855.2 | E938.5 | E950.4 | E962.0 | E980.4 |
| nerve block (peripheral) (plexus) | 968.6 | E855.2 | E938.6 | E950.4 | E962.0 | E980.4 |
| **Chloroptic** | 976.5 | E858.7 | E946.5 | E950.4 | E962.0 | E980.4 |
| **Chloropurine** | 963.1 | E858.1 | E933.1 | E950.4 | E962.0 | E980.4 |
| **Chloroquine** (hydrochloride) (phosphate) | 961.4 | E857 | E931.4 | E950.4 | E962.0 | E980.4 |
| **Chlorothen** | 963.0 | E858.1 | E933.0 | E950.4 | E962.0 | E980.4 |
| **Chlorothiazide** | 974.3 | E858.5 | E944.3 | E950.4 | E962.0 | E980.4 |
| **Chlorotrianisene** | 962.2 | E858.0 | E932.2 | E950.4 | E962.0 | E980.4 |
| **Chlorovinyldichloroarsine** | 985.1 | E866.3 | — | E950.8 | E962.1 | E980.8 |
| **Chloroxylenol** | 976.0 | E858.7 | E946.0 | E950.4 | E962.0 | E980.4 |
| **Chlorphenesin** (carbamate) | 968.0 | E855.1 | E938.0 | E950.4 | E962.0 | E980.4 |
| topical (antifungal) | 976.0 | E858.7 | E946.0 | E950.4 | E962.0 | E980.4 |
| **Chlorpheniramine** | 963.0 | E858.1 | E933.0 | E950.4 | E962.0 | E980.4 |
| **Chlorphenoxamine** | 966.4 | E855.0 | E936.4 | E950.4 | E962.0 | E980.4 |
| **Chlorphentermine** | 977.0 | E858.8 | E947.0 | E950.4 | E962.0 | E980.4 |
| **Chlorproguanil** | 961.4 | E857 | E931.4 | E950.4 | E962.0 | E980.4 |
| **Chlorpromazine** | 969.1 | E853.0 | E939.1 | E950.3 | E962.0 | E980.3 |
| **Chlorpropamide** | 962.3 | E858.0 | E932.3 | E950.4 | E962.0 | E980.4 |
| **Chlorprothixene** | 969.3 | E853.8 | E939.3 | E950.3 | E962.0 | E980.3 |
| **Chlorquinaldol** | 976.0 | E858.7 | E946.0 | E950.4 | E962.0 | E980.4 |
| **Chlortetracycline** | 960.4 | E856 | E930.4 | E950.4 | E962.0 | E980.4 |
| **Chlorthalidone** | 974.4 | E858.5 | E944.4 | E950.4 | E962.0 | E980.4 |
| **Chlortrianisene** | 962.2 | E858.0 | E932.2 | E950.4 | E962.0 | E980.4 |
| **Chlor-Trimeton** | 963.0 | E858.1 | E933.0 | E950.4 | E962.0 | E980.4 |
| **Chlorzoxazone** | 968.0 | E855.1 | E938.0 | E950.4 | E962.0 | E980.4 |
| **Choke damp** | 987.8 | E869.8 | — | E952.8 | E962.2 | E982.8 |
| **Cholebrine** | 977.8 | E858.8 | E947.8 | E950.4 | E962.0 | E980.4 |
| **Cholera vaccine** | 978.2 | E858.8 | E948.2 | E950.4 | E962.0 | E980.4 |
| **Cholesterol-lowering agents** | 972.2 | E858.3 | E942.2 | E950.4 | E962.0 | E980.4 |
| **Cholestyramine** (resin) | 972.2 | E858.3 | E942.2 | E950.4 | E962.0 | E980.4 |
| **Cholic acid** | 973.4 | E858.4 | E943.4 | E950.4 | E962.0 | E980.4 |
| **Choline** | | | | | | |
| dihydrogen citrate | 977.1 | E858.8 | E947.1 | E950.4 | E962.0 | E980.4 |
| salicylate | 965.1 | E850.3 | E935.3 | E950.0 | E962.0 | E980.0 |
| theophyllinate | 974.1 | E858.5 | E944.1 | E950.4 | E962.0 | E980.4 |
| **Cholinergics** | 971.0 | E855.3 | E941.0 | E950.4 | E962.0 | E980.4 |
| **Cholografin** | 977.8 | E858.8 | E947.8 | E950.4 | E962.0 | E980.4 |
| **Chorionic gonadotropin** | 962.4 | E858.0 | E932.4 | E950.4 | E962.0 | E980.4 |
| **Chromates** | 983.9 | E864.3 | — | E950.7 | E962.1 | E980.6 |
| dust or mist | 987.8 | E869.8 | — | E952.8 | E962.2 | E982.8 |
| lead | 984.0 | E866.0 | — | E950.9 | E962.1 | E980.9 |
| paint | 984.0 | E861.5 | — | E950.9 | E962.1 | E980.9 |
| **Chromic acid** | 983.9 | E864.3 | — | E950.7 | E962.1 | E980.6 |
| dust or mist | 987.8 | E869.8 | — | E952.8 | E962.2 | E982.8 |
| **Chromium** | 985.6 | E866.4 | — | E950.9 | E962.1 | E980.9 |
| compounds — see Chromates | | | | | | |
| **Chromonar** | 972.4 | E858.3 | E942.4 | E950.4 | E962.0 | E980.4 |
| **Chromyl chloride** | 983.9 | E864.3 | — | E950.7 | E962.1 | E980.6 |
| **Chrysarobin** (ointment) | 976.4 | E858.7 | E946.4 | E950.4 | E962.0 | E980.4 |
| **Chrysazin** | 973.1 | E858.4 | E943.1 | E950.4 | E962.0 | E980.4 |
| **Chymar** | 963.4 | E858.1 | E933.4 | E950.4 | E962.0 | E980.4 |
| ophthalmic preparation | 976.5 | E858.7 | E946.5 | E950.4 | E962.0 | E980.4 |
| **Chymotrypsin** | 963.4 | E858.1 | E933.4 | E950.4 | E962.0 | E980.4 |
| ophthalmic preparation | 976.5 | E858.7 | E946.5 | E950.4 | E962.0 | E980.4 |
| **Cicuta maculata or virosa** | 988.2 | E865.4 | — | E950.9 | E962.1 | E980.9 |
| **Cigarette lighter fluid** | 981 | E862.1 | — | E950.9 | E962.1 | E980.9 |
| **Cinchocaine** (spinal) | 968.7 | E855.2 | E938.7 | E950.4 | E962.0 | E980.4 |
| topical (surface) | 968.5 | E855.2 | E938.5 | E950.4 | E962.0 | E980.4 |
| **Cinchona** | 961.4 | E857 | E931.4 | E950.4 | E962.0 | E980.4 |
| **Cinchonine alkaloids** | 961.4 | E857 | E931.4 | E950.4 | E962.0 | E980.4 |
| **Cinchophen** | 974.7 | E858.5 | E944.7 | E950.4 | E962.0 | E980.4 |
| **Cinnarizine** | 963.0 | E858.1 | E933.0 | E950.4 | E962.0 | E980.4 |
| **Citanest** | 968.9 | E855.2 | E938.9 | E950.4 | E962.0 | E980.4 |

☑ Additional Digit Required — Refer to the Tabular List for Digit Selection     ⓦ Subterms under main terms may continue to next column or page

| | | External Cause (E-Code) | | | | |
|---|---|---|---|---|---|---|
| | Poisoning | Accident | Therapeutic Use | Suicide Attempt | Assault | Undetermined |
| **Citanest** — *continued* | | | | | | |
| infiltration (subcutaneous) | 968.5 | E855.2 | E938.5 | E950.4 | E962.0 | E980.4 |
| nerve block (peripheral) | | | | | | |
| (plexus) | 968.6 | E855.2 | E938.6 | E950.4 | E962.0 | E980.4 |
| **Citric acid** | 989.89 | E866.8 | — | E950.9 | E962.1 | E980.9 |
| **Citrovorum factor** | 964.1 | E858.2 | E934.1 | E950.4 | E962.0 | E980.4 |
| **Claviceps purpurea** | 988.2 | E865.4 | — | E950.9 | E962.1 | E980.9 |
| **Cleaner, cleansing agent** | | | | | | |
| **NEC** | 989.89 | E861.3 | — | E950.9 | E962.1 | E980.9 |
| of paint or varnish | 982.8 | E862.9 | — | E950.9 | E962.1 | E980.9 |
| **Clematis vitalba** | 988.2 | E865.4 | — | E950.9 | E962.1 | E980.9 |
| **Clemizole** | 963.0 | E858.1 | E933.0 | E950.4 | E962.0 | E980.4 |
| penicillin | 960.0 | E856 | E930.0 | E950.4 | E962.0 | E980.4 |
| **Clidinium** | 971.1 | E855.4 | E941.1 | E950.4 | E962.0 | E980.4 |
| **Clindamycin** | 960.8 | E856 | E930.8 | E950.4 | E962.0 | E980.4 |
| **Cliradon** | 965.09 | E850.2 | E935.2 | E950.0 | E962.0 | E980.0 |
| **Clocortolone** | 962.0 | E858.0 | E932.0 | E950.4 | E962.0 | E980.4 |
| **Clofedanol** | 975.4 | E858.6 | E945.4 | E950.4 | E962.0 | E980.4 |
| **Clofibrate** | 972.2 | E858.3 | E942.2 | E950.4 | E962.0 | E980.4 |
| **Clomethiazole** | 967.1 | E852.0 | E937.1 | E950.2 | E962.0 | E980.2 |
| **Clomiphene** | 977.8 | E858.8 | E947.8 | E950.4 | E962.0 | E980.4 |
| **Clonazepam** | 969.4 | E853.2 | E939.4 | E950.3 | E962.0 | E980.3 |
| **Clonidine** | 972.6 | E858.3 | E942.6 | E950.4 | E962.0 | E980.4 |
| **Clopamide** | 974.3 | E858.5 | E944.3 | E950.4 | E962.0 | E980.4 |
| **Clorazepate** | 969.4 | E853.2 | E939.4 | E950.3 | E962.0 | E980.3 |
| **Clorexolone** | 974.4 | E858.5 | E944.4 | E950.4 | E962.0 | E980.4 |
| **Clorox** (bleach) | 983.9 | E864.3 | — | E950.7 | E962.1 | E980.6 |
| **Clortermine** | 977.0 | E858.8 | E947.0 | E950.4 | E962.0 | E980.4 |
| **Clotrimazole** | 976.0 | E858.7 | E946.0 | E950.4 | E962.0 | E980.4 |
| **Cloxacillin** | 960.0 | E856 | E930.0 | E950.4 | E962.0 | E980.4 |
| **Coagulants NEC** | 964.5 | E858.2 | E934.5 | E950.4 | E962.0 | E980.4 |
| **Coal** (carbon monoxide from) — | | | | | | |
| *see also* Carbon, monoxide, | | | | | | |
| coal | | | | | | |
| oil — *see* Kerosene | | | | | | |
| tar NEC | 983.0 | E864.0 | — | E950.7 | E962.1 | E980.6 |
| fumes | 987.8 | E869.8 | — | E952.8 | E962.2 | E982.8 |
| medicinal (ointment) | 976.4 | E858.7 | E946.4 | E950.4 | E962.0 | E980.4 |
| analgesics NEC | 965.5 | E850.5 | E935.5 | E950.0 | E962.0 | E980.0 |
| naphtha (solvent) | 981 | E862.0 | — | E950.9 | E962.1 | E980.9 |
| **Cobalt** (fumes) (industrial) | 985.8 | E866.4 | — | E950.9 | E962.1 | E980.9 |
| **Cobra** (venom) | 989.5 | E905.0 | — | E950.9 | E962.1 | E980.9 |
| **Coca** (leaf) | 970.8 | E854.3 | E940.8 | E950.4 | E962.0 | E980.4 |
| **Cocaine** (hydrochloride) | | | | | | |
| (salt) | 970.8 | E854.3 | E940.8 | E950.4 | E962.0 | E980.4 |
| topical anesthetic | 968.5 | E855.2 | E938.5 | E950.4 | E962.0 | E980.4 |
| **Coccidioidin** | 977.8 | E858.8 | E947.8 | E950.4 | E962.0 | E980.4 |
| **Cocculus indicus** | 988.2 | E865.3 | — | E950.9 | E962.1 | E980.9 |
| **Cochineal** | 989.89 | E866.8 | — | E950.9 | E962.1 | E980.9 |
| medicinal products | 977.4 | E858.8 | E947.4 | E950.4 | E962.0 | E980.4 |
| **Codeine** | 965.09 | E850.2 | E935.2 | E950.0 | E962.0 | E980.0 |
| **Coffee** | 989.89 | E866.8 | — | E950.9 | E962.1 | E980.9 |
| **Cogentin** | 971.1 | E855.4 | E941.1 | E950.4 | E962.0 | E980.4 |
| **Coke fumes or gas** (carbon | | | | | | |
| monoxide) | 986 | E868.3 | — | E952.1 | E962.2 | E982.1 |
| industrial use | 986 | E868.8 | — | E952.1 | E962.2 | E982.1 |
| **Colace** | 973.2 | E858.4 | E943.2 | E950.4 | E962.0 | E980.4 |
| **Colchicine** | 974.7 | E858.5 | E944.7 | E950.4 | E962.0 | E980.4 |
| **Colchicum** | 988.2 | E865.3 | — | E950.9 | E962.1 | E980.9 |
| **Cold cream** | 976.3 | E858.7 | E946.3 | E950.4 | E962.0 | E980.4 |
| **Colestipol** | 972.2 | E858.3 | E942.2 | E950.4 | E962.0 | E980.4 |
| **Colistimethate** | 960.8 | E856 | E930.8 | E950.4 | E962.0 | E980.4 |
| **Colistin** | 960.8 | E856 | E930.8 | E950.4 | E962.0 | E980.4 |
| **Collagen** | 977.8 | E866.8 | E947.8 | E950.9 | E962.1 | E980.9 |
| **Collagenase** | 976.8 | E858.7 | E946.8 | E950.4 | E962.0 | E980.4 |
| **Collodion** (flexible) | 976.3 | E858.7 | E946.3 | E950.4 | E962.0 | E980.4 |
| **Colocynth** | 973.1 | E858.4 | E943.1 | E950.4 | E962.0 | E980.4 |
| **Coloring matter** — *see* Dye(s) | | | | | | |
| **Combustion gas** — *see* Carbon, monoxide | | | | | | |
| **Compazine** | 969.1 | E853.0 | E939.1 | E950.3 | E962.0 | E980.3 |
| **Compound** | | | | | | |
| 42 (warfarin) | 989.4 | E863.7 | — | E950.6 | E962.1 | E980.7 |
| 269 (endrin) | 989.2 | E863.0 | — | E950.6 | E962.1 | E980.7 |
| 497 (dieldrin) | 989.2 | E863.0 | — | E950.6 | E962.1 | E980.7 |
| 1080 (sodium | | | | | | |
| fluoroacetate) | 989.4 | E863.7 | — | E950.6 | E962.1 | E980.7 |
| 3422 (parathion) | 989.3 | E863.1 | — | E950.6 | E962.1 | E980.7 |
| 3911 (phorate) | 989.3 | E863.1 | — | E950.6 | E962.1 | E980.7 |
| 3956 (toxaphene) | 989.2 | E863.0 | — | E950.6 | E962.1 | E980.7 |
| 4049 (malathion) | 989.3 | E863.1 | — | E950.6 | E962.1 | E980.7 |

| | | External Cause (E-Code) | | | | |
|---|---|---|---|---|---|---|
| | Poisoning | Accident | Therapeutic Use | Suicide Attempt | Assault | Undetermined |
| **Compound** — *continued* | | | | | | |
| 4124 (dicapthon) | 989.4 | E863.4 | — | E950.6 | E962.1 | E980.7 |
| E (cortisone) | 962.0 | E858.0 | E932.0 | E950.4 | E962.0 | E980.4 |
| F (hydrocortisone) | 962.0 | E858.0 | E932.0 | E950.4 | E962.0 | E980.4 |
| **Congo red** | 977.8 | E858.8 | E947.8 | E950.4 | E962.0 | E980.4 |
| **Coniine, conine** | 965.7 | E850.7 | E935.7 | E950.0 | E962.0 | E980.0 |
| **Conium** (maculatum) | 988.2 | E865.4 | — | E950.9 | E962.1 | E980.9 |
| **Conjugated estrogens** | | | | | | |
| (equine) | 962.2 | E858.0 | E932.2 | E950.4 | E962.0 | E980.4 |
| **Contac** | 975.6 | E858.6 | E945.6 | E950.4 | E962.0 | E980.4 |
| **Contact lens solution** | 976.5 | E858.7 | E946.5 | E950.4 | E962.0 | E980.4 |
| **Contraceptives** (oral) | 962.2 | E858.0 | E932.2 | E950.4 | E962.0 | E980.4 |
| vaginal | 976.8 | E858.7 | E946.8 | E950.4 | E962.0 | E980.4 |
| **Contrast media** | | | | | | |
| (roentgenographic) | 977.8 | E858.8 | E947.8 | E950.4 | E962.0 | E980.4 |
| **Convallaria majalis** | 988.2 | E865.4 | — | E950.9 | E962.1 | E980.9 |
| **Copper** (dust) (fumes) (salts) | | | | | | |
| **NEC** | 985.8 | E866.4 | — | E950.9 | E962.1 | E980.9 |
| arsenate, arsenite | 985.1 | E866.3 | — | E950.8 | E962.1 | E980.8 |
| insecticide | 985.1 | E863.4 | — | E950.8 | E962.1 | E980.8 |
| emetic | 973.6 | E858.4 | E943.6 | E950.4 | E962.0 | E980.4 |
| fungicide | 985.8 | E863.6 | — | E950.6 | E962.1 | E980.7 |
| insecticide | 985.8 | E863.4 | — | E950.6 | E962.1 | E980.7 |
| oleate | 976.0 | E858.7 | E946.0 | E950.4 | E962.0 | E980.4 |
| sulfate | 983.9 | E864.3 | — | E950.7 | E962.1 | E980.6 |
| cupric | 973.6 | E858.4 | E943.6 | E950.4 | E962.0 | E980.4 |
| cuprous | 983.9 | E864.3 | — | E950.7 | E962.1 | E980.6 |
| fungicide | 983.9 | E863.6 | — | E950.7 | E962.1 | E980.6 |
| **Copperhead snake** (bite) | | | | | | |
| (venom) | 989.5 | E905.0 | — | E950.9 | E962.1 | E980.9 |
| **Coral** (sting) | 989.5 | E905.6 | — | E950.9 | E962.1 | E980.9 |
| snake (bite) (venom) | 989.5 | E905.0 | — | E950.9 | E962.1 | E980.9 |
| **Cordran** | 976.0 | E858.7 | E946.0 | E950.4 | E962.0 | E980.4 |
| **Corn cures** | 976.4 | E858.7 | E946.4 | E950.4 | E962.0 | E980.4 |
| **Cornhusker's lotion** | 976.3 | E858.7 | E946.3 | E950.4 | E962.0 | E980.4 |
| **Corn starch** | 976.3 | E858.7 | E946.3 | E950.4 | E962.0 | E980.4 |
| **Corrosive** | 983.9 | E864.4 | — | E950.7 | E962.1 | E980.6 |
| acids NEC | 983.1 | E864.1 | — | E950.7 | E962.1 | E980.6 |
| aromatics | 983.0 | E864.0 | — | E950.7 | E962.1 | E980.6 |
| disinfectant | 983.0 | E861.4 | — | E950.7 | E962.1 | E980.6 |
| fumes NEC | 987.9 | E869.9 | — | E952.9 | E962.2 | E982.9 |
| specified NEC | 983.9 | E864.3 | — | E950.7 | E962.1 | E980.6 |
| sublimate — *see* Mercury, chloride | | | | | | |
| **Cortate** | 962.0 | E858.0 | E932.0 | E950.4 | E962.0 | E980.4 |
| **Cort-Dome** | 962.0 | E858.0 | E932.0 | E950.4 | E962.0 | E980.4 |
| ENT agent | 976.6 | E858.7 | E946.6 | E950.4 | E962.0 | E980.4 |
| ophthalmic preparation | 976.5 | E858.7 | E946.5 | E950.4 | E962.0 | E980.4 |
| topical NEC | 976.0 | E858.7 | E946.0 | E950.4 | E962.0 | E980.4 |
| **Cortef** | 962.0 | E858.0 | E932.0 | E950.4 | E962.0 | E980.4 |
| ENT agent | 976.6 | E858.7 | E946.6 | E950.4 | E962.0 | E980.4 |
| ophthalmic preparation | 976.5 | E858.7 | E946.5 | E950.4 | E962.0 | E980.4 |
| topical NEC | 976.0 | E858.7 | E946.0 | E950.4 | E962.0 | E980.4 |
| **Corticosteroids** | | | | | | |
| (fluorinated) | 962.0 | E858.0 | E932.0 | E950.4 | E962.0 | E980.4 |
| ENT agent | 976.6 | E858.7 | E946.6 | E950.4 | E962.0 | E980.4 |
| ophthalmic preparation | 976.5 | E858.7 | E946.5 | E950.4 | E962.0 | E980.4 |
| topical NEC | 976.0 | E858.7 | E946.0 | E950.4 | E962.0 | E980.4 |
| **Corticotropin** | 962.4 | E858.0 | E932.4 | E950.4 | E962.0 | E980.4 |
| **Cortisol** | 962.0 | E858.0 | E932.0 | E950.4 | E962.0 | E980.4 |
| ENT agent | 976.6 | E858.7 | E946.6 | E950.4 | E962.0 | E980.4 |
| ophthalmic preparation | 976.5 | E858.7 | E946.5 | E950.4 | E962.0 | E980.4 |
| topical NEC | 976.0 | E858.7 | E946.0 | E950.4 | E962.0 | E980.4 |
| **Cortisone derivatives** | | | | | | |
| (acetate) | 962.0 | E858.0 | E932.0 | E950.4 | E962.0 | E980.4 |
| ENT agent | 976.6 | E858.7 | E946.6 | E950.4 | E962.0 | E980.4 |
| ophthalmic preparation | 976.5 | E858.7 | E946.5 | E950.4 | E962.0 | E980.4 |
| topical NEC | 976.0 | E858.7 | E946.0 | E950.4 | E962.0 | E980.4 |
| **Cortogen** | 962.0 | E858.0 | E932.0 | E950.4 | E962.0 | E980.4 |
| ENT agent | 976.6 | E858.7 | E946.6 | E950.4 | E962.0 | E980.4 |
| ophthalmic preparation | 976.5 | E858.7 | E946.5 | E950.4 | E962.0 | E980.4 |
| **Cortone** | 962.0 | E858.0 | E932.0 | E950.4 | E962.0 | E980.4 |
| ENT agent | 976.6 | E858.7 | E946.6 | E950.4 | E962.0 | E980.4 |
| ophthalmic preparation | 976.5 | E858.7 | E946.5 | E950.4 | E962.0 | E980.4 |
| **Cortril** | 962.0 | E858.0 | E932.0 | E950.4 | E962.0 | E980.4 |
| ENT agent | 976.6 | E858.7 | E946.6 | E950.4 | E962.0 | E980.4 |
| ophthalmic preparation | 976.5 | E858.7 | E946.5 | E950.4 | E962.0 | E980.4 |
| topical NEC | 976.0 | E858.7 | E946.0 | E950.4 | E962.0 | E980.4 |
| **Cosmetics** | 989.89 | E866.7 | — | E950.9 | E962.1 | E980.9 |
| **Cosyntropin** | 977.8 | E858.8 | E947.8 | E950.4 | E962.0 | E980.4 |
| **Cotarnine** | 964.5 | E858.2 | E934.5 | E950.4 | E962.0 | E980.4 |

☑ Additional Digit Required — Refer to the Tabular List for Digit Selection  ▲ Subterms under main terms may continue to next column or page

**2008 ICD-9-CM**  ▶◀ Revised Text  ● New Line  ▲ Revised Code  **Volume 2 — 311**

|  | Poisoning | Accident | Therapeutic Use | Suicide Attempt | Assault | Undetermined |
|---|---|---|---|---|---|---|
| Cottonseed oil | 976.3 | E858.7 | E946.3 | E950.4 | E962.0 | E980.4 |
| Cough mixtures |  |  |  |  |  |  |
| (antitussives) | 975.4 | E858.6 | E945.4 | E950.4 | E962.0 | E980.4 |
| containing opiates | 965.09 | E850.2 | E935.2 | E950.0 | E962.0 | E980.0 |
| expectorants | 975.5 | E858.6 | E945.5 | E950.4 | E962.0 | E980.4 |
| Coumadin | 964.2 | E858.2 | E934.2 | E950.4 | E962.0 | E980.4 |
| rodenticide | 989.4 | E863.7 | — | E950.6 | E962.1 | E980.7 |
| Coumarin | 964.2 | E858.2 | E934.2 | E950.4 | E962.0 | E980.4 |
| Coumetarol | 964.2 | E858.2 | E934.2 | E950.4 | E962.0 | E980.4 |
| Cowbane | 988.2 | E865.4 | — | E950.9 | E962.1 | E980.9 |
| Cozyme | 963.5 | E858.1 | E933.5 | E950.4 | E962.0 | E980.4 |
| Crack | 970.8 | E854.3 | E940.8 | E950.4 | E962.0 | E980.4 |
| Creolin | 983.0 | E864.0 | — | E950.7 | E962.1 | E980.6 |
| disinfectant | 983.0 | E861.4 | — | E950.7 | E962.1 | E980.6 |
| Creosol (compound) | 983.0 | E864.0 | — | E950.7 | E962.1 | E980.6 |
| Creosote (beechwood) (coal |  |  |  |  |  |  |
| tar) | 983.0 | E864.0 | — | E950.7 | E962.1 | E980.6 |
| medicinal (expectorant) | 975.5 | E858.6 | E945.5 | E950.4 | E962.0 | E980.4 |
| syrup | 975.5 | E858.6 | E945.5 | E950.4 | E962.0 | E980.4 |
| Cresol | 983.0 | E864.0 | — | E950.7 | E962.1 | E980.6 |
| disinfectant | 983.0 | E861.4 | — | E950.7 | E962.1 | E980.6 |
| Cresylic acid | 983.0 | E864.0 | — | E950.7 | E962.1 | E980.6 |
| Cropropamide | 965.7 | E850.7 | E935.7 | E950.0 | E962.0 | E980.0 |
| with crotethamide | 970.0 | E854.3 | E940.0 | E950.4 | E962.0 | E980.4 |
| Crotamiton | 976.0 | E858.7 | E946.0 | E950.4 | E962.0 | E980.4 |
| Crotethamide | 965.7 | E850.7 | E935.7 | E950.0 | E962.0 | E980.0 |
| with cropropamide | 970.0 | E854.3 | E940.0 | E950.4 | E962.0 | E980.4 |
| Croton (oil) | 973.1 | E858.4 | E943.1 | E950.4 | E962.0 | E980.4 |
| chloral | 967.1 | E852.0 | E937.1 | E950.2 | E962.0 | E980.2 |
| Crude oil | 981 | E862.1 | — | E950.9 | E962.1 | E980.9 |
| Cryogenine | 965.8 | E850.8 | E935.8 | E950.0 | E962.0 | E980.0 |
| Cryolite (pesticide) | 989.4 | E863.4 | — | E950.6 | E962.1 | E980.7 |
| Cryptenamine | 972.6 | E858.3 | E942.6 | E950.4 | E962.0 | E980.4 |
| Crystal violet | 976.0 | E858.7 | E946.0 | E950.4 | E962.0 | E980.4 |
| Cuckoopint | 988.2 | E865.4 | — | E950.9 | E962.1 | E980.9 |
| Cumetharol | 964.2 | E858.2 | E934.2 | E950.4 | E962.0 | E980.4 |
| Cupric sulfate | 973.6 | E858.4 | E943.6 | E950.4 | E962.0 | E980.4 |
| Cuprous sulfate | 983.9 | E864.3 | — | E950.7 | E962.1 | E980.6 |
| Curare, curarine | 975.2 | E858.6 | E945.2 | E950.4 | E962.0 | E980.4 |
| Cyanic acid — see Cyanide(s) |  |  |  |  |  |  |
| Cyanide(s) (compounds) |  |  |  |  |  |  |
| (hydrogen) (potassium) |  |  |  |  |  |  |
| (sodium) NEC | 989.0 | E866.8 | — | E950.9 | E962.1 | E980.9 |
| dust or gas (inhalation) |  |  |  |  |  |  |
| NEC | 987.7 | E869.8 | — | E952.8 | E962.2 | E982.8 |
| fumigant | 989.0 | E863.8 | — | E950.6 | E962.1 | E980.7 |
| mercuric — see Mercury |  |  |  |  |  |  |
| pesticide (dust) (fumes) | 989.0 | E863.4 | — | E950.6 | E962.1 | E980.7 |
| Cyanocobalamin | 964.1 | E858.2 | E934.1 | E950.4 | E962.0 | E980.4 |
| Cyanogen (chloride) (gas) |  |  |  |  |  |  |
| NEC | 987.8 | E869.8 | — | E952.8 | E962.2 | E982.8 |
| Cyclaine | 968.5 | E855.2 | E938.5 | E950.4 | E962.0 | E980.4 |
| Cyclamen europaeum | 988.2 | E865.4 | — | E950.9 | E962.1 | E980.9 |
| Cyclandelate | 972.5 | E858.3 | E942.5 | E950.4 | E962.0 | E980.4 |
| Cyclazocine | 965.09 | E850.2 | E935.2 | E950.0 | E962.0 | E980.0 |
| Cyclizine | 963.0 | E858.1 | E933.0 | E950.4 | E962.0 | E980.4 |
| Cyclobarbital, |  |  |  |  |  |  |
| cyclobarbitone | 967.0 | E851 | E937.0 | E950.1 | E962.0 | E980.1 |
| Cycloguanil | 961.4 | E857 | E931.4 | E950.4 | E962.0 | E980.4 |
| Cyclohexane | 982.0 | E862.4 | — | E950.9 | E962.1 | E980.9 |
| Cyclohexanol | 980.8 | E860.8 | — | E950.9 | E962.1 | E980.9 |
| Cyclohexanone | 982.8 | E862.4 | — | E950.9 | E962.1 | E980.9 |
| Cyclomethycaine | 968.5 | E855.2 | E938.5 | E950.4 | E962.0 | E980.4 |
| Cyclopentamine | 971.2 | E855.5 | E941.2 | E950.4 | E962.0 | E980.4 |
| Cyclopenthiazide | 974.3 | E858.5 | E944.3 | E950.4 | E962.0 | E980.4 |
| Cyclopentolate | 971.1 | E855.4 | E941.1 | E950.4 | E962.0 | E980.4 |
| Cyclophosphamide | 963.1 | E858.1 | E933.1 | E950.4 | E962.0 | E980.4 |
| Cyclopropane | 968.2 | E855.1 | E938.2 | E950.4 | E962.0 | E980.4 |
| Cycloserine | 960.6 | E856 | E930.6 | E950.4 | E962.0 | E980.4 |
| Cyclothiazide | 974.3 | E858.5 | E944.3 | E950.4 | E962.0 | E980.4 |
| Cycrimine | 966.4 | E855.0 | E936.4 | E950.4 | E962.0 | E980.4 |
| Cymarin | 972.1 | E858.3 | E942.1 | E950.4 | E962.0 | E980.4 |
| Cyproheptadine | 963.0 | E858.1 | E933.0 | E950.4 | E962.0 | E980.4 |
| Cyprolidol | 969.0 | E854.0 | E939.0 | E950.3 | E962.0 | E980.3 |
| Cytarabine | 963.1 | E858.1 | E933.1 | E950.4 | E962.0 | E980.4 |
| Cytisus |  |  |  |  |  |  |
| laburnum | 988.2 | E865.4 | — | E950.9 | E962.1 | E980.9 |
| scoparius | 988.2 | E865.4 | — | E950.9 | E962.1 | E980.9 |
| Cytomel | 962.7 | E858.0 | E932.7 | E950.4 | E962.0 | E980.4 |
| Cytosine (antineoplastic) | 963.1 | E858.1 | E933.1 | E950.4 | E962.0 | E980.4 |
| Cytoxan | 963.1 | E858.1 | E933.1 | E950.4 | E962.0 | E980.4 |

|  | Poisoning | Accident | Therapeutic Use | Suicide Attempt | Assault | Undetermined |
|---|---|---|---|---|---|---|
| Dacarbazine | 963.1 | E858.1 | E933.1 | E950.4 | E962.0 | E980.4 |
| Dactinomycin | 960.7 | E856 | E930.7 | E950.4 | E962.0 | E980.4 |
| DADPS | 961.8 | E857 | E931.8 | E950.4 | E962.0 | E980.4 |
| Dakin's solution (external) | 976.0 | E858.7 | E946.0 | E950.4 | E962.0 | E980.4 |
| Dalmane | 969.4 | E853.2 | E939.4 | E950.3 | E962.0 | E980.3 |
| DAM | 977.2 | E858.8 | E947.2 | E950.4 | E962.0 | E980.4 |
| Danilone | 964.2 | E858.2 | E934.2 | E950.4 | E962.0 | E980.4 |
| Danthron | 973.1 | E858.4 | E943.1 | E950.4 | E962.0 | E980.4 |
| Dantrolene | 975.2 | E858.6 | E945.2 | E950.4 | E962.0 | E980.4 |
| Daphne (gnidium) |  |  |  |  |  |  |
| (mezereum) | 988.2 | E865.4 | — | E950.9 | E962.1 | E980.9 |
| berry | 988.2 | E865.3 | — | E950.9 | E962.1 | E980.9 |
| Dapsone | 961.8 | E857 | E931.8 | E950.4 | E962.0 | E980.4 |
| Daraprim | 961.4 | E857 | E931.4 | E950.4 | E962.0 | E980.4 |
| Darnel | 988.2 | E865.3 | — | E950.9 | E962.1 | E980.9 |
| Darvon | 965.8 | E850.8 | E935.8 | E950.0 | E962.0 | E980.0 |
| Daunorubicin | 960.7 | E856 | E930.7 | E950.4 | E962.0 | E980.4 |
| DBI | 962.3 | E858.0 | E932.3 | E950.4 | E962.0 | E980.4 |
| D-Con (rodenticide) | 989.4 | E863.7 | — | E950.6 | E962.1 | E980.7 |
| DDS | 961.8 | E857 | E931.8 | E950.4 | E962.0 | E980.4 |
| DDT | 989.2 | E863.0 | — | E950.6 | E962.1 | E980.7 |
| Deadly nightshade | 988.2 | E865.4 | — | E950.9 | E962.1 | E980.9 |
| berry | 988.2 | E865.3 | — | E950.9 | E962.1 | E980.9 |
| Deanol | 969.7 | E854.2 | E939.7 | E950.3 | E962.0 | E980.3 |
| Debrisoquine | 972.6 | E858.3 | E942.6 | E950.4 | E962.0 | E980.4 |
| Decaborane | 989.89 | E866.8 | — | E950.9 | E962.1 | E980.9 |
| fumes | 987.8 | E869.8 | — | E952.8 | E962.2 | E982.8 |
| Decadron | 962.0 | E858.0 | E932.0 | E950.4 | E962.0 | E980.4 |
| ENT agent | 976.6 | E858.7 | E946.6 | E950.4 | E962.0 | E980.4 |
| ophthalmic preparation | 976.5 | E858.7 | E946.5 | E950.4 | E962.0 | E980.4 |
| topical NEC | 976.0 | E858.7 | E946.0 | E950.4 | E962.0 | E980.4 |
| Decahydronaphthalene | 982.0 | E862.4 | — | E950.9 | E962.1 | E980.9 |
| Decalin | 982.0 | E862.4 | — | E950.9 | E962.1 | E980.9 |
| Decamethonium | 975.2 | E858.6 | E945.2 | E950.4 | E962.0 | E980.4 |
| Decholin | 973.4 | E858.4 | E943.4 | E950.4 | E962.0 | E980.4 |
| sodium (diagnostic) | 977.8 | E858.8 | E947.8 | E950.4 | E962.0 | E980.4 |
| Declomycin | 960.4 | E856 | E930.4 | E950.4 | E962.0 | E980.4 |
| Deferoxamine | 963.8 | E858.1 | E933.8 | E950.4 | E962.0 | E980.4 |
| Dehydrocholic acid | 973.4 | E858.4 | E943.4 | E950.4 | E962.0 | E980.4 |
| DeKalin | 982.0 | E862.4 | — | E950.9 | E962.1 | E980.9 |
| Delalutin | 962.2 | E858.0 | E932.2 | E950.4 | E962.0 | E980.4 |
| Delphinium | 988.2 | E865.3 | — | E950.9 | E962.1 | E980.9 |
| Deltasone | 962.0 | E858.0 | E932.0 | E950.4 | E962.0 | E980.4 |
| Deltra | 962.0 | E858.0 | E932.0 | E950.4 | E962.0 | E980.4 |
| Delvinal | 967.0 | E851 | E937.0 | E950.1 | E962.0 | E980.1 |
| Demecarium (bromide) | 971.0 | E855.3 | E941.0 | E950.4 | E962.0 | E980.4 |
| Demeclocycline | 960.4 | E856 | E930.4 | E950.4 | E962.0 | E980.4 |
| Demecolcine | 963.1 | E858.1 | E933.1 | E950.4 | E962.0 | E980.4 |
| Demelanizing agents | 976.8 | E858.7 | E946.8 | E950.4 | E962.0 | E980.4 |
| Demerol | 965.09 | E850.2 | E935.2 | E950.0 | E962.0 | E980.0 |
| Demethylchlortetracycline | 960.4 | E856 | E930.4 | E950.4 | E962.0 | E980.4 |
| Demethyltetracycline | 960.4 | E856 | E930.4 | E950.4 | E962.0 | E980.4 |
| Demeton | 989.3 | E863.1 | — | E950.6 | E962.1 | E980.7 |
| Demulcents | 976.3 | E858.7 | E946.3 | E950.4 | E962.0 | E980.4 |
| Demulen | 962.2 | E858.0 | E932.2 | E950.4 | E962.0 | E980.4 |
| Denatured alcohol | 980.0 | E860.1 | — | E950.9 | E962.1 | E980.9 |
| Dendrid | 976.5 | E858.7 | E946.5 | E950.4 | E962.0 | E980.4 |
| Dental agents, topical | 976.7 | E858.7 | E946.7 | E950.4 | E962.0 | E980.4 |
| Deodorant spray (feminine |  |  |  |  |  |  |
| hygiene) | 976.8 | E858.7 | E946.8 | E950.4 | E962.0 | E980.4 |
| Deoxyribonuclease | 963.4 | E858.1 | E933.4 | E950.4 | E962.0 | E980.4 |
| Depressants |  |  |  |  |  |  |
| appetite, central | 977.0 | E858.8 | E947.0 | E950.4 | E962.0 | E980.4 |
| cardiac | 972.0 | E858.3 | E942.0 | E950.4 | E962.0 | E980.4 |
| central nervous system |  |  |  |  |  |  |
| (anesthetic) | 968.4 | E855.1 | E938.4 | E950.4 | E962.0 | E980.4 |
| psychotherapeutic | 969.5 | E853.9 | E939.5 | E950.3 | E962.0 | E980.3 |
| Dequalinium | 976.0 | E858.7 | E946.0 | E950.4 | E962.0 | E980.4 |
| Dermolate | 976.2 | E858.7 | E946.2 | E950.4 | E962.0 | E980.4 |
| DES | 962.2 | E858.0 | E932.2 | E950.4 | E962.0 | E980.4 |
| Desenex | 976.0 | E858.7 | E946.0 | E950.4 | E962.0 | E980.4 |
| Deserpidine | 972.6 | E858.3 | E942.6 | E950.4 | E962.0 | E980.4 |
| Desipramine | 969.0 | E854.0 | E939.0 | E950.3 | E962.0 | E980.3 |
| Deslanoside | 972.1 | E858.3 | E942.1 | E950.4 | E962.0 | E980.4 |
| Desocodeine | 965.09 | E850.2 | E935.2 | E950.0 | E962.0 | E980.0 |
| Desomorphine | 965.09 | E850.2 | E935.2 | E950.0 | E962.0 | E980.0 |
| Desonide | 976.0 | E858.7 | E946.0 | E950.4 | E962.0 | E980.4 |
| Desoxycorticosterone |  |  |  |  |  |  |
| derivatives | 962.0 | E858.0 | E932.0 | E950.4 | E962.0 | E980.4 |
| Desoxyephedrine | 969.7 | E854.2 | E939.7 | E950.3 | E962.0 | E980.3 |
| DET | 969.6 | E854.1 | E939.6 | E950.3 | E962.0 | E980.3 |

---

☑ Additional Digit Required — Refer to the Tabular List for Digit Selection             ▽ Subterms under main terms may continue to next column or page

| | Poisoning | External Cause (E-Code) Accident | Therapeutic Use | Suicide Attempt | Assault | Undetermined |
|---|---|---|---|---|---|---|
| **Detergents** (ingested) | | | | | | |
| (synthetic) | 989.6 | E861.0 | — | E950.9 | E962.1 | E980.9 |
| ENT agent | 976.6 | E858.7 | E946.6 | E950.4 | E962.0 | E980.4 |
| external medication | 976.2 | E858.7 | E946.2 | E950.4 | E962.0 | E980.4 |
| ophthalmic preparation | 976.5 | E858.7 | E946.5 | E950.4 | E962.0 | E980.4 |
| topical NEC | 976.0 | E858.7 | E946.0 | E950.4 | E962.0 | E980.4 |
| **Deterrent, alcohol** | 977.3 | E858.8 | E947.3 | E950.4 | E962.0 | E980.4 |
| **Detrothyronine** | 962.7 | E858.0 | E932.7 | E950.4 | E962.0 | E980.4 |
| **Dettol** (external medication) | 976.0 | E858.7 | E946.0 | E950.4 | E962.0 | E980.4 |
| **Dexamethasone** | 962.0 | E858.0 | E932.0 | E950.4 | E962.0 | E980.4 |
| **Dexamphetamine** | 969.7 | E854.2 | E939.7 | E950.3 | E962.0 | E980.3 |
| **Dexedrine** | 969.7 | E854.2 | E939.7 | E950.3 | E962.0 | E980.3 |
| **Dexpanthenol** | 963.5 | E858.1 | E933.5 | E950.4 | E962.0 | E980.4 |
| **Dextran** | 964.8 | E858.2 | E934.8 | E950.4 | E962.0 | E980.4 |
| **Dextriferron** | 964.0 | E858.2 | E934.0 | E950.4 | E962.0 | E980.4 |
| **Dextroamphetamine** | 969.7 | E854.2 | E939.7 | E950.3 | E962.0 | E980.3 |
| **Dextro calcium** | | | | | | |
| pantothenate | 963.5 | E858.1 | E933.5 | E950.4 | E962.0 | E980.4 |
| **Dextromethorphan** | 975.4 | E858.6 | E945.4 | E950.4 | E962.0 | E980.4 |
| **Dextromoramide** | 965.09 | E850.2 | E935.2 | E950.0 | E962.0 | E980.0 |
| **Dextro pantothenyl** | | | | | | |
| alcohol | 963.5 | E858.1 | E933.5 | E950.4 | E962.0 | E980.4 |
| topical | 976.8 | E858.7 | E946.8 | E950.4 | E962.0 | E980.4 |
| **Dextropropoxyphene** | | | | | | |
| (hydrochloride) | 965.8 | E850.8 | E935.8 | E950.0 | E962.0 | E980.0 |
| **Dextrorphan** | 965.09 | E850.2 | E935.2 | E950.0 | E962.0 | E980.0 |
| **Dextrose NEC** | 974.5 | E858.5 | E944.5 | E950.4 | E962.0 | E980.4 |
| **Dextrothyroxin** | 962.7 | E858.0 | E932.7 | E950.4 | E962.0 | E980.4 |
| **DFP** | 971.0 | E855.3 | E941.0 | E950.4 | E962.0 | E980.4 |
| **DHE-45** | 972.9 | E858.3 | E942.9 | E950.4 | E962.0 | E980.4 |
| **Diabinese** | 962.3 | E858.0 | E932.3 | E950.4 | E962.0 | E980.4 |
| **Diacetyl monoxime** | 977.2 | E858.8 | E947.2 | E950.4 | E962.0 | E980.4 |
| **Diacetylmorphine** | 965.01 | E850.0 | E935.0 | E950.0 | E962.0 | E980.0 |
| **Diagnostic agents** | 977.8 | E858.8 | E947.8 | E950.4 | E962.0 | E980.4 |
| **Dial** (soap) | 976.2 | E858.7 | E946.2 | E950.4 | E962.0 | E980.4 |
| sedative | 967.0 | E851 | E937.0 | E950.1 | E962.0 | E980.1 |
| **Diallylbarbituric acid** | 967.0 | E851 | E937.0 | E950.1 | E962.0 | E980.1 |
| **Diaminodiphenylsulfone** | 961.8 | E857 | E931.8 | E950.4 | E962.0 | E980.4 |
| **Diamorphine** | 965.01 | E850.0 | E935.0 | E950.0 | E962.0 | E980.0 |
| **Diamox** | 974.2 | E858.5 | E944.2 | E950.4 | E962.0 | E980.4 |
| **Diamthazole** | 976.0 | E858.7 | E946.0 | E950.4 | E962.0 | E980.4 |
| **Diaphenylsulfone** | 961.8 | E857 | E931.8 | E950.4 | E962.0 | E980.4 |
| **Diasone** (sodium) | 961.8 | E857 | E931.8 | E950.4 | E962.0 | E980.4 |
| **Diazepam** | 969.4 | E853.2 | E939.4 | E950.3 | E962.0 | E980.3 |
| **Diazinon** | 989.3 | E863.1 | — | E950.6 | E962.1 | E980.7 |
| **Diazomethane** (gas) | 987.8 | E869.8 | — | E952.8 | E962.2 | E982.8 |
| **Diazoxide** | 972.5 | E858.3 | E942.5 | E950.4 | E962.0 | E980.4 |
| **Dibenamine** | 971.3 | E855.6 | E941.3 | E950.4 | E962.0 | E980.4 |
| **Dibenzheptropine** | 963.0 | E858.1 | E933.0 | E950.4 | E962.0 | E980.4 |
| **Dibenzyline** | 971.3 | E855.6 | E941.3 | E950.4 | E962.0 | E980.4 |
| **Diborane** (gas) | 987.8 | E869.8 | — | E952.8 | E962.2 | E982.8 |
| **Dibromomannitol** | 963.1 | E858.1 | E933.1 | E950.4 | E962.0 | E980.4 |
| **Dibucaine** (spinal) | 968.7 | E855.2 | E938.7 | E950.4 | E962.0 | E980.4 |
| topical (surface) | 968.5 | E855.2 | E938.5 | E950.4 | E962.0 | E980.4 |
| **Dibunate sodium** | 975.4 | E858.6 | E945.4 | E950.4 | E962.0 | E980.4 |
| **Dibutoline** | 971.1 | E855.4 | E941.1 | E950.4 | E962.0 | E980.4 |
| **Dicapthon** | 989.4 | E863.4 | — | E950.6 | E962.1 | E980.7 |
| **Dichloralphenazone** | 967.1 | E852.0 | E937.1 | E950.2 | E962.0 | E980.2 |
| **Dichlorodifluoromethane** | 987.4 | E869.2 | — | E952.8 | E962.2 | E982.8 |
| **Dichloroethane** | 982.3 | E862.4 | — | E950.9 | E962.1 | E980.9 |
| **Dichloroethylene** | 982.3 | E862.4 | — | E950.9 | E962.1 | E980.9 |
| **Dichloroethyl sulfide** | 987.8 | E869.8 | — | E952.8 | E962.2 | E982.8 |
| **Dichlorohydrin** | 982.3 | E862.4 | — | E950.9 | E962.1 | E980.9 |
| **Dichloromethane** (solvent) | | | | | | |
| (vapor) | 982.3 | E862.4 | — | E950.9 | E962.1 | E980.9 |
| **Dichlorophen(e)** | 961.6 | E857 | E931.6 | E950.4 | E962.0 | E980.4 |
| **Dichlorphenamide** | 974.2 | E858.5 | E944.2 | E950.4 | E962.0 | E980.4 |
| **Dichlorvos** | 989.3 | E863.1 | — | E950.6 | E962.1 | E980.7 |
| **Diclofenac sodium** | 965.69 | E850.6 | E935.6 | E950.0 | E962.0 | E980.0 |
| **Dicoumarin, dicumarol** | 964.2 | E858.2 | E934.2 | E950.4 | E962.0 | E980.4 |
| **Dicyanogen** (gas) | 987.8 | E869.8 | — | E952.8 | E962.2 | E982.8 |
| **Dicyclomine** | 971.1 | E855.4 | E941.1 | E950.4 | E962.0 | E980.4 |
| **Dieldrin** (vapor) | 989.2 | E863.0 | — | E950.6 | E962.1 | E980.7 |
| **Dienestrol** | 962.2 | E858.0 | E932.2 | E950.4 | E962.0 | E980.4 |
| **Dietetics** | 977.0 | E858.8 | E947.0 | E950.4 | E962.0 | E980.4 |
| **Diethazine** | 966.4 | E855.0 | E936.4 | E950.4 | E962.0 | E980.4 |
| **Diethyl** | | | | | | |
| barbituric acid | 967.0 | E851 | E937.0 | E950.1 | E962.0 | E980.1 |
| carbamazine | 961.6 | E857 | E931.6 | E950.4 | E962.0 | E980.4 |
| carbinol | 980.8 | E860.8 | — | E950.9 | E962.1 | E980.9 |
| carbonate | 982.8 | E862.4 | — | E950.9 | E962.1 | E980.9 |
| **Diethyl** — continued | | | | | | |
| dioxide | 982.8 | E862.4 | — | E950.9 | E962.1 | E980.9 |
| ether (vapor) — see ther(s) | | | | | | |
| glycol (monoacetate) (monoethyl ether) | 982.8 | E862.4 | — | E950.9 | E962.1 | E980.9 |
| propion | 977.0 | E858.8 | E947.0 | E950.4 | E962.0 | E980.4 |
| stilbestrol | 962.2 | E858.0 | E932.2 | E950.4 | E962.0 | E980.4 |
| **Diethylene** | | | | | | |
| **Diethylsulfone-diethylmethane** | 967.8 | E852.8 | E937.8 | E950.2 | E962.0 | E980.2 |
| **Difencloxazine** | 965.09 | E850.2 | E935.2 | E950.0 | E962.0 | E980.0 |
| **Diffusin** | 963.4 | E858.1 | E933.4 | E950.4 | E962.0 | E980.4 |
| **Diflos** | 971.0 | E855.3 | E941.0 | E950.4 | E962.0 | E980.4 |
| **Digestants** | 973.4 | E858.4 | E943.4 | E950.4 | E962.0 | E980.4 |
| **Digitalin(e)** | 972.1 | E858.3 | E942.1 | E950.4 | E962.0 | E980.4 |
| **Digitalis glycosides** | 972.1 | E858.3 | E942.1 | E950.4 | E962.0 | E980.4 |
| **Digitoxin** | 972.1 | E858.3 | E942.1 | E950.4 | E962.0 | E980.4 |
| **Digoxin** | 972.1 | E858.3 | E942.1 | E950.4 | E962.0 | E980.4 |
| **Dihydrocodeine** | 965.09 | E850.2 | E935.2 | E950.0 | E962.0 | E980.0 |
| **Dihydrocodeinone** | 965.09 | E850.2 | E935.2 | E950.0 | E962.0 | E980.0 |
| **Dihydroergocristine** | 972.9 | E858.3 | E942.9 | E950.4 | E962.0 | E980.4 |
| **Dihydroergotamine** | 972.9 | E858.3 | E942.9 | E950.4 | E962.0 | E980.4 |
| **Dihydroergotoxine** | 972.9 | E858.3 | E942.9 | E950.4 | E962.0 | E980.4 |
| **Dihydrohydroxycodeinone** | 965.09 | E850.2 | E935.2 | E950.0 | E962.0 | E980.0 |
| **Dihydrohydroxymorphinone** | 965.09 | E850.2 | E935.2 | E950.0 | E962.0 | E980.0 |
| **Dihydroisocodeine** | 965.09 | E850.2 | E935.2 | E950.0 | E962.0 | E980.0 |
| **Dihydromorphine** | 965.09 | E850.2 | E935.2 | E950.0 | E962.0 | E980.0 |
| **Dihydromorphinone** | 965.09 | E850.2 | E935.2 | E950.0 | E962.0 | E980.0 |
| **Dihydrostreptomycin** | 960.6 | E856 | E930.6 | E950.4 | E962.0 | E980.4 |
| **Dihydrotachysterol** | 962.6 | E858.0 | E932.6 | E950.4 | E962.0 | E980.4 |
| **Dihydroxyanthraquinone** | 973.1 | E858.4 | E943.1 | E950.4 | E962.0 | E980.4 |
| **Dihydroxycodeinone** | 965.09 | E850.2 | E935.2 | E950.0 | E962.0 | E980.0 |
| **Diiodohydroxyquin** | 961.3 | E857 | E931.3 | E950.4 | E962.0 | E980.4 |
| topical | 976.0 | E858.7 | E946.0 | E950.4 | E962.0 | E980.4 |
| **Diiodohydroxyquinoline** | 961.3 | E857 | E931.3 | E950.4 | E962.0 | E980.4 |
| **Dilantin** | 966.1 | E855.0 | E936.1 | E950.4 | E962.0 | E980.4 |
| **Dilaudid** | 965.09 | E850.2 | E935.2 | E950.0 | E962.0 | E980.0 |
| **Diloxanide** | 961.5 | E857 | E931.5 | E950.4 | E962.0 | E980.4 |
| **Dimefline** | 970.0 | E854.3 | E940.0 | E950.4 | E962.0 | E980.4 |
| **Dimenhydrinate** | 963.0 | E858.1 | E933.0 | E950.4 | E962.0 | E980.4 |
| **Dimercaprol** | 963.8 | E858.1 | E933.8 | E950.4 | E962.0 | E980.4 |
| **Dimercaptopropanol** | 963.8 | E858.1 | E933.8 | E950.4 | E962.0 | E980.4 |
| **Dimetane** | 963.0 | E858.1 | E933.0 | E950.4 | E962.0 | E980.4 |
| **Dimethicone** | 976.3 | E858.7 | E946.3 | E950.4 | E962.0 | E980.4 |
| **Dimethindene** | 963.0 | E858.1 | E933.0 | E950.4 | E962.0 | E980.4 |
| **Dimethisoquin** | 968.5 | E855.2 | E938.5 | E950.4 | E962.0 | E980.4 |
| **Dimethisterone** | 962.2 | E858.0 | E932.2 | E950.4 | E962.0 | E980.4 |
| **Dimethoxanate** | 975.4 | E858.6 | E945.4 | E950.4 | E962.0 | E980.4 |
| **Dimethyl** | | | | | | |
| arsine, arsinic acid — see Arsenic | | | | | | |
| carbinol | 980.2 | E860.3 | — | E950.9 | E962.1 | E980.9 |
| diguanide | 962.3 | E858.0 | E932.3 | E950.4 | E962.0 | E980.4 |
| ketone | 982.8 | E862.4 | — | E950.9 | E962.1 | E980.9 |
| vapor | 987.8 | E869.8 | — | E952.8 | E962.2 | E982.8 |
| meperidine | 965.09 | E850.2 | E935.2 | E950.0 | E962.0 | E980.0 |
| parathion | 989.3 | E863.1 | — | E950.6 | E962.1 | E980.7 |
| polysiloxane | 973.8 | E858.4 | E943.8 | E950.4 | E962.0 | E980.4 |
| sulfate (fumes) | 987.8 | E869.8 | — | E952.8 | E962.2 | E982.8 |
| liquid | 983.9 | E864.3 | — | E950.7 | E962.1 | E980.6 |
| sulfoxide NEC | 982.8 | E862.4 | — | E950.9 | E962.1 | E980.9 |
| medicinal | 976.4 | E858.7 | E946.4 | E950.4 | E962.0 | E980.4 |
| triptamine | 969.6 | E854.1 | E939.6 | E950.3 | E962.0 | E980.3 |
| tubocurarine | 975.2 | E858.6 | E945.2 | E950.4 | E962.0 | E980.4 |
| **Dindevan** | 964.2 | E858.2 | E934.2 | E950.4 | E962.0 | E980.4 |
| **Dinitrobenzene** | 983.0 | E864.0 | — | E950.7 | E962.1 | E980.6 |
| vapor | 987.8 | E869.8 | — | E952.8 | E962.2 | E982.8 |
| **Dinitro (-ortho-) cresol** | | | | | | |
| (herbicide) (spray) | 989.4 | E863.5 | — | E950.6 | E962.1 | E980.7 |
| insecticide | 989.4 | E863.4 | — | E950.6 | E962.1 | E980.7 |
| **Dinitro-orthocresol** | | | | | | |
| (herbicide) | 989.4 | E863.5 | — | E950.6 | E962.1 | E980.7 |
| insecticide | 989.4 | E863.4 | — | E950.6 | E962.1 | E980.7 |
| **Dinitrophenol** (herbicide) | | | | | | |
| (spray) | 989.4 | E863.5 | — | E950.6 | E962.1 | E980.7 |
| insecticide | 989.4 | E863.4 | — | E950.6 | E962.1 | E980.7 |
| **Dinoprost** | 975.0 | E858.6 | E945.0 | E950.4 | E962.0 | E980.4 |
| **Dioctyl sulfosuccinate** (calcium) | | | | | | |
| (sodium) | 973.2 | E858.4 | E943.2 | E950.4 | E962.0 | E980.4 |
| **Diodoquin** | 961.3 | E857 | E931.3 | E950.4 | E962.0 | E980.4 |
| **Dione derivatives NEC** | 966.3 | E855.0 | E936.3 | E950.4 | E962.0 | E980.4 |
| **Dionin** | 965.09 | E850.2 | E935.2 | E950.0 | E962.0 | E980.0 |

✓ Additional Digit Required — Refer to the Tabular List for Digit Selection

Subterms under main terms may continue to next column or page

| | Poisoning | Accident | Therapeutic Use | Suicide Attempt | Assault | Undetermined |
|---|---|---|---|---|---|---|
| **Dioxane** | 982.8 | E862.4 | — | E950.9 | E962.1 | E980.9 |
| **Dioxin** — *see* Herbicide | | | | | | |
| **Dioxyline** | 972.5 | E858.3 | E942.5 | E950.4 | E962.0 | E980.4 |
| **Dipentene** | 982.8 | E862.4 | — | E950.9 | E962.1 | E980.9 |
| **Diphemanil** | 971.1 | E855.4 | E941.1 | E950.4 | E962.0 | E980.4 |
| **Diphenadione** | 964.2 | E858.2 | E934.2 | E950.4 | E962.0 | E980.4 |
| **Diphenhydramine** | 963.0 | E858.1 | E933.0 | E950.4 | E962.0 | E980.4 |
| **Diphenidol** | 963.0 | E858.1 | E933.0 | E950.4 | E962.0 | E980.4 |
| **Diphenoxylate** | 973.5 | E858.4 | E943.5 | E950.4 | E962.0 | E980.4 |
| **Diphenylchloroarsine** | 985.1 | E866.3 | — | E950.8 | E962.1 | E980.8 |
| **Diphenylhydantoin** | | | | | | |
| (sodium) | 966.1 | E855.0 | E936.1 | E950.4 | E962.0 | E980.4 |
| **Diphenylpyraline** | 963.0 | E858.1 | E933.0 | E950.4 | E962.0 | E980.4 |
| **Diphtheria** | | | | | | |
| antitoxin | 979.9 | E858.8 | E949.9 | E950.4 | E962.0 | E980.4 |
| toxoid | 978.5 | E858.8 | E948.5 | E950.4 | E962.0 | E980.4 |
| with tetanus toxoid | 978.9 | E858.8 | E948.9 | E950.4 | E962.0 | E980.4 |
| with pertussis component | 978.6 | E858.8 | E948.6 | E950.4 | E962.0 | E980.4 |
| vaccine | 978.5 | E858.8 | E948.5 | E950.4 | E962.0 | E980.4 |
| **Dipipanone** | 965.09 | E850.2 | E935.2 | E950.0 | E962.0 | E980.0 |
| **Diplovax** | 979.5 | E858.8 | E949.5 | E950.4 | E962.0 | E980.4 |
| **Diprophylline** | 975.1 | E858.6 | E945.1 | E950.4 | E962.0 | E980.4 |
| **Dipyridamole** | 972.4 | E858.3 | E942.4 | E950.4 | E962.0 | E980.4 |
| **Dipyrone** | 965.5 | E850.5 | E935.5 | E950.0 | E962.0 | E980.0 |
| **Diquat** | 989.4 | E863.5 | — | E950.6 | E962.1 | E980.7 |
| **Disinfectant NEC** | 983.9 | E861.4 | — | E950.7 | E962.1 | E980.6 |
| alkaline | 983.2 | E861.4 | — | E950.7 | E962.1 | E980.6 |
| aromatic | 983.0 | E861.4 | — | E950.7 | E962.1 | E980.6 |
| **Disipal** | 966.4 | E855.0 | E936.4 | E950.4 | E962.0 | E980.4 |
| **Disodium edetate** | 963.8 | E858.1 | E933.8 | E950.4 | E962.0 | E980.4 |
| **Disulfamide** | 974.4 | E858.5 | E944.4 | E950.4 | E962.0 | E980.4 |
| **Disulfanilamide** | 961.0 | E857 | E931.0 | E950.4 | E962.0 | E980.4 |
| **Disulfiram** | 977.3 | E858.8 | E947.3 | E950.4 | E962.0 | E980.4 |
| **Dithiazanine** | 961.6 | E857 | E931.6 | E950.4 | E962.0 | E980.4 |
| **Dithioglycerol** | 963.8 | E858.1 | E933.8 | E950.4 | E962.0 | E980.4 |
| **Dithranol** | 976.4 | E858.7 | E946.4 | E950.4 | E962.0 | E980.4 |
| **Diucardin** | 974.3 | E858.5 | E944.3 | E950.4 | E962.0 | E980.4 |
| **Diupres** | 974.3 | E858.5 | E944.3 | E950.4 | E962.0 | E980.4 |
| **Diuretics NEC** | 974.4 | E858.5 | E944.4 | E950.4 | E962.0 | E980.4 |
| carbonic acid anhydrase inhibitors | 974.2 | E858.5 | E944.2 | E950.4 | E962.0 | E980.4 |
| mercurial | 974.0 | E858.5 | E944.0 | E950.4 | E962.0 | E980.4 |
| osmotic | 974.4 | E858.5 | E944.4 | E950.4 | E962.0 | E980.4 |
| purine derivatives | 974.1 | E858.5 | E944.1 | E950.4 | E962.0 | E980.4 |
| saluretic | 974.3 | E858.5 | E944.3 | E950.4 | E962.0 | E980.4 |
| **Diuril** | 974.3 | E858.5 | E944.3 | E950.4 | E962.0 | E980.4 |
| **Divinyl ether** | 968.2 | E855.1 | E938.2 | E950.4 | E962.0 | E980.4 |
| **D-lysergic acid diethylamide** | 969.6 | E854.1 | E939.6 | E950.3 | E962.0 | E980.3 |
| **DMCT** | 960.4 | E856 | E930.4 | E950.4 | E962.0 | E980.4 |
| **DMSO** | 982.8 | E862.4 | — | E950.9 | E962.1 | E980.9 |
| **DMT** | 969.6 | E854.1 | E939.6 | E950.3 | E962.0 | E980.3 |
| **DNOC** | 989.4 | E863.5 | — | E950.6 | E962.1 | E980.7 |
| **DOCA** | 962.0 | E858.0 | E932.0 | E950.4 | E962.0 | E980.4 |
| **Dolophine** | 965.02 | E850.1 | E935.1 | E950.0 | E962.0 | E980.0 |
| **Doloxene** | 965.8 | E850.8 | E935.8 | E950.0 | E962.0 | E980.0 |
| **DOM** | 969.6 | E854.1 | E939.6 | E950.3 | E962.0 | E980.3 |
| **Domestic gas** — *see* Gas, utility | | | | | | |
| **Domiphen** (bromide) (lozenges) | 976.6 | E858.7 | E946.6 | E950.4 | E962.0 | E980.4 |
| **Dopa** (levo) | 966.4 | E855.0 | E936.4 | E950.4 | E962.0 | E980.4 |
| **Dopamine** | 971.2 | E855.5 | E941.2 | E950.4 | E962.0 | E980.4 |
| **Doriden** | 967.5 | E852.4 | E937.5 | E950.2 | E962.0 | E980.2 |
| **Dormiral** | 967.0 | E851 | E937.0 | E950.1 | E962.0 | E980.1 |
| **Dormison** | 967.8 | E852.8 | E937.8 | E950.2 | E962.0 | E980.2 |
| **Dornase** | 963.4 | E858.1 | E933.4 | E950.4 | E962.0 | E980.4 |
| **Dorsacaine** | 968.5 | E855.2 | E938.5 | E950.4 | E962.0 | E980.4 |
| **Dothiepin hydrochloride** | 969.0 | E854.0 | E939.0 | E950.3 | E962.0 | E980.3 |
| **Doxapram** | 970.0 | E854.3 | E940.0 | E950.4 | E962.0 | E980.4 |
| **Doxepin** | 969.0 | E854.0 | E939.0 | E950.3 | E962.0 | E980.3 |
| **Doxorubicin** | 960.7 | E856 | E930.7 | E950.4 | E962.0 | E980.4 |
| **Doxycycline** | 960.4 | E856 | E930.4 | E950.4 | E962.0 | E980.4 |
| **Doxylamine** | 963.0 | E858.1 | E933.0 | E950.4 | E962.0 | E980.4 |
| **Dramamine** | 963.0 | E858.1 | E933.0 | E950.4 | E962.0 | E980.4 |
| **Drano** (drain cleaner) | 983.2 | E864.2 | — | E950.7 | E962.1 | E980.6 |
| **Dromoran** | 965.09 | E850.2 | E935.2 | E950.0 | E962.0 | E980.0 |
| **Dromostanolone** | 962.1 | E858.0 | E932.1 | E950.4 | E962.0 | E980.4 |
| **Droperidol** | 969.2 | E853.1 | E939.2 | E950.3 | E962.0 | E980.3 |
| **Drotrecogin alfa** | 964.2 | E858.2 | E934.2 | E950.4 | E962.0 | E980.4 |
| **Drug** | 977.9 | E858.9 | E947.9 | E950.5 | E962.0 | E980.5 |

| | Poisoning | Accident | Therapeutic Use | Suicide Attempt | Assault | Undetermined |
|---|---|---|---|---|---|---|
| **Drug** — *continued* | | | | | | |
| AHFS List | | | | | | |
| 4:00 antihistamine drugs | 963.0 | E858.1 | E933.0 | E950.4 | E962.0 | E980.4 |
| 8:04 amebacides | 961.5 | E857 | E931.5 | E950.4 | E962.0 | E980.4 |
| arsenical anti-infectives | 961.1 | E857 | E931.1 | E950.4 | E962.0 | E980.4 |
| quinoline derivatives | 961.3 | E857 | E931.3 | E950.4 | E962.0 | E980.4 |
| 8:08 anthelmintics | 961.6 | E857 | E931.6 | E950.4 | E962.0 | E980.4 |
| quinoline derivatives | 961.3 | E857 | E931.3 | E950.4 | E962.0 | E980.4 |
| 8:12.04 antifungal antibiotics | 960.1 | E856 | E930.1 | E950.4 | E962.0 | E980.4 |
| 8:12.06 cephalosporins | 960.5 | E856 | E930.5 | E950.4 | E962.0 | E980.4 |
| 8:12.08 chloramphenicol | 960.2 | E856 | E930.2 | E950.4 | E962.0 | E980.4 |
| 8:12.12 erythromycins | 960.3 | E856 | E930.3 | E950.4 | E962.0 | E980.4 |
| 8:12.16 penicillins | 960.0 | E856 | E930.0 | E950.4 | E962.0 | E980.4 |
| 8:12.20 streptomycins | 960.6 | E856 | E930.6 | E950.4 | E962.0 | E980.4 |
| 8:12.24 tetracyclines | 960.4 | E856 | E930.4 | E950.4 | E962.0 | E980.4 |
| 8:12.28 other antibiotics | 960.8 | E856 | E930.8 | E950.4 | E962.0 | E980.4 |
| antimycobacterial | 960.6 | E856 | E930.6 | E950.4 | E962.0 | E980.4 |
| macrolides | 960.3 | E856 | E930.3 | E950.4 | E962.0 | E980.4 |
| 8:16 antituberculars | 961.8 | E857 | E931.8 | E950.4 | E962.0 | E980.4 |
| antibiotics | 960.6 | E856 | E930.6 | E950.4 | E962.0 | E980.4 |
| 8:18 antivirals | 961.7 | E857 | E931.7 | E950.4 | E962.0 | E980.4 |
| 8:20 plasmodicides (antimalarials) | 961.4 | E857 | E931.4 | E950.4 | E962.0 | E980.4 |
| 8:24 sulfonamides | 961.0 | E857 | E931.0 | E950.4 | E962.0 | E980.4 |
| 8:26 sulfones | 961.8 | E857 | E931.8 | E950.4 | E962.0 | E980.4 |
| 8:28 treponemicides | 961.2 | E857 | E931.2 | E950.4 | E962.0 | E980.4 |
| 8:32 trichomonacides | 961.5 | E857 | E931.5 | E950.4 | E962.0 | E980.4 |
| nitrofuran derivatives | 961.9 | E857 | E931.9 | E950.4 | E962.0 | E980.4 |
| quinoline derivatives | 961.3 | E857 | E931.3 | E950.4 | E962.0 | E980.4 |
| 8:36 urinary germicides | 961.9 | E857 | E931.9 | E950.4 | E962.0 | E980.4 |
| quinoline derivatives | 961.3 | E857 | E931.3 | E950.4 | E962.0 | E980.4 |
| 8:40 other anti-infectives | 961.9 | E857 | E931.9 | E950.4 | E962.0 | E980.4 |
| 10:00 antineoplastic agents | 963.1 | E858.1 | E933.1 | E950.4 | E962.0 | E980.4 |
| antibiotics | 960.7 | E856 | E930.7 | E950.4 | E962.0 | E980.4 |
| progestogens | 962.2 | E858.0 | E932.2 | E950.4 | E962.0 | E980.4 |
| 12:04 parasympathomimetic (cholinergic) agents | 971.0 | E855.3 | E941.0 | E950.4 | E962.0 | E980.4 |
| 12:08 parasympatholytic (cholinergic-blocking) agents | 971.1 | E855.4 | E941.1 | E950.4 | E962.0 | E980.4 |
| 12:12 Sympathomimetic (adrenergic) agents | 971.2 | E855.5 | E941.2 | E950.4 | E962.0 | E980.4 |
| 12:16 sympatholytic (adrenergic-blocking) agents | 971.3 | E855.6 | E941.3 | E950.4 | E962.0 | E980.4 |
| 12:20 skeletal muscle relaxants central nervous system muscle-tone depressants | 968.0 | E855.1 | E938.0 | E950.4 | E962.0 | E980.4 |
| myoneural blocking agents | 975.2 | E858.6 | E945.2 | E950.4 | E962.0 | E980.4 |
| 16:00 blood derivatives | 964.7 | E858.2 | E934.7 | E950.4 | E962.0 | E980.4 |
| 20:04.04 iron preparations | 964.0 | E858.2 | E934.0 | E950.4 | E962.0 | E980.4 |
| 20:04.08 liver and stomach preparations | 964.1 | E858.2 | E934.1 | E950.4 | E962.0 | E980.4 |
| 20:04 antianemia drugs | 964.1 | E858.2 | E934.1 | E950.4 | E962.0 | E980.4 |
| 20:12.04 anticoagulants | 964.2 | E858.2 | E934.2 | E950.4 | E962.0 | E980.4 |
| 20:12.08 antiheparin agents | 964.5 | E858.2 | E934.5 | E950.4 | E962.0 | E980.4 |
| 20:12.12 coagulants | 964.5 | E858.2 | E934.5 | E950.4 | E962.0 | E980.4 |
| 20:12.16 hemostatics NEC | 964.5 | E858.2 | E934.5 | E950.4 | E962.0 | E980.4 |
| capillary active drugs | 972.8 | E858.3 | E942.8 | E950.4 | E962.0 | E980.4 |
| 24:04 cardiac drugs | 972.9 | E858.3 | E942.9 | E950.4 | E962.0 | E980.4 |
| cardiotonic agents | 972.1 | E858.3 | E942.1 | E950.4 | E962.0 | E980.4 |
| rhythm regulators | 972.0 | E858.3 | E942.0 | E950.4 | E962.0 | E980.4 |
| 24:06 antilipemic agents | 972.2 | E858.3 | E942.2 | E950.4 | E962.0 | E980.4 |
| thyroid derivatives | 962.7 | E858.0 | E932.7 | E950.4 | E962.0 | E980.4 |
| 24:08 hypotensive agents | 972.6 | E858.3 | E942.6 | E950.4 | E962.0 | E980.4 |
| adrenergic blocking agents | 971.3 | E855.6 | E941.3 | E950.4 | E962.0 | E980.4 |
| ganglion blocking agents | 972.3 | E858.3 | E942.3 | E950.4 | E962.0 | E980.4 |
| vasodilators | 972.5 | E858.3 | E942.5 | E950.4 | E962.0 | E980.4 |
| 24:12 vasodilating agents NEC | 972.5 | E858.3 | E942.5 | E950.4 | E962.0 | E980.4 |
| coronary | 972.4 | E858.3 | E942.4 | E950.4 | E962.0 | E980.4 |
| nicotinic acid derivatives | 972.2 | E858.3 | E942.2 | E950.4 | E962.0 | E980.4 |
| 24:16 sclerosing agents | 972.7 | E858.3 | E942.7 | E950.4 | E962.0 | E980.4 |
| 28:04 general anesthetics | 968.4 | E855.1 | E938.4 | E950.4 | E962.0 | E980.4 |
| gaseous anesthetics | 968.2 | E855.1 | E938.2 | E950.4 | E962.0 | E980.4 |
| halothane | 968.1 | E855.1 | E938.1 | E950.4 | E962.0 | E980.4 |

☑ Additional Digit Required — Refer to the Tabular List for Digit Selection

    ▶◀ Revised Text     ● New Line     ▲ Revised Code     ☜ Subterms under main terms may continue to next column or page    

| Drug — continued | Poisoning | Accident | Therapeutic Use | Suicide Attempt | Assault | Undetermined |
|---|---|---|---|---|---|---|
| 28:04 general anesthetics — continued | | | | | | |
|   intravenous anesthetics | 968.3 | E855.1 | E938.3 | E950.4 | E962.0 | E980.4 |
| 28:08 analgesics and antipyretics | 965.9 | E850.9 | E935.9 | E950.0 | E962.0 | E980.0 |
|   antirheumatics | 965.69 | E850.6 | E935.6 | E950.0 | E962.0 | E980.0 |
|   aromatic analgesics | 965.4 | E850.4 | E935.4 | E950.0 | E962.0 | E980.0 |
|   non-narcotic NEC | 965.7 | E850.7 | E935.7 | E950.0 | E962.0 | E980.0 |
|   opium alkaloids | 965.00 | E850.2 | E935.2 | E950.0 | E962.0 | E980.0 |
|     heroin | 965.01 | E850.0 | E935.0 | E950.0 | E962.0 | E980.0 |
|     methadone | 965.02 | E850.1 | E935.1 | E950.0 | E962.0 | E980.0 |
|     specified type NEC | 965.09 | E850.2 | E935.2 | E950.0 | E962.0 | E980.0 |
|   pyrazole derivatives | 965.5 | E850.5 | E935.5 | E950.0 | E962.0 | E980.0 |
|   salicylates | 965.1 | E850.3 | E935.3 | E950.0 | E962.0 | E980.0 |
|   specified NEC | 965.8 | E850.8 | E935.8 | E950.0 | E962.0 | E980.0 |
| 28:10 narcotic antagonists | 970.1 | E854.3 | E940.1 | E950.4 | E962.0 | E980.4 |
| 28:12 anticonvulsants | 966.3 | E855.0 | E936.3 | E950.4 | E962.0 | E980.4 |
|   barbiturates | 967.0 | E851 | E937.0 | E950.1 | E962.0 | E980.1 |
|   benzodiazepine-based tranquilizers | 969.4 | E853.2 | E939.4 | E950.3 | E962.0 | E980.3 |
|   bromides | 967.3 | E852.2 | E937.3 | E950.2 | E962.0 | E980.2 |
|   hydantoin derivatives | 966.1 | E855.0 | E936.1 | E950.4 | E962.0 | E980.4 |
|   oxazolidine (derivatives) | 966.0 | E855.0 | E936.0 | E950.4 | E962.0 | E980.4 |
|   succinimides | 966.2 | E855.0 | E936.2 | E950.4 | E962.0 | E980.4 |
| 28:16.04 antidepressants | 969.0 | E854.0 | E939.0 | E950.3 | E962.0 | E980.3 |
| 28:16.08 tranquilizers | 969.5 | E853.9 | E939.5 | E950.3 | E962.0 | E980.3 |
|   benzodiazepine-based | 969.4 | E853.2 | E939.4 | E950.3 | E962.0 | E980.3 |
|   butyrophenone-based | 969.2 | E853.1 | E939.2 | E950.3 | E962.0 | E980.3 |
|   major NEC | 969.3 | E853.8 | E939.3 | E950.3 | E962.0 | E980.3 |
|   phenothiazine-based | 969.1 | E853.0 | E939.1 | E950.3 | E962.0 | E980.3 |
| 28:16.12 other psychotherapeutic agents | 969.8 | E855.8 | E939.8 | E950.3 | E962.0 | E980.3 |
| 28:20 respiratory and cerebral stimulants | 970.9 | E854.3 | E940.9 | E950.4 | E962.0 | E980.4 |
|   analeptics | 970.0 | E854.3 | E940.0 | E950.4 | E962.0 | E980.4 |
|   anorexigenic agents | 977.0 | E858.8 | E947.0 | E950.4 | E962.0 | E980.4 |
|   psychostimulants | 969.7 | E854.2 | E939.7 | E950.3 | E962.0 | E980.3 |
|   specified NEC | 970.8 | E854.3 | E940.8 | E950.4 | E962.0 | E980.4 |
| 28:24 sedatives and hypnotics | 967.9 | E852.9 | E937.9 | E950.2 | E962.0 | E980.2 |
|   barbiturates | 967.0 | E851 | E937.0 | E950.1 | E962.0 | E980.1 |
|   benzodiazepine-based tranquilizers | 969.4 | E853.2 | E939.4 | E950.3 | E962.0 | E980.3 |
|   chloral hydrate (group) | 967.1 | E852.0 | E937.1 | E950.2 | E962.0 | E980.2 |
|   glutethamide group | 967.5 | E852.4 | E937.5 | E950.2 | E962.0 | E980.2 |
|   intravenous anesthetics | 968.3 | E855.1 | E938.3 | E950.4 | E962.0 | E980.4 |
|   methaqualone (compounds) | 967.4 | E852.3 | E937.4 | E950.2 | E962.0 | E980.2 |
|   paraldehyde | 967.2 | E852.1 | E937.2 | E950.2 | E962.0 | E980.2 |
|   phenothiazine-based tranquilizers | 969.1 | E853.0 | E939.1 | E950.3 | E962.0 | E980.3 |
|   specified NEC | 967.8 | E852.8 | E937.8 | E950.2 | E962.0 | E980.2 |
|   thiobarbiturates | 968.3 | E855.1 | E938.3 | E950.4 | E962.0 | E980.4 |
|   tranquilizer NEC | 969.5 | E853.9 | E939.5 | E950.3 | E962.0 | E980.3 |
| 36:04 to 36:88 diagnostic agents | 977.8 | E858.8 | E947.8 | E950.4 | E962.0 | E980.4 |
| 40:00 electrolyte, caloric, and water balance agents NEC | 974.5 | E858.5 | E944.5 | E950.4 | E962.0 | E980.4 |
| 40:04 acidifying agents | 963.2 | E858.1 | E933.2 | E950.4 | E962.0 | E980.4 |
| 40:08 alkalinizing agents | 963.3 | E858.1 | E933.3 | E950.4 | E962.0 | E980.4 |
| 40:10 ammonia detoxicants | 974.5 | E858.5 | E944.5 | E950.4 | E962.0 | E980.4 |
| 40:12 replacement solutions | 974.5 | E858.5 | E944.5 | E950.4 | E962.0 | E980.4 |
|   plasma expanders | 964.8 | E858.2 | E934.8 | E950.4 | E962.0 | E980.4 |
| 40:16 sodium-removing resins | 974.5 | E858.5 | E944.5 | E950.4 | E962.0 | E980.4 |
| 40:18 potassium-removing resins | 974.5 | E858.5 | E944.5 | E950.4 | E962.0 | E980.4 |
| 40:20 caloric agents | 974.5 | E858.5 | E944.5 | E950.4 | E962.0 | E980.4 |
| 40:24 salt and sugar substitutes | 974.5 | E858.5 | E944.5 | E950.4 | E962.0 | E980.4 |
| 40:28 diuretics NEC | 974.4 | E858.5 | E944.4 | E950.4 | E962.0 | E980.4 |
|   carbonic acid anhydrase inhibitors | 974.2 | E858.5 | E944.2 | E950.4 | E962.0 | E980.4 |
|   mercurials | 974.0 | E858.5 | E944.0 | E950.4 | E962.0 | E980.4 |
|   purine derivatives | 974.1 | E858.5 | E944.1 | E950.4 | E962.0 | E980.4 |
|   saluretics | 974.3 | E858.5 | E944.3 | E950.4 | E962.0 | E980.4 |
|   thiazides | 974.3 | E858.5 | E944.3 | E950.4 | E962.0 | E980.4 |
| 40:36 irrigating solutions | 974.5 | E858.5 | E944.5 | E950.4 | E962.0 | E980.4 |

| Drug — continued | Poisoning | Accident | Therapeutic Use | Suicide Attempt | Assault | Undetermined |
|---|---|---|---|---|---|---|
| 40:40 uricosuric agents | 974.7 | E858.5 | E944.7 | E950.4 | E962.0 | E980.4 |
| 44:00 enzymes | 963.4 | E858.1 | E933.4 | E950.4 | E962.0 | E980.4 |
|   fibrinolysis-affecting agents | 964.4 | E858.2 | E934.4 | E950.4 | E962.0 | E980.4 |
|   gastric agents | 973.4 | E858.4 | E943.4 | E950.4 | E962.0 | E980.4 |
| 48:00 expectorants and cough preparations | | | | | | |
|   antihistamine agents | 963.0 | E858.1 | E933.0 | E950.4 | E962.0 | E980.4 |
|   antitussives | 975.4 | E858.6 | E945.4 | E950.4 | E962.0 | E980.4 |
|   codeine derivatives | 965.09 | E850.2 | E935.2 | E950.0 | E962.0 | E980.0 |
|   expectorants | 975.5 | E858.6 | E945.5 | E950.4 | E962.0 | E980.4 |
|   narcotic agents NEC | 965.09 | E850.2 | E935.2 | E950.0 | E962.0 | E980.0 |
| 52:04.04 antibiotics (EENT) | | | | | | |
|   ENT agent | 976.6 | E858.7 | E946.6 | E950.4 | E962.0 | E980.4 |
|   ophthalmic preparation | 976.5 | E858.7 | E946.5 | E950.4 | E962.0 | E980.4 |
| 52:04.06 antivirals (EENT) | | | | | | |
|   ENT agent | 976.6 | E858.7 | E946.6 | E950.4 | E962.0 | E980.4 |
|   ophthalmic preparation | 976.5 | E858.7 | E946.5 | E950.4 | E962.0 | E980.4 |
| 52:04.08 sulfonamides (EENT) | | | | | | |
|   ENT agent | 976.6 | E858.7 | E946.6 | E950.4 | E962.0 | E980.4 |
|   ophthalmic preparation | 976.5 | E858.7 | E946.5 | E950.4 | E962.0 | E980.4 |
| 52:04.12 miscellaneous anti-infectives (EENT) | | | | | | |
|   ENT agent | 976.6 | E858.7 | E946.6 | E950.4 | E962.0 | E980.4 |
|   ophthalmic preparation | 976.5 | E858.7 | E946.5 | E950.4 | E962.0 | E980.4 |
| 52:04 anti-infectives (EENT) | | | | | | |
|   ENT agent | 976.6 | E858.7 | E946.6 | E950.4 | E962.0 | E980.4 |
|   ophthalmic preparation | 976.5 | E858.7 | E946.5 | E950.4 | E962.0 | E980.4 |
| 52:08 anti-inflammatory agents (EENT) | | | | | | |
|   ENT agent | 976.6 | E858.7 | E946.6 | E950.4 | E962.0 | E980.4 |
|   ophthalmic preparation | 976.5 | E858.7 | E946.5 | E950.4 | E962.0 | E980.4 |
| 52:10 carbonic anhydrase inhibitors | 974.2 | E858.5 | E944.2 | E950.4 | E962.0 | E980.4 |
| 52:12 contact lens solutions | 976.5 | E858.7 | E946.5 | E950.4 | E962.0 | E980.4 |
| 52:16 local anesthetics (EENT) | 968.5 | E855.2 | E938.5 | E950.4 | E962.0 | E980.4 |
| 52:20 miotics | 971.0 | E855.3 | E941.0 | E950.4 | E962.0 | E980.4 |
| 52:24 mydriatics | | | | | | |
|   adrenergics | 971.2 | E855.5 | E941.2 | E950.4 | E962.0 | E980.4 |
|   anticholinergics | 971.1 | E855.4 | E941.1 | E950.4 | E962.0 | E980.4 |
|   antimuscarinics | 971.1 | E855.4 | E941.1 | E950.4 | E962.0 | E980.4 |
|   parasympatholytics | 971.1 | E855.4 | E941.1 | E950.4 | E962.0 | E980.4 |
|   spasmolytics | 971.1 | E855.4 | E941.1 | E950.4 | E962.0 | E980.4 |
|   sympathomimetics | 971.2 | E855.5 | E941.2 | E950.4 | E962.0 | E980.4 |
| 52:28 mouth washes and gargles | 976.6 | E858.7 | E946.6 | E950.4 | E962.0 | E980.4 |
| 52:32 vasoconstrictors (EENT) | 971.2 | E855.5 | E941.2 | E950.4 | E962.0 | E980.4 |
| 52:36 unclassified agents (EENT) | | | | | | |
|   ENT agent | 976.6 | E858.7 | E946.6 | E950.4 | E962.0 | E980.4 |
|   ophthalmic preparation | 976.5 | E858.7 | E946.5 | E950.4 | E962.0 | E980.4 |
| 56:04 antacids and adsorbents | 973.0 | E858.4 | E943.0 | E950.4 | E962.0 | E980.4 |
| 56:08 antidiarrhea agents | 973.5 | E858.4 | E943.5 | E950.4 | E962.0 | E980.4 |
| 56:10 antiflatulents | 973.8 | E858.4 | E943.8 | E950.4 | E962.0 | E980.4 |
| 56:12 cathartics NEC | 973.3 | E858.4 | E943.3 | E950.4 | E962.0 | E980.4 |
|   emollients | 973.2 | E858.4 | E943.2 | E950.4 | E962.0 | E980.4 |
|   irritants | 973.1 | E858.4 | E943.1 | E950.4 | E962.0 | E980.4 |
| 56:16 digestants | 973.4 | E858.4 | E943.4 | E950.4 | E962.0 | E980.4 |
| 56:20 emetics and antiemetics | | | | | | |
|   antiemetics | 963.0 | E858.1 | E933.0 | E950.4 | E962.0 | E980.4 |
|   emetics | 973.6 | E858.4 | E943.6 | E950.4 | E962.0 | E980.4 |
| 56:24 lipotropic agents | 977.1 | E858.8 | E947.1 | E950.4 | E962.0 | E980.4 |
| 56:40 miscellaneous G.I. drugs | 973.8 | E858.4 | E943.8 | E950.4 | E962.0 | E980.4 |
| 60:00 gold compounds | 965.69 | E850.6 | E935.6 | E950.0 | E962.0 | E980.0 |
| 64:00 heavy metal antagonists | 963.8 | E858.1 | E933.8 | E950.4 | E962.0 | E980.4 |
| 68:04 adrenals | 962.0 | E858.0 | E932.0 | E950.4 | E962.0 | E980.4 |
| 68:08 androgens | 962.1 | E858.0 | E932.1 | E950.4 | E962.0 | E980.4 |
| 68:12 contraceptives, oral | 962.2 | E858.0 | E932.2 | E950.4 | E962.0 | E980.4 |
| 68:16 estrogens | 962.2 | E858.0 | E932.2 | E950.4 | E962.0 | E980.4 |
| 68:18 gonadotropins | 962.4 | E858.0 | E932.4 | E950.4 | E962.0 | E980.4 |
| 68:20.08 insulins | 962.3 | E858.0 | E932.3 | E950.4 | E962.0 | E980.4 |
| 68:20 insulins and antidiabetic agents | 962.3 | E858.0 | E932.3 | E950.4 | E962.0 | E980.4 |
| 68:24 parathyroid | 962.6 | E858.0 | E932.6 | E950.4 | E962.0 | E980.4 |
| 68:28 pituitary (posterior) | 962.5 | E858.0 | E932.5 | E950.4 | E962.0 | E980.4 |
|   anterior | 962.4 | E858.0 | E932.4 | E950.4 | E962.0 | E980.4 |

☑ Additional Digit Required — Refer to the Tabular List for Digit Selection      ⁜ Subterms under main terms may continue to next column or page

| | Poisoning | Accident | Therapeutic Use | Suicide Attempt | Assault | Undetermined |
|---|---|---|---|---|---|---|
| **External Cause (E-Code)** | | | | | | |
| **Drug** — *continued* | | | | | | |
| 68:32 progestogens | 962.2 | E858.0 | E932.2 | E950.4 | E962.0 | E980.4 |
| 68:34 other corpus luteum hormones NEC | 962.2 | E858.0 | E932.2 | E950.4 | E962.0 | E980.4 |
| 68:36 thyroid and antithyroid | | | | | | |
| antithyroid | 962.8 | E858.0 | E932.8 | E950.4 | E962.0 | E980.4 |
| thyroid (derivatives) | 962.7 | E858.0 | E932.7 | E950.4 | E962.0 | E980.4 |
| 72:00 local anesthetics | | | | | | |
| NEC | 968.9 | E855.2 | E938.9 | E950.4 | E962.0 | E980.4 |
| infiltration (intradermal) (subcutaneous) (submucosal) | 968.5 | E855.2 | E938.5 | E950.4 | E962.0 | E980.4 |
| nerve blocking (peripheral) (plexus) (regional) | 968.6 | E855.2 | E938.6 | E950.4 | E962.0 | E980.4 |
| spinal | 968.7 | E855.2 | E938.7 | E950.4 | E962.0 | E980.4 |
| topical (surface) | 968.5 | E855.2 | E938.5 | E950.4 | E962.0 | E980.4 |
| 76:00 oxytocics | 975.0 | E858.6 | E945.0 | E950.4 | E962.0 | E980.4 |
| 78:00 radioactive agents | 990 | — | — | — | — | — |
| 80:04 serums NEC | 979.9 | E858.8 | E949.9 | E950.4 | E962.0 | E980.4 |
| immune gamma globulin (human) | 964.6 | E858.2 | E934.6 | E950.4 | E962.0 | E980.4 |
| 80:08 toxoids NEC | 978.8 | E858.8 | E948.8 | E950.4 | E962.0 | E980.4 |
| diphtheria | 978.5 | E858.8 | E948.5 | E950.4 | E962.0 | E980.4 |
| and diphtheria | 978.9 | E858.8 | E948.9 | E950.4 | E962.0 | E980.4 |
| with pertussis component | 978.6 | E858.8 | E948.6 | E950.4 | E962.0 | E980.4 |
| and tetanus | 978.9 | E858.8 | E948.9 | E950.4 | E962.0 | E980.4 |
| with pertussis component | 978.6 | E858.8 | E948.6 | E950.4 | E962.0 | E980.4 |
| tetanus | 978.4 | E858.8 | E948.4 | E950.4 | E962.0 | E980.4 |
| 80:12 vaccines | 979.9 | E858.8 | E949.9 | E950.4 | E962.0 | E980.4 |
| bacterial NEC | 978.8 | E858.8 | E948.8 | E950.4 | E962.0 | E980.4 |
| with other bacterial components | 978.9 | E858.8 | E948.9 | E950.4 | E962.0 | E980.4 |
| pertussis component | 978.6 | E858.8 | E948.6 | E950.4 | E962.0 | E980.4 |
| viral and rickettsial components | 979.7 | E858.8 | E949.7 | E950.4 | E962.0 | E980.4 |
| rickettsial NEC | 979.6 | E858.8 | E949.6 | E950.4 | E962.0 | E980.4 |
| with bacterial component | 979.7 | E858.8 | E949.7 | E950.4 | E962.0 | E980.4 |
| pertussis component | 978.6 | E858.8 | E948.6 | E950.4 | E962.0 | E980.4 |
| viral component | 979.7 | E858.8 | E949.7 | E950.4 | E962.0 | E980.4 |
| viral NEC | 979.6 | E858.8 | E949.6 | E950.4 | E962.0 | E980.4 |
| with bacterial component | 979.7 | E858.8 | E949.7 | E950.4 | E962.0 | E980.4 |
| pertussis component | 978.6 | E858.8 | E948.6 | E950.4 | E962.0 | E980.4 |
| rickettsial component | 979.7 | E858.8 | E949.7 | E950.4 | E962.0 | E980.4 |
| 84:04.04 antibiotics (skin and mucous membrane) | 976.0 | E858.7 | E946.0 | E950.4 | E962.0 | E980.4 |
| 84:04.08 fungicides (skin and mucous membrane) | 976.0 | E858.7 | E946.0 | E950.4 | E962.0 | E980.4 |
| 84:04.12 scabicides and pediculicides (skin and mucous membrane) | 976.0 | E858.7 | E946.0 | E950.4 | E962.0 | E980.4 |
| 84:04.16 miscellaneous local anti-infectives (skin and mucous membrane) | 976.0 | E858.7 | E946.0 | E950.4 | E962.0 | E980.4 |
| 84:06 anti-inflammatory agents (skin and mucous membrane) | 976.0 | E858.7 | E946.0 | E950.4 | E962.0 | E980.4 |
| 84:08 antipruritics and local anesthetics | | | | | | |
| antipruritics | 976.1 | E858.7 | E946.1 | E950.4 | E962.0 | E980.4 |
| local anesthetics | 968.5 | E855.2 | E938.5 | E950.4 | E962.0 | E980.4 |
| 84:12 astringents | 976.2 | E858.7 | E946.2 | E950.4 | E962.0 | E980.4 |
| 84:16 cell stimulants and proliferants | 976.8 | E858.7 | E946.8 | E950.4 | E962.0 | E980.4 |
| 84:20 detergents | 976.2 | E858.7 | E946.2 | E950.4 | E962.0 | E980.4 |
| 84:24 emollients, demulcents, and protectants | 976.3 | E858.7 | E946.3 | E950.4 | E962.0 | E980.4 |
| 84:28 keratolytic agents | 976.4 | E858.7 | E946.4 | E950.4 | E962.0 | E980.4 |
| 84:32 keratoplastic agents | 976.4 | E858.7 | E946.4 | E950.4 | E962.0 | E980.4 |
| 84:36 miscellaneous agents (skin and mucous membrane) | 976.8 | E858.7 | E946.8 | E950.4 | E962.0 | E980.4 |

| | Poisoning | Accident | Therapeutic Use | Suicide Attempt | Assault | Undetermined |
|---|---|---|---|---|---|---|
| **External Cause (E-Code)** | | | | | | |
| **Drug** — *continued* | | | | | | |
| 86:00 spasmolytic agents | 975.1 | E858.6 | E945.1 | E950.4 | E962.0 | E980.4 |
| antiasthmatics | 975.7 | E858.6 | E945.7 | E950.4 | E962.0 | E980.4 |
| papaverine | 972.5 | E858.3 | E942.5 | E950.4 | E962.0 | E980.4 |
| theophylline | 974.1 | E858.5 | E944.1 | E950.4 | E962.0 | E980.4 |
| 88:04 vitamin A | 963.5 | E858.1 | E933.5 | E950.4 | E962.0 | E980.4 |
| 88:08 vitamin B complex | 963.5 | E858.1 | E933.5 | E950.4 | E962.0 | E980.4 |
| hematopoietic vitamin | 964.1 | E858.2 | E934.1 | E950.4 | E962.0 | E980.4 |
| nicotinic acid derivatives | 972.2 | E858.3 | E942.2 | E950.4 | E962.0 | E980.4 |
| 88:12 vitamin C | 963.5 | E858.1 | E933.5 | E950.4 | E962.0 | E980.4 |
| 88:16 vitamin D | 963.5 | E858.1 | E933.5 | E950.4 | E962.0 | E980.4 |
| 88:20 vitamin E | 963.5 | E858.1 | E933.5 | E950.4 | E962.0 | E980.4 |
| 88:24 vitamin K activity | 964.3 | E858.2 | E934.3 | E950.4 | E962.0 | E980.4 |
| 88:28 multivitamin preparations | 963.5 | E858.1 | E933.5 | E950.4 | E962.0 | E980.4 |
| 92:00 unclassified therapeutic agents | 977.8 | E858.8 | E947.8 | E950.4 | E962.0 | E980.4 |
| specified NEC | 977.8 | E858.8 | E947.8 | E950.4 | E962.0 | E980.4 |
| **Duboisine** | 971.1 | E855.4 | E941.1 | E950.4 | E962.0 | E980.4 |
| **Dulcolax** | 973.1 | E858.4 | E943.1 | E950.4 | E962.0 | E980.4 |
| **Duponol** (C) (EP) | 976.2 | E858.7 | E946.2 | E950.4 | E962.0 | E980.4 |
| **Durabolin** | 962.1 | E858.0 | E932.1 | E950.4 | E962.0 | E980.4 |
| **Dyclone** | 968.5 | E855.2 | E938.5 | E950.4 | E962.0 | E980.4 |
| **Dyclonine** | 968.5 | E855.2 | E938.5 | E950.4 | E962.0 | E980.4 |
| **Dydrogesterone** | 962.2 | E858.0 | E932.2 | E950.4 | E962.0 | E980.4 |
| **Dyes** NEC | 989.89 | E866.8 | — | E950.9 | E962.1 | E980.9 |
| diagnostic agents | 977.8 | E858.8 | E947.8 | E950.4 | E962.0 | E980.4 |
| pharmaceutical NEC | 977.4 | E858.8 | E947.4 | E950.4 | E962.0 | E980.4 |
| **Dyfols** | 971.0 | E855.3 | E941.0 | E950.4 | E962.0 | E980.4 |
| **Dymelor** | 962.3 | E858.0 | E932.3 | E950.4 | E962.0 | E980.4 |
| **Dynamite** | 989.89 | E866.8 | — | E950.9 | E962.1 | E980.9 |
| fumes | 987.8 | E869.8 | — | E952.8 | E962.2 | E982.8 |
| **Dyphylline** | 975.1 | E858.6 | E945.1 | E950.4 | E962.0 | E980.4 |
| **Ear preparations** | 976.6 | E858.7 | E946.6 | E950.4 | E962.0 | E980.4 |
| **Echothiopate, ecothiopate** | 971.0 | E855.3 | E941.0 | E950.4 | E962.0 | E980.4 |
| **Ecstasy** | 969.7 | E854.2 | E939.7 | E950.3 | E962.0 | E980.3 |
| **Ectylurea** | 967.8 | E852.8 | E937.8 | E950.2 | E962.0 | E980.2 |
| **Edathamil disodium** | 963.8 | E858.1 | E933.8 | E950.4 | E962.0 | E980.4 |
| **Edecrin** | 974.4 | E858.5 | E944.4 | E950.4 | E962.0 | E980.4 |
| **Edetate, disodium** (calcium) | 963.8 | E858.1 | E933.8 | E950.4 | E962.0 | E980.4 |
| **Edrophonium** | 971.0 | E855.3 | E941.0 | E950.4 | E962.0 | E980.4 |
| **Elase** | 976.8 | E858.7 | E946.8 | E950.4 | E962.0 | E980.4 |
| **Elaterium** | 973.1 | E858.4 | E943.1 | E950.4 | E962.0 | E980.4 |
| **Elder** | 988.2 | E865.4 | — | E950.9 | E962.1 | E980.9 |
| berry (unripe) | 988.2 | E865.3 | — | E950.9 | E962.1 | E980.9 |
| **Electrolytes** NEC | 974.5 | E858.5 | E944.5 | E950.4 | E962.0 | E980.4 |
| **Electrolytic agent** NEC | 974.5 | E858.5 | E944.5 | E950.4 | E962.0 | E980.4 |
| **Embramine** | 963.0 | E858.1 | E933.0 | E950.4 | E962.0 | E980.4 |
| **Emetics** | 973.6 | E858.4 | E943.6 | E950.4 | E962.0 | E980.4 |
| **Emetine** (hydrochloride) | 961.5 | E857 | E931.5 | E950.4 | E962.0 | E980.4 |
| **Emollients** | 976.3 | E858.7 | E946.3 | E950.4 | E962.0 | E980.4 |
| **Emylcamate** | 969.5 | E853.8 | E939.5 | E950.3 | E962.0 | E980.3 |
| **Encyprate** | 969.0 | E854.0 | E939.0 | E950.3 | E962.0 | E980.3 |
| **Endocaine** | 968.5 | E855.2 | E938.5 | E950.4 | E962.0 | E980.4 |
| **Endrin** | 989.2 | E863.0 | — | E950.6 | E962.1 | E980.7 |
| **Enflurane** | 968.2 | E855.1 | E938.2 | E950.4 | E962.0 | E980.4 |
| **Enovid** | 962.2 | E858.0 | E932.2 | E950.4 | E962.0 | E980.4 |
| **ENT preparations** (anti-infectives) | 976.6 | E858.7 | E946.6 | E950.4 | E962.0 | E980.4 |
| **Enzodase** | 963.4 | E858.1 | E933.4 | E950.4 | E962.0 | E980.4 |
| **Enzymes** NEC | 963.4 | E858.1 | E933.4 | E950.4 | E962.0 | E980.4 |
| **Epanutin** | 966.1 | E855.0 | E936.1 | E950.4 | E962.0 | E980.4 |
| **Ephedra** (tincture) | 971.2 | E855.5 | E941.2 | E950.4 | E962.0 | E980.4 |
| **Ephedrine** | 971.2 | E855.5 | E941.2 | E950.4 | E962.0 | E980.4 |
| **Epiestriol** | 962.2 | E858.0 | E932.2 | E950.4 | E962.0 | E980.4 |
| **Epilim** — see Sodium valproate | | | | | | |
| **Epinephrine** | 971.2 | E855.5 | E941.2 | E950.4 | E962.0 | E980.4 |
| **Epsom salt** | 973.3 | E858.4 | E943.3 | E950.4 | E962.0 | E980.4 |
| **Equanil** | 969.5 | E853.8 | E939.5 | E950.3 | E962.0 | E980.3 |
| **Equisetum** (diuretic) | 974.4 | E858.5 | E944.4 | E950.4 | E962.0 | E980.4 |
| **Ergometrine** | 975.0 | E858.6 | E945.0 | E950.4 | E962.0 | E980.4 |
| **Ergonovine** | 975.0 | E858.6 | E945.0 | E950.4 | E962.0 | E980.4 |
| **Ergot** NEC | 988.2 | E865.4 | — | E950.9 | E962.1 | E980.9 |
| medicinal (alkaloids) | 975.0 | E858.6 | E945.0 | E950.4 | E962.0 | E980.4 |
| **Ergotamine** (tartrate) (for migraine) NEC | 972.9 | E858.3 | E942.9 | E950.4 | E962.0 | E980.4 |
| **Ergotrate** | 975.0 | E858.6 | E945.0 | E950.4 | E962.0 | E980.4 |
| **Erythrityl tetranitrate** | 972.4 | E858.3 | E942.4 | E950.4 | E962.0 | E980.4 |
| **Erythrol tetranitrate** | 972.4 | E858.3 | E942.4 | E950.4 | E962.0 | E980.4 |
| **Erythromycin** | 960.3 | E856 | E930.3 | E950.4 | E962.0 | E980.4 |
| ophthalmic preparation | 976.5 | E858.7 | E946.5 | E950.4 | E962.0 | E980.4 |

| | Poisoning | Accident | Therapeutic Use | Suicide Attempt | Assault | Undetermined |
|---|---|---|---|---|---|---|
| **Erythromycin** — *continued* | | | | | | |
| topical NEC | 976.0 | E858.7 | E946.0 | E950.4 | E962.0 | E980.4 |
| **Eserine** | 971.0 | E855.3 | E941.0 | E950.4 | E962.0 | E980.4 |
| **Eskabarb** | 967.0 | E851 | E937.0 | E950.1 | E962.0 | E980.1 |
| **Eskalith** | 969.8 | E855.8 | E939.8 | E950.3 | E962.0 | E980.3 |
| **Estradiol** (cypionate) (dipropionate) | | | | | | |
| (valerate) | 962.2 | E858.0 | E932.2 | E950.4 | E962.0 | E980.4 |
| **Estriol** | 962.2 | E858.0 | E932.2 | E950.4 | E962.0 | E980.4 |
| **Estrogens** (with | | | | | | |
| progestogens) | 962.2 | E858.0 | E932.2 | E950.4 | E962.0 | E980.4 |
| **Estrone** | 962.2 | E858.0 | E932.2 | E950.4 | E962.0 | E980.4 |
| **Etafedrine** | 971.2 | E855.5 | E941.2 | E950.4 | E962.0 | E980.4 |
| **Ethacrynate sodium** | 974.4 | E858.5 | E944.4 | E950.4 | E962.0 | E980.4 |
| **Ethacrynic acid** | 974.4 | E858.5 | E944.4 | E950.4 | E962.0 | E980.4 |
| **Ethambutol** | 961.8 | E857 | E931.8 | E950.4 | E962.0 | E980.4 |
| **Ethamide** | 974.2 | E858.5 | E944.2 | E950.4 | E962.0 | E980.4 |
| **Ethamivan** | 970.0 | E854.3 | E940.0 | E950.4 | E962.0 | E980.4 |
| **Ethamsylate** | 964.5 | E858.2 | E934.5 | E950.4 | E962.0 | E980.4 |
| **Ethanol** | 980.0 | E860.1 | — | E950.9 | E962.1 | E980.9 |
| beverage | 980.0 | E860.0 | — | E950.9 | E962.1 | E980.9 |
| **Ethchlorvynol** | 967.8 | E852.8 | E937.8 | E950.2 | E962.0 | E980.2 |
| **Ethebenecid** | 974.7 | E858.5 | E944.7 | E950.4 | E962.0 | E980.4 |
| **Ether(s)** (diethyl) (ethyl) | | | | | | |
| (vapor) | 987.8 | E869.8 | — | E952.8 | E962.2 | E982.8 |
| anesthetic | 968.2 | E855.1 | E938.2 | E950.4 | E962.0 | E980.4 |
| petroleum — *see* Ligroin | | | | | | |
| solvent | 982.8 | E862.4 | — | E950.9 | E962.1 | E980.9 |
| **Ethidine chloride** (vapor) | 987.8 | E869.8 | — | E952.8 | E962.2 | E982.8 |
| liquid (solvent) | 982.3 | E862.4 | — | E950.9 | E962.1 | E980.9 |
| **Ethinamate** | 967.8 | E852.8 | E937.8 | E950.2 | E962.0 | E980.2 |
| **Ethinylestradiol** | 962.2 | E858.0 | E932.2 | E950.4 | E962.0 | E980.4 |
| **Ethionamide** | 961.8 | E857 | E931.8 | E950.4 | E962.0 | E980.4 |
| **Ethisterone** | 962.2 | E858.0 | E932.2 | E950.4 | E962.0 | E980.4 |
| **Ethobral** | 967.0 | E851 | E937.0 | E950.1 | E962.0 | E980.1 |
| **Ethocaine** (infiltration) | | | | | | |
| (topical) | 968.5 | E855.2 | E938.5 | E950.4 | E962.0 | E980.4 |
| nerve block (peripheral) | | | | | | |
| (plexus) | 968.6 | E855.2 | E938.6 | E950.4 | E962.0 | E980.4 |
| spinal | 968.7 | E855.2 | E938.7 | E950.4 | E962.0 | E980.4 |
| **Ethoheptazine** (citrate) | 965.7 | E850.7 | E935.7 | E950.0 | E962.0 | E980.0 |
| **Ethopropazine** | 966.4 | E855.0 | E936.4 | E950.4 | E962.0 | E980.4 |
| **Ethosuximide** | 966.2 | E855.0 | E936.2 | E950.4 | E962.0 | E980.4 |
| **Ethotoin** | 966.1 | E855.0 | E936.1 | E950.4 | E962.0 | E980.4 |
| **Ethoxazene** | 961.9 | E857 | E931.9 | E950.4 | E962.0 | E980.4 |
| **Ethoxzolamide** | 974.2 | E858.5 | E944.2 | E950.4 | E962.0 | E980.4 |
| **Ethyl** | | | | | | |
| acetate (vapor) | 982.8 | E862.4 | — | E950.9 | E962.1 | E980.9 |
| alcohol | 980.0 | E860.1 | — | E950.9 | E962.1 | E980.9 |
| beverage | 980.0 | E860.0 | — | E950.9 | E962.1 | E980.9 |
| aldehyde (vapor) | 987.8 | E869.8 | — | E952.8 | E962.2 | E982.8 |
| liquid | 989.89 | E866.8 | — | E950.9 | E962.1 | E980.9 |
| aminobenzoate | 968.5 | E855.2 | E938.5 | E950.4 | E962.0 | E980.4 |
| biscoumacetate | 964.2 | E858.2 | E934.2 | E950.4 | E962.0 | E980.4 |
| bromide (anesthetic) | 968.2 | E855.1 | E938.2 | E950.4 | E962.0 | E980.4 |
| carbamate (antineoplastic) | 963.1 | E858.1 | E933.1 | E950.4 | E962.0 | E980.4 |
| carbinol | 980.3 | E860.4 | — | E950.9 | E962.1 | E980.9 |
| chaulmoograte | 961.8 | E857 | E931.8 | E950.4 | E962.0 | E980.4 |
| chloride (vapor) | 987.8 | E869.8 | — | E952.8 | E962.2 | E982.8 |
| anesthetic (local) | 968.5 | E855.2 | E938.5 | E950.4 | E962.0 | E980.4 |
| inhaled | 968.2 | E855.1 | E938.2 | E950.4 | E962.0 | E980.4 |
| solvent | 982.3 | E862.4 | — | E950.9 | E962.1 | E980.9 |
| estranol | 962.1 | E858.0 | E932.1 | E950.4 | E962.0 | E980.4 |
| ether — *see* Ether(s) | | | | | | |
| formate (solvent) NEC | 982.8 | E862.4 | — | E950.9 | E962.1 | E980.9 |
| iodoacetate | 987.5 | E869.3 | — | E952.8 | E962.2 | E982.8 |
| lactate (solvent) NEC | 982.8 | E862.4 | — | E950.9 | E962.1 | E980.9 |
| methylcarbinol | 980.8 | E860.8 | — | E950.9 | E962.1 | E980.9 |
| morphine | 965.09 | E850.2 | E935.2 | E950.0 | E962.0 | E980.0 |
| **Ethylene** (gas) | 987.1 | E869.8 | — | E952.8 | E962.2 | E982.8 |
| anesthetic (general) | 968.2 | E855.1 | E938.2 | E950.4 | E962.0 | E980.4 |
| chlorohydrin (vapor) | 982.3 | E862.4 | — | E950.9 | E962.1 | E980.9 |
| dichloride (vapor) | 982.3 | E862.4 | — | E950.9 | E962.1 | E980.9 |
| glycol(s) (any) (vapor) | 982.8 | E862.4 | — | E950.9 | E962.1 | E980.9 |
| **Ethylidene** | | | | | | |
| chloride NEC | 982.3 | E862.4 | — | E950.9 | E962.1 | E980.9 |
| diethyl ether | 982.8 | E862.4 | — | E950.9 | E962.1 | E980.9 |
| **Ethynodiol** | 962.2 | E858.0 | E932.2 | E950.4 | E962.0 | E980.4 |
| **Etidocaine** | 968.9 | E855.2 | E938.9 | E950.4 | E962.0 | E980.4 |
| infiltration (subcutaneous) | 968.5 | E855.2 | E938.5 | E950.4 | E962.0 | E980.4 |
| nerve (peripheral) (plexus) | 968.6 | E855.2 | E938.6 | E950.4 | E962.0 | E980.4 |
| **Etilfen** | 967.0 | E851 | E937.0 | E950.1 | E962.0 | E980.1 |

| | Poisoning | Accident | Therapeutic Use | Suicide Attempt | Assault | Undetermined |
|---|---|---|---|---|---|---|
| **Etomide** | 965.7 | E850.7 | E935.7 | E950.0 | E962.0 | E980.0 |
| **Etorphine** | 965.09 | E850.2 | E935.2 | E950.0 | E962.0 | E980.0 |
| **Etoval** | 967.0 | E851 | E937.0 | E950.1 | E962.0 | E980.1 |
| **Etryptamine** | 969.0 | E854.0 | E939.0 | E950.3 | E962.0 | E980.3 |
| **Eucaine** | 968.5 | E855.2 | E938.5 | E950.4 | E962.0 | E980.4 |
| **Eucalyptus** (oil) NEC | 975.5 | E858.6 | E945.5 | E950.4 | E962.0 | E980.4 |
| **Eucatropine** | 971.1 | E855.4 | E941.1 | E950.4 | E962.0 | E980.4 |
| **Eucodal** | 965.09 | E850.2 | E935.2 | E950.0 | E962.0 | E980.0 |
| **Euneryl** | 967.0 | E851 | E937.0 | E950.1 | E962.0 | E980.1 |
| **Euphthalmine** | 971.1 | E855.4 | E941.1 | E950.4 | E962.0 | E980.4 |
| **Eurax** | 976.0 | E858.7 | E946.0 | E950.4 | E962.0 | E980.4 |
| **Euresol** | 976.4 | E858.7 | E946.4 | E950.4 | E962.0 | E980.4 |
| **Euthroid** | 962.7 | E858.0 | E932.7 | E950.4 | E962.0 | E980.4 |
| **Evans blue** | 977.8 | E858.8 | E947.8 | E950.4 | E962.0 | E980.4 |
| **Evipal** | 967.0 | E851 | E937.0 | E950.1 | E962.0 | E980.1 |
| sodium | 968.3 | E855.1 | E938.3 | E950.4 | E962.0 | E980.4 |
| **Evipan** | 967.0 | E851 | E937.0 | E950.1 | E962.0 | E980.1 |
| sodium | 968.3 | E855.1 | E938.3 | E950.4 | E962.0 | E980.4 |
| **Exalgin** | 965.4 | E850.4 | E935.4 | E950.0 | E962.0 | E980.0 |
| **Excipients,** | | | | | | |
| **pharmaceutical** | 977.4 | E858.8 | E947.4 | E950.4 | E962.0 | E980.4 |
| **Exhaust gas** — *see* Carbon, monoxide | | | | | | |
| **Ex-Lax** (phenolphthalein) | 973.1 | E858.4 | E943.1 | E950.4 | E962.0 | E980.4 |
| **Expectorants** | 975.5 | E858.6 | E945.5 | E950.4 | E962.0 | E980.4 |
| **External medications** (skin) | | | | | | |
| (mucous membrane) | 976.9 | E858.7 | E946.9 | E950.4 | E962.0 | E980.4 |
| dental agent | 976.7 | E858.7 | E946.7 | E950.4 | E962.0 | E980.4 |
| ENT agent | 976.6 | E858.7 | E946.6 | E950.4 | E962.0 | E980.4 |
| ophthalmic preparation | 976.5 | E858.7 | E946.5 | E950.4 | E962.0 | E980.4 |
| specified NEC | 976.8 | E858.7 | E946.8 | E950.4 | E962.0 | E980.4 |
| **Eye agents** (anti-infective) | 976.5 | E858.7 | E946.5 | E950.4 | E962.0 | E980.4 |
| **Factor IX complex** (human) | 964.5 | E858.2 | E934.5 | E950.4 | E962.0 | E980.4 |
| **Fecal softeners** | 973.2 | E858.4 | E943.2 | E950.4 | E962.0 | E980.4 |
| **Fenbutrazate** | 977.0 | E858.8 | E947.0 | E950.4 | E962.0 | E980.4 |
| **Fencamfamin** | 970.8 | E854.3 | E940.8 | E950.4 | E962.0 | E980.4 |
| **Fenfluramine** | 977.0 | E858.8 | E947.0 | E950.4 | E962.0 | E980.4 |
| **Fenoprofen** | 965.61 | E850.6 | E935.6 | E950.0 | E962.0 | E980.0 |
| **Fentanyl** | 965.09 | E850.2 | E935.2 | E950.0 | E962.0 | E980.0 |
| **Fentazin** | 969.1 | E853.0 | E939.1 | E950.3 | E962.0 | E980.3 |
| **Fenticlor, fentichlor** | 976.0 | E858.7 | E946.0 | E950.4 | E962.0 | E980.4 |
| **Fer de lance** (bite) (venom) | 989.5 | E905.0 | — | E950.9 | E962.1 | E980.9 |
| **Ferric** — *see* Iron | | | | | | |
| **Ferrocholinate** | 964.0 | E858.2 | E934.0 | E950.4 | E962.0 | E980.4 |
| **Ferrous fumerate, gluconate,** lactate, salt NEC, sulfate | | | | | | |
| (medicinal) | 964.0 | E858.2 | E934.0 | E950.4 | E962.0 | E980.4 |
| **Ferrum** — *see* Iron | | | | | | |
| **Fertilizers NEC** | 989.89 | E866.5 | — | E950.9 | E962.1 | E980.9 |
| with herbicide mixture | 989.4 | E863.5 | — | E950.6 | E962.1 | E980.7 |
| **Fibrinogen** (human) | 964.7 | E858.2 | E934.7 | E950.4 | E962.0 | E980.4 |
| **Fibrinolysin** | 964.4 | E858.2 | E934.4 | E950.4 | E962.0 | E980.4 |
| **Fibrinolysis-affecting** | | | | | | |
| **agents** | 964.4 | E858.2 | E934.4 | E950.4 | E962.0 | E980.4 |
| **Filix mas** | 961.6 | E857 | E931.6 | E950.4 | E962.0 | E980.4 |
| **Fiorinal** | 965.1 | E850.3 | E935.3 | E950.0 | E962.0 | E980.0 |
| **Fire damp** | 987.1 | E869.8 | — | E952.8 | E962.2 | E982.8 |
| **Fish, nonbacterial or** | | | | | | |
| **noxious** | 988.0 | E865.2 | — | E950.9 | E962.1 | E980.9 |
| shell | 988.0 | E865.1 | — | E950.9 | E962.1 | E980.9 |
| **Flagyl** | 961.5 | E857 | E931.5 | E950.4 | E962.0 | E980.4 |
| **Flavoxate** | 975.1 | E858.6 | E945.1 | E950.4 | E962.0 | E980.4 |
| **Flaxedil** | 975.2 | E858.6 | E945.2 | E950.4 | E962.0 | E980.4 |
| **Flaxseed** (medicinal) | 976.3 | E858.7 | E946.3 | E950.4 | E962.0 | E980.4 |
| **Flomax** ● | 971.3 | E855.6 | E941.3 | E950.4 | E962.0 | E980.4 |
| **Florantyrone** | 973.4 | E858.4 | E943.4 | E950.4 | E962.0 | E980.4 |
| **Floraquin** | 961.3 | E857 | E931.3 | E950.4 | E962.0 | E980.4 |
| **Florinef** | 962.0 | E858.0 | E932.0 | E950.4 | E962.0 | E980.4 |
| ENT agent | 976.6 | E858.7 | E946.6 | E950.4 | E962.0 | E980.4 |
| ophthalmic preparation | 976.5 | E858.7 | E946.5 | E950.4 | E962.0 | E980.4 |
| topical NEC | 976.0 | E858.7 | E946.0 | E950.4 | E962.0 | E980.4 |
| **Flowers of sulfur** | 976.4 | E858.7 | E946.4 | E950.4 | E962.0 | E980.4 |
| **Floxuridine** | 963.1 | E858.1 | E933.1 | E950.4 | E962.0 | E980.4 |
| **Flucytosine** | 961.9 | E857 | E931.9 | E950.4 | E962.0 | E980.4 |
| **Fludrocortisone** | 962.0 | E858.0 | E932.0 | E950.4 | E962.0 | E980.4 |
| ENT agent | 976.6 | E858.7 | E946.6 | E950.4 | E962.0 | E980.4 |
| ophthalmic preparation | 976.5 | E858.7 | E946.5 | E950.4 | E962.0 | E980.4 |
| topical NEC | 976.0 | E858.7 | E946.0 | E950.4 | E962.0 | E980.4 |
| **Flumethasone** | 976.0 | E858.7 | E946.0 | E950.4 | E962.0 | E980.4 |
| **Flumethiazide** | 974.3 | E858.5 | E944.3 | E950.4 | E962.0 | E980.4 |
| **Flumidin** | 961.7 | E857 | E931.7 | E950.4 | E962.0 | E980.4 |

☑ Additional Digit Required — Refer to the Tabular List for Digit Selection

Subterms under main terms may continue to next column or page

| | Poisoning | Accident | Therapeutic Use | Suicide Attempt | Assault | Undeter-mined |
|---|---|---|---|---|---|---|
| | | **External Cause (E-Code)** | | | | |
| Flunitrazepam | 969.4 | E853.2 | E939.4 | E950.3 | E962.0 | E980.3 |
| Fluocinolone | 976.0 | E858.7 | E946.0 | E950.4 | E962.0 | E980.4 |
| Fluocortolone | 962.0 | E858.0 | E932.0 | E950.4 | E962.0 | E980.4 |
| Fluohydrocortisone | 962.0 | E858.0 | E932.0 | E950.4 | E962.0 | E980.4 |
| ENT agent | 976.6 | E858.7 | E946.6 | E950.4 | E962.0 | E980.4 |
| ophthalmic preparation | 976.5 | E858.7 | E946.5 | E950.4 | E962.0 | E980.4 |
| topical NEC | 976.0 | E858.7 | E946.0 | E950.4 | E962.0 | E980.4 |
| Fluonid | 976.0 | E858.7 | E946.0 | E950.4 | E962.0 | E980.4 |
| Fluopromazine | 969.1 | E853.0 | E939.1 | E950.3 | E962.0 | E980.3 |
| Fluoracetate | 989.4 | E863.7 | — | E950.6 | E962.1 | E980.7 |
| Fluorescein (sodium) | 977.8 | E858.8 | E947.8 | E950.4 | E962.0 | E980.4 |
| **Fluoride(s) (pesticides) (sodium)** | | | | | | |
| NEC | 989.4 | E863.4 | — | E950.6 | E962.1 | E980.7 |
| hydrogen — see Hydrofluoric acid | | | | | | |
| medicinal | 976.7 | E858.7 | E946.7 | E950.4 | E962.0 | E980.4 |
| not pesticide NEC | 983.9 | E864.4 | — | E950.7 | E962.1 | E980.6 |
| stannous | 976.7 | E858.7 | E946.7 | E950.4 | E962.0 | E980.4 |
| **Fluorinated corticosteroids** | 962.0 | E858.0 | E932.0 | E950.4 | E962.0 | E980.4 |
| Fluorine (compounds) (gas) | 987.8 | E869.8 | — | E952.8 | E962.2 | E982.8 |
| salt — see Fluoride(s) | | | | | | |
| Fluoristan | 976.7 | E858.7 | E946.7 | E950.4 | E962.0 | E980.4 |
| Fluoroacetate | 989.4 | E863.7 | — | E950.6 | E962.1 | E980.7 |
| Fluorodeoxyuridine | 963.1 | E858.1 | E933.1 | E950.4 | E962.0 | E980.4 |
| **Fluorometholone (topical)** | | | | | | |
| NEC | 976.0 | E858.7 | E946.0 | E950.4 | E962.0 | E980.4 |
| ophthalmic preparation | 976.5 | E858.7 | E946.5 | E950.4 | E962.0 | E980.4 |
| Fluorouracil | 963.1 | E858.1 | E933.1 | E950.4 | E962.0 | E980.4 |
| Fluothane | 968.1 | E855.1 | E938.1 | E950.4 | E962.0 | E980.4 |
| Fluoxetine hydrochloride | 969.0 | E854.0 | E939.0 | E950.3 | E962.0 | E980.3 |
| Fluoxymesterone | 962.1 | E858.0 | E932.1 | E950.4 | E962.0 | E980.4 |
| Fluphenazine | 969.1 | E853.0 | E939.1 | E950.3 | E962.0 | E980.3 |
| Fluprednisolone | 962.0 | E858.0 | E932.0 | E950.4 | E962.0 | E980.4 |
| Flurandrenolide | 976.0 | E858.7 | E946.0 | E950.4 | E962.0 | E980.4 |
| Flurazepam (hydrochloride) | 969.4 | E853.2 | E939.4 | E950.3 | E962.0 | E980.3 |
| Flurbiprofen | 965.61 | E850.6 | E935.6 | E950.0 | E962.0 | E980.0 |
| Flurobate | 976.0 | E858.7 | E946.0 | E950.4 | E962.0 | E980.4 |
| Flurothyl | 969.8 | E855.8 | E939.8 | E950.3 | E962.0 | E980.3 |
| Fluroxene | 968.2 | E855.1 | E938.2 | E950.4 | E962.0 | E980.4 |
| Folacin | 964.1 | E858.2 | E934.1 | E950.4 | E962.0 | E980.4 |
| Folic acid | 964.1 | E858.2 | E934.1 | E950.4 | E962.0 | E980.4 |
| **Follicle stimulating hormone** | 962.4 | E858.0 | E932.4 | E950.4 | E962.0 | E980.4 |
| **Food, foodstuffs, nonbacterial or noxious** | 988.9 | E865.9 | — | E950.9 | E962.1 | E980.9 |
| berries, seeds | 988.2 | E865.3 | — | E950.9 | E962.1 | E980.9 |
| fish | 988.0 | E865.2 | — | E950.9 | E962.1 | E980.9 |
| mushrooms | 988.1 | E865.5 | — | E950.9 | E962.1 | E980.9 |
| plants | 988.2 | E865.9 | — | E950.9 | E962.1 | E980.9 |
| specified type NEC | 988.2 | E865.4 | — | E950.9 | E962.1 | E980.9 |
| shellfish | 988.0 | E865.1 | — | E950.9 | E962.1 | E980.9 |
| specified NEC | 988.8 | E865.8 | — | E950.9 | E962.1 | E980.9 |
| Fool's parsley | 988.2 | E865.4 | — | E950.9 | E962.1 | E980.9 |
| Formaldehyde (solution) | 989.89 | E861.4 | — | E950.9 | E962.1 | E980.9 |
| fungicide | 989.4 | E863.6 | — | E950.6 | E962.1 | E980.7 |
| gas or vapor | 987.8 | E869.8 | — | E952.8 | E962.2 | E982.8 |
| Formalin | 989.89 | E861.4 | — | E950.9 | E962.1 | E980.9 |
| fungicide | 989.4 | E863.6 | — | E950.6 | E962.1 | E980.7 |
| vapor | 987.8 | E869.8 | — | E952.8 | E962.2 | E982.8 |
| Formic acid | 983.1 | E864.1 | — | E950.7 | E962.1 | E980.6 |
| automobile | 981 | E862.1 | — | E950.9 | E962.1 | E980.9 |
| exhaust gas, not in transit | 986 | E868.2 | — | E952.0 | E962.2 | E982.0 |
| vapor NEC | 987.1 | E869.8 | — | E952.8 | E962.2 | E982.8 |
| gas (domestic use) (see also Carbon, monoxide, fuel) | | | | | | |
| utility | 987.1 | E868.1 | — | E951.8 | E962.2 | E981.8 |
| incomplete combustion of — see Carbon, monoxide, fuel, utility | | | | | | |
| in mobile container | 987.0 | E868.0 | — | E951.1 | E962.2 | E981.1 |
| piped (natural) | 987.1 | E867 | — | E951.0 | E962.2 | E981.0 |
| industrial, incomplete combustion | 986 | E868.3 | — | E952.1 | E962.2 | E982.1 |
| vapor | 987.8 | E869.8 | — | E952.8 | E962.2 | E982.8 |
| Fowler's solution | 985.1 | E866.3 | — | E950.8 | E962.1 | E980.8 |
| Foxglove | 988.2 | E865.4 | — | E950.9 | E962.1 | E980.9 |
| Fox green | 977.8 | E858.8 | E947.8 | E950.4 | E962.0 | E980.4 |
| Framycetin | 960.8 | E856 | E930.8 | E950.4 | E962.0 | E980.4 |
| Frangula (extract) | 973.1 | E858.4 | E943.1 | E950.4 | E962.0 | E980.4 |

| | Poisoning | Accident | Therapeutic Use | Suicide Attempt | Assault | Undeter-mined |
|---|---|---|---|---|---|---|
| | | **External Cause (E-Code)** | | | | |
| Frei antigen | 977.8 | E858.8 | E947.8 | E950.4 | E962.0 | E980.4 |
| Freons | 987.4 | E869.2 | — | E952.8 | E962.2 | E982.8 |
| Fructose | 974.5 | E858.5 | E944.5 | E950.4 | E962.0 | E980.4 |
| Frusemide | 974.4 | E858.5 | E944.4 | E950.4 | E962.0 | E980.4 |
| FSH | 962.4 | E858.0 | E932.4 | E950.4 | E962.0 | E980.4 |
| **Fuel** | | | | | | |
| Fugillin | 960.8 | E856 | E930.8 | E950.4 | E962.0 | E980.4 |
| Fulminate of mercury | 985.0 | E866.1 | — | E950.9 | E962.1 | E980.9 |
| Fulvicin | 960.1 | E856 | E930.1 | E950.4 | E962.0 | E980.4 |
| Fumadil | 960.8 | E856 | E930.8 | E950.4 | E962.0 | E980.4 |
| Fumagillin | 960.8 | E856 | E930.8 | E950.4 | E962.0 | E980.4 |
| **Fumes** (from) | 987.9 | E869.9 | — | E952.9 | E962.2 | E982.9 |
| carbon monoxide — see Carbon, monoxide | | | | | | |
| charcoal (domestic use) | 986 | E868.3 | — | E952.1 | E962.2 | E982.1 |
| chloroform — see Chloroform | | | | | | |
| coke (in domestic stoves, fireplaces) | 986 | E868.3 | — | E952.1 | E962.2 | E982.1 |
| corrosive NEC | 987.8 | E869.8 | — | E952.8 | E962.2 | E982.8 |
| ether — see Ether(s) | | | | | | |
| freons | 987.4 | E869.2 | — | E952.8 | E962.2 | E982.8 |
| hydrocarbons | 987.1 | E869.8 | — | E952.8 | E962.2 | E982.8 |
| petroleum (liquefied) | 987.0 | E868.0 | — | E951.1 | E962.2 | E981.1 |
| distributed through pipes (pure or mixed with air) | 987.0 | E867 | — | E951.0 | E962.2 | E981.0 |
| lead — see Lead | | | | | | |
| metals — see specified metal | | | | | | |
| nitrogen dioxide | 987.2 | E869.0 | — | E952.8 | E962.2 | E982.8 |
| pesticides — see Pesticides | | | | | | |
| petroleum (liquefied) | 987.0 | E868.0 | — | E951.1 | E962.2 | E981.1 |
| distributed through pipes (pure or mixed with air) | 987.0 | E867 | — | E951.0 | E962.2 | E981.0 |
| polyester | 987.8 | E869.8 | — | E952.8 | E962.2 | E982.8 |
| specified, source other (see also substance specified) | 987.8 | E869.8 | — | E952.8 | E962.2 | E982.8 |
| sulfur dioxide | 987.3 | E869.1 | — | E952.8 | E962.2 | E982.8 |
| **Fumigants** | 989.4 | E863.8 | — | E950.6 | E962.1 | E980.7 |
| **Fungicides** — see also Antifungals | 989.4 | E863.6 | — | E950.6 | E962.1 | E980.7 |
| **Fungi, noxious, used as food** | 988.1 | E865.5 | — | E950.9 | E962.1 | E980.9 |
| Fungizone | 960.1 | E856 | E930.1 | E950.4 | E962.0 | E980.4 |
| topical | 976.0 | E858.7 | E946.0 | E950.4 | E962.0 | E980.4 |
| Furacin | 976.0 | E858.7 | E946.0 | E950.4 | E962.0 | E980.4 |
| Furadantin | 961.9 | E857 | E931.9 | E950.4 | E962.0 | E980.4 |
| Furadantin | 961.9 | E857 | E931.9 | E950.4 | E962.0 | E980.4 |
| Furazolidone | 961.9 | E857 | E931.9 | E950.4 | E962.0 | E980.4 |
| **Furnace** (coal burning) (domestic), gas from | 986 | E868.3 | — | E952.1 | E962.2 | E982.1 |
| industrial | 986 | E868.8 | — | E952.1 | E962.2 | E982.1 |
| Furniture polish | 989.89 | E861.2 | — | E950.9 | E962.1 | E980.9 |
| Furosemide | 974.4 | E858.5 | E944.4 | E950.4 | E962.0 | E980.4 |
| Furoxone | 961.9 | E857 | E931.9 | E950.4 | E962.0 | E980.4 |
| **Fusel oil** (amyl) (butyl) (propyl) | 980.3 | E860.4 | — | E950.9 | E962.1 | E980.9 |
| Fusidic acid | 960.8 | E856 | E930.8 | E950.4 | E962.0 | E980.4 |
| Gallamine | 975.2 | E858.6 | E945.2 | E950.4 | E962.0 | E980.4 |
| Gallotannic acid | 976.2 | E858.7 | E946.2 | E950.4 | E962.0 | E980.4 |
| Gamboge | 973.1 | E858.4 | E943.1 | E950.4 | E962.0 | E980.4 |
| Gamimune | 964.6 | E858.2 | E934.6 | E950.4 | E962.0 | E980.4 |
| **Gamma-benzene hexachloride** (vapor) | 989.2 | E863.0 | — | E950.6 | E962.1 | E980.7 |
| Gamma globulin | 964.6 | E858.2 | E934.6 | E950.4 | E962.0 | E980.4 |
| **Gamma hydroxy butyrate** (GHB) | 968.4 | E855.1 | E938.4 | E950.4 | E962.0 | E980.4 |
| Gamulin | 964.6 | E858.2 | E934.6 | E950.4 | E962.0 | E980.4 |
| **Ganglionic blocking agents** | 972.3 | E858.3 | E942.3 | E950.4 | E962.0 | E980.4 |
| Ganja | 969.6 | E854.1 | E939.6 | E950.3 | E962.0 | E980.3 |
| Garamycin | 960.8 | E856 | E930.8 | E950.4 | E962.0 | E980.4 |
| ophthalmic preparation | 976.5 | E858.7 | E946.5 | E950.4 | E962.0 | E980.4 |
| topical NEC | 976.0 | E858.7 | E946.0 | E950.4 | E962.0 | E980.4 |
| Gardenal | 967.0 | E851 | E937.0 | E950.1 | E962.0 | E980.1 |
| Gardepanyl | 967.0 | E851 | E937.0 | E950.1 | E962.0 | E980.1 |
| **Gas** | 987.9 | E869.9 | — | E952.9 | E962.2 | E982.9 |
| acetylene | 987.1 | E868.1 | — | E951.8 | E962.2 | E981.8 |
| incomplete combustion of — see Carbon, monoxide, fuel, utility | | | | | | |
| air contaminants, source or type not specified | 987.9 | E869.9 | — | E952.9 | E962.2 | E982.9 |

---

☑ Additional Digit Required — Refer to the Tabular List for Digit Selection

▽ Subterms under main terms may continue to next column or page

| | Poisoning | Accident | Therapeutic Use | Suicide Attempt | Assault | Undetermined |
|---|---|---|---|---|---|---|
| **Gas** — *continued* | | | | | | |
| anesthetic (general) NEC | 968.2 | E855.1 | E938.2 | E950.4 | E962.0 | E980.4 |
| blast furnace | 986 | E868.8 | — | E952.1 | E962.2 | E982.1 |
| butane — see Butane | | | | | | |
| carbon monoxide — see Carbon, monoxide | | | | | | |
| chlorine | 987.6 | E869.8 | — | E952.8 | E962.2 | E982.8 |
| coal — see Carbon, monoxide, coal | | | | | | |
| cyanide | 987.7 | E869.8 | — | E952.8 | E962.2 | E982.8 |
| dicyanogen | 987.8 | E869.8 | — | E952.8 | E962.2 | E982.8 |
| domestic — see Gas, utility | | | | | | |
| exhaust — see Carbon, monoxide, exhaust gas | | | | | | |
| from wood- or coal-burning stove or fireplace | 986 | E868.3 | — | E952.1 | E962.2 | E982.1 |
| fuel (domestic use) (*see also* Carbon, monoxide, fuel) | | | | | | |
| industrial use | 986 | E868.8 | — | E952.1 | E962.2 | E982.1 |
| utility | 987.1 | E868.1 | — | E951.8 | E962.2 | E981.8 |
| incomplete combustion of — see Carbon, monoxide, fuel, utility | | | | | | |
| in mobile container | 987.0 | E868.0 | — | E951.1 | E962.2 | E981.1 |
| piped (natural) | 987.1 | E867 | — | E951.0 | E962.2 | E981.0 |
| garage | 986 | E868.2 | — | E952.0 | E962.2 | E982.0 |
| hydrocarbon NEC | 987.1 | E869.8 | — | E952.8 | E962.2 | E982.8 |
| incomplete combustion of — see Carbon, monoxide, fuel, utility | | | | | | |
| liquefied (mobile container) | 987.0 | E868.0 | — | E951.1 | E962.2 | E981.1 |
| piped | 987.0 | E867 | — | E951.0 | E962.2 | E981.0 |
| hydrocyanic acid | 987.7 | E869.8 | — | E952.8 | E962.2 | E982.8 |
| illuminating — see Gas, utility | | | | | | |
| incomplete combustion, any — see Carbon, monoxide | | | | | | |
| kiln | 986 | E868.8 | — | E952.1 | E962.2 | E982.1 |
| lacrimogenic | 987.5 | E869.3 | — | E952.8 | E962.2 | E982.8 |
| marsh | 987.1 | E869.8 | — | E952.8 | E962.2 | E982.8 |
| motor exhaust, not in transit | 986 | E868.8 | — | E952.1 | E962.2 | E982.1 |
| mustard — see Mustard, gas | | | | | | |
| natural | 987.1 | E867 | — | E951.0 | E962.2 | E981.0 |
| nerve (war) | 987.9 | E869.9 | — | E952.9 | E962.2 | E982.9 |
| oils | 981 | E862.1 | — | E950.9 | E961.1 | E980.9 |
| petroleum (liquefied) (distributed in mobile containers) | 987.0 | E868.0 | — | E951.1 | E962.2 | E981.1 |
| piped (pure or mixed with air) | 987.0 | E867 | — | E951.1 | E962.2 | E981.1 |
| piped (manufactured) (natural) NEC | 987.1 | E867 | — | E951.0 | E962.2 | E981.0 |
| producer | 986 | E868.8 | — | E952.1 | E962.2 | E982.1 |
| propane — see Propane | | | | | | |
| refrigerant (freon) | 987.4 | E869.2 | — | E952.8 | E962.2 | E982.8 |
| not freon | 987.9 | E869.9 | — | E952.9 | E962.2 | E982.9 |
| sewer | 987.8 | E869.8 | — | E952.8 | E962.2 | E982.8 |
| specified source NEC (see also substance specified) | 987.8 | E869.8 | — | E952.8 | E962.2 | E982.8 |
| stove — see Gas, utility | | | | | | |
| tear | 987.5 | E869.3 | — | E952.8 | E962.2 | E982.8 |
| utility (for cooking, heating, or lighting) (piped) NEC | 987.1 | E868.1 | — | E951.8 | E962.2 | E981.8 |
| incomplete combustion of — see Carbon, monoxide, fuel, utilty | | | | | | |
| in mobile container | 987.0 | E868.0 | — | E951.1 | E962.2 | E981.1 |
| piped (natural) | 987.1 | E867 | — | E951.0 | E962.2 | E981.0 |
| water | 987.1 | E868.1 | — | E951.8 | E962.2 | E981.8 |
| incomplete combustion of — see Carbon, monoxide, fuel, utility | | | | | | |
| **Gaseous substance** — see Gas | | | | | | |
| **Gasoline, gasolene** | 981 | E862.1 | — | E950.9 | E961.1 | E980.9 |
| vapor | 987.1 | E869.8 | — | E952.8 | E962.2 | E982.8 |
| **Gastric enzymes** | 973.4 | E858.4 | E943.4 | E950.4 | E962.0 | E980.4 |
| **Gastrografin** | 977.8 | E858.8 | E947.8 | E950.4 | E962.0 | E980.4 |
| **Gastrointestinal agents** | 973.9 | E858.4 | E943.9 | E950.4 | E962.0 | E980.4 |
| specified NEC | 973.8 | E858.4 | E943.8 | E950.4 | E962.0 | E980.4 |
| **Gaultheria procumbens** | 988.2 | E865.4 | — | E950.9 | E961.1 | E980.9 |
| **Gelatin** (intravenous) | 964.8 | E858.2 | E934.8 | E950.4 | E962.0 | E980.4 |
| absorbable (sponge) | 964.5 | E858.2 | E934.5 | E950.4 | E962.0 | E980.4 |

| | Poisoning | Accident | Therapeutic Use | Suicide Attempt | Assault | Undetermined |
|---|---|---|---|---|---|---|
| **Gelfilm** | 976.8 | E858.7 | E946.8 | E950.4 | E962.0 | E980.4 |
| **Gelfoam** | 964.5 | E858.2 | E934.5 | E950.4 | E962.0 | E980.4 |
| **Gelsemine** | 970.8 | E854.3 | E940.8 | E950.4 | E962.0 | E980.4 |
| **Gelsemium** (sempervirens) | 988.2 | E865.4 | — | E950.9 | E962.1 | E980.9 |
| **Gemonil** | 967.0 | E851 | E937.0 | E950.1 | E962.0 | E980.1 |
| **Gentamicin** | 960.8 | E856 | E930.8 | E950.4 | E962.0 | E980.4 |
| ophthalmic preparation | 976.5 | E858.7 | E946.5 | E950.4 | E962.0 | E980.4 |
| topical NEC | 976.0 | E858.7 | E946.0 | E950.4 | E962.0 | E980.4 |
| **Gentian violet** | 976.0 | E858.7 | E946.0 | E950.4 | E962.0 | E980.4 |
| **Gexane** | 976.0 | E858.7 | E946.0 | E950.4 | E962.0 | E980.4 |
| **Gila monster** (venom) | 989.5 | E905.0 | — | E950.9 | E962.1 | E980.9 |
| **Ginger, Jamaica** | 989.89 | E866.8 | — | E950.9 | E962.1 | E980.9 |
| **Gitalin** | 972.1 | E858.3 | E942.1 | E950.4 | E962.0 | E980.4 |
| **Gitoxin** | 972.1 | E858.3 | E942.1 | E950.4 | E962.0 | E980.4 |
| **Glandular extract (medicinal) NEC** | 977.9 | E858.9 | E947.9 | E950.5 | E962.0 | E980.5 |
| **Glaucarubin** | 961.5 | E857 | E931.5 | E950.4 | E962.0 | E980.4 |
| **Globin zinc insulin** | 962.3 | E858.0 | E932.3 | E950.4 | E962.0 | E980.4 |
| **Glucagon** | 962.3 | E858.0 | E932.3 | E950.4 | E962.0 | E980.4 |
| **Glucochloral** | 967.1 | E852.0 | E937.1 | E950.2 | E962.0 | E980.2 |
| **Glucocorticoids** | 962.0 | E858.0 | E932.0 | E950.4 | E962.0 | E980.4 |
| **Glucose** | 974.5 | E858.5 | E944.5 | E950.4 | E962.0 | E980.4 |
| oxidase reagent | 977.8 | E858.8 | E947.8 | E950.4 | E962.0 | E980.4 |
| **Glucosulfone sodium** | 961.8 | E857 | E931.8 | E950.4 | E962.0 | E980.4 |
| **Glue(s)** | 989.89 | E866.6 | — | E950.9 | E962.1 | E980.9 |
| **Glutamic acid** (hydrochloride) | 973.4 | E858.4 | E943.4 | E950.4 | E962.0 | E980.4 |
| **Glutaraldehyde** | 989.89 | E861.4 | — | E950.9 | E962.1 | E980.9 |
| **Glutathione** | 963.8 | E858.1 | E933.8 | E950.4 | E962.0 | E980.4 |
| **Glutethimide** (group) | 967.5 | E852.4 | E937.5 | E950.2 | E962.0 | E980.2 |
| **Glycerin** (lotion) | 976.3 | E858.7 | E946.3 | E950.4 | E962.0 | E980.4 |
| **Glycerol** (topical) | 976.3 | E858.7 | E946.3 | E950.4 | E962.0 | E980.4 |
| **Glyceryl** | | | | | | |
| guaiacolate | 975.5 | E858.6 | E945.5 | E950.4 | E962.0 | E980.4 |
| triacetate (topical) | 976.0 | E858.7 | E946.0 | E950.4 | E962.0 | E980.4 |
| trinitrate | 972.4 | E858.3 | E942.4 | E950.4 | E962.0 | E980.4 |
| **Glycine** | 974.5 | E858.5 | E944.5 | E950.4 | E962.0 | E980.4 |
| **Glycobiarsol** | 961.1 | E857 | E931.1 | E950.4 | E962.0 | E980.4 |
| **Glycols** (ether) | 982.8 | E862.4 | — | E950.9 | E962.1 | E980.9 |
| **Glycopyrrolate** | 971.1 | E855.4 | E941.1 | E950.4 | E962.0 | E980.4 |
| **Glymidine** | 962.3 | E858.0 | E932.3 | E950.4 | E962.0 | E980.4 |
| **Gold** (compounds) (salts) | 965.69 | E850.6 | E935.6 | E950.0 | E962.0 | E980.0 |
| **Golden sulfide of antimony** | 985.4 | E866.2 | — | E950.9 | E962.1 | E980.9 |
| **Goldylocks** | 988.2 | E865.4 | — | E950.9 | E962.1 | E980.9 |
| **Gonadal tissue extract** | 962.9 | E858.0 | E932.9 | E950.4 | E962.0 | E980.4 |
| beverage | 980.0 | E860.0 | — | E950.9 | E962.1 | E980.9 |
| female | 962.2 | E858.0 | E932.2 | E950.4 | E962.0 | E980.4 |
| male | 962.1 | E858.0 | E932.1 | E950.4 | E962.0 | E980.4 |
| **Gonadotropin** | 962.4 | E858.0 | E932.4 | E950.4 | E962.0 | E980.4 |
| **Grain alcohol** | 980.0 | E860.1 | — | E950.9 | E962.1 | E980.9 |
| **Gramicidin** | 960.8 | E856 | E930.8 | E950.4 | E962.0 | E980.4 |
| **Gratiola officinalis** | 988.2 | E865.4 | — | E950.9 | E962.1 | E980.9 |
| **Grease** | 989.89 | E866.8 | — | E950.9 | E962.1 | E980.9 |
| **Green hellebore** | 988.2 | E865.4 | — | E950.9 | E962.1 | E980.9 |
| **Green soap** | 976.2 | E858.7 | E946.2 | E950.4 | E962.0 | E980.4 |
| **Grifulvin** | 960.1 | E856 | E930.1 | E950.4 | E962.0 | E980.4 |
| **Griseofulvin** | 960.1 | E856 | E930.1 | E950.4 | E962.0 | E980.4 |
| **Growth hormone** | 962.4 | E858.0 | E932.4 | E950.4 | E962.0 | E980.4 |
| **Guaiacol** | 975.5 | E858.6 | E945.5 | E950.4 | E962.0 | E980.4 |
| **Guaiac reagent** | 977.8 | E858.8 | E947.8 | E950.4 | E962.0 | E980.4 |
| **Guaifenesin** | 975.5 | E858.6 | E945.5 | E950.4 | E962.0 | E980.4 |
| **Guaiphenesin** | 975.5 | E858.6 | E945.5 | E950.4 | E962.0 | E980.4 |
| **Guanatol** | 961.4 | E857 | E931.4 | E950.4 | E962.0 | E980.4 |
| **Guanethidine** | 972.6 | E858.3 | E942.6 | E950.4 | E962.0 | E980.4 |
| **Guano** | 989.89 | E866.5 | — | E950.9 | E962.1 | E980.9 |
| **Guanochlor** | 972.6 | E858.3 | E942.6 | E950.4 | E962.0 | E980.4 |
| **Guanoctine** | 972.6 | E858.3 | E942.6 | E950.4 | E962.0 | E980.4 |
| **Guanoxan** | 972.6 | E858.3 | E942.6 | E950.4 | E962.0 | E980.4 |
| **Hair treatment agent NEC** | 976.4 | E858.7 | E946.4 | E950.4 | E962.0 | E980.4 |
| **Halcinonide** | 976.0 | E858.7 | E946.0 | E950.4 | E962.0 | E980.4 |
| **Halethazole** | 976.0 | E858.7 | E946.0 | E950.4 | E962.0 | E980.4 |
| **Hallucinogens** | 969.6 | E854.1 | E939.6 | E950.3 | E962.0 | E980.3 |
| **Haloperidol** | 969.2 | E853.1 | E939.2 | E950.3 | E962.0 | E980.3 |
| **Haloprogin** | 976.0 | E858.7 | E946.0 | E950.4 | E962.0 | E980.4 |
| **Halotex** | 976.0 | E858.7 | E946.0 | E950.4 | E962.0 | E980.4 |
| **Halothane** | 968.1 | E855.1 | E938.1 | E950.4 | E962.0 | E980.4 |
| **Halquinols** | 976.0 | E858.7 | E946.0 | E950.4 | E962.0 | E980.4 |
| **Harmonyl** | 972.6 | E858.3 | E942.6 | E950.4 | E962.0 | E980.4 |
| **Hartmann's solution** | 974.5 | E858.5 | E944.5 | E950.4 | E962.0 | E980.4 |
| **Hashish** | 969.6 | E854.1 | E939.6 | E950.3 | E962.0 | E980.3 |

☑ Additional Digit Required — Refer to the Tabular List for Digit Selection

▽ Subterms under main terms may continue to next column or page

| | | External Cause (E-Code) | | | | |
|---|---|---|---|---|---|---|
| | Poisoning | Accident | Therapeutic Use | Suicide Attempt | Assault | Undetermined |
| **Hawaiian wood rose seeds** | 969.6 | E854.1 | E939.6 | E950.3 | E962.0 | E980.3 |
| **Headache cures, drugs, powders NEC** | 977.9 | E858.9 | E947.9 | E950.5 | E962.0 | E980.9 |
| **Heavenly Blue** (morning glory) | 969.6 | E854.1 | E939.6 | E950.3 | E962.0 | E980.3 |
| **Heavy metal antagonists** | 963.8 | E858.1 | E933.8 | E950.4 | E962.0 | E980.4 |
| anti-infectives | 961.2 | E857 | E931.2 | E950.4 | E962.0 | E980.4 |
| **Hedaquinium** | 976.0 | E858.7 | E946.0 | E950.4 | E962.0 | E980.4 |
| **Hedge hyssop** | 988.2 | E865.4 | — | E950.9 | E962.1 | E980.9 |
| **Heet** | 976.8 | E858.7 | E946.8 | E950.4 | E962.0 | E980.4 |
| **Helenin** | 961.6 | E857 | E931.6 | E950.4 | E962.0 | E980.4 |
| **Hellebore** (black) (green) (white) | 988.2 | E865.4 | — | E950.9 | E962.1 | E980.9 |
| **Hemlock** | 988.2 | E865.4 | — | E950.9 | E962.1 | E980.9 |
| **Hemostatics** | 964.5 | E858.2 | E934.5 | E950.4 | E962.0 | E980.4 |
| capillary active drugs | 972.8 | E858.3 | E942.8 | E950.4 | E962.0 | E980.4 |
| **Henbane** | 988.2 | E865.4 | — | E950.9 | E962.1 | E980.9 |
| **Heparin** (sodium) | 964.2 | E858.2 | E934.2 | E950.4 | E962.0 | E980.4 |
| **Heptabarbital, heptabarbitone** | 967.0 | E851 | E937.0 | E950.1 | E962.0 | E980.1 |
| **Heptachlor** | 989.2 | E863.0 | — | E950.6 | E962.1 | E980.7 |
| **Heptalgin** | 965.09 | E850.2 | E935.2 | E950.0 | E962.0 | E980.0 |
| **Herbicides** | 989.4 | E863.5 | — | E950.6 | E962.1 | E980.7 |
| **Heroin** | 965.01 | E850.0 | E935.0 | E950.0 | E962.0 | E980.0 |
| **Herplex** | 976.5 | E858.7 | E946.5 | E950.4 | E962.0 | E980.4 |
| **HES** | 964.8 | E858.2 | E934.8 | E950.4 | E962.0 | E980.4 |
| **Hetastarch** | 964.8 | E858.2 | E934.8 | E950.4 | E962.0 | E980.4 |
| **Hexachlorocyclohexane** | 989.2 | E863.0 | — | E950.6 | E962.1 | E980.7 |
| **Hexachlorophene** | 976.2 | E858.7 | E946.2 | E950.4 | E962.0 | E980.4 |
| **Hexadimethrine** (bromide) | 964.5 | E858.2 | E934.5 | E950.4 | E962.0 | E980.4 |
| **Hexafluorenium** | 975.2 | E858.6 | E945.2 | E950.4 | E962.0 | E980.4 |
| **Hexa-germ** | 976.2 | E858.7 | E946.2 | E950.4 | E962.0 | E980.4 |
| **Hexahydrophenol** | 980.8 | E860.8 | — | E950.9 | E962.1 | E980.9 |
| **Hexalin** | 980.8 | E860.8 | — | E950.9 | E962.1 | E980.9 |
| **Hexamethonium** | 972.3 | E858.3 | E942.3 | E950.4 | E962.0 | E980.4 |
| **Hexamethyleneamine** | 961.9 | E857 | E931.9 | E950.4 | E962.0 | E980.4 |
| **Hexamine** | 961.9 | E857 | E931.9 | E950.4 | E962.0 | E980.4 |
| **Hexanone** | 982.8 | E862.4 | — | E950.9 | E962.1 | E980.9 |
| **Hexapropymate** | 967.8 | E852.8 | E937.8 | E950.2 | E962.0 | E980.2 |
| **Hexestrol** | 962.2 | E858.0 | E932.2 | E950.4 | E962.0 | E980.4 |
| **Hexethal** (sodium) | 967.0 | E851 | E937.0 | E950.1 | E962.0 | E980.1 |
| **Hexetidine** | 976.0 | E858.7 | E946.0 | E950.4 | E962.0 | E980.4 |
| **Hexobarbital, hexobarbitone** | 967.0 | E851 | E937.0 | E950.1 | E962.0 | E980.1 |
| sodium (anesthetic) | 968.3 | E855.1 | E938.3 | E950.4 | E962.0 | E980.4 |
| soluble | 968.3 | E855.1 | E938.3 | E950.4 | E962.0 | E980.4 |
| **Hexocyclium** | 971.1 | E855.4 | E941.1 | E950.4 | E962.0 | E980.4 |
| **Hexoestrol** | 962.2 | E858.0 | E932.2 | E950.4 | E962.0 | E980.4 |
| **Hexone** | 982.8 | E862.4 | — | E950.9 | E962.1 | E980.9 |
| **Hexylcaine** | 968.5 | E855.2 | E938.5 | E950.4 | E962.0 | E980.4 |
| **Hexylresorcinol** | 961.6 | E857 | E931.6 | E950.4 | E962.0 | E980.4 |
| **Hinkle's pills** | 973.1 | E858.4 | E943.1 | E950.4 | E962.0 | E980.4 |
| **Histalog** | 977.8 | E858.8 | E947.8 | E950.4 | E962.0 | E980.4 |
| **Histamine** (phosphate) | 972.5 | E858.3 | E942.5 | E950.4 | E962.0 | E980.4 |
| **Histoplasmin** | 977.8 | E858.8 | E947.8 | E950.4 | E962.0 | E980.4 |
| **Holly berries** | 988.2 | E865.3 | — | E950.9 | E962.1 | E980.9 |
| **Homatropine** | 971.1 | E855.4 | E941.1 | E950.4 | E962.0 | E980.4 |
| **Homo-tet** | 964.6 | E858.2 | E934.6 | E950.4 | E962.0 | E980.4 |
| **Hormones** (synthetic substitute) | | | | | | |
| NEC | 962.9 | E858.0 | E932.9 | E950.4 | E962.0 | E980.4 |
| adrenal cortical steroids | 962.0 | E858.0 | E932.0 | E950.4 | E962.0 | E980.4 |
| antidiabetic agents | 962.3 | E858.0 | E932.3 | E950.4 | E962.0 | E980.4 |
| follicle stimulating | 962.4 | E858.0 | E932.4 | E950.4 | E962.0 | E980.4 |
| gonadotropic | 962.4 | E858.0 | E932.4 | E950.4 | E962.0 | E980.4 |
| growth | 962.4 | E858.0 | E932.4 | E950.4 | E962.0 | E980.4 |
| ovarian (substitutes) | 962.2 | E858.0 | E932.2 | E950.4 | E962.0 | E980.4 |
| parathyroid (derivatives) | 962.6 | E858.0 | E932.6 | E950.4 | E962.0 | E980.4 |
| pituitary (posterior) | 962.5 | E858.0 | E932.5 | E950.4 | E962.0 | E980.4 |
| anterior | 962.4 | E858.0 | E932.4 | E950.4 | E962.0 | E980.4 |
| thyroid (derivative) | 962.7 | E858.0 | E932.7 | E950.4 | E962.0 | E980.4 |
| **Hornet** (sting) | 989.5 | E905.3 | — | E950.9 | E962.1 | E980.9 |
| **Horticulture agent NEC** | 989.4 | E863.9 | — | E950.6 | E962.1 | E980.7 |
| **Hyaluronidase** | 963.4 | E858.1 | E933.4 | E950.4 | E962.0 | E980.4 |
| **Hyazyme** | 963.4 | E858.1 | E933.4 | E950.4 | E962.0 | E980.4 |
| **Hycodan** | 965.09 | E850.2 | E935.2 | E950.0 | E962.0 | E980.0 |
| **Hydantoin derivatives** | 966.1 | E855.0 | E936.1 | E950.4 | E962.0 | E980.4 |
| **Hydeltra** | 962.0 | E858.0 | E932.0 | E950.4 | E962.0 | E980.4 |
| **Hydergine** | 971.3 | E855.6 | E941.3 | E950.4 | E962.0 | E980.4 |
| **Hydrabamine penicillin** | 960.0 | E856 | E930.0 | E950.4 | E962.0 | E980.4 |
| **Hydralazine, hydrallazine** | 972.6 | E858.3 | E942.6 | E950.4 | E962.0 | E980.4 |
| **Hydrargaphen** | 976.0 | E858.7 | E946.0 | E950.4 | E962.0 | E980.4 |
| **Hydrazine** | 983.9 | E864.3 | — | E950.7 | E962.1 | E980.6 |
| **Hydriodic acid** | 975.5 | E858.6 | E945.5 | E950.4 | E962.0 | E980.4 |
| **Hydrocarbon gas** | 987.1 | E869.8 | — | E952.8 | E962.2 | E982.8 |
| incomplete combustion of — see Carbon, monoxide, fuel, utility | | | | | | |
| liquefied (mobile container) | 987.0 | E868.0 | — | E951.1 | E962.2 | E981.1 |
| piped (natural) | 987.0 | E867 | — | E951.0 | E962.2 | E981.0 |
| **Hydrochloric acid** (liquid) | 983.1 | E864.1 | — | E950.7 | E962.1 | E980.6 |
| medicinal | 973.4 | E858.4 | E943.4 | E950.4 | E962.0 | E980.4 |
| vapor | 987.8 | E869.8 | — | E952.8 | E962.2 | E982.8 |
| **Hydrochlorothiazide** | 974.3 | E858.5 | E944.3 | E950.4 | E962.0 | E980.4 |
| **Hydrocodone** | 965.09 | E850.2 | E935.2 | E950.0 | E962.0 | E980.0 |
| **Hydrocortisone** | 962.0 | E858.0 | E932.0 | E950.4 | E962.0 | E980.4 |
| ENT agent | 976.6 | E858.7 | E946.6 | E950.4 | E962.0 | E980.4 |
| ophthalmic preparation | 976.5 | E858.7 | E946.5 | E950.4 | E962.0 | E980.4 |
| topical NEC | 976.0 | E858.7 | E946.0 | E950.4 | E962.0 | E980.4 |
| **Hydrocortone** | 962.0 | E858.0 | E932.0 | E950.4 | E962.0 | E980.4 |
| ENT agent | 976.6 | E858.7 | E946.6 | E950.4 | E962.0 | E980.4 |
| ophthalmic preparation | 976.5 | E858.7 | E946.5 | E950.4 | E962.0 | E980.4 |
| topical NEC | 976.0 | E858.7 | E946.0 | E950.4 | E962.0 | E980.4 |
| **Hydrocyanic acid** — see Cyanide(s) | | | | | | |
| **Hydroflumethiazide** | 974.3 | E858.5 | E944.3 | E950.4 | E962.0 | E980.4 |
| **Hydrofluoric acid** (liquid) | 983.1 | E864.1 | — | E950.7 | E962.1 | E980.6 |
| vapor | 987.8 | E869.8 | — | E952.8 | E962.2 | E982.8 |
| **Hydrogen** | 987.8 | E869.8 | — | E952.8 | E962.2 | E982.8 |
| arsenide | 985.1 | E866.3 | -- | E950.8 | E962.1 | E980.8 |
| arseniureted | 985.1 | E866.3 | | E950.8 | E962.1 | E980.8 |
| cyanide (salts) | 989.0 | E866.8 | — | E950.9 | E962.1 | E980.9 |
| gas | 987.7 | E869.8 | — | E952.8 | E962.2 | E982.8 |
| fluoride (liquid) | 983.1 | E864.1 | — | E950.7 | E962.1 | E980.6 |
| vapor | 987.8 | E869.8 | — | E952.8 | E962.2 | E982.8 |
| peroxide (solution) | 976.6 | E858.7 | E946.6 | E950.4 | E962.0 | E980.4 |
| phosphureted | 987.8 | E869.8 | — | E952.8 | E962.2 | E982.8 |
| sulfide (gas) | 987.8 | E869.8 | — | E952.8 | E962.2 | E982.8 |
| arseniureted | 985.1 | E866.3 | — | E950.8 | E962.1 | E980.8 |
| sulfureted | 987.8 | E869.8 | — | E952.8 | E962.2 | E982.8 |
| **Hydromorphinol** | 965.09 | E850.2 | E935.2 | E950.0 | E962.0 | E980.0 |
| **Hydromorphinone** | 965.09 | E850.2 | E935.2 | E950.0 | E962.0 | E980.0 |
| **Hydromorphone** | 965.09 | E850.2 | E935.2 | E950.0 | E962.0 | E980.0 |
| **Hydromox** | 974.3 | E858.5 | E944.3 | E950.4 | E962.0 | E980.4 |
| **Hydrophilic lotion** | 976.3 | E858.7 | E946.3 | E950.4 | E962.0 | E980.4 |
| **Hydroquinone** | 983.0 | E864.0 | — | E950.7 | E962.1 | E980.6 |
| vapor | 987.8 | E869.8 | — | E952.8 | E962.2 | E982.8 |
| **Hydrosulfuric acid** (gas) | 987.8 | E869.8 | — | E952.8 | E962.2 | E982.8 |
| **Hydrous wool fat** (lotion) | 976.3 | E858.7 | E946.3 | E950.4 | E962.0 | E980.4 |
| **Hydroxide, caustic** | 983.2 | E864.2 | — | E950.7 | E962.1 | E980.6 |
| **Hydroxocobalamin** | 964.1 | E858.2 | E934.1 | E950.4 | E962.0 | E980.4 |
| **Hydroxyamphetamine** | 971.2 | E855.5 | E941.2 | E950.4 | E962.0 | E980.4 |
| **Hydroxychloroquine** | 961.4 | E857 | E931.4 | E950.4 | E962.0 | E980.4 |
| **Hydroxydihydrocodeinone** | 965.09 | E850.2 | E935.2 | E950.0 | E962.0 | E980.0 |
| **Hydroxyethyl starch** | 964.8 | E858.2 | E934.8 | E950.4 | E962.0 | E980.4 |
| **Hydroxyphenamate** | 969.5 | E853.8 | E939.5 | E950.3 | E962.0 | E980.3 |
| **Hydroxyphenylbutazone** | 965.5 | E850.5 | E935.5 | E950.0 | E962.0 | E980.0 |
| **Hydroxyprogesterone** | 962.2 | E858.0 | E932.2 | E950.4 | E962.0 | E980.4 |
| **Hydroxyquinoline derivatives** | 961.3 | E857 | E931.3 | E950.4 | E962.0 | E980.4 |
| **Hydroxystilbamidine** | 961.5 | E857 | E931.5 | E950.4 | E962.0 | E980.4 |
| **Hydroxyurea** | 963.1 | E858.1 | E933.1 | E950.4 | E962.0 | E980.4 |
| **Hydroxyzine** | 969.5 | E853.8 | E939.5 | E950.3 | E962.0 | E980.3 |
| **Hyoscine** (hydrobromide) | 971.1 | E855.4 | E941.1 | E950.4 | E962.0 | E980.4 |
| **Hyoscyamine** | 971.1 | E855.4 | E941.1 | E950.4 | E962.0 | E980.4 |
| **Hyoscyamus** (albus)(niger) | 988.2 | E865.4 | — | E950.9 | E962.1 | E980.9 |
| **Hypaque** | 977.8 | E858.8 | E947.8 | E950.4 | E962.0 | E980.4 |
| **Hypertussis** | 964.6 | E858.2 | E934.6 | E950.4 | E962.0 | E980.4 |
| **Hypnotics NEC** | 967.9 | E852.9 | E937.9 | E950.2 | E962.0 | E980.2 |
| **Hypochlorites** — see Sodium, hypochlorite | | | | | | |
| **Hypotensive agents NEC** | 972.6 | E858.3 | E942.6 | E950.4 | E962.0 | E980.4 |
| **Ibufenac** | 965.69 | E850.6 | E935.6 | E950.0 | E962.0 | E980.0 |
| **Ibuprofen** | 965.61 | E850.6 | E935.6 | E950.0 | E962.0 | E980.0 |
| **ICG** | 977.8 | E858.8 | E947.8 | E950.4 | E962.0 | E980.4 |
| **Ichthammol** | 976.4 | E858.7 | E946.4 | E950.4 | E962.0 | E980.4 |
| **Ichthyol** | 976.4 | E858.7 | E946.4 | E950.4 | E962.0 | E980.4 |
| **Idoxuridine** | 976.5 | E858.7 | E946.5 | E950.4 | E962.0 | E980.4 |
| **IDU** | 976.5 | E858.7 | E946.5 | E950.4 | E962.0 | E980.4 |
| **Iletin** | 962.3 | E858.0 | E932.3 | E950.4 | E962.0 | E980.4 |
| **Ilex** | 988.2 | E865.4 | — | E950.9 | E962.1 | E980.9 |

☑ Additional Digit Required — Refer to the Tabular List for Digit Selection

▽ Subterms under main terms may continue to next column or page

▶◀ Revised Text    ● New Line    ▲ Revised Code

*2008 ICD-9-CM*

| | Poisoning | Accident (E-Code) | Therapeutic Use | Suicide Attempt | Assault | Undetermined |
|---|---|---|---|---|---|---|
| **Illuminating gas** — see Gas, utility | | | | | | |
| **Ilopan** | 963.5 | E858.1 | E933.5 | E950.4 | E962.0 | E980.4 |
| **Ilotycin** | 960.3 | E856 | E930.3 | E950.4 | E962.0 | E980.4 |
|   ophthalmic preparation | 976.5 | E858.7 | E946.5 | E950.4 | E962.0 | E980.4 |
|   topical NEC | 976.0 | E858.7 | E946.0 | E950.4 | E962.0 | E980.4 |
| **Imipramine** | 969.0 | E854.0 | E939.0 | E950.3 | E962.0 | E980.3 |
| **Immu-G** | 964.6 | E858.2 | E934.6 | E950.4 | E962.0 | E980.4 |
| **Immuglobin** | 964.6 | E858.2 | E934.6 | E950.4 | E962.0 | E980.4 |
| **Immune serum globulin** | 964.6 | E858.2 | E934.6 | E950.4 | E962.0 | E980.4 |
| **Immunosuppressive agents** | 963.1 | E858.1 | E933.1 | E950.4 | E962.0 | E980.4 |
| **Immu-tetanus** | 964.6 | E858.2 | E934.6 | E950.4 | E962.0 | E980.4 |
| **Indandione** (derivatives) | 964.2 | E858.2 | E934.2 | E950.4 | E962.0 | E980.4 |
| **Inderal** | 972.0 | E858.3 | E942.0 | E950.4 | E962.0 | E980.4 |
| **Indian** | | | | | | |
|   hemp | 969.6 | E854.1 | E939.6 | E950.3 | E962.0 | E980.3 |
|   tobacco | 988.2 | E865.4 | — | E950.9 | E962.1 | E980.9 |
| **Indigo carmine** | 977.8 | E858.8 | E947.8 | E950.4 | E962.0 | E980.4 |
| **Indocin** | 965.69 | E850.6 | E935.6 | E950.0 | E962.0 | E980.0 |
| **Indocyanine green** | 977.8 | E858.8 | E947.8 | E950.4 | E962.0 | E980.4 |
| **Indomethacin** | 965.69 | E850.6 | E935.6 | E950.0 | E962.0 | E980.0 |
| **Industrial** | | | | | | |
|   alcohol | 980.9 | E860.9 | — | E950.9 | E962.1 | E980.9 |
|   fumes | 987.8 | E869.8 | — | E952.8 | E962.2 | E982.8 |
|   solvents (fumes) (vapors) | 982.8 | E862.9 | — | E950.9 | E962.1 | E980.9 |
| **Influenza vaccine** | 979.6 | E858.8 | E949.6 | E950.4 | E962.0 | E982.8 |
| **Ingested substances NEC** | 989.9 | E866.9 | — | E950.9 | E962.1 | E980.9 |
| **INH** (isoniazid) | 961.8 | E857 | E931.8 | E950.4 | E962.0 | E980.4 |
| **Inhalation, gas** (noxious) — see Gas | | | | | | |
| **Ink** | 989.89 | E866.8 | — | E950.9 | E962.1 | E980.9 |
| **Innovar** | 967.6 | E852.5 | E937.6 | E950.2 | E962.0 | E980.2 |
| **Inositol niacinate** | 972.2 | E858.3 | E942.2 | E950.4 | E962.0 | E980.4 |
| **Inproquone** | 963.1 | E858.1 | E933.1 | E950.4 | E962.0 | E980.4 |
| **Insecticides** — see also Pesticides | 989.4 | E863.4 | — | E950.6 | E962.1 | E980.7 |
|   chlorinated | 989.2 | E863.0 | — | E950.6 | E962.1 | E980.7 |
|   mixtures | 989.4 | E863.3 | — | E950.6 | E962.1 | E980.7 |
|   organochlorine (compounds) | 989.2 | E863.0 | — | E950.6 | E962.1 | E980.7 |
|   organophosphorus (compounds) | 989.3 | E863.1 | — | E950.6 | E962.1 | E980.7 |
| **Insect (sting), venomous** | 989.5 | E905.5 | — | E950.9 | E962.1 | E980.9 |
| **Insular tissue extract** | 962.3 | E858.0 | E932.3 | E950.4 | E962.0 | E980.4 |
| **Insulin** (amorphous) (globin) (isophane) (Lente) (NPH) (protamine) (Semilente) (Ultralente) (zinc) | 962.3 | E858.0 | E932.3 | E950.4 | E962.0 | E980.4 |
| **Intranarcon** | 968.3 | E855.1 | E938.3 | E950.4 | E962.0 | E980.4 |
| **Inulin** | 977.8 | E858.8 | E947.8 | E950.4 | E962.0 | E980.4 |
| **Invert sugar** | 974.5 | E858.5 | E944.5 | E950.4 | E962.0 | E980.4 |
| **Inza** — see Naproxen | | | | | | |
| **Iodide NEC** — see also Iodine | | | | | | |
|   Iodine | 976.0 | E858.7 | E946.0 | E950.4 | E962.0 | E980.4 |
|   mercury (ointment) | 976.0 | E858.7 | E946.0 | E950.4 | E962.0 | E980.4 |
|   methylate | 976.0 | E858.7 | E946.0 | E950.4 | E962.0 | E980.4 |
|   potassium (expectorant) NEC | 975.5 | E858.6 | E945.5 | E950.4 | E962.0 | E980.4 |
| **Iodinated glycerol** | 975.5 | E858.6 | E945.5 | E950.4 | E962.0 | E980.4 |
| **Iodine** (antiseptic, external) (tincture) NEC | 976.0 | E858.7 | E946.0 | E950.4 | E962.0 | E980.4 |
|   diagnostic | 977.8 | E858.8 | E947.8 | E950.4 | E962.0 | E980.4 |
|   for thyroid conditions (antithyroid) | 962.8 | E858.0 | E932.8 | E950.4 | E962.0 | E980.4 |
|   vapor | 987.8 | E869.8 | — | E952.8 | E962.2 | E982.8 |
| **Iodized oil** | 977.8 | E858.8 | E947.8 | E950.4 | E962.0 | E980.4 |
| **Iodobismitol** | 961.2 | E857 | E931.2 | E950.4 | E962.0 | E980.4 |
| **Iodochlorhydroxyquin** | 961.3 | E857 | E931.3 | E950.4 | E962.0 | E980.4 |
|   topical | 976.0 | E858.7 | E946.0 | E950.4 | E962.0 | E980.4 |
| **Iodoform** | 976.0 | E858.7 | E946.0 | E950.4 | E962.0 | E980.4 |
| **Iodopanoic acid** | 977.8 | E858.8 | E947.8 | E950.4 | E962.0 | E980.4 |
| **Iodophthalein** | 977.8 | E858.8 | E947.8 | E950.4 | E962.0 | E980.4 |
| **Ion exchange resins** | 974.5 | E858.5 | E944.5 | E950.4 | E962.0 | E980.4 |
| **Iopanoic acid** | 977.8 | E858.8 | E947.8 | E950.4 | E962.0 | E980.4 |
| **Iophendylate** | 977.8 | E858.8 | E947.8 | E950.4 | E962.0 | E980.4 |
| **Iothiouracil** | 962.8 | E858.0 | E932.8 | E950.4 | E962.0 | E980.4 |
| **Ipecac** | 973.6 | E858.4 | E943.6 | E950.4 | E962.0 | E980.4 |
| **Ipecacuanha** | 973.6 | E858.4 | E943.6 | E950.4 | E962.0 | E980.4 |
| **Ipodate** | 977.8 | E858.8 | E947.8 | E950.4 | E962.0 | E980.4 |
| **Ipral** | 967.0 | E851 | E937.0 | E950.1 | E962.0 | E980.1 |
| **Ipratropium** | 975.1 | E858.6 | E945.1 | E950.4 | E962.0 | E980.4 |
| **Iproniazid** | 969.0 | E854.0 | E939.0 | E950.3 | E962.0 | E980.3 |
| **Iron** (compounds) (medicinal) (preparations) | 964.0 | E858.2 | E934.0 | E950.4 | E962.0 | E980.4 |
|   dextran | 964.0 | E858.2 | E934.0 | E950.4 | E962.0 | E980.4 |
|   nonmedicinal (dust) (fumes) NEC | 985.8 | E866.4 | — | E950.9 | E962.1 | E980.9 |
| **Irritant drug** | 977.9 | E858.9 | E947.9 | E950.5 | E962.0 | E980.5 |
| **Ismelin** | 972.6 | E858.3 | E942.6 | E950.4 | E962.0 | E980.4 |
| **Isoamyl nitrite** | 972.4 | E858.3 | E942.4 | E950.4 | E962.0 | E980.4 |
| **Isobutyl acetate** | 982.8 | E862.4 | — | E950.9 | E962.1 | E980.9 |
| **Isocarboxazid** | 969.0 | E854.0 | E939.0 | E950.3 | E962.0 | E980.3 |
| **Isoephedrine** | 971.2 | E855.5 | E941.2 | E950.4 | E962.0 | E980.4 |
| **Isoetharine** | 971.2 | E855.5 | E941.2 | E950.4 | E962.0 | E980.4 |
| **Isofluorophate** | 971.0 | E855.3 | E941.0 | E950.4 | E962.0 | E980.4 |
| **Isoniazid** (INH) | 961.8 | E857 | E931.8 | E950.4 | E962.0 | E980.4 |
| **Isopentaquine** | 961.4 | E857 | E931.4 | E950.4 | E962.0 | E980.4 |
| **Isophane insulin** | 962.3 | E858.0 | E932.3 | E950.4 | E962.0 | E980.4 |
| **Isopregnenone** | 962.2 | E858.0 | E932.2 | E950.4 | E962.0 | E980.4 |
| **Isoprenaline** | 971.2 | E855.5 | E941.2 | E950.4 | E962.0 | E980.4 |
| **Isopropamide** | 971.1 | E855.4 | E941.1 | E950.4 | E962.0 | E980.4 |
| **Isopropanol** | 980.2 | E860.3 | — | E950.9 | E962.1 | E980.9 |
|   topical (germicide) | 976.0 | E858.7 | E946.0 | E950.4 | E962.0 | E980.4 |
| **Isopropyl** | | | | | | |
|   acetate | 982.8 | E862.4 | — | E950.9 | E962.1 | E980.9 |
|   alcohol | 980.2 | E860.3 | — | E950.9 | E962.1 | E980.9 |
|    topical (germicide) | 976.0 | E858.7 | E946.0 | E950.4 | E962.0 | E980.4 |
|   ether | 982.8 | E862.4 | — | E950.9 | E962.1 | E980.9 |
| **Isoproterenol** | 971.2 | E855.5 | E941.2 | E950.4 | E962.0 | E980.4 |
| **Isosorbide dinitrate** | 972.4 | E858.3 | E942.4 | E950.4 | E962.0 | E980.4 |
| **Isothipendyl** | 963.0 | E858.1 | E933.0 | E950.4 | E962.0 | E980.4 |
| **Isoxazolyl penicillin** | 960.0 | E856 | E930.0 | E950.4 | E962.0 | E980.4 |
| **Isoxsuprine hydrochloride** | 972.5 | E858.3 | E942.5 | E950.4 | E962.0 | E980.4 |
| **I-thyroxine sodium** | 962.7 | E858.0 | E932.7 | E950.4 | E962.0 | E980.4 |
| **Jaborandi** (pilocarpus) (extract) | 971.0 | E855.3 | E941.0 | E950.4 | E962.0 | E980.4 |
| **Jalap** | 973.1 | E858.4 | E943.1 | E950.4 | E962.0 | E980.4 |
| **Jamaica** | | | | | | |
|   dogwood (bark) | 965.7 | E850.7 | E935.7 | E950.0 | E962.0 | E980.0 |
|   ginger | 989.89 | E866.8 | — | E950.9 | E962.1 | E980.9 |
| **Jatropha** | 988.2 | E865.4 | — | E950.9 | E962.1 | E980.9 |
|   curcas | 988.2 | E865.3 | — | E950.9 | E962.1 | E980.9 |
| **Jectofer** | 964.0 | E858.2 | E934.0 | E950.4 | E962.0 | E980.4 |
| **Jellyfish** (sting) | 989.5 | E905.6 | — | E950.9 | E962.1 | E980.9 |
| **Jequirity** (bean) | 988.2 | E865.3 | — | E950.9 | E962.1 | E980.9 |
| **Jimson weed** | 988.2 | E865.4 | — | E950.9 | E962.1 | E980.9 |
|   seeds | 988.2 | E865.3 | — | E950.9 | E962.1 | E980.9 |
| **Juniper tar** (oil) (ointment) | 976.4 | E858.7 | E946.4 | E950.4 | E962.0 | E980.4 |
| **Kallikrein** | 972.5 | E858.3 | E942.5 | E950.4 | E962.0 | E980.4 |
| **Kanamycin** | 960.6 | E856 | E930.6 | E950.4 | E962.0 | E980.4 |
| **Kantrex** | 960.6 | E856 | E930.6 | E950.4 | E962.0 | E980.4 |
| **Kaolin** | 973.5 | E858.4 | E943.5 | E950.4 | E962.0 | E980.4 |
| **Karaya** (gum) | 973.3 | E858.4 | E943.3 | E950.4 | E962.0 | E980.4 |
| **Kemithal** | 968.3 | E855.1 | E938.3 | E950.4 | E962.0 | E980.4 |
| **Kenacort** | 962.0 | E858.0 | E932.0 | E950.4 | E962.0 | E980.4 |
| **Keratolytics** | 976.4 | E858.7 | E946.4 | E950.4 | E962.0 | E980.4 |
| **Keratoplastics** | 976.4 | E858.7 | E946.4 | E950.4 | E962.0 | E980.4 |
| **Kerosene, kerosine (fuel) (solvent) NEC** | 981 | E862.1 | — | E950.9 | E962.1 | E980.9 |
|   insecticide | 981 | E863.4 | — | E950.6 | E962.1 | E980.7 |
|   vapor | 987.1 | E869.8 | — | E952.8 | E962.2 | E982.8 |
| **Ketamine** | 968.3 | E855.1 | E938.3 | E950.4 | E962.0 | E980.4 |
| **Ketobemidone** | 965.09 | E850.2 | E935.2 | E950.0 | E962.0 | E980.0 |
| **Ketols** | 982.8 | E862.4 | — | E950.9 | E962.1 | E980.9 |
| **Ketone oils** | 982.8 | E862.4 | — | E950.9 | E962.1 | E980.9 |
| **Ketoprofen** | 965.61 | E850.6 | E935.6 | E950.0 | E962.0 | E980 |
| **Kiln gas or vapor** (carbon monoxide) | 986 | E868.8 | — | E952.1 | E962.2 | E982.1 |
| **Konsyl** | 973.3 | E858.4 | E943.3 | E950.4 | E962.0 | E980.4 |
| **Kosam seed** | 988.2 | E865.3 | — | E950.9 | E962.1 | E980.9 |
| **Krait** (venom) | 989.5 | E905.0 | — | E950.9 | E962.1 | E980.9 |
| **Kwell** (insecticide) | 989.2 | E863.0 | — | E950.6 | E962.1 | E980.7 |
|   anti-infective (topical) | 976.0 | E858.7 | E946.0 | E950.4 | E962.0 | E980.4 |
| **Laburnum** (flowers) (seeds) | 988.2 | E865.3 | — | E950.9 | E962.1 | E980.9 |
|   leaves | 988.2 | E865.4 | — | E950.9 | E962.1 | E980.9 |
| **Lacquers** | 989.89 | E861.6 | — | E950.9 | E962.1 | E980.9 |
| **Lacrimogenic gas** | 987.5 | E869.3 | — | E952.8 | E962.2 | E982.8 |
| **Lactic acid** | 983.1 | E864.1 | — | E950.7 | E962.1 | E980.6 |
| **Lactobacillus acidophilus** | 973.5 | E858.4 | E943.5 | E950.4 | E962.0 | E980.4 |
| **Lactoflavin** | 963.5 | E858.1 | E933.5 | E950.4 | E962.0 | E980.4 |
| **Lactuca** (virosa) (extract) | 967.8 | E852.8 | E937.8 | E950.2 | E962.0 | E980.2 |

☑ Additional Digit Required — Refer to the Tabular List for Digit Selection
▶◀ Revised Text    ● New Line    ▲ Revised Code
▽ Subterms under main terms may continue to next column or page

| | Poisoning | Accident | Therapeutic Use | Suicide Attempt | Assault | Undetermined |
|---|---|---|---|---|---|---|
| **External Cause (E-Code)** | | | | | | |
| Lactucarium | 967.8 | E852.8 | E937.8 | E950.2 | E962.0 | E980.2 |
| Laevulose | 974.5 | E858.5 | E944.5 | E950.4 | E962.0 | E980.4 |
| Lanatoside (C) | 972.1 | E858.3 | E942.1 | E950.4 | E962.0 | E980.4 |
| Lanolin (lotion) | 976.3 | E858.7 | E946.3 | E950.4 | E962.0 | E980.4 |
| Largactil | 969.1 | E853.0 | E939.1 | E950.3 | E962.0 | E980.3 |
| Larkspur | 988.2 | E865.3 | — | E950.9 | E962.1 | E980.9 |
| Laroxyl | 969.0 | E854.0 | E939.0 | E950.3 | E962.0 | E980.3 |
| Lasix | 974.4 | E858.5 | E944.4 | E950.4 | E962.0 | E980.4 |
| Latex | 989.82 | E866.8 | — | E950.9 | E962.1 | E980.9 |
| Lathyrus (seed) | 988.2 | E865.3 | — | E950.9 | E962.1 | E980.9 |
| Laudanum | 965.09 | E850.2 | E935.2 | E950.0 | E962.0 | E980.0 |
| Laudexium | 975.2 | E858.6 | E945.2 | E950.4 | E962.0 | E980.4 |
| Laurel, black or cherry | 988.2 | E865.4 | — | E950.9 | E962.1 | E980.9 |
| Laurolinium | 976.0 | E858.7 | E946.0 | E950.4 | E962.0 | E980.4 |
| Lauryl sulfoacetate | 976.2 | E858.7 | E946.2 | E950.4 | E962.0 | E980.4 |
| Laxatives NEC | 973.3 | E858.4 | E943.3 | E950.4 | E962.0 | E980.4 |
| emollient | 973.2 | E858.4 | E943.2 | E950.4 | E962.0 | E980.4 |
| L-dopa | 966.4 | E855.0 | E936.4 | E950.4 | E962.0 | E980.4 |
| **Lead** (dust) (fumes) (vapor) **NEC** | 984.9 | E866.0 | — | E950.9 | E962.1 | E980.9 |
| acetate (dust) | 984.1 | E866.0 | — | E950.9 | E962.1 | E980.9 |
| anti-infectives | 961.2 | E857 | E931.2 | E950.4 | E962.0 | E980.4 |
| antiknock compound (tetraethyl) | 984.1 | E862.1 | — | E950.9 | E962.1 | E980.9 |
| arsenate, arsenite (dust) (insecticide) (vapor) | 985.1 | E863.4 | — | E950.8 | E962.1 | E980.8 |
| herbicide | 985.1 | E863.5 | — | E950.8 | E962.1 | E980.8 |
| carbonate | 984.0 | E866.0 | — | E950.9 | E962.1 | E980.9 |
| paint | 984.0 | E861.5 | — | E950.9 | E962.1 | E980.9 |
| chromate | 984.0 | E866.0 | — | E950.9 | E962.1 | E980.9 |
| paint | 984.0 | E861.5 | — | E950.9 | E962.1 | E980.9 |
| dioxide | 984.0 | E866.0 | — | E950.9 | E962.1 | E980.9 |
| inorganic (compound) | 984.0 | E866.0 | — | E950.9 | E962.1 | E980.9 |
| paint | 984.0 | E861.5 | — | E950.9 | E962.1 | E980.9 |
| iodide | 984.0 | E866.0 | — | E950.9 | E962.1 | E980.9 |
| pigment (paint) | 984.0 | E861.5 | — | E950.9 | E962.1 | E980.9 |
| monoxide (dust) | 984.0 | E866.0 | — | E950.9 | E962.1 | E980.9 |
| paint | 984.0 | E861.5 | — | E950.9 | E962.1 | E980.9 |
| organic | 984.1 | E866.0 | — | E950.9 | E962.1 | E980.9 |
| oxide | 984.0 | E866.0 | — | E950.9 | E962.1 | E980.9 |
| paint | 984.0 | E861.5 | — | E950.9 | E962.1 | E980.9 |
| paint | 984.0 | E861.5 | — | E950.9 | E962.1 | E980.9 |
| salts | 984.0 | E866.0 | — | E950.9 | E962.1 | E980.9 |
| specified compound NEC | 984.8 | E866.0 | — | E950.9 | E962.1 | E980.9 |
| tetra-ethyl | 984.1 | E862.1 | — | E950.9 | E962.1 | E980.9 |
| Lebanese red | 969.6 | E854.1 | E939.6 | E950.3 | E962.0 | E980.3 |
| Lente Iletin (insulin) | 962.3 | E858.0 | E932.3 | E950.4 | E962.0 | E980.4 |
| Leptazol | 970.0 | E854.3 | E940.0 | E950.4 | E962.0 | E980.4 |
| Leritine | 965.09 | E850.2 | E935.2 | E950.0 | E962.0 | E980.0 |
| Letter | 962.7 | E858.0 | E932.7 | E950.4 | E962.0 | E980.4 |
| Lettuce opium | 967.8 | E852.8 | E937.8 | E950.2 | E962.0 | E980.2 |
| Leucovorin (factor) | 964.1 | E858.2 | E934.1 | E950.4 | E962.0 | E980.4 |
| Leukeran | 963.1 | E858.1 | E933.1 | E950.4 | E962.0 | E980.4 |
| Levalbuterol | 975.7 | E858.6 | E945.7 | E950.4 | E962.0 | E980.4 |
| Levallorphan | 970.1 | E854.3 | E940.1 | E950.4 | E962.0 | E980.4 |
| Levanil | 967.8 | E852.8 | E937.8 | E950.2 | E962.0 | E980.2 |
| Levarterenol | 971.2 | E855.5 | E941.2 | E950.4 | E962.0 | E980.4 |
| Levodopa | 966.4 | E855.0 | E936.4 | E950.4 | E962.0 | E980.4 |
| Levo-dromoran | 965.09 | E850.2 | E935.2 | E950.0 | E962.0 | E980.0 |
| Levoid | 962.7 | E858.0 | E932.7 | E950.4 | E962.0 | E980.4 |
| Levo-iso-methadone | 965.02 | E850.1 | E935.1 | E950.0 | E962.0 | E980.0 |
| Levomepromazine | 967.8 | E852.8 | E937.8 | E950.2 | E962.0 | E980.2 |
| Levoprome | 967.8 | E852.8 | E937.8 | E950.2 | E962.0 | E980.2 |
| Levopropoxyphene | 975.4 | E858.6 | E945.4 | E950.4 | E962.0 | E980.4 |
| Levorphan, levorphanol | 965.09 | E850.2 | E935.2 | E950.0 | E962.0 | E980.0 |
| Levothyroxine (sodium) | 962.7 | E858.0 | E932.7 | E950.4 | E962.0 | E980.4 |
| Levsin | 971.1 | E855.4 | E941.1 | E950.4 | E962.0 | E980.4 |
| Levulose | 974.5 | E858.5 | E944.5 | E950.4 | E962.0 | E980.4 |
| Lewisite (gas) | 985.1 | E866.3 | — | E950.8 | E962.1 | E980.8 |
| Librium | 969.4 | E853.2 | E939.4 | E950.3 | E962.0 | E980.3 |
| Lidex | 976.0 | E858.7 | E946.0 | E950.4 | E962.0 | E980.4 |
| **Lidocaine** (infiltration) (topical) | 968.5 | E855.2 | E938.5 | E950.4 | E962.0 | E980.4 |
| nerve block (peripheral) (plexus) | 968.6 | E855.2 | E938.6 | E950.4 | E962.0 | E980.4 |
| spinal | 968.7 | E855.2 | E938.7 | E950.4 | E962.0 | E980.4 |
| Lighter fluid | 981 | E862.1 | — | E950.9 | E962.1 | E980.9 |
| **Lignocaine** (infiltration) (topical) | 968.5 | E855.2 | E938.5 | E950.4 | E962.0 | E980.4 |
| nerve block (peripheral) (plexus) | 968.6 | E855.2 | E938.6 | E950.4 | E962.0 | E980.4 |

| | Poisoning | Accident | Therapeutic Use | Suicide Attempt | Assault | Undetermined |
|---|---|---|---|---|---|---|
| **External Cause (E-Code)** | | | | | | |
| **Lignocaine** — continued | | | | | | |
| spinal | 968.7 | E855.2 | E938.7 | E950.4 | E962.0 | E980.4 |
| Ligroin(e) (solvent) | 981 | E862.0 | — | E950.9 | E962.1 | E980.9 |
| vapor | 987.1 | E869.8 | — | E952.8 | E962.2 | E982.8 |
| Ligustrum vulgare | 988.2 | E865.3 | — | E950.9 | E962.1 | E980.9 |
| Lily of the valley | 988.2 | E865.4 | — | E950.9 | E962.1 | E980.9 |
| Lime (chloride) | 983.2 | E864.2 | — | E950.7 | E962.1 | E980.6 |
| solution, sulferated | 976.4 | E858.7 | E946.4 | E950.4 | E962.0 | E980.4 |
| Limonene | 982.8 | E862.4 | — | E950.9 | E962.1 | E980.9 |
| Lincomycin | 960.8 | E856 | E930.8 | E950.4 | E962.0 | E980.4 |
| Lindane (insecticide) (vapor) | 989.2 | E863.0 | — | E950.6 | E962.1 | E980.7 |
| anti-infective (topical) | 976.0 | E858.7 | E946.0 | E950.4 | E962.0 | E980.4 |
| Liniments NEC | 976.9 | E858.7 | E946.9 | E950.4 | E962.0 | E980.4 |
| Linoleic acid | 972.2 | E858.3 | E942.2 | E950.4 | E962.0 | E980.4 |
| Liothyronine | 962.7 | E858.0 | E932.7 | E950.4 | E962.0 | E980.4 |
| Liotrix | 962.7 | E858.0 | E932.7 | E950.4 | E962.0 | E980.4 |
| Lipancreatin | 973.4 | E858.4 | E943.4 | E950.4 | E962.0 | E980.4 |
| Lipo-Lutin | 962.2 | E858.0 | E932.2 | E950.4 | E962.0 | E980.4 |
| Lipotropic agents | 977.1 | E858.8 | E947.1 | E950.4 | E962.0 | E980.4 |
| **Liquefied petroleum gases** | 987.0 | E868.0 | — | E951.1 | E962.2 | E981.1 |
| piped (pure or mixed with air) | 987.0 | E867 | — | E951.0 | E962.2 | E981.0 |
| Liquid petrolatum | 973.2 | E858.4 | E943.2 | E950.4 | E962.0 | E980.4 |
| substance | 989.9 | E866.9 | — | E950.9 | E962.1 | E980.9 |
| specified NEC | 989.89 | E866.8 | — | E950.9 | E962.1 | E980.9 |
| Lirugen | 979.4 | E858.8 | E949.4 | E950.4 | E962.0 | E980.4 |
| Lithane | 969.8 | E855.8 | E939.8 | E950.3 | E962.0 | E980.3 |
| Lithium | 985.8 | E866.4 | — | E950.9 | E962.1 | E980.9 |
| carbonate | 969.8 | E855.8 | E939.8 | E950.3 | E962.0 | E980.3 |
| Lithonate | 969.8 | E855.8 | E939.8 | E950.3 | E962.0 | E980.3 |
| **Liver** (extract) (injection) (preparations) | 964.1 | E858.2 | E934.1 | E950.4 | E962.0 | E980.4 |
| Lizard (bite) (venom) | 989.5 | E905.0 | — | E950.9 | E962.1 | E980.9 |
| LMD | 964.8 | E858.2 | E934.8 | E950.4 | E962.0 | E980.4 |
| Lobelia | 988.2 | E865.4 | — | E950.9 | E962.1 | E980.9 |
| Lobeline | 970.0 | E854.3 | E940.0 | E950.4 | E962.0 | E980.4 |
| Locorten | 976.0 | E858.7 | E946.0 | E950.4 | E962.0 | E980.4 |
| Lolium temulentum | 988.2 | E865.3 | — | E950.9 | E962.1 | E980.9 |
| Lomotil | 973.5 | E858.4 | E943.5 | E950.4 | E962.0 | E980.4 |
| Lomustine | 963.1 | E858.1 | E933.1 | E950.4 | E962.0 | E980.4 |
| Lophophora williamsii | 969.6 | E854.1 | E939.6 | E950.3 | E962.0 | E980.3 |
| Lorazepam | 969.4 | E853.2 | E939.4 | E950.3 | E962.0 | E980.3 |
| Lotions NEC | 976.9 | E858.7 | E946.9 | E950.4 | E962.0 | E980.4 |
| Lotronex | 973.8 | E858.4 | E943.8 | E950.4 | E962.0 | E980.4 |
| Lotusate | 967.0 | E851 | E937.0 | E950.1 | E962.0 | E980.1 |
| Lowila | 976.2 | E858.7 | E946.2 | E950.4 | E962.0 | E980.4 |
| Loxapine | 969.3 | E853.8 | E939.3 | E950.3 | E962.0 | E980.3 |
| Lozenges (throat) | 976.6 | E858.7 | E946.6 | E950.4 | E962.0 | E980.4 |
| LSD (25) | 969.6 | E854.1 | E939.6 | E950.3 | E962.0 | E980.3 |
| L-Tryptophan — see amino acid | | | | | | |
| Lubricating oil NEC | 981 | E862.2 | — | E950.9 | E962.1 | E980.9 |
| Lucanthone | 961.6 | E857 | E931.6 | E950.4 | E962.0 | E980.4 |
| Luminal | 967.0 | E851 | E937.0 | E950.1 | E962.0 | E980.1 |
| Lung irritant (gas) NEC | 987.9 | E869.9 | — | E952.9 | E962.2 | E982.9 |
| Lutocylol | 962.2 | E858.0 | E932.2 | E950.4 | E962.0 | E980.4 |
| Lutromone | 962.2 | E858.0 | E932.2 | E950.4 | E962.0 | E980.4 |
| Lututrin | 975.0 | E858.6 | E945.0 | E950.4 | E962.0 | E980.4 |
| Lye (concentrated) | 983.2 | E864.2 | — | E950.7 | E962.1 | E980.6 |
| Lygranum (skin test) | 977.8 | E858.8 | E947.8 | E950.4 | E962.0 | E980.4 |
| Lymecycline | 960.4 | E856 | E930.4 | E950.4 | E962.0 | E980.4 |
| **Lymphogranuloma venereum antigen** | 977.8 | E858.8 | E947.8 | E950.4 | E962.0 | E980.4 |
| Lynestrenol | 962.2 | E858.0 | E932.2 | E950.4 | E962.0 | E980.4 |
| Lyovac Sodium Edecrin | 974.4 | E858.5 | E944.4 | E950.4 | E962.0 | E980.4 |
| Lypressin | 962.5 | E858.0 | E932.5 | E950.4 | E962.0 | E980.4 |
| **Lysergic acid** (amide) (diethylamide) | 969.6 | E854.1 | E939.6 | E950.3 | E962.0 | E980.3 |
| Lysergide | 969.6 | E854.1 | E939.6 | E950.3 | E962.0 | E980.3 |
| Lysine vasopressin | 962.5 | E858.0 | E932.5 | E950.4 | E962.0 | E980.4 |
| Lysol | 983.0 | E864.0 | — | E950.7 | E962.1 | E980.6 |
| Lytta (vitatta) | 976.8 | E858.7 | E946.8 | E950.4 | E962.0 | E980.4 |
| Mace | 987.5 | E869.3 | — | E952.8 | E962.2 | E982.8 |
| Macrolides (antibiotics) | 960.3 | E856 | E930.3 | E950.4 | E962.0 | E980.4 |
| Mafenide | 976.0 | E858.7 | E946.0 | E950.4 | E962.0 | E980.4 |
| Magaldrate | 973.0 | E858.4 | E943.0 | E950.4 | E962.0 | E980.4 |
| Magic mushroom | 969.6 | E854.1 | E939.6 | E950.3 | E962.0 | E980.3 |
| Magnamycin | 960.8 | E856 | E930.8 | E950.4 | E962.0 | E980.4 |
| Magnesia magma | 973.0 | E858.4 | E943.0 | E950.4 | E962.0 | E980.4 |
| **Magnesium (compounds) (fumes) NEC** | 985.8 | E866.4 | — | E950.9 | E962.1 | E980.9 |

☑ Additional Digit Required — Refer to the Tabular List for Digit Selection

322 — Volume 2    ►◄ Revised Text    ● New Line    ▲ Revised Code    Subterms under main terms may continue to next column or page    *2008 ICD-9-CM*

| | Poisoning | Accident | Therapeutic Use | Suicide Attempt | Assault | Undetermined |
|---|---|---|---|---|---|---|
| **Magnesium (compounds) (fumes)** — continued | | | | | | |
| antacid | 973.0 | E858.4 | E943.0 | E950.4 | E962.0 | E980.4 |
| carbonate | 973.0 | E858.4 | E943.0 | E950.4 | E962.0 | E980.4 |
| cathartic | 973.3 | E858.4 | E943.3 | E950.4 | E962.0 | E980.4 |
| citrate | 973.3 | E858.4 | E943.3 | E950.4 | E962.0 | E980.4 |
| hydroxide | 973.0 | E858.4 | E943.0 | E950.4 | E962.0 | E980.4 |
| oxide | 973.0 | E858.4 | E943.0 | E950.4 | E962.0 | E980.4 |
| sulfate (oral) | 973.3 | E858.4 | E943.3 | E950.4 | E962.0 | E980.4 |
| intravenous | 966.3 | E855.0 | E936.3 | E950.4 | E962.0 | E980.4 |
| trisilicate | 973.0 | E858.4 | E943.0 | E950.4 | E962.0 | E980.4 |
| **Malathion** (insecticide) | 989.3 | E863.1 | — | E950.6 | E962.1 | E980.7 |
| **Male fern** (oleoresin) | 961.6 | E857 | E931.6 | E950.4 | E962.0 | E980.4 |
| **Mandelic acid** | 961.9 | E857 | E931.9 | E950.4 | E962.0 | E980.4 |
| **Manganese compounds** (fumes) NEC | 985.2 | E866.4 | — | E950.9 | E962.1 | E980.9 |
| **Mannitol (diuretic) (medicinal) NEC** | 974.4 | E858.5 | E944.4 | E950.4 | E962.0 | E980.4 |
| hexanitrate | 972.4 | E858.3 | E942.4 | E950.4 | E962.0 | E980.4 |
| mustard | 963.1 | E858.1 | E933.1 | E950.4 | E962.0 | E980.4 |
| **Mannomustine** | 963.1 | E858.1 | E933.1 | E950.4 | E962.0 | E980.4 |
| **MAO inhibitors** | 969.0 | E854.0 | E939.0 | E950.3 | E962.0 | E980.3 |
| **Mapharsen** | 961.1 | E857 | E931.1 | E950.4 | E962.0 | E980.4 |
| **Marcaine** | 968.9 | E855.2 | E938.9 | E950.4 | E962.0 | E980.4 |
| infiltration (subcutaneous) | 968.5 | E855.2 | E938.5 | E950.4 | E962.0 | E980.4 |
| nerve block (peripheral) (plexus) | 968.6 | E855.2 | E938.6 | E950.4 | E962.0 | E980.4 |
| **Marezine** | 963.0 | E858.1 | E933.0 | E950.4 | E962.0 | E980.4 |
| **Marihuana, marijuana** (derivatives) | 969.6 | E854.1 | E939.6 | E950.3 | E962.0 | E980.3 |
| **Marine animals or plants** (sting) | 989.5 | E905.6 | — | E950.9 | E962.1 | E980.9 |
| **Marplan** | 969.0 | E854.0 | E939.0 | E950.3 | E962.0 | E980.3 |
| **Marsh gas** | 987.1 | E869.8 | — | E952.8 | E962.2 | E982.8 |
| **Marsilid** | 969.0 | E854.0 | E939.0 | E950.3 | E962.0 | E980.3 |
| **Matulane** | 963.1 | E858.1 | E933.1 | E950.4 | E962.0 | E980.4 |
| **Mazindol** | 977.0 | E858.8 | E947.0 | E950.4 | E962.0 | E980.4 |
| **MDMA** | 969.7 | E854.2 | E939.7 | E950.3 | E962.0 | E980.3 |
| **Meadow saffron** | 988.2 | E865.3 | — | E950.9 | E962.1 | E980.9 |
| **Measles vaccine** | 979.4 | E858.8 | E949.4 | E950.4 | E962.0 | E980.4 |
| **Meat, noxious or nonbacterial** | 988.8 | E865.0 | — | E950.9 | E962.1 | E980.9 |
| **Mebanazine** | 969.0 | E854.0 | E939.0 | E950.3 | E962.0 | E980.3 |
| **Mebaral** | 967.0 | E851 | E937.0 | E950.1 | E962.0 | E980.1 |
| **Mebendazole** | 961.6 | E857 | E931.6 | E950.4 | E962.0 | E980.4 |
| **Mebeverine** | 975.1 | E858.6 | E945.1 | E950.4 | E962.0 | E980.4 |
| **Mebhydroline** | 963.0 | E858.1 | E933.0 | E950.4 | E962.0 | E980.4 |
| **Mebrophenhydramine** | 963.0 | E858.1 | E933.0 | E950.4 | E962.0 | E980.4 |
| **Mebutamate** | 969.5 | E853.8 | E939.5 | E950.3 | E962.0 | E980.3 |
| **Mecamylamine** (chloride) | 972.3 | E858.3 | E942.3 | E950.4 | E962.0 | E980.4 |
| **Mechlorethamine hydrochloride** | 963.1 | E858.1 | E933.1 | E950.4 | E962.0 | E980.4 |
| **Meclizene** (hydrochloride) | 963.0 | E858.1 | E933.0 | E950.4 | E962.0 | E980.4 |
| **Meclofenoxate** | 970.0 | E854.3 | E940.0 | E950.4 | E962.0 | E980.4 |
| **Meclozine** (hydrochloride) | 963.0 | E858.1 | E933.0 | E950.4 | E962.0 | E980.4 |
| **Medazepam** | 969.4 | E853.2 | E939.4 | E950.3 | E962.0 | E980.3 |
| **Medicine, medicinal substance** | 977.9 | E858.9 | E947.9 | E950.5 | E962.0 | E980.5 |
| specified NEC | 977.8 | E858.8 | E947.8 | E950.4 | E962.0 | E980.4 |
| **Medinal** | 967.0 | E851 | E937.0 | E950.1 | E962.0 | E980.1 |
| **Medomin** | 967.0 | E851 | E937.0 | E950.1 | E962.0 | E980.1 |
| **Medroxyprogesterone** | 962.2 | E858.0 | E932.2 | E950.4 | E962.0 | E980.4 |
| **Medrysone** | 976.5 | E858.7 | E946.5 | E950.4 | E962.0 | E980.4 |
| **Mefenamic acid** | 965.7 | E850.7 | E935.7 | E950.0 | E962.0 | E980.0 |
| **Megahallucinogen** | 969.6 | E854.1 | E939.6 | E950.3 | E962.0 | E980.3 |
| **Megestrol** | 962.2 | E858.0 | E932.2 | E950.4 | E962.0 | E980.4 |
| **Meglumine** | 977.8 | E858.8 | E947.8 | E950.4 | E962.0 | E980.4 |
| **Meladinin** | 976.3 | E858.7 | E946.3 | E950.4 | E962.0 | E980.4 |
| **Melanizing agents** | 976.3 | E858.7 | E946.3 | E950.4 | E962.0 | E980.4 |
| **Melarsoprol** | 961.1 | E857 | E931.1 | E950.4 | E962.0 | E980.4 |
| **Melia azedarach** | 988.2 | E865.3 | — | E950.9 | E962.1 | E980.9 |
| **Mellaril** | 969.1 | E853.0 | E939.1 | E950.3 | E962.0 | E980.3 |
| **Meloxine** | 976.3 | E858.7 | E946.3 | E950.4 | E962.0 | E980.4 |
| **Melphalan** | 963.1 | E858.1 | E933.1 | E950.4 | E962.0 | E980.4 |
| **Menadiol sodium diphosphate** | 964.3 | E858.2 | E934.3 | E950.4 | E962.0 | E980.4 |
| **Menadione** (sodium bisulfite) | 964.3 | E858.2 | E934.3 | E950.4 | E962.0 | E980.4 |
| **Menaphthone** | 964.3 | E858.2 | E934.3 | E950.4 | E962.0 | E980.4 |
| **Meningococcal vaccine** | 978.8 | E858.8 | E948.8 | E950.4 | E962.0 | E980.4 |
| **Menningovax-C** | 978.8 | E858.8 | E948.8 | E950.4 | E962.0 | E980.4 |
| **Menotropins** | 962.4 | E858.0 | E932.4 | E950.4 | E962.0 | E980.4 |
| **Menthol NEC** | 976.1 | E858.7 | E946.1 | E950.4 | E962.0 | E980.4 |
| **Mepacrine** | 961.3 | E857 | E931.3 | E950.4 | E962.0 | E980.4 |
| **Meparfynol** | 967.8 | E852.8 | E937.8 | E950.2 | E962.0 | E980.2 |
| **Mepazine** | 969.1 | E853.0 | E939.1 | E950.3 | E962.0 | E980.3 |
| **Mepenzolate** | 971.1 | E855.4 | E941.1 | E950.4 | E962.0 | E980.4 |
| **Meperidine** | 965.09 | E850.2 | E935.2 | E950.0 | E962.0 | E980.0 |
| **Mephenamin(e)** | 966.4 | E855.0 | E936.4 | E950.4 | E962.0 | E980.4 |
| **Mephenesin** (carbamate) | 968.0 | E855.1 | E938.0 | E950.4 | E962.0 | E980.4 |
| **Mephenoxalone** | 969.5 | E853.8 | E939.5 | E950.3 | E962.0 | E980.3 |
| **Mephentermine** | 971.2 | E855.4 | E941.2 | E950.4 | E962.0 | E980.4 |
| **Mephenytoin** | 966.1 | E855.0 | E936.1 | E950.4 | E962.0 | E980.4 |
| **Mephobarbital** | 967.0 | E851 | E937.0 | E950.1 | E962.0 | E980.1 |
| **Mepiperphenidol** | 971.1 | E855.4 | E941.1 | E950.4 | E962.0 | E980.4 |
| **Mepivacaine** | 968.9 | E855.2 | E938.9 | E950.4 | E962.0 | E980.4 |
| infiltration (subcutaneous) | 968.5 | E855.2 | E938.5 | E950.4 | E962.0 | E980.4 |
| nerve block (peripheral) (plexus) | 968.6 | E855.2 | E938.6 | E950.4 | E962.0 | E980.4 |
| topical (surface) | 968.5 | E855.2 | E938.5 | E950.4 | E962.0 | E980.4 |
| **Meprednisone** | 962.0 | E858.0 | E932.0 | E950.4 | E962.0 | E980.4 |
| **Meprobam** | 969.5 | E853.8 | E939.5 | E950.3 | E962.0 | E980.3 |
| **Meprobamate** | 969.5 | E853.8 | E939.5 | E950.3 | E962.0 | E980.3 |
| **Mepyramine** (maleate) | 963.0 | E858.1 | E933.0 | E950.4 | E962.0 | E980.4 |
| **Meralluride** | 974.0 | E858.5 | E944.0 | E950.4 | E962.0 | E980.4 |
| **Merbaphen** | 974.0 | E858.5 | E944.0 | E950.4 | E962.0 | E980.4 |
| **Merbromin** | 976.0 | E858.7 | E946.0 | E950.4 | E962.0 | E980.4 |
| **Mercaptomerin** | 974.0 | E858.5 | E944.0 | E950.4 | E962.0 | E980.4 |
| **Mercaptopurine** | 963.1 | E858.1 | E933.1 | E950.4 | E962.0 | E980.4 |
| **Mercumatilin** | 974.0 | E858.5 | E944.0 | E950.4 | E962.0 | E980.4 |
| **Mercuramide** | 974.0 | E858.5 | E944.0 | E950.4 | E962.0 | E980.4 |
| **Mercuranin** | 976.0 | E858.7 | E946.0 | E950.4 | E962.0 | E980.4 |
| **Mercurochrome** | 976.0 | E858.7 | E946.0 | E950.4 | E962.0 | E980.4 |
| **Mercury, mercuric, mercurous** (compounds) (cyanide) (fumes) (nonmedicinal) (vapor) NEC | 985.0 | E866.1 | — | E950.9 | E962.1 | E980.9 |
| ammoniated | 976.0 | E858.7 | E946.0 | E950.4 | E962.0 | E980.4 |
| anti-infective | 961.2 | E857 | E931.2 | E950.4 | E962.0 | E980.4 |
| topical | 976.0 | E858.7 | E946.0 | E950.4 | E962.0 | E980.4 |
| chloride (antiseptic) NEC | 976.0 | E858.7 | E946.0 | E950.4 | E962.0 | E980.4 |
| fungicide | 985.0 | E863.6 | | E950.6 | E962.1 | E980.7 |
| diuretic compounds | 974.0 | E858.5 | E944.0 | E950.4 | E962.0 | E980.4 |
| fungicide | 985.0 | E863.6 | — | E950.6 | E962.1 | E980.7 |
| organic (fungicide) | 985.0 | E863.6 | — | E950.6 | E962.1 | E980.7 |
| **Merethoxylline** | 974.0 | E858.5 | E944.0 | E950.4 | E962.0 | E980.4 |
| **Mersalyl** | 974.0 | E858.5 | E944.0 | E950.4 | E962.0 | E980.4 |
| **Merthiolate** (topical) | 976.0 | E858.7 | E946.0 | E950.4 | E962.0 | E980.4 |
| ophthalmic preparation | 976.5 | E858.7 | E946.5 | E950.4 | E962.0 | E980.4 |
| **Meruvax** | 979.4 | E858.8 | E949.4 | E950.4 | E962.0 | E980.4 |
| **Mescal buttons** | 969.6 | E854.1 | E939.6 | E950.3 | E962.0 | E980.3 |
| **Mescaline** (salts) | 969.6 | E854.1 | E939.6 | E950.3 | E962.0 | E980.3 |
| **Mesoridazine besylate** | 969.1 | E853.0 | E939.1 | E950.3 | E962.0 | E980.3 |
| **Mestanolone** | 962.1 | E858.0 | E932.1 | E950.4 | E962.0 | E980.4 |
| **Mestranol** | 962.2 | E858.0 | E932.2 | E950.4 | E962.0 | E980.4 |
| **Metacresylacetate** | 976.0 | E858.7 | E946.0 | E950.4 | E962.0 | E980.4 |
| **Metaldehyde** (snail killer) NEC | 989.4 | E863.4 | — | E950.6 | E962.1 | E980.7 |
| **Metals (heavy) (nonmedicinal) NEC** | 985.9 | E866.4 | — | E950.9 | E962.1 | E980.9 |
| dust, fumes, or vapor NEC | 985.9 | E866.4 | — | E950.9 | E962.1 | E980.9 |
| light NEC | 985.9 | E866.4 | — | E950.9 | E962.1 | E980.9 |
| dust, fumes, or vapor NEC | 985.9 | E866.4 | — | E950.9 | E962.1 | E980.9 |
| pesticides (dust) (vapor) | 985.9 | E863.4 | — | E950.6 | E962.1 | E980.7 |
| **Metamucil** | 973.3 | E858.4 | E943.3 | E950.4 | E962.0 | E980.4 |
| **Metaphen** | 976.0 | E858.7 | E946.0 | E950.4 | E962.0 | E980.4 |
| **Metaproterenol** | 975.1 | E858.6 | E945.1 | E950.4 | E962.0 | E980.4 |
| **Metaraminol** | 972.8 | E858.3 | E942.8 | E950.4 | E962.0 | E980.4 |
| **Metaxalone** | 968.0 | E855.1 | E938.0 | E950.4 | E962.0 | E980.4 |
| **Metformin** | 962.3 | E858.0 | E932.3 | E950.4 | E962.0 | E980.4 |
| **Methacycline** | 960.4 | E856 | E930.4 | E950.4 | E962.0 | E980.4 |
| **Methadone** | 965.02 | E850.1 | E935.1 | E950.0 | E962.0 | E980.0 |
| **Methallenestril** | 962.2 | E858.0 | E932.2 | E950.4 | E962.0 | E980.4 |
| **Methamphetamine** | 969.7 | E854.2 | E939.7 | E950.3 | E962.0 | E980.3 |
| **Methandienone** | 962.1 | E858.0 | E932.1 | E950.4 | E962.0 | E980.4 |
| **Methandriol** | 962.1 | E858.0 | E932.1 | E950.4 | E962.0 | E980.4 |
| **Methandrostenolone** | 962.1 | E858.0 | E932.1 | E950.4 | E962.0 | E980.4 |
| **Methane gas** | 987.1 | E869.8 | — | E952.8 | E962.2 | E982.8 |
| **Methanol** | 980.1 | E860.2 | — | E950.9 | E962.1 | E980.9 |
| vapor | 987.8 | E869.8 | — | E952.8 | E962.2 | E982.8 |
| **Methantheline** | 971.1 | E855.4 | E941.1 | E950.4 | E962.0 | E980.4 |

☑ Additional Digit Required — Refer to the Tabular List for Digit Selection

Subterms under main terms may continue to next column or page

| | Poisoning | Accident | Therapeutic Use | Suicide Attempt | Assault | Undetermined |
|---|---|---|---|---|---|---|
| Methaphenilene | 963.0 | E858.1 | E933.0 | E950.4 | E962.0 | E980.4 |
| Methapyrilene | 963.0 | E858.1 | E933.0 | E950.4 | E962.0 | E980.4 |
| Methaqualone (compounds) | 967.4 | E852.3 | E937.4 | E950.2 | E962.0 | E980.2 |
| Metharbital, metharbitone | 967.0 | E851 | E937.0 | E950.1 | E962.0 | E980.1 |
| Methazolamide | 974.2 | E858.5 | E944.2 | E950.4 | E962.0 | E980.4 |
| Methdilazine | 963.0 | E858.1 | E933.0 | E950.4 | E962.0 | E980.4 |
| Methedrine | 969.7 | E854.2 | E939.7 | E950.3 | E962.0 | E980.3 |
| Methenamine (mandelate) | 961.9 | E857 | E931.9 | E950.4 | E962.0 | E980.4 |
| Methenolone | 962.1 | E858.0 | E932.1 | E950.4 | E962.0 | E980.4 |
| Methergine | 975.0 | E858.6 | E945.0 | E950.4 | E962.0 | E980.4 |
| Methiacil | 962.8 | E858.0 | E932.8 | E950.4 | E962.0 | E980.4 |
| Methicillin (sodium) | 960.0 | E856 | E930.0 | E950.4 | E962.0 | E980.4 |
| Methimazole | 962.8 | E858.0 | E932.8 | E950.4 | E962.0 | E980.4 |
| Methionine | 977.1 | E858.8 | E947.1 | E950.4 | E962.0 | E980.4 |
| Methisazone | 961.7 | E857 | E931.7 | E950.4 | E962.0 | E980.4 |
| Methitural | 967.0 | E851 | E937.0 | E950.1 | E962.0 | E980.1 |
| Methixene | 971.1 | E855.4 | E941.1 | E950.4 | E962.0 | E980.4 |
| Methobarbital, methobarbitone | 967.0 | E851 | E937.0 | E950.1 | E962.0 | E980.1 |
| Methocarbamol | 968.0 | E855.1 | E938.0 | E950.4 | E962.0 | E980.4 |
| Methohexital, methohexitone (sodium) | 968.3 | E855.1 | E938.3 | E950.4 | E962.0 | E980.4 |
| Methoin | 966.1 | E855.0 | E936.1 | E950.4 | E962.0 | E980.4 |
| Methopholine | 965.7 | E850.7 | E935.7 | E950.0 | E962.0 | E980.0 |
| Methorate | 975.4 | E858.6 | E945.4 | E950.4 | E962.0 | E980.4 |
| Methoserpidine | 972.6 | E858.3 | E942.6 | E950.4 | E962.0 | E980.4 |
| Methotrexate | 963.1 | E858.1 | E933.1 | E950.4 | E962.0 | E980.4 |
| Methotrimeprazine | 967.8 | E852.8 | E937.8 | E950.2 | E962.0 | E980.2 |
| Methoxa-Dome | 976.3 | E858.7 | E946.3 | E950.4 | E962.0 | E980.4 |
| Methoxamine | 971.2 | E855.5 | E941.2 | E950.4 | E962.0 | E980.4 |
| Methoxsalen | 976.3 | E858.7 | E946.3 | E950.4 | E962.0 | E980.4 |
| Methoxybenzyl penicillin | 960.0 | E856 | E930.0 | E950.4 | E962.0 | E980.4 |
| Methoxychlor | 989.2 | E863.0 | — | E950.6 | E962.1 | E980.7 |
| Methoxyflurane | 968.2 | E855.1 | E938.2 | E950.4 | E962.0 | E980.4 |
| Methoxyphenamine | 971.2 | E855.5 | E941.2 | E950.4 | E962.0 | E980.4 |
| Methoxypromazine | 969.1 | E853.0 | E939.1 | E950.3 | E962.0 | E980.3 |
| Methoxypsoralen | 976.3 | E858.7 | E946.3 | E950.4 | E962.0 | E980.4 |
| Methscopolamine (bromide) | 971.1 | E855.4 | E941.1 | E950.4 | E962.0 | E980.4 |
| Methsuximide | 966.2 | E855.0 | E936.2 | E950.4 | E962.0 | E980.4 |
| Methyclothiazide | 974.3 | E858.5 | E944.3 | E950.4 | E962.0 | E980.4 |
| **Methyl** | | | | | | |
| acetate | 982.8 | E862.4 | — | E950.9 | E962.1 | E980.9 |
| acetone | 982.8 | E862.4 | — | E950.9 | E962.1 | E980.9 |
| alcohol | 980.1 | E860.2 | — | E950.9 | E962.1 | E980.9 |
| amphetamine | 969.7 | E854.2 | E939.7 | E950.3 | E962.0 | E980.3 |
| androstanolone | 962.1 | E858.0 | E932.1 | E950.4 | E962.0 | E980.4 |
| atropine | 971.1 | E855.4 | E941.1 | E950.4 | E962.0 | E980.4 |
| benzene | 982.0 | E862.4 | — | E950.9 | E962.1 | E980.9 |
| bromide (gas) | 987.8 | E869.8 | — | E952.8 | E962.2 | E982.8 |
| fumigant | 987.8 | E863.8 | — | E950.6 | E962.2 | E980.7 |
| butanol | 980.8 | E860.8 | — | E950.9 | E962.1 | E980.9 |
| carbinol | 980.1 | E860.2 | — | E950.9 | E962.1 | E980.9 |
| cellosolve | 982.8 | E862.4 | — | E950.9 | E962.1 | E980.9 |
| cellulose | 973.3 | E858.4 | E943.3 | E950.4 | E962.0 | E980.4 |
| chloride (gas) | 987.8 | E869.8 | — | E952.8 | E962.2 | E982.8 |
| cyclohexane | 982.8 | E862.4 | — | E950.9 | E962.1 | E980.9 |
| cyclohexanone | 982.8 | E862.4 | — | E950.9 | E962.1 | E980.9 |
| dihydromorphinone | 965.09 | E850.2 | E935.2 | E950.0 | E962.0 | E980.0 |
| ergometrine | 975.0 | E858.6 | E945.0 | E950.4 | E962.0 | E980.4 |
| ergonovine | 975.0 | E858.6 | E945.0 | E950.4 | E962.0 | E980.4 |
| ethyl ketone | 982.8 | E862.4 | — | E950.9 | E962.1 | E980.9 |
| hydrazine | 983.9 | E864.3 | — | E950.7 | E962.1 | E980.6 |
| isobutyl ketone | 982.8 | E862.4 | — | E950.9 | E962.1 | E980.9 |
| morphine NEC | 965.09 | E850.2 | E935.2 | E950.0 | E962.0 | E980.0 |
| parafynol | 967.8 | E852.8 | E937.8 | E950.2 | E962.0 | E980.2 |
| parathion | 989.3 | E863.1 | — | E950.6 | E962.1 | E980.7 |
| pentynol NEC | 967.8 | E852.8 | E937.8 | E950.2 | E962.0 | E980.2 |
| peridol | 969.2 | E853.1 | E939.2 | E950.3 | E962.0 | E980.3 |
| phenidate | 969.7 | E854.2 | E939.7 | E950.3 | E962.0 | E980.3 |
| prednisolone | 962.0 | E858.0 | E932.0 | E950.4 | E962.0 | E980.4 |
| ENT agent | 976.6 | E858.7 | E946.6 | E950.4 | E962.0 | E980.4 |
| ophthalmic preparation | 976.5 | E858.7 | E946.5 | E950.4 | E962.0 | E980.4 |
| topical NEC | 976.0 | E858.7 | E946.0 | E950.4 | E962.0 | E980.4 |
| propylcarbinol | 980.8 | E860.8 | — | E950.9 | E962.1 | E980.9 |
| rosaniline NEC | 976.0 | E858.7 | E946.0 | E950.4 | E962.0 | E980.4 |
| salicylate NEC | 976.3 | E858.7 | E946.3 | E950.4 | E962.0 | E980.4 |
| sulfate (fumes) | 987.8 | E869.8 | — | E952.8 | E962.2 | E982.8 |
| liquid | 983.9 | E864.3 | — | E950.7 | E962.1 | E980.6 |
| sulfonal | 967.8 | E852.8 | E937.8 | E950.2 | E962.0 | E980.2 |
| testosterone | 962.1 | E858.0 | E932.1 | E950.4 | E962.0 | E980.4 |

| | Poisoning | Accident | Therapeutic Use | Suicide Attempt | Assault | Undetermined |
|---|---|---|---|---|---|---|
| **Methyl** — *continued* | | | | | | |
| thiouracil | 962.8 | E858.0 | E932.8 | E950.4 | E962.0 | E980.4 |
| Methylated spirit | 980.0 | E860.1 | — | E950.9 | E962.1 | E980.9 |
| Methyldopa | 972.6 | E858.3 | E942.6 | E950.4 | E962.0 | E980.4 |
| **Methylene** | | | | | | |
| blue | 961.9 | E857 | E931.9 | E950.4 | E962.0 | E980.4 |
| chloride or dichloride (solvent) NEC | 982.3 | E862.4 | — | E950.9 | E962.1 | E980.9 |
| Methylhexabital | 967.0 | E851 | E937.0 | E950.1 | E962.0 | E980.1 |
| Methylparaben (ophthalmic) | 976.5 | E858.7 | E946.5 | E950.4 | E962.0 | E980.4 |
| Methyprylon | 967.5 | E852.4 | E937.5 | E950.2 | E962.0 | E980.2 |
| Methysergide | 971.3 | E855.6 | E941.3 | E950.4 | E962.0 | E980.4 |
| Metoclopramide | 963.0 | E858.1 | E933.0 | E950.4 | E962.0 | E980.4 |
| Metofoline | 965.7 | E850.7 | E935.7 | E950.0 | E962.0 | E980.0 |
| Metopon | 965.09 | E850.2 | E935.2 | E950.0 | E962.0 | E980.0 |
| Metronidazole | 961.5 | E857 | E931.5 | E950.4 | E962.0 | E980.4 |
| Metycaine | 968.9 | E855.2 | E938.9 | E950.4 | E962.0 | E980.4 |
| infiltration (subcutaneous) | 968.5 | E855.2 | E938.5 | E950.4 | E962.0 | E980.4 |
| nerve block (peripheral) (plexus) | 968.6 | E855.2 | E938.6 | E950.4 | E962.0 | E980.4 |
| topical (surface) | 968.5 | E855.2 | E938.5 | E950.4 | E962.0 | E980.4 |
| Metyrapone | 977.8 | E858.8 | E947.8 | E950.4 | E962.0 | E980.4 |
| Mevinphos | 989.3 | E863.1 | — | E950.6 | E962.1 | E980.7 |
| Mezereon (berries) | 988.2 | E865.3 | — | E950.9 | E962.1 | E980.9 |
| Micatin | 976.0 | E858.7 | E946.0 | E950.4 | E962.0 | E980.4 |
| Miconazole | 976.0 | E858.7 | E946.0 | E950.4 | E962.0 | E980.4 |
| Midol | 965.1 | E850.3 | E935.3 | E950.0 | E962.0 | E980.0 |
| Mifepristone | 962.9 | E858.0 | E932.9 | E950.4 | E962.0 | E980.4 |
| Milk of magnesia | 973.0 | E858.4 | E943.0 | E950.4 | E962.0 | E980.4 |
| Millipede (tropical) (venomous) | 989.5 | E905.4 | — | E950.9 | E962.1 | E980.9 |
| Miltown | 969.5 | E853.8 | E939.5 | E950.3 | E962.0 | E980.3 |
| **Mineral** | | | | | | |
| oil (medicinal) | 973.2 | E858.4 | E943.2 | E950.4 | E962.0 | E980.4 |
| nonmedicinal | 981 | E862.1 | — | E950.9 | E962.1 | E980.9 |
| topical | 976.3 | E858.7 | E946.3 | E950.4 | E962.0 | E980.4 |
| salts NEC | 974.6 | E858.5 | E944.6 | E950.4 | E962.0 | E980.4 |
| spirits | 981 | E862.0 | — | E950.9 | E962.1 | E980.9 |
| Minocycline | 960.4 | E856 | E930.4 | E950.4 | E962.0 | E980.4 |
| Mithramycin (antineoplastic) | 960.7 | E856 | E930.7 | E950.4 | E962.0 | E980.4 |
| Mitobronitol | 963.1 | E858.1 | E933.1 | E950.4 | E962.0 | E980.4 |
| Mitomycin (antineoplastic) | 960.7 | E856 | E930.7 | E950.4 | E962.0 | E980.4 |
| Mitotane | 963.1 | E858.1 | E933.1 | E950.4 | E962.0 | E980.4 |
| Moderil | 972.6 | E858.3 | E942.6 | E950.4 | E962.0 | E980.4 |
| Mogadon — *see* Nitrazepam | | | | | | |
| Molindone | 969.3 | E853.8 | E939.3 | E950.3 | E962.0 | E980.3 |
| Monistat | 976.0 | E858.7 | E946.0 | E950.4 | E962.0 | E980.4 |
| Monkshood | 988.2 | E865.4 | — | E950.9 | E962.1 | E980.9 |
| Monoamine oxidase inhibitors | 969.0 | E854.0 | E939.0 | E950.3 | E962.0 | E980.3 |
| Monochlorobenzene | 982.0 | E862.4 | — | E950.9 | E962.1 | E980.9 |
| Monosodium glutamate | 989.89 | E866.8 | — | E950.9 | E962.1 | E980.9 |
| Monoxide, carbon — *see* Carbon, monoxide | | | | | | |
| Moperone | 969.2 | E853.1 | E939.2 | E950.3 | E962.0 | E980.3 |
| Morning glory seeds | 969.6 | E854.1 | E939.6 | E950.3 | E962.0 | E980.3 |
| Moroxydine (hydrochloride) | 961.7 | E857 | E931.7 | E950.4 | E962.0 | E980.4 |
| Morphazinamide | 961.8 | E857 | E931.8 | E950.4 | E962.0 | E980.4 |
| Morphinans | 965.09 | E850.2 | E935.2 | E950.0 | E962.0 | E980.0 |
| **Morphine NEC** | 965.09 | E850.2 | E935.2 | E950.0 | E962.0 | E980.0 |
| antagonists | 970.1 | E854.3 | E940.1 | E950.4 | E962.0 | E980.4 |
| Morpholinylethylmorphine | 965.09 | E850.2 | E935.2 | E950.0 | E962.0 | E980.0 |
| Morrhuate sodium | 972.7 | E858.3 | E942.7 | E950.4 | E962.0 | E980.4 |
| **Moth balls** — *see also* Pesticides | 989.4 | E863.4 | — | E950.6 | E962.1 | E980.7 |
| naphthalene | 983.0 | E863.4 | — | E950.7 | E962.1 | E980.6 |
| Motor exhaust gas — *see* Carbon, monoxide, exhaust gas | | | | | | |
| Mouth wash | 976.6 | E858.7 | E946.6 | E950.4 | E962.0 | E980.4 |
| Mucolytic agent | 975.5 | E858.6 | E945.5 | E950.4 | E962.0 | E980.4 |
| Mucomyst | 975.5 | E858.6 | E945.5 | E950.4 | E962.0 | E980.4 |
| Mucous membrane agents (external) | 976.9 | E858.7 | E946.9 | E950.4 | E962.0 | E980.4 |
| specified NEC | 976.8 | E858.7 | E946.8 | E950.4 | E962.0 | E980.4 |
| **Mumps** | | | | | | |
| immune globulin (human) | 964.6 | E858.2 | E934.6 | E950.4 | E962.0 | E980.4 |
| skin test antigen | 977.8 | E858.8 | E947.8 | E950.4 | E962.0 | E980.4 |
| vaccine | 979.6 | E858.8 | E949.6 | E950.4 | E962.0 | E980.4 |

☑ Additional Digit Required — Refer to the Tabular List for Digit Selection

324 — Volume 2          ►◄ Revised Text          ● New Line          ▲ Revised Code          Subterms under main terms may continue to next column or page          *2008 ICD-9-CM*

| | Poisoning | Accident | Therapeutic Use | Suicide Attempt | Assault | Undetermined |
|---|---|---|---|---|---|---|
| **Mumpsvax** | 979.6 | E858.8 | E949.6 | E950.4 | E962.0 | E980.4 |
| **Muriatic acid** — *see* Hydrochloric acid | | | | | | |
| **Muscarine** | 971.0 | E855.3 | E941.0 | E950.4 | E962.0 | E980.4 |
| **Muscle affecting agents** | | | | | | |
| NEC | 975.3 | E858.6 | E945.3 | E950.4 | E962.0 | E980.4 |
| oxytocic | 975.0 | E858.6 | E945.0 | E950.4 | E962.0 | E980.4 |
| relaxants | 975.3 | E858.6 | E945.3 | E950.4 | E962.0 | E980.4 |
| central nervous system | 968.0 | E855.1 | E938.0 | E950.4 | E962.0 | E980.4 |
| skeletal | 975.2 | E858.6 | E945.2 | E950.4 | E962.0 | E980.4 |
| smooth | 975.1 | E858.6 | E945.1 | E950.4 | E962.0 | E980.4 |
| **Mushrooms, noxious** | 988.1 | E865.5 | — | E950.9 | E962.1 | E980.9 |
| **Mussel, noxious** | 988.0 | E865.1 | — | E950.9 | E962.1 | E980.9 |
| **Mustard** (emetic) | 973.6 | E858.4 | E943.6 | E950.4 | E962.0 | E980.4 |
| gas | 987.8 | E869.8 | — | E952.8 | E962.2 | E982.8 |
| nitrogen | 963.1 | E858.1 | E933.1 | E950.4 | E962.0 | E980.4 |
| **Mustine** | 963.1 | E858.1 | E933.1 | E950.4 | E962.0 | E980.4 |
| **M-vac** | 979.4 | E858.8 | E949.4 | E950.4 | E962.0 | E980.4 |
| **Mycifradin** | 960.8 | E856 | E930.8 | E950.4 | E962.0 | E980.4 |
| topical | 976.0 | E858.7 | E946.0 | E950.4 | E962.0 | E980.4 |
| **Mycitracin** | 960.8 | E856 | E930.8 | E950.4 | E962.0 | E980.4 |
| ophthalmic preparation | 976.5 | E858.7 | E946.5 | E950.4 | E962.0 | E980.4 |
| **Mycostatin** | 960.1 | E856 | E930.1 | E950.4 | E962.0 | E980.4 |
| topical | 976.0 | E858.7 | E946.0 | E950.4 | E962.0 | E980.4 |
| **Mydriacyl** | 971.1 | E855.4 | E941.1 | E950.4 | E962.0 | E980.4 |
| **Myelobromal** | 963.1 | E858.1 | E933.1 | E950.4 | E962.0 | E980.4 |
| **Myleran** | 963.1 | E858.1 | E933.1 | E950.4 | E962.0 | E980.4 |
| **Myochrysin(e)** | 965.69 | E850.6 | E935.6 | E950.0 | E962.0 | E980.0 |
| **Myoneural blocking agents** | 975.2 | E858.6 | E945.2 | E950.4 | E962.0 | E980.4 |
| **Myristica fragrans** | 988.2 | E865.3 | — | E950.9 | E962.1 | E980.9 |
| **Myristicin** | 988.2 | E865.3 | — | E950.9 | E962.1 | E980.9 |
| **Mysoline** | 966.3 | E855.0 | E936.3 | E950.4 | E962.0 | E980.4 |
| **Nafcillin** (sodium) | 960.0 | E856 | E930.0 | E950.4 | E962.0 | E980.4 |
| **Nail polish remover** | 982.8 | E862.4 | — | E950.9 | E962.1 | E908.9 |
| **Nalidixic acid** | 961.9 | E857 | E931.9 | E950.4 | E962.0 | E980.4 |
| **Nalorphine** | 970.1 | E854.3 | E940.1 | E950.4 | E962.0 | E980.4 |
| **Naloxone** | 970.1 | E854.3 | E940.1 | E950.4 | E962.0 | E980.4 |
| **Nandrolone** (decanoate) (phenproprioate) | 962.1 | E858.0 | E932.1 | E950.4 | E962.0 | E980.4 |
| **Naphazoline** | 971.2 | E855.5 | E941.2 | E950.4 | E962.0 | E980.4 |
| **Naphtha** (painter's) (petroleum) | 981 | E862.0 | — | E950.9 | E962.1 | E980.9 |
| solvent | 981 | E862.0 | — | E950.9 | E962.1 | E980.9 |
| vapor | 987.1 | E869.8 | — | E952.8 | E962.2 | E982.8 |
| **Naphthalene** (chlorinated) | 983.0 | E864.0 | — | E950.7 | E962.1 | E980.6 |
| insecticide or moth repellent | 983.0 | E863.4 | — | E950.7 | E962.1 | E980.6 |
| vapor | 987.8 | E869.8 | — | E952.8 | E962.2 | E982.8 |
| **Naphthol** | 983.0 | E864.0 | — | E950.7 | E962.1 | E980.6 |
| **Naphthylamine** | 983.0 | E864.0 | — | E950.7 | E962.1 | E980.6 |
| **Naprosyn** — *see* Naproxen | | | | | | |
| **Naproxen** | 965.61 | E850.6 | E935.6 | E950.0 | E962.0 | E980.0 |
| **Narcotic** (drug) | 967.9 | E852.9 | E937.9 | E950.2 | E962.0 | E980.2 |
| analgesic NEC | 965.8 | E850.8 | E935.8 | E950.0 | E962.0 | E980.0 |
| antagonist | 970.1 | E854.3 | E940.1 | E950.4 | E962.0 | E980.4 |
| specified NEC | 967.8 | E852.8 | E937.8 | E950.2 | E962.0 | E980.2 |
| **Narcotine** | 975.4 | E858.6 | E945.4 | E950.4 | E962.0 | E980.4 |
| **Nardil** | 969.0 | E854.0 | E939.0 | E950.3 | E962.0 | E980.3 |
| **Natrium cyanide** — *see* Cyanide(s) | | | | | | |
| **Natural** | | | | | | |
| blood (product) | 964.7 | E858.2 | E934.7 | E950.4 | E962.0 | E980.4 |
| gas (piped) | 987.1 | E867 | — | E951.0 | E962.2 | E981.0 |
| incomplete combustion | 986 | E867 | — | E951.0 | E962.2 | E981.0 |
| **Nealbarbital, nealbarbitone** | 967.0 | E851 | E937.0 | E950.1 | E962.0 | E980.1 |
| **Nectadon** | 975.4 | E858.6 | E945.4 | E950.4 | E962.0 | E980.4 |
| **Nematocyst** (sting) | 989.5 | E905.6 | — | E950.9 | E962.1 | E980.9 |
| **Nembutal** | 967.0 | E851 | E937.0 | E950.1 | E962.0 | E980.1 |
| **Neoarsphenamine** | 961.1 | E857 | E931.1 | E950.4 | E962.0 | E980.4 |
| **Neocinchophen** | 974.7 | E858.5 | E944.7 | E950.4 | E962.0 | E980.4 |
| **Neomycin** | 960.8 | E856 | E930.8 | E950.4 | E962.0 | E980.4 |
| ENT agent | 976.6 | E858.7 | E946.6 | E950.4 | E962.0 | E980.4 |
| ophthalmic preparation | 976.5 | E858.7 | E946.5 | E950.4 | E962.0 | E980.4 |
| topical NEC | 976.0 | E858.7 | E946.0 | E950.4 | E962.0 | E980.4 |
| **Neonal** | 967.0 | E851 | E937.0 | E950.1 | E962.0 | E980.1 |
| **Neoprontosil** | 961.0 | E857 | E931.0 | E950.4 | E962.0 | E980.4 |
| **Neosalvarsan** | 961.1 | E857 | E931.1 | E950.4 | E962.0 | E980.4 |
| **Neosilversalvarsan** | 961.1 | E857 | E931.1 | E950.4 | E962.0 | E980.4 |
| **Neosporin** | 960.8 | E856 | E930.8 | E950.4 | E962.0 | E980.4 |
| **Neosporin** — *continued* | | | | | | |
| ENT agent | 976.6 | E858.7 | E946.6 | E950.4 | E962.0 | E980.4 |
| opthalmic preparation | 976.5 | E858.7 | E946.5 | E950.4 | E962.0 | E980.4 |
| topical NEC | 976.0 | E858.7 | E946.0 | E950.4 | E962.0 | E980.4 |
| **Neostigmine** | 971.0 | E855.3 | E941.0 | E950.4 | E962.0 | E980.4 |
| **Neraval** | 967.0 | E851 | E937.0 | E950.1 | E962.0 | E980.1 |
| **Neravan** | 967.0 | E851 | E937.0 | E950.1 | E962.0 | E980.1 |
| **Nerium oleander** | 988.2 | E865.4 | — | E950.9 | E962.1 | E980.9 |
| **Nerve gases** (war) | 987.9 | E869.9 | — | E952.9 | E962.2 | E982.9 |
| **Nesacaine** | 968.9 | E855.2 | E938.9 | E950.4 | E962.0 | E980.4 |
| infiltration (subcutaneous) | 968.5 | E855.2 | E938.5 | E950.4 | E962.0 | E980.4 |
| nerve block (peripheral) (plexus) | 968.6 | E855.2 | E938.6 | E950.4 | E962.0 | E980.4 |
| **Neurobarb** | 967.0 | E851 | E937.0 | E950.1 | E962.0 | E980.1 |
| **Neuroleptics NEC** | 969.3 | E853.8 | E939.3 | E950.3 | E962.0 | E980.3 |
| **Neuroprotective agent** | 977.8 | E858.8 | E947.8 | E950.4 | E962.0 | E980.4 |
| **Neutral spirits** | 980.0 | E860.1 | — | E950.9 | E962.1 | E980.9 |
| beverage | 980.0 | E860.0 | — | E950.9 | E962.1 | E980.9 |
| **Niacin, niacinamide** | 972.2 | E858.3 | E942.2 | E950.4 | E962.0 | E980.4 |
| **Nialamide** | 969.0 | E854.0 | E939.0 | E950.3 | E962.0 | E980.3 |
| **Nickle** (carbonyl) (compounds) (fumes) (tetracarbonyl) (vapor) | 985.8 | E866.4 | — | E950.9 | E962.1 | E980.9 |
| **Niclosamide** | 961.6 | E857 | E931.6 | E950.4 | E962.0 | E980.4 |
| **Nicomorphine** | 965.09 | E850.2 | E935.2 | E950.0 | E962.0 | E980.0 |
| **Nicotinamide** | 972.2 | E858.3 | E942.2 | E950.4 | E962.0 | E980.4 |
| **Nicotine** (insecticide) (spray) (sulfate) NEC | 989.4 | E863.4 | — | E950.6 | E962.1 | E980.7 |
| not insecticide | 989.89 | E866.8 | — | E950.9 | E962.1 | E980.9 |
| **Nicotinic acid** (derivatives) | 972.2 | E858.3 | E942.2 | E950.4 | E962.0 | E980.4 |
| **Nicotinyl alcohol** | 972.2 | E858.3 | E942.2 | E950.4 | E962.0 | E980.4 |
| **Nicoumalone** | 964.2 | E858.2 | E934.2 | E950.4 | E962.0 | E980.4 |
| **Nifenazone** | 965.5 | E850.5 | E935.5 | E950.0 | E962.0 | E980.0 |
| **Nifuraldezone** | 961.9 | E857 | E931.9 | E950.4 | E962.0 | E980.4 |
| **Nightshade** (deadly) | 988.2 | E865.4 | — | E950.9 | E962.1 | E980.9 |
| **Nikethamide** | 970.0 | E854.3 | E940.0 | E950.4 | E962.0 | E980.4 |
| **Nilstat** | 960.1 | E856 | E930.1 | E950.4 | E962.0 | E980.4 |
| topical | 976.0 | E858.7 | E946.0 | E950.4 | E962.0 | E980.4 |
| **Nimodipine** | 977.8 | E858.8 | E947.8 | E950.4 | E962.0 | E980.4 |
| **Niridazole** | 961.6 | E857 | E931.6 | E950.4 | E962.0 | E980.4 |
| **Nisentil** | 965.09 | E850.2 | E935.2 | E950.0 | E962.0 | E980.0 |
| **Nitrates** | 972.4 | E858.3 | E942.4 | E950.4 | E962.0 | E980.4 |
| **Nitrazepam** | 969.4 | E853.2 | E939.4 | E950.3 | E962.0 | E980.3 |
| **Nitric** | | | | | | |
| acid (liquid) | 983.1 | E864.1 | — | E950.7 | E962.1 | E980.6 |
| vapor | 987.8 | E869.8 | — | E952.8 | E962.2 | E982.8 |
| oxide (gas) | 987.2 | E869.0 | — | E952.8 | E962.2 | E982.8 |
| **Nitrite, amyl** (medicinal) (vapor) | 972.4 | E858.3 | E942.4 | E950.4 | E962.0 | E980.4 |
| **Nitroaniline** | 983.0 | E864.0 | — | E950.7 | E962.1 | E980.6 |
| vapor | 987.8 | E869.8 | — | E952.8 | E962.2 | E982.8 |
| **Nitrobenzene, nitrobenzol** | 983.0 | E864.0 | — | E950.7 | E962.1 | E980.6 |
| vapor | 987.8 | E869.8 | — | E952.8 | E962.2 | E982.8 |
| **Nitrocellulose** | 976.3 | E858.7 | E946.3 | E950.4 | E962.0 | E980.4 |
| **Nitrofuran derivatives** | 961.9 | E857 | E931.9 | E950.4 | E962.0 | E980.4 |
| **Nitrofurantoin** | 961.9 | E857 | E931.9 | E950.4 | E962.0 | E980.4 |
| **Nitrofurazone** | 976.0 | E858.7 | E946.0 | E950.4 | E962.0 | E980.4 |
| **Nitrogen** (dioxide) (gas) (oxide) | 987.2 | E869.0 | — | E952.8 | E962.2 | E982.8 |
| mustard (antineoplastic) | 963.1 | E858.1 | E933.1 | E950.4 | E962.0 | E980.4 |
| nonmedicinal | 989.89 | E866.8 | — | E950.9 | E962.1 | E980.9 |
| fumes | 987.8 | E869.8 | — | E952.8 | E962.2 | E982.8 |
| **Nitroglycerin, nitroglycerol** (medicinal) | 972.4 | E858.3 | E942.4 | E950.4 | E962.0 | E980.4 |
| **Nitrohydrochloric acid** | 983.1 | E864.1 | — | E950.7 | E962.1 | E980.6 |
| **Nitromersol** | 976.0 | E858.7 | E946.0 | E950.4 | E962.0 | E980.4 |
| **Nitronaphthalene** | 983.0 | E864.0 | — | E950.7 | E962.2 | E980.6 |
| **Nitrophenol** | 983.0 | E864.0 | — | E950.7 | E962.2 | E980.6 |
| **Nitrothiazol** | 961.6 | E857 | E931.6 | E950.4 | E962.0 | E980.4 |
| **Nitrotoluene, nitrotoluol** | 983.0 | E864.0 | — | E950.7 | E962.1 | E980.6 |
| vapor | 987.8 | E869.8 | — | E952.8 | E962.2 | E982.8 |
| **Nitrous** | 968.2 | E855.1 | E938.2 | E950.4 | E962.0 | E980.4 |
| acid (liquid) | 983.1 | E864.1 | — | E950.7 | E962.1 | E980.6 |
| fumes | 987.2 | E869.0 | — | E952.8 | E962.2 | E982.8 |
| oxide (anesthetic) NEC | 968.2 | E855.1 | E938.2 | E950.4 | E962.0 | E980.4 |
| **Nitrozone** | 976.0 | E858.7 | E946.0 | E950.4 | E962.0 | E980.4 |
| **Noctec** | 967.1 | E852.0 | E937.1 | E950.2 | E962.0 | E980.2 |
| **Noludar** | 967.5 | E852.4 | E937.5 | E950.2 | E962.0 | E980.2 |
| **Noptil** | 967.0 | E851 | E937.0 | E950.1 | E962.0 | E980.1 |
| **Noradrenalin** | 971.2 | E855.5 | E941.2 | E950.4 | E962.0 | E980.4 |
| **Noramidopyrine** | 965.5 | E850.5 | E935.5 | E950.0 | E962.0 | E980.0 |

| | Poisoning | Accident | Therapeutic Use | Suicide Attempt | Assault | Undetermined |
|---|---|---|---|---|---|---|
| **Norepinephrine** | 971.2 | E855.5 | E941.2 | E950.4 | E962.0 | E980.4 |
| **Norethandrolone** | 962.1 | E858.0 | E932.1 | E950.4 | E962.0 | E980.4 |
| **Norethindrone** | 962.2 | E858.0 | E932.2 | E950.4 | E962.0 | E980.4 |
| **Norethisterone** | 962.2 | E858.0 | E932.2 | E950.4 | E962.0 | E980.4 |
| **Norethynodrel** | 962.2 | E858.0 | E932.2 | E950.4 | E962.0 | E980.4 |
| **Norlestrin** | 962.2 | E858.0 | E932.2 | E950.4 | E962.0 | E980.4 |
| **Norlutin** | 962.2 | E858.0 | E932.2 | E950.4 | E962.0 | E980.4 |
| **Normison** — see Benzodiazepines | | | | | | |
| **Normorphine** | 965.09 | E850.2 | E935.2 | E950.0 | E962.0 | E980.0 |
| **Nortriptyline** | 969.0 | E854.0 | E939.0 | E950.3 | E962.0 | E980.3 |
| **Noscapine** | 975.4 | E858.6 | E945.4 | E950.4 | E962.0 | E980.4 |
| **Nose preparations** | 976.6 | E858.7 | E946.6 | E950.4 | E962.0 | E980.4 |
| **Novobiocin** | 960.8 | E856 | E930.8 | E950.4 | E962.0 | E980.4 |
| **Novocain** (infiltration) (topical) | 968.5 | E855.2 | E938.5 | E950.4 | E962.0 | E980.4 |
| nerve block (peripheral) (plexus) | 968.6 | E855.2 | E938.6 | E950.4 | E962.0 | E980.4 |
| spinal | 968.7 | E855.2 | E938.7 | E950.4 | E962.0 | E980.4 |
| **Noxythiolin** | 961.9 | E857 | E931.9 | E950.4 | E962.0 | E980.4 |
| **NPH Iletin** (insulin) | 962.3 | E858.0 | E932.3 | E950.4 | E962.0 | E980.4 |
| **Numorphan** | 965.09 | E850.2 | E935.2 | E950.0 | E962.0 | E980.0 |
| **Nunol** | 967.0 | E851 | E937.0 | E950.1 | E962.0 | E980.1 |
| **Nupercaine** (spinal anesthetic) | 968.7 | E855.2 | E938.7 | E950.4 | E962.0 | E980.4 |
| topical (surface) | 968.5 | E855.2 | E938.5 | E950.4 | E962.0 | E980.4 |
| **Nutmeg oil** (liniment) | 976.3 | E858.7 | E946.3 | E950.4 | E962.0 | E980.4 |
| **Nux vomica** | 989.1 | E863.7 | — | E950.6 | E962.1 | E980.7 |
| **Nydrazid** | 961.8 | E857 | E931.8 | E950.4 | E962.0 | E980.4 |
| **Nylidrin** | 971.2 | E855.5 | E941.2 | E950.4 | E962.0 | E980.4 |
| **Nystatin** | 960.1 | E856 | E930.1 | E950.4 | E962.0 | E980.4 |
| topical | 976.0 | E858.7 | E946.0 | E950.4 | E962.0 | E980.4 |
| **Nytol** | 963.0 | E858.1 | E933.0 | E950.4 | E962.0 | E980.4 |
| **Oblivion** | 967.8 | E852.8 | E937.8 | E950.2 | E962.0 | E980.2 |
| **Octyl nitrite** | 972.4 | E858.3 | E942.4 | E950.4 | E962.0 | E980.4 |
| **Oestradiol** (cypionate) (dipropionate) (valerate) | 962.2 | E858.0 | E932.2 | E950.4 | E962.0 | E980.4 |
| **Oestriol** | 962.2 | E858.0 | E932.2 | E950.4 | E962.0 | E980.4 |
| **Oestrone** | 962.2 | E858.0 | E932.2 | E950.4 | E962.0 | E980.4 |
| **Oil (of) NEC** | 989.89 | E866.8 | — | E950.9 | E962.1 | E980.9 |
| bitter almond | 989.0 | E866.8 | — | E950.9 | E962.1 | E980.9 |
| camphor | 976.1 | E858.7 | E946.1 | E950.4 | E962.0 | E980.4 |
| colors | 989.89 | E861.6 | — | E950.9 | E962.1 | E980.9 |
| fumes | 987.8 | E869.8 | — | E952.8 | E962.2 | E982.8 |
| lubricating | 981 | E862.2 | — | E950.9 | E962.1 | E980.9 |
| specified source, other — see substance specified | | | | | | |
| vitriol (liquid) | 983.1 | E864.1 | — | E950.7 | E962.1 | E980.6 |
| fumes | 987.8 | E869.8 | — | E952.8 | E962.2 | E982.8 |
| wintergreen (bitter) NEC | 976.3 | E858.7 | E946.3 | E950.4 | E962.0 | E980.4 |
| **Ointments NEC** | 976.9 | E858.7 | E946.9 | E950.4 | E962.0 | E980.4 |
| **Oleander** | 988.2 | E865.4 | — | E950.9 | E962.1 | E980.9 |
| **Oleandomycin** | 960.3 | E856 | E930.3 | E950.4 | E962.0 | E980.4 |
| **Oleovitamin A** | 963.5 | E858.1 | E933.5 | E950.4 | E962.0 | E980.4 |
| **Oleum ricini** | 973.1 | E858.4 | E943.1 | E950.4 | E962.0 | E980.4 |
| **Olive oil (medicinal) NEC** | 973.2 | E858.4 | E943.2 | E950.4 | E962.0 | E980.4 |
| **OMPA** | 989.3 | E863.1 | — | E950.6 | E962.1 | E980.7 |
| **Oncovin** | 963.1 | E858.1 | E933.1 | E950.4 | E962.0 | E980.4 |
| **Ophthaine** | 968.5 | E855.2 | E938.5 | E950.4 | E962.0 | E980.4 |
| **Ophthetic** | 968.5 | E855.2 | E938.5 | E950.4 | E962.0 | E980.4 |
| **Opiates, opioids, opium NEC** | 965.00 | E850.2 | E935.2 | E950.0 | E962.0 | E980.0 |
| antagonists | 970.1 | E854.3 | E940.1 | E950.4 | E962.0 | E980.4 |
| **Oracon** | 962.2 | E858.0 | E932.2 | E950.4 | E962.0 | E980.4 |
| **Oragrafin** | 977.8 | E858.8 | E947.8 | E950.4 | E962.0 | E980.4 |
| **Oral contraceptives** | 962.2 | E858.0 | E932.2 | E950.4 | E962.0 | E980.4 |
| **Orciprenaline** | 975.1 | E858.6 | E945.1 | E950.4 | E962.0 | E980.4 |
| **Organidin** | 975.5 | E858.6 | E945.5 | E950.4 | E962.0 | E980.4 |
| **Organophosphates** | 989.3 | E863.1 | — | E950.6 | E962.1 | E980.7 |
| **Orimune** | 979.5 | E858.8 | E949.5 | E950.4 | E962.0 | E980.4 |
| **Orinase** | 962.3 | E858.0 | E932.3 | E950.4 | E962.0 | E980.4 |
| **Orphenadrine** | 966.4 | E855.0 | E936.4 | E950.4 | E962.0 | E980.4 |
| **Ortal** (sodium) | 967.0 | E851 | E937.0 | E950.1 | E962.0 | E980.1 |
| **Orthoboric acid** | 976.0 | E858.7 | E946.0 | E950.4 | E962.0 | E980.4 |
| ENT agent | 976.6 | E858.7 | E946.6 | E950.4 | E962.0 | E980.4 |
| ophthalmic preparation | 976.5 | E858.7 | E946.5 | E950.4 | E962.0 | E980.4 |
| **Orthocaine** | 968.5 | E855.2 | E938.5 | E950.4 | E962.0 | E980.4 |
| **Ortho-Novum** | 962.2 | E858.0 | E932.2 | E950.4 | E962.0 | E980.4 |
| **Orthotolidine** (reagent) | 977.8 | E858.8 | E947.8 | E950.4 | E962.0 | E980.4 |
| **Osmic acid** (liquid) | 983.1 | E864.1 | — | E950.7 | E962.1 | E980.6 |
| fumes | 987.8 | E869.8 | — | E952.8 | E962.2 | E982.8 |
| **Osmotic diuretics** | 974.4 | E858.5 | E944.4 | E950.4 | E962.0 | E980.4 |
| **Ouabain** | 972.1 | E858.3 | E942.1 | E950.4 | E962.0 | E980.4 |
| **Ovarian hormones** (synthetic substitutes) | 962.2 | E858.0 | E932.2 | E950.4 | E962.0 | E980.4 |
| **Ovral** | 962.2 | E858.0 | E932.2 | E950.4 | E962.0 | E980.4 |
| **Ovulation suppressants** | 962.2 | E858.0 | E932.2 | E950.4 | E962.0 | E980.4 |
| **Ovulen** | 962.2 | E858.0 | E932.2 | E950.4 | E962.0 | E980.4 |
| **Oxacillin** (sodium) | 960.0 | E856 | E930.0 | E950.4 | E962.0 | E980.4 |
| **Oxalic acid** | 983.1 | E864.1 | — | E950.7 | E962.1 | E980.6 |
| **Oxanamide** | 969.5 | E853.8 | E939.5 | E950.3 | E962.0 | E980.3 |
| **Oxandrolone** | 962.1 | E858.0 | E932.1 | E950.4 | E962.0 | E980.4 |
| **Oxaprozin** | 965.61 | E850.6 | E935.6 | E950.0 | E962.0 | E980.0 |
| **Oxazepam** | 969.4 | E853.2 | E939.4 | E950.3 | E962.0 | E980.3 |
| **Oxazolidine derivatives** | 966.0 | E855.0 | E936.0 | E950.4 | E962.0 | E980.4 |
| **Ox bile extract** | 973.4 | E858.4 | E943.4 | E950.4 | E962.0 | E980.4 |
| **Oxedrine** | 971.2 | E855.5 | E941.2 | E950.4 | E962.0 | E980.4 |
| **Oxeladin** | 975.4 | E858.6 | E945.4 | E950.4 | E962.0 | E980.4 |
| **Oxethazaine NEC** | 968.5 | E855.2 | E938.5 | E950.4 | E962.0 | E980.4 |
| **Oxidizing agents NEC** | 983.9 | E864.3 | — | E950.7 | E962.1 | E980.6 |
| **Oxolinic acid** | 961.3 | E857 | E931.3 | E950.4 | E962.0 | E980.4 |
| **Oxophenarsine** | 961.1 | E857 | E931.1 | E950.4 | E962.0 | E980.4 |
| **Oxsoralen** | 976.3 | E858.7 | E946.3 | E950.4 | E962.0 | E980.4 |
| **Oxtriphylline** | 975.7 | E858.6 | E945.7 | E950.4 | E962.0 | E980.4 |
| **Oxybuprocaine** | 968.5 | E855.2 | E938.5 | E950.4 | E962.0 | E980.4 |
| **Oxybutynin** | 975.1 | E858.6 | E945.1 | E950.4 | E962.0 | E980.4 |
| **Oxycodone** | 965.09 | E850.2 | E935.2 | E950.0 | E962.0 | E980.0 |
| **Oxygen** | 987.8 | E869.8 | — | E952.8 | E962.2 | E982.8 |
| **Oxylone** | 976.0 | E858.7 | E946.0 | E950.4 | E962.0 | E980.4 |
| ophthalmic preparation | 976.5 | E858.7 | E946.5 | E950.4 | E962.0 | E980.4 |
| **Oxymesterone** | 962.1 | E858.0 | E932.1 | E950.4 | E962.0 | E980.4 |
| **Oxymetazoline** | 971.2 | E855.5 | E941.2 | E950.4 | E962.0 | E980.4 |
| **Oxymetholone** | 962.1 | E858.0 | E932.1 | E950.4 | E962.0 | E980.4 |
| **Oxymorphone** | 965.09 | E850.2 | E935.2 | E950.0 | E962.0 | E980.0 |
| **Oxypertine** | 969.0 | E854.0 | E939.0 | E950.3 | E962.0 | E980.3 |
| **Oxyphenbutazone** | 965.5 | E850.5 | E935.5 | E950.0 | E962.0 | E980.0 |
| **Oxyphencyclimine** | 971.1 | E855.4 | E941.1 | E950.4 | E962.0 | E980.4 |
| **Oxyphenisatin** | 973.1 | E858.4 | E943.1 | E950.4 | E962.0 | E980.4 |
| **Oxyphenonium** | 971.1 | E855.4 | E941.1 | E950.4 | E962.0 | E980.4 |
| **Oxyquinoline** | 961.3 | E857 | E931.3 | E950.4 | E962.0 | E980.4 |
| **Oxytetracycline** | 960.4 | E856 | E930.4 | E950.4 | E962.0 | E980.4 |
| **Oxytocics** | 975.0 | E858.6 | E945.0 | E950.4 | E962.0 | E980.4 |
| **Oxytocin** | 975.0 | E858.6 | E945.0 | E950.4 | E962.0 | E980.4 |
| **Ozone** | 987.8 | E869.8 | — | E952.8 | E962.2 | E982.8 |
| **PABA** | 976.3 | E858.7 | E946.3 | E950.4 | E962.0 | E980.4 |
| **Packed red cells** | 964.7 | E858.2 | E934.7 | E950.4 | E962.0 | E980.4 |
| **Paint NEC** | 989.89 | E861.6 | — | E950.9 | E962.1 | E980.9 |
| cleaner | 982.8 | E862.9 | — | E950.9 | E962.1 | E980.9 |
| fumes NEC | 987.8 | E869.8 | — | E952.8 | E962.1 | E982.8 |
| lead (fumes) | 984.0 | E861.5 | — | E950.9 | E962.1 | E980.9 |
| solvent NEC | 982.8 | E862.9 | — | E950.9 | E962.1 | E980.9 |
| stripper | 982.8 | E862.9 | — | E950.9 | E962.1 | E980.9 |
| **Palfium** | 965.09 | E850.2 | E935.2 | E950.0 | E962.0 | E980.0 |
| **Palivizumab** | 979.9 | E858.8 | E949.6 | E950.4 | E962.0 | E980.4 |
| **Paludrine** | 961.4 | E857 | E931.4 | E950.4 | E962.0 | E980.4 |
| **PAM** | 977.2 | E855.8 | E947.2 | E950.4 | E962.0 | E980.4 |
| **Pamaquine** (naphthoate) | 961.4 | E857 | E931.4 | E950.4 | E962.0 | E980.4 |
| **Pamprin** | 965.1 | E850.3 | E935.3 | E950.0 | E962.0 | E980.0 |
| **Panadol** | 965.4 | E850.4 | E935.4 | E950.0 | E962.0 | E980.0 |
| **Pancreatic dornase** (mucolytic) | 963.4 | E858.1 | E933.4 | E950.4 | E962.0 | E980.4 |
| **Pancreatin** | 973.4 | E858.4 | E943.4 | E950.4 | E962.0 | E980.4 |
| **Pancrelipase** | 973.4 | E858.4 | E943.4 | E950.4 | E962.0 | E980.4 |
| **Pangamic acid** | 963.5 | E858.1 | E933.5 | E950.4 | E962.0 | E980.4 |
| **Panthenol** | 963.5 | E858.1 | E933.5 | E950.4 | E962.0 | E980.4 |
| topical | 976.8 | E858.7 | E946.8 | E950.4 | E962.0 | E980.4 |
| **Pantopaque** | 977.8 | E858.8 | E947.8 | E950.4 | E962.0 | E980.4 |
| **Pantopon** | 965.00 | E850.2 | E935.2 | E950.0 | E962.0 | E980.0 |
| **Pantothenic acid** | 963.5 | E858.1 | E933.5 | E950.4 | E962.0 | E980.4 |
| **Panwarfin** | 964.2 | E858.2 | E934.2 | E950.4 | E962.0 | E980.4 |
| **Papain** | 973.4 | E858.4 | E943.4 | E950.4 | E962.0 | E980.4 |
| **Papaverine** | 972.5 | E858.3 | E942.5 | E950.4 | E962.0 | E980.4 |
| **Para-aminobenzoic acid** | 976.3 | E858.7 | E946.3 | E950.4 | E962.0 | E980.4 |
| **Para-aminophenol derivatives** | 965.4 | E850.4 | E935.4 | E950.0 | E962.0 | E980.0 |
| **Para-aminosalicylic acid** (derivatives) | 961.8 | E857 | E931.8 | E950.4 | E962.0 | E980.4 |
| **Paracetaldehyde** (medicinal) | 967.2 | E852.1 | E937.2 | E950.2 | E962.0 | E980.2 |
| **Paracetamol** | 965.4 | E850.4 | E935.4 | E950.0 | E962.0 | E980.0 |
| **Paracodin** | 965.09 | E850.2 | E935.2 | E950.0 | E962.0 | E980.0 |
| **Paradione** | 966.0 | E855.0 | E936.0 | E950.4 | E962.0 | E980.4 |

☑ Additional Digit Required — Refer to the Tabular List for Digit Selection

▽ Subterms under main terms may continue to next column or page

▶◀ Revised Text    ● New Line    ▲ Revised Code

2008 ICD-9-CM

| | Poisoning | Accident | Therapeutic Use | Suicide Attempt | Assault | Undetermined |
|---|---|---|---|---|---|---|
| **Paraffin(s)** (wax) | 981 | E862.3 | — | E950.9 | E962.1 | E980.9 |
| liquid (medicinal) | 973.2 | E858.4 | E943.2 | E950.4 | E962.0 | E980.4 |
| nonmedicinal (oil) | 981 | E962.1 | — | E950.9 | E962.1 | E980.9 |
| **Paraldehyde** (medicinal) | 967.2 | E852.1 | E937.2 | E950.2 | E962.0 | E980.2 |
| **Paramethadione** | 966.0 | E855.0 | E936.0 | E950.4 | E962.0 | E980.4 |
| **Paramethasone** | 962.0 | E858.0 | E932.0 | E950.4 | E962.0 | E980.4 |
| **Paraquat** | 989.4 | E863.5 | — | E950.6 | E962.1 | E980.7 |
| **Parasympatholytics** | 971.1 | E855.4 | E941.1 | E950.4 | E962.0 | E980.4 |
| **Parasympathomimetics** | 971.0 | E855.3 | E941.0 | E950.4 | E962.0 | E980.4 |
| **Parathion** | 989.3 | E863.1 | — | E950.6 | E962.1 | E980.7 |
| **Parathormone** | 962.6 | E858.0 | E932.6 | E950.4 | E962.0 | E980.4 |
| **Parathyroid** (derivatives) | 962.6 | E858.0 | E932.6 | E950.4 | E962.0 | E980.4 |
| **Paratyphoid vaccine** | 978.1 | E858.8 | E948.1 | E950.4 | E962.0 | E980.4 |
| **Paredrine** | 971.2 | E855.5 | E941.2 | E950.4 | E962.0 | E980.4 |
| **Paregoric** | 965.00 | E850.2 | E935.2 | E950.0 | E962.0 | E980.0 |
| **Pargyline** | 972.3 | E858.3 | E942.3 | E950.4 | E962.0 | E980.4 |
| **Paris green** | 985.1 | E866.3 | — | E950.8 | E962.1 | E980.8 |
| insecticide | 985.1 | E863.4 | — | E950.8 | E962.1 | E980.8 |
| **Parnate** | 969.0 | E854.0 | E939.0 | E950.3 | E962.0 | E980.3 |
| **Paromomycin** | 960.8 | E856 | E930.8 | E950.4 | E962.0 | E980.4 |
| **Paroxypropione** | 963.1 | E858.1 | E933.1 | E950.4 | E962.0 | E980.4 |
| **Parzone** | 965.09 | E850.2 | E935.2 | E950.0 | E962.0 | E980.0 |
| **PAS** | 961.8 | E857 | E931.8 | E950.4 | E962.0 | E980.4 |
| **PCBs** | 981 | E862.3 | — | E950.9 | E962.1 | E980.9 |
| **PCP** (pentachlorophenol) | 989.4 | E863.6 | — | E950.6 | E962.1 | E980.7 |
| herbicide | 989.4 | E863.5 | — | E950.6 | E962.1 | E980.7 |
| insecticide | 989.4 | E863.4 | — | E950.6 | E962.1 | E980.7 |
| phencyclidine | 968.3 | E855.1 | E938.3 | E950.4 | E962.0 | E980.4 |
| **Peach kernel oil** (emulsion) | 973.2 | E858.4 | E943.2 | E950.4 | E962.0 | E980.4 |
| **Peanut oil** (emulsion) NEC | 973.2 | E858.4 | E943.2 | E950.4 | E962.0 | E980.4 |
| topical | 976.3 | E858.7 | E946.3 | E950.4 | E962.0 | E980.4 |
| **Pearly Gates** (morning glory | | | | | | |
| seeds) | 969.6 | E854.1 | E939.6 | E950.3 | E962.0 | E980.3 |
| **Pecazine** | 969.1 | E853.0 | E939.1 | E950.3 | E962.0 | E980.3 |
| **Pecilocin** | 960.1 | E856 | E930.1 | E950.4 | E962.0 | E980.4 |
| **Pectin** (with kaolin) NEC | 973.5 | E858.4 | E943.5 | E950.4 | E962.0 | E980.4 |
| **Pelletierine tannate** | 961.6 | E857 | E931.6 | E950.4 | E962.0 | E980.4 |
| **Pemoline** | 969.7 | E854.2 | E939.7 | E950.3 | E962.0 | E980.3 |
| **Pempidine** | 972.3 | E858.3 | E942.3 | E950.4 | E962.0 | E980.4 |
| **Penamecillin** | 960.0 | E856 | E930.0 | E950.4 | E962.0 | E980.4 |
| **Penethamate hydriodide** | 960.0 | E856 | E930.0 | E950.4 | E962.0 | E980.4 |
| **Penicillamine** | 963.8 | E858.1 | E933.8 | E950.4 | E962.0 | E980.4 |
| **Penicillin** (any type) | 960.0 | E856 | E930.0 | E950.4 | E962.0 | E980.4 |
| **Penicillinase** | 963.4 | E858.1 | E933.4 | E950.4 | E962.0 | E980.4 |
| **Pentachlorophenol** | | | | | | |
| (fungicide) | 989.4 | E863.6 | — | E950.6 | E962.1 | E980.7 |
| herbicide | 989.4 | E863.5 | — | E950.6 | E962.1 | E980.7 |
| insecticide | 989.4 | E863.4 | — | E950.6 | E962.1 | E980.7 |
| **Pentaerythritol** | 972.4 | E858.3 | E942.4 | E950.4 | E962.0 | E980.4 |
| chloral | 967.1 | E852.0 | E937.1 | E950.2 | E962.0 | E980.2 |
| tetranitrate NEC | 972.4 | E858.3 | E942.4 | E950.4 | E962.0 | E980.4 |
| **Pentagastrin** | 977.8 | E858.8 | E947.8 | E950.4 | E962.0 | E980.4 |
| **Pentalin** | 982.3 | E862.4 | — | E950.9 | E962.1 | E980.9 |
| **Pentamethonium** (bromide) | 972.3 | E858.3 | E942.3 | E950.4 | E962.0 | E980.4 |
| **Pentamidine** | 961.5 | E857 | E931.5 | E950.4 | E962.0 | E980.4 |
| **Pentanol** | 980.8 | E860.8 | — | E950.9 | E962.1 | E980.9 |
| **Pentaquine** | 961.4 | E857 | E931.4 | E950.4 | E962.0 | E980.4 |
| **Pentazocine** | 965.8 | E850.8 | E935.8 | E950.0 | E962.0 | E980.0 |
| **Penthienate** | 971.1 | E855.4 | E941.1 | E950.4 | E962.0 | E980.4 |
| **Pentobarbital, pentobarbitone** | | | | | | |
| (sodium) | 967.0 | E851 | E937.0 | E950.1 | E962.0 | E980.1 |
| **Pentolinium** (tartrate) | 972.3 | E858.3 | E942.3 | E950.4 | E962.0 | E980.4 |
| **Pentothal** | 968.3 | E855.1 | E938.3 | E950.4 | E962.0 | E980.4 |
| **Pentylenetetrazol** | 970.0 | E854.3 | E940.0 | E950.4 | E962.0 | E980.4 |
| **Pentylsalicylamide** | 961.8 | E857 | E931.8 | E950.4 | E962.0 | E980.4 |
| **Pepsin** | 973.4 | E858.4 | E943.4 | E950.4 | E962.0 | E980.4 |
| **Peptavlon** | 977.8 | E858.8 | E947.8 | E950.4 | E962.0 | E980.4 |
| **Percaine** (spinal) | 968.7 | E855.2 | E938.7 | E950.4 | E962.0 | E980.4 |
| topical (surface) | 968.5 | E855.2 | E938.5 | E950.4 | E962.0 | E980.4 |
| **Perchloroethylene** (vapor) | 982.3 | E862.4 | — | E950.9 | E962.1 | E980.9 |
| medicinal | 961.6 | E857 | E931.6 | E950.4 | E962.0 | E980.4 |
| **Percodan** | 965.09 | E850.2 | E935.2 | E950.0 | E962.0 | E980.0 |
| **Percogesic** | 965.09 | E850.2 | E935.2 | E950.0 | E962.0 | E980.0 |
| **Percorten** | 962.0 | E858.0 | E932.0 | E950.4 | E962.0 | E980.4 |
| **Pergonal** | 962.4 | E858.0 | E932.4 | E950.4 | E962.0 | E980.4 |
| **Perhexiline** | 972.4 | E858.3 | E942.4 | E950.4 | E962.0 | E980.4 |
| **Periactin** | 963.0 | E858.1 | E933.0 | E950.4 | E962.0 | E980.4 |
| **Periclor** | 967.1 | E852.0 | E937.1 | E950.2 | E962.0 | E980.2 |
| **Pericyazine** | 969.1 | E853.0 | E939.1 | E950.3 | E962.0 | E980.3 |
| **Peritrate** | 972.4 | E858.3 | E942.4 | E950.4 | E962.0 | E980.4 |
| **Permanganates NEC** | 983.9 | E864.3 | — | E950.7 | E962.1 | E980.6 |

| | Poisoning | Accident | Therapeutic Use | Suicide Attempt | Assault | Undetermined |
|---|---|---|---|---|---|---|
| **Permanganates** — *continued* | | | | | | |
| potassium (topical) | 976.0 | E858.7 | E946.0 | E950.4 | E962.0 | E980.4 |
| **Pernocton** | 967.0 | E851 | E937.0 | E950.1 | E962.0 | E980.1 |
| **Pernoston** | 967.0 | E851 | E937.0 | E950.1 | E962.0 | E980.1 |
| **Peronin(e)** | 965.09 | E850.2 | E935.2 | E950.0 | E962.0 | E980.0 |
| **Perphenazine** | 969.1 | E853.0 | E939.1 | E950.3 | E962.0 | E980.3 |
| **Pertofrane** | 969.0 | E854.0 | E939.0 | E950.3 | E962.0 | E980.3 |
| **Pertussis** | | | | | | |
| immune serum (human) | 964.6 | E858.2 | E934.6 | E950.4 | E962.0 | E980.4 |
| vaccine (with diphtheria toxoid) | | | | | | |
| (with tetanus toxoid) | 978.6 | E858.8 | E948.6 | E950.4 | E962.0 | E980.4 |
| **Peruvian balsam** | 976.8 | E858.7 | E946.8 | E950.4 | E962.0 | E980.4 |
| **Pesticides** (dust) (fumes) | | | | | | |
| (vapor) | 989.4 | E863.4 | — | E950.6 | E962.1 | E980.7 |
| arsenic | 985.1 | E863.4 | — | E950.8 | E962.1 | E980.8 |
| chlorinated | 989.2 | E863.0 | — | E950.6 | E962.1 | E980.7 |
| cyanide | 989.0 | E863.4 | — | E950.6 | E962.1 | E980.7 |
| kerosene | 981 | E863.4 | — | E950.6 | E962.1 | E980.7 |
| mixture (of compounds) | 989.4 | E863.3 | — | E950.6 | E962.1 | E980.7 |
| naphthalene | 983.0 | E863.4 | — | E950.7 | E962.1 | E980.6 |
| organochlorine | | | | | | |
| (compounds) | 989.2 | E863.0 | — | E950.6 | E962.1 | E980.7 |
| petroleum (distillate) (products) | | | | | | |
| NEC | 981 | E863.4 | — | E950.6 | E962.1 | E980.7 |
| specified ingredient NEC | 989.4 | E863.4 | — | E950.6 | E962.1 | E980.7 |
| strychnine | 989.1 | E863.4 | — | E950.6 | E962.1 | E980.7 |
| thallium | 985.8 | E863.7 | — | E950.6 | E962.1 | E980.7 |
| **Pethidine** (hydrochloride) | 965.09 | E850.2 | E935.2 | E950.0 | E962.0 | E980.0 |
| **Petrichloral** | 967.1 | E852.0 | E937.1 | E950.2 | E962.0 | E980.2 |
| **Petrol** | 981 | E862.1 | — | E950.9 | E962.1 | E980.9 |
| vapor | 987.1 | E869.8 | — | E952.8 | E962.2 | E982.8 |
| **Petrolatum** (jelly) (ointment) | 976.3 | E858.7 | E946.3 | E950.4 | E962.0 | E980.4 |
| hydrophilic | 976.3 | E858.7 | E946.3 | E950.4 | E962.0 | E980.4 |
| liquid | 973.2 | E858.4 | E943.2 | E950.4 | E962.0 | E980.4 |
| topical | 976.3 | E858.7 | E946.3 | E950.4 | E962.0 | E980.4 |
| nonmedicinal | 981 | E862.1 | — | E950.9 | E962.1 | E980.9 |
| **Petroleum** (cleaners) (fuels) | | | | | | |
| (products) NEC | 981 | E862.1 | — | E950.9 | E962.1 | E980.9 |
| benzin(e) — see Ligroin | | | | | | |
| ether — see Ligroin | | | | | | |
| jelly — see Petrolatum | | | | | | |
| naphtha — see Ligroin | | | | | | |
| pesticide | 981 | E863.4 | — | E950.6 | E962.1 | E980.7 |
| solids | 981 | E862.3 | — | E950.9 | E962.1 | E980.9 |
| solvents | 981 | E862.0 | — | E950.9 | E962.1 | E980.9 |
| vapor | 987.1 | E869.8 | — | E952.8 | E962.2 | E982.8 |
| **Peyote** | 969.6 | E854.1 | E939.6 | E950.3 | E962.0 | E980.3 |
| **Phanodorm, phanodorn** | 967.0 | E851 | E937.0 | E950.1 | E962.0 | E980.1 |
| **Phanquinone, phanquone** | 961.5 | E857 | E931.5 | E950.4 | E962.0 | E980.4 |
| **Pharmaceutical excipient or** | | | | | | |
| **adjunct** | 977.4 | E858.8 | E947.4 | E950.4 | E962.0 | E980.4 |
| **Phenacemide** | 966.3 | E855.0 | E936.3 | E950.4 | E962.0 | E980.4 |
| **Phenacetin** | 965.4 | E850.4 | E935.4 | E950.0 | E962.0 | E980.0 |
| **Phenadoxone** | 965.09 | E850.2 | E935.2 | E950.0 | E962.0 | E980.0 |
| **Phenaglycodol** | 969.5 | E853.8 | E939.5 | E950.3 | E962.0 | E980.3 |
| **Phenantoin** | 966.1 | E855.0 | E936.1 | E950.4 | E962.0 | E980.4 |
| **Phenaphthazine reagent** | 977.8 | E858.8 | E947.8 | E950.4 | E962.0 | E980.4 |
| **Phenazocine** | 965.09 | E850.2 | E935.2 | E950.0 | E962.0 | E980.0 |
| **Phenazone** | 965.5 | E850.5 | E935.5 | E950.0 | E962.0 | E980.0 |
| **Phenazopyridine** | 976.1 | E858.7 | E946.1 | E950.4 | E962.0 | E980.4 |
| **Phenbenicillin** | 960.0 | E856 | E930.0 | E950.4 | E962.0 | E980.4 |
| **Phenbutrazate** | 977.0 | E858.8 | E947.0 | E950.4 | E962.0 | E980.4 |
| **Phencyclidine** | 968.3 | E855.1 | E938.3 | E950.4 | E962.0 | E980.4 |
| **Phendimetrazine** | 977.0 | E858.8 | E947.0 | E950.4 | E962.0 | E980.4 |
| **Phenelzine** | 969.0 | E854.0 | E939.0 | E950.3 | E962.0 | E980.3 |
| **Phenergan** | 967.8 | E852.8 | E937.8 | E950.2 | E962.0 | E980.2 |
| **Phenethicillin** (potassium) | 960.0 | E856 | E930.0 | E950.4 | E962.0 | E980.4 |
| **Phenetsal** | 965.1 | E850.3 | E935.3 | E950.0 | E962.0 | E980.0 |
| **Pheneturide** | 966.3 | E855.0 | E936.3 | E950.4 | E962.0 | E980.4 |
| **Phenformin** | 962.3 | E858.0 | E932.3 | E950.4 | E962.0 | E980.4 |
| **Phenglutarimide** | 971.1 | E855.4 | E941.1 | E950.4 | E962.0 | E980.4 |
| **Phenicarbazide** | 965.8 | E850.8 | E935.8 | E950.0 | E962.0 | E980.0 |
| **Phenindamine** (tartrate) | 963.0 | E858.1 | E933.0 | E950.4 | E962.0 | E980.4 |
| **Phenindione** | 964.2 | E858.2 | E934.2 | E950.4 | E962.0 | E980.4 |
| **Pheniprazine** | 969.0 | E854.0 | E939.0 | E950.3 | E962.0 | E980.3 |
| **Pheniramine** (maleate) | 963.0 | E858.1 | E933.0 | E950.4 | E962.0 | E980.4 |
| **Phenmetrazine** | 977.0 | E858.8 | E947.0 | E950.4 | E962.0 | E980.4 |
| **Phenobal** | 967.0 | E851 | E937.0 | E950.1 | E962.0 | E980.1 |
| **Phenobarbital** | 967.0 | E851 | E937.0 | E950.1 | E962.0 | E980.1 |
| **Phenobarbitone** | 967.0 | E851 | E937.0 | E950.1 | E962.0 | E980.1 |
| **Phenoctide** | 976.0 | E858.7 | E946.0 | E950.4 | E962.0 | E980.4 |

| | Poisoning | Accident | Therapeutic Use | Suicide Attempt | Assault | Undetermined |
|---|---|---|---|---|---|---|
| **Phenol** (derivatives) NEC | 983.0 | E864.0 | — | E950.7 | E962.1 | E980.6 |
| disinfectant | 983.0 | E864.0 | — | E950.7 | E962.1 | E980.6 |
| pesticide | 989.4 | E863.4 | — | E950.6 | E962.1 | E980.7 |
| red | 977.8 | E858.8 | E947.8 | E950.4 | E962.0 | E980.4 |
| **Phenolphthalein** | 973.1 | E858.4 | E943.1 | E950.4 | E962.0 | E980.4 |
| **Phenolsulfonphthalein** | 977.8 | E858.8 | E947.8 | E950.4 | E962.0 | E980.4 |
| **Phenomorphan** | 965.09 | E850.2 | E935.2 | E950.0 | E962.0 | E980.0 |
| **Phenonyl** | 967.0 | E851 | E937.0 | E950.1 | E962.0 | E980.1 |
| **Phenoperidine** | 965.09 | E850.2 | E935.2 | E950.0 | E962.0 | E980.0 |
| **Phenoquin** | 974.7 | E858.5 | E944.7 | E950.4 | E962.0 | E980.4 |
| **Phenothiazines (tranquilizers)** | | | | | | |
| **NEC** | 969.1 | E853.0 | E939.1 | E950.3 | E962.0 | E980.3 |
| insecticide | 989.3 | E863.4 | — | E950.6 | E962.1 | E980.7 |
| **Phenoxybenzamine** | 971.3 | E855.6 | E941.3 | E950.4 | E962.0 | E980.4 |
| **Phenoxymethyl penicillin** | 960.0 | E856 | E930.0 | E950.4 | E962.0 | E980.4 |
| **Phenprocoumon** | 964.2 | E858.2 | E934.2 | E950.4 | E962.0 | E980.4 |
| **Phensuximide** | 966.2 | E855.0 | E936.2 | E950.4 | E962.0 | E980.4 |
| **Phentermine** | 977.0 | E858.8 | E947.0 | E950.4 | E962.0 | E980.4 |
| **Phentolamine** | 971.3 | E855.6 | E941.3 | E950.4 | E962.0 | E980.4 |
| **Phenyl** | | | | | | |
| butazone | 965.5 | E850.5 | E935.5 | E950.0 | E962.0 | E980.0 |
| enediamine | 983.0 | E864.0 | — | E950.7 | E962.1 | E980.6 |
| hydrazine | 983.0 | E864.0 | — | E950.7 | E962.1 | E980.6 |
| antineoplastic | 963.1 | E858.1 | E933.1 | E950.4 | E962.0 | E980.4 |
| mercuric compounds — see Mercury | | | | | | |
| salicylate | 976.3 | E858.7 | E946.3 | E950.4 | E962.0 | E980.4 |
| **Phenylephrin** | 971.2 | E855.5 | E941.2 | E950.4 | E962.0 | E980.4 |
| **Phenylethylbiguanide** | 962.3 | E858.0 | E932.3 | E950.4 | E962.0 | E980.4 |
| **Phenylpropanolamine** | 971.2 | E855.5 | E941.2 | E950.4 | E962.0 | E980.4 |
| **Phenylsulfthion** | 989.3 | E863.1 | — | E950.6 | E962.1 | E980.7 |
| **Phenyramidol,** | | | | | | |
| **phenyramidon** | 965.7 | E850.7 | E935.7 | E950.0 | E962.0 | E980.0 |
| **Phenytoin** | 966.1 | E855.0 | E936.1 | E950.4 | E962.0 | E980.4 |
| **pHisoHex** | 976.2 | E858.7 | E946.2 | E950.4 | E962.0 | E980.4 |
| **Pholcodine** | 965.09 | E850.2 | E935.2 | E950.0 | E962.0 | E980.0 |
| **Phorate** | 989.3 | E863.1 | — | E950.6 | E962.1 | E980.7 |
| **Phosdrin** | 989.3 | E863.1 | — | E950.6 | E962.1 | E980.7 |
| **Phosgene** (gas) | 987.8 | E869.8 | — | E952.8 | E962.2 | E982.8 |
| **Phosphate** (tricresyl) | 989.89 | E866.8 | — | E950.9 | E962.1 | E980.9 |
| organic | 989.3 | E863.1 | — | E950.6 | E962.1 | E980.7 |
| solvent | 982.8 | E862.4 | — | E950.9 | E926.1 | E980.9 |
| **Phosphine** | 987.8 | E869.8 | — | E952.8 | E962.2 | E982.8 |
| fumigant | 987.8 | E863.8 | — | E950.6 | E962.2 | E980.7 |
| **Phospholine** | 971.0 | E855.3 | E941.0 | E950.4 | E962.0 | E980.4 |
| **Phosphoric acid** | 983.1 | E864.1 | — | E950.7 | E962.1 | E980.6 |
| **Phosphorus (compounds)** | | | | | | |
| **NEC** | 983.9 | E864.3 | — | E950.7 | E962.1 | E980.6 |
| rodenticide | 983.9 | E863.7 | — | E950.7 | E962.1 | E980.6 |
| **Phthalimidoglutarimide** | 967.8 | E852.8 | E937.8 | E950.2 | E962.0 | E980.2 |
| **Phthalylsulfathiazole** | 961.0 | E857 | E931.0 | E950.4 | E962.0 | E980.4 |
| **Phylloquinone** | 964.3 | E858.2 | E934.3 | E950.4 | E962.0 | E980.4 |
| **Physeptone** | 965.02 | E850.1 | E935.1 | E950.0 | E962.0 | E980.0 |
| **Physostigma venenosum** | 988.2 | E865.4 | — | E950.9 | E962.1 | E980.9 |
| **Physostigmine** | 971.0 | E855.3 | E941.0 | E950.4 | E962.0 | E980.4 |
| **Phytolacca decandra** | 988.2 | E865.4 | — | E950.9 | E962.1 | E980.9 |
| **Phytomenadione** | 964.3 | E858.2 | E934.3 | E950.4 | E962.0 | E980.4 |
| **Phytonadione** | 964.3 | E858.2 | E934.3 | E950.4 | E962.0 | E980.4 |
| **Picric** (acid) | 983.0 | E864.0 | — | E950.7 | E962.1 | E980.6 |
| **Picrotoxin** | 970.0 | E854.3 | E940.0 | E950.4 | E962.0 | E980.4 |
| **Pilocarpine** | 971.0 | E855.3 | E941.0 | E950.4 | E962.0 | E980.4 |
| **Pilocarpus (jaborandi)** | | | | | | |
| **extract** | 971.0 | E855.3 | E941.0 | E950.4 | E962.0 | E980.4 |
| **Pimaricin** | 960.1 | E856 | E930.1 | E950.4 | E962.0 | E980.4 |
| **Pimonidine** | 965.09 | E850.2 | E935.2 | E950.0 | E962.0 | E980.0 |
| **Pine oil, pinesol** | | | | | | |
| **(disinfectant)** | 983.9 | E861.4 | — | E950.7 | E962.1 | E980.6 |
| **Pinkroot** | 961.6 | E857 | E931.6 | E950.4 | E962.0 | E980.4 |
| **Pipadone** | 965.09 | E850.2 | E935.2 | E950.0 | E962.0 | E980.0 |
| **Pipamazine** | 963.0 | E858.1 | E933.0 | E950.4 | E962.0 | E980.4 |
| **Pipazethate** | 975.4 | E858.6 | E945.4 | E950.4 | E962.0 | E980.4 |
| **Pipenzolate** | 971.1 | E855.4 | E941.1 | E950.4 | E962.0 | E980.4 |
| **Piperacetazine** | 969.1 | E853.0 | E939.1 | E950.3 | E962.0 | E980.3 |
| **Piperazine NEC** | 961.6 | E857 | E931.6 | E950.4 | E962.0 | E980.4 |
| estrone sulfate | 962.2 | E858.0 | E932.2 | E950.4 | E962.0 | E980.4 |
| **Piper cubeba** | 988.2 | E865.4 | — | E950.9 | E962.1 | E980.9 |
| **Piperidione** | 975.4 | E858.6 | E945.4 | E950.4 | E962.0 | E980.4 |
| **Piperidolate** | 971.1 | E855.4 | E941.1 | E950.4 | E962.0 | E980.4 |
| **Piperocaine** | 968.9 | E855.2 | E938.9 | E950.4 | E962.0 | E980.4 |
| infiltration (subcutaneous) | 968.5 | E855.2 | E938.5 | E950.4 | E962.0 | E980.4 |

| | Poisoning | Accident | Therapeutic Use | Suicide Attempt | Assault | Undetermined |
|---|---|---|---|---|---|---|
| **Piperocaine** — *continued* | | | | | | |
| nerve block (peripheral) | | | | | | |
| (plexus) | 968.6 | E855.2 | E938.6 | E950.4 | E962.0 | E980.4 |
| topical (surface) | 968.5 | E855.2 | E938.5 | E950.4 | E962.0 | E980.4 |
| **Pipobroman** | 963.1 | E858.1 | E933.1 | E950.4 | E962.0 | E980.4 |
| **Pipradrol** | 970.8 | E854.3 | E940.8 | E950.4 | E962.0 | E980.4 |
| **Piscidia** (bark) (erythrina) | 965.7 | E850.7 | E935.7 | E950.0 | E962.0 | E980.0 |
| **Pitch** | 983.0 | E864.0 | — | E950.7 | E962.1 | E980.6 |
| **Pitkin's solution** | 968.7 | E855.2 | E938.7 | E950.4 | E962.0 | E980.4 |
| **Pitocin** | 975.0 | E858.6 | E945.0 | E950.4 | E962.0 | E980.4 |
| **Pitressin** (tannate) | 962.5 | E858.0 | E932.5 | E950.4 | E962.0 | E980.4 |
| **Pituitary extracts** | | | | | | |
| (posterior) | 962.5 | E858.0 | E932.5 | E950.4 | E962.0 | E980.4 |
| anterior | 962.4 | E858.0 | E932.4 | E950.4 | E962.0 | E980.4 |
| **Pituitrin** | 962.5 | E858.0 | E932.5 | E950.4 | E962.0 | E980.4 |
| **Placental extract** | 962.9 | E858.0 | E932.9 | E950.4 | E962.0 | E980.4 |
| **Placidyl** | 967.8 | E852.8 | E937.8 | E950.2 | E962.0 | E980.2 |
| **Plague vaccine** | 978.3 | E858.8 | E948.3 | E950.4 | E962.0 | E980.4 |
| **Plant foods or fertilizers** | | | | | | |
| **NEC** | 989.89 | E866.5 | — | E950.9 | E962.1 | E980.9 |
| mixed with herbicides | 989.4 | E863.5 | — | E950.6 | E962.1 | E980.7 |
| **Plants, noxious, used as** | | | | | | |
| **food** | 988.2 | E865.9 | — | E950.9 | E962.1 | E980.9 |
| berries and seeds | 988.2 | E865.3 | — | E950.9 | E962.1 | E980.9 |
| specified type NEC | 988.2 | E865.4 | — | E950.9 | E962.1 | E980.9 |
| **Plasma** (blood) | 964.7 | E858.2 | E934.7 | E950.4 | E962.0 | E980.4 |
| expanders | 964.8 | E858.2 | E934.8 | E950.4 | E962.0 | E980.4 |
| **Plasmanate** | 964.7 | E858.2 | E934.7 | E950.4 | E962.0 | E980.4 |
| **Plegicil** | 969.1 | E853.0 | E939.1 | E950.3 | E962.0 | E980.3 |
| **Podophyllin** | 976.4 | E858.7 | E946.4 | E950.4 | E962.0 | E980.4 |
| **Podophyllum resin** | 976.4 | E858.7 | E946.4 | E950.4 | E962.0 | E980.4 |
| **Poison NEC** | 989.9 | E866.9 | — | E950.9 | E962.1 | E980.9 |
| **Poisonous berries** | 988.2 | E865.3 | — | E950.9 | E962.1 | E980.9 |
| **Pokeweed** (any part) | 988.2 | E865.4 | — | E950.9 | E962.1 | E980.9 |
| **Poldine** | 971.1 | E855.4 | E941.1 | E950.4 | E962.0 | E980.4 |
| **Poliomyelitis vaccine** | 979.5 | E858.8 | E949.5 | E950.4 | E962.0 | E980.4 |
| **Poliovirus vaccine** | 979.5 | E858.8 | E949.5 | E950.4 | E962.0 | E980.4 |
| **Polish** (car) (floor) (furniture) | | | | | | |
| (metal) (silver) | 989.89 | E861.2 | — | E950.9 | E962.1 | E980.9 |
| abrasive | 989.89 | E861.3 | — | E950.9 | E962.1 | E980.9 |
| porcelain | 989.89 | E861.3 | — | E950.9 | E962.1 | E980.9 |
| **Poloxalkol** | 973.2 | E858.4 | E943.2 | E950.4 | E962.0 | E980.4 |
| **Polyaminostyrene resins** | 974.5 | E858.5 | E944.5 | E950.4 | E962.0 | E980.4 |
| **Polychlorinated biphenyl** — *see* PCBs | | | | | | |
| **Polycycline** | 960.4 | E856 | E930.4 | E950.4 | E962.0 | E980.4 |
| **Polyester resin hardener** | 982.8 | E862.4 | — | E950.9 | E962.1 | E980.9 |
| fumes | 987.8 | E869.8 | — | E952.8 | E962.2 | E982.8 |
| **Polyestradiol** (phosphate) | 962.2 | E858.0 | E932.2 | E950.4 | E962.0 | E980.4 |
| **Polyethanolamine alkyl** | | | | | | |
| **sulfate** | 976.2 | E858.7 | E946.2 | E950.4 | E962.0 | E980.4 |
| **Polyethylene glycol** | 976.3 | E858.7 | E946.3 | E950.4 | E962.0 | E980.4 |
| **Polyferose** | 964.0 | E858.2 | E934.0 | E950.4 | E962.0 | E980.4 |
| **Polymyxin B** | 960.8 | E856 | E930.8 | E950.4 | E962.0 | E980.4 |
| ENT agent | 976.6 | E858.7 | E946.6 | E950.4 | E962.0 | E980.4 |
| ophthalmic preparation | 976.5 | E858.7 | E946.5 | E950.4 | E962.0 | E980.4 |
| topical NEC | 976.0 | E858.7 | E946.0 | E950.4 | E962.0 | E980.4 |
| **Polynoxylin(e)** | 976.0 | E858.7 | E946.0 | E950.4 | E962.0 | E980.4 |
| **Polyoxymethyleneurea** | 976.0 | E858.7 | E946.0 | E950.4 | E962.0 | E980.4 |
| **Polytetrafluoroethylene** | | | | | | |
| (inhaled) | 987.8 | E869.8 | — | E952.8 | E962.2 | E982.8 |
| **Polythiazide** | 974.3 | E858.5 | E944.3 | E950.4 | E962.0 | E980.4 |
| **Polyvinylpyrrolidone** | 964.8 | E858.2 | E934.8 | E950.4 | E962.0 | E980.4 |
| **Pontocaine** (hydrochloride) | | | | | | |
| (infiltration) (topical) | 968.5 | E855.2 | E938.5 | E950.4 | E962.0 | E980.4 |
| nerve block (peripheral) | | | | | | |
| (plexus) | 968.6 | E855.2 | E938.6 | E950.4 | E962.0 | E980.4 |
| spinal | 968.7 | E855.2 | E938.7 | E950.4 | E962.0 | E980.4 |
| **Pot** | 969.6 | E854.1 | E939.6 | E950.3 | E962.0 | E980.3 |
| **Potash** (caustic) | 983.2 | E864.2 | — | E950.7 | E962.1 | E980.6 |
| **Potassic saline injection** | | | | | | |
| (lactated) | 974.5 | E858.5 | E944.5 | E950.4 | E962.0 | E980.4 |
| **Potassium (salts) NEC** | 974.5 | E858.5 | E944.5 | E950.4 | E962.0 | E980.4 |
| aminosalicylate | 961.8 | E857 | E931.8 | E950.4 | E962.0 | E980.4 |
| arsenite (solution) | 985.1 | E866.3 | — | E950.8 | E962.1 | E980.8 |
| bichromate | 983.9 | E864.3 | — | E950.7 | E962.1 | E980.6 |
| bisulfate | 983.9 | E864.3 | — | E950.7 | E962.1 | E980.6 |
| bromide (medicinal) NEC | 967.3 | E852.2 | E937.3 | E950.2 | E962.0 | E980.2 |
| carbonate | 983.2 | E864.2 | — | E950.7 | E962.1 | E980.6 |
| chlorate NEC | 983.9 | E864.3 | — | E950.7 | E962.1 | E980.6 |
| cyanide — see Cyanide | | | | | | |

☑ Additional Digit Required — Refer to the Tabular List for Digit Selection
▽ Subterms under main terms may continue to next column or page
328 — Volume 2　　　▶◀ Revised Text　　　● New Line　　　▲ Revised Code　　　**2008 ICD-9-CM**

| | Poisoning | External Cause (E-Code) | | | | |
|---|---|---|---|---|---|---|
| | | Accident | Therapeutic Use | Suicide Attempt | Assault | Undetermined |
| **Potassium (salts)** — *continued* | | | | | | |
| hydroxide | 983.2 | E864.2 | — | E950.7 | E962.1 | E980.6 |
| iodide (expectorant) NEC | 975.5 | E858.6 | E945.5 | E950.4 | E962.0 | E980.4 |
| nitrate | 989.89 | E866.8 | — | E950.9 | E962.1 | E980.9 |
| oxalate | 983.9 | E864.3 | — | E950.7 | E962.1 | E980.6 |
| perchlorate NEC | 977.8 | E858.8 | E947.8 | E950.4 | E962.0 | E980.4 |
| antithyroid | 962.8 | E858.0 | E932.8 | E950.4 | E962.0 | E980.4 |
| permanganate | 976.0 | E858.7 | E946.0 | E950.4 | E962.0 | E980.4 |
| nonmedicinal | 983.9 | E864.3 | — | E950.7 | E962.1 | E980.6 |
| **Povidone-iodine** (anti-infective) NEC | 976.0 | E858.7 | E946.0 | E950.4 | E962.0 | E980.4 |
| **Practolol** | 972.0 | E858.3 | E942.0 | E950.4 | E962.0 | E980.4 |
| **Pralidoxime** (chloride) | 977.2 | E858.8 | E947.2 | E950.4 | E962.0 | E980.4 |
| **Pramoxine** | 968.5 | E855.2 | E938.5 | E950.4 | E962.0 | E980.4 |
| **Prazosin** | 972.6 | E858.3 | E942.6 | E950.4 | E962.0 | E980.4 |
| **Prednisolone** | 962.0 | E858.0 | E932.0 | E950.4 | E962.0 | E980.4 |
| ENT agent | 976.6 | E858.7 | E946.6 | E950.4 | E962.0 | E980.4 |
| ophthalmic preparation | 976.5 | E858.7 | E946.5 | E950.4 | E962.0 | E980.4 |
| topical NEC | 976.0 | E858.7 | E946.0 | E950.4 | E962.0 | E980.4 |
| **Prednisone** | 962.0 | E858.0 | E932.0 | E950.4 | E962.0 | E980.4 |
| **Pregnanediol** | 962.2 | E858.0 | E932.2 | E950.4 | E962.0 | E980.4 |
| **Pregneninolone** | 962.2 | E858.0 | E932.2 | E950.4 | E962.0 | E980.4 |
| **Preludin** | 977.0 | E858.8 | E947.0 | E950.4 | E962.0 | E980.4 |
| **Premarin** | 962.2 | E858.0 | E932.2 | E950.4 | E962.0 | E980.4 |
| **Prenylamine** | 972.4 | E858.3 | E942.4 | E950.4 | E962.0 | E980.4 |
| **Preparation H** | 976.8 | E858.7 | E946.8 | E950.4 | E962.0 | E980.4 |
| **Preservatives** | 989.89 | E866.8 | — | E950.9 | E962.1 | E980.9 |
| **Pride of China** | 988.2 | E865.3 | — | E950.9 | E962.1 | E980.9 |
| **Prilocaine** | 968.9 | E855.2 | E938.9 | E950.4 | E962.0 | E980.4 |
| infiltration (subcutaneous) | 968.5 | E855.2 | E938.5 | E950.4 | E962.0 | E980.4 |
| nerve block (peripheral) (plexus) | 968.6 | E855.2 | E938.6 | E950.4 | E962.0 | E980.4 |
| **Primaquine** | 961.4 | E857 | E931.4 | E950.4 | E962.0 | E980.4 |
| **Primidone** | 966.3 | E855.0 | E936.3 | E950.4 | E962.0 | E980.4 |
| **Primula** (veris) | 988.2 | E865.4 | — | E950.9 | E962.1 | E980.9 |
| **Prinadol** | 965.09 | E850.2 | E935.2 | E950.0 | E962.0 | E980.0 |
| **Priscol, Priscoline** | 971.3 | E855.6 | E941.3 | E950.4 | E962.0 | E980.4 |
| **Privet** | 988.2 | E865.4 | — | E950.9 | E962.1 | E980.9 |
| **Privine** | 971.2 | E855.5 | E941.2 | E950.4 | E962.0 | E980.4 |
| **Pro-Banthine** | 971.1 | E855.4 | E941.1 | E950.4 | E962.0 | E980.4 |
| **Probarbital** | 967.0 | E851 | E937.0 | E950.1 | E962.0 | E980.1 |
| **Probenecid** | 974.7 | E858.5 | E944.7 | E950.4 | E962.0 | E980.4 |
| **Procainamide** (hydrochloride) | 972.0 | E858.3 | E942.0 | E950.4 | E962.0 | E980.4 |
| **Procaine** (hydrochloride) (infiltration) (topical) | 968.5 | E855.2 | E938.5 | E950.4 | E962.0 | E980.4 |
| nerve block (peripheral) (plexus) | 968.6 | E855.2 | E938.6 | E950.4 | E962.0 | E980.4 |
| penicillin G | 960.0 | E856 | E930.0 | E950.4 | E962.0 | E980.4 |
| spinal | 968.7 | E855.2 | E938.7 | E950.4 | E962.0 | E980.4 |
| **Procalmidol** | 969.5 | E853.8 | E939.5 | E950.3 | E962.0 | E980.3 |
| **Procarbazine** | 963.1 | E858.1 | E933.1 | E950.4 | E962.0 | E980.4 |
| **Prochlorperazine** | 969.1 | E853.0 | E939.1 | E950.3 | E962.0 | E980.3 |
| **Procyclidine** | 966.4 | E855.0 | E936.4 | E950.4 | E962.0 | E980.4 |
| **Producer gas** | 986 | E868.8 | — | E952.1 | E962.2 | E982.1 |
| **Profenamine** | 966.4 | E855.0 | E936.4 | E950.4 | E962.0 | E980.4 |
| **Profenil** | 975.1 | E858.6 | E945.1 | E950.4 | E962.0 | E980.4 |
| **Progesterones** | 962.2 | E858.0 | E932.2 | E950.4 | E962.0 | E980.4 |
| **Progestin** | 962.2 | E858.0 | E932.2 | E950.4 | E962.0 | E980.4 |
| **Progestogens** (with estrogens) | 962.2 | E858.0 | E932.2 | E950.4 | E962.0 | E980.4 |
| **Progestone** | 962.2 | E858.0 | E932.2 | E950.4 | E962.0 | E980.4 |
| **Proguanil** | 961.4 | E857 | E931.4 | E950.4 | E962.0 | E980.4 |
| **Prolactin** | 962.4 | E858.0 | E932.4 | E950.4 | E962.0 | E980.4 |
| **Proloid** | 962.7 | E858.0 | E932.7 | E950.4 | E962.0 | E980.4 |
| **Proluton** | 962.2 | E858.0 | E932.2 | E950.4 | E962.0 | E980.4 |
| **Promacetin** | 961.8 | E857 | E931.8 | E950.4 | E962.0 | E980.4 |
| **Promazine** | 969.1 | E853.0 | E939.1 | E950.3 | E962.0 | E980.3 |
| **Promedol** | 965.09 | E850.2 | E935.2 | E950.0 | E962.0 | E980.0 |
| **Promethazine** | 967.8 | E852.8 | E937.8 | E950.2 | E962.0 | E980.2 |
| **Promin** | 961.8 | E857 | E931.8 | E950.4 | E962.0 | E980.4 |
| **Pronestyl** (hydrochloride) | 972.0 | E858.3 | E942.0 | E950.4 | E962.0 | E980.4 |
| **Pronetalol, pronethalol** | 972.0 | E858.3 | E942.0 | E950.4 | E962.0 | E980.4 |
| **Prontosil** | 961.0 | E857 | E931.0 | E950.4 | E962.0 | E980.4 |
| **Propamidine isethionate** | 961.5 | E857 | E931.5 | E950.4 | E962.0 | E980.4 |
| **Propanal** (medicinal) | 967.8 | E852.8 | E937.8 | E950.2 | E962.0 | E980.2 |
| **Propane** (gas) (distributed in mobile container) | 987.0 | E868.0 | — | E951.1 | E962.2 | E981.1 |
| distributed through pipes | 987.0 | E867 | — | E951.0 | E962.2 | E981.0 |
| incomplete combustion of — see Carbon monoxide, Propane | | | | | | |

| | Poisoning | External Cause (E-Code) | | | | |
|---|---|---|---|---|---|---|
| | | Accident | Therapeutic Use | Suicide Attempt | Assault | Undetermined |
| **Propanidid** | 968.3 | E855.1 | E938.3 | E950.4 | E962.0 | E980.4 |
| **Propanol** | 980.3 | E860.4 | — | E950.9 | E962.1 | E980.9 |
| **Propantheline** | 971.1 | E855.4 | E941.1 | E950.4 | E962.0 | E980.4 |
| **Proparacaine** | 968.5 | E855.2 | E938.5 | E950.4 | E962.0 | E980.4 |
| **Propatyl nitrate** | 972.4 | E858.3 | E942.4 | E950.4 | E962.0 | E980.4 |
| **Propicillin** | 960.0 | E856 | E930.0 | E950.4 | E962.0 | E980.4 |
| **Propiolactone** (vapor) | 987.8 | E869.8 | — | E952.8 | E962.2 | E982.8 |
| **Propiomazine** | 967.8 | E852.8 | E937.8 | E950.2 | E962.0 | E980.2 |
| **Propionaldehyde** (medicinal) | 967.8 | E852.8 | E937.8 | E950.2 | E962.0 | E980.2 |
| **Propionate compound** | 976.0 | E858.7 | E946.0 | E950.4 | E962.0 | E980.4 |
| **Propion gel** | 976.0 | E858.7 | E946.0 | E950.4 | E962.0 | E980.4 |
| **Propitocaine** | 968.9 | E855.2 | E938.9 | E950.4 | E962.0 | E980.4 |
| infiltration (subcutaneous) | 968.5 | E855.2 | E938.5 | E950.4 | E962.0 | E980.4 |
| nerve block (peripheral) (plexus) | 968.6 | E855.2 | E938.6 | E950.4 | E962.0 | E980.4 |
| **Propoxur** | 989.3 | E863.2 | — | E950.6 | E962.1 | E980.7 |
| **Propoxycaine** | 968.9 | E855.2 | E938.9 | E950.4 | E962.0 | E980.4 |
| infiltration (subcutaneous) | 968.5 | E855.2 | E938.5 | E950.4 | E962.0 | E980.4 |
| nerve block (peripheral) (plexus) | 968.6 | E855.2 | E938.6 | E950.4 | E962.0 | E980.4 |
| topical (surface) | 968.5 | E855.2 | E938.5 | E950.4 | E962.0 | E980.4 |
| **Propoxyphene** (hydrochloride) | 965.8 | E850.8 | E935.8 | E950.0 | E962.0 | E980.0 |
| **Propranolol** | 972.0 | E858.3 | E942.0 | E950.4 | E962.0 | E980.4 |
| **Propyl** | | | | | | |
| alcohol | 980.3 | E860.4 | — | E950.9 | E962.1 | E980.9 |
| carbinol | 980.3 | E860.4 | — | E950.9 | E962.1 | E980.9 |
| hexadrine | 971.2 | E855.5 | E941.2 | E950.4 | E962.0 | E980.4 |
| iodone | 977.8 | E858.8 | E947.8 | E950.4 | E962.0 | E980.4 |
| thiouracil | 962.8 | E858.0 | E932.8 | E950.4 | E962.0 | E980.4 |
| **Propylene** | 987.1 | E869.8 | — | E952.8 | E962.2 | E982.8 |
| **Propylparaben** (ophthalmic) | 976.5 | E858.7 | E946.5 | E950.4 | E962.0 | E980.4 |
| **Proscillaridin** | 972.1 | E858.3 | E942.1 | E950.4 | E962.0 | E980.4 |
| **Prostaglandins** | 975.0 | E858.6 | E945.0 | E950.4 | E962.0 | E980.4 |
| **Prostigmin** | 971.0 | E855.3 | E941.0 | E950.4 | E962.0 | E980.4 |
| **Protamine** (sulfate) | 964.5 | E858.2 | E934.5 | E950.4 | E962.0 | E980.4 |
| zinc insulin | 962.3 | E858.0 | E932.3 | E950.4 | E962.0 | E980.4 |
| **Protectants** (topical) | 976.3 | E858.7 | E946.3 | E950.4 | E962.0 | E980.4 |
| **Protein hydrolysate** | 974.5 | E858.5 | E944.5 | E950.4 | E962.0 | E980.4 |
| **Prothiaden** — *see* Dothiepin hydrochloride | | | | | | |
| **Prothionamide** | 961.8 | E857 | E931.8 | E950.4 | E962.0 | E980.4 |
| **Prothipendyl** | 969.5 | E853.8 | E939.5 | E950.3 | E962.0 | E980.3 |
| **Protokylol** | 971.2 | E855.5 | E941.2 | E950.4 | E962.0 | E980.4 |
| **Protopam** | 977.2 | E858.8 | E947.2 | E950.4 | E962.0 | E980.4 |
| **Protoveratrine(s) (A) (B)** | 972.6 | E858.3 | E942.6 | E950.4 | E962.0 | E980.4 |
| **Protriptyline** | 969.0 | E854.0 | E939.0 | E950.3 | E962.0 | E980.3 |
| **Provera** | 962.2 | E858.0 | E932.2 | E950.4 | E962.0 | E980.4 |
| **Provitamin A** | 963.5 | E858.1 | E933.5 | E950.4 | E962.0 | E980.4 |
| **Proxymetacaine** | 968.5 | E855.2 | E938.5 | E950.4 | E962.0 | E980.4 |
| **Proxyphylline** | 975.1 | E858.6 | E945.1 | E950.4 | E962.0 | E980.4 |
| **Prozac** — *see* Fluoxetine hydrochloride | | | | | | |
| **Prunus** | | | | | | |
| laurocerasus | 988.2 | E865.4 | — | E950.9 | E962.1 | E980.9 |
| virginiana | 988.2 | E865.4 | — | E950.9 | E962.1 | E980.9 |
| **Prussic acid** | 989.0 | E866.8 | — | E950.9 | E962.1 | E980.9 |
| vapor | 987.7 | E869.8 | — | E952.8 | E962.2 | E982.8 |
| **Pseudoephedrine** | 971.2 | E855.5 | E941.2 | E950.4 | E962.0 | E980.4 |
| **Psilocin** | 969.6 | E854.1 | E939.6 | E950.3 | E962.0 | E980.3 |
| **Psilocybin** | 969.6 | E854.1 | E939.6 | E950.3 | E962.0 | E980.3 |
| **PSP** | 977.8 | E858.8 | E947.8 | E950.4 | E962.0 | E980.4 |
| **Psychedelic agents** | 969.6 | E854.1 | E939.6 | E950.3 | E962.0 | E980.3 |
| **Psychodysleptics** | 969.6 | E854.1 | E939.6 | E950.3 | E962.0 | E980.3 |
| **Psychostimulants** | 969.7 | E854.2 | E939.7 | E950.3 | E962.0 | E980.3 |
| **Psychotherapeutic agents** | 969.9 | E855.9 | E939.9 | E950.3 | E962.0 | E980.3 |
| antidepressants | 969.0 | E854.0 | E939.0 | E950.3 | E962.0 | E980.3 |
| specified NEC | 969.8 | E855.8 | E939.8 | E950.3 | E962.0 | E980.3 |
| tranquilizers NEC | 969.5 | E853.9 | E939.5 | E950.3 | E962.0 | E980.3 |
| **Psychotomimetic agents** | 969.6 | E854.1 | E939.6 | E950.3 | E962.0 | E980.3 |
| **Psychotropic agents** | 969.9 | E854.8 | E939.9 | E950.3 | E962.0 | E980.3 |
| specified NEC | 969.8 | E854.8 | E939.8 | E950.3 | E962.0 | E980.3 |
| **Psyllium** | 973.3 | E858.4 | E943.3 | E950.4 | E962.0 | E980.4 |
| **Pteroylglutamic acid** | 964.1 | E858.2 | E934.1 | E950.4 | E962.0 | E980.4 |
| **Pteroyltriglutamate** | 963.1 | E858.1 | E933.1 | E950.4 | E962.0 | E980.4 |
| **PTFE** | 987.8 | E869.8 | — | E952.8 | E962.2 | E982.8 |
| **Pulsatilla** | 988.2 | E865.4 | — | E950.9 | E962.1 | E980.9 |
| **Purex** (bleach) | 983.9 | E864.3 | — | E950.7 | E962.1 | E980.6 |
| **Purine diuretics** | 974.1 | E858.5 | E944.1 | E950.4 | E962.0 | E980.4 |

| | Poisoning | Accident | Therapeutic Use | Suicide Attempt | Assault | Undetermined |
|---|---|---|---|---|---|---|
| Purinethol | 963.1 | E858.1 | E933.1 | E950.4 | E962.0 | E980.4 |
| PVP | 964.8 | E858.2 | E934.8 | E950.4 | E962.0 | E980.4 |
| Pyrabital | 965.7 | E850.7 | E935.7 | E950.0 | E962.0 | E980.0 |
| Pyramidon | 965.5 | E850.5 | E935.5 | E950.0 | E962.0 | E980.0 |
| Pyrantel (pamoate) | 961.6 | E857 | E931.6 | E950.4 | E962.0 | E980.4 |
| Pyrathiazine | 963.0 | E858.1 | E933.0 | E950.4 | E962.0 | E980.4 |
| Pyrazinamide | 961.8 | E857 | E931.8 | E950.4 | E962.0 | E980.4 |
| Pyrazinoic acid (amide) | 961.8 | E857 | E931.8 | E950.4 | E962.0 | E980.4 |
| Pyrazole (derivatives) | 965.5 | E850.5 | E935.5 | E950.0 | E962.0 | E980.0 |
| Pyrazolone (analgesics) | 965.5 | E850.5 | E935.5 | E950.0 | E962.0 | E980.0 |
| Pyrethrins, pyrethrum | 989.4 | E863.4 | — | E950.6 | E962.1 | E980.7 |
| Pyribenzamine | 963.0 | E858.1 | E933.0 | E950.4 | E962.0 | E980.4 |
| Pyridine (liquid) (vapor) | 982.0 | E862.4 | — | E950.9 | E962.1 | E980.9 |
| aldoxime chloride | 977.2 | E858.8 | E947.2 | E950.4 | E962.0 | E980.4 |
| Pyridium | 976.1 | E858.7 | E946.1 | E950.4 | E962.0 | E980.4 |
| Pyridostigmine | 971.0 | E855.3 | E941.0 | E950.4 | E962.0 | E980.4 |
| Pyridoxine | 963.5 | E858.1 | E933.5 | E950.4 | E962.0 | E980.4 |
| Pyrilamine | 963.0 | E858.1 | E933.0 | E950.4 | E962.0 | E980.4 |
| Pyrimethamine | 961.4 | E857 | E931.4 | E950.4 | E962.0 | E980.4 |
| Pyrogallic acid | 983.0 | E864.0 | — | E950.7 | E962.1 | E980.6 |
| Pyroxylin | 976.3 | E858.7 | E946.3 | E950.4 | E962.0 | E980.4 |
| Pyrrobutamine | 963.0 | E858.1 | E933.0 | E950.4 | E962.0 | E980.4 |
| Pyrrocitine | 968.5 | E855.2 | E938.5 | E950.4 | E962.0 | E980.4 |
| Pyrvinium (pamoate) | 961.6 | E857 | E931.6 | E950.4 | E962.0 | E980.4 |
| PZI | 962.3 | E858.0 | E932.3 | E950.4 | E962.0 | E980.4 |
| Quaalude | 967.4 | E852.3 | E937.4 | E950.2 | E962.0 | E980.2 |
| Quaternary ammonium derivatives | 971.1 | E855.4 | E941.1 | E950.4 | E962.0 | E980.4 |
| Quicklime | 983.2 | E864.2 | — | E950.7 | E962.1 | E980.6 |
| Quinacrine | 961.3 | E857 | E931.3 | E950.4 | E962.0 | E980.4 |
| Quinaglute | 972.0 | E858.3 | E942.0 | E950.4 | E962.0 | E980.4 |
| Quinalbarbitone | 967.0 | E851 | E937.0 | E950.1 | E962.0 | E980.1 |
| Quinestradiol | 962.2 | E858.0 | E932.2 | E950.4 | E962.0 | E980.4 |
| Quinethazone | 974.3 | E858.5 | E944.3 | E950.4 | E962.0 | E980.4 |
| Quinidine (gluconate) (polygalacturonate) (salts) (sulfate) | 972.0 | E858.3 | E942.0 | E950.4 | E962.0 | E980.4 |
| Quinine | 961.4 | E857 | E931.4 | E950.4 | E962.0 | E980.4 |
| Quiniobine | 961.3 | E857 | E931.3 | E950.4 | E962.0 | E980.4 |
| Quinolines | 961.3 | E857 | E931.3 | E950.4 | E962.0 | E980.4 |
| Quotane | 968.5 | E855.2 | E938.5 | E950.4 | E962.0 | E980.4 |
| Rabies | | | | | | |
| immune globulin (human) | 964.6 | E858.2 | E934.6 | E950.4 | E962.0 | E980.4 |
| vaccine | 979.1 | E858.8 | E949.1 | E950.4 | E962.0 | E980.4 |
| Racemoramide | 965.09 | E850.2 | E935.2 | E950.0 | E962.0 | E980.0 |
| Racemorphan | 965.09 | E850.2 | E935.2 | E950.0 | E962.0 | E980.0 |
| Radiator alcohol | 980.1 | E860.2 | — | E950.9 | E962.1 | E980.9 |
| Radio-opaque (drugs) (materials) | 977.8 | E858.8 | E947.8 | E950.4 | E962.0 | E980.4 |
| Ranunculus | 988.2 | E865.4 | — | E950.9 | E962.1 | E980.9 |
| Rat poison | 989.4 | E863.7 | — | E950.6 | E962.1 | E980.7 |
| Rattlesnake (venom) | 989.5 | E905.0 | — | E950.9 | E962.1 | E980.9 |
| Raudixin | 972.6 | E858.3 | E942.6 | E950.4 | E962.0 | E980.4 |
| Rautensin | 972.6 | E858.3 | E942.6 | E950.4 | E962.0 | E980.4 |
| Rautina | 972.6 | E858.3 | E942.6 | E950.4 | E962.0 | E980.4 |
| Rautotal | 972.6 | E858.3 | E942.6 | E950.4 | E962.0 | E980.4 |
| Rauwiloid | 972.6 | E858.3 | E942.6 | E950.4 | E962.0 | E980.4 |
| Rauwoldin | 972.6 | E858.3 | E942.6 | E950.4 | E962.0 | E980.4 |
| Rauwolfia (alkaloids) | 972.6 | E858.3 | E942.6 | E950.4 | E962.0 | E980.4 |
| Realgar | 985.1 | E866.3 | — | E950.8 | E962.1 | E980.8 |
| Red cells, packed | 964.7 | E858.2 | E934.7 | E950.4 | E962.0 | E980.4 |
| Reducing agents, industrial NEC | 983.9 | E864.3 | — | E950.7 | E962.1 | E980.6 |
| Refrigerant gas (freon) | 987.4 | E869.2 | — | E952.8 | E962.2 | E982.8 |
| central nervous system | 968.0 | E855.1 | E938.0 | E950.4 | E962.0 | E980.4 |
| not freon | 987.9 | E869.9 | — | E952.9 | E962.2 | E982.9 |
| Regroton | 974.4 | E858.5 | E944.4 | E950.4 | E962.0 | E980.4 |
| Rela | 968.0 | E855.1 | E938.0 | E950.4 | E962.0 | E980.4 |
| Relaxants, skeletal muscle (autonomic) | 975.2 | E858.6 | E945.2 | E950.4 | E962.0 | E980.4 |
| Renese | 974.3 | E858.5 | E944.3 | E950.4 | E962.0 | E980.4 |
| Renografin | 977.8 | E858.8 | E947.8 | E950.4 | E962.0 | E980.4 |
| Replacement solutions | 974.5 | E858.5 | E944.5 | E950.4 | E962.0 | E980.4 |
| Rescinnamine | 972.6 | E858.3 | E942.6 | E950.4 | E962.0 | E980.4 |
| Reserpine | 972.6 | E858.3 | E942.6 | E950.4 | E962.0 | E980.4 |
| Resorcin, resorcinol | 976.4 | E858.7 | E946.4 | E950.4 | E962.0 | E980.4 |
| Respaire | 975.5 | E858.6 | E945.5 | E950.4 | E962.0 | E980.4 |
| Respiratory agents NEC | 975.8 | E858.6 | E945.8 | E950.4 | E962.0 | E980.4 |
| Retinoic acid | 976.8 | E858.7 | E946.8 | E950.4 | E962.0 | E980.4 |
| Retinol | 963.5 | E858.1 | E933.5 | E950.4 | E962.0 | E980.4 |
| Rh (D) immune globulin (human) | 964.6 | E858.2 | E934.6 | E950.4 | E962.0 | E980.4 |
| Rhodine | 965.1 | E850.3 | E935.3 | E950.0 | E962.0 | E980.0 |
| RhoGAM | 964.6 | E858.2 | E934.6 | E950.4 | E962.0 | E980.4 |
| Riboflavin | 963.5 | E858.1 | E933.5 | E950.4 | E962.0 | E980.4 |
| Ricin | 989.89 | E866.8 | — | E950.9 | E962.1 | E980.9 |
| Ricinus communis | 988.2 | E865.3 | — | E950.9 | E962.1 | E980.9 |
| Rickettsial vaccine NEC | 979.6 | E858.8 | E949.6 | E950.4 | E962.0 | E980.4 |
| with viral and bacterial vaccine | 979.7 | E858.8 | E949.7 | E950.4 | E962.0 | E980.4 |
| Rifampin | 960.6 | E856 | E930.6 | E950.4 | E962.0 | E980.4 |
| Rimifon | 961.8 | E857 | E931.8 | E950.4 | E962.0 | E980.4 |
| Ringer's injection (lactated) | 974.5 | E858.5 | E944.5 | E950.4 | E962.0 | E980.4 |
| Ristocetin | 960.8 | E856 | E930.8 | E950.4 | E962.0 | E980.4 |
| Ritalin | 969.7 | E854.2 | E939.7 | E950.3 | E962.0 | E980.3 |
| Roach killers — *see* Pesticides | | | | | | |
| Rocky Mountain spotted fever vaccine | 979.6 | E858.8 | E949.6 | E950.4 | E962.0 | E980.4 |
| Rodenticides | 989.4 | E863.7 | — | E950.6 | E962.1 | E980.7 |
| Rohypnol | 969.4 | E853.2 | E939.4 | E950.3 | E962.0 | E980.3 |
| Rolaids | 973.0 | E858.4 | E943.0 | E950.4 | E962.0 | E980.4 |
| Rolitetracycline | 960.4 | E856 | E930.4 | E950.4 | E962.0 | E980.4 |
| Romilar | 975.4 | E858.6 | E945.4 | E950.4 | E962.0 | E980.4 |
| Rose water ointment | 976.3 | E858.7 | E946.3 | E950.4 | E962.0 | E980.4 |
| Rosuvastatin calcium | 972.1 | E858.3 | E942.2 | E950.4 | E962.0 | E980.4 |
| Rotenone | 989.4 | E863.7 | — | E950.6 | E962.1 | E980.7 |
| Rotoxamine | 963.0 | E858.1 | E933.0 | E950.4 | E962.0 | E980.4 |
| Rough-on-rats | 989.4 | E863.7 | — | E950.6 | E962.1 | E980.7 |
| RU486 | 962.9 | E858.0 | E932.9 | E950.4 | E962.0 | E980.4 |
| Rubbing alcohol | 980.2 | E860.3 | — | E950.9 | E962.1 | E980.9 |
| Rubella virus vaccine | 979.4 | E858.8 | E949.4 | E950.4 | E962.0 | E980.4 |
| Rubelogen | 979.4 | E858.8 | E949.4 | E950.4 | E962.0 | E980.4 |
| Rubeovax | 979.4 | E858.8 | E949.4 | E950.4 | E962.0 | E980.4 |
| Rubidomycin | 960.7 | E856 | E930.7 | E950.4 | E962.0 | E980.4 |
| Rue | 988.2 | E865.4 | — | E950.9 | E962.1 | E980.9 |
| Ruta | 988.2 | E865.4 | — | E950.9 | E962.1 | E980.9 |
| Sabadilla (medicinal) | 976.0 | E858.7 | E946.0 | E950.4 | E962.0 | E980.4 |
| pesticide | 989.4 | E863.4 | — | E950.6 | E962.1 | E980.7 |
| Sabin oral vaccine | 979.5 | E858.8 | E949.5 | E950.4 | E962.0 | E980.4 |
| Saccharated iron oxide | 964.0 | E858.2 | E934.0 | E950.4 | E962.0 | E980.4 |
| Saccharin | 974.5 | E858.5 | E944.5 | E950.4 | E962.0 | E980.4 |
| Safflower oil | 972.2 | E858.3 | E942.2 | E950.4 | E962.0 | E980.4 |
| Salbutamol sulfate | 975.7 | E858.6 | E945.7 | E950.4 | E962.0 | E980.4 |
| Salicylamide | 965.1 | E850.3 | E935.3 | E950.0 | E962.0 | E980.0 |
| Salicylate(s) | 965.1 | E850.3 | E935.3 | E950.0 | E962.0 | E980.0 |
| methyl | 976.3 | E858.7 | E946.3 | E950.4 | E962.0 | E980.4 |
| theobromine calcium | 974.1 | E858.5 | E944.1 | E950.4 | E962.0 | E980.4 |
| Salicylazosulfapyridine | 961.0 | E857 | E931.0 | E950.4 | E962.0 | E980.4 |
| Salicylhydroxamic acid | 976.0 | E858.7 | E946.0 | E950.4 | E962.0 | E980.4 |
| Salicylic acid (keratolytic) NEC | 976.4 | E858.7 | E946.4 | E950.4 | E962.0 | E980.4 |
| congeners | 965.1 | E850.3 | E935.3 | E950.0 | E962.0 | E980.0 |
| salts | 965.1 | E850.3 | E935.3 | E950.0 | E962.0 | E980.0 |
| Saliniazid | 961.8 | E857 | E931.8 | E950.4 | E962.0 | E980.4 |
| Salol | 976.3 | E858.7 | E946.3 | E950.4 | E962.0 | E980.4 |
| Salt (substitute) NEC | 974.5 | E858.5 | E944.5 | E950.4 | E962.0 | E980.4 |
| Saluretics | 974.3 | E858.5 | E944.3 | E950.4 | E962.0 | E980.4 |
| Saluron | 974.3 | E858.5 | E944.3 | E950.4 | E962.0 | E980.4 |
| Salvarsan 606 (neosilver) (silver) | 961.1 | E857 | E931.1 | E950.4 | E962.0 | E980.4 |
| Sambucus canadensis | 988.2 | E865.4 | — | E950.9 | E962.1 | E980.9 |
| berry | 988.2 | E865.3 | — | E950.9 | E962.1 | E980.9 |
| Sandril | 972.6 | E858.3 | E942.6 | E950.4 | E962.0 | E980.4 |
| Sanguinaria canadensis | 988.2 | E865.4 | — | E950.9 | E962.1 | E980.9 |
| Saniflush (cleaner) | 983.9 | E861.3 | — | E950.7 | E962.1 | E980.6 |
| Santonin | 961.6 | E857 | E931.6 | E950.4 | E962.0 | E980.4 |
| Santyl | 976.8 | E858.7 | E946.8 | E950.4 | E962.0 | E980.4 |
| Sarkomycin | 960.7 | E856 | E930.7 | E950.4 | E962.0 | E980.4 |
| Saroten | 969.0 | E854.0 | E939.0 | E950.3 | E962.0 | E980.3 |
| Saturnine — *see* Lead | | | | | | |
| Savin (oil) | 976.4 | E858.7 | E946.4 | E950.4 | E962.0 | E980.4 |
| Scammony | 973.1 | E858.4 | E943.1 | E950.4 | E962.0 | E980.4 |
| Scarlet red | 976.8 | E858.7 | E946.8 | E950.4 | E962.0 | E980.4 |
| Scheele's green | 985.1 | E866.3 | — | E950.8 | E962.1 | E980.8 |
| insecticide | 985.1 | E863.4 | — | E950.8 | E962.1 | E980.8 |
| Schradan | 989.3 | E863.1 | — | E950.6 | E962.1 | E980.7 |
| Schweinfurt(h) green | 985.1 | E866.3 | — | E950.8 | E962.1 | E980.8 |
| insecticide | 985.1 | E863.4 | — | E950.8 | E962.1 | E980.8 |
| Scilla — *see* Squill | | | | | | |
| Sclerosing agents | 972.7 | E858.3 | E942.7 | E950.4 | E962.0 | E980.4 |

☑ Additional Digit Required — Refer to the Tabular List for Digit Selection

▽ Subterms under main terms may continue to next column or page

| | Poisoning | Accident | Therapeutic Use | Suicide Attempt | Assault | Undetermined |
|---|---|---|---|---|---|---|
| Scopolamine | 971.1 | E855.4 | E941.1 | E950.4 | E962.0 | E980.4 |
| Scouring powder | 989.89 | E861.3 | — | E950.9 | E962.1 | E980.9 |
| Sea | | | | | | |
| anemone (sting) | 989.5 | E905.6 | — | E950.9 | E962.1 | E980.9 |
| cucumber (sting) | 989.5 | E905.6 | — | E950.9 | E962.1 | E980.9 |
| snake (bite) (venom) | 989.5 | E905.0 | — | E950.9 | E962.1 | E980.9 |
| urchin spine (puncture) | 989.5 | E905.6 | — | E950.9 | E962.1 | E980.9 |
| Secbutabarbital | 967.0 | E851 | E937.0 | E950.1 | E962.0 | E980.1 |
| Secbutabarbitone | 967.0 | E851 | E937.0 | E950.1 | E962.0 | E980.1 |
| Secobarbital | 967.0 | E851 | E937.0 | E950.1 | E962.0 | E980.1 |
| Seconal | 967.0 | E851 | E937.0 | E950.1 | E962.0 | E980.1 |
| Secretin | 977.8 | E858.8 | E947.8 | E950.4 | E962.0 | E980.4 |
| Sedatives, nonbarbiturate | 967.9 | E852.9 | E937.9 | E950.2 | E962.0 | E980.2 |
| specified NEC | 967.8 | E852.8 | E937.8 | E950.2 | E962.0 | E980.2 |
| Sedormid | 967.8 | E852.8 | E937.8 | E950.2 | E962.0 | E980.2 |
| Seed (plant) | 988.2 | E865.3 | — | E950.9 | E962.1 | E980.9 |
| disinfectant or dressing | 989.89 | E866.5 | — | E950.9 | E962.1 | E980.9 |
| Selenium (fumes) NEC | 985.8 | E866.4 | — | E950.9 | E962.1 | E980.9 |
| disulfide or sulfide | 976.4 | E858.7 | E946.4 | E950.4 | E962.0 | E980.4 |
| Selsun | 976.4 | E858.7 | E946.4 | E950.4 | E962.0 | E980.4 |
| Senna | 973.1 | E858.4 | E943.1 | E950.4 | E962.0 | E980.4 |
| Septisol | 976.2 | E858.7 | E946.2 | E950.4 | E962.0 | E980.4 |
| Serax | 969.4 | E853.2 | E939.4 | E950.3 | E962.0 | E980.3 |
| Serenesil | 967.8 | E852.8 | E937.8 | E950.2 | E962.0 | E980.2 |
| Serenium (hydrochloride) | 961.9 | E857 | E931.9 | E950.4 | E962.0 | E980.4 |
| Serepax — see Oxazepam | | | | | | |
| Sernyl | 968.3 | E855.1 | E938.3 | E950.4 | E962.0 | E980.4 |
| Serotonin | 977.8 | E858.8 | E947.8 | E950.4 | E962.0 | E980.4 |
| Serpasil | 972.6 | E858.3 | E942.6 | E950.4 | E962.0 | E980.4 |
| Sewer gas | 987.8 | E869.8 | — | E952.8 | E962.2 | E982.8 |
| Shampoo | 989.6 | E861.0 | — | E950.9 | E962.1 | E980.9 |
| Shellfish, nonbacterial or noxious | 988.0 | E865.1 | — | E950.9 | E962.1 | E980.9 |
| Silicones NEC | 989.83 | E866.8 | E947.8 | E950.9 | E962.1 | E980.9 |
| Silvadene | 976.0 | E858.7 | E946.0 | E950.4 | E962.0 | E980.4 |
| Silver (compound) (medicinal) | | | | | | |
| NEC | 976.0 | E858.7 | E946.0 | E950.4 | E962.0 | E980.4 |
| anti-infectives | 976.0 | E858.7 | E946.0 | E950.4 | E962.0 | E980.4 |
| arsphenamine | 961.1 | E857 | E931.1 | E950.4 | E962.0 | E980.4 |
| nitrate | 976.0 | E858.7 | E946.0 | E950.4 | E962.0 | E980.4 |
| ophthalmic preparation | 976.5 | E858.7 | E946.5 | E950.4 | E962.0 | E980.4 |
| toughened (keratolytic) | 976.4 | E858.7 | E946.4 | E950.4 | E962.0 | E980.4 |
| nonmedicinal (dust) | 985.8 | E866.4 | — | E950.9 | E962.1 | E980.9 |
| protein (mild) (strong) | 976.0 | E858.7 | E946.0 | E950.4 | E962.0 | E980.4 |
| salvarsan | 961.1 | E857 | E931.1 | E950.4 | E962.0 | E980.4 |
| Simethicone | 973.8 | E858.4 | E943.8 | E950.4 | E962.0 | E980.4 |
| Sinequan | 969.0 | E854.0 | E939.0 | E950.3 | E962.0 | E980.3 |
| Singoserp | 972.6 | E858.3 | E942.6 | E950.4 | E962.0 | E980.4 |
| Sintrom | 964.2 | E858.2 | E934.2 | E950.4 | E962.0 | E980.4 |
| Sitosterols | 972.2 | E858.3 | E942.2 | E950.4 | E962.0 | E980.4 |
| Skeletal muscle relaxants | 975.2 | E858.6 | E945.2 | E950.4 | E962.0 | E980.4 |
| Skin | | | | | | |
| agents (external) | 976.9 | E858.7 | E946.9 | E950.4 | E962.0 | E980.4 |
| specified NEC | 976.8 | E858.7 | E946.8 | E950.4 | E962.0 | E980.4 |
| test antigen | 977.8 | E858.8 | E947.8 | E950.4 | E962.0 | E980.4 |
| Sleep-eze | 963.0 | E858.1 | E933.0 | E950.4 | E962.0 | E980.4 |
| Sleeping draught (drug) (pill) (tablet) | 967.9 | E852.9 | E937.9 | E950.2 | E962.0 | E980.2 |
| Smallpox vaccine | 979.0 | E858.8 | E949.0 | E950.4 | E962.0 | E980.4 |
| Smelter fumes NEC | 985.9 | E866.4 | — | E950.9 | E962.1 | E980.9 |
| Smog | 987.3 | E869.1 | — | E952.8 | E962.2 | E982.8 |
| Smoke NEC | 987.9 | E869.9 | — | E952.9 | E962.2 | E982.9 |
| Smooth muscle relaxant | 975.1 | E858.6 | E945.1 | E950.4 | E962.0 | E980.4 |
| Snail killer | 989.4 | E863.4 | — | E950.6 | E962.1 | E980.7 |
| Snake (bite) (venom) | 989.5 | E905.0 | — | E950.9 | E962.1 | E980.9 |
| Snuff | 989.89 | E866.8 | — | E950.9 | E962.1 | E980.9 |
| Soap (powder) (product) | 989.6 | E861.1 | — | E950.9 | E962.1 | E980.9 |
| bicarb | 963.3 | E858.1 | E933.3 | E950.4 | E962.0 | E980.4 |
| chlorinated — see Sodium, hypochlorite | | | | | | |
| medicinal, soft | 976.2 | E858.7 | E946.2 | E950.4 | E962.0 | E980.4 |
| Soda (caustic) | 983.2 | E864.2 | — | E950.7 | E962.1 | E980.6 |
| Sodium | | | | | | |
| acetosulfone | 961.8 | E857 | E931.8 | E950.4 | E962.0 | E980.4 |
| acetrizoate | 977.8 | E858.8 | E947.8 | E950.4 | E962.0 | E980.4 |
| amytal | 967.0 | E851 | E937.0 | E950.1 | E962.0 | E980.1 |
| arsenate — see Arsenic | | | | | | |
| bicarbonate | 963.3 | E858.1 | E933.3 | E950.4 | E962.0 | E980.4 |
| bichromate | 983.9 | E864.3 | — | E950.7 | E962.1 | E980.6 |
| biphosphate | 963.2 | E858.1 | E933.2 | E950.4 | E962.0 | E980.4 |
| bisulfate | 983.9 | E864.3 | — | E950.7 | E962.1 | E980.6 |
| **Sodium** — continued | | | | | | |
| borate (cleanser) | 989.6 | E861.3 | — | E950.9 | E962.1 | E980.9 |
| bromide NEC | 967.3 | E852.2 | E937.3 | E950.2 | E962.0 | E980.2 |
| cacodylate (nonmedicinal) | | | | | | |
| NEC | 978.8 | E858.8 | E948.8 | E950.4 | E962.0 | E980.4 |
| anti-infective | 961.1 | E857 | E931.1 | E950.4 | E962.0 | E980.4 |
| herbicide | 989.4 | E863.5 | — | E950.6 | E962.1 | E980.7 |
| calcium edetate | 963.8 | E858.1 | E933.8 | E950.4 | E962.0 | E980.4 |
| carbonate NEC | 983.2 | E864.2 | — | E950.7 | E962.1 | E980.6 |
| chlorate NEC | 983.9 | E864.3 | — | E950.7 | E962.1 | E980.6 |
| herbicide | 983.9 | E863.5 | — | E950.7 | E962.1 | E980.6 |
| chloride NEC | 974.5 | E858.5 | E944.5 | E950.4 | E962.0 | E980.4 |
| chromate | 983.9 | E864.3 | — | E950.7 | E962.1 | E980.6 |
| citrate | 963.3 | E858.1 | E933.3 | E950.4 | E962.0 | E980.4 |
| cyanide — see Cyanide(s) | | | | | | |
| cyclamate | 974.5 | E858.5 | E944.5 | E950.4 | E962.0 | E980.4 |
| diatrizoate | 977.8 | E858.8 | E947.8 | E950.4 | E962.0 | E980.4 |
| dibunate | 975.4 | E858.6 | E945.4 | E950.4 | E962.0 | E980.4 |
| dioctyl sulfosuccinate | 973.2 | E858.4 | E943.2 | E950.4 | E962.0 | E980.4 |
| edetate | 963.8 | E858.1 | E933.8 | E950.4 | E962.0 | E980.4 |
| ethacrynate | 974.4 | E858.5 | E944.4 | E950.4 | E962.0 | E980.4 |
| fluoracetate (dust) (rodenticide) | 989.4 | E863.7 | — | E950.6 | E962.1 | E980.7 |
| fluoride — see Fluoride(s) | | | | | | |
| free salt | 974.5 | E858.5 | E944.5 | E950.4 | E962.0 | E980.4 |
| glucosulfone | 961.8 | E857 | E931.8 | E950.4 | E962.0 | E980.4 |
| hydroxide | 983.2 | E864.2 | — | E950.7 | E962.1 | E980.6 |
| hypochlorite (bleach) NEC | 983.9 | E864.3 | — | E950.7 | E962.1 | E980.6 |
| disinfectant | 983.9 | E861.4 | — | E950.7 | E962.1 | E980.6 |
| medicinal (anti-infective) (external) | 976.0 | E858.7 | E946.0 | E950.4 | E962.0 | E980.4 |
| vapor | 987.8 | E869.8 | — | E952.8 | E962.2 | E982.8 |
| hyposulfite | 976.0 | E858.7 | E946.0 | E950.4 | E962.0 | E980.4 |
| indigotindisulfonate | 977.8 | E858.8 | E947.8 | E950.4 | E962.0 | E980.4 |
| iodide | 977.8 | E858.8 | E947.8 | E950.4 | E962.0 | E980.4 |
| iothalamate | 977.8 | E858.8 | E947.8 | E950.4 | E962.0 | E980.4 |
| iron edetate | 964.0 | E858.2 | E934.0 | E950.4 | E962.0 | E980.4 |
| lactate | 963.3 | E858.1 | E933.3 | E950.4 | E962.0 | E980.4 |
| lauryl sulfate | 976.2 | E858.7 | E946.2 | E950.4 | E962.0 | E980.4 |
| L-triiodothyronine | 962.7 | E858.0 | E932.7 | E950.4 | E962.0 | E980.4 |
| metrizoate | 977.8 | E858.8 | E947.8 | E950.4 | E962.0 | E980.4 |
| monofluoracetate (dust) (rodenticide) | 989.4 | E863.7 | — | E950.6 | E962.1 | E980.7 |
| morrhuate | 972.7 | E858.3 | E942.7 | E950.4 | E962.0 | E980.4 |
| nafcillin | 960.0 | E856 | E930.0 | E950.4 | E962.0 | E980.4 |
| nitrate (oxidizing agent) | 983.9 | E864.3 | — | E950.7 | E962.1 | E980.6 |
| nitrite (medicinal) | 972.4 | E858.3 | E942.4 | E950.4 | E962.0 | E980.4 |
| nitroferricyanide | 972.6 | E858.3 | E942.6 | E950.4 | E962.0 | E980.4 |
| nitroprusside | 972.6 | E858.3 | E942.6 | E950.4 | E962.0 | E980.4 |
| para-aminohippurate | 977.8 | E858.8 | E947.8 | E950.4 | E962.0 | E980.4 |
| perborate (nonmedicinal) | | | | | | |
| NEC | 989.89 | E866.8 | — | E950.9 | E962.1 | E980.9 |
| medicinal | 976.6 | E858.7 | E946.6 | E950.4 | E962.0 | E980.4 |
| soap | 989.6 | E861.1 | — | E950.9 | E962.1 | E980.9 |
| percarbonate — see Sodium, perborate | | | | | | |
| phosphate | 973.3 | E858.4 | E943.3 | E950.4 | E962.0 | E980.4 |
| polystyrene sulfonate | 974.5 | E858.5 | E944.5 | E950.4 | E962.0 | E980.4 |
| propionate | 976.0 | E858.7 | E946.0 | E950.4 | E962.0 | E980.4 |
| psylliate | 972.7 | E858.3 | E942.7 | E950.4 | E962.0 | E980.4 |
| removing resins | 974.5 | E858.5 | E944.5 | E950.4 | E962.0 | E980.4 |
| salicylate | 965.1 | E850.3 | E935.3 | E950.0 | E962.0 | E980.0 |
| sulfate | 973.3 | E858.4 | E943.3 | E950.4 | E962.0 | E980.4 |
| sulfoxone | 961.8 | E857 | E931.8 | E950.4 | E962.0 | E980.4 |
| tetradecyl sulfate | 972.7 | E858.3 | E942.7 | E950.4 | E962.0 | E980.4 |
| thiopental | 968.3 | E855.1 | E938.3 | E950.4 | E962.0 | E980.4 |
| thiosalicylate | 965.1 | E850.3 | E935.3 | E950.0 | E962.0 | E980.0 |
| thiosulfate | 976.0 | E858.7 | E946.0 | E950.4 | E962.0 | E980.4 |
| tolbutamide | 977.8 | E858.8 | E947.8 | E950.4 | E962.0 | E980.4 |
| tyropanoate | 977.8 | E858.8 | E947.8 | E950.4 | E962.0 | E980.4 |
| valproate | 966.3 | E855.0 | E936.3 | E950.4 | E962.0 | E980.4 |
| Solanine | 977.8 | E858.8 | E947.8 | E950.4 | E962.0 | E980.4 |
| Solanum dulcamara | 988.2 | E865.4 | — | E950.9 | E962.1 | E980.9 |
| Solapsone | 961.8 | E857 | E931.8 | E950.4 | E962.0 | E980.4 |
| Solasulfone | 961.8 | E857 | E931.8 | E950.4 | E962.0 | E980.4 |
| Soldering fluid | 983.1 | E864.1 | — | E950.7 | E962.1 | E980.6 |
| Solid substance | 989.9 | E866.9 | — | E950.9 | E962.1 | E980.9 |
| specified NEC | 989.9 | E866.8 | — | E950.9 | E962.1 | E980.9 |
| Solvents, industrial | 982.8 | E862.9 | — | E950.9 | E962.1 | E980.9 |
| naphtha | 981 | E862.0 | — | E950.9 | E962.1 | E980.9 |
| petroleum | 981 | E862.0 | — | E950.9 | E962.1 | E980.9 |
| specified NEC | 982.8 | E862.4 | — | E950.9 | E962.1 | E980.9 |

| | Poisoning | Accident | Therapeutic Use | Suicide Attempt | Assault | Undetermined |
|---|---|---|---|---|---|---|
| **Soma** | 968.0 | E855.1 | E938.0 | E950.4 | E962.0 | E980.4 |
| **Somatotropin** | 962.4 | E858.0 | E932.4 | E950.4 | E962.0 | E980.4 |
| **Sominex** | 963.0 | E858.1 | E933.0 | E950.4 | E962.0 | E980.4 |
| **Somnos** | 967.1 | E852.0 | E937.1 | E950.2 | E962.0 | E980.2 |
| **Somonal** | 967.0 | E851 | E937.0 | E950.1 | E962.0 | E980.1 |
| **Soneryl** | 967.0 | E851 | E937.0 | E950.1 | E962.0 | E980.1 |
| **Soothing syrup** | 977.9 | E858.9 | E947.9 | E950.5 | E962.0 | E980.5 |
| **Sopor** | 967.4 | E852.3 | E937.4 | E950.2 | E962.0 | E980.2 |
| **Soporific drug** | 967.9 | E852.9 | E937.9 | E950.2 | E962.0 | E980.2 |
|   specified type NEC | 967.8 | E852.8 | E937.8 | E950.2 | E962.0 | E980.2 |
| **Sorbitol NEC** | 977.4 | E858.8 | E947.4 | E950.4 | E962.0 | E980.4 |
| **Sotradecol** | 972.7 | E858.3 | E942.7 | E950.4 | E962.0 | E980.4 |
| **Spacoline** | 975.1 | E858.6 | E945.1 | E950.4 | E962.0 | E980.4 |
| **Spanish fly** | 976.8 | E858.7 | E946.8 | E950.4 | E962.0 | E980.4 |
| **Sparine** | 969.1 | E853.0 | E939.1 | E950.3 | E962.0 | E980.3 |
| **Sparteine** | 975.0 | E858.6 | E945.0 | E950.4 | E962.0 | E980.4 |
| **Spasmolytics** | 975.1 | E858.6 | E945.1 | E950.4 | E962.0 | E980.4 |
|   anticholinergics | 971.1 | E855.4 | E941.1 | E950.4 | E962.0 | E980.4 |
| **Spectinomycin** | 960.8 | E856 | E930.8 | E950.4 | E962.0 | E980.4 |
| **Speed** | 969.7 | E854.2 | E939.7 | E950.3 | E962.0 | E980.3 |
| **Spermicides** | 976.8 | E858.7 | E946.8 | E950.4 | E962.0 | E980.4 |
| **Spider** (bite) (venom) | 989.5 | E905.1 | — | E950.9 | E962.1 | E980.9 |
|   antivenin | 979.9 | E858.8 | E949.9 | E950.4 | E962.0 | E980.4 |
| **Spigelia** (root) | 961.6 | E857 | E931.6 | E950.4 | E962.0 | E980.4 |
| **Spiperone** | 969.2 | E853.1 | E939.2 | E950.3 | E962.0 | E980.3 |
| **Spiramycin** | 960.3 | E856 | E930.3 | E950.4 | E962.0 | E980.4 |
| **Spirilene** | 969.5 | E853.8 | E939.5 | E950.3 | E962.0 | E980.3 |
| **Spirit(s)** (neutral) NEC | 980.0 | E860.1 | — | E950.9 | E962.1 | E980.9 |
|   beverage | 980.0 | E860.0 | — | E950.9 | E962.1 | E980.9 |
|   industrial | 980.9 | E860.9 | — | E950.9 | E962.1 | E980.9 |
|   mineral | 981 | E862.0 | — | E950.9 | E962.1 | E980.9 |
|   of salt — see Hydrochloric acid | | | | | | |
|   surgical | 980.9 | E860.9 | — | E950.9 | E962.1 | E980.9 |
| **Spironolactone** | 974.4 | E858.5 | E944.4 | E950.4 | E962.0 | E980.4 |
| **Sponge, absorbable** (gelatin) | 964.5 | E858.2 | E934.5 | E950.4 | E962.0 | E980.4 |
| **Sporostacin** | 976.0 | E858.7 | E946.0 | E950.4 | E962.0 | E980.4 |
| **Sprays** (aerosol) | 989.89 | E866.8 | — | E950.9 | E962.1 | E980.9 |
|   cosmetic | 989.89 | E866.7 | — | E950.9 | E962.1 | E980.9 |
|   medicinal NEC | 977.9 | E858.9 | E947.9 | E950.5 | E962.0 | E980.5 |
|   pesticides — see Pesticides | | | | | | |
|   specified content — see substance specified | | | | | | |
| **Spurge flax** | 988.2 | E865.4 | — | E950.9 | E962.1 | E980.9 |
| **Spurges** | 988.2 | E865.4 | — | E950.9 | E962.1 | E980.9 |
| **Squill** (expectorant) NEC | 975.5 | E858.6 | E945.5 | E950.4 | E962.0 | E980.4 |
|   rat poison | 989.4 | E863.7 | — | E950.6 | E962.1 | E980.7 |
| **Squirting cucumber** (cathartic) | 973.1 | E858.4 | E943.1 | E950.4 | E962.0 | E980.4 |
| **Stains** | 989.89 | E866.8 | — | E950.9 | E962.1 | E980.9 |
| **Stannous** — see also Tin | | | | | | |
|   fluoride | 976.7 | E858.7 | E946.7 | E950.4 | E962.0 | E980.4 |
| **Stanolone** | 962.1 | E858.0 | E932.1 | E950.4 | E962.0 | E980.4 |
| **Stanozolol** | 962.1 | E858.0 | E932.1 | E950.4 | E962.0 | E980.4 |
| **Staphisagria or stavesacre** (pediculicide) | 976.0 | E858.7 | E946.0 | E950.4 | E962.0 | E980.4 |
| **Stelazine** | 969.1 | E853.0 | E939.1 | E950.3 | E962.0 | E980.3 |
| **Stemetil** | 969.1 | E853.0 | E939.1 | E950.3 | E962.0 | E980.3 |
| **Sterculia** (cathartic) (gum) | 973.3 | E858.4 | E943.3 | E950.4 | E962.0 | E980.4 |
| **Sternutator gas** | 987.8 | E869.8 | — | E952.8 | E962.2 | E982.8 |
| **Steroids NEC** | 962.0 | E858.0 | E932.0 | E950.4 | E962.0 | E980.4 |
|   ENT agent | 976.6 | E858.7 | E946.6 | E950.4 | E962.0 | E980.4 |
|   ophthalmic preparation | 976.5 | E858.7 | E946.5 | E950.4 | E962.0 | E980.4 |
|   topical NEC | 976.0 | E858.7 | E946.0 | E950.4 | E962.0 | E980.4 |
| **Stibine** | 985.8 | E866.4 | — | E950.9 | E962.1 | E980.9 |
| **Stibophen** | 961.2 | E857 | E931.2 | E950.4 | E962.0 | E980.4 |
| **Stilbamide, stilbamidine** | 961.5 | E857 | E931.5 | E950.4 | E962.0 | E980.4 |
| **Stilbestrol** | 962.2 | E858.0 | E932.2 | E950.4 | E962.0 | E980.4 |
| **Stimulants** (central nervous system) | 970.9 | E854.3 | E940.9 | E950.4 | E962.0 | E980.4 |
|   analeptics | 970.0 | E854.3 | E940.0 | E950.4 | E962.0 | E980.4 |
|   opiate antagonist | 970.1 | E854.3 | E940.1 | E950.4 | E962.0 | E980.4 |
|   psychotherapeutic NEC | 969.0 | E854.0 | E939.0 | E950.3 | E962.0 | E980.3 |
|   specified NEC | 970.8 | E854.3 | E940.8 | E950.4 | E962.0 | E980.4 |
| **Storage batteries** (acid) (cells) | 983.1 | E864.1 | — | E950.7 | E962.1 | E980.6 |
| **Stovaine** | 968.9 | E855.2 | E938.9 | E950.4 | E962.0 | E980.4 |
|   infiltration (subcutaneous) | 968.5 | E855.2 | E938.5 | E950.4 | E962.0 | E980.4 |
|   nerve block (peripheral) (plexus) | 968.6 | E855.2 | E938.6 | E950.4 | E962.0 | E980.4 |
|   spinal | 968.7 | E855.2 | E938.7 | E950.4 | E962.0 | E980.4 |

| | Poisoning | Accident | Therapeutic Use | Suicide Attempt | Assault | Undetermined |
|---|---|---|---|---|---|---|
| **Stovaine** — continued | | | | | | |
|   topical (surface) | 968.5 | E855.2 | E938.5 | E950.4 | E962.0 | E980.4 |
| **Stovarsal** | 961.1 | E857 | E931.1 | E950.4 | E962.0 | E980.4 |
| **Stove gas** — see Gas, utility | | | | | | |
| **Stoxil** | 976.5 | E858.7 | E946.5 | E950.4 | E962.0 | E980.4 |
| **STP** | 969.6 | E854.1 | E939.6 | E950.3 | E962.0 | E980.3 |
| **Stramonium** (medicinal) NEC | 971.1 | E855.4 | E941.1 | E950.4 | E962.0 | E980.4 |
|   natural state | 988.2 | E865.4 | — | E950.9 | E962.1 | E980.9 |
| **Streptodornase** | 964.4 | E858.2 | E934.4 | E950.4 | E962.0 | E980.4 |
| **Streptoduocin** | 960.6 | E856 | E930.6 | E950.4 | E962.0 | E980.4 |
| **Streptokinase** | 964.4 | E858.2 | E934.4 | E950.4 | E962.0 | E980.4 |
| **Streptomycin** | 960.6 | E856 | E930.6 | E950.4 | E962.0 | E980.4 |
| **Streptozocin** | 960.7 | E856 | E930.7 | E950.4 | E962.0 | E980.4 |
| **Stripper** (paint) (solvent) | 982.8 | E862.9 | — | E950.9 | E962.1 | E980.9 |
| **Strobane** | 989.2 | E863.0 | — | E950.6 | E962.1 | E980.7 |
| **Strophanthin** | 972.1 | E858.3 | E942.1 | E950.4 | E962.0 | E980.4 |
| **Strophanthus hispidus or kombe** | 988.2 | E865.4 | — | E950.9 | E962.1 | E980.9 |
| **Strychnine** (rodenticide) (salts) | 989.1 | E863.7 | — | E950.6 | E962.1 | E980.7 |
|   medicinal NEC | 970.8 | E854.3 | E940.8 | E950.4 | E962.0 | E980.4 |
| **Strychnos** (ignatii) — see Strychnine | | | | | | |
| **Styramate** | 968.0 | E855.1 | E938.0 | E950.4 | E962.0 | E980.4 |
| **Styrene** | 983.0 | E864.0 | — | E950.7 | E962.1 | E980.6 |
| **Succinimide** (anticonvulsant) | 966.2 | E855.0 | E936.2 | E950.4 | E962.0 | E980.4 |
|   mercuric — see Mercury | | | | | | |
| **Succinylcholine** | 975.2 | E858.6 | E945.2 | E950.4 | E962.0 | E980.4 |
| **Succinylsulfathiazole** | 961.0 | E857 | E931.0 | E950.4 | E962.0 | E980.4 |
| **Sucrose** | 974.5 | E858.5 | E944.5 | E950.4 | E962.0 | E980.4 |
| **Sulfacetamide** | 961.0 | E857 | E931.0 | E950.4 | E962.0 | E980.4 |
|   ophthalmic preparation | 976.5 | E858.7 | E946.5 | E950.4 | E962.0 | E980.4 |
| **Sulfachlorpyridazine** | 961.0 | E857 | E931.0 | E950.4 | E962.0 | E980.4 |
| **Sulfacytine** | 961.0 | E857 | E931.0 | E950.4 | E962.0 | E980.4 |
| **Sulfadiazine** | 961.0 | E857 | E931.0 | E950.4 | E962.0 | E980.4 |
|   silver (topical) | 976.0 | E858.7 | E946.0 | E950.4 | E962.0 | E980.4 |
| **Sulfadimethoxine** | 961.0 | E857 | E931.0 | E950.4 | E962.0 | E980.4 |
| **Sulfadimidine** | 961.0 | E857 | E931.0 | E950.4 | E962.0 | E980.4 |
| **Sulfaethidole** | 961.0 | E857 | E931.0 | E950.4 | E962.0 | E980.4 |
| **Sulfafurazole** | 961.0 | E857 | E931.0 | E950.4 | E962.0 | E980.4 |
| **Sulfaguanidine** | 961.0 | E857 | E931.0 | E950.4 | E962.0 | E980.4 |
| **Sulfamerazine** | 961.0 | E857 | E931.0 | E950.4 | E962.0 | E980.4 |
| **Sulfameter** | 961.0 | E857 | E931.0 | E950.4 | E962.0 | E980.4 |
| **Sulfamethizole** | 961.0 | E857 | E931.0 | E950.4 | E962.0 | E980.4 |
| **Sulfamethoxazole** | 961.0 | E857 | E931.0 | E950.4 | E962.0 | E980.4 |
| **Sulfamethoxydiazine** | 961.0 | E857 | E931.0 | E950.4 | E962.0 | E980.4 |
| **Sulfamethoxypyridazine** | 961.0 | E857 | E931.0 | E950.4 | E962.0 | E980.4 |
| **Sulfamethylthiazole** | 961.0 | E857 | E931.0 | E950.4 | E962.0 | E980.4 |
| **Sulfamylon** | 976.0 | E858.7 | E946.0 | E950.4 | E962.0 | E980.4 |
| **Sulfan blue** (diagnostic dye) | 977.8 | E858.8 | E947.8 | E950.4 | E962.0 | E980.4 |
| **Sulfanilamide** | 961.0 | E857 | E931.0 | E950.4 | E962.0 | E980.4 |
| **Sulfanilylguanidine** | 961.0 | E857 | E931.0 | E950.4 | E962.0 | E980.4 |
| **Sulfaphenazole** | 961.0 | E857 | E931.0 | E950.4 | E962.0 | E980.4 |
| **Sulfaphenylthiazole** | 961.0 | E857 | E931.0 | E950.4 | E962.0 | E980.4 |
| **Sulfaproxyline** | 961.0 | E857 | E931.0 | E950.4 | E962.0 | E980.4 |
| **Sulfapyridine** | 961.0 | E857 | E931.0 | E950.4 | E962.0 | E980.4 |
| **Sulfapyrimidine** | 961.0 | E857 | E931.0 | E950.4 | E962.0 | E980.4 |
| **Sulfarsphenamine** | 961.1 | E857 | E931.1 | E950.4 | E962.0 | E980.4 |
| **Sulfasalazine** | 961.0 | E857 | E931.0 | E950.4 | E962.0 | E980.4 |
| **Sulfasomizole** | 961.0 | E857 | E931.0 | E950.4 | E962.0 | E980.4 |
| **Sulfasuxidine** | 961.0 | E857 | E931.0 | E950.4 | E962.0 | E980.4 |
| **Sulfinpyrazone** | 974.7 | E858.5 | E944.7 | E950.4 | E962.0 | E980.4 |
| **Sulfisoxazole** | 961.0 | E857 | E931.0 | E950.4 | E962.0 | E980.4 |
|   ophthalmic preparation | 976.5 | E858.7 | E946.5 | E950.4 | E962.0 | E980.4 |
| **Sulfomyxin** | 960.8 | E856 | E930.8 | E950.4 | E962.0 | E980.4 |
| **Sulfonal** | 967.8 | E852.8 | E937.8 | E950.2 | E962.0 | E980.2 |
| **Sulfonamides** (mixtures) | 961.0 | E857 | E931.0 | E950.4 | E962.0 | E980.4 |
| **Sulfones** | 961.8 | E857 | E931.8 | E950.4 | E962.0 | E980.4 |
| **Sulfonethylmethane** | 967.8 | E852.8 | E937.8 | E950.2 | E962.0 | E980.2 |
| **Sulfonmethane** | 967.8 | E852.8 | E937.8 | E950.2 | E962.0 | E980.2 |
| **Sulfonphthal, sulfonphthol** | 977.8 | E858.8 | E947.8 | E950.4 | E962.0 | E980.4 |
| **Sulfonylurea derivatives, oral** | 962.3 | E858.0 | E932.3 | E950.4 | E962.0 | E980.4 |
| **Sulfoxone** | 961.8 | E857 | E931.8 | E950.4 | E962.0 | E980.4 |
| **Sulfur, sulfureted, sulfuric, sulfurous, sulfuryl** (compounds) NEC | 989.89 | E866.8 | — | E950.9 | E962.1 | E980.9 |
|   acid | 983.1 | E864.1 | — | E950.7 | E962.1 | E980.6 |
|   dioxide | 987.3 | E869.1 | — | E952.8 | E962.2 | E982.8 |

☑ Additional Digit Required — Refer to the Tabular List for Digit Selection

Subterms under main terms may continue to next column or page

▶◀ Revised Text     ● New Line     ▲ Revised Code     *2008 ICD-9-CM*

| Substance | Poisoning | Accident | Therapeutic Use | Suicide Attempt | Assault | Undetermined |
|---|---|---|---|---|---|---|
| Sulfur, sulfureted, sulfuric, sulfurous, sulfuryl (compounds) — continued | | | | | | |
| ether — see Ether(s) | | | | | | |
| hydrogen | 987.8 | E869.8 | — | E952.8 | E962.2 | E982.8 |
| medicinal (keratolytic)(ointment) | | | | | | |
| NEC | 976.4 | E858.7 | E946.4 | E950.4 | E962.0 | E980.4 |
| pesticide (vapor) | 989.4 | E863.4 | | E950.6 | E962.1 | E980.7 |
| vapor NEC | 987.8 | E869.8 | — | E952.8 | E962.2 | E982.8 |
| Sulkowitch's reagent | 977.8 | E858.8 | E947.8 | E950.4 | E962.0 | E980.4 |
| Sulphadione | 961.8 | E857 | E931.8 | E950.4 | E962.0 | E980.4 |
| Sulph — see also Sulf- | | | | | | |
| Sulthiame, sultiame | 966.3 | E855.0 | E936.3 | E950.4 | E962.0 | E980.4 |
| Superinone | 975.5 | E858.6 | E945.5 | E950.4 | E962.0 | E980.4 |
| Suramin | 961.5 | E857 | E931.5 | E950.4 | E962.0 | E980.4 |
| Surfacaine | 968.5 | E855.2 | E938.5 | E950.4 | E962.0 | E980.4 |
| Surital | 968.3 | E855.1 | E938.3 | E950.4 | E962.0 | E980.4 |
| Sutilains | 976.8 | E858.7 | E946.8 | E950.4 | E962.0 | E980.4 |
| Suxamethonium (bromide)(chloride)(iodide) | 975.2 | E858.6 | E945.2 | E950.4 | E962.0 | E980.4 |
| Suxethonium (bromide) | 975.2 | E858.6 | E945.2 | E950.4 | E962.0 | E980.4 |
| Sweet oil (birch) | 976.3 | E858.7 | E946.3 | E950.4 | E962.0 | E980.4 |
| Sym-dichloroethyl ether | 982.3 | E862.4 | — | E950.9 | E962.1 | E980.9 |
| Sympatholytics | 971.3 | E855.6 | E941.3 | E950.4 | E962.0 | E980.4 |
| Sympathomimetics | 971.2 | E855.5 | E941.2 | E950.4 | E962.0 | E980.4 |
| Synagis | 979.6 | E858.8 | E949.6 | E950.4 | E962.0 | E980.4 |
| Synalar | 976.0 | E858.7 | E946.0 | E950.4 | E962.0 | E980.4 |
| Synthroid | 962.7 | E858.0 | E932.7 | E950.4 | E962.0 | E980.4 |
| Syntocinon | 975.0 | E858.6 | E945.0 | E950.4 | E962.0 | E980.4 |
| Syrosingopine | 972.6 | E858.3 | E942.6 | E950.4 | E962.0 | E980.4 |
| Systemic agents (primarily) | 963.9 | E858.1 | E933.9 | E950.4 | E962.0 | E980.4 |
| specified NEC | 963.8 | E858.1 | E933.8 | E950.4 | E962.0 | E980.4 |
| Tablets — see also specified substance | 977.9 | E858.9 | E947.9 | E950.5 | E962.0 | E980.5 |
| Tace | 962.2 | E858.0 | E932.2 | E950.4 | E962.0 | E980.4 |
| Tacrine | 971.0 | E855.3 | E941.0 | E950.4 | E962.0 | E980.4 |
| Talbutal | 967.0 | E851 | E937.0 | E950.1 | E962.0 | E980.1 |
| Talc | 976.3 | E858.7 | E946.3 | E950.4 | E962.0 | E980.4 |
| Talcum | 976.3 | E858.7 | E946.3 | E950.4 | E962.0 | E980.4 |
| Tamsulosin ● | 971.3 | E855.6 | E941.3 | E950.4 | E962.0 | E980.4 |
| Tandearil, tanderil | 965.5 | E850.5 | E935.5 | E950.0 | E962.0 | E980.0 |
| Tannic acid | 983.1 | E864.1 | — | E950.7 | E962.1 | E980.6 |
| medicinal (astringent) | 976.2 | E858.7 | E946.2 | E950.4 | E962.0 | E980.4 |
| Tannin — see Tannic acid | | | | | | |
| Tansy | 988.2 | E865.4 | — | E950.9 | E962.1 | E980.9 |
| TAO | 960.3 | E856 | E930.3 | E950.4 | E962.0 | E980.4 |
| Tapazole | 962.8 | E858.0 | E932.8 | E950.4 | E962.0 | E980.4 |
| Tar NEC | 983.0 | E864.0 | — | E950.7 | E962.1 | E980.6 |
| camphor — see Naphthalene | | | | | | |
| fumes | 987.8 | E869.8 | — | E952.8 | E962.2 | E982.8 |
| Taractan | 969.3 | E853.8 | E939.3 | E950.3 | E962.0 | E980.3 |
| Tarantula (venomous) | 989.5 | E905.1 | — | E950.9 | E962.1 | E980.9 |
| Tartar emetic (anti-infective) | 961.2 | E857 | E931.2 | E950.4 | E962.0 | E980.4 |
| Tartaric acid | 983.1 | E864.1 | — | E950.7 | E962.1 | E980.6 |
| Tartrated antimony (anti-infective) | 961.2 | E857 | E931.2 | E950.4 | E962.0 | E980.4 |
| TCA — see Trichloroacetic acid | | | | | | |
| TDI | 983.0 | E864.0 | | E950.7 | E962.1 | E980.6 |
| vapor | 987.8 | E869.8 | — | E952.8 | E962.2 | E982.8 |
| Tear gas | 987.5 | E869.3 | — | E952.8 | E962.2 | E982.8 |
| Teclothiazide | 974.3 | E858.5 | E944.3 | E950.4 | E962.0 | E980.4 |
| Tegretol | 966.3 | E855.0 | E936.3 | E950.4 | E962.0 | E980.4 |
| Telepaque | 977.8 | E858.8 | E947.8 | E950.4 | E962.0 | E980.4 |
| Tellurium | 985.8 | E866.4 | — | E950.9 | E962.1 | E980.9 |
| fumes | 985.8 | E866.4 | — | E950.9 | E962.1 | E980.9 |
| TEM | 963.1 | E858.1 | E933.1 | E950.4 | E962.0 | E980.4 |
| Temazepan — see Benzodiazepines | | | | | | |
| TEPA | 963.1 | E858.1 | E933.1 | E950.4 | E962.0 | E980.4 |
| TEPP | 989.3 | E863.1 | — | E950.6 | E962.1 | E980.7 |
| Terbutaline | 971.2 | E855.5 | E941.2 | E950.4 | E962.0 | E980.4 |
| Teroxalene | 961.6 | E857 | E931.6 | E950.4 | E962.0 | E980.4 |
| Terpin hydrate | 975.5 | E858.6 | E945.5 | E950.4 | E962.0 | E980.4 |
| Terramycin | 960.4 | E856 | E930.4 | E950.4 | E962.0 | E980.4 |
| Tessalon | 975.4 | E858.6 | E945.4 | E950.4 | E962.0 | E980.4 |
| Testosterone | 962.1 | E858.0 | E932.1 | E950.4 | E962.0 | E980.4 |
| Tetanus (vaccine) | 978.4 | E858.8 | E948.4 | E950.4 | E962.0 | E980.4 |
| antitoxin | 979.9 | E858.8 | E949.9 | E950.4 | E962.0 | E980.4 |
| immune globulin (human) | 964.6 | E858.2 | E934.6 | E950.4 | E962.0 | E980.4 |
| toxoid | 978.4 | E858.8 | E948.4 | E950.4 | E962.0 | E980.4 |

| Substance | Poisoning | Accident | Therapeutic Use | Suicide Attempt | Assault | Undetermined |
|---|---|---|---|---|---|---|
| Tetanus — continued | | | | | | |
| toxoid — continued | | | | | | |
| with diphtheria toxoid | 978.9 | E858.8 | E948.9 | E950.4 | E962.0 | E980.4 |
| with pertussis | 978.6 | E858.8 | E948.6 | E950.4 | E962.0 | E980.4 |
| Tetrabenazine | 969.5 | E853.8 | E939.5 | E950.3 | E962.0 | E980.3 |
| Tetracaine (infiltration)(topical) | 968.5 | E855.2 | E938.5 | E950.4 | E962.0 | E980.4 |
| nerve block (peripheral)(plexus) | 968.6 | E855.2 | E938.6 | E950.4 | E962.0 | E980.4 |
| spinal | 968.7 | E855.2 | E938.7 | E950.4 | E962.0 | E980.4 |
| Tetrachlorethylene — see Tetrachloroethylene | | | | | | |
| Tetrachlormethiazide | 974.3 | E858.5 | E944.3 | E950.4 | E962.0 | E980.4 |
| Tetrachloroethane (liquid) | | | | | | |
| (vapor) | 982.3 | E862.4 | — | E950.9 | E962.1 | E980.9 |
| paint or varnish | 982.3 | E861.6 | — | E950.9 | E962.1 | E980.9 |
| Tetrachloroethylene (liquid) | | | | | | |
| (vapor) | 982.3 | E862.4 | — | E950.9 | E962.1 | E980.9 |
| medicinal | 961.6 | E857 | E931.6 | E950.4 | E962.0 | E980.4 |
| Tetrachloromethane — see Carbon, tetrachloride | | | | | | |
| Tetracycline | 960.4 | E856 | E930.4 | E950.4 | E962.0 | E980.4 |
| ophthalmic preparation | 976.5 | E858.7 | E946.5 | E950.4 | E962.0 | E980.4 |
| topical NEC | 976.0 | E858.7 | E946.0 | E950.4 | E962.0 | E980.4 |
| Tetraethylammonium chloride | 972.3 | E858.3 | E942.3 | E950.4 | E962.0 | E980.4 |
| Tetraethyl lead (antiknock compound) | 984.1 | E862.1 | — | E950.9 | E962.1 | E980.9 |
| Tetraethyl pyrophosphate | 989.3 | E863.1 | — | E950.6 | E962.1 | E980.7 |
| Tetraethylthiuram disulfide | 977.3 | E858.8 | E947.3 | E950.4 | E962.0 | E980.4 |
| Tetrahydroaminoacridine | 971.0 | E855.3 | E941.0 | E950.4 | E962.0 | E980.4 |
| Tetrahydrocannabinol | 969.6 | E854.1 | E939.6 | E950.3 | E962.0 | E980.3 |
| Tetrahydronaphthalene | 982.0 | E862.4 | — | E950.9 | E962.1 | E980.9 |
| Tetrahydrozoline | 971.2 | E855.5 | E941.2 | E950.4 | E962.0 | E980.4 |
| Tetralin | 982.0 | E862.4 | — | E950.9 | E962.1 | E980.9 |
| Tetramethylthiuram (disulfide) | | | | | | |
| NEC | 989.4 | E863.6 | — | E950.6 | E962.1 | E980.7 |
| medicinal | 976.2 | E858.7 | E946.2 | E950.4 | E962.0 | E980.4 |
| Tetronal | 967.8 | E852.8 | E937.8 | E950.2 | E962.0 | E980.2 |
| Tetryl | 983.0 | E864.0 | — | E950.7 | E962.1 | E980.6 |
| Thalidomide | 967.8 | E852.8 | E937.8 | E950.2 | E962.0 | E980.2 |
| Thallium (compounds)(dust) | | | | | | |
| NEC | 985.8 | E866.4 | — | E950.9 | E962.1 | E980.9 |
| pesticide (rodenticide) | 985.8 | E863.7 | — | E950.6 | E962.1 | E980.7 |
| THC | 969.6 | E854.1 | E939.6 | E950.3 | E962.0 | E980.3 |
| Thebacon | 965.09 | E850.2 | E935.2 | E950.0 | E962.0 | E980.0 |
| Thebaine | 965.09 | E850.2 | E935.2 | E950.0 | E962.0 | E980.0 |
| Theobromine (calcium salicylate) | 974.1 | E858.5 | E944.1 | E950.4 | E962.0 | E980.4 |
| Theophylline (diuretic) | 974.1 | E858.5 | E944.1 | E950.4 | E962.0 | E980.4 |
| ethylenediamine | 975.7 | E858.6 | E945.7 | E950.4 | E962.0 | E980.4 |
| Thiabendazole | 961.6 | E857 | E931.6 | E950.4 | E962.0 | E980.4 |
| Thialbarbital, thialbarbitone | 968.3 | E855.1 | E938.3 | E950.4 | E962.0 | E980.4 |
| Thiamine | 963.5 | E858.1 | E933.5 | E950.4 | E962.0 | E980.4 |
| Thiamylal (sodium) | 968.3 | E855.1 | E938.3 | E950.4 | E962.0 | E980.4 |
| Thiazesim | 969.0 | E854.0 | E939.0 | E950.3 | E962.0 | E980.3 |
| Thiazides (diuretics) | 974.3 | E858.5 | E944.3 | E950.4 | E962.0 | E980.4 |
| Thiethylperazine | 963.0 | E858.1 | E933.0 | E950.4 | E962.0 | E980.4 |
| Thimerosal (topical) | 976.0 | E858.7 | E946.0 | E950.4 | E962.0 | E980.4 |
| ophthalmic preparation | 976.5 | E858.7 | E946.5 | E950.4 | E962.0 | E980.4 |
| Thioacetazone | 961.8 | E857 | E931.8 | E950.4 | E962.0 | E980.4 |
| Thiobarbiturates | 968.3 | E855.1 | E938.3 | E950.4 | E962.0 | E980.4 |
| Thiobismol | 961.2 | E857 | E931.2 | E950.4 | E962.0 | E980.4 |
| Thiocarbamide | 962.8 | E858.0 | E932.8 | E950.4 | E962.0 | E980.4 |
| Thiocarbarsone | 961.1 | E857 | E931.1 | E950.4 | E962.0 | E980.4 |
| Thiocarlide | 961.8 | E857 | E931.8 | E950.4 | E962.0 | E980.4 |
| Thioguanine | 963.1 | E858.1 | E933.1 | E950.4 | E962.0 | E980.4 |
| Thiomercaptomerin | 974.0 | E858.5 | E944.0 | E950.4 | E962.0 | E980.4 |
| Thiomerin | 974.0 | E858.5 | E944.0 | E950.4 | E962.0 | E980.4 |
| Thiopental, thiopentone (sodium) | 968.3 | E855.1 | E938.3 | E950.4 | E962.0 | E980.4 |
| Thiopropazate | 969.1 | E853.0 | E939.1 | E950.3 | E962.0 | E980.3 |
| Thioproperazine | 969.1 | E853.0 | E939.1 | E950.3 | E962.0 | E980.3 |
| Thioridazine | 969.1 | E853.0 | E939.1 | E950.3 | E962.0 | E980.3 |
| Thio-TEPA, thiotepa | 963.1 | E858.1 | E933.1 | E950.4 | E962.0 | E980.4 |
| Thiothixene | 969.3 | E853.8 | E939.3 | E950.3 | E962.0 | E980.3 |
| Thiouracil | 962.8 | E858.0 | E932.8 | E950.4 | E962.0 | E980.4 |
| Thiourea | 962.8 | E858.0 | E932.8 | E950.4 | E962.0 | E980.4 |
| Thiphenamil | 971.1 | E855.4 | E941.1 | E950.4 | E962.0 | E980.4 |

☑ Additional Digit Required — Refer to the Tabular List for Digit Selection

Subterms under main terms may continue to next column or page

| | Poisoning | Accident | Therapeutic Use | Suicide Attempt | Assault | Undetermined |
|---|---|---|---|---|---|---|
| Thiram NEC | 989.4 | E863.6 | — | E950.6 | E962.1 | E980.7 |
| medicinal | 976.2 | E858.7 | E946.2 | E950.4 | E962.0 | E980.4 |
| Thonzylamine | 963.0 | E858.1 | E933.0 | E950.4 | E962.0 | E980.4 |
| Thorazine | 969.1 | E853.0 | E939.1 | E950.3 | E962.0 | E980.3 |
| Thornapple | 988.2 | E865.4 | — | E950.9 | E962.1 | E980.9 |
| Throat preparation (lozenges) | | | | | | |
| NEC | 976.6 | E858.7 | E946.6 | E950.4 | E962.0 | E980.4 |
| Thrombin | 964.5 | E858.2 | E934.5 | E950.4 | E962.0 | E980.4 |
| Thrombolysin | 964.4 | E858.2 | E934.4 | E950.4 | E962.0 | E980.4 |
| Thymol | 983.0 | E864.0 | — | E950.7 | E962.1 | E980.6 |
| Thymus extract | 962.9 | E858.0 | E932.9 | E950.4 | E962.0 | E980.4 |
| Thyroglobulin | 962.7 | E858.0 | E932.7 | E950.4 | E962.0 | E980.4 |
| Thyroid (derivatives) | | | | | | |
| (extract) | 962.7 | E858.0 | E932.7 | E950.4 | E962.0 | E980.4 |
| Thyrolar | 962.7 | E858.0 | E932.7 | E950.4 | E962.0 | E980.4 |
| Thyrothrophin, thyrotropin | 977.8 | E858.8 | E947.8 | E950.4 | E962.0 | E980.4 |
| Thyroxin(e) | 962.7 | E858.0 | E932.7 | E950.4 | E962.0 | E980.4 |
| Tigan | 963.0 | E858.1 | E933.0 | E950.4 | E962.0 | E980.4 |
| Tigloidine | 968.0 | E855.1 | E938.0 | E950.4 | E962.0 | E980.4 |
| Tin (chloride) (dust) (oxide) | | | | | | |
| NEC | 985.8 | E866.4 | — | E950.9 | E962.1 | E980.9 |
| anti-infectives | 961.2 | E857 | E931.2 | E950.4 | E962.0 | E980.4 |
| Tinactin | 976.0 | E858.7 | E946.0 | E950.4 | E962.0 | E980.4 |
| Tincture, iodine — see Iodine | | | | | | |
| Tindal | 969.1 | E853.0 | E939.1 | E950.3 | E962.0 | E980.3 |
| Titanium (compounds) | | | | | | |
| (vapor) | 985.8 | E866.4 | — | E950.9 | E962.1 | E980.9 |
| ointment | 976.3 | E858.7 | E946.3 | E950.4 | E962.0 | E980.4 |
| Titroid | 962.7 | E858.0 | E932.7 | E950.4 | E962.0 | E980.4 |
| TMTD — see Tetramethylthiuram disulfide | | | | | | |
| TNT | 989.89 | E866.8 | — | E950.9 | E962.1 | E980.9 |
| fumes | 987.8 | E869.8 | — | E952.8 | E962.2 | E982.8 |
| Toadstool | 988.1 | E865.5 | — | E950.9 | E962.1 | E980.9 |
| Tobacco NEC | 989.84 | E866.8 | — | E950.9 | E962.1 | E980.9 |
| Indian | 988.2 | E865.4 | — | E950.9 | E962.1 | E980.9 |
| smoke, second-hand | 987.8 | E869.4 | — | — | — | — |
| Tocopherol | 963.5 | E858.1 | E933.5 | E950.4 | E962.0 | E980.4 |
| Tocosamine | 975.0 | E858.6 | E945.0 | E950.4 | E962.0 | E980.4 |
| Tofranil | 969.0 | E854.0 | E939.0 | E950.3 | E962.0 | E980.3 |
| Toilet deodorizer | 989.89 | E866.8 | — | E950.9 | E962.1 | E980.9 |
| Tolazamide | 962.3 | E858.0 | E932.3 | E950.4 | E962.0 | E980.4 |
| Tolazoline | 971.3 | E855.6 | E941.3 | E950.4 | E962.0 | E980.4 |
| Tolbutamide | 962.3 | E858.0 | E932.3 | E950.4 | E962.0 | E980.4 |
| sodium | 977.8 | E858.8 | E947.8 | E950.4 | E962.0 | E980.4 |
| Tolmetin | 965.69 | E850.6 | E935.6 | E950.0 | E962.0 | E980.0 |
| Tolnaftate | 976.0 | E858.7 | E946.0 | E950.4 | E962.0 | E980.4 |
| Tolpropamine | 976.1 | E858.7 | E946.1 | E950.4 | E962.0 | E980.4 |
| Tolserol | 968.0 | E855.1 | E938.0 | E950.4 | E962.0 | E980.4 |
| Toluene (liquid) (vapor) | 982.0 | E862.4 | — | E950.9 | E962.1 | E980.9 |
| diisocyanate | 983.0 | E864.0 | — | E950.7 | E962.1 | E980.6 |
| Toluidine | 983.0 | E864.0 | — | E950.7 | E962.1 | E980.6 |
| vapor | 987.8 | E869.8 | — | E952.8 | E962.2 | E982.8 |
| Toluol (liquid) (vapor) | 982.0 | E862.4 | — | E950.9 | E962.1 | E980.9 |
| Tolylene-2, 4-diisocyanate | 983.0 | E864.0 | — | E950.7 | E962.1 | E980.6 |
| Tonics, cardiac | 972.1 | E858.3 | E942.1 | E950.4 | E962.0 | E980.4 |
| Toxaphene (dust) (spray) | 989.2 | E863.0 | — | E950.6 | E962.1 | E980.7 |
| Toxoids NEC | 978.8 | E858.8 | E948.8 | E950.4 | E962.0 | E980.4 |
| Tractor fuel NEC | 981 | E862.1 | — | E950.9 | E962.1 | E980.9 |
| Tragacanth | 973.3 | E858.4 | E943.3 | E950.4 | E962.0 | E980.4 |
| Tramazoline | 971.2 | E855.5 | E941.2 | E950.4 | E962.0 | E980.4 |
| Tranquilizers | 969.5 | E853.9 | E939.5 | E950.3 | E962.0 | E980.3 |
| benzodiazepine-based | 969.4 | E853.2 | E939.4 | E950.3 | E962.0 | E980.3 |
| butyrophenone-based | 969.2 | E853.1 | E939.2 | E950.3 | E962.0 | E980.3 |
| major NEC | 969.3 | E853.8 | E939.3 | E950.3 | E962.0 | E980.3 |
| phenothiazine-based | 969.1 | E853.0 | E939.1 | E950.3 | E962.0 | E980.3 |
| specified NEC | 969.5 | E853.8 | E939.5 | E950.3 | E962.0 | E980.3 |
| Trantoin | 961.9 | E857 | E931.9 | E950.4 | E962.0 | E980.4 |
| Tranxene | 969.4 | E853.2 | E939.4 | E950.3 | E962.0 | E980.3 |
| Tranylcypromine (sulfate) | 969.0 | E854.0 | E939.0 | E950.3 | E962.0 | E980.3 |
| Trasentine | 975.1 | E858.6 | E945.1 | E950.4 | E962.0 | E980.4 |
| Travert | 974.5 | E858.5 | E944.5 | E950.4 | E962.0 | E980.4 |
| Trecator | 961.8 | E857 | E931.8 | E950.4 | E962.0 | E980.4 |
| Tretinoin | 976.8 | E858.7 | E946.8 | E950.4 | E962.0 | E980.4 |
| Triacetin | 976.0 | E858.7 | E946.0 | E950.4 | E962.0 | E980.4 |
| Triacetyloleandomycin | 960.3 | E856 | E930.3 | E950.4 | E962.0 | E980.4 |
| Triamcinolone | 962.0 | E858.0 | E932.0 | E950.4 | E962.0 | E980.4 |
| ENT agent | 976.6 | E858.7 | E946.6 | E950.4 | E962.0 | E980.4 |
| medicinal (keratolytic) | 976.4 | E858.7 | E946.4 | E950.4 | E962.0 | E980.4 |
| ophthalmic preparation | 976.5 | E858.7 | E946.5 | E950.4 | E962.0 | E980.4 |
| Triamcinolone — continued | | | | | | |
| topical NEC | 976.0 | E858.7 | E946.0 | E950.4 | E962.0 | E980.4 |
| Triamterene | 974.4 | E858.5 | E944.4 | E950.4 | E962.0 | E980.4 |
| Triaziquone | 963.1 | E858.1 | E933.1 | E950.4 | E962.0 | E980.4 |
| Tribromacetaldehyde | 967.3 | E852.2 | E937.3 | E950.2 | E962.0 | E980.2 |
| Tribromoethanol | 968.2 | E855.1 | E938.2 | E950.4 | E962.0 | E980.4 |
| Tribromomethane | 967.3 | E852.2 | E937.3 | E950.2 | E962.0 | E980.2 |
| Trichlorethane | 982.3 | E862.4 | — | E950.9 | E962.1 | E980.9 |
| Trichlormethiazide | 974.3 | E858.5 | E944.3 | E950.4 | E962.0 | E980.4 |
| Trichloroacetic acid | 983.1 | E864.1 | — | E950.7 | E962.1 | E980.6 |
| Trichloroethane | 967.1 | E852.0 | E937.1 | E950.2 | E962.0 | E980.2 |
| Trichloroethylene (liquid) | | | | | | |
| (vapor) | 982.3 | E862.4 | — | E950.9 | E962.1 | E980.9 |
| anesthetic (gas) | 968.2 | E855.1 | E938.2 | E950.4 | E962.0 | E980.4 |
| Trichloroethyl phosphate | 967.1 | E852.0 | E937.1 | E950.2 | E962.0 | E980.2 |
| Trichlorofluoromethane NEC | 987.4 | E869.2 | — | E952.8 | E962.2 | E982.8 |
| Trichlorotriethylamine | 963.1 | E858.1 | E933.1 | E950.4 | E962.0 | E980.4 |
| Trichomonacides NEC | 961.5 | E857 | E931.5 | E950.4 | E962.0 | E980.4 |
| Trichomycin | 960.1 | E856 | E930.1 | E950.4 | E962.0 | E980.4 |
| Triclofos | 967.1 | E852.0 | E937.1 | E950.2 | E962.0 | E980.2 |
| Tricresyl phosphate | 989.89 | E866.8 | — | E950.9 | E962.1 | E980.9 |
| solvent | 982.8 | E862.4 | — | E950.9 | E962.1 | E980.9 |
| Tricyclamol | 966.4 | E855.0 | E936.4 | E950.4 | E962.0 | E980.4 |
| Tridesilon | 976.0 | E858.7 | E946.0 | E950.4 | E962.0 | E980.4 |
| Tridihexethyl | 971.1 | E855.4 | E941.1 | E950.4 | E962.0 | E980.4 |
| Tridione | 966.0 | E855.0 | E936.0 | E950.4 | E962.0 | E980.4 |
| Triethanolamine NEC | 983.2 | E864.2 | — | E950.7 | E962.1 | E980.6 |
| detergent | 983.2 | E861.0 | — | E950.7 | E962.1 | E980.6 |
| trinitrate | 972.4 | E858.3 | E942.4 | E950.4 | E962.0 | E980.4 |
| Triethanomelamine | 963.1 | E858.1 | E933.1 | E950.4 | E962.0 | E980.4 |
| Triethylene melamine | 963.1 | E858.1 | E933.1 | E950.4 | E962.0 | E980.4 |
| Triethylenephosphoramide | 963.1 | E858.1 | E933.1 | E950.4 | E962.0 | E980.4 |
| Triethylenethiophosphoramide | 963.1 | E858.1 | E933.1 | E950.4 | E962.0 | E980.4 |
| Trifluoperazine | 969.1 | E853.0 | E939.1 | E950.3 | E962.0 | E980.3 |
| Trifluperidol | 969.2 | E853.1 | E939.2 | E950.3 | E962.0 | E980.3 |
| Triflupromazine | 969.1 | E853.0 | E939.1 | E950.3 | E962.0 | E980.3 |
| Trihexyphenidyl | 971.1 | E855.4 | E941.1 | E950.4 | E962.0 | E980.4 |
| Triiodothyronine | 962.7 | E858.0 | E932.7 | E950.4 | E962.0 | E980.4 |
| Trilene | 968.2 | E855.1 | E938.2 | E950.4 | E962.0 | E980.4 |
| Trimeprazine | 963.0 | E858.1 | E933.0 | E950.4 | E962.0 | E980.4 |
| Trimetazidine | 972.4 | E858.3 | E942.4 | E950.4 | E962.0 | E980.4 |
| Trimethadione | 966.0 | E855.0 | E936.0 | E950.4 | E962.0 | E980.4 |
| Trimethaphan | 972.3 | E858.3 | E942.3 | E950.4 | E962.0 | E980.4 |
| Trimethidinium | 972.3 | E858.3 | E942.3 | E950.4 | E962.0 | E980.4 |
| Trimethobenzamide | 963.0 | E858.1 | E933.0 | E950.4 | E962.0 | E980.4 |
| Trimethylcarbinol | 980.8 | E860.8 | — | E950.9 | E962.1 | E980.9 |
| Trimethylpsoralen | 976.3 | E858.7 | E946.3 | E950.4 | E962.0 | E980.4 |
| Trimeton | 963.0 | E858.1 | E933.0 | E950.4 | E962.0 | E980.4 |
| Trimipramine | 969.0 | E854.0 | E939.0 | E950.3 | E962.0 | E980.3 |
| Trimustine | 963.1 | E858.1 | E933.1 | E950.4 | E962.0 | E980.4 |
| Trinitrin | 972.4 | E858.3 | E942.4 | E950.4 | E962.0 | E980.4 |
| Trinitrophenol | 983.0 | E864.0 | — | E950.7 | E962.1 | E980.6 |
| Trinitrotoluene | 989.89 | E866.8 | — | E950.9 | E962.1 | E980.9 |
| fumes | 987.8 | E869.8 | — | E952.8 | E962.2 | E982.8 |
| Trional | 967.8 | E852.8 | E937.8 | E950.2 | E962.0 | E980.2 |
| Trioxide of arsenic — see Arsenic | | | | | | |
| Trioxsalen | 976.3 | E858.7 | E946.3 | E950.4 | E962.0 | E980.4 |
| Tripelennamine | 963.0 | E858.1 | E933.0 | E950.4 | E962.0 | E980.4 |
| Triperidol | 969.2 | E853.1 | E939.2 | E950.3 | E962.0 | E980.3 |
| Triprolidine | 963.0 | E858.1 | E933.0 | E950.4 | E962.0 | E980.4 |
| Trisoralen | 976.3 | E858.7 | E946.3 | E950.4 | E962.0 | E980.4 |
| Troleandomycin | 960.3 | E856 | E930.3 | E950.4 | E962.0 | E980.4 |
| Trolnitrate (phosphate) | 972.4 | E858.3 | E942.4 | E950.4 | E962.0 | E980.4 |
| Trometamol | 963.3 | E858.1 | E933.3 | E950.4 | E962.0 | E980.4 |
| Tromethamine | 963.3 | E858.1 | E933.3 | E950.4 | E962.0 | E980.4 |
| Tronothane | 968.5 | E855.2 | E938.5 | E950.4 | E962.0 | E980.4 |
| Tropicamide | 971.1 | E855.4 | E941.1 | E950.4 | E962.0 | E980.4 |
| Troxidone | 966.0 | E855.0 | E936.0 | E950.4 | E962.0 | E980.4 |
| Tryparsamide | 961.1 | E857 | E931.1 | E950.4 | E962.0 | E980.4 |
| Trypsin | 963.4 | E858.1 | E933.4 | E950.4 | E962.0 | E980.4 |
| Tryptizol | 969.0 | E854.0 | E939.0 | E950.3 | E962.0 | E980.3 |
| Tuaminoheptane | 971.2 | E855.5 | E941.2 | E950.4 | E962.0 | E980.4 |
| Tuberculin (old) | 977.8 | E858.8 | E947.8 | E950.4 | E962.0 | E980.4 |
| Tubocurare | 975.2 | E858.6 | E945.2 | E950.4 | E962.0 | E980.4 |
| Tubocurarine | 975.2 | E858.6 | E945.2 | E950.4 | E962.0 | E980.4 |
| Turkish green | 969.6 | E854.1 | E939.6 | E950.3 | E962.0 | E980.3 |
| Turpentine (spirits of) (liquid) | | | | | | |
| (vapor) | 982.8 | E862.4 | — | E950.9 | E962.1 | E980.9 |
| Tybamate | 969.5 | E853.8 | E939.5 | E950.3 | E962.0 | E980.3 |

☑ Additional Digit Required — Refer to the Tabular List for Digit Selection

Subterms under main terms may continue to next column or page

| | Poisoning | Accident | Therapeutic Use | Suicide Attempt | Assault | Undetermined |
|---|---|---|---|---|---|---|
| Tyloxapol | 975.5 | E858.6 | E945.5 | E950.4 | E962.0 | E980.4 |
| Tymazoline | 971.2 | E855.5 | E941.2 | E950.4 | E962.0 | E980.4 |
| Typhoid vaccine | 978.1 | E858.8 | E948.1 | E950.4 | E962.0 | E980.4 |
| Typhus vaccine | 979.2 | E858.8 | E949.2 | E950.4 | E962.0 | E980.4 |
| Tyrothricin | 976.0 | E858.7 | E946.0 | E950.4 | E962.0 | E980.4 |
| ENT agent | 976.6 | E858.7 | E946.6 | E950.4 | E962.0 | E980.4 |
| ophthalmic preparation | 976.5 | E858.7 | E946.5 | E950.4 | E962.0 | E980.4 |
| Undecenoic acid | 976.0 | E858.7 | E946.0 | E950.4 | E962.0 | E980.4 |
| Undecylenic acid | 976.0 | E858.7 | E946.0 | E950.4 | E962.0 | E980.4 |
| Unna's boot | 976.3 | E858.7 | E946.3 | E950.4 | E962.0 | E980.4 |
| Uracil mustard | 963.1 | E858.1 | E933.1 | E950.4 | E962.0 | E980.4 |
| Uramustine | 963.1 | E858.1 | E933.1 | E950.4 | E962.0 | E980.4 |
| Urari | 975.2 | E858.6 | E945.2 | E950.4 | E962.0 | E980.4 |
| Urea | 974.4 | E858.5 | E944.4 | E950.4 | E962.0 | E980.4 |
| topical | 976.8 | E858.7 | E946.8 | E950.4 | E962.0 | E980.4 |
| Urethan(e) (antineoplastic) | 963.1 | E858.1 | E933.1 | E950.4 | E962.0 | E980.4 |
| Urginea (maritima) (scilla) — see Squill | | | | | | |
| Uric acid metabolism agents NEC | 974.7 | E858.5 | E944.7 | E950.4 | E962.0 | E980.4 |
| Urokinase | 964.4 | E858.2 | E934.4 | E950.4 | E962.0 | E980.4 |
| Urokon | 977.8 | E858.8 | E947.8 | E950.4 | E962.0 | E980.4 |
| Urotropin | 961.9 | E857 | E931.9 | E950.4 | E962.0 | E980.4 |
| Urtica | 988.2 | E865.4 | — | E950.9 | E962.1 | E980.9 |
| Utility gas — see Gas, utility | | | | | | |
| Vaccine NEC | 979.9 | E858.8 | E949.9 | E950.4 | E962.0 | E980.4 |
| bacterial NEC | 978.8 | E858.8 | E948.8 | E950.4 | E962.0 | E980.4 |
| with | | | | | | |
| other bacterial component | 978.9 | E858.8 | E948.9 | E950.4 | E962.0 | E980.4 |
| pertussis component | 978.6 | E858.8 | E948.6 | E950.4 | E962.0 | E980.4 |
| viral-rickettsial component | 979.7 | E858.8 | E949.7 | E950.4 | E962.0 | E980.4 |
| mixed NEC | 978.9 | E858.8 | E948.9 | E950.4 | E962.0 | E980.4 |
| BCG | 978.0 | E858.8 | E948.0 | E950.4 | E962.0 | E980.4 |
| cholera | 978.2 | E858.8 | E948.2 | E950.4 | E962.0 | E980.4 |
| diphtheria | 978.5 | E858.8 | E948.5 | E950.4 | E962.0 | E980.4 |
| influenza | 979.6 | E858.8 | E949.6 | E950.4 | E962.0 | E980.4 |
| measles | 979.4 | E858.8 | E949.4 | E950.4 | E962.0 | E980.4 |
| meningococcal | 978.8 | E858.8 | E948.8 | E950.4 | E962.0 | E980.4 |
| mumps | 979.6 | E858.8 | E949.6 | E950.4 | E962.0 | E980.4 |
| paratyphoid | 978.1 | E858.8 | E948.1 | E950.4 | E962.0 | E980.4 |
| pertussis (with diphtheria toxoid) (with tetanus toxoid) | 978.6 | E858.8 | E948.6 | E950.4 | E962.0 | E980.4 |
| plague | 978.3 | E858.8 | E948.3 | E950.4 | E962.0 | E980.4 |
| poliomyelitis | 979.5 | E858.8 | E949.5 | E950.4 | E962.0 | E980.4 |
| poliovirus | 979.5 | E858.8 | E949.5 | E950.4 | E962.0 | E980.4 |
| rabies | 979.1 | E858.8 | E949.1 | E950.4 | E962.0 | E980.4 |
| respiratory syncytial virus | 979.6 | E858.8 | E949.6 | E950.4 | E962.0 | E980.4 |
| rickettsial NEC | 979.6 | E858.8 | E949.6 | E950.4 | E962.0 | E980.4 |
| with | | | | | | |
| bacterial component | 979.7 | E858.8 | E949.7 | E950.4 | E962.0 | E980.4 |
| pertussis component | 978.6 | E858.8 | E948.6 | E950.4 | E962.0 | E980.4 |
| viral component | 979.7 | E858.8 | E949.7 | E950.4 | E962.0 | E980.4 |
| Rocky mountain spotted fever | 979.6 | E858.8 | E949.6 | E950.4 | E962.0 | E980.4 |
| rotavirus | 979.6 | E858.8 | E949.6 | E950.4 | E962.0 | E980.4 |
| rubella virus | 979.4 | E858.8 | E949.4 | E950.4 | E962.0 | E980.4 |
| sabin oral | 979.5 | E858.8 | E949.5 | E950.4 | E962.0 | E980.4 |
| smallpox | 979.0 | E858.8 | E949.0 | E950.4 | E962.0 | E980.4 |
| tetanus | 978.4 | E858.8 | E948.4 | E950.4 | E962.0 | E980.4 |
| typhoid | 978.1 | E858.8 | E948.1 | E950.4 | E962.0 | E980.4 |
| typhus | 979.2 | E858.8 | E949.2 | E950.4 | E962.0 | E980.4 |
| viral NEC | 979.6 | E858.8 | E949.6 | E950.4 | E962.0 | E980.4 |
| with | | | | | | |
| bacterial component | 979.7 | E858.8 | E949.7 | E950.4 | E962.0 | E980.4 |
| pertussis component | 978.6 | E858.8 | E948.6 | E950.4 | E962.0 | E980.4 |
| rickettsial component | 979.7 | E858.8 | E949.7 | E950.4 | E962.0 | E980.4 |
| yellow fever | 979.3 | E858.8 | E949.3 | E950.4 | E962.0 | E980.4 |
| Vaccinia immune globulin (human) | 964.6 | E858.2 | E934.6 | E950.4 | E962.0 | E980.4 |
| Vaginal contraceptives | 976.8 | E858.7 | E946.8 | E950.4 | E962.0 | E980.4 |
| Valethamate | 971.1 | E855.4 | E941.1 | E950.4 | E962.0 | E980.4 |
| Valisone | 976.0 | E858.7 | E946.0 | E950.4 | E962.0 | E980.4 |
| Valium | 969.4 | E853.2 | E939.4 | E950.3 | E962.0 | E980.3 |
| Valmid | 967.8 | E852.8 | E937.8 | E950.2 | E962.0 | E980.2 |
| Vanadium | 985.8 | E866.4 | — | E950.9 | E962.1 | E980.9 |
| Vancomycin | 960.8 | E856 | E930.8 | E950.4 | E962.0 | E980.4 |
| Vapor — see also Gas | 987.9 | E869.9 | — | E952.9 | E962.2 | E982.9 |
| kiln (carbon monoxide) | 986 | E868.8 | — | E952.1 | E962.2 | E982.1 |
| lead — see Lead | | | | | | |

| | Poisoning | Accident | Therapeutic Use | Suicide Attempt | Assault | Undetermined |
|---|---|---|---|---|---|---|
| Vapor — see also Gas — continued | | | | | | |
| specified source NEC (see also specific substance) | 987.8 | E869.8 | — | E952.8 | E962.2 | E982.8 |
| Varidase | 964.4 | E858.2 | E934.4 | E950.4 | E962.0 | E980.4 |
| Varnish | 989.89 | E861.6 | — | E950.9 | E962.1 | E980.9 |
| cleaner | 982.8 | E862.9 | — | E950.9 | E962.1 | E980.9 |
| Vaseline | 976.3 | E858.7 | E946.3 | E950.4 | E962.0 | E980.4 |
| Vasodilan | 972.5 | E858.3 | E942.5 | E950.4 | E962.0 | E980.4 |
| Vasodilators NEC | 972.5 | E858.3 | E942.5 | E950.4 | E962.0 | E980.4 |
| coronary | 972.4 | E858.3 | E942.4 | E950.4 | E962.0 | E980.4 |
| Vasopressin | 962.5 | E858.0 | E932.5 | E950.4 | E962.0 | E980.4 |
| Vasopressor drugs | 962.5 | E858.0 | E932.5 | E950.4 | E962.0 | E980.4 |
| Venom, venomous (bite) (sting) | 989.5 | E905.9 | — | E950.9 | E962.1 | E980.9 |
| arthropod NEC | 989.5 | E905.5 | — | E950.9 | E962.1 | E980.9 |
| bee | 989.5 | E905.3 | — | E950.9 | E962.1 | E980.9 |
| centipede | 989.5 | E905.4 | — | E950.9 | E962.1 | E980.9 |
| hornet | 989.5 | E905.3 | — | E950.9 | E962.1 | E980.9 |
| lizard | 989.5 | E905.0 | — | E950.9 | E962.1 | E980.9 |
| marine animals or plants | 989.5 | E905.6 | — | E950.9 | E962.1 | E980.9 |
| millipede (tropical) | 989.5 | E905.4 | — | E950.9 | E962.1 | E980.9 |
| plant NEC | 989.5 | E905.7 | — | E950.9 | E962.1 | E980.9 |
| marine | 989.5 | E905.6 | — | E950.9 | E962.1 | E980.9 |
| scorpion | 989.5 | E905.2 | — | E950.9 | E962.1 | E980.9 |
| snake | 989.5 | E905.0 | — | E950.9 | E962.1 | E980.9 |
| specified NEC | 989.5 | E905.8 | — | E950.9 | E962.1 | E980.9 |
| spider | 989.5 | E905.1 | — | E950.9 | E962.1 | E980.9 |
| wasp | 989.5 | E905.3 | — | E950.9 | E962.1 | E980.9 |
| Ventolin — see Salbutamol sulfate | | | | | | |
| Veramon | 967.0 | E851 | E937.0 | E950.1 | E962.0 | E980.1 |
| Veratrum | | | | | | |
| album | 988.2 | E865.4 | — | E950.9 | E962.1 | E980.9 |
| alkaloids | 972.6 | E858.3 | E942.6 | E950.4 | E962.0 | E980.4 |
| viride | 988.2 | E865.4 | — | E950.9 | E962.1 | E980.9 |
| Verdigris — see also Copper | 985.8 | E866.4 | — | E950.9 | E962.1 | E980.9 |
| Veronal | 967.0 | E851 | E937.0 | E950.1 | E962.0 | E980.1 |
| Veroxil | 961.6 | E857 | E931.6 | E950.4 | E962.0 | E980.4 |
| Versidyne | 965.7 | E850.7 | E935.7 | E950.0 | E962.0 | E980.0 |
| Viagra | 972.5 | E858.3 | E942.5 | E950.4 | E962.0 | E980.4 |
| Vienna | | | | | | |
| green | 985.1 | E866.3 | — | E950.8 | E962.1 | E980.8 |
| insecticide | 985.1 | E863.4 | — | E950.6 | E962.1 | E980.7 |
| red | 989.89 | E866.8 | — | E950.9 | E962.1 | E980.9 |
| pharmaceutical dye | 977.4 | E858.8 | E947.4 | E950.4 | E962.0 | E980.4 |
| Vinbarbital, vinbarbitone | 967.0 | E851 | E937.0 | E950.1 | E962.0 | E980.1 |
| Vinblastine | 963.1 | E858.1 | E933.1 | E950.4 | E962.0 | E980.4 |
| Vincristine | 963.1 | E858.1 | E933.1 | E950.4 | E962.0 | E980.4 |
| Vinesthene, vinethene | 968.2 | E855.1 | E938.2 | E950.4 | E962.0 | E980.4 |
| Vinyl | | | | | | |
| bital | 967.0 | E851 | E937.0 | E950.1 | E962.0 | E980.1 |
| ether | 968.2 | E855.1 | E938.2 | E950.4 | E962.0 | E980.4 |
| Vioform | 961.3 | E857 | E931.3 | E950.4 | E962.0 | E980.4 |
| topical | 976.0 | E858.7 | E946.0 | E950.4 | E962.0 | E980.4 |
| Viomycin | 960.6 | E856 | E930.6 | E950.4 | E962.0 | E980.4 |
| Viosterol | 963.5 | E858.1 | E933.5 | E950.4 | E962.0 | E980.4 |
| Viper (venom) | 989.5 | E905.0 | — | E950.9 | E962.1 | E980.9 |
| Viprynium (embonate) | 961.6 | E857 | E931.6 | E950.4 | E962.0 | E980.4 |
| Virugon | 961.7 | E857 | E931.7 | E950.4 | E962.0 | E980.4 |
| Visine | 976.5 | E858.7 | E946.5 | E950.4 | E962.0 | E980.4 |
| Vitamins NEC | 963.5 | E858.1 | E933.5 | E950.4 | E962.0 | E980.4 |
| B$_{12}$ | 964.1 | E858.2 | E934.1 | E950.4 | E962.0 | E980.4 |
| hematopoietic | 964.1 | E858.2 | E934.1 | E950.4 | E962.0 | E980.4 |
| K | 964.3 | E858.2 | E934.3 | E950.4 | E962.0 | E980.4 |
| Vleminckx's solution | 976.4 | E858.7 | E946.4 | E950.4 | E962.0 | E980.4 |
| Voltaren — see Diclofenac sodium | | | | | | |
| Warfarin (potassium) (sodium) | 964.2 | E858.2 | E934.2 | E950.4 | E962.0 | E980.4 |
| rodenticide | 989.4 | E863.7 | — | E950.6 | E962.1 | E980.7 |
| Wasp (sting) | 989.5 | E905.3 | — | E950.9 | E962.1 | E980.9 |
| Water | | | | | | |
| balance agents NEC | 974.5 | E858.5 | E944.5 | E950.4 | E962.0 | E980.4 |
| gas | 987.1 | E868.1 | — | E951.8 | E962.2 | E981.8 |
| incomplete combustion of — see Carbon, monoxide, fuel, utility | | | | | | |
| hemlock | 988.2 | E865.4 | — | E950.9 | E962.1 | E980.9 |
| moccasin (venom) | 989.5 | E905.0 | — | E950.9 | E962.1 | E980.9 |

| | | External Cause (E-Code) | | | | |
|---|---|---|---|---|---|---|
| | Poisoning | Accident | Therapeutic Use | Suicide Attempt | Assault | Undetermined |
| **Wax** (paraffin) (petroleum) | 981 | E862.3 | — | E950.9 | E962.1 | E980.9 |
| automobile | 989.89 | E861.2 | — | E950.9 | E962.1 | E980.9 |
| floor | 981 | E862.0 | — | E950.9 | E962.1 | E980.9 |
| **Weed killers NEC** | 989.4 | E863.5 | — | E950.6 | E962.1 | E980.7 |
| **Welldorm** | 967.1 | E852.0 | E937.1 | E950.2 | E962.0 | E980.2 |
| **White** | | | | | | |
| arsenic — see Arsenic | | | | | | |
| hellebore | 988.2 | E865.4 | — | E950.9 | E962.1 | E980.9 |
| lotion (keratolytic) | 976.4 | E858.7 | E946.4 | E950.4 | E962.0 | E980.4 |
| spirit | 981 | E862.0 | — | E950.9 | E962.1 | E980.9 |
| **Whitewashes** | 989.89 | E861.6 | — | E950.9 | E962.1 | E980.9 |
| **Whole blood** | 964.7 | E858.2 | E934.7 | E950.4 | E962.0 | E980.4 |
| **Wild** | | | | | | |
| black cherry | 988.2 | E865.4 | — | E950.9 | E962.1 | E980.9 |
| poisonous plants NEC | 988.2 | E865.4 | — | E950.9 | E962.1 | E980.9 |
| **Window cleaning fluid** | 989.89 | E861.3 | — | E950.9 | E962.1 | E980.9 |
| **Wintergreen** (oil) | 976.3 | E858.7 | E946.3 | E950.4 | E962.0 | E980.4 |
| **Witch hazel** | 976.2 | E858.7 | E946.2 | E950.4 | E962.0 | E980.4 |
| **Wood** | | | | | | |
| alcohol | 980.1 | E860.2 | — | E950.9 | E962.1 | E980.9 |
| spirit | 980.1 | E860.2 | — | E950.9 | E962.1 | E980.9 |
| **Woorali** | 975.2 | E858.6 | E945.2 | E950.4 | E962.0 | E980.4 |
| **Wormseed, American** | 961.6 | E857 | E931.6 | E950.4 | E962.0 | E980.4 |
| **Xanthine diuretics** | 974.1 | E858.5 | E944.1 | E950.4 | E962.0 | E980.4 |
| **Xanthocillin** | 960.0 | E856 | E930.0 | E950.4 | E962.0 | E980.4 |
| **Xanthotoxin** | 976.3 | E858.7 | E946.3 | E950.4 | E962.0 | E980.4 |
| **Xigris** | 964.2 | E858.2 | E934.2 | E950.4 | E962.0 | E980.4 |
| **Xylene** (liquid) (vapor) | 982.0 | E862.4 | — | E950.9 | E962.1 | E980.9 |
| **Xylocaine** (infiltration) | | | | | | |
| (topical) | 968.5 | E855.2 | E938.5 | E950.4 | E962.0 | E980.4 |
| nerve block (peripheral) | | | | | | |
| (plexus) | 968.6 | E855.2 | E938.6 | E950.4 | E962.0 | E980.4 |
| spinal | 968.7 | E855.2 | E938.7 | E950.4 | E962.0 | E980.4 |
| **Xylol** (liquid) (vapor) | 982.0 | E862.4 | — | E950.9 | E962.1 | E980.9 |
| **Xylometazoline** | 971.2 | E855.5 | E941.2 | E950.4 | E962.0 | E980.4 |
| **Yellow** | | | | | | |
| fever vaccine | 979.3 | E858.8 | E949.3 | E950.4 | E962.0 | E980.4 |
| jasmine | 988.2 | E865.4 | — | E950.9 | E962.1 | E980.9 |
| **Yew** | 988.2 | E865.4 | — | E950.9 | E962.1 | E980.9 |
| **Zactane** | 965.7 | E850.7 | E935.7 | E950.0 | E962.0 | E980.0 |
| **Zaroxolyn** | 974.3 | E858.5 | E944.3 | E950.4 | E962.0 | E980.4 |
| **Zephiran** (topical) | 976.0 | E858.7 | E946.0 | E950.4 | E962.0 | E980.4 |
| ophthalmic preparation | 976.5 | E858.7 | E946.5 | E950.4 | E962.0 | E980.4 |
| **Zerone** | 980.1 | E860.2 | — | E950.9 | E962.1 | E980.9 |
| **Zinc** (compounds) (fumes) (salts) | | | | | | |
| (vapor) NEC | 985.8 | E866.4 | — | E950.9 | E962.1 | E980.9 |
| anti-infectives | 976.0 | E858.7 | E946.0 | E950.4 | E962.0 | E980.4 |
| antivaricose | 972.7 | E858.3 | E942.7 | E950.4 | E962.0 | E980.4 |
| bacitracin | 976.0 | E858.7 | E946.0 | E950.4 | E962.0 | E980.4 |
| chloride | 976.2 | E858.7 | E946.2 | E950.4 | E962.0 | E980.4 |
| gelatin | 976.3 | E858.7 | E946.3 | E950.4 | E962.0 | E980.4 |
| oxide | 976.3 | E858.7 | E946.3 | E950.4 | E962.0 | E980.4 |
| peroxide | 976.0 | E858.7 | E946.0 | E950.4 | E962.0 | E980.4 |
| pesticides | 985.8 | E863.4 | — | E950.6 | E962.1 | E980.7 |
| phosphide (rodenticide) | 985.8 | E863.7 | — | E950.6 | E962.1 | E980.7 |
| stearate | 976.3 | E858.7 | E946.3 | E950.4 | E962.0 | E980.4 |
| sulfate (antivaricose) | 972.7 | E858.3 | E942.7 | E950.4 | E962.0 | E980.4 |
| ENT agent | 976.6 | E858.7 | E946.6 | E950.4 | E962.0 | E980.4 |
| ophthalmic solution | 976.5 | E858.7 | E946.5 | E950.4 | E962.0 | E980.4 |
| topical NEC | 976.0 | E858.7 | E946.0 | E950.4 | E962.0 | E980.4 |
| undecylenate | 976.0 | E858.7 | E946.0 | E950.4 | E962.0 | E980.4 |
| **Zovant** | 964.2 | E858.2 | E934.2 | E950.4 | E962.0 | E980.4 |
| **Zoxazolamine** | 968.0 | E855.1 | E938.0 | E950.4 | E962.0 | E980.4 |
| **Zygadenus** (venenosus) | 988.2 | E865.4 | — | E950.9 | E962.1 | E980.9 |

☑ Additional Digit Required — Refer to the Tabular List for Digit Selection　　　　　　　▽ Subterms under main terms may continue to next column or page

**336 — Volume 2**　　　　　▶◀ Revised Text　　　● New Line　　　▲ Revised Code　　　*2008 ICD-9-CM*

# SECTION 3

## Alphabetic Index to External Causes of Injury and Poisoning (E Code)

This section contains the index to the codes which classify environmental events, circumstances, and other conditions as the cause of injury and other adverse effects. Where a code from the section Supplementary Classification of External Causes of Injury and Poisoning (E800-E999) is applicable, it is intended that the E code shall be used in addition to a code from the main body of the classification, Chapters 1 to 17.

The alphabetic index to the E codes is organized by main terms which describe the accident, circumstance, event, or specific agent which caused the injury or other adverse effect.

*Note — Transport accidents (E800-E848) include accidents involving:*

> *aircraft and spacecraft (E840-E845)*
>
> *watercraft (E830-E838)*
>
> *motor vehicle (E810-E825)*
>
> *railway (E800-E807)*
>
> *other road vehicles (E826-E829)*

*For definitions and examples related to transport accidents — see Volume 1 code categories E800-E848.*

*The fourth-digit subdivisions for use with categories E800-E848 to identify the injured person are found at the end of this section.*

*For identifying the place in which an accident or poisoning occurred (circumstances classifiable to categories E850-E869 and E880-E928) — see the listing in this section under "Accident, occurring."*

See the Table of Drugs and Chemicals (Section 2 of this volume) for identifying the specific agent involved in drug overdose or a wrong substance given or taken in error, and for intoxication or poisoning by a drug or other chemical substance.

The specific adverse effect, reaction, or localized toxic effect to a correct drug or substance properly administered in therapeutic or prophylactic dosage should be classified according to the nature of the adverse effect (e.g., allergy, dermatitis, tachycardia) listed in Section 1 of this volume.

☑ Additional Digit Required — Refer to the Tabular List for Digit Selection
**2008 ICD-9-CM**      ▶◀ Revised Text      ● New Line      ▲ Revised Code

▽ Subterms under main terms may continue to next column or page
**Volume 2 — 337**

## A

**Abandonment**
  causing exposure to weather conditions — *see* Exposure
  child, with intent to injure or kill E968.4
  helpless person, infant, newborn E904.0
    with intent to injure or kill E968.4

**Abortion, criminal, injury to child** E968.8

**Abuse** (alleged) (suspected)
  adult
    by
        child E967.4
        ex-partner E967.3
        ex-spouse E967.3
        father E967.0
        grandchild E967.7
        grandparent E967.6
        mother E967.2
        non-related caregiver E967.8
        other relative E967.7
        other specified person E967.1
        partner E967.3
        sibling E967.5
        spouse E967.3
        stepfather E967.0
        stepmother E967.2
        unspecified person E967.9
  child
    by
        boyfriend of parent or guardian E967.0
        child E967.4
        father E967.0
        female partner of parent or guardian E967.2
        girlfriend of parent or guardian E967.2
        grandchild E967.7
        grandparent E967.6
        male partner of parent or guardian E967.0
        mother E967.2
        non-related caregiver E967.8
        other relative E967.7
        other specified person(s) E967.1
        sibling E967.5
        stepfather E967.0
        stepmother E967.2
        unspecified person E967.9

**Accident (to)** E928.9
  aircraft (in transit) (powered) E841 ☑
    at landing, take-off E840 ☑
    due to, caused by cataclysm — *see* categories E908 ☑, E909 ☑
    late effect of E929.1
    unpowered (*see also* Collision, aircraft, unpowered) E842 ☑
    while alighting, boarding E843 ☑
  amphibious vehicle
    on
        land — *see* Accident, motor vehicle
        water — *see* Accident, watercraft
  animal-drawn vehicle NEC E827 ☑
  animal, ridden NEC E828 ☑
  balloon (*see also* Collision, aircraft, unpowered) E842 ☑
  caused by, due to
    abrasive wheel (metalworking) E919.3
    animal NEC E906.9
      being ridden (in sport or transport) E828 ☑
    avalanche NEC E909.2
    band saw E919.4
    bench saw E919.4
    bore, earth-drilling or mining (land) (seabed) E919.1
    bulldozer E919.7

**Accident (to)** — *continued*
  caused by, due to — *continued*
    cataclysmic
      earth surface movement or eruption E909.9
      storm E908.9
    chain
      hoist E919.2
        agricultural operations E919.0
        mining operations E919.1
      saw E920.1
    circular saw E919.4
    cold (excessive) (*see also* Cold, exposure to) E901.9
    combine E919.0
    conflagration — *see* Conflagration
    corrosive liquid, substance NEC E924.1
    cotton gin E919.8
    crane E919.2
      agricultural operations E919.0
      mining operations E919.1
    cutting or piercing instrument (*see also* Cut) E920.9
    dairy equipment E919.8
    derrick E919.2
      agricultural operations E919.0
      mining operations E919.1
    drill E920.1
      earth (land) (seabed) E919.1
      hand (powered) E920.1
        not powered E920.4
      metalworking E919.3
      woodworking E919.4
    earth(-)
      drilling machine E919.1
      moving machine E919.7
      scraping machine E919.7
    electric
      current (*see also* Electric shock) E925.9
      motor (*see also* Accident, machine, by type of machine)
        current (of) — *see* Electric shock
    elevator (building) (grain) E919.2
      agricultural operations E919.0
      mining operations E919.1
    environmental factors NEC E928.9
    excavating machine E919.7
    explosive material (*see also* Explosion) E923.9
    farm machine E919.0
    firearm missile — *see* Shooting
    fire, flames (*see also* Fire)
      conflagration — *see* Conflagration
    forging (metalworking) machine E919.3
    forklift (truck) E919.2
      agricultural operations E919.0
      mining operations E919.1
    gas turbine E919.5
    harvester E919.0
    hay derrick, mower, or rake E919.0
    heat (excessive) (*see also* Heat) E900.9
    hoist (*see also* Accident, caused by, due to, lift) E919.2
      chain — *see* Accident, caused by, due to, chain
      shaft E919.1
    hot
      liquid E924.0
        caustic or corrosive E924.1
      object (not producing fire or flames) E924.8
      substance E924.9
        caustic or corrosive E924.1
        liquid (metal) NEC E924.0
        specified type NEC E924.8
    human bite E928.3
    ignition — *see* Ignition
    internal combustion engine E919.5
    landslide NEC E909.2

**Accident (to)** — *continued*
  caused by, due to — *continued*
    lathe (metalworking) E919.3
      turnings E920.8
      woodworking E919.4
    lift, lifting (appliances) E919.2
      agricultural operations E919.0
      mining operations E919.1
      shaft E919.1
    lightning NEC E907
    machine, machinery (*see also* Accident, machine)
      drilling, metal E919.3
      manufacturing, for manufacture of
        beverages E919.8
        clothing E919.8
        foodstuffs E919.8
        paper E919.8
        textiles E919.8
      milling, metal E919.3
      moulding E919.4
      power press, metal E919.3
      printing E919.8
      rolling mill, metal E919.3
      sawing, metal E919.3
      specified type NEC E919.8
      spinning E919.8
      weaving E919.8
    natural factor NEC E928.9
    overhead plane E919.4
    plane E920.4
      overhead E919.4
    powered
      hand tool NEC E920.1
      saw E919.4
        hand E920.1
    printing machine E919.8
    pulley (block) E919.2
      agricultural operations E919.0
      mining operations E919.1
      transmission E919.6
    radial saw E919.4
    radiation — *see* Radiation
    reaper E919.0
    road scraper E919.7
      when in transport under its own power — *see* categories E810-E825 ☑
    roller coaster E919.8
    sander E919.4
    saw E920.4
      band E919.4
      bench E919.4
      chain E920.1
      circular E919.4
      hand E920.4
        powered E920.1
      powered, except hand E919.4
      radial E919.4
    sawing machine, metal E919.3
    shaft
      hoist E919.1
      lift E919.1
      transmission E919.6
    shears E920.4
      hand E920.4
        powered E920.1
      mechanical E919.3
    shovel E920.4
      steam E919.7
    spinning machine E919.8
    steam (*see also* Burning, steam)
      engine E919.5
      shovel E919.7
    thresher E919.0
    thunderbolt NEC E907
    tractor E919.0
      when in transport under its own power — *see* categories E810-E825 ☑
    transmission belt, cable, chain, gear, pinion, pulley, shaft E919.6
    turbine (gas) (water driven) E919.5
    under-cutter E919.1

**Accident (to)** — *continued*
  caused by, due to — *continued*
    weaving machine E919.8
    winch E919.2
      agricultural operations E919.0
      mining operations E919.1
  diving E883.0
    with insufficient air supply E913.2
  glider (hang) (*see also* Collision, aircraft, unpowered) E842 ☑
  hovercraft
    on
        land — *see* Accident, motor vehicle
        water — *see* Accident, watercraft
  ice yacht (*see also* Accident, vehicle NEC) E848
  in
    medical, surgical procedure
      as, or due to misadventure — *see* Misadventure
      causing an abnormal reaction or later complication without mention of misadventure — *see* Reaction, abnormal
  kite carrying a person (*see also* Collision, involving aircraft, unpowered) E842 ☑
  land yacht (*see also* Accident, vehicle NEC) E848
  late effect of — *see* Late effect
  launching pad E845 ☑
  machine, machinery (*see also* Accident, caused by, due to, by specific type of machine) E919.9
    agricultural including animal-powered E919.0
    earth-drilling E919.1
    earth moving or scraping E919.7
    excavating E919.7
    involving transport under own power on highway or transport vehicle — *see* categories E810-E825 ☑, E840-E845 ☑
    lifting (appliances) E919.2
    metalworking E919.3
    mining E919.1
    prime movers, except electric motors E919.5
      electric motors — *see* Accident, machine, by specific type of machine
    recreational E919.8
    specified type NEC E919.8
    transmission E919.6
    watercraft (deck) (engine room) (galley) (laundry) (loading) E836 ☑
    woodworking or forming E919.4
  motor vehicle (on public highway) (traffic) E819 ☑
    due to cataclysm — *see* categories E908 ☑, E909 ☑
    involving
      collision (*see also* Collision, motor vehicle) E812 ☑
      nontraffic, not on public highway — *see* categories E820-E825 ☑
      not involving collision — *see* categories E816-E819 ☑
  nonmotor vehicle NEC E829 ☑
    nonroad — *see* Accident, vehicle NEC
    road, except pedal cycle, animal-drawn vehicle, or animal being ridden E829 ☑
  nonroad vehicle NEC — *see* Accident, vehicle NEC
  not elsewhere classifiable involving
    cable car (not on rails) E847
      on rails E829 ☑
    coal car in mine E846

## Accident (to) — continued

not elsewhere classifiable involving — continued

hand truck — see Accident, vehicle NEC

logging car E846

sled(ge), meaning snow or ice vehicle E848

tram, mine or quarry E846

truck

mine or quarry E846

self-propelled, industrial E846

station baggage E846

tub, mine or quarry E846

vehicle NEC E848

snow and ice E848

used only on industrial premises E846

wheelbarrow E848

occurring (at) (in)

apartment E849.0

baseball field, diamond E849.4

construction site, any E849.3

dock E849.8

yard E849.3

dormitory E849.7

factory (building) (premises) E849.3

farm E849.1

buildings E849.1

house E849.0

football field E849.4

forest E849.8

garage (place of work) E849.3

private (home) E849.0

gravel pit E849.2

gymnasium E849.4

highway E849.5

home (private) (residential) E849.0

institutional E849.7

hospital E849.7

hotel E849.6

house (private) (residential) E849.0

movie E849.6

public E849.6

institution, residential E849.7

jail E849.7

mine E849.2

motel E849.6

movie house E849.6

office (building) E849.6

orphanage E849.7

park (public) E849.4

mobile home E849.8

trailer E849.8

parking lot or place E849.8

place

industrial NEC E849.3

parking E849.8

public E849.5

specified place NEC E849.5

recreational NEC E849.4

sport NEC E849.4

playground (park) (school) E849.4

prison E849.6

public building NEC E849.6

quarry E849.2

railway

line NEC E849.8

yard E849.3

residence

home (private) E849.0

resort (beach) (lake) (mountain) (seashore) (vacation) E849.4

restaurant E849.6

sand pit E849.2

school (building) (private) (public) (state) E849.6

reform E849.7

riding E849.4

seashore E849.8

resort E849.4

shop (place of work) E849.3

commercial E849.6

skating rink E849.4

sports palace E849.4

stadium E849.4

## Accident (to) — continued

occurring — continued

store E849.6

street E849.5

swimming pool (public) E849.4

private home or garden E849.0

tennis court, public E849.4

theatre, theater E849.6

trailer court E849.8

tunnel E849.8

under construction E849.2

warehouse E849.3

yard

dock E849.3

industrial E849.3

private (home) E849.0

railway E849.3

off-road type motor vehicle (not on public highway) NEC E821 ☑

on public highway — see categories E810-E819 ☑

pedal cycle E826 ☑

railway E807 ☑

due to cataclysm — see categories E908 ☑, E909 ☑

involving

avalanche E909.2

burning by engine, locomotive, train (see also Explosion, railway engine) E803 ☑

collision (see also Collision, railway) E800 ☑

derailment (see also Derailment, railway) E802 ☑

explosion (see also Explosion, railway engine) E803 ☑

fall (see also Fall, from, railway rolling stock) E804 ☑

fire (see also Explosion, railway engine) E803 ☑

hitting by, being struck by object falling in, on, from, rolling stock, train, vehicle E806 ☑

rolling stock, train, vehicle E805 ☑

overturning, railway rolling stock, train, vehicle (see also Derailment, railway) E802 ☑

running off rails, railway (see also Derailment, railway) E802 ☑

specified circumstances NEC E806 ☑

train or vehicle hit by

avalanche E909.2

falling object (earth, rock, tree) E806 ☑

due to cataclysm — see categories E908 ☑, E909 ☑

landslide E909.2

roller skate E885.1

scooter (nonmotorized) E885.0

skateboard E885.2

ski(ing) E885.3

jump E884.9

lift or tow (with chair or gondola) E847

snowboard E885.4

snow vehicle, motor driven (not on public highway) E820 ☑

on public highway — see categories E810-E819 ☑

spacecraft E845 ☑

specified cause NEC E928.8

street car E829 ☑

traffic NEC E819 ☑

vehicle NEC (with pedestrian) E848

battery powered

airport passenger vehicle E846

truck (baggage) (mail) E846

## Accident (to) — continued

vehicle — continued

powered commercial or industrial (with other vehicle or object within commercial or industrial premises) E846

watercraft E838 ☑

with

drowning or submersion resulting from

accident other than to watercraft E832 ☑

accident to watercraft E830 ☑

injury, except drowning or submersion, resulting from accident other than to watercraft — see categories E833-E838 ☑

accident to watercraft E831 ☑

due to, caused by cataclysm — see categories E908 ☑, E909 ☑

machinery E836 ☑

**Acid throwing** E961

**Acosta syndrome** E902.0

**Aeroneurosis** E902.1

**Aero-otitis media** — see Effects of, air pressure

**Aerosinusitis** — see Effects of, air pressure

**After-effect, late** — see Late effect

**Air**

blast

in

terrorism E979.2

war operations E993

embolism (traumatic) NEC E928.9

in

infusion or transfusion E874.1

perfusion E874.2

sickness E903

**Alpine sickness** E902.0

**Altitude sickness** — see Effects of, air pressure

**Anaphylactic shock, anaphylaxis** — see also Table of Drugs and Chemicals E947.9

due to bite or sting (venomous) — see Bite, venomous

**Andes disease** E902.0

**Apoplexy**

heat — see Heat

**Arachnidism** E905.1

**Arson** E968.0

**Asphyxia, asphyxiation**

by

chemical

in

terrorism E979.7

war operations E997.2

explosion — see Explosion

food (bone) (regurgitated food) (seed) E911

foreign object, except food E912

fumes

in

terrorism (chemical weapons) E979.7

war operations E997.2

gas (see also Table of Drugs and Chemicals)

in

terrorism E979.7

war operations E997.2

legal

execution E978

intervention (tear) E972

tear E972

mechanical means (see also Suffocation) E913.9

from

conflagration — see Conflagration

fire (see also Fire) E899

in

terrorism E979.3

## Asphyxia, asphyxiation — continued

from — continued

fire (see also Fire) — continued

in — continued

war operations E990.9

ignition — see Ignition

**Aspiration**

foreign body — see Foreign body, aspiration

mucus, not of newborn (with asphyxia, obstruction respiratory passage, suffocation) E912

phlegm (with asphyxia, obstruction respiratory passage, suffocation) E912

vomitus (with asphyxia, obstruction respiratory passage, suffocation) (see also Foreign body, aspiration, food) E911

**Assassination** (attempt) — see also Assault E968.9

**Assault** (homicidal) (by) (in) E968.9

acid E961

swallowed E962.1

air gun E968.6

BB gun E968.6

bite NEC E968.8

of human being E968.7

bomb ((placed in) car or house) E965.8

antipersonnel E965.5

letter E965.7

petrol E965.6

brawl (hand) (fists) (foot) E960.0

burning, burns (by fire) E968.0

acid E961

swallowed E962.1

caustic, corrosive substance E961

swallowed E962.1

chemical from swallowing caustic, corrosive substance NEC E962.1

hot liquid E968.3

scalding E968.3

vitriol E961

swallowed E962.1

caustic, corrosive substance E961

swallowed E962.1

cut, any part of body E966

dagger E966

drowning E964

explosive(s) E965.9

bomb (see also Assault, bomb) E965.8

dynamite E965.8

fight (hand) (fists) (foot) E960.0

with weapon E968.9

blunt or thrown E968.2

cutting or piercing E966

firearm — see Shooting, homicide

fire E968.0

firearm(s) — see Shooting, homicide

garrotting E963

gunshot (wound) — see Shooting, homicide

hanging E963

injury NEC E968.9

knife E966

late effect of E969

ligature E963

poisoning E962.9

drugs or medicinals E962.0

gas(es) or vapors, except drugs and medicinals E962.2

solid or liquid substances, except drugs and medicinals E962.1

puncture, any part of body E966

pushing

before moving object, train, vehicle E968.5

from high place E968.1

rape E960.1

scalding E968.3

shooting — see Shooting, homicide

sodomy E960.1

stab, any part of body E966

---

☑ Additional Digit Required — Refer to the Tabular List for Digit Selection

🔲 Subterms under main terms may continue to next column or page

**Assault** — *continued*
strangulation E963
submersion E964
suffocation E963
transport vehicle E968.5
violence NEC E968.9
vitriol E961
swallowed E962.1
weapon E968.9
blunt or thrown E968.2
cutting or piercing E966
firearm — *see* Shooting, homicide
wound E968.9
cutting E966
gunshot — *see* Shooting, homicide
knife E966
piercing E966
puncture E966
stab E966
**Attack by animal** NEC E906.9
**Avalanche** E909.2
falling on or hitting
motor vehicle (in motion) (on public highway) E909.2
railway train E909.2
**Aviators' disease** E902.1

## B

**Barotitis, barodontalgia, barosinusitis, barotrauma** (otitic) (sinus) — *see* Effects of, air pressure
**Battered**
baby or child (syndrome) — *see* Abuse, child; category E967 ☑
person other than baby or child — *see* Assault
**Bayonet wound** — *see also* Cut, by bayonet E920.3
in
legal intervention E974
terrorism E979.8
war operations E995
**Bean in nose** E912
**Bed set on fire** NEC E898.0
**Beheading** (by guillotine)
homicide E966
legal execution E978
**Bending, injury in** E927
**Bends** E902.0
**Bite**
animal NEC E906.5
other specified (except arthropod) E906.3
venomous NEC E905.9
arthropod (nonvenomous) NEC E906.4
venomous — *see* Sting
black widow spider E905.1
cat E906.3
centipede E905.4
cobra E905.0
copperhead snake E905.0
coral snake E905.0
dog E906.0
fer de lance E905.0
gila monster E905.0
human being
accidental E928.3
assault E968.7
insect (nonvenomous) E906.4
venomous — *see* Sting
krait E905.0
late effect of — *see* Late effect
lizard E906.2
venomous E905.0
mamba E905.0
marine animal
nonvenomous E906.3
snake E906.2
venomous E905.6
snake E905.0
millipede E906.4
venomous E905.4
moray eel E906.3
rat E906.1
rattlesnake E905.0
rodent, except rat E906.3

**Bite** — *continued*
serpent — *see* Bite, snake
shark E906.3
snake (venomous) E905.0
nonvenomous E906.2
sea E905.0
spider E905.1
nonvenomous E906.4
tarantula (venomous) E905.1
venomous NEC E905.9
by specific animal — *see category* E905 ☑
viper E905.0
water moccasin E905.0
**Blast** (air)
from nuclear explosion E996
in
terrorism E979.2
from nuclear explosion E979.5
underwater E979.0
war operations E993
from nuclear explosion E996
underwater E992
**Blizzard** E908.3
**Blow** E928.9
by law-enforcing agent, police (on duty) E975
with blunt object (baton) (nightstick) (stave) (truncheon) E973
**Blowing up** — *see also* Explosion E923.9
**Brawl** (hand) (fists) (foot) E960.0
**Breakage** (accidental)
cable of cable car not on rails E847
ladder (causing fall) E881.0
part (any) of
animal-drawn vehicle E827 ☑
ladder (causing fall) E881.0
motor vehicle
in motion (on public highway) E818 ☑
not on public highway E825 ☑
nonmotor road vehicle, except animal-drawn vehicle or pedal cycle E829 ☑
off-road type motor vehicle (not on public highway) NEC E821 ☑
on public highway E818 ☑
pedal cycle E826 ☑
scaffolding (causing fall) E881.1
snow vehicle, motor-driven (not on public highway) E820 ☑
on public highway E818 ☑
vehicle NEC — *see* Accident, vehicle
**Broken**
glass
fall on E888.0
injury by E920.8
power line (causing electric shock) E925.1
**Bumping against, into** (accidentally)
object (moving) E917.9
caused by crowd E917.1
with subsequent fall E917.6
furniture E917.3
with subsequent fall E917.7
in
running water E917.2
sports E917.0
with subsequent fall E917.5
stationary E917.4
with subsequent fall E917.8
person(s) E917.9
with fall E886.9
in sports E886.0
as, or caused by, a crowd E917.1
with subsequent fall E917.6
in sports E917.0
with fall E886.0
**Burning, burns** (accidental) (by) (from) (on) E899
acid (any kind) E924.1
swallowed — *see* Table of Drugs and Chemicals

**Burning, burns** — *continued*
bedclothes (*see also* Fire, specified NEC) E898.0
blowlamp (*see also* Fire, specified NEC) E898.1
blowtorch (*see also* Fire, specified NEC) E898.1
boat, ship, watercraft — *see* categories E830 ☑, E831 ☑, E837 ☑
bonfire (controlled) E897
uncontrolled E892
candle (*see also* Fire, specified NEC) E898.1
caustic liquid, substance E924.1
swallowed — *see* Table of Drugs and Chemicals
chemical E924.1
from swallowing caustic, corrosive substance — *see* Table of Drugs and Chemicals
in
terrorism E979.7
war operations E997.2
cigar(s) or cigarette(s) (*see also* Fire, specified NEC) E898.1
clothes, clothing, nightdress — *see* Ignition, clothes
with conflagration — *see* Conflagration
conflagration — *see* Conflagration
corrosive liquid, substance E924.1
swallowed — *see* Table of Drugs and Chemicals
electric current (*see also* Electric shock) E925.9
fire, flames (*see also* Fire) E899
flare, Verey pistol E922.8
heat
from appliance (electrical) E924.8
in local application, or packing during medical or surgical procedure E873.5
homicide (attempt) (*see also* Assault, burning) E968.0
hot
liquid E924.0
caustic or corrosive E924.1
object (not producing fire or flames) E924.8
substance E924.9
caustic or corrosive E924.1
liquid (metal) NEC E924.0
specified type NEC E924.8
tap water E924.2
ignition (*see also* Ignition)
clothes, clothing, nightdress (*see also* Ignition, clothes)
with conflagration — *see* Conflagration
highly inflammable material (benzine) (fat) (gasoline) (kerosene) (paraffin) (petrol) E894
in
terrorism E979.3
from nuclear explosion E979.5
petrol bomb E979.3
war operations (from fire-producing device or conventional weapon) E990.9
from nuclear explosion E996
petrol bomb E990.0
inflicted by other person
stated as
homicidal, intentional (*see also* Assault, burning) E968.0
undetermined whether accidental or intentional (*see also* Burn, stated as undetermined whether accidental or intentional) E988.1
internal, from swallowed caustic, corrosive liquid, substance — *see* Table of Drugs and Chemicals
lamp (*see also* Fire, specified NEC) E898.1

**Burning, burns** — *continued*
late effect of NEC E929.4
lighter (cigar) (cigarette) (*see also* Fire, specified NEC) E898.1
lightning E907
liquid (boiling) (hot) (molten) E924.0
caustic, corrosive (external) E924.1
swallowed — *see* Table of Drugs and Chemicals
local application of externally applied substance in medical or surgical care E873.5
machinery — *see* Accident, machine
matches (*see also* Fire, specified NEC) E898.1
medicament, externally applied E873.5
metal, molten E924.0
object (hot) E924.8
producing fire or flames — *see* Fire
oven (electric) (gas) E924.8
pipe (smoking) (*see also* Fire, specified NEC) E898.1
radiation — *see* Radiation
railway engine, locomotive, train (*see also* Explosion, railway engine) E803 ☑
self-inflicted (unspecified whether accidental or intentional) E988.1
caustic or corrosive substance NEC E988.7
stated as intentional, purposeful E958.1
caustic or corrosive substance NEC E958.7
stated as undetermined whether accidental or intentional E988.1
caustic or corrosive substance NEC E988.7
steam E924.0
pipe E924.8
substance (hot) E924.9
boiling or molten E924.0
caustic, corrosive (external) E924.1
swallowed — *see* Table of Drugs and Chemicals
suicidal (attempt) NEC E958.1
caustic substance E958.7
late effect of E959
tanning bed E926.2
therapeutic misadventure
overdose of radiation E873.2
torch, welding (*see also* Fire, specified NEC) E898.1
trash fire (*see also* Burning, bonfire) E897
vapor E924.0
vitriol E924.1
x-rays E926.3
in medical, surgical procedure — *see* Misadventure, failure, in dosage, radiation
**Butted by animal** E906.8

## C

**Cachexia, lead or saturnine** E866.0
from pesticide NEC (*see also* Table of Drugs and Chemicals) E863.4
**Caisson disease** E902.2
**Capital punishment** (any means) E978
**Car sickness** E903
**Casualty** (not due to war) NEC E928.9
terrorism E979.8
war (*see also* War operations) E995
**Cat**
bite E906.3
scratch E906.8
**Cataclysmic** (any injury)
earth surface movement or eruption E909.9
specified type NEC E909.8
storm or flood resulting from storm E908.9
specified type NEC E909.8
**Catching fire** — *see* Ignition

---

☑ Additional Digit Required — Refer to the Tabular List for Digit Selection          ⁀ Subterms under main terms may continue to next column or page

340 — Volume 2               ▶◀ Revised Text          ● New Line     ▲ Revised Code                      *2008 ICD-9-CM*

## Caught

between
  objects (moving) (stationary and
    moving) E918
    and machinery — *see* Accident,
      machine
by cable car, not on rails E847
in
  machinery (moving parts of) — *see*,
    Accident, machine
  object E918

**Cave-in** (causing asphyxia, suffocation
  (by pressure)) — *see also* Suffocation, due to, cave-in E913.3
  with injury other than asphyxia or
    suffocation E916
    with asphyxia or suffocation (*see
      also* Suffocation, due to,
      cave-in) E913.3
  struck or crushed by E916
    with asphyxia or suffocation (*see
      also* Suffocation, due to,
      cave-in) E913.3

**Change(s) in air pressure —** *see also*
  Effects of, air pressure
  sudden, in aircraft (ascent) (descent)
    (causing aeroneurosis or avia-
    tors' disease) E902.1

**Chilblains** E901.0
  due to manmade conditions E901.1

**Choking** (on) (any object except food or
  vomitus) E912
  apple E911
  bone E911
  food, any type (regurgitated) E911
  mucus or phlegm E912
  seed E911

**Civil insurrection —** *see* War operations

**Cloudburst** E908.8

**Cold, exposure to** (accidental) (excessive)
  (extreme) (place) E901.9
  causing chilblains or immersion foot
    E901.0
  due to
    manmade conditions E901.1
    specified cause NEC E901.8
    weather (conditions) E901.0
  late effect of NEC E929.5
  self-inflicted (undetermined whether
    accidental or intentional)
    E988.3
    suicidal E958.3
  suicide E958.3

**Colic, lead, painter's, or saturnine —**
  *see* category E866 ☑

**Collapse**
  building E916
    burning (uncontrolled fire) E891.8
      in terrorism E979.3
      private E890.8
  dam E909.3
  due to heat — *see* Heat
  machinery — *see* Accident, machine
    or vehicle
  man-made structure E909.3
  postoperative NEC E878.9
  structure
    burning (uncontrolled fire) NEC
      E891.8
      in terrorism E979.3

## Collision (accidental)

*Note — In the case of collisions between
different types of vehicles, persons and
objects, priority in classification is in the
following order:*

> *Aircraft*
>
> *Watercraft*
>
> *Motor vehicle*
>
> *Railway vehicle*
>
> *Pedal cycle*
>
> *Animal-drawn vehicle*
>
> *Animal being ridden*
>
> *Streetcar or other nonmotor road
> vehicle*
>
> *Other vehicle*
>
> *Pedestrian or person using
> pedestrian conveyance*
>
> *Object (except where falling from
> or set in motion by vehicle etc.
> listed above)*

*In the listing below, the combinations
are listed only under the vehicle etc.
having priority. For definitions, see
Supplementary Classification of External Causes of Injury and Poisoning
(E800–E999).*

aircraft (with object or vehicle) (fixed)
  (movable) (moving) E841 ☑
  with
    person (while landing, taking
      off) (without accident to
      aircraft) E844 ☑
    powered (in transit) (with unpow-
      ered aircraft) E841 ☑
      while landing, taking off E840 ☑
    unpowered E842 ☑
    while landing, taking off E840 ☑
animal being ridden (in sport or
  transport) E828 ☑
  and
    animal (being ridden) (herded)
      (unattended) E828 ☑
    nonmotor road vehicle, except
      pedal cycle or animal-
      drawn vehicle E828 ☑
    object (fallen) (fixed) (movable)
      (moving) not falling from
      or set in motion by vehicle
      of higher priority E828 ☑
    pedestrian (conveyance or vehi-
      cle) E828 ☑
animal-drawn vehicle E827 ☑
  and
    animal (being ridden) (herded)
      (unattended) E827 ☑
    nonmotor road vehicle, except
      pedal cycle E827 ☑
    object (fallen) (fixed) (movable)
      (moving) not falling from
      or set in motion by vehicle
      of higher priority E827 ☑
    pedestrian (conveyance or vehi-
      cle) E827 ☑
    streetcar E827 ☑
motor vehicle (on public highway)
  (traffic accident) E812 ☑
  after leaving, running off, public
    highway (without antecedent
    collision) (without re-entry)
    E816 ☑
    with antecedent collision on
      public highway — *see*
      categories E810–E815 ☑
    with re-entrance collision with
      another motor vehicle
      E811 ☑
  and
    abutment (bridge) (overpass)
      E815 ☑

## Collision — *continued*

motor vehicle — *continued*
  and — *continued*
    animal (herded) (unattended)
      E815 ☑
    carrying person, property
      E813 ☑
    animal-drawn vehicle E813 ☑
    another motor vehicle (aban-
      doned) (disabled) (parked)
      (stalled) (stopped) E812 ☑
    with, involving re-entrance
      (on same roadway)
      (across median strip)
      E811 ☑
    any object, person, or vehicle off
      the public highway result-
      ing from a noncollision
      motor vehicle nontraffic
      accident E816 ☑
    avalanche, fallen or not moving
      E815 ☑
      falling E909.2
    boundary fence E815 ☑
    culvert E815 ☑
    fallen
      stone E815 ☑
      tree E815 ☑
    guard post or guard rail E815 ☑
    inter-highway divider E815 ☑
    landslide, fallen or not moving
      E815 ☑
      moving E909 ☑
    machinery (road) E815 ☑
    nonmotor road vehicle NEC
      E813 ☑
    object (any object, person, or
      vehicle off the public
      highway resulting from a
      noncollision motor vehicle
      nontraffic accident)
      E815 ☑
    off, normally not on, public
      highway resulting from
      a noncollision motor
      vehicle traffic accident
      E816 ☑
    pedal cycle E813 ☑
    pedestrian (conveyance) E814 ☑
    person (using pedestrian con-
      veyance) E814 ☑
    post or pole (lamp) (light) (signal)
      (telephone) (utility)
      E815 ☑
    railway rolling stock, train, vehi-
      cle E810 ☑
    safety island E815 ☑
    street car E813 ☑
    traffic signal, sign, or marker
      (temporary) E815 ☑
    tree E815 ☑
    tricycle E813 ☑
    wall of cut made for road
      E815 ☑
  due to cataclysm — *see* categories
    E908 ☑, E909 ☑
  not on public highway, nontraffic
    accident E822 ☑
    and
      animal (carrying person,
        property) (herded)
        (unattended) E822 ☑
      animal-drawn vehicle
        E822 ☑
      another motor vehicle (mov-
        ing), except off-road
        motor vehicle E822 ☑
        stationary E823 ☑
      avalanche, fallen, not moving
        E823 ☑
        moving E909.2
      landslide, fallen, not moving
        E823 ☑
        moving E909.2

## Collision — *continued*

motor vehicle — *continued*
  not on public highway, nontraffic
    accident — *continued*
    and — *continued*
      nonmotor vehicle (moving)
        E822 ☑
        stationary E823 ☑
      object (fallen) (normally)
        (fixed) (movable but not
        in motion) (stationary)
        E823 ☑
        moving, except when
          falling from, set in
          motion by, aircraft
          or cataclysm
          E822 ☑
      pedal cycle (moving) E822 ☑
        stationary E823 ☑
      pedestrian (conveyance)
        E822 ☑
      person (using pedestrian
        conveyance) E822 ☑
      railway rolling stock, train,
        vehicle (moving)
        E822 ☑
        stationary E823 ☑
      road vehicle (any) (moving)
        E822 ☑
        stationary E823 ☑
      tricycle (moving) E822 ☑
        stationary E823 ☑
    off-road type motor vehicle (not on
      public highway) E821 ☑
    and
      animal (being ridden) (-drawn
        vehicle) E821 ☑
      another off-road motor vehicle,
        except snow vehicle
        E821 ☑
      other motor vehicle, not on
        public highway E821 ☑
      other object or vehicle NEC,
        fixed or movable, not set
        in motion by aircraft, mo-
        tor vehicle on highway, or
        snow vehicle, motor driv-
        en E821 ☑
      pedal cycle E821 ☑
      pedestrian (conveyance) E821 ☑
      railway train E821 ☑
    on public highway — *see* Collision,
      motor vehicle
pedal cycle E826 ☑
  and
    animal (carrying person, proper-
      ty) (herded) (unherded)
      E826 ☑
    animal-drawn vehicle E826 ☑
    another pedal cycle E826 ☑
    nonmotor road vehicle E826 ☑
    object (fallen) (fixed) (movable)
      (moving) not falling from
      or set in motion by air-
      craft, motor vehicle, or
      railway train NEC E826 ☑
    pedestrian (conveyance) E826 ☑
    person (using pedestrian con-
      veyance) E826 ☑
    street car E826 ☑
pedestrian(s) (conveyance) E917.9
  with fall E886.9
    in sports E886.0
  and
    crowd, human stampede E917.1
      with subsequent fall E917.6
    furniture E917.3
      with subsequent fall E917.7
    machinery — *see* Accident, ma-
      chine
    object (fallen) (moving) not
      falling from NEC, fixed or
      set in motion by any vehi-
      cle classifiable to
      E800–E848 ☑, E917.9

**Collision** — *continued*

pedestrian(s) — *continued*

and — *continued*

object not falling from, fixed or set in motion by any vehicle classifiable to — *continued*

with subsequent fall E917.6

caused by a crowd E917.1

with subsequent fall E917.6

furniture E917.3

with subsequent fall E917.7

in

running water E917.2

with drowning or submersion — *see* Submersion

sports E917.0

with subsequent fall E917.5

stationary E917.4

with subsequent fall E917.8

vehicle, nonmotor, nonroad E848

in

running water E917.2

with drowning or submersion — *see* Submersion

sports E917.0

with fall E886.0

person(s) (using pedestrian conveyance) (*see also* Collision, pedestrian) E917.9

railway (rolling stock) (train) (vehicle) (with (subsequent) derailment, explosion, fall or fire) E800 ☑

with antecedent derailment E802 ☑

and

animal (carrying person) (herded) (unattended) E801 ☑

another railway train or vehicle E800 ☑

buffers E801 ☑

fallen tree on railway E801 ☑

farm machinery, nonmotor (in transport) (stationary) E801 ☑

gates E801 ☑

nonmotor vehicle E801 ☑

object (fallen) (fixed) (movable) (moving) not falling from, set in motion by, aircraft or motor vehicle NEC E801 ☑

pedal cycle E801 ☑

pedestrian (conveyance) E805 ☑

person (using pedestrian conveyance) E805 ☑

platform E801 ☑

rock on railway E801 ☑

street car E801 ☑

snow vehicle, motor-driven (not on public highway) E820 ☑

and

animal (being ridden) (-drawn vehicle) E820 ☑

another off-road motor vehicle E820 ☑

other motor vehicle, not on public highway E820 ☑

other object or vehicle NEC, fixed or movable, not set in motion by aircraft or motor vehicle on highway E820 ☑

pedal cycle E820 ☑

pedestrian (conveyance) E820 ☑

railway train E820 ☑

on public highway — *see* Collision, motor vehicle

street car(s) E829 ☑

**Collision** — *continued*

street car(s) — *continued*

and

animal, herded, not being ridden, unattended E829 ☑

nonmotor road vehicle NEC E829 ☑

object (fallen) (fixed) (movable) (moving) not falling from or set in motion by aircraft, animal-drawn vehicle, animal being ridden, motor vehicle, pedal cycle, or railway train E829 ☑

pedestrian (conveyance) E829 ☑

person (using pedestrian conveyance) E829 ☑

vehicle

animal-drawn — *see* Collision, animal-drawn vehicle

motor — *see* Collision, motor vehicle

nonmotor

nonroad E848

and

another nonmotor, nonroad vehicle E848

object (fallen) (fixed) (movable) (moving) not falling from or set in motion by aircraft, animal-drawn vehicle, animal being ridden, motor vehicle, pedal cycle, railway train, or streetcar E848

road, except animal being ridden, animal-drawn vehicle, or pedal cycle E829 ☑

and

animal, herded, not being ridden, unattended E829 ☑

another nonmotor road vehicle, except animal being ridden, animal-drawn vehicle, or pedal cycle E829 ☑

object (fallen) (fixed) (movable) (moving) not falling from or set in motion by, aircraft, animal-drawn vehicle, animal being ridden, motor vehicle, pedal cycle, or railway train E829 ☑

pedestrian (conveyance) E829 ☑

person (using pedestrian conveyance) E829 ☑

vehicle, nonmotor, nonroad E829 ☑

watercraft E838 ☑

and

person swimming or water skiing E838 ☑

causing

drowning, submersion E830 ☑

injury except drowning, submersion E831 ☑

**Combustion, spontaneous** — *see* Ignition

**Complication of medical or surgical procedure or treatment**

as an abnormal reaction — *see* Reaction, abnormal

delayed, without mention of misadventure — *see* Reaction, abnormal

due to misadventure — *see* Misadventure

**Compression**

divers' squeeze E902.2

trachea by

food E911

foreign body, except food E912

**Conflagration**

building or structure, except private dwelling (barn) (church) (convalescent or residential home) (factory) (farm outbuilding) (hospital) (hotel) (institution) (educational) (domitory) (residential) (school) (shop) (store) (theater) E891.9

with or causing (injury due to)

accident or injury NEC E891.9

specified circumstance NEC E891.8

burns, burning E891.3

carbon monoxide E891.2

fumes E891.2

polyvinylchloride (PVC) or similar material E891.1

smoke E891.2

causing explosion E891.0

in terrorism E979.3

not in building or structure E892

private dwelling (apartment) (boarding house) (camping place) (caravan) (farmhouse) (home (private)) (house) (lodging house) (private garage) (rooming house) (tenement) E890.9

with or causing (injury due to)

accident or injury NEC E890.9

specified circumstance NEC E890.8

burns, burning E890.3

carbon monoxide E890.2

fumes E890.2

polyvinylchloride (PVC) or similar material E890.1

smoke E890.2

causing explosion E890.0

**Constriction, external**

caused by

hair E928.4

other object E928.5

**Contact with**

dry ice E901.1

liquid air, hydrogen, nitrogen E901.1

**Cramp(s)**

Heat — *see* Heat

swimmers (*see also* category E910 ) E910.2

not in recreation or sport E910.3

**Cranking** (car) (truck) (bus) (engine), injury by E917.9

**Crash**

aircraft (in transit) (powered) E841 ☑

at landing, take-off E840 ☑

in

terrorism E979.1

war operations E994

on runway NEC E840 ☑

stated as

homicidal E968.8

suicidal E958.6

undetermined whether accidental or intentional E988.6

unpowered E842 ☑

glider E842 ☑

motor vehicle (*see also* Accident, motor vehicle)

homicidal E968.5

suicidal E958.5

undetermined whether accidental or intentional E988.5

**Crushed** (accidentally) E928.9

between

boat(s), ship(s), watercraft (and dock or pier) (without accident to watercraft) E838 ☑

**Crushed** — *continued*

between — *continued*

boat(s), ship(s), watercraft — *continued*

after accident to, or collision, watercraft E831 ☑

objects (moving) (stationary and moving) E918

by

avalanche NEC E909.2

boat, ship, watercraft after accident to, collision, watercraft E831 ☑

cave-in E916

with asphyxiation or suffocation (*see also* Suffocation, due to, cave-in) E913.3

crowd, human stampede E917.1

falling

aircraft (*see also* Accident, aircraft) E841 ☑

in

terrorism E979.1

war operations E994

earth, material E916

with asphyxiation or suffocation (*see also* Suffocation, due to, cave-in) E913.3

object E916

on ship, watercraft E838 ☑

while loading, unloading watercraft E838 ☑

landslide NEC E909.2

lifeboat after abandoning ship E831 ☑

machinery — *see* Accident, machine

railway rolling stock, train, vehicle (part of) E805 ☑

street car E829 ☑

vehicle NEC — *see* Accident, vehicle NEC

in

machinery — *see* Accident, machine

object E918

transport accident — *see* categories E800-E848 ☑

late effect of NEC E929.9

**Cut, cutting** (any part of body) (accidental) E920.9

by

arrow E920.8

axe E920.4

bayonet (*see also* Bayonet wound) E920.3

blender E920.2

broken glass E920.8

following fall E888.0

can opener E920.4

powered E920.2

chisel E920.4

circular saw E919.4

cutting or piercing instrument (*see also* category) E920 ☑

following fall E888.0

late effect of E929.8

dagger E920.3

dart E920.8

drill — *see* Accident, caused by drill

edge of stiff paper E920.8

electric

beater E920.2

fan E920.2

knife E920.2

mixer E920.2

fork E920.4

garden fork E920.4

hand saw or tool (not powered) E920.4

powered E920.1

hedge clipper E920.4

powered E920.1

hoe E920.4

**Cut, cutting** — *continued*
  by — *continued*
    ice pick E920.4
    knife E920.3
      electric E920.2
    lathe turnings E920.8
    lawn mower E920.4
      powered E920.0
      riding E919.8
    machine — *see* Accident, machine
    meat
      grinder E919.8
      slicer E919.8
    nails E920.8
    needle E920.4
      hypodermic E920.5
    object, edged, pointed, sharp — *see*
      category E920 ☑
    following fall E888.0
    paper cutter E920.4
    piercing instrument (*see also* category) E920 ☑
      late effect of E929.8
    pitchfork E920.4
    powered
      can opener E920.2
      garden cultivator E920.1
        riding E919.8
      hand saw E920.1
      hand tool NEC E920.1
      hedge clipper E920.1
      household appliance or implement E920.2
      lawn mower (hand) E920.0
        riding E919.8
      rivet gun E920.1
      staple gun E920.1
    rake E920.4
    saw
      circular E919.4
      hand E920.4
    scissors E920.4
    screwdriver E920.4
    sewing machine (electric) (powered) E920.2
      not powered E920.4
    shears E920.4
    shovel E920.4
    spade E920.4
    splinters E920.8
    sword E920.3
    tin can lid E920.8
    wood slivers E920.8
  homicide (attempt) E966
  inflicted by other person
    stated as
      intentional, homicidal E966
      undetermined whether accidental or intentional E986
  late effect of NEC E929.8
  legal
    execution E978
    intervention E974
  self-inflicted (unspecified whether accidental or intentional) E986
    stated as intentional, purposeful E956
  stated as undetermined whether accidental or intentional E986
  suicidal (attempt) E956
  terrorism E979.8
  war operations E995
**Cyclone** E908.1

### D

**Death due to injury occurring one year or more previous** — *see* Late effect
**Decapitation** (accidental circumstances) NEC E928.9
  homicidal E966
  legal execution (by guillotine) E978
**Deprivation** — *see also* Privation
  homicidal intent E968.4

**Derailment** (accidental)
  railway (rolling stock) (train) (vehicle) (with subsequent collision) E802 ☑
    with
      collision (antecedent) (*see also* Collision, railway) E800 ☑
      explosion (subsequent) (without antecedent collision) E802 ☑
        antecedent collision E803 ☑
      fall (without collision (antecedent)) E802 ☑
      fire (without collision (antecedent)) E802 ☑
    street car E829 ☑
**Descent**
  parachute (voluntary) (without accident to aircraft) E844 ☑
    due to accident to aircraft — *see* categories E840-E842 ☑
**Desertion**
  child, with intent to injure or kill E968.4
  helpless person, infant, newborn E904.0
    with intent to injure or kill E968.4
**Destitution** — *see* Privation
**Disability, late effect or sequela of injury** — *see* Late effect
**Disease**
  Andes E902.0
  aviators' E902.1
  caisson E902.2
  range E902.0
**Divers' disease, palsy, paralysis, squeeze** E902.0
**Dog bite** E906.0
**Dragged by**
  cable car (not on rails) E847
    on rails E829 ☑
  motor vehicle (on highway) E814 ☑
    not on highway, nontraffic accident E825 ☑
  street car E829 ☑
**Drinking poison** (accidental) — *see* Table of Drugs and Chemicals
**Drowning** — *see* Submersion
**Dust in eye** E914

### E

**Earth falling** (on) (with asphyxia or suffocation (by pressure)) — *see also* Suffocation, due to, cave-in E913.3
  as, or due to, a cataclysm (involving any transport vehicle) — *see* categories E908 ☑, E909
  not due to cataclysmic action E913.3
    motor vehicle (in motion) (on public highway) E813 ☑
      not on public highway E825 ☑
    nonmotor road vehicle NEC E829 ☑
    pedal cycle E826 ☑
    railway rolling stock, train, vehicle E806 ☑
    street car E829 ☑
  struck or crushed by E916
    with asphyxiation or suffocation E913.3
    with injury other than asphyxia, suffocation E916
**Earthquake** (any injury) E909.0
**Effect(s) (adverse) of**
  air pressure E902.9
    at high altitude E902.9
      in aircraft E902.1
    residence or prolonged visit (causing conditions classifiable to E902.0) E902.0
    due to
      diving E902.2
      specified cause NEC E902.8
    in aircraft E902.1

**Effect(s) (adverse) of** — *continued*
  cold, excessive (exposure to) (*see also* Cold, exposure to) E901.9
  heat (excessive) (*see also* Heat) E900.9
  hot
    place — *see* Heat
    weather E900.0
  insulation — *see* Heat
  late — *see* Late effect of
  motion E903
  nuclear explosion or weapon
    in
      terrorism E979.5
      war operations (blast) (fireball) (heat) (radiation) (direct) (secondary) E996
  radiation — *see* Radiation
  terrorism, secondary E979.9
  travel E903
**Electric shock, electrocution** (accidental) (from exposed wire, faulty appliance, high voltage cable, live rail, open socket) (by) (in) E925.9
  appliance or wiring
    domestic E925.0
    factory E925.2
    farm (building) E925.8
    house E925.0
    home E925.0
    industrial (conductor) (control apparatus) (transformer) E925.2
    outdoors E925.8
    public building E925.8
    residential institution E925.8
    school E925.8
    specified place NEC E925.8
  caused by other person
    stated as
      intentional, homicidal E968.8
      undetermined whether accidental or intentional E988.4
  electric power generating plant, distribution station E925.1
  homicidal (attempt) E968.8
  legal execution E978
  lightning E907
  machinery E925.9
    domestic E925.0
    factory E925.2
    farm E925.8
    home E925.0
  misadventure in medical or surgical procedure
    in electroshock therapy E873.4
  self-inflicted (undetermined whether accidental or intentional) E988.4
    stated as intentional E958.4
  stated as undetermined whether accidental or intentional E988.4
  suicidal (attempt) E958.4
  transmission line E925.1
**Electrocution** — *see* Electric shock
**Embolism**
  air (traumatic) NEC — *see* Air, embolism
**Encephalitis**
  lead or saturnine E866.0
    from pesticide NEC E863.4
**Entanglement**
  in
    bedclothes, causing suffocation E913.0
    wheel of pedal cycle E826 ☑
**Entry of foreign body, material, any** — *see* Foreign body
**Execution, legal** (any method) E978
**Exhaustion**
  cold — *see* Cold, exposure to
  due to excessive exertion E927
  heat — *see* Heat
**Explosion** (accidental) (in) (of) (on) E923.9
  acetylene E923.2
  aerosol can E921.8

**Explosion** — *continued*
  aircraft (in transit) (powered) E841 ☑
    at landing, take-off E840 ☑
    in
      terrorism E979.1
      war operations E994
    unpowered E842 ☑
  air tank (compressed) (in machinery) E921.1
  anesthetic gas in operating theatre E923.2
  automobile tire NEC E921.8
    causing transport accident — *see* categories E810-E825 ☑
  blasting (cap) (materials) E923.1
  boiler (machinery), not on transport vehicle E921.0
    steamship — *see* Explosion, watercraft
  bomb E923.8
    in
      terrorism E979.2
      war operations E993
        after cessation of hostilities E998
        atom, hydrogen or nuclear E996
        injury by fragments from E991.9
          antipersonnel bomb E991.3
  butane E923.2
  caused by
    other person
      stated as
        intentional, homicidal — *see* Assault, explosive
        undetermined whether accidental or homicidal E985.5
  coal gas E923.2
  detonator E923.1
  dynamite E923.1
  explosive (material) NEC E923.9
    gas(es) E923.2
    missile E923.8
      in
        terrorism E979.2
        war operations E993
          injury by fragments from E991.9
            antipersonnel bomb E991.3
    used in blasting operations E923.1
  fire-damp E923.2
  fireworks E923.0
  gas E923.2
    cylinder (in machinery) E921.1
    pressure tank (in machinery) E921.1
  gasoline (fumes) (tank) not in moving motor vehicle E923.2
  grain store (military) (munitions) E923.8
  grenade E923.8
    in
      terrorism E979.2
      war operations E993
        injury by fragments from E991.9
  homicide (attempt) — *see* Assault, explosive
  hot water heater, tank (in machinery) E921.0
  in mine (of explosive gases) NEC E923.2
  late effect of NEC E929.8
  machinery (*see also* Accident, machine)
    pressure vessel — *see* Explosion, pressure vessel
  methane E923.2
  missile E923.8
    in
      terrorism E979.2
      war operations E993

---

☑ Additional Digit Required — Refer to the Tabular List for Digit Selection

⌐⌐ Subterms under main terms may continue to next column or page

**Explosion** — *continued*
missile — *continued*
in — *continued*
war operations — *continued*
injury by fragments from E991.9
motor vehicle (part of)
in motion (on public highway) E818 ✓
not on public highway E825 ✓
munitions (dump) (factory) E923.8
in
terrorism E979.2
war operations E993
of mine E923.8
in
terrorism
at sea or in harbor E979.0
land E979.2
marine E979.0
war operations
after cessation of hostilities E998
at sea or in harbor E992
land E993
after cessation of hostilities E998
injury by fragments from E991.9
marine E992
own weapons
in
terrorism (*see also* Suicide) E979.2
war operations E993
injury by fragments from E991.9
antipersonnel bomb E991.3
pressure
cooker E921.8
gas tank (in machinery) E921.1
vessel (in machinery) E921.9
on transport vehicle — *see* categories E800-E848 ✓
specified type NEC E921.8
propane E923.2
railway engine, locomotive, train (boiler) (with subsequent collision, derailment, fall) E803 ✓
with
collision (antecedent) (*see also* Collision, railway) E800 ✓
derailment (antecedent) E802 ✓
fire (without antecedent collision or derailment) E803 ✓
secondary fire resulting from — *see* Fire
self-inflicted (unspecified whether accidental or intentional) E985.5
stated as intentional, purposeful E955.5
shell (artillery) E923.8
in
terrorism E979.2
war operations E993
injury by fragments from E991.9
stated as undetermined whether caused accidentally or purposely inflicted E985.5
steam or water lines (in machinery) E921.0
suicide (attempted) E955.5
terrorism — *see* Terrorism, explosion
torpedo E923.8
in
terrorism E979.0
war operations E992
transport accident — *see* categories E800-E848 ✓
war operations — *see* War operations, explosion
watercraft (boiler) E837 ✓

**Explosion** — *continued*
watercraft — *continued*
causing drowning, submersion (after jumping from watercraft) E830 ✓
**Exposure** (weather) (conditions) (rain) (wind) E904.3
with homicidal intent E968.4
environmental ●
to ●
algae bloom E928.6 ●
blue-green algae bloom E928.6 ●
brown tide E928.6 ●
cyanobacteria bloom E928.6 ●
Florida red tide E928.6 ●
harmful alage ●
and toxins E928.6 ●
bloom E928.6 ●
pfisteria piscicida E928.6 ●
red tide E928.6 ●
excessive E904.3
cold (*see also* Cold, exposure to) E901.9
self-inflicted — *see* Cold, exposure to, self-inflicted
heat (*see also* Heat) E900.9
helpless person, infant, newborn due to abandonment or neglect E904.0
noise E928.1
prolonged in deep-freeze unit or refrigerator E901.1
radiation — *see* Radiation
resulting from transport accident — *see* categories E800-E848 ✓
smoke from, due to
fire — *see* Fire
tobacco, second-hand E869.4
vibration E928.2

## F

**Fallen on by**
animal (horse) (not being ridden) E906.8
being ridden (in sport or transport) E828 ✓
**Fall, falling** (accidental) E888.9
building E916
burning E891.8
private E890.8
down
escalator E880.0
ladder E881.0
in boat, ship, watercraft E833 ✓
staircase E880.9
stairs, steps — *see* Fall, from, stairs
earth (with asphyxia or suffocation (by pressure)) (*see also* Earth, falling) E913.3
from, off
aircraft (at landing, take-off) (in-transit) (while alighting, boarding) E843 ✓
resulting from accident to aircraft — *see* categories E840-E842 ✓
animal (in sport or transport) E828 ✓
animal-drawn vehicle E827 ✓
balcony E882
bed E884.4
bicycle E826 ✓
boat, ship, watercraft (into water) E832 ✓
after accident to, collision, fire on E830 ✓
and subsequently struck by (part of) boat E831 ✓
and subsequently struck by (part of) while alighting, boat E831 ✓
burning, crushed, sinking E830 ✓

**Fall, falling** — *continued*
from, off — *continued*
boat, ship, watercraft — *continued*
burning, crushed, sinking — *continued*
and subsequently struck by (part of) boat E831 ✓
bridge E882
building E882
burning (uncontrolled fire) E891.8
in terrorism E979.3
private E890.8
bunk in boat, ship, watercraft E834 ✓
due to accident to watercraft E831 ✓
cable car (not on rails) E847
on rails E829 ✓
car — *see* Fall from motor vehicle
chair E884.2
cliff E884.1
commode E884.6
curb (sidewalk) E880.1
elevation aboard ship E834 ✓
due to accident to ship E831 ✓
embankment E884.9
escalator E880.0
fire escape E882
flagpole E882
furniture NEC E884.5
gangplank (into water) (*see also* Fall, from, boat) E832 ✓
to deck, dock E834 ✓
hammock on ship E834 ✓
due to accident to watercraft E831 ✓
haystack E884.9
high place NEC E884.9
stated as undetermined whether accidental or intentional — *see* Jumping, from, high place
horse (in sport or transport) E828 ✓
in-line skates E885.1
ladder E881.0
in boat, ship, watercraft E833 ✓
due to accident to watercraft E831 ✓
machinery (*see also* Accident, machine)
not in operation E884.9
motor vehicle (in motion) (on public highway) E818 ✓
not on public highway E825 ✓
stationary, except while alighting, boarding, entering, leaving E884.9
while alighting, boarding, entering, leaving E824 ✓
stationary, except while alighting, boarding, entering, leaving E884.9
while alighting, boarding, entering, leaving, except off-road type motor vehicle E817 ✓
off-road type — *see* Fall, from, off-road type motor vehicle
nonmotor road vehicle (while alighting, boarding) NEC E829 ✓
stationary, except while alighting, boarding, entering, leaving E884.9
off road type motor vehicle (not on public highway) NEC E821 ✓
on public highway E818 ✓
while alighting, boarding, entering, leaving E817 ✓

**Fall, falling** — *continued*
from, off — *continued*
off road type motor vehicle — *continued*
snow vehicle — *see* Fall from snow vehicle, motor-driven
one
deck to another on ship E834 ✓
due to accident to ship E831 ✓
level to another NEC E884.9
boat, ship, or watercraft E834 ✓
due to accident to watercraft E831 ✓
pedal cycle E826 ✓
playground equipment E884.0
railway rolling stock, train, vehicle (while alighting, boarding) E804 ✓
with
collision (*see also* Collision, railway) E800 ✓
derailment (*see also* Derailment, railway) E802 ✓
explosion (*see also* Explosion, railway engine) E803 ✓
rigging (aboard ship) E834 ✓
due to accident to watercraft E831 ✓
roller skates E885.1
scaffolding E881.1
scooter (nonmotorized) E885.0
sidewalk (curb) E880.1
moving E885.9
skateboard E885.2
skis E885.3
snowboard E885.4
snow vehicle, motor-driven (not on public highway) E820 ✓
on public highway E818 ✓
while alighting, boarding, entering, leaving E817 ✓
stairs, steps E880.9
boat, ship, watercraft E833 ✓
due to accident to watercraft E831 ✓
motor bus, motor vehicle — *see* Fall, from, motor vehicle, while alighting, boarding
street car E829 ✓
stationary vehicle NEC E884.9
stepladder E881.0
street car (while boarding, alighting) E829 ✓
stationary, except while boarding or alighting E884.9
structure NEC E882
burning (uncontrolled fire) E891.8
in terrorism E979.3
table E884.9
toilet E884.6
tower E882
tree E884.9
turret E882
vehicle NEC (*see also* Accident, vehicle NEC)
stationary E884.9
viaduct E882
wall E882
wheelchair E884.3
window E882
in, on
aircraft (at landing, take-off) (in-transit) E843 ✓
resulting from accident to aircraft — *see* categories E840-E842 ✓
boat, ship, watercraft E835 ✓
due to accident to watercraft E831 ✓

✓ Additional Digit Required — Refer to the Tabular List for Digit Selection    Subterms under main terms may continue to next column or page

344 — Volume 2 · October 2007    ▶◀ Revised Text    ● New Line    ▲ Revised Code    *2008 ICD-9-CM*

☑ Additional Digit Required — Refer to the Tabular List for Digit Selection    ▽ Subterms under main terms may continue to next column or page

**2008 ICD-9-CM**    ▶◀ Revised Text    ● New Line    ▲ Revised Code    **Volume 2 — 345**

**Foreign body, object or material —**
*continued*
   larynx — *see* Foreign body, air pas-
      sage
   late effect of NEC E929.8
   lung — *see* Foreign body, air passage
   mouth — *see* Foreign body, alimentary
      canal, mouth
   nasal passage — *see* Foreign body, air
      passage, nose
   nose — *see* Foreign body, air passage,
      nose
   ocular muscle E914
   operation wound (left in) — *see* Misad-
      venture, foreign object
   orbit E914
   pharynx — *see* Foreign body, alimen-
      tary canal, pharynx
   rectum (causing injury or obstruction)
      E915
   stomach (hairball) (causing injury or
      obstruction) E915
   tear ducts or glands E914
   trachea — *see* Foreign body, air pas-
      sage
   urethra (causing injury or obstruction)
      E915
   vagina (causing injury or obstruction)
      E915
**Found dead, injured**
   from exposure (to) — *see* Exposure
   on
      public highway E819 ☑
      railway right of way E807 ☑
**Fracture** (circumstances unknown or
      unspecified) E887
   due to specified external means — *see*
      manner of accident
   late effect of NEC E929.3
   occurring in water transport NEC
      E835 ☑
**Freezing** — *see* Cold, exposure to
**Frostbite** E901.0
   due to manmade conditions E901.1
**Frozen** — *see* Cold, exposure to

**G**

**Garrotting, homicidal** (attempted) E963
**Gored** E906.8
**Gunshot wound** — *see also* Shooting
   E922.9

**H**

**Hailstones, injury by** E904.3
**Hairball** (stomach) (with obstruction)
   E915
**Hanged himself** — *see also* Hanging,
   self-inflicted E983.0
**Hang gliding** E842 ☑
**Hanging** (accidental) E913.8
   caused by other person
      in accidental circumstances
         E913.8
      stated as
         intentional, homicidal E963
         undetermined whether acciden-
            tal or intentional E983.0
   homicide (attempt) E963
   in bed or cradle E913.0
   legal execution E978
   self-inflicted (unspecified whether ac-
      cidental or intentional) E983.0
      in accidental circumstances
         E913.8
      stated as intentional, purposeful
         E953.0
   stated as undetermined whether acci-
      dental or intentional E983.0
   suicidal (attempt) E953.0
**Heat** (apoplexy) (collapse) (cramps) (ef-
      fects of) (excessive) (exhaustion)
      (fever) (prostration) (stroke) E900.9

**Heat** — *continued*
   due to
      manmade conditions (as listed in
         E900.1, except boat, ship,
         watercraft) E900.1
      weather (conditions) E900.0
   from
      electric heating appartus causing
         burning E924.8
      nuclear explosion
         in
            terrorism E979.5
            war operations E996
   generated in, boiler, engine, evapora-
      tor, fire room of boat, ship, wa-
      tercraft E838 ☑
   inappropriate in local application or
      packing in medical or surgical
      procedure E873.5
   late effect of NEC E989
**Hemorrhage**
   delayed following medical or surgical
      treatment without mention of
      misadventure — *see* Reaction,
      abnormal
   during medical or surgical treatment
      as misadventure — *see* Misad-
      venture, cut
**High**
   altitude, effects E902.9
   level of radioactivity, effects — *see*
      Radiation
   pressure effects (*see also* Effects of,
      air pressure)
      from rapid descent in water (caus-
         ing caisson or divers' disease,
         palsy, or paralysis) E902.2
   temperature, effects — *see* Heat
**Hit, hitting** (accidental) by
   aircraft (propeller) (without accident
      to aircraft) E844 ☑
      unpowered E842 ☑
   avalanche E909.2
   being thrown against object in or part
      of
      motor vehicle (in motion) (on public
         highway) E818 ☑
         not on public highway E825 ☑
      nonmotor road vehicle NEC
         E829 ☑
      street car E829 ☑
   boat, ship, watercraft
      after fall from watercraft E838 ☑
      damaged, involved in accident
         E831 ☑
      while swimming, water skiing
         E838 ☑
   bullet (*see also* Shooting) E922.9
      from air gun E922.4
      in
         terrorism E979.4
         war operations E991.2
            rubber E991.0
   flare, Verey pistol (*see also* Shooting)
      E922.8
   hailstones E904.3
   landslide E909.2
   law-enforcing agent (on duty) E975
      with blunt object (baton) (night
         stick) (stave) (truncheon)
         E973
   machine — *see* Accident, machine
   missile
      firearm (*see also* Shooting) E922.9
         in
            terrorism — *see* Terrorism,
               missile
            war operations — *see* War oper-
               ations, missile
      motor vehicle (on public highway)
         (traffic accident) E814 ☑
         not on public highway, nontraffic
            accident E822 ☑
      nonmotor road vehicle NEC E829 ☑
   object
      falling E916

**Hit, hitting** by — *continued*
   object — *continued*
      falling — *continued*
         from, in, on
            aircraft E844 ☑
               due to accident to aircraft
                  — *see* categories
                  E840-E842 ☑
               unpowered E842 ☑
            boat, ship, watercraft
               E838 ☑
               due to accident to water-
                  craft E831 ☑
            building E916
               burning (uncontrolled fire)
                  E891.8
                  in terrorism E979.3
                  private E890.8
            cataclysmic
               earth surface movement
                  or eruption E909.9
               storm E908.9
            cave-in E916
               'with asphyxiation or suffo-
                  cation (*see also* Suf-
                  focation, due to,
                  cave-in) E913.3
            earthquake E909.0
            motor vehicle (in motion) (on
               public highway)
               E818 ☑
               not on public highway
                  E825 ☑
                  stationary E916
            nonmotor road vehicle NEC
               E829 ☑
            pedal cycle E826 ☑
            railway rolling stock, train,
               vehicle E806 ☑
            street car E829 ☑
            structure, burning NEC
               E891.8
            vehicle, stationary E916
      moving NEC — *see* Striking
         against, object
      projected NEC — *see* Striking
         against, object
      set in motion by
         compressed air or gas, spring,
            striking, throwing — *see*
            Striking against, object
         explosion — *see* Explosion
      thrown into, on, or towards
         motor vehicle (in motion) (on
            public highway) E818 ☑
            not on public highway
               E825 ☑
         nonmotor road vehicle NEC
            E829 ☑
         pedal cycle E826 ☑
         street car E829 ☑
   off-road type motor vehicle (not on
      public highway) E821 ☑
      on public highway E814 ☑
   other person(s) E917.9
      with blunt or thrown object E917.9
         in sports E917.0
            with subsequent fall E917.5
         intentionally, homicidal E968.2
      as, or caused by, a crowd E917.1
         with subsequent fall E917.6
      in sports E917.0
   pedal cycle E826 ☑
   police (on duty) E975
      with blunt object (baton) (night-
         stick) (stave) (truncheon)
         E973
   railway, rolling stock, train, vehicle
      (part of) E805 ☑
   shot — *see* Shooting
   snow vehicle, motor-driven (not on
      public highway) E820 ☑
      on public highway E814 ☑
   street car E829 ☑
   vehicle NEC — *see* Accident, vehicle
      NEC

**Homicide, homicidal** (attempt) (justifiable) — *see also* Assault E968.9
**Hot**
   liquid, object, substance, accident
      caused by (*see also* Accident,
      caused by, hot, by type of sub-
      stance)
      late effect of E929.8
   place, effects — *see* Heat
   weather, effects E900.0
**Humidity, causing problem** E904.3
**Hunger** E904.1
   resulting from
      abandonment or neglect E904.0
      transport accident — *see* categories
         E800-E848 ☑
**Hurricane** (any injury) E908.0
**Hypobarism, hypobaropathy** — *see*
   Effects of, air pressure
**Hypothermia** — *see* Cold, exposure to

**I**

**Ictus**
   caloris — *see* Heat
   solaris E900.0
**Ignition** (accidental)
   anesthetic gas in operating theatre
      E923.2
   bedclothes
      with
         conflagration — *see* Conflagra-
            tion
         ignition (of)
            clothing — *see* Ignition,
               clothes
            highly inflammable material
               (benzine) (fat) (gasoline)
               (kerosene) (paraffin)
               (petrol) E894
   benzine E894
   clothes, clothing (from controlled fire)
      (in building) E893.9
      with conflagration — *see* Conflagra-
         tion
      from
         bonfire E893.2
         highly inflammable material
            E894
         sources or material as listed in
            E893.8
         trash fire E893.2
         uncontrolled fire — *see* Confla-
            gration
      in
         private dwelling E893.0
         specified building or structure,
            except private dwelling
            E893.1
      not in building or structure E893.2
   explosive material — *see* Explosion
   fat E894
   gasoline E894
   kerosene E894
   material
      explosive — *see* Explosion
      highly inflammable E894
         with conflagration — *see* Confla-
            gration
         with explosion E923.2
   nightdress — *see* Ignition, clothes
   paraffin E894
   petrol E894
**Immersion** — *see* Submersion
**Implantation of quills of porcupine**
   E906.8
**Inanition** (from) E904.9
   hunger — *see* Lack of, food
   resulting from homicidal intent
      E968.4
   thirst — *see* Lack of, water
**Inattention after, at birth** E904.0
   homicidal, infanticidal intent E968.4
**Infanticide** — *see also* Assault

**Ingestion**
foreign body (causing injury) (with obstruction) — see Foreign body, alimentary canal
poisonous substance NEC — see Table of Drugs and Chemicals

**Inhalation**
excessively cold substance, manmade E901.1
foreign body — see Foreign body, aspiration
liquid air, hydrogen, nitrogen E901.1
mucus, not of newborn (with asphyxia, obstruction respiratory passage, suffocation) E912
phlegm (with asphyxia, obstruction respiratory passage, suffocation) E912
poisonous gas — see Table of Drugs and Chemicals
smoke from, due to
  fire — see Fire
  tobacco, second-hand E869.4
vomitus (with asphyxia, obstruction respiratory passage, suffocation) E911

**Injury, injured** (accidental(ly)) NEC E928.9
by, caused by, from
  air rifle (BB gun) E922.4
  animal (not being ridden) NEC E906.9
    being ridden (in sport or transport) E828 ☑
  assault (see also Assault) E968.9
  avalanche E909.2
  bayonet (see also Bayonet wound) E920.3
  being thrown against some part of, or object in
    motor vehicle (in motion) (on public highway) E818 ☑
      not on public highway E825 ☑
    nonmotor road vehicle NEC E829 ☑
    off-road motor vehicle NEC E821 ☑
    railway train E806 ☑
    snow vehicle, motor-driven E820 ☑
    street car E829 ☑
  bending E927
  bite, human E928.3
  broken glass E920.8
  bullet — see Shooting
  cave-in (see also Suffocation, due to, cave-in) E913.3
    without asphyxiation or suffocation E916
  earth surface movement or eruption E909.9
    storm E908.9
  cloudburst E908.8
  cutting or piercing instrument (see also Cut) E920.9
  cyclone E908.1
  earthquake E909.0
  earth surface movement or eruption E909.9
  electric current (see also Electric shock) E925.9
  explosion (see also Explosion) E923.9
  fire — see Fire
  flare, Verey pistol E922.8
  flood E908.2
  foreign body — see Foreign body
  hailstones E904.3
  hurricane E908.0
  landslide E909.2
  law-enforcing agent, police, in course of legal intervention — see Legal intervention
  lightning E907

**Injury, injured** — continued
by, caused by, from — continued
  live rail or live wire — see Electric shock
  machinery (see also Accident, machine)
    aircraft, without accident to aircraft E844 ☑
    boat, ship, watercraft (deck) (engine room) (galley) (laundry) (loading) E836 ☑
  missile
    explosive E923.8
    firearm — see Shooting
    in
      terrorism — see Terrorism, missile
      war operations — see War operations, missile
  moving part of motor vehicle (in motion) (on public highway) E818 ☑
    not on public highway, nontraffic accident E825 ☑
    while alighting, boarding, entering, leaving — see Fall, from, motor vehicle, while alighting, boarding
  nail E920.8
  needle (sewing) E920.4
    hypodermic E920.5
  noise E928.1
  object
    fallen on
      motor vehicle (in motion) (on public highway) E818 ☑
      not on public highway E825 ☑
    falling — see Hit by, object, falling
  paintball gun E922.5
  radiation — see Radiation
  railway rolling stock, train, vehicle (part of) E805 ☑
    door or window E806 ☑
  rotating propeller, aircraft E844 ☑
  rough landing of off-road type motor vehicle (after leaving ground or rough terrain) E821 ☑
    snow vehicle E820 ☑
  saber (see also Wound, saber) E920.3
  shot — see Shooting
  sound waves E928.1
  splinter or sliver, wood E920.8
  straining E927
  street car (door) E829 ☑
  suicide (attempt) E958.9
  sword E920.3
  terrorism — see Terrorism
  third rail — see Electric shock
  thunderbolt E907
  tidal wave E909.4
    caused by storm E908.0
  tornado E908.1
  torrential rain E908.2
  twisting E927
  vehicle NEC — see Accident, vehicle NEC
  vibration E928.2
  volcanic eruption E909.1
  weapon burst, in war operations E993
  weightlessness (in spacecraft, real or simulated) E928.0
  wood splinter or sliver E920.8
due to
  civil insurrection — see War operations
    occurring after cessation of hostilities E998
  terrorism — see Terrorism

**Injury, injured** — continued
due to — continued
  war operations — see War operations
    occurring after cessation of hostilities E998
  homicidal (see also Assault) E968.9
inflicted (by)
  in course of arrest (attempted), suppression of disturbance, maintenance of order, by law enforcing agents — see Legal intervention
  law-enforcing agent (on duty) — see Legal intervention
  other person
    stated as
      accidental E928.9
      homicidal, intentional — see Assault
      undetermined whether accidental or intentional — see Injury, stated as undetermined
  police (on duty) — see Legal intervention
in, on
  civil insurrection — see War operations
  fight E960.0
  parachute descent (voluntary) (without accident to aircraft) E844 ☑
    with accident to aircraft — see categories E840-E842 ☑
  public highway E819 ☑
  railway right of way E807 ☑
  terrorism — see Terrorism
  war operations — see War operations
late effect of E929.9
purposely (inflicted) by other person(s) — see Assault
self-inflicted (unspecified whether accidental or intentional) E988.9
  stated as
    accidental E928.9
    intentionally, purposely E958.9
specified cause NEC E928.8
stated as
  hanging E983.0
  knife E986
  late effect of E989
  puncture (any part of body) E986
  shooting — see Shooting, stated as undetermined whether accidental or intentional
  specified means NEC E988.8
  stab (any part of body) E986
  strangulation — see Suffocation, stated as undetermined whether accidental or intentional
  submersion E984
  suffocation — see Suffocation, stated as undetermined whether accidental or intentional
  undetermined whether accidentally or purposely inflicted (by) E988.9
    cut (any part of body) E986
    cutting or piercing instrument (classifiable to E920) E986
    drowning E984
    explosive(s) (missile) E985.5
    falling from high place E987.9
      manmade structure, except residential E987.1
    natural site E987.2
    residential premises E987.0
  to child due to criminal abortion E968.8

**Insufficient nourishment** — see also Lack of, food

**Insufficient nourishment** — see also Lack of, food — continued
  homicidal intent E968.4
**Insulation, effects** — see Heat
**Interruption of respiration by**
  food lodged in esophagus E911
  foreign body, except food, in esophagus E912
**Intervention, legal** — see Legal intervention
**Intoxication, drug or poison** — see Table of Drugs and Chemicals
**Irradiation** — see Radiation

### J

**Jammed** (accidentally)
  between objects (moving) (stationary and moving) E918
  in object E918
**Jumped or fell from high place, so stated** — see Jumping, from, high place, stated as
  in undetermined circumstances
**Jumping**
  before train, vehicle or other moving object (unspecified whether accidental or intentional) E988.0
    stated as
      intentional, purposeful E958.0
      suicidal (attempt) E958.0
  from
    aircraft
      by parachute (voluntarily) (without accident to aircraft) E844 ☑
      due to accident to aircraft — see categories E840-E842 ☑
    boat, ship, watercraft (into water)
      after accident to, fire on, watercraft E830 ☑
        and subsequently struck by (part of) boat E831 ☑
      burning, crushed, sinking E830 ☑
        and subsequently struck by (part of) boat E831 ☑
      voluntarily, without accident (to boat) with injury other than drowning or submersion E883.0
    building (see also Jumping, from, high place)
      burning (uncontrolled fire) E891.8
        in terrorism E979.3
        private E890.8
    cable car (not on rails) E847
      on rails E829 ☑
    high place
      in accidental circumstances or in sport — see categories E880-E884 ☑
      stated as
        with intent to injure self E957.9
          man-made structures NEC E957.1
          natural sites E957.2
          residential premises E957.0
        in undetermined circumstances E987.9
          man-made structures NEC E987.1
          natural sites E987.2
          residential premises E987.0
        suicidal (attempt) E957.9
          man-made structures NEC E957.1
          natural sites E957.1
          residential premises E957.0
    motor vehicle (in motion) (on public highway) — see Fall, from, motor vehicle

---

☑ Additional Digit Required — Refer to the Tabular List for Digit Selection          ▽ Subterms under main terms may continue to next column or page

*2008 ICD-9-CM*          ▶◀ Revised Text          ● New Line          ▲ Revised Code          **Volume 2 — 347**

**Index**

**Jumping — Misadventure(s) to patient(s)**

**Jumping** — *continued*
  from — *continued*
    nonmotor road vehicle NEC
      E829 ☑
    street car E829 ☑
    structure (*see also* Jumping, from,
      high place)
      burning NEC (uncontrolled fire)
        E891.8
      in terrorism E979.3
    into water
      with injury other than drowning or
        submersion E883.0
      drowning or submersion — *see*
        Submersion
    from, off, watercraft — *see* Jump-
      ing, from, boat
**Justifiable homicide** — *see* Assault

### K

**Kicked by**
  animal E906.8
  person(s) (accidentally) E917.9
    with intent to injure or kill E960.0
    as, or caused by a crowd E917.1
      with subsequent fall E917.6
    in fight E960.0
    in sports E917.0
      with subsequent fall E917.5
**Kicking against**
  object (moving) E917.9
    in sports E917.0
      with subsequent fall E917.5
    stationary E917.4
      with subsequent fall E917.8
  person — *see* Striking against, person
**Killed, killing** (accidentally) NEC — *see
  also* Injury E928.9
  in
    action — *see* War operations
    brawl, fight (hand) (fists) (foot)
      E960.0
      by weapon (*see also* Assault)
        cutting, piercing E966
        firearm — *see* Shooting,
          homicide
    self
      stated as
        accident E928.9
        suicide — *see* Suicide
      unspecified whether accidental or
        suicidal E988.9
**Knocked down** (accidentally) (by) NEC
  E928.9
  animal (not being ridden) E906.8
    being ridden (in sport or transport)
      E828 ☑
  blast from explosion (*see also* Explo-
    sion) E923.9
  crowd, human stampede E917.6
  late effect of — *see* Late effect
  person (accidentally) E917.9
    in brawl, fight E960.0
    in sports E917.5
  transport vehicle — *see* vehicle in-
    volved under Hit by
  while boxing E917.5

### L

**Laceration NEC** E928.9
**Lack of**
  air (refrigerator or closed place), suffo-
    cation by E913.2
  care (helpless person) (infant) (new-
    born) E904.0
    homicidal intent E968.4
  food except as result of transport acci-
    dent E904.1
  helpless person, infant, newborn
    due to
      abandonment or neglect E904.0
  water except as result of transport
    accident E904.2

**Lack of** — *continued*
  water except as result of transport ac-
    cident — *continued*
    helpless person, infant, newborn
      due to
        abandonment or neglect E904.0
**Landslide** E909.2
  falling on, hitting
    motor vehicle (any) (in motion) (on
      or off public highway) E909.2
    railway rolling stock, train, vehicle
      E909.2
**Late effect of**
  accident NEC (accident classifiable to
    E928.9) E929.9
    specified NEC (accident classifiable
      to E910–E928.8) E929.8
  assault E969
  fall, accidental (accident classifiable
    to E880–E888) E929.3
  fire, accident caused by (accident
    classifiable to E890–E899)
    E929.4
  homicide, attempt (any means) E969
  injury due to terrorism E999.1
  injury undetermined whether acciden-
    tally or purposely inflicted (in-
    jury classifiable to E980–E988)
    E989
  legal intervention (injury classifiable
    to E970–E976) E977
  medical or surgical procedure, test or
    therapy
    as, or resulting in, or from
      abnormal or delayed reaction or
        complication — *see* Reac-
        tion, abnormal
      misadventure — *see* Misadven-
        ture
  motor vehicle accident (accident clas-
    sifiable to E810–E825) E929.0
  natural or environmental factor, acci-
    dent due to (accident classifiable
    to E900–E909) E929.5
  poisoning, accidental (accident classi-
    fiable to E850–E858,
    E860–E869) E929.2
  suicide, attempt (any means) E959
  transport accident NEC (accident
    classifiable to E800–E807,
    E826–E838, E840–E848)
    E929.1
  war operations, injury due to (injury
    classifiable to E990–E998)
    E999.0
**Launching pad accident** E845 ☑
**Legal**
  execution, any method E978
  intervention (by) (injury from) E976
    baton E973
    bayonet E974
    blow E975
    blunt object (baton) (nightstick)
      (stave) (truncheon) E973
    cutting or piercing instrument
      E974
    dynamite E971
    execution, any method E973
    explosive(s) (shell) E971
    firearm(s) E970
    gas (asphyxiation) (poisoning) (tear)
      E972
    grenade E971
    late effect of E977
    machine gun E970
    manhandling E975
    mortar bomb E971
    nightstick E973
    revolver E970
    rifle E970
    specified means NEC E975
    stabbing E974
    stave E973
    truncheon E973
**Lifting, injury in** E927

**Lightning** (shock) (stroke) (struck by)
  E907
**Liquid** (noncorrosive) in eye E914
  corrosive E924.1
**Loss of control**
  motor vehicle (on public highway)
    (without antecedent collision)
    E816 ☑
    with
      antecedent collision on public
        highway — *see* Collision,
        motor vehicle
      involving any object, person
        or vehicle not on public
        highway E816 ☑
      not on public highway, non-
        traffic accident E825 ☑
        with antecedent collision
          — *see* Collision,
          motor vehicle, not
          on public highway
      on public highway — *see*
        Collision, motor vehicle
    off-road type motor vehicle (not on
      public highway) E821 ☑
      on public highway — *see* Loss of
        control, motor vehicle
    snow vehicle, motor-driven (not on
      public highway) E820 ☑
      on public highway — *see* Loss of
        control, motor vehicle
**Lost at sea** E832 ☑
  with accident to watercraft E830 ☑
  in war operations E995
**Low**
  pressure, effects — *see* Effects of, air
    pressure
  temperature, effects — *see* Cold, expo-
    sure to
**Lying before train, vehicle or other
  moving object** (unspecified
    whether accidental or intentional)
    E988.0
  stated as intentional, purposeful, sui-
    cidal (attempt) E958.0
**Lynching** — *see also* Assault E968.9

### M

**Malfunction, atomic power plant in
  water transport** E838 ☑
**Mangled** (accidentally) NEC E928.9
**Manhandling** (in brawl, fight) E960.0
  legal intervention E975
**Manslaughter** (nonaccidental) — *see*
  Assault
**Marble in nose** E912
**Mauled by animal** E906.8
**Medical procedure, complication of**
  delayed or as an abnormal reaction
    without mention of misadventure
      — *see* Reaction, abnormal
  due to or as a result of misadventure
    — *see* Misadventure
**Melting of fittings and furniture in
  burning**
  in terrorism E979.3
**Minamata disease** E865.2
**Misadventure(s) to patient(s) during
  surgical or medical care** E876.9
  contaminated blood, fluid, drug or bi-
    ological substance (presence of
    agents and toxins as listed in
    E875) E875.9
    administered (by) NEC E875.9
      infusion E875.0
      injection E875.1
      specified means NEC E875.2
      transfusion E875.0
      vaccination E875.1
  cut, cutting, puncture, perforation or
    hemorrhage (accidental) (inad-
    vertent) (inappropriate) (during)
    E870.9
    aspiration of fluid or tissue (by
      puncture or catheterization,
      except heart) E870.5

**Misadventure(s) to patient(s) during
  surgical or medical care** —
  *continued*
  cut, cutting, puncture, perforation or
    hemorrhage — *continued*
    biopsy E870.8
      needle (aspirating) E870.5
    blood sampling E870.5
    catheterization E870.5
      heart E870.6
    dialysis (kidney) E870.2
    endoscopic examination E870.4
    enema E870.7
    infusion E870.1
    injection E870.3
    lumbar puncture E870.5
    needle biopsy E870.5
    paracentesis, abdominal E870.5
    perfusion E870.2
    specified procedure NEC E870.8
    surgical operation E870.0
    thoracentesis E870.5
    transfusion E870.1
    vaccination E870.3
  excessive amount of blood or other
    fluid during transfusion or infu-
    sion E873.0
  failure
    in dosage E873.9
      electroshock therapy E873.4
      inappropriate temperature (too
        hot or too cold) in local
        application and packing
        E873.5
      infusion
        excessive amount of fluid
          E873.0
        incorrect dilution of fluid
          E873.1
      insulin-shock therapy E873.4
      nonadministration of necessary
        drug or medicinal E873.6
      overdose (*see also* Overdose)
        radiation, in therapy E873.2
      radiation
        inadvertent exposure of pa-
          tient (receiving radia-
          tion for test or therapy)
          E873.3
        not receiving radiation for
          test or therapy —
          *see* Radiation
      overdose E873.2
    specified procedure NEC E873.8
    transfusion
      excessive amount of blood
        E873.0
  mechanical, of instrument or appa-
    ratus (during procedure)
    E874.9
    aspiration of fluid or tissue (by
      puncture or catheteriza-
      tion, except of heart)
      E874.4
    biopsy E874.8
      needle (aspirating) E874.4
    blood sampling E874.4
    catheterization E874.4
      heart E874.5
    dialysis (kidney) E874.2
    endoscopic examination E874.3
    enema E874.8
    infusion E874.1
    injection E874.8
    lumbar puncture E874.4
    needle biopsy E874.4
    paracentesis, abdominal E874.4
    perfusion E874.2
    specified procedure NEC E874.8
    surgical operation E874.0
    thoracentesis E874.4
    transfusion E874.1
    vaccination E874.8
  sterile precautions (during proce-
    dure) E872.9

☑ Additional Digit Required — Refer to the Tabular List for Digit Selection      Subterms under main terms may continue to next column or page

348 — Volume 2      ▶◀ Revised Text      ● New Line      ▲ Revised Code      *2008 ICD-9-CM*

**Misadventure(s) to patient(s) during surgical or medical care —** *continued*
failure — *continued*
sterile precautions — *continued*
aspiration of fluid or tissue (by puncture or catheterization, except heart) E872.5
biopsy E872.8
needle (aspirating) E872.5
blood sampling E872.5
catheterization E872.5
heart E872.6
dialysis (kidney) E872.2
endoscopic examination E872.4
enema E872.8
infusion E872.1
injection E872.3
lumbar puncture E872.5
needle biopsy E872.5
paracentesis, abdominal E872.5
perfusion E872.2
removal of catheter or packing E872.8
specified procedure NEC E872.8
surgical operation E872.0
thoracentesis E872.5
transfusion E872.1
vaccination E872.3
suture or ligature during surgical procedure E876.2
to introduce or to remove tube or instrument E876.4
foreign object left in body — *see* Misadventure, foreign object
foreign object left in body (during procedure) E871.9
aspiration of fluid or tissue (by puncture or catheterization, except heart) E871.5
biopsy E871.8
needle (aspirating) E871.5
blood sampling E871.5
catheterization E871.5
heart E871.6
dialysis (kidney) E871.2
endoscopic examination E871.4
enema E871.8
infusion E871.1
injection E871.3
lumbar puncture E871.5
needle biopsy E871.5
paracentesis, abdominal E871.5
perfusion E871.2
removal of catheter or packing E871.7
specified procedure NEC E871.8
surgical operation E871.0
thoracentesis E871.5
transfusion E871.1
vaccination E871.3
hemorrhage — *see* Misadventure, cut
inadvertent exposure of patient to radiation (being received for test or therapy) E873.3
inappropriate
operation performed E876.5
temperature (too hot or too cold) in local application or packing E873.5
infusion (*see also* Misadventure, by specific type, infusion)
excessive amount of fluid E873.0
incorrect dilution of fluid E873.1
wrong fluid E876.1
mismatched blood in transfusion E876.0
nonadministration of necessary drug or medicinal E873.6
overdose (*see also* Overdose)
radiation, in therapy E873.2
perforation — *see* Misadventure, cut
performance of inappropriate operation E876.5
puncture — *see* Misadventure, cut

**Misadventure(s) to patient(s) during surgical or medical care —** *continued*
specified type NEC E876.8
failure
suture or ligature during surgical operation E876.2
to introduce or to remove tube or instrument E876.4
foreign object left in body E871.9
infusion of wrong fluid E876.1
performance of inappropriate operation E876.5
transfusion of mismatched blood E876.0
wrong
fluid in infusion E876.1
placement of endotracheal tube during anesthetic procedure E876.3
transfusion (*see also* Misadventure, by specific type, transfusion)
excessive amount of blood E873.0
mismatched blood E876.0
wrong
drug given in error — *see* Table of Drugs and Chemicals
fluid in infusion E876.1
placement of endotracheal tube during anesthetic procedure E876.3
**Motion** (effects) E903
sickness E903
**Mountain sickness** E902.0
**Mucus aspiration or inhalation, not of newborn** (with asphyxia, obstruction respiratory passage, suffocation) E912
**Mudslide of cataclysmic nature** E909.2
**Murder (attempt)** — *see also* Assault E968.9

N

**Nail, injury by** E920.8
**Needlestick** (sewing needle) E920.4
hypodermic E920.5
**Neglect** — *see also* Privation
criminal E968.4
homicidal intent E968.4
**Noise** (causing injury) (pollution) E928.1

O

**Object**
falling
from, in, on, hitting
aircraft E844 ☑
due to accident to aircraft — *see* categories E840-E842 ☑
machinery (*see also* Accident, machine)
not in operation E916
motor vehicle (in motion) (on public highway) E818 ☑
not on public highway E825 ☑
stationary E916
nonmotor road vehicle NEC E829 ☑
pedal cycle E826 ☑
person E916
railway rolling stock, train, vehicle E806 ☑
street car E829 ☑
watercraft E838 ☑
due to accident to watercraft E831 ☑
set in motion by
accidental explosion of pressure vessel — *see* category E921 ☑
firearm — *see* category E922 ☑
machine(ry) — *see* Accident, machine

**Object** — *continued*
set in motion by — *continued*
transport vehicle — *see* categories E800-E848 ☑
thrown from, in, on, towards
aircraft E844 ☑
cable car (not on rails) E847
on rails E829
motor vehicle (in motion) (on public highway) E818 ☑
not on public highway E825 ☑
nonmotor road vehicle NEC E829 ☑
pedal cycle E826 ☑
street car E829 ☑
vehicle NEC — *see* Accident, vehicle NEC
**Obstruction**
air passages, larynx, respiratory passages
by
external means NEC — *see* Suffocation
food, any type (regurgitated) (vomited) E911
material or object, except food E912
mucus E912
phlegm E912
vomitus E911
digestive tract, except mouth or pharynx
by
food, any type E915
foreign body (any) E915
esophagus
without asphyxia or obstruction of respiratory passage E915
food E911
foreign body, except food E912
mouth or pharynx
by
food, any type E911
material or object, except food E912
respiration — *see* Obstruction, air passages
**Oil in eye** E914
**Overdose**
anesthetic (drug) — *see* Table of Drugs and Chemicals
drug — *see* Table of Drugs and Chemicals
**Overexertion** (lifting) (pulling) (pushing) E927
**Overexposure** (accidental) (to)
cold (*see also* Cold, exposure to) E901.9
due to manmade conditions E901.1
heat (*see also* Heat) E900.9
radiation — *see* Radiation
radioactivity — *see* Radiation
sun, except sunburn E900.0
weather — *see* Exposure
wind — *see* Exposure
**Overheated** — *see also* Heat E900.9
**Overlaid** E913.0
**Overturning** (accidental)
animal-drawn vehicle E827 ☑
boat, ship, watercraft
causing
drowning, submersion E830 ☑
injury except drowning, submersion E831 ☑
machinery — *see* Accident, machine
motor vehicle (*see also* Loss of control, motor vehicle) E816 ☑
with antecedent collision on public highway — *see* Collision, motor vehicle
not on public highway, nontraffic accident E825 ☑
with antecedent collision — *see* Collision, motor vehicle, not on public highway
nonmotor road vehicle NEC E829 ☑

**Overturning** — *continued*
off-road type motor vehicle — *see* Loss of control, off-road type motor vehicle
pedal cycle E826 ☑
railway rolling stock, train, vehicle (*see also* Derailment, railway) E802 ☑
street car E829 ☑
vehicle NEC — *see* Accident, vehicle NEC

P

**Palsy, divers'** E902.2
**Parachuting** (voluntary) (without accident to aircraft) E844 ☑
due to accident to aircraft — *see* categories E840-E842 ☑
**Paralysis**
divers' E902.2
lead or saturnine E866.0
from pesticide NEC E863.4
**Pecked by bird** E906.8
**Phlegm aspiration or inhalation** (with asphyxia, obstruction respiratory passage, suffocation) E912
**Piercing** — *see also* Cut E920.9
**Pinched**
between objects (moving) (stationary and moving) E918
in object E918
**Pinned under**
machine(ry) — *see* Accident, machine
**Place of occurrence of accident** — *see* Accident (to), occurring (at) (in)
**Plumbism** E866.0
from insecticide NEC E863.4
**Poisoning** (accidental) (by) — *see also* Table of Drugs and Chemicals
carbon monoxide
generated by
aircraft in transit E844 ☑
motor vehicle
in motion (on public highway) E818 ☑
not on public highway E825 ☑
watercraft (in transit) (not in transit) E838 ☑
caused by injection of poisons or toxins into or through skin by plant thorns, spines, or other mechanism E905.7
marine or sea plants E905.6
fumes or smoke due to
conflagration — *see* Conflagration
explosion or fire — *see* Fire
ignition — *see* Ignition
gas
in legal intervention E972
legal execution, by E978
on watercraft E838 ☑
used as anesthetic — *see* Table of Drugs and Chemicals
in
terrorism (chemical weapons) E979.7
war operations E997.2
execution E978
intervention
by gas E972
late effect of — *see* Late effect
legal
**Pressure, external, causing asphyxia, suffocation** — *see also* Suffocation E913.9
**Privation** E904.9
food (*see also* Lack of, food) E904.1
helpless person, infant, newborn due to abandonment or neglect E904.0
late effect of NEC E929.5
resulting from transport accident — *see* categories E800-E848 ☑
water (*see also* Lack of, water) E904.2

☑ Additional Digit Required — Refer to the Tabular List for Digit Selection
▽ Subterms under main terms may continue to next column or page
**2008 ICD-9-CM**
▶◀ Revised Text
● New Line
▲ Revised Code
**Volume 2 — 349**

**Projected objects, striking against or struck by** — *see* Striking against, object

**Prolonged stay in**
  high altitude (causing conditions as listed in E902.0) E902.0
  weightless environment E928.0

**Prostration**
  heat — *see* Heat

**Pulling, injury in** E927

**Puncture, puncturing** — *see also* Cut E920.9
  by
    plant thorns or spines E920.8
      toxic reaction E905.7
        marine or sea plants E905.6
    sea-urchin spine E905.6

**Pushing** (injury in) (overexertion) E927
  by other person(s) (accidental) E917.9
    with fall E886.9
      in sports E886.0
    as, or caused by, a crowd, human stampede E917.1
      with subsequent fall E917.6
    before moving vehicle or object
      stated as
        intentional, homicidal E968.5
        undetermined whether accidental or intentional E988.8
    from
      high place
        in accidental circum-stances — *see* categories E880-E884 ☑
        stated as
          intentional, homicidal E968.1
          undetermined whether accidental or intentional E987.9
          man-made structure, except residential E987.1
          natural site E987.2
          residential E987.0
      motor vehicle (*see also* Fall, from, motor vehicle) E818 ☑
        stated as
          intentional, homicidal E968.5
          undetermined whether accidental or intentional E988.8
    in sports E917.0
      with fall E886.0

### R

**Radiation** (exposure to) E926.9
  abnormal reaction to medical test or therapy E879.2
  arc lamps E926.2
  atomic power plant (malfunction) NEC E926.9
    in water transport E838 ☑
  electromagnetic, ionizing E926.3
  gamma rays E926.3
  in
    terrorism (from or following nuclear explosion) (direct) (secondary) E979.5
      laser E979.8
    war operations (from or following nuclear explosion) (direct) (secondary) E996
      laser(s) E997.0
    water transport E838 ☑
  inadvertent exposure of patient (receiving test or therapy) E873.3
  infrared (heaters and lamps) E926.1
    excessive heat from E900.1
  ionized, ionizing (particles, artificially accelerated) E926.8
    electromagnetic E926.3

**Radiation** — *continued*
  isotopes, radioactive — *see* Radiation, radioactive isotopes
  laser(s) E926.4
    in
      terrorism E979.8
      war operations E997.0
    misadventure in medical care — *see* Misadventure, failure, in dosage, radiation
  late effect of NEC E929.8
    excessive heat from — *see* Heat
  light sources (visible) (ultraviolet) E926.2
  misadventure in medical or surgical procedure — *see* Misadventure, failure, in dosage, radiation
  overdose (in medical or surgical procedure) E873.2
  radar E926.0
  radioactive isotopes E926.5
    atomic power plant malfunction E926.5
      in water transport E838 ☑
    misadventure in medical or surgical treatment — *see* Misadventure, failure, in dosage, radiation
  radiobiologicals — *see* Radiation, radioactive isotopes
  radiofrequency E926.0
  radiopharmaceuticals — *see* Radiation, radioactive isotopes
  radium NEC E926.9
  sun E926.2
    excessive heat from E900.0
  tanning bed E926.2
  welding arc or torch E926.2
    excessive heat from E900.1
  x-rays (hard) (soft) E926.3
    misadventure in medical or surgical treatment — *see* Misadventure, failure, in dosage, radiation

**Rape** E960.1

**Reaction, abnormal to or following** (medical or surgical procedure) E879.9
  amputation (of limbs) E878.5
  anastomosis (arteriovenous) (blood vessel) (gastrojejunal) (skin) (tendon) (natural, artificial material, tissue) E878.2
    external stoma, creation of E878.3
  aspiration (of fluid) E879.4
    tissue E879.8
  biopsy E879.8
  blood
    sampling E879.7
    transfusion
      procedure E879.8
  bypass — *see* Reaction, abnormal, anastomosis
  catheterization
    cardiac E879.0
    urinary E879.6
  colostomy E878.3
  cystostomy E878.3
  dialysis (kidney) E879.1
  drugs or biologicals — *see* Table of Drugs and Chemicals
  duodenostomy E878.3
  electroshock therapy E879.3
  formation of external stoma E878.3
  gastrostomy E878.3
  graft — *see* Reaction, abnormal, anastomosis
  hypothermia E879.8
  implant, implantation (of)
    artificial
      internal device (cardiac pacemaker) (electrodes in brain) (heart valve prosthesis) (orthopedic) E878.1
      material or tissue (for anastomosis or bypass) E878.2

**Reaction, abnormal to or following** — *continued*
  implant, implantation — *continued*
    artificial — *continued*
      material or tissue — *continued*
        with creation of external stoma E878.3
      natural tissues (for anastomosis or bypass) E878.2
        with creation of external stoma E878.3
      as transplantation — *see* Reaction, abnormal, transplant
  infusion
    procedure E879.8
  injection
    procedure E879.8
      specific type of procedure) E879.9
  insertion of gastric or duodenal sound E879.5
  insulin-shock therapy E879.3
  lumbar puncture E879.4
  perfusion E879.1
  procedures other than surgical operation (*see also* Reaction, abnormal, by
    specified procedure NEC E879.8
  radiological procedure or therapy E879.2
  removal of organ (partial) (total) NEC E878.6
    with
      anastomosis, bypass or graft E878.2
      formation of external stoma E878.3
      implant of artificial internal device E878.1
      transplant(ation)
        partial organ E878.4
        whole organ E878.0
  sampling
    blood E879.7
    fluid NEC E879.4
    tissue E879.8
  shock therapy E879.3
  surgical operation (*see also* Reaction, abnormal, by specified type of operation) E878.9
    restorative NEC E878.4
      with
        anastomosis, bypass or graft E878.2
        fomation of external stoma E878.3
        implant(ation) — *see* Reaction, abnormal, implant
        transplant(ation) — *see* Reaction, abnormal, transplant
    specified operation NEC E878.8
  thoracentesis E879.4
  transfusion
    procedure E879.8
  transplant, transplantation (heart) (kidney) (liver) E878.0
    partial organ E878.4
  ureterostomy E878.3
  vaccination E879.8

**Reduction in**
  atmospheric pressure (*see also* Effects of, air pressure)
    while surfacing from
      deep water diving causing caisson or divers' disease, palsy or paralysis E902.2
      underground E902.8

**Residual** (effect) — *see* Late effect

**Rock falling on or hitting** (accidentally)
  motor vehicle (in motion) (on public highway) E818 ☑
    not on public highway E825 ☑
  nonmotor road vehicle NEC E829 ☑

**Rock falling on or hitting** — *continued*
  pedal cycle E826 ☑
  person E916
  railway rolling stock, train, vehicle E806 ☑

**Running off, away**
  animal (being ridden) (in sport or transport) E828 ☑
    not being ridden E906.8
  animal-drawn vehicle E827 ☑
  rails, railway (*see also* Derailment) E802 ☑
  roadway
    motor vehicle (without antecedent collision) E816 ☑
      with
        antecedent collision — *see* Collision motor vehicle
        subsequent collision
          involving any object, person or vehicle not on public highway E816 ☑
          on public highway E811 ☑
      nontraffic accident E825 ☑
        with antecedent collision — *see* Collision, motor vehicle, not on public highway
    nonmotor road vehicle NEC E829 ☑
    pedal cycle E826 ☑

**Run over** (accidentally) (by)
  animal (not being ridden) E906.8
    being ridden (in sport or transport) E828 ☑
  animal-drawn vehicle E827 ☑
  machinery — *see* Accident, machine
  motor vehicle (on public highway) — *see* Hit by, motor vehicle
  nonmotor road vehicle NEC E829 ☑
  railway train E805 ☑
  street car E829 ☑
  vehicle NEC E848

### S

**Saturnism** E866.0
  from insecticide NEC E863.4

**Scald, scalding** (accidental) (by) (from) (in) E924.0
  acid — *see* Scald, caustic
  boiling tap water E924.2
  caustic or corrosive liquid, substance E924.1
    swallowed — *see* Table of Drugs and Chemicals
  homicide (attempt) — *see* Assault, burning
  inflicted by other person
    stated as
      intentional or homicidal E968.3
      undetermined whether accidental or intentional E988.2
  late effect of NEC E929.8
  liquid (boiling) (hot) E924.0
  local application of externally applied substance in medical or surgical care E873.5
  molten metal E924.0
  self-inflicted (unspecified whether accidental or intentional) E988.2
    stated as intentional, purposeful E958.2
  stated as undetermined whether accidental or intentional E988.2
  steam E924.0
  tap water (boiling) E924.2
  transport accident — *see* categories E800-E848 ☑
  vapor E924.0

**Scratch, cat** E906.8

**Sea**
  sickness E903

☑ Additional Digit Required — Refer to the Tabular List for Digit Selection    ᵛ Subterms under main terms may continue to next column or page

350 — Volume 2    ▶◀ Revised Text    ● New Line    ▲ Revised Code    *2008 ICD-9-CM*

**Self-mutilation** — *see* Suicide
**Sequelae (of)**
  in
    terrorism E999.1
    war operations E999.0
**Shock**
  anaphylactic (*see also* Table of Drugs
    and Chemicals) E947.9
    due to
      bite (venomous) — *see* Bite,
        venomous NEC
      sting — *see* Sting
  electric (*see also* Electric shock)
    E925.9
  from electric appliance or current (*see*
    *also* Electric shock) E925.9
**Shooting, shot** (accidental(ly)) E922.9
  air gun E922.4
  BB gun E922.4
  hand gun (pistol) (revolver) E922.0
  himself (*see also* Shooting, self-inflict-
    ed) E985.4
    hand gun (pistol) (revolver) E985.0
    military firearm, except hand gun
      E985.3
      hand gun (pistol) (revolver)
        E985.0
    rifle (hunting) E985.2
      military E985.3
    shotgun (automatic) E985.1
    specified firearm NEC E985.4
    Verey pistol E985.4
  homicide (attempt) E965.4
    air gun E968.6
    BB gun E968.6
    hand gun (pistol) (revolver) E965.0
    military firearm, except hand gun
      E965.3
      hand gun (pistol) (revolver)
        E965.0
    paintball gun E965.4
    rifle (hunting) E965.2
      military E965.3
    shotgun (automatic) E965.1
    specified firearm NEC E965.4
    Verey pistol E965.4
  in
    terrorism — *see* Terrorism, shoot-
      ing
    war operations — *see* War opera-
      tions, shooting
  inflicted by other person
    in accidental circumstances
      E922.9
      hand gun (pistol) (revolver)
        E922.0
      military firearm, except hand
        gun E922.3
        hand gun (pistol) (revolver)
          E922.0
      rifle (hunting) E922.2
        military E922.3
      shotgun (automatic) E922.1
      specified firearm NEC E922.8
      Verey pistol E922.8
    stated as
      intentional, homicidal E965.4
        hand gun (pistol) (revolver)
          E965.0
        military firearm, except hand
          gun E965.3
          hand gun (pistol) (re-
            volver) E965.0
        paintball gun E965.4
        rifle (hunting) E965.2
          military E965.3
        shotgun (automatic) E965.1
        specified firearm E965.4
        Verey pistol E965.4
      undetermined whether acciden-
        tal or intentional E985.4
        air gun E985.6
        BB gun E985.6
        hand gun (pistol) (revolver)
          E985.0

**Shooting, shot** — *continued*
  inflicted by other person — *contin-*
    *ued*
    stated as — *continued*
      undetermined whether acciden-
        tal or intentional — *contin-*
        *ued*
        military firearm, except hand
          gun E985.3
          hand gun (pistol) (re-
            volver) E985.0
        paintball gun E985.7
        rifle (hunting) E985.2
        shotgun (automatic) E985.1
        specified firearm NEC E985.4
        Verey pistol E985.4
  legal
    execution E978
    intervention E970
  military firearm, except hand gun
    E922.3
    hand gun (pistol) (revolver) E922.0
  paintball gun E922.5
  rifle (hunting) E922.2
    military E922.3
  self-inflicted (unspecified whether ac-
    cidental or intentional) E985.4
    air gun E985.6
    BB gun E985.6
    hand gun (pistol) (revolver) E985.0
    military firearm, except hand gun
      E985.3
      hand gun (pistol) (revolver)
        E985.0
    paintball gun E985.7
    rifle (hunting) E985.2
      military E985.3
    shotgun (automatic) E985.1
    specified firearm NEC E985.4
    stated as
      accidental E922.9
        hand gun (pistol) (revolver)
          E922.0
        military firearm, except hand
          gun E922.3
          hand gun (pistol) (re-
            volver) E922.0
        paintball gun E922.5
        rifle (hunting) E922.2
          military E922.3
        shotgun (automatic) E922.1
        specified firearm NEC E922.8
        Verey pistol E922.8
      intentional, purposeful E955.4
        hand gun (pistol) (revolver)
          E955.0
        military firearm, except hand
          gun E955.3
          hand gun (pistol) (re-
            volver) E955.0
        paintball gun E955.7
        rifle (hunting) E955.2
          military E955.3
        shotgun (automatic) E955.1
        specified firearm NEC E955.4
        Verey pistol E955.4
    shotgun (automatic) E922.1
    specified firearm NEC E922.8
    stated as undetermined whether acci-
      dental or intentional E985.4
    hand gun (pistol) (revolver) E985.0
    military firearm, except hand gun
      E985.3
      hand gun (pistol) (revolver)
        E985.0
    paintball gun E985.7
    rifle (hunting) E985.2
      military E985.3
    shotgun (automatic) E985.1
    specified firearm NEC E985.4
    Verey pistol E985.4
  suicidal (attempt) E955.4
    air gun E955.6
    BB gun E955.6
    hand gun (pistol) (revolver) E955.0

**Shooting, shot** — *continued*
  suicidal — *continued*
    military firearm, except hand gun
      E955.3
      hand gun (pistol) (revolver)
        E955.0
    paintball gun E955.7
    rifle (hunting) E955.2
      military E955.3
    shotgun (automatic) E955.1
    specified firearm NEC E955.4
    Verey pistol E955.4
  Verey pistol E922.8
**Shoving** (accidentally) by other person
  — *see also* Pushing by other person
  E917.9
**Sickness**
  air E903
  alpine E902.0
  car E903
  motion E903
  mountain E902.0
  sea E903
  travel E903
**Sinking** (accidental)
  boat, ship, watercraft (causing
    drowning, submersion) E830 ☑
    causing injury except drowning,
      submersion E831 ☑
**Siriasis** E900.0
**Skydiving** E844 ☑
**Slashed wrists** — *see also* Cut, self-in-
  flicted E986
**Slipping** (accidental)
  on
    deck (of boat, ship, watercraft) (icy)
      (oily) (wet) E835 ☑
    ice E885.9
    ladder of ship E833 ☑
      due to accident to watercraft
        E831 ☑
    mud E885.9
    oil E885.9
    snow E885.9
    stairs of ship E833 ☑
      due to accident to watercraft
        E831 ☑
    surface
      slippery E885 ☑
      wet E885 ☑
**Sliver, wood, injury by** E920.8
**Smothering, smothered** — *see also*
  Suffocation E913.9
**Smouldering building or structure in**
  **terrorism** E979.3
**Sodomy** (assault) E960.1
**Solid substance in eye (any part) or**
  **adnexa** E914
**Sound waves** (causing injury) E928.1
**Splinter, injury by** E920.8
**Stab, stabbing** E966
  accidental — *see* Cut
**Starvation** E904.1
  helpless person, infant, newborn —
    *see* Lack of food
  homicidal intent E968.4
  late effect of NEC E929.5
  resulting from accident connected
    with transport — *see* categories
    E800-E848 ☑
**Stepped on**
  by
    animal (not being ridden) E906.8
      being ridden (in sport or trans-
        port) E828 ☑
    crowd E917.1
    person E917.9
      in sports E917.0
  in sports E917.0
**Stepping on**
  object (moving) E917.9
    in sports E917.0
      with subsequent fall E917.5
    stationary E917.4
      with subsequent fall E917.8
  person E917.9

**Stepping on** — *continued*
  person — *continued*
    as, or caused by a crowd E917.1
      with subsequent fall E917.6
    in sports E917.0
**Sting** E905.9
  ant E905.5
  bee E905.3
  caterpillar E905.5
  coral E905.6
  hornet E905.3
  insect NEC E905.5
  jellyfish E905.6
  marine animal or plant E905.6
  nematocysts E905.6
  scorpion E905.2
  sea anemone E905.6
  sea cucumber E905.6
  wasp E905.3
  yellow jacket E905.3
**Storm** E908.9
  specified type NEC E908.8
**Straining, injury in** E927
**Strangling** — *see* Suffocation
**Strangulation** — *see* Suffocation
**Strenuous movements** (in recreational
  or other activities) E927
**Striking against**
  bottom (when jumping or diving into
    water) E883.0
  object (moving) E917.9
    caused by crowd E917.1
      with subsequent fall E917.6
    furniture E917.3
      with subsequent fall E917.7
    in
      running water E917.2
        with drowning or submersion
          — *see* Submersion
      sports E917.0
        with subsequent fall E917.5
      stationary E917.4
        with subsequent fall E917.8
  person(s) E917.9
    with fall E886.9
      in sports E886.0
    as, or caused by, a crowd E917.1
      with subsequent fall E917.6
    in sports E917.0
      with fall E886.0
**Stroke**
  heat — *see* Heat
  lightning E907
**Struck by** — *see also* Hit by
  bullet
    in
      terrorism E979.4
      war operations E991.2
        rubber E991.0
  lightning E907
  missile
    in terrorism — *see* Terrorism, mis-
      sile
  object
    falling
      from, in, on
        building
          burning (uncontrolled fire)
            in terrorism E979.3
  thunderbolt E907
**Stumbling over animal, carpet, curb,**
  **rug or (small) object (with fall)**
  E885.9
  without fall — *see* Striking against,
    object
**Submersion (accidental)** E910.8
  boat, ship, watercraft (causing
    drowning, submersion) E830 ☑
    causing injury except drowning,
      submersion E831 ☑
  by other person
    in accidental circumstances — *see*
      category E910 ☑
    intentional, homicidal E964

---

☑ Additional Digit Required — Refer to the Tabular List for Digit Selection      ▽ Subterms under main terms may continue to next column or page

**Terrorism** — *continued*
　exposure to ionizing radiation from
　　nuclear explosion E979.5
　falling aircraft E979.1
　firearms E979.4
　fireball effects from nuclear explosion
　　E979.5
　fire or fire-producing device E979.3
　fragments from artillery shell, bomb
　　NEC, grenade, guided missile,
　　land-mine, rocket, shell, shrap-
　　nel E979.2
　gas or fumes E979.7
　grenade (explosion) (fragments)
　　E979.2
　guided missile (explosion) (fragments)
　　E979.2
　　nuclear E979.5
　heat from nuclear explosion E979.5
　hot substances E979.3
　hydrogen cyanide E979.7
　land-mine (explosion) (fragments)
　　E979.2
　laser(s) E979.8
　late effect of E999.1
　lewisite E979.7
　lung irritant (chemical) (fumes) (gas)
　　E979.7
　marine mine E979.0
　mine E979.2
　　at sea E979.0
　　in harbor E979.0
　　land (explosion) (fragments) E979.2
　　marine E979.0
　missile (explosion) (fragments) (guided)
　　E979.2
　　marine E979.0
　　nuclear weapons E979.5
　mortar bomb (explosion) (fragments)
　　E979.2
　mustard gas E979.7
　nerve gas E979.7
　nuclear weapons E979.5
　pellets (shotgun) E979.4
　petrol bomb E979.3
　phosgene E979.7
　piercing object E979.8
　poisoning (chemical) (fumes) (gas)
　　E979.7
　radiation, ionizing from nuclear explo-
　　sion E979.5
　rocket (explosion) (fragments) E979.2
　saber, sabre E979.8
　sarin E979.7
　screening smoke E979.7
　sequelae effect (of) E999.1
　shell (aircraft) (artillery) (cannon)
　　(land-based) (explosion) (frag-
　　ments) E979.2
　　sea-based E979.0
　shooting E979.4
　　bullet(s) E979.4
　　pellet(s) (rifle) (shotgun) E979.4
　shrapnel E979.2
　smallpox E979.7
　stabbing object(s) E979.8
　submersion E979.8
　torpedo E979.0
　underwater blast E979.0
　vesicant (chemical) (fumes) (gas)
　　E979.7
　weapon burst E979.2
**Thermic fever** E900.9
**Thermoplegia** E900.9
**Thirst** — *see also* Lack of water
　resulting from accident connected
　　with transport — *see* categories
　　E800-E848 ☑
**Thrown** (accidentally)
　against object in or part of vehicle
　　by motion of vehicle
　　　aircraft E844 ☑
　　　boat, ship, watercraft E838 ☑
　　　motor vehicle (on public high-
　　　　way) E818 ☑

**Thrown** — *continued*
　against object in or part of vehicle —
　　*continued*
　　by motion of vehicle — *contin-
　　　ued*
　　　motor vehicle — *continued*
　　　　not on public highway
　　　　　E825 ☑
　　　　off-road type (not on public
　　　　　highway) E821 ☑
　　　　on public highway
　　　　　E818 ☑
　　　　snow vehicle E820 ☑
　　　　　on public highway
　　　　　　E818 ☑
　　　nonmotor road vehicle NEC
　　　　E829 ☑
　　　railway rolling stock, train, vehicle
　　　　E806 ☑
　　　street car E829 ☑
　from
　　animal (being ridden) (in sport or
　　　transport) E828 ☑
　　high place, homicide (attempt)
　　　E968.1
　　machinery — *see* Accident, ma-
　　　chine
　　vehicle NEC — *see* Accident, vehi-
　　　cle NEC
　off — *see* Thrown, from
　overboard (by motion of boat, ship,
　　watercraft) E832 ☑
　　by accident to boat, ship, water-
　　　craft E830 ☑
**Thunderbolt** NEC E907
**Tidal wave** (any injury) E909.4
　caused by storm E908.0
**Took**
　overdose of drug — *see* Table of Drugs
　　and Chemicals
　poison — *see* Table of Drugs and
　　Chemicals
**Tornado** (any injury) E908.1
**Torrential rain** (any injury) E908.2
**Traffic accident NEC** E819 ☑
**Trampled by animal** E906.8
　being ridden (in sport or transport)
　　E828 ☑
**Trapped** (accidentally)
　between
　　objects (moving) (stationary and
　　　moving) E918
　by
　　door of
　　　elevator E918
　　　motor vehicle (on public high-
　　　　way) (while alighting,
　　　　boarding) — *see* Fall,
　　　　from, motor vehicle, while
　　　　alighting
　　　railway train (underground)
　　　　E806 ☑
　　　street car E829 ☑
　　　subway train E806 ☑
　in object E918
**Travel** (effects) E903
　sickness E903
**Tree**
　falling on or hitting E916
　　motor vehicle (in motion) (on public
　　　highway) E818 ☑
　　　not on public highway E825 ☑
　　nonmotor road vehicle NEC
　　　E829 ☑
　　pedal cycle E826 ☑
　　person E916
　　railway rolling stock, train, vehicle
　　　E806 ☑
　　street car E829 ☑
**Trench foot** E901.0
**Tripping over animal, carpet, curb,
　rug, or small object** (with fall)
　E885 ☑
　without fall — *see* Striking against,
　　object
**Tsunami** E909.4

**Twisting, injury in** E927

## V

**Violence, nonaccidental** — *see also* As-
　sault E968.9
**Volcanic eruption** (any injury) E909.1
**Vomitus in air passages** (with asphyxia,
　obstruction or suffocation) E911

## W

**War operations** (during hostilities) (in-
　jury) (by) (in) E995
　after cessation of hostilities, injury
　　due to E998
　air blast E993
　aircraft burned, destroyed, exploded,
　　shot down E994
　asphyxia from
　　chemical E997.2
　　fire, conflagration (caused by fire
　　　producing device or conven-
　　　tional weapon) E990.9
　　　from nuclear explosion E996
　　　petrol bomb E990.0
　　fumes E997.2
　　gas E997.2
　battle wound NEC E995
　bayonet E995
　biological warfare agents E997.1
　blast (air) (effects) E993
　　from nuclear explosion E996
　　underwater E992
　bomb (mortar) (explosion) E993
　　after cessation of hostilities E998
　　fragments, injury by E991.9
　　　antipersonnel E991.3
　bullet(s) (from carbine, machine gun,
　　pistol, rifle, shotgun) E991.2
　　rubber E991.0
　burn from
　　chemical E997.2
　　fire, conflagration (caused by fire-
　　　producing device or conven-
　　　tional weapon) E990.9
　　　from nuclear explosion E996
　　　petrol bomb E990.0
　　gas E997.2
　burning aircraft E994
　chemical E997.2
　chlorine E997.2
　conventional warfare, specified form
　　NEC E995
　crushing by falling aircraft E994
　depth charge E992
　destruction of aircraft E994
　disability as sequela one year or more
　　after injury E999.0
　drowning E995
　effect (direct) (secondary) nuclear
　　weapon E996
　explosion (artillery shell) (breech
　　block) (cannon shell) E993
　　after cessation of hostilities of
　　　bomb, mine placed in war
　　　E998
　　aircraft E994
　　bomb (mortar) E993
　　　atom E996
　　　hydrogen E996
　　　injury by fragments from
　　　　E991.9
　　　　antipersonnel E991.3
　　　nuclear E996
　　depth charge E992
　　injury by fragments from E991.9
　　　antipersonnel E991.3
　　marine weapon E992
　　mine
　　　at sea or in harbor E992
　　　land E993
　　　　injury by fragments from
　　　　　E991.9
　　　marine E992
　　munitions (accidental) (being used
　　　in war) (dump) (factory) E993

**War operations** — *continued*
　explosion — *continued*
　　nuclear (weapon) E996
　　own weapons (accidental) E993
　　　injury by fragments from
　　　　E991.9
　　　　antipersonnel E991.3
　　sea-based artillery shell E992
　　torpedo E992
　exposure to ionizing radiation from
　　nuclear explosion E996
　falling aircraft E994
　fireball effects from nuclear explosion
　　E996
　fire or fire-producing device E990.9
　　petrol bomb E990.0
　fragments from
　　antipersonnel bomb E991.3
　　artillery shell, bomb NEC, grenade,
　　　guided missile, land mine,
　　　rocket, shell, shrapnel
　　　E991.9
　fumes E997.2
　gas E997.2
　grenade (explosion) E993
　　fragments, injury by E991.9
　guided missile (explosion) E993
　　fragments, injury by E991.9
　　nuclear E996
　heat from nuclear explosion E996
　injury due to, but occurring after ces-
　　sation of hostilities E998
　lacrimator (gas) (chemical) E997.2
　land mine (explosion) E993
　　after cessation of hostilities E998
　　fragments, injury by E991.9
　laser(s) E997.0
　late effect of E999.0
　lewisite E997.2
　lung irritant (chemical) (fumes) (gas)
　　E997.2
　marine mine E992
　mine
　　after cessation of hostilities E998
　　at sea E992
　　in harbor E992
　　land (explosion) E993
　　　fragments, injury by E991.9
　　marine E992
　missile (guided) (explosion) E993
　　fragments, injury by E991.9
　　marine E992
　　nuclear E996
　mortar bomb (explosion) E993
　　fragments, injury by E991.9
　mustard gas E997.2
　nerve gas E997.2
　phosgene E997.2
　poisoning (chemical) (fumes) (gas)
　　E997.2
　radiation, ionizing from nuclear explo-
　　sion E996
　rocket (explosion) E993
　　fragments, injury by E991.9
　saber, sabre E995
　screening smoke E997.8
　shell (aircraft) (artillery) (cannon) (land
　　based) (explosion) E993
　　fragments, injury by E991.9
　　sea-based E992
　shooting E991.2
　　after cessation of hostilities E998
　　bullet(s) E991.2
　　　rubber E991.0
　　pellet(s) (rifle) E991.1
　　shrapnel E991.9
　　submersion E995
　　torpedo E992
　unconventional warfare, except by
　　nuclear weapon E997.9
　　biological (warfare) E997.1
　　gas, fumes, chemicals E997.2
　　laser(s) E997.0
　　specified type NEC E997.8
　underwater blast E992

Terrorism — War operations

☑ Additional Digit Required — Refer to the Tabular List for Digit Selection　　　　　▽ Subterms under main terms may continue to next column or page

*2008 ICD-9-CM*　　　▶◀ Revised Text　　　● New Line　　　▲ Revised Code　　　**Volume 2 — 353**

**War operations** — *continued*
vesicant (chemical) (fumes) (gas) E997.2
weapon burst E993

**Washed**
away by flood — *see* Flood
away by tidal wave — *see* Tidal wave
off road by storm (transport vehicle) E908.9

**Washed** — *continued*
overboard E832 ☑

**Weather exposure** — *see also* Exposure
cold E901.0
hot E900.0

**Weightlessness** (causing injury) (effects of) (in spacecraft, real or simulated) E928.0

**Wound** (accidental) NEC — *see also* Injury E928.9
battle (*see also* War operations) E995
bayonet E920.3
in
legal intervention E974
war operations E995
gunshot — *see* Shooting
incised — *see* Cut

**Wound** — *see also* Injury — *continued*
saber, sabre E920.3
in war operations E995

---

## Railway Accidents (E800-E807)

The following fourth-digit subdivisions are for use with categories E800-E807 to identify the injured person:

**.0 Railway employee**
Any person who by virtue of his employment in connection with a railway, whether by the railway company or not, is at increased risk of involvement in a railway accident, such as:
catering staff on train
postal staff on train
driver
railway fireman
guard
shunter
porter
sleeping car attendant

**.1 Passenger on railway**
Any authorized person traveling on a train, except a railway employee
EXCLUDES    intending passenger waiting at station (.8)
unauthorized rider on railway vehicle (.8)

**.2 Pedestrian** See definition (r), E-Codes-2

**.3 Pedal cyclist** See definition (p), E-Codes-2

**.8 Other specified person** Intending passenger waiting at station
Unauthorized rider on railway vehicle

**.9 Unspecified person**

## Motor Vehicle Traffic and Nontraffic Accidents (E810-E825)

The following fourth-digit subdivisions are for use with categories E810-E819 and E820-E825 to identify the injured person:

**.0 Driver of motor vehicle other than motorcycle** See definition (1), E-Codes-2

**.1 Passenger in motor vehicle other than motorcycle** See definition (1), E-Codes-2

**.2 Motorcyclist** See definition (1), E-Codes-2

**.3 Passenger on motorcycle** See definition (1), E-Codes-2

**.4 Occupant of streetcar**

**.5 Rider of animal; occupant of animal-drawn vehicle**

**.6 Pedal cyclist** See definition (p), E-Codes-2

**.7 Pedestrian** See definition (r), E-Codes-2

**.8 Other specified person**
Occupant of vehicle other than above
Person in railway train involved in accident
Unauthorized rider of motor vehicle

**.9 Unspecified person**

### Other Road Vehicle Accidents (E826-E829)
**(animal-drawn vehicle, streetcar, pedal cycle, and other nonmotor road vehicle accidents)**

The following fourth-digit subdivisions are for use with categories E826-E829 to identify the injured person:

**.0 Pedestrian** See definition (r), E-Codes-2

**.1 Pedal cyclist** (does not apply to codes E827, E828, E829) See definition (p), E-Codes-2

**.2 Rider of animal** (does not apply to code E829)

**.3 Occupant of animal-drawn vehicle** (does not apply to codes E828, E829)

**.4 Occupant of streetcar**

**.8 Other specified person**

**.9 Unspecified person**

---

## Water Transport Accidents (E830-E838)

The following fourth-digit subdivisions are for use with categories E830-E838 to identify the injured person:

**.0 Occupant of small boat, unpowered**

**.1 Occupant of small boat, powered** See definition (t), E-Codes-2
EXCLUDES    water skier (.4)

**.2 Occupant of other watercraft — crew**
Persons:
engaged in operation of watercraft
providing passenger services [cabin attendants, ship's physician, catering personnel]
working on ship during voyage in other capacity [musician in band, operators of shops and beauty parlors]

**.3 Occupant of other watercraft — other than crew**
Passenger
Occupant of lifeboat, other than crew, after abandoning ship

**.4 Water skier**

**.5 Swimmer**

**.6 Dockers, stevedores**
Longshoreman employed on the dock in loading and unloading ships

**.8 Other specified person**
Immigration and custom officials on board ship
Persons:
accompanying passenger or member of crew visiting boat
Pilot (guiding ship into port)

**.9 Unspecified person**

### Air and Space Transport Accidents (E840-E845)

The following fourth-digit subdivisions are for use with categories E840-E845 to identify the injured person:

**.0 Occupant of spacecraft**
Crew
Passenger (civilian)          in military aircraft [air force]
(military)          [army] [national guard] [navy]
Troops

**.1 Occupant of military aircraft, any**
EXCLUDES    occupants of aircraft operated under jurisdiction of police departments (.5) parachutist (.7)

**.2 Crew of commercial aircraft (powered) in surface to surface transport**

**.3 Other occupant of commercial aircraft (powered) in surface to surface transport**
Flight personnel:
not part of crew
on familiarization flight Passenger on aircraft

**.4 Occupant of commercial aircraft (powered) in surface to air transport**
Occupant [crew] [passenger] of aircraft (powered) engaged in activities, such as:
air drops of emergency supplies
air drops of parachutists, except from military craft
crop dusting
lowering of construction material [bridge or telephone pole]
sky writing

**.5 Occupant of other powered aircraft**
Occupant [crew] [passenger] of aircraft (powered) engaged in activities, such as:
aerial spraying (crops)(fire retardants)
aerobatic flying
aircraft racing
rescue operation
storm surveillance
traffic suveillance
Occupant of private plane NOS

**.6 Occupant of unpowered aircraft, except parachutist**
Occupant of aircraft classifiable to E842

**.7 Parachutist (military)(other)**
Person making voluntary descent
person making descent after accident to aircraft (.1-.6)

**.8 Ground crew, airline employee**
Persons employed at airfields (civil)(military) or launching pads, not occupants of aircraft

**.9 Other person**

---

☑ Additional Digit Required — Refer to the Tabular List for Digit Selection

ᵂ Subterms under main terms may continue to next column or page

# 1. INFECTIOUS AND PARASITIC DISEASES (001-139)

Note: Categories for "late effects" of infectious and parasitic diseases are to be found at 137-139.

INCLUDES   diseases generally recognized as communicable or transmissible as well as a few diseases of unknown but possibly infectious origin

EXCLUDES   acute respiratory infections (460-466)
carrier or suspected carrier of infectious organism (V02.0-V02.9)
certain localized infections
influenza ►(487.0-487.8, 488)◄

## INTESTINAL INFECTIOUS DISEASES (001-009)

EXCLUDES   helminthiases (120.0-129)

### √4th 001 Cholera

DEF: An acute infectious enteritis caused by a potent enterotoxin elaborated by *Vibrio cholerae*; the vibrio produces a toxin in the intestinal tract that changes the permeability of the mucosa leading to diarrhea and dehydration.

**001.0 Due to Vibrio cholerae** CC
CC Excl: 001.0-001.9

**001.1 Due to Vibrio cholerae el tor** CC
CC Excl: See code: 001.0

**001.9 Cholera, unspecified** CC
CC Excl: See code: 001.0

### √4th 002 Typhoid and paratyphoid fevers

DEF: Typhoid fever: an acute generalized illness caused by *Salmonella typhi*; notable clinical features are fever, headache, abdominal pain, cough, toxemia, leukopenia, abnormal pulse, rose spots on the skin, bacteremia, hyperplasia of intestinal lymph nodes, mesenteric lymphadenopathy, and Peyer's patches in the intestines.

DEF: Paratyphoid fever: a prolonged febrile illness, much like typhoid but usually less severe; caused by salmonella serotypes other than *S. typhi*, especially *S. enteritidis* serotypes paratyphi A and B and *S. choleraesuis*.

**002.0 Typhoid fever** CC
Typhoid (fever) (infection) [any site]
CC Excl: 002.0-002.9

**002.1 Paratyphoid fever A** CC
CC Excl: See code: 002.0

**002.2 Paratyphoid fever B** CC
CC Excl: See code: 002.0

**002.3 Paratyphoid fever C** CC
CC Excl: See code: 002.0

**002.9 Paratyphoid fever, unspecified** CC
CC Excl: See code: 002.0

### √4th 003 Other salmonella infections

INCLUDES   infection or food poisoning by Salmonella [any serotype]

DEF: Infections caused by a genus of gram-negative, anaerobic bacteria of the family *Enterobacteriaceae*; affecting warm-blooded animals, like humans; major symptoms are enteric fevers, acute gastroenteritis and septicemia.

**003.0 Salmonella gastroenteritis** CC
Salmonellosis
CC Excl: 002.0, 0 02.9-003.0, 004.9-005.2, 007.5, 008.00-009.0, 040.41-040.42, 536.8, 558.2-558.9, 564.1, 567.21, 567.23, 567.31-567.39, 567.89, 777.5, 777.8

**003.1 Salmonella septicemia** MCC HIV
CC Excl: 003.1, 020.2, 022.3, 036.2, 038.0-038.9, 040.89-041.85, 041.89-041.9, 054.5, 139.8, 771.81, 771.83-771.89, 995.90-995.94, V09.0-V09.91

### √5th 003.2 Localized salmonella infections

**003.20 Localized salmonella infection, unspecified** HIV

**003.21 Salmonella meningitis** MCC HIV
CC Excl: 003.21, 013.00-013.16, 036.0, 047.0-047.9, 049.0-049.1, 072.1, 078.88-078.89, 079.81, 079.88-079.99, 090.42, 091.81, 094.2, 098.89, 100.81, 112.83, 114.2, 115.01, 115.11, 115.91, 130.0, 139.8, 320.0-322.9, 349.89-349.9

**003.22 Salmonella pneumonia** MCC HIV
CC Excl: 003.22, 011.00-012.16, 012.80-012.86, 017.90-017.96, 020.3-020.5, 021.3, 022.1, 031.0, 039.1, 073.0, 115.05, 115.15, 115.95, 122.1, 130.4, 136.3, 480.0-480.2, 480.8-487.1, 488, 495.0-495.7, 500, 502-508.9, 517.1, 517.8, 518.89, 519.8-519.9

**003.23 Salmonella arthritis** CC HIV
CC Excl: 003.23, 015.80-015.96, 036.82, 056.71, 098.50-098.51, 098.59, 098.89, 711.00-714.0, 715.00, 715.09-715.10, 715.18-716.99, 718.00-718.08, 719.00-719.10, 719.18-719.69, 719.80-719.99

**003.24 Salmonella osteomyelitis** CC HIV
CC Excl: 003.24, 015.50-015.56, 015.70-015.76, 015.90-015.96, 730.00-730.39, 730.80-730.99

**003.29 Other** CC HIV
CC Excl: 003.29

**003.8 Other specified salmonella infections** CC HIV
CC Excl: 003.8

**003.9 Salmonella infection, unspecified** CC HIV
CC Excl: 003.9

### √4th 004 Shigellosis

INCLUDES   bacillary dysentery

DEF: Acute infectious dysentery caused by the genus *Shigella*, of the family *Enterobacteriaceae*; affecting the colon causing the release of blood-stained stools with accompanying tenesmus, abdominal cramps and fever.

**004.0 Shigella dysenteriae** CC
Infection by group A Shigella (Schmitz) (Shiga)
CC Excl: 001.1, 002.0, 002.9-003.0, 004.0, 004.9-005.2, 006.0-006.2, 006.9, 007.1-007.9, 008.1-008.3, 008.5, 008.8-009.0, 014.80-014.86, 040.41-040.42, 112.85, 129, 487.8, 536.3, 536.8, 555.0-557.9, 558.2-558.9, 564.1, 775.0-775.7, 775.9, 777.5, 777.8

**004.1 Shigella flexneri**
Infection by group B Shigella

**004.2 Shigella boydii**
Infection by group C Shigella

**004.3 Shigella sonnei**
Infection by group D Shigella

**004.8 Other specified Shigella infections**

**004.9 Shigellosis, unspecified**

### √4th 005 Other food poisoning (bacterial)

EXCLUDES   salmonella infections (003.0-003.9)
toxic effect of:
    food contaminants (989.7)
    noxious foodstuffs (988.0-988.9)

DEF: Enteritis caused by ingesting contaminated foods and characterized by diarrhea, abdominal pain, vomiting; symptoms may be mild or life threatening.

**005.0 Staphylococcal food poisoning** CC
Staphylococcal toxemia specified as due to food
CC Excl: 001.0-009.3, 040.41-040.42

▲ **005.1 Botulism food poisoning** CC
►Botulism NOS◄
Food poisoning due to Clostridium botulinum
EXCLUDES   ► infant botulism (040.41)
    wound botulism (040.42)◄
CC Excl: 005.0-005.2, 008.45-008.46, 040.41-040.42

**005.2 Food poisoning due to Clostridium perfringens** CC
**[C. welchii]**
Enteritis necroticans
CC Excl: 003.0, 004.9-005.2, 007.5, 008.00-009.0, 040.41-040.42, 487.8, 536.3, 536.8, 558.2-558.9, 564.1, 567.21, 567.23, 567.31-567.39, 567.89, 777.5, 777.8

---

√4th Additional Digit Required     Unacceptable PDx     Manifestation Code     ►◄ Revised Text     ● New Code     ▲ Revised Code Title

**005.3 Food poisoning due to other Clostridia** `CC`
**CC Excl:** See code: 005.0

**005.4 Food poisoning due to Vibrio parahaemolyticus** `CC`
**CC Excl:** See code: 005.0

√5th **005.8 Other bacterial food poisoning**
**EXCLUDES** *salmonella food poisoning (003.0-003.9)*

**005.81 Food poisoning due to Vibrio vulnificus** `CC`
**CC Excl:** See code: 005.0

**005.89 Other bacterial food poisoning** `CC`
Food poisoning due to Bacillus cereus
**CC Excl:** See code: 005.0

**005.9 Food poisoning, unspecified**

√4th **006 Amebiasis**
**INCLUDES** infection due to Entamoeba histolytica
**EXCLUDES** *amebiasis due to organisms other than Entamoeba histolytica (007.8)*
**DEF:** Infection of the large intestine caused by *Entamoeba histolytica*; usually asymptomatic but symptoms may range from mild diarrhea to profound life-threatening dysentery. Extraintestinal complications include hepatic abscess, which may rupture into the lung, pericardium or abdomen, causing life-threatening infections.

**006.0 Acute amebic dysentery without mention of abscess** `CC`
Acute amebiasis
**CC Excl:** 006.0-006.1, 007.5
**DEF:** Sudden, severe *Entamoeba histolytica* infection causing bloody stools.

**006.1 Chronic intestinal amebiasis without mention of abscess** `CC`
Chronic:
amebiasis
amebic dysentery
**CC Excl:** See code: 006.0

**006.2 Amebic nondysenteric colitis** `CC`
**CC Excl:** 003.0, 004.9-005.0, 005.2, 006.0-006.2, 006.9, 007.1-009.0, 129, 487.8, 536.3, 536.8, 555.0-557.9, 558.2-558.9, 564.1, 777.5, 777.8
**DEF:** *Entamoeba histolytica* infection with inflamed colon but no dysentery.

**006.3 Amebic liver abscess** `MCC`
Hepatic amebiasis
**CC Excl:** 006.3, 572.0

**006.4 Amebic lung abscess** `MCC`
Amebic abscess of lung (and liver)
**CC Excl:** 006.4, 513.0

**006.5 Amebic brain abscess** `MCC`
Amebic abscess of brain (and liver) (and lung)
**CC Excl:** 006.5, 324.0

**006.6 Amebic skin ulceration**
Cutaneous amebiasis

**006.8 Amebic infection of other sites** `CC`
Amebic: Ameboma
appendicitis
balanitis
**EXCLUDES** *specific infections by free-living amebae (136.2)*
**CC Excl:** 006.0-006.5, 006.8

**006.9 Amebiasis, unspecified**
Amebiasis NOS

√4th **007 Other protozoal intestinal diseases**
**INCLUDES** protozoal:
colitis
diarrhea
dysentery

**007.0 Balantidiasis**
Infection by Balantidium coli

**007.1 Giardiasis** `CC`
Infection by Giardia lamblia  Lambliasis
**CC Excl:** 003.0, 004.9-005.0, 005.2, 006.0-006.2, 006.9, 007.1-009.0, 129, 487.8, 536.3, 536.8, 558.2-558.9, 564.1

**007.2 Coccidiosis** `CC` `HIV`
Infection by Isospora belli and Isospora hominis
Isosporiasis
**CC Excl:** See code: 007.1

**007.3 Intestinal trichomoniasis**
**DEF:** Colitis, diarrhea, or dysentery caused by the protozoa *Trichomonas*.

**007.4 Cryptosporidiosis** `CC`
**CC Excl:** See code: 007.1
**AHA:** 4Q, '97, 30
**DEF:** An intestinal infection by protozoan parasites causing intractable diarrhea in patients with AIDS and other immunosuppressed individuals.

**007.5 Cyclosporiasis** `CC`
**CC Excl:** 003.0, 004.9-005.0, 005.2, 006.0-006.2, 006.9, 007.1-009.0, 129, 487.8, 536.3, 536.8, 558.2-558.9, 564.1, 567.21, 567.23, 567.31-567.39, 567.89
**AHA:** 4Q, '00, 38
**DEF:** An infection of the small intestine by the protozoal organism, *Cyclospora caytenanesis*, spread to humans though ingestion of contaminated water or food. Symptoms include watery diarrhea with frequent explosive bowel movements, loss of appetite, loss of weight, bloating, increased gas, stomach cramps, nausea, vomiting, muscle aches, low grade fever, and fatigue.

**007.8 Other specified protozoal intestinal diseases** `CC`
Amebiasis due to organisms other than Entamoeba histolytica
**CC Excl:** See code: 007.1

**007.9 Unspecified protozoal intestinal disease** `CC`
Flagellate diarrhea
Protozoal dysentery NOS
**CC Excl:** See code: 007.1

√4th **008 Intestinal infections due to other organisms**
**INCLUDES** any condition classifiable to 009.0-009.3 with mention of the responsible organisms
**EXCLUDES** *food poisoning by these organisms (005.0-005.9)*

√5th **008.0 Escherichia coli [E. coli]**
**AHA:** 4Q, '92, 17

**008.00 E. coli, unspecified** `CC`
E. coli enteritis NOS
**CC Excl:** 003.0, 004.9-005.0, 005.2, 007.5, 008.00-009.0, 487.8, 536.3, 536.8, 558.2-558.9, 564.1, 567.21, 567.23, 567.31-567.39, 567.89, 777.5, 777.8

**008.01 Enteropathogenic E. coli** `CC`
**CC Excl:** See code: 008.00
**DEF:** *E. coli* causing inflammation of intestines.

**008.02 Enterotoxigenic E. coli** `CC`
**CC Excl:** See code: 008.00
**DEF:** A toxic reaction to *E. coli* of the intestinal mucosa, causing voluminous watery secretions.

**008.03 Enteroinvasive E. coli** `CC`
**CC Excl:** See code: 008.00
**DEF:** *E. coli* infection penetrating intestinal mucosa.

**008.04 Enterohemorrhagic E. coli** `CC`
**CC Excl:** See code: 008.00
**DEF:** *E. coli* infection penetrating the intestinal mucosa, producing microscopic ulceration and bleeding.

`N` Newborn Age: 0    `P` Pediatric Age: 0-17    `M` Maternity Age: 12-55    `A` Adult Age: 15-124    `CC` CC Condition    `MCC` Major CC Condition    `HIV` HIV Related Dx

2 — Volume 1 • October 2007

© *2007 Ingenix*

**008.09 Other intestinal E. coli infections** CC
  CC Excl: See code: 008.00

**008.1 Arizona group of paracolon bacilli** CC
  CC Excl: See code: 008.00

**008.2 Aerobacter aerogenes** CC
  Enterobacter aeogenes
  CC Excl: See code: 008.00

**008.3 Proteus (mirabilis) (morganii)** CC
  CC Excl: See code: 008.00

✓5th **008.4 Other specified bacteria**
  AHA: 4Q, '92, 18

  **008.41 Staphylococcus** CC
    Staphylococcal enterocolitis
    CC Excl: 001.1, 002.0, 002.9-003.0, 004.9-005.2, 006.0-006.2, 006.9, 007.1-009.0, 014.80-014.86, 040.41-040.42, 112.85, 129, 487.8, 536.3, 536.8, 555.0-557.9, 558.2-558.9, 564.1, 775.0-775.7, 775.9, 777.5, 777.8

  **008.42 Pseudomonas** CC
    CC Excl: See code: 008.41
    AHA: 2Q, '89, 10

  **008.43 Campylobacter** CC
    CC Excl: See code 008.41

  **008.44 Yersinia enterocolitica** CC
    CC Excl: See code 008.41

  **008.45 Clostridium difficile** CC
    Pseudomembranous colitis
    CC Excl: See code 008.41

    DEF: An overgrowth of a species of bacterium that is a part of the normal colon flora in human infants and sometimes in adults; produces a toxin that causes pseudomembranous enterocolitis.; typically is seen in patients undergoing antibiotic therapy.

  **008.46 Other anaerobes** CC
    Anaerobic enteritis NOS
    Bacteroides (fragilis)
    Gram-negative anaerobes
    CC Excl: See code 008.41

  **008.47 Other gram-negative bacteria** CC
    Gram-negative enteritis NOS
    EXCLUDES   gram-negative anaerobes (008.46)
    CC Excl: See code 008.41

  **008.49 Other** CC
    CC Excl: See code 008.41
    AHA: 2Q, '89, 10; 1Q, '88, 6

**008.5 Bacterial enteritis, unspecified** CC
  CC Excl: 001.1, 002.0, 002.9-003.0, 004.9-005.0, 005.2, 006.0-006.2, 006.9, 007.1-009.0, 014.80-014.86, 112.85, 129, 487.8, 536.3, 536.8, 558.2-558.9, 564.1, 567.21, 567.23, 567.31-567.39, 567.89, 777.5, 777.8

✓5th **008.6 Enteritis due to specified virus**
  AHA: 4Q, '92, 18

  **008.61 Rotavirus** CC
    CC Excl: 003.0, 004.9-005.0, 005.2, 006.0-006.2, 006.9, 007.1-009.0, 014.80-014.86, 112.85, 129, 487.8, 536.3, 536.8, 558.2-558.9, 564.1, 567.21, 567.23, 567.31-567.39, 567.89, 777.5, 777.8

  **008.62 Adenovirus** CC
    CC Excl: See code: 008.61

  **008.63 Norwalk virus** CC
    Norwalk-like agent
    CC Excl: See code: 008.61

**008.64 Other small round viruses [SRVs]** CC
  Small round virus NOS
  CC Excl: See code: 008.61

**008.65 Calicivirus** CC
  CC Excl: See code: 008.61
  DEF: Enteritis due to a subgroup of *Picornaviruses*.

**008.66 Astrovirus** CC
  CC Excl: See code: 008.61

**008.67 Enterovirus NEC** CC
  Coxsackie virus        Echovirus
    EXCLUDES   poliovirus (045.0-045.9)
  CC Excl: See code: 008.61

**008.69 Other viral enteritis** CC
  Torovirus
  CC Excl: See code: 008.61
  AHA: 1Q, '03, 10

**008.8 Other organism, not elsewhere classified**
  Viral:               Viral:
    enteritis NOS        gastroenteritis
    EXCLUDES   influenza with involvement of gastrointestinal tract (487.8)

✓4th **009 Ill-defined intestinal infections**
    EXCLUDES   diarrheal disease or intestinal infection due to specified organism (001.0-008.8)
      diarrhea following gastrointestinal surgery (564.4)
      intestinal malabsorption (579.0-579.9)
      ischemic enteritis (557.0-557.9)
      other noninfectious gastroenteritis and colitis (558.1-558.9)
      regional enteritis (555.0-555.9)
      ulcerative colitis (556)

**009.0 Infectious colitis, enteritis, and gastroenteritis** CC
  Colitis  ⎫
  Enteritis ⎬ septic
  Gastroenteritis ⎭

  Dysentery:           Dysentery:
    NOS                  hemorrhagic
    catarrhal
  CC Excl: 001.0-009.3, 040.41-040.42
  AHA: 3Q, '99, 4

  DEF: Colitis: An inflammation of mucous membranes of the colon.
  DEF: Enteritis: An inflammation of mucous membranes of the small intestine.
  DEF: Gastroenteritis: An inflammation of mucous membranes of stomach and intestines.

**009.1 Colitis, enteritis, and gastroenteritis of presumed infectious origin** CC
    EXCLUDES   colitis NOS (558.9)
      enteritis NOS (558.9)
      gastroenteritis NOS (558.9)
  CC Excl: 009.1
  AHA: 3Q, '99, 6

**009.2 Infectious diarrhea** CC
  Diarrhea:
    dysenteric
    epidemic
  Infectious diarrheal disease NOS
  CC Excl: See code: 009.0

**009.3 Diarrhea of presumed infectious origin** CC
    EXCLUDES   diarrhea NOS (787.91)
  CC Excl: 009.3
  AHA: N-D, '87, 7

---

✓4th
✓5th  Additional Digit Required          Unacceptable PDx          Manifestation Code          ▶◀ Revised Text          ● New Code          ▲ Revised Code Title

## TUBERCULOSIS (010-018)

INCLUDES    infection by Mycobacterium tuberculosis (human) (bovine)

EXCLUDES    *congenital tuberculosis (771.2)*
*late effects of tuberculosis (137.0-137.4)*

The following fifth-digit subclassification is for use with categories 010-018:

0 **unspecified**
1 **bacteriological or histological examination not done**
2 **bacteriological or histological examination unknown (at present)**
3 **tubercle bacilli found (in sputum) by microscopy**
4 **tubercle bacilli not found (in sputum) by microscopy, but found by bacterial culture**
5 **tubercle bacilli not found by bacteriological examination, but tuberculosis confirmed histologically**
6 **tubercle bacilli not found by bacteriological or histological examination but tuberculosis confirmed by other methods [inoculation of animals]**

DEF: An infection by *Mycobacterium tuberculosis* causing the formation of small, rounded nodules, called tubercles, that can disseminate throughout the body via lymph and blood vessels. Localized tuberculosis is most often seen in the lungs.

√4ᵗʰ **010 Primary tuberculous infection**

DEF: Tuberculosis of the lungs occurring when the patient is first infected.

§ √5ᵗʰ **010.0    Primary tuberculous infection**    CC HIV
EXCLUDES    *nonspecific reaction to tuberculin skin test without active tuberculosis (795.5)*
*positive PPD (795.5)*
*positive tuberculin skin test without active tuberculosis (795.5)*
**CC Excl:** 010.00-018.96

DEF: Hilar or paratracheal lymph node enlargement in pulmonary tuberculosis.

§ √5ᵗʰ **010.1    Tuberculous pleurisy in primary progressive tuberculosis**    CC HIV
**CC Excl:** See code: 010.0

DEF: Inflammation and exudation in the lining of the tubercular lung.

§ √5ᵗʰ **010.8    Other primary progressive tuberculosis**    CC HIV
EXCLUDES    *tuberculous erythema nodosum (017.1)*
**CC Excl:** See code: 010.0

§ √5ᵗʰ **010.9    Primary tuberculous infection, unspecified**    CC HIV
**CC Excl:** See code: 010.0

√4ᵗʰ **011 Pulmonary tuberculosis**    HIV
Use additional code to identify any associated silicosis (502)

§ √5ᵗʰ **011.0    Tuberculosis of lung, infiltrative**    CC HIV
**CC Excl:** 011.00-012.86, 017.90-018.96, 031.0, 031.2-031.9, 041.81-041.9, 137.0, 139.8, 480.0-480.2, 480.8-487.1, 488, 494.0-508.9, 517.1, 518.89

§ √5ᵗʰ **011.1    Tuberculosis of lung, nodular**    CC HIV
**CC Excl:** See code: 011.0

§ √5ᵗʰ **011.2    Tuberculosis of lung with cavitation**    CC HIV
**CC Excl:** See code: 011.0

§ √5ᵗʰ **011.3    Tuberculosis of bronchus**    CC HIV
EXCLUDES    *isolated bronchial tuberculosis (012.2)*
**CC Excl:** See code: 011.0

§ √5ᵗʰ **011.4    Tuberculous fibrosis of lung**    CC HIV
**CC Excl:** See code: 011.0

§ √5ᵗʰ **011.5    Tuberculous bronchiectasis**    CC HIV
**CC Excl:** See code: 011.0

§ √5ᵗʰ **011.6    Tuberculous pneumonia [any form]**    MCC HIV
**CC Excl:** For codes 011.60-011.65: See code 011.0; For code 011.66: 011.66, 139.8, 480.0-480.2, 480.8-487.1, 488, 494.0-508.9, 517.1, 518.89

DEF: Inflammatory pulmonary reaction to tuberculous cells.

§ √5ᵗʰ **011.7    Tuberculous pneumothorax**    CC HIV
**CC Excl:** See code: 011.0

DEF: Spontaneous rupture of damaged tuberculous pulmonary tissue.

§ √5ᵗʰ **011.8    Other specified pulmonary tuberculosis**    CC HIV
**CC Excl:** See code: 011.0

§ √5ᵗʰ **011.9    Pulmonary tuberculosis, unspecified**    CC HIV
Respiratory tuberculosis NOS
Tuberculosis of lung NOS
**CC Excl:** See code: 011.0

√4ᵗʰ **012 Other respiratory tuberculosis**
EXCLUDES    *respiratory tuberculosis, unspecified (011.9)*

§ √5ᵗʰ **012.0    Tuberculous pleurisy**    CC HIV
Tuberculosis of pleura
Tuberculous empyema
Tuberculous hydrothorax
EXCLUDES    *pleurisy with effusion without mention of cause (511.9)*
*tuberculous pleurisy in primary progressive tuberculosis (010.1)*
**CC Excl:** 011.00-012.86, 017.90-018.96, 031.0, 031.2-031.9, 041.81-041.9, 137.0, 139.8, 480.0-480.2, 480.8-487.1, 488, 494.0-508.9, 517.1, 518.89

DEF: Inflammation and exudation in the lining of the tubercular lung.

§ √5ᵗʰ **012.1    Tuberculosis of intrathoracic lymph nodes**    CC HIV
Tuberculosis of lymph nodes:
hilar
mediastinal
tracheobronchial
Tuberculous tracheobronchial adenopathy
EXCLUDES    *that specified as primary (010.0-010.9)*
**CC Excl:** See code: 012.0

§ √5ᵗʰ **012.2    Isolated tracheal or bronchial tuberculosis**    CC HIV
**CC Excl:** 010.00-014.86, 018.00-018.96

§ √5ᵗʰ **012.3    Tuberculous laryngitis**    CC HIV
Tuberculosis of glottis
**CC Excl:** See code: 012.2

§ √5ᵗʰ **012.8    Other specified respiratory tuberculosis**    CC HIV
Tuberculosis of:        Tuberculosis of:
mediastinum        nose (septum)
nasopharynx        sinus [any nasal]
**CC Excl:** See code: 012.2

√4ᵗʰ **013 Tuberculosis of meninges and central nervous system**

§ √5ᵗʰ **013.0    Tuberculous meningitis**    MCC HIV
Tuberculosis of meninges (cerebral) (spinal)
Tuberculous:
leptomeningitis
meningoencephalitis
EXCLUDES    *tuberculoma of meninges (013.1)*
**CC Excl:** 003.21, 013.00-013.16, 013.40-013.56, 013.80-013.96, 017.90-017.96, 031.2-031.9, 036.0, 041.81-041.9, 047.0-047.9, 049.0-049.1, 053.0, 054.72, 072.1, 090.42, 091.81, 094.2, 098.89, 100.81, 112.83, 114.2, 115.01, 115.11, 115.91, 130.0, 137.1, 139.8, 320.0-322.9, 349.89-349.9, 357.0

§ √5ᵗʰ **013.1    Tuberculoma of meninges**    MCC HIV
**CC Excl:** See code: 013.0

---

§    Requires fifth-digit. See beginning of section 010-018 for codes and definitions.

N Newborn Age: 0    P Pediatric Age: 0-17    M Maternity Age: 12-55    A Adult Age: 15-124    CC CC Condition    MCC Major CC Condition    HIV HIV Related Dx

4 — Volume 1 • October 2007    © 2007 Ingenix

§ ✓5ᵗʰ **013.2** **Tuberculoma of brain** `MCC` `HIV`
Tuberculosis of brain (current disease)
**CC Excl:** 013.20-013.36, 013.60-013.96, 017.90-017.96, 031.2-031.9, 041.81-041.9, 137.1, 139.8

§ ✓5ᵗʰ **013.3** **Tuberculous abscess of brain** `MCC` `HIV`
**CC Excl:** See code: 013.2

§ ✓5ᵗʰ **013.4** **Tuberculoma of spinal cord** `MCC` `HIV`
**CC Excl:** 013.00-013.16, 013.40-013.56, 013.80-013.96, 017.90-017.96, 031.2-031.9, 041.81-041.9, 137.1, 139.8

§ ✓5ᵗʰ **013.5** **Tuberculous abscess of spinal cord** `MCC` `HIV`
**CC Excl:** See code: 013.4

§ ✓5ᵗʰ **013.6** **Tuberculous encephalitis or myelitis** `MCC` `HIV`
**CC Excl:** See code: 013.2

§ ✓5ᵗʰ **013.8** **Other specified tuberculosis of central** `MCC` `HIV`
**nervous system**
**CC Excl:** 013.80-013.96, 017.90-017.96, 031.2-031.9, 041.81-041.9, 137.1, 139.8

§ ✓5ᵗʰ **013.9** **Unspecified tuberculosis of central nervous** `MCC` `HIV`
**system**
Tuberculosis of central nervous system NOS
**CC Excl:** See code: 013.8

✓4ᵗʰ **014 Tuberculosis of intestines, peritoneum, and mesenteric glands**

§ ✓5ᵗʰ **014.0** **Tuberculous peritonitis** `MCC` `HIV`
Tuberculous ascites
**CC Excl:** 014.00-014.86, 017.90-017.96, 031.2-031.9, 041.81-041.9, 139.8

**DEF:** Tuberculous inflammation of the membrane lining the abdomen.

§ ✓5ᵗʰ **014.8** **Other** `CC` `HIV`
Tuberculosis (of):
anus
intestine (large) (small)
mesenteric glands
rectum
retroperitoneal (lymph nodes)
Tuberculous enteritis
**CC Excl: For codes 014.80, 014.82-014.86:** 014.00-014.86, 017.90-017.96, 031.2-031.9, 041.81-041.9, 139.8; **For code 014.81:** 014.81, 139.8

✓4ᵗʰ **015 Tuberculosis of bones and joints**
Use additional code to identify manifestation, as:
tuberculous:
arthropathy (711.4)
necrosis of bone (730.8)
osteitis (730.8)
osteomyelitis (730.8)
synovitis (727.01)
tenosynovitis (727.01)

§ ✓5ᵗʰ **015.0** **Vertebral column** `CC` `HIV`
Pott's disease
Use additional code to identify manifestation, as:
curvature of spine [Pott's] (737.4)
kyphosis (737.4)
spondylitis (720.81)
**CC Excl:** 015.00-015.06

§ ✓5ᵗʰ **015.1** **Hip** `CC` `HIV`
**CC Excl:** 015.10-015.16

§ ✓5ᵗʰ **015.2** **Knee** `CC` `HIV`
**CC Excl:** 015.20-015.26

§ ✓5ᵗʰ **015.5** **Limb bones** `CC` `HIV`
Tuberculous dactylitis
**CC Excl:** 015.10-015.56

§ ✓5ᵗʰ **015.6** **Mastoid** `CC` `HIV`
Tuberculous mastoiditis
**CC Excl:** 015.60-015.66

§ ✓5ᵗʰ **015.7** **Other specified bone** `CC` `HIV`
**CC Excl: For code 015.70:** 015.00-015.70; **For code 015.71:** 015.00-015.66, 015.71; **For code 015.72:** 015.00-015.66, 015.72; **For code 015.73:** 015.00-015.66, 015.73; **For code 015.74:** 015.00-015.66, 015.74; **For code 015.75:** 015.00-015.66, 015.75; **For code 015.76:** 015.00-015.66, 015.76

§ ✓5ᵗʰ **015.8** **Other specified joint** `CC` `HIV`
**CC Excl:** 015.80-015.86

§ ✓5ᵗʰ **015.9** **Tuberculosis of unspecified bones and joints** `CC` `HIV`
**CC Excl: For codes 015.90, 015.92-015.96:** 015.00-015.66, 015.80-015.96; **For codes 015.91:** 015.00-015.66, 015.80-015.93, 015.95-015.96

✓4ᵗʰ **016 Tuberculosis of genitourinary system**

§ ✓5ᵗʰ **016.0** **Kidney** `CC` `HIV`
Renal tuberculosis
Use additional code to identify manifestation, as:
tuberculous:
nephropathy (583.81)
pyelitis (590.81)
pyelonephritis (590.81)
**CC Excl:** 016.00-016.36, 016.90-016.96, 017.90-017.96, 031.2-031.9, 041.81-041.9, 137.2, 139.8

§ ✓5ᵗʰ **016.1** **Bladder** `CC` `HIV`
**CC Excl:** See code: 016.0

§ ✓5ᵗʰ **016.2** **Ureter** `CC` `HIV`
**CC Excl:** See code: 016.0

§ ✓5ᵗʰ **016.3** **Other urinary organs** `CC` `HIV`
**CC Excl:** See code: 016.0

§ ✓5ᵗʰ **016.4** **Epididymis** `CC` `HIV` ♂
**CC Excl:** 016.40-016.56, 016.90-016.96, 017.90-017.96, 031.2-031.9, 041.81-041.9, 137.2, 139.8

§ ✓5ᵗʰ **016.5** **Other male genital organs** `CC` `HIV` ♂
Use additional code to identify manifestation, as:
tuberculosis of:
prostate (601.4)
seminal vesicle (608.81)
testis (608.81)
**CC Excl:** See code: 016.4

§ ✓5ᵗʰ **016.6** **Tuberculous oophoritis and salpingitis** `CC` `HIV` ♀
**CC Excl:** 016.60-016.96, 017.90-017.96, 031.2-031.9, 041.81-041.9, 137.2, 139.8

§ ✓5ᵗʰ **016.7** **Other female genital organs** `CC` `HIV` ♀
Tuberculous:
cervicitis
endometritis
**CC Excl:** See code: 016.6

§ ✓5ᵗʰ **016.9** **Genitourinary tuberculosis, unspecified** `CC` `HIV`
**CC Excl:** 016.90-016.96, 017.90-017.96, 031.2-031.9, 041.81-041.9, 137.2, 139.8

✓4ᵗʰ **017 Tuberculosis of other organs**

§ ✓5ᵗʰ **017.0** **Skin and subcutaneous cellular tissue** `CC` `HIV`

| Lupus: | Tuberculosis: |
|---|---|
| exedens | cutis |
| vulgaris | lichenoides |
| Scrofuloderma | papulonecrotica |
| Tuberculosis: | verrucosa cutis |
| colliquativa | |

**EXCLUDES** *lupus erythematosus (695.4)*
*disseminated (710.0)*
*lupus NOS (710.0)*
*nonspecific reaction to tuberculin skin test without active tuberculosis (795.5)*
*positive PPD (795.5)*
*positive tuberculin skin test without active tuberculosis (795.5)*

**CC Excl:** 010.00-018.96

§ Requires fifth-digit. See beginning of section 010-018 for codes and definitions.

---

✓4ᵗʰ / ✓5ᵗʰ Additional Digit Required     Unacceptable PDx     Manifestation Code     ◄► Revised Text     ● New Code     ▲ Revised Code Title

§ ✓5ᵗʰ **017.1 Erythema nodosum with hypersensitivity reaction in tuberculosis** `HIV`

Bazin's disease
Erythema: Erythema:
induratum nodosum, tuberculous
Tuberculosis indurativa

**EXCLUDES** erythema nodosum NOS (695.2)

DEF: Tender, inflammatory, bilateral nodules appearing on the shins and thought to be an allergic reaction to tuberculotoxin.

§ ✓5ᵗʰ **017.2 Peripheral lymph nodes** `CC` `HIV`

Scrofula Tuberculous adenitis
Scrofulous abscess

**EXCLUDES** tuberculosis of lymph nodes:
bronchial and mediastinal (012.1)
mesenteric and retroperitoneal (014.8)
tuberculous tracheobronchial adenopathy (012.1)

CC Excl: 017.20-017.26, 017.90-017.96, 031.2-031.9, 041.81-041.9, 139.8

DEF: Scrofula: Old name for tuberculous cervical lymphadenitis.

§ ✓5ᵗʰ **017.3 Eye** `CC` `HIV`

Use additional code to identify manifestation, as:
tuberculous:
chorioretinitis, disseminated (363.13)
episcleritis (379.09)
interstitial keratitis (370.59)
iridocyclitis, chronic (364.11)
keratoconjunctivitis (phlyctenular) (370.31)

CC Excl: 017.30-017.36, 017.90-017.96, 031.2-031.9, 041.81-041.9, 139.8

§ ✓5ᵗʰ **017.4 Ear** `CC` `HIV`

Tuberculosis of ear
Tuberculous otitis media

**EXCLUDES** tuberculous mastoiditis (015.6)

CC Excl: 017.40-017.46, 017.90-017.96, 031.2-031.9, 041.81-041.9, 139.8

§ ✓5ᵗʰ **017.5 Thyroid gland** `CC` `HIV`

CC Excl: 017.50-017.56, 017.90-017.96, 031.2-031.9, 041.81-041.9, 139.8

§ ✓5ᵗʰ **017.6 Adrenal glands** `CC` `HIV`

Addison's disease, tuberculous

CC Excl: 017.60-017.66, 017.90-017.96, 031.2-031.9, 041.81-041.9, 139.8

§ ✓5ᵗʰ **017.7 Spleen** `CC` `HIV`

CC Excl: 017.70-017.76, 017.90-017.96, 031.2-031.9, 041.81-041.9, 139.8

§ ✓5ᵗʰ **017.8 Esophagus** `CC` `HIV`

CC Excl: 017.80-017.96, 031.2-031.9, 041.81-041.9, 139.8

§ ✓5ᵗʰ **017.9 Other specified organs** `CC` `HIV`

Use additional code to identify manifestation, as:
tuberculosis of:
endocardium [any valve] (424.91)
myocardium (422.0)
pericardium (420.0)

CC Excl: 017.90-017.96, 031.2-031.9, 041.81-041.9, 139.8

✓4ᵗʰ **018 Miliary tuberculosis**

**INCLUDES** tuberculosis:
disseminated
generalized
miliary, whether of a single specified site, multiple sites, or unspecified site
polyserositis

DEF: A form of tuberculosis caused by caseous material carried through the bloodstream planting seedlike tubercles in various body organs.

§ ✓5ᵗʰ **018.0 Acute miliary tuberculosis** `MCC` `HIV`

CC Excl: 017.90-018.96, 031.2-031.9, 041.81-041.9, 139.8

§ ✓5ᵗʰ **018.8 Other specified miliary tuberculosis** `MCC` `HIV`

CC Excl: See code: 018.0

§ ✓5ᵗʰ **018.9 Miliary tuberculosis, unspecified** `MCC` `HIV`

CC Excl: See code: 018.0

## ZOONOTIC BACTERIAL DISEASES (020-027)

✓4ᵗʰ **020 Plague**

**INCLUDES** infection by Yersinia [Pasteurella] pestis

**020.0 Bubonic** `MCC`

CC Excl: 020.0-020.9

DEF: Most common acute and severe form of plague characterized by lymphadenopathy (buboes), chills, fever and headache.

**020.1 Cellulocutaneous** `MCC`

CC Excl: See code: 020.0

DEF: Plague characterized by inflammation and necrosis of skin.

**020.2 Septicemic** `MCC`

CC Excl: 020.0-020.9, 771.81, 771.83-771.89, 995.90-995.94

DEF: Plague characterized by massive infection in the bloodstream.

**020.3 Primary pneumonic** `MCC`

CC Excl: 011.00-012.16, 012.80-012.86, 017.90-017.96, 020.0-020.9, 021.3, 022.1, 031.0, 039.1, 073.0, 115.05, 115.15, 115.95, 122.1, 130.4, 136.3, 480.0-487.1, 488, 495.0-495.9, 500-502

DEF: Plague characterized by massive pulmonary infection.

**020.4 Secondary pneumonic** `MCC`

CC Excl: 011.73-011.93, 480.3

DEF: Lung infection as a secondary complication of plague.

**020.5 Pneumonic, unspecified** `MCC`

CC Excl: 020.5, 480.3

**020.8 Other specified types of plague** `MCC`

Abortive plague
Ambulatory plague
Pestis minor

CC Excl: 020.8

**020.9 Plague, unspecified** `MCC`

CC Excl: 020.9

✓4ᵗʰ **021 Tularemia**

**INCLUDES** deerfly fever
infection by Francisella [Pasteurella] tularensis
rabbit fever

DEF: A febrile disease transmitted by the bites of deer flies, fleas and ticks, by inhalations of aerosolized *F. tularensis* or by ingestion of contaminated food or water; patients quickly develop fever, chills, weakness, headache, backache and malaise.

**021.0 Ulceroglandular tularemia** `CC`

CC Excl: 021.0

DEF: Lesions occur at the site *Francisella tularensis* organism enters body, usually the fingers or hands.

**021.1 Enteric tularemia** `CC`

Tularemia: Tularemia:
cryptogenic typhoidal
intestinal

CC Excl: 021.1

**021.2 Pulmonary tularemia** `CC`

Bronchopneumonic tularemia

CC Excl: 482.49-487.1, 488, 495.0-495.9, 500-508.9, 517.1, 517.8, 518.89, 519.8-519.9

**021.3 Oculoglandular tularemia** `CC`

CC Excl: 021.3, 480.3

DEF: Painful conjunctival infection by *Francisella tularensis* organism with possible corneal, preauricular lymph, or lacrimal involvement.

**021.8 Other specified tularemia** `CC`

Tularemia: Tularemia:
generalized or disseminated glandular

CC Excl: 021.0-021.9

**021.9 Unspecified tularemia** `CC`

CC Excl: See code: 021.8

§ Requires fifth-digit. See beginning of section 010-018 for codes and definitions.

`N` Newborn Age: 0 `P` Pediatric Age: 0-17 `M` Maternity Age: 12-55 `A` Adult Age: 15-124 `CC` CC Condition `MCC` Major CC Condition `HIV` HIV Related Dx

**6 — Volume 1 • October 2007**

© 2007 Ingenix

## ✓4ᵗʰ 022 Anthrax

AHA: 4Q '02, 70

DEF: An infectious bacterial disease usually transmitted by contact with infected animals or their discharges or products; it is classified by primary routes of inoculation as cutaneous, gastrointestinal and by inhalation.

**022.0 Cutaneous anthrax**    `CC`
Malignant pustule
CC Excl: 022.0

**022.1 Pulmonary anthrax**    `MCC`
Respiratory anthrax
Wool-sorters' disease
CC Excl: 011.00-012.16, 012.80-012.86, 017.90-017.96, 020.3-020.5, 021.3, 022.1, 031.0, 039.1, 073.0, 115.05, 115.15, 115.95, 122.1, 130.4, 136.3, 480.0-487.1, 488, 494.0-495.9, 500-508.9, 517.1, 517.8, 518.89, 519.8-519.9

**022.2 Gastrointestinal anthrax**    `CC`
CC Excl: 022.2

**022.3 Anthrax septicemia**    `MCC`
CC Excl: 003.1, 020.2, 022.3, 036.2, 038.0-038.9, 040.89-041.9, 054.5, 139.8, 771.81, 771.83-771.89, 995.90-995.94, V09.0-V09.91

**022.8 Other specified manifestations of anthrax**    `CC`
CC Excl: 022.8

**022.9 Anthrax, unspecified**    `CC`
CC Excl: 022.0-022.9

## ✓4ᵗʰ 023 Brucellosis

INCLUDES   fever:
Malta
Mediterranean
undulant

DEF: An infectious disease caused by gram-negative, aerobic coccobacilli organisms; it is transmitted to humans through contact with infected tissue or dairy products; fever, sweating, weakness and aching are symptoms.

**023.0 Brucella melitensis**
DEF: Infection from direct or indirect contact with infected sheep or goats.

**023.1 Brucella abortus**
DEF: Infection from direct or indirect contact with infected cattle.

**023.2 Brucella suis**
DEF: Infection from direct or indirect contact with infected swine.

**023.3 Brucella canis**
DEF: Infection from direct or indirect contact with infected dogs.

**023.8 Other brucellosis**    `CC`
Infection by more than one organism
CC Excl: 023.0-023.9

**023.9 Brucellosis, unspecified**    `CC`
CC Excl: See code: 023.8

## 024 Glanders    `CC`

Infection by:
Actinobacillus mallei
Malleomyces mallei
Pseudomonas mallei

Infection by:
Farcy
Malleus

CC Excl: 024

DEF: Equine infection causing mucosal inflammation and skin ulcers in humans.

## 025 Melioidosis    `CC`

Infection by:
Malleomyces pseudomallei
Pseudomonas pseudomallei

Infection by:
Pseudoglanders
Whitmore's bacillus

CC Excl: 025

DEF: Rare infection caused by *Pseudomonas pseudomallei*; clinical symptoms range from localized infection to fatal septicemia.

## ✓4ᵗʰ 026 Rat-bite fever

**026.0 Spirillary fever**    `CC`
Rat-bite fever due to Spirillum minor [S. minus]
Sodoku
CC Excl: 026.0-026.9

**026.1 Streptobacillary fever**    `CC`
Epidemic arthritic erythema
Haverhill fever
Rat-bite fever due to Streptobacillus moniliformis
CC Excl: See code: 026.0

**026.9 Unspecified rat-bite fever**    `CC`
CC Excl: See code: 026.0

## ✓4ᵗʰ 027 Other zoonotic bacterial diseases

**027.0 Listeriosis**    `CC`
Infection ⎫
Septicemia ⎬ by Listeria monocytogenes

Use additional code to identify manifestation, as meningitis (320.7)
EXCLUDES   congenital listeriosis (771.2)
CC Excl: 027.0-027.9

**027.1 Erysipelothrix infection**
Erysipeloid (of Rosenbach)
Infection ⎫ by Erysipelothrix insidiosa
Septicemia ⎬ [E. rhusiopathiae]

DEF: Usually associated with handling of fish, meat, or poultry; symptoms range from localized inflammation to septicemia.

**027.2 Pasteurellosis**    `CC`
Pasteurella pseudotuberculosis infection
Mesenteric adenitis ⎫ by Pasteurella multocida
Septic infection (cat ⎬ [P. septica]
bite) (dog bite) ⎭

EXCLUDES   infection by:
Francisella [Pasteurella] tularensis (021.0-021.9)
Yersinia [Pasteurella] pestis (020.0-020.9)

CC Excl: See code: 027.0

DEF: Swelling, abscesses, or septicemia from *Pasteurella multocida*, commonly transmitted to humans by a dog or cat scratch.

**027.8 Other specified zoonotic bacterial diseases**    `CC`
CC Excl: See code: 027.0

**027.9 Unspecified zoonotic bacterial disease**    `CC`
CC Excl: See code: 027.0

## OTHER BACTERIAL DISEASES (030-041)

EXCLUDES   bacterial venereal diseases (098.0-099.9)
bartonellosis (088.0)

## ✓4ᵗʰ 030 Leprosy

INCLUDES   Hansen's disease
infection by Mycobacterium leprae

**030.0 Lepromatous [type L]**    `CC`
Lepromatous leprosy (macular) (diffuse) (infiltrated) (nodular) (neuritic)
CC Excl: 030.0

DEF: Infectious, disseminated leprosy bacilli with lesions and deformities.

**030.1 Tuberculoid [type T]**    `CC`
Tuberculoid leprosy (macular) (maculoanesthetic) (major) (minor) (neuritic)
CC Excl: 030.1

DEF: Relatively benign, self-limiting leprosy with neuralgia and scales.

**Infectious and Parasitic Diseases**

**030.2–036.0**

**030.2  Indeterminate [group I]**  `CC`
Indeterminate [uncharacteristic] leprosy (macular)
(neuritic)
**CC Excl:** 030.2

DEF: Uncharacteristic leprosy, frequently an early manifestation.

**030.3  Borderline [group B]**  `CC`
Borderline or dimorphous leprosy (infiltrated)
(neuritic)
**CC Excl:** 030.3

DEF: Transitional form of leprosy, neither lepromatous nor tuberculoid.

**030.8  Other specified leprosy**  `CC`
**CC Excl:** 030.8

**030.9  Leprosy, unspecified**  `CC`
**CC Excl:** 030.9

`√4ᵗʰ` **031  Diseases due to other mycobacteria**

**031.0  Pulmonary**  `CC`
Battey disease
Infection by Mycobacterium:
avium
intracellulare [Battey bacillus]
kansasii
**CC Excl:** 011.00-012.86, 017.90-017.96, 031.0, 031.2-031.9, 041.81-041.9, 137.0, 139.8, 480.0-480.2, 480.8-487.1, 488, 494.0-508.9, 517.1, 518.89

**031.1  Cutaneous**  `CC`
Buruli ulcer
Infection by Mycobacterium:
marinum [M. balnei]
ulcerans
**CC Excl:** 031.0-031.9

**031.2  Disseminated**  `CC` `HIV`
Disseminated mycobacterium avium-intracellulare
complex (DMAC)
Mycobacterium avium-intracellulare complex (MAC)
bacteremia
**CC Excl:** See code: 031.1

AHA: 4Q, '97, 31

DEF: Disseminated mycobacterium avium-intracellulare complex (DMAC): A serious systemic form of MAC commonly observed in patients in the late course of AIDS.

DEF: Mycobacterium avium-intracellulare complex (MAC) bacterium: Human pulmonary disease, lymphadenitis in children and systemic disease in immunocompromised individuals caused by a slow growing, gram-positive, aerobic organism.

**031.8  Other specified mycobacterial diseases**  `CC` `HIV`
**CC Excl:** See code: 031.1

**031.9  Unspecified diseases due to mycobacteria**  `CC` `HIV`
Atypical mycobacterium infection NOS
**CC Excl:** See code: 031.1

`√4ᵗʰ` **032  Diphtheria**
`INCLUDES`  infection by Corynebacterium diphtheriae

**032.0  Faucial diphtheria**  `CC`
Membranous angina, diphtheritic
**CC Excl:** 032.0-032.9

DEF: Diphtheria of the throat.

**032.1  Nasopharyngeal diphtheria**  `CC`
**CC Excl:** See code: 032.0

**032.2  Anterior nasal diphtheria**  `CC`
**CC Excl:** See code: 032.0

**032.3  Laryngeal diphtheria**  `CC`
Laryngotracheitis, diphtheritic
**CC Excl:** See code: 032.0

`√5ᵗʰ` **032.8  Other specified diphtheria**

**032.81  Conjunctival diphtheria**  `CC`
Pseudomembranous diphtheritic
conjunctivitis
**CC Excl:** See code: 032.0

**032.82  Diphtheritic myocarditis**  `CC`
**CC Excl:** 032.82, 074.20, 074.22-074.23, 093.82, 390, 391.2-391.9, 398.0-398.90, 398.99, 422.0-422.99, 429.0, 429.71-429.79, 459.89-459.9

**032.83  Diphtheritic peritonitis**  `CC`
**CC Excl:** 014.00-014.06, 032.83, 090.0, 095.2, 098.86, 099.56, 540.0-540.1, 567.0-567.1, 567.22, 567.29, 567.81, 567.9, 569.89-569.9, 577.8, 614.5-614.7, 639.0, 670.00-670.04, 777.6, 998.7

**032.84  Diphtheritic cystitis**  `CC`
**CC Excl:** See code: 032.0

**032.85  Cutaneous diphtheria**  `CC`
**CC Excl:** See code: 032.0

**032.89  Other**  `CC`
**CC Excl:** See code: 032.0

**032.9  Diphtheria, unspecified**  `CC`
**CC Excl:** See code: 032.0

`√4ᵗʰ` **033  Whooping cough**
`INCLUDES`  pertussis
Use additional code to identify any associated pneumonia
(484.3)

DEF: An acute, highly contagious respiratory tract infection caused by *Bordetella pertussis* and *B. bronchiseptica*; characteristic paroxysmal cough.

**033.0  Bordetella pertussis [B. pertussis]**  `CC`
**CC Excl:** 033.0-033.9

**033.1  Bordetella parapertussis [B. parapertussis]**  `CC`
**CC Excl:** See code: 033.0

**033.8  Whooping cough due to other specified organism**  `CC`
Bordetella bronchiseptica [B. bronchiseptica]
**CC Excl:** See code: 033.0

**033.9  Whooping cough, unspecified organism**  `CC`
**CC Excl:** See code: 033.0

`√4ᵗʰ` **034  Streptococcal sore throat and scarlet fever**

**034.0  Streptococcal sore throat**
Septic:                    Streptococcal:
angina                    laryngitis
sore throat              pharyngitis
Streptococcal:           tonsillitis
angina

**034.1  Scarlet fever**  `CC`
Scarlatina
`EXCLUDES`  *parascarlatina (057.8)*
**CC Excl:** 034.0-035

DEF: Streptococcal infection and fever with red rash spreading from trunk.

**035  Erysipelas**
`EXCLUDES`  *postpartum or puerperal erysipelas (670)*
DEF: An acute superficial cellulitis involving the dermal lymphatics; it is often caused by group A streptococci.

`√4ᵗʰ` **036  Meningococcal infection**

**036.0  Meningococcal meningitis**  `MCC`
Cerebrospinal fever (meningococcal)
Meningitis:
cerebrospinal
epidemic
**CC Excl:** 003.21, 013.00-013.16, 036.0, 036.89-036.9, 041.81-041.9, 047.0-047.9, 049.0-049.1, 053.0, 054.72, 072.1, 090.42, 091.81, 094.2, 098.89, 100.81, 112.83, 114.2, 115.01, 115.11, 115.91, 130.0, 139.8, 320.0-322.9, 349.89-349.9, 357.0

---

`N` Newborn Age: 0     `P` Pediatric Age: 0-17     `M` Maternity Age: 12-55     `A` Adult Age: 15-124     `CC` CC Condition     `MCC` Major CC Condition     `HIV` HIV Related Dx

**036.1**   **Meningococcal encephalitis**    `MCC`
CC Excl: 036.1, 036.89-036.9, 041.81-041.9, 139.8

**036.2**   **Meningococcemia**    `MCC`
Meningococcal septicemia
CC Excl: 003.1, 020.2, 036.2, 036.89-036.9, 038.0-038.9, 041.81-041.9, 054.5, 139.8, 995.90-995.94

**036.3**   **Waterhouse-Friderichsen syndrome,**    `MCC`
**meningococcal**
Meningococcal hemorrhagic adrenalitis
Meningococcic adrenal syndrome
Waterhouse-Friderichsen syndrome NOS
CC Excl: 036.3, 036.89-036.9, 041.81-041.9, 139.8

√5ᵗʰ **036.4**   **Meningococcal carditis**
   **036.40 Meningococcal carditis, unspecified**    `MCC`
     CC Excl: 036.40, 036.89-036.9, 041.81-041.9, 139.8

   **036.41 Meningococcal pericarditis**    `MCC`
     CC Excl: 036.41, 036.89-036.9, 041.81-041.9, 139.8

     DEF: Meningococcal infection of the outer membrane of the heart.

   **036.42 Meningococcal endocarditis**    `MCC`
     CC Excl: 036.42, 036.89-036.9, 041.81-041.9, 139.8

     DEF: Meningococcal infection of the membranes lining the cavities of the heart.

   **036.43 Meningococcal myocarditis**    `MCC`
     CC Excl: 036.43, 041.81-041.9, 139.8

     DEF: Meningococcal infection of the muscle of the heart.

√5ᵗʰ **036.8**   **Other specified meningococcal infections**
   **036.81 Meningococcal optic neuritis**    `CC`
     CC Excl: 036.81, 036.89-036.9, 041.81-041.9, 139.8

   **036.82 Meningococcal arthropathy**    `CC`
     CC Excl: 036.82-036.9, 041.81-041.9, 139.8

   **036.89 Other**    `CC`
     CC Excl: 036.89-036.9, 041.81-041.9, 139.8

**036.9**   **Meningococcal infection, unspecified**    `CC`
Meningococcal infection NOS
CC Excl: See code: 036.89

**037 Tetanus**    `MCC`
   `EXCLUDES`   tetanus:
     complicating:
       abortion (634-638 with .0, 639.0)
       ectopic or molar pregnancy (639.0)
     neonatorum (771.3)
     puerperal (670)

CC Excl: 037, 139.8

DEF: An acute, often fatal, infectious disease caused by the anaerobic, spore-forming bacillus *Clostridium tetani*; the bacillus most often enters the body through a contaminated wound, burns, surgical wounds, or cutaneous ulcers. Symptoms include lockjaw, spasms, seizures, and paralysis.

√4ᵗʰ **038 Septicemia**
Use additional code for systemic inflammatory response syndrome (SIRS) (995.91-995.92)
   `EXCLUDES`   bacteremia (790.7)
     during labor (659.3)
     following ectopic or molar pregnancy (639.0)
     following infusion, injection, transfusion, or
       vaccination (999.3)
     postpartum, puerperal (670)
     septicemia (sepsis) of newborn (771.81)
     that complicating abortion (634-638
       with .0, 639.0)

AHA: 2Q, '04, 16; 4Q, '88, 10; 3Q, '88, 12

DEF: A systemic disease associated with the presence and persistence of pathogenic microorganisms or their toxins in the blood.

**038.0**   **Streptococcal septicemia**    `MCC` `HIV`
CC Excl: 003.1, 020.2, 036.2, 038.0-038.9, 040.82-041.9, 054.5, 139.8, 995.90-995.94, V09.0-V09.91

AHA: 4Q, '03, 79; 2Q, '96, 5

√5ᵗʰ **038.1**   **Staphylococcal septicemia**
AHA: 4Q, '97, 32

   **038.10 Staphylococcal septicemia,**    `MCC` `HIV`
**unspecified**
     CC Excl: See code: 038.0

   **038.11 Staphylococcus aureus septicemia**   `MCC` `HIV`
     CC Excl: See code: 038.0

     AHA: 1Q, '05, 7; 2Q, '00, 5; 4Q, '98, 42

   **038.19 Other staphylococcal septicemia**   `MCC` `HIV`
     CC Excl: See code: 038.0

     AHA: 2Q, '00, 5

**038.2**   **Pneumococcal septicemia [Streptococcus**   `MCC` `HIV`
**pneumoniae septicemia]**
CC Excl: See code 038.0

AHA: 2Q, '96, 5; 1Q, '91, 13

**038.3**   **Septicemia due to anaerobes**    `MCC` `HIV`
Septicemia due to bacteroides
   `EXCLUDES`   gas gangrene (040.0)
     that due to anaerobic streptococci
     (038.0)

CC Excl: See code 038.0

√5ᵗʰ **038.4**   **Septicemia due to other gram-negative organisms**
DEF: Infection of blood by microorganisms categorized as gram-negative by Gram's method of staining for identification of bacteria.

   **038.40 Gram-negative organism,**    `MCC` `HIV`
**unspecified**
     Gram-negative septicemia NOS
     CC Excl: See code 038.0

   **038.41 Hemophilus influenzae**    `MCC` `HIV`
**[H. influenzae]**
     CC Excl: See code 038.0

   **038.42 Escherichia coli [E. coli]**    `MCC` `HIV`
     CC Excl: See code 038.0

     AHA: 4Q, '03, 73

   **038.43 Pseudomonas**    `MCC` `HIV`
     CC Excl: See code 038.0

   **038.44 Serratia**    `MCC` `HIV`
     CC Excl: See code 038.0

   **038.49 Other**    `MCC` `HIV`
     CC Excl: See code 038.0

**038.8**   **Other specified septicemias**    `MCC` `HIV`
   `EXCLUDES`   septicemia (due to):
     anthrax (022.3)
     gonococcal (098.89)
     herpetic (054.5)
     meningococcal (036.2)
     septicemic plague (020.2)

CC Excl: See code 038.0

**038.9**   **Unspecified septicemia**    `MCC` `HIV`
Septicemia NOS
   `EXCLUDES`   bacteremia NOS (790.7)

CC Excl: See code 038.0

AHA: 2Q, '05, 18-19; 2Q, '04, 16; 4Q, '03, 79; 2Q, '00, 3; 3Q, '99, 5, 9; 1Q, '98, 5; 3Q, '96, 16; 2Q, '96, 6

√4ᵗʰ
√5ᵗʰ Additional Digit Required     Unacceptable PDx     Manifestation Code     ◄► Revised Text     ● New Code     ▲ Revised Code Title

**Infectious and Parasitic Diseases**

**039–041.84**

✓4ᵗʰ **039 Actinomycotic infections**

> INCLUDES   actinomycotic mycetoma
> infection by Actinomycetales, such as species
> of Actinomyces, Actinomadura, Nocardia,
> Streptomyces
> maduromycosis (actinomycotic)
> schizomycetoma (actinomycotic)

DEF: Inflammatory lesions and abscesses at site of infection by *Actinomyces israelii.*

**039.0   Cutaneous**    CC HIV
Erythrasma
Trichomycosis axillaris
CC Excl: 039.0, 039.8-039.9

**039.1   Pulmonary**    CC HIV
Thoracic actinomycosis
CC Excl: 039.1, 039.8-039.9, 480.3

**039.2   Abdominal**    CC HIV
CC Excl: 039.2, 039.8-039.9

**039.3   Cervicofacial**    CC
CC Excl: 039.3, 039.8-039.9

**039.4   Madura foot**    CC HIV
> EXCLUDES   madura foot due to mycotic infection
> (117.4)

CC Excl: 039.4-039.9

**039.8   Of other specified sites**    CC HIV
CC Excl: 039.0-039.9

**039.9   Of unspecified site**    CC HIV
Actinomycosis NOS
Maduromycosis NOS
Nocardiosis NOS
CC Excl: See code: 039.8

✓4ᵗʰ **040 Other bacterial diseases**

> EXCLUDES   bacteremia NOS (790.7)
> bacterial infection NOS (041.9)

**040.0   Gas gangrene**    MCC
Gas bacillus infection or gangrene
Infection by Clostridium:
histolyticum
oedematiens
perfringens [welchii]
septicum
sordellii
Malignant edema
Myonecrosis, clostridial
Myositis, clostridial
CC Excl: 040.0, 139.8

AHA: 1Q, '95, 11

**040.1   Rhinoscleroma**
DEF: Growths on the nose and nasopharynx caused by *Klebsiella rhinoscleromatis.*

**040.2   Whipple's disease**    CC
Intestinal lipodystrophy
CC Excl: 040.2

**040.3   Necrobacillosis**    CC
CC Excl: 040.3
DEF: Infection with *Fusobacterium necrophorum* causing abscess or necrosis.

● ✓5ᵗʰ **040.4   Other specified botulism**
Non-foodborne intoxication due to toxins of
Clostridium botulinum [C. botulinum]
> EXCLUDES   botulism NOS (005.1)
> food poisoning due to toxins of
> Clostridium botulinum (005.1)

● **040.41 Infant botulism**    CC
CC Excl: 005.0-005.2, 008.45-008.46, 040.41-040.42

● **040.42 Wound botulism**    CC
Non-foodborne botulism NOS
Use additional code to identify complicated
open wound
CC Excl: See code 040.41

✓5ᵗʰ **040.8   Other specified bacterial diseases**

**040.81 Tropical pyomyositis**    CC
CC Excl: 040.81, 040.89

**040.82 Toxic shock syndrome**    MCC
Use additional code to identify the organism
CC Excl: 040.82, 338.0-338.4, 780.91-780.99, 785.50-785.59,
785.9, 799.81-799.89

AHA: 4Q, '02, 44
DEF: Syndrome caused by staphylococcal exotoxin that
may rapidly progress to severe and intractable shock;
symptoms include characteristic sunburn-like rash with
peeling of skin on palms and soles, sudden onset high
fever, vomiting, diarrhea, myalgia, and hypotension.

**040.89 Other**
AHA: N-D, '86, 7

✓4ᵗʰ **041 Bacterial infection in conditions classified elsewhere and of unspecified site**
Note: This category is provided to be used as an additional
code to identify the bacterial agent in diseases classified elsewhere. This category will also be used to classify bacterial infections of unspecified nature or site.

> EXCLUDES   septicemia (038.0-038.9)

AHA: 2Q, '01, 12; J-A, '84, 19

✓5ᵗʰ **041.0   Streptococcus**

**041.00 Streptococcus, unspecified**

**041.01 Group A**
AHA: 1Q, '02, 3

**041.02 Group B**

**041.03 Group C**

**041.04 Group D [Enterococcus]**

**041.05 Group G**

**041.09 Other Streptococcus**

✓5ᵗʰ **041.1   Staphylococcus**

**041.10 Staphylococcus, unspecified**
AHA: 2Q, '06, 15

**041.11 Staphylococcus aureus**
AHA: 2Q, '06, 16; 4Q, '03, 104, 106; 2Q, '01, 11;
4Q, '98, 42, 54; 4Q, '97, 32

**041.19 Other Staphylococcus**

**041.2   Pneumococcus**

**041.3   Friedländer's bacillus**
Infection by Klebsiella pneumoniae

**041.4   Escherichia coli [E. coli]**

**041.5   Hemophilus influenzae [H. influenzae]**

**041.6   Proteus (mirabilis) (morganii)**

**041.7   Pseudomonas**
AHA: 4Q, '02, 45

✓5ᵗʰ **041.8   Other specified bacterial infections**

**041.81 Mycoplasma**
Eaton's agent
Pleuropneumonia-like organisms [PPLO]

**041.82 Bacteroides fragilis**
DEF: Anaerobic gram-negative bacilli of the
gastrointestinal tract; frequently implicated in intra-
abdominal infection; commonly resistant to antibiotics.

**041.83 Clostridium perfringens**

**041.84 Other anaerobes**
Gram-negative anaerobes
> EXCLUDES   Helicobacter pylori (041.86)

N Newborn Age: 0    P Pediatric Age: 0-17    M Maternity Age: 12-55    A Adult Age: 15-124    CC CC Condition    MCC Major CC Condition    HIV HIV Related Dx

10 — Volume 1 • October 2007

© 2007 Ingenix

**041.85  Other gram-negative organisms**
Aerobacter aerogenes
Gram-negative bacteria NOS
Mima polymorpha
Serratia
> EXCLUDES    *gram-negative anaerobes (041.84)*

AHA: 1Q, '95, 18

**041.86  Helicobacter pylori [H. pylori]**
AHA: 4Q, '95, 60

**041.89  Other specified bacteria**
AHA: 2Q, '06, 7; 2Q, '03, 7

**041.9  Bacterial infection, unspecified**
AHA: 2Q, '91, 9

## HUMAN IMMUNODEFICIENCY VIRUS (HIV) INFECTION (042)

**042  Human immunodeficiency virus [HIV] disease**          MCC
Acquired immune deficiency syndrome
Acquired immunodeficiency syndrome
AIDS
AIDS-like syndrome
AIDS-related complex
ARC
HIV infection, symptomatic
Use additional code(s) to identify all manifestations of HIV
Use additional code to identify HIV-2 infection (079.53)
> EXCLUDES    *asymptomatic HIV infection status  (V08)*
> *exposure to HIV virus (V01.79)*
> *nonspecific serologic evidence of HIV (795.71)*

**CC Excl:** 042, 139.8

AHA:   3Q, '06, 15; 1Q, '05, 7; 2Q, '04, 11; 1Q, '04, 5; 1Q, '03, 15; 1Q, '99, 14;
       4Q, '97, 30, 31; 1Q, '93, 21; 2Q, '92, 11; 3Q, '90, 17; J-A, '87, 8

## POLIOMYELITIS AND OTHER NON-ARTHROPOD-BORNE VIRAL DISEASES OF CENTRAL NERVOUS SYSTEM (045-049)

**045  Acute poliomyelitis**
> EXCLUDES    *late effects of acute poliomyelitis (138)*

The following fifth-digit subclassification is for use with category 045:
    **0  poliovirus, unspecified type**
    **1  poliovirus type I**
    **2  poliovirus type II**
    **3  poliovirus type III**

**045.0  Acute paralytic poliomyelitis specified as bulbar**          MCC
Infantile paralysis (acute)  }
Poliomyelitis (acute) (anterior)  } specified as bulbar

Polioencephalitis (acute) (bulbar)
Polioencephalomyelitis (acute) (anterior) (bulbar)

**CC Excl:** 045.00-045.13

DEF: Acute paralytic infection occurring where the brain merges with the spinal cord; affecting breathing, swallowing, and heart rate.

**045.1  Acute poliomyelitis with other paralysis**          MCC
Paralysis:                     Paralysis:
  acute atrophic, spinal         infantile, paralytic
Poliomyelitis (acute)  }
  anterior            } with paralysis except
  epidemic            } bulbar

**CC Excl:** See code: 045.0

DEF: Paralytic infection affecting peripheral or spinal nerves.

**045.2  Acute nonparalytic poliomyelitis**
Poliomyelitis (acute)  }
  anterior            } specified as nonparalytic
  epidemic

DEF: Nonparalytic infection causing pain, stiffness, and paresthesias.

**045.9  Acute poliomyelitis, unspecified**
Infantile paralysis  }
Poliomyelitis (acute)  } unspecified whether
  anterior            } paralytic or
  epidemic            } nonparalytic

**046  Slow virus infection of central nervous system**
**046.0  Kuru**          CC
**CC Excl:** 046.0-046.9

DEF:  A chronic, progressive, fatal nervous system disorder; clinical symptoms include cerebellar ataxia, trembling, spasticity and progressive dementia.

**046.1  Jakob-Creutzfeldt disease**          CC
Subacute spongiform encephalopathy
**CC Excl:** 013.60-013.66, 046.0-046.9, 048-049.0, 049.8, 052.0, 052.2, 054.3, 054.74, 056.01, 057.8-058.29, 062.0-064, 066.2-066.3, 072.2, 073.7, 079.99, 081.9, 083.9, 090.41, 094.81, 117.5, 124, 130.0, 290.12, 323.01-323.9, 341.1, 487.8, 771.2, 984.9

DEF:  Communicable, progressive spongiform encephalopathy thought to be caused by an infectious particle known as a "prion" (proteinaceous infection particle). This is a progressive, fatal disease manifested principally by mental deterioration.

**046.2  Subacute sclerosing panencephalitis**          CC
Dawson's inclusion body encephalitis
Van Bogaert's sclerosing leukoencephalitis
**CC Excl:** 046.2, 139.8

DEF:  Progressive viral infection causing cerebral dysfunction, blindness, dementia, and death (SSPE).

**046.3  Progressive multifocal leukoencephalopathy**          CC HIV
Multifocal leukoencephalopathy NOS
**CC Excl:** 013.60-013.66, 046.0-046.9, 048-049.0, 049.8, 052.0, 052.2, 054.3, 054.74, 056.01, 057.8-058.29, 062.0-064, 066.2-066.3, 072.2, 073.7, 075, 081.9, 083.9, 090.41, 094.81, 117.5, 124, 130.0, 290.12, 323.01-323.9, 341.1, 487.8, 771.2, 984.9

DEF: Infection affecting cerebral cortex in patients with weakened immune systems.

**046.8  Other specified slow virus infection of central nervous system**          CC HIV
**CC Excl:** 046.0-046.9, 066.40-066.49, 079.82

**046.9  Unspecified slow virus infection of central nervous system**          CC HIV
**CC Excl:** See code: 046.0

**047  Meningitis due to enterovirus**
> INCLUDES    meningitis:          meningitis:
>   abacterial            viral
>   aseptic

> EXCLUDES    *meningitis due to:*
> *adenovirus (049.1)*
> *arthropod-borne virus (060.0-066.9)*
> *leptospira (100.81)*
> *virus of:*
> *herpes simplex (054.72)*
> *herpes zoster (053.0)*
> *lymphocytic choriomeningitis (049.0)*
> *mumps (072.1)*
> *poliomyelitis (045.0-045.9)*
> *any other infection specifically classified elsewhere*

AHA: J-F, '87, 6

**047.0  Coxsackie virus**          CC
**CC Excl:** 003.21, 013.00-013.16, 036.0, 047.0-047.9, 049.0-049.1, 072.1, 078.88-078.89, 079.81, 079.88-079.99, 090.42, 091.81, 094.2, 098.89, 100.81, 112.83, 114.2, 115.01, 115.11, 115.91, 130.0, 139.8, 320.0-322.9, 349.89-349.9, 357.0

**047.1  ECHO virus**          CC
Meningo-eruptive syndrome
**CC Excl:** See code: 047.0

**047.8  Other specified viral meningitis**          CC
**CC Excl:** See code: 047.0

**047.9  Unspecified viral meningitis**          CC
Viral meningitis NOS
**CC Excl:** See code: 047.0

---

Additional Digit Required          Unacceptable PDx          Manifestation Code          ◄► Revised Text          ● New Code          ▲ Revised Code Title

**048 Other enterovirus diseases of central nervous system** `CC`
Boston exanthem

CC Excl: 013.60-013.66, 046.2, 046.8, 048-049.0, 049.8, 052.0, 052.2, 054.3, 054.74, 056.01, 057.8-058.29, 062.0-064, 066.2-066.49, 072.2, 073.7, 075, 079.82, 079.99, 081.9, 083.9, 090.41, 094.81, 117.5, 124, 130.0, 290.12, 323.01-323.9, 341.1, 487.8, 771.2, 984.9

`✓4ᵗʰ` **049 Other non-arthropod-borne viral diseases of central nervous system**

> EXCLUDES  late effects of viral encephalitis (139.0)

**049.0 Lymphocytic choriomeningitis** `CC`
Lymphocytic:
   meningitis (serous) (benign)
   meningoencephalitis (serous) (benign)

CC Excl: 003.21, 013.00-013.16, 036.0, 047.0-047.9, 049.0-049.1, 066.40-066.49, 072.1, 078.88-078.89, 079.81-079.82, 079.88-079.99, 090.42, 091.81, 094.2, 098.89, 100.81, 112.83, 114.2, 115.01, 115.11, 115.91, 130.0, 139.8, 320.0-322.9, 349.89-349.9, 357.0

**049.1 Meningitis due to adenovirus** `CC`

CC Excl: 003.21, 013.00-013.16, 036.0, 047.0-047.9, 049.0-049.1, 072.1, 078.88-078.89, 079.81, 079.88-079.99, 090.42, 091.81, 094.2, 098.89, 100.81, 112.83, 114.2, 115.01, 115.11, 115.91, 130.0, 139.8, 320.0-322.9, 349.89-349.9, 357.0

DEF: Inflammation of lining of brain caused by Arenaviruses and usually occurring in adults in fall and winter months.

**049.8 Other specified non-arthropod-borne viral diseases of central nervous system** `CC` `HIV`
Encephalitis:          Encephalitis:
   acute:                 lethargica
      inclusion body      Rio Bravo
      necrotizing         von Economo's disease
      epidemic

> EXCLUDES ▶ human herpesvirus 6 encephalitis (058.21)
> other human herpesvirus encephalitis (058.29)◄

CC Excl: 013.60-013.66, 046.2, 046.8, 048-049.0, 049.8, 052.0, 052.2, 054.3, 054.74, 056.01, 057.8-058.29, 062.0-064, 066.2-066.49, 072.2, 073.7, 075, 079.82, 079.99, 081.9, 083.9, 090.41, 094.81, 117.5, 124, 130.0, 290.12, 323.01-323.9, 341.1, 382.4, 487.8, 710.0, 771.2, 984.9

**049.9 Unspecified non-arthropod-borne viral diseases of central nervous system** `CC` `HIV`
Viral encephalitis NOS

CC Excl: 013.60-013.66, 046.2, 046.8, 048-049.0, 049.8-049.9, 052.0, 052.2, 054.3, 054.74, 056.01, 057.8-058.29, 062.0-064, 066.2-066.3, 072.2, 073.7, 075, 079.99, 081.9, 083.9, 090.41, 094.81, 117.5, 124, 130.0, 290.12, 323.01-323.9, 341.1, 382.4, 487.8, 710.0, 771.2, 984.9

## VIRAL DISEASES ACCOMPANIED BY EXANTHEM (050-058)

> EXCLUDES  arthropod-borne viral diseases (060.0-066.9)
> Boston exanthem (048)

`✓4ᵗʰ` **050 Smallpox**

**050.0 Variola major** `CC`
Hemorrhagic (pustular) smallpox
Malignant smallpox
Purpura variolosa

CC Excl: 050.0-052.9

DEF: Form of smallpox known for its high mortality; exists only in laboratories.

**050.1 Alastrim** `CC`
Variola minor

CC Excl: See code: 050.0

DEF: Mild form of smallpox known for its low mortality rate.

**050.2 Modified smallpox** `CC`
Varioloid

CC Excl: See code: 050.0

DEF: Mild form occurring in patients with history of infection or vaccination.

**050.9 Smallpox, unspecified** `CC`

CC Excl: See code: 050.0

`✓4ᵗʰ` **051 Cowpox and paravaccinia**

**051.0 Cowpox**
Vaccinia not from vaccination

> EXCLUDES  vaccinia (generalized) (from vaccination) (999.0)

DEF: A disease contracted by milking infected cows; vesicles usually appear on the fingers, may spread to hands and adjacent areas and usually disappear without scarring; other associated features of the disease may include local edema, lymphangitis and regional lymphadenitis with or without fever.

**051.1 Pseudocowpox**
Milkers' node

DEF: Hand lesions and mild fever in dairy workers caused by exposure to paravaccinia.

**051.2 Contagious pustular dermatitis**
Ecthyma contagiosum          Orf

DEF: Skin eruptions caused by exposure to poxvirus-infected sheep or goats.

**051.9 Paravaccinia, unspecified**

`✓4ᵗʰ` **052 Chickenpox**
DEF: Contagious infection by Varicella-zoster virus causing rash with pustules and fever.

**052.0 Postvaricella encephalitis** `MCC`
Postchickenpox encephalitis

CC Excl: 051.9-052.0, 052.2-052.9, 078.88-078.89, 079.81, 079.88-079.99, 139.8

**052.1 Varicella (hemorrhagic) pneumonitis** `MCC`

CC Excl: 051.9, 052.1-052.9, 078.88-078.89, 079.81, 079.88-079.99, 139.8

**052.2 Postvaricella myelitis** `MCC`
Postchickenpox myelitis

CC Excl: 051.9, 052.2-052.9, 053.14, 054.74, 078.88-078.89, 079.81, 079.88-079.99, 139.8, 323.01-323.02, 323.41-323.82, 341.20-341.22

AHA: 4Q, '06, 58-63

**052.7 With other specified complications** `CC`

CC Excl: 051.9, 052.2-052.9, 078.88-078.89, 079.81, 079.88-079.99, 139.8

AHA: 1Q, '02, 3

**052.8 With unspecified complication** `CC`

CC Excl: See code: 052.7

**052.9 Varicella without mention of complication** `CC`
Chickenpox NOS          Varicella NOS

CC Excl: See code: 052.7

`✓4ᵗʰ` **053 Herpes zoster**

> INCLUDES  shingles
> zona

DEF: Self-limiting infection by varicella-zoster virus causing unilateral eruptions and neuralgia along affected nerves.

**053.0 With meningitis** `MCC` `HIV`

CC Excl: 003.21, 013.00-013.16, 036.0, 047.0-047.9, 049.0-049.1, 053.0-053.19, 053.79-053.9, 054.72, 054.74-054.9, 058.81-058.89, 072.1, 078.88-078.89, 079.81, 079.88-079.99, 090.42, 091.81, 094.2, 098.89, 100.81, 112.83, 114.2, 115.01, 115.11, 115.91, 130.0, 139.8, 320.0-322.9, 349.89-349.9, 357.0

DEF: Varicella-zoster virus infection causing inflammation of the lining of the brain and/or spinal cord.

`✓5ᵗʰ` **053.1 With other nervous system complications**

**053.10 With unspecified nervous system complication** `CC` `HIV`

CC Excl: 053.0-053.19, 053.79-053.9, 054.72, 054.74-054.9, 058.81-058.89, 078.88-078.89, 079.81, 079.88-079.99, 139.8

**053.11 Geniculate herpes zoster** `CC` `HIV`
Herpetic geniculate ganglionitis

CC Excl: See code: 053.10

DEF: Unilateral eruptions and neuralgia along the facial nerve geniculum affecting face and outer and middle ear.

---

`N` Newborn Age: 0   `P` Pediatric Age: 0-17   `M` Maternity Age: 12-55   `A` Adult Age: 15-124   `CC` CC Condition   `MCC` Major CC Condition   `HIV` HIV Related Dx

**053.12 Postherpetic trigeminal neuralgia** `CC` `HIV`
CC Excl: See code: 053.10

DEF: Severe oral or nasal pain following a herpes zoster infection.

**053.13 Postherpetic polyneuropathy** `CC` `HIV`
CC Excl: See code: 053.10

DEF: Multiple areas of pain following a herpes zoster infection.

**053.14 Herpes zoster myelitis** `MCC`
CC Excl: 052.2, 053.0-053.19, 053.79-053.9, 054.72, 054.74-054.9, 058.81-058.89, 078.88-078.89, 079.81, 079.88-079.99, 139.8, 323.01-323.02, 323.41-323.82, 341.20-341.22

AHA: 4Q, '06, 58-63

**053.19 Other** `CC` `HIV`
CC Excl: See code: 053.10

√5ᵗʰ **053.2 With ophthalmic complications**
**053.20 Herpes zoster dermatitis of eyelid** `CC` `HIV`
Herpes zoster ophthalmicus
CC Excl: 053.20-053.29

**053.21 Herpes zoster keratoconjunctivitis** `CC` `HIV`
CC Excl: See code: 053.20

**053.22 Herpes zoster iridocyclitis** `CC` `HIV`
CC Excl: See code: 053.20

**053.29 Other** `CC` `HIV`
CC Excl: See code: 053.20

√5ᵗʰ **053.7 With other specified complications**
**053.71 Otitis externa due to herpes zoster** `CC` `HIV`
CC Excl: 053.71

**053.79 Other** `CC` `HIV`
CC Excl: 053.0-054.71, 054.73-054.9, 058.21-058.89, 078.88-078.89, 079.81, 079.88-079.99, 139.8

**053.8 With unspecified complication** `CC` `HIV`
CC Excl: See code: 053.79

**053.9 Herpes zoster without mention of complication** `HIV`
Herpes zoster NOS

√4ᵗʰ **054 Herpes simplex**
EXCLUDES congenital herpes simplex (771.2)

**054.0 Eczema herpeticum** `HIV`
Kaposi's varicelliform eruption
DEF: Herpes simplex virus invading site of preexisting skin inflammation.

√5ᵗʰ **054.1 Genital herpes**
AHA: J-F, '87, 15, 16

**054.10 Genital herpes, unspecified** `HIV`
Herpes progenitalis
**054.11 Herpetic vulvovaginitis** `HIV` ♀
**054.12 Herpetic ulceration of vulva** `HIV` ♀
**054.13 Herpetic infection of penis** `HIV` ♂
**054.19 Other** `HIV`
**054.2 Herpetic gingivostomatitis** `CC` `HIV`
CC Excl: 054.2

**054.3 Herpetic meningoencephalitis** `MCC` `HIV`
Herpes encephalitis
Simian B disease
EXCLUDES ▶ human herpesvirus 6 encephalitis (058.21)
other human herpesvirus encephalitis (058.29)◀

CC Excl: 054.3, 054.74-054.9, 058.21-058.89, 139.8

DEF: Inflammation of the brain and its lining, caused by infection of herpes simplex 1 in adults and simplex 2 in newborns.

√5ᵗʰ **054.4 With ophthalmic complications**
**054.40 With unspecified ophthalmic complication** `CC` `HIV`
CC Excl: 054.40-054.49, 054.79-054.9, 058.81-058.89

**054.41 Herpes simplex dermatitis of eyelid** `CC` `HIV`
CC Excl: See code: 054.40

**054.42 Dendritic keratitis** `CC` `HIV`
CC Excl: See code: 054.40

**054.43 Herpes simplex disciform keratitis** `CC` `HIV`
CC Excl: See code: 054.40

**054.44 Herpes simplex iridocyclitis** `CC` `HIV`
CC Excl: See code: 054.40

**054.49 Other** `CC` `HIV`
CC Excl: See code: 054.40

**054.5 Herpetic septicemia** `MCC` `HIV`
CC Excl: 003.1, 020.2, 036.2, 038.0-038.9, 054.5, 054.74-054.9, 058.81-058.89, 139.8, 995.90-995.94

AHA: 2Q, '00, 5

**054.6 Herpetic whitlow** `HIV`
Herpetic felon
DEF: A primary infection of the terminal segment of a finger by herpes simplex; intense itching and pain start the disease, vesicles form, and tissue ultimately is destroyed.

√5ᵗʰ **054.7 With other specified complications**
**054.71 Visceral herpes simplex** `CC` `HIV`
CC Excl: 054.71-054.72, 054.74-054.9, 058.81-058.89, 139.8

**054.72 Herpes simplex meningitis** `MCC` `HIV`
CC Excl: 003.21, 013.00-013.16, 036.0, 047.0-047.9, 049.0-049.1, 053.0, 054.72, 054.74-054.9, 058.81-058.89, 072.1, 090.42, 091.81, 094.2, 098.89, 100.81, 112.83, 114.2, 115.01, 115.11, 115.91, 130.0, 139.8, 320.0-322.9, 349.89-349.9, 357.0

**054.73 Herpes simplex otitis externa** `MCC`
**054.74 Herpes simplex myelitis**
CC Excl: 052.2, 053.14, 054.74-054.9, 058.81-058.89, 078.88-078.89, 079.81, 079.88-079.99, 139.8, 323.01-323.02, 323.41-323.82, 341.20-341.22

AHA: 4Q, '06, 58-63

**054.79 Other** `CC` `HIV`
CC Excl: 054.74-054.9, 058.81-058.89, 078.88-078.89, 079.81, 079.88-079.99, 139.8

**054.8 With unspecified complication** `HIV`
**054.9 Herpes simplex without mention of complication** `HIV`

√4ᵗʰ **055 Measles**
INCLUDES morbilli      rubeola
**055.0 Postmeasles encephalitis** `MCC`
CC Excl: 055.0, 055.79-055.9, 078.88-078.89, 079.81, 079.88-079.99, 139.8

**055.1 Postmeasles pneumonia** `MCC`
CC Excl: 055.1, 055.79-055.9, 078.88-078.89, 079.81, 079.88-079.99, 139.8

**055.2 Postmeasles otitis media**
√5ᵗʰ **055.7 With other specified complications**
**055.71 Measles keratoconjunctivitis** `CC`
Measles keratitis
CC Excl: 055.71-055.9, 078.88-078.89, 079.81, 079.88-079.99, 139.8

**055.79 Other** `CC`
CC Excl: 055.79-055.9, 078.88-078.89, 079.81, 079.88--079.99, 139.8

**055.8 With unspecified complication**
**055.9 Measles without mention of complication**

---

√4ᵗʰ √5ᵗʰ Additional Digit Required  Unacceptable PDx  Manifestation Code  ▶◀ Revised Text  ● New Code  ▲ Revised Code Title

**√4ᵗʰ 056 Rubella**

INCLUDES German measles

EXCLUDES congenital rubella (771.0)

DEF: Acute but usually benign togavirus infection causing fever, sore throat, and rash; associated with complications to fetus as a result of maternal infection.

**√5ᵗʰ 056.0 With neurological complications**

**056.00 With unspecified neurological complication** CC

CC Excl: 056.00-056.09, 056.79-056.9, 078.88-078.89, 079.81, 079.88-079.99, 139.8

**056.01 Encephalomyelitis due to rubella** MCC

Encephalitis
Meningoencephalitis } due to rubella

CC Excl: See code: 056.00

**056.09 Other** CC

CC Excl: See code: 056.00

**√5ᵗʰ 056.7 With other specified complications**

**056.71 Arthritis due to rubella** CC

CC Excl: 056.71-056.9, 078.88-078.89, 079.81, 079.88-079.99, 139.8

**056.79 Other** CC

CC Excl: 056.00-056.09, 056.79-056.9, 078.88-078.89, 079.81, 079.88-079.99, 139.8

**056.8 With unspecified complications**

**056.9 Rubella without mention of complication**

**√4ᵗʰ 057 Other viral exanthemata**

DEF: Skin eruptions or rashes and fever caused by viruses, including poxviruses.

**057.0 Erythema infectiosum [fifth disease]** CC

CC Excl: 057.0, 079.83

DEF: A moderately contagious, benign, epidemic disease, usually seen in children, and of probable viral etiology; a red macular rash appears on the face and may spread to the limbs and trunk.

**057.8 Other specified viral exanthemata**

Dukes (-Filatow) disease
Fourth disease
Parascarlatina
Pseudoscarlatina

EXCLUDES ► exanthema subitum [sixth disease] (058.10-058.12)

roseola infantum (058.10-058.12) ◄

**057.9 Viral exanthem, unspecified**

**►OTHER HUMAN HERPESVIRUS (058)◄**

**√4ᵗʰ 058 Other human herpesvirus**

EXCLUDES congenital herpes (771.2)
cytomegalovirus (078.5)
Epstein-Barr virus (075)
herpes NOS (054.0-054.9)
herpes simplex (054.0-054.9)
herpes zoster (053.0-053.9)
human herpesvirus NOS (054.0-054.9)
human herpesvirus 1 (054.0-054.9)
human herpesvirus 2 (054.0-054.9)
human herpesvirus 3 (052.0-053.9)
human herpesvirus 4 (075)
human herpesvirus 5 (078.5)
varicella (052.0-052.9)
varicella-zoster virus (052.0-053.9)

**√5ᵗʰ 058.1 Roseola infantum**

Exanthema subitum [sixth disease]

**058.10 Roseola infantum, unspecified**

Exanthema subitum [sixth disease], unspecified

**058.11 Roseola infantum due to human herpesvirus 6**

Exanthema subitum [sixth disease] due to human herpesvirus 6

**058.12 Roseola infantum due to human herpesvirus 7**

Exanthema subitum [sixth disease] due to human herpesvirus 7

**√5ᵗʰ 058.2 Other human herpesvirus encephalitis**

EXCLUDES herpes encephalitis NOS (054.3)
herpes simplex encephalitis (054.3)
human herpesvirus encephalitis NOS (054.3)
simian B herpesvirus encephalitis (054.3)

**058.21 Human herpesvirus 6 encephalitis** MCC HIV

CC Excl: 054.3, 054.74-054.9, 058.21-058.89, 139.8

**058.29 Other human herpesvirus encephalitis** MCC HIV

Human herpesvirus 7 encephalitis

CC Excl: See code: 058.21

**√5ᵗʰ 058.8 Other human herpesvirus infections**

**058.81 Human herpesvirus 6 infection**

**058.82 Human herpesvirus 7 infection**

**058.89 Other human herpesvirus infection**

Human herpesvirus 8 infection
Kaposi's sarcoma-associated herpesvirus infection

**ARTHROPOD-BORNE VIRAL DISEASES (060-066)**

Use additional code to identify any associated meningitis (321.2)

EXCLUDES late effects of viral encephalitis (139.0)

**√4ᵗʰ 060 Yellow fever**

DEF: Fever and jaundice from infection by mosquito-borne virus of genus Flavivirus.

**060.0 Sylvatic** CC

Yellow fever: jungle
Yellow fever: sylvan

CC Excl: 060.0-060.9

DEF: Yellow fever transmitted from animal to man, via mosquito.

**060.1 Urban** CC

CC Excl: See code: 060.0

DEF: Yellow fever transmitted from man to man, via mosquito.

**060.9 Yellow fever, unspecified** CC

CC Excl: See code: 060.0

**061 Dengue** CC

Breakbone fever

EXCLUDES hemorrhagic fever caused by dengue virus (065.4)

CC Excl: 061

DEF: Acute, self-limiting infection by mosquito-borne virus characterized by fever and generalized aches.

**√4ᵗʰ 062 Mosquito-borne viral encephalitis**

**062.0 Japanese encephalitis** MCC

Japanese B encephalitis

CC Excl: 013.60-013.66, 046.2, 046.8, 048-049.0, 049.8, 052.0, 052.2, 054.3, 054.74, 056.01, 057.8-058.29, 062.0-064, 066.2-066.49, 072.2, 073.7, 075, 079.82, 079.99, 081.9, 083.9, 090.41, 094.81, 117.5, 124, 130.0, 290.12, 323.01-323.9, 341.1, 487.8, 771.2, 984.9

DEF: Flavivirus causing inflammation of the brain, with a wide range of clinical manifestations.

**062.1 Western equine encephalitis** MCC

CC Excl: See code: 062.0

DEF: Alphavirus WEE infection causing inflammation of the brain, found in areas west of the Mississippi; transmitted horse to mosquito to man.

N Newborn Age: 0   P Pediatric Age: 0-17   M Maternity Age: 12-55   A Adult Age: 15-124   CC CC Condition   MCC Major CC Condition   HIV HIV Related Dx

14 — Volume 1 • October 2007

© 2007 Ingenix

**062.2   Eastern equine encephalitis** `MCC`

> EXCLUDES   *Venezuelan equine encephalitis (066.2)*

**CC Excl:** See code: 062.0

DEF: Alphavirus EEE causing inflammation of the brain and spinal cord, found as far north as Canada and south into South America and Mexico; transmitted horse to mosquito to man.

**062.3   St. Louis encephalitis** `MCC`

**CC Excl:** See code: 062.0

DEF: Epidemic form caused by Flavivirus and transmitted by mosquito, and characterized by fever, difficulty in speech, and headache.

**062.4   Australian encephalitis** `MCC`

     Australian arboencephalitis     Murray Valley
     Australian X disease            encephalitis

**CC Excl:** See code: 062.0

DEF: Flavivirus causing inflammation of the brain, occurring in Australia and New Guinea.

**062.5   California virus encephalitis** `MCC`

     Encephalitis:           Tahyna fever
        California
        La Crosse

**CC Excl:** See code: 062.0

DEF: Bunyamwere virus causing inflammation of the brain.

**062.8   Other specified mosquito-borne viral encephalitis** `MCC`

     Encephalitis by Ilheus virus

> EXCLUDES   *West Nile virus (066.40-066.49)*

**CC Excl:** See code: 062.0

**062.9   Mosquito-borne viral encephalitis, unspecified** `MCC`

**CC Excl:** See code: 062.0

√4th **063   Tick-borne viral encephalitis**

> INCLUDES   diphasic meningoencephalitis

**063.0   Russian spring-summer [taiga] encephalitis** `MCC`

**CC Excl:** See code: 062.0

**063.1   Louping ill** `MCC`

**CC Excl:** See code: 062.0

DEF: Inflammation of brain caused by virus transmitted sheep to tick to man; incidence usually limited to British Isles.

**063.2   Central European encephalitis** `MCC`

**CC Excl:** See code: 062.0

DEF: Inflammation of brain caused by virus transmitted by tick; limited to central Europe and presenting with two distinct phases.

**063.8   Other specified tick-borne viral encephalitis** `MCC`

     Langat encephalitis
     Powassan encephalitis

**CC Excl:** See code: 062.0

**063.9   Tick-borne viral encephalitis, unspecified** `MCC`

**CC Excl:** See code: 062.0

**064   Viral encephalitis transmitted by other and unspecified arthropods** `MCC`

     Arthropod-borne viral encephalitis, vector unknown
     Negishi virus encephalitis

> EXCLUDES   *viral encephalitis NOS (049.9)*

**CC Excl:** See code: 062.0

√4th **065   Arthropod-borne hemorrhagic fever**

**065.0   Crimean hemorrhagic fever [CHF Congo virus]** `CC`

     Central Asian hemorrhagic fever

**CC Excl:** 065.0-066.9

**065.1   Omsk hemorrhagic fever** `CC`

**CC Excl:** See code: 065.0

**065.2   Kyasanur Forest disease** `CC`

**CC Excl:** See code: 065.0

**065.3   Other tick-borne hemorrhagic fever** `CC`

**CC Excl:** See code: 065.0

**065.4   Mosquito-borne hemorrhagic fever** `CC`

     Chikungunya hemorrhagic fever
     Dengue hemorrhagic fever

> EXCLUDES   *Chikungunya fever (066.3)*
> *dengue (061)*
> *yellow fever (060.0-060.9)*

**CC Excl:** See code: 065.0

**065.8   Other specified arthropod-borne hemorrhagic fever** `CC`

     Mite-borne hemorrhagic fever

**CC Excl:** See code: 065.0

**065.9   Arthropod-borne hemorrhagic fever, unspecified** `CC`

     Arbovirus hemorrhagic fever NOS

**CC Excl:** See code: 065.0

√4th **066   Other arthropod-borne viral diseases**

**066.0   Phlebotomus fever** `CC`

     Changuinola fever        Sandfly fever

**CC Excl:** See code: 065.0

DEF: Sandfly-borne viral infection occurring in Asia, Mideast and South America.

**066.1   Tick-borne fever** `CC`

     Nairobi sheep disease     Tick fever:
     Tick fever:               Kemerovo
        American mountain    Quaranfil
        Colorado

**CC Excl:** See code: 065.0

**066.2   Venezuelan equine fever** `CC`

     Venezuelan equine encephalitis

**CC Excl:** 013.60-013.66, 046.2, 046.8, 048-049.0, 049.8, 052.0, 052.2, 054.3, 054.74, 056.01, 057.8-058.29, 062.0-066.9, 072.2, 073.7, 075, 079.82, 079.99, 081.9, 083.9, 090.41, 094.81, 117.5, 124, 130.0, 290.12, 323.01-323.9, 341.1, 487.8, 771.2, 984.9

DEF: Alphavirus VEE infection causing inflammation of the brain, usually limited to South America, Mexico, and Florida; transmitted horse to mosquito to man

**066.3   Other mosquito-borne fever** `CC`

     Fever (viral):          Fever (viral):
        Bunyamwera         Oropouche
        Bwamba             Pixuna
        Chikungunya       Rift valley
        Guama              Ross river
        Mayaro            Wesselsbron
        Mucambo          Zika
        O'Nyong-Nyong

> EXCLUDES   *dengue (061)*
> *yellow fever (060.0-060.9)*

**CC Excl:** See code: 066.2

√5th **066.4   West Nile fever**

**AHA:** 4Q, '02, 44

DEF: Mosquito-borne fever causing fatal inflammation of the brain, the lining of the brain, or of the lining of the brain and spinal cord.

**066.40   West Nile fever, unspecified** `MCC`

     West Nile fever NOS
     West Nile fever without complications
     West Nile virus NOS

**CC Excl:** 013.60-013.66, 046.2, 046.8, 048-049.0, 049.8, 052.0, 052.2, 054.3, 054.74, 056.01, 057.8-058.29, 062.0-066.3, 066.8-066.9, 072.2, 073.7, 075, 079.99, 081.9, 083.9, 090.41, 094.81, 117.5, 124, 130.0, 323.01-323.9, 341.1, 487.8, 771.2

**066.41   West Nile fever with encephalitis** `MCC`

     West Nile encephalitis
     West Nile encephalomyelitis

**CC Excl:** See code: 066.40

**AHA:** 4Q, '04, 51

---

√4th   Additional Digit Required        Unacceptable PDx        Manifestation Code        ◄► Revised Text        ● New Code        ▲ Revised Code Title
√5th

Infectious and Parasitic Diseases

066.42 – 072.2

**066.42** **West Nile fever with other neurologic** `MCC`
**manifestation**
Use additional code to specify the neurologic
manifestation
CC Excl: See code: 066.40

AHA: 4Q, '04, 51

**066.49** **West Nile fever with other** `MCC`
**complications**
Use additional code to specify the other
conditions
CC Excl: See code: 066.40

**066.8** **Other specified arthropod-borne viral diseases** `CC`
Chandipura fever
Piry fever
CC Excl: 065.0-066.9

**066.9** **Arthropod-borne viral disease, unspecified** `CC`
Arbovirus infection NOS
CC Excl: 065.0-066.9

## OTHER DISEASES DUE TO VIRUSES AND CHLAMYDIAE (070-079)

✓4ᵗʰ **070 Viral hepatitis**

`INCLUDES`   viral hepatitis (acute) (chronic)

`EXCLUDES`   *cytomegalic inclusion virus hepatitis (078.5)*

The following fifth-digit subclassification is for use with
categories 070.2 and 070.3:
   **0 acute or unspecified, without mention of**
     **hepatitis delta**
   **1 acute or unspecified, with hepatitis delta**
   **2 chronic, without mention of hepatitis delta**
   **3 chronic, with hepatitis delta**

AHA: ▶2Q,'07, 5◀

DEF: Hepatitis A : HAV infection is self-limiting with flulike symptoms;
transmission, fecal-oral.

DEF: Hepatitis B: HBV infection can be chronic and systemic; transmission,
bodily fluids.

DEF: Hepatitis C: HCV infection can be chronic and systemic; transmission,
blood transfusion and unidentified agents.

DEF: Hepatitis D (delta): HDV occurs only in the presence of hepatitis B virus.

DEF: Hepatitis E: HEV is epidemic form; transmission and nature under
investigation.

**070.0** **Viral hepatitis A with hepatic coma** `MCC`
CC Excl: 070.0-070.9, 078.88-078.89, 079.81, 079.88-079.99, 139.8

**070.1** **Viral hepatitis A without mention of hepatic** `CC`
**coma**
Infectious hepatitis
CC Excl: See code: 070.0

✓5ᵗʰ **070.2** **Viral hepatitis B with hepatic coma** `MCC`
CC Excl: See code: 070.0

AHA: 4Q, '91, 28; **For code 070.20:** ▶2Q, '07, 6◀

✓5ᵗʰ **070.3** **Viral hepatitis B without mention of hepatic** `CC`
**coma**
Serum hepatitis
CC Excl: See code: 070.0

AHA: 1Q, '93, 28; 4Q, '91, 28

✓5ᵗʰ **070.4** **Other specified viral hepatitis with hepatic coma**
AHA: 4Q, '91, 28

**070.41** **Acute hepatitis C with hepatic coma** `MCC`
CC Excl: See code: 070.0

**070.42** **Hepatitis delta without mention of** `MCC`
**active hepatitis B disease with**
**hepatic coma**
Hepatitis delta with hepatitis B carrier state
CC Excl: See code: 070.0

**070.43** **Hepatitis E with hepatic coma** `MCC`
CC Excl: See code: 070.0

**070.44** **Chronic hepatitis C with hepatic** `MCC`
**coma**
CC Excl: See code: 070.0

AHA: ▶2Q,'07, 5◀

**070.49** **Other specified viral hepatitis with** `MCC`
**hepatic coma**
CC Excl: See code: 070.0

✓5ᵗʰ **070.5** **Other specified viral hepatitis without mention of**
**hepatic coma**
AHA: 4Q, '91, 28

**070.51** **Acute hepatitis C without mention** `CC`
**of hepatic coma**
CC Excl: See code: 070.0

**070.52** **Hepatitis delta without mention of** `CC`
**active hepatititis B disease or hepatic coma**
CC Excl: See code: 070.0

**070.53** **Hepatitis E without mention of** `CC`
**hepatic coma**
CC Excl: See code: 070.0

**070.54** **Chronic hepatitis C without mention** `CC`
**of hepatic coma**
AHA: 2Q, '06, 13

**070.59** **Other specified viral hepatitis** `CC`
**without mention of hepatic coma**
CC Excl: See code: 070.0

**070.6** **Unspecified viral hepatitis with hepatic coma** `MCC`
`EXCLUDES`   *unspecified viral hepatitis C with*
*hepatic coma (070.71)*
CC Excl: See code: 070.0

✓5ᵗʰ **070.7** **Unspecified viral hepatitis C**

**070.70** **Unspecified viral hepatitis C without**
**hepatic coma**
Unspecified viral hepatitis C NOS
AHA: 4Q, '04, 52

**070.71** **Unspecified viral hepatitis C with** `MCC`
**hepatic coma**
CC Excl: See code: 070.0

AHA: 4Q, '04, 52

**070.9** **Unspecified viral hepatitis without mention** `CC`
**of hepatic coma**
Viral hepatitis NOS
`EXCLUDES`   *unspecified viral hepatitis C without*
*hepatic coma (070.70)*
CC Excl: See code: 070.0

**071 Rabies** `CC`
Hydrophobia
Lyssa
CC Excl: 071

DEF: Acute infectious disease of the CNS caused by a rhabdovirus; usually
spread by virus-laden saliva from bites by infected animals; it progresses
from fever, restlessness, and extreme excitability, to hydrophobia, seizures,
confusion and death.

✓4ᵗʰ **072 Mumps**
DEF: Acute infectious disease caused by paramyxovirus; usually seen in
children less than 15 years of age; salivary glands are typically enlarged, and
other organs, such as testes, pancreas and meninges, are often involved.

**072.0** **Mumps orchitis** `CC` ♂
CC Excl: 072.0, 072.79-072.9, 078.88-078.89, 079.81, 079.88-079.99, 139.8

**072.1** **Mumps meningitis** `MCC`
CC Excl: 003.21, 013.00-013.16, 036.0, 047.0-047.9, 049.0-049.1, 053.0,
054.72, 072.1, 072.79-072.9, 078.88-078.89, 079.81, 079.88-079.99, 090.42,
091.81, 094.2, 098.89, 100.81, 112.83, 114.2, 115.01, 115.11, 115.91, 130.0,
139.8, 320.0-322.9, 349.89-349.9, 357.0

**072.2** **Mumps encephalitis** `MCC`
Mumps meningoencephalitis
CC Excl: 072.2, 072.79-072.9, 078.88-078.89, 079.81, 079.88-079.99, 139.8

---

`N` Newborn Age: 0    `P` Pediatric Age: 0-17    `M` Maternity Age: 12-55    `A` Adult Age: 15-124    `CC` CC Condition    `MCC` Major CC Condition    `HIV` HIV Related Dx

**072.3**    **Mumps pancreatitis**    `CC`
CC Excl: 072.3, 072.79-072.9, 078.88-078.89, 079.81, 079.88-079.99, 139.8

✓5ᵗʰ **072.7**    **Mumps with other specified complications**
    **072.71 Mumps hepatitis**    `CC`
      CC Excl: 072.71, 072.79-072.9, 078.88-078.89, 079.81, 079.88-079.99, 139.8

    **072.72 Mumps polyneuropathy**    `CC`
      CC Excl: 072.72-072.9, 078.88-078.89, 079.81, 079.88-079.99, 139.8

    **072.79 Other**    `CC`
      CC Excl: 072.79-072.9, 078.88-078.89, 079.81, 079.88-079.99, 139.8

**072.8**    **Mumps with unspecified complication**    `CC`
CC Excl: 072.79-072.9, 078.88-078.89, 079.81, 079.88-079.99

**072.9**    **Mumps without mention of complication**
    Epidemic parotitis
    Infectious parotitis

✓4ᵗʰ **073 Ornithosis**
   INCLUDES   parrot fever
          psittacosis
   DEF: *Chlamydia psittaci* infection often transmitted from birds to humans.

**073.0**    **With pneumonia**    `MCC`
    Lobular pneumonitis due to ornithosis
    CC Excl: 011.00-012.16, 012.80-012.86, 017.90-017.96, 020.3-020.5, 021.3, 022.1, 031.0, 039.1, 073.0, 073.8-073.9, 115.05, 115.15, 115.95, 122.1, 130.4, 136.3, 480.0-487.1, 488, 495.0-495.9, 500-508.9, 517.1, 517.8, 518.89, 519.8-519.9

**073.7**    **With other specified complications**    `CC`
    CC Excl: 013.60-013.66, 046.2, 046.8, 048-049.0, 049.8, 052.0, 052.2, 054.3, 054.74, 056.01, 057.8-058.29, 062.0-064, 066.2-066.49, 072.2, 073.0-073.9, 079.82, 079.99, 081.9, 083.9, 090.41, 094.81, 117.5, 124, 130.0, 290.12, 323.01-323.9, 341.1, 487.8, 771.2, 984.9

**073.8**    **With unspecified complication**    `CC`
    CC Excl: 073.0, 073.8-073.9

**073.9**    **Ornithosis, unspecified**    `CC`
    CC Excl: See code: 073.8

✓4ᵗʰ **074 Specific diseases due to Coxsackie virus**
   EXCLUDES   Coxsackie virus:
            infection NOS (079.2)
            meningitis (047.0)

**074.0**    **Herpangina**
    Vesicular pharyngitis
    DEF: Acute infectious coxsackie virus infection causing throat lesions, fever, and vomiting; generally affects children in summer.

**074.1**    **Epidemic pleurodynia**
    Bornholm disease       Epidemic:
    Devil's grip            myalgia
                       myositis
    DEF: Paroxysmal pain in chest, accompanied by fever and usually limited to children and young adults; caused by coxsackie virus.

✓5ᵗʰ **074.2**    **Coxsackie carditis**
    **074.20 Coxsackie carditis, unspecified**    `CC`
      CC Excl: 074.20, 074.22-074.23, 093.82, 390, 391.2-391.9, 398.0-398.90, 398.99, 422.0-422.99, 429.0, 429.71-429.79, 459.89-459.9

    **074.21 Coxsackie pericarditis**    `CC`
      CC Excl: 074.21, 093.81, 391.0, 393, 420.0-420.99, 423.3-423.9, 459.89-459.9
      DEF: Coxsackie infection of the outer lining of the heart.

    **074.22 Coxsackie endocarditis**    `CC`
      CC Excl: 002.0, 036.42, 074.22, 083.0, 093.20-093.24, 098.84, 112.81, 115.94, 116.0, 390, 391.1, 391.8-392.0, 394.0-395.9, 396.9-397.9, 398.90, 398.99, 421.0-421.9, 424.0-424.99, 425.3, 459.89-459.9, 746.09, 746.89, 996.61
      DEF: Coxsackie infection within the heart's cavities.

**074.23 Coxsackie myocarditis**    `CC`
    Aseptic myocarditis of newborn
    CC Excl: See code: 074.20
    DEF: Coxsackie infection of the muscle of the heart.

**074.3**    **Hand, foot, and mouth disease**
    Vesicular stomatitis and exanthem
    DEF: Mild coxsackie infection causing lesions on hands, feet and oral mucosa, most commonly seen in preschool children.

**074.8**    **Other specified diseases due to Coxsackie virus**
    Acute lymphonodular pharyngitis

**075 Infectious mononucleosis**
    Glandular fever          Pfeiffer's disease
    Monocytic angina
    AHA: 3Q, '01, 13; M-A, '87, 8
    DEF: Acute infection by Epstein-Barr virus causing fever, sore throat, enlarged lymph glands and spleen, and fatigue; usually seen in teens and young adults.

✓4ᵗʰ **076 Trachoma**
   EXCLUDES   late effect of trachoma (139.1)
   DEF: A chronic infectious disease of the cornea and conjunctiva caused by a strain of the bacteria *Chlamydia trachomatis*; the infection can cause photophobia, pain, excessive tearing and sometimes blindness.

**076.0**    **Initial stage**
    Trachoma dubium

**076.1**    **Active stage**
    Granular conjunctivitis (trachomatous)
    Trachomatous:
      follicular conjunctivitis
      pannus

**076.9**    **Trachoma, unspecified**
    Trachoma NOS

✓4ᵗʰ **077 Other diseases of conjunctiva due to viruses and Chlamydiae**
   EXCLUDES   ophthalmic complications of viral diseases classified elsewhere

**077.0**    **Inclusion conjunctivitis**
    Paratrachoma       Swimming pool conjunctivitis
    EXCLUDES   inclusion blennorrhea (neonatal) (771.6)
    DEF: Pus in conjunctiva caused by *Chlamydiae trachomatis*.

**077.1**    **Epidemic keratoconjunctivitis**
    Shipyard eye
    DEF: Highly contagious corneal or conjunctival infection caused by adenovirus type 8; symptoms include inflammation and corneal infiltrates.

**077.2**    **Pharyngoconjunctival fever**
    Viral pharyngoconjunctivitis

**077.3**    **Other adenoviral conjunctivitis**
    Acute adenoviral follicular conjunctivitis

**077.4**    **Epidemic hemorrhagic conjunctivitis**
    Apollo:
      conjunctivitis
      disease
    Conjunctivitis due to enterovirus type 70
    Hemorrhagic conjunctivitis (acute) (epidemic)

**077.8**    **Other viral conjunctivitis**
    Newcastle conjunctivitis

✓5ᵗʰ **077.9**    **Unspecified diseases of conjunctiva due to viruses and Chlamydiae**
    **077.98 Due to Chlamydiae**
    **077.99 Due to viruses**
      Viral conjunctivitis NOS

✓4ᵗʰ **078 Other diseases due to viruses and Chlamydiae**
   EXCLUDES   viral infection NOS (079.0-079.9)
            viremia NOS (790.8)

**078.0**    **Molluscum contagiosum**
    DEF: Benign poxvirus infection causing small bumps on the skin or conjunctiva; transmitted by close contact.

---

✓4ᵗʰ / ✓5ᵗʰ Additional Digit Required     Unacceptable PDx     Manifestation Code     ◄► Revised Text     ● New Code     ▲ Revised Code Title

**Infectious and Parasitic Diseases**

**078.1–079.81**

√5th **078.1 Viral warts**
Viral warts due to human papilloma virus
**AHA:** 2Q, '97, 9; 4Q, '93, 22

DEF: A keratotic papilloma of the epidermis caused by the human papilloma virus; the superficial vegetative lesions last for varying durations and eventually regress spontaneously.

**078.10 Viral warts, unspecified**
Condyloma NOS    Verruca:
Verruca:        Vulgaris
    NOS        Warts (infectious)

**078.11 Condyloma acuminatum**
DEF: Clusters of mucosa or epidermal lesions on external genitalia; viral infection is sexually transmitted.

**078.19 Other specified viral warts**
Genital warts NOS    Verruca:
Verruca:        plantaris
   plana

**078.2 Sweating fever**
Miliary fever        Sweating disease
DEF: A viral infection characterized by profuse sweating; various papular, vesicular and other eruptions cause the blockage of sweat glands.

**078.3 Cat-scratch disease**    `CC`
Benign lymphoreticulosis (of inoculation)
Cat-scratch fever
**CC Excl:** 078.3, 079.82

**078.4 Foot and mouth disease**
Aphthous fever      Epizootic:
Epizootic:        stomatitis
   aphthae
DEF: Ulcers on oral mucosa, legs, and feet after exposure to infected animal.

**078.5 Cytomegaloviral disease**    `CC` `HIV`
Cytomegalic inclusion disease
Salivary gland virus disease
Use additional code to identify manifestation, as:
   cytomegalic inclusion virus:
     hepatitis (573.1)
     pneumonia (484.1)
EXCLUDES   *congenital cytomegalovirus infection (771.1)*
**CC Excl:** 078.5-078.7, 078.89-079.50, 079.59, 079.81-079.82, 079.89, 079.99

**AHA:** 1Q, '03, 10; 3Q, '98, 4; 2Q, '93, 11; 1Q, '89, 9

DEF: A herpesvirus inclusion associated with serious disease morbidity including fever, leukopenia, pneumonia, retinitis, hepatitis and organ transplant; often leads to syndromes such as hepatomegaly, splenomegaly and thrombocytopenia; a common post-transplant complication for organ transplant recipients.

**078.6 Hemorrhagic nephrosonephritis**    `CC`
Hemorrhagic fever:    Hemorrhagic fever:
   epidemic        Russian
   Korean        with renal syndrome
**CC Excl:** 016.00-016.06, 016.30-016.36, 016.90-016.96, 017.90-017.96, 078.6, 079.82, 098.10, 098.19, 098.30-098.31, 098.89, 112.2, 131.00, 131.8-131.9, 250.40-250.43, 250.80-250.93, 274.10, 274.19, 580.0-584.9, 586-591, 593.0-593.2, 593.89-593.9, 599.7-599.9

DEF: Viral infection causing kidney dysfunction and bleeding disorders.

**078.7 Arenaviral hemorrhagic fever**    `CC`
Hemorrhagic fever:    Hemorrhagic fever:
   Argentine        Junin virus
   Bolivian        Machupo virus
**CC Excl:** 078.5-079.82, 079.88-079.99

√5th **078.8 Other specified diseases due to viruses and Chlamydiae**
EXCLUDES   *epidemic diarrhea (009.2)*
*lymphogranuloma venereum (099.1)*

**078.81 Epidemic vertigo**
**078.82 Epidemic vomiting syndrome**
Winter vomiting disease
**078.88 Other specified diseases due to Chlamydiae**
**AHA:** 4Q, '96, 22

**078.89 Other specified diseases due to viruses**
Epidemic cervical myalgia
Marburg disease
Tanapox

√4th **079 Viral and chlamydial infection in conditions classified elsewhere and of unspecified site**
Note: This category is provided to be used as an additional code to identify the viral agent in diseases classifiable elsewhere. This category will also be used to classify virus infection of unspecified nature or site.

**079.0 Adenovirus**
**079.1 ECHO virus**
DEF: An "orphan" enteric RNA virus, certain serotypes of which are associated with human disease, especially aseptic meningitis.

**079.2 Coxsackie virus**
DEF: A heterogenous group of viruses associated with aseptic meningitis, myocarditis, pericarditis, and acute onset juvenile diabetes.

**079.3 Rhinovirus**
DEF: Rhinoviruses affect primarily the upper respiratory tract. Over 100 distinct types infect humans.

**079.4 Human papillomavirus**
**AHA:** 2Q, '97, 9; 4Q, '93, 22

DEF: Viral infection caused by the genus *Papillomavirus* causing cutaneous and genital warts, including verruca vulgaris and condyloma acuminatum; certain types are associated with cervical dysplasia, cancer and other genital malignancies.

√5th **079.5 Retrovirus**
EXCLUDES   *human immunodeficiency virus, type 1 [HIV-1] (042)*
*human T-cell lymphotrophic virus, type III [HTLV-III] (042)*
*lymphadenopathy-associated virus [LAV] (042)*
**AHA:** 4Q, '93, 22, 23

DEF: A large group of RNA viruses that carry reverse transcriptase and include the leukoviruses and lentiviruses.

**079.50 Retrovirus, unspecified**
**079.51 Human T-cell lymphotrophic virus, type I [HTLV-I]**    `CC`
**CC Excl:** 079.51-079.59, 079.81-079.82, 079.88-079.99

**079.52 Human T-cell lymphotrophic virus, type II [HTLV-II]**    `CC`
**CC Excl:** 079.50-079.59, 079.81-079.82, 079.88-079.99

**079.53 Human immunodeficiency virus, type 2 [HIV-2]**    `CC`
**CC Excl:** 042, 079.50-079.59, 079.81-079.82, 079.88-079.99

**079.59 Other specified retrovirus**
**079.6 Respiratory syncytial virus (RSV)**
**AHA:** 4Q, '96, 27, 28

DEF: The major respiratory pathogen of young children, causing severe bronchitis and bronchopneumonia, and minor infection in adults.

√5th **079.8 Other specified viral and chlamydial infections**
**AHA:** 1Q, '88, 12

**079.81 Hantavirus**    `CC`
**CC Excl:** 070.70-070.71, 078.5-079.82, 079.88-079.99
**AHA:** 4Q, '95, 60

DEF: An infection caused by the Muerto Canyon virus whose primary rodent reservoir is the deer mouse Peromyscus maniculatus; commonly characterized by fever, myalgias, headache, cough and rapid decline.

---

`N` Newborn Age: 0     `P` Pediatric Age: 0-17     `M` Maternity Age: 12-55     `A` Adult Age: 15-124     `CC` CC Condition     `MCC` Major CC Condition     `HIV` HIV Related Dx

18 — Volume 1 • October 2007                                 © 2007 Ingenix

079.82 **SARS-associated coronavirus**  `CC`
**CC Excl:** 011.00-012.16, 012.80-012.86, 017.90-017.96, 021.2, 031.0, 039.1, 079.82, 079.89, 115.05, 115.15, 115.95, 122.1, 130.4, 136.3, 480.0-480.2, 480.8-487.1, 488, 494.0-508.9, 517.1, 517.8, 518.89, 519.8-519.9, 748.61

**AHA:** 4Q, '03, 46

**DEF:** A life-threatening respiratory disease described as severe acute respiratory syndrome (SARS); etiology coronavirus; most common presenting symptoms may range from mild to more severe forms of flu-like conditions; fever, chills, cough, headache, myalgia; diagnosis of SARS is based upon clinical, laboratory, and epidemiological criteria.

• 079.83 **Parvovirus B19**  `CC`
Human parvovirus
Parvovirus NOS
**EXCLUDES** erythema infectiosum [fifth disease] (057.0)

**CC Excl:** 057.0, 079.83

079.88 **Other specified chlamydial infection**
079.89 **Other specified viral infection**
√5ᵗʰ 079.9 **Unspecified viral and chlamydial infections**
**EXCLUDES** viremia NOS (790.8)

**AHA:** 2Q, '91, 8

079.98 **Unspecified chlamydial infection**
Chlamydial infections NOS
079.99 **Unspecified viral infection**
Viral infections NOS

## RICKETTSIOSES AND OTHER ARTHROPOD-BORNE DISEASES (080-088)

**EXCLUDES** arthropod-borne viral diseases (060.0-066.9)

080 **Louse-borne [epidemic] typhus**  `CC`
Typhus (fever):    Typhus (fever):
  classical        exanthematic NOS
  epidemic       louse-borne
**CC Excl:** 080-083.9, 085.0-088.9
**DEF:** *Rickettsia prowazekii*; causes severe headache, rash, high fever.

√4ᵗʰ 081 **Other typhus**
081.0 **Murine [endemic] typhus**  `CC`
Typhus (fever):    Typhus (fever):
  endemic       flea-borne
**CC Excl:** See code: 080
**DEF:** Milder typhus caused by *Rickettsia typhi (mooseri)*; transmitted by rat flea.

081.1 **Brill's disease**  `CC`
Brill-Zinsser disease
Recrudescent typhus (fever)
**CC Excl:** See code: 080

081.2 **Scrub typhus**  `CC`
Japanese river fever   Mite-borne typhus
Kedani fever        Tsutsugamushi
**CC Excl:** See code: 080

081.9 **Typhus, unspecified**  `CC`
Typhus (fever) NOS
**CC Excl:** 013.60-013.66, 046.2, 046.8, 048-049.0, 049.8, 052.0, 052.2, 054.3, 054.74, 056.01, 057.8-058.29, 062.0-064, 066.2-066.49, 072.2, 073.7, 079.82, 079.99-084.0, 085.0-088.9, 090.41, 094.81, 117.5, 124, 130.0, 290.12, 323.01-323.9, 341.1, 487.8, 771.2, 984.9

√4ᵗʰ 082 **Tick-borne rickettsioses**
082.0 **Spotted fevers**  `CC`
Rocky mountain spotted fever
Sao Paulo fever
**CC Excl:** See code: 080

082.1 **Boutonneuse fever**  `CC`
African tick typhus   Marseilles fever
India tick typhus    Mediterranean tick fever
Kenya tick typhus
**CC Excl:** See code: 080

082.2 **North Asian tick fever**  `CC`
Siberian tick typhus
**CC Excl:** See code: 080

082.3 **Queensland tick typhus**  `CC`
**CC Excl:** See code: 080

√5ᵗʰ 082.4 **Ehrlichiosis**
**AHA:** 3Q, '06, 11; 4Q, '00, 38

082.40 **Ehrlichiosis, unspecified**  `CC`
**CC Excl:** See code: 080

082.41 **Ehrlichiosis chaffeensis [E. chaffeensis]**  `CC`
**CC Excl:** See code: 080

**DEF:** A febrile illness caused by bacterial infection, also called human monocytic ehrlichiosis (HME). Causal organism is *Ehrlichia chaffeensis*, transmitted by the Lone Star tick, *Amblyomma americanum*. Symptoms include fever, chills, myalgia, nausea, vomiting, diarrhea, confusion, and severe headache occurring one week after a tick bite. Clinical findings are lymphadenopathy, rash, thrombocytopenia, leukopenia, and abnormal liver function tests.

082.49 **Other ehrlichiosis**  `CC`
**CC Excl:** See code: 080

082.8 **Other specified tick-borne rickettsioses**  `CC`
Lone star fever
**CC Excl:** See code: 080
**AHA:** 4Q, '99, 19

082.9 **Tick-borne rickettsiosis, unspecified**  `CC`
Tick-borne typhus NOS
**CC Excl:** See code: 080

√4ᵗʰ 083 **Other rickettsioses**
083.0 **Q fever**  `CC`
**CC Excl:** See code: 080
**DEF:** Infection of *Coxiella burnettii* usually acquired through airborne organisms.

083.1 **Trench fever**  `CC`
Quintan fever
Wolhynian fever
**CC Excl:** See code: 080

083.2 **Rickettsialpox**  `CC`
Vesicular rickettsiosis
**CC Excl:** 082.0-083.9
**DEF:** Infection of *Rickettsia akari* usually acquired through a mite bite.

083.8 **Other specified rickettsioses**  `CC`
**CC Excl:** See code: 083.2

083.9 **Rickettsiosis, unspecified**  `CC`
**CC Excl:** See code: 083.2

√4ᵗʰ 084 **Malaria**
Note: Subcategories 084.0-084.6 exclude the listed conditions with mention of pernicious complications (084.8-084.9).
**EXCLUDES** congenital malaria (771.2)
**DEF:** Mosquito-borne disease causing high fever and prostration and cataloged by species of *Plasmodium: P. falciparum, P. malariae, P. ovale,* and *P. vivax.*

084.0 **Falciparum malaria [malignant tertian]**  `MCC`
Malaria (fever):
  by Plasmodium falciparum
  subtertian
**CC Excl:** 084.0-086.9

---

√4ᵗʰ / √5ᵗʰ Additional Digit Required    Unacceptable PDx    Manifestation Code    ▶◀ Revised Text    ● New Code    ▲ Revised Code Title

**Infectious and Parasitic Diseases**

**084.1–087.1**

**084.1**    **Vivax malaria [benign tertian]**    `CC`
Malaria (fever) by Plasmodium vivax
**CC Excl:** 084.0-088.9

**084.2**    **Quartan malaria**    `CC`
Malaria (fever) by Plasmodium malariae
Malariae malaria
**CC Excl:** See code: 084.0

**084.3**    **Ovale malaria**    `CC`
Malaria (fever) by Plasmodium ovale
**CC Excl:** See code: 084.0

**084.4**    **Other malaria**    `CC`
Monkey malaria
**CC Excl:** See code: 084.0

**084.5**    **Mixed malaria**    `CC`
Malaria (fever) by more than one parasite
**CC Excl:** See code: 084.0

**084.6**    **Malaria, unspecified**    `CC`
Malaria (fever) NOS
**CC Excl:** 079.82, 084.0-086.9

**084.7**    **Induced malaria**    `CC`
Therapeutically induced malaria
**EXCLUDES** accidental infection from syringe, blood transfusion, etc. (084.0-084.6, above, according to parasite species)
transmission from mother to child during delivery (771.2)
**CC Excl:** 084.1-086.9

**084.8**    **Blackwater fever**    `CC`
Hemoglobinuric:    Malarial hemoglobinuria
fever (bilious)
malaria
**CC Excl:** See code: 084.0

**DEF:** Severe hemic and renal complication of *Plasmodium falciparum* infection.

**084.9**    **Other pernicious complications of malaria**    `CC`
Algid malaria
Cerebral malaria
Use additional code to identify complication, as:
malarial:
hepatitis (573.2)
nephrosis (581.81)
**CC Excl:** See code: 084.0

**√4ᵗʰ**   **085 Leishmaniasis**

**085.0**    **Visceral [kala-azar]**    `CC`
Dumdum fever    Leishmaniasis:
Infection by Leishmania:    dermal, post-kala-azar
donovani    Mediterranean
infantum    visceral (Indian)
**CC Excl:** 080-088.9

**085.1**    **Cutaneous, urban**    `CC`
Aleppo boil    Leishmaniasis, cutaneous:
Baghdad boil    dry form
Delhi boil    late
Infection by Leishmania    recurrent
tropica (minor)    ulcerating
   Oriental sore
**CC Excl:** See code: 085.0

**085.2**    **Cutaneous, Asian desert**    `CC`
Infection by Leishmania tropica major
Leishmaniasis, cutaneous:
acute necrotizing
rural
wet form
zoonotic form
**CC Excl:** See code: 085.0

**085.3**    **Cutaneous, Ethiopian**    `CC`
Infection by Leishmania ethiopica
Leishmaniasis, cutaneous:
diffuse
lepromatous
**CC Excl:** See code: 085.0

**085.4**    **Cutaneous, American**    `CC`
Chiclero ulcer
Infection by Leishmania mexicana
Leishmaniasis tegumentaria diffusa
**CC Excl:** See code: 085.0

**085.5**    **Mucocutaneous (American)**    `CC`
Espundia
Infection by Leishmania braziliensis
Uta
**CC Excl:** See code: 085.0

**085.9**    **Leishmaniasis, unspecified**    `CC`
**CC Excl:** See code: 085.0

**√4ᵗʰ**   **086 Trypanosomiasis**
Use additional code to identify manifestations, as:
trypanosomiasis:
encephalitis (323.2)
meningitis (321.3)

**086.0**    **Chagas' disease with heart involvement**    `CC`
American trypanosomiasis ⎫ with heart
Infection by Trypanosoma cruzi ⎬ involvement
Any condition classifiable to 086.2 with heart involvement
**CC Excl:** 086.0, 139.8

**086.1**    **Chagas' disease with other organ involvement**    `CC`
American trypanosomiasis ⎫ with involvement of
Infection by Trypanosoma ⎬ organ other
cruzi ⎭ than heart
Any condition classifiable to 086.2 with involvement of organ other than heart
**CC Excl:** 080-088.9

**086.2**    **Chagas' disease without mention of organ involvement**    `CC`
American trypanosomiasis
Infection by Trypanosoma cruzi
**CC Excl:** See code: 086.1

**086.3**    **Gambian trypanosomiasis**    `CC`
Gambian sleeping sickness
Infection by Trypanosoma gambiense
**CC Excl:** See code: 086.1

**086.4**    **Rhodesian trypanosomiasis**    `CC`
Infection by Trypanosoma rhodesiense
Rhodesian sleeping sickness
**CC Excl:** See code: 086.1

**086.5**    **African trypanosomiasis, unspecified**    `CC`
Sleeping sickness NOS
**CC Excl:** See code: 086.1

**086.9**    **Trypanosomiasis, unspecified**    `CC`
**CC Excl:** 013.60-013.66, 046.2, 046.8, 048-049.0, 049.8, 052.0, 052.2, 054.3, 054.74, 056.01, 057.8-058.29, 062.0-064, 066.2-066.3, 072.2, 073.7, 075, 078.3, 079.99-088.9, 090.41, 094.81, 117.5, 124, 130.0, 290.12, 323.01-323.9, 341.1, 382.4, 487.8, 771.2, 984.9

**√4ᵗʰ**   **087 Relapsing fever**
**INCLUDES** recurrent fever
**DEF:** Infection of *Borrelia;* symptoms are episodic and include fever and arthralgia.

**087.0**    **Louse-borne**    `CC`
**CC Excl:** 080-083.9, 085.0-088.9

**087.1**    **Tick-borne**    `CC`
**CC Excl:** See code: 087.0

---

`N` Newborn Age: 0    `P` Pediatric Age: 0-17    `M` Maternity Age: 12-55    `A` Adult Age: 15-124    `CC` CC Condition    `MCC` Major CC Condition    `HIV` HIV Related Dx

**087.9 Relapsing fever, unspecified** `CC`
    **CC Excl:** See code: 087.0

√4th **088 Other arthropod-borne diseases**
  **088.0 Bartonellosis** `CC`
    Carrión's disease     Verruga peruana
    Oroya fever
    **CC Excl:** See code: 087.0

√5th **088.8 Other specified arthropod-borne diseases**
  **088.81 Lyme disease** `CC`
    Erythema chronicum migrans
    **CC Excl:** See code: 087.0

    **AHA:** 4Q, '91, 15; 3Q, '90, 14; 2Q, '89, 10

    **DEF:** A recurrent multisystem disorder caused by the spirochete *Borrelia burgdorferi* with the carrier being the tick *Ixodes dammini*; the disease begins with lesions of erythema chronicum migrans; it is followed by arthritis of the large joints, myalgia, malaise, and neurological and cardiac manifestations.

  **088.82 Babesiosis** `CC`
    Babesiasis
    **CC Excl:** 080-088.9

    **AHA:** 4Q, '93, 23

    **DEF:** A tick-borne disease caused by infection of *Babesia*, characterized by fever, malaise, listlessness, severe anemia and hemoglobinuria.

  **088.89 Other**
  **088.9 Arthropod-borne disease, unspecified**

## SYPHILIS AND OTHER VENEREAL DISEASES (090-099)

    **EXCLUDES**   *nonvenereal endemic syphilis (104.0)*
                *urogenital trichomoniasis (131.0)*

√4th **090 Congenital syphilis**
    **DEF:** Infection by spirochete *Treponema pallidum* acquired in utero from the infected mother.

  **090.0 Early congenital syphilis, symptomatic** `CC`
    Congenital syphilitic:    Congenital syphilitic:
      choroiditis          splenomegaly
      coryza (chronic)   Syphilitic (congenital):
      hepatomegaly       epiphysitis
      mucous patches     osteochondritis
      periostitis          pemphigus
    Any congenital syphilitic condition specified as early or manifest less than two years after birth
    **CC Excl:** 090.0-097.9

  **090.1 Early congenital syphilis, latent**
    Congenital syphilis without clinical manifestations, with positive serological reaction and negative spinal fluid test, less than two years after birth

  **090.2 Early congenital syphilis, unspecified** `CC`
    Congenital syphilis NOS, less than two years after birth
    **CC Excl:** 090.0-099.9, 139.8

  **090.3 Syphilitic interstitial keratitis** `CC`
    Syphilitic keratitis:    Syphilitic keratitis:
      parenchymatous     punctata profunda
    **EXCLUDES**   *interstitial keratitis NOS (370.50)*
    **CC Excl:** See code: 090.0

√5th **090.4 Juvenile neurosyphilis**
    Use additional code to identify any associated mental disorder
    **DEF:** *Treponema pallidum* infection involving the nervous system.

  **090.40 Juvenile neurosyphilis, unspecified** `CC`
    Congenital neurosyphilis
    Dementia paralytica juvenilis
    Juvenile:
      general paresis
      tabes
      taboparesis
    **CC Excl:** 090.0-097.9, 099.40-099.9, 139.8

  **090.41 Congenital syphilitic encephalitis** `MCC`
    **CC Excl:** See code: 090.40

    **DEF:** Congenital *Treponema pallidum* infection involving the brain.

  **090.42 Congenital syphilitic meningitis** `MCC`
    **CC Excl:** 003.21, 013.00-013.16, 036.0, 047.0-047.9, 049.0-049.1, 053.0, 054.72, 072.1, 090.0-097.9, 098.89, 099.40-099.9, 100.81, 112.83, 114.2, 115.01, 115.11, 115.91, 130.0, 139.8, 320.0-322.9, 349.89-349.9, 357.0

    **DEF:** Congenital *Treponema pallidum* infection involving the lining of the brain and/or spinal cord.

  **090.49 Other** `CC`
    **CC Excl:** See code: 090.40

  **090.5 Other late congenital syphilis, symptomatic** `CC`
    Gumma due to congenital syphilis
    Hutchinson's teeth
    Syphilitic saddle nose
    Any congenital syphilitic condition specified as late or manifest two years or more after birth
    **CC Excl:** 090.0-097.9

  **090.6 Late congenital syphilis, latent**
    Congenital syphilis without clinical manifestations, with positive serological reaction and negative spinal fluid test, two years or more after birth

  **090.7 Late congenital syphilis, unspecified**
    Congenital syphilis NOS, two years or more after birth

  **090.9 Congenital syphilis, unspecified**

√4th **091 Early syphilis, symptomatic**
    **EXCLUDES**   *early cardiovascular syphilis (093.0-093.9)*
                *early neurosyphilis (094.0-094.9)*

  **091.0 Genital syphilis (primary)**
    Genital chancre
    **DEF:** Genital lesion at the site of initial infection by *Treponema pallidum*.

  **091.1 Primary anal syphilis**
    **DEF:** Anal lesion at the site of initial infection by *Treponema pallidum*.

  **091.2 Other primary syphilis**
    Primary syphilis of:    Primary syphilis of:
      breast            lip
      fingers          tonsils
    **DEF:** Lesion at the site of initial infection by *Treponema pallidum*.

  **091.3 Secondary syphilis of skin or mucous membranes** `CC`
    Condyloma latum    Secondary syphilis of:
    Secondary syphilis of:    skin
      anus             tonsils
      mouth           vulva
      pharynx
    **CC Excl:** 090.0-097.9

    **DEF:** Transitory or chronic lesions following initial syphilis infection.

  **091.4 Adenopathy due to secondary syphilis** `CC`
    Syphilitic adenopathy (secondary)
    Syphilitic lymphadenitis (secondary)
    **CC Excl:** 090.0-097.9

**Infectious and Parasitic Diseases**

**091.5–094.81**

√5ᵗʰ **091.5　Uveitis due to secondary syphilis**
　**091.50　Syphilitic uveitis, unspecified** CC
　　CC Excl: 090.0-097.9

　**091.51　Syphilitic chorioretinitis (secondary)** CC
　　CC Excl: 090.0-097.9

　　DEF: Inflammation of choroid and retina as a secondary infection.

　**091.52　Syphilitic iridocyclitis (secondary)** CC
　　CC Excl: 090.0-097.9

　　DEF: Inflammation of iris and ciliary body as a secondary infection.

√5ᵗʰ **091.6　Secondary syphilis of viscera and bone**
　**091.61　Secondary syphilitic periostitis** CC
　　CC Excl: 015.90-015.96, 090.0-099.9, 102.6, 730.10-730.19, 730.30-730.39, 733.99

　　DEF: Inflammation of outer layers of bone as a secondary infection.

　**091.62　Secondary syphilitic hepatitis** CC
　　Secondary syphilis of liver
　　CC Excl: 090.0-099.9, 571.49-571.9, 573.1-573.3, 573.8-573.9

　**091.69　Other viscera** CC
　　CC Excl: 090.0-099.9, 139.8

　**091.7　Secondary syphilis, relapse** CC
　　Secondary syphilis, relapse (treated) (untreated)
　　CC Excl: 090.0-099.9, 139.8

　　DEF: Return of symptoms of syphilis following asymptomatic period.

√5ᵗʰ **091.8　Other forms of secondary syphilis**
　**091.81　Acute syphilitic meningitis (secondary)** MCC
　　CC Excl: 003.21, 013.00-013.16, 036.0, 047.0-047.9, 049.0-049.1, 072.1, 078.88-078.89, 079.81, 079.88-079.99, 090.0-099.9, 100.81, 112.83, 114.2, 115.01, 115.11, 115.91, 130.0, 139.8, 320.0-322.9, 349.89-349.9, 357.0

　　DEF: Sudden, severe inflammation of the lining of the brain and/or spinal cord as a secondary infection.

　**091.82　Syphilitic alopecia** CC
　　CC Excl: 090.0-099.9

　　DEF: Hair loss following initial syphillis infection.

　**091.89　Other** CC
　　CC Excl: 090.0-099.9, 139.8

　**091.9　Unspecified secondary syphilis** CC
　　CC Excl: 090.0-099.9, 139.8

√4ᵗʰ **092　Early syphilis, latent**
　INCLUDES　syphilis (acquired) without clinical manifestations, with positive serological reaction and negative spinal fluid test, less than two years after infection

　**092.0　Early syphilis, latent, serological relapse after treatment**
　**092.9　Early syphilis, latent, unspecified**

√4ᵗʰ **093　Cardiovascular syphilis**
　**093.0　Aneurysm of aorta, specified as syphilitic** CC
　　Dilatation of aorta, specified as syphilitic
　　CC Excl: 090.0-097.9, 099.40-099.9, 139.8

　**093.1　Syphilitic aortitis** CC
　　CC Excl: See code: 093.0

　　DEF: Inflammation of the aorta – the main artery leading from the heart.

√5ᵗʰ **093.2　Syphilitic endocarditis**
　　DEF: Inflammation of the tissues lining the cavities of the heart.

　**093.20　Valve, unspecified** CC
　　Syphilitic ostial coronary disease
　　CC Excl: See code: 093.0

　**093.21　Mitral valve** CC
　　CC Excl: See code: 093.0

　**093.22　Aortic valve** CC
　　Syphilitic aortic incompetence or stenosis
　　CC Excl: See code: 093.0

　**093.23　Tricuspid valve** CC
　　CC Excl: See code: 093.0

　**093.24　Pulmonary valve** CC
　　CC Excl: See code: 093.0

√5ᵗʰ **093.8　Other specified cardiovascular syphilis**
　**093.81　Syphilitic pericarditis** CC
　　CC Excl: See code: 093.0

　　DEF: Inflammation of the outer lining of the heart.

　**093.82　Syphilitic myocarditis** CC
　　CC Excl: See code: 093.0

　　DEF: Inflammation of the muscle of the heart.

　**093.89　Other** CC
　　CC Excl: See code: 093.0

　**093.9　Cardiovascular syphilis, unspecified** CC
　　CC Excl: See code: 093.0

√4ᵗʰ **094　Neurosyphilis**
　　Use additional code to identify any associated mental disorder
　**094.0　Tabes dorsalis** CC
　　Locomotor ataxia (progressive)
　　Posterior spinal sclerosis (syphilitic)
　　Tabetic neurosyphilis
　　Use additional code to identify manifestation, as:
　　　neurogenic arthropathy [Charcot's joint disease] (713.5)
　　CC Excl: 090.0-097.9, 099.40-099.9, 139.8

　　DEF: Progressive degeneration of nerves associated with long-term syphilis; causing pain, wasting away, incontinence, and ataxia.

　**094.1　General paresis** CC
　　Dementia paralytica
　　General paralysis (of the insane) (progressive)
　　Paretic neurosyphilis
　　Taboparesis
　　CC Excl: 090.0-097.9, 099.40-099.9, 139.8

　　DEF: Degeneration of brain associated with long-term syphilis, causing loss of brain function, progressive dementia, and paralysis.

　**094.2　Syphilitic meningitis** MCC
　　Meningovascular syphilis
　　EXCLUDES　acute syphilitic meningitis (secondary) (091.81)
　　CC Excl: 003.21, 013.00-013.16, 036.0, 047.0-047.9, 049.0-049.1, 053.0, 054.72, 072.1, 090.0-097.9, 098.89, 099.40-099.9, 100.81, 112.83, 114.2, 115.01, 115.11, 115.91, 130.0, 139.8, 320.0-322.9, 349.89-349.9, 357.0

　　DEF: Inflammation of the lining of the brain and/or spinal cord.

　**094.3　Asymptomatic neurosyphilis** CC
　　CC Excl: 090.0-097.9, 099.40-099.9, 139.8

√5ᵗʰ **094.8　Other specified neurosyphilis**
　**094.81　Syphilitic encephalitis** MCC
　　CC Excl: 090.0-097.9, 099.40-099.9, 139.8

---

N Newborn Age: 0　　P Pediatric Age: 0-17　　M Maternity Age: 12-55　　A Adult Age: 15-124　　CC CC Condition　　MCC Major CC Condition　　HIV HIV Related Dx

**094.82  Syphilitic Parkinsonism**  `CC`
CC Excl: 090.0-099.9, 332.0-333.0

DEF: Decreased motor function, tremors, and muscular rigidity.

**094.83  Syphilitic disseminated retinochoroiditis** `CC`
CC Excl: 017.30-017.36, 090.0-099.9, 115.02, 115.12, 362.01, 362.12-362.13, 362.29, 362.41, 362.52, 362.76, 363.00, 363.05-363.10, 363.13-363.15, 646.80-646.84

DEF: Inflammation of retina and choroid due to neurosyphilis.

**094.84  Syphilitic optic atrophy**  `CC`
CC Excl: 003.21, 013.00-013.16, 036.0, 047.0-047.9, 049.0-049.1, 072.1, 078.88-078.89, 079.81, 079.88-079.99, 090.0-099.9, 100.81, 112.83, 114.2, 115.01, 115.11, 115.91, 130.0, 139.8, 320.0-322.9, 349.89-349.9, 357.0

DEF: Degeneration of the eye and its nerves due to neurosyphilis.

**094.85  Syphilitic retrobulbar neuritis**  `CC`
CC Excl: 090.0-099.9, 377.32

DEF: Inflammation of the posterior optic nerve to neurosyphilis.

**094.86  Syphilitic acoustic neuritis**  `CC`
CC Excl: 090.0-099.9, 388.5

DEF: Inflammation of acoustic nerve due to neurosyphilis.

**094.87  Syphilitic ruptured cerebral aneurysm**  `MCC`
CC Excl: 090.0-097.9, 099.40-099.9, 139.8

**094.89  Other**  `CC`
CC Excl: 090.0-097.9, 099.40-099.9, 139.8

**094.9  Neurosyphilis, unspecified**  `CC`
Gumma (syphilitic)
Syphilis (early) (late)  } of central nervous system NOS
Syphiloma

CC Excl: 090.0-097.9, 099.40-099.9, 139.8

**√4th  095  Other forms of late syphilis, with symptoms**
INCLUDES  gumma (syphilitic)
syphilis, late, tertiary, or unspecified stage

**095.0  Syphilitic episcleritis**  `CC`
CC Excl: 017.30-017.36, 090.0-099.9, 379.00-379.02, 379.09

**095.1  Syphilis of lung**  `CC`
CC Excl: 090.0-099.9

**095.2  Syphilitic peritonitis**  `CC`
CC Excl: 014.00-014.06, 032.83, 090.0-099.9, 540.0-540.1, 567.0-567.1, 567.22, 567.29, 567.81, 567.9, 569.89-569.9, 577.8, 614.5-614.7, 639.0, 670.00-670.04, 777.6, 998.7

**095.3  Syphilis of liver**  `CC`
CC Excl: 090.0-099.9

**095.4  Syphilis of kidney**  `CC`
CC Excl: 090.0-099.9

**095.5  Syphilis of bone**  `CC`
CC Excl: 090.0-099.9

**095.6  Syphilis of muscle**  `CC`
Syphilitic myositis
CC Excl: 090.0-099.9

**095.7  Syphilis of synovium, tendon, and bursa**  `CC`
Syphilitic:        Syphilitic:
bursitis          synovitis
CC Excl: 090.0-099.9

**095.8  Other specified forms of late symptomatic syphilis**  `CC`
EXCLUDES  cardiovascular syphilis (093.0-093.9)
neurosyphilis (094.0-094.9)
CC Excl: 090.0-099.9

**095.9  Late symptomatic syphilis, unspecified**  `CC`
CC Excl: 090.0-099.9

**096  Late syphilis, latent**
Syphilis (acquired) without clinical manifestations, with positive serological reaction and negative spinal fluid test, two years or more after infection

**√4th  097  Other and unspecified syphilis**
**097.0  Late syphilis, unspecified**
**097.1  Latent syphilis, unspecified**
Positive serological reaction for syphilis
**097.9  Syphilis, unspecified**
Syphilis (acquired) NOS
EXCLUDES  syphilis NOS causing death under two years of age (090.9)

**√4th  098  Gonococcal infections**
DEF: *Neisseria gonorrhoeae* infection generally acquired in utero or in sexual congress.

**098.0  Acute, of lower genitourinary tract**  `CC`
Gonococcal:            Gonorrhea (acute):
Bartholinitis (acute)    NOS
urethritis (acute)       genitourinary (tract) NOS
vulvovaginitis (acute)
CC Excl: 098.0-098.39, 098.89, 099.40-099.9, 139.8

**√5th  098.1  Acute, of upper genitourinary tract**
**098.10  Gonococcal infection (acute) of upper genitourinary tract, site unspecified**  `CC`
CC Excl: See code: 098.0

**098.11  Gonococcal cystitis (acute)**  `CC`
Gonorrhea (acute) of bladder
CC Excl: See code: 098.0

**098.12  Gonococcal prostatitis (acute)**  `CC` ♂
CC Excl: See code: 098.0

**098.13  Gonococcal epididymo-orchitis (acute)** `CC` ♂
Gonococcal orchitis (acute)
CC Excl: See code: 098.0

DEF: Acute inflammation of the testes.

**098.14  Gonococcal seminal vesiculitis (acute)** `CC` ♂
Gonorrhea (acute) of seminal vesicle
CC Excl: See code: 098.0

**098.15  Gonococcal cervicitis (acute)**  `CC` ♀
Gonorrhea (acute) of cervix
CC Excl: See code: 098.0

**098.16  Gonococcal endometritis (acute)**  `CC` ♀
Gonorrhea (acute) of uterus
CC Excl: See code: 098.0

**098.17  Gonococcal salpingitis, specified as acute**  `CC` ♀
CC Excl: See code: 098.0

DEF: Acute inflammation of the fallopian tubes.

**098.19  Other**  `CC`
CC Excl: See code: 098.0

Infectious and Parasitic Diseases

094.82–098.19

**Infectious and Parasitic Diseases**

**098.2–099.0**

**098.2   Chronic, of lower genitourinary tract**

Gonococcal:
  Bartholinitis
  urethritis      }   specified as chronic
  vulvovaginitis        or with
Gonorrhea:            duration of
  NOS            two months
  genitourinary (tract)    or more

Any condition classifiable to 098.0 specified as
  chronic or with duration of two months or more

**√5ᵗʰ 098.3   Chronic, of upper genitourinary tract**

**INCLUDES**   any condition classifiable to 098.1
              stated as chronic or with a
              duration of two months or more

**098.30 Chronic gonococcal infection of upper**
        **genitourinary tract, site unspecified**

**098.31 Gonococcal cystitis, chronic**
        Any condition classifiable to 098.11,
          specified as chronic
        Gonorrhea of bladder, chronic

**098.32 Gonococcal prostatitis, chronic**     ♂
        Any condition classifiable to 098.12,
          specified as chronic

**098.33 Gonococcal epididymo-orchitis, chronic**   ♂
        Any condition classifiable to 098.13,
          specified as chronic
        Chronic gonococcal orchitis

DEF: Chronic inflammation of the testes.

**098.34 Gonococcal seminal vesiculitis, chronic**   ♂
        Any condition classifiable to 098.14,
          specified as chronic
        Gonorrhea of seminal vesicle, chronic

**098.35 Gonococcal cervicitis, chronic**     ♀
        Any condition classifiable to 098.15,
          specified as chronic
        Gonorrhea of cervix, chronic

**098.36 Gonococcal endometritis, chronic**     ♀
        Any condition classifiable to 098.16,
          specified as chronic

DEF: Chronic inflammation of the uterus.

**098.37 Gonococcal salpingitis (chronic)**     ♀

DEF: Chronic inflammation of the fallopian tubes.

**098.39 Other**

**√5ᵗʰ 098.4   Gonococcal infection of eye**

**098.40 Gonococcal conjunctivitis (neonatorum)** `CC`
        Gonococcal ophthalmia (neonatorum)
        CC Excl: 090.0-099.9

DEF: Infection of conjunctiva present at birth.

**098.41 Gonococcal iridocyclitis**     `CC`
        CC Excl: 090.0-099.9

DEF: Inflammation and infection of iris and ciliary body.

**098.42 Gonococcal endophthalmia**     `CC`
        CC Excl: 090.0-099.9

DEF: Inflammation and infection of contents of eyeball.

**098.43 Gonococcal keratitis**     `CC`
        CC Excl: 090.0-099.9

DEF: Inflammation and infection of the cornea.

**098.49 Other**     `CC`
        CC Excl: 090.0-099.9

**√5ᵗʰ 098.5   Gonococcal infection of joint**

**098.50 Gonococcal arthritis**     `CC`
        Gonococcal infection of joint NOS
        CC Excl: 003.23, 015.80-015.96, 017.90-017.96, 036.82,
        056.71, 090.0-099.9, 711.00-714.0, 715.00, 715.09-715.10,
        715.18-716.99, 718.00-718.08, 719.00-719.10, 719.18-719.69,
        719.80-719.99

**098.51 Gonococcal synovitis and tenosynovitis** `CC`
        CC Excl: See code: 098.50

**098.52 Gonococcal bursitis**     `CC`
        CC Excl: See code: 098.50

DEF: Inflammation of the sac-like cavities in a joint.

**098.53 Gonococcal spondylitis**     `CC`
        CC Excl: See code: 098.50

**098.59 Other**     `CC`
        Gonococcal rheumatism
        CC Excl: See code: 098.50

**098.6   Gonococcal infection of pharynx**

**098.7   Gonococcal infection of anus and rectum**
        Gonococcal proctitis

**√5ᵗʰ 098.8   Gonococcal infection of other specified sites**

**098.81 Gonococcal keratosis (blennorrhagica)** `CC`
        CC Excl: 098.40-098.49, 098.81

DEF: Pustular skin lesions caused by *Neisseria
gonorrhoeae*.

**098.82 Gonococcal meningitis**     `MCC`
        CC Excl: 003.21, 013.00-013.16, 036.0, 047.0-047.9, 049.0-
        049.1, 072.1, 078.88-078.89, 079.81, 079.88-079.99, 090.0-
        099.9, 100.81, 112.83, 114.2, 115.01, 115.11, 115.91, 130.0,
        139.8, 320.0-322.9, 349.89-349.9, 357.0

DEF: Inflammation of lining of brain and/or spinal cord.

**098.83 Gonococcal pericarditis**     `MCC`
        CC Excl: 074.21, 090.0-099.9, 391.0, 393, 420.0-420.99, 423.3-
        423.9, 459.89-459.9

DEF: Inflammation of the outer lining of the heart.

**098.84 Gonococcal endocarditis**     `MCC`
        CC Excl: 002.0, 036.42, 074.22, 083.0, 090.0-099.9, 112.81,
        115.94, 116.0, 390, 391.1, 391.8-392.0, 394.0-395.9, 396.9-
        397.9, 398.90, 398.99, 421.0-421.9, 424.0-424.99, 425.3,
        459.89-459.9, 711.00, 711.08-711.09, 746.09, 746.89, 996.61

DEF: Inflammation of tissues lining the cavities of heart.

**098.85 Other gonococcal heart disease**     `CC`
        CC Excl: 002.0, 036.42, 074.20, 074.22-074.23, 083.0, 090.0-
        099.9, 112.81, 115.94, 116.0, 390, 391.1-392.0, 394.0-395.9,
        396.9-398.90, 398.99, 421.0-422.99, 424.0-424.99, 425.3, 429.0,
        429.71-429.79, 459.89-459.9, 711.00, 711.08-711.09, 746.09,
        746.89, 996.61

**098.86 Gonococcal peritonitis**     `CC`
        CC Excl: 014.00-014.06, 032.83, 090.0-099.9, 540.0-540.1,
        567.0-567.1, 567.22, 567.29, 567.81, 567.9, 569.89-569.9,
        577.8, 614.5-614.7, 639.0, 670.00-670.04, 777.6, 998.7

DEF: Inflammation of the membrane lining the abdomen.

**098.89 Other**     `CC`
        Gonococcemia
        CC Excl: 090.0-099.9, 588.81-588.89

**√4ᵗʰ 099   Other venereal diseases**

**099.0   Chancroid**
        Bubo (inguinal):       Chancre:
          chancroidal          Ducrey's
          due to Hemophilus     simple
            ducreyi           soft
                     Ulcus molle (cutis) (skin)

DEF: A sexually transmitted disease caused by *Haemophilus
ducreyi*; it is identified by a painful primary ulcer at the site of
inoculation (usually external genitalia) with related lymphadenitis.

`N` Newborn Age: 0    `P` Pediatric Age: 0-17    `M` Maternity Age: 12-55    `A` Adult Age: 15-124    `CC` CC Condition    `MCC` Major CC Condition    `HIV` HIV Related Dx

24 — Volume 1 • October 2007            © 2007 Ingenix

**099.1 Lymphogranuloma venereum**
Climatic or tropical bubo
(Durand-) Nicolas-Favre disease
Esthiomene
Lymphogranuloma inguinale
DEF: Sexually transmitted infection of *Chlamydia trachomatis* causing skin lesions.

**099.2 Granuloma inguinale**
Donovanosis      Granuloma venereum
Granuloma pudendi    Pudendal ulcer
(ulcerating)
DEF: Chronic, sexually transmitted infection of *Calymmatobacterium granulomatis* causing progressive, anogenital skin ulcers.

**099.3 Reiter's disease**
Reiter's syndrome
Use additional code for associated:
arthropathy (711.1)
conjunctivitis (372.33)
DEF: A symptom complex of unknown etiology consisting of urethritis, conjunctivitis, arthritis and myocutaneous lesions. It occurs most commonly in young men and patients with HIV and may precede or follow AIDS. Also a form of reactive arthritis.

√5th **099.4 Other nongonococcal urethritis [NGU]**
**099.40 Unspecified**
Nonspecific urethritis

**099.41 Chlamydia trachomatis**

**099.49 Other specified organism**

√5th **099.5 Other venereal diseases due to Chlamydia trachomatis**
EXCLUDES   *Chlamydia trachomatis infection of conjunctiva (076.0-076.9, 077.0, 077.9)*
*Lymphogranuloma venereum (099.1)*
DEF: Venereal diseases caused by *Chlamydia trachomatis* at other sites besides the urethra (e.g., pharynx, anus and rectum, conjunctiva and peritoneum).

**099.50 Unspecified site**

**099.51 Pharynx**

**099.52 Anus and rectum**

**099.53 Lower genitourinary sites**
Use additional code to specify site of infection, such as:
bladder (595.4)
cervix (616.0)
vagina and vulva (616.11)
EXCLUDES   *urethra (099.41)*

**099.54 Other genitourinary sites**
Use additional code to specify site of infection, such as:
pelvic inflammatory disease NOS (614.9)
testis and epididymis (604.91)

**099.55 Unspecified genitourinary site**

**099.56 Peritoneum**    CC
Perihepatitis
CC Excl: 014.00-014.06, 032.83, 090.0-099.9, 540.0-540.1, 567.0-567.1, 567.22, 567.29, 567.81, 567.9, 569.89-569.9, 577.8, 614.5-614.7, 639.0, 670.00-670.04, 777.6, 998.7

**099.59 Other specified site**

**099.8 Other specified venereal diseases**

**099.9 Venereal disease, unspecified**

## OTHER SPIROCHETAL DISEASES (100-104)

√4th **100 Leptospirosis**
DEF: An infection of any spirochete of the genus Leptospire in blood. This zoonosis is transmitted to humans most often by exposure with contaminated animal tissues or water and less often by contact with urine. Patients present with flulike symptoms, the most common being muscle aches involving the thighs and low back. Treatment is with hydration and antibiotics.

**100.0 Leptospirosis icterohemorrhagica**    CC
Leptospiral or spirochetal jaundice (hemorrhagic)
Weil's disease
CC Excl: 100.0-100.9

√5th **100.8 Other specified leptospiral infections**
**100.81 Leptospiral meningitis (aseptic)**    MCC
CC Excl: 003.21, 013.00-013.16, 036.0, 047.0-047.9, 049.0-049.1, 072.1, 078.88-078.89, 079.81, 079.88-079.99, 090.42, 091.81, 094.2, 098.89, 100.0-100.9, 112.83, 114.2, 115.01, 115.11, 115.91, 130.0, 139.8, 320.0-322.9, 349.89-349.9, 357.0

**100.89 Other**    CC
Fever:      Infection by Leptospira:
Fort Bragg    australis
pretibial      bataviae
swamp      pyrogenes
CC Excl: See code: 100.0

**100.9 Leptospirosis, unspecified**    CC
CC Excl: See code: 100.0

**101 Vincent's angina**    CC
Acute necrotizing ulcerative:    Trench mouth
gingivitis      Vincent's:
stomatitis      gingivitis
Fusospirochetal pharyngitis    infection [any site]
Spirochetal stomatitis
CC Excl: 101
DEF: Painful ulceration with edema and hypermic patches of the oropharyngeal and throat membranes; it is caused by spreading of acute ulcerative gingivitis.

√4th **102 Yaws**
INCLUDES   frambesia
pian
DEF: An infectious, endemic, tropical disease caused by *Treponema pertenue*; it usually affects persons 15 years old or younger; a primary cutaneous lesion develops, then a granulomatous skin eruption, and occasionally lesions that destroy skin and bone.

**102.0 Initial lesions**
Chancre of yaws
Frambesia, initial or primary
Initial frambesial ulcer
Mother yaw

**102.1 Multiple papillomata and wet crab yaws**
Butter yaws      Plantar or palmar
Frambesioma      papilloma of yaws
Pianoma

**102.2 Other early skin lesions**
Cutaneous yaws, less than five years after infection
Early yaws (cutaneous) (macular) (papular) (maculopapular) (micropapular)
Frambeside of early yaws

**102.3 Hyperkeratosis**
Ghoul hand
Hyperkeratosis, palmar or plantar (early) (late) due to yaws
Worm-eaten soles
DEF: Overgrowth of skin of palm of bottoms of feet, due to yaws.

**102.4 Gummata and ulcers**
Gummatous frambeside
Nodular late yaws (ulcerated)
DEF: Rubbery lesions and areas of dead skin caused by yaws.

**102.5 Gangosa**
Rhinopharyngitis mutilans
DEF: Massive, mutilating lesions of the nose and oral cavity caused by yaws.

**102.6 Bone and joint lesions**
Goundou
Gumma, bone  } of yaws (late)
Gummatous osteitis or periostitis

Hydrarthrosis
Osteitis  } of yaws (early) (late)
Periostitis (hypertrophic)

**102.7 Other manifestations**
Juxta-articular nodules of yaws
Mucosal yaws

**102.8 Latent yaws**
Yaws without clinical manifestations, with positive serology

**102.9 Yaws, unspecified**

**✓4ᵗʰ 103 Pinta**
DEF: A chronic form of treponematosis, endemic in areas of tropical America; it is identified by the presence of red, violet, blue, coffee-colored or white spots on the skin.

**103.0 Primary lesions**
Chancre (primary)
Papule (primary)  } of pinta [carate]
Pintid

**103.1 Intermediate lesions**
Erythematous plaques
Hyperchromic lesions  } of pinta [carate]
Hyperkeratosis

**103.2 Late lesions**
Cardiovascular lesions
Skin lesions:
  achromic
  cicatricial  } of pinta [carate]
  dyschromic
Vitiligo

**103.3 Mixed lesions**
Achromic and hyperchromic skin lesions of pinta [carate]

**103.9 Pinta, unspecified**

**✓4ᵗʰ 104 Other spirochetal infection**
**104.0 Nonvenereal endemic syphilis**
Bejel
Njovera
DEF: *Treponema pallidum, T. pertenue,* or *T. caroteum* infection transmitted non-sexually, causing lesions on mucosa and skin.

**104.8 Other specified spirochetal infections**
EXCLUDES  relapsing fever (087.0-087.9)
syphilis (090.0-097.9)

**104.9 Spirochetal infection, unspecified**

### MYCOSES (110-118)
Use additional code to identify manifestation as:
arthropathy (711.6)
meningitis (321.0-321.1)
otitis externa (380.15)
EXCLUDES  infection by Actinomycetales, such as species of Actinomyces, Actinomadura, Nocardia, Streptomyces (039.0-039.9)

**✓4ᵗʰ 110 Dermatophytosis**
INCLUDES  infection by species of Epidermophyton, Microsporum, and Trichophyton tinea, any type except those in 111
DEF: Superficial infection of the skin caused by a parasitic fungus.

**110.0 Of scalp and beard**
Kerion
Sycosis, mycotic
Trichophytic tinea [black dot tinea], scalp

**110.1 Of nail**
Dermatophytic onychia
Onychomycosis
Tinea unguium

**110.2 Of hand**
Tinea manuum

**110.3 Of groin and perianal area**
Dhobie itch
Eczema marginatum
Tinea cruris

**110.4 Of foot**
Athlete's foot
Tinea pedis

**110.5 Of the body**
Herpes circinatus
Tinea imbricata [Tokelau]

**110.6 Deep seated dermatophytosis**
Granuloma trichophyticum
Majocchi's granuloma

**110.8 Of other specified sites**

**110.9 Of unspecified site**
Favus NOS
Microsporic tinea NOS
Ringworm NOS

**✓4ᵗʰ 111 Dermatomycosis, other and unspecified**
**111.0 Pityriasis versicolor**
Infection by Malassezia [Pityrosporum] furfur
Tinea flava
Tinea versicolor

**111.1 Tinea nigra**
Infection by Cladosporium species
Keratomycosis nigricans
Microsporosis nigra
Pityriasis nigra
Tinea palmaris nigra

**111.2 Tinea blanca**
Infection by Trichosporon (beigelii) cutaneum
White piedra

**111.3 Black piedra**
Infection by Piedraia hortai

**111.8 Other specified dermatomycoses**

**111.9 Dermatomycosis, unspecified**

**✓4ᵗʰ 112 Candidiasis**
INCLUDES  infection by Candida species
moniliasis
EXCLUDES  neonatal monilial infection (771.7)
DEF: Fungal infection caused by Candida; usually seen in mucous membranes or skin.

**112.0 Of mouth**  CC HIV
Thrush (oral)
CC Excl: 112.0-112.9, 117.9, 139.8

**112.1 Of vulva and vagina**  ♀
Candidal vulvovaginitis
Monilial vulvovaginitis

**112.2 Of other urogenital sites**  CC
Candidal balanitis
CC Excl: 112.2, 112.4-112.9, 588.81-588.89
AHA: 4Q, '03, 105; 4Q, '96, 33

**112.3 Of skin and nails**  HIV
Candidal intertrigo
Candidal onychia
Candidal perionyxis [paronychia]

**112.4 Of lung**  MCC HIV
Candidal pneumonia
CC Excl: See code: 112.0
AHA: 2Q, '98, 7

**112.5 Disseminated**  MCC HIV
Systemic candidiasis
CC Excl: See code: 112.0
AHA: 2Q, '00, 5; 2Q, '89, 10

---

N Newborn Age: 0    P Pediatric Age: 0-17    M Maternity Age: 12-55    A Adult Age: 15-124    CC CC Condition    MCC Major CC Condition    HIV HIV Related Dx

√5ᵗʰ **112.8 Of other specified sites**

**112.81 Candidal endocarditis** `MCC` `HIV`
CC Excl: See code: 112.0

**112.82 Candidal otitis externa** `CC` `HIV`
Otomycosis in moniliasis
CC Excl: See code: 112.0

**112.83 Candidal meningitis** `MCC` `HIV`
CC Excl: 003.21, 013.00-013.16, 036.0, 047.0-047.9, 049.0-049.1, 053.0, 054.72, 072.1, 090.42, 091.81, 094.2, 098.89, 100.81, 112.0-112.9, 114.2, 115.01, 115.11, 115.91, 117.9, 130.0, 139.8, 320.0-322.9, 349.89-349.9, 357.0

**112.84 Candidal esophagitis** `CC` `HIV`
CC Excl: See code: 112.0

AHA: 4Q, '92, 19

**112.85 Candidal enteritis** `CC` `HIV`
CC Excl: See code: 112.0

AHA: 4Q, '92, 19

**112.89 Other** `CC`
CC Excl: 112.4-112.9

AHA: 1Q, '92, 17; 3Q, '91, 20

**112.9 Of unspecified site** `HIV`

√4ᵗʰ **114 Coccidioidomycosis**
`INCLUDES` infection by Coccidioides (immitis)
Posada-Wernicke disease

AHA: 4Q, '93, 23

DEF: A fungal disease caused by inhalation of dust particles containing arthrospores of *Coccidiodes immitis*; a self-limited respiratory infection; the primary form is known as San Joaquin fever, desert fever or valley fever.

**114.0 Primary coccidioidomycosis (pulmonary)** `CC` `HIV`
Acute pulmonary coccidioidomycosis
Coccidioidomycotic pneumonitis
Desert rheumatism
Pulmonary coccidioidomycosis
San Joaquin Valley fever
CC Excl: 114.0, 114.3-114.9, 117.9, 139.8

DEF: Acute, self-limiting *Coccidioides immitis* infection of the lung.

**114.1 Primary extrapulmonary coccidioidomycosis** `CC` `HIV`
Chancriform syndrome
Primary cutaneous coccidioidomycosis
CC Excl: 114.0-114.9

DEF: Acute, self-limiting *Coccidioides immitis* infection in nonpulmonary site.

**114.2 Coccidioidal meningitis** `MCC` `HIV`
CC Excl: 003.21, 013.00-013.16, 036.0, 047.0-047.9, 049.0-049.1, 053.0, 054.72, 072.1, 090.42, 091.81, 094.2, 098.89, 100.81, 112.83, 114.2-114.3, 114.9, 115.01, 115.11, 115.91, 117.9, 130.0, 139.8, 320.0-322.9, 349.89-349.9, 357.0

DEF: *Coccidioides immitis* infection of the lining of the brain and/or spinal cord.

**114.3 Other forms of progressive coccidioidomycosis** `CC` `HIV`
Coccidioidal granuloma
Disseminated coccidioidomycosis
CC Excl: 114.3, 114.9, 117.9, 139.8

**114.4 Chronic pulmonary coccidioidomycosis** `CC` `HIV`
CC Excl: 114.0-115.99

**114.5 Pulmonary coccidioidomycosis, unspecified** `CC` `HIV`
CC Excl: See code: 114.4

**114.9 Coccidioidomycosis, unspecified** `CC` `HIV`
CC Excl: See code: 114.3

√4ᵗʰ **115 Histoplasmosis**
The following fifth-digit subclassification is for use with category 115:
 **0 without mention of manifestation**
 **1 meningitis**
 **2 retinitis**
 **3 pericarditis**
 **4 endocarditis**
 **5 pneumonia**
 **9 other**

√5ᵗʰ **115.0 Infection by Histoplasma capsulatum**
American histoplasmosis
Darling's disease
Reticuloendothelial cytomycosis
Small form histoplasmosis
CC Excl: For code **115.01**: 003.21, 013.00-013.16, 036.0, 047.0-047.9, 049.0-049.1, 053.0, 054.72, 072.1, 090.42, 091.81, 094.2, 098.89, 100.81, 112.83, 114.2, 115.00-115.01, 115.09, 115.11, 115.90-115.91, 115.99, 117.9, 130.0, 139.8, 320.0-322.9, 349.89-349.9, 357.0; For code **115.02**: 115.00, 115.02, 115.09, 115.90, 115.92, 115.99, 117.9, 139.8; For code **115.03**: 115.00, 115.03, 115.09, 115.90, 115.93, 115.99, 117.9, 139.8; For code **115.04**:115.00, 115.04, 115.09, 115.90, 115.94, 115.99, 117.9, 139.8; For code **115.05**: 115.00, 115.05-115.09, 115.90, 115.95-115.99, 117.9, 139.8, 480.0-480.2, 480.8-487.1, 488, 494.0-508.9, 517.1, 518.89; For code **115.09**: 114.0-115.09

√5ᵗʰ **115.1 Infection by Histoplasma duboisii**
African histoplasmosis
Large form histoplasmosis
CC Excl: For code **115.11**: 003.21, 013.00-013.16, 036.0, 047.0-047.9, 049.0-049.1, 053.0, 054.72, 072.1, 090.42, 091.81, 094.2, 098.89, 100.81, 112.83, 114.2, 115.00-115.01, 115.09, 115.11, 115.90-115.91, 115.99, 117.9, 130.0, 139.8, 320.0-322.9, 349.89-349.9, 357.0; For code **115.12**: 115.10, 115.12, 115.19-115.90, 115.92, 115.99, 117.9, 139.8; For code **115.13**: 115.10, 115.13, 115.19-115.90, 115.93, 115.99, 117.9, 139.8; For code **115.14**:115.10, 115.14, 115.19-115.90, 115.94, 115.99, 117.9, 139.8; For code **115.15**: 115.05, 115.10, 115.15-115.90, 115.95-115.99, 117.9, 139.8, 480.0-480.2, 480.8-487.1, 488, 494.0-508.9, 517.1, 518.89; For code **115.19**:115.10, 115.19-115.90, 115.99, 117.9, 139.8

√5ᵗʰ **115.9 Histoplasmosis, unspecified** `MCC 1, 3-5` `CC 2` `HIV`

Histoplasmosis NOS
CC Excl: For code **115.91**: 003.21, 013.00-013.16, 036.0, 047.0-047.9, 049.0-049.1, 053.0, 054.72, 072.1, 090.42, 091.81, 094.2, 098.89, 100.81, 112.83, 114.2, 115.01, 115.11, 115.91, 115.99, 117.9, 130.0, 139.8, 320.0-322.9, 349.89-349.9, 357.0; For code **115.92**:115.92, 115.99, 117.9, 139.8; For code **115.93**: 115.93, 115.99, 117.9, 139.8; For code **115.94**: 115.94, 115.99, 117.9, 139.8; For code **115.95**:115.05, 115.15, 115.95-115.99, 117.9, 139.8

√4ᵗʰ **116 Blastomycotic infection**

**116.0 Blastomycosis** `CC`
Blastomycotic dermatitis
Chicago disease
Cutaneous blastomycosis
Disseminated blastomycosis
Gilchrist's disease
Infection by Blastomyces [Ajellomyces] dermatitidis
North American blastomycosis
Primary pulmonary blastomycosis
CC Excl: 116.0, 117.9, 139.8

**116.1 Paracoccidioidomycosis** `CC`
Brazilian blastomycosis
Infection by Paracoccidioides [Blastomyces] brasiliensis
Lutz-Splendore-Almeida disease
Mucocutaneous-lymphangitic paracoccidioidomycosis
Pulmonary paracoccidioidomycosis
South American blastomycosis
Visceral paracoccidioidomycosis
CC Excl: 116.1, 117.9, 139.8

---

√4ᵗʰ
√5ᵗʰ Additional Digit Required    Unacceptable PDx    `Manifestation Code`    ◄► Revised Text    ● New Code    ▲ Revised Code Title

**Infectious and Parasitic Diseases**

**116.2–121.5**

**116.2 Lobomycosis**
Infections by Loboa [Blastomyces] loboi
Keloidal blastomycosis
Lobo's disease

☑4ᵗʰ **117 Other mycoses**

**117.0 Rhinosporidiosis**
Infection by Rhinosporidium seeberi

**117.1 Sporotrichosis**
Cutaneous sporotrichosis
Disseminated sporotrichosis
Infection by Sporothrix [Sporotrichum] schenckii
Lymphocutaneous sporotrichosis
Pulmonary sporotrichosis
Sporotrichosis of the bones

**117.2 Chromoblastomycosis**
Chromomycosis
Infection by Cladosporidium carrionii, Fonsecaea
compactum, Fonsecaea pedrosoi, Phialophora
verrucosa

**117.3 Aspergillosis**   `CC`
Infection by Aspergillus species, mainly A.
fumigatus, A. flavus group, A. terreus group

**CC Excl:** 117.3, 117.9, 139.8

**AHA:** 4Q, '97, 40

**117.4 Mycotic mycetomas**   `CC`
Infection by various genera and species of
Ascomycetes and Deuteromycetes, such as
Acremonium [Cephalosporium] falciforme,
Neotestudina rosatii, Madurella grisea,
Madurella mycetomii, Pyrenochaeta romeroi,
Zopfia [Leptosphaeria] senegalensis
Madura foot, mycotic
Maduromycosis, mycotic
    **EXCLUDES**   *actinomycotic mycetomas (039.0-039.9)*

**CC Excl:** 117.4, 117.9, 139.8

**117.5 Cryptococcosis**   `CC` `HIV`
Busse-Buschke's disease
European cryptococcosis
Infection by Cryptococcus neoformans
Pulmonary cryptococcosis
Systemic cryptococcosis
Torula

**CC Excl:** 117.5, 117.9, 139.8

**117.6 Allescheriosis [Petriellidosis]**   `CC`
Infections by Allescheria [Petriellidium] boydii
[Monosporium apiospermum]
    **EXCLUDES**   *mycotic mycetoma (117.4)*

**CC Excl:** 117.6, 117.9, 139.8

**117.7 Zygomycosis [Phycomycosis or**   `MCC`
**Mucormycosis]**
Infection by species of Absidia, Basidiobolus,
Conidiobolus, Cunninghamella,
Entomophthora, Mucor, Rhizopus, Saksenaea

**CC Excl:** 117.7, 117.9, 139.8

**117.8 Infection by dematiacious fungi,**   `CC`
**[Phaehyphomycosis]**
Infection by dematiacious fungi, such as
Cladosporium trichoides [bantianum],
Dreschlera hawaiiensis, Phialophora
gougerotii, Phialophora jeanselmi

**CC Excl:** 117.8-117.9

**117.9 Other and unspecified mycoses**   `CC`
**CC Excl:** See code: 117.8

**118 Opportunistic mycoses**   `CC` `HIV`
Infection of skin, subcutaneous tissues, and/or organs by a
wide variety of fungi generally considered to be
pathogenic to compromised hosts only (e.g., infection
by species of Alternaria, Dreschlera, Fusarium)

**CC Excl:** 117.9-118, 139.8

**HELMINTHIASES (120-129)**

☑4ᵗʰ **120 Schistosomiasis [bilharziasis]**
**DEF:** Infection caused by *Schistosoma*, a genus of flukes or trematode
parasites.

**120.0 Schistosoma haematobium**   `CC`
Vesical schistosomiasis NOS
**CC Excl:** 120.0-120.9

**120.1 Schistosoma mansoni**   `CC`
Intestinal schistosomiasis NOS
**CC Excl:** See code: 120.0

**120.2 Schistosoma japonicum**   `CC`
Asiatic schistosomiasis NOS
Katayama disease or fever
**CC Excl:** See code: 120.0

**120.3 Cutaneous**   `CC`
Cercarial dermatitis
Infection by cercariae of Schistosoma
Schistosome dermatitis
Swimmers' itch
**CC Excl:** See code: 120.0

**120.8 Other specified schistosomiasis**   `CC`
Infection by Schistosoma:
bovis
intercalatum
mattheii
spindale
Schistosomiasis chestermani
**CC Excl:** See code: 120.0

**120.9 Schistosomiasis, unspecified**   `CC`
Blood flukes NOS
Hemic distomiasis
**CC Excl:** See code: 120.0

☑4ᵗʰ **121 Other trematode infections**

**121.0 Opisthorchiasis**   `CC`
Infection by:
cat liver fluke
Opisthorchis (felineus) (tenuicollis) (viverrini)
**CC Excl:** 121.0-121.9

**121.1 Clonorchiasis**   `CC`
Biliary cirrhosis due to clonorchiasis
Chinese liver fluke disease
Hepatic distomiasis due to Clonorchis sinensis
Oriental liver fluke disease
**CC Excl:** See code: 121.0

**121.2 Paragonimiasis**   `CC`
Infection by Paragonimus
Lung fluke disease (oriental)
Pulmonary distomiasis
**CC Excl:** See code: 121.0

**121.3 Fascioliasis**   `CC`
Infection by Fasciola:
gigantica
hepatica
Liver flukes NOS
Sheep liver fluke infection
**CC Excl:** See code: 121.0

**121.4 Fasciolopsiasis**   `CC`
Infection by Fasciolopsis (buski)
Intestinal distomiasis
**CC Excl:** See code: 121.0

**121.5 Metagonimiasis**   `CC`
Infection by Metagonimus yokogawai
**CC Excl:** See code: 121.0

---

`N` Newborn Age: 0    `P` Pediatric Age: 0-17    `M` Maternity Age: 12-55    `A` Adult Age: 15-124    `CC` CC Condition    `MCC` Major CC Condition    `HIV` HIV Related Dx

**121.6**   **Heterophyiasis**   `CC`
     Infection by:
         Heterophyes heterophyes
         Stellantchasmus falcatus
     **CC Excl:** See code: 121.0

**121.8**   **Other specified trematode infections**   `CC`
     Infection by:
         Dicrocoelium dendriticum
         Echinostoma ilocanum
         Gastrodiscoides hominis
     **CC Excl:** See code: 121.0

**121.9**   **Trematode infection, unspecified**
     Distomiasis NOS
     Fluke disease NOS

**✓4ᵗʰ 122 Echinococcosis**
     **INCLUDES**   echinococciasis
                  hydatid disease
                  hydatidosis
     **DEF:** Infection caused by larval forms of tapeworms of the genus
     *Echinococcus.*

**122.0**   **Echinococcus granulosus infection of liver**   `CC`
     **CC Excl:** 122.0, 122.8-122.9

**122.1**   **Echinococcus granulosus infection of lung**   `CC`
     **CC Excl:** 122.1, 122.8-122.9, 480.3

**122.2**   **Echinococcus granulosus infection of thyroid**   `CC`
     **CC Excl:** 122.2, 122.8-122.9

**122.3**   **Echinococcus granulosus infection, other**   `CC`
     **CC Excl:** 122.3, 122.8-122.9

**122.4**   **Echinococcus granulosus infection,**   `CC`
     **unspecified**
     **CC Excl:** 122.4, 122.8-122.9

**122.5**   **Echinococcus multilocularis infection of liver**   `CC`
     **CC Excl:** 122.5, 122.8-122.9

**122.6**   **Echinococcus multilocularis infection, other**   `CC`
     **CC Excl:** 122.6, 122.8-122.9

**122.7**   **Echinococcus multilocularis infection,**   `CC`
     **unspecified**
     **CC Excl:** 122.7-122.9

**122.8**   **Echinococcosis, unspecified, of liver**   `CC`
     **CC Excl:** 122.8-122.9

**122.9**   **Echinococcosis, other and unspecified**   `CC`
     **CC Excl:** See code: 122.8

**✓4ᵗʰ 123 Other cestode infection**

**123.0**   **Taenia solium infection, intestinal form**   `CC`
     Pork tapeworm (adult) (infection)
     **CC Excl:** 001.1, 002.0, 002.9-003.0, 004.9-005.2, 006.0-006.2, 006.9,
     007.1-009.0, 014.80-014.86, 040.41-040.42, 112.85, 123.0-123.9, 129,
     487.8, 536.3, 536.8, 558.2-558.9, 564.1, 777.5, 777.8

**123.1**   **Cysticercosis**   `CC`
     Cysticerciasis
     Infection by Cysticercus cellulosae [larval form of
         Taenia solium]
     **CC Excl:** 123.0-123.9
     **AHA:** 2Q, '97, 8

**123.2**   **Taenia saginata infection**   `CC`
     Beef tapeworm (infection)
     Infection by Taeniarhynchus saginatus
     **CC Excl:** See code: 123.1

**123.3**   **Taeniasis, unspecified**   `CC`
     **CC Excl:** See code: 123.1

**123.4**   **Diphyllobothriasis, intestinal**   `CC`
     Diphyllobothrium (adult) (latum) (pacificum)
         infection
     Fish tapeworm (infection)
     **CC Excl:** See code: 123.1

**123.5**   **Sparganosis [larval diphyllobothriasis]**   `CC`
     Infection by:
         Diphyllobothrium larvae
         Sparganum (mansoni) (proliferum)
         Spirometra larvae
     **CC Excl:** See code: 123.1

**123.6**   **Hymenolepiasis**   `CC`
     Dwarf tapeworm (infection)
     Hymenolepis (diminuta) (nana) infection
     Rat tapeworm (infection)
     **CC Excl:** See code: 123.1

**123.8**   **Other specified cestode infection**   `CC`
     Diplogonoporus (grandis) ⎫
     Dipylidium (caninum)   ⎬ infection
     Dog tapeworm (infection)
     **CC Excl:** See code: 123.1

**123.9**   **Cestode infection, unspecified**
     Tapeworm (infection) NOS

**124 Trichinosis**   `CC`
     Trichinella spiralis infection
     Trichinellosis
     Trichiniasis
     **CC Excl:** 013.60-013.66, 046.2, 046.8, 048-049.0, 049.8, 052.0, 052.2, 054.3, 054.74,
     056.01, 057.8-058.29, 062.0-064, 066.2-066.49, 072.2, 073.7, 079.82, 079.99, 081.9,
     083.9, 090.41, 094.81, 117.5, 124, 130.0, 290.12, 323.01-323.9, 341.1, 487.8, 771.2,
     984.9
     **DEF:** Infection by *Trichinella spiralis*, the smallest of the parasitic nematodes.

**✓4ᵗʰ 125 Filarial infection and dracontiasis**

**125.0**   **Bancroftian filariasis**   `CC`
     Chyluria        ⎫
     Elephantiasis  ⎪
     Infection        ⎬ due to Wuchereria bancrofti
     Lymphadenitis ⎪
     Lymphangitis   ⎭
     Wuchereriasis
     **CC Excl:** 125.0-125.9

**125.1**   **Malayan filariasis**   `CC`
     Brugia filariasis ⎫
     Chyluria       ⎪
     Elephantiasis  ⎬ due to Brugia
     Infection       ⎪   [Wuchereria]
     Lymphadenitis ⎪   malayi
     Lymphangitis  ⎭
     **CC Excl:** See code: 125.0

**125.2**   **Loiasis**   `CC`
     Eyeworm disease of Africa
     Loa loa infection
     **CC Excl:** See code: 125.0

**125.3**   **Onchocerciasis**   `CC`
     Onchocerca volvulus infection
     Onchocercosis
     **CC Excl:** See code: 125.0

**125.4**   **Dipetalonemiasis**   `CC`
     Infection by:
         Acanthocheilonema perstans
         Dipetalonema perstans
     **CC Excl:** See code: 125.0

**125.5**   **Mansonella ozzardi infection**   `CC`
     Filariasis ozzardi
     **CC Excl:** See code: 125.0

---

✓4ᵗʰ
✓5ᵗʰ   Additional Digit Required      Unacceptable PDx      Manifestation Code      ◄► Revised Text      ● New Code      ▲ Revised Code Title

**Infectious and Parasitic Diseases**

**121.6–125.5**

**125.6    Other specified filariasis**    `CC`
     Dirofilaria infection
     Infection by:
       Acanthocheilonema streptocerca
       Dipetalonema streptocerca
     **CC Excl:** See code: 125.0

**125.7    Dracontiasis**    `CC`
     Guinea-worm infection
     Infection by Dracunculus medinensis
     **CC Excl:** See code: 125.0

**125.9    Unspecified filariasis**    `CC`
     **CC Excl:** See code: 125.0

√4ᵗʰ **126 Ancylostomiasis and necatoriasis**
     `INCLUDES`    cutaneous larva migrans due to Ancylostoma
                 hookworm (disease) (infection)
                 uncinariasis

**126.0    Ancylostoma duodenale**    `CC`
     **CC Excl:** 126.0-126.9

**126.1    Necator americanus**    `CC`
     **CC Excl:** See code: 126.0

**126.2    Ancylostoma braziliense**    `CC`
     **CC Excl:** See code: 126.0

**126.3    Ancylostoma ceylanicum**    `CC`
     **CC Excl:** See code: 126.0

**126.8    Other specified Ancylostoma**    `CC`
     **CC Excl:** See code: 126.0

**126.9    Ancylostomiasis and necatoriasis,**    `CC`
     **unspecified**
     Creeping eruption NOS
     Cutaneous larva migrans NOS
     **CC Excl:** See code: 126.0

√4ᵗʰ **127 Other intestinal helminthiases**

**127.0    Ascariasis**    `CC`
     Ascaridiasis
     Infection by Ascaris lumbricoides
     Roundworm infection
     **CC Excl:** 127.0-127.9

**127.1    Anisakiasis**    `CC`
     Infection by Anisakis larva
     **CC Excl:** See code: 127.0

**127.2    Strongyloidiasis**    `CC` `HIV`
     Infection by Strongyloides stercoralis
     `EXCLUDES`    *trichostrongyliasis (127.6)*
     **CC Excl:** See code: 127.0

**127.3    Trichuriasis**    `CC`
     Infection by Trichuris trichiuria
     Trichocephaliasis
     Whipworm (disease) (infection)
     **CC Excl:** See code: 127.0

**127.4    Enterobiasis**    `CC`
     Infection by Enterobius vermicularis
     Oxyuriasis
     Oxyuris vermicularis infection
     Pinworm (disease) (infection)
     Threadworm infection
     **CC Excl:** See code: 127.0

**127.5    Capillariasis**    `CC`
     Infection by Capillaria philippinensis
     `EXCLUDES`    *infection by Capillaria hepatica (128.8)*
     **CC Excl:** See code: 127.0

**127.6    Trichostrongyliasis**    `CC`
     Infection by Trichostrongylus species
     **CC Excl:** See code: 127.0

**127.7    Other specified intestinal helminthiasis**    `CC`
     Infection by:
       Oesophagostomum apiostomum and related
          species
       Ternidens diminutus
       other specified intestinal helminth
     Physalopteriasis
     **CC Excl:** 127.0-129

**127.8    Mixed intestinal helminthiasis**    `CC`
     Infection by intestinal helminths classified to more
       than one of the categories 120.0-127.7
     Mixed helminthiasis NOS
     **CC Excl:** See code: 127.7

**127.9    Intestinal helminthiasis, unspecified**    `CC`
     **CC Excl:** See code: 127.7

√4ᵗʰ **128 Other and unspecified helminthiases**

**128.0    Toxocariasis**
     Larva migrans visceralis
     Toxocara (canis) (cati) infection
     Visceral larva migrans syndrome

**128.1    Gnathostomiasis**
     Infection by Gnathostoma spinigerum and related
       species

**128.8    Other specified helminthiasis**
     Infection by:
       Angiostrongylus cantonensis
       Capillaria hepatica
       other specified helminth

**128.9    Helminth infection, unspecified**
     Helminthiasis NOS      Worms NOS

**129 Intestinal parasitism, unspecified**

## OTHER INFECTIOUS AND PARASITIC DISEASES (130–136)

√4ᵗʰ **130 Toxoplasmosis**
     `INCLUDES`    infection by toxoplasma gondii
                 toxoplasmosis (acquired)
     `EXCLUDES`    *congenital toxoplasmosis (771.2)*

**130.0    Meningoencephalitis due to toxoplasmosis**    `MCC` `HIV`
     Encephalitis due to acquired toxoplasmosis
     **CC Excl:** 130.0, 130.7-130.9, 139.8

**130.1    Conjunctivitis due to toxoplasmosis**    `CC` `HIV`
     **CC Excl:** 130.1, 130.7-130.9, 139.8

**130.2    Chorioretinitis due to toxoplasmosis**    `CC` `HIV`
     Focal retinochoroiditis due to acquired
       toxoplasmosis
     **CC Excl:** 130.2, 130.7-130.9, 139.8

**130.3    Myocarditis due to toxoplasmosis**    `MCC` `HIV`
     **CC Excl:** 130.3, 130.7-130.9, 139.8

**130.4    Pneumonitis due to toxoplasmosis**    `MCC` `HIV`
     **CC Excl:** 130.4, 130.7-130.9, 139.8, 480.0-480.2, 480.8-487.1, 488, 494.0-
     508.9, 517.1, 518.89

**130.5    Hepatitis due to toxoplasmosis**    `CC` `HIV`
     **CC Excl:** 130.5-130.9, 139.8

**130.7    Toxoplasmosis of other specified sites**    `CC` `HIV`
     **CC Excl:** 130.7-130.9, 139.8

**130.8    Multisystemic disseminated**    `MCC` `HIV`
     **toxoplasmosis**
     Toxoplasmosis of multiple sites
     **CC Excl:** See code: 130.7

**130.9    Toxoplasmosis, unspecified**    `CC` `HIV`
     **CC Excl:** 130.9

---

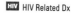

`N` Newborn Age: 0     `P` Pediatric Age: 0-17     `M` Maternity Age: 12-55     `A` Adult Age: 15-124     `CC` CC Condition     `MCC` Major CC Condition     `HIV` HIV Related Dx

✓4ᵗʰ **131 Trichomoniasis**
> INCLUDES   infection due to Trichomonas (vaginalis)

✓5ᵗʰ **131.0 Urogenital trichomoniasis**

**131.00 Urogenital trichomoniasis, unspecified**
> Fluor (vaginalis)     ⎱ trichomonal or due to
> Leukorrhea     ⎰ Trichomonas
> (vaginalis)     (vaginalis)

> DEF: *Trichomonas vaginalis* infection of reproductive and urinary organs, transmitted through coitus.

**131.01 Trichomonal vulvovaginitis**     ♀
> Vaginitis, trichomonal or due to Trichomonas (vaginalis)

> DEF: *Trichomonas vaginalis* infection of vulva and vagina; often asymptomatic, transmitted through coitus.

**131.02 Trichomonal urethritis**
> DEF: *Trichomonas vaginalis* infection of the urethra.

**131.03 Trichomonal prostatitis**     ♂
> DEF: *Trichomonas vaginalis* infection of the prostate.

**131.09 Other**

**131.8 Other specified sites**
> EXCLUDES   intestinal (007.3)

**131.9 Trichomoniasis, unspecified**

✓4ᵗʰ **132 Pediculosis and phthirus infestation**

**132.0 Pediculus capitis [head louse]**

**132.1 Pediculus corporis [body louse]**

**132.2 Phthirus pubis [pubic louse]**
> Pediculus pubis

**132.3 Mixed infestation**
> Infestation classifiable to more than one of the categories 132.0-132.2

**132.9 Pediculosis, unspecified**

✓4ᵗʰ **133 Acariasis**

**133.0 Scabies**
> Infestation by Sarcoptes scabiei
> Norwegian scabies
> Sarcoptic itch

**133.8 Other acariasis**
> Chiggers     Infestation by:
> Infestation by:     Trombicula
>     Demodex folliculorum

**133.9 Acariasis, unspecified**
> Infestation by mites NOS

✓4ᵗʰ **134 Other infestation**

**134.0 Myiasis**
> Infestation by:     Infestation by:
>     Dermatobia (hominis)     maggots
>     fly larvae     Oestrus ovis
>     Gasterophilus (intestinalis)

**134.1 Other arthropod infestation**
> Infestation by:     Jigger disease
>     chigoe     Scarabiasis
>     sand flea     Tungiasis
>     Tunga penetrans

**134.2 Hirudiniasis**
> Hirudiniasis (external) (internal)
> Leeches (aquatic) (land)

**134.8 Other specified infestations**

**134.9 Infestation, unspecified**
> Infestation (skin) NOS
> Skin parasites NOS

**135 Sarcoidosis**
> Besnier-Boeck-Schaumann disease
> Lupoid (miliary) of Boeck
> Lupus pernio (Besnier)
> Lymphogranulomatosis, benign (Schaumann's)
> Sarcoid (any site):
>     NOS
>     Boeck
>     Darier-Roussy
> Uveoparotid fever

> DEF: A chronic, granulomatous reticulosis (abnormal increase in cells), affecting any organ or tissue; acute form has high rate of remission; chronic form is progressive.

✓4ᵗʰ **136 Other and unspecified infectious and parasitic diseases**

**136.0 Ainhum**
> Dactylolysis spontanea

> DEF: A disease affecting the toes, especially the fifth digit, and sometimes the fingers, especially seen in black adult males; it is characterized by a linear constriction around the affected digit leading to spontaneous amputation of the distal part of the digit.

**136.1 Behçet's syndrome**
> DEF: A chronic inflammatory disorder of unknown etiology involving the small blood vessels; it is characterized by recurrent aphthous ulceration of the oral and pharyngeal mucous membranes and the genitalia, skin lesions, severe uvetis, retinal vascularitis and optic atrophy.

**136.2 Specific infections by free-living amebae**   MCC
> Meningoencephalitis due to Naegleria

> CC Excl: 136.0-136.9

**136.3 Pneumocystosis**   MCC   HIV
> Pneumonia due to Pneumocystis carinii
> Pneumonia due to Pneumocystis jiroveci

> CC Excl: 136.3, 139.8, 480.0-480.2, 480.8-487.1, 488, 494.0-508.9, 517.1, 518.89

> AHA: 1Q, '05, 7; 1Q, '03, 15; N-D, '87, 5-6

> DEF: *Pneumocystis carinii* fungus causing pneumonia in immunocompromised patients; a leading cause of death among AIDS patients.

**136.4 Psorospermiasis**   CC
> CC Excl: See code: 136.2

**136.5 Sarcosporidiosis**   CC
> Infection by Sarcocystis lindemanni

> CC Excl: See code: 136.2

> DEF: *Sarcocystis* infection causing muscle cysts of intestinal inflammation.

**136.8 Other specified infectious and parasitic diseases** HIV
> Candiru infestation

**136.9 Unspecified infectious and parasitic diseases**
> Infectious disease NOS     Parasitic disease NOS

> AHA: 2Q, '91, 8

## LATE EFFECTS OF INFECTIOUS AND PARASITIC DISEASES (137-139)

✓4ᵗʰ **137 Late effects of tuberculosis**
> Note: This category is to be used to indicate conditions classifiable to 010-018 as the cause of late effects, which are themselves classified elsewhere. The "late effects" include those specified as such, as sequelae, or as due to old or inactive tuberculosis, without evidence of active disease.

**137.0 Late effects of respiratory or unspecified tuberculosis**

**137.1 Late effects of central nervous system tuberculosis**

**137.2 Late effects of genitourinary tuberculosis**

**137.3 Late effects of tuberculosis of bones and joints**

**137.4 Late effects of tuberculosis of other specified organs**

**138 Late effects of acute poliomyelitis**

> Note: This category is to be used to indicate conditions classifiable to 045 as the cause of late effects, which are themselves classified elsewhere. The "late effects" include conditions specified as such, or as sequelae, or as due to old or inactive poliomyelitis, without evidence of active disease.

✓4ᵗʰ **139 Late effects of other infectious and parasitic diseases**

> Note: This category is to be used to indicate conditions classifiable to categories 001-009, 020-041, 046-136 as the cause of late effects, which are themselves classified elsewhere. The "late effects" include conditions specified as such; they also include sequela of diseases classifiable to the above categories if there is evidence that the disease itself is no longer present.

**139.0 Late effects of viral encephalitis**

> Late effects of conditions classifiable to 049.8-049.9, 062-064

**139.1 Late effects of trachoma**

> Late effects of conditions classifiable to 076

**139.8 Late effects of other and unspecified infectious and parasitic diseases**

> **AHA:** 2Q, '06, 17; 4Q, '91, 15; 3Q, '90, 14; M-A, '87, 8

---

N Newborn Age: 0    P Pediatric Age: 0-17    M Maternity Age: 12-55    A Adult Age: 15-124    CC CC Condition    MCC Major CC Condition    HIV HIV Related Dx

**Neoplasms**

## 2. NEOPLASMS (140-239)

Notes:

1. Content

This chapter contains the following broad groups:

| | |
|---|---|
| 140-195 | Malignant neoplasms, stated or presumed to be primary, of specified sites, except of lymphatic and hematopoietic tissue |
| 196-198 | Malignant neoplasms, stated or presumed to be secondary, of specified sites |
| 199 | Malignant neoplasms, without specification of site |
| 200-208 | Malignant neoplasms, stated or presumed to be primary, of lymphatic and hematopoietic tissue |
| 210-229 | Benign neoplasms |
| 230-234 | Carcinoma in situ |
| 235-238 | Neoplasms of uncertain behavior [see Note, above category 235] |
| 239 | Neoplasms of unspecified nature |

2. Functional activity

All neoplasms are classified in this chapter, whether or not functionally active. An additional code from Chapter 3 may be used to identify such functional activity associated with any neoplasm, e.g.:

> catecholamine-producing malignant pheochromocytoma of adrenal:
>> code 194.0, additional code 255.6

> basophil adenoma of pituitary with Cushing's syndrome:
>> code 227.3, additional code 255.0

3. Morphology [Histology]

For those wishing to identify the histological type of neoplasms, a comprehensive coded nomenclature, which comprises the morphology rubrics of the ICD-Oncology, is given in Appendix A.

4. Malignant neoplasms overlapping site boundaries

Categories 140-195 are for the classification of primary malignant neoplasms according to their point of origin. A malignant neoplasm that overlaps two or more subcategories within a three-digit rubric and whose point of origin cannot be determined should be classified to the subcategory .8 "Other."

For example, "carcinoma involving tip and ventral surface of tongue" should be assigned to 141.8. On the other hand, "carcinoma of tip of tongue, extending to involve the ventral surface" should be coded to 141.2, as the point of origin, the tip, is known. Three subcategories (149.8, 159.8, 165.8) have been provided for malignant neoplasms that overlap the boundaries of three-digit rubrics within certain systems.

Overlapping malignant neoplasms that cannot be classified as indicated above should be assigned to the appropriate subdivision of category 195 (Malignant neoplasm of other and ill-defined sites).

**AHA:** 2Q, '90, 7

**DEF:** An abnormal growth, such as a tumor. Morphology determines behavior, i.e., whether it will remain intact (benign) or spread to adjacent tissue (malignant). The term mass is not synonymous with neoplasm, as it is often used to describe cysts and thickenings such as those occurring with hematoma or infection.

### MALIGNANT NEOPLASM OF LIP, ORAL CAVITY, AND PHARYNX (140-149)

> **EXCLUDES**   carcinoma in situ (230.0)

**√4ᵗʰ 140 Malignant neoplasm of lip**
> **EXCLUDES**   skin of lip (173.0)

**140.0**   **Upper lip, vermilion border**
> Upper lip:      Upper lip:
> NOS             lipstick area
> external

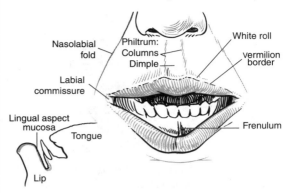

**Lip**

**140.1**   **Lower lip, vermilion border**
> Lower lip:      Lower lip:
> NOS             lipstick area
> external

**140.3**   **Upper lip, inner aspect**
> Upper lip:      Upper lip:
> buccal aspect    mucosa
> frenulum       oral aspect

**140.4**   **Lower lip, inner aspect**
> Lower lip:      Lower lip:
> buccal aspect    mucosa
> frenulum       oral aspect

**140.5**   **Lip, unspecified, inner aspect**
> Lip, not specified whether upper or lower:
> buccal aspect
> frenulum
> mucosa
> oral aspect

**140.6**   **Commissure of lip**
> Labial commissure

**140.8**   **Other sites of lip**
> Malignant neoplasm of contiguous or overlapping sites of lip whose point of origin cannot be determined

**140.9**   **Lip, unspecified, vermilion border**
> Lip, not specified as upper or lower:
> NOS
> external
> lipstick area

**√4ᵗʰ 141 Malignant neoplasm of tongue**
**141.0**   **Base of tongue**
> Dorsal surface of base of tongue
> Fixed part of tongue NOS
>
> **AHA:** 4Q, '06, 90

**141.1**   **Dorsal surface of tongue**
> Anterior two-thirds of tongue, dorsal surface
> Dorsal tongue NOS
> Midline of tongue
> **EXCLUDES**   dorsal surface of base of tongue (141.0)

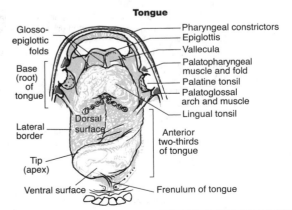

**Tongue**

**√4ᵗʰ / √5ᵗʰ** Additional Digit Required    Unacceptable PDx    Manifestation Code    ►◄ Revised Text    ● New Code    ▲ Revised Code Title

© 2007 Ingenix          October 2007 • Volume 1 — 33

**Neoplasms**

**141.2–146.7**

**Main Salivary Glands**

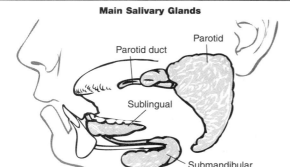

**141.2 Tip and lateral border of tongue**

**141.3 Ventral surface of tongue**
  Anterior two-thirds of tongue, ventral surface
  Frenulum linguae

**141.4 Anterior two-thirds of tongue, part unspecified**
  Mobile part of tongue NOS

**141.5 Junctional zone**
  Border of tongue at junction of fixed and mobile parts at insertion of anterior tonsillar pillar

**141.6 Lingual tonsil**

**141.8 Other sites of tongue**
  Malignant neoplasm of contiguous or overlapping sites of tongue whose point of origin cannot be determined

**141.9 Tongue, unspecified**
  Tongue NOS

✓4th **142 Malignant neoplasm of major salivary glands**
  **INCLUDES** salivary ducts
  **EXCLUDES** malignant neoplasm of minor salivary glands:
    NOS (145.9)
    buccal mucosa (145.0)
    soft palate (145.3)
    tongue (141.0-141.9)
    tonsil, palatine (146.0)

**142.0 Parotid gland**

**142.1 Submandibular gland**
  Submaxillary gland

**142.2 Sublingual gland**

**142.8 Other major salivary glands**
  Malignant neoplasm of contiguous or overlapping sites of salivary glands and ducts whose point of origin cannot be determined

**142.9 Salivary gland, unspecified**
  Salivary gland (major) NOS

✓4th **143 Malignant neoplasm of gum**
  **INCLUDES** alveolar (ridge) mucosa
    gingiva (alveolar) (marginal)
    interdental papillae
  **EXCLUDES** malignant odontogenic neoplasms (170.0-170.1)

**143.0 Upper gum**

**143.1 Lower gum**

**143.8 Other sites of gum**
  Malignant neoplasm of contiguous or overlapping sites of gum whose point of origin cannot be determined

**143.9 Gum, unspecified**

✓4th **144 Malignant neoplasm of floor of mouth**

**144.0 Anterior portion**
  Anterior to the premolar-canine junction

**144.1 Lateral portion**

**144.8 Other sites of floor of mouth**
  Malignant neoplasm of contiguous or overlapping sites of floor of mouth whose point of origin cannot be determined

**144.9 Floor of mouth, part unspecified**

✓4th **145 Malignant neoplasm of other and unspecified parts of mouth**
  **EXCLUDES** mucosa of lips (140.0-140.9)

**145.0 Cheek mucosa**
  Buccal mucosa
  Cheek, inner aspect

**145.1 Vestibule of mouth**
  Buccal sulcus (upper) (lower)
  Labial sulcus (upper) (lower)

**145.2 Hard palate**

**145.3 Soft palate**
  **EXCLUDES** nasopharyngeal [posterior] [superior] surface of soft palate (147.3)

**145.4 Uvula**

**145.5 Palate, unspecified**
  Junction of hard and soft palate     Roof of mouth

**145.6 Retromolar area**

**145.8 Other specified parts of mouth**
  Malignant neoplasm of contiguous or overlapping sites of mouth whose point of origin cannot be determined

**145.9 Mouth, unspecified**
  Buccal cavity NOS
  Minor salivary gland, unspecified site
  Oral cavity NOS

✓4th **146 Malignant neoplasm of oropharynx**

**146.0 Tonsil**
  Tonsil:
    NOS
    faucial
    palatine
  **EXCLUDES** lingual tonsil (141.6)
    pharyngeal tonsil (147.1)

  **AHA:** S-O, '87, 8

**146.1 Tonsillar fossa**

**146.2 Tonsillar pillars (anterior) (posterior)**
  Faucial pillar     Palatoglossal arch
  Glossopalatine fold    Palatopharyngeal arch

**146.3 Vallecula**
  Anterior and medial surface of the pharyngoepiglottic fold

**146.4 Anterior aspect of epiglottis**
  Epiglottis, free border [margin]
  Glossoepiglottic fold(s)
  **EXCLUDES** epiglottis:
    NOS (161.1)
    suprahyoid portion (161.1)

**146.5 Junctional region**
  Junction of the free margin of the epiglottis, the aryepiglottic fold, and the pharyngoepiglottic fold

**146.6 Lateral wall of oropharynx**

**146.7 Posterior wall of oropharynx**

**Mouth**

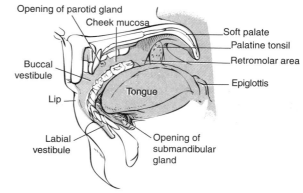

---

| N | Newborn Age: 0 | P | Pediatric Age: 0-17 | M | Maternity Age: 12-55 | A | Adult Age: 15-124 | CC | CC Condition | MCC | Major CC Condition | HIV | HIV Related Dx |

34 — Volume 1 • October 2007

© 2007 Ingenix

**Oropharynx**

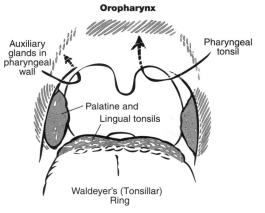

**146.8**   **Other specified sites of oropharynx**
Branchial cleft
Malignant neoplasm of contiguous or overlapping sites of oropharynx whose point of origin cannot be determined

**146.9**   **Oropharynx, unspecified**
**AHA:** 2Q, '02, 6

✓4th **147 Malignant neoplasm of nasopharynx**

**147.0**   **Superior wall**
Roof of nasopharynx

**147.1**   **Posterior wall**
Adenoid      Pharyngeal tonsil

**147.2**   **Lateral wall**
Fossa of Rosenmüller   Pharyngeal recess
Opening of auditory tube

**147.3**   **Anterior wall**
Floor of nasopharynx
Nasopharyngeal [posterior] [superior] surface of soft palate
Posterior margin of nasal septum and choanae

**147.8**   **Other specified sites of nasopharynx**
Malignant neoplasm of contiguous or overlapping sites of nasopharynx whose point of origin cannot be determined

**147.9**   **Nasopharynx, unspecified**
Nasopharyngeal wall NOS

✓4th **148 Malignant neoplasm of hypopharynx**

**148.0**   **Postcricoid region**

**148.1**   **Pyriform sinus**
Pyriform fossa

**148.2**   **Aryepiglottic fold, hypopharyngeal aspect**
Aryepiglottic fold or interarytenoid fold:
NOS
marginal zone
> **EXCLUDES**   *aryepiglottic fold or interarytenoid fold, laryngeal aspect (161.1)*

**Nasopharynx**

**Hypopharynx**

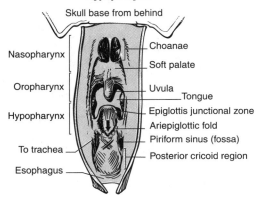

**148.3**   **Posterior hypopharyngeal wall**

**148.8**   **Other specified sites of hypopharynx**
Malignant neoplasm of contiguous or overlapping sites of hypopharynx whose point of origin cannot be determined

**148.9**   **Hypopharynx, unspecified**
Hypopharyngeal wall NOS
Hypopharynx NOS

✓4th **149 Malignant neoplasm of other and ill-defined sites within the lip, oral cavity, and pharynx**

**149.0**   **Pharynx, unspecified**

**149.1**   **Waldeyer's ring**

**149.8**   **Other**
Malignant neoplasms of lip, oral cavity, and pharynx whose point of origin cannot be assigned to any one of the categories 140-148
> **EXCLUDES**   *"book leaf" neoplasm [ventral surface of tongue and floor of mouth] (145.8)*

**149.9**   **Ill-defined**

## MALIGNANT NEOPLASM OF DIGESTIVE ORGANS AND PERITONEUM (150-159)
> **EXCLUDES**   *carcinoma in situ (230.1-230.9)*

✓4th **150 Malignant neoplasm of esophagus**

**150.0**   **Cervical esophagus**   `CC`
**CC Excl:** 150.0-150.9, 159.0, 159.8-159.9, 176.3, 195.8, 199.0-199.1, 239.0, 239.8-239.9

**150.1**   **Thoracic esophagus**   `CC`
**CC Excl:** See code: 150.0

**150.2**   **Abdominal esophagus**   `CC`
> **EXCLUDES**   *adenocarcinoma (151.0)*
> *cardio-esophageal junction (151.0)*

**CC Excl:** See code 150.0

**150.3**   **Upper third of esophagus**   `CC`
**CC Excl:** See code 150.0

Proximal third of esophagus

**150.4**   **Middle third of esophagus**   `CC`
**CC Excl:** See code 150.0

---

Neoplasms

150.5–154.1

**150.5  Lower third of esophagus**  `CC`
Distal third of esophagus
**EXCLUDES**  *adenocarcinoma (151.0)*
*cardio-esophageal junction (151.0)*
CC Excl: See code 150.0

**150.8  Other specified part**  `CC`
Malignant neoplasm of contiguous or overlapping sites of esophagus whose point of origin cannot be determined
CC Excl: See code 150.0

**150.9  Esophagus, unspecified**  `CC`
CC Excl: See code 150.0

✓4th **151  Malignant neoplasm of stomach**
**EXCLUDES**  *malignant stromal tumor of stomach (171.5)*

**151.0  Cardia**  `CC`
Cardiac orifice
Cardio-esophageal junction
**EXCLUDES**  *squamous cell carcinoma (150.2, 150.5)*
CC Excl: 151.0-151.9, 159.0, 159.8-159.9, 176.3, 195.8, 199.0-199.1, 239.0, 239.8-239.9

**151.1  Pylorus**  `CC`
Prepylorus          Pyloric canal
CC Excl: See code 151.0

**151.2  Pyloric antrum**  `CC`
Antrum of stomach NOS
CC Excl: See code 151.0

**151.3  Fundus of stomach**  `CC`
CC Excl: See code 151.0

**151.4  Body of stomach**  `CC`
CC Excl: See code 151.0

**151.5  Lesser curvature, unspecified**  `CC`
Lesser curvature, not classifiable to 151.1-151.4
CC Excl: See code 151.0

**151.6  Greater curvature, unspecified**  `CC`
Greater curvature, not classifiable to 151.0-151.4
CC Excl: See code 151.0

**151.8  Other specified sites of stomach**  `CC`
Anterior wall, not classifiable to 151.0-151.4
Posterior wall, not classifiable to 151.0-151.4
Malignant neoplasm of contiguous or overlapping sites of stomach whose point of origin cannot be determined
CC Excl: See code 151.0

**151.9  Stomach, unspecified**  `CC`
Carcinoma ventriculi   Gastric cancer
CC Excl: See code 151.0

AHA: 2Q, '01, 17

✓4th **152  Malignant neoplasm of small intestine, including duodenum**
**EXCLUDES**  *malignant stromal tumor of small intestine (171.5)*

**152.0  Duodenum**  `CC`
CC Excl: 152.0, 152.8-152.9, 159.0, 159.8-159.9, 176.3, 195.8, 199.0-199.1, 239.0, 239.8-239.9

**152.1  Jejunum**  `CC`
CC Excl: 152.1, 152.8-152.9, 159.0, 159.8-159.9, 176.3, 195.8, 199.0-199.1, 239.0, 239.8-239.9

**152.2  Ileum**  `CC`
**EXCLUDES**  *ileocecal valve (153.4)*
CC Excl: 152.2, 152.8-152.9, 159.0, 159.8-159.9, 176.3, 195.8, 199.0-199.1, 239.0, 239.8-239.9

**152.3  Meckel's diverticulum**  `CC`
CC Excl: 152.3-152.9, 159.0, 159.8-159.9, 176.3, 195.8, 199.0-199.1, 239.0, 239.8-239.9

**152.8  Other specified sites of small intestine**  `CC`
Duodenojejunal junction
Malignant neoplasm of contiguous or overlapping sites of small intestine whose point of origin cannot be determined
CC Excl: 152.8-152.9, 159.0, 159.8-159.9, 176.3, 195.8, 199.0-199.1, 239.0, 239.8-239.9

**152.9  Small intestine, unspecified**  `CC`
CC Excl: See code 152.8

✓4th **153  Malignant neoplasm of colon**

**153.0  Hepatic flexure**  `CC`
CC Excl: 153.0, 153.8-153.9, 159.0, 159.8-159.9, 176.3, 195.8, 199.0-199.1, 239.0, 239.8-239.9

**153.1  Transverse colon**  `CC`
CC Excl: 153.1, 153.8-153.9, 159.0, 159.8-159.9, 176.3, 195.8, 199.0-199.1, 239.0, 239.8-239.9

**153.2  Descending colon**  `CC`
Left colon
CC Excl: 153.2, 153.8-153.9, 159.0, 159.8-159.9, 176.3, 195.8, 199.0-199.1, 239.0, 239.8-239.9

**153.3  Sigmoid colon**  `CC`
Sigmoid (flexure)
**EXCLUDES**  *rectosigmoid junction (154.0)*
CC Excl: 153.3, 153.8-153.9, 159.0, 159.8-159.9, 176.3, 195.8, 199.0-199.1, 239.0, 239.8-239.9

**153.4  Cecum**  `CC`
Ileocecal valve
CC Excl: 153.4, 153.8-153.9, 159.0, 159.8-159.9, 176.3, 195.8, 199.0-199.1, 239.0, 239.8-239.9

**153.5  Appendix**  `CC`
CC Excl: 153.5, 153.8-153.9, 159.0, 159.8-159.9, 176.3, 195.8, 199.0-199.1, 239.0, 239.8-239.9

**153.6  Ascending colon**  `CC`
Right colon
CC Excl: 153.6, 153.8-153.9, 159.0, 159.8-159.9, 176.3, 195.8, 199.0-199.1, 239.0, 239.8-239.9

**153.7  Splenic flexure**  `CC`
CC Excl: 153.7-153.9, 159.0, 159.8-159.9, 176.3, 195.8, 199.0-199.1, 239.0, 239.8-239.9

**153.8  Other specified sites of large intestine**  `CC`
Malignant neoplasm of contiguous or overlapping sites of colon whose point of origin cannot be determined
**EXCLUDES**  *ileocecal valve (153.4)*
*rectosigmoid junction (154.0)*
CC Excl: 153.8-153.9, 159.0, 159.8-159.9, 176.3, 195.8, 199.0-199.1, 239.0, 239.8-239.9

**153.9  Colon, unspecified**  `CC`
Large intestine NOS
CC Excl: See code: 153.8

✓4th **154  Malignant neoplasm of rectum, rectosigmoid junction, and anus**

**154.0  Rectosigmoid junction**  `CC`
Colon with rectum
Rectosigmoid (colon)
CC Excl: 154.0, 154.8, 159.0, 159.8-159.9, 176.3, 195.8, 199.0-199.1, 239.0, 239.8-239.9

**154.1  Rectum**  `CC`
Rectal ampulla
CC Excl: 154.1, 154.8, 159.0, 159.8-159.9, 176.3, 195.8, 199.0-199.1, 239.0, 239.8-239.9

---

`N` Newborn Age: 0     `P` Pediatric Age: 0-17     `M` Maternity Age: 12-55     `A` Adult Age: 15-124     `CC` CC Condition     `MCC` Major CC Condition     `HIV` HIV Related Dx

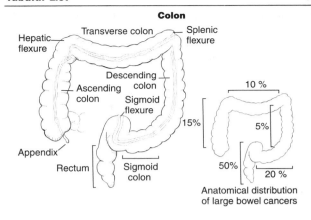

**Colon**

Anatomical distribution of large bowel cancers

**154.2 Anal canal**    `cc`
Anal sphincter
> EXCLUDES   *skin of anus (172.5, 173.5)*

CC Excl: 154.2-154.8, 159.0, 159.8-159.9, 176.3, 195.8, 199.0-199.1, 239.0, 239.8-239.9

AHA: 1Q, '01, 8

**154.3 Anus, unspecified**    `cc`
> EXCLUDES   *anus:*
>      *margin (172.5, 173.5)*
>      *skin (172.5, 173.5)*
>      *perianal skin (172.5, 173.5)*

CC Excl: See code: 154.2

**154.8 Other**    `cc`
Anorectum
Cloacogenic zone
Malignant neoplasm of contiguous or overlapping sites of rectum, rectosigmoid junction, and anus whose point of origin cannot be determined

CC Excl: 154.8, 159.0, 159.8-159.9, 176.3, 195.8, 199.0-199.1, 239.0, 239.8-239.9

✓4ᵗʰ **155 Malignant neoplasm of liver and intrahepatic bile ducts**

**155.0 Liver, primary**    `cc`
Carcinoma:
   liver, specified as primary
   hepatocellular
   liver cell
Hepatoblastoma

CC Excl: 155.0-155.2, 159.0, 159.8-159.9, 176.3, 195.8, 199.0-199.1, 239.0, 239.8-239.9

**155.1 Intrahepatic bile ducts**    `cc`
Canaliculi biliferi    Intrahepatic:
Interlobular:      biliary passages
   bile ducts      canaliculi
   biliary canals    gall duct
> EXCLUDES   *hepatic duct (156.1)*

CC Excl: See code 155.0

**155.2 Liver, not specified as primary or secondary**    `cc`
CC Excl: See code 155.0

✓4ᵗʰ **156 Malignant neoplasm of gallbladder and extrahepatic bile ducts**

**156.0 Gallbladder**    `cc`
CC Excl: 156.0, 156.8-156.9, 159.0, 159.8-159.9, 176.3, 195.8, 199.0-199.1, 239.0, 239.8-239.9

**156.1 Extrahepatic bile ducts**    `cc`
Biliary duct or passage NOS
Common bile duct
Cystic duct
Hepatic duct
Sphincter of Oddi

CC Excl: 156.1, 156.8-156.9, 159.0, 159.8-159.9, 176.3, 195.8, 199.0-199.1, 239.0, 239.8-239.9

**156.2 Ampulla of Vater**    `cc`
CC Excl: 156.2-156.9, 159.0, 159.8-159.9, 176.3, 195.8, 199.0-199.1, 239.0, 239.8-239.9

DEF: Malignant neoplasm in the area of dilation at the juncture of the common bile and pancreatic ducts near the opening into the lumen of the duodenum.

**156.8 Other specified sites of gallbladder and extrahepatic bile ducts**    `cc`
Malignant neoplasm of contiguous or overlapping sites of gallbladder and extrahepatic bile ducts whose point of origin cannot be determined

CC Excl: 156.8-156.9, 159.0, 159.8-159.9, 176.3, 195.8, 199.0-199.1, 239.0, 239.8-239.9

**156.9 Biliary tract, part unspecified**    `cc`
Malignant neoplasm involving both intrahepatic and extrahepatic bile ducts

CC Excl: See code: 156.8

✓4ᵗʰ **157 Malignant neoplasm of pancreas**

**157.0 Head of pancreas**    `cc`
CC Excl: 157.0-157.9, 159.0, 159.8-159.9, 176.3, 195.8, 199.0-199.1, 239.0, 239.8-239.9

AHA: 2Q, '05, 9; 4Q, '00, 40

**157.1 Body of pancreas**    `cc`
CC Excl: See code 157.0

**157.2 Tail of pancreas**    `cc`
CC Excl: See code 157.0

**157.3 Pancreatic duct**    `cc`
Duct of:
   Santorini
   Wirsung

CC Excl: See code 157.0

**157.4 Islets of Langerhans**    `cc`
Islets of Langerhans, any part of pancreas
Use additional code to identify any functional activity

CC Excl: See code 157.0

DEF: Malignant neoplasm within the structures of the pancreas that produce insulin, somatostatin and glucagon.

**157.8 Other specified sites of pancreas**    `cc`
Ectopic pancreatic tissue
Malignant neoplasm of contiguous or overlapping sites of pancreas whose point of origin cannot be determined

CC Excl: See code 157.0

**157.9 Pancreas, part unspecified**    `cc`
CC Excl: See code 157.0

AHA: 4Q, '89, 11

✓4ᵗʰ **158 Malignant neoplasm of retroperitoneum and peritoneum**

**158.0 Retroperitoneum**    `cc`
Periadrenal tissue    Perirenal tissue
Perinephric tissue    Retrocecal tissue

CC Excl: 158.0, V58.0

Neoplasms

154.2–158.0

**Neoplasms**

**158.8–162.0**

### Retroperitoneum and Peritoneum

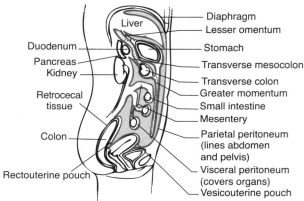

Diaphragm
Liver
Lesser omentum
Duodenum
Stomach
Pancreas
Transverse mesocolon
Kidney
Transverse colon
Retrocecal tissue
Greater momentum
Small intestine
Mesentery
Colon
Parietal peritoneum (lines abdomen and pelvis)
Visceral peritoneum (covers organs)
Rectouterine pouch
Vesicouterine pouch

**158.8 Specified parts of peritoneum** `CC`

Cul-de-sac (of Douglas)
Mesentery
Mesocolon
Omentum
Peritoneum:
  parietal
  pelvic
Rectouterine pouch
Malignant neoplasm of contiguous or overlapping sites of retroperitoneum and peritoneum whose point of origin cannot be determined

**CC Excl:** 158.0-158.9, V58.0

**158.9 Peritoneum, unspecified** `CC`

**CC Excl:** See code: 158.8

√4th **159 Malignant neoplasm of other and ill-defined sites within the digestive organs and peritoneum**

**159.0 Intestinal tract, part unspecified**
Intestine NOS

**159.1 Spleen, not elsewhere classified**
Angiosarcoma
Fibrosarcoma } of spleen

> **EXCLUDES** Hodgkin's disease (201.0-201.9)
> lymphosarcoma (200.1)
> reticulosarcoma (200.0)

**159.8 Other sites of digestive system and intra-abdominal organs**
Malignant neoplasm of digestive organs and peritoneum whose point of origin cannot be assigned to any one of the categories 150-158

> **EXCLUDES** anus and rectum (154.8)
> cardio-esophageal junction (151.0)
> colon and rectum (154.0)

**159.9 Ill-defined**
Alimentary canal or tract NOS
Gastrointestinal tract NOS

> **EXCLUDES** abdominal NOS (195.2)
> intra-abdominal NOS (195.2)

### MALIGNANT NEOPLASM OF RESPIRATORY AND INTRATHORACIC ORGANS (160-165)

> **EXCLUDES** carcinoma in situ (231.0-231.9)

√4th **160 Malignant neoplasm of nasal cavities, middle ear, and accessory sinuses**

**160.0 Nasal cavities**
Cartilage of nose
Septum of nose
Conchae, nasal
Vestibule of nose
Internal nose

> **EXCLUDES** nasal bone (170.0)
> nose NOS (195.0)
> olfactory bulb (192.0)
> posterior margin of septum and choanae (147.3)
> skin of nose (172.3, 173.3)
> turbinates (170.0)

**160.1 Auditory tube, middle ear, and mastoid air cells**
Antrum tympanicum
Tympanic cavity
Eustachian tube

> **EXCLUDES** auditory canal (external) (172.2, 173.2)
> bone of ear (meatus) (170.0)
> cartilage of ear (171.0)
> ear (external) (skin) (172.2, 173.2)

**160.2 Maxillary sinus**
Antrum (Highmore) (maxillary)

**160.3 Ethmoidal sinus**

**160.4 Frontal sinus**

**160.5 Sphenoidal sinus**

**160.8 Other**
Malignant neoplasm of contiguous or overlapping sites of nasal cavities, middle ear, and accessory sinuses whose point of origin cannot be determined

**160.9 Accessory sinus, unspecified**

√4th **161 Malignant neoplasm of larynx**

**161.0 Glottis**
Intrinsic larynx
Laryngeal commissure (anterior) (posterior)
True vocal cord
Vocal cord NOS

**161.1 Supraglottis**
Aryepiglottic fold or interarytenoid fold, laryngeal aspect
Epiglottis (suprahyoid portion) NOS
Extrinsic larynx
False vocal cords
Posterior (laryngeal) surface of epiglottis
Ventricular bands

> **EXCLUDES** anterior aspect of epiglottis (146.4)
> aryepiglottic fold or interarytenoid fold:
> NOS (148.2)
> hypopharyngeal aspect (148.2)
> marginal zone (148.2)

**161.2 Subglottis**

**161.3 Laryngeal cartilages**
Cartilage:
  arytenoid
  cricoid
Cartilage:
  cuneiform
  thyroid

**161.8 Other specified sites of larynx**
Malignant neoplasm of contiguous or overlapping sites of larynx whose point of origin cannot be determined

**161.9 Larynx, unspecified**

√4th **162 Malignant neoplasm of trachea, bronchus, and lung**

**162.0 Trachea** `CC`
Cartilage
Mucosa } of trachea

**CC Excl:** 162.0-162.9, 165.8-165.9, 176.4, 195.1, 195.8, 197.0-197.1, 197.3, 199.0-199.1, 239.1, 239.8-239.9

N Newborn Age: 0    P Pediatric Age: 0-17    M Maternity Age: 12-55    A Adult Age: 15-124    CC CC Condition    MCC Major CC Condition    HIV HIV Related Dx

38 — Volume 1 • October 2007

© 2007 Ingenix

**Neoplasms**

**162.2 Main bronchus** `CC`
Carina
Hilus of lung
**CC Excl:** 162.2, 162.8-162.9, 165.8-165.9, 176.4, 195.8, 199.0-199.1, 239.1, 239.8-239.9

**162.3 Upper lobe, bronchus or lung** `CC`
**CC Excl:** 162.3, 162.8-162.9, 165.8-165.9, 176.4, 195.8, 199.0-199.1, 239.1, 239.8-239.9

**AHA:** 1Q, '04, 4

**162.4 Middle lobe, bronchus or lung** `CC`
**CC Excl:** 162.4, 162.8-162.9, 165.8-165.9, 176.4, 195.8, 199.0-199.1, 239.1, 239.8-239.9

**162.5 Lower lobe, bronchus or lung** `CC`
**CC Excl:** 162.5-162.9, 165.8-165.9, 176.4, 195.8, 199.0-199.1, 239.1, 239.8-239.9

**162.8 Other parts of bronchus or lung** `CC`
Malignant neoplasm of contiguous or overlapping sites of bronchus or lung whose point of origin cannot be determined
**CC Excl:** 162.8-162.9, 165.8-165.9, 176.4, 195.8, 199.0-199.1, 239.1, 239.8-239.9

**AHA:** 3Q, '06, 7

**162.9 Bronchus and lung, unspecified** `CC`
**CC Excl:** See code: 162.8

**AHA:** 3Q, '06, 14-15; 2Q, '97, 3; 4Q, '96, 48

**√4ᵗʰ 163 Malignant neoplasm of pleura**
**163.0 Parietal pleura** `CC`
**CC Excl:** 163.0-163.9, 165.8-165.9, 195.8, 199.0-199.1, 239.1, 239.8-239.9

**163.1 Visceral pleura** `CC`
**CC Excl:** See code 163.0

**163.8 Other specified sites of pleura** `CC`
Malignant neoplasm of contiguous or overlapping sites of pleura whose point of origin cannot be determined
**CC Excl:** See code 163.0

**163.9 Pleura, unspecified** `CC`
**CC Excl:** See code 163.0

**√4ᵗʰ 164 Malignant neoplasm of thymus, heart, and mediastinum**
**164.0 Thymus** `CC`
**CC Excl:** 164.0

**164.1 Heart** `CC`
Endocardium    Myocardium
Epicardium     Pericardium
**EXCLUDES** *great vessels (171.4)*
**CC Excl:** 164.1

**164.2 Anterior mediastinum** `CC`
**CC Excl:** 164.2-164.9, 165.8-165.9, 195.8, 199.0-199.1, 239.1, 239.8-239.9

**164.3 Posterior mediastinum** `CC`
**CC Excl:** See code 164.2

**164.8 Other** `CC`
Malignant neoplasm of contiguous or overlapping sites of thymus, heart, and mediastinum whose point of origin cannot be determined
**CC Excl:** See code 164.2

**164.9 Mediastinum, part unspecified** `CC`
**CC Excl:** See code 164.2

**√4ᵗʰ 165 Malignant neoplasm of other and ill-defined sites within the respiratory system and intrathoracic organs**
**165.0 Upper respiratory tract, part unspecified**
**165.8 Other**
Malignant neoplasm of respiratory and intrathoracic organs whose point of origin cannot be assigned to any one of the categories 160-164

**165.9 Ill-defined sites within the respiratory system**
Respiratory tract NOS
**EXCLUDES** *intrathoracic NOS (195.1)*
*thoracic NOS (195.1)*

## MALIGNANT NEOPLASM OF BONE, CONNECTIVE TISSUE, SKIN, AND BREAST (170-176)

**EXCLUDES** *carcinoma in situ:*   *carcinoma in situ:*
*breast (233.0)*      *skin (232.0-232.9)*

**√4ᵗʰ 170 Malignant neoplasm of bone and articular cartilage**
**INCLUDES** cartilage (articular) (joint)
periosteum
**EXCLUDES** *bone marrow NOS (202.9)*
*cartilage:*
*ear (171.0)*
*eyelid (171.0)*
*larynx (161.3)*
*nose (160.0)*
*synovia (171.0-171.9)*

**AHA:** 4Q, '06, 103

**170.0 Bones of skull and face, except mandible** `CC`
Bone:          Bone:
ethmoid       sphenoid
frontal        temporal
malar         zygomatic
nasal         Maxilla (superior)
occipital     Turbinate
orbital       Upper jaw bone
parietal      Vomer
**EXCLUDES** *carcinoma, any type except intraosseous or odontogenic:*
*maxilla, maxillary (sinus) (160.2)*
*upper jaw bone (143.0)*
*jaw bone (lower) (170.1)*
**CC Excl:** 170.0, 170.9, V58.0

**170.1 Mandible** `CC`
Inferior maxilla
Jaw bone NOS
Lower jaw bone
**EXCLUDES** *carcinoma, any type except intraosseous or odontogenic:*
*jaw bone NOS (143.9)*
*lower (143.1)*
*upper jaw bone (170.0)*
**CC Excl:** 170.1, 170.9, V58.0

**170.2 Vertebral column, excluding sacrum and coccyx** `CC`
Spinal column    Vertebra
Spine
**EXCLUDES** *sacrum and coccyx (170.6)*
**CC Excl:** 170.2, 170.9, V58.0

**Skull**

Orbital rim — Frontal — Roof — Zygoma (malar) — Ethmoid — Zygomatic arch — Lacrimal — Nasal — Condylar process — Maxilla — Palate — Coronoid process — Alveolar margins — Ramus — Mandible — Body — Angle — Symphysis

---

**Neoplasms**

**170.3–172.4**

**170.3 Ribs, sternum, and clavicle** `CC`
Costal cartilage
Costovertebral joint
Xiphoid process
**CC Excl:** 170.3, 170.9, V58.0

**170.4 Scapula and long bones of upper limb** `CC`
Acromion        Radius
Bones NOS of upper limb    Ulna
Humerus
**CC Excl:** 170.4, 170.9, V58.0

**AHA:** 2Q, '99, 9

**170.5 Short bones of upper limb** `CC`
Carpal            Scaphoid (of hand)
Cuneiform, wrist    Semilunar or lunate
Metacarpal       Trapezium
Navicular, of hand   Trapezoid
Phalanges of hand   Unciform
Pisiform
**CC Excl:** 170.5, 170.9, V58.0

**170.6 Pelvic bones, sacrum, and coccyx** `CC`
Coccygeal vertebra    Pubic bone
Ilium            Sacral vertebra
Ischium
**CC Excl:** 170.6, 170.9, V58.0

**170.7 Long bones of lower limb** `CC`
Bones NOS of lower limb
Femur
Fibula
Tibia
**CC Excl:** 170.7, 170.9, V58.0

**170.8 Short bones of lower limb** `CC`
Astragalus [talus]    Navicular (of ankle)
Calcaneus        Patella
Cuboid          Phalanges of foot
Cuneiform, ankle   Tarsal
Metatarsal
**CC Excl:** 170.8-170.9, V58.0

**170.9 Bone and articular cartilage, site unspecified** `CC`
**CC Excl:** 170.0-170.9, V58.0

`√4th` **171 Malignant neoplasm of connective and other soft tissue**
`INCLUDES`   blood vessel
bursa
fascia
fat
ligament, except uterine
malignant stromal tumors
muscle
peripheral, sympathetic, and parasympathetic
     nerves and ganglia
synovia
tendon (sheath)
`EXCLUDES`   *cartilage (of):*
    *articular (170.0-170.9)*
    *larynx (161.3)*
    *nose (160.0)*
*connective tissue:*
    *breast (174.0-175.9)*
    *internal organs (except stromal tumors)—*
       *code to malignant neoplasm of the site*
       *[e.g., leiomyosarcoma of stomach, 151.9]*
*heart (164.1)*
*uterine ligament (183.4)*

**171.0 Head, face, and neck** `CC`
Cartilage of:        Cartilage of:
   ear                 eyelid
**CC Excl:** V58.0

**AHA:** 2Q, '99, 6

**171.2 Upper limb, including shoulder** `CC`
Arm           Forearm
Finger        Hand
**CC Excl:** See code: 171.0

**171.3 Lower limb, including hip** `CC`
Foot          Thigh
Leg           Toe
Popliteal space
**CC Excl:** See code: 171.0

**171.4 Thorax** `CC`
Axilla         Great vessels
Diaphragm
`EXCLUDES`   *heart (164.1)*
           *mediastinum (164.2-164.9)*
           *thymus (164.0)*
**CC Excl:** See code: 171.0

**171.5 Abdomen** `CC`
Abdominal wall     Hypochondrium
`EXCLUDES`   *peritoneum (158.8)*
           *retroperitoneum (158.0)*
**CC Excl:** See code: 171.0

**171.6 Pelvis** `CC`
Buttock        Inguinal region
Groin          Perineum
`EXCLUDES`   *pelvic peritoneum (158.8)*
           *retroperitoneum (158.0)*
           *uterine ligament, any (183.3-183.5)*
**CC Excl:** See code: 171.0

**171.7 Trunk, unspecified** `CC`
Back NOS        Flank NOS
**CC Excl:** See code: 171.0

**171.8 Other specified sites of connective and other soft tissue** `CC`
Malignant neoplasm of contiguous or overlapping
    sites of connective tissue whose point of origin
    cannot be determined
**CC Excl:** See code: 171.0

**171.9 Connective and other soft tissue, site unspecified** `CC`
**CC Excl:** See code: 171.0

`√4th` **172 Malignant melanoma of skin**
`INCLUDES`   melanocarcinoma
melanoma (skin) NOS
`EXCLUDES`   *skin of genital organs (184.0-184.9, 187.1-187.9)*
*sites other than skin—code to malignant*
     *neoplasm of the site*

**DEF:** Malignant neoplasm of melanocytes; most common in skin, may involve
oral cavity, esophagus, anal canal, vagina, leptomeninges, or conjunctiva.

**172.0 Lip**
`EXCLUDES`   *vermilion border of lip (140.0-140.1,*
           *140.9)*

**172.1 Eyelid, including canthus**

**172.2 Ear and external auditory canal**
Auricle (ear)
Auricular canal, external
External [acoustic] meatus
Pinna

**172.3 Other and unspecified parts of face**
Cheek (external)    Forehead
Chin            Nose, external
Eyebrow        Temple

**172.4 Scalp and neck**

---

| `N` Newborn Age: 0 | `P` Pediatric Age: 0-17 | `M` Maternity Age: 12-55 | `A` Adult Age: 15-124 | `CC` CC Condition | `MCC` Major CC Condition | `HIV` HIV Related Dx |
|---|---|---|---|---|---|---|

**172.5 Trunk, except scrotum**

| | |
|---|---|
| Axilla | Perianal skin |
| Breast | Perineum |
| Buttock | Umbilicus |
| Groin | |

EXCLUDES   anal canal (154.2)
         anus NOS (154.3)
         scrotum (187.7)

**172.6 Upper limb, including shoulder**

| | |
|---|---|
| Arm | Forearm |
| Finger | Hand |

**172.7 Lower limb, including hip**

| | |
|---|---|
| Ankle | Leg |
| Foot | Popliteal area |
| Heel | Thigh |
| Knee | Toe |

**172.8 Other specified sites of skin**
Malignant melanoma of contiguous or overlapping sites of skin whose point of origin cannot be determined

**172.9 Melanoma of skin, site unspecified**

√4th **173 Other malignant neoplasm of skin**

INCLUDES   malignant neoplasm of:
         sebaceous glands
         sudoriferous, sudoriparous glands
         sweat glands

EXCLUDES   Kaposi's sarcoma (176.0-176.9)
         malignant melanoma of skin (172.0-172.9)
         skin of genital organs (184.0-184.9, 187.1-187.9)

AHA: 1Q, '00, 18; 2Q, '96, 12

**173.0 Skin of lip**
EXCLUDES   vermilion border of lip (140.0-140.1, 140.9)

**173.1 Eyelid, including canthus**
EXCLUDES   cartilage of eyelid (171.0)

**173.2 Skin of ear and external auditory canal**

| | |
|---|---|
| Auricle (ear) | External meatus |
| Auricular canal, external | Pinna |

EXCLUDES   cartilage of ear (171.0)

**173.3 Skin of other and unspecified parts of face**

| | |
|---|---|
| Cheek, external | Forehead |
| Chin | Nose, external |
| Eyebrow | Temple |

AHA: 1Q, '00, 3

**173.4 Scalp and skin of neck**

**173.5 Skin of trunk, except scrotum**

| | |
|---|---|
| Axillary fold | Skin of: |
| Perianal skin |   buttock |
| Skin of: |   chest wall |
|   abdominal wall |   groin |
|   anus |   perineum |
|   back |   Umbilicus |
|   breast | |

EXCLUDES   anal canal (154.2)
         anus NOS (154.3)
         skin of scrotum (187.7)

AHA: 1Q, '01, 8

**Female Breast**

**173.6 Skin of upper limb, including shoulder**

| | |
|---|---|
| Arm | Forearm |
| Finger | Hand |

**173.7 Skin of lower limb, including hip**

| | |
|---|---|
| Ankle | Leg |
| Foot | Popliteal area |
| Heel | Thigh |
| Knee | Toe |

**173.8 Other specified sites of skin**
Malignant neoplasm of contiguous or overlapping sites of skin whose point of origin cannot be determined

**173.9 Skin, site unspecified**

√4th **174 Malignant neoplasm of female breast**
Use additional code to identify estrogen receptor status (V86.0, V86.1)

INCLUDES   breast (female)    Paget's disease of:
         connective tissue    breast
         soft parts    nipple

EXCLUDES   skin of breast (172.5, 173.5)

AHA: 3Q, '97, 8; 4Q, '89, 11

| | | |
|---|---|---|
| **174.0** | **Nipple and areola** | ♀ |
| **174.1** | **Central portion** | ♀ |
| **174.2** | **Upper-inner quadrant** | ♀ |
| **174.3** | **Lower-inner quadrant** | ♀ |
| **174.4** | **Upper-outer quadrant** | ♀ |

AHA: 1Q, '04, 3

| | | |
|---|---|---|
| **174.5** | **Lower-outer quadrant** | ♀ |
| **174.6** | **Axillary tail** | ♀ |
| **174.8** | **Other specified sites of female breast** | ♀ |

| | |
|---|---|
| Ectopic sites | Midline of breast |
| Inner breast | Outer breast |
| Lower breast | Upper breast |

Malignant neoplasm of contiguous or overlapping sites of breast whose point of origin cannot be determined

| | | |
|---|---|---|
| **174.9** | **Breast (female), unspecified** | ♀ |

AHA: 3Q, '05, 11

√4th **175 Malignant neoplasm of male breast**
Use additional code to identify estrogen receptor status (V86.0, V86.1)
EXCLUDES   skin of breast (172.5, 173.5)

| | | |
|---|---|---|
| **175.0** | **Nipple and areola** | ♂ |
| **175.9** | **Other and unspecified sites of male breast** | ♂ |

Ectopic breast tissue, male

√4th **176 Kaposi's sarcoma**

AHA: 4Q, '91, 24

| | | |
|---|---|---|
| **176.0** | **Skin** | CC HIV |

CC Excl: 176.0, 176.8-176.9, V58.0

| | | |
|---|---|---|
| **176.1** | **Soft tissue** | CC HIV |

| | |
|---|---|
| Blood vessel | Ligament |
| Connective tissue | Lymphatic(s) NEC |
| Fascia | Muscle |

EXCLUDES   lymph glands and nodes (176.5)
CC Excl: 176.1, 176.8-176.9, V58.0

| | | |
|---|---|---|
| **176.2** | **Palate** | CC HIV |

CC Excl: 176.2, 176.8-176.9, V58.0

| | | |
|---|---|---|
| **176.3** | **Gastrointestinal sites** | CC HIV |

CC Excl: 176.3, 176.8-176.9, V58.0

| | | |
|---|---|---|
| **176.4** | **Lung** | CC HIV |

CC Excl: 162.8-162.9, 165.8-165.9, 176.4, 195.8, 199.0-199.1, 239.1, 239.8-239.9

| | | |
|---|---|---|
| **176.5** | **Lymph nodes** | CC HIV |

CC Excl: 176.5, 195.8-196.9, 199.0-199.1, 239.8-239.9

| | | |
|---|---|---|
| **176.8** | **Other specified sites** | CC HIV |

Oral cavity NEC
CC Excl: 176.0-176.9, V58.0

| | | |
|---|---|---|
| **176.9** | **Unspecified** | CC HIV |

Viscera NOS
CC Excl: 176.0-192.9, 195.0-199.1, 230.0-233.2, 233.30-237.6, 237.9-238.3, 238.8-239.9, V58.0

## MALIGNANT NEOPLASM OF GENITOURINARY ORGANS (179-189)

| EXCLUDES | *carcinoma in situ (233.1-233.9)* |

**179 Malignant neoplasm of uterus, part unspecified** ♀

**√4ᵗʰ 180 Malignant neoplasm of cervix uteri**

| INCLUDES | invasive malignancy [carcinoma] |
| EXCLUDES | *carcinoma in situ (233.1)* |

**180.0 Endocervix** ♀
Cervical canal NOS    Endocervical gland
Endocervical canal

**180.1 Exocervix** ♀

**180.8 Other specified sites of cervix** ♀
Cervical stump
Squamocolumnar junction of cervix
Malignant neoplasm of contiguous or overlapping
sites of cervix uteri whose point of origin
cannot be determined

**180.9 Cervix uteri, unspecified** ♀

**181 Malignant neoplasm of placenta** ♀
Choriocarcinoma NOS
Chorioepithelioma NOS

| EXCLUDES | *chorioadenoma (destruens) (236.1)* |
| | *hydatidiform mole (630)* |
| | *malignant (236.1)* |
| | *invasive mole (236.1)* |
| | *male choriocarcinoma NOS (186.0-186.9)* |

**√4ᵗʰ 182 Malignant neoplasm of body of uterus**

| EXCLUDES | *carcinoma in situ (233.2)* |

**182.0 Corpus uteri, except isthmus** ♀
Cornu      Fundus
Endometrium      Myometrium

**182.1 Isthmus** ♀
Lower uterine segment

**182.8 Other specified sites of body of uterus** ♀
Malignant neoplasm of contiguous or overlapping
sites of body of uterus whose point of origin
cannot be determined

| EXCLUDES | *uterus NOS (179)* |

**√4ᵗʰ 183 Malignant neoplasm of ovary and other uterine adnexa**

| EXCLUDES | *Douglas' cul-de-sac (158.8)* |

**183.0 Ovary** CC ♀
Use additional code to identify any functional
activity
CC Excl: 183.0-183.9, 195.3, 198.6, 199.0-199.1

**183.2 Fallopian tube** ♀
Oviduct      Uterine tube

**183.3 Broad ligament** ♀
Mesovarium      Parovarian region

**183.4 Parametrium** ♀
Uterine ligament NOS   Uterosacral ligament

**183.5 Round ligament** ♀
AHA: 3Q, '99, 5

**183.8 Other specified sites of uterine adnexa** ♀
Tubo-ovarian
Utero-ovarian
Malignant neoplasm of contiguous or overlapping
sites of ovary and other uterine adnexa whose
point of origin cannot be determined

**183.9 Uterine adnexa, unspecified** ♀

**√4ᵗʰ 184 Malignant neoplasm of other and unspecified female genital organs**

| EXCLUDES | *carcinoma in situ ▶(233.30-233.39)◀* |

**184.0 Vagina** ♀
Gartner's duct      Vaginal vault

**184.1 Labia majora** ♀
Greater vestibular [Bartholin's] gland

**184.2 Labia minora** ♀

**184.3 Clitoris** ♀

**184.4 Vulva, unspecified** ♀
External female genitalia NOS
Pudendum

**184.8 Other specified sites of female genital organs** ♀
Malignant neoplasm of contiguous or overlapping
sites of female genital organs whose point of
origin cannot be determined

**184.9 Female genital organ, site unspecified** ♀
Female genitourinary tract NOS

**185 Malignant neoplasm of prostate** ♂

| EXCLUDES | *seminal vesicles (187.8)* |

AHA: 3Q, '03, 13; 3Q, '99, 5; 3Q, '92, 7

**√4ᵗʰ 186 Malignant neoplasm of testis**
Use additional code to identify any functional activity

**186.0 Undescended testis** ♂
Ectopic testis      Retained testis

**186.9 Other and unspecified testis** ♂
Testis:      Testis:
   NOS        scrotal
   descended

**√4ᵗʰ 187 Malignant neoplasm of penis and other male genital organs** ♂

**187.1 Prepuce** ♂
Foreskin

**187.2 Glans penis** ♂

**187.3 Body of penis** ♂
Corpus cavernosum

**187.4 Penis, part unspecified** ♂
Skin of penis NOS

**187.5 Epididymis** ♂

**187.6 Spermatic cord** ♂
Vas deferens

**187.7 Scrotum** ♂
Skin of scrotum

**187.8 Other specified sites of male genital organs** ♂
Seminal vesicle
Tunica vaginalis
Malignant neoplasm of contiguous or overlapping
sites of penis and other male genital organs
whose point of origin cannot be determined

**187.9 Male genital organ, site unspecified** ♂
Male genital organ or tract NOS

**√4ᵗʰ 188 Malignant neoplasm of bladder**

| EXCLUDES | *carcinoma in situ (233.7)* |

**188.0 Trigone of urinary bladder**

**188.1 Dome of urinary bladder**

**188.2 Lateral wall of urinary bladder**

**188.3 Anterior wall of urinary bladder**

**188.4 Posterior wall of urinary bladder**

**188.5 Bladder neck**
Internal urethral orifice

**188.6 Ureteric orifice**

**188.7 Urachus**

**188.8 Other specified sites of bladder**
Malignant neoplasm of contiguous or overlapping
sites of bladder whose point of origin cannot be
determined

**188.9 Bladder, part unspecified**
Bladder wall NOS
AHA: 1Q, '00, 5

**√4ᵗʰ 189 Malignant neoplasm of kidney and other and unspecified urinary organs**

**189.0 Kidney, except pelvis** CC
Kidney NOS      Kidney parenchyma
CC Excl: 189.0-189.1, 189.8-189.9, 195.8, 199.0-199.1, 239.5, 239.8-239.9
AHA: 2Q, '05, 4; 2Q, '04, 4

**189.1 Renal pelvis** CC
Renal calyces      Ureteropelvic junction
CC Excl: See code: 189.0

**189.2 Ureter** CC

| EXCLUDES | *ureteric orifice of bladder (188.6)* |

CC Excl: 189.2, 189.8-189.9, 195.8, 199.0-199.1, 239.5, 239.8-239.9

N Newborn Age: 0    P Pediatric Age: 0-17    M Maternity Age: 12-55    A Adult Age: 15-124    CC CC Condition    MCC Major CC Condition    HIV HIV Related Dx

42 — Volume 1 • October 2007        © 2007 Ingenix

**189.3** **Urethra** `CC`
> EXCLUDES urethral orifice of bladder (188.5)

CC Excl: 189.3-189.9, 198.82

**189.4** **Paraurethral glands** `CC`
CC Excl: See code: 189.3

**189.8** **Other specified sites of urinary organs** `CC`
> Malignant neoplasm of contiguous or overlapping sites of kidney and other urinary organs whose point of origin cannot be determined

CC Excl: 189.0-189.9, 195.3, 198.0-198.1

**189.9** **Urinary organ, site unspecified** `CC`
> Urinary system NOS

CC Excl: See code: 189.8

## MALIGNANT NEOPLASM OF OTHER AND UNSPECIFIED SITES (190-199)
> EXCLUDES carcinoma in situ (234.0-234.9)

√4ᵗʰ **190 Malignant neoplasm of eye**
> EXCLUDES carcinoma in situ (234.0)
> eyelid (skin) (172.1, 173.1)
> cartilage (171.0)
> optic nerve (192.0)
> orbital bone (170.0)

**190.0** **Eyeball, except conjunctiva, cornea, retina, and choroid**
> Ciliary body          Sclera
> Crystalline lens      Uveal tract
> Iris

**190.1** **Orbit**
> Connective tissue of orbit
> Extraocular muscle
> Retrobulbar
> EXCLUDES bone of orbit (170.0)

**190.2** **Lacrimal gland**

**190.3** **Conjunctiva**

**190.4** **Cornea**

**190.5** **Retina**

**190.6** **Choroid**

**190.7** **Lacrimal duct**
> Lacrimal sac          Nasolacrimal duct

**190.8** **Other specified sites of eye**
> Malignant neoplasm of contiguous or overlapping sites of eye whose point of origin cannot be determined

**190.9** **Eye, part unspecified**

√4ᵗʰ **191 Malignant neoplasm of brain**
> EXCLUDES cranial nerves (192.0)
> retrobulbar area (190.1)

**191.0** **Cerebrum, except lobes and ventricles** `CC`
> Basal ganglia        Globus pallidus
> Cerebral cortex      Hypothalamus
> Corpus striatum      Thalamus

CC Excl: 191.0-192.1, 192.8-192.9, 195.8, 199.0-199.1, 239.6-239.9

**191.1** **Frontal lobe** `CC`
CC Excl: See code 191.0

AHA: 4Q, '05, 118

**191.2** **Temporal lobe** `CC`
> Hippocampus          Uncus

CC Excl: See code 191.0

AHA: 4Q, '06, 123

**Brain and Meninges**

Fourth ventricle — Cerebrum — Corpus callosum — Thalamus — Hypothalamus — Hypophysis — Pons — Cerebellum — Medulla oblongata

**Midsagittal Section (between hemispheres)**

**191.3** **Parietal lobe** `CC`
CC Excl: See code 191.0

**191.4** **Occipital lobe** `CC`
CC Excl: See code 191.0

**191.5** **Ventricles** `CC`
> Choroid plexus        Floor of ventricle

CC Excl: See code 191.0

**191.6** **Cerebellum NOS** `CC`
> Cerebellopontine angle

CC Excl: See code 191.0

**191.7** **Brain stem** `CC`
> Cerebral peduncle    Midbrain
> Medulla oblongata    Pons

CC Excl: See code 191.0

**191.8** **Other parts of brain** `CC`
> Corpus callosum
> Tapetum
> Malignant neoplasm of contiguous or overlapping sites of brain whose point of origin cannot be determined

CC Excl: See code 191.0

**191.9** **Brain, unspecified** `CC`
> Cranial fossa NOS

CC Excl: See code 191.0

√4ᵗʰ **192 Malignant neoplasm of other and unspecified parts of nervous system**
> EXCLUDES peripheral, sympathetic, and parasympathetic nerves and ganglia (171.0-171.9)

**192.0** **Cranial nerves** `CC`
> Olfactory bulb

CC Excl: 192.0, 192.8-192.9, 195.8, 199.0-199.1, 239.6-239.9

**192.1** **Cerebral meninges** `CC`
> Dura (mater)          Meninges NOS
> Falx (cerebelli) (cerebri)  Tentorium

CC Excl: 192.1, 192.8-192.9, 195.8, 199.0-199.1, 239.6-239.9

**192.2** **Spinal cord** `CC`
> Cauda equina

CC Excl: 192.2, 192.8-192.9, 195.8, 199.0-199.1, 239.6-239.9

**192.3** **Spinal meninges** `CC`
CC Excl: 192.3-192.9, 195.8, 199.0-199.1, 239.6-239.9

**192.8** **Other specified sites of nervous system** `CC`
> Malignant neoplasm of contiguous or overlapping sites of other parts of nervous system whose point of origin cannot be determined

CC Excl: 191.0-192.9, 195.8, 199.0-199.1, 239.6-239.9

**192.9** **Nervous system, part unspecified** `CC`
> Nervous system (central) NOS
> EXCLUDES meninges NOS (192.1)

CC Excl: 191.0-192.9, 195.8, 198.3-198.4, 199.0-199.1, 239.6-239.9

---

√4ᵗʰ Additional Digit Required     Unacceptable PDx     Manifestation Code     ◄► Revised Text     ● New Code     ▲ Revised Code Title
√5ᵗʰ

**Neoplasms**

**193–196.9**

**193 Malignant neoplasm of thyroid gland**
Thyroglossal duct
Use additional code to identify any functional activity

√4ᵗʰ **194 Malignant neoplasm of other endocrine glands and related structures**
Use additional code to identify any functional activity

EXCLUDES    *islets of Langerhans (157.4)*
*ovary (183.0)*
*testis (186.0-186.9)*
*thymus (164.0)*

**194.0 Adrenal gland**    CC
Adrenal cortex      Suprarenal gland
Adrenal medulla
CC Excl: 194.0, 194.9, 195.2, 195.8, 198.7, 199.0-199.1

**194.1 Parathyroid gland**    CC
CC Excl: 194.1, 194.8-194.9

**194.3 Pituitary gland and craniopharyngeal duct**    CC
Craniobuccal pouch      Rathke's pouch
Hypophysis      Sella turcica
CC Excl: 194.3, V58.0

AHA: J-A, '85, 9

**194.4 Pineal gland**    CC
CC Excl: 194.4, V58.0

**194.5 Carotid body**    CC
CC Excl: 194.5, 194.8-194.9

**194.6 Aortic body and other paraganglia**    CC
Coccygeal body      Para-aortic body
Glomus jugulare
CC Excl: 194.5-194.9

**194.8 Other**    CC
Pluriglandular involvement NOS
Note: If the sites of multiple involvements are known, they should be coded separately.
CC Excl: 194.0-194.9

**194.9 Endocrine gland, site unspecified**    CC
CC Excl: See code: 194.8

√4ᵗʰ **195 Malignant neoplasm of other and ill-defined sites**
INCLUDES    malignant neoplasms of contiguous sites, not elsewhere classified, whose point of origin cannot be determined

EXCLUDES    *malignant neoplasm:*
*lymphatic and hematopoietic tissue (200.0-208.9)*
*secondary sites (196.0-198.8)*
*unspecified site (199.0-199.1)*

**195.0 Head, face, and neck**
Cheek NOS      Nose NOS
Jaw NOS      Supraclavicular region NOS
AHA: 4Q, '03, 107

**195.1 Thorax**
Axilla      Intrathoracic NOS
Chest (wall) NOS

**195.2 Abdomen**
Intra-abdominal NOS
AHA: 2Q, '97, 3

**195.3 Pelvis**
Groin
Inguinal region NOS
Presacral region
Sacrococcygeal region
Sites overlapping systems within pelvis, as:
rectovaginal (septum)
rectovesical (septum)

**195.4 Upper limb**
**195.5 Lower limb**
**195.8 Other specified sites**
Back NOS      Trunk NOS
Flank NOS

√4ᵗʰ **196 Secondary and unspecified malignant neoplasm of lymph nodes**
EXCLUDES    *any malignant neoplasm of lymph nodes, specified as primary (200.0-202.9)*
*Hodgkin's disease (201.0-201.9)*
*lymphosarcoma (200.1)*
*other forms of lymphoma (202.0-202.9)*
*reticulosarcoma (200.0)*

**196.0 Lymph nodes of head, face, and neck**    CC
Cervical      Scalene
Cervicofacial      Supraclavicular
CC Excl: 176.5, 195.8, 196.0-196.9, 199.0-199.1, 239.8-239.9

**196.1 Intrathoracic lymph nodes**    CC
Bronchopulmonary      Mediastinal
Intercostal      Tracheobronchial
CC Excl: See code 196.0

AHA: 3Q, '06, 7

**196.2 Intra-abdominal lymph nodes**    CC
Intestinal      Retroperitoneal
Mesenteric
CC Excl: See code 196.0

AHA: 4Q, '03, 111

**196.3 Lymph nodes of axilla and upper limb**    CC
Brachial      Infraclavicular
Epitrochlear      Pectoral
CC Excl: See code 196.0

**196.5 Lymph nodes of inguinal region and lower limb**    CC
Femoral      Popliteal
Groin      Tibial
CC Excl: See code 196.0

**196.6 Intrapelvic lymph nodes**    CC
Hypogastric      Obturator
Iliac      Parametrial
CC Excl: See code 196.0

**196.8 Lymph nodes of multiple sites**    CC
CC Excl: See code 196.0

**196.9 Site unspecified**    CC
Lymph nodes NOS
CC Excl: See code 196.0

**Lymph Nodes**

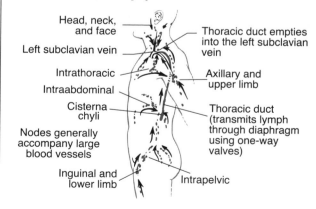

Head, neck, and face
Left subclavian vein
Intrathoracic
Intraabdominal
Cisterna chyli
Nodes generally accompany large blood vessels
Inguinal and lower limb
Thoracic duct empties into the left subclavian vein
Axillary and upper limb
Thoracic duct (transmits lymph through diaphragm using one-way valves)
Intrapelvic

---

N Newborn Age: 0    P Pediatric Age: 0-17    M Maternity Age: 12-55    A Adult Age: 15-124    CC CC Condition    MCC Major CC Condition    HIV HIV Related Dx

44 — Volume 1 • October 2007

© 2007 Ingenix

√4ᵗʰ **197 Secondary malignant neoplasm of respiratory and digestive systems**

> **EXCLUDES**   *lymph node metastasis (196.0-196.9)*

**AHA:** M-J, '85, 3

**197.0**   **Lung**     CC
      Bronchus
      **CC Excl:** 195.8, 197.0, 197.3, 198.89-199.1, 239.8-239.9

      **AHA:** 1Q, '06, 4; 2Q, '99, 9

**197.1**   **Mediastinum**     CC
      **CC Excl:** 195.8, 197.1, 197.3, 198.89-199.1, 239.8-239.9

      **AHA:** 3Q, '06, 7

**197.2**   **Pleura**     CC
      **CC Excl:** 195.8, 197.2-197.3, 198.89-199.1, 239.8-239.9

      **AHA:** 4Q, '03, 110; 4Q, '89, 11

**197.3**   **Other respiratory organs**     CC
      Trachea
      **CC Excl:** 195.8, 197.0-197.3, 198.89-199.1, 239.8-239.9

**197.4**   **Small intestine, including duodenum**     CC
      **CC Excl:** 195.8, 197.4, 197.8, 198.89-199.1, 239.8-239.9

**197.5**   **Large intestine and rectum**     CC
      **CC Excl:** 195.8, 197.5, 197.8, 198.89-199.1, 239.8-239.9

**197.6**   **Retroperitoneum and peritoneum**     CC
      **CC Excl:** 195.8, 197.6, 197.8, 198.89-199.1, 239.8-239.9

      **AHA:** 2Q, '04, 4; 4Q, '89, 11

**197.7**   **Liver, specified as secondary**     CC
      **CC Excl:** 195.8, 197.7-197.8, 198.89-199.1, 239.8-239.9

      **AHA:** 1Q, '06, 4; 2Q, '05, 9

**197.8**   **Other digestive organs and spleen**     CC
      **CC Excl:** 195.8, 197.4-197.8, 198.89-199.1, 239.8-239.9

      **AHA:** 2Q, '97, 3; 2Q, '92, 3

√4ᵗʰ **198 Secondary malignant neoplasm of other specified sites**

> **EXCLUDES**   *lymph node metastasis (196.0-196.9)*

**AHA:** M-J, '85, 3

**198.0**   **Kidney**     CC
      **CC Excl:** 195.8, 198.0-198.1, 198.89-199.1, 239.8-239.9

**198.1**   **Other urinary organs**     CC
      **CC Excl:** See code: 198.0

**198.2**   **Skin**     CC
      Skin of breast
      **CC Excl:** 195.8, 198.2, 198.89-199.1, 239.8-239.9

**198.3**   **Brain and spinal cord**     CC
      **CC Excl:** 195.8, 198.3, 198.89-199.1, 239.8-239.9

      **AHA:** 3Q, '99, 7

**198.4**   **Other parts of nervous system**     CC
      Meninges (cerebral) (spinal)
      **CC Excl:** 195.8, 198.4, 198.89-199.1, 239.8-239.9

      **AHA:** J-F, '87, 7

**198.5**   **Bone and bone marrow**     CC
      **CC Excl:** 195.8, 198.5, 198.89-199.1, 239.8-239.9

      **AHA:** ▶1Q, '07, 6;◀ 4Q, '03, 110; 3Q, '99, 5; 2Q, '92, 3; 1Q, '91, 16; 4Q, '89, 10

**198.6**   **Ovary**     CC ♀
      **CC Excl:** 195.8, 198.6, 198.89-199.1, 239.8-239.9

**198.7**   **Adrenal gland**     CC
      Suprarenal gland
      **CC Excl:** 195.8, 198.7, 198.89-199.1, 239.8-239.9

√5ᵗʰ **198.8**   **Other specified sites**

**198.81**   **Breast**     CC

> **EXCLUDES**   *skin of breast (198.2)*

      **CC Excl:** 195.8, 198.81, 198.89-199.1, 239.8-239.9

**198.82**   **Genital organs**     CC
      **CC Excl:** 195.8, 198.82-199.1, 239.8-239.9

**198.89**   **Other**     CC

> **EXCLUDES**   *retroperitoneal lymph nodes (196.2)*

      **CC Excl:** 195.8, 198.89-199.1, 239.8-239.9

      **AHA:** 2Q, '05, 4; 2Q, '97, 4

√4ᵗʰ **199 Malignant neoplasm without specification of site**

**199.0**   **Disseminated**     CC

| Carcinomatosis | |
| Generalized: | unspecified site |
|   cancer | (primary) |
|   malignancy | (secondary) |
| Multiple cancer | |

      **CC Excl:** See code 198.89

      **AHA:** 4Q, '89, 10

**199.1**   **Other**

| Cancer | |
| Carcinoma | unspecified site (primary) |
| Malignancy | (secondary) |

      **AHA:** 3Q, '06, 14-15; 1Q, '06, 4

## MALIGNANT NEOPLASM OF LYMPHATIC AND HEMATOPOIETIC TISSUE (200-208)

> **EXCLUDES**   *secondary neoplasm of:*
>      *bone marrow (198.5)*
>      *spleen (197.8)*
>    *secondary and unspecified neoplasm of lymph*
>      *nodes (196.0-196.9)*

The following fifth-digit subclassification is for use with categories 200-202:

   0   **unspecified site, extranodal and solid organ sites**
   1   **lymph nodes of head, face, and neck**
   2   **intrathoracic lymph nodes**
   3   **intra-abdominal lymph nodes**
   4   **lymph nodes of axilla and upper limb**
   5   **lymph nodes of inguinal region and lower limb**
   6   **intrapelvic lymph nodes**
   7   **spleen**
   8   **lymph nodes of multiple sites**

▲ √4ᵗʰ **200 Lymphosarcoma and reticulosarcoma and other specified malignant tumors of lymphatic tissue**

      **AHA:** 2Q, '92, 3; N-D, '86, 5

√5ᵗʰ **200.0**   **Reticulosarcoma**     CC HIV

      Lymphoma (malignant):
        histiocytic (diffuse):
          nodular
          pleomorphic cell type
        reticulum cell type
      Reticulum cell sarcoma:
        NOS
        pleomorphic cell type

      **CC Excl: For code 200.00:** 200.00-200.08, 239.8-239.9; **For code 200.01:** 200.00-200.01, 200.08, 239.8-239.9; **For code 200.02:** 200.00, 200.02, 200.08, 239.8-239.9 **For code 200.03:** 200.00, 200.03, 200.08, 239.8-239.9; **For code 200.04:** 200.00, 200.04, 200.08, 239.8-239.9; **For code 200.05:** 200.00, 200.05, 200.08, 239.8-239.9; **For code 200.06:** 200.00, 200.06, 200.08, 239.8-239.9; **For code 200.07:** 200.00, 200.07-200.08, 239.8-239.9; **For code 200.08:** 200.00-200.08, 239.8-239.9

      **AHA: For Code 200.03:** 3Q, '01, 12

      **DEF:** Malignant lymphoma of primarily histolytic cells; commonly originates in reticuloendothelium of lymph nodes.

---

√4ᵗʰ Additional Digit Required      Unacceptable PDx      Manifestation Code      ▶◀ Revised Text      ● New Code      ▲ Revised Code Title
√5ᵗʰ

**Neoplasms**

**200.1–200.6**

§ ✓5th **200.1** **Lymphosarcoma**   CC

Lymphoblastoma (diffuse)
Lymphoma (malignant):
   lymphoblastic (diffuse)
   lymphocytic (cell type)
     (diffuse)
   lymphocytic (diffuse)
   prolymphocytic

Lymphosarcoma:
  NOS
  diffuse NOS
  lymphoblastic
   (diffuse)
  lymphosarcoma type

**EXCLUDES**   lymphosarcoma:
    follicular or nodular (202.0)
    mixed cell type (200.8)
    lymphosarcoma cell leukemia (207.8)

CC Excl: For code **200.10:** 200.10-200.18, 239.8-239.9; For code **200.11:** 200.10-200.11, 200.18, 239.8-239.9; For code **200.12:** 200.10, 200.12, 200.18, 239.8-239.9; For code **200.13:** 200.10, 200.13, 200.18, 239.8-239.9; For code **200.14:** 200.10, 200.14, 200.18, 239.8-239.9; For code **200.15:** 200.10, 200.15, 200.18, 239.8-239.9; For code **200.16:** 200.10, 200.16, 200.18, 239.8-239.9; For code **200.17:** 200.10, 200.17-200.18, 239.8-239.9; For code **200.18:** 200.10-200.18, 239.8-239.9

DEF: Malignant lymphoma created from anaplastic lymphoid cells resembling lymphocytes or lymphoblasts.

§ ✓5th **200.2** **Burkitt's tumor or lymphoma**   CC HIV

Malignant lymphoma, Burkitt's type

CC Excl: For code **200.20:** 200.20-200.28, 239.8-239.9; For code **200.21:** 200.20-200.21, 200.28, 239.8-239.9; For code **200.22:** 200.20, 200.22, 200.28, 239.8-239.9; For code **200.23:** 200.20, 200.23, 200.28, 239.8-239.9; For code **200.24:** 200.20, 200.24, 200.28, 239.8-239.9; For code **200.25:**200.20, 200.25, 200.28, 239.8-239.9; For code **200.26:** 200.20, 200.26, 200.28, 239.8-239.9; For code **200.27:** 200.20, 200.27-200.28, 239.8-239.9; For code **200.28:** 200.20-200.28, 239.8-239.9

DEF: Large osteolytic lesion most common in jaw or as abdominal mass; usually found in central Africa but reported elsewhere.

● § ✓5th **200.3** **Marginal zone lymphoma**   CC HIV

Extranodal marginal zone B-cell lymphoma
Mucosa associated lymphoid tissue [MALT]
Nodal marginal zone B-cell lymphoma
Splenic marginal zone B-cell lymphoma

CC Excl: For code **200.30:** 200.30-200.78, 202.70-202.90, 239.8-239.9; For code **200.31:** 200.30-200.31, 200.38-200.41, 200.48-200.51, 200.58-200.61, 200.68-200.71, 200.78, 202.70-202.71, 202.78-202.81, 202.88, 202.91, 239.8-239.9; For code **200.32:** 200.30, 200.32, 200.38-200.40, 200.42, 200.48-200.50, 200.52, 200.58-200.60, 200.62, 200.68-200.70, 200.72, 200.78, 202.70, 202.72, 202.78-202.80, 202.82, 202.88, 202.92, 239.8-239.9; For code **200.33:** 200.30, 200.33, 200.38-200.40, 200.43, 200.48-200.50, 200.53, 200.58-200.60, 200.63, 200.68-200.70, 200.73, 200.78, 202.70, 202.73, 202.78-202.80, 202.83, 202.88, 202.93, 239.8-239.9; For code **200.34:** 200.30, 200.34, 200.38-200.40, 200.44, 200.48-200.50, 200.54, 200.58-200.60, 200.64, 200.68-200.70, 200.74, 200.78, 202.70, 202.74, 202.78-202.80, 202.84, 202.88, 202.94, 239.8-239; For code **200.35:** 200.30, 200.35, 200.38-200.40, 200.45, 200.48-200.50, 200.55, 200.58-200.60, 200.65, 200.68-200.70, 200.75, 200.78, 202.70, 202.75, 202.78-202.80, 202.85, 202.88, 202.95, 239.8-239.9; For code **200.36:** 200.30, 200.36, 200.38-200.40, 200.46, 200.48-200.50, 200.56, 200.58-200.60, 200.66, 200.68-200.70, 200.76, 200.78, 202.70, 202.76, 202.78-202.80, 202.86, 202.88, 202.96, 239.8-239.9; For code **200.37:** 200.30, 200.37-200.40, 200.47-200.50, 200.57-200.60, 200.67-200.70, 200.77-200.78, 202.70, 202.77-202.80, 202.87-202.88, 202.97, 239.8-239.9; For code **200.38:** 200.30-200.78, 202.70-202.88, 202.98, 239.8-239.9

● § ✓5th **200.4** **Mantle cell lymphoma**   CC HIV

CC Excl: For code **200.40:** 200.30-200.78, 202.70-202.90, 239.8-239.9; For code **200.41:** 200.30-200.31, 200.38-200.41, 200.48-200.51, 200.58-200.61, 200.68-200.71, 200.78, 202.70-202.71, 202.78-202.81, 202.88, 202.91, 239.8-239.9; For code **200.42:** 200.30, 200.32, 200.38-200.40, 200.42, 200.48-200.50, 200.52, 200.58-200.60, 200.62, 200.68-200.70, 200.72, 200.78, 202.70, 202.72, 202.78-202.80, 202.82, 202.88, 202.92, 239.8-239.9; For code **200.43:** 200.30, 200.33, 200.38-200.40, 200.43, 200.48-200.50, 200.53, 200.58-200.60, 200.63, 200.68-200.70, 200.73, 200.78, 202.70, 202.73, 202.78-202.80, 202.83, 202.88, 202.93, 239.8-239.9; For code **200.44:** 200.30, 200.34, 200.38-200.40, 200.44, 200.48-200.50, 200.54, 200.58-200.60, 200.64, 200.68-200.70, 200.74, 200.78, 202.70, 202.74, 202.78-202.80, 202.84, 202.88, 202.94, 239.8-239.9; For code **200.45:** 200.30, 200.35, 200.38-200.40, 200.45, 200.48-200.50, 200.55, 200.58-200.60, 200.65, 200.68-200.70, 200.75, 200.78, 202.70, 202.75, 202.78-202.80, 202.85, 202.88, 202.95, 239.8-239.9; For code **200.46:** 200.30, 200.36, 200.38-200.40, 200.46, 200.48-200.50, 200.56, 200.58-200.60, 200.66, 200.68-200.70, 200.76, 200.78, 202.70, 202.76, 202.78-202.80, 202.86, 202.88, 202.96, 239.8-239.9; For code **200.47:** 200.30, 200.37-200.40, 200.47-200.50, 200.57-200.60, 200.67-200.70, 200.77-200.78, 202.70, 202.77-202.80, 202.87-202.88, 202.97, 239.8-239.9; For code **200.48:** 200.30-200.78, 202.70-202.90, 202.98, 239.8-239.9

● § ✓5th **200.5** **Primary central nervous system lymphoma**   CC HIV

CC Excl: For code **200.50:** 200.30-200.78, 202.70-202.90, 239.8-239.9; For code **200.51:** 200.30-200.31, 200.38-200.41, 200.48-200.51, 200.58-200.61, 200.68-200.71, 200.78, 202.70-202.71, 202.78-202.81, 202.88, 202.91, 239.8-239.9; For code **200.52:** 200.30, 200.32, 200.38-200.40, 200.42, 200.48-200.50, 200.52, 200.58-200.60, 200.62, 200.68-200.70, 200.72, 200.78, 202.70, 202.72, 202.78-202.80, 202.82, 202.88, 202.92, 239.8-239.9; For code **200.53:** 200.30, 200.33, 200.38-200.40, 200.43, 200.48-200.50, 200.53, 200.58-200.60, 200.63, 200.68-200.70, 200.73, 200.78, 202.70, 202.73, 202.78-202.80, 202.83, 202.88, 202.93, 239.8-239.9; For code **200.54:** 200.30, 200.34, 200.38-200.40, 200.44, 200.48-200.50, 200.54, 200.58-200.60, 200.64, 200.68-200.70, 200.74, 200.78, 202.70, 202.74, 202.78-202.80, 202.84, 202.88, 202.94, 239.8-239.9; For code **200.55:** 200.30, 200.35, 200.38-200.40, 200.45, 200.48-200.50, 200.55, 200.58-200.60, 200.65, 200.68-200.70, 200.75, 200.78, 202.70, 202.75, 202.78-202.80, 202.85, 202.88, 202.95, 239.8-239.9; For code **200.56:** 200.30, 200.36, 200.38-200.40, 200.46, 200.48-200.50, 200.56, 200.58-200.60, 200.66, 200.68-200.70, 200.76, 200.78, 202.70, 202.76, 202.78-202.80, 202.86, 202.88, 202.96, 239.8-239.9; For code **200.57:** 200.30, 200.37-200.40, 200.47-200.50, 200.57-200.60, 200.67-200.70, 200.77-200.78, 202.70, 202.77-202.80, 202.87-202.88, 202.97, 239.8-239.9; For code **200.58:** 200.30-200.78, 202.70-202.90, 202.98, 239.8-239.9

● § ✓5th **200.6** **Anaplastic large cell lymphoma**   CC HIV

CC Excl: For code **200.60:** 200.30-200.78, 202.70-202.90, 239.8-239.9; For code **200.61:** 200.30-200.31, 200.38-200.41, 200.48-200.51, 200.58-200.61, 200.68-200.71, 200.78, 202.70-202.71, 202.78-202.81, 202.88, 202.91, 239.8-239.9; For code **200.62:** 200.30, 200.32, 200.38-200.40, 200.42, 200.48-200.50, 200.52, 200.58-200.60, 200.62, 200.68-200.70, 200.72, 200.78, 202.70, 202.72, 202.78-202.80, 202.82, 202.88, 202.92, 239.8-239.9; For code **200.63:** 200.30, 200.33, 200.38-200.40, 200.43, 200.48-200.50, 200.53, 200.58-200.60, 200.63, 200.68-200.70, 200.73, 200.78, 202.70, 202.73, 202.78-202.80, 202.83, 202.88, 202.93, 239.8-239.9; For code **200.64:** 200.30, 200.34, 200.38-200.40, 200.44, 200.48-200.50, 200.54, 200.58-200.60, 200.64, 200.68-200.70, 200.74, 200.78, 202.70, 202.74, 202.78-202.80, 202.84, 202.88, 202.94, 239.8-239.9; For code **200.65:** 200.30, 200.35, 200.38-200.40, 200.45, 200.48-200.50, 200.55, 200.58-200.60, 200.65, 200.68-200.70, 200.75, 200.78, 202.70, 202.75, 202.78-202.80, 202.85, 202.88, 202.95, 239.8-239.9; For code **200.66:** 200.30, 200.36, 200.38-200.40, 200.46, 200.48-200.50, 200.56, 200.58-200.60, 200.66, 200.68-200.70, 200.76, 200.78, 202.70, 202.76, 202.78-202.80, 202.86, 202.88, 202.96, 239.8-239.9; For code **200.67:** 200.30, 200.37-200.40, 200.47-200.50, 200.57-200.60, 200.67-200.70, 200.77-200.78, 202.70, 202.77-202.80, 202.87-202.88, 202.97, 239.8-239.9; For code **200.68:** 200.30-200.78, 202.70-202.90, 202.98, 239.8-239.9

---

§ Requires fifth-digit. See beginning of section 200–208 for codes and definitions.

N Newborn Age: 0    P Pediatric Age: 0-17    M Maternity Age: 12-55    A Adult Age: 15-124    CC CC Condition    MCC Major CC Condition    HIV HIV Related Dx

§ ✓5ᵗʰ **200.7 Large cell lymphoma** `CC` `HIV`

CC Excl: For code **200.70**: 200.30-200.78, 202.70-202.90, 239.8-239.9; For code **200.71**: 200.30-200.31, 200.38-200.41, 200.48-200.51, 200.58-200.61, 200.68-200.71, 200.78, 202.70-202.71, 202.78-202.81, 202.88, 202.91, 239.8-239.9; For code **200.72**: 200.30, 200.32, 200.38-200.40, 200.42, 200.48-200.50, 200.52, 200.58-200.60, 200.62, 200.68-200.70, 200.72, 200.78, 202.70, 202.72, 202.78-202.80, 202.82, 202.88, 202.92, 239.8-239.9; For code **200.73**: 200.30, 200.33, 200.38-200.40, 200.43, 200.48-200.50, 200.53, 200.58-200.60, 200.63, 200.68-200.70, 200.73, 200.78, 202.70, 202.73, 202.78-202.80, 202.83, 202.88, 202.93, 239.8-239.9; For code **200.74**: 200.30, 200.34, 200.38-200.40, 200.44, 200.48-200.50, 200.54, 200.58-200.60, 200.64, 200.68-200.70, 200.74, 200.78, 202.70, 202.74, 202.78-202.80, 202.84, 202.88, 202.94, 239.8-239.9; For code **200.75**: 200.30, 200.35, 200.38-200.40, 200.45, 200.48-200.50, 200.55, 200.58-200.60, 200.65, 200.68-200.70, 200.75, 200.78, 202.70, 202.75, 202.78-202.80, 202.85, 202.88, 202.95, 239.8-239.9; For code **200.76**: 200.30, 200.36, 200.38-200.40, 200.46, 200.48-200.50, 200.56, 200.58-200.60, 200.66, 200.68-200.70, 200.76, 200.78, 202.70, 202.76, 202.78-202.80, 202.86, 202.88, 202.96, 239.8-239.9; For code **200.77**: 200.30, 200.37-200.40, 200.47-200.50, 200.57-200.60, 200.67-200.70, 200.77-200.78, 202.70, 202.77-202.80, 202.87-202.88, 202.97, 239.8-239.9; For code **200.78**: 200.30-200.78, 202.70-202.88, 202.98, 239.98, 239.8-239.9

§ ✓5ᵗʰ **200.8 Other named variants** `CC` `HIV`

Lymphoma (malignant):
   lymphoplasmacytoid type
   mixed lymphocytic-histiocytic (diffuse)
Lymphosarcoma, mixed cell type (diffuse)
Reticulolymphosarcoma (diffuse)

CC Excl: For code **200.80**: 200.80-200.88, 239.8-239.9; For code **200.81**: 200.80-200.81, 200.88, 239.8-239.9; For code **200.82**: 200.80, 200.82, 200.88, 239.8-239.9; For code **200.83**: 200.80, 200.83, 200.88, 239.8-239.9; For code **200.84**: 200.80, 200.84, 200.88, 239.8-239.9; For code **200.85**: 200.80, 200.85, 200.88, 239.8-239.9; For code **200.86**: 200.80, 200.86, 200.88, 239.8-239.9; For code **200.87**: 200.80, 200.87-200.88, 239.8-239.9; For code **200.88**: 200.80-200.88, 239.8-239.9

✓4ᵗʰ **201 Hodgkin's disease**

AHA: 2Q, '92, 3; N-D, '86, 5

DEF: Painless, progressive enlargement of lymph nodes, spleen and general lymph tissue; symptoms include anorexia, lassitude, weight loss, fever, pruritis, night sweats, anemia.

§ ✓5ᵗʰ **201.0 Hodgkin's paragranuloma** `CC`

CC Excl: For code **201.00**: 201.00-201.08, 201.90, 239.8-239.9; For code **201.01**: 201.00-201.01, 201.08, 201.90-201.91, 239.8-239.9; For code **201.02**: 201.00, 201.02, 201.08, 201.90, 201.92, 239.8-239.9; For code **201.03**: 201.00, 201.03, 201.08, 201.90, 201.93, 239.8-239.9; For code **201.04**: 201.00, 201.04, 201.08, 201.90, 201.94, 239.8-239.9; For code **201.05**: 201.00, 201.05, 201.08, 201.90, 201.95, 239.8-239.9; For code **201.06**: 201.00, 201.06, 201.08, 201.90, 201.96, 239.8-239.9; For code **201.07**: 201.00, 201.07-201.08, 201.90, 201.97, 239.8-239.9; For code **201.08**: 201.00-201.08, 201.90, 201.98, 239.8-239.9

§ ✓5ᵗʰ **201.1 Hodgkin's granuloma** `CC`

CC Excl: For code **201.10**: 201.10-201.18, 201.90, 201.98, 239.8-239.9; For code **201.11**: 201.10-201.11, 201.18, 201.90-201.91, 201.98, 239.8-239.9; For code **201.12**: 201.10, 201.12, 201.18, 201.90, 201.92, 201.98, 239.8-239.9; For code **201.13**: 201.10, 201.13, 201.18, 201.90, 201.93, 201.98, 239.8-239.9; For code **201.14**: 201.10, 201.14, 201.18, 201.90, 201.94, 201.98, 239.8-239.9; For code **201.15**: 201.10, 201.15, 201.18, 201.90, 201.95, 201.98, 239.8-239.9; For code **201.16**: 201.10, 201.16, 201.18, 201.90, 201.96, 201.98, 239.8-239.9; For code **201.17**: 201.10, 201.17-201.18, 201.90, 201.97-201.98, 239.8-239.9; For code **201.18**: 201.10-201.18, 201.90, 201.98, 239.8-239.9

AHA: 2Q, '99, 7

§ ✓5ᵗʰ **201.2 Hodgkin's sarcoma** `CC`

CC Excl: For code **201.20**: 201.20-201.28, 201.90, 201.98, 239.8-239.9; For code **201.21**: 201.20-201.21, 201.28, 201.90-201.91, 201.98, 239.8-239.9; For code **201.22**: 201.20, 201.22, 201.28, 201.90, 201.92, 201.98, 239.8-239.9; For code **201.23**: 201.20, 201.23, 201.28, 201.90, 201.93, 201.98, 239.8-239.9; For code **201.24**: 201.20, 201.24, 201.28, 201.90, 201.94, 201.98, 239.8-239.9; For code **201.25**: 201.20, 201.25, 201.28, 201.90, 201.95, 201.98, 239.8-239.9; For code **201.26**: 201.20, 201.26, 201.28, 201.90, 201.96, 201.98, 239.8-239.9; For code **201.27**: 201.20, 201.27-201.28, 201.90, 201.97-201.98, 239.8-239.9; For code **201.28**: 201.20-201.28, 201.90, 201.98, 239.8-239.9

§ ✓5ᵗʰ **201.4 Lymphocytic-histiocytic predominance** `CC`

CC Excl: For code **201.40**: 201.40-201.48, 201.90, 201.98, 239.8-239.9; For code **201.41**: 201.40-201.41, 201.48, 201.90-201.91, 201.98, 239.8-239.9; For code **201.42**: 201.40, 201.42, 201.48, 201.90, 201.92, 201.98, 239.8-239.9; For code **201.43**: 201.40, 201.43, 201.48, 201.90, 201.93, 201.98, 239.8-239.9; For code **201.44**: 201.40, 201.45, 201.48, 201.90, 201.95, 201.98, 239.8-239.9; For code **201.45**: 201.40, 201.45, 201.48, 201.90, 201.95, 201.98, 239.8-239.9; For code **201.46**: 201.40, 201.46, 201.48, 201.90, 201.96, 201.98, 239.8-239.9; For code **201.47**: 201.40, 201.47-201.48, 201.90, 201.97-201.98, 239.8-239.9; For code **201.48**: 201.40-201.48, 201.90, 201.98, 239.8-239.9

§ ✓5ᵗʰ **201.5 Nodular sclerosis** `CC`

Hodgkin's disease, nodular sclerosis:
   NOS
   cellular phase

CC Excl: For code **201.50**: 201.50-201.58, 201.90, 201.98, 239.8-239.9; For code **201.51**: 201.50-201.51, 201.58, 201.90-201.91, 201.98, 239.8-239.9; For code **201.52**: 201.50, 201.52, 201.58, 201.90, 201.92, 201.98, 239.8-239.9; For code **201.53**: 201.50, 201.53, 201.58, 201.90, 201.93, 201.98, 239.8-239.9; For code **201.54**: 201.50, 201.54, 201.58, 201.90, 201.94, 201.98, 239.8-239.9; For code **201.55**: 201.50, 201.55, 201.58, 201.90, 201.95, 201.98, 239.8-239.9; For code **201.56**: 201.50, 201.56, 201.58, 201.90, 201.96, 201.98, 239.8-239.9; For code **201.57**: 201.50, 201.57-201.58, 201.90, 201.97-201.98, 239.8-239.9; For code **201.58**: 201.50-201.58, 201.90, 201.98, 239.8-239.9

§ ✓5ᵗʰ **201.6 Mixed cellularity** `CC`

CC Excl: For code **201.60**: 201.60-201.68, 201.90, 201.98, 239.8-239.9; For code **201.61**: 201.60-201.61, 201.68, 201.90-201.91, 201.98, 239.8-239.9; For code **201.62**: 201.60, 201.62, 201.68, 201.90, 201.92, 201.98, 239.8-239.9; For code **201.63**: 201.60, 201.63, 201.68, 201.90, 201.93, 201.98, 239.8-239.9; For code **201.64**: 201.60, 201.64, 201.68, 201.90, 201.94, 201.98, 239.8-239.9; For code **201.65**: 201.60, 201.65, 201.68, 201.90, 201.95, 201.98, 239.8-239.9; For code **201.66**: 201.60, 201.66, 201.68, 201.90, 201.96, 201.98, 239.8-239.9; For code **201.67**: 201.60, 201.67-201.68, 201.90, 201.97-201.98, 239.8-239.9; For code **201.68**: 201.60-201.68, 201.90, 201.98, 239.8-239.9

§ ✓5ᵗʰ **201.7 Lymphocytic depletion** `CC`

Hodgkin's disease, lymphocytic depletion:
   NOS
   diffuse fibrosis
   reticular type

CC Excl: For code **201.70**: 201.70-201.90, 201.98, 239.8-239.9; For code **201.71**: 201.70-201.71, 201.78, 201.91, 201.98, 239.8-239.9; For code **201.72**: 201.70, 201.72, 201.78, 201.92, 201.98, 239.8-239.9; For code **201.73**: 201.70, 201.73, 201.78, 201.93, 201.98, 239.8-239.9; For code **201.74**: 201.70, 201.74, 201.78, 201.94, 201.98, 239.8-239.9; For code **201.75**: 201.70, 201.75, 201.78, 201.95, 201.98, 239.8-239.9; For code **201.76**: 201.70, 201.76, 201.78, 201.96, 201.98, 239.8-239.9; For code **201.77**: 201.70, 201.77-201.78, 201.97-201.98, 239.8-239.9; For code **201.78**: 201.70-201.78, 201.98, 239.8-239.9

§ ✓5ᵗʰ **201.9 Hodgkin's disease, unspecified** `CC`

Hodgkin's:        Malignant:
   disease NOS       lymphogranuloma
   lymphoma NOS     lymphogranulomatosis

CC Excl: For code **201.90**: 201.90-201.98, 239.8-239.9; For code **201.91**: 201.90-201.91, 201.98, 239.8-239.9; For code **201.92**: 201.90, 201.92, 201.98, 239.8-239.9; For code **201.93**: 201.90, 201.93, 201.98, 239.8-239.9; For code **201.94**: 201.90, 201.94, 201.98, 239.8-239.9; For code **201.95**: 201.90, 201.95, 201.98, 239.8-239.9; For code **201.96**: 201.90, 201.96, 201.98, 239.8-239.9; For code **201.97**: 201.90, 201.97-201.98, 239.8-239.9; For code **201.98**: 201.90-201.98, 239.8-239.9

---

§ Requires fifth-digit. See beginning of section 200–208 for codes and definitions.

✓4ᵗʰ Additional Digit Required     Unacceptable PDx     Manifestation Code     ▶◀ Revised Text     ● New Code     ▲ Revised Code Title
✓5ᵗʰ

**Neoplasms**

**202– 202.5**

**✓4ᵗʰ 202 Other malignant neoplasms of lymphoid and histiocytic tissue**
AHA: 2Q, '92, 3; N-D, '86, 5

§ ✓5ᵗʰ **202.0 Nodular lymphoma**    CC
Brill-Symmers disease    Lymphosarcoma:
Lymphoma:          follicular (giant)
   follicular (giant)      nodular
   lymphocytic, nodular

CC Excl: For code **202.00**: 200.30, 200.40, 200.50, 200.60, 200.70, 202.00-202.08, 202.70, 202.80, 202.90, 239.8-239.9; For code **202.01**: 200.31, 200.41, 200.51, 200.61, 200.71, 202.00-202.01, 202.08, 202.71, 202.81, 202.91, 239.8-239.9; For code **202.02**: ; For code **202.03**: 200.32, 200.42, 200.52, 200.62, 200.72, 202.00, 202.02, 202.08, 202.72, 202.82, 202.92, 239.8-239.9; For code **202.04**: 200.34, 200.44, 200.54, 200.64, 200.74, 202.00, 202.04, 202.08, 202.74, 202.84, 202.94, 239.8-239.9; For code **202.05**: 200.35, 200.45, 200.55, 200.65, 200.75, 202.00, 202.05, 202.08, 202.75, 202.85, 202.95, 239.8-239.9; For code **202.06**: 200.36, 200.46, 200.56, 200.66, 200.76, 202.00, 202.06, 202.08, 202.76, 202.86, 202.96, 239.8-239.9; For code **202.07**: 200.37, 200.47, 200.57, 200.67, 200.77, 202.00, 202.07-202.08, 202.77, 202.87, 202.97, 239.8-239.9; For code **202.08**: 200.38, 200.48, 200.58, 200.68, 200.78, 202.00-202.08, 202.78, 202.88, 202.98, 239.8-239.9

DEF: Lymphomatous cells clustered into nodules within the lymph node; usually occurs in older adults and may involve all nodes and possibly extranodal sites.

§ ✓5ᵗʰ **202.1 Mycosis fungoides**    CC
CC Excl: For code **202.10**: 200.30, 200.40, 200.50, 200.60, 200.70, 202.10-202.18, 202.70, 202.80, 202.90, 239.8-239.9; For code **202.11**: 200.31, 200.41, 200.51, 200.61, 200.71, 202.10-202.11, 202.18, 202.71, 202.81, 202.91, 239.8-239.9; For code **202.12**: 200.32, 200.42, 200.52, 200.62, 200.72, 202.10, 202.12, 202.18, 202.72, 202.82, 202.92, 239.8-239.9; For code **202.13**: 200.33, 200.43, 200.53, 200.63, 200.73, 202.10, 202.13, 202.18, 202.73, 202.83, 202.93, 239.8-239.9; For code **202.14**: 200.34, 200.44, 200.54, 200.64, 200.74, 202.10, 202.14, 202.18, 202.74, 202.84, 202.94, 239.8-239.9; For code **202.15**: 200.35, 200.45, 200.55, 200.65, 200.75, 202.10, 202.15, 202.18, 202.75, 202.85, 202.95, 239.8-239.9; For code **202.16**: 200.36, 200.46, 200.56, 200.66, 200.76, 202.10, 202.16, 202.18, 202.76, 202.86, 202.96, 239.8-239.9; For code **202.17**: 200.37, 200.47, 200.57, 200.67, 200.77, 202.10, 202.17-202.18, 202.77, 202.87, 202.97, 239.8-239.9; For code **202.18**: 200.38, 200.48, 200.58, 200.68, 200.78, 202.10-202.18, 202.78, 202.88, 202.98, 239.8-239.9

AHA: 2Q, '92, 4

DEF: Type of cutaneous T-cell lymphoma; may evolve into generalized lymphoma; formerly thought to be of fungoid origin.

§ ✓5ᵗʰ **202.2 Sézary's disease**    CC
CC Excl: For code **202.20**: 200.30, 200.40, 200.50, 200.60, 200.70, 202.20-202.28, 202.70, 202.80, 202.90, 239.8-239.9; For code **202.21**: 200.31, 200.41, 200.51, 200.61, 200.71, 202.20-202.21, 202.28, 202.71, 202.81, 202.91, 239.8-239.9; For code **202.22**: 200.32, 200.42, 200.52, 200.62, 200.72, 202.20, 202.22, 202.28, 202.72, 202.82, 202.92, 239.8-239.9; For code **202.23**: 200.33, 200.43, 200.53, 200.63, 200.73, 202.20, 202.23, 202.28, 202.73, 202.83, 202.93, 239.8-239.9; For code **202.24**: 200.34, 200.44, 200.54, 200.64, 200.74, 202.20, 202.24, 202.28, 202.74, 202.84, 202.94, 239.8-239.9; For code **202.25**: 200.35, 200.45, 200.55, 200.65, 200.75, 202.20, 202.25, 202.28, 202.75, 202.85, 202.95, 239.8-239.9; For code **202.26**: 200.36, 200.46, 200.56, 200.66, 200.76, 202.20, 202.26, 202.28, 202.76, 202.86, 202.96, 239.8-239.9; For code **202.27**: 200.37, 200.47, 200.57, 200.67, 200.77, 202.20, 202.27-202.28, 202.77, 202.87, 202.97, 239.8-239.9; For code **202.28**: 200.38, 200.48, 200.58, 200.68, 200.78, 202.20-202.28, 202.78, 202.88, 202.98, 239.8-239.9

AHA: 2Q, '99, 7

DEF: Type of cutaneous T-cell lymphoma with erythroderma, intense pruritus, peripheral lymphadenopathy, abnormal hyperchromatic mononuclear cells in skin, lymph nodes and peripheral blood.

§ ✓5ᵗʰ **202.3 Malignant histiocytosis**    CC
Histiocytic medullary reticulosis
Malignant:
   reticuloendotheliosis
   reticulosis

CC Excl: For code **202.30**: 200.30, 200.40, 200.50, 200.60, 200.70, 202.30-202.38, 202.70, 202.80, 202.90, 239.8-239.9; For code **202.31**: 200.31, 200.41, 200.51, 200.61, 200.71, 202.30-202.31, 202.38, 202.71, 202.81, 202.91, 239.8-239.9; For code **202.32**: 200.32, 200.42, 200.52, 200.62, 200.72, 202.30, 202.32, 202.38, 202.72, 202.82, 202.92, 239.8-239.9; For code **202.33**: 200.33, 200.43, 200.53, 200.63, 200.73, 202.30, 202.33, 202.38, 202.73, 202.83, 202.93, 239.8-239.9; For code **202.34**: 200.34, 200.44, 200.54, 200.64, 200.74, 202.30, 202.34, 202.38, 202.74, 202.84, 202.94, 239.8-239.9; For code **202.35**: 200.35, 200.45, 200.55, 200.65, 200.75, 202.30, 202.35, 202.38, 202.75, 202.85, 202.95, 239.8-239.9; For code **202.36**: 200.36, 200.46, 200.56, 200.66, 200.76, 202.30, 202.36, 202.38, 202.76, 202.86, 202.96, 239.8-239.9; For code **202.37**: 200.37, 200.47, 200.57, 200.67, 200.77, 202.30, 202.37-202.38, 202.77, 202.87, 202.97, 239.8-239.9; For code **202.38**: 200.38, 200.48, 200.58, 200.68, 200.78, 202.30-202.38, 202.78, 202.88, 202.98, 239.8-239.9

§ ✓5ᵗʰ **202.4 Leukemic reticuloendotheliosis**    CC
Hairy-cell leukemia

CC Excl: For code **202.40**: 200.30, 200.40, 200.50, 200.60, 200.70, 202.40-202.48, 202.70, 202.80, 202.90, 239.8-239.9; For code **202.41**: 200.31, 200.41, 200.51, 200.61, 200.71, 202.40-202.41, 202.48, 202.71, 202.81, 202.91, 239.8-239.9; For code **202.42**: 200.32, 200.42, 200.52, 200.62, 200.72, 202.40, 202.42, 202.48, 202.72, 202.82, 202.92, 239.8-239.9; For code **202.43**: 200.33, 200.43, 200.53, 200.63, 200.73, 202.40, 202.43, 202.48, 202.73, 202.83, 202.93, 239.8-239.9; For code **202.44**: 200.34, 200.44, 200.54, 200.64, 200.74, 202.40, 202.44, 202.48, 202.74, 202.84, 202.94, 239.8-239.9; For code **202.45**: 200.35, 200.45, 200.55, 200.65, 200.75, 202.40, 202.45, 202.48, 202.75, 202.85, 202.95, 239.8-239.9; For code **202.46**: 200.36, 200.46, 200.56, 200.66, 200.76, 202.40, 202.46, 202.48, 202.76, 202.86, 202.96, 239.8-239.9; For code **202.47**: 200.37, 200.47, 200.57, 200.67, 200.77, 202.40, 202.47-202.48, 202.77, 202.87, 202.97, 239.8-239.9; For code **202.48**: 200.38, 200.48, 200.58, 200.68, 200.78, 202.40-202.48, 202.78, 202.88, 202.98, 239.8-239.9

DEF: Chronic leukemia with large, mononuclear cells with "hairy" appearance in marrow, spleen, liver, blood.

§ ✓5ᵗʰ **202.5 Letterer-Siwe disease**    CC
Acute:
   differentiated progressive histiocytosis
   histiocytosis X (progressive)
   infantile reticuloendotheliosis
   reticulosis of infancy
   **EXCLUDES**   *Hand-Schüller-Christian disease (277.89)*
              *histiocytosis (acute) (chronic) (277.89)*
              *histiocytosis X (chronic) (277.89)*

CC Excl: For code **202.50**: 200.30, 200.40, 200.50, 200.60, 200.70, 202.50-202.58, 202.70, 202.80, 202.90, 239.8-239.9; For code **202.51**: 200.31, 200.41, 200.51, 200.61, 200.71, 202.50-202.51, 202.58, 202.71, 202.81, 202.91, 239.8-239.9; For code **202.52**: 200.32, 200.42, 200.52, 200.62, 200.72, 202.50, 202.52, 202.58, 202.72, 202.82, 202.92, 239.8-239.9; For code **202.53**: 200.33, 200.43, 200.53, 200.63, 200.73, 202.50, 202.53, 202.58, 202.73, 202.83, 202.93, 239.8-239.9; For code **202.54**: 200.34, 200.44, 200.54, 200.64, 200.74, 202.50, 202.54, 202.58, 202.74, 202.84, 202.94, 239.8-239.9; For code **202.55**: 200.35, 200.45, 200.55, 200.65, 200.75, 202.50, 202.55, 202.58, 202.75, 202.85, 202.95, 239.8-239.9; For code **202.56**: 200.36, 200.46, 200.56, 200.66, 200.76, 202.50, 202.56, 202.58, 202.76, 202.86, 202.96, 239.8-239.9; For code **202.57**: 200.37, 200.47, 200.57, 200.67, 200.77, 202.50, 202.57-202.58, 202.77, 202.87, 202.97, 239.8-239.9; For code **202.58**: 200.38, 200.48, 200.58, 200.68, 200.78, 202.50-202.58, 202.78, 202.88, 202.98, 239.8-239.9

DEF: A recessive reticuloendotheliosis of early childhood, with a hemorrhagic tendency, eczema-like skin eruption, hepatosplenomegaly, including lymph node enlargement, and progressive anemia; it is often a fatal disease with no established cause.

---

§   Requires fifth-digit. See beginning of section 200–208 for codes and definitions.

N Newborn Age: 0    P Pediatric Age: 0-17    M Maternity Age: 12-55    A Adult Age: 15-124    CC CC Condition    MCC Major CC Condition    HIV HIV Related Dx

**Neoplasms**

**202.6–204.9**

§ ✓5th **202.6   Malignant mast cell tumors**   CC

Malignant:     Mast cell sarcoma
   mastocytoma     Systemic tissue mast
   mastocytosis       cell disease

EXCLUDES   *mast cell leukemia (207.8)*

CC Excl: For code **202.60:** 200.30, 200.40, 200.50, 200.60, 200.70, 202.60-202.70, 202.80, 202.90, 239.8-239.9; **For code 202.61:** 200.31, 200.41, 200.51, 200.61, 200.71, 202.60-202.61, 202.68, 202.71, 202.81, 202.91, 239.8-239.9; **For code 202.62:** 200.32, 200.42, 200.52, 200.62, 200.72, 202.60, 202.62, 202.68, 202.72, 202.82, 202.92, 239.8-239.9; **For code 202.63:** 200.33, 200.43, 200.53, 200.63, 200.73, 202.60, 202.63, 202.68, 202.73, 202.83, 202.93, 239.8-239.9; **For code 202.64:** 200.34, 200.44, 200.54, 200.64, 200.74, 202.60, 202.64, 202.68, 202.74, 202.84, 202.94, 239.8-239.9; **For code 202.65:** 200.35, 200.45, 200.55, 200.65, 200.75, 202.60, 202.65, 202.68, 202.75, 202.85, 202.95, 239.8-239.9; **For code 202.66:** 200.36, 200.46, 200.56, 200.66, 200.76, 202.60, 202.66, 202.68, 202.76, 202.86, 202.96, 239.8-239.9; **For code 202.67:** 200.37, 200.47, 200.57, 200.67, 200.77, 202.60, 202.67-202.68, 202.77, 202.87, 202.97, 239.8-239.9; **For code 202.68:** 200.38, 200.48, 200.58, 200.68, 200.78, 202.60-202.68, 202.78, 202.98, 239.8-239.9

● § ✓5th **202.7   Peripheral T-cell lymphoma**   CC HIV

CC Excl: For code **202.70:** 200.30-200.78, 202.70-202.90, 239.8-239.9; **For code 202.71:** 200.30-200.31, 200.38-200.41, 200.48-200.51, 200.58-200.61, 200.68-200.71, 200.78, 202.70-202.71, 202.78-202.81, 202.88, 202.91, 239.8-239.9; **For code 202.72:** 200.30, 200.32, 200.38-200.40, 200.42, 200.48-200.50, 200.52, 200.58-200.60, 200.62, 200.68-200.70, 200.72, 200.78, 202.70, 202.72, 202.78-202.80, 202.82, 202.88, 202.92, 239.8-239.9; **For code 202.73:** 200.30, 200.33, 200.38-200.40, 200.43, 200.48-200.50, 200.53, 200.58-200.60, 200.63, 200.68-200.70, 200.73, 200.78, 202.70, 202.73, 202.78-202.80, 202.83, 202.88, 202.93, 239.8-239.9; **For code 202.74:** 200.30, 200.34, 200.38-200.40, 200.44, 200.48-200.50, 200.54, 200.58-200.60, 200.64, 200.68-200.70, 200.74, 200.78, 202.70, 202.74, 202.78-202.80, 202.84, 202.88, 202.94, 239.8-239; **For code 202.75:** 200.30, 200.35, 200.38-200.40, 200.45, 200.48-200.50, 200.55, 200.58-200.60, 200.65, 200.68-200.70, 200.75, 200.78, 202.70, 202.75, 202.78-202.80, 202.85, 202.88, 202.95, 239.8-239.9; **For code 202.76:** 200.30, 200.36, 200.38-200.40, 200.46, 200.48-200.50, 200.56, 200.58-200.60, 200.66, 200.68-200.70, 200.76, 200.78, 202.70, 202.76, 202.78-202.80, 202.86, 202.88, 202.96, 239.8-239.9; **For code 202.77:** 200.30, 200.37-200.40, 200.47-200.50, 200.57-200.60, 200.67-200.70, 200.77-200.78, 202.70, 202.77-202.80, 202.87-202.88, 202.97, 239.8-239.9; **For code 202.78:** 200.30-200.78, 202.70-202.88, 202.98, 239.8-239.9

§ ✓5th **202.8   Other lymphomas**   CC HIV

Lymphoma (malignant):
   NOS
   diffuse

EXCLUDES   *benign lymphoma (229.0)*

CC Excl: For code **202.80:** 200.30-200.78, 202.70-202.90, 239.8-239.9; **For code 202.81:** 200.30-200.31, 200.38-200.41, 200.48-200.51, 200.58-200.61, 200.68-200.71, 200.78, 202.70-202.71, 202.78-202.81, 202.88, 202.91, 239.8-239.9; **For code 202.82:** 200.30, 200.32, 200.38-200.40, 200.42, 200.48-200.50, 200.52, 200.58-200.60, 200.62, 200.68-200.70, 200.72, 200.78, 202.70, 202.72, 202.78-202.80, 202.82, 202.88, 202.92, 239.8-239.9; **For code 202.83:** 200.30, 200.33, 200.38-200.40, 200.43, 200.48-200.50, 200.53, 200.58-200.60, 200.63, 200.68-200.70, 200.73, 200.78, 202.70, 202.73, 202.78-202.80, 202.83, 202.88, 202.93, 239.8-239.9; **For code 202.84:** 200.30, 200.34, 200.38-200.40, 200.44, 200.48-200.50, 200.54, 200.58-200.60, 200.64, 200.68-200.70, 200.74, 200.78, 202.70, 202.74, 202.78-202.80, 202.84, 202.88, 202.94, 239.8-239; **For code 202.85:** 200.30, 200.35, 200.38-200.40, 200.45, 200.48-200.50, 200.55, 200.58-200.60, 200.65, 200.68-200.70, 200.75, 200.78, 202.70, 202.75, 202.78-202.80, 202.85, 202.88, 202.95, 239.8-239.9; **For code 202.86:** 200.30, 200.36, 200.38-200.40, 200.46, 200.48-200.50, 200.56, 200.58-200.60, 200.66, 200.68-200.70, 200.76, 200.78, 202.70, 202.76, 202.78-202.80, 202.86, 202.88, 202.96, 239.8-239.9; **For code 202.87:** 200.30, 200.37-200.40, 200.47-200.50, 200.57-200.60, 200.67-200.70, 200.77-200.78, 202.70, 202.77-202.80, 202.87-202.88, 202.97, 239.8-239.9; **For code 202.88:** 200.30-200.78, 202.70-202.88, 202.98, 239.8-239.9

AHA: 4Q, '06, 135; 2Q, '06, 20-21; 2Q, '92, 4

§ ✓5th **202.9   Other and unspecified malignant neoplasms of lymphoid and histiocytic tissue**   CC

Follicular dendritic cell sarcoma
Interdigitating dendritic cell sarcoma
Langerhans cell sarcoma
Malignant neoplasm of bone marrow NOS

CC Excl: For code **202.90:** 202.90-202.98, 239.8-239.9; **For code 202.91:** 202.90-202.91, 202.98, 239.8-239.9; **For code 202.92:** 202.90, 202.92, 202.98, 239.8-239.9; **For code 202.93:** 202.90, 202.93, 202.98, 239.8-239.9; **For code 202.94:** 202.90, 202.94, 202.98, 239.8-239.9; **For code 202.95:** 202.90, 202.95, 202.98, 239.8-239.9; **For code 202.96:** 202.90, 202.96, 202.98, 239.8-239.9; **For code 202.97:** 202.90, 202.97-202.98, 239.8-239.9; **For code 202.98:** 202.90-202.98, 239.8-239.9

✓4th **203   Multiple myeloma and immunoproliferative neoplasms**

AHA: 4Q, '91, 26

The following fifth-digit subclassification is for use with category 203:
   **0   without mention of remission**
   **1   in remission**

✓5th **203.0   Multiple myeloma**   CC

Kahler's disease     Myelomatosis

EXCLUDES   *solitary myeloma (238.6)*

CC Excl: 203.00-208.91, 239.8-239.9

AHA: 1Q, '96, 16; 4Q, '89, 10; For code **203.00:** ▶2Q,'07, 8◀

✓5th **203.1   Plasma cell leukemia**   CC

Plasmacytic leukemia

CC Excl: See code 203.0

AHA: 4Q, '91, 26

✓5th **203.8   Other immunoproliferative neoplasms**   CC

CC Excl: See code 203.0

AHA: 4Q, '90, 26; S-O, '86, 12

✓4th **204   Lymphoid leukemia**

INCLUDES   leukemia:
    lymphatic
    lymphoblastic
    lymphocytic
    lymphogenous

AHA: 3Q, '93, 4

The following fifth-digit subclassification is for use with category 204:
   **0   without mention of remission**
   **1   in remission**

✓5th **204.0   Acute**   CC

EXCLUDES   *acute exacerbation of chronic lymphoid leukemia (204.1)*

CC Excl: 203.00-208.91, 239.8-239.9

AHA: 3Q, '99, 6

✓5th **204.1   Chronic**   CC

CC Excl: See code: 204.0

✓5th **204.2   Subacute**   CC

CC Excl: See code: 204.0

✓5th **204.8   Other lymphoid leukemia**   CC

Aleukemic leukemia:    Aleukemic leukemia:
   lymphatic         lymphoid
   lymphocytic

CC Excl: See code: 204.0

✓5th **204.9   Unspecified lymphoid leukemia**   CC

CC Excl: See code: 204.0

§   Requires fifth-digit. See beginning of section 200–208 for codes and definitions.

✓4th ✓5th Additional Digit Required       Unacceptable PDx       Manifestation Code       ▶◀ Revised Text       ● New Code       ▲ Revised Code Title

**Neoplasms**

**205–210.1**

√4ᵗʰ **205 Myeloid leukemia**

INCLUDES   leukemia:     leukemia:
        granulocytic     myelomonocytic
        myeloblastic     myelosclerotic
        myelocytic     myelosis
        myelogenous

AHA: 3Q, '93, 3; 4Q, '91, 26; 4Q, '90, 3; M-J, '85, 18

The following fifth-digit subclassification is for use with category 205:
    0   **without mention of remission**
    1   **in remission**

√5ᵗʰ **205.0 Acute**         CC
    Acute promyelocytic leukemia
    EXCLUDES   *acute exacerbation of chronic myeloid leukemia (205.1)*
    CC Excl: 203.00-208.91, 239.8-239.9
    AHA: 2Q, '06, 20-21

√5ᵗʰ **205.1 Chronic**         CC
    Eosinophilic leukemia     Neutrophilic leukemia
    CC Excl: See code: 205.0
    AHA: 1Q, '00, 6; J-A, '85, 13

√5ᵗʰ **205.2 Subacute**         CC
    CC Excl: See code: 205.0

√5ᵗʰ **205.3 Myeloid sarcoma**         CC
    Chloroma        Granulocytic sarcoma
    CC Excl: See code: 205.0

√5ᵗʰ **205.8 Other myeloid leukemia**         CC
    Aleukemic leukemia:   Aleukemic leukemia:
        granulocytic     myeloid
        myelogenous     Aleukemic myelosis
    CC Excl: See code: 205.0

√5ᵗʰ **205.9 Unspecified myeloid leukemia**         CC
    CC Excl: See code: 205.0

√4ᵗʰ **206 Monocytic leukemia**

INCLUDES   leukemia:
        histiocytic
        monoblastic
        monocytoid

The following fifth-digit subclassification is for use with category 206:
    0   **without mention of remission**
    1   **in remission**

√5ᵗʰ **206.0 Acute**         CC
    EXCLUDES   *acute exacerbation of chronic monocytic leukemia (206.1)*
    CC Excl: 203.00-208.91, 239.8-239.9

√5ᵗʰ **206.1 Chronic**         CC
    CCC Excl: See code: 206.0

√5ᵗʰ **206.2 Subacute**         CC
    CC Excl: See code: 206.0

√5ᵗʰ **206.8 Other monocytic leukemia**         CC
    Aleukemic:
        monocytic leukemia
        monocytoid leukemia
    CC Excl: See code: 206.0

√5ᵗʰ **206.9 Unspecified monocytic leukemia**         CC
    CC Excl: See code: 206.0

√4ᵗʰ **207 Other specified leukemia**

EXCLUDES   *leukemic reticuloendotheliosis (202.4)*
        *plasma cell leukemia (203.1)*

The following fifth-digit subclassification is for use with category 207:
    0   **without mention of remission**
    1   **in remission**

√5ᵗʰ **207.0 Acute erythremia and erythroleukemia**         CC
    Acute erythremic myelosis
    Di Guglielmo's disease
    Erythremic myelosis
    CC Excl: 203.00-208.91, 239.8-239.9
    DEF: Erythremia: polycythemia vera.
    DEF: Erythroleukemia: a malignant blood dyscrasia (a myeloproliferative disorder).

√5ᵗʰ **207.1 Chronic erythremia**         CC
    Heilmeyer-Schöner disease
    CC Excl: See code: 207.0

√5ᵗʰ **207.2 Megakaryocytic leukemia**         CC
    Megakaryocytic myelosis   Thrombocytic leukemia
    CC Excl: See code: 207.0

√5ᵗʰ **207.8 Other specified leukemia**         CC
    Lymphosarcoma cell leukemia
    CC Excl: See code: 207.0

√4ᵗʰ **208 Leukemia of unspecified cell type**

The following fifth-digit subclassification is for use with category 208:
    0   **without mention of remission**
    1   **in remission**

√5ᵗʰ **208.0 Acute**         CC
    Acute leukemia NOS   Stem cell leukemia
    Blast cell leukemia
    EXCLUDES   *acute exacerbation of chronic unspecified leukemia (208.1)*
    CC Excl: 203.00-208.91, 239.8-239.9

√5ᵗʰ **208.1 Chronic**         CC
    Chronic leukemia NOS
    CC Excl: See code: 208.0

√5ᵗʰ **208.2 Subacute**         CC
    Subacute leukemia NOS
    CC Excl: See code: 208.0

√5ᵗʰ **208.8 Other leukemia of unspecified cell type**         CC
    CC Excl: See code: 208.0

√5ᵗʰ **208.9 Unspecified leukemia**         CC
    Leukemia NOS
    CC Excl: See code: 208.0

## BENIGN NEOPLASMS (210-229)

√4ᵗʰ **210 Benign neoplasm of lip, oral cavity, and pharynx**

EXCLUDES   *cyst (of):*
        *jaw (526.0-526.2, 526.89)*
        *oral soft tissue (528.4)*
        *radicular (522.8)*

**210.0 Lip**
    Frenulum labii
    Lip (inner aspect) (mucosa) (vermilion border)
    EXCLUDES   *labial commissure (210.4)*
        *skin of lip (216.0)*

**210.1 Tongue**
    Lingual tonsil

---

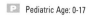 Newborn Age: 0    P Pediatric Age: 0-17    M Maternity Age: 12-55    A Adult Age: 15-124    CC CC Condition    MCC Major CC Condition    HIV HIV Related Dx

**210.2** **Major salivary glands**

Gland:      Gland:

parotid        submandibular

sublingual

> **EXCLUDES** *benign neoplasms of minor salivary*
> *glands:*
> *NOS (210.4)*
> *buccal mucosa (210.4)*
> *lips (210.0)*
> *palate (hard) (soft) (210.4)*
> *tongue (210.1)*
> *tonsil, palatine (210.5)*

**210.3** **Floor of mouth**

**210.4** **Other and unspecified parts of mouth**

Gingiva      Oral mucosa

Gum (upper) (lower)    Palate (hard) (soft)

Labial commissure    Uvula

Oral cavity NOS

> **EXCLUDES** *benign odontogenic neoplasms of bone*
> *(213.0-213.1)*
> *developmental odontogenic cysts (526.0)*
> *mucosa of lips (210.0)*
> *nasopharyngeal [posterior] [superior]*
> *surface of soft palate (210.7)*

**210.5** **Tonsil**

Tonsil (faucial) (palatine)

> **EXCLUDES** *lingual tonsil (210.1)*
> *pharyngeal tonsil (210.7)*
> *tonsillar:*
> *fossa (210.6)*
> *pillars (210.6)*

**210.6** **Other parts of oropharynx**

Branchial cleft or vestiges    Tonsillar:

Epiglottis, anterior aspect      fossa

Fauces NOS          pillars

Mesopharynx NOS     Vallecula

> **EXCLUDES** *epiglottis:*
> *NOS (212.1)*
> *suprahyoid portion (212.1)*

**210.7** **Nasopharynx**

Adenoid tissue      Pharyngeal tonsil

Lymphadenoid tissue    Posterior nasal septum

**210.8** **Hypopharynx**

Arytenoid fold      Postcricoidregion

Laryngopharynx     Pyriform fossa

**210.9** **Pharynx, unspecified**

Throat NOS

**√4ᵗʰ** **211** **Benign neoplasm of other parts of digestive system**

> **EXCLUDES** *benign stromal tumors of digestive system*
> *(215.5)*

**211.0** **Esophagus**

**211.1** **Stomach**

Body    ⎫

Cardia   ⎬ of stomach

Fundus   ⎭

Cardiac orifice

Pylorus

**211.2** **Duodenum, jejunum, and ileum**

Small intestine NOS

> **EXCLUDES** *ampulla of Vater (211.5)*
> *ileocecal valve (211.3)*

**211.3** **Colon**

Appendix      Ileocecal valve

Cecum        Large intestine NOS

> **EXCLUDES** *rectosigmoid junction (211.4)*

**AHA:** 3Q, '05, 17; 2Q, '05, 16; 4Q, '01, 56

**211.4** **Rectum and anal canal**

Anal canal or sphincter    Rectosigmoid junction

Anus NOS

> **EXCLUDES** *anus:*
> *margin (216.5)*
> *skin (216.5)*
> *perianal skin (216.5)*

**211.5** **Liver and biliary passages**

Ampulla of Vater     Gallbladder

Common bile duct    Hepatic duct

Cystic duct        Sphincter of Oddi

**211.6** **Pancreas, except islets of Langerhans**

**211.7** **Islets of Langerhans**

Islet cell tumor

Use additional code to identify any functional
activity

**211.8** **Retroperitoneum and peritoneum**

Mesentery      Omentum

Mesocolon      Retroperitoneal tissue

**211.9** **Other and unspecified site**

Alimentary tract NOS

Digestive system NOS

Gastrointestinal tract NOS

Intestinal tract NOS

Intestine NOS

Spleen, not elsewhere classified

**√4ᵗʰ** **212** **Benign neoplasm of respiratory and intrathoracic organs**

**212.0** **Nasal cavities, middle ear, and accessory sinuses**

Cartilage of nose     Sinus:

Eustachian tube       ethmoidal

Nares           frontal

Septum of nose      maxillary

                   sphenoidal

> **EXCLUDES** *auditory canal (external) (216.2)*
> *bone of:*
> *ear (213.0)*
> *nose [turbinates] (213.0)*
> *cartilage of ear (215.0)*
> *ear (external) (skin) (216.2)*
> *nose NOS (229.8)*
> *skin (216.3)*
> *olfactory bulb (225.1)*
> *polyp of:*
> *accessory sinus (471.8)*
> *ear (385.30-385.35)*
> *nasal cavity (471.0)*
> *posterior margin of septum and*
> *choanae (210.7)*

**212.1** **Larynx**

Cartilage:       Epiglottis (suprahyoid portion) NOS

arytenoid      Glottis

cricoid        Vocal cords (false) (true)

cuneiform

thyroid

> **EXCLUDES** *epiglottis, anterior aspect (210.6)*
> *polyp of vocal cord or larynx (478.4)*

**212.2** **Trachea**

**212.3** **Bronchus and lung**

Carina           Hilus of lung

**212.4** **Pleura**

**212.5** **Mediastinum**

**212.6** **Thymus**

**212.7** **Heart**

> **EXCLUDES** *great vessels (215.4)*

**212.8** **Other specified sites**

**212.9** **Site unspecified**

Respiratory organ NOS

Upper respiratory tract NOS

> **EXCLUDES** *intrathoracic NOS (229.8)*
> *thoracic NOS (229.8)*

**√4ᵗʰ** **213** **Benign neoplasm of bone and articular cartilage**

> **INCLUDES** cartilage (articular) (joint)
> periosteum

> **EXCLUDES** *cartilage of:*      *cartilage of:*
> *ear (215.0)*         *nose (212.0)*
> *eyelid (215.0)*      *exostosis NOS (726.91)*
> *larynx (212.1)*      *synovia (215.0-215.9)*

**213.0** **Bones of skull and face**

> **EXCLUDES** *lower jaw bone (213.1)*

**210.2–213.0**

**Neoplasms**

**213.1–219.9**

213.1    **Lower jaw bone**

213.2    **Vertebral column, excluding sacrum and coccyx**

213.3    **Ribs, sternum, and clavicle**

213.4    **Scapula and long bones of upper limb**

213.5    **Short bones of upper limb**

213.6    **Pelvic bones, sacrum, and coccyx**

213.7    **Long bones of lower limb**

213.8    **Short bones of lower limb**

213.9    **Bone and articular cartilage, site unspecified**

✓4ᵗʰ **214 Lipoma**

INCLUDES   angiolipoma
fibrolipoma
hibernoma
lipoma (fetal) (infiltrating) (intramuscular)
myelolipoma
myxolipoma

DEF: Benign tumor frequently composed of mature fat cells; may occasionally be composed of fetal fat cells.

214.0    **Skin and subcutaneous tissue of face**

214.1    **Other skin and subcutaneous tissue**

214.2    **Intrathoracic organs**

214.3    **Intra-abdominal organs**

214.4    **Spermatic cord**         ♂

214.8    **Other specified sites**
AHA: 3Q, '94, 7

214.9    **Lipoma, unspecified site**

✓4ᵗʰ **215 Other benign neoplasm of connective and other soft tissue**

INCLUDES   blood vessel
bursa
fascia
ligament
muscle
peripheral, sympathetic, and parasympathetic
     nerves and ganglia
synovia
tendon (sheath)

EXCLUDES   *cartilage:*
     *articular (213.0-213.9)*
     *larynx (212.1)*
     *nose (212.0)*
*connective tissue of:*
     *breast (217)*
     *internal organ, except lipoma and*
       *hemangioma—code to benign neoplasm*
       *of the site*
*lipoma (214.0-214.9)*

215.0    **Head, face, and neck**

215.2    **Upper limb, including shoulder**

215.3    **Lower limb, including hip**

215.4    **Thorax**
EXCLUDES   *heart (212.7)*
     *mediastinum (212.5)*
     *thymus (212.6)*

215.5    **Abdomen**
Abdominal wall
Benign stromal tumors of abdomen
Hypochondrium

215.6    **Pelvis**
Buttock           Inguinal region
Groin             Perineum
EXCLUDES   *uterine:*
     *leiomyoma (218.0-218.9)*
     *ligament, any (221.0)*

215.7    **Trunk, unspecified**
Back NOS          Flank NOS

215.8    **Other specified sites**

215.9    **Site unspecified**

✓4ᵗʰ **216 Benign neoplasm of skin**

INCLUDES   blue nevus        pigmented nevus
dermatofibroma    syringoadenoma
hydrocystoma      syringoma

EXCLUDES   *skin of genital organs (221.0-222.9)*

AHA: 1Q, '00, 21

216.0    **Skin of lip**
EXCLUDES   *vermilion border of lip (210.0)*

216.1    **Eyelid, including canthus**
EXCLUDES   *cartilage of eyelid (215.0)*

216.2    **Ear and external auditory canal**
Auricle (ear)          External meatus
Auricular canal, external   Pinna
EXCLUDES   *cartilage of ear (215.0)*

216.3    **Skin of other and unspecified parts of face**
Cheek, external       Nose, external
Eyebrow             Temple

216.4    **Scalp and skin of neck**
AHA: 3Q, '91, 12

216.5    **Skin of trunk, except scrotum**
Axillary fold         Skin of:
Perianal skin         buttock
Skin of:              chest wall
   abdominal wall      groin
   anus               perineum
   back               Umbilicus
   breast
EXCLUDES   *anal canal (211.4)*
     *anus NOS (211.4)*
     *skin of scrotum (222.4)*

216.6    **Skin of upper limb, including shoulder**

216.7    **Skin of lower limb, including hip**

216.8    **Other specified sites of skin**

216.9    **Skin, site unspecified**

**217 Benign neoplasm of breast**
Breast (male) (female):      Breast (male) (female):
   connective tissue         soft parts
   glandular tissue
EXCLUDES   *adenofibrosis (610.2)*
     *benign cyst of breast (610.0)*
     *fibrocystic disease (610.1)*
     *skin of breast (216.5)*

AHA: 1Q, '00, 4

✓4ᵗʰ **218 Uterine leiomyoma**

INCLUDES   fibroid (bleeding) (uterine)
uterine:
   fibromyoma
   myoma

DEF: Benign tumor primarily derived from uterine smooth muscle tissue; may contain fibrous, fatty, or epithelial tissue; also called uterine fibroid or myoma.

218.0    **Submucous leiomyoma of uterus**    ♀

218.1    **Intramural leiomyoma of uterus**    ♀
Interstitial leiomyoma of uterus

218.2    **Subserous leiomyoma of uterus**    ♀

218.9    **Leiomyoma of uterus, unspecified**    ♀
AHA: 1Q, '03, 4

✓4ᵗʰ **219 Other benign neoplasm of uterus**

219.0    **Cervix uteri**    ♀

219.1    **Corpus uteri**    ♀
Endometrium       Myometrium
Fundus

219.8    **Other specified parts of uterus**    ♀

219.9    **Uterus, part unspecified**    ♀

---

N Newborn Age: 0    P Pediatric Age: 0-17    M Maternity Age: 12-55    A Adult Age: 15-124    CC CC Condition    MCC Major CC Condition    HIV HIV Related Dx

**Types of Uterine Fibroids**

Cornual — Pedunculated
Uterine cavity — Intramural
Subserosal — Submucosal
— Cervical

**Types of Uterine Fibroids**

**Eyeball**

Posterior segment
Vitreous
Optic nerve
Optic disc
Choroid
Sclera
Retina
Pars plana
Lens
Iris
Conjunctiva
Sclera
Cornea
Anterior chamber

## 220 Benign neoplasm of ovary ♀
Use additional code to identify any functional activity (256.0-256.1)

**EXCLUDES** cyst:
    corpus albicans (620.2)
    corpus luteum (620.1)
    endometrial (617.1)
    follicular (atretic) (620.0)
    graafian follicle (620.0)
    ovarian NOS (620.2)
    retention (620.2)

## ✓4th 221 Benign neoplasm of other female genital organs
**INCLUDES** adenomatous polyp
    benign teratoma

**EXCLUDES** cyst:
    epoophoron (752.11)
    fimbrial (752.11)
    Gartner's duct (752.11)
    parovarian (752.11)

  **221.0 Fallopian tube and uterine ligaments** ♀
    Oviduct
    Parametruim
    Uterine ligament (broad) (round) (uterosacral)
    Uterine tube

  **221.1 Vagina** ♀
  **221.2 Vulva** ♀
    Clitoris
    External female genitalia NOS
    Greater vestibular [Bartholin's] gland
    Labia (majora) (minora)
    Pudendum
    **EXCLUDES** Bartholin's (duct) (gland) cyst (616.2)

  **221.8 Other specified sites of female genital organs** ♀
  **221.9 Female genital organ, site unspecified** ♀
    Female genitourinary tract NOS

## ✓4th 222 Benign neoplasm of male genital organs
  **222.0 Testis** ♂
    Use additional code to identify any functional activity

  **222.1 Penis** ♂
    Corpus cavernosum   Prepuce
    Glans penis

  **222.2 Prostate** ♂
    **EXCLUDES** adenomatous hyperplasia of prostate (600.20-600.21)
    prostatic:
      adenoma (600.20-600.21)
      enlargement (600.00-600.01)
      hypertrophy (600.00-600.01)

  **222.3 Epididymis** ♂
  **222.4 Scrotum** ♂
    Skin of scrotum
  **222.8 Other specified sites of male genital organs** ♂
    Seminal vesicle
    Spermatic cord
  **222.9 Male genital organ, site unspecified** ♂
    Male genitourinary tract NOS

## ✓4th 223 Benign neoplasm of kidney and other urinary organs
  **223.0 Kidney, except pelvis**
    Kidney NOS
    **EXCLUDES** renal:
      calyces (223.1)
      pelvis (223.1)

  **223.1 Renal pelvis**
  **223.2 Ureter**
    **EXCLUDES** ureteric orifice of bladder (223.3)
  **223.3 Bladder**
  **✓5th 223.8 Other specified sites of urinary organs**
    **223.81 Urethra**
      **EXCLUDES** urethral orifice of bladder (223.3)
    **223.89 Other**
      Paraurethral glands
  **223.9 Urinary organ, site unspecified**
    Urinary system NOS

## ✓4th 224 Benign neoplasm of eye
**EXCLUDES** cartilage of eyelid (215.0)
    eyelid (skin) (216.1)
    optic nerve (225.1)
    orbital bone (213.0)

  **224.0 Eyeball, except conjunctiva, cornea, retina, and choroid**
    Ciliary body     Sclera
    Iris          Uveal tract

  **224.1 Orbit**
    **EXCLUDES** bone of orbit (213.0)
  **224.2 Lacrimal gland**
  **224.3 Conjunctiva**
  **224.4 Cornea**
  **224.5 Retina**
    **EXCLUDES** hemangioma of retina (228.03)
  **224.6 Choroid**
  **224.7 Lacrimal duct**
    Lacrimal sac     Nasolacrimal duct
  **224.8 Other specified parts of eye**
  **224.9 Eye, part unspecified**

## ✓4th 225 Benign neoplasm of brain and other parts of nervous system
**EXCLUDES** hemangioma (228.02)
    neurofibromatosis (237.7)
    peripheral, sympathetic, and parasympathetic nerves and ganglia (215.0-215.9)
    retrobulbar (224.1)

  **225.0 Brain**
  **225.1 Cranial nerves**
    Acoustic neuroma
    **AHA:** 4Q, '04, 113
  **225.2 Cerebral meninges**
    Meninges NOS    Meningioma (cerebral)
  **225.3 Spinal cord**
    Cauda equina

---

**Neoplasms**

**225.4–231.9**

**225.4 Spinal meninges**
Spinal meningioma

**225.8 Other specified sites of nervous system**

**225.9 Nervous system, part unspecified**
Nervous system (central) NOS
> EXCLUDES   meninges NOS (225.2)

**226 Benign neoplasm of thyroid glands**
Use additional code to identify any functional activity

✓4ᵗʰ **227 Benign neoplasm of other endocrine glands and related structures**
Use additional code to identify any functional activity
> EXCLUDES   ovary (220)      testis (222.0)
> pancreas (211.6)

**227.0 Adrenal gland**
Suprarenal gland

**227.1 Parathyroid gland**

**227.3 Pituitary gland and craniopharyngeal duct (pouch)**
Craniobuccal pouch    Rathke's pouch
Hypophysis    Sella turcica

**227.4 Pineal gland**
Pineal body

**227.5 Carotid body**

**227.6 Aortic body and other paraganglia**
Coccygeal body    Para-aortic body
Glomus jugulare
AHA: N-D, '84, 17

**227.8 Other**

**227.9 Endocrine gland, site unspecified**

✓4ᵗʰ **228 Hemangioma and lymphangioma, any site**
> INCLUDES   angioma (benign) (cavernous) (congenital) NOS
> cavernous nevus
> glomus tumor
> hemangioma (benign) (congenital)
> EXCLUDES   benign neoplasm of spleen, except hemangioma
> and lymphangioma (211.9)
> glomus jugulare (227.6)
> nevus:
> NOS (216.0-216.9)
> blue or pigmented (216.0-216.9)
> vascular (757.32)

AHA: 1Q, '00, 21

✓5ᵗʰ **228.0 Hemangioma, any site**
AHA: J-F, '85, 19
DEF: A common benign tumor usually occurring in infancy; composed of newly formed blood vessels due to malformation of angioblastic tissue.

**228.00 Of unspecified site**

**228.01 Of skin and subcutaneous tissue**

**228.02 Of intracranial structures**

**228.03 Of retina**

**228.04 Of intra-abdominal structures**
Peritoneum    Retroperitoneal tissue

**228.09 Of other sites**
Systemic angiomatosis
AHA: 3Q, '91, 20

**228.1 Lymphangioma, any site**
Congenital lymphangioma    Lymphatic nevus

✓4ᵗʰ **229 Benign neoplasm of other and unspecified sites**

**229.0 Lymph nodes**
> EXCLUDES   lymphangioma (228.1)

**229.8 Other specified sites**
Intrathoracic NOS    Thoracic NOS

**229.9 Site unspecified**

## CARCINOMA IN SITU (230-234)

> INCLUDES   Bowen's disease
> erythroplasia
> Queyrat's erythroplasia
> EXCLUDES   leukoplakia—see Alphabetic Index

DEF: A neoplastic type; with tumor cells confined to epithelium of origin; without further invasion.

✓4ᵗʰ **230 Carcinoma in situ of digestive organs**

**230.0 Lip, oral cavity, and pharynx**
Gingiva    Oropharynx
Hypopharynx    Salivary gland or duct
Mouth [any part]    Tongue
Nasopharynx
> EXCLUDES   aryepiglottic fold or interarytenoid fold,
> laryngeal aspect (231.0)
> epiglottis:
> NOS (231.0)
> suprahyoid portion (231.0)
> skin of lip (232.0)

**230.1 Esophagus**

**230.2 Stomach**
Body ⎫
Cardia ⎬ of stomach
Fundus ⎭
Cardiac orifice    Pylorus

**230.3 Colon**
Appendix    Ileocecal valve
Cecum    Large intestine NOS
> EXCLUDES   rectosigmoid junction (230.4)

**230.4 Rectum**
Rectosigmoid junction

**230.5 Anal canal**
Anal sphincter

**230.6 Anus, unspecified**
> EXCLUDES   anus:
> margin (232.5)
> skin (232.5)
> perianal skin (232.5)

**230.7 Other and unspecified parts of intestine**
Duodenum    Jejunum
Ileum    Small intestine NOS
> EXCLUDES   ampulla of Vater (230.8)

**230.8 Liver and biliary system**
Ampulla of Vater    Gallbladder
Common bile duct    Hepatic duct
Cystic duct    Sphincter of Oddi

**230.9 Other and unspecified digestive organs**
Digestive organ NOS    Pancreas
Gastrointestinal tract NOS    Spleen

✓4ᵗʰ **231 Carcinoma in situ of respiratory system**

**231.0 Larynx**
Cartilage:    Epiglottis:
arytenoid    NOS
cricoid    posterior surface
cuneiform    suprahyoid portion
thyroid    Vocal cords (false) (true)
> EXCLUDES   aryepiglottic fold or interarytenoid fold:
> NOS (230.0)
> hypopharyngeal aspect (230.0)
> marginal zone (230.0)

**231.1 Trachea**

**231.2 Bronchus and lung**
Carina
Hilus of lung

**231.8 Other specified parts of respiratory system**
Accessory sinuses    Nasal cavities
Middle ear    Pleura
> EXCLUDES   ear (external) (skin) (232.2)
> nose NOS (234.8)
> skin (232.3)

**231.9 Respiratory system, part unspecified**
Respiratory organ NOS

Ⓝ Newborn Age: 0    Ⓟ Pediatric Age: 0-17    Ⓜ Maternity Age: 12-55    Ⓐ Adult Age: 15-124    CC CC Condition    MCC Major CC Condition    HIV HIV Related Dx

54 — Volume 1 • October 2007

© 2007 Ingenix

√4th **232 Carcinoma in situ of skin**

    INCLUDES  pigment cells

    **232.0 Skin of lip**
        EXCLUDES  *vermilion border of lip (230.0)*

    **232.1 Eyelid, including canthus**

    **232.2 Ear and external auditory canal**

    **232.3 Skin of other and unspecified parts of face**

    **232.4 Scalp and skin of neck**

    **232.5 Skin of trunk, except scrotum**

        Anus, margin      Skin of:
        Axillary fold        breast
        Perianal skin       buttock
        Skin of:           chest wall
          abdominal wall   groin
          anus           perineum
          back           Umbilicus
        EXCLUDES  *anal canal (230.5)*
                     *anus NOS (230.6)*
                     *skin of genital organs* ▶*(233.30-233.39, 233.5-233.6)*◀

    **232.6 Skin of upper limb, including shoulder**

    **232.7 Skin of lower limb, including hip**

    **232.8 Other specified sites of skin**

    **232.9 Skin, site unspecified**

√4th **233 Carcinoma in situ of breast and genitourinary system**

    **233.0 Breast**
        EXCLUDES  *Paget's disease (174.0-174.9)*
                     *skin of breast (232.5)*

    **233.1 Cervix uteri**             ♀
       ▶Adenocarcinoma in situ of cervix◀
       Cervical intraepithelial glandular neoplasia
       Cervical intraepithelial neoplasia III [CIN III]
       Severe dysplasia of cervix
       EXCLUDES  *cervical intraepithelial neoplasia II [CIN II] (622.12)*
                    *cytologic evidence of malignancy without histologic confirmation (795.06)*
                    *high grade squamous intraepithelial lesion (HGSIL) (795.04)*
                    *moderate dysplasia of cervix (622.12)*
       **AHA:** 3Q, '92, 7; 3Q, '92, 8; 1Q, '91, 11

    **233.2 Other and unspecified parts of uterus**    ♀

√5th **233.3 Other and unspecified female genital organs**  ♀

      • **233.30 Unspecified female genital organ**  ♀

      • **233.31 Vagina**  ♀
          Severe dysplasia of vagina
          Vaginal intraepithelial neoplasia III [VAIN III]

      • **233.32 Vulva**  ♀
          Severe dysplasia of vulva
          Vulvar intraepithelial neoplasia III [VIN III]

      • **233.39 Other female genital organ**  ♀

    **233.4 Prostate**  ♂

    **233.5 Penis**  ♂

    **233.6 Other and unspecified male genital organs**  ♂

    **233.7 Bladder**

    **233.9 Other and unspecified urinary organs**

√4th **234 Carcinoma in situ of other and unspecified sites**

    **234.0 Eye**
        EXCLUDES  *cartilage of eyelid (234.8)*
                     *eyelid (skin) (232.1)*
                     *optic nerve (234.8)*
                     *orbital bone (234.8)*

    **234.8 Other specified sites**
       Endocrine gland [any]

    **234.9 Site unspecified**
       Carcinoma in situ NOS

## NEOPLASMS OF UNCERTAIN BEHAVIOR (235-238)

Note: Categories 235–238 classify by site certain histomorphologically well-defined neoplasms, the subsequent behavior of which cannot be predicted from the present appearance.

√4th **235 Neoplasm of uncertain behavior of digestive and respiratory systems**
    EXCLUDES  *stromal tumors of uncertain behavior of digestive system (238.1)*

    **235.0 Major salivary glands**
       Gland:           Gland:
         parotid         submandibular
         sublingual
       EXCLUDES  *minor salivary glands (235.1)*

    **235.1 Lip, oral cavity, and pharynx**
       Gingiva           Nasopharynx
       Hypopharynx     Oropharynx
       Minor salivary glands  Tongue
       Mouth
       EXCLUDES  *aryepiglottic fold or interarytenoid fold, laryngeal aspect (235.6)*
                     *epiglottis:*
                       *NOS (235.6)*
                       *suprahyoid portion (235.6)*
                     *skin of lip (238.2)*

    **235.2 Stomach, intestines, and rectum**

    **235.3 Liver and biliary passages**
       Ampulla of Vater     Gallbladder
       Bile ducts [any]      Liver

    **235.4 Retroperitoneum and peritoneum**

    **235.5 Other and unspecified digestive organs**
       Anal:           Esophagus
         canal          Pancreas
         sphincter     Spleen
       Anus NOS
       EXCLUDES  *anus:*
                     *margin (238.2)*
                     *skin (238.2)*
                     *perianal skin (238.2)*

    **235.6 Larynx**
       EXCLUDES  *aryepiglottic fold or interarytenoid fold:*
                     *NOS (235.1)*
                     *hypopharyngeal aspect (235.1)*
                     *marginal zone (235.1)*

    **235.7 Trachea, bronchus, and lung**

    **235.8 Pleura, thymus, and mediastinum**

    **235.9 Other and unspecified respiratory organs**
       Accessory sinuses    Nasal cavities
       Middle ear         Respiratory organ NOS
       EXCLUDES  *ear (external) (skin) (238.2)*
                     *nose (238.8)*
                     *skin (238.2)*

√4th **236 Neoplasm of uncertain behavior of genitourinary organs**

    **236.0 Uterus**  ♀

    **236.1 Placenta**  ♀
       Chorioadenoma (destruens)
       Invasive mole
       Malignant hydatid(iform) mole

    **236.2 Ovary**  ♀
       Use additional code to identify any functional activity

    **236.3 Other and unspecified female genital organs**  ♀

    **236.4 Testis**  ♂
       Use additional code to identify any functional activity

    **236.5 Prostate**  ♂

    **236.6 Other and unspecified male genital organs**  ♂

    **236.7 Bladder**

√5th **236.9 Other and unspecified urinary organs**

      **236.90 Urinary organ, unspecified**

      **236.91 Kidney and ureter**

      **236.99 Other**

---

**Neoplasms**

**237–238.75**

✓4th **237 Neoplasm of uncertain behavior of endocrine glands and nervous system**

**237.0 Pituitary gland and craniopharyngeal duct**
Use additional code to identify any functional activity

**237.1 Pineal gland**

**237.2 Adrenal gland**
Suprarenal gland
Use additional code to identify any functional activity

**237.3 Paraganglia**
Aortic body      Coccygeal body
Carotid body      Glomus jugulare
**AHA:** N-D, '84, 17

**237.4 Other and unspecified endocrine glands**
Parathyroid gland      Thyroid gland

**237.5 Brain and spinal cord**

**237.6 Meninges**
Meninges:      Meninges:
NOS             spinal
cerebral

✓5th **237.7 Neurofibromatosis**
von Recklinghausen's disease
**DEF:** An inherited condition with developmental changes in the nervous system, muscles, bones and skin; multiple soft tumors (neurofibromas) distributed over the entire body.

**237.70 Neurofibromatosis, unspecified**

**237.71 Neurofibromatosis, type 1 [von Recklinghausen's disease]**

**237.72 Neurofibromatosis, type 2 [acoustic neurofibromatosis]**
**DEF:** Inherited condition with cutaneous lesions, benign tumors of peripheral nerves and bilateral 8th nerve masses.

**237.9 Other and unspecified parts of nervous system**
Cranial nerves
**EXCLUDES** *peripheral, sympathetic, and parasympathetic nerves and ganglia (238.1)*

✓4th **238 Neoplasm of uncertain behavior of other and unspecified sites and tissues**

**238.0 Bone and articular cartilage**
**EXCLUDES** *cartilage:*
*ear (238.1)*
*eyelid (238.1)*
*larynx (235.6)*
*nose (235.9)*
*synovia (238.1)*
**AHA:** 4Q, '04, 128

**238.1 Connective and other soft tissue**
Peripheral, sympathetic, and parasympathetic nerves and ganglia
Stromal tumors of digestive system
**EXCLUDES** *cartilage (of):*
*articular (238.0)*
*larynx (235.6)*
*nose (235.9)*
*connective tissue of breast (238.3)*

**238.2 Skin**
**EXCLUDES** *anus NOS (235.5)*
*skin of genital organs (236.3, 236.6)*
*vermilion border of lip (235.1)*

**238.3 Breast**
**EXCLUDES** *skin of breast (238.2)*

**238.4 Polycythemia vera**
**DEF:** Abnormal proliferation of all bone marrow elements, increased red cell mass and total blood volume; unknown etiology, frequently associated with splenomegaly, leukocytosis, and thrombocythemia.

**238.5 Histiocytic and mast cells**    CC
Mast cell tumor NOS
Mastocytoma NOS
**CC Excl:** 238.4-238.79, 289.83, V58.0

**238.6 Plasma cells**    CC
Plasmacytoma NOS
Solitary myeloma
**CC Excl:** See code: 238.5

✓5th **238.7 Other lymphatic and hematopoietic tissues**
**EXCLUDES** *acute myelogenous leukemia (205.0)*
*chronic myelomonocytic leukemia (205.1)*
*myelofibrosis (289.83)*
*myelosclerosis NOS (289.89)*
*myelosis:*
*NOS (205.9)*
*megakaryocytic (207.2)*
**AHA:** 3Q, '01, 13; 1Q, '97, 5; 2Q, '89, 8

**238.71 Essential thrombocythemia**
Essential hemorrhagic thrombocythemia
Essential thrombocytosis
Idiopathic (hemorrhagic) thrombocythemia
Primary thrombocytosis
**AHA:** 4Q, '06, 63-66

**238.72 Low grade myelodysplastic syndrome lesions**
Refractory anemia (RA)
Refractory anemia with ringed sideroblasts (RARS)
Refractory cytopenia with multilineage dysplasia (RCMD)
Refractory cytopenia with multilineage dysplasia and ringed sideroblasts (RCMD-RS)
**AHA:** 4Q, '06, 63-66

**DEF:** Refractory anemia (RA): Form of bone marrow disorder (myelodysplastic syndrome) that interferes with red blood cell production in the bone marrow; malignancy unresponsive to hematinics; characteristic normal or hypercellular marrow with abnormal erythrocyte development and reticulocytopenia.

**238.73 High grade myelodysplastic syndrome lesions**    CC
Refractory anemia with excess blasts-1 (RAEB-1)
Refractory anemia with excess blasts-2 (RAEB-2)
**CC Excl:** 202.40-202.48, 203.10-208.91, 238.4-238.9
**AHA:** 4Q, '06, 63-66

**238.74 Myelodysplastic syndrome with 5q deletion**    CC
5q minus syndrome NOS
**EXCLUDES** *constitutional 5q deletion (758.39)*
*high grade myelodysplastic syndrome with 5q deletion (238.73)*
**CC Excl:** See code: 238.73
**AHA:** 4Q, '06, 63-66

**238.75 Myelodysplastic syndrome, unspecified**
**AHA:** 4Q, '06, 63-66

---

N Newborn Age: 0    P Pediatric Age: 0-17    M Maternity Age: 12-55    A Adult Age: 15-124    CC CC Condition    MCC Major CC Condition    HIV HIV Related Dx

**238.76 Myelofibrosis with myeloid metaplasia** CC
Agnogenic myeloid metaplasia
Idiopathic myelofibrosis (chronic)
Myelosclerosis with myeloid metaplasia
Primary myelofibrosis
EXCLUDES  myelofibrosis NOS (289.83)
myelophthisic anemia (284.2)
myelophthisis (284.2)
secondary myelofibrosis (289.83)

CC Excl: See code: 238.73

AHA: 4Q, '06, 63-66

**238.79 Other lymphatic and hematopoietic tissues** CC
Lymphoproliferative disease (chronic) NOS
Megakaryocytic myelosclerosis
Myeloproliferative disease (chronic) NOS
Panmyelosis (acute)

CC Excl: See code: 238.73

AHA: 4Q, '06, 63-66

**238.8 Other specified sites**
Eye              Heart
EXCLUDES  eyelid (skin) (238.2)
cartilage (238.1)

**238.9 Site unspecified**

## NEOPLASMS OF UNSPECIFIED NATURE (239)

**239 Neoplasms of unspecified nature**
Note: Category 239 classifies by site neoplasms of unspecified morphology and behavior. The term "mass,"unless otherwise stated, is not to be regarded as a neoplastic growth.
INCLUDES  "growth" NOS        new growth NOS
neoplasm NOS        tumor NOS

**239.0 Digestive system**
EXCLUDES  anus:
margin (239.2)
skin (239.2)
perianal skin (239.2)

**239.1 Respiratory system**

**239.2 Bone, soft tissue, and skin**
EXCLUDES  anal canal (239.0)
anus NOS (239.0)
bone marrow (202.9)
cartilage:
larynx (239.1)
nose (239.1)
connective tissue of breast (239.3)
skin of genital organs (239.5)
vermilion border of lip (239.0)

**239.3 Breast**
EXCLUDES  skin of breast (239.2)

**239.4 Bladder**

**239.5 Other genitourinary organs**

**239.6 Brain**
EXCLUDES  cerebral meninges (239.7)
cranial nerves (239.7)

**239.7 Endocrine glands and other parts of nervous system**
EXCLUDES  peripheral, sympathetic, and parasympathetic nerves and ganglia (239.2)

**239.8 Other specified sites**
EXCLUDES  eyelid (skin) (239.2)
cartilage (239.2)
great vessels (239.2)
optic nerve (239.7)

**239.9 Site unspecified**

# 3. ENDOCRINE, NUTRITIONAL AND METABOLIC DISEASES, AND IMMUNITY DISORDERS (240-279)

**EXCLUDES** *endocrine and metabolic disturbances specific to the fetus and newborn (775.0-775.9)*

Note: All neoplasms, whether functionally active or not, are classified in Chapter 2. Codes in Chapter 3 (i.e., 242.8, 246.0, 251-253, 255-259) may be used to identify such functional activity associated with any neoplasm, or by ectopic endocrine tissue.

## DISORDERS OF THYROID GLAND (240-246)

### √4ᵗʰ 240 Simple and unspecified goiter
DEF: An enlarged thyroid gland often caused by an inadequate dietary intake of iodine.

**240.0 Goiter, specified as simple**
Any condition classifiable to 240.9, specified as simple

**240.9 Goiter, unspecified**
Enlargement of thyroid
Goiter or struma:
　NOS
　diffuse colloid
　endemic
Goiter or struma:
　hyperplastic
　nontoxic (diffuse)
　parenchymatous
　sporadic
**EXCLUDES** *congenital (dyshormonogenic) goiter (246.1)*

### √4ᵗʰ 241 Nontoxic nodular goiter
**EXCLUDES** *adenoma of thyroid (226)*
*cystadenoma of thyroid (226)*

**241.0 Nontoxic uninodular goiter**
Thyroid nodule　　Uninodular goiter (nontoxic)
DEF: Enlarged thyroid, commonly due to decreased thyroid production, with single nodule; no clinical hypothyroidism.

**241.1 Nontoxic multinodular goiter**
Multinodular goiter (nontoxic)
DEF: Enlarged thyroid, commonly due to decreased thyroid production with multiple nodules; no clinical hypothyroidism.

**241.9 Unspecified nontoxic nodular goiter**
Adenomatous goiter
Nodular goiter (nontoxic) NOS
Struma nodosa (simplex)

### √4ᵗʰ 242 Thyrotoxicosis with or without goiter
**EXCLUDES** *neonatal thyrotoxicosis (775.3)*
DEF: A condition caused by excess quantities of thyroid hormones being introduced into the tissues

The following fifth-digit subclassification is for use with category 242:
　0　without mention of thyrotoxic crisis or storm
　1　with mention of thyrotoxic crisis or storm

### √5ᵗʰ 242.0 Toxic diffuse goiter　　　`MCC 1`
Basedow's disease
Exophthalmic or toxic goiter NOS
Graves' disease
Primary thyroid hyperplasia
**CC Excl:** 017.50-017.56, 017.90-017.96, 240.0-246.9, 259.5-259.9

DEF: Diffuse thyroid enlargement accompanied by hyperthyroidism, bulging eyes, and dermatopathy.

### √5ᵗʰ 242.1 Toxic uninodular goiter　　`MCC 1`
Thyroid nodule　}　toxic or with
Uninodular goiter　}　hyperthyroidism
**CC Excl:** See code 242.0

DEF: Symptomatic hyperthyroidism with a single nodule on the enlarged thyroid gland. Abrupt onset of symptoms; including extreme nervousness, insomnia, weight loss, tremors, and psychosis or coma.

### √5ᵗʰ 242.2 Toxic multinodular goiter　　`MCC 1`
Secondary thyroid hyperplasia
**CC Excl:** See code 242.0

DEF: Symptomatic hyperthyroidism with multiple nodules on the enlarged thyroid gland. Abrupt onset of symptoms; including extreme nervousness, insomnia, weight loss, tremors, and psychosis or coma

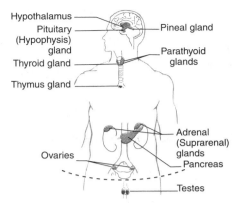
**The Endocrine System**

Hypothalamus
Pituitary (Hypophysis) gland
Thyroid gland
Thymus gland
Pineal gland
Parathyroid glands
Adrenal (Suprarenal) glands
Ovaries
Pancreas
Testes

### √5ᵗʰ 242.3 Toxic nodular goiter, unspecified　　`MCC 1`
Adenomatous goiter
Nodular goiter
Struma nodosa
}　toxic or with hyperthyroidism

Any condition classifiable to 241.9 specified as toxic or with hyperthyroidism
**CC Excl:** See code 242.0

### √5ᵗʰ 242.4 Thyrotoxicosis from ectopic thyroid nodule　`MCC 1`
**CC Excl:** See code 242.0

### √5ᵗʰ 242.8 Thyrotoxicosis of other specified origin　`MCC 1`
Overproduction of thyroid-stimulating hormone [TSH]
Thyrotoxicosis:
　factitia from ingestion of excessive thyroid material
Use additional E code to identify cause, if drug-induced
**CC Excl:** See code 242.0

### √5ᵗʰ 242.9 Thyrotoxicosis without mention of goiter or other cause　`MCC 1`
Hyperthyroidism NOS
Thyrotoxicosis NOS
**CC Excl:** See code 242.0

### 243 Congenital hypothyroidism
Congenital thyroid insufficiency
Cretinism (athyrotic) (endemic)
Use additional code to identify associated mental retardation
**EXCLUDES** *congenital (dyshormonogenic) goiter (246.1)*
DEF: Underproduction of thyroid hormone present from birth.

### √4ᵗʰ 244 Acquired hypothyroidism
**INCLUDES**　athyroidism (acquired)
　hypothyroidism (acquired)
　myxedema (adult) (juvenile)
　thyroid (gland) insufficiency (acquired)

**244.0 Postsurgical hypothyroidism**
DEF: Underproduction of thyroid hormone due to surgical removal of all or part of the thyroid gland.

**244.1 Other postablative hypothyroidism**
Hypothyroidism following therapy, such as irradiation

**244.2 Iodine hypothyroidism**
Hypothyroidism resulting from administration or ingestion of iodide
Use additional E code to identify drug

**244.3 Other iatrogenic hypothyroidism**
Hypothyroidism resulting from:
　P-aminosalicylic acid [PAS]
　Phenylbutazone
　Resorcinol
Iatrogenic hypothyroidism NOS
Use additional E code to identify drug

**244.8 Other specified acquired hypothyroidism**
Secondary hypothyroidism NEC
**AHA:** J-A, '85, 9

---

√4ᵗʰ √5ᵗʰ Additional Digit Required　　　Unacceptable PDx　　　Manifestation Code　　　►◄ Revised Text　　　● New Code　　　▲ Revised Code Title

**Endocrine, Nutritional and Metabolic, Immunity**

**244.9–250.3**

**244.9    Unspecified hypothyroidism**

Hypothyroidism  
Myxedema     } primary or NOS

**AHA:** 3Q, '99, 19; 4Q, '96, 29

**√4th 245   Thyroiditis**

**245.0    Acute thyroiditis**     **CC**

Abscess of thyroid     Thyroiditis:  
Thyroiditis:     pyogenic  
   nonsuppurative, acute     suppurative  
Use additional code to identify organism

**CC Excl:** 245.0-245.9

**DEF:** Inflamed thyroid caused by infection, with abscess and liquid puris.

**245.1    Subacute thyroiditis**

Thyroiditis:     Thyroiditis:  
  de Quervain's     granulomatous  
  giant cell     viral

**DEF:** Inflammation of the thyroid, characterized by fever and painful enlargement of the thyroid gland, with granulomas in the gland.

**245.2    Chronic lymphocytic thyroiditis**

Hashimoto's disease  
Struma lymphomatosa  
Thyroiditis:  
  autoimmune  
  lymphocytic (chronic)

**DEF:** Autoimmune disease of thyroid; lymphocytes infiltrate the gland and thyroid antibodies are produced; women more often affected.

**245.3    Chronic fibrous thyroiditis**

Struma fibrosa     Thyroiditis:  
Thyroiditis:     ligneous  
  invasive (fibrous)     Riedel's

**DEF:** Persistent fibrosing inflammation of thyroid with adhesions to nearby structures; rare condition

**245.4    Iatrogenic thyroiditis**

Use additional code to identify cause  
**DEF:** Thyroiditis resulting from treatment or intervention by physician or in a patient intervention setting.

**245.8    Other and unspecified chronic thyroiditis**

Chronic thyroiditis:  
  NOS  
  nonspecific

**245.9    Thyroiditis, unspecified**

Thyroiditis NOS

**√4th 246   Other disorders of thyroid**

**246.0    Disorders of thyrocalcitonin secretion**

Hypersecretion of calcitonin or thyrocalcitonin

**246.1    Dyshormonogenic goiter**

Congenital (dyshormonogenic) goiter  
Goiter due to enzyme defect in synthesis of thyroid hormone  
Goitrous cretinism (sporadic)

**246.2    Cyst of thyroid**

**EXCLUDES**   cystadenoma of thyroid (226)

**246.3    Hemorrhage and infarction of thyroid**     **CC**

**CC Excl:** 246.3

**246.8    Other specified disorders of thyroid**

Abnormality of thyroid-binding globulin  
Atrophy of thyroid  
Hyper-TBG-nemia  
Hypo-TBG-nemia

**AHA:** 2Q, '06, 5

**246.9    Unspecified disorder of thyroid**

## DISEASES OF OTHER ENDOCRINE GLANDS (250-259)

**√4th 250   Diabetes mellitus**

**EXCLUDES**   gestational diabetes (648.8)  
     hyperglycemia NOS ▶(790.29)◀  
     neonatal diabetes mellitus (775.1)  
     nonclinical diabetes (790.29)

The following fifth-digit subclassification is for use with category 250:

**0 type II or unspecified type, not stated as uncontrolled**  
Fifth-digit 0 is for use for type II patients, even if the patient requires insulin  
Use additional code, if applicable, for associated long-term (current) insulin use V58.67

**1 type I [juvenile type], not stated as uncontrolled**

**2 type II or unspecified type, uncontrolled**  
Fifth-digit 2 is for use for type II patients, even if the patient requires insulin  
Use additional code, if applicable, for associated long-term (current) insulin use V58.67

**3 type I [juvenile type], uncontrolled**

**AHA:** 4Q, '04, 56; 2Q, '04, 17; 2Q, '02, 13; 2Q,'01, 16; 2Q,'98, 15; 4Q, '97, 32; 2Q, '97, 14; 3Q, '96, 5; 4Q, '93, 19; 2Q, '92, 5; 3Q, '91, 3; 2Q, '90, 22; N-D, '85, 11

**DEF:** Diabetes mellitus: Inability to metabolize carbohydrates, proteins, and fats with insufficient secretion of insulin. Symptoms may be unremarkable, with long-term complications, involving kidneys, nerves, blood vessels, and eyes.

**DEF:** Uncontrolled diabetes: A nonspecific term indicating that the current treatment regimen does not keep the blood sugar level of a patient within acceptable levels.

[7] **√5th 250.0   Diabetes mellitus without mention of complication**

Diabetes mellitus without mention of complication or manifestation classifiable to 250.1-250.9  
Diabetes (mellitus) NOS

**AHA:** 1Q, '06, 14; 4Q, '97, 32; 3Q, '91, 3, 12; N-D, '85, 11; **For code 250.00:** 1Q, '05, 15; 4Q, '04, 55; 4Q, '03, 105, 108; 2Q, '03, 16; 1Q, '02, 7, 11; **For code 250.01:** 4Q, '04, 55; 4Q, '03, 110; 2Q, '03, 6; **For code 250.02:** 1Q, '03, 5

**√5th 250.1   Diabetes with ketoacidosis**     **MCC**

Diabetic:  
  acidosis     }  
  ketosis     } without mention of coma

**CC Excl: For code 250.10:** 250.00-251.3, 259.8-259.9; **For code 250.11-250.13:** 250.00-251.3, 259.5-259.9

**AHA:** 3Q, '91, 6; **For code 250.11:** 2Q, '06, 19-20; 4Q, '03, 82; **For code 250.13:** 2Q, '06, 19-20

**DEF:** Diabetic hyperglycemic crisis causing ketone presence in body fluids.

**√5th 250.2   Diabetes with hyperosmolarity**     **MCC**

Hyperosmolar (nonketotic) coma

**CC Excl: For code 250.20:** 250.00-251.3, 259.8-259.9; **For code 250.21-250.23:** 250.00-251.3, 259.5-259.9

**AHA:** 4Q, '93, 19; 3Q, '91, 7

**√5th 250.3   Diabetes with other coma**     **MCC**

Diabetic coma (with ketoacidosis)  
Diabetic hypoglycemic coma  
Insulin coma NOS  
**EXCLUDES**   diabetes with hyperosmolar coma (250.2)

**CC Excl: For code 250.30:** 250.00-251.3, 259.8-259.9; **For code 250.31-250.33:** 250.00-251.3, 259.5-259.9

**AHA:** 3Q, '91, 7, 12

**DEF:** Coma (not hyperosmolar) caused by hyperglycemia or hypoglycemia as complication of diabetes.

---

[7]   Questionable admission = 0

**N** Newborn Age: 0    **P** Pediatric Age: 0-17    **M** Maternity Age: 12-55    **A** Adult Age: 15-124    **CC** CC Condition    **MCC** Major CC Condition    **HIV** HIV Related Dx

**60 — Volume 1 • October 2007**      © **2007 Ingenix**

§ ✓5ᵗʰ **250.4　Diabetes with renal manifestations**
　　　Use additional code to identify manifestation, as:
　　　　chronic kidney disease (585.1-585.9)
　　　　diabetic:
　　　　　nephropathy NOS (583.81)
　　　　　nephrosis (581.81)
　　　　　intercapillary glomerulosclerosis (581.81)
　　　　　Kimmelstiel-Wilson syndrome (581.81)
　　　**AHA:** 3Q, '91, 8, 12; S-O, '87, 9; S-O, '84, 3; **For code 250.40:** 1Q, '03, 20

§ ✓5ᵗʰ **250.5　Diabetes with ophthalmic manifestations**
　　　Use additional code to identify manifestation, as:
　　　　diabetic:
　　　　　blindness (369.00-369.9)
　　　　　cataract (366.41)
　　　　　glaucoma (365.44)
　　　　　macular edema (362.07)
　　　　　retinal edema (362.07)
　　　　　retinopathy (362.01-362.07)
　　　**AHA:**4Q, '05, 65; 3Q, '91, 8; S-O, '85, 11; **For code 250.50:** 4Q, '05, 67

§ ✓5ᵗʰ **250.6　Diabetes with neurological manifestations**
　　　Use additional code to identify manifestation, as:
　　　　diabetic:
　　　　　amyotrophy ▶(353.1)◀
　　　　　gastroparalysis (536.3)
　　　　　gastroparesis (536.3)
　　　　　mononeuropathy (354.0-355.9)
　　　　　neurogenic arthropathy (713.5)
　　　　　peripheral autonomic neuropathy (337.1)
　　　　　polyneuropathy (357.2)
　　　**AHA:** 2Q, '93, 6; 2Q, '92, 15; 3Q, '91, 9; N-D, '84, 9; **For code 250.60:**
　　　　4Q, '03, 105; **For code 250.61:** 2Q, '04, 7

§ ✓5ᵗʰ **250.7　Diabetes with peripheral circulatory disorders**
　　　　Use additional code to identify manifestation, as:
　　　　　diabetic:
　　　　　　gangrene (785.4)
　　　　　　peripheral angiopathy (443.81)
　　　**AHA:** 1Q, '96, 10; 3Q, '94, 5; 2Q, '94, 17; 3Q, '91, 10, 12; 3Q, '90, 15;
　　　　**For code 250.70:** 1Q, '04, 14

　　　**DEF:** Blood vessel damage or disease, usually in the feet, legs, or hands, as a complication of diabetes.

§ ✓5ᵗʰ **250.8　Diabetes with other specified manifestations**
　　　　Diabetic hypoglycemia
　　　　Hypoglycemic shock
　　　　Use additional code to identify manifestation, as:
　　　　　any associated ulceration (707.10-707.9)
　　　　　diabetic bone changes (731.8)
　　　　Use additional E code to identify cause, if drug-induced
　　　**AHA:** 4Q, '00, 44; 4Q, '97, 43; 2Q, '97, 16; 4Q, '93, 20; 3Q, '91, 10;
　　　　**For code 250.80:** 1Q, '04, 14

§ ✓5ᵗʰ **250.9　Diabetes with unspecified complication**
　　　**AHA:** 2Q, '92, 15; 3Q, '91, 7, 12

✓4ᵗʰ **251　Other disorders of pancreatic internal secretion**
　　**251.0　Hypoglycemic coma**　　　　　　　　　　　**cc**
　　　　Iatrogenic hyperinsulinism
　　　　Non-diabetic insulin coma
　　　　Use additional E code to identify cause, if drug-induced
　　　　　**EXCLUDES**　hypoglycemic coma in diabetes mellitus
　　　　　　　　　　　　(250.3)
　　　**CC Excl:** 250.00-251.3, 259.5-259.9

　　　**AHA:** M-A, '85, 8
　　　**DEF:** Coma induced by low blood sugar in non-diabetic patient.

**251.1　Other specified hypoglycemia**
　　Hyperinsulinism:　　　Hyperplasia of pancreatic
　　　NOS　　　　　　　　　　islet beta cells NOS
　　　ectopic
　　　functional
　　　**EXCLUDES**　hypoglycemia:
　　　　　　　　　　in diabetes mellitus (250.8)
　　　　　　　　　　in infant of diabetic mother (775.0)
　　　　　　　　hypoglycemic coma (251.0)
　　　　　　　　neonatal hypoglycemia (775.6)
　　　Use additional E code to identify cause, if drug-induced.
　　**AHA:** 1Q, '03, 10
　　**DEF:** Excessive production of insulin by the pancreas; associated with obesity and insulin-producing tumors.

**251.2　Hypoglycemia, unspecified**
　　Hypoglycemia:　　　Hypoglycemia:
　　　NOS　　　　　　　　spontaneous
　　　reactive
　　　**EXCLUDES**　hypoglycemia:
　　　　　　　　　　with coma (251.0)
　　　　　　　　　　in diabetes mellitus (250.8)
　　　　　　　　　　leucine-induced (270.3)
　　**AHA:** M-A, '85, 8

**251.3　Postsurgical hypoinsulinemia**　　　　　**cc**
　　Hypoinsulinemia following complete or partial pancreatectomy
　　Postpancreatectomy hyperglycemia
　　**CC Excl:** See code: 251.0
　　**AHA:** 3Q, '91, 6

**251.4　Abnormality of secretion of glucagon**
　　Hyperplasia of pancreatic islet alpha cells with glucagon excess
　　**DEF:** Production malfunction of a pancreatic hormone secreted by cells of the islets of Langerhans.

**251.5　Abnormality of secretion of gastrin**
　　Hyperplasia of pancreatic alpha cells with gastrin excess
　　Zollinger-Ellison syndrome

**251.8　Other specified disorders of pancreatic internal secretion**
　　**AHA:** 2Q, '98, 15; 3Q, '91, 6

**251.9　Unspecified disorder of pancreatic internal secretion**
　　Islet cell hyperplasia NOS

✓4ᵗʰ **252　Disorders of parathyroid gland**
✓5ᵗʰ **252.0　Hyperparathyroidism**
　　　**EXCLUDES**　ectopic hyperparathyroidism (259.3)
　　**DEF:** Abnormally high secretion of parathyroid hormones causing bone deterioration, reduced renal function, kidney stones.

　　**252.00　Hyperparathyroidism, unspecified**
　　**252.01　Primary hyperparathyroidism**
　　　　Hyperplasia of parathyroid
　　　**DEF:** Parathyroid dysfunction commonly caused by hyperplasia of two or more glands; characteristic hypercalcemia and increased parathyroid hormone levels.

**Dorsal View of Parathyroid Glands**

Pharynx　　　　　　　　　Thyroid gland

Parathyroid glands

Trachea　　　　　　　　　Esophagus

Parathyroid glands
Parathyroid hormone (PTH)
Calcium in bones ──────── Calcium in blood

---

§　Requires fifth-digit.　See beginning of category 250 for codes and definitions.

✓4ᵗʰ ✓5ᵗʰ Additional Digit Required　　　Unacceptable PDx　　　Manifestation Code　　　▶◀ Revised Text　　　● New Code　　　▲ Revised Code Title

**Endocrine, Nutritional and Metabolic, Immunity**

**252.02–254.9**

**252.02 Secondary hyperparathyroidism, non-renal**

> **EXCLUDES**    secondary hyperpara-
> thyroidism (of renal
> origin) (588.81)

**AHA:** 4Q, '04, 57-59

**DEF:** Underlying disease of nonrenal origin decreases blood levels of calcium causing the parathyroid to release increased levels of parathyroid hormone; parathyroid hormone levels return to normal once underlying condition is treated and blood calcium levels are normal.

**252.08 Other hyperparathyroidism**

Tertiary hyperparathyroidism

**DEF:** Tertiary hyperparathyroidism: chronic secondary hyperparathyroidism leads to adenomatous parathyroid causing irreversible abnormal production of parathyroid hormone (PTH); PTH remains high after the serum calcium levels are brought under control.

**252.1 Hypoparathyroidism**

Parathyroiditis (autoimmune)
Tetany:
    parathyroid
    parathyroprival

> **EXCLUDES**    pseudohypoparathyroidism (275.4)
> pseudopseudohypoparathyroidism (275.4)
> tetany NOS (781.7)
> transitory neonatal
> hypoparathyroidism (775.4)

**DEF:** Abnormally low secretion of parathyroid hormones which causes decreased calcium and increased phosphorus in the blood. Resulting in muscle cramps, tetany, urinary frequency and cataracts.

**252.8 Other specified disorders of parathyroid gland**

Cyst ⎫
Hemorrhage ⎬ of parathyroid gland

**252.9 Unspecified disorder of parathyroid gland**

√4ᵗʰ **253 Disorders of the pituitary gland and its hypothalamic control**

> **INCLUDES**    the listed conditions whether the disorder is in the pituitary or the hypothalamus
> **EXCLUDES**    Cushing's syndrome (255.0)

**253.0 Acromegaly and gigantism**

Overproduction of growth hormone

**DEF:** Acromegaly: chronic, beginning in middle age; caused by hypersecretion of the pituitary growth hormone; produces enlarged parts of skeleton, especially the nose, ears, jaws, fingers and toes.

**DEF:** Gigantism: pituitary gigantism caused by excess growth of short flat bones; men may grow 78 to 80 inches tall.

**253.1 Other and unspecified anterior pituitary hyperfunction**    `CC`

Forbes-Albright syndrome

> **EXCLUDES**    overproduction of:
> ACTH (255.3)
> thyroid-stimulating hormone [TSH] (242.8)

**CC Excl:** 253.1, 253.4, 253.6

**AHA:** J-A, '85, 9

**DEF:** Spontaneous galactorrhea-amenorrhea syndrome unrelated to pregnancy; usually related to presence of pituitary tumor.

**253.2 Panhypopituitarism**    `CC`

Cachexia, pituitary
Necrosis of pituitary (postpartum)
Pituitary insufficiency NOS
Sheehan's syndrome
Simmonds' disease

> **EXCLUDES**    iatrogenic hypopituitarism (253.7)

**CC Excl:** 253.0-253.9, 259.5-259.9

**DEF:** Damage to or absence of pituitary gland leading to impaired sexual function, weight loss, fatigue, bradycardia, hypotension, pallor, depression, and impaired growth in children; called Simmonds' disease if cachexia is prominent.

**253.3 Pituitary dwarfism**

Isolated deficiency of (human) growth hormone [HGH]
Lorain-Levi dwarfism

**DEF:** Dwarfism with infantile physical characteristics due to abnormally low secretion of growth hormone and gonadotropin deficiency.

**253.4 Other anterior pituitary disorders**

Isolated or partial deficiency of an anterior pituitary hormone, other than growth hormone
Prolactin deficiency

**AHA:** J-A, '85, 9

**253.5 Diabetes insipidus**    `CC`

Vasopressin deficiency

> **EXCLUDES**    nephrogenic diabetes insipidus (588.1)

**CC Excl:** 253.1-253.2, 253.4-253.9, 259.5-259.9

**DEF:** Metabolic disorder causing insufficient antidiuretic hormone release; symptoms include frequent urination, thirst, ravenous hunger, loss of weight, fatigue.

**253.6 Other disorders of neurohypophysis**    `CC`

Syndrome of inappropriate secretion of antidiuretic hormone [ADH]

> **EXCLUDES**    ectopic antidiuretic hormone secretion (259.3)

**CC Excl:** 253.0-253.9, 259.8-259.9

**253.7 Iatrogenic pituitary disorders**

Hypopituitarism:      Hypopituitarism:
  hormone-induced      postablative
  hypophysectomy-induced    radiotherapy-induced
Use additional E code to identify cause

**DEF:** Pituitary dysfunction that results from drug therapy, radiation therapy, or surgery, causing mild to severe symptoms.

**253.8 Other disorders of the pituitary and other syndromes of diencephalohypophyseal origin**

Abscess of pituitary      Cyst of Rathke's pouch
Adiposogenital dystrophy    Fröhlich's syndrome

> **EXCLUDES**    craniopharyngioma (237.0)

**253.9 Unspecified**

Dyspituitarism

√4ᵗʰ **254 Diseases of thymus gland**

> **EXCLUDES**    aplasia or dysplasia with immunodeficiency (279.2)
> hypoplasia with immunodeficiency (279.2)
> myasthenia gravis (358.00-358.01)

**254.0 Persistent hyperplasia of thymus**

Hypertrophy of thymus

**DEF:** Continued abnormal growth of the twin lymphoid lobes that produce T lymphocytes.

**254.1 Abscess of thymus**    `CC`

**CC Excl:** 254.0-254.9, 259.5-259.9

**254.8 Other specified diseases of thymus gland**

Atrophy ⎫
Cyst ⎬ of thymus

> **EXCLUDES**    thymoma (212.6)

**254.9 Unspecified disease of thymus gland**

---

| ⓝ Newborn Age: 0 | ⓟ Pediatric Age: 0-17 | ⓜ Maternity Age: 12-55 | ⓐ Adult Age: 15-124 | `CC` CC Condition | `MCC` Major CC Condition | `HIV` HIV Related Dx |

**✓4th 255 Disorders of adrenal glands**

INCLUDES    the listed conditions whether the basic disorder is in the adrenals or is pituitary-induced

**255.0 Cushing's syndrome**   CC
Adrenal hyperplasia due to excess ACTH
Cushing's syndrome:
NOS
iatrogenic
idiopathic
pituitary-dependent
Ectopic ACTH syndrome
Iatrogenic syndrome of excess cortisol
Overproduction of cortisol
Use additional E code to identify cause, if drug-induced
EXCLUDES   *congenital adrenal hyperplasia (255.2)*

CC Excl: 255.0-255.2, 259.5-259.9

DEF: Due to adrenal cortisol oversecretion or glucocorticoid medications; may cause fatty tissue of the face, neck and body; osteoporosis and curvature of spine, hypertension, diabetes mellitus, female genitourinary problems, male impotence, degeneration of muscle tissues, weakness.

**✓5th 255.1 Hyperaldosteronism**
AHA: 4Q, '03, 48
DEF: Oversecretion of aldosterone causing fluid retention, hypertension.

**255.10 Hyperaldosteronism, unspecified**
Aldosteronism NOS
Primary aldosteronism, unspecified
EXCLUDES   *Conn's syndrome (255.12)*

**255.11 Glucocorticoid-remediable aldosteronism**
Familial aldosteronism type I
EXCLUDES   *Conn's syndrome (255.12)*
DEF: A rare autosomal dominant familial form of primary aldosteronism in which the secretion of aldosterone is under the influence of adrenocortiotrophic hormone (ACTH) rather than the renin-angiotensin mechanism; characterized by moderate hypersecretion of aldosterone and suppressed plasma renin activity rapidly reversed by administration of glucosteroids; symptoms include hypertension and mild hypokalemia.

**255.12 Conn's syndrome**
DEF: A type of primary aldosteronism caused by an adenoma of the glomerulosa cells in the adrenal cortex; presence of hypertension.

**255.13 Bartter's syndrome**
DEF: A cluster of symptoms caused by a defect in the ability of the kidney to reabsorb potassium; signs include alkalosis (hypokalemic alkalosis), increased aldosterone, increased plasma renin, and normal blood pressure; symptoms include muscle cramping, weakness, constipation, frequency of urination, and failure to grow; also known as urinary potassium wasting or juxtaglomerular cell hyperplasia.

**255.14 Other secondary aldosteronism**
AHA: 3Q, '06, 24

**255.2 Adrenogenital disorders**
Achard-Thiers syndrome
Adrenogenital syndromes, virilizing or feminizing, whether acquired or associated with congenital adrenal hyperplasia consequent on inborn enzyme defects in hormone synthesis
Congenital adrenal hyperplasia
Female adrenal pseudohermaphroditism
Male:
macrogenitosomia praecox
sexual precocity with adrenal hyperplasia
Virilization (female) (suprarenal)
EXCLUDES   *adrenal hyperplasia due to excess ACTH (255.0)*
*isosexual virilization (256.4)*

**255.3 Other corticoadrenal overactivity**   CC
Acquired benign adrenal androgenic overactivity
Overproduction of ACTH
CC Excl: 017.60-017.66, 017.90-017.96, 255.3, 255.41-255.9, 259.5-259.9

**✓5th 255.4 Corticoadrenal insufficiency**
EXCLUDES   *tuberculous Addison's disease (017.6)*
AHA: 3Q, '06, 24
DEF: Underproduction of adrenal hormones causing low blood pressure.

**255.41 Glucocorticoid deficiency**   CC
Addisonian crisis
Addison's disease NOS
Adrenal atrophy (autoimmune)
Adrenal calcification
Adrenal crisis
Adrenal hemorrhage
Adrenal infarction
Adrenal insufficiency NOS
Combined glucocorticoid and mineralocorticoid deficiency
Corticoadrenal insufficiency NOS
CC Excl: See code: 255.3

**255.42 Mineralocorticoid deficiency**   CC
Hypoaldosteronism
EXCLUDES   *combined glucocorticoid and mineralocorticoid deficiency (255.41)*
CC Excl: See code: 255.3

**255.5 Other adrenal hypofunction**   CC
Adrenal medullary insufficiency
EXCLUDES   *Waterhouse-Friderichsen syndrome (meningococcal) (036.3)*
CC Excl: See code 255.3

**255.6 Medulloadrenal hyperfunction**   CC
Catecholamine secretion by pheochromocytoma
CC Excl: See code 255.3

**255.8 Other specified disorders of adrenal glands**
Abnormality of cortisol-binding globulin

**255.9 Unspecified disorder of adrenal glands**

**✓4th 256 Ovarian dysfunction**
AHA: 4Q, '00, 51

**256.0 Hyperestrogenism**   ♀
DEF: Excess secretion of estrogen by the ovaries; characterized by ovaries containing multiple follicular cysts filled with serous fluid.

**256.1 Other ovarian hyperfunction**   ♀
Hypersecretion of ovarian androgens
AHA: 3Q, '95, 15

**256.2 Postablative ovarian failure**   ♀
Ovarian failure:    Ovarian failure:
iatrogenic      postsurgical
postirradiation
Use additional code for states associated with artificial menopause (627.4)
EXCLUDES   *acquired absence of ovary (V45.77)*
*asymptomatic age-related (natural) postmenopausal status (V49.81)*
AHA: 2Q, '02, 12
DEF: Failed ovarian function after medical or surgical intervention.

**✓5th 256.3 Other ovarian failure**
Use additional code for states associated with natural menopause (627.2)
EXCLUDES   *asymptomatic age-related (natural) postmenopausal status (V49.81)*
AHA: 4Q, '01, 41

**256.31 Premature menopause**   A ♀
DEF: Permanent cessation of ovarian function before the age of 40 occuring naturally of unknown cause.

**256.39 Other ovarian failure**   ♀
Delayed menarche
Ovarian hypofunction
Primary ovarian failure NOS

**256.4 Polycystic ovaries**   ♀
Isosexual virilization    Stein-Leventhal syndrome
DEF: Multiple serous filled cysts of ovary; symptoms of infertility, hirsutism, oligomenorrhea or amenorrhea.

---

✓4th ✓5th Additional Digit Required     Unacceptable PDx     Manifestation Code     ►◄ Revised Text     ● New Code     ▲ Revised Code Title

**256.8** Other ovarian dysfunction ♀

**256.9** Unspecified ovarian dysfunction ♀

✓4ᵗʰ **257 Testicular dysfunction**

**257.0** Testicular hyperfunction ♂
Hypersecretion of testicular hormones

**257.1** Postablative testicular hypofunction ♂
Testicular hypofunction: Testicular hypofunction:
iatrogenic                        postsurgical
postirradiation

**257.2** Other testicular hypofunction
Defective biosynthesis of testicular androgen
Eunuchoidism:
NOS
hypogonadotropic
Failure:
Leydig's cell, adult
seminiferous tubule, adult
Testicular hypogonadism
EXCLUDES *azoospermia (606.0)*

**257.8** Other testicular dysfunction
EXCLUDES *androgen insensitivity syndrome (259.5)*

**257.9** Unspecified testicular dysfunction ♂

✓4ᵗʰ **258 Polyglandular dysfunction and related disorders**

✓5ᵗʰ **258.0** Polyglandular activity in multiple endocrine adenomatosis
▶Multiple endocrine neoplasia [MEN] syndromes
Use additional codes to identify any malignancies and other conditions associated with the syndromes◀

● **258.01 Multiple endocrine neoplasia [MEN] type I**
Wermer's syndrome
DEF: Wermer's syndrome: A rare hereditary condition characterized by the presence of adenomas or hyperplasia in more than one endocrine gland causing premature aging.

● **258.02 Multiple endocrine neoplasia [MEN] type IIA**
Sipple's syndrome

● **258.03 Multiple endocrine neoplasia [MEN] type IIB**

**258.1** Other combinations of endocrine dysfunction
Lloyd's syndrome
Schmidt's syndrome

**258.8** Other specified polyglandular dysfunction

**258.9** Polyglandular dysfunction, unspecified

✓4ᵗʰ **259 Other endocrine disorders**

**259.0** Delay in sexual development and puberty, not elsewhere classified
Delayed puberty

**259.1** Precocious sexual development and puberty, not elsewhere classified ℙ
Sexual precocity:   Sexual precocity:
NOS                    cryptogenic
constitutional          idiopathic

**259.2** Carcinoid syndrome CC
Hormone secretion by carcinoid tumors
CC Excl: 259.2-259.3, 259.5-259.9

DEF: Presence of carcinoid tumors that spread to liver; characterized by cyanotic flushing of skin, diarrhea, bronchospasm, acquired tricuspid and pulmonary stenosis, sudden drops in blood pressure, edema, ascites.

**259.3** Ectopic hormone secretion, not elsewhere classified
Ectopic:
antidiuretic hormone secretion [ADH]
hyperparathyroidism
EXCLUDES *ectopic ACTH syndrome (255.0)*
AHA: N-D, '85, 4

**259.4** Dwarfism, not elsewhere classified
Dwarfism:
NOS
constitutional
EXCLUDES *dwarfism:*
*achondroplastic (756.4)*
*intrauterine (759.7)*
*nutritional (263.2)*
*pituitary (253.3)*
*renal (588.0)*
*progeria (259.8)*

**259.5** Androgen insensitivity syndrome
Partial androgen insensitivity
Reifenstein syndrome
AHA: 4Q, '05, 53
DEF: X chromosome abnormality that prohibits the body from recognizing androgen; XY genotype with ambiguous genitalia; also called testicular feminization.

**259.8** Other specified endocrine disorders
Pineal gland dysfunction   Werner's syndrome
Progeria

**259.9** Unspecified endocrine disorder
Disturbance:          Infantilism NOS
endocrine NOS
hormone NOS

## NUTRITIONAL DEFICIENCIES (260-269)
EXCLUDES *deficiency anemias (280.0-281.9)*

**260 Kwashiorkor** MCC
Nutritional edema with dyspigmentation of skin and hair
CC Excl: 260-263.9

DEF: Syndrome, particularly of children; excessive carbohydrate with inadequate protein intake, inhibited growth potential, anomalies in skin and hair pigmentation, edema and liver disease.

**261 Nutritional marasmus** MCC
Nutritional atrophy
Severe calorie deficiency
Severe malnutrition NOS
CC Excl: See code 260

AHA: 3Q, '06, 14; 2Q, '06, 12

DEF: Protein-calorie malabsorption or malnutrition of children; characterized by tissue wasting, dehydration, and subcutaneous fat depletion; may occur with infectious disease; also called infantile atrophy.

**262 Other severe, protein-calorie malnutrition** MCC
Nutritional edema without mention of dyspigmentation of skin and hair
CC Excl: See code 260

AHA: 4Q, '92, 24; J-A, '85, 12

✓4ᵗʰ **263 Other and unspecified protein-calorie malnutrition**
AHA: 4Q, '92, 24

**263.0** Malnutrition of moderate degree
AHA: J-A, '85, 1
DEF: Malnutrition characterized by biochemical changes in electrolytes, lipids, blood plasma.

**263.1** Malnutrition of mild degree
AHA: J-A, '85, 1

**263.2** Arrested development following protein-calorie malnutrition CC
Nutritional dwarfism
Physical retardation due to malnutrition
CC Excl: See code 260

**263.8** Other protein-calorie malnutrition CC
CC Excl: See code 260

**263.9** Unspecified protein-calorie malnutrition CC
Dystrophy due to malnutrition
Malnutrition (calorie) NOS
EXCLUDES *nutritional deficiency NOS (269.9)*
CC Excl: See code 260

AHA: 4Q, '03, 109; N-D, '84, 19

---

Ⓝ Newborn Age: 0    ℙ Pediatric Age: 0-17    Ⓜ Maternity Age: 12-55    Ⓐ Adult Age: 15-124    CC CC Condition    MCC Major CC Condition    HIV HIV Related Dx

✓4ᵗʰ **264 Vitamin A deficiency**

**264.0 With conjunctival xerosis**
DEF: Vitamin A deficiency with conjunctival dryness.

**264.1 With conjunctival xerosis and Bitot's spot**
Bitot's spot in the young child
DEF: Vitamin A deficiency with conjunctival dryness, superficial spots of keratinized epithelium.

**264.2 With corneal xerosis**
DEF: Vitamin A deficiency with corneal dryness.

**264.3 With corneal ulceration and xerosis**
DEF: Vitamin A deficiency with corneal dryness, epithelial ulceration.

**264.4 With keratomalacia**
DEF: Vitamin A deficiency creating corneal dryness; progresses to corneal insensitivity, softness, necrosis; usually bilateral.

**264.5 With night blindness**
DEF: Vitamin A deficiency causing vision failure in dim light.

**264.6 With xerophthalmic scars of cornea**
DEF: Vitamin A deficiency with corneal scars from dryness.

**264.7 Other ocular manifestations of vitamin A deficiency**
Xerophthalmia due to vitamin A deficiency

**264.8 Other manifestations of vitamin A deficiency**
Follicular keratosis ⎫ due to vitamin A
Xeroderma ⎬ deficiency

**264.9 Unspecified vitamin A deficiency**
Hypovitaminosis A NOS

✓4ᵗʰ **265 Thiamine and niacin deficiency states**

**265.0 Beriberi**      **cc**
CC Excl: 265.0-266.9, 269.1-269.9

DEF: Inadequate vitamin B$_1$ (thiamine) intake, affects heart and peripheral nerves; individual may become edematous and develop cardiac disease due to the excess fluid; alcoholics and people with a diet of excessive polished rice prone to the disease.

**265.1 Other and unspecified manifestations of**  **cc**
**thiamine deficiency**
Other vitamin B$_1$ deficiency states
CC Excl: See code: 265.0

**265.2 Pellagra**
Deficiency:      Deficiency:
niacin (-tryptophan)   vitamin PP
nicotinamide       Pellagra (alcoholic)
nicotinic acid
DEF: Niacin deficiency causing dermatitis, inflammation of mucous membranes, diarrhea, and psychic disturbances.

✓4ᵗʰ **266 Deficiency of B-complex components**

**266.0 Ariboflavinosis**      **cc**
Riboflavin [vitamin B$_2$] deficiency
CC Excl: See code: 265.0

AHA: S-O, '86, 10
DEF: Vitamin B$_2$ (riboflavin) deficiency marked by swollen lips and tongue fissures, corneal vascularization, scaling lesions, and anemia.

**266.1 Vitamin B$_6$ deficiency**
Deficiency:      Deficiency:
pyridoxal        pyridoxine
pyridoxamine    Vitamin B$_6$ deficiency
             syndrome
EXCLUDES   *vitamin B$_6$-responsive sideroblastic anemia (285.0)*
DEF: Vitamin B$_6$ deficiency causing skin, lip, and tongue disturbances, peripheral neuropathy; and convulsions in infants.

**266.2 Other B-complex deficiencies**
Deficiency:      Deficiency:
cyanocobalamin   vitamin B$_{12}$
folic acid
EXCLUDES   *combined system disease with anemia (281.0-281.1)*
*deficiency anemias (281.0-281.9)*
*subacute degeneration of spinal cord with anemia (281.0-281.1)*

**266.9 Unspecified vitamin B deficiency**

**267 Ascorbic acid deficiency**
Deficiency of vitamin C    Scurvy
EXCLUDES   *scorbutic anemia (281.8)*
DEF: Vitamin C deficiency causing swollen gums, myalgia, weight loss, and weakness.

✓4ᵗʰ **268 Vitamin D deficiency**
EXCLUDES   *vitamin D-resistant:*
*osteomalacia (275.3)*
*rickets (275.3)*

**268.0 Rickets, active**      **cc**
EXCLUDES   *celiac rickets (579.0)*
*renal rickets (588.0)*

CC Excl: 268.0-269.9

DEF: Inadequate vitamin D intake, usually in pediatrics, that affects bones most involved with muscular action; may cause nodules on ends and sides of bones; delayed closure of fontanels in infants; symptoms may include muscle soreness, and profuse sweating.

**268.1 Rickets, late effect**
Any condition specified as due to rickets and stated to be a late effect or sequela of rickets
▶Code first the nature of late effect◀
DEF: Distorted or demineralized bones as a result of vitamin D deficiency.

**268.2 Osteomalacia, unspecified**
DEF: Softening of bones due to decrease in calcium; marked by pain, tenderness, muscular weakness, anorexia, and weight loss.

**268.9 Unspecified vitamin D deficiency**
Avitaminosis D

✓4ᵗʰ **269 Other nutritional deficiencies**

**269.0 Deficiency of vitamin K**
EXCLUDES   *deficiency of coagulation factor due to vitamin K deficiency (286.7)*
*vitamin K deficiency of newborn (776.0)*

**269.1 Deficiency of other vitamins**
Deficiency:      Deficiency:
vitamin E       vitamin P

**269.2 Unspecified vitamin deficiency**
Multiple vitamin deficiency NOS

**269.3 Mineral deficiency, not elsewhere classified**
Deficiency:      Deficiency:
calcium, dietary   iodine
EXCLUDES   *deficiency:*
*calcium NOS (275.4)*
*potassium (276.8)*
*sodium (276.1)*

**269.8 Other nutritional deficiency**
EXCLUDES   *adult failure to thrive (783.7)*
*failure to thrive in childhood (783.41)*
*feeding problems (783.3)*
*newborn (779.3)*

**269.9 Unspecified nutritional deficiency**

## OTHER METABOLIC AND IMMUNITY DISORDERS (270-279)
Use additional code to identify any associated mental retardation

✓4ᵗʰ **270 Disorders of amino-acid transport and metabolism**
EXCLUDES   *abnormal findings without manifest disease (790.0-796.9)*
*disorders of purine and pyrimidine metabolism (277.1-277.2)*
*gout (274.0-274.9)*

**270.0 Disturbances of amino-acid transport**  **cc**
Cystinosis      Glycinuria (renal)
Cystinuria      Hartnup disease
Fanconi (-de Toni) (-Debré) syndrome
CC Excl: 270.0-273.3, 273.8-273.9

**270.1 Phenylketonuria [PKU]**    **cc**
Hyperphenylalaninemia
CC Excl: See code: 270.0

DEF: Inherited metabolic condition causing excess phenylpyruvic and other acids in urine; results in mental retardation, neurological manifestations, including spasticity and tremors, light pigmentation, eczema, and mousy odor.

**Endocrine, Nutritional and Metabolic, Immunity**

**270.2–272.1**

**270.2** **Other disturbances of aromatic amino-acid** `CC`
**metabolism**

Albinism     Hypertyrosinemia
Alkaptonuria     Indicanuria
Alkaptonuric ochronosis     Kynureninase defects
Disturbances of metabolism   Oasthouse urine disease
   of tyrosine and     Ochronosis
   tryptophan     Tyrosinosis
Homogentisic acid defects   Tyrosinuria
Hydroxykynureninuria    Waardenburg syndrome

**EXCLUDES** *vitamin B₆-deficiency syndrome (266.1)*

*vitamin $B_6$-deficiency syndrome (266.1)*

**CC Excl:** See code: 270.0

**AHA:** 3Q, '99, 20

**270.3** **Disturbances of branched-chain amino-acid** `CC`
**metabolism**

Disturbances of metabolism of leucine, isoleucine,
   and valine
Hypervalinemia
Intermittent branched-chain ketonuria
Leucine-induced hypoglycemia
Leucinosis
Maple syrup urine disease

**CC Excl:** See code: 270.0

**AHA:** 3Q, '00, 8

**270.4** **Disturbances of sulphur-bearing amino-acid** `CC`
**metabolism**

Cystathioninemia
Cystathioninuria
Disturbances of metabolism of methionine,
   homocystine, and cystathionine
Homocystinuria
Hypermethioninemia
Methioninemia

**CC Excl:** See code: 270.0

**AHA:** ▶2Q, '07, 7;◀1Q, '04, 6

**270.5** **Disturbances of histidine metabolism** `CC`

Carnosinemia     Hyperhistidinemia
Histidinemia     Imidazole aminoaciduria

**CC Excl:** See code: 270.0

**270.6** **Disorders of urea cycle metabolism** `CC`

Argininosuccinic aciduria
Citrullinemia
Disorders of metabolism of ornithine, citrulline,
   argininosuccinic acid, arginine, and ammonia
Hyperammonemia
Hyperomithinemia

**CC Excl:** See code: 270.0

**270.7** **Other disturbances of straight-chain** `CC`
**amino-acid metabolism**

Glucoglycinuria
Glycinemia (with methyl-malonic acidemia)
Hyperglycinemia
Hyperlysinemia
Other disturbances of metabolism of glycine,
   threonine, serine, glutamine, and lysine
Pipecolic acidemia
Saccharopinuria

**CC Excl:** See code: 270.0

**AHA:** 3Q, '00, 8

**Lipid Metabolism**

**270.8** **Other specified disorders of amino-acid** `CC`
**metabolism**

Alaninemia     Iminoacidopathy
Ethanolaminuria    Prolinemia
Glycoprolinuria     Prolinuria
Hydroxyprolinemia   Sarcosinemia
Hyperprolinemia

**CC Excl:** See code: 270.0

**270.9** **Unspecified disorder of amino-acid metabolism** `CC`

**CC Excl:** See code: 270.0

✓4ᵗʰ **271 Disorders of carbohydrate transport and metabolism**

**EXCLUDES** *abnormality of secretion of glucagon (251.4)*
*diabetes mellitus (250.0-250.9)*
*hypoglycemia NOS (251.2)*
*mucopolysaccharidosis (277.5)*

**271.0** **Glycogenosis** `CC`

Amylopectinosis
Glucose-6-phosphatase deficiency
Glycogen storage disease
McArdle's disease
Pompe's disease
von Gierke's disease

**CC Excl:** 270.0-273.3, 273.8-273.9

**AHA:** 1Q, '98, 5

**271.1** **Galactosemia** `CC`

Galactose-1-phosphate uridyl transferase deficiency
Galactosuria

**CC Excl:** See code: 271.0

**DEF:** Any of three genetic disorders due to defective galactose
metabolism; symptoms include failure to thrive in infancy, jaundice,
liver and spleen damage, cataracts, and mental retardation.

**271.2** **Hereditary fructose intolerance**

Essential benign fructosuria    Fructosemia
**DEF:** Chromosome recessive disorder of carbohydrate metabolism;
in infants, occurs after dietary sugar introduced; characterized by
enlarged spleen, yellowish cast to skin, and progressive inability
to thrive.

**271.3** **Intestinal disaccharidase deficiencies and**
**disaccharide malabsorption**

Intolerance or malabsorption (congenital) (of):
   glucose-galactose
   lactose
   sucrose-isomaltose

**271.4** **Renal glycosuria**

Renal diabetes
**DEF:** Persistent abnormal levels of glucose in urine, with normal
blood glucose levels; caused by failure of the renal tubules to
reabsorb glucose.

**271.8** **Other specified disorders of carbohydrate** `CC`
**transport and metabolism**

Essential benign pentosuria   Mannosidosis
Fucosidosis     Oxalosis
Glycolic aciduria    Xylosuria
Hyperoxaluria (primary)   Xylulosuria

**CC Excl:** See code: 271.0

**271.9** **Unspecified disorder of carbohydrate transport**
**and metabolism**

✓4ᵗʰ **272 Disorders of lipid metabolism**

**EXCLUDES** *localized cerebral lipidoses (330.1)*

**272.0** **Pure hypercholesterolemia**

Familial hypercholesterolemia
Fredrickson Type IIa hyperlipoproteinemia
Hyperbetalipoproteinemia
Hyperlipidemia, Group A
Low-density-lipoid-type [LDL] hyperlipoproteinemia

**AHA:** 4Q, '05, 71

**272.1** **Pure hyperglyceridemia**

Endogenous hyperglyceridemia
Fredrickson Type IV hyperlipoproteinemia
Hyperlipidemia, Group B
Hyperprebetalipoproteinemia
Hypertriglyceridemia, essential
Very-low-density-lipoid-type [VLDL]
   hyperlipoproteinemia

---

`N` Newborn Age: 0    `P` Pediatric Age: 0-17    `M` Maternity Age: 12-55    `A` Adult Age: 15-124    `CC` CC Condition    `MCC` Major CC Condition    `HIV` HIV Related Dx

**272.2   Mixed hyperlipidemia**
Broad- or floating-betalipoproteinemia
Fredrickson Type IIb or III hyperlipoproteinemia
Hypercholesterolemia with endogenous
hyperglyceridemia
Hyperbetalipoproteinemia with
prebetalipoproteinemia
Tubo-eruptive xanthoma
Xanthoma tuberosum
DEF: Elevated levels of lipoprotein, a complex of fats and proteins,
in blood due to inherited metabolic disorder.

**272.3   Hyperchylomicronemia**
Bürger-Grütz syndrome
Fredrickson type I or V hyperlipoproteinemia
Hyperlipidemia, Group D
Mixed hyperglyceridemia

**272.4   Other and unspecified hyperlipidemia**
Alpha-lipoproteinemia
Combined hyperlipidemia
Hyperlipidemia NOS
Hyperlipoproteinemia NOS

**AHA:** 1Q, '05, 17

DEF: Hyperlipoproteinemia: elevated levels of transient
chylomicrons in the blood which are a form of lipoproteins which
transport dietary cholesterol and triglycerides from the small
intestine to the blood.

**272.5   Lipoprotein deficiencies**
Abetalipoproteinemia
Bassen-Kornzweig syndrome
High-density lipoid deficiency
Hypoalphalipoproteinemia
Hypobetalipoproteinemia (familial)
DEF: Abnormally low levels of lipoprotein, a complex of fats and
protein, in the blood.

**272.6   Lipodystrophy**
Barraquer-Simons disease
Progressive lipodystrophy
Use additional E code to identify cause, if iatrogenic
*EXCLUDES*   intestinal lipodystrophy (040.2)
DEF: Disturbance of fat metabolism resulting in loss of fatty tissue
in some areas of the body.

**272.7   Lipidoses**
Chemically-induced lipidosis
Disease:
Anderson's
Fabry's
Gaucher's
I cell [mucolipidosis I]
lipoid storage NOS
Niemann-Pick
pseudo-Hurler's or mucolipdosis III
triglyceride storage, Type I or II
Wolman's or triglyceride storage, Type III
Mucolipidosis II
Primary familial xanthomatosis
*EXCLUDES*   cerebral lipidoses (330.1)
Tay-Sachs disease (330.1)
DEF: Lysosomal storage diseases marked by an abnormal amount of
lipids in reticuloendothelial cells.

**272.8   Other disorders of lipoid metabolism**
Hoffa's disease or liposynovitis prepatellaris
Launois-Bensaude's lipomatosis
Lipoid dermatoarthritis

**272.9   Unspecified disorder of lipoid metabolism**

✓4th **273   Disorders of plasma protein metabolism**
*EXCLUDES*   agammaglobulinemia and
hypogammaglobulinemia (279.0-279.2)
coagulation defects (286.0-286.9)
hereditary hemolytic anemias (282.0-282.9)

**273.0   Polyclonal hypergammaglobulinemia**
Hypergammaglobulinemic purpura:
benign primary
Waldenström's
DEF: Elevated blood levels of gamma globulins, frequently found in
patients with chronic infectious diseases.

**273.1   Monoclonal paraproteinemia**
Benign monoclonal hypergammaglobulinemia [BMH]
Monoclonal gammopathy:
NOS
associated with lymphoplasmacytic dyscrasias
benign
Paraproteinemia:
benign (familial)
secondary to malignant or inflammatory disease

**273.2   Other paraproteinemias**
Cryoglobulinemic:   Mixed cryoglobulinemia
purpura
vasculitis

**273.3   Macroglobulinemia**
Macroglobulinemia (idiopathic) (primary)
Waldenström's macroglobulinemia
DEF: Elevated blood levels of macroglobulins (plasma globulins of
high weight); characterized by malignant neoplasms of bone
marrow, spleen, liver, or lymph nodes; symptoms include
weakness, fatigue, bleeding disorders, and vision problems.

**273.4   Alpha-1-antitrypsin deficiency**
AAT deficiency
DEF: Disorder of plasma protein metabolism that results in a
deficiency of Alpha-1-antitrypsin, an acute-phase reactive protein,
released into the blood in response to infection or injury to protect
tissue against the harmful effect of enzymes.

**273.8   Other disorders of plasma protein metabolism**
Abnormality of transport protein
Bisalbuminemia
**AHA:** 2Q, '98, 11

**273.9   Unspecified disorder of plasma protein metabolism**

✓4th **274   Gout**
*EXCLUDES*   lead gout (984.0-984.9)

**AHA:** 2Q, '95, 4

DEF: Purine and pyrimidine metabolic disorders; manifested by hyperuricemia
and recurrent acute inflammatory arthritis; monosodium urate or monohydrate
crystals may be deposited in and around the joints, leading to joint
destruction, and severe crippling.

**274.0   Gouty arthropathy**
✓5th **274.1   Gouty nephropathy**
**274.10   Gouty nephropathy, unspecified**
**AHA:** N-D, '85, 15

**274.11   Uric acid nephrolithiasis**   CC
**CC Excl:** 016.00-016.06, 016.30-016.36, 016.90-016.96,
017.90-017.96, 078.6, 098.10, 098.19, 098.30-098.31, 098.89,
112.2, 131.00, 131.8-131.9, 250.40-250.43, 250.80-250.93,
274.10-274.19, 274.89, 580.0-584.9, 586-588.1, 588.9-591,
593.0-593.2, 593.89-593.9, 599.60-599.9

DEF:  Sodium urate stones in the kidney.

**274.19   Other**
✓5th **274.8   Gout with other specified manifestations**
**274.81   Gouty tophi of ear**
DEF: Chalky sodium urate deposit in the ear due to gout;
produces chronic inflammation of external ear.

**274.82   Gouty tophi of other sites**
Gouty tophi of heart
**274.89   Other**
Use additional code to identify
manifestations, as:
gouty:
iritis (364.11)
neuritis (357.4)

**274.9   Gout, unspecified**

✓4th **275   Disorders of mineral metabolism**
*EXCLUDES*   abnormal findings without manifest disease
(790.0-796.9)

**275.0   Disorders of iron metabolism**
Bronzed diabetes    Pigmentary cirrhosis (of liver)
Hemochromatosis
*EXCLUDES*   anemia:
iron deficiency (280.0-280.9)
sideroblastic (285.0)

**AHA:** 2Q, '97, 11

**275.1  Disorders of copper metabolism**
Hepatolenticular degeneration
Wilson's disease

**275.2  Disorders of magnesium metabolism**
Hypermagnesemia    Hypomagnesemia

**275.3  Disorders of phosphorus metabolism**
Familial hypophosphatemia  Vitamin D-resistant:
Hypophosphatasia        osteomalacia
                                      rickets

✓5th **275.4  Disorders of calcium metabolism**
EXCLUDES  *parathyroid disorders (252.00-252.9)*
*vitamin D deficiency (268.0-268.9)*

**AHA:** 4Q, '97, 33

**275.40  Unspecified disorder of calcium metabolism**
**275.41  Hypocalcemia**
**DEF:** Abnormally decreased blood calcium level; symptoms include hyperactive deep tendon reflexes, muscle, abdominal cramps, and carpopedal spasm.

**275.42  Hypercalcemia**
**AHA:** 4Q, '03, 110

**DEF:** Abnormally increased blood calcium level; symptoms include muscle weakness, fatigue, nausea, depression, and constipation.

**275.49  Other disorders of calcium metabolism**
Nephrocalcinosis
Pseudohypoparathyroidism
Pseudopseudohypoparathyroidism
**DEF:** Nephrocalcinosis: calcium phosphate deposits in the tubules of the kidney with resultant renal insufficiency.

**DEF:** Pseudohypoparathyroidism: inherited disorder with signs and symptoms of hypoparathyroidism; caused by inadequate response to parathyroid hormone, not hormonal deficiency. Symptoms include muscle cramps, tetany, urinary frequency, blurred vision due to cataracts, and dry scaly skin.

**DEF:** Pseudopseudohypoparathyroidism: clinical manifestations of hypoparathyroidism without affecting blood calcium levels.

**275.8  Other specified disorders of mineral metabolism**
**275.9  Unspecified disorder of mineral metabolism**
✓4th **276 Disorders of fluid, electrolyte, and acid-base balance**
EXCLUDES  *diabetes insipidus (253.5)*
*familial periodic paralysis (359.3)*

**276.0  Hyperosmolality and/or hypernatremia**  CC
Sodium [Na] excess    Sodium [Na] overload
**CC Excl:** 276.0-276.9

**276.1  Hyposmolality and/or hyponatremia**  CC
Sodium [Na] deficiency
**CC Excl:** See code: 276.0

**276.2  Acidosis**  CC
Acidosis:       Acidosis:
  NOS             metabolic
  lactic          respiratory
EXCLUDES  *diabetic acidosis (250.1)*
**CC Excl:** See code 276.0
**AHA:** J-F, '87, 15
**DEF:** Disorder involves decrease of pH (hydrogen ion) concentration in blood and cellular tissues; caused by increase in acid and decrease in bicarbonate.

**276.3  Alkalosis**  CC
Alkalosis:      Alkalosis:
  NOS             respiratory
  metabolic
**CC Excl:** See code: 276.0
**DEF:** Accumulation of base (non-acid part of salt), or loss of acid without relative loss of base in body fluids; caused by increased arterial plasma bicarbonate concentration or loss of carbon dioxide due to hyperventilation.

**276.4  Mixed acid-base balance disorder**  CC
Hypercapnia with mixed acid-base disorder
**CC Excl:** See code 276.0

✓5th **276.5  Volume depletion**
EXCLUDES  *hypovolemic shock:*
*postoperative (998.0)*
*traumatic (958.4)*
**AHA:** 4Q, '05, 54; 2Q, '05, 9; 1Q, '03, 5, 22; 3Q, '02, 21; 4Q, '97, 30; 2Q, '88, 9

**276.50  Volume depletion, unspecified**
**DEF:** Depletion of total body water (dehydration) and/or contraction of total intravascular plasma (hypovolemia).

**276.51  Dehydration**
**DEF:** Depletion of total body water; blood volume may be normal while fluid is pulled from other tissues.

**276.52  Hypovolemia**
Depletion of volume of plasma
**DEF:** Depletion of volume plasma; depletion of total blood volume.

**276.6  Fluid overload**
Fluid retention
EXCLUDES  *ascites* ▶*(789.51-789.59)*◄
*localized edema (782.3)*
**AHA:** 4Q, '06, 136

**276.7  Hyperpotassemia**
Hyperkalemia        Potassium [K]:
Potassium [K]:        intoxication
  excess              overload
**AHA:** 1Q, '05, 9; 2Q,'01, 12
**DEF:** Elevated blood levels of potassium; symptoms include abnormal EKG readings, weakness; related to defective renal excretion.

**276.8  Hypopotassemia**
Hypokalemia      Potassium [K] deficiency
**DEF:** Decreased blood levels of potassium; symptoms include neuromuscular disorders.

**276.9  Electrolyte and fluid disorders not elsewhere classified**
Electrolyte imbalance  Hypochloremia
Hyperchloremia
EXCLUDES  *electrolyte imbalance:*
*associated with hyperemesis*
*gravidarum (643.1)*
*complicating labor and delivery (669.0)*
*following abortion and ectopic or molar pregnancy (634-638 with .4, 639.4)*

**AHA:** J-F, '87, 15
✓4th **277 Other and unspecified disorders of metabolism**
✓5th **277.0  Cystic fibrosis**
Fibrocystic disease of the pancreas
Mucoviscidosis
**AHA:** 4Q, '90, 16; 3Q, '90, 18

**DEF:** Generalized, genetic disorder of infants, children, and young adults marked by exocrine gland dysfunction; characterized by chronic pulmonary disease with excess mucus production, pancreatic deficiency, high levels of electrolytes in the sweat.

**277.00  Without mention of meconium ileus**  CC
Cystic fibrosis NOS
**CC Excl:** 277.00-277.09
**AHA:** 2Q, '03, 12

**277.01  With meconium ileus**  MCC N
Meconium:
ileus (of newborn)
obstruction of intestine in mucoviscidosis
**CC Excl:** See code 277.00

**277.02  With pulmonary manifestations**  MCC
Cystic fibrosis with pulmonary exacerbation
Use additional code to identify any
infectious organism present, such as:
pseudomonas (041.7)
**CC Excl:** See code 277.00

---

N  Newborn Age: 0    P  Pediatric Age: 0-17    M  Maternity Age: 12-55    A  Adult Age: 15-124    CC  CC Condition    MCC  Major CC Condition    HIV  HIV Related Dx

68 — Volume 1 • October 2007

© 2007 Ingenix

**277.03 With gastrointestinal manifestations** `CC`

> **EXCLUDES** *with meconium ileus (277.01)*

**CC Excl:** See code 277.00

**AHA:** 4Q, '02, 45

**277.09 With other manifestations** `CC`

**CC Excl:** See code 277.00

**277.1 Disorders of porphyrin metabolism** `CC`

Hematoporphyria
Hematoporphyrinuria
Hereditary coproporphyria
Porphyria
Porphyrinuria
Protocoproporphyria
Protoporphyria
Pyrroloporphyria

**CC Excl:** 277.1-277.2, 277.4-277.7

**277.2 Other disorders of purine and pyrimidine metabolism** `CC`

Hypoxanthine-guanine-phosphoribosyltransferase deficiency [HG-PRT deficiency]
Lesch-Nyhan syndrome
Xanthinuria

> **EXCLUDES** *gout (274.0-274.9)*
> *orotic aciduric anemia (281.4)*

**CC Excl:** See code: 277.1

**√5ᵗʰ 277.3 Amyloidosis**

**AHA:** 1Q, '96, 16

**DEF:** Conditions of diverse etiologies characterized by the accumulation of insoluble fibrillar proteins (amyloid) in various organs and tissues of the body, compromising vital functions.

**277.30 Amyloidosis, unspecified** `CC`

Amyloidosis NOS

**CC Excl:** 277.30-277.39, 277.7

**AHA:** 4Q, '06, 66

**277.31 Familial Mediterranean fever** `CC`

Benign paroxysmal peritonitis
Hereditary amyloid nephropathy
Periodic familial polyserositis
Recurrent polyserositis

**CC Excl:** See code: 277.30

**AHA:** 4Q, '06, 66

**DEF:** Childhood or early-life onset of recurrent attacks characterized by high fevers with pain and inflammation of chest and abdominal cavities, skin and joints, also rash or vasculitis. Underlying cause is unknown, or possibly genetic, but may be precipitated by stress, trauma or exertion.

**277.39 Other amyloidosis** `CC`

Hereditary cardiac amyloidosis
Inherited systemic amyloidosis
Neuropathic (Portuguese) (Swiss) amyloidosis
Secondary amyloidosis

**CC Excl:** See code: 277.30

**AHA:** 4Q, '06, 66

**277.4 Disorders of bilirubin excretion**

Hyperbilirubinemia:
  congenital
  constitutional
Syndrome:
  Crigler-Najjar
Syndrome:
  Dubin-Johnson
  Gilbert's
  Rotor's

> **EXCLUDES** *hyperbilirubinemias specific to the perinatal period (774.0-774.7)*

**277.5 Mucopolysaccharidosis** `CC`

Gargoylism
Hunter's syndrome
Hurler's syndrome
Lipochondrodystrophy
Maroteaux-Lamy syndrome
Morquio-Brailsford disease
Osteochondrodystrophy
Sanfilippo's syndrome
Scheie's syndrome

**CC Excl:** 277.1-277.31, 277.4-277.7

**DEF:** Metabolism disorders evidenced by excretion of various mucopolysaccharides in urine and infiltration of these substances into connective tissue, with resulting various defects of bone, cartilage and connective tissue.

**277.6 Other deficiencies of circulating enzymes**

Hereditary angioedema

**277.7 Dysmetabolic syndrome X**

Use additional code for associated manifestation, such as:
  cardiovascular disease (414.00-414.07)
  obesity (278.00-278.01)

**AHA:** 4Q, '01, 42

**DEF:** A specific group of metabolic disorders that are related to the state of insulin resistance (decreased cellular response to insulin) without elevated blood sugars; often related to elevated cholesterol and triglycerides, obesity, cardiovascular disease, and high blood pressure.

**√5ᵗʰ 277.8 Other specified disorders of metabolism**

**AHA:** 4Q, '03, 50; 2Q, '01, 18; S-O, '87, 9

**277.81 Primary carnitine deficiency**

**277.82 Carnitine deficiency due to inborn errors of metabolism**

**277.83 Iatrogenic carnitine deficiency**

Carnitine deficiency due to:
  hemodialysis
  valproic acid therapy

**277.84 Other secondary carnitine deficiency**

**277.85 Disorders of fatty acid oxidation** `CC`

Carnitine palmitoyltransferase deficiencies (CPT1, CPT2)
Glutaric aciduria type II (type IIA, IIB, IIC)
Long chain 3-hydroxyacyl CoA dehydrogenase deficiency (LCHAD)
Long chain/very long chain acyl CoA dehydrogenase deficiency (LCAD, VLCAD)
Medium chain acyl CoA dehydrogenase deficiency (MCAD)
Short chain acyl CoA dehydrogenase deficiency (SCAD)

> **EXCLUDES** *primary carnitine deficiency (277.81)*

**CC Excl:** 277.81-277.84, 277.86-277.89

**277.86 Peroxisomal disorders** `CC`

Adrenomyeloneuropathy
Neonatal adrenoleukodystrophy
Rhizomelic chrondrodysplasia punctata
X-linked adrenoleukodystrophy
Zellweger syndrome

> **EXCLUDES** *infantile Refsum disease (356.3)*

**CC Excl:** 277.4, 277.81-277.85, 277.87-277.89

**277.87 Disorders of mitochondrial metabolism** `CC`

Kearns-Sayre syndrome
Mitochondrial Encephalopathy, Lactic Acidosis and Stroke-like episodes (MELAS syndrome)
Mitochondrial Neurogastrointestinal Encephalopathy syndrome (MNGIE)
Myoclonus with Epilepsy and with Ragged Red Fibers (MERRF syndrome)
Neuropathy, Ataxia and Retinitis Pigmentosa (NARP syndrome)
Use additional code for associated conditions

> **EXCLUDES** *disorders of pyruvate metabolism (271.8)*
> *Leber's optic atrophy (377.16)*
> *Leigh's subacute necrotizing encephalopathy (330.8)*
> *Reye's syndrome (331.81)*

**CC Excl:** 277.4, 277.81-277.86, 277.89

**AHA:** 4Q, '04, 62

**277.89 Other specified disorders of metabolism** `CC`

Hand-Schüller-Christian disease
Histiocytosis (acute) (chronic)
Histiocytosis X (chronic)

> **EXCLUDES** *histiocytosis:*
> *acute differentiated progressive (202.5)*
> *X, acute (progressive) (202.5)*

**CC Excl:** 277.4, 277.81-277.87

---

√4ᵗʰ / √5ᵗʰ Additional Digit Required    Unacceptable PDx    Manifestation Code    ◄► Revised Text    ● New Code    ▲ Revised Code Title

**277.9**   **Unspecified disorder of metabolism**
Enzymopathy NOS

✓4th **278 Overweight, obesity and other hyperalimentation**
EXCLUDES   *hyperalimentation NOS (783.6)*
*poisoning by vitamins NOS (963.5)*
*polyphagia (783.6)*

✓5th **278.0**   **Overweight and obesity**
Use additional code to identify Body Mass Index (BMI), if known (V85.0-V85.54)
EXCLUDES   *adiposogenital dystrophy (253.8)*
*obesity of endocrine origin NOS (259.9)*
AHA: 4Q, '05, 97

**278.00**   **Obesity, unspecified**
Obesity NOS
AHA: 4Q, '01, 42; 1Q, '99, 5, 6
DEF: BMI (body mass index) between 30.0 and 38.9.

**278.01**   **Morbid obesity**
Severe obesity
AHA: 2Q, '06, 5-6; 3Q, '03, 6-8
DEF: Increased weight beyond limits of skeletal and physical requirements (125 percent or more over ideal body weight), as a result of excess fat in subcutaneous connective tissues.
DEF: BMI (body mass index) greater than 39.

**278.02**   **Overweight**
AHA: 4Q, '05, 55
DEF: BMI (body mass index) between 25 and 29.9.

**278.1**   **Localized adiposity**
Fat pad
AHA: 2Q, '06, 10

**278.2**   **Hypervitaminosis A**

**278.3**   **Hypercarotinemia**
DEF: Elevated blood carotene level due to ingesting excess carotenoids or the inability to convert carotenoids to vitamin A.

**278.4**   **Hypervitaminosis D**
DEF: Weakness, fatigue, loss of weight, and other symptoms resulting from ingesting excessive amounts of vitamin D.

**278.8**   **Other hyperalimentation**

✓4th **279 Disorders involving the immune mechanism**

✓5th **279.0**   **Deficiency of humoral immunity**
DEF: Inadequate immune response to bacterial infections with potential reinfection by viruses due to lack of circulating immunoglobulins (acquired antibodies).

**279.00**   **Hypogammaglobulinemia, unspecified**   CC
Agammaglobulinemia NOS
CC Excl: 279.00-279.9

**279.01**   **Selective IgA immunodeficiency**   CC
CC Excl: See code: 279.00

**279.02**   **Selective IgM immunodeficiency**   CC
CC Excl: 279.02-279.9

**279.03**   **Other selective immunoglobulin deficiencies**   CC
Selective deficiency of IgG
CC Excl: See code: 279.02

**279.04**   **Congenital hypogammaglobulinemia**   CC
Agammaglobulinemia:
Bruton's type
X-linked
CC Excl: See code 279.02

**279.05**   **Immunodeficiency with increased IgM**   CC
Immunodeficiency with hyper-IgM:
autosomal recessive
X-linked
CC Excl: See code 279.02

**279.06**   **Common variable immunodeficiency**   CC
Dysgammaglobulinemia (acquired) (congenital) (primary)
Hypogammaglobulinemia:
acquired primary
congenital non-sex-linked
sporadic
CC Excl: See code 279.02

**279.09**   **Other**   CC
Transient hypogammaglobulinemia of infancy
CC Excl: See code 279.02

✓5th **279.1**   **Deficiency of cell-mediated immunity**
**279.10**   **Immunodeficiency with predominant T-cell defect, unspecified**   CC
CC Excl: See code 279.02
AHA: S-O, '87, 10

**279.11**   **DiGeorge's syndrome**   CC
Pharyngeal pouch syndrome
Thymic hypoplasia
CC Excl: See code 279.02

DEF: Congenital disorder due to defective development of the third and fourth pharyngeal pouches; results in hypoplasia or aplasia of the thymus, parathyroid glands; related to congenital heart defects, anomalies of the great vessels, esophageal atresia, and abnormalities of facial structures.

**279.12**   **Wiskott-Aldrich syndrome**   CC
CC Excl: See code 279.02

DEF: A disease characterized by chronic conditions, such as eczema, suppurative otitis media and anemia; it results from an X-linked recessive gene and is classified as an immune deficiency syndrome.

**279.13**   **Nezelof's syndrome**   CC
Cellular immunodeficiency with abnormal immunoglobulin deficiency
CC Excl: See code 279.02

DEF: Immune system disorder characterized by a pathological deficiency in cellular immunity and humoral antibodies resulting in inability to fight infectious diseases.

**279.19**   **Other**   CC
EXCLUDES   *ataxia-telangiectasia (334.8)*
CC Excl: See code 279.02

**279.2**   **Combined immunity deficiency**   CC
Agammaglobulinemia:
autosomal recessive
Swiss-type
x-linked recessive
Severe combined immunodeficiency [SCID]
Thymic:
alymophoplasia
aplasia or dysplasia with immunodeficiency
EXCLUDES   *thymic hypoplasia (279.11)*
CC Excl: See code 279.02
DEF: Agammaglobulinemia: No immunoglobulins in the blood.
DEF: Thymic alymphoplasia: Severe combined immunodeficiency; result of failed lymphoid tissue development.

**279.3**   **Unspecified immunity deficiency**   CC
CC Excl: See code 279.02

**279.4**   **Autoimmune disease, not elsewhere classified**
Autoimmune disease NOS
EXCLUDES   *transplant failure or rejection (996.80-996.89)*

**279.8**   **Other specified disorders involving the immune mechanism**
Single complement [$C_1$-$C_9$] deficiency or dysfunction

**279.9**   **Unspecified disorder of immune mechanism**
AHA: 3Q, '92, 13

---

N Newborn Age: 0    P Pediatric Age: 0-17    M Maternity Age: 12-55    A Adult Age: 15-124    CC CC Condition    MCC Major CC Condition    HIV HIV Related Dx

## 4. DISEASES OF THE BLOOD AND BLOOD-FORMING ORGANS (280-289)

> **EXCLUDES** *anemia complicating pregnancy or the puerperium (648.2)*

### ✓4th 280 Iron deficiency anemias

> **INCLUDES** anemia:
> asiderotic
> hypochromic-microcytic
> sideropenic
>
> **EXCLUDES** *familial microcytic anemia (282.49)*

**280.0 Secondary to blood loss (chronic)**
Normocytic anemia due to blood loss
> **EXCLUDES** *acute posthemorrhagic anemia (285.1)*

**AHA:** 4Q, '93, 34

**280.1 Secondary to inadequate dietary iron intake**

**280.8 Other specified iron deficiency anemias**
Paterson-Kelly syndrome
Plummer-Vinson syndrome
Sideropenic dysphagia

**280.9 Iron deficiency anemia, unspecified**
Anemia:
achlorhydric
chlorotic
idiopathic hypochromic
iron [Fe] deficiency NOS

### ✓4th 281 Other deficiency anemias

**281.0 Pernicious anemia**
Anemia:
Addison's
Biermer's
congenital pernicious
Congenital intrinsic factor [Castle's] deficiency
> **EXCLUDES** *combined system disease without mention of anemia (266.2)*
> *subacute degeneration of spinal cord without mention of anemia (266.2)*

**AHA:** N-D, '84, 1; S-O, '84, 16

**DEF:** Chronic progressive anemia due to Vitamin B12 malabsorption; caused by lack of a secretion known as intrinsic factor, which is produced by the gastric mucosa of the stomach.

**281.1 Other vitamin $B_{12}$ deficiency anemia**
Anemia:
vegan's
vitamin $B_{12}$ deficiency (dietary)
due to selective vitamin $B_{12}$ malabsorption with proteinuria
Syndrome:
Imerslund's
Imerslund-Gräsbeck
> **EXCLUDES** *combined system disease without mention of anemia (266.2)*
> *subacute degeneration of spinal cord without mention of anemia (266.2)*

**281.2 Folate-deficiency anemia**
Congenital folate malabsorption
Folate or folic acid deficiency anemia:
NOS
dietary
drug-induced
Goat's milk anemia
Nutritional megaloblastic anemia (of infancy)
Use additional E code to identify drug
**DEF:** Macrocytic anemia resembles pernicious anemia but without absence of hydrochloric acid secretions; responsive to folic acid therapy.

**281.3 Other specified megaloblastic anemias not elsewhere classified**
Combined $B_{12}$ and folate-deficiency anemia
Refractory megaloblastic anemia
**DEF:** Megaloblasts predominant in bone marrow with few normoblasts; rare familial type associated with proteinuria and genitourinary tract anomalies.

**281.4 Protein-deficiency anemia**
Amino-acid-deficiency anemia

**281.8 Anemia associated with other specified nutritional deficiency**
Scorbutic anemia

**281.9 Unspecified deficiency anemia**
Anemia:     Anemia:
dimorphic     nutritional NOS
macrocytic     simple chronic
megaloblastic NOS

### ✓4th 282 Hereditary hemolytic anemias

**DEF:** Escalated rate of erythrocyte destruction; similar to all anemias, occurs when imbalance exists between blood loss and blood production.

**282.0 Hereditary spherocytosis**
Acholuric (familial) jaundice
Congenital hemolytic anemia (spherocytic)
Congenital spherocytosis
Minkowski-Chauffard syndrome
Spherocytosis (familial)
> **EXCLUDES** *hemolytic anemia of newborn (773.0-773.5)*

**DEF:** Hereditary, chronic illness marked by abnormal red blood cell membrane; symptoms include enlarged spleen, jaundice; and anemia in severe cases.

**282.1 Hereditary elliptocytosis**
Elliptocytosis (congenital)
Ovalocytosis (congenital) (hereditary)
**DEF:** Genetic hemolytic anemia characterized by malformed, elliptical erythrocytes; there is increased destruction of red cells with resulting anemia.

**282.2 Anemias due to disorders of glutathione metabolism**
Anemia:
6-phosphogluconic dehydrogenase deficiency
enzyme deficiency, drug-induced
erythrocytic glutathione deficiency
glucose-6-phosphate dehydrogenase [G-6-PD] deficiency
glutathione-reductase deficiency
hemolytic nonspherocytic (hereditary), type I
Disorder of pentose phosphate pathway
Favism

**282.3 Other hemolytic anemias due to enzyme deficiency**
Anemia:
hemolytic nonspherocytic (hereditary), type II
hexokinase deficiency
pyruvate kinase [PK] deficiency
triosephosphate isomerase deficiency

### ✓5th 282.4 Thalassemias
> **EXCLUDES** *sickle-cell:*
> *disease (282.60-282.69)*
> *trait (282.5)*

**AHA:** 4Q, '03, 51

**DEF:** A group of inherited hemolytic disorders characterized by decreased production of at least one of the four polypeptide globin chains which results in defective hemoglobin synthesis; symptoms include severe anemia, expanded marrow spaces, transfusional and absorptive iron overload, impaired growth rate, thickened cranial bones, and pathologic fractures.

---

✓4th / ✓5th Additional Digit Required    Unacceptable PDx    Manifestation Code    ▶◀ Revised Text    ● New Code    ▲ Revised Code Title

© 2007 Ingenix

October 2007 • Volume 1 — 71

**Blood and Blood Forming Organs**

**282.41–283.11**

**282.41 Sickle-cell thalassemia without crisis**
Sickle-cell thalassemia NOS
Thalassemia Hb-S disease without crisis

**282.42 Sickle-cell thalassemia with crisis** `MCC`
Sickle-cell thalassemia with vaso-occlusive pain
Thalassemia Hb-S disease with crisis
Use additional code for type of crisis, such as:
  acute chest syndrome (517.3)
  splenic sequestration (289.52)

CC Excl: 280.0-284.2, 284.81-285.9, 289.81-289.9, 517.3

**282.49 Other thalassemia**
Cooley's anemia
Hb-Bart's disease
Hereditary leptocytosis
Mediterranean anemia (with other hemoglobinopathy)
Microdrepanocytosis
Thalassemia (alpha) (beta) (intermedia) (major) (minima) (minor) (mixed) (trait) (with other hemoglobinopathy)
Thalassemia NOS

**282.5 Sickle-cell trait**
Hb-AS genotype        Heterozygous:
Hemoglobin S [Hb-S] trait    hemoglobin S
                     Hb-S
     **EXCLUDES** *that with other hemoglobinopathy (282.60-282.69)*
                   *that with thalassemia (282.49)*
DEF: Heterozygous genetic makeup characterized by one gene for normal hemoglobin and one for sickle-cell hemoglobin; clinical disease rarely present.

√5ᵗʰ **282.6 Sickle-cell disease**
Sickle-cell anemia
     **EXCLUDES** *sickle-cell thalassemia (282.41-282.42)*
                   *sickle-cell trait (282.5)*
DEF: Inherited blood disorder; sickle-shaped red blood cells are hard and pointed, clogging blood flow; anemia characterized by, periodic episodes of pain, acute abdominal discomfort, skin ulcerations of the legs, increased infections; occurs primarily in persons of African descent.

**282.60 Sickle-cell disease, unspecified**
Sickle-cell anemia NOS
AHA: 2Q, '97, 11

**282.61 Hb-SS disease without crisis**

**282.62 Hb-SS disease with crisis** `MCC`
Hb-SS disease with vaso-occlusive pain
Sickle-cell crisis NOS
Use additional code for type of crisis, such as:
  acute chest syndrome (517.3)
  splenic sequestration (289.52)

CC Excl: See code: 282.42

AHA: 4Q, '03, 56; 2Q, '98, 8; 2Q, '91, 15

**282.63 Sickle-cell/Hb-C disease without crisis**
Hb-S/Hb-C disease without crisis

**282.64 Sickle-cell/Hb-C disease with crisis** `MCC`
Hb-S/Hb-C disease with crisis
Sickle-cell/Hb-C disease with vaso-occlusive pain
Use additional code for type of crisis, such as:
  acute chest syndrome (517.3)
  splenic sequestration (289.52)

CC Excl: See code: 282.42

AHA: 4Q, '03, 51

**282.68 Other sickle-cell disease without crisis**
Hb-S/Hb-D
Hb-S/Hb-E      } disease without crisis
Sickle-cell/Hb-D
Sickle-cell/Hb-E

AHA: 4Q, '03, 51

**282.69 Other sickle-cell disease with crisis** `MCC`
Hb-S/Hb-D
Hb-S/Hb-E      } disease with crisis
Sickle-cell/Hb-D
Sickle-cell/Hb-E
Other sickle-cell disease with vaso-occlusive pain
Use additional code for type of crisis, such as:
  acute chest syndrome (517.3)
  splenic sequestration (289.52)

CC Excl: 280.0-285.9, 289.81-289.9, 517.3

**282.7 Other hemoglobinopathies**
Abnormal hemoglobin NOS
Congenital Heinz-body anemia
Disease:
  hemoglobin C [Hb-C]
  hemoglobin D [Hb-D]
  hemoglobin E [Hb-E]
  hemoglobin Zurich [Hb-Zurich]
Hemoglobinopathy NOS
Hereditary persistence of fetal hemoglobin [HPFH]
Unstable hemoglobin hemolytic disease
     **EXCLUDES** *familial polycythemia (289.6)*
                   *hemoglobin M [Hb-M] disease (289.7)*
                   *high-oxygen-affinity hemoglobin (289.0)*
DEF: Any disorder of hemoglobin due to alteration of molecular structure; may include overt anemia.

**282.8 Other specified hereditary hemolytic anemias** `CC`
Stomatocytosis
CC Excl: 280.0-284.2, 284.81-285.9, 289.9, 517.3, 776.5-776.6

**282.9 Hereditary hemolytic anemia, unspecified** `CC`
Hereditary hemolytic anemia NOS
CC Excl: See code: 282.8

√4ᵗʰ **283 Acquired hemolytic anemias**
DEF: Non-hereditary anemia characterized by premature destruction of red blood cells; caused by infectious organisms, poisons, and physical agents
AHA: N-D, '84, 1

**283.0 Autoimmune hemolytic anemias** `CC`
Autoimmune hemolytic disease (cold type) (warm type)
Chronic cold hemagglutinin disease
Cold agglutinin disease or hemoglobinuria
Hemolytic anemia:
  cold type (secondary) (symptomatic)
  drug-induced
  warm type (secondary) (symptomatic)
Use additional E code to identify cause, if drug-induced
     **EXCLUDES** *Evans' syndrome (287.32)*
                   *hemolytic disease of newborn (773.0-773.5)*
CC Excl: 280.0-284.2, 284.81-285.9, 289.81-289.9, 517.3

√5ᵗʰ **283.1 Non-autoimmune hemolytic anemias**
Use additional E code to identify cause
DEF: Hemolytic anemia and thrombocytopenia with acute renal failure; relatively rare condition; 50 percent of patients require renal dialysis.
AHA: 4Q, '93, 25

**283.10 Non-autoimmune hemolytic anemia, unspecified** `CC`
CC Excl: See code: 283.0

**283.11 Hemolytic-uremic syndrome** `MCC`
CC Excl: See code: 283.0

---

`N` Newborn Age: 0    `P` Pediatric Age: 0-17    `M` Maternity Age: 12-55    `A` Adult Age: 15-124    `CC` CC Condition    `MCC` Major CC Condition    `HIV` HIV Related Dx

**283.19 Other non-autoimmune hemolytic**    `CC`
    **anemias**

      Hemolytic anemia:      Hemolytic anemia:
        mechanical          toxic
        microangiopathic

      **CC Excl:** See code: 283.0

**283.2 Hemoglobinuria due to hemolysis from**
    **external causes**

      Acute intravascular hemolysis
      Hemoglobinuria:
        from exertion
        march
        paroxysmal (cold) (nocturnal)
        due to other hemolysis
      Marchiafava-Micheli syndrome
      Use additional E code to identify cause

**283.9 Acquired hemolytic anemia, unspecified**    `CC`

      Acquired hemolytic anemia NOS
      Chronic idiopathic hemolytic anemia

      **CC Excl:** See code: 283.0

√4ᵗʰ **284 Aplastic anemia and other bone marrow failure syndromes**
    **AHA:** 1Q, '91, 14; N-D, '84, 1; S-O, '84, 16

    **DEF:** Bone marrow failure to produce the normal amount of blood components; generally non-responsive to usual therapy.

√5ᵗʰ **284.0 Constitutional aplastic anemia**
    **AHA:** 1Q, '91, 14

    **284.01 Constitutional red blood cell aplasia**    `CC`

      Aplasia, (pure) red cell:
        congenital
        of infants
        primary
      Blackfan-Diamond syndrome
      Familial hypoplastic anemia

      **CC Excl:** 280.0-284.09, 284.81-285.9, 289.9, 776.5-776.6

      **AHA:** 4Q, '06, 67-69

    **284.09 Other constitutional aplastic anemia**    `CC`

      Fanconi's anemia
      Pancytopenia with malformations

      **CC Excl:** 280.0-284.09, 284.81-285.9, 287.30-287.39, 289.9, 776.5-776.6

      **AHA:** 4Q, '06, 67-69

**284.1 Pancytopenia**    `CC`

      `EXCLUDES`   *pancytopenia (due to) (with):*
        *aplastic anemia NOS (284.9)*
        *bone marrow infiltration (284.2)*
        *constitutional red blood cell aplasia (284.01)*
        *drug induced ▶(284.89)◀*
        *hairy cell leukemia (202.4)*
        *human immunodeficiency virus disease (042)*
        *leukoerythroblastic anemia (284.2)*
        *malformations (284.09)*
        *myelodysplastic syndromes (238.72-238.75)*
        *myeloproliferative disease (238.79)*
        *other constitutional aplastic anemia (284.09)*

      **CC Excl:** 284.2, 284.81-285.9, 288.00-288.09, 288.4-288.62, 288.66-288.69, 289.9, 776.6

      **AHA:** 4Q, '06, 67-69

**284.2 Myelophthisis**    `CC`

      Leukoerythroblastic anemia
      Myelophthisic anemia
      *Code first the underlying disorder, such as:*
        malignant neoplasm of breast (174.0-174.9, 175.0-175.9)
        tuberculosis (015.0-015.9)

      `EXCLUDES`   *idiopathic myelofibrosis (238.76)*
        *myelofibrosis NOS (289.83)*
        *myelofibrosis with myeloid metaplasia (238.76)*
        *primary myelofibrosis (238.76)*
        *secondary myelofibrosis (289.83)*

      **CC Excl:** 284.1-284.2, 284.81-285.9, 288.00-288.09, 288.4-288.62, 288.66-288.69, 289.9, 776.6

      **AHA:** 4Q, '06, 67-69

      **DEF:** A secondary disease process involving replacement of normal hematopoeitic tissue in the bone marrow with abnormal tissue, such as fibrous tissue or tumors. Occurs with advanced-stage neoplasms, granulomatous diseases such as miliary tuberculosis, and other inflammatory or infectious diseases or in countries where access to medical care is not readily available.

√5ᵗʰ **284.8 Other specified aplastic anemias**
    **AHA:** 3Q, '05, 11; 1Q, '97, 5; 1Q, '92, 15; 1Q, '91, 14

  ●   **284.81 Red cell aplasia (acquired) (adult)**    `MCC`
      **(with thymoma)**
      Red cell aplasia NOS

      **CC Excl:** 280.0-284.2, 284.81-285.9, 289.81-289.9, 517.3

  ●   **284.89 Other specified aplastic anemias**    `MCC`

      Aplastic anemia (due to):
        chronic systemic disease
        drugs
        infection
        radiation
        toxic (paralytic)
      Use additional E code to identify cause

      **CC Excl:** See code: 284.81

**284.9 Aplastic anemia, unspecified**    `CC`

      Anemia:
        aplastic (idiopathic) NOS
        aregenerative
        hypoplastic NOS
        nonregenerative
      Medullary hypoplasia

      `EXCLUDES`   *refractory anemia (238.72)*

      **CC Excl:** See code: 284.81

√4ᵗʰ **285 Other and unspecified anemias**
    **AHA:** 1Q, '91, 14; N-D, '84, 1

**285.0 Sideroblastic anemia**

      Anemia:
        hypochromic with iron loading
        sideroachrestic
        sideroblastic:      sideroblastic:
          acquired        secondary (drug-induced)
          congenital          (due to disease)
          hereditary      sex-linked hypochromic
          primary         vitamin B6-responsive
      Pyridoxine-responsive (hypochromic) anemia
      Use additional E code to identify cause, if drug induced

      `EXCLUDES`   *refractory sideroblastic anemia (238.72)*

      **DEF:** Characterized by a disruption of final heme synthesis; results in iron overload of reticuloendothelial tissues.

**285.1 Acute posthemorrhagic anemia**    `CC`

      Anemia due to acute blood loss

      `EXCLUDES`   *anemia due to chronic blood loss (280.0)*
        *blood loss anemia NOS (280.0)*

      **CC Excl:** 280.0-285.9, 289.81-289.9, 517.3, 958.2

      **AHA:** ▶1Q. '07, 19;◀ 2Q, '92, 15

**Blood and Blood Forming Organs**

**285.2–286.5**

✓5th **285.2**   **Anemia of chronic disease**
     Anemia in chronic illness
     **AHA:** 4Q, '00, 39

     **285.21 Anemia in chronic kidney disease**
         Anemia in end stage renal disease
         Erythropoietin-resistant anemia (EPO resistant anemia)

     **285.22 Anemia in neoplastic disease**

     **285.29 Anemia of other chronic disease**
         Anemia in other chronic illness

**285.8**   **Other specified anemias**
     Anemia:
         dyserythropoietic (congenital)
         dyshematopoietic (congenital)
         von Jaksch's
     Infantile pseudoleukemia
     **AHA:** 1Q, '91, 16

**285.9**   **Anemia, unspecified**
     Anemia:          Anemia:
       NOS            profound
       essential        progressive
       normocytic, not due    secondary
         to blood loss   Oligocythemia

     **EXCLUDES**   *anemia (due to):*
            *blood loss:*
              *acute (285.1)*
              *chronic or unspecified (280.0)*
            *iron deficiency (280.0-280.9)*

     **AHA:** ▶1Q. '07, 19;◀ 1Q, '02, 14; 2Q, '92, 16; M-A, '85, 13; N-D, '84, 1

✓4th **286**   **Coagulation defects**
     **AHA:** 2Q, '06, 17

**286.0**   **Congenital factor VIII disorder**    MCC
     Antihemophilic globulin   Hemophilia:
       [AHG] deficiency        A
     Factor VIII (functional)    classical
       deficiency           familial
     Hemophilia:          hereditary
       NOS             Subhemophilia
     **EXCLUDES**   *factor VIII deficiency with vascular defect (286.4)*

     **CC Excl:** 286.0-287.9, 289.81-289.9

     **DEF:** Hereditary, sex-linked, results in missing antihemophilic globulin (AHG) (factor VIII); causes abnormal coagulation characterized by increased tendency to bleeding, large bruises of skin, soft tissue; may also be bleeding in mouth, nose, gastrointestinal tract; after childhood, hemorrhages in joints, resulting in swelling and impaired function.

**286.1**   **Congenital factor IX disorder**    MCC
     Christmas disease
     Deficiency:
       factor IX (functional)
       plasma thromboplastin component [PTC]
     Hemophilia B

     **CC Excl:** See code: 286.0

     **DEF:** Deficiency of plasma thromboplastin component (PTC) (factor IX) and plasma thromboplastin antecedent (PTA); PTC deficiency clinically indistinguishable from classical hemophilia; PTA deficiency found in both sexes.

**286.2**   **Congenital factor XI deficiency**    CC
     Hemophilia C
     Plasma thromboplastin antecedent [PTA] deficiency
     Rosenthal's disease

     **CC Excl:** See code: 286.0

**286.3**   **Congenital deficiency of other clotting factors**    CC
     Congenital afibrinogenemia
     Deficiency:
       AC globulin factor:
         I [fibrinogen]
         II [prothrombin]
         V [labile]
         VII [stable]
         X [Stuart-Prower]
         XII [Hageman]
         XIII [fibrin stabilizing]
       Laki-Lorand factor
       proaccelerin
     Disease
       Owren's
       Stuart-Prower
     Dysfibrinogenemia (congenital)
     Dysprothrombinemia (constitutional)
     Hypoproconvertinemia
     Hypoprothrmbinemia (hereditary)
     Parahemophilia

     **CC Excl:** See code: 286.0

**286.4**   **von Willebrand's disease**    CC
     Angiohemophilia (A) (B)
     Constitutional thrombopathy
     Factor VIII deficiency with vascular defect
     Pseudohemophilia type B
     Vascular hemophilia
     von Willebrand's (-Jürgens') disease
     **EXCLUDES**   *factor VIII deficiency:*
            *NOS (286.0)*
            *with functional defect (286.0)*
            *hereditary capillary fragility (287.8)*

     **CC Excl:** See code: 286.0

     **DEF:** Abnormal blood coagulation caused by deficient blood Factor VII; congenital; symptoms include excess or prolonged bleeding, such as hemorrhage during menstruation, following birthing, or after surgical procedure.

**286.5**   **Hemorrhagic disorder due to intrinsic circulating anticoagulants**    CC
     Antithrombinemia
     Antithromboplastinemia
     Antithromboplastino-genemia
     Hyperheparinemia
     Increase in:
       anti-VIIIa
       anti-IXa
       anti-Xa
       anti-XIa
       antithrombin
     Secondary hemophilia
     Systemic lupus erythematosus [SLE] inhibitor

     **CC Excl:** See code: 286.0

     **AHA:** 3Q, '04, 7; No.5, '93, 16; 3Q, '92, 15; 3Q, '90, 14

---

N Newborn Age: 0    P Pediatric Age: 0-17    M Maternity Age: 12-55    A Adult Age: 15-124    CC CC Condition    MCC Major CC Condition    HIV HIV Related Dx

74 — Volume 1 • October 2007          © 2007 Ingenix

**286.6  Defibrination syndrome**    `MCC`
  Afibrinogenemia, acquired
  Consumption coagulopathy
  Diffuse or disseminated intravascular coagulation
    [DIC syndrome]
  Fibrinolytic hemorrhage, acquired
  Hemorrhagic fibrinogenolysis
  Pathologic fibrinolysis
  Purpura:
    fibrinolytic
    fulminans
    `EXCLUDES`  *that complicating:*
            *abortion (634-638 with .1, 639.1)*
            *pregnancy or the puerperium (641.3,*
              *666.3)*
            *disseminated intravascular coagulation*
              *in newborn (776.2)*

  **CC Excl:** See code: 286.0

  **AHA:** 4Q, '93, 29

  DEF: Characterized by destruction of circulating fibrinogen; often
  precipitated by other conditions, such as injury, causing release of
  thromboplastic particles in blood stream.

**286.7  Acquired coagulation factor deficiency**    `CC`
  Deficiency of coagulation factor due to:
    liver disease
    vitamin K deficiency
  Hypoprothrombinemia, acquired
  Use additional E code to identify cause, if drug
    induced
    `EXCLUDES`  *vitamin K deficiency of newborn*
            *(776.0)*

  **CC Excl:** See code: 286.0

  **AHA:** 4Q, '93, 29

**286.9  Other and unspecified coagulation defects**    `CC`
  Defective coagulation NOS
  Deficiency, coagulation factor NOS
  Delay, coagulation
  Disorder:
    coagulation
    hemostasis
    `EXCLUDES`  *abnormal coagulation profile (790.92)*
            *hemorrhagic disease of newborn*
              *(776.0)*
            *that complicating:*
              *abortion (634-638 with .1, 639.1)*
              *pregnancy or the puerperium (641.3,*
                *666.3)*

  **CC Excl:** See code: 286.0

  **AHA:**  4Q, '99, 22; 4Q, '93, 29

√4ᵗʰ **287  Purpura and other hemorrhagic conditions**
    `EXCLUDES`  *hemorrhagic thrombocythemia (238.79)*
            *purpura fulminans (286.6)*

  **AHA:** 1Q, '91, 14

**287.0  Allergic purpura**    `CC`
  Peliosis rheumatica       Purpura:
  Purpura:                    rheumatica
    anaphylactoid             Schönlein-Henoch
    autoimmune                vascular
    Henoch's                Vasculitis, allergic
    nonthrombocytopenic:
      hemorrhagic
      idiopathic
    `EXCLUDES`  *hemorrhagic purpura (287.39)*
            *purpura annularis telangiectodes*
              *(709.1)*

  **CC Excl:** See code: 286.0

  DEF: Any hemorrhagic condition, thrombocytic or
  nonthrombocytopenic in origin, caused by a presumed allergic
  reaction.

**287.1  Qualitative platelet defects**
  Thrombasthenia (hemorrhagic) (hereditary)
  Thrombocytasthenia
  Thrombocytopathy (dystrophic)
  Thrombopathy (Bernard-Soulier)
    `EXCLUDES`  *von Willebrand's disease (286.4)*

**287.2  Other nonthrombocytopenic purpuras**
  Purpura:
    NOS
    senile
    simplex

√5ᵗʰ **287.3  Primary thrombocytopenia**
    `EXCLUDES`  *thrombotic thrombocytopenic purpura*
              *(446.6)*
            *transient thrombocytopenia of newborn*
              *(776.1)*

  **AHA:** 4Q, '05, 56

  DEF: Decrease in number of blood platelets in circulating blood and
  purpural skin hemorrhages.

  **287.30  Primary thrombocytopenia, unspecified**
    Megakaryocytic hypoplasia

  **287.31  Immune thrombocytopenic purpura**    `CC`
    Idiopathic thrombocytopenic purpura
    Tidal platelet dysgenesis
    **CC Excl:** See code: 286.0

    **AHA:** 4Q, '05, 57

    DEF: Tidal platelet dysgenesis: Platelet counts fluctuate
    from normal to very low within periods of 20 to 40 days
    and may involve autoimmune platelet destruction.

  **287.32  Evans' syndrome**    `CC`
    **CC Excl:** See code: 286.0

    DEF: Combination of immunohemolytic anemia and
    autoimmune hemolytic anemia, sometimes with
    neutropenia.

  **287.33  Congenital and hereditary**    `CC`
       **thrombocytopenic purpura**
    Congenital and hereditary
      thrombocytopenia
    Thrombocytopenia with absent radii (TAR)
      syndrome
      `EXCLUDES`  *Wiskott-Aldrich syndrome*
              *(279.12)*

    **CC Excl:** See code: 286.0

    DEF: Thrombocytopenia with absent radii (TAR)
    syndrome: autosomal recessive syndrome characterized
    by thrombocytopenia and bilateral radial aplasia;
    manifestations include skeletal, gastrointestinal,
    hematologic, and cardiac system abnormalities.

  **287.39  Other primary thrombocytopenia**

**287.4  Secondary thrombocytopenia**
  Posttransfusion purpura
  Thrombocytopenia (due to):
    dilutional
    drugs
    extracorporeal circulation of blood
    massive blood transfusion
    platelet alloimmunization
  Use additional E code to identify cause
    `EXCLUDES`  *transient thrombocytopenia of newborn*
              *(776.1)*

  **AHA:** M-A, '85, 14

  DEF: Reduced number of platelets in circulating blood as
  consequence of an underlying disease or condition.

**287.5  Thrombocytopenia, unspecified**
**287.8  Other specified hemorrhagic conditions**
  Capillary fragility (hereditary)
  Vascular pseudohemophilia
**287.9  Unspecified hemorrhagic conditions**
  Hemorrhagic diathesis (familial)

**Blood and Blood Forming Organs**

**288–288.9**

√4ᵗʰ **288 Diseases of white blood cells**
     EXCLUDES    leukemia (204.0-208.9)
   **AHA:** 4Q, '06, 69; 1Q, '91, 14

√5ᵗʰ **288.0 Neutropenia**
     Decreased absolute neutrophil count [ANC]
     ▶Use additional code for any associated:
       fever (780.6)
       mucositis (478.11, 528.00-528.09, 538, 616.81)◀
     EXCLUDES   neutropenic splenomegaly (289.53)
              transitory neonatal neutropenia (776.7)
   **AHA:** 4Q, '06, 69-73; 3Q, '05, 11; 3Q, '99, 6; 2Q, '99, 9; 3Q, '96, 16;
          2Q, '96, 6

   **DEF:** Sudden, severe condition characterized by reduced number of
   white blood cells; results in sores in the throat, stomach or skin;
   symptoms include chills, fever; some drugs can bring on condition.

     **288.00 Neutropenia, unspecified**
         **AHA:** 4Q, '06, 69-73

     **288.01 Congenital neutropenia**
         Congenital agranulocytosis
         Infantile genetic agranulocytosis
         Kostmann's syndrome
         **AHA:** 4Q, '06, 69-73

     **288.02 Cyclic neutropenia**
         Cyclic hematopoiesis
         Periodic neutropenia
         **AHA:** 4Q, '06, 69-73

     **288.03 Drug induced neutropenia**
         Use additional E code to identify drug
         **AHA:** 4Q, '06, 69-73

     **288.04 Neutropenia due to infection**
         **AHA:** 4Q, '06, 69-73

     **288.09 Other neutropenia**
         Agranulocytosis
         Neutropenia:
           immune
           toxic
         **AHA:** 4Q, '06, 69-73

**288.1 Functional disorders of polymorphonuclear neutrophils**
     Chronic (childhood) granulomatous disease
     Congenital dysphagocytosis
     Job's syndrome
     Lipochrome histiocytosis (familial)
     Progressive septic granulomatosis

**288.2 Genetic anomalies of leukocytes**
     Anomaly (granulation) (granulocyte) or syndrome:
       Alder's (-Reilly)
       Chédiak-Steinbrinck (-Higashi)
       Jordan's
       May-Hegglin
       Pelger-Huet
     Hereditary:
       hypersegmentation
       hyposegmentation
       leukomelanopathy

**288.3 Eosinophilia**
     Eosinophilia:        Eosinophilia:
       allergic            secondary
       hereditary       Eosinophilic leukocytosis
       idiopathic
     EXCLUDES   Löffler's syndrome (518.3)
              pulmonary eosinophilia (518.3)
   **AHA:** 3Q, '00, 11

   **DEF:** Elevated number of eosinophils in the blood; characteristic of
   allergic states and various parasitic infections.

**288.4 Hemophagocytic syndromes**    CC
     Familial hemophagocytic lymphohistiocytosis
     Familial hemophagocytic reticulosis
     Hemophagocytic syndrome, infection-associated
     Histiocytic syndromes
     Macrophage activation syndrome
   **CC Excl:** 284.1-284.2, 284.81-284.9, 286.6, 287.30-288.09, 288.50, 288.59,
     289.9

   **AHA:** 4Q, '06, 69-73

√5ᵗʰ **288.5 Decreased white blood cell count**
     EXCLUDES    neutropenia (288.01-288.09)

     **288.50 Leukocytopenia, unspecified**
         Decreased leukocytes, unspecified
         Decreased white blood cell count,
           unspecified
         Leukopenia NOS
         **AHA:** 4Q, '06, 69-73

     **288.51 Lymphocytopenia**
         Decreased lymphocytes
         **AHA:** 4Q, '06, 69-73

     **288.59 Other decreased white blood cell count**
         Basophilic leukopenia
         Eosinophilic leukopenia
         Monocytopenia
         Plasmacytopenia
         **AHA:** 4Q, '06, 69-73

√5ᵗʰ **288.6 Elevated white blood cell count**
     EXCLUDES    eosinophilia (288.3)

     **288.60 Leukocytosis, unspecified**
         Elevated leukocytes, unspecified
         Elevated white blood cell count, unspecified
         **AHA:** 4Q, '06, 69-73

     **288.61 Lymphocytosis (symptomatic)**
         Elevated lymphocytes
         **AHA:** 4Q, '06, 69-73

     **288.62 Leukemoid reaction**
         Basophilic leukemoid reaction
         Lymphocytic leukemoid reaction
         Monocytic leukemoid reaction
         Myelocytic leukemoid reaction
         Neutrophilic leukemoid reaction
         **AHA:** 4Q, '06, 69-73

     **288.63 Monocytosis (symptomatic)**
         EXCLUDES   infectious mononucleosis (075)
         **AHA:** 4Q, '06, 69-73

     **288.64 Plasmacytosis**
         **AHA:** 4Q, '06, 69-73

     **288.65 Basophilia**
         **AHA:** 4Q, '06, 69-73

     **288.66 Bandemia**
         Bandemia without diagnosis of specific
           infection
         EXCLUDES   confirmed infection—code to
                 infection
                 leukemia (204.00-208.9)

     **288.69 Other elevated white blood cell count**
         **AHA:** 4Q, '06, 69-73

**288.8 Other specified disease of white blood cells**
     EXCLUDES   decreased white blood cell counts
              (288.50-288.59)
           elevated white blood cell counts
              (288.60-288.69)
           immunity disorders (279.0-279.9)
   **AHA:** M-A, '87, 12

**288.9 Unspecified disease of white blood cells**

N Newborn Age: 0    P Pediatric Age: 0-17    M Maternity Age: 12-55    A Adult Age: 15-124    CC CC Condition    MCC Major CC Condition    HIV HIV Related Dx

76 — Volume 1 • October 2007           © 2007 Ingenix

✓4ᵗʰ **289 Other diseases of blood and blood-forming organs**

**289.0 Polycythemia, secondary**

High-oxygen-affinity
hemoglobin
Polycythemia:
acquired
benign
due to:
fall in plasma volume
high altitude

Polycythemia:
emotional
erythropoietin
hypoxemic
nephrogenous
relative
spurious
stress

EXCLUDES　polycythemia:
neonatal (776.4)
primary (238.4)
vera (238.4)

DEF: Elevated number of red blood cells in circulating blood as result of reduced oxygen supply to the tissues.

**289.1 Chronic lymphadenitis**

Chronic:
adenitis
lymphadenitis 〕 any lymph node, except mesenteric

EXCLUDES　acute lymphadenitis (683)
mesenteric (289.2)
enlarged glands NOS (785.6)

DEF: Persistent inflammation of lymph node tissue; origin of infection is usually elsewhere.

**289.2 Nonspecific mesenteric lymphadenitis**

Mesenteric lymphadenitis (acute) (chronic)

DEF: Inflammation of the lymph nodes in peritoneal fold that encases abdominal organs; disease resembles acute appendicitis; unknown etiology.

**289.3 Lymphadenitis, unspecified, except mesenteric**

AHA: 2Q, '92, 8

**289.4 Hypersplenism**

"Big spleen" syndrome　　Hypersplenia
Dyssplenism

EXCLUDES　primary splenic neutropenia (289.53)

DEF: An overactive spleen; it causes a deficiency of the peripheral blood components, an increase in bone marrow cells and sometimes a notable increase in the size of the spleen.

✓5ᵗʰ **289.5 Other diseases of spleen**

**289.50 Disease of spleen, unspecified**

**289.51 Chronic congestive splenomegaly**

**289.52 Splenic sequestration**

Code first sickle-cell disease in crisis
(282.42, 282.62, 282.64, 282.69)

AHA: 4Q, '03, 51

DEF: Blood is entrapped in the spleen due to vessel occlusion; most often associated with sickle-cell disease; spleen becomes enlarged and there is a sharp drop in hemoglobin.

**289.53 Neutropenic splenomegaly**

AHA: 4Q, '06, 73

**289.59 Other**

Lien migrans
Perisplenitis
Splenic:
abscess
atrophy
cyst

Splenic:
fibrosis
infarction
rupture, nontraumatic
Splenitis
Wandering spleen

EXCLUDES　bilharzial splenic fibrosis
(120.0-120.9)
hepatolienal fibrosis (571.5)
splenomegaly NOS (789.2)

**289.6 Familial polycythemia**

Familial:
benign polycythemia
erythrocytosis

DEF: Elevated number of red blood cells.

**289.7 Methemoglobinemia**　　　CC

Congenital NADH [DPNH]-methemoglobin-reductase
deficiency
Hemoglobin M [Hb-M] disease
Methemoglobinemia:
NOS
acquired (with sulfhemoglobinemia)
hereditary
toxic
Stokvis' disease
Sulfhemoglobinemia
Use additional E code to identify cause

CC Excl: 282.7-283.10, 283.19-283.9, 285.8-285.9, 289.7, 289.9

DEF: Presence in the blood of methemoglobin, a chemically altered form of hemoglobin; causes cyanosis, headache, dizziness, ataxia dyspnea, tachycardia, nausea, stupor, coma, and, rarely, death.

✓5ᵗʰ **289.8 Other specified diseases of blood and blood-forming organs**

AHA: 4Q, '03, 56; 1Q, '02, 16; 2Q, '89, 8; M-A, '87, 12

DEF: Hypercoagulable states: a group of inherited or acquired abnormalities of specific proteins and anticoagulant factors; also called thromboembolic states or thrombotic disorders, these disorders result in the abnormal development of blood clots.

**289.81 Primary hypercoagulable state**　　CC

Activated protein C resistance
Antithrombin III deficiency
Factor V Leiden mutation
Lupus anticoagulant
Protein C deficiency
Protein S deficiency
Prothrombin gene mutation

CC Excl: 288.00-288.9, 289.53, 289.81-289.9

DEF: Activated protein C resistance: decreased effectiveness of protein C to degrade factor V, necessary to inhibit clotting cascade; also called Factor V Leiden mutation.

DEF: Antithrombin III deficiency: deficiency in plasma antithrombin III one of six naturally occurring antithrombins that limit coagulation.

DEF: Factor V Leiden mutation: also called activated protein C resistance.

DEF: Lupus anticoagulant: deficiency in a circulating anticoagulant that inhibits the conversion of prothrombin into thrombin; autoimmune antibodies induce procoagulant surfaces on platelets; also called anti-phospholipid syndrome.

DEF: Protein C deficiency: deficiency of activated protein C which functions to bring the blood-clotting process into balance; same outcome as factor V Leiden mutation.

DEF: Protein S deficiency: similar to protein C deficiency; protein S is a vitamin K dependent cofactor in the activation of protein C.

DEF: Prothrombin gene mutation: increased levels of prothrombin, or factor II, a plasma protein that is converted to thrombin, which acts upon fibrinogen to form the fibrin.

**289.82 Secondary hypercoagulable state**　　CC

CC Excl: See code: 289.81

**289.83 Myelofibrosis** CC

Myelofibrosis NOS

Secondary myelofibrosis

*Code first the underlying disorder, such as:*

malignant neoplasm of breast (174.0-174.9, 175.0-175.9)

EXCLUDES *idiopathic myelofibrosis (238.76)*

*leukoerythroblastic anemia (284.2)*

*myelofibrosis with myeloid metaplasia (238.76)*

*myelophthisic anemia (284.2)*

*myelophthisis (284.2)*

*primary myelofibrosis (238.76)*

**CC Excl:** 202.40-202.48, 203.10-208.91, 238.4-238.9

**AHA:** 4Q, '06, 73

**DEF:** A progressive bone marrow disease characterized by the replacement of bone marrow with the overgrowth of neoplastic stem cells and fibrotic tissue, also progressive anemia and enlarged spleen.

**289.89 Other specified diseases of blood and blood-forming organs**

Hypergammaglobulinemia

Pseudocholinesterase deficiency

**289.9 Unspecified diseases of blood and blood-forming organs**

Blood dyscrasia NOS

Erythroid hyperplasia

**AHA:** M-A, '85, 14

---

N Newborn Age: 0    P Pediatric Age: 0-17    M Maternity Age: 12-55    A Adult Age: 15-124    CC CC Condition    MCC Major CC Condition    HIV HIV Related Dx

## 5. MENTAL DISORDERS (290-319)

### PSYCHOSES (290-299)

> **EXCLUDES** mental retardation (317-319)

### ORGANIC PSYCHOTIC CONDITIONS (290-294)

> **INCLUDES** psychotic organic brain syndrome
>
> **EXCLUDES** nonpsychotic syndromes of organic etiology (310.0-310.9)
> psychoses classifiable to 295-298 and without impairment of orientation, comprehension, calculation, learning capacity, and judgment, but associated with physical disease, injury, or condition affecting the brain [eg., following childbirth] (295.0-298.8)

✓4th **290 Dementias**

Code first the associated neurological condition

> **EXCLUDES** dementia due to alcohol (291.0-291.2)
> dementia due to drugs (292.82)
> dementia not classified as senile, presenile, or arteriosclerotic (294.10-294.11)
> psychoses classifiable to 295-298 occurring in the senium without dementia or delirium (295.0-298.8)
> senility with mental changes of nonpsychotic severity (310.1)
> transient organic psychotic conditions (293.0-293.9)

**290.0 Senile dementia, uncomplicated** `A`

Senile dementia:
NOS
simple type

> **EXCLUDES** mild memory disturbances, not amounting to dementia, associated with senile brain disease (310.1)
> senile dementia with:
> delirium or confusion (290.3)
> delusional [paranoid] features (290.20)
> depressive features (290.21)

**AHA:** 4Q, '99, 4

✓5th **290.1 Presenile dementia**

Brain syndrome with presenile brain disease

> **EXCLUDES** arteriosclerotic dementia (290.40-290.43)
> dementia associated with other cerebral conditions (294.10-294.11)

**AHA:** N-D, '84, 20

**290.10 Presenile dementia, uncomplicated** `A` `HIV`

Presenile dementia:
NOS
simple type

**290.11 Presenile dementia with delirium** `CC` `A` `HIV`

Presenile dementia with acute confusional state

**CC Excl:** 290.0-290.12, 290.20-290.3, 290.8-290.9, 292.81, 293.0, V62.84

**AHA:** 1Q, '88, 3

**290.12 Presenile dementia with delusional features** `CC` `A` `HIV`

Presenile dementia, paranoid type

**CC Excl:** 079.82, 290.0-290.12, 290.20-290.3, 290.8-290.9, 292.81, 293.0

**290.13 Presenile dementia with depressive features** `CC` `A` `HIV`

Presenile dementia, depressed type

**CC Excl:** 290.0, 290.13-290.3, 296.21-296.24, 296.30-296.34, 296.43-296.44, 296.53-296.54, 296.63-296.64

✓5th **290.2 Senile dementia with delusional or depressive features**

> **EXCLUDES** senile dementia:
> NOS (290.0)
> with delirium and/or confusion (290.3)

**290.20 Senile dementia with delusional features** `CC` `A`

Senile dementia, paranoid type
Senile psychosis NOS

**CC Excl:** 290.0-290.20, 290.3

**290.21 Senile dementia with depressive features** `CC` `A`

**CC Excl:** 290.13, 290.21

**290.3 Senile dementia with delirium** `CC` `A`

Senile dementia with acute confusional state

> **EXCLUDES** senile:
> dementia NOS (290.0)
> psychosis NOS (290.20)

**CC Excl:** 290.10-290.20, 290.3, V62.84

✓5th **290.4 Vascular dementia**

Multi-infarct dementia or psychosis
Use additional code to identify cerebral atherosclerosis (437.0)

> **EXCLUDES** suspected cases with no clear evidence of arteriosclerosis (290.9)

**AHA:** 1Q, '88, 3

**290.40 Vascular dementia, uncomplicated** `A`

Arteriosclerotic dementia:
NOS
simple type

**290.41 Vascular dementia with delirium** `CC` `A`

Arteriosclerotic dementia with acute confusional state

**CC Excl:** 290.11-290.12, 290.20, 290.3, 290.41

**290.42 Vascular dementia with delusions** `CC` `A`

Arteriosclerotic dementia, paranoid type

**CC Excl:** 290.42

**290.43 Vascular dementia with depressed mood** `CC` `A`

Arteriosclerotic dementia, depressed type

**CC Excl:** 290.43

**290.8 Other specified senile psychotic conditions** `CC`

Presbyophrenic psychosis

**CC Excl:** 290.8-291.0, 292.11, 292.81-292.82, 295.00-295.04, 295.10-295.14, 295.21-295.24, 295.31, 295.33-295.34, 295.40-295.44, 295.53-295.54, 295.63-295.64, 295.71, 295.73-295.74, 295.80-295.84, 295.91, 295.93-295.94, 296.21-296.24, 296.30-296.34

**290.9 Unspecified senile psychotic condition** `CC` `A`

**CC Excl:** See code: 290.8

✓4th **291 Alcohol induced mental disorders**

> **EXCLUDES** alcoholism without psychosis (303.0-303.9)

**AHA:** 1Q, '88, 3; S-O, '86, 3

**291.0 Alcohol withdrawal delirium** `CC`

Alcoholic delirium    Delirium tremens

> **EXCLUDES** alcohol withdrawal (291.81)

**CC Excl:** 291.0-294.9, 303.00-305.03, 305.20-305.93, 790.3

**AHA:** 2Q, '91, 11

✓4th ✓5th Additional Digit Required      Unacceptable PDx      `Manifestation Code`      ▶◀ Revised Text      ● New Code      ▲ Revised Code Title

© **2007 Ingenix**      October 2007 • Volume 1 — **79**

**Mental Disorders**

**291.1–292.9**

**291.1 Alcohol induced persisting amnestic disorder**
Alcoholic polyneuritic psychosis
Korsakoff's psychosis, alcoholic
Wernicke-Korsakoff syndrome (alcoholic)
**AHA:** 1Q, '88, 3

**DEF:** Prominent and lasting reduced memory span, disordered time appreciation and confabulation, occurring in alcoholics, as sequel to acute alcoholic psychosis.

**291.2 Alcohol induced persisting dementia**    `CC`
Alcoholic dementia NOS
Alcoholism associated with dementia NOS
Chronic alcoholic brain syndrome
**CC Excl:** See code: 291.0

**291.3 Alcohol induced psychotic disorder with hallucinations**    `CC`
Alcoholic:      Alcoholic:
hallucinosis (acute)    psychosis with hallucinosis
**EXCLUDES** *alcohol withdrawal with delirium (291.0)*
*schizophrenia (295.0-295.9) and paranoid states (297.0-297.9) taking the form of chronic hallucinosis with clear consciousness in an alcoholic*
**CC Excl:** See code: 291.0
**AHA:** 2Q, '91, 11

**DEF:** Psychosis lasting less than six months with slight or no clouding of consciousness in which auditory hallucinations predominate.

**291.4 Idiosyncratic alcohol intoxication**
Pathologic:      Pathologic:
alcohol intoxication    drunkenness
**EXCLUDES** *acute alcohol intoxication (305.0)*
*in alcoholism (303.0)*
*simple drunkenness (305.0)*

**DEF:** Unique behavioral patterns, like belligerence, after intake of relatively small amounts of alcohol; behavior not due to excess consumption.

**291.5 Alcohol induced psychotic disorder with delusions**
Alcoholic:      Alcoholic:
paranoia      psychosis, paranoid type
**EXCLUDES** *nonalcoholic paranoid states (297.0-297.9)*
*schizophrenia, paranoid type (295.3)*

√5ᵗʰ **291.8 Other specified alcohol induced mental disorders**
**AHA:** 3Q, '94, 13; J-A, '85, 10

**291.81 Alcohol withdrawal**    `CC`
Alcohol:
abstinence syndrome or symptoms
withdrawal syndrome or symptoms
**EXCLUDES** *alcohol withdrawal:*
*delirium (291.0)*
*hallucinosis (291.3)*
*delirium tremens (291.0)*
**CC Excl:** See code: 291.0
**AHA:** 4Q, '96, 28; 2Q, '91, 11

**291.82 Alcohol induced sleep disorders**
Alcohol induced circadian rhythm sleep disorders
Alcohol induced hypersomnia
Alcohol induced insomnia
Alcohol induced parasomnia

**291.89 Other**    `CC`
Alcohol induced anxiety disorder
Alcohol induced mood disorder
Alcohol induced sexual dysfunction
**CC Excl:** See code: 291.0

**291.9 Unspecified alcohol induced mental disorders**    `CC`
Alcoholic:
mania NOS
psychosis NOS
Alcoholism (chronic) with psychosis
Alcohol related disorder NOS
**CC Excl:** See code: 291.0

√4ᵗʰ **292 Drug induced mental disorders**
`INCLUDES` organic brain syndrome associated with consumption of drugs
Use additional code for any associated drug dependence (304.0-304.9)
Use additional E code to identify drug
**AHA:** 3Q, '04, 8; 2Q, '91, 11; S-O, '86, 3

**292.0 Drug withdrawal**    `CC`
Drug:
abstinence syndrome or symptoms
withdrawal syndrome or symptoms
**CC Excl:** See code: 291.0
**AHA:** 1Q, '97, 12; 1Q, '88, 3

√5ᵗʰ **292.1 Drug induced psychotic disorders**
**292.11 Drug induced psychotic disorder with delusions**    `CC`
Paranoid state induced by drugs
**CC Excl:** See code: 291.0

**292.12 Drug induced psychotic disorder with hallucinations**    `CC`
Hallucinatory state induced by drugs
**EXCLUDES** *states following LSD or other hallucinogens, lasting only a few days or less ["bad trips"] (305.3)*
**CC Excl:** See code: 291.0

**292.2 Pathological drug intoxication**
Drug reaction:
NOS     ⎫ resulting in brief
idiosyncratic   ⎬ psychotic states
pathologic    ⎭
**EXCLUDES** *expected brief psychotic reactions to hallucinogens ["bad trips"] (305.3)*
*physiological side-effects of drugs (e.g., dystonias)*

√5ᵗʰ **292.8 Other specified drug induced mental disorders**
**292.81 Drug induced delirium**    `CC`
**CC Excl:** 291.0-294.9, 303.00-305.03, 305.20-305.93, 790.3
**AHA:** 1Q, '88, 3

**292.82 Drug induced persisting dementia**    `CC`
**CC Excl:** See code: 292.81

**292.83 Drug induced persisting amnestic disorder**

**292.84 Drug induced mood disorder**
Depressive state induced by drugs

**292.85 Drug induced sleep disorders**
Drug induced circadian rhythm sleep disorder
Drug induced hypersomnia
Drug induced insomnia
Drug induced parasomnia

**292.89 Other**
Drug induced anxiety disorder
Drug induced organic personality syndrome
Drug induced sexual dysfunction
Drug intoxication

**292.9 Unspecified drug induced mental disorder**
Drug related disorder NOS
Organic psychosis NOS due to or associated with drugs

---

N Newborn Age: 0     P Pediatric Age: 0-17     M Maternity Age: 12-55     A Adult Age: 15-124     `CC` CC Condition     `MCC` Major CC Condition     `HIV` HIV Related Dx

         © *2007 Ingenix*

☑4ᵗʰ **293 Transient mental disorders due to conditions classified elsewhere**

INCLUDES  transient organic mental disorders not associated with alcohol or drugs

Code first the associated physical or neurological condition

EXCLUDES  confusional state or delirium superimposed on senile dementia (290.3)
dementia due to:
   alcohol (291.0-291.9)
   arteriosclerosis (290.40-290.43)
   drugs (292.82)
   senility (290.0)

**293.0 Delirium due to conditions classified elsewhere** CC
Acute:
   confusional state
   infective psychosis
   organic reaction
   posttraumatic organic psychosis
   psycho-organic syndrome
Acute psychosis associated with endocrine, metabolic, or cerebrovascular disorder
Epileptic:
   confusional state
   twilight state

CC Excl: 290.11, 290.3, 293.0, V62.84

AHA: 1Q, '88, 3

**293.1 Subacute delirium** CC
Subacute:
   confusional state
   infective psychosis
   organic reaction
   posttraumatic organic psychosis
   psycho-organic syndrome
   psychosis associated with endocrine or metabolic disorder

CC Excl: 293.0-293.1, 293.89-293.9

☑5ᵗʰ **293.8 Other specified transient mental disorders due to conditions classified elsewhere**

**293.81 Psychotic disorder with delusions in conditions classified elsewhere** CC
Transient organic psychotic condition, paranoid type

CC Excl: 291.0-294.9, 303.00-305.03, 305.20-305.93, 790.3

**293.82 Psychotic disorder with hallucinations in conditions classified elsewhere** CC
Transient organic psychotic condition, hallucinatory type

CC Excl: See code: 293.81

**293.83 Mood disorder in conditions classified elsewhere**
Transient organic psychotic condition, depressive type

**293.84 Anxiety disorder in conditions classified elsewhere**
AHA: 4Q, '96, 29

**293.89 Other**
Catatonic disorder in conditions classified elsewhere

**293.9 Unspecified transient mental disorder in conditions classified elsewhere** CC
Organic psychosis:
   infective NOS
   posttraumatic NOS
   transient NOS
Psycho-organic syndrome

CC Excl: See code: 293.81

☑4ᵗʰ **294 Persistent mental disorders due to conditions classified elsewhere**

INCLUDES  organic psychotic brain syndromes (chronic), not elsewhere classified

AHA: M-A, '85, 12

**294.0 Amnestic disorder in conditions classified elsewhere**
Korsakoff's psychosis or syndrome (nonalcoholic)
Code first underlying condition

EXCLUDES  alcoholic:
   amnestic syndrome (291.1)
   Korsakoff's psychosis (291.1)

☑5ᵗʰ **294.1 Dementia in conditions classified elsewhere**
Dementia of the Alzheimer's type
Code first any underlying physical condition, as:
dementia in:
   Alzheimer's disease (331.0)
   cerebral lipidoses (330.1)
   dementia with Lewy bodies (331.82)
   dementia with Parkinsonism (331.82)
   epilepsy (345.0-345.9)
   frontal dementia (331.19)
   frontotemporal dementia (331.19)
   general paresis [syphilis] (094.1)
   hepatolenticular degeneration (275.1)
   Huntington's chorea (333.4)
   Jakob-Creutzfeldt disease (046.1)
   multiple sclerosis (340)
   Pick's disease of the brain (331.11)
   polyarteritis nodosa (446.0)
   syphilis (094.1)

EXCLUDES  dementia:
   arteriosclerotic (290.40-290.43)
   presenile (290.10-290.13)
   senile (290.0)
   epileptic psychosis NOS (294.8)

AHA: 4Q, '00, 40; 1Q, '99, 14; N-D, '85, 5

**294.10 Dementia in conditions classified elsewhere without behavioral disturbance**
Dementia in conditions classified elsewhere NOS

**294.11 Dementia in conditions classified elsewhere with behavioral disturbance** CC
Aggressive behavior
Combative behavior
Violent behavior
Wandering off

CC Excl: 294.11

AHA: 4Q, '00, 41

**294.8 Other persistent mental disorders due to conditions classified elsewhere**
Amnestic disorder NOS
Dementia NOS
Epileptic psychosis NOS
Mixed paranoid and affective organic psychotic states
Use additional code for associated epilepsy (345.0-345.9)

EXCLUDES  mild memory disturbances, not amounting to dementia (310.1)

AHA: 3Q, '03, 14; 1Q, '88, 5

**294.9 Unspecified persistent mental disorders due to conditions classified elsewhere** HIV
Cognitive disorder NOS
Organic psychosis (chronic)
AHA: ►2Q, '07, 4◄

**Mental Disorders**

**295–296**

## OTHER PSYCHOSES (295-299)

Use additional code to identify any associated physical disease, injury, or condition affecting the brain with psychoses classifiable to 295-298

√4th **295 Schizophrenic disorders**

INCLUDES    schizophrenia of the types described in 295.0-295.9 occurring in children

EXCLUDES    *childhood type schizophrenia (299.9)*
*infantile autism (299.0)*

The following fifth-digit subclassification is for use with category 295:

  0  **unspecified**
  1  **subchronic**
  2  **chronic**
  3  **subchronic with acute exacerbation**
  4  **chronic with acute exacerbation**
  5  **in remission**

DEF: Group of disorders with disturbances in thought (delusions, hallucinations), mood (blunted, flattened, inappropriate affect), sense of self, relationship to world; also bizarre, purposeless behavior, repetitive activity, or inactivity.

√5th **295.0 Simple type**    CC 0-4
Schizophrenia simplex
EXCLUDES    *latent schizophrenia (295.5)*

CC Excl: For codes 295.00-295.04: 295.00-301.9, 306.0-319, 388.45

√5th **295.1 Disorganized type**    CC 0-4
Hebephrenia
Hebephrenic type schizophrenia

CC Excl: For codes 295.10-295.14: 295.00-301.9, 306.0-319, 388.45

DEF: Inappropriate behavior; results in extreme incoherence and disorganization of time, place and sense of social appropriateness; withdrawal from routine social interaction may occur.

√5th **295.2 Catatonic type**    CC 0-4
Catatonic (schizophrenia):    Schizophrenic:
   agitation            catalepsy
   excitation          catatonia
   excited type       flexibilitas cerea
   stupor
   withdrawn type

CC Excl: For codes 295.20-295.24: 295.00-301.9, 306.0-319, 388.45

DEF: Extreme changes in motor activity; one extreme is decreased response or reaction to the environment and the other is spontaneous activity.

√5th **295.3 Paranoid type**    CC 0-4
Paraphrenic schizophrenia
EXCLUDES    *involutional paranoid state (297.2)*
*paranoia (297.1)*
*paraphrenia (297.2)*

CC Excl: For codes 295.30-295.34: 295.00-301.9, 306.0-319, 388.45

DEF: Preoccupied with delusional suspicions and auditory hallucinations related to single theme; usually hostile, grandiose, overly religious, occasionally hypochondriacal.

√5th **295.4 Schizophreniform disorder**    CC 0-4
Oneirophrenia        Schizophreniform:
Schizophreniform:      psychosis, confusional type
   attack
EXCLUDES    *acute forms of schizophrenia of:*
*catatonic type (295.2)*
*hebephrenic type (295.1)*
*paranoid type (295.3)*
*simple type (295.0)*
*undifferentiated type (295.8)*

CC Excl: For codes 295.40-295.44: 295.00-301.9, 306.0-319, 388.45

√5th **295.5 Latent schizophrenia**    CC 3-4
Latent schizophrenic reaction
Schizophrenia:
   borderline
   incipient
   prepsychotic
   prodromal
   pseudoneurotic
   pseudopsychopathic
EXCLUDES    *schizoid personality (301.20-301.22)*

CC Excl: For code 295.53-295.54: 295.00-295.04, 295.10-295.14, 295.21-295.24, 295.31, 295.33-295.34, 295.40-295.44, 295.53-295.54, 295.63-295.64, 295.71, 295.73-295.74, 295.80-295.84, 295.91, 295.93-295.94

AHA: For code 295.50: 1Q, '06, 10

√5th **295.6 Residual type**    CC 0-4
Chronic undifferentiated schizophrenia
Restzustand (schizophrenic)
Schizophrenic residual state

CC Excl: For codes 295.60-295.64: 295.00-301.9, 306.0-319, 388.45

AHA: For code 295.62: 4Q, '06, 78

√5th **295.7 Schizoaffective disorder**    CC 1-4
Cyclic schizophrenia
Mixed schizophrenic and affective psychosis
Schizo-affective psychosis
Schizophreniform psychosis, affective type

CC Excl: For codes 295.71-295.74: 295.00-301.9, 306.0-319, 388.45

√5th **295.8 Other specified types of schizophrenia**    CC 0-4
Acute (undifferentiated) schizophrenia
Atypical schizophrenia
Cenesthopathic schizophrenia
EXCLUDES    *infantile autism (299.0)*

CC Excl: For codes 295.80-295.84: 295.00-301.9, 306.0-319, 388.45

√5th **295.9 Unspecified schizophrenia**    CC 1-4
Schizophrenia:
   NOS
   mixed NOS
   undifferentiated NOS
   undifferentiated type
Schizophrenic reaction NOS
Schizophreniform psychosis NOS

CC Excl: For codes 295.91-295.94: 295.00-301.9, 306.0-319, 388.45

AHA: 3Q, '95, 6

√4th **296 Episodic mood disorders**

INCLUDES    episodic affective disorders
EXCLUDES    *neurotic depression (300.4)*
*reactive depressive psychosis (298.0)*
*reactive excitation (298.1)*

The following fifth-digit subclassification is for use with categories 296.0-296.6:

  0  **unspecified**
  1  **mild**
  2  **moderate**
  3  **severe, without mention of psychotic behavior**
  4  **severe, specified as with psychotic behavior**
  5  **in partial or unspecified remission**
  6  **in full remission**

AHA: M-A, '85, 14

---

N Newborn Age: 0     P Pediatric Age: 0-17     M Maternity Age: 12-55     A Adult Age: 15-124     CC CC Condition     MCC Major CC Condition     HIV HIV Related Dx

§ ✓5th **296.0** **Bipolar I disorder, single manic episode** `CC 0-4`

Hypomania (mild) NOS
Hypomanic psychosis
Mania (monopolar) NOS
Manic-depressive psychosis
or reaction:
hypomanic
manic
} single episode or unspecified

**EXCLUDES** *circular type, if there was a previous attack of depression (296.4)*

**CC Excl: For codes 296.00-296.02:** 295.00-301.9, 306.0-319, 388.45; **For codes 296.03:** 296.03-296.04, 296.13-296.14, 296.43-296.44, 296.53-296.54, 296.63-296.64; **For codes 296.04:** 295.00-301.9, 306.0-319, 388.45

**DEF:** Mood disorder identified by hyperactivity; may show extreme agitation or exaggerated excitability; speech and thought processes may be accelerated.

§ ✓5th **296.1** **Manic disorder, recurrent episode** `CC 0-4`

Any condition classifiable to 296.0, stated to be recurrent

**EXCLUDES** *circular type, if there was a previous attack of depression (296.4)*

**CC Excl: For codes 296.10-296.12:** 295.00-301.9, 306.0-319, 388.45; **For codes 296.13:** 296.13-296.14, 296.43-296.44, 296.53-296.54, 296.63-296.64; **For codes 296.14:** 295.00-301.9, 306.0-319, 388.45

§ ✓5th **296.2** **Major depressive disorder, single episode** `CC 0-4`

Depressive psychosis
Endogenous depression
Involutional melancholia
Manic-depressive psychosis or
reaction, depressed type
Monopolar depression
Psychotic depression
} single episode or unspecified

**EXCLUDES** *circular type, if previous attack was of manic type (296.5)*
*depression NOS (311)*
*reactive depression (neurotic) (300.4)*
*psychotic (298.0)*

**CC Excl: For code 296.20:** 295.00-301.9, 306.0-319, 388.45; **For codes 296.21-296.24:** 296.21-296.24, 296.30-296.34

**DEF:** Mood disorder that produces depression; may exhibit as sadness, low self-esteem, or guilt feelings; other manifestations may be withdrawal from friends and family; interrupted sleep.

§ ✓5th **296.3** **Major depressive disorder, recurrent episode** `CC 0-4`

Any condition classifiable to 296.2, stated to be recurrent

**EXCLUDES** *circular type, if previous attack was of manic type (296.5)*
*depression NOS (311)*
*reactive depression (neurotic) (300.4)*
*psychotic (298.0)*

**CC Excl: For codes 296.30-296.33:** 296.21-296.24, 296.30-296.34; **For codes 296.34:** 295.00-301.9, 306.0-319, 388.45

§ ✓5th **296.4** **Bipolar I disorder, most recent episode (or current) manic** `CC 0-4`

Bipolar disorder, now manic
Manic-depressive psychosis, circular type but currently manic

**EXCLUDES** *brief compensatory or rebound mood swings (296.99)*

**CC Excl: For codes 296.40-296.42 and 296.44:** 295.00-301.9, 306.0-319, 388.45; **For code 296.43:** 296.43-296.44, 296.63-296.64

§ ✓5th **296.5** **Bipolar I disorder, most recent episode (or current) depressed** `CC 0-4`

Bipolar disorder, now depressed
Manic-depressive psychosis, circular type but currently depressed

**EXCLUDES** *brief compensatory or rebound mood swings (296.99)*

**CC Excl: For codes 296.50-296.52 and 296.54:** 295.00-301.9, 306.0-319, 388.45; **For code 296.53:** 296.43-296.44, 296.53-296.54, 296.63-296.64

§ ✓5th **296.6** **Bipolar I disorder, most recent episode (or current) mixed** `CC 0-4`

Manic-depressive psychosis, circular type, mixed

**CC Excl: For codes 296.60-296.62 and 296.64:** 295.00-301.9, 306.0-319, 388.45; **For code 296.63:** 296.43-296.44, 296.53-296.54, 296.63-296.64

**296.7** **Bipolar I disorder, most recent episode (or current) unspecified**

Atypical bipolar affective disorder NOS
Manic-depressive psychosis, circular type, current condition not specified as either manic or depressive

**DEF:** Manic-depressive disorder referred to as bipolar because of the mood range from manic to depressive.

✓5th **296.8** **Other and unspecified bipolar disorders**

**296.80** **Bipolar disorder, unspecified**

Bipolar disorder NOS
Manic-depressive:
reaction NOS
syndrome NOS

**296.81** **Atypical manic disorder**

**296.82** **Atypical depressive disorder**

**296.89** **Other** `CC`

Bipolar II disorder
Manic-depressive psychosis, mixed type

**CC Excl:** 295.00-301.9, 306.0-319, 388.45

✓5th **296.9** **Other and unspecified episodic mood disorder**

**EXCLUDES** *psychogenic affective psychoses (298.0-298.8)*

**296.90** **Unspecified episodic mood disorder**

Affective psychosis NOS
Melancholia NOS
Mood disorder NOS

**AHA:** M-A, '85, 14

**296.99** **Other specified episodic mood disorder** `CC`

Mood swings:
brief compensatory
rebound

**CC Excl:** 295.00-301.9, 306.0-319, 388.45

✓4th **297** **Delusional disorders**

**INCLUDES** paranoid disorders
**EXCLUDES** *acute paranoid reaction (298.3)*
*alcoholic jealousy or paranoid state (291.5)*
*paranoid schizophrenia (295.3)*

**297.0** **Paranoid state, simple**

**297.1** **Delusional disorder**

Chronic paranoid psychosis
Sander's disease
Systematized delusions

**EXCLUDES** *paranoid personality disorder (301.0)*

**297.2** **Paraphrenia**

Involutional paranoid state
Late paraphrenia
Paraphrenia (involutional)

**DEF:** Paranoid schizophrenic disorder that persists over a prolonged period but does not distort personality despite persistent delusions.

---

§ Requires fifth-digit. See category 296 for codes and definitions.

**Mental Disorders**

**297.3–300.00**

**297.3 Shared psychotic disorder**
Folie à deux
Induced psychosis or paranoid disorder
**DEF:** Mental disorder two people share; first person with the delusional disorder convinces second person because of a close relationship and shared experiences to accept the delusions.

**297.8 Other specified paranoid states**
Paranoia querulans
Sensitiver Beziehungswahn
　　EXCLUDES　*acute paranoid reaction or state (298.3)*
　　　　　　　*senile paranoid state (290.20)*

**297.9 Unspecified paranoid state**
Paranoid:　　　　　　　Paranoid:
　disorder NOS　　　　　reaction NOS
　psychosis NOS　　　　state NOS
**AHA:** J-A, '85, 9

√4th **298 Other nonorganic psychoses**
　　INCLUDES　psychotic conditions due to or provoked by:
　　　　　emotional stress
　　　　　environmental factors as major part of
　　　　　etiology

**298.0 Depressive type psychosis**　　　CC
Psychogenic depressive psychosis
Psychotic reactive depression
Reactive depressive psychosis
　　EXCLUDES　*manic-depressive psychosis, depressed type (296.2-296.3)*
　　　　　　　*neurotic depression (300.4)*
　　　　　　　*reactive depression NOS (300.4)*
**CC Excl:** 295.00-301.9, 306.0-319, 388.45

**298.1 Excitative type psychosis**　　　CC
Acute hysterical psychosis　Reactive excitation
Psychogenic excitation
　　EXCLUDES　*manic-depressive psychosis, manic type (296.0-296.1)*
**CC Excl:** See code: 298.0

**DEF:** Affective disorder similar to manic-depressive psychosis, in the manic phase, seemingly brought on by stress.

**298.2 Reactive confusion**
Psychogenic confusion　Psychogenic twilight state
　　EXCLUDES　*acute confusional state (293.0)*
**DEF:** Confusion, disorientation, cloudiness in consciousness; brought on by severe emotional upheaval.

**298.3 Acute paranoid reaction**　　　CC
Acute psychogenic paranoid psychosis
Bouffée délirante
　　EXCLUDES　*paranoid states (297.0-297.9)*
**CC Excl:** See code: 298.0

**298.4 Psychogenic paranoid psychosis**　　　CC
Protracted reactive paranoid psychosis
**CC Excl:** See code: 298.0

**298.8 Other and unspecified reactive psychosis**
Brief psychotic disorder
Brief reactive psychosis NOS
Hysterical psychosis
Psychogenic psychosis NOS
Psychogenic stupor
　　EXCLUDES　*acute hysterical psychosis (298.1)*

**298.9 Unspecified psychosis**　　　HIV
Atypical psychosis
Psychosis NOS
Psychotic disorder NOS
**AHA:** 3Q, '06, 22

√4th **299 Pervasive developmental disorders**
　　EXCLUDES　*adult type psychoses occurring in childhood, as:*
　　　　*affective disorders (296.0-296.9)*
　　　　*manic-depressive disorders (296.0-296.9)*
　　　　*schizophrenia (295.0-295.9)*

The following fifth-digit subclassification is for use with category 299:
　**0　current or active state**
　**1　residual state**

√5th **299.0 Autistic disorder**　　　CC
Childhood autism
Infantile psychosis
Kanner's syndrome
　　EXCLUDES　*disintegrative psychosis (299.1)*
　　　　　　　*Heller's syndrome (299.1)*
　　　　　　　*schizophrenic syndrome of childhood (299.9)*
**CC Excl:** 295.00-301.9, 306.0-319, 388.45

**DEF:** Severe mental disorder of children, results in impaired social behavior; abnormal development of communicative skills, appears to be unaware of the need for emotional support and offers little emotional response to family members.

√5th **299.1 Childhood disintegrative disorder**　　　CC
Heller's syndrome
Use additional code to identify any associated neurological disorder
　　EXCLUDES　*infantile autism (299.0)*
　　　　　　　*schizophrenic syndrome of childhood (299.9)*
**CC Excl:** See code: 299.0

**DEF:** Mental disease of children identified by impaired development of reciprocal social skills, verbal and nonverbal communication skills, imaginative play.

√5th **299.8 Other specified pervasive developmental disorders**　　　CC
Asperger's disorder
Atypical childhood psychosis
Borderline psychosis of childhood
　　EXCLUDES　*simple stereotypes without psychotic disturbance (307.3)*
**CC Excl:** See code: 299.0

√5th **299.9 Unspecified pervasive developmental disorder**　　　CC
Child psychosis NOS
Pervasive developmental disorder NOS
Schizophrenia, childhood type NOS
Schizophrenic syndrome of childhood NOS
　　EXCLUDES　*schizophrenia of adult type occurring in childhood (295.0-295.9)*
**CC Excl:** See code: 299.0

## NEUROTIC DISORDERS, PERSONALITY DISORDERS, AND OTHER NONPSYCHOTIC MENTAL DISORDERS (300-316)

√4th **300 Anxiety, dissociative and somatoform disorders**
√5th **300.0 Anxiety states**
　　EXCLUDES　*anxiety in:*
　　　　*acute stress reaction (308.0)*
　　　　*transient adjustment reaction (309.24)*
　　　　*neurasthenia (300.5)*
　　　　*psychophysiological disorders (306.0-306.9)*
　　　　*separation anxiety (309.21)*
**DEF:** Mental disorder characterized by anxiety and avoidance behavior not particularly related to any specific situation or stimulus; symptoms include emotional instability, apprehension, fatigue.

**300.00 Anxiety state, unspecified**
Anxiety:　　　　　　Anxiety:
　neurosis　　　　　　state (neurotic)
　reaction　　　　　Atypical anxiety disorder
**AHA:** 1Q, '02, 6

N Newborn Age: 0　P Pediatric Age: 0-17　M Maternity Age: 12-55　A Adult Age: 15-124　CC CC Condition　MCC Major CC Condition　HIV HIV Related Dx

84 — Volume 1 • October 2007

© 2007 Ingenix

✓5th **300.01 Panic disorder without agoraphobia**

Panic:                   Panic:
    attack                   state

EXCLUDES    *panic disorder with*
                *agoraphobia (300.21)*

DEF: Neurotic disorder characterized by recurrent panic or anxiety, apprehension, fear or terror; symptoms include shortness of breath, palpitations, dizziness, faintness or shakiness; fear of dying may persist or fear of other morbid consequences.

**300.02 Generalized anxiety disorder**

**300.09 Other**

✓5th **300.1 Dissociative, conversion and factitious disorders**

EXCLUDES    *adjustment reaction (309.0-309.9)*
                *anorexia nervosa (307.1)*
                *gross stress reaction (308.0-308.9)*
                *hysterical personality (301.50-301.59)*
                *psychophysiologic disorders (306.0-*
                    *306.9)*

**300.10 Hysteria, unspecified**

**300.11 Conversion disorder**

Astasia-abasia,          Hysterical:
    hysterical               blindness
Conversion hysteria      deafness
    or reaction              paralysis

AHA: N-D, '85, 15

DEF: Mental disorder that impairs physical functions with no physiological basis; sensory motor symptoms include seizures, paralysis, temporary blindness; increase in stress or avoidance of unpleasant responsibilities may precipitate.

**300.12 Dissociative amnesia**

Hysterical amnesia

**300.13 Dissociative fugue**

Hysterical fugue

DEF: Dissociative hysteria; identified by loss of memory, flight from familiar surroundings; conscious activity is not associated with perception of surroundings, no later memory of episode.

**300.14 Dissociative identity disorder**

**300.15 Dissociative disorder or reaction, unspecified**

DEF: Hysterical neurotic episode; sudden but temporary changes in perceived identity, memory, consciousness, segregated memory patterns exist separate from dominant personality.

**300.16 Factitious disorder with predominantly psychological signs and symptoms**

Compensation neurosis
Ganser's syndrome, hysterical

DEF: A disorder characterized by the purposeful assumption of mental illness symptoms; the symptoms are not real, possibly representing what the patient imagines mental illness to be like, and are acted out more often when another person is present.

**300.19 Other and unspecified factitious illness**

Factitious disorder (with combined psychological and physical signs and symptoms) (with predominantly physical signs and symptoms) NOS

EXCLUDES    *multiple operations or hospital*
                *addiction syndrome*
                *(301.51)*

✓5th **300.2 Phobic disorders**

EXCLUDES    *anxiety state not associated with a*
                *specific situation or object*
                *(300.00-300.09)*
                *obsessional phobias (300.3)*

**300.20 Phobia, unspecified**

Anxiety-hysteria NOS
Phobia NOS

**300.21 Agoraphobia with panic disorder**

Fear of:
    open spaces  ⎫
    streets        ⎬  with panic attacks
    travel        ⎭

Panic disorder with agoraphobia

EXCLUDES    *agoraphobia without panic*
                *disorder (300.22)*
                *panic disorder without*
                    *agoraphobia (300.01)*

**300.22 Agoraphobia without mention of panic attacks**

Any condition classifiable to 300.21 without mention of panic attacks

**300.23 Social phobia**

Fear of:                 Fear of:
    eating in public         washing in public
    public speaking

**300.29 Other isolated or specific phobias**

Acrophobia           Claustrophobia
Animal phobias       Fear of crowds

**300.3 Obsessive-compulsive disorders**

Anancastic neurosis      Obsessional phobia [any]
Compulsive neurosis

EXCLUDES    *obsessive-compulsive symptoms*
                *occurring in:*
                *endogenous depression (296.2-*
                    *296.3)*
                *organic states (eg., encephalitis)*
                *schizophrenia (295.0-295.9)*

**300.4 Dysthymic disorder**

Anxiety depression       Neurotic depressive state
Depression with anxiety  Reactive depression
Depressive reaction

EXCLUDES    *adjustment reaction with depressive*
                *symptoms (309.0-309.1)*
                *depression NOS (311)*
                *manic-depressive psychosis, depressed*
                    *type (296.2-296.3)*
                *reactive depressive psychosis (298.0)*

DEF: Depression without psychosis; less severe depression related to personal change or unexpected circumstances; also referred to as "reactional depression."

**300.5 Neurasthenia**

Fatigue neurosis         Psychogenic:
Nervous debility             general fatigue
Psychogenic:
    asthenia
Use additional code to identify any associated
    physical disorder

EXCLUDES    *anxiety state (300.00-300.09)*
                *neurotic depression (300.4)*
                *psychophysiological disorders (306.0-*
                    *306.9)*
                *specific nonpsychotic mental disorders*
                    *following organic brain damage*
                    *(310.0-310.9)*

DEF: Physical and mental symptoms caused primarily by what is known as mental exhaustion; symptoms include chronic weakness, fatigue.

**300.6 Depersonalization disorder**

Derealization (neurotic)
Neurotic state with depersonalization episode

EXCLUDES    *depersonalization associated with:*
                *anxiety (300.00-300.09)*
                *depression (300.4)*
                *manic-depressive disorder or*
                    *psychosis (296.0-296.9)*
                *schizophrenia (295.0-295.9)*

DEF: Dissociative disorder characterized by feelings of strangeness about self or body image; symptoms include dizziness, anxiety, fear of insanity, loss of reality of surroundings.

**300.7 Hypochondriasis**
　Body dysmorphic disorder
　**EXCLUDES** *hypochondriasis in:*
　　　　*hysteria (300.10-300.19)*
　　　　*manic-depressive psychosis,*
　　　　　*depressed type (296.2-296.3)*
　　　　*neurasthenia (300.5)*
　　　　*obsessional disorder (300.3)*
　　　　*schizophrenia (295.0-295.9)*

✓5ᵗʰ **300.8 Somatoform disorders**

　**300.81 Somatization disorder**
　　Briquet's disorder
　　Severe somatoform disorder

　**300.82 Undifferentiated somatoform disorder**
　　Atypical somatoform disorder
　　Somatoform disorder NOS
　　**AHA:** 4Q, '96, 29

　　**DEF:** Disorders in which patients have symptoms that suggest an organic disease but no evidence of physical disorder after repeated testing.

　**300.89 Other somatoform disorders**
　　Occupational neurosis, including writers' cramp
　　Psychasthenia
　　Psychasthenic neurosis

**300.9 Unspecified nonpsychotic mental disorder**
　Psychoneurosis NOS

✓4ᵗʰ **301 Personality disorders**
　**INCLUDES** character neurosis
　Use additional code to identify any associated neurosis or psychosis, or physical condition
　**EXCLUDES** *nonpsychotic personality disorder associated with organic brain syndromes (310.0-310.9)*

**301.0 Paranoid personality disorder**
　Fanatic personality
　Paranoid personality (disorder)
　Paranoid traits
　**EXCLUDES** *acute paranoid reaction (298.3)*
　　　　*alcoholic paranoia (291.5)*
　　　　*paranoid schizophrenia (295.3)*
　　　　*paranoid states (297.0-297.9)*
　**AHA:** J-A, '85, 9

✓5ᵗʰ **301.1 Affective personality disorder**
　**EXCLUDES** *affective psychotic disorders (296.0-296.9)*
　　　　*neurasthenia (300.5)*
　　　　*neurotic depression (300.4)*

　**301.10 Affective personality disorder, unspecified**
　**301.11 Chronic hypomanic personality disorder**
　　Chronic hypomanic disorder
　　Hypomanic personality
　**301.12 Chronic depressive personality disorder**
　　Chronic depressive disorder
　　Depressive character or personality
　**301.13 Cyclothymic disorder**
　　Cycloid personality
　　Cyclothymia
　　Cyclothymic personality

✓5ᵗʰ **301.2 Schizoid personality disorder**
　**EXCLUDES** *schizophrenia (295.0-295.9)*
　**301.20 Schizoid personality disorder, unspecified**
　**301.21 Introverted personality**
　**301.22 Schizotypal personality disorder**

**301.3 Explosive personality disorder**
　Aggressive:　　　　Emotional instability
　　personality　　　　(excessive)
　　reaction　　　　Pathological emotionality
　Aggressiveness　　Quarrelsomeness
　**EXCLUDES** *dyssocial personality (301.7)*
　　　　*hysterical neurosis (300.10-300.19)*

**301.4 Obsessive-compulsive personality disorder**
　Anancastic personality
　Obsessional personality
　**EXCLUDES** *obsessive-compulsive disorder (300.3)*
　　　　*phobic state (300.20-300.29)*

✓5ᵗʰ **301.5 Histrionic personality disorder**
　**EXCLUDES** *hysterical neurosis (300.10-300.19)*
　**DEF:** Extreme emotional behavior, often theatrical; often concerned about own appeal; may demand attention, exhibit seductive behavior.

　**301.50 Histrionic personality disorder, unspecified**
　　Hysterical personality NOS
　**301.51 Chronic factitious illness with**　　**cc**
　　**physical symptoms**
　　Hospital addiction syndrome
　　Multiple operations syndrome
　　Munchausen syndrome
　　**CC Excl:** 295.00-301.9, 306.0-319, 388.45

　**301.59 Other histrionic personality disorder**
　　Personality:　　　　Personality:
　　　emotionally unstable　　psychoinfantile
　　　labile

**301.6 Dependent personality disorder**
　Asthenic personality
　Inadequate personality
　Passive personality
　**EXCLUDES** *neurasthenia (300.5)*
　　　　*passive-aggressive personality (301.84)*
　**DEF:** Overwhelming feeling of helplessness; fears of abandonment may persist; difficulty in making personal decisions without confirmation by others; low self-esteem due to irrational sensitivity to criticism.

**301.7 Antisocial personality disorder**
　Amoral personality
　Asocial personality
　Dyssocial personality
　Personality disorder with predominantly sociopathic or asocial manifestation
　**EXCLUDES** *disturbance of conduct without specifiable personality disorder (312.0-312.9)*
　　　　*explosive personality (301.3)*
　**AHA:** S-O, '84, 16
　**DEF:** Continuous antisocial behavior that violates rights of others; social traits include extreme aggression, total disregard for traditional social rules.

✓5ᵗʰ **301.8 Other personality disorders**
　**301.81 Narcissistic personality disorder**
　　**DEF:** Grandiose fantasy or behavior, lack of social empathy, hypersensitive to the lack of others' judgment, exploits others; also sense of entitlement to have expectations met, need for continual admiration.

　**301.82 Avoidant personality disorder**
　　**DEF:** Personality disorder marked by feelings of social inferiority; sensitivity to criticism, emotionally restrained due to fear of rejection.

　**301.83 Borderline personality disorder**
　　**DEF:** Personality disorder characterized by unstable moods, self-image, and interpersonal relationships; uncontrolled anger, impulsive and self-destructive acts, fears of abandonment, feelings of emptiness and boredom, recurrent suicide threats or self-mutilation.

　**301.84 Passive-aggressive personality**
　　**DEF:** Pattern of procrastination and refusal to meet standards; introduce own obstacles to success and exploit failure.

---

**N** Newborn Age: 0　　**P** Pediatric Age: 0-17　　**M** Maternity Age: 12-55　　**A** Adult Age: 15-124　　**CC** CC Condition　　**MCC** Major CC Condition　　**HIV** HIV Related Dx

### 301.89 Other
Personality:     Personality:
  eccentric       masochistic
  "haltlose" type    psychoneurotic
  immature
> **EXCLUDES**    *psychoinfantile personality*
> *(301.59)*

### 301.9 Unspecified personality disorder
Pathological personality NOS
Personality disorder NOS
Psychopathic:
  constitutional state
  personality (disorder)

### ✓4th 302 Sexual and gender identity disorders
> **EXCLUDES**    *sexual disorder manifest in:*
> *organic brain syndrome (290.0-294.9,*
> *310.0-310.9)*
> *psychosis (295.0-298.9)*

### 302.0 Ego-dystonic sexual orientation
Ego-dystonic lesbianism
Sexual orientation conflict disorder
> **EXCLUDES**    *homosexual pedophilia (302.2)*

### 302.1 Zoophilia
Bestiality
DEF: A sociodeviant disorder marked by engaging in sexual intercourse with animals.

### 302.2 Pedophilia
DEF: A sociodeviant condition of adults characterized by sexual activity with children.

### 302.3 Transvestic fetishism
> **EXCLUDES**    *trans-sexualism (302.5)*

DEF: The desire to dress in clothing of opposite sex.

### 302.4 Exhibitionism
DEF: Sexual deviant behavior; exposure of genitals to strangers; behavior prompted by intense sexual urges and fantasies.

### ✓5th 302.5 Trans-sexualism
▶Sex reassignment surgery status◀
> **EXCLUDES**    *transvestism (302.3)*

DEF: Gender identity disturbance; overwhelming desire to change anatomic sex, due to belief that individual is a member of the opposite sex.

### 302.50 With unspecified sexual history
### 302.51 With asexual history
### 302.52 With homosexual history
### 302.53 With heterosexual history
### 302.6 Gender identity disorder in children
Feminism in boys
Gender identity disorder NOS
> **EXCLUDES**    *gender identity disorder in adult*
> *(302.85)*
> *trans-sexualism (302.50-302.53)*
> *transvestism (302.3)*

### ✓5th 302.7 Psychosexual dysfunction
> **EXCLUDES**    *impotence of organic origin (607.84)*
> *normal transient symptoms from*
> *ruptured hymen*
> *transient or occasional failures of*
> *erection due to fatigue, anxiety,*
> *alcohol, or drugs*

### 302.70 Psychosexual dysfunction, unspecified
Sexual dysfunction NOS
### 302.71 Hypoactive sexual desire disorder
> **EXCLUDES**    *decreased sexual desire NOS*
> *(799.81)*

### 302.72 With inhibited sexual excitement
Female sexual arousal disorder
Frigidity
Impotence
Male erectile disorder
### 302.73 Female orgasmic disorder ♀
### 302.74 Male orgasmic disorder ♂

### 302.75 Premature ejaculation ♂
### 302.76 Dyspareunia, psychogenic ♀
DEF: Difficult or painful sex due to psychosomatic state.

### 302.79 With other specified psychosexual dysfunctions
Sexual aversion disorder

### ✓5th 302.8 Other specified psychosexual disorders
### 302.81 Fetishism
DEF: Psychosexual disorder noted for intense sexual urges and arousal precipitated by fantasies; use of inanimate objects, such as clothing, to stimulate sexual arousal, orgasm.

### 302.82 Voyeurism
DEF: Psychosexual disorder characterized by uncontrollable impulse to observe others, without their knowledge, who are nude or engaged in sexual activity.

### 302.83 Sexual masochism
DEF: Psychosexual disorder noted for need to achieve sexual gratification through humiliating or hurtful acts inflicted on self.

### 302.84 Sexual sadism
DEF: Psychosexual disorder noted for need to achieve sexual gratification through humiliating or hurtful acts inflicted on someone else.

### 302.85 Gender identity disorder in adolescents or adults
▶Use additional code to identify sex reassignment surgery status (302.5)◀
> **EXCLUDES**    *gender identity disorder NOS*
> *(302.6)*
> *gender identity disorder in*
> *children (302.6)*

### 302.89 Other
Frotteurism
Nymphomania
Satyriasis

### 302.9 Unspecified psychosexual disorder
Paraphilia NOS
Pathologic sexuality NOS
Sexual deviation NOS
Sexual disorder NOS

### ✓4th 303 Alcohol dependence syndrome
Use additional code to identify any associated condition, as:
  alcoholic psychoses (291.0-291.9)
  drug dependence (304.0-304.9)
  physical complications of alcohol, such as:
    cerebral degeneration (331.7)
    cirrhosis of liver (571.2)
    epilepsy (345.0-345.9)
    gastritis (535.3)
    hepatitis (571.1)
    liver damage NOS (571.3)
> **EXCLUDES**    *drunkenness NOS (305.0)*

The following fifth-digit subclassification is for use with category 303:

| 0 unspecified | 2 episodic |
|---|---|
| 1 continuous | 3 in remission |

AHA: 3Q, '95, 6; 2Q, '91, 9; 4Q, '88, 8; S-O, '86, 3

### ✓5th 303.0 Acute alcoholic intoxication
Acute drunkenness in alcoholism

### ✓5th 303.9 Other and unspecified alcohol dependence
Chronic alcoholism      Dipsomania
AHA: 2Q, '02, 4; 2Q, '89, 9 ; For code 303.90: ▶2Q, '07, 6◀

---

**Mental Disorders**

**304-305.9**

☑4th **304 Drug dependence**

> **EXCLUDES** *nondependent abuse of drugs (305.1-305.9)*

The following fifth-digit subclassification is for use with category 304:

| | |
|---|---|
| 0   unspecified | 2   episodic |
| 1   continuous | 3   in remission |

**AHA:** 2Q, '91, 10; 4Q, '88, 8; S-O, '86, 3

☑5th **304.0   Opioid type dependence**    `CC 1`

| | |
|---|---|
| Heroin | Opium alkaloids and their |
| Meperidine |    derivatives |
| Methadone | Synthetics with morphine-like |
| Morphine |    effects |
| Opium | |

**CC Excl:** For code **304.01:** 291.0-292.9, 303.00-305.03, 305.20-305.93, 790.3

**AHA:** 2Q, '06, 7

☑5th **304.1   Sedative, hypnotic or anxiolytic dependence**    `CC 1`

Barbiturates
Nonbarbiturate sedatives and tranquilizers with a
   similar effect:

| | |
|---|---|
| chlordiazepoxide | meprobamate |
| diazepam | methaqualone |
| glutethimide | |

**CC Excl:** For code **304.11:** 291.0-292.9, 303.00-305.03, 305.20-305.93, 790.3

☑5th **304.2   Cocaine dependence**    `CC 1`

Coca leaves and derivatives

**CC Excl:** For code **304.21:** 291.0-292.9, 303.00-305.03, 305.20-305.93, 790.3

☑5th **304.3   Cannabis dependence**

| | |
|---|---|
| Hashish | Marihuana |
| Hemp | |

☑5th **304.4   Amphetamine and other psychostimulant dependence**    `CC 1`

| | |
|---|---|
| Methylphenidate | Phenmetrazine |

**CC Excl:** For code **304.41:** 291.0-292.9, 303.00-305.03, 305.20-305.93, 790.3

☑5th **304.5   Hallucinogen dependence**    `CC 1`

Dimethyltryptamine [DMT]
Lysergic acid diethylamide [LSD] and derivatives
Mescaline
Psilocybin

**CC Excl:** For code **304.51:** 291.0-292.9, 303.00-305.03, 305.20-305.93, 790.3

☑5th **304.6   Other specified drug dependence**    `CC 1`

Absinthe addiction
Glue sniffing
Inhalant dependence
Phencyclidine dependence

> **EXCLUDES** *tobacco dependence (305.1)*

**CC Excl:** For code **304.61:** 291.0-292.9, 303.00-305.03, 305.20-305.93, 790.3

☑5th **304.7   Combinations of opioid type drug with any other**    `CC 1`

**CC Excl:** For code **304.71:** 291.0-292.9, 303.00-305.03, 305.20-305.93, 790.3

**AHA:** M-A, '86, 12

☑5th **304.8   Combinations of drug dependence excluding opioid type drug**    `CC 1`

**CC Excl:** For code **304.81:** 291.0-292.9, 303.00-305.03, 305.20-305.93, 790.3

**AHA:** M-A, '86, 12

☑5th **304.9   Unspecified drug dependence**    `CC 1`

Drug addiction NOS    Drug dependence NOS

**CC Excl:** For code **304.91:** 291.0-292.9, 303.00-305.03, 305.20-305.93, 790.3

**AHA:** For code **304.90:** 4Q, '03, 103

☑4th **305 Nondependent abuse of drugs**

Note: Includes cases where a person, for whom no other diagnosis is possible, has come under medical care because of the maladaptive effect of a drug on which he is not dependent and that he has taken on his own initiative to the detriment of his health or social functioning.

> **EXCLUDES** *alcohol dependence syndrome (303.0-303.9)*
> *drug dependence (304.0-304.9)*
> *drug withdrawal syndrome (292.0)*
> *poisoning by drugs or medicinal substances (960.0-979.9)*

The following fifth-digit subclassification is for use with codes 305.0, 305.2-305.9:

| | |
|---|---|
| 0   unspecified | 2   episodic |
| 1   continuous | 3   in remission |

**AHA:** 2Q, '91, 10; 4Q, '88, 8; S-O, '86, 3

☑5th **305.0   Alcohol abuse**

Drunkenness NOS
Excessive drinking of alcohol NOS
"Hangover" (alcohol)
Inebriety NOS

> **EXCLUDES** *acute alcohol intoxication in alcoholism (303.0)*
> *alcoholic psychoses (291.0-291.9)*

**AHA:** 3Q, '96, 16

**305.1   Tobacco use disorder**

Tobacco dependence

> **EXCLUDES** *history of tobacco use (V15.82)*
> *smoking complicating pregnancy (649.0)*
> *tobacco use disorder complicating pregnancy (649.0)*

**AHA:** 2Q, '96, 10; N-D, '84, 12

☑5th **305.2   Cannabis abuse**

☑5th **305.3   Hallucinogen abuse**

Acute intoxication from hallucinogens ["bad trips"]
LSD reaction

☑5th **305.4   Sedative, hypnotic or anxiolytic abuse**

☑5th **305.5   Opioid abuse**

☑5th **305.6   Cocaine abuse**

**AHA:** For code **305.60:** 1Q, '05, 6; 1Q, '93, 25

☑5th **305.7   Amphetamine or related acting sympathomimetic abuse**

**AHA:** For code **305.70:** 2Q, '03, 10–11

☑5th **305.8   Antidepressant type abuse**

☑5th **305.9   Other, mixed, or unspecified drug abuse**

Caffeine intoxication
Inhalant abuse
"Laxative habit"
Misuse of drugs NOS
Nonprescribed use of drugs or patent medicinals
Phencyclidine abuse

**AHA:** 3Q, '99, 20

---

 Newborn Age: 0     Pediatric Age: 0-17     Maternity Age: 12-55     Adult Age: 15-124     `CC` CC Condition    `MCC` Major CC Condition    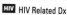 `HIV` HIV Related Dx

**✓4ᵗʰ 306 Physiological malfunction arising from mental factors**

INCLUDES   psychogenic:

| physical symptoms | not involving |
|---|---|
| physiological manifestations } | tissue damage |

EXCLUDES   *hysteria (300.11-300.19)*
*physical symptoms secondary to a psychiatric disorder classified elsewhere*
*psychic factors associated with physical conditions involving tissue damage classified elsewhere (316)*
*specific nonpsychotic mental disorders following organic brain damage (310.0-310.9)*

DEF: Functional disturbances or interruptions due to mental or psychological causes; no tissue damage sustained in these conditions.

**306.0    Musculoskeletal**
Psychogenic paralysis
Psychogenic torticollis

EXCLUDES   *Gilles de la Tourette's syndrome (307.23)*
*paralysis as hysterical or conversion reaction (300.11)*
*tics (307.20-307.22)*

**306.1    Respiratory**

| Psychogenic: | Psychogenic: |
|---|---|
| air hunger | hyperventilation |
| cough | yawning |
| hiccough | |

EXCLUDES   *psychogenic asthma (316 and 493.9)*

**306.2    Cardiovascular**
Cardiac neurosis
Cardiovascular neurosis
Neurocirculatory asthenia
Psychogenic cardiovascular disorder

EXCLUDES   *psychogenic paroxysmal tachycardia (316 and 427.2)*

**AHA:** J-A, '85, 14

DEF: Neurocirculatory asthenia: functional nervous and circulatory irregularities with palpitations, dyspnea, fatigue, rapid pulse, precordial pain, fear of effort, discomfort during exercise, anxiety; also called DaCosta's syndrome, Effort syndrome, Irritable or Soldier's Heart.

**306.3    Skin**
Psychogenic pruritus

EXCLUDES   *psychogenic:*
*alopecia (316 and 704.00)*
*dermatitis (316 and 692.9)*
*eczema (316 and 691.8 or 692.9)*
*urticaria (316 and 708.0-708.9)*

**306.4    Gastrointestinal**
Aerophagy
Cyclical vomiting, psychogenic
Diarrhea, psychogenic
Nervous gastritis
Psychogenic dyspepsia

EXCLUDES   *cyclical vomiting NOS (536.2)*
*globus hystericus (300.11)*
*mucous colitis (316 and 564.9)*
*psychogenic:*
*cardiospasm (316 and 530.0)*
*duodenal ulcer (316 and 532.0-532.9)*
*gastric ulcer (316 and 531.0-531.9)*
*peptic ulcer NOS (316 and 533.0-533.9)*
*vomiting NOS (307.54)*

**AHA:** 2Q, '89, 11

DEF: Aerophagy: excess swallowing of air, usually unconscious; related to anxiety; results in distended abdomen or belching, often interpreted by the patient as a physical disorder.

**✓5ᵗʰ 306.5    Genitourinary**

EXCLUDES   *enuresis, psychogenic (307.6)*
*frigidity (302.72)*
*impotence (302.72)*
*psychogenic dyspareunia (302.76)*

**306.50   Psychogenic genitourinary malfunction, unspecified**

**306.51   Psychogenic vaginismus** ♀
Functional vaginismus

DEF: Psychogenic response resulting in painful contractions of vaginal canal muscles; can be severe enough to prevent sexual intercourse.

**306.52   Psychogenic dysmenorrhea** ♀

**306.53   Psychogenic dysuria**

**306.59   Other**
**AHA:** M-A, '87, 11

**306.6    Endocrine**

**306.7    Organs of special sense**

EXCLUDES   *hysterical blindness or deafness (300.11)*
*psychophysical visual disturbances (368.16)*

**306.8    Other specified psychophysiological malfunction**

| Bruxism | Teeth grinding |
|---|---|

**306.9    Unspecified psychophysiological malfunction**
Psychophysiologic disorder NOS
Psychosomatic disorder NOS

**✓4ᵗʰ 307 Special symptoms or syndromes, not elsewhere classified**

Note: This category is intended for use if the psychopathology is manifested by a single specific symptom or group of symptoms which is not part of an organic illness or other mental disorder classifiable elsewhere.

EXCLUDES   *those due to mental disorders classified elsewhere*
*those of organic origin*

**307.0    Stuttering**

EXCLUDES   *dysphasia (784.5)*
*lisping or lalling (307.9)*
*retarded development of speech (315.31-315.39)*

**307.1    Anorexia nervosa**    CC

EXCLUDES   *eating disturbance NOS (307.50)*
*feeding problem (783.3)*
*of nonorganic origin (307.59)*
*loss of appetite (783.0)*
*of nonorganic origin (307.59)*

**CC Excl:** 306.4, 306.8-306.9, 307.1, 307.50-307.59, 309.22

**AHA:** 2Q, '06, 12; 4Q, '89, 11

**✓5ᵗʰ 307.2    Tics**

EXCLUDES   *nail-biting or thumb-sucking (307.9)*
*stereotypes occurring in isolation (307.3)*
*tics of organic origin (333.3)*

DEF: Involuntary muscle response usually confined to the face, shoulders.

**307.20   Tic disorder, unspecified**
Tic disorder NOS

**307.21   Transient tic disorder**

**307.22   Chronic motor or vocal tic disorder**

**307.23   Tourette's disorder**
Motor-verbal tic disorder

DEF: Syndrome of facial and vocal tics in childhood; progresses to spontaneous or involuntary jerking, obscene utterances, other uncontrollable actions considered inappropriate.

**307.3    Stereotypic movement disorder**

| Body-rocking | Spasmus nutans |
|---|---|
| Head banging | Stereotypes NOS |

EXCLUDES   *tics (307.20-307.23)*
*of organic origin (333.3)*

√5ᵗʰ **307.4 Specific disorders of sleep of nonorganic origin**
EXCLUDES narcolepsy (347.00-347.11)
organic hypersomnia (327.10-327.19)
organic insomnia (327.00-327.09)
those of unspecified cause (780.50-780.59)

**307.40 Nonorganic sleep disorder, unspecified**

**307.41 Transient disorder of initiating or maintaining sleep**
Adjustment insomnia
Hyposomnia ⎫ associated with inter-
Insomnia ⎬ mittent emotional
Sleeplessness ⎭ reactions or conflicts

**307.42 Persistent disorder of initiating or maintaining sleep**
Hyposomnia, insomnia, or sleeplessness associated with:
anxiety
conditioned arousal
depression (major) (minor)
psychosis
Idiopathic insomnia
Paradoxical insomnia
Primary insomnia
Psychophysiological insomnia

**307.43 Transient disorder of initiating or maintaining wakefulness**
Hypersomnia associated with acute or intermittent emotional reactions or conflicts

**307.44 Persistent disorder of initiating or maintaining wakefulness**
Hypersomnia associated with depression (major) (minor)
Insufficient sleep syndrome
Primary hypersomnia
EXCLUDES sleep deprivation (V69.4)

**307.45 Circadian rhythm sleep disorder of nonorganic origin**

**307.46 Sleep arousal disorder**
Night terror disorder
Night terrors
Sleep terror disorder
Sleepwalking
Somnambulism
DEF: Sleepwalking marked by extreme terror, panic, screaming, confusion; no recall of event upon arousal; term may refer to simply the act of sleepwalking.

**307.47 Other dysfunctions of sleep stages or arousal from sleep**
Nightmare disorder
Nightmares:
NOS
REM-sleep type
Sleep drunkenness

**307.48 Repetitive intrusions of sleep**
Repetitive intrusion of sleep with:
atypical polysomnographic features
environmental disturbances
repeated REM-sleep interruptions

**307.49 Other**
"Short-sleeper"
Subjective insomnia complaint

√5ᵗʰ **307.5 Other and unspecified disorders of eating**
EXCLUDES anorexia:
nervosa (307.1)
of unspecified cause (783.0)
overeating, of unspecified cause (783.6)
vomiting:
NOS (787.0)
cyclical (536.2)
psychogenic (306.4)

**307.50 Eating disorder, unspecified**
Eating disorder NOS

**307.51 Bulimia nervosa** CC
Overeating of nonorganic origin
CC Excl: 307.1, 307.50-307.51, 307.53-307.59
DEF: Mental disorder commonly characterized by binge eating followed by self-induced vomiting; perceptions of being fat; and fear the inability to stop eating voluntarily.

**307.52 Pica**
Perverted appetite of nonorganic origin
DEF: Compulsive eating disorder characterized by craving for substances, other than food; such as paint chips or dirt.

**307.53 Rumination disorder**
Regurgitation, of nonorganic origin, of food with reswallowing
EXCLUDES obsessional rumination (300.3)

**307.54 Psychogenic vomiting**

**307.59 Other**
Feeding disorder of infancy or early childhood of nonorganic origin
Infantile feeding ⎫
disturbances ⎬ of nonorganic
Loss of appetite ⎭ origin

**307.6 Enuresis**
Enuresis (primary) (secondary) of nonorganic origin
EXCLUDES enuresis of unspecified cause (788.3)
DEF: Involuntary urination past age of normal control; also called bedwetting; no trace to biological problem; focus on psychological issues.

**307.7 Encopresis**
Encopresis (continuous) (discontinuous) of nonorganic origin
EXCLUDES encopresis of unspecified cause (787.6)
DEF: Inability to control bowel movements; cause traced to psychological, not biological, problems.

√5ᵗʰ **307.8 Pain disorders related to psychological factors**

**307.80 Psychogenic pain, site unspecified**

**307.81 Tension headache**
EXCLUDES headache:
NOS (784.0)
migraine (346.0-346.9)
AHA: N-D, '85, 16

**307.89 Other**
Code first to type or site of pain
EXCLUDES pain disorder exclusively attributed to psychological factors (307.80)
psychogenic pain (307.80)

**307.9 Other and unspecified special symptoms or syndromes, not elsewhere classified**
Communication disorder NOS
Hair plucking
Lalling
Lisping
Masturbation
Nail-biting
Thumb-sucking

√4ᵗʰ **308 Acute reaction to stress**
INCLUDES catastrophic stress
combat fatigue
gross stress reaction (acute)
transient disorders in response to exceptional physical or mental stress which usually subside within hours or days
EXCLUDES adjustment reaction or disorder (309.0-309.9)
chronic stress reaction (309.1-309.9)

**308.0 Predominant disturbance of emotions**
Anxiety ⎫ as acute reaction to
Emotional crisis ⎬ exceptional
Panic state ⎭ [gross] stress

N Newborn Age: 0  P Pediatric Age: 0-17  M Maternity Age: 12-55  A Adult Age: 15-124  CC CC Condition  MCC Major CC Condition  HIV HIV Related Dx

90 — Volume 1 • October 2007

© 2007 Ingenix

**308.1 Predominant disturbance of consciousness**
Fugues as acute reaction to exceptional [gross] stress

**308.2 Predominant psychomotor disturbance**
Agitation states ⎤ as acute reaction to exceptional
Stupor ⎦ [gross] stress

**308.3 Other acute reactions to stress**
Acute situational disturbance
Acute stress disorder
> EXCLUDES *prolonged posttraumatic emotional disturbance (309.81)*

**308.4 Mixed disorders as reaction to stress**

**308.9 Unspecified acute reaction to stress**

√4th **309 Adjustment reaction**
> INCLUDES adjustment disorders
> reaction (adjustment) to chronic stress
> EXCLUDES *acute reaction to major stress (308.0-308.9)*
> *neurotic disorders (300.0-300.9)*

**309.0 Adjustment disorder with depressed mood**
Grief reaction
> EXCLUDES *affective psychoses (296.0-296.9)*
> *neurotic depression (300.4)*
> *prolonged depressive reaction (309.1)*
> *psychogenic depressive psychosis (298.0)*

**309.1 Prolonged depressive reaction**
> EXCLUDES *affective psychoses (296.0-296.9)*
> *brief depressive reaction (309.0)*
> *neurotic depression (300.4)*
> *psychogenic depressive psychosis (298.0)*

√5th **309.2 With predominant disturbance of other emotions**
**309.21 Separation anxiety disorder**
DEF: Abnormal apprehension by a child when physically separated from support environment; byproduct of abnormal symbiotic child-parent relationship.

**309.22 Emancipation disorder of adolescence and early adult life**
DEF: Adjustment reaction of late adolescence; conflict over independence from parental supervision; symptoms include difficulty in making decisions, increased reliance on parental advice, deliberate adoption of values in opposition of parents.

**309.23 Specific academic or work inhibition**

**309.24 Adjustment disorder with anxiety**

**309.28 Adjustment disorder with mixed anxiety and depressed mood**
Adjustment reaction with anxiety and depression

**309.29 Other**
Culture shock

**309.3 Adjustment disorder with disturbance of conduct**
Conduct disturbance ⎤ as adjustment reaction
Destructiveness ⎦
> EXCLUDES *destructiveness in child (312.9)*
> *disturbance of conduct NOS (312.9)*
> *dyssocial behavior without manifest psychiatric disorder (V71.01-V71.02)*
> *personality disorder with predominantly sociopathic or asocial manifestations (301.7)*

**309.4 Adjustment disorder with mixed disturbance of emotions and conduct**

√5th **309.8 Other specified adjustment reactions**
**309.81 Posttraumatic stress disorder**
Chronic posttraumatic stress disorder
Concentration camp syndrome
Posttraumatic stress disorder NOS
Post-traumatic stress disorder (PTSD)
> EXCLUDES *acute stress disorder (308.3)*
> *posttraumatic brain syndrome:*
> *nonpsychotic (310.2)*
> *psychotic (293.0-293.9)*

DEF: Preoccupation with traumatic events beyond normal experience; events such as rape, personal assault, combat, natural disasters, accidents, torture precipitate disorder; also recurring flashbacks of trauma; symptoms include difficulty remembering, sleeping, or concentrating, and guilt feelings for surviving.

**309.82 Adjustment reaction with physical symptoms**

**309.83 Adjustment reaction with withdrawal**
Elective mutism as adjustment reaction
Hospitalism (in children) NOS

**309.89 Other**

**309.9 Unspecified adjustment reaction**
Adaptation reaction NOS
Adjustment reaction NOS

√4th **310 Specific nonpsychotic mental disorders due to brain damage**
> EXCLUDES *neuroses, personality disorders, or other nonpsychotic conditions occurring in a form similar to that seen with functional disorders but in association with a physical condition (300.0-300.9, 301.0-301.9)*

**310.0 Frontal lobe syndrome**
Lobotomy syndrome
Postleucotomy syndrome [state]
> EXCLUDES *postcontusion syndrome (310.2)*

**310.1 Personality change due to conditions classified elsewhere**
Cognitive or personality change of other type, of nonpsychotic severity
Organic psychosyndrome of nonpsychotic severity
Presbyophrenia NOS
Senility with mental changes of nonpsychotic severity
> EXCLUDES *memory loss of unknown cause (780.93)*

AHA: 2Q, '05, 6

DEF: Personality disorder caused by organic factors, such as brain lesions, head trauma, or cerebrovascular accident (CVA).

**310.2 Postconcussion syndrome**
Postcontusion syndrome or encephalopathy
Posttraumatic brain syndrome, nonpsychotic
Status postcommotio cerebri
> EXCLUDES *frontal lobe syndrome (310.0)*
> *postencephalitic syndrome (310.8)*
> *any organic psychotic conditions following head injury (293.0-294.0)*

AHA: 4Q, '90, 24

DEF: Nonpsychotic disorder due to brain trauma, causes symptoms unrelated to any disease process; symptoms include amnesia, serial headaches, rapid heartbeat, fatigue, disrupted sleep patterns, inability to concentrate.

**310.8 Other specified nonpsychotic mental disorders following organic brain damage**
Mild memory disturbance
Postencephalitic syndrome
Other focal (partial) organic psychosyndromes

**310.9 Unspecified nonpsychotic mental disorder following organic brain damage** HIV
AHA: 4Q, '03, 103

√4th ⎯ Additional Digit Required
√5th

Unacceptable PDx     Manifestation Code     ►◄ Revised Text     ● New Code     ▲ Revised Code Title

**Mental Disorders**

**311–314.00**

## 311 Depressive disorder, not elsewhere classified

Depressive disorder NOS    Depression NOS
Depressive state NOS

**EXCLUDES**    *acute reaction to major stress with depressive symptoms (308.0)*
*affective personality disorder (301.10-301.13)*
*affective psychoses (296.0-296.9)*
*brief depressive reaction (309.0)*
*depressive states associated with stressful events (309.0-309.1)*
*disturbance of emotions specific to childhood and adolescence, with misery and unhappiness (313.1)*
*mixed adjustment reaction with depressive symptoms (309.4)*
*neurotic depression (300.4)*
*prolonged depressive adjustment reaction (309.1)*
*psychogenic depressive psychosis (298.0)*

**AHA:** 4Q, '03, 75

## ✓4th 312 Disturbance of conduct, not elsewhere classified

**EXCLUDES**    *adjustment reaction with disturbance of conduct (309.3)*
*drug dependence (304.0-304.9)*
*dyssocial behavior without manifest psychiatric disorder (V71.01-V71.02)*
*personality disorder with predominantly sociopathic or asocial manifestations (301.7)*
*sexual deviations (302.0-302.9)*

The following fifth-digit subclassification is for use with categories 312.0-312.2:

0   unspecified
1   mild
2   moderate
3   severe

### ✓5th 312.0 Undersocialized conduct disorder, aggressive type

Aggressive outburst    Unsocialized aggressive
Anger reaction            disorder

**DEF:** Mental condition identified by behaviors disrespectful of others' rights and of age-appropriate social norms or rules; symptoms include bullying, vandalism, verbal and physical abusiveness, lying, stealing, defiance.

### ✓5th 312.1 Undersocialized conduct disorder, unaggressive type

Childhood truancy, unsocialized
Solitary stealing
Tantrums

### ✓5th 312.2 Socialized conduct disorder

Childhood truancy, socialized   Group delinquency

**EXCLUDES**    *gang activity without manifest psychiatric disorder (V71.01)*

### ✓5th 312.3 Disorders of impulse control, not elsewhere classified

312.30 Impulse control disorder, unspecified
312.31 Pathological gambling
312.32 Kleptomania
312.33 Pyromania
312.34 Intermittent explosive disorder
312.35 Isolated explosive disorder
312.39 Other
   Trichotillomania

### 312.4 Mixed disturbance of conduct and emotions

Neurotic delinquency

**EXCLUDES**    *compulsive conduct disorder (312.3)*

### ✓5th 312.8 Other specified disturbances of conduct, not elsewhere classified

312.81 Conduct disorder, childhood onset type
312.82 Conduct disorder, adolescent onset type
312.89 Other conduct disorder
   Conduct disorder of unspecified onset

### 312.9 Unspecified disturbance of conduct

Delinquency (juvenile)
Disruptive behavior disorder NOS

## ✓4th 313 Disturbance of emotions specific to childhood and adolescence

**EXCLUDES**    *adjustment reaction (309.0-309.9)*
*emotional disorder of neurotic type (300.0-300.9)*
*masturbation, nail-biting, thumbsucking, and other isolated symptoms (307.0-307.9)*

### 313.0 Overanxious disorder

Anxiety and fearfulness } of childhood and
Overanxious disorder        adolescence

**EXCLUDES**    *abnormal separation anxiety (309.21)*
*anxiety states (300.00-300.09)*
*hospitalism in children (309.83)*
*phobic state (300.20-300.29)*

### 313.1 Misery and unhappiness disorder

**EXCLUDES**    *depressive neurosis (300.4)*

### ✓5th 313.2 Sensitivity, shyness, and social withdrawal disorder

**EXCLUDES**    *infantile autism (299.0)*
*schizoid personality (301.20-301.22)*
*schizophrenia (295.0-295.9)*

313.21 Shyness disorder of childhood
   Sensitivity reaction of childhood or adolescence

313.22 Introverted disorder of childhood
   Social withdrawal } of childhood or
   Withdrawal        adolescence
   reaction

313.23 Selective mutism
   **EXCLUDES**    *elective mutism as adjustment reaction (309.83)*

### 313.3 Relationship problems

Sibling jealousy

**EXCLUDES**    *relationship problems associated with aggression, destruction, or other forms of conduct disturbance (312.0-312.9)*

### ✓5th 313.8 Other or mixed emotional disturbances of childhood or adolescence

313.81 Oppositional defiant disorder
   **DEF:** Mental disorder of children noted for pervasive opposition, defiance of authority.

313.82 Identity disorder
   Identity problem
   **DEF:** Distress of adolescents caused by inability to form acceptable self-identity; uncertainty about career choice, sexual orientation, moral values.

313.83 Academic underachievement disorder

313.89 Other    **P**
   Reactive attachment disorder of infancy or early childhood

### 313.9 Unspecified emotional disturbance of childhood or adolescence    **P**

Mental disorder of infancy, childhood or adolescence NOS

## ✓4th 314 Hyperkinetic syndrome of childhood

**EXCLUDES**    *hyperkinesis as symptom of underlying disorder—code the underlying disorder*

### ✓5th 314.0 Attention deficit disorder

Adult
Child

**DEF:** A behavioral disorder usually diagnosed at an early age; characterized by the inability to focus attention for a normal period of time.

314.00 Without mention of hyperactivity
   Predominantly inattentive type
   **AHA:** 1Q, '97, 8

**N** Newborn Age: 0    **P** Pediatric Age: 0-17    **M** Maternity Age: 12-55    **A** Adult Age: 15-124    **CC** CC Condition    **MCC** Major CC Condition    **HIV** HIV Related Dx

92 — Volume 1

© 2007 Ingenix

**314.01  With hyperactivity**
Combined type
Overactivity NOS
Predominantly hyperactive/impulsive type
Simple disturbance of attention with
overactivity
**AHA:** 1Q, '97, 8

**314.1  Hyperkinesis with developmental delay**
Developmental disorder of hyperkinesis
Use additional code to identify any associated
neurological disorder

**314.2  Hyperkinetic conduct disorder**
Hyperkinetic conduct disorder without
developmental delay
**EXCLUDES** *hyperkinesis with significant delays in
specific skills (314.1)*

**314.8  Other specified manifestations of hyperkinetic
syndrome**

**314.9  Unspecified hyperkinetic syndrome**
Hyperkinetic reaction of childhood or adolescence
NOS
Hyperkinetic syndrome NOS

√4th **315  Specific delays in development**
**EXCLUDES** *that due to a neurological disorder (320.0-389.9)*

√5th **315.0  Specific reading disorder**
**315.00  Reading disorder, unspecified**
**315.01  Alexia**
**DEF:** Lack of ability to understand written language;
manifestation of aphasia.

**315.02  Developmental dyslexia**
**DEF:** Serious impairment of reading skills unexplained in
relation to general intelligence and teaching processes;
it can be inherited or congenital.

**315.09  Other**
Specific spelling difficulty

**315.1  Mathematics disorder**
Dyscalculia

**315.2  Other specific learning difficulties**
Disorder of written expression
**EXCLUDES** *specific arithmetical disorder (315.1)
specific reading disorder (315.00-
315.09)*

√5th **315.3  Developmental speech or language disorder**
**315.31  Expressive language disorder**
Developmental aphasia
Word deafness
**EXCLUDES** *acquired aphasia (784.3)
elective mutism (309.83,
313.0, 313.23)*

**315.32  Mixed receptive-expressive language
disorder**
▶Central auditory processing disorder◀
**EXCLUDES** ▶*acquired auditory processing
disorder (388.45)*◀
**AHA:** 2Q, '05, 5; 4Q, '96, 30

**315.34  Speech and language developmental delay
due to hearing loss**
Use additional code to identify type of
hearing loss (389.00-389.9)

**315.39  Other**
Developmental articulation disorder
Dyslalia
Phonological disorder
**EXCLUDES** *lisping and lalling (307.9)
stammering and stuttering
(307.0)*

**315.4  Developmental coordination disorder**
Clumsiness syndrome
Dyspraxia syndrome
Specific motor development disorder

**315.5  Mixed development disorder**
**AHA:** 2Q, '02, 11

**315.8  Other specified delays in development**

**315.9  Unspecified delay in development**
Developmental disorder NOS
Learning disorder NOS

**316  Psychic factors associated with diseases classified
elsewhere**
Psychologic factors in physical conditions classified elsewhere
Use additional code to identify the associated physical
condition, as:
psychogenic:
asthma (493.9)
dermatitis (692.9)
duodenal ulcer (532.0-532.9)
eczema (691.8, 692.9)
gastric ulcer (531.0-531.9)
mucous colitis (564.9)
paroxysmal tachycardia (427.2)
ulcerative colitis (556)
urticaria (708.0-708.9)
psychosocial dwarfism (259.4)
**EXCLUDES** *physical symptoms and physiological
malfunctions, not involving tissue damage,
of mental origin (306.0-306.9)*

### MENTAL RETARDATION (317-319)
Use additional code(s) to identify any associated psychiatric
or physical condition(s)

**317  Mild mental retardation**
High-grade defect
IQ 50-70
Mild mental subnormality

√4th **318  Other specified mental retardation**
**318.0  Moderate mental retardation**
IQ 35-49
Moderate mental subnormality

**318.1  Severe mental retardation**    CC
IQ 20-34
Severe mental subnormality
**CC Excl:** 318.1-318.2

**318.2  Profound mental retardation**    CC
IQ under 20
Profound mental subnormality
**CC Excl:** See code: 318.1

**319  Unspecified mental retardation**
Mental deficiency NOS
Mental subnormality NOS

## 6. DISEASES OF THE NERVOUS SYSTEM AND SENSE ORGANS (320-389)

## INFLAMMATORY DISEASES OF THE CENTRAL NERVOUS SYSTEM (320-326)

✓4ᵗʰ **320 Bacterial meningitis**

INCLUDES
arachnoiditis
leptomeningitis
meningitis            } bacterial
meningoencephalitis
meningomyelitis
pachymeningitis

**AHA:** J-F, '87, 6

**DEF:** Bacterial infection causing inflammation of the lining of the brain and/or spinal cord.

**320.0 Hemophilus meningitis**　　MCC
Meningitis due to Hemophilus influenzae [H. influenzae]
**CC Excl:** 003.21, 013.00-013.16, 036.0, 047.0-047.9, 049.0-049.1, 053.0, 054.72, 072.1, 090.42, 091.81, 094.2, 098.89, 100.81, 112.83, 114.2, 115.01, 115.11, 115.91, 130.0, 250.60-250.63, 250.80-250.93, 320.0-322.9, 349.89-349.9, 357.0

**320.1 Pneumococcal meningitis**　　MCC
**CC Excl:** See code: 320.0

**320.2 Streptococcal meningitis**　　MCC
**CC Excl:** See code: 320.0

**320.3 Staphylococcal meningitis**　　MCC
**CC Excl:** See code: 320.0

**320.7 _Meningitis in other bacterial diseases classified elsewhere_**　　MCC
_Code first underlying disease, as:_
actinomycosis (039.8)
listeriosis (027.0)
typhoid fever (002.0)
whooping cough (033.0-033.9)
EXCLUDES _meningitis (in):_
_epidemic (036.0)_
_gonococcal (098.82)_
_meningococcal (036.0)_
_salmonellosis (003.21)_
_syphilis:_
_NOS (094.2)_
_congenital (090.42)_
_meningovascular (094.2)_
_secondary (091.81)_
_tuberculous (013.0)_
**CC Excl:** See code: 320.0

✓5ᵗʰ **320.8 Meningitis due to other specified bacteria**
**320.81 Anaerobic meningitis**　　MCC
Bacteroides (fragilis)
Gram-negative anaerobes
**CC Excl:** See code 320.0

**320.82 Meningitis due to gram-negative bacteria, not elsewhere classified**　　MCC
Aerobacter aerogenes pneumoniae
Escherichia coli [E. coli]
Friedländer bacillus
Klebsiella
Proteus morganii
Pseudomonas
EXCLUDES _gram-negative anaerobes (320.81)_
**CC Excl:** See code: 320.0

**320.89 Meningitis due to other specified bacteria**　　MCC
Bacillus pyocyaneus
**CC Excl:** See code: 320.0

**320.9 Meningitis due to unspecified bacterium**　　MCC
Meningitis:　　　　Meningitis:
bacterial NOS　　pyogenic NOS
purulent NOS　　 suppurative NOS
**CC Excl:** See code: 320.0

✓4ᵗʰ **321 Meningitis due to other organisms**

INCLUDES
arachnoiditis
leptomeningitis } due to organisms
meningitis        other than
pachymeningitis  bacteria

**AHA:** J-F, '87, 6

**DEF:** Infection causing inflammation of the lining of the brain and/or spinal cord, due to organisms other than bacteria.

**321.0 _Cryptococcal meningitis_**　　MCC
_Code first underlying disease (117.5)_
**CC Excl:** See code: 320.0

**321.1 _Meningitis in other fungal diseases_**　　MCC
_Code first underlying disease (110.0-118)_
EXCLUDES _meningitis in:_
_candidiasis (112.83)_
_coccidioidomycosis (114.2)_
_histoplasmosis (115.01, 115.11, 115.91)_
**CC Excl:** See code: 320.0

**321.2 _Meningitis due to viruses not elsewhere classified_**　　MCC
_Code first underlying disease, as:_
meningitis due to arbovirus (060.0-066.9)
EXCLUDES _meningitis (due to):_
_abacterial (047.0-047.9)_
_adenovirus (049.1)_
_aseptic NOS (047.9)_
_Coxsackie (virus)(047.0)_
_ECHO virus (047.1)_
_enterovirus (047.0-047.9)_
_herpes simplex virus (054.72)_
_herpes zoster virus (053.0)_
_lymphocytic choriomeningitis virus (049.0)_
_mumps (072.1)_
_viral NOS (047.9)_
_meningo-eruptive syndrome (047.1)_
**CC Excl:** 003.21, 013.00-013.16, 036.0, 047.0-047.9, 049.0-049.1, 053.0, 054.72, 072.1, 090.42, 091.81, 094.2, 098.89, 100.81, 112.83, 114.2, 115.01, 115.11, 115.91, 130.0, 320.0-322.9, 349.89-349.9, 357.0

**AHA:** 4Q, '04, 51

**321.3 _Meningitis due to trypanosomiasis_**　　MCC
_Code first underlying disease (086.0-086.9)_
**CC Excl:** See code: 321.2

**321.4 _Meningitis in sarcoidosis_**　　MCC
_Code first underlying disease (135)_
**CC Excl:** See code: 321.2

**321.8 _Meningitis due to other nonbacterial organisms classified elsewhere_**　　MCC
_Code first underlying disease_
EXCLUDES _leptospiral meningitis (100.81)_
**CC Excl:** See code: 321.2

✓4ᵗʰ **322 Meningitis of unspecified cause**

INCLUDES
arachnoiditis
leptomeningitis } with no organism
meningitis        specified as
pachymeningitis  cause

**AHA:** J-F, '87, 6

**DEF:** Infection causing inflammation of the lining of the brain and/or spinal cord, due to unspecified cause.

**322.0 Nonpyogenic meningitis**　　MCC
Meningitis with clear cerebrospinal fluid
**CC Excl:** See code: 321.2

**322.1 Eosinophilic meningitis**　　MCC
**CC Excl:** See code: 321.2

**322.2 Chronic meningitis**　　CC
**CC Excl:** See code: 321.2

✓4ᵗʰ / ✓5ᵗʰ Additional Digit Required　　Unacceptable PDx　　Manifestation Code　　◄► Revised Text　　● New Code　　▲ Revised Code Title

**Nervous System and Sense Organs**

**320-322.2**

**Nervous System and Sense Organs**

**322.9–323.61**

**322.9   Meningitis, unspecified**    MCC
CC Excl: See code: 321.2

√4ᵗʰ **323 Encephalitis, myelitis, and encephalomyelitis**

INCLUDES   acute disseminated encephalomyelitis
meningoencephalitis, except bacterial
meningomyelitis, except bacterial
myelitis:
    ascending
    transverse

EXCLUDES   *acute transverse myelitis NOS (341.20)*
*acute transverse myelitis in conditions classified*
*   elsewhere (341.21)*
*bacterial:*
*   meningoencephalitis (320.0-320.9)*
*   meningomyelitis (320.0-320.9)*
*idiopathic transverse myelitis (341.22)*

DEF: Encephalitis: inflammation of brain tissues.
DEF: Myelitis: inflammation of the spinal cord.
DEF: Encephalomyelitis: inflammation of brain and spinal cord.

√5ᵗʰ **323.0   Encephalitis, myelitis, and encephalomyelitis
    in viral diseases classified elsewhere**
*Code first underlying disease, as:*
   cat-scratch disease (078.3)
   infectious mononucleosis (075)
   ornithosis (073.7)

**323.01 *Encephalitis and encephalomyelitis***   MCC
***in viral diseases classified elsewhere***
EXCLUDES   *encephalitis (in):*
*   arthropod-borne viral*
*    (062.0-064)*
*   herpes simplex (054.3)*
*   mumps (072.2)*
*   other viral diseases of*
*    central nervous*
*    system (049.8-049.9)*
*   poliomyelitis (045.0-045.9)*
*   rubella (056.01)*
*   slow virus infections of*
*    central nervous*
*    system (046.0-046.9)*
*   viral NOS (049.9)*
*   West Nile (066.41)*

CC Excl: 003.21, 013.00-013.16, 013.60-013.66, 036.0, 046.2,
046.8, 047.0-049.8, 051.9-052.0, 052.7-053.13, 053.19, 053.79-
053.9, 054.3, 054.72, 054.79-054.9, 056.01, 057.8-058.89,
062.0-064, 066.2-066.49, 072.1-072.2, 073.7, 075, 078.89,
079.81-079.82, 079.89, 079.99, 090.41-090.42, 091.81, 094.2,
094.81, 098.89, 100.81, 112.83, 114.2, 115.01, 115.11, 115.91,
130.0, 139.8, 290.12, 320.0-323.9, 341.1, 349.89-349.9, 357.0,
487.8, 771.2

AHA: 4Q, '06, 58-63

**323.02 *Myelitis in viral diseases classified***   MCC
***elsewhere***
EXCLUDES   *myelitis (in):*
*   herpes simplex (054.74)*
*   herpes zoster (053.14)*
*   poliomyelitis (045.0-045.9)*
*   rubella (056.01)*
*   other viral diseases of*
*    central nervous*
*    system (049.8-049.9)*

AHA: 4Q, '06, 58-63

CC Excl: See code: 323.01

**323.1 *Encephalitis, myelitis, and encephalomyelitis***   MCC
***in rickettsial diseases classified elsewhere***
*Code first underlying disease (080-083.9)*
DEF: Inflammation of the brain caused by rickettsial disease
carried by louse, tick, or mite.

CC Excl: 013.60-013.66, 046.2, 046.8, 048-049.0, 049.8, 052.0, 052.2,
054.3, 054.74, 056.01, 057.8-058.29, 062.0-064, 066.2-066.49, 072.2, 073.7,
079.82, 079.99, 081.9, 083.9, 090.41, 094.81, 117.5, 124, 130.0, 290.12,
323.01-323.9, 341.1, 487.8, 771.2, 984.9

**323.2 *Encephalitis, myelitis, and encephalomyelitis***   MCC
***in protozoal diseases classified elsewhere***
*Code first underlying disease, as:*
   malaria (084.0-084.9)
   trypanosomiasis (086.0-086.9)
DEF: Inflammation of the brain caused by protozoal disease carried
by mosquitoes and flies.

CC Excl: 013.60-013.66, 046.2, 046.8, 048-049.0, 049.8, 052.0, 052.2,
054.3, 054.74, 056.01, 057.8-058.29, 062.0-064, 066.2-066.49, 072.2, 073.7,
079.82, 079.99, 081.9, 083.9, 084.6, 090.41, 094.81, 117.5, 124, 130.0,
290.12, 323.01-323.9, 341.1, 487.8, 771.2, 984.9

√5ᵗʰ **323.4   Other encephalitis, myelitis, and encephalomyelitis
    due to infection classified elsewhere**
*Code first underlying disease*

**323.41 *Other encephalitis and***   MCC
***encephalomyelitis due to infection***
***classified elsewhere***
EXCLUDES   *encephalitis (in):*
*   meningococcal (036.1)*
*   syphilis:*
*    NOS (094.81)*
*    congenital (090.41)*
*   toxoplasmosis (130.0)*
*   tuberculosis (013.6)*
*   meningoencephalitis due to*
*    free-living ameba*
*    [Naegleria] (136.2)*

CC Excl: See code: 323.01

AHA: 4Q, '06, 58-63

**323.42 *Other myelitis due to infection***   MCC
***classified elsewhere***
EXCLUDES   *myelitis (in):*
*   syphilis (094.89)*
*   tuberculosis (013.6)*

CC Excl: See code: 323.01

AHA: 4Q, '06, 58-63

√5ᵗʰ **323.5   Encephalitis, myelitis, and encephalomyelitis
    following immunization procedures**
*Use additional E code to identify vaccine*

**323.51 Encephalitis and encephalomyelitis**   MCC
**following immunization procedures**
Encephalitis postimmunization or
    postvaccinal
Encephalomyelitis postimmunization or
    postvaccinal

CC Excl: See code: 323.01

AHA: 4Q, '06, 58-63

**323.52 Myelitis following immunization**   MCC
**procedures**
Myelitis postimmunization or postvaccinal

CC Excl: See code: 323.01

AHA: 4Q, '06, 58-63

√5ᵗʰ **323.6   Postinfectious encephalitis, myelitis, and
    encephalomyelitis**
*Code first underlying disease*
DEF: Infection, inflammation of brain several weeks following the
outbreak of a systemic infection.

**323.61 *Infectious acute disseminated***   MCC
***encephalomyelitis [ADEM]***
Acute necrotizing hemorrhagic
    encephalopathy
EXCLUDES   *noninfectious acute*
*   disseminated*
*   encephalomyelitis*
*   (ADEM) (323.81)*

CC Excl: See code: 323.01

AHA: 4Q, '06, 58-63

---

N Newborn Age: 0    P Pediatric Age: 0-17    M Maternity Age: 12-55    A Adult Age: 15-124    CC CC Condition    MCC Major CC Condition    HIV HIV Related Dx

**323.62** *Other postinfectious encephalitis and encephalomyelitis*   `MCC`

> `EXCLUDES` encephalitis:
> postchickenpox (052.0)
> postmeasles (055.0)

**CC Excl:** See code: 323.01

**AHA:** 4Q, '06, 58-63

**323.63** *Postinfectious myelitis*   `MCC`

> `EXCLUDES` postchickenpox myelitis (052.2)
> herpes simplex myelitis (054.74)
> herpes zoster myelitis (053.14)

**CC Excl:** See code: 323.01

**AHA:** 4Q, '06, 58-63

√5th **323.7** **Toxic encephalitis, myelitis, and encephalomyelitis**

> *Code first underlying cause, as:*
> carbon tetrachloride (982.1)
> hydroxyquinoline derivatives (961.3)
> lead (984.0-984.9)
> mercury (985.0)
> thallium (985.8)

**AHA:** 2Q, '97, 8

**323.71** *Toxic encephalitis and encephalomyelitis*   `MCC`

**CC Excl:** See code: 323.01

**AHA:** 4Q, '06, 58-63

**323.72** *Toxic myelitis*   `MCC`

**CC Excl:** See code: 323.01

**AHA:** 4Q, '06, 58-63

√5th **323.8** **Other causes of encephalitis, myelitis, and encephalomyelitis**

**323.81** **Other causes of encephalitis and encephalomyelitis**   `MCC` `HIV`

> Noninfectious acute disseminated encephalomyelitis (ADEM)

**CC Excl:** See code: 323.01

**AHA:** 4Q, '06, 58-63

**323.82** **Other causes of myelitis**   `MCC` `HIV`

> Transverse myelitis NOS

**CC Excl:** See code: 323.01

**AHA:** 4Q, '06, 58-63

**323.9** **Unspecified cause of encephalitis, myelitis, and encephalomyelitis**   `MCC` `HIV`

**CC Excl:** 013.60-013.66, 046.2, 046.8, 048-049.0, 049.8, 052.0, 052.2, 054.3, 054.74, 056.01, 057.8-058.29, 062.0-064, 066.2-066.49, 072.2, 073.7, 075, 078.3, 079.82, 079.99, 081.9, 083.9, 084.6, 090.41, 094.81, 117.5, 124, 130.0, 290.12, 323.01-323.9, 341.1, 382.4, 487.8, 710.0, 771.2, 984.9

**AHA:** 1Q, '06, 8

√4th **324** **Intracranial and intraspinal abscess**

**324.0** **Intracranial abscess**   `MCC`

> Abscess (embolic):
> cerebellar
> cerebral
>
> Abscess (embolic) of brain [any part]:
> epidural
> extradural
> otogenic
> subdural

> `EXCLUDES` tuberculous (013.3)

**CC Excl:** 006.5, 013.20-013.36, 250.60-250.63, 250.80-250.93, 324.0-325, 348.8-348.9

**324.1** **Intraspinal abscess**   `MCC`

> Abscess (embolic) of spinal cord [any part]:
> epidural
> extradural
> subdural

> `EXCLUDES` tuberculous (013.5)

**CC Excl:** 006.5, 013.20-013.36, 250.60-250.63, 250.80-250.93, 324.1

**324.9** **Of unspecified site**   `MCC`

> Extradural or subdural abscess NOS

**CC Excl:** 006.5, 013.20-013.36, 250.60-250.63, 250.80-250.93, 324.0-325

**325** **Phlebitis and thrombophlebitis of intracranial venous sinuses**   `MCC`

> Embolism
> Endophlebitis
> Phlebitis, septic or suppurative
> Thrombophlebitis
> Thrombosis
>
> } of cavernous, lateral, or other intracranial or unspecified intracranial venous sinus

> `EXCLUDES` *that specified as:*
> *complicating pregnancy, childbirth, or the puerperium (671.5)*
> *of nonpyogenic origin (437.6)*

**CC Excl:** See code: 324.9

**DEF:** Inflammation and formation of blood clot in a vein within the brain or its lining.

**326** **Late effects of intracranial abscess or pyogenic infection**

> Note: This category is to be used to indicate conditions whose primary classification is to 320-325 [excluding 320.7, 321.0-321.8, 323.01-323.42, 323.6-323.7] as the cause of late effects, themselves classifiable elsewhere. The "late effects" include conditions specified as such, or as sequelae, which may occur at any time after the resolution of the causal condition.
> Use additional code to identify condition, as:
> hydrocephalus (331.4)
> paralysis (342.0-342.9, 344.0-344.9)

## ORGANIC SLEEP DISORDERS (327)

√4th **327** **Organic sleep disorders**

**AHA:** 4Q, '05, 59-64

√5th **327.0** **Organic disorders of initiating and maintaining sleep [Organic insomnia]**

> `EXCLUDES` insomnia NOS (780.52)
> insomnia not due to a substance or known physiological condition (307.41-307.42)
> insomnia with sleep apnea NOS (780.51)

**327.00** **Organic insomnia, unspecified**

**327.01** *Insomnia due to medical condition classified elsewhere*

> *Code first underlying condition*
> `EXCLUDES` insomnia due to mental disorder (327.02)

**327.02** *Insomnia due to mental disorder*

> *Code first mental disorder*
> `EXCLUDES` alcohol induced insomnia (291.82)
> drug induced insomnia (292.85)

**327.09** **Other organic insomnia**

√5th **327.1** **Organic disorder of excessive somnolence [Organic hypersomnia]**

> `EXCLUDES` hypersomnia NOS (780.54)
> hypersomnia not due to a substance or known physiological condition (307.43-307.44)
> hypersomnia with sleep apnea NOS (780.53)

**327.10** **Organic hypersomnia, unspecified**

**327.11** **Idiopathic hypersomnia with long sleep time**

**327.12** **Idiopathic hypersomnia without long sleep time**

**327.13** **Recurrent hypersomnia**

> Kleine-Levin syndrome
> Menstrual related hypersomnia

---

**Nervous System and Sense Organs**

**327.14– 330.9**

**327.14 Hypersomnia due to medical condition classified elsewhere**
Code first underlying condition
EXCLUDES hypersomnia due to mental disorder (327.15)

**327.15 Hypersomnia due to mental disorder**
Code first mental disorder
EXCLUDES alcohol induced hypersomnia (291.82)
drug induced hypersomnia (292.85)

**327.19 Other organic hypersomnia**

✓5ᵗʰ **327.2 Organic sleep apnea**
EXCLUDES Cheyne-Stokes breathing (786.04)
hypersomnia with sleep apnea NOS (780.53)
insomnia with sleep apnea NOS (780.51)
sleep apnea in newborn (770.81-770.82)
sleep apnea NOS (780.57)

**327.20 Organic sleep apnea, unspecified**
**327.21 Primary central sleep apnea**
**327.22 High altitude periodic breathing**
**327.23 Obstructive sleep apnea (adult) (pediatric)**
**327.24 Idiopathic sleep related nonobstructive alveolar hypoventilation**
Sleep related hypoxia
**327.25 Congenital central alveolar hypoventilation syndrome**
**327.26 Sleep related hypoventilation/hypoxemia in conditions classifiable elsewhere**
Code first underlying condition
**327.27 Central sleep apnea in conditions classified elsewhere**
Code first underlying condition
**327.29 Other organic sleep apnea**

✓5ᵗʰ **327.3 Circadian rhythm sleep disorder**
Organic disorder of sleep wake cycle
Organic disorder of sleep wake schedule
EXCLUDES alcohol induced circadian rhythm sleep disorder (291.82)
circadian rhythm sleep disorder of nonorganic origin (307.45)
disruption of 24 hour sleep wake cycle NOS (780.55)
drug induced circadian rhythm sleep disorder (292.85)

**327.30 Circadian rhythm sleep disorder, unspecified**
**327.31 Circadian rhythm sleep disorder, delayed sleep phase type**
**327.32 Circadian rhythm sleep disorder, advanced sleep phase type**
**327.33 Circadian rhythm sleep disorder, irregular sleep-wake type**
**327.34 Circadian rhythm sleep disorder, free-running type**
**327.35 Circadian rhythm sleep disorder, jet lag type**
**327.36 Circadian rhythm sleep disorder, shift work type**
**327.37 Circadian rhythm sleep disorder in conditions classified elsewhere**
Code first underlying condition
**327.39 Other circadian rhythm sleep disorder**

✓5ᵗʰ **327.4 Organic parasomnia**
EXCLUDES alcohol induced parasomnia (291.82)
drug induced parasomnia (292.85)
parasomnia not due to a known physiological condition (307.47)
**327.40 Organic parasomnia, unspecified**
**327.41 Confusional arousals**
**327.42 REM sleep behavior disorder**
**327.43 Recurrent isolated sleep paralysis**

**327.44 Parasomnia in conditions classified elsewhere**
Code first underlying condition
**327.49 Other organic parasomnia**

✓5ᵗʰ **327.5 Organic sleep related movement disorders**
EXCLUDES restless legs syndrome (333.94)
sleep related movement disorder NOS (780.58)
**327.51 Periodic limb movement disorder**
Periodic limb movement sleep disorder
**327.52 Sleep related leg cramps**
**327.53 Sleep related bruxism**
**327.59 Other organic sleep related movement disorders**
**327.8 Other organic sleep disorders**
AHA: ▶2Q, '07, 6◀

## HEREDITARY AND DEGENERATIVE DISEASES OF THE CENTRAL NERVOUS SYSTEM (330-337)

EXCLUDES hepatolenticular degeneration (275.1)
multiple sclerosis (340)
other demyelinating diseases of central nervous system (341.0-341.9)

✓4ᵗʰ **330 Cerebral degenerations usually manifest in childhood**
Use additional code to identify associated mental retardation

**330.0 Leukodystrophy** CC
Krabbe's disease    Pelizaeus-Merzbacher
Leukodystrophy:      disease
   NOS      Sulfatide lipidosis
   globoid cell
   metachromatic
   sudanophilic
CC Excl: 330.0-330.9, 331.7, 348.8-348.9, 349.89-349.9
DEF: Hereditary disease of arylsulfatase or cerebroside sulfatase; characterized by a diffuse loss of myelin in CNS; infantile form causes blindness, motor disturbances, rigidity, mental deterioration and, occasionally, convulsions.

**330.1 Cerebral lipidoses** CC
Amaurotic (familial) idiocy    Disease:
Disease:      Spielmeyer-Vogt
   Batten      Tay-Sachs
   Jansky-Bielschowsky    Gangliosidosis
   Kufs'
CC Excl: 330.1-331.2, 331.7, 331.83-331.9
DEF: Genetic disorder causing abnormal lipid accumulation in the reticuloendothelial cells of the brain.

**330.2 Cerebral degeneration in generalized lipidoses** CC
Code first underlying disease, as:
Fabry's disease (272.7)
Gaucher's disease (272.7)
Niemann-Pick disease (272.7)
sphingolipidosis (272.7)
CC Excl: See code: 330.1

**330.3 Cerebral degeneration of childhood in other diseases classified elsewhere** CC
Code first underlying disease, as:
Hunter's disease (277.5)
mucopolysaccharidosis (277.5)
CC Excl: See code: 330.1

**330.8 Other specified cerebral degenerations in childhood** CC
Alpers' disease or gray-matter degeneration
Infantile necrotizing encephalomyelopathy
Leigh's disease
Subacute necrotizing encephalopathy or encephalomyelopathy
CC Excl: See code: 330.1
AHA: N-D, '85, 5

**330.9 Unspecified cerebral degeneration in childhood** CC
CC Excl: See code: 330.1

---

N Newborn Age: 0    P Pediatric Age: 0-17    M Maternity Age: 12-55    A Adult Age: 15-124    CC CC Condition    MCC Major CC Condition    HIV HIV Related Dx

√4ᵗʰ **331 Other cerebral degenerations**
▶Use additional code, where applicable, to identify:
   with behavioral disturbance (294.11)
   without behavioral disturbance (294.10)◀

**331.0 Alzheimer's disease**
**AHA:** 4Q, '00, 41; 4Q, '99, 7; N-D, '84, 20
**DEF:** Diffuse atrophy of cerebral cortex; causing a progressive decline in intellectual and physical functions, including memory loss, personality changes and profound dementia.

√5ᵗʰ **331.1 Frontotemporal dementia**
**AHA:** 4Q, '03, 57
**DEF:** Rare, progressive degenerative brain disease, similar to Alzheimer's; cortical atrophy affects the frontal and temporal lobes.

   **331.11 Pick's disease**
   **DEF:** A less common form of progressive frontotemporal dementia with asymmetrical atrophy of the frontal and temporal regions of the cerebral cortex including abnormal rounded brain cells called Pick cells together with the presence of abnormal staining of protein (called tau) within the cells, called Pick bodies; symptoms include prominent apathy, deterioration of social skills, behavioral changes such as disinhibition and restlessness, echolalia, impairment of language, memory, and intellect, increased carelessness, poor personal hygiene, and decreased attention span.

   **331.19 Other frontotemporal dementia**
   Frontal dementia

**331.2 Senile degeneration of brain**
   **EXCLUDES** senility NOS (797)

**331.3 Communicating hydrocephalus** CC
▶Secondary normal pressure hydrocephalus◀
   **EXCLUDES** ▶congenital hydrocephalus (742.3)
     idiopathic normal pressure
       hydrocephalus (331.5)
     normal pressure hydrocephalus (331.5)
     spina bifida with hydrocephalus
       (741.0)◀
   **CC Excl:** 331.3-331.5
   **AHA:** S-O, '85, 12
   **DEF:** Subarachnoid hemorrhage and meningitis causing excess buildup of cerebrospinal fluid in cavities due to nonabsorption of fluid back through fluid pathways.

**331.4 Obstructive hydrocephalus** CC
Acquired hydrocephalus NOS
   **EXCLUDES** ▶congenital hydrocephalus (742.3)
     idiopathic normal pressure
       hydrocephalus (331.5)
     normal pressure hydrocephalus (331.5)
     spina bifida with hydrocephalus
       (741.0)◀
   **CC Excl:** 250.60-250.63, 250.80-250.93, 331.3-331.7, 331.82-331.9, 348.8-348.9, 741.00-741.03, 742.3-742.4, 742.59-742.9
   **AHA:** 4Q, '03, 106; 1Q, '99, 9
   **DEF:** Obstruction of cerebrospinal fluid passage from brain into spinal canal.

● **331.5 Idiopathic normal pressure hydrocephalus [INPH]** CC
Normal pressure hydrocephalus NOS
   **EXCLUDES** congenital hydrocephalus (742.3)
     secondary normal pressure
       hydrocephalus (331.3)
     spina bifida with hydrocephalus
       (741.0)
   **CC Excl:** See code: 331.3

**331.7 Cerebral degeneration in diseases classified elsewhere**
*Code first underlying disease, as:*
   alcoholism (303.0-303.9)
   beriberi (265.0)
   cerebrovascular disease (430-438)
   congenital hydrocephalus (741.0, 742.3)
   myxedema (244.0-244.9)
   neoplastic disease (140.0-239.9)
   vitamin $B_{12}$ deficiency (266.2)
   **EXCLUDES** cerebral degeneration in:
     Jakob-Creutzfeldt disease (046.1)
     progressive multifocal
       leukoencephalopathy (046.3)
     subacute spongiform
       encephalopathy (046.1)

√5ᵗʰ **331.8 Other cerebral degeneration**
**331.81 Reye's syndrome** MCC P
   **CC Excl:** 331.81
   **DEF:** Rare childhood illness, often developed after a bout of viral upper respiratory infection; characterized by vomiting, elevated serum transaminase, changes in liver and other viscera; symptoms may be followed by an encephalopathic phase with brain swelling, disturbances of consciousness and seizures; can be fatal.

**331.82 Dementia with Lewy bodies**
   Dementia with Parkinsonism
   Lewy body dementia
   Lewy body disease
   **AHA:** 4Q, '03, 57
   **DEF:** A cerebral dementia with neurophysiologic changes including increased hippocampal volume, hypoperfusion in the occipital lobes, and beta amyloid deposits with neurofibrillarity tangles, atrophy of cortex and brainstem, hallmark neuropsychologic characteristics are fluctuating cognition with pronounced variation in attention and alertness; recurrent hallucinations; and parkinsonism.

**331.83 Mild cognitive impairment, so stated**
   **EXCLUDES** altered mental status (780.97)
     cerebral degeneration (331.0-331.9)
     change in mental status (780.97)
     cognitive deficits following (late effects of) cerebral hemorrhage or infarction (438.0)
     cognitive impairment due to intracranial or head injury (850-854, 959.01)
     cognitive impairment due to late effect of intracranial injury (907.0)
     dementia (290.0-290.43, 294.8)
     mild memory disturbance (310.8)
     neurologic neglect syndrome (781.8)
     personality change, nonpsychotic (310.1)
   **AHA:** 4Q, '06, 75

**331.89 Other**
   Cerebral ataxia

**331.9 Cerebral degeneration, unspecified**

√4ᵗʰ **332 Parkinson's disease**
   **EXCLUDES** dementia with Parkinsonism (331.82)0

**332.0 Paralysis agitans**
   Parkinsonism or Parkinson's disease:
     NOS
     idiopathic
     primary
   **AHA:** M-A, '87, 7
   **DEF:** Form of parkinsonism; progressive, occurs in senior years; characterized by masklike facial expression; condition affects ability to stand erect, walk smoothly; weakened muscles, also tremble and involuntarily movement.

---

**Nervous System and Sense Organs**

**332.1–333.93**

**332.1 Secondary Parkinsonism** `CC`
Neuroleptic-induced Parkinsonism
Parkinsonism due to drugs
Use additional E code to identify drug, if drug-induced
> **EXCLUDES** *Parkinsonism (in):*
> *Huntington's disease (333.4)*
> *progressive supranuclear palsy*
> *(333.0)*
> *Shy-Drager syndrome (333.0)*
> *syphilitic (094.82)*

**CC Excl:** 332.0-332.1

✓4th **333 Other extrapyramidal disease and abnormal movement disorders**
> **INCLUDES** other forms of extrapyramidal, basal ganglia, or striatopallidal disease
> **EXCLUDES** *abnormal movements of head NOS (781.0)*
> *sleep related movement disorders*
> *(327.51-327.59)*

**333.0 Other degenerative diseases of the basal ganglia** `CC`
Atrophy or degeneration:
olivopontocerebellar [Déjérine-Thomas syndrome]
pigmentary pallidal [Hallervorden-Spatz disease]
striatonigral
Parkinsonian syndrome associated with:
idiopathic orthostatic hypotension
symptomatic orthostatic hypotension
Progressive supranuclear ophthalmoplegia
Shy-Drager syndrome

**CC Excl:** 332.0-332.1, 335.23, 337.0, 348.30-348.39
**AHA:** 3Q, '96, 8

**333.1 Essential and other specified forms of tremor**
Benign essential tremor
Familial tremor
Medication-induced postural tremor
Use additional E code to identify drug, if drug-induced
> **EXCLUDES** *tremor NOS (781.0)*

**333.2 Myoclonus**
Familial essential myoclonus
Progressive myoclonic epilepsy
Unverricht-Lundborg disease
Use additional E code to identify drug, if drug-induced
**AHA:** 3Q, '97, 4; M-A, '87, 12
**DEF:** Spontaneous movements or contractions of muscles.

**333.3 Tics of organic origin**
Use additional E code to identify drug, if drug-induced
> **EXCLUDES** *Gilles de la Tourette's syndrome (307.23)*
> *habit spasm (307.22)*
> *tic NOS (307.20)*

**333.4 Huntington's chorea** `CC`
**CC Excl:** 332.0-332.1, 340-341.1, 341.8-341.9, 343.0-344.2, 348.1, 348.30-348.9, 349.1, 349.82-349.9
**DEF:** Genetic disease characterized by chronic progressive mental deterioration; dementia and death within 15 years of onset.

**333.5 Other choreas**
Hemiballism(us)    Paroxysmal choreo-athetosis
Use additional E code to identify drug, if drug-induced
> **EXCLUDES** *Sydenham's or rheumatic chorea*
> *(392.0-392.9)*

**333.6 Genetic torsion dystonia**
Dystonia:    (Schwalbe-) Ziehen-
deformans progressiva    Oppenheim disease
musculorum deformans
**DEF:** Sustained muscular contractions, causing twisting and repetitive movements that result in abnormal postures of trunk and limbs; etiology unknown.

✓5th **333.7 Acquired torsion dystonia**
**333.71 Athetoid cerebral palsy** `CC`
Double athetosis (syndrome)
Vogt's disease
> **EXCLUDES** *infantile cerebral palsy (343.0-343.9)*

**CC Excl:** 332.0-332.1, 333.71, 333.90, 333.99, 343.0-343.9, 348.30-348.39
**AHA:** 4Q, '06, 76-78

**333.72 Acute dystonia due to drugs** `CC`
Acute dystonic reaction due to drugs
Neuroleptic induced acute dystonia
Use additional E code to identify drug
> **EXCLUDES** *blepharospasm due to drugs*
> *(333.85)*
> *orofacial dyskinesia due to*
> *drugs (333.85)*
> *secondary Parkinsonism*
> *(332.1)*
> *subacute dyskinesia due to*
> *drugs (333.85)*
> *tardive dyskinesia (333.85)*

**CC Excl:** 332.0-332.1, 333.71, 333.90, 333.99, 348.30-348.39
**AHA:** 4Q, '06, 76-78

**333.79 Other acquired torsion dystonia** `CC`
**CC Excl:** See code: 333.72
**AHA:** 4Q, '06, 76-78

✓5th **333.8 Fragments of torsion dystonia**
Use additional E code to identify drug, if drug-induced
**333.81 Blepharospasm**
> **EXCLUDES** *blepharospasm due to drugs*
> *(333.85)*

**DEF:** Uncontrolled winking or blinking due to orbicularis oculi muscle spasm.
**333.82 Orofacial dyskinesia**
> **EXCLUDES** *orofacial dyskinesia due to*
> *drugs (333.85)*

**DEF:** Uncontrolled movement of mouth or facial muscles.
**333.83 Spasmodic torticollis**
> **EXCLUDES** *torticollis:*
> *NOS (723.5)*
> *hysterical (300.11)*
> *psychogenic (306.0)*

**DEF:** Uncontrolled movement of head due to spasms of neck muscle.
**333.84 Organic writers' cramp**
> **EXCLUDES** *pychogenic (300.89)*

**333.85 Subacute dyskinesia due to drugs**
Blepharospasm due to drugs
Orofacial dyskinesia due to drugs
Tardive dyskinesia
Use additional E code to identify drug
> **EXCLUDES** *acute dystonia due to drugs*
> *(333.72)*
> *acute dystonic reaction due to*
> *drugs (333.72)*
> *secondary Parkinsonism (332.1)*

**AHA:** 4Q, '06, 76-78

**333.89 Other**
**Other and unspecified extrapyramidal diseases and abnormal movement disorders**
✓5th **333.9**
**333.90 Unspecified extrapyramidal disease** `CC`
**and abnormal movement disorder**
Medication-induced movement disorders NOS
Use additional E code to identify drug, if drug-induced
**CC Excl:** 332.0-332.1, 333.1-333.83, 333.85-333.93, 333.99, 335.22-335.23, 340-341.1, 341.8-341.9, 343.0-344.2, 348.1, 348.30-348.9, 349.1, 349.82-349.9

**333.91 Stiff-man syndrome** `CC`
**CC Excl:** See code: 333.90

**333.92 Neuroleptic malignant syndrome** `MCC`
Use additional E code to identify drug
> **EXCLUDES** *neuroleptic induced Parkinsonism (332.1)*

**CC Excl:** 333.0-333.93, 333.99, 342.00-342.92, 348.2-348.39
**AHA:** 4Q, '94, 37

**333.93 Benign shuddering attacks**
**AHA:** 4Q, '94, 37

---

`N` Newborn Age: 0     `P` Pediatric Age: 0-17     `M` Maternity Age: 12-55     `A` Adult Age: 15-124     `CC` CC Condition     `MCC` Major CC Condition     `HIV` HIV Related Dx

**333.94　Restless legs syndrome [RLS]**

AHA: 4Q, '06, 79

DEF: Neurological disorder of unknown etiology with an irresistible urge to move the legs, which may temporarily relieve the symptoms, is accompanied by motor restlessness and sensations of pain, burning, prickling, or tingling.

**333.99　Other**

Neuroleptic-induced acute akathisia
Use additional E code to identify drug, if drug-induced

AHA: 4Q, '04, 95; 2Q, '04, 12; 4Q, '94, 37

√4th **334　Spinocerebellar disease**

　EXCLUDES　olivopontocerebellar degeneration (333.0)
　　　　　peroneal muscular atrophy (356.1)

**334.0　Friedreich's ataxia**　CC

CC Excl: 334.0-334.9, 348.30-348.39

DEF: Genetic recessive disease of children; sclerosis of dorsal, lateral spinal cord columns; characterized by ataxia, speech impairment, swaying and irregular movements, with muscle paralysis, especially of lower limbs.

**334.1　Hereditary spastic paraplegia**　CC

CC Excl: 333.0-333.93, 333.99-337.9, 340-344.9, 348.1, 348.30-348.39, 348.8-349.2, 349.82-349.9

**334.2　Primary cerebellar degeneration**　CC

Cerebellar ataxia:
　Marie's
　Sanger-Brown
Dyssynergia cerebellaris myoclonica
Primary cerebellar degeneration:
　NOS
　hereditary
　sporadic

CC Excl: 333.0-333.93, 333.99-337.9, 340-344.9, 348.0-348.1, 348.30-348.39, 348.8-348.9, 349.82-349.9

AHA: M-A, '87, 9

**334.3　Other cerebellar ataxia**　CC

Cerebellar ataxia NOS
Use additional E code to identify drug, if drug-induced

CC Excl: See code: 334.2

**334.4　Cerebellar ataxia in diseases classified elsewhere**　CC

Code first underlying disease, as:
　alcoholism (303.0-303.9)
　myxedema (244.0-244.9)
　neoplastic disease (140.0-239.9)

CC Excl: See code: 334.2

**334.8　Other spinocerebellar diseases**　CC

Ataxia-telangiectasia [Louis-Bar syndrome]
Corticostriatal-spinal degeneration

CC Excl: See code: 334.2

**334.9　Spinocerebellar disease, unspecified**　CC

CC Excl: 334.0-334.9

√4th **335　Anterior horn cell disease**

**335.0　Werdnig-Hoffmann disease**　CC

Infantile spinal muscular atrophy
Progressive muscular atrophy of infancy

CC Excl: 250.60-250.63, 250.80-250.93, 334.8-337.9, 349.89-349.9

DEF: Spinal muscle atrophy manifested in prenatal period or shortly after birth; symptoms include hypotonia, atrophy of skeletal muscle; death occurs in infancy.

√5th **335.1　Spinal muscular atrophy**

**335.10　Spinal muscular atrophy, unspecified**　CC

CC Excl: See code: 335.0

**335.11　Kugelberg-Welander disease**　CC

Spinal muscular atrophy:
　familial　　　juvenile

CC Excl: See code: 335.0

DEF: Hereditary; juvenile muscle atrophy; appears during first two decades of life; due to lesions of anterior horns of spinal cord; includes wasting, diminution of lower body muscles and twitching.

**335.19　Other**　CC

Adult spinal muscular atrophy

CC Excl: See code: 335.0

√5th **335.2　Motor neuron disease**

**335.20　Amyotrophic lateral sclerosis**　CC  A

Motor neuron disease (bulbar) (mixed type)

CC Excl: See code: 335.0

AHA: 4Q, '95, 81

**335.21　Progressive muscular atrophy**　CC

Duchenne-Aran muscular atrophy
Progressive muscular atrophy (pure)

CC Excl: See code: 335.0

**335.22　Progressive bulbar palsy**　CC

CC Excl: See code: 335.0

**335.23　Pseudobulbar palsy**　CC

CC Excl: See code: 335.0

**335.24　Primary lateral sclerosis**　CC

CC Excl: See code: 335.0

**335.29　Other**　CC

CC Excl: See code: 335.0

**335.8　Other anterior horn cell diseases**　CC

CC Excl: See code: 335.0

**335.9　Anterior horn cell disease, unspecified**　CC

CC Excl: See code: 335.0

√4th **336　Other diseases of spinal cord**

**336.0　Syringomyelia and syringobulbia**　CC

CC Excl: 334.8-337.9, 340-344.9, 348.30-348.39, 348.8-349.2, 349.89-349.9

AHA: 1Q, '89, 10

**336.1　Vascular myelopathies**　MCC

Acute infarction of spinal cord (embolic) (nonembolic)
Arterial thrombosis of spinal cord
Edema of spinal cord
Hematomyelia
Subacute necrotic myelopathy

CC Excl: 250.60-250.63, 334.8-337.9, 340-344.9, 348.1, 348.30-348.39, 349.0-349.2, 349.89-349.9

**336.2　Subacute combined degeneration of spinal cord in diseases classified elsewhere**　CC

Code first underlying disease, as:
　pernicious anemia (281.0)
　other vitamin $B_{12}$ deficiency anemia (281.1)
　vitamin $B_{12}$ deficiency (266.2)

CC Excl: 334.8-337.9, 340-344.9, 348.1, 348.30-348.39, 349.0-349.2, 349.89-349.9

**336.3　Myelopathy in other diseases classified elsewhere**　CC

Code first underlying disease, as:
　myelopathy in neoplastic disease (140.0-239.9)

　EXCLUDES　myelopathy in:
　　　intervertebral disc disorder
　　　　(722.70-722.73)
　　　spondylosis (721.1, 721.41-721.42,
　　　　721.91)

CC Excl: See code: 336.1

AHA: 3Q, '99, 5

**336.8　Other myelopathy**　CC

Myelopathy:　　　　　Myelopathy:
　drug-induced　　　　radiation-induced
Use additonal E code to identify cause

CC Excl: See code: 336.1

**336.9　Unspecified disease of spinal cord**　CC  HIV

Cord compression NOS　　Myelopathy NOS
　EXCLUDES　myelitis (323.02, 323.1, 323.2, 323.42,
　　　　　323.52, 323.63, 323.72, 323.82,
　　　　　323.9)
　　　　　spinal (canal) stenosis (723.0, 724.00-
　　　　　724.09)

CC Excl: 250.60-250.63, 334.1, 334.8-337.9, 340-344.9, 348.1, 348.30-348.39, 349.0-349.2, 349.89-349.9

---

**Nervous System and Sense Organs**

**337–341.21**

√4th **337 Disorders of the autonomic nervous system**

INCLUDES   disorders of peripheral autonomic, sympathetic, parasympathetic, or vegetative system

EXCLUDES   *familial dysautonomia [Riley-Day syndrome] (742.8)*

**337.0 Idiopathic peripheral autonomic neuropathy**   CC
Carotid sinus syncope or syndrome
Cervical sympathetic dystrophy or paralysis
CC Excl: 250.60-250.63, 334.8-337.9, 340-344.9, 348.1, 348.30-348.39, 349.0-349.2, 349.89-349.9

**337.1 *Peripheral autonomic neuropathy in***   CC
***disorders classified elsewhere***
*Code first underlying disease, as:*
amyloidosis (277.30-277.39)
diabetes (250.6)
CC Excl: 337.0-337.29, 337.9, 348.30-348.39
AHA: 2Q, '93, 6; 3Q, '91, 9; N-D, '84, 9

√5th **337.2 Reflex sympathetic dystrophy**
AHA: 4Q, '93, 24

DEF: Disturbance of the sympathetic nervous system evidenced by sweating, pain, pallor and edema following injury to nerves or blood vessels.

**337.20 Reflex sympathetic dystrophy, unspecified** CC
CC Excl: 337.20-337.29

**337.21 Reflex sympathetic dystrophy of**   CC
**the upper limb**
CC Excl: See code: 337.0

**337.22 Reflex sympathetic dystrophy of**   CC
**the lower limb**
CC Excl: See code: 337.0

**337.29 Reflex sympathetic dystrophy of other**   CC
**specified site**
CC Excl: See code: 337.0

**337.3 Autonomic dysreflexia**
Use additional code to identify the cause, such as:
decubitus ulcer (707.00-707.09)
fecal impaction (560.39)
urinary tract infection (599.0)
AHA: 4Q, '98, 37

DEF: Noxious stimuli evokes paroxysmal hypertension, bradycardia, excess sweating, headache, pilomotor responses, facial flushing, and nasal congestion due to uncontrolled parasympathetic nerve response; usually occurs in patients with spinal cord injury above major sympathetic outflow tract ($T_6$).

**337.9 Unspecified disorder of autonomic nervous system**

### PAIN (338)

√4th **338 Pain, not elsewhere classified**
Use additional code to identify:
pain associated with psychological factors (307.89)

EXCLUDES   *generalized pain (780.96)*
*localized pain, unspecified type—code to pain by site*
*pain disorder exclusively attributed to psychological factors (307.80)*

AHA: ▶2Q, '07, 12◀

**338.0 Central pain syndrome**
Déjérine-Roussy syndrome
Myelopathic pain syndrome
Thalamic pain syndrome (hyperesthetic)
AHA: 4Q, '06, 79-81

√5th **338.1 Acute pain**
**338.11 Acute pain due to trauma**
AHA: ▶1Q, '07, 7;◀ 4Q, '06, 79-81

**338.12 Acute post-thoracotomy pain**
Post-thoracotomy pain NOS
AHA: 4Q, '06, 79-81

**338.18 Other acute postoperative pain**
Postoperative pain NOS
AHA: 4Q, '06, 79-81

**338.19 Other acute pain**
EXCLUDES   *neoplasm related acute pain (338.3)*
AHA: ▶2Q, '07, 11;◀ 4Q, '06, 79-81

√5th **338.2 Chronic pain**
EXCLUDES   *causalgia (355.9)*
*lower limb (355.71)*
*upper limb (354.4)*
*chronic pain syndrome (338.4)*
*myofascial pain syndrome (729.1)*
*neoplasm related chronic pain (338.3)*
*reflex sympathetic dystrophy (337.20-337.29)*

**338.21 Chronic pain due to trauma**
AHA: 4Q, '06, 79-81

**338.22 Chronic post-thoracotomy pain**
AHA: 4Q, '06, 79-81

**338.28 Other chronic postoperative pain**
AHA: 4Q, '06, 79-81

**338.29 Other chronic pain**
AHA: 4Q, '06, 79-81

**338.3 Neoplasm related pain (acute) (chronic)**
Cancer associated pain
Pain due to malignancy (primary) (secondary)
Tumor associated pain
AHA: ▶2Q, '07, 11;◀ 4Q, '06, 79-81

**338.4 Chronic pain syndrome**
Chronic pain associated with significant psychosocial dysfunction
AHA: ▶2Q, '07, 11;◀ 4Q, '06, 79-81

### OTHER DISORDERS OF THE CENTRAL NERVOUS SYSTEM (340-349)

**340 Multiple sclerosis**
Disseminated or multiple sclerosis:
NOS     cord
brain stem     generalized
CC Excl: 250.60-250.63, 250.80-250.93, 340, 341.8-341.9

√4th **341 Other demyelinating diseases of central nervous system**

**341.0 Neuromyelitis optica**   CC
CC Excl: 341.0, 348.30-348.39

**341.1 Schilder's disease**   CC
Baló's concentric sclerosis    Encephalitis periaxialis:
Encephalitis periaxialis:      diffusa [Schilder's]
concentrica [Baló's]
CC Excl: 066.40-066.49, 079.82, 348.30-348.39

DEF: Chronic leukoencephalopathy of children and adolescents; symptoms include blindness, deafness, bilateral spasticity and progressive mental deterioration.

√5th **341.2 Acute (transverse) myelitis**
EXCLUDES   *acute (transverse) myelitis (in) (due to):*
*following immunization procedures (323.52)*
*infection classified elsewhere (323.42)*
*postinfectious (323.63)*
*protozoal diseases classified elsewhere (323.2)*
*rickettsial diseases classified elsewhere (323.1)*
*toxic (323.72)*
*viral diseases classified elsewhere (323.02)*
*transverse myelitis NOS (323.82)*

**341.20 Acute (transverse) myelitis NOS**   CC
CC Excl: 003.21, 013.00-013.16, 036.0, 047.0-047.9, 049.0-049.1, 053.0-053.13, 053.19, 053.79-053.9, 054.72, 054.79-054.9, 058.81-058.89, 072.1, 078.89, 079.81, 079.89, 079.99, 090.42, 091.81, 094.2, 098.89, 100.81, 112.83, 114.2, 115.01, 115.11, 115.91, 130.0, 139.8, 250.60-250.63, 320.0-322.9, 334.8-337.9, 340-341.1, 341.8-344.9, 348.1, 348.30-348.39, 349.0-349.2, 349.89-349.9, 357.0
AHA: 4Q, '06, 58-63

**341.21 *Acute (transverse) myelitis in***   CC
***conditions classified elsewhere***
*Code first underlying condition*
CC Excl: See code: 341.20
AHA: 4Q, '06, 58-63

N Newborn Age: 0    P Pediatric Age: 0-17    M Maternity Age: 12-55    A Adult Age: 15-124    CC CC Condition    MCC Major CC Condition    HIV HIV Related Dx

102 — Volume 1 • October 2007

© 2007 Ingenix

341.22 **Idiopathic transverse myelitis**    `CC`
    **CC Excl:** See code: 341.20
    **AHA:** 4Q, '06, 58-63

341.8 **Other demyelinating diseases of central nervous system**    `CC`
    Central demyelination of corpus callosum
    Central pontine myelinosis
    Marchiafava (-Bignami) disease
    **CC Excl:** 333.1-333.93, 333.99-337.9, 340-344.9, 348.30-348.39, 348.8-348.9, 349.82-349.9
    **AHA:** N-D, '87, 6

341.9 **Demyelinating disease of central nervous system, unspecified**    `CC` `HIV`
    **CC Excl:** See code: 341.8

√4ᵗʰ 342 **Hemiplegia and hemiparesis**
    Note: This category is to be used when hemiplegia (complete) (incomplete) is reported without further specification, or is stated to be old or long-standing but of unspecified cause. The category is also for use in multiple coding to identify these types of hemiplegia resulting from any cause.
    **EXCLUDES** *congenital (343.1)*
               *hemiplegia due to late effect of cerebrovascular accident (438.20-438.22)*
               *infantile NOS (343.4)*

    The following fifth-digits are for use with codes 342.0-342.9:
      **0  affecting unspecified side**
      **1  affecting dominant side**
      **2  affecting nondominant side**

    **AHA:** 4Q, '94, 38

√5ᵗʰ 342.0 **Flaccid hemiplegia**    `CC`
    **CC Excl:** 334.0-337.9, 340-344.9, 348.30-348.39, 348.8-348.9, 349.82-349.9

√5ᵗʰ 342.1 **Spastic hemiplegia**    `CC`
    **CC Excl:** See code: 342.0

√5ᵗʰ 342.8 **Other specified hemiplegia**    `CC`
    **CC Excl:** See code: 342.0

√5ᵗʰ 342.9 **Hemiplegia, unspecified**    `CC`
    **CC Excl:** See code: 342.0
    **AHA:** 3Q, '06, 5; 4Q, '98, 87

√4ᵗʰ 343 **Infantile cerebral palsy**
    **INCLUDES**  cerebral:
               palsy NOS
               spastic infantile paralysis
        congenital spastic paralysis (cerebral)
        Little's disease
        paralysis (spastic) due to birth injury:
               intracranial
               spinal
    **EXCLUDES** *athetoid cerebral palsy (333.71)*
               *hereditary cerebral paralysis, such as:*
                 *hereditary spastic paraplegia (334.1)*
                 *Vogt's disease (333.71)*
               *spastic paralysis specified as noncongenital or noninfantile (344.0-344.9)*

343.0 **Diplegic**    `CC`
    Congenital diplegia
    Congenital paraplegia
    **CC Excl:** 343.0, 348.30-348.39
    **DEF:** Paralysis affecting both sides of the body simultaneously.

343.1 **Hemiplegic**    `CC`
    Congenital hemiplegia
    **EXCLUDES** *infantile hemiplegia NOS (343.4)*
    **CC Excl:** 343.1, 348.30-348.39

343.2 **Quadriplegic**    `MCC`
    Tetraplegic
    **CC Excl:** 250.60-250.63, 250.80-250.93, 342.00-344.9, 348.8-348.9, 349.89-349.9, 742.59-742.9

343.3 **Monoplegic**

343.4 **Infantile hemiplegia**    `CC`
    Infantile hemiplegia (postnatal) NOS
    **CC Excl:** See code: 342.0

343.8 **Other specified infantile cerebral palsy**

343.9 **Infantile cerebral palsy, unspecified**
    Cerebral palsy NOS
    **AHA:** 4Q, '05, 89

√4ᵗʰ 344 **Other paralytic syndromes**
    Note: This category is to be used when the listed conditions are reported without further specification or are stated to be old or long-standing but of unspecified cause. The category is also for use in multiple coding to identify these conditions resulting from any cause.
    **INCLUDES**  paralysis (complete) (incomplete), except as classifiable to 342 and 343
    **EXCLUDES** *congenital or infantile cerebral palsy (343.0-343.9)*
               *hemiplegia (342.0-342.9)*
               *congenital or infantile (343.1, 343.4)*

√5ᵗʰ 344.0 **Quadriplegia and quadriparesis**
    344.00 **Quadriplegia unspecified**    `MCC`
        **CC Excl:** See code: 343.2
        **AHA:** 4Q, '03, 103; 4Q, '98, 38

    344.01 **C₁-C₄ complete**    `MCC`
        **CC Excl:** See code: 343.2

    344.02 **C₁-C₄ incomplete**    `MCC`
        **CC Excl:** See code: 343.2

    344.03 **C₅-C₇ complete**    `MCC`
        **CC Excl:** See code: 343.2

    344.04 **C₅-C₇ incomplete**    `MCC`
        **CC Excl:** See code: 343.2

    344.09 **Other**    `MCC`
        **CC Excl:** See code: 343.2
        **AHA:** 1Q, '01, 12; 4Q, '98, 39

344.1 **Paraplegia**    `CC`
    Paralysis of both lower limbs    Paraplegia (lower)
    **CC Excl:** See code: 342.0
    **AHA:** 4Q, '03, 110; M-A, '87, 10

344.2 **Diplegia of upper limbs**    `CC`
    Diplegia (upper)
    Paralysis of both upper limbs
    **CC Excl:** 344.00-344.09, 344.2, 344.81-344.9, 349.89-349.9

√5ᵗʰ 344.3 **Monoplegia of lower limb**
    Paralysis of lower limb
    **EXCLUDES** *monoplegia of lower limb due to late effect of cerebrovascular accident (438.40-438.42)*
    344.30 **Affecting unspecified side**
    344.31 **Affecting dominant side**
    344.32 **Affecting nondominant side**

√5ᵗʰ 344.4 **Monoplegia of upper limb**
    Paralysis of upper limb
    **EXCLUDES** *monoplegia of upper limb due to late effect of cerebrovascular accident (438.30-438.32)*
    344.40 **Affecting unspecified side**
    344.41 **Affecting dominant side**
    344.42 **Affecting nondominant side**

344.5 **Unspecified monoplegia**

√5ᵗʰ 344.6 **Cauda equina syndrome**
    **DEF:** Dull pain and paresthesias in sacrum, perineum and bladder due to compression of spinal nerve roots; pain radiates down buttocks, back of thigh, calf of leg and into foot with prickling, burning sensations.
    344.60 **Without mention of neurogenic bladder**  `CC`
        **CC Excl:** 344.00-344.1, 344.30-344.32, 344.60-344.9, 349.89-349.9

---

√4ᵗʰ **Additional Digit Required**          **Unacceptable PDx**          **Manifestation Code**          ►◄ Revised Text          ● New Code          ▲ Revised Code Title
√5ᵗʰ

**344.61 With neurogenic bladder** `CC`
Acontractile bladder
Autonomic hyperreflexia of bladder
Cord bladder
Detrusor hyperreflexia

**CC Excl:** 334.0-337.9, 340-344.9, 348.30-348.39, 348.8-348.9, 349.82-349.9, 599.60-599.69

**AHA:** M-J, '87, 12; M-A, '87, 10

√5th **344.8 Other specified paralytic syndromes**
**344.81 Locked-in state** `MCC`

**CC Excl:** 342.00-344.9, 348.30-348.39, 348.8-348.9, 349.82-349.9

**AHA:** 4Q, '93, 24

**DEF:** State of consciousness where patients are paralyzed and unable to respond to environmental stimuli; patients have eye movements, and stimuli can enter the brain but patients cannot respond to stimuli.

**344.89 Other specified paralytic syndrome**
**AHA:** 2Q, '99, 4

**344.9 Paralysis, unspecified**

√4th **345 Epilepsy and recurrent seizures**
The following fifth-digit subclassification is for use with categories 345.0, .1, .4-.9:
**0 without mention of intractable epilepsy**
**1 with intractable epilepsy**

**EXCLUDES** progressive myoclonic epilepsy (333.2)
**AHA:** 1Q, '93, 24; 2Q, '92, 8; 4Q, '92, 23

**DEF:** Brain disorder characterized by electrical-like disturbances; may include occasional impairment or loss of consciousness, abnormal motor phenomena and psychic or sensory disturbances.

√5th **345.0 Generalized nonconvulsive epilepsy** `CC 1`
Absences:   Pykno-epilepsy
atonic    Seizures:
typical    akinetic
Minor epilepsy   atonic
Petit mal

**CC Excl:** For code **345.01:** 250.60-250.63, 345.00-345.91, 348.8-348.9, 349.89, 349.9

**AHA:** For code **345.00:** 1Q, '04, 18

√5th **345.1 Generalized convulsive epilepsy** `CC 1`
Epileptic seizures:  Epileptic seizures:
clonic    tonic-clonic
myoclonic   Grand mal
tonic    Major epilepsy
**EXCLUDES** convulsions:
NOS (780.39)
infantile (780.39)
newborn (779.0)
infantile spasms (345.6)

**CC Excl:** For code **345.11:** See code 345.01

**AHA:** 3Q, '97, 4

**DEF:** Convulsive seizures with tension of limbs (tonic) or rhythmic contractions (clonic).

**345.2 Petit mal status** `MCC`
Epileptic absence status

**CC Excl:** 250.60-250.63, 250.80-250.93, 345.00-345.91, 348.8-348.9, 349.89-349.9

**DEF:** Minor myoclonic spasms and sudden momentary loss of consciousness in epilepsy.

**345.3 Grand mal status** `MCC`
Status epilepticus NOS
**EXCLUDES** epilepsia partialis continua (345.7)
status:
psychomotor (345.7)
temporal lobe (345.7)

**CC Excl:** See code: 345.2

**AHA:** 3Q, '05, 12

**DEF:** Sudden loss of consciousness followed by generalized convulsions in epilepsy.

√5th **345.4 Localization-related (focal) (partial) epilepsy** `CC`
**and epileptic syndromes with complex partial seizures**
Epilepsy:
limbic system
partial:
secondarily generalized
with impairment of consciousness
with memory and ideational disturbances
psychomotor
psychosensory
temporal lobe
Epileptic automatism

**CC Excl:** For code **345.40:** 345.00-345.91, 348.30-348.39, 348.9, 349.89-349.9; For code **345.41:** 250.60-250.63, 345.00-345.91, 348.8-348.9, 349.89-349.9

√5th **345.5 Localization-related (focal) (partial) epilepsy** `CC`
**and epileptic syndromes with simple partial seizures**
Epilepsy:
Bravais-Jacksonian NOS
focal (motor) NOS
Jacksonian NOS
motor partial
partial NOS:
without impairment of consciousness
sensory-induced
somatomotor
somatosensory
visceral
visual

**CC Excl:** For code **345.50:** 345.00-345.91, 348.30-348.39, 348.9, 349.89-349.9; For code **345.51:** 250.60-250.63, 345.00-345.91, 348.8-348.9, 349.89-349.9

√5th **345.6 Infantile spasms** `CC`
Hypsarrhythmia   Salaam attacks
Lightning spasms
**EXCLUDES** salaam tic (781.0)

**CC Excl:** For code **345.60:** 345.00-345.91, 348.30-348.39, 348.9, 349.89-349.9; For code **345.61:** 250.60-250.63, 345.00-345.91, 348.8-348.9, 349.89-349.9

**AHA:** N-D, '84, 12

√5th **345.7 Epilepsia partialis continua** `CC 0` `MCC 1`
Kojevnikov's epilepsy

**CC Excl:** 250.60-250.63, 345.00-345.91, 348.8-348.9, 349.89-349.9

**DEF:** Continuous muscle contractions and relaxation; result of abnormal neural discharge.

√5th **345.8 Other forms of epilepsy and recurrent seizures** `CC`
Epilepsy:    Epilepsy:
cursive [running]  gelastic

**CC Excl:** 250.60-250.63, 345.00-345.91, 348.8-348.9, 349.89-349.9

√5th **345.9 Epilepsy, unspecified** `CC 1`
Epileptic convulsions, fits, or seizures NOS
Recurrent seizures NOS
Seizure disorder NOS
**EXCLUDES** convulsion (convulsive) disorder (780.39)
convulsive seizure or fit NOS (780.39)
recurrent convulsions (780.39)

**CC Excl:** For code **345.91:** 250.60-250.63, 345.00-345.91, 348.8-348.9, 349.89-349.9

**AHA:** N-D, '87, 12

`N` Newborn Age: 0  `P` Pediatric Age: 0-17  `M` Maternity Age: 12-55  `A` Adult Age: 15-124  `CC` CC Condition  `MCC` Major CC Condition  `HIV` HIV Related Dx

104 — Volume 1 • October 2007   © 2007 Ingenix

√4ᵗʰ **346 Migraine**

The following fifth-digit subclassification is for use with category 346:

  **0**  without mention of intractable migraine
  **1**  with intractable migraine, so stated

DEF: Benign vascular headache of extreme pain; commonly associated with irritability, nausea, vomiting and often photophobia; premonitory visual hallucination of a crescent in the visual field (scotoma).

√5ᵗʰ **346.0**  **Classical migraine**
    Migraine preceded or accompanied by transient focal neurological phenomena
    Migraine with aura

√5ᵗʰ **346.1**  **Common migraine**
    Atypical migraine      Sick headache

√5ᵗʰ **346.2**  **Variants of migraine**
    Cluster headache     Migraine:
    Histamine cephalgia     lower half
    Horton's neuralgia     retinal
    Migraine:           Neuralgia:
      abdominal      ciliary
      basilar       migrainous

√5ᵗʰ **346.8**  **Other forms of migraine**
    Migraine:          Migraine:
      hemiplegic      ophthalmoplegic

√5ᵗʰ **346.9**  **Migraine, unspecified**
    AHA: N-D, '85, 16

√4ᵗʰ **347 Cataplexy and narcolepsy**
    DEF: Cataplexy: Sudden onset of muscle weakness with loss of tone and strength; caused by aggressive or spontaneous emotions.
    DEF: Narcolepsy: Brief, recurrent, uncontrollable episodes of sound sleep.

√5ᵗʰ **347.0**  **Narcolepsy**
    **347.00 Without cataplexy**
       Narcolepsy NOS
    **347.01 With cataplexy**

√5ᵗʰ **347.1**  **Narcolepsy in conditions classified elsewhere**
    *Code first underlying condition*
    **347.10**  *Without cataplexy*
    **347.11**  *With cataplexy*

√4ᵗʰ **348 Other conditions of brain**

  **348.0**  **Cerebral cysts**
    Arachnoid cyst      Porencephaly, acquired
    Porencephalic cyst    Pseudoporencephaly
    **EXCLUDES**  *porencephaly (congenital) (742.4)*

  **348.1**  **Anoxic brain damage**     CC
    **EXCLUDES**  *that occurring in:*
      *abortion (634-638 with .7, 639.8)*
      *ectopic or molar pregnancy (639.8)*
      *labor or delivery (668.2, 669.4)*
      *that of newborn (767.0, 768.0-768.9,*
        *772.1-772.2)*
    Use additional E code to identify cause
    CC Excl: 250.60-250.63, 250.80-250.93, 348.1-348.2, 349.89-349.9
    DEF: Brain injury due to lack of oxygen, other than birth trauma.

  **348.2**  **Benign intracranial hypertension**
    Pseudotumor cerebri
    **EXCLUDES**  *hypertensive encephalopathy (437.2)*
    DEF: Elevated pressure in brain due to fluid retention in brain cavities.

√5ᵗʰ **348.3**  **Encephalopathy, not elsewhere classified**
    AHA: 4Q, '03, 58; 3Q, '97, 4
    **348.30 Encephalopathy, unspecified**    MCC   HIV
       CC Excl: 333.92, 344.81, 348.31-348.39
    **348.31 Metabolic encephalopathy**    MCC   HIV
       Septic encephalopathy
       **EXCLUDES**  *toxic metabolic encepha-
         lopathy (349.82)*
       CC Excl: 333.92, 344.81, 348.30, 348.39

---

  **348.39 Other encephalopathy**    MCC   HIV
    **EXCLUDES**  *encephalopathy:*
      *alcoholic (291.2)*
      *hepatic (572.2)*
      *hypertensive (437.2)*
      *toxic (349.82)*
    CC Excl: 333.92, 344.81, 348.30-348.31

  **348.4**  **Compression of brain**    MCC
    Compression ⎫
    Herniation   ⎬ brain (stem)
    Posterior fossa compression syndrome
    CC Excl: 342.90
    AHA: 4Q, '94, 37
    DEF: Elevated pressure in brain due to blood clot, tumor, fracture, abscess, other condition.

  **348.5**  **Cerebral edema**    MCC
    CC Excl: 348.5
    DEF: Elevated pressure in the brain due to fluid retention in brain tissues.

  **348.8**  **Other conditions of brain**
    Cerebral:         Cerebral:
      calcification      fungus
    AHA: S-O, '87, 9

  **348.9**  **Unspecified condition of brain**    HIV

√4ᵗʰ **349 Other and unspecified disorders of the nervous system**

  **349.0**  **Reaction to spinal or lumbar puncture**
    Headache following lumbar puncture
    AHA: 2Q, '99, 9; 3Q, '90, 18

  **349.1**  **Nervous system complications from surgically implanted device**    CC
    **EXCLUDES**  *immediate postoperative complications (997.00-997.09)*
      *mechanical complications of nervous system device (996.2)*
    CC Excl: 250.60-250.63, 250.80-250.93, 349.1, 349.89-349.9

  **349.2**  **Disorders of meninges, not elsewhere classified**
    Adhesions, meningeal (cerebral) (spinal)
    Cyst, spinal meninges
    Meningocele, acquired
    Pseudomeningocele, acquired
    AHA: 1Q, '06, 15; 2Q, '98, 18; 3Q, '94, 4

√5ᵗʰ **349.8**  **Other specified disorders of nervous system**
    **349.81 Cerebrospinal fluid rhinorrhea**    CC
       **EXCLUDES**  *cerebrospinal fluid otorrhea (388.61)*
       CC Excl: 250.60-250.63, 250.80-250.93, 349.81, 349.89-349.9
       DEF: Cerebrospinal fluid discharging from the nose; caused by fracture of frontal bone with tearing of dura mater and arachnoid.

**Cranial Nerves**

Olfactory bulb (I)
Optic nerve (II)
Oculomotor nerve (III)
Trochlear nerve (IV)
Trigeminal nerve (V)
Abducens nerve (VI)
Facial nerve (VII)
Vestibulocochlear nerve (VIII)
Glossopharyngeal nerve (IX)
Vagus nerve (X)
Accessory nerve (XI)
Hypoglossal nerve (XII)

Pons

---

**Peripheral Nervous System**

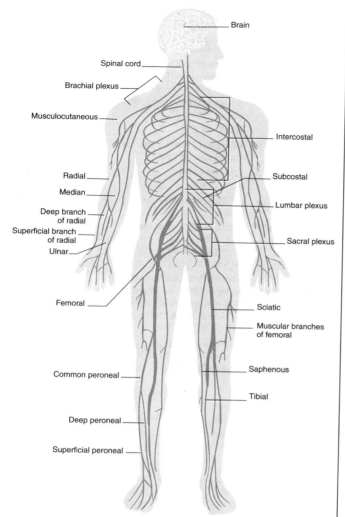

Brain
Spinal cord
Brachial plexus
Musculocutaneous
Intercostal
Radial
Subcostal
Median
Lumbar plexus
Deep branch of radial
Superficial branch of radial
Ulnar
Sacral plexus
Femoral
Sciatic
Muscular branches of femoral
Common peroneal
Saphenous
Tibial
Deep peroneal
Superficial peroneal

**349.82   Toxic encephalopathy**    `MCC`

Toxic metabolic encephalopathy
Use additional E code to identify cause

**CC Excl:** 013.60-013.66, 017.90-017.96, 036.1, 049.8-049.9, 052.0, 054.3, 058.21-058.29, 062.0-063.9, 072.2, 090.41, 094.81, 130.0, 250.60-250.63, 250.80-250.93, 323.01-323.9, 341.20-341.22, 348.30-348.39, 348.8-348.9, 349.82-349.9

**AHA** 4Q, '93, 29

*DEF: Brain tissue degeneration due to toxic substance.*

**349.89   Other**

**349.9    Unspecified disorders of nervous system**    `HIV`

Disorder of nervous system (central) NOS

## DISORDERS OF THE PERIPHERAL NERVOUS SYSTEM (350-359)

> **EXCLUDES**   *diseases of:*
> *acoustic [8th] nerve (388.5)*
> *oculomotor [3rd, 4th, 6th] nerves (378.0-378.9)*
> *optic [2nd] nerve (377.0-377.9)*
> *peripheral autonomic nerves (337.0-337.9)*
> *neuralgia*
> *neuritis*  } *NOS or "rheumatic" (729.2)*
> *radiculitis*
> *peripheral neuritis in pregnancy (646.4)*

**✓4ᵗʰ 350 Trigeminal nerve disorders**

> **INCLUDES**   disorders of 5th cranial nerve

**350.1   Trigeminal neuralgia**

Tic douloureux     Trigeminal neuralgia NOS
Trifacial neuralgia

> **EXCLUDES**   *postherpetic (053.12)*

**350.2   Atypical face pain**

**350.8   Other specified trigeminal nerve disorders**

**350.9   Trigeminal nerve disorder, unspecified**

**✓4ᵗʰ 351 Facial nerve disorders**

> **INCLUDES**   disorders of 7th cranial nerve
> **EXCLUDES**   *that in newborn (767.5)*

**351.0   Bell's palsy**

Facial palsy

*DEF: Unilateral paralysis of face due to lesion on facial nerve; produces facial distortion.*

**351.1   Geniculate ganglionitis**

Geniculate ganglionitis NOS

> **EXCLUDES**   *herpetic (053.11)*

*DEF: Inflammation of tissue at bend in facial nerve.*

**351.8   Other facial nerve disorders**

Facial myokymia     Melkersson's syndrome

**AHA:** 3Q, '02, 13

**351.9   Facial nerve disorder, unspecified**

**✓4ᵗʰ 352 Disorders of other cranial nerves**

**352.0   Disorders of olfactory [lst] nerve**

**352.1   Glossopharyngeal neuralgia**

**AHA:** 2Q, '02, 8

*DEF: Pain between throat and ear along petrosal and jugular ganglia.*

**352.2   Other disorders of glossopharyngeal [9th] nerve**

**352.3   Disorders of pneumogastric [10th] nerve**

Disorders of vagal nerve

> **EXCLUDES**   *paralysis of vocal cords or larynx (478.30-478.34)*

*DEF: Nerve disorder affecting ear, tongue, pharynx, larynx, esophagus, viscera and thorax.*

**352.4   Disorders of accessory [11th] nerve**

*DEF: Nerve disorder affecting palate, pharynx, larynx, thoracic viscera, sternocleidomastoid and trapezius muscles.*

**352.5   Disorders of hypoglossal [12th] nerve**

*DEF: Nerve disorder affecting tongue muscles.*

**352.6   Multiple cranial nerve palsies**

Collet-Sicard syndrome    Polyneuritis cranialis

**352.9   Unspecified disorder of cranial nerves**

**✓4ᵗʰ 353 Nerve root and plexus disorders**

> **EXCLUDES**   *conditions due to:*
> *intervertebral disc disorders (722.0-722.9)*
> *spondylosis (720.0-721.9)*
> *vertebrogenic disorders (723.0-724.9)*

**353.0   Brachial plexus lesions**

Cervical rib syndrome
Costoclavicular syndrome
Scalenus anticus syndrome
Thoracic outlet syndrome

> **EXCLUDES**   *brachial neuritis or radiculitis NOS (723.4)*
> *that in newborn (767.6)*

**AHA:** 3Q, '06, 12

*DEF: Acquired disorder in tissue along nerves in shoulder; causes corresponding motor and sensory dysfunction.*

---

`N` Newborn Age: 0    `P` Pediatric Age: 0-17    `M` Maternity Age: 12-55    `A` Adult Age: 15-124    `CC` CC Condition    `MCC` Major CC Condition    `HIV` HIV Related Dx

**Trigeminal and Facial Nerve Branches**

Temporal branches

Zygomatic branches

Buccal branches

Mandibular branch

Cervical branch

**Branches of Facial Nerve (above)**

Maxillary (V2)

**Divisions of Trigeminal Nerve (below)**

Ophthalmic (V1)

Trigeminal nerve (CN V)

Mandibulary (V3)

**353.1**   **Lumbosacral plexus lesions**
▶Code first, if applicable, associated diabetes mellitus (250.6)◀

DEF: Acquired disorder in tissue along nerves in lower back; causes corresponding motor and sensory dysfunction.

**353.2**   **Cervical root lesions, not elsewhere classified**

**353.3**   **Thoracic root lesions, not elsewhere classified**

**353.4**   **Lumbosacral root lesions, not elsewhere classified**

**353.5**   **Neuralgic amyotrophy**
Parsonage-Aldren-Turner syndrome

**353.6**   **Phantom limb (syndrome)**

DEF: Abnormal tingling or a burning sensation, transient aches, and intermittent or continuous pain perceived as originating in the absent limb.

**353.8**   **Other nerve root and plexus disorders**

**353.9**   **Unspecified nerve root and plexus disorder**

√4th **354 Mononeuritis of upper limb and mononeuritis multiplex**

DEF: Inflammation of a single nerve; known as mononeuritis multiplex when several nerves in unrelated body areas are affected.

**354.0**   **Carpal tunnel syndrome**
Median nerve entrapment
Partial thenar atrophy

DEF: Compression of median nerve by tendons; causes pain, tingling, numbness and burning sensation in hand.

**354.1**   **Other lesion of median nerve**
Median nerve neuritis

**354.2**   **Lesion of ulnar nerve**
Cubital tunnel syndrome
Tardy ulnar nerve palsy

**354.3**   **Lesion of radial nerve**
Acute radial nerve palsy

AHA: N-D, '87, 6

**354.4**   **Causalgia of upper limb**

EXCLUDES   causalgia:
NOS (355.9)
lower limb (355.71)

DEF: Peripheral nerve damage, upper limb; usually due to injury; causes burning sensation and trophic skin changes.

**354.5**   **Mononeuritis multiplex**
Combinations of single conditions classifiable to 354 or 355

**354.8**   **Other mononeuritis of upper limb**

**354.9**   **Mononeuritis of upper limb, unspecified**

√4th **355 Mononeuritis of lower limb**

**355.0**   **Lesion of sciatic nerve**

EXCLUDES   sciatica NOS (724.3)

AHA: 2Q, '89, 12

DEF: Acquired disorder of sciatic nerve; causes motor and sensory dysfunction in back, buttock and leg.

**355.1**   **Meralgia paresthetica**
Lateral cutaneous femoral nerve of thigh compression or syndrome

DEF: Inguinal ligament entraps lateral femoral cutaneous nerve; causes tingling, pain and numbness along outer thigh.

**355.2**   **Other lesion of femoral nerve**

**355.3**   **Lesion of lateral popliteal nerve**
Lesion of common peroneal nerve

**355.4**   **Lesion of medial popliteal nerve**

**355.5**   **Tarsal tunnel syndrome**

DEF: Compressed, entrapped posterior tibial nerve; causes tingling, pain and numbness in sole of foot.

**355.6**   **Lesion of plantar nerve**
Morton's metatarsalgia, neuralgia, or neuroma

√5th **355.7**   **Other mononeuritis of lower limb**
**355.71**   **Causalgia of lower limb**

EXCLUDES   causalgia:
NOS (355.9)
upper limb (354.4)

DEF: Dysfunction of lower limb peripheral nerve, usually due to injury; causes burning pain and trophic skin changes.

**355.79**   **Other mononeuritis of lower limb**

**355.8**   **Mononeuritis of lower limb, unspecified**

**355.9**   **Mononeuritis of unspecified site**
Causalgia NOS

EXCLUDES   causalgia:
lower limb (355.71)
upper limb (354.4)

√4th **356 Hereditary and idiopathic peripheral neuropathy**

**356.0**   **Hereditary peripheral neuropathy**
Déjérine-Sottas disease

**356.1**   **Peroneal muscular atrophy**
Charcôt-Marie-Tooth disease
Neuropathic muscular atrophy

DEF: Genetic disorder, in muscles innervated by peroneal nerves; symptoms include muscle wasting in lower limbs and locomotor difficulties.

**356.2**   **Hereditary sensory neuropathy**

DEF: Inherited disorder in dorsal root ganglia, optic nerve, and cerebellum, causing sensory losses, shooting pains, and foot ulcers.

**356.3**   **Refsum's disease**    CC
Heredopathia atactica polyneuritiformis

CC Excl: 350.1-357.9

DEF: Genetic disorder of lipid metabolism; causes persistent, painful inflammation of nerves and retinitis pigmentosa.

**356.4**   **Idiopathic progressive polyneuropathy**

**356.8**   **Other specified idiopathic peripheral neuropathy**
Supranuclear paralysis

**356.9**   **Unspecified**

√4th **357 Inflammatory and toxic neuropathy**

**357.0**   **Acute infective polyneuritis**    CC
Guillain-Barré syndrome   Postinfectious polyneuritis

CC Excl: 003.21, 013.00-013.16, 036.0, 036.89-036.9, 041.81-041.9, 047.0-047.9, 049.0-049.1, 053.0, 054.72, 072.1, 090.42, 091.81, 094.2, 098.89, 100.81, 112.83, 114.2, 115.01, 115.11, 115.91, 130.0, 139.8, 320.0-322.9, 349.89-349.9, 357.0

AHA: 2Q, '98, 12

DEF: Guillain-Barré syndrome: acute demyelinaty polyneuropathy preceded by viral illness (i.e., herpes, cytomegalovirus [CMV], Epstein-Barr virus [EBV]) or a bacterial illness; areflexic motor paralysis with mild sensory disturbance and acellular rise in spinal fluid protein.

**357.1**   *Polyneuropathy in collagen vascular disease*
Code first underlying disease, as:
disseminated lupus erythematosus (710.0)
polyarteritis nodosa (446.0)
rheumatoid arthritis (714.0)

**357.2**   *Polyneuropathy in diabetes*
Code first underlying disease (250.6)
AHA: 4Q, '03, 105; 2Q, '92, 15; 3Q, '91, 9

**357.3**   *Polyneuropathy in malignant disease*
Code first underlying disease (140.0-208.9)

**Nervous System and Sense Organs**

**357.4–359.4**

**357.4　Polyneuropathy in other diseases classified elsewhere**

*Code first underlying disease, as:*
  amyloidosis (277.30-277.39)
  beriberi (265.0)
  chronic uremia (585.9)
  deficiency of B vitamins (266.0-266.9)
  diphtheria (032.0-032.9)
  hypoglycemia (251.2)
  pellagra (265.2)
  porphyria (277.1)
  sarcoidosis (135)
  uremia NOS (586)

  **EXCLUDES**　*polyneuropathy in:*
  　*herpes zoster (053.13)*
  　*mumps (072.72)*

AHA: 2Q, '98, 15

**357.5　Alcoholic polyneuropathy**

**357.6　Polyneuropathy due to drugs**
  Use additional E code to identify drug

**357.7　Polyneuropathy due to other toxic agents**
  Use additional E code to identify toxic agent

✓5ᵗʰ **357.8　Other**
  AHA: 4Q, '02, 47; 2Q, '98, 12

　**357.81　Chronic inflammatory demyelinating polyneuritis**　**CC**
  　CC Excl: 351.0-353.5, 353.8-356.9, 357.81-357.89
  　DEF: Inflammation of peripheral nerves resulting in destruction of myelin sheath; associated with diabetes mellitus, dys-proteinemias, renal failure and malnutrition; symptoms in-clude tingling, numbness, burning pain, diminished tendon reflexes, weakness, and atrophy in lower extremities.

　**357.82　Critical illness polyneuropathy**　**CC**
  　Acute motor neuropathy
  　CC Excl: 351.0-353.5, 353.8-356.9, 357.81-357.9
  　AHA: 4Q, '03, 111

  　DEF: An acute axonal neuropathy, both sensory and motor, that is associated with Systemic Inflammatory Response Syndrome (SIRS).

　**357.89　Other inflammatory and toxic neuropathy**

**357.9　Unspecified**

✓4ᵗʰ **358　Myoneural disorders**

✓5ᵗʰ **358.0　Myasthenia gravis**
  AHA: 4Q, '03, 59
  DEF: Autoimmune disorder of acetylcholine at neuromuscular junction; causing fatigue of voluntary muscles.

　**358.00　Myasthenia gravis without (acute) exacerbation**
  　Myasthenia gravis NOS

　**358.01　Myasthenia gravis with (acute) exacerbation**　**MCC**
  　Myasthenia gravis in crisis
  　CC Excl: 250.60-250.63, 250.80-250.93, 349.89-349.9, 358.00-358.1
  　AHA: 1Q, '05, 4; 4Q, '04, 139

**358.1　Myasthenic syndromes in diseases classified elsewhere**　**CC**
  Eaton-Lambert syndrome from stated cause classified elsewhere
  *Code first underlying disease, as:*
  　botulism (005.1)
  　hypothyroidism (244.0-244.9)
  　malignant neoplasm (140.0-208.9)
  　pernicious anemia (281.0)
  　thyrotoxicosis (242.0-242.9)
  CC Excl: See code: 358.01

**358.2　Toxic myoneural disorders**
  Use additional E code to identify toxic agent

**358.8　Other specified myoneural disorders**

**358.9　Myoneural disorders, unspecified**
  AHA: 2Q, '02, 16

✓4ᵗʰ **359　Muscular dystrophies and other myopathies**
  **EXCLUDES**　*idiopathic polymyositis (710.4)*

**359.0　Congenital hereditary muscular dystrophy**　**CC**
  Benign congenital myopathy　　Myotubular myopathy
  Central core disease　　　　　Nemaline body disease
  Centronuclear myopathy
  　**EXCLUDES**　*arthrogryposis multiplex congenita (754.89)*
  CC Excl: 250.60-250.63, 250.80-250.93, 349.89-349.9, 359.0-359.1
  DEF: Genetic disorder; causing progressive or nonprogressive muscle weakness.

**359.1　Hereditary progressive muscular dystrophy**　**CC**
  Muscular dystrophy:　　　Muscular dystrophy:
  　NOS　　　　　　　　　　Gower's
  　distal　　　　　　　　　Landouzy-Déjérine
  　Duchenne　　　　　　　limb-girdle
  　Erb's　　　　　　　　　ocular
  　fascioscapulohumeral　　oculopharyngeal
  CC Excl: See code: 359.0
  DEF: Genetic degenerative, muscle disease; causes progressive weakness, wasting of muscle with no nerve involvement.

✓5ᵗʰ **359.2　Myotonic disorders**
  　**EXCLUDES**　▶*periodic paralysis (359.3)*◀
  DEF: Impaired movement due to spasmatic, rigid muscles.

　**359.21　Myotonic muscular dystrophy**
  　Dystrophia myotonica
  　Myotonia atrophica
  　Myotonic dystrophy
  　Proximal myotonic myopathy [PROMM]
  　Steinert's disease

　**359.22　Myotonia congenita**
  　Acetazolamide responsive myotonia congenita
  　Dominant form [Thomsen's disease]
  　Recessive form [Becker's disease]

　**359.23　Myotonic chondrodystrophy**
  　Congenital myotonic chondrodystrophy
  　Schwartz-Jampel disease

　**359.24　Drug induced myotonia**
  　Use additional E code to identify drug

　**359.29　Other specified myotonic disorder**
  　Myotonia fluctuans
  　Myotonia levior
  　Myotonia permanens
  　Paramyotonia congenita (of von Eulenburg)

**359.3　Periodic paralysis**
  ▶Familial periodic paralysis◀
  Hypokalemic familial periodic paralysis
  ▶Hyperkalemic periodic paralysis
  Hypokalemic periodic paralysis
  Potassium sensitive periodic paralysis◀
  　**EXCLUDES**　▶*paramyotonia congenita (of von Eulenburg) (359.29)*◀
  DEF: Genetic disorder; characterized by rapidly progressive flaccid paralysis; attacks often occur after exercise or exposure to cold or dietary changes.

**359.4　Toxic myopathy**　**CC**
  Use additional E code to identify toxic agent
  CC Excl: 349.89-349.9, 358.00-359.1, 359.21-359.9
  AHA: 1Q, '88, 5
  DEF: Muscle disorder caused by toxic agent.

---

**N** Newborn Age: 0　　**P** Pediatric Age: 0-17　　**M** Maternity Age: 12-55　　**A** Adult Age: 15-124　　**CC** CC Condition　　**MCC** Major CC Condition　　**HIV** HIV Related Dx

108 — Volume 1 • October 2007　　　　　　　　　　　　　　　　　　　© 2007 Ingenix

**359.5 Myopathy in endocrine diseases classified elsewhere**

Code first underlying disease, as:
Addison's disease ▶(255.41)◀
Cushing's syndrome (255.0)
hypopituitarism (253.2)
myxedema (244.0-244.9)
thyrotoxicosis (242.0-242.9)

DEF: Muscle disorder secondary to dysfunction in hormone secretion.

**359.6 Symptomatic inflammatory myopathy in diseases classified elsewhere**   CC

Code first underlying disease, as:
amyloidosis (277.30-277.39)
disseminated lupus erythematosus (710.0)
malignant neoplasm (140.0-208.9)
polyarteritis nodosa (446.0)
rheumatoid arthritis (714.0)
sarcoidosis (135)
scleroderma (710.1)
Sjögren's disease (710.2)

CC Excl: 250.60-250.63, 250.80-250.93, 349.89-349.9, 358.00-359.1, 359.21-359.9

√5ᵗʰ **359.8 Other myopathies**

AHA: 4Q, '02, 47; 3Q, '90, 17

**359.81 Critical illness myopathy**   CC
Acute necrotizing myopathy
Acute quadriplegic myopathy
Intensive care (ICU) myopathy
Myopathy of critical illness

CC Excl: 358.1-359.1, 359.21-359.9

**359.89 Other myopathies**
**359.9 Myopathy, unspecified**

## DISORDERS OF THE EYE AND ADNEXA (360-379)

√4ᵗʰ **360 Disorders of the globe**

INCLUDES   disorders affecting multiple structures of eye

√5ᵗʰ **360.0 Purulent endophthalmitis**

EXCLUDES   bleb associated endophthalmitis (379.63)

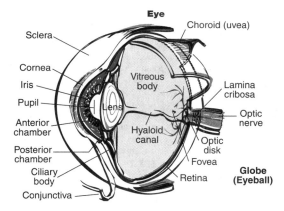

**Eye**

Sclera
Cornea
Iris
Pupil
Anterior chamber
Posterior chamber
Ciliary body
Conjunctiva
Choroid (uvea)
Vitreous body
Lens
Hyaloid canal
Lamina cribosa
Optic nerve
Optic disk
Fovea
Retina

**Globe (Eyeball)**

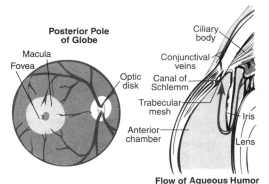

**Posterior Pole of Globe**

Macula
Fovea
Optic disk
Ciliary body
Conjunctival veins
Canal of Schlemm
Trabecular mesh
Anterior chamber
Iris
Lens

**Flow of Aqueous Humor**

**Adnexa**

Upper eyelid
Orbicularis oculi muscle
Orbital septum
Tarsal plate (cartilage)
Conjunctival fornix
Lower eyelid
Tarsal plate
Orbital septum
Orbital floor
Orbital roof
Levator palpebri muscle
Müller's muscle
Globe (eyeball)
Optic nerve
Fascia bulbi (Tenon's capsule)
Retrobulbar space
Extraocular muscle

**360.00 Purulent endophthalmitis, unspecified**   CC
CC Excl: 360.00-360.04, 360.13, 360.19, 364.05

**360.01 Acute endophthalmitis**   CC
CC Excl: See code 360.00

**360.02 Panophthalmitis**   CC
CC Excl: See code 360.00

**360.03 Chronic endophthalmitis**
**360.04 Vitreous abscess**   CC
CC Excl: 360.00-360.19

√5ᵗʰ **360.1 Other endophthalmitis**

EXCLUDES   bleb associated endophthalmitis (379.63)

**360.11 Sympathetic uveitis**   CC
CC Excl: 360.11-360.12

DEF: Inflammation of vascular layer of uninjured eye; follows injury to other eye.

**360.12 Panuveitis**   CC
CC Excl: 360.11-360.12

DEF: Inflammation of entire vascular layer of eye, including choroid, iris and ciliary body.

**360.13 Parasitic endophthalmitis NOS**   CC
CC Excl: 360.00-360.04, 360.13, 360.19, 364.05

DEF: Parasitic infection causing inflammation of the entire eye.

**360.14 Ophthalmia nodosa**
DEF: Conjunctival inflammation caused by embedded hairs.

**360.19 Other**   CC
Phacoanaphylactic endophthalmitis
CC Excl: 360.00-360.04, 360.13, 360.19, 364.05

√5ᵗʰ **360.2 Degenerative disorders of globe**

AHA: 3Q, '91, 3

**360.20 Degenerative disorder of globe, unspecified**
**360.21 Progressive high (degenerative) myopia**
Malignant myopia

DEF: Severe, progressive nearsightedness in adults, complicated by serious disease of the choroid; leads to retinal detachment and blindness.

**360.23 Siderosis**
DEF: Iron pigment deposits within tissue of eyeball; caused by high iron content of blood.

**360.24 Other metallosis**
Chalcosis
DEF: Metal deposits, other than iron, within eyeball tissues.

**360.29 Other**
EXCLUDES   xerophthalmia (264.7)

√5ᵗʰ **360.3 Hypotony of eye**

**360.30 Hypotony, unspecified**
DEF: Low osmotic pressure causing lack of tone, tension and strength.

**360.31 Primary hypotony**
**360.32 Ocular fistula causing hypotony**
DEF: Low intraocular pressure due to leak through abnormal passage.

**Nervous System and Sense Organs**

**360.33–362.01**

**360.33 Hypotony associated with other ocular disorders**

**360.34 Flat anterior chamber**
DEF: Low pressure behind cornea, causing compression.

✓5th **360.4 Degenerated conditions of globe**

**360.40 Degenerated globe or eye, unspecified**

**360.41 Blind hypotensive eye**
Atrophy of globe
Phthisis bulbi
DEF: Vision loss due to extremely low intraocular pressure.

**360.42 Blind hypertensive eye**
Absolute glaucoma
DEF: Vision loss due to painful, high intraocular pressure.

**360.43 Hemophthalmos, except current injury**
EXCLUDES   traumatic (871.0-871.9, 921.0-921.9)
DEF: Pool of blood within eyeball, not from current injury.

**360.44 Leucocoria**
DEF: Whitish mass or reflex in the pupil behind lens; also called cat's eye reflex; often indicative of retinoblastoma.

✓5th **360.5 Retained (old) intraocular foreign body, magnetic**
EXCLUDES   current penetrating injury with magnetic foreign body (871.5)
retained (old) foreign body of orbit (376.6)

**360.50 Foreign body, magnetic, intraocular, unspecified**

**360.51 Foreign body, magnetic, in anterior chamber**

**360.52 Foreign body, magnetic, in iris or ciliary body**

**360.53 Foreign body, magnetic, in lens**

**360.54 Foreign body, magnetic, in vitreous**

**360.55 Foreign body, magnetic, in posterior wall**

**360.59 Foreign body, magnetic, in other or multiple sites**

✓5th **360.6 Retained (old) intraocular foreign body, nonmagnetic**
Retained (old) foreign body:
NOS
nonmagnetic
EXCLUDES   current penetrating injury with (nonmagnetic) foreign body (871.6)
retained (old) foreign body in orbit (376.6)

**360.60 Foreign body, intraocular, unspecified**

**360.61 Foreign body in anterior chamber**

**360.62 Foreign body in iris or ciliary body**

**360.63 Foreign body in lens**

**360.64 Foreign body in vitreous**

**360.65 Foreign body in posterior wall**

**360.69 Foreign body in other or multiple sites**

✓5th **360.8 Other disorders of globe**

**360.81 Luxation of globe**
DEF: Displacement of eyeball.

**360.89 Other**

**360.9 Unspecified disorder of globe**

✓4th **361 Retinal detachments and defects**
DEF: Light-sensitive layer at back of eye, separates from blood supply; disrupting vision.

✓5th **361.0 Retinal detachment with retinal defect**
Rhegmatogenous retinal detachment
EXCLUDES   detachment of retinal pigment epithelium (362.42-362.43)
retinal detachment (serous) (without defect) (361.2)

**361.00 Retinal detachment with retinal defect, unspecified**

**361.01 Recent detachment, partial, with single defect**

**361.02 Recent detachment, partial, with multiple defects**

**361.03 Recent detachment, partial, with giant tear**

**361.04 Recent detachment, partial, with retinal dialysis**
Dialysis (juvenile) of retina (with detachment)

**361.05 Recent detachment, total or subtotal**

**361.06 Old detachment, partial**
Delimited old retinal detachment

**361.07 Old detachment, total or subtotal**

✓5th **361.1 Retinoschisis and retinal cysts**
EXCLUDES   juvenile retinoschisis (362.73)
microcystoid degeneration of retina (362.62)
parasitic cyst of retina (360.13)

**361.10 Retinoschisis, unspecified**
DEF: Separation of retina due to degenerative process of aging; should not be confused with acute retinal detachment.

**361.11 Flat retinoschisis**
DEF: Slow, progressive split of retinal sensory layers

**361.12 Bullous retinoschisis**
DEF: Fluid retention between split retinal sensory layers.

**361.13 Primary retinal cysts**

**361.14 Secondary retinal cysts**

**361.19 Other**
Pseudocyst of retina

**361.2 Serous retinal detachment**   CC
Retinal detachment without retinal defect
EXCLUDES   central serous retinopathy (362.41)
retinal pigment epithelium detachment (362.42-362.43)
CC Excl: 361.00-361.9, 362.40-362.43

✓5th **361.3 Retinal defects without detachment**
EXCLUDES   chorioretinal scars after surgery for detachment (363.30-363.35)
peripheral retinal degeneration without defect (362.60-362.66)

**361.30 Retinal defect, unspecified**
Retinal break(s) NOS

**361.31 Round hole of retina without detachment**

**361.32 Horseshoe tear of retina without detachment**
Operculum of retina without mention of detachment

**361.33 Multiple defects of retina without detachment**

✓5th **361.8 Other forms of retinal detachment**

**361.81 Traction detachment of retina**   CC
Traction detachment with vitreoretinal organization
CC Excl: 361.00-361.9, 362.40-362.43

**361.89 Other**   CC
CC Excl: 361.00-361.9, 362.40-362.43
AHA: 3Q, '99, 12

**361.9 Unspecified retinal detachment**   CC
CC Excl: 361.00-361.9, 362.40-362.43
AHA: N-D, '87, 10

✓4th **362 Other retinal disorders**
EXCLUDES   chorioretinal scars (363.30-363.35)
chorioretinitis (363.0-363.2)

✓5th **362.0 Diabetic retinopathy**
*Code first diabetes (250.5)*
DEF: Retinal changes in diabetes of long duration; causes hemorrhages, microaneurysms, waxy deposits and proliferative noninflammatory degenerative disease of retina.
AHA: 4Q, '05, 65; 3Q, '91, 8

*362.01 Background diabetic retinopathy*
Diabetic retinal microaneurysms
Diabetic retinopathy NOS

---

N Newborn Age: 0    P Pediatric Age: 0-17    M Maternity Age: 12-55    A Adult Age: 15-124    CC CC Condition    MCC Major CC Condition    HIV HIV Related Dx

110 — Volume 1 • October 2007          © 2007 Ingenix

**362.02 Proliferative diabetic retinopathy**
AHA: 3Q, '96, 5

DEF: Occurrence of the ischemic effects of vessel blockages result in neovascularization; new blood vessels begin to form to compensate for restricted blood flow; multiple areas of the retina and inner vitreous may be affected.

**362.03 Nonproliferative diabetic retinopathy NOS**
**362.04 Mild nonproliferative diabetic retinopathy**

DEF: Early stages of degenerative condition of the retina due to diabetes; microaneurysm formation; small balloon-like swelling of the retinal vessels.

**362.05 Moderate nonproliferative diabetic retinopathy**

DEF: Stage of degenerative condition of the retina due to diabetes with pronounced microaneurysms; vessel blockages can occur.

**362.06 Severe nonproliferative diabetic retinopathy**
AHA: 4Q, '05, 67

DEF: Stage of degenerative condition of the retina due to diabetes in which vascular breakdown in the retina results in multiple vascular blockages, or "beadings," intraretinal hemorrhages can be numerous.

**362.07 Diabetic macular edema**
Note: Code 362.07 must be used with a code for diabetic retinopathy (362.01-362.06)
Diabetic retinal edema

DEF: Leakage from retinal blood vessels causes swelling of the macula and impaired vision; exudates or plaques may develop in the posterior pole of the retina due to the breakdown of retinal vasculature.

**√5ᵗʰ 362.1 Other background retinopathy and retinal vascular changes**
**362.10 Background retinopathy, unspecified**
AHA: 1Q, '06, 12

**362.11 Hypertensive retinopathy**
AHA: 3Q, '90, 3

DEF: Retinal irregularities caused by systemic hypertension.

**362.12 Exudative retinopathy**
Coats' syndrome
AHA: 3Q, '99, 12

**362.13 Changes in vascular appearance**
Vascular sheathing of retina
Use additional code for any associated atherosclerosis (440.8)

**362.14 Retinal microaneurysms NOS**
DEF: Microscopic dilation of retinal vessels in nondiabetic.

**362.15 Retinal telangiectasia**
DEF: Dilation of blood vessels of the retina.

**362.16 Retinal neovascularization NOS**
Neovascularization:
choroidal
subretinal
DEF: New and abnormal vascular growth in the retina.

**362.17 Other intraretinal microvascular abnormalities**
Retinal sclerosis     Retinal varices

**362.18 Retinal vasculitis**
Eales' disease     Retinal:
Retinal:     perivasculitis
arteritis     phlebitis
endarteritis
DEF: Inflammation of retinal blood vessels.

**√5ᵗʰ 362.2 Other proliferative retinopathy**
**362.21 Retrolental fibroplasia**
DEF: Fibrous tissue in vitreous, from retina to lens, causing blindness; associated with premature infants requiring high amounts of oxygen.

**362.29 Other nondiabetic proliferative retinopathy**
AHA: 3Q, '96, 5

**√5ᵗʰ 362.3 Retinal vascular occlusion**
DEF: Obstructed blood flow to and from retina.

**362.30 Retinal vascular occlusion, unspecified** CC
CC Excl: 362.30-362.37

**362.31 Central retinal artery occlusion** CC
CC Excl: See code: 362.30

**362.32 Arterial branch occlusion** CC
CC Excl: See code: 362.30

**362.33 Partial arterial occlusion** CC
Hollenhorst plaque     Retinal microembolism
CC Excl: See code: 362.30

**362.34 Transient arterial occlusion** CC
Amaurosis fugax
CC Excl: See code: 362.30
AHA: 1Q, '00, 16

**362.35 Central retinal vein occlusion** CC
CC Excl: See code: 362.30
AHA: 2Q, '93, 6

**362.36 Venous tributary (branch) occlusion**
**362.37 Venous engorgement**
Occlusion:
incipient ⎫ of retinal vein
partial ⎭

**√5ᵗʰ 362.4 Separation of retinal layers**
EXCLUDES     retinal detachment (serous) (361.2)
rhegmatogenous (361.00-361.07)

**362.40 Retinal layer separation, unspecified** CC
CC Excl: 361.00-361.9, 362.40-362.43

**362.41 Central serous retinopathy**
DEF: Serous-filled blister causing detachment of retina from pigment epithelium.

**362.42 Serous detachment of retinal pigment epithelium** CC
Exudative detachment of retinal pigment epithelium
CC Excl: See code: 362.40
DEF: Blister of fatty fluid causing detachment of retina from pigment epithelium.

**362.43 Hemorrhagic detachment of retinal pigment epithelium** CC
CC Excl: See code: 362.40
DEF: Blood-filled blister causing detachment of retina from pigment epithelium.

**√5ᵗʰ 362.5 Degeneration of macula and posterior pole**
EXCLUDES     degeneration of optic disc (377.21-377.24)
hereditary retinal degeneration [dystrophy] (362.70-362.77)

**362.50 Macular degeneration (senile), unspecified**
**362.51 Nonexudative senile macular degeneration**
Senile macular degeneration:
atrophic
dry

**362.52 Exudative senile macular degeneration**
Kuhnt-Junius degeneration
Senile macular degeneration:
disciform
wet
DEF: Leakage in macular blood vessels with loss of visual acuity.

**362.53 Cystoid macular degeneration**
Cystoid macular edema
DEF: Retinal swelling and cyst formation in macula.

---

**362.54 Macular cyst, hole, or pseudohole**
**362.55 Toxic maculopathy**
> Use additional E code to identify drug, if drug induced

**362.56 Macular puckering**
> Preretinal fibrosis

**362.57 Drusen (degenerative)**
> DEF: White, hyaline deposits on Bruch's membrane (lamina basalis choroideae).

✓5ᵗʰ **362.6 Peripheral retinal degenerations**
> EXCLUDES   hereditary retinal degeneration [dystrophy] (362.70-362.77)
> retinal degeneration with retinal defect (361.00-361.07)

**362.60 Peripheral retinal degeneration, unspecified**
**362.61 Paving stone degeneration**
> DEF: Degeneration of peripheral retina; causes thinning through which choroid is visible.

**362.62 Microcystoid degeneration**
> Blessig's cysts    Iwanoff's cysts

**362.63 Lattice degeneration**
> Palisade degeneration of retina
> DEF: Degeneration of retina; often bilateral, usually benign; characterized by lines intersecting at irregular intervals in peripheral retina; retinal thinning and retinal holes may occur.

**362.64 Senile reticular degeneration**
> DEF: Net-like appearance of retina; sign of degeneration.

**362.65 Secondary pigmentary degeneration**
> Pseudoretinitis pigmentosa

**362.66 Secondary vitreoretinal degenerations**

✓5ᵗʰ **362.7 Hereditary retinal dystrophies**
> DEF: Genetically induced progressive changes in retina.

**362.70 Hereditary retinal dystrophy, unspecified**
**362.71 *Retinal dystrophy in systemic or cerebroretinal lipidoses***
> Code first underlying disease, as:
> cerebroretinal lipidoses (330.1)
> systemic lipidoses (272.7)

**362.72 *Retinal dystrophy in other systemic disorders and syndromes***
> Code first underlying disease, as:
> Bassen-Kornzweig syndrome (272.5)
> Refsum's disease (356.3)

**362.73 Vitreoretinal dystrophies**
> Juvenile retinoschisis

**362.74 Pigmentary retinal dystrophy**
> Retinal dystrophy, albipunctate
> Retinitis pigmentosa

**362.75 Other dystrophies primarily involving the sensory retina**
> Progressive cone(-rod) dystrophy
> Stargardt's disease

**362.76 Dystrophies primarily involving the retinal pigment epithelium**
> Fundus flavimaculatus
> Vitelliform dystrophy

**362.77 Dystrophies primarily involving Bruch's membrane**
> Dystrophy:
> hyaline
> pseudoinflammatory foveal
> Hereditary drusen

✓5ᵗʰ **362.8 Other retinal disorders**
> EXCLUDES   chorioretinal inflammations (363.0-363.2)
> chorioretinal scars (363.30-363.35)

**362.81 Retinal hemorrhage**
> Hemorrhage:
> preretinal
> retinal (deep) (superficial)
> subretinal
> **AHA:** 4Q, '96, 43

**362.82 Retinal exudates and deposits**
**362.83 Retinal edema**
> Retinal:
> cotton wool spots
> edema (localized) (macular) (peripheral)
> DEF: Retinal swelling due to fluid accumulation.

**362.84 Retinal ischemia**    CC
> CC Excl: 362.81-362.89
> DEF: Reduced retinal blood supply.

**362.85 Retinal nerve fiber bundle defects**
**362.89 Other retinal disorders**
**362.9 Unspecified retinal disorder**

✓4ᵗʰ **363 Chorioretinal inflammations, scars, and other disorders of choroid**

✓5ᵗʰ **363.0 Focal chorioretinitis and focal retinochoroiditis**
> EXCLUDES   focal chorioretinitis or retinochoroiditis in:
> histoplasmosis (115.02, 115.12, 115.92)
> toxoplasmosis (130.2)
> congenital infection (771.2)

**363.00 Focal chorioretinitis, unspecified**
> Focal:
> choroiditis or chorioretinitis NOS
> retinitis or retinochoroiditis NOS

**363.01 Focal choroiditis and chorioretinitis, juxtapapillary**
**363.03 Focal choroiditis and chorioretinitis of other posterior pole**
**363.04 Focal choroiditis and chorioretinitis, peripheral**
**363.05 Focal retinitis and retinochoroiditis, juxtapapillary**
> Neuroretinitis

**363.06 Focal retinitis and retinochoroiditis, macular or paramacular**
**363.07 Focal retinitis and retinochoroiditis of other posterior pole**
**363.08 Focal retinitis and retinochoroiditis, peripheral**

✓5ᵗʰ **363.1 Disseminated chorioretinitis and disseminated retinochoroiditis**
> EXCLUDES   disseminated choroiditis or chorioretinitis in secondary syphilis (091.51)
> neurosyphilitic disseminated retinitis or retinochoroiditis (094.83)
> retinal (peri)vasculitis (362.18)

**363.10 Disseminated chorioretinitis, unspecified**    CC
> Disseminated:
> choroiditis or chorioretinitis NOS
> retinitis or retinochoroiditis NOS
> CC Excl: 363.00-363.22

**363.11 Disseminated choroiditis and chorioretinitis, posterior pole**    CC
> CC Excl: See code: 363.10

**363.12 Disseminated choroiditis and chorioretinitis, peripheral**    CC
> CC Excl: See code: 363.10

**363.13 Disseminated choroiditis and chorioretinitis, generalized**    CC
> Code first any underlying disease, as:
> tuberculosis (017.3)
> CC Excl: See code: 363.10

**363.14 Disseminated retinitis and retinochoroiditis, metastatic**    CC
> CC Excl: See code: 363.10

**363.15 Disseminated retinitis and retinochoroiditis, pigment epitheliopathy**    CC
> Acute posterior multifocal placoid pigment epitheliopathy
> CC Excl: See code: 363.10
> DEF: Widespread inflammation of retina and choroid; characterized by pigmented epithelium involvement.

N Newborn Age: 0    P Pediatric Age: 0-17    M Maternity Age: 12-55    A Adult Age: 15-124    CC CC Condition    MCC Major CC Condition    HIV HIV Related Dx

112 — Volume 1 • October 2007

© 2007 Ingenix

**363.2 Other and unspecified forms of chorioretinitis and retinochoroiditis**

> EXCLUDES    panophthalmitis (360.02)
> sympathetic uveitis (360.11)
> uveitis NOS (364.3)

**363.20 Chorioretinitis, unspecified**    CC

Choroiditis NOS
Retinitis NOS
Uveitis, posterior NOS

**CC Excl:** See code: 363.10

**363.21 Pars planitis**

Posterior cyclitis

DEF: Inflammation of peripheral retina and ciliary body; characterized by bands of white cells.

**363.22 Harada's disease**

DEF: Retinal detachment and bilateral widespread exudative choroiditis; symptoms include headache, vomiting, increased lymphocytes in cerebrospinal fluid; and temporary or permanent deafness may occur.

**363.3 Chorioretinal scars**

Scar (postinflammatory) (postsurgical) (posttraumatic):
   choroid
   retina

**363.30 Chorioretinal scar, unspecified**

**363.31 Solar retinopathy**

DEF: Retinal scarring caused by solar radiation.

**363.32 Other macular scars**

**363.33 Other scars of posterior pole**

**363.34 Peripheral scars**

**363.35 Disseminated scars**

**363.4 Choroidal degenerations**

**363.40 Choroidal degeneration, unspecified**

Choroidal sclerosis NOS

**363.41 Senile atrophy of choroid**

DEF: Wasting away of choroid; due to aging.

**363.42 Diffuse secondary atrophy of choroid**

DEF: Wasting away of choroid in systemic disease.

**363.43 Angioid streaks of choroid**

DEF: Degeneration of choroid; characterized by dark brown steaks radiating from optic disk; occurs with pseudoxanthoma, elasticum or Paget's disease.

**363.5 Hereditary choroidal dystrophies**

Hereditary choroidal atrophy:
   partial [choriocapillaris]
   total [all vessels]

**363.50 Hereditary choroidal dystrophy or atrophy, unspecified**

**363.51 Circumpapillary dystrophy of choroid, partial**

**363.52 Circumpapillary dystrophy of choroid, total**

Helicoid dystrophy of choroid

**363.53 Central dystrophy of choroid, partial**

Dystrophy, choroidal:
   central areolar
   circinate

**363.54 Central choroidal atrophy, total**

Dystrophy, choroidal:
   central gyrate
   serpiginous

**363.55 Choroideremia**

DEF: Hereditary choroid degeneration, occurs in first decade; characterized by constricted visual field and ultimately blindness in males; less debilitating in females.

**363.56 Other diffuse or generalized dystrophy, partial**

Diffuse choroidal sclerosis

**363.57 Other diffuse or generalized dystrophy, total**

Generalized gyrate atrophy, choroid

**363.6 Choroidal hemorrhage and rupture**

**363.61 Choroidal hemorrhage, unspecified**

**363.62 Expulsive choroidal hemorrhage**

**363.63 Choroidal rupture**    CC

**CC Excl:** 363.61-363.9

**363.7 Choroidal detachment**

**363.70 Choroidal detachment, unspecified**    CC

**CC Excl:** See code: 363.63

**363.71 Serous choroidal detachment**    CC

**CC Excl:** See code: 363.63

DEF: Detachment of choroid from sclera; due to blister of serous fluid.

**363.72 Hemorrhagic choroidal detachment**    CC

**CC Excl:** See code: 363.63

DEF: Detachment of choroid from sclera; due to blood-filled blister.

**363.8 Other disorders of choroid**

**AHA:** 1Q, '06, 12

**363.9 Unspecified disorder of choroid**

**364 Disorders of iris and ciliary body**

**364.0 Acute and subacute iridocyclitis**

Anterior uveitis
Cyclitis     } acute,
Iridocyclitis    } subacute
Iritis

> EXCLUDES    gonococcal (098.41)
> herpes simplex (054.44)
> herpes zoster (053.22)

**364.00 Acute and subacute iridocyclitis, unspecified**    CC

**CC Excl:** 364.00-364.3

**364.01 Primary iridocyclitis**    CC

**CC Excl:** See code: 364.00

**364.02 Recurrent iridocyclitis**    CC

**CC Excl:** See code: 364.00

**364.03 Secondary iridocyclitis, infectious**    CC

**CC Excl:** See code: 364.00

**364.04 Secondary iridocyclitis, noninfectious**

Aqueous:      Aqueous:
   cells          flare
   fibrin

**364.05 Hypopyon**

DEF: Accumulation of white blood cells between cornea and lens.

**364.1 Chronic iridocyclitis**

> EXCLUDES    posterior cyclitis (363.21)

**364.10 Chronic iridocyclitis, unspecified**

**364.11 Chronic iridocyclitis in diseases classified elsewhere**

Code first underlying disease, as:
   sarcoidosis (135)
   tuberculosis (017.3)

> EXCLUDES    syphilitic iridocyclitis (091.52)

DEF: Persistent inflammation of iris and ciliary body; due to underlying disease or condition.

**364.2 Certain types of iridocyclitis**

> EXCLUDES    posterior cyclitis (363.21)
> sympathetic uveitis (360.11)

**364.21 Fuchs' heterochromic cyclitis**

DEF: Chronic cyclitis characterized by differences in the color of the two irises; the lighter iris appears in the inflamed eye.

**364.22 Glaucomatocyclitic crises**    CC

**CC Excl:** See code: 364.00

DEF: One-sided form of secondary open angle glaucoma; recurrent, uncommon and of short duration; causes high intraocular pressure, rarely damage.

---

| 4th / 5th Additional Digit Required | Unacceptable PDx | Manifestation Code | ►◄ Revised Text | ● New Code | ▲ Revised Code Title |

**364.23 Lens-induced iridocyclitis**
DEF: Inflammation of iris; due to immune reaction to proteins in lens following trauma or other lens abnormality.

**364.24 Vogt-Koyanagi syndrome**
DEF: Uveomeningitis with exudative iridocyclitis and choroiditis; causes depigmentation of hair and skin, detached retina; tinnitus and loss of hearing may occur.

**364.3 Unspecified iridocyclitis** `CC`
Uveitis NOS

CC Excl: See code: 364.00-364.3

√5ᵗʰ **364.4 Vascular disorders of iris and ciliary body**
**364.41 Hyphema**
Hemorrhage of iris or ciliary body
DEF: Hemorrhage in anterior chamber; also called hyphemia or "blood shot" eyes.

**364.42 Rubeosis iridis**
Neovascularization of iris or ciliary body
DEF: Blood vessel and connective tissue formation on surface of iris; symptomatic of diabetic retinopathy, central retinal vein occlusion and retinal detachment.

√5ᵗʰ **364.5 Degenerations of iris and ciliary body**
**364.51 Essential or progressive iris atrophy**
**364.52 Iridoschisis**
DEF: Splitting of the iris into two layers.

**364.53 Pigmentary iris degeneration**
Acquired heterochromia
Pigment dispersion syndrome } of iris
Translucency

**364.54 Degeneration of pupillary margin**
Atrophy of sphincter
Ectropion of pigment epithelium } of iris

**364.55 Miotic cysts of pupillary margin**
DEF: Serous-filled sacs in pupillary margin of iris.

**364.56 Degenerative changes of chamber angle**
**364.57 Degenerative changes of ciliary body**
**364.59 Other iris atrophy**
Iris atrophy (generalized) (sector shaped)

√5ᵗʰ **364.6 Cysts of iris, ciliary body, and anterior chamber**
EXCLUDES    miotic pupillary cyst (364.55)
parasitic cyst (360.13)
**364.60 Idiopathic cysts**
DEF: Fluid-filled sacs in iris or ciliary body; unknown etiology.

**364.61 Implantation cysts**
Epithelial down-growth, anterior chamber
Implantation cysts (surgical) (traumatic)
**364.62 Exudative cysts of iris or anterior chamber**
**364.63 Primary cyst of pars plana**
DEF: Fluid-filled sacs of outermost ciliary ring.

**364.64 Exudative cyst of pars plana**
DEF: Protein, fatty-filled sacs of outermost ciliary ring; due to fluid lead from blood vessels.

√5ᵗʰ **364.7 Adhesions and disruptions of iris and ciliary body**
EXCLUDES    flat anterior chamber (360.34)
**364.70 Adhesions of iris, unspecified**
Synechiae (iris) NOS
**364.71 Posterior synechiae**
DEF: Adhesion binding iris to lens.

**364.72 Anterior synechiae**
DEF: Adhesion binding the iris to cornea.

**364.73 Goniosynechiae**
Peripheral anterior synechiae
DEF: Adhesion binding iris to cornea at the angle of the anterior chamber.

**364.74 Pupillary membranes**
Iris bombé          Pupillary:
Pupillary:              seclusion
occlusion
DEF: Membrane traversing the pupil and blocking vision.

**364.75 Pupillary abnormalities**
Deformed pupil   Rupture of sphincter, pupil
Ectopic pupil

**364.76 Iridodialysis**
DEF: Separation of the iris from the ciliary body base; due to trauma or surgical accident.

**364.77 Recession of chamber angle**
DEF: Receding of anterior chamber angle of the eye; restricts vision.

√5ᵗʰ **364.8 Other disorders of iris and ciliary body**
AHA: ▶2Q, '07, 9◀

**364.81 Floppy iris syndrome**
Intraoperative floppy iris syndrome [IFIS]
Use additional E code to identify cause,
such as:
sympatholytics [antiadrenergics] causing
adverse effect in therapeutic use
(E941.3)

**364.89 Other disorders of iris and ciliary body**
Prolapse of iris NOS
EXCLUDES    prolapse of iris in recent
wound (871.1)

**364.9 Unspecified disorder of iris and ciliary body**

√4ᵗʰ **365 Glaucoma**
EXCLUDES    blind hypertensive eye [absolute glaucoma]
(360.42)
congenital glaucoma (743.20-743.22)
DEF: Rise in intraocular pressure which restricts blood flow; multiple causes.

√5ᵗʰ **365.0 Borderline glaucoma [glaucoma suspect]**
AHA: 1Q, '90, 8

**365.00 Preglaucoma, unspecified**
**365.01 Open angle with borderline findings**
Open angle with:
borderline intraocular pressure
cupping of optic discs
DEF: Minor block of aqueous outflow from eye.

**365.02 Anatomical narrow angle**
**365.03 Steroid responders**
**365.04 Ocular hypertension**
DEF: High fluid pressure within eye; no apparent cause.

√5ᵗʰ **365.1 Open-angle glaucoma**
**365.10 Open-angle glaucoma, unspecified**
Wide-angle glaucoma NOS
**365.11 Primary open angle glaucoma**
Chronic simple glaucoma
DEF: High intraocular pressure, despite free flow of aqueous.

**365.12 Low tension glaucoma**
**365.13 Pigmentary glaucoma**
DEF: High intraocular pressure; due to iris pigment granules blocking aqueous flow.

**365.14 Glaucoma of childhood**
Infantile or juvenile glaucoma
**365.15 Residual stage of open angle glaucoma**
√5ᵗʰ **365.2 Primary angle-closure glaucoma**
**365.20 Primary angle-closure glaucoma, unspecified**
**365.21 Intermittent angle-closure glaucoma**
Angle-closure glaucoma:
interval
subacute
DEF: Recurring attacks of high intraocular pressure; due to blocked aqueous flow.

**365.22 Acute angle-closure glaucoma** `CC`
CC Excl: See code: 365.22
DEF: Sudden, severe rise in intraocular pressure due to blockage in aqueous drainage.

**365.23 Chronic angle-closure glaucoma**
AHA: 2Q, '98, 16

**365.24 Residual stage of angle-closure glaucoma**

N Newborn Age: 0    P Pediatric Age: 0-17    M Maternity Age: 12-55    A Adult Age: 15-124    CC CC Condition    MCC Major CC Condition    HIV HIV Related Dx

114 — Volume 1 • October 2007                                        © 2007 Ingenix

✓5ᵗʰ **365.3    Corticosteroid-induced glaucoma**

**DEF:** Elevated intraocular pressure; due to long-term corticosteroid therapy.

**365.31 Glaucomatous stage**

**365.32 Residual stage**

✓5ᵗʰ **365.4    Glaucoma associated with congenital anomalies, dystrophies, and systemic syndromes**

**365.41 Glaucoma associated with chamber angle anomalies**

Code first associated disorder, as:
Axenfeld's anomaly (743.44)
Rieger's anomaly or syndrome (743.44)

**365.42 Glaucoma associated with anomalies of iris**

Code first associated disorder, as:
aniridia (743.45)
essential iris atrophy (364.51)

**365.43 Glaucoma associated with other anterior segment anomalies**

Code first associated disorder, as:
microcornea (743.41)

**365.44 Glaucoma associated with systemic syndromes**

Code first associated disease, as
neurofibromatosis (237.7)
Sturge-Weber (-Dimitri) syndrome (759.6)

✓5ᵗʰ **365.5    Glaucoma associated with disorders of the lens**

**365.51 Phacolytic glaucoma**

Use additional code for associated hypermature cataract (366.18)

**DEF:** Elevated intraocular pressure; due to lens protein blocking aqueous flow.

**365.52 Pseudoexfoliation glaucoma**

Use additional code for associated pseudoexfoliation of capsule (366.11)

**DEF:** Glaucoma characterized by small grayish particles deposited on the lens.

**365.59 Glaucoma associated with other lens disorders**

Use additional code for associated disorder, as:
dislocation of lens (379.33-379.34)
spherophakia (743.36)

✓5ᵗʰ **365.6    Glaucoma associated with other ocular disorders**

**365.60 Glaucoma associated with unspecified ocular disorder**

**365.61 Glaucoma associated with pupillary block**

Use additional code for associated disorder, as:
seclusion of pupil [iris bombé] (364.74)

**DEF:** Acute, open-angle glaucoma caused by mature cataract; aqueous flow is blocked by lens material and macrophages.

**365.62 Glaucoma associated with ocular inflammations**

Use additional code for associated disorder, as:
glaucomatocyclitic crises (364.22)
iridocyclitis (364.0-364.3)

**365.63 Glaucoma associated with vascular disorders**

Use additional code for associated disorder, as:
central retinal vein occlusion (362.35)
hyphema (364.41)

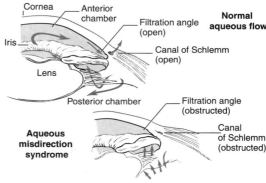

**Aqueous Misdirection Syndrome**

Cornea — Anterior chamber — Filtration angle (open) — **Normal aqueous flow**

Iris — Canal of Schlemm (open)

Lens

Posterior chamber — Filtration angle (obstructed)

**Aqueous misdirection syndrome** — Canal of Schlemm (obstructed)

**365.64 Glaucoma associated with tumors or cysts**

Use additional code for associated disorder, as:
benign neoplasm (224.0-224.9)
epithelial down-growth (364.61)
malignant neoplasm (190.0-190.9)

**365.65 Glaucoma associated with ocular trauma**

Use additional code for associated condition, as:
contusion of globe (921.3)
recession of chamber angle (364.77)

✓5ᵗʰ **365.8    Other specified forms of glaucoma**

**365.81 Hypersecretion glaucoma**

**365.82 Glaucoma with increased episcleral venous pressure**

**365.83 Aqueous misdirection**

Malignant glaucoma

**AHA:** 4Q, '02, 48

**DEF:** A form of glaucoma that occurs when aqueous humor flows into the posterior chamber of the eye (vitreous) rather than through the normal recycling channels into the anterior chamber.

**365.89 Other specified glaucoma**

**AHA:** 2Q, '98, 16

**365.9    Unspecified glaucoma**

**AHA:** 3Q, '03, 14; 2Q, '01, 16

✓4ᵗʰ **366 Cataract**

**DEF:** A variety of conditions that create a cloudy, or calcified lens that obstructs vision.

**EXCLUDES**   congenital cataract (743.30-743.34)

✓5ᵗʰ **366.0    Infantile, juvenile, and presenile cataract**

**366.00 Nonsenile cataract, unspecified**

**366.01 Anterior subcapsular polar cataract**

**DEF:** Defect within the front, center lens surface.

**366.02 Posterior subcapsular polar cataract**

**DEF:** Defect within the rear, center lens surface.

**366.03 Cortical, lamellar, or zonular cataract**

**DEF:** Opacities radiating from center to edge of lens; appear as thin, concentric layers of lens.

**366.04 Nuclear cataract**

**366.09 Other and combined forms of nonsenile cataract**

✓5ᵗʰ **366.1    Senile cataract**

**AHA:** 3Q, '91, 9; S-O, '85, 10

**366.10 Senile cataract, unspecified**    Ⓐ

**AHA:** 1Q, '03, 5

**366.11 Pseudoexfoliation of lens capsule**    Ⓐ

**366.12 Incipient cataract**    Ⓐ

Cataract:          Cataract:
coronary            punctate
immature NOS   Water clefts

**DEF:** Minor disorders of lens not affecting vision; due to aging.

**Cataract**

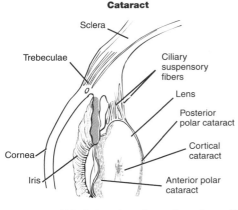

Sclera
Trebeculae
Ciliary suspensory fibers
Lens
Posterior polar cataract
Cortical cataract
Cornea
Iris
Anterior polar cataract

**366.13 Anterior subcapsular polar senile cataract**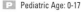

**366.14 Posterior subcapsular polar senile cataract** A

**366.15 Cortical senile cataract** A

**366.16 Nuclear sclerosis** A
     Cataracta brunescens
     Nuclear cataract

**366.17 Total or mature cataract** A

**366.18 Hypermature cataract** A
     Morgagni cataract

**366.19 Other and combined forms of senile cataract** A

✓5th **366.2 Traumatic cataract**

**366.20 Traumatic cataract, unspecified**

**366.21 Localized traumatic opacities**
     Vossius' ring

**366.22 Total traumatic cataract**

**366.23 Partially resolved traumatic cataract**

✓5th **366.3 Cataract secondary to ocular disorders**

**366.30 Cataracta complicata, unspecified**

**366.31 Glaucomatous flecks (subcapsular)**
     Code first underlying glaucoma
       (365.0-365.9)

**366.32 Cataract in inflammatory disorders**
     Code first underlying condition, as:
       chronic choroiditis (363.0-363.2)

**366.33 Cataract with neovascularization**
     Code first underlying condition, as:
       chronic iridocyclitis (364.10)

**366.34 Cataract in degenerative disorders**
     Sunflower cataract
     Code first underlying condition, as:
       chalcosis (360.24)
       degenerative myopia (360.21)
       pigmentary retinal dystrophy (362.74)

✓5th **366.4 Cataract associated with other disorders**

**366.41 _Diabetic cataract_**
     _Code first diabetes (250.5)_
     **AHA:** 3Q, '91, 9; S-O, '85, 11

**366.42 _Tetanic cataract_**
     _Code first underlying disease, as:_
       calcinosis (275.4)
       hypoparathyroidism (252.1)

**366.43 _Myotonic cataract_**
     _Code first underlying disorder_ ▶(359.21-
       359.29)◀

**366.44 _Cataract associated with other syndromes_**
     _Code first underlying condition, as:_
       craniofacial dysostosis (756.0)
       galactosemia (271.1)

**366.45 Toxic cataract**
     Drug-induced cataract
     Use additional E code to identify drug or
       other toxic substance

**366.46 Cataract associated with radiation and other physical influences**
     Use additional E code to identify cause

✓5th **366.5 After-cataract**

**366.50 After-cataract, unspecified**
     Secondary cataract NOS

**366.51 Soemmering's ring**
     **DEF:** A donut-shaped lens remnant and a capsule behind
     the pupil as a result of cataract surgery or trauma.

**366.52 Other after-cataract, not obscuring vision**

**366.53 After-cataract, obscuring vision**

**366.8 Other cataract**
     Calcification of lens

**366.9 Unspecified cataract**

✓4th **367 Disorders of refraction and accommodation**

**367.0 Hypermetropia**
     Far-sightedness      Hyperopia
     **DEF:** Refraction error, called also hyperopia, focal point is posterior
     to retina; abnormally short anteroposterior diameter or subnormal
     refractive power; causes farsightedness.

**367.1 Myopia**
     Near-sightedness
     **DEF:** Refraction error, focal point is anterior to retina; causes near-
     sightedness.

✓5th **367.2 Astigmatism**

**367.20 Astigmatism, unspecified**

**367.21 Regular astigmatism**

**367.22 Irregular astigmatism**

✓5th **367.3 Anisometropia and aniseikonia**

**367.31 Anisometropia**
     **DEF:** Eyes with refractive powers that differ by at least
     one diopter.

**367.32 Aniseikonia**
     **DEF:** Eyes with unequal retinal imaging; usually due to
     refractive error.

**367.4 Presbyopia**
     **DEF:** Loss of crystalline lens elasticity; causes errors of
     accommodation; due to aging.

✓5th **367.5 Disorders of accommodation**

**367.51 Paresis of accommodation**
     Cycloplegia
     **DEF:** Partial paralysis of ciliary muscle; causing focus
     problems.

**367.52 Total or complete internal ophthalmoplegia**
     **DEF:** Total paralysis of ciliary muscle; large pupil
     incapable of focus.

**367.53 Spasm of accommodation**
     **DEF:** Abnormal contraction of ciliary muscle; causes
     focus problems.

✓5th **367.8 Other disorders of refraction and accommodation**

**367.81 Transient refractive change**

**367.89 Other**
     Drug-induced ⎫ disorders of refraction
     Toxic ⎭ and accommodation

**367.9 Unspecified disorder of refraction and accommodation**

✓4th **368 Visual disturbances**
     **EXCLUDES**   electrophysiological disturbances
       (794.11-794.14)

✓5th **368.0 Amblyopia ex anopsia**
     **DEF:** Vision impaired due to disuse; esotropia often cause.

**368.00 Amblyopia, unspecified**

**368.01 Strabismic amblyopia**
     Suppression amblyopia

**368.02 Deprivation amblyopia**
     **DEF:** Decreased vision associated with suppressed
     retinal image of one eye.

**368.03 Refractive amblyopia**

✓5th **368.1 Subjective visual disturbances**

**368.10 Subjective visual disturbance, unspecified**

**368.11 Sudden visual loss**   CC
     **CC Excl:** 368.10-368.12, 368.16

**368.12 Transient visual loss**   CC
     Concentric fading    Scintillating scotoma
     **CC Excl:** See code: 368.11

N Newborn Age: 0     P Pediatric Age: 0-17     M Maternity Age: 12-55     A Adult Age: 15-124     CC CC Condition     MCC Major CC Condition     HIV HIV Related Dx

116 — Volume 1 • October 2007          © 2007 Ingenix

**368.13 Visual discomfort**
Asthenopia          Photophobia
Eye strain

**368.14 Visual distortions of shape and size**
Macropsia           Micropsia
Metamorphopsia

**368.15 Other visual distortions and entoptic phenomena**
Photopsia            Refractive:
Refractive:              polyopia
  diplopia             Visual halos

**368.16 Psychophysical visual disturbances**
Visual:              Visual:
  agnosia              hallucinations
  disorientation       syndrome

**368.2    Diplopia**
Double vision

**☑5ᵗʰ 368.3    Other disorders of binocular vision**
**368.30 Binocular vision disorder, unspecified**
**368.31 Suppression of binocular vision**
**368.32 Simultaneous visual perception without fusion**
**368.33 Fusion with defective stereopsis**
DEF: Faulty depth perception though normal ability to focus.
**368.34 Abnormal retinal correspondence**

**☑5ᵗʰ 368.4    Visual field defects**
**368.40 Visual field defect, unspecified**
**368.41 Scotoma involving central area**
Scotoma:             Scotoma:
  central              paracentral
  centrocecal
DEF: Vision loss (blind spot) in central five degrees of visual field.
**368.42 Scotoma of blind spot area**
Enlarged:            Paracecal scotoma
  angioscotoma
  blind spot
**368.43 Sector or arcuate defects**
Scotoma:             Scotoma:
  arcuate              Seidel
  Bjerrum
DEF: Arc-shaped blind spot caused by retinal nerve damage.
**368.44 Other localized visual field defect**
Scotoma:             Visual field defect:
  NOS                  nasal step
  ring                 peripheral
**368.45 Generalized contraction or constriction**
**368.46 Homonymous bilateral field defects**
Hemianopsia (altitudinal) (homonymous)
Quadrant anopia
DEF: Disorders found in the corresponding vertical halves of the visual fields of both eyes.
**368.47 Heteronymous bilateral field defects**
Hemianopsia:         Hemianopsia:
  binasal              bitemporal
DEF: Disorders in the opposite halves of the visual fields of both eyes.

**☑5ᵗʰ 368.5    Color vision deficiencies**
Color blindness
**368.51 Protan defect**
Protanomaly          Protanopia
DEF: Mild difficulty distinguishing green and red hues with shortened spectrum; sex-linked affecting one percent of males.
**368.52 Deutan defect**
Deuteranomaly  Deuteranopia
DEF: Male-only disorder; difficulty in distinguishing green and red, no shortened spectrum.

**368.53 Tritan defect**
Tritanomaly          Tritanopia
DEF: Difficulty in distinguishing blue and yellow; occurs often due to drugs, retinal detachment and central nervous system diseases.
**368.54 Achromatopsia**
Monochromatism (cone) (rod)
DEF: Complete color blindness; caused by disease, injury to retina, optic nerve or pathway.
**368.55 Acquired color vision deficiencies**
**368.59 Other color vision deficiencies**

**☑5ᵗʰ 368.6    Night blindness**
Nyctalopia
DEF: Nyctalopia: disorder of vision in dim light or night blindness.
**368.60 Night blindness, unspecified**
**368.61 Congenital night blindness**
Hereditary night blindness
Oguchi's disease
**368.62 Acquired night blindness**
**EXCLUDES**   that due to vitamin A deficiency (264.5)
**368.63 Abnormal dark adaptation curve**
Abnormal threshold ⎫ of cones or
Delayed adaptation  ⎬ rods
**368.69 Other night blindness**

**368.8    Other specified visual disturbances**
Blurred vision NOS
AHA: 4Q, '02, 56

**368.9    Unspecified visual disturbance**
AHA: 3Q, '06, 22; 1Q, '04, 15

**☑4ᵗʰ 369   Blindness and low vision**
Note: Visual impairment refers to a functional limitation of the eye (e.g., limited visual acuity or visual field). It should be distinguished from visual disability, indicating a limitation of the abilities of the individual (e.g., limited reading skills, vocational skills), and from visual handicap, indicating a limitation of personal and socioeconomic independence (e.g., limited mobility, limited employability).
The levels of impairment defined in the table on the next page are based on the recommendations of the WHO Study Group on Prevention of Blindness (Geneva, November 6–10, 1972; WHO Technical Report Series 518), and of the International Council of Ophthalmology (1976).
Note that definitions of blindness vary in different settings.
For international reporting WHO defines blindness as profound impairment. This definition can be applied to blindness of one eye (369.1, 369.6) and to blindness of the individual (369.0).
For determination of benefits in the U.S.A., the definition of legal blindness as severe impairment is often used. This definition applies to blindness of the individual only.
**EXCLUDES**   correctable impaired vision due to refractive errors (367.0-367.9)

**☑5ᵗʰ 369.0    Profound impairment, both eyes**
**369.00 Impairment level not further specified**
Blindness:
  NOS according to WHO definition
  both eyes
**369.01 Better eye: total impairment; lesser eye: total impairment**
**369.02 Better eye: near-total impairment; lesser eye: not further specified**
**369.03 Better eye: near-total impairment; lesser eye: total impairment**
**369.04 Better eye: near-total impairment; lesser eye: near-total impairment**
**369.05 Better eye: profound impairment; lesser eye: not further specified**

369.06 **Better eye: profound impairment; lesser eye: total impairment**

369.07 **Better eye: profound impairment; lesser eye: near-total impairment**

369.08 **Better eye: profound impairment; lesser eye: profound impairment**

√4ᵗʰ 369.1 **Moderate or severe impairment, better eye, profound impairment lesser eye**

369.10 **Impairment level not further specified**
　　Blindness, one eye, low vision other eye

369.11 **Better eye: severe impairment; lesser eye: blind, not further specified**

369.12 **Better eye: severe impairment; lesser eye: total impairment**

369.13 **Better eye: severe impairment; lesser eye: near-total impairment**

369.14 **Better eye: severe impairment; lesser eye: profound impairment**

369.15 **Better eye: moderate impairment; lesser eye: blind, not further specified**

369.16 **Better eye: moderate impairment; lesser eye: total impairment**

369.17 **Better eye: moderate impairment; lesser eye: near-total impairment**

369.18 **Better eye: moderate impairment; lesser eye: profound impairment**

√5ᵗʰ 369.2 **Moderate or severe impairment, both eyes**

369.20 **Impairment level not further specified**
　　Low vision, both eyes NOS

369.21 **Better eye: severe impairment; lesser eye: not further specified**

369.22 **Better eye: severe impairment; lesser eye: severe impairment**

369.23 **Better eye: moderate impairment; lesser eye: not further specified**

369.24 **Better eye: moderate impairment; lesser eye: severe impairment**

369.25 **Better eye: moderate impairment; lesser eye: moderate impairment**

369.3 **Unqualified visual loss, both eyes**
　　**EXCLUDES**　*blindness NOS:*
　　　　*legal [U.S.A. definition] (369.4)*
　　　　*WHO definition (369.00)*

369.4 **Legal blindness, as defined in U.S.A.**
　　Blindness NOS according to U.S.A. definition
　　**EXCLUDES**　*legal blindness with specification of impairment level (369.01-369.08, 369.11-369.14, 369.21-369.22)*

√5ᵗʰ 369.6 **Profound impairment, one eye**

369.60 **Impairment level not further specified**
　　Blindness, one eye

369.61 **One eye: total impairment; other eye: not specified**

369.62 **One eye: total impairment; other eye: near normal vision**

369.63 **One eye: total impairment; other eye: normal vision**

369.64 **One eye: near-total impairment; other eye: not specified**

369.65 **One eye: near-total impairment; other eye: near-normal vision**

369.66 **One eye: near-total impairment; other eye: normal vision**

369.67 **One eye: profound impairment; other eye: not specified**

369.68 **One eye: profound impairment; other eye: near-normal vision**

369.69 **One eye: profound impairment; other eye: normal vision**

√5ᵗʰ 369.7 **Moderate or severe impairment, one eye**

369.70 **Impairment level not further specified**
　　Low vision, one eye

369.71 **One eye: severe impairment; other eye: not specified**

| Classification | | LEVELS OF VISUAL IMPAIRMENT | Additional descriptors which may be encountered |
|---|---|---|---|
| "legal" | WHO | Visual acuity and/or visual field limitation (whichever is worse) | |
| | (N E A R -) N O R M A L V I S I O N | RANGE OF NORMAL VISION<br>20/10  20/13  20/16  20/20  20/25<br>2.0    1.6    1.25   1.0   0.8 | |
| | | NEAR-NORMAL VISION<br>20/30  20/40  20/50  20/60<br>0.7    0.6    0.5    0.4   0.3 | |
| | L O W   V I S I O N | MODERATE VISUAL IMPAIRMENT<br>20/70  20/80  20/100  20/125<br>20/160<br>0.25  0.20  0.16  0.12 | Moderate low vision |
| L E G A L   B L I N D N E S S   (U.S.A.) both eyes | | SEVERE VISUAL IMPAIRMENT<br>20/200  20/250  20/320  20/400<br>0.10   0.08   0.06   0.05<br>Visual field:  20 degrees or less | Severe low vision, "Legal" blindness |
| | B L I N D N E S S (WHO) one or both eyes | PROFOUND VISUAL IMPAIRMENT<br>20/500  20/630  20/800  20/1000<br>0.04   0.03   0.025  0.02<br>Count fingers at:  less than 3m<br>　　　　　　　　(10 ft.)<br>Visual field:  10 degrees or less | Profound low vision, Moderate blindness |
| | | NEAR-TOTAL VISUAL IMPAIRMENT<br>Visual acuity:  less than 0.02 (20/1000)<br>Count fingers at:  1m (3 ft.) or less<br>Hand movements:  5m (15 ft.) or less<br>Light projection, light perception<br>Visual field:  5 degrees or less | Severe blindness, Near-total blindness |
| | | TOTAL VISUAL IMPAIRMENT<br>No light perception (NLP) | Total blindness |

Visual acuity refers to best achievable acuity with correction.
Non-listed Snellen fractions may be classified by converting to the nearest decimal
　equivalent, e.g. 10/200 = 0.05, 6/30 = 0.20.
CF (count fingers) without designation of distance, may be classified to profound
　impairment.
HM (hand motion) without designation of distance, may be classified to near-total
　impairment.
Visual field measurements refer to the largest field diameter for a 1/100 white test
　object.

369.72 **One eye: severe impairment; other eye: near-normal vision**

369.73 **One eye: severe impairment; other eye: normal vision**

369.74 **One eye: moderate impairment; other eye: not specified**

369.75 **One eye: moderate impairment; other eye: near-normal vision**

369.76 **One eye: moderate impairment; other eye: normal vision**

369.8 **Unqualified visual loss, one eye**

369.9 **Unspecified visual loss**
　　**AHA:** 4Q, '02, 114; 3Q, '02, 20

√4ᵗʰ **370 Keratitis**

√5ᵗʰ 370.0 **Corneal ulcer**
　　**EXCLUDES**　*that due to vitamin A deficiency (264.3)*

370.00 **Corneal ulcer, unspecified**

370.01 **Marginal corneal ulcer**

370.02 **Ring corneal ulcer**

370.03 **Central corneal ulcer**

370.04 **Hypopyon ulcer**
　　Serpiginous ulcer
　　**DEF:** Corneal ulcer with an accumulation of pus in the eye's anterior chamber..

Ⓝ Newborn Age: 0　　Ⓟ Pediatric Age: 0-17　　Ⓜ Maternity Age: 12-55　　Ⓐ Adult Age: 15-124　　**CC** CC Condition　　**MCC** Major CC Condition　　**HIV** HIV Related Dx

**118 — Volume 1 • October 2007**　　　　　　　　　　　　　　　　　　　　　　　　　　© **2007 Ingenix**

**370.05 Mycotic corneal ulcer**
DEF: Fungal infection causing corneal tissue loss.

**370.06 Perforated corneal ulcer**
DEF: Tissue loss through all layers of cornea.

**370.07 Mooren's ulcer**
DEF: Tissue loss, with chronic inflammation, at junction of cornea and sclera; seen in elderly.

√5th **370.2 Superficial keratitis without conjunctivitis**
EXCLUDES   dendritic [herpes simplex] keratitis (054.42)

**370.20 Superficial keratitis, unspecified**
**370.21 Punctate keratitis**
Thygeson's superficial punctate keratitis

DEF: Formation of cellular and fibrinous deposits (keratic precipitates) on posterior surface; deposits develop after injury or iridocyclitis.

**370.22 Macular keratitis**
Keratitis:          Keratitis:
areolar          stellate
nummular          striate

**370.23 Filamentary keratitis**
DEF: Keratitis characterized by twisted filaments of mucoid material on the cornea's surface.

**370.24 Photokeratitis**
Snow blindness
Welders' keratitis
AHA: 3Q, '96, 6

DEF: Painful, inflamed cornea; due to extended exposure to ultraviolet light.

√5th **370.3 Certain types of keratoconjunctivitis**
**370.31 Phlyctenular keratoconjunctivitis**
Phlyctenulosis
Use additional code for any associated tuberculosis (017.3)

DEF: Miniature blister on conjunctiva or cornea; associated with tuberculosis and malnutrition disorders.

**370.32 Limbar and corneal involvement in vernal conjunctivitis**
Use additional code for vernal conjunctivitis (372.13)

DEF: Corneal itching and inflammation in conjunctivitis; often limited to lining of eyelids.

**370.33 Keratoconjunctivitis sicca, not specified as Sjögren's**
EXCLUDES   Sjögren's syndrome (710.2)

DEF: Inflammation of conjunctiva and cornea; characterized by "horny" looking tissue and excess blood in these areas; decreased flow of lacrimal (tear) is a contributing factor.

**370.34 Exposure keratoconjunctivitis**
AHA: 3Q, '96, 6

DEF: Incomplete closure of eyelid causing dry, inflamed eye.

**370.35 Neurotrophic keratoconjunctivitis**
√5th **370.4 Other and unspecified keratoconjunctivitis**
**370.40 Keratoconjunctivitis, unspecified**
Superficial keratitis with conjunctivitis NOS

**370.44 Keratitis or keratoconjunctivitis in exanthema**
Code first underlying condition (050.0-052.9)
EXCLUDES   herpes simplex (054.43)
herpes zoster (053.21)
measles (055.71)

**370.49 Other**
EXCLUDES   epidemic keratoconjunctivitis (077.1)

√5th **370.5 Interstitial and deep keratitis**
**370.50 Interstitial keratitis, unspecified**
**370.52 Diffuse interstitial keratitis**
Cogan's syndrome
DEF: Inflammation of cornea; with deposits in middle corneal layers; may obscure vision.

**370.54 Sclerosing keratitis**
DEF: Chronic corneal inflammation leading to opaque scarring.

**370.55 Corneal abscess**
DEF: Pocket of pus and inflammation on the cornea.

**370.59 Other**
EXCLUDES   disciform herpes simplex keratitis (054.43)
syphilitic keratitis (090.3)

√5th **370.6 Corneal neovascularization**
**370.60 Corneal neovascularization, unspecified**
**370.61 Localized vascularization of cornea**
DEF: Limited infiltration of cornea by new blood vessels.

**370.62 Pannus (corneal)**
AHA: 3Q, '02, 20

DEF: Buildup of superficial vascularization and granulated tissue under epithelium of cornea.

**370.63 Deep vascularization of cornea**
DEF: Deep infiltration of cornea by new blood vessels.

**370.64 Ghost vessels (corneal)**
**370.8 Other forms of keratitis**
AHA: 3Q, '94, 5

**370.9 Unspecified keratitis**
√4th **371 Corneal opacity and other disorders of cornea**
√5th **371.0 Corneal scars and opacities**
EXCLUDES   that due to vitamin A deficiency (264.6)
**371.00 Corneal opacity, unspecified**
Corneal scar NOS
**371.01 Minor opacity of cornea**
Corneal nebula
**371.02 Peripheral opacity of cornea**
Corneal macula not interfering with central vision
**371.03 Central opacity of cornea**
Corneal:
leucoma ⎤ interfering with central
macula ⎦ vision
**371.04 Adherent leucoma**
DEF: Dense, opaque corneal growth adhering to the iris; also spelled as leukoma.

**371.05 Phthisical cornea**
Code first underlying tuberculosis (017.3)
√5th **371.1 Corneal pigmentations and deposits**
**371.10 Corneal deposit, unspecified**
**371.11 Anterior pigmentations**
Stähli's lines
**371.12 Stromal pigmentations**
Hematocornea
**371.13 Posterior pigmentations**
Krukenberg spindle
**371.14 Kayser-Fleischer ring**
DEF: Copper deposits forming ring at outer edge of cornea; seen in Wilson's disease and other liver disorders.

**371.15 Other deposits associated with metabolic disorders**
**371.16 Argentous deposits**
DEF: Silver deposits in cornea.

√5th **371.2 Corneal edema**
**371.20 Corneal edema, unspecified**

√4th / √5th Additional Digit Required          Unacceptable PDx          Manifestation Code          ◄► Revised Text          ● New Code          ▲ Revised Code Title

© 2007 Ingenix

October 2007 • Volume 1 — 119

**371.21 Idiopathic corneal edema**

DEF: Corneal swelling and fluid retention of unknown cause.

**371.22 Secondary corneal edema**

DEF: Corneal swelling and fluid retention caused by an underlying disease, injury, or condition.

**371.23 Bullous keratopathy**

DEF: Corneal degeneration; characterized by recurring, rupturing epithelial "blisters;" ruptured blebs expose corneal nerves, cause great pain; occurs in glaucoma, iridocyclitis and Fuchs' epithelial dystrophy.

**371.24 Corneal edema due to wearing of contact lenses**

✓5th **371.3 Changes of corneal membranes**

**371.30 Corneal membrane change, unspecified**
**371.31 Folds and rupture of Bowman's membrane**
**371.32 Folds in Descemet's membrane**
**371.33 Rupture in Descemet's membrane**

✓5th **371.4 Corneal degenerations**

**371.40 Corneal degeneration, unspecified**
**371.41 Senile corneal changes**

Arcus senilis      Hassall-Henle bodies

**371.42 Recurrent erosion of cornea**

EXCLUDES    Mooren's ulcer (370.07)

**371.43 Band-shaped keratopathy**

DEF: Horizontal bands of superficial corneal calcium deposits.

**371.44 Other calcerous degenerations of cornea**
**371.45 Keratomalacia NOS**

EXCLUDES    that due to vitamin A
deficiency (264.4)

DEF: Destruction of the cornea by keratinization of the epithelium with ulceration and perforation of the cornea; seen in cases of vitamin A deficiency.

**371.46 Nodular degeneration of cornea**

Salzmann's nodular dystrophy

**371.48 Peripheral degenerations of cornea**

Marginal degeneration of cornea [Terrien's]

**371.49 Other**

Discrete colliquative keratopathy

✓5th **371.5 Hereditary corneal dystrophies**

DEF: Genetic disorder; leads to opacities, edema or lesions of cornea.

**371.50 Corneal dystrophy, unspecified**
**371.51 Juvenile epithelial corneal dystrophy**
**371.52 Other anterior corneal dystrophies**

Corneal dystrophy:      Corneal dystrophy:
microscopic cystic      ring-like

**371.53 Granular corneal dystrophy**
**371.54 Lattice corneal dystrophy**
**371.55 Macular corneal dystrophy**
**371.56 Other stromal corneal dystrophies**

Crystalline corneal dystrophy

**371.57 Endothelial corneal dystrophy**

Combined corneal dystrophy
Cornea guttata
Fuchs' endothelial dystrophy

**371.58 Other posterior corneal dystrophies**

Polymorphous corneal dystrophy

✓5th **371.6 Keratoconus**

DEF: Bilateral bulging protrusion of anterior cornea; often due to noninflammatory thinning.

**371.60 Keratoconus, unspecified**
**371.61 Keratoconus, stable condition**
**371.62 Keratoconus, acute hydrops**

✓5th **371.7 Other corneal deformities**

**371.70 Corneal deformity, unspecified**
**371.71 Corneal ectasia**

DEF: Bulging protrusion of thinned, scarred cornea.

**371.72 Descemetocele**

DEF: Protrusion of Descemet's membrane into cornea.

**371.73 Corneal staphyloma**

DEF: Protrusion of cornea into adjacent tissue.

✓5th **371.8 Other corneal disorders**

**371.81 Corneal anesthesia and hypoesthesia**

DEF: Decreased or absent sensitivity of cornea.

**371.82 Corneal disorder due to contact lens**

EXCLUDES    corneal edema due to contact
lens (371.24)

DEF: Contact lens wear causing cornea disorder, excluding swelling.

**371.89 Other**

AHA: 3Q, '99, 12

**371.9 Unspecified corneal disorder**

✓4th **372 Disorders of conjunctiva**

EXCLUDES    keratoconjunctivitis (370.3-370.4)

✓5th **372.0 Acute conjunctivitis**

**372.00 Acute conjunctivitis, unspecified**
**372.01 Serous conjunctivitis, except viral**

EXCLUDES    viral conjunctivitis NOS (077.9)

**372.02 Acute follicular conjunctivitis**

Conjunctival folliculosis NOS

EXCLUDES    conjunctivitis:
adenoviral (acute follicular)
(077.3)
epidemic hemorrhagic
(077.4)
inclusion (077.0)
Newcastle (077.8)
epidemic keratoconjunctivitis
(077.1)
pharyngoconjunctival fever
(077.2)

DEF: Severe conjunctival inflammation with dense infiltrations of lymphoid tissues of inner eyelids; may be traced to a viral or chlamydial etiology.

**372.03 Other mucopurulent conjunctivitis**

Catarrhal conjunctivitis

EXCLUDES    blennorrhea neonatorum
(gonococcal) (098.40)
neonatal conjunctivitis(771.6)
ophthalmia neonatorum NOS
(771.6)

**372.04 Pseudomembranous conjunctivitis**

Membranous conjunctivitis

EXCLUDES    diphtheritic conjunctivitis
(032.81)

DEF: Severe inflammation of conjunctiva; false membrane develops on inner surface of eyelid; membrane can be removed without harming epithelium, due to bacterial infections, toxic and allergic factors, and viral infections.

**372.05 Acute atopic conjunctivitis**

DEF: Sudden, severe conjunctivitis due to allergens.

✓5th **372.1 Chronic conjunctivitis**

**372.10 Chronic conjunctivitis, unspecified**
**372.11 Simple chronic conjunctivitis**
**372.12 Chronic follicular conjunctivitis**

DEF: Persistent conjunctival inflammation with dense, localized infiltrations of lymphoid tissues of inner eyelids.

**372.13 Vernal conjunctivitis**

AHA: 3Q, '96, 8

**372.14 Other chronic allergic conjunctivitis**

AHA: 3Q, '96, 8

**372.15 Parasitic conjunctivitis**

Code first underlying disease, as:
filariasis (125.0-125.9)
mucocutaneous leishmaniasis (085.5)

✓5th **372.2 Blepharoconjunctivitis**

**372.20 Blepharoconjunctivitis, unspecified**
**372.21 Angular blepharoconjunctivitis**

DEF: Inflammation at junction of upper and lower eyelids; may block lacrimal secretions.

**372.22 Contact blepharoconjunctivitis**

N Newborn Age: 0    P Pediatric Age: 0-17    M Maternity Age: 12-55    A Adult Age: 15-124    CC CC Condition    MCC Major CC Condition    HIV HIV Related Dx

120 — Volume 1 • October 2007

© 2007 Ingenix

✓5th **372.3 Other and unspecified conjunctivitis**
    **372.30 Conjunctivitis, unspecified**
    **372.31** *Rosacea conjunctivitis*
        *Code first underlying rosacea dermatitis*
        *(695.3)*
    **372.33** *Conjunctivitis in mucocutaneous disease*
        *Code first underlying disease, as:*
        erythema multiforme (695.1)
        Reiter's disease (099.3)
        **EXCLUDES** *ocular pemphigoid (694.61)*
    **372.39 Other**
        **AHA:** ▶2Q, '07, 9◀

✓5th **372.4 Pterygium**
        **EXCLUDES** *pseudopterygium (372.52)*
    **DEF:** Wedge-shaped, conjunctival thickening that advances from
    the inner corner of the eye toward the cornea.
    **372.40 Pterygium, unspecified**
    **372.41 Peripheral pterygium, stationary**
    **372.42 Peripheral pterygium, progressive**
    **372.43 Central pterygium**
    **372.44 Double pterygium**
    **372.45 Recurrent pterygium**

✓5th **372.5 Conjunctival degenerations and deposits**
    **372.50 Conjunctival degeneration, unspecified**
    **372.51 Pinguecula**
        **DEF:** Proliferative spot on the bulbar conjunctiva located
        near the sclerocorneal junction, usually on the nasal
        side; it is seen in elderly people.
    **372.52 Pseudopterygium**
        **DEF:** Conjunctival scar joined to the cornea; it looks like
        a pterygium but is not attached to the tissue.
    **372.53 Conjunctival xerosis**
        **EXCLUDES** *conjunctival xerosis due to*
        *vitamin A deficiency*
        *(264.0, 264.1, 264.7)*
        **DEF:** Dry conjunctiva due to vitamin A deficiency; related
        to Bitot's spots; may develop into xerophthalmia and
        keratomalacia.
    **372.54 Conjunctival concretions**
        **DEF:** Calculus or deposit on conjunctiva.
    **372.55 Conjunctival pigmentations**
        Conjunctival argyrosis
        **DEF:** Color deposits in conjunctiva.
    **372.56 Conjunctival deposits**

✓5th **372.6 Conjunctival scars**
    **372.61 Granuloma of conjunctiva**
    **372.62 Localized adhesions and strands of**
        **conjunctiva**
        **DEF:** Abnormal fibrous connections in conjunctiva.
    **372.63 Symblepharon**
        Extensive adhesions of conjunctiva
        **DEF:** Adhesion of the eyelids to the eyeball.
    **372.64 Scarring of conjunctiva**
        Contraction of eye socket (after enucleation)

✓5th **372.7 Conjunctival vascular disorders and cysts**
    **372.71 Hyperemia of conjunctiva**
        **DEF:** Conjunctival blood vessel congestion causing eye
        redness.
    **372.72 Conjunctival hemorrhage**
        Hyposphagma
        Subconjunctival hemorrhage
    **372.73 Conjunctival edema**
        Chemosis of conjunctiva
        Subconjunctival edema
        **DEF:** Fluid retention and swelling in conjunctival
        tissue.
    **372.74 Vascular abnormalities of conjunctiva**
        Aneurysm(ata) of conjunctiva
    **372.75 Conjunctival cysts**
        **DEF:** Abnormal sacs of fluid in conjunctiva.

✓5th **372.8 Other disorders of conjunctiva**
    **372.81 Conjunctivochalasis**
        **AHA:** 4Q, '00, 41
        **DEF:** Bilateral condition of redundant conjunctival tissue
        between globe and lower eyelid margin; may cover
        lower punctum, interferring with normal tearing.
    **372.89 Other disorders of conjunctiva**
    **372.9 Unspecified disorder of conjunctiva**

✓4th **373 Inflammation of eyelids**
✓5th **373.0 Blepharitis**
        **EXCLUDES** *blepharoconjunctivitis (372.20-372.22)*
    **373.00 Blepharitis, unspecified**
    **373.01 Ulcerative blepharitis**
    **373.02 Squamous blepharitis**

✓5th **373.1 Hordeolum and other deep inflammation of eyelid**
    **DEF:** Purulent, localized, staphylococcal infection in sebaceous
    glands of eyelids.
    **373.11 Hordeolum externum**
        Hordeolum NOS Stye
        **DEF:** Infection of the oil glands in the eyelash follicles.
    **373.12 Hordeolum internum**
        Infection of meibomian gland
        **DEF:** Infection of the oil gland of the eyelid margin.
    **373.13 Abscess of eyelid**
        Furuncle of eyelid
        **DEF:** Inflamed pocket of pus on the eyelid.

    **373.2 Chalazion**
        Meibomian (gland) cyst
        **EXCLUDES** *infected meibomian gland (373.12)*
        **DEF:** Chronic inflammation of the meibomian gland, causing an
        eyelid mass.

✓5th **373.3 Noninfectious dermatoses of eyelid**
    **373.31 Eczematous dermatitis of eyelid**
    **373.32 Contact and allergic dermatitis of eyelid**
    **373.33 Xeroderma of eyelid**
    **373.34 Discoid lupus erythematosus of eyelid**

    **373.4** *Infective dermatitis of eyelid of types resulting in*
    *deformity*
        *Code first underlying disease, as:*
        leprosy (030.0-030.9)
        lupus vulgaris (tuberculous) (017.0)
        yaws (102.0-102.9)

    **373.5** *Other infective dermatitis of eyelid*
        *Code first underlying disease, as:*
        actinomycosis (039.3)
        impetigo (684)
        mycotic dermatitis (110.0-111.9)
        vaccinia (051.0)
        postvaccination (999.0)
        **EXCLUDES** *herpes:*
        *simplex (054.41)*
        *zoster (053.20)*

**Entropion and Ectropion**

Normal eyelashes · Entropion · Ectropion

✓4th / ✓5th **Additional Digit Required**    **Unacceptable PDx**    **Manifestation Code**    ▶◀ Revised Text    ● New Code    ▲ Revised Code Title

**October 2007 • Volume 1 — 121**

**Nervous System and Sense Organs**

**373.6–375.31**

**373.6** *Parasitic infestation of eyelid*
Code first underlying disease, as:
leishmaniasis (085.0-085.9)
loiasis (125.2)
onchocerciasis (125.3)
pediculosis (132.0)

**373.8** **Other inflammations of eyelids**
**373.9** **Unspecified inflammation of eyelid**
√4th **374 Other disorders of eyelids**
√5th **374.0** **Entropion and trichiasis of eyelid**
DEF: Entropion: turning inward of eyelid edge toward eyeball.
DEF: Trichiasis: ingrowing eyelashes marked by irritation with possible distortion of sight.
**374.00 Entropion, unspecified**
**374.01 Senile entropion** A
**374.02 Mechanical entropion**
**374.03 Spastic entropion**
**374.04 Cicatricial entropion**
**374.05 Trichiasis without entropion**
√5th **374.1** **Ectropion**
DEF: Turning outward (eversion) of eyelid edge; exposes palpebral conjunctiva; dryness irritation result.
**374.10 Ectropion, unspecified**
**374.11 Senile ectropion** A
**374.12 Mechanical ectropion**
**374.13 Spastic ectropion**
**374.14 Cicatricial ectropion**
√5th **374.2** **Lagophthalmos**
DEF: Incomplete closure of eyes; causes dry eye and other complications.
**374.20 Lagophthalmos, unspecified**
**374.21 Paralytic lagophthalmos**
**374.22 Mechanical lagophthalmos**
**374.23 Cicatricial lagophthalmos**
√5th **374.3** **Ptosis of eyelid**
**374.30 Ptosis of eyelid, unspecified**
AHA: 2Q, '96, 11
**374.31 Paralytic ptosis**
DEF: Drooping of upper eyelid due to nerve disorder.
**374.32 Myogenic ptosis**
DEF: Drooping of upper eyelid due to muscle disorder.
**374.33 Mechanical ptosis**
DEF: Outside force causes drooping of upper eyelid.
**374.34 Blepharochalasis**
Pseudoptosis
DEF: Loss of elasticity, thickened or indurated skin of eyelids associated with recurrent episodes of idiopathic edema causing intracellular tissue atrophy.
√5th **374.4** **Other disorders affecting eyelid function**
EXCLUDES     blepharoclonus (333.81)
blepharospasm (333.81)
facial nerve palsy (351.0)
third nerve palsy or paralysis (378.51-378.52)
tic (psychogenic) (307.20-307.23)
organic (333.3)
**374.41 Lid retraction or lag**
**374.43 Abnormal innervation syndrome**
Jaw-blinking
Paradoxical facial movements
**374.44 Sensory disorders**
**374.45 Other sensorimotor disorders**
Deficient blink reflex
**374.46 Blepharophimosis**
Ankyloblepharon
DEF: Narrowing of palpebral fissure horizontally; caused by laterally displaced inner canthi; either acquired or congenital.
√5th **374.5** **Degenerative disorders of eyelid and periocular area**
**374.50 Degenerative disorder of eyelid, unspecified**
**374.51** *Xanthelasma*
Xanthoma (planum) (tuberosum) of eyelid
Code first underlying condition (272.0-272.9)
DEF: Fatty tumors of the eyelid linked to high fat content of blood.

**374.52 Hyperpigmentation of eyelid**
Chloasma          Dyspigmentation
DEF: Excess pigment of eyelid.
**374.53 Hypopigmentation of eyelid**
Vitiligo of eyelid
DEF: Lack of color pigment of the eyelid.
**374.54 Hypertrichosis of eyelid**
DEF: Excessive eyelash growth.
**374.55 Hypotrichosis of eyelid**
Madarosis of eyelid
DEF: Less than normal, or absent, eyelashes.
**374.56 Other degenerative disorders of skin affecting eyelid**
√5th **374.8 Other disorders of eyelid**
**374.81 Hemorrhage of eyelid**
EXCLUDES     black eye (921.0)
**374.82 Edema of eyelid**
Hyperemia of eyelid
DEF: Swelling and fluid retention in eyelid.
**374.83 Elephantiasis of eyelid**
DEF: Filarial disease causing dermatitis and enlargement of eyelid.
**374.84 Cysts of eyelids**
Sebaceous cyst of eyelid
**374.85 Vascular anomalies of eyelid**
**374.86 Retained foreign body of eyelid**
**374.87 Dermatochalasis**
DEF: Acquired form of connective tissue disorder associated with decreased elastic tissue and abnormal elastin formation resulting in loss of elasticity of the skin of the eyelid, generally associated with aging.
**374.89 Other disorders of eyelid**
**374.9 Unspecified disorder of eyelid**
√4th **375 Disorders of lacrimal system**
√5th **375.0 Dacryoadenitis**
**375.00 Dacryoadenitis, unspecified**
**375.01 Acute dacryoadenitis**
DEF: Severe, sudden inflammation of the lacrimal gland.
**375.02 Chronic dacryoadenitis**
DEF: Persistent inflammation of the lacrimal gland.
**375.03 Chronic enlargement of lacrimal gland**
√5th **375.1 Other disorders of lacrimal gland**
**375.11 Dacryops**
DEF: Overproduction and constant flow of tears; may cause distended lacrimal duct.
**375.12 Other lacrimal cysts and cystic degeneration**
**375.13 Primary lacrimal atrophy**
**375.14 Secondary lacrimal atrophy**
DEF: Wasting away of the lacrimal gland due to another disease.
**375.15 Tear film insufficiency, unspecified**
Dry eye syndrome
AHA: 3Q, '96, 6
DEF: Eye dryness and irritation from insufficient tear production.
**375.16 Dislocation of lacrimal gland**
√5th **375.2 Epiphora**
DEF: Abnormal development of tears due to stricture of lacrimal passages.
**375.20 Epiphora, unspecified as to cause**
**375.21 Epiphora due to excess lacrimation**
DEF: Tear overflow due to overproduction.
**375.22 Epiphora due to insufficient drainage**
DEF: Tear overflow due to blocked drainage.
√5th **375.3 Acute and unspecified inflammation of lacrimal passages**
EXCLUDES     neonatal dacryocystitis (771.6)
**375.30 Dacryocystitis, unspecified**
**375.31 Acute canaliculitis, lacrimal**

N Newborn Age: 0    P Pediatric Age: 0-17    M Maternity Age: 12-55    A Adult Age: 15-124    CC CC Condition    MCC Major CC Condition    HIV HIV Related Dx

122 — Volume 1 • October 2007

© 2007 Ingenix

**375.32　Acute dacryocystitis**
　　　Acute peridacryocystitis
**375.33　Phlegmonous dacryocystitis**
　　　DEF: Infection of the tear sac with pockets of pus.

√5th **375.4　Chronic inflammation of lacrimal passages**
　　**375.41　Chronic canaliculitis**
　　**375.42　Chronic dacryocystitis**
　　**375.43　Lacrimal mucocele**
√5th **375.5　Stenosis and insufficiency of lacrimal passages**
　　**375.51　Eversion of lacrimal punctum**
　　　　DEF: Abnormal turning outward of the tear duct.
　　**375.52　Stenosis of lacrimal punctum**
　　　　DEF: Abnormal narrowing of the tear duct.
　　**375.53　Stenosis of lacrimal canaliculi**
　　**375.54　Stenosis of lacrimal sac**
　　　　DEF: Abnormal narrowing of the tear sac.
　　**375.55　Obstruction of nasolacrimal duct, neonatal**
　　　　**EXCLUDES**　congenital anomaly of
　　　　　　　　　nasolacrimal duct
　　　　　　　　　(743.65)
　　　　DEF: Acquired, abnormal obstruction of tear drainage
　　　　system from the eye to the nose; in an infant.
　　**375.56　Stenosis of nasolacrimal duct, acquired**
　　**375.57　Dacryolith**
　　　　DEF: Concretion or stone anywhere in lacrimal system.
√5th **375.6　Other changes of lacrimal passages**
　　**375.61　Lacrimal fistula**
　　　　DEF: Abnormal communication from the lacrimal system.
　　**375.69　Other**
√5th **375.8　Other disorders of lacrimal system**
　　**375.81　Granuloma of lacrimal passages**
　　　　DEF: Abnormal nodules within lacrimal system.
　　**375.89　Other**
　**375.9　Unspecified disorder of lacrimal system**
√4th **376　Disorders of the orbit**
√5th **376.0　Acute inflammation of orbit**
　　**376.00　Acute inflammation of orbit, unspecified**
　　**376.01　Orbital cellulitis**　　　　　　**cc**
　　　　Abscess of orbit
　　　　**CC Excl:** 376.00-376.04
　　　　DEF: Infection of tissue between the orbital bone and
　　　　eyeball.
　　**376.02　Orbital periostitis**　　　　　**cc**
　　　　**CC Excl:** 003.24, 015.50-015.56, 015.70-015.76, 015.90-015.96,
　　　　017.90-017.96, 376.02, 730.00-730.39, 730.80-730.99
　　　　DEF: Inflammation of connective tissue covering the
　　　　orbital bone.
　　**376.03　Orbital osteomyelitis**　　　　**cc**
　　　　**CC Excl:** 003.24, 015.50-015.56, 015.70-015.76, 015.90-015.96,
　　　　017.90-017.96, 376.03, 730.00-730.39, 730.80-730.99
　　　　DEF: Inflammation of the orbital bone.

**Lacrimal System**

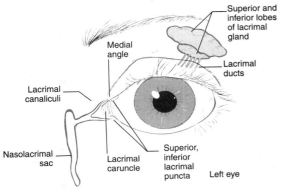

**376.04　Tenonitis**
√5th **376.1　Chronic inflammatory disorders of orbit**
　　**376.10　Chronic inflammation of orbit, unspecified**
　　**376.11　Orbital granuloma**
　　　　Pseudotumor (inflammatory) of orbit
　　　　DEF: Abnormal nodule between orbital bone and eyeball.
　　**376.12　Orbital myositis**
　　　　DEF: Painful inflammation of the muscles of the eye.
　　**376.13　*Parasitic infestation of orbit***
　　　　*Code first underlying disease, as:*
　　　　　hydatid infestation of orbit (122.3, 122.6,
　　　　　　122.9)
　　　　　myiasis of orbit (134.0)
√5th **376.2　Endocrine exophthalmos**
　　　*Code first underlying thyroid disorder (242.0-242.9)*
　　**376.21　*Thyrotoxic exophthalmos***
　　　　DEF: Painful inflammation of eye muscles.
　　**376.22　*Exophthalmic ophthalmoplegia***
　　　　DEF: Inability to rotate eye as a result of bulging eyes.
√5th **376.3　Other exophthalmic conditions**
　　**376.30　Exophthalmos, unspecified**
　　　　DEF: Abnormal protrusion of eyeball.
　　**376.31　Constant exophthalmos**
　　　　DEF: Continuous, abnormal protrusion or bulging of
　　　　eyeball.
　　**376.32　Orbital hemorrhage**
　　　　DEF: Bleeding behind the eyeball, causing it to bulge
　　　　forward.
　　**376.33　Orbital edema or congestion**
　　　　DEF: Fluid retention behind eyeball, causing forward
　　　　bulge.
　　**376.34　Intermittent exophthalmos**
　　**376.35　Pulsating exophthalmos**
　　　　DEF: Bulge or protrusion; associated with a carotid-
　　　　cavernous fistula.
　　**376.36　Lateral displacement of globe**
　　　　DEF: Abnormal displacement of the eyeball away from
　　　　nose, toward temple.
√5th **376.4　Deformity of orbit**
　　**376.40　Deformity of orbit, unspecified**
　　**376.41　Hypertelorism of orbit**
　　　　DEF: Abnormal increase in interorbital distance;
　　　　associated with congenital facial deformities; may be
　　　　accompanied by mental deficiency.
　　**376.42　Exostosis of orbit**
　　　　DEF: Abnormal bony growth of orbit.
　　**376.43　Local deformities due to bone disease**
　　　　DEF: Acquired abnormalities of orbit; due to bone
　　　　disease.
　　**376.44　Orbital deformities associated with
　　　　craniofacial deformities**
　　**376.45　Atrophy of orbit**
　　　　DEF: Wasting away of bone tissue of orbit.
　　**376.46　Enlargement of orbit**
　　**376.47　Deformity due to trauma or surgery**
√5th **376.5　Enophthalmos**
　　　DEF: Recession of eyeball deep into eye socket.
　　**376.50　Enophthalmos, unspecified as to cause**
　　**376.51　Enophthalmos due to atrophy of orbital
　　　　tissue**
　　**376.52　Enophthalmos due to trauma or surgery**
　**376.6　Retained (old) foreign body following penetrating
　　　wound of orbit**
　　　Retrobulbar foreign body
√5th **376.8　Other orbital disorders**
　　**376.81　Orbital cysts**
　　　　Encephalocele of orbit
　　　　**AHA:** 3Q, '99, 13
　　**376.82　Myopathy of extraocular muscles**
　　　　DEF: Disease in the muscles that control eyeball
　　　　movement.

**Nervous System and Sense Organs**

**376.89–378.04**

376.89 **Other**

376.9 **Unspecified disorder of orbit**

✓4th 377 **Disorders of optic nerve and visual pathways**

✓5th 377.0 **Papilledema**

377.00 **Papilledema, unspecified** CC

CC Excl: 017.30-017.36, 017.90-017.96, 036.81, 250.50-250.53, 250.80-250.93, 377.00-377.03, 377.14, 377.24, 379.60-379.90, 379.99, 743.8-743.9

377.01 **Papilledema associated with increased intracranial pressure** CC

CC Excl: See code: 377.00

377.02 **Papilledema associated with decreased ocular pressure**

377.03 **Papilledema associated with retinal disorder**

377.04 **Foster-Kennedy syndrome**

DEF: Retrobulbar optic neuritis, central scotoma and optic atrophy; caused by tumors in frontal lobe of brain that press downward.

✓5th 377.1 **Optic atrophy**

377.10 **Optic atrophy, unspecified**

377.11 **Primary optic atrophy**

EXCLUDES neurosyphilitic optic atrophy (094.84)

377.12 **Postinflammatory optic atrophy**

DEF: : Adverse effect of inflammation causing wasting away of eye.

377.13 **Optic atrophy associated with retinal dystrophies**

DEF: Progressive changes in retinal tissue due to metabolic disorder causing wasting away of eye.

377.14 **Glaucomatous atrophy [cupping] of optic disc**

377.15 **Partial optic atrophy**

Temporal pallor of optic disc

377.16 **Hereditary optic atrophy**

Optic atrophy:     Optic atrophy:
   dominant hereditary     Leber's

✓5th 377.2 **Other disorders of optic disc**

377.21 **Drusen of optic disc**

377.22 **Crater-like holes of optic disc**

377.23 **Coloboma of optic disc**

DEF: Ocular malformation caused by the failure of fetal fissure of optic stalk to close.

377.24 **Pseudopapilledema**

✓5th 377.3 **Optic neuritis**

EXCLUDES meningococcal optic neuritis (036.81)

377.30 **Optic neuritis, unspecified** CC

CC Excl: 377.30-377.39

377.31 **Optic papillitis** CC

CC Excl: See code: 377.30

DEF: Swelling and inflammation of the optic disc.

377.32 **Retrobulbar neuritis (acute)** CC

EXCLUDES syphilitic retrobulbar neuritis (094.85)

CC Excl: See code: 377.30

DEF: Inflammation of optic nerve immediately behind the eyeball.

377.33 **Nutritional optic neuropathy**

DEF: Malnutrition causing optic nerve disorder.

377.34 **Toxic optic neuropathy**

Toxic amblyopia

DEF: Toxic substance causing optic nerve disorder.

377.39 **Other** CC

EXCLUDES ischemic optic neuropathy (377.41)

CC Excl: See code: 377.30

✓5th 377.4 **Other disorders of optic nerve**

377.41 **Ischemic optic neuropathy**

DEF: Decreased blood flow affecting optic nerve.

377.42 **Hemorrhage in optic nerve sheaths**

DEF: Bleeding in meningeal lining of optic nerve.

377.43 **Optic nerve hypoplasia**

AHA: 4Q, '06, 81

377.49 **Other**

Compression of optic nerve

✓5th 377.5 **Disorders of optic chiasm**

377.51 **Associated with pituitary neoplasms and disorders** CC

CC Excl: 377.51-377.63

DEF: Abnormal pituitary growth causing disruption in nerve chain from retina to brain.

377.52 **Associated with other neoplasms** CC

CC Excl: See code: 377.51

DEF: Abnormal growth, other than pituitary, causing disruption in nerve chain from retina to brain.

377.53 **Associated with vascular disorders** CC

CC Excl: See code: 377.51

DEF: Vascular disorder causing disruption in nerve chain from retina to brain.

377.54 **Associated with inflammatory disorders** CC

CC Excl: See code: 377.51

DEF: Inflammatory disease causing disruption in nerve chain from retina to brain.

✓5th 377.6 **Disorders of other visual pathways**

377.61 **Associated with neoplasms** CC

CC Excl: See code: 377.51

377.62 **Associated with vascular disorders** CC

CC Excl: See code: 377.51

377.63 **Associated with inflammatory disorders** CC

CC Excl: See code: 377.51

✓5th 377.7 **Disorders of visual cortex**

EXCLUDES visual:
   agnosia (368.16)
   hallucinations (368.16)
   halos (368.15)

377.71 **Associated with neoplasms** CC

CC Excl: 377.71-377.9

377.72 **Associated with vascular disorders** CC

CC Excl: See code: 377.71

377.73 **Associated with inflammatory disorders** CC

CC Excl: See code: 377.71

377.75 **Cortical blindness**

DEF: Blindness due to brain disorder, rather than eye disorder.

377.9 **Unspecified disorder of optic nerve and visual pathways**

✓4th 378 **Strabismus and other disorders of binocular eye movements**

EXCLUDES nystagmus and other irregular eye movements (379.50-379.59)

DEF: Misalignment of the eyes due to imbalance in extraocular muscles.

✓5th 378.0 **Esotropia**

Convergent concomitant strabismus

EXCLUDES intermittent esotropia (378.20-378.22)

DEF: Visual axis deviation created by one eye fixing upon an image and the other eye deviating inward.

378.00 **Esotropia, unspecified**

378.01 **Monocular esotropia**

378.02 **Monocular esotropia with A pattern**

378.03 **Monocular esotropia with V pattern**

378.04 **Monocular esotropia with other noncomitancies**

Monocular esotropia with X or Y pattern

N Newborn Age: 0    P Pediatric Age: 0-17    M Maternity Age: 12-55    A Adult Age: 15-124    CC CC Condition    MCC Major CC Condition    HIV HIV Related Dx

124 — Volume 1 • October 2007

© 2007 Ingenix

378.05  Alternating esotropia
378.06  Alternating esotropia with A pattern
378.07  Alternating esotropia with V pattern
378.08  Alternating esotropia with other noncomitancies
Alternating esotropia with X or Y pattern

√5ᵗʰ  378.1  Exotropia
Divergent concomitant strabismus
**EXCLUDES**  *intermittent exotropia (378.20, 378.23-378.24)*
DEF: Visual axis deviation created by one eye fixing upon an image and the other eye deviating outward.

378.10  Exotropia, unspecified
378.11  Monocular exotropia
378.12  Monocular exotropia with A pattern
378.13  Monocular exotropia with V pattern
378.14  Monocular exotropia with other noncomitancies
Monocular exotropia with X or Y pattern
378.15  Alternating exotropia
378.16  Alternating exotropia with A pattern
378.17  Alternating exotropia with V pattern
378.18  Alternating exotropia with other noncomitancies
Alternating exotropia with X or Y pattern

√5ᵗʰ  378.2  Intermittent heterotropia
**EXCLUDES**  *vertical heterotropia (intermittent) (378.31)*
DEF: Deviation of eyes seen only at intervals; it is also called strabismus.

378.20  Intermittent heterotropia, unspecified
Intermittent:          Intermittent:
esotropia NOS        exotropia NOS
378.21  Intermittent esotropia, monocular
378.22  Intermittent esotropia, alternating
378.23  Intermittent exotropia, monocular
378.24  Intermittent exotropia, alternating

√5ᵗʰ  378.3  Other and unspecified heterotropia
378.30  Heterotropia, unspecified
378.31  Hypertropia
Vertical heterotropia (constant) (intermittent)
378.32  Hypotropia
378.33  Cyclotropia
378.34  Monofixation syndrome
Microtropia
378.35  Accommodative component in esotropia

√5ᵗʰ  378.4  Heterophoria
DEF: Deviation occurring only when the other eye is covered.
378.40  Heterophoria, unspecified
378.41  Esophoria
378.42  Exophoria
378.43  Vertical heterophoria
378.44  Cyclophoria
378.45  Alternating hyperphoria

√5ᵗʰ  378.5  Paralytic strabismus
DEF:  Deviation of the eye due to nerve paralysis affecting muscle.

### Eye Musculature

Muscles and actions (right eye)

R.          L.
Monocular
(one eye only)
esotropia (inward)

Monocular exotropia
(outward)

Monocular hypertropia
(upward)

378.50  Paralytic strabismus, unspecified
378.51  Third or oculomotor nerve palsy, partial
**AHA:** 3Q, '91, 9
378.52  Third or oculomotor nerve palsy, total
**AHA:** 2Q, '89, 12
378.53  Fourth or trochlear nerve palsy
**AHA:** 2Q, '01, 21
378.54  Sixth or abducens nerve palsy
**AHA:** 2Q, '89, 12
378.55  External ophthalmoplegia
378.56  Total ophthalmoplegia

√5ᵗʰ  378.6  Mechanical strabismus
DEF:  Deviation of the eye due to an outside force upon the extraocular muscles.
378.60  Mechanical strabismus, unspecified
378.61  Brown's (tendon) sheath syndrome
DEF: Congenital or acquired shortening of the anterior sheath of the superior oblique muscle; the eye is unable to move upward and inward; it is usually unilateral.
378.62  Mechanical strabismus from other musculofascial disorders
378.63  Limited duction associated with other conditions

√5ᵗʰ  378.7  Other specified strabismus
378.71  Duane's syndrome
DEF: Congenital, affects one eye; due to abnormal fibrous bands attached to rectus muscle; inability to abduct affected eye with retraction of globe.
378.72  Progressive external ophthalmoplegia
DEF:  Paralysis progressing from one eye muscle to another.
378.73  Strabismus in other neuromuscular disorders

√5ᵗʰ  378.8  Other disorders of binocular eye movements
**EXCLUDES**  *nystagmus (379.50-379.56)*
378.81  Palsy of conjugate gaze
DEF: Paralysis progressing from one eye muscle to another.
378.82  Spasm of conjugate gaze
DEF: Muscle contractions impairing parallel movement of eye.
378.83  Convergence insufficiency or palsy
378.84  Convergence excess or spasm
378.85  Anomalies of divergence
378.86  Internuclear ophthalmoplegia
DEF: Eye movement anomaly due to brainstem lesion.
378.87  Other dissociated deviation of eye movements
Skew deviation

378.9  Unspecified disorder of eye movements
Ophthalmoplegia NOS     Strabismus NOS
**AHA:** 2Q, '01, 21

√4ᵗʰ  379  Other disorders of eye
√5ᵗʰ  379.0  Scleritis and episcleritis
**EXCLUDES**  *syphilitic episcleritis (095.0)*
379.00  Scleritis, unspecified
Episcleritis NOS
379.01  Episcleritis periodica fugax
DEF: Hyperemia (engorgement) of the sclera and overlying conjunctiva characterized by a sudden onset and short duration.
379.02  Nodular episcleritis
DEF: Inflammation of the outermost layer of the sclera, with formation of nodules.
379.03  Anterior scleritis
379.04  Scleromalacia perforans
DEF: Scleral thinning, softening and degeneration; seen with rheumatoid arthritis.
379.05  Scleritis with corneal involvement
Scleroperikeratitis

√4ᵗʰ  Additional Digit Required
√5ᵗʰ
Unacceptable PDx     Manifestation Code     ►◄ Revised Text     ● New Code     ▲ Revised Code Title

**379.06 Brawny scleritis**
DEF: Severe scleral inflammation with thickening corneal margins.

**379.07 Posterior scleritis**
Sclerotenonitis

**379.09 Other**
Scleral abscess

√5ᵗʰ **379.1 Other disorders of sclera**
EXCLUDES blue sclera (743.47)

**379.11 Scleral ectasia**
Scleral staphyloma NOS
DEF: Protrusion of the contents of the eyeball where the sclera has thinned.

**379.12 Staphyloma posticum**
DEF: Ring-shaped protrusion or bulging of sclera and uveal tissue at posterior pole of eye.

**379.13 Equatorial staphyloma**
DEF: Ring-shaped protrusion or bulging of sclera and uveal tissue midway between front and back of eye.

**379.14 Anterior staphyloma, localized**
**379.15 Ring staphyloma**
**379.16 Other degenerative disorders of sclera**
**379.19 Other**

√5ᵗʰ **379.2 Disorders of vitreous body**
DEF: Disorder of clear gel that fills space between retina and lens.

**379.21 Vitreous degeneration**
Vitreous:            Vitreous:
  cavitation          liquefaction
  detachment

**379.22 Crystalline deposits in vitreous**
Asteroid hyalitis    Synchysis scintillans

**379.23 Vitreous hemorrhage**
AHA: 3Q, '91, 15

**379.24 Other vitreous opacities**
Vitreous floaters

**379.25 Vitreous membranes and strands**
**379.26 Vitreous prolapse**
DEF: Slipping of vitreous from normal position.

**379.29 Other disorders of vitreous**
EXCLUDES vitreous abscess (360.04)
AHA: 1Q, '99, 11

√5ᵗʰ **379.3 Aphakia and other disorders of lens**
EXCLUDES after-cataract (366.50-366.53)

**379.31 Aphakia**
EXCLUDES cataract extraction status (V45.61)
DEF: Absence of eye's crystalline lens.

**379.32 Subluxation of lens**
**379.33 Anterior dislocation of lens**
DEF: Lens displaced toward iris.

**379.34 Posterior dislocation of lens**
DEF: Lens displaced backward toward vitreous.

### Ear and Mastoid Process

**379.39 Other disorders of lens**

√5ᵗʰ **379.4 Anomalies of pupillary function**
**379.40 Abnormal pupillary function, unspecified**
**379.41 Aniscoria**
DEF: Unequal pupil diameter.

**379.42 Miosis (persistent), not due to miotics**
DEF: Abnormal contraction of pupil less than 2 millimeters.

**379.43 Mydriasis (persistent), not due to mydriatics**
DEF: Morbid dilation of pupil.

**379.45 Argyll Robertson pupil, atypical**
Argyll Robertson phenomenon or pupil, nonsyphilitic
EXCLUDES Argyll Robertson pupil (syphilitic) (094.89)
DEF: Failure of pupil to respond to light; affects both eyes; may be caused by diseases such as syphilis of the central nervous system or miosis.

**379.46 Tonic pupillary reaction**
Adie's pupil or syndrome

**379.49 Other**
Hippus            Pupillary paralysis

√5ᵗʰ **379.5 Nystagmus and other irregular eye movements**
**379.50 Nystagmus, unspecified**
AHA: 4Q, '02, 68; 2Q, '01, 21

DEF: Involuntary, rapid, rhythmic movement of eyeball; vertical, horizontal, rotatory or mixed; cause may be congenital, acquired, physiological, neurological, myopathic, or due to ocular diseases.

**379.51 Congenital nystagmus**
**379.52 Latent nystagmus**
**379.53 Visual deprivation nystagmus**
**379.54 Nystagmus associated with disorders of the vestibular system**
**379.55 Dissociated nystagmus**
**379.56 Other forms of nystagmus**
**379.57 Deficiencies of saccadic eye movements**
Abnormal optokinetic response
DEF: Saccadic eye movements; small, rapid, involuntary movements by both eyes simultaneously, due to changing point of fixation on visualized object.

**379.58 Deficiencies of smooth pursuit movements**
**379.59 Other irregularities of eye movements**
Opsoclonus

√5ᵗʰ **379.6 Inflammation (infection) of postprocedural bleb**
Postprocedural blebitis
**379.60 Inflammation (infection) of postprocedural bleb, unspecified**
AHA: 4Q, '06, 82

**379.61 Inflammation (infection) of postprocedural bleb, stage 1**
AHA: 4Q, '06, 82

**379.62 Inflammation (infection) of postprocedural bleb, stage 2**
AHA: 4Q, '06, 82

**379.63 Inflammation (infection) of postprocedural bleb, stage 3**
Bleb associated endophthalmitis
AHA: 4Q, '06, 82

**379.8 Other specified disorders of eye and adnexa**
√5ᵗʰ **379.9 Unspecified disorder of eye and adnexa**
**379.90 Disorder of eye, unspecified**
**379.91 Pain in or around eye**
**379.92 Swelling or mass of eye**
**379.93 Redness or discharge of eye**
**379.99 Other ill-defined disorders of eye**
EXCLUDES blurred vision NOS (368.8)

N Newborn Age: 0    P Pediatric Age: 0-17    M Maternity Age: 12-55    A Adult Age: 15-124    CC CC Condition    MC Major Complication    CD Complex Dx    HIV HIV Related Dx

126 — Volume 1 • October 2007                                                                            2007 ICD•9•CM

## DISEASES OF THE EAR AND MASTOID PROCESS (380-389)

√4ᵗʰ **380 Disorders of external ear**

√5ᵗʰ **380.0 Perichondritis and chondritis of pinna**

Chondritis of auricle
Perichondritis of auricle

**380.00 Perichondritis of pinna, unspecified**
**380.01 Acute perichondritis of pinna**
**380.02 Chronic perichondritis of pinna**
**380.03 Chondritis of pinna**
AHA: 4Q, '04, 76
DEF: Infection that has progressed into the cartilage; presents as indurated and edematous skin over the pinna; vascular compromise occurs with tissue necrosis and deformity.

√5ᵗʰ **380.1 Infective otitis externa**

**380.10 Infective otitis externa, unspecified**
Otitis externa (acute):   Otitis externa (acute):
NOS                         hemorrhagica
circumscribed              infective NOS
diffuse

**380.11 Acute infection of pinna**
EXCLUDES   furuncular otitis externa (680.0)

**380.12 Acute swimmers' ear**
Beach ear    Tank ear
DEF: Otitis externa due to swimming.

**380.13 Other acute infections of external ear**
Code first underlying disease, as:
erysipelas (035)
impetigo (684)
seborrheic dermatitis (690.10-690.18)
EXCLUDES   herpes simplex (054.73)
herpes zoster (053.71)

**380.14 Malignant otitis externa**   CC
CC Excl: 380.14, 383.00-383.1
DEF: Severe necrotic otitis externa; due to bacteria.

**380.15 Chronic mycotic otitis externa**
Code first underlying disease, as:
aspergillosis (117.3)
otomycosis NOS (111.9)
EXCLUDES   candidal otitis externa (112.82)

**380.16 Other chronic infective otitis externa**
Chronic infective otitis externa NOS

√5ᵗʰ **380.2 Other otitis externa**

**380.21 Cholesteatoma of external ear**
Keratosis obturans of external ear (canal)
EXCLUDES   cholesteatoma NOS (385.30-385.35)
postmastoidectomy (383.32)
DEF: Cystlike mass filled with debris, including cholesterol; rare, congenital condition.

**380.22 Other acute otitis externa**
Acute otitis externa:   Acute otitis externa:
actinic                   eczematoid
chemical                  reactive
contact

**380.23 Other chronic otitis externa**
Chronic otitis externa NOS

√5ᵗʰ **380.3 Noninfectious disorders of pinna**

**380.30 Disorder of pinna, unspecified**
**380.31 Hematoma of auricle or pinna**
**380.32 Acquired deformities of auricle or pinna**
EXCLUDES   cauliflower ear (738.7)
AHA: 3Q, '03, 12

**380.39 Other**
EXCLUDES   gouty tophi of ear (274.81)

**380.4 Impacted cerumen**
Wax in ear

√5ᵗʰ **380.5 Acquired stenosis of external ear canal**
Collapse of external ear canal

**380.50 Acquired stenosis of external ear canal, unspecified as to cause**
**380.51 Secondary to trauma**
DEF: Narrowing of the external ear canal; due to trauma.

**380.52 Secondary to surgery**
DEF: Postsurgical narrowing of the external ear canal.

**380.53 Secondary to inflammation**
DEF: Narrowing of the external ear canal; due to chronic inflammation.

√5ᵗʰ **380.8 Other disorders of external ear**
**380.81 Exostosis of external ear canal**
**380.89 Other**

**380.9 Unspecified disorder of external ear**

√4ᵗʰ **381 Nonsuppurative otitis media and Eustachian tube disorders**

√5ᵗʰ **381.0 Acute nonsuppurative otitis media**
Acute tubotympanic catarrh
Otitis media, acute or subacute:
catarrhal
exudative
transudative
with effusion
EXCLUDES   otitic barotrauma (993.0)

**381.00 Acute nonsuppurative otitis media, unspecified**
**381.01 Acute serous otitis media**
Acute or subacute secretory otitis media
DEF: Sudden, severe infection of the middle ear.

**381.02 Acute mucoid otitis media**
Acute or subacute seromucinous otitis media
Blue drum syndrome
DEF: Sudden, severe infection of the middle ear, with mucous.

**381.03 Acute sanguinous otitis media**
DEF: Sudden, severe infection of the middle ear, with blood.

**381.04 Acute allergic serous otitis media**
**381.05 Acute allergic mucoid otitis media**
**381.06 Acute allergic sanguinous otitis media**

√5ᵗʰ **381.1 Chronic serous otitis media**
Chronic tubotympanic catarrh
**381.10 Chronic serous otitis media, simple or unspecified**
DEF: Persistent infection of the middle ear, without pus.

**381.19 Other**
Serosanguinous chronic otitis media

√5ᵗʰ **381.2 Chronic mucoid otitis media**
Glue ear
EXCLUDES   adhesive middle ear disease (385.10-385.19)
DEF: Chronic condition; characterized by viscous fluid in middle ear; due to obstructed Eustachian tube.

**381.20 Chronic mucoid otitis media, simple or unspecified**
**381.29 Other**
Mucosanguinous chronic otitis media

**381.3 Other and unspecified chronic nonsuppurative otitis media**
Otitis media, chronic:   Otitis media, chronic:
allergic                  seromucinous
exudative                 transudative
secretory                 with effusion

**381.4 Nonsuppurative otitis media, not specified as acute or chronic**
Otitis media:   Otitis media:
allergic        seromucinous
catarrhal       serous
exudative       transudative
mucoid          with effusion
secretory

√4ᵗʰ Additional Digit Required   Unacceptable PDx   Manifestation Code   ►◄ Revised Text   ● New Code   ▲ Revised Code Title
√5ᵗʰ

√5th **381.5   Eustachian salpingitis**
    **381.50   Eustachian salpingitis, unspecified**
    **381.51   Acute Eustachian salpingitis**
      DEF: Sudden, severe inflammation of the Eustachian tube.
    **381.52   Chronic Eustachian salpingitis**
      DEF: Persistent inflammation of the Eustachian tube.

√5th **381.6   Obstruction of Eustachian tube**
    Stenosis
    Stricture  } of Eustachian tube
    **381.60   Obstruction of Eustachian tube, unspecified**
    **381.61   Osseous obstruction of Eustachian tube**
      Obstruction of Eustachian tube from cholesteatoma, polyp, or other osseous lesion
    **381.62   Intrinsic cartilaginous obstruction of Eustachian tube**
      DEF: Blockage of Eustachian tube; due to cartilage overgrowth.
    **381.63   Extrinsic cartilaginous obstruction of Eustachian tube**
      Compression of Eustachian tube

    **381.7   Patulous Eustachian tube**
      DEF: Distended, oversized Eustachian tube.

√5th **381.8   Other disorders of Eustachian tube**
    **381.81   Dysfunction of Eustachian tube**
    **381.89   Other**

    **381.9   Unspecified Eustachian tube disorder**

√4th **382   Suppurative and unspecified otitis media**

√5th **382.0   Acute suppurative otitis media**
    Otitis media, acute:     Otitis media, acute:
      necrotizing NOS       purulent
    **382.00   Acute suppurative otitis media without spontaneous rupture of ear drum**
      DEF: Sudden, severe inflammation of middle ear, with pus.
    **382.01   Acute suppurative otitis media with spontaneous rupture of ear drum**
      DEF: Sudden, severe inflammation of middle ear, with pressure tearing ear drum tissue.
    **382.02   *Acute suppurative otitis media in diseases classified elsewhere***
      *Code first underlying disease, as:*
      influenza (487.8)
      scarlet fever (034.1)
      **EXCLUDES**   *postmeasles otitis (055.2)*

    **382.1   Chronic tubotympanic suppurative otitis media**
    Benign chronic
      suppurative otitis     (with anterior
      media       perforation of
    Chronic tubotympanic       ear drum)
      disease
    DEF: Inflammation of tympanic cavity and auditory tube; with pus formation.

    **382.2   Chronic atticoantral suppurative otitis media**
    Chronic atticoantral
      disease     (with posterior or superior
    Persistent mucosal       marginal perforation
      disease       of ear drum)
    DEF: Inflammation of upper tympanic membrane and mastoid antrum with pus formation.

    **382.3   Unspecified chronic suppurative otitis media**
    Chronic purulent otitis media
        **EXCLUDES**   *tuberculous otitis media (017.4)*

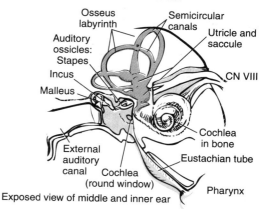

**Middle and Inner Ear**

Osseous labyrinth
Semicircular canals
Auditory ossicles:
Stapes
Incus
Malleus
Utricle and saccule
CN VIII
Cochlea in bone
Eustachian tube
External auditory canal
Cochlea (round window)
Pharynx

Exposed view of middle and inner ear

    **382.4   Unspecified suppurative otitis media**
    Purulent otitis media NOS

    **382.9   Unspecified otitis media**
    Otitis media:     Otitis media:
      NOS       chronic NOS
      acute NOS
    **AHA:** N-D, '84, 16

√4th **383   Mastoiditis and related conditions**

√5th **383.0   Acute mastoiditis**
    Abscess of mastoid     Empyema of mastoid
    **383.00   Acute mastoiditis without complications** CC
      **CC Excl:** 015.60-015.66, 017.40-017.46, 017.90-017.96, 383.00-383.9, 388.71-388.9, 744.00, 744.02, 744.09, 744.29-744.3
      DEF: Sudden, severe inflammation of mastoid air cells.
    **383.01   Subperiosteal abscess of mastoid**   CC
      **CC Excl:** See code: 383.00
      DEF: Pocket of pus within the mastoid bone.
    **383.02   Acute mastoiditis with other**   CC
        **complications**
      Gradenigo's syndrome
      **CC Excl:** See code: 383.00

    **383.1   Chronic mastoiditis**
    Caries of mastoid
    Fistula of mastoid
        **EXCLUDES**   *tuberculous mastoiditis (015.6)*
    DEF: Persistent inflammation of the mastoid air cells.

√5th **383.2   Petrositis**
    Coalescing osteitis
    Inflammation  } of petrous bone
    Osteomyelitis
    **383.20   Petrositis, unspecified**
    **383.21   Acute petrositis**
      DEF: Sudden, severe inflammation of dense bone behind the ear.
    **383.22   Chronic petrositis**
      DEF: Persistent inflammation of dense bone behind the ear.

√5th **383.3   Complications following mastoidectomy**
    **383.30   Postmastoidectomy complication, unspecified**
    **383.31   Mucosal cyst of postmastoidectomy cavity**
      DEF: Mucous-lined cyst cavity following removal of mastoid bone.
    **383.32   Recurrent cholesteatoma of postmastoidectomy cavity**
      DEF: Cystlike mass of cell debris in cavity following removal of mastoid bone.

---

N Newborn Age: 0     P Pediatric Age: 0-17     M Maternity Age: 12-55     A Adult Age: 15-124     CC CC Condition     MCC Major CC Condition     HIV HIV Related Dx

**383.33** **Granulations of postmastoidectomy cavity**
Chronic inflammation of postmastoidectomy cavity

DEF: Granular tissue in cavity following removal of mastoid bone.

√5th **383.8** **Other disorders of mastoid**
**383.81** **Postauricular fistula**
DEF: Abnormal passage behind mastoid cavity.

**383.89** **Other**

**383.9** **Unspecified mastoiditis**

√4th **384 Other disorders of tympanic membrane**

√5th **384.0** **Acute myringitis without mention of otitis media**
**384.00** **Acute myringitis, unspecified**
Acute tympanitis NOS
DEF: Sudden, severe inflammation of ear drum.

**384.01** **Bullous myringitis**
Myringitis bullosa hemorrhagica
DEF: Type of viral otitis media characterized by the appearance of serous or hemorrhagic blebs on the tympanic membrane.

**384.09** **Other**

**384.1** **Chronic myringitis without mention of otitis media**
Chronic tympanitis
DEF: Persistent inflammation of ear drum; with no evidence of middle ear infection.

√5th **384.2** **Perforation of tympanic membrane**
Perforation of ear drum:   Perforation of ear drum:
NOS                                    postinflammatory
persistent posttraumatic

EXCLUDES   *otitis media with perforation of tympanic membrane (382.00-382.9)*
*traumatic perforation [current injury] (872.61)*

**384.20** **Perforation of tympanic membrane, unspecified**

**384.21** **Central perforation of tympanic membrane**

**384.22** **Attic perforation of tympanic membrane**
Pars flaccida

**384.23** **Other marginal perforation of tympanic membrane**

**384.24** **Multiple perforations of tympanic membrane**

**384.25** **Total perforation of tympanic membrane**

√5th **384.8** **Other specified disorders of tympanic membrane**
**384.81** **Atrophic flaccid tympanic membrane**
Healed perforation of ear drum

**384.82** **Atrophic nonflaccid tympanic membrane**

**384.9** **Unspecified disorder of tympanic membrane**

√4th **385 Other disorders of middle ear and mastoid**
EXCLUDES   *mastoiditis (383.0-383.9)*

√5th **385.0** **Tympanosclerosis**
**385.00** **Tympanosclerosis, unspecified as to involvement**

**385.01** **Tympanosclerosis involving tympanic membrane only**
DEF: Tough, fibrous tissue impeding functions of ear drum.

**385.02** **Tympanosclerosis involving tympanic membrane and ear ossicles**
DEF: Tough, fibrous tissue impeding functions of middle ear bones (stapes, malleus, incus).

**385.03** **Tympanosclerosis involving tympanic membrane, ear ossicles, and middle ear**
DEF: Tough, fibrous tissue impeding functions of ear drum, middle ear bones and middle ear canal.

**385.09** **Tympanosclerosis involving other combination of structures**

**Cholesteatoma**
Middle ear chamber

Cholesteatoma        Ear drum
sac

√5th **385.1** **Adhesive middle ear disease**
Adhesive otitis           Otitis media:
Otitis media:                    fibrotic
chronic adhesive
EXCLUDES   *glue ear (381.20-381.29)*
DEF: Adhesions of middle ear structures.

**385.10** **Adhesive middle ear disease, unspecified as to involvement**

**385.11** **Adhesions of drum head to incus**

**385.12** **Adhesions of drum head to stapes**

**385.13** **Adhesions of drum head to promontorium**

**385.19** **Other adhesions and combinations**

√5th **385.2** **Other acquired abnormality of ear ossicles**
**385.21** **Impaired mobility of malleus**
Ankylosis of malleus

**385.22** **Impaired mobility of other ear ossicles**
Ankylosis of ear ossicles, except malleus

**385.23** **Discontinuity or dislocation of ear ossicles**
DEF: Disruption in auditory chain; created by malleus, incus and stapes.

**385.24** **Partial loss or necrosis of ear ossicles**
DEF: Tissue loss in malleus, incus and stapes.

√5th **385.3** **Cholesteatoma of middle ear and mastoid**
Cholesterosis
Epidermosis         of (middle) ear
Keratosis
Polyp

EXCLUDES   *cholesteatoma:*
*external ear canal (380.21)*
*recurrent of postmastoidectomy cavity (383.32)*

DEF: Cystlike mass of middle ear and mastoid antrum filled with debris, including cholesterol.

**385.30** **Cholesteatoma, unspecified**

**385.31** **Cholesteatoma of attic**

**385.32** **Cholesteatoma of middle ear**

**385.33** **Cholesteatoma of middle ear and mastoid**
AHA: 3Q, '00, 10

DEF: Cystlike mass of cell debris in middle ear and mastoid air cells behind ear.

**385.35** **Diffuse cholesteatosis**

√5th **385.8** **Other disorders of middle ear and mastoid**
**385.82** **Cholesterin granuloma**
DEF: Granuloma formed of fibrotic tissue; contains cholesterol crystals surrounded by foreign-body cells; found in the middle ear and mastoid area.

**385.83** **Retained foreign body of middle ear**
AHA: 3Q, '94, 7; N-D, '87, 9

**385.89** **Other**

**385.9** **Unspecified disorder of middle ear and mastoid**

**Nervous System and Sense Organs**

**383.33–385.9**

√4th **386 Vertiginous syndromes and other disorders of vestibular system**

EXCLUDES    vertigo NOS (780.4)

AHA: M-A, '85, 12

√5th **386.0 Ménière's disease**
Endolymphatic hydrops
Lermoyez's syndrome
Ménière's syndrome or vertigo

DEF: Distended membranous labyrinth of middle ear from endolymphatic hydrops; causes ischemia, failure of nerve function; hearing and balance dysfunction; symptoms include fluctuating deafness, ringing in ears and dizziness.

**386.00 Ménière's disease, unspecified**
Ménière's disease (active)

**386.01 Active Ménière's disease, cochleovestibular**

**386.02 Active Ménière's disease, cochlear**

**386.03 Active Ménière's disease, vestibular**

**386.04 Inactive Ménière's disease**
Ménière's disease in remission

√5th **386.1 Other and unspecified peripheral vertigo**

EXCLUDES    epidemic vertigo (078.81)

**386.10 Peripheral vertigo, unspecified**

**386.11 Benign paroxysmal positional vertigo**
Benign paroxysmal positional nystagmus

**386.12 Vestibular neuronitis**
Acute (and recurrent) peripheral vestibulopathy

DEF: Transient benign vertigo, unknown cause; characterized by response to caloric stimulation on one side, nystagmus with rhythmic movement of eyes; normal auditory function present; occurs in young adults.

**386.19 Other**
Aural vertigo
Otogenic vertigo

**386.2 Vertigo of central origin**
Central positional nystagmus
Malignant positional vertigo

√5th **386.3 Labyrinthitis**

**386.30 Labyrinthitis, unspecified**

**386.31 Serous labyrinthitis**
Diffuse labyrinthitis

DEF: Inflammation of labyrinth; with fluid buildup.

**386.32 Circumscribed labyrinthitis**
Focal labyrinthitis

**386.33 Suppurative labyrinthitis**
Purulent labyrinthitis

DEF: Inflammation of labyrinth; with pus.

**386.34 Toxic labyrinthitis**

DEF: Inflammation of labyrinth; due to toxic reaction.

**386.35 Viral labyrinthitis**

√5th **386.4 Labyrinthine fistula**

**386.40 Labyrinthine fistula, unspecified**

**386.41 Round window fistula**

**386.42 Oval window fistula**

**386.43 Semicircular canal fistula**

**386.48 Labyrinthine fistula of combined sites**

√5th **386.5 Labyrinthine dysfunction**

**386.50 Labyrinthine dysfunction, unspecified**

**386.51 Hyperactive labyrinth, unilateral**

DEF: Abnormal increased sensitivity of labyrinth to stimuli such as sound, pressure or gravitational change, affecting one ear.

**386.52 Hyperactive labyrinth, bilateral**

DEF: Abnormal increased sensitivity of labyrinth to stimuli such as sound, pressure or gravitational change, affecting both ears.

**386.53 Hypoactive labyrinth, unilateral**

DEF: Abnormal decreased sensitivity of labyrinth to stimuli such as sound, pressure or gravitational change, affecting one ear.

**386.54 Hypoactive labyrinth, bilateral**

DEF: Abnormal decreased sensitivity of labyrinth to stimuli such as sound, pressure or gravitational change, affecting both ears.

**386.55 Loss of labyrinthine reactivity, unilateral**

DEF: Decreased function of the labyrinth sensors, affecting one ear

**386.56 Loss of labyrinthine reactivity, bilateral**

DEF: Decreased function of the labyrinth sensors, affecting both ears

**386.58 Other forms and combinations**

**386.8 Other disorders of labyrinth**

**386.9 Unspecified vertiginous syndromes and labyrinthine disorders**

√4th **387 Otosclerosis**

INCLUDES    otospongiosis

DEF: Synonym for otospongiosis, spongy bone formation in the labyrinth bones of the ear; it causes progressive hearing impairment.

**387.0 Otosclerosis involving oval window, nonobliterative**

DEF: Tough, fibrous tissue impeding functions of oval window.

**387.1 Otosclerosis involving oval window, obliterative**

DEF: Tough, fibrous tissue blocking oval window.

**387.2 Cochlear otosclerosis**
Otosclerosis involving:    Otosclerosis involving:
otic capsule            round window

DEF: Tough, fibrous tissue impeding functions of cochlea.

**387.8 Other otosclerosis**

**387.9 Otosclerosis, unspecified**

√4th **388 Other disorders of ear**

√5th **388.0 Degenerative and vascular disorders of ear**

**388.00 Degenerative and vascular disorders, unspecified**

**388.01 Presbyacusis**

DEF: Progressive, bilateral perceptive hearing loss caused by advancing age; it is also known as presbycusis.

**388.02 Transient ischemic deafness**

DEF: Restricted blood flow to auditory organs causing temporary hearing loss.

√5th **388.1 Noise effects on inner ear**

**388.10 Noise effects on inner ear, unspecified**

**388.11 Acoustic trauma (explosive) to ear**
Otitic blast injury

**388.12 Noise-induced hearing loss**

**388.2 Sudden hearing loss, unspecified**

√5th **388.3 Tinnitus**

DEF: Abnormal noises in ear; may be heard by others beside the affected individual; noises include ringing, clicking, roaring and buzzing.

**388.30 Tinnitus, unspecified**

**388.31 Subjective tinnitus**

**388.32 Objective tinnitus**

√5th **388.4 Other abnormal auditory perception**

**388.40 Abnormal auditory perception, unspecified**

**388.41 Diplacusis**

DEF: Perception of a single auditory sound as two sounds at two different levels of intensity.

**388.42 Hyperacusis**

DEF: Exceptionally acute sense of hearing caused by such conditions as Bell's palsy; this term may also refer to painful sensitivity to sounds.

**388.43 Impairment of auditory discrimination**

DEF: Impaired ability to distinguish tone of sound.

**388.44 Recruitment**

DEF: Perception of abnormally increased loudness caused by a slight increase in sound intensity; it is a term used in audiology.

---

N Newborn Age: 0    P Pediatric Age: 0-17    M Maternity Age: 12-55    A Adult Age: 15-124    CC CC Condition    MCC Major CC Condition    HIV HIV Related Dx

**388.45 Acquired auditory processing disorder**
Auditory processing disorder NOS
> EXCLUDES   *central auditory processing disorder (315.32)*

**388.5 Disorders of acoustic nerve**
Acoustic neuritis
Degeneration ⎫
Disorder      ⎬ of acoustic or eighth nerve

> EXCLUDES   *acoustic neuroma (225.1)*
> *syphilitic acoustic neuritis (094.86)*

**AHA:** M-A, '87, 8

✓5ᵗʰ **388.6 Otorrhea**
    **388.60 Otorrhea, unspecified**
      Discharging ear NOS
    **388.61 Cerebrospinal fluid otorrhea**   CC
> EXCLUDES   *cerebrospinal fluid rhinorrhea (349.81)*

    **CC Excl:** 388.61-388.69

    **DEF:** Spinal fluid leakage from ear.

    **388.69 Other**
      Otorrhagia

✓5ᵗʰ **388.7 Otalgia**
    **388.70 Otalgia, unspecified**
      Earache NOS
    **388.71 Otogenic pain**
    **388.72 Referred pain**

**388.8 Other disorders of ear**
**388.9 Unspecified disorder of ear**

✓4ᵗʰ **389 Hearing loss**
✓5ᵗʰ **389.0 Conductive hearing loss**
    Conductive deafness
> EXCLUDES ▶ *mixed conductive and sensorineural hearing loss (389.20-389.22)*◀

**AHA:** 4Q, '89, 5

**DEF:** Dysfunction in sound-conducting structures of external or middle ear causing hearing loss.

    **389.00 Conductive hearing loss, unspecified**
    **389.01 Conductive hearing loss, external ear**
    **389.02 Conductive hearing loss, tympanic membrane**
    **389.03 Conductive hearing loss, middle ear**
    **389.04 Conductive hearing loss, inner ear**
    **389.05 Conductive hearing loss, unilateral**
    **389.06 Conductive hearing loss, bilateral**
    **389.08 Conductive hearing loss of combined types**

✓5ᵗʰ **389.1 Sensorineural hearing loss**
    Perceptive hearing loss or deafness
> EXCLUDES   *abnormal auditory perception (388.40-388.44)*
> ▶ *mixed conductive and sensorineural hearing loss (389.20-389.22)*◀
> *psychogenic deafness (306.7)*

**AHA:** 4Q, '89, 5

**DEF:** Nerve conduction causing hearing loss.

    **389.10 Sensorineural hearing loss, unspecified**
      **AHA:** 1Q, '93, 29

    **389.11 Sensory hearing loss, bilateral**
    **389.12 Neural hearing loss, bilateral**
    **389.13 Neural hearing loss, unilateral**
    **389.14 Central hearing loss**
    **389.15 Sensorineural hearing loss, unilateral**
      **AHA:** 4Q, '06, 84

    **389.16 Sensorineural hearing loss, asymmetrical**
      **AHA:** 4Q, '06, 84

    **389.17 Sensory hearing loss, unilateral**
    **389.18 Sensorineural hearing loss, bilateral**
      **AHA:** 4Q, '06, 84

✓5ᵗʰ **389.2 Mixed conductive and sensorineural hearing loss**
    Deafness or hearing loss of type classifiable to ▶389.00-389.08 with type classifiable to 389.10-389.18◀
    **389.20 Mixed hearing loss, unspecified**
    **389.21 Mixed hearing loss, unilateral**
    **389.22 Mixed hearing loss, bilateral**
**389.7 Deaf, non-speaking, not elsewhere classifiable**
**389.8 Other specified forms of hearing loss**
**389.9 Unspecified hearing loss**
    Deafness NOS
    **AHA:** 1Q, '04, 15

---

✓4ᵗʰ
✓5ᵗʰ Additional Digit Required     Unacceptable PDx     Manifestation Code     ▶◀ Revised Text     ● New Code     ▲ Revised Code Title

## 7. DISEASES OF THE CIRCULATORY SYSTEM (390-459)

### ACUTE RHEUMATIC FEVER (390-392)

**DEF:** Febrile disease occurs mainly in children or young adults following throat infection by group A *streptococci*; symptoms include fever, joint pain, lesions of heart, blood vessels and joint connective tissue, abdominal pain, skin changes, and chorea.

**390 Rheumatic fever without mention of heart involvement**
     Arthritis, rheumatic, acute or subacute
     Rheumatic fever (active) (acute)
     Rheumatism, articular, acute or subacute
     **EXCLUDES**    *that with heart involvement (391.0-391.9)*

**√4ᵗʰ 391 Rheumatic fever with heart involvement**
     **EXCLUDES**    *chronic heart diseases of rheumatic origin (398.0-398.9) unless rheumatic fever is also present or there is evidence of recrudescence or activity of the rheumatic process*

   **391.0 Acute rheumatic pericarditis**    `CC`
     Rheumatic:
       fever (active) (acute) with pericarditis
       pericarditis (acute)
     Any condition classifiable to 390 with pericarditis
     **EXCLUDES**   *that not specified as rheumatic (420.0-420.9)*

     **CC Excl:** 074.21, 093.81, 391.0, 393, 420.0-420.99, 423.3-423.9, 459.89-459.9

     **DEF:** Sudden, severe inflammation of heart lining due to rheumatic fever.

   **391.1 Acute rheumatic endocarditis**    `CC`
     Rheumatic:
       endocarditis, acute
       fever (active) (acute) with endocarditis or valvulitis
       valvulitis acute
     Any condition classifiable to 390 with endocarditis or valvulitis

     **CC Excl:** 002.0, 036.42, 074.22, 083.0, 093.20-093.24, 098.84, 112.81, 115.94, 390, 391.1, 391.8-392.0, 394.0-395.9, 396.9-397.9, 398.90, 398.99, 421.0-421.9, 424.0-424.99, 425.3, 459.89-459.9, 746.09, 746.89, 996.61

     **DEF:** Sudden, severe inflammation of heart cavities due to rheumatic fever.

   **391.2 Acute rheumatic myocarditis**    `CC`
     Rheumatic fever (active) (acute) with myocarditis
     Any condition classifiable to 390 with myocarditis

     **CC Excl:** 074.20, 074.22-074.23, 093.82, 390, 391.2-391.9, 398.0-398.90, 398.99, 422.0-422.99, 429.0, 429.71-429.79, 459.89-459.9

     **DEF:** Sudden, severe inflammation of heart muscles due to rheumatic fever.

   **391.8 Other acute rheumatic heart disease**    `CC`
     Rheumatic:
       fever (active) (acute) with other or multiple types of heart involvement
       pancarditis, acute
     Any condition classifiable to 390 with other or multiple types of heart involvement

     **CC Excl:** 391.0-398.99, 428.20-428.43

   **391.9 Acute rheumatic heart disease, unspecified**    `CC`
     Rheumatic:
       carditis, acute
       fever (active) (acute) with unspecified type of heart involvement
       heart disease, active or acute
     Any condition classifiable to 390 with unspecified type of heart involvement

     **CC Excl:** 391.0-398.99

**√4ᵗʰ 392 Rheumatic chorea**
     **INCLUDES**    Sydenham's chorea
     **EXCLUDES**    *chorea:*
         *NOS (333.5)*
         *Huntington's (333.4)*

     **DEF:** Childhood disease linked with rheumatic fever and streptococcal infections; symptoms include spasmodic, involuntary movements of limbs or facial muscles, psychic symptoms, and irritability.

   **392.0 With heart involvement**    `CC`
     Rheumatic chorea with heart involvement of any type classifiable to 391

     **CC Excl:** See code: 391.8

   **392.9 Without mention of heart involvement**    `CC`
     **CC Excl:** See code: 391.9

### CHRONIC RHEUMATIC HEART DISEASE (393-398)

**393 Chronic rheumatic pericarditis**    `CC`
     Adherent pericardium, rheumatic
     Chronic rheumatic:
       mediastinopericarditis
       myopericarditis
     **EXCLUDES**    *pericarditis NOS or not specified as rheumatic (423.0-423.9)*

     **CC Excl:** 074.21, 093.81, 391.0, 393, 420.0-420.99, 423.3-423.9, 459.89-459.9

     **DEF:** Persistent inflammation of heart lining due to rheumatic heart disease.

**√4ᵗʰ 394 Diseases of mitral valve**
     **EXCLUDES**    *that with aortic valve involvement (396.0-396.9)*

   **394.0 Mitral stenosis**
     Mitral (valve):         Mitral (valve):
       obstruction (rheumatic)    stenosis NOS

     **DEF:** Narrowing, of mitral valve between left atrium and left ventricle; due to rheumatic heart disease.

   **394.1 Rheumatic mitral insufficiency**
     Rheumatic mitral:      Rheumatic mitral:
       incompetence        regurgitation
     **EXCLUDES**    *that not specified as rheumatic (424.0)*

     **AHA:** 2Q, '05, 14

     **DEF:** Malfunction of mitral valve between left atrium and left ventricle; due to rheumatic heart disease.

   **394.2 Mitral stenosis with insufficiency**
     Mitral stenosis with incompetence or regurgitation

     **AHA:** ►1Q, '07, 11◄

     **DEF:** A narrowing or stricture of the mitral valve situated between the left atrium and left ventricle. The stenosis interferes with blood flow from the atrium into the ventricle. If the valve does not completely close, it becomes insufficient (inadequate) and cannot prevent regurgitation (abnormal backward flow) into the atrium when the left ventricle contracts. This abnormal function is also called incompetence.

   **394.9 Other and unspecified mitral valve diseases**
     Mitral (valve):
       disease (chronic)
       failure

**√4ᵗʰ 395 Diseases of aortic valve**
     **EXCLUDES**    *that not specified as rheumatic (424.1)*
                *that with mitral valve involvement (396.0-396.9)*

   **395.0 Rheumatic aortic stenosis**
     Rheumatic aortic (valve) obstruction

     **AHA:** 4Q, '88, 8

     **DEF:** Narrowing of the aortic valve; results in backflow into ventricle; due to rheumatic heart disease.

   **395.1 Rheumatic aortic insufficiency**
     Rheumatic aortic:
       incompetence
       regurgitation

     **DEF:** Malfunction of the aortic valve; results in backflow into left ventricle; due to rheumatic heart disease.

---

√4ᵗʰ
√5ᵗʰ   Additional Digit Required      Unacceptable PDx      Manifestation Code      ►◄ Revised Text      ● New Code      ▲ Revised Code Title

**395.2 Rheumatic aortic stenosis with insufficiency**
Rheumatic aortic stenosis with incompetence or regurgitation
DEF: Malfunction and narrowing, of the aortic valve; results in backflow into left ventricle; due to rheumatic heart disease.

**395.9 Other and unspecified rheumatic aortic diseases**
Rheumatic aortic (valve) disease

✓4ᵗʰ **396 Diseases of mitral and aortic valves**
INCLUDES    involvement of both mitral and aortic valves, whether specified as rheumatic or not
AHA: N-D, '87, 8

**396.0 Mitral valve stenosis and aortic valve stenosis**
Atypical aortic (valve) stenosis
Mitral and aortic (valve) obstruction (rheumatic)

**396.1 Mitral valve stenosis and aortic valve insufficiency**

**396.2 Mitral valve insufficiency and aortic valve stenosis**
AHA: 2Q, '00, 16

**396.3 Mitral valve insufficiency and aortic valve insufficiency**
Mitral and aortic (valve):
incompetence
regurgitation

**396.8 Multiple involvement of mitral and aortic valves**
Stenosis and insufficiency of mitral or aortic valve with stenosis or insufficiency, or both, of the other valve

**396.9 Mitral and aortic valve diseases, unspecified**

✓4ᵗʰ **397 Diseases of other endocardial structures**

**397.0 Diseases of tricuspid valve**
Tricuspid (valve)              Tricuspid (valve)
(rheumatic):                    (rheumatic):
disease                         regurgitation
insufficiency                   stenosis
obstruction
AHA: 3Q, '06, 7; 2Q, '00, 16
DEF: Malfunction of the valve between right atrium and right ventricle; due to rheumatic heart disease.

**397.1 Rheumatic diseases of pulmonary valve**
EXCLUDES    that not specified as rheumatic (424.3)

**397.9 Rheumatic diseases of endocardium, valve unspecified**
Rheumatic:
endocarditis (chronic)
valvulitis (chronic)
EXCLUDES    that not specified as rheumatic (424.90-424.99)

✓4ᵗʰ **398 Other rheumatic heart disease**

**398.0 Rheumatic myocarditis**    CC
Rheumatic degeneration of myocardium
EXCLUDES    myocarditis not specified as rheumatic (429.0)
CC Excl: 390, 391.2-391.9, 398.0-398.90, 398.99, 422.0-422.99, 429.0, 429.71-429.79, 459.89-459.9
DEF: Chronic inflammation of heart muscle; due to rheumatic heart disease.

✓5ᵗʰ **398.9 Other and unspecified rheumatic heart diseases**
**398.90 Rheumatic heart disease, unspecified**
Rheumatic:
carditis
heart disease NOS
EXCLUDES    carditis not specified as rheumatic (429.89)
heart disease NOS not specified as rheumatic (429.9)

**398.91 Rheumatic heart failure (congestive)**    CC
Rheumatic left ventricular failure
CC Excl: 398.90-398.99, 402.01, 402.11, 402.91, 428.0-428.9, 459.89-459.9
AHA: 2Q, '05, 14; 1Q, '95, 6; 3Q, '88, 3
DEF: Decreased cardiac output, edema and hypertension; due to rheumatic heart disease.

**398.99 Other**

## HYPERTENSIVE DISEASE (401-405)
EXCLUDES    that complicating pregnancy, childbirth, or the puerperium (642.0-642.9)
that involving coronary vessels (410.00-414.9)
AHA: 3Q, '90, 3; 2Q, '89, 12; S-O, '87, 9; J-A, '84, 11

✓4ᵗʰ **401 Essential hypertension**
INCLUDES    high blood pressure
hyperpiesia
hyperpiesis
hypertension (arterial) (essential) (primary) (systemic)
hypertensive vascular:
degeneration
disease
EXCLUDES    elevated blood pressure without diagnosis of hypertension (796.2)
pulmonary hypertension (416.0-416.9)
that involving vessels of:
brain (430-438)
eye (362.11)
AHA: 2Q, '92, 5
DEF: Hypertension that occurs without apparent organic cause; idiopathic.

**401.0 Malignant**    CC
CC Excl: 401.0-405.99, 459.89-459.9
AHA: M-J, '85, 19
DEF: Severe high arterial blood pressure; results in necrosis in kidney, retina, etc.; hemorrhages occur and death commonly due to uremia or rupture of cerebral vessel.

**401.1 Benign**
DEF: Mildly elevated arterial blood pressure.

**401.9 Unspecified**
AHA: 4Q, '05, 71; 3Q, '05, 8; 4Q, '04, 78; 4Q, '03, 105, 108, 111; 3Q, '03, 14; 2Q, '03, 16; 4Q, '97, 37

✓4ᵗʰ **402 Hypertensive heart disease**
INCLUDES    hypertensive:
cardiomegaly
cardiopathy
cardiovascular disease
heart (disease) (failure)
any condition classifiable to 429.0-429.3, 429.8, 429.9 due to hypertension
Use additional code to specify type of heart failure (428.0-428.43), if known
AHA: 4Q, '02, 49; 2Q, '93, 9; N-D, '84, 18

✓5ᵗʰ **402.0 Malignant**
**402.00 Without heart failure**    CC
CC Excl: See code: 401.0

**402.01 With heart failure**    CC
CC Excl: 398.91, 401.0-405.99, 428.0-428.9, 459.89-459.9

✓5ᵗʰ **402.1 Benign**
**402.10 Without heart failure**
**402.11 With heart failure**

✓5ᵗʰ **402.9 Unspecified**
**402.90 Without heart failure**
**402.91 With heart failure**
AHA: 4Q, '02, 52; 1Q, '93, 19; 2Q, '89, 12

---

N Newborn Age: 0    P Pediatric Age: 0-17    M Maternity Age: 12-55    A Adult Age: 15-124    CC CC Condition    MCC Major CC Condition    HIV HIV Related Dx

134 — Volume 1 • October 2007

© 2007 Ingenix

✓4ᵗʰ **403 Hypertensive chronic kidney disease**

> **INCLUDES**    arteriolar nephritis
> arteriosclerosis of:
> > kidney
> > renal arterioles
>
> arteriosclerotic nephritis (chronic) (interstitial)
> hypertensive:
> > nephropathy
> > renal failure
> > uremia (chronic)
>
> nephrosclerosis
> renal sclerosis with hypertension
> any condition classifiable to 585, 586, or 587
> > with any condition classifiable to 401

> **EXCLUDES**    *acute renal failure (584.5-584.9)*
> *renal disease stated as not due to hypertension*
> *renovascular hypertension (405.0-405.9 with*
> > *fifth-digit 1)*

The following fifth-digit subclassification is for use with category 403:

> **0**   **with chronic kidney disease stage I through stage IV, or unspecified**
> > Use additional code to identify the stage of chronic kidney disease (585.1-585.4, 585.9)
>
> **1**   **with chronic kidney disease stage V or end stage renal disease**
> > Use additional code to identify the stage of chronic kidney disease (585.5, 585.6)

**AHA:** 4Q, '06, 84-86; 4Q, '05, 68; 4Q, '92, 22; 2Q, '92, 5

✓5ᵗʰ **403.0**   **Malignant**    `CC`
> **CC Excl:** 401.0-405.99, 459.89-459.9

✓5ᵗʰ **403.1**   **Benign**    `CC 1`
> **CC Excl: For code 403.11:** See code 403.0

✓5ᵗʰ **403.9**   **Unspecified**    `CC 1`
> **CC Excl:** 401.0-415.99, 459.89-459.9

> **AHA: For code 403.90:** ▶2Q, '07, 3;◀ 4Q, '06, 86; **For code 403.91:** 4Q, '05, 69; 1Q, '04, 14; 1Q, '03, 20; 2Q, '01, 11; 3Q, '91, 8

✓4ᵗʰ **404 Hypertensive heart and chronic kidney disease**

> **INCLUDES**    disease:
> > cardiorenal
> > cardiovascular renal
> > any condition classifiable to 402 with any condition classifiable to 403
>
> Use additional code to specify type of heart failure (428.0-428.43), if known

The following fifth-digit subclassification is for use with category 404:

> **0**   **without heart failure and with chronic kidney disease stage I through stage IV, or unspecified**
> > Use additional code to identify the stage of chronic kidney disease (585.1-585.4, 585.9)
>
> **1**   **with heart failure and with chronic kidney disease stage I through stage IV, or unspecified**
> > Use additional code to identify the stage of chronic kidney disease (585.1-585.4, 585.9)
>
> **2**   **without heart failure and with chronic kidney disease stage V or end stage renal disease**
> > Use additional code to identify the stage of chronic kidney disease (585.5, 585.6)
>
> **3**   **with heart failure and chronic kidney disease stage V or end stage renal disease**
> > Use additional code to identify the stage of chronic kidney disease (585.5-585.6)

**AHA:** 4Q, '06, 84-86; 4Q, '05, 68; 4Q, '02, 49; 3Q, '90, 3; J-A, '84, 14

✓5ᵗʰ **404.0**   **Malignant**    `CC`
> **CC Excl:** 401.0-405.99, 459.89-459.9

✓5ᵗʰ **404.1**   **Benign**    `CC 1-3`
> **CC Excl: For codes 404.11-404.13:** 401.0-405.99, 459.89-459.9

✓5ᵗʰ **404.9**   **Unspecified**    `CC 1-3`
> **CC Excl: For codes 404.91-404.93:** 401.0-405.99, 459.89-459.9

✓4ᵗʰ **405 Secondary hypertension**

> **AHA:** 3Q, '90, 3; S-O, '87, 9, 11; J-A, '84, 14
>
> **DEF:** High arterial blood pressure due to or with a variety of primary diseases, such as renal disorders, CNS disorders, endocrine, and vascular diseases.

✓5ᵗʰ **405.0**   **Malignant**
> **405.01 Renovascular**    `CC`
> > **CC Excl:** See code: 404.0
>
> **405.09 Other**    `CC`
> > **CC Excl:** See code: 404.0

✓5ᵗʰ **405.1**   **Benign**
> **405.11 Renovascular**
> **405.19 Other**

✓5ᵗʰ **405.9**   **Unspecified**
> **405.91 Renovascular**
> **405.99 Other**
> > **AHA:** 3Q, '00, 4

## ISCHEMIC HEART DISEASE (410-414)

> **INCLUDES**    that with mention of hypertension
> Use additional code to identify presence of hypertension (401.0-405.9)

**AHA:** 3Q, '91, 10; J-A, '84, 5

✓4ᵗʰ **410 Acute myocardial infarction**

> **INCLUDES**    cardiac infarction
> coronary (artery):
> > embolism
> > occlusion
> > rupture
> > thrombosis
>
> infarction of heart, myocardium, or ventricle
> rupture of heart, myocardium, or ventricle
> ST elevation (STEMI) and non-ST elevation (NSTEMI) myocardial infarction
> any condition classifiable to 414.1-414.9
> > specified as acute or with a stated duration of 8 weeks or less

The following fifth-digit subclassification is for use with category 410:

> **0**   **episode of care unspecified**
> > Use when the source document does not contain sufficient information for the assignment of fifth digit 1 or 2.
>
> **1**   **initial episode of care**
> > Use fifth-digit 1 to designate the first episode of care (regardless of facility site) for a newly diagnosed myocardial infarction. The fifth-digit 1 is assigned regardless of the number of times a patient may be transferred during the initial episode of care.
>
> **2**   **subsequent episode of care**
> > Use fifth-digit 2 to designate an episode of care following the initial episode when the patient is admitted for further observation, evaluation or treatment for a myocardial infarction that has received initial treatment, but is still less than 8 weeks old.

**AHA:** 2Q, '06, 9; 4Q, '05, 69; 3Q, '01, 21; 3Q, '98, 15; 4Q, '97, 37; 3Q, '95, 9; 4Q, 92, 24; 1Q, '92, 10; 3Q, '91, 18; 1Q, '91, 14; 3Q, '89, 3

**DEF:** A sudden insufficiency of blood supply to an area of the heart muscle; usually due to a coronary artery occlusion.

---

✓4ᵗʰ / ✓5ᵗʰ Additional Digit Required     Unacceptable PDx     Manifestation Code     ▶◀ Revised Text     ● New Code     ▲ Revised Code Title

**© 2007 Ingenix**       **October 2007 • Volume 1 — 135**

**Acute Myocardial Infarction**

Anatomic Sites

Anterolateral 410.0

Anteroseptal 410.1

Inferoposterior 410.3

Apical 410.1

Other and septum 410.4

Other lateral 410.5

Posterobasal 410.6

Postero-lateral 410.5

Atrium only 410.8

Septum only

Papillary muscle

§ ✓5th **410.0**   **Of anterolateral wall**    MCC 1

ST elevation myocardial infarction (STEMI) of anterolateral wall

**CC Excl: For code 410.01:** 410.00-410.92, 459.89-459.9

§ ✓5th **410.1**   **Of other anterior wall**    MCC 1

Infarction:

anterior (wall) NOS    (with contiguous portion
anteroapical    of intraventricular
anteroseptal    septum)

ST elevation myocardial infarction (STEMI) of other anterior wall

**CC Excl: For code 410.11:** See code 410.0

**AHA: For code 410.11:** 3Q, '03, 10

§ ✓5th **410.2**   **Of inferolateral wall**    MCC 1

ST elevation myocardial infarction (STEMI) of inferolateral wall

**CC Excl: For code 410.21:** See code 410.0

§ ✓5th **410.3**   **Of inferoposterior wall**    MCC 1

ST elevation myocardial infarction (STEMI) of inferoposterior wall

**CC Excl: For code 410.31:** See code 410.0

§ ✓5th **410.4**   **Of other inferior wall**    MCC 1

Infarction:

diaphragmatic wall    (with contiguous portion
NOS    of intraventricular
inferior (wall) NOS    septum)

ST elevation myocardial infarction (STEMI) of other inferior wall

**CC Excl: For code 410.41:** See code 410.0

**AHA:** 1Q, '00, 7, 26; 4Q, '99, 9; 3Q, '97, 10; **For code 410.41:** 2Q, '01, 8, 9

§ ✓5th **410.5**   **Of other lateral wall**    MCC 1

Infarction:

apical-lateral
basal-lateral
high lateral
posterolateral

ST elevation myocardial infarction (STEMI) of other lateral wall

**CC Excl: For code 410.51:** See code 410.0

§ ✓5th **410.6**   **True posterior wall infarction**    MCC 1

Infarction:

posterobasal
strictly posterior

ST elevation myocardial infarction (STEMI) of true posterior wall

**CC Excl: For code 410.61:** See code 410.0

§ ✓5th **410.7**   **Subendocardial infarction**    MCC 1

Non-ST elevation myocardial infarction (NSTEMI)
Nontransmural infarction

**CC Excl: For code 410.71:** See code 410.0

**AHA:** 1Q, '00, 7; **For code 410.71:** 4Q, '05, 71; 2Q, '05, 19

§   Requires fifth-digit. See category 410 for codes and definitions.

§ ✓5th **410.8**   **Of other specified sites**    MCC 1

Infarction of:
atrium
papillary muscle
septum alone
ST elevation myocardial infarction (STEMI) of other specified sites

**CC Excl: For code 410.81:** See code 410.0

§ ✓5th **410.9**   **Unspecified site**    MCC 1

Acute myocardial infarction NOS
Coronary occlusion NOS
Myocardial infarction NOS

**CC Excl: For code 410.91:** See code 410.0

**AHA:** 1Q, '96, 17; 1Q, '92, 9; **For code 410.91:** 2Q, '05, 18; 3Q, '02, 5

✓4th **411 Other acute and subacute forms of ischemic heart disease**

**AHA:** 4Q, '94, 55; 3Q, '91, 24

**411.0**   **Postmyocardial infarction syndrome**    CC

Dressler's syndrome

**CC Excl:** 411.0, 411.81-411.89, 459.89-459.9

**DEF:** Complication developing several days/weeks after myocardial infarction; symptoms include fever, leukocytosis, chest pain, evidence of pericarditis, pleurisy, and pneumonitis; tendency to recur.

**411.1**   **Intermediate coronary syndrome**    CC

Impending infarction    Preinfarction syndrome
Preinfarction angina    Unstable angina

**EXCLUDES**   angina (pectoris) (413.9)
         decubitus (413.0)

**CC Excl:** 398.91, 402.01, 402.11, 402.91, 404.01, 404.03, 404.11, 404.13, 404.91, 404.93, 410.00-410.92, 411.1-411.89, 413.0-414.00, 414.2-414.9, 428.0-428.1, 428.9, 459.89-459.9, 785.50-785.51

**AHA:** 4Q, '05, 105; 2Q, '04, 3; 1Q, '03, 12; 3Q, '01, 15; 2Q, '01, 7, 9; 4Q, '98, 86; 2Q, '96, 10; 3Q, '91, 24; 1Q, '91, 14; 3Q, '90, 6; 4Q, '89, 10

**DEF:** A condition representing an intermediate stage between angina of effort and acute myocardial infarction. It is often documented by the physician as "unstable angina."

✓5th **411.8**   **Other**

**AHA:** 3Q, '91, 18; 3Q, '89, 4

**411.81 Acute coronary occlusion without myocardial infarction**    CC

Acute coronary (artery):
embolism    without or not
obstruction    resulting in
occlusion    myocardial
thrombosis    infarction

**EXCLUDES**   obstruction without infarction
due to atherosclerosis
(414.00-414.07)
occlusion without infarction
due to atherosclerosis
(414.00-414.07)

**CC Excl:** 410.00-411.89, 413.0-413.9, 414.8-414.9, 459.89-459.9

**AHA:** 3Q, '91, 24; 1Q, '91, 14

**DEF:** Interrupted blood flow to a portion of the heart; without tissue death.

**411.89 Other**    CC

Coronary insufficiency (acute)
Subendocardial ischemia

**CC Excl:** See code: 411.81

**AHA:** 3Q, '01, 14; 1Q, '92, 9

**412 Old myocardial infarction**

Healed myocardial infarction
Past myocardial infarction diagnosed on ECG [EKG] or other special investigation, but currently presenting no symptoms

**AHA:** 2Q, '03, 10; 2Q, '01, 9; 3Q, '98, 15; 2Q, '91, 22; 3Q, '90, 7

N Newborn Age: 0    P Pediatric Age: 0-17    M Maternity Age: 12-55    A Adult Age: 15-124    CC CC Condition    MCC Major CC Condition    HIV HIV Related Dx

136 — Volume 1 • October 2007

© 2007 Ingenix

**Circulatory System**

**✓4th 413 Angina pectoris**

DEF: Severe constricting pain in the chest, often radiating from the precordium to the left shoulder and down the arm, due to ischemia of the heart muscle; usually caused by coronary disease; pain is often precipitated by effort or excitement.

**413.0 Angina decubitus**                **CC**

Nocturnal angina

**CC Excl:** 410.00-410.92, 411.1-411.89, 413.0-413.9, 414.8-414.9, 459.89-459.9

DEF: Angina occurring only in the recumbent position.

**413.1 Prinzmetal angina**                **CC**

Variant angina pectoris

**CC Excl:** See code: 413.0

**AHA:** 3Q, '06, 23

DEF Angina occurring when patient is recumbent; associated with ST-segment elevations.

**413.9 Other and unspecified angina pectoris**

Angina:                    Anginal syndrome
NOS                        Status anginosus
cardiac                    Stenocardia
of effort                  Syncope anginosa
    **EXCLUDES**   *preinfarction angina (411.1)*

**AHA:** 3Q, '02, 4; 3Q, '91, 16; 3Q, '90, 6

**✓4th 414 Other forms of chronic ischemic heart disease**

**EXCLUDES**   *arteriosclerotic cardiovascular disease [ASCVD] (429.2)*
*cardiovascular:*
*arteriosclerosis or sclerosis (429.2)*
*degeneration or disease (429.2)*

**✓5th 414.0 Coronary atherosclerosis**

Arteriosclerotic heart disease [ASHD]
Atherosclerotic heart disease
Coronary (artery):
    arteriosclerosis
    arteritis or endarteritis
    atheroma
    sclerosis
    stricture
▶Use additional code, if applicable, to identify chronic total occlusion of coronary artery (414.2)◀
    **EXCLUDES**   *embolism of graft (996.72)*
*occlusion NOS of graft (996.72)*
*thrombus of graft (996.72)*

**AHA:** 2Q, '97, 13; 2Q, '95, 17; 4Q, '94, 49; 2Q, '94, 13; 1Q, '94, 6; 3Q, '90, 7

DEF: A chronic condition marked by thickening and loss of elasticity of the coronary artery; caused by deposits of plaque containing cholesterol, lipoid material and lipophages.

**414.00 Of unspecified type of vessel, native or graft**                **A**

**AHA:** 1Q, '04, 24; 2Q, '03, 16; 3Q, '01, 15; 4Q, '99, 4; 3Q, '97, 15; 4Q, '96, 31

**414.01 Of native coronary artery**                **A**

**AHA:** 3Q, '06, 25; 4Q, '05, 71; 2Q, '04, 3; 4Q, '03, 108; 3Q, '03, 9, 14; 3Q, '02, 4-9; 3Q, '01, 15; 2Q, '01, 8, 9; 3Q, '97, 15; 2Q, '96, 10; 4Q, '96, 31

DEF: Plaque deposits in natural heart vessels.

**414.02 Of autologous vein bypass graft**                **CC A**

**CC Excl:** 414.00-414.05, 414.07, 414.2

DEF: Plaque deposit in grafted vein originating within patient.

**414.03 Of nonautologous biological bypass graft**                **CC A**

**CC Excl:** See code: 414.02

DEF: Plaque deposits in grafted vessel originating outside patient.

**414.04 Of artery bypass graft**                **CC A**

Internal mammary artery

**CC Excl:** See code: 414.02

**AHA:** 4Q, '96, 31

DEF: Plaque deposits in grafted artery originating within patient.

**Arteries of the Heart**

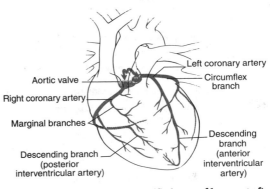

Aortic valve
Right coronary artery
Marginal branches
Descending branch (posterior interventricular artery)
Left coronary artery
Circumflex branch
Descending branch (anterior interventricular artery)

**414.05 Of unspecified type of bypass graft**                **A**

Bypass graft NOS

**AHA:** 3Q, '97, 15; 4Q, '96, 31

**414.06 Of native coronary artery of transplanted heart**                **CC**

**CC Excl:** 414.00-414.07, 414.2

**AHA:** 4Q, '03, 60; 4Q, '02, 53

**414.07 Of bypass graft (artery) (vein) of transplanted heart**                **CC A**

**CC Excl:** 414.00-414.06, 414.2

**✓5th 414.1 Aneurysm and dissection of heart**

**AHA:** 4Q, '02, 54

**414.10 Aneurysm of heart (wall)**                **CC**

Aneurysm (arteriovenous):
    mural
    ventricular

**CC Excl:** 414.10-414.11, 414.19

**414.11 Aneurysm of coronary vessels**

Aneurysm (arteriovenous) of coronary vessels

**AHA:** 3Q, '03, 10; 1Q, '99, 17

DEF: Dilatation of all three-vessel wall layers forming a sac filled with blood.

**414.12 Dissection of coronary artery**                **MCC**

**CC Excl:** 414.12, 443.29, 447.2, 447.5-447.9

DEF: A tear in the intimal arterial wall of a coronary artery resulting in the sudden intrusion of blood within the layers of the wall.

**414.19 Other aneurysm of heart**                **CC**

Arteriovenous fistula, acquired, of heart

**CC Excl:** See code: 414.10

**● 414.2 Chronic total occlusion of coronary artery**

Complete occlusion of coronary artery
Total occlusion of coronary artery
Code first coronary atherosclerosis (414.00-414.07)
    **EXCLUDES**   *acute coronary occlusion with myocardial infarction (410.00-410.92)*
*acute coronary occlusion without myocardial infarction (411.81)*

**414.8 Other specified forms of chronic ischemic heart disease**

Chronic coronary insufficiency
Ischemia, myocardial (chronic)
Any condition classifiable to 410 specified as chronic, or presenting with symptoms after 8 weeks from date of infarction
    **EXCLUDES**   *coronary insufficiency (acute) (411.89)*

**AHA:** 3Q, '01, 15; 1Q, '92, 10; 3Q, '90, 7, 15; 2Q, '90, 19

**414.9 Chronic ischemic heart disease, unspecified**

Ischemic heart disease NOS

---

✓4th / ✓5th  Additional Digit Required        Unacceptable PDx        Manifestation Code        ▶◀ Revised Text        ● New Code        ▲ Revised Code Title

© **2007 Ingenix**

413–414.9

## DISEASES OF PULMONARY CIRCULATION (415-417)

**✓4th 415 Acute pulmonary heart disease**

**415.0 Acute cor pulmonale** MCC

EXCLUDES cor pulmonale NOS (416.9)

CC Excl: 415.0, 416.8-416.9, 459.89-459.9

DEF: A heart-lung disease marked by dilation and failure of the right side of heart; due to pulmonary embolism; ventilatory function is impaired and pulmonary hypertension results within hours.

**✓5th 415.1 Pulmonary embolism and infarction**

Pulmonary (artery) (vein):
apoplexy
embolism
infarction (hemorrhagic)
thrombosis

EXCLUDES that complicating:
abortion (634-638 with .6, 639.6)
ectopic or molar pregnancy (639.6)
pregnancy, childbirth, or the
puerperium (673.0-673.8)

AHA: 4Q, '90, 25

DEF: Embolism: Closure of the pulmonary artery or branch; due to thrombosis (blood clot).

DEF: Infarction: Necrosis of lung tissue; due to obstructed arterial blood supply, most often by pulmonary embolism.

**415.11 Iatrogenic pulmonary embolism and infarction** MCC

CC Excl: 415.11-415.19, 459.89-459.9

AHA: 4Q, '95, 58

**415.12 Septic pulmonary embolism** MCC

Septic embolism NOS
Code first underlying infection, such as:
septicemia (038.0-038.9)

EXCLUDES septic arterial embolism (449)

CC Excl: See code: 415.11

**415.19 Other** MCC

CC Excl: See code: 415.11

**✓4th 416 Chronic pulmonary heart disease**

**416.0 Primary pulmonary hypertension** CC

Idiopathic pulmonary arteriosclerosis
Pulmonary hypertension (essential) (idiopathic) (primary)

CC Excl: 416.0, 416.8-416.9, 417.8-417.9, 459.89-459.9

DEF: A rare increase in pulmonary circulation, often resulting in right ventricular failure or fatal syncope.

**416.1 Kyphoscoliotic heart disease** CC

CC Excl: 416.0-416.9

DEF: High blood pressure within the lungs as a result of curvature of the spine.

**416.8 Other chronic pulmonary heart diseases**

Pulmonary hypertension, secondary

**416.9 Chronic pulmonary heart disease, unspecified**

Chronic cardiopulmonary disease
Cor pulmonale (chronic) NOS

**✓4th 417 Other diseases of pulmonary circulation**

**417.0 Arteriovenous fistula of pulmonary vessels** CC

EXCLUDES congenital arteriovenous fistula (747.3)

CC Excl: 417.0-417.9

DEF: Abnormal communication between blood vessels within lung.

**417.1 Aneurysm of pulmonary artery** CC

EXCLUDES congenital aneurysm (747.3)

CC Excl: See code: 417.0

**417.8 Other specified diseases of pulmonary circulation**

Pulmonary:                      Pulmonary:
arteritis                       endarteritis
Rupture  }
Stricture } of pulmonary vessel

**417.9 Unspecified disease of pulmonary circulation**

## OTHER FORMS OF HEART DISEASE (420-429)

**✓4th 420 Acute pericarditis**

INCLUDES acute:
mediastinopericarditis
myopericarditis
pericardial effusion
pleuropericarditis
pneumopericarditis

EXCLUDES acute rheumatic pericarditis (391.0)
postmyocardial infarction syndrome [Dressler's] (411.0)

DEF: Inflammation of the pericardium (heart sac); pericardial friction rub results from this inflammation and is heard as a scratchy or leathery sound.

**420.0 Acute pericarditis in diseases classified elsewhere** CC

Code first underlying disease, as:
actinomycosis (039.8)
amebiasis (006.8)
chronic uremia (585.9)
nocardiosis (039.8)
tuberculosis (017.9)
uremia NOS (586)

EXCLUDES pericarditis (acute) (in):
Coxsackie (virus) (074.21)
gonococcal (098.83)
histoplasmosis (115.0-115.9 with fifth-digit 3)
meningococcal infection (036.41)
syphilitic (093.81)

CC Excl: 391.0, 393, 420.0-420.99, 423.3-423.9, 459.89-459.9

**Anatomy**

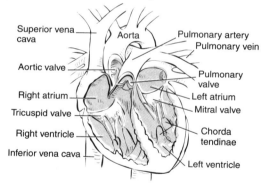

Superior vena cava
Aorta
Pulmonary artery
Pulmonary vein
Aortic valve
Pulmonary valve
Right atrium
Left atrium
Tricuspid valve
Mitral valve
Right ventricle
Chorda tendinae
Inferior vena cava
Left ventricle

**Blood Flow**

N Newborn Age: 0    P Pediatric Age: 0-17    M Maternity Age: 12-55    A Adult Age: 15-124    CC CC Condition    MCC Major CC Condition    HIV HIV Related Dx

138 — Volume 1 • October 2007

© 2007 Ingenix

√5ᵗʰ **420.9   Other and unspecified acute pericarditis**

**420.90 Acute pericarditis, unspecified**  `CC`

| Pericarditis (acute): | Pericarditis (acute): |
|---|---|
| NOS | sicca |
| infective NOS | |

**CC Excl:** See code: 420.0

**AHA:** 2Q, '89, 12

**420.91 Acute idiopathic pericarditis**  `CC`

| Pericarditis, acute: | Pericarditis, acute: |
|---|---|
| benign | viral |
| nonspecific | |

**CC Excl:** See code: 420.0

**420.99 Other**  `CC`

| Pericarditis (acute): | Pericarditis (acute): |
|---|---|
| pneumococcal | suppurative |
| purulent | Pneumopyopericardium |
| staphylococcal | Pyopericardium |
| streptococcal | |

> **EXCLUDES** pericarditis in diseases classified elsewhere (420.0)

**CC Excl:** See code: 420.0

√4ᵗʰ **421   Acute and subacute endocarditis**

**DEF:** Bacterial inflammation of the endocardium (intracardiac area); major symptoms include fever, fatigue, heart murmurs, splenomegaly, embolic episodes and areas of infarction.

**421.0   Acute and subacute bacterial endocarditis**  `MCC` `HIV`

| Endocarditis (acute) | Endocarditis (acute) |
|---|---|
| (chronic) (subacute): | (chronic) (subacute): |
| bacterial | ulcerative |
| infective NOS | vegetative |
| lenta | Infective aneurysm |
| malignant | Subacute bacterial |
| purulent | endocarditis [SBE] |
| septic | |

Use additional code to identify infectious organism [e.g., Streptococcus 041.0, Staphylococcus 041.1]

**CC Excl:** 391.1, 397.9, 421.0-421.9, 424.90-424.99, 459.89-459.9

**AHA:** 1Q, '99, 12; 1Q, '91, 15

**421.1   Acute and subacute infective endocarditis in diseases classified elsewhere**  `MCC`

Code first underlying disease, as:
  blastomycosis (116.0)
  Q fever (083.0)
  typhoid (fever) (002.0)

> **EXCLUDES** endocarditis (in):
>   Coxsackie (virus) (074.22)
>   gonococcal (098.84)
>   histoplasmosis (115.0-115.9 with fifth-digit 4)
>   meningococcal infection (036.42)
>   monilial (112.81)

**CC Excl:** See code: 421.0

**421.9   Acute endocarditis, unspecified**  `MCC` `HIV`

| Endocarditis | |
|---|---|
| Myoendocarditis | } acute or subacute |
| Periendocarditis | |

> **EXCLUDES** acute rheumatic endocarditis (391.1)

**CC Excl:** See code: 421.0

√4ᵗʰ **422   Acute myocarditis**

> **EXCLUDES** acute rheumatic myocarditis (391.2)

**DEF:** Acute inflammation of the muscular walls of the heart (myocardium).

**422.0   Acute myocarditis in diseases classified elsewhere**  `MCC`

Code first underlying disease, as:
  myocarditis (acute):
    influenzal (487.8)
    tuberculous (017.9)

> **EXCLUDES** myocarditis (acute) (due to):
>   aseptic, of newborn (074.23)
>   Coxsackie (virus) (074.23)
>   diphtheritic (032.82)
>   meningococcal infection (036.43)
>   syphilitic (093.82)
>   toxoplasmosis (130.3)

**CC Excl:** 391.2, 398.0, 422.0-422.99, 429.0, 429.71-429.79, 459.89-459.9

√5ᵗʰ **422.9   Other and unspecified acute myocarditis**

**422.90 Acute myocarditis, unspecified**  `MCC` `HIV`

Acute or subacute (interstitial) myocarditis

**CC Excl:** See code: 422.0

**422.91 Idiopathic myocarditis**  `MCC` `HIV`

Myocarditis (acute or subacute):
  Fiedler's
  giant cell
  isolated (diffuse) (granulomatous)
  nonspecific granulomatous

**CC Excl:** See code: 422.0

**422.92 Septic myocarditis**  `MCC` `HIV`

Myocarditis, acute or subacute:
  pneumococcal
  staphylococcal

Use additional code to identify infectious organism [e.g., Staphylococcus 041.1]

> **EXCLUDES** myocarditis, acute or subacute:
>   in bacterial diseases classified elsewhere (422.0)
>   streptococcal (391.2)

**CC Excl:** See code 422.0

**422.93 Toxic myocarditis**  `MCC` `HIV`

**CC Excl:** See code: 422.0

**DEF:** Inflammation of the heart muscle due to an adverse reaction to certain drugs or chemicals reaching the heart through the bloodstream.

**422.99 Other**  `MCC` `HIV`

**CC Excl:** See code: 422.0

√4ᵗʰ **423   Other diseases of pericardium**

> **EXCLUDES** that specified as rheumatic (393)

**423.0   Hemopericardium**  `CC`

**CC Excl:** 423.0-423.9, 459.89-459.9

**DEF:** Blood in the pericardial sac (pericardium).

**423.1   Adhesive pericarditis**  `CC`

| Adherent pericardium | Pericarditis: |
|---|---|
| Fibrosis of pericardium | adhesive |
| Milk spots | obliterative |
| | Soldiers' patches |

**CC Excl:** See code: 423.0

**DEF:** Two layers of serous pericardium adhere to each other by fibrous adhesions.

**423.2   Constrictive pericarditis**  `CC`

Concato's disease   Pick's disease of heart (and liver)

**CC Excl:** See code: 423.0

**DEF:** Inflammation identified by a rigid, thickened and sometimes calcified pericardium; ventricles of the heart cannot be adequately filled and congestive heart failure may result.

● 　　**423.3　Cardiac tamponade** 　　　　　　　　　　CC
　　　　　Code first the underlying cause
　　　　　**CC Excl:** 074.21, 093.81, 391.0, 393, 420.0-420.99, 423.3-423.9, 459.89-459.9

　　**423.8　Other specified diseases of pericardium** 　　CC
　　　　　Calcification
　　　　　Fistula 　　　} of pericardium

　　　　　**CC Excl:** See code: 423.3

　　　　　**AHA:** 2Q, '89, 12

　　**423.9　Unspecified disease of pericardium** 　　　CC
　　　　　**CC Excl:** See code: 423.3

　　　　　**AHA:** ▶1Q, '07, 11◀

✓4ᵗʰ **424　Other diseases of endocardium**
　　　　　EXCLUDES 　*bacterial endocarditis (421.0-421.9)*
　　　　　　　　　　　*rheumatic endocarditis (391.1, 394.0-397.9)*
　　　　　　　　　　　*syphilitic endocarditis (093.20-093.24)*

　　**424.0　Mitral valve disorders**
　　　　　Mitral (valve):
　　　　　　incompetence
　　　　　　insufficiency 　} NOS of specified cause,
　　　　　　regurgitation 　　　except rheumatic

　　　　　EXCLUDES 　*mitral (valve):*
　　　　　　　　　　　*disease (394.9)*
　　　　　　　　　　　*failure (394.9)*
　　　　　　　　　　　*stenosis (394.0)*
　　　　　　　　　　*the listed conditions:*
　　　　　　　　　　　*specified as rheumatic (394.1)*
　　　　　　　　　　　*unspecified as to cause but with*
　　　　　　　　　　　　*mention of:*
　　　　　　　　　　　　*diseases of aortic valve (396.0-*
　　　　　　　　　　　　　*396.9)*
　　　　　　　　　　　　*mitral stenosis or obstruction*
　　　　　　　　　　　　　*(394.2)*

　　　　　**AHA:** 3Q, '06, 7; 2Q, '00, 16; 3Q, '98, 11; N-D, '87, 8; N-D, '84, 8

　　**424.1　Aortic valve disorders**
　　　　　Aortic (valve):
　　　　　　incompetence
　　　　　　insufficiency 　} NOS of specified
　　　　　　regurgitation 　　　cause, except
　　　　　　stenosis 　　　　　　rheumatic

　　　　　EXCLUDES 　*hypertrophic subaortic stenosis (425.1)*
　　　　　　　　　　　*that specified as rheumatic (395.0-395.9)*
　　　　　　　　　　　*that of unspecified cause but with*
　　　　　　　　　　　*mention of diseases of mitral*
　　　　　　　　　　　*valve (396.0-396.9)*

　　　　　**AHA:** 4Q, '88, 8; N-D, '87, 8

　　**424.2　Tricuspid valve disorders, specified as nonrheumatic**
　　　　　Tricuspid valve:
　　　　　　incompetence
　　　　　　insufficiency 　} of specified cause,
　　　　　　regurgitation 　　　except
　　　　　　stenosis 　　　　　　rheumatic

　　　　　EXCLUDES 　*rheumatic or of unspecified cause (397.0)*

　　**424.3　Pulmonary valve disorders**
　　　　　Pulmonic:
　　　　　　incompetence NOS
　　　　　　insufficiency NOS
　　　　　　regurgitation NOS
　　　　　　stenosis NOS
　　　　　EXCLUDES 　*that specified as rheumatic (397.1)*

✓5ᵗʰ **424.9　Endocarditis, valve unspecified**
　　**424.90　Endocarditis, valve unspecified, unspecified cause** 　　　　　　CC
　　　　　Endocarditis (chronic):
　　　　　　NOS
　　　　　　nonbacterial thrombotic
　　　　　Valvular:
　　　　　　incompetence
　　　　　　insufficiency 　} of unspecified
　　　　　　regurgitation 　　valve,
　　　　　　stenosis 　　　　　unspecified
　　　　　　　　　　　　　　　cause

　　　　　Valvulitis (chronic)
　　　　　**CC Excl:** 424.90-424.99, 459.89-459.9

　　**424.91　Endocarditis in diseases classified elsewhere** 　　　　　　CC
　　　　　Code first underlying disease as:
　　　　　　atypical verrucous endocarditis [Libman-Sacks] (710.0)
　　　　　　disseminated lupus erythematosus (710.0)
　　　　　　tuberculosis (017.9)
　　　　　EXCLUDES 　*syphilitic (093.20-093.24)*

　　　　　**CC Excl:** See code: 424.90

　　**424.99　Other** 　　　　　　　　　　　　　CC
　　　　　Any condition classifiable to 424.90 with specified cause, except rheumatic
　　　　　EXCLUDES 　*endocardial fibroelastosis (425.3)*
　　　　　　　　　　　*that specified as rheumatic (397.9)*

　　　　　**CC Excl:** See code: 424.90

✓4ᵗʰ **425　Cardiomyopathy**
　　　　　INCLUDES 　myocardiopathy
　　　　　**AHA:** J-A, '85, 15

　　**425.0　Endomyocardial fibrosis** 　　　　　CC
　　　　　**CC Excl:** 398.91, 402.01, 402.11, 402.91, 404.01, 404.03, 404.11, 404.13, 404.91, 404.93, 414.00-414.07, 414.2-414.9, 425.0-425.9, 426.10-426.13, 426.50-426.54, 426.81-426.89, 427.31-427.42, 427.60-427.89, 428.0-428.1, 428.9, 459.89-459.9, 746.86, 785.0-785.1, 785.50-785.51

**Heart Valve Disorders**

Valve stenosis
(trouble opening)

Incompetent valve
(trouble closing)

causes regurgitation
(backflow of blood)

Insuficient valve
(unable to close completely)

Shortened, fused
chorda tendinae

Ventricular hypertrophy

**Normal Heart Valve Function**

Atrium contracts
Valve leaflet (cusp)
Chorda tendinae
Papillary muscle
Ventricle fills
Great artery (aorta or pulmonary artery)

Atrium fills
Ventricle contracts
Great vein (vena cava or pulmonary vein)
Great artery (blood to body or lungs)

---

N Newborn Age: 0 　　P Pediatric Age: 0-17 　　M Maternity Age: 12-55 　　A Adult Age: 15-124 　　CC CC Condition 　　MCC Major CC Condition 　　HIV HIV Related Dx

140 — Volume 1 • October 2007

**425.1 Hypertrophic obstructive cardiomyopathy** `CC`

Hypertrophic subaortic stenosis (idiopathic)

**CC Excl:** See code: 425.0

DEF: Cardiomyopathy marked by left ventricle hypertrophy, enlarged septum; results in obstructed blood flow.

**425.2 Obscure cardiomyopathy of Africa** `CC`

Becker's disease

Idiopathic mural endomyocardial disease

**CC Excl:** See code: 425.0

**425.3 Endocardial fibroelastosis** `CC`

Elastomyofibrosis

**CC Excl:** See code: 425.0

DEF: A condition marked by left ventricle hypertrophy and conversion of the endocardium into a thick fibroelastic coat; capacity of the ventricle may be reduced, but is often increased.

**425.4 Other primary cardiomyopathies** `CC`

Cardiomyopathy:
NOS
congestive
constrictive
familial
hypertrophic

Cardiomyopathy:
idiopathic
nonobstructive
obstructive
restrictive
Cardiovascular collagenosis

**CC Excl:** See code: 425.0

**AHA:** ▶1Q, '07, 20;◀ 2Q, '05, 14; 1Q, '00, 22; 4Q, '97, 55; 2Q, '90, 19

**425.5 Alcoholic cardiomyopathy** `CC`

**CC Excl:** See code: 425.0

**AHA:** S-O, '85, 15

DEF: Heart disease as result of excess alcohol consumption.

**425.7 Nutritional and metabolic cardiomyopathy** `CC`

Code first underlying disease, as:
amyloidosis (277.30-277.39)
beriberi (265.0)
cardiac glycogenosis (271.0)
mucopolysaccharidosis (277.5)
thyrotoxicosis (242.0-242.9)

**EXCLUDES**   gouty tophi of heart (274.82)

**CC Excl:** See code 425.0

**425.8 Cardiomyopathy in other diseases classified elsewhere** `CC`

Code first underlying disease, as:
Friedreich's ataxia (334.0)
myotonia atrophica ▶(359.21)◀
progressive muscular dystrophy (359.1)
sarcoidosis (135)

**EXCLUDES**   cardiomyopathy in Chagas' disease (086.0)

**CC Excl:** See code: 425.0

**AHA:** 2Q, '93, 9

**425.9 Secondary cardiomyopathy, unspecified** `CC`

**CC Excl:** See code: 425.0

√4th **426 Conduction disorders**

DEF: Disruption or disturbance in the electrical impulses that regulate heartbeats.

**426.0 Atrioventricular block, complete** `CC`

Third degree atrioventricular block

**CC Excl:** 426.0-427.5, 427.89, 459.89-459.9

**AHA:** 2Q, '06, 14

√5th **426.1 Atrioventricular block, other and unspecified**

**426.10 Atrioventricular block, unspecified**

Atrioventricular [AV] block (incomplete) (partial)

**AHA:** 2Q, '06, 14

**426.11 First degree atrioventricular block**

Incomplete atrioventricular block, first degree
Prolonged P-R interval NOS

**Nerve Conduction of the Heart**

Sinoatrial node (pacemaker)
Internodal tracts:
Anterior
Middle
Posterior
Atrioventricular node
Common bundle (of His)
Atrioventricular block
Accessory bundle (of Kent)
Right bundle branch
Right bundle branch block
Moderator band
Bachmann's bundle
Left bundle branch block
Left bundle branch:
Anterior fascicle
Posterior fascicle
Left bundle branch hemiblock
Purkinje fibers

**426.12 Mobitz (type) II atrioventricular block** `CC`

Incomplete atrioventricular block:
Mobitz (type) II
second degree, Mobitz (type) II

**CC Excl:** See code: 426.0

DEF: Impaired conduction of excitatory impulse from cardiac atrium to ventricle through AV node.

**426.13 Other second degree atrioventricular block**

Incomplete atrioventricular block:
Mobitz (type) I [Wenckebach's]
second degree:
NOS
Mobitz (type) I
with 2:1 atrioventricular response [block]
Wenckebach's phenomenon

DEF: Wenckebach's phenomenon: impulses generated at constant rate to sinus node, P-R interval lengthens; results in cycle of ventricular inadequacy and shortened P-R interval; second-degree A-V block commonly called "Mobitz type 1."

**426.2 Left bundle branch hemiblock**

Block:
left anterior fascicular
left posterior fascicular

**426.3 Other left bundle branch block**

Left bundle branch block:
NOS
anterior fascicular with posterior fascicular
complete
main stem

**426.4 Right bundle branch block**

**AHA:** 3Q, '00, 3

√5th **426.5 Bundle branch block, other and unspecified**

**426.50 Bundle branch block, unspecified**

**426.51 Right bundle branch block and left posterior fascicular block**

**426.52 Right bundle branch block and left anterior fascicular block**

**426.53 Other bilateral bundle branch block** `CC`

Bifascicular block NOS
Bilateral bundle branch block NOS
Right bundle branch with left bundle branch block (incomplete) (main stem)

**CC Excl:** 426.0-427.5, 427.89, 459.89-459.9

**426.54 Trifascicular block** `CC`

**CC Excl:** 426.0-427.5, 427.89, 459.89-459.9

**426.6 Other heart block**

Intraventricular block:
NOS
diffuse
myofibrillar

Sinoatrial block
Sinoauricular block

Normal and Long QT Electrocardiogram

**426.7 Anomalous atrioventricular excitation**
Atrioventricular conduction:
accelerated
accessory
pre-excitation
Ventricular pre-excitation
Wolff-Parkinson-White syndrome
**DEF:** Wolff-Parkinson-White: normal conduction pathway is bypassed; results in short P-R interval on EKG; tendency to supraventricular tachycardia.

**✓5ᵗʰ 426.8 Other specified conduction disorders**
**426.81 Lown-Ganong-Levine syndrome**
Syndrome of short P-R interval, normal QRS complexes, and supraventricular tachycardias
**426.82 Long QT syndrome**
**AHA:** 4Q, '05, 72
**DEF:** Condition characterized by recurrent syncope, malignant arrhythmias, and sudden death; characteristic prolonged Q-T interval on electrocardiogram.
**426.89 Other** `CC`
Dissociation:
atrioventricular [AV]
interference
isorhythmic
Nonparoxysmal AV nodal tachycardia
**CC Excl:** 426.0-426.5, 427.89, 459.89-459.9

**426.9 Conduction disorder, unspecified**
Heart block NOS
Stokes-Adams syndrome

**✓4ᵗʰ 427 Cardiac dysrhythmias**
**EXCLUDES** *that complicating:*
*abortion (634-638 with .7, 639.8)*
*ectopic or molar pregnancy (639.8)*
*labor or delivery (668.1, 669.4)*
**AHA:** J-A, '85, 15
**DEF:** Disruption or disturbance in the rhythm of heartbeats.

**427.0 Paroxysmal supraventricular tachycardia** `CC`
Paroxysmal tachycardia:     Paroxysmal tachycardia:
atrial [PAT]                junctional
atrioventricular [AV]       nodal
**CC Excl:** See code: 426.89
**DEF:** Rapid atrial rhythm.

**427.1 Paroxysmal ventricular tachycardia** `CC`
Ventricular tachycardia (paroxysmal)
**CC Excl:** See code: 426.89
**AHA:** 2Q, '06, 15-16; 3Q, '95, 9; M-A, '86, 11
**DEF:** Rapid ventricular rhythm.

**427.2 Paroxysmal tachycardia, unspecified**
Bouveret-Hoffmann syndrome
Paroxysmal tachycardia:
essential
NOS

**✓5ᵗʰ 427.3 Atrial fibrillation and flutter**
**427.31 Atrial fibrillation**
**AHA:** 3Q, '05, 8; 4Q, '04, 78, 121; 3Q, '04, 7; 4Q, '03, 95, 105; 1Q, '03, 8; 2Q, '99, 17; 3Q, '95, 8
**DEF:** Irregular, rapid atrial contractions.
**427.32 Atrial flutter** `CC`
**CC Excl:** See code: 426.89
**AHA:** 4Q, '03, 94
**DEF:** Regular, rapid atrial contractions.

**✓5ᵗʰ 427.4 Ventricular fibrillation and flutter**
¹ **427.41 Ventricular fibrillation** `MCC`
**CC Excl:** See code: 426.89
**AHA:** 3Q, '02, 5
**DEF:** Irregular, rapid ventricular contractions.
**427.42 Ventricular flutter** `MCC`
**CC Excl:** See code: 426.89
**DEF:** Regular, rapid, ventricular contractions.

¹ **427.5 Cardiac arrest** `MCC`
Cardiorespiratory arrest
**CC Excl:** 427.0-427.5, 459.89-459.9
**AHA:** 3Q,'02, 5; 2Q, '00, 12; 3Q, '95, 8; 2Q, '88, 8

**✓5ᵗʰ 427.6 Premature beats**
**427.60 Premature beats, unspecified**
Ectopic beats          Premature contractions
Extrasystoles          or systoles NOS
Extrasystolic arrhythmia
**427.61 Supraventricular premature beats**
Atrial premature beats, contractions, or systoles
**427.69 Other**
Ventricular premature beats, contractions, or systoles
**AHA:** 4Q, '93, 42

**✓5ᵗʰ 427.8 Other specified cardiac dysrhythmias**
**427.81 Sinoatrial node dysfunction**
Sinus bradycardia:   Syndrome:
persistent           sick sinus
severe               tachycardia-
bradycardia
**EXCLUDES** *sinus bradycardia NOS (427.89)*
**AHA:** 3Q, '00, 8
**DEF:** Complex cardiac arrhythmia; appears as severe sinus bradycardia, sinus bradycardia with tachycardia, or sinus bradycardia with atrioventricular block.
**427.89 Other**
Rhythm disorder:    Rhythm disorder:
coronary sinus      nodal
ectopic             Wandering (atrial)
pacemaker
**EXCLUDES** *carotid sinus syncope (337.0)*
*neonatal bradycardia (779.81)*
*neonatal tachycardia (779.82)*
*reflex bradycardia (337.0)*
*tachycardia NOS (785.0)*

**427.9 Cardiac dysrhythmia, unspecified**
Arrhythmia (cardiac) NOS
**AHA:** 2Q, '89, 10

**✓4ᵗʰ 428 Heart failure**
Code, if applicable, heart failure due to hypertension first (402.0-402.9, with fifth-digit 1 or 404.0-404.9 with fifth-digit 1 or 3)
**EXCLUDES** *following cardiac surgery (429.4)*
*rheumatic (398.91)*
*that complicating:*
*abortion (634-638 with .7, 639.8)*
*ectopic or molar pregnancy (639.8)*
*labor or delivery (668.1, 669.4)*
**AHA:** 4Q, '02, 49; 3Q, '98, 5; 2Q, '90, 16; 2Q, '90, 19; 2Q, '89, 10; 3Q, '88, 3

¹ MCC=Only if patient is discharged alive.

**N** Newborn Age: 0     **P** Pediatric Age: 0-17     **M** Maternity Age: 12-55     **A** Adult Age: 15-124     `CC` CC Condition     `MCC` Major CC Condition     `HIV` HIV Related Dx

142 — Volume 1 • October 2007

© 2007 Ingenix

**Echocardiography of Heart Failure**

Four-chamber echocardiograms, two-dimensional views.
LV: Left ventricle
RV: Right ventricle
RA: Right atrium
LA: Left atrium

Systolic dysfunction with dilated LV

Diastolic dysfunction with LV hypertrophy

**428.0  Congestive heart failure, unspecified**
Congestive heart disease
Right heart failure (secondary to left heart failure)
**EXCLUDES**    *fluid overload NOS (276.6)*

AHA:▶1Q, 07, 20;◀ 3Q, '06, 7; 4Q, '05, 120; 3Q, '05, 8; 1Q, '05, 5, 9; 1Q, '05, 5, 9; 4Q, '04, 140; 3Q, '04, 7;4Q, '03, 109; 1Q, '03, 9; 4Q, '02, 52; 2Q, '01, 13; 4Q, '00, 48; 2Q, '00, 16; 1Q, '00, 22; 4Q, '99, 4; 1Q, '99, 11; 4Q, '97, 55; 3Q, '97, 10; 3Q, '96, 9; 3Q, '91, 18; 3Q, '91, 19; 2Q, '89, 12

DEF: Mechanical inadequacy; caused by inability of heart to pump and circulate blood; results in fluid collection in lungs, hypertension, congestion and edema of tissue.

**428.1  Left heart failure**    `CC`
Acute edema of lung ⎫ with heart disease NOS
Acute pulmonary edema ⎭ or heart failure
Cardiac asthma
Left ventricular failure
CC Excl: 398.91, 402.01, 402.11, 402.91, 428.0-428.9, 459.89-459.9

DEF: Mechanical inadequacy of left ventricle; causing fluid in lungs.

√5ᵗʰ **428.2  Systolic heart failure**
**EXCLUDES**    *combined systolic and diastolic heart failure (428.40-428.43)*

DEF: Heart failure due to a defect in expulsion of blood caused by an abnormality in systolic function, or ventricular contractile dysfunction.

**428.20  Unspecified**    `CC`
CC Excl: 398.91, 402.01, 402.11, 402.91, 428.0-428.9, 459.89-459.9, 518.4

**428.21  Acute**    `MCC`
CC Excl: See code: 428.20

**428.22  Chronic**    `CC`
CC Excl: See code: 428.20

AHA: 4Q, '05, 120

**428.23  Acute on chronic**    `MCC`
CC Excl: See code: 428.20

AHA: 1Q, '03, 9

√5ᵗʰ **428.3  Diastolic heart failure**
**EXCLUDES**    *combined systolic and diastolic heart failure (428.40-428.43)*

DEF: Heart failure due to resistance to ventricular filling caused by an abnormality in the diastolic function.

**428.30  Unspecified**    `CC`
CC Excl: See code: 428.20

AHA: 4Q, '02, 52

**428.31  Acute**    `MCC`
CC Excl: See code: 428.20

**428.32  Chronic**    `CC`
CC Excl: See code: 428.20

**428.33  Acute on chronic**    `MCC`
CC Excl: See code: 428.20

AHA: ▶1Q, '07, 20◀

√5ᵗʰ **428.4  Combined systolic and diastolic heart failure**
**428.40  Unspecified**    `CC`
CC Excl: See code: 428.20

**428.41  Acute**    `MCC`
CC Excl: See code: 428.20

AHA: 4Q, '04, 140

**428.42  Chronic**    `CC`
CC Excl: See code: 428.20

**428.43  Acute on chronic**    `MCC`
CC Excl: See code: 428.20

AHA: 3Q, '06, 7; 4Q, '02, 52

**428.9  Heart failure, unspecified**
Cardiac failure NOS      Myocardial failure NOS
Heart failure NOS        Weak heart
AHA: 2Q, '89, 10; N-D, '85, 14

√4ᵗʰ **429  Ill-defined descriptions and complications of heart disease**
**429.0  Myocarditis, unspecified**
Myocarditis:
NOS                    ⎫
chronic (interstitial) ⎬ (with mention of
fibroid                ⎪   arteriosclerosis)
senile                 ⎭

Use additional code to identify presence of arteriosclerosis
**EXCLUDES**    *acute or subacute (422.0-422.9)*
*rheumatic (398.0)*
*acute (391.2)*
*that due to hypertension (402.0-402.9)*

**429.1  Myocardial degeneration**
Degeneration of heart or
myocardium:            ⎫
fatty                  ⎪
mural                  ⎬ (with mention of
muscular               ⎪   arteriosclerosis)
Myocardial:            ⎪
degeneration           ⎪
disease                ⎭

Use additional code to identify presence of arteriosclerosis
**EXCLUDES**    *that due to hypertension (402.0-402.9)*

**429.2  Cardiovascular disease, unspecified**
Arteriosclerotic cardiovascular disease [ASCVD]
Cardiovascular arteriosclerosis
Cardiovascular:
degeneration    ⎫
disease         ⎬ (with mention of
sclerosis       ⎭   arteriosclerosis)

Use additional code to identify presence of arteriosclerosis
**EXCLUDES**    *that due to hypertension (402.0-402.9)*

**429.3  Cardiomegaly**
Cardiac:              Ventricular dilatation
dilatation
hypertrophy
**EXCLUDES**    *that due to hypertension (402.0-402.9)*

**429.4  Functional disturbances following cardiac surgery**
Cardiac insufficiency ⎫ following cardiac surgery
Heart failure         ⎭ or due to prosthesis
Postcardiotomy syndrome
Postvalvulotomy syndrome
**EXCLUDES**    *cardiac failure in the immediate postoperative period (997.1)*
AHA: 2Q, '02, 12; N-D, '85, 6

**429.5  Rupture of chordae tendineae**    `MCC`
CC Excl: 429.5, 429.71-429.79, 459.89-459.9

DEF: Torn tissue, between heart valves and papillary muscles.

**429.6  Rupture of papillary muscle**    `MCC`
CC Excl: 429.6-429.81, 459.89-459.9

DEF: Torn muscle, between chordae tendineae and heart wall.

✓5ᵗʰ **429.7 Certain sequelae of myocardial infarction, not elsewhere classified**

Use additional code to identify the associated myocardial infarction:

with onset of 8 weeks or less (410.00-410.92)

with onset of more than 8 weeks (414.8)

EXCLUDES    *congenital defects of heart (745, 746)*
*coronary aneurysm (414.11)*
*disorders of papillary muscle (429.6, 429.81)*
*postmyocardial infarction syndrome (411.0)*
*rupture of chordae tendineae (429.5)*

AHA: 3Q, '89, 5

**429.71 Acquired cardiac septal defect**   CC   A

EXCLUDES    *acute septal infarction (410.00-410.92)*

CC Excl: 422.0-422.99, 429.0, 429.4-429.82, 459.89-459.9, 745.0-745.9, 746.89-746.9, 747.83-747.9, 759.7-759.89

DEF: Abnormal communication, between opposite heart chambers; due to defect of septum; not present at birth.

**429.79 Other**   CC   A

Mural thrombus (atrial) (ventricular), acquired, following myocardial infarction

CC Excl: See code: 429.71

AHA: 1Q, '92, 10

✓5ᵗʰ **429.8 Other ill-defined heart diseases**

**429.81 Other disorders of papillary muscle**   CC

Papillary muscle:    Papillary muscle:
atrophy             incompetence
degeneration        incoordination
dysfunction         scarring

CC Excl: 429.6-429.81, 459.89-459.9

**429.82 Hyperkinetic heart disease**   CC

CC Excl: 429.71-429.79, 429.82, 459.89-459.9

DEF: Condition of unknown origin in young adults; marked by increased cardiac output at rest, increased rate of ventricular ejection; may lead to heart failure.

**429.83 Takotsubo syndrome**   CC

Broken heart syndrome
Reversible left ventricular dysfunction following sudden emotional stress
Stress induced cardiomyopathy
Transient left ventricular apical ballooning syndrome

CC Excl: 398.91, 402.01, 402.11, 402.91, 428.0-428.9, 429.83, 429.9, 459.89-459.9

AHA: 4Q, '06, 87

**429.89 Other**

Carditis

EXCLUDES    *that due to hypertension (402.0-402.9)*

AHA: 2Q, '06, 18; 3Q, '05, 14; 1Q, '92, 10

**429.9 Heart disease, unspecified**

Heart disease (organic) NOS    Morbus cordis NOS

EXCLUDES    *that due to hypertension (402.0-402.9)*

AHA: 1Q, '93, 19

## CEREBROVASCULAR DISEASE (430-438)

INCLUDES    with mention of hypertension (conditions classifiable to 401-405)

Use additional code to identify presence of hypertension

EXCLUDES    *any condition classifiable to 430-434, 436, 437 occurring during pregnancy, childbirth, or the puerperium, or specified as puerperal (674.0)*
*iatrogenic cerebrovascular infarction or hemorrhage (997.02)*

AHA: 1Q, '93, 27; 3Q, '91, 10; 3Q, '90, 3; 2Q, '89, 8; M-A, '85, 6

**430 Subarachnoid hemorrhage**   MCC

Meningeal hemorrhage    Ruptured:
Ruptured:               (congenital) cerebral
   berry aneurysm        aneurysm NOS

EXCLUDES    *syphilitic ruptured cerebral aneurysm (094.87)*

CC Excl: 430-432.9, 459.89-459.9, 780.01-780.09, 800.00-801.99, 803.00-804.96, 850.0-852.19, 852.21-854.19

AHA: 4Q, '04, 77

DEF: Bleeding in space between brain and lining.

**431 Intracerebral hemorrhage**   MCC

Hemorrhage (of):      Hemorrhage (of):
   basilar              internal capsule
   bulbar              intrapontine
   cerebellar         pontine
   cerebral           subcortical
   cerebromeningeal   ventricular
   cortical           Rupture of blood vessel in brain

CC Excl: See code: 430

AHA: 4Q, '04, 77

DEF: Bleeding within the brain.

✓4ᵗʰ **432 Other and unspecified intracranial hemorrhage**

AHA: 4Q, '04, 7

**432.0 Nontraumatic extradural hemorrhage**   MCC

Nontraumatic epidural hemorrhage

CC Excl: See code: 430

DEF: Bleeding, nontraumatic, between skull and brain lining.

**432.1 Subdural hemorrhage**   MCC

Subdural hematoma, nontraumatic

CC Excl: See code: 430

DEF: Bleeding, between outermost and other layers of brain lining.

**432.9 Unspecified intracranial hemorrhage**   CC

Intracranial hemorrhage NOS

CC Excl: See code: 430

✓4ᵗʰ **433 Occlusion and stenosis of precerebral arteries**

INCLUDES    embolism
narrowing         } of basilar, carotid, and
obstruction            vertebral arteries
thrombosis

EXCLUDES    *insufficiency NOS of precerebral arteries (435.0-435.9)*

The following fifth-digit subclassification is for use with category 433:

   **0 without mention of cerebral infarction**
   **1 with cerebral infarction**

AHA: 2Q, '95, 14; 3Q, '90, 16

DEF: Blockage, stricture, arteries branching into brain.

✓5ᵗʰ **433.0 Basilar artery**   MCC 1

CC Excl: For code **433.01:** 250.70-250.93, 433.00-433.91, 435.0, 459.89-459.9

✓5ᵗʰ **433.1 Carotid artery**   MCC 1

CC Excl: For code **433.11:** 250.70-250.93, 433.00-433.91, 459.89-459.9

AHA: 1Q, '00, 16; For code **433.10:** 1Q, '06, 17; 1Q, '02, 7, 10

✓5ᵗʰ **433.2 Vertebral artery**   MCC 1

CC Excl: For code **433.21:** 250.70-250.93, 433.00-433.91, 435.1, 459.89-459.9

---

N Newborn Age: 0    P Pediatric Age: 0-17    M Maternity Age: 12-55    A Adult Age: 15-124    CC CC Condition    MCC Major CC Condition    HIV HIV Related Dx

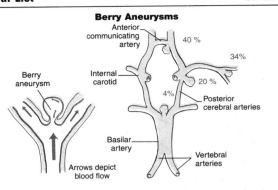

**Berry Aneurysms**

Anterior communicating artery 40 %
34%
Berry aneurysm
Internal carotid 20 %
4%
Posterior cerebral arteries
Basilar artery
Vertebral arteries
Arrows depict blood flow

√5ᵗʰ **433.3**    **Multiple and bilateral**    `MCC 1`

CC Excl: For code 433.31: 250.70-250.93, 433.00-433.91, 459.89-459.9

AHA: 2Q, '02, 19

√5ᵗʰ **433.8**    **Other specified precerebral artery**    `MCC 1`

CC Excl: For code 433.81: 250.70-250.93, 433.00-433.91, 435.0, 459.89-459.9

√5ᵗʰ **433.9**    **Unspecified precerebral artery**    `MCC 1`
Precerebral artery NOS

CC Excl: For code 433.91: 250.70-250.93, 433.00-433.91, 435.0, 459.89-459.9

√4ᵗʰ **434 Occlusion of cerebral arteries**

The following fifth-digit subclassification is for use with category 434:
        **0  without mention of cerebral infarction**
        **1  with cerebral infarction**

AHA: 2Q, '95, 14

√5ᵗʰ **434.0**    **Cerebral thrombosis**    `MCC 1`
Thrombosis of cerebral arteries

CC Excl: For code 434.01: 250.70-250.93, 434.00-434.91, 436, 459.89-459.9

AHA: For code 434.01: 4Q, '04, 77

√5ᵗʰ **434.1**    **Cerebral embolism**    `MCC 1`

CC Excl: For code 434.11: 250.70-250.93, 434.00-434.91, 436, 459.89-459.9

AHA: For code 434.11: 4Q, '04, 77; 3Q, '97, 11

√5ᵗʰ **434.9**    **Cerebral artery occlusion, unspecified**    `MCC 1`

CC Excl: For code 434.91: 250.70-250.93, 434.00-434.91, 436, 459.89-459.9

AHA: For code 434.91: ▶1Q, '07, 23;◀ 4Q, '04, 77-78; 4Q, '98, 87

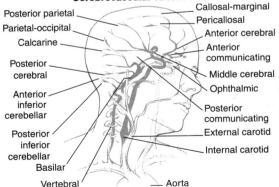

**Cerebrovascular Arteries**

Posterior parietal
Parietal-occipital
Calcarine
Posterior cerebral
Anterior inferior cerebellar
Posterior inferior cerebellar
Basilar
Vertebral
Callosal-marginal
Pericallosal
Anterior cerebral
Anterior communicating
Middle cerebral
Ophthalmic
Posterior communicating
External carotid
Internal carotid
Aorta

√4ᵗʰ **435 Transient cerebral ischemia**

`INCLUDES`    cerebrovascular insufficiency (acute) with transient focal neurological signs and symptoms
insufficiency of basilar, carotid, and vertebral arteries
spasm of cerebral arteries

`EXCLUDES`    *acute cerebrovascular insufficiency NOS (437.1)*
*that due to any condition classifiable to 433 (433.0-433.9)*

**435.0**    **Basilar artery syndrome**    `CC`
CC Excl: 250.70-250.93, 433.00-433.91, 435.0-435.9, 459.89-459.9

**435.1**    **Vertebral artery syndrome**    `CC`
CC Excl: See code: 435.0

**435.2**    **Subclavian steal syndrome**    `CC`
CC Excl: See code: 435.0

DEF: Cerebrovascular insufficiency, due to occluded subclavian artery; symptoms include pain in mastoid and posterior head regions, flaccid paralysis of arm and diminished or absent radial pulse on affected side.

**435.3**    **Vertebrobasilar artery syndrome**    `CC`
CC Excl: See code: 435.0

AHA: 4Q, '95, 60

DEF: Transient ischemic attack; due to brainstem dysfunction; symptoms include confusion, vertigo, binocular blindness, diplopia, unilateral or bilateral weakness and paresthesis of extremities.

**435.8**    **Other specified transient cerebral ischemias**    `CC`
CC Excl: See code: 435.0

**435.9**    **Unspecified transient cerebral ischemia**    `CC`
Impending cerebrovascular accident
Intermittent cerebral ischemia
Transient ischemic attack [TIA]

CC Excl: See code: 435.0

AHA: N-D, '85, 12

**436 Acute, but ill-defined, cerebrovascular disease**    `CC`

Apoplexy, apoplectic:        Apoplexy, apoplectic:
  NOS                              seizure
  attack                         Cerebral seizure
  cerebral

`EXCLUDES`    *any condition classifiable to categories 430-435*
*cerebrovascular accident (434.91)*
*CVA (ischemic) (434.91)*
    *embolic (434.11)*
    *hemorrhagic (430, 431, 432.0-432.9)*
    *thrombotic (434.01)*
*postoperative cerebrovascular accident (997.02)*
*stroke (ischemic) (434.91)*
    *embolic (434.11)*
    *hemorrhagic (430, 431, 432.0-432.9)*
    *thrombotic (434.01)*

CC Excl: 250.70-250.93, 430-432.9, 434.00-434.91, 436, 459.89-459.9, 780.01-780.09, 800.00-801.99, 803.00-804.96, 850.0-852.19, 852.21-854.19

AHA: 4Q, '04, 77; 4Q, '99, 3

√4ᵗʰ **437 Other and ill-defined cerebrovascular disease**

**437.0**    **Cerebral atherosclerosis**    `A`
Atheroma of cerebral arteries
Cerebral arteriosclerosis

**437.1**    **Other generalized ischemic cerebrovascular disease**    `CC`
Acute cerebrovascular insufficiency NOS
Cerebral ischemia (chronic)

CC Excl: 250.70-250.93, 430-432.9, 434.00-436, 437.1, 459.89-459.9

**437.2**    **Hypertensive encephalopathy**    `CC`
CC Excl: 250.70-250.93, 437.2, 459.89-459.9

AHA: J-A, '84, 14

DEF: Cerebral manifestations (such as visual disturbances and headache) due to high blood pressure.

√4ᵗʰ √5ᵗʰ Additional Digit Required    `Unacceptable PDx`    `Manifestation Code`    ▶◀ Revised Text    ● New Code    ▲ Revised Code Title

© 2007 Ingenix                                        October 2007 • Volume 1 — 145

## Map of Major Arteries

**Branches of Abdominal Aorta**

 Newborn Age: 0    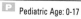 Pediatric Age: 0-17    M Maternity Age: 12-55    A Adult Age: 15-124    CC CC Condition    MCC Major CC Condition    HIV HIV Related Dx

146 — Volume 1

© 2007 Ingenix

**437.3** **Cerebral aneurysm, nonruptured**
Internal carotid artery, intracranial portion
Internal carotid artery NOS
EXCLUDES *congenital cerebral aneurysm,*
*nonruptured (747.81)*
*internal carotid artery, extracranial*
*portion (442.81)*

**437.4** **Cerebral arteritis** `CC`
CC Excl: 250.70-250.93, 437.4, 459.89-459.9

AHA: 4Q, '99, 21
DEF: Inflammation of a cerebral artery or arteries.

**437.5** **Moyamoya disease** `CC`
CC Excl: 250.70-250.93, 437.5, 459.89-459.9

DEF: Cerebrovascular ischemia; vessels occlude and rupture
causing tiny hemorrhages at base of brain; predominantly affects
Japanese.

**437.6** **Nonpyogenic thrombosis of intracranial** `CC`
**venous sinus**
EXCLUDES *pyogenic (325)*
CC Excl: 250.70-250.93, 437.6, 459.89-459.9

**437.7** **Transient global amnesia**
AHA: 4Q, '92, 20
DEF: Episode of short-term memory loss, not often recurrent;
pathogenesis unknown; with no signs or symptoms of neurological
disorder.

**437.8** **Other**
**437.9** **Unspecified**
Cerebrovascular disease or lesion NOS

✓4ᵗʰ **438 Late effects of cerebrovascular disease**
Note: This category is to be used to indicate conditions in
430-437 as the cause of late effects. The "late effects"
include conditions specified as such, as sequelae,
which may occur at any time after the onset of the
causal condition.
EXCLUDES ► *personal history of:*
*cerebral infarction without residual deficits*
*(V12.54)*
*PRIND [Prolonged reversible ischemic*
*neurologic deficit] (V12.54)*
*RIND [Reversible ischemic neurological*
*deficit] (V12.54)*
*transient ischemic attack [TIA] (V12.54)◄*

AHA: 3Q, '06, 3-4; 4Q, '99, 4, 6, 7; 4Q, '98, 39, 88; 4Q, '97, 35, 37;
4Q, '92, 21;N-D,'86, 12; M-A, '86, 7

**438.0** **Cognitive deficits**
✓5ᵗʰ **438.1** **Speech and language deficits**
**438.10** **Speech and language deficit, unspecified**
**438.11** **Aphasia**
AHA: 4Q, '03, 105; 4Q, '97, 36
DEF: Impairment or absence of the ability to
communicate by speech, writing or signs or to
comprehend the spoken or written language due to
disease or injury to the brain. Total aphasia is the loss of
function of both sensory and motor areas of the brain.

**438.12** **Dysphasia**
AHA: 4Q, '99, 3, 9
DEF: Impaired speech; marked by inability to sequence
language.

**438.19** **Other speech and language deficits**
✓5ᵗʰ **438.2** **Hemiplegia/hemiparesis**
DEF: Paralysis of one side of the body.
**438.20** **Hemiplegia affecting unspecified side** `CC`
CC Excl: 438.20

AHA: 4Q, '03, 105; 4Q, '99, 3, 9

**438.21** **Hemiplegia affecting dominant side** `CC`
CC Excl: 438.21

**438.22** **Hemiplegia affecting nondominant side** `CC`
CC Excl: 438.22

AHA: 4Q, '03, 105; 1Q, '02, 16

✓5ᵗʰ **438.3** **Monoplegia of upper limb**
DEF: Paralysis of one limb or one muscle group.
**438.30** **Monoplegia of upper limb affecting**
**unspecified side**
**438.31** **Monoplegia of upper limb affecting**
**dominant side**
**438.32** **Monoplegia of upper limb affecting**
**nondominant side**

✓5ᵗʰ **438.4** **Monoplegia of lower limb**
**438.40** **Monoplegia of lower limb affecting**
**unspecified side**
**438.41** **Monoplegia of lower limb affecting**
**dominant side**
**438.42** **Monoplegia of lower limb affecting**
**nondominant side**

✓5ᵗʰ **438.5** **Other paralytic syndrome**
Use additional code to identify type of paralytic
syndrome, such as:
locked-in state (344.81)
quadriplegia (344.00-344.09)
EXCLUDES *late effects of cerebrovascular accident*
*with:*
*hemiplegia/hemiparesis (438.20-*
*438.22)*
*monoplegia of lower limb (438.40-*
*438.42)*
*monoplegia of upper limb (438.30-*
*438.32)*

**438.50** **Other paralytic syndrome affecting**
**unspecified side**
**438.51** **Other paralytic syndrome affecting**
**dominant side**
**438.52** **Other paralytic syndrome affecting**
**nondominant side**
**438.53** **Other paralytic syndrome, bilateral**
AHA: 4Q, '98, 39

**438.6** **Alterations of sensations**
Use additional code to identify the altered sensation
**438.7** **Disturbances of vision**
Use additional code to identify the visual disturbance
AHA: 4Q, '02, 56

✓5ᵗʰ **438.8** **Other late effects of cerebrovascular disease**
**438.81** **Apraxia**
DEF: Inability to activate learned movements; no known
sensory or motor impairment.

**438.82** **Dysphagia**
►Use additional code to identify the type of
dysphagia, if known (787.20-787.29)◄
DEF: Inability or difficulty in swallowing.

**438.83** **Facial weakness**
Facial droop
**438.84** **Ataxia**
AHA: 4Q, '02, 56

**438.85** **Vertigo**
**438.89** **Other late effects of cerebrovascular disease**
Use additional code to identify the late effect
AHA: 1Q, '05, 13; 4Q, '98, 39

**438.9** **Unspecified late effects of cerebrovascular disease**

---

✓4ᵗʰ ✓5ᵗʰ Additional Digit Required | Unacceptable PDx | Manifestation Code | ►◄ Revised Text | ● New Code | ▲ Revised Code Title

© 2007 Ingenix | October 2007 • Volume 1 — 147

## DISEASES OF ARTERIES, ARTERIOLES, AND CAPILLARIES ▶(440-449)◀

✓4ᵗʰ **440 Atherosclerosis**

INCLUDES
- arteriolosclerosis
- arteriosclerosis (obliterans) (senile)
- arteriosclerotic vascular disease
- atheroma
- degeneration:
  - arterial
  - arteriovascular
  - vascular
- endarteritis deformans or obliterans
- senile:
  - arteritis
  - endarteritis

EXCLUDES     *atheroembolism (445.01-445.89)*
*atherosclerosis of bypass graft of the extremities (440.30-440.32)*

DEF: Stricture and reduced elasticity of an artery; due to plaque deposits.

**440.0   Of aorta**   A
    **AHA:** 2Q, '93, 7; 2Q, '93, 8; 4Q, '88, 8

**440.1   Of renal artery**   A
    EXCLUDES   *atherosclerosis of renal arterioles (403.00-403.91)*

✓5ᵗʰ **440.2   Of native arteries of the extremities**
    ▶Use additional code, if applicable, to identify chronic total occlusion of artery of the extremities (440.4)◀

    EXCLUDES   *atherosclerosis of bypass graft of the extremities (440.30-440.32)*

    **AHA:** 4Q, '94, 49; 4Q, '93, 27; 4Q, '92, 25; 3Q, '90, 15; M-A, '87, 6

**440.20   Atherosclerosis of the extremities, unspecified**   A

**440.21   Atherosclerosis of the extremities with intermittent claudication**   A
    DEF: Atherosclerosis; marked by pain, tension and weakness after walking; no symptoms while at rest.

**440.22   Atherosclerosis of the extremities with rest pain**   A
    INCLUDES   any condition classifiable to 440.21
    DEF: Atherosclerosis, marked by pain, tension and weakness while at rest.

**440.23   Atherosclerosis of the extremities with ulceration**   A
    INCLUDES   any condition classifiable to 440.21 and 440.22
    Use additional code for any associated ulceration (707.10-707.9)
    **AHA:** 4Q, '00, 44

**440.24   Atherosclerosis of the extremities with gangrene**   CC
    INCLUDES   any condition classifiable to 440.21, 440.22, and 440.23 with ischemic gangrene 785.4
    Use additional code for any associated ulceration (707.10-707.9)
    EXCLUDES   *gas gangrene (040.0)*
    **CC Excl:** 338.0-338.4, 440.24, 780.91-780.99, 785.4, 799.81-799.89
    **AHA:** 4Q, '03, 109; 3Q, '03, 14; 4Q, '95, 54; 1Q, '95, 11

**440.29   Other**   A

✓5ᵗʰ **440.3   Of bypass graft of extremities**
    EXCLUDES   *atherosclerosis of native arteries of the extremities (440.21-440.24)*
*embolism [occlusion NOS] [thrombus] of graft (996.74)*
    **AHA:** 4Q, '94, 49

**440.30   Of unspecified graft**   A
**440.31   Of autologous vein bypass graft**   A
**440.32   Of nonautologous biological bypass graft**   A

● **440.4   Chronic total occlusion of artery of the extremities**
    Complete occlusion of artery of the extremities
    Total occlusion of artery of the extremities
    Code first atherosclerosis of arteries of the extremities (440.20-440.29, 440.30-440.32)
    EXCLUDES   *acute occlusion of artery of extremity (444.21-444.22)*

**440.8   Of other specified arteries**   A
    EXCLUDES
- *basilar (433.0)*
- *carotid (433.1)*
- *cerebral (437.0)*
- *coronary (414.00-414.07)*
- *mesenteric (557.1)*
- *precerebral (433.0-433.9)*
- *pulmonary (416.0)*
- *vertebral (433.2)*

**440.9   Generalized and unspecified atherosclerosis**   A
    Arteriosclerotic vascular disease NOS
    EXCLUDES   *arteriosclerotic cardiovascular disease [ASCVD] (429.2)*

✓4ᵗʰ **441 Aortic aneurysm and dissection**
    EXCLUDES   *syphilitic aortic aneurysm (093.0)*
*traumatic aortic aneurysm (901.0, 902.0)*

✓5ᵗʰ **441.0   Dissection of aorta**
    **AHA:** 4Q, '89, 10
    DEF: Dissection or splitting of wall of the aorta; due to blood entering through intimal tear or interstitial hemorrhage.

**441.00   Unspecified site**   MCC
    **CC Excl:** 250.70-250.93, 441.00-441.9, 459.89-459.9

**441.01   Thoracic**   MCC
    **CC Excl:** See code: 441.00

**441.02   Abdominal**   MCC
    **CC Excl:** See code: 441.00

**441.03   Thoracoabdominal**   MCC
    **CC Excl:** See code: 441.00

**441.1   Thoracic aneurysm, ruptured**   MCC
    **CC Excl:** See code: 441.00

**441.2   Thoracic aneurysm without mention of rupture**
    **AHA:** 3Q, '92, 10

**441.3   Abdominal aneurysm, ruptured**   MCC
    **CC Excl:** See code: 441.00

**441.4   Abdominal aneurysm without mention of rupture**
    **AHA:** 4Q, '00, 64; 1Q, '99, 15, 16, 17; 3Q, '92, 10

**441.5   Aortic aneurysm of unspecified site, ruptured**   MCC
    Rupture of aorta NOS
    **CC Excl:** See code: 441.00

**441.6   Thoracoabdominal aneurysm, ruptured**   MCC
    **CC Excl:** See code: 441.00

### Thoracic and Abdominal Aortic Aneurysm

Thoracic aneurysm

Abdominal aneurysm

Aorta

N Newborn Age: 0    P Pediatric Age: 0-17    M Maternity Age: 12-55    A Adult Age: 15-124     CC CC Condition    MCC Major CC Condition    HIV HIV Related Dx

148 — Volume 1 • October 2007

© 2007 Ingenix

**441.7**   **Thoracoabdominal aneurysm, without mention of rupture**
AHA: 2Q, '06, 16

**441.9**   **Aortic aneurysm of unspecified site without mention of rupture**
Aneurysm
Dilatation         } of aorta
Hyaline necrosis

√4th **442 Other aneurysm**
INCLUDES   aneurysm (ruptured) (cirsoid) (false) (varicose)
aneurysmal varix
EXCLUDES   *arteriovenous aneurysm or fistula:*
*acquired (447.0)*
*congenital (747.60-747.69)*
*traumatic (900.0-904.9)*

DEF: Dissection or splitting of arterial wall; due to blood entering through intimal tear or interstitial hemorrhage.

**442.0**   **Of artery of upper extremity**
**442.1**   **Of renal artery**
**442.2**   **Of iliac artery**
AHA: 1Q, '99, 16, 17

**442.3**   **Of artery of lower extremity**
Aneurysm:
femoral      } artery
popliteal
AHA: 3Q, '02, 24-26; 1Q, '99, 16

√5th **442.8**   **Of other specified artery**
**442.81 Artery of neck**
Aneurysm of carotid artery (common) (external) (internal, extracranial portion)
EXCLUDES   *internal carotid artery, intra-cranial portion (437.3)*

**442.82 Subclavian artery**
**442.83 Splenic artery**
**442.84 Other visceral artery**
Aneurysm:
celiac
gastroduodenal
gastroepiploic
hepatic                    } artery
pancreaticoduodenal
superior mesenteric

**442.89 Other**
Aneurysm:
mediastinal   } artery
spinal
EXCLUDES   *cerebral (nonruptured) (437.3)*
*congenital (747.81)*
*ruptured (430)*
*coronary (414.11)*
*heart (414.10)*
*pulmonary (417.1)*

**442.9**   **Of unspecified site**

√4th **443 Other peripheral vascular disease**
**443.0**   **Raynaud's syndrome**
Raynaud's:          Raynaud's:
disease             phenomenon (secondary)
Use additional code to identify gangrene (785.4)
DEF: Constriction of the arteries, due to cold or stress; bilateral ischemic attacks of fingers, toes, nose or ears; symptoms include pallor, paresthesia and pain; more common in females.

**443.1**   **Thromboangiitis obliterans [Buerger's disease]**
Presenile gangrene
DEF: Inflammatory disease of extremity blood vessels, mainly the lower; occurs primarily in young men and leads to tissue ischemia and gangrene.

√5th **443.2**   **Other arterial dissection**
EXCLUDES   *dissection of aorta (441.00-441.03)*
*dissection of coronary arteries (414.12)*
AHA: 4Q, '02, 54

**443.21 Dissection of carotid artery**        MCC
CC Excl: 447.2, 447.5-447.9

**443.22 Dissection of iliac artery**          MCC
CC Excl: See code: 443.21

**443.23 Dissection of renal artery**          MCC
CC Excl: See code: 443.21

**443.24 Dissection of vertebral artery**      MCC
CC Excl: See code: 443.21

**443.29 Dissection of other artery**          MCC
CC Excl: See code: 443.21

√5th **443.8**   **Other specified peripheral vascular diseases**
**443.81 *Peripheral angiopathy in diseases classified elsewhere***
*Code first underlying disease, as:*
diabetes mellitus (250.7)
AHA: 1Q, '04, 14; 3Q, '91, 10

**443.82 Erythromelalgia**
AHA: 4Q, '05, 73
DEF: Rare syndrome of paroxysmal vasodilation; maldistribution of blood flow causes redness, pain, increased skin temperature, and burning sensations in various parts of the body.

**443.89 Other**
Acrocyanosis            Erythrocyanosis
Acroparesthesia:
simple [Schultze's type]
vasomotor [Nothnagel's type]
EXCLUDES   *chilblains (991.5)*
*frostbite (991.0-991.3)*
*immersion foot (991.4)*

**443.9**   **Peripheral vascular disease, unspecified**
Intermittent claudication NOS
Peripheral:
angiopathy NOS
vascular disease NOS
Spasm of artery
EXCLUDES   *atherosclerosis of the arteries of the extremities (440.20-440.22)*
*spasm of cerebral artery (435.0-435.9)*
AHA: 4Q, '92, 25; 3Q, '91, 10

√4th **444 Arterial embolism and thrombosis**
INCLUDES   infarction:
embolic
thrombotic
occlusion
EXCLUDES   *atheroembolism (445.01-445.89)*
*that complicating:*
*abortion (634-638 with .6, 639.6)*
*ectopic or molar pregnancy (639.6)*
*pregnancy, childbirth, or the pueperium (673.0-673.8)*
►*septic arterial embolism (449)*◄
AHA: 2Q, '92, 11; 4Q, '90, 27

**444.0**   **Of abdominal aorta**              CC
Aortic bifurcation syndrome     Leriche's syndrome
Aortoiliac obstruction          Saddle embolus
CC Excl: 250.70-250.93, 444.0, 444.89-444.9, 449, 459.89-459.9
AHA: 2Q, '93, 7; 4Q, '90, 27

**444.1**   **Of thoracic aorta**              CC
Embolism or thrombosis of aorta (thoracic)
CC Excl: 250.70-250.93, 444.1, 444.89-444.9, 449, 459.89-459.9

---

√4th Additional Digit Required
√5th
© 2007 Ingenix

Unacceptable PDx          Manifestation Code          ◄► Revised Text          ● New Code          ▲ Revised Code Title

**Map of Major Veins**

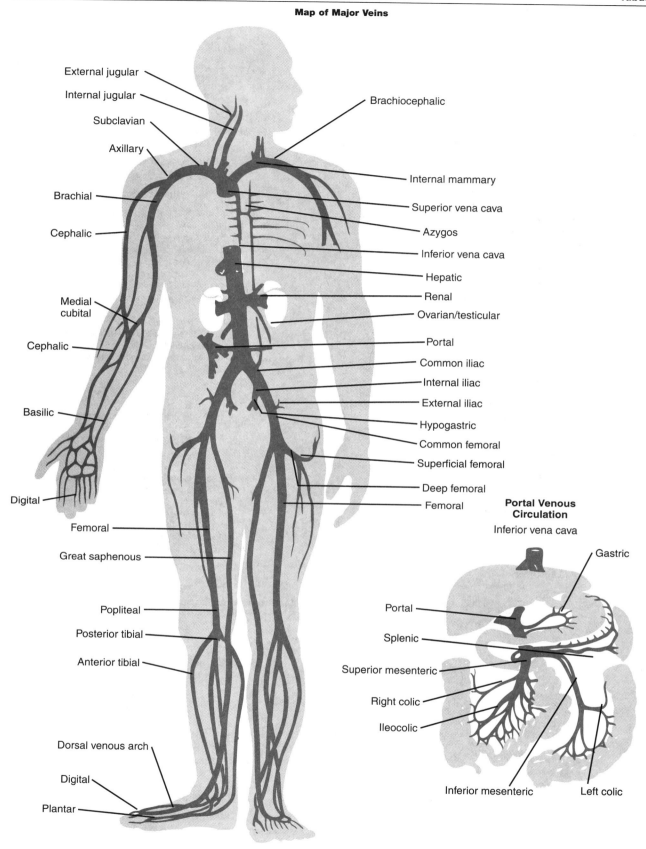

Portal Venous
Circulation

### Arterial Diseases and Disorders

Lipids
Calcium deposits

Intimal proliferation

Atherosclerosis narrowing lumen

Thrombus (clot) forming in lumen

Organization of thrombus and recanalization

Embolus (from elsewhere) occluding lumen

Aneurysm bypasses lumen or...

...bulges from arterial wall

Arteriovenous fistula

√5ᵗʰ **444.2 Of arteries of the extremities**
AHA: M-A, '87, 6

  **444.21 Upper extremity** `CC`
    CC Excl: 250.70-250.93, 444.21, 444.89-444.9, 449, 459.89-459.9

  **444.22 Lower extremity** `CC`
    Arterial embolism or thrombosis:
      femoral
      peripheral NOS
      popliteal
    *EXCLUDES*   *iliofemoral (444.81)*
    CC Excl: 250.70-250.93, 444.22, 444.89-444.9, 449, 459.89-459.9

    AHA: 3Q, '03, 10; 1Q, '03, 17; 3Q, '90, 16

√5ᵗʰ **444.8 Of other specified artery**
  **444.81 Iliac artery** `CC`
    CC Excl: 250.70-250.93, 444.81-444.9, 449, 459.89-459.9
    AHA: 1Q, '03, 16

  **444.89 Other** `CC`
    *EXCLUDES*   *basilar (433.0)*
                *carotid (433.1)*
                *cerebral (434.0-434.9)*
                *coronary (410.00-410.92)*
                *mesenteric (557.0)*
                *ophthalmic (362.30-362.34)*
                *precerebral (433.0-433.9)*
                *pulmonary (415.19)*
                *renal (593.81)*
                *retinal (362.30-362.34)*
                *vertebral (433.2)*
    CC Excl: 250.70-250.93, 444.89-444.9, 449, 459.89-459.9

**444.9 Of unspecified artery** `CC`
  CC Excl: See code: 444.89

√4ᵗʰ **445 Atheroembolism**
  *INCLUDES*   atherothrombotic microembolism
                  cholesterol embolism
  AHA: 4Q, '02, 57

√5ᵗʰ **445.0 Of extremities**
  **445.01 Upper extremity** `CC`
    CC Excl: 250.70-250.93, 444.89-445.01, 449, 459.89-459.9

  **445.02 Lower extremity** `CC`
    CC Excl: 250.70-250.93, 444.89-444.9, 445.02, 449, 459.89-459.9

√5ᵗʰ **445.8 Of other sites**
  **445.81 Kidney** `CC`
    Use additional code for any associated acute renal failure or chronic kidney disease (584, 585)
    CC Excl: 250.70-250.93, 444.89-444.9, 445.81, 449, 459.89-459.9

  **445.89 Other site** `CC`
    CC Excl: 250.70-250.93, 444.89-444.9, 445.89, 449, 459.89-459.9

√4ᵗʰ **446 Polyarteritis nodosa and allied conditions**
  **446.0 Polyarteritis nodosa** `CC`
    Disseminated necrotizing periarteritis
    Necrotizing angiitis
    Panarteritis (nodosa)
    Periarteritis (nodosa)
    CC Excl: 250.70-250.93, 446.0-446.7, 459.89-459.9

    DEF: Inflammation of small and mid-size arteries; symptoms related to involved arteries in kidneys, muscles, gastrointestinal tract and heart; results in tissue death.

  **446.1 Acute febrile mucocutaneous lymph node syndrome [MCLS]** `CC`
    Kawasaki disease
    CC Excl: 446.0-446.29, 446.4-446.7, 459.89-459.9

    DEF: Acute febrile disease of children; marked by erythema of conjunctiva and mucous membranes of upper respiratory tract, skin eruptions and edema.

√5ᵗʰ **446.2 Hypersensitivity angiitis**
    *EXCLUDES*   *antiglomerular basement membrane disease without pulmonary hemorrhage (583.89)*

  **446.20 Hypersensitivity angiitis, unspecified** `CC`
    CC Excl: See code: 446.0

  **446.21 Goodpasture's syndrome** `CC`
    Antiglomerular basement membrane antibody-mediated nephritis with pulmonary hemorrhage
    Use additional code to identify renal disease (583.81)
    CC Excl: See code: 446.0

    DEF: Glomerulonephritis associated with hematuria, progresses rapidly; results in death from renal failure.

  **446.29 Other specified hypersensitivity angiitis** `CC`
    CC Excl: See code: 446.0

    AHA: 1Q, '95, 3

  **446.3 Lethal midline granuloma** `CC`
    Malignant granuloma of face
    CC Excl: See code: 446.0

    DEF: Granulomatous lesion; in nose or paranasal sinuses; often fatal; occurs chiefly in males.

  **446.4 Wegener's granulomatosis** `CC`
    Necrotizing respiratory granulomatosis
    Wegener's syndrome
    CC Excl: See code: 446.0

    AHA: 3Q, '00, 11

    DEF: A disease occurring mainly in men; marked by necrotizing granulomas and ulceration of the upper respiratory tract; underlying condition is a vasculitis affecting small vessels and is possibly due to an immune disorder.

  **446.5 Giant cell arteritis**
    Bagratuni's syndrome     Horton's disease
    Cranial arteritis         Temporal arteritis
    DEF: Inflammation of arteries; due to giant cells affecting carotid artery branches, resulting in occlusion; symptoms include fever, headache and neurological problems; occurs in elderly.

  **446.6 Thrombotic microangiopathy** `MCC`
    Moschcowitz's syndrome
    Thrombotic thrombocytopenic purpura
    CC Excl: See code: 446.0

    DEF: Blockage of small blood vessels; due to hyaline deposits; symptoms include purpura, CNS disorders; results in protracted disease or rapid death.

√4ᵗʰ √5ᵗʰ Additional Digit Required     Unacceptable PDx     Manifestation Code     ►◄ Revised Text     ● New Code     ▲ Revised Code Title

**446.7** **Takayasu's disease** `CC`
Aortic arch arteritis    Pulseless disease
**CC Excl:** See code: 446.0

DEF: Progressive obliterative arteritis of brachiocephalic trunk, left subclavian, and left common carotid arteries above aortic arch; results in ischemia in brain, heart and arm; pulses impalpable in head, neck and arms; more common in young adult females.

√4ᵗʰ **447 Other disorders of arteries and arterioles**

**447.0** **Arteriovenous fistula, acquired**
Arteriovenous aneurysm, acquired
**EXCLUDES** cerebrovascular (437.3)
coronary (414.19)
pulmonary (417.0)
surgically created arteriovenous shunt
or fistula:
complication (996.1, 996.61-996.62)
status or presence (V45.1)
traumatic (900.0-904.9)

DEF: Communication between an artery and vein caused by error in healing.

**447.1** **Stricture of artery**
**AHA:** 2Q, '93, 8; M-A, '87, 6

**447.2** **Rupture of artery** `CC`
Erosion
Fistula, except arteriovenous } of artery
Ulcer
**EXCLUDES** traumatic rupture of artery (900.0-904.9)
**CC Excl:** 414.12, 443.22-443.29, 447.2

**447.3** **Hyperplasia of renal artery**
Fibromuscular hyperplasia of renal artery
DEF: Overgrowth of cells in muscular lining of renal artery.

**447.4** **Celiac artery compression syndrome** `CC`
Celiac axis syndrome
Marable's syndrome
**CC Excl:** 447.4

**447.5** **Necrosis of artery** `CC`
**CC Excl:** 447.5

**447.6** **Arteritis, unspecified**
Aortitis NOS
Endarteritis NOS
**EXCLUDES** arteritis, endarteritis:
aortic arch (446.7)
cerebral (437.4)
coronary (414.00-414.07)
deformans (440.0-440.9)
obliterans (440.0-440.9)
pulmonary (417.8)
senile (440.0-440.9)
polyarteritis NOS (446.0)
syphilitic aortitis (093.1)
**AHA:** 1Q, '95, 3

**447.8** **Other specified disorders of arteries and arterioles**
Fibromuscular hyperplasia of arteries, except renal

**447.9** **Unspecified disorders of arteries and arterioles**

√4ᵗʰ **448 Disease of capillaries**

**448.0** **Hereditary hemorrhagic telangiectasia**
Rendu-Osler-Weber disease
DEF: Genetic disease with onset after puberty; results in multiple telangiectases, dilated venules on skin and mucous membranes; recurrent bleeding may occur.

**448.1** **Nevus, non-neoplastic**
Nevus:
araneus
senile
spider
stellar
**EXCLUDES** neoplastic (216.0-216.9)
port wine (757.32)
strawberry (757.32)

DEF: Enlarged or malformed blood vessels of skin; results in reddish swelling, skin patch, or birthmark.

**448.9** **Other and unspecified capillary diseases**
Capillary:
hemorrhage
hyperpermeability
thrombosis
**EXCLUDES** capillary fragility (hereditary) (287.8)

● **449 Septic arterial embolism** `CC`
Code first underlying infection, such as:
infective endocarditis (421.0)
lung abscess (513.0)
Use additional code to identify the site of the embolism (433.0-433.9, 444.0-444.9)
**EXCLUDES** septic pulmonary embolism (415.12)
**CC Excl:** 250.70-250.93, 444.89-444.9, 449, 459.89-459.9

## DISEASES OF VEINS AND LYMPHATICS, AND OTHER DISEASES OF CIRCULATORY SYSTEM (451-459)

√4ᵗʰ **451 Phlebitis and thrombophlebitis**
**INCLUDES** endophlebitis
inflammation, vein
periphlebitis
suppurative phlebitis
Use additional E code to identify drug, if drug-induced
**EXCLUDES** that complicating:
abortion (634-638 with .7, 639.8)
ectopic or molar pregnancy (639.8)
pregnancy, childbirth, or the puerperium
(671.0-671.9)
that due to or following:
implant or catheter device (996.61-996.62)
infusion, perfusion, or transfusion (999.2)
**AHA:** 1Q, '92, 16

DEF: Inflammation of a vein (phlebitis) with formation of a thrombus (thrombophlebitis).

**451.0** **Of superficial vessels of lower extremities**
Saphenous vein (greater) (lesser)
**AHA:** 3Q, '91, 16

√5ᵗʰ **451.1** **Of deep vessels of lower extremities**
**AHA:** 3Q, '91, 16

**451.11** **Femoral vein (deep) (superficial)** `CC`
**CC Excl:** 250.70-250.93, 451.0-451.9, 459.89-459.9

**451.19** **Other** `CC`
Femoropopliteal vein
Popliteal vein
Tibial vein
**CC Excl:** 250.70-250.93, 451.0-451.9, 459.89-459.9

**451.2** **Of lower extremities, unspecified**
**AHA:** 4Q, '04, 80

√5ᵗʰ **451.8** **Of other sites**
**EXCLUDES** intracranial venous sinus (325)
nonpyogenic (437.6)
portal (vein) (572.1)

**451.81** **Iliac vein** `CC`
**CC Excl:** See code: 451.19

**451.82** **Of superficial veins of upper extremities**
Antecubital vein
Basilic vein
Cephalic vein

---

N Newborn Age: 0    P Pediatric Age: 0-17    M Maternity Age: 12-55    A Adult Age: 15-124    `CC` CC Condition    `MCC` Major CC Condition    `HIV` HIV Related Dx

**451.83  Of deep veins of upper extremities**  `CC`
Brachial vein
Radial vein
Ulnar vein
**CC Excl:** 451.0-451.2, 451.83, 451.89-451.9

**451.84  Of upper extremities, unspecified**
**451.89  Other**  `CC`
Axillary vein
Jugular vein
Subclavian vein
Thrombophlebitis of breast (Mondor's disease)
**CC Excl:** 451.0-451.2, 451.89-451.9

**451.9  Of unspecified site**

**452  Portal vein thrombosis**  `MCC`
Portal (vein) obstruction
> **EXCLUDES**  hepatic vein thrombosis (453.0)
> phlebitis of portal vein (572.1)

**CC Excl:** 250.70-250.93, 452, 453.40-453.9, 459.89-459.9

**DEF:** Formation of a blood clot in main vein of liver.

**453  Other venous embolism and thrombosis**  ✓4th
> **EXCLUDES**  that complicating:
> abortion (634-638 with .7, 639.8)
> ectopic or molar pregnancy (639.8)
> pregnancy, childbirth, or the puerperium
> (671.0-671.9)
> that with inflammation, phlebitis, and
> thrombophlebitis (451.0-451.9)

**AHA:** 1Q, '92, 16

**453.0  Budd-Chiari syndrome**  `MCC`
Hepatic vein thrombosis
**CC Excl:** 250.70-250.93, 453.0, 453.40-453.9, 459.89-459.9

**DEF:** Thrombosis or other obstruction of hepatic vein; symptoms include enlarged liver, extensive collateral vessels, intractable ascites and severe portal hypertension.

**453.1  Thrombophlebitis migrans**  `CC`
**CC Excl:** 250.70-250.93, 453.1, 453.40-453.9, 459.89-459.9

**DEF:** Slow, advancing thrombophlebitis; appearing first in one vein then another.

**453.2  Of vena cava**  `MCC`
**CC Excl:** 250.70-250.93, 453.2, 453.40-453.9, 459.89-459.9

**453.3  Of renal vein**  `CC`
**CC Excl:** 250.70-250.93, 453.3-453.9, 459.89-459.9

**453.4  Venous embolism and thrombosis of deep vessels of lower extremity**  ✓5th
**453.40  Venous embolism and thrombosis of unspecified deep vessels of lower extremity**  `CC`
Deep vein thrombosis NOS
DVT NOS
**CC Excl:** 250.70-250.93, 453.40-453.9, 459.89-459.9

**453.41  Venous embolism and thrombosis of deep vessels of proximal lower extremity**  `CC`
Femoral        Thigh
Iliac          Upper leg NOS
Popliteal
**CC Excl:** See code: 453.40

**AHA:** 4Q, '04, 79

**453.42  Venous embolism and thrombosis of deep vessels of distal lower extremity**  `CC`
Calf
Lower leg NOS
Peroneal
Tibial
**CC Excl:** See code: 453.40

**453.8  Of other specified veins**  `CC`
> **EXCLUDES**  cerebral (434.0-434.9)
> coronary (410.00-410.92)
> intracranial venous sinus (325)
> nonpyogenic (437.6)
> mesenteric (557.0)
> portal (452)
> precerebral (433.0-433.9)
> pulmonary (415.19)

**CC Excl:** See code: 453.40

**AHA:** 3Q, '91, 16; M-A, '87, 6

**453.9  Of unspecified site**  `CC`
Embolism of vein
Thrombosis (vein)
**CC Excl:** See code: 453.40

**454  Varicose veins of lower extremities**  ✓4th
> **EXCLUDES**  that complicating pregnancy, childbirth, or the
> puerperium (671.0)

**AHA:** 2Q, '91, 20

**DEF:** Dilated leg veins; due to incompetent vein valves that allow reversed blood flow and cause tissue erosion or weakness of wall; may be painful.

**454.0  With ulcer**  `A`
Varicose ulcer (lower extremity, any part)
Varicose veins with ulcer of lower extremity [any part] or of unspecified site
Any condition classifiable to 454.9 with ulcer or specified as ulcerated

**AHA:** 4Q, '99, 18

**454.1  With inflammation**  `A`
Stasis dermatitis
Varicose veins with inflammation of lower extremity [any part] or of unspecified site
Any condition classifiable to 454.9 with inflammation or specified as inflamed

**454.2  With ulcer and inflammation**  `CC` `A`
Varicose veins with ulcer and inflammation of lower extremity [any part] or of unspecified site
Any condition classifiable to 454.9 with ulcer and inflammation
**CC Excl:** 454.0-454.2, 454.9

**454.8  With other complications**
Edema          Swelling
Pain
**AHA:** 4Q, '02, 58

**454.9  Asymptomatic varicose veins**  `A`
Phlebectasia ⎫
Varicose veins ⎬ of lower extremity [any part]
Varix ⎭ or of unspecified site
Varicose veins NOS

**AHA:** 4Q, '02, 58

**455  Hemorrhoids**  ✓4th
> **INCLUDES**  hemorrhoids (anus) (rectum)
> piles
> varicose veins, anus or rectum

> **EXCLUDES**  that complicating pregnancy, childbirth, or the
> puerperium (671.8)

**DEF:** Varicose condition of external hemorrhoidal veins causing painful swellings at the anus.

**455.0  Internal hemorrhoids without mention of complication**
**AHA:** 3Q, '05, 17

**455.1  Internal thrombosed hemorrhoids**

**455.2  Internal hemorrhoids with other complication**
Internal hemorrhoids:     Internal hemorrhoids:
bleeding                  strangulated
prolapsed                 ulcerated
**AHA:** 3Q, '05, 17; 1Q, '03, 8

**Circulatory System**

**455.3–458.9**

**455.3 External hemorrhoids without mention of complication**
AHA: ▶1Q, '07, 13;◀ 3Q, '05, 17

**455.4 External thrombosed hemorrhoids**

**455.5 External hemorrhoids with other complication**
External hemorrhoids:     External hemorrhoids:
  bleeding                  strangulated
  prolapsed                 ulcerated
AHA: 3Q, '05, 17; 1Q, '03, 8

**455.6 Unspecified hemorrhoids without mention of complication**
Hemorrhoids NOS

**455.7 Unspecified thrombosed hemorrhoids**
Thrombosed hemorrhoids, unspecified whether internal or external

**455.8 Unspecified hemorrhoids with other complication**
Hemorrhoids, unspecified whether internal or external:
  bleeding
  prolapsed
  strangulated
  ulcerated

**455.9 Residual hemorrhoidal skin tags**
Skin tags, anus or rectum

**√4ᵗʰ 456 Varicose veins of other sites**

**456.0 Esophageal varices with bleeding** `MCC`
CC Excl: 251.5, 456.0, 456.20, 459.89-459.9, 530.20-530.21, 530.7, 530.82, 530.85, 531.00-534.91, 535.01, 535.11, 535.21, 535.31, 535.41, 535.51, 535.61, 537.83, 562.02-562.03, 562.12-562.13, 569.3, 569.85, 578.0-578.9

DEF: Distended, tortuous, veins of lower esophagus, usually due to portal hypertension.

**456.1 Esophageal varices without mention of bleeding** `CC`
CC Excl: 251.5, 456.0-456.20, 459.89-459.9, 530.7, 530.82, 531.00-534.91, 535.01, 535.11, 535.21, 535.31, 535.41, 535.51, 535.61, 537.83, 578.0-578.9

**√5ᵗʰ 456.2 Esophageal varices in diseases classified elsewhere**
Code first underlying cause, as:
  cirrhosis of liver (571.0-571.9)
  portal hypertension (572.3)

  **456.20 With bleeding** `MCC`
  CC Excl: 456.0, 456.20, 459.89-459.9, 530.82
  AHA: N-D, '85, 14

  **456.21 Without mention of bleeding** `CC`
  CC Excl: 251.5, 456.0, 456.20-456.21, 459.89-459.9, 530.7, 530.82, 531.00-534.91, 535.01, 535.11, 535.21, 535.31, 535.41, 535.51, 535.61, 537.83, 578.0-578.9
  AHA: 3Q, '05, 15; 2Q, '02, 4

**456.3 Sublingual varices**
DEF: Distended, tortuous veins beneath tongue.

**456.4 Scrotal varices** ♂
Varicocele

**456.5 Pelvic varices**
Varices of broad ligament

**456.6 Vulval varices** ♀
Varices of perineum
  EXCLUDES that complicating pregnancy, childbirth, or the puerperium (671.1)

**456.8 Varices of other sites**
Varicose veins of nasal septum (with ulcer)
  EXCLUDES placental varices (656.7)
  retinal varices (362.17)
  varicose ulcer of unspecified site (454.0)
  varicose veins of unspecified site (454.9)
AHA: 2Q, '02, 4

**√4ᵗʰ 457 Noninfectious disorders of lymphatic channels**

**457.0 Postmastectomy lymphedema syndrome** `A`
Elephantiasis
Obliteration of lymphatic vessel } due to mastectomy

AHA: 2Q, '02, 12
DEF: Reduced lymphatic circulation following mastectomy; symptoms include swelling of the arm on the operative side.

**457.1 Other lymphedema**
Elephantiasis          Lymphedema:
  (nonfilarial) NOS    praecox
Lymphangiectasis       secondary
Lymphedema:            Obliteration, lymphatic vessel
  acquired (chronic)
  EXCLUDES elephantiasis (nonfilarial):
    congenital (757.0)
    eyelid (374.83)
    vulva (624.8)

AHA: 3Q, '04, 5
DEF: Fluid retention due to reduced lymphatic circulation; due to other than mastectomy.

**457.2 Lymphangitis**
Lymphangitis:
  NOS
  chronic
  subacute
  EXCLUDES acute lymphangitis (682.0-682.9)

**457.8 Other noninfectious disorders of lymphatic channels**
Chylocele (nonfilarial)  Lymph node or vessel:
Chylous:                 fistula
  ascites               infarction
  cyst                  rupture
  EXCLUDES chylocele:
    filarial (125.0-125.9)
    tunica vaginalis (nonfilarial) (608.84)

AHA: 1Q, '04, 5; 3Q, '03, 17

**457.9 Unspecified noninfectious disorder of lymphatic channels**

**√4ᵗʰ 458 Hypotension**
  INCLUDES hypopiesis
  EXCLUDES cardiovascular collapse (785.50)
    maternal hypotension syndrome (669.2)
    shock (785.50-785.59)
    Shy-Drager syndrome (333.0)

**458.0 Orthostatic hypotension**
Hypotension:
  orthostatic (chronic)
  postural
AHA: 3Q, '00, 8; 3Q, '91, 9
DEF: Low blood pressure; occurs when standing.

**458.1 Chronic hypotension**
Permanent idiopathic hypotension
DEF: Persistent low blood pressure.

**√5ᵗʰ 458.2 Iatrogenic hypotension**
AHA: 4Q, '03, 60; 3Q, '02, 12; 4Q, '95, 57
DEF: Abnormally low blood pressure; due to medical treatment.

  **458.21 Hypotension of hemodialysis**
  Intra-dialytic hypotension
  AHA: 4Q, '03, 61

  **458.29 Other iatrogenic hypotension**
  Postoperative hypotension

**458.8 Other specified hypotension**
AHA: 4Q, '97, 37

**458.9 Hypotension, unspecified**
Hypotension (arterial) NOS

---

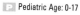

`N` Newborn Age: 0  `P` Pediatric Age: 0-17  `M` Maternity Age: 12-55  `A` Adult Age: 15-124  `CC` CC Condition  `MCC` Major CC Condition  `HIV` HIV Related Dx

**√4ᵗʰ 459 Other disorders of circulatory system**

**459.0 Hemorrhage, unspecified**
Rupture of blood vessel NOS
Spontaneous hemorrhage NEC

EXCLUDES hemorrhage:
gastrointestinal NOS (578.9)
in newborn NOS (772.9)
secondary or recurrent following
trauma (958.2)
traumatic rupture of blood vessel
(900.0-904.9)

AHA: 4Q, '90, 26

**√5ᵗʰ 459.1 Postphlebitic syndrome**
Chronic venous hypertension due to deep vein
thrombosis

EXCLUDES chronic venous hypertension without
deep vein thrombosis (459.30-
459.39)

AHA: 4Q, '02, 58; 2Q, '91, 20

DEF: Various conditions following deep vein thrombosis; including
edema, pain, stasis dermatitis, cellulitis, varicose veins and
ulceration of the lower leg.

**459.10 Postphlebitic syndrome without
complications**
Asymptomatic postphlebitic syndrome
Postphlebitic syndrome NOS

**459.11 Postphlebitic syndrome with ulcer** CC
CC Excl: 451.0-451.9

**459.12 Postphlebitic syndrome with inflammation**

**459.13 Postphlebitic syndrome with ulcer** CC
**and inflammation**
CC Excl: See code: 459.11

**459.19 Postphlebitic syndrome with other
complication**

**459.2 Compression of vein** CC
Stricture of vein
Vena cava syndrome (inferior) (superior)
CC Excl: 459.2

**√5ᵗʰ 459.3 Chronic venous hypertension (idiopathic)**
Stasis edema

EXCLUDES chronic venous hypertension due to
deep vein thrombosis
(459.10-459.9)
varicose veins (454.0-454.9)

AHA: 4Q, '02, 59

**459.30 Chronic venous hypertension without
complications**
Asymptomatic chronic venous hypertension
Chronic venous hypertension NOS

**459.31 Chronic venous hypertension** CC
**with ulcer**
CC Excl: 454.0-454.2, 454.9, 459.81-459.9

AHA: 4Q, '02, 43

**459.32 Chronic venous hypertension with
inflammation**

**459.33 Chronic venous hypertension with** CC
**ulcer and inflammation**
CC Excl: See code: 459.31

**459.39 Chronic venous hypertension with other
complication**

**√5ᵗʰ 459.8 Other specified disorders of circulatory system**
**459.81 Venous (peripheral) insufficiency,
unspecified**
Chronic venous insufficiency NOS
Use additional code for any associated
ulceration (707.10-707.9)

AHA: 3Q, '04, 5; 2Q, '91, 20; M-A, '87, 6

DEF: Insufficient drainage, venous blood, any part of
body, results in edema or dermatosis.

**459.89 Other**
Collateral circulation (venous), any site
Phlebosclerosis
Venofibrosis

**459.9 Unspecified circulatory system disorder**

# 8. DISEASES OF THE RESPIRATORY SYSTEM (460-519)

Use additional code to identify infectious organism

## ACUTE RESPIRATORY INFECTIONS (460-466)

**EXCLUDES** *pneumonia and influenza* ▶*(480.0-488)*◀

### 460 Acute nasopharyngitis [common cold]

Coryza (acute)
Nasal catarrh, acute
Nasopharyngitis:
  NOS
  acute
Nasopharyngitis:
  infective NOS
Rhinitis:
  acute
  infective

**EXCLUDES** *nasopharyngitis, chronic (472.2)*
*pharyngitis:*
  *acute or unspecified (462)*
  *chronic (472.1)*
*rhinitis:*
  *allergic (477.0-477.9)*
  *chronic or unspecified (472.0)*
*sore throat:*
  *acute or unspecified (462)*
  *chronic (472.1)*

**AHA:** 1Q, '88, 12

**DEF:** Acute inflammation of mucous membranes; extends from nares to pharynx.

### ✓4th 461 Acute sinusitis

**INCLUDES**
abscess
empyema
infection
inflammation
suppuration
} acute, of sinus
(accessory)
(nasal)

**EXCLUDES** *chronic or unspecified sinusitis (473.0-473.9)*

**461.0 Maxillary**
  Acute antritis
**461.1 Frontal**
**461.2 Ethmoidal**
**461.3 Sphenoidal**
**461.8 Other acute sinusitis**
  Acute pansinusitis
**461.9 Acute sinusitis, unspecified**
  Acute sinusitis NOS

### 462 Acute pharyngitis

Acute sore throat NOS
Pharyngitis (acute):
  NOS
  gangrenous
  infective
  phlegmonous
  pneumococcal
Pharyngitis (acute):
  staphylococcal
  suppurative
  ulcerative
Sore throat (viral) NOS
Viral pharyngitis

**EXCLUDES** *abscess:*
  *peritonsillar [quinsy] (475)*
  *pharyngeal NOS (478.29)*
  *retropharyngeal (478.24)*
*chronic pharyngitis (472.1)*
*infectious mononucleosis (075)*
*that specified as (due to):*
  *Coxsackie (virus) (074.0)*
  *gonococcus (098.6)*
  *herpes simplex (054.79)*
  *influenza (487.1)*
  *septic (034.0)*
  *streptococcal (034.0)*

**AHA:** 4Q, '99, 26; S-O, '85, 8

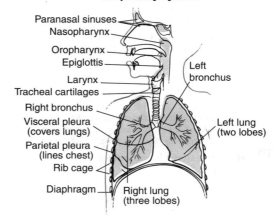

**Respiratory System**

### 463 Acute tonsillitis

Tonsillitis (acute):
  NOS
  follicular
  gangrenous
  infective
  pneumococcal
Tonsillitis (acute):
  septic
  staphylococcal
  suppurative
  ulcerative
  viral

**EXCLUDES** *chronic tonsillitis (474.0)*
*hypertrophy of tonsils (474.1)*
*peritonsillar abscess [quinsy] (475)*
*sore throat:*
  *acute or NOS (462)*
  *septic (034.0)*
*streptococcal tonsillitis (034.0)*

**AHA:** N-D, '84, 16

### ✓4th 464 Acute laryngitis and tracheitis

**EXCLUDES** *that associated with influenza (487.1)*
*that due to Streptococcus (034.0)*

#### ✓5th 464.0 Acute laryngitis

Laryngitis (acute):
  NOS
  edematous
  Hemophilus influenzae [H. influenzae]
  pneumococcal
  septic
  suppurative
  ulcerative

**EXCLUDES** *chronic laryngitis (476.0-476.1)*
*influenzal laryngitis (487.1)*

**464.00 Without mention of obstruction**
**464.01 With obstruction** `MCC`
  **CC Excl:** 012.20-012.86, 464.00-464.31, 579.8-519.9

#### ✓5th 464.1 Acute tracheitis

Tracheitis (acute):
  NOS
  catarrhal
Tracheitis (acute):
  viral

**EXCLUDES** *chronic tracheitis (491.8)*

**464.10 Without mention of obstruction**
**464.11 With obstruction** `MCC`
  **CC Excl:** 012.20-012.86, 017.90-017.96, 464.00-464.31, 519.8-519.9

#### ✓5th 464.2 Acute laryngotracheitis

Laryngotracheitis (acute)
Tracheitis (acute) with laryngitis (acute)

**EXCLUDES** *chronic laryngotracheitis (476.1)*

**464.20 Without mention of obstruction**
**464.21 With obstruction** `MCC`
  **CC Excl:** See code 464.11

---

**Respiratory System**

**464.3–472.2**

√5th **464.3  Acute epiglottitis**
Viral epiglottitis
EXCLUDES  *epiglottitis, chronic (476.1)*

**464.30  Without mention of obstruction**  CC
CC Excl: 464.01, 464.30-464.31, 464.51

**464.31  With obstruction**  MCC
CC Excl: See code 464.11

**464.4  Croup**
Croup syndrome
DEF: Acute laryngeal obstruction due to allergy, foreign body or infection; symptoms include barking cough, hoarseness and harsh, persistent high-pitched respiratory sound.

√5th **464.5  Supraglottitis, unspecified**
AHA: 4Q, '01, 42

DEF: A rapidly advancing generalized upper respiratory infection of the lingual tonsillar area, epiglottic folds, false vocal cords, and the epiglottis; seen most commonly in children, but can affect people of any age.

**464.50  Without mention of obstruction**
AHA: 4Q, '01, 43

**464.51  With obstruction**  MCC
CC Excl: 012.20-012.86, 017.90-017.96, 464.00-464.31, 519.8-519.9

√4th **465  Acute upper respiratory infections of multiple or unspecified sites**
EXCLUDES  *upper respiratory infection due to:*
*influenza (487.1)*
*Streptococcus (034.0)*

**465.0  Acute laryngopharyngitis**
DEF: Acute infection of the vocal cords and pharynx.

**465.8  Other multiple sites**
Multiple URI

**465.9  Unspecified site**
Acute URI NOS
Upper respiratory infection (acute)

√4th **466  Acute bronchitis and bronchiolitis**
INCLUDES  that with:
bronchospasm
obstruction

**466.0  Acute bronchitis**

Bronchitis, acute
or subacute:
fibrinous
membranous
pneumococcal
purulent
septic

Bronchitis, acute
or subacute:
viral
with tracheitis
Croupous bronchitis
Tracheobronchitis, acute

EXCLUDES  *acute bronchitis with chronic obstructive pulmonary disease (491.22)*

AHA: 4Q, '04, 137; 1Q, '04, 3; 4Q, '02, 46; 4Q, '96, 28; 4Q, '91, 24; 1Q, '88, 12

DEF: Acute inflammation of main branches of bronchial tree due to infectious or irritant agents; symptoms include cough with a varied production of sputum, fever, substernal soreness, and lung rales.

√5th **466.1  Acute bronchiolitis**
Bronchiolitis (acute)   Capillary pneumonia
DEF: Acute inflammation of finer subdivisions of bronchial tree due to infectious or irritant agents; symptoms include cough with a varied production of sputum, fever, substernal soreness, and lung rales.

**466.11  Acute bronchiolitis due to respiratory syncytial virus (RSV)**  CC
CC Excl: 466.11

AHA: 1Q, '05, 10; 4Q, '96, 27

**466.19  Acute bronchiolitis due to other infectious organisms**  CC
Use additional code to identify organism
CC Excl: 466.0-466.19

## OTHER DISEASES OF THE UPPER RESPIRATORY TRACT (470-478)

**470  Deviated nasal septum**
Deflected septum (nasal) (acquired)
EXCLUDES  *congenital (754.0)*

√4th **471  Nasal polyps**
EXCLUDES  *adenomatous polyps (212.0)*

**471.0  Polyp of nasal cavity**
Polyp:                    Polyp:
choanal                nasopharyngeal

**471.1  Polypoid sinus degeneration**
Woakes' syndrome or ethmoiditis

**471.8  Other polyp of sinus**
Polyp of sinus:
accessory
ethmoidal
maxillary
sphenoidal

**471.9  Unspecified nasal polyp**
Nasal polyp NOS

√4th **472  Chronic pharyngitis and nasopharyngitis**
**472.0  Chronic rhinitis**

Ozena                    Rhinitis:
Rhinitis:                    hypertrophic
NOS                    obstructive
atrophic                    purulent
granulomatous        ulcerative

EXCLUDES  *allergic rhinitis (477.0-477.9)*
DEF: Persistent inflammation of mucous membranes of nose.

**472.1  Chronic pharyngitis**
Chronic sore throat      Pharyngitis:
Pharyngitis:                    granular (chronic)
atrophic                    hypertrophic

**472.2  Chronic nasopharyngitis**
EXCLUDES  *acute or unspecified nasopharyngitis (460)*
DEF: Persistent inflammation of mucous membranes extending from nares to pharynx.

**Upper Respiratory System**

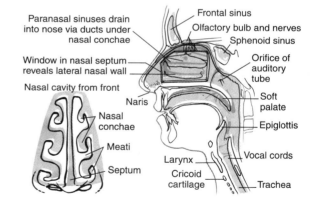

Paranasal sinuses drain into nose via ducts under nasal conchae

Window in nasal septum reveals lateral nasal wall

Nasal cavity from front

Naris

Nasal conchae

Meati

Septum

Frontal sinus

Olfactory bulb and nerves

Sphenoid sinus

Orifice of auditory tube

Soft palate

Epiglottis

Vocal cords

Larynx

Cricoid cartilage

Trachea

---

N Newborn Age: 0    P Pediatric Age: 0-17    M Maternity Age: 12-55    A Adult Age: 15-124    CC CC Condition    MCC Major CC Condition    HIV HIV Related Dx

158 — Volume 1 • October 2007                                            © 2007 *Ingenix*

**Paranasal Sinuses**

Frontal
Ethmoid
Sphenoid
Maxillary

Frontal
Ethmoid
Sphenoid

Maxillary

√4th **473 Chronic sinusitis**

INCLUDES  abscess
empyema
infection
suppuration  (chronic) of sinus
(accessory) (nasal)

EXCLUDES  acute sinusitis (461.0-461.9)

473.0 **Maxillary**
Antritis (chronic)
473.1 **Frontal**
473.2 **Ethmoidal**
EXCLUDES  Woakes' ethmoiditis (471.1)
473.3 **Sphenoidal**
473.8 **Other chronic sinusitis**
Pansinusitis (chronic)
473.9 **Unspecified sinusitis (chronic)**
Sinusitis (chronic) NOS

√4th **474 Chronic disease of tonsils and adenoids**
√5th 474.0 **Chronic tonsillitis and adenoiditis**
EXCLUDES  acute or unspecified tonsillitis (463)

AHA: 4Q, '97, 38

474.00 **Chronic tonsillitis**
474.01 **Chronic adenoiditis**
474.02 **Chronic tonsillitis and adenoiditis**
√5th 474.1 **Hypertrophy of tonsils and adenoids**
Enlargement
Hyperplasia  of tonsils or adenoids
Hypertrophy

EXCLUDES  that with:
adenoiditis (474.01)
adenoiditis and tonsillitis (474.02)
tonsillitis (474.00)

474.10 **Tonsils with adenoids**
AHA: 2Q, '05, 16

474.11 **Tonsils alone**
474.12 **Adenoids alone**
474.2 **Adenoid vegetations**
DEF: Fungus-like growth of lymph tissue between the nares and pharynx.

474.8 **Other chronic disease of tonsils and adenoids**
Amygdalolith          Tonsillar tag
Calculus, tonsil       Ulcer, tonsil
Cicatrix of tonsil (and adenoid)
474.9 **Unspecified chronic disease of tonsils and adenoids**
Disease (chronic) of tonsils (and adenoids)
475 **Peritonsillar abscess**    CC
Abscess of tonsil          Quinsy
Peritonsillar cellulitis
EXCLUDES  tonsillitis:
acute or NOS (463)
chronic (474.0)

CC Excl: 475, 519.8-519.9

√4th **476 Chronic laryngitis and laryngotracheitis**
476.0 **Chronic laryngitis**
Laryngitis:          Laryngitis:
catarrhal            sicca
hypertrophic
476.1 **Chronic laryngotracheitis**
Laryngitis, chronic, with tracheitis (chronic)
Tracheitis, chronic, with laryngitis
EXCLUDES  chronic tracheitis (491.8)
laryngitis and tracheitis, acute or
unspecified (464.00-464.51)

√4th **477 Allergic rhinitis**
INCLUDES  allergic rhinitis (nonseasonal) (seasonal)
hay fever
spasmodic rhinorrhea
EXCLUDES  allergic rhinitis with asthma (bronchial) (493.0)
DEF: True immunoglobulin E (IgE)-mediated allergic reaction of nasal mucosa;
seasonal (typical hay fever) or perennial (year-round allergens: dust, food,
dander).

477.0 **Due to pollen**
Pollinosis
477.1 **Due to food**
AHA: 4Q, '00, 42

477.2 **Due to animal (cat) (dog) hair and dander**
477.8 **Due to other allergen**
477.9 **Cause unspecified**
AHA: 2Q, '97, 9

√4th **478 Other diseases of upper respiratory tract**
478.0 **Hypertrophy of nasal turbinates**
DEF: Overgrowth, enlargement of shell-shaped bones, in nasal cavity.

√5th 478.1 **Other diseases of nasal cavity and sinuses**
EXCLUDES  varicose ulcer of nasal septum (456.8)
478.11 **Nasal mucositis (ulcerative)**
Use additional E code to identify adverse
effects of therapy, such as:
antineoplastic and immunosuppressive
drugs (E930.7, E933.1)
radiation therapy (E879.2)
AHA: 4Q, '06, 88-90

478.19 **Other diseases of nasal cavity and sinuses**
Abscess
Necrosis  of nose (septum)
Ulcer

Cyst or mucocele of sinus (nasal)
Rhinolith
AHA: 4Q, '06, 88-90

√5th 478.2 **Other diseases of pharynx, not elsewhere classified**
478.20 **Unspecified disease of pharynx**
478.21 **Cellulitis of pharynx or nasopharynx**    CC
CC Excl: 478.20-478.24, 519.8-519.9

478.22 **Parapharyngeal abscess**    CC
CC Excl: See code: 478.21

478.24 **Retropharyngeal abscess**    CC
CC Excl: See code 478.21

DEF: Purulent infection, behind pharynx and front of
precerebral fascia.

478.25 **Edema of pharynx or nasopharynx**
478.26 **Cyst of pharynx or nasopharynx**
478.29 **Other**
Abscess of pharynx or nasopharynx
EXCLUDES  ulcerative pharyngitis (462)

√5th 478.3 **Paralysis of vocal cords or larynx**
DEF: Loss of motor ability of vocal cords or larynx; due to nerve or
muscle damage.

478.30 **Paralysis, unspecified**
Laryngoplegia    Paralysis of glottis

**Respiratory System**

478.31 Unilateral, partial
478.32 Unilateral, complete
478.33 Bilateral, partial
478.34 Bilateral, complete   `CC`

**CC Excl:** 478.30-478.34, 478.5, 478.70, 519.8-519.9

**478.4 Polyp of vocal cord or larynx**

`EXCLUDES`   adenomatous polyps (212.1)

**478.5 Other diseases of vocal cords**

Abscess
Cellulitis
Granuloma  } of vocal cords
Leukoplakia

Chorditis (fibrinous) (nodosa) (tuberosa)
Singers' nodes

**478.6 Edema of larynx**

Edema (of):       Edema (of):
glottis           supraglottic
subglottic

**√5ᵗʰ 478.7 Other diseases of larynx, not elsewhere classified**

**478.70 Unspecified disease of larynx**

**478.71 Cellulitis and perichondritis of larynx**   `CC`

**CC Excl:** 478.70-478.71, 478.79

**DEF:** Inflammation of deep soft tissues or lining of bone of the larynx.

**478.74 Stenosis of larynx**

**478.75 Laryngeal spasm**

Laryngismus (stridulus)

**DEF:** Involuntary muscle contraction of the larynx.

**478.79 Other**

Abscess
Necrosis
Obstruction  } of larynx
Pachyderma
Ulcer

`EXCLUDES`   ulcerative laryngitis (464.00-464.01)

**AHA:** 3Q, '91, 20

**478.8 Upper respiratory tract hypersensitivity reaction, site unspecified**

`EXCLUDES`   hypersensitivity reaction of lower respiratory tract, as:
extrinsic allergic alveolitis (495.0-495.9)
pneumoconiosis (500-505)

**478.9 Other and unspecified diseases of upper respiratory tract**

Abscess
Cicatrix  } of trachea

**Lungs**

Right Lung (Three Lobes) — Trachea — Left Lung (Two Lobes)
Bronchopulmonary segments: — Primary bronchus
Upper lobe — Secondary bronchus
Middle lobe — S1 S3 — S1,2 — S3/S4/S5 Upper lobe
Lower lobe — S2 — S5 — S4 — S6 — S7,8 Lower lobe
Diaphragm — S8 — S9 S10 S7 S10 — S9

---

**PNEUMONIA AND INFLUENZA ▶(480-488)◀**

`EXCLUDES`   pneumonia:
allergic or eosinophilic (518.3)
aspiration:
NOS (507.0)
newborn (770.18)
solids and liquids (507.0-507.8)
congenital (770.0)
lipoid (507.1)
passive (514)
rheumatic (390)

**√4ᵗʰ 480 Viral pneumonia**

**480.0 Pneumonia due to adenovirus**   `MCC`

**CC Excl:** 011.00-012.16, 012.80-012.86, 017.90-017.96, 020.3-020.5, 021.3, 022.1, 031.0, 039.1, 073.0, 115.05, 115.15, 115.95, 122.1, 130.4, 136.3, 480.0-487.1, 488, 495.0-495.9, 500-508.9, 517.1, 517.8, 518.89, 519.8-519.9

**480.1 Pneumonia due to respiratory syncytial virus**   `MCC`

**CC Excl:** See code: 480.0

**AHA:** 4Q, '96, 28; 1Q, '88, 12

**480.2 Pneumonia due to parainfluenza virus**   `MCC`

**CC Excl:** See code: 480.0

**480.3 Pneumonia due to SARS-associated coronavirus**   `MCC`

**CC Excl:** 011.00-012.16, 012.80-012.86, 017.90-017.96, 021.2, 031.0, 039.1, 115.05, 115.15, 115.95, 122.1, 130.4, 136.3, 480.0-487.1, 488, 494.0-508.9, 517.1, 517.8, 518.89, 519.8-519.9, 748.61

**AHA:** 4Q, '03, 46-47

**DEF:** A severe adult respiratory syndrome caused by the coronavirus, specified as inflammation of the lungs with consolidation.

**480.8 Pneumonia due to other virus not elesewhere classified**   `MCC` `HIV`

`EXCLUDES`   congenital rubella pneumonitis (771.0)
influenza with pneumonia, any form (487.0)
pneumonia complicating viral diseases classified elsewhere (484.1-484.8)

**CC Excl:** See code: 480.0

**480.9 Viral pneumonia, unspecified**   `MCC` `HIV`

**CC Excl:** See code: 480.0

**AHA:** 3Q, '98, 5

**481 Pneumococcal pneumonia [Streptococcus pneumoniae pneumonia]**   `MCC` `HIV`

Lobar pneumonia, organism unspecified

**CC Excl:** 011.00-012.16, 012.80-012.86, 017.90-017.96, 021.2, 031.0, 039.1, 115.05, 115.15, 115.95, 122.1, 130.4, 136.3, 480.0-480.2, 480.8-487.1, 488, 494.0-508.9, 517.1, 517.8, 518.89, 519.8-519.9, 748.61

**AHA:** 2Q, '98, 7; 4Q, '92, 19; 1Q, '92, 18; 1Q, '91, 13; 1Q, '88, 13; M-A, '85, 6

**√4ᵗʰ 482 Other bacterial pneumonia**

**AHA:** 4Q, '93, 39

**482.0 Pneumonia due to Klebsiella pneumoniae**   `MCC` `HIV`

**CC Excl:** See code 481

**482.1 Pneumonia due to Pseudomonas**   `MCC` `HIV`

**CC Excl:** See code 481

**482.2 Pneumonia due to Hemophilus influenzae [H. influenzae]**   `MCC` `HIV`

**CC Excl:** See code 481

**AHA:** 2Q, '05, 19

**√5ᵗʰ 482.3 Pneumonia due to Streptococcus**

`EXCLUDES`   Streptococcus pneumoniae (481)

**AHA:** 1Q, '88, 13

**482.30 Streptococcus, unspecified**   `MCC` `HIV`

**CC Excl:** See code 481

---

`N` Newborn Age: 0    `P` Pediatric Age: 0-17    `M` Maternity Age: 12-55    `A` Adult Age: 15-124    `CC` CC Condition    `MCC` Major CC Condition    `HIV` HIV Related Dx

282.31 **Group A** `MCC` `HIV`
CC Excl: See code 481

482.32 **Group B** `MCC` `HIV`
CC Excl: See code 481

482.39 **Other Streptococcus** `MCC` `HIV`
CC Excl: See code 481

√5ᵗʰ 482.4 **Pneumonia due to Staphylococcus**
AHA: 3Q, '91, 16

482.40 **Pneumonia due to Staphylococcus, unspecified** `MCC` `HIV`
CC Excl: See code 481

482.41 **Pneumonia due to Staphylococcus aureus** `MCC` `HIV`
CC Excl: See code 481

482.49 **Other Staphylococcus pneumonia** `MCC` `HIV`
CC Excl: See code 481

√5ᵗʰ 482.8 **Pneumonia due to other specified bacteria**
**EXCLUDES** *pneumonia, complicating infectious disease classified elsewhere (484.1-484.8)*

AHA: 3Q, '88, 11

482.81 **Anaerobes** `MCC` `HIV`
Bacteroides (melaninogenicus)
Gram-negative anaerobes
CC Excl: See code 481

482.82 **Escherichia coli [E. coli]** `MCC` `HIV`
CC Excl: See code 481

482.83 **Other gram-negative bacteria** `MCC` `HIV`
Gram-negative pneumonia NOS
Proteus
Serratia marcescens
**EXCLUDES** *gram-negative anaerobes (482.81)*
*Legionnaires' disease (482.84)*

CC Excl: See code 481

AHA: 2Q, '98, 5; 3Q, '94, 9

482.84 **Legionnaires' disease** `MCC` `HIV`
CC Excl: See code 481

AHA: 4Q, '97, 38

DEF: Severe and often fatal infection by Legionella pneumophilia; symptoms include high fever, gastrointestinal pain, headache, myalgia, dry cough, and pneumonia; transmitted airborne via air conditioning systems, humidifiers, water faucets, shower heads; not person-to-person contact.

482.89 **Other specified bacteria** `MCC` `HIV`
CC Excl: See code 481

AHA: 2Q, '97, 6

482.9 **Bacterial pneumonia unspecified** `MCC` `HIV`
CC Excl: See code 481

AHA: 2Q, '98, 6; 2Q, '97, 6; 1Q, '94, 17

√4ᵗʰ 483 **Pneumonia due to other specified organism**
AHA: N-D, '87, 5

483.0 **Mycoplasma pneumoniae** `MCC`
Eaton's agent
Pleuropneumonia-like organism [PPLO]
CC Excl: See code 481

483.1 **Chlamydia** `MCC`
CC Excl: See code 481

AHA: 4Q, '96, 31

483.8 **Other specified organism** `MCC`
CC Excl: See code 481

√4ᵗʰ 484 **Pneumonia in infectious diseases classified elsewhere**
**EXCLUDES** *influenza with pneumonia, any form (487.0)*

484.1 *Pneumonia in cytomegalic inclusion disease* `MCC`
*Code first underlying disease (078.5)*
CC Excl: See code 481

484.3 *Pneumonia in whooping cough* `MCC`
*Code first underlying disease (033.0-033.9)*
CC Excl: See code 481

484.5 *Pneumonia in anthrax* `MCC`
*Code first underlying disease (022.1)*
CC Excl: See code 481

484.6 *Pneumonia in aspergillosis* `MCC`
*Code first underlying disease (117.3)*
CC Excl: See code 481

AHA: 4Q, '97, 40

484.7 *Pneumonia in other systemic mycoses* `MCC`
*Code first underlying disease*
**EXCLUDES** *pneumonia in:*
*candidiasis (112.4)*
*coccidioidomycosis (114.0)*
*histoplasmosis (115.0-115.9 with fifth-digit 5)*

CC Excl: See code 481

484.8 *Pneumonia in other infectious diseases classified elsewhere* `MCC`
*Code first underlying disease, as:*
Q fever (083.0)
typhoid fever (002.0)
**EXCLUDES** *pneumonia in:*
*actinomycosis (039.1)*
*measles (055.1)*
*nocardiosis (039.1)*
*ornithosis (073.0)*
*Pneumocystis carinii (136.3)*
*salmonellosis (003.22)*
*toxoplasmosis (130.4)*
*tuberculosis (011.6)*
*tularemia (021.2)*
*varicella (052.1)*

CC Excl: See code 481

485 **Bronchopneumonia, organism unspecified** `MCC`
Bronchopneumonia:  Pneumonia:
hemorrhagic  lobular
terminal  segmental
Pleurobronchopneumonia
**EXCLUDES** *bronchiolitis (acute) (466.11-466.19)*
*chronic (491.8)*
*lipoid pneumonia (507.1)*
CC Excl: See code 481

√4ᵗʰ √5ᵗʰ Additional Digit Required      Unacceptable PDx      Manifestation Code      ►◄ Revised Text      ● New Code      ▲ Revised Code Title

**Respiratory System**

**486–491.9**

**486 Pneumonia, organism unspecified** `MCC` `HIV`

EXCLUDES   *hypostatic or passive pneumonia (514)*
*influenza with pneumonia, any form (487.0)*
*inhalation or aspiration pneumonia due to*
*    foreign materials (507.0-507.8)*
*pneumonitis due to fumes and vapors (506.0)*

**CC Excl:** 011.00-012.16, 012.80-012.86, 017.90-017.96, 021.2, 031.0, 039.1, 115.05, 115.15, 115.95, 122.1, 130.4, 136.3, 480.0-480.2, 480.8-487.1, 488, 494.0-508.9, 517.1, 517.8, 518.89, 519.8-519.9, 748.61

**AHA:** 4Q, '99, 6; 3Q, '99, 9; 3Q, '98, 7; 2Q, '98, 4, 5; 1Q, '98, 8; 3Q, '97, 9;
    3Q, '94, 10; 3Q, '88, 11

✓4ᵗʰ **487 Influenza**

EXCLUDES   *Hemophilus influenzae [H. influenzae]:*
*    infection NOS (041.5)*
*▶influenza due to identified avian influenza*
*    virus (488)◀*
*laryngitis (464.00-464.01)*
*meningitis (320.0)*

**487.0   With pneumonia** `MCC`
Influenza with pneumonia, any form
Influenzal:
  bronchopneumonia
  pneumonia
Use additional code to identify the type of
    pneumonia (480.0-480.9, 481, 482.0-482.9,
    483.0-483.8, 485)

**CC Excl:** See code 486

**AHA:** 1Q, '06, 18; 2Q, '05, 18

**487.1   With other respiratory manifestations**
Influenza NOS
Influenzal:
  laryngitis
  pharyngitis
  respiratory infection (upper) (acute)

**AHA:** 1Q, '06, 18; 2Q, '05, 18; 4Q, '99, 26

**487.8   With other manifestations**
Encephalopathy due to influenza
Influenza with involvement of gastrointestinal tract

EXCLUDES   *"intestinal flu" [viral gastroenteritis]*
*    (008.8)*

● **488 Influenza due to identified avian influenza virus**
Note: Influenza caused by influenza viruses that normally
    infect only birds and, less commonly, other animals

EXCLUDES   *influenza caused by other influenza viruses*
*    (487)*

## CHRONIC OBSTRUCTIVE PULMONARY DISEASE AND ALLIED CONDITIONS (490-496)

**AHA:** 3Q, '88, 5

**490 Bronchitis, not specified as acute or chronic**
Bronchitis NOS:         Tracheobronchitis NOS
  catarrhal
  with tracheitis NOS

EXCLUDES   *bronchitis:*
*    allergic NOS (493.9)*
*    asthmatic NOS (493.9)*
*    due to fumes and vapors (506.0)*

**Bronchioli and Alveoli**

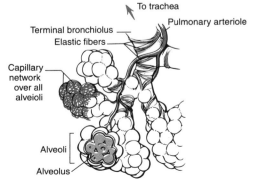

To trachea
Pulmonary arteriole
Terminal bronchiolus
Elastic fibers
Capillary network over all alveioli
Alveoli
Alveolus

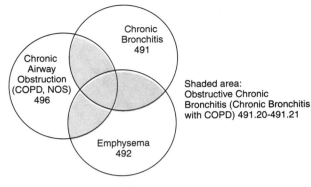

**Interrelationship Between Chronic Airway Obstruction, Chronic Bronchitis, and Emphysema**

Chronic Bronchitis 491

Chronic Airway Obstruction (COPD, NOS) 496

Emphysema 492

Shaded area:
Obstructive Chronic
Bronchitis (Chronic Bronchitis
with COPD) 491.20-491.21

✓4ᵗʰ **491 Chronic bronchitis**

EXCLUDES   *chronic obstructive asthma (493.2)*

**491.0   Simple chronic bronchitis**
Catarrhal bronchitis, chronic
Smokers' cough

**491.1   Mucopurulent chronic bronchitis**
Bronchitis (chronic) (recurrent):
  fetid
  mucopurulent
  purulent

**AHA:** 3Q, '88, 12

**DEF:** Chronic bronchial infection characterized by both mucus and
pus secretions in the bronchial tree; recurs after asymptomatic
periods; signs are coughing, expectoration and secondary changes
in the lung.

✓5ᵗʰ **491.2   Obstructive chronic bronchitis**
Bronchitis:
  emphysematous
  obstructive (chronic) (diffuse)
Bronchitis with:
  chronic airway obstruction
  emphysema

EXCLUDES   *asthmatic bronchitis (acute) NOS*
*    (493.9)*
*chronic obstructive asthma (493.2)*

**AHA:** 3Q, '97, 9; 4Q, '91, 25; 2Q, '91, 21

**491.20   Without exacerbation**
Emphysema with chronic bronchitis

**AHA:** 3Q, '97, 9

**491.21   With (acute) exacerbation** `CC`
Acute exacerbation of chronic obstructive
    pulmonary disease [COPD]
Decompensated chronic obstructive
    pulmonary disease [COPD]
Decompensated chronic obstructive
    pulmonary disease [COPD] with
    exacerbation

EXCLUDES   *chronic obstructive asthma*
*    with acute exacerbation*
*    (493.22)*

**CC Excl:** 491.1-491.9, 493.20-493.21

**AHA:** 1Q, '04, 3; 3Q, '02, 18, 19; 4Q, '01, 43; 2Q, '96, 10

**491.22   With acute bronchitis** `CC`
**CC Excl:** See code 491.21

**AHA:** 3Q, '06, 20; 4Q, '04, 82

**491.8   Other chronic bronchitis**
Chronic:
  tracheitis
  tracheobronchitis

**491.9   Unspecified chronic bronchitis**

---

`N` Newborn Age: 0     `P` Pediatric Age: 0-17     `M` Maternity Age: 12-55     `A` Adult Age: 15-124     `CC` CC Condition     `MCC` Major CC Condition     `HIV` HIV Related Dx

√4ᵗʰ **492 Emphysema**
AHA: 2Q, '91, 21

**492.0 Emphysematous bleb**
Giant bullous emphysema
Ruptured emphysematous bleb
Tension pneumatocele
Vanishing lung
AHA: 2Q, '93, 3

DEF: Formation of vesicle or bulla in emphysematous lung, more than one millimeter; contains serum or blood.

**492.8 Other emphysema**

Emphysema (lung or pulmonary):
NOS
centriacinar
centrilobular
obstructive
panacinar
panlobular

Emphysema (lung or pulmonary):
unilateral
vesicular
MacLeod's syndrome
Swyer-James syndrome
Unilateral hyperlucent lung

EXCLUDES   emphysema:
  with chronic bronchitis (491.20-491.22)
  compensatory (518.2)
  due to fumes and vapors (506.4)
  interstitial (518.1)
    newborn (770.2)
  mediastinal (518.1)
  surgical (subcutaneous) (998.81)
  traumatic (958.7)

AHA: 1Q, '05, 4; 4Q, '93, 41; J-A, '84, 17

√4ᵗʰ **493 Asthma**
EXCLUDES   wheezing NOS (786.07)

The following fifth-digit subclassification is for use with codes 493.0-493.2, 493.9:
  **0 unspecified**
  **1 with status asthmaticus**
  **2 with (acute) exacerbation**

AHA: 4Q, '04, 137; 4Q, '03, 62; 4Q, '01, 43; 4Q, '00, 42; 1Q, '91, 13; 3Q, '88, 9; J-A, '85, 8; N-D, '84, 17

DEF: Status asthmaticus: severe, intractable episode of asthma unresponsive to normal therapeutic measures.

√5ᵗʰ **493.0 Extrinsic asthma**    CC 1-2

Asthma:
allergic with
  stated cause
atopic
childhood

Asthma:
hay
platinum
Hay fever with asthma

EXCLUDES   asthma:
  allergic NOS (493.9)
  detergent (507.8)
  miners' (500)
  wood (495.8)

CC Excl: For code 493.01 and 493.02: 493.00-493.92, 517.8, 518.89, 519.8-519.9

DEF: Transient stricture of airway diameters of bronchi; due to environmental factor; also called allergic (bronchial) asthma.

√5ᵗʰ **493.1 Intrinsic asthma**    CC 1-2
Late-onset asthma
CC Excl: For code 493.11 and 493.12: See code 493.01

AHA: 3Q, '88, 9; M-A, '85, 7

DEF: Transient stricture, of airway diameters of bronchi; due to pathophysiological disturbances.

√5ᵗʰ **493.2 Chronic obstructive asthma**    CC 1-2
Asthma with chronic obstructive pulmonary disease [COPD]
Chronic asthmatic bronchitis
EXCLUDES   acute bronchitis (466.0)
  chronic obstructive bronchitis (491.20-491.22)

CC Excl: For code 493.21: 491.1-493.92, 517.8, 518.89, 519.8-519.9; For code 493.22: 493.00-493.92, 517.8, 518.89, 519.8-519.9

AHA: 2Q, '91, 21; 2Q, '90, 20; For code 493.20: 4Q, '03, 108; For code 493.22: 3Q, '06, 20

DEF: Persistent narrowing of airway diameters in the bronchial tree, restricting airflow and causing constant labored breathing.

√5ᵗʰ **493.8 Other forms of asthma**
AHA: 4Q, '03, 62

**493.81 Exercise induced bronchospasm**
**493.82 Cough variant asthma**

√5ᵗʰ **493.9 Asthma, unspecified**    CC 1-2
Asthma (bronchial) (allergic NOS)
Bronchitis:
  allergic
  asthmatic

CC Excl: For code 493.91 and 493.92: 493.00-493.92, 517.8, 518.89, 519.8-519.9

AHA: 4Q, '97, 40, For code 493.90: 4Q, '04, 137; 4Q, '03, 108; 4Q, '99, 25; 1Q, '97, 7; For code 493.91: 1Q, '05, 5; For code 493.92: 1Q, '03, 9

√4ᵗʰ **494 Bronchiectasis**
Bronchiectasis (fusiform) (postinfectious) (recurrent)
Bronchiolectasis
EXCLUDES   congenital (748.61)
  tuberculous bronchiectasis (current disease) (011.5)

AHA: 4Q, '00, 42

DEF: Dilation of bronchi; due to infection or chronic conditions; causes decreased lung capacity and recurrent infections of lungs.

**494.0 Bronchiectasis without acute exacerbation**
**494.1 Bronchiectasis with acute exacerbation**    CC
CC Excl: 017.90-017.96, 487.1, 488, 494.1, 496, 506.1, 506.4-506.9, 748.61

√4ᵗʰ **495 Extrinsic allergic alveolitis**
INCLUDES   allergic alveolitis and pneumonitis due to inhaled organic dust particles of fungal, thermophilic actinomycete, or other origin

DEF: Pneumonitis due to particles inhaled into lung, often at workplace; symptoms include cough, chills, fever, increased heart and respiratory rates; develops within hours of exposure.

**495.0 Farmers' lung**
**495.1 Bagassosis**
**495.2 Bird-fanciers' lung**
Budgerigar-fanciers' disease or lung
Pigeon-fanciers' disease or lung
**495.3 Suberosis**
Cork-handlers' disease or lung
**495.4 Malt workers' lung**
Alveolitis due to Aspergillus clavatus
**495.5 Mushroom workers' lung**
**495.6 Maple bark-strippers' lung**
Alveolitis due to Cryptostroma corticale

---

**Respiratory System**

**495.7-508.8**

**495.7 "Ventilation" pneumonitis** `CC`

Allergic alveolitis due to fungal, thermophilic actinomycete, and other organisms growing in ventilation [air conditioning] systems

CC Excl: 011.00-012.16, 012.80-012.86, 017.90-017.96, 021.2, 031.0, 039.1, 115.05, 115.15, 115.95, 122.1, 130.4, 136.3, 480.0-480.2, 480.8-487.1, 488, 494.0-508.9, 517.1, 517.8, 518.89, 519.8-519.9, 748.61

**495.8 Other specified allergic alveolitis and pneumonitis** `CC`

Cheese-washers' lung
Coffee workers' lung
Fish-meal workers' lung
Furriers' lung
Grain-handlers' disease or lung
Pituitary snuff-takers' disease
Sequoiosis or red-cedar asthma
Wood asthma

CC Excl: See code 495.7

**495.9 Unspecified allergic alveolitis and pneumonitis** `CC`

Alveolitis, allergic (extrinsic)
Hypersensitivity pneumonitis

CC Excl: See code 495.7

**496 Chronic airway obstruction, not elsewhere classified**

Note: This code is not to be used with any code from categories 491-493

Chronic:
nonspecific lung disease
obstructive lung disease
obstructive pulmonary disease [COPD] NOS

EXCLUDES *chronic obstructive lung disease [COPD]*
*specified (as) (with):*
*allergic alveolitis (495.0-495.9)*
*asthma (493.20-493.22)*
*bronchiectasis (494.0-494.1)*
*bronchitis (491.20-491.22)*
*with emphysema (491.20-491.22)*
*decompensated (491.21)*
*emphysema (492.0-492.8)*

AHA: 4Q, '03, 109; 2Q, '00, 15; 2Q, '92, 16; 2Q, '91, 21; 3Q, '88, 56

## PNEUMOCONIOSES AND OTHER LUNG DISEASES DUE TO EXTERNAL AGENTS (500-508)

DEF: Permanent deposits of particulate matter, within lungs; due to occupational or environmental exposure; results in chronic induration and fibrosis. (See specific listings in 500-508 code range)

**500 Coal workers' pneumoconiosis** `A`

Anthracosilicosis     Coal workers' lung
Anthracosis     Miner's asthma
Black lung disease

**501 Asbestosis** `A`

**502 Pneumoconiosis due to other silica or silicates**

Pneumoconiosis due to talc
Silicotic fibrosis (massive) of lung
Silicosis (simple) (complicated)

**503 Pneumoconiosis due to other inorganic dust**

Aluminosis (of lung)     Graphite fibrosis (of lung)
Baritosis     Siderosis
Bauxite fibrosis (of lung)     Stannosis
Berylliosis

**504 Pneumonopathy due to inhalation of other dust**

Byssinosis     Flax-dressers' disease
Cannabinosis

EXCLUDES *allergic alveolitis (495.0-495.9)*
*asbestosis (501)*
*bagassosis (495.1)*
*farmers' lung (495.0)*

**505 Pneumoconiosis, unspecified**

**506 Respiratory conditions due to chemical fumes and vapors** ✓4th

Use additional E code to identify cause

**506.0 Bronchitis and pneumonitis due to fumes and vapors** `CC`

Chemical bronchitis (acute)

CC Excl: 011.00-012.16, 012.80-012.86, 017.90-017.96, 021.2, 031.0, 039.1, 115.05, 115.15, 115.95, 122.1, 130.4, 136.3, 480.0-480.2, 480.8-487.1, 488, 494.0-508.9, 517.1, 517.8, 518.89, 519.8-519.9, 748.61

**506.1 Acute pulmonary edema due to fumes and vapors** `MCC`

Chemical pulmonary edema (acute)

EXCLUDES *acute pulmonary edema NOS (518.4)*
*chronic or unspecified pulmonary edema (514)*

CC Excl: See code 506.0

AHA: 3Q, '88, 4

**506.2 Upper respiratory inflammation due to fumes and vapors**

AHA: 3Q, '05, 10

**506.3 Other acute and subacute respiratory conditions due to fumes and vapors**

**506.4 Chronic respiratory conditions due to fumes and vapors**

Emphysema (diffuse) (chronic)
Obliterative bronchiolitis (chronic) (subacute)
Pulmonary fibrosis (chronic)
   } due to inhalation of chemical fumes and vapors

**506.9 Unspecified respiratory conditions due to fumes and vapors**

Silo-fillers' disease

**507 Pneumonitis due to solids and liquids** ✓4th

EXCLUDES *fetal aspiration pneumonitis (770.18)*

AHA: 3Q, '91, 16

**507.0 Due to inhalation of food or vomitus** `MCC`

Aspiration pneumonia (due to):
NOS
food (regurgitated)
gastric secretions
milk
saliva
vomitus

CC Excl: See code 506.0

AHA: 1Q, '89, 10

**507.1 Due to inhalation of oils and essences** `MCC`

Lipoid pneumonia (exogenous)

EXCLUDES *endogenous lipoid pneumonia (516.8)*

CC Excl: See code 506.0

**507.8 Due to other solids and liquids** `MCC`

Detergent asthma

CC Excl: See code 506.0

**508 Respiratory conditions due to other and unspecified external agents** ✓4th

Use additional E code to identify cause

**508.0 Acute pulmonary manifestations due to radiation** `CC`

Radiation pneumonitis

CC Excl: See code 506.0

AHA: 2Q, '88, 4

**508.1 Chronic and other pulmonary manifestations due to radiation** `CC`

Fibrosis of lung following radiation

CC Excl: See code 506.0

**508.8 Respiratory conditions due to other specified external agents**

---

| `N` Newborn Age: 0 | `P` Pediatric Age: 0-17 | `M` Maternity Age: 12-55 | `A` Adult Age: 15-124 | `CC` CC Condition | `MCC` Major CC Condition | `HIV` HIV Related Dx |

**508.9**   **Respiratory conditions due to unspecified external agent**

## OTHER DISEASES OF RESPIRATORY SYSTEM (510-519)

✓4ᵗʰ **510 Empyema**

Use additional code to identify infectious organism (041.0-041.9)

> **EXCLUDES**   abscess of lung (513.0)

DEF: Purulent infection; within pleural space.

**510.0**   **With fistula**                      `MCC`

Fistula:
  bronchocutaneous
  bronchopleural
  hepatopleural
  mediastinal
  pleural
  thoracic
Any condition classifiable to 510.9 with fistula

**CC Excl:** 510.0-510.9, 517.8, 518.89, 519.8-519.9

DEF: Purulent infection of respiratory cavity; with communication from cavity to another structure.

**510.9**   **Without mention of fistula**       `MCC`

Abscess:              Pleurisy:
  pleura                 septic
  thorax                 seropurulent
Empyema (chest) (lung)   suppurative
  (pleura)             Pyopneumothorax
Fibrinopurulent pleurisy Pyothorax
Pleurisy:
  purulent

**CC Excl:** See code: 510.0

**AHA:** 3Q, '94, 6

✓4ᵗʰ **511 Pleurisy**

> **EXCLUDES**   malignant pleural effusion (197.2)
> pleurisy with mention of tuberculosis,
> current disease (012.0)

DEF: Inflammation of serous membrane of lungs and lining of thoracic cavity; causes exudation in cavity or membrane surface.

**511.0**   **Without mention of effusion or current tuberculosis**

Adhesion, lung or pleura Pleurisy:
Calcification of pleura      NOS
Pleurisy (acute) (sterile):  pneumococcal
  diaphragmatic              staphylococcal
  fibrinous                  streptococcal
  interlobar                 Thickening of pleura

**AHA:** 3Q, '94, 5

**511.1**   **With effusion, with mention of a bacterial**   `MCC`
**cause other than tuberculosis**

Pleurisy with effusion (exudative) (serous):
  pneumococcal
  staphylococcal
  streptococcal
  other specified nontuberculous bacterial cause

**CC Excl:** 011.00-012.16, 012.80-012.86, 017.90-017.96, 511.0-511.9, 517.8, 518.89, 519.8-519.9

**511.8**   **Other specified forms of effusion,**   `MCC`
**except tuberculous**

Encysted pleurisy
Hemopneumothorax
Hemothorax
Hydropneumothorax
Hydrothorax

> **EXCLUDES**   traumatic (860.2-860.5, 862.29,
> 862.39)

**CC Excl:** See code: 511.1

**AHA:** 1Q, '97, 10

**511.9**   **Unspecified pleural effusion**       `CC`

Pleural effusion NOS
Pleurisy:
  exudative
  serofibrinous
  serous
  with effusion NOS

**CC Excl:** See code 511.1

**AHA:** 2Q, '03, 7; 3Q, '91, 19; 4Q, '89, 11

✓4ᵗʰ **512 Pneumothorax**

DEF: Collapsed lung; due to gas or air in pleural space.

**512.0**   **Spontaneous tension pneumothorax**   `MCC`

**CC Excl:** 512.0-512.8, 517.8, 518.89, 519.8-519.9

**AHA:** 3Q, '94, 5

DEF: Leaking air from lung into lining causing collapse.

**512.1**   **Iatrogenic pneumothorax**           `CC`

Postoperative pneumothorax

**CC Excl:** See code 512.0

**AHA:** 4Q, '94, 40

DEF: Air trapped in the lining of the lung following surgery.

**512.8**   **Other spontaneous pneumothorax**    `CC`

Pneumothorax:
  NOS
  acute
  chronic

> **EXCLUDES**   pneumothorax:
> congenital (770.2)
> traumatic (860.0-860.1, 860.4-
> 860.5)
> tuberculous, current disease (011.7)

**CC Excl:** See code 512.0

**AHA:** 2Q, '93, 3

✓4ᵗʰ **513 Abscess of lung and mediastinum**

**513.0**   **Abscess of lung**                   `MCC`

Abscess (multiple) of lung
Gangrenous or necrotic pneumonia
Pulmonary gangrene or necrosis

**CC Excl:** 006.4, 011.00-012.16, 012.80-012.86, 017.90-017.96, 513.0, 519.8-519.9

**AHA:** 2Q, '98, 7

**513.1**   **Abscess of mediastinum**            `MCC`

**CC Excl:** 513.1, 519.8-519.9

**514 Pulmonary congestion and hypostasis**      `CC`

Hypostatic:                Pulmonary edema:
  bronchopneumonia           NOS
  pneumonia                  chronic
Passive pneumonia
Pulmonary congestion
  (chronic) (passive)

> **EXCLUDES**   acute pulmonary edema:
> NOS (518.4)
> with mention of heart disease or failure
> (428.1)
> hypostatic pneumonia due to or specified as a
> specific type of pneumonia—code to the
> type of pneumonia (480.0-480.9, 481,
> 482.0-482.49, 483.0-483.8, 485, 486,
> 487.0)

**CC Excl:** 514, 517.8, 518.89, 519.8-519.9

**AHA:** 2Q, '98, 6; 3Q, '88, 5

DEF: Excessive retention of interstitial fluid in the lungs and pulmonary vessels; due to poor circulation.

✓4ᵗʰ / ✓5ᵗʰ Additional Digit Required     Unacceptable PDx     `Manifestation Code`     ▶◀ Revised Text     ● New Code     ▲ Revised Code Title

© 2007 Ingenix                                October 2007 • Volume 1 — 165

**Respiratory System**

**508.9–514**

**Respiratory System**

**515–518.4**

**515 Postinflammatory pulmonary fibrosis**

Cirrhosis of lung
Fibrosis of lung (atrophic)
(confluent) (massive)
(perialveolar)     chronic or unspecified
(peribronchial)
Induration of lung

**DEF:** Fibrosis and scarring of the lungs due to inflammatory reaction.

**✓4ᵗʰ 516 Other alveolar and parietoalveolar pneumonopathy**

**516.0 Pulmonary alveolar proteinosis**   `CC`

**CC Excl:** 011.00-012.16, 012.80-012.86, 017.90-017.96, 494.0-508.9, 515-516.9, 517.2, 517.8, 518.89, 519.8-519.9, 748.61

**DEF:** Reduced ventilation; due to proteinaceous deposits on alveoli; symptoms include dyspnea, cough, chest pain, weakness, weight loss, and hemoptysis.

**516.1 *Idiopathic pulmonary hemosiderosis***   `CC`

*Code first underlying disease (275.0)*
Essential brown induration of lung

**CC Excl:** See code: 516.0

**DEF:** Fibrosis of alveolar walls; marked by abnormal amounts hemosiderin in lungs; primarily affects children; symptoms include anemia, fluid in lungs, and blood in sputum; etiology unknown.

**516.2 Pulmonary alveolar microlithiasis**   `CC`

**CC Excl:** See code: 516.0

**DEF:** Small calculi in pulmonary alveoli resembling sand-like particles on x-ray.

**516.3 Idiopathic fibrosing alveolitis**   `CC`

Alveolar capillary block
Diffuse (idiopathic) (interstitial) pulmonary fibrosis
Hamman-Rich syndrome

**CC Excl:** See code: 516.0

**516.8 Other specified alveolar and parietoalveolar pneumonopathies**   `CC`

Endogenous lipoid pneumonia
Interstitial pneumonia (desquamative) (lymphoid)

EXCLUDES   *lipoid pneumonia, exogenous or unspecified (507.1)*

**CC Excl:** See code: 516.0

**AHA:** 2Q, '06, 20; 1Q, '92, 12

**516.9 Unspecified alveolar and parietoalveolar pneumonopathy**   `CC`

**CC Excl:** See code: 516.0

**✓4ᵗʰ 517 Lung involvement in conditions classified elsewhere**

EXCLUDES   *rheumatoid lung (714.81)*

**517.1 *Rheumatic pneumonia***   `CC`

*Code first underlying disease (390)*

**CC Excl:** 011.00-012.16, 012.80-012.86, 017.90-017.96, 480.0-480.2, 480.8-487.1, 488, 494.0-508.9, 515-517.2, 517.8, 518.89, 519.8-519.9, 748.61

**517.2 *Lung involvement in systemic sclerosis***   `CC`

*Code first underlying disease (710.1)*

**CC Excl:** 011.00-012.16, 012.80-012.86, 017.90-017.96, 494.0-508.9, 515-516.9, 517.2, 517.8, 518.89, 519.8-519.9, 748.61

**517.3 *Acute chest syndrome***   `CC`

*Code first sickle-cell disease in crisis (282.42, 282.62, 282.64, 282.69)*

**CC Excl:** 280.0-282.3, 282.5-282.63, 282.69-284.2, 284.81-285.9, 289.9, 776.5-776.6

**AHA:** 4Q, '03, 51, 56

**517.8 *Lung involvement in other diseases classified elsewhere***

*Code first underlying disease, as:*
amyloidosis (277.30-277.39)
polymyositis (710.4)
sarcoidosis (135)
Sjögren's disease (710.2)
systemic lupus erythematosus (710.0)

EXCLUDES   *syphilis (095.1)*

**AHA:** 2Q, '03, 7

**✓4ᵗʰ 518 Other diseases of lung**

**518.0 Pulmonary collapse**   `CC`

Atelectasis
Collapse of lung
Middle lobe syndrome

EXCLUDES   *atelectasis:*
*congenital (partial) (770.5)*
*primary (770.4)*
*tuberculous, current disease (011.8)*

**CC Excl:** 518.0, 519.8-519.9

**AHA:** 4Q, '90, 25

**518.1 Interstitial emphysema**

Mediastinal emphysema

EXCLUDES   *surgical (subcutaneous) emphysema (998.81)*
*that in fetus or newborn (770.2)*
*traumatic emphysema (958.7)*

**DEF:** Escaped air from the alveoli trapped in the interstices of the lung; trauma or cough may cause the disease.

**518.2 Compensatory emphysema**

**DEF:** Distention of all or part of the lung caused by disease processes or surgical intervention that decreased volume in another part of the lung; overcompensation reaction to the loss of capacity in another part of the lung.

**518.3 Pulmonary eosinophilia**   `CC`

Eosinophilic asthma
Löffler's syndrome
Pneumonia:
allergic
eosinophilic
Tropical eosinophilia

**CC Excl:** 011.00-012.16, 012.80-012.86, 017.90-017.96, 020.3-020.5, 021.3, 022.1, 031.0, 039.1, 073.0, 115.05, 115.15, 115.95, 122.1, 130.4, 136.3, 480.0-480.2, 480.8-487.1, 488, 494.0-495.9, 500-508.9, 517.1, 517.8, 518.3, 518.89, 519.8-519.9, 748.61

**DEF:** Infiltration, into pulmonary parenchyma of eosinophilia; results in cough, fever, and dyspnea.

**518.4 Acute edema of lung, unspecified**   `MCC`

Acute pulmonary edema NOS
Pulmonary edema, postoperative

EXCLUDES   *pulmonary edema:*
*acute, with mention of heart disease or failure (428.1)*
*chronic or unspecified (514)*
*due to external agents (506.0-508.9)*

**CC Excl:** 398.91, 428.0-428.9, 518.4, 519.8-519.9

**DEF:** Severe, sudden fluid retention within lung tissues.

---

`N` Newborn Age: 0    `P` Pediatric Age: 0-17    `M` Maternity Age: 12-55    `A` Adult Age: 15-124    `CC` CC Condition    `MCC` Major CC Condition    `HIV` HIV Related Dx

**518.5** **Pulmonary insufficiency following trauma and surgery** `MCC`
> Adult respiratory distress syndrome
> Pulmonary insufficiency following:
>> shock
>> surgery
>> trauma
> Shock lung

> EXCLUDES adult respiratory distress syndrome associated with other conditions (518.82)
>> pneumonia:
>>> aspiration (507.0)
>>> hypostatic (514)
>> respiratory failure in other conditions (518.81, 518.83-518.84)

**CC Excl:** 518.5, 519.8-519.9

**AHA:** 4Q, '04, 139; 3Q, '88, 3; 3Q, '88, 7; S-O, '87, 1

**518.6** **Allergic bronchopulmonary aspergillosis** `CC`

**CC Excl:** 518.6, 519.8-519.9

**AHA:** 4Q, '97, 39

**DEF:** Noninvasive hypersensitive reaction; due to allergic reaction to *Aspergillus fumigatus* (mold).

**518.7** **Transfusion related acute lung injury [TRALI]** `CC`

**CC Excl:** 518.7, 997.3, 997.91-997.99, 998.81, 998.83-998.9

**AHA:** 4Q, '06, 91

**DEF:** A relatively rare, but serious pulmonary complication of blood transfusion, with acute respiratory distress, noncardiogenic pulmonary edema, cyanosis, hypoxemia, hypotension, fever and chills.

√5ᵗʰ **518.8** **Other diseases of lung**

**518.81 Acute respiratory failure** `MCC`
> Respiratory failure NOS

> EXCLUDES acute and chronic respiratory failure (518.84)
>> acute respiratory distress (518.82)
>> chronic respiratory failure (518.83)
>> respiratory arrest (799.1)
>> respiratory failure, newborn (770.84)

**CC Excl:** 518.81-518.84, 519.8-519.9, 799.1

**AHA:** 2Q, '06, 25; 4Q, '05, 96; 2Q, '05, 19; 1Q, '05, 3-8; 1Q, '05, 3–8; 4Q, '04, 139; 1Q, '03, 15; 4Q, '98, 41; 3Q, '91, 14; 2Q, '91, 3; 4Q, '90, 25; 2Q, '90, 20; 3Q, '88, 7; 3Q, '88, 10; S-O, '87, 1

**518.82 Other pulmonary insufficiency, not elsewhere classified** `CC`
> Acute respiratory distress
> Acute respiratory insufficiency
> Adult respiratory distress syndrome NEC

> EXCLUDES adult respiratory distress syndrome associated with trauma and surgery (518.5)
>> pulmonary insufficiency following trauma and surgery (518.5)
>> respiratory distress:
>>> NOS (786.09)
>>> newborn (770.89)
>>> syndrome, newborn (769)
>> shock lung (518.5)

**CC Excl:** See code: 518.81

**AHA:** 4Q, '03, 105; 2Q, '91, 21; 3Q, '88, 7

**518.83 Chronic respiratory failure** `CC`

**CC Excl:** See code: 518.81

**AHA:** 4Q, '05, 96; 4Q, '03, 103, 111

**518.84 Acute and chronic respiratory failure** `MCC`
> Acute on chronic respiratory failure

**CC Excl:** See code: 518.81

**518.89 Other diseases of lung, not elsewhere classified**
> Broncholithiasis          Lung disease NOS
> Calcification of lung      Pulmolithiasis

**AHA:** 3Q, '90, 18; 4Q, '88, 6

**DEF:** Broncholithiasis: calculi in lumen of transbronchial tree.

**DEF:** Pulmolithiasis: calculi in lung.

√4ᵗʰ **519** **Other diseases of respiratory system**

√5ᵗʰ **519.0** **Tracheostomy complications**

**519.00 Tracheostomy complication, unspecified** `CC`

**CC Excl:** 519.00-519.19, 519.8-519.9

**519.01 Infection of tracheostomy** `CC`
> Use additional code to identify type of infection, such as:
>> abscess or cellulitis of neck (682.1)
>> septicemia (038.0-038.9)
> Use additional code to identify organism (041.00-041.9)

**CC Excl:** See code 519.00

**AHA:** 4Q, '98, 41

**519.02 Mechanical complication of tracheostomy** `CC`
> Tracheal stenosis due to tracheostomy

**CC Excl:** See code 519.00

**519.09 Other tracheostomy complications** `CC`
> Hemorrhage due to tracheostomy
> Tracheoesophageal fistula due to tracheostomy

**CC Excl:** See code 519.00

√5ᵗʰ **519.1** **Other diseases of trachea and bronchus, not elsewhere classified**

**AHA:** 3Q, '02, 18; 3Q, '88, 6

**519.11 Acute bronchospasm**
> Bronchospasm NOS

> EXCLUDES acute bronchitis with bronchospasm (466.0)
>> asthma (493.00-493.92)
>> exercise induced bronchospasm (493.81)

**AHA:** 4Q, '06, 92

**519.19 Other diseases of trachea and bronchus**
> Calcification ⎫
> Stenosis     ⎬ of bronchus or trachea
> Ulcer        ⎭

**AHA:** 4Q, '06, 92

**519.2** **Mediastinitis** `MCC`

**CC Excl:** 519.2-519.3, 519.8-519.9

**DEF:** Inflammation of tissue between organs behind sternum.

**519.3** **Other diseases of mediastinum, not elsewhere classified**
> Fibrosis  ⎫
> Hernia    ⎬ of mediastinum
> Retraction ⎭

**519.4** **Disorders of diaphragm**
> Diaphragmitis          Relaxation of diaphragm
> Paralysis of diaphragm

> EXCLUDES congenital defect of diaphragm (756.6)
>> diaphragmatic hernia (551-553 with .3)
>> congenital (756.6)

**519.8** **Other diseases of respiratory system, not elsewhere classified**

**AHA:** 4Q, '89, 12

**519.9** **Unspecified disease of respiratory system**
> Respiratory disease (chronic) NOS

√4ᵗʰ
√5ᵗʰ Additional Digit Required          Unacceptable PDx          Manifestation Code          ►◄ Revised Text          ● New Code          ▲ Revised Code Title

## 9. DISEASES OF THE DIGESTIVE SYSTEM (520-579)

### DISEASES OF ORAL CAVITY, SALIVARY GLANDS, AND JAWS (520-529)

✓4ᵗʰ **520 Disorders of tooth development and eruption**

**520.0 Anodontia**
Absence of teeth (complete) (congenital) (partial)
Hypodontia
Oligodontia
EXCLUDES    *acquired absence of teeth (525.10-525.19)*

**520.1 Supernumerary teeth**
Distomolar
Fourth molar
Mesiodens
Paramolar
Supplemental teeth
EXCLUDES    *supernumerary roots (520.2)*

**520.2 Abnormalities of size and form**
Concrescence ⎫
Fusion     ⎬ of teeth
Gemination ⎭

Dens evaginatus     Microdontia
Dens in dente       Peg-shaped [conical] teeth
Dens invaginatus    Supernumerary roots
Enamel pearls       Taurodontism
Macrodontia        Tuberculum paramolare
EXCLUDES    *that due to congenital syphilis (090.5)*
*tuberculum Carabelli, which is regarded as a normal variation*

**520.3 Mottled teeth**
Mottling of enamel
Dental fluorosis     Nonfluoride enamel opacities

**Digestive System**

**The Oral Cavity**

**Teeth**

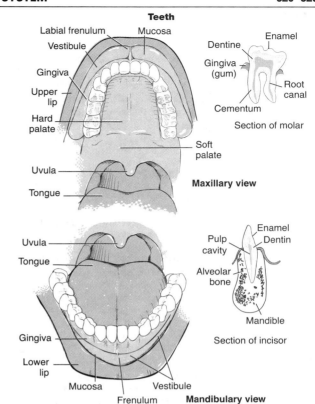

Section of molar

Maxillary view

Section of incisor

Mandibulary view

**520.4 Disturbances of tooth formation**
Aplasia and hypoplasia of cementum
Dilaceration of tooth
Enamel hypoplasia (neonatal) (postnatal) (prenatal)
Horner's teeth
Hypocalcification of teeth
Regional odontodysplasia
Turner's tooth
EXCLUDES    *Hutchinson's teeth and mulberry molars in congenital syphilis (090.5)*
*mottled teeth (520.3)*

**520.5 Hereditary disturbances in tooth structure, not elsewhere classified**
Amelogenesis ⎫
Dentinogenesis ⎬ imperfecta
Odontogenesis ⎭

Dentinal dysplasia
Shell teeth

**520.6 Disturbances in tooth eruption**
Teeth:           Tooth eruption:
   embedded       late
   impacted        obstructed
   natal            premature
   neonatal
   prenatal
   primary [deciduous]:
     persistent
     shedding, premature
EXCLUDES    *exfoliation of teeth (attributable to disease of surrounding tissues) (525.0-525.19)*

AHA: 1Q, '06, 18; 2Q, '05, 15

**520.7 Teething syndrome**

**520.8 Other specified disorders of tooth development and eruption**
Color changes during tooth formation
Pre-eruptive color changes
EXCLUDES    *posteruptive color changes (521.7)*

**520.9 Unspecified disorder of tooth development and eruption**

√4th **521 Diseases of hard tissues of teeth**

√5th **521.0 Dental caries**
  **AHA:** 4Q, '01, 44

  **521.00 Dental caries, unspecified**

  **521.01 Dental caries limited to enamel**
    Initial caries      White spot lesion

  **521.02 Dental caries extending into dentine**

  **521.03 Dental caries extending into pulp**

  **521.04 Arrested dental caries**

  **521.05 Odontoclasia**
    Infantile melanodontia
    Melanodontoclasia

    **EXCLUDES** *internal and external resorption of teeth (521.40-521.49)*

    **DEF:** A pathological dental condition described as stained areas, loss of tooth substance, and hypoplasia linked to nutritional deficiencies during tooth development and to cariogenic oral conditions; synonyms are melanodontoclasia and infantile melanodontia.

  **521.06 Dental caries pit and fissure**
    Primary dental caries, pit and fissure origin

  **521.07 Dental caries of smooth surface**
    Primary dental caries, smooth surface origin

  **521.08 Dental caries of root surface**
    Primary dental caries, root surface

  **521.09 Other dental caries**
    **AHA:** 3Q, '02, 14

√5th **521.1 Excessive attrition (approximal wear) (occlusal wear)**

  **521.10 Excessive attrition, unspecified**

  **521.11 Excessive attrition, limited to enamel**

  **521.12 Excessive attrition, extending into dentine**

  **521.13 Excessive attrition, extending into pulp**

  **521.14 Excessive attrition, localized**

  **521.15 Excessive attrition, generalized**

√5th **521.2 Abrasion**
    Abrasion:
      dentifrice
      habitual
      occupational        } of teeth
      ritual
      traditional
    Wedge defect NOS

  **521.20 Abrasion, unspecified**

  **521.21 Abrasion, limited to enamel**

  **521.22 Abrasion, extending into dentine**

  **521.23 Abrasion, extending into pulp**

  **521.24 Abrasion, localized**

  **521.25 Abrasion, generalized**

√5th **521.3 Erosion**
    Erosion of teeth:        Erosion of teeth:
      NOS                      idiopathic
      due to:                  occupational
        medicine
        persistent vomiting

  **521.30 Erosion, unspecified**

  **521.31 Erosion, limited to enamel**

  **521.32 Erosion, extending into dentine**

  **521.33 Erosion, extending into pulp**

  **521.34 Erosion, localized**

  **521.35 Erosion, generalized**

√5th **521.4 Pathological resorption**
    **DEF:** Loss of dentin and cementum due to disease process.

  **521.40 Pathological resorption, unspecified**

  **521.41 Pathological resorption, internal**

  **521.42 Pathological resorption, external**

  **521.49 Other pathological resorption**
    Internal granuloma of pulp

**521.5 Hypercementosis**
    Cementation hyperplasia
    **DEF:** Excess deposits of cementum, on tooth root. Primary dental caries, root surface

**521.6 Ankylosis of teeth**
    **DEF:** Adhesion of tooth to surrounding bone.

**521.7 Intrinsic posteruptive color changes**
    Staining [discoloration] of teeth:
      NOS
      due to:
        drugs
        metals
        pulpal bleeding

    **EXCLUDES** *accretions [deposits] on teeth (523.6)*
      *extrinsic color changes (523.6)*
      *pre-eruptive color changes (520.8)*

√5th **521.8 Other specified diseases of hard tissues of teeth**
    **521.81 Cracked tooth**
      **EXCLUDES** *asymptomatic craze lines in enamel—omit code*
        *broken tooth due to trauma (873.63, 873.73)*
        *fractured tooth due to trauma (873.63, 873.73)*

    **521.89 Other specified diseases of hard tissues of teeth**
      Irradiated enamel
      Sensitive dentin

**521.9 Unspecified disease of hard tissues of teeth**

√4th **522 Diseases of pulp and periapical tissues**

**522.0 Pulpitis**                                         **CC**
    Pulpal:                  Pulpitis:
      abscess                  chronic (hyperplastic)
      polyp                      (ulcerative)
    Pulpitis:                  suppurative
      acute
    **CC Excl:** 520.0-525.9

**522.1 Necrosis of the pulp**
    Pulp gangrene
    **DEF:** Death of pulp tissue.

**522.2 Pulp degeneration**
    Denticles                Pulp stones
    Pulp calcifications

**522.3 Abnormal hard tissue formation in pulp**
    Secondary or irregular dentin

**522.4 Acute apical periodontitis of pulpal origin**      **CC**
    **CC Excl:** See code: 522.0

    **DEF:** Severe inflammation of periodontal ligament due to pulpal inflammation or necrosis.

**522.5 Periapical abscess without sinus**
    Abscess:                 Abscess:
      dental                   dentoalveolar
    **EXCLUDES** *periapical abscess with sinus (522.7)*

**522.6 Chronic apical periodontitis**
    Apical or periapical granuloma
    Apical periodontitis NOS

**522.7 Periapical abscess with sinus**
    Fistula:                 Fistula:
      alveolar process         dental

**522.8 Radicular cyst**
    Cyst:                    Cyst:
      apical (periodontal)     radiculodental
      periapical               residual radicular
    **EXCLUDES** *lateral developmental or lateral periodontal cyst (526.0)*
    **DEF:** Cyst in tissue around tooth apex due to chronic infection of granuloma around root.

**522.9 Other and unspecified diseases of pulp and periapical tissues**

| **N** Newborn Age: 0 | **P** Pediatric Age: 0-17 | **M** Maternity Age: 12-55 | **A** Adult Age: 15-124 | **CC** CC Condition | **MCC** Major CC Condition | **HIV** HIV Related Dx |

√4th **523 Gingival and periodontal diseases**

√5th **523.0 Acute gingivitis**

> EXCLUDES    acute necrotizing ulcerative gingivitis (101)
> herpetic gingivostomatitis (054.2)

**523.00 Acute gingivitis, plaque induced**
Acute gingivitis NOS

**523.01 Acute gingivitis, non-plaque induced**

√5th **523.1 Chronic gingivitis**
Gingivitis (chronic):     Gingivitis (chronic):
   desquamative        simple marginal
   hyperplastic         ulcerative

> EXCLUDES   herpetic gingivostomatitis (054.2)

**523.10 Chronic gingivitis, plaque induced**
Chronic gingivitis NOS
Gingivitis NOS

**523.11 Chronic gingivitis, non-plaque induced**

√5th **523.2 Gingival recession**
Gingival recession (postinfective) (postoperative)

**523.20 Gingival recession, unspecified**

**523.21 Gingival recession, minimal**

**523.22 Gingival recession, moderate**

**523.23 Gingival recession, severe**

**523.24 Gingival recession, localized**

**523.25 Gingival recession, generalized**

√5th **523.3 Aggressive and acute periodontitis**
Acute:
   pericementitis
   pericoronitis

> EXCLUDES   acute apical periodontitis (522.4)
> periapical abscess (522.5, 522.7)

DEF: Severe inflammation, of tissues supporting teeth.

**523.30 Aggressive periodontitis, unspecified**

**523.31 Aggressive periodontitis, localized**
Periodontal abscess

**523.32 Aggressive periodontitis, generalized**

**523.33 Acute periodontitis**

√5th **523.4 Chronic periodontitis**
Chronic pericoronitis     Periodontitis:
Pericementitis (chronic)    complex
                           simplex
                           NOS

> EXCLUDES   chronic apical periodontitis (522.6)

**523.40 Chronic periodontitis, unspecified**

**523.41 Chronic periodontitis, localized**

**523.42 Chronic periodontitis, generalized**

**523.5 Periodontosis**

**523.6 Accretions on teeth**
Dental calculus:      Deposits on teeth:
   subgingival         soft
   supragingival       tartar
Deposits on teeth:     tobacco
   betel        Extrinsic discoloration of teeth
   materia alba

> EXCLUDES   intrinsic discoloration of teeth (521.7)

DEF: Foreign material on tooth surface, usually plaque or calculus.

**523.8 Other specified periodontal diseases**
Giant cell:
   epulis
   peripheral granuloma
Gingival:
   cysts
   enlargement NOS
   fibromatosis
Gingival polyp
Periodontal lesions due to traumatic occlusion
Peripheral giant cell granuloma

> EXCLUDES   leukoplakia of gingiva (528.6)

**523.9 Unspecified gingival and periodontal disease**
AHA: 3Q ,'02, 14

√4th **524 Dentofacial anomalies, including malocclusion**

√5th **524.0 Major anomalies of jaw size**

> EXCLUDES   hemifacial atrophy or hypertrophy (754.0)
> unilateral condylar hyperplasia or hypoplasia of mandible (526.89)

**524.00 Unspecified anomaly**
DEF: Unspecified deformity of jaw size.

**524.01 Maxillary hyperplasia**
DEF: Overgrowth or over development of upper jaw bone.

**524.02 Mandibular hyperplasia**
DEF: Overgrowth or over development of lower jaw bone.

**524.03 Maxillary hypoplasia**
DEF: Incomplete or underdeveloped, upper jaw bone.

**524.04 Mandibular hypoplasia**
DEF: Incomplete or underdeveloped, lower jaw bone.

**524.05 Macrogenia**
DEF: Enlarged, jaw, especially chin; affects bone, soft tissue, or both.

**524.06 Microgenia**
DEF: Underdeveloped mandible, characterized by an extremely small chin.

**524.07 Excessive tuberosity of jaw**
Entire maxillary tuberosity

**524.09 Other specified anomaly**

√5th **524.1 Anomalies of relationship of jaw to cranial base**

**524.10 Unspecified anomaly**
Prognathism      Retrognathism
DEF: Prognathism: protrusion of lower jaw.
DEF: Retrognathism: jaw is located posteriorly to a normally positioned jaw; backward position of mandible.

**524.11 Maxillary asymmetry**
DEF: Absence of symmetry of maxilla.

**524.12 Other jaw asymmetry**

**524.19 Other specified anomaly**

√5th **524.2 Anomalies of dental arch relationship**
Anomaly of dental arch

> EXCLUDES   hemifacial atrophy or hypertrophy (754.0)
> soft tissue impingement (524.81-524.82)
> unilateral condylar hyperplasia or hypoplasia of mandible (526.89)

**524.20 Unspecified anomaly of dental arch relationship**

**524.21 Malocclusion, Angle's class I**
Neutro-occlusion

**524.22 Malocclusion, Angle's class II**
Disto-occlusion Division I
Disto-occlusion Division II

**524.23 Malocclusion, Angle's class III**
Mesio-occlusion

**524.24 Open anterior occlusal relationship**
Anterior open bite

**524.25 Open posterior occlusal relationship**
Posterior open bite

**524.26 Excessive horizontal overlap**
Excessive horizontal overjet

**524.27 Reverse articulation**
Anterior articulation
Crossbite
Posterior articulation

**524.28 Anomalies of interarch distance**
Excessive interarch distance
Inadequate interarch distance

**524.29 Other anomalies of dental arch relationship**
Other anomalies of dental arch

---

√4th √5th   Additional Digit Required      Unacceptable PDx      Manifestation Code      ►◄ Revised Text      ● New Code      ▲ Revised Code Title

**Digestive System**

**524.3–525.41**

**Angle's Classification of Malocclusion**

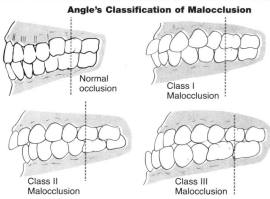

Normal occlusion

Class I Malocclusion

Class II Malocclusion

Class III Malocclusion

√5ᵗʰ **524.3 Anomalies of tooth position of fully erupted teeth**

    **EXCLUDES**   *impacted or embedded teeth with abnormal position of such teeth or adjacent teeth (520.6)*

    **524.30 Unspecified anomaly of tooth position**
       Diastema of teeth NOS
       Displacement of teeth NOS
       Transposition of teeth NOS

    **524.31 Crowding of teeth**

    **524.32 Excessive spacing of teeth**

    **524.33 Horizontal displacement of teeth**
       Tipped teeth
       Tipping of teeth

    **524.34 Vertical displacement of teeth**
       Extruded tooth
       Infraeruption of teeth
       Intruded tooth
       Supraeruption of teeth

    **524.35 Rotation of tooth/teeth**

    **524.36 Insufficient interocclusal distance of teeth (ridge)**
       Lack of adequate intermaxillary vertical dimension

    **524.37 Excessive interocclusal distance of teeth**
       Excessive intermaxillary vertical dimension
       Loss of occlusal vertical dimension

    **524.39 Other anomalies of tooth position**

  **524.4 Malocclusion, unspecified**

    DEF: Malposition of top and bottom teeth; interferes with chewing.

√5ᵗʰ **524.5 Dentofacial functional abnormalities**

    **524.50 Dentofacial functional abnormality, unspecified**

    **524.51 Abnormal jaw closure**

    **524.52 Limited mandibular range of motion**

    **524.53 Deviation in opening and closing of the mandible**

    **524.54 Insufficient anterior guidance**
       Insufficient anterior occlusal guidance

    **524.55 Centric occlusion maximum intercuspation discrepancy**
       Centric occlusion of teeth discrepancy

    **524.56 Non-working side interference**
       Balancing side interference

    **524.57 Lack of posterior occlusal support**

    **524.59 Other dentofacial functional abnormalities**
       Abnormal swallowing   Sleep postures
       Mouth breathing     Tongue, lip, or finger habits

√5ᵗʰ **524.6 Temporomandibular joint disorders**

    **EXCLUDES**   *current temporomandibular joint: dislocation (830.0-830.1) strain (848.1)*

    **524.60 Temporomandibular joint disorders, unspecified**
       Temporomandibular joint-pain-dysfunction syndrome [TMJ]

    **524.61 Adhesions and ankylosis (bony or fibrous)**
       DEF: Stiffening or union of temporomandibular joint due to bony or fibrous union across joint.

    **524.62 Arthralgia of temporomandibular joint**
       DEF: Pain in temporomandibular joint; not inflammatory in nature.

    **524.63 Articular disc disorder (reducing or non-reducing)**

    **524.64 Temporomandibular joint sounds on opening and/or closing the jaw**

    **524.69 Other specified temporomandibular joint disorders**

√5ᵗʰ **524.7 Dental alveolar anomalies**

    **524.70 Unspecified alveolar anomaly**

    **524.71 Alveolar maxillary hyperplasia**
       DEF: Excessive tissue formation in the dental alveoli of upper jaw.

    **524.72 Alveolar mandibular hyperplasia**
       DEF: Excessive tissue formation in the dental alveoli of lower jaw.

    **524.73 Alveolar maxillary hypoplasia**
       DEF: Incomplete or underdeveloped, alveolar tissue of upper jaw.

    **524.74 Alveolar mandibular hypoplasia**
       DEF: Incomplete or underdeveloped, alveolar tissue of lower jaw.

    **524.75 Vertical displacement of alveolus and teeth**
       Extrusion of alveolus and teeth

    **524.76 Occlusal plane deviation**

    **524.79 Other specified alveolar anomaly**

√5ᵗʰ **524.8 Other specified dentofacial anomalies**

    **524.81 Anterior soft tissue impingement**

    **524.82 Posterior soft tissue impingement**

    **524.89 Other specified dentofacial anomalies**

  **524.9 Unspecified dentofacial anomalies**

√4ᵗʰ **525 Other diseases and conditions of the teeth and supporting structures**

  **525.0 Exfoliation of teeth due to systemic causes**
    DEF: Deterioration of teeth and surrounding structures due to systemic disease.

√5ᵗʰ **525.1 Loss of teeth due to trauma, extraction, or periodontal disease**
       *Code first class of edentulism (525.40-525.44, 525.50-525.54)*
    AHA: 4Q, '05, 74; 4Q, '01, 44

    *525.10 Acquired absence of teeth, unspecified*
       Tooth extraction status, NOS

    *525.11 Loss of teeth due to trauma*

    *525.12 Loss of teeth due to periodontal disease*

    *525.13 Loss of teeth due to caries*

    *525.19 Other loss of teeth*

√5ᵗʰ **525.2 Atrophy of edentulous alveolar ridge**

    **525.20 Unspecified atrophy of edentulous alveolar ridge**
       Atrophy of the mandible NOS
       Atrophy of the maxilla NOS

    **525.21 Minimal atrophy of the mandible**

    **525.22 Moderate atrophy of the mandible**

    **525.23 Severe atrophy of the mandible**

    **525.24 Minimal atrophy of the maxilla**

    **525.25 Moderate atrophy of the maxilla**

    **525.26 Severe atrophy of the maxilla**

  **525.3 Retained dental root**

√5ᵗʰ **525.4 Complete edentulism**
       Use additional code to identify cause of edentulism (525.10-525.19)
    AHA: 4Q, '05, 74

    **525.40 Complete edentulism, unspecified**
       Edentulism NOS

    **525.41 Complete edentulism, class I**

---

  **N** Newborn Age: 0     **P** Pediatric Age: 0-17     **M** Maternity Age: 12-55     **A** Adult Age: 15-124     **CC** CC Condition     **MCC** Major CC Condition     **HIV** HIV Related Dx

**525.42 Complete edentulism, class II**
**525.43 Complete edentulism, class III**
**525.44 Complete edentulism, class IV**

√5ᵗʰ **525.5 Partial edentulism**
    Use additional code to identify cause of edentulism
    (525.10-525.19)

    **AHA:** 4Q, '05, 74

**525.50 Partial edentulism, unspecified**
**525.51 Partial edentulism, class I**
**525.52 Partial edentulism, class II**
**525.53 Partial edentulism, class III**
**525.54 Partial edentulism, class IV**

√5ᵗʰ **525.6 Unsatisfactory restoration of tooth**
    Defective bridge, crown, fillings
    Defective dental restoration
        **EXCLUDES** *dental restoration status (V45.84)*
            *unsatisfactory endodontic treatment*
            *(526.61-526.69)*

**525.60 Unspecified unsatisfactory restoration of tooth**
    Unspecified defective dental restoration

**525.61 Open restoration margins**
    Dental restoration failure of marginal
        integrity
    Open margin on tooth restoration

**525.62 Unrepairable overhanging of dental restorative materials**
    Overhanging of tooth restoration

**525.63 Fractured dental restorative material without loss of material**
        **EXCLUDES** *cracked tooth (521.81)*
            *fractured tooth (873.63,*
                *873.73)*

**525.64 Fractured dental restorative material with loss of material**
        **EXCLUDES** *cracked tooth (521.81)*
            *fractured tooth (873.63,*
                *873.73)*

**525.65 Contour of existing restoration of tooth biologically incompatible with oral health**
    Dental restoration failure of periodontal
        anatomical integrity
    Unacceptable contours of existing
        restoration
    Unacceptable morphology of existing
        restoration

**525.66 Allergy to existing dental restorative material**
    Use additional code to identify the specific
        type of allergy

**525.67 Poor aesthetics of existing restoration**
    Dental restoration aesthetically inadequate
        or displeasing

**525.69 Other unsatisfactory restoration of existing tooth**

● √5ᵗʰ **525.7 Endosseous dental implant failure**
● **525.71 Osseointegration failure of dental implant**
    Hemorrhagic complications of dental
        implant placement
    Iatrogenic osseointegration failure of dental
        implant
    Osseointegration failure of dental implant
        due to complications of systemic
        disease
    Osseointegration failure of dental implant
        due to poor bone quality
    Pre-integration failure of dental implant
        NOS
    Pre-osseointegration failure of dental
        implant

● **525.72 Post-osseointegration biological failure of dental implant**
    Failure of dental implant due to lack of
        attached gingiva
    Failure of dental implant due to occlusal
        trauma (caused by poor prosthetic
        design)
    Failure of dental implant due to
        parafunctional habits
    Failure of dental implant due to periodontal
        infection (peri-implantitis)
    Failure of dental implant due to poor oral
        hygiene
    Iatrogenic post-osseointegration failure of
        dental implant
    Post-osseointegration failure of dental
        implant due to complications of
        systemic disease

● **525.73 Post-osseointegration mechanical failure of dental implant**
    Failure of dental prosthesis causing loss of
        dental implant
    Fracture of dental implant
        **EXCLUDES** *cracked tooth (521.81)*
            *fractured dental restorative*
                *material with loss of*
                *material (525.64)*
            *fractured dental restorative*
                *material without loss of*
                *material (525.63)*
            *fractured tooth (873.63,*
                *873.73)*

● **525.79 Other endosseous dental implant failure**
    Dental implant failure NOS

**525.8 Other specified disorders of the teeth and supporting structures**
    Enlargement of alveolar ridge NOS
    Irregular alveolar process

**525.9 Unspecified disorder of the teeth and supporting structures**

√4ᵗʰ **526 Diseases of the jaws**

**526.0 Developmental odontogenic cysts**
    Cyst:                    Cyst:
        dentigerous              lateral periodontal
        eruption                 primordial
        follicular               Keratocyst
        lateral developmental
        **EXCLUDES** *radicular cyst (522.8)*

**526.1 Fissural cysts of jaw**
    Cyst:                          Cyst:
        globulomaxillary               median palatal
        incisor canal                  nasopalatine
        median anterior maxillary  palatine of papilla
        **EXCLUDES** *cysts of oral soft tissues (528.4)*

**526.2 Other cysts of jaws**
    Cyst of jaw:          Cyst of jaw:
        NOS                   hemorrhagic
        aneurysmal            traumatic

**526.3 Central giant cell (reparative) granuloma**
        **EXCLUDES** *peripheral giant cell granuloma (523.8)*

**526.4 Inflammatory conditions**
    Abscess
    Osteitis                        } of jaw (acute) (chronic)
    Osteomyelitis (neonatal)        } (suppurative)
    Periostitis

    Sequestrum of jaw bone
        **EXCLUDES** *alveolar osteitis (526.5)*
            ▶*osteonecrosis of jaw (733.45)*◀

**526.5 Alveolitis of jaw**
    Alveolar osteitis          Dry socket
    **DEF:** Inflammation, of alveoli or tooth socket.

√5ᵗʰ **526.6 Periradicular pathology associated with previous endodontic treatment**
    **526.61 Perforation of root canal space**
    **526.62 Endodontic overfill**
    **526.63 Endodontic underfill**

---

√4ᵗʰ / √5ᵗʰ  Additional Digit Required     Unacceptable PDx     **Manifestation Code**     ▶◀ Revised Text     ● New Code     ▲ Revised Code Title

© 2007 Ingenix                                                                    **October 2007 • Volume 1 — 173**

**526.69 Other periradicular pathology associated with previous endodontic treatment**

✓5ᵗʰ **526.8 Other specified diseases of the jaws**

**526.81 Exostosis of jaw**
Torus mandibularis    Torus palatinus
DEF: Spur or bony outgrowth on the jaw.

**526.89 Other**
Cherubism
Fibrous dysplasia
Latent bone cyst     } of jaw(s)
Osteoradionecrosis

Unilateral condylar hyperplasia or hypoplasia of mandible

**526.9 Unspecified disease of the jaws**

✓4ᵗʰ **527 Diseases of the salivary glands**

**527.0 Atrophy**
DEF: Wasting away, necrosis of salivary gland tissue.

**527.1 Hypertrophy**
DEF: Overgrowth or overdeveloped salivary gland tissue.

**527.2 Sialoadenitis**
Parotitis:           Sialoangitis
    NOS              Sialodochitis
    allergic
    toxic
EXCLUDES    epidemic or infectious parotitis (072.0-072.9)
            uveoparotid fever (135)
DEF: Inflammation of salivary gland.

**527.3 Abscess**  CC
CC Excl: 527.0-527.9, 537.89-538

**527.4 Fistula**  CC
EXCLUDES    congenital fistula of salivary gland (750.24)
CC Excl: See code: 527.3

**527.5 Sialolithiasis**
Calculus  }
Stone     } of salivary gland or duct
Sialodocholithiasis

**527.6 Mucocele**
Mucous:
    extravasation cyst of salivary gland
    retention cyst of salivary gland
Ranula
DEF: Dilated salivary gland cavity filled with mucous.

**527.7 Disturbance of salivary secretion**
Hyposecretion      Sialorrhea
Ptyalism           Xerostomia

**527.8 Other specified diseases of the salivary glands**
Benign lymphoepithelial lesion of salivary gland
Sialectasia
Sialosis
Stenosis   }
Stricture  } of salivary duct

**527.9 Unspecified disease of the salivary glands**

✓4ᵗʰ **528 Diseases of the oral soft tissues, excluding lesions specific for gingiva and tongue**

✓5ᵗʰ **528.0 Stomatitis and mucositis (ulcerative)**
EXCLUDES    cellulitis and abscess of mouth (528.3)
            diphtheritic stomatitis (032.0)
            epizootic stomatitis (078.4)
            gingivitis (523.0-523.1)
            oral thrush (112.0)
            Stevens-Johnson syndrome (695.1)
            stomatitis:
                acute necrotizing ulcerative (101)
                aphthous (528.2)
                gangrenous (528.1)
                herpetic (054.2)
                Vincent's (101)
AHA: 2Q, '99, 9
DEF: Stomatitis: Inflammation of oral mucosa; labial and buccal mucosa, tongue, palate, floor of the mouth, and gingivae.

**528.00 Stomatitis and mucositis, unspecified**
Mucositis NOS
Ulcerative mucositis NOS
Ulcerative stomatitis NOS
Vesicular stomatitis NOS
AHA: 4Q, '06, 88-90

**528.01 Mucositis (ulcerative) due to antineoplastic therapy**
Use additional E code to identify adverse effects of therapy, such as:
    antineoplastic and immunosuppressive drugs (E930.7, E933.1)
    radiation therapy (E879.2)
AHA: 4Q, '06, 88-90

**528.02 Mucositis (ulcerative) due to other drugs**
Use additional E code to identify drug
AHA: 4Q, '06, 88-90

**528.09 Other stomatitis and mucositis (ulcerative)**
AHA: 4Q, '06, 88-90

**528.1 Cancrum oris**
Gangrenous stomatitis    Noma
DEF: A severely gangrenous lesion of mouth due to fusospirochetal infection; destroys buccal, labial and facial tissues; can be fatal; found primarily in debilitated and malnourished children.

**528.2 Oral aphthae**
Aphthous stomatitis       Recurrent aphthous ulcer
Canker sore               Stomatitis herpetiformis
Periadenitis mucosa
    necrotica recurrens
EXCLUDES    herpetic stomatitis (054.2)
DEF: Small oval or round ulcers of the mouth marked by a grayish exudate and a red halo effect.

**528.3 Cellulitis and abscess**  CC
Cellulitis of mouth (floor)    Oral fistula
Ludwig's angina
EXCLUDES    abscess of tongue (529.0)
            cellulitis or abscess of lip (528.5)
            fistula (of):
                dental (522.7)
                lip (528.5)
            gingivitis (523.00-523.11)
CC Excl: 528.00-528.09, 528.3, 529.0, 529.2

**528.4 Cysts**
Dermoid cyst
Epidermoid cyst
Epstein's pearl          }
Lymphoepithelial cyst    } of mouth
Nasoalveolar cyst
Nasolabial cyst
EXCLUDES    cyst:                cyst:
                gingiva (523.8)      tongue (529.8)

**528.5 Diseases of lips**
Abscess
Cellulitis   }
Fistula      } of lip(s)
Hypertrophy
Cheilitis:               Cheilodynia
    NOS                  Cheilosis
    angular
EXCLUDES    actinic cheilitis (692.79)
            congenital fistula of lip (750.25)
            leukoplakia of lips (528.6)
AHA: S-O, '86, 10

**528.6 Leukoplakia of oral mucosa, including tongue**
Leukokeratosis of oral    Leukoplakia of:
    mucosa                    gingiva
                              lips
                              tongue
EXCLUDES    carcinoma in situ (230.0, 232.0)
            leukokeratosis nicotina palati (528.79)
DEF: Thickened white patches of epithelium on mucous membranes of mouth.

N Newborn Age: 0    P Pediatric Age: 0-17    M Maternity Age: 12-55    A Adult Age: 15-124    CC CC Condition    MCC Major CC Condition    HIV HIV Related Dx

174 — Volume 1 • October 2007

© 2007 Ingenix

√5th **528.7 Other disturbances of oral epithelium, including tongue**

> EXCLUDES   carcinoma in situ (230.0, 232.0)
> leukokeratosis NOS ▶(702.8)◀

**528.71 Minimal keratinized residual ridge mucosa**
Minimal keratinization of alveolar ridge mucosa

**528.72 Excessive keratinized residual ridge mucosa**
Excessive keratinization of alveolar ridge mucosa

**528.79 Other disturbances of oral epithelium, including tongue**
Erythroplakia of mouth or tongue
Focal epithelial hyperplasia of mouth or tongue
Leukoedema of mouth or tongue
Leukokeratosis nicotina palate
Other oral epithelium disturbances

**528.8 Oral submucosal fibrosis, including of tongue**

**528.9 Other and unspecified diseases of the oral soft tissues**
Cheek and lip biting    Melanoplakia
Denture sore mouth    Papillary hyperplasia of palate
Denture stomatitis

Eosinophilic granuloma ⎫
Irritative hyperplasia   ⎬ of oral mucosa
Pyogenic granuloma    ⎪
Ulcer (traumatic)     ⎭

√4th **529 Diseases and other conditions of the tongue**

**529.0 Glossitis**
Abscess ⎫
Ulceration (traumatic) ⎬ of tongue

> EXCLUDES   glossitis:
> benign migratory (529.1)
> Hunter's (529.4)
> median rhomboid (529.2)
> Moeller's (529.4)

**529.1 Geographic tongue**
Benign migratory glossitis
Glossitis areata exfoliativa
DEF: Chronic glossitis; marked by filiform papillae atrophy and inflammation; no known etiology.

**529.2 Median rhomboid glossitis**
DEF: A noninflammatory, congenital disease characterized by rhomboid-like lesions at the middle third of the tongue's dorsal surface.

**529.3 Hypertrophy of tongue papillae**
Black hairy tongue    Hypertrophy of foliate papillae
Coated tongue    Lingua villosa nigra

**529.4 Atrophy of tongue papillae**
Bald tongue    Glossitis:
Glazed tongue     Moeller's
Glossitis:      Glossodynia exfoliativa
Hunter's      Smooth atrophic tongue

**529.5 Plicated tongue**
Fissured ⎫
Furrowed ⎬ tongue
Scrotal   ⎭

> EXCLUDES   fissure of tongue, congenital (750.13)
DEF: Cracks, fissures or furrows, on dorsal surface of tongue.

**529.6 Glossodynia**
Glossopyrosis    Painful tongue
> EXCLUDES   glossodynia exfoliativa (529.4)

**529.8 Other specified conditions of the tongue**
Atrophy   ⎫
Crenated   ⎬
Enlargement ⎬ (of) tongue
Hypertrophy ⎭

Glossocele
Glossoptosis
> EXCLUDES   erythroplasia of tongue (528.79)
> leukoplakia of tongue (528.6)
> macroglossia (congenital) (750.15)
> microglossia (congenital) (750.16)
> oral submucosal fibrosis (528.8)

**529.9 Unspecified condition of the tongue**

## DISEASES OF ESOPHAGUS, STOMACH, AND DUODENUM
## (530-538)

√4th **530 Diseases of esophagus**
> EXCLUDES   esophageal varices (456.0-456.2)

**530.0 Achalasia and cardiospasm**
Achalasia (of cardia)    Megaesophagus
Aperistalsis of esophagus
> EXCLUDES   congenital cardiospasm (750.7)
DEF: Failure of smooth muscle fibers to relax, at gastrointestinal junctures; such as esophagogastric sphincter when swallowing.

√5th **530.1 Esophagitis**
Abscess of esophagus    Esophagitis:
Esophagitis:      peptic
   NOS       postoperative
   chemical      regurgitant
Use additional E code to identify cause, if induced by chemical
> EXCLUDES   tuberculous esophagitis (017.8)
AHA: 4Q, '93, 27; 1Q, '92, 17; 3Q, '91, 20

**530.10 Esophagitis, unspecified**
AHA: 3Q, '05, 17

**530.11 Reflux esophagitis**
AHA: 4Q, '95, 82
DEF: Inflammation of lower esophagus; due to regurgitated gastric acid.

**530.12 Acute esophagitis**    **CC**
CC Excl: 530.10-530.21, 530.4, 530.7, 530.82, 530.85-530.89
AHA: 4Q, '01, 45
DEF: An acute inflammation of the mucous lining or submucosal coat of the esophagus.

**530.19 Other esophagitis**
AHA: 3Q, '01, 10

√5th **530.2 Ulcer of esophagus**
Ulcer of esophagus:    Ulcer of esophagus:
   fungal      peptic
Ulcer of esophagus due to ingestion of:
   aspirin      chemicals
   medicines
Use additional E code to identify cause, if induced by chemical or drug
AHA: 4Q, '03, 63

**530.20 Ulcer of esophagus without bleeding**    **CC**
Ulcer of esophagus NOS
CC Excl: 530.21, 530.89-530.9, 537.84

**530.21 Ulcer of esophagus with bleeding**    **MCC**
> EXCLUDES   bleeding esophageal varices (456.0, 456.20)
CC Excl: 251.5, 456.0, 530.20-530.21, 530.7, 530.82, 530.85, 531.00-534.91, 535.01, 535.11, 535.21, 535.31, 535.41, 535.51, 535.61, 537.83, 537.89-538, 562.02-562.03, 562.12-562.13, 569.3, 569.85, 578.0-578.9

**530.3 Stricture and stenosis of esophagus**
Compression of esophagus
Obstruction of esophagus
> EXCLUDES   congenital stricture of esophagus (750.3)
AHA: 2Q, '01, 4; 2Q, '97, 3; 1Q, '88, 13

**530.4 Perforation of esophagus**    **MCC**
Rupture of esophagus
> EXCLUDES   traumatic perforation of esophagus (862.22, 862.32, 874.4-874.5)
CC Excl: 530.4, 530.7-530.81, 530.83-530.84, 530.89-530.9

**530.5 Dyskinesia of esophagus**
Corkscrew esophagus    Esophagospasm
Curling esophagus    Spasm of esophagus
> EXCLUDES   cardiospasm (530.0)
AHA: 1Q, '88, 13; N-D, '84, 19
DEF: Difficulty performing voluntary esophageal movements.

**Esophagus**

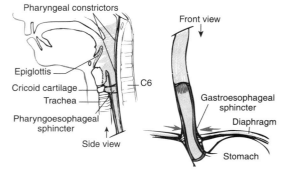

### 530.6    Diverticulum of esophagus, acquired

Diverticulum, acquired:   Diverticulum, acquired:
   epiphrenic             traction
   pharyngoesophageal    Zenker's
   pulsion              (hypopharyngeal)
   subdiaphragmatic     Esophageal pouch, acquired
                       Esophagocele, acquired

**EXCLUDES**   *congenital diverticulum of esophagus (750.4)*

**AHA:** J-F, '85, 3

### 530.7    Gastroesophageal laceration-hemorrhage syndrome   MCC

Mallory-Weiss syndrome

**CC Excl:** 251.5, 456.0, 530.20-530.21, 530.4, 530.7-530.85, 530.89-534.91, 535.01, 535.11, 535.21, 535.31, 535.41, 535.51, 535.61, 537.83, 562.02-562.03, 562.12-562.13, 569.3, 569.85, 578.0-578.9

**DEF:** Laceration of distal esophagus and proximal stomach due to vomiting, hiccups or other sustained activity.

### √5th 530.8    Other specified disorders of esophagus

#### 530.81    Esophageal reflux

Gastroesophageal reflux

**EXCLUDES**   *reflux esophagitis (530.11)*

**AHA:** 2Q, '01, 4; 1Q, '95, 7; 4Q, '92, 27

**DEF:** Regurgitation of the gastric contents into esophagus and possibly pharynx; where aspiration may occur between the vocal cords and down into the trachea.

#### 530.82    Esophageal hemorrhage   MCC

**EXCLUDES**   *hemorrhage due to esophageal varices (456.0-456.2)*

**CC Excl:** 251.5, 456.0, 456.20, 459.89-459.9, 530.20-530.21, 530.7, 530.82, 530.85, 531.00-534.91, 535.01, 535.11, 535.21, 535.31, 535.41, 535.51, 535.61, 537.83, 562.02-562.03, 562.12-562.13, 569.3, 569.85, 578.0-578.9

**AHA:** 1Q, '05, 17

#### 530.83    Esophageal leukoplakia

#### 530.84    Tracheoesophageal fistula   MCC

**EXCLUDES**   *congenital tracheoesophageal fistula (750.3)*

**CC Excl:** 530.4, 530.7-530.81, 530.83-530.84, 530.89-530.9

#### 530.85    Barrett's esophagus

**AHA:** 4Q, '03, 63

**DEF:** A metaplastic disorder in which specialized columnar epithelial cells replace the normal squamous epithelial cells; an acquired condition secondary to chronic gastroesophageal reflux damage to the mucosa; associated with increased risk of developing adenocarcinoma.

#### 530.86    Infection of esophagostomy   CC

Use additional code to specify infection

**CC Excl:** 530.86-530.87, 536.40-536.49, 997.4, 997.71, 997.91-997.99, 998.81, 998.83-998.9

#### 530.87    Mechanical complication of esophagostomy   CC

Malfunction of esophagostomy

**CC Excl:** See code: 530.86

#### 530.89    Other

**EXCLUDES**   *Paterson-Kelly syndrome (280.8)*

### 530.9    Unspecified disorder of esophagus

### √4th 531    Gastric ulcer

**INCLUDES**   ulcer (peptic):
              prepyloric
              pylorus
              stomach

Use additional E code to identify drug, if drug-induced

**EXCLUDES**   *peptic ulcer NOS (533.0-533.9)*

The following fifth-digit subclassification is for use with category 531:

   **0  without mention of obstruction**
   **1  with obstruction**

**AHA:** 1Q, '91, 15; 4Q, '90, 27

**DEF:** Destruction of tissue in lumen of stomach due to action of gastric acid and pepsin on gastric mucosa decreasing resistance to ulcers.

#### √5th 531.0    Acute with hemorrhage   MCC

**CC Excl:** 251.5, 456.0, 530.20-530.21, 530.7, 530.82, 530.85, 531.00-534.91, 535.01, 535.11, 535.21, 535.31, 535.41, 535.51, 535.61, 537.83, 537.89-538, 562.02-562.03, 562.12-562.13, 569.3, 569.85, 578.0-578.9

**AHA:** N-D, '84, 15

#### √5th 531.1    Acute with perforation   MCC

**CC Excl:** See code 531.0

#### √5th 531.2    Acute with hemorrhage and perforation   MCC

**CC Excl:** See code 531.0

#### √5th 531.3    Acute without mention of hemorrhage or perforation   MCC 1  CC 0

**CC Excl:** See code 531.0

#### √5th 531.4    Chronic or unspecified with hemorrhage   MCC

**CC Excl:** See code 531.0

**AHA:** 4Q, '90, 22

#### √5th 531.5    Chronic or unspecified with perforation   MCC

**CC Excl:** See code 531.0

#### √5th 531.6    Chronic or unspecified with hemorrhage and perforation   MCC

**CC Excl:** See code 531.0

#### √5th 531.7    Chronic without mention of hemorrhage or perforation   MCC 1

**CC Excl:** For code 531.71: see code 531.0

#### √5th 531.9    Unspecified as acute or chronic, without mention of hemorrhage or perforation   MCC 1

**CC Excl:** For code 531.91: see code 531.0

### √4th 532    Duodenal ulcer

**INCLUDES**   erosion (acute) of duodenum
             ulcer (peptic):
                duodenum
                postpyloric

Use additional E code to identify drug, if drug-induced

**EXCLUDES**   *peptic ulcer NOS (533.0-533.9)*

The following fifth-digit subclassification is for use with category 532:

   **0  without mention of obstruction**
   **1  with obstruction**

**AHA:** 4Q, '90, 27; 1Q, '91, 15

**DEF:** Ulcers in duodenum due to action of gastric acid and pepsin on mucosa decreasing resistance to ulcers.

**Stomach**

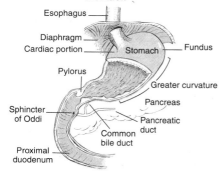

---

§ ✓5ᵗʰ **532.0** **Acute with hemorrhage**   `MCC`
CC Excl: 251.5, 456.0, 530.20-530.21, 530.7, 530.82, 530.85, 531.00-534.91, 535.01, 535.11, 535.21, 535.31, 535.41, 535.51, 535.61, 537.3, 537.83, 537.89-538, 562.02-562.03, 562.12-562.13, 569.3, 569.85, 578.0-578.9

AHA: 4Q, '90, 22

§ ✓5ᵗʰ **532.1** **Acute with perforation**   `MCC`
CC Excl: See code 532.0

§ ✓5ᵗʰ **532.2** **Acute with hemorrhage and perforation**   `MCC`
CC Excl: See code 532.0

§ ✓5ᵗʰ **532.3** **Acute without mention of hemorrhage** `MCC 1` `CC 0`
**or perforation**
CC Excl: For code 532.30: 251.5, 456.0, 530.7, 530.82, 531.00-534.91, 535.01, 535.11, 535.21, 535.31, 535.41, 535.51, 535.61, 537.3, 537.83-538, 562.02-562.03, 562.12-562.13, 569.3, 569.85, 578.0-578.9;
For code 532.31: 251.5, 456.0, 530.20-530.21, 530.7, 530.82, 530.85, 531.00-534.91, 535.01, 535.11, 535.21, 535.31, 535.41, 535.51, 535.61, 537.3, 537.83, 537.89-538, 562.02-562.03, 562.12-562.13, 569.3, 569.85, 578.0-578.9

§ ✓5ᵗʰ **532.4** **Chronic or unspecified with hemorrhage**   `MCC`
CC Excl: See code 532.0

§ ✓5ᵗʰ **532.5** **Chronic or unspecified with perforation**   `MCC`
CC Excl: See code 532.0

§ ✓5ᵗʰ **532.6** **Chronic or unspecified with hemorrhage and**   `MCC`
**perforation**
CC Excl: See code 532.0

§ ✓5ᵗʰ **532.7** **Chronic without mention of hemorrhage or** `MCC 1`
**perforation**
CC Excl: For code 532.71: See code 532.0

§ ✓5ᵗʰ **532.9** **Unspecified as acute or chronic, without** `MCC 1`
**mention of hemorrhage or perforation**
CC Excl: For code 532.91: See code 532.0

✓4ᵗʰ **533 Peptic ulcer, site unspecified**
`INCLUDES`   gastroduodenal ulcer NOS   stress ulcer NOS
peptic ulcer NOS
Use additional E code to identify drug, if drug-induced
`EXCLUDES`   peptic ulcer:
*duodenal (532.0-532.9)*
*gastric (531.0-531.9)*

The following fifth-digit subclassification is for use with category 533:
    0 **without mention of obstruction**
    1 **with obstruction**

AHA: 1Q, '91, 15; 4Q, '90, 27
DEF: Ulcer of mucous membrane of esophagus, stomach or duodenum due to gastric acid secretion.

✓5ᵗʰ **533.0** **Acute with hemorrhage**   `MCC`
CC Excl: See code 532.0

✓5ᵗʰ **533.1** **Acute with perforation**   `MCC`
CC Excl: See code 533.0

✓5ᵗʰ **533.2** **Acute with hemorrhage and perforation**   `MCC`
CC Excl: See code 533.0

✓5ᵗʰ **533.3** **Acute without mention of hemorrhage** `MCC 1` `CC 0`
**and perforation**
CC Excl: See code: 533.0

✓5ᵗʰ **533.4** **Chronic or unspecified with hemorrhage**   `MCC`
CC Excl: See code 533.0

✓5ᵗʰ **533.5** **Chronic or unspecified with perforation**   `MCC`
CC Excl: See code 533.0

✓5ᵗʰ **533.6** **Chronic or unspecified with hemorrhage and**   `MCC`
**perforation**
CC Excl: See code 533.0

✓5ᵗʰ **533.7** **Chronic without mention of hemorrhage or** `MCC 1`
**perforation**
CC Excl: For code 533.71: See code 533.0
AHA: 2Q, '89, 16

✓5ᵗʰ **533.9** **Unspecified as acute or chronic, without** `MCC 1`
**mention of hemorrhage or perforation**
CC Excl: For code 533.91: See code 533.0

✓4ᵗʰ **534 Gastrojejunal ulcer**
`INCLUDES`   ulcer (peptic) or erosion:   ulcer (peptic) or erosion:
    anastomotic            jejunal
    gastrocolic            marginal
    gastrointestinal      stomal
    gastrojejunal
`EXCLUDES`   *primary ulcer of small intestine (569.82)*

The following fifth-digit subclassification is for use with category 534:
    0 **without mention of obstruction**
    1 **with obstruction**

AHA: 1Q, '91, 15; 4Q, '90, 27

✓5ᵗʰ **534.0** **Acute with hemorrhage**   `MCC`
CC Excl: 251.5, 456.0, 530.20-530.21, 530.7, 530.82, 530.85, 531.00-534.91, 535.01, 535.11, 535.21, 535.31, 535.41, 535.51, 535.61, 537.83, 537.89-538, 562.02-562.03, 562.12-562.13, 569.3, 569.85, 578.0-578.9

✓5ᵗʰ **534.1** **Acute with perforation**   `MCC`
CC Excl: See code 534.0

✓5ᵗʰ **534.2** **Acute with hemorrhage and perforation**   `MCC`
CC Excl: See code 534.0

✓5ᵗʰ **534.3** **Acute without mention of hemorrhage** `MCC 1` `CC 0`
**or perforation**
CC Excl:: See code 534.0

✓5ᵗʰ **534.4** **Chronic or unspecified with hemorrhage**   `MCC`
CC Excl: See code 534.0

✓5ᵗʰ **534.5** **Chronic or unspecified with perforation**   `MCC`
CC Excl: See code 534.0

✓5ᵗʰ **534.6** **Chronic or unspecified with hemorrhage and**   `MCC`
**perforation**
CC Excl: See code 534.0

✓5ᵗʰ **534.7** **Chronic without mention of hemorrhage or** `MCC 1`
**perforation**
CC Excl: For code 534.71: See code 534.0

✓5ᵗʰ **534.9** **Unspecified as acute or chronic, without** `MCC 1`
**mention of hemorrhage or perforation**
CC Excl: For code 534.91: See code 534.0

✓4ᵗʰ **535 Gastritis and duodenitis**
The following fifth-digit subclassification is for use with category 535:
    0 **without mention of hemorrhage**
    1 **with hemorrhage**

AHA: 2Q, '92, 9; 4Q, '91, 25

✓5ᵗʰ **535.0** **Acute gastritis**   `MCC 1`
CC Excl: For code 535.01: 251.5, 456.0, 530.20-530.21, 530.7, 530.82, 530.85, 531.00-534.91, 535.01, 535.11, 535.21, 535.31, 535.41, 535.51, 535.61, 537.83, 562.02-562.03, 562.12-562.13, 569.3, 569.85, 578.0-578.9

AHA: 2Q, '92, 8; N-D, '86, 9

✓5ᵗʰ **535.1** **Atrophic gastritis**   `MCC 1`
    Gastritis:            Gastritis:
    atrophic-hyperplastic     chronic (atrophic)
CC Excl: For code 535.11: See code 535.01
AHA: 1Q, '94, 18
DEF: Inflammation of stomach, with mucous membrane atrophy and peptic gland destruction.

✓5ᵗʰ **535.2** **Gastric mucosal hypertrophy**   `MCC 1`
    Hypertrophic gastritis
CC Excl: For code 535.21: See code 535.01

✓5ᵗʰ **535.3** **Alcoholic gastritis**   `MCC 1`
CC Excl: For code 535.31: See code 535.01

✓5ᵗʰ **535.4** **Other specified gastritis**   `MCC 1`
    Gastritis:            Gastritis:
    allergic             superficial
    bile induced        toxic
    irritant
CC Excl: For code 535.41: See code 535.01
AHA: 4Q, '90, 27

---

§   Requires fifth digit. See category 532 for codes and definitions.

✓4ᵗʰ / ✓5ᵗʰ Additional Digit Required     Unacceptable PDx     Manifestation Code     ▶◀ Revised Text     ● New Code     ▲ Revised Code Title

**Digestive System**

**535.5–537.84**

§ ✓5ᵗʰ **535.5 Unspecified gastritis and gastroduodenitis** [MCC 1]
CC Excl: For code 535.51: See code 535.01
AHA: For code 535.50: 3Q, '05, 17; 4Q, '99, 25

§ ✓5ᵗʰ **535.6 Duodenitis** [MCC 1]
CC Excl: For code 535.61: See code 535.01
AHA: For code 535.60: 3Q, '05, 17
DEF: Inflammation of intestine, between pylorus and jejunum.

✓4ᵗʰ **536 Disorders of function of stomach**
[EXCLUDES] *functional disorders of stomach specified as psychogenic (306.4)*

**536.0 Achlorhydria**
DEF: Absence of gastric acid due to gastric mucosa atrophy; unresponsive to histamines; also known as gastric anacidity.

**536.1 Acute dilatation of stomach** [CC]
Acute distention of stomach
CC Excl: 536.1

**536.2 Persistent vomiting**
Habit vomiting    Uncontrollable vomiting
Persistent vomiting [not of pregnancy]
[EXCLUDES] *excessive vomiting in pregnancy (643.0-643.9)*
*vomiting NOS (787.0)*

**536.3 Gastroparesis**
Gastroparalysis
▶Code first underlying disease, such as:
diabetes mellitus (250.6)◀
AHA: 2Q, '04, 7; 2Q, '01, 4; 4Q, '94, 42
DEF: Slight degree of paralysis within muscular coat of stomach.

✓5ᵗʰ **536.4 Gastrostomy complications**
AHA: 4Q, '98, 42

**536.40 Gastrostomy complication, unspecified**

**536.41 Infection of gastrostomy** [CC]
Use additional code to specify type of infection, such as:
abscess or cellulitis of abdomen (682.2)
septicemia (038.0-038.9)
Use additional code to identify organism (041.00-041.9)
CC Excl: 530.86-530.87, 536.40-536.49, 997.4, 997.71, 997.91-997.99, 998.81, 998.83-998.9
AHA: 4Q, '98, 42

**536.42 Mechanical complication of gastrostomy** [CC]
CC Excl: See code 536.41

**536.49 Other gastrostomy complications**
AHA: 4Q, '98, 42

**536.8 Dyspepsia and other specified disorders of function of stomach**
Achylia gastrica    Hyperchlorhydria
Hourglass contraction    Hypochlorhydria
of stomach    Indigestion
Hyperacidity    Tachygastria
[EXCLUDES] *achlorhydria (536.0)*
*heartburn (787.1)*
AHA: 2Q, '93, 6; 2Q, '89, 16; N-D, '84, 9

**536.9 Unspecified functional disorder of stomach**
Functional gastrointestinal:
disorder
disturbance
irritation

✓4ᵗʰ **537 Other disorders of stomach and duodenum**

**537.0 Acquired hypertrophic pyloric stenosis** [CC]
Constriction
Obstruction } of pylorus, acquired or adult
Stricture
[EXCLUDES] *congenital or infantile pyloric stenosis (750.5)*
CC Excl: 536.3, 536.8-537.0, 537.3, 750.5, 750.8-750.9, 751.1, 751.5
AHA: 2Q, '01, 4; J-F, '85, 14

**537.1 Gastric diverticulum**
[EXCLUDES] *congenital diverticulum of stomach (750.7)*
AHA: J-F, '85, 4
DEF: Herniated sac or pouch, within stomach or duodenum.

**537.2 Chronic duodenal ileus**
DEF: Persistent obstruction between pylorus and jejunum.

**537.3 Other obstruction of duodenum** [CC]
Cicatrix
Stenosis
Stricture } of duodenum
Volvulus
[EXCLUDES] *congenital obstruction of duodenum (751.1)*
CC Excl: 537.3, 750.8-750.9, 751.1, 751.5

**537.4 Fistula of stomach or duodenum** [CC]
Gastrocolic fistula    Gastrojejunocolic fistula
CC Excl: 537.4, 750.8-750.9, 751.5

**537.5 Gastroptosis**
DEF: Downward displacement of stomach.

**537.6 Hourglass stricture or stenosis of stomach**
Cascade stomach
[EXCLUDES] *congenital hourglass stomach (750.7)*
*hourglass contraction of stomach (536.8)*

✓5ᵗʰ **537.8 Other specified disorders of stomach and duodenum**
AHA: 4Q, '91, 25

**537.81 Pylorospasm**
[EXCLUDES] *congenital pylorospasm (750.5)*
DEF: Spasm of the pyloric sphincter.

**537.82 Angiodysplasia of stomach and duodenum (without mention of hemorrhage)**
AHA: ▶2Q, '07, 7;◀3Q, '96, 10; 4Q, '90, 4

**537.83 Angiodysplasia of stomach and duodenum with hemorrhage** [MCC]
CC Excl: 251.5, 456.0, 530.20-530.21, 530.7, 530.82, 530.85, 531.00-534.91, 535.01, 535.11, 535.21, 535.31, 535.41, 535.51, 535.61, 537.83, 562.02-562.03, 562.12-562.13, 569.3, 569.85, 578.0-578.9
AHA: ▶2Q, '07, 7◀
DEF: Bleeding of stomach and duodenum due to vascular abnormalities.

**537.84 Dieulafoy lesion (hemorrhagic) of stomach and duodenum** [MCC]
CC Excl: 251.5, 456.0, 530.20-530.21, 530.7, 530.82, 530.85, 531.00-534.91, 535.01, 535.11, 535.21, 535.31, 535.41, 535.51, 535.61, 537.83-537.84, 562.02-562.03, 562.12-562.13, 569.3, 569.85, 578.0-578.9
AHA: 4Q, '02, 60
DEF: An abnormally large and convoluted submucosal artery protruding through a defect in the mucosa in the stomach or intestines that can erode the epithelium causing hemorrhaging; also called Dieulafoy's vascular malformation.

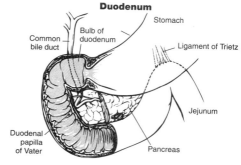

§ Requires fifth digit. See category 535 for codes and definitions.

[N] Newborn Age: 0    [P] Pediatric Age: 0-17    [M] Maternity Age: 12-55    [A] Adult Age: 15-124    [CC] CC Condition    [MCC] Major CC Condition    [HIV] HIV Related Dx

**537.89  Other**
Gastric or duodenal:
prolapse
rupture
Intestinal metaplasia of gastric mucosa
Passive congestion of stomach

> EXCLUDES    *diverticula of duodenum (562.00-562.01)*
> *gastrointestinal hemorrhage (578.0-578.9)*

AHA: 3Q, '05, 15; N-D, '84, 7

**537.9  Unspecified disorder of stomach and duodenum**

**538  Gastrointestinal mucositis (ulcerative)**    `CC`
Use additional E code to identify adverse effects of therapy, such as:
antineoplastic and immunosuppressive drugs (E930.7, E933.1)
radiation therapy (E879.2)

> EXCLUDES    *mucositis (ulcerative) of mouth and oral soft tissue (528.00- 528.09)*

CC Excl: 251.5, 456.0, 530.20-530.21, 530.7, 530.82, 530.85, 531.00-534.91, 535.01, 535.11, 535.21, 535.31, 535.41, 535.51, 535.61, 537.83, 537.89-538, 562.02-562.03, 562.12-562.13, 569.3, 569.85, 578.0-578.9

AHA: 4Q, '06, 88-90

## APPENDICITIS (540-543)

**✓4th 540  Acute appendicitis**
AHA: N-D, '84, 19
DEF: Inflammation of vermiform appendix due to fecal obstruction, neoplasm or foreign body of appendiceal lumen; causes infection, edema and infarction of appendiceal wall; may result in mural necrosis, and perforation.

**540.0  With generalized peritonitis**    `MCC`
Appendicitis (acute):
fulminating
gangrenous   } with:
obstructive        perforation
Cecitis (acute)    peritonitis (generalized)
                          rupture
Rupture of appendix

> EXCLUDES    *acute appendicitis with peritoneal abscess (540.1)*

CC Excl: 537.89-543.9

**540.1  With peritoneal abscess**    `MCC`
Abscess of appendix
With generalized peritonitis
CC Excl: See code 540.0
AHA: N-D, '84, 19

**540.9  Without mention of peritonitis**    `CC`
Acute:
appendicitis:
fulminating
gangrenous      without mention of
inflamed            perforation,
obstructive        peritonitis, or rupture
cecitis

CC Excl: See code 540.0
AHA: 1Q, '01, 15; 4Q, '97, 52

**Appendix**

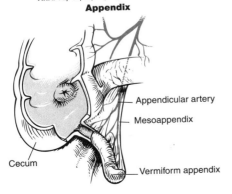

Appendicular artery
Mesoappendix
Cecum
Vermiform appendix

**541  Appendicitis, unqualified**
AHA: 2Q, '90, 26

**542  Other appendicitis**
Appendicitis:              Appendicitis:
chronic                        relapsing
recurrent                     subacute

> EXCLUDES    *hyperplasia (lymphoid) of appendix (543.0)*

AHA: 1Q, '01, 15

**✓4th 543  Other diseases of appendix**
**543.0  Hyperplasia of appendix (lymphoid)**
DEF: Proliferation of cells in appendix tissue.

**543.9  Other and unspecified diseases of appendix**
Appendicular or appendiceal:
colic
concretion
fistula
Diverticulum
Fecalith
Intussusception   } of appendix
Mucocele
Stercolith

## HERNIA OF ABDOMINAL CAVITY (550-553)

> INCLUDES    hernia:
> acquired
> congenital, except diaphragmatic or hiatal

**✓4th 550  Inguinal hernia**    `CC`

> INCLUDES    bubonocele
> inguinal hernia (direct) (double) (indirect) (oblique) (sliding)
> scrotal hernia

The following fifth-digit subclassification is for use with category 550:
**0  unilateral or unspecified (not specified as recurrent)**
Unilateral NOS
**1  unilateral or unspecified, recurrent**
**2  bilateral (not specified as recurrent)**
Bilateral NOS
**3  bilateral, recurrent**

CC Excl: 537.89-538, 550.00-550.93, 552.8-552.9, 553.8-553.9

AHA: N-D, '85, 12
DEF: Hernia protrusion of an abdominal organ or tissue through inguinal canal.
DEF: Indirect inguinal hernia: (external or oblique) leaves abdomen through deep inguinal ring, passes through inguinal canal lateral to the inferior epigastric artery.
DEF: Direct inguinal hernia: (internal) emerges between inferior epigastric artery and rectus muscle edge.

**✓5th 550.0  Inguinal hernia, with gangrene**    `MCC`
Inguinal hernia with gangrene (and obstruction)
CC Excl: 537.89-538, 550.00-550.93, 552.8-552.9, 553.8-553.9

**✓5th 550.1  Inguinal hernia, with obstruction, without mention of gangrene**    `CC`
Inguinal hernia with mention of incarceration, irreducibility, or strangulation
CC Excl: See code 550.0

**✓5th 550.9  Inguinal hernia, without mention of obstruction or gangrene**
Inguinal hernia NOS
AHA: For code 550.91: 3Q, '03, 10; 1Q, '03, 4

**✓4th 551  Other hernia of abdominal cavity, with gangrene**
> INCLUDES    that with gangrene (and obstruction)

**✓5th 551.0  Femoral hernia with gangrene**
**551.00  Unilateral or unspecified (not specified as recurrent)**    `MCC`
Femoral hernia NOS with gangrene
CC Excl: 537.89-538, 551.00-551.03, 552.8-553.03, 553.8-553.9

**551.01  Unilateral or unspecified, recurrent**    `MCC`
CC Excl: See code 551.00

**551.02 Bilateral (not specified as recurrent)** `MCC`
CC Excl: See code 551.00

**551.03 Bilateral, recurrent** `MCC`
CC Excl: See code 551.00

**551.1 Umbilical hernia with gangrene** `MCC`
Parumbilical hernia specified as gangrenous
CC Excl: 537.89-538, 551.1-551.29, 552.1-552.29, 552.8-552.9, 553.1-553.29, 553.8-553.9

√5ᵗʰ **551.2 Ventral hernia with gangrene**

**551.20 Ventral, unspecified, with gangrene** `MCC`
CC Excl: See code 551.1

**551.21 Incisional, with gangrene** `MCC`
Hernia:
postoperative
recurrent, ventral } specified as gangrenous
CC Excl: See code 551.1

**551.29 Other** `MCC`
Epigastric hernia specified as gangrenous
CC Excl: See code 551.1

**551.3 Diaphragmatic hernia with gangrene** `MCC`
Hernia:
hiatal (esophageal) (sliding)
paraesophageal
Thoracic stomach } specified as gangrenous

EXCLUDES *congenital diaphragmatic hernia (756.6)*
CC Excl: 551.3, 552.3-552.9, 553.3-553.9

**Inguinal Hernias**

**Femoral Hernia**

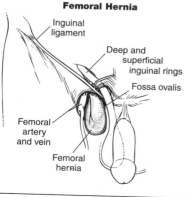

**551.8 Hernia of other specified sites, with gangrene** `MCC`
Any condition classifiable to 553.8 if specified as gangrenous
CC Excl: 537.89-538, 550.00-553.9

**551.9 Hernia of unspecified site, with gangrene** `MCC`
Any condition classifiable to 553.9 if specified as gangrenous
CC Excl: See code 551.8

√4ᵗʰ **552 Other hernia of abdominal cavity, with obstruction, but without mention of gangrene**
EXCLUDES *that with mention of gangrene (551.0-551.9)*

√5ᵗʰ **552.0 Femoral hernia with obstruction**
Femoral hernia specified as incarcerated, irreducible, strangulated, or causing obstruction

**552.00 Unilateral or unspecified (not specified as recurrent)** `CC`
CC Excl: 537.89-538, 551.00-551.03, 552.00-552.03, 552.8-553.03, 553.8-553.9

**552.01 Unilateral or unspecified, recurrent** `CC`
CC Excl: See code 552.00

**552.02 Bilateral (not specified as recurrent)** `CC`
CC Excl: See code 552.00

**552.03 Bilateral, recurrent** `CC`
CC Excl: See code 552.00

**552.1 Umbilical hernia with obstruction** `CC`
Parumbilical hernia specified as incarcerated, irreducible, strangulated, or causing obstruction
CC Excl: 551.1-551.29, 552.1-552.29, 552.8-552.9, 553.8-553.9

√5ᵗʰ **552.2 Ventral hernia with obstruction**
Ventral hernia specified as incarcerated, irreducible, strangulated, or causing obstruction

**552.20 Ventral, unspecified, with obstruction** `CC`
CC Excl: See code 552.1

**552.21 Incisional, with obstruction** `CC`
Hernia:
postoperative
recurrent,
ventral } specified as incarcerated, irreducible, strangulated, or causing obstruction
CC Excl: See code 552.1
AHA: 3Q, '03, 11

**552.29 Other** `CC`
Epigastric hernia specified as incarcerated, irreducible, strangulated, or causing obstruction
CC Excl: See code 552.1

**Hernias of Abdominal Cavity**

`N` Newborn Age: 0   `P` Pediatric Age: 0-17   `M` Maternity Age: 12-55   `A` Adult Age: 15-124   `CC` CC Condition   `MCC` Major CC Condition   `HIV` HIV Related Dx

180 — Volume 1 • October 2007

© 2007 Ingenix

**552.3  Diaphragmatic hernia with obstruction**  `CC`
Hernia:
hiatal (esophageal) (sliding) ⎤ specified as incarcerated,
paraesophageal ⎬ irreducible,
Thoracic stomach ⎭ strangulated, or causing obstruction

**EXCLUDES**  *congenital diaphragmatic hernia (756.6)*

CC Excl: 551.3, 552.3-552.9, 553.3-553.9

**552.8  Hernia of other specified sites, with obstruction** `CC`
Any condition classifiable to 553.8 if specified as incarcerated, irreducible, strangulated, or causing obstruction

**EXCLUDES**  *hernia due to adhesion with obstruction (560.81)*

CC Excl: 550.00-553.9

AHA: 1Q, '04, 10

**552.9  Hernia of unspecified site, with obstruction** `CC`
Any condition classifiable to 553.9 if specified as incarcerated, irreducible, strangulated, or causing obstruction

CC Excl: See code: 552.8

√4ᵗʰ **553  Other hernia of abdominal cavity without mention of obstruction or gangrene**
**EXCLUDES**  *the listed conditions with mention of:*
*gangrene (and obstruction) (551.0-551.9)*
*obstruction (552.0-552.9)*

√5ᵗʰ **553.0  Femoral hernia**
**553.00  Unilateral or unspecified (not specified as recurrent)**
Femoral hernia NOS

**553.01  Unilateral or unspecified, recurrent**

**553.02  Bilateral (not specified as recurrent)**

**553.03  Bilateral, recurrent**

**553.1  Umbilical hernia**
Parumbilical hernia

√5ᵗʰ **553.2  Ventral hernia**
**553.20  Ventral, unspecified**
AHA: 2Q, '06, 10; 3Q, '03, 6

**553.21  Incisional**
Hernia:                   Hernia:
postoperative       recurrent, ventral
AHA: 3Q, '03, 6

**553.29  Other**
Hernia:              Hernia:
epigastric        spigelian

**553.3  Diaphragmatic hernia**
Hernia:
hiatal (esophageal) (sliding)
paraesophageal
Thoracic stomach
**EXCLUDES**  *congenital:*
*diaphragmatic hernia (756.6)*
*hiatal hernia (750.6)*
*esophagocele (530.6)*

AHA: 2Q, '01, 6; 1Q, '00, 6

### Diaphragmatic Hernias

Esophagus

Gastroesophageal junction (remains in place)

Stomach

Diaphragm

Gastroesophageal junction (slides up and down)

**Paraesophageal Hiatal Hernia**

**Sliding Hiatal Hernia**

**553.8  Hernia of other specified sites**
Hernia:              Hernia:
ischiatic          pudendal
ischiorectal      retroperitoneal
lumbar            sciatic
obturator         Other abdominal hernia of specified site

**EXCLUDES**  *vaginal enterocele (618.6)*

**553.9  Hernia of unspecified site**
Enterocele          Hernia:
Epiplocele          intestinal
Hernia:              intra-abdominal
NOS               Rupture (nontraumatic)
interstitial        Sarcoepiplocele

## NONINFECTIOUS ENTERITIS AND COLITIS (555-558)

√4ᵗʰ **555  Regional enteritis**
**INCLUDES**  Crohn's disease
Granulomatous enteritis
**EXCLUDES**  *ulcerative colitis (556)*

DEF: Inflammation of intestine; classified to site.

**555.0  Small intestine**  `CC`
Ileitis:                    Regional enteritis or
regional                   Crohn's disease of:
segmental              duodenum
terminal                ileum
                            jejunum

CC Excl: 555.0-556.9

**555.1  Large intestine**  `CC`
Colitis:                   Regional enteritis or
granulmatous          Crohn's disease of:
regional                colon
transmural             large bowel
                            rectum

CC Excl: See code: 555.0
AHA: 3Q, '99, 8

**555.2  Small intestine with large intestine**  `CC`
Regional ileocolitis
CC Excl: See code: 555.0

AHA: 1Q, '03, 18

**555.9  Unspecified site**  `CC`
Crohn's disease NOS      Regional enteritis NOS
CC Excl: 555.0-555.9

AHA: 2Q, '05, 11; 3Q, '99, 8; 4Q, '97, 42; 2Q, '97, 3

√4ᵗʰ **556  Ulcerative colitis**
AHA: 3Q, '99, 8

DEF: Chronic inflammation of mucosal lining of intestinal tract; may be single area or entire colon.

**556.0  Ulcerative (chronic) enterocolitis**  `CC`
CC Excl: 555.0-556.9

**556.1  Ulcerative (chronic) ileocolitis**  `CC`
CC Excl: 555.0-556.9

**556.2  Ulcerative (chronic) proctitis**  `CC`
CC Excl: 555.0-556.9

**556.3  Ulcerative (chronic) proctosigmoiditis**  `CC`
CC Excl: 555.0-556.9

**556.4  Pseudopolyposis of colon**  `CC`
CC Excl: 555.0-556.9

**556.5  Left-sided ulcerative (chronic) colitis**  `CC`
CC Excl: 555.0-556.9

**556.6  Universal ulcerative (chronic) colitis**  `CC`
Pancolitis
CC Excl: 555.0-556.9

**556.8  Other ulcerative colitis**  `CC`
CC Excl: 555.0-556.9

Digestive System

552.3–556.8

**Digestive System**

**556.9–560.39**

**Large Intestine**

**556.9**    **Ulcerative colitis, unspecified**    `CC`
Ulcerative enteritis NOS

**CC Excl:** 555.0-556.9

**AHA:** 1Q, '03, 10

**✓4ᵗʰ 557 Vascular insufficiency of intestine**
**EXCLUDES**   *necrotizing enterocolitis of the newborn (777.5)*

**DEF:** Inadequacy of intestinal vessels.

**557.0**    **Acute vascular insufficiency of intestine**    `MCC`
Acute:
hemorrhagic enterocolitis
ischemic colitis, enteritis, or enterocolitis
massive necrosis of intestine
Bowel infarction
Embolism of mesenteric artery
Fulminant enterocolitis
Hemorrhagic necrosis of intestine
Infarction of appendices epiploicae
Intestinal gangrene
Intestinal infarction (acute) (agnogenic)
(hemorrhagic) (nonocclusive)
Mesenteric infarction (embolic) (thrombotic)
Necrosis of intestine
Terminal hemorrhagic enteropathy
Thrombosis of mesenteric artery

**CC Excl:** 557.0-557.1

**AHA:** 4Q, '01, 53

**557.1**    **Chronic vascular insufficiency of intestine**    `CC`
Angina, abdominal
Chronic ischemic colitis, enteritis, or enterocolitis
Ischemic stricture of intestine
Mesenteric:
angina
artery syndrome (superior)
vascular insufficiency

**CC Excl:** 557.0-557.9

**AHA:** 3Q, '96, 9; 4Q, '90, 4; N-D, '86, 11; N-D, '84, 7

**557.9**    **Unspecified vascular insufficiency of intestine**    `CC`
Alimentary pain due to vascular insufficiency
Ischemic colitis, enteritis, or enterocolitis NOS

**CC Excl:** 557.0-557.9

**✓4ᵗʰ 558 Other and unspecified noninfectious gastroenteritis and colitis**

**EXCLUDES**   *infectious:*
*colitis, enteritis, or gastroenteritis (009.0-009.1)*
*diarrhea (009.2-009.3)*

**558.1**    **Gastroenteritis and colitis due to radiation**    `CC`
Radiation enterocolitis

**CC Excl:** 558.1

**558.2**    **Toxic gastroenteritis and colitis**    `CC`
Use additional E code to identify cause

**CC Excl:** 558.2

**558.3**    **Allergic gastroenteritis and colitis**
Use additional code to identify type of food allergy
(V15.01-V15.05)

**AHA:** 1Q, '03, 12; 4Q, '00, 42

**DEF:** True immunoglobulin E (IgE)-mediated allergic reaction of the lining of the stomach, intestines, or colon to food proteins; causes nausea, vomiting, diarrhea, and abdominal cramping.

**558.9**    **Other and unspecified noninfectious gastroenteritis and colitis**

Colitis
Enteritis
Gastroenteritis      } NOS, dietetic, or
Ileitis                      noninfectious
Jejunitis
Sigmoiditis

**AHA:** 3Q, '99, 4, 6; N-D, '87, 7

## OTHER DISEASES OF INTESTINES AND PERITONEUM (560-569)

**✓4ᵗʰ 560 Intestinal obstruction without mention of hernia**
**EXCLUDES**   *duodenum (537.2-537.3)*
*inguinal hernia with obstruction (550.1)*
*intestinal obstruction complicating hernia*
*(552.0-552.9)*
*mesenteric:*
*embolism (557.0)*
*infarction (557.0)*
*thrombosis (557.0)*
*neonatal intestinal obstruction (277.01, 777.1-*
*777.2, 777.4)*

**560.0**    **Intussusception**    `CC`
Intussusception (colon) (intestine) (rectum)
Invagination of intestine or colon
**EXCLUDES**   *intussusception of appendix (543.9)*

**CC Excl:** 560.0-560.9, 569.89-569.9

**AHA:** 4Q, '98, 82

**DEF:** Prolapse of a bowel section into adjacent section; occurs primarily in children; symptoms include paroxysmal pain, vomiting, presence of lower abdominal tumor and blood, and mucous passage from rectum.

**560.1**    **Paralytic ileus**    `CC`
Adynamic ileus
Ileus (of intestine) (of bowel) (of colon)
Paralysis of intestine or colon
**EXCLUDES**   *gallstone ileus (560.31)*

**CC Excl:** See code 560.0

**AHA:** J-F, '87, 13

**DEF:** Obstruction of ileus due to inhibited bowel motility.

**560.2**    **Volvulus**    `MCC`
Knotting
Strangulation     } of intestine, bowel, or
Torsion                colon
Twist

**CC Excl:** See code 560.0

**DEF:** Entanglement of bowel; causes obstruction; may compromise bowel circulation.

**✓5ᵗʰ 560.3**    **Impaction of intestine**
**560.30 Impaction of intestine, unspecified**    `CC`
Impaction of colon
**CC Excl:** See code 560.0

**560.31 Gallstone ileus**    `CC`
Obstruction of intestine by gallstone
**CC Excl:** See code 560.0

**560.39 Other**    `CC`
Concretion of intestine
Enterolith
Fecal impaction
**CC Excl:** See code 560.0

**AHA:** 4Q, '98, 38

---

`N` Newborn Age: 0    `P` Pediatric Age: 0-17    `M` Maternity Age: 12-55    `A` Adult Age: 15-124    `CC` CC Condition    `MCC` Major CC Condition    `HIV` HIV Related Dx

**Volvulus and Diverticulitis**

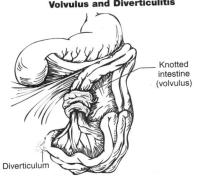

Knotted intestine (volvulus)

Diverticulum

✓5th **560.8 Other specified intestinal obstruction**

**560.81 Intestinal or peritoneal adhesions with obstruction (postoperative) (postinfection)** `CC`

> EXCLUDES   adhesions without obstruction (568.0)

CC Excl: See code 560.0

AHA: 4Q, '95, 55; 3Q, '95, 6; N-D, '87, 9

DEF: Obstruction of peritoneum or intestine due to abnormal union of tissues.

**560.89 Other** `CC`

Acute pseudo-obstruction of intestine
Mural thickening causing obstruction

> EXCLUDES   ischemic stricture of intestine (557.1)

CC Excl: See code 560.0

AHA: 2Q, '97, 3; 1Q, '88, 6

**560.9 Unspecified intestinal obstruction** `CC`

Enterostenosis
Obstruction ⎤
Occlusion    ⎥ of intestine or colon
Stenosis     ⎥
Stricture    ⎦

> EXCLUDES   congenital stricture or stenosis of intestine (751.1-751.2)

CC Excl: See code 560.0

✓4th **562 Diverticula of intestine**

Use additional code to identify any associated:
peritonitis (567.0-567.9)

> EXCLUDES   congenital diverticulum of colon (751.5)
> diverticulum of appendix (543.9)
> Meckel's diverticulum (751.0)

AHA: 4Q, '91, 25; J-F, '85, 1

✓5th **562.0 Small intestine**

**562.00 Diverticulosis of small intestine (without mention of hemorrhage)**

Diverticulosis:
duodenum ⎤
ileum      ⎥ without mention of
jejunum   ⎦ diverticulitis

DEF: Saclike herniations of mucous lining of small intestine.

**562.01 Diverticulitis of small intestine (without mention of hemorrhage)** `CC`

Diverticulitis (with diverticulosis):
duodenum
ileum
jejunum
small intestine

CC Excl: 562.00-562.03

DEF: Inflamed saclike herniations of mucous lining of small intestine

**562.02 Diverticulosis of small intestine with hemorrhage** `MCC`

CC Excl: 251.5, 456.0, 530.20-530.21, 530.7, 530.82, 530.85, 531.00-534.91, 535.01, 535.11, 535.21, 535.31, 535.41, 535.51, 535.61, 537.83, 562.02-562.03, 562.12-562.13, 569.3, 569.85, 578.0-578.9

**562.03 Diverticulitis of small intestine with hemorrhage** `MCC`

CC Excl: See code 562.02

✓5th **562.1 Colon**

**562.10 Diverticulosis of colon (without mention of hemorrhage)**

Diverticulosis: ⎤
NOS              ⎥ without mention
intestine (large) ⎥ of
Diverticular disease ⎥ diverticulitis
(colon)          ⎦

AHA: 3Q, '05, 17; 3Q, '02, 15; 4Q, '90, 21; J-F, '85, 5

DEF: Saclike herniations of mucous lining of large intestine.

**562.11 Diverticulitis of colon (without mention of hemorrhage)** `CC`

Diverticulitis (with diverticulosis):
NOS
colon
intestine (large)

CC Excl: 562.10-562.13

AHA: 1Q, '96, 14; J-F, '85, 5

DEF: Inflamed saclike herniations of mucosal lining of large intestine.

**562.12 Diverticulosis of colon with hemorrhage** `MCC`

CC Excl: See code 562.02

**562.13 Diverticulitis of colon with hemorrhage** `MCC`

CC Excl: See code 562.02

✓4th **564 Functional digestive disorders, not elsewhere classified**

> EXCLUDES   functional disorders of stomach (536.0-536.9)
> those specified as psychogenic (306.4)

✓5th **564.0 Constipation**

AHA: 4Q, '01, 45

**564.00 Constipation, unspecified**

**564.01 Slow transit constipation**

DEF:  Delay in the transit of fecal material through the colon secondary to smooth muscle dysfunction or decreased peristaltic contractions along the colon:  also called colonic inertia or delayed transit.

**564.02 Outlet dysfunction constipation**

DEF:  Failure to relax the paradoxical contractions of the striated pelvic floor muscles during the attempted defecation.

**564.09 Other constipation**

**564.1 Irritable bowel syndrome**

Irritable colon
Spastic colon

AHA: 1Q, '88, 6

DEF: Functional gastrointestinal disorder (FGID); symptoms following meals include diarrhea, constipation, abdominal pain; other symptoms include bloating, gas, distended abdomen, nausea, vomiting, appetite loss, emotional distress, and depression.

**564.2 Postgastric surgery syndromes**

Dumping syndrome      Postgastrectomy syndrome
Jejunal syndrome      Postvagotomy syndrome

> EXCLUDES   malnutrition following gastrointestinal surgery (579.3)
> postgastrojejunostomy ulcer (534.0-534.9)

AHA: 1Q, '95, 11

**564.3 Vomiting following gastrointestinal surgery**

Vomiting (bilious) following gastrointestinal surgery

✓4th ✓5th  Additional Digit Required

Unacceptable PDx

Manifestation Code

▶◀ Revised Text      ● New Code      ▲ Revised Code Title

**October 2007 • Volume 1 — 183**

© 2007 Ingenix

**Digestive System**

**564.4–567.31**

### Anal Fistula and Abscess

Urethra
Fistula
Bladder
Abscess
Rectum

### Psoas Muscle Abscess

Psoas minor muscle
Psoas major muscle
Small intestine (ilium)
Peritoneal cavity
Small intestine (jejunum)
**Abscess**
Ascending colon
Ascending colon
Psoas major muscle
Pelvic bone
Psoas major muscle
Spinous process of L4
Erector spinae muscles

**564.4 Other postoperative functional disorders**
Diarrhea following gastrointestinal surgery
**EXCLUDES**   *colostomy and enterostomy complications (569.60-569.69)*

**564.5 Functional diarrhea**
**EXCLUDES**   *diarrhea:*
*NOS (787.91)*
*psychogenic (306.4)*

DEF: Diarrhea with no detectable organic cause.

**564.6 Anal spasm**
Proctalgia fugax

**564.7 Megacolon, other than Hirschsprung's**    **CC**
Dilatation of colon
**EXCLUDES**   *megacolon:*
*congenital [Hirschsprung's] (751.3)*
*toxic (556)*

CC Excl: 564.1-564.9

DEF: Enlarged colon; congenital or acquired; can occur acutely or become chronic.

**√5ᵗʰ 564.8 Other specified functional disorders of intestine**
**EXCLUDES**   *malabsorption (579.0-579.9)*
AHA: 1Q, '88, 6

**564.81 Neurogenic bowel**    **CC**
CC Excl: See code: 564.7
AHA: 1Q, '01, 12; 4Q, '98, 45

DEF: Disorder of bowel due to spinal cord lesion above conus medullaris; symptoms include precipitous micturition, nocturia, catheter intolerance, headache, sweating, nasal obstruction and spastic contractions.

**564.89 Other functional disorders of intestine**
Atony of colon

**564.9 Unspecified functional disorder of intestine**

**√4ᵗʰ 565 Anal fissure and fistula**

**565.0 Anal fissure**
**EXCLUDES**   ▶*anal sphincter tear (healed) (non-traumatic) (old) (569.43)*◀
*traumatic (863.89, 863.99)*

DEF: Ulceration of cleft at anal mucosa; causes pain, itching, bleeding, infection, and sphincter spasm; may occur with hemorrhoids.

**565.1 Anal fistula**
Fistula:       Fistula:
anorectal      rectum to skin
rectal
**EXCLUDES**   *fistula of rectum to internal organs—see Alphabetic Index*
*ischiorectal fistula (566)*
*rectovaginal fistula (619.1)*

AHA: ▶1Q, '07, 13◀

DEF: Abnormal opening on cutaneous surface near anus; may lack connection with rectum.

**566 Abscess of anal and rectal regions**    **CC**
Abscess:              Cellulitis:
ischiorectal         anal
perianal            perirectal
perirectal          rectal
                     Ischiorectal fistula

CC Excl: 566

**√4ᵗʰ 567 Peritonitis and retroperitoneal infections**
**EXCLUDES**   *peritonitis:*
*benign paroxysmal (277.31)*
*pelvic, female (614.5, 614.7)*
*periodic familial (277.31)*
*puerperal (670)*
*with or following:*
*abortion (634-638 with .0, 639.0)*
*appendicitis (540.0-540.1)*
*ectopic or molar pregnancy (639.0)*

DEF: Inflammation of the peritoneal cavity.

**567.0 *Peritonitis in infectious diseases classified elsewhere***    **MCC**
*Code first underlying disease*
**EXCLUDES**   *peritonitis:*
*gonococcal (098.86)*
*syphilitic (095.2)*
*tuberculous (014.0)*

CC Excl: 567.0-567.29, 567.38-567.9, 569.89-569.9

**567.1 Pneumococcal peritonitis**    **MCC**
CC Excl: See code: 567.0

**√5ᵗʰ 567.2 Other suppurative peritonitis**
AHA: 4Q, '05, 74; 2Q, '01, 11, 12; 3Q, '99, 9; 2Q, '98, 19

**567.21 Peritonitis (acute) generalized**    **MCC**
Pelvic peritonitis, male
CC Excl: See code 567.0

**567.22 Peritoneal abscess**    **MCC**
Abscess (of):        Abscess (of):
abdominopelvic     retrocecal
mesenteric          subdiaphragmatic
omentum            subhepatic
peritoneum         subphrenic
CC Excl: See code 567.0

**567.23 Spontaneous bacterial peritonitis**    **MCC**
**EXCLUDES**   *bacterial peritonitis NOS (567.29)*
CC Excl: See code 567.0

**567.29 Other suppurative peritonitis**    **MCC**
Subphrenic peritonitis
CC Excl: See code 567.0

**√5ᵗʰ 567.3 Retroperitoneal infections**
AHA: 4Q, '05, 74

**567.31 Psoas muscle abscess**    **MCC**
CC Excl: 567.31, 728.0, 728.11-728.3, 728.81, 728.86

DEF: Infection that extends into or around the psoas muscle that connects the lumbar vertebrae to the femur.

---

**N** Newborn Age: 0    **P** Pediatric Age: 0-17    **M** Maternity Age: 12-55    **A** Adult Age: 15-124    **CC** CC Condition    **MCC** Major CC Condition    **HIV** HIV Related Dx

184 — Volume 1 • October 2007                                       © 2007 Ingenix

### 567.38 Other retroperitoneal abscess `MCC`
AHA: 4Q, '05, 77

CC Excl: See code 567.0

### 567.39 Other retroperitoneal infections `MCC`
CC Excl: See code 567.0

## √5th 567.8 Other specified peritonitis
AHA: 4Q, '05, 74

### 567.81 Choleperitonitis `MCC`
Peritonitis due to bile

CC Excl: See code 567.0

DEF: Inflammation or infection due to presence of bile in the peritoneum resulting from rupture of the bile passages or gallbladder.

### 567.82 Sclerosing mesenteritis `CC`
Fat necrosis of peritoneum
(Idiopathic) sclerosing mesenteric fibrosis
Mesenteric lipodystrophy
Mesenteric panniculitis
Retractile mesenteritis

CC Excl: See code 567.0

AHA: 4Q, '05, 77

DEF: Inflammatory processes involving the mesenteric fat; progresses to fibrosis and necrosis of tissue.

### 567.89 Other specified peritonitis `MCC`
Chronic proliferative peritonitis
Mesenteric saponification
Peritonitis due to urine

CC Excl: See code 567.0

## 567.9 Unspecified peritonitis `MCC`
Peritonitis NOS
Peritonitis of unspecified cause

CC Excl: See code 567.0

AHA: 1Q, '04, 10

## √4th 568 Other disorders of peritoneum

### 568.0 Peritoneal adhesions (postoperative) (postinfection)
Adhesions (of):          Adhesions (of):
  abdominal (wall)         mesenteric
  diaphragm                omentum
  intestine                stomach
  male pelvis              Adhesive bands

EXCLUDES    adhesions:
              pelvic, female (614.6)
              with obstruction:
                duodenum (537.3)
                intestine (560.81)

AHA: 3Q, '03, 7, 11; 4Q, '95, 55; 3Q, '95, 7; S-O, '85, 11

DEF: Abnormal union of tissues in peritoneum.

## √5th 568.8 Other specified disorders of peritoneum

### 568.81 Hemoperitoneum (nontraumatic) `MCC`
CC Excl: 568.81

### 568.82 Peritoneal effusion (chronic) `CC`
EXCLUDES    ascites NOS ▶(789.51-
              789.59)◀

CC Excl: 568.82

DEF: Persistent leakage of fluid within peritoneal cavity.

### 568.89 Other
Peritoneal:          Peritoneal:
  cyst                 granuloma

## 568.9 Unspecified disorder of peritoneum

## √4th 569 Other disorders of intestine

### 569.0 Anal and rectal polyp
Anal and rectal polyp NOS

EXCLUDES    adenomatous anal and rectal polyp
              (211.4)

---

**Rectum and Anus**

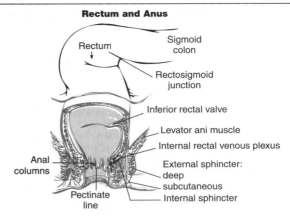

### 569.1 Rectal prolapse
Procidentia:          Prolapse:
  anus (sphincter)      anal canal
  rectum (sphincter)    rectal mucosa
Proctoptosis

EXCLUDES    prolapsed hemorrhoids (455.2, 455.5)

### 569.2 Stenosis of rectum and anus
Stricture of anus (sphincter)

### 569.3 Hemorrhage of rectum and anus `CC`
EXCLUDES    gastrointestinal bleeding NOS (578.9)
              melena (578.1)

CC Excl: 251.5, 456.0, 530.20-530.21, 530.7, 530.82, 530.85, 531.00-534.91, 535.01, 535.11, 535.21, 535.31, 535.41, 535.51, 535.61, 537.83, 562.02-562.03, 562.12-562.13, 569.3, 569.85, 578.0-578.9

AHA: 3Q, '05, 17

## √5th 569.4 Other specified disorders of rectum and anus

### 569.41 Ulcer of anus and rectum `CC`
Solitary ulcer  } of anus (sphincter) or
Stercoral ulcer }   rectum (sphincter)

CC Excl: 569.41

### 569.42 Anal or rectal pain
AHA: 1Q, '03, 8; 1Q, '96, 13

### 569.43 Anal sphincter tear (healed) (old)
Tear of anus, nontraumatic
Use additional code for any associated fecal
  incontinence (787.6)

EXCLUDES    anal fissure (565.0)
              anal sphincter tear (healed)
              (old) complicating
              delivery (654.8)

### 569.49 Other
Granuloma } of rectum (sphincter)
Rupture   }

Hypertrophy of anal papillae
Proctitis NOS

EXCLUDES    fistula of rectum to:
              internal organs—see
                Alphabetic Index
              skin (565.1)
              hemorrhoids (455.0-455.9)
              incontinence of sphincter ani
                (787.6)

### 569.5 Abscess of intestine `CC`
EXCLUDES    appendiceal abscess (540.1)

CC Excl: 569.5

## √5th 569.6 Colostomy and enterostomy complications
AHA: 4Q, '95, 58

DEF: Complication in a surgically created opening, from intestine to surface skin.

### 569.60 Colostomy and enterostomy
complication, unspecified

---

**569.61 Infection of colostomy or enterostomy** `CC`
Use additional code to identify organism (041.00-041.9)
Use additional code to specify type of infection, such as:
abscess or cellulitis of abdomen (682.2)
septicemia (038.0-038.9)

CC Excl: 569.60-569.69

**569.62 Mechanical complication of colostomy** `CC`
**and enterostomy**
Malfunction of colostomy and enterostomy

CC Excl: 530.86-530.87, 536.40-536.49, 569.60-569.69, 997.4, 997.71, 997.91-997.99, 998.81, 998.83-998.9

AHA: 2Q, '05, 11 ; 1Q, '03, 10; 4Q, '98, 44

**569.69 Other complication** `CC`
Fistula          Prolapse
Hernia

CC Excl: See code: 569.61

AHA: 3Q, '98, 16

✓5ᵗʰ **569.8 Other specified disorders of intestine**
AHA: 4Q, '91, 25

**569.81 Fistula of intestine, excluding** `CC`
**rectum and anus**
Fistula:                    Fistula:
abdominal wall         enteroenteric
enterocolic             ileorectal

**EXCLUDES** fistula of intestine to internal organs—see Alphabetic Index
persistent postoperative fistula (998.6)

CC Excl: 569.81

AHA: 3Q, '99, 8

**569.82 Ulceration of intestine** `CC`
Primary ulcer of intestine
Ulceration of colon

**EXCLUDES** that with perforation (569.83)

CC Excl: 569.82

**569.83 Perforation of intestine** `MCC`
CC Excl: 569.83

**569.84 Angiodysplasia of intestine (without**
**mention of hemorrhage)**
AHA: 3Q, '96, 10; 4Q, '90, 4; 4Q, '90, 21

DEF: Small vascular abnormalities of the intestinal tract without bleeding problems.

**569.85 Angiodysplasia of intestine with** `MCC`
**hemorrhage**
CC Excl: 251.5, 456.0, 530.20-530.21, 530.7, 530.82, 530.85, 531.00-534.91, 535.01, 535.11, 535.21, 535.31, 535.41, 535.51, 535.61, 537.83, 562.02-562.03, 562.12-562.13, 569.3, 569.85, 578.0-578.9

AHA: 3Q, '96, 9

DEF: Small vascular abnormalities of the intestinal tract with bleeding problems.

**569.86 Dieulafoy lesion (hemorrhagic)** `MCC`
**of intestine**
CC Excl: 251.5, 456.0, 530.20-530.21, 530.7, 530.82, 530.85, 531.00-534.91, 535.01, 535.11, 535.21, 535.31, 535.41, 535.51, 535.61, 537.83, 562.02-562.03, 562.12-562.13, 569.3, 569.85-569.86, 578.0-578.9

AHA: 4Q, '02, 60-61

**569.89 Other**
Enteroptosis
Granuloma      } of intestine
Prolapse
Pericolitis
Perisigmoiditis
Visceroptosis

**EXCLUDES** gangrene of intestine, mesentery, or omentum (557.0)
hemorrhage of intestine NOS (578.9)
obstruction of intestine (560.0-560.9)

AHA: 3Q, '96, 9

**569.9 Unspecified disorder of intestine**

## OTHER DISEASES OF DIGESTIVE SYSTEM (570-579)

**570 Acute and subacute necrosis of liver** `MCC`
Acute hepatic failure
Acute or subacute hepatitis, not specified as infective
Necrosis of liver (acute) (diffuse) (massive) (subacute)
Parenchymatous degeneration of liver
Yellow atrophy (liver) (acute) (subacute)

**EXCLUDES** icterus gravis of newborn (773.0-773.2)
serum hepatitis (070.2-070.3)
that with:
abortion (634-638 with .7, 639.8)
ectopic or molar pregnancy (639.8)
pregnancy, childbirth, or the puerperium (646.7)
viral hepatitis (070.0-070.9)

CC Excl: 570, 573.4-573.9

AHA: 2Q, '05, 9; 1Q, '00, 22

✓4ᵗʰ **571 Chronic liver disease and cirrhosis**
**571.0 Alcoholic fatty liver**
**571.1 Acute alcoholic hepatitis** `A`
Acute alcoholic liver disease

AHA: 2Q, '02, 4

**571.2 Alcoholic cirrhosis of liver** `A`
Florid cirrhosis
Laennec's cirrhosis (alcoholic)
AHA: ▶2Q, '07, 6;◄ 2Q, '02, 4; 1Q, '02, 3; N-D, '85, 14

DEF: Fibrosis and dysfunction, of liver; due to alcoholic liver disease.

**571.3 Alcoholic liver damage, unspecified** `A`
✓5ᵗʰ **571.4 Chronic hepatitis**

**EXCLUDES** viral hepatitis (acute) (chronic) (070.0-070.9)

**571.40 Chronic hepatitis, unspecified**
**571.41 Chronic persistent hepatitis**

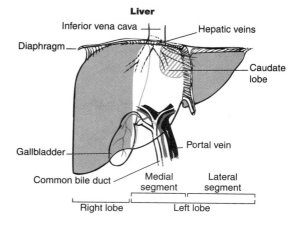

**Liver**
Inferior vena cava
Hepatic veins
Diaphragm
Caudate lobe
Portal vein
Gallbladder
Common bile duct
Medial segment
Lateral segment
Right lobe
Left lobe

`N` Newborn Age: 0   `P` Pediatric Age: 0-17   `M` Maternity Age: 12-55   `A` Adult Age: 15-124   `CC` CC Condition   `MCC` Major CC Condition   `HIV` HIV Related Dx

186 — Volume 1 • October 2007

© 2007 Ingenix

**571.49  Other**
Chronic hepatitis:
active
aggressive
Recurrent hepatitis
**AHA:** 3Q, '99, 19; N-D, '85, 14

**571.5  Cirrhosis of liver without mention of alcohol**
Cirrhosis of liver:    Cirrhosis of liver:
NOS                          postnecrotic
cryptogenic             Healed yellow atrophy
macronodular               (liver)
micronodular          Portal cirrhosis
posthepatitic
**AHA:** ▶2Q, '07, 5◀

**DEF:** Fibrosis and dysfunction of liver; not alcohol related.

**571.6  Biliary cirrhosis**
Chronic nonsuppurative destructive cholangitis
Cirrhosis:
cholangitic
cholestatic

**571.8  Other chronic nonalcoholic liver disease**
Chronic yellow atrophy (liver)
Fatty liver, without mention of alcohol
**AHA:** 2Q, '96, 12

**571.9  Unspecified chronic liver disease without mention of alcohol**

**√4ᵗʰ 572  Liver abscess and sequelae of chronic liver disease**

**572.0  Abscess of liver**   `MCC`
**EXCLUDES**  amebic liver abscess (006.3)
**CC Excl:** 006.3, 572.0-572.1, 573.8-573.9

**572.1  Portal pyemia**   `MCC`
Phlebitis of portal vein    Pylephlebitis
Portal thrombophlebitis   Pylethrombophlebitis
**CC Excl:** See code 572.0

**DEF:** Inflammation of portal vein or branches; may be due to intestinal disease; symptoms include fever, chills, jaundice, sweating, and abscess in various body parts.

**572.2  Hepatic coma**   `MCC`
Hepatic encephalopathy
Hepatocerebral intoxication
Portal-systemic encephalopathy
**EXCLUDES** ▶ hepatic coma associated with viral hepatitis—see category 070◀
**CC Excl:** 572.2, 573.8-573.9
**AHA:** ▶2Q, '07, 5;◀ 2Q, '05, 9; 1Q, '02, 3; 3Q, '95, 14

**572.3  Portal hypertension**   `CC`
**CC Excl:** 572.2-572.3, 573.8-573.9
**AHA:** 3Q, '05, 15
**DEF:** Abnormally high blood pressure in the portal vein.

**572.4  Hepatorenal syndrome**   `MCC`
**EXCLUDES**  that following delivery (674.8)
**CC Excl:** 572.4, 573.8-573.9
**AHA:** 3Q, '93, 15
**DEF:** Hepatic and renal failure characterized by cirrhosis with ascites or obstructive jaundice, oliguria, and low sodium concentration.

**572.8  Other sequelae of chronic liver disease**

**√4ᵗʰ 573  Other disorders of liver**
**EXCLUDES**  amyloid or lardaceous degeneration of liver (277.39)
congenital cystic disease of liver (751.62)
glycogen infiltration of liver (271.0)
hepatomegaly NOS (789.1)
portal vein obstruction (452)

**573.0  Chronic passive congestion of liver**
**DEF:** Blood accumulation in liver tissue.

**573.1  *Hepatitis in viral diseases classified elsewhere***   `CC`
*Code first underlying disease as:*
Coxsackie virus disease (074.8)
cytomegalic inclusion virus disease (078.5)
infectious mononucleosis (075)
**EXCLUDES**  *hepatitis (in):*
*mumps (072.71)*
*viral (070.0-070.9)*
*yellow fever (060.0-060.9)*
**CC Excl:** 573.1-573.3, 573.8-573.9

**573.2  *Hepatitis in other infectious diseases classified elsewhere***   `CC`
*Code first underlying disease, as:*
malaria (084.9)
**EXCLUDES**  *hepatitis in:*
*late syphilis (095.3)*
*secondary syphilis (091.62)*
*toxoplasmosis (130.5)*
**CC Excl:** See code: 573.1

**573.3  Hepatitis, unspecified**
Toxic (noninfectious) hepatitis
Use additional E code to identify cause
**AHA:** 3Q, '98, 3, 4; 4Q, '90, 26

**573.4  Hepatic infarction**   `MCC`
**CC Excl:** 570, 573.4-573.9

**573.8  Other specified disorders of liver**
Hepatoptosis

**573.9  Unspecified disorder of liver**

**√4ᵗʰ 574  Cholelithiasis**
The following fifth-digit subclassification is for use with category 574:
**0  without mention of obstruction**
**1  with obstruction**

**√5ᵗʰ 574.0  Calculus of gallbladder with acute cholecystitis**   `CC`
Biliary calculus
Calculus of cystic duct  } with acute cholecystitis
Cholelithiasis

Any condition classifiable to 574.2 with acute cholecystitis
**CC Excl: For code 574.00:** 574.00-574.21, 574.40, 574.60-574.61, 574.80-574.81, 575.0-575.12, 575.9, 576.8-576.9; **For code 574.01:** 574.00-574.21, 574.60-574.61, 574.80-574.81, 575.0-575.12, 575.9, 576.8-576.9
**AHA:** 4Q, '96, 32

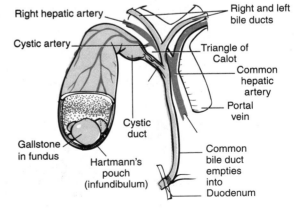

**Gallbladder and Bile Ducts**

Right hepatic artery
Right and left bile ducts
Cystic artery
Triangle of Calot
Common hepatic artery
Portal vein
Cystic duct
Gallstone in fundus
Hartmann's pouch (infundibulum)
Common bile duct empties into Duodenum

**√4ᵗʰ √5ᵗʰ** Additional Digit Required    Unacceptable PDx    Manifestation Code    ▶◀ Revised Text    ● New Code    ▲ Revised Code Title

© 2007 Ingenix    **October 2007 • Volume 1 — 187**

**Digestive System**

**574.1–575.6**

§ ✓5ᵗʰ **574.1** **Calculus of gallbladder with other cholecystitis**    `CC`

> Biliary calculus
> Calculus of cystic duct } with cholecystitis
> Cholelithiasis

Cholecystitis with cholelithiasis NOS
Any condition classifiable to 574.2 with cholecystitis (chronic)

**CC Excl:** See code 574.01

**AHA:** 3Q, '99, 9; 4Q, '96, 32, 69; 2Q, '96, 13; **For code 574.10:** 1Q, '03, 5

§ ✓5ᵗʰ **574.2** **Calculus of gallbladder without mention of cholecystitis**    `CC 1`

> Biliary:           Cholelithiasis NOS
>   calculus NOS     Colic (recurrent) of
>   colic NOS          gallbladder
> Calculus of cystic duct   Gallstone (impacted)

**CC Excl: For code 574.21:** See code 574.01

**AHA: For code 574.20:** 1Q, '88, 14

§ ✓5ᵗʰ **574.3** **Calculus of bile duct with acute cholecystitis**    `CC`

> Calculus of bile
>   duct [any]     } with acute
> Choledocholithiasis   cholecystitis

Any condition classifiable to 574.5 with acute cholecystitis

**CC Excl:** 574.30-575.12, 576.8-576.9

§ ✓5ᵗʰ **574.4** **Calculus of bile duct with other cholecystitis**    `CC`

> Calculus of bile duct
>   [any]          } with cholecystitis
> Choledocholithiasis   (chronic)

Any condition classifiable to 574.5 with cholecystitis (chronic)

**CC Excl:** See code 574.3

§ ✓5ᵗʰ **574.5** **Calculus of bile duct without mention of cholecystitis**    `CC 1`

> Calculus of:        Choledocholithiasis
>   bile duct [any]  Hepatic:
>   common duct        colic (recurrent)
>   hepatic duct       lithiasis

**CC Excl: For code 574.51:** 574.30-575.12, 576.8-576.9

**AHA:** 3Q, '94, 11

§ ✓5ᵗʰ **574.6** **Calculus of gallbladder and bile duct with acute cholecystitis**    `CC`

Any condition classifiable to 574.0 and 574.3

**CC Excl:** 574.60-574.61, 575.0-575.12, 575.9, 576.8-576.9

**AHA:** 4Q, '96, 32

§ ✓5ᵗʰ **574.7** **Calculus of gallbladder and bile duct with other cholecystitis**    `CC`

Any condition classifiable to 574.1 and 574.4

**CC Excl:** 574.30-575.12, 576.8-576.9

**AHA:** 4Q, '96, 32

§ ✓5ᵗʰ **574.8** **Calculus of gallbladder and bile duct with acute and chronic cholecystitis**    `MCC1` `CC 0`

Any condition classifiable to 574.6 and 574.7

**CC Excl:** 574.80-574.81, 575.0-575.12, 575.9, 576.8-576.9

**AHA:** 4Q, '96, 32

§ ✓5ᵗʰ **574.9** **Calculus of gallbladder and bile duct without cholecystitis**    `CC 1`

Any condition classifiable to 574.2 and 574.5

**CC Excl: For code 574.91:** 574.30-575.12, 576.8-576.9

**AHA:** 4Q, '96, 32

✓4ᵗʰ **575 Other disorders of gallbladder**

**575.0** **Acute cholecystitis**    `CC`

> Abscess of gallbladder
> Angiocholecystitis
> Cholecystitis:
>   emphysematous (acute) } without mention
>   gangrenous             of calculus
>   suppurative
> Empyema of gallbladder
> Gangrene of gallbladder

**EXCLUDES** *that with:*
> *acute and chronic cholecystitis (575.12)*
> *choledocholithiasis (574.3)*
> *choledocholithiasis and cholelithiasis (574.6)*
> *cholelithiasis (574.0)*

**CC Excl:** 574.60-574.61, 574.80-574.81, 575.0-575.12, 575.9, 576.8-576.9

**AHA:** 3Q, '91, 17

✓5ᵗʰ **575.1** **Other cholecystitis**

> Cholecystitis:
>   NOS      } without mention
>   chronic    of calculus

**EXCLUDES** *that with:*
> *choledocholithiasis (574.4)*
> *choledocholithiasis and cholelithiasis (574.8)*
> *cholelithiasis (574.1)*

**AHA:** 4Q, '96, 32

**575.10** **Cholecystitis, unspecified**
> Cholecystitis NOS

**575.11** **Chronic cholecystitis**

**575.12** **Acute and chronic cholecystitis**    `CC`

**CC Excl:** 575.0-575.12, 575.9, 576.8-576.9

**AHA:** 4Q, '97, 52; 4Q, '96, 32

**575.2** **Obstruction of gallbladder**    `CC`

> Occlusion
> Stenosis   } of cystic duct or gallbladder without
> Stricture    mention of calculus

**EXCLUDES** *that with calculus (574.0-574.2 with fifth-digit 1)*

**CC Excl:** 575.2-575.9, 576.8-576.9

**575.3** **Hydrops of gallbladder**    `CC`
> Mucocele of gallbladder

**CC Excl:** See code 575.2

**AHA:** 2Q, '89, 13

**DEF:** Serous fluid accumulation in bladder.

**575.4** **Perforation of gallbladder**    `MCC`
> Rupture of cystic duct or gallbladder

**CC Excl:** See code 575.2

**575.5** **Fistula of gallbladder**    `CC`
> Fistula:              Fistula:
>   cholecystoduodenal    cholecystoenteric

**CC Excl:** See code 575.2

**575.6** **Cholesterolosis of gallbladder**
> Strawberry gallbladder

**AHA:** 4Q, '90, 17

**DEF:** Cholesterol deposits in gallbladder tissue.

---

§ Requires fifth digit. See category 574 for codes and definitions.

 Newborn Age: 0     Pediatric Age: 0-17    `M` Maternity Age: 12-55    `A` Adult Age: 15-124    `CC` CC Condition    `MC` Major Complication    `CD` Complex Dx    `HIV` HIV Related Dx

 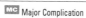

**575.8 Other specified disorders of gallbladder**

Adhesions
Atrophy
Cyst
Hypertrophy } (of) cystic duct or
Nonfunctioning    gallbladder
Ulcer

Biliary dyskinesia

**EXCLUDES**   Hartmann's pouch of intestine (V44.3)
     nonvisualization of gallbladder (793.3)

**AHA:** 4Q, '90, 26; 2Q, '89, 13

**575.9 Unspecified disorder of gallbladder**

✓4ᵗʰ **576 Other disorders of biliary tract**

**EXCLUDES**   that involving the:
     cystic duct (575.0-575.9)
     gallbladder (575.0-575.9)

**576.0 Postcholecystectomy syndrome**

**AHA:** 1Q, '88, 10

**DEF:** Jaundice or abdominal pain following cholecystectomy.

**576.1 Cholangitis**     **CC**

Cholangitis:       Cholangitis:
   NOS           recurrent
   acute          sclerosing
   ascending      secondary
   chronic        stenosing
   primary       suppurative

**CC Excl:** 576.1, 576.8-576.9

**AHA:** 2Q, '99, 13

**576.2 Obstruction of bile duct**     **MCC**

Occlusion } of bile duct, except cystic
Stenosis      duct, without mention
Stricture      of calculus

**EXCLUDES**   congenital (751.61)
     that with calculus (574.3-574.5 with
       fifth-digit 1)

**CC Excl:** 574.31, 574.41, 574.51, 576.2, 576.8-576.9, 751.61

**AHA:** 3Q, '03, 17-18; 1Q, '01, 8; 2Q, '99, 13

**576.3 Perforation of bile duct**     **MCC**

Rupture of bile duct, except cystic duct

**CC Excl:** 576.3-576.4, 576.8-576.9

**576.4 Fistula of bile duct**     **CC**

Choledochoduodenal fistula

**CC Excl:** See code: 576.3

**576.5 Spasm of sphincter of Oddi**

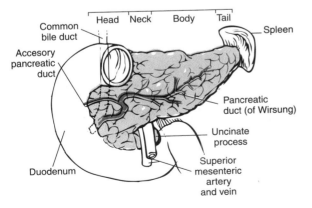

**Pancreas**

Head   Neck   Body   Tail

Common bile duct
Accesory pancreatic duct
Duodenum
Spleen
Pancreatic duct (of Wirsung)
Uncinate process
Superior mesenteric artery and vein

**576.8 Other specified disorders of biliary tract**

Adhesions
Atrophy
Cyst
Hypertrophy } of bile duct [any]
Stasis
Ulcer

**EXCLUDES**   congenital choledochal cyst (751.69)

**AHA:** 3Q, '03, 17; 2Q, '99, 14

**576.9 Unspecified disorder of biliary tract**

✓4ᵗʰ **577 Diseases of pancreas**

**577.0 Acute pancreatitis**     **MCC**

Abscess of pancreas    Pancreatitis:
Necrosis of pancreas:     acute (recurrent)
   acute             apoplectic
   infective         hemorrhagic
Pancreatitis:         subacute
   NOS            suppurative

**EXCLUDES**   mumps pancreatitis (072.3)

**CC Excl:** 577.0-577.1, 577.8-577.9

**AHA:** 3Q, '99, 9; 2Q, '98, 19; 2Q, '96, 13; 2Q, '89, 9

**577.1 Chronic pancreatitis**     **CC**

Chronic pancreatitis:    Pancreatitis:
   NOS             painless
   infectious        recurrent
   interstitial       relapsing

**CC Excl:** 251.8, 577.0-577.9

**AHA:** 1Q, '01, 8; 2Q, '96, 13; 3Q, '94, 11

**577.2 Cyst and pseudocyst of pancreas**     **CC**

**CC Excl:** 577.2-577.9

**577.8 Other specified diseases of pancreas**

Atrophy
Calculus
Cirrhosis } of pancreas
Fibrosis

Pancreatic:
  infantilism
  necrosis:
   NOS
   aseptic
   fat
Pancreatolithiasis

**EXCLUDES**   fibrocystic disease of pancreas
     (277.00-277.09)
     islet cell tumor of pancreas (211.7)
     pancreatic steatorrhea (579.4)

**AHA:** 1Q, '01, 8

**577.9 Unspecified disease of pancreas**

✓4ᵗʰ **578 Gastrointestinal hemorrhage**

**EXCLUDES**   that with mention of:
     angiodysplasia of stomach and duodenum
       (537.83)
     angiodysplasia of intestine (569.85)
     diverticulitis, intestine:
       large (562.13)
       small (562.03)
     diverticulosis, intestine:
       large (562.12)
       small (562.02)
     gastritis and duodenitis (535.0-535.6)
     ulcer:
       duodenal, gastric, gastrojejuunal or peptic
       (531.00-534.91)

**AHA:** 2Q, '92, 9; 4Q, '90, 20

**578.0 Hematemesis**     **CC**

Vomiting of blood

**CC Excl:** 251.5, 456.0, 530.20-530.21, 530.7, 530.82, 530.85, 531.00-534.91, 535.01, 535.11, 535.21, 535.31, 535.41, 535.51, 535.61, 537.83, 562.02-562.03, 562.12-562.13, 569.3, 569.85, 578.0-578.9

**AHA:** 2Q, '02, 4

✓4ᵗʰ / ✓5ᵗʰ Additional Digit Required     Unacceptable PDx     Manifestation Code     ▶◀ Revised Text     ● New Code     ▲ Revised Code Title

**October 2007 • Volume 1 — 189**

© 2007 Ingenix

**Digestive System**

**578.1–579.9**

**578.1   Blood in stool**   `CC`
Melena
> **EXCLUDES**   melena of the newborn (772.4, 777.3)
> occult blood (792.1)

**CC Excl:** See code 578.0

**AHA:** 2Q, '06, 17; 2Q, '92, 8

**578.9   Hemorrhage of gastrointestinal tract, unspecified**   `CC`
Gastric hemorrhage
Intestinal hemorrhage

**CC Excl:** See code 578.0

**AHA:** 4Q, '06, 91;  3Q, '05, 17; N-D, '86, 9

✓4ᵗʰ **579   Intestinal malabsorption**

**579.0   Celiac disease**
Celiac:              Gee (-Herter) disease
  crisis            Gluten enteropathy
  infantilism       Idiopathic steatorrhea
  rickets           Nontropical sprue

**DEF:** Malabsorption syndrome due to gluten consumption; symptoms include fetid, bulky, frothy, oily stools; distended abdomen, gas, weight loss, asthenia, electrolyte depletion and vitamin B, D and K deficiency.

**579.1   Tropical sprue**   `CC`
Sprue:              Tropical steatorrhea
  NOS
  tropical

**CC Excl:** 277.03, 579.0-579.9

**DEF:** Diarrhea, occurs in tropics; may be due to enteric infection and malnutrition.

**579.2   Blind loop syndrome**   `CC`
Postoperative blind loop syndrome

**CC Excl:** See code: 579.1

**DEF:** Obstruction or impaired passage in small intestine due to alterations, from strictures or surgery; causes stasis, abnormal bacterial flora, diarrhea, weight loss, multiple vitamin deficiency, and megaloblastic anemia.

**579.3   Other and unspecified postsurgical nonabsorption**   `CC`
Hypoglycemia   } following gastrointestinal
Malnutrition   }   surgery

**CC Excl:** 579.3-579.9

**AHA:** 4Q, '03, 104

**579.4   Pancreatic steatorrhea**   `CC`
**CC Excl:** See code: 579.1

**DEF:** Excess fat in feces due to absence of pancreatic juice in intestine.

**579.8   Other specified intestinal malabsorption**   `CC`
Enteropathy:         Steatorrhea (chronic)
  exudative
  protein-losing

**CC Excl:** See code: 579.1

**AHA:** 1Q, '88, 6

**579.9   Unspecified intestinal malabsorption**   `CC`
Malabsorption syndrome NOS

**CC Excl:** See code: 579.1

**AHA:** 4Q, '04, 59

---

N Newborn Age: 0     P Pediatric Age: 0-17     M Maternity Age: 12-55     A Adult Age: 15-124     `CC` CC Condition     `MCC` Major CC Condition     `HIV` HIV Related Dx

## 10. DISEASES OF THE GENITOURINARY SYSTEM (580-629)

**Kidney**

**Nephron**

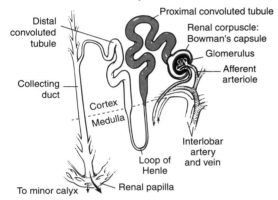

### NEPHRITIS, NEPHROTIC SYNDROME, AND NEPHROSIS (580-589)

| EXCLUDES | *hypertensive chronic kidney disease (403.00-403.91, 404.00-404.93)* |
|---|---|

✓4ᵗʰ **580 Acute glomerulonephritis**

| INCLUDES | acute nephritis |
|---|---|

**DEF:** Acute, severe inflammation in tuft of capillaries that filter the kidneys.

**580.0　With lesion of proliferative glomerulonephritis** MCC

Acute (diffuse) proliferative glomerulonephritis
Acute poststreptococcal glomerulonephritis

**CC Excl:** 016.00-016.06, 016.30-016.36, 016.90-016.96, 017.90-017.96, 098.10, 098.19, 098.30-098.31, 098.89, 112.2, 131.00, 131.8-131.9, 250.40-250.43, 250.80-250.93, 274.10, 274.19, 580.0-591, 593.0-593.2, 593.89-593.9, 599.7-599.9

**580.4　With lesion of rapidly progressive glomerulonephritis** MCC

Acute nephritis with lesion of necrotizing glomerulitis

**CC Excl:** See code 580.0

**DEF:** Acute glomerulonephritis; progresses to ESRD with diffuse epithelial proliferation.

✓5ᵗʰ **580.8　With other specified pathological lesion in kidney**

**580.81　*Acute glomerulonephritis in diseases classified elsewhere*** MCC

*Code first underlying disease, as:*
infectious hepatitis (070.0-070.9)
mumps (072.79)
subacute bacterial endocarditis (421.0)
typhoid fever (002.0)

**CC Excl:** See code 580.0

**580.89　Other** MCC

Glomerulonephritis, acute, with lesion of:
exudative nephritis
interstitial (diffuse) (focal) nephritis

**CC Excl:** 016.00-016.06, 016.30-016.36, 016.90-016.96, 017.90-017.96, 098.10, 098.19, 098.30-098.31, 098.89, 112.2, 131.00, 131.8-131.9, 274.10, 274.19, 580.0-591, 593.0-593.2, 593.89-593.9, 599.7-599.9

**580.9　Acute glomerulonephritis with unspecified pathological lesion in kidney** MCC

Glomerulonephritis:　⎫
　NOS　　　　　　⎬ specified as acute
　hemorrhagic　　⎪
Nephritis　　　　 ⎪
Nephropathy　　　⎭

**CC Excl:** See code: 580.0

✓4ᵗʰ **581 Nephrotic syndrome**

**DEF:** Disease process marked by symptoms such as; extensive edema, notable proteinuria, hypoalbuminemia, and susceptibility to intercurrent infections.

**581.0　With lesion of proliferative glomerulonephritis** CC

**CC Excl:** 016.00-016.06, 016.30-016.36, 016.90-016.96, 017.90-017.96, 098.10, 098.19, 098.30-098.31, 098.89, 112.2, 131.00, 131.8-131.9, 250.40-250.43, 250.80-250.93, 274.10, 274.19, 580.0-591, 593.0-593.2, 593.89-593.9, 599.7-599.9

**581.1　With lesion of membranous glomerulonephritis** CC

Epimembranous nephritis
Idiopathic membranous glomerular disease
Nephrotic syndrome with lesion of:
　focal glomerulosclerosis
　sclerosing membranous glomerulonephritis
　segmental hyalinosis

**CC Excl:** See code: 581.0

**581.2　With lesion of membranoproliferative glomerulonephritis** CC

Nephrotic syndrome with lesion (of):
　endothelial　　　　　　　⎫
　hypocomplementemic　　 ⎪
　　persistent　　　　　　 ⎬ glomerulonephritis
　lobular　　　　　　　　　⎪
　mesangiocapillary　　　 ⎪
　mixed membranous and　 ⎪
　　proliferative　　　　　⎭

**CC Excl:** See code: 581.0

**DEF:** Glomerulonephritis combined with clinical features of nephrotic syndrome; characterized by uneven thickening of glomerular capillary walls and mesangial cell increase; slowly progresses to ESRD.

**581.3　With lesion of minimal change glomerulonephritis** CC

Foot process disease
Lipoid nephrosis
Minimal change:
　glomerular disease
　glomerulitis
　nephrotic syndrome

**CC Excl:** See code: 581.0

**AHA:** ▶1Q, '07, 23◀

✓4ᵗʰ **581.8　With other specified pathological lesion in kidney**

**581.81　*Nephrotic syndrome in diseases classified elsewhere*** CC

*Code first underlying disease, as:*
amyloidosis (277.30-277.39)
diabetes mellitus (250.4)
malaria (084.9)
polyarteritis (446.0)
systemic lupus erythematosus (710.0)

| EXCLUDES | *nephrosis in epidemic hemorrhagic fever (078.6)* |
|---|---|

**CC Excl:** See code: 581.0

**AHA:** 3Q, '91, 8, 12; S-O, '85, 3

**581.89　Other** CC

Glomerulonephritis with edema and lesion of:
exudative nephritis
interstitial (diffuse) (focal) nephritis

**CC Excl:** See code: 581.0

✓4ᵗʰ / ✓5ᵗʰ Additional Digit Required　　　　Unacceptable PDx　　　　Manifestation Code　　　▶◀ Revised Text　　　● New Code　　　▲ Revised Code Title

© 2007 Ingenix　　　　　　　　　　　　　　　　　　　　　　　　　　　　　　**October 2007 • Volume 1 — 191**

**581.9   Nephrotic syndrome with unspecified pathological lesion in kidney** `CC`
Glomerulonephritis with edema NOS
Nephritis:
   nephrotic NOS
   with edema NOS
Nephrosis NOS
Renal disease with edema NOS
**CC Excl:** See code 581.0

√4ᵗʰ **582   Chronic glomerulonephritis**
   `INCLUDES`   chronic nephritis

**DEF:** Slow progressive type of nephritis characterized by inflammation of the capillary loops in the glomeruli of the kidney, which leads to renal failure.

**582.0   With lesion of proliferative glomerulonephritis** `CC`
Chronic (diffuse) proliferative glomerulonephritis
**CC Excl:** 016.00-016.06, 016.30-016.36, 016.90-016.96, 017.90-017.96, 078.6, 098.10, 098.19, 098.30-098.31, 098.89, 112.2, 131.00, 131.8-131.9, 250.40-250.43, 250.80-250.93, 274.10, 274.19, 580.0-584.9, 586-591, 593.0-593.2, 593.89-593.9, 599.7-599.9

**582.1   With lesion of membranous glomerulonephritis** `CC`
Chronic glomerulonephritis:
   membranous
   sclerosing
Focal glomerulosclerosis
Segmental hyalinosis
**CC Excl:** See code: 582.0

**AHA:** S-O, '84, 16

**582.2   With lesion of membranoproliferative glomerulonephritis** `CC`
Chronic glomerulonephritis:
   endothelial
   hypocomplementemic persistent
   lobular
   membranoproliferative
   mesangiocapillary
   mixed membranous and proliferative
**CC Excl:** See code: 582.0

**DEF:** Chronic glomerulonephritis with mesangial cell proliferation.

**582.4   With lesion of rapidly progressive glomerulonephritis** `CC`
Chronic nephritis with lesion of necrotizing glomerulitis
**CC Excl:** See code: 582.0

**DEF:** Chronic glomerulonephritis rapidly progresses to ESRD; marked by diffuse epithelial proliferation.

√5ᵗʰ **582.8   With other specified pathological lesion in kidney**
  **582.81   *Chronic glomerulonephritis in diseases classified elsewhere*** `CC`
    *Code first underlying disease, as:*
     amyloidosis (277.30-277.39)
     systemic lupus erythematosus (710.0)
    **CC Excl:** See code: 582.0

  **582.89   Other** `CC`
    Chronic glomerulonephritis with lesion of:
     exudative nephritis
     interstitial (diffuse) (focal) nephritis
    **CC Excl:** See code: 582.0

**582.9   Chronic glomerulonephritis with unspecified pathological lesion in kidney** `CC`
Glomerulonephritis:
   NOS
   hemorrhagic   } specified as chronic
Nephritis
Nephropathy
**CC Excl:** See code: 582.0

**AHA:** 2Q, '01, 12

√4ᵗʰ **583   Nephritis and nephropathy, not specified as acute or chronic**
   `INCLUDES`   "renal disease" so stated, not specified as acute or chronic but with stated pathology or cause

**583.0   With lesion of proliferative glomerulonephritis** `CC`
Proliferative:      Proliferative:
  glomerulonephritis    nephritis NOS
   (diffuse) NOS     nephropathy NOS
**CC Excl:** See code: 582.0

**583.1   With lesion of membranous glomerulonephritis** `CC`
Membranous:
   glomerulonephritis NOS
   nephritis NOS
Membranous nephropathy NOS
**CC Excl:** See code: 582.0

**DEF:** Kidney inflammation or dysfunction with deposits on glomerular capillary basement membranes.

**583.2   With lesion of membranoproliferative glomerulonephritis** `CC`
Membranoproliferative:
   glomerulonephritis NOS
   nephritis NOS
   nephropathy NOS
Nephritis NOS, with lesion of:
   hypocomplementemic ⎤
    persistent       ⎥
   lobular           } glomerulonephritis
   mesangiocapillary   ⎥
   mixed membranous  ⎥
    and proliferative ⎦
**CC Excl:** See code: 582.0

**DEF:** Kidney inflammation or dysfunction with mesangial cell proliferation.

**583.4   With lesion of rapidly progressive glomerulonephritis** `MCC`
Necrotizing or rapidly progressive:
   glomerulitis NOS
   glomerulonephritis NOS
   nephritis NOS
   nephropathy NOS
Nephritis, unspecified, with lesion of necrotizing glomerulitis
**CC Excl:** 016.00-016.06, 016.30-016.36, 016.90-016.96, 017.90-017.96, 098.10, 098.19, 098.30-098.31, 098.89, 112.2, 131.00, 131.8-131.9, 250.40-250.43, 250.80-250.93, 274.10, 274.19, 580.0-591, 593.0-593.2, 593.89-593.9, 599.7-599.9

**DEF:** Kidney inflammation or dysfunction; rapidly progresses to ESRD marked by diffuse epithelial proliferation.

**583.6   With lesion of renal cortical necrosis** `MCC`
Nephritis NOS    } with (renal) cortical
Nephropathy NOS }    necrosis
Renal cortical necrosis NOS
**CC Excl:** 583.6, 588.81-588.89

**583.7   With lesion of renal medullary necrosis** `CC`
Nephritis NOS    } with (renal) medullary
Nephropathy NOS }    [papillary] necrosis
**CC Excl:** 583.7, 588.81-588.89

√5ᵗʰ **583.8   With other specified pathological lesion in kidney**
  **583.81   *Nephritis and nephropathy, not specified as acute or chronic, in diseases classified elsewhere***
    *Code first underlying disease, as:*
     amyloidosis (277.30-277.39)
     diabetes mellitus (250.4)
     gonococcal infection (098.19)
     Goodpasture's syndrome (446.21)
     systemic lupus erythematosus (710.0)
     tuberculosis (016.0)
    `EXCLUDES`   gouty nephropathy (274.10)
                  syphilitic nephritis (095.4)
    **AHA:** 2Q, '03, 7; 3Q, '91, 8; S-O, '85, 3

---

`N` Newborn Age: 0    `P` Pediatric Age: 0-17    `M` Maternity Age: 12-55    `A` Adult Age: 15-124    `CC` CC Condition    `MCC` Major CC Condition    `HIV` HIV Related Dx

**583.89 Other**

| | |
|---|---|
| Glomerulitis | with lesion of: |
| Glomerulonephritis | exudative |
| Nephritis | nephritis |
| Nephropathy | interstitial |
| Renal disease | nephritis |

**583.9 With unspecified pathological lesion in kidney**

Glomerulitis
Glomerulonephritis } NOS
Nephritis
Nephropathy

> **EXCLUDES** *nephropathy complicating pregnancy, labor, or the puerperium (642.0-642.9, 646.2)*
> *renal disease NOS with no stated cause (593.9)*

### ✓4ᵗʰ 584 Acute renal failure

> **EXCLUDES** *following labor and delivery (669.3)*
> *posttraumatic (958.5)*
> *that complicating:*
> *abortion (634-638 with .3, 639.3)*
> *ectopic or molar pregnancy (639.3)*

**AHA:** 1Q, '93, 18; 2Q, '92, 5; 4Q, '92, 22

**DEF:** State resulting from increasing urea and related substances from the blood (azotemia), often with urine output of less than 500 ml per day.

**584.5 With lesion of tubular necrosis**   `MCC`

Lower nephron nephrosis
Renal failure with (acute) tubular necrosis
Tubular necrosis:
   NOS
   acute

**CC Excl:** 250.40-250.43, 250.80-250.93, 274.10, 274.19, 580.0-591, 593.0-593.2, 593.89-593.9, 599.7-599.9, 753.0-753.3, 753.9

**DEF:** Acute decline in kidney efficiency with destruction of tubules.

**584.6 With lesion of renal cortical necrosis**   `MCC`

**CC Excl:** See code: 584.5

**DEF:** Acute decline in kidney efficiency with destruction of renal tissues that filter blood.

**584.7 With lesion of renal medullary [papillary] necrosis**   `MCC`

Necrotizing renal papillitis

**CC Excl:** See code: 584.5

**DEF:** Acute decline in kidney efficiency with destruction of renal tissues that collect urine.

**584.8 With other specified pathological lesion in kidney**   `MCC`

**CC Excl:** 250.40-250.43, 250.80-250.93, 274.10, 274.19, 580.0-591, 593.0-593.2, 593.89-593.9, 599.7-599.9

**AHA:** N-D, '85, 1

**584.9 Acute renal failure, unspecified**   `MCC`

**CC Excl:** See code: 584.5

**AHA:** 2Q, '05, 18; 2Q, '03, 7; 1Q, '03, 22; 3Q, '02, 21, 28; 2Q, '01, 14; 1Q, '00, 22; 3Q, '96, 9; 4Q, '88, 1

### ✓4ᵗʰ 585 Chronic kidney disease [CKD]

Chronic uremia
Code first hypertensive chronic kidney disease, if applicable, (403.00-403.91, ▶404.00-404.93◀)
Use additional code to identify kidney transplant status, if applicable (V42.0)
Use additional code to identify manifestation as:
  uremic:
    neuropathy (357.4)
    pericarditis (420.0)

**AHA:** 4Q, '06, 84-86; 4Q, '05, 68, 77; 1Q, '04, 5; 4Q, '03, 61, 111; 2Q, '03, 7; 2Q, '01, 12, 13; 1Q, '01, 3; 4Q, '98, 55; 3Q, '98, 6, 7; 2Q, '98, 20; 3Q, '96, 9; 1Q, '93, 18; 3Q, '91, 8; 4Q, '89, 1; N-D, '85, 15; S-O, '84, 3

**585.1 Chronic kidney disease, Stage I**

**DEF:** Some kidney damage; normal or slightly increased GFR (> 90).

**585.2 Chronic kidney disease, Stage II (mild)**

**DEF:** Kidney damage with mild decrease in GFR (60–89).

**585.3 Chronic kidney disease, Stage III (moderate)**

**AHA:** 4Q, '05, 69

**DEF:** Kidney damage with moderate decrease in GFR (30–59).

**585.4 Chronic kidney disease, Stage IV (severe)**   `CC`

**CC Excl:** See code: 584.5

**DEF:** Kidney damage with severe decrease in GFR (15–29).

**585.5 Chronic kidney disease, Stage V**   `CC`

> **EXCLUDES** *chronic kidney disease, stage V requiring chronic dialysis (585.6)*

**CC Excl:** See code 584.5

**DEF:** Kidney failure with GFR value of less than 15.

**585.6 End stage renal disease**   `MCC`

Chronic kidney disease requiring chronic dialysis

**CC Excl:** See code 584.5

**AHA:** 4Q, '06, 136; 4Q, '05, 79

**DEF:** Federal government indicator of a stage V CKD patient undergoing treatment by dialysis or transplantation.

**585.9 Chronic kidney disease, unspecified**

Chronic renal disease
Chronic renal failure NOS
Chronic renal insufficiency

**AHA:** ▶2Q, '07, 3;◀ 4Q, '06, 86; 4Q, '05, 79

### 586 Renal failure, unspecified

Uremia NOS

> **EXCLUDES** *following labor and delivery (669.3)*
> *posttraumatic renal failure (958.5)*
> *that complicating:*
> *abortion (634-638 with .3, 639.3)*
> *ectopic or molar pregnancy (639.3)*
> *uremia:*
> *extrarenal (788.9)*
> *prerenal (788.9)*
> *with any condition classifiable to 401 (403.0-403.9 with fifth-digit 1)*

**AHA:** 3Q, '98, 6; 1Q, '93, 18; 1Q, '88, 3

**DEF:** Renal failure: kidney functions cease; malfunction may be due to inability to excrete metabolized substances or retain level of electrolytes.

**DEF:** Uremia: excess urea, creatinine and other nitrogenous products of protein and amino acid metabolism in blood due to reduced excretory function in bilateral kidney disease; also called azotemia.

### 587 Renal sclerosis, unspecified

| | |
|---|---|
| Atrophy of kidney | Renal: |
| Contracted kidney | cirrhosis |
| | fibrosis |

> **EXCLUDES** *nephrosclerosis (arteriolar) (arteriosclerotic) (403.00-403.91)*
> *with hypertension (403.00-403.91)*

### ✓4ᵗʰ 588 Disorders resulting from impaired renal function

**588.0 Renal osteodystrophy**

Azotemic osteodystrophy
Phosphate-losing tubular disorders
Renal:
  dwarfism      infantilism
  rickets

**DEF:** Bone disorder that results in various bone diseases such as osteomalacia, osteoporosis or osteosclerosis; caused by impaired renal function, an abnormal level of phosphorus in the blood and impaired stimulation of the parathyroid.

**588.1 Nephrogenic diabetes insipidus**   `CC`

> **EXCLUDES** *diabetes insipidus NOS (253.5)*

**CC Excl:** 016.00-016.06, 016.30-016.36, 016.90-016.96, 017.90-017.96, 078.6, 098.10, 098.19, 098.30-098.31, 098.89, 112.2, 131.00, 131.8-131.9, 250.40-250.43, 250.80-250.93, 274.10, 274.19, 580.0-584.9, 585.3-585.6, 586-591, 593.0-593.2, 593.89-593.9, 599.7-599.9

**DEF:** Type of diabetes due to renal tubules inability to reabsorb water; not responsive to vasopressin; may develop into chronic renal insufficiency.

---

✓4ᵗʰ ✓5ᵗʰ Additional Digit Required     Unacceptable PDx     `Manifestation Code`     ▶◀ Revised Text     ● New Code     ▲ Revised Code Title

© 2007 Ingenix      October 2007 • Volume 1 — 193

**✓5ᵗʰ 588.8 Other specified disorders resulting from impaired renal function**

> **EXCLUDES** *secondary hypertension (405.0-405.9)*

**588.81 Secondary hyperparathyroidism (of renal origin)** `CC`

Secondary hyperparathyroidism NOS

**CC Excl:** 016.00-016.06, 016.30-016.36, 016.90-016.96, 017.90-017.96, 078.6, 098.10, 098.19, 098.30-098.31, 098.89, 112.2, 131.00, 131.8-131.9, 250.40-250.43, 250.80-250.93, 274.10, 274.19, 580.0-584.9, 586-588.1, 588.89-591, 593.0-593.2, 593.89-593.9, 599.7-599.9

**AHA:** 4Q, '04, 58-59

**DEF:** Parathyroid dysfunction caused by chronic renal failure; phosphate clearance is impaired, phosphate is released from bone, vitamin D is not produced, intestinal calcium absorption is low, and blood levels of calcium are lowered causing excessive production of parathyroid hormone.

**588.89 Other specified disorders resulting from impaired renal function**

Hypokalemic nephropathy

**588.9 Unspecified disorder resulting from impaired renal function**

**✓4ᵗʰ 589 Small kidney of unknown cause**

**589.0 Unilateral small kidney**

**589.1 Bilateral small kidneys**

**589.9 Small kidney, unspecified**

## OTHER DISEASES OF URINARY SYSTEM (590-599)

**✓4ᵗʰ 590 Infections of kidney**

Use additional code to identify organism, such as Escherichia coli [E. coli] (041.4)

**✓5ᵗʰ 590.0 Chronic pyelonephritis**

Chronic pyelitis
Chronic pyonephrosis
Code if applicable, any casual condition first

**590.00 Without lesion of renal medullary necrosis**

**590.01 With lesion of renal medullary necrosis** `CC`

**CC Excl:** 016.00-016.06, 016.30-016.36, 016.90-016.96, 017.90-017.96, 078.6, 098.10, 098.19, 098.30-098.31, 098.89, 112.2, 131.00, 131.8-131.9, 250.40-250.43, 250.80-250.93, 274.10, 274.19, 580.0-584.9, 586-591, 593.0-593.2, 593.89-593.9, 599.7-599.9, 646.61-646.64

**✓5ᵗʰ 590.1 Acute pyelonephritis**

Acute pyelitis          Acute pyonephrosis

**590.10 Without lesion of renal medullary necrosis** `CC`

**CC Excl:** 016.00-016.06, 016.30-016.36, 016.90-016.96, 017.90-017.96, 098.10, 098.19, 098.30-098.31, 098.89, 112.2, 131.00, 131.8-131.9, 250.40-250.43, 250.80-250.93, 274.10, 274.19, 580.0-591, 593.0-593.2, 593.89-593.9, 599.0, 599.7-599.9

**590.11 With lesion of renal medullary necrosis** `MCC`

**CC Excl:** See code 590.10

**590.2 Renal and perinephric abscess** `MCC`

Abscess:          Abscess:
  kidney            perirenal
  nephritic        Carbuncle of kidney

**CC Excl:** See code 590.10

**590.3 Pyeloureteritis cystica** `CC`

Infection of renal pelvis and ureter
Ureteritis cystica

**CC Excl:** 016.00-016.06, 016.30-016.36, 016.90-016.96, 017.90-017.96, 098.10, 098.19, 098.30-098.31, 098.89, 112.2, 131.00, 131.8-131.9, 274.10, 274.19, 580.0-591, 593.0-593.2, 593.89-593.9, 599.0, 599.7-599.9

**DEF:** Inflammation and formation of submucosal cysts in the kidney, pelvis, and ureter.

**Genitourinary System**

Inferior vena cava — Aorta — Left kidney — Right kidney — Ureter — Anterior division of internal iliac artery — Ovarian or testicular artery and vein — Superior and Inferior vesicular arteries — Urinary bladder — Ureteral orifice — Urethra — Urogenital diaphragm

**✓5ᵗʰ 590.8 Other pyelonephritis or pyonephrosis, not specified as acute or chronic**

**590.80 Pyelonephritis, unspecified** `CC`

Pyelitis NOS
Pyelonephritis NOS

**CC Excl:** See code 590.3

**AHA:** 1Q, '98, 10; 4Q, '97, 40

**590.81 *Pyelitis or pyelonephritis in diseases classified elsewhere*** `CC`

*Code first underlying disease, as:*
    tuberculosis (016.0)

**CC Excl:** See code 590.3

**590.9 Infection of kidney, unspecified**

> **EXCLUDES** *urinary tract infection NOS (599.0)*

**591 Hydronephrosis** `CC`

Hydrocalycosis          Hydroureteronephrosis
Hydronephrosis

> **EXCLUDES** *congenital hydronephrosis (753.29)*
> *hydroureter (593.5)*

**CC Excl:** See code 590.3

**AHA:** 2Q, '98, 9

**DEF:** Distention of kidney and pelvis, with urine build-up due to ureteral obstruction; pyonephrosis may result.

**✓4ᵗʰ 592 Calculus of kidney and ureter**

> **EXCLUDES** *nephrocalcinosis (275.4)*

**592.0 Calculus of kidney**

Nephrolithiasis NOS          Staghorn calculus
Renal calculus or stone      Stone in kidney

> **EXCLUDES** *uric acid nephrolithiasis (274.11)*

**AHA:** 1Q, '00, 4

**592.1 Calculus of ureter** `CC`

Ureteric stone
Ureterolithiasis

**CC Excl:** 592.0-592.9, 593.3-593.5, 593.89-594.9, 599.60-599.9

**AHA:** 2Q, '98, 9; 1Q, '98, 10; 1Q, '91, 11

**592.9 Urinary calculus, unspecified**

**AHA:** 1Q, '98, 10; 4Q, '97, 40

**✓4ᵗʰ 593 Other disorders of kidney and ureter**

**593.0 Nephroptosis**

Floating kidney          Mobile kidney

**593.1 Hypertrophy of kidney**

**593.2 Cyst of kidney, acquired**

Cyst (multiple) (solitary) of kidney, not congenital
Peripelvic (lymphatic) cyst

> **EXCLUDES** *calyceal or pyelogenic cyst of kidney (591)*
> *congenital cyst of kidney (753.1)*
> *polycystic (disease of) kidney (753.1)*

**AHA:** 4Q, '90, 3

**DEF:** Abnormal, fluid-filled sac in the kidney, not present at birth.

---

`N` Newborn Age: 0     `P` Pediatric Age: 0-17     `M` Maternity Age: 12-55     `A` Adult Age: 15-124     `CC` CC Condition     `MCC` Major CC Condition     `HIV` HIV Related Dx

**593.3  Stricture or kinking of ureter**

Angulation ⎫
Constriction ⎭ of ureter (post-operative)

Stricture of pelviureteric junction

**AHA:** 2Q, '98, 9

**DEF:** Stricture or knot in tube connecting kidney to bladder.

**593.4  Other ureteric obstruction**                    `CC`

Idiopathic retroperitoneal fibrosis
Occlusion NOS of ureter

**EXCLUDES**   *that due to calculus (592.1)*

**CC Excl:** 593.3-593.5, 593.89-593.9, 595.0-595.9, 596.8-596.9, 599.0, 599.60-599.9, 753.4-753.5, 753.9, V45.74

**AHA:** 2Q, '97, 4

**593.5  Hydroureter**                              `CC`

**EXCLUDES**   *congenital hydroureter (753.22)*
*hydroureteronephrosis (591)*

**CC Excl:** 593.3-593.5, 593.89-593.9, 595.0-595.9, 596.8-596.9, 599.0, 599.60-599.9, 753.4-753.5, 753.9

**593.6  Postural proteinuria**

Benign postural proteinuria
Orthostatic proteinuria

**EXCLUDES**   *proteinuria NOS (791.0)*

**DEF:** Excessive amounts of serum protein in the urine caused by the body position, e.g., orthostatic and lordotic.

**✓5ᵗʰ 593.7  Vesicoureteral reflux**

**AHA:** 4Q, '94, 42

**DEF:** Backflow of urine, from bladder into ureter due to obstructed bladder neck.

**593.70  Unspecified or without reflux nephropathy**
**593.71  With reflux nephropathy, unilateral**
**593.72  With reflux nephropathy, bilateral**
**593.73  With reflux nephropathy NOS**

**✓5ᵗʰ 593.8  Other specified disorders of kidney and ureter**

**593.81  Vascular disorders of kidney**          `CC`

Renal (artery):      Renal (artery):
  embolism         thrombosis
  hemorrhage       Renal infarction

**CC Excl:** 593.70-593.81, 593.9

**593.82  Ureteral fistula**                       `CC`

Intestinoureteral fistula

**EXCLUDES**   *fistula between ureter and*
*female genital tract*
*(619.0)*

**CC Excl:** 593.82-593.9

**DEF:** Abnormal communication, between tube connecting kidney to bladder and another structure.

**593.89  Other**

Adhesions, kidney   Polyp of ureter
  or ureter        Pyelectasia
Periureteritis      Ureterocele

**EXCLUDES**   *tuberculosis of ureter (016.2)*
*ureteritis cystica (590.3)*

**593.9  Unspecified disorder of kidney and ureter**

Acute renal disease
Acute renal insufficiency
Renal disease NOS
Salt-losing nephritis or syndrome

**EXCLUDES**   *chronic renal insufficiency (585.9)*
*cystic kidney disease (753.1)*
*nephropathy, so stated (583.0-583.9)*
*renal disease:*
*arising in pregnancy or the*
*puerperium (642.1-642.2,*
*642.4-642.7, 646.2)*
*not specified as acute or chronic, but*
*with stated pathology or cause*
*(583.0-583.9)*

**AHA:** 4Q, '05, 79; 1Q, '93, 17

**✓4ᵗʰ 594  Calculus of lower urinary tract**

**594.0  Calculus in diverticulum of bladder**

**DEF:** Stone or mineral deposit in abnormal sac on the bladder wall.

**594.1  Other calculus in bladder**

Urinary bladder stone

**EXCLUDES**   *staghorn calculus (592.0)*

**DEF:** Stone or mineral deposit in bladder.

**594.2  Calculus in urethra**

**DEF:** Stone or mineral deposit in tube that empties urine from bladder.

**594.8  Other lower urinary tract calculus**

**AHA:** J-F, '85, 16

**594.9  Calculus of lower urinary tract, unspecified**

**EXCLUDES**   *calculus of urinary tract NOS (592.9)*

**✓4ᵗʰ 595  Cystitis**

**EXCLUDES**   *prostatocystitis (601.3)*

Use additional code to identify organism, such as Escherichia coli [E. coli] (041.4)

**595.0  Acute cystitis**                          `CC`

**EXCLUDES**   *trigonitis (595.3)*

**CC Excl:** 016.10-016.16, 016.30-016.36, 016.90-016.96, 017.90-017.96, 098.0, 098.11, 098.2, 098.39, 098.89, 112.2, 131.00, 131.8-131.9, 593.3-593.5, 593.89-593.9, 595.0-595.9, 596.8-596.9, 599.0, 599.60-599.9

**AHA:** 2Q, '99, 15

**DEF:** Acute inflammation of bladder.

**595.1  Chronic interstitial cystitis**

Hunner's ulcer          Submucous cystitis
Panmural fibrosis of bladder

**DEF:** Inflamed lesion affecting bladder wall; symptoms include urinary frequency, pain on bladder filling, nocturia, and distended bladder.

**595.2  Other chronic cystitis**

Chronic cystitis NOS      Subacute cystitis

**EXCLUDES**   *trigonitis (595.3)*

**DEF:** Persistent inflammation of bladder.

**595.3  Trigonitis**

Follicular cystitis        Urethrotrigonitis
Trigonitis (acute) (chronic)

**DEF:** Inflammation of the triangular area of the bladder called the trigonum vesicae.

**595.4  *Cystitis in diseases classified elsewhere***

*Code first underlying disease, as:*
actinomycosis (039.8)
amebiasis (006.8)
bilharziasis (120.0-120.9)
Echinococcus infestation (122.3, 122.6)

**EXCLUDES**   *cystitis:*
*diphtheritic (032.84)*
*gonococcal (098.11, 098.31)*
*monilial (112.2)*
*trichomonal (131.09)*
*tuberculous (016.1)*

**✓5ᵗʰ 595.8  Other specified types of cystitis**

**595.81  Cystitis cystica**

**DEF:** Inflammation of the bladder characterized by formation of multiple cysts.

**595.82  Irradiation cystitis**                   `CC`

Use additional E code to identify cause

**CC Excl:** see code 595.0

**DEF:** Inflammation of the bladder due to effects of radiation.

**595.89  Other**

Abscess of bladder   Cystitis:
Cystitis:              emphysematous
  bullous            glandularis

**595.9  Cystitis, unspecified**

---

**Bladder**
**Anterior View**

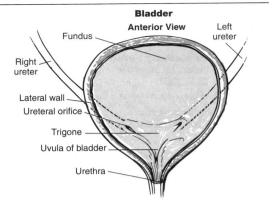

Fundus

Left ureter

Right ureter

Lateral wall

Ureteral orifice

Trigone

Uvula of bladder

Urethra

**Lateral View**

Urachus

Left ureter

Peritoneum

Pubic bone

Urogenital diaphragm

### ✓4ᵗʰ 596 Other disorders of bladder

Use additional code to identify urinary incontinence (625.6, 788.30-788.39)

**AHA:** M-A, '87, 10

#### 596.0 Bladder neck obstruction

Contracture (acquired) ⎱ of bladder neck or
Obstruction (acquired) ⎰ vesicourethral
Stenosis (acquired) orifice

> **EXCLUDES** *congenital (753.6)*

**AHA:** 3Q, '02, 28; 2Q, '01, 14; N-D, '86, 10

**DEF:** Bladder outlet and vesicourethral obstruction; occurs more often in males as a consequence of benign prostatic hypertrophy or prostatic cancer; may also occur in either sex due to strictures, following radiation, cystoscopy, catheterization, injury, infection, blood clots, bladder cancer, impaction or disease compressing bladder neck.

#### 596.1 Intestinovesical fistula    `CC`

Fistula:     Fistula:
   enterovesical      vesicoenteric
   vesicocolic       vesicorectal

**CC Excl:** 098.0, 098.2, 098.39, 098.89, 596.1-596.2, 596.8-596.9, 599.7-599.9, 788.1

**DEF:** Abnormal communication, between intestine and bladder.

#### 596.2 Vesical fistula, not elsewhere classified    `CC`

Fistula:     Fistula:
   bladder NOS     vesicocutaneous
   urethrovesical    vesicoperineal

> **EXCLUDES** *fistula between bladder and female genital tract (619.0)*

**CC Excl:** See code: 596.1

**DEF:** Abnormal communication between bladder and another structure.

#### 596.3 Diverticulum of bladder

Diverticulitis ⎱ of bladder
Diverticulum (acquired) (false) ⎰

> **EXCLUDES** *that with calculus in diverticulum of bladder (594.0)*

**DEF:** Abnormal pouch in bladder wall.

#### 596.4 Atony of bladder

High compliance bladder
Hypotonicity ⎱ of bladder
Inertia ⎰

> **EXCLUDES** *neurogenic bladder (596.54)*

**DEF:** Distended, bladder with loss of expulsive force; linked to CNS disease.

### ✓5ᵗʰ 596.5 Other functional disorders of bladder

> **EXCLUDES** *cauda equina syndrome with neurogenic bladder (344.61)*

#### 596.51 Hypertonicity of bladder

Hyperactivity
Overactive bladder

**DEF:** Abnormal tension of muscular wall of bladder; may appear after surgery of voluntary nerve.

#### 596.52 Low bladder compliance

**DEF:** Low bladder capacity; causes increased pressure and frequent urination.

#### 596.53 Paralysis of bladder

**DEF:** Impaired bladder motor function due to nerve or muscle damage.

#### 596.54 Neurogenic bladder NOS

**AHA:** 1Q, '01, 12

**DEF:** Unspecified dysfunctional bladder due to lesion of central, peripheral nervous system; may result in incontinence, residual urine retention, urinary infection, stones and renal failure.

#### 596.55 Detrusor sphincter dyssynergia

**DEF:** Instability of the urinary bladder sphincter muscle associated with urinary incontinence..

#### 596.59 Other functional disorder of bladder

Detrusor instability

**DEF:** Detrusor instability: instability of bladder; marked by uninhibited contractions often leading to incontinence.

#### 596.6 Rupture of bladder, nontraumatic    `MCC`

**CC Excl:** 596.6-596.9, 599.7-599.9, 788.1

#### 596.7 Hemorrhage into bladder wall    `CC`

Hyperemia of bladder

> **EXCLUDES** *acute hemorrhagic cystitis (595.0)*

**CC Excl:** See code: 596.6

#### 596.8 Other specified disorders of bladder

Bladder:       Bladder:
   calcified        hemorrhage
   contracted     hypertrophy

> **EXCLUDES** *cystocele, female (618.01-618.02, 618.09, 618.2-618.4)*
> *hernia or prolapse of bladder, female (618.01-618.02, 618.09, 618.2-618.4)*

**AHA:** J-F, '85, 8

#### 596.9 Unspecified disorder of bladder

**AHA:** J-F, '85, 8

### ✓4ᵗʰ 597 Urethritis, not sexually transmitted, and urethral syndrome

> **EXCLUDES** *nonspecific urethritis, so stated (099.4)*

#### 597.0 Urethral abscess    `CC`

Abscess:        Abscess of:
   periurethral       Cowper's gland
   urethral (gland)    Littré's gland
Abscess of:       Periurethral cellulitis
   bulbourethral gland

> **EXCLUDES** *urethral caruncle (599.3)*

**CC Excl:** 098.0, 098.2, 098.39, 098.89, 099.40-099.49, 112.2, 131.00, 131.02, 131.8-131.9, 597.0-598.01, 598.8-599.0, 599.60-599.9, 607.1-607.83, 607.85-607.9, 608.4-608.81, 608.85, 608.87-608.89, 752.61-752.69, 752.81-752.9, 753.6-753.9, 788.1

**DEF:** Pocket of pus in tube that empties urine from the bladder.

**N** Newborn Age: 0    **P** Pediatric Age: 0-17    **M** Maternity Age: 12-55    **A** Adult Age: 15-124    **CC** CC Condition    **MCC** Major CC Condition    **HIV** HIV Related Dx

196 — Volume 1 • October 2007          © 2007 Ingenix

√5th **597.8 Other urethritis**

**597.80 Urethritis, unspecified**

**597.81 Urethral syndrome NOS**

**597.89 Other**

Adenitis, Skene's glands
Cowperitis
Meatitis, urethral
Ulcer, urethra (meatus)
Verumontanitis

> **EXCLUDES** *trichomonal (131.02)*

√4th **598 Urethral stricture**

Use additional code to identify urinary incontinence (625.6, 788.30-788.39)

> **INCLUDES** pinhole meatus
> stricture of urinary meatus

> **EXCLUDES** *congenital stricture of urethra and urinary meatus (753.6)*

DEF: Narrowing of tube that empties urine from bladder.

√5th **598.0 Urethral stricture due to infection**

**598.00 Due to unspecified infection**

**598.01 Due to infective diseases classified elsewhere**

Code first underlying disease, as:
gonococcal infection (098.2)
schistosomiasis (120.0-120.9)
syphilis (095.8)

**598.1 Traumatic urethral stricture**

Stricture of urethra:    Stricture of urethra:
late effect of injury    postobstetric

> **EXCLUDES** *postoperative following surgery on genitourinary tract (598.2)*

**598.2 Postoperative urethral stricture**

Postcatheterization stricture of urethra

AHA: 3Q, '97, 6

**598.8 Other specified causes of urethral stricture**

AHA: N-D, '84, 9

**598.9 Urethral stricture, unspecified**

√4th **599 Other disorders of urethra and urinary tract**

**599.0 Urinary tract infection, site not specified**   **CC**

> **EXCLUDES** *candidiasis of urinary tract (112.2)*
> *urinary tract infection of newborn (771.82)*

Use additional code to identify organism, such as Escherichia coli [E. coli] (041.4)

CC Excl: 098.2, 098.39, 098.89, 099.40-099.49, 112.2, 131.00, 131.8-131.9, 590.10-591, 593.89-593.9, 595.0-595.9, 599.0, 599.60-599.89, 788.1, 996.64

AHA: 3Q, '05, 12; 2Q, '04, 13; 4Q, '03, 79; 4Q, '99, 6; 2Q, '99, 15; 1Q, '98, 5; 2Q, '96, 7; 4Q, '96, 33; 2Q, '95, 7; 1Q, '92, 13

**599.1 Urethral fistula**   **CC**

Fistula:
urethroperineal
urethrorectal
Urinary fistula NOS

> **EXCLUDES** *fistula:*
> *urethroscrotal (608.89)*
> *urethrovaginal (619.0)*
> *urethrovesicovaginal (619.0)*

CC Excl: 597.0-598.9, 599.1-599.9, 607.1-607.83, 607.85-607.9, 608.4-608.81, 608.85, 608.87-608.89, 752.61-752.69, 752.81-752.9, 753.9, 788.1

AHA: 3Q, '97, 6

**599.2 Urethral diverticulum**

DEF: Abnormal pouch in urethral wall.

**599.3 Urethral caruncle**

Polyp of urethra

**599.4 Urethral false passage**

DEF: Abnormal opening in urethra due to surgery; trauma or disease.

**599.5 Prolapsed urethral mucosa**

Prolapse of urethra
Urethrocele

> **EXCLUDES** *urethrocele, female (618.03, 618.09, 618.2-618.4)*

√5th **599.6 Urinary obstruction**

Use additional code to identify urinary incontinence (625.6, 788.30-788.39)

> **EXCLUDES** *obstructive nephropathy NOS (593.89)*

AHA: 4Q, '05, 80

**599.60 Urinary obstruction, unspecified**

Obstructive uropathy NOS
Urinary (tract) obstruction NOS

**599.69 Urinary obstruction, not elsewhere classified**

Code, if applicable, any causal condition first, such as:
hyperplasia of prostate (600.0-600.9 with fifth-digit 1)

AHA: 4Q, '06, 93

**599.7 Hematuria**

Hematuria (benign) (essential)

> **EXCLUDES** *hemoglobinuria (791.2)*

AHA: 1Q, '00, 5; 3Q, '95, 8

DEF: Blood in urine.

√5th **599.8 Other specified disorders of urethra and urinary tract**

Use additional code to identify urinary incontinence (625.6, 788.30-788.39), if present

> **EXCLUDES** *symptoms and other conditions classifiable to 788.0-788.2, 788.4-788.9, 791.0-791.9*

**599.81 Urethral hypermobility**

DEF: Hyperactive urethra.

**599.82 Intrinsic (urethral) spincter deficiency [ISD]**

AHA: 2Q, '96, 15

DEF: Malfunctioning urethral sphincter.

**599.83 Urethral instability**

DEF: Inconsistent functioning of urethra.

**599.84 Other specified disorders of urethra**

Rupture of urethra (nontraumatic)
Urethral:
cyst
granuloma

DEF: Rupture of urethra due to herniation or breaking down of tissue; not due to trauma.

DEF: Urethral cyst: abnormal sac in urethra; usually fluid filled.

DEF: Granuloma: inflammatory cells forming small nodules in urethra.

**599.89 Other specified disorders of urinary tract**

**599.9 Unspecified disorder of urethra and urinary tract**

**Genitourinary System**

**600–601.3**

## DISEASES OF MALE GENITAL ORGANS (600-608)

☑4ᵗʰ **600 Hyperplasia of prostate**

INCLUDES   enlarged prostate

**AHA:** 3Q, '05, 20; 4Q, '00, 43; 3Q, '94, 12; 3Q, '92, 7; N-D, '86, 10

DEF: Fibrostromal proliferation in periurethral glands, causes blood in urine; etiology unknown.

☑5ᵗʰ **600.0 Hypertrophy (benign) of prostate**
Benign prostatic hypertrophy
Enlargement of prostate
Smooth enlarged prostate
Soft enlarged prostate

**AHA:** 4Q, '06, 93-95; 3Q, '05, 20; 4Q, '03, 63; 1Q, '03, 6; 3Q, '02, 28; 2Q, '01, 14

**600.00 Hypertrophy (benign) of prostate** A ♂
**without urinary obstruction and other lower urinary tract symptoms [LUTS]**
Hypertrophy (benign) of prostate NOS

**600.01 Hypertrophy (benign) of prostate** A ♂
**with urinary obstruction and other urinary tract symptoms [LUTS]**
Hypertrophy (benign) of prostate with urinary retention
Use additional code to identify symptoms:
incomplete bladder emptying (788.21)
nocturia (788.43)
straining on urination (788.65)
urinary frequency (788.41)
urinary hesitancy (788.64)
urinary incontinence (788.30-788.39)
urinary obstruction (599.69)
urinary retention (788.20)
urinary urgency (788.63)
weak urinary stream (788.62)

**AHA:** 4Q, '06, 93-95; 4Q, '03, 64

☑5ᵗʰ **600.1 Nodular prostate**
Hard, firm prostate
Multinodular prostate
EXCLUDES   malignant neoplasm of prostate (185)

**AHA:** 4Q, '03, 63

DEF: Hard, firm nodule in prostate.

**600.10 Nodular prostate without urinary** A ♂
**obstruction**
Nodular prostate NOS

**600.11 Nodular prostate with urinary** A ♂
**obstruction**
Nodular prostate with urinary retention

☑5ᵗʰ **600.2 Benign localized hyperplasia of prostate**
Adenofibromatous hypertrophy of prostate
Adenoma of prostate
Fibroadenoma of prostate
Fibroma of prostate
Myoma of prostate
Polyp of prostate
EXCLUDES   benign neoplasms of prostate (222.2)
hypertrophy of prostate (600.00-600.01)
malignant neoplasm of prostate (185)

**AHA:** 4Q, '06, 93-95; 4Q, '03, 63

DEF: Benign localized hyperplasia is a clearly defined epithelial tumor. Other terms used for this condition are adenofibromatous hypertrophy of prostate, adenoma of prostate, fibroadenoma of prostate, fibroma of prostate, myoma of prostate, and polyp of prostate.

**600.20 Benign localized hyperplasia of** A ♂
**prostate without urinary obstruction and other lower urinary tract symptoms [LUTS]**
Benign localized hyperplasia of prostate NOS

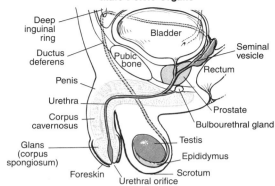

**Male Pelvic Organs**

Deep inguinal ring · Ductus deferens · Penis · Urethra · Corpus cavernosus · Glans (corpus spongiosum) · Foreskin · Bladder · Pubic bone · Seminal vesicle · Rectum · Prostate · Bulbourethral gland · Testis · Epididymus · Scrotum · Urethral orifice

**600.21 Benign localized hyperplasia of** A ♂
**prostate with urinary obstruction and other lower urinary tract symptoms [LUTS]**
Benign localized hyperplasia of prostate with urinary retention
Use additional code to identify symptoms:
incomplete bladder emptying (788.21)
nocturia (788.43)
straining on urination (788.65)
urinary frequency (788.41)
urinary hesitancy (788.64)
urinary incontinence (788.30-788.39)
urinary obstruction (599.69)
urinary retention (788.20)
urinary urgency (788.63)
weak urinary stream (788.62)

**600.3 Cyst of prostate** A ♂
DEF: Sacs of fluid, which differentiate this from either nodular or adenomatous tumors.

☑5ᵗʰ **600.9 Hyperplasia of prostate, unspecified**
Median bar
Prostatic obstruction NOS
**AHA:** 4Q, '06, 93-95; 4Q, '03, 63

**600.90 Hyperplasia of prostate, unspecified,** A ♂
**without urinary obstruction and other lower urinary tract symptoms [LUTS]**
Hyperplasia of prostate NOS

**600.91 Hyperplasia of prostate, unspecified** A ♂
**with urinary obstruction and other lower urinary tract symptoms [LUTS]**
Hyperplasia of prostate, unspecified, with urinary retention
Use additional code to identify symptoms:
incomplete bladder emptying (788.21)
nocturia (788.43)
straining on urination (788.65)
urinary frequency (788.41)
urinary hesitancy (788.64)
urinary incontinence (788.30-788.39)
urinary obstruction (599.69)
urinary retention (788.20)
urinary urgency (788.63)
weak urinary stream (788.62)

☑4ᵗʰ **601 Inflammatory diseases of prostate**
Use additional code to identify organism, such as Staphylococcus (041.1), or Streptococcus (041.0)

**601.0 Acute prostatitis** CC A ♂
**CC Excl:** 098.12, 098.32, 098.89, 112.2, 131.00, 131.03, 131.8-131.9, 600.00-602.9

**601.1 Chronic prostatitis** A ♂

**601.2 Abscess of prostate** CC A ♂
**CC Excl:** See code: 601.0

**601.3 Prostatocystitis** A ♂

---

N Newborn Age: 0    P Pediatric Age: 0-17    M Maternity Age: 12-55    A Adult Age: 15-124    CC CC Condition    MCC Major CC Condition    HIV HIV Related Dx

**601.4** *Prostatitis in diseases classified elsewhere*  A ♂
    *Code first underlying disease, as:*
        actinomycosis (039.8)
        blastomycosis (116.0)
        syphilis (095.8)
        tuberculosis (016.5)
    **EXCLUDES** *prostatitis:*
            *gonococcal (098.12, 098.32)*
            *monilial (112.2)*
            *trichomonal (131.03)*

**601.8** **Other specified inflammatory diseases of prostate**  A ♂
        Prostatitis:            Prostatitis:
          cavitary                granulomatous
          diverticular

**601.9** **Prostatitis, unspecified**  A ♂
        Prostatitis NOS

✓4ᵗʰ **602 Other disorders of prostate**

**602.0** **Calculus of prostate**  A ♂
        Prostatic stone
        DEF: Stone or mineral deposit in prostate.

**602.1** **Congestion or hemorrhage of prostate**  A ♂
        DEF: Bleeding or fluid collection in prostate.

**602.2** **Atrophy of prostate**  A ♂

**602.3** **Dysplasia of prostate**  ♂
        Prostatic intraepithelial neoplasia I (PIN I)
        Prostatic intraepithelial neoplasia II (PIN II)
        **EXCLUDES** *prostatic intraepithelial neoplasia III*
                *(PIN III) (233.4)*

        AHA: 4Q, '01, 46

        DEF: Abnormality of shape and size of the intraepithelial tissues of
        the prostate; pre-malignant condition characterized by stalks and
        absence of a basilar cell layer; synonyms are intraductal dysplasia,
        large acinar atypical hyperplasia, atypical primary hyperplasia,
        hyperplasia with malignant changes, marked atypia, or duct-acinar
        dysplasia.

**602.8** **Other specified disorders of prostate**  A ♂
        Fistula     ⎫
        Infarction  ⎬ of prostate
        Stricture   ⎭
        Periprostatic adhesions

**602.9** **Unspecified disorder of prostate**  A ♂

✓4ᵗʰ **603 Hydrocele**
        **INCLUDES** hydrocele of spermatic cord, testis, or tunica
                    vaginalis
        **EXCLUDES** *congenital (778.6)*
    DEF: Circumscribed collection of fluid in tunica vaginalis, spermatic cord or
    testis.

**603.0** **Encysted hydrocele**

**603.1** **Infected hydrocele**  CC
        Use additional code to identify organism
        CC Excl: 112.2, 131.00, 131.8-131.9, 603.0-603.9

**603.8** **Other specified types of hydrocele**

**603.9** **Hydrocele, unspecified**

✓4ᵗʰ **604 Orchitis and epididymitis**
        Use additional code to identify organism, such as Escherichia
        coli [E. coli] (041.4), Staphylococcus (041.1), or
        Streptococcus (041.0)

**604.0** **Orchitis, epididymitis, and epididymo-orchitis, with abscess**  CC ♂
        Abscess of epididymis or testis
        CC Excl: 072.0, 098.13-098.14, 098.33-098.34, 098.89, 112.2, 131.00,
        131.8-131.9, 604.0-604.99

✓5ᵗʰ **604.9** **Other orchitis, epididymitis, and epididymo-orchitis, without mention of abscess**
        **604.90 Orchitis and epididymitis, unspecified**  ♂

**Common Inguinal Canal Anomalies**

**604.91** *Orchitis and epididymitis in diseases classified elsewhere*  ♂
        *Code first underlying disease, as:*
            diphtheria (032.89)
            filariasis (125.0-125.9)
            syphilis (095.8)
        **EXCLUDES** *orchitis:*
                *gonococcal (098.13, 098.33)*
                *mumps (072.0)*
                *tuberculous (016.5)*
                *tuberculous epididymitis*
                    *(016.4)*

        **604.99 Other**  ♂

**605 Redundant prepuce and phimosis**  ♂
        Adherent prepuce        Phimosis (congenital)
        Paraphimosis            Tight foreskin
        DEF: Constriction of preputial orifice causing inability of the prepuce to be
        drawn back over the glans; it may be congenital or caused by infection.

✓4ᵗʰ **606 Infertility, male**
        AHA: 2Q, '96, 9

**606.0** **Azoospermia**  A ♂
        Absolute infertility      Infertility due to:
        Infertility due to:          spermatogenic arrest
          germinal (cell) aplasia     (complete)
        DEF: Absence of spermatozoa in the semen or inability to produce
        spermatozoa.

**606.1** **Oligospermia**  A ♂
        Infertility due to:
          germinal cell desquamation
          hypospermatogenesis
          incomplete spermatogenic arrest
        DEF: Insufficient number of sperm in semen.

**606.8** **Infertility due to extratesticular causes**  A ♂
        Infertility due to:       Infertility due to:
          drug therapy              radiation
          infection                 systemic disease
          obstruction of efferent
            ducts

**606.9** **Male infertility, unspecified**  A ♂

✓4ᵗʰ **607 Disorders of penis**
        **EXCLUDES** *phimosis (605)*

**607.0** **Leukoplakia of penis**  ♂
        Kraurosis of penis
        **EXCLUDES** *carcinoma in situ of penis (233.5)*
                *erythroplasia of Queyrat (233.5)*
        DEF: White, thickened patches on glans penis.

**607.1** **Balanoposthitis**  ♂
        Balanitis
        Use additional code to identify organism
        DEF: Inflammation of glans penis and prepuce.

**607.2** **Other inflammatory disorders of penis**  ♂
        Abscess    ⎫
        Boil       ⎬ of corpus cavernosum
        Carbuncle  ⎭   or penis
        Cellulitis
        Cavernitis (penis)
        Use additional code to identify organism
        **EXCLUDES** *herpetic infection (054.13)*

**Genitourinary System**

607.3–608.84

**607.3 Priapism** `CC` ♂
     Painful erection
**CC Excl:** 607.0-607.9
DEF: Prolonged penile erection without sexual stimulation.

✓5th **607.8 Other specified disorders of penis**

     **607.81 Balanitis xerotica obliterans** ♂
         Induratio penis plastica
         DEF: Inflammation of the glans penis, caused by stricture of the opening of the prepuce.

     **607.82 Vascular disorders of penis** `CC` ♂
         Embolism
         Hematoma } of corpus
            (nontraumatic)   cavernosum
         Hemorrhage   or penis
         Thrombosis
         **CC Excl:** 607.82-607.83

     **607.83 Edema of penis** ♂
         DEF: Fluid retention within penile tissues.

     **607.84 Impotence of organic origin** `A` ♂
         **EXCLUDES** nonorganic (302.72)
         **AHA:** 3Q, '91, 11
         DEF: Physiological cause interfering with erection.

     **607.85 Peyronie's disease** ♂
         **AHA:** 4Q, '03, 64
         DEF: A severe curvature of the erect penis due to fibrosis of the cavernous sheaths.

     **607.89 Other** ♂
         Atrophy
         Fibrosis } of corpus cavernosum
         Hypertrophy   or penis
         Ulcer (chronic)

**607.9 Unspecified disorder of penis** ♂

✓4th **608 Other disorders of male genital organs**

     **608.0 Seminal vesiculitis** ♂
         Abscess } of seminal vesicle
         Cellulitis
         Vesiculitis (seminal)
         Use additional code to identify organism
         **EXCLUDES** gonococcal infection (098.14, 098.34)
         DEF: Inflammation of seminal vesicle.

     **608.1 Spermatocele** ♂
         DEF: Cystic enlargement of the epididymis or the testis; the cysts contain spermatozoa.

✓5th **608.2 Torsion of testis**
     DEF: Twisted or rotated testis; may compromise blood flow.

     **608.20 Torsion of testis, unspecified** `CC` ♂
         **CC Excl:** 608.20-608.24
         **AHA:** 4Q, '06, 95

     **608.21 Extravaginal torsion of spermatic cord** `CC` ♂
         **CC Excl:** See code: 608.20
         **AHA:** 4Q, '06, 95
         DEF: Torsion of the spermatic cord just below the tunica vaginalis attachments. Often manifests in the neonatal period after having developed in utero. This type of torsion accounts for approximately 5% of all torsions. It is usually associated with high birth weight.

     **608.22 Intravaginal torsion of spermatic cord** `CC` ♂
         ▶Torsion of spermatic cord NOS◀
         **CC Excl:** See code: 608.20
         **AHA:** 4Q, '06, 95
         DEF: Torsion within the tunica vaginalis also called the "bell-clapper" anomaly. It usually occurs in older children, with peak incidence occurring at approximately 13 years of age. This type of torsion accounts for roughly 16% emergency room torsion encounters. Of note, the left testis is most frequently affected, with only 2% cases presenting as bilateral torsions.

     **608.23 Torsion of appendix testis** `CC` ♂
         **CC Excl:** See code: 608.20
         **AHA:** 4Q, '06, 95
         DEF: Torsion of small solid projection of tissue on the upper outer surface of the testis (hydatid of Morgagni); a remnant of the embryologic mullerian duct.

     **608.24 Torsion of appendix epididymis** `CC` ♂
         **CC Excl:** See code: 608.20
         **AHA:** 4Q, '06, 95
         DEF: Torsion of small stalked appendage of the head of the epididymis (pedunculated hydatid); a detached embryologic efferent duct.

**608.3 Atrophy of testis** ♂

**608.4 Other inflammatory disorders of male genital organs** ♂
     Abscess
     Boil } of scrotum, spermatic cord, testis
     Carbuncle   [except abscess], tunica
     Cellulitis   vaginalis, or vas deferens
     Vasitis
     Use additional code to identify organism
     **EXCLUDES** abscess of testis (604.0)

✓5th **608.8 Other specified disorders of male genital organs**

     **608.81 Disorders of male genital organs in diseases classified elsewhere** ♂
         *Code first underlying disease, as:*
            filariasis (125.0-125.9)
            tuberculosis (016.5)

     **608.82 Hematospermia** ♂
         **AHA:** 4Q, '01, 46
         DEF: Presence of blood in the ejaculate; relatively common, affecting men of any age after puberty; cause is often difficult to determine since the semen originates in several organs, often the result of a viral or bacterial infection and inflammation.

     **608.83 Vascular disorders** ♂
         Hematoma
         (non- } of seminal vesicle,
            traumatic)   spermatic cord,
         Hemorrhage   testis, scrotum,
         Thrombosis   tunica vaginalis,
            or vas deferens
         Hematocele NOS, male
         **AHA:** 4Q, '03, 110

     **608.84 Chylocele of tunica vaginalis** ♂
         DEF: Chylous effusion into tunica vaginalis; due to infusion of lymphatic fluids.

**Torsion of the Testis**

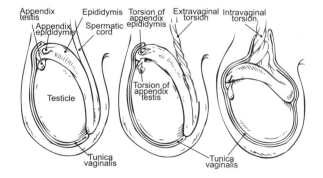

Appendix testis   Epididymis   Torsion of appendix   Extravaginal torsion   Intravaginal torsion
Appendix epididymis   Spermatic cord   Torsion of appendix epididymis
Testicle   Torsion of appendix testis
Tunica vaginalis   Tunica vaginalis

N Newborn Age: 0    P Pediatric Age: 0-17    M Maternity Age: 12-55    A Adult Age: 15-124    CC CC Condition    MCC Major CC Condition    HIV HIV Related Dx

200 — Volume 1 • October 2007       © 2007 Ingenix

**608.85 Stricture** ♂
Stricture of:                  Stricture of:
spermatic cord            vas deferens
tunica vaginalis

**608.86 Edema** ♂

**608.87 Retrograde ejaculation** ♂
AHA: 4Q, '01, 46

DEF: Condition where the semen travels to the bladder
rather than out through the urethra due to damaged
nerves causing the bladder neck to remain open during
ejaculation.

**608.89 Other** ♂
Atrophy        ⎫ of seminal vesicle, sperm-
Fibrosis       ⎬ atic cord, testis, scro-
Hypertrophy    ⎪ tum, tunica vaginalis,
Ulcer          ⎭ or vas deferens

EXCLUDES   *atrophy of testis (608.3)*

**608.9 Unspecified disorder of male genital organs** ♂

## DISORDERS OF BREAST (610-611)

4ᵗʰ **610 Benign mammary dysplasias**

**610.0 Solitary cyst of breast**
Cyst (solitary) of breast

**610.1 Diffuse cystic mastopathy** A
Chronic cystic mastitis    Fibrocystic disease of
Cystic breast                      breast

AHA: 2Q, '06, 10

DEF: Extensive formation of nodular cysts in breast tissue;
symptoms include tenderness, change in size and hyperplasia of
ductal epithelium.

**610.2 Fibroadenosis of breast**
Fibroadenosis of breast:   Fibroadenosis of breast:
NOS                                  diffuse
chronic                              periodic
cystic                               segmental

DEF: Non-neoplastic nodular condition of breast.

**610.3 Fibrosclerosis of breast**
DEF: Fibrous tissue in breast.

**610.4 Mammary duct ectasia**
Comedomastitis          Mastitis:
Duct ectasia                    periductal
plasma cell

DEF: Atrophy of duct epithelium; causes distended collecting ducts
of mammary gland; drying up of breast secretion, intraductal
inflammation and periductal and interstitial chronic inflammatory
reaction.

**610.8 Other specified benign mammary dysplasias**
Mazoplasia              Sebaceous cyst of breast

**610.9 Benign mammary dysplasia, unspecified**

4ᵗʰ **611 Other disorders of breast**

EXCLUDES   *that associated with lactation or the puerperium
(675.0-676.9)*

**611.0 Inflammatory disease of breast**
Abscess (acute) (chronic)   Mastitis (acute) (subacute)
(nonpuerperal) of:                (nonpuerperal):
areola                                   NOS
breast                                   infective
Mammillary fistula                retromammary
submammary

EXCLUDES   *carbuncle of breast (680.2)*
*chronic cystic mastitis (610.1)*
*neonatal infective mastitis (771.5)*
*thrombophlebitis of breast [Mondor's
disease] (451.89)*

**611.1 Hypertrophy of breast**
Gynecomastia            Hypertrophy of breast:
NOS
massive pubertal

**611.2 Fissure of nipple**

**611.3 Fat necrosis of breast**
Fat necrosis (segmental) of breast

DEF: Splitting of neutral fats in adipose tissue cells as a result of
trauma; a firm circumscribed mass is then formed in the breast.

**611.4 Atrophy of breast**

**611.5 Galactocele**

**611.6 Galactorrhea not associated with childbirth**

5ᵗʰ **611.7 Signs and symptoms in breast**

**611.71 Mastodynia**
Pain in breast

**611.72 Lump or mass in breast**
AHA: 2Q, '03, 4-5

**611.79 Other**
Induration of breast    Nipple discharge
Inversion of nipple     Retraction of nipple

**611.8 Other specified disorders of breast**
Hematoma (nontraumatic)  ⎫ of breast
Infarction                            ⎭

Occlusion of breast duct
Subinvolution of breast (postlactational) (postpartum)

**611.9 Unspecified breast disorder**

## INFLAMMATORY DISEASE OF FEMALE PELVIC ORGANS (614-616)

Use additional code to identify organism, such as
Staphylococcus (041.1), or Streptococcus (041.0)

EXCLUDES   *that associated with pregnancy, abortion,
childbirth, or the puerperium (630-676.9)*

4ᵗʰ **614 Inflammatory disease of ovary, fallopian tube, pelvic
cellular tissue, and peritoneum**

EXCLUDES   *endometritis (615.0-615.9)*
*major infection following delivery (670)*
*that complicating:*
*abortion (634-638 with .0, 639.0)*
*ectopic or molar pregnancy (639.0)*
*pregnancy or labor (646.6)*

**614.0 Acute salpingitis and oophoritis** CC ♀
Any condition classifiable to 614.2, specified as
acute or subacute

CC Excl: 016.60-016.96, 017.90-017.96, 098.15-098.17, 098.35-098.37,
098.89, 112.2, 131.00, 131.8-131.9, 614.0-615.9, 616.81-616.9, 625.8-
625.9, 629.20-629.81, 629.89-629.9, 752.81-752.9

DEF: Acute inflammation, of ovary and fallopian tube.

**614.1 Chronic salpingitis and oophoritis** ♀
Hydrosalpinx             Salpingitis:
Salpingitis:                  isthmica nodosa
follicularis
Any condition classifiable to 614.2, specified as
chronic

DEF: Persistent inflammation of ovary and fallopian tube.

**614.2 Salpingitis and oophoritis not specified as
acute, subacute, or chronic** ♀
Abscess (of):             Pyosalpinx
fallopian tube          Perisalpingitis
ovary                       Salpingitis
tubo-ovarian           Salpingo-oophoritis
Oophoritis                Tubo-ovarian inflammatory
Perioophoritis               disease

EXCLUDES   *gonococcal infection (chronic) (098.37)*
*acute (098.17)*
*tuberculous (016.6)*

AHA: 2Q, '91, 5

**614.3 Acute parametritis and pelvic cellulitis** CC ♀
Acute inflammatory pelvic disease
Any condition classifiable to 614.4, specified as
acute

CC Excl: See code 614.0

DEF: Parametritis: inflammation of the parametrium; pelvic
cellulitis is a synonym for parametritis.

**Genitourinary System**

**614.4–616.8**

**Female Genitourinary System**

Diagram labels: Uterine (fallopian) tube, Ovary, Rectouterine pouch (of Douglas), Uterus (fundus), Cervix, Bladder, Rectum, Pubic bone, Clitoris, Urogenital diaphragm, Urethral orifice (meatus), Labia minora, Labia majora, Anus, Vaginal canal

**614.4  Chronic or unspecified parametritis and pelvic cellulitis**  ♀

Abscess (of):
broad ligament ⎤
parametrium ⎥
pelvis, female ⎬ chronic or NOS
pouch of Douglas ⎦

Chronic inflammatory pelvic disease
Pelvic cellulitis, female
**EXCLUDES** *tuberculous (016.7)*

**614.5  Acute or unspecified pelvic peritonitis, female**  MCC ♀

**CC Excl:** See code 614.0

**AHA:** 4Q, '05, 74

**614.6  Pelvic peritoneal adhesions, female (postoperative) (postinfection)**  ♀

Adhesions:          Adhesions:
peritubal            tubo-ovarian
Use additional code to identify any associated infertility (628.2)
**AHA:** 3Q, '03, 6; 1Q, '03, 4; 3Q, '95, 7; 3Q, '94, 12

DEF: Fibrous scarring abnormally joining structures within abdomen.

**614.7  Other chronic pelvic peritonitis, female**  CC ♀
**EXCLUDES** *tuberculous(016.7)*

**CC Excl:** See code: 614.0

**614.8  Other specified inflammatory disease of female pelvic organs and tissues**  ♀

**614.9  Unspecified inflammatory disease of female pelvic organs and tissues**  ♀

Pelvic infection or inflammation, female NOS
Pelvic inflammatory disease [PID]

√4ᵗʰ **615 Inflammatory diseases of uterus, except cervix**
**EXCLUDES** *following delivery (670)*
*hyperplastic endometritis (621.30-621.33)*
*that complicating:*
*abortion (634-638 with .0, 639.0)*
*ectopic or molar pregnancy (639.0)*
*pregnancy or labor (646.6)*

**615.0  Acute**  CC ♀

Any condition classifiable to 615.9, specified as acute or subacute
**CC Excl:** 016.60-016.96, 017.90-017.96, 098.15-098.17, 098.35-098.37, 098.89, 112.2, 131.00, 131.8-131.9, 614.0-616.0, 616.81-616.9, 621.8-621.9, 625.8-625.9, 629.20-629.81, 629.89-629.9, 752.81-752.9

**615.1  Chronic**  ♀

Any condition classifiable to 615.9, specified as chronic

**615.9  Unspecified inflammatory disease of uterus**  ♀

Endometritis          Myometritis
Endomyometritis       Perimetritis
Intrauterine infection  Pyometra
Metritis              Uterine abscess

√4ᵗʰ **616 Inflammatory disease of cervix, vagina, and vulva**
**EXCLUDES** *that complicating:*
*abortion (634-638 with .0, 639.0)*
*ectopic or molar pregnancy (639.0)*
*pregnancy, childbirth, or the puerperium (646.6)*

**616.0  Cervicitis and endocervicitis**  ♀

Cervicitis ⎤ with or without mention of
Endocervicitis ⎦ erosion or ectropion
Nabothian (gland) cyst or follicle
**EXCLUDES** *erosion or ectropion without mention of cervicitis (622.0)*

√5ᵗʰ **616.1  Vaginitis and vulvovaginitis**

DEF: Inflammation or infection of vagina or external female genitalia.

**616.10  Vaginitis and vulvovaginitis, unspecified**  ♀
Vaginitis:
NOS
postirradiation
Vulvitis NOS
Vulvovaginitis NOS
Use additional code to identify organism, such as Escherichia coli [E. coli] (041.4), Staphylococcus (041.1), or Streptococcus (041.0)
**EXCLUDES** *noninfective leukorrhea (623.5)*
*postmenopausal or senile vaginitis (627.3)*

**616.11  Vaginitis and vulvovaginitis in diseases classified elsewhere**  ♀
Code first underlying disease, as:
pinworm vaginitis (127.4)
**EXCLUDES** *herpetic vulvovaginitis (054.11)*
*monilial vulvovaginitis (112.1)*
*trichomonal vaginitis or vulvovaginitis (131.01)*

**616.2  Cyst of Bartholin's gland**  ♀
Bartholin's duct cyst
DEF: Fluid-filled sac within gland of vaginal orifice.

**616.3  Abscess of Bartholin's gland**  CC ♀
Vulvovaginal gland abscess
**CC Excl:** 016.70-016.96, 017.90-017.96, 112.1-112.2, 131.00-131.01, 131.8-131.9, 616.10-616.9, 624.3-624.9, 625.8-625.9, 629.20-629.81, 629.89-629.9, 752.81-752.9

**616.4  Other abscess of vulva**  CC ♀
Abscess ⎤
Carbuncle ⎬ of vulva
Furuncle ⎦
**CC Excl:** See code 616.3

√5ᵗʰ **616.5  Ulceration of vulva**

**616.50  Ulceration of vulva, unspecified**  ♀
Ulcer NOS of vulva

**616.51  Ulceration of vulva in diseases classified elsewhere**  ♀
Code first underlying disease, as:
Behçet's syndrome (136.1)
tuberculosis (016.7)
**EXCLUDES** *vulvar ulcer (in):*
*gonococcal (098.0)*
*herpes simplex (054.12)*
*syphilitic (091.0)*

√5ᵗʰ **616.8  Other specified inflammatory diseases of cervix, vagina, and vulva**
**EXCLUDES** *noninflammatory disorders of:*
*cervix (622.0-622.9)*
*vagina (623.0-623.9)*
*vulva (624.0-624.9)*

N Newborn Age: 0   P Pediatric Age: 0-17   M Maternity Age: 12-55   A Adult Age: 15-124   CC CC Condition   MCC Major CC Condition   HIV HIV Related Dx

202 — Volume 1 • October 2007

© 2007 Ingenix

**616.81 Mucositis (ulcerative) of cervix, vagina, and vulva** `cc` ♀

Use additional E code to identify adverse effects of therapy, such as:
antineoplastic and immunosuppressive drugs (E930.7, E933.1)
radiation therapy (E879.2)

CC Excl: 616.0, 616.81-616.9

AHA: 4Q, '06, 88-90

**616.89 Other inflammatory disease of cervix, vagina and vulva** ♀

Caruncle, vagina or labium
Ulcer, vagina

AHA: 4Q, '06, 88-90

**616.9 Unspecified inflammatory disease of cervix, vagina, and vulva** ♀

## OTHER DISORDERS OF FEMALE GENITAL TRACT (617-629)

√4ᵗʰ **617 Endometriosis**

**617.0 Endometriosis of uterus** ♀

Adenomyosis
Endometriosis:
  cervix

Endometriosis:
  internal
  myometrium

EXCLUDES *stromal endometriosis (236.0)*

AHA: 3Q, '92, 7

DEF: Aberrant uterine mucosal tissue; creating products of menses and inflamed uterine tissues.

**617.1 Endometriosis of ovary** ♀

Chocolate cyst of ovary
Endometrial cystoma of ovary

DEF: Aberrant uterine tissue; creating products of menses and inflamed ovarian tissues.

**617.2 Endometriosis of fallopian tube** ♀

DEF: Aberrant uterine tissue; creating products of menses and inflamed tissues of fallopian tubes.

**617.3 Endometriosis of pelvic peritoneum** ♀

Endometriosis:
  broad ligament
  cul-de-sac (Douglas')

Endometriosis:
  parametrium
  round ligament

DEF: Aberrant uterine tissue; creating products of menses and inflamed peritoneum tissues.

**617.4 Endometriosis of rectovaginal septum and vagina** ♀

DEF: Aberrant uterine tissue; creating products of menses and inflamed tissues in and behind vagina.

**617.5 Endometriosis of intestine** ♀

Endometriosis:
  appendix
  colon

Endometriosis:
  rectum

DEF: Aberrant uterine tissue; creating products of menses and inflamed intestinal tissues.

**617.6 Endometriosis in scar of skin** ♀

**617.8 Endometriosis of other specified sites** ♀

Endometriosis:
  bladder
  lung

Endometriosis:
  umbilicus
  vulva

**617.9 Endometriosis, site unspecified** ♀

√4ᵗʰ **618 Genital prolapse**

Use additional code to identify urinary incontinence (625.6, 788.31, 788.33-788.39)

EXCLUDES *that complicating pregnancy, labor, or delivery (654.4)*

√5ᵗʰ **618.0 Prolapse of vaginal walls without mention of uterine prolapse**

EXCLUDES *that with uterine prolapse (618.2-618.4)*
*enterocele (618.6)*
*vaginal vault prolapse following hysterectomy (618.5)*

**618.00 Unspecified prolapse of vaginal walls** ♀

Vaginal prolapse NOS

**618.01 Cystocele, midline** ♀

Cystocele NOS

DEF: Defect in the pubocervical fascia, the supportive layer of the bladder, causing bladder drop and herniated into the vagina along the midline.

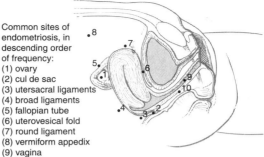

**Common Sites of Endometriosis**

Common sites of endometriosis, in descending order of frequency:
(1) ovary
(2) cul de sac
(3) utersacral ligaments
(4) broad ligaments
(5) fallopian tube
(6) uterovesical fold
(7) round ligament
(8) vermiform appedix
(9) vagina
(10) rectovaginal septum

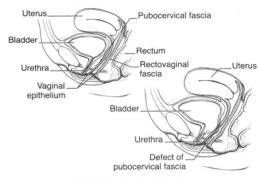

**Vaginal Midline Cystocele**

Normal vaginal support

**618.02 Cystocele, lateral** ♀

Paravaginal

DEF: Loss of support of the lateral attachment of the vagina at the arcus tendinous results in bladder drop; bladder herniates into the vagina laterally; also called paravaginal defect.

**618.03 Urethrocele** ♀

**618.04 Rectocele** ♀

Proctocele

**618.05 Perineocele** ♀

**618.09 Other prolapse of vaginal walls without mention of uterine prolapse** ♀

Cystourethrocele

**618.1 Uterine prolapse without mention of vaginal wall prolapse** ♀

Descensus uteri
Uterine prolapse:
  NOS
  complete

Uterine prolapse:
  first degree
  second degree
  third degree

EXCLUDES *that with mention of cystocele, urethrocele, or rectocele (618.2-618.4)*

**618.2 Uterovaginal prolapse, incomplete** ♀

DEF: Downward displacement of uterus downward into vagina.

**618.3 Uterovaginal prolapse, complete** ♀

DEF: Downward displacement of uterus exposed within external genitalia.

**618.4 Uterovaginal prolapse, unspecified** ♀

**618.5 Prolapse of vaginal vault after hysterectomy** ♀

**618.6 Vaginal enterocele, congenital or acquired** ♀

Pelvic enterocele, congenital or acquired

DEF: Vaginal vault hernia formed by the loop of the small intestine protruding into the rectal vaginal pouch; can also accompany uterine prolapse or follow hysterectomy.

**618.7 Old laceration of muscles of pelvic floor** ♀

Genitourinary System

616.81-618.7

**Vaginal Lateral Cystocele**

Normal vaginal support

Symphysis pubis — Cooper's ligament

Bladder — Arcus tendineus, Pubocervical fascia

Arcus tendineus defect

Lateral cystocele

**Types of Vaginal Hernias**

Urethrocele
Uterus, Bladder, Rectum, Urethra, Vaginal canal, Urethrocele

Cystocele
Uterus, Bladder, Rectum, Urethra, Vaginal canal, Cystocele

Rectocele
Uterus, Bladder, Rectum, Urethra, Vaginal canal, Rectocele

Enterocele
Uterus, Bladder, Rectum, Urethra, Vaginal canal, Terminal ileum

✓5th **618.8** **Other specified genital prolapse**

**618.81 Incompetence or weakening of pubocervical tissue** ♀

**618.82 Incompetence or weakening of rectovaginal tissue** ♀

**618.83 Pelvic muscle wasting** ♀
Disuse atrophy of pelvic muscles and anal sphincter

**618.84 Cervical stump prolapse** ♀
**AHA:** 4Q, '06, 97

**618.89 Other specified genital prolapse** ♀

**618.9 Unspecified genital prolapse** ♀

✓4th **619 Fistula involving female genital tract**
EXCLUDES *vesicorectal and intestinovesical fistula (596.1)*

**619.0 Urinary-genital tract fistula, female** CC ♀
Fistula:               Fistula:
cervicovesical      uteroureteric
ureterovaginal      uterovesical
urethrovaginal      vesicocervicovaginal
urethrovesicovaginal  vesicovaginal
**CC Excl:** 619.0-619.9

**619.1 Digestive-genital tract fistula, female** CC ♀
Fistula:               Fistula:
intestinouterine    rectovulval
intestinovaginal    sigmoidovaginal
rectovaginal        uterorectal
**CC Excl:** See code: 619.0

**619.2 Genital tract-skin fistula, female** CC ♀
Fistula:               Fistula:
uterus to abdominal wall  vaginoperineal
**CC Excl:** See code: 619.0

**619.8 Other specified fistulas involving female genital tract** CC ♀
Fistula:               Fistula:
cervix              uterus
cul-de-sac (Douglas')  vagina
**CC Excl:** See code: 619.0

**619.9 Unspecified fistula involving female genital tract** CC ♀
**CC Excl:** see code 619.0

✓4th **620 Noninflammatory disorders of ovary, fallopian tube, and broad ligament**
EXCLUDES *hydrosalpinx (614.1)*

**620.0 Follicular cyst of ovary** ♀
Cyst of graafian follicle
**DEF:** Fluid-filled, encapsulated cyst due to occluded follicle duct that secretes hormones into ovaries.

**620.1 Corpus luteum cyst or hematoma** ♀
Corpus luteum hemorrhage or rupture
Lutein cyst
**DEF:** Fluid-filled cyst due to serous developing from corpus luteum or clotted blood.

**620.2 Other and unspecified ovarian cyst** ♀
Cyst:
  NOS
  corpus albicans
  retention NOS       } of ovary
  serous
  theca-lutein
Simple cystoma of ovary
EXCLUDES *cystadenoma (benign) (serous) (220)*
*developmental cysts (752.0)*
*neoplastic cysts (220)*
*polycystic ovaries (256.4)*
*Stein-Leventhal syndrome (256.4)*

**620.3 Acquired atrophy of ovary and fallopian tube** ♀
Senile involution of ovary

**620.4 Prolapse or hernia of ovary and fallopian tube** ♀
Displacement of ovary and fallopian tube
Salpingocele

**620.5 Torsion of ovary, ovarian pedicle, or fallopian tube** CC ♀
Torsion:               Torsion:
accessory tube      hydatid of Morgagni
**CC Excl:** 620.0-620.9

**620.6 Broad ligament laceration syndrome** ♀
Masters-Allen syndrome

**620.7 Hematoma of broad ligament** ♀
Hematocele, broad ligament
**DEF:** Blood within peritoneal fold that supports uterus.

**620.8 Other noninflammatory disorders of ovary, fallopian tube, and broad ligament** ♀
Cyst
Polyp } of broad ligament or fallopian tube

Infarction
Rupture } of ovary or fallopian tube

Hematosalpinx
EXCLUDES *hematosalpinx in ectopic pregnancy (639.2)*
*peritubal adhesions (614.6)*
*torsion of ovary, ovarian pedicle, or fallopian tube (620.5)*

**Uterus and Ovaries**

Fundus of uterus, Mesosalpinx, Mesovarium, Suspensory ligaments, Uterine (fallopian tube), Ligament of ovary, Body, Ovary, Uterosacral ligament, Cervix, Vagina, Ovary, Broad ligament, Fimbria

---

**620.9** **Unspecified noninflammatory disorder of ovary, fallopian tube, and broad ligament** ♀

√4ᵗʰ **621 Disorders of uterus, not elsewhere classified**

**621.0** **Polyp of corpus uteri** ♀
Polyp:                    Polyp:
endometrium          uterus NOS
**EXCLUDES** *cervical polyp NOS (622.7)*

**621.1** **Chronic subinvolution of uterus** ♀
**EXCLUDES** *puerperal (674.8)*
**AHA:** 1Q, '91, 11
**DEF:** Abnormal size of uterus after delivery; the uterus does not return to its normal size after the birth of a child.

**621.2** **Hypertrophy of uterus** ♀
Bulky or enlarged uterus
**EXCLUDES** *puerperal (674.8)*

√5ᵗʰ **621.3** **Endometrial hyperplasia**
Hyperplasia (adenomatous) (cystic) (glandular) of endometrium
**DEF:** Abnormal cystic overgrowth of endometrial tissue.

**621.30** **Endometrial hyperplasia, unspecified** ♀
Endometrial hyperplasia NOS

**621.31** **Simple endometrial hyperplasia without atypia** ♀

**621.32** **Complex endometrial hyperplasia without atypia** ♀

**621.33** **Endometrial hyperplasia with atypia** ♀

**621.4** **Hematometra** ♀
Hemometra
**EXCLUDES** *that in congenital anomaly (752.2-752.3)*
**DEF:** Accumulated blood in uterus.

**621.5** **Intrauterine synechiae** ♀
Adhesions of uterus     Band(s) of uterus

**621.6** **Malposition of uterus** ♀
Anteversion
Retroflexion ⎫ of uterus
Retroversion ⎭
**EXCLUDES** *malposition complicating pregnancy, labor, or delivery (654.3-654.4)*

**621.7** **Chronic inversion of uterus** ♀
**EXCLUDES** *current obstetrical trauma (665.2)
prolapse of uterus (618.1-618.4)*

**621.8** **Other specified disorders of uterus, not elsewhere classified** ♀
Atrophy, acquired ⎫
Cyst                        ⎪
Fibrosis NOS            ⎬ of uterus
Old laceration (postpartum) ⎪
Ulcer                        ⎭
**EXCLUDES** *bilharzial fibrosis (120.0-120.9)
endometriosis (617.0)
fistulas (619.0-619.8)
inflammatory diseases (615.0-615.9)*

**621.9** **Unspecified disorder of uterus** ♀

√4ᵗʰ **622 Noninflammatory disorders of cervix**
**EXCLUDES** *abnormality of cervix complicating pregnancy, labor, or delivery (654.5-654.6)
fistula (619.0-619.8)*

**622.0** **Erosion and ectropion of cervix** ♀
Eversion ⎫ of cervix
Ulcer     ⎭
**EXCLUDES** *that in chronic cervicitis (616.0)*
**DEF:** Ulceration or turning outward of uterine cervix.

√5ᵗʰ **622.1** **Dysplasia of cervix (uteri)**
**EXCLUDES** *abnormal results from cervical cytologic examination without histologic confirmation (795.00-795.09)
carcinoma in situ of cervix (233.1)
cervical intraepithelial neoplasia III [CIN III] (233.1)*
**AHA:** 1Q, '91, 11
**DEF:** Abnormal cell structures in portal between uterus and vagina.

**622.10** **Dysplasia of cervix, unspecified** ♀
Anaplasia of cervix     Cervical dysplasia
Cervical atypism         NOS

**622.11** **Mild dysplasia of cervix** ♀
Cervical intraepithelial neoplasia I [CIN I]

**622.12** **Moderate dysplasia of cervix** ♀
Cervical intraepithelial neoplasia II [CIN II]
**EXCLUDES** *carcinoma in situ of cervix (233.1)
cervical intraepithelial neoplasia III [CIN III] (233.1)
severe dysplasia (233.1)*

**622.2** **Leukoplakia of cervix (uteri)** ♀
**EXCLUDES** *carcinoma in situ of cervix (233.1)*
**DEF:** Thickened, white patches on portal between uterus and vagina.

**622.3** **Old laceration of cervix** ♀
Adhesions ⎫
Band(s)     ⎬ of cervix
Cicatrix (postpartum) ⎭
**EXCLUDES** *current obstetrical trauma (665.3)*
**DEF:** Scarring or other evidence of old wound on cervix.

**622.4** **Stricture and stenosis of cervix** ♀
Atresia (acquired) ⎫
Contracture           ⎬ of cervix
Occlusion             ⎭
Pinpoint os uteri
**EXCLUDES** *congenital (752.49)
that complicating labor (654.6)*

**622.5** **Incompetence of cervix** ♀
**EXCLUDES** *complicating pregnancy (654.5)
that affecting fetus or newborn (761.0)*
**DEF:** Inadequate functioning of cervix; marked by abnormal widening during pregnancy; causing miscarriage.

**622.6** **Hypertrophic elongation of cervix** ♀
**DEF:** Overgrowth of cervix tissues extending down into vagina.

**622.7** **Mucous polyp of cervix** ♀
Polyp NOS of cervix
**EXCLUDES** *adenomatous polyp of cervix (219.0)*

**622.8** **Other specified noninflammatory disorders of cervix** ♀
Atrophy (senile) ⎫
Cyst                 ⎪
Fibrosis            ⎬ of cervix
Hemorrhage      ⎭
**EXCLUDES** *endometriosis (617.0)
fistula (619.0-619.8)
inflammatory diseases (616.0)*

**622.9** **Unspecified noninflammatory disorder of cervix** ♀

√4ᵗʰ **623 Noninflammatory disorders of vagina**
**EXCLUDES** *abnormality of vagina complicating pregnancy, labor, or delivery (654.7)
congenital absence of vagina (752.49)
congenital diaphragm or bands (752.49)
fistulas involving vagina (619.0-619.8)*

**623.0** **Dysplasia of vagina** ♀
▶Vaginal intraepithelial neoplasia I and II [VAIN I and II]◀
**EXCLUDES** ▶ *carcinoma in situ of vagina (233.31)
severe dysplasia of vagina (233.31)
vaginal intraepithelial neoplasia III [VAIN III] (233.31)*◀

**Genitourinary System**

**623.1–626.3**

**623.1　Leukoplakia of vagina** ♀
DEF: Thickened white patches on vaginal canal.

**623.2　Stricture or atresia of vagina** ♀
Adhesions (postoperative) (postradiation) of vagina
Occlusion of vagina
Stenosis, vagina
Use additional E code to identify any external cause
**EXCLUDES** congenital atresia or stricture (752.49)

**623.3　Tight hymenal ring** ♀
Rigid hymen
Tight hymenal ring } acquired or congenital
Tight introitus
**EXCLUDES** imperforate hymen (752.42)

**623.4　Old vaginal laceration** ♀
**EXCLUDES** old laceration involving muscles of pelvic floor (618.7)
DEF: Scarring or other evidence of old wound on vagina.

**623.5　Leukorrhea, not specified as infective** ♀
Leukorrhea NOS of vagina
Vaginal discharge NOS
**EXCLUDES** trichomonal (131.00)
DEF: Viscid whitish discharge, from vagina.

**623.6　Vaginal hematoma** ♀
**EXCLUDES** current obstetrical trauma (665.7)

**623.7　Polyp of vagina** ♀

**623.8　Other specified noninflammatory disorders of vagina** ♀
Cyst
Hemorrhage } of vagina

**623.9　Unspecified noninflammatory disorder of vagina** ♀

√4ᵗʰ **624　Noninflammatory disorders of vulva and perineum**
**EXCLUDES** abnormality of vulva and perineum complicating pregnancy, labor, or delivery (654.8)
condyloma acuminatum (078.1)
fistulas involving:
perineum — see Alphabetic Index
vulva (619.0-619.8)
vulval varices (456.6)
vulvar involvement in skin conditions (690-709.9)

√5ᵗʰ **624.0　Dystrophy of vulva**
**EXCLUDES** ▶ carcinoma in situ of vulva (233.32)
severe dysplasia of vulva (233.32)
vulvar intraepithelial neoplasia III [VIN III] (233.32)◀

● **624.01　Vulvar intraepithelial neoplasia I [VIN I]** ♀
Mild dysplasia of vulva

● **624.02　Vulvar intraepithelial neoplasia II [VIN II]** ♀
Moderate dysplasia of vulva

● **624.09　Other dystrophy of vulva** ♀
Kraurosis of vulva
Leukoplakia of vulva

**624.1　Atrophy of vulva** ♀

**624.2　Hypertrophy of clitoris** ♀
**EXCLUDES** that in endocrine disorders (255.2, 256.1)

**624.3　Hypertrophy of labia** ♀
Hypertrophy of vulva NOS
DEF: Overgrowth of fleshy folds on either side of vagina.

**624.4　Old laceration or scarring of vulva** ♀
DEF: Scarring or other evidence of old wound on external female genitalia.

**624.5　Hematoma of vulva** ♀
**EXCLUDES** that complicating delivery (664.5)
DEF: Blood in tissue of external genitalia.

**624.6　Polyp of labia and vulva** ♀

**624.8　Other specified noninflammatory disorders of vulva and perineum** ♀
Cyst
Edema } of vulva
Stricture
**AHA:** 1Q, '03, 13; 1Q, '95, 8

**624.9　Unspecified noninflammatory disorder of vulva and perineum** ♀

√4ᵗʰ **625　Pain and other symptoms associated with female genital organs**

**625.0　Dyspareunia** ♀
**EXCLUDES** psychogenic dyspareunia (302.76)
DEF: Difficult or painful sexual intercourse.

**625.1　Vaginismus** ♀
Colpospasm　　　Vulvismus
**EXCLUDES** psychogenic vaginismus (306.51)
DEF: Vaginal spasms; due to involuntary contraction of musculature; prevents intercourse.

**625.2　Mittelschmerz** ♀
Intermenstrual pain　　Ovulation pain
DEF: Pain occurring between menstrual periods.

**625.3　Dysmenorrhea** ♀
Painful menstruation
**EXCLUDES** psychogenic dysmenorrhea (306.52)
**AHA:** 2Q, '94, 12

**625.4　Premenstrual tension syndromes** ♀
Menstrual:　　　　Premenstrual dysphoric disorder
　migraine　　　　Premenstrual syndrome
　molimen　　　　Premenstrual tension NOS
**AHA:** 4Q, '03, 116

**625.5　Pelvic congestion syndrome** ♀
Congestion-fibrosis syndrome　Taylor's syndrome
DEF: Excessive accumulation of blood in vessels of pelvis; may occur after orgasm; causes abnormal menstruation, lower back pain and vaginal discharge.

**625.6　Stress incontinence, female** ♀
**EXCLUDES** mixed incontinence (788.33)
stress incontinence, male (788.32)
DEF: Involuntary leakage of urine due to insufficient sphincter control; occurs upon sneezing, laughing, coughing, sudden movement or lifting.

**625.8　Other specified symptoms associated with female genital organs** ♀
**AHA:** N-D, '85, 16

**625.9　Unspecified symptom associated with female genital organs** ♀
**AHA:** 4Q, '06, 110

√4ᵗʰ **626　Disorders of menstruation and other abnormal bleeding from female genital tract**
**EXCLUDES** menopausal and premenopausal bleeding (627.0)
pain and other symptoms associated with menstrual cycle (625.2-625.4)
postmenopausal bleeding (627.1)

**626.0　Absence of menstruation** ♀
Amenorrhea (primary) (secondary)

**626.1　Scanty or infrequent menstruation** ♀
Hypomenorrhea　　　Oligomenorrhea

**626.2　Excessive or frequent menstruation** ♀
Heavy periods　　　Menorrhagia
Menometrorrhagia　　Plymenorrhea
**EXCLUDES** premenopausal (627.0)
that in puberty (626.3)

**626.3　Puberty bleeding** ♀
Excessive bleeding associated with onset of menstrual periods
Pubertal menorrhagia

---

🄽 Newborn Age: 0　　🄿 Pediatric Age: 0-17　　🄼 Maternity Age: 12-55　　🄰 Adult Age: 15-124　　**CC** CC Condition　　**MCC** Major CC Condition　　**HIV** HIV Related Dx

**626.4  Irregular menstrual cycle** ♀
Irregular:                Irregular:
bleeding NOS          periods
menstruation

**626.5  Ovulation bleeding** ♀
Regular intermenstrual bleeding

**626.6  Metrorrhagia** ♀
Bleeding unrelated to menstrual cycle
Irregular intermenstrual bleeding

**626.7  Postcoital bleeding** ♀
DEF: Bleeding from vagina after sexual intercourse.

**626.8  Other** ♀
Dysfunctional or functional uterine hemorrhage
NOS
Menstruation:
retained
suppression of

**626.9  Unspecified** ♀

√4ᵗʰ **627  Menopausal and postmenopausal disorders**
EXCLUDES  *asymptomatic age-related (natural) postmenopausal status (V49.81)*

**627.0  Premenopausal menorrhagia** ♀
Excessive bleeding associated with onset of
menopause
Menorrhagia:
climacteric
menopausal
preclimacteric

**627.1  Postmenopausal bleeding** ♀
**627.2  Symptomatic menopausal or female climacteric** ♀
**states**
Symptoms, such as flushing, sleeplessness,
headache, lack of concentration, associated
with the menopause

**627.3  Postmenopausal atrophic vaginitis** ♀
Senile (atrophic) vaginitis

**627.4  Symptomatic states associated with artificial** ♀
**menopause**
Postartificial menopause syndromes
Any condition classifiable to 627.1, 627.2, or 627.3
which follows induced menopause
DEF: Conditions arising after hysterectomy.

**627.8  Other specified menopausal and** ♀
**postmenopausal disorders**
EXCLUDES  *premature menopause NOS (256.31)*

**627.9  Unspecified menopausal and postmenopausal** ♀
**disorder**

√4ᵗʰ **628  Infertility, female**
INCLUDES  primary and secondary sterility
AHA: 2Q, '96, 9; 1Q, '95, 7

DEF: Infertility: inability to conceive for at least one year with regular
intercourse.

DEF: Primary infertility: occurring in patients who have never conceived.

DEF: Secondary infertility: occurring in patients who have previously
conceived.

**628.0  Associated with anovulation** ♀
Anovulatory cycle
Use additional code for any associated Stein-
Leventhal syndrome (256.4)

**628.1  Of pituitary-hypothalamic origin** ♀
*Code first underlying cause, as:*
adiposogenital dystrophy (253.8)
anterior pituitary disorder (253.0-253.4)

**628.2  Of tubal origin** ♀
Infertility associated with congenital anomaly of tube
Tubal:
block
occlusion
stenosis
Use additional code for any associated peritubal
adhesions (614.6)

**628.3  Of uterine origin** ♀
Infertility associated with congenital anomaly of
uterus
Nonimplantation
Use additional code for any associated tuberculous
endometritis (016.7)

**628.4  Of cervical or vaginal origin** ♀
Infertility associated with:
anomaly of cervical mucus
congenital structural anomaly
dysmucorrhea

**628.8  Of other specified origin** ♀
**628.9  Of unspecified origin** ♀

√4ᵗʰ **629  Other disorders of female genital organs**
**629.0  Hematocele, female, not elsewhere classified** ♀
EXCLUDES  *hematocele or hematoma:*
*broad ligament (620.7)*
*fallopian tube (620.8)*
*that associated with ectopic*
*pregnancy (633.00-633.91)*
*uterus (621.4)*
*vagina (623.6)*
*vulva (624.5)*

**629.1  Hydrocele, canal of Nuck** ♀
Cyst of canal of Nuck (acquired)
EXCLUDES  *congenital (752.41)*

√5ᵗʰ **629.2  Female genital mutilation status**
Female circumcision status
Female genital cutting
AHA: 4Q, '04, 88

**629.20  Female genital mutilation status,** ♀
**unspecified**
Female genital cutting status, unspecified
Female genital mutilation status NOS

**629.21  Female genital mutilation Type I** ♀
**status**
Clitorectomy status
Female genital cutting Type I status
DEF: Female genital mutilation involving clitorectomy,
with part or all of the clitoris removed.

**629.22  Female genital mutilation Type II** ♀
**status**
Clitorectomy with excision of labia
minora status
Female genital cutting Type II status
AHA: 4Q, '04, 90

DEF: Female genital mutilation involving clitoris and the
labia minora amputation.

**629.23  Female genital mutilation Type III** ♀
**status**
Female genital cutting Type III status
Infibulation status
AHA: 4Q, '04, 90

DEF: Female genital mutilation involving removal, most or
all of the labia minora excised, labia majora incised
which is then made into a hood of skin over the urethral
and vaginal opening.

**629.29  Other female genital mutilation status** ♀
Female genital cutting Type IV status
Female genital mutilation Type IV status
Other female genital cutting status
AHA: 4Q, '06, 97

---

√4ᵗʰ / √5ᵗʰ  Additional Digit Required          Unacceptable PDx          Manifestation Code          ►◄ Revised Text          ● New Code          ▲ Revised Code Title

**√5ᵗʰ 629.8   Other specified disorders of female genital organs**

  **629.81   Habitual aborter without current pregnancy**   ♀

         **EXCLUDES**   *habitual aborter with current pregnancy (646.3)*

         **AHA:** 4Q, '06, 98

  **629.89   Other specified disorders of female genital organs**   ♀

         **AHA:** 4Q, '06, 98

**629.9   Unspecified disorder of female genital organs**   ♀

---

**N** Newborn Age: 0    **P** Pediatric Age: 0-17    **M** Maternity Age: 12-55    **A** Adult Age: 15-124    **CC** CC Condition    **MCC** Major CC Condition    **HIV** HIV Related Dx

## 11. COMPLICATIONS OF PREGNANCY, CHILDBIRTH, AND THE PUERPERIUM (630-677)

### ECTOPIC AND MOLAR PREGNANCY (630-633)

Use additional code from category 639 to identify any complications

**630 Hydatidiform mole**　　M♀

Trophoblastic disease NOS　　Vesicular mole

> **EXCLUDES** chorioadenoma (destruens) (236.1)
> chorionepithelioma (181)
> malignant hydatidiform mole (236.1)

DEF: Abnormal product of pregnancy; marked by mass of cysts resembling bunch of grapes due to chorionic villi proliferation, and dissolution; must be surgically removed.

**631 Other abnormal product of conception**　　M♀

Blighted ovum　　Mole:
Mole:　　　　　　fleshy
　NOS　　　　　　stone
　carneous

**632 Missed abortion**　　M♀

Early fetal death before completion of 22 weeks' gestation with retention of dead fetus

Retained products of conception, not following spontaneous or induced abortion or delivery

> **EXCLUDES** failed induced abortion (638.0-638.9)
> fetal death (intrauterine) (late) (656.4)
> missed delivery (656.4)
> that with abnormal product of conception (630, 631)

**AHA:** 1Q, '01, 5

**√4ᵗʰ 633 Ectopic pregnancy**

> **INCLUDES** ruptured ectopic pregnancy

**AHA:** 4Q, '02, 61

DEF: Fertilized egg develops outside uterus.

**√5ᵗʰ 633.0　Abdominal pregnancy**

Intraperitoneal pregnancy

**633.00 Abdominal pregnancy without**　　CC M♀
**intrauterine pregnancy**
CC Excl: 633.01, 633.11-633.91

**633.01 Abdominal pregnancy with**　　CC M♀
**intrauterine pregnancy**
CC Excl: 633.00-633.91

**√5ᵗʰ 633.1　Tubal pregnancy**

Fallopian pregnancy
Rupture of (fallopian) tube due to pregnancy
Tubal abortion

**AHA:** 2Q, '90, 27

**633.10 Tubal pregnancy without**　　CC M♀
**intrauterine pregnancy**
CC Excl: See code: 633.01

**633.11 Tubal pregnancy with**　　CC M♀
**intrauterine pregnancy**
CC Excl: See code: 633.01

**√5ᵗʰ 633.2　Ovarian pregnancy**

**633.20 Ovarian pregnancy without**　　CC M♀
**intrauterine pregnancy**
CC Excl: See code: 633.01

**633.21 Ovarian pregnancy with**　　CC M♀
**intrauterine pregnancy**
CC Excl: See code: 633.01

**√5ᵗʰ 633.8　Other ectopic pregnancy**

Pregnancy:　　　　Pregnancy:
　cervical　　　　　intraligamentous
　combined　　　　mesometric
　cornual　　　　　mural

**633.80 Other ectopic pregnancy without**　　CC M♀
**intrauterine pregnancy**
CC Excl: See code: 633.01

**633.81 Other ectopic pregnancy with**　　CC M♀
**intrauterine pregnancy**
CC Excl: See code: 633.01

**√5ᵗʰ 633.9　Unspecified ectopic pregnancy**

**633.90 Unspecified ectopic pregnancy**　　CC M♀
**without intrauterine pregnancy**
CC Excl: See code: 633.01

**633.91 Unspecified ectopic pregnancy**　　CC M♀
**with intrauterine pregnancy**
CC Excl: See code: 633.01

### OTHER PREGNANCY WITH ABORTIVE OUTCOME (634-639)

The following fourth-digit subdivisions are for use with categories 634-638:

**.0 Complicated by genital tract and pelvic infection**
　Endometritis
　Salpingo-oophoritis
　Sepsis NOS
　Septicemia NOS
　Any condition classifiable to 639.0, with condition classifiable to 634-638

> **EXCLUDES** urinary tract infection (634-638 with .7)

**.1 Complicated by delayed or excessive hemorrhage**
　Afibrinogenemia
　Defibrination syndrome
　Intravascular hemolysis
　Any condition classifiable to 639.1, with condition classifiable to 634-638

**.2 Complicated by damage to pelvic organs and tissues**
　Laceration, perforation, or tear of:
　　bladder
　　uterus
　Any condition classifiable to 639.2, with condition classifiable to 634-638

**.3 Complicated by renal failure**
　Oliguria
　Uremia
　Any condition classifiable to 639.3, with condition classifiable to 634-638

**.4 Complicated by metabolic disorder**
　Electrolyte imbalance with conditions classifiable to 634-638

**.5 Complicated by shock**
　Circulatory collapse
　Shock (postoperative) (septic)
　Any condition classifiable to 639.5, with condition classifiable to 634-638

**.6 Complicated by embolism**
　Embolism:
　　NOS
　　amniotic fluid
　　pulmonary
　Any condition classifiable to 639.6, with condition classifiable to 634-638

**.7 With other specified complications**
　Cardiac arrest or failure
　Urinary tract infection
　Any condition classifiable to 639.8, with condition classifiable to 634-638

**.8 With unspecified complication**

**.9 Without mention of complication**

---

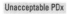

**Complications of Pregnancy, Childbirth & Puerperium**

**634–636.5**

**Ectopic Pregnancy Sites**

§ ✓4th **634 Spontaneous abortion**

Requires fifth-digit to identify stage:

    **0 unspecified**
    **1 incomplete**
    **2 complete**

INCLUDES   miscarriage
         spontaneous abortion

**AHA:** 2Q, '91, 16

**DEF:** Spontaneous premature expulsion of the products of conception from the uterus.

✓5th **634.0 Complicated by genital tract and pelvic infection**   CC M ♀
    **CC Excl:** 634.00-638.9, 640.00-641.23, 646.80-646.93, 648.90-650, 669.40-669.44, 669.80-669.94

✓5th **634.1 Complicated by delayed or excessive hemorrhage**   M ♀
    **AHA:** For Code 634.11: 1Q, '03, 6

✓5th **634.2 Complicated by damage to pelvic organs or tissues**   CC M ♀
    **CC Excl:** See code: 634.0

✓5th **634.3 Complicated by renal failure**   MCC M ♀
    **CC Excl:** See code: 634.0

✓5th **634.4 Complicated by metabolic disorder**   CC M ♀
    **CC Excl:** See code: 634.0

✓5th **634.5 Complicated by shock**   MCC M ♀
    **CC Excl:** See code: 634.0

✓5th **634.6 Complicated by embolism**   MCC 1-2 CC 0 M ♀
    **CC Excl:** See code: 634.0

✓5th **634.7 With other specified complications**   CC M ♀
    **CC Excl:** See code: 634.0

✓5th **634.8 With unspecified complication**   CC M ♀
    **CC Excl:** See code: 634.0

✓5th **634.9 Without mention of complication**   M ♀

§ ✓4th **635 Legally induced abortion**

Requires fifth-digit to identify stage:

    **0 unspecified**
    **1 incomplete**
    **2 complete**

INCLUDES   abortion or termination of pregnancy:
         elective
         legal
         therapeutic

EXCLUDES   *menstrual extraction or regulation (V25.3)*

**AHA:** 2Q, '94, 14

**DEF:** Intentional expulsion of products of conception from uterus performed by medical professionals inside boundaries of law.

§   See beginning of section 634-639 for fourth-digit definitions.

---

✓5th **635.0 Complicated by genital tract and pelvic infection**   CC M ♀
    **CC Excl:** 634.00-635.02, 635.20-635.22, 635.70-638.9, 640.00-641.23, 646.80-646.93, 648.90-650, 669.40-669.44, 669.80-669.94

✓5th **635.1 Complicated by delayed or excessive hemorrhage**   M ♀

✓5th **635.2 Complicated by damage to pelvic organs or tissues**   CC M ♀
    **CC Excl:** For code 635.20: 634.00-638.9, 640.00-641.23, 646.80-646.93, 648.90-650, 669.40-669.44, 669.80-669.94; For code 635.21: 634.00-635.62, 638.5-638.9, 640.00-641.00; For code 635.22: 635.22

✓5th **635.3 Complicated by renal failure**   MCC M ♀
    **CC Excl:** For code 635.30: 635.30-635.32; For code 635.31: 635.30-635.32, 637.11-638.9, 640.00-641.23, 646.80-646.93, 648.90-650, 669.40-669.44, 669.80-669.94; For code 635.32: 634.00-634.92, 635.30-635.32, 635.70-638.9, 640.00-641.23, 646.80-646.93, 648.90-650, 669.40-669.44, 669.80-669.94

✓5th **635.4 Complicated by metabolic disorder**   CC M ♀
    **CC Excl:** 634.00-638.9, 640.00-641.23, 646.80-646.93, 648.90-650, 669.40-669.44, 669.80-669.94

✓5th **635.5 Complicated by shock**   MCC M ♀
    **CC Excl:** 634.00-634.92, 635.50-635.52, 635.70-638.9, 640.00-641.23, 646.80-646.93, 648.90-650, 669.40-669.44, 669.80-669.94

✓5th **635.6 Complicated by embolism**   MCC M ♀
    **CC Excl:** 634.00-634.92, 635.60-638.9, 640.00-641.23, 646.80-646.93, 648.90-650, 669.40-669.44, 669.80-669.94

✓5th **635.7 With other specified complications**   CC M ♀
    **CC Excl:** 634.00-638.9, 640.00-641.23, 646.80-646.93, 648.90-650, 669.40-669.44, 669.80-669.94

✓5th **635.8 With unspecified complication**   CC M ♀
    **CC Excl:** 634.00-638.9, 640.00-641.23, 646.80-646.93, 648.90-650, 669.40-669.44, 669.80-669.94

✓5th **635.9 Without mention of complication**   M ♀
    **AHA:** For code 635.92: 2Q, '94, 14

§ ✓4th **636 Illegally induced abortion**

Requires fifth-digit to identify stage:

    **0 unspecified**
    **1 incomplete**
    **2 complete**

INCLUDES   abortion:
         criminal
         illegal
         self-induced

**DEF:** Intentional expulsion of products of conception from uterus; outside boundaries of law.

✓5th **636.0 Complicated by genital tract and pelvic infection**   CC M ♀
    **CC Excl:** 634.00-636.02, 636.70-638.9, 640.00-641.23, 646.80-646.93, 648.90-650, 669.40-669.44, 669.80-669.94

✓5th **636.1 Complicated by delayed or excessive hemorrhage**   M ♀

✓5th **636.2 Complicated by damage to pelvic organs or tissues**   CC M ♀
    **CC Excl:** 634.00-638.9, 640.00-641.23, 646.80-646.93, 648.90-650, 669.40-669.44, 669.80-669.94

✓5th **636.3 Complicated by renal failure**   MCC M ♀
    **CC Excl:** 634.00-635.92, 636.30-636.32, 636.70-638.9, 640.00-641.23, 646.80-646.93, 648.90-650, 669.40-669.44, 669.80-669.94

✓5th **636.4 Complicated by metabolic disorder**   CC M ♀
    **CC Excl:** See code: 636.2

✓5th **636.5 Complicated by shock**   MCC M ♀
    **CC Excl:** For codes 636.50 and 636.51: 634.00-635.92, 636.50-636.52, 636.70-638.9, 640.00-641.23, 646.80-646.93, 648.90-650, 669.40-669.44, 669.80-669.94; For code 636.52: 634.00-635.92, 636.50-636.52, 636.70-636.92, 637.50-637.52, 637.70-637.92, 638.5, 638.7-638.9, 640.00-641.23, 646.80-646.93, 648.90-650, 669.40-669.44, 669.80-669.94

---

N Newborn Age: 0    P Pediatric Age: 0-17    M Maternity Age: 12-55    A Adult Age: 15-124    CC CC Condition    MCC Major CC Condition    HIV HIV Related Dx

210 — Volume 1 • October 2007          © 2007 Ingenix

✓5ᵗʰ **636.6  Complicated by embolism**    MCC M ♀
CC Excl: 634.00-635.92, 636.60-638.9, 640.00-641.23, 646.80-646.93, 648.90-650, 669.40-669.44, 669.80-669.94

✓5ᵗʰ **636.7  With other specified complications**    CC M ♀
CC Excl: See code: 636.2

✓5ᵗʰ **636.8  With unspecified complication**    CC M ♀
CC Excl: See code: 636.2

✓5ᵗʰ **636.9  Without mention of complication**    M ♀

§ ✓4ᵗʰ **637  Unspecified abortion**
Requires fifth-digit to identify stage:
0  **unspecified**
1  **incomplete**
2  **complete**

INCLUDES    abortion NOS
retained products of conception following abortion, not classifiable elsewhere

✓5ᵗʰ **637.0  Complicated by genital tract and pelvic infection**    CC M ♀
CC Excl: 634.00-637.02, 637.70-638.9, 640.00-641.23, 646.80-646.93, 648.90-650, 669.40-669.44, 669.80-669.94

✓5ᵗʰ **637.1  Complicated by delayed or excessive hemorrhage**    M ♀

✓5ᵗʰ **637.2  Complicated by damage to pelvic organs or tissues**    CC M ♀
CC Excl: 634.00-638.9, 640.00-641.23, 646.80-646.93, 648.90-650, 669.40-669.44, 669.80-669.94

✓5ᵗʰ **637.3  Complicated by renal failure**    MCC M ♀
CC Excl: 634.00-636.92, 637.30-637.32, 637.70-638.9, 640.00-641.23, 646.80-646.93, 648.90-650, 669.40-669.44, 669.80-669.94

✓5ᵗʰ **637.4  Complicated by metabolic disorder**    CC M ♀
CC Excl: See code: 637.2

✓5ᵗʰ **637.5  Complicated by shock**    MCC M ♀
CC Excl: 634.00-636.92, 637.50-637.52, 637.70-638.9, 640.00-641.23, 646.80-646.93, 648.90-650, 669.40-669.44, 669.80-669.94

✓5ᵗʰ **637.6  Complicated by embolism**    MCC M ♀
CC Excl: For codes 637.60 and 637.61: 634.00-636.92, 637.60-638.9, 640.00-641.23, 646.80-646.93, 648.90-650, 669.40-669.44, 669.80-669.94; For code 637.62: 634.00-636.02, 636.11-636.92, 637.60-638.9, 640.00-641.23, 646.80-646.93, 648.90-650, 669.40-669.44, 669.80-669.94

✓5ᵗʰ **637.7  With other specified complications**    CC M ♀
CC Excl: See code: 637.2

✓5ᵗʰ **637.8  With unspecified complication**    CC M ♀
CC Excl: For codes 637.80 and 637.82: 634.00-638.9, 640.00-641.23, 646.80-646.93, 648.90-650, 669.40-669.44, 669.80-669.94; For code 637.81: 634.00-635.32, 635.41-638.9, 640.00-641.23, 648.90-650, 669.40-669.44, 669.80-669.94

✓5ᵗʰ **637.9  Without mention of complication**    M ♀

§ ✓4ᵗʰ **638  Failed attempted abortion**
INCLUDES    failure of attempted induction of (legal) abortion
EXCLUDES    incomplete abortion (634.0-637.9)
**DEF: Continued pregnancy despite an attempted legal abortion.**

**638.0  Complicated by genital tract and pelvic infection**    CC M ♀
CC Excl: 634.00-638.0, 638.7-638.9, 640.00-641.23, 646.80-646.93, 648.90-650, 669.40-669.44, 669.80-669.94

**638.1  Complicated by delayed or excessive hemorrhage**    CC M ♀
CC Excl: 634.00-637.92, 638.1, 638.7-638.9, 640.00-641.23, 646.80-646.93, 648.90-650, 669.40-669.44, 669.80-669.94

**638.2  Complicated by damage to pelvic organs or tissues**    CC M ♀
CC Excl: 634.00-637.92, 638.2, 638.7-638.9, 640.00-641.23, 646.80-646.93, 648.90-650, 669.40-669.44, 669.80-669.94

**638.3  Complicated by renal failure**    MCC M ♀
CC Excl: 634.00-637.92, 638.3, 638.7-638.9, 640.00-641.23, 646.80-646.93, 648.90-650, 669.40-669.44, 669.80-669.94

**638.4  Complicated by metabolic disorder**    CC M ♀
CC Excl: 634.00-638.9, 640.00-641.23, 646.80-646.93, 648.90-650, 669.40-669.44, 669.80-669.94

**638.5  Complicated by shock**    MCC M ♀
CC Excl: 634.00-637.12, 637.21-637.92, 638.4-638.5, 638.7-638.9, 640.00-641.23, 646.80-646.93, 648.90-650, 669.40-669.44, 669.80-669.94

**638.6  Complicated by embolism**    MCC M ♀
CC Excl: 634.00-637.92, 638.6-638.9, 640.00-641.23, 646.80-646.93, 648.90-650, 669.40-669.44, 669.80-669.94

**638.7  With other specified complications**    CC M ♀
CC Excl: See code: 638.4

**638.8  With unspecified complication**    CC M ♀
CC Excl: See code: 638.4

**638.9  Without mention of complication**    M ♀

✓4ᵗʰ **639  Complications following abortion and ectopic and molar pregnancies**
Note: This category is provided for use when it is required to classify separately the complications classifiable to the fourth-digit level in categories 634-638; for example:
a)  when the complication itself was responsible for an episode of medical care, the abortion, ectopic or molar pregnancy itself having been dealt with at a previous episode
b)  when these conditions are immediate complications of ectopic or molar pregnancies classifiable to 630-633 where they cannot be identified at fourth-digit level.

**639.0  Genital tract and pelvic infection**    CC M ♀
Endometritis
Parametritis
Pelvic peritonitis
Salpingitis    } following conditions classifiable to 630-638
Salpingo-oophoritis
Sepsis NOS
Septicemia NOS

EXCLUDES    urinary tract infection (639.8)
CC Excl: 639.0, 639.2-641.23, 646.80-646.93, 648.90-650, 669.40-669.44, 669.80-669.94

**639.1  Delayed or excessive hemorrhage**    CC M ♀
Afibrinogenemia
Defibrination syndrome    } following conditions classifiable to 630-638
Intravascular hemolysis

CC Excl: 639.1-641.23, 646.80-646.93, 648.90-650, 669.40-669.44, 669.80-669.94

**639.2  Damage to pelvic organs and tissues**    CC M ♀
Laceration, perforation, or tear of:
bladder
bowel
broad ligament    } following conditions classifiable to 630-638
cervix
periurethral tissue
uterus
vagina

CC Excl: 639.2-641.23, 646.80-646.93, 648.90-650, 669.40-669.44, 669.80-669.94

**639.3  Renal failure**    MCC M ♀
Oliguria
Renal:
failure (acute)    } following conditions classifiable to 630-638
shutdown
tubular necrosis
Uremia

CC Excl: See code: 639.2

§  See beginning of section 634-639 for fourth-digit definitions.

---

✓4ᵗʰ ✓5ᵗʰ  Additional Digit Required    Unacceptable PDx    Manifestation Code    ◄► Revised Text    ● New Code    ▲ Revised Code Title

**639.4** **Metabolic disorders** `CC` `M` ♀

Electrolyte imbalance following conditions classifiable to 630-638

**CC Excl:** See code: 639.2

**639.5** **Shock** `MCC` `M` ♀

Circulatory collapse
Shock (postoperative) } following conditions classifiable to 630-638
(septic)

**CC Excl:** See code: 639.2

**639.6** **Embolism** `MCC` `M` ♀

Embolism:
NOS
air
amniotic fluid
blood-clot } following conditions classifiable to 630-638
fat
pulmonary
pyemic
septic
soap

**CC Excl:** See code: 639.2

**639.8** **Other specified complications following abortion or ectopic and molar pregnancy** `CC` `M` ♀

Acute yellow atrophy or necrosis of liver
Cardiac arrest or failure } following conditions classifiable to 630-638
Cerebral anoxia
Urinary tract infection

**CC Excl:** See code: 639.2

**639.9** **Unspecified complication following abortion or ectopic and molar pregnancy** `CC` `M` ♀

Complication(s) not further specified following conditions classifiable to 630-638

**CC Excl:** See code: 639.2

## COMPLICATIONS MAINLY RELATED TO PREGNANCY (640-649)

INCLUDES the listed conditions even if they arose or were present during labor, delivery, or the puerperium

**AHA:** 2Q, '90, 11

The following fifth-digit subclassification is for use with categories 640-649 to denote the current episode of care. Valid fifth-digits are in [brackets] under each code.

**0 unspecified as to episode of care or not applicable**

**1 delivered, with or without mention of antepartum condition**
Antepartum condition with delivery
Delivery NOS (with mention of antepartum complication during current episode of care)
Intrapartum obstetric condition (with mention of antepartum complication during current episode of care)
Pregnancy, delivered (with mention of antepartum complication during current episode of care)

**2 delivered, with mention of postpartum complication**
Delivery with mention of puerperal complication during current episode of care

**3 antepartum condition or complication**
Antepartum obstetric condition, not delivered during the current episode of care

**4 postpartum condition or complication**
Postpartum or puerperal obstetric condition or complication following delivery that occurred:
during previous episode of care
outside hospital, with subsequent admission for observation or care

**Placenta Previa**

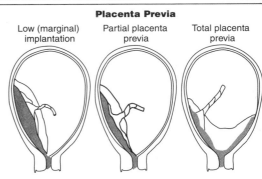

Low (marginal) implantation    Partial placenta previa    Total placenta previa

√4ᵗʰ **640 Hemorrhage in early pregnancy**

INCLUDES hemorrhage before completion of 22 weeks' gestation

§ √5ᵗʰ **640.0** **Threatened abortion** `CC 1,3` `M` ♀
[0,1,3] **CC Excl:** For codes 640.01 and 640.03: 640.00-641.13, 646.80-646.93, 648.90-650, 669.80-669.94

DEF: Bloody discharge during pregnancy; cervix may be dilated and pregnancy is threatened, but the pregnancy is not terminated.

§ √5ᵗʰ **640.8** **Other specified hemorrhage in early** `M` ♀
[0,1,3] **pregnancy**

§ √5ᵗʰ **640.9** **Unspecified hemorrhage in early** `CC 3` `M` ♀
[0,1,3] **pregnancy**
**CC Excl:** For code 640.93: 640.00-641.13, 646.80-646.93, 648.90-650, 669.40-669.44, 669.80-669.94

√4ᵗʰ **641 Antepartum hemorrhage, abruptio placentae, and placenta previa**

§ √5ᵗʰ **641.0** **Placenta previa without hemorrhage** `CC 1,3` `M` ♀
[0,1,3]
Low impantation of placenta
Placenta previa noted: } without hemorrhage
during pregnancy
before labor (and delivered by caesarean delivery.)

**CC Excl:** For codes 641.01 and 641.03: 640.00-641.13, 646.80-646.93, 648.90-650, 669.40-669.44, 669.80-669.94

DEF: Placenta implanted in lower segment of uterus; commonly causes hemorrhage in the last trimester of pregnancy.

§ √5ᵗʰ **641.1** **Hemorrhage from placenta previa** `MCC 1,3` `M` ♀
[0,1,3]
Low-lying placenta
Placenta previa } NOS or with hemorrhage (intrapartum)
incomplete
marginal
partial
total

EXCLUDES *hemorrhage from vasa previa (663.5)*

**CC Excl:** For codes 641.11 and 641.13: 640.00-641.13, 646.80-646.93, 648.90-650, 669.40-669.44, 669.80-669.94

§ √5ᵗʰ **641.2** **Premature separation of placenta** `MCC 1` `CC 3` `M` ♀
[0,1,3]
Ablatio placentae
Abruptio placentae
Accidental antepartum hemorrhage
Couvelaire uterus
Detachment of placenta (premature)
Premature separation of normally implanted placenta

**CC Excl:** For code 641.21: 640.00-641.13, 641.21, 646.80-646.93, 648.90-650, 669.40-669.44, 669.80-669.94; For code 641.23: 640.00-641.13, 641.23, 646.80-646.93, 648.90-650, 669.40-669.44, 669.80-669.94

DEF: Abruptio placentae: premature detachment of the placenta, characterized by shock, oliguria and decreased fibrinogen.

---

**§** Requires fifth-digit. Valid digits are in [brackets] under each code. See beginning of section 640-649 for codes and definitions.

`N` Newborn Age: 0    `P` Pediatric Age: 0-17    `M` Maternity Age: 12-55    `A` Adult Age: 15-124    `CC` CC Condition    `MCC` Major CC Condition    `HIV` HIV Related Dx

**212 — Volume 1 • October 2007**                                                                 © *2007 Ingenix*

**Abruptio Placentae**

| (concealed bleeding) | (apparent hemorrhage) | (concealed hemorrhage) |
| --- | --- | --- |

§ ✓5ᵗʰ **641.3 Antepartum hemorrhage associated** MCC 1,3 M ♀
[0,1,3]　**with coagulation defects**

Antepartum or intrapartum hemorrhage associated with:
　afibrinogenemia
　hyperfibrinolysis
　hypofibrinogenemia

EXCLUDES　*coagulation defects not associated with antepartum hemorrhage (649.3)*

CC Excl: For codes 641.31 and 641.33: 641.30-641.93, 646.80-646.93, 648.90-650, 669.40-669.44, 669.80-669.94

DEF: Uterine hemorrhage prior to delivery.

§ ✓5ᵗʰ **641.8 Other antepartum hemorrhage** M ♀
[0,1,3]

Antepartum or intrapartum hemorrhage associated with:
　trauma
　uterine leiomyoma

§ ✓5ᵗʰ **641.9 Unspecified antepartum hemorrhage** M ♀
[0,1,3]

| Hemorrhage: | Hemorrhage: |
| --- | --- |
| antepartum NOS | of pregnancy NOS |
| intrapartum NOS | |

✓4ᵗʰ **642 Hypertension complicating pregnancy, childbirth, and the puerperium**

§ ✓5ᵗʰ **642.0 Benign essential hypertension** CC 1-3 M ♀
[0-4]　**complicating pregnancy, childbirth, and the puerperium**

| Hypertension: | specified as complicating, |
| --- | --- |
| benign essential | or as a reason for |
| chronic NOS | obstetric care during |
| essential | pregnancy, childbirth, |
| pre-existing NOS | or the puerperium |

CC Excl: For codes 642.01, 642.02, 642.03: 642.00-642.94, 646.10-646.14, 646.80-646.93, 648.90-650, 669.40-669.44, 669.80-669.94

§ ✓5ᵗʰ **642.1 Hypertension secondary to** MCC 1-2 CC 3-4 M ♀
[0-4]　**renal disease, complicating pregnancy, childbirth, and the puerperium**

Hypertension secondary to renal disease, specified as complicating, or as a reason for obstetric care during pregnancy, childbirth, or the puerperium

CC Excl: For codes 642.11-642.14: See code: 642.01

§ ✓5ᵗʰ **642.2 Other pre-existing hypertension complicating** M ♀
[0-4]　**pregnancy, childbirth, and the puerperium**

| Hypertensive: | specified as |
| --- | --- |
| chronic kidney disease | complicating, or as a reason for |
| heart and chronic kidney disease | obstetric care during pregnancy, childbirth, or the |
| heart disease | puerperium |
| Malignant hypertension | |

§ ✓5ᵗʰ **642.3 Transient hypertension of pregnancy** CC 1-2 M ♀
[0-4]

Gestational hypertension
Transient hypertension, so described, in pregnancy, childbirth, or the puerperium

CC Excl: For codes 642.31, 642.32: See code: 642.01

AHA: 3Q, '90, 4

§ ✓5ᵗʰ **642.4 Mild or unspecified pre-eclampsia** MCC 2 CC 1,3,4
[0-4]　M ♀

Hypertension in pregnancy, childbirth, or the puerperium, not specified as pre-existing, with either albuminuria or edema, or both; mild or unspecified

| Pre-eclampsia: | Toxemia (pre-eclamptic): |
| --- | --- |
| NOS | NOS |
| mild | mild |

EXCLUDES　*albuminuria in pregnancy, without mention of hypertension (646.2)*
*edema in pregnancy, without mention of hypertension (646.1)*

CC Excl: For codes 642.41-642.44: See code: 642.01

§ ✓5ᵗʰ **642.5 Severe pre-eclampsia** MCC 1-4 M ♀
[0-4]

Hypertension in pregnancy, childbirth, or the puerperium, not specified as pre-existing, with either albuminuria or edema, or both; specified as severe
Pre-eclampsia, severe
Toxemia (pre-eclamptic), severe

CC Excl: For codes 642.51-642.54: See code: 642.01

AHA: N-D, '85, 3

§ ✓5ᵗʰ **642.6 Eclampsia** MCC 1-4 M ♀
[0-4]

Toxemia:
　eclamptic
　with convulsions

CC Excl: For codes 642.61-642.64: See code: 642.01

§ ✓5ᵗʰ **642.7 Pre-eclampsia or eclampsia** MCC 1-4 M ♀
[0-4]　**superimposed on pre-existing hypertension**

Conditions classifiable to 642.4-642.6, with conditions classifiable to 642.0-642.2

CC Excl: For codes 642.71-642.74: See code: 642.01

§ ✓5ᵗʰ **642.9 Unspecified hypertension complicating** CC 1-4 M ♀
[0-4]　**pregnancy, childbirth, or the puerperium**

Hypertension NOS, without mention of albuminuria or edema, complicating pregnancy, childbirth, or the puerperium

CC Excl: For codes 642.91, 642.92, 642.94: 642.00-642.94, 646.10-646.14, 646.80-646.93, 648.90-650, 669.40-669.44, 669.80-669.94; For codes 642.93: 642.01-642.44, 642.61-642.94

✓4ᵗʰ **643 Excessive vomiting in pregnancy**

INCLUDES
| hyperemesis vomiting: | arising during |
| --- | --- |
| persistent | pregnancy |
| vicious | |

hyperemesis gravidarum

§ ✓5ᵗʰ **643.0 Mild hyperemesis gravidarum** M ♀
[0,1,3]

Hyperemesis gravidarum, mild or unspecified, starting before the end of the 22nd week of gestation

DEF: Detrimental vomiting and nausea.

§ ✓5ᵗʰ **643.1 Hyperemesis gravidarum with metabolic** M ♀
[0,1,3]　**disturbance**

Hyperemesis gravidarum, starting before the end of the 22nd week of gestation, with metabolic disturbance, such as:
　carbohydrate depletion
　dehydration
　electrolyte imbalance

§　Requires fifth-digit. Valid digits are in [brackets] under each code. See beginning of section 640-649 for codes and definitions.

| ✓4ᵗʰ ✓5ᵗʰ Additional Digit Required | Unacceptable PDx | Manifestation Code | ◄►◄ Revised Text | ● New Code | ▲ Revised Code Title |
| --- | --- | --- | --- | --- | --- |

© 2007 Ingenix　　　　　　　　　　　　　　　　　　　　　　　　　**October 2007 • Volume 1 — 213**

**Complications of Pregnancy, Childbirth & Puerperium**

**643.2–647.3**

§ ✓5ᵗʰ **643.2 Late vomiting of pregnancy** M ♀
[0,1,3] Excessive vomiting starting after 22 completed weeks of gestation

§ ✓5ᵗʰ **643.8 Other vomiting complicating pregnancy** M ♀
[0,1,3] Vomiting due to organic disease or other cause, specified as complicating pregnancy, or as a reason for obstetric care during pregnancy
Use additional code to specify cause

§ ✓5ᵗʰ **643.9 Unspecified vomiting of pregnancy** M ♀
[0,1,3] Vomiting as a reason for care during pregnancy, length of gestation unspecified

✓4ᵗʰ **644 Early or threatened labor**

§ ✓5ᵗʰ **644.0 Threatened premature labor** MCC 3 M ♀
[0,3] Premature labor after 22 weeks, but before 37 completed weeks of gestation without delivery
EXCLUDES *that occurring before 22 completed weeks of gestation (640.0)*

CC Excl: For code 644.03: 644.00-644.21, 646.80-646.93, 648.90-650, 669.40-669.44, 669.80-669.94

§ ✓5ᵗʰ **644.1 Other threatened labor** CC 3 M ♀
[0,3] False labor:
NOS
after 37 completed weeks of gestation } without delivery
Threatened labor NOS

CC Excl: For code 644.13: See code 644.03

§ ✓5ᵗʰ **644.2 Early onset of delivery** MCC 1 CC 0 M ♀
[0,1] Onset (spontaneous) of delivery
Premature labor with onset of delivery } before 37 completed weeks of gestation

CC Excl: See code: 644.03

AHA: 2Q, '91, 16

✓4ᵗʰ **645 Late pregnancy**
AHA: 4Q, '00, 43; 4Q, '91, 26

§ ✓5ᵗʰ **645.1 Post term pregnancy** M ♀
[0,1,3] Pregnancy over 40 completed weeks to 42 completed weeks gestation

§ ✓5ᵗʰ **645.2 Prolonged pregnancy** M ♀
[0,1,3] Pregnancy which has advanced beyond 42 completed weeks gestation

✓4ᵗʰ **646 Other complications of pregnancy, not elsewhere classified**
Use additional code(s) to further specify complication
AHA: 4Q, '95, 59

§ ✓5ᵗʰ **646.0 Papyraceous fetus** M ♀
[0,1,3]

DEF: Fetus that dies in the second trimester of pregnancy and is retained in the uterus, with subsequent atrophy and mummification; commonly occurs in twin pregnancy, nonviable fetus becomes compressed by growth of living twin and exhibits parchment-like skin.

§ ✓5ᵗʰ **646.1 Edema or excessive weight gain in pregnancy,** M ♀
[0-4] **without mention of hypertension**
Gestational edema
Maternal obesity syndrome
EXCLUDES *that with mention of hypertension (642.0-642.9)*

§ ✓5ᵗʰ **646.2 Unspecified renal disease in pregnancy,** CC 1-4 M ♀
[0-4] **without mention of hypertension**
Albuminuria
Nephropathy NOS
Renal disease NOS
Uremia } in pregnancy or the puerperium, without mention of hypertension

Gestational proteinuria
EXCLUDES *that with mention of hypertension (642.0-642.9)*

CC Excl: For codes 646.21- 646.24: 646.21-646.24

§ ✓5ᵗʰ **646.3 Habitual aborter** CC 1 M ♀
[0,1,3] EXCLUDES *with current abortion (634.0-634.9)*
*without current pregnancy ▶(629.81)◀*

CC Excl: For code 646.31: 646.31

DEF: Three or more consecutive spontaneous abortions.

§ ✓5ᵗʰ **646.4 Peripheral neuritis in pregnancy** M ♀
[0-4]

§ ✓5ᵗʰ **646.5 Asymptomatic bacteriuria in pregnancy** M ♀
[0-4]

§ ✓5ᵗʰ **646.6 Infections of genitourinary tract in** CC 1-4 M ♀
[0-4] **pregnancy**
Conditions classifiable to 590, 595, 597, 599.0, 616 complicating pregnancy, childbirth, or the puerperium
Conditions classifiable to 614.0-614.5, 614.7-614.9, 615 complicating pregnancy or labor
EXCLUDES *major puerperal infection (670)*

CC Excl: For code 646.61-646.64: 646.60-646.64, 646.80-646.93, 648.90-650, 669.40-669.44, 669.80-669.94

AHA: For code 646.63: 4Q, '04, 90

§ ✓5ᵗʰ **646.7 Liver disorders in pregnancy** CC 1,3 M ♀
[0,1,3] Acute yellow atrophy of liver (obstetric) (true)
Icterus gravis
Necrosis of liver } of pregnancy

EXCLUDES *hepatorenal syndrome following delivery (674.8)*
*viral hepatitis (647.6)*

CC Excl: For code 646.71, 646.73: 646.70-646.93, 648.90-650, 669.40-669.44, 669.80-669.94

§ ✓5ᵗʰ **646.8 Other specified complications of pregnancy** M ♀
[0-4] Fatigue during pregnancy
Herpes gestationis
Insufficient weight gain of pregnancy
AHA: 3Q, '98, 16; J-F, '85, 15

§ ✓5ᵗʰ **646.9 Unspecified complication of pregnancy** M ♀
[0,1,3]

✓4ᵗʰ **647 Infectious and parasitic conditions in the mother classifiable elsewhere, but complicating pregnancy, childbirth, or the puerperium**
INCLUDES *the listed conditions when complicating the pregnant state, aggravated by the pregnancy, or when a main reason for obstetric care*
EXCLUDES *those conditions in the mother known or suspected to have affected the fetus (655.0-655.9)*
Use additional code(s) to further specify complication

§ ✓5ᵗʰ **647.0 Syphilis** CC 1-4 M ♀
[0-4] Conditions classifiable to 090-097

CC Excl: For code 647.01- 647.04: 646.81-647.24

§ ✓5ᵗʰ **647.1 Gonorrhea** CC 1-4 M ♀
[0-4] Conditions classifiable to 098

CC Excl: For code 647.11-647.14: See code: 647.01

§ ✓5ᵗʰ **647.2 Other venereal diseases** CC 1-4 M ♀
[0-4] Conditions classifiable to 099

CC Excl: For code 647.21-647.24: See code: 647.01

§ ✓5ᵗʰ **647.3 Tuberculosis** CC 1-4 M ♀
[0-4] Conditions classifiable to 010-018

CC Excl: For code 647.31-647.34: 646.80-646.93, 647.30-647.34, 648.90-650, 669.40-669.44, 669.80-669.94

§ Requires fifth-digit. Valid digits are in [brackets] under each code. See beginning of section 640-649 for codes and definitions.

N Newborn Age: 0    P Pediatric Age: 0-17    M Maternity Age: 12-55    A Adult Age: 15-124    CC CC Condition    MCC Major CC Condition    HIV HIV Related Dx

§ ✓5ᵗʰ **647.4 Malaria**   CC 1-4   M ♀
[0-4]     Conditions classifiable to 084
**CC Excl:** For code 647.41-647.44: 646.80-646.93, 647.40-647.44, 648.90-650, 669.40-669.44, 669.80-669.94

§ ✓5ᵗʰ **647.5 Rubella**   CC 1-4   M ♀
[0-4]     Conditions classifiable to 056
**CC Excl:** For code 647.51-647.54: 647.51-647.94

§ ✓5ᵗʰ **647.6 Other viral diseases**   CC 1-4   M ♀
[0-4]     Conditions classifiable to 042 and 050-079,
       except 056
**CC Excl:** For code 647.61-647.64: See code 647.51

**AHA:** J-F, '85, 15

§ ✓5ᵗʰ **647.8 Other specified infectious and parasitic**   CC 1-4   M ♀
[0-4] **diseases**
**CC Excl:** For code 647.81-647.84: See code 647.51

§ ✓5ᵗʰ **647.9 Unspecified infection or infestation**   CC 1-4   M ♀
[0-4]   **CC Excl:** For code 647.91-647.94: See code 647.51

✓4ᵗʰ **648 Other current conditions in the mother classifiable elsewhere, but complicating pregnancy, childbirth, or the puerperium**
> **INCLUDES**   the listed conditions when complicating the pregnant state, aggravated by the pregnancy, or when a main reason for obstetric care
>
> **EXCLUDES**   *those conditions in the mother known or suspected to have affected the fetus (655.0-665.9)*

Use additional code(s) to identify the condition

§ ✓5ᵗʰ **648.0 Diabetes mellitus**   MCC 1,2   CC 0,3,4   M ♀
[0-4]     Conditions classifiable to 250
> **EXCLUDES**   *gestational diabetes (648.8)*

**CC Excl:** 646.80-646.93, 648.00-648.04, 648.90-650, 669.40-669.44, 669.80-669.94

**AHA:** 3Q, '91, 5, 11

§ ✓5ᵗʰ **648.1 Thyroid dysfunction**   M ♀
[0-4]     Conditions classifiable to 240-246

§ ✓5ᵗʰ **648.2 Anemia**   M ♀
[0-4]     Conditions classifiable to 280-285
**AHA:** For Code 648.22: 1Q, '02, 14

§ ✓5ᵗʰ **648.3 Drug dependence**   CC 1-4   M ♀
[0-4]     Conditions classifiable to 304
**CC Excl:** For code 648.31-648.34: 646.80-646.93, 648.30-648.34, 648.90-650, 669.40-669.44, 669.80-669.94

**AHA:** 2Q, '98, 13; 4Q, '88, 8

§ ✓5ᵗʰ **648.4 Mental disorders**   M ♀
[0-4]     Conditions classifiable to 290-303, 305.0, 305.2-
       305.9, 306-316, 317-319
**AHA:** 2Q, '98, 13; 4Q, '95, 63

§ ✓5ᵗʰ **648.5 Congenital cardiovascular disorders**   CC 1-4   M ♀
[0-4]     Conditions classifiable to 745-747
**CC Excl:** For code 648.51, 648.52, 648.53, 648.54: 646.80-646.93, 648.50-648.64, 648.90-650, 669.40-669.44, 669.80-669.94

§ ✓5ᵗʰ **648.6 Other cardiovascular diseases**   CC 1-4   M ♀
[0-4]     Conditions classifiable to 390-398, 410-429
> **EXCLUDES**   *cerebrovascular disorders in the puerperium (674.0)*
> *peripartum cardiomyopathy (674.5)*
> *venous complications (671.0-671.9)*

**CC Excl:** For code 648.61, 648.62, 648.63, 648.64: See code 648.51

**AHA:** 3Q, '98, 11

§ ✓5ᵗʰ **648.7 Bone and joint disorders of back, pelvis,**   CC 1-4   M ♀
[0-4] **and lower limbs**
    Conditions classifiable to 720-724, and those
       classifiable to 711-719 or 725-738, specified as
       affecting the lower limbs
**CC Excl:** For code 648.71, 648.72, 648.73, 648.74: 648.71-648.74

§ ✓5ᵗʰ **648.8 Abnormal glucose tolerance**   M ♀
[0-4]     Conditions classifiable to 790.21-790.29
    Gestational diabetes
    Use additional code, if applicable, for associated
       long-term (current) insulin use (V58.67)
**AHA:** 3Q, '91, 5; For code 648.83: 4Q, '04, 56

**DEF:** Glucose intolerance arising in pregnancy, resolving at end of pregnancy.

§ ✓5ᵗʰ **648.9 Other current conditions classifiable**   M ♀
[0-4] **elsewhere**
    Conditions classifiable to 440-459
    Nutritional deficiencies [conditions classifiable to
       260-269]
**AHA:** 3Q, '06, 14; 4Q, '04, 88; N-D, '87, 10; For code 648.91: 1Q, '02, 14; For code 648.93: 4Q, '04, 90

✓4ᵗʰ **649 Other conditions or status of the mother complicating pregnancy, childbirth, or the puerperium**
**AHA:** 4Q, '06, 99

§ ✓5ᵗʰ **649.0 Tobacco use disorder complicating pregnancy,**   M ♀
[0-4] **childbirth, or the puerperium**
    Smoking complicating pregnancy, childbirth, or the
       puerperium
**AHA:** 4Q, '06, 99

§ ✓5ᵗʰ **649.1 Obesity complicating pregnancy, childbirth,**   M ♀
[0-4] **or the puerperium**
    Use additional code to identify the obesity (278.00,
       278.01)
**AHA:** 4Q, '06, 99

§ ✓5ᵗʰ **649.2 Bariatric surgery status complicating**   M ♀
[0-4] **pregnancy, childbirth, or the puerperium**
    Gastric banding status complicating pregnancy,
       childbirth, or the puerperium
    Gastric bypass status for obesity complicating
       pregnancy, childbirth, or the puerperium
    Obesity surgery status complicating pregnancy,
       childbirth, or the puerperium
**AHA:** 4Q, '06, 99, 118

§ ✓5ᵗʰ **649.3 Coagulation defects complicating**   CC   M ♀
[0-4] **pregnancy, childbirth, or the puerperium**
    Conditions classifiable to 286
    Use additional code to identify the specific
       coagulation defect (286.0-286.9)
> **EXCLUDES**   *coagulation defects causing antepartum hemorrhage (641.3)*
> *postpartum coagulation defects (666.3)*

**CC Excl:** For code 649.30: 648.90; For codes 649.31, 649.32, 649.33, 649.34: 648.91-648.94

**AHA:** 4Q, '06, 99

§ ✓5ᵗʰ **649.4 Epilepsy complicating pregnancy,**   CC 1-4   M ♀
[0-4] **childbirth, or the puerperium**
    Conditions classifiable to 345
    Use additional code to identify the specific type of
       epilepsy (345.00-345.91)
> **EXCLUDES**   *eclampsia (642.6)*

**CC Excl:** For codes 649.41, 649.42, 649.43, 649.44: 648.91-648.94

**AHA:** 4Q, '06, 99

§ ✓5ᵗʰ **649.5 Spotting complicating pregnancy**   M ♀
[0,1,3]   **EXCLUDES**   *antepartum hemorrhage (641.0-641.9)*
        *hemorrhage in early pregnancy (640.0-*
        *640.9)*

**AHA:** 4Q, '06, 99

§ ✓5ᵗʰ **649.6 Uterine size date discrepancy**   M ♀
[0-4]

**AHA:** 4Q, '06, 99

---

§ Requires fifth-digit. Valid digits are in [brackets] under each code. See beginning of section 640-649 for codes and definitions.

---

✓4ᵗʰ / ✓5ᵗʰ Additional Digit Required     Unacceptable PDx     Manifestation Code     ►◄ Revised Text     ● New Code     ▲ Revised Code Title

## NORMAL DELIVERY, AND OTHER INDICATIONS FOR CARE IN PREGNANCY, LABOR, AND DELIVERY (650–659)

The following fifth-digit subclassification is for use with categories 651-659 to denote the current episode of care. Valid fifth-digits are in [brackets] under each code.

   0   unspecified as to episode of care or not applicable
   1   delivered, with or without mention of antepartum condition
   2   delivered, with mention of postpartum complication
   3   antepartum condition or complication
   4   postpartum condition or complication

**650 Normal delivery**    M ♀
    Delivery requiring minimal or no assistance, with or without episiotomy, without fetal manipulation [e.g., rotation version] or instrumentation [forceps] of spontaneous, cephalic, vaginal, full-term, single, live-born infant. This code is for use as a single diagnosis code and is not to be used with any other code in the range 630-676.

    **EXCLUDES**   *breech delivery (assisted) (spontaneous) NOS (652.2)*
          *delivery by vacuum extractor, forceps, cesarean section, or breech extraction, without specified complication (669.5-669.7)*

    Use additional code to indicate outcome of delivery (V27.0)
    AHA: 2Q, '02, 10; 3Q, '01, 12; 3Q, '00, 5; 4Q, '95, 28, 59

✓4ᵗʰ **651 Multiple gestation**
§ ✓5ᵗʰ **651.0 Twin pregnancy**    CC 1 M ♀
   [0,1,3]
    CC Excl: For code 651.01: 650-651.63, 651.71-652.20, 652.23-652.93
    AHA: 3Q, '06, 16

§ ✓5ᵗʰ **651.1 Triplet pregnancy**    CC 1,3 ♀
   [0,1,3]
    CC Excl: For code 651.11, 651.13: 650-651.63, 651.71-652.93

§ ✓5ᵗʰ **651.2 Quadruplet pregnancy**    CC 1,3 M ♀
   [0,1,3]
    CC Excl: For code 651.21, 651.23: See code 651.11

§ ✓5ᵗʰ **651.3 Twin pregnancy with fetal loss and retention of one fetus**    M ♀
   [0,1,3]

§ ✓5ᵗʰ **651.4 Triplet pregnancy with fetal loss and retention of one or more fetus(es)**    CC 1,3 M ♀
   [0,1,3]
    CC Excl: For code 651.41, 651.43: See code 651.11

§ ✓5ᵗʰ **651.5 Quadruplet pregnancy with fetal loss and retention of one or more fetus(es)**    CC 1,3 M ♀
   [0,1,3]
    CC Excl: For code 651.51, 651.53: See code 651.11

§ ✓5ᵗʰ **651.6 Other multiple pregnancy with fetal loss and retention of one or more fetus(es)**    M ♀
   [0,1,3]

§ ✓5ᵗʰ **651.7 Multiple gestation following (elective) fetal reduction**    M ♀
   [0,1,3]
    Fetal reduction of multiple fetuses reduced to single fetus
    AHA: 3Q, '06, 18; For code 651.71: 4Q, '05, 81

### Malposition and Malpresentation

Breech

Shoulder (arm prolapse)

Mother's pelvis

Face (mentum)

Compound (extremity together with head)

Oblique

---

### Cephalopelvic Disproportion

Pubic symphysis

Ischial tuberosity

Contraction of pelvic outlet (from below)

Cephalopelvic disproportion due to: Contraction of pelvic inlet, or large fetus, or hydrocephalus

Pubic symphysis

Pelvic inlet from above

§ ✓5ᵗʰ **651.8 Other specified multiple gestation**    CC 1,3 M ♀
   [0,1,3]
    CC Excl: For code 651.81, 651.83: See code 651.11

§ ✓5ᵗʰ **651.9 Unspecified multiple gestation**    M ♀
   [0,1,3]

✓4ᵗʰ **652 Malposition and malpresentation of fetus**
    Code first any associated obstructed labor (660.0)

§ ✓5ᵗʰ **652.0 Unstable lie**    M ♀
   [0,1,3]
    **DEF:** Changing fetal position.

§ ✓5ᵗʰ **652.1 Breech or other malpresentation successfully converted to cephalic presentation**    M ♀
   [0,1,3]
    Cephalic version NOS
    **DEF:** Fetal presentation of buttocks or feet at birth canal.

§ ✓5ᵗʰ **652.2 Breech presentation without mention of version**    M ♀
   [0,1,3]
    Breech delivery (assisted) (spontaneous) NOS
    Buttocks presentation
    Complete breech
    Frank breech
    **EXCLUDES** *footling presentation (652.8)*
           *incomplete breech (652.8)*

§ ✓5ᵗʰ **652.3 Transverse or oblique presentation**    M ♀
   [0,1,3]
    Oblique lie        Transverse lie
    **EXCLUDES** *transverse arrest of fetal head (660.3)*

§ ✓5ᵗʰ **652.4 Face or brow presentation**    M ♀
   [0,1,3]
    Mentum presentation

§ ✓5ᵗʰ **652.5 High head at term**    M ♀
   [0,1,3]
    Failure of head to enter pelvic brim

§ ✓5ᵗʰ **652.6 Multiple gestation with malpresentation of one fetus or more**    M ♀
   [0,1,3]

§ ✓5ᵗʰ **652.7 Prolapsed arm**    M ♀
   [0,1,3]

§ ✓5ᵗʰ **652.8 Other specified malposition or malpresentation**    M ♀
   [0,1,3]
    Compound presentation

§ ✓5ᵗʰ **652.9 Unspecified malposition or malpresentation**    M ♀
   [0,1,3]

✓4ᵗʰ **653 Disproportion**
    Code first any associated obstructed labor (660.1)

§ ✓5ᵗʰ **653.0 Major abnormality of bony pelvis, not further specified**    M ♀
   [0,1,3]
    Pelvic deformity NOS

§ ✓5ᵗʰ **653.1 Generally contracted pelvis**    M ♀
   [0,1,3]
    Contracted pelvis NOS

§ ✓5ᵗʰ **653.2 Inlet contraction of pelvis**    M ♀
   [0,1,3]
    Inlet contraction (pelvis)

§ ✓5ᵗʰ **653.3 Outlet contraction of pelvis**    M ♀
   [0,1,3]
    Outlet contraction (pelvis)

§ ✓5ᵗʰ **653.4 Fetopelvic disproportion**    M ♀
   [0,1,3]
    Cephalopelvic disproportion NOS
    Disproportion of mixed maternal and fetal origin, with normally formed fetus

§ ✓5ᵗʰ **653.5 Unusually large fetus causing disproportion**    M ♀
   [0,1,3]
    Disproportion of fetal origin with normally formed fetus
    Fetal disproportion NOS
    **EXCLUDES** *that when the reason for medical care was concern for the fetus (656.6)*

---

§   Requires fifth-digit. Valid digits are in [brackets] under each code. See beginning of section 640-649 for codes and definitions.

N Newborn Age: 0    P Pediatric Age: 0-17    M Maternity Age: 12-55    A Adult Age: 15-124    CC CC Condition    MCC Major CC Condition    HIV HIV Related Dx

§ ✓5ᵗʰ **653.6 Hydrocephalic fetus causing disproportion** Ⓜ ♀
[0,1,3] EXCLUDES *that when the reason for medical care was concern for the fetus (655.0)*

§ ✓5ᵗʰ **653.7 Other fetal abnormality causing disproportion** Ⓜ ♀
[0,1,3] Conjoined twins Fetal:
Fetal: myelomeningocele
ascites sacral teratoma
hydrops tumor

§ ✓5ᵗʰ **653.8 Disproportion of other origin** Ⓜ ♀
[0,1,3] EXCLUDES *shoulder (girdle) dystocia (660.4)*

§ ✓5ᵗʰ **653.9 Unspecified disproportion** Ⓜ ♀
[0,1,3]

✓4ᵗʰ **654 Abnormality of organs and soft tissues of pelvis**
INCLUDES the listed conditions during pregnancy, childbirth, or the puerperium
Code first any associated obstructed labor (660.2)
EXCLUDES ▶ *trauma to perineum and vulva complicating current delivery (664.0-664.9)◀*

§ ✓5ᵗʰ **654.0 Congenital abnormalities of uterus** Ⓜ ♀
[0-4] Double uterus
Uterus bicornis

§ ✓5ᵗʰ **654.1 Tumors of body of uterus** Ⓜ ♀
[0-4] Uterine fibroids

§ ✓5ᵗʰ **654.2 Previous cesarean delivery** Ⓜ ♀
[0,1,3] Uterine scar from previous cesarean delivery
AHA: 1Q, '92, 8

§ ✓5ᵗʰ **654.3 Retroverted and incarcerated gravid uterus** Ⓜ ♀
[0-4]
DEF: Retroverted: tilted back uterus; no change in angle of longitudinal axis.
DEF: Incarcerated: immobile, fixed uterus.

§ ✓5ᵗʰ **654.4 Other abnormalities in shape or position of** Ⓜ ♀
[0-4] **gravid uterus and of neighboring structures**
Cystocele
Pelvic floor repair
Pendulous abdomen
Prolapse of gravid uterus
Rectocele
Rigid pelvic floor

§ ✓5ᵗʰ **654.5 Cervical incompetence** MCC 1-4 Ⓜ ♀
[0-4] Presence of Shirodkar suture with or without mention of cervical incompetence
CC Excl: For code 654.51-654.54: 654.51-654.54
DEF: Abnormal cervix; tendency to dilate in second trimester; causes premature fetal expulsion.
DEF: Shirodkar suture: purse-string suture used to artificially close incompetent cervix.

§ ✓5ᵗʰ **654.6 Other congenital or acquired abnormality of** Ⓜ ♀
[0-4] **cervix**
Cicatricial cervix
Polyp of cervix
Previous surgery to cervix
Rigid cervix (uteri)
Stenosis or stricture of cervix
Tumor of cervix

§ ✓5ᵗʰ **654.7 Congenital or acquired abnormality of vagina** Ⓜ ♀
[0-4] Previous surgery to vagina
Septate vagina
Stenosis of vagina (acquired) (congenital)
Stricture of vagina
Tumor of vagina

§ ✓5ᵗʰ **654.8 Congenital or acquired abnormality of vulva** Ⓜ ♀
[0-4] ▶Anal sphincter tear (healed) (old) complicating delivery◀
Fibrosis of perineum
Persistent hymen
Previous surgery to perineum or vulva
Rigid perineum
Tumor of vulva
EXCLUDES ▶ *anal sphincter tear (healed) (old) not associated with delivery (569.43)◀*
*varicose veins of vulva (671.1)*
AHA: 1Q, '03, 14

§ ✓5ᵗʰ **654.9 Other and unspecified** Ⓜ ♀
[0-4] Uterine scar NEC

✓4ᵗʰ **655 Known or suspected fetal abnormality affecting management of mother**
INCLUDES the listed conditions in the fetus as a reason for observation or obstetrical care of the mother, or for termination of pregnancy
AHA: 3Q, '90, 4

§ ✓5ᵗʰ **655.0 Central nervous system malformation in fetus** Ⓜ ♀
[0,1,3] Fetal or suspected fetal:
anencephaly
hydrocephalus
spina bifida (with myelomeningocele)

§ ✓5ᵗʰ **655.1 Chromosomal abnormality in fetus** Ⓜ ♀
[0,1,3]

§ ✓5ᵗʰ **655.2 Hereditary disease in family possibly** Ⓜ ♀
[0,1,3] **affecting fetus**

§ ✓5ᵗʰ **655.3 Suspected damage to fetus from viral** Ⓜ ♀
[0,1,3] **disease in the mother**
Suspected damage to fetus from maternal rubella

§ ✓5ᵗʰ **655.4 Suspected damage to fetus from other** Ⓜ ♀
[0,1,3] **disease in the mother**
Suspected damage to fetus from maternal:
alcohol addiction
listeriosis
toxoplasmosis

§ ✓5ᵗʰ **655.5 Suspected damage to fetus from drugs** Ⓜ ♀
[0,1,3]

§ ✓5ᵗʰ **655.6 Suspected damage to fetus from radiation** Ⓜ ♀
[0,1,3]

§ ✓5ᵗʰ **655.7 Decreased fetal movements** Ⓜ ♀
[0,1,3] AHA: 4Q, '97, 41

§ ✓5ᵗʰ **655.8 Other known or suspected fetal abnormality,** Ⓜ ♀
[0,1,3] **not elsewhere classified**
Suspected damage to fetus from:
environmental toxins
intrauterine contraceptive device
AHA: 3Q, '06, 16, 18

§ ✓5ᵗʰ **655.9 Unspecified** Ⓜ ♀
[0,1,3]

✓4ᵗʰ **656 Other fetal and placental problems affecting management of mother**

§ ✓5ᵗʰ **656.0 Fetal-maternal hemorrhage** Ⓜ ♀
[0,1,3] Leakage (microscopic) of fetal blood into maternal circulation

§ ✓5ᵗʰ **656.1 Rhesus isoimmunization** CC 3 Ⓜ ♀
[0,1,3] Anti-D [Rh] antibodies
Rh incompatibility
CC Excl: For code 656.13: 656.11-656.13
DEF: Antibodies developing against Rh factor; mother with Rh negative develops antibodies against Rh positive fetus.

§ ✓5ᵗʰ **656.2 Isoimmunization from other and unspecified** Ⓜ ♀
[0,1,3] **blood-group incompatibility**
ABO isoimmunization.
AHA: 4Q, '06, 135

§ ✓5ᵗʰ **656.3 Fetal distress** CC 1 Ⓜ ♀
[0,1,3] Fetal metabolic acidemia
EXCLUDES *abnormal fetal acid-base balance (656.8)*
*abnormality in fetal heart rate or rhythm (659.7)*
*fetal bradycardia (659.7)*
*fetal tachycardia (659.7)*
*meconium in liquor (656.8)*
CC Excl: For code 656.31: 656.31-656.33, 659.71, 763.82
AHA: N-D, '86, 4
DEF: Life-threatening disorder; fetal anoxia, hemolytic disease and other miscellaneous diseases cause fetal distress.

§ Requires fifth-digit. Valid digits are in [brackets] under each code. See beginning of section 640-649 for codes and definitions.

✓4ᵗʰ / ✓5ᵗʰ Additional Digit Required   Unacceptable PDx   Manifestation Code   ▶◀ Revised Text   ● New Code   ▲ Revised Code Title

**Complications of Pregnancy, Childbirth & Puerperium**

**656.4–660**

§ ✓5th **656.4** **Intrauterine death**    CC 1, 3   M♀
[0,1,3]   Fetal death:
    NOS
    after completion of 22 weeks' gestation
    late
   Missed delivery
   EXCLUDES    *missed abortion (632)*
   CC Excl: For code **656.41**: 656.41-656.43; For code **656.43**: 656.43

§ ✓5th **656.5** **Poor fetal growth**    CC 1   M♀
[0,1,3]   "Light-for-dates"
   "Placental insufficiency"
   "Small-for-dates"
   CC Excl: For code **656.51**: 656.51-656.53

§ ✓5th **656.6** **Excessive fetal growth**    M♀
[0,1,3]   "Large-for-dates"

§ ✓5th **656.7** **Other placental conditions**    M♀
[0,1,3]   Abnormal placenta
   Placental infarct
   EXCLUDES    *placental polyp (674.4)*
               *placentitis (658.4)*

§ ✓5th **656.8** **Other specified fetal and placental problems**    M♀
[0,1,3]   Abnormal acid-base balance
   Intrauterine acidosis
   Lithopedian
   Meconium in liquor
   DEF: Lithopedion: Calcified fetus; not expelled by mother.

§ ✓5th **656.9** **Unspecified fetal and placental problem**    M♀
[0,1,3]

✓4th **657 Polyhydramnios**    CC 1   M♀
[0,1,3]
§ ✓5th Use 0 as fourth-digit for this category
   Hydramnios
   CC Excl: For code **657.01**: 657.01-657.03

   AHA: 3Q, '06, 16; 4Q, '91, 26

   DEF: Excess amniotic fluid.

✓4th **658 Other problems associated with amniotic cavity and membranes**
   EXCLUDES    *amniotic fluid embolism (673.1)*

§ ✓5th **658.0** **Oligohydramnios**    CC 1,3   M♀
[0,1,3]   Oligohydramnios without mention of rupture of
     membranes
   CC Excl: For code **658.01, 658.03**: 658.01-658.03

   AHA: 3Q, '06, 16

   DEF: Deficient amount of amniotic fluid.

§ ✓5th **658.1** **Premature rupture of membranes**    M♀
[0,1,3]   Rupture of amniotic sac less than 24 hours prior to
     the onset of labor
   AHA: For code **658.13**: 1Q, '01, 5; 4Q, '98, 77

§ ✓5th **658.2** **Delayed delivery after spontaneous or unspecified rupture of membranes**    M♀
[0,1,3]   Prolonged rupture of membranes NOS
   Rupture of amniotic sac 24 hours or more prior to
     the onset of labor

§ ✓5th **658.3** **Delayed delivery after artificial rupture of membranes**    M♀
[0,1,3]

§ ✓5th **658.4** **Infection of amniotic cavity**    MCC 1,3   M♀
[0,1,3]   Amnionitis
   Chorioamnionitis
   Membranitis
   Placentitis
   CC Excl: For code **658.41, 658.43**: 658.41-658.43

§ ✓5th **658.8** **Other**    CC 1   M♀
[0,1,3]   Amnion nodosum
   Amniotic cyst
   CC Excl: For code **658.81**: 658.81

§ ✓5th **658.9** **Unspecified**    M♀
[0,1,3]

---

✓4th **659 Other indications for care or intervention related to labor and delivery, not elsewhere classified**

§ ✓5th **659.0** **Failed mechanical induction**    M♀
[0,1,3]   Failure of induction of labor by surgical or other
     instrumental methods

§ ✓5th **659.1** **Failed medical or unspecified induction**    M♀
[0,1,3]   Failed induction NOS
   Failure of induction of labor by medical methods,
     such as oxytocic drugs

§ ✓5th **659.2** **Maternal pyrexia during labor, unspecified**    CC 1   M♀
[0,1,3]
   CC Excl: For code **659.21**: 659.21-659.23

   DEF: Fever during labor.

§ ✓5th **659.3** **Generalized infection during labor**    MCC 1,3   M♀
[0,1,3]   Septicemia during labor
   CC Excl: For code **659.31, 659.33**: 646.80-646.93, 648.90-650,
   659.30-659.33, 669.40-669.44, 669.80-669.94

§ ✓5th **659.4** **Grand multiparity**    M♀
[0,1,3]   EXCLUDES    *supervision only, in pregnancy (V23.3)*
                *without current pregnancy (V61.5)*

   DEF: Having borne six or more children previously.

§ ✓5th **659.5** **Elderly primigravida**    M♀
[0,1,3]   First pregnancy in a woman who will be 35 years of
     age or older at expected date of delivery
   EXCLUDES    *supervision only, in pregnancy (V23.81)*

   AHA: 3Q, '01, 12

§ ✓5th **659.6** **Elderly multigravida**    M♀
[0,1,3]   Second or more pregnancy in a woman who will
     be 35 years of age or older at expected date
     of delivery
   EXCLUDES    *elderly primigravida 659.5*
               *supervision only, in pregnancy (V23.82)*

   AHA: 3Q, '01, 12

§ ✓5th **659.7** **Abnormality in fetal heart rate or rhythm**    M♀
[0,1,3]   Depressed fetal heart tones
   Fetal:
     bradycardia
     tachycardia
   Fetal heart rate decelerations
   Non-reassuring fetal heart rate or rhythm
   AHA: 4Q, '98, 48

§ ✓5th **659.8** **Other specified indications for care or intervention related to labor and delivery**    M♀
[0,1,3]   Pregnancy in a female less than 16 years old at
     expected date of delivery
   Very young maternal age
   AHA: 3Q, '01, 12

§ ✓5th **659.9** **Unspecified indication for care or intervention**    M♀
[0,1,3] **related to labor and delivery**

### COMPLICATIONS OCCURRING MAINLY IN THE COURSE OF LABOR AND DELIVERY (660-669)

The following fifth-digit subclassification is for use with
categories 660-669 to denote the current episode of care. Valid
fifth-digits are in [brackets] under each code.

   **0** **unspecified as to episode of care or not applicable**
   **1** **delivered, with or without mention of antepartum condition**
   **2** **delivered, with mention of postpartum complication**
   **3** **antepartum condition or complication**
   **4** **postpartum condition or complication**

✓4th **660 Obstructed labor**
   AHA: 3Q, '95, 10

---

§   Requires fifth-digit. Valid digits are in [brackets] under each code. See beginning of section 640-649 for codes and definitions.

---

N Newborn Age: 0    P Pediatric Age: 0-17    M Maternity Age: 12-55    A Adult Age: 15-124    CC CC Condition    MCC Major CC Condition    HIV HIV Related Dx

§ ✓5ᵗʰ **660.0** **Obstruction caused by malposition of** `CC 3` M ♀
[0,1,3] **fetus at onset of labor**
Any condition classifiable to 652, causing
obstruction during labor
Use additional code from 652.0-652.9 to identify
condition
**CC Excl: For code 660.03:** 646.80-646.93, 648.90-650, 655.70-655.73,
660.03, 665.00-665.11, 665.50-665.54, 665.80-665.94, 669.40-669.44,
669.80-669.94

§ ✓5ᵗʰ **660.1** **Obstruction by bony pelvis** M ♀
[0,1,3] Any condition classifiable to 653, causing
obstruction during labor
Use additional code from 653.0-653.9 to identify
condition

§ ✓5ᵗʰ **660.2** **Obstruction by abnormal pelvic soft tissues** M ♀
[0,1,3] Prolapse of anterior lip of cervix
Any condition classifiable to 654, causing
obstruction during labor
Use additional code from 654.0-654.9 to identify
condition

§ ✓5ᵗʰ **660.3** **Deep transverse arrest and persistent** M ♀
[0,1,3] **occipitoposterior position**

§ ✓5ᵗʰ **660.4** **Shoulder (girdle) dystocia** M ♀
[0,1,3] Impacted shoulders
**DEF: Obstructed labor due to impacted fetal shoulders.**

§ ✓5ᵗʰ **660.5** **Locked twins** M ♀
[0,1,3]

§ ✓5ᵗʰ **660.6** **Failed trial of labor, unspecified** M ♀
[0,1,3] Failed trial of labor, without mention of
condition or suspected condition

§ ✓5ᵗʰ **660.7** **Failed forceps or vacuum extractor,** M ♀
[0,1,3] **unspecified**
Application of ventouse or forceps, without
mention of condition

§ ✓5ᵗʰ **660.8** **Other causes of obstructed labor** M ♀
[0,1,3] Use additional code to identify condition
**AHA: 4Q, '04, 88**

§ ✓5ᵗʰ **660.9** **Unspecified obstructed labor** M ♀
[0,1,3] Dystocia:      Dystocia:
NOS            maternal NOS
fetal NOS

✓4ᵗʰ **661** **Abnormality of forces of labor**

§ ✓5ᵗʰ **661.0** **Primary uterine inertia** M ♀
[0,1,3] Failure of cervical dilation
Hypotonic uterine dysfunction, primary
Prolonged latent phase of labor
**DEF: Lack of efficient contractions during labor causing prolonged
labor.**

§ ✓5ᵗʰ **661.1** **Secondary uterine inertia** M ♀
[0,1,3] Arrested active phase of labor
Hypotonic uterine dysfunction, secondary

§ ✓5ᵗʰ **661.2** **Other and unspecified uterine inertia** M ♀
[0,1,3] ▶Atony of uterus without hemorrhage◀
Desultory labor
Irregular labor
Poor contractions
Slow slope active phase of labor
     `EXCLUDES` ▶ *atony of uterus with hemorrhage*
*(666.1)*
*postpartum atony of uterus without*
*hemorrhage (669.8)◀*

§ ✓5ᵗʰ **661.3** **Precipitate labor** M ♀
[0,1,3] **DEF: Rapid labor and delivery.**

§ ✓5ᵗʰ **661.4** **Hypertonic, incoordinate, or prolonged** M ♀
[0,1,3] **uterine contractions**
Cervical spasm
Contraction ring (dystocia)
Dyscoordinate labor
Hourglass contraction of uterus
Hypertonic uterine dysfunction
Incoordinate uterine action
Retraction ring (Bandl's) (pathological)
Tetanic contractions
Uterine dystocia NOS
Uterine spasm

§ ✓5ᵗʰ **661.9** **Unspecified abnormality of labor** M ♀
[0,1,3]

✓4ᵗʰ **662** **Long labor**

§ ✓5ᵗʰ **662.0** **Prolonged first stage** M ♀
[0,1,3]

§ ✓5ᵗʰ **662.1** **Prolonged labor, unspecified** `CC 1` M ♀
[0,1,3]
**CC Excl: For code 662.11:** 646.80-646.93, 648.90-650, 655.70-655.73,
662.11, 665.00-665.11, 665.50-665.54, 665.80-665.94, 669.40-669.44,
669.80-669.94

§ ✓5ᵗʰ **662.2** **Prolonged second stage** M ♀
[0,1,3]

§ ✓5ᵗʰ **662.3** **Delayed delivery of second twin, triplet, etc.** M ♀
[0,1,3]

✓4ᵗʰ **663** **Umbilical cord complications**

§ ✓5ᵗʰ **663.0** **Prolapse of cord** M ♀
[0,1,3] Presentation of cord
**DEF: Abnormal presentation of fetus; marked by protruding
umbilical cord during labor; can cause fetal death.**

§ ✓5ᵗʰ **663.1** **Cord around neck, with compression** M ♀
[0,1,3] Cord tightly around neck

§ ✓5ᵗʰ **663.2** **Other and unspecified cord entanglement,** M ♀
[0,1,3] **with compression**
Entanglement of cords of twins in mono-amniotic
sac
Knot in cord (with compression)

§ ✓5ᵗʰ **663.3** **Other and unspecified cord entanglement,** M ♀
[0,1,3] **without mention of compression**
**AHA: For code 663.31: 2Q, '03, 9**

§ ✓5ᵗʰ **663.4** **Short cord** M ♀
[0,1,3]

§ ✓5ᵗʰ **663.5** **Vasa previa** M ♀
[0,1,3]
**DEF: Abnormal presentation of fetus marked by blood vessels of
umbilical cord in front of fetal head.**

§ ✓5ᵗʰ **663.6** **Vascular lesions of cord** M ♀
[0,1,3] Bruising of cord
Hematoma of cord
Thrombosis of vessels of cord

§ ✓5ᵗʰ **663.8** **Other umbilical cord complications** M ♀
[0,1,3] Velamentous insertion of umbilical cord

§ ✓5ᵗʰ **663.9** **Unspecified umbilical cord complication** M ♀
[0,1,3]

✓4ᵗʰ **664** **Trauma to perineum and vulva during delivery**
     `INCLUDES`      damage from instruments
that from extension of episiotomy
**AHA: 1Q, '92, 11; N-D, '84, 10**

§ ✓5ᵗʰ **664.0** **First-degree perineal laceration** M ♀
[0,1,4] Perineal laceration, rupture, or tear involving:
fourchette
hymen
labia
skin
vagina
vulva

---

§ Requires fifth-digit. Valid digits are in [brackets] under each code. See beginning of section 640-649 for codes and definitions.

✓4ᵗʰ Additional Digit Required      Unacceptable PDx      Manifestation Code      ▶◀ Revised Text      ● New Code      ▲ Revised Code Title
✓5ᵗʰ

© 2007 Ingenix                

**Complications of Pregnancy, Childbirth & Puerperium**

**664.1–666.1**

**Perineal Lacerations**

First degree

Second degree

Anus

Third degree

Fourth degree

§ ✓5th **664.1** **Second-degree perineal laceration** Ⓜ♀
[0,1,4]      Perineal laceration, rupture, or tear (following
              episiotomy) involving:
                  pelvic floor
                  perineal muscles
                  vaginal muscles
          **EXCLUDES** *that involving anal sphincter (664.2)*

§ ✓5th **664.2** **Third-degree perineal laceration** CC 1 Ⓜ♀
[0,1,4]      Perineal laceration, rupture, or tear (following
              episiotomy) involving:
                  anal sphincter
                  rectovaginal septum
                  sphincter NOS
          **EXCLUDES** ▶*anal sphincter tear during delivery not
              associated with third-degree
              perineal laceration (664.6)*◀
              *that with anal or rectal mucosal
              laceration (664.3)*
          **CC Excl: For code 664.21:** 646.80-646.93, 648.90-650, 655.70-655.73,
          664.21, 664.61, 665.00-665.11, 665.50-665.54, 665.80-665.94, 669.40-
          669.44, 669.80-669.94

§ ✓5th **664.3** **Fourth-degree perineal laceration** CC 1 Ⓜ♀
[0,1,4]      Perineal laceration, rupture, or tear as classifiable to
              664.2 and involving also:
                  anal mucosa
                  rectal mucosa
          **CC Excl: For code 664.31:** 646.80-646.93, 648.90-650, 655.70-655.73,
          664.31, 665.00-665.11, 665.50-665.54, 665.80-665.94, 669.40-669.44,
          669.80-669.94

§ ✓5th **664.4** **Unspecified perineal laceration** Ⓜ♀
[0,1,4]      Central laceration
          **AHA:** 1Q, '92, 8

§ ✓5th **664.5** **Vulval and perineal hematoma** Ⓜ♀
[0,1,4]      **AHA:** N-D, '84, 10

● § ✓5th **664.6** **Anal sphincter tear complicating delivery,** CC 1, 4
[0,1,4]      **not associated with third-degree perineal** Ⓜ♀
          **laceration**
          **EXCLUDES** *third-degree perineal laceration (664.2)*
          **CC Excl: For code 664.61, 664.64:** 646.80-646.93, 648.90-650, 655.70-
          655.73, 664.21, 664.60-664.64, 665.00-665.11, 665.50-665.54, 665.80-
          665.94, 669.40-669.44, 669.80-669.94

§ ✓5th **664.8** **Other specified trauma to perineum and vulva** Ⓜ♀
[0,1,4]

§ ✓5th **664.9** **Unspecified trauma to perineum and vulva** Ⓜ♀
[0,1,4]

✓4th **665** **Other obstetrical trauma**
          **INCLUDES** damage from instruments

§ ✓5th **665.0** **Rupture of uterus before onset of** MCC 1,3 Ⓜ♀
[0,1,3]      **labor**
          **CC Excl: For code 665.01, 665.03:** 646.80-646.93, 648.90-650, 655.70-
          655.73, 665.00-665.11, 665.50-665.54, 665.80-665.94, 669.40-669.44,
          669.80-669.94

§ ✓5th **665.1** **Rupture of uterus during labor** MCC 1 Ⓜ♀
[0,1]       Rupture of uterus NOS
          **CC Excl: For code 665.11:** See code 665.01

§ ✓5th **665.2** **Inversion of uterus** CC 2 Ⓜ♀
[0,2,4]
          **CC Excl: For code 665.22:** 646.80-646.93, 648.90-650, 655.70-655.73,
          665.00-665.11, 665.22, 665.50-665.54, 665.80-665.94, 669.40-669.44,
          669.80-669.94

§ ✓5th **665.3** **Laceration of cervix** CC 1 Ⓜ♀
[0,1,4]
          **CC Excl: For code 665.31:** 646.80-646.93, 648.90-650, 655.70-655.73,
          665.00-665.11, 665.31, 665.50-665.54, 665.80-665.94, 669.40-669.44,
          669.80-669.94

§ ✓5th **665.4** **High vaginal laceration** CC 1 Ⓜ♀
[0,1,4]      Laceration of vaginal wall or sulcus without
              mention of perineal laceration
          **CC Excl: For code 665.41:** 646.80-646.93, 648.90-650, 655.70-655.73,
          665.00-665.11, 665.41, 665.50-665.54, 665.80-665.94, 669.40-669.44,
          669.80-669.94

§ ✓5th **665.5** **Other injury to pelvic organs** CC 1 Ⓜ♀
[0,1,4]      Injury to:              Injury to:
                  bladder                urethra
          **CC Excl: For code 665.51:** See code 665.01
          **AHA:** M-A, '87, 10

§ ✓5th **665.6** **Damage to pelvic joints and ligaments** CC 1 Ⓜ♀
[0,1,4]      Avulsion of inner symphyseal cartilage
              Damage to coccyx
              Separation of symphysis (pubis)
          **CC Excl: For code 665.61:** 646.80-646.93, 648.90-650, 655.70-655.73,
          665.00-665.11, 665.50-665.54, 665.61, 665.80-665.94, 669.40-669.44,
          669.80-669.94
          **AHA:** N-D, '84, 12

§ ✓5th **665.7** **Pelvic hematoma** CC 1,2 Ⓜ♀
[0,1,2,4]    Hematoma of vagina
          **CC Excl: For code 665.71:** 646.80-646.93, 648.90-650, 655.70-655.73,
          665.00-665.11, 665.50-665.54, 665.71, 665.80-665.94, 669.40-669.44,
          669.80-669.94; **For code 665.72:** 646.80-646.93, 648.90-650, 655.70-
          655.73, 665.00-665.11, 665.50-665.54, 665.72, 665.80-665.94, 669.40-
          669.44, 669.80-669.94

§ ✓5th **665.8** **Other specified obstetrical trauma** Ⓜ♀
[0-4]

§ ✓5th **665.9** **Unspecified obstetrical trauma** Ⓜ♀
[0-4]

✓4th **666** **Postpartum hemorrhage**
          **AHA:** 1Q, '88, 14

§ ✓5th **666.0** **Third-stage hemorrhage** CC 2,4 Ⓜ♀
[0,2,4]      Hemorrhage associated with retained, trapped, or
              adherent placenta
              Retained placenta NOS
          **CC Excl: For code 666.02:** 646.80-646.93, 648.90-650, 655.70-655.73,
          665.00-665.11, 665.50-665.54, 665.80-665.94, 666.02, 669.40-669.44,
          669.80-669.94; **For code 666.04:** 646.80-646.93, 648.90-650, 655.70-
          655.73, 665.00-665.11, 665.50-665.54, 665.80-665.94, 666.04, 669.40-
          669.44, 669.80-669.94

§ ✓5th **666.1** **Other immediate postpartum** CC 2,4 Ⓜ♀
[0,2,4]      **hemorrhage**
              Atony of uterus with hemorrhage
              Hemorrhage within the first 24 hours following
                  delivery of placenta
              ▶Postpartum atony of uterus with hemorrhage◀
              Postpartum hemorrhage (atonic) NOS
          **EXCLUDES** *atony of uterus without hemorrhage*
              ▶*(661.2)*
              *postpartum atony of uterus without
              hemorrhage (669.8)*◀
          **CC Excl: For code 666.12:** 646.80-646.93, 648.90-650, 655.70-655.73,
          665.00-665.11, 665.50-665.54, 665.80-665.94, 666.12, 669.40-669.44,
          669.80-669.94; **For code 666.14:** 666.10-666.14

§ Requires fifth-digit. Valid digits are in [brackets] under each code. See beginning of section 640-649 for codes and definitions.

Ⓝ Newborn Age: 0    Ⓟ Pediatric Age: 0-17    Ⓜ Maternity Age: 12-55    Ⓐ Adult Age: 15-124    CC CC Condition    MCC Major CC Condition    HIV HIV Related Dx

§ ✓5ᵗʰ **666.2 Delayed and secondary postpartum**   `CC 2,4` `M` ♀
[0,2,4] **hemorrhage**
    Hemorrhage:
      after the first 24 hours following delivery
      associated with retained portions of placenta or
        membranes
    Postpartum hemorrhage specified as delayed or
      secondary
    Retained products of conception NOS, following
      delivery

    **CC Excl: For code 666.22:** 646.80-646.93, 648.90-650, 655.70-655.73,
    665.00-665.11, 665.50-665.54, 665.80-665.94, 666.22, 669.40-669.44,
    669.80-669.94; **For code 666.24:** 666.20-666.24

§ ✓5ᵗʰ **666.3 Postpartum coagulation defects**   `CC 2` `M` ♀
[0,2,4]     Postpartum:       Postpartum:
      afibrinogenemia       fibrinolysis

    **CC Excl: For code 666.32:** 646.80-646.93, 648.90-650, 666.00-666.34,
    669.40-669.44, 669.80-669.94

✓4ᵗʰ **667 Retained placenta or membranes, without hemorrhage**
    **AHA:** 1Q, '88, 14

    **DEF:** Postpartum condition resulting from failure to expel placental membrane
    tissues due to failed contractions of uterine wall.

§ ✓5ᵗʰ **667.0 Retained placenta without hemorrhage**   `M` ♀
[0,2,4]     Placenta accreta
    Retained placenta:  ⎫ without
      NOS         ⎬ hemorrhage
      total        ⎭

§ ✓5ᵗʰ **667.1 Retained portions of placenta or membranes,**   `M` ♀
[0,2,4] **without hemorrhage**
    Retained products of conception following delivery,
      without hemorrhage

✓4ᵗʰ **668 Complications of the administration of anesthetic or other**
**sedation in labor and delivery**
    `INCLUDES` complications arising from the administration
      of a general or local anesthetic, analgesic,
      or other sedation in labor and delivery
    `EXCLUDES` *reaction to spinal or lumbar puncture (349.0)*
      *spinal headache (349.0)*
    Use additional code(s) to further specify complication

§ ✓5ᵗʰ **668.0 Pulmonary complications**   `M` ♀
[0-4]     Inhalation [aspiration] of  ⎫
      stomach contents    ⎬ following anesthesia
      or secretions        ⎬ or other
    Mendelson's syndrome   ⎬ sedation in labor
    Pressure collapse of lung ⎭ or delivery

§ ✓5ᵗʰ **668.1 Cardiac complications**   `M` ♀
[0-4]     Cardiac arrest or failure following anesthesia or
      other sedation in labor and delivery

§ ✓5ᵗʰ **668.2 Central nervous system complications**   `M` ♀
[0-4]     Cerebral anoxia following anesthesia or other
      sedation in labor and delivery

§ ✓5ᵗʰ **668.8 Other complications of anesthesia or**   `M` ♀
[0-4] **other sedation in labor and delivery**
    **AHA:** 2Q, '99, 9

§ ✓5ᵗʰ **668.9 Unspecified complication of anesthesia**   `M` ♀
[0-4] **and other sedation**

✓4ᵗʰ **669 Other complications of labor and delivery, not elsewhere**
**classified**

§ ✓5ᵗʰ **669.0 Maternal distress**   `M` ♀
[0-4]     Metabolic disturbance in labor and delivery

§ ✓5ᵗʰ **669.1 Shock during or following labor and**   `MCC 1-4` `M` ♀
[0-4] **delivery**
    Obstetric shock

    **CC Excl: For codes 669.11-669.14:** 646.80-646.93, 648.90-650, 669.10-
    669.14, 669.40-669.44, 669.80-669.94

§ ✓5ᵗʰ **669.2 Maternal hypotension syndrome**   `MCC 1-2` `CC 4`
[0-4]                              `M` ♀

    **CC Excl: For code 669.21:** 646.80-646.93, 648.90-650, 669.10-669.14,
    669.21, 669.40-669.44, 669.80-669.94; **For code 669.22:** 646.80-646.93,
    648.90-650, 669.10-669.14, 669.22, 669.40-669.44, 669.80-669.94; **For**
    **code 669.24:** 646.80-646.93, 648.90-650, 669.10-669.14, 669.24, 669.40-
    669.44, 669.80-669.94

    **DEF:** Low arterial blood pressure, in mother, during labor and
    delivery.

§ ✓5ᵗʰ **669.3 Acute renal failure following labor and**   `MCC 2,4`
[0,2,4] **delivery**                             `M` ♀
    **CC Excl: For codes 669.32, 669.34:** 646.80-646.93, 648.90-650, 669.30-
    669.44, 669.80-669.94

§ ✓5ᵗʰ **669.4 Other complications of obstetrical surgery**   `M` ♀
[0-4] **and procedures**
    Cardiac:    ⎫ following cesarean or other
      arrest    ⎬ obstetrical surgery or
      failure    ⎬ procedure, including
    Cerebral anoxia ⎭ delivery NOS

    `EXCLUDES` *complications of obstetrical surgical*
      *wounds (674.1-674.3)*

§ ✓5ᵗʰ **669.5 Forceps or vacuum extractor delivery**   `M` ♀
[0,1] **without mention of indication**
    Delivery by ventouse, without mention of indication

§ ✓5ᵗʰ **669.6 Breech extraction, without mention of**   `M` ♀
[0,1] **indication**
    `EXCLUDES` *breech delivery NOS (652.2)*

§ ✓5ᵗʰ **669.7 Cesarean delivery, without mention of**   `M` ♀
[0,1] **indication**
    **AHA: For code 669.71:** 1Q, '01, 11

§ ✓5ᵗʰ **669.8 Other complications of labor and delivery**   `M` ♀
[0-4]

    **AHA:** 4Q, '06, 135

§ ✓5ᵗʰ **669.9 Unspecified complication of labor and delivery** `M` ♀
[0-4]

---

§ Requires fifth-digit. Valid digits are in [brackets] under each code. See beginning of section 640-649 for codes and definitions.

✓4ᵗʰ
✓5ᵗʰ Additional Digit Required     Unacceptable PDx     `Manifestation Code`     ▶◀ Revised Text     ● New Code     ▲ Revised Code Title

 © **2007 Ingenix**          **October 2007 • Volume 1 — 221**

**Complications of Pregnancy, Childbirth & Puerperium**

**670–674.2**

## COMPLICATIONS OF THE PUERPERIUM (670-677)

Note: Categories 671 and 673-676 include the listed conditions even if they occur during pregnancy or childbirth.

The following fifth-digit subclassification is for use with categories 670-676 to denote the current episode of care. Valid fifth-digits are in [brackets] under each code.

0 unspecified as to episode of care or not applicable
1 delivered, with or without mention of antepartum condition
2 delivered, with mention of postpartum complication
3 antepartum condition or complication
4 postpartum condition or complication

✓4ᵗʰ **670 Major puerperal infection** MCC 2,4 M ♀
[0,2,4]
§ ✓5ᵗʰ Use 0 as fourth-digit for this category

Puerperal:                    Puerperal:
  endometritis                  peritonitis
  fever (septic)                pyemia
  pelvic:                       salpingitis
    cellulitis                  septicemia
  sepsis

EXCLUDES    infection following abortion (639.0)
            minor genital tract infection following delivery (646.6)
            puerperal pyrexia NOS (672)
            puerperal fever NOS (672)
            puerperal pyrexia of unknown origin (672)
            urinary tract infection following delivery (646.6)

CC Excl: For code 670.02, 670.04: 646.80-646.93, 648.90-650, 669.40-669.44, 669.80-670.04

AHA: 4Q, '91, 26; 2Q, '91, 7

DEF: Infection and inflammation, following childbirth.

✓4ᵗʰ **671 Venous complications in pregnancy and the puerperium**
§ ✓5ᵗʰ **671.0 Varicose veins of legs** M ♀
[0-4]        Varicose veins NOS
             DEF: Distended, tortuous veins on legs associated with pregnancy.

§ ✓5ᵗʰ **671.1 Varicose veins of vulva and perineum** M ♀
[0-4]
             DEF: Distended, tortuous veins on external female genitalia associated with pregnancy.

§ ✓5ᵗʰ **671.2 Superficial thrombophlebitis** CC M ♀
[0-4]        Thrombophlebitis (superficial)
             CC Excl: 646.80-646.93, 648.90-650, 669.40-669.44, 669.80-669.94, 671.20-671.94

§ ✓5ᵗʰ **671.3 Deep phlebothrombosis, antepartum** MCC 1,3 CC 0
[0,1,3]      Deep vein thrombosis antepartum        M ♀
             CC Excl: See code: 671.2

§ ✓5ᵗʰ **671.4 Deep phlebothrombosis, postpartum** MCC 2,4
[0,2,4]      Deep-vein thrombosis, postpartum       CC 0 M ♀
             Pelvic thrombophlebitis, postpartum
             Phlegmasia alba dolens (puerperal)
             CC Excl: See code: 671.2

§ ✓5ᵗʰ **671.5 Other phlebitis and thrombosis** CC M ♀
[0-4]        Cerebral venous thrombosis
             Thrombosis of intracranial venous sinus
             CC Excl: See code: 671.2

§ ✓5ᵗʰ **671.8 Other venous complications** CC M ♀
[0-4]        Hemorrhoids
             CC Excl: For codes 671.80-671.83: 646.80-646.93, 648.90-650, 669.40-669.44, 669.80-669.94, 671.20-671.94; For code 671.84: 671.80-671.84

§ ✓5ᵗʰ **671.9 Unspecified venous complication** CC 0-2 M ♀
[0-4]        Phlebitis NOS
             Thrombosis NOS
             CC Excl: For code 671.90-671.92: 646.80-646.93, 648.90-650, 669.40-669.44, 669.80-669.94, 671.20-671.94

✓4ᵗʰ **672 Pyrexia of unknown origin during the puerperium** CC 2,4
[0,2,4]                                                         M ♀
§ ✓5ᵗʰ Use 0 as fourth-digit for this category

Postpartum fever NOS
Puerperal fever NOS
Puerperal pyrexia NOS

CC Excl: For code 672.02: 646.80-646.93, 648.90-650, 669.40-669.44, 669.80-669.94, 671.20, 671.23-671.30, 671.33-671.40, 671.50, 671.53-671.80, 671.83-671.90, 671.93-671.94, 672.02; For code 672.04: 672.02-672.04

AHA: 4Q, '91, 26

DEF: Fever of unknown origin experienced by the mother after childbirth.

✓4ᵗʰ **673 Obstetrical pulmonary embolism**
INCLUDES   pulmonary emboli in pregnancy, childbirth, or the puerperium, or specified as puerperal
EXCLUDES   embolism following abortion (639.6)

§ ✓5ᵗʰ **673.0 Obstetrical air embolism** MCC 1-4 M ♀
[0-4]
             CC Excl: 646.80-646.93, 648.90-650, 669.40-669.44, 669.80-669.94, 673.00-673.84
             DEF: Sudden blocking of pulmonary artery with air or nitrogen bubbles during puerperium.

§ ✓5ᵗʰ **673.1 Amniotic fluid embolism** MCC 1-4 M ♀
[0-4]        CC Excl: For code 673.11-673.14: See code: 673.0
             DEF: Sudden onset of pulmonary artery blockage from amniotic fluid entering the mother's circulation near the end of pregnancy due to strong uterine contractions.

§ ✓5ᵗʰ **673.2 Obstetrical blood-clot embolism** MCC 1-4 M ♀
[0-4]        Puerperal pulmonary embolism NOS
             CC Excl: For code 673.21-673.24: See code: 673.0
             AHA: For code 673.24: 1Q, '05, 6
             DEF: Blood clot blocking artery in the lung; associated with pregnancy.

§ ✓5ᵗʰ **673.3 Obstetrical pyemic and septic embolism** MCC 1-4
[0-4]        CC Excl: See code: 673.0                         CC 0 M ♀

§ ✓5ᵗʰ **673.8 Other pulmonary embolism** MCC 1-4 M ♀
[0-4]        Fat embolism
             CC Excl: For code 673.81-673.84: See code: 673.0

✓4ᵗʰ **674 Other and unspecified complications of the puerperium, not elsewhere classified**
§ ✓5ᵗʰ **674.0 Cerebrovascular disorders in the** MCC 1
[0-4]        **puerperium**                          CC 2-4 M ♀
             Any condition classifiable to 430-434, 436-437 occurring during pregnancy, childbirth, or the puerperium, or specified as puerperal
             EXCLUDES    intracranial venous sinus thrombosis (671.5)
             CC Excl: For code 674.01-674.04: 646.80-646.93, 648.90-650, 669.40-669.44, 669.80-669.94, 674.00-674.04, 674.50-674.54

§ ✓5ᵗʰ **674.1 Disruption of cesarean wound** M ♀
[0,2,4]      Dehiscence or disruption of uterine wound
             EXCLUDES    uterine rupture before onset of labor (665.0)
                         uterine rupture during labor (665.1)

§ ✓5ᵗʰ **674.2 Disruption of perineal wound** M ♀
[0,2,4]      Breakdown of perineum
             Disruption of wound of:
               episiotomy
               perineal laceration
             Secondary perineal tear
             AHA: For code 674.24: 1Q, '97, 9

§ Requires fifth-digit. Valid digits are in [brackets] under each code. See beginning of section 640-649 for codes and definitions.

N Newborn Age: 0    P Pediatric Age: 0-17    M Maternity Age: 12-55    A Adult Age: 15-124    CC CC Condition    MCC Major CC Condition    HIV HIV Related Dx

§ ✓5ᵗʰ **674.3 Other complications of obstetrical surgical** Ⓜ ♀
  [0,2,4]   **wounds**

Hematoma ⎫
Hemorrhage ⎬ of cesarean section or perineal
Infection ⎭      wound

**EXCLUDES**   damage from instruments in delivery
           (664.0-665.9)

**AHA:** 2Q, '91, 7

§ ✓5ᵗʰ **674.4 Placental polyp** Ⓜ ♀
  [0,2,4]

§ ✓5ᵗʰ **674.5 Peripartum cardiomyopathy** MCC Ⓜ ♀
  [0-4]      Postpartum cardiomyopathy

**CC Excl:** See code: 674.01

**AHA:** 4Q, '03, 65

**DEF:** Any structural or functional abnormality of the ventricular
myocardium, non-inflammatory disease of obscure or unknown
etiology with onset during the postpartum period.

§ ✓5ᵗʰ **674.8 Other** Ⓜ ♀
  [0,2,4]     Hepatorenal syndrome, following delivery
          Postpartum:
            subinvolution of uterus
            uterine hypertrophy

**AHA:** 3Q, '98, 16

§ ✓5ᵗʰ **674.9 Unspecified** Ⓜ ♀
  [0,2,4]     Sudden death of unknown cause during the
           puerperium

✓4ᵗʰ **675 Infections of the breast and nipple associated with**
**childbirth**

**INCLUDES**   the listed conditions during pregnancy,
           childbirth, or the puerperium

§ ✓5ᵗʰ **675.0 Infections of nipple** Ⓜ ♀
  [0-4]    Abscess of nipple

§ ✓5ᵗʰ **675.1 Abscess of breast** CC 1,2 Ⓜ ♀
  [0-4]     Abscess:
          mammary
          subareolar
          submammary
          purulent
          retromammary
          submammary

**CC Excl:** For codes 675.11-675.12: 646.80-646.93, 648.90-650, 669.40-
669.44, 669.80-669.94, 675.00-675.94

§ ✓5ᵗʰ **675.2 Nonpurulent mastitis** Ⓜ ♀
  [0-4]     Lymphangitis of breast
          Mastitis:
            NOS
            interstitial
            parenchymatous

§ ✓5ᵗʰ **675.8 Other specified infections of the breast and** Ⓜ ♀
  [0-4]   **nipple**

§ ✓5ᵗʰ **675.9 Unspecified infection of the breast and nipple** Ⓜ ♀
  [0-4]

✓4ᵗʰ **676 Other disorders of the breast associated with childbirth and**
**disorders of lactation**

**INCLUDES**   the listed conditions during pregnancy, the
           puerperium, or lactation

**Lactation Process: Ejection Reflex Arc**

§ ✓5ᵗʰ **676.0 Retracted nipple** Ⓜ ♀
  [0-4]

§ ✓5ᵗʰ **676.1 Cracked nipple** Ⓜ ♀
  [0-4]    Fissure of nipple

§ ✓5ᵗʰ **676.2 Engorgement of breasts** Ⓜ ♀
  [0-4]

**DEF:** Abnormal accumulation of milk in ducts of breast.

§ ✓5ᵗʰ **676.3 Other and unspecified disorder of breast** Ⓜ ♀
  [0-4]

§ ✓5ᵗʰ **676.4 Failure of lactation** Ⓜ ♀
  [0-4]    Agalactia

**DEF:** Abrupt ceasing of milk secretion by breast.

§ ✓5ᵗʰ **676.5 Suppressed lactation** Ⓜ ♀
  [0-4]

§ ✓5ᵗʰ **676.6 Galactorrhea** Ⓜ ♀
  [0-4]     **EXCLUDES**   galactorrhea not associated with
               childbirth (611.6)

**DEF:** Excessive or persistent milk secretion by breast; may be in
absence of nursing.

§ ✓5ᵗʰ **676.8 Other disorders of lactation** Ⓜ ♀
  [0-4]    Galactocele

**DEF:** Galactocele: Obstructed mammary gland, creating retention
cyst, results in milk-filled cysts enlarging mammary gland.

§ ✓5ᵗʰ **676.9 Unspecified disorder of lactation** Ⓜ ♀
  [0-4]

**677 Late effect of complication of pregnancy, childbirth,** ♀
**and the puerperium**

**Note:** This category is to be used to indicate conditions in
632-648.9 and 651-676.9 as the cause of the late
effect, themselves classifiable elsewhere. The "late
effects" include conditions specified as such, or as
sequelae, which may occur at any time after
puerperium.
**Code first** any sequelae

**AHA:** 1Q, '97, 9; 4Q, '94, 42

§   Requires fifth-digit. Valid digits are in [brackets] under each code. See beginning of section 640-649 for codes and definitions.

# 12. DISEASES OF THE SKIN AND SUBCUTANEOUS TISSUE
## (680-709)

**Skin and Subcutaneous Layer**

## INFECTIONS OF SKIN AND SUBCUTANEOUS TISSUE (680-686)

> EXCLUDES   *certain infections of skin classified under "Infectious and Parasitic Diseases," such as:*
> *erysipelas (035)*
> *erysipeloid of Rosenbach (027.1)*
> *herpes:*
> *simplex (054.0-054.9)*
> *zoster (053.0-053.9)*
> *molluscum contagiosum (078.0)*
> *viral warts (078.1)*

### ✓4th 680 Carbuncle and furuncle

> INCLUDES   boil
> furunculosis

**DEF:** Carbuncle: necrotic boils in skin and subcutaneous tissue of neck or back mainly due to staphylococcal infection.

**DEF:** Furuncle: circumscribed inflammation of corium and subcutaneous tissue due to staphylococcal infection.

#### 680.0   Face
Ear [any part]
Face [any part, except eye]
Nose (septum)
Temple (region)
> EXCLUDES   *eyelid (373.13)*
> *lacrimal apparatus (375.31)*
> *orbit (376.01)*

#### 680.1   Neck
#### 680.2   Trunk
Abdominal wall
Back [any part, except buttocks]
Breast
Chest wall
Flank
Groin
Pectoral region
Perineum
Umbilicus
> EXCLUDES   *buttocks (680.5)*
> *external genital organs:*
> *female (616.4)*
> *male (607.2, 608.4)*

#### 680.3   Upper arm and forearm
Arm [any part, except hand]
Axilla
Shoulder
#### 680.4   Hand
Finger [any]
Thumb
Wrist
#### 680.5   Buttock
Anus
Gluteal region
#### 680.6   Leg, except foot
Ankle            Knee
Hip              Thigh
#### 680.7   Foot
Heel
Toe
#### 680.8   Other specified sites
Head [any part, except face]
Scalp
> EXCLUDES   *external genital organs:*
> *female (616.4)*
> *male (607.2, 608.4)*

#### 680.9   Unspecified site
Boil NOS              Furuncle NOS
Carbuncle NOS

### ✓4th 681 Cellulitis and abscess of finger and toe
> INCLUDES   that with lymphangitis
Use additional code to identify organism, such as Staphylococcus (041.1)

**AHA:** 2Q, '91, 5; J-F, '87, 12

**DEF:** Acute suppurative inflammation and edema in subcutaneous tissue or muscle of finger or toe.

#### ✓5th 681.0   Finger
##### 681.00   Cellulitis and abscess, unspecified
##### 681.01   Felon
Pulp abscess        Whitlow
> EXCLUDES   *herpetic whitlow (054.6)*

**DEF:** Painful abscess of fingertips caused by infection in the closed space of terminal phalanx.

##### 681.02   Onychia and paronychia of finger
Panaritium  } of finger
Perionychia }

**DEF:** Onychia: inflammation of nail matrix; causes nail loss.

**DEF:** Paronychia: inflammation of tissue folds around nail.

#### ✓5th 681.1   Toe
##### 681.10   Cellulitis and abscess, unspecified
**AHA:** 1Q, '05, 14

##### 681.11   Onychia and paronychia of toe
Panaritium  } of toe
Perionychia }

**Skin and Subcutaneous Tissue**

**681.9—684**

**681.9**    **Cellulitis and abscess of unspecified digit**
Infection of nail NOS

✓4ᵗʰ **682** **Other cellulitis and abscess**

| INCLUDES | abscess (acute) | (with lymphangitis) |
|---|---|---|
| | cellulitis (diffuse) | except of |
| | lymphangitis, acute | finger or toe |

Use additional code to identify organism, such as
Staphylococcus (041.1)

**EXCLUDES**   *lymphangitis (chronic) (subacute) (457.2)*

**AHA:** 2Q, '91, 5; J-F, '87, 12; S-O, '85, 10

**DEF:** Cellulitis: Acute suppurative inflammation of deep subcutaneous tissue and sometimes muscle due to infection of wound, burn or other lesion.

**682.0**    **Face**      `CC`

| Cheek, external | Nose, external |
|---|---|
| Chin | Submandibular |
| Forehead | Temple (region) |

**EXCLUDES**   *ear [any part] (380.10-380.16)*
*eyelid (373.13)*
*lacrimal apparatus (375.31)*
*lip (528.5)*
*mouth (528.3)*
*nose (internal) (478.1)*
*orbit (376.01)*

**CC Excl:** 017.00-017.06, 017.90-017.96, 040.82-041.9, 682.0, 682.8-682.9, 686.00-686.9, 705.83, 709.8, V09.0-V09.91

**682.1**    **Neck**      `CC`

**CC Excl:** 017.00-017.06, 017.90-017.96, 040.82-041.9, 682.1, 682.8-682.9, 686.00-686.9, 705.83, 709.8, V09.0-V09.91

**682.2**    **Trunk**      `CC`

| Abdominal wall | Groin |
|---|---|
| Back [any part, except | Pectoral region |
| buttock] | Perineum |
| Chest wall | Umbilicus, except newborn |
| Flank | |

**EXCLUDES**   *anal and rectal regions (566)*
*breast:*
  *NOS (611.0)*
  *puerperal (675.1)*
*external genital organs:*
  *female (616.3-616.4)*
  *male (604.0, 607.2, 608.4)*
*umbilicus, newborn (771.4)*

**CC Excl:** 017.00-017.06, 017.90-017.96, 040.82-041.9, 682.2, 682.8-682.9, 686.00-686.9, 705.83, 709.8, V09.0-V09.91

**AHA:** 4Q, '98, 42

**682.3**    **Upper arm and forearm**      `CC`
Arm [any part, except hand]
Axilla
Shoulder

**EXCLUDES**   *hand (682.4)*

**CC Excl:** 017.00-017.06, 017.90-017.96, 040.82-041.9, 682.3, 682.8-682.9, 686.00-686.9, 705.83, 709.8, V09.0-V09.91

**AHA:** 2Q, '03, 7

**682.4**    **Hand, except fingers and thumb**      `CC`
Wrist

**EXCLUDES**   *finger and thumb (681.00-681.02)*

**CC Excl:** 017.00-017.06, 017.90-017.96, 040.82-041.9, 682.4, 682.8-682.9, 686.00-686.9, 705.83, 709.8, V09.0-V09.91

**682.5**    **Buttock**      `CC`
Gluteal region

**EXCLUDES**   *anal and rectal regions (566)*

**CC Excl:** 017.00-017.06, 017.90-017.96, 040.82-041.9, 682.5, 682.8-682.9, 686.00-686.9, 705.83, 709.8, V09.0-V09.91

**682.6**    **Leg, except foot**      `CC`

| Ankle | Knee |
|---|---|
| Hip | Thigh |

**CC Excl:** 017.00-017.06, 017.90-017.96, 040.82-041.9, 682.6, 682.8-682.9, 686.00-686.9, 705.83, 709.8, V09.0-V09.91

**AHA:** 3Q, '04, 5; 4Q, '03, 108

**682.7**    **Foot, except toes**      `CC`
Heel

**EXCLUDES**   *toe (681.10-681.11)*

**CC Excl:** 017.00-017.06, 017.90-017.96, 040.82-041.9, 682.7-682.9, 686.00-686.9, 705.83, 709.8, V09.0-V09.91

**682.8**    **Other specified sites**      `CC`
Head [except face]
Scalp

**EXCLUDES**   *face (682.0)*

**CC Excl:** 017.00-017.06, 017.90-017.96, 040.82-041.9, 682.8-682.9, 686.00-686.9, 705.83, 709.8, V09.0-V09.91

**682.9**    **Unspecified site**      `CC`

| Abscess NOS | Lymphangitis, acute NOS |
|---|---|
| Cellulitis NOS | |

**EXCLUDES**   *lymphangitis NOS (457.2)*

**CC Excl:** See code: 682.8

**683 Acute lymphadenitis**

| Abscess (acute) | lymph gland or node, |
|---|---|
| Adenitis, acute | except mesenteric |
| Lymphadenitis, acute | |

Use additional code to identify organism, such as
Staphylococcus (041.1)

**EXCLUDES**   *enlarged glands NOS (785.6)*
*lymphadenitis:*
  *chronic or subacute, except mesenteric*
   *(289.1)*
  *mesenteric (acute) (chronic) (subacute)*
   *(289.2)*
  *unspecified (289.3)*

**DEF:** Acute inflammation of lymph nodes due to primary infection located elsewhere in the body.

**684 Impetigo**
Impetiginization of other dermatoses
Impetigo (contagiosa) [any site] [any organism]:
  bullous
  circinate
  neonatorum
  simplex
Pemphigus neonatorum

**EXCLUDES**   *impetigo herpetiformis (694.3)*

**DEF:** Infectious skin disease commonly occurring in children; caused by group A streptococci or *Staphylococcus aureus*; skin lesions usually appear on the face and consist of subcorneal vesicles and bullae that burst and form yellow crusts.

**Lymphatic System of Head and Neck**

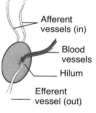

Afferent vessels (in)
Blood vessels
Hilum
Efferent vessel (out)
Schematic of lymph node
Jugulodigastric
Submental
Submandibular
Jugulomyohyoid
Anterior cervical
Superficial parotid
Occipital

**Lymphatic drainage of the head, neck, and face**

| N | Newborn Age: 0 | P | Pediatric Age: 0-17 | M | Maternity Age: 12-55 | A | Adult Age: 15-124 | `CC` CC Condition | `MCC` Major CC Condition | `HIV` HIV Related Dx |

**226 — Volume 1 • October 2007**      **© 2007 Ingenix**

### Stages of Pilonidal Disease

- Normal follicle
- Stretched follicle
- Infected follicle
- Acute abscess
- Chronic abscess
- Epithelial tube

✓4th **685 Pilonidal cyst**

INCLUDES   fistula } coccygeal or pilonidal
sinus

DEF: Hair-containing cyst or sinus in the tissues of the sacrococcygeal area; often drains through opening at the postanal dimple.

**685.0 With abscess** CC
CC Excl: 685.0-685.1, 709.8

**685.1 Without mention of abscess**

✓4th **686 Other local infections of skin and subcutaneous tissue**
Use additional code to identify any infectious organism (041.0-041.8)

✓5th **686.0 Pyoderma**
Dermatitis:       Dermatitis:
purulent          suppurative
septic

DEF: Nonspecific purulent skin disease related most to furuncles, pustules, or possibly carbuncles.

**686.00 Pyoderma, unspecified**

**686.01 Pyoderma gangrenosum** CC
CC Excl: 686.00-686.09

AHA: 4Q, '97, 42

DEF: Persistent debilitating skin disease, characterized by irregular, boggy, blue-red ulcerations, with central healing and undermined edges.

**686.09 Other pyoderma**

**686.1 Pyogenic granuloma**
Granuloma:
septic
suppurative
telangiectaticum
EXCLUDES   *pyogenic granuloma of oral mucosa (528.9)*

DEF: Solitary polypoid capillary hemangioma often asociated with local irritation, trauma, and superimposed inflammation; located on the skin and gingival or oral mucosa.

**686.8 Other specified local infections of skin and subcutaneous tissue**
Bacterid (pustular)       Ecthyma
Dermatitis vegetans       Perlèche
EXCLUDES   *dermatitis infectiosa eczematoides (690.8)*
*panniculitis (729.30-729.39)*

**686.9 Unspecified local infection of skin and subcutaneous tissue**
Fistula of skin NOS
Skin infection NOS
EXCLUDES   *fistula to skin from internal organs — see Alphabetic Index*

## OTHER INFLAMMATORY CONDITIONS OF SKIN AND SUBCUTANEOUS TISSUE (690-698)
EXCLUDES   *panniculitis (729.30-729.39)*

✓4th **690 Erythematosquamous dermatosis**
EXCLUDES   *eczematous dermatitis of eyelid (373.31)*
*parakeratosis variegata (696.2)*
*psoriasis (696.0-696.1)*
*seborrheic keratosis (702.11-702.19)*

✓5th **690.1 Seborrheic dermatitis**
AHA: 4Q, '95, 58

**690.10 Seborrheic dermatitis, unspecified**
Seborrheic dermatitis NOS

**690.11 Seborrhea capitis** P
Cradle cap

**690.12 Seborrheic infantile dermatitis** P

**690.18 Other seborrheic dermatitis**

**690.8 Other erythematosquamous dermatosis**

✓4th **691 Atopic dermatitis and related conditions**
DEF: Atopic dermatitis: chronic, pruritic, inflammatory skin disorder found on the face and antecubital and popliteal fossae; noted in persons with a hereditary predisposition to pruritus, and often accompanied by allergic rhinitis, hay fever, asthma, and extreme itching; also called allergic dermatitis, allergic or atopic eczema, or disseminated neurodermatitis.

**691.0 Diaper or napkin rash**
Ammonia dermatitis       Diaper or napkin:
Diaper or napkin:          rash
dermatitis             Psoriasiform napkin eruption
erythema

**691.8 Other atopic dermatitis and related conditions**
Atopic dermatitis       Eczema:
Besnier's prurigo          intrinsic (allergic)
Eczema:                 Neurodermatitis:
atopic                 atopic
flexural               diffuse (of Brocq)

✓4th **692 Contact dermatitis and other eczema**
INCLUDES   dermatitis:       eczema (acute) (chronic):
NOS                NOS
contact            allergic
occupational       erythematous
venenata           occupational
EXCLUDES   *allergy NOS (995.3)*
*contact dermatitis of eyelids (373.32)*
*dermatitis due to substances taken internally (693.0-693.9)*
*eczema of external ear (380.22)*
*perioral dermatitis (695.3)*
*urticarial reactions (708.0-708.9, 995.1)*

DEF: Contact dermatitis: acute or chronic dermatitis caused by initial irritant effect of a substance, or by prior sensitization to a substance coming once again in contact with skin.

**692.0 Due to detergents**

**692.1 Due to oils and greases**

**692.2 Due to solvents**
Dermatitis due to solvents of:
chlorocompound
cyclohexane
ester                  } group
glycol
hydrocarbon
ketone

**692.3 Due to drugs and medicines in contact with skin**

Dermatitis (allergic) (contact) due to:
- arnica
- fungicides
- iodine
- keratolytics
- mercurials

Dermatitis (allergic) (contact) due to:
- neomycin
- pediculocides
- phenols
- scabicides
- any drug applied to skin

Dermatitis medicamentosa due to drug applied to skin

Use additional E code to identify drug

EXCLUDES  allergy NOS due to drugs (995.27)
dermatitis due to ingested drugs (693.0)
dermatitis medicamentosa NOS (693.0)

**692.4 Due to other chemical products**

Dermatitis due to:
- acids
- adhesive plaster
- alkalis
- caustics
- dichromate
- insecticide
- nylon
- plastic
- rubber

AHA: 2Q, '89, 16

**692.5 Due to food in contact with skin**

Dermatitis, contact, due to:
- cereals
- fish
- flour

Dermatitis, contact, due to:
- fruit
- meat
- milk

EXCLUDES  dermatitis due to:
dyes (692.89)
ingested foods (693.1)
preservatives (692.89)

**692.6 Due to plants [except food]**

Dermatitis due to:
- lacquer tree [Rhus verniciflua]
- poison:
  - ivy [Rhus toxicodendron]
  - oak [Rhus diversiloba]
  - sumac [Rhus venenata]
  - vine [Rhus radicans]
- primrose [Primula]
- ragweed [Senecio jacobae]
- other plants in contact with the skin

EXCLUDES  allergy NOS due to pollen (477.0)
nettle rash (708.8)

**√5ᵗʰ 692.7 Due to solar radiation**

EXCLUDES  sunburn due to other ultraviolet radiation exposure (692.82)

**692.70 Unspecified dermatitis due to sun**

**692.71 Sunburn**

First degree sunburn
Sunburn NOS

AHA: 4Q, '01, 47

**692.72 Acute dermatitis due to solar radiation**

Acute solar skin damage NOS
Berloque dermatitis
Photoallergic response
Phototoxic response
Polymorphus light eruption

EXCLUDES  sunburn (692.71, 692.76-692.77)

Use additional E code to identify drug, if drug induced

DEF: Berloque dermatitis: Phytophotodermatitis due to sun exposure after use of a product containing bergamot oil; causes red patches, which may turn brown.

DEF: Photoallergic response: Dermatitis due to hypersensitivity to the sun; causes papulovesicular, eczematous or exudative eruptions.

DEF: Phototoxic response: Chemically induced sensitivity to sun causes burn-like reaction, occasionally vesiculation and subsequent hyperpigmentation.

DEF: Polymorphous light eruption: Inflammatory skin eruptions due to sunlight exposure; eruptions differ in size and shape.

DEF: Acute solar skin damage (NOS): Rapid, unspecified injury to skin from sun.

**692.73 Actinic reticuloid and actinic granuloma**

DEF: Actinic reticuloid: Dermatosis aggravated by light, causes chronic eczema-like eruption on exposed skin which extends to other unexposed surfaces; occurs in the eldery.

DEF: Actinic granuloma: Inflammatory response of skin to sun causing small nodule of microphages.

**692.74 Other chronic dermatitis due to solar radiation**

Chronic solar skin damage NOS
Solar elastosis

EXCLUDES  actinic [solar] keratosis (702.0)

DEF: Solar elastosis: Premature aging of skin of light-skinned people; causes inelasticity, thinning or thickening, wrinkling, dryness, scaling and hyperpigmentation.

DEF: Chronic solar skin damage (NOS): Chronic skin impairment due to exposure to the sun, not otherwise specified.

**692.75 Disseminated superficial actinic porokeratosis [DSAP]**

DEF: Autosomal dominant skin condition occurring in skin that has been overexposed to the sun. Primarily affects women over the age of 16; characterized by numerous superficial annular, keratotic, brownish-red spots or thickenings with depressed centers and sharp, ridged borders. High risk that condition will evolve into squamous cell carcinoma.

AHA: 4Q, '00, 43

**692.76 Sunburn of second degree**

AHA: 4Q, '01, 47

**692.77 Sunburn of third degree**

AHA: 4Q, '01, 47

**692.79 Other dermatitis due to solar radiation**

Hydroa aestivale
Photodermatitis
Photosensitiveness } (due to sun)
Solar skin damage NOS

**√5ᵗʰ 692.8 Due to other specified agents**

**692.81 Dermatitis due to cosmetics**

**692.82 Dermatitis due to other radiation**

Infrared rays
Light, except from sun
Radiation NOS
Tanning bed
Ultraviolet rays, except from sun
X-rays

EXCLUDES  solar radiation (692.70-692.79)

AHA: 4Q, '01, 47; 3Q, '00, 5

**692.83 Dermatitis due to metals**

Jewelry

N Newborn Age: 0   P Pediatric Age: 0-17   M Maternity Age: 12-55   A Adult Age: 15-124   CC CC Condition   MCC Major CC Condition   HIV HIV Related Dx

228 — Volume 1

© 2007 Ingenix

**692.84 Due to animal (cat) (dog) dander**
Due to animal (cat) (dog) hair

**692.89 Other**
Dermatitis due to:    Dermatitis due to:
cold weather        hot weather
dyes              preservatives
EXCLUDES    *allergy (NOS) (rhinitis) due to*
*animal hair or dander*
*(477.2)*
*allergy to dust (477.8)*
*sunburn (692.71, 692.76-*
*692.77)*

**692.9    Unspecified cause**
Dermatitis:
NOS
contact NOS
venenata NOS
Eczema NOS

**√4ᵗʰ 693    Dermatitis due to substances taken internally**
EXCLUDES    *adverse effect NOS of drugs and medicines*
*(995.20)*
*allergy NOS (995.3)*
*contact dermatitis (692.0-692.9)*
*urticarial reactions (708.0-708.9, 995.1)*

DEF: Inflammation of skin due to ingested substance.

**693.0    Due to drugs and medicines**
Dermatitis medicamentosa NOS
Use additional E code to identify drug
EXCLUDES    *that due to drugs in contact with skin*
*(692.3)*

AHA: ▶2Q, '07, 8◀

**693.1    Due to food**
**693.8    Due to other specified substances taken internally**
**693.9    Due to unspecified substance taken internally**
EXCLUDES    *dermatitis NOS (692.9)*

**√4ᵗʰ 694    Bullous dermatoses**
**694.0    Dermatitis herpetiformis**
Dermatosis herpetiformis
Duhring's disease
Hydroa herpetiformis
EXCLUDES    *herpes gestationis (646.8)*
*dermatitis herpetiformis:*
*juvenile (694.2)*
*senile (694.5)*

DEF: Chronic, relapsing multisystem disease manifested most in the cutaneous system; seen as an extremely pruritic eruption of various combinations of lesions that frequently heal leaving hyperpigmentation or hypopigmentation and occasionally scarring; usually associated with an asymptomatic gluten-sensitive enteropathy, and immunogenic factors are believed to play a role in its origin.

**694.1    Subcorneal pustular dermatosis**
Sneddon-Wilkinson disease or syndrome

DEF: Chronic relapses of sterile pustular blebs beneath the horny skin layer of the trunk and skin folds; resembles dermatitis herpetiformis.

**694.2    Juvenile dermatitis herpetiformis**
Juvenile pemphigoid

**694.3    Impetigo herpetiformis**

DEF: Rare dermatosis associated with pregnancy; marked by itching pustules in third trimester, hypocalcemia, tetany, fever and lethargy; may result in maternal or fetal death.

**694.4    Pemphigus**    CC
Pemphigus:        Pemphigus:
NOS            malignant
erythematosus     vegetans
foliaceus         vulgaris
EXCLUDES    *pemphigus neonatorum (684)*

CC Excl: 694.4-694.9, 709.8

DEF: Chronic, relapsing, sometimes fatal skin diseases; causes vesicles, bullae; autoantibodies against intracellular connections cause acantholysis.

**694.5    Pemphigoid**    CC
Benign pemphigus NOS
Bullous pemphigoid
Herpes circinatus bullosus
Senile dermatitis herpetiformis

CC Excl: See code 694.4

**√5ᵗʰ 694.6    Benign mucous membrane pemphigoid**
Cicatricial pemphigoid
Mucosynechial atrophic bullous dermatitis

**694.60    Without mention of ocular involvement**
**694.61    With ocular involvement**
Ocular pemphigus

DEF: Mild self-limiting, subepidermal blistering of mucosa including the conjunctiva, seen predominantly in the elderly. It produces adhesions and scarring.

**694.8    Other specified bullous dermatoses**
EXCLUDES    *herpes gestationis (646.8)*

**694.9    Unspecified bullous dermatoses**

**√4ᵗʰ 695    Erythematous conditions**
**695.0    Toxic erythema**    CC
Erythema venenatum

CC Excl: 695.0-695.4, 709.8

**695.1    Erythema multiforme**    CC
Erythema iris
Herpes iris
Lyell's syndrome
Scalded skin syndrome
Stevens-Johnson syndrome
Toxic epidermal necrolysis

CC Excl: 695.0-695.9, 709.8

DEF: Symptom complex with a varied skin eruption pattern of macular, bullous, papular, nodose, or vesicular lesions on the neck, face, and legs; gastritis and rheumatic pains are also noticeable, first-seen symptoms; complex is secondary to a number of factors, including infections, ingestants, physical agents, malignancy and pregnancy.

**695.2    Erythema nodosum**
EXCLUDES    *tuberculous erythema nodosum (017.1)*

DEF: Panniculitis (an inflammatory reaction of the subcutaneous fat) of women, usually seen as a hypersensitivity reaction to various infections, drugs, sarcoidosis, and specific enteropathies; the acute stage is often associated with other symptoms, including fever, malaise, and arthralgia; the lesions are pink to blue in color, appear in crops as tender nodules and are found on the front of the legs below the knees.

**695.3    Rosacea**
Acne:
erythematosa
rosacea
Perioral dermatitis
Rhinophyma

DEF: Chronic skin disease, usually of the face, characterized by persistent erythema and sometimes by telangiectasis with acute episodes of edema, engorgement papules, and pustules.

**695.4    Lupus erythematosus**
Lupus:
erythematodes (discoid)
erythematosus (discoid), not disseminated
EXCLUDES    *lupus (vulgaris) NOS (017.0)*
*systemic [disseminated] lupus*
*erythematosus (710.0)*

DEF: Group of connective tissue disorders occurring as various cutaneous diseases of unknown origin; it primarily affects women between the ages of 20 and 40.

**√5ᵗʰ 695.8    Other specified erythematous conditions**
**695.81    Ritter's disease**
Dermatitis exfoliativa neonatorum

DEF: Infectious skin disease of infants and young children marked by eruptions ranging from a localized bullous type to widespread development of easily ruptured fine vesicles and bullae; results in exfoliation of large planes of skin and leaves raw areas; also called staphylococcal scalded skin syndrome.

**Skin and Subcutaneous Tissue**

**695.89–701.0**

**695.89 Other**
Erythema intertrigo
Intertrigo
Pityriasis rubra (Hebra)
EXCLUDES *mycotic intertrigo (111.0-111.9)*

AHA:: S-O, '86, 10

**695.9 Unspecified erythematous condition**
Erythema NOS        Erythroderma (secondary)

√4th **696 Psoriasis and similar disorders**

**696.0 Psoriatic arthropathy**
DEF: Psoriasis associated with inflammatory arthritis; often involves interphalangeal joints.

**696.1 Other psoriasis**
Acrodermatitis continua        Psoriasis:
Dermatitis repens                      NOS
                                                  any type, except
                                                    arthropathic
EXCLUDES *psoriatic arthropathy (696.0)*

**696.2 Parapsoriasis**
Parakeratosis variegata
Parapsoriasis lichenoides chronica
Pityriasis lichenoides et varioliformis
DEF: Erythrodermas similar to lichen, planus and psoriasis; symptoms include redness and itching; resistant to treatment.

**696.3 Pityriasis rosea**
Pityriasis circinata (et maculata)
DEF: Common, self-limited rash of unknown etiology marked by a solitary erythematous, salmon or fawn-colored herald plaque on the trunk, arms or thighs; followed by development of papular or macular lesions that tend to peel and form a scaly collarette.

**696.4 Pityriasis rubra pilaris**
Devergie's disease        Lichen ruber acuminatus
EXCLUDES *pityriasis rubra (Hebra) (695.89)*
DEF: Inflammatory disease of hair follicles; marked by firm, red lesions topped by horny plugs; may form patches; occurs on fingers elbows, knees.

**696.5 Other and unspecified pityriasis**
Pityriasis:        Pityriasis:
NOS                    streptogenes
alba
EXCLUDES *pityriasis:*
*simplex (690.18)*
*versicolor (111.0)*

**696.8 Other**

√4th **697 Lichen**
EXCLUDES *lichen:*
*obtusus corneus (698.3)*
*pilaris (congenital) (757.39)*
*ruber acuminatus (696.4)*
*sclerosus et atrophicus (701.0)*
*scrofulosus (017.0)*
*simplex chronicus (698.3)*
*spinulosus (congenital) (757.39)*
*urticatus (698.2)*

**697.0 Lichen planus**
Lichen:        Lichen:
planopilaris        ruber planus
DEF: Inflammatory, pruritic skin disease; marked by angular, flat-top, violet-colored papules; may be acute and widespread or chronic and localized.

**697.1 Lichen nitidus**
Pinkus' disease
DEF: Chronic, inflammatory, usually asymptomatic skin disorder, characterized by numerous glistening, flat-topped, discrete, smooth, skin-colored micropapules most often on penis, lower abdomen, inner thighs, wrists, forearms, breasts and buttocks.

**697.8 Other lichen, not elsewhere classified**
Lichen:        Lichen:
ruber moniliforme        striata

**697.9 Lichen, unspecified**

√4th **698 Pruritus and related conditions**
EXCLUDES *pruritus specified as psychogenic (306.3)*
DEF: Pruritus: Intense, persistent itching due to irritation of sensory nerve endings from organic or psychogenic causes.

**698.0 Pruritus ani**
Perianal itch

**698.1 Pruritus of genital organs**

**698.2 Prurigo**
Lichen urticatus        Prurigo:
Prurigo:                        mitis
NOS                            simplex
Hebra's                    Urticaria papulosa (Hebra)
EXCLUDES *prurigo nodularis (698.3)*

**698.3 Lichenification and lichen simplex chronicus**
Hyde's disease
Neurodermatitis (circumscripta) (local)
Prurigo nodularis
EXCLUDES *neurodermatitis, diffuse (of Brocq) (691.8)*
DEF: Lichenification: thickening of skin due to prolonged rubbing or scratching.

DEF: Lichen simplex chronicus: eczematous dermatitis, of face, neck, extremities, scrotum, vulva, and perianal region due to repeated itching, rubbing and scratching; spontaneous or evolves with other dermatoses.

**698.4 Dermatitis factitia [artefacta]**
Dermatitis ficta
Neurotic excoriation
Use additional code to identify any associated mental disorder
DEF: Various types of self-inflicted skin lesions characterized in appearance as an erythema to a gangrene.

**698.8 Other specified pruritic conditions**
Pruritus:        Winter itch
hiemalis
senilis

**698.9 Unspecified pruritic disorder**
Itch NOS        Pruritus NOS

## OTHER DISEASES OF SKIN AND SUBCUTANEOUS TISSUE (700-709)

EXCLUDES *conditions confined to eyelids (373.0-374.9)*
*congenital conditions of skin, hair, and nails (757.0-757.9)*

**700 Corns and callosities**
Callus        Clavus
DEF: Corns: Conical or horny thickening of skin on toes, due to friction, pressure from shoes and hosiery; pain and inflammation may develop.

DEF: Callosities: Localized overgrowth (hyperplasia) of the horny epidermal layer due to pressure or friction.

√4th **701 Other hypertrophic and atrophic conditions of skin**
EXCLUDES *dermatomyositis (710.3)*
*hereditary edema of legs (757.0)*
*scleroderma (generalized) (710.1)*

**701.0 Circumscribed scleroderma**
Addison's keloid
Dermatosclerosis, localized        Morphea
Lichen sclerosus                        Scleroderma, circum-
et atrophicus                            scribed or localized
DEF: Thickened, hardened, skin and subcutaneous tissue; may involve musculoskeletal system.

---

N Newborn Age: 0    P Pediatric Age: 0-17    M Maternity Age: 12-55    A Adult Age: 15-124    CC CC Condition    MCC Major CC Condition    HIV HIV Related Dx

**701.1  Keratoderma, acquired**

Acquired:
  ichthyosis
  keratoderma palmaris et plantaris
Elastosis perforans serpiginosa
Hyperkeratosis:
  NOS
  follicularis in cutem penetrans
  palmoplantaris climacterica
Keratoderma:
  climactericum
  tylodes, progressive
Keratosis (blennorrhagica)

> **EXCLUDES**  Darier's disease [keratosis follicularis]
> (congenital) (757.39)
> keratosis:
>   arsenical (692.4)
>   gonococcal (098.81)

**AHA:** 4Q, '94, 48

**701.2  Acquired acanthosis nigricans**

Keratosis nigricans

**DEF:** Diffuse velvety hyperplasia of the spinous skin layer of the axilla and other body folds marked by gray, brown, or black pigmentation; in adult form it is often associated with an internal carcinoma (malignant acanthosis nigricans) in a benign, nevoid form it is relatively generalized; benign juvenile form with obesity is sometimes caused by an endocrine disturbance.

**701.3  Striae atrophicae**

Atrophic spots of skin
Atrophoderma maculatum
Atrophy blanche (of Milian)
Degenerative colloid atrophy
Senile degenerative atrophy
Striae distensae

**DEF:** Bands of atrophic, depressed, wrinkled skin associated with stretching of skin from pregnancy, obesity, or rapid growth during puberty.

**701.4  Keloid scar**

Cheloid
Hypertrophic scar
Keloid

**DEF:** Overgrowth of scar tissue due to excess amounts of collagen during connective tissue repair; occurs mainly on upper trunk, face.

**701.5  Other abnormal granulation tissue**

Excessive granulation

**701.8  Other specified hypertrophic and atrophic conditions of skin**

Acrodermatitis atrophicans chronica
Atrophia cutis senilis
Atrophoderma neuriticum
Confluent and reticulate papillomatosis
Cutis laxa senilis
Elastosis senilis
Folliculitis ulerythematosa reticulata
Gougerot-Carteaud syndrome or disease

**701.9  Unspecified hypertrophic and atrophic conditions of skin**

Skin tag          Atrophoderma

√4th **702  Other dermatoses**

> **EXCLUDES**  carcinoma in situ (232.0-232.9)

**702.0  Actinic keratosis**

**AHA:** 1Q, '92, 18

**DEF:** Wart-like growth, red or skin-colored; may form a cutaneous horn.

√5th **702.1  Seborrheic keratosis**

**DEF:** Common, benign, lightly pigmented, warty growth composed of basaloid cells.

**702.11  Inflamed seborrheic keratosis**

**AHA:** 4Q, '94, 48

**702.19  Other seborrheic keratosis**

Seborrheic keratosis NOS

**702.8  Other specified dermatoses**

√4th **703  Diseases of nail**

> **EXCLUDES**  congenital anomalies (757.5)
> onychia and paronychia (681.02, 681.11)

**703.0  Ingrowing nail**

Ingrowing nail with infection    Unguis incarnatus

> **EXCLUDES**  infection, nail NOS (681.9)

**703.8  Other specified diseases of nail**

Dystrophia unguium          Onychauxis
Hypertrophy of nail          Onychogryposis
Koilonychia                  Onycholysis
Leukonychia (punctata) (striata)

**703.9  Unspecified disease of nail**

√4th **704  Diseases of hair and hair follicles**

> **EXCLUDES**  congenital anomalies (757.4)

√5th **704.0  Alopecia**

> **EXCLUDES**  madarosis (374.55)
> syphilitic alopecia (091.82)

**DEF:** Lack of hair, especially on scalp; often called baldness; may be partial or total; occurs at any age.

**704.00  Alopecia, unspecified**

Baldness
Loss of hair

**704.01  Alopecia areata**

Ophiasis

**DEF:** Alopecia areata: usually reversible, inflammatory, patchy hair loss found in beard or scalp.

**DEF:** Ophiasis: alopecia areata of children; marked by band around temporal and occipital scalp margins.

**704.02  Telogen effluvium**

**DEF:** Shedding of hair from premature telogen development in follicles due to stress, including shock, childbirth, surgery, drugs or weight loss.

**704.09  Other**

Folliculitis decalvans
Hypotrichosis:
  NOS
  postinfectional NOS
Pseudopelade

**704.1  Hirsutism**

Hypertrichosis:          Polytrichia
  NOS
  lanuginosa, acquired

> **EXCLUDES**  hypertrichosis of eyelid (374.54)

**DEF:** Excess hair growth; often in unexpected places and amounts.

**704.2  Abnormalities of the hair**

Atrophic hair          Trichiasis:
Clastothrix              NOS
Fragilitas crinium       cicatrical
                         Trichorrhexis (nodosa)

> **EXCLUDES**  trichiasis of eyelid (374.05)

**704.3  Variations in hair color**

Canities (premature)    Poliosis:
Grayness, hair (premature)   NOS
Heterochromia of hair    circumscripta, acquired

**704.8  Other specified diseases of hair and hair follicles**

Folliculitis:            Sycosis:
  NOS                     NOS
  abscedens et suffodiens  barbae [not parasitic]
  pustular                lupoid
Perifolliculitis:         vulgaris
  NOS
  capitis abscedens et suffodiens
  scalp

**704.9  Unspecified disease of hair and hair follicles**

√4th **705  Disorders of sweat glands**

**705.0  Anhidrosis**

Hypohidrosis          Oligohidrosis

**DEF:** Lack or deficiency of ability to sweat.

√4th / √5th Additional Digit Required    Unacceptable PDx    Manifestation Code    ▶◀ Revised Text    ● New Code    ▲ Revised Code Title

**October 2007 • Volume 1 — 231**

© 2007 Ingenix

**705.1   Prickly heat**
Heat rash     Sudamina
Miliaria rubra (tropicalis)

√5ᵗʰ **705.2 Focal hyperhidrosis**

EXCLUDES   generalized (secondary) hyperhidrosis (780.8)

**705.21   Primary focal hyperhidrosis**
Focal hyperhidrosis NOS     Hyperhidrosis of:
Hyperhidrosis NOS     axilla
    face
    palms
    soles

**AHA:** 4Q, '04, 91

DEF: A rare condition that is a disorder of the sweat glands resulting in excessive production of sweat; occurs in the absence of any underlying or causative condition and is almost always focal, confined to one or more specific areas of the body.

**705.22   Secondary focal hyperhidrosis**
Frey's syndrome

**AHA:** 4Q, '04, 91

DEF: Secondary focal hyperhidrosis: a symptom of an underlying disease process resulting in excessive sweating beyond what the body requires to maintain thermal control, confined to one or more specific areas of the body.
DEF: Frey's syndrome: an auriculotemporal syndrome due to lesion on the parotid gland; characteristic redness and excessive sweating on the cheek in connection with eating.

√5ᵗʰ **705.8   Other specified disorders of sweat glands**

**705.81   Dyshidrosis**
Cheiropompholyx     Pompholyx
DEF: Vesicular eruption, on hands, feet causing itching and burning.

**705.82   Fox-Fordyce disease**
DEF: Chronic, usually pruritic disease chiefly of women evidenced by small follicular papular eruptions, especially in the axillary and pubic areas; develops from the closure and rupture of the affected apocrine glands' intraepidermal portion of the ducts.

**705.83   Hidradenitis**
Hidradenitis suppurativa
DEF: Inflamed sweat glands.

**705.89   Other**
Bromhidrosis     Granulosis rubra nasi
Chromhidrosis     Urhidrosis

EXCLUDES   generalized hyperhidrosis (780.8)
    hidrocystoma (216.0-216.9)

DEF: Bromhidrosis: foul-smelling axillary sweat due to decomposed bacteria.
DEF: Chromhidrosis: secretion of colored sweat.
DEF: Granulosis rubra nasi: ideopathic condition of children; causes redness, sweating around nose, face and chin; tends to end by puberty.
DEF: Urhidrosis: urinous substance, such as uric acid, in sweat; occurs in uremia.

**705.9   Unspecified disorder of sweat glands**
Disorder of sweat glands NOS

√4ᵗʰ **706 Diseases of sebaceous glands**

**706.0   Acne varioliformis**
Acne:     Acne:
  frontalis     necrotica
DEF: Rare form of acne characterized by persistent brown papulo-pustules usually on the brow and temporoparietal part of the scalp.

**706.1   Other acne**
Acne:     Acne:
  NOS     vulgaris
  conglobata     Blackhead
  cystic     Comedo
  pustular

EXCLUDES   acne rosacea (695.3)

**Four Stages of Decubitus Ulcers**

**First Stage**
Nonblanchable erythema

**Second Stage**
Partial thickness skin loss involving epidermis, dermis, or both

**Third Stage**
Full thickness skin loss extending through subcutaneous tissue

**Fourth Stage**
Full thickness skin loss extending to muscle and bone

**706.2   Sebaceous cyst**
Atheroma, skin     Wen
Keratin cyst
DEF: Benign epidermal cyst, contains sebum and keratin; presents as firm, circumscribed nodule.

**706.3   Seborrhea**

EXCLUDES   seborrhea:
    capitis (690.11)
    sicca (690.18)
  seborrheic
    dermatitis (690.10)
    keratosis (702.11-702.19)

DEF: Seborrheic dermatitis marked by excessive secretion of sebum; the sebum forms an oily coating, crusts, or scales on the skin; it is also called hypersteatosis.

**706.8   Other specified diseases of sebaceous glands**
Asteatosis (cutis)
Xerosis cutis

**706.9   Unspecified disease of sebaceous glands**

√4ᵗʰ **707 Chronic ulcer of skin**

INCLUDES   non-infected sinus of skin
    non-healing ulcer

EXCLUDES   specific infections classified under "Infectious and Parasitic Diseases" (001.0-136.9)
    varicose ulcer (454.0, 454.2)

**AHA:** 4Q, '04, 92

√5ᵗʰ **707.0   Decubitus ulcer**
Bed sore     Plaster ulcer
Decubitus ulcer [any site]     Pressure ulcer

**AHA:** 1Q, '04, 14; 4Q, '03, 110; 4Q, '99, 20; 1Q, '96, 15; 3Q, '90, 15; N-D, '87, 9

**707.00   Unspecified site**     `CC`
**CC Excl:** 707.00-707.09, 707.8-707.9, 709.8

**707.01   Elbow**     `CC`
**CC Excl:** See code 707.00

**707.02   Upper back**     `MCC`
Shoulder blades
**CC Excl:** See code 707.00

**707.03   Lower back**     `MCC`
Sacrum
**CC Excl:** See code 707.00
**AHA:** 1Q, '05, 16

**707.04   Hip**     `MCC`
**CC Excl:** See code 707.00

**707.05   Buttock**     `MCC`
**CC Excl:** See code 707.00

**707.06   Ankle**     `MCC`
**CC Excl:** See code 707.00

**707.07   Heel**     `MCC`
**CC Excl:** See code 707.00
**AHA:** 1Q, '05, 16

**707.09   Other site**     `CC`
Head
**CC Excl:** See code 707.00

---

N Newborn Age: 0    P Pediatric Age: 0-17    M Maternity Age: 12-55    A Adult Age: 15-124    CC CC Condition    MCC Major CC Condition    HIV HIV Related Dx

232 — Volume 1 • October 2007

© 2007 Ingenix

✓5ᵗʰ **707.1 Ulcer of lower limbs, except decubitus**

Ulcer, chronic:
neurogenic ⎫
trophic ⎬ of lower limb

Code, if applicable, any causal condition first:
atherosclerosis of the extremities with ulceration (440.23)
chronic venous hypertension with ulcer (459.31)
chronic venous hypertension with ulcer and inflammation (459.33)
diabetes mellitus (250.80-250.83)
postphlebitic syndrome with ulcer (459.11)
postphlebitic syndrome with ulcer and inflammation (459.13)

**AHA:** 4Q, '00, 44; 4Q, '99, 15

**707.10 Ulcer of lower limb, unspecified** `CC`
**CC Excl:** 440.23, 707.10-707.9, 709.8

**AHA:** 3Q, '04, 5; 4Q, '02, 43

**707.11 Ulcer of thigh** `CC`
**CC Excl:** See code 707.10

**707.12 Ulcer of calf** `CC`
**CC Excl:** See code 707.10

**707.13 Ulcer of ankle** `CC`
**CC Excl:** See code 707.10

**707.14 Ulcer of heel and midfoot** `CC`
Plantar surface of midfoot
**CC Excl:** See code 707.10

**707.15 Ulcer of other part of foot**
Toes

**707.19 Ulcer of other part of lower limb** `CC`
**CC Excl:** See code 707.10

**707.8 Chronic ulcer of other specified sites**

Ulcer, chronic:
neurogenic ⎫
trophic ⎬ of other specified sites

**707.9 Chronic ulcer of unspecified site**
Chronic ulcer NOS
Trophic ulcer NOS
Tropical ulcer NOS
Ulcer of skin NOS

✓4ᵗʰ **708 Urticaria**

`EXCLUDES` edema:
*angioneurotic (995.1)*
*Quincke's (995.1)*
*hereditary angioedema (277.6)*
*urticaria:*
*giant (995.1)*
*papulosa (Hebra) (698.2)*
*pigmentosa (juvenile) (congenital) (757.33)*

**DEF:** Skin disorder marked by raised edematous patches of skin or mucous membrane with intense itching; also called hives.

**708.0 Allergic urticaria**

**708.1 Idiopathic urticaria**

**708.2 Urticaria due to cold and heat**
Thermal urticaria

**708.3 Dermatographic urticaria**
Dermatographia      Factitial urticaria

**708.4 Vibratory urticaria**

**708.5 Cholinergic urticaria**

**708.8 Other specified urticaria**
Nettle rash      Urticaria:
Urticaria:      recurrent periodic
chronic

**708.9 Urticaria, unspecified**
Hives NOS

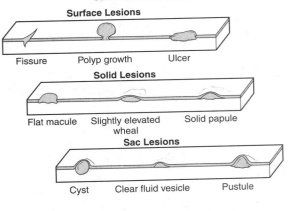

**Cutaneous Lesions**

**Surface Lesions**
Fissure    Polyp growth    Ulcer

**Solid Lesions**
Flat macule    Slightly elevated wheal    Solid papule

**Sac Lesions**
Cyst    Clear fluid vesicle    Pustule

✓4ᵗʰ **709 Other disorders of skin and subcutaneous tissue**

✓5ᵗʰ **709.0 Dyschromia**

`EXCLUDES` *albinism (270.2)*
*pigmented nevus (216.0-216.9)*
*that of eyelid (374.52-374.53)*

**DEF:** Pigment disorder of skin or hair.

**709.00 Dyschromia, unspecified**

**709.01 Vitiligo**
**DEF:** Persistent, progressive development of nonpigmented white patches on otherwise normal skin.

**709.09 Other**

**709.1 Vascular disorders of skin**
Angioma serpiginosum
Purpura (primary)annularis telangiectodes

**709.2 Scar conditions and fibrosis of skin**
Adherent scar (skin)      Fibrosis, skin NOS
Cicatrix      Scar NOS
Disfigurement (due to scar)
`EXCLUDES` *keloid scar (701.4)*

**AHA:** N-D, '84, 19

**709.3 Degenerative skin disorders**
Calcinosis:      Degeneration, skin
circumscripta      Deposits, skin
cutis      Senile dermatosis NOS
Colloid milium      Subcutaneous calcification

**709.4 Foreign body granuloma of skin and subcutaneous tissue**
`EXCLUDES` *residual foreign body without granuloma of skin and subcutaneous tissue (729.6)*
*that of muscle (728.82)*

**709.8 Other specified disorders of skin**
Epithelial hyperplasia
Menstrual dermatosis
Vesicular eruption

**AHA:** N-D, '87, 6

**DEF:** Epithelial hyperplasia: increased number of epitheleal cells.

**DEF:** Vesicular eruption: liquid-filled structures appearing through skin.

**709.9 Unspecified disorder of skin and subcutaneous tissue**
Dermatosis NOS

---

# 13. DISEASES OF THE MUSCULOSKELETAL SYSTEM AND CONNECTIVE TISSUE (710-739)

## Joint Structures

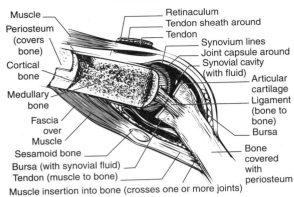

Muscle
Periosteum (covers bone)
Cortical bone
Medullary bone
Fascia over Muscle
Sesamoid bone
Bursa (with synovial fluid)
Tendon (muscle to bone)
Muscle insertion into bone (crosses one or more joints)

Retinaculum
Tendon sheath around
Tendon
Synovium lines
Joint capsule around
Synovial cavity (with fluid)
Articular cartilage
Ligament (bone to bone)
Bursa
Bone covered with periosteum

---

The following fifth-digit subclassification is for use with categories 711-712, 715-716, 718-719, and 730:

**0 site unspecified**

**1 shoulder region**
     Acromioclavicular joint(s)
     Clavicle
     Glenohumeral joint(s)
     Scapula
     Sternoclavicular joint(s)

**2 upper arm**
     Elbow joint
     Humerus

**3 forearm**
     Radius
     Ulna
     Wrist joint

**4 hand**
     Carpus
     Metacarpus
     Phalanges [fingers]

**5 pelvic region and thigh**
     Buttock
     Femur
     Hip (joint)

**6 lower leg**
     Fibula      Patella
     Knee joint      Tibia

**7 ankle and foot**
     Ankle joint      Phalanges, foot
     Digits [toes]      Tarsus
     Metatarsus      Other joints in foot

**8 other specified sites**
     Head      Skull
     Neck      Trunk
     Ribs      Vertebral column

**9 multiple sites**

## ARTHROPATHIES AND RELATED DISORDERS (710-719)

     **EXCLUDES** *disorders of spine (720.0-724.9)*

**✓4th 710 Diffuse diseases of connective tissue**
     **INCLUDES** all collagen diseases whose effects are not mainly confined to a single system
     **EXCLUDES** *those affecting mainly the cardiovascular system, i.e., polyarteritis nodosa and allied conditions (446.0-446.7)*

---

**710.0 Systemic lupus erythematosus**
     Disseminated lupus erythematosus
     Libman-Sacks disease
     Use additional code to identify manifestation, as:
     endocarditis (424.91)
     nephritis (583.81)
       chronic (582.81)
     nephrotic syndrome (581.81)
     **EXCLUDES** *lupus erythematosus (discoid) NOS (695.4)*

**AHA:** 2Q, '03, 7-8; 2Q, '97, 8

**DEF:** A chronic multisystemic inflammatory disease affecting connective tissue; marked by anemia, leukopenia, muscle and joint pains, fever, rash of a butterfly pattern around cheeks and forehead area; of unknown etiology.

**710.1 Systemic sclerosis**
     Acrosclerosis      Progressive systemic sclerosis
     CRST syndrome      Scleroderma
     Use additional code to identify manifestation, as:
     lung involvement (517.2)
     myopathy (359.6)
     **EXCLUDES** *circumscribed scleroderma (701.0)*

**AHA:** 1Q, '88, 6

**DEF:** Systemic disease, involving excess fibrotic collagen build-up; symptoms include thickened skin; fibrotic degenerative changes in various organs; and vascular abnomalities; condition occurs more often in females.

**710.2 Sicca syndrome**
     Keratoconjunctivitis sicca      Sjögren's disease

**DEF:** Autoimmune disease; associated with keratoconjunctivitis, laryngopharyngitis, rhinitis, dry mouth, enlarged parotid gland, and chronic polyarthritis.

**710.3 Dermatomyositis**      `CC`
     Poikilodermatomyositis
     Polymyositis with skin involvement

**CC Excl:** 710.3

**DEF:** Polymyositis associated with flat-top purple papules on knuckles; marked by upper eyelid rash, edema of eyelids and orbit area, red rash on forehead, neck, shoulders, trunk and arms; symptoms include fever, weight loss aching muscles; visceral cancer (in individuals older than 40).

**710.4 Polymyositis**      `CC`

**CC Excl:** 710.4

**DEF:** Chronic, progressive, inflammatory skeletal muscle disease; causes weakness of limb girdles, neck, pharynx; may precede or follow scleroderma, Sjogren's disease, systemic lupus erythematosus, arthritis, or malignancy.

**710.5 Eosinophilia myalgia syndrome**      `CC`
     Toxic oil syndrome
     Use additional E code to identify drug, if drug induced

**CC Excl:** 292.0-293.9, 710.5

**AHA:** 4Q, '92, 21

**DEF:** Eosinophilia myalgia syndrome (EMS): inflammatory, multisystem fibrosis; associated with ingesting elementary L-tryptophan; symptoms include myalgia, weak limbs and bulbar muscles, distal sensory loss, areflexia, arthralgia, cough, fever, fatigue, skin rashes, myopathy, and eosinophil counts greater than 1000/microliter.

**DEF:** Toxic oil syndrome: syndrome similar to EMS due to ingesting contaminated cooking oil.

---

✓4th / ✓5th Additional Digit Required      Unacceptable PDx      Manifestation Code      ▶◀ Revised Text      ● New Code      ▲ Revised Code Title

710.8   **Other specified diffuse diseases of connective** `CC` **tissue**
> Multifocal fibrosclerosis (idiopathic) NEC
> Systemic fibrosclerosing syndrome

**CC Excl:** 710.8

**AHA:** M-A, '87, 12

710.9   **Unspecified diffuse connective tissue disease**
> Collagen disease NOS

√4ᵗʰ **711 Arthropathy associated with infections**

INCLUDES   arthritis
                arthropathy     }   associated with
                polyarthritis        conditions
                polyarthropathy }   classifiable below

EXCLUDES   *rheumatic fever (390)*

The following fifth-digit subclassification is for use with category 711; valid digits are in [brackets] under each code. See list at beginning of chapter for definitions.

    **0 site unspecified**
    **1 shoulder region**
    **2 upper arm**
    **3 forearm**
    **4 hand**
    **5 pelvic region and thigh**
    **6 lower leg**
    **7 ankle and foot**
    **8 other specified sites**
    **9 multiple sites**

**AHA:** 1Q, '92, 17

§ √5ᵗʰ **711.0 Pyogenic arthritis**     `CC`
[0-9]
> Arthritis or polyarthritis (due to):
>     coliform [Escherichia coli]
>     Hemophilus influenzae [H. influenzae]
>     pneumococcal
>     Pseudomonas
>     staphylococcal
>     streptococcal
> Pyarthrosis
> Use additional code to identify infectious organism
>     (041.0-041.8)

**CC Excl: For codes 711.00, 711.08-711.09:** 015.80-015.96, 017.90-017.96, 036.82, 056.71, 098.50-098.51, 098.59, 098.89, 711.00-714.0, 715.00, 715.09-715.10, 715.18-716.99, 718.00-718.08, 719.00-719.10, 719.18-719.99; **For code 711.01:** 015.80-015.96, 017.90-017.96, 036.82, 056.71, 098.50-098.51, 098.59, 098.89, 711.00-711.01, 711.08-711.11, 711.18-711.21, 711.28-711.31, 711.38-711.41, 711.48-711.51, 711.58-711.61, 711.68-711.71, 711.78-711.81, 711.88-711.91, 711.98-712.11, 712.18-712.21, 712.28-712.31, 712.38-712.81, 712.88-712.91, 712.98-714.0, 715.00, 715.09-715.11, 715.18-715.21, 715.28-715.31, 715.38-715.91, 715.98-716.01, 716.08-716.11, 716.18-716.21, 716.28-716.31, 716.38-716.41, 716.48-716.51, 716.58-716.61, 716.68-716.81, 716.88-716.91, 716.98-716.99, 718.00-718.01, 718.08, 719.00-719.01, 719.08-719.11, 719.18-719.21, 719.28-719.31, 719.38-719.41, 719.48-719.51, 719.58-719.61, 719.68-719.81, 719.88-719.91, 719.98-719.99; **For code 711.02:** 015.80-015.96, 017.90-017.96, 036.82, 056.71, 098.50-098.51, 098.59, 098.89, 711.00, 711.02, 711.08-711.10, 711.12, 711.18-711.20, 711.22, 711.28-711.30, 711.32, 711.38-711.40, 711.42, 711.48-711.50, 711.52, 711.58-711.60, 711.62, 711.68-711.70, 711.72, 711.78-711.80, 711.82, 711.88-711.90, 711.92, 711.98-712.10, 712.12, 712.18-712.20, 712.22, 712.28-712.30, 712.32, 712.38-712.80, 712.82, 712.88-712.90, 712.92, 712.98-714.0, 715.00, 715.09-715.10, 715.12, 715.18-715.20, 715.22, 715.28-715.30, 715.32, 715.38-715.90, 715.92, 715.98-716.00, 716.02, 716.08-716.10, 716.12, 716.18-716.20, 716.22, 716.28-716.30, 716.32, 716.38-716.40, 716.42, 716.48-716.50, 716.52, 716.58-716.60, 716.62, 716.68-716.80, 716.82, 716.88-716.90, 716.92, 716.98-716.99, 718.00, 718.02, 718.08, 719.00, 719.02, 719.08-719.10, 719.12, 719.18-719.20, 719.22, 719.28-719.30, 719.32, 719.38-719.40, 719.42, 719.48-719.50, 719.52, 719.58-719.60, 719.62, 719.68-719.80, 719.82, 719.88-719.90, 719.92, 719.98-719.99; **For code 711.03:** 015.80-015.96, 017.90-017.96, 036.82, 056.71, 098.50-098.51, 098.59, 098.89, 711.00, 711.03, 711.08-711.10, 711.13, 711.18-711.20, 711.23, 711.28-711.30, 711.33, 711.38-711.40, 711.43, 711.48-711.50, 711.53, 711.58-711.60, 711.63, 711.68-

---

711.70, 711.73, 711.78-711.80, 711.83, 711.88-711.90, 711.93, 711.98-712.10, 712.13, 712.18-712.20, 712.23, 712.28-712.30, 712.33, 712.38-712.80, 712.83, 712.88-712.90, 712.93, 712.98-714.0, 715.00, 715.09-715.10, 715.13, 715.18-715.20, 715.23, 715.28-715.30, 715.33, 715.38-715.90, 715.93, 715.98-716.00, 716.03, 716.08-716.10, 716.13, 716.18-716.20, 716.23, 716.28-716.30, 716.33, 716.38-716.40, 716.43, 716.48-716.50, 716.53, 716.58-716.60, 716.63, 716.68-716.80, 716.83, 716.88-716.90, 716.93, 716.98-716.99, 718.00, 718.03, 718.08, 719.00, 719.03, 719.08-719.10, 719.13, 719.18-719.20, 719.23, 719.28-719.30, 719.33, 719.38-719.40, 719.43, 719.48-719.50, 719.53, 719.58-719.60, 719.63, 719.68-719.80, 719.83, 719.88-719.90, 719.93, 719.98-719.99; **For code 711.04:** 015.80-015.96, 017.90-017.96, 036.82, 056.71, 098.50-098.51, 098.59, 098.89, 711.00, 711.04, 711.08-711.10, 711.14, 711.18-711.20, 711.24, 711.28-711.30, 711.34, 711.38-711.40, 711.44, 711.48-711.50, 711.54, 711.58-711.60, 711.64, 711.68-711.70, 711.74, 711.78-711.80, 711.84, 711.88-711.90, 711.94, 711.98-712.10, 712.14, 712.18-712.20, 712.24, 712.28-712.30, 712.34, 712.38-712.80, 712.84, 712.88-712.90, 712.94, 712.98-714.0, 715.00-715.10, 715.14, 715.18-715.20, 715.24, 715.28-715.30, 715.34, 715.38-715.90, 715.94, 715.98-716.00, 716.04, 716.08-716.10, 716.14, 716.18-716.20, 716.24, 716.28-716.30, 716.34, 716.38-716.40, 716.44, 716.48-716.50, 716.54, 716.58-716.60, 716.64, 716.68-716.80, 716.84, 716.88-716.90, 716.94, 716.98-716.99, 718.00, 718.04, 718.08, 719.00, 719.04, 719.08-719.10, 719.14, 719.18-719.20, 719.24, 719.28-719.30, 719.34, 719.38-719.40, 719.44, 719.48-719.50, 719.54, 719.58-719.60, 719.64, 719.68-719.80, 719.84, 719.88-719.90, 719.94, 719.98-719.99; **For code 711.05:** 015.80-015.96, 017.90-017.96, 036.82, 056.71, 098.50-098.51, 098.59, 098.89, 711.00, 711.05, 711.08-711.10, 711.15, 711.18-711.20, 711.25, 711.28-711.30, 711.35, 711.38-711.40, 711.45, 711.48-711.50, 711.55, 711.58-711.60, 711.65, 711.68-711.70, 711.75, 711.78-711.80, 711.85, 711.88-711.90, 711.95, 711.98-712.10, 712.15, 712.18-712.20, 712.25, 712.28-712.30, 712.35, 712.38-712.80, 712.85, 712.88-712.90, 712.95, 712.98-714.0, 715.00, 715.09-715.10, 715.15, 715.18-715.20, 715.25, 715.28-715.30, 715.35, 715.38-715.90, 715.95, 715.98-716.00, 716.05, 716.08-716.10, 716.15, 716.18-716.20, 716.25, 716.28-716.30, 716.35, 716.38-716.40, 716.45, 716.48-716.50, 716.55, 716.58-716.60, 716.65, 716.68-716.80, 716.85, 716.88-716.90, 716.95, 716.98-716.99, 718.00, 718.05, 718.08, 719.00, 719.05, 719.08-719.10, 719.15, 719.18-719.20, 719.25, 719.28-719.30, 719.35, 719.38-719.40, 719.45, 719.48-719.50, 719.55, 719.58-719.60, 719.65, 719.68-719.80, 719.85, 719.88-719.90, 719.95, 719.98-719.99; **For code 711.06:** 015.80-015.96, 017.90-017.96, 036.82, 056.71, 098.50-098.51, 098.59, 098.89, 711.00, 711.06, 711.08-711.10, 711.16, 711.18-711.20, 711.26, 711.28-711.30, 711.36, 711.38-711.40, 711.46, 711.48-711.50, 711.56, 711.58-711.60, 711.66, 711.68-711.70, 711.76, 711.78-711.80, 711.86, 711.88-711.90, 711.96, 711.98-712.10, 712.16, 712.18-712.20, 712.26, 712.28-712.30, 712.36, 712.38-712.80, 712.86, 712.88-712.90, 712.96, 712.98-714.0, 715.00, 715.09-715.10, 715.16, 715.18-715.20, 715.26, 715.28-715.30, 715.36, 715.38-715.90, 715.96, 715.98-716.00, 716.06, 716.08-716.10, 716.16, 716.18-716.20, 716.26, 716.28-716.30, 716.36, 716.38-716.40, 716.46, 716.48-716.50, 716.56, 716.58-716.60, 716.66, 716.68-716.80, 716.86, 716.88-716.90, 716.96, 716.98-716.99, 718.00, 718.08, 719.00, 719.06, 719.08-719.10, 719.16, 719.18-719.20, 719.26, 719.28-719.30, 719.36, 719.38-719.40, 719.46, 719.48-719.50, 719.56, 719.58-719.60, 719.66, 719.68-719.80, 719.86, 719.88-719.90, 719.96, 719.98-719.99; **For code 711.07:** 015.80-015.96, 017.90-017.96, 036.82, 056.71, 098.50-098.51, 098.59, 098.89, 711.00, 711.07-711.10, 711.17-711.20, 711.27-711.30, 711.37-711.40, 711.47-711.50, 711.57-711.60, 711.67-711.70, 711.77-711.80, 711.87-711.90, 711.97-712.10, 712.17-712.20, 712.27-712.30, 712.37-712.80, 712.87-712.90, 712.97-714.0, 715.00, 715.09-715.10, 715.17-715.20, 715.27-715.30, 715.37-715.90, 715.97-716.00, 716.07-716.10, 716.17-716.20, 716.27-716.30, 716.37-716.40, 716.47-716.50, 716.57-716.60, 716.67-716.80, 716.87-716.90, 716.97-716.99, 718.00, 718.07-718.08, 719.00, 719.07-719.10, 719.17-719.20, 719.27-719.30, 719.37-719.40, 719.47-719.50, 719.57-719.60, 719.67-719.80, 719.87-719.90, 719.97-719.99

**AHA:** 1Q, '92, 16; 1Q, '91, 15

**DEF:** Infectious arthritis caused by various bacteria; marked by inflamed synovial membranes, and purulent effusion in joints.

---

§   Requires fifth-digit. Valid digits are in [brackets] under each code. See beginning of section 710-739 for codes and definitions.

N Newborn Age: 0    P Pediatric Age: 0-17    M Maternity Age: 12-55    A Adult Age: 15-124    CC CC Condition    MCC Major CC Condition    HIV HIV Related Dx

236 — Volume 1 • October 2007

§ ✓5ᵗʰ **711.1**   ***Arthropathy associated with Reiter's disease***   `CC`
[0-9]   ***and nonspecific urethritis***

     *Code first underlying disease as:*
       nonspecific urethritis (099.4)
       Reiter's disease (099.3)

**CC Excl:** 003.23, 015.80-015.96, 017.90-017.96, 036.82, 056.71, 098.50-098.51, 098.59, 098.89, 711.00-714.0, 715.00, 715.09-715.10, 715.18-716.99, 718.00-718.08, 719.00-719.10, 719.18-719.69, 719.80-719.99

**DEF:** Reiter's disease: joint disease marked by diarrhea, urethritis, conjunctivitis, keratosis and arthritis; of unknown etiology; affects young males.

**DEF:** Urethritis: inflamed urethra.

§ ✓5ᵗʰ **711.2**   ***Arthropathy in Behçet's syndrome***   `CC`
[0-9]   *Code first underlying disease (136.1)*

**CC Excl:** 003.23, 015.80-015.96, 017.90-017.96, 036.82, 056.71, 098.50-098.51, 098.59, 098.89, 711.00-714.0, 715.00, 715.09-715.10, 715.18-716.99, 718.00-718.08, 719.00-719.10, 719.18-719.69, 719.80-719.99

**DEF:** Behçet's syndrome: Chronic inflammatory disorder, of unknown etiology; affects small blood vessels; causes ulcers of oral and pharyngeal mucous membranes and genitalia, skin lesions, retinal vasculitis, optic atrophy and severe uveitis.

§ ✓5ᵗʰ **711.3**   ***Postdysenteric arthropathy***   `CC`
[0-9]   *Code first underlying disease as:*
       dysentery (009.0)
       enteritis, infectious (008.0-009.3)
       paratyphoid fever (002.1-002.9)
       typhoid fever (002.0)
     **EXCLUDES**   *salmonella arthritis (003.23)*

**CC Excl: For codes 711.30-711.35, 711.37, and 711.39:** 003.23, 015.80-015.96, 017.90-017.96, 036.82, 056.71, 098.50-098.51, 098.59, 098.89, 711.00-714.0, 715.00, 715.09-715.10, 715.18-716.99, 718.00-718.08, 719.00-719.10, 719.18-719.69, 719.80-719.99; **For code 711.36:** 003.23, 015.80-015.96, 017.90-017.96, 036.82, 056.71, 098.50-098.51, 098.59, 098.89, 711.00-714.0, 715.00, 715.09-715.10, 715.18-716.07, 716.09-716.99, 718.00-718.08, 719.00-719.10, 719.18-719.69, 719.80-719.99; **For code 711.38:** 003.23, 015.80-015.96, 017.90-017.96, 036.82, 056.71, 098.50-098.51, 098.59, 098.89, 711.00-714.0, 715.00, 715.09-715.10, 715.18-716.57, 716.59-716.99, 718.00-718.08, 719.00-719.10, 719.18-719.69, 719.80-719.99

§ ✓5ᵗʰ **711.4**   ***Arthropathy associated with other bacterial***   `CC`
[0-9]   ***diseases***

     *Code first underlying disease as:*
       diseases classifiable to 010-040, 090-099, except
         as in 711.1, 711.3, and 713.5
       leprosy (030.0-030.9)
       tuberculosis (015.0-015.9)
     **EXCLUDES**   *gonococcal arthritis (098.50)*
                    *meningococcal arthritis (036.82)*

**CC Excl: For codes 711.40, 711.42-711.49:** 003.23, 015.80-015.96, 017.90-017.96, 036.82, 056.71, 098.50-098.51, 098.59, 098.89, 711.00-714.0, 715.00, 715.09-715.10, 715.18-716.99, 718.00-718.08, 719.00-719.10, 719.18-719.69, 719.80-719.99; **For code 711.41:** 003.23, 015.80-015.96, 017.90-017.96, 036.82, 056.71, 098.50-098.51, 098.59, 098.89, 711.00-714.0, 715.00, 715.09-715.10, 715.18-716.99, 718.00-718.08, 719.00-719.10, 719.18-719.39, 719.41-719.69, 719.80-719.99

§ ✓5ᵗʰ **711.5**   ***Arthropathy associated with other viral***   `CC`
[0-9]   ***diseases***

     *Code first underlying disease as:*
       diseases classifiable to 045-049, 050-079, 480,
         487
       O'nyong nyong (066.3)
     **EXCLUDES**   *that due to rubella (056.71)*

**CC Excl:** 003.23, 015.80-015.96, 017.90-017.96, 036.82, 056.71, 098.50-098.51, 098.59, 098.89, 711.00-714.0, 715.00, 715.09-715.10, 715.18-716.99, 718.00-718.08, 719.00-719.10, 719.18-719.69, 719.80-719.99

§ ✓5ᵗʰ **711.6**   ***Arthropathy associated with mycoses***   `CC`
[0-9]   *Code first underlying disease (110.0-118)*

**CC Excl: For codes 711.60, 711.68-711.69:** 015.80-015.96, 017.90-017.96, 036.82, 056.71, 098.50-098.51, 098.59, 098.89, 711.00-714.0, 715.00, 715.09-715.10, 715.18-716.99, 718.00-718.08, 719.00-719.10, 719.18-719.99; **For code 711.61:** 015.80-015.96, 017.90-017.96, 036.82, 056.71, 098.50-098.51, 098.59, 098.89, 711.00-714.0, 715.00, 715.09-715.10, 715.18-716.99, 718.00-718.08, 719.00-719.10, 719.18-719.99; **For code 711.62:** 015.80-015.96, 017.90-017.96, 036.82, 056.71, 098.50-098.51, 098.59, 098.89, 711.00-711.01, 711.08-711.11, 711.18-711.21, 711.28-711.31, 711.38-711.41, 711.48-711.51, 711.58-711.61, 711.68-711.71, 711.78-711.81, 711.88-711.91, 711.98-712.11, 712.18-712.21, 712.28-712.31, 712.38-712.81, 712.88-712.91, 712.98-714.0, 715.00, 715.09-715.11, 715.18-715.21, 715.28-715.31, 715.38-715.91, 715.98-716.01, 716.08-716.11, 716.18-716.21, 716.28-716.31, 716.38-716.41, 716.48-716.51, 716.58-716.61, 716.68-716.81, 716.88-716.91, 716.98-716.99, 718.00-718.01, 718.08, 719.00-719.01, 719.08-719.11, 719.18-719.21, 719.28-719.31, 719.38-719.41, 719.48-719.51, 719.58-719.61, 719.68-719.81, 719.88-719.91, 719.98-719.99; **For code 711.63:** 015.80-015.96, 017.90-017.96, 036.82, 056.71, 098.50-098.51, 098.59, 098.89, 711.00, 711.02, 711.08-711.10, 711.12, 711.18-711.20, 711.22, 711.28-711.30, 711.32, 711.38-711.40, 711.42, 711.48-711.50, 711.52, 711.58-711.60, 711.62, 711.68-711.70, 711.72, 711.78-711.80, 711.82, 711.88-711.90, 711.92, 711.98-712.10, 712.12, 712.18-712.20, 712.22, 712.28-712.30, 712.32, 712.38-712.80, 712.82, 712.88-712.90, 712.92, 712.98-714.0, 715.00, 715.09-715.10, 715.12, 715.18-715.20, 715.22, 715.28-715.30, 715.32, 715.38-715.90, 715.92, 715.98-716.00, 716.02, 716.08-716.10, 716.12, 716.18-716.20, 716.22, 716.28-716.30, 716.32, 716.38-716.40, 716.42, 716.48-716.50, 716.52, 716.58-716.60, 716.62, 716.68-716.80, 716.82, 716.88-716.90, 716.92, 716.98-716.99, 718.00, 718.02, 718.08, 719.00, 719.02, 719.08-719.10, 719.12, 719.18-719.20, 719.22, 719.28-719.30, 719.32, 719.38-719.40, 719.42, 719.48-719.50, 719.52, 719.58-719.60, 719.62, 719.68-719.80, 719.82, 719.88-719.90, 719.92, 719.98-719.99; **For code 711.64:** 015.80-015.96, 017.90-017.96, 036.82, 056.71, 098.50-098.51, 098.59, 098.89, 711.00, 711.03, 711.08-711.10, 711.13, 711.18-711.20, 711.23, 711.28-711.30, 711.33, 711.38-711.40, 711.43, 711.48-711.50, 711.53, 711.58-711.60, 711.63, 711.68-711.70, 711.73, 711.78-711.80, 711.83, 711.88-711.90, 711.93, 711.98-712.10, 712.13, 712.18-712.20, 712.23, 712.28-712.30, 712.33, 712.38-712.80, 712.83, 712.88-712.90, 712.93, 712.98-714.0, 715.00, 715.09-715.10, 715.13, 715.18-715.20, 715.23, 715.28-715.30, 715.33, 715.38-715.90, 715.93, 715.98-716.00, 716.03, 716.08-716.10, 716.13, 716.18-716.20, 716.23, 716.28-716.30, 716.33, 716.38-716.40, 716.43, 716.48-716.50, 716.53, 716.58-716.60, 716.63, 716.68-716.80, 716.83, 716.88-716.90, 716.93, 716.98-716.99, 718.00, 718.03, 718.08, 719.00, 719.03, 719.08-719.10, 719.13, 719.18-719.20, 719.23, 719.28-719.30, 719.33, 719.38-719.40, 719.43, 719.48-719.50, 719.53, 719.58-719.60, 719.63, 719.68-719.80, 719.83, 719.88-719.90, 719.93, 719.98-719.99; **For code 711.65:** 015.80-015.96, 017.90-017.96, 036.82, 056.71, 098.50-098.51, 098.59, 098.89, 711.00, 711.04, 711.08-711.10, 711.14, 711.18-711.20, 711.24, 711.28-711.30, 711.34, 711.38-711.40, 711.44, 711.48-711.50, 711.54, 711.58-711.60, 711.64, 711.68-711.70, 711.74, 711.78-711.80, 711.84, 711.88-711.90, 711.94, 711.98-712.10, 712.14, 712.18-712.20, 712.24, 712.28-712.30, 712.34, 712.38-712.80, 712.84, 712.88-712.90, 712.94, 712.98-714.0, 715.00-715.10, 715.14, 715.18-715.20, 715.24, 715.28-715.30, 715.34, 715.38-715.90, 715.94, 715.98-716.00, 716.04, 716.08-716.10, 716.14, 716.18-716.20, 716.24, 716.28-716.30, 716.34, 716.38-716.40, 716.44, 716.48-716.50, 716.54, 716.58-716.60, 716.64, 716.68-716.80, 716.84, 716.88-716.90, 716.94, 716.98-716.99, 718.00, 718.04, 718.08, 719.00, 719.04, 719.08-719.10, 719.14, 719.18-719.20, 719.24, 719.28-719.30, 719.34, 719.38-719.40, 719.44, 719.48-719.50, 719.54, 719.58-719.60, 719.64, 719.68-719.80, 719.84, 719.88-719.90, 719.94, 719.98-719.99; **For code 711.66:** 015.80-015.96, 017.90-017.96, 036.82, 056.71, 098.50-098.51, 098.59, 098.89, 711.00, 711.05, 711.08-711.10, 711.15, 711.18-711.20, 711.25, 711.28-711.30, 711.35, 711.38-711.40, 711.45, 711.48-711.50, 711.55, 711.58-711.60, 711.65, 711.68-711.70, 711.75, 711.78-711.80, 711.85, 711.88-711.90, 711.95, 711.98-712.10, 712.15, 712.18-712.20, 712.25, 712.28-712.30, 712.35, 712.38-712.80, 712.85, 712.88-712.90, 712.95, 712.98-714.0, 715.00, 715.09-715.10, 715.15, 715.18-715.20, 715.25, 715.28-715.30, 715.35, 715.38-715.90, 715.95, 715.98-716.00, 716.05, 716.08-716.10, 716.15, 716.18-716.20, 716.25, 716.28-716.30, 716.35, 716.38-716.40, 716.45, 716.48-716.50, 716.55, 716.58-716.60, 716.65, 716.68-716.80, 716.85, 716.88-716.90, 716.95, 716.98-716.99, 718.00, 718.05, 718.08, 719.00, 719.05, 719.08-719.10, 719.15, 719.18-719.20, 719.25, 719.28-719.30, 719.35, 719.38-719.40, 719.45, 719.48-719.50, 719.55, 719.58-719.60, 719.65, 719.68-719.80,

---

§   Requires fifth-digit. Valid digits are in [brackets] under each code. See beginning of section 710-739 for codes and definitions.

| ▨4ᵗʰ   Additional Digit Required | Unacceptable PDx | Manifestation Code | ▶◀ Revised Text | ● New Code | ▲ Revised Code Title |
|---|---|---|---|---|---|
| ▨5ᵗʰ | | | | | |

**Musculoskeletal and Connective Tissue**

**711.6–713.1**

719.85, 719.88-719.90, 719.95, 719.98-719.99; **For code 711.67:** 015.80-015.96, 017.90-017.96, 036.82, 056.71, 098.50-098.51, 098.59, 098.89, 711.00, 711.06, 711.08-711.10, 711.16, 711.18-711.20, 711.26, 711.28-711.30, 711.36, 711.38-711.40, 711.46, 711.48-711.50, 711.56, 711.58-711.60, 711.66, 711.68-711.70, 711.76, 711.78-711.80, 711.86, 711.88-711.90, 711.96, 711.98-712.10, 712.16, 712.18-712.20, 712.26, 712.28-712.30, 712.36, 712.38-712.80, 712.86, 712.88-712.90, 712.96, 712.98-714.0, 715.00, 715.09-715.10, 715.16, 715.18-715.20, 715.26, 715.28-715.30, 715.36, 715.38-715.90, 715.96, 715.98-716.00, 716.06, 716.08-716.10, 716.16, 716.18-716.20, 716.26, 716.28-716.30, 716.36, 716.38-716.40, 716.46, 716.48-716.50, 716.56, 716.58-716.60, 716.66, 716.68-716.80, 716.86, 716.88-716.90, 716.96, 716.98-716.99, 718.00, 718.08, 719.00, 719.06, 719.08-719.10, 719.16, 719.18-719.20, 719.26, 719.28-719.30, 719.36, 719.38-719.40, 719.46, 719.48-719.50, 719.56, 719.58-719.60, 719.66, 719.68-719.80, 719.86, 719.88-719.90, 719.96, 719.98-719.99 **For code 711.68:** 015.80-015.96, 017.90-017.96, 036.82, 056.71, 098.50-098.51, 098.59, 098.89, 711.00-711.99, 712.10-712.99, 713.0-713.8, 714.0, 715.00, 715.09-715.10, 715.18-715.98, 716.00-716.99, 718.00-718.08, 719.00-719.10, 719.18-719.99 **For code 711.69:** See code 711.68

**§**   ✓5ᵗʰ   **711.7**   *Arthropathy associated with helminthiasis*   **CC**
[0-9]      *Code first underlying disease as:*
       filariasis (125.0-125.9)
**CC Excl: For codes 711.70-711.74, 711.76, 711.78-711.79:** 003.23, 015.80-015.96, 017.90-017.96, 036.82, 056.71, 098.50-098.51, 098.59, 098.89, 711.00-714.0, 715.00, 715.09-715.10, 715.18-716.99, 718.00-718.08, 719.00-719.10, 719.18-719.69, 719.80-719.99; **For code 711.75:** 003.23, 015.80-015.96, 017.90-017.96, 036.82, 056.71, 098.50-098.51, 098.59, 098.89, 711.00-714.0, 715.00, 715.09-715.10, 715.18-716.99, 718.00-718.08, 719.00-719.10, 719.18-719.43, 719.45-719.69, 719.80-719.99; **For code 711.77:** 003.23, 015.80-015.96, 017.90-017.96, 036.82, 056.71, 098.50-098.51, 098.59, 098.89, 711.00-714.0, 715.00, 715.09-715.10, 715.18-716.99, 718.00-718.08, 719.00-719.10, 719.18-719.69, 719.80-719.97, 719.99

**§**   ✓5ᵗʰ   **711.8**   *Arthropathy associated with other infectious*   **CC**
[0-9]    *and parasitic diseases*
     *Code first underlying disease as:*
       diseases classifiable to 080-088, 100-104, 130-136
     **EXCLUDES**   *arthropathy associated with sarcoidosis (713.7)*
**CC Excl: For codes 711.80, 711.82-711.89:** 003.23, 015.80-015.96, 017.90-017.96, 036.82, 056.71, 098.50-098.51, 098.59, 098.89, 711.00-714.0, 715.00, 715.09-715.10, 715.18-716.99, 718.00-718.08, 719.00-719.10, 719.18-719.69, 719.80-719.99; **For code 711.81:** 003.23, 015.80-015.96, 017.90-017.96, 036.82, 056.71, 098.50-098.51, 098.59, 098.89, 711.00-711.41, 711.43-714.0, 715.00, 715.09-715.10, 715.18-716.99, 718.00-718.08, 719.00-719.10, 719.18-719.69, 719.80-719.99

**AHA:** 4Q, '91, 15; 3Q, '90, 14

**§**   ✓5ᵗʰ   **711.9**   **Unspecified infective arthritis**   **CC**
[0-9]      Infective arthritis or polyarthritis (acute) (chronic) (subacute) NOS
**CC Excl:** 003.23, 015.80-015.96, 017.90-017.96, 036.82, 056.71, 098.50-098.51, 098.59, 098.89, 711.00-714.0, 715.00, 715.09-715.10, 715.18-716.99, 718.00-718.08, 719.00-719.10, 719.18-719.69, 719.80-719.99

✓4ᵗʰ   **712**   **Crystal arthropathies**
     **INCLUDES**   crystal-induced arthritis and synovitis
     **EXCLUDES**   *gouty arthropathy (274.0)*
**DEF:** Joint disease due to urate crystal deposit in joints or synovial membranes.

The following fifth-digit subclassification is for use with category 712; valid digits are in [brackets] under each code. See list at beginning of chapter for definitions.

   0   **site unspecified**
   1   **shoulder region**
   2   **upper arm**
   3   **forearm**
   4   **hand**
   5   **pelvic region and thigh**
   6   **lower leg**
   7   **ankle and foot**
   8   **other specified sites**
   9   **multiple sites**

**§**   ✓5ᵗʰ   **712.1**   *Chondrocalcinosis due to dicalcium phosphate*
[0-9]    *crystals*
     Chondrocalcinosis due to dicalcium phosphate crystals (with other crystals)
     *Code first underlying disease (275.4)*

**§**   ✓5ᵗʰ   **712.2**   *Chondrocalcinosis due to pyrophosphate crystals*
[0-9]      *Code first underlying disease (275.4)*

**§**   ✓5ᵗʰ   **712.3**   *Chondrocalcinosis, unspecified*
[0-9]      *Code first underlying disease (275.4)*

**§**   ✓5ᵗʰ   **712.8**   **Other specified crystal arthropathies**
[0-9]

**§**   ✓5ᵗʰ   **712.9**   **Unspecified crystal arthropathy**
[0-9]

✓4ᵗʰ   **713**   **Arthropathy associated with other disorders classified elsewhere**
     **INCLUDES**   arthritis
                  arthropathy     associated with
                  polyarthritis     conditions
                  polyarthropathy     classifiable below

     **713.0**   *Arthropathy associated with other endocrine and metabolic disorders*
       *Code first underlying disease as:*
         acromegaly (253.0)
         hemochromatosis (275.0)
         hyperparathyroidism (252.00-252.08)
         hypogammaglobulinemia (279.00-279.09)
         hypothyroidism (243-244.9)
         lipoid metabolism disorder (272.0-272.9)
         ochronosis (270.2)
       **EXCLUDES**   *arthropathy associated with:*
            *amyloidosis (713.7)*
            *crystal deposition disorders, except gout (712.1-712.9)*
            *diabetic neuropathy (713.5)*
            *gouty arthropathy (274.0)*

     **713.1**   *Arthropathy associated with gastrointestinal conditions other than infections*
       *Code first underlying disease as:*
         regional enteritis (555.0-555.9)
         ulcerative colitis (556)

---

**§**   Requires fifth-digit. Valid digits are in [brackets] under each code. See beginning of section 710-739 for codes and definitions.

**N** Newborn Age: 0    **P** Pediatric Age: 0-17    **M** Maternity Age: 12-55    **A** Adult Age: 15-124    **CC** CC Condition    **MCC** Major CC Condition    **HIV** HIV Related Dx

**713.2  Arthropathy associated with hematological disorders**

Code first underlying disease as:
hemoglobinopathy (282.4-282.7)
hemophilia (286.0-286.2)
leukemia (204.0-208.9)
malignant reticulosis (202.3)
multiple myelomatosis (203.0)

> EXCLUDES    arthropathy associated with Henoch-Schönlein purpura (713.6)

**713.3  Arthropathy associated with dermatological disorders**

Code first underlying disease as:
erythema multiforme (695.1)
erythema nodosum (695.2)

> EXCLUDES    psoriatic arthropathy (696.0)

**713.4  Arthropathy associated with respiratory disorders**

Code first underlying disease as:
diseases classifiable to 490-519

> EXCLUDES    arthropathy associated with respiratory infections (711.0, 711.4-711.8)

**713.5  Arthropathy associated with neurological disorders**

Charcôt's arthropathy ⎫ associated with diseases
Neuropathic arthritis ⎬ classifiable elsewhere

Code first underlying disease as:
neuropathic joint disease [Charcôt's joints]:
NOS (094.0)
diabetic (250.6)
syringomyelic (336.0)
tabetic [syphilitic] (094.0)

**713.6  Arthropathy associated with hypersensitivity reaction**

Code first underlying disease as:
Henoch (-Schönlein) purpura (287.0)
serum sickness (999.5)

> EXCLUDES    allergic arthritis NOS (716.2)

**713.7  Other general diseases with articular involvement**

Code first underlying disease as:
amyloidosis (277.30-277.39)
familial Mediterranean fever (277.31)
sarcoidosis (135)

**AHA:** 2Q, '97, 12

**713.8  Arthropathy associated with other condition classifiable elsewhere**

Code first underlying disease as:
conditions classifiable elsewhere except as in 711.1-711.8, 712, and 713.0-713.7

✓4ᵗʰ **714  Rheumatoid arthritis and other inflammatory polyarthropathies**

> EXCLUDES    rheumatic fever (390)
> rheumatoid arthritis of spine NOS (720.0)

**AHA:** 2Q, '95, 3

**714.0  Rheumatoid arthritis**

Arthritis or polyarthritis:
atrophic
rheumatic (chronic)
Use additional code to identify manifestation, as:
myopathy (359.6)
polyneuropathy (357.1)

> EXCLUDES    juvenile rheumatoid arthritis NOS (714.30)

**AHA:** 2Q, '06, 20; 1Q, '90, 5

**DEF:** Chronic systemic disease principally of joints, manifested by inflammatory changes in articular structures and synovial membranes, atrophy, and loss in bone density.

**714.1  Felty's syndrome**
Rheumatoid arthritis with splenoadenomegaly and leukopenia

**DEF:** Syndrome marked by rheumatoid arthritis, splenomegaly, leukopenia, pigmented spots on lower extremity skin, anemia, and thrombocytopenia.

**714.2  Other rheumatoid arthritis with visceral or systemic involvement**
Rheumatoid carditis

✓5ᵗʰ **714.3  Juvenile chronic polyarthritis**

**DEF:** Rheumatoid arthritis of more than one joint; lasts longer than six weeks in age 17 or younger; symptoms include fever, erythematous rash, weight loss, lymphadenopathy, hepatosplenomegaly and pericarditis.

**714.30  Polyarticular juvenile rheumatoid arthritis, chronic or unspecified**
Juvenile rheumatoid arthritis NOS
Still's disease

**714.31  Polyarticular juvenile rheumatoid arthritis, acute**    CC

**CC Excl:** 036.82, 056.71, 711.00-714.4, 715.00, 715.09-715.10, 715.18-716.99, 718.00-718.08, 719.00-719.10, 719.18-719.99

**714.32  Pauciarticular juvenile rheumatoid arthritis**

**714.33  Monoarticular juvenile rheumatoid arthritis**

**714.4  Chronic postrheumatic arthropathy**
Chronic rheumatoid nodular fibrositis
Jaccoud's syndrome

**DEF:** Persistent joint disorder; follows previous rheumatic infection.

✓5ᵗʰ **714.8  Other specified inflammatory polyarthropathies**
**714.81  Rheumatoid lung**
Caplan's syndrome
Diffuse interstitial rheumatoid disease of lung
Fibrosing alveolitis, rheumatoid

**DEF:** Lung disorders associated with rheumatoid arthritis.

**714.89  Other**

**714.9  Unspecified inflammatory polyarthropathy**
Inflammatory polyarthropathy or polyarthritis NOS

> EXCLUDES    polyarthropathy NOS (716.5)

**Musculoskeletal and Connective Tissue**

**715–717.5**

✓4th **715 Osteoarthrosis and allied disorders**

Note: Localized, in the subcategories below, includes bilateral involvement of the same site.

INCLUDES   arthritis or polyarthritis:
> degenerative
> hypertrophic
> degenerative joint disease
> osteoarthritis

EXCLUDES   *Marie-Strümpell spondylitis (720.0)*
> *osteoarthrosis [osteoarthritis] of spine (721.0-721.9)*

The following fifth-digit subclassification is for use with category 715; valid digits are in [brackets] under each code. See list at beginning of chapter for definitions.

- 0   site unspecified
- 1   shoulder region
- 2   upper arm
- 3   forearm
- 4   hand
- 5   pelvic region and thigh
- 6   lower leg
- 7   ankle and foot
- 8   other specified sites
- 9   multiple sites

§ ✓5th **715.0 Osteoarthrosis, generalized**
[0,4,9]   Degenerative joint disease, involving multiple joints
> Primary generalized hypertrophic osteoarthrosis

**DEF:** Chronic noninflammatory arthritis; marked by degenerated articular cartilage and enlarged bone; symptoms include pain and stiffness with activity; occurs among elderly.

§ ✓5th **715.1 Osteoarthrosis, localized, primary**
[0-8]   Localized osteoarthropathy, idiopathic

§ ✓5th **715.2 Osteoarthrosis, localized, secondary**
[0-8]   Coxae malum senilis

§ ✓5th **715.3 Osteoarthrosis, localized, not specified whether primary or secondary**
[0-8]   Otto's pelvis

**AHA:** For code 715.35: 3Q, '04, 12; 2Q, '04, 15; For code 715.36: 4Q, '03, 118; 2Q, '95, 5

§ ✓5th **715.8 Osteoarthrosis involving, or with mention of more than one site, but not specified as generalized**
[0,9]

§ ✓5th **715.9 Osteoarthrosis, unspecified whether generalized or localized**
[0-8]

**AHA:** For code 715.90: 2Q, '97, 12

✓4th **716 Other and unspecified arthropathies**

EXCLUDES   *cricoarytenoid arthropathy (478.79)*

The following fifth-digit subclassification is for use with category 716; valid digits are in [brackets] under each code. See list at beginning of chapter for definitions.

- 0   site unspecified
- 1   shoulder region
- 2   upper arm
- 3   forearm
- 4   hand
- 5   pelvic region and thigh
- 6   lower leg
- 7   ankle and foot
- 8   other specified sites
- 9   multiple sites

**AHA:** 2Q, '95, 3

§ ✓5th **716.0 Kaschin-Beck disease**
[0-9]   Endemic polyarthritis

**DEF:** Chronic degenerative disease of spine and peripheral joints; occurs in eastern Siberian, northern Chinese, and Korean youth; may be a mycotoxicosis caused by eating cereals infected with fungus.

§ ✓5th **716.1 Traumatic arthropathy**
[0-9]   **AHA:** For Code 716.11: 1Q, '02, 9

§ ✓5th **716.2 Allergic arthritis**
[0-9]   EXCLUDES   *arthritis associated with Henoch-Schönlein purpura or serum sickness (713.6)*

§ ✓5th **716.3 Climacteric arthritis**   ♀
[0-9]   Menopausal arthritis

**DEF:** Ovarian hormone deficiency; causes pain in small joints, shoulders, elbows or knees; affects females at menopause; also called arthropathia ovaripriva.

§ ✓5th **716.4 Transient arthropathy**
[0-9]   EXCLUDES   *palindromic rheumatism (719.3)*

§ ✓5th **716.5 Unspecified polyarthropathy or polyarthritis**
[0-9]

§ ✓5th **716.6 Unspecified monoarthritis**
[0-8]   Coxitis

§ ✓5th **716.8 Other specified arthropathy**
[0-9]

§ ✓5th **716.9 Arthropathy, unspecified**
[0-9]   Arthritis
> Arthropathy } (acute) (chronic) (subacute)
>
> Articular rheumatism (chronic)
> Inflammation of joint NOS

✓4th **717 Internal derangement of knee**

INCLUDES   degeneration
> rupture, old } of articular cartilage or meniscus of knee
> tear, old

EXCLUDES   *acute derangement of knee (836.0-836.6)*
> *ankylosis (718.5)*
> *contracture (718.4)*
> *current injury (836.0-836.6)*
> *deformity (736.4-736.6)*
> *recurrent dislocation (718.3)*

**717.0 Old bucket handle tear of medial meniscus**
> Old bucket handle tear of unspecified cartilage

**717.1 Derangement of anterior horn of medial meniscus**

**717.2 Derangement of posterior horn of medial meniscus**

**717.3 Other and unspecified derangement of medial meniscus**
> Degeneration of internal semilunar cartilage

✓5th **717.4 Derangement of lateral meniscus**

> **717.40 Derangement of lateral meniscus, unspecified**

> **717.41 Bucket handle tear of lateral meniscus**

> **717.42 Derangement of anterior horn of lateral meniscus**

> **717.43 Derangement of posterior horn of lateral meniscus**

> **717.49 Other**

**717.5 Derangement of meniscus, not elsewhere classified**
> Congenital discoid meniscus
> Cyst of semilunar cartilage
> Derangement of semilunar cartilage NOS

**Disruption and Tears of Meniscus**

Bucket-handle

Flap-type

Radial
Peripheral

Horizontal cleavage

Vertical

Congenital discoid meniscus

§   Requires fifth-digit. Valid digits are in [brackets] under each code. See beginning of section 710-739 for codes and definitions.

N Newborn Age: 0    P Pediatric Age: 0-17    M Maternity Age: 12-55    A Adult Age: 15-124    CC CC Condition    MCC Major CC Condition    HIV HIV Related Dx

**Internal Derangements of Knee**

Disruptions of Cruciate Ligament

Anterior

Posterior

Chondromalacia of Patella

"Kissing" lesion of femur

**717.6    Loose body in knee**
> Joint mice, knee
> Rice bodies, knee (joint)
>
> **DEF:** The presence in the joint synovial area of a small, frequently calcified, loose body created from synovial membrane, organized fibrin fragments of articular cartilage or arthritis osteophytes.

**717.7    Chondromalacia of patella**
> Chondromalacia patellae
> Degeneration [softening] of articular cartilage of patella
>
> **AHA:** M-A, '85, 14; N-D, '84, 9
>
> **DEF:** Softened patella cartilage.

✓5ᵗʰ **717.8    Other internal derangement of knee**
     **717.81   Old disruption of lateral collateral ligament**
     **717.82   Old disruption of medial collateral ligament**
     **717.83   Old disruption of anterior cruciate ligament**
     **717.84   Old disruption of posterior cruciate ligament**
     **717.85   Old disruption of other ligaments of knee**
         Capsular ligament of knee
     **717.89   Other**
         Old disruption of ligaments NOS

**717.9    Unspecified internal derangement of knee**
> Derangement NOS of knee

✓4ᵗʰ **718 Other derangement of joint**
> **EXCLUDES**   current injury (830.0-848.9)
>                  jaw (524.60-524.69)

> The following fifth-digit subclassification is for use with category 718; valid digits are in [brackets] under each code. See list at beginning of chapter for definitions.
>     0   site unspecified
>     1   shoulder region
>     2   upper arm
>     3   forearm
>     4   hand
>     5   pelvic region and thigh
>     6   lower leg
>     7   ankle and foot
>     8   other specified sites
>     9   multiple sites

§ ✓5ᵗʰ **718.0    Articular cartilage disorder**
> [0-5,7-9]    Meniscus:         Meniscus:
>             disorder          tear, old
>             rupture, old    Old rupture of ligament(s) of joint NOS
>         **EXCLUDES**   articular cartilage disorder:
>                           in ochronosis (270.2)
>                           knee (717.0-717.9)
>                   chondrocalcinosis (275.4)
>                   metastatic calcification (275.4)

§ ✓5ᵗʰ **718.1    Loose body in joint**
> [0-5,7-9]    Joint mice
>       **EXCLUDES**   knee (717.6)
>
> **AHA:** For code 718.17: 2Q, '01, 15
>
> **DEF:** Calcified loose bodies in synovial fluid; due to arthritic osteophytes.

§ ✓5ᵗʰ **718.2    Pathological dislocation**
> [0-9]    Dislocation or displacement of joint, not recurrent and not current injury
>       Spontaneous dislocation (joint)

§ ✓5ᵗʰ **718.3    Recurrent dislocation of joint**
> [0-9]    **AHA:** N-D, '87, 7

§ ✓5ᵗʰ **718.4    Contracture of joint**
> [0-9]    **AHA:** 4Q, '98, 40

§ ✓5ᵗʰ **718.5    Ankylosis of joint**
> [0-9]    Ankylosis of joint (fibrous) (osseous)
>       **EXCLUDES**   spine (724.9)
>                     stiffness of joint without mention of ankylosis (719.5)
>
> **DEF:** Immobility and solidification, of joint; due to disease, injury or surgical procedure.

§ ✓5ᵗʰ **718.6    Unspecified intrapelvic protrusion of acetabulum**
> [0,5]    Protrusio acetabuli, unspecified
>
> **DEF:** Sinking of the floor of acetabulum; causing femoral head to protrude, limits hip movement; of unknown etiology.

§ ✓5ᵗʰ **718.7    Developmental dislocation of joint**
> [0-9]    **EXCLUDES**   congenital dislocation of joint (754.0-755.8)
>                          traumatic dislocation of joint (830-839)
>
> **AHA:** 4Q, '01, 48

§ ✓5ᵗʰ **718.8    Other joint derangement, not elsewhere classified**
> [0-9]    Flail joint (paralytic)       Instability of joint
>       **EXCLUDES**   deformities classifiable to 736 (736.0-736.9)
>
> **AHA:** For code 718.81: 2Q, '00, 14

§ ✓5ᵗʰ **718.9    Unspecified derangement of joint**
> [0-5,7-9]   **EXCLUDES**   knee (717.9)

✓4ᵗʰ **719 Other and unspecified disorders of joint**
> **EXCLUDES**   jaw (524.60-524.69)

> The following fifth-digit subclassification is for use with codes 719.0-719.6, 719.8-719.9; valid digits are in [brackets] under each code. See list at beginning of chapter for definitions.
>     0   site unspecified
>     1   shoulder region
>     2   upper arm
>     3   forearm
>     4   hand
>     5   pelvic region and thigh
>     6   lower leg
>     7   ankle and foot
>     8   other specified sites
>     9   multiple sites

§ ✓5ᵗʰ **719.0    Effusion of joint**
> [0-9]    Hydrarthrosis
>       Swelling of joint, with or without pain
>       **EXCLUDES**   intermittent hydrarthrosis (719.3)

§ ✓5ᵗʰ **719.1    Hemarthrosis**          **CC**
> [0-9]    **EXCLUDES**   current injury (840.0-848.9)
>
> **CC Excl:** For codes: **719.10, 719.15, 719.18-719.19:** 719.10-719.19, 958.91-958.92; **For code 719.11:** 719.10-719.13, 719.18-719.19, 958.91; **For code 719.12:** 719.10-719.12, 719.18-719.19, 958.91; **For code 719.13:** 719.10, 719.12-719.14, 719.18-719.19, 958.91; **For code 719.14:** 719.10, 719.13-719.14, 719.18-719.19, 958.91; **For code 719.16-719.17:** 719.10, 719.16-719.19, 958.92

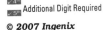
✓4ᵗʰ / ✓5ᵗʰ Additional Digit Required     Unacceptable PDx     Manifestation Code     ▶◀ Revised Text     ● New Code     ▲ Revised Code Title

Musculoskeletal and Connective Tissue

717.6–719.1

*Musculoskeletal and Connective Tissue*

*719.2–721.91*

### Joint Derangements and Disorders

Loose body in joint

Dislocation of joint

Joint contracture

Ankylosis of joint

Synovial effusion (fluid)

Hemarthrosis (blood)

§ ✓5ᵗʰ **719.2** **Villonodular synovitis**
[0-9]

DEF: Overgrowth of synovial tissue, especially at knee joint; due to macrophage infiltration of giant cells in synovial villi and fibrous nodules.

§ ✓5ᵗʰ **719.3** **Palindromic rheumatism**
[0-9]
  Hench-Rosenberg syndrome
  Intermittent hydrarthrosis

DEF: Recurrent episodes of afebrile arthritis and periarthritis marked by their complete disappearance after a few days or hours; causes swelling, redness, and disability usually affecting only one joint; no known cause; affects adults of either sex.

§ ✓5ᵗʰ **719.4** **Pain in joint**
[0-9]
  Arthralgia
  **AHA: For code 719.46:** 1Q, '01, 3

§ ✓5ᵗʰ **719.5** **Stiffness of joint, not elsewhere classified**
[0-9]

§ ✓5ᵗʰ **719.6** **Other symptoms referable to joint**
[0-9]
  Joint crepitus          Snapping hip
  **AHA:** 1Q, '94, 15; **For code 719.66:** ▶2Q, '07, 6◀

**719.7** **Difficulty in walking**
  **EXCLUDES** *abnormality of gait (781.2)*
  **AHA:** 2Q, '04, 15; 4Q, '03, 66

§ ✓5ᵗʰ **719.8** **Other specified disorders of joint**
[0-9]
  Calcification of joint       Fistula of joint
  **EXCLUDES** *temporomandibular joint-pain-dysfunction syndrome [Costen's syndrome] (524.60)*

§ ✓5ᵗʰ **719.9** **Unspecified disorder of joint**
[0-9]

### DORSOPATHIES (720-724)
  **EXCLUDES** *curvature of spine (737.0-737.9)*
  *osteochondrosis of spine (juvenile) (732.0)*
  *adult (732.8)*

✓4ᵗʰ **720** **Ankylosing spondylitis and other inflammatory spondylopathies**

**720.0** **Ankylosing spondylitis**
  Rheumatoid arthritis of spine NOS
  Spondylitis:
    Marie-Strümpell
    rheumatoid

DEF: Rheumatoid arthritis of spine and sacroiliac joints; fusion and deformity in spine follows; affects mainly males; cause unknown.

**720.1** **Spinal enthesopathy**
  Disorder of peripheral ligamentous or muscular attachments of spine
  Romanus lesion

DEF: Tendinous or muscular vertebral bone attachment abnormality.

**720.2** **Sacroiliitis, not elsewhere classified**
  Inflammation of sacroiliac joint NOS
  DEF: Pain due to inflammation in joint, at juncture of sacrum and hip.

✓5ᵗʰ **720.8** **Other inflammatory spondylopathies**
  **720.81** *Inflammatory spondylopathies in diseases classified elsewhere*
    Code first underlying disease as:
      tuberculosis (015.0)
  **720.89** **Other**

**720.9** **Unspecified inflammatory spondylopathy**
  Spondylitis NOS

✓4ᵗʰ **721** **Spondylosis and allied disorders**
  **AHA:** 2Q, '89, 14

DEF: Degenerative changes in spinal joint.

**721.0** **Cervical spondylosis without myelopathy**
  Cervical or cervicodorsal:   Cervical or cervicodorsal:
    arthritis                    spondylarthritis
    osteoarthritis

**721.1** **Cervical spondylosis with myelopathy**   CC
  Anterior spinal artery compression syndrome
  Spondylogenic compression of cervical spinal cord
  Vertebral artery compression syndrome
  **CC Excl:** 721.0-721.1

**721.2** **Thoracic spondylosis without myelopathy**
  Thoracic:              Thoracic:
    arthritis              spondylarthritis
    osteoarthritis

**721.3** **Lumbosacral spondylosis without myelopathy**
  Lumbar or lumbosacral:   Lumbar or lumbosacral:
    arthritis                spondylarthritis
    osteoarthritis
  **AHA:** 4Q, '02, 107

✓5ᵗʰ **721.4** **Thoracic or lumbar spondylosis with myelopathy**
  **721.41** **Thoracic region**   CC
    Spondylogenic compression of thoracic spinal cord
    **CC Excl:** 721.41

  **721.42** **Lumbar region**   CC
    Spondylogenic compression of lumbar spinal cord
    **CC Excl:** 721.3, 721.42, 722.10, 722.2, 722.32, 722.52-722.70, 722.73, 722.83-722.90, 722.93

**721.5** **Kissing spine**
  Baastrup's syndrome
  DEF: Compression of spinous processes of adjacent vertebrae; due to mutual contact.

**721.6** **Ankylosing vertebral hyperostosis**
**721.7** **Traumatic spondylopathy**   CC
  Kümmell's disease or spondylitis
  **CC Excl:** 721.7

**721.8** **Other allied disorders of spine**
✓5ᵗʰ **721.9** **Spondylosis of unspecified site**
  **721.90** **Without mention of myelopathy**
    Spinal:
      arthritis (deformans) (degenerative) (hypertrophic)
      osteoarthritis NOS
    Spondylarthrosis NOS
  **721.91** **With myelopathy**   CC
    Spondylogenic compression of spinal cord NOS
    **CC Excl:** 721.0-721.91

---

§  Requires fifth-digit. Valid digits are in [brackets] under each code. See beginning of section 710-739 for codes and definitions.

Ⓝ Newborn Age: 0   Ⓟ Pediatric Age: 0-17   Ⓜ Maternity Age: 12-55   Ⓐ Adult Age: 15-124   CC CC Condition   MCC Major CC Condition   HIV HIV Related Dx

### Normal Anatomy of Vertebral Disc

### Derangement of Vertebral Disc

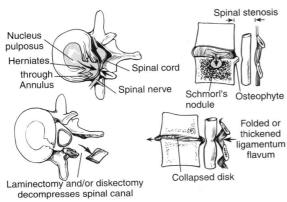

√4ᵗʰ **722 Intervertebral disc disorders**
    **AHA:** 1Q, '88, 10

    **722.0**   **Displacement of cervical intervertebral disc without myelopathy**
       Neuritis (brachial) or radiculitis due to displacement or rupture of cervical intervertebral disc
       Any condition classifiable to 722.2 of the cervical or cervicothoracic intervertebral disc

√5ᵗʰ **722.1**   **Displacement of thoracic or lumbar intervertebral disc without myelopathy**

       **722.10 Lumbar intervertebral disc without myelopathy**
          Lumbago or sciatica due to displacement of intervertebral disc
          Neuritis or radiculitis due to displacement or rupture of lumbar intervertebral disc
          Any condition classifiable to 722.2 of the lumbar or lumbosacral intervertebral disc
          **AHA:** ▶1Q, '07, 9;◀ 3Q, '03, 12; 1Q, '03, 7; 4Q, '02, 107

       **722.11 Thoracic intervertebral disc without myelopathy**
          Any condition classifiable to 722.2 of thoracic intervertebral disc

    **722.2**   **Displacement of intervertebral disc, site unspecified, without myelopathy**
       Discogenic syndrome NOS
       Herniation of nucleus pulposus NOS
       Intervertebral disc NOS:
          extrusion
          prolapse
          protrusion
          rupture
       Neuritis or radiculitis due to displacement or rupture of intervertebral disc

√5ᵗʰ **722.3**   **Schmorl's nodes**
       **DEF:** Irregular bone defect in the margin of the vertebral body; causes herniation into end plate of vertebral body.

       **722.30 Unspecified region**
       **722.31 Thoracic region**
       **722.32 Lumbar region**
       **722.39 Other**

    **722.4**   **Degeneration of cervical intervertebral disc**
       Degeneration of cervicothoracic intervertebral disc

√5ᵗʰ **722.5**   **Degeneration of thoracic or lumbar intervertebral disc**
       **722.51 Thoracic or thoracolumbar intervertebral disc**
       **722.52 Lumbar or lumbosacral intervertebral disc**
          **AHA:** 2Q, '06, 18; 4Q, '04, 133

    **722.6**   **Degeneration of intervertebral disc, site unspecified**
       Degenerative disc disease NOS
       Narrowing of intervertebral disc or space NOS

√5ᵗʰ **722.7**   **Intervertebral disc disorder with myelopathy**
       **722.70 Unspecified region**
       **722.71 Cervical region**     `CC`
          **CC Excl:** 722.0, 722.71

       **722.72 Thoracic region**     `CC`
          **CC Excl:** 722.11, 722.72

       **722.73 Lumbar region**     `CC`
          **CC Excl:** 722.11, 722.73

√5ᵗʰ **722.8**   **Postlaminectomy syndrome**
       **AHA:** J-F, '87, 7

       **DEF:** Spinal disorder due to spinal laminectomy surgery.

       **722.80 Unspecified region**
       **722.81 Cervical region**
       **722.82 Thoracic region**
       **722.83 Lumbar region**
          **AHA:** 2Q, '97, 15

√5ᵗʰ **722.9**   **Other and unspecified disc disorder**
       Calcification of intervertebral cartilage or disc
       Discitis
       **722.90 Unspecified region**
          **AHA:** N-D, '84, 19

       **722.91 Cervical region**
       **722.92 Thoracic region**
       **722.93 Lumbar region**

√4ᵗʰ **723 Other disorders of cervical region**
       **EXCLUDES**   *conditions due to:*
          *intervertebral disc disorders (722.0-722.9)*
          *spondylosis (721.0-721.9)*
    **AHA:** 3Q, '94, 14; 2Q, '89, 14

    **723.0**   **Spinal stenosis in cervical region**
       **AHA:** 4Q, '03, 101

    **723.1**   **Cervicalgia**
       Pain in neck
       **DEF:** Pain in cervical spine or neck region.

    **723.2**   **Cervicocranial syndrome**
       Barré-Liéou syndrome
       Posterior cervical sympathetic syndrome
       **DEF:** Neurologic disorder of upper cervical spine and nerve roots.

**Spinal Stenosis in Cervical Region**

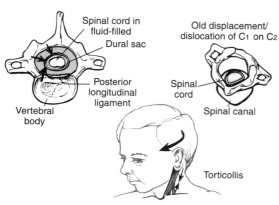

Spinal cord in fluid-filled Dural sac
Old displacement/dislocation of C₁ on C₂
Posterior longitudinal ligament
Spinal cord
Vertebral body
Spinal canal
Torticollis

**723.3   Cervicobrachial syndrome (diffuse)**
AHA: N-D, '85, 12

DEF: Complex of symptoms due to scalenus anterior muscle compressing the brachial plexus; pain radiates from shoulder to arm or back of neck.

**723.4   Brachial neuritis or radiculitis NOS**
Cervical radiculitis
Radicular syndrome of upper limbs

**723.5   Torticollis, unspecified**
Contracture of neck
EXCLUDES     congenital (754.1)
due to birth injury (767.8)
hysterical (300.11)
ocular torticollis (781.93)
psychogenic (306.0)
spasmodic (333.83)
traumatic, current (847.0)
AHA: 2Q, '01, 21; 1Q, '95, 7

DEF: Abnormally positioned neck relative to head; due to cervical muscle or fascia contractions; also called wryneck.

**723.6   Panniculitis specified as affecting neck**
DEF: Inflammation of the panniculus adiposus (subcutaneous fat) in the neck.

**723.7   Ossification of posterior longitudinal ligament in cervical region**

**723.8   Other syndromes affecting cervical region**
Cervical syndrome NEC
Klippel's disease
Occipital neuralgia
AHA: 1Q, '00, 7

**723.9   Unspecified musculoskeletal disorders and symptoms referable to neck**
Cervical (region) disorder NOS

✓4ᵗʰ **724 Other and unspecified disorders of back**
EXCLUDES     collapsed vertebra (code to cause, e.g., osteoporosis, 733.00-733.09)
conditions due to:
intervertebral disc disorders (722.0-722.9)
spondylosis (721.0-721.9)
AHA: 2Q, '89, 14

✓5ᵗʰ **724.0   Spinal stenosis, other than cervical**
**724.00  Spinal stenosis, unspecified region**
**724.01  Thoracic region**
**724.02  Lumbar region**
AHA: ▶1Q, '07, 10, 20;◀ 4Q, '99, 13

**724.09  Other**
**724.1   Pain in thoracic spine**

**724.2   Lumbago**
Low back pain          Lumbalgia
Low back syndrome
AHA: ▶2Q, '07, 11;◀ N-D, '85, 12

**724.3   Sciatica**
Neuralgia or neuritis of sciatic nerve
EXCLUDES     specified lesion of sciatic nerve (355.0)
AHA: 2Q, '89, 12

**724.4   Thoracic or lumbosacral neuritis or radiculitis, unspecified**
Radicular syndrome of lower limbs
AHA: 2Q, '99, 3

**724.5   Backache, unspecified**
Vertebrogenic (pain) syndrome NOS

**724.6   Disorders of sacrum**
Ankylosis
Instability          } lumbosacral or sacroiliac (joint)

✓5ᵗʰ **724.7   Disorders of coccyx**
**724.70  Unspecified disorder of coccyx**
**724.71  Hypermobility of coccyx**
**724.79  Other**
Coccygodynia

**724.8   Other symptoms referable to back**
Ossification of posterior longitudinal ligament NOS
Panniculitis specified as sacral or affecting back

**724.9   Other unspecified back disorders**
Ankylosis of spine NOS
Compression of spinal nerve root NEC
Spinal disorder NOS
EXCLUDES     sacroiliitis (720.2)

## RHEUMATISM, EXCLUDING THE BACK (725-729)
INCLUDES     disorders of muscles and tendons and their attachments, and of other soft tissues

**725 Polymyalgia rheumatica**
DEF: Joint and muscle pain, pelvis, and shoulder girdle stiffness, high sedimentation rate and temporal arteritis; occurs in elderly.

✓4ᵗʰ **726 Peripheral enthesopathies and allied syndromes**
Note: Enthesopathies are disorders of peripheral ligamentous or muscular attachments.
EXCLUDES     spinal enthesopathy (720.1)

**726.0   Adhesive capsulitis of shoulder**

✓5ᵗʰ **726.1   Rotator cuff syndrome of shoulder and allied disorders**
**726.10  Disorders of bursae and tendons in shoulder region, unspecified**
Rotator cuff syndrome NOS
Supraspinatus syndrome NOS
AHA: 2Q, '01, 11

**726.11  Calcifying tendinitis of shoulder**
**726.12  Bicipital tenosynovitis**
**726.19  Other specified disorders**
EXCLUDES     complete rupture of rotator cuff, nontraumatic (727.61)

**726.2   Other affections of shoulder region, not elsewhere classified**
Periarthritis of shoulder
Scapulohumeral fibrositis

✓5ᵗʰ **726.3   Enthesopathy of elbow region**
**726.30  Enthesopathy of elbow, unspecified**
**726.31  Medial epicondylitis**
**726.32  Lateral epicondylitis**
Epicondylitis NOS   Tennis elbow
Golfers' elbow

**726.33  Olecranon bursitis**
Bursitis of elbow

**726.39  Other**

N Newborn Age: 0   P Pediatric Age: 0-17   M Maternity Age: 12-55   A Adult Age: 15-124   CC CC Condition   MCC Major CC Condition   HIV HIV Related Dx

244 — Volume 1 • October 2007

© 2007 Ingenix

**726.4 Enthesopathy of wrist and carpus**
Bursitis of hand or wrist
Periarthritis of wrist

**726.5 Enthesopathy of hip region**
Bursitis of hip      Psoas tendinitis
Gluteal tendinitis      Trochanteric tendinitis
Iliac crest spur

√5th **726.6 Enthesopathy of knee**

**726.60 Enthesopathy of knee, unspecified**
Bursitis of knee NOS

**726.61 Pes anserinus tendinitis or bursitis**
DEF: Inflamed tendons of sartorius, gracilis and
semitendinosus muscles of medial aspect of knee.

**726.62 Tibial collateral ligament bursitis**
Pellegrini-Stieda syndrome

**726.63 Fibular collateral ligament bursitis**

**726.64 Patellar tendinitis**

**726.65 Prepatellar bursitis**
AHA: 2Q, '06, 15

**726.69 Other**
Bursitis:
infrapatellar
subpatellar

√5th **726.7 Enthesopathy of ankle and tarsus**

**726.70 Enthesopathy of ankle and tarsus,
unspecified**
Metatarsalgia NOS
EXCLUDES   *Morton's metatarsalgia (355.6)*

**726.71 Achilles bursitis or tendinitis**

**726.72 Tibialis tendinitis**
Tibialis (anterior) (posterior) tendinitis

**726.73 Calcaneal spur**
DEF: Overgrowth of calcaneous bone; causes pain on
walking; due to chronic avulsion injury of plantar fascia
from calcaneus.

**726.79 Other**
Peroneal tendinitis

**726.8 Other peripheral enthesopathies**

√5th **726.9 Unspecified enthesopathy**

**726.90 Enthesopathy of unspecified site**
Capsulitis NOS
Periarthritis NOS
Tendinitis NOS

**726.91 Exostosis of unspecified site**
Bone spur NOS
AHA: 2Q, '01, 15

√4th **727 Other disorders of synovium, tendon, and bursa**

√5th **727.0 Synovitis and tenosynovitis**

**727.00 Synovitis and tenosynovitis, unspecified**
Synovitis NOS
Tenosynovitis NOS

**Bunion**

Normal
metatarsophalangeal
joint

Exostosis

**Ganglia**

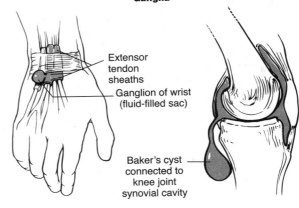

Extensor
tendon
sheaths
Ganglion of wrist
(fluid-filled sac)

Baker's cyst
connected to
knee joint
synovial cavity

**727.01 *Synovitis and tenosynovitis in diseases
classified elsewhere***
*Code first underlying disease as:*
tuberculosis (015.0-015.9)
EXCLUDES   *crystal-induced (275.4)*
*gonococcal (098.51)*
*gouty (274.0)*
*syphilitic (095.7)*

**727.02 Giant cell tumor of tendon sheath**

**727.03 Trigger finger (acquired)**
DEF: Stenosing tenosynovitis or nodule in flexor tendon;
cessation of flexion or extension movement in finger,
followed by snapping into place.

**727.04 Radial styloid tenosynovitis**
de Quervain's disease

**727.05 Other tenosynovitis of hand and wrist**

**727.06 Tenosynovitis of foot and ankle**

**727.09 Other**

**727.1 Bunion**
DEF: Enlarged first metatarsal head due to inflamed bursa; results
in laterally displaced great toe.

**727.2 Specific bursitides often of occupational origin**
Beat:      Miners':
elbow      elbow
hand      knee
knee
Chronic crepitant synovitis of wrist

**727.3 Other bursitis**
Bursitis NOS
EXCLUDES   *bursitis:*
*gonococcal (098.52)*
*subacromial (726.19)*
*subcoracoid (726.19)*
*subdeltoid (726.19)*
*syphilitic (095.7)*
*"frozen shoulder" (726.0)*

√5th **727.4 Ganglion and cyst of synovium, tendon, and bursa**

**727.40 Synovial cyst, unspecified**
EXCLUDES   *that of popliteal space (727.51)*
AHA: 2Q, '97, 6

**727.41 Ganglion of joint**

**727.42 Ganglion of tendon sheath**

**727.43 Ganglion, unspecified**

**727.49 Other**
Cyst of bursa

**Musculoskeletal and Connective Tissue**

**727.5–728.86**

√5ᵗʰ **727.5 Rupture of synovium**

**727.50 Rupture of synovium, unspecified**

**727.51 Synovial cyst of popliteal space**
Baker's cyst (knee)

**727.59 Other**

√5ᵗʰ **727.6 Rupture of tendon, nontraumatic**

**727.60 Nontraumatic rupture of unspecified tendon**

**727.61 Complete rupture of rotator cuff**

**727.62 Tendons of biceps (long head)**

**727.63 Extensor tendons of hand and wrist**

**727.64 Flexor tendons of hand and wrist**

**727.65 Quadriceps tendon**

**727.66 Patellar tendon**

**727.67 Achilles tendon**

**727.68 Other tendons of foot and ankle**

**727.69 Other**

√5ᵗʰ **727.8 Other disorders of synovium, tendon, and bursa**

**727.81 Contracture of tendon (sheath)**
Short Achilles tendon (acquired)

**727.82 Calcium deposits in tendon and bursa**
Calcification of tendon NOS
Calcific tendinitis NOS

> EXCLUDES    peripheral ligamentous or
> muscular attachments
> (726.0-726.9)

**727.83 Plica syndrome**
Plica knee
AHA: 4Q, '00, 44
DEF: A fold in the synovial tissue that begins to form before birth, creating a septum between two pockets of synovial tissue; two most common plicae are the medial patellar plica and the suprapatellar plica. Plica syndrome, or plica knee, refers to symptomatic plica. Experienced by females more commonly than males.

**727.89 Other**
Abscess of bursa or tendon

> EXCLUDES    xanthomatosis localized to
> tendons (272.7)

AHA: 2Q, '89, 15

**727.9 Unspecified disorder of synovium, tendon, and bursa**

√4ᵗʰ **728 Disorders of muscle, ligament, and fascia**

> EXCLUDES    enthesopathies (726.0-726.9)
> muscular dystrophies (359.0-359.1)
> myoneural disorders (358.00-358.9)
> myopathies (359.2-359.9)
> old disruption of ligaments of knee (717.81-
> 717.89)

**728.0 Infective myositis** CC
Myositis:
purulent
suppurative

> EXCLUDES    myositis:
> epidemic (074.1)
> interstitial (728.81)
> syphilitic (095.6)
> tropical (040.81)

CC Excl: 567.31, 728.0, 728.11-728.3, 728.81, 728.86

DEF: Inflamed connective septal tissue of muscle.

√5ᵗʰ **728.1 Muscular calcification and ossification**

**728.10 Calcification and ossification, unspecified**
Massive calcification (paraplegic)

**728.11 Progressive myositis ossificans**
DEF: Progressive myositic disease; marked by bony tissue formed by voluntary muscle; occurs among very young.

**728.12 Traumatic myositis ossificans**
Myositis ossificans (circumscripta)

**728.13 Postoperative heterotopic calcification**
DEF: Abnormal formation of calcium deposits in muscular tissue after surgery, marked by a corresponding loss of muscle tone and tension.

**728.19 Other**
Polymyositis ossificans

**728.2 Muscular wasting and disuse atrophy, not elsewhere classified**
Amyotrophia NOS
Myofibrosis

> EXCLUDES    neuralgic amyotrophy (353.5)
> pelvic muscle wasting and disuse
> atrophy (618.83)
> progressive muscular atrophy
> (335.0-335.9)

**728.3 Other specific muscle disorders**
Arthrogryposis
Immobility syndrome (paraplegic)

> EXCLUDES    arthrogryposis multiplex congenita
> (754.89)
> stiff-man syndrome (333.91)

**728.4 Laxity of ligament**

**728.5 Hypermobility syndrome**

**728.6 Contracture of palmar fascia** A
Dupuytren's contracture
DEF: Dupuytren's contracture: flexion deformity of finger, due to shortened, thickened fibrosing of palmar fascia; cause unknown; associated with long-standing epilepsy; occurs more often in males.

√5ᵗʰ **728.7 Other fibromatoses**

**728.71 Plantar fascial fibromatosis**
Contracture of plantar fascia
Plantar fasciitis (traumatic)
DEF: Plantar fascia fibromatosis; causes nodular swelling and pain; not associated with contractures.

**728.79 Other**
Garrod's or knuckle pads
Nodular fasciitis
Pseudosarcomatous fibromatosis
(proliferative) (subcutaneous)
DEF: Knuckle pads: Pea-size nodules on dorsal surface of interphalangeal joints; new growth of fibrous tissue with thickened dermis and epidermis.

√5ᵗʰ **728.8 Other disorders of muscle, ligament, and fascia**

**728.81 Interstitial myositis**
DEF: Inflammation of septal connective parts of muscle tissue.

**728.82 Foreign body granuloma of muscle**
Talc granuloma of muscle

**728.83 Rupture of muscle, nontraumatic**

**728.84 Diastasis of muscle**
Diastasis recti (abdomen)

> EXCLUDES    diastasis recti complicating
> pregnancy, labor, and
> delivery (665.8)

DEF: Muscle separation, such as recti abdominis after repeated pregnancies.

**728.85 Spasm of muscle**

**728.86 Necrotizing fasciitis** MCC
Use additional code to identify:
infectious organism (041.00-041.89)
gangrene (785.4), if applicable
CC Excl: 567.31, 728.0, 728.11-728.3, 728.81, 728.86

AHA: 4Q, '95, 54

DEF: Fulminating infection begins with extensive cellulitis, spreads to superficial and deep fascia; causes thrombosis of subcutaneous vessels, and gangrene of underlying tissue.

---

N Newborn Age: 0    P Pediatric Age: 0-17    M Maternity Age: 12-55    A Adult Age: 15-124    CC CC Condition    MCC Major CC Condition    HIV HIV Related Dx

© 2007 Ingenix

**728.87 Muscle weakness (generalized)**
> *EXCLUDES* generalized weakness (780.79)

AHA: 1Q, '05, 13; 4Q, '03, 66

**728.88 Rhabdomyolysis** [CC]
CC Excl: 567.31, 728.0, 728.11-728.3, 728.81, 728.86, 728.88

AHA: 4Q, '03, 66

DEF: A disintegration or destruction of muscle; an acute disease characterized by the excretion of myoglobin into the urine.

**728.89 Other**
Eosinophilic fasciitis
Use additional E code to identify drug, if drug induced

AHA: 3Q, '06, 13; 3Q, '02, 28; 2Q, '01, 14, 15

DEF: Eosinophilic fasciitis: inflammation of fascia of extremities associated with eosinophilia, edema, and swelling; occurs alone or as part of myalgia syndrome.

**728.9 Unspecified disorder of muscle, ligament, and fascia**

AHA: 4Q, '88, 11

√4th **729 Other disorders of soft tissues**
> *EXCLUDES* acroparesthesia (443.89)
> carpal tunnel syndrome (354.0)
> disorders of the back (720.0-724.9)
> entrapment syndromes (354.0-355.9)
> palindromic rheumatism (719.3)
> periarthritis (726.0-726.9)
> psychogenic rheumatism (306.0)

**729.0 Rheumatism, unspecified and fibrositis**
DEF: General term describes diseases of muscle, tendon, nerve, joint, or bone; symptoms include pain and stiffness.

**729.1 Myalgia and myositis, unspecified**
Fibromyositis NOS
DEF: Myalgia: muscle pain.
DEF: Myositis: inflamed voluntary muscle.
DEF: Fibromyositis: inflamed fibromuscular tissue.

**729.2 Neuralgia, neuritis, and radiculitis, unspecified**
> *EXCLUDES* brachial radiculitis (723.4)
> cervical radiculitis (723.4)
> lumbosacral radiculitis (724.4)
> mononeuritis (354.0-355.9)
> radiculitis due to intervertebral disc involvement (722.0-722.2, 722.7)
> sciatica (724.3)

DEF: Neuralgia: paroxysmal pain along nerve; symptoms include brief pain and tenderness at point nerve exits.
DEF: Neuritis: inflamed nerve, symptoms include paresthesia, paralysis and loss of reflexes at nerve site.
DEF: Radiculitis: inflamed nerve root.

√5th **729.3 Panniculitis, unspecified**
DEF: Inflammatory reaction of subcutaneous fat; causes nodules; often develops in abdominal region.

**729.30 Panniculitis, unspecified site**
Weber-Christian disease
DEF: Febrile, nodular, nonsuppurative, relapsing inflammation of subcutaneous fat.

**729.31 Hypertrophy of fat pad, knee**
Hypertrophy of infrapatellar fat pad

**729.39 Other site**
> *EXCLUDES* panniculitis specified as (affecting):
> back (724.8)
> neck (723.6)
> sacral (724.8)

**729.4 Fasciitis, unspecified**
> *EXCLUDES* necrotizing fasciitis (728.86)
> nodular fasciitis (728.79)

AHA: 2Q, '94, 13

**729.5 Pain in limb**
AHA: ▶2Q, '07, 11◀

**729.6 Residual foreign body in soft tissue**
> *EXCLUDES* foreign body granuloma:
> muscle (728.82)
> skin and subcutaneous tissue (709.4)

√5th **729.7 Nontraumatic compartment syndrome**
> *EXCLUDES* compartment syndrome NOS (958.90)
> traumatic compartment syndrome (958.90-958.99)

DEF: Compression of nerves and blood vessels within an enclosed space, leading to impaired blood flow and muscle and nerve damage.

**729.71 Nontraumatic compartment syndrome** [CC]
**of upper extremity**
Nontraumatic compartment syndrome of shoulder, arm, forearm, wrist, hand, and fingers
CC Excl: 729.81, 729.89-729.9, 903.8, 904.9

AHA: 4Q, '06, 100-102

**729.72 Nontraumatic compartment syndrome** [CC]
**of lower extremity**
Nontraumatic compartment syndrome of hip, buttock, thigh, leg, foot, and toes
CC Excl: 729.81, 729.89-729.9, 904.7, 904.9

AHA: 4Q, '06, 100-102

**729.73 Nontraumatic compartment syndrome** [CC]
**of abdomen**
CC Excl: 863.0-867.3,867.5-868.14,869.0-869.1,879.2-879.9,929.0-929.9, 958.8, 959.8-959.9

AHA: 4Q, '06, 100-102

**729.79 Nontraumatic compartment syndrome** [CC]
**of other sites**
CC Excl: 868.03-868.10, 868.13-869.1

AHA: 4Q, '06, 100-102

√5th **729.8 Other musculoskeletal symptoms referable to limbs**
**729.81 Swelling of limb**
AHA: 4Q, '88, 6

**729.82 Cramp**
**729.89 Other**
> *EXCLUDES* abnormality of gait (781.2)
> tetany (781.7)
> transient paralysis of limb (781.4)

AHA: 4Q, '88, 12

**729.9 Other and unspecified disorders of soft tissue**
Polyalgia

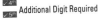

√4th
√5th Additional Digit Required

Unacceptable PDx

Manifestation Code

▶◀ Revised Text

● New Code

▲ Revised Code Title

**October 2007 • Volume 1 — 247**

© 2007 Ingenix

## OSTEOPATHIES, CHONDROPATHIES, AND ACQUIRED MUSCULOSKELETAL DEFORMITIES (730-739)

✓4th **730 Osteomyelitis, periostitis, and other infections involving bone**

> **EXCLUDES**    jaw (526.4-526.5)
>    petrous bone (383.2)

Use additional code to identify organism, such as Staphylococcus (041.1)

The following fifth-digit subclassification is for use with category 730; valid digits are in [brackets] under each code. See list at beginning of chapter for definitions.

   0   site unspecified
   1   shoulder region
   2   upper arm
   3   forearm
   4   hand
   5   pelvic region and thigh
   6   lower leg
   7   ankle and foot
   8   other specified sites
   9   multiple sites

**AHA:** 4Q, '97, 43

DEF: Osteomyelitis: bacterial inflammation of bone tissue and marrow.

DEF: Periostitis: inflammation of specialized connective tissue; causes swelling of bone and aching pain.

✓5th **730.0  Acute osteomyelitis**    `CC`
[0-9]
>   Abscess of any bone except accessory sinus, jaw, or mastoid
>   Acute or subacute osteomyelitis, with or without mention of periostitis
>   Use additional code to identify major osseous defect, if applicable (731.3)

**CC Excl: For code 730.00:** 015.50-015.56, 015.70-015.76, 015.90-015.96, 017.90-017.96, 730.00-730.39, 730.80-730.99 **For code 730.01:** 015.50-015.56, 015.70-015.76, 015.90-015.96, 017.90-017.96, 730.00, 730.08-730.11, 730.18-730.21, 730.28-730.31, 730.38-730.39, 730.80-730.81, 730.88-730.91, 730.98-730.99 **For code 730.02:** 015.50-015.56, 015.70-015.76, 015.90-015.96, 017.90-017.96, 730.00, 730.08-730.10, 730.12, 730.18-730.20, 730.22, 730.28-730.30, 730.32, 730.38-730.39, 730.80, 730.82, 730.88-730.90, 730.92, 730.98-730.99 **For code 730.03:** 015.50-015.56, 015.70-015.76, 015.90-015.96, 017.90-017.96, 730.00, 730.08-730.10, 730.13, 730.18-730.20, 730.23, 730.28-730.30, 730.33, 730.38-730.39, 730.80, 730.83, 730.88-730.90, 730.93, 730.98-730.99 **For code 730.04:** 015.50-015.56, 015.70-015.76, 015.90-015.96, 017.90-017.96, 730.00, 730.08-730.10, 730.14, 730.18-730.20, 730.24, 730.28-730.30, 730.34, 730.38-730.39, 730.80, 730.84, 730.88-730.90, 730.94, 730.98-730.99 **For code 730.05:** 015.10-015.16, 015.50-015.56, 015.70-015.76, 015.90-015.96, 017.90-017.96, 730.00, 730.08-730.10, 730.15, 730.18-730.20, 730.25, 730.28-730.30, 730.35, 730.38-730.39, 730.80, 730.85, 730.88-730.90, 730.95, 730.98-730.99; **For code 730.06:** 015.20-015.56, 015.70-015.76, 015.90-015.96, 017.90-017.96, 730.00, 730.08-730.10, 730.16, 730.18-730.20, 730.26, 730.28-730.30, 730.36, 730.38-730.39, 730.80, 730.86, 730.88-730.90, 730.96, 730.98-730.99 **For code 730.07:** 015.50-015.56, 015.70-015.76, 015.90-015.96, 017.90-017.96, 730.00, 730.08-730.10, 730.17-730.20, 730.27-730.30, 730.37-730.39, 730.80, 730.87-730.90, 730.97-730.99 **For code 730.08:** 015.00-015.06, 015.50-015.56, 015.70-015.76, 015.90-015.96, 017.90-017.96, 730.00-730.39, 730.80-730.99 **For code 730.09:** 015.50-015.56, 015.70-015.76, 015.90-015.96, 017.90-017.96, 730.00-730.39, 730.80-730.99

**AHA:** 4Q, '06, 103; **For code 730.06:** 1Q, '02, 4; **For code 730.07:** 1Q, '04, 14

✓5th **730.1  Chronic osteomyelitis**    `CC`
[0-9]
>   Brodie's abscess
>   Chronic or old osteomyelitis, with or without mention of periostitis
>   Sequestrum of bone
>   Sclerosing osteomyelitis of Garré
>   Use additional code to identify major osseous defect, if applicable (731.3)

> **EXCLUDES**    aseptic necrosis of bone (733.40-733.49)

**CC Excl: For code 730.10:** 730.10-730.39, 730.80-731.1; **For codes 730.11-730.19:** 003.24, 015.50-015.56, 015.70-015.76, 015.90-015.96, 017.90-017.96, 730.00-730.39, 730.80-730.99

**AHA:** 4Q, '06, 103; **For code 730.17:** 3Q, '00, 4

✓5th **730.2  Unspecified osteomyelitis**    `CC`
[0-9]
>   Osteitis or osteomyelitis NOS, with or without mention of periostitis
>   Use additional code to identify major osseous defect, if applicable (731.3)

**CC Excl: For code 730.20:** 730.10-730.39, 730.80-731.1; **For codes 730.21-730.29:** 003.24, 015.50-015.56, 015.70-015.76, 015.90-015.96, 017.90-017.96, 730.00-730.39, 730.80-730.99

**AHA:** 4Q, '06, 103;

✓5th **730.3  Periostitis without mention of osteomyelitis**
[0-9]
>   Abscess of periosteum ⎱ without mention of
>   Periostosis              ⎰ osteomyelitis

> **EXCLUDES**    that in secondary syphilis (091.61)

✓5th **730.7  *Osteopathy resulting from poliomyelitis***
[0-9]
>   Code first underlying disease (045.0-045.9)

✓5th **730.8  *Other infections involving bone in diseases classified elsewhere***    `CC`
[0-9]
>   Code first underlying disease as:
>     tuberculosis (015.0-015.9)
>     typhoid fever (002.0)

> **EXCLUDES**    syphilis of bone NOS (095.5)

**CC Excl: For codes 730.80, 730.89:** 015.50-015.56, 015.70-015.76, 015.90-015.96, 017.90-017.96, 730.00-730.39, 730.80-730.99; **For code 730.81:** 015.50-015.56, 015.70-015.76, 015.90-015.96, 017.90-017.96, 730.00-730.01, 730.08-730.11, 730.18-730.21, 730.28-730.31, 730.38-730.39, 730.80, 730.88-730.91, 730.98-730.99; **For code 730.82:** 015.50-015.56, 015.70-015.76, 015.90-015.96, 017.90-017.96, 730.00, 730.02, 730.08-730.10, 730.12, 730.18-730.20, 730.22, 730.28-730.30, 730.32, 730.38-730.39, 730.80, 730.88-730.90, 730.92, 730.98-730.99; **For code 730.83:** 015.50-015.56, 015.70-015.76, 015.90-015.96, 017.90-017.96, 730.00, 730.03, 730.08-730.10, 730.13, 730.18-730.20, 730.23, 730.28-730.30, 730.33, 730.38-730.39, 730.80, 730.88-730.90, 730.93, 730.98-730.99; **For code 730.84:** 015.50-015.56, 015.70-015.76, 015.90-015.96, 017.90-017.96, 730.00, 730.04, 730.08-730.10, 730.14, 730.18-730.20, 730.24, 730.28-730.30, 730.34, 730.38-730.39, 730.80, 730.88-730.90, 730.94, 730.98-730.99; **For code 730.85:** 015.10-015.16, 015.50-015.56, 015.70-015.76, 015.90-015.96, 017.90-017.96, 730.00, 730.05, 730.08-730.10, 730.15, 730.18-730.20, 730.25, 730.28-730.30, 730.35, 730.38-730.39, 730.80, 730.88-730.90, 730.95, 730.98-730.99; **For code 730.86:** 015.20-015.56, 015.70-015.76, 015.90-015.96, 017.90-017.96, 730.00, 730.06, 730.08-730.10, 730.16, 730.18-730.20, 730.26, 730.28-730.30, 730.36, 730.38-730.39, 730.80, 730.88-730.90, 730.96, 730.98-730.99; **For code 730.87:** 015.50-015.56, 015.70-015.76, 015.90-015.96, 017.90-017.96, 730.00, 730.07-730.10, 730.17-730.20, 730.27-730.30, 730.37-730.39, 730.80, 730.88-730.90, 730.97-730.99; **For code 730.88:** 015.00-015.06, 015.50-015.56, 015.70-015.76, 015.90-015.96, 017.90-017.96, 730.00-730.39, 730.80-730.99

**AHA:** 2Q, '97, 16; 3Q, '91, 10

✓5th **730.9  Unspecified infection of bone**    `CC`
[0-9]
**CC Excl: For codes 730.90, 730.99:** 015.50-015.56, 015.70-015.76, 015.90-015.96, 017.90-017.96, 730.00-730.39, 730.80-730.99; **For code 730.91:** 015.50-015.56, 015.70-015.76, 015.90-015.96, 017.90-017.96, 730.00-730.01, 730.08-730.11, 730.18-730.21, 730.28-730.31, 730.38-730.39, 730.80-730.81, 730.88-730.90, 730.98-730.99; **For code 730.92:** 015.50-015.56, 015.70-015.76, 015.90-015.96, 017.90-017.96, 730.00, 730.02, 730.08-730.10, 730.12, 730.18-730.20, 730.22, 730.28-730.30, 730.32, 730.38-730.39, 730.80, 730.82, 730.88-730.90, 730.98-730.99; **For code 730.93:** 015.50-015.56, 015.70-015.76, 015.90-015.96, 017.90-017.96, 730.00, 730.03, 730.08-730.10, 730.13, 730.18-730.20, 730.23, 730.28-730.30, 730.33, 730.38-730.39, 730.80, 730.83, 730.88-730.90, 730.98-730.99; **For code 730.94:** 015.50-015.56, 015.70-015.76, 015.90-015.96, 017.90-017.96, 730.00, 730.04, 730.08-730.10, 730.14, 730.18-730.20, 730.24, 730.28-730.30, 730.34, 730.38-730.39, 730.80, 730.84, 730.88-730.90, 730.98-730.99; **For code 730.95:** 015.10-015.16, 015.50-015.56, 015.70-015.76, 015.90-015.96, 017.90-017.96, 730.00, 730.05, 730.08-730.10, 730.15, 730.18-730.20, 730.25, 730.28-730.30, 730.35, 730.38-730.39, 730.80, 730.85, 730.88-730.90, 730.98-730.99; **For code 730.96:** 015.20-015.56, 015.70-015.76, 015.90-015.96, 017.90-017.96, 730.00, 730.06, 730.08-730.10, 730.16, 730.18-730.20, 730.26, 730.28-730.30, 730.36, 730.38-730.39, 730.80, 730.86, 730.88-730.90, 730.98-730.99; **For code 730.97:** 015.50-015.56, 015.70-015.76, 015.90-015.96, 017.90-017.96, 730.00, 730.07, 730.08-730.10, 730.17-730.20, 730.27-730.30, 730.37-730.39, 730.80, 730.87-730.90, 730.98-730.99; **For code 730.98:** 0015.00-015.06, 015.50-015.56, 015.70-015.76, 015.90-015.96, 017.90-017.96, 730.00-730.39, 730.80-730.99

**N** Newborn Age: 0   **P** Pediatric Age: 0-17   **M** Maternity Age: 12-55   **A** Adult Age: 15-124   `CC` CC Condition   `MCC` Major CC Condition   `HIV` HIV Related Dx

© 2007 Ingenix

**Slipped Femoral Epiphysis**

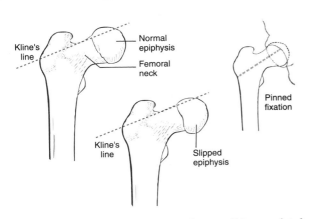

**✓4ᵗʰ 731.1 Osteitis deformans and osteopathies associated with other disorders classified elsewhere**

DEF: Osteitis deformans: Bone disease marked by episodes of increased bone loss, excessive repair attempts follow; causes weakened, deformed bones with increased mass, bowed long bones, deformed flat bones, pain and pathological fractures; may be fatal if associated with congestive heart failure, giant cell tumors or bone sarcoma; also called Paget's disease.

**731.0 Osteitis deformans without mention of bone tumor**
Paget's disease of bone

**731.1 *Osteitis deformans in diseases classified elsewhere***
*Code first underlying disease as:*
malignant neoplasm of bone (170.0-170.9)

**731.2 Hypertrophic pulmonary osteoarthropathy**
Bamberger-Marie disease

DEF: Clubbing, of fingers and toes; related to enlarged ends of long bones; due to chronic lung and heart disease.

**731.3 Major osseous defects**
Code first underlying disease, if known, such as:
aseptic necrosis (733.40-733.49)
malignant neoplasm of bone (170.0-170.9)
osteomyelitis (730.00-730.29)
osteoporosis (733.00-733.09)
peri-prosthetic osteolysis (996.45)

AHA: 4Q, '06, 103

**731.8 *Other bone involvement in diseases classified elsewhere***
*Code first underlying disease as:*
diabetes mellitus (250.8)
Use additional code to specify bone condition, such as:
acute osteomyelitis (730.00-730.09)

AHA: 1Q, '04, 14; 4Q, '97, 43; 2Q, '97, 16

**✓4ᵗʰ 732 Osteochondropathies**

DEF: Conditions related to both bone and cartilage, or conditions in which cartilage is converted to bone (enchondral ossification).

**732.0 Juvenile osteochondrosis of spine**
Juvenile osteochondrosis (of):
marginal or vertebral epiphysis (of Scheuermann)
spine NOS
Vertebral epiphysitis
**EXCLUDES** *adolescent postural kyphosis (737.0)*

**732.1 Juvenile osteochondrosis of hip and pelvis**
Coxa plana
Ischiopubic synchondrosis (of van Neck)
Osteochondrosis (juvenile) of:
acetabulum
head of femur (of Legg-Calvé-Perthes)
iliac crest (of Buchanan)
symphysis pubis (of Pierson)
Pseudocoxalgia

**732.2 Nontraumatic slipped upper femoral epiphysis**
Slipped upper femoral epiphysis NOS

**732.3 Juvenile osteochondrosis of upper extremity**
Osteochondrosis (juvenile) of:
capitulum of humerus (of Panner)
carpal lunate (of Kienbock)
hand NOS
head of humerus (of Haas)
heads of metacarpals (of Mauclaire)
lower ulna (of Burns)
radial head (of Brailsford)
upper extremity NOS

**732.4 Juvenile osteochondrosis of lower extremity, excluding foot**
Osteochondrosis (juvenile) of:
lower extremity NOS
primary patellar center (of Köhler)
proximal tibia (of Blount)
secondary patellar center (of Sinding-Larsen)
tibial tubercle (of Osgood-Schlatter)
Tibia vara

**732.5 Juvenile osteochondrosis of foot**
Calcaneal apophysitis
Epiphysitis, os calcis
Osteochondrosis (juvenile) of:
astragalus (of Diaz)
calcaneum (of Sever)
foot NOS
metatarsal
second (of Freiberg)
fifth (of Iselin)
os tibiale externum (of Haglund)
tarsal navicular (of Köhler)

**732.6 Other juvenile osteochondrosis**
Apophysitis ⎫
Epiphysitis ⎬ specified as juvenile,
Osteochondritis ⎪ of other site,
Osteochondrosis ⎭ or site NOS

**732.7 Osteochondritis dissecans**

**732.8 Other specified forms of osteochondropathy**
Adult osteochondrosis of spine

**732.9 Unspecified osteochondropathy**
Apophysitis ⎫ NOS
Epiphysitis ⎬ not specified as adult
Osteochondritis ⎪ or juvenile, of
Osteochondrosis ⎭ unspecified site

**✓4ᵗʰ 733 Other disorders of bone and cartilage**
**EXCLUDES** *bone spur (726.91)*
*cartilage of, or loose body in, joint (717.0-717.9, 718.0-718.9)*
*giant cell granuloma of jaw (526.3)*
*osteitis fibrosa cystica generalisata (252.01)*
*osteomalacia (268.2)*
*polyostotic fibrous dysplasia of bone (756.54)*
*prognathism, retrognathism (524.1)*
*xanthomatosis localized to bone (272.7)*

**✓5ᵗʰ 733.0 Osteoporosis**
Use additional code to identify major osseous defect, if applicable (731.3)

AHA: 4Q, '06, 103

DEF: Bone mass reduction that ultimately results in fractures after minimal trauma; dorsal kyphosis or loss of height often occur.

**733.00 Osteoporosis, unspecified**
Wedging of vertebra NOS
AHA: ▶1Q, '07, 22;◀3Q, '01, 19; 2Q, '98, 12

**733.01 Senile osteoporosis**
Postmenopausal osteoporosis
AHA: ▶1Q, '07, 5, 6◀

**733.02 Idiopathic osteoporosis**

**733.03 Disuse osteoporosis**

**733.09 Other**
Drug-induced osteoporosis
Use additional E code to identify drug
AHA: 4Q, '03, 108

---

✓4ᵗʰ / ✓5ᵗʰ Additional Digit Required    Unacceptable PDx    Manifestation Code    ▶◀ Revised Text    ● New Code    ▲ Revised Code Title

© 2007 Ingenix

**Musculoskeletal and Connective Tissue**

**733.1–733.99**

✓5ᵗʰ **733.1 Pathologic fracture**
Spontaneous fracture
**EXCLUDES** stress fracture (733.93-733.95)
traumatic fracture (800-829)
**AHA:** ▶1Q, '07, 3-4;◀ 4Q, '93, 25; N-D, '86, 10; N-D, '85, 16
**DEF:** Fracture due to bone structure weakening by pathological processes (e.g., osteoporosis, neoplasms and osteomalacia).

**733.10 Pathologic fracture, unspecified site** CC
**CC Excl:** 733.10-733.19, 733.93-733.95

**733.11 Pathologic fracture of humerus** CC
**CC Excl:** See code 733.10

**733.12 Pathologic fracture of distal radius and ulna** CC
Wrist NOS
**CC Excl:** See code 733.10

**733.13 Pathologic fracture of vertebrae** CC
Collapse of vertebra NOS
**CC Excl:** See code 733.10
**AHA:** ▶1Q, '07, 5, 6, 22;◀ 3Q, '99, 5

**733.14 Pathologic fracture of neck of femur** CC
Femur NOS     Hip NOS
**CC Excl:** See code 733.10
**AHA:** 1Q, '01, 1; 1Q, '96, 16

**733.15 Pathologic fracture of other specified part of femur** CC
**CC Excl:** See code 733.10
**AHA:** 2Q, '98, 12

**733.16 Pathologic fracture of tibia or fibula** CC
Ankle NOS
**CC Excl:** See code 733.10

**733.19 Pathologic fracture of other specified site** CC
**CC Excl:** See code 733.10
**AHA:** ▶1Q, '07, 20◀

✓4ᵗʰ **733.2 Cyst of bone**
**733.20 Cyst of bone (localized), unspecified**
**733.21 Solitary bone cyst**
Unicameral bone cyst
**733.22 Aneurysmal bone cyst**
**DEF:** Solitary bone lesion, bulges into periosteum; marked by calcified rim.

**733.29 Other**
Fibrous dysplasia (monostotic)
**EXCLUDES** cyst of jaw (526.0-526.2, 526.89)
osteitis fibrosa cystica (252.01)
polyostotic fibrousdyplasia of bone (756.54)

**733.3 Hyperostosis of skull**
Hyperostosis interna frontalis
Leontiasis ossium
**DEF:** Abnormal bone growth on inner aspect of cranial bones.

✓5ᵗʰ **733.4 Aseptic necrosis of bone**
**EXCLUDES** osteochondropathies (732.0-732.9)
Use additional code to identify major osseous defect, if applicable (731.3)
**AHA:** 4Q, '06, 103
**DEF:** Infarction of bone tissue due to a nonfectious etiology, such as a fracture, ischemic disorder or administration of immunosuppressive drugs; leads to degenerative joint disease or nonunion of fractures.

**733.40 Aseptic necrosis of bone, site unspecified** CC
**CC Excl:** 733.40-733.49

**733.41 Head of humerus** CC
**CC Excl:** 733.40-733.41, 733.45-733.49

**733.42 Head and neck of femur** CC
Femur NOS
**EXCLUDES** Legg-Calvé-Perthes disease (732.1)
**CC Excl:** 733.40, 733.42, 733.45-733.49

**733.43 Medial femoral condyle** CC
**CC Excl:** 733.40, 733.43, 733.45-733.49

**733.44 Talus** CC
**CC Excl:** 733.40, 733.44-733.49

**733.45 Jaw** CC
Use additional E code to identify drug, if drug-induced
**EXCLUDES** osteoradionecrosis of jaw (526.89)
**CC Excl:** See code: 733.40

**733.49 Other** CC
**CC Excl:** See code: 733.40

**733.5 Osteitis condensans**
Piriform sclerosis of ilium
**DEF:** Idiopathic condition marked by low back pain; associated with oval or triangular sclerotic, opaque bone next to sacroiliac joints in the ileum.

**733.6 Tietze's disease**
Costochondral junction syndrome
Costochondritis
**DEF:** Painful, idiopathic, nonsuppurative, swollen costal cartilage sometimes confused with cardiac symptoms because the anterior chest pain resembles that of coronary artery disease.

**733.7 Algoneurodystrophy**
Disuse atrophy of bone     Sudeck's atrophy
**DEF:** Painful, idiopathic.

✓5ᵗʰ **733.8 Malunion and nonunion of fracture**
**AHA:** 2Q, '94, 5

**733.81 Malunion of fracture** CC
**CC Excl:** 733.81-733.82

**733.82 Nonunion of fracture** CC
Pseudoarthrosis (bone)
**CC Excl:** See code: 733.81

✓5ᵗʰ **733.9 Other unspecified disorders of bone and cartilage**
**733.90 Disorder of bone and cartilage**
**733.91 Arrest of bone development or growth**
Epiphyseal arrest
**733.92 Chondromalacia**
Chondromalacia:
NOS
localized, except patella
systemic
tibial plateau
**EXCLUDES** chondromalacia of patella (717.7)
**DEF:** Articular cartilage softening.

**733.93 Stress fracture of tibia or fibula**
Stress reaction of tibia or fibula
**AHA:** 4Q, '01, 48

**733.94 Stress fracture of the metatarsals**
Stress reaction of metatarsals
**AHA:** 4Q, '01, 48

**733.95 Stress fracture of other bone**
Stress reaction of other bone
**AHA:** 4Q, '01, 48

**733.99 Other**
Diaphysitis
Hypertrophy of bone
Relapsing polychondritis
**AHA:** J-F, '87, 14

---

N Newborn Age: 0    P Pediatric Age: 0-17    M Maternity Age: 12-55    A Adult Age: 15-124    CC CC Condition    MCC Major CC Condition    HIV HIV Related Dx

**734 Flat foot**
Pes planus (acquired)
Talipes planus (acquired)
> EXCLUDES   congenital (754.61)
> rigid flat foot (754.61)
> spastic (everted) flat foot (754.61)

**√4th 735 Acquired deformities of toe**
> EXCLUDES   congenital (754.60-754.69, 755.65-755.66)

**735.0 Hallux valgus (acquired)**
DEF: Angled displacement of the great toe, causing it to ride over or under other toes.

**735.1 Hallux varus (acquired)**
DEF: Angled displacement of the great toe toward the body midline, away from the other toes.

**735.2 Hallux rigidus**
DEF: Limited flexion movement at metatarsophalangeal joint of great toe; due to degenerative joint disease.

**735.3 Hallux malleus**
DEF: Extended proximal phalanx, flexed distal phalanges, of great toe; foot resembles claw or hammer.

**735.4 Other hammer toe (acquired)**
**735.5 Claw toe (acquired)**
DEF: Hyperextended proximal phalanges, flexed middle and distal phalanges.

**735.8 Other acquired deformities of toe**
**735.9 Unspecified acquired deformity of toe**

**√4th 736 Other acquired deformities of limbs**
> EXCLUDES   congenital (754.3-755.9)

**√5th 736.0 Acquired deformities of forearm, excluding fingers**
**736.00 Unspecified deformity**
Deformity of elbow, forearm, hand, or wrist (acquired) NOS

**736.01 Cubitus valgus (acquired)**
DEF: Deviation of the elbow away from the body midline upon extension; it occurs when the palm is turning outward.

**736.02 Cubitus varus (acquired)**
DEF: Elbow joint displacement angled laterally; when the forearm is extended, it is deviated toward the midline of the body; also called "gun stock" deformity.

**736.03 Valgus deformity of wrist (acquired)**
DEF: Abnormal angulation away from the body midline.

**736.04 Varus deformity of wrist (acquired)**
DEF: Abnormal angulation toward the body midline.

**736.05 Wrist drop (acquired)**
DEF: Inability to extend the hand at the wrist due to extensor muscle paralysis

**736.06 Claw hand (acquired)**
DEF: Flexion and atrophy of the hand and fingers; found in ulnar nerve lesions, syringomyelia, and leprosy.

**736.07 Club hand, acquired**
DEF: Twisting of the hand out of shape or position; caused by the congenital absence of the ulna or radius.

**736.09 Other**
**736.1 Mallet finger**
DEF: Permanently flexed distal phalanx.

**√5th 736.2 Other acquired deformities of finger**
**736.20 Unspecified deformity**
Deformity of finger (acquired) NOS

**736.21 Boutonniere deformity**
DEF: A deformity of the finger caused by flexion of the proximal interphalangeal joint and hyperextension of the distal joint; also called buttonhole deformity.

**736.22 Swan-neck deformity**
DEF: Flexed distal and hyperextended proximal interphalangeal joint.

**736.29 Other**
> EXCLUDES   trigger finger (727.03)
AHA: 2Q, '05, 7; 2Q, '89, 13

**√5th 736.3 Acquired deformities of hip**
**736.30 Unspecified deformity**
Deformity of hip (acquired) NOS

**736.31 Coxa valga (acquired)**
DEF: Increase of at least 140 degrees in the angle formed by the axis of the head and the neck of the femur, and the axis of its shaft.

**736.32 Coxa vara (acquired)**
DEF: The bending downward of the neck of the femur: causing difficulty in movement; a right angle or less may be formed by the axis of the head and neck of the femur, and the axis of its shaft.

**736.39 Other**
AHA: 2Q, '91, 18

**√5th 736.4 Genu valgum or varum (acquired)**
**736.41 Genu valgum (acquired)**
DEF: Abnormally close together and an abnormally large space between the ankles; also called "knock-knees."

**736.42 Genu varum (acquired)**
DEF: Abnormally separated knees and the inward bowing of the legs; it is also called "bowlegs."

**736.5 Genu recurvatum (acquired)**
DEF: Hyperextended knees; also called "backknee."

**Acquired Deformities of Toe**

Hallux valgus

Hallux varus

Hallux malleus (hammer of big toe)

Hammertoe

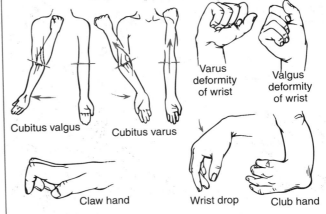

**Acquired Deformities of Forearm**

Cubitus valgus

Cubitus varus

Varus deformity of wrist

Valgus deformity of wrist

Claw hand

Wrist drop

Club hand

**736.6 Other acquired deformities of knee**
Deformity of knee (acquired) NOS

√5ᵗʰ **736.7 Other acquired deformities of ankle and foot**
> **EXCLUDES**   *deformities of toe (acquired) (735.0-735.9)*
> *pes planus (acquired) (734)*

**736.70 Unspecified deformity of ankle and foot, acquired**

**736.71 Acquired equinovarus deformity**
Clubfoot, acquired
> **EXCLUDES**   *clubfoot not specified as acquired (754.5-754.7)*

**736.72 Equinus deformity of foot, acquired**
DEF: A plantar flexion deformity that forces people to walk on their toes.

**736.73 Cavus deformity of foot**
> **EXCLUDES**   *that with claw foot (736.74)*

DEF: Abnormally high longitudinal arch of the foot.

**736.74 Claw foot, acquired**
DEF: High foot arch with hyperextended toes at metatarsophalangeal joint and flexed toes at distal joints; also called "main en griffe."

**736.75 Cavovarus deformity of foot, acquired**
DEF: Inward turning of the heel from the midline of the leg and an abnormally high longitudinal arch.

**736.76 Other calcaneus deformity**

**736.79 Other**
Acquired:
pes
talipes } not elsewhere classified

√5ᵗʰ **736.8 Acquired deformities of other parts of limbs**

**736.81 Unequal leg length (acquired)**

**736.89 Other**
Deformity (acquired):
arm or leg, not elsewhere classified
shoulder

**736.9 Acquired deformity of limb, site unspecified**

√4ᵗʰ **737 Curvature of spine**
> **EXCLUDES**   *congenital (754.2)*

**737.0 Adolescent postural kyphosis**
> **EXCLUDES**   *osteochondrosis of spine (juvenile) (732.0)*
> *adult (732.8)*

**Acquired Deformities of Hip**

Genu valga (knock-knee)    Normal angle    Coxa valga    Coxa vara    Genu vara (bowleg)

**Acquired Deformities of Lower Limb**

Cavus deformity

Equinovarus    Cavovarus

Genu recurvatum

**Axis of Deformity (may be multiple)**
Dorsal
Valgus   Varus
Plantar
Equinus Calcaneus

√5ᵗʰ **737.1 Kyphosis (acquired)**

**737.10 Kyphosis (acquired) (postural)**

**737.11 Kyphosis due to radiation**

**737.12 Kyphosis, postlaminectomy**
AHA: J-F, '87, 7

**737.19 Other**
> **EXCLUDES**   *that associated with conditions classifiable elsewhere (737.41)*

AHA: ▶1Q, '07, 20◀

√5ᵗʰ **737.2 Lordosis (acquired)**
DEF: Swayback appearance created by an abnormally increased spinal curvature; it is also referred to as "hollow back" or "saddle back."

**737.20 Lordosis (acquired) (postural)**

**737.21 Lordosis, postlaminectomy**

**737.22 Other postsurgical lordosis**

**737.29 Other**
> **EXCLUDES**   *that associated with conditions classifiable elsewhere (737.42)*

√5ᵗʰ **737.3 Kyphoscoliosis and scoliosis**
DEF: Kyphoscoliosis: backward and lateral curvature of the spinal column; it is found in vertebral osteochondrosis.

DEF: Scoliosis: an abnormal deviation of the spine to the left or right of the midline

**737.30 Scoliosis [and kyphoscoliosis], idiopathic**
AHA: 3Q, '03, 19

**737.31 Resolving infantile idiopathic scoliosis**

**737.32 Progressive infantile idiopathic scoliosis**
AHA: 3Q, '02, 12

**737.33 Scoliosis due to radiation**

**737.34 Thoracogenic scoliosis**

**737.39 Other**
> **EXCLUDES**   *that associated with conditions classifiable elsewhere (737.43)*
> *that in kyphoscoliotic heart disease (416.1)*

AHA: 2Q, '02, 16

---

**N** Newborn Age: 0    **P** Pediatric Age: 0-17    **M** Maternity Age: 12-55    **A** Adult Age: 15-124    **CC** CC Condition    **MCC** Major CC Condition    **HIV** HIV Related Dx

√5ᵗʰ **737.4  Curvature of spine associated with other conditions**
Code first associated condition as:
  Charcôt-Marie-Tooth disease (356.1)
  mucopolysaccharidosis (277.5)
  neurofibromatosis (237.7)
  osteitis deformans (731.0)
  osteitis fibrosa cystica (252.01)
  osteoporosis (733.00-733.09)
  poliomyelitis (138)
  tuberculosis [Pott's curvature] (015.0)

**737.40** *Curvature of spine, unspecified*

**737.41** *Kyphosis*

**737.42** *Lordosis*

**737.43** *Scoliosis*

**737.8  Other curvatures of spine**

**737.9  Unspecified curvature of spine**
Curvature of spine (acquired) (idiopathic) NOS
Hunchback, acquired
  **EXCLUDES**  deformity of spine NOS (738.5)

√4ᵗʰ **738 Other acquired deformity**
  **EXCLUDES**  congenital (754.0-756.9, 758.0-759.9)
    dentofacial anomalies (524.0-524.9)

**738.0  Acquired deformity of nose**
Deformity of nose (acquired)
Overdevelopment of nasal bones
  **EXCLUDES**  deflected or deviated nasal septum (470)

√5ᵗʰ **738.1  Other acquired deformity of head**

**738.10  Unspecified deformity**

**738.11  Zygomatic hyperplasia**
DEF: Abnormal enlargement of the zygoma (processus zygomaticus temporalis).

**738.12  Zygomatic hypoplasia**
DEF: Underdevelopment of the zygoma (processus zygomaticus temporalis).

**738.19  Other specified deformity**
AHA: 1Q, '06, 6; 2Q, '03, 13

**738.2  Acquired deformity of neck**

**738.3  Acquired deformity of chest and rib**
Deformity:                  Pectus:
  chest (acquired)           carinatum, acquired
  rib (acquired)             excavatum, acquired

**738.4  Acquired spondylolisthesis**
Degenerative spondylolisthesis
Spondylolysis, acquired
  **EXCLUDES**  congenital (756.12)

AHA: ▶1Q, '07, 10◀

DEF: Vertebra displaced forward over another; due to bilateral defect in vertebral arch, eroded articular surface of posterior facts and elongated pedicle between fifth lumbar vertebra and sacrum.

**Kyphosis and Lordosis**

Kyphosis (hump)

Lordosis (concave)

**Scoliosis and Kyphoscoliosis**

Scoliosis                  Kyphoscoliosis

**738.5  Other acquired deformity of back or spine**
Deformity of spine NOS
  **EXCLUDES**  curvature of spine (737.0-737.9)

**738.6  Acquired deformity of pelvis**
Pelvic obliquity
  **EXCLUDES**  intrapelvic protrusion of acetabulum (718.6)
    that in relation to labor and delivery (653.0-653.4, 653.8-653.9)

DEF: Pelvic obliquity: slanting or inclination of the pelvis at an angle between 55 and 60 degrees between the plane of the pelvis and the horizontal plane.

**738.7  Cauliflower ear**
DEF: Abnormal external ear; due to injury, subsequent perichondritis.

**738.8  Acquired deformity of other specified site**
Deformity of clavicle
AHA: 2Q, '01, 15

**738.9  Acquired deformity of unspecified site**

√4ᵗʰ **739 Nonallopathic lesions, not elsewhere classified**
  **INCLUDES**  segmental dysfunction
    somatic dysfunction

DEF: Disability, loss of function or abnormality of a body part that is neither classifiable to a particular system nor brought about therapeutically to counteract another disease.

**739.0  Head region**
Occipitocervical region

**739.1  Cervical region**
Cervicothoracic region

**739.2  Thoracic region**
Thoracolumbar region

**739.3  Lumbar region**
Lumbosacral region

**739.4  Sacral region**
Sacrococcygeal region  Sacroiliac region

**739.5  Pelvic region**
Hip region            Pubic region

**739.6  Lower extremities**

**739.7  Upper extremities**
Acromioclavicular region
Sternoclavicular region

**739.8  Rib cage**
Costochondral region  Sternochondral region
Costovertebral region

**739.9  Abdomen and other**
AHA: 2Q, '89, 14

## 14. CONGENITAL ANOMALIES (740-759)

✓4th **740 Anencephalus and similar anomalies**

**740.0 Anencephalus** `MCC`

Acrania                Hemicephaly
Amyelencephalus        Hemianencephaly

**CC Excl:** 740.0-740.2

**DEF:** Fetus without cerebrum, cerebellum and flat bones of skull.

**740.1 Craniorachischisis** `MCC`
**CC Excl:** See code: 740.0

**DEF:** Congenital slit in cranium and vertebral column

**740.2 Iniencephaly** `MCC`
**CC Excl:** See code: 740.0

**DEF:** Spinal cord passes through enlarged occipital bone (foramen magnum); absent vertebral bone layer and spinal processes; resulting in both reduction in number and proper fusion of the vertebrae.

✓4th **741 Spina bifida**

**EXCLUDES**    spina bifida occulta (756.17)

The following fifth-digit subclassification is for use with category 741:

**0** unspecified region
**1** cervical region
**2** dorsal [thoracic] region
**3** lumbar region

**AHA:** 3Q, '94, 7

**DEF:** Lack of closure of spinal cord's bony encasement; marked by cord protrusion into lumbosacral area; evident by elevated alpha-fetoprotein of amniotic fluid

✓5th **741.0 With hydrocephalus** `CC`

Arnold-Chiari syndrome, type II
Any condition classifiable to 741.9 with any condition classifiable to 742.3
Chiari malformation, type II

**CC Excl:** 741.00-741.93, 742.59-742.9, 759.7-759.89

**AHA:** 4Q, '97, 51; 4Q, '94, 37; S-O, '87, 10

✓5th **741.9 Without mention of hydrocephalus**

Hydromeningocele (spinal)   Myelocystocele
Hydromyelocele              Rachischisis
Meningocele (spinal)        Spina bifida (aperta)
Meningomyelocele            Syringomyelocele
Myelocele

✓4th **742 Other congenital anomalies of nervous system**

**EXCLUDES**    congenital central alveolar hypoventilation syndrome (327.25)

**742.0 Encephalocele** `CC`

Encephalocystocele
Encephalomyelocele
Hydroencephalocele
Hydromeningocele, cranial
Meningocele, cerebral
Meningoencephalocele

**CC Excl:** 742.0-742.2, 742.4

**AHA:** 4Q, '94, 37

**DEF:** Brain tissue protrudes through skull defect.

**Spina Bifida**

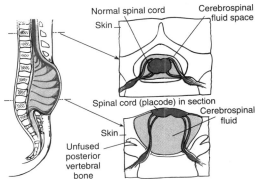

Normal spinal cord
Skin
Cerebrospinal fluid space
Spinal cord (placode) in section
Skin
Cerebrospinal fluid
Unfused posterior vertebral bone

**Normal Ventricles and Hydrocephalus**

Cerebrospinal fluid in ventricles    **Normal Ventricles**
Third ventricle (III)
Choroid plexus produces Cerebrospinal fluid (CSF)
Lateral ventricles (I and II)
Fourth ventricle (IV)
Foramen of Luschka
Foramen of Monro
Cerebral aqueduct (Sylvius)
Foramen of Magendie

**Hydrocephalus**

Enlarged ventricles
Blockage of any CSF passage increases pressure in skull, which may push tissue through the Incisura tentorii or through the Foramen magnum

**742.1 Microcephalus**

Hydromicrocephaly
Micrencephaly

**DEF:** Extremely small head or brain.

**742.2 Reduction deformities of brain** `MCC`

Absence
Agenesis        } of part of brain
Aplasia
Hypoplasia

Agyria          Holoprosencephaly
Arhinencephaly  Microgyria

**CC Excl:** See code 742.0

**AHA:** 3Q, '03, 15; 4Q, '94, 37

**742.3 Congenital hydrocephalus**

Aqueduct of Sylvius:
anomaly
obstruction, congenital
stenosis
Atresia of foramina of Magendie and Luschka
Hydrocephalus in newborn

**EXCLUDES**    hydrocephalus:
acquired (331.3-331.4)
due to congenital toxoplasmosis (771.2)
with any condition classifiable to 741.9 (741.0)

**AHA:** 4Q, '05, 83

**DEF:** Fluid accumulation within the skull; involves subarachnoid (external) or ventricular (internal) brain spaces.

**742.4 Other specified anomalies of brain** `CC`

Congenital cerebral cyst   Multiple anomalies of brain
Macroencephaly             NOS
Macrogyria                 Porencephaly
Megalencephaly             Ulegyria

**CC Excl:** See code: 742.4

**AHA:** 1Q, '99, 9; 3Q, '92, 12

✓5th **742.5 Other specified anomalies of spinal cord**

**742.51 Diastematomyelia**

**DEF:** Congenital anomaly often associated with spina bifida; the spinal cord is separated into halves by a bony tissue resembling a "spike" (a spicule), each half surrounded by a dural sac.

Additional Digit Required    Unacceptable PDx    Manifestation Code    `MCV` Major Cardiovascular Condition    ▶◀ Revised Text    ● New Code    ▲ Revised Code Title

October 2007 • Volume 1 — 255

© 2007 Ingenix

**Congenital Anomalies**

**742.53 Hydromyelia**
Hydrorhachis

DEF: Dilated central spinal cord canal; characterized by increased fluid accumulation.

**742.59 Other**
Amyelia
Atelomyelia
Congenital anomaly of spinal meninges
Defective development of cauda equina
Hypoplasia of spinal cord
Myelatelia
Myelodysplasia

AHA: 2Q, '91, 14; 1Q, '89, 10

**742.8 Other specified anomalies of nervous system**
Agenesis of nerve
Displacement of brachial plexus
Familial dysautonomia
Jaw-winking syndrome
Marcus-Gunn syndrome
Riley-Day syndrome

**EXCLUDES** *neurofibromatosis (237.7)*

**742.9 Unspecified anomaly of brain, spinal cord, and nervous system**

Anomaly
Congenital:
  disease     of:   { brain
  lesion         nervous system
Deformity         spinal cord

✓4th **743 Congenital anomalies of eye**

✓5th **743.0 Anophthalmos**

DEF: Complete absence of the eyes or the presence of vestigial eyes.

**743.00 Clinical anophthalmos, unspecified**
Agenesis
Congenital absence   } of eye
Anophthalmos NOS

**743.03 Cystic eyeball, congenital**

**743.06 Cryptophthalmos**
DEF: Eyelids continue over eyeball, results in apparent absence of eyelids.

✓5th **743.1 Microphthalmos**
Dysplasia
Hypoplasia   } of eye
Rudimentary eye

DEF: Abnormally small eyeballs, may be opacities of cornea and lens, scarring of choroid and retina.

**743.10 Microphthalmos, unspecified**

**743.11 Simple microphthalmos**

**743.12 Microphthalmos associated with other anomalies of eye and adnexa**

✓5th **743.2 Buphthalmos**
Glaucoma:        Hydrophthalmos
  congenital
  newborn

**EXCLUDES** *glaucoma of childhood (365.14)*
*traumatic glaucoma due to birth injury (767.8)*

DEF: Distended, enlarged fibrous coats of eye; due to intraocular pressure of congenital glaucoma.

**743.20 Buphthalmos, unspecified**

**743.21 Simple buphthalmos**

**743.22 Buphthalmos associated with other ocular anomalies**

Keratoglobus, congenital   } associated with
Megalocornea            buphthalmos

✓5th **743.3 Congenital cataract and lens anomalies**
**EXCLUDES** *infantile cataract (366.00-366.09)*
DEF: Opaque eye lens.

**743.30 Congenital cataract, unspecified**

**743.31 Capsular and subcapsular cataract**

**743.32 Cortical and zonular cataract**

**743.33 Nuclear cataract**

**743.34 Total and subtotal cataract, congenital**

**743.35 Congenital aphakia**
Congenital absence of lens

**743.36 Anomalies of lens shape**
Microphakia       Spherophakia

**743.37 Congenital ectopic lens**

**743.39 Other**

✓5th **743.4 Coloboma and other anomalies of anterior segment**
DEF: Coloboma: ocular tissue defect associated with defect of ocular fetal intraocular fissure; may cause small pit on optic disk, major defects of iris, ciliary body, choroid, and retina.

**743.41 Anomalies of corneal size and shape**
Microcornea
**EXCLUDES** *that associated with buphthalmos (743.22)*

**743.42 Corneal opacities, interfering with vision, congenital**

**743.43 Other corneal opacities, congenital**

**743.44 Specified anomalies of anterior chamber, chamber angle, and related structures**
Anomaly:        Anomaly:
  Axenfeld's      Rieger's
  Peters'

**743.45 Aniridia**
AHA: 3Q, '02, 20
DEF: Incompletely formed or absent iris; affects both eyes; dominant trait; also called congenital hyperplasia of iris.

**743.46 Other specified anomalies of iris and ciliary body**
Anisocoria, congenital    Coloboma of iris
Atresia of pupil          Corectopia

**743.47 Specified anomalies of sclera**

**743.48 Multiple and combined anomalies of anterior segment**

**743.49 Other**

✓5th **743.5 Congenital anomalies of posterior segment**

**743.51 Vitreous anomalies**
Congenital vitreous opacity

**743.52 Fundus coloboma**
DEF: Absent retinal and choroidal tissue; occurs in lower fundus; a bright white ectatic zone of exposed sclera extends into and changes the optic disk.

**743.53 Chorioretinal degeneration, congenital**

**743.54 Congenital folds and cysts of posterior segment**

**743.55 Congenital macular changes**

**743.56 Other retinal changes, congenital**
AHA: 3Q, '99, 12

**743.57 Specified anomalies of optic disc**
Coloboma of optic disc (congenital)

**743.58 Vascular anomalies**
Congenital retinal aneurysm

**743.59 Other**

N Newborn Age: 0    P Pediatric Age: 0-17    M Maternity Age: 12-55    A Adult Age: 15-124    CC CC Condition    MCC Major CC Condition    HIV HIV Related Dx

256 — Volume 1 • October 2007

© 2007 Ingenix

√5th **743.6 Congenital anomalies of eyelids, lacrimal system, and orbit**

**743.61 Congenital ptosis**
DEF: Drooping of eyelid.

**743.62 Congenital deformities of eyelids**
Ablepharon
Absence of eyelid
Accessory eyelid
Congenital:
ectropion
entropion
AHA: 1Q, '00, 22

**743.63 Other specified congenital anomalies of eyelid**
Absence, agenesis, of cilia

**743.64 Specified congenital anomalies of lacrimal gland**

**743.65 Specified congenital anomalies of lacrimal passages**
Absence, agenesis of:
lacrimal apparatus
punctum lacrimale
Accessory lacrimal canal

**743.66 Specified congenital anomalies of orbit**

**743.69 Other**
Accessory eye muscles

**743.8 Other specified anomalies of eye**
EXCLUDES   *congenital nystagmus (379.51)*
*ocular albinism (270.2)*
*optic nerve hypoplasia (377.43)*
*retinitis pigmentosa (362.74)*

**743.9 Unspecified anomaly of eye**
Congenital:
anomaly NOS } of eye [any part]
deformity NOS

√4th **744 Congenital anomalies of ear, face, and neck**
EXCLUDES   *anomaly of:*
*cervical spine (754.2, 756.10-756.19)*
*larynx (748.2-748.3)*
*nose (748.0-748.1)*
*parathyroid gland (759.2)*
*thyroid gland (759.2)*
*cleft lip (749.10-749.25)*

√5th **744.0 Anomalies of ear causing impairment of hearing**
EXCLUDES   *congenital deafness without mention of cause (389.0-389.9)*

**744.00 Unspecified anomaly of ear with impairment of hearing**

**744.01 Absence of external ear**
Absence of:
auditory canal (external)
auricle (ear) (with stenosis or atresia of auditory canal)

**744.02 Other anomalies of external ear with impairment of hearing**
Atresia or stricture of auditory canal (external)

**744.03 Anomaly of middle ear, except ossicles**
Atresia or stricture of osseous meatus (ear)

**744.04 Anomalies of ear ossicles**
Fusion of ear ossicles

**744.05 Anomalies of inner ear**
Congenital anomaly of:
membranous labyrinth
organ of Corti

**744.09 Other**
Absence of ear, congenital

**744.1 Accessory auricle**
Accessory tragus      Supernumerary:
Polyotia                 ear
Preauricular appendage    lobule
DEF: Redundant tissue or structures of ear.

√5th **744.2 Other specified anomalies of ear**
EXCLUDES   *that with impairment of hearing (744.00-744.09)*

**744.21 Absence of ear lobe, congenital**

**744.22 Macrotia**
DEF: Abnormally large pinna of ear.

**744.23 Microtia**
DEF: Hypoplasia of pinna; associated with absent or closed auditory canal.

**744.24 Specified anomalies of Eustachian tube**
Absence of Eustachian tube

**744.29 Other**
Bat ear           Prominence of auricle
Darwin's tubercle   Ridge ear
Pointed ear
EXCLUDES   *preauricular sinus (744.46)*

**744.3 Unspecified anomaly of ear**
Congenital:
anomaly NOS } of ear, not elsewhere
deformity NOS    classified

√5th **744.4 Branchial cleft cyst or fistula; preauricular sinus**

**744.41 Branchial cleft sinus or fistula**
Branchial:
sinus (external) (internal)
vestige
DEF: Cyst due to failed closure of embryonic branchial cleft.

**744.42 Branchial cleft cyst**

**744.43 Cervical auricle**

**744.46 Preauricular sinus or fistula**

**744.47 Preauricular cyst**

**744.49 Other**
Fistula (of):         Fistula (of):
auricle, congenital    cervicoaural

**744.5 Webbing of neck**
Pterygium colli
DEF: Thick, triangular skinfold, stretches from lateral side of neck across shoulder; associated with Turner's and Noonan's syndromes.

√5th **744.8 Other specified anomalies of face and neck**

**744.81 Macrocheilia**
Hypertrophy of lip, congenital
DEF: Abnormally large lips.

**744.82 Microcheilia**
DEF: Abnormally small lips.

**744.83 Macrostomia**
DEF: Bilateral or unilateral anomaly, of mouth due to malformed maxillary and mandibular processes; results in mouth extending toward ear.

**744.84 Microstomia**
DEF: Abnormally small mouth.

**744.89 Other**
EXCLUDES   *congenital fistula of lip (750.25)*
*musculoskeletal anomalies (754.0-754.1, 756.0)*

**744.9 Unspecified anomalies of face and neck**
Congenital:
anomaly NOS } of face [any part] or
deformity NOS   neck [any part]

**Heart Defects**

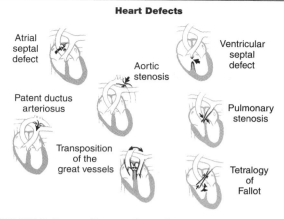

Atrial septal defect

Ventricular septal defect

Aortic stenosis

Patent ductus arteriosus

Pulmonary stenosis

Transposition of the great vessels

Tetralogy of Fallot

√4th **745 Bulbus cordis anomalies and anomalies of cardiac septal closure**

**745.0 Common truncus**  `MCC`

Absent septum } between aorta and
Communication (abnormal) } pulmonary artery

Aortic septal defect
Common aortopulmonary trunk
Persistent truncus arteriosus

CC Excl: 429.71-429.79, 745.0-745.9, 746.89-746.9, 747.83-747.9, 759.7-759.89

√5th **745.1 Transposition of great vessels**

**745.10 Complete transposition of great vessels**  `MCC`

Transposition of great vessels:
NOS
classical

CC Excl: See code 745.0

**745.11 Double outlet right ventricle**  `MCC`

Dextratransposition of aorta
Incomplete transposition of great vessels
Origin of both great vessels from right ventricle
Taussig-Bing syndrome or defect

CC Excl: See code 745.0

**745.12 Corrected transposition of great vessels** `CC`
CC Excl: See code 745.0

**745.19 Other**  `MCC`
CC Excl: See code 745.0

**745.2 Tetralogy of Fallot**  `MCC`

Fallot's pentalogy
Ventricular septal defect with pulmonary stenosis or atresia, dextraposition of aorta, and hypertrophy of right ventricle

**EXCLUDES**  Fallot's triad (746.09)

CC Excl: See code 745.0

DEF: Obstructed cardiac outflow causes pulmonary stenosis, interventricular septal defect and right ventricular hypertrophy.

**745.3 Common ventricle**  `MCC`

Cor triloculare biatriatum
Single ventricle

CC Excl: See code 745.0

**745.4 Ventricular septal defect**  `CC`

Eisenmenger's defect or complex
Gerbo dedefect
Interventricular septal defect
Left ventricular-right atrial communication
Roger's disease

**EXCLUDES**  common atrioventricular canal type (745.69)
single ventricle (745.3)

CC Excl: See code 745.0

**745.5 Ostium secundum type atrial septal defect**  `CC`

Defect:                    Patent or persistent:
atrium secundum           foramen ovale
fossa ovalis              ostium secundum
Lutembacher's syndrome

CC Excl: 429.71-429.79, 745.0-745.3, 745.5-745.9, 746.89-746.9, 747.89-747.9, 759.7, 759.89

DEF: Opening in atrial septum due to failure of the septum secundum and the endocardial cushions to fuse; there is a rim of septum surrounding the defect.

√5th **745.6 Endocardial cushion defects**

DEF: Atrial and/or ventricular septal defects causing abnormal fusion of cushions in atrioventricular canal.

**745.60 Endocardial cushion defect, unspecified type**  `CC`

CC Excl: See code 745.0

DEF: Septal defect due to imperfect fusion of endocardial cushions.

**745.61 Ostium primum defect**  `CC`

Persistent ostium primum

CC Excl: See code: 745.0

DEF: Opening in low, posterior septum primum; causes cleft in basal portion of atrial septum; associated with cleft mitral valve.

**745.69 Other**  `CC`

Absence of atrial septum
Atrioventricular canal type ventricular septal defect
Common atrioventricular canal
Common atrium

CC Excl: See code 745.0

**745.7 Cor biloculare**  `MCC`

Absence of atrial and ventricular septa

CC Excl: See code 745.0

DEF: Atrial and ventricular septal defect; marked by heart with two cardiac chambers (one atrium, one ventricle), and one atrioventricular valve.

**745.8 Other**

**745.9 Unspecified defect of septal closure**

Septal defect NOS

√4th **746 Other congenital anomalies of heart**

**EXCLUDES**  endocardial fibroelastosis (425.3)

√5th **746.0 Anomalies of pulmonary valve**

**EXCLUDES**  infundibular or subvalvular pulmonic stenosis (746.83)
tetralogy of Fallot (745.2)

**746.00 Pulmonary valve anomaly, unspecified**  `CC`

CC Excl: 746.00-746.09, 746.89-746.9, 747.89-747.9, 759.7, 759.89

**746.01 Atresia, congenital**  `MCC`

Congenital absence of pulmonary valve

CC Excl: 746.00-746.09, 746.89-746.9, 747.89-747.9, 759.7, 759.89

**746.02 Stenosis, congenital**  `CC`

CC Excl: See code 746.01

AHA: 1Q, '04, 16

DEF: Stenosis of opening between pulmonary artery and right ventricle; causes obstructed blood outflow from right ventricle.

**746.09 Other**  `CC`

Congenital insufficiency of pulmonary valve
Fallot's triad or trilogy

CC Excl: See code: 746.00

Newborn Age: 0   Pediatric Age: 0-17   Maternity Age: 12-55   Adult Age: 15-124   `CC` CC Condition   `MCC` Major CC Condition   `HIV` HIV Related Dx

**746.1 Tricuspid atresia and stenosis, congenital** `MCC`
Absence of tricuspid valve
**CC Excl:** 746.1-746.7, 746.89-746.9, 747.83-747.9, 759.7-759.89

**746.2 Ebstein's anomaly** `MCC`
**CC Excl:** See code 746.1
DEF: Malformation of the tricuspid valve characterized by septal and posterior leaflets attaching to the wall of the right ventricle; causing the right ventricle to fuse with the atrium producing a large right atrium and a small ventricle; causes a malfunction of the right ventricle with accompanying complications such as heart failure and abnormal cardiac rhythm.

**746.3 Congenital stenosis of aortic valve** `CC`
Congenital aortic stenosis
**EXCLUDES** congenital:
subaortic stenosis (746.81)
supravalvular aortic stenosis (747.22)
**CC Excl:** See code 746.1
**AHA:** 4Q, '88, 8
DEF: Stenosis of orifice of aortic valve; obstructs blood outflow from left ventricle.

**746.4 Congenital insufficiency of aortic valve** `CC`
Bicuspid aortic valve
Congenital aortic insufficiency
**CC Excl:** See code 746.1
DEF: Impaired functioning of aortic valve due to incomplete closure; causes backflow (regurgitation) of blood from aorta to left ventricle.

**746.5 Congenital mitral stenosis** `CC`
Fused commissure
Parachute deformity } of mitral valve
Supernumerary cusps
**CC Excl:** See code 746.1
DEF: Stenosis of left atrioventricular orifice.

**746.6 Congenital mitral insufficiency** `CC`
**CC Excl:** See code 746.1
DEF: Impaired functioning of mitral valve due to incomplete closure; causes backflow of blood from left ventricle to left atrium.

**746.7 Hypoplastic left heart syndrome** `MCC`
Atresia, or marked hypoplasia, of aortic orifice or valve, with hypoplasia of ascending aorta and defective development of left ventricle (with mitral valve atresia)
**CC Excl:** See code 746.1

**√5ᵗʰ 746.8 Other specified anomalies of heart**

    **746.81 Subaortic stenosis** `MCC`
    **CC Excl:** 746.81-746.84, 746.89-746.9, 747.83-747.9, 759.7-759.89
    DEF: Stenosis, of left ventricular outflow tract due to fibrous tissue ring or septal hypertrophy below aortic valve.

    **746.82 Cor triatriatum** `MCC`
    **CC Excl:** See code 746.81
    DEF: Transverse septum divides left atrium due to failed resorption of embryonic common pulmonary vein; results in three atrial chambers.

    **746.83 Infundibular pulmonic stenosis** `CC`
    Subvalvular pulmonic stenosis
    **CC Excl:** See code 746.81
    DEF: Stenosis of right ventricle outflow tract within infundibulum due to fibrous diaphragm below valve or long, narrow fibromuscular channel.

    **746.84 Obstructive anomalies of heart, not elsewhere classified** `MCC`
    Uhl's disease
    **CC Excl:** See code: 746.81

    **746.85 Coronary artery anomaly** `CC`
    Anomalous origin or communication of coronary artery
    Arteriovenous malformation of coronary artery
    Coronary artery:
      absence
      arising from aorta or pulmonary trunk
      single
    **CC Excl:** 746.85, 746.89-746.9
    **AHA:** N-D, '85, 3

    **746.86 Congenital heart block** `MCC`
    Complete or incomplete atrioventricular [AV] block
    **CC Excl:** 746.86, 746.89-746.9, 747.83-747.9, 759.7-759.89
    DEF: Impaired conduction of electrical impulses; due to maldeveloped junctional tissue.

    **746.87 Malposition of heart and cardiac apex** `CC`
    Abdominal heart    Levocardia (isolated)
    Dextrocardia    Mesocardia
    Ectopia cordis
    **EXCLUDES** dextrocardia with complete transposition of viscera (759.3)
    **CC Excl:** 746.81-746.84, 746.87-746.9, 747.89-747.9, 759.7, 759.89

    **746.89 Other**
    Atresia
    Hypoplasia } of cardiac vein
    Congenital:      Congenital:
      cardiomegaly    pericardial defect
      diverticulum, left ventricle
    **AHA:** 3Q, '00, 3; 1Q, '99, 11; J-F, '85, 3

**746.9 Unspecified anomaly of heart**
Congenital:
  anomaly of heart NOS
  heart disease NOS

**√4ᵗʰ 747 Other congenital anomalies of circulatory system**

    **747.0 Patent ductus arteriosus** `CC`
    Patent ductus Botalli
    Persistent ductus arteriosus
    **CC Excl:** 747.0, 747.89
    DEF: Open lumen in ductus arteriosus causes arterial blood recirculation in lungs; inhibits blood supply to aorta; symptoms such as shortness of breath more noticeable upon activity.

    **√5ᵗʰ 747.1 Coarctation of aorta**
    DEF: Localized deformity of aortic media seen as a severe constriction of the vessel lumen; major symptom is high blood pressure in the arms and low pressure in the legs; a CVA, rupture of the aorta, bacterial endocarditis or congestive heart failure can follow if left untreated.

      **747.10 Coarctation of aorta (preductal) (postductal)** `CC`
      Hypoplasia of aortic arch
      **CC Excl:** 747.10-747.22, 747.89-747.9, 759.7, 759.89
      **AHA:** 1Q, '99, 11; 4Q, '88, 8

      **747.11 Interruption of aortic arch** `MCC`
      **CC Excl:** 747.10-747.22, 747.83-747.9, 759.7-759.89

**Congenital Anomalies**

**747.2–747.83**

√5th **747.2 Other anomalies of aorta**

**747.20 Anomaly of aorta, unspecified** `CC`
**CC Excl:** 747.10-747.22, 747.89-747.9, 759.7, 759.89

**747.21 Anomalies of aortic arch** `CC`
Anomalous origin, right subclavian artery
Dextraposition of aorta
Double aortic arch
Kommerell's diverticulum
Overriding aorta
Persistent:
    convolutions, aortic arch
    right aortic arch
Vascular ring
> **EXCLUDES** *hypoplasia of aortic arch (747.10)*

**CC Excl:** See code: 747.20
**AHA:** 1Q, '03, 15

**747.22 Atresia and stenosis of aorta** `CC`
Absence ⎫
Aplasia ⎬ of aorta
Hypoplasia ⎪
Stricture ⎭
Supra (valvular)-aortic stenosis
> **EXCLUDES** *congenital aortic (valvular) stenosis or stricture, so stated (746.3)*
> *hypoplasia of aorta in hypoplastic left heart syndrome (746.7)*

**CC Excl:** 747.10-747.22, 747.83-747.9, 759.7-759.89

**747.29 Other** `CC`
Aneurysm of sinus of Valsalva
Congenital:
    aneurysm ⎫
    dilation ⎬ of aorta

**CC Excl:** 747.10-747.29, 747.89-747.9, 759.7, 759.89

**747.3 Anomalies of pulmonary artery** `MCC`
Agenesis ⎫
Anomaly ⎪
Atresia ⎬ of pulmonary artery
Coarctation ⎪
Hypoplasia ⎪
Stenosis ⎭
Pulmonary arteriovenous aneurysm

**CC Excl:** 747.3, 747.89-747.9

**AHA:** 1Q, '04, 16; 1Q, '94, 15; 4Q, '88, 8

√5th **747.4 Anomalies of great veins**

**747.40 Anomaly of great veins, unspecified** `CC`
Anomaly NOS of:    Anomaly NOS of:
    pulmonary veins     vena cava

**CC Excl:** 747.40, 747.89-747.9

**747.41 Total anomalous pulmonary venous connection** `CC`
Total anomalous pulmonary venous return [TAPVR]:
    subdiaphragmatic
    supradiaphragmatic

**CC Excl:** 747.41, 747.89-747.9

**747.42 Partial anomalous pulmonary venous connection** `CC`
Partial anomalous pulmonary venous return

**CC Excl:** 747.42, 747.89-747.9

**747.49 Other anomalies of great veins** `CC`
Absence ⎫ of vena cava
Congenital stenosis ⎬ (inferior)
    ⎭ (superior)
Persistent:
    left posterior cardinal vein
    left superior vena cava
Scimitar syndrome
Transposition of pulmonary veins NOS

**CC Excl:** 747.49, 747.89-747.9

**747.5 Absence or hypoplasia of umbilical artery**
Single umbilical artery

√5th **747.6 Other anomalies of peripheral vascular system**
Absence ⎫
Anomaly ⎬ of artery or vein, NEC
Atresia ⎭
Arteriovenous aneurysm (peripheral)
Arteriovenous malformation of the peripheral vascular system
Congenital:
    aneurysm (peripheral)    stricture, artery
    phlebectasia      varix
Multiple renal arteries
> **EXCLUDES** *anomalies of:*
> *cerebral vessels (747.81)*
> *pulmonary artery (747.3)*
> *congenital retinal aneurysm (743.58)*
> *hemangioma (228.00-228.09)*
> *lymphangioma (228.1)*

**747.60 Anomaly of the peripheral vascular system, unspecified site**

**747.61 Gastrointestinal vessel anomaly**
**AHA:** 3Q, '96, 10

**747.62 Renal vessel anomaly**

**747.63 Upper limb vessel anomaly**

**747.64 Lower limb vessel anomaly**

**747.69 Anomalies of other specified sites of peripheral vascular system**

√5th **747.8 Other specified anomalies of circulatory system**

**747.81 Anomalies of cerebrovascular system** `MCC`
Arteriovenous malformation of brain
Cerebral arteriovenous aneurysm, congenital
Congenital anomalies of cerebral vessels
> **EXCLUDES** *ruptured cerebral (arteriovenous) aneurysm (430)*

**CC Excl:** 747.81, 747.89-747.9

**747.82 Spinal vessel anomaly** `CC`
Arteriovenous malformation of spinal vessel
**CC Excl:** 747.82, 747.89-747.9

**AHA:** 3Q, '95, 5

**747.83 Persistent fetal circulation** `MCC` `N`
Persistent pulmonary hypertension
Primary pulmonary hypertension of newborn
**CC Excl:** 416.0, 416.8-416.9

**AHA:** 4Q, '02, 62

**DEF:** A return to fetal-type circulation due to constriction of pulmonary arterioles and opening of the ductus arteriosus and foramen ovale, right-to-left shunting occurs, oxygenation of the blood does not occur, and the lungs remain constricted after birth; PFC is seen in term or post-term infants causes include asphyxiation, meconium aspiration syndrome, acidosis, sepsis, and developmental immaturity.

---

`N` Newborn Age: 0    `P` Pediatric Age: 0-17    `M` Maternity Age: 12-55    `A` Adult Age: 15-124    `CC` CC Condition    `MCC` Major CC Condition    `HIV` HIV Related Dx

**260 — Volume 1 • October 2007**

© 2007 Ingenix

**Persistent Fetal Circulation**

**747.89 Other** `CC`

    Aneurysm, congenital, specified site not elsewhere classified

    **EXCLUDES** *congenital aneurysm:*
      *coronary (746.85)*
      *peripheral (747.6)*
      *pulmonary (747.3)*
      *retinal (743.58)*

    **CC Excl:** 745.0-745.9, 747.89

    **AHA:** 4Q, '02, 63

**747.9   Unspecified anomaly of circulatory system** `CC`
    **CC Excl:** 745.0-747.82, 747.89-747.9

✓4ᵗʰ **748 Congenital anomalies of respiratory system**

    **EXCLUDES** *congenital central alveolar hypoventilation syndrome (327.25)*
      *congenital defect of diaphragm (756.6)*

**748.0   Choanal atresia**

    Atresia }  of nares (anterior)
    Congenital stenosis }   (posterior)

    **DEF:** Occluded posterior nares (choana), bony or membranous due to failure of embryonic bucconasal membrane to rupture.

**748.1   Other anomalies of nose**

    Absent nose        Congenital:
    Accessory nose        notching of tip of nose
    Cleft nose            perforation of wall of
    Congenital:             nasal sinus
      deformity of nose    Deformity of wall of nasal
                         sinus

    **EXCLUDES** *congenital deviation of nasal septum (754.0)*

**748.2   Web of larynx**

    Web of larynx:       Web of larynx:
      NOS                  subglottic
      glottic

    **DEF:** Malformed larynx; marked by thin, translucent, or thick, fibrotic spread between vocal folds; affects speech.

**748.3   Other anomalies of larynx, trachea, and bronchus** `CC`

    Absence or agenesis of:    Congenital:
      bronchus                dilation, trachea
      larynx                 stenosis:
      trachea                 larynx
    Anomaly (of):           trachea
      cricoid cartilage      tracheocele
      epiglottis        Diverticulum:
      thyroid cartilage      bronchus
      tracheal cartilage     trachea
    Atresia (of):         Fissure of epiglottis
      epiglottis        Laryngocele
      glottis          Posterior cleft of cricoid
      larynx            cartilage (congenital)
      trachea         Rudimentary tracheal
    Cleft thyroid, cartilage,     bronchus
      congenital      Stridor, laryngeal, congenital

    **CC Excl:** 493.81, 519.19, 748.3, 748.8-748.9

    **AHA:** 1Q, '99, 14

**748.4   Congenital cystic lung** `CC`

    Disease, lung:       Honeycomb lung, congenital
      cystic, congenital
      polycystic, congenital
      **EXCLUDES** *acquired or unspecified cystic lung (518.89)*

    **CC Excl:** 748.4-748.9
    **DEF:** Enlarged air spaces of lung parenchyma.

**748.5   Agenesis, hypoplasia, and dysplasia of lung** `MCC`

    Absence of lung (fissures) (lobe)
      (lobe)             Hypoplasia of lung
    Aplasia of lung       Sequestration of lung

    **CC Excl:** See code 748.4

✓5ᵗʰ **748.6   Other anomalies of lung**

    **748.60 Anomaly of lung, unspecified**

    **748.61 Congenital bronchiectasis** `CC`

      **CC Excl:** 494.0-494.1, 496, 506.1,506.4-506.9, 748.61

    **748.69 Other**

      Accessory lung (lobe)
      Azygos lobe (fissure), lung

**748.8   Other specified anomalies of respiratory system**

    Abnormal communication between pericardial and pleural sacs
    Anomaly, pleural folds
    Atresia of nasopharynx
    Congenital cyst of mediastinum

**748.9   Unspecified anomaly of respiratory system**

    Anomaly of respiratory system NOS

✓4ᵗʰ **749 Cleft palate and cleft lip**

✓5ᵗʰ **749.0   Cleft palate**

    **749.00 Cleft palate, unspecified**

    **749.01 Unilateral, complete**

    **749.02 Unilateral, incomplete**
      Cleft uvula

    **749.03 Bilateral, complete**

    **749.04 Bilateral, incomplete**

✓5ᵗʰ **749.1   Cleft lip**

    Cheiloschisis        Harelip
    Congenital fissure of lip    Labium leporinum

    **749.10 Cleft lip, unspecified**

    **749.11 Unilateral, complete**

    **749.12 Unilateral, incomplete**

    **749.13 Bilateral, complete**

    **749.14 Bilateral, incomplete**

✓5ᵗʰ **749.2   Cleft palate with cleft lip**
    Cheilopalatoschisis

    **749.20 Cleft palate with cleft lip, unspecified**

    **749.21 Unilateral, complete**

    **749.22 Unilateral, incomplete**

    **749.23 Bilateral, complete**
      **AHA:** 1Q, '96, 14

    **749.24 Bilateral, incomplete**

    **749.25 Other combinations**

✓4ᵗʰ **750 Other congenital anomalies of upper alimentary tract**

    **EXCLUDES** *dentofacial anomalies (524.0-524.9)*

**750.0   Tongue tie**

    Ankyloglossia

    **DEF:** Restricted tongue movement due to lingual frenum extending toward tip of tongue. Tongue may be fused to mouth floor affecting speech.

**Congenital Anomalies**

**750.1–751.2**

**Cleft Lip and Palate**

Unilateral cleft lip     Cleft lip with cleft alveolar ridge

No cleft palate     No cleft palate

Unilateral cleft lip and cleft palate

Alveolar ridge

Cleft palate

Prolabium

Bilateral cleft lip and cleft palate

Isolated cleft palate

✓5ᵗʰ **750.1 Other anomalies of tongue**

**750.10 Anomaly of tongue, unspecified**

**750.11 Aglossia**
DEF: Absence of tongue.

**750.12 Congenital adhesions of tongue**

**750.13 Fissure of tongue**
Bifid tongue     Double tongue

**750.15 Macroglossia**
Congenital hypertrophy of tongue

**750.16 Microglossia**
Hypoplasia of tongue

**750.19 Other**

✓5ᵗʰ **750.2 Other specified anomalies of mouth and pharynx**

**750.21 Absence of salivary gland**

**750.22 Accessory salivary gland**

**750.23 Atresia, salivary duct**
Imperforate salivary duct

**750.24 Congenital fistula of salivary gland**

**750.25 Congenital fistula of lip**
Congenital (mucus) lip pits

**750.26 Other specified anomalies of mouth**
Absence of uvula

**750.27 Diverticulum of pharynx**
Pharyngeal pouch

**750.29 Other specified anomalies of pharynx**
Imperforate pharynx

**750.3 Tracheoesophageal fistula, esophageal atresia and stenosis** `MCC`
Absent esophagus     Congenital fistula:
Atresia of esophagus     esophagobronchial
Congenital:     esophagotracheal
   esophageal ring     Imperforate esophagus
   stenosis of esophagus     Webbed esophagus
   stricture of esophagus
CC Excl: 530.84, 750.3-750.4, 751.8-751.9

**750.4 Other specified anomalies of esophagus** `CC`
Dilatation, congenital
Displacement, congenital
Diverticulum     } (of) esophagus
Duplication
Giant
Esophageal pouch
**EXCLUDES** *congenital hiatus hernia (750.6)*
CC Excl: 750.4, 751.8-751.9

AHA: J-F, '85, 3

**750.5 Congenital hypertrophic pyloric stenosis**
Congenital or infantile:
   constriction
   hypertrophy
   spasm     } of pylorus
   stenosis
   stricture

DEF: Obstructed pylorus due to overgrowth of pyloric muscle.

**750.6 Congenital hiatus hernia**
Displacement of cardia through esophageal hiatus
**EXCLUDES** *congenital diaphragmatic hernia (756.6)*

**750.7 Other specified anomalies of stomach**
Congenital:
   cardiospasm
   hourglass stomach
Displacement of stomach
Diverticulum of stomach, congenital
Duplication of stomach
Megalogastria
Microgastria
Transposition of stomach

**750.8 Other specified anomalies of upper alimentary tract**

**750.9 Unspecified anomaly of upper alimentary tract**
Congenital:
   anomaly NOS     } of upper alimentary tract [any
   deformity NOS     part, except tongue]

✓4ᵗʰ **751 Other congenital anomalies of digestive system**

**751.0 Meckel's diverticulum**
Meckel's diverticulum (displaced) (hypertrophic)
Persistent:
   omphalomesenteric duct
   vitelline duct

AHA: 1Q, '04, 10

DEF: Malformed sacs or appendages of ileum of small intestine; can cause strangulation, volvulus and intussusception.

**751.1 Atresia and stenosis of small intestine** `CC` `P`
Atresia of:     Atresia of:
   duodenum     intestine NOS
   ileum
Congenital:
   absence     }
   obstruction    of small intestine or
   stenosis     intestine NOS
   stricture     }
Imperforate jejunum
CC Excl: 751.1, 751.8-751.9

**751.2 Atresia and stenosis of large intestine rectum, and anal canal** `CC` `P`
Absence:     Congenital or infantile:
   anus (congenital)     obstruction of large
   appendix, congenital     intestine
   large intestine, congenital     occlusion of anus
   rectum     stricture of anus
Atresia of:     Imperforate:
   anus     anus
   colon     rectum
   rectum     Stricture of rectum,
       congenital
CC Excl: 751.2, 751.8-751.9

AHA: 2Q, '98, 16

`N` Newborn Age: 0    `P` Pediatric Age: 0-17    `M` Maternity Age: 12-55    `A` Adult Age: 15-124    `CC` CC Condition    `MCC` Major CC Condition    `HIV` HIV Related Dx

262 — Volume 1 • October 2007

© 2007 Ingenix

**751.3**   **Hirschsprung's disease and other congenital functional disorders of colon** `CC`

     Aganglionosis      Congenital megacolon

     Congenital dilation of colon      Macrocolon

     **CC Excl:** 751.3, 751.8-751.9

     **DEF:** Hirschsprung's disease: enlarged or dilated colon (megacolon), with absence of ganglion cells in the narrowed wall distally; causes inability to defecate.

**751.4**   **Anomalies of intestinal fixation** `CC`

     Congenital adhesions:      Rotation of cecum or colon:

       omental, anomalous      failure of

       peritoneal      incomplete

       Jackson's membrane      insufficient

       Malrotation of colon      Universal mesentery

     **CC Excl:** 751.4-751.5

**751.5**   **Other anomalies of intestine** `CC`

     Congenital diverticulum, colon      Megaloappendix

     Dolichocolon      Megaloduodenum

     Duplication of:      Microcolon

       anus      Persistent cloaca

       appendix      Transposition of:

       cecum        appendix

       intestine        colon

     Ectopic anus        intestine

     **CC Excl:** 751.0-751.5

     **AHA:** 3Q, '02, 11; 3Q, '01, 8

**751.6**   **Anomalies of gallbladder, bile ducts, and liver** √5th

     **751.60 Unspecified anomaly of gallbladder, bile ducts, and liver** `CC`

       **CC Excl:** 751.60

     **751.61 Biliary atresia** `MCC` `P`

       Congenital:

         absence

         hypoplasia    } of bile duct (common)

         obstruction      or passage

         stricture

       **CC Excl:** 751.61, 751.8-751.9

       **AHA:** S-O, '87, 8

     **751.62 Congenital cystic disease of liver** `CC`

       Congenital polycystic disease of liver

       Fibrocystic disease of liver

       **CC Excl:** 751.62-751.69

     **751.69 Other anomalies of gallbladder, bile ducts, and liver** `CC`

       Absence of:      Duplication of:

         gallbladder, congenital    biliary duct

         liver (lobe)      cystic duct

       Accessory:      gallbladder

         hepatic ducts      liver

         liver      Floating:

       Congenital:        gallbladder

         choledochal cyst      liver

         hepatomegaly      Intrahepatic

                           gallbladder

       **CC Excl:** 751.60-751.69

       **AHA:** S-O, '87, 8

**751.7**   **Anomalies of pancreas** `CC`

     Absence

     Accessory

     Agenesis    } (of) pancreas

     Annular

     Hypoplasia

     Ectopic pancreatic tissue      Pancreatic heterotopia

     **EXCLUDES**    *diabetes mellitus:*

         *congenital (250.0-250.9)*

         *neonatal (775.1)*

       *fibrocystic disease of pancreas*

         *(277.00-277.09)*

     **CC Excl:** 751.7-751.9

**751.8**   **Other specified anomalies of digestive system**

     Absence (complete) (partial) of alimentary tract NOS

     Duplication

     Malposition, congenital    } of digestive organs NOS

     **EXCLUDES**    *congenital diaphragmatic hernia*

         *(756.6)*

       *congenital hiatus hernia (750.6)*

**751.9**   **Unspecified anomaly of digestive system**

     Congenital:

       anomaly NOS

       deformity NOS    } of digestive system NOS

√4th **752 Congenital anomalies of genital organs**

     **EXCLUDES**    *syndromes associated with anomalies in the*

         *number and form of chromosomes (758.0-*

         *758.9)*

       *testicular feminization syndrome (259.5)*

**752.0**   **Anomalies of ovaries** ♀

     Absence, congenital

     Accessory

     Ectopic    } (of) ovary

     Streak

√5th **752.1 Anomalies of fallopian tubes and broad ligaments**

     **752.10 Unspecified anomaly of fallopian tubes and broad ligaments** ♀

     **752.11 Embryonic cyst of fallopian tubes and broad ligaments** ♀

       Cyst:

         epoophoron

         fimbrial

         parovarian

       **AHA:** S-O, '85, 13

     **752.19 Other** ♀

       Absence

       Accessory    } (of) fallopian tube or

       Atresia        broad ligament

**752.2**   **Doubling of uterus** ♀

     Didelphic uterus

     Doubling of uterus [any degree] (associated with doubling of cervix and vagina)

**752.3**   **Other anomalies of uterus** ♀

     Absence, congenital

     Agenesis

     Aplasia    } (of) uterus

     Bicornuate

     Uterus unicornis

     Uterus with only one functioning horn

     **AHA:** 3Q, '06, 18

√5th **752.4 Anomalies of cervix, vagina, and external female genitalia**

     **752.40 Unspecified anomaly of cervix, vagina, and external female genitalia** ♀

     **752.41 Embryonic cyst of cervix, vagina, and external female genitalia** ♀

       Cyst of:

         canal of Nuck, congenital

         Gartner's duct

         vagina, embryonal

         vulva, congenital

       **DEF:** Embryonic fluid-filled cysts, of cervix, vagina or external female genitalia.

     **752.42 Imperforate hymen** ♀

       **DEF:** Complete closure of membranous fold around external opening of vagina.

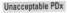

**Congenital Anomalies**

**752.49–753.20**

### Hypospadias and Epispadias

Glans penis
Glandular hypospadias
Penile hypospadias
Penile raphe
Scrotal hypospadias
Scrotum
Scrotal raphe

Normal external urethral orifice
Glans penis
Foreskin (retracted)
Epispadias

**Hypospadias (ventral view)**

**Epispadias (dorsal view)**

**752.49 Other anomalies of cervix, vagina, and external female genitalia** ♀

Absence ⎫ of cervix, clitoris, vagina,
Agenesis ⎭    or vulva

Congenital stenosis or stricture of:
   cervical canal
   vagina

**EXCLUDES**   double vagina associated with total duplication (752.2)

**AHA:** 3Q, '06, 18

**√5th** **752.5** **Undescended and retractile testicle**

**AHA:** 4Q, '96, 33

**752.51 Undescended testis** ♂
   Cryptorchism
   Ectopic testis

**752.52 Retractile testis** ♂

**√5th** **752.6** **Hypospadias and epispadias and other penile anomalies**

**AHA:** 4Q, '96, 34, 35

**752.61 Hypospadias** ♂

**AHA:** 4Q, '03, 67-68; 3Q, '97, 6

DEF: Abnormal opening of urethra on the ventral surface of the penis or perineum; also a rare defect of vagina.

**752.62 Epispadias** ♂
   Anaspadias

DEF: Urethra opening on dorsal surface of penis; in females appears as a slit in the upper wall of urethra.

**752.63 Congenital chordee** ♂

DEF: Ventral bowing of penis due to fibrous band along corpus spongiosum; occurs with hypospadias.

**752.64 Micropenis** ♂

**752.65 Hidden penis** ♂

**752.69 Other penile anomalies** ♂

**752.7** **Indeterminate sex and pseudohermaphroditism**

Gynandrism    Pseudohermaphroditism
Hermaphroditism    (male) (female)
Ovotestis    Pure gonadal dysgenesis

**EXCLUDES**   pseudohermaphroditism:
   female, with adrenocortical disorder (255.2)
   male, with gonadal disorder (257.8)
   with specified chromosomal anomaly (758.0-758.9)
   testicular feminization syndrome (259.5)

DEF: Pseudohermaphroditism: presence of gonads of one sex and external genitalia of other sex.

**√5th** **752.8** **Other specified anomalies of genital organs**

**EXCLUDES**   congenital hydrocele (778.6)
   penile anomalies (752.61-752.69)
   phimosis or paraphimosis (605)

**752.81 Scrotal transposition** ♂

**AHA:** 4Q, '03, 67-68

**752.89 Other specified anomalies of genital organs**

Absence of:    Fusion of testes
   prostate    Hypoplasia of testis
   spermatic cord    Monorchism
   vas deferens    Polyorchism
Anorchism
Aplasia (congenital) of:
   prostate
   round ligament
   testicle
Atresia of:
   ejaculatory duct
   vas deferens

**752.9** **Unspecified anomaly of genital organs**

Congenital:
   anomaly NOS ⎫ of genital organ,
   deformity NOS ⎭   not elsewhere classified

**√4th** **753** **Congenital anomalies of urinary system**

**753.0** **Renal agenesis and dysgenesis** CC

Atrophy of kidney:    Atrophy of kidney:
   congenital    infantile
Congenital absence of kidney(s)
Hypoplasia of kidney(s)

**CC Excl:** 599.60-599.69, 753.0

**√5th** **753.1** **Cystic kidney disease**

**EXCLUDES**   acquired cyst of kidney (593.2)

**AHA:** 4Q, '90, 3

**753.10 Cystic kidney disease, unspecified** CC
**CC Excl:** 599.60-599.69, 753.10

**753.11 Congenital single renal cyst** CC
**CC Excl:** 599.60-599.69, 753.11

**753.12 Polycystic kidney, unspecified type** CC
**CC Excl:** 599.60-599.69, 753.12-753.14

**753.13 Polycystic kidney, autosomal dominant** CC
**CC Excl:** See code: 753.12

DEF: Slow progressive disease characterized by bilateral cysts causing increased kidney size and impaired function.

**753.14 Polycystic kidney, autosomal recessive** CC
**CC Excl:** See code: 753.12

DEF: Rare disease characterized by multiple cysts involving kidneys and liver, producing renal and hepatic failure in childhood or adolescence.

**753.15 Renal dysplasia** CC
**CC Excl:** 599.60-599.69, 753.15

**753.16 Medullary cystic kidney** CC
   Nephronopthisis
**CC Excl:** 599.60-599.69, 753.16-753.19

DEF: Diffuse kidney disease results in uremia onset prior to age 20.

**753.17 Medullary sponge kidney** CC
**CC Excl:** See code: 753.16

DEF: Dilated collecting tubules; usually asymptomatic but calcinosis in tubules may cause renal insufficiency.

**753.19 Other specified cystic kidney disease** CC
   Multicystic kidney
**CC Excl:** See code: 753.16

**√5th** **753.2** **Obstructive defects of renal pelvis and ureter**

**AHA:** 4Q, '96, 35

**753.20 Unspecified obstructive defect of renal pelvis and ureter** CC
**CC Excl:** 599.60-599.69, 753.20-753.22, 753.29

N Newborn Age: 0    P Pediatric Age: 0-17    M Maternity Age: 12-55    A Adult Age: 15-124    CC CC Condition    MCC Major CC Condition    HIV HIV Related Dx

264 — Volume 1 • October 2007      © 2007 Ingenix

**753.21 Congenital obstruction of ureteropelvic** `CC` **junction**

CC Excl: See code: 753.20

DEF: Stricture at junction of ureter and renal pelvis.

**753.22 Congenital obstruction of ureterovesical** `CC` **junction**

Adynamic ureter    Congenital hydroureter

CC Excl: See code: 753.20

DEF: Stricture at junction of ureter and bladder.

**753.23 Congenital ureterocele**      `CC`

CC Excl: See code: 753.20

**753.29 Other**      `CC`

CC Excl: See code: 753.20

**753.3 Other specified anomalies of kidney**

| | |
|---|---|
| Accessory kidney | Fusion of kidneys |
| Congenital: | Giant kidney |
|   calculus of kidney | Horseshoe kidney |
|   displaced kidney | Hyperplasia of kidney |
| Discoid kidney | Lobulation of kidney |
| Double kidney with | Malrotation of kidney |
|   double pelvis | Trifid kidney (pelvis) |
| Ectopic kidney | |

AHA: ▶1Q, '07, 23◀

**753.4 Other specified anomalies of ureter**

| | |
|---|---|
| Absent ureter | Double ureter |
| Accessory ureter | Ectopic ureter |
| Deviation of ureter | Implantation, anomalous |
| Displaced ureteric |   of ureter |
|   orifice | |

**753.5 Exstrophy of urinary bladder**      `CC`

Ectopia vesicae
Extroversion of bladder

CC Excl: 599.60-599.69, 753.5, 753.9

DEF: Absence of lower abdominal and anterior bladder walls with posterior bladder wall protrusion.

**753.6 Atresia and stenosis of urethra and bladder** `CC` **neck**

| | |
|---|---|
| Congenital obstruction: | Imperforate urinary |
|   bladder neck |   meatus |
|   urethra | Impervious urethra |
| Congenital stricture of: | Urethral valve formation |
|   urethra (valvular) | |
|   urinary meatus | |
|   vesicourethral orifice | |

CC Excl: 599.60-599.69, 753.6, 753.9

**753.7 Anomalies of urachus**

Cyst ⎫
Fistula ⎬ (of) urachussinus
Patent ⎭

Persistent umbilical sinus

**753.8 Other specified anomalies of bladder and urethra**

| | |
|---|---|
| Absence, congenital of: | Congenital urethrorectal |
|   bladder |   fistula |
|   urethra | Congenital prolapse of: |
| Accessory: |   bladder (mucosa) |
|   bladder |   urethra |
|   urethra | Double: |
| Congenital: |   urethra |
|   diverticulum of bladder |   urinary meatus |
|   hernia of bladder | |

**753.9 Unspecified anomaly of urinary system**

Congenital:
  anomaly NOS ⎫ of urinary system [any part,
  deformity NOS ⎬   except urachus]

`✓4ᵗʰ` **754 Certain congenital musculoskeletal deformities**

`INCLUDES` nonteratogenic deformities which are considered to be due to intrauterine malposition and pressure

**754.0 Of skull, face, and jaw**

| | |
|---|---|
| Asymmetry of face | Dolichocephaly |
| Compression facies | Plagiocephaly |
| Depressions in skull | Potter's facies |
| Deviation of nasal | Squashed or bent nose, |
|   septum, congenital |   congenital |

`EXCLUDES` *dentofacial anomalies (524.0-524.9)*
*syphilitic saddle nose (090.5)*

**754.1 Of sternocleidomastoid muscle**

Congenital sternomastoid torticollis
Congenital wryneck
Contracture of sternocleidomastoid (muscle)
Sternomastoid tumor

**754.2 Of spine**      `CC`

Congenital postural:
  lordosis        scoliosis

CC Excl: 754.2

`✓5ᵗʰ` **754.3 Congenital dislocation of hip**

**754.30 Congenital dislocation of hip, unilateral**
Congenital dislocation of hip NOS

**754.31 Congenital dislocation of hip, bilateral**

**754.32 Congenital subluxation of hip, unilateral**
Congenital flexion deformity, hip or thigh
Predislocation status of hip at birth
Preluxation of hip, congenital

**754.33 Congenital subluxation of hip, bilateral**

**754.35 Congenital dislocation of one hip with subluxation of other hip**

`✓5ᵗʰ` **754.4 Congenital genu recurvatum and bowing of long bones of leg**

**754.40 Genu recurvatum**
DEF: Backward curving of knee joint.

**754.41 Congenital dislocation of knee (with genu recurvatum)**

**754.42 Congenital bowing of femur**

**754.43 Congenital bowing of tibia and fibula**

**754.44 Congenital bowing of unspecified long bones of leg**

`✓5ᵗʰ` **754.5 Varus deformities of feet**
`EXCLUDES` *acquired (736.71, 736.75, 736.79)*

**754.50 Talipes varus**
Congenital varus deformity of foot, unspecified
Pes varus

DEF: Inverted foot marked by outer sole resting on ground.

**754.51 Talipes equinovarus**
Equinovarus (congenital)

DEF: Elevated, outward rotation of heel; also called clubfoot.

**754.52 Metatarsus primus varus**
DEF: Malformed first metatarsal bone, with bone angled toward body.

**754.53 Metatarsus varus**

**754.59 Other**
Talipes calcaneovarus

`✓5ᵗʰ` **754.6 Valgus deformities of feet**
`EXCLUDES` *valgus deformity of foot (acquired) (736.79)*

**754.60 Talipes valgus**
Congenital valgus deformity of foot, unspecified

**754.61 Congenital pes planus**
Congenital rocker bottom flat foot
Flat foot, congenital
`EXCLUDES` *pes planus (acquired) (734)*

Unacceptable PDx     Manifestation Code     ▶◀ Revised Text     ● New Code     ▲ Revised Code Title

**754.62 Talipes calcaneovalgus**

**754.69 Other**
Talipes:          Talipes:
equinovalgus    planovalgus

✓5th **754.7 Other deformities of feet**
EXCLUDES   acquired (736.70-736.79)

**754.70 Talipes, unspecified**
Congenital deformity of foot NOS

**754.71 Talipes cavus**
Cavus foot (congenital)

**754.79 Other**
Asymmetric talipes
Talipes:
calcaneus
equinus

✓5th **754.8 Other specified nonteratogenic anomalies**

**754.81 Pectus excavatum**
Congenital funnel chest

**754.82 Pectus carinatum**
Congenital pigeon chest [breast]

**754.89 Other**   CC
Club hand (congenital)
Congenital:
deformity of chest wall
dislocation of elbow
Generalized flexion contractures of lower
limb joints, congenital
Spade-like hand (congenital)
CC Excl: 754.81-754.89

✓4th **755 Other congenital anomalies of limbs**
EXCLUDES   those deformities classifiable to 754.0-754.8

✓5th **755.0 Polydactyly**

**755.00 Polydactyly, unspecified digits**
Supernumerary digits

**755.01 Of fingers**
Accessory fingers

**755.02 Of toes**
Accessory toes

✓5th **755.1 Syndactyly**
Symphalangy          Webbing of digits

**755.10 Of multiple and unspecified sites**

**755.11 Of fingers without fusion of bone**

**755.12 Of fingers with fusion of bone**

**755.13 Of toes without fusion of bone**

**755.14 Of toes with fusion of bone**

✓5th **755.2 Reduction deformities of upper limb**

**755.20 Unspecified reduction deformity of upper
limb**
Ectromelia NOS  ⎫
Hemimelia NOS   ⎬ of upper limb

Shortening of arm, congenital

**755.21 Transverse deficiency of upper limb**
Amelia of upper limb
Congenital absence of:
fingers, all (complete or partial)
forearm, including hand and fingers
upper limb, complete
Congenital amputation of upper limb
Transverse hemimelia of upper limb

**755.22 Longitudinal deficiency of upper limb, not
elsewhere classified**
Phocomelia NOS of upper limb
Rudimentary arm

**755.23 Longitudinal deficiency, combined,
involving humerus, radius, and ulna
(complete or incomplete)**
Congenital absence of arm and forearm
(complete or incomplete) with or
without metacarpal deficiency and/or
phalangeal deficiency, incomplete
Phocomelia, complete, of upper limb

**755.24 Longitudinal deficiency, humeral, complete
or partial (with or without distal
deficiencies, incomplete)**
Congenital absence of humerus (with or
without absence of some [but not all]
distal elements)
Proximal phocomelia of upper limb

**755.25 Longitudinal deficiency, radioulnar,
complete or partial (with or without distal
deficiencies, incomplete)**
Congenital absence of radius and ulna (with
or without absence of some [but not
all] distal elements)
Distal phocomelia of upper limb

**755.26 Longitudinal deficiency, radial, complete or
partial (with or without distal deficiencies,
incomplete)**
Agenesis of radius
Congenital absence of radius (with or
without absence of some [but not all]
distal elements)

**755.27 Longitudinal deficiency, ulnar, complete or
partial (with or without distal deficiencies,
incomplete)**
Agenesis of ulna
Congenital absence of ulna (with or without
absence of some [but not all] distal
elements)

**755.28 Longitudinal deficiency, carpals or
metacarpals, complete or partial (with or
without incomplete phalangeal deficiency)**

**755.29 Longitudinal deficiency, phalanges,
complete or partial**
Absence of finger, congenital
Aphalangia of upper limb, terminal,
complete or partial
EXCLUDES   terminal deficiency of all five
digits (755.21)
transverse deficiency of
phalanges (755.21)

✓5th **755.3 Reduction deformities of lower limb**

**755.30 Unspecified reduction deformity of lower
limb**
Ectromelia NOS  ⎫
Hemimelia NOS   ⎬ of lower limb

Shortening of leg, congenital

**755.31 Transverse deficiency of lower limb**
Amelia of lower limb
Congenital absence of:
foot
leg, including foot and toes
lower limb, complete
toes, all, complete
Transverse hemimelia of lower limb

**755.32 Longitudinal deficiency of lower limb, not
elsewhere classified**
Phocomelia NOS of lower limb

**755.33 Longitudinal deficiency, combined,
involving femur, tibia, and fibula (complete
or incomplete)**
Congenital absence of thigh and (lower) leg
(complete or incomplete) with or
without metacarpal deficiency and/or
phalangeal deficiency, incomplete
Phocomelia, complete, of lower limb

N Newborn Age: 0   P Pediatric Age: 0-17   M Maternity Age: 12-55   A Adult Age: 15-124   CC CC Condition   MCC Major CC Condition   HIV HIV Related Dx

266 — Volume 1 • October 2007

© 2007 Ingenix

**755.34 Longitudinal deficiency, femoral, complete or partial (with or without distal deficiencies, incomplete)**
> Congenital absence of femur (with or without absence of some [but not all] distal elements)
> Proximal phocomelia of lower limb

**755.35 Longitudinal deficiency, tibiofibular, complete or partial (with or without distal deficiencies, incomplete)**
> Congenital absence of tibia and fibula (with or without absence of some [but not all] distal elements)
> Distal phocomelia of lower limb

**755.36 Longitudinal deficiency, tibia, complete or partial (with or without distal deficiencies, incomplete)**
> Agenesis of tibia
> Congenital absence of tibia (with or without absence of some [but not all] distal elements)

**755.37 Longitudinal deficiency, fibular, complete or partial (with or without distal deficiencies, incomplete)**
> Agenesis of fibula
> Congenital absence of fibula (with or without absence of some [but not all] distal elements)

**755.38 Longitudinal deficiency, tarsals or metatarsals, complete or partial (with or without incomplete phalangeal deficiency)**

**755.39 Longitudinal deficiency, phalanges, complete or partial**
> Absence of toe, congenital
> Aphalangia of lower limb, terminal, complete or partial
> > **EXCLUDES**  terminal deficiency of all five digits (755.31)
> > transverse deficiency of phalanges (755.31)

**755.4 Reduction deformities, unspecified limb**
> Absence, congenital (complete or partial) of limb NOS
> Amelia
> Ectromelia  } of unspecified limb
> Hemimelia
> Phocomelia

√5th **755.5 Other anomalies of upper limb, including shoulder girdle**

**755.50 Unspecified anomaly of upper limb**

**755.51 Congenital deformity of clavicle**

**755.52 Congenital elevation of scapula**
> Sprengel's deformity

**755.53 Radioulnar synostosis**
> DEF: Osseous adhesion of radius and ulna.

**755.54 Madelung's deformity**
> DEF: Distal ulnar overgrowth or radial shortening; also called carpus curvus.

**755.55 Acrocephalosyndactyly**  MCC
> Apert's syndrome
> **CC Excl:** 755.50, 755.55, 755.59
>
> DEF: Premature cranial suture fusion (craniostenosis); marked by cone-shaped or pointed (acrocephaly) head and webbing of the fingers (syndactyly); it is very similar to craniofacial dysostosis.

**755.56 Accessory carpal bones**

**755.57 Macrodactylia (fingers)**
> DEF: Abnormally large fingers, toes.

**755.58 Cleft hand, congenital**
> Lobster-claw hand
> DEF: Extended separation between fingers into metacarpus; also may refer to large fingers and absent middle fingers of hand.

**755.59 Other**
> Cleidocranial dysostosis
> Cubitus:
> > valgus, congenital
> > varus, congenital
> > **EXCLUDES**  club hand (congenital) (754.89)
> > congenital dislocation of elbow (754.89)

√5th **755.6 Other anomalies of lower limb, including pelvic girdle**

**755.60 Unspecified anomaly of lower limb**

**755.61 Coxa valga, congenital**
> DEF: Abnormally wide angle between the neck and shaft of the femur.

**755.62 Coxa vara, congenital**
> DEF: Diminished angle between neck and shaft of femur.

**755.63 Other congenital deformity of hip (joint)**
> Congenital anteversion of femur (neck)
> > **EXCLUDES**  congenital dislocation of hip (754.30-754.35)
>
> **AHA:** 1Q, '94, 15; S-O, '84, 15

**755.64 Congenital deformity of knee (joint)**
> Congenital:
> > absence of patella
> > genu valgum [knock-knee]
> > genu varum [bowleg]
> Rudimentary patella

**755.65 Macrodactylia of toes**
> DEF: Abnormally large toes.

**755.66 Other anomalies of toes**
> Congenital:        Congenital:
> > hallux valgus    hammer toe
> > hallux varus

**755.67 Anomalies of foot, not elsewhere classified**
> Astragaloscaphoid synostosis
> Calcaneonavicular bar
> Coalition of calcaneus
> Talonavicular synostosis
> Tarsal coalitions

**755.69 Other**
> Congenital:
> > angulation of tibia
> > deformity (of):
> > > ankle (joint)
> > > sacroiliac (joint)
> > fusion of sacroiliac joint

**755.8 Other specified anomalies of unspecified limb**

**755.9 Unspecified anomaly of unspecified limb**
> Congenital:
> > anomaly NOS  } of unspecified limb
> > deformity NOS
> > **EXCLUDES**  reduction deformity of unspecified limb (755.4)

**Congenital Anomalies**

**756–756.79**

√4th **756 Other congenital musculoskeletal anomalies**

> EXCLUDES   *those deformities classifiable to 754.0-754.8*

**756.0 Anomalies of skull and face bones**

| | |
|---|---|
| Absence of skull bones | Imperfect fusion of skull |
| Acrocephaly | Oxycephaly |
| Congenital deformity | Platybasia |
| of forehead | Premature closure of |
| Craniosynostosis | cranial sutures |
| Crouzon's disease | Tower skull |
| Hypertelorism | Trigonocephaly |

> EXCLUDES   *acrocephalosyndactyly [Apert's syndrome] (755.55)*
> *dentofacial anomalies (524.0-524.9)*
> *skull defects associated with brain anomalies, such as:*
> *anencephalus (740.0)*
> *encephalocele (742.0)*
> *hydrocephalus (742.3)*
> *microcephalus (742.1)*

AHA: 3Q, '98, 9; 3Q, '96, 15

√5th **756.1 Anomalies of spine**

**756.10 Anomaly of spine, unspecified**

**756.11 Spondylolysis, lumbosacral region**
Prespondylolisthesis (lumbosacral)

DEF: Bilateral or unilateral defect through the pars interarticularis of a vertebra causes spondylolisthesis.

**756.12 Spondylolisthesis**

DEF: Downward slipping of lumbar vertebra over next vertebra; usually related to pelvic deformity.

**756.13 Absence of vertebra, congenital**    CC

CC Excl: 756.10-756.19

**756.14 Hemivertebra**

DEF: Incomplete development of one side of a vertebra.

**756.15 Fusion of spine [vertebra], congenital**

**756.16 Klippel-Feil syndrome**

DEF: Short, wide neck; limits range of motion due to abnormal number of cervical vertebra or fused hemivertebrae.

**756.17 Spina bifida occulta**

> EXCLUDES   *spina bifida (aperta) (741.0-741.9)*

DEF: Spina bifida marked by a bony spinal canal defect without a protrusion of the cord or meninges; it is diagnosed by radiography and has no symptoms.

**756.19 Other**
Platyspondylia     Supernumerary vertebra

**756.2 Cervical rib**
Supernumerary rib in the cervical region

DEF: Costa cervicalis: extra rib attached to cervical vertebra.

**756.3 Other anomalies of ribs and sternum**    CC

| | |
|---|---|
| Congenital absence of: | Congenital: |
| rib | fissure of sternum |
| sternum | fusion of ribs |
| | Sternum bifidum |

> EXCLUDES   *nonteratogenic deformity of chest wall (754.81-754.89)*

CC Excl: 756.2-756.3

**756.4 Chondrodystrophy**

| | |
|---|---|
| Achondroplasia | Enchondromatosis |
| Chondrodystrophia (fetalis) | Ollier's disease |
| Dyschondroplasia | |

> EXCLUDES ▶ *congenital myotonic chondrodystrophy (359.23)*◀
> *lipochondrodystrophy [Hurler's syndrome] (277.5)*
> *Morquio's disease (277.5)*

AHA: 2Q, '02, 16; S-O, '87, 10

DEF: Abnormal development of cartilage.

√5th **756.5 Osteodystrophies**

**756.50 Osteodystrophy, unspecified**

**756.51 Osteogenesis imperfecta**    CC
Fragilitas ossium     Osteopsathyrosis

CC Excl: 756.50-756.59

DEF: A collagen disorder commonly characterized by brittle, osteoporotic, easily fractured bones, hypermobility of joints, blue sclerae, and a tendency to hemorrhage.

**756.52 Osteopetrosis**    CC

CC Excl: See code: 756.51

DEF: Abnormally dense bone, optic atrophy, hepatosplenomegaly, deafness; sclerosing depletes bone marrow and nerve foramina of skull; often fatal.

**756.53 Osteopoikilosis**

DEF: Multiple sclerotic foci on ends of long bones, stippling in round, flat bones; identified by x-ray.

**756.54 Polyostotic fibrous dysplasia of bone**

DEF: Fibrous tissue displaces bone results in segmented ragged-edge café-au-lait spots; occurs in girls of early puberty.

**756.55 Chondroectodermal dysplasia**
Ellis-van Creveld syndrome

DEF: Inadequate enchondral bone formation; impaired development of hair and teeth, polydactyly, and cardiac septum defects.

**756.56 Multiple epiphyseal dysplasia**

**756.59 Other**
Albright (-McCune)-Sternberg syndrome

**756.6 Anomalies of diaphragm**    MCC

| | |
|---|---|
| Absence of diaphragm | Eventration of diaphragm |
| Congenital hernia: | |
| diaphragmatic | |
| foramen of Morgagni | |

> EXCLUDES   *congenital hiatus hernia (750.6)*

CC Excl: 750.6, 756.6

√5th **756.7 Anomalies of abdominal wall**

**756.70 Anomaly of abdominal wall, unspecified**    MCC

CC Excl: 756.70-756.79

**756.71 Prune belly syndrome**    MCC
Eagle-Barrett syndrome
Prolapse of bladder mucosa

CC Excl: See code: 756.70

AHA: 4Q, '97, 44

DEF: Prune belly syndrome: absence of lower rectus abdominis muscle and lower and medial oblique muscles; results in dilated bladder and ureters, dysplastic kidneys and hydronephrosis; more common in male infants with undescended testicles.

**756.79 Other congenital anomalies of abdominal wall**    MCC

| | |
|---|---|
| Exomphalos | Omphalocele |
| Gastroschisis | |

> EXCLUDES   *umbilical hernia (551-553 with .1)*

CC Excl: See code: 756.70

DEF: Exomphalos: umbilical hernia prominent navel.

DEF: Gastroschisis: fissure of abdominal wall, results in protruding small or large intestine.

DEF: Omphalocele: hernia of umbilicus due to impaired abdominal wall; results in membrane-covered intestine protruding through peritoneum and amnion.

N Newborn Age: 0    P Pediatric Age: 0-17    M Maternity Age: 12-55    A Adult Age: 15-124    CC CC Condition    MCC Major CC Condition    HIV HIV Related Dx

268 — Volume 1 • October 2007

© 2007 Ingenix

√5ᵗʰ **756.8 Other specified anomalies of muscle, tendon, fascia, and connective tissue**

**756.81 Absence of muscle and tendon**
Absence of muscle (pectoral)

**756.82 Accessory muscle**

**756.83 Ehlers-Danlos syndrome**    CC
CC Excl: 756.83-756.89

DEF: Danlos syndrome: connective tissue disorder causes hyperextended skin and joints; results in fragile blood vessels with bleeding, poor wound healing and subcutaneous pseudotumors.

**756.89 Other**
Amyotrophia congenita
Congenital shortening of tendon
AHA: 3Q, '99, 16

**756.9 Other and unspecified anomalies of musculoskeletal system**
Congenital:
  anomaly NOS } of musculoskeletal system,
  deformity NOS }    not elsewhere classified

√4ᵗʰ **757 Congenital anomalies of the integument**
INCLUDES   anomalies of skin, subcutaneous tissue, hair, nails, and breast
EXCLUDES   hemangioma (228.00-228.09)
     pigmented nevus (216.0-216.9)

**757.0 Hereditary edema of legs**
Congenital lymphedema
Hereditary trophedema
Milroy's disease

**757.1 Ichthyosis congenita**
Congenital ichthyosis
Harlequin fetus
Ichthyosiform erythroderma
DEF: Overproduction of skin cells causes scaling of skin; may result in stillborn fetus or death soon after birth.

**757.2 Dermatoglyphic anomalies**
Abnormal palmar creases
DEF: Abnormal skin-line patterns of fingers, palms, toes and soles; initial finding of possible chromosomal abnormalities.

√5ᵗʰ **757.3 Other specified anomalies of skin**

**757.31 Congenital ectodermal dysplasia**
DEF: Tissues and structures originate in embryonic ectoderm; includes anhidrotic and hidrotic ectodermal dysplasia and EEC syndrome.

**757.32 Vascular hamartomas**
Birthmarks      Strawberry nevus
Port-wine stain
DEF: Benign tumor of blood vessels; due to malformed angioblastic tissues.

**757.33 Congenital pigmentary anomalies of skin**
Congenital poikiloderma
Urticaria pigmentosa
Xeroderma pigmentosum
EXCLUDES   albinism (270.2)

**757.39 Other**
Accessory skin tags, congenital
Congenital scar
Epidermolysis bullosa
Keratoderma (congenital)
EXCLUDES   pilonidal cyst (685.0-685.1)

**757.4 Specified anomalies of hair**
Congenital:      Congenital:
  alopecia        hypertrichosis
  atrichosis       monilethrix
  beaded hair     Persistent lanugo

**757.5 Specified anomalies of nails**
Anonychia      Congenital:
Congenital:     leukonychia
  clubnail       onychauxis
  koilonychia     pachyonychia

**757.6 Specified anomalies of breast**
Absent
Accessory      } breast or nipple
Supernumerary }

Hypoplasia of breast
EXCLUDES   absence of pectoral muscle (756.81)

**757.8 Other specified anomalies of the integument**

**757.9 Unspecified anomaly of the integument**
Congenital:
  anomaly NOS } of integument
  deformity NOS }

√4ᵗʰ **758 Chromosomal anomalies**
INCLUDES   syndromes associated with anomalies in the number and form of chromosomes
Use additional codes for conditions associated with the chromosomal anomalies

**758.0 Down's syndrome**
Mongolism      Trisomy:
Translocation Down's   21 or 22
  syndrome       G

**758.1 Patau's syndrome**    CC
Trisomy:      Trisomy:
  13          $D_1$
CC Excl: 758.0-758.9

DEF: Trisomy of 13th chromosome; characteristic failure to thrive, severe mental impairment, seizures, abnormal eyes, low-set ears and sloped forehead.

**758.2 Edwards' syndrome**    CC
Trisomy:      Trisomy:
  18          $E_3$
CC Excl: See code: 758.1

DEF: Trisomy of 18th chromosome; characteristic mental and physical impairments; mainly affects females.

√5ᵗʰ **758.3 Autosomal deletion syndromes**

**758.31 Cri-du-chat syndrome**    CC
Deletion 5p
CC Excl: 758.0-758.2, 758.32-758.9

DEF: Hereditary congenital syndrome caused by a microdeletion of short arm of chromosome 5; characterized by catlike cry in newborn, microencephaly, severe mental deficiency, and hypertelorism.

**758.32 Velo-cardio-facial syndrome**    MCC
Deletion 22q11.2
CC Excl: 758.0-758.31, 758.33-758.9

DEF: Microdeletion syndrome affecting multiple organs; characteristic cleft palate, heart defects, elongated face with almond-shaped eyes, wide nose, small ears, weak immune systems, weak musculature, hypothyroidism, short stature, and scoliosis; deletion at q11.2 on the long arm of the chromosome 22.

**758.33 Other microdeletions**    CC
Miller-Dieker syndrome
Smith-Magenis syndrome
CC Excl: 758.0-758.32, 758.39-758.9

DEF: Miller-Dieker syndrome: deletion from the short arm of chromosome 17; characteristic mental retardation, speech and motor development delays, neurological complications, and multiple abnormalities affecting the kidneys, heart, gastrointestinal tract, and other organ; death in infancy or early childhood.
DEF: Smith-Magenis syndrome: deletion in a certain area of chromosome 17 that results in craniofacial changes, speech delay, hoarse voice, hearing loss in many, and behavioral problems, such as self-destructive head banging, wrist biting, and tearing at nails.

---

√4ᵗʰ √5ᵗʰ Additional Digit Required      Unacceptable PDx      Manifestation Code      ►◄ Revised Text      ● New Code      ▲ Revised Code Title

**Congenital Anomalies**

**758.39–759.9**

**758.39 Other autosomal deletions** `CC`
CC Excl: 758.0-758.33, 758.4-758.9

**758.4 Balanced autosomal translocation in normal individual**

**758.5 Other conditions due to autosomal anomalies**
Accessory autosomes NEC

**758.6 Gonadal dysgenesis**
Ovarian dysgenesis     XO syndrome
Turner's syndrome
*EXCLUDES*   pure gonadal dysgenesis (752.7)

**758.7 Klinefelter's syndrome** ♂
XXY syndrome

DEF: Impaired embryonic development of seminiferous tubes; results in small testes, azoospermia, infertility and enlarged mammary glands.

√5ᵗʰ **758.8 Other conditions due to chromosome anomalies**
**758.81 Other conditions due to sex chromosome anomalies**
**758.89 Other**

**758.9 Conditions due to anomaly of unspecified chromosome**

√4ᵗʰ **759 Other and unspecified congenital anomalies**

**759.0 Anomalies of spleen** `CC`
Aberrant
Absent  } spleen
Accessory
Congenital splenomegaly
Ectopic spleen
Lobulation of spleen
CC Excl: 759.0, 759.9

**759.1 Anomalies of adrenal gland**
Aberrant
Absent  } adrenal gland
Accessory
*EXCLUDES*   adrenogenital disorders (255.2)
congenital disorders of steroid metabolism (255.2)

**759.2 Anomalies of other endocrine glands**
Absent parathyroid gland    Persistent thyroglossal
Accessory thyroid gland      or thyrolingual duct
Thyroglossal (duct) cyst
*EXCLUDES*   congenital:
goiter (246.1)
hypothyroidism (243)

**759.3 Situs inversus** `CC`
Situs inversus or transversus:   Transposition of
abdominalis              viscera:
thoracis               abdominal
thoracic
*EXCLUDES*   dextrocardia without mention of complete transposition (746.87)
CC Excl: 759.3, 759.7, 759.9

DEF: Laterally transposed thoracic and abdominal viscera.

**759.4 Conjoined twins** `MCC`
Craniopagus      Thoracopagus
Dicephalus       Xiphopagus
Pygopagus
CC Excl: 759.4, 759.7, 759.9

**759.5 Tuberous sclerosis** `CC`
Bourneville's disease    Epiloia
CC Excl: 759.5-759.7, 759.9

DEF: Hamartomas of brain, retina and viscera, impaired mental ability, seizures and adenoma sebaceum.

**759.6 Other hamartoses, not elsewhere classified** `CC`
Syndrome:          Syndrome:
Peutz-Jeghers      von Hippel-Lindau
Sturge-Weber (-Dimitri)
*EXCLUDES*   neurofibromatosis (237.7)
CC Excl: 759.6, 759.9

AHA: 3Q, '92, 12
DEF: Peutz-Jeghers: hereditary syndrome characterized by hamartomas of small intestine.
DEF: Sturge-Weber: congenital syndrome characterized by unilateral port-wine stain over trigeminal nerve, underlying meninges and cerebral cortex.
DEF: von Hipple-Lindau: hereditary syndrome of congenital angiomatosis of the retina and cerebellum.

**759.7 Multiple congenital anomalies, so described** `CC`
Congenital:           Congenital:
anomaly, multiple NOS    deformity, multiple
NOS
CC Excl: See code: 759.3

√5ᵗʰ **759.8 Other specified anomalies**
AHA: S-O, '87, 9; S-O, '85, 11
**759.81 Prader-Willi syndrome** `CC`
CC Excl: 759.6-759.9

**759.82 Marfan syndrome** `CC`
CC Excl: See code: 759.81

AHA: 3Q, '93, 11
**759.83 Fragile X syndrome**
AHA: 4Q, '94, 41

**759.89 Other** `CC`
Congenital malformation syndromes affecting multiple systems, not elsewhere classified
Laurence-Moon-Biedl syndrome
CC Excl: 759.81-759.89

AHA: 3Q, '06, 21; 2Q, '05, 17; 2Q, '04, 12; 1Q, '01, 3; 3Q, '99, 17, 18; 3Q, '98, 8

**759.9 Congenital anomaly, unspecified**

---

N Newborn Age: 0     P Pediatric Age: 0-17     M Maternity Age: 12-55     A Adult Age: 15-124     `CC` CC Condition     `MCC` Major CC Condition     `HIV` HIV Related Dx

## 15. CERTAIN CONDITIONS ORIGINATING IN THE PERINATAL PERIOD (760-779)

INCLUDES    conditions which have their origin in the perinatal period, before birth through the first 28 days after birth, even though death or morbidity occurs later
Use additional code(s) to further specify condition

### MATERNAL CAUSES OF PERINATAL MORBIDITY AND MORTALITY (760-763)

AHA: 2Q, '89, 14; 3Q, '90, 5

✓4th **760 Fetus or newborn affected by maternal conditions which may be unrelated to present pregnancy**

INCLUDES    the listed maternal conditions only when specified as a cause of mortality or morbidity of the fetus or newborn

EXCLUDES    *maternal endocrine and metabolic disorders affecting fetus or newborn (775.0-775.9)*

AHA: 1Q, '94, 8; 2Q, '92, 12; N-D, '84, 11

**760.0 Maternal hypertensive disorders**
Fetus or newborn affected by maternal conditions classifiable to 642

**760.1 Maternal renal and urinary tract diseases**
Fetus or newborn affected by maternal conditions classifiable to 580-599

**760.2 Maternal infections**
Fetus or newborn affected by maternal infectious disease classifiable to 001-136 and 487, but fetus or newborn not manifesting that disease

EXCLUDES    *congenital infectious diseases (771.0-771.8)*
*maternal genital tract and other localized infections (760.8)*

**760.3 Other chronic maternal circulatory and respiratory diseases**
Fetus or newborn affected by chronic maternal conditions classifiable to 390-459, 490-519, 745-748

**760.4 Maternal nutritional disorders**
Fetus or newborn affected by:
maternal disorders classifiable to 260-269
maternal malnutrition NOS

EXCLUDES    *fetal malnutrition (764.10-764.29)*

**760.5 Maternal injury**
Fetus or newborn affected by maternal conditions classifiable to 800-995

**760.6 Surgical operation on mother**

EXCLUDES    *cesarean section for present delivery (763.4)*
*damage to placenta from amniocentesis, cesarean section, or surgical induction (762.1)*
*previous surgery to uterus or pelvic organs (763.89)*

✓5th **760.7 Noxious influences affecting fetus or newborn via placenta or breast milk**
Fetus or newborn affected by noxious substance transmitted via placenta or breast milk

EXCLUDES    *anesthetic and analgesic drugs administered during labor and delivery (763.5)*
*drug withdrawal syndrome in newborn (779.5)*

AHA: 3Q, '91, 21

**760.70 Unspecified noxious substance**
Fetus or newborn affected by:
Drug NEC

**760.71 Alcohol**
Fetal alcohol syndrome

**760.72 Narcotics**

**760.73 Hallucinogenic agents**

**760.74 Anti-infectives**
Antibiotics
Antifungals

**760.75 Cocaine**
AHA: 3Q, '94, 6; 2Q, '92, 12; 4Q, '91, 26

**760.76 Diethylstilbestrol [DES]**
AHA: 4Q, '94, 45

**760.77 Anticonvulsants**    N
Carbamazepine    Phenytoin
Phenobarbital    Valproic acid
AHA: 4Q, '05, 82

**760.78 Antimetabolic agents**    N
Methotrexate    Statins
Retinoic acid
AHA: 4Q, '05, 82-83

**760.79 Other**
Fetus or newborn affected by:
immune sera
medicinal agents    transmitted via placenta
NEC    or breast
toxic substance NEC

**760.8 Other specified maternal conditions affecting fetus or newborn**
Maternal genital tract and other localized infection affecting fetus or newborn, but fetus or newborn not manifesting that disease

EXCLUDES    *maternal urinary tract infection affecting fetus or newborn (760.1)*

**760.9 Unspecified maternal condition affecting fetus or newborn**

✓4th **761 Fetus or newborn affected by maternal complications of pregnancy**

INCLUDES    the listed maternal conditions only when specified as a cause of mortality or morbidity of the fetus or newborn

**761.0 Incompetent cervix**
DEF: Inadequate functioning of uterine cervix.

**761.1 Premature rupture of membranes**

**761.2 Oligohydramnios**
EXCLUDES    *that due to premature rupture of membranes (761.1)*
DEF: Deficient amniotic fluid.

**761.3 Polyhydramnios**
Hydramnios (acute) (chronic)
DEF: Excess amniotic fluid.

**761.4 Ectopic pregnancy**
Pregnancy:    Pregnancy:
abdominal    tubal
intraperitoneal

**761.5 Multiple pregnancy**
Triplet (pregnancy)    Twin (pregnancy)

**761.6 Maternal death**

**761.7 Malpresentation before labor**
Breech presentation
External version
Oblique lie    before labor
Transverse lie
Unstable lie

**761.8 Other specified maternal complications of pregnancy affecting fetus or newborn**
Spontaneous abortion, fetus

**761.9 Unspecified maternal complication of pregnancy affecting fetus or newborn**

**Conditions in the Perinatal Period**

**762–763.9**

✓4ᵗʰ **762 Fetus or newborn affected by complications of placenta, cord, and membranes**

> INCLUDES the listed maternal conditions only when specified as a cause of mortality or morbidity in the fetus or newborn

**AHA:** 1Q, '94, 8

**762.0 Placenta previa** N

> DEF: Placenta developed in lower segment of uterus; causes hemorrhaging in last trimester.

**762.1 Other forms of placental separation and hemorrhage** N

> Abruptio placentae
> Antepartum hemorrhage
> Damage to placenta from amniocentesis, cesarean section, or surgical induction
> Maternal blood loss
> Premature separation of placenta
> Rupture of marginal sinus

**762.2 Other and unspecified morphological and functional abnormalities of placenta** N

> Placental:
>     dysfunction
>     infarction
>     insufficiency

**762.3 Placental transfusion syndromes** N

> Placental and cord abnormality resulting in twin-to-twin or other transplacental transfusion
> Use additional code to indicate resultant condition in fetus or newborn:
>     fetal blood loss (772.0)
>     polycythemia neonatorum (776.4)

**762.4 Prolapsed cord** N

> Cord presentation

**762.5 Other compression of umbilical cord** N

> Cord around neck
> Entanglement of cord
> Knot in cord
> Torsion of cord

**AHA:** 2Q, '03, 9

**762.6 Other and unspecified conditions of umbilical cord** N

> Short cord
> Thrombosis ⎤
> Varices     ⎬ of umbilical cord
> Velamentous insertion ⎟
> Vasa previa ⎦

> EXCLUDES infection of umbilical cord (771.4)
> single umbilical artery (747.5)

**762.7 Chorioamnionitis** N

> Amnionitis
> Membranitis
> Placentitis

> DEF: Inflamed fetal membrane.

**762.8 Other specified abnormalities of chorion and amnion** N

**762.9 Unspecified abnormality of chorion and amnion** N

✓4ᵗʰ **763 Fetus or newborn affected by other complications of labor and delivery**

> INCLUDES the listed conditions only when specified as a cause of mortality or morbidity in the fetus or newborn

**AHA:** 1Q, '94, 8

**763.0 Breech delivery and extraction** N

**763.1 Other malpresentation, malposition, and disproportion during labor and delivery** N

> Fetus or newborn affected by:
>     abnormality of bony pelvis
>     contracted pelvis
>     persistent occipitoposterior position
>     shoulder presentation
>     transverse lie
>     conditions classifiable to 652, 653, and 660

**763.2 Forceps delivery** N

> Fetus or newborn affected by forceps extraction

**763.3 Delivery by vacuum extractor** N

**763.4 Cesarean delivery** N

> EXCLUDES placental separation or hemorrhage from cesarean section (762.1)

**763.5 Maternal anesthesia and analgesia**

> Reactions and intoxications from maternal opiates and tranquilizers during labor and delivery

> EXCLUDES drug withdrawal syndrome in newborn (779.5)

**763.6 Precipitate delivery** N

> Rapid second stage

**763.7 Abnormal uterine contractions** N

> Fetus or newborn affected by:
>     contraction ring
>     hypertonic labor
>     hypotonic uterine dysfunction
>     uterine inertia or dysfunction
>     conditions classifiable to 661, except 661.3

✓5ᵗʰ **763.8 Other specified complications of labor and delivery affecting fetus or newborn**

**AHA:** 4Q, '98, 46

**763.81 Abnormality in fetal heart rate or rhythm before the onset of labor** N

**763.82 Abnormality in fetal heart rate or rhythm during labor** N

> **AHA:** 4Q, '98, 46

**763.83 Abnormality in fetal heart rate or rhythm, unspecified as to time of onset** N

**763.84 Meconium passage during delivery** N

> EXCLUDES meconium aspiration (770.11, 770.12)
> meconium staining (779.84)

> **AHA:** 4Q, '05, 83

> DEF: Fetal intestinal activity that increases in response to a distressed state during delivery; anal sphincter relaxes, and meconium is passed into the amniotic fluid.

**763.89 Other specified complications of labor and delivery affecting fetus or newborn** N

> Fetus or newborn affected by:
>     abnormality of maternal soft tissues
>     destructive operation on live fetus to facilitate delivery
>     induction of labor (medical)
>     previous surgery to uterus or pelvic organs
>     other conditions classifiable to 650-669
>     other procedures used in labor and delivery

**763.9 Unspecified complication of labor and delivery affecting fetus or newborn** N

---

N Newborn Age: 0    P Pediatric Age: 0-17    M Maternity Age: 12-55    A Adult Age: 15-124    CC CC Condition    MCC Major CC Condition    HIV HIV Related Dx

272 — Volume 1 • October 2007

© 2007 Ingenix

## OTHER CONDITIONS ORIGINATING IN THE PERINATAL PERIOD (764-779)

The following fifth-digit subclassification is for use with category 764 and codes 765.0-765.1 to denote birthweight:

   0   unspecified [weight]
   1   less than 500 grams
   2   500-749 grams
   3   750-999 grams
   4   1,000-1,249 grams
   5   1,250-1,499 grams
   6   1,500-1,749 grams
   7   1,750-1,999 grams
   8   2,000-2,499 grams
   9   2,500 grams and over

✓4th **764 Slow fetal growth and fetal malnutrition**
    AHA: 3Q, '04, 4; 4Q, '02, 63; 1Q, "94, 8; 2Q, '91, 19; 2Q, '89, 15

✓5th **764.0 "Light-for-dates" without mention of fetal malnutrition**
    Infants underweight for gestational age
    "Small-for-dates"

✓5th **764.1 "Light-for-dates" with signs of fetal malnutrition**
    Infants "light-for-dates" classifiable to 764.0, who in addition show signs of fetal malnutrition, such as dry peeling skin and loss of subcutaneous tissue

✓5th **764.2 Fetal malnutrition without mention of "light-for-dates"**
    Infants, not underweight for gestational age, showing signs of fetal malnutrition, such as dry peeling skin and loss of subcutaneous tissue
    Intrauterine malnutrition

✓5th **764.9 Fetal growth retardation, unspecified**
    Intrauterine growth retardation
    AHA: For code 764.97: 1Q, '97, 6

✓4th **765 Disorders relating to short gestation and low birthweight**
    **INCLUDES**   the listed conditions, without further specification, as causes of mortality, morbidity, or additional care, in fetus or newborn
    AHA: 1Q, '97, 6; 1Q, '94, 8; 2Q, '91, 19; 2Q, '89, 15

✓5th **765.0 Extreme immaturity**
    Note: Usually implies a birthweight of less than 1000 grams.
    Use additional code for weeks of gestation (765.20-765.29)
    AHA: 3Q, '04, 4; 4Q, '02, 63; For code 765.03: 4Q, '01, 51

✓5th **765.1 Other preterm infants**
    Note: Usually implies a birthweight of 1000-2499 grams.
    Prematurity NOS
    Prematurity or small size, not classifiable to 765.0 or as "light-for-dates" in 764
    Use additional code for weeks of gestation (765.20-765.29)
    AHA: 3Q, '04, 4; 4Q, '02, 63; For code 765.10: 1Q, '94, 14; For code 765.17: 1Q, '97, 6; For code 765.18: 4Q, '02, 64

✓5th **765.2 Weeks of gestation**
    AHA: 3Q, '04, 4; 4Q, '02, 63

    **765.20 Unspecified weeks of gestation**
    **765.21 Less than 24 completed weeks of gestation**
    **765.22 24 completed weeks of gestation**
    **765.23 25-26 completed weeks of gestation**
    **765.24 27-28 completed weeks of gestation**
    **765.25 29-30 completed weeks of gestation**
    **765.26 31-32 completed weeks of gestation**
    **765.27 33-34 completed weeks of gestation**

    **765.28 35-36 completed weeks of gestation**
    AHA: 4Q, '02, 64

    **765.29 37 or more completed weeks of gestation**

✓4th **766 Disorders relating to long gestation and high birthweight**
    **INCLUDES**   the listed conditions, without further specification, as causes of mortality, morbidity, or additional care, in fetus or newborn

    **766.0 Exceptionally large baby**
    Note: Usually implies a birthweight of 4500 grams or more.

    **766.1 Other "heavy-for-dates" infants**
    Other fetus or infant "heavy-" or "large-for-dates" regardless of period of gestation

✓5th **766.2 Late infant, not "heavy-for-dates"**
    AHA: 2Q, '06, 12

    **766.21 Post-term infant**
    Infant with gestation period over 40 completed weeks to 42 completed weeks
    AHA: 4Q, '03, 69

    **766.22 Prolonged gestation of infant**
    Infant with gestation period over 42 completed weeks
    Postmaturity NOS

✓4th **767 Birth trauma**
    **767.0 Subdural and cerebral hemorrhage**   MCC
    Subdural and cerebral hemorrhage, whether described as due to birth trauma or to intrapartum anoxia or hypoxia
    Subdural hematoma (localized)
    Tentorial tear
    Use additional code to identify cause
    **EXCLUDES**   intraventricular hemorrhage (772.10-772.14)
          subarachnoid hemorrhage (772.2)
    CC Excl: 767.0, 767.8-767.9, 779.81-779.84, 779.89

✓5th **767.1 Injuries to scalp**
    AHA: 4Q, '03, 69

    **767.11 Epicranial subaponeurotic hemorrhage (massive)**   CC
    Subgaleal hemorrhage
    CC Excl: 767.0-767.11, 767.8-767.9, 779.81-779.84, 779.89

    DEF: A hemorrhage that occurs within the space between the galea aponeurotica, or epicranial aponeurosis, a thin tendinous structure that is attached to the skull laterally and provides an insertion site for the occipitalis posteriorly and the frontalis muscle anteriorly, and the periosteum of the skull.

    **767.19 Other injuries to scalp**
    Caput succedaneum
    Cephalhematoma
    Chignon (from vacuum extraction)

    **767.2 Fracture of clavicle**

**Epicranial Subaponeurosis**

 ✓4th / ✓5th Additional Digit Required     Unacceptable PDx     Manifestation Code     ▶◀ Revised Text     ● New Code     ▲ Revised Code Title

© 2007 Ingenix         October 2007 • Volume 1 — 273

**Conditions in the Perinatal Period**

**767.3–770.15**

**767.3 Other injuries to skeleton**   N
Fracture of:
long bones
skull
> **EXCLUDES** *congenital dislocation of hip*
> *(754.30-754.35)*
> *fracture of spine, congenital (767.4)*

**767.4 Injury to spine and spinal cord**   N
Dislocation ⎫
Fracture ⎬ of spine or spinal cord
Laceration ⎪ due to birth trauma
Rupture ⎭

**767.5 Facial nerve injury**   N
Facial palsy

**767.6 Injury to brachial plexus**   N
Palsy or paralysis:
brachial
Erb (-Duchenne)
Klumpke (-Déjérine)

**767.7 Other cranial and peripheral nerve injuries**   N
Phrenic nerve paralysis

**767.8 Other specified birth trauma**   N
Eye damage     Rupture of:
Hematoma of:     liver
liver (subcapsular)     spleen
testes     Scalpel wound
vulva     Traumatic glaucoma
> **EXCLUDES** *hemorrhage classifiable to 772.0-772.9*

**767.9 Birth trauma, unspecified**   N
Birth injury NOS

✓4ᵗʰ **768 Intrauterine hypoxia and birth asphyxia**
Use only when associated with newborn morbidity
classifiable elsewhere
> **EXCLUDES** *acidemia NOS of newborn (775.81)*
> *acidosis NOS of newborn (775.81)*
> *cerebral ischemia NOS (779.2)*
> *hypoxia NOS of newborn (770.88)*
> *mixed metabolic and respiratory acidosis of*
> *newborn (775.81)*
> *respiratory arrest of newborn (770.87)*

**AHA:** 4Q, '92, 20

**DEF:** Oxygen intake insufficiency due to interrupted placental circulation or premature separation of placenta.

**768.0 Fetal death from asphyxia or anoxia before**   N
**onset of labor or at unspecified time**

**768.1 Fetal death from asphyxia or anoxia during**   N
**labor**

**768.2 Fetal distress before onset of labor, in liveborn**   N
**infant**
Fetal metabolic acidemia before onset of labor, in liveborn infant

**768.3 Fetal distress first noted during labor and**   N
**delivery, in liveborn infant**
Fetal metabolic acidemia first noted during labor and delivery, in liveborn infant

**768.4 Fetal distress, unspecified as to time of onset,**   N
**in liveborn infant**
Fetal metabolic acidemia unspecified as to time of onset, in liveborn infant
**AHA:** N-D, '86, 10

**768.5 Severe birth asphyxia**   MCC N
Birth asphyxia with neurologic involvement
> **EXCLUDES** *hypoxic-ischemic encephalopathy [HIE]*
> *(768.7)*

**CC Excl:** 768.5-768.6, 768.9-770.86, 770.89-770.9, 779.81-779.84, 779.89

**AHA:** N-D, '86, 3

**768.6 Mild or moderate birth asphyxia**   N
Birth asphyxia (without mention of neurologic involvement)
> **EXCLUDES** *hypoxic-ischemic encephalopathy [HIE]*
> *(768.7)*

**AHA:** N-D, '86, 3

**768.7 Hypoxic-ischemic encephalopathy [HIE]**   MCC N
**CC Excl:** 768.5-768.6, 768.9

**AHA:** 4Q, '06, 104

**768.9 Unspecified birth asphyxia in liveborn infant**   N
Anoxia ⎫
Asphyxia ⎬ NOS, in liveborn infant

**769 Respiratory distress syndrome**   MCC N
Cardiorespiratory distress syndrome of newborn
Hyaline membrane disease (pulmonary)
Idiopathic respiratory distress syndrome [IRDS or RDS] of newborn
Pulmonary hypoperfusion syndrome
> **EXCLUDES** *transient tachypnea of newborn (770.6)*

**CC Excl:** 768.5-768.6, 768.9-770.86, 770.89-770.9, 779.81-779.84, 779.89

**AHA:** 1Q, '89, 10; N-D, '86, 6

**DEF:** Severe chest contractions upon air intake and expiratory grunting; infant appears blue due to oxygen deficiency and has rapid respiratory rate; formerly called hyaline membrane disease.

✓4ᵗʰ **770 Other respiratory conditions of fetus and newborn**
**770.0 Congenital pneumonia**   MCC N
Infective pneumonia acquired prenatally
> **EXCLUDES** *pneumonia from infection acquired*
> *after birth (480.0-486)*

**CC Excl:** 768.5-768.6, 768.9-770.86, 770.89-770.9, 779.81-779.84, 779.89

**AHA:** 1Q, '05, 10

✓5ᵗʰ **770.1 Fetal and newborn aspiration**
> **EXCLUDES** *aspiration of postnatal stomach*
> *contents (770.85, 770.86)*
> *meconium passage during delivery*
> *(763.84)*
> *meconium staining (779.84)*

**AHA:** 4Q, '05, 83

**770.10 Fetal and newborn aspiration,**   N
**unspecified**

**770.11 Meconium aspiration without**   N
**respiratory symptoms**
Meconium aspiration NOS

**770.12 Meconium aspiration with**   MCC N
**respiratory symptoms**
Meconium aspiration pneumonia
Meconium aspiration pneumonitis
Meconium aspiration syndrome NOS
Use additional code to identify any
secondary pulmonary hypertension
(416.8), if applicable

**CC Excl:** See code: 770.0

**DEF:** Meconium aspiration syndrome: aspiration of fetal intestinal material during or prior to delivery, usually a complication of placental insufficiency, causing pneumonitis and bronchial obstruction (inflammatory reaction of lungs).

**770.13 Aspiration of clear amniotic fluid**   N
**without respiratory symptoms**
Aspiration of clear amniotic fluid NOS

**770.14 Aspiration of clear amniotic fluid**   MCC N
**with respiratory symptoms**
Aspiration of clear amniotic fluid with
pneumonia
Aspiration of clear amniotic fluid with
pneumonitis
Use additional code to identify any
secondary pulmonary hypertension
(416.8), if applicable

**CC Excl:** See code: 770.0

**770.15 Aspiration of blood without**   N
**respiratory symptoms**
Aspiration of blood NOS

---

N Newborn Age: 0    P Pediatric Age: 0-17    M Maternity Age: 12-55    A Adult Age: 15-124    CC CC Condition    MCC Major CC Condition    HIV HIV Related Dx

**770.16 Aspiration of blood with respiratory symptoms** `MCC` `N`
Aspiration of blood with pneumonia
Aspiration of blood with pneumonitis
Use additional code to identify any secondary pulmonary hypertension (416.8), if applicable
**CC Excl:** See code: 770.0

**770.17 Other fetal and newborn aspiration without respiratory symptoms** `N`

**770.18 Other fetal and newborn aspiration with respiratory symptoms** `MCC` `N`
Other aspiration pneumonia
Other aspiration pneumonitis
Use additional code to identify any secondary pulmonary hypertension (416.8), if applicable
**CC Excl:** See code: 770.0

**770.2 Interstitial emphysema and related conditions** `MCC` `N`
Pneumomediastinum ⎫
Pneumopericardium ⎬ originating in the
Pneumothorax ⎭ perinatal period

**CC Excl:** See code: 770.0

**770.3 Pulmonary hemorrhage** `MCC` `N`
Hemorrhage:
alveolar (lung) ⎫
intra-alveolar (lung) ⎬ originating in the
massive pulmonary ⎭ perinatal period

**CC Excl:** See code: 770.0

**770.4 Primary atelectasis** `CC` `N`
Pulmonary immaturity NOS
**CC Excl:** See code: 770.0

**DEF:** Alveoli fail to expand causing insufficient air intake by newborn.

**770.5 Other and unspecified atelectasis** `CC` `N`
Atelectasis:
NOS ⎫
partial ⎬ originating in the
secondary ⎭ perinatal period
Pulmonary collapse

**CC Excl:** See code: 770.0

**770.6 Transitory tachypnea of newborn** `N`
Idiopathic tachypnea of newborn
Wet lung syndrome
**EXCLUDES** respiratory distress syndrome (769)
**AHA:** 4Q, '95, 4; 1Q, '94, 12; 3Q, '93, 7; 1Q, '89, 10; N-D, '86, 6
**DEF:** Quick, shallow breathing of newborn; short-term problem.

**770.7 Chronic respiratory disease arising in the perinatal period** `MCC`
Bronchopulmonary dysplasia
Interstitial pulmonary fibrosis of prematurity
Wilson-Mikity syndrome
**CC Excl:** See code: 770.0

**AHA:** 2Q, '91, 19; N-D, '86, 11

√5ᵗʰ **770.8 Other respiratory problems after birth**
**EXCLUDES** mixed metabolic and respiratory acidosis of newborn (775.81)
**AHA:** 4Q, '02, 65; 2Q, '98, 10; 2Q, '96, 10

**770.81 Primary apnea of newborn** `CC` `N`
Apneic spells of newborn NOS
Essential apnea of newborn
Sleep apnea of newborn
**CC Excl:** 770.82-770.83, 770.87-770.9, 786.03

**DEF:** Cessation of breathing when a neonate makes no respiratory effort for 15 seconds, resulting in cyanosis and bradycardia.

**770.82 Other apnea of newborn** `CC` `N`
Obstructive apnea of newborn
**CC Excl:** 770.81-770.83, 770.87-770.9, 786.03

**770.83 Cyanotic attacks of newborn** `CC` `N`
**CC Excl:** 770.81-770.83, 770.87-770.9, 782.5, 786.03

**770.84 Respiratory failure of newborn** `MCC` `N`
**EXCLUDES** respiratory distress syndrome (769)
**CC Excl:** 768.5-768.6, 768.9-770.86, 770.89-770.9, 779.81-779.84, 779.89

**770.85 Aspiration of postnatal stomach contents without respiratory symptoms** `N`
Aspiration of postnatal stomach contents NOS
**AHA:** 4Q, '05, 83

**770.86 Aspiration of postnatal stomach contents with respiratory symptoms** `MCC` `N`
Aspiration of postnatal stomach contents with pneumonia
Aspiration of postnatal stomach contents with pneumonitis
Use additional code to identify any secondary pulmonary hypertension (416.8), if applicable
**CC Excl:** See code: 770.84

**AHA:** 4Q, '05, 83

**770.87 Respiratory arrest of newborn** `MCC` `N`
**CC Excl:** 770.11, 770.13, 770.15, 770.17, 770.6, 770.81-770.85, 770.88-770.9, 779.85, 786.03, 799.1

**AHA:** 4Q, '06, 104-106

**770.88 Hypoxemia of newborn** `N`
Hypoxia NOS of newborn
**AHA:** 4Q, '06, 104-106

**770.89 Other respiratory problems after birth** `N`

**770.9 Unspecified respiratory condition of fetus and newborn** `N`

√4ᵗʰ **771 Infections specific to the perinatal period**
`INCLUDES` infections acquired before or during birth or via the umbilicus or during the first 28 days after birth
`EXCLUDES` congenital pneumonia (770.0)
congenital syphilis (090.0-090.9)
▶infant botulism (040.41)◀
maternal infectious disease as a cause of mortality or morbidity in fetus or newborn, but fetus or newborn not manifesting the disease (760.2)
ophthalmia neonatorum due to gonococcus (098.40)
other infections not specifically classified to this category

**AHA:** N-D, '85, 4

**771.0 Congenital rubella** `CC` `N`
Congenital rubella pneumonitis
**CC Excl:** 771.0-771.2, 779.81-779.84, 779.89

**771.1 Congenital cytomegalovirus infection** `MCC` `N`
Congenital cytomegalic inclusion disease
**CC Excl:** See code: 771.0

**771.2 Other congenital infections** `MCC` `N`
Congenital: ⎪ Congenital:
herpes simplex ⎪ toxoplasmosis
listeriosis ⎪ tuberculosis
malaria
**CC Excl:** 013.60-013.66, 046.2, 046.8, 048-049.0, 049.8, 052.0, 052.2, 054.3, 054.74, 056.01, 057.8-058.29, 062.0-064, 066.2-066.49, 072.2, 073.7, 075, 078.3, 079.82, 079.99, 081.9, 083.9, 084.6, 090.41, 094.81, 117.5, 124, 130.0, 290.12, 323.01-323.9, 341.1, 382.4, 487.8, 710.0, 771.2, 984.9

**771.3 Tetanus neonatorum** `MCC` `N`
Tetanus omphalitis
**EXCLUDES** hypocalcemic tetany (775.4)
**CC Excl:** 771.3, 779.81-779.84, 779.89

**DEF:** Severe infection of central nervous system; due to exotoxin of tetanus bacillus from navel infection prompted by nonsterile technique during umbilical ligation.

**771.4 Omphalitis of the newborn** `CC` `N`
Infection: ⎪ Infection:
navel cord ⎪ umbilical stump
**EXCLUDES** tetanus omphalitis (771.3)
**CC Excl:** 771.89

**DEF:** Inflamed umbilicus.

√4ᵗʰ / √5ᵗʰ Additional Digit Required    Unacceptable PDx    `Manifestation Code`    ▶◀ Revised Text    ● New Code    ▲ Revised Code Title

October 2007 • Volume 1 — 275

© 2007 Ingenix

**Conditions in the Perinatal Period**

**771.5–774.0**

**771.5**   **Neonatal infective mastitis**   `CC` `N`
> **EXCLUDES**   *noninfective neonatal mastitis (778.7)*
> **CC Excl:** See code: 771.4

**771.6**   **Neonatal conjunctivitis and dacryocystitis**   `N`
> Ophthalmia neonatorum NOS
> **EXCLUDES**   *ophthalmia neonatorum due to gonococcus (098.40)*

**771.7**   **Neonatal Candida infection**   `N`
> Neonatal moniliasis
> Thrush in newborn

✓5th **771.8**   **Other infection specific to the perinatal period**   `N`
> Use additional code to identify organism (041.00-041.9)
> **AHA:** 4Q, '02, 66

     **771.81**   **Septicemia [sepsis] of newborn**   `MCC` `N`
>      **CC Excl:** 771.4-771.89, 776.0-776.9, 779.81-779.84, 779.89

     **771.82**   **Urinary tract infection of newborn**   `CC` `N`
>      **CC Excl:** 041.9, 590.00-590.9, 593.89-593.9, 595.0-595.81, 595.89-595.9, 599.0, 599.9, 771.89, 788.1, 996.64

     **771.83**   **Bacteremia of newborn**   `CC` `N`
>      **CC Excl:** See code: 771.81

     **771.89**   **Other infections specific to the perinatal period**   `CC` `N`
>      Intra-amniotic infection of fetus NOS
>      Infection of newborn NOS
>      **CC Excl:** 003.1, 020.2, 022.3, 036.2, 038.0-038.9, 040.89-041.9, 054.5, 139.8, 771.82-771.89, 779.9, 790.7

✓4th **772 Fetal and neonatal hemorrhage**
> **EXCLUDES**   *hematological disorders of fetus and newborn (776.0-776.9)*

**772.0**   **Fetal blood loss**   `N`
> Fetal blood loss from:
>     cut end of co-twin's cord
>     placenta
>     ruptured cord
>     vasa previa
> Fetal exsanguination
> Fetal hemorrhage into:
>     co-twin
>     mother's circulation

✓5th **772.1**   **Intraventricular hemorrhage**
> Intraventricular hemorrhage from any perinatal cause
> **AHA:** 4Q, '01, 49; 3Q, '92, 8; 4Q, '88, 8

     **772.10**   **Unspecified grade**   `CC` `N`
>      **CC Excl:** 772.0-772.2, 772.8-772.9, 776.0-776.9, 779.81-779.84, 779.89

     **772.11**   **Grade I**   `CC` `N`
>      Bleeding into germinal matrix
>      **CC Excl:** See code: 772.10

     **772.12**   **Grade II**   `CC` `N`
>      Bleeding into ventricle
>      **CC Excl:** See code 772.10

     **772.13**   **Grade III**   `MCC` `N`
>      Bleeding with enlargement of ventricle
>      **CC Excl:** See code 772.10
>      **AHA:** 4Q, '01, 51

     **772.14**   **Grade IV**   `MCC` `N`
>      Bleeding into cerebral cortex
>      **CC Excl:** See code 772.10

**772.2**   **Subarachnoid hemorrhage**   `MCC` `N`
> Subarachnoid hemorrhage from any perinatal cause
> **EXCLUDES**   *subdural and cerebral hemorrhage (767.0)*
> **CC Excl:** 772.0-772.2, 772.8-772.9, 776.0-776.9, 779.7-779.84, 779.89

**772.3**   **Umbilical hemorrhage after birth**   `N`
> Slipped umbilical ligature

**772.4**   **Gastrointestinal hemorrhage**   `MCC` `N`
> **EXCLUDES**   *swallowed maternal blood (777.3)*
> **CC Excl:** 772.0, 772.4-772.5, 772.8-772.9, 776.0-776.9, 779.81-779.84, 779.89

**772.5**   **Adrenal hemorrhage**   `CC` `N`
> **CC Excl:** See code: 772.4

**772.6**   **Cutaneous hemorrhage**   `N`
> Bruising
> Ecchymoses     } in fetus or newborn
> Petechiae
> Superficial hematoma

**772.8**   **Other specified hemorrhage of fetus or newborn**   `N`
> **EXCLUDES**   *hemorrhagic disease of newborn (776.0)*
>                    *pulmonary hemorrhage (770.3)*

**772.9**   **Unspecified hemorrhage of newborn**   `N`

✓4th **773 Hemolytic disease of fetus or newborn, due to isoimmunization**
> **DEF:** Hemolytic anemia of fetus or newborn due to maternal antibody formation against fetal erythrocytes; infant blood contains nonmaternal antigen.

**773.0**   **Hemolytic disease due to Rh isoimmunization**   `N`
> Anemia                        } due to RH:
> Erythroblastosis (fetalis)        antibodies
> Hemolytic disease (fetus)       isoimmunization
>     (newborn)              maternal/fetal
> Jaundice                   incompatibility
> Rh hemolytic disease
> Rh isoimmunization

**773.1**   **Hemolytic disease due to ABO isoimmumization**   `N`
> ABO hemolytic disease    ABO isoimmunization
> Anemia                     } due to ABO:
> Erythroblastosis (fetalis)     antibodies
> Hemolytic disease (fetus)   isoimmunization
>     (newborn)          maternal/fetal
> Jaundice              incompatibility
> **AHA:** 3Q, '92, 8
>
> **DEF:** Incompatible Rh fetal-maternal blood grouping; prematurely destroys red blood cells; detected by Coombs test.

**773.2**   **Hemolytic disease due to other and unspecified isoimmunization**   `N`
> Eythroblastosis (fetalis) (neonatorum) NOS
> Hemolytic disease (fetus) (newborn) NOS
> Jaundice or anemia due to other and unspecified blood-group incompatibility
> **AHA:** 1Q, '94, 13

**773.3**   **Hydrops fetalis due to isoimmunization**   `MCC` `N`
> Use additional code to identify type of isoimmunization (773.0-773.2)
> **CC Excl:** 773.0-773.5, 779.81-779.84, 779.89
>
> **DEF:** Massive edema of entire body and severe anemia; may result in fetal death or stillbirth.

**773.4**   **Kernicterus due to isoimmunization**   `MCC` `N`
> Use additional code to identify type of isoimmunization (773.0-773.2)
> **CC Excl:** See code: 773.3
>
> **DEF:** Complication of erythroblastosis fetalis associated with severe neural symptoms, high blood bilirubin levels and nerve cell destruction; results in bilirubin-pigmented gray matter of central nervous system.

**773.5**   **Late anemia due to isoimmunization**   `N`

✓4th **774 Other perinatal jaundice**

**774.0**   ***Perinatal jaundice from hereditary hemolytic anemias***   `N`
> *Code first underlying disease (282.0-282.9)*

---

`N` Newborn Age: 0     `P` Pediatric Age: 0-17     `M` Maternity Age: 12-55     `A` Adult Age: 15-124     `CC` CC Condition     `MCC` Major CC Condition     `HIV` HIV Related Dx

**774.1 Perinatal jaundice from other excessive hemolysis**    N

Fetal or neonatal jaundice from:
- bruising
- drugs or toxins transmitted from mother
- infection
- polycythemia
- swallowed maternal blood

Use additional code to identify cause

EXCLUDES   *jaundice due to isoimmunization (773.0-773.2)*

**774.2 Neonatal jaundice associated with preterm delivery**    N

Hyperbilirubinemia of prematurity
Jaundice due to delayed conjugation associated with preterm delivery

AHA: 3Q, '91, 21

✓5ᵗʰ **774.3 Neonatal jaundice due to delayed conjugation from other causes**

**774.30 Neonatal jaundice due to delayed conjugation, cause unspecified**    N

DEF: Jaundice of newborn with abnormal bilirubin metabolism; causes excess accumulated unconjugated bilirubin in blood.

**774.31 Neonatal jaundice due to delayed conjugation in diseases classified elsewhere**    N

Code first underlying diseases as:
- congenital hypothyroidism (243)
- Crigler-Najjar syndrome (277.4)
- Gilbert's syndrome (277.4)

**774.39 Other**    N

Jaundice due to delayed conjugation from causes, such as:
- breast milk inhibitors
- delayed development of conjugating system

**774.4 Perinatal jaundice due to hepatocellular damage**    MCC   N

Fetal or neonatal hepatitis
Giant cell hepatitis
Inspissated bile syndrome

CC Excl: 774.0-774.7, 779.81-779.84, 779.89

**774.5 Perinatal jaundice from other causes**    N

Code first underlying cause as:
- congenital obstruction of bile duct (751.61)
- galactosemia (271.1)
- mucoviscidosis (277.00-277.09)

**774.6 Unspecified fetal and neonatal jaundice**    N

Icterus neonatorum
Neonatal hyperbilirubinemia (transient)
Physiologic jaundice NOS in newborn

EXCLUDES   *that in preterm infants (774.2)*

AHA: 1Q, '94, 13; 2Q, '89, 15

**774.7 Kernicterus not due to isoimmunization**    MCC   N

Bilirubin encephalopathy
Kernicterus of newborn NOS

EXCLUDES   *kernicterus due to isoimmunization (773.4)*

CC Excl: See code: 774.4

✓4ᵗʰ **775 Endocrine and metabolic disturbances specific to the fetus and newborn**

INCLUDES   transitory endocrine and metabolic disturbances caused by the infant's response to maternal endocrine and metabolic factors, its removal from them, or its adjustment to extrauterine existence

**775.0 Syndrome of "infant of a diabetic mother"**    N

Maternal diabetes mellitus affecting fetus or newborn (with hypoglycemia)

AHA: 1Q, '04, 7-8; 3Q, '91, 5

**775.1 Neonatal diabetes mellitus**    CC   N

Diabetes mellitus syndrome in newborn infant

CC Excl: 775.0-775.7, 775.9, 779.81-779.84, 779.89

AHA: 3Q, '91, 6

**775.2 Neonatal myasthenia gravis**    CC   N

CC Excl: See code: 775.1

**775.3 Neonatal thyrotoxicosis**    CC   N

Neonatal hyperthyroidism (transient)

CC Excl: See code 775.1

**775.4 Hypocalcemia and hypomagnesemia of newborn**    CC   N

Cow's milk hypocalcemia
Hypocalcemic tetany, neonatal
Neonatal hypoparathyroidism
Phosphate-loading hypocalcemia

CC Excl: See code 775.1

**775.5 Other transitory neonatal electrolyte disturbances**    N

Dehydration, neonatal

AHA: 1Q, '05, 9

**775.6 Neonatal hypoglycemia**    N

EXCLUDES   *infant of mother with diabetes mellitus (775.0)*

AHA: 1Q, '94, 8

**775.7 Late metabolic acidosis of newborn**    MCC   N

CC Excl: See code 775.1

**775.8 Other neonatal endocrine and metabolic disturbances**

**775.81 Other acidosis of newborn**    CC   N

Acidemia NOS of newborn
Acidosis of newborn NOS
Mixed metabolic and respiratory acidosis of newborn

CC Excl: 775.5, 775.7, 775.9

AHA: 4Q, '06, 104-106

**775.89 Other neonatal endocrine and metabolic disturbances**    CC   N

Amino-acid metabolic disorders described as transitory

CC Excl: 775.0-775.7, 775.9

AHA: 4Q, '06, 104-106

**775.9 Unspecified endocrine and metabolic disturbances specific to the fetus and newborn**    N

✓4ᵗʰ **776 Hematological disorders of fetus and newborn**

INCLUDES   disorders specific to the fetus or newborn

**776.0 Hemorrhagic disease of newborn**    CC   N

Hemorrhagic diathesis of newborn
Vitamin K deficiency of newborn

EXCLUDES   *fetal or neonatal hemorrhage (772.0-772.9)*

CC Excl: 776.0-776.9, 779.81-779.84, 779.89

**776.1 Transient neonatal thrombocytopenia**    MCC   N

Neonatal thrombocytopenia due to:
- exchange transfusion
- idiopathic maternal thrombocytopenia
- isoimmunization

CC Excl: See code 776.0

DEF: Temporary decrease in blood platelets of newborn.

**Conditions in the Perinatal Period**

**776.2–779.3**

**776.2** **Disseminated intravascular coagulation in** `MCC` `N`
**newborn**
CC Excl: See code 776.0

DEF: Disseminated intravascular coagulation of newborn: clotting disorder due to excess thromboplastic agents in blood as a result of disease or trauma; causes blood clotting within vessels and reduces available elements necessary for blood coagulation.

**776.3** **Other transient neonatal disorders of** `CC` `N`
**coagulation**
Transient coagulation defect, newborn
CC Excl: See code 776.0

**776.4** **Polycythemia neonatorum** `N`
Plethora of newborn    Polycythemia due to:
Polycythemia due to:     maternal-fetal transfusion
   donor twin transfusion
DEF: Abnormal increase of total red blood cells of newborn.

**776.5** **Congenital anemia** `CC` `N`
Anemia following fetal blood loss
`EXCLUDES`   anemia due to isoimmunization (773.0-773.2, 773.5)
          hereditary hemolytic anemias (282.0-282.9)
CC Excl: 280.0-282.3, 282.5-284.2, 284.81-285.9, 289.9, 517.3, 776.5-776.6

**776.6** **Anemia of prematurity** `CC` `N`
CC Excl: See code: 776.5

**776.7** **Transient neonatal neutropenia** `MCC` `N`
Isoimmune neutropenia
Maternal transfer neutropenia
`EXCLUDES`   congenital neutropenia (nontransient) (288.01)
CC Excl: 280.1-281.9, 282.5-282.63, 282.69-282.7, 283.0, 283.11, 284.01-284.2, 284.81-285.0, 285.21-285.9, 289.9, 776.7-776.9

DEF: Decreased neutrophilic leukocytes in blood of newborn.

**776.8** **Other specified transient hematological** `N`
**disorders**

**776.9** **Unspecified hematological disorder specific** `N`
**to fetus or newborn**

`✓4ᵗʰ` **777 Perinatal disorders of digestive system**
`INCLUDES`   disorders specific to the fetus and newborn
`EXCLUDES`   intestinal obstruction classifiable to 560.0-560.9

**777.1** **Meconium obstruction** `N`
Congenital fecaliths      Meconium ileus NOS
Delayed passage of meconium   Meconium plug
                         syndrome
`EXCLUDES`   meconium ileus in cystic fibrosis (277.01)
DEF: Meconium blocked digestive tract of newborn.

**777.2** **Intestinal obstruction due to inspissated** `N`
**milk**

**777.3** **Hematemesis and melena due to swallowed** `N`
**maternal blood**
Swallowed blood syndrome in newborn
`EXCLUDES`   that not due to swallowed maternal blood (772.4)

**777.4** **Transitory ileus of newborn** `CC` `N`
`EXCLUDES`   Hirschsprung's disease (751.3)
CC Excl: 777.1-777.9

**777.5** **Necrotizing enterocolitis in fetus or** `MCC` `N`
**newborn**
Pseudomembranous enterocolitis in newborn
CC Excl: 777.1-777.9, 779.81-779.84, 779.89

DEF: Acute inflammation of small intestine due to pseudomembranous plaque over ulceration; may be due to aggressive antibiotic therapy.

**777.6** **Perinatal intestinal perforation** `MCC` `N`
Meconium peritonitis
CC Excl: See code: 777.5

**777.8** **Other specified perinatal disorders of digestive** `N`
**system**

**777.9** **Unspecified perinatal disorder of digestive** `N`
**system**

`✓4ᵗʰ` **778 Conditions involving the integument and temperature**
**regulation of fetus and newborn**

**778.0** **Hydrops fetalis not due to** `MCC` `N`
**isoimmunization**
Idiopathic hydrops
`EXCLUDES`   hydrops fetalis due to isoimmunization (773.3)
CC Excl: 778.0, 779.81-779.84, 779.89

DEF: Edema of entire body, unrelated to immune response.

**778.1** **Sclerema neonatorum** `CC` `N`
Subcutaneous fat necrosis
CC Excl: 778.1, 778.5

DEF: Diffuse, rapidly progressing white, waxy, nonpitting hardening of tissue, usually of legs and feet, life-threatening; found in preterm or debilitated infants; unknown etiology.

**778.2** **Cold injury syndrome of newborn** `N`
**778.3** **Other hypothermia of newborn** `N`
**778.4** **Other disturbances of temperature regulation** `N`
**of newborn**
Dehydration fever in newborn
Environmentally-induced pyrexia
Hyperthermia in newborn
Transitory fever of newborn

**778.5** **Other and unspecified edema of newborn** `CC` `N`
Edema neonatorum
CC Excl: 778.1-778.5

**778.6** **Congenital hydrocele** `N`
Congenital hydrocele of tunica vaginalis

**778.7** **Breast engorgement in newborn** `N`
Noninfective mastitis of newborn
`EXCLUDES`   infective mastitis of newborn (771.5)

**778.8** **Other specified conditions involving the** `N`
**integument of fetus and newborn**
Urticaria neonatorum
`EXCLUDES`   impetigo neonatorum (684)
          pemphigus neonatorum (684)

**778.9** **Unspecified condition involving the** `N`
**integument and temperature regulation of**
**fetus and newborn**

`✓4ᵗʰ` **779 Other and ill-defined conditions originating in the perinatal**
**period**

**779.0** **Convulsions in newborn** `MCC` `N`
Fits }
Seizures } in newborn
CC Excl: 779.0-779.1, 779.81-779.84, 779.89
AHA: N-D, '94, 11

**779.1** **Other and unspecified cerebral irritability** `N`
**in newborn**

**779.2** **Cerebral depression, coma, and other** `MCC` `N`
**abnormal cerebral signs**
Cerebral ischemia NOS of newborn
CNS dysfunction in newborn NOS
`EXCLUDES`   cerebral ischemia due to birth trauma (767.0)
          intrauterine cerebral ischemia (768.2-768.9)
          intraventricular hemorrhage (772.10-772.14)
CC Excl: 779.0-779.2

**779.3** **Feeding problems in newborn** `N`
Regurgitation of food
Slow feeding     } in newborn
Vomiting
AHA: 2Q, '89, 15

N Newborn Age: 0    P Pediatric Age: 0-17    M Maternity Age: 12-55    A Adult Age: 15-124    CC CC Condition    MC Major Complication    CD Complex Dx    HIV HIV Related Dx

278 — Volume 1 • October 2007                           ©2007 Ingenix

**779.4 Drug reactions and intoxications specific to newborn** `CC` `N`

Gray syndrome from chloramphenicol administration in newborn

**EXCLUDES** *fetal alcohol syndrome (760.71)*
*reactions and intoxications from maternal opiates and tranquilizers (763.5)*

CC Excl: 779.4-779.5

**779.5 Drug withdrawal syndrome in newborn** `CC` `N`

Drug withdrawal syndrome in infant of dependent mother

**EXCLUDES** *fetal alcohol syndrome (760.71)*

CC Excl: See code: 779.4

AHA: 3Q, '94, 6

**779.6 Termination of pregnancy (fetus)** `N`

Fetal death due to:
induced abortion
termination of pregnancy

**EXCLUDES** *spontaneous abortion (fetus) (761.8)*

**779.7 Periventricular leukomalacia** `MCC`

CC Excl: 772.0-772.2, 772.8-772.9, 776.0-776.9, 779.7-779.84, 779.89

AHA: 4Q, '01, 50, 51

DEF: Necrosis of white matter adjacent to lateral ventricles with the formation of cysts; cause of PVL has not been firmly established, but thought to be related to inadequate blood flow in certain areas of the brain.

`✓5th` **779.8 Other specified conditions originating in the perinatal period**

AHA: 4Q, '02, 67; 1Q, '94, 15

**779.81 Neonatal bradycardia** `N`

**EXCLUDES** *abnormality in fetal heart rate or rhythm complicating labor and delivery (763.81-763.83)*
*bradycardia due to birth asphyxia (768.5-768.9)*

**779.82 Neonatal tachycardia** `N`

**EXCLUDES** *abnormality in fetal heart rate or rhythm complicating labor and delivery (763.81-763.83)*

**779.83 Delayed separation of umbilical cord** `N`

AHA: 4Q, '03, 71

**779.84 Meconium staining** `N`

**EXCLUDES** *meconium aspiration (770.11, 770.12)*
*meconium passage during delivery (763.84)*

AHA: 4Q, '05, 83, 88

**779.85 Cardiac arrest of newborn** `MCC` `N`

CC Excl: 779.85

AHA: 4Q, '06, 104-106

**779.89 Other specified conditions originating in the perinatal period** `N`

Use additional code to specify condition

AHA: 1Q, '06, 18; 2Q, '05, 15; 1Q, '05, 9

**779.9 Unspecified condition originating in the perinatal period** `N`

Congenital debility NOS
Stillbirth NEC

`✓4th` `✓5th` Additional Digit Required    Unacceptable PDx    Manifestation Code    ►◄ Revised Text    ● New Code    ▲ Revised Code Title

© 2007 Ingenix     October 2007 • Volume 1 — 279

## 16. SYMPTOMS, SIGNS, AND ILL-DEFINED CONDITIONS
### (780-799)

This section includes symptoms, signs, abnormal results of laboratory or other investigative procedures, and ill-defined conditions regarding which no diagnosis classifiable elsewhere is recorded.

Signs and symptoms that point rather definitely to a given diagnosis are assigned to some category in the preceding part of the classification. In general, categories 780-796 include the more ill-defined conditions and symptoms that point with perhaps equal suspicion to two or more diseases or to two or more systems of the body, and without the necessary study of the case to make a final diagnosis. Practically all categories in this group could be designated as "not otherwise specified," or as "unknown etiology," or as "transient." The Alphabetic Index should be consulted to determine which symptoms and signs are to be allocated here and which to more specific sections of the classification; the residual subcategories numbered .9 are provided for other relevant symptoms which cannot be allocated elsewhere in the classification.

The conditions and signs or symptoms included in categories 780-796 consist of: (a) cases for which no more specific diagnosis can be made even after all facts bearing on the case have been investigated; (b) signs or symptoms existing at the time of initial encounter that proved to be transient and whose causes could not be determined; (c) provisional diagnoses in a patient who failed to return for further investigation or care; (d) cases referred elsewhere for investigation or treatment before the diagnosis was made; (e) cases in which a more precise diagnosis was not available for any other reason; (f) certain symptoms which represent important problems in medical care and which it might be desired to classify in addition to a known cause.

### SYMPTOMS (780-789)
**AHA:** 1Q, '91, 12; 2Q, '90, 3; 2Q, '90, 5; 2Q, '90, 15; M-A, '85, 3

**√4ᵗʰ 780 General symptoms**

**√5ᵗʰ 780.0 Alteration of consciousness**

> **EXCLUDES** coma:
> diabetic (250.2-250.3)
> hepatic (572.2)
> originating in the perinatal period
> (779.2)

**AHA:** 4Q, '92, 20

**780.01 Coma** [MCC]

**CC Excl:** 070.0-070.9, 250.00-251.3, 338.0-338.4, 348.8-348.9, 349.89-349.9, 430-432.9, 572.2, 780.01-780.09, 780.2, 780.4, 780.91-780.99, 799.81-799.89, 800.0-801.99, 803.00-804.96, 850.0-852.19, 852.21-854.19

**AHA:** 3Q, '96, 16

**DEF:** State of unconsciousness from which the patient cannot be awakened.

**780.02 Transient alteration of awareness**

**DEF:** Temporary, recurring spells of reduced consciousness.

**780.03 Persistent vegetative state** [CC]

**CC Excl:** See code: 780.01

**DEF:** Persistent wakefulness without consciousness due to nonfunctioning cerebral cortex.

**780.09 Other**

Drowsiness    Stupor
Semicoma    Unconsciousness
Somnolence

**780.1 Hallucinations** [CC]

Hallucinations:    Hallucinations:
NOS            olfactory
auditory       tactile
gustatory

> **EXCLUDES** those associated with mental disorders, as functional psychoses (295.0-298.9)
> organic brain syndromes (290.0-294.9, 310.0-310.9)
> visual hallucinations (368.16)

**CC Excl:** 338.0-338.4, 780.1, 780.4, 780.91-780.99, 799.81-799.89

**DEF:** Perception of external stimulus in absence of stimulus; inability to distinguish between real and imagined.

**780.2 Syncope and collapse**

Blackout      (Near) (Pre) syncope
Fainting       Vasovagal attack

> **EXCLUDES** carotid sinus syncope (337.0)
> heat syncope (992.1)
> neurocirculatory asthenia (306.2)
> orthostatic hypotension (458.0)
> shock NOS (785.50)

**AHA:** 1Q, '02, 6; 3Q, '00, 12; 3Q, '95, 14; N-D, '85, 12

**DEF:** Sudden unconsciousness due to reduced blood flow to brain.

**√5ᵗʰ 780.3 Convulsions**

> **EXCLUDES** convulsions:
> epileptic (345.10-345.91)
> in newborn (779.0)

**AHA:** 2Q, '97, 8; 1Q, '97, 12; 3Q, '94, 9; 1Q, '93, 24; 4Q, '92, 23; N-D, '87, 12

**DEF:** Sudden, involuntary contractions of the muscles.

**780.31 Febrile convulsions (simple), unspecified** [CC]

Febrile seizure NOS

**CC Excl:** 338.0-338.4, 345.00-345.91, 348.8-348.9, 349.89-349.9, 779.0-779.1, 780.31-780.39, 780.91-780.99, 799.81-799.89

**AHA:** 4Q, '97, 45

**780.32 Complex febrile convulsions** [CC]

Febrile seizure:
atypical
complex
complicated

> **EXCLUDES** status epilepticus (345.3)

**CC Excl:** See code: 780.31

**AHA:** 4Q, '06, 106

**780.39 Other convulsions**

Convulsive disorder NOS
Fit NOS
Recurrent convulsions NOS
Seizure NOS

**AHA:** 3Q, '06, 22; 4Q, '04, 51; 1Q, '03, 7; 2Q, '99, 17; 4Q, '98, 39

**780.4 Dizziness and giddiness**

Light-headedness    Vertigo NOS

> **EXCLUDES** Ménière's disease and other specified vertiginous syndromes (386.0-386.9)

**AHA:** 2Q, '03, 11; 3Q, '00, 12; 2Q, '97, 9; 2Q, '91, 17

**DEF:** Whirling sensations in head with feeling of falling.

**√5ᵗʰ 780.5 Sleep disturbances**

> **EXCLUDES** circadian rhythm sleep disorders (327.30-327.39)
> organic hypersomnia (327.10-327.19)
> organic insomnia (327.00-327.09)
> organic sleep apnea (327.20-327.29)
> organic sleep related movement disorders (327.51-327.59)
> parasomnias (327.40-327.49)
> that of nonorganic origin (307.40-307.49)

**AHA:** 4Q, '05, 59

**780.50 Sleep disturbance, unspecified**

**780.51 Insomnia with sleep apnea, unspecified**

**DEF:** Transient cessation of breathing disturbing sleep.

**780.52 Insomnia, unspecified**

**DEF:** Inability to maintain adequate sleep cycle.

**780.53 Hypersomnia with sleep apnea, unspecified**

**AHA:** 1Q, '93, 28; N-D, '85, 4

**DEF:** Autonomic response inhibited during sleep; causes insufficient oxygen intake, acidosis and pulmonary hypertension.

**780.54 Hypersomnia, unspecified**

**DEF:** Prolonged sleep cycle.

**780.55 Disruptions of 24 hour sleep wake cycle, unspecified**

**780.56 Dysfunctions associated with sleep stages or arousal from sleep**

**780.57 Unspecified sleep apnea**
AHA: 1Q, '01, 6 ; 1Q, '97, 5; 1Q, '93, 28

**780.58 Sleep related movement disorder, unspecified**
> EXCLUDES    restless legs syndrome (333.94)

AHA: 4Q, '04, 95

**780.59 Other**

**780.6 Fever**

| | |
|---|---|
| Chills with fever | Hyperpyrexia NOS |
| Fever NOS | Pyrexia |
| Fever of unknown origin (FUO) | Pyrexia of unknown origin |

Code first underlying condition when associated fever is present, such as with:
    leukemia (codes from categories 204-208)
    neutropenia (288.00-288.09)
    sickle-cell disease (282.60-282.69)
> EXCLUDES    pyrexia of unknown origin (during):
>     in newborn (778.4)
>     labor (659.2)
>     the puerperium (672)

AHA: 3Q, '05, 16; 3Q, '00,13; 4Q, '99, 26; 2Q, '91, 8

DEF: Elevated body temperature; no known cause.

**√5ᵗʰ 780.7 Malaise and fatigue**
> EXCLUDES    debility, unspecified (799.3)
>     fatigue (during):
>       combat (308.0-308.9)
>       heat (992.6)
>       pregnancy (646.8)
>     neurasthenia (300.5)
>     senile asthenia (797)

AHA: 4Q, '88, 12; M-A, '87, 8

**780.71 Chronic fatigue syndrome**
AHA: 4Q, '98, 48

DEF: Persistent fatigue, symptoms include weak muscles, sore throat, lymphadenitis, headache, depression and mild fever; no known cause; also called chronic mononucleosis, benign myalgic encephalomyelitis, Iceland disease and neurosthenia.

**780.79 Other malaise and fatigue**

| | |
|---|---|
| Asthenia NOS | Postviral (asthenic) syndrome |
| Lethargy | Tiredness |

AHA: 4Q, '04, 78; 1Q, '00, 6; 4Q, '99, 26

DEF: Asthenia: Any weakness, lack of strength or loss of energy, especially neuromuscular.
DEF: Lethargy: Listlessness, drowsiness, stupor and apathy.
DEF: Malaise: Vague feeling of debility or lack of good health.
DEF: Postviral (asthenic) syndrome: Listlessness, drowsiness, stupor and apathy; follows acute viral infection.
DEF: Tiredness: General exhaustion or fatigue.

**780.8 Generalized hyperhidrosis**
Diaphoresis
Excessive sweating
Secondary hyperhidrosis
> EXCLUDES    focal (localized) (primary) (secondary)
>     hyperhidrosis (705.21-705.22)
>     Frey's syndrome (705.22)

DEF: Excessive sweating, appears as droplets on skin; general or localized.

**√5ᵗʰ 780.9 Other general symptoms**
> EXCLUDES    hypothermia:
>     NOS (accidental) (991.6)
>     due to anesthesia (995.89)
>     of newborn (778.2-778.3)
>     memory disturbance as part of a
>       pattern of mental disorder

AHA: 4Q, '02, 67; 4Q, '99, 10; 3Q, '93, 11; N-D, '85, 12

**780.91 Fussy infant (baby)**    P

**780.92 Excessive crying of infant (baby)**    N
> EXCLUDES    excessive crying of child, adolescent or adult (780.95)

**780.93 Memory loss**
Amnesia (retrograde)
Memory loss NOS
> EXCLUDES    mild memory disturbance due to organic brain damage (310.1)
>     transient global amnesia (437.7)

AHA: 4Q, '03, 71

**780.94 Early satiety**
AHA: 4Q, '03, 72

DEF: The premature feeling of being full; mechanism of satiety is mutlifactorial.

**780.95 Excessive crying of child, adolescent, or adult**
> EXCLUDES    excessive crying of infant (baby) (780.92)

AHA: 4Q, '05, 89

**780.96 Generalized pain**
Pain NOS
AHA: 4Q, '06, 79-81

**780.97 Altered mental status**
Change in mental status
> EXCLUDES    altered level of consciousness (780.01-780.09)
>     altered mental status due to known condition—code to condition
>     delirium NOS (780.09)

AHA: 4Q, '06, 107

**780.99 Other general symptoms**
Chill(s) NOS
Hypothermia, not associated with low environmental temperature
AHA: 4Q, '03, 103

**√4ᵗʰ 781 Symptoms involving nervous and musculoskeletal systems**
> EXCLUDES    depression NOS (311)
>     disorders specifically relating to:
>       back (724.0-724.9)
>       hearing (388.0-389.9)
>       joint (718.0-719.9)
>       limb (729.0-729.9)
>       neck (723.0-723.9)
>       vision (368.0-369.9)
>     pain in limb (729.5)

**781.0 Abnormal involuntary movements**

| | |
|---|---|
| Abnormal head movements | Spasms NOS |
| Fasciculation | Tremor NOS |

> EXCLUDES    abnormal reflex (796.1)
>     chorea NOS (333.5)
>     infantile spasms (345.60-345.61)
>     spastic paralysis (342.1, 343.0-344.9)
>     specified movement disorders
>       classifiable to 333 (333.0-333.9)
>     that of nonorganic origin (307.2-307.3)

N Newborn Age: 0    P Pediatric Age: 0-17    M Maternity Age: 12-55    A Adult Age: 15-124    CC CC Condition    MCC Major CC Condition    HIV HIV Related Dx

282 — Volume 1 • October 2007

© 2007 Ingenix

**781.1 Disturbances of sensation of smell and taste**
Anosmia          Parosmia
Parageusia
DEF: Anosmia: loss of sense of smell due to organic factors, including loss of olfactory nerve conductivity, cerebral disease, nasal fossae formation and peripheral olfactory nerve diseases; can also be psychological disorder.
DEF: Parageusia: distorted sense of taste, or bad taste in mouth.
DEF: Parosmia: distorted sense of smell.

**781.2 Abnormality of gait**
Gait:              Gait:
ataxic               spastic
paralytic            staggering
EXCLUDES  *ataxia:*
*NOS (781.3)*
*locomotor (progressive) (094.0)*
*difficulty in walking (719.7)*
AHA: 2Q, '05, 6; 2Q, '04, 15
DEF: Abnormal, asymmetric gait.

**781.3 Lack of coordination**
Ataxia NOS          Muscular incoordination
EXCLUDES  *ataxic gait (781.2)*
*cerebellar ataxia (334.0-334.9)*
*difficulty in walking (719.7)*
*vertigo NOS (780.4)*
AHA: 4Q, '04, 51; 3Q, '97, 12

**781.4 Transient paralysis of limb**  `CC`
Monoplegia, transient NOS
EXCLUDES  *paralysis (342.0-344.9)*
CC Excl: 781.4, 781.94

**781.5 Clubbing of fingers**
DEF: Enlarged soft tissue of distal fingers.

**781.6 Meningismus**  `CC`
Dupré's syndrome          Meningism
CC Excl: 781.4, 781.94
AHA: 3Q, '00,13; J-F, '87, 7
DEF: Condition with signs and symptoms that resemble meningeal irritation; it is associated with febrile illness and dehydration with no evidence of infection.

**781.7 Tetany**  `CC`
Carpopedal spasm
EXCLUDES  *tetanus neonatorum (771.3)*
*tetany:*
*hysterical (300.11)*
*newborn (hypocalcemic) (775.4)*
*parathyroid (252.1)*
*psychogenic (306.0)*
CC Excl: 037, 332.0-333.93, 333.99-334.4, 338.0-338.4, 342.10-342.12, 771.3, 780.91-780.99, 781.7, 799.81-799.89
DEF: Nerve and muscle hyperexcitability; symptoms include muscle spasms, twitching, cramps, laryngospasm with inspiratory stridor, hyperreflexia and choreiform movements.

**781.8 Neurologic neglect syndrome**  `CC`
Asomatognosia          Left-sided neglect
Hemi-akinesia          Sensory extinction
Hemi-inattention          Sensory neglect
Hemispatial neglect          Visuospatial neglect
CC Excl: 781.8-781.92, 781.94-781.99
AHA: 4Q, '94, 37

`✓5th` **781.9 Other symptoms involving nervous and musculoskeletal systems**
AHA: 4Q, '00, 45

**781.91 Loss of height**
EXCLUDES  *osteoporosis (733.00-733.09)*

**781.92 Abnormal posture**

**781.93 Ocular torticollis**
AHA: 4Q, '02, 68
DEF: Abnormal head posture as a result of a contracted state of cervical muscles to correct a visual disturbance; either double vision or a visual field defect.

**781.94 Facial weakness**
Facial droop
EXCLUDES  *facial weakness due to late effect of cerebrovascular accident (438.83)*
AHA: 4Q, '03, 72

**781.99 Other symptoms involving nervous and musculoskeletal systems**

`✓4th` **782 Symptoms involving skin and other integumentary tissue**
EXCLUDES  *symptoms relating to breast (611.71-611.79)*

**782.0 Disturbance of skin sensation**
Anesthesia of skin          Numbness
Burning or prickling sensation          Paresthesia
Hyperesthesia          Tingling
Hypoesthesia

**782.1 Rash and other nonspecific skin eruption**
Exanthem
EXCLUDES  *vesicular eruption (709.8)*

**782.2 Localized superficial swelling, mass, or lump**
Subcutaneous nodules
EXCLUDES  *localized adiposity (278.1)*

**782.3 Edema**
Anasarca
Dropsy
Localized edema NOS
EXCLUDES  *ascites* ▶*(789.51-789.59)*◄
*edema of:*
*newborn NOS (778.5)*
*pregnancy (642.0-642.9, 646.1)*
*fluid retention (276.6)*
*hydrops fetalis (773.3, 778.0)*
*hydrothorax (511.8)*
*nutritional edema (260, 262)*
AHA: 2Q, '00, 18
DEF: Edema: excess fluid in intercellular body tissue.
DEF: Anasarca: massive edema in all body tissues.
DEF: Dropsy: serous fluid accumulated in body cavity or cellular tissue.
DEF: Localized edema: edema in specific body areas.

**782.4 Jaundice, unspecified, not of newborn**  `CC`
Cholemia NOS
Icterus NOS
EXCLUDES  *jaundice in newborn (774.0-774.7)*
*due to isoimmunization (773.0-773.2, 773.4)*
CC Excl: 774.0-774.7, 782.4, 782.9
DEF: Bilirubin deposits of skin, causing yellow cast.

**782.5 Cyanosis**
EXCLUDES  *newborn (770.83)*
DEF: Deficient oxygen of blood; causes blue cast to skin.

`✓5th` **782.6 Pallor and flushing**
**782.61 Pallor**
**782.62 Flushing**
Excessive blushing

**782.7 Spontaneous ecchymoses**
Petechiae
EXCLUDES  *ecchymosis in fetus or newborn (772.6)*
*purpura (287.0-287.9)*
DEF: Hemorrhagic spots of skin; resemble freckles.

**782.8 Changes in skin texture**
Induration } of skin
Thickening
**782.9 Other symptoms involving skin and integumentary tissues**

`✓4th` **783 Symptoms concerning nutrition, metabolism, and development**
**783.0 Anorexia**
Loss of appetite
EXCLUDES  *anorexia nervosa (307.1)*
*loss of appetite of nonorganic origin (307.59)*

`✓4th` `✓5th` Additional Digit Required          Unacceptable PDx          Manifestation Code          ►◄ Revised Text          ● New Code          ▲ Revised Code Title

**Symptoms, Signs, and Ill-Defined Conditions**

**783.1–785.2**

**783.1   Abnormal weight gain**

> EXCLUDES   *excessive weight gain in pregnancy (646.1)*
> *obesity (278.00)*
> *morbid (278.01)*

✓5ᵗʰ **783.2   Abnormal loss of weight and underweight**

Use additional code to identify Body Mass Index (BMI), if known (V85.0-V85.54)

AHA: 4Q, '00, 45

**783.21   Loss of weight**

AHA: 4Q, '05, 96

**783.22   Underweight**

AHA: 4Q, '05, 96

**783.3   Feeding difficulties and mismanagement**

Feeding problem (elderly) (infant)

> EXCLUDES   *feeding disturbance or problems:*
> *in newborn (779.3)*
> *of nonorganic origin (307.50-307.59)*

AHA: 3Q, '97, 12

✓5ᵗʰ **783.4   Lack of expected normal physiological development in childhood**

> EXCLUDES   *delay in sexual development and puberty (259.0)*
> *gonadal dysgenesis (758.6)*
> *pituitary dwarfism (253.3)*
> *slow fetal growth and fetal malnutrition (764.00-764.99)*
> *specific delays in mental development (315.0-315.9)*

AHA: 4Q, '00, 45; 3Q, '97, 4

**783.40   Lack of normal physiological development, unspecified**

Inadequate development
Lack of development

**783.41   Failure to thrive**    P

Failure to gain weight

AHA: 1Q, '03, 12

DEF: Organic failure to thrive: acute or chronic illness that interferes with nutritional intake, absorption, metabolism excretion and energy requirements. Nonorganic FTT is symptom of neglect or abuse.

**783.42   Delayed milestones**    P

Late talker      Late walker

**783.43   Short stature**

Growth failure      Lack of growth
Growth retardation    Physical retardation

DEF: Constitutional short stature: stature inconsistent with chronological age. Genetic short stature is when skeletal maturation matches chronological age.

**783.5   Polydipsia**

Excessive thirst

**783.6   Polyphagia**

Excessive eating      Hyperalimentation NOS

> EXCLUDES   *disorders of eating of nonorganic origin (307.50-307.59)*

**783.7   Adult failure to thrive**    A

**783.9   Other symptoms concerning nutrition, metabolism, and development**

Hypometabolism

> EXCLUDES   *abnormal basal metabolic rate (794.7)*
> *dehydration (276.51)*
> *other disorders of fluid, electrolyte, and acid-base balance (276.0-276.9)*

AHA: 2Q, '04, 3

✓4ᵗʰ **784   Symptoms involving head and neck**

> EXCLUDES   *encephalopathy NOS (348.30)*
> *specific symptoms involving neck classifiable to 723 (723.0-723.9)*

**784.0   Headache**

Facial pain      Pain in head NOS

> EXCLUDES   *atypical face pain (350.2)*
> *migraine (346.0-346.9)*
> *tension headache (307.81)*

AHA: 3Q, '06, 22; 2Q, '06, 17; 3Q, '00, 13; 1Q, '90, 4; 3Q, '92, 14

**784.1   Throat pain**

> EXCLUDES   *dysphagia ▶(787.20-787.29)◀*
> *neck pain (723.1)*
> *sore throat (462)*
> *chronic (472.1)*

**784.2   Swelling, mass, or lump in head and neck**

Space-occupying lesion, intracranial NOS

AHA: 1Q, '03, 8

**784.3   Aphasia**    CC

> EXCLUDES   *aphasia due to late effects of cerebrovascular disease (438.11)*
> *developmental aphasia (315.31)*

CC Excl: 315.31, 432.0-434.91, 436, 784.3-784.5

AHA: 4Q, '04, 78; 4Q, '98, 87; 3Q, '97, 12

DEF: Inability to communicate through speech, written word, or sign language.

✓5ᵗʰ **784.4   Voice disturbance**

**784.40   Voice disturbance, unspecified**

**784.41   Aphonia**

Loss of voice

**784.49   Other**

Change in voice    Hypernasality
Dysphonia      Hyponasality
Hoarseness

**784.5   Other speech disturbance**

Dysarthria      Slurred speech
Dysphasia

> EXCLUDES   *stammering and stuttering (307.0)*
> *that of nonorganic origin (307.0, 307.9)*

✓5ᵗʰ **784.6   Other symbolic dysfunction**

> EXCLUDES   *developmental learning delays (315.0-315.9)*

**784.60   Symbolic dysfunction, unspecified**

**784.61   Alexia and dyslexia**

Alexia (with agraphia)

DEF: Alexia: Inability to understand written word due to central brain lesion.

DEF: Dyslexia: Ability to recognize letters but inability to read, spell, and write words; genetic.

**784.69   Other**

Acalculia      Agraphia NOS
Agnosia      Apraxia

**784.7   Epistaxis**

Hemorrhage from nose    Nosebleed

AHA: 3Q, '04, 7

**784.8   Hemorrhage from throat**

> EXCLUDES   *hemoptysis (786.3)*

✓5ᵗʰ **784.9   Other symptoms involving head and neck**

**784.91   Postnasal drip**

AHA: 4Q, '06, 108

**784.99   Other symptoms involving head and neck**

Choking sensation
▶Feeling of foreign body in throat◀
Halitosis
Mouth breathing
Sneezing

> EXCLUDES   *▶ foreign body in throat (933.0)◀*

AHA: 4Q, '06, 108

✓4ᵗʰ **785   Symptoms involving cardiovascular system**

> EXCLUDES   *heart failure NOS (428.9)*

**785.0   Tachycardia, unspecified**

Rapid heart beat

> EXCLUDES   *neonatal tachycardia (779.82)*
> *paroxysmal tachycardia (427.0-427.2)*

AHA: 2Q, '03, 11

DEF: Excessively rapid heart rate.

**785.1   Palpitations**

Awareness of heart beat

> EXCLUDES   *specified dysrhythmias (427.0-427.9)*

**785.2   Undiagnosed cardiac murmurs**

Heart murmurs NOS

AHA: 4Q, '92, 16

---

N Newborn Age: 0    P Pediatric Age: 0-17    M Maternity Age: 12-55    A Adult Age: 15-124    CC CC Condition    MCC Major CC Condition    HIV HIV Related Dx

785.3   **Other abnormal heart sounds**
          Cardiac dullness, increased or decreased
          Friction fremitus, cardiac
          Precordial friction

785.4   **Gangrene**                                                    `CC`
          Gangrene:
            NOS
            spreading cutaneous
          Gangrenous cellulitis
          Phagedena
          Code first any associated underlying condition
            EXCLUDES    *gangrene of certain sites — see*
                          *Alphabetic Index*
                        *gangrene with atherosclerosis of the*
                          *extremities (440.24)*
                        *gas gangrene (040.0*
          CC Excl: 338.0-338.4, 440.24, 780.91-780.99, 785.4, 799.81-799.89

          AHA: 1Q, '04, 14; 3Q, '91, 12; 3Q, '90, 15; M-A, '86, 12
          DEF: Gangrene: necrosis of skin tissue due to bacterial infection,
          diabetes, embolus and vascular supply loss.
          DEF: Gangrenous cellulitis: group A streptococcal infection; begins
          with severe cellulitis, spreads to superficial and deep fascia;
          produces gangrene of underlying tissues.

√5ᵗʰ  785.5   **Shock without mention of trauma**
          785.50   **Shock, unspecified**                               `CC`
                    Failure of peripheral circulation
                    CC Excl: 338.0-338.4, 780.91-780.99, 785.50-785.59, 785.9,
                    799.81-799.89

                    AHA: 2Q, '96, 10
                    DEF: Peripheral circulatory failure due to heart
                    insufficiencies.

      ¹  785.51   **Cardiogenic shock**                                 `MCC`
                    CC Excl: See code: 785.50

                    AHA: 3Q, '05, 14

                    DEF: Shock syndrome: associated with myocardial
                    infarction, cardiac tamponade and massive pulmonary
                    embolism; symptoms include mental confusion, reduced
                    blood pressure, tachycardia, pallor and cold, clammy
                    skin.

          785.52   *Septic shock*                                       `MCC`
                    Shock:
                      endotoxic
                      gram-negative
                    Code first:
                      systemic inflammatory response
                        syndrome due to infectious process
                        with organ dysfunction (995.92)
                    CC Excl: See code 785.50
                    AHA: 4Q, '06, 113; 2Q, '05, 18-19; 4Q, '03, 73, 79

      ¹  785.59   **Other**                                            `MCC`
                    Shock:
                      hypovolemic
                      EXCLUDES    *shock (due to):*
                                    *anesthetic (995.4)*
                                    *anaphylactic (995.0)*
                                    *due to serum (999.4)*
                                    *electric (994.8)*
                                    *following abortion (639.5)*
                                    *lightning (994.0)*
                                    *obstetrical (669.1)*
                                    *postoperative (998.0)*
                                    *traumatic (958.4)*

                    CC Excl: see code 785.50
                    AHA: 2Q, '00, 3

785.6   **Enlargement of lymph nodes**
          Lymphadenopathy          "Swollen glands"
            EXCLUDES    *lymphadenitis (chronic) (289.1-289.3)*
                          *acute (683)*

785.9   **Other symptoms involving cardiovascular system**
          Bruit (arterial)          Weak pulse

√4ᵗʰ  786   **Symptoms involving respiratory system and other chest
          symptoms**
      √5ᵗʰ  786.0   **Dyspnea and respiratory abnormalities**
                    786.00  **Respiratory abnormality, unspecified**

786.01  **Hyperventilation**
          EXCLUDES    *hyperventilation, psychogenic*
                        *(306.1)*
          DEF: Rapid breathing causes carbon dioxide loss from
          blood.

786.02  **Orthopnea**
          DEF: Difficulty breathing except in upright position.

786.03  **Apnea**
          EXCLUDES    *apnea of newborn (770.81,*
                        *770.82)*
                      *sleep apnea (780.51, 780.53,*
                        *780.57)*
          AHA: 4Q, '98, 50
          DEF: Cessation of breathing.

786.04  **Cheyne-Stokes respiration**                                   `CC`
          CC Excl: 518.81-518.84, 519.8-519.9, 786.03-786.04, 799.1
          AHA: 4Q, '98, 50
          DEF: Rhythmic increase of depth and frequency of
          breathing with apnea; occurs in frontal lobe and
          diencephalic dysfunction.

786.05  **Shortness of breath**
          AHA: 4Q, '99, 25; 1Q, '99, 6; 4Q, '98, 50
          DEF: Inability to take in sufficient oxygen.

786.06  **Tachypnea**
          EXCLUDES    *transitory tachypnea of*
                        *newborn (770.6)*
          AHA: 4Q, '98, 50
          DEF: Abnormal rapid respiratory rate; called
          hyperventilation.

786.07  **Wheezing**
          EXCLUDES    *asthma (493.00-493.92)*
          AHA: 4Q, '98, 50
          DEF: Stenosis of respiratory passageway; causes
          whistling sound; due to asthma, coryza, croup,
          emphysema, hay fever, edema, and pleural effusion.

786.09  **Other**
          Respiratory:          Respiratory:
            distress              insufficiency
          EXCLUDES    *respiratory distress:*
                        *following trauma and*
                          *surgery (518.5)*
                        *newborn (770.89)*
                        *syndrome (newborn) (769)*
                          *adult (518.5)*
                        *respiratory failure (518.81,*
                          *518.83-518.84)*
                          *newborn (770.84)*
          AHA: 4Q, '05, 90; 2Q, '98, 10; 1Q, '97, 7; 1Q, '90, 9

786.1   **Stridor**
          EXCLUDES    *congenital laryngeal stridor (748.3)*
          DEF: Obstructed airway causes harsh sound.

786.2   **Cough**
          EXCLUDES    *cough:*
                        *psychogenic (306.1)*
                        *smokers' (491.0)*
                        *with hemorrhage (786.3)*
          AHA: 4Q, '99, 26

786.3   **Hemoptysis**                                                  `CC`
          Cough with hemorrhage
          Pulmonary hemorrhage NOS
          EXCLUDES    *pulmonary hemorrhage of newborn*
                        *(770.3)*
          CC Excl: 338.0-338.4, 780.91-780.99, 786.3-786.4, 786.9, 799.81-799.89
          AHA: 2Q, '06, 17; 4Q, '90, 26
          DEF: Coughing up blood or blood-stained sputum.

786.4   **Abnormal sputum**
          Abnormal:
            amount
            color        } (of) sputum
            odor
          Excessive

Symptoms, Signs, and Ill-Defined Conditions

786.5–788.29

✓5ᵗʰ **786.5　Chest pain**
　　**786.50　Chest pain, unspecified**
　　　　AHA:▶1Q, '07, 19;◄ 2Q, '06, 7; 1Q, '03, 6; 1Q, '02, 4;
　　　　4Q, '99, 25
　　**786.51　Precordial pain**
　　　　DEF: Chest pain over heart and lower thorax.
　　**786.52　Painful respiration**
　　　　Pain:
　　　　　anterior chest wall
　　　　　pleuritic
　　　　Pleurodynia
　　　　**EXCLUDES**　epidemic pleurodynia (074.1)
　　　　AHA: N-D, '84, 17
　　**786.59　Other**
　　　　Discomfort ⎫
　　　　Pressure　⎬ in chest
　　　　Tightness ⎭
　　　　**EXCLUDES**　pain in breast (611.71)
　　　　AHA: 1Q, '02, 6

**786.6　Swelling, mass, or lump in chest**
　　**EXCLUDES**　lump in breast (611.72)
**786.7　Abnormal chest sounds**
　　Abnormal percussion, chest　　Rales
　　Friction sounds, chest　　　　Tympany, chest
　　**EXCLUDES**　wheezing (786.07)
**786.8　Hiccough**
　　**EXCLUDES**　psychogenic hiccough (306.1)
**786.9　Other symptoms involving respiratory system and chest**
　　Breath-holding spell

✓4ᵗʰ **787　Symptoms involving digestive system**
　　**EXCLUDES**　constipation (564.00-564.09)
　　　　　pylorospasm (537.81)
　　　　　congenital (750.5)

✓5ᵗʰ **787.0　Nausea and vomiting**
　　Emesis
　　**EXCLUDES**　hematemesis NOS (578.0)
　　　　vomiting:
　　　　　bilious, following gastrointestinal
　　　　　　surgery (564.3)
　　　　　cyclical (536.2)
　　　　　　psychogenic (306.4)
　　　　　excessive, in pregnancy (643.0-
　　　　　　643.9)
　　　　　habit (536.2)
　　　　　of newborn (779.3)
　　　　　psychogenic NOS (307.54)
　　AHA: M-A, '85, 11

　　**787.01　Nausea with vomiting**
　　　　AHA: 1Q, '03, 5
　　**787.02　Nausea alone**
　　　　AHA: 3Q, '00, 12; 2Q, '97, 9
　　**787.03　Vomiting alone**

**787.1　Heartburn**
　　Pyrosis　　　　Waterbrash
　　**EXCLUDES**　dyspepsia or indigestion (536.8)
　　AHA: 2Q, '01, 6

✓5ᵗʰ **787.2　Dysphagia**
　　▶Code first, if applicable, dysphagia due to late effect
　　　of cerebrovascular accident (438.82)◄
　　AHA: 4Q, '03, 103, 109; 2Q, '01, 4

● 　　**787.20　Dysphagia, unspecified**
　　　　Difficulty in swallowing NOS
● 　　**787.21　Dysphagia, oral phase**
● 　　**787.22　Dysphagia, oropharyngeal phase**
● 　　**787.23　Dysphagia, pharyngeal phase**
● 　　**787.24　Dysphagia, pharyngoesophageal phase**
● 　　**787.29　Other dysphagia**
　　　　Cervical dysphagia
　　　　Neurogenic dysphagia

**787.3　Flatulence, eructation, and gas pain**
　　Abdominal distention (gaseous)
　　Bloating
　　Tympanites (abdominal) (intestinal)
　　**EXCLUDES**　aerophagy (306.4)
　　DEF: Flatulence: excess air or gas in intestine or stomach.
　　DEF: Eructation: belching, expelling gas through mouth.
　　DEF: Gas pain: gaseous pressure affecting gastrointestinal system.
**787.4　Visible peristalsis**
　　Hyperperistalsis
　　DEF: Increase in involuntary movements of intestines.
**787.5　Abnormal bowel sounds**
　　Absent bowel sounds　　　Hyperactive bowel sounds
**787.6　Incontinence of feces**
　　Encopresis NOS
　　Incontinence of sphincter ani
　　**EXCLUDES**　that of nonorganic origin (307.7)
　　AHA: 1Q, '97, 9
**787.7　Abnormal feces**
　　Bulky stools
　　**EXCLUDES**　abnormal stool content (792.1)
　　　　melena:
　　　　　NOS (578.1)
　　　　　newborn (772.4, 777.3)

✓5ᵗʰ **787.9　Other symptoms involving digestive system**
　　**EXCLUDES**　gastrointestinal hemorrhage (578.0-
　　　　　578.9)
　　　　intestinal obstruction (560.0-560.9)
　　　　specific functional digestive disorders:
　　　　　esophagus (530.0-530.9)
　　　　　stomach and duodenum (536.0-
　　　　　　536.9)
　　　　those not elsewhere classified
　　　　　(564.00-564.9)

　　**787.91　Diarrhea**
　　　　Diarrhea NOS
　　　　AHA: 4Q, '95, 54
　　**787.99　Other**
　　　　Change in bowel habits
　　　　Tenesmus (rectal)
　　　　DEF: Tenesmus: Painful, ineffective straining at the
　　　　rectum with limited passage of fecal matter.

✓4ᵗʰ **788　Symptoms involving urinary system**
　　**EXCLUDES**　hematuria (599.7)
　　　　nonspecific findings on examination of the urine
　　　　　(791.0-791.9)
　　　　small kidney of unknown cause (589.0-589.9)
　　　　uremia NOS (586)
　　　　urinary obstruction (599.60, 599.69)

**788.0　Renal colic**
　　Colic (recurrent) of:　Colic (recurrent) of:
　　　kidney　　　　　　　ureter
　　AHA: 3Q, '04, 8
　　DEF: Kidney pain.
**788.1　Dysuria**
　　Painful urination　　　Strangury
✓5ᵗʰ **788.2　Retention of urine**
　　Code, if applicable, any causal condition first,
　　　such as:
　　　　hyperplasia of prostate (600.0-600.9 with fifth-
　　　　　digit 1)
　　DEF: Accumulation of urine in the bladder due to inability to void

　　**788.20　Retention of urine, unspecified**
　　　　AHA: 4Q, '06, 93, 95; 2Q, '04, 18; 3Q, '03, 12-13;
　　　　1Q, '03, 6; 3Q, '96, 10
　　**788.21　Incomplete bladder emptying**
　　　　AHA: 4Q, '06, 93
　　**788.29　Other specified retention of urine**

---

ℕ Newborn Age: 0　　ℙ Pediatric Age: 0-17　　𝕄 Maternity Age: 12-55　　𝔸 Adult Age: 15-124　　 CC Condition　　 Major CC Condition　　 HIV Related Dx

286 — Volume 1 • October 2007

© 2007 Ingenix

√5ᵗʰ **788.3 Urinary incontinence**
Code, if applicable, any causal condition first,
such as:
congenital ureterocele (753.23)
genital prolapse (618.00-618.9)
hyperplasia of prostate (600.0-600.9 with fifth-
digit 1)
**EXCLUDES** *that of nonorganic origin (307.6)*
AHA: 4Q, '06, 93; 4Q, '92, 22

**788.30 Urinary incontinence, unspecified**
Enuresis NOS

**788.31 Urge incontinence**
AHA: 1Q, '00, 19
DEF: Inability to control urination, upon urge to urinate.

**788.32 Stress incontinence, male** ♂
**EXCLUDES** *stress incontinence, female (625.6)*
DEF: Inability to control urination associated with weak sphincter in males.

**788.33 Mixed incontinence, (male) (female)**
Urge and stress
DEF: Urge, stress incontinence: involuntary discharge of urine due to anatomic displacement.

**788.34 Incontinence without sensory awareness**
DEF: Involuntary discharge of urine without sensory warning.

**788.35 Post-void dribbling**
DEF: Involuntary discharge of residual urine after voiding.

**788.36 Nocturnal enuresis**
DEF: Involuntary discharge of urine during the night.

**788.37 Continuous leakage**
DEF: Continuous, involuntary urine seepage.

**788.38 Overflow incontinence**
DEF: Leakage caused by pressure of retained urine in the bladder after the bladder has fully contracted due to weakened bladder muscles or an obstruction of the urethra.

**788.39 Other urinary incontinence**

√5ᵗʰ **788.4 Frequency of urination and polyuria**
Code, if applicable, any causal condition first,
such as:
hyperplasia of prostate (600.0-600.9 with fifth-
digit 1)

**788.41 Urinary frequency**
Frequency of micturition
AHA: 4Q, '06, 93

**788.42 Polyuria**
DEF: Excessive urination.

**788.43 Nocturia**
AHA: 4Q, '06, 93
DEF: Urination affecting sleep patterns.

**788.5 Oliguria and anuria**
Deficient secretion of urine
Suppression of urinary secretion
**EXCLUDES** *that complicating:*
*abortion (634-638 with .3, 639.3)*
*ectopic or molar pregnancy (639.3)*
*pregnancy, childbirth, or the puerp-
erium (642.0-642.9, 646.2)*
DEF: Oliguria: diminished urinary secretion related to fluid intake.
DEF: Anuria: lack of urinary secretion due to renal failure or obstructed urinary tract.

√5ᵗʰ **788.6 Other abnormality of urination**
Code, if applicable, any causal condition first,
such as:
hyperplasia of prostate (600.0-600.9 with fifth-
digit 1)

**788.61 Splitting of urinary stream**
Intermittent urinary stream

**788.62 Slowing of urinary stream**
Weak stream
AHA: 4Q, '06, 93

**788.63 Urgency of urination**
**EXCLUDES** *urge incontinence (788.31, 788.33)*
AHA: 4Q, '06, 93; 4Q, '03, 74
DEF: Feeling of intense need to urinate; abrupt sensation of imminent urination.

**788.64 Urinary hesitancy**
AHA: 4Q, '06, 93, 109

**788.65 Straining on urination**
AHA: 4Q, '06, 93, 109

**788.69 Other**

**788.7 Urethral discharge**
Penile discharge          Urethrorrhea

**788.8 Extravasation of urine**          **CC**
CC Excl: 788.8-788.9
DEF: Leaking or infiltration of urine into tissues.

**788.9 Other symptoms involving urinary system**
Extrarenal uremia          Vesical:
Vesical:                        tenesmus
pain
AHA: 1Q, '05, 12; 4Q, '88, 1

√4ᵗʰ **789 Other symptoms involving abdomen and pelvis**
**EXCLUDES** *symptoms referable to genital organs:*
*female (625.0-625.9)*
*male (607.0-608.9)*
*psychogenic (302.70-302.79)*

The following fifth-digit subclassification is to be used for codes 789.0, 789.3, 789.4, 789.6:
**0** unspecified site
**1** right upper quadrant
**2** left upper quadrant
**3** right lower quadrant
**4** left lower quadrant
**5** periumbilic
**6** epigastric
**7** generalized
**9** other specified site
Multiple sites

√5ᵗʰ **789.0 Abdominal pain**
Colic:                        Colic:
NOS                          infantile
Cramps, abdominal
**EXCLUDES** *renal colic (788.0)*
AHA: 1Q, '95, 3; For code 789.06: 1Q, '02, 5

**789.1 Hepatomegaly**
Enlargement of liver

**789.2 Splenomegaly**
Enlargement of spleen

√5ᵗʰ **789.3 Abdominal or pelvic swelling, mass, or lump**
Diffuse or generalized swelling or mass:
abdominal NOS
umbilical
**EXCLUDES** *abdominal distention (gaseous) (787.3)*
*ascites ▶(789.51-789.59)◀*

√5ᵗʰ **789.4 Abdominal rigidity**

√5ᵗʰ **789.5 Ascites**
Fluid in peritoneal cavity
AHA: 2Q, '05, 8; 4Q, '89, 11
DEF: Serous fluid effusion and accumulation in abdominal cavity.

**789.51 Malignant ascites**          **CC**
Code first malignancy, such as:
malignant neoplasm of ovary (183.0)
secondary malignant neoplasm of
retroperitoneum and peritoneum
(197.6)
CC Excl: 338.0-338.4, 780.91-780.99, 789.30-789.49, 789.51-
789.59, 789.9, 799.81-799.89

**789.59 Other ascites**          **CC**
CC Excl: See code: 789.51

---

√4ᵗʰ **Additional Digit Required**          **Unacceptable PDx**          **Manifestation Code**          ◄► Revised Text          ● New Code          ▲ Revised Code Title
√5ᵗʰ

© 2007 Ingenix                                                  **October 2007 • Volume 1 — 287**

√5th **789.6 Abdominal tenderness**
Rebound tenderness

**789.9 Other symptoms involving abdomen and pelvis**
Umbilical:            Umbilical:
  bleeding              discharge

## NONSPECIFIC ABNORMAL FINDINGS (790-796)
AHA: 2Q, '90, 16

√4th **790 Nonspecific findings on examination of blood**
EXCLUDES   abnormality of:
  platelets (287.0-287.9)
  thrombocytes (287.0-287.9)
  white blood cells (288.00-288.9)

√5th **790.0 Abnormality of red blood cells**
EXCLUDES   anemia:
  congenital (776.5)
  newborn, due to isoimmunization
    (773.0-773.2, 773.5)
  of premature infant (776.6)
  other specified types (280.0-285.9)
hemoglobin disorders (282.5-282.7)
polycythemia:
  familial (289.6)
  neonatorum (776.4)
  secondary (289.0)
  vera (238.4)

AHA: 4Q, '00, 46

**790.01 Precipitous drop in hematocrit**   CC
Drop in hematocrit
**CC Excl:** 285.1, 285.8-285.9

**790.09 Other abnormality of red blood cells**
Abnormal red cell morphology NOS
Abnormal red cell volume NOS
Anisocytosis
Poikilocytosis

**790.1 Elevated sedimentation rate**

√5th **790.2 Abnormal glucose**
EXCLUDES   diabetes mellitus (250.00-250.93)
dysmetabolic syndrome X (277.7)
gestational diabetes (648.8)
glycosuria (791.5)
hypoglycemia (251.2)
that complicating pregnancy, childbirth,
  or puerperium (648.8)

AHA: 4Q, '03, 74; 3Q, '91, 5

**790.21 Impaired fasting glucose**
Elevated fasting glucose

**790.22 Impaired glucose tolerance test (oral)**
Elevated glucose tolerance test

**790.29 Other abnormal glucose**
Abnormal glucose NOS
Abnormal non-fasting glucose
Hyperglycemia NOS
Pre-diabetes NOS
**AHA:** 2Q, '05, 21

**790.3 Excessive blood level of alcohol**
Elevated blood-alcohol
AHA: S-O, '86, 3

**790.4 Nonspecific elevation of levels of transaminase or lactic acid dehydrogenase [LDH]**

**790.5 Other nonspecific abnormal serum enzyme levels**
Abnormal serum level of:
  acid phosphatase
  alkaline phosphatase
  amylase
  lipase
EXCLUDES   deficiency of circulating enzymes (277.6)

**790.6 Other abnormal blood chemistry**
Abnormal blood level of:   Abnormal blood level of:
  cobalt                       lithium
  copper                       magnesium
  iron                         mineral
  lead                         zinc
EXCLUDES   abnormality of electrolyte or acid-base
    balance (276.0-276.9)
hypoglycemia NOS (251.2)
lead poisoning (984.0-984.9)
specific finding indicating abnormality
  of:
  amino-acid transport and
    metabolism (270.0-270.9)
  carbohydrate transport and
    metabolism (271.0-271.9)
  lipid metabolism (272.0-272.9)
uremia NOS (586)

AHA: 4Q, '88, 1

**790.7 Bacteremia**   CC
EXCLUDES   bacteremia of newborn (771.83)
septicemia (038)
Use additional code to identify organism (041)
**CC Excl:** 338.0-338.4, 780.91-780.99, 790.7-790.99, 799.81-799.89

AHA: 2Q, '03, 7; 4Q, '93, 29; 3Q, '88, 12
**DEF:** Laboratory finding of bacteria in the blood in the absence of two or more signs of sepsis; transient in nature, progresses to septicemia with severe infectious process.

**790.8 Viremia, unspecified**
AHA: 4Q, '88, 10
**DEF:** Presence of a virus in the blood stream.

√5th **790.9 Other nonspecific findings on examination of blood**
AHA: 4Q, '93, 29

**790.91 Abnormal arterial blood gases**
**790.92 Abnormal coagulation profile**
Abnormal or prolonged:
  bleeding time
  coagulation time
  partial thromboplastin time [PTT]
  prothrombin time [PT]
EXCLUDES   coagulation (hemorrhagic)
    disorders (286.0-286.9)

**790.93 Elevated prostate specific antigen, [PSA]**   A ♂

**790.94 Euthyroid sick syndrome**
AHA: 4Q, '97, 45
**DEF:** Transient alteration of thyroid hormone metabolism due to nonthyroid illness or stress.

**790.95 Elevated C-reactive protein [CRP]**
**DEF:** Inflammation in an arterial wall results in elevated C-reactive protein (CRP) in the blood; CRP is a recognized risk factor in cardiovascular disease.

**790.99 Other**
AHA: 2Q, '03, 14

√4th **791 Nonspecific findings on examination of urine**
EXCLUDES   hematuria NOS (599.7)
specific findings indicating abnormality of:
  amino-acid transport and metabolism (270.0-270.9)
  carbohydrate transport and metabolism (271.0-271.9)

**791.0 Proteinuria**
Albuminuria
Bence-Jones proteinuria
EXCLUDES   postural proteinuria (593.6)
that arising during pregnancy or the
  puerperium (642.0-642.9, 646.2)

AHA: 3Q, '91, 8
**DEF:** Excess protein in urine.

N Newborn Age: 0     P Pediatric Age: 0-17     M Maternity Age: 12-55     A Adult Age: 15-124     CC CC Condition     MCC Major CC Condition     HIV HIV Related Dx

**288 — Volume 1 • October 2007**

© 2007 Ingenix

**791.1 Chyluria**   `CC`
> EXCLUDES   *filarial (125.0-125.9)*

**CC Excl:** 338.0-338.4, 780.91-780.99, 791.1, 791.9, 799.81-799.89

DEF: Excess chyle in urine.

**791.2 Hemoglobinuria**

DEF: Free hemoglobin in blood due to rapid hemolysis of red blood cells.

**791.3 Myoglobinuria**   `CC`

**CC Excl:** 338.0-338.4, 780.91-780.99, 791.2-791.3, 791.9, 799.81-799.89

DEF: Myoglobin (oxygen-transporting pigment) in urine.

**791.4 Biliuria**

DEF: Bile pigments in urine.

**791.5 Glycosuria**
> EXCLUDES   *renal glycosuria (271.4)*

DEF: Sugar in urine.

**791.6 Acetonuria**
Ketonuria

DEF: Excess acetone in urine.

**791.7 Other cells and casts in urine**

**791.9 Other nonspecific findings on examination of urine**
| | |
|---|---|
| Crystalluria | Elevated urine levels of: |
| Elevated urine levels of: | indolacetic acid |
| 17-ketosteroids | vanillylmandelic acid [VMA] |
| catecholamines | Melanuria |

**AHA:** 1Q, '05, 12

**✓4ᵗʰ 792 Nonspecific abnormal findings in other body substances**
> EXCLUDES   *that in chromosomal analysis (795.2)*

**792.0 Cerebrospinal fluid**

**792.1 Stool contents**
| | |
|---|---|
| Abnormal stool color | Occult stool |
| Fat in stool | Pus in stool |
| Mucus in stool | |

> EXCLUDES   *blood in stool [melena] (578.1)*
>          *newborn (772.4, 777.3)*

**AHA:** 2Q, '92, 9

**792.2 Semen**   ♂
Abnormal spermatozoa
> EXCLUDES   *azoospermia (606.0)*
>          *oligospermia (606.1)*

**792.3 Amniotic fluid**   `M` ♀
**AHA:** N-D, '86, 4
DEF: Nonspecific abnormal findings in amniotic fluid.

**792.4 Saliva**
> EXCLUDES   *that in chromosomal analysis (795.2)*

**792.5 Cloudy (hemodialysis) (peritoneal) dialysis effluent**
**AHA:** 4Q, '00, 46

**792.9 Other nonspecific abnormal findings in body substances**
| | |
|---|---|
| Peritoneal fluid | Synovial fluid |
| Pleural fluid | Vaginal fluids |

**✓4ᵗʰ 793 Nonspecific abnormal findings on radiological and other examination of body structure**
> INCLUDES   nonspecific abnormal findings of:
>      thermography
>      ultrasound examination [echogram]
>      x-ray examination
> EXCLUDES   *abnormal results of function studies and*
>          *radioisotope scans (794.0-794.9)*

**793.0 Skull and head**
> EXCLUDES   *nonspecific abnormal*
>          *echoencephalogram (794.01)*

**AHA:** 3Q, '06, 22

**793.1 Lung field**
Coin lesion  ⎫
Shadow     ⎬ (of) lung

DEF: Coin lesion of lung: coin-shaped, solitary pulmonary nodule.

**793.2 Other intrathoracic organ**
| Abnormal: | Abnormal: |
|---|---|
| echocardiogram | ultrasound cardiogram |
| heart shadow | Mediastinal shift |

**793.3 Biliary tract**
Nonvisualization of gallbladder

**793.4 Gastrointestinal tract**

**793.5 Genitourinary organs**
| Filling defect: | Filling defect: |
|---|---|
| bladder | ureter |
| kidney | |

**793.6 Abdominal area, including retroperitoneum**

**793.7 Musculoskeletal system**

**✓5ᵗʰ 793.8 Breast**
**AHA:** 4Q, '01, 51

**793.80 Abnormal mammogram, unspecified**

**793.81 Mammographic microcalcification**
> EXCLUDES   *mammographic calcification (793.89)*
>          *mammographic calculus (793.89)*

DEF: Calcium and cellular debris deposits in the breast that cannot be felt but can be detected on a mammogram; can be a sign of cancer, benign conditions, or changes in the breast tissue as a result of inflammation, injury, or obstructed duct.

**793.89 Other abnormal findings on radiological examination of breast**
Mammographic calcification
Mammographic calculus

**✓5ᵗʰ 793.9 Other**
> EXCLUDES   *abnormal finding by radioisotope*
>          *localization of placenta (794.9)*

**793.91 Image test inconclusive due to excess body fat**
Use additional code to identify Body Mass Index (BMI), if known (V85.0-V85.54)
**AHA:** 4Q, '06, 109

**793.99 Other nonspecific abnormal findings on radiological and other examinations of body structure**
Abnormal:
     placental finding by x-ray or ultrasound method
     radiological findings in skin and subcutaneous tissue
**AHA:** 4Q, '06, 109

**✓4ᵗʰ 794 Nonspecific abnormal results of function studies**
> INCLUDES   radioisotope:
>      scans
>      uptake studies
>      scintiphotography

**✓5ᵗʰ 794.0 Brain and central nervous system**
**794.00 Abnormal function study, unspecified**
**794.01 Abnormal echoencephalogram**
**794.02 Abnormal electroencephalogram [EEG]**
**794.09 Other**
Abnormal brain scan

**✓5ᵗʰ 794.1 Peripheral nervous system and special senses**
**794.10 Abnormal response to nerve stimulation, unspecified**
**794.11 Abnormal retinal function studies**
Abnormal electroretinogram [ERG]
**794.12 Abnormal electro-oculogram [EOG]**
**794.13 Abnormal visually evoked potential**
**794.14 Abnormal oculomotor studies**
**794.15 Abnormal auditory function studies**
**AHA:** 1Q, '04, 15-16
**794.16 Abnormal vestibular function studies**
**794.17 Abnormal electromyogram [EMG]**
> EXCLUDES   *that of eye (794.14)*

**794.19 Other**

---

| ✓4ᵗʰ ✓5ᵗʰ Additional Digit Required | Unacceptable PDx | Manifestation Code | ►◄ Revised Text | ● New Code | ▲ Revised Code Title |
|---|---|---|---|---|---|

**Symptoms, Signs, and Ill-Defined Conditions**

**794.2–795.71**

**794.2 Pulmonary**
Abnormal lung scan
Reduced:
　ventilatory capacity
Reduced:
　vital capacity

√5ᵗʰ **794.3 Cardiovascular**

**794.30 Abnormal function study, unspecified**

**794.31 Abnormal electrocardiogram [ECG] [EKG]**
　EXCLUDES　long QT syndrome (426.82)

**794.39 Other**
Abnormal:
　ballistocardiogram
　phonocardiogram
Abnormal:
　vectorcardiogram

**794.4 Kidney**
Abnormal renal function test

**794.5 Thyroid**
Abnormal thyroid:
　scan
Abnormal thyroid:
　uptake

**794.6 Other endocrine function study**

**794.7 Basal metabolism**
Abnormal basal metabolic rate [BMR]

**794.8 Liver**
Abnormal liver scan

**794.9 Other**
Bladder
Pancreas
Placenta
Spleen

√4ᵗʰ **795 Other and nonspecific abnormal cytological, histological, immunological and DNA test findings**
　EXCLUDES　nonspecific abnormalities of red blood cells (790.01-790.09)

√5ᵗʰ **795.0 Abnormal Papanicolaou smear of cervix and cervical HPV**
Abnormal thin preparation smear of cervix
Abnormal cervical cytology
　EXCLUDES　carcinoma in-situ of cervix (233.1)
　　　　　　cervical intraepithelial neoplasia I (CIN I) (622.11)
　　　　　　cervical intraepithelial neoplasia II (CIN II) (622.12)
　　　　　　cervical intraepithelial neoplasia III (CIN III) (233.1)
　　　　　　dysplasia (histologically confirmed) of cervix (uteri) NOS (622.10)
　　　　　　mild dysplasia (histologically confirmed) (622.11)
　　　　　　moderate dysplasia (histologically confirmed) (622.12)
　　　　　　severe dysplasia (histologically confirmed) (233.1)
AHA: 4Q, '02, 69

**795.00 Abnormal glandular Papanicolaou smear of cervix**　♀
Atypical endocervical cells NOS
Atypical endometrial cells NOS
Atypical glandular cells NOS

**795.01 Papanicolaou smear of cervix with atypical squamous cells of undetermined significance [ASC-US]**　♀
AHA: 2Q, '06, 4

**795.02 Papanicolaou smear of cervix with atypical squamous cells cannot exclude high grade squamous intraepithelial lesion [ASC-H]**　♀

**795.03 Papanicolaou smear of cervix with low grade squamous intraepithelial lesion [LGSIL]**　♀

**795.04 Papanicolaou smear of cervix with high grade squamous intraepithelial lesion [HGSIL]**　♀

**795.05 Cervical high risk human papillomavirus [HPV] DNA test positive**　♀

**795.06 Papanicolaou smear of cervix with cytologic evidence of malignancy**　♀
AHA: 4Q, '06, 110

**795.08 Unsatisfactory smear**　♀
Inadequate sample
AHA: 2Q, '06, 4

**795.09 Other abnormal Papanicolaou smear of cervix and cervical HPV**　♀
Cervical low risk human papillomavirus (HPV) DNA test positive
Use additional code for associated human papillomavirus (079.4)
　EXCLUDES　encounter for Papanicolaou cervical smear to confirm findings of recent normal smear following initial abnormal smear (V72.32)

**795.1 Nonspecific abnormal Papanicolaou smear of other site**

**795.2 Nonspecific abnormal findings on chromosomal analysis**
Abnormal karyotype

√5ᵗʰ **795.3 Nonspecific positive culture findings**
Positive culture findings in:
　nose
　sputum
　throat
　wound
　EXCLUDES　that of:
　　　　　　blood (790.7-790.8)
　　　　　　urine (791.9)

**795.31 Nonspecific positive findings for anthrax**
Positive findings by nasal swab
AHA: 4Q, '02, 70

**795.39 Other nonspecific positive culture findings**

**795.4 Other nonspecific abnormal histological findings**

**795.5 Nonspecific reaction to tuberculin skin test without active tuberculosis**
Abnormal result of
　Mantoux test
PPD positive
Tuberculin (skin test):
　positive
　reactor

**795.6 False positive serological test for syphilis**
False positive Wassermann reaction

√5ᵗʰ **795.7 Other nonspecific immunological findings**
　EXCLUDES　abnormal tumor markers (795.81-795.89)
　　　　　　elevated prostate specific antigen [PSA] (790.93)
　　　　　　elevated tumor associated antigens (795.81-795.89)
　　　　　　isoimmunization, in pregnancy (656.1-656.2)
　　　　　　　affecting fetus or newborn (773.0-773.2)
AHA: 2Q, '93, 6

**795.71 Nonspecific serologic evidence of human immunodeficiency virus [HIV]**
Inclusive human immunodeficiency [HIV] test (adult) (infant)
Note: This code is **only** to be used when a test finding is reported as nonspecific. Asymptomatic positive findings are coded to V08. If any HIV infection symptom or condition is present, see code 042. Negative findings are not coded.
　EXCLUDES　acquired immunodeficiency syndrome [AIDS] (042)
　　　　　　asymptomatic human immuno-deficiency virus, [HIV] infection status (V08)
　　　　　　HIV infection, symptomatic (042)
　　　　　　human immunodeficiency virus [HIV] disease (042)
　　　　　　positive (status) NOS (V08)
AHA: 2Q, '04, 11; 1Q, '93, 21; 1Q, '93, 22; 2Q, '92, 11; J-A, '87, 24

 Newborn Age: 0　　 Pediatric Age: 0-17　　 Maternity Age: 12-55　　 Adult Age: 15-124　　CC CC Condition　　MCC Major CC Condition　　HIV HIV Related Dx

**795.79 Other and unspecified nonspecific immunological findings**
Raised antibody titer
Raised level of immunoglobulins

√5ᵗʰ **795.8 Abnormal tumor markers**
Elevated tumor associated antigens [TAA]
Elevated tumor specific antigens [TSA]
**EXCLUDES** *elevated prostate specific antigen [PSA] (790.93)*

**795.81 Elevated carcinoembryonic antigen [CEA]**
AHA: 4Q, '06, 111

**795.82 Elevated cancer antigen 125 [CA 125]** ♀
AHA: 4Q, '06, 111

**795.89 Other abnormal tumor markers**
AHA: 4Q, '06, 111

√4ᵗʰ **796 Other nonspecific abnormal findings**

**796.0 Nonspecific abnormal toxicological findings**
Abnormal levels of heavy metals or drugs in blood, urine, or other tissue
**EXCLUDES** *excessive blood level of alcohol (790.3)*
AHA: 1Q, '97, 16

**796.1 Abnormal reflex**

**796.2 Elevated blood pressure reading without diagnosis of hypertension**
Note: This category is to be used to record an episode of elevated blood pressure in a patient in whom no formal diagnosis of hypertension has been made, or as an incidental finding.
AHA: 2Q, '03, 11; 3Q, '90, 4; J-A, '84, 12

**796.3 Nonspecific low blood pressure reading**

**796.4 Other abnormal clinical findings**
AHA: 1Q, '97, 16

**796.5 Abnormal finding on antenatal screening** ♀ Ⓜ
AHA: 4Q, '97, 46

**796.6 Abnormal findings on neonatal screening** Ⓝ
**EXCLUDES** *nonspecific serologic evidence of human immunodeficiency virus [HIV] (795.71)*
AHA: 4Q, '04, 99

**796.9 Other**

## ILL-DEFINED AND UNKNOWN CAUSES OF MORBIDITY AND MORTALITY (797-799)

**797 Senility without mention of psychosis**
Old age     Senile:
Senescence     debility
Senile asthenia     exhaustion
**EXCLUDES** *senile psychoses (290.0-290.9)*

√4ᵗʰ **798 Sudden death, cause unknown**

**798.0 Sudden infant death syndrome** Ⓟ
Cot death     Sudden death of nonspecific
Crib death     cause in infancy
DEF: Death of infant under age one due to nonspecific cause.

**798.1 Instantaneous death**
**798.2 Death occurring in less than 24 hours from onset of symptoms, not otherwise explained**
Death known not to be violent or instantaneous, for which no cause could be discovered
Died without sign of disease

**798.9 Unattended death**
Death in circumstances where the body of the deceased was found and no cause could be discovered
Found dead

√4ᵗʰ **799 Other ill-defined and unknown causes of morbidity and mortality**

√5ᵗʰ **799.0 Asphyxia and hypoxemia**
**EXCLUDES** *asphyxia and hypoxemia (due to):*
*carbon monoxide (986)*
*hypercapnia (786.09)*
*inhalation of food or foreign body (932-934.9)*
*newborn (768.0-768.9)*
*traumatic (994.7)*

**799.01 Asphyxia** ᶜᶜ
CC Excl: 338.0-338.4, 518.81-518.84, 780.91-780.99, 798.0, 799.01-799.1, 799.81-799.89
AHA: 4Q, '05, 90
DEF: Lack of oxygen in inspired air, causing a deficiency of oxygen in tissues (hypoxia) and elevated levels of arterial carbon dioxide (hypercapnia).

**799.02 Hypoxemia**
AHA: 2Q, '06, 24, 25; 4Q, '05, 90
DEF: Deficient oxygenation of the blood.

¹ **799.1 Respiratory arrest** ᴹᶜᶜ
Cardiorespiratory failure
**EXCLUDES** *cardiac arrest (427.5)*
*failure of peripheral circulation (785.50)*
*respiratory distress:*
*NOS (786.09)*
*acute (518.82)*
*following trauma and surgery (518.5)*
*newborn (770.89)*
*syndrome (newborn) (769)*
*adult (following trauma and surgery) (518.5)*
*other (518.82)*
*respiratory failure (518.81, 518.83-518.84)*
*newborn (770.84)*
*respiratory insufficiency (786.09)*
*acute (518.82)*
CC Excl: See code: 799.01

**799.2 Nervousness**
"Nerves"

**799.3 Debility, unspecified**
**EXCLUDES** *asthenia (780.79)*
*nervous debility (300.5)*
*neurasthenia (300.5)*
*senile asthenia (797)*

**799.4 Cachexia** ᶜᶜ
Wasting disease
Code first underlying condition, if known
CC Excl: 338.0-338.4, 780.91-780.99, 799.3-799.89
AHA: 3Q, '06, 14, 15; 3Q, '90, 17
DEF: General ill health and poor nutrition.

√5ᵗʰ **799.8 Other ill-defined conditions**
**799.81 Decreased libido** Ⓐ
Decreased sexual desire
**EXCLUDES** *psychosexual dysfunction with inhibited sexual desire (302.71)*
AHA: 4Q, '03, 75

**799.89 Other ill-defined conditions**
**799.9 Other unknown and unspecified cause**
Undiagnosed disease, not specified as to site or system involved
Unknown cause of morbidity or mortality
AHA: 1Q, '98,.4; 1Q, '90, 20

¹ MCC= Only if patient is discharged alive.

√4ᵗʰ √5ᵗʰ Additional Digit Required     Unacceptable PDx     Manifestation Code     ►◄ Revised Text     ● New Code     ▲ Revised Code Title

## 17. INJURY AND POISONING (800-999)

Use E code(s) to identify the cause and intent of the injury or poisoning (E800-E999)

Note:

1. The principle of multiple coding of injuries should be followed wherever possible. Combination categories for multiple injuries are provided for use when there is insufficient detail as to the nature of the individual conditions, or for primary tabulation purposes when it is more convenient to record a single code; otherwise, the component injuries should be coded separately.

   Where multiple sites of injury are specified in the titles, the word "with" indicates involvement of both sites, and the word "and" indicates involvement of either or both sites. The word "finger" includes thumb.

2. Categories for "late effect" of injuries are to be found at 905-909.

### FRACTURES (800-829)

**EXCLUDES**
- malunion (733.81)
- nonunion (733.82)
- pathological or spontaneous fracture (733.10-733.19)
- stress fractures (733.93-733.95)

The terms "condyle," "coronoid process," "ramus," and "symphysis" indicate the portion of the bone fractured, not the name of the bone involved.

The descriptions "closed" and "open" used in the fourth-digit subdivisions include the following terms:

closed (with or without delayed healing):

| | |
|---|---|
| comminuted | impacted |
| depressed | linear |
| elevated | simple |
| fissured | slipped epiphysis |
| fracture NOS | spiral |
| greenstick | |

open (with or without delayed healing):

| | |
|---|---|
| compound | puncture |
| infected | with foreign body |
| missile | |

A fracture not indicated as closed or open should be classified as closed.

**AHA:** ▶1Q, '07, 3-4;◀ 4Q, '90, 26; 3Q, '90, 5; 3Q, '90, 13; 2Q, '90, 7; 2Q, '89, 15, S-O, '85, 3

### FRACTURE OF SKULL (800-804)

The following fifth-digit subclassification is for use with the appropriate codes in categories 800, 801, 803, and 804:

- **0** unspecified state of consciousness
- **1** with no loss of consciousness
- **2** with brief [less than one hour] loss of consciousness
- **3** with moderate [1-24 hours] loss of consciousness
- **4** with prolonged [more than 24 hours] loss of consciousness and return to pre-existing conscious level
- **5** with prolonged [more than 24 hours] loss of consciousness, without return to pre-existing conscious level

  Use fifth-digit 5 to designate when a patient is unconscious and dies before regaining consciousness, regardless of the duration of the loss of consciousness

- **6** with loss of consciousness of unspecified duration
- **9** with concussion, unspecified

√4th **800 Fracture of vault of skull**

    **INCLUDES**   frontal bone
                       parietal bone

    **AHA:** 4Q,'96, 36

    **DEF:** Fracture of bone that forms skull dome and protects brain.

**Fractures**

√5th **800.0** **Closed without mention of intracranial injury**    MCC 3-5   CC 0-2, 6, 9
    **CC Excl:** 800.00-801.99, 803.00-804.99, 829.0-829.1, 850.0-852.19, 852.21-854.19, 873.8-873.9, 879.8-879.9, 905.0,925.1-925.2,929.0-929.9,958.8-959.09, 959.8-959.9

√5th **800.1** **Closed with cerebral laceration and contusion**    MCC
    **CC Excl:** See code 800.0

√5th **800.2** **Closed with subarachnoid, subdural, and extradural hemorrhage**    MCC
    **CC Excl:** See code 800.0

√5th **800.3** **Closed with other and unspecified intracranial hemorrhage**    MCC
    **CC Excl:** See code 800.0

√5th **800.4** **Closed with intracranial injury of other and unspecified nature**   MCC 3-5   CC 0-2, 6, 9
    **CC Excl:** See code 800.0

√5th **800.5** **Open without mention of intracranial injury**    MCC
    **CC Excl:** See code 800.0

√5th **800.6** **Open with cerebral laceration and contusion**    MCC
    **CC Excl:** See code 800.0

√5th **800.7** **Open with subarachnoid, subdural, and extradural hemorrhage**    MCC
    **CC Excl:** See code 800.0

√5th **800.8** **Open with other and unspecified intracranial hemorrhage**    MCC
    **CC Excl:** See code 800.0

√5th **800.9** **Open with intracranial injury of other and unspecified nature**    MCC
    **CC Excl:** See code 800.0

**Skull**

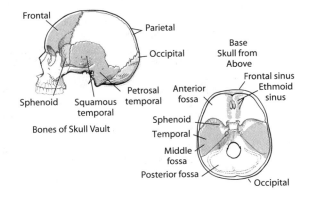

**Injury and Poisoning**

**801–802.6**

✓4th **801 Fracture of base of skull**

| INCLUDES | fossa: | sinus: |
|---|---|---|
| | anterior | ethmoid |
| | middle | frontal |
| | posterior | sphenoid bone |
| | occiput bone | temporal bone |
| | orbital roof | |

**AHA:** 4Q, '96, 36

**DEF:** Fracture of bone that forms skull floor.

§ ✓5th **801.0 Closed without mention of intracranial injury**    MCC 3-5   CC 0-2, 6, 9
**CC Excl:** 800.00-801.99, 803.00-804.99, 829.0-829.1, 850.0-852.19, 852.21-854.19, 873.8-873.9, 879.8-879.9, 905.0,925.1-925.2,929.0-929.9,958.8-959.09, 959.8-959.9

§ ✓5th **801.1 Closed with cerebral laceration and contusion**    MCC
**CC Excl:** See code: 801.0

**AHA:** 4Q, '96, 36

§ ✓5th **801.2 Closed with subarachnoid, subdural, and extradural hemorrhage**    MCC
**CC Excl:** See code: 801.0

§ ✓5th **801.3 Closed with other and unspecified intracranial hemorrhage**    MCC
**CC Excl:** See code: 801.0

§ ✓5th **801.4 Closed with intracranial injury of other and unspecified nature**    MCC 3-5   CC 0-2, 6, 9
**CC Excl:** See code 801.0

§ ✓5th **801.5 Open without mention of intracranial injury**    MCC
**CC Excl:** See code: 801.0

§ ✓5th **801.6 Open with cerebral laceration and contusion**    MCC
**CC Excl:** See code: 801.0

§ ✓5th **801.7 Open with subarachnoid, subdural, and extradural hemorrhage**    MCC
**CC Excl:** See code: 801.0

§ ✓5th **801.8 Open with other and unspecified intracranial hemorrhage**    MCC
**CC Excl:** See code: 801.0

§ ✓5th **801.9 Open with intracranial injury of other and unspecified nature**    MCC
**CC Excl:** See code: 801.0

✓4th **802 Fracture of face bones**

**AHA:** 4Q, '96, 36

**802.0 Nasal bones, closed**
**802.1 Nasal bones, open**    CC
**CC Excl:** 800.00-802.1, 803.00-804.99, 829.0-829.1, 850.0-852.19, 852.21-854.19, 873.8-873.9, 879.8-879.9, 905.0,925.1-925.2,929.0-929.9,958.8-959.09, 959.8-959.9

✓5th **802.2 Mandible, closed**
Inferior maxilla    Lower jaw (bone)

    **802.20 Unspecified site**    CC
    **CC Excl:** 800.00-801.99, 802.20-802.5, 803.00-804.99, 829.0-830.1, 850.0-852.19, 852.21-854.19, 873.8-873.9, 879.8-879.9, 905.0,925.1-925.2,929.0-929.9,958.8-959.09, 959.8-959.9

    **802.21 Condylar process**    CC
    **CC Excl:** See code 802.20

    **802.22 Subcondylar**    CC
    **CC Excl:** See code 802.20

    **802.23 Coronoid process**    CC
    **CC Excl:** See code 802.20

**Facial Fractures**

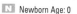

**LeFort Fracture Types**

Frontal bone, Nasal bone, Orbital floor, Zygomatic bone (malar) and arch, Subcondylar, Body, Angle, Maxilla, Symphysis, Parasymphysis

Type III, Type II, Type I

**Common Fracture Sites of Mandible**

    **802.24 Ramus, unspecified**    CC
    **CC Excl:** See code 802.20

    **802.25 Angle of jaw**    CC
    **CC Excl:** See code 802.20

    **802.26 Symphysis of body**    CC
    **CC Excl:** See code 802.20

    **802.27 Alveolar border of body**    CC
    **CC Excl:** See code 802.20

    **802.28 Body, other and unspecified**    CC
    **CC Excl:** See code 802.20

    **802.29 Multiple sites**    CC
    **CC Excl:** See code 802.20

✓5th **802.3 Mandible, open**
    **802.30 Unspecified site**    CC
    **CC Excl:** See code 802.20

    **802.31 Condylar process**    CC
    **CC Excl:** See code 802.20

    **802.32 Subcondylar**    CC
    **CC Excl:** See code 802.20

    **802.33 Coronoid process**    CC
    **CC Excl:** See code 802.20

    **802.34 Ramus, unspecified**    CC
    **CC Excl:** See code 802.20

    **802.35 Angle of jaw**    CC
    **CC Excl:** See code 802.20

    **802.36 Symphysis of body**    CC
    **CC Excl:** See code 802.20

    **802.37 Alveolar border of body**    CC
    **CC Excl:** See code 802.20

    **802.38 Body, other and unspecified**    CC
    **CC Excl:** See code 802.20

    **802.39 Multiple sites**    CC
    **CC Excl:** See code 802.20

**802.4 Malar and maxillary bones, closed**    CC
Superior maxilla    Zygoma
Upper jaw (bone)    Zygomatic arch
**CC Excl:** See code 802.20

**802.5 Malar and maxillary bones, open**    CC
**CC Excl:** See code 802.20

**802.6 Orbital floor (blow-out), closed**    CC
**CC Excl:** 800.00-801.99, 802.6-804.99, 829.0-829.1, 850.0-852.19, 852.21-854.19, 873.8-873.9, 879.8-879.9, 905.0,925.1-925.2,929.0-929.9,958.8-959.09, 959.8-959.9

§   Requires fifth-digit. See beginning of section 800-804 for codes and definitions.

 Newborn Age: 0     Pediatric Age: 0-17    M Maternity Age: 12-55    A Adult Age: 15-124    CC CC Condition    MCC Major CC Condition     HIV HIV Related Dx

294 — Volume 1 • October 2007       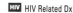 © 2007 Ingenix

802.7　**Orbital floor (blow-out), open**　　`CC`
CC Excl: See code 802.6

802.8　**Other facial bones, closed**　　`CC`
　　Alveolus　　　　　　Palate
　　Orbit:
　　　NOS
　　　part other than roof or floor
　　`EXCLUDES`　*orbital:*
　　　　　　　　*floor (802.6)*
　　　　　　　　*roof (801.0-801.9)*
CC Excl: See code 802.6

802.9　**Other facial bones, open**　　`CC`
CC Excl: See code 802.6

`✓4ᵗʰ` **803　Other and unqualified skull fractures**
　　`INCLUDES`　skull NOS　　　skull multiple NOS
　　**AHA:** 4Q, '96, 36

§ `✓5ᵗʰ` 803.0　**Closed without mention of**　`MCC 3-5` `CC 0-2, 6, 9`
　　　　**intracranial injury**
CC Excl: 800.00-801.99, 803.00-804.99, 829.0-829.1, 850.0-852.19,
852.21-854.19, 873.8-873.9, 879.8-879.9, 905.0,925.1-925.2,929.0-
929.9,958.8-959.09, 959.8-959.9

§ `✓5ᵗʰ` 803.1　**Closed with cerebral laceration and**　`MCC`
　　　　**contusion**
CC Excl: See code 803.0

§ `✓5ᵗʰ` 803.2　**Closed with subarachnoid, subdural, and**　`MCC`
　　　　**extradural hemorrhage**
CC Excl: See code 803.0

§ `✓5ᵗʰ` 803.3　**Closed with other and unspecified**　`MCC`
　　　　**intracranial hemorrhage**
CC Excl: See code 803.0

§ `✓5ᵗʰ` 803.4　**Closed with intracranial injury**　`MCC 3-5` `CC 0-2, 6, 9`
　　　　**of other and unspecified nature**
CC Excl: See code 803.0

§ `✓5ᵗʰ` 803.5　**Open without mention of intracranial injury**　`MCC`
CC Excl: See code 803.0

§ `✓5ᵗʰ` 803.6　**Open with cerebral laceration and contusion**　`MCC`
CC Excl: See code 803.0

§ `✓5ᵗʰ` 803.7　**Open with subarachnoid, subdural, and**　`MCC`
　　　　**extradural hemorrhage**
CC Excl: See code 803.0

§ `✓5ᵗʰ` 803.8　**Open with other and unspecified**　`MCC`
　　　　**intracranial hemorrhage**
CC Excl: See code 803.0

§ `✓5ᵗʰ` 803.9　**Open with intracranial injury of other and**　`MCC`
　　　　**unspecified nature**
CC Excl: See code 803.0

`✓4ᵗʰ` **804　Multiple fractures involving skull or face with other bones**
　　**AHA:** 4Q, '96, 36

§ `✓5ᵗʰ` 804.0　**Closed without mention of**　`MCC 3-5` `CC 0-2, 6, 9`
　　　　**intracranial injury**
CC Excl: 800.00-801.99, 803.00-804.99, 829.0-829.1, 850.0-852.19,
852.21-854.19, 873.8-873.9, 879.8-879.9, 905.0,925.1-925.2,929.0-
929.9,958.8-959.09, 959.8-959.9

§ `✓5ᵗʰ` 804.1　**Closed with cerebral laceration and**　`MCC`
　　　　**contusion**
CC Excl: See code: 804.0
　　**AHA:** For code 804.10: 1Q, '06, 6

§ `✓5ᵗʰ` 804.2　**Closed with subarachnoid, subdural, and**　`MCC`
　　　　**extradural hemorrhage**
CC Excl: See code: 804.0

§ `✓5ᵗʰ` 804.3　**Closed with other and unspecified**　`MCC`
　　　　**intracranial hemorrhage**
CC Excl: See code: 804.0

§ `✓5ᵗʰ` 804.4　**Closed with intracranial injury**　`MCC 3-5` `CC 0-2, 6, 9`
　　　　**of other and unspecified nature**
CC Excl: See code: 804.0

§ `✓5ᵗʰ` 804.5　**Open without mention of**　`MCC 3-5` `CC 0-2, 6, 9`
　　　　**intracranial injury**
CC Excl: See code: 804.0

§ `✓5ᵗʰ` 804.6　**Open with cerebral laceration and**　`MCC`
　　　　**contusion**
CC Excl: See code: 804.0

§ `✓5ᵗʰ` 804.7　**Open with subarachnoid, subdural, and**　`MCC`
　　　　**extradural hemorrage**
CC Excl: See code: 804.0

§ `✓5ᵗʰ` 804.8　**Open with other and unspecified**　`MCC`
　　　　**intracranial hemorrhage**
CC Excl: See code: 804.0

§ `✓5ᵗʰ` 804.9　**Open with intracranial injury of**　`MCC 3-5` `CC 0-2, 6, 9`
　　　　**other and unspecified nature**
CC Excl: See code: 804.0

## FRACTURE OF NECK AND TRUNK (805-809)

`✓4ᵗʰ` **805　Fracture of vertebral column without mention of spinal cord injury**
　　`INCLUDES`　neural arch　　　transverse process
　　　　　　　　spine　　　　　vertebra
　　　　　　　　spinous process

The following fifth-digit subclassification is for use with codes 805.0-805.1:
　　0　cervical vertebra, unspecified level
　　1　first cervical vertebra
　　2　second cervical vertebra
　　3　third cervical vertebra
　　4　fourth cervical vertebra
　　5　fifth cervical vertebra
　　6　sixth cervical vertebra
　　7　seventh cervical vertebra
　　8　multiple cervical vertebrae

`✓5ᵗʰ` 805.0　**Cervical, closed**　　`CC`
　　　　Atlas　　　　　　Axis
CC Excl: 805.00-805.18, 805.8-806.19, 806.8-806.9, 829.0-829.1, 839.00-
839.18, 839.40, 839.49-839.50, 839.59, 839.69, 839.79-839.9, 847.0, 847.9,
848.8-848.9, 879.8-879.9, 905.1, 926.11,929.0-929.9,952.00-952.09,952.8-
952.9,958.8-958.99,959.11-959.19, 959.8-959.9

`✓5ᵗʰ` 805.1　**Cervical, open**　　`MCC`
CC Excl: See code 805.0

805.2　**Dorsal [thoracic], closed**　　`CC`
CC Excl: 805.2-805.3, 805.8-805.9, 806.20-806.39, 806.8-806.9, 829.0-
829.1, 839.21, 839.31-839.40, 839.49-839.50, 839.59, 839.69, 839.79-839.9,
847.1, 847.9, 848.8-848.9, 879.8-879.9, 905.1, 926.11,929.0-929.9,952.10-
952.19,952.8-952.9,958.8-958.99,959.11-959.19, 959.8-959.9

805.3　**Dorsal [thoracic], open**　　`MCC`
CC Excl: See code 805.2

805.4　**Lumbar, closed**　　`CC`
CC Excl: 805.4-805.5, 805.8-805.9, 806.4-806.5, 806.8-806.9, 829.0-829.1,
839.20, 839.30, 839.40, 839.49-839.50, 839.59, 839.69, 839.79-839.9,
847.2, 847.9, 848.8-848.9, 879.8-879.9, 905.1, 926.11,929.0-929.9,
952.2,952.8-952.9,958.8-958.99,959.11-959.19, 959.8-959.9

　　**AHA:** ▶1Q, '07, 7;◀ 4Q, '99, 12

805.5　**Lumbar, open**　　`MCC`
CC Excl: See code 805.4

805.6　**Sacrum and coccyx, closed**　　`CC`
CC Excl: 805.6-805.9, 806.60-806.9, 829.0-829.1, 839.40-839.59, 839.69,
839.79-839.9, 846.0-846.9, 847.3-847.9, 848.5-848.9, 879.8-879.9, 905.1,
926.11,929.0-929.9,952.3-952.9,958.8-958.99,959.11-959.19, 959.8-959.9

§　Requires fifth-digit. See beginning of section 800-804 for codes and definitions.

`✓4ᵗʰ`／`✓5ᵗʰ` Additional Digit Required　　　　Unacceptable PDx　　　Manifestation Code　　　▶◀ Revised Text　　　● New Code　　　▲ Revised Code Title

© 2007 Ingenix　　　　　　　　　　　　　　　　　　　　　　　October 2007 • Volume 1 — 295

## Vertebral Column

**805.7** **Sacrum and coccyx, open** `MCC`
CC Excl: See code 805.6

**805.8** **Unspecified, closed** `CC`
CC Excl: 733.10-733.19, 733.93-733.95, 805.00-806.9, 829.0-829.1, 839.00-839.59, 839.69, 839.79-839.9, 846.0-847.9, 848.5-848.9, 879.8-879.9, 905.1, 926.11,929.0-929.9,952.00-952.9,958.8-958.99,959.11-959.19, 959.8-959.9

**805.9** **Unspecified, open** `MCC`
CC Excl: See code 805.8

✓4ᵗʰ **806 Fracture of vertebral column with spinal cord injury**

INCLUDES any condition classifiable to 805 with:
complete or incomplete transverse lesion (of cord)
hematomyelia
injury to:
    cauda equina
    nerve
paralysis
paraplegia
quadriplegia
spinal concussion

✓5ᵗʰ **806.0** **Cervical, closed**

**806.00** **$C_1$-$C_4$ level with unspecified spinal** `MCC`
**cord injury**
Cervical region NOS with spinal cord injury NOS
CC Excl: 733.10-733.19, 733.93-733.95, 805.00-805.18, 805.8-806.19, 806.8-806.9, 829.0-829.1, 839.00-839.18, 839.40, 839.49-839.50, 839.59, 839.69, 839.79-839.9, 847.9, 848.8-848.9, 879.8-879.9, 905.1, 926.11,929.0-929.9,952.00-952.09,952.8-952.9,958.8-958.99,959.11-959.19, 959.8-959.9

**806.01** **$C_1$-$C_4$ level with complete lesion of** `MCC`
**cord**
CC Excl: See code 806.00

**806.02** **$C_1$-$C_4$ level with anterior cord** `MCC`
**syndrome**
CC Excl: See code 806.00

**806.03** **$C_1$-$C_4$ level with central cord** `MCC`
**Syndrome**
CC Excl: See code 806.00

**806.04** **$C_1$-$C_4$ level with other specified** `MCC`
**spinal cord injury**
$C_1$-$C_4$ level with:
incomplete spinal cord lesion NOS
posterior cord syndrome
CC Excl: See code 806.00

**806.05** **$C_5$-$C_7$ level with unspecified spinal** `MCC`
**cord injury**
CC Excl: See code 806.00

**806.06** **$C_5$-$C_7$ level with complete lesion of** `MCC`
**cord**
CC Excl: See code 806.00

**806.07** **$C_5$-$C_7$ level with anterior cord** `MCC`
**syndrome**
CC Excl: See code 806.00

**806.08** **$C_5$-$C_7$ level with central cord** `MCC`
**syndrome**
CC Excl: See code 806.00

**806.09** **$C_5$-$C_7$ level with other specified** `MCC`
**spinal cord injury**
$C_5$-$C_7$ level with:
incomplete spinal cord lesion NOS
posterior cord syndrome
CC Excl: See code 806.00

✓5ᵗʰ **806.1** **Cervical, open**

**806.10** **$C_1$-$C_4$ level with unspecified spinal** `MCC`
**cord injury**
CC Excl: See code 806.00

**806.11** **$C_1$-$C_4$ level with complete lesion of** `MCC`
**cord**
CC Excl: See code 806.00

**806.12** **$C_1$-$C_4$ level with anterior cord** `MCC`
**syndrome**
CC Excl: See code 806.00

**806.13** **$C_1$-$C_4$ level with central cord** `MCC`
**syndrome**
CC Excl: See code 806.00

**806.14** **$C_1$-$C_4$ level with other specified** `MCC`
**spinal cord injury**
$C_1$-$C_4$ level with:
incomplete spinal cord lesion NOS
posterior cord syndrome
CC Excl: See code 806.00

**806.15** **$C_5$-$C_7$ level with unspecified spinal** `MCC`
**cord injury**
CC Excl: See code 806.00

**806.16** **$C_5$-$C_7$ level with complete lesion of** `MCC`
**cord**
CC Excl: See code 806.00

**806.17** **$C_5$-$C_7$ level with anterior cord** `MCC`
**syndrome**
CC Excl: See code 806.00

**806.18** **$C_5$-$C_7$ level with central cord** `MCC`
**syndrome**
CC Excl: See code 806.00

**806.19** **$C_5$-$C_7$ level with other specified** `MCC`
**spinal cord injury**
$C_5$-$C_7$ level with:
incomplete spinal cord lesion NOS
posterior cord syndrome
CC Excl: See code 806.00

 Newborn Age: 0   P Pediatric Age: 0-17   M Maternity Age: 12-55   A Adult Age: 15-124   CC CC Condition   MCC Major CC Condition   HIV HIV Related Dx

296 — Volume 1 • October 2007                                                                   © 2007 Ingenix

√5th **806.2**   **Dorsal [thoracic], closed**

**806.20**   $T_1$-$T_6$ level with unspecified spinal cord injury    `MCC`

     Thoracic region NOS with spinal cord injury NOS

     **CC Excl:** 733.10-733.19, 733.93-733.95, 805.2-805.3, 805.8-805.9, 806.20-806.39, 806.8-806.9, 829.0-829.1, 839.21, 839.31-839.40, 839.49-839.50, 839.59, 839.69, 839.79-839.9, 847.1, 847.9, 848.8-848.9, 879.8-879.9, 905.1, 926.11,929.0-929.9,952.10-952.19,952.8-952.9,958.8-958.99,959.11-959.19, 959.8-959.9

**806.21**   $T_1$-$T_6$ level with complete lesion of cord    `MCC`

     **CC Excl:** See code 806.20

**806.22**   $T_1$-$T_6$ level with anterior cord syndrome    `MCC`

     **CC Excl:** See code 806.20

**806.23**   $T_1$-$T_6$ level with central cord syndrome    `MCC`

     **CC Excl:** See code 806.20

**806.24**   $T_1$-$T_6$ level with other specified spinal cord injury    `MCC`

     $T_1$-$T_6$ level with:
       incomplete spinal cord lesion NOS
       posterior cord syndrome

     **CC Excl:** See code 806.20

**806.25**   $T_7$-$T_{12}$ level with unspecified spinal cord injury    `MCC`

     **CC Excl:** See code 806.20

**806.26**   $T_7$-$T_{12}$ level with complete lesion of cord    `MCC`

     **CC Excl:** See code 806.20

**806.27**   $T_7$-$T_{12}$ level with anterior cord syndrome    `MCC`

     **CC Excl:** See code 806.20

**806.28**   $T_7$-$T_{12}$ level with central cord syndrome    `MCC`

     **CC Excl:** See code 806.20

**806.29**   $T_7$-$T_{12}$ level with other specified spinal cord injury    `MCC`

     $T_7$-$T_{12}$ level with:
       incomplete spinal cord lesion NOS
       posterior cord syndrome

     **CC Excl:** See code 806.20

√5th **806.3**   **Dorsal [thoracic], open**

**806.30**   $T_1$-$T_6$ level with unspecified spinal cord injury    `MCC`

     **CC Excl:** See code 806.20

**806.31**   $T_1$-$T_6$ level with complete lesion of cord    `MCC`

     **CC Excl:** See code 806.20

**806.32**   $T_1$-$T_6$ level with anteriorr cord syndrome    `MCC`

     **CC Excl:** See code 806.20

**806.33**   $T_1$-$T_6$ level with centralr cord syndrome    `MCC`

     **CC Excl:** See code 806.20

**806.34**   $T_1$-$T_6$ level with other specified spinal cord injury    `MCC`

     $T_1$-$T_6$ level with:
       incomplete spinal cord lesion NOS
       posterior cord syndrome

     **CC Excl:** See code 806.20

**806.35**   $T_7$-$T_{12}$ level with unspecified spinal cord injury    `MCC`

     **CC Excl:** See code 806.20

**806.36**   $T_7$-$T_{12}$ level with complete lesion of cord    `MCC`

     **CC Excl:** See code 806.20

**806.37**   $T_7$-$T_{12}$ level with anterior cord syndrome    `MCC`

     **CC Excl:** See code 806.20

**806.38**   $T_7$-$T_{12}$ level with central cord syndrome    `MCC`

     **CC Excl:** See code 806.20

**806.39**   $T_7$-$T_{12}$ level with other specified spinal cord injury    `MCC`

     $T_7$-$T_{12}$ level with:
       incomplete spinal cord lesion NOS
       posterior cord syndrome

     **CC Excl:** See code 806.20

**806.4**   **Lumbar, closed**    `MCC`

     **CC Excl:** 733.10-733.19, 733.93-733.95, 805.4-805.5, 805.8-805.9, 806.4-806.5, 806.8-806.9, 829.0-829.1, 839.20, 839.30, 839.40, 839.49-839.50, 839.59, 839.69, 839.79-839.9, 847.2, 847.9, 848.8-848.9, 879.8-879.9, 905.1, 926.11,929.0-929.9, 952.2,952.8-952.9,958.8-958.99,959.11-959.19, 959.8-959.9

     **AHA:** 4Q, '99, 11, 13

**806.5**   **Lumbar, open**    `MCC`

     **CC Excl:** See code 806.4

√5th **806.6**   **Sacrum and coccyx, closed**

**806.60**   With unspecified spinal cord injury    `MCC`

     **CC Excl:** 733.10-733.19, 733.93-733.95, 805.6-805.9, 806.60-806.9, 829.0-829.1, 839.40-839.59, 839.69, 839.79-839.9, 846.0-847.0, 847.3-847.9, 848.5-848.9, 879.8-879.9, 905.1, 926.11,929.0-929.9,952.3-952.9,958.8-958.99,959.11-959.19, 959.8-959.9

**806.61**   With complete cauda equina lesion    `MCC`

     **CC Excl:** See code 806.60

**806.62**   With other cauda equina injury    `MCC`

     **CC Excl:** See code 806.60

**806.69**   With other spinal cord injury    `MCC`

     **CC Excl:** See code 806.60

√5th **806.7**   **Sacrum and coccyx, open**

**806.70**   With unspecified spinal cord injury    `MCC`

     **CC Excl:** See code 806.60

**806.71**   With complete cauda equina lesion    `MCC`

     **CC Excl:** See code 806.60

**806.72**   With other cauda equina injury    `MCC`

     **CC Excl:** See code 806.60

**806.79**   With other spinal cord injury    `MCC`

     **CC Excl:** See code 806.60

**806.8**   **Unspecified, closed**    `MCC`

     **CC Excl:** 733.10-733.19, 733.93-733.95, 805.00-806.9, 829.0-829.1, 839.00-839.59, 839.69, 839.79-839.9, 846.0-847.9, 848.5-848.9, 879.8-879.9, 905.1, 926.11,929.0-929.9,952.00-952.9,958.8-958.99,959.11-959.19, 959.8-959.9

**806.9**   **Unspecified, open**    `MCC`

     **CC Excl:** See code 806.8

**Injury and Poisoning**

**807–809.0**

✓4th **807 Fracture of rib(s), sternum, larynx, and trachea**

The following fifth-digit subclassification is for use with codes 807.0-807.1:

0   rib(s), unspecified
1   one rib
2   two ribs
3   three ribs
4   four ribs
5   five ribs
6   six ribs
7   seven ribs
8   eight or more ribs
9   multiple ribs, unspecified

✓5th **807.0 Rib(s), closed** `CC`
CC Excl: **For codes 807.00-807.02:** 807.00-807.4, 819.0-819.1, 828.0-829.1, 848.8-848.9, 879.8-879.9,929.0-929.9,958.8-958.99, 959.8-959.9; **For code 807.03:** 807.00-807.19, 807.4, 819.0-819.1, 828.0-829.1, 848.8-848.9, 879.8-879.9,929.0-929.9, 958.8, 959.8-959.9; **For codes 807.04-807.09:** 807.00-807.19, 807.4, 819.0-819.1, 828.0-829.1, 848.8-848.9, 879.8-879.9,929.0-929.9,958.8-958.99, 959.8-959.9

✓5th **807.1 Rib(s), open** `MCC`
CC Excl: 807.00-807.19, 807.4, 819.0-819.1, 828.0-829.1, 848.8-848.9, 879.8-879.9,929.0-929.9,958.8-958.99, 959.8-959.9

**807.2 Sternum, closed** `CC`
CC Excl: 807.2-807.4, 829.0-829.1, 848.8-848.9, 879.8-879.9,929.0-929.9,958.8-958.99, 959.8-959.9

DEF: Break in flat bone (breast bone) in anterior thorax.

**807.3 Sternum, open** `MCC`
CC Excl: See code: 807.2

DEF: Break, with open wound, in flat bone in mid anterior thorax.

**807.4 Flail chest** `MCC`
CC Excl: 807.00-807.4, 829.0-829.1, 848.8-848.9, 879.8-879.9,929.0-929.9,958.8-958.99, 959.8-959.9

**807.5 Larynx and trachea, closed** `MCC`
Hyoid bone      Trachea
Thyroid cartilage
CC Excl: 807.5-807.6, 829.0-829.1, 848.8-848.9, 879.8-879.9,929.0-929.9,958.8-958.99, 959.8-959.9

**807.6 Larynx and trachea, open** `MCC`
CC Excl: See code 807.5

✓4th **808 Fracture of pelvis**

**808.0 Acetabulum, closed** `MCC`
CC Excl: 733.10-733.19, 733.93-733.95, 808.0-808.1, 808.43-808.49, 808.53-809.1, 829.0-829.1, 835.00-835.13, 843.0-843.9, 846.0-846.9, 848.5-848.9, 879.8-879.9,929.0-929.9,958.8-958.99, 959.6, 959.8-959.9

**808.1 Acetabulum, open** `MCC`
CC Excl: 808.0-808.1, 808.43-808.49, 808.53-809.1, 829.0-829.1, 835.00-835.13, 843.0-843.9, 846.0-846.9, 848.5-848.9, 879.8-879.9,929.0-929.9,958.8-958.99, 959.6, 959.8-959.9

**808.2 Pubis, closed** `CC`
CC Excl: 733.10-733.19, 733.93-733.95, 808.2-808.3, 808.43-808.49, 808.53-809.1, 829.0-829.1, 835.00-835.13, 843.0-843.9, 846.0-846.9, 848.5-848.9, 879.8-879.9,929.0-929.9,958.8-958.99, 959.6, 959.8-959.9

**808.3 Pubis, open** `MCC`
CC Excl: See code 808.2

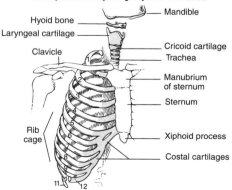

**Ribs, Sternum, Larynx, and Trachea**

Hyoid bone
Laryngeal cartilage
Clavicle
Rib cage
Mandible
Cricoid cartilage
Trachea
Manubrium of sternum
Sternum
Xiphoid process
Costal cartilages

**Pelvis and Pelvic Fractures**

Fractures Disrupting Pelvic Circle

Pelvic circle
Stable

Unstable (two-place fracture)

Iliac crest
Anterior superior iliac spine
Ischial spine
Acetabulum
Ilium
L5
Sacrum
Coccyx
Pubis
Femur
Ischial tuberosity
Pubic symphysis

Pelvic Bones

Acetabular Fractures
Posterior pillar
Transverse

✓5th **808.4 Other specified part, closed**
**808.41 Ilium** `CC`
CC Excl: 733.10, 733.19, 808.0-809.1, 829.0-829.1, 835.00-835.13, 843.0-843.9, 846.0-846.9, 848.5-848.9, 879.8-879.9,929.0-929.9, 958.8, 958.99, 959.6, 959.8-959.9

**808.42 Ischium** `CC`
CC Excl: 808.42

**808.43 Multiple pelvic fractures with disruption of pelvic circle** `CC`
CC Excl: 733.10-733.19, 733.93-733.95, 808.0-809.1, 829.0-829.1, 835.00-835.13, 843.0-843.9, 846.0-846.9, 848.5-848.9, 879.8-879.9,929.0-929.9,958.8-958.99, 959.6, 959.8-959.9

**808.49 Other** `CC`
Innominate bone
Pelvic rim
CC Excl: See code: 808.43

✓5th **808.5 Other specified part, open**
**808.51 Ilium** `MCC`
CC Excl: 733.10-733.19, 733.93-733.95, 808.41, 808.43-808.51, 808.53-809.1, 829.0-829.1, 835.00-835.13, 843.0-843.9, 846.0-846.9, 848.5-848.9, 879.8-879.9,929.0-929.9,958.8-958.99, 959.6, 959.8-959.9

**808.52 Ischium** `MCC`
CC Excl: 733.10-733.19, 733.93-733.95, 808.42-808.49, 808.52-809.1, 829.0-829.1, 835.00-835.13, 843.0-843.9, 846.0-846.9, 848.5-848.9, 879.8-879.9,929.0-929.9,958.8-958.99, 959.6, 959.8-959.9

**808.53 Multiple pelvic fractures with disruption of pelvic circle** `MCC`
CC Excl: See code: 808.43

**808.59 Other** `MCC`
CC Excl: See code: 808.43

**808.8 Unspecified, closed** `CC`
CC Excl: See code: 808.43

**808.9 Unspecified, open** `MCC`
CC Excl: See code: 808.43

✓4th **809 Ill-defined fractures of bones of trunk**
`INCLUDES` bones of trunk with other bones except those of skull and face
multiple bones of trunk
`EXCLUDES` *multiple fractures of:*
*pelvic bones alone (808.0-808.9)*
*ribs alone (807.0-807.1, 807.4)*
*ribs or sternum with limb bones (819.0-819.1, 828.0-828.1)*
*skull or face with other bones (804.0-804.9)*

**809.0 Fracture of bones of trunk, closed** `CC`
CC Excl: 733.10, 733.19, 808.0-809.1, 829.0-829.1, 835.00-835.13, 843.0-843.9, 846.0-846.9, 848.5-848.9, 879.8-879.9,929.0-929.9, 958.8, 958.99, 959.6, 959.8-959.9

`N` Newborn Age: 0    `P` Pediatric Age: 0-17    `M` Maternity Age: 12-55    `A` Adult Age: 15-124    `CC` CC Condition    `MCC` Major CC Condition    `HIV` HIV Related Dx

**809.1**    **Fracture of bones of trunk, open**    `MCC`
CC Excl: See code: 809.0

## FRACTURE OF UPPER LIMB (810-819)

✓4th **810 Fracture of clavicle**

INCLUDES    collar bone
interligamentous part of clavicle

The following fifth-digit subclassification is for use with category 810:

   **0 unspecified part**
     Clavicle NOS
   **1 sternal end of clavicle**
   **2 shaft of clavicle**
   **3 acromial end of clavicle**

✓5th **810.0 Closed**
✓5th **810.1 Open**    `CC`
CC Excl: 810.00-810.13, 818.0-819.1

✓4th **811 Fracture of scapula**

INCLUDES    shoulder blade

The following fifth-digit subclassification is for use with category 811:

   **0 unspecified part**
   **1 acromial process**
     Acromion (process)
   **2 coracoid process**
   **3 glenoid cavity and neck of scapula**
   **9 other**

✓5th **811.0 Closed**
✓5th **811.1 Open**    `CC`
CC Excl: 811.00-811.19, 818.0-819.1

✓4th **812 Fracture of humerus**
   ✓5th **812.0 Upper end, closed**

     **812.00 Upper end, unspecified part**    `CC`
       Proximal end      Shoulder
     CC Excl: 812.00-812.59, 819.0-819.1

     **812.01 Surgical neck**    `CC`
       Neck of humerus NOS
     CC Excl: See code: 812.00

     **812.02 Anatomical neck**    `CC`
     CC Excl: See code: 812.00

     **812.03 Greater tuberosity**    `CC`
     CC Excl: See code: 812.00

     **812.09 Other**    `CC`
       Head        Upper epiphysis
       Lesser tuberosity
     CC Excl: See code: 812.00

   ✓5th **812.1 Upper end, open**
     **812.10 Upper end, unspecified part**    `MCC`
     CC Excl: 812.10-812.59, 818.0-819.1

     **812.11 Surgical neck**    `MCC`
     CC Excl: See code: 812.10

     **812.12 Anatomical neck**    `MCC`
     CC Excl: See code: 812.10

     **812.13 Greater tuberosity**    `MCC`
     CC Excl: See code: 812.10

     **812.19 Other**    `MCC`
     CC Excl: See code: 812.10

   ✓5th **812.2 Shaft or unspecified part, closed**
     **812.20 Unspecified part of humerus**    `CC`
       Humerus NOS      Upper arm NOS
       Lesser tuberosity
     CC Excl: See code: 812.00

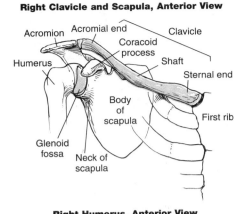

**Right Clavicle and Scapula, Anterior View**

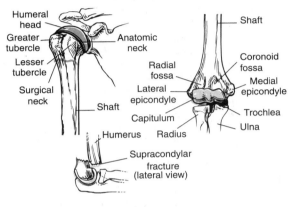

**Right Humerus, Anterior View**

     **812.21 Shaft of humerus**    `CC`
     CC Excl: 812.21

     AHA: 4Q, '05, 129; 3Q, '99, 14

✓5th **812.3 Shaft or unspecified part, open**
     **812.30 Unspecified part of humerus**    `MCC`
     CC Excl: See code: 812.10

     **812.31 Shaft of humerus**    `MCC`
     CC Excl: See code: 812.10

✓5th **812.4 Lower end, closed**
     Distal end of humerus      Elbow
     **812.40 Lower end, unspecified part**    `CC`
     CC Excl: 812.00-812.59, 819.0-819.1

     **812.41 Supracondylar fracture of humerus**    `CC`
     CC Excl: See code: 812.40

     **812.42 Lateral condyle**    `CC`
       External condyle
     CC Excl: See code: 812.40

     **812.43 Medial condyle**    `CC`
       Internal epicondyle
     CC Excl: See code: 812.40

     **812.44 Condyle(s), unspecified**    `CC`
       Articular process NOS
       Lower epiphysis NOS
     CC Excl: See code: 812.40

     **812.49 Other**    `CC`
       Multiple fractures of lower end
       Trochlea
     CC Excl: See code: 812.40

✓5th **812.5 Lower end, open**
     **812.50 Lower end, unspecified part**    `MCC`
     CC Excl: 812.00-812.59, 819.0-819.1

---

✓4th ✓5th Additional Digit Required      Unacceptable PDx      Manifestation Code      ▶◀ Revised Text      ● New Code      ▲ Revised Code Title

**Injury and Poisoning**

**812.51–813.52**

**812.51 Supracondylar fracture of humerus** `MCC`
CC Excl: See code: 812.50

**812.52 Lateral condyle** `MCC`
CC Excl: See code: 812.50

**812.53 Medial condyle** `MCC`
CC Excl: See code: 812.50

**812.54 Condyle(s), unspecified** `MCC`
CC Excl: See code: 812.50

**812.59 Other** `MCC`
CC Excl: See code: 812.50

√4th **813 Fracture of radius and ulna**
√5th **813.0 Upper end, closed**
Proximal end
**813.00 Upper end of forearm, unspecified**
**813.01 Olecranon process of ulna**
**813.02 Coronoid process of ulna**
**813.03 Monteggia's fracture**
DEF: Fracture near the head of the ulnar shaft, causing dislocation of the radial head.
**813.04 Other and unspecified fractures of proximal end of ulna (alone)**
Multiple fractures of ulna, upper end
**813.05 Head of radius**
**813.06 Neck of radius**
**813.07 Other and unspecified fractures of proximal end of radius (alone)**
Multiple fractures of radius, upper end
**813.08 Radius with ulna, upper end [any part]**
√5th **813.1 Upper end, open**
**813.10 Upper end of forearm, unspecified** `MCC`
CC Excl: 813.10-813.44, 813.50-813.93, 818.0-819.1

**813.11 Olecranon process of ulna** `MCC`
CC Excl: 813.10-813.40, 813.42-813.44, 813.50-813.93, 818.0-819.1

**813.12 Coronoid process of ulna** `MCC`
CC Excl: See code: 813.10

**813.13 Monteggia's fracture** `MCC`
CC Excl: See code: 813.10

**813.14 Other and unspecified fractures of proximal end of ulna (alone)** `MCC`
CC Excl: See code: 813.10

**813.15 Head of radius** `MCC`
CC Excl: See code: 813.10

**813.16 Neck of radius** `MCC`
CC Excl: See code: 813.10

**Right Radius and Ulna, Anterior View**

Olecranon process
Coronoid process
Radius
Ulna
Radius
Colles' fracture
Shafts
Radial styloid process
Ulnar styloid process
Humerus (lateral view)
Radius dislocated
Monteggia's fracture-dislocation

**813.17 Other and unspecified fractures of proximal end of radius (alone)** `MCC`
CC Excl: See code: 813.10

**813.18 Radius with ulna, upper end [any part]** `MCC`
CC Excl: See code: 813.10

√5th **813.2 Shaft, closed**
**813.20 Shaft, unspecified** `CC`
CC Excl: 813.00-813.93, 819.0-819.1

**813.21 Radius (alone)** `CC`
CC Excl: See code: 813.20

**813.22 Ulna (alone)** `CC`
CC Excl: See code: 813.20

**813.23 Radius with ulna** `CC`
CC Excl: See code: 813.20

√5th **813.3 Shaft, open**
**813.30 Shaft, unspecified** `MCC`
CC Excl: 813.10-813.44, 813.50-813.93, 818.0-819.1

**813.31 Radius (alone)** `MCC`
CC Excl: See code: 813.30

**813.32 Ulna (alone)** `MCC`
CC Excl: See code: 813.30

**813.33 Radius with ulna** `MCC`
CC Excl: See code: 813.30

√5th **813.4 Lower end, closed**
Distal end
**813.40 Lower end of forearm, unspecified** `CC`
CC Excl: 813.00-813.93, 819.0-819.1

**813.41 Colles' fracture** `CC`
Smith's fracture
CC Excl: See code: 813.40

DEF: Break of lower end of radius; associated with backward movement of the radius lower section.
**813.42 Other fractures of distal end of radius (alone)** `CC`
Dupuytren's fracture, radius
Radius, lower end
CC Excl: See code: 813.40

DEF: Dupuytren's fracture: fracture and dislocation of the forearm; the fracture is of the radius above the wrist, and the dislocation is of the ulna at the lower end.
**813.43 Distal end of ulna (alone)** `CC`
Ulna:
head                lower epiphysis
lower end           styloid process
CC Excl: See code: 813.40

**813.44 Radius with ulna, lower end** `CC`
CC Excl: See code: 813.40
AHA: ▶1Q, '07, 7◀

**813.45 Torus fracture of radius** `CC`
CC Excl: See code: 813.40
AHA: 4Q, '02, 70

√5th **813.5 Lower end, open**
**813.50 Lower end of forearm, unspecified** `MCC`
CC Excl: 813.10-813.44, 813.50-813.93, 818.0-819.1

**813.51 Colles' fracture** `MCC`
CC Excl: See code: 813.50

**813.52 Other fractures of distal end of radius (alone)** `MCC`
CC Excl: See code: 813.50

| | | | | | |
|---|---|---|---|---|---|
| `N` Newborn Age: 0 | `P` Pediatric Age: 0-17 | `M` Maternity Age: 12-55 | `A` Adult Age: 15-124 | `CC` CC Condition | `MCC` Major CC Condition | `HIV` HIV Related Dx |

**Hand Fractures**

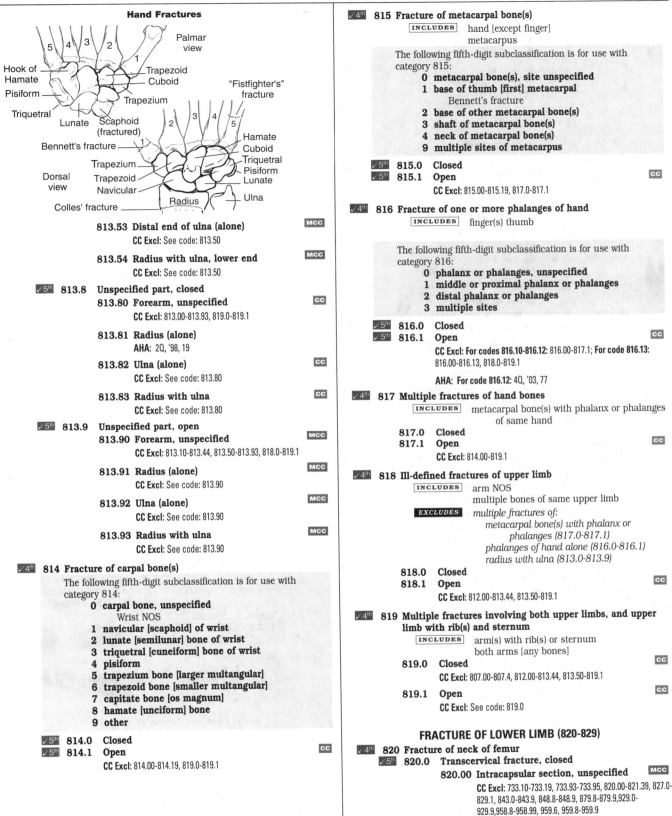

813.53 **Distal end of ulna (alone)** `MCC`
CC Excl: See code: 813.50

813.54 **Radius with ulna, lower end** `MCC`
CC Excl: See code: 813.50

√5ᵗʰ 813.8 **Unspecified part, closed**
813.80 **Forearm, unspecified** `CC`
CC Excl: 813.00-813.93, 819.0-819.1

813.81 **Radius (alone)**
AHA: 2Q, '98, 19

813.82 **Ulna (alone)** `CC`
CC Excl: See code: 813.80

813.83 **Radius with ulna** `CC`
CC Excl: See code: 813.80

√5ᵗʰ 813.9 **Unspecified part, open**
813.90 **Forearm, unspecified** `MCC`
CC Excl: 813.10-813.44, 813.50-813.93, 818.0-819.1

813.91 **Radius (alone)** `MCC`
CC Excl: See code: 813.90

813.92 **Ulna (alone)** `MCC`
CC Excl: See code: 813.90

813.93 **Radius with ulna** `MCC`
CC Excl: See code: 813.90

√4ᵗʰ 814 **Fracture of carpal bone(s)**
The following fifth-digit subclassification is for use with category 814:
 0 carpal bone, unspecified
  Wrist NOS
 1 navicular [scaphoid] of wrist
 2 lunate [semilunar] bone of wrist
 3 triquetral [cuneiform] bone of wrist
 4 pisiform
 5 trapezium bone [larger multangular]
 6 trapezoid bone [smaller multangular]
 7 capitate bone [os magnum]
 8 hamate [unciform] bone
 9 other

√5ᵗʰ 814.0 **Closed**
√5ᵗʰ 814.1 **Open** `CC`
CC Excl: 814.00-814.19, 819.0-819.1

√4ᵗʰ 815 **Fracture of metacarpal bone(s)**
`INCLUDES` hand [except finger]
metacarpus
The following fifth-digit subclassification is for use with category 815:
 0 metacarpal bone(s), site unspecified
 1 base of thumb [first] metacarpal
  Bennett's fracture
 2 base of other metacarpal bone(s)
 3 shaft of metacarpal bone(s)
 4 neck of metacarpal bone(s)
 9 multiple sites of metacarpus

√5ᵗʰ 815.0 **Closed**
√5ᵗʰ 815.1 **Open** `CC`
CC Excl: 815.00-815.19, 817.0-817.1

√4ᵗʰ 816 **Fracture of one or more phalanges of hand**
`INCLUDES` finger(s) thumb

The following fifth-digit subclassification is for use with category 816:
 0 phalanx or phalanges, unspecified
 1 middle or proximal phalanx or phalanges
 2 distal phalanx or phalanges
 3 multiple sites

√5ᵗʰ 816.0 **Closed**
√5ᵗʰ 816.1 **Open** `CC`
CC Excl: For codes 816.10-816.12: 816.00-817.1; For code 816.13: 816.00-816.13, 818.0-819.1

AHA: For code 816.12: 4Q, '03, 77

√4ᵗʰ 817 **Multiple fractures of hand bones**
`INCLUDES` metacarpal bone(s) with phalanx or phalanges of same hand
817.0 **Closed**
817.1 **Open** `CC`
CC Excl: 814.00-819.1

√4ᵗʰ 818 **Ill-defined fractures of upper limb**
`INCLUDES` arm NOS
multiple bones of same upper limb
`EXCLUDES` *multiple fractures of:*
  *metacarpal bone(s) with phalanx or*
   *phalanges (817.0-817.1)*
  *phalanges of hand alone (816.0-816.1)*
  *radius with ulna (813.0-813.9)*
818.0 **Closed**
818.1 **Open** `CC`
CC Excl: 812.00-813.44, 813.50-819.1

√4ᵗʰ 819 **Multiple fractures involving both upper limbs, and upper limb with rib(s) and sternum**
`INCLUDES` arm(s) with rib(s) or sternum
both arms [any bones]
819.0 **Closed** `CC`
CC Excl: 807.00-807.4, 812.00-813.44, 813.50-819.1
819.1 **Open** `CC`
CC Excl: See code: 819.0

**FRACTURE OF LOWER LIMB (820-829)**

√4ᵗʰ 820 **Fracture of neck of femur**
√5ᵗʰ 820.0 **Transcervical fracture, closed**
820.00 **Intracapsular section, unspecified** `MCC`
CC Excl: 733.10-733.19, 733.93-733.95, 820.00-821.39, 827.0-829.1, 843.0-843.9, 848.8-848.9, 879.8-879.9, 929.0-929.9, 958.8-958.99, 959.6, 959.8-959.9

820.01 **Epiphysis (separation) (upper)** `MCC`
Transepiphyseal
CC Excl: See code 820.00

√4ᵗʰ
√5ᵗʰ **Additional Digit Required**   Unacceptable PDx   Manifestation Code   ▶◀ Revised Text   ● New Code   ▲ Revised Code Title

© 2007 Ingenix                                                    October 2007 • Volume 1 — 301

**820.02 Midcervical section** `MCC`
Transcervical NOS
**CC Excl:** See code 820.00
**AHA:** 3Q, '03, 12

**820.03 Base of neck** `MCC`
Cervicotrochanteric section
**CC Excl:** See code 820.00

**820.09 Other** `MCC`
Head of femur
Subcapital
**CC Excl:** See code 820.00

√5th **820.1 Transcervical fracture, open**

**820.10 Intracapsular section, unspecified** `MCC`
**CC Excl:** See code 820.00

**820.11 Epiphysis (separation) (upper)** `MCC`
**CC Excl:** See code 820.00

**820.12 Midcervical section** `MCC`
**CC Excl:** See code 820.00

**820.13 Base of neck** `MCC`
**CC Excl:** See code 820.00

**820.19 Other** `MCC`
**CC Excl:** See code 820.00

√5th **820.2 Pertrochanteric fracture, closed**

**820.20 Trochanteric section, unspecified** `MCC`
Trochanter:     Trochanter:
    NOS           lesser
    greater
**CC Excl:** See code 820.00

**820.21 Intertrochanteric section** `MCC`
**CC Excl:** See code 820.00

**820.22 Subtrochanteric section** `MCC`
**CC Excl:** See code 820.00

√5th **820.3 Pertrochanteric fracture, open**

**820.30 Trochanteric section, unspecified** `MCC`
**CC Excl:** See code 820.00

**820.31 Intertrochanteric section** `MCC`
**CC Excl:** See code 820.00

**820.32 Subtrochanteric section** `MCC`
**CC Excl:** See code 820.00

**820.8 Unspecified part of neck of femur, closed** `MCC`
Hip NOS        Neck of femur NOS
**CC Excl:** See code 820.00

**820.9 Unspecified part of neck of femur, open** `MCC`
**CC Excl:** See code 820.00

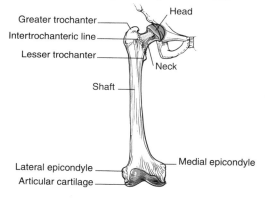

**Right Femur, Anterior View**

Greater trochanter
Intertrochanteric line
Lesser trochanter
Head
Neck
Shaft
Lateral epicondyle
Articular cartilage
Medial epicondyle

√4th **821 Fracture of other and unspecified parts of femur**
√5th **821.0 Shaft or unspecified part, closed**

**821.00 Unspecified part of femur** `MCC`
Thigh        Upper leg
**EXCLUDES**    hip NOS (820.8)
**CC Excl:** 733.10-733.19, 733.93-733.95, 820.00-821.39, 827.0-
829.1, 843.0-843.9, 848.8-848.9, 879.8-879.9,929.0-
929.9,958.8-958.99, 959.6, 959.8-959.9

**821.01 Shaft** `MCC`
**CC Excl:** See code: 821.00
**AHA:** ▶1Q, '07, 4;◀ 1Q, '99, 5

√5th **821.1 Shaft or unspecified part, open**

**821.10 Unspecified part of femur** `MCC`
**CC Excl:** See code: 821.00

**821.11 Shaft** `MCC`
**CC Excl:** See code: 821.00

√5th **821.2 Lower end, closed**
Distal end

**821.20 Lower end, unspecified part** `CC`
**CC Excl:** 733.10, 733.14-733.15, 733.19, 820.00-821.39,
827.0-829.1, 843.0-843.9, 848.8-848.9, 879.8-879.9,929.0-
929.9, 958.8, 958.99, 959.6, 959.8-959.9

**821.21 Condyle, femoral** `CC`
**CC Excl:** See code: 821.20

**821.22 Epiphysis, lower (separation)** `CC`
**CC Excl:** See code: 821.20

**821.23 Supracondylar fracture of femur** `CC`
**CC Excl:** See code: 821.20

**821.29 Other** `CC`
Multiple fractures of lower end
**CC Excl:** See code: 821.20

√5th **821.3 Lower end, open**

**821.30 Lower end, unspecified part** `MCC`
**CC Excl:** See code: 821.20

**821.31 Condyle, femoral** `MCC`
**CC Excl:** See code: 821.20

**821.32 Epiphysis, lower (separation)** `MCC`
**CC Excl:** See code: 821.20

**821.33 Supracondylar fracture of femur** `MCC`
**CC Excl:** See code: 821.20

**821.39 Other** `MCC`
**CC Excl:** 733.10, 733.14-733.15, 733.19, 821.39-822.1, 827.0-
829.1, 843.0-843.9, 848.8-848.9, 879.8-879.9,929.0-929.9,
958.8, 958.99, 959.6, 959.8-959.9

√4th **822 Fracture of patella**

**822.0 Closed** `CC`
**CC Excl:** 822.0-822.1, 828.0-828.1

**822.1 Open** `CC`
**CC Excl:** 733.10, 733.19, 822.1-823.32, 823.80-823.92, 827.0-829.1, 843.0-
843.9, 848.8-848.9, 879.8-879.9,929.0-929.9, 958.8, 958.99, 959.6, 959.8-
959.9

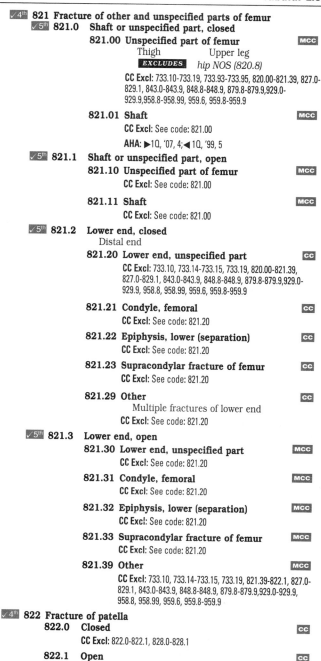

**Right Tibia and Fibula, Anterior View**

Patella
Tibial plateau
Tibial tubercle
Shaft of fibula
Tibia
Lateral (fibular) malleolus
Medial (tibial) malleolus

Pott's fracture

`N` Newborn Age: 0    `P` Pediatric Age: 0-17    `M` Maternity Age: 12-55    `A` Adult Age: 15-124    `CC` CC Condition    `MCC` Major CC Condition    `HIV` HIV Related Dx

302 — Volume 1 • October 2007

© 2007 Ingenix

✓4ᵗʰ **823 Fracture of tibia and fibula**

  **EXCLUDES**   *Dupuytren's fracture (824.4-824.5)*
                  *ankle (824.4-824.5)*
                  *radius (813.42, 813.52)*
                  *Pott's fracture (824.4-824.5)*
                  *that involving ankle (824.0-824.9)*

The following fifth-digit subclassification is for use with category 823:

    **0**  tibia alone
    **1**  fibula alone
    **2**  fibula with tibia

✓5ᵗʰ **823.0**  **Upper end, closed**     `CC 0, 2`
      Head                 Tibia:
      Proximal end        condyles
                      tuberosity
    **CC Excl:** For codes **823.00, 823.02:**733.10, 733.16-733.19, 823.00-823.32, 823.80-823.92, 827.0-829.1, 843.0-843.9, 848.8-848.9, 879.8-879.9,929.0-929.9, 958.8, 958.99, 959.6, 959.8-959.9

✓5ᵗʰ **823.1**  **Upper end, open**     `MCC`
    **CC Excl:** See code: 823.00

✓5ᵗʰ **823.2**  **Shaft, closed**     `CC 0, 2`
    **CC Excl:** See code: 823.00

✓5ᵗʰ **823.3**  **Shaft, open**     `MCC`
    **CC Excl:** See code: 823.00

✓5ᵗʰ **823.4**  **Torus fracture**     `CC 0, 2`
    **CC Excl:** See code: 823.00

    **AHA:** 4Q, '02, 70

    **DEF:** A bone deformity in children, occurring commonly in the tibia and fibula, in which the bone bends and buckles but does not fracture.

✓5ᵗʰ **823.8**  **Unspecified part, closed**     `CC 0, 2`
      Lower leg NOS
    **CC Excl:** For code **823.80:** 823.00-823.92; For code **823.82:** 733.10, 733.16-733.19, 823.00-823.32, 823.80-823.92, 827.0-829.1, 843.0-843.9, 848.8-848.9, 879.8-879.9,929.0-929.9, 958.8, 958.99, 959.6, 959.8-959.9

    **AHA:** For code 823.82: 1Q, '97, 8

✓5ᵗʰ **823.9**  **Unspecified part, open**     `MCC`
    **CC Excl:** See code: 823.00

✓4ᵗʰ **824 Fracture of ankle**

    **824.0**  **Medial malleolus, closed**
        Tibia involving:       Tibia involving:
          ankle                  malleolus
      **AHA:** 1Q, '04, 9

    **824.1**  **Medial malleolus, open**     `CC`
      **CC Excl:** 733.10, 733.16-733.19, 824.1-824.9, 827.0-829.1, 843.0-843.9, 848.8-848.9, 879.8-879.9,929.0-929.9, 958.8, 958.99, 959.6, 959.8-959.9

    **824.2**  **Lateral malleolus, closed**
        Fibula involving:
          ankle
          malleolus
      **AHA:** 2Q, '02, 3

    **824.3**  **Lateral malleolus, open**     `CC`
      **CC Excl:** See code: 824.1

    **824.4**  **Bimalleolar, closed**
        Dupuytren's fracture, fibula     Pott's fracture
      **DEF:** Bimalleolar, closed: Breaking of both nodules (malleoli) on either side of ankle joint, without an open wound.

      **DEF:** Dupuytren's fracture (Pott's fracture): The breaking of the farthest end of the lower leg bone (fibula), with injury to the farthest end joint of the other lower leg bone (tibia).

    **824.5**  **Bimalleolar, open**     `CC`
      **CC Excl:** See code: 824.1

    **824.6**  **Trimalleolar, closed**
        Lateral and medial malleolus with anterior or posterior lip of tibia

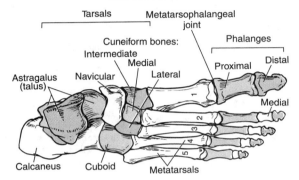

**Torus Fracture**

Fibula — Tibia — Diaphysis — Direction of force — Torus, bulging, fracture

Anterior views of torus compression fracture

**Right Foot, Dorsal**

Tarsals — Metatarsophalangeal joint — Cuneiform bones: Intermediate, Medial, Lateral — Phalanges — Proximal, Distal — Astragalus (talus) — Navicular — Medial — Calcaneus — Cuboid — Metatarsals

    **824.7**  **Trimalleolar, open**     `CC`
      **CC Excl:** See code: 824.1

    **824.8**  **Unspecified, closed**
      Ankle NOS
      **AHA:** 3Q, '00, 12

    **824.9**  **Unspecified, open**     `CC`
      **CC Excl:** See code: 824.1

✓4ᵗʰ **825 Fracture of one or more tarsal and metatarsal bones**

    **825.0**  **Fracture of calcaneus, closed**
      Heel bone       Os calcis

    **825.1**  **Fracture of calcaneus, open**     `CC`
      **CC Excl:** 733.10, 733.16-733.19, 825.1-825.39, 827.0-829.1, 843.0-843.9, 848.8-848.9, 879.8-879.9,929.0-929.9, 958.8, 958.99, 959.6, 959.8-959.9

✓5ᵗʰ **825.2**  **Fracture of other tarsal and metatarsal bones, closed**
    **825.20**  **Unspecified bone(s) of foot [except toes]**
        Instep
    **825.21**  **Astragalus**
        Talus
    **825.22**  **Navicular [scaphoid], foot**
    **825.23**  **Cuboid**
    **825.24**  **Cuneiform, foot**
    **825.25**  **Metatarsal bone(s)**
    **825.29**  **Other**
        Tarsal with metatarsal bone(s) only
        **EXCLUDES**   *calcaneus (825.0)*

✓5ᵗʰ **825.3**  **Fracture of other tarsal and metatarsal bones, open**
    **825.30**  **Unspecified bone(s) of foot [except toes]** `CC`
      **CC Excl:** 825.0-826.1

    **825.31**  **Astragalus**     `CC`
      **CC Excl:** 733.10, 733.19, 825.1-825.39, 827.0-829.1, 843.0-843.9, 848.8-848.9, 879.8-879.9,929.0-929.9, 958.8, 958.99, 959.6, 959.8-959.9

825.32 **Navicular [scaphoid], foot**    `CC`
CC Excl: See code: 825.31

825.33 **Cuboid**    `CC`
CC Excl: See code: 825.31

825.34 **Cuneiform, foot**    `CC`
CC Excl: See code: 825.31

825.35 **Metatarsal bone(s)**    `CC`
CC Excl: See code: 825.31

825.39 **Other**    `CC`
CC Excl: See code: 825.0-826.1

✓4ᵗʰ 826 **Fracture of one or more phalanges of foot**
`INCLUDES` toe(s)

826.0    **Closed**
826.1    **Open**

✓4ᵗʰ 827 **Other, multiple, and ill-defined fractures of lower limb**
`INCLUDES`    leg NOS
multiple bones of same lower limb
`EXCLUDES`    *multiple fractures of:*
*ankle bones alone (824.4-824.9)*
*phalanges of foot alone (826.0-826.1)*
*tarsal with metatarsal bones (825.29,*
*825.39)*
*tibia with fibula (823.0-823.9 with*
*fifth-digit 2)*

827.0    **Closed**
827.1    **Open**    `CC`
CC Excl: 820.00-823.32, 823.80-829.1

✓4ᵗʰ 828 **Multiple fractures involving both lower limbs, lower with upper limb, and lower limb(s) with rib(s) and sternum**
`INCLUDES`    arm(s) with leg(s) [any bones]
both legs [any bones]
leg(s) with rib(s) or sternum

828.0    **Closed**    `MCC`
CC Excl: See code: 827.1

828.1    **Open**    `MCC`
CC Excl: See code: 827.1

✓4ᵗʰ 829 **Fracture of unspecified bones**
829.0    **Unspecified bone, closed**
829.1    **Unspecified bone, open**

### DISLOCATION (830-839)

`INCLUDES`    displacement
subluxation
`EXCLUDES`    *congenital dislocation (754.0-755.8)*
*pathological dislocation (718.2)*
*recurrent dislocation (718.3)*

The descriptions "closed" and "open," used in the fourth-digit subdivisions, include the following terms:

closed:                  open:
complete               compound
dislocation NOS      infected
partial                   with foreign body
simple
uncomplicated
A dislocation not indicated as closed or open should be classified as closed.

**AHA:** 3Q, '90, 12

✓4ᵗʰ 830 **Dislocation of jaw**
`INCLUDES`    jaw (cartilage) (meniscus)
mandible
maxilla (inferior)
temporomandibular (joint)

830.0    **Closed dislocation**
830.1    **Open dislocation**    `CC`
CC Excl: 830.0-830.1, 839.69, 839.79-839.9

✓4ᵗʰ 831 **Dislocation of shoulder**
`EXCLUDES`    *sternoclavicular joint (839.61, 839.71)*
*sternum (839.61, 839.71)*

The following fifth-digit subclassification is for use with category 831:
0    **shoulder, unspecified**
Humerus NOS
1    **anterior dislocation of humerus**
2    **posterior dislocation of humerus**
3    **inferior dislocation of humerus**
4    **acromioclavicular (joint)**
Clavicle
9    **other**
Scapula

✓5ᵗʰ 831.0    **Closed dislocation**
✓5ᵗʰ 831.1    **Open dislocation**    `CC`
CC Excl: For code 831.10: 831.10, 839.69, 839.79-839.9;
For code 831.11: 831.11, 839.69, 839.79-839.9; For code 831.12,
839.69, 839.79-839.9; For code 831.13: 831.13, 839.69, 839.79-839.9;
For code 831.14: 831.14, 839.69, 839.79-839.9; For code 831.19: 831.19,
839.69, 839.79-839.9

✓4ᵗʰ 832 **Dislocation of elbow**
The following fifth-digit subclassification is for use with category 832:
0    **elbow unspecified**
1    **anterior dislocation of elbow**
2    **posterior dislocation of elbow**
3    **medial dislocation of elbow**
4    **lateral dislocation of elbow**
9    **other**

✓5ᵗʰ 832.0    **Closed dislocation**
✓5ᵗʰ 832.1    **Open dislocation**    `CC`
CC Excl: For code 832.10: 832.10; For code 832.11: 832.11;
For code 832.12: 832.12; For code 832.13: 832.13;
For code 832.14: 832.14; For code 832.19: 832.19

✓4ᵗʰ 833 **Dislocation of wrist**
The following fifth-digit subclassification is for use with category 833:
0    **wrist, unspecified part**
Carpal (bone)
Radius, distal end
1    **radioulnar (joint), distal**
2    **radiocarpal (joint)**
3    **midcarpal (joint)**
4    **carpometacarpal (joint)**
5    **metacarpal (bone), proximal end**
9    **other**
Ulna, distal end

✓5ᵗʰ 833.0    **Closed dislocation**
✓5ᵗʰ 833.1    **Open dislocation**    `CC`
CC Excl: For codes 833.10, 833.13-833.19: 833.00-833.19;
For code 833.11: 833.11; For code 833.12: 833.12

✓4ᵗʰ 834 **Dislocation of finger**
`INCLUDES`    finger(s)            thumb
phalanx of hand

The following fifth-digit subclassification is for use with category 834:
0    **finger, unspecified part**
1    **metacarpophalangeal (joint)**
Metacarpal (bone), distal end
2    **interphalangeal (joint), hand**

✓5ᵗʰ 834.0    **Closed dislocation**
✓5ᵗʰ 834.1    **Open dislocation**

---

 Newborn Age: 0     Pediatric Age: 0-17     Maternity Age: 12-55     Adult Age: 15-124     CC Condition    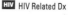 Major CC Condition    HIV HIV Related Dx

304 — Volume 1 • October 2007    © 2007 Ingenix

√4ᵗʰ **835 Dislocation of hip**

The following fifth-digit subclassification is for use with category 835:

    **0 dislocation of hip, unspecified**
    **1 posterior dislocation**
    **2 obturator dislocation**
    **3 other anterior dislocation**

√5ᵗʰ **835.0 Closed dislocation** `CC`
    **CC Excl: For code 835.00:** 835.00, 839.69, 839.79-839.9;
    **For code 835.01:** 835.01, 839.69, 839.79-839.9; **For code 835.02:** 835.02,
    839.69, 839.79-839.9; **For code 835.03:** 835.03, 839.69, 839.79-839.9

√5ᵗʰ **835.1 Open dislocation** `MCC`
    **CC Excl: For code 835.10:** 835.10, 839.69, 839.79-839.9;
    **For code 835.11:** 835.11, 839.69, 839.79-839.9; **For code 835.12:** 835.12,
    839.69, 839.79-839.9; **For code 835.13:** 835.13, 839.69, 839.79-839.9

√4ᵗʰ **836 Dislocation of knee**

    `EXCLUDES`  dislocation of knee:
        old or pathological (718.2)
        recurrent (718.3)
        internal derangement of knee joint (717.0-717.5,
          717.8-717.9)
        old tear of cartilage or meniscus of knee (717.0-
          717.5, 717.8-717.9)

**836.0 Tear of medial cartilage or meniscus of knee, current**
    Bucket handle tear:
      NOS     ⎫
             ⎬ current injury
      medial meniscus ⎭

**836.1 Tear of lateral cartilage or meniscus of knee, current**

**836.2 Other tear of cartilage or meniscus of knee, current**
    Tear of:
      cartilage    ⎫
      (semilunar) ⎬ current injury, not specified
      meniscus   ⎭ as medial or lateral

**836.3 Dislocation of patella, closed**
**836.4 Dislocation of patella, open** `CC`
    **CC Excl:** 836.3-836.4

√5ᵗʰ **836.5 Other dislocation of knee, closed**
    **836.50 Dislocation of knee, unspecified**
    **836.51 Anterior dislocation of tibia, proximal end**
        Posterior dislocation of femur, distal end
    **836.52 Posterior dislocation of tibia, proximal end**
        Anterior dislocation of femur, distal end
    **836.53 Medial dislocation of tibia, proximal end**
    **836.54 Lateral dislocation of tibia, proximal end**
    **836.59 Other**

√5ᵗʰ **836.6 Other dislocation of knee, open**
    **836.60 Dislocation of knee, unspecified** `CC`
        **CC Excl:** 717.0-717.9, 718.26, 718.36, 836.60, 839.69,
        839.79-839.9

    **836.61 Anterior dislocation of tibia, proximal end** `CC`
        **CC Excl:** 836.61, 839.69, 839.79-839.9

    **836.62 Posterior dislocation of tibia, proximal end** `CC`
        **CC Excl:** 836.62, 839.69, 839.79-839.9

    **836.63 Medial dislocation of tibia, proximal end** `CC`
        **CC Excl:** 836.63, 839.69, 839.79-839.9

    **836.64 Lateral dislocation of tibia, proximal end** `CC`
        **CC Excl:** 836.64, 839.69, 839.79-839.9

    **836.69 Other** `CC`
        **CC Excl:** 836.69, 839.69, 839.79-839.9

√4ᵗʰ **837 Dislocation of ankle**

    `INCLUDES`  astragalus
               fibula, distal end
               navicular, foot
               scaphoid, foot
               tibia, distal end

    **837.0 Closed dislocation**
    **837.1 Open dislocation** `CC`
        **CC Excl:** 837.1, 839.69, 839.79-839.9

√4ᵗʰ **838 Dislocation of foot**

The following fifth-digit subclassification is for use with category 838:

    **0 foot, unspecified**
    **1 tarsal (bone), joint unspecified**
    **2 midtarsal (joint)**
    **3 tarsometatarsal (joint)**
    **4 metatarsal (bone), joint unspecified**
    **5 metatarsophalangeal (joint)**
    **6 interphalangeal (joint), foot**
    **9 other**
        Phalanx of foot
        Toe(s)

√5ᵗʰ **838.0 Closed dislocation**
√5ᵗʰ **838.1 Open dislocation**

√4ᵗʰ **839 Other, multiple, and ill-defined dislocations**
√5ᵗʰ **839.0 Cervical vertebra, closed**
    Cervical spine        Neck

    **839.00 Cervical vertebra, unspecified** `CC`
        **CC Excl:** 805.00-805.18, 806.00-806.19, 806.8-806.9, 839.00-
        839.18, 847.0, 848.8-848.9, 879.8-879.9,929.0-929.9,952.00-
        952.09,958.8-958.99, 959.8-959.9

    **839.01 First cervical vertebra** `CC`
        **CC Excl:** See code 839.00

    **839.02 Second cervical vertebra** `CC`
        **CC Excl:** See code 839.00

    **839.03 Third cervical vertebra** `CC`
        **CC Excl:** See code 839.00

    **839.04 Fourth cervical vertebra** `CC`
        **CC Excl:** See code 839.00

    **839.05 Fifth cervical vertebra** `CC`
        **CC Excl:** See code 839.00

    **839.06 Sixth cervical vertebra** `CC`
        **CC Excl:** See code 839.00

    **839.07 Seventh cervical vertebra** `CC`
        **CC Excl:** See code 839.00

    **839.08 Multiple cervical vertebrae** `CC`
        **CC Excl:** See code 839.00

√5ᵗʰ **839.1 Cervical vertebra, open**
    **839.10 Cervical vertebra, unspecified** `MCC`
        **CC Excl:** See code 839.00

    **839.11 First cervical vertebra** `MCC`
        **CC Excl:** See code 839.00

    **839.12 Second cervical vertebra** `MCC`
        **CC Excl:** See code 839.00

    **839.13 Third cervical vertebra** `MCC`
        **CC Excl:** See code 839.00

    **839.14 Fourth cervical vertebra** `MCC`
        **CC Excl:** See code 839.00

    **839.15 Fifth cervical vertebra** `MCC`
        **CC Excl:** See code 839.00

    **839.16 Sixth cervical vertebra** `MCC`
        **CC Excl:** See code 839.00

    **839.17 Seventh cervical vertebra** `MCC`
        **CC Excl:** See code 839.00

    **839.18 Multiple cervical vertebrae** `MCC`
        **CC Excl:** See code 839.00

√5ᵗʰ **839.2  Thoracic and lumbar vertebra, closed**
   **839.20  Lumbar vertebra**
   **839.21  Thoracic vertebra**
         Dorsal [thoracic] vertebra
√5ᵗʰ **839.3  Thoracic and lumbar vertebra, open**
   **839.30  Lumbar vertebra**                                    `MCC`
         CC Excl: 839.30

   **839.31  Thoracic vertebra**                                   `MCC`
         CC Excl: 839.21, 839.31

√5ᵗʰ **839.4  Other vertebra, closed**
   **839.40  Vertebra, unspecified site**
         Spine NOS
   **839.41  Coccyx**
   **839.42  Sacrum**
         Sacroiliac (joint)
   **839.49  Other**
√5ᵗʰ **839.5  Other vertebra, open**
   **839.50  Vertebra, unspecified site**                          `MCC`
         CC Excl: 839.10-839.18, 839.30-839.31, 839.50-839.59,
         839.79, 839.9

   **839.51  Coccyx**                                              `CC`
         CC Excl: 839.51

   **839.52  Sacrum**                                              `CC`
         CC Excl: 839.52

   **839.59  Other**                                               `MCC`
         CC Excl: See code: 839.50

√5ᵗʰ **839.6  Other location, closed**
   **839.61  Sternum**                                             `CC`
         Sternoclavicular joint
         CC Excl: 839.61, 839.71

   **839.69  Other**
         Pelvis
√5ᵗʰ **839.7  Other location, open**
   **839.71  Sternum**                                             `MCC`
         CC Excl: See code: 839.61

   **839.79  Other**                                               `CC`
         CC Excl: 830.1, 831.10-831.19, 832.10-832.19, 833.10-833.19,
         834.10-834.12, 835.10-835.13, 836.4, 836.60-836.69, 837.1,
         838.10-838.19, 839.10-839.18, 839.30-839.31, 839.50-839.59,
         839.71-839.79, 839.9

**839.8  Multiple and ill-defined, closed**
      Arm
      Back
      Hand
      Multiple locations, except fingers or toes alone
      Other ill-defined locations
      Unspecified location
**839.9  Multiple and ill-defined, open**
   CC Excl: See code: 839.79                                       `CC`

## SPRAINS AND STRAINS OF JOINTS AND ADJACENT MUSCLES
### (840-848)

| INCLUDES | avulsion | |
|---|---|---|
| | hemarthrosis | of: |
| | laceration | joint capsule |
| | rupture | ligament |
| | sprain | muscle |
| | strain | tendon |
| | tear | |

`EXCLUDES`  *laceration of tendon in open wounds (880-884
and 890-894 with .2)*

√4ᵗʰ **840  Sprains and strains of shoulder and upper arm**
   **840.0  Acromioclavicular (joint) (ligament)**
   **840.1  Coracoclavicular (ligament)**
   **840.2  Coracohumeral (ligament)**
   **840.3  Infraspinatus (muscle) (tendon)**

**840.4  Rotator cuff (capsule)**
   `EXCLUDES`  *complete rupture of rotator cuff,
                    nontraumatic (727.61)*
**840.5  Subscapularis (muscle)**
**840.6  Supraspinatus (muscle) (tendon)**
**840.7  Superior glenoid labrum lesion**
      SLAP lesion
   AHA: 4Q,'01, 52

   DEF:  Detachment injury of the superior aspect of the glenoid
   labrum which is the ring of fibrocartilage attached to the rim of the
   glenoid cavity of the scapula.

**840.8  Other specified sites of shoulder and upper arm**
**840.9  Unspecified site of shoulder and upper arm**
      Arm NOS                    Shoulder NOS
√4ᵗʰ **841  Sprains and strains of elbow and forearm**
   **841.0  Radial collateral ligament**
   **841.1  Ulnar collateral ligament**
   **841.2  Radiohumeral (joint)**
   **841.3  Ulnohumeral (joint)**
   **841.8  Other specified sites of elbow and forearm**
   **841.9  Unspecified site of elbow and forearm**
         Elbow NOS
√4ᵗʰ **842  Sprains and strains of wrist and hand**
   √5ᵗʰ **842.0  Wrist**
      **842.00  Unspecified site**
      **842.01  Carpal (joint)**
      **842.02  Radiocarpal (joint) (ligament)**
      **842.09  Other**
            Radioulnar joint, distal
   √5ᵗʰ **842.1  Hand**
      **842.10  Unspecified site**
      **842.11  Carpometacarpal (joint)**
      **842.12  Metacarpophalangeal (joint)**
      **842.13  Interphalangeal (joint)**
      **842.19  Other**
            Midcarpal (joint)
√4ᵗʰ **843  Sprains and strains of hip and thigh**
   **843.0  Iliofemoral (ligament)**
   **843.1  Ischiocapsular (ligament)**
   **843.8  Other specified sites of hip and thigh**
   **843.9  Unspecified site of hip and thigh**
         Hip NOS                    Thigh NOS
√4ᵗʰ **844  Sprains and strains of knee and leg**
   **844.0  Lateral collateral ligament of knee**
   **844.1  Medial collateral ligament of knee**
   **844.2  Cruciate ligament of knee**
   **844.3  Tibiofibular (joint) (ligament), superior**
   **844.8  Other specified sites of knee and leg**
   **844.9  Unspecified site of knee and leg**
         Knee NOS                    Leg NOS
√4ᵗʰ **845  Sprains and strains of ankle and foot**
   √5ᵗʰ **845.0  Ankle**
      **845.00  Unspecified site**
            AHA: 2Q, '02, 3

      **845.01  Deltoid (ligament), ankle**
            Internal collateral (ligament), ankle
      **845.02  Calcaneofibular (ligament)**
      **845.03  Tibiofibular (ligament), distal**
            AHA: 1Q, '04, 9

      **845.09  Other**
            Achilles tendon
   √5ᵗʰ **845.1  Foot**
      **845.10  Unspecified site**
      **845.11  Tarsometatarsal (joint) (ligament)**
      **845.12  Metatarsophalangeal (joint)**
      **845.13  Interphalangeal (joint), toe**
      **845.19  Other**
√4ᵗʰ **846  Sprains and strains of sacroiliac region**
   **846.0  Lumbosacral (joint) (ligament)**
   **846.1  Sacroiliac ligament**

---

**N** Newborn Age: 0    **P** Pediatric Age: 0-17    **M** Maternity Age: 12-55    **A** Adult Age: 15-124    `CC` CC Condition    `MCC` Major CC Condition    `HIV` HIV Related Dx

846.2    Sacrospinatus (ligament)
846.3    Sacrotuberous (ligament)
846.8    Other specified sites of sacroiliac region
846.9    Unspecified site of sacroiliac region

✓4th **847**   **Sprains and strains of other and unspecified parts of back**
    `EXCLUDES`   *lumbosacral (846.0)*

847.0    **Neck**
      Anterior longitudinal (ligament), cervical
      Atlanto-axial (joints)
      Atlanto-occipital (joints)
      Whiplash injury
      `EXCLUDES`   *neck injury NOS (959.0)*
                 *thyroid region (848.2)*

847.1    **Thoracic**
847.2    **Lumbar**
847.3    **Sacrum**
      Sacrococcygeal (ligament)
847.4    **Coccyx**
847.9    **Unspecified site of back**
      Back NOS

✓4th **848**   **Other and ill-defined sprains and strains**
848.0    **Septal cartilage of nose**
848.1    **Jaw**
      Temporomandibular (joint) (ligament)
848.2    **Thyroid region**
      Cricoarytenoid (joint) (ligament)
      Cricothyroid (joint) (ligament)
      Thyroid cartilage
848.3    **Ribs**
      Chondrocostal   } without mention of
       (joint)       } injury to
      Costal cartilage } sternum

✓5th **848.4**
      **Sternum**
      **848.40 Unspecified site**
      **848.41 Sternoclavicular (joint) (ligament)**
      **848.42 Chondrosternal (joint)**
      **848.49 Other**
           Xiphoid cartilage
848.5    **Pelvis**
      Symphysis pubis
      `EXCLUDES`   *that in childbirth (665.6)*
848.8    **Other specified sites of sprains and strains**
848.9    **Unspecified site of sprain and strain**

## INTRACRANIAL INJURY, EXCLUDING THOSE WITH SKULL FRACTURE (850-854)

    `EXCLUDES`   *intracranial injury with skull fracture (800-801 and 803-804, except .0 and .5)*
                   *open wound of head without intracranial injury (870.0-873.9)*
                   *skull fracture alone (800-801 and 803-804 with .0, .5)*

The description "with open intracranial wound," used in the fourth-digit subdivisions, includes those specified as open or with mention of infection or foreign body.

The following fifth-digit subclassification is for use with categories 851-854:

0   **unspecified state of consciousness**
1   **with no loss of consciousness**
2   **with brief [less than one hour] loss of consciousness**
3   **with moderate [1-24 hours] loss of consciousness**
4   **with prolonged [more than 24 hours] loss of consciousness and return to pre-existing conscious level**
5   **with prolonged [more than 24 hours] loss of consciousness, without return to pre-existing conscious level**
     Use fifth-digit 5 to designate when a patient is unconscious and dies before regaining consciousness, regardless of the duration of the loss of consciousness
6   **with loss of consciousness of unspecified duration**
9   **with concussion, unspecified**

**AHA:** 1Q, '93, 22

✓4th **850**   **Concussion**
    `INCLUDES`   commotio cerebri
    `EXCLUDES`   *concussion with:*
           *cerebral laceration or contusion (851.0-851.9)*
           *cerebral hemorrhage (852-853)*
           *head injury NOS (959.01)*

    **AHA:** 2Q, '96, 6; 4Q, '90, 24

850.0    **With no loss of consciousness**
      Concussion with mental confusion or disorientation, without loss of consciousness

✓5th **850.1**   **With brief loss of consciousness**
      Loss of consciousness for less than one hour
    **AHA:** 4Q, '03, 76; 1Q, '99, 10; 2Q, '92, 5

      **850.11 With loss of consciousness of 30 minutes or less**   `CC`
           **CC Excl:** 800.00-801.99, 803.00-804.99, 850.0-852.19, 852.21-854.19, 873.8-873.9, 879.8-879.9, 905.0,925.1-925.2,929.0-929.9,958.8-959.09, 959.8-959.9

      **850.12 With loss of consciousness from 31 to 59 minutes**   `CC`
           **CC Excl:** See code: 850.11

850.2    **With moderate loss of consciousness**   `CC`
      Loss of consciousness for 1-24 hours
      **CC Excl:** See code: 850.11

850.3    **With prolonged loss of consciousness and return to pre-existing conscious level**   `CC`
      Loss of consciousness for more than 24 hours with complete recovery
      **CC Excl:** See code: 850.11

850.4    **With prolonged loss of consciousness, without return to pre-existing conscious level**   `MCC`
      **CC Excl:** See code: 850.11

850.5    **With loss of consciousness of unspecified duration**   `CC`
      **CC Excl:** See code: 850.11

850.9    **Concussion, unspecified**

**Brain**

Corpus callosum
Cerebrum
Hypothalamus
Interventricular foramen
Fornix
Third ventricle
Pineal body
Optic chiasm
Corpora quadrigemina
Cerebral aqueduct
Vermis
Hypophysis
Pons
Fourth ventricle
Median aperture
Mamillary body
Peduncle
Spinal cord
Medulla oblangata

Precentral gyrus (motor)
Central sulcus
Postcentral gyrus (sensory)
Anterior horn of lateral ventricle
Body and posterior horn of lateral ventricle
Intraventricular foramen
Third ventricle
Lateral sulcus
Inferior horn of lateral ventricle
Cerebral aqueduct
Lateral aperture
Fourth ventricle
Median aperture

✓4th / ✓5th   Additional Digit Required      Unacceptable PDx      `Manifestation Code`      ▶◀ Revised Text      ● New Code      ▲ Revised Code Title

© 2007 Ingenix                             **October 2007 • Volume 1 — 307**

**Injury and Poisoning**

**851–860**

√4th **851 Cerebral laceration and contusion**
AHA: 4Q, '96, 36; 1Q, '93, 22; 4Q, '90, 24

§ √5th **851.0 Cortex (cerebral) contusion withou mention of open intracranial wound** `MCC 5` `CC 2-4, 6`
CC Excl: For codes 851.02-851.06: 800.0-801.99, 803.00-804.99, 850.0-852.19, 852.21-854.19, 873.8-873.9, 879.8-879.9, 905.0,925.1-925.2,929.0-929.9,958.8-959.09, 959.8-959.9

§ √5th **851.1 Cortex (cerebral) contusion with open intracranial wound** `MCC`
CC Excl: 800.00-801.99, 803.00-804.99, 850.0-852.19, 852.21-854.19, 873.8-873.9, 879.8-879.9, 905.0,925.1-925.2,929.0-929.9,958.8-959.09, 959.8-959.9

AHA: 1Q, '92, 9

§ √5th **851.2 Cortex (cerebral) laceration without mention of open intracranial wound** `MCC`
CC Excl: See code: 851.1

§ √5th **851.3 Cortex (cerebral) laceration with open intracranial wound** `MCC`
CC Excl: See code: 851.1

§ √5th **851.4 Cerebellar or brain stem contusion without mention of open intracranial wound** `MCC 5` `CC 2-4, 6`
CC Excl: For codes 851.42-851.46: 800.00-801.99, 803.00-804.99, 850.0-852.19, 852.21-854.19, 873.8-873.9, 879.8-879.9, 905.0, 925.1-925.2,929.0-929.9,958.8-959.09, 959.8-959.9

§ √5th **851.5 Cerebellar or brain stem contusion with open intracranial wound** `MCC`
CC Excl: See code: 851.1

§ √5th **851.6 Cerebellar or brain stem laceration without mention of open intracranial wound** `MCC`
CC Excl: See code: 851.1

§ √5th **851.7 Cerebellar or brain stem laceration with open intracranial wound** `MCC`
CC Excl: See code: 851.1

§ √5th **851.8 Other and unspecified cerebral laceration and contusion, without mention of open intracranial wound** `MCC`
Brain (membrane) NOS
CC Excl: See code: 851.1

AHA: 4Q, '96, 37

§ √5th **851.9 Other and unspecified cerebral laceration and contusion, with open intracranial wound** `MCC`
CC Excl: See code: 851.1

√4th **852 Subarachnoid, subdural, and extradural hemorrhage, following injury**
EXCLUDES Cerebral contusion or laceration (with hemorrhage) (851.0-851.9)

DEF: Bleeding from lining of brain; due to injury.

§ √5th **852.0 Subarachnoid hemorrhage following injury without mention of open intracranial wound** `MCC`
Middle meningeal hemorrhage following injury
CC Excl: 800.00-801.99, 803.00-804.99, 850.0-852.19, 852.21-854.19, 873.8-873.9, 879.8-879.9, 905.0,925.1-925.2,929.0-929.9,958.8-959.09, 959.8-959.9

§ √5th **852.1 Subarachnoid hemorrhage following injury with open intracranial wound** `MCC`
CC Excl: See code: 852.0

§ √5th **852.2 Subdural hemorrhage following injury without mention of open intracranial wound** `MCC`
CC Excl: For code 852.20: 800.00-801.99, 803.00-804.99, 850.0-854.19, 873.8-873.9, 879.8-879.9, 905.0,925.1-925.2,929.0-929.9,958.8-959.09, 959.8-959.9; For codes 852.21-852.29: 800.00-801.99, 803.00-804.99, 850.0-852.19, 852.21-854.19, 873.8-873.9, 879.8-879.9, 905.0,925.1-925.2,929.0-929.9,958.8-959.09, 959.8-959.9

AHA: 4Q, '96, 43

§ √5th **852.3 Subdural hemorrhage following injury with open intracranial wound** `MCC`
CC Excl: See code: 852.0

§ √5th **852.4 Extradural hemorrhage following injury without mention of open intracranial wound** `MCC`
Epidural hematoma following injury
CC Excl: See code: 852.0

§ √5th **852.5 Extradural hemorrhage following injury with open intracranial wound** `MCC`
CC Excl: See code: 852.0

√4th **853 Other and unspecified intracranial hemorrhage following injury**

§ √5th **853.0 Without mention of open intracranial wound** `MCC`
Cerebral compression due to injury
Intracranial hematoma following injury
Traumatic cerebral hemorrhage
CC Excl: 800.00-801.99, 803.00-804.99, 850.0-852.19, 852.21-854.19, 873.8-873.9, 879.8-879.9, 905.0,925.1-925.2,929.0-929.9,958.8-959.09, 959.8-959.9

AHA: 3Q, '90, 14

§ √5th **853.1 With open intracranial wound** `MCC`
CC Excl: See code: 853.0

√4th **854 Intracranial injury of other and unspecified nature**
INCLUDES brain injury NOS
cavernous sinus
intracranial injury
EXCLUDES any condition classifiable to 850-853
head injury NOS (959.01)

AHA: 1Q, '99, 10; 2Q, '92, 6

§ √5th **854.0 Without mention of open intracranial wound** `MCC 5` `CC 2-4, 6`
CC Excl: For codes 854.02-854.06: 800.00-801.99, 803.00-804.99, 850.0-852.19, 852.21-854.19, 873.8-873.9, 879.8-879.9, 905.0,925.1-925.2,929.0-929.9,958.8-959.09, 959.8-959.9

AHA: For code 854.00: 2Q, '05, 6

§ √5th **854.1 With open intracranial wound** `MCC`
CC Excl: 800.00-801.99, 803.00-804.99, 850.0-852.19, 852.21-854.19, 873.8-873.9, 879.8-879.9, 905.0,925.1-925.2,929.0-929.9,958.8-959.09, 959.8-959.9

## INTERNAL INJURY OF THORAX, ABDOMEN, AND PELVIS (860-869)

INCLUDES blast injuries
blunt trauma
bruise
concussion injuries (except cerebral)
crushing
hematoma          of internal organs
laceration
puncture
tear
traumatic rupture

EXCLUDES concussion NOS (850.0-850.9)
flail chest (807.4)
foreign body entering through orifice (930.0-939.9)
injury to blood vessels (901.0-902.9)
The description "with open wound," used in the fourth-digit subdivisions, includes those with mention of infection or foreign body.

√4th **860 Traumatic pneumothorax and hemothorax**
AHA: 2Q, '93, 4

DEF: Traumatic pneumothorax: air or gas leaking into pleural space of lung due to trauma.

DEF: Traumatic hemothorax: blood buildup in pleural space of lung due to trauma.

§ Requires fifth digit. See beginning of section 850-854 for codes and definitions.

N Newborn Age: 0    P Pediatric Age: 0-17    M Maternity Age: 12-55    A Adult Age: 15-124    `CC` CC Condition    `MCC` Major CC Condition    `HIV` HIV Related Dx

**860.0  Pneumothorax without mention of open wound into thorax** `CC`

CC Excl: 860.0-860.5, 861.20-861.32, 862.29, 862.39-862.9, 875.0-875.1, 879.8-879.9,929.0-929.9,958.7-958.99, 959.8-959.9

**860.1  Pneumothorax with open wound into thorax** `MCC`

CC Excl: See code 860.0

**860.2  Hemothorax without mention of open wound into thorax** `MCC`

CC Excl: See code 860.0

**860.3  Hemothorax with open wound into thorax** `MCC`

CC Excl: See code 860.0

**860.4  Pneumohemothorax without mention of open wound into thorax** `MCC`

CC Excl: See code 860.0

**860.5  Pneumohemothorax with open wound into thorax** `MCC`

CC Excl: See code 860.0

✓4th **861  Injury to heart and lung**

> EXCLUDES  *injury to blood vessels of thorax (901.0-901.9)*

✓5th **861.0  Heart, without mention of open wound into thorax**

AHA: 1Q, '92, 9

**861.00  Unspecified injury** `CC`

CC Excl: 861.00-861.13, 862.29, 862.39-862.9, 959.9

**861.01  Contusion** `CC`

Cardiac contusion  Myocardial contusion

CC Excl: 861.00-861.13, 862.29, 862.39-862.9, 875.0-875.1, 879.8-879.9,929.0-929.9,958.7-958.99, 959.8-959.9

DEF: Bruising within the pericardium with no mention of open wound.

**861.02  Laceration without penetration of heart chambers** `MCC`

CC Excl: See code 861.01

DEF: Tearing injury of heart tissue, without penetration of chambers; no open wound.

**861.03  Laceration with penetration of heart chambers** `MCC`

CC Excl: See code 861.01

✓5th **861.1  Heart, with open wound into thorax**

**861.10  Unspecified injury** `MCC`

CC Excl: See code 861.01

**861.11  Contusion** `MCC`

CC Excl: See code 861.01

**861.12  Laceration without penetration of heart chambers** `MCC`

CC Excl: See code 861.01

**861.13  Laceration with penetration of heart chambers** `MCC`

CC Excl: See code 861.01

✓5th **861.2  Lung, without mention of open wound into thorax**

**861.20  Unspecified injury** `CC`

CC Excl: 861.20-861.32, 862.29, 862.39-862.9, 875.0-875.1, 879.8-879.9,929.0-929.9,958.7-958.8, 958.99, 959.8-959.9

**861.21  Contusion** `CC`

CC Excl: See code: 861.20

DEF: Bruising of lung without mention of open wound.

**861.22  Laceration** `MCC`

CC Excl: 861.20-861.32, 862.29, 862.39-862.9, 875.0-875.1, 879.8-879.9,929.0-929.9,958.7-958.99, 959.8-959.9

✓5th **861.3  Lung, with open wound into thorax**

**861.30  Unspecified injury** `MCC`

CC Excl: See code 861.22

**861.31  Contusion** `MCC`

CC Excl: See code 861.22

**861.32  Laceration** `MCC`

CC Excl: See code 861.22

✓4th **862  Injury to other and unspecified intrathoracic organs**

> EXCLUDES  *injury to blood vessels of thorax (901.0-901.9)*

**862.0  Diaphragm, without mention of open wound into cavity** `CC`

CC Excl: 862.0-862.1, 862.29, 862.39-862.9, 875.0-875.1, 879.8-879.9,929.0-929.9,958.7-958.8, 958.99, 959.8-959.9

**862.1  Diaphragm, with open wound into cavity** `MCC`

CC Excl: 862.0-862.1, 862.29, 862.39-862.9, 875.0-875.1, 879.8-879.9,929.0-929.9,958.7-958.99, 959.8-959.9

✓5th **862.2  Other specified intrathoracic organs, without mention of open wound into cavity**

**862.21  Bronchus** `MCC`

CC Excl: 862.21, 862.29-862.31, 862.39-862.9, 875.0-875.1, 879.8-879.9,929.0-929.9,958.7-958.99, 959.8-959.9

**862.22  Esophagus** `MCC`

CC Excl: 862.22-862.29, 862.32-862.9, 875.0-875.1, 879.8-879.9,929.0-929.9,958.7-958.99, 959.8-959.9

**862.29  Other** `CC`

Pleura
Thymus gland

CC Excl: 862.29, 862.39-862.9, 875.0-875.1, 879.8-879.9,929.0-929.9,958.7-958.99, 959.8-959.9

✓5th **862.3  Other specified intrathoracic organs, with open wound into cavity**

**862.31  Bronchus** `MCC`

CC Excl: See code: 862.21

**862.32  Esophagus** `MCC`

CC Excl: See code: 862.22

**862.39  Other** `MCC`

CC Excl: See code: 862.29

**862.8  Multiple and unspecified intrathoracic organs, without mention of open wound into cavity** `CC`

Crushed chest
Multiple intrathoracic organs

CC Excl: 862.29, 862.39-862.9, 875.0-875.1, 879.8-879.9,929.0-929.9,958.7-958.8,958.93-958.99, 959.8-959.9

**862.9  Multiple and unspecified intrathoracic organs, with open wound into cavity** `MCC`

CC Excl: See code: 862.29

✓4th **863  Injury to gastrointestinal tract**

> EXCLUDES  *anal sphincter laceration during delivery (664.2)*
> *bile duct (868.0-868.1 with fifth-digit 2)*
> *gallbladder (868.0-868.1 with fifth-digit 2)*

**863.0  Stomach, without mention of open wound into cavity** `CC`

CC Excl: 729.73, 863.0-863.1, 863.80, 863.89-863.90, 863.99, 868.00, 868.03-868.10, 868.13-869.1, 879.2-879.9,929.0-929.9, 958.8,958.93-958.99, 959.8-959.9

**863.1  Stomach, with open wound into cavity** `MCC`

CC Excl: 863.0-863.1, 863.80, 863.89-863.90, 863.99, 868.00, 868.03-868.10, 868.13-869.1, 879.2-879.9,929.0-929.9,958.8-958.99, 959.8-959.9

✓5th **863.2  Small intestine, without mention of open wound into cavity**

**863.20  Small intestine, unspecified site** `CC`

CC Excl: 729.73, 863.20-863.39, 863.80, 863.89-863.90, 863.99, 868.00, 868.03-868.10, 868.13-869.1, 879.2-879.9,929.0-929.9, 958.8,958.93-958.99, 959.8-959.9

**863.21  Duodenum** `CC`

CC Excl: See code: 863.20

**863.29  Other** `CC`

CC Excl: See code: 863.20

✓4th / ✓5th  Additional Digit Required       Unacceptable PDx       Manifestation Code       ▶◀ Revised Text       ● New Code       ▲ Revised Code Title

© 2007 Ingenix                                                                    October 2007 • Volume 1 — 309

**Injury and Poisoning**

**860.0–863.29**

✓5ᵗʰ **863.3** **Small intestine, with open wound into cavity**
　**863.30** **Small intestine, unspecified site** `MCC`
　　CC Excl: 863.20-863.39, 863.80, 863.89-863.90, 863.99,
　　868.00, 868.03-868.10, 868.13-869.1, 879.2-879.9,929.0-
　　929.9,958.8-958.99, 959.8-959.9

　**863.31** **Duodenum** `MCC`
　　CC Excl: 863.21, 863.31-863.39, 863.80, 863.89-863.90,
　　863.99, 868.00, 868.03-868.10, 868.13-869.1, 879.2-
　　879.9,929.0-929.9,958.8-958.99, 959.8-959.9

　**863.39** **Other** `MCC`
　　CC Excl: See code: 863.30

✓5ᵗʰ **863.4** **Colon or rectum, without mention of open wound into cavity**
　**863.40** **Colon, unspecified site** `CC`
　　CC Excl: 729.73, 863.40-863.80, 863.89-863.90, 863.99,
　　868.00, 868.03-868.10, 868.13-869.1, 879.2-879.9,929.0-929.9,
　　958.8,958.93-958.99, 959.8-959.9

　**863.41** **Ascending [right] colon** `CC`
　　CC Excl: See code: 863.40

　**863.42** **Transverse colon** `CC`
　　CC Excl: See code: 863.40

　**863.43** **Descending [left] colon** `CC`
　　CC Excl: See code: 863.40

　**863.44** **Sigmoid colon** `CC`
　　CC Excl: See code: 863.40

　**863.45** **Rectum** `CC`
　　CC Excl: See code: 863.40

　**863.46** **Multiple sites in colon and rectum** `CC`
　　CC Excl: See code: 863.40

　**863.49** **Other** `CC`
　　CC Excl: See code: 863.40

✓5ᵗʰ **863.5** **Colon or rectum, with open wound into cavity**
　**863.50** **Colon, unspecified site** `MCC`
　　CC Excl: 863.40-863.80, 863.89-863.90, 863.99, 868.00,
　　868.03-868.10, 868.13-869.1, 879.2-879.9,929.0-929.9,
　　958.8-958.99, 959.8-959.9

　**863.51** **Ascending [right] colon** `MCC`
　　CC Excl: See code 863.50

　**863.52** **Transverse colon** `MCC`
　　CC Excl: See code 863.50

　**863.53** **Descending [left] colon** `MCC`
　　CC Excl: See code 863.50

　**863.54** **Sigmoid colon** `MCC`
　　CC Excl: See code 863.50

　**863.55** **Rectum** `MCC`
　　CC Excl: See code 863.50

　**863.56** **Multiple sites in colon and rectum** `MCC`
　　CC Excl: See code 863.50

　**863.59** **Other** `MCC`
　　CC Excl: See code 863.50

✓5ᵗʰ **863.8** **Other and unspecified gastrointestinal sites, without mention of open wound into cavity**
　**863.80** **Gastrointestinal tract, unspecified site** `CC`
　　CC Excl: 729.73, 863.0-863.80, 863.89-863.90, 863.99, 868.00,
　　868.03-868.10, 868.13-869.1, 879.2-879.9,929.0-929.9,
　　958.8,958.93-958.99, 959.8-959.9

　**863.81** **Pancreas, head** `CC`
　　CC Excl: 729.73, 863.80-863.84, 863.91-863.94, 863.99,
　　868.00, 868.03-868.10, 868.13-869.1, 879.2-879.9,929.0-929.9,
　　958.8,958.93-958.99, 959.8-959.9

　**863.82** **Pancreas, body** `CC`
　　CC Excl: See code: 863.81

　**863.83** **Pancreas, tail** `CC`
　　CC Excl: See code: 863.81

　**863.84** **Pancreas, multiple and unspecified sites** `CC`
　　CC Excl: See code: 863.81

　**863.85** **Appendix** `CC`
　　CC Excl: 729.73, 863.40-863.80, 863.85-863.90, 863.99,
　　868.00, 868.03-868.10, 868.13-869.1, 879.2-879.9,929.0-929.9,
　　958.8,958.93-958.99, 959.8-959.9

　**863.89** **Other** `CC`
　　Intestine NOS
　　CC Excl: 729.73, 863.0-863.84, 863.89-863.94, 863.99, 868.00,
　　868.03-868.10, 868.13-869.1, 879.2-879.9,929.0-929.9,958.8-
　　958.90,958.93-958.99, 959.8-959.9

✓5ᵗʰ **863.9** **Other and unspecified gastrointestinal sites, with open wound into cavity**
　**863.90** **Gastrointestinal tract, unspecified site** `MCC`
　　CC Excl: 863.80-863.84, 863.89-863.94, 863.99, 868.00,
　　868.03-868.10, 868.13-869.1, 879.2-879.9,929.0-929.9,958.8-
　　958.99, 959.8-959.9

　**863.91** **Pancreas, head** `MCC`
　　CC Excl: 863.80-863.84, 863.91-863.94, 863.99, 868.00,
　　868.03-868.10, 868.13-869.1, 879.2-879.9,929.0-929.9,958.8-
　　958.99, 959.8-959.9

　**863.92** **Pancreas, body** `MCC`
　　CC Excl: See code 863.91

　**863.93** **Pancreas, tail** `MCC`
　　CC Excl: See code 863.91

　**863.94** **Pancreas, multiple and unspecified sites** `MCC`
　　CC Excl: See code 863.91

　**863.95** **Appendix** `MCC`
　　CC Excl: 863.80, 863.85, 863.95-863.99, 868.00, 868.03-
　　868.10, 868.13-869.1, 879.2-879.9,929.0-929.9,958.8-958.99,
　　959.8-959.9

　**863.99** **Other** `MCC`
　　CC Excl: 863.80, 863.99, 868.00, 868.03-868.10, 868.13-869.1,
　　879.2-879.9,929.0-929.9,958.8-958.99, 959.8-959.9

✓4ᵗʰ **864** **Injury to liver**
　The following fifth-digit subclassification is for use with category 864:
　　**0** **unspecified injury**
　　**1** **hematoma and contusion**
　　**2** **laceration, minor**
　　　Laceration involving capsule only, or without significant involvement of hepatic parenchyma [i.e., less than 1 cm deep]
　　**3** **laceration, moderate**
　　　Laceration involving parenchyma but without major disruption of parenchyma [i.e., less than 10 cm long and less than 3 cm deep]
　　**4** **laceration, major**
　　　Laceration with significant disruption of hepatic parenchyma [i.e., 10 cm long and 3 cm deep]
　　　Multiple moderate lacerations, with or without hematoma
　　　Stellate lacerations of liver
　　**5** **laceration, unspecified**
　　**9** **other**

✓5ᵗʰ **864.0** **Without mention of open wound into cavity** `MCC 3,4` `CC 0-2, 5,9`
　　CC Excl: 863.80, 863.99-864.19, 868.00, 868.03-868.10, 868.13-869.1,
　　879.2-879.9,929.0-929.9,958.8-958.99, 959.8-959.9

✓5ᵗʰ **864.1** **With open wound into cavity** `MCC`
　　CC Excl: See code 864.0

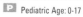 Newborn Age: 0　　　P Pediatric Age: 0-17　　　M Maternity Age: 12-55　　　A Adult Age: 15-124　　　CC CC Condition　　　MCC Major CC Condition　　　HIV HIV Related Dx

310 — Volume 1 • October 2007　　　　　　　　　　　　　　　　　　　　　　　© 2007 Ingenix

√4ᵗʰ **865 Injury to spleen**

The following fifth-digit subclassification is for use with category 865:

    0 unspecified injury
    1 hematoma without rupture of capsule
    2 capsular tears, without major disruption of parenchyma
    3 laceration extending into parenchyma
    4 massive parenchymal disruption
    9 other

√5ᵗʰ **865.0 Without mention of wound into cavity**    `MCC 3,4` `CC 0-2, 9`

CC Excl: 865.00-865.19, 868.00, 868.03-868.10, 868.13-869.1, 879.2-879.9,929.0-929.9,958.8-958.99, 959.8-959.9

√5ᵗʰ **865.1 With open wound into cavity**    `MCC`

CC Excl: See code 865.0

√4ᵗʰ **866 Injury to kidney**

The following fifth-digit subclassification is for use with category 866:

    0 unspecified injury
    1 hematoma without rupture of capsule
    2 laceration
    3 complete disruption of kidney parenchyma

√5ᵗʰ **866.0 Without mention of open wound into cavity**    `MCC 3` `CC 0-2`

CC Excl: 866.00-866.13, 868.00, 868.03-868.10, 868.13-869.1, 879.2-879.9,929.0-929.9,958.8-958.99, 959.8-959.9

√5ᵗʰ **866.1 With open wound into cavity**    `MCC`

CC Excl: See code 866.0

√4ᵗʰ **867 Injury to pelvic organs**

    `EXCLUDES` injury during delivery (664.0-665.9)

**867.0 Bladder and urethra, without mention of open wound into cavity**    `CC`

CC Excl: 867.0-867.1, 867.6-868.00, 868.03-868.10, 868.13-869.1, 879.2-879.9,929.0-929.9,958.8-958.99, 959.8-959.9

AHA: N-D, '85, 15

**867.1 Bladder and urethra, with open wound into cavity**    `MCC`

CC Excl: See code 867.0

**867.2 Ureter, without mention of open wound into cavity**    `CC`

CC Excl: 867.2-867.3, 867.6-868.00, 868.03-868.10, 868.13-869.1, 879.2-879.9,929.0-929.9,958.8-958.99, 959.8-959.9

**867.3 Ureter, with open wound into cavity**    `MCC`

CC Excl: See code 867.2

**867.4 Uterus, without mention of open wound intocavity**    `CC` ♀

CC Excl: 867.4-868.00, 868.03-868.10, 868.13-869.1, 879.2-879.9,929.0-929.9,958.8-958.99, 959.8-959.9

**867.5 Uterus, with open wound into cavity**    `MCC` ♀

CC Excl: See code 867.4

**867.6 Other specified pelvic organs, without mention of open wound into cavity**    `CC`

    Fallopian tube     Seminal vesicle
    Ovary     Vas deferens
    Prostate

CC Excl: 867.6-868.00, 868.03-868.10, 868.13-869.1, 879.2-879.9,929.0-929.9,958.8-958.99, 959.8-959.9

**867.7 Other specified pelvic organs, with open wound into cavity**    `MCC`

CC Excl: See code 867.6

**867.8 Unspecified pelvic organ, without mention of open wound into cavity**    `CC`

CC Excl: See code 867.6

**867.9 Unspecified pelvic organ, with open wound into cavity**    `MCC`

CC Excl: See code 867.6

√4ᵗʰ **868 Injury to other intra-abdominal organs**

The following fifth-digit subclassification is for use with category 868:

    0 unspecified intra-abdominal organ
    1 adrenal gland
    2 bile duct and gallbladder
    3 peritoneum
    4 retroperitoneum
    9 other and multiple intra-abdominal organs

√5ᵗʰ **868.0 Without mention of open wound into cavity**    `CC`

CC Excl: For codes 868.00, **868.03-863.09:** 868.00, 868.03-868.10, 868.13-869.1, 879.2-879.9,929.0-929.9,958.8-958.99, 959.8-959.9; **For code 868.01:** 868.00-868.01, 868.03-868.11, 868.13-869.1, 879.2-879.9,929.0-929.9,958.8-958.99, 959.8-959.9; **For code 868.02:** 868.00, 868.02-868.10, 868.13-869.1, 879.2-879.9,929.0-929.9,958.8-958.99, 959.8-959.9

√5ᵗʰ **868.1 With open wound into cavity**    `MCC`

CC Excl: For codes **868.10, 868.13-868.19:** 868.00, 868.03-868.10, 868.13-869.1, 879.2-879.9,929.0-929.9,958.8-958.99, 959.8-959.9; **For code 868.11:** 868.00-868.01, 868.03-868.11, 868.13-869.1, 879.2-879.9,929.0-929.9,958.8-958.99, 959.8-959.9; **For code 868.12:** 868.00, 868.03-868.10, 868.12-869.1, 879.2-879.9,929.0-929.9,958.8-958.99, 959.8-959.9

√4ᵗʰ **869 Internal injury to unspecified or ill-defined organs**

    `INCLUDES` internal injury NOS
               multiple internal injury NOS

**869.0 Without mention of open wound into cavity**    `CC`

CC Excl: 868.00, 868.03-868.10, 868.13-869.1, 879.2-879.9,929.0-929.9,958.8-958.99, 959.8-959.9

**869.1 With open wound into cavity**    `MCC`

CC Excl: See code: 869.0

AHA: 2Q, '89, 15

### OPEN WOUND (870-897)

    `INCLUDES` animal bite
              avulsion
              cut
              laceration
              puncture wound
              traumatic amputation

    `EXCLUDES` burn (940.0-949.5)
              crushing (925-929.9)
              puncture of internal organs (860.0-869.1)
              superficial injury (910.0-919.9)
              that incidental to:
                 dislocation (830.0-839.9)
                 fracture (800.0-829.1)
                 internal injury (860.0-869.1)
                 intracranial injury (851.0-854.1)

Note: The description "complicated" used in the fourth-digit subdivisions includes those with mention of delayed healing, delayed treatment, foreign body, or infection. Use additional code to identify infection

AHA: 4Q, '01, 52

### OPEN WOUND OF HEAD, NECK, AND TRUNK (870-879)

√4ᵗʰ **870 Open wound of ocular adnexa**

**870.0 Laceration of skin of eyelid and periocular area**

**870.1 Laceration of eyelid, full-thickness, not involving lacrimal passages**

**870.2 Laceration of eyelid involving lacrimal passages** `CC`

CC Excl: 870.0-871.9, 879.8-879.9,929.0-929.9, 958.8, 959.8-959.9

**870.3 Penetrating wound of orbit, without mention of foreign body** `CC`

CC Excl: 870.0-871.9, 879.8-879.9,929.0-929.9,958.8-958.99, 959.8-959.9

**870.4 Penetrating wound of orbit with foreign body** `CC`

    `EXCLUDES` retained (old) foreign body in orbit (376.6)

CC Excl: See code 870.3

**Injury and Poisoning**

**870.8–873.61**

**870.8**   **Other specified open wounds of ocular adnexa** `CC`
CC Excl: See code 870.3

**870.9**   **Unspecified open wound of ocular adnexa** `CC`
CC Excl: See code 870.3

√4ᵗʰ **871 Open wound of eyeball**
EXCLUDES   *2nd cranial nerve [optic] injury (950.0-950.9)*
*3rd cranial nerve [oculomotor] injury (951.0)*

**871.0**   **Ocular laceration without prolapse of intraocular tissue** `CC`
CC Excl: See code 870.3
AHA: 3Q, '96, 7
DEF: Tear in ocular tissue without displacing structures.

**871.1**   **Ocular laceration with prolapse or exposure of intraocular tissue** `CC`
CC Excl: See code 870.3

**871.2**   **Rupture of eye with partial loss of intraocular tissue** `CC`
CC Excl: See code 870.3
DEF: Forcible tearing of eyeball, with tissue loss.

**871.3**   **Avulsion of eye** `CC`
Traumatic enucleation
CC Excl: See code 870.3
DEF: Traumatic extraction of eyeball from socket.

**871.4**   **Unspecified laceration of eye**

**871.5**   **Penetration of eyeball with magnetic foreign body** `CC`
EXCLUDES   *retained (old) magnetic foreign body in globe (360.50-360.59)*
CC Excl: 870.0-871.9, 879.8-879.9, 929.0-929.9, 958.8, 959.8-959.9

**871.6**   **Penetration of eyeball with (nonmagnetic) foreign body** `CC`
EXCLUDES   *retained (old) (nonmagnetic) foreign body in globe (360.60-360.69)*
CC Excl: 870.0-871.9, 879.8-879.9, 929.0-929.9, 958.8, 959.8-959.9

**871.7**   **Unspecified ocular penetration**

**871.9**   **Unspecified open wound of eyeball** `CC`
CC Excl: See code: 870.3

√4ᵗʰ **872 Open wound of ear**

√5ᵗʰ **872.0**   **External ear, without mention of complication**
**872.00** External ear, unspecified site
**872.01** Auricle, ear
Pinna
DEF: Open wound of fleshy, outer ear.
**872.02** Auditory canal
DEF: Open wound of passage from external ear to eardrum.

√5ᵗʰ **872.1**   **External ear, complicated**
**872.10** External ear, unspecified site
**872.11** Auricle, ear
**872.12** Auditory canal `CC`
CC Excl: 872.00-872.9, 879.8-879.9, 929.0-929.9, 958.8, 959.8-959.9

√5ᵗʰ **872.6**   **Other specified parts of ear, without mention of complication**
**872.61** Ear drum `CC`
Drumhead     Tympanic membrane
CC Excl: See code: 872.12
**872.62** Ossicles `CC`
CC Excl: See code: 872.12
**872.63** Eustachian tube `CC`
CC Excl: See code: 872.12
DEF: Open wound of channel between nasopharynx and tympanic cavity.

**872.64** Cochlea `CC`
CC Excl: See code: 872.12
DEF: Open wound of snail shell shaped tube of inner ear.

**872.69** Other and multiple sites `CC`
CC Excl: See code 872.12

√5ᵗʰ **872.7**   **Other specified parts of ear, complicated**
**872.71** Ear drum `CC`
CC Excl: See code: 872.12
**872.72** Ossicles `CC`
CC Excl: 872.00-872.9, 879.8-879.9, 929.0-929.9, 958.8-958.99, 959.8-959.9
**872.73** Eustachian tube `CC`
CC Excl: See code 872.72
**872.74** Cochlea `CC`
CC Excl: See code 872.72
**872.79** Other and multiple sites `CC`
CC Excl: See code: 872.12

**872.8**   **Ear, part unspecified, without mention of complication**
Ear NOS

**872.9**   **Ear, part unspecified, complicated**

√4ᵗʰ **873 Other open wound of head**
**873.0**   **Scalp, without mention of complication**
**873.1**   **Scalp, complicated**

√5ᵗʰ **873.2**   **Nose, without mention of complication**
**873.20** Nose, unspecified site
**873.21** Nasal septum
DEF: Open wound between nasal passages.
**873.22** Nasal cavity
DEF: Open wound of nostrils.
**873.23** Nasal sinus `CC`
CC Excl: 873.20-873.39, 879.8-879.9, 929.0-929.9, 958.8, 959.8-959.9
DEF: Open wound of mucous-lined respiratory cavities.
**873.29** Multiple sites

√5ᵗʰ **873.3**   **Nose, complicated**
**873.30** Nose, unspecified site
**873.31** Nasal septum
**873.32** Nasal cavity
**873.33** Nasal sinus `CC`
CC Excl: 873.20-873.39, 879.8-879.9, 929.0-929.9, 958.8-958.99, 959.8-959.9
**873.39** Multiple sites

√5ᵗʰ **873.4**   **Face, without mention of complication**
**873.40** Face, unspecified site
**873.41** Cheek
**873.42** Forehead
Eyebrow
AHA: 4Q, '96, 43
**873.43** Lip
**873.44** Jaw
**873.49** Other and multiple sites

√5ᵗʰ **873.5**   **Face, complicated**
**873.50** Face, unspecified site
**873.51** Cheek
**873.52** Forehead
**873.53** Lip
**873.54** Jaw
**873.59** Other and multiple sites

√5ᵗʰ **873.6**   **Internal structures of mouth, without mention of complication**
**873.60** Mouth, unspecified site
**873.61** Buccal mucosa
DEF: Open wound of inside of cheek.

---

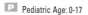 **N** Newborn Age: 0    **P** Pediatric Age: 0-17    **M** Maternity Age: 12-55    **A** Adult Age: 15-124    **CC** CC Condition    **MCC** Major CC Condition    **HIV** HIV Related Dx

**873.62** Gum (alveolar process)

**873.63** Tooth (broken) (fractured) (due to trauma)

> EXCLUDES    cracked tooth (521.81)

AHA: 1Q, '04, 17

**873.64** Tongue and floor of mouth

**873.65** Palate

DEF: Open wound of roof of mouth.

**873.69** Other and multiple sites

✓5th **873.7** Internal structures of mouth, complicated

**873.70** Mouth, unspecified site

**873.71** Buccal mucosa

**873.72** Gum (alveolar process)

**873.73** Tooth (broken) (fractured) (due to trauma)

> EXCLUDES    cracked tooth (521.81)

AHA: 1Q, '04, 17

**873.74** Tongue and floor of mouth

**873.75** Palate

**873.79** Other and multiple sites

**873.8** Other and unspecified open wound of head without mention of complication

Head NOS

**873.9** Other and unspecified open wound of head, complicated

✓4th **874** Open wound of neck

✓5th **874.0** Larynx and trachea, without mention of complication

**874.00** Larynx with trachea    MCC

CC Excl: 847.0, 874.00-874.12, 874.8-874.9, 879.8-879.9,929.0-929.9,958.8-958.99, 959.8-959.9

**874.01** Larynx    MCC

CC Excl: See code 874.00

**874.02** Trachea    MCC

CC Excl: See code 874.00

✓5th **874.1** Larynx and trachea, complicated

**874.10** Larynx with trachea    MCC

CC Excl: See code 874.00

**874.11** Larynx    MCC

CC Excl: See code 874.00

**874.12** Trachea    MCC

CC Excl: See code 874.00

**874.2** Thyroid gland, without mention of complication CC

CC Excl: 847.0, 874.2-874.3, 874.8-874.9, 879.8-879.9,929.0-929.9, 958.8, 959.8-959.9

**874.3** Thyroid gland, complicated    CC

CC Excl: 847.0, 874.2-874.3, 874.8-874.9, 879.8-879.9, 929.0-929.9,958.8-958.99, 959.8-959.9

**874.4** Pharynx, without mention of complication    CC

Cervical esophagus

CC Excl: 847.0, 874.4-874.9, 879.8-879.9,929.0-929.9, 958.8, 959.8-959.9

**874.5** Pharynx, complicated    CC

CC Excl: 847.0, 874.4-874.9, 879.8-879.9,929.0-929.9,958.8-958.99, 959.8-959.9

**874.8** Other and unspecified parts, without mention of complication

Nape of neck    Throat NOS
Supraclavicular region

**874.9** Other and unspecified parts, complicated

✓4th **875** Open wound of chest (wall)

> EXCLUDES    open wound into thoracic cavity (860.0-862.9)
> traumatic pneumothorax and hemothorax
> (860.1, 860.3, 860.5)

AHA: 3Q, '93, 17

**875.0** Without mention of complication    CC

CC Excl: 847.1, 862.29, 862.39-862.9, 875.0-875.1, 879.8-879.9,929.0-929.9,958.7-958.99, 959.8-959.9

**875.1** Complicated    CC

CC Excl: See code 875.0

✓4th **876** Open wound of back

> INCLUDES    loin
> lumbar region

> EXCLUDES    open wound into thoracic cavity (860.0-862.9)
> traumatic pneumothorax and hemothorax
> (860.1, 860.3, 860.5)

**876.0** Without mention of complication

**876.1** Complicated

✓4th **877** Open wound of buttock

> INCLUDES    sacroiliac region

**877.0** Without mention of complication

**877.1** Complicated

✓4th **878** Open wound of genital organs (external), including traumatic amputation

> EXCLUDES    injury during delivery (664.0-665.9)
> internal genital organs (867.0-867.9)

**878.0** Penis, without mention of complication    ♂

**878.1** Penis, complicated    ♂

**878.2** Scrotum and testes, without mention of complication    ♂

**878.3** Scrotum and testes, complicated    ♂

**878.4** Vulva, without mention of complication    ♀

Labium (majus) (minus)

**878.5** Vulva, complicated    ♀

**878.6** Vagina, without mention of complication    ♀

**878.7** Vagina, complicated    ♀

**878.8** Other and unspecified parts, without mention of complication

**878.9** Other and unspecified parts, complicated

✓4th **879** Open wound of other and unspecified sites, except limbs

**879.0** Breast, without mention of complication

**879.1** Breast, complicated

**879.2** Abdominal wall, anterior, without mention of complication

Abdominal wall NOS    Pubic region
Epigastric region    Umbilical region
Hypogastric region

AHA: 2Q, '91, 22

**879.3** Abdominal wall, anterior, complicated

**879.4** Abdominal wall, lateral, without mention of complication

Flank    Iliac (region)
Groin    Inguinal region
Hypochondrium

**879.5** Abdominal wall, lateral, complicated

**879.6** Other and unspecified parts of trunk, without mention of complication

Pelvic region    Trunk NOS
Perineum

**879.7** Other and unspecified parts of trunk, complicated

**879.8** Open wound(s) (multiple) of unspecified site(s) without mention of complication

Multiple open wounds NOS    Open wound NOS

**879.9** Open wound(s) (multiple) of unspecified site(s), complicated

## OPEN WOUND OF UPPER LIMB (880-887)

AHA: N-D, '85, 5

✓4th **880** Open wound of shoulder and upper arm

The following fifth-digit subclassification is for use with category 880:

   0 shoulder region
   1 scapular region
   2 axillary region
   3 upper arm
   9 multiple sites

✓5th **880.0** Without mention of complication

✓5th **880.1** Complicated

AHA: 2Q, '06, 7

✓5th **880.2** With tendon involvement    CC

CC Excl: 880.00-880.29

---

√4ᵗʰ **881 Open wound of elbow, forearm, and wrist**
  The following fifth-digit subclassification is for use with
  category 881:
  **0 forearm**
  **1 elbow**
  **2 wrist**

√5ᵗʰ **881.0 Without mention of complication**
√5ᵗʰ **881.1 Complicated**
√5ᵗʰ **881.2 With tendon involvement**    `CC`
    CC Excl: 881.00-881.22

√4ᵗʰ **882 Open wound of hand except finger(s) alone**
  **882.0 Without mention of complication**
  **882.1 Complicated**
  **882.2 With tendon involvement**    `CC`
    CC Excl: 882.0-882.2

√4ᵗʰ **883 Open wound of finger(s)**
  INCLUDES  fingernail
      thumb (nail)
  **883.0 Without mention of complication**
  **883.1 Complicated**
  **883.2 With tendon involvement**    `CC`
    CC Excl: 883.0-883.2

√4ᵗʰ **884 Multiple and unspecified open wound of upper limb**
  INCLUDES  arm NOS
      multiple sites of one upper limb
      upper limb NOS
  **884.0 Without mention of complication**
  **884.1 Complicated**
  **884.2 With tendon involvement**    `CC`
    CC Excl: 884.0-884.2

√4ᵗʰ **885 Traumatic amputation of thumb (complete) (partial)**
  INCLUDES  thumb(s) (with finger(s) of either hand)
  **885.0 Without mention of complication**
    AHA: 1Q, '03, 7
  **885.1 Complicated**

√4ᵗʰ **886 Traumatic amputation of other finger(s) (complete) (partial)**
  INCLUDES  finger(s) of one or both hands, without mention
      of thumb(s)
  **886.0 Without mention of complication**
  **886.1 Complicated**

√4ᵗʰ **887 Traumatic amputation of arm and hand (complete) (partial)**
  **887.0 Unilateral, below elbow, without mention**    `CC`
    **of complication**
    CC Excl: 880.00-887.7,929.0-929.9,958.8-958.99, 959.8-959.9
  **887.1 Unilateral, below elbow, complicated**    `CC`
    CC Excl: See code 887.0
  **887.2 Unilateral, at or above elbow, without**    `CC`
    **mention of complication**
    CC Excl: See code 887.0
  **887.3 Unilateral, at or above elbow, complicated**    `CC`
    CC Excl: See code 887.0
  **887.4 Unilateral, level not specified, without**    `CC`
    **mention of complication**
    CC Excl: See code 887.0
  **887.5 Unilateral, level not specified, complicated**    `CC`
    CC Excl: See code 887.0
  **887.6 Bilateral [any level], without mention of**    `MCC`
    **complication**
      One hand and other arm
    CC Excl: See code 887.0
  **887.7 Bilateral [any level], complicated**    `MCC`
    CC Excl: See code 887.0

## OPEN WOUND OF LOWER LIMB (890-897)
  AHA: N-D, '85, 5

√4ᵗʰ **890 Open wound of hip and thigh**
  **890.0 Without mention of complication**
  **890.1 Complicated**
  **890.2 With tendon involvement**    `CC`
    CC Excl: 890.0-890.2

√4ᵗʰ **891 Open wound of knee, leg [except thigh], and ankle**
  INCLUDES  leg NOS
      multiple sites of leg, except thigh
  EXCLUDES  *that of thigh (890.0-890.2)*
      *with multiple sites of lower limb (894.0-894.2)*
  **891.0 Without mention of complication**
  **891.1 Complicated**
  **891.2 With tendon involvement**    `CC`
    CC Excl: 891.0-891.2

√4ᵗʰ **892 Open wound of foot except toe(s) alone**
  INCLUDES  heel
  **892.0 Without mention of complication**
  **892.1 Complicated**
  **892.2 With tendon involvement**    `CC`
    CC Excl: 892.0-892.2

√4ᵗʰ **893 Open wound of toe(s)**
  INCLUDES  toenail
  **893.0 Without mention of complication**
  **893.1 Complicated**
  **893.2 With tendon involvement**    `CC`
    CC Excl: 893.0-893.2

√4ᵗʰ **894 Multiple and unspecified open wound of lower limb**
  INCLUDES  lower limb NOS
      multiple sites of one lower limb, with thigh
  **894.0 Without mention of complication**
  **894.1 Complicated**
  **894.2 With tendon involvement**    `CC`
    CC Excl: 894.0-894.2

√4ᵗʰ **895 Traumatic amputation of toe(s) (complete) (partial)**
  INCLUDES  toe(s) of one or both feet
  **895.0 Without mention of complication**
  **895.1 Complicated**

√4ᵗʰ **896 Traumatic amputation of foot (complete) (partial)**
  **896.0 Unilateral, without mention of complication**    `CC`
    CC Excl: 890.0-897.7,929.0-929.9,958.8-958.99, 959.8-959.9
  **896.1 Unilateral, complicated**    `CC`
    CC Excl: See code 896.0
  **896.2 Bilateral, without mention of complication**    `MCC`
    EXCLUDES  *one foot and other leg (897.6-897.7)*
    CC Excl: See code 896.0
  **896.3 Bilateral, complicated**    `MCC`
    CC Excl: See code 896.0

√4ᵗʰ **897 Traumatic amputation of leg(s) (complete) (partial)**
  **897.0 Unilateral, below knee, without mention of**    `CC`
    **complication**
    CC Excl: See code 896.0
  **897.1 Unilateral, below knee, complicated**    `CC`
    CC Excl: See code 896.0
  **897.2 Unilateral, at or above knee, without**    `CC`
    **mention of complication**
    CC Excl: See code 896.0
  **897.3 Unilateral, at or above knee, complicated**    `CC`
    CC Excl: See code 896.0
  **897.4 Unilateral, level not specified, without**    `CC`
    **mention of complication**
    CC Excl: See code 896.0
  **897.5 Unilateral, level not specified, complicated**    `CC`
    CC Excl: See code 896.0
  **897.6 Bilateral [any level], without mention of**    `MCC`
    **complication**
      One foot and other leg
    CC Excl: See code 896.0
  **897.7 Bilateral [any level], complicated**    `MCC`
    CC Excl: See code 896.0
    AHA: 3Q, '90, 5

N Newborn Age: 0   P Pediatric Age: 0-17   M Maternity Age: 12-55   A Adult Age: 15-124   CC CC Condition   MCC Major CC Condition   HIV HIV Related Dx

314 — Volume 1 • October 2007                                                     © 2007 Ingenix

## INJURY TO BLOOD VESSELS (900-904)

| INCLUDES | arterial hematoma | of blood vessel, |
| --- | --- | --- |
| | avulsion | secondary to |
| | cut | other injuries |
| | laceration | e.g., fracture |
| | rupture | or open |
| | traumatic aneurysm | wound |
| | or fistula (arteri- | |
| | ovenous) | |

| EXCLUDES | accidental puncture or laceration during medical procedure (998.2) |
| --- | --- |
| | intracranial hemorrhage following injury (851.0-854.1) |

**AHA:** 3Q, '90, 5

✓4ᵗʰ **900 Injury to blood vessels of head and neck**

✓5ᵗʰ **900.0 Carotid artery**

**900.00 Carotid artery, unspecified** `CC`
CC Excl: 900.00,900.82-900.9, 904.9,929.0-929.9, 958.8-958.99, 959.8-959.9

**900.01 Common carotid artery** `CC`
CC Excl: See code 900.00

**900.02 External carotid artery** `CC`
CC Excl: See code 900.00

**900.03 Internal carotid artery** `CC`
CC Excl: See code 900.00

**900.1 Internal jugular vein** `CC`
CC Excl: 900.82-900.9, 904.9,929.0-929.9,958.8-958.99, 959.8-959.9

✓5ᵗʰ **900.8 Other specified blood vessels of head and neck**

**900.81 External jugular vein** `CC`
Jugular vein NOS
CC Excl: See code 900.1

**900.82 Multiple blood vessels of head and neck** `CC`
CC Excl: See code 900.1

**900.89 Other** `CC`
CC Excl: See code 900.1

**900.9 Unspecified blood vessel of head and neck** `CC`
CC Excl: See code 900.1

✓4ᵗʰ **901 Injury to blood vessels of thorax**

| EXCLUDES | traumatic hemothorax (860.2-860.5) |
| --- | --- |

**901.0 Thoracic aorta** `MCC`
CC Excl: 901.0, 904.9,929.0-929.9,958.8-958.99, 959.8-959.9

**901.1 Innominate and subclavian arteries** `MCC`
CC Excl: 901.1, 904.9,929.0-929.9,958.8-958.99, 959.8-959.9

**901.2 Superior vena cava** `MCC`
CC Excl: 901.2, 904.9,929.0-929.9,958.8-958.99, 959.8-959.9

**901.3 Innominate and subclavian veins** `MCC`
CC Excl: 901.3, 904.9,929.0-929.9,958.8-958.99, 959.8-959.9

✓5ᵗʰ **901.4 Pulmonary blood vessels**

**901.40 Pulmonary vessel(s), unspecified** `MCC`
CC Excl: 901.40-901.41, 904.9,929.0-929.9,958.8-958.90, 958.99, 959.8-959.9

**901.41 Pulmonary artery** `MCC`
CC Excl: 901.40-901.41, 904.9,929.0-929.9,958.8-958.99, 959.8-959.9

**901.42 Pulmonary vein** `MCC`
CC Excl: 901.40, 901.42, 904.9,929.0-929.9,958.8-958.99, 959.8-959.9

✓5ᵗʰ **901.8 Other specified blood vessels of thorax**

**901.81 Intercostal artery or vein** `CC`
CC Excl: 901.81, 901.83-901.89

**901.82 Internal mammary artery or vein** `CC`
CC Excl: 901.82-901.89

**901.83 Multiple blood vessels of thorax** `MCC`
CC Excl: 904.9,929.0-929.9,958.8-958.99, 959.8-959.9

**901.89 Other** `CC`
Azygos vein
Hemiazygos vein
CC Excl: 901.0-901.9

**901.9 Unspecified blood vessel of thorax** `CC`
CC Excl: See code: 901.89

✓4ᵗʰ **902 Injury to blood vessels of abdomen and pelvis**

**902.0 Abdominal aorta** `MCC`
CC Excl: 902.0,902.87-902.9, 904.9,929.0-929.9,958.8-958.99, 959.8-959.9

✓5ᵗʰ **902.1 Inferior vena cava**

**902.10 Inferior vena cava, unspecified** `MCC`
CC Excl: 902.10,902.87-902.9, 904.9,929.0-929.9, 958.8-958.99, 959.8-959.9

**902.11 Hepatic veins** `MCC`
CC Excl: 902.11,902.87-902.9, 904.9,929.0-929.9, 958.8-958.99, 959.8-959.9

**902.19 Other** `MCC`
CC Excl: 902.19,902.87-902.9, 904.9,929.0-929.9, 958.8-958.99, 959.8-959.9

✓5ᵗʰ **902.2 Celiac and mesenteric arteries**

**902.20 Celiac and mesenteric arteries, unspecified** `MCC`
CC Excl: 902.20,902.87-902.9, 904.9,929.0-929.9, 958.8-958.99, 959.8-959.9

**902.21 Gastric artery** `MCC`
CC Excl: 902.21,902.87-902.9, 904.9,929.0-929.9, 958.8-958.90,958.93-958.99, 959.8-959.9

**902.22 Hepatic artery** `MCC`
CC Excl: 902.22,902.87-902.9, 904.9,929.0-929.9, 958.8-958.99, 959.8-959.9

**902.23 Splenic artery** `MCC`
CC Excl: 902.23,902.87-902.9, 904.9,929.0-929.9, 958.8-958.99, 959.8-959.9

**902.24 Other specified branches of celiac axis** `MCC`
CC Excl: 902.24,902.87-902.9, 904.9,929.0-929.9, 958.8-958.99, 959.8-959.9

**902.25 Superior mesenteric artery (trunk)** `MCC`
CC Excl: 902.25,902.87-902.9, 904.9,929.0-929.9, 958.8-958.99, 959.8-959.9

**902.26 Primary branches of superior mesenteric artery** `MCC`
Ileocolic artery
CC Excl: 902.26,902.87-902.9, 904.9,929.0-929.9, 958.8-958.99, 959.8-959.9

**902.27 Inferior mesenteric artery** `MCC`
CC Excl: 902.27,902.87-902.9, 904.9,929.0-929.9, 958.8-958.99, 959.8-959.9

**902.29 Other** `MCC`
CC Excl: 902.29,902.87-902.9, 904.9,929.0-929.9, 958.8-958.99, 959.8-959.9

✓5ᵗʰ **902.3 Portal and splenic veins**

**902.31 Superior mesenteric vein and primary subdivisions** `MCC`
Ileocolic vein
CC Excl: 902.31,902.87-902.9, 904.9,929.0-929.9, 958.8-958.99, 959.8-959.9

**902.32 Inferior mesenteric vein** `MCC`
CC Excl: 902.32,902.87-902.9, 904.9,929.0-929.9, 958.8-958.99, 959.8-959.9

---

✓4ᵗʰ / ✓5ᵗʰ Additional Digit Required | Unacceptable PDx | Manifestation Code | ◄► Revised Text | ● New Code | ▲ Revised Code Title

**Injury and Poisoning**

**902.33–904.6**

**902.33 Portal vein** `MCC`
CC Excl: 902.33,902.87-902.9, 904.9,929.0-929.9, 958.8-958.99, 959.8-959.9

**902.34 Splenic vein** `MCC`
CC Excl: 902.34,902.87-902.9, 904.9,929.0-929.9, 958.8-958.99, 959.8-959.9

**902.39 Other** `MCC`
Cystic vein      Gastric vein
CC Excl: 902.39,902.87-902.9, 904.9,929.0-929.9, 958.8-958.99, 959.8-959.9

√5th **902.4 Renal blood vessels**
**902.40 Renal vessel(s), unspecified** `MCC`
CC Excl: 902.40,902.87-902.9, 904.9,929.0-929.9, 958.8-958.99, 959.8-959.9

**902.41 Renal artery** `MCC`
CC Excl: 902.41,902.87-902.9, 904.9,929.0-929.9, 958.8-958.99, 959.8-959.9

**902.42 Renal vein** `MCC`
CC Excl: 902.42,902.87-902.9, 904.9,929.0-929.9, 958.8-958.99, 959.8-959.9

**902.49 Other** `MCC`
Suprarenal arteries
CC Excl: 902.49,902.87-902.9, 904.9,929.0-929.9, 958.8-958.99, 959.8-959.9

√5th **902.5 Iliac blood vessels**
**902.50 Iliac vessel(s), unspecified** `MCC`
CC Excl: 902.50,902.53-902.54, 902.59,902.87-902.9, 904.9,929.0-929.9,958.8-958.99, 959.8-959.9

**902.51 Hypogastric artery** `MCC`
CC Excl: 902.51,902.87-902.9, 904.9,929.0-929.9, 958.8-958.99, 959.8-959.9

**902.52 Hypogastric vein** `MCC`
CC Excl: 902.52,902.87-902.9, 904.9,929.0-929.9, 958.8-958.99, 959.8-959.9

**902.53 Iliac artery** `MCC`
CC Excl: 902.50, 902.53, 902.59,902.87-902.9, 904.9, 929.0-929.9,958.8-958.99, 959.8-959.9

**902.54 Iliac vein** `MCC`
CC Excl: 902.50, 902.54, 902.59,902.87-902.9, 904.9, 929.0-929.9,958.8-958.99, 959.8-959.9

**902.55 Uterine artery** `CC`♀
CC Excl: 902.55, 902.59,902.87-902.9, 904.9,929.0-929.9,958.8-958.90,958.93-958.99, 959.8-959.9

**902.56 Uterine vein** `CC`♀
CC Excl: 902.56-902.59,902.87-902.9, 904.9,929.0-929.9,958.8-958.90,958.93-958.99, 959.8-959.9

**902.59 Other** `MCC`
CC Excl: See code: 902.50

√5th **902.8 Other specified blood vessels of abdomen and pelvis**
**902.81 Ovarian artery** `CC`♀
CC Excl: 902.81,902.87-902.9, 904.9,929.0-929.9,958.8-958.90,958.93-958.99, 959.8-959.9

**902.82 Ovarian vein** `CC`♀
CC Excl: 902.82-902.9, 904.9,929.0-929.9,958.8-958.90,958.93-958.99, 959.8-959.9

**902.87 Multiple blood vessels of abdomen and pelvis** `MCC`
CC Excl: 902.87-902.9, 904.9,929.0-929.9,958.8-958.99, 959.8-959.9

**902.89 Other** `CC`
CC Excl: 902.87-902.9, 904.9,929.0-929.9,958.8-958.90,958.93-958.99, 959.8-959.9

**902.9 Unspecified blood vessel of abdomen and pelvis** `CC`
CC Excl: 902.0-902.9, 904.9,929.0-929.9,958.8-958.90,958.93-958.99, 959.8-959.9

√4th **903 Injury to blood vessels of upper extremity**
√5th **903.0 Axillary blood vessels**
**903.00 Axillary vessel(s), unspecified** `MCC`
CC Excl: 903.00-903.02,903.8-903.9, 904.9

**903.01 Axillary artery** `MCC`
CC Excl: 903.00-903.01,903.8-903.9, 904.9

**903.02 Axillary vein** `MCC`
CC Excl: 903.00, 903.02,903.8-903.9, 904.9

**903.1 Brachial blood vessels** `CC`
CC Excl: 903.1, 903.8-903.9, 904.9

**903.2 Radial blood vessels** `CC`
CC Excl: 903.2, 903.8-903.9, 904.9

**903.3 Ulnar blood vessels** `CC`
CC Excl: 903.3, 903.8-903.9, 904.9

**903.4 Palmar artery** `CC`
CC Excl: 903.4, 903.8-903.9, 904.9

**903.5 Digital blood vessels** `CC`
CC Excl: 903.5-903.9, 904.9

**903.8 Other specified blood vessels of upper extremity** `CC`
Multiple blood vessels of upper extremity
CC Excl: 903.3-903.9, 904.9

**903.9 Unspecified blood vessel of upper extremity** `CC`
CC Excl: See code: 903.8

√4th **904 Injury to blood vessels of lower extremity and unspecified sites**
**904.0 Common femoral artery** `MCC`
Femoral artery above profunda origin
CC Excl: 904.0, 904.7-904.9

**904.1 Superficial femoral artery** `MCC`
CC Excl: 904.1, 904.7-904.9

**904.2 Femoral veins** `MCC`
CC Excl: 904.2, 904.7-904.9

**904.3 Saphenous veins** `CC`
Saphenous vein (greater) (lesser)
CC Excl: 904.3, 904.7-904.9

√5th **904.4 Popliteal blood vessels**
**904.40 Popliteal vessel(s), unspecified** `MCC`
CC Excl: 904.40, 904.7-904.9

**904.41 Popliteal artery** `MCC`
CC Excl: 904.41, 904.7-904.9

**904.42 Popliteal vein** `MCC`
CC Excl: 904.42, 904.7-904.9

√5th **904.5 Tibial blood vessels**
**904.50 Tibial vessel(s), unspecified** `CC`
CC Excl: 904.50, 904.7-904.9

**904.51 Anterior tibial artery** `CC`
CC Excl: 904.51, 904.7-904.9

**904.52 Anterior tibial vein** `CC`
CC Excl: 904.52, 904.7-904.9

**904.53 Posterior tibial artery** `CC`
CC Excl: 904.53, 904.7-904.9

**904.54 Posterior tibial vein** `CC`
CC Excl: 904.54, 904.7-904.9

**904.6 Deep plantar blood vessels** `CC`
CC Excl: 904.6-904.9

---

N Newborn Age: 0    P Pediatric Age: 0-17    M Maternity Age: 12-55    A Adult Age: 15-124    `CC` CC Condition    `MCC` Major CC Condition    HIV HIV Related Dx

© 2007 Ingenix

**904.7**   **Other specified blood vessels of lower extremity** [CC]
Multiple blood vessels of lower extremity
**CC Excl:** 729.72, 904.0-904.9

**904.8**   **Unspecified blood vessel of lower extremity** [CC]
**CC Excl:** See code: 904.7

**904.9**   **Unspecified site** [CC]
Injury to blood vessel NOS
**CC Excl:** 729.71-729.72, 900.00-904.9

## LATE EFFECTS OF INJURIES, POISONINGS, TOXIC EFFECTS, AND OTHER EXTERNAL CAUSES (905-909)

Note: These categories are to be used to indicate conditions classifiable to 800-999 as the cause of late effects, which are themselves classified elsewhere. The "late effects" include those specified as such, or as sequelae, which may occur at any time after the acute injury.

√4ᵗʰ **905 Late effects of musculoskeletal and connective tissue injuries**
**AHA:** 1Q, '95, 10; 2Q, '94, 3

**905.0**   **Late effect of fracture of skull and face bones**
Late effect of injury classifiable to 800-804
**AHA:** 3Q, '97, 12

**905.1**   **Late effect of fracture of spine and trunk without mention of spinal cord lesion**
Late effect of injury classifiable to 805, 807-809
**AHA:** ▶1Q, '07, 20◀

**905.2**   **Late effect of fracture of upper extremities**
Late effect of injury classifiable to 810-819

**905.3**   **Late effect of fracture of neck of femur**
Late effect of injury classifiable to 820

**905.4**   **Late effect of fracture of lower extremities**
Late effect of injury classifiable to 821-827

**905.5**   **Late effect of fracture of multiple and unspecified bones**
Late effect of injury classifiable to 828-829

**905.6**   **Late effect of dislocation**
Late effect of injury classifiable to 830-839

**905.7**   **Late effect of sprain and strain without mention of tendon injury**
Late effect of injury classifiable to 840-848, except tendon injury

**905.8**   **Late effect of tendon injury**
Late effect of tendon injury due to:
open wound [injury classifiable to 880-884 with .2, 890-894 with .2]
sprain and strain [injury classifiable to 840-848]
**AHA:** 2Q, '89, 13; 2Q, '89, 15

**905.9**   **Late effect of traumatic amputation**
Late effect of injury classifiable to 885-887, 895-897
**EXCLUDES**   late amputation stump complication (997.60-997.69)

√4ᵗʰ **906 Late effects of injuries to skin and subcutaneous tissues**

**906.0**   **Late effect of open wound of head, neck, and trunk**
Late effect of injury classifiable to 870-879

**906.1**   **Late effect of open wound of extremities without mention of tendon injury**
Late effect of injury classifiable to 880-884, 890-894 except .2

**906.2**   **Late effect of superficial injury**
Late effect of injury classifiable to 910-919

**906.3**   **Late effect of contusion**
Late effect of injury classifiable to 920-924

**906.4**   **Late effect of crushing**
Late effect of injury classifiable to 925-929

**906.5**   **Late effect of burn of eye, face, head, and neck**
Late effect of injury classifiable to 940-941
**AHA:** 4Q, '04, 76

**906.6**   **Late effect of burn of wrist and hand**
Late effect of injury classifiable to 944
**AHA:** 4Q, '94, 22

**906.7**   **Late effect of burn of other extremities**
Late effect of injury classifiable to 943 or 945
**AHA:** 4Q, '94, 22

**906.8**   **Late effect of burns of other specified sites**
Late effect of injury classifiable to 942, 946-947
**AHA:** 4Q, '94, 22

**906.9**   **Late effect of burn of unspecified site**
Late effect of injury classifiable to 948-949
**AHA:** 4Q, '94, 22

√4ᵗʰ **907 Late effects of injuries to the nervous system**

**907.0**   **Late effect of intracranial injury without mention of skull fracture**
Late effect of injury classifiable to 850-854
**AHA:** 4Q, '03, 103; 3Q, '90, 14

**907.1**   **Late effect of injury to cranial nerve**
Late effect of injury classifiable to 950-951

**907.2**   **Late effect of spinal cord injury**
Late effect of injury classifiable to 806, 952
**AHA:** 4Q, '03, 103; 4Q, '98, 38

**907.3**   **Late effect of injury to nerve root(s), spinal plexus(es), and other nerves of trunk**
Late effect of injury classifiable to 953-954
**AHA:** ▶2Q, '07, 11◀

**907.4**   **Late effect of injury to peripheral nerve of shoulder girdle and upper limb**
Late effect of injury classifiable to 955

**907.5**   **Late effect of injury to peripheral nerve of pelvic girdle and lower limb**
Late effect of injury classifiable to 956

**907.9**   **Late effect of injury to other and unspecified nerve**
Late effect of injury classifiable to 957

√4ᵗʰ **908 Late effects of other and unspecified injuries**

**908.0**   **Late effect of internal injury to chest**
Late effect of injury classifiable to 860-862

**908.1**   **Late effect of internal injury to intra-abdominal organs**
Late effect of injury classifiable to 863-866, 868

**908.2**   **Late effect of internal injury to other internal organs**
Late effect of injury classifiable to 867 or 869

**908.3**   **Late effect of injury to blood vessel of head, neck, and extremities**
Late effect of injury classifiable to 900, 903-904

**908.4**   **Late effect of injury to blood vessel of thorax, abdomen, and pelvis**
Late effect of injury classifiable to 901-902

**908.5**   **Late effect of foreign body in orifice**
Late effect of injury classifiable to 930-939

**908.6**   **Late effect of certain complications of trauma**
Late effect of complications classifiable to 958

**908.9**   **Late effect of unspecified injury**
Late effect of injury classifiable to 959
**AHA:** 3Q, '00, 4

√4ᵗʰ **909 Late effects of other and unspecified external causes**

**909.0**   **Late effect of poisoning due to drug, medicinal or biological substance**
Late effect of conditions classifiable to 960-979
**EXCLUDES**   late effect of adverse effect of drug, medicinal or biological substance (909.5)
**AHA:** 4Q, '03, 103

**909.1**   **Late effect of toxic effects of nonmedical substances**
Late effect of conditions classifiable to 980-989

**909.2**   **Late effect of radiation**
Late effect of conditions classifiable to 990

**909.3**   **Late effect of complications of surgical and medical care**
Late effect of conditions classifiable to 996-999
**AHA:** 1Q, '93, 29

**909.4**   **Late effect of certain other external causes**
Late effect of conditions classifiable to 991-994

**Injury and Poisoning**

**909.5–916.3**

**909.5 Late effect of adverse effect of drug, medical or biological substance**

> **EXCLUDES** *late effect of poisoning due to drug, medicinal or biological substance (909.0)*

**AHA:** 4Q, '94, 48

**909.9 Late effect of other and unspecified external causes**

## SUPERFICIAL INJURY (910-919)

> **EXCLUDES** *burn (blisters) (940.0-949.5)*
> *contusion (920-924.9)*
> *foreign body:*
>    *granuloma (728.82)*
>    *inadvertently left in operative wound (998.4)*
>    *residual in soft tissue (729.6)*
> *insect bite, venomous (989.5)*
> *open wound with incidental foreign body (870.0-897.7)*

**AHA:** 2Q, '89, 15

✓4ᵗʰ **910 Superficial injury of face, neck, and scalp except eye**

> **INCLUDES**    cheek      lip
>                ear       nose
>                gum     throat

> **EXCLUDES** *eye and adnexa (918.0-918.9)*

**910.0 Abrasion or friction burn without mention of infection**

**910.1 Abrasion or friction burn, infected**

**910.2 Blister without mention of infection**

**910.3 Blister, infected**

**910.4 Insect bite, nonvenomous, without mention of infection**

**910.5 Insect bite, nonvenomous, infected**

**910.6 Superficial foreign body (splinter) without major open wound and without mention of infection**

**910.7 Superficial foreign body (splinter) without major open wound, infected**

**910.8 Other and unspecified superficial injury of face, neck, and scalp without mention of infection**

**910.9 Other and unspecified superficial injury of face, neck, and scalp, infected**

✓4ᵗʰ **911 Superficial injury of trunk**

> **INCLUDES**   abdominal wall      interscapular region
>                anus              labium (majus) (minus)
>                back              penis
>                breast           perineum
>                buttock         scrotum
>                chest wall      testis
>                flank            vagina
>                groin            vulva

> **EXCLUDES** *hip (916.0-916.9)*
> *scapular region (912.0-912.9)*

**911.0 Abrasion or friction burn without mention of infection**

**AHA:** 3Q, '01, 10

**911.1 Abrasion or friction burn, infected**

**911.2 Blister without mention of infection**

**911.3 Blister, infected**

**911.4 Insect bite, nonvenomous, without mention of infection**

**911.5 Insect bite, nonvenomous, infected**

**911.6 Superficial foreign body (splinter) without major open wound and without mention of infection**

**911.7 Superficial foreign body (splinter) without major open wound, infected**

**911.8 Other and unspecified superficial injury of trunk without mention of infection**

**911.9 Other and unspecified superficial injury of trunk, infected**

✓4ᵗʰ **912 Superficial injury of shoulder and upper arm**

> **INCLUDES**   axilla               scapular region

**912.0 Abrasion or friction burn without mention of infection**

**912.1 Abrasion or friction burn, infected**

**912.2 Blister without mention of infection**

**912.3 Blister, infected**

**912.4 Insect bite, nonvenomous, without mention of infection**

**912.5 Insect bite, nonvenomous, infected**

**912.6 Superficial foreign body (splinter) without major open wound and without mention of infection**

**912.7 Superficial foreign body (splinter) without major open wound, infected**

**912.8 Other and unspecified superficial injury of shoulder and upper arm without mention of infection**

**912.9 Other and unspecified superficial injury of shoulder and upper arm, infected**

✓4ᵗʰ **913 Superficial injury of elbow, forearm, and wrist**

**913.0 Abrasion or friction burn without mention of infection**

**913.1 Abrasion or friction burn, infected**

**913.2 Blister without mention of infection**

**913.3 Blister, infected**

**913.4 Insect bite, nonvenomous, without mention of infection**

**913.5 Insect bite, nonvenomous, infected**

**913.6 Superficial foreign body (splinter) without major open wound and without mention of infection**

**913.7 Superficial foreign body (splinter) without major open wound, infected**

**913.8 Other and unspecified superficial injury of elbow, forearm, and wrist without mention of infection**

**913.9 Other and unspecified superficial injury of elbow, forearm, and wrist, infected**

✓4ᵗʰ **914 Superficial injury of hand(s) except finger(s) alone**

**914.0 Abrasion or friction burn without mention of infection**

**914.1 Abrasion or friction burn, infected**

**914.2 Blister without mention of infection**

**914.3 Blister, infected**

**914.4 Insect bite, nonvenomous, without mention of infection**

**914.5 Insect bite, nonvenomous, infected**

**914.6 Superficial foreign body (splinter) without major open wound and without mention of infection**

**914.7 Superficial foreign body (splinter) without major open wound, infected**

**914.8 Other and unspecified superficial injury of hand without mention of infection**

**914.9 Other and unspecified superficial injury of hand, infected**

✓4ᵗʰ **915 Superficial injury of finger(s)**

> **INCLUDES**   fingernail           thumb (nail)

**915.0 Abrasion or friction burn without mention of infection**

**915.1 Abrasion or friction burn, infected**

**915.2 Blister without mention of infection**

**915.3 Blister, infected**

**915.4 Insect bite, nonvenomous, without mention of infection**

**915.5 Insect bite, nonvenomous, infected**

**915.6 Superficial foreign body (splinter) without major open wound and without mention of infection**

**915.7 Superficial foreign body (splinter) without major open wound, infected**

**915.8 Other and unspecified superficial injury of fingers without mention of infection**

**AHA:** 3Q, '01, 10

**915.9 Other and unspecified superficial injury of fingers, infected**

✓4ᵗʰ **916 Superficial injury of hip, thigh, leg, and ankle**

**916.0 Abrasion or friction burn without mention of infection**

**916.1 Abrasion or friction burn, infected**

**916.2 Blister without mention of infection**

**916.3 Blister, infected**

**N** Newborn Age: 0    **P** Pediatric Age: 0-17    **M** Maternity Age: 12-55    **A** Adult Age: 15-124    **CC** CC Condition    **MCC** Major CC Condition    **HIV** HIV Related Dx

318 — Volume 1 • October 2007                  © 2007 Ingenix

916.4 Insect bite, nonvenomous, without mention of infection

916.5 Insect bite, nonvenomous, infected

916.6 Superficial foreign body (splinter) without major open wound and without mention of infection

916.7 Superficial foreign body (splinter) without major open wound, infected

916.8 Other and unspecified superficial injury of hip, thigh, leg, and ankle without mention of infection

916.9 Other and unspecified superficial injury of hip, thigh, leg, and ankle, infected

√4ᵗʰ **917 Superficial injury of foot and toe(s)**

INCLUDES  heel  toenail

917.0 Abrasion or friction burn without mention of infection

917.1 Abrasion or friction burn, infected

917.2 Blister without mention of infection

917.3 Blister, infected

917.4 Insect bite, nonvenomous, without mention of infection

917.5 Insect bite, nonvenomous, infected

917.6 Superficial foreign body (splinter) without major open wound and without mention of infection

917.7 Superficial foreign body (splinter) without major open wound, infected

917.8 Other and unspecified superficial injury of foot and toes without mention of infection

AHA: 1Q, '03, 13

917.9 Other and unspecified superficial injury of foot and toes, infected

AHA: 1Q, '03, 13

√4ᵗʰ **918 Superficial injury of eye and adnexa**

EXCLUDES  burn (940.0-940.9)
foreign body on external eye (930.0-930.9)

918.0 Eyelids and periocular area

Abrasion            Superficial foreign body
Insect bite          (splinter)

918.1 Cornea

Corneal abrasion      Superficial laceration
EXCLUDES  corneal injury due to contact lens (371.82)

918.2 Conjunctiva

918.9 Other and unspecified superficial injuries of eye

Eye (ball) NOS

√4ᵗʰ **919 Superficial injury of other, multiple, and unspecified sites**

EXCLUDES  multiple sites classifiable to the same three-digit category (910.0-918.9)

919.0 Abrasion or friction burn without mention of infection

919.1 Abrasion or friction burn, infected

919.2 Blister without mention of infection

919.3 Blister, infected

919.4 Insect bite, nonvenomous, without mention of infection

919.5 Insect bite, nonvenomous, infected

919.6 Superficial foreign body (splinter) without major open wound and without mention of infection

919.7 Superficial foreign body (splinter) without major open wound, infected

919.8 Other and unspecified superficial injury without mention of infection

919.9 Other and unspecified superficial injury, infected

## CONTUSION WITH INTACT SKIN SURFACE (920-924)

INCLUDES  bruise      } without fracture or open
hematoma    }  wound

EXCLUDES  concussion (850.0-850.9)
hemarthrosis (840.0-848.9)
internal organs (860.0-869.1)
that incidental to:
crushing injury (925-929.9)
dislocation (830.0-839.9)
fracture (800.0-829.1)
internal injury (860.0-869.1)
intracranial injury (850.0-854.1)
nerve injury (950.0-957.9)
open wound (870.0-897.7)

920 Contusion of face, scalp, and neck except eye(s)

Cheek              Mandibular joint area
Ear (auricle)      Nose
Gum                Throat
Lip

√4ᵗʰ **921 Contusion of eye and adnexa**

921.0 Black eye, not otherwise specified

921.1 Contusion of eyelids and periocular area

921.2 Contusion of orbital tissues

921.3 Contusion of eyeball

AHA: J-A, '85, 16

921.9 Unspecified contusion of eye

Injury of eye NOS

√4ᵗʰ **922 Contusion of trunk**

922.0 Breast

922.1 Chest wall

922.2 Abdominal wall

Flank              Groin

√5ᵗʰ 922.3 Back

AHA: 4Q, '96, 39

922.31 Back

EXCLUDES  interscapular region (922.33)

AHA: 3Q, '99, 14

922.32 Buttock

922.33 Interscapular region

922.4 Genital organs

Labium (majus) (minus)  Vulva
Penis                    Vagina
Perineum                 Testis
Scrotum

922.8 Multiple sites of trunk

922.9 Unspecified part

Trunk NOS

√4ᵗʰ **923 Contusion of upper limb**

√5ᵗʰ 923.0 Shoulder and upper arm

923.00 Shoulder region

923.01 Scapular region

923.02 Axillary region

923.03 Upper arm

923.09 Multiple sites

√5ᵗʰ 923.1 Elbow and forearm

923.10 Forearm

923.11 Elbow

√5ᵗʰ 923.2 Wrist and hand(s), except finger(s) alone

923.20 Hand(s)

923.21 Wrist

923.3 Finger

Fingernail          Thumb (nail)

923.8 Multiple sites of upper limb

923.9 Unspecified part of upper limb

Arm NOS

√4ᵗʰ **924 Contusion of lower limb and of other and unspecified sites**

√5ᵗʰ 924.0 Hip and thigh

924.00 Thigh

924.01 Hip

√5ᵗʰ 924.1 Knee and lower leg

924.10 Lower leg

924.11 Knee

---

√4ᵗʰ / √5ᵗʰ  Additional Digit Required          Unacceptable PDx          Manifestation Code          ▶◀ Revised Text          ● New Code          ▲ Revised Code Title

**Injury and Poisoning**

**924.2–938**

√5ᵗʰ **924.2 Ankle and foot, excluding toe(s)**
     **924.20 Foot**
         Heel
     **924.21 Ankle**
**924.3 Toe**
     Toenail
**924.4 Multiple sites of lower limb**
**924.5 Unspecified part of lower limb**
     Leg NOS
**924.8 Multiple sites, not elsewhere classified**
     AHA: 1Q, '03, 7
**924.9 Unspecified site**

### CRUSHING INJURY (925-929)
Use additional code to identify any associated injuries,
     such as:
     fractures (800-829)
     internal injuries (860.0-869.1)
     intracranial injuries (850.0-854.1)

AHA: 4Q, '03, 77; 2Q, '93, 7

√4ᵗʰ **925 Crushing injury of face, scalp, and neck**
     Cheek            Pharynx
     Ear              Throat
     Larynx
     **925.1 Crushing injury of face and scalp** `CC`
         Cheek            Ear
         CC Excl: 873.8-873.9, 905.0,925.1-925.2,929.0-929.9,958.8-959.09,
         959.8-959.9

     **925.2 Crushing injury of neck** `CC`
         Larynx           Throat
         Pharynx
         CC Excl: See code: 925.1

√4ᵗʰ **926 Crushing injury of trunk**
     **926.0 External genitalia**
         Labium (majus) (minus)    Testis
         Penis                 Vulva
         Scrotum
   √5ᵗʰ **926.1 Other specified sites**
         **926.11 Back**
         **926.12 Buttock**
         **926.19 Other**
            Breast
     **926.8 Multiple sites of trunk**
     **926.9 Unspecified site**
         Trunk NOS

√4ᵗʰ **927 Crushing injury of upper limb**
   √5ᵗʰ **927.0 Shoulder and upper arm**
         **927.00 Shoulder region**
         **927.01 Scapular region**
         **927.02 Axillary region**
         **927.03 Upper arm**
         **927.09 Multiple sites**
   √5ᵗʰ **927.1 Elbow and forearm**
         **927.10 Forearm**
         **927.11 Elbow**
   √5ᵗʰ **927.2 Wrist and hand(s), except finger(s) alone**
         **927.20 Hand(s)**
         **927.21 Wrist**
     **927.3 Finger(s)**
         AHA: 4Q, '03, 77
     **927.8 Multiple sites of upper limb**
     **927.9 Unspecified site**
         Arm NOS

√4ᵗʰ **928 Crushing injury of lower limb**
   √5ᵗʰ **928.0 Hip and thigh**
         **928.00 Thigh** `CC`
            CC Excl: 928.00, 928.8-929.9
         **928.01 Hip** `CC`
            CC Excl: 928.01, 928.8-929.9

√5ᵗʰ **928.1 Knee and lower leg**
     **928.10 Lower leg**
     **928.11 Knee**
√5ᵗʰ **928.2 Ankle and foot, excluding toe(s) alone**
     **928.20 Foot**
         Heel
     **928.21 Ankle**
**928.3 Toe(s)**
**928.8 Multiple sites of lower limb**
**928.9 Unspecified site**
     Leg NOS
√4ᵗʰ **929 Crushing injury of multiple and unspecified sites**
**929.0 Multiple sites, not elsewhere classified**
**929.9 Unspecified site**

### EFFECTS OF FOREIGN BODY ENTERING THROUGH ORIFICE (930-939)
     **EXCLUDES** *foreign body:*
         *granuloma (728.82)*
         *inadvertently left in operative wound (998.4,*
            *998.7)*
         *in open wound (800-839, 851-897)*
         *residual in soft tissues (729.6)*
         *superficial without major open wound (910-*
            *919 with .6 or .7)*
√4ᵗʰ **930 Foreign body on external eye**
     **EXCLUDES** *foreign body in penetrating wound of:*
         *eyeball (871.5-871.6)*
            *retained (old) (360.5-360.6)*
         *ocular adnexa (870.4)*
            *retained (old) (376.6)*
     **930.0 Corneal foreign body**
     **930.1 Foreign body in conjunctival sac**
     **930.2 Foreign body in lacrimal punctum**
     **930.8 Other and combined sites**
     **930.9 Unspecified site**
         External eye NOS
**931 Foreign body in ear**
     Auditory canal           Auricle
**932 Foreign body in nose**
     Nasal sinus             Nostril
√4ᵗʰ **933 Foreign body in pharynx and larynx**
     **933.0 Pharynx**
         Nasopharynx       Throat NOS
     **933.1 Larynx**
         Asphyxia due to foreign body
         Choking due to:
            food (regurgitated)
            phlegm
√4ᵗʰ **934 Foreign body in trachea, bronchus, and lung**
     **934.0 Trachea** `CC`
         CC Excl: 934.0
     **934.1 Main bronchus** `CC`
         CC Excl: 934.0-934.9
         AHA: 3Q, '02, 18
     **934.8 Other specified parts** `CC`
         Bronchioles         Lung
         CC Excl: See code: 934.1
     **934.9 Respiratory tree, unspecified**
         Inhalation of liquid or vomitus, lower respiratory
            tract NOS
√4ᵗʰ **935 Foreign body in mouth, esophagus, and stomach**
     **935.0 Mouth**
     **935.1 Esophagus**
         AHA: 1Q, '88, 13
     **935.2 Stomach**
**936 Foreign body in intestine and colon**
**937 Foreign body in anus and rectum**
     Rectosigmoid (junction)
**938 Foreign body in digestive system, unspecified**
     Alimentary tract NOS
     Swallowed foreign body

---

`N` Newborn Age: 0    `P` Pediatric Age: 0-17    `M` Maternity Age: 12-55    `A` Adult Age: 15-124    `CC` CC Condition    `MC` Major Complication    `CD` Complex Dx    `HIV` HIV Related Dx

√4th **939 Foreign body in genitourinary tract**

     939.0    **Bladder and urethra**

     939.1    **Uterus, any part**                  ♀

              EXCLUDES    *intrauterine contraceptive device:*
                           *complications from (996.32, 996.65)*
                           *presence of (V45.51)*

     939.2    **Vulva and vagina**                 ♂

     939.3    **Penis**

     939.9    **Unspecified site**

## BURNS (940-949)

INCLUDES    burns from:
                  electrical heating appliance
                  electricity
                  flame
                  hot object
                  lightning
                  radiation
             chemical burns (external) (internal)
             scalds

EXCLUDES    *friction burns (910-919 with .0, .1)*
                  *sunburn (692.71, 692.76-692.77)*

AHA: 4Q, 94, 22; 2Q, '90, 7; 4Q, '88, 3; M-A, '86, 9

√4th **940 Burn confined to eye and adnexa**

     940.0    **Chemical burn of eyelids and periocular area**

     940.1    **Other burns of eyelids and periocular area**

     940.2    **Alkaline chemical burn of cornea and conjunctival sac**

     940.3    **Acid chemical burn of cornea and conjunctival sac**

     940.4    **Other burn of cornea and conjunctival sac**

     940.5    **Burn with resulting rupture and destruction**    CC
              **of eyeball**
              CC Excl:

     940.9    **Unspecified burn of eye and adnexa**

√4th **941 Burn of face, head, and neck**

              EXCLUDES    *mouth (947.0)*

The following fifth-digit subclassification is for use with category 941:

     0    face and head, unspecified site

     1    ear [any part]

     2    eye (with other parts of face, head, and neck)

     3    lip(s)

     4    chin

     5    nose (septum)

     6    scalp [any part]
            Temple (region)

     7    forehead and cheek

     8    neck

     9    multiple sites [except with eye] of face, head, and neck

AHA: 4Q, '94, 22; M-A, '86, 9

√5th   941.0    **Unspecified degree**

√5th   941.1    **Erythema [first degree]**
              AHA: For code 941.19: 3Q, '05, 10

√5th   941.2    **Blisters, epidermal loss [second degree]**

√5th   941.3    **Full-thickness skin loss [third degree NOS]**   CC
              CC Excl: For code 941.30: 941.30, 941.39; For code 941.31: 941.31, 941.39; For code 941.32: 941.32, 941.39; For code 941.33: 941.33, 941.39; For code 941.34: 941.34, 941.39; For code 941.35: 941.35, 941.39; For code 941.36: 941.36, 941.39; For code 941.37: 941.37, 941.39; For code 941.38: 941.38-941.39; For code 941.39: 941.30-941.39

√5th   941.4    **Deep necrosis of underlying tissues [deep third degree] without mention of loss of a body part**   CC
              CC Excl: For code 941.40, 941.49: 941.40, 941.49; For code 941.41: 941.40-941.41, 941.49; For code 941.42: 941.40, 941.42, 941.49; For code 941.43: 941.40, 941.43, 941.49; For code 941.44: 941.40, 941.44, 941.49; For code 941.45: 941.40, 941.45, 941.49; For code 941.46: 941.40, 941.46, 941.49; For code 941.47: 941.40, 941.47, 941.49; For code 941.48: 941.40, 941.48-941.49

√5th   941.5    **Deep necrosis of underlying tissues [deep third degree] with loss of a body part**   CC
              CC Excl: For code 941.50, 941.59: 941.50, 941.59; For code 941.51: 941.50-941.51, 941.59; For code 941.52: 941.50, 941.52, 941.59; For code 941.53: 941.50, 941.53, 941.59; For code 941.54: 941.50, 941.54, 941.59; For code 941.55: 941.50, 941.55, 941.59; For code 941.56: 941.50, 941.56, 941.59; For code 941.57: 941.50, 941.57, 941.59; For code 941.58: 941.50, 941.58-941.59

√4th **942 Burn of trunk**

              EXCLUDES    *scapular region (943.0-943.5 with fifth-digit 6)*

The following fifth-digit subclassification is for use with category 942:

     0    trunk, unspecified site

     1    breast

     2    chest wall, excluding breast and nipple

     3    abdominal wall
            Flank                  Groin

     4    back [any part]
            Buttock
            Interscapular region

     5    genitalia
            Labium (majus) (minus)        Scrotum
            Penis                   Testis
            Perineum              Vulva

     9    other and multiple sites of trunk

AHA: 4Q, '94, 22; M-A, '86, 9

√5th   942.0    **Unspecified degree**

√5th   942.1    **Erythema [first degree]**

√5th   942.2    **Blisters, epidermal loss [second degree]**

√5th   942.3    **Full-thickness skin loss [third degree NOS]**   CC
              CC Excl: For code 942.30, 942.39: 942.30, 942.39; For code 942.31: 942.30-942.31, 942.39; For code 942.32: 942.30, 942.32, 942.39; For code 942.33: 942.30, 942.33, 942.39; For code 942.34: 942.30, 942.34, 942.39; For code 942.35: 942.30, 942.35-942.39

√5th   942.4    **Deep necrosis of underlying tissues [deep third degree] without mention of loss of a body part**   CC
              CC Excl: For code 942.40: 942.40, 942.49; For code 942.41: 942.40-942.41, 942.49; For code 942.42: 942.40, 942.42, 942.49; For code 942.43: 942.40, 942.43, 942.49; For code 942.44: 942.40, 942.44, 942.49; For code 942.45: 942.40, 942.45-942.49; For code 942.49: 942.40-942.49

√5th   942.5    **Deep necrosis of underlying tissues [deep third degree] with loss of a body part**   CC
              CC Excl: For code 942.50: 942.50, 942.59; For code 942.51: 942.50-942.51, 942.59; For code 942.52: 942.50, 942.52, 942.59; For code 942.53: 942.50, 942.53, 942.59; For code 942.54: 942.50, 942.54, 942.59; For code 942.55: 942.50, 942.55-942.59; For code 942.59: 942.50, 942.59

√4th **943 Burn of upper limb, except wrist and hand**

The following fifth-digit subclassification is for use with category 943:

     0    upper limb, unspecified site

     1    forearm

     2    elbow

     3    upper arm

     4    axilla

     5    shoulder

     6    scapular region

     9    multiple sites of upper limb, except wrist and hand

AHA: 4Q, '94, 22; M-A, '86, 9

√5th   943.0    **Unspecified degree**

√5th   943.1    **Erythema [first degree]**

√5th   943.2    **Blisters, epidermal loss [second degree]**

√5th   943.3    **Full-thickness skin loss [third degree NOS]**   CC
              CC Excl: For code 943.30, 943.39: 943.30, 943.39; For code 943.31: 943.30-943.31, 943.39; For code 943.32: 943.30, 943.32, 943.39; For code 943.33: 943.30, 943.33, 943.39; For code 943.34: 943.30, 943.34, 943.39; For code 943.35: 943.30, 943.35, 943.39; For code 943.36: 943.30, 943.36-943.39

---

√4th √5th Additional Digit Required      Unacceptable PDx      Manifestation Code      MCV Major Cardiovascular Condition      ◄► Revised Text      ● New Code      ▲ Revised Code Title

©2007 Ingenix                                            **October 2007 • Volume 1 — 321**

**Injury and Poisoning**

**943.4–948**

§ ✓5th **943.4** **Deep necrosis of underlying tissues [deep third degree] without mention of loss of a body part** `CC`
CC Excl: For code **943.40**, **943.49**: 943.40, 943.49; For code **943.41**: 943.40-943.41, 943.49; **For code 943.42**: 943.40, 943.42, 943.49; **For code 943.43**: 943.40, 943.43, 943.49; **For code 943.44**: 943.40, 943.44, 943.49; **For code 943.45**: 943.40, 943.45, 943.49; **For code 943.46**: 943.40, 943.46-943.49

§ ✓5th **943.5** **Deep necrosis of underlying tissues [deep third degree] with loss of a body part** `CC`
CC Excl: For code **943.50**, **943.59**: 943.50, 943.59; For code **943.51**: 943.50-943.51, 943.59; **For code 943.52**: 943.50, 943.52, 943.59; **For code 943.53**: 943.50, 943.53, 943.59; **For code 943.54**: 943.50, 943.54, 943.59; **For code 943.55**: 943.50, 943.55, 943.59; **For code 943.56**: 943.50, 943.56-943.59

✓4th **944** **Burn of wrist(s) and hand(s)**

The following fifth-digit subclassification is for use with category 944:
   **0** hand, unspecified site
   **1** single digit [finger (nail)] other than thumb
   **2** thumb (nail)
   **3** two or more digits, not including thumb
   **4** two or more digits including thumb
   **5** palm
   **6** back of hand
   **7** wrist
   **8** multiple sites of wrist(s) and hand(s)

✓5th **944.0** **Unspecified degree**
✓5th **944.1** **Erythema [first degree]**
✓5th **944.2** **Blisters, epidermal loss [second degree]**
✓5th **944.3** **Full-thickness skin loss [third degree NOS]** `CC`
CC Excl: For code **944.30**, **944.38**: 944.30, 944.38; **For code 944.31**: 944.30-944.31, 944.38; **For code 944.32**: 944.30, 944.32, 944.38; **For code 944.33**: 944.30, 944.33, 944.38; **For code 944.34**: 944.30, 944.34, 944.38; **For code 944.35**: 944.30, 944.35, 944.38; **For code 944.36**: 944.30, 944.36, 944.38; **For code 944.37**: 944.37-944.38

✓5th **944.4** **Deep necrosis of underlying tissues [deep third degree] without mention of loss of a body part** `CC`
CC Excl: For code **944.40**, **944.48**: 944.40, 944.48; **For code 944.41**: 944.40-944.41, 944.48; **For code 944.42**: 944.40, 944.42, 944.48; **For code 944.43**: 944.40, 944.43, 944.48; **For code 944.44**: 944.40, 944.44, 944.48; **For code 944.45**: 944.40, 944.45, 944.48; **For code 944.46**: 944.40, 944.46, 944.48; **For code 944.47**: 944.47-944.48

✓5th **944.5** **Deep necrosis of underlying tissues [deep third degree] with loss of a body part** `CC`
CC Excl: For code **944.50**, **944.58**: 944.50, 944.58; **For code 944.51**: 944.50-944.51, 944.58; **For code 944.52**: 944.50, 944.52, 944.58; **For code 944.53**: 944.50, 944.53, 944.58; **For code 944.54**: 944.50, 944.54, 944.58; **For code 944.55**: 944.50, 944.55, 944.58; **For code 944.56**: 944.50, 944.56, 944.58; **For code 944.57**: 944.57-944.58

✓4th **945** **Burn of lower limb(s)**

The following fifth-digit subclassification is for use with category 945:
   **0** lower limb [leg], unspecified site
   **1** toe(s) (nail)
   **2** foot
   **3** ankle
   **4** lower leg
   **5** knee
   **6** thigh [any part]
   **9** multiple sites of lower limb(s)

AHA: 4Q, '94, 22; M-A, '86, 9

✓5th **945.0** **Unspecified degree**
✓5th **945.1** **Erythema [first degree]**
✓5th **945.2** **Blisters, epidermal loss [second degree]**

✓5th **945.3** **Full-thickness skin loss [third degree NOS]** `CC`
CC Excl: For code **945.30**, **945.39**: 945.30, 945.39; **For code 945.31**: 945.30-945.31, 945.39; **For code 945.32**: 945.30, 945.32, 945.39; **For code 945.33**: 945.30, 945.33, 945.39; **For code 945.34**: 945.30, 945.34, 945.39; **For code 945.35**: 945.30, 945.35, 945.39; **For code 945.36**: 945.30, 945.36-945.39

✓5th **945.4** **Deep necrosis of underlying tissues [deep third degree] without mention of loss of a body part** `CC`
CC Excl: For code **945.40**, **945.49**: 945.40, 945.49; **For code 945.41**: 945.40-945.41, 945.49; **For code 945.42**: 945.40, 945.42, 945.49; **For code 945.43**: 945.40, 945.43, 945.49; **For code 945.44**: 945.40, 945.44, 945.49; **For code 945.45**: 945.40, 945.45, 945.49; **For code 945.46**: 945.40, 945.46-945.49

✓5th **945.5** **Deep necrosis of underlying tissues [deep third degree] with loss of a body part** `CC`
CC Excl: For code **945.50**, **945.59**: 945.50, 945.59; **For code 945.51**: 945.50-945.51, 945.59; **For code 945.52**: 945.50, 945.52, 945.59; **For code 945.53**: 945.50, 945.53, 945.59; **For code 945.54**: 945.50, 945.54, 945.59; **For code 945.55**: 945.50, 945.55, 945.59; **For code 945.56**: 945.50, 945.56-945.59

✓4th **946** **Burns of multiple specified sites**
   `INCLUDES` burns of sites classifiable to more than one three-digit category in 940-945
   `EXCLUDES` multiple burns NOS (949.0-949.5)
AHA: 4Q, '94, 22; M-A, '86, 9

  **946.0** **Unspecified degree**
  **946.1** **Erythema [first degree]**
  **946.2** **Blisters, epidermal loss [second degree]**
  **946.3** **Full-thickness skin loss [third degree NOS]** `CC`
CC Excl: 946.3

  **946.4** **Deep necrosis of underlying tissues [deep third degree] without mention of loss of a body part** `CC`
CC Excl: 946.4

  **946.5** **Deep necrosis of underlying tissues [deep third degree] with loss of a body part** `CC`
CC Excl: 946.5

✓4th **947** **Burn of internal organs**
   `INCLUDES` burns from chemical agents (ingested)
AHA: 4Q, '94, 22; M-A, '86, 9

  **947.0** **Mouth and pharynx**
     Gum         Tongue
  **947.1** **Larynx, trachea, and lung** `CC`
CC Excl: 947.1, 947.8-947.9

  **947.2** **Esophagus** `CC`
CC Excl: 947.2, 947.8-947.9

  **947.3** **Gastrointestinal tract** `CC`
     Colon         Small intestine
     Rectum       Stomach
CC Excl: 947.3, 947.8-947.9

  **947.4** **Vagina and uterus** `CC` ♀
CC Excl: 947.4-947.9

  **947.8** **Other specified sites**
  **947.9** **Unspecified site**

✓4th **948** **Burns classified according to extent of body surface involved**
   Note: This category is to be used when the site of the burn is unspecified, or with categories 940-947 when the site is specified.
   `EXCLUDES` sunburn (692.71, 692.76-692.77)

The following fifth-digit subclassification is for use with category 948 to indicate the percent of body surface with third degree burn; valid digits are in [brackets] under each code:
   **0** less than 10 percent or unspecified
   **1** 10-19%
   **2** 20-29%
   **3** 30-39%
   **4** 40-49%
   **5** 50-59%
   **6** 60-69%
   **7** 70-79%
   **8** 80-89%
   **9** 90% or more of body surface

AHA: 4Q, '94, 22; 4Q, '88, 3; M-A, '86, 9; N-D, '84, 13

§ Requires fifth-digit. See category 943 for codes and definitions.

`N` Newborn Age: 0    `P` Pediatric Age: 0-17    `M` Maternity Age: 12-55    `A` Adult Age: 15-124    `CC` CC Condition    `MCC` Major CC Condition    `HIV` HIV Related Dx

§ ✓5th **948.0** **Burn [any degree] involving less than 10 percent of**
[0]    **body surface**

§ ✓5th **948.1** **10-19 percent of body surface**    `CC 0-1`
[0-1]

     **CC Excl:** 948.00-948.99

§ ✓5th **948.2** **20-29 percent of body surface**    `MCC 1,2` `CC 0`
[0-2]

     **CC Excl:** See code: 948.1

§ ✓5th **948.3** **30-39 percent of body surface**    `MCC 1-3` `CC 0`
[0-3]

     **CC Excl:** See code: 948.1

§ ✓5th **948.4** **40-49 percent of body surface**    `MCC 1-4` `CC 0`
[0-4]

     **CC Excl:** See code: 948.1

§ ✓5th **948.5** **50-59 percent of body surface**    `MCC 1-5` `CC 0`
[0-5]

     **CC Excl:** See code: 948.1

§ ✓5th **948.6** **60-69 percent of body surface**    `MCC 1-6` `CC 0`
[0-6]

     **CC Excl:** See code: 948.1

§ ✓5th **948.7** **70-79 percent of body surface**    `MCC 1-7` `CC 0`
[0-7]

     **CC Excl:** See code: 948.1

§ ✓5th **948.8** **80-89 percent of body surface**    `MCC 1-8` `CC 0`
[0-8]

     **CC Excl:** See code: 948.1

§ ✓5th **948.9** **90 percent or more of body surface**    `MCC 1-9` `CC 0`
[0-9]

     **CC Excl:** See code: 948.1

✓4th **949 Burn, unspecified**

     **INCLUDES**   burn NOS     multiple burns NOS

     **EXCLUDES**   *burn of unspecified site but with statement of*
        *the extent of body surface involved (948.0-*
        *948.9)*

     **AHA:** 4Q, '94, 22; M-A, '86, 9

     **949.0**   **Unspecified degree**
     **949.1**   **Erythema [first degree]**
     **949.2**   **Blisters, epidermal loss [second degree]**

### Burns

#### Degrees of Burns

First (redness)    Second (blistering)    Third (fill thickness)    Deep Third (deep necrosis)    Eschar

#### Rule of Nines
#### Estimation of Total Body Surface Burned

Head and neck 9%
Each arm 9%
Posterior trunk 18%
Anterior trunk 18%
Genitalia 1%
Anterior leg 9%
Posterior leg 9%

**949.3** **Full-thickness skin loss [third degree NOS]** `CC`

     **CC Excl:** 941.30-941.39,942.30-942.39,944.30-944.38,945.30-945.39,
     946.3, 949.3

**949.4** **Deep necrosis of underlying tissues [deep third** `CC`
     **degree] without mention of loss of a body part**

     **CC Excl:** 941.40-941.49,942.40-942.49,944.40-944.48,945.40-945.49,
     946.4, 949.4

**949.5** **Deep necrosis of underlying tissues [deep third** `CC`
     **degree] with loss of a body part**

     **CC Excl:** 946.5, 949.5

## INJURY TO NERVES AND SPINAL CORD (950-957)

     **INCLUDES**    division of nerve
                  lesion in continuity    (with open
                  traumatic neuroma    wound)
                  traumatic transient paralysis

     **EXCLUDES**   *accidental puncture or laceration during medical*
               *procedure (998.2)*

✓4th **950 Injury to optic nerve and pathways**

     **950.0**   **Optic nerve injury**    `CC`
          Second cranial nerve

          **CC Excl:** 950.0-950.9, 951.8-951.9

     **950.1**   **Injury to optic chiasm**    `CC`
          **CC Excl:** See code: 950.0

     **950.2**   **Injury to optic pathways**    `CC`
          **CC Excl:** See code: 950.0

     **950.3**   **Injury to visual cortex**    `CC`
          **CC Excl:** See code: 950.0

     **950.9**   **Unspecified**    `CC`
          Traumatic blindness NOS

          **CC Excl:** See code: 950.0

✓4th **951 Injury to other cranial nerve(s)**

     **951.0**   **Injury to oculomotor nerve**    `CC`
          Third cranial nerve

          **CC Excl:** 951.0, 951.8-951.9

     **951.1**   **Injury to trochlear nerve**    `CC`
          Fourth cranial nerve

          **CC Excl:** 951.1, 951.8-951.9

     **951.2**   **Injury to trigeminal nerve**    `CC`
          Fifth cranial nerve

          **CC Excl:** 951.2, 951.8-951.9

     **951.3**   **Injury to abducens nerve**    `CC`
          Sixth cranial nerve

          **CC Excl:** 951.3, 951.8-951.9

     **951.4**   **Injury to facial nerve**    `CC`
          Seventh cranial nerve

          **CC Excl:** 951.4, 951.8-951.9

     **951.5**   **Injury to acoustic nerve**    `CC`
          Auditory nerve
          Eighth cranial nerve
          Traumatic deafness NOS

          **CC Excl:** 951.5, 951.8-951.9

     **951.6**   **Injury to accessory nerve**    `CC`
          Eleventh cranial nerve

          **CC Excl:** 951.6, 951.8-951.9

     **951.7**   **Injury to hypoglossal nerve**    `CC`
          Twelfth cranial nerve

          **CC Excl:** 951.7-951.9

     **951.8**   **Injury to other specified cranial nerves**    `CC`
          Glossopharyngeal [9th cranial] nerve
          Olfactory [1st cranial] nerve
          Pneumogastric [10th cranial] nerve
          Traumatic anosmia NOS
          Vagus [10th cranial] nerve

          **CC Excl:** 951.8-951.9

---

§ Requires fifth-digit. Valid digits are in [brackets] under each code. See category 948 for code and definitions.

✓4th / ✓5th Additional Digit Required      Unacceptable PDx      Manifestation Code      ▶◀ Revised Text      ● New Code      ▲ Revised Code Title

© 2007 Ingenix

**Spinal Nerve Roots**

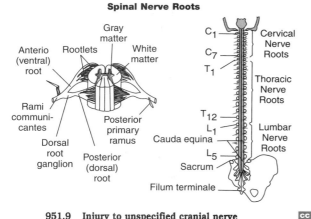

**951.9** Injury to unspecified cranial nerve `CC`
CC Excl: See code: 951.8

√4th **952** Spinal cord injury without evidence of spinal bone injury
√5th **952.0** Cervical

**952.00** $C_1$-$C_4$ level with unspecified spinal cord injury `MCC`
Spinal cord injury, cervical region NOS
CC Excl: 805.00-805.18, 805.8-806.19, 806.8-806.9, 839.00-839.18, 839.40, 839.49-839.50, 839.59, 839.69, 839.79-839.9, 847.9, 905.1, 926.11,952.00-952.09,952.8-952.9,958.8-958.99,959.11-959.19, 959.8-959.9

**952.01** $C_1$-$C_4$ level with complete lesion of spinal cord `MCC`
CC Excl: See code 952.00

**952.02** $C_1$-$C_4$ level with anterior cord syndrome `MCC`
CC Excl: See code 952.00

**952.03** $C_1$-$C_4$ level with central cord syndrome `MCC`
CC Excl: See code 952.00

**952.04** $C_1$-$C_4$ level with other specified spinal cord injury `MCC`
Incomplete spinal cord lesion at $C_1$-$C_4$ level:
NOS
with posterior cord syndrome
CC Excl: See code 952.00

**952.05** $C_5$-$C_7$ level with unspecified spinal cord injury `MCC`
CC Excl: See code 952.00

**952.06** $C_5$-$C_7$ level with complete lesion of spinal cord `MCC`
CC Excl: See code 952.00

**952.07** $C_5$-$C_7$ level with anterior cord syndrome `MCC`
CC Excl: See code 952.00

**952.08** $C_5$-$C_7$ level with central cord syndrome `MCC`
CC Excl: See code 952.00

**952.09** $C_5$-$C_7$ level with other specified spinal cord injury `MCC`
Incomplete spinal cord lesion at $C_5$-$C_7$ level:
NOS
with posterior cord syndrome
CC Excl: See code 952.00

√5th **952.1** Dorsal [thoracic]
**952.10** $T_1$-$T_6$ level with unspecified spinal cord injury `MCC`
Spinal cord injury, thoracic region NOS
CC Excl: 805.8-805.9, 806.20-806.39, 839.40, 839.49-839.50, 839.59, 839.69, 839.79-839.9, 847.9, 905.1, 926.11,952.10-952.19,952.8-952.9,958.8-958.99,959.11-959.19, 959.8-959.9

**952.11** $T_1$-$T_6$ level with complete lesion of spinal cord `MCC`
CC Excl: See code 952.10

**952.12** $T_1$-$T_6$ level with anterior cord syndrome `MCC`
CC Excl: See code 952.10

**952.13** $T_1$-$T_6$ level with central cord syndrome `MCC`
CC Excl: See code 952.10

**952.14** $T_1$-$T_6$ level with other specified spinal cord injury `MCC`
Incomplete spinal cord lesion at $T_1$-$T_6$ level:
NOS
with posterior cord syndrome
CC Excl: See code 952.10

**952.15** $T_7$-$T_{12}$ level with unspecified spinal cord injury `MCC`
CC Excl: See code 952.10

**952.16** $T_7$-$T_{12}$ level with complete lesion of spinal cord `MCC`
CC Excl: See code 952.10

**952.17** $T_7$-$T_{12}$ level with anterior cord syndrome `MCC`
CC Excl: See code 952.10

**952.18** $T_7$-$T_{12}$ level with central cord syndrome `MCC`
CC Excl: See code 952.10

**952.19** $T_7$-$T_{12}$ level with other specified spinal cord injury `MCC`
Incomplete spinal cord lesion at $T_7$-$T_{12}$ level:
NOS
with posterior cord syndrome
CC Excl: See code 952.10

**952.2** Lumbar `MCC`
CC Excl: 805.8-805.9, 806.4-806.5, 839.40, 839.49-839.50, 839.59, 839.69, 839.79-839.9, 847.9, 905.1, 926.11, 952, 952.8-952.9, 958.8-958.99,959.11-959.19, 959.8-959.9

**952.3** Sacral `MCC`
CC Excl: 805.8-805.9, 806.60-806.79, 839.40, 839.49-839.50, 839.59, 839.69, 839.79-839.9, 847.9, 905.1, 926.11, 952.3-952.9, 958.8-958.99,959.11-959.19, 959.8-959.9

**952.4** Cauda equina `MCC`
CC Excl: See code 952.3

**952.8** Multiple sites of spinal cord `MCC`
CC Excl: 805.8-805.9, 839.40, 839.49-839.50, 839.59, 839.69, 839.79-839.9, 847.9, 905.1, 926.11, 952.8-952.9, 958.8-958.99, 959.11-959.19, 959.8-959.9

**952.9** Unspecified site of spinal cord

√4th **953** Injury to nerve roots and spinal plexus
**953.0** Cervical root
**953.1** Dorsal root
**953.2** Lumbar root
**953.3** Sacral root
**953.4** Brachial plexus
**953.5** Lumbosacral plexus
**953.8** Multiple sites
**953.9** Unspecified site

√4th **954** Injury to other nerve(s) of trunk, excluding shoulder and pelvic girdles
**954.0** Cervical sympathetic
**954.1** Other sympathetic
Celiac ganglion or plexus          Splanchnic nerve(s)
Inferior mesenteric plexus      Stellate ganglion
**954.8** Other specified nerve(s) of trunk
**954.9** Unspecified nerve of trunk

√4th **955** Injury to peripheral nerve(s) of shoulder girdle and upper limb
**955.0** Axillary nerve
**955.1** Median nerve
**955.2** Ulnar nerve
**955.3** Radial nerve
**955.4** Musculocutaneous nerve
**955.5** Cutaneous sensory nerve, upper limb

---

`N` Newborn Age: 0     `P` Pediatric Age: 0-17     `M` Maternity Age: 12-55     `A` Adult Age: 15-124     `CC` CC Condition     `MCC` Major CC Condition     `HIV` HIV Related Dx

955.6   **Digital nerve**
955.7   **Other specified nerve(s) of shoulder girdle and upper limb**
955.8   **Multiple nerves of shoulder girdle and upper limb**
955.9   **Unspecified nerve of shoulder girdle and upper limb**

√4th **956 Injury to peripheral nerve(s) of pelvic girdle and lower limb**
956.0   **Sciatic nerve**
956.1   **Femoral nerve**
956.2   **Posterior tibial nerve**
956.3   **Peroneal nerve**
956.4   **Cutaneous sensory nerve, lower limb**
956.5   **Other specified nerve(s) of pelvic girdle and lower limb**
956.8   **Multiple nerves of pelvic girdle and lower limb**
956.9   **Unspecified nerve of pelvic girdle and lower limb**

√4th **957 Injury to other and unspecified nerves**
957.0   **Superficial nerves of head and neck**
957.1   **Other specified nerve(s)**
957.8   **Multiple nerves in several parts**
     Multiple nerve injury NOS
957.9   **Unspecified site**
     Nerve injury NOS

## CERTAIN TRAUMATIC COMPLICATIONS AND UNSPECIFIED INJURIES (958-959)

√4th **958 Certain early complications of trauma**
   **EXCLUDES**   *adult respiratory distress syndrome (518.5)*
      *flail chest (807.4)*
      *shock lung (518.5)*
      *that occurring during or following medical procedures (996.0-999.9)*

958.0   **Air embolism**    `MCC`
     Pneumathemia
   **EXCLUDES**   *that complicating:*
      *abortion (634-638 with .6, 639.6)*
      *ectopic or molar pregnancy (639.6)*
      *pregnancy, childbirth, or the puerperium (673.0)*

   **CC Excl:** 958.0, 958.8-958.99, 959.8-959.9, 997.91-997.99, 998.81, 998.83-998.9, 999.1

   **DEF:** Arterial obstruction due to introduction of air bubbles into the veins following surgery or trauma.

958.1   **Fat embolism**    `MCC`
   **EXCLUDES**   *that complicating:*
      *abortion (634-638 with .6, 639.6)*
      *pregnancy, childbirth, or the puerperium (673.8)*

   **CC Excl:** 958.1, 958.8-958.99, 959.8-959.9, 997.91-997.99, 998.81, 998.83-998.9

   **DEF:** Arterial blockage due to the entrance of fat in circulatory system, after fracture of large bones or administration of corticosteroids.

958.2   **Secondary and recurrent hemorrhage**    `CC`
   **CC Excl:** 958.2, 958.8-958.99, 959.8-959.9, 997.91-997.99, 998.81, 998.83-998.9

958.3   **Posttraumatic wound infection, not elsewhere classified**    `CC`
   **EXCLUDES**   *infected open wounds–code to complicated open wound of site*

   **CC Excl:** 958.3, 958.8-958.99, 959.8-959.9, 997.91-997.99, 998.81, 998.83-998.9

   **AHA:** 4Q, '01, 53; S-O, '85, 10

958.4   **Traumatic shock**    `MCC`
     Shock (immediate) (delayed) following injury
   **EXCLUDES**   *shock:*
      *anaphylactic (995.0)*
       *due to serum (999.4)*
      *anesthetic (995.4)*
      *electric (994.8)*
      *following abortion (639.5)*
      *lightning (994.0)*
      *nontraumatic NOS (785.50)*
      *obstetric (669.1)*
      *postoperative (998.0)*

   **CC Excl:** 958.4, 958.8-958.99, 959.8-959.9, 997.91-997.99, 998.81, 998.83-998.9

   **DEF:** Shock, immediate or delayed following injury.

958.5   **Traumatic anuria**    `MCC`
     Crush syndrome
     Renal failure following crushing
   **EXCLUDES**   *that due to a medical procedure (997.5)*

   **CC Excl:** 958.5, 958.8-958.99, 959.8-959.9, 995.4, 997.91-998.13, 998.81, 998.83-998.9

   **DEF:** Complete suppression of urinary secretion by kidneys due to trauma.

958.6   **Volkmann's ischemic contracture**
     Posttraumatic muscle contracture
   **DEF:** Muscle deterioration due to loss of blood supply from injury or tourniquet; causes muscle contraction and results in inability to extend the muscles fully.

958.7   **Traumatic subcutaneous emphysema**    `CC`
   **EXCLUDES**   *subcutaneous emphysema resulting from a procedure (998.81)*

   **CC Excl:** 860.0-860.5, 861.20-862.1, 862.29-862.9, 875.0-875.1, 958.7-958.99, 959.8-959.9, 997.91-997.99, 998.81, 998.83-998.9

958.8   **Other early complications of trauma**
   **AHA:** 2Q, '92, 13

√5th **958.9 Traumatic compartment syndrome**
   **EXCLUDES**   *nontraumatic compartment syndrome (729.71-729.79)*

   **DEF:** Compression of nerves and blood vessels within an enclosed space due to previous trauma, which leads to impaired blood flow and muscle and nerve damage.

958.90   **Compartment syndrome, unspecified**    `CC`
   **CC Excl:** 868.03-868.10, 868.13-869.1

   **AHA:** 4Q, '06, 100-102

958.91   **Traumatic compartment syndrome of upper extremity**    `CC`
     Traumatic compartment syndrome of shoulder, arm, forearm, wrist, hand, and fingers
   **CC Excl:** 729.81, 729.89-729.9

   **AHA:** 4Q, '06, 100-102

958.92   **Traumatic compartment syndrome of lower extremity**    `CC`
     Traumatic compartment syndrome of hip, buttock, thigh, leg, foot, and toes
   **CC Excl:** See code: 958.91

   **AHA:** 4Q, '06, 100-102

958.93   **Traumatic compartment syndrome of abdomen**    `CC`
   **CC Excl:** 863.0-867.3, 867.5-869.1, 879.2-879.9, 929.0-929.9, 958.8, 959.8-959.9

   **AHA:** 4Q, '06, 100-102

958.99   **Traumatic compartment syndrome of other sites**    `CC`
   **CC Excl:** 868.03-868.10, 868.13-869.1

   **AHA:** 4Q, '06, 100-102

√4th **959 Injury, other and unspecified**
   **INCLUDES**   injury NOS
   **EXCLUDES**   *injury NOS of:*
      *blood vessels (900.0-904.9)*
      *eye (921.0-921.9)*
      *internal organs (860.0-869.1)*
      *intracranial sites (854.0-854.1)*
      *nerves (950.0-951.9, 953.0-957.9)*
      *spinal cord (952.0-952.9)*

**Injury and Poisoning**

**959.0–962.1**

√5th **959.0 Head, face and neck**

    **959.01 Head injury, unspecified**

      EXCLUDES  *concussion (850.1-850.9)*
        *with head injury NOS*
        *(850.1-850.9)*
        *head injury NOS with loss of*
        *consciousness (850.1-*
        *850.5)*
        *specified intracranial injuries*
        *(850.0-854.1)*

      **AHA:** 4Q, '97, 46

    **959.09 Injury of face and neck**

| Cheek | Mouth |
|---|---|
| Ear | Nose |
| Eyebrow | Throat |
| Lip | |

      **AHA:** 4Q, '97, 46

√5th **959.1 Trunk**

    EXCLUDES  *scapular region (959.2)*

  **AHA:** 4Q, '03, 78; 1Q, '99, 10

    **959.11 Other injury of chest wall**

    **959.12 Other injury of abdomen**

    **959.13 Fracture of corpus cavernosum penis** ♂

    **959.14 Other injury of external genitals**

    **959.19 Other injury of other sites of trunk**
      Injury of trunk NOS

**959.2 Shoulder and upper arm**

| Axilla | Scapular region |
|---|---|

**959.3 Elbow, forearm, and wrist**

  **AHA:** 1Q, '97, 8

**959.4 Hand, except finger**

**959.5 Finger**

| Fingernail | Thumb (nail) |
|---|---|

**959.6 Hip and thigh**
  Upper leg

**959.7 Knee, leg, ankle, and foot**

**959.8 Other specified sites, including multiple**

    EXCLUDES  *multiple sites classifiable to the same*
      *four-digit category (959.0-959.7)*

**959.9 Unspecified site**

## POISONING BY DRUGS, MEDICINAL AND BIOLOGICAL SUBSTANCES (960-979)

INCLUDES  overdose of these substances
    wrong substance given or taken in error

EXCLUDES  *adverse effects ["hypersensitivity," "reaction,"*
  *etc.] of correct substance properly*
  *administered. Such cases are to be*
  *classified according to the nature of the*
  *adverse effect, such as:*
  *adverse effect NOS (995.20)*
  *allergic lymphadenitis (289.3)*
  *aspirin gastritis (535.4)*
  *blood disorders (280.0-289.9)*
  *dermatitis:*
    *contact (692.0-692.9)*
    *due to ingestion (693.0-693.9)*
  *nephropathy (583.9)*
  *[The drug giving rise to the adverse effect may*
  *be identified by use of categories E930-*
  *E949.]*
  *drug dependence (304.0-304.9)*
  *drug reaction and poisoning affecting the*
  *newborn (760.0-779.9)*
  *nondependent abuse of drugs (305.0-305.9)*
  *pathological drug intoxication (292.2)*
  Use additional code to specify the effects of the poisoning

  **AHA:** 2Q, '90, 11

√4th **960 Poisoning by antibiotics**

    EXCLUDES  *antibiotics:*
      *ear, nose, and throat (976.6)*
      *eye (976.5)*
      *local (976.0)*

**960.0 Penicillins**

| Ampicillin | Cloxacillin |
|---|---|
| Carbenicillin | Penicillin G |

**960.1 Antifungal antibiotics**

| Amphotericin B | Nystatin |
|---|---|
| Griseofulvin | Trichomycin |

    EXCLUDES  *preparations intended for topical use*
      *(976.0-976.9)*

**960.2 Chloramphenicol group**

| Chloramphenicol | Thiamphenicol |
|---|---|

**960.3 Erythromycin and other macrolides**

| Oleandomycin | Spiramycin |
|---|---|

**960.4 Tetracycline group**

| Doxycycline | Oxytetracycline |
|---|---|
| Minocycline | |

**960.5 Cephalosporin group**

| Cephalexin | Cephaloridine |
|---|---|
| Cephaloglycin | Cephalothin |

**960.6 Antimycobacterial antibiotics**

| Cycloserine | Rifampin |
|---|---|
| Kanamycin | Streptomycin |

**960.7 Antineoplastic antibiotics**
  Actinomycin such as:

| Bleomycin | Daunorubicin |
|---|---|
| Cactinomycin | Mitomycin |
| Dactinomycin | |

**960.8 Other specified antibiotics**

**960.9 Unspecified antibiotic**

√4th **961 Poisoning by other anti-infectives**

    EXCLUDES  *anti-infectives:*
      *ear, nose, and throat (976.6)*
      *eye (976.5)*
      *local (976.0)*

**961.0 Sulfonamides**

| Sulfadiazine | Sulfamethoxazole |
|---|---|
| Sulfafurazole | |

**961.1 Arsenical anti-infectives**

**961.2 Heavy metal anti-infectives**

| Compounds of: | Compounds of: |
|---|---|
| antimony | lead |
| bismuth | mercury |

    EXCLUDES  *mercurial diuretics (974.0)*

**961.3 Quinoline and hydroxyquinoline derivatives**

| Chiniofon | Diiodohydroxyquin |
|---|---|

    EXCLUDES  *antimalarial drugs (961.4)*

**961.4 Antimalarials and drugs acting on other blood protozoa**

| Chloroquine | Proguanil [chloroguanide] |
|---|---|
| Cycloguanil | Pyrimethamine |
| Primaquine | Quinine |

**961.5 Other antiprotozoal drugs**
  Emetine

**961.6 Anthelmintics**

| Hexylresorcinol | Thiabendazole |
|---|---|
| Piperazine | |

**961.7 Antiviral drugs**
  Methisazone

    EXCLUDES  *amantadine (966.4)*
      *cytarabine (963.1)*
      *idoxuridine (976.5)*

**961.8 Other antimycobacterial drugs**

| Ethambutol | Para-aminosalicylic acid |
|---|---|
| Ethionamide | derivatives |
| Isoniazid | Sulfones |

**961.9 Other and unspecified anti-infectives**
  Flucytosine
  Nitrofuran derivatives

√4th **962 Poisoning by hormones and synthetic substitutes**

    EXCLUDES  *oxytocic hormones (975.0)*

**962.0 Adrenal cortical steroids**

| Cortisone derivatives | Fluorinated corticosteroids |
|---|---|
| Desoxycorticosterone derivatives | |

**962.1 Androgens and anabolic congeners**

| Methandriol | Oxymetholone |
|---|---|
| Nandrolone | Testosterone |

N Newborn Age: 0   P Pediatric Age: 0-17   M Maternity Age: 12-55   A Adult Age: 15-124   CC CC Condition   MCC Major CC Condition   HIV HIV Related Dx

326 — Volume 1 • October 2007

© 2007 Ingenix

**962.2 Ovarian hormones and synthetic substitutes**
Contraceptives, oral
Estrogens
Estrogens and progestogens, combined
Progestogens

**962.3 Insulins and antidiabetic agents**
Acetohexamide
Biguanide derivatives, oral
Chlorpropamide
Glucagon
Insulin
Phenformin
Sulfonylurea derivatives, oral
Tolbutamide

**AHA:** M-A, '85, 8

**962.4 Anterior pituitary hormones**
Corticotropin
Gonadotropin
Somatotropin [growth hormone]

**962.5 Posterior pituitary hormones**
Vasopressin
**EXCLUDES** *oxytocic hormones (975.0)*

**962.6 Parathyroid and parathyroid derivatives**

**962.7 Thyroid and thyroid derivatives**
Dextrothyroxin
Levothyroxine sodium
Liothyronine
Thyroglobulin

**962.8 Antithyroid agents**
Iodides
Thiouracil
Thiourea

**962.9 Other and unspecified hormones and synthetic substitutes**

✓4ᵗʰ **963 Poisoning by primarily systemic agents**
**963.0 Antiallergic and antiemetic drugs**
Antihistamines
Chlorpheniramine
Diphenhydramine
Diphenylpyraline
Thonzylamine
Tripelennamine
**EXCLUDES** *phenothiazine-based tranquilizers (969.1)*

**963.1 Antineoplastic and immunosuppressive drugs**
Azathioprine
Busulfan
Chlorambucil
Cyclophosphamide
Cytarabine
Fluorouracil
Mercaptopurine
thio-TEPA
**EXCLUDES** *antineoplastic antibiotics (960.7)*

**963.2 Acidifying agents**
**963.3 Alkalizing agents**
**963.4 Enzymes, not elsewhere classified**
Penicillinase
**963.5 Vitamins, not elsewhere classified**
Vitamin A
Vitamin D
**EXCLUDES** *nicotinic acid (972.2)*
*vitamin K (964.3)*

**963.8 Other specified systemic agents**
Heavy metal antagonists
**963.9 Unspecified systemic agent**

✓4ᵗʰ **964 Poisoning by agents primarily affecting blood constituents**
**964.0 Iron and its compounds**
Ferric salts
Ferrous sulfate and other ferrous salts
**964.1 Liver preparations and other antianemic agents**
Folic acid
**964.2 Anticoagulants**
Coumarin
Heparin
Phenindione
Warfarin sodium
**AHA:** 1Q, '94, 22

**964.3 Vitamin K [phytonadione]**
**964.4 Fibrinolysis-affecting drugs**
Aminocaproic acid
Streptodornase
Streptokinase
Urokinase
**964.5 Anticoagulant antagonists and other coagulants**
Hexadimethrine
Protamine sulfate
**964.6 Gamma globulin**
**964.7 Natural blood and blood products**
Blood plasma
Human fibrinogen
Packed red cells
Whole blood
**EXCLUDES** *transfusion reactions (999.4-999.8)*

**964.8 Other specified agents affecting blood constituents**
Macromolecular blood substitutes
Plasma expanders
**964.9 Unspecified agent affecting blood constituents**

✓4ᵗʰ **965 Poisoning by analgesics, antipyretics, and antirheumatics**
**EXCLUDES** *drug dependence (304.0-304.9)*
*nondependent abuse (305.0-305.9)*

✓5ᵗʰ **965.0 Opiates and related narcotics**
**965.00 Opium (alkaloids), unspecified**
**965.01 Heroin**
Diacetylmorphine
**965.02 Methadone**
**965.09 Other**
Codeine [methylmorphine]
Meperidine [pethidine]
Morphine

**965.1 Salicylates**
Acetylsalicylic acid [aspirin]
Salicylic acid salts
**AHA:** N-D, '94, 15

**965.4 Aromatic analgesics, not elsewhere classified**
Acetanilid
Paracetamol [acetaminophen]
Phenacetin [acetophenetidin]

**965.5 Pyrazole derivatives**
Aminophenazone [aminopyrine]
Phenylbutazone

✓5ᵗʰ **965.6 Antirheumatics [antiphlogistics]**
**EXCLUDES** *salicylates (965.1)*
*steroids (962.0-962.9)*
**AHA:** 4Q, '98, 50

**965.61 Propionic acid derivatives**
Fenoprofen
Flurbiprofen
Ibuprofen
Ketoprofen
Naproxen
Oxaprozin
**AHA:** 4Q, '98, 50

**965.69 Other antirheumatics**
Gold salts
Indomethacin
**965.7 Other non-narcotic analgesics**
Pyrabital
**965.8 Other specified analgesics and antipyretics**
Pentazocine
**965.9 Unspecified analgesic and antipyretic**

✓4ᵗʰ **966 Poisoning by anticonvulsants and anti-Parkinsonism drugs**
**966.0 Oxazolidine derivatives**
Paramethadione
Trimethadione
**966.1 Hydantoin derivatives**
Phenytoin
**966.2 Succinimides**
Ethosuximide
Phensuximide
**966.3 Other and unspecified anticonvulsants**
Primidone
**EXCLUDES** *barbiturates (967.0)*
*sulfonamides (961.0)*

**966.4 Anti-Parkinsonism drugs**
Amantadine
Ethopropazine [profenamine]
Levodopa [L-dopa]

✓4ᵗʰ **967 Poisoning by sedatives and hypnotics**
**EXCLUDES** *drug dependence (304.0-304.9)*
*nondependent abuse (305.0-305.9)*

**967.0 Barbiturates**
Amobarbital [amylobarbitone]
Barbital [barbitone]
Butabarbital [butabarbitone]
Pentobarbital [pentobarbitone]
Phenobarbital [phenobarbitone]
Secobarbital [quinalbarbitone]
**EXCLUDES** *thiobarbiturate anesthetics (968.3)*

**967.1 Chloral hydrate group**
**967.2 Paraldehyde**

**Injury and Poisoning**

**967.3–973.9**

**967.3**    **Bromine compounds**
     Bromide
     Carbromal (derivatives)

**967.4**    **Methaqualone compounds**

**967.5**    **Glutethimide group**

**967.6**    **Mixed sedatives, not elsewhere classified**

**967.8**    **Other sedatives and hypnotics**

**967.9**    **Unspecified sedative or hypnotic**
     Sleeping:
       drug ⎫
       pill  ⎬ NOS
       tablet ⎭

✓4th **968 Poisoning by other central nervous system depressants and anesthetics**

    **EXCLUDES**   *drug dependence (304.0-304.9)*
               *nondependent abuse (305.0-305.9)*

**968.0**    **Central nervous system muscle-tone depressants**
     Chlorphenesin (carbamate)    Methocarbamol
     Mephenesin

**968.1**    **Halothane**

**968.2**    **Other gaseous anesthetics**
     Ether
     Halogenated hydrocarbon derivatives, except
       halothane
     Nitrous oxide

**968.3**    **Intravenous anesthetics**
     Ketamine
     Methohexital [methohexitone]
     Thiobarbiturates, such as thiopental sodium

**968.4**    **Other and unspecified general anesthetics**

**968.5**    **Surface [topical] and infiltration anesthetics**
     Cocaine             Procaine
     Lidocaine [lignocaine]    Tetracaine
     **AHA:** 1Q, '93, 25

**968.6**    **Peripheral nerve- and plexus-blocking anesthetics**

**968.7**    **Spinal anesthetics**

**968.9**    **Other and unspecified local anesthetics**

✓4th **969 Poisoning by psychotropic agents**

    **EXCLUDES**   *drug dependence (304.0-304.9)*
               *nondependent abuse (305.0-305.9)*

**969.0**    **Antidepressants**
     Amitriptyline
     Imipramine
     Monoamine oxidase [MAO] inhibitors

**969.1**    **Phenothiazine-based tranquilizers**
     Chlorpromazine      Prochlorperazine
     Fluphenazine        Promazine

**969.2**    **Butyrophenone-based tranquilizers**
     Haloperidol         Trifluperidol
     Spiperone

**969.3**    **Other antipsychotics, neuroleptics, and major tranquilizers**

**969.4**    **Benzodiazepine-based tranquilizers**
     Chlordiazepoxide    Lorazepam
     Diazepam         Medazepam
     Flurazepam       Nitrazepam

**969.5**    **Other tranquilizers**
     Hydroxyzine
                    Meprobamate

**969.6**    **Psychodysleptics [hallucinogens]**
     Cannabis (derivatives)    Mescaline
     Lysergide [LSD]       Psilocin
     Marihuana (derivatives)   Psilocybin

**969.7**    **Psychostimulants**
     Amphetamine
     Caffeine
     **EXCLUDES**   *central appetite depressants (977.0)*
     **AHA:** 2Q, '03, 11

**969.8**    **Other specified psychotropic agents**

**969.9**    **Unspecified psychotropic agent**

✓4th **970 Poisoning by central nervous system stimulants**

**970.0**    **Analeptics**
     Lobeline
                   Nikethamide

**970.1**    **Opiate antagonists**
     Levallorphan
                   Naloxone
     Nalorphine

**970.8**    **Other specified central nervous system stimulants**
     **AHA:** 1Q, '05, 6

**970.9**    **Unspecified central nervous system stimulant**

✓4th **971 Poisoning by drugs primarily affecting the autonomic nervous system**

**971.0**    **Parasympathomimetics [cholinergics]**
     Acetylcholine       Pilocarpine
     Anticholinesterase:
       organophosphorus
       reversible

**971.1**    **Parasympatholytics [anticholinergics and antimuscarinics] and spasmolytics**
     Atropine         Quaternary ammonium
     Homatropine       derivatives
     Hyoscine [scopolamine]
     **EXCLUDES**   *papaverine (972.5)*

**971.2**    **Sympathomimetics [adrenergics]**
     Epinephrine [adrenalin]   Levarterenol [noradrenalin]

**971.3**    **Sympatholytics [antiadrenergics]**
     Phenoxybenzamine    Tolazolinehydrochloride

**971.9**    **Unspecified drug primarily affecting autonomic nervous system**

✓4th **972 Poisoning by agents primarily affecting the cardiovascular system**

**972.0**    **Cardiac rhythm regulators**
     Practolol         Propranolol
     Procainamide      Quinidine
     **EXCLUDES**   *lidocaine (968.5)*

**972.1**    **Cardiotonic glycosides and drugs of similar action**
     Digitalis glycosides    Strophanthins
     Digoxin

**972.2**    **Antilipemic and antiarteriosclerotic drugs**
     Clofibrate        Nicotinic acid derivatives

**972.3**    **Ganglion-blocking agents**
     Pentamethonium bromide

**972.4**    **Coronary vasodilators**
     Dipyridamole      Nitrites
     Nitrates [nitroglycerin]

**972.5**    **Other vasodilators**
     Cyclandelate      Papaverine
     Diazoxide
     **EXCLUDES**   *nicotinic acid (972.2)*

**972.6**    **Other antihypertensive agents**
     Clonidine        Rauwolfia alkaloids
     Guanethidine      Reserpine

**972.7**    **Antivaricose drugs, including sclerosing agents**
     Sodium morrhuate    Zinc salts

**972.8**    **Capillary-active drugs**
     Adrenochrome derivatives   Metaraminol

**972.9**    **Other and unspecified agents primarily affecting the cardiovascular system**

✓4th **973 Poisoning by agents primarily affecting the gastrointestinal system**

**973.0**    **Antacids and antigastric secretion drugs**
     Aluminum hydroxide   Magnesium trisilicate
     **AHA:** 1Q, '03, 19

**973.1**    **Irritant cathartics**
     Bisacodyl        Phenolphthalein
     Castor oil

**973.2**    **Emollient cathartics**
     Dioctyl sulfosuccinates

**973.3**    **Other cathartics, including intestinal atonia drugs**
     Magnesium sulfate

**973.4**    **Digestants**
     Pancreatin       Pepsin
     Papain

**973.5**    **Antidiarrheal drugs**
     Kaolin          Pectin
     **EXCLUDES**   *anti-infectives (960.0-961.9)*

**973.6**    **Emetics**

**973.8**    **Other specified agents primarily affecting the gastrointestinal system**

**973.9**    **Unspecified agent primarily affecting the gastrointestinal system**

---

**N** Newborn Age: 0    **P** Pediatric Age: 0-17    **M** Maternity Age: 12-55    **A** Adult Age: 15-124    **CC** CC Condition    **MCC** Major CC Condition    **HIV** HIV Related Dx

328 — Volume 1 • October 2007          © 2007 Ingenix

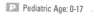

✓4ᵗʰ **974 Poisoning by water, mineral, and uric acid metabolism drugs**
     **974.0 Mercurial diuretics**
         Chlormerodrin       Mersalyl
         Mercaptomerin
     **974.1 Purine derivative diuretics**
         Theobromine       Theophylline
         EXCLUDES   *aminophylline [theophylline*
                         *ethylenediamine] (975.7)*
                         *caffeine (969.7)*
     **974.2 Carbonic acid anhydrase inhibitors**
         Acetazolamide
     **974.3 Saluretics**
         Benzothiadiazides     Chlorothiazide group
     **974.4 Other diuretics**
         Ethacrynic acid      Furosemide
     **974.5 Electrolytic, caloric, and water-balance agents**
     **974.6 Other mineral salts, not elsewhere classified**
     **974.7 Uric acid metabolism drugs**
         Allopurinol         Probenecid
         Colchicine

✓4ᵗʰ **975 Poisoning by agents primarily acting on the smooth and skeletal muscles and respiratory system**
     **975.0 Oxytocic agents**
         Ergot alkaloids      Prostaglandins
         Oxytocin
     **975.1 Smooth muscle relaxants**
         Adiphenine      Metaproterenol [orciprenaline]
         EXCLUDES   *papaverine (972.5)*
     **975.2 Skeletal muscle relaxants**
     **975.3 Other and unspecified drugs acting on muscles**
     **975.4 Antitussives**
         Dextromethorphan    Pipazethate
     **975.5 Expectorants**
         Acetylcysteine      Terpin hydrate
         Guaifenesin
     **975.6 Anti-common cold drugs**
     **975.7 Antiasthmatics**
         Aminophylline [theophylline ethylenediamine]
     **975.8 Other and unspecified respiratory drugs**

✓4ᵗʰ **976 Poisoning by agents primarily affecting skin and mucous membrane, ophthalmological, otorhinolaryngological, and dental drugs**
     **976.0 Local anti-infectives and anti-inflammatory drugs**
     **976.1 Antipruritics**
     **976.2 Local astringents and local detergents**
     **976.3 Emollients, demulcents, and protectants**
     **976.4 Keratolytics, keratoplastics, other hair treatment drugs and preparations**
     **976.5 Eye anti-infectives and other eye drugs**
         Idoxuridine
     **976.6 Anti-infectives and other drugs and preparations for ear, nose, and throat**
     **976.7 Dental drugs topically applied**
         EXCLUDES   *anti-infectives (976.0)*
                    *local anesthetics (968.5)*
     **976.8 Other agents primarily affecting skin and mucous membrane**
         Spermicides [vaginal contraceptives]
     **976.9 Unspecified agent primarily affecting skin and mucous membrane**

✓4ᵗʰ **977 Poisoning by other and unspecified drugs and medicinal substances**
     **977.0 Dietetics**
         Central appetite depressants
     **977.1 Lipotropic drugs**
     **977.2 Antidotes and chelating agents, not elsewhere classified**
     **977.3 Alcohol deterrents**
     **977.4 Pharmaceutical excipients**
         Pharmaceutical adjuncts
     **977.8 Other specified drugs and medicinal substances**
         Contrast media used for diagnostic x-ray procedures
         Diagnostic agents and kits
     **977.9 Unspecified drug or medicinal substance**

✓4ᵗʰ **978 Poisoning by bacterial vaccines**
     **978.0 BCG**
     **978.1 Typhoid and paratyphoid**
     **978.2 Cholera**
     **978.3 Plague**
     **978.4 Tetanus**
     **978.5 Diphtheria**
     **978.6 Pertussis vaccine, including combinations with a pertussis component**
     **978.8 Other and unspecified bacterial vaccines**
     **978.9 Mixed bacterial vaccines, except combinations with a pertussis component**

✓4ᵗʰ **979 Poisoning by other vaccines and biological substances**
     EXCLUDES   *gamma globulin (964.6)*
     **979.0 Smallpox vaccine**
     **979.1 Rabies vaccine**
     **979.2 Typhus vaccine**
     **979.3 Yellow fever vaccine**
     **979.4 Measles vaccine**
     **979.5 Poliomyelitis vaccine**
     **979.6 Other and unspecified viral and rickettsial vaccines**
         Mumps vaccine
     **979.7 Mixed viral-rickettsial and bacterial vaccines, except combinations with a pertussis component**
         EXCLUDES   *combinations with a pertussis*
                    *component (978.6)*
     **979.9 Other and unspecified vaccines and biological substances**

## TOXIC EFFECTS OF SUBSTANCES CHIEFLY NONMEDICINAL AS TO SOURCE (980-989)

     EXCLUDES   *burns from chemical agents (ingested) (947.0-947.9)*
                *localized toxic effects indexed elsewhere (001.0-799.9)*
                *respiratory conditions due to external agents (506.0-508.9)*
     Use additional code to specify the nature of the toxic effect

✓4ᵗʰ **980 Toxic effect of alcohol**
     **980.0 Ethyl alcohol**
         Denatured alcohol     Grain alcohol
         Ethanol
         Use additional code to identify any associated:
            acute alcohol intoxication (305.0)
              in alcoholism (303.0)
            drunkenness (simple) (305.0)
            pathological (291.4)
         **AHA:** 3Q, '96, 16
     **980.1 Methyl alcohol**
         Methanol         Wood alcohol
     **980.2 Isopropyl alcohol**
         Dimethyl carbinol    Rubbing alcohol
         Isopropanol
     **980.3 Fusel oil**
         Alcohol:         Alcohol:
          amyl            propyl
          butyl
     **980.8 Other specified alcohols**
     **980.9 Unspecified alcohol**

     **981 Toxic effect of petroleum products**
         Benzine           Petroleum:
         Gasoline         ether
         Kerosene        naphtha
         Paraffin wax     spirit

✓4ᵗʰ **982 Toxic effect of solvents other than petroleum-based**
     **982.0 Benzene and homologues**
     **982.1 Carbon tetrachloride**
     **982.2 Carbon disulfide**
         Carbon bisulfide
     **982.3 Other chlorinated hydrocarbon solvents**
         Tetrachloroethylene    Trichloroethylene
         EXCLUDES   *chlorinated hydrocarbon preparations other than solvents (989.2)*
     **982.4 Nitroglycol**
     **982.8 Other nonpetroleum-based solvents**
         Acetone

Injury and Poisoning

---

✓4ᵗʰ Additional Digit Required     Unacceptable PDx     Manifestation Code     ▶◀ Revised Text     ● New Code     ▲ Revised Code Title
✓5ᵗʰ

√4th **983 Toxic effect of corrosive aromatics, acids, and caustic alkalis**

    983.0 **Corrosive aromatics**
       Carbolic acid or phenol
       Cresol

    983.1 **Acids**
       Acid:        Acid:
         hydrochloric      sulfuric
         nitric

    983.2 **Caustic alkalis**
       Lye        Sodium hydroxide
       Potassium hydroxide

    983.9 **Caustic, unspecified**

√4th **984 Toxic effect of lead and its compounds (including fumes)**

    INCLUDES    that from all sources except medicinal substances

    984.0 **Inorganic lead compounds**
       Lead dioxide      Lead salts

    984.1 **Organic lead compounds**
       Lead acetate
       Tetraethyl lead

    984.8 **Other lead compounds**

    984.9 **Unspecified lead compound**

√4th **985 Toxic effect of other metals**

    INCLUDES    that from all sources except medicinal substances

    985.0 **Mercury and its compounds**
       Minamata disease

    985.1 **Arsenic and its compounds**

    985.2 **Manganese and its compounds**

    985.3 **Beryllium and its compounds**

    985.4 **Antimony and its compounds**

    985.5 **Cadmium and its compounds**

    985.6 **Chromium**

    985.8 **Other specified metals**
       Brass fumes      Iron compounds
       Copper salts      Nickel compounds
       AHA: 1Q, '88, 5

    985.9 **Unspecified metal**

   **986 Toxic effect of carbon monoxide**
       Carbon monoxide from any source

√4th **987 Toxic effect of other gases, fumes, or vapors**

    987.0 **Liquefied petroleum gases**
       Butane      Propane

    987.1 **Other hydrocarbon gas**

    987.2 **Nitrogen oxides**
       Nitrogen dioxide      Nitrous fumes

    987.3 **Sulfur dioxide**

    987.4 **Freon**
       Dichloromonofluoromethane

    987.5 **Lacrimogenic gas**
       Bromobenzyl cyanide   Ethyliodoacetate
       Chloroacetophenone

    987.6 **Chlorine gas**

    987.7 **Hydrocyanic acid gas**

    987.8 **Other specified gases, fumes, or vapors**
       Phosgene      Polyester fumes

    987.9 **Unspecified gas, fume, or vapor**
       AHA: 3Q, '05, 10

√4th **988 Toxic effect of noxious substances eaten as food**

    EXCLUDES   *allergic reaction to food, such as:*
       *gastroenteritis (558.3)*
       *rash (692.5, 693.1)*
       *food poisoning (bacterial) (005.0-005.9)*
       *toxic effects of food contaminants, such as:*
         *aflatoxin and other mycotoxin (989.7)*
         *mercury (985.0)*

    988.0 **Fish and shellfish**

    988.1 **Mushrooms**

    988.2 **Berries and other plants**

    988.8 **Other specified noxious substances eaten as food**

    988.9 **Unspecified noxious substance eaten as food**

√4th **989 Toxic effect of other substances, chiefly nonmedicinal as to source**

    989.0 **Hydrocyanic acid and cyanides**
       Potassium cyanide    Sodium cyanide
       EXCLUDES   *gas and fumes (987.7)*

    989.1 **Strychnine and salts**

    989.2 **Chlorinated hydrocarbons**
       Aldrin      DDT
       Chlordane      Dieldrin
       EXCLUDES   *chlorinated hydrocarbon solvents (982.0-982.3)*

    989.3 **Organophosphate and carbamate**
       Carbaryl      Parathion
       Dichlorvos      Phorate
       Malathion      Phosdrin

    989.4 **Other pesticides, not elsewhere classified**
       Mixtures of insecticides

    989.5 **Venom**
       Bites of venomous snakes, lizards, and spiders
       Tick paralysis

    989.6 **Soaps and detergents**

    989.7 **Aflatoxin and other mycotoxin [food contaminants]**

√5th   989.8 **Other substances, chiefly nonmedicinal as to source**
       AHA: 4Q, '95, 60

       989.81 **Asbestos**
         EXCLUDES   *asbestosis (501)*
           *exposure to asbestos (V15.84)*

       989.82 **Latex**

       989.83 **Silicone**
         EXCLUDES   *silicone used in medical devices, implants and grafts (996.00-996.79)*

       989.84 **Tobacco**

       989.89 **Other**

    989.9 **Unspecified substance, chiefly nonmedicinal as to source**

## OTHER AND UNSPECIFIED EFFECTS OF EXTERNAL CAUSES (990-995)

   **990 Effects of radiation, unspecified**
       Complication of:      Radiation sickness
         phototherapy
         radiation therapy
       EXCLUDES   *specified adverse effects of radiation. Such conditions are to be classified according to the nature of the adverse effect, as:*
         *burns (940.0-949.5)*
         *dermatitis (692.7-692.8)*
         *leukemia (204.0-208.9)*
         *pneumonia (508.0)*
         *sunburn (692.71, 692.76-692.77)*
         *[The type of radiation giving rise to the adverse effect may be identified by use of the E codes.]*

√4th **991 Effects of reduced temperature**

    991.0 **Frostbite of face**    CC
       CC Excl: 991.0, 991.3

    991.1 **Frostbite of hand**    CC
       CC Excl: 991.1, 991.3

    991.2 **Frostbite of foot**    CC
       CC Excl: 991.2-991.3

    991.3 **Frostbite of other and unspecified sites**    CC
       CC Excl: 991.0-991.4

    991.4 **Immersion foot**    CC
       Trench foot
       CC Excl: 991.3-991.4

       DEF: Paresthesia, edema, blotchy cyanosis of foot, the skin is soft (macerated), pale and wrinkled, and the sole is swollen with surface ridging and following sustained immersion in water.

---

N Newborn Age: 0     P Pediatric Age: 0-17     M Maternity Age: 12-55     A Adult Age: 15-124     CC CC Condition     MCC Major CC Condition     HIV HIV Related Dx

**991.5 Chilblains**
Erythema pernio     Perniosis
DEF: Red, swollen, itchy skin; follows damp cold exposure; also associated with pruritus and a burning feeling, in hands, feet, ears, and face in children, legs and toes in women, and hands and fingers in men.

**991.6 Hypothermia**
Hypothermia (accidental)
EXCLUDES   hypothermia following anesthesia (995.89)
    hypothermia not associated with low environmental temperature (780.99)
DEF: Reduced body temperature due to low environmental temperatures.

**991.8 Other specified effects of reduced temperature**
**991.9 Unspecified effect of reduced temperature**
Effects of freezing or excessive cold NOS

**√4th 992 Effects of heat and light**
EXCLUDES   burns (940.0-949.5)
    diseases of sweat glands due to heat (705.0-705.9)
    malignant hyperpyrexia following anesthesia (995.86)
    sunburn (692.71, 692.76-692.77)

**992.0 Heat stroke and sunstroke**   CC
Heat apoplexy    Siriasis
Heat pyrexia    Thermoplegia
Ictus solaris
CC Excl: 992.0-992.9
DEF: Headache, vertigo, cramps and elevated body temperature due to high environmental temperatures.

**992.1 Heat syncope**
Heat collapse
**992.2 Heat cramps**
**992.3 Heat exhaustion, anhydrotic**
Heat prostration due to water depletion
EXCLUDES   that associated with salt depletion (992.4)
**992.4 Heat exhaustion due to salt depletion**
Heat prostration due to salt (and water) depletion
**992.5 Heat exhaustion, unspecified**
Heat prostration NOS
**992.6 Heat fatigue, transient**
**992.7 Heat edema**
DEF: Fluid retention due to high environmental temperatures.
**992.8 Other specified heat effects**
**992.9 Unspecified**

**√4th 993 Effects of air pressure**
**993.0 Barotrauma, otitic**
Aero-otitis media
Effects of high altitude on ears
DEF: Ringing ears, deafness, pain and vertigo due to air pressure changes.
**993.1 Barotrauma, sinus**
Aerosinusitis
Effects of high altitude on sinuses
**993.2 Other and unspecified effects of high altitude**
Alpine sickness    Hypobaropathy
Andes disease    Mountain sickness
Anoxia due to high altitude
AHA: 3Q, '88, 4
**993.3 Caisson disease**   CC
Bends    Decompression sickness
Compressed-air disease   Divers' palsy or paralysis
CC Excl: 993.3-993.9
DEF: Rapid reduction in air pressure while breathing compressed air; symptoms include skin lesions, joint pains, respiratory and neurological problems.
**993.4 Effects of air pressure caused by explosion**

**993.8 Other specified effects of air pressure**
**993.9 Unspecified effect of air pressure**
**√4th 994 Effects of other external causes**
EXCLUDES   certain adverse effects not elsewhere classified (995.0-995.8)
**994.0 Effects of lightning**
Shock from lightning   Struck by lightning NOS
EXCLUDES   burns (940.0-949.5)
**994.1 Drowning and nonfatal submersion**   CC
Bathing cramp
Immersion
CC Excl: 994.1
AHA: 3Q, '88, 4
**994.2 Effects of hunger**
Deprivation of food
Starvation
**994.3 Effects of thirst**
Deprivation of water
**994.4 Exhaustion due to exposure**
**994.5 Exhaustion due to excessive exertion**
Overexertion
**994.6 Motion sickness**
Air sickness
Seasickness
Travel sickness
**994.7 Asphyxiation and strangulation**   CC
Suffocation (by):
bedclothes
cave-in
constriction
mechanical
plastic bag
pressure
strangulation
EXCLUDES   asphyxia from:
carbon monoxide (986)
inhalation of food or foreign body (932-934.9)
other gases, fumes, and vapors (987.0-987.9)
CC Excl: 994.7
**994.8 Electrocution and nonfatal effects of electric current**
Shock from electric current
EXCLUDES   electric burns (940.0-949.5)
**994.9 Other effects of external causes**
Effects of:
abnormal gravitational [G] forces or states
weightlessness
**√4th 995 Certain adverse effects not elsewhere classified**
EXCLUDES   complications of surgical and medical care (996.0-999.9)
**995.0 Other anaphylactic shock**   CC
Allergic shock
Anaphylactic reaction
Anaphylaxis
} NOS or due to adverse effect of correct medicinal substance properly administered
Use additional E code to identify external cause, such as:
adverse effects of correct medicinal substance properly administered [E930-E949]
EXCLUDES   anaphylactic reaction to serum (999.4)
anaphylactic shock due to adverse food reaction (995.60-995.69)
CC Excl: 995.60-995.69
AHA: 4Q, '93, 30
DEF: Immediate sensitivity response after exposure to specific antigen; results in life-threatening respiratory distress; usually followed by vascular collapse, shock, urticaria, angioedema and pruritus.

**Injury and Poisoning**

**995.1–995.8**

**995.1 Angioneurotic edema**
Giant urticaria
> EXCLUDES    urticaria:
>> due to serum (999.5)
>> other specified (698.2, 708.0-708.9, 757.33)

DEF: Circulatory response of deep dermis, subcutaneous or submucosal tissues; causes localized edema and wheals.

✓5th **995.2 Other and unspecified adverse effect of drug, medicinal and biological substance**

Adverse effect
Allergic reaction  } (due) to correct medicinal
Hypersensitivity     substance properly
Idiosyncrasy     administered

Drug:            Drug:
   hypersensitivity NOS      reaction NOS
> EXCLUDES    pathological drug intoxication (292.2)

AHA: 2Q, '97, 12; 3Q, '95, 13; 3Q, '92, 16

**995.20 Unspecified adverse effect of unspecified drug, medicinal and biological substance**
AHA: 4Q, '06, 112

**995.21 Arthus phenomenon**
Arthus reaction
AHA: 4Q, '06, 112

**995.22 Unspecified adverse effect of anesthesia**
AHA: 4Q, '06, 112

**995.23 Unspecified adverse effect of insulin**
AHA: 4Q, '06, 112

**995.27 Other drug allergy**
Drug allergy NOS
Drug hypersensitivity NOS
AHA: 4Q, '06, 112

**995.29 Unspecified adverse effect of other drug, medicinal and biological substance**
AHA: 4Q, '06, 112

**995.3 Allergy, unspecified**
Allergic reaction NOS      Idiosyncrasy NOS
Hypersensitivity NOS
> EXCLUDES    allergic reaction NOS to correct medicinal substance properly administered (995.27)
>> allergy to existing dental restorative materials (525.66)
>> specific types of allergic reaction, such as:
>>> allergic diarrhea (558.3)
>>> dermatitis (691.0-693.9)
>>> hayfever (477.0-477.9)

**995.4 Shock due to anesthesia**    CC
Shock due to anesthesia in which the correct substance was properly administered
> EXCLUDES    complications of anesthesia in labor or delivery (668.0-668.9)
>> overdose or wrong substance given (968.0-969.9)
>> postoperative shock NOS (998.0)
>> specified adverse effects of anesthesia classified elsewhere, such as:
>>> anoxic brain damage (348.1)
>>> hepatitis (070.0-070.9), etc.
>> unspecified adverse effect of anesthesia (995.22)

CC Excl: 958.4, 995.4, 997.91-998.13, 998.81, 998.83-998.9

✓5th **995.5 Child maltreatment syndrome**
Use additional code(s), if applicable, to identify any associated injuries
Use additional E code to identify:
   nature of abuse (E960-E968)
   perpetrator (E967.0-E967.9)
AHA: 1Q, '98, 11

**995.50 Child abuse, unspecified**    CC   P
CC Excl: 995.50-995.59, 995.80-995.85

**995.51 Child emotional/psychological abuse**   CC   P
CC Excl: See code: 995.50
AHA: 4Q, '96, 38, 40

**995.52 Child neglect (nutritional)**    CC   P
CC Excl: See code: 995.50
AHA: 4Q, '96, 38, 40

**995.53 Child sexual abuse**    CC   P
CC Excl: See code: 995.50
AHA: 4Q, '96, 39, 40

**995.54 Child physical abuse**    CC   P
Battered baby or child syndrome
> EXCLUDES    shaken infant syndrome (995.55)

CC Excl: See code: 995.50
AHA: 3Q, '99, 14; 4Q, '96, 39, 40

**995.55 Shaken infant syndrome**    CC   P
Use additional code(s) to identify any associated injuries
CC Excl: See code: 995.50
AHA: 4Q, '96, 40, 43

**995.59 Other child abuse and neglect**   CC   P
Multiple forms of abuse
CC Excl: See code: 995.50

✓5th **995.6 Anaphylactic shock due to adverse food reaction**
Anaphylactic shock due to nonpoisonous foods
AHA: 4Q, '93, 30

**995.60 Due to unspecified food**    CC
CC Excl: 995.60-995.69

**995.61 Due to peanuts**    CC
CC Excl: See code: 995.60

**995.62 Due to crustaceans**    CC
CC Excl: See code: 995.60

**995.63 Due to fruits and vegetables**    CC
CC Excl: See code: 995.60

**995.64 Due to tree nuts and seeds**    CC
CC Excl: See code: 995.60

**995.65 Due to fish**    CC
CC Excl: See code: 995.60

**995.66 Due to food additives**    CC
CC Excl: See code: 995.60

**995.67 Due to milk products**    CC
CC Excl: See code: 995.60

**995.68 Due to eggs**    CC
CC Excl: See code: 995.60

**995.69 Due to other specified food**    CC
CC Excl: See code: 995.60

**995.7 Other adverse food reactions, not elsewhere classified**
Use additional code to identify the type of reaction, such as:
   hives (708.0)      wheezing (786.07)
> EXCLUDES    anaphylactic shock due to adverse food reaction (995.60-995.69)
>> asthma (493.0, 493.9)
>> dermatitis due to food (693.1)
>>> in contact with skin (692.5)
>> gastroenteritis and colitis due to food (558.3)
>> rhinitis due to food (477.1)

✓5th **995.8 Other specified adverse effects, not elsewhere classified**

N Newborn Age: 0    P Pediatric Age: 0-17    M Maternity Age: 12-55    A Adult Age: 15-124    CC CC Condition    MCC Major CC Condition    HIV HIV Related Dx

332 — Volume 1 • October 2007          © 2007 Ingenix

**995.80 Adult maltreatment, unspecified** `CC` `A`
Abused person NOS
Use additional code to identify:
   any associated injury
   perpetrator (E967.0-E967.9)
**CC Excl:** 995.80

**AHA:** 4Q, '96, 41, 43

**995.81 Adult physical abuse** `CC` `A`
Battered:                    Battered:
   person syndrome NEC          spouse
   man                          woman
Use additional code to identify:
   any association injury
   nature of abuse (E960-E968)
   perpetrator (E967.0-E967.9)
**CC Excl:** 995.50-995.59, 995.80-995.85

**AHA:** 4Q, '96, 42, 43

**995.82 Adult emotional/psychological abuse** `A`
Use additional E code to identify perpetrator
(E967.0-E967.9)

**995.83 Adult sexual abuse** `CC` `A`
Use additional code(s) to identify:
   any associated injury
   perpetrator (E967.0-E967.9)
**CC Excl:** See code: 995.81

**995.84 Adult neglect (nutritional)** `CC` `A`
Use additional code(s) to identify:
   intent of neglect (E904.0, E968.4)
   perpetrator (E967.0-E967.9)
**CC Excl:** See code: 995.81

**995.85 Other adult abuse and neglect** `CC` `A`
Multiple forms of abuse and neglect
Use additional code(s) to identify
   any associated injury
   intent of neglect (E904.0, E968.4)
   nature of abuse (E960-E968)
   perpetrator (E967.0-E967.9)
**CC Excl:** See code: 995.81

**995.86 Malignant hyperthermia** `CC`
Malignant hyperpyrexia due to anesthesia
**CC Excl:** 958.4, 995.4, 995.86, 997.91-998.13, 998.81, 998.83-998.9

**AHA:** 4Q, '98, 51

**995.89 Other**
Hypothermia due to anesthesia
**AHA:** 2Q, '04, 18; 3Q, '03, 12

`√5ᵗʰ` **995.9   Systemic inflammatory response syndrome (SIRS)**
**AHA:** 4Q, '06, 113-116; 2Q, '04, 16; 4Q, '02, 71

**DEF:** Clinical response to infection or trauma that can trigger an
acute inflammatory reaction and progresses to coagulation,
impaired fibrinolysis, and organ failure; manifested by two or more
of the following symptoms: fever, tachycardia, tachypnea,
leukocytosis or leukopenia.

**995.90 Systemic inflammatory response** `CC`
**syndrome, unspecified**
SIRS NOS
**CC Excl:** 003.1, 020.2, 036.2, 038.0-038.9, 040.82-041.9, 054.5,
139.8, 995.90-995.94, V09.0-V09.91

**Continuum of Illness Due to Infection**

Bacteremia ➡ Septicemia ➡ Sepsis
Severe Sepsis ⬅ Severe Sepsis ⬅
with Septic Shock
⬇
MODS ➡ Death
(Multiple Organ
Dysfunction Syndrome)

**995.91 Sepsis** `MCC`
Systemic inflammatory response syndrome
   due to infectious process without
   acute organ dysfunction
Code first underlying infection
`EXCLUDES`  *sepsis with acute organ*
             *dysfunction (995.92)*
             *sepsis with multiple organ*
             *dysfunction (995.92)*
             *severe sepsis (995.92)*
**CC Excl:** See code 995.90

**AHA:** 4Q, '06, 113-116; 2Q, '04, 16; 4Q, '03, 79

**995.92 Severe sepsis** `MCC`
Sepsis with acute organ dysfunction
Sepsis with multiple organ dysfunction
   (MOD)
Systemic inflammatory response syndrome
   due to infectious process with acute
   organ dysfunction
Code first underlying infection
Use additional code to specify acuteorgan
   dysfunction, such as:
   acute renal failure (584.5-584.9)
   acute respiratory failure (518.81)
   critical illness myopathy (359.81)
   critical illness polyneuropathy (357.82)
   disseminated intravascular coagulopathy
      [DIC] (286.6)
   encephalopathy (348.31)
   hepatic failure (570)
   septic shock (785.52)
**CC Excl:** See code 995.90

**AHA:** 4Q, '06, 113-116; 2Q, '05, 18-19; 1Q, '05, 7; 1Q, '05, 7;
2Q, '04, 16; 4Q, '03, 73, 79

**995.93 Systemic inflammatory response** `CC`
**syndrome due to noninfectious process**
**without acute organ dysfunction**
Code first underlying conditions, such as:
   acute pancreatitis (577.0)
   trauma
`EXCLUDES`  *systemic inflammatory*
             *response syndrome due*
             *to noninfectious process*
             *with acute organ*
             *dysfunction (995.94)*
**CC Excl:** See code 995.90

**AHA:** 4Q, '06, 113-116

**995.94 Systemic inflammatory response** `MCC`
**syndrome due to noninfectious process**
**with acute organ dysfunction**
Code first underlying conditions, such
   as:
   acute pancreatitis (577.0)
   trauma
Use additional code to specify acute organ
   dysfunction, such as:
   acute renal failure (584.5-584.9)
   acute respiratory failure (518.81)
   critical illness myopathy (359.81)
   critical illness polyneuropathy (357.82)
   disseminated intravascular coagulopathy
      [DIC] syndrome (286.6)
   encephalopathy (348.31)
   hepatic failure (570)
`EXCLUDES`  *severe sepsis (995.92)*
**CC Excl:** See code 995.90
**AHA:** 4Q, '06, 113-116; 4Q, '03, 79

**Injury and Poisoning**

**995.80–995.94**

---

`√4ᵗʰ` `√5ᵗʰ` Additional Digit Required    Unacceptable PDx    Manifestation Code    ◄► Revised Text    ● New Code    ▲ Revised Code Title

## COMPLICATIONS OF SURGICAL AND MEDICAL CARE, NOT ELSEWHERE CLASSIFIED (996-999)

EXCLUDES    *adverse effects of medicinal agents (001.0-799.9, 995.0-995.8)*
*burns from local applications and irradiation (940.0-949.5)*
*complications of:*
  *conditions for which the procedure was performed*
  *surgical procedures during abortion, labor, and delivery (630-676.9)*
*poisoning and toxic effects of drugs and chemicals (960.0-989.9)*
*postoperative conditions in which no complications are present, such as:*
  *artificial opening status (V44.0-V44.9)*
  *closure of external stoma (V55.0-V55.9)*
  *fitting of prosthetic device (V52.0-V52.9)*
*specified complications classified elsewhere*
  *anesthetic shock (995.4)*
  *electrolyte imbalance (276.0-276.9)*
  *postlaminectomy syndrome (722.80-722.83)*
  *postmastectomy lymphedema syndrome (457.0)*
  *postoperative psychosis (293.0-293.9)*
  *any other condition classified elsewhere in the Alphabetic Index when described as due to a procedure*

√4ᵗʰ **996 Complications peculiar to certain specified procedures**

INCLUDES    *complications, not elsewhere classified, in the use of artificial substitutes [e.g., Dacron, metal, Silastic, Teflon] or natural sources [e.g., bone] involving:*
  *anastomosis (internal)*
  *graft (bypass) (patch)*
  *implant*
  *internal device:*
    *catheter*        *fixation*
    *electronic*      *prosthetic*
  *reimplant*
  *transplant*

EXCLUDES    *accidental puncture or laceration during procedure (998.2)*
*complications of internal anastomosis of:*
  *gastrointestinal tract (997.4)*
  *urinary tract (997.5)*
▶*endosseous dental implant failures (525.71-525.79)*
*intraoperative floppy iris syndrome [IFIS] (364.81)*◀
*mechanical complication of respirator (V46.14)*
*other specified complications classified elsewhere, such as:*
  *hemolytic anemia (283.1)*
  *functional cardiac disturbances (429.4)*
  *serum hepatitis (070.2-070.3)*

AHA: 1Q, '94, 3

√5ᵗʰ **996.0 Mechanical complication of cardiac device, implant, and graft**

Breakdown (mechanical)    Obstruction, mechanical
Displacement              Perforation
Leakage                   Protrusion

AHA: 2Q, '93, 9

**996.00 Unspecified device, implant, and graft**    CC
CC Excl: 996.00, 996.04, 996.61-996.62, 996.70-996.74, 997.91-997.99, 998.81, 998.83-998.9

**996.01 Due to cardiac pacemaker (electrode)**    CC
CC Excl: 996.01, 997.91-997.99, 998.81, 998.83-998.9
AHA: 2Q, '06, 15; 2Q, '99, 11

**996.02 Due to heart valve prosthesis**    CC
CC Excl: 996.02, 997.91-997.99, 998.81, 998.83-998.9

**996.03 Due to coronary bypass graft**    CC
EXCLUDES    *atherosclerosis of graft (414.02, 414.03)*
*embolism [occlusion NOS] [thrombus] of graft (996.72)*
CC Excl: 996.03, 997.91-997.99, 998.81, 998.83-998.9
AHA: 2Q, '95, 17; N-D, '86, 5

**996.04 Due to automatic implantable cardiac defibrillator**    CC
CC Excl: 996.04, 997.91-997.99, 998.81, 998.83-998.9
AHA: 2Q, '05, 3

**996.09 Other**    CC
CC Excl: 996.09, 997.91-997.99, 998.81, 998.83-998.9
AHA: 2Q, '93, 9

**996.1 Mechanical complication of other vascular device, implant, and graft**    CC
Mechanical complications involving:
  aortic (bifurcation) graft (replacement)
  arteriovenous:
    dialysis catheter  ⎫
    fistula            ⎬  surgically created
    shunt              ⎭
  balloon (counterpulsation) device, intra-aortic
  carotid artery bypass graft
  femoral-popliteal bypass graft
  umbrella device, vena cava
EXCLUDES    *atherosclerosis of biological graft (440.30-440.32)*
*embolism [occlusion NOS] [thrombus] of (biological) (synthetic) graft (996.74)*
*peritoneal dialysis catheter (996.56)*
CC Excl: 996.1, 997.91-997.99, 998.81, 998.83-998.9
AHA: 1Q, '06, 10; 2Q, '05, 8; 1Q, '02, 13; 1Q, '95, 3

**996.2 Mechanical complication of nervous system device, implant, and graft**    CC
Mechanical complications involving:
  dorsal column stimulator
  electrodes implanted in brain [brain "pacemaker"]
  peripheral nerve graft
  ventricular (communicating) shunt
CC Excl: 996.2, 996.63, 996.75, 997.91-997.99, 998.81, 998.83-998.9
AHA: 2Q, '99, 4; S-O, '87, 10

√5ᵗʰ **996.3 Mechanical complication of genitourinary device, implant, and graft**
AHA: 3Q, '01, 13; S-O, '85, 3

**996.30 Unspecified device, implant, and graft**    CC
CC Excl: 996.30, 996.64-996.65, 996.76, 997.91-997.99, 998.81, 998.83-998.9

**996.31 Due to urethral [indwelling] catheter**

**996.32 Due to intrauterine contraceptive device**    ♀

**996.39 Other**    CC
Cystostomy catheter
Prosthetic reconstruction of vas deferens
Repair (graft) of ureter without mention of resection
EXCLUDES    *complications due to:*
  *external stoma of urinary tract (997.5)*
  *internal anastomosis of urinary tract (997.5)*
CC Excl: 996.39, 996.64-996.65, 996.76, 997.91-997.99, 998.81, 998.83-998.9

---

N Newborn Age: 0    P Pediatric Age: 0-17    M Maternity Age: 12-55    A Adult Age: 15-124    CC CC Condition    MC Major Complication    CD Complex Dx    HIV HIV Related Dx

©2007 Ingenix

**Injury and Poisoning**

**996.4–996.61**

√5th **996.4** **Mechanical complication of internal orthopedic device, implant, and graft**
Mechanical complications involving:
external (fixation) device utilizing internal screw(s), pin(s) or other methods of fixation
grafts of bone, cartilage, muscle, or tendon
internal (fixation) device such as nail, plate, rod, etc.
Use additional code to identify prosthetic joint with mechanical complication (V43.60-V43.69)
**EXCLUDES** complications of external orthopedic device, such as:
pressure ulcer due to cast (707.00-707.09)
**AHA:** 4Q, '05, 91; 2Q, '99, 10; 2Q, '98, 19; 2Q, '96, 11; 3Q, '95, 16; N-D, '85, 11

**996.40** **Unspecified mechanical complication of internal orthopedic device, implant, and graft** `CC`
**CC Excl:** 996.40-996.49, 996.66-996.67, 996.77-996.78, 997.91-997.99, 998.81, 998.83-998.9

**996.41** **Mechanical loosening of prosthetic joint** `CC`
Aseptic loosening
**CC Excl:** See code: 996.40
**AHA:** 4Q, '05, 112

**996.42** **Dislocation of prosthetic joint** `CC`
Instability of prosthetic joint
Subluxation of prosthetic joint
**CC Excl:** See code 996.40

**996.43** **Prosthetic joint implant failure** `CC`
Breakage (fracture) of prosthetic joint
**CC Excl:** See code 996.40

**996.44** **Peri-prosthetic fracture around prosthetic joint** `CC`
**CC Excl:** See code 996.40
**AHA:** 4Q, '05, 93

**996.45** **Peri-prosthetic osteolysis** `CC`
Use additional code to identify major osseous defect, if applicable (731.3)
**CC Excl:** See code 996.40
**AHA:** 4Q, '06, 103

**996.46** **Articular bearing surface wear of prosthetic joint** `CC`
**CC Excl:** See code 996.40

**996.47** **Other mechanical complication of prosthetic joint implant** `CC`
Mechanical complication of prosthetic joint NOS
**CC Excl:** See code 996.40

**996.49** **Other mechanical complication of other internal orthopedic device, implant, and graft** `CC`
**EXCLUDES** mechanical complication of prosthetic joint implant (996.41-996.47)
**CC Excl:** See code 996.40

√5th **996.5** **Mechanical complication of other specified prosthetic device, implant, and graft**
Mechanical complications involving:
prosthetic implant in:
bile duct      chin
breast      orbit of eye
nonabsorbable surgical material NOS
other graft, implant, and internal device, not elsewhere classified
**AHA:** 1Q, '98, 11

**996.51** **Due to corneal graft** `CC`
**CC Excl:** 996.51, 997.91-997.99

**996.52** **Due to graft of other tissue, not elsewhere classified** `CC`
Skin graft failure or rejection
**EXCLUDES** failure of artificial skin graft (996.55)
failure of decellularized allodermis (996.55)
sloughing of temporary skin allografts or xenografts (pigskin)—omit code
**CC Excl:** 996.52, 996.55, 997.91-997.99
**AHA:** 1Q, '96, 10

**996.53** **Due to ocular lens prosthesis** `CC`
**EXCLUDES** contact lenses—code to condition
**CC Excl:** 996.53, 997.91-997.99
**AHA:** 1Q, '00, 9

**996.54** **Due to breast prosthesis** `CC`
Breast capsule (prosthesis)
Mammary implant
**CC Excl:** 996.54, 997.91-997.99
**AHA:** 2Q, '98, 14; 3Q, '92, 4

**996.55** **Due to artificial skin graft and decellularized allodermis** `CC`
Dislodgement      Non-adherence
Displacement      Poor incorporation
Failure      Shearing
**CC Excl:** 996.52, 996.55-996.60, 996.68-996.70, 996.79, 997.91-997.99
**AHA:** 4Q, '98, 52

**996.56** **Due to peritoneal dialysis catheter** `CC`
**EXCLUDES** mechanical complication of arteriovenous dialysis catheter (996.1)
**CC Excl:** 996.56-996.60, 996.68-996.70, 996.79, 997.91-997.99
**AHA:** 4Q, '98, 54

**996.57** **Due to insulin pump** `CC`
**CC Excl:** 996.00-996.30, 996.39-996.79, 997.91-997.99, 998.81, 998.83-998.9
**AHA:** 4Q, '03, 81-82

**996.59** **Due to other implant and internal device, not elsewhere classified** `CC`
Nonabsorbable surgical material NOS
Prosthetic implant in:
bile duct
chin
orbit of eye
**CC Excl:** See code: 996.56
**AHA:** 2Q, '99, 13; 3Q, '94, 7

√5th **996.6** **Infection and inflammatory reaction due to internal prosthetic device, implant, and graft**
Infection (causing obstruction) ⎤ due to (presence of) any device, implant, and graft classi-
Inflammation ⎦ fiable to 996.0-996.5
Use additional code to identify specified infections
**AHA:** 2Q, '89, 16; J-F, '87, 14

**996.60** **Due to unspecified device, implant, and graft** `CC`
**CC Excl:** See code: 996.57

**996.61** **Due to cardiac device, implant, and graft** `CC`
Cardiac pacemaker or defibrillator:
electrode(s), lead(s)
pulse generator
subcutaneous pocket
Coronary artery bypass graft
Heart valve prosthesis
**CC Excl:** 996.00-996.1, 996.52, 996.55-996.62, 996.68-996.74, 996.79, 997.91-997.99, 998.81, 998.83-998.9

**996.62 Due to other vascular device, implant, and graft** `CC`
Arterial graft
Arteriovenous fistula or shunt
Infusion pump
Vascular catheter (arterial) (dialysis)
▶(peripheral venous)◄
**EXCLUDES** ▶ infection due to:
central venous catheter
(999.31)
Hickman catheter (999.31)
peripherally inserted
central catheter [PICC]
(999.31)
triple lumen catheter
(999.31)◄
**CC Excl:** See code 996.61
**AHA:** 2Q, '04, 16; 1Q, '04, 5; 4Q, '03, 107, 111; 2Q, '03, 7;
2Q, '94, 13

**996.63 Due to nervous system device, implant,** `CC` **and graft**
Electrodes implanted in brain
Peripheral nerve graft
Spinal canal catheter
Ventricular (communicating) shunt (catheter)
**CC Excl:** 996.2, 996.52, 996.55-996.60, 996.63, 996.68-996.70,
996.75, 996.79, 997.91-997.99, 998.81, 998.83-998.9

**996.64 Due to indwelling urinary catheter** `CC`
Use additional code to identify specified
infections, such as:
Cystitis (595.0-595.9)
Sepsis (038.0-038.9)
**CC Excl:** 599.0, 996.30, 996.39, 996.56-996.60, 996.64-996.65,
996.68-996.70, 996.76, 996.79, 997.91-997.99, 998.81,
998.83-998.9
**AHA:** 3Q, '93, 6

**996.65 Due to other genitourinary device, implant, and graft** `CC`
Intrauterine contraceptive device
**CC Excl:** 996.30, 996.39, 996.52, 996.55-996.60, 996.64-
996.65, 996.68-996.70, 996.76, 996.79, 997.91-997.99,
998.81, 998.83-998.9
**AHA:** 1Q, '00, 15

**996.66 Due to internal joint prosthesis** `CC`
Use additional code to identify infected
prosthetic joint (V43.60-V43.69)
**CC Excl:** 996.40-996.49, 996.52, 996.55-996.60, 996.66-996.70,
996.77-996.79, 997.91-997.99, 998.81, 998.83-998.9
**AHA:** ▶2Q, '07, 7;◄ '05, 91, 113; 2Q, '91, 18

**996.67 Due to other internal orthopedic device,** `CC` **implant, and graft**
Bone growth stimulator (electrode)
Internal fixation device (pin) (rod) (screw)
**CC Excl:** See code: 996.66

**996.68 Due to peritoneal dialysis catheter** `CC`
Exit-site infection or inflammation
**CC Excl:** 996.56-996.60, 996.68-996.70, 996.79, 997.91-997.99
**AHA:** 4Q, '98, 54

**996.69 Due to other internal prosthetic device,** `CC` **implant, and graft**
Breast prosthesis          Prosthetic orbital
Ocular lens prosthesis       implant
**CC Excl:** 996.00-996.30, 996.39-996.79, 997.91-997.99, 998.81,
998.83-998.9
**AHA:** 4Q, '03, 108; 4Q, '98, 52

√5th **996.7 Other complications of internal (biological) (synthetic) prosthetic device, implant, and graft**
Complication NOS ⎫
occlusion NOS  ⎪
Embolism     ⎪  due to (presence of) any
Fibrosis     ⎬  device, implant, and
Hemorrhage   ⎪  graft classifiable to
Pain       ⎪  996.0-996.5
Stenosis     ⎪
Thrombus     ⎭
Use additional code to identify complication,
such as:
pain due to presence of device, implant or graft
(338.18-338.19, 338.28-338.29)
**EXCLUDES** transplant rejection (996.8)
**AHA:** ▶2Q, '07, 12;◄ 4Q, '05, 94; 1Q, '89, 9; N-D, '86, 5

**996.70 Due to unspecified device, implant, and graft**

**996.71 Due to heart valve prosthesis** `CC`
**CC Excl:** 996.00, 996.02, 996.09-996.1, 996.52, 996.55-996.62,
996.68-996.74, 996.79, 997.91-997.99, 998.81, 998.83-998.9

**996.72 Due to other cardiac device, implant, and graft** `CC`
Cardiac pacemaker or defibrillator:
electrode(s), lead(s)
subcutaneous pocket
Coronary artery bypass (graft)
**EXCLUDES** occlusion due to athero-
sclerosis (414.02-414.06)
**CC Excl:** 996.00-996.02, 996.04-996.1, 996.52, 996.55-996.62,
996.68-996.74, 996.79, 997.91-997.99, 998.81, 998.83-998.9
**AHA:** 3Q, '06, 8, 25; 3Q, '01, 20

**996.73 Due to renal dialysis device, implant, and graft** `CC`
**CC Excl:** 996.1, 996.52, 996.55-996.60, 996.68-996.70,
996.73, 996.79, 997.91-997.99, 998.81, 998.83-998.9
**AHA:** 2Q, '91, 18

**996.74 Due to other vascular device, implant, and graft** `CC`
**EXCLUDES** occlusion of biological graft
due to atherosclerosis
(440.30-440.32)
**CC Excl:** 996.00-996.1, 996.52, 996.55-996.62, 996.68-996.74,
996.79, 997.91-997.99, 998.81, 998.83-998.9
**AHA:** 1Q, '03, 16, 17

**996.75 Due to nervous system device, implant,** `CC` **and graft**
**CC Excl:** 996.2, 996.52, 996.55-996.60, 996.63, 996.68-996.70,
996.75, 996.79, 997.91-997.99, 998.81, 998.83-998.9

**996.76 Due to genitourinary device, implant, and graft** `CC`
**CC Excl:** 996.30, 996.39, 996.52, 996.55-996.60,
996.64-996.65, 996.68-996.70, 996.76, 996.79, 997.91-997.99,
998.81, 998.83-998.9
**AHA:** 1Q, '00, 15

**996.77 Due to internal joint prosthesis** `CC`
▶Use additional code to identify prosthetic
joint (V43.60-V43.69)◄
**CC Excl:** 996.40-996.49, 996.52, 996.55-996.60, 996.66-996.70,
996.77-996.79, 997.91-997.99, 998.81, 998.83-998.9
**AHA:** 4Q, '05, 91

**996.78 Due to other internal orthopedic device, implant, and graft** `CC`
**CC Excl:** 996.40-996.49, 996.52, 996.55-996.60, 996.66-996.70,
996.77-996.79, 997.91-997.99, 998.81, 998.83-998.9
**AHA:** 2Q, '03, 14

---

`N` Newborn Age: 0  `P` Pediatric Age: 0-17  `M` Maternity Age: 12-55  `A` Adult Age: 15-124  `CC` CC Condition  `MC` Major Complication  `CD` Complex Dx  `HIV` HIV Related Dx

**996.79 Due to other internal prosthetic device, implant, and graft** `CC`

CC Excl: 996.00-996.30, 996.39-996.79, 997.91-997.99, 998.81, 998.83-998.9

AHA: 2Q, '04, 7; 1Q,'01, 8; 3Q, '95, 14; 3Q, '92, 4

✓5ᵗʰ **996.8 Complications of transplanted organ**

Transplant failure or rejection
Use additional code to identify nature of complication, such as:
    Cytomegalovirus (CMV) infection (078.5)

AHA: 3Q, '01, 12; 3Q, '93, 3, 4; 2Q, '93, 11; 1Q, '93, 24

**996.80 Transplanted organ, unspecified** `CC`

CC Excl: 996.80, 996.87, 997.91-997.99

**996.81 Kidney** `CC`

CC Excl: 996.81, 997.91-997.99

AHA: 3Q, '03, 16; 3Q, '98, 6, 7; 3Q, '94, 8; 2Q, '94, 9; 1Q, '93, 24

**996.82 Liver** `CC`

CC Excl: 996.82, 997.91-997.99

AHA: 3Q, '03, 17; 3Q, '98, 3, 4

**996.83 Heart** `CC`

CC Excl: 996.83, 997.91-997.99

AHA: 3Q, '03, 16; 4Q, '02, 53; 3Q, '98, 5

**996.84 Lung** `CC`

CC Excl: 996.84, 997.91-997.99

AHA: 2Q, '03, 12; 3Q, '98, 5

**996.85 Bone marrow** `CC`

Graft-versus-host disease (acute) (chronic)

CC Excl: 996.85, 997.91-997.99

AHA: 4Q, '90, 4

**996.86 Pancreas** `CC`

CC Excl: 996.86, 997.91-997.99

**996.87 Intestine** `CC`

CC Excl: 996.80, 996.87, 997.91-997.99

**996.89 Other specified transplanted organ** `CC`

CC Excl: 996.89, 997.91-997.99

AHA: 3Q, '94, 5

✓5ᵗʰ **996.9 Complications of reattached extremity or body part**

**996.90 Unspecified extremity** `CC`

CC Excl: 996.90, 997.91-997.99, 998.81, 998.83-998.9

**996.91 Forearm** `CC`

CC Excl: 996.91, 997.91-997.99, 998.81, 998.83-998.9

**996.92 Hand** `CC`

CC Excl: 996.92, 997.91-997.99, 998.81, 998.83-998.9

**996.93 Finger(s)** `CC`

CC Excl: 996.93, 997.91-997.99, 998.81, 998.83-998.9

**996.94 Upper extremity, other and unspecified** `CC`

CC Excl: 996.94, 997.91-997.99, 998.81, 998.83-998.9

**996.95 Foot and toe(s)** `CC`

CC Excl: 996.95, 997.91-997.99, 998.81, 998.83-998.9

**996.96 Lower extremity, other and unspecified** `CC`

CC Excl: 996.96, 997.91-997.99, 998.81, 998.83-998.9

**996.99 Other specified body part** `CC`

CC Excl: 996.99, 997.91-997.99, 998.81, 998.83-998.9

✓4ᵗʰ **997 Complications affecting specified body systems, not elsewhere classified**

Use additional code to identify complications

EXCLUDES   *the listed conditions when specified as:*
    *causing shock (998.0)*
    *complications of:*
      *anesthesia:*
        *adverse effect (001.0-799.9, 995.0-995.8)*
        *in labor or delivery (668.0-668.9)*
        *poisoning (968.0-969.9)*
      *implanted device or graft (996.0-996.9)*
      *obstetrical procedures (669.0-669.4)*
      *reattached extremity (996.90-996.96)*
      *transplanted organ (996.80-996.89)*

AHA: 1Q, '94, 4; 1Q, '93, 26

✓5ᵗʰ **997.0 Nervous system complications**

**997.00 Nervous system complication, unspecified**

**997.01 Central nervous system complication** `CC`

Anoxic brain damage
Cerebral hypoxia

EXCLUDES   *cerebrovascular hemorrhage or infarction (997.02)*

CC Excl: 997.00-997.09, 997.91-997.99, 998.81, 998.83-998.9

AHA: ►1Q, '07, 22;◄ 1Q, '06, 15

**997.02 Iatrogenic cerebrovascular infarction or hemorrhage** `CC`

Postoperative stroke

CC Excl: See code: 997.01

AHA: 3Q, '06, 6; 2Q, '04, 8; 4Q, '95, 57

**997.09 Other nervous system complications** `CC`

CC Excl: See code: 997.01

**997.1 Cardiac complications** `CC`

Cardiac:
  arrest        ⎫
  insufficiency   ⎬ during or resulting
Cardiorespiratory failure ⎪  from a procedure
Heart failure      ⎭

EXCLUDES   *the listed conditions as long-term effects of cardiac surgery or due to the presence of cardiac prosthetic device (429.4)*

CC Excl: 997.1, 997.91-997.99, 998.81, 998.83-998.9

AHA: 2Q, '02, 12

**997.2 Peripheral vascular complications** `CC`

Phlebitis or thrombophlebitis during or resulting from a procedure

EXCLUDES   *the listed conditions due to:*
    *implant or catheter device (996.62)*
    *infusion, perfusion, or transfusion (999.2)*
    *complications affecting blood vessels (997.71-997.79)*

CC Excl: 997.2, 997.79-997.99, 998.81, 998.83-998.9

AHA: 1Q, '03, 6; 3Q, '02, 24-26

**Injury and Poisoning**

**997.3–998.0**

**997.3**   **Respiratory complications**   `CC`

Mendelson's syndrome ⎱ resulting from a
Pneumonia (aspiration) ⎰   procedure

> **EXCLUDES**   *iatrogenic [postoperative] pneumothorax (512.1)*
> *iatrogenic pulmonary embolism (415.11)*
> *Mendelson's syndrome in labor and delivery (668.0)*
> *specified complications classified elsewhere, such as:*
> *adult respiratory distress syndrome (518.5)*
> *pulmonary edema, postoperative (518.4)*
> *respiratory insufficiency, acute, postoperative (518.5)*
> *shock lung (518.5)*
> *tracheostomy complications (519.00-519.09)*
> *transfusion related acute lung injury [TRALI] (518.7)*

**CC Excl:** 518.7, 997.3, 997.91-997.99, 998.81, 998.83-998.9

**AHA:** 1Q, '97, 10; 2Q, '93, 3; 2Q, '93, 9; 4Q, '90, 25

**DEF:** Mendelson's syndrome: acid pneumonitis due to aspiration of gastric acids, may occur after anesthesia or sedation.

**997.4**   **Digestive system complications**   `CC`

Complications of:
intestinal (internal) anastomosis and bypass, not elsewhere classified; except that involving urinary tract

Hepatic failure ⎱
Hepatorenal syndrome ⎰ specified as due to
Intestinal obstruction NOS ⎰ a procedure

> **EXCLUDES**   *gastrostomy complications (536.40-536.49)*
> *specified gastrointestinal complications classified elsewhere, such as:*
> *blind loop syndrome (579.2)*
> *colostomy and enterostomy complications (569.60-569.69)*
> *gastrojejunal ulcer (534.0-534.9)*
> *infection of esophagostomy (530.86)*
> *infection of external stoma (569.61)*
> *mechanical complication of esophagostomy (530.87)*
> *pelvic peritoneal adhesions, female (614.6)*
> *peritoneal adhesions (568.0)*
> *peritoneal adhesions with obstruction (560.81)*
> *postcholecystectomy syndrome (576.0)*
> *postgastric surgery syndromes (564.2)*
> *vomiting following gastrointestinal surgery (564.3)*

**CC Excl:** 530.86-530.87, 536.40-536.49, 997.4, 997.71, 997.91-997.99, 998.81, 998.83-998.9

**AHA:** 2Q, '01, 4-6; 3Q, '99, 4; 2Q, '99, 14; 3Q, '97, 7; 1Q, '97, 11; 2Q, '95, 7; 1Q, '93, 26; 3Q, '92, 15; 2Q, '89, 15; 1Q, '88, 14

**997.5**   **Urinary complications**

Complications of:
external stoma of urinary tract
internal anastomosis and bypass of urinary tract, including that involving intestinal tract

Oliguria or anuria ⎱
Renal: ⎰
   failure (acute) ⎰ specified as due to
   insufficiency (acute) ⎰ procedure
Tubular necrosis (acute) ⎰

> **EXCLUDES**   *specified complications classified elsewhere, such as:*
> *postoperative stricture of:*
> *ureter (593.3)*
> *urethra (598.2)*

**AHA:** 3Q, '03, 13; 3Q, '96, 10, 15; 4Q, '95, 73; 1Q, '92, 13; 2Q, '89, 16; M-A, '87, 10; S-O, '85, 3

✓5ᵗʰ **997.6**   **Amputation stump complication**

> **EXCLUDES**   *admission for treatment for a current traumatic amputation — code to complicated traumatic amputation*
> *phantom limb (syndrome) (353.6)*

**AHA:** 4Q, '95, 82

**997.60**   **Unspecified complication**

**997.61**   **Neuroma of amputation stump**

**DEF:** Hyperplasia generated nerve cell mass following amputation.

**997.62**   **Infection (chronic)**   `CC`

Use additional code to identify the organism

**CC Excl:** 997.60, 997.62-997.69, 997.91-997.99, 998.81, 998.83-998.9

**AHA:** 1Q, '05, 15 4Q, '96, 46

**997.69**   **Other**

**AHA:** 1Q, '05, 15

✓5ᵗʰ **997.7**   **Vascular complications of other vessels**

> **EXCLUDES**   *peripheral vascular complications (997.2)*

**997.71**   **Vascular complications of mesenteric artery**   `CC`

**CC Excl:** 997.2, 997.71-997.99, 998.81, 998.83-998.9

**AHA:** 4Q, '01, 53

**997.72**   **Vascular complications of renal artery**   `CC`

**CC Excl:** See code 997.71

**997.79**   **Vascular complications of other vessels**   `CC`

**CC Excl:** See code 997.71

✓5ᵗʰ **997.9**   **Complications affecting other specified body systems, not elsewhere classified**

> **EXCLUDES**   *specified complications classified elsewhere, such as:*
> *broad ligament laceration syndrome (620.6)*
> *postartificial menopause syndrome (627.4)*
> *postoperative stricture of vagina (623.2)*

**997.91**   **Hypertension**

> **EXCLUDES**   *essential hypertension (401.0-401.9)*

**AHA:** 4Q, '95, 57

**997.99**   **Other**   `CC`

Vitreous touch syndrome

**CC Excl:** 997.91-997.99, 998.81, 998.83-998.9

**AHA:** 2Q, '94, 12; 1Q, '94, 17

**DEF:** Vitreous touch syndrome: vitreous protruding through pupil and attaches to corneal epithelium; causes aqueous fluid in vitreous body; marked by corneal edema, loss of lucidity; complication of cataract surgery.

✓4ᵗʰ **998**   **Other complications of procedures, not elsewhere classified**

**AHA:** 1Q, '94, 4

**998.0**   **Postoperative shock**   `CC`

Collapse NOS ⎱ during or resulting
Shock (endotoxic) (hypo- ⎰ from a surgical
   volemic) (septic) ⎰ procedure

> **EXCLUDES**   *shock:*
> *anaphylactic due to serum (999.4)*
> *anesthetic (995.4)*
> *electric (994.8)*
> *following abortion (639.5)*
> *obstetric (669.1)*
> *traumatic (958.4)*

**CC Excl:** 958.4, 995.4, 997.91-998.13, 998.81, 998.83-998.9

---

N Newborn Age: 0    P Pediatric Age: 0-17    M Maternity Age: 12-55    A Adult Age: 15-124    `CC` CC Condition    `MCC` Major CC Condition    `HIV` HIV Related Dx

**338 — Volume 1 • October 2007**          © *2007 Ingenix*

√5th **998.1** **Hemorrhage or hematoma or seroma complicating a procedure**

　　EXCLUDES　*hemorrhage, hematoma, or seroma:*
　　　　　*complicating cesarean section or*
　　　　　*puerperal perineal wound*
　　　　　*(674.3)*
　　　　　*due to implanted device or graft*
　　　　　*(996.70-996.79)*

**998.11** **Hemorrhage complicating a procedure** `CC`
　　**CC Excl:** 456.0, 456.20, 530.81-530.83, 530.89, 531.00-531.01, 531.20-531.21, 531.40-531.41, 531.60-531.61, 532.00-532.01, 532.20-532.21, 532.40-532.41, 532.60-532.61, 533.00-533.01, 533.20-533.21, 533.40-533.41, 533.60-533.61, 534.00-534.01, 534.20-534.21, 534.40-534.41, 534.60-534.61, 535.01, 535.11, 535.21, 535.31, 535.41, 535.51, 535.61, 537.83, 562.02-562.03, 562.12-562.13, 569.3, 569.85, 578.0-578.9, 772.4, 997.91-998.13, 998.81, 998.89-998.9

　　**AHA:** 3Q, '03, 13; 1Q, '03, 4; 4Q, '97, 52; 1Q, '97, 10

**998.12** **Hematoma complicating a procedure** `CC`
　　**CC Excl:** see code 998.11

　　**AHA:** 3Q, '06, 12; 1Q, '03, 6; 3Q, '02, 24, 26

**998.13** **Seroma complicating a procedure** `CC`
　　**CC Excl:** See code 998.11

　　**AHA:** 4Q, '96, 46; 1Q, '93, 26; 2Q, '92, 15; S-O, '87, 8

**998.2** **Accidental puncture or laceration during a procedure** `CC`
　　Accidental perforation by catheter or other
　　　　instrument during a procedure on:
　　　　blood vessel
　　　　nerve
　　　　organ
　　　　EXCLUDES　*iatrogenic [postoperative] pneumothorax*
　　　　　　*(512.1)*
　　　　　*puncture or laceration caused by*
　　　　　　*implanted device intentionally left*
　　　　　　*in operation wound (996.0-996.5)*
　　　　　*specified complications classified*
　　　　　　*elsewhere, such as:*
　　　　　　*broad ligament laceration syndrome*
　　　　　　*(620.6)*
　　　　　*trauma from instruments during*
　　　　　　*delivery (664.0-665.9)*

　　**CC Excl:** 997.91-997.99, 998.2, 998.81, 998.83-998.9

　　**AHA:** ▶2Q, '07, 9;◀ 1Q, '06, 15; 3Q, '02, 24, 26; 3Q, '94, 6; 3Q, '90, 17; 3Q, '90, 18

√5th **998.3** **Disruption of operation wound**
　　Dehiscence ⎫
　　Rupture　　⎬ of operation wound
　　　　EXCLUDES　*disruption of:*
　　　　　*cesarean wound (674.1)*
　　　　　*perineal wound, puerperal (674.2)*

　　**AHA:** 4Q, '02, 73; 1Q, '93, 19

**998.31** **Disruption of internal operation wound** `CC`
　　**CC Excl:** 997.91-997.99, 998.31, 998.32, 998.81-998.89, 998.9

**998.32** **Disruption of external operation wound** `CC`
　　Disruption of operation wound NOS

　　**CC Excl:** See code: 998.31

　　**AHA:** 1Q, '06, 8; 1Q, '05, 11; 4Q, '03, 104, 106

**998.4** **Foreign body accidentally left during a procedure** `CC`
　　Adhesions　　⎫ due to foreign body accidentally left
　　Obstruction　⎬　in operative wound or body
　　Perforation　⎭　cavity during a procedure
　　　　EXCLUDES　*obstruction or perforation caused by*
　　　　　*implanted device intentionally left*
　　　　　*in body (996.0-996.5)*

　　**CC Excl:** 997.91-997.99, 998.4, 998.81, 998.83-998.9

　　**AHA:** 1Q, '89, 9

√5th **998.5** **Postoperative infection**
　　　　EXCLUDES　*bleb associated endophthalmitis*
　　　　　*(379.63)*
　　　　　*infection due to:*
　　　　　　*implanted device (996.60-996.69)*
　　　　　　*infusion, perfusion, or transfusion*
　　　　　　▶*(999.31-999.39)*◀
　　　　　*postoperative obstetrical wound*
　　　　　　*infection (674.3)*

**998.51** **Infected postoperative seroma** `CC`
　　Use additional code to identify organism
　　**CC Excl:** 997.91-997.99, 998.51-998.59, 998.81, 998.89-998.9

　　**AHA:** 4Q, '96, 46

**998.59** **Other postoperative infection** `CC`
　　Abscess:　　　⎫
　　　intra-abdominal ⎪
　　　stitch　　　　 ⎪
　　　subphrenic　　⎬ postoperative
　　　wound　　　　 ⎪
　　Septicemia　　　⎭
　　Use additional code to identify infection
　　**CC Excl:** See code: 998.51

　　**AHA:** 2Q, '06, 23; 4Q, '04, 76; 4Q, '03, 104, 106-107; 3Q, '98, 3; 3Q, '95, 5; 2Q, '95, 7; 3Q, '94, 6; 1Q, '93, 19; J-F, '87, 14

**998.6** **Persistent postoperative fistula** `CC`
　　**CC Excl:** 997.91-997.99, 998.6, 998.81, 998.83-998.9

　　**AHA:** J-F, '87, 14

**998.7** **Acute reaction to foreign substance accidentally left during a procedure** `CC`
　　Peritonitis:　　　　Peritonitis:
　　　aseptic　　　　　　chemical
　　**CC Excl:** 997.91-997.99, 998.7-998.81, 998.83-998.9

√5th **998.8** **Other specified complications of procedures, not elsewhere classified**
　　**AHA:** 4Q, '94, 46; 1Q, '89, 9

**998.81** **Emphysema (subcutaneous) (surgical) resulting from a procedure**

**998.82** **Cataract fragments in eye following cataract surgery**

**998.83** **Non-healing surgical wound** `CC`
　　**CC Excl:** 997.91-997.99, 998.81, 998.83-998.9

　　**AHA:** 4Q, '96, 47

**998.89** **Other specified complications**
　　**AHA:** 3Q, '06, 9; 3Q, '05, 16; 3Q, '99, 13; 2Q, '98, 16

**998.9** **Unspecified complication of procedure, not elsewhere classified**
　　Postoperative complication NOS
　　　　EXCLUDES　*complication NOS of obstetrical, surgery*
　　　　　*or procedure (669.4)*

　　**AHA:** 4Q, '93, 37

**999 Complications of medical care, not elsewhere classified** ✓4ᵗʰ

INCLUDES complications, not elsewhere classified, of:
- dialysis (hemodialysis) (peritoneal) (renal)
- extracorporeal circulation
- hyperalimentation therapy
- immunization
- infusion
- inhalation therapy
- injection
- inoculation
- perfusion
- transfusion
- vaccination
- ventilation therapy

▶Use additional code, where applicable, to identify specific complication◀

EXCLUDES specified complications classified elsewhere such as:
- complications of implanted device (996.0-996.9)
- contact dermatitis due to drugs (692.3)
- dementia dialysis (294.8)
  - transient (293.9)
- dialysis disequilibrium syndrome (276.0-276.9)
- poisoning and toxic effects of drugs and chemicals (960.0-989.9)
- postvaccinal encephalitis (323.51)
- water and electrolyte imbalance (276.0-276.9)

**999.0 Generalized vaccinia** CC
CC Excl: 999.0

DEF: Skin eruption, self-limiting; follows vaccination; due to transient viremia with virus localized in skin.

**999.1 Air embolism** MCC
Air embolism to any site following infusion, perfusion, or transfusion

EXCLUDES embolism specified as:
- complicating:
  - abortion (634-638 with .6, 639.6)
  - ectopic or molar pregnancy (639.6)
  - pregnancy, childbirth, or the puerperium (673.0)
- due to implanted device (996.7)
- traumatic (958.0)

CC Excl: 958.0, 999.1

**999.2 Other vascular complications** CC
Phlebitis / Thromboembolism / Thrombophlebitis } following infusion, perfusion, or transfusion

EXCLUDES the listed conditions when specified as:
- due to implanted device (996.61-996.62. 996.72-996.74)
- postoperative NOS (997.2, 997.71-997.79)

CC Excl: 999.2
AHA: 2Q, '97, 5

**999.3 Other infection** ✓5ᵗʰ
Infection / Sepsis / Septicemia } following infusion, injection, transfusion, or vaccination

▶Use additional code to identify the specified infection, such as:
- septicemia (038.0-038.9)◀

EXCLUDES the listed conditions when specified as:
- due to implanted device (996.60-996.69)
- postoperative NOS (998.51-998.59)

AHA: 2Q, '01, 11, 12; 2Q, '97, 5; J-F, '87, 14

**999.31 Infection due to central venous catheter** CC
Catheter-related bloodstream infection [CRBSI]
Infection due to:
- Hickman catheter
- Peripherally inserted central catheter [PICC]
- Triple lumen catheter

EXCLUDES infection due to:
- arterial catheter (996.62)
- catheter NOS (996.69)
- peripheral venous catheter (996.62)
- urinary catheter (996.64)

CC Excl: 996.62, 999.31-999.39

**999.39 Infection following other infusion, injection, transfusion, or vaccination** CC
CC Excl: 996.62, 999.31-999.39

**999.4 Anaphylactic shock due to serum** CC
EXCLUDES shock:
- allergic NOS (995.0)
- anaphylactic:
  - NOS (995.0)
  - due to drugs and chemicals (995.0)

CC Excl: 999.4

DEF: Life-threatening hypersensitivity to foreign serum; causes respiratory distress, vascular collapse, and shock.

**999.5 Other serum reaction** CC
Intoxication by serum / Serum sickness
Protein sickness / Urticaria due to serum
Serum rash

EXCLUDES serum hepatitis (070.2-070.3)

CC Excl: 999.5

DEF: Serum sickness: Hypersensitivity to foreign serum; causes fever, hives, swelling, and lymphadenopathy.

**999.6 ABO incompatibility reaction** CC
Incompatible blood transfusion
Reaction to blood group incompatibility in infusion or transfusion

CC Excl: 999.6

**999.7 Rh incompatibility reaction** CC
Elevation of Rh titer
Reactions due to Rh factor in infusion or transfusion

CC Excl: 999.7

**999.8 Other transfusion reaction** CC
Septic shock due to transfusion
Transfusion reaction NOS

EXCLUDES postoperative shock (998.0)
transfusion related acute lung injury [TRALI] (518.7)

CC Excl: 999.8
AHA: 3Q, '00, 9

**999.9 Other and unspecified complications of medical care, not elsewhere classified**
Complications, not elsewhere classified, of:
- electroshock
- inhalation } therapy
- ultrasound
- ventilation

Unspecified misadventure of medical care

EXCLUDES unspecified complication of:
- phototherapy (990)
- radiation therapy (999)

AHA: 3Q, '06, 25; 1Q, '03, 19; 2Q, '97, 5

# SUPPLEMENTARY CLASSIFICATION OF FACTORS INFLUENCING HEALTH STATUS AND CONTACT WITH HEALTH SERVICES (V01-V86)

This classification is provided to deal with occasions when circumstances other than a disease or injury classifiable to categories 001-999 (the main part of ICD) are recorded as "diagnoses" or "problems." This can arise mainly in three ways:

a) When a person who is not currently sick encounters the health services for some specific purpose, such as to act as a donor of an organ or tissue, to receive prophylactic vaccination, or to discuss a problem which is in itself not a disease or injury. This will be a fairly rare occurrence among hospital inpatients, but will be relatively more common among hospital outpatients and patients of family practitioners, health clinics, etc.

b) When a person with a known disease or injury, whether it is current or resolving, encounters the health care system for a specific treatment of that disease or injury (e.g., dialysis for renal disease; chemotherapy for malignancy; cast change).

c) When some circumstance or problem is present which influences the person's health status but is not in itself a current illness or injury. Such factors may be elicited during population surveys, when the person may or may not be currently sick, or be recorded as an additional factor to be borne in mind when the person is receiving care for some current illness or injury classifiable to categories 001-999.

In the latter circumstances the V code should be used only as a supplementary code and should not be the one selected for use in primary, single cause tabulations. Examples of these circumstances are a personal history of certain diseases, or a person with an artificial heart valve in situ.

AHA: J-F, '87, 8

## PERSONS WITH POTENTIAL HEALTH HAZARDS RELATED TO COMMUNICABLE DISEASES (V01-V06)

> **EXCLUDES**   family history of infectious and parasitic diseases (V18.8)
> personal history of infectious and parasitic diseases (V12.0)

√4ᵗʰ **V01 Contact with or exposure to communicable diseases**

   **V01.0 Cholera**
      Conditions classifiable to 001

   **V01.1 Tuberculosis**
      Conditions classifiable to 010-018

   **V01.2 Poliomyelitis**
      Conditions classifiable to 045

   **V01.3 Smallpox**
      Conditions classifiable to 050

   **V01.4 Rubella**
      Conditions classifiable to 056

   **V01.5 Rabies**
      Conditions classifiable to 071

   **V01.6 Venereal diseases**
      Conditions classifiable to 090-099

√5ᵗʰ **V01.7 Other viral diseases**
      Conditions classifiable to 042-078 and V08, except as above
      AHA: 2Q, '92, 11
    ² **V01.71 Varicella**
    ² **V01.79 Other viral diseases**

√5ᵗʰ **V01.8 Other communicable diseases**
      Conditions classifiable to 001-136, except as above
      AHA: J-A, '87, 24
    **V01.81 Anthrax**
      AHA: 4Q, '02, 70, 78
    ² **V01.82 Exposure to SARS-associated coronavirus**
      AHA: 4Q, '03, 46-47
    ² **V01.83 Escherichia coli (E. coli)**
    ² **V01.84 Meningococcus**
    **V01.89 Other communicable diseases**

   **V01.9 Unspecified communicable disease**

---

√4ᵗʰ **V02 Carrier or suspected carrier of infectious diseases**
   AHA: 3Q, '95, 18; 3Q, '94, 4

   **V02.0 Cholera**
   **V02.1 Typhoid**
   **V02.2 Amebiasis**
   **V02.3 Other gastrointestinal pathogens**
   **V02.4 Diphtheria**

√5ᵗʰ **V02.5 Other specified bacterial diseases**
    **V02.51 Group B streptococcus**
      AHA: 3Q, '06, 14; 1Q, '02, 14; 4Q, '98, 56
    **V02.52 Other streptococcus**
    **V02.59 Other specified bacterial diseases**
      Meningococcal   Staphylococcal

√5ᵗʰ **V02.6 Viral hepatitis**
     Hepatitis Australian-antigen [HAA] [SH] carrier
     Serum hepatitis carrier
    **V02.60 Viral hepatitis carrier, unspecified**
      AHA: 4Q, '97, 47
    **V02.61 Hepatitis B carrier**
      AHA: 4Q, '97, 47
    **V02.62 Hepatitis C carrier**
      AHA: 4Q, '97, 47
    **V02.69 Other viral hepatitis carrier**
      AHA: 4Q, '97, 47

   **V02.7 Gonorrhea**
   **V02.8 Other venereal diseases**
   **V02.9 Other specified infectious organism**
      AHA: 3Q, '95, 18; 1Q, '93, 22; J-A, '87, 24

√4ᵗʰ **V03 Need for prophylactic vaccination and inoculation against bacterial diseases**
> **EXCLUDES**   vaccination not carried out (V64.00-V64.09)
> vaccines against combinations of diseases (V06.0-V06.9)

   **V03.0 Cholera alone**
   **V03.1 Typhoid-paratyphoid alone [TAB]**
   **V03.2 Tuberculosis [BCG]**
   **V03.3 Plague**
   **V03.4 Tularemia**
   **V03.5 Diphtheria alone**
   **V03.6 Pertussis alone**
   **V03.7 Tetanus toxoid alone**

√5ᵗʰ **V03.8 Other specified vaccinations against single bacterial diseases**
    **V03.81 Hemophilus influenza, type B [Hib]**
    **V03.82 Streptococcus pneumoniae [pneumococcus]**
    **V03.89 Other specified vaccination**
      AHA: 2Q, '00, 9

   **V03.9 Unspecified single bacterial disease**

√4ᵗʰ **V04 Need for prophylactic vaccination and inoculation against certain viral diseases**
> **EXCLUDES**   vaccines against combinations of diseases (V06.0-V06.9)

   **V04.0 Poliomyelitis**
   **V04.1 Smallpox**
   **V04.2 Measles alone**
   **V04.3 Rubella alone**
   **V04.4 Yellow fever**
   **V04.5 Rabies**
   **V04.6 Mumps alone**
   **V04.7 Common cold**

√5ᵗʰ **V04.8 Other viral diseases**
      AHA: 4Q, '03, 83
    **V04.81 Influenza**
    **V04.82 Respiratory syncytial virus (RSV)**
    **V04.89 Other viral diseases**
      AHA: ▶2Q, '07, 9◀

---

² These V codes may be used as principal diagnosis on Medicare patients.

√4ᵗʰ √5ᵗʰ Additional Digit Required     Unacceptable PDx     Manifestation Code     ▶◀ Revised Text     ● New Code     ▲ Revised Code Title

**V Codes**

**V05–V09.91**

√4th **V05 Need for other prophylactic vaccination and inoculation against single diseases**

> EXCLUDES   *vaccines against combinations of diseases (V06.0-V06.9)*

V05.0 **Athropod-borne viral encephalitis**

V05.1 **Other arthropod-borne viral diseases**

V05.2 **Leishmaniasis**

V05.3 **Viral hepatitis**

V05.4 **Varicella**
> Chickenpox

V05.8 **Other specified disease**
> AHA: 1Q, '01, 4; 3Q, '91, 20

V05.9 **Unspecified single disease**

√4th **V06 Need for prophylactic vaccination and inoculation against combinations of diseases**

> Note: Use additional single vaccination codes from categories V03-V05 to identify any vaccinations not included in a combination code.

V06.0 **Cholera with typhoid-paratyphoid [cholera+TAB]**

V06.1 **Diphtheria-tetanus-pertussis, combined [DTP] [DTaP]**
> AHA: 4Q, '03, 83; 3Q, '98, 13

V06.2 **Diphtheria-tetanus-pertussis with typhoid-paratyphoid [DTP+TAB]**

V06.3 **Diphtheria-tetanus-pertussis with poliomyelitis [DTP+polio]**

V06.4 **Measles-mumps-rubella [MMR]**

V06.5 **Tetanus-diphtheria [Td] [DT]**
> AHA: 4Q, '03, 83

V06.6 **Streptococcus pneumoniae [pneumococcus] and influenza**

V06.8 **Other combinations**
> EXCLUDES   *multiple single vaccination codes (V03.0-V05.9)*
> AHA: 1Q, '94, 19

V06.9 **Unspecified combined vaccine**

## PERSONS WITH NEED FOR ISOLATION, OTHER POTENTIAL HEALTH HAZARDS AND PROPHYLACTIC MEASURES (V07-V09)

√4th **V07 Need for isolation and other prophylactic measures**

> EXCLUDES   *prophylactic organ removal (V50.41-V50.49)*

² V07.0 **Isolation**
> Admission to protect the individual from his surroundings or for isolation of individual after contact with infectious diseases

V07.1 **Desensitization to allergens**

V07.2 **Prophylactic immunotherapy**
> Administration of:
> antivenin
> immune sera [gamma globulin]
> RhoGAM
> tetanus antitoxin

√5th V07.3 **Other prophylactic chemotherapy**

> V07.31 **Prophylactic fluoride administration**

> ² V07.39 **Other prophylactic chemotherapy**
> > EXCLUDES   *maintenance chemotherapy following disease (V58.11)*

V07.4 **Hormone replacement therapy (postmenopausal)** ♀

² V07.8 **Other specified prophylactic measure**
> AHA: 1Q, '92, 11

V07.9 **Unspecified prophylactic measure**

**V08 Asymptomatic human immunodeficiency virus [HIV] infection status**
> HIV positive NOS
> Note: This code is *only* to be used when no HIV infection symptoms or conditions are present. If any HIV infection symptoms or conditions are present, see code 042.
> > EXCLUDES   *AIDS (042)*
> > *human immunodeficiency virus [HIV] disease (042)*
> > *exposure to HIV (V01.79)*
> > *nonspecific serologic evidence of HIV (795.71)*
> > *symptomatic human immunodeficiency virus [HIV] infection (042)*
> AHA: 2Q, '04, 11; 2Q, '99, 8; 3Q, '95, 18

√4th **V09 Infection with drug-resistant microorganisms**

> Note: This category is intended for use as an additional code for infectious conditions classified elsewhere to indicate the presence of drug-resistance of the infectious organism.
> AHA: 3Q, '94, 4; 4Q, '93, 22

V09.0 **Infection with microorganisms resistant to penicillins**
> Methicillin-resistant staphylococcus aureus (MRSA)
> AHA: ▶2Q, '06, 16;◀4Q, '03, 104, 106

V09.1 **Infection with microorganisms resistant to cephalosporins and other B-lactam antibiotics**

V09.2 **Infection with microorganisms resistant to macrolides**

V09.3 **Infection with microorganisms resistant to tetracyclines**

V09.4 **Infection with microorganisms resistant to aminoglycosides**

√5th V09.5 **Infection with microorganisms resistant to quinolones and fluoroquinolones**

> V09.50 **Without mention of resistance to multiple quinolones and fluoroquinoles**

> V09.51 **With resistance to multiple quinolones and fluoroquinoles**

V09.6 **Infection with microorganisms resistant to sulfonamides**

√5th V09.7 **Infection with microorganisms resistant to other specified antimycobacterial agents**
> > EXCLUDES   *Amikacin (V09.4)*
> > *Kanamycin (V09.4)*
> > *Streptomycin [SM] (V09.4)*

> V09.70 **Without mention of resistance to multiple antimycobacterial agents**

> V09.71 **With resistance to multiple antimycobacterial agents**

√5th V09.8 **Infection with microorganisms resistant to other specified drugs**
> Vancomycin (glycopeptide) intermediate staphylococcus aureus (VISA/GISA)
> Vancomycin (glycopeptide) resistant enterococcus (VRE)
> Vancomycin (glycopeptide) resistant staphylococcus aureus (VRSA/GRSA)

> V09.80 **Without mention of resistance to multiple drugs**

> V09.81 **With resistance to multiple drugs**

√5th V09.9 **Infection with drug-resistant microorganisms, unspecified**
> Drug resistance, NOS

> V09.90 **Without mention of multiple drug resistance**

> V09.91 **With multiple drug resistance**
> > Multiple drug resistance NOS

---

² These V codes may be used as principal diagnosis on Medicare patients.

N Newborn Age: 0    P Pediatric Age: 0-17    M Maternity Age: 12-55    A Adult Age: 15-124    CC CC Condition    MCC Major CC Condition    HIV HIV Related Dx

**PERSONS WITH POTENTIAL HEALTH HAZARDS RELATED TO PERSONAL AND FAMILY HISTORY (V10-V19)**

> **EXCLUDES** *obstetric patients where the possibility that the fetus might be affected is the reason for observation or management during pregnancy (655.0-655.9)*

AHA: J-F, '87, 1

✓4th **V10 Personal history of malignant neoplasm**
AHA: 4Q, '02, 80; 4Q, '98, 69; 1Q, '95, 4; 3Q, '92, 5; M-J, '85, 10; 2Q, '90, 9

✓5th **V10.0 Gastrointestinal tract**
History of conditions classifiable to 140-159

**V10.00 Gastrointestinal tract, unspecified**

**V10.01 Tongue**

**V10.02 Other and unspecified oral cavity and pharynx**

**V10.03 Esophagus**

**V10.04 Stomach**

**V10.05 Large intestine**
AHA: 3Q, '99, 7; 1Q, '95, 4

**V10.06 Rectum, rectosigmoid junction, and anus**

**V10.07 Liver**

**V10.09 Other**
AHA: 4Q, '03, 111

✓5th **V10.1 Trachea, bronchus, and lung**
History of conditions classifiable to 162

**V10.11 Bronchus and lung**

**V10.12 Trachea**

✓5th **V10.2 Other respiratory and intrathoracic organs**
History of conditions classifiable to 160, 161, 163-165

**V10.20 Respiratory organ, unspecified**

**V10.21 Larynx**
AHA: 4Q, '03, 108, 110

**V10.22 Nasal cavities, middle ear, and accessory sinuses**

**V10.29 Other**

**V10.3 Breast**
History of conditions classifiable to 174 and 175
AHA: ▶1Q, '07, 6; ◀ 2Q, '03, 5; 4Q, '01, 66; 4Q, '98, 65; 4Q, '97, 50; 1Q, '91, 16; 1Q, '90, 21

✓5th **V10.4 Genital organs**
History of conditions classifiable to 179-187

**V10.40 Female genital organ, unspecified** ♀

**V10.41 Cervix uteri** ♀

**V10.42 Other parts of uterus** ♀

**V10.43 Ovary** ♀

**V10.44 Other female genital organs** ♀

**V10.45 Male genital organ, unspecified** ♂

**V10.46 Prostate** ♂

**V10.47 Testis** ♂

**V10.48 Epididymis** ♂

**V10.49 Other male genital organs** ♂

✓5th **V10.5 Urinary organs**
History of conditions classifiable to 188 and 189

**V10.50 Urinary organ, unspecified**

**V10.51 Bladder**

**V10.52 Kidney**
AHA: 2Q, '04, 4

> **EXCLUDES** *renal pelvis (V10.53)*

**V10.53 Renal pelvis**
AHA: 4Q, '01, 55

**V10.59 Other**

✓5th **V10.6 Leukemia**
Conditions classifiable to 204-208

> **EXCLUDES** *leukemia in remission (204-208)*

AHA: 2Q, '92, 13; 4Q, '91, 26; 4Q, '90, 3

**V10.60 Leukemia, unspecified**

**V10.61 Lymphoid leukemia**

**V10.62 Myeloid leukemia**

**V10.63 Monocytic leukemia**

**V10.69 Other**

✓5th **V10.7 Other lymphatic and hematopoietic neoplasms**
Conditions classifiable to 200-203

> **EXCLUDES** *listed conditions in 200-203 in remission*

AHA: M-J, '85, 18

**V10.71 Lymphosarcoma and reticulosarcoma**

**V10.72 Hodgkin's disease**

**V10.79 Other**

✓5th **V10.8 Personal history of malignant neoplasm of other sites**
History of conditions classifiable to 170-173, 190-195

**V10.81 Bone**
AHA: 2Q, '03, 13

**V10.82 Malignant melanoma of skin**

**V10.83 Other malignant neoplasm of skin**

**V10.84 Eye**

**V10.85 Brain**
AHA: 1Q, '01, 6

**V10.86 Other parts of nervous system**

> **EXCLUDES** *peripheral sympathetic, and parasympathetic nerves (V10.89)*

**V10.87 Thyroid**

**V10.88 Other endocrine glands and related structures**

**V10.89 Other**

**V10.9 Unspecified personal history of malignant neoplasm**

✓4th **V11 Personal history of mental disorder**

**V11.0 Schizophrenia**

> **EXCLUDES** *that in remission (295.0-295.9 with fifth-digit 5)*

**V11.1 Affective disorders**
Personal history of manic-depressive psychosis

> **EXCLUDES** *that in remission (296.0-296.6 with fifth-digit 5, 6)*

**V11.2 Neurosis**

**V11.3 Alcoholism**

**V11.8 Other mental disorders**

**V11.9 Unspecified mental disorder**

✓4th **V12 Personal history of certain other diseases**
AHA: 3Q, '92, 11

✓5th **V12.0 Infectious and parasitic diseases**

> **EXCLUDES** *personal history of infectious diseases specific to a body system*

**V12.00 Unspecified infectious and parasitic disease**
**V12.01 Tuberculosis**
**V12.02 Poliomyelitis**
**V12.03 Malaria**
**V12.09 Other**

**V12.1 Nutritional deficiency**

**V12.2 Endocrine, metabolic, and immunity disorders**

> **EXCLUDES** *history of allergy (V14.0-V14.9, V15.01-V15.09)*

**V12.3 Diseases of blood and blood-forming organs**

✓5th **V12.4 Disorders of nervous system and sense organs**

**V12.40 Unspecified disorder of nervous system and sense organs**

**V12.41 Benign neoplasm of the brain**
AHA: 4Q, '97, 48

**V12.42 Infections of the central nervous system**
Encephalitis    Meningitis
AHA: 4Q, '05, 95

**V12.49 Other disorders of nervous system and sense organs**
AHA: 4Q, '98, 59

✓5th **V12.5 Diseases of circulatory system**
AHA: 4Q, '95, 61

> **EXCLUDES** *old myocardial infarction (412) postmyocardial infarction syndrome (411.0)*

**V12.50 Unspecified circulatory disease**

| ✓4th ✓5th Additional Digit Required | Unacceptable PDx | Manifestation Code | ▶◀ Revised Text | ● New Code | ▲ Revised Code Title |

**V12.51 Venous thrombosis and embolism**
Pulmonary embolism
AHA: 3Q, '06, 12; 4Q, '03, 108; 1Q, '02, 15

**V12.52 Thrombophlebitis**

**V12.53 Sudden cardiac arrest**
Sudden cardiac death successfully resuscitated

**V12.54 Transient ischemic attack [TIA], and cerebral infarction without residual deficits**
Prolonged reversible ischemic neurological deficit [PRIND]
Reversible ischemic neurologic deficit [RIND]
Stroke NOS without residual deficits
**EXCLUDES** *late effects of cerebrovascular disease (438.0-438.9)*

**V12.59 Other**
AHA: ▶2Q, '07, 3;◀ 4Q, '99, 4; 4Q, '98, 88; 4Q, '97, 37

√5th **V12.6 Diseases of respiratory system**
**EXCLUDES** *tuberculosis (V12.01)*

**V12.60 Unspecified disease of respiratory system**

**V12.61 Pneumonia (recurrent)**
AHA: 4Q, '05, 95

**V12.69 Other diseases of respiratory system**

√5th **V12.7 Diseases of digestive system**
AHA: 1Q, '95, 3; 2Q, '89, 16

**V12.70 Unspecified digestive disease**

**V12.71 Peptic ulcer disease**

**V12.72 Colonic polyps**
AHA: 3Q, '02, 15

**V12.79 Other**

√4th **V13 Personal history of other diseases**

√5th **V13.0 Disorders of urinary system**

**V13.00 Unspecified urinary disorder**

**V13.01 Urinary calculi**

**V13.02 Urinary (tract) infection**
AHA: 4Q, '05, 95

**V13.03 Nephrotic syndrome**
AHA: 4Q, '05, 95

**V13.09 Other**

**V13.1 Trophoblastic disease** ♀
**EXCLUDES** *supervision during a current pregnancy (V23.1)*

√5th **V13.2 Other genital system and obstetric disorders**
**EXCLUDES** *supervision during a current pregnancy of a woman with poor obstetric history (V23.0-V23.9)*
*habitual aborter (646.3)*
*without current pregnancy ▶(629.81)◀*

**V13.21 Personal history of pre-term labor** ♀
**EXCLUDES** *current pregnancy with history of pre-term labor (V23.41)*
AHA: 4Q, '02, 78

**V13.22 Personal history of cervical dysplasia** ♀
Personal history of conditions classifiable to 622.10-622.12
**EXCLUDES** *personal history of malignant neoplasm of cervix uteri (V10.41)*

**V13.29 Other genital system and obstetric disorders** ♀

**V13.3 Diseases of skin and subcutaneous tissue**

**V13.4 Arthritis**

**V13.5 Other musculoskeletal disorders**

√5th **V13.6 Congenital malformations**
AHA: 4Q, '98, 63

**V13.61 Hypospadias** ♂

**V13.69 Other congenital malformations**
AHA: 1Q, '04, 16

**V13.7 Perinatal problems**
**EXCLUDES** *low birth weight status (V21.30-V21.35)*

**V13.8 Other specified diseases**

**V13.9 Unspecified disease**
AHA: 4Q, '06, 117

√4th **V14 Personal history of allergy to medicinal agents**

**V14.0 Penicillin**

**V14.1 Other antibiotic agent**

**V14.2 Sulfonamides**

**V14.3 Other anti-infective agent**

**V14.4 Anesthetic agent**

**V14.5 Narcotic agent**

**V14.6 Analgesic agent**

**V14.7 Serum or vaccine**

**V14.8 Other specified medicinal agents**

**V14.9 Unspecified medicinal agent**

√4th **V15 Other personal history presenting hazards to health**

√5th **V15.0 Allergy, other than to medicinal agents**
**EXCLUDES** *allergy to food substance used as base for medicinal agent (V14.0-V14.9)*
AHA: 4Q, '00, 42, 49

**V15.01 Allergy to peanuts**

**V15.02 Allergy to milk products**
**EXCLUDES** *lactose intolerance (271.3)*
AHA: 1Q, '03, 12

**V15.03 Allergy to eggs**

**V15.04 Allergy to seafood**
Seafood (octopus) (squid) ink
Shellfish

**V15.05 Allergy to other foods**
Food additives    Nuts other than peanuts

**V15.06 Allergy to insects**
Bugs
Insect bites and stings
Spiders

**V15.07 Allergy to latex**
Latex sensitivity

**V15.08 Allergy to radiographic dye**
Contrast media used for diagnostic x-ray procedures

**V15.09 Other allergy, other than to medicinal agents**

**V15.1 Surgery to heart and great vessels**
**EXCLUDES** *replacement by transplant or other means (V42.1-V42.2, V43.2-V43.4)*
AHA: 1Q, '04, 16

**V15.2 Surgery to other major organs**
**EXCLUDES** *replacement by transplant or other means (V42.0-V43.8)*

**V15.3 Irradiation**
Previous exposure to therapeutic or other ionizing radiation

√5th **V15.4 Psychological trauma**
**EXCLUDES** *history of condition classifiable to 290-316 (V11.0-V11.9)*

**V15.41 History of physical abuse**
Rape
AHA: 3Q, '99, 15

**V15.42 History of emotional abuse**
Neglect
AHA: 3Q, '99, 15

**V15.49 Other**
AHA: 3Q, '99, 15

**V15.5 Injury**

**V15.6 Poisoning**

**V15.7 Contraception**
**EXCLUDES** *current contraceptive management (V25.0-V25.4)*
*presence of intrauterine contraceptive device as incidental finding (V45.5)*

---

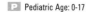 N Newborn Age: 0    P Pediatric Age: 0-17    M Maternity Age: 12-55    A Adult Age: 15-124    CC CC Condition    MCC Major CC Condition    HIV HIV Related Dx

 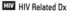

✓5ᵗʰ **V15.8** **Other specified personal history presenting hazards to health**
AHA: 4Q, '95, 62

**V15.81** **Noncompliance with medical treatment**
AHA: 4Q, '06, 136; 2Q, '03, 7; 2Q, '01, 11, 12, 13; 2Q, '99, 17; 2Q, '97, 11; 1Q, '97, 12; 3Q, '96, 9

**V15.82** **History of tobacco use**
EXCLUDES   *tobacco dependence (305.1)*

**V15.84** **Exposure to asbestos**

**V15.85** **Exposure to potentially hazardous body fluids**

**V15.86** **Exposure to lead**

**V15.87** **History of extracorporeal membrane oxygenation [ECMO]**
AHA: 4Q, '03, 84

**V15.88** **History of fall**
At risk for falling
AHA: 4Q, '05, 95

**V15.89** **Other**
AHA: 1Q, '90, 21; N-D, '84, 12

**V15.9** **Unspecified personal history presenting hazards to health**

✓4ᵗʰ **V16 Family history of malignant neoplasm**

**V16.0** **Gastrointestinal tract**
Family history of condition classifiable to 140-159
AHA: 1Q, '99, 4

**V16.1** **Trachea, bronchus, and lung**
Family history of condition classifiable to 162

**V16.2** **Other respiratory and intrathoracic organs**
Family history of condition classifiable to 160-161, 163-165

**V16.3** **Breast**
Family history of condition classifiable to 174
AHA: 4Q, '04, 107; 2Q, '03, 4; 2Q, '00, 8; 1Q, '92, 11

✓5ᵗʰ **V16.4** **Genital organs**
Family history of condition classifiable to 179-187
AHA: 4Q, '97, 48

**V16.40** **Genital organ, unspecified**

**V16.41** **Ovary**

**V16.42** **Prostate**

**V16.43** **Testis**

**V16.49** **Other**
AHA: 2Q, '06, 2

✓5ᵗʰ **V16.5** **Urinary organs**
Family history of condition classifiable to ▶188-189◀

**V16.51** **Kidney**

**V16.52** **Bladder**

**V16.59** **Other**

**V16.6** **Leukemia**
Family history of condition classifiable to 204-208

**V16.7** **Other lymphatic and hematopoietic neoplasms**
Family history of condition classifiable to 200-203

**V16.8** **Other specified malignant neoplasm**
Family history of other condition classifiable to 140-199

**V16.9** **Unspecified malignant neoplasm**

✓4ᵗʰ **V17 Family history of certain chronic disabling diseases**

**V17.0** **Psychiatric condition**
EXCLUDES   *family history of mental retardation (V18.4)*

**V17.1** **Stroke (cerebrovascular)**

**V17.2** **Other neurological diseases**
Epilepsy      Huntington's chorea

**V17.3** **Ischemic heart disease**

✓5ᵗʰ **V17.4** **Other cardiovascular diseases**
AHA: 1Q, '04, 6

**V17.41** **Family history of sudden cardiac death [SCD]**
EXCLUDES   *family history of ischemic heart disease (V17.3)*
*family history of myocardial infarction (V17.3)*

**V17.49** **Family history of other cardiovascular diseases**
Family history of cardiovascular disease NOS

**V17.5** **Asthma**

**V17.6** **Other chronic respiratory conditions**

**V17.7** **Arthritis**

✓5ᵗʰ **V17.8** **Other musculoskeletal diseases**

**V17.81** **Osteoporosis**
AHA: 4Q, '05, 95

**V17.89** **Other musculoskeletal diseases**

✓4ᵗʰ **V18 Family history of certain other specific conditions**

**V18.0** **Diabetes mellitus**
AHA: 1Q, '04, 8

✓5ᵗʰ **V18.1** **Other endocrine and metabolic diseases**

**V18.11** **Multiple endocrine neoplasia [MEN] syndrome**

**V18.19** **Other endocrine and metabolic diseases**

**V18.2** **Anemia**

**V18.3** **Other blood disorders**

**V18.4** **Mental retardation**

✓5ᵗʰ **V18.5** **Digestive disorders**

**V18.51** **Colonic polyps**
EXCLUDES   *family history of malignant neoplasm of gastro-intestinal tract (V16.0)*
AHA: 4Q, '06, 117

**V18.59** **Other digestive disorders**

✓5ᵗʰ **V18.6** **Kidney diseases**

**V18.61** **Polycystic kidney**

**V18.69** **Other kidney diseases**

**V18.7** **Other genitourinary diseases**

**V18.8** **Infectious and parasitic diseases**

**V18.9** **Genetic disease carrier**
AHA: 4Q, '05, 95

✓4ᵗʰ **V19 Family history of other conditions**

**V19.0** **Blindness or visual loss**

**V19.1** **Other eye disorders**

**V19.2** **Deafness or hearing loss**

**V19.3** **Other ear disorders**

**V19.4** **Skin conditions**

**V19.5** **Congenital anomalies**

**V19.6** **Allergic disorders**

**V19.7** **Consanguinity**

**V19.8** **Other condition**

## PERSONS ENCOUNTERING HEALTH SERVICES IN CIRCUMSTANCES RELATED TO REPRODUCTION AND DEVELOPMENT (V20-V29)

✓4ᵗʰ **V20 Health supervision of infant or child**

2 **V20.0** **Foundling**   P

**V20.1** **Other healthy infant or child receiving care**   P
Medical or nursing care supervision of healthy infant in cases of:
maternal illness, physical or psychiatric
socioeconomic adverse condition at home
too many children at home preventing or interfering with normal care
AHA: 1Q, '00, 25; 3Q, '89, 14

---

2   These V codes may be used as principal diagnosis on Medicare patients.

---

✓4ᵗʰ
✓5ᵗʰ   Additional Digit Required      Unacceptable PDx      Manifestation Code      ▶◀ Revised Text      ● New Code      ▲ Revised Code Title

**V Codes**

**V20.2–V25.3**

**V20.2** **Routine infant or child health check** [P]
Developmental testing of infant or child
Immunizations appropriate for age
Initial and subsequent routine newborn check
Routine vision and hearing testing
Use additional code(s) to identify:
special screening examination(s) performed
(V73.0-V82.9)
**EXCLUDES** *special screening for developmental handicaps (V79.3)*

**AHA:** 1Q, '04, 15

✓4ᵗʰ **V21 Constitutional states in development**

**V21.0** **Period of rapid growth in childhood**
**V21.1** **Puberty**
**V21.2** **Other adolescence**
✓5ᵗʰ **V21.3** **Low birth weight status**
**EXCLUDES** *history of perinatal problems*
**AHA:** 4Q, '00, 51

**V21.30** **Low birth weight status, unspecified**
**V21.31** **Low birth weight status, less than 500 grams**
**V21.32** **Low birth weight status, 500-999 grams**
**V21.33** **Low birth weight status, 1000-1499 grams**
**V21.34** **Low birth weight status, 1500-1999 grams**
**V21.35** **Low birth weight status, 2000-2500 grams**

**V21.8** **Other specified constitutional states in development**
**V21.9** **Unspecified constitutional state in development**

✓4ᵗʰ **V22 Normal pregnancy**
**EXCLUDES** *pregnancy examination or test, pregnancy unconfirmed (V72.40)*

**V22.0** **Supervision of normal first pregnancy** ♀
**AHA:** 3Q, '99, 16

**V22.1** **Supervision of other normal pregnancy** ♀
**AHA:** 3Q, '99, 16

**V22.2** **Pregnant state, incidental** ♀
Pregnant state NOS

✓4ᵗʰ **V23 Supervision of high-risk pregnancy**
**AHA:** 1Q, '90, 10

**V23.0** **Pregnancy with history of infertility** [M] ♀
**V23.1** **Pregnancy with history of trophoblastic disease** [M] ♀
Pregnancy with history of:
hydatidiform mole          vesicular mole
**EXCLUDES** *that without current pregnancy (V13.1)*

**V23.2** **Pregnancy with history of abortion** [M] ♀
Pregnancy with history of conditions classifiable to 634-638
**EXCLUDES** *habitual aborter:*
*care during pregnancy (646.3)*
*that without current pregnancy*
▶*(629.81)*◀

**V23.3** **Grand multiparity** [M] ♀
**EXCLUDES** *care in relation to labor and delivery (659.4)*
*that without current pregnancy (V61.5)*

✓5ᵗʰ **V23.4** **Pregnancy with other poor obstetric history**
Pregnancy with history of other conditions classifiable to 630-676

**V23.41** **Pregnancy with history of pre-term labor** [M] ♀
**AHA:** 4Q, '02, 79

**V23.49** **Pregnancy with other poor obstetric history** [M] ♀

**V23.5** **Pregnancy with other poor reproductive history** [M] ♀
Pregnancy with history of stillbirth or neonatal death

**V23.7** **Insufficient prenatal care** [M] ♀
History of little or no prenatal care

✓5ᵗʰ **V23.8** **Other high-risk pregnancy**
**AHA:** 4Q, '98, 56, 63

**V23.81** **Elderly primigravida** [M] ♀
First pregnancy in a woman who will be 35 years of age or older at expected date of delivery
**EXCLUDES** *elderly primigravida complicating pregnancy (659.5)*

**V23.82** **Elderly multigravida** [M] ♀
Second or more pregnancy in a woman who will be 35 years of age or older at expected date of delivery
**EXCLUDES** *elderly multigravida complicating pregnancy (659.6)*

**V23.83** **Young primigravida** [M] ♀
First pregnancy in a female less than 16 years old at expected date of delivery
**EXCLUDES** *young primigravida complicating pregnancy (659.8)*

**V23.84** **Young multigravida** [M] ♀
Second or more pregnancy in a female less than 16 years old at expected date of delivery
**EXCLUDES** *young multigravida complicating pregnancy (659.8)*

**V23.89** **Other high-risk pregnancy** [M] ♀
**AHA:** 3Q, '06, 14

**V23.9** **Unspecified high-risk pregnancy** [M] ♀

✓4ᵗʰ **V24 Postpartum care and examination**
² **V24.0** **Immediately after delivery** [M] ♀
Care and observation in uncomplicated cases
**AHA:** 3Q, '06, 11

**V24.1** **Lactating mother** ♀
Supervision of lactation

**V24.2** **Routine postpartum follow-up** ♀

✓4ᵗʰ **V25 Encounter for contraceptive management**
**AHA:** 4Q, '92, 24

✓5ᵗʰ **V25.0** **General counseling and advice**
**V25.01** **Prescription of oral contraceptives** ♀
**V25.02** **Initiation of other contraceptive measures**
Fitting of diaphragm
Prescription of foams, creams, or other agents
**AHA:** 3Q, '97, 7

**V25.03** **Encounter for emergency contraceptive counseling and prescription**
Encounter for postcoital contraceptive counseling and prescription
**AHA:** 4Q, '03, 84

**V25.04** **Counseling and instruction in natural family planning to avoid pregnancy**

**V25.09** **Other**
Family planning advice

**V25.1** **Insertion of intrauterine contraceptive device** ♀
² **V25.2** **Sterilization**
Admission for interruption of fallopian tubes or vas deferens

² **V25.3** **Menstrual extraction** ♀
Menstrual regulation

---

² These V codes may be used as principal diagnosis on Medicare patients.

[N] Newborn Age: 0    [P] Pediatric Age: 0-17    [M] Maternity Age: 12-55    [A] Adult Age: 15-124    [CC] CC Condition    [MCC] Major CC Condition    [HIV] HIV Related Dx

✓5th **V25.4** **Surveillance of previously prescribed contraceptive methods**
Checking, reinsertion, or removal of contraceptive device
Repeat prescription for contraceptive method
Routine examination in connection with contraceptive maintenance

**EXCLUDES** *presence of intrauterine contraceptive device as incidental finding (V45.5)*

**V25.40** **Contraceptive surveillance, unspecified**
**V25.41** **Contraceptive pill** ♀
**V25.42** **Intrauterine contraceptive device** ♀
Checking, reinsertion, or removal of intrauterine device
**V25.43** **Implantable subdermal contraceptive** ♀
**V25.49** **Other contraceptive method**
AHA: 3Q, '97, 7

**V25.5** **Insertion of implantable subdermal contraceptive** ♀
AHA: 3Q, '92, 9

**V25.8** **Other specified contraceptive management**
Postvasectomy sperm count

**EXCLUDES** *sperm count following sterilization reversal (V26.22)*
*sperm count for fertility testing (V26.21)*

AHA: 3Q, '96, 9

**V25.9** **Unspecified contraceptive management**

✓4th **V26** **Procreative management**
2 **V26.0** **Tuboplasty or vasoplasty after previous sterilization**
AHA: 2Q, '95, 10

**V26.1** **Artificial insemination** ♀

✓5th **V26.2** **Investigation and testing**
**EXCLUDES** *postvasectomy sperm count (V25.8)*
AHA: 4Q, '00, 56

**V26.21** **Fertility testing**
Fallopian insufflation
Sperm count for fertility testing
**EXCLUDES** *genetic counseling and testing (V26.31-V26.39)*

**V26.22** **Aftercare following sterilization reversal**
Fallopian insufflation following sterilization reversal
Sperm count following sterilization reversal

**V26.29** **Other investigation and testing**
AHA: 2Q, '96, 9; N-D, '85, 15

✓5th **V26.3** **Genetic counseling and testing**
**EXCLUDES** *fertility testing (V26.21)*
*nonprocreative genetic screening (V82.71, V82.79)*

AHA: 4Q, '05, 96

**V26.31** **Testing of female for genetic disease carrier status** ♀
AHA: 4Q, '06, 117

**V26.32** **Other genetic testing of female** ♀
Use additional code to identify habitual aborter (629.81, 646.3)
AHA: 4Q, '06, 117

**V26.33** **Genetic counseling**
**V26.34** **Testing of male for genetic disease carrier status** ♂
AHA: 4Q, '06, 117

**V26.35** **Encounter for testing of male partner of habitual aborter** ♂
AHA: 4Q, '06, 117

**V26.39** **Other genetic testing of male** ♂
AHA: 4Q, '06, 117

✓5th **V26.4** **General counseling and advice**
● **V26.41** **Procreative counseling and advice using natural family planning**
● **V26.49** **Other procreative management, counseling and advice**

✓5th **V26.5** **Sterilization status**
**V26.51** **Tubal ligation status** ♀
**EXCLUDES** *infertility not due to previous tubal ligation (628.0-628.9)*

**V26.52** **Vasectomy status** ♂

✓5th **V26.8** **Other specified procreative management**
**V26.81** **Encounter for assisted reproductive fertility procedure cycle**
Patient undergoing in vitro fertilization cycle
Use additional code to identify the type of infertility
**EXCLUDES** *pre-cycle diagnosis and testing—code to reason for encounter*

● **V26.89** **Other specified procreative management**
**V26.9** **Unspecified procreative management**

✓4th **V27** **Outcome of delivery**
Note: This category is intended for the coding of the outcome of delivery on the mother's record.
AHA: 2Q, '91, 16

**V27.0** **Single liveborn** Ⓜ♀
AHA: 4Q, '05, 81; 2Q, '03, 9; 2Q, '02, 10; 1Q, '01, 10; 3Q, '00, 5; 4Q, '98, 77; 4Q, '95, 59; 1Q, '92, 9

**V27.1** **Single stillborn** Ⓜ♀
**V27.2** **Twins, both liveborn** Ⓜ♀
**V27.3** **Twins, one liveborn and one stillborn** Ⓜ♀
**V27.4** **Twins, both stillborn** Ⓜ♀
**V27.5** **Other multiple birth, all liveborn** Ⓜ♀
**V27.6** **Other multiple birth, some liveborn** Ⓜ♀
**V27.7** **Other multiple birth, all stillborn** Ⓜ♀
**V27.9** **Unspecified outcome of delivery** Ⓜ♀

Single birth ⎫
Multiple birth ⎬ outcome to infant unspecified

✓4th **V28** **Encounter for antenatal screening of mother**
**EXCLUDES** *abnormal findings on screening — code to findings*
*routine prenatal care (V22.0-V23.9)*

AHA: 4Q, '06, 117; 1Q, '04, 11

**V28.0** **Screening for chromosomal anomalies by amniocentesis** Ⓜ♀
**V28.1** **Screening for raised alpha-fetoprotein levels in amniotic fluid** Ⓜ♀
**V28.2** **Other screening based on amniocentesis** Ⓜ♀
**V28.3** **Screening for malformation using ultrasonics** ♀
**V28.4** **Screening for fetal growth retardation using ultrasonics** ♀
**V28.5** **Screening for isoimmunization** ♀
**V28.6** **Screening for Streptococcus B** Ⓜ♀
AHA: 4Q, '97, 46

**V28.8** **Other specified antenatal screening** ♀
AHA: 3Q, '99, 16

**V28.9** **Unspecified antenatal screening** ♀

2 These V codes may be used as principal diagnosis on Medicare patients.

✓4ᵗʰ **V29 Observation and evaluation of newborns and infants for suspected condition not found**

Note: This category is to be used for newborns, within the neonatal period, (the first 28 days of life) who are suspected of having an abnormal condition resulting from exposure from the mother or the birth process, but without signs or symptoms, and, which after examination and observation, is found not to exist.

AHA: 1Q, '00, 25; 4Q, '94, 47; 1Q, '94, 9; 4Q, '92, 21

² **V29.0 Observation for suspected infectious condition** N
AHA: 1Q, '01, 10

² **V29.1 Observation for suspected neurological condition** N

² **V29.2 Observation for suspected respiratory condition** N

**V29.3 Observation for suspected genetic or metabolic condition** N
AHA: 2Q, '05, 21; 4Q, '98, 59, 68

² **V29.8 Observation for other specified suspected condition** N
AHA: 2Q, '03, 15

**V29.9 Observation for unspecified suspected condition** N
AHA: 1Q, '02, 6

## LIVEBORN INFANTS ACCORDING TO TYPE OF BIRTH (V30-V39)

Note: These categories are intended for the coding of liveborn infants who are consuming health care [e.g., crib or bassinet occupancy].

The following fourth-digit subdivisions are for use with categories V30-V39:

✓5ᵗʰ **0 Born in hospital** N
**1 Born before admission to hospital** N
**2 Born outside hospital and not hospitalized**

The following two fifth-digits are for use with the fourth-digit .0, Born in hospital:

**0 delivered without mention of cesarean delivery**
**1 delivered by cesarean delivery**

AHA: 1Q, '01, 10

³ ✓4ᵗʰ **V30 Single liveborn**
AHA: 2Q, '03, 9; 4Q, '98, 46, 59; 1Q, '94, 9; For code V30.00: 1Q, '04, 8, 16; 4Q, '03, 68; For code V30.01: 4Q, '05, 88; For code V30.10: 3Q, '06, 10

³ ✓4ᵗʰ **V31 Twin, mate liveborn**
AHA: 3Q, '92, 10

³ ✓4ᵗʰ **V32 Twin, mate stillborn**

³ ✓4ᵗʰ **V33 Twin, unspecified**

³ ✓4ᵗʰ **V34 Other multiple, mates all liveborn**

³ ✓4ᵗʰ **V35 Other multiple, mates all stillborn**

³ ✓4ᵗʰ **V36 Other multiple, mates live and stillborn**

³ ✓4ᵗʰ **V37 Other multiple, unspecified**

⁴ ✓4ᵗʰ **V39 Unspecified**

## PERSONS WITH A CONDITION INFLUENCING THEIR HEALTH STATUS (V40-V49)

Note: These categories are intended for use when these conditions are recorded as "diagnoses" or "problems."

✓4ᵗʰ **V40 Mental and behavioral problems**
**V40.0 Problems with learning**
**V40.1 Problems with communication [including speech]**
**V40.2 Other mental problems**
**V40.3 Other behavioral problems**
**V40.9 Unspecified mental or behavioral problem**

✓4ᵗʰ **V41 Problems with special senses and other special functions**
**V41.0 Problems with sight**
**V41.1 Other eye problems**
**V41.2 Problems with hearing**
**V41.3 Other ear problems**
**V41.4 Problems with voice production**
**V41.5 Problems with smell and taste**
**V41.6 Problems with swallowing and mastication**

**V41.7 Problems with sexual function**
EXCLUDES   *marital problems (V61.10)*
*psychosexual disorders (302.0-302.9)*

**V41.8 Other problems with special functions**

**V41.9 Unspecified problem with special functions**

✓4ᵗʰ **V42 Organ or tissue replaced by transplant**
INCLUDES   homologous or heterologous (animal) (human) transplant organ status

AHA: 3Q, '98, 3, 4

**V42.0 Kidney** CC
CC Excl: 996.80-996.81, 996.87, V42.0, V42.89-V42.9
AHA: 1Q, '03, 10; 3Q, '01, 12

**V42.1 Heart** CC
CC Excl: 996.80, 996.83, 996.87, V42.1, V42.89-V42.9
AHA: 3Q, '03, 16; 3Q, '01, 13

**V42.2 Heart valve**

**V42.3 Skin**

**V42.4 Bone**

**V42.5 Cornea**

**V42.6 Lung** CC
CC Excl: 996.80, 996.84, 996.87, V42.6, V42.89-V42.9

**V42.7 Liver** CC
CC Excl: 996.80, 996.82, 996.87, V42.7, V42.89-V42.9

✓5ᵗʰ **V42.8 Other specified organ or tissue**
AHA: 4Q, '98, 64; 4Q, '97, 49

**V42.81 Bone marrow** CC
CC Excl: 996.80, 996.85, 996.87, V42.9

**V42.82 Peripheral stem cells** CC
CC Excl: 996.80, 996.87, V42.9

**V42.83 Pancreas** CC
CC Excl: 996.80, 996.86-996.87, V42.83, V42.9
AHA: 1Q, '03, 10; 2Q, '01, 16

**V42.84 Intestines** CC
CC Excl: 996.80, 996.89, V42.84-V42.9
AHA: 4Q, '00, 48, 50

**V42.89 Other**

**V42.9 Unspecified organ or tissue**

✓4ᵗʰ **V43 Organ or tissue replaced by other means**
INCLUDES   organ or tissue assisted by other means
replacement of organ by:
   artificial device
   mechanical device
   prosthesis
EXCLUDES   *cardiac pacemaker in situ (V45.01)*
*fitting and adjustment of prosthetic device (V52.0-V52.9)*
*renal dialysis status (V45.1)*

**V43.0 Eye globe**

**V43.1 Lens**
Pseudophakos
AHA: 4Q, '98, 65

✓5ᵗʰ **V43.2 Heart**
AHA: 4Q, '03, 85

**V43.21 Heart assist device** CC
CC Excl: 996.80, 996.83, 996.87, V42.1, V43.21-V43.22

**V43.22 Fully implantable artificial heart** CC
CC Excl: See code: V43.21

**V43.3 Heart valve**
AHA: 3Q, '06, 7; 3Q, '02, 13, 14

**V43.4 Blood vessel**

**V43.5 Bladder**

✓5ᵗʰ **V43.6 Joint**
AHA: 4Q, '05, 91

---

² These V codes may be used as principal diagnosis on Medicare patients.
     codes with the fourth digit of 0 or 1 may be used as a principal diagnosis for Medicare patients.
     codes with fourth digit of 0 may be used as a principal diagnosis for Medicare patients.

orn Age: 0    P Pediatric Age: 0-17    M Maternity Age: 12-55    A Adult Age: 15-124    CC CC Condition    MC Major Complication    CD Complex Dx    HIV HIV Related Dx

Volume 1 • October 2007                                        ©2007 Ingenix

**V43.60 Unspecified joint**
**V43.61 Shoulder**
**V43.62 Elbow**
**V43.63 Wrist**
**V43.64 Hip**
    AHA: 3Q, '06, 4, 5; 4Q, '05, 93, 112; 2Q, '04, 15

**V43.65 Knee**
    AHA: 3Q, '06, 5

**V43.66 Ankle**
**V43.69 Other**
**V43.7 Limb**
√5th **V43.8 Other organ or tissue**
**V43.81 Larynx**
    AHA: 4Q, '95, 55

**V43.82 Breast**
    AHA: 4Q, '95, 55

**V43.83 Artificial skin**
**V43.89 Other**

√4th **V44 Artificial opening status**
> *EXCLUDES*   artificial openings requiring attention or management (V55.0-V55.9)

**V44.0 Tracheostomy**
    AHA: 4Q, '03, 103, 107, 111; 1Q, '01, 6

**V44.1 Gastrostomy**
    AHA: 4Q, '03, 103, 107-108, 110; 1Q, '01, 12; 3Q, '97, 12; 1Q, '93, 26

**V44.2 Ileostomy**
**V44.3 Colostomy**
    AHA: 4Q, '03, 110

**V44.4 Other artificial opening of gastrointestinal tract**
√5th **V44.5 Cystostomy**
**V44.50 Cystostomy, unspecified**
**V44.51 Cutaneous-vesicostomy**
**V44.52 Appendico-vesicostomy**
**V44.59 Other cystostomy**

**V44.6 Other artificial opening of urinary tract**
    Nephrostomy      Urethrostomy
    Ureterostomy

**V44.7 Artificial vagina**
**V44.8 Other artificial opening status**
**V44.9 Unspecified artificial opening status**

√4th **V45 Other postprocedural states**
> *EXCLUDES*   aftercare management (V51-V58.9)
> malfunction or other complication — code to condition

    AHA: 4Q, '03, 85

√5th **V45.0 Cardiac device in situ**
> *EXCLUDES*   artificial heart (V43.22)
> heart assist device (V43.21)

**V45.00 Unspecified cardiac device**
**V45.01 Cardiac pacemaker**
**V45.02 Automatic implantable cardiac defibrillator**
**V45.09 Other specified cardiac device**
    Carotid sinus pacemaker in situ

**V45.1 Renal dialysis status**
    Hemodialysis status
    Patient requiring intermittent renal dialysis
    Peritoneal dialysis status
    Presence of arterial-venous shunt (for dialysis)
> *EXCLUDES*   admission for dialysis treatment or session (V56.0)

    AHA: 4Q, '06, 136; 4Q, '05, 96; 2Q, '03, 7; 2Q, '01, 12, 13

**V45.2 Presence of cerebrospinal fluid drainage device**
    Cerebral ventricle (communicating) shunt, valve, or device in situ
> *EXCLUDES*   malfunction (996.2)

    AHA: 4Q, '03, 106

**V45.3 Intestinal bypass or anastomosis status**
> *EXCLUDES*   bariatric surgery status (V45.86)
> gastric bypass status (V45.86)
> obesity surgery status (V45.86)

**V45.4 Arthrodesis status**
    AHA: N-D, '84, 18

√5th **V45.5 Presence of contraceptive device**
> *EXCLUDES*   checking, reinsertion, or removal of device (V25.42)
> complication from device (996.32)
> insertion of device (V25.1)

**V45.51 Intrauterine contraceptive device**   ♀
**V45.52 Subdermal contraceptive implant**
**V45.59 Other**

√5th **V45.6 States following surgery of eye and adnexa**
    Cataract extraction     ⎫
    Filtering bleb     ⎬ state following eye surgery
    Surgical eyelid adhesion ⎭
> *EXCLUDES*   aphakia (379.31)
> artificial eye globe (V43.0)

    AHA: 4Q, '98, 65; 4Q, '97, 49

**V45.61 Cataract extraction status**
    Use additional code for associated artificial lens status (V43.1)

**V45.69 Other states following surgery of eye and adnexa**
    AHA: 2Q, '01, 16; 1Q, '98, 10; 4Q, '97, 19

√5th **V45.7 Acquired absence of organ**
    AHA: 4Q, '98, 65; 4Q, '97, 50

2 **V45.71 Acquired absence of breast**
    AHA: 4Q, '01, 66; 4Q, '97, 50

**V45.72 Acquired absence of intestine (large) (small)**
**V45.73 Acquired absence of kidney**
**V45.74 Other parts of urinary tract**
    Bladder
    AHA: 4Q, '00, 51

**V45.75 Stomach**
    AHA: 4Q, '00, 51

**V45.76 Lung**
    AHA: 4Q, '00, 51

**V45.77 Genital organs**
> *EXCLUDES*   female genital mutilation status (629.20-629.29)

    AHA: 1Q, '03, 13, 14; 4Q, '00, 51

**V45.78 Eye**
    AHA: 4Q, '00, 51

**V45.79 Other acquired absence of organ**
    AHA: 4Q, '00, 51

√5th **V45.8 Other postprocedural status**
**V45.81 Aortocoronary bypass status**
    AHA: 4Q, '03, 105; 3Q, '01, 15; 3Q, '97, 16

**V45.82 Percutaneous transluminal coronary angioplasty status**
**V45.83 Breast implant removal status**
    AHA: 4Q, '95, 55

**V45.84 Dental restoration status**
    Dental crowns status
    Dental fillings status
    AHA: 4Q, '01, 54

**V45.85 Insulin pump status**
**V45.86 Bariatric surgery status**
    Gastric banding status
    Gastric bypass status for obesity
    Obesity surgery status
> *EXCLUDES*   bariatric surgery status complicating pregnancy, childbirth or the puerperium (649.2)
> intestinal bypass or anastomosis status (V45.3)

    AHA: 4Q, '06, 118

---

2   These V codes may be used as principal diagnosis on Medicare patients.

√4th
√5th Additional Digit Required      Unacceptable PDx      Manifestation Code      ◄► Revised Text      ● New Code      ▲ Revised Code Title

**V Codes**

**V45.89–V50.0**

**V45.89 Other**
Presence of neuropacemaker or other electronic device

> **EXCLUDES** artificial heart valve in situ (V43.3)
> vascular prosthesis in situ (V43.4)

AHA: 1Q, '95, 11

√4ᵗʰ **V46 Other dependence on machines**

**V46.0 Aspirator**

√5ᵗʰ **V46.1 Respirator [Ventilator]**
Iron lung
AHA: 4Q, '05, 96; 4Q, '03, 103; 1Q, '01, 12; J-F, '87, 7 3

² **V46.11 Dependence on respirator, status** `CC`
CC Excl: V46.0-V46.9
AHA: 4Q, '04, 100

² **V46.12 Encounter for respirator dependence during power failure** `CC`
CC Excl: See code V46.11
AHA: 4Q, '04, 100

² **V46.13 Encounter for weaning from respirator [ventilator]** `CC`
CC Excl: See code V46.11

² **V46.14 Mechanical complication of respirator [ventilator]** `CC`
Mechanical failure of respirator [ventilator]
CC Excl: See code V46.11

**V46.2 Supplemental oxygen**
Long-term oxygen therapy
AHA: 4Q, '03, 108; 4Q, '02, 79

**V46.8 Other enabling machines**
Hyperbaric chamber
Possum [Patient-Operated-Selector-Mechanism]

> **EXCLUDES** cardiac pacemaker (V45.0)
> kidney dialysis machine (V45.1)

**V46.9 Unspecified machine dependence**
AHA: 4Q, '06, 117

√4ᵗʰ **V47 Other problems with internal organs**

**V47.0 Deficiencies of internal organs**

**V47.1 Mechanical and motor problems with internal organs**

**V47.2 Other cardiorespiratory problems**
Cardiovascular exercise intolerance with pain (with):
at rest
less than ordinary activity
ordinary activity

**V47.3 Other digestive problems**

**V47.4 Other urinary problems**

**V47.5 Other genital problems**

**V47.9 Unspecified**

√4ᵗʰ **V48 Problems with head, neck, and trunk**

**V48.0 Deficiencies of head**

> **EXCLUDES** deficiencies of ears, eyelids, and nose (V48.8)

**V48.1 Deficiencies of neck and trunk**

**V48.2 Mechanical and motor problems with head**

**V48.3 Mechanical and motor problems with neck and trunk**

**V48.4 Sensory problem with head**

**V48.5 Sensory problem with neck and trunk**

**V48.6 Disfigurements of head**

**V48.7 Disfigurements of neck and trunk**

**V48.8 Other problems with head, neck, and trunk**

**V48.9 Unspecified problem with head, neck, or trunk**

√4ᵗʰ **V49 Other conditions influencing health status**

**V49.0 Deficiencies of limbs**

**V49.1 Mechanical problems with limbs**

**V49.2 Motor problems with limbs**

**V49.3 Sensory problems with limbs**

**V49.4 Disfigurements of limbs**

**V49.5 Other problems of limbs**

√5ᵗʰ **V49.6 Upper limb amputation status**
AHA: 4Q, '05, 94; 4Q, '98, 42; 4Q, '94, 39

**V49.60 Unspecified level**

**V49.61 Thumb**

**V49.62 Other finger(s)**
AHA: 2Q, '05, 7

**V49.63 Hand**

**V49.64 Wrist**
Disarticulation of wrist

**V49.65 Below elbow**

**V49.66 Above elbow**
Disarticulation of elbow

**V49.67 Shoulder**
Disarticulation of shoulder

√5ᵗʰ **V49.7 Lower limb amputation status**
AHA: 3Q, '06, 5; 4Q, '05, 94; 4Q, '98, 42; 4Q, '94, 39

**V49.70 Unspecified level**

**V49.71 Great toe**

**V49.72 Other toe(s)**

**V49.73 Foot**

**V49.74 Ankle**
Disarticulation of ankle

**V49.75 Below knee**

**V49.76 Above knee**
Disarticulation of knee
AHA: 2Q, '05, 14

**V49.77 Hip**
Disarticulation of hip

√5ᵗʰ **V49.8 Other specified conditions influencing health status**
AHA: 4Q, '00, 51

**V49.81 Asymptomatic postmenopausal status (age-related) (natural)** `A` ♀

> **EXCLUDES** menopausal and premenopausal disorder (627.0-627.9)
> postsurgical menopause (256.2)
> premature menopause (256.31)
> symptomatic menopause (627.0-627.9)

AHA: 4Q, '02, 79; 4Q, '00, 54

**V49.82 Dental sealant status**
AHA: 4Q, '01, 54

**V49.83 Awaiting organ transplant status**

**V49.84 Bed confinement status**
AHA: 4Q, '05, 96

**V49.85 Dual sensory impairment**
Blindness with deafness
Combined visual hearing impairment
Code first:
hearing impairment (389.00-389.9)
visual impairment (369.00-369.9)

**V49.89 Other specified conditions influencing health status**
AHA: 4Q, '05, 94

**V49.9 Unspecified**

## PERSONS ENCOUNTERING HEALTH SERVICES FOR SPECIFIC PROCEDURES AND AFTERCARE (V50-V59)

Note: Categories V51-V58 are intended for use to indicate a reason for care in patients who may have already been treated for some disease or injury not now present, or who are receiving care to consolidate the treatment, to deal with residual states, or to prevent recurrence.

> **EXCLUDES** follow-up examination for medical surveillance following treatment (V67.0-V67.9)

√4ᵗʰ **V50 Elective surgery for purposes other than remedying health states**

² **V50.0 Hair transplant**

V codes may be used as principal diagnosis on Medicare patients.

| n Age: 0 | `P` Pediatric Age: 0-17 | `M` Maternity Age: 12-55 | `A` Adult Age: 15-124 | `CC` CC Condition | `MCC` Major CC Condition | `HIV` HIV Related Dx |

2  **V50.1  Other plastic surgery for unacceptable cosmetic appearance**
  Breast augmentation or reduction
  Face-lift
  > EXCLUDES *plastic surgery following healed injury or operation (V51)*

2  **V50.2  Routine or ritual circumcision** ♂
  Circumcision in the absence of significant medical indication

**V50.3  Ear piercing**

✓5ᵗʰ  **V50.4  Prophylactic organ removal**
  > EXCLUDES *organ donations (V59.0-V59.9)*
  > *therapeutic organ removal — code to condition*
  **AHA:** 4Q, '94, 44

2  **V50.41  Breast**
  **AHA:** 4Q, '04, 107

2  **V50.42  Ovary** ♀
2  **V50.49  Other**

**V50.8  Other**

**V50.9  Unspecified**

2  **V51  Aftercare involving the use of plastic surgery**
  Plastic surgery following healed injury or operation
  > EXCLUDES *cosmetic plastic surgery (V50.2)*
  > *plastic surgery as treatment for current injury — code to condition*
  > *repair of scarred tissue — code to scar*

✓4ᵗʰ  **V52  Fitting and adjustment of prosthetic device and implant**
  > INCLUDES removal of device
  > EXCLUDES *malfunction or complication of prosthetic device (996.0-996.7)*
  > *status only, without need for care (V43.0-V43.8)*
  **AHA:** 4Q, '05, 94; 4Q, '95, 55 ; 1Q, '90, 7

2  **V52.0  Artificial arm (complete) (partial)**
2  **V52.1  Artificial leg (complete) (partial)**
2  **V52.2  Artificial eye**
2  **V52.3  Dental prosthetic device**
2  **V52.4  Breast prosthesis and implant** ♀
  > EXCLUDES *admission for implant insertion (V50.1)*
  **AHA:** 4Q, '95, 80, 81

2  **V52.8  Other specified prosthetic device**
  **AHA:** 2Q, '02, 12, 16

**V52.9  Unspecified prosthetic device**

✓4ᵗʰ  **V53  Fitting and adjustment of other device**
  > INCLUDES removal of device
  > replacement of device
  > EXCLUDES *status only, without need for care (V45.0-V45.8)*

✓5ᵗʰ  **V53.0  Devices related to nervous system and special senses**
  **AHA:** 4Q, '98, 66; 4Q, '97, 51

2  **V53.01  Fitting and adjustment of cerebral ventricular (communicating) shunt**
  **AHA:** 4Q, '97, 51

2  **V53.02  Neuropacemaker (brain) (peripheral nerve) (spinal cord)**

2  **V53.09  Fitting and adjustment of other devices related to nervous system and special senses**
  Auditory substitution device
  Visual substitution device
  **AHA:** 2Q, '99, 4

**V53.1  Spectacles and contact lenses**

**V53.2  Hearing aid**

✓5ᵗʰ  **V53.3  Cardiac device**
  Reprogramming
  **AHA:** 3Q, '92, 3; 1Q, '90, 7; M-J, '87, 8 ; N-D, '84, 18

**V53.31  Cardiac pacemaker**
  > EXCLUDES *mechanical complication of cardiac pacemaker (996.01)*
  **AHA:** 1Q, '02, 3

**V53.32  Automatic implantable cardiac defibrillator**
  **AHA:** 3Q, '05, 8

**V53.39  Other cardiac device**
  **AHA:** ▶1Q, '07, 20◀

**V53.4  Orthodontic devices**

**V53.5  Other intestinal appliance**
  > EXCLUDES *colostomy (V55.3)*
  > *ileostomy (V55.2)*
  > *other artificial opening of digestive tract (V55.4)*

**V53.6  Urinary devices**
  Urinary catheter
  > EXCLUDES *cystostomy (V55.5)*
  > *nephrostomy (V55.6)*
  > *ureterostomy (V55.6)*
  > *urethrostomy (V55.6)*

**V53.7  Orthopedic devices**
  Orthopedic:     Orthopedic:
     brace          corset
     cast           shoes
  > EXCLUDES *other orthopedic aftercare (V54)*

**V53.8  Wheelchair**

✓5ᵗʰ  **V53.9  Other and unspecified device**
  **AHA:** 2Q, '03, 6

**V53.90  Unspecified device**

**V53.91  Fitting and adjustment of insulin pump**
  Insulin pump titration

**V53.99  Other device**

✓4ᵗʰ  **V54  Other orthopedic aftercare**
  > EXCLUDES *fitting and adjustment of orthopedic devices (V53.7)*
  > *malfunction of internal orthopedic device (996.40-996.49)*
  > *other complication of nonmechanical nature (996.60-996.79)*
  **AHA:** ▶1Q, '07, 3-4;◀ 3Q, '95, 3

✓5ᵗʰ  **V54.0  Aftercare involving internal fixation device**
  > EXCLUDES *malfunction of internal orthopedic device (996.40-996.49)*
  > *other complication of nonmechanical nature (996.60-996.79)*
  > *removal of external fixation device (V54.89 )*
  **AHA:** 4Q, '03, 87

2  **V54.01  Encounter for removal of internal fixation device**

2  **V54.02  Encounter for lengthening/adjustment of growth rod**

2  **V54.09  Other aftercare involving internal fixation device**

✓5ᵗʰ  **V54.1  Aftercare for healing traumatic fracture**
  > EXCLUDES *aftercare for amputation stump (V54.89)*
  **AHA:** 4Q, '02, 80

2  **V54.10  Aftercare for healing traumatic fracture of arm, unspecified**

2  **V54.11  Aftercare for healing traumatic fracture of upper arm**

2  **V54.12  Aftercare for healing traumatic fracture of lower arm**
  **AHA:** ▶1Q, '07, 7◀

2  **V54.13  Aftercare for healing traumatic fracture of hip**
  **AHA:** 4Q, '03, 103, 105; 2Q, '03, 16

2  **V54.14  Aftercare for healing traumatic fracture of leg, unspecified**

2  **V54.15  Aftercare for healing traumatic fracture of upper leg**
  > EXCLUDES *aftercare for healing traumatic fracture of hip (V54.13)*
  **AHA:** 3Q, '06, 6

---

2  These V codes may be used as principal diagnosis on Medicare patients.

**V Codes**

**V54.16–V58.0**

² V54.16 **Aftercare for healing traumatic fracture of lower leg**

² V54.17 **Aftercare for healing traumatic fracture of vertebrae**

² V54.19 **Aftercare for healing traumatic fracture of other bone**
AHA: 1Q, '05, 13; 4Q, '02, 80

√5th V54.2 **Aftercare for healing pathologic fracture**
AHA: 4Q, '02, 80

² V54.20 **Aftercare for healing pathologic fracture of arm, unspecified**

² V54.21 **Aftercare for healing pathologic fracture of upper arm**

² V54.22 **Aftercare for healing pathologic fracture of lower arm**

² V54.23 **Aftercare for healing pathologic fracture of hip**

² V54.24 **Aftercare for healing pathologic fracture of leg, unspecified**

² V54.25 **Aftercare for healing pathologic fracture of upper leg**
EXCLUDES  *aftercare for healing pathologic fracture of hip (V54.23)*

² V54.26 **Aftercare for healing pathologic fracture of lower leg**

² V54.27 **Aftercare for healing pathologic fracture of vertebrae**
AHA: ▶1Q, '07, 6;◀ 4Q, '03, 108

² V54.29 **Aftercare for healing pathologic fracture of other bone**
AHA: 4Q, '02, 80

√5th V54.8 **Other orthopedic aftercare**
AHA: 3Q, '01, 19; 4Q, '99, 5

² V54.81 **Aftercare following joint replacement**
Use additional code to identify joint replacement site (V43.60-V43.69)
AHA: 3Q, '06, 4; 2Q, '04, 15; 4Q, '02, 80

² V54.89 **Other orthopedic aftercare**
Aftercare for healing fracture NOS

V54.9 **Unspecified orthopedic aftercare**

√4th V55 **Attention to artificial openings**
INCLUDES  adjustment or repositioning of catheter
closure
passage of sounds or bougies
reforming
removal or replacement of catheter
toilet or cleansing
EXCLUDES  *complications of external stoma (519.00-519.09, 569.60-569.69, 997.4, 997.5)*
*status only, without need for care (V44.0-V44.9)*

² V55.0 **Tracheostomy**

² V55.1 **Gastrostomy**                                    CC
CC Excl: V55.1
AHA: 4Q, '99, 9; 3Q, '97, 7, 8; 1Q, '96, 14; 3Q, '95, 13

² V55.2 **Ileostomy**

² V55.3 **Colostomy**
AHA: 2Q, '05, 4; 3Q, '97, 9

² V55.4 **Other artificial opening of digestive tract**
AHA: 2Q, '05, 14; 1Q, '03, 10

² V55.5 **Cystostomy**

² V55.6 **Other artificial opening of urinary tract**
Nephrostomy          Urethrostomy
Ureterostomy

² V55.7 **Artificial vagina**

² V55.8 **Other specified artificial opening**

V55.9 **Unspecified artificial opening**

√4th V56 **Encounter for dialysis and dialysis catheter care**
Use additional code to identify the associated condition
EXCLUDES  *dialysis preparation — code to condition*
AHA: 4Q, '98, 66; 1Q, '93, 29

² V56.0 **Extracorporeal dialysis**
Dialysis (renal) NOS
EXCLUDES  *dialysis status (V45.1)*
AHA: 4Q, '05, 79; 1Q, '04, 23; 4Q, '00, 40; 3Q, '98, 6; 2Q, '98, 20

V56.1 **Fitting and adjustment of extracorporeal dialysis catheter**
Removal or replacement of catheter
Toilet or cleansing
Use additional code for any concurrent extracorporeal dialysis (V56.0)
AHA: 2Q, '98, 20

V56.2 **Fitting and adjustment of peritoneal dialysis catheter**
Use additional code for any concurrent peritoneal dialysis (V56.8)
AHA: 4Q, '98, 55

√5th V56.3 **Encounter for adequacy testing for dialysis**
AHA: 4Q, '00, 55

V56.31 **Encounter for adequacy testing for hemodialysis**

V56.32 **Encounter for adequacy testing for peritoneal dialysis**
Peritoneal equilibration test

² V56.8 **Other dialysis**
Peritoneal dialysis
AHA: 4Q, '98, 55

√4th V57 **Care involving use of rehabilitation procedures**
Use additional code to identify underlying condition
AHA: 3Q, '06, 3; 1Q, '02, 19; 3Q, '97, 12; 1Q, '90, 6; S-O, '86, 3

V57.0 **Breathing exercises**

⁵ V57.1 **Other physical therapy**
Therapeutic and remedial exercises, except breathing
AHA: 3Q, '06, 4; 2Q, '04, 15; 4Q, '02, 56; 4Q, '99, 5

√5th V57.2 **Occupational therapy and vocational rehabilitation**

⁵ V57.21 **Encounter for occupational therapy**
AHA: 4Q, '99, 7

⁵ V57.22 **Encounter for vocational therapy**

⁵ V57.3 **Speech therapy**
AHA: 4Q, '97, 36

V57.4 **Orthoptic training**

√5th V57.8 **Other specified rehabilitation procedure**

V57.81 **Orthotic training**
Gait training in the use of artificial limbs

⁵ V57.89 **Other**
Multiple training or therapy
AHA: 3Q, '06, 6; 4Q, '03, 105-106, 108; 2Q, '03, 16; 1Q '02, 16; 3Q, '01, 21; 3Q, '97, 11, 12; S-O, '86, 4

⁵ V57.9 **Unspecified rehabilitation procedure**

√4th V58 **Encounter for other and unspecified procedures and aftercare**
EXCLUDES  *convalescence and palliative care (V66)*

² V58.0 **Radiotherapy**
Encounter or admission for radiotherapy
EXCLUDES  *encounter for radioactive implant — code to condition*
*radioactive iodine therapy — code to condition*
AHA: 3Q, '92, 5; 2Q, '90, 7; J-F, '87, 13

codes may be used as principal diagnosis on Medicare patients.
tation codes acceptable as a principal diagnosis when accompanied by a secondary diagnosis reflecting the condition treated.

n Age: 0    P Pediatric Age: 0-17    M Maternity Age: 12-55    A Adult Age: 15-124    CC CC Condition    MCC Major CC Condition    HIV HIV Related Dx

ume 1 • October 2007    © 2007 Ingenix

✓5ᵗʰ **V58.1 Encounter for antineoplastic chemotherapy and immunotherapy**

Encounter or admission for chemotherapy

> **EXCLUDES** *chemotherapy and immunotherapy for nonneoplastic conditions — code to condition*
> *prophylactic chemotherapy against disease which has never been present (V03.0-V07.9)*

AHA: 1Q, '04, 13; 2Q, '03, 16; 3Q, '93, 4; 2Q, '92, 6; 2Q, '91, 17; 2Q, '90, 7; S-O, '84, 5

² **V58.11 Encounter for antineoplastic chemotherapy**
AHA: 2Q, '06, 20-21; 4Q, '05, 98

² **V58.12 Encounter for antineoplastic immunotherapy**
AHA: 4Q, '05, 98

**V58.2 Blood transfusion, without reported diagnosis**

✓5ᵗʰ **V58.3 Attention to dressings and sutures**

Change or removal of wound packing

> **EXCLUDES** *attention to drains (V58.49)*
> *planned postoperative wound closure (V58.41)*

AHA: 2Q, '05, 14

**V58.30 Encounter for change or removal of nonsurgical wound dressing**
Encounter for change or removal of wound dressing NOS
AHA: 4Q, '06, 117

**V58.31 Encounter for change or removal of surgical wound dressing**
AHA: 4Q, '06, 117

**V58.32 Encounter for removal of sutures**
Encounter for removal of staples
AHA: 4Q, '06, 117

✓5ᵗʰ **V58.4 Other aftercare following surgery**

Note: Codes from this subcategory should be used in conjunction with other aftercare codes to fully identify the reason for the aftercare encounter

> **EXCLUDES** *aftercare following sterilization reversal surgery (V26.22)*
> *attention to artificial openings (V55.0-V55.9)*
> *orthopedic aftercare (V54.0-V54.9)*

AHA: 4Q, '99, 9; N-D, '87, 9

⁶ **V58.41 Encounter for planned postoperative wound closure**

> **EXCLUDES** *disruption of operative wound (998.3)*
> *encounter for dressings and suture aftercare (V58.30-V58.32)*

AHA: 4Q, '99, 15

⁶ **V58.42 Aftercare following surgery for neoplasm**
Conditions classifiable to 140-239
AHA: 4Q, '02, 80

⁶ **V58.43 Aftercare following surgery for injury and trauma**
Conditions classifiable to 800-999

> **EXCLUDES** *aftercare for healing traumatic fracture (V54.10-V54.19)*

AHA: 4Q, '02, 80

⁶ **V58.44 Aftercare following organ transplant**
Use additional code to identify the organ transplanted (V42.0-V42.9)
AHA: 4Q, '04, 101

⁶ **V58.49 Other specified aftercare following surgery**
Change or removal of drains
AHA: 1Q, '96, 8, 9

⁶ **V58.5 Orthodontics**

> **EXCLUDES** *fitting and adjustment of orthodontic device (V53.4)*

✓5ᵗʰ **V58.6 Long-term (current) drug use**

> **EXCLUDES** *drug abuse (305.00-305.93)*
> *drug dependence (304.00-304.93)*
> *hormone replacement therapy (postmenopausal) (V07.4)*

AHA: 4Q, '03, 85; 4Q, '02, 84; 3Q, '02, 15; 4Q, '95, 61

⁶ **V58.61 Long-term (current) use of anticoagulants**

> **EXCLUDES** *long-term (current) use of aspirin (V58.66)*

AHA: 3Q, '06, 13; 3Q, '04, 7; 4Q, '03, 108; 3Q, '02, 13-16; 1Q, '02, 15, 16

**V58.62 Long-term (current) use of antibiotics**
AHA: 4Q, '98, 59

**V58.63 Long-term (current) use of antiplatelets/antithrombotics**

> **EXCLUDES** *long-term (current) use of aspirin (V58.66)*

**V58.64 Long-term (current) use of non-steroidal anti-inflammatories (NSAID)**

> **EXCLUDES** *long-term (current) use of aspirin (V58.66)*

**V58.65 Long-term (current) use of steroids**

**V58.66 Long-term (current) use of aspirin**
AHA: 4Q, '04, 102

**V58.67 Long-term (current) use of insulin**
AHA: 4Q, '04, 55-56, 103

⁶ **V58.69 Long-term (current) use of other medications**
▶Other high-risk medications◀
AHA: 2Q, '04, 10; 1Q, '04, 13; 1Q, '03, 11; 2Q, '00, 8; 3Q, '99, 13; 2Q, '99, 17; 1Q, '97, 12; 2Q, '96, 7

✓5ᵗʰ **V58.7 Aftercare following surgery to specified body systems, not elsewhere classified**

Note: Codes from this subcategory should be used in conjunction with other aftercare codes to fully identify the reason for the aftercare encounter

> **EXCLUDES** *aftercare following organ transplant (V58.44)*
> *aftercare following surgery for neoplasm (V58.42)*

AHA: 4Q, '03, 104; 4Q, '02, 80

⁶ **V58.71 Aftercare following surgery of the sense organs, NEC**
Conditions classifiable to 360-379, 380-389

⁶ **V58.72 Aftercare following surgery of the nervous system, NEC**
Conditions classifiable to 320-359

> **EXCLUDES** *aftercare following surgery of the sense organs, NEC (V58.71)*

⁶ **V58.73 Aftercare following surgery of the circulatory system, NEC**
Conditions classifiable to 390-459
AHA: 4Q, '03, 105

⁶ **V58.74 Aftercare following surgery of the respiratory system, NEC**
Conditions classifiable to 460-519

⁶ **V58.75 Aftercare following surgery of the teeth, oral cavity and digestive system, NEC**
Conditions classifiable to 520-579
AHA: 2Q, '05, 14

⁶ **V58.76 Aftercare following surgery of the genitourinary system, NEC**
Conditions classifiable to 580-629

> **EXCLUDES** *aftercare following sterilization reversal (V26.22)*

AHA: 1Q, '05, 11-12

⁶ **V58.77 Aftercare following surgery of the skin and subcutaneous tissue, NEC**
Conditions classifiable to 680-709

⁶ **V58.78 Aftercare following surgery of the musculoskeletal system, NEC**
Conditions classifiable to 710-739

> **EXCLUDES** ▶*orthopedic aftercare (V54.01-V54.9)*◀

---

² These V codes may be used as principal diagnosis on Medicare patients.
⁶ These V codes are acceptable as principal diagnosis and group to DRGs 949-950.

---

✓4ᵗʰ
✓5ᵗʰ Additional Digit Required    Unacceptable PDx    Manifestation Code    ▶◀ Revised Text    ● New Code    ▲ Revised Code Title

**V Codes**

**V58.8–V61.22**

☑5ᵗʰ **V58.8 Other specified procedures and aftercare**
AHA: 4Q, '94, 45; 2Q, '94, 8

  6 **V58.81 Fitting and adjustment of vascular catheter**
Removal or replacement of catheter
Toilet or cleansing
**EXCLUDES** *complication of renal dialysis (996.73)*
*complication of vascular catheter (996.74)*
*dialysis preparation — code to condition*
*encounter for dialysis (V56.0-V56.8)*
*fitting and adjustment of dialysis catheter (V56.1)*

  6 **V58.82 Fitting and adjustment of nonvascular catheter, NEC**
Removal or replacement of catheter
Toilet or cleansing
**EXCLUDES** *fitting and adjustment of peritoneal dialysis catheter (V56.2)*
*fitting and adjustment of urinary catheter (V53.6)*

  6 **V58.83 Encounter for therapeutic drug monitoring**
Use additional code for any associated long-term (current) drug use (V58.61-V58.69)
**EXCLUDES** *blood-drug testing for medicolegal reasons (V70.4)*
AHA: 2Q, '04, 10; 1Q, '04, 13;4Q, '03, 85; 4Q, '02, 84; 3Q, '02, 13-16

DEF: Drug monitoring: Measurement of the level of a specific drug in the body or measurement of a specific function to assess effectiveness of a drug.

  **V58.89 Other specified aftercare**
AHA: 4Q, '98, 59

  6 **V58.9 Unspecified aftercare**

☑4ᵗʰ **V59 Donors**
**EXCLUDES** *examination of potential donor (V70.8)*
*self-donation of organ or tissue — code to condition*
AHA: 4Q, '95, 62; 1Q, '90, 10; N-D, '84, 8

☑5ᵗʰ **V59.0 Blood**
  **V59.01 Whole blood**
  **V59.02 Stem cells**
  **V59.09 Other**

2 **V59.1 Skin**
2 **V59.2 Bone**
2 **V59.3 Bone marrow**
2 **V59.4 Kidney**
2 **V59.5 Cornea**
2 **V59.6 Liver**

☑5ᵗʰ **V59.7 Egg (oocyte) (ovum)**
AHA: 4Q, '05, 99

  **V59.70 Egg (oocyte) (ovum) donor, unspecified** ♀
  **V59.71 Egg (oocyte) (ovum) donor, under age 35, anonymous recipient** ♀
Egg donor, under age 35 NOS
  **V59.72 Egg (oocyte) (ovum) donor, under age 35, designated recipient** ♀
  **V59.73 Egg (oocyte) (ovum) donor, age 35 and over, anonymous recipient** ♀
Egg donor, age 35 and over NOS
  **V59.74 Egg (oocyte) (ovum) donor, age 35 and over, designated recipient** ♀

2 **V59.8 Other specified organ or tissue**
AHA: 3Q, '02, 20

2 **V59.9 Unspecified organ or tissue**

## PERSONS ENCOUNTERING HEALTH SERVICES IN OTHER CIRCUMSTANCES (V60-V69)

☑4ᵗʰ **V60 Housing, household, and economic circumstances**

**V60.0 Lack of housing**
Hobos    Transients
Social migrants    Vagabonds
Tramps

**V60.1 Inadequate housing**
Lack of heating    Technical defects in
Restriction of space    home preventing adequate care

**V60.2 Inadequate material resources**
Economic problem    Poverty NOS

**V60.3 Person living alone**

**V60.4 No other household member able to render care**
Person requiring care (has) (is):
family member too handicapped, ill, or otherwise unsuited to render care
partner temporarily away from home
temporarily away from usual place of abode
**EXCLUDES** *holiday relief care (V60.5)*

**V60.5 Holiday relief care**
Provision of health care facilities to a person normally cared for at home, to enable relatives to take a vacation

**V60.6 Person living in residential institution**
Boarding school resident

**V60.8 Other specified housing or economic circumstances**

**V60.9 Unspecified housing or economic circumstance**

☑4ᵗʰ **V61 Other family circumstances**
**INCLUDES** when these circumstances or fear of them, affecting the person directly involved or others, are mentioned as the reason, justified or not, for seeking or receiving medical advice or care
AHA: 1Q, '90, 9

**V61.0 Family disruption**
Divorce    Estrangement

☑5ᵗʰ **V61.1 Counseling for marital and partner problems**
**EXCLUDES** *problems related to: psychosexual disorders (302.0-302.9) sexual function (V41.7)*

  **V61.10 Counseling for marital and partner problems, unspecified**
Marital conflict
Marital relationship problem
Partner conflict
Partner relationship problem

  **V61.11 Counseling for victim of spousal and partner abuse**
**EXCLUDES** *encounter for treatment of current injuries due to abuse (995.80-995.85)*

  **V61.12 Counseling for perpetrator of spousal and partner abuse**

☑5ᵗʰ **V61.2 Parent-child problems**

  **V61.20 Counseling for parent-child problem, unspecified**
Concern about behavior of child
Parent-child conflict
Parent-child relationship problem

  2 **V61.21 Counseling for victim of child abuse**
Child battering    Child neglect
**EXCLUDES** *current injuries due to abuse (995.50-995.59)*

  **V61.22 Counseling for perpetrator of parental child abuse**
**EXCLUDES** *counseling for non-parental abuser (V62.83)*

---

2 These V codes may be used as principal diagnosis on Medicare patients.
6 These V codes are acceptable as principal diagnosis and group to DRGs 949-950.

N Newborn Age: 0    P Pediatric Age: 0-17    M Maternity Age: 12-55    A Adult Age: 15-124    CC CC Condition    MCC Major CC Condition    HIV HIV Related Dx

**V61.29 Other**
    Problem concerning adopted or foster child
    AHA: 3Q, '99, 16

**V61.3 Problems with aged parents or in-laws**
✓5th **V61.4 Health problems within family**
    **V61.41 Alcoholism in family**
    **V61.49 Other**
        Care of ⎫ sick or handicapped person
        Presence of ⎬ in family or household

**V61.5 Multiparity**
**V61.6 Illegitimacy or illegitimate pregnancy** M ♀
**V61.7 Other unwanted pregnancy** M ♀
**V61.8 Other specified family circumstances**
    Problems with family members NEC
    Sibling relationship problem
**V61.9 Unspecified family circumstance**

✓4th **V62 Other psychosocial circumstances**
    INCLUDES those circumstances or fear of them, affecting
        the person directly involved or others,
        mentioned as the reason, justified or not,
        for seeking or receiving medical advice or
        care
    EXCLUDES previous psychological trauma (V15.41-V15.49)

**V62.0 Unemployment**
    EXCLUDES circumstances when main problem is
        economic inadequacy or poverty
        (V60.2)

**V62.1 Adverse effects of work environment**
**V62.2 Other occupational circumstances or maladjustment**
    Career choice problem
    Dissatisfaction with employment
    Occupational problem

**V62.3 Educational circumstances**
    Academic problem
    Dissatisfaction with school environment
    Educational handicap

**V62.4 Social maladjustment**
    Acculturation problem    Social:
    Cultural deprivation        isolation
    Political, religious, or     persecution
        sex discrimination

**V62.5 Legal circumstances**
    Imprisonment    Litigation
    Legal investigation    Prosecution

**V62.6 Refusal of treatment for reasons of religion or conscience**

✓5th **V62.8 Other psychological or physical stress, not elsewhere classified**

    **V62.81 Interpersonal problems, not elsewhere classified**
        Relational problem NOS

    **V62.82 Bereavement, uncomplicated**
        EXCLUDES bereavement as adjustment
            reaction (309.0)

    **V62.83 Counseling for perpetrator of physical/sexual abuse**
        EXCLUDES counseling for perpetrator of
            parental child abuse
            (V61.22)
            counseling for perpetrator of
            spousal and partner
            abuse (V61.12)

    **V62.84 Suicidal ideation** CC
        EXCLUDES suicidal tendencies (300.9)
        CC Excl: 290.11, 290.3, 293.0
        AHA: 4Q, '05, 96
        DEF: Thoughts of committing suicide; no actual attempt of
        suicide has been made.

**V62.89 Other**
    Borderline intellectual functioning
    Life circumstance problems
    Phase of life problems
    Religious or spiritual problem

**V62.9 Unspecified psychosocial circumstance**

✓5th **V63 Unavailability of other medical facilities for care**
    AHA: 1Q, '91, 21

**V63.0 Residence remote from hospital or other health care facility**

**V63.1 Medical services in home not available**
    EXCLUDES no other household member able to
        render care (V60.4)
    AHA: 4Q, '01, 67; 1Q, '01, 12

**V63.2 Person awaiting admission to adequate facility elsewhere**

**V63.8 Other specified reasons for unavailability of medical facilities**
    Person on waiting list undergoing social agency
        investigation

**V63.9 Unspecified reason for unavailability of medical facilities**

✓4th **V64 Persons encountering health services for specific procedures, not carried out**

✓5th **V64.0 Vaccination not carried out**
    AHA: 4Q, '05, 99

    **V64.00 Vaccination not carried out, unspecified reason**
    **V64.01 Vaccination not carried out because of acute illness**
    **V64.02 Vaccination not carried out because of chronic illness or condition**
    **V64.03 Vaccination not carried out because of immune compromised state**
    **V64.04 Vaccination not carried out because of allergy to vaccine or component**
    **V64.05 Vaccination not carried out because of caregiver refusal**
        ►Guardian refusal
        Parent refusal◄
        AHA: ►1Q, '07, 12◄

    **V64.06 Vaccination not carried out because of patient refusal**
    **V64.07 Vaccination not carried out for religious reasons**
    **V64.08 Vaccination not carried out because patient had disease being vaccinated against**
    **V64.09 Vaccination not carried out for other reason**

**V64.1 Surgical or other procedure not carried out because of contraindication**

**V64.2 Surgical or other procedure not carried out because of patient's decision**
    AHA: 2Q, '01, 8

**V64.3 Procedure not carried out for other reasons**

✓5th **V64.4 Closed surgical procedure converted to open procedure**
    AHA: 4Q, '03, 87; 4Q, '98, 68; 4Q, '97, 52

    **V64.41 Laparoscopic surgical procedure converted to open procedure**
    **V64.42 Thoracoscopic surgical procedure converted to open procedure**
    **V64.43 Arthroscopic surgical procedure converted to open procedure**

✓4th **V65 Other persons seeking consultation**
    2 **V65.0 Healthy person accompanying sick person**
        Boarder

✓5th **V65.1 Person consulting on behalf of another person**
    Advice or treatment for nottending third party
    EXCLUDES concern (normal) about sick person in
        family (V61.41-V61.49)
    AHA: 4Q, '03, 84

    **V65.11 Pediatric pre-birth visit for expectant mother** M ♀

---

2   These V codes may be used as principal diagnosis on Medicare patients.

**V65.19 Other person consulting on behalf of another person**

² **V65.2 Person feigning illness**
　　Malingerer　　　　　　Peregrinating patient
　　AHA: 3Q, '99, 20

**V65.3 Dietary surveillance and counseling**
　　Dietary surveillance and counseling (in):
　　　NOS　　　　　　　gastritis
　　　colitis　　　　　　hypercholesterolemia
　　　diabetes mellitus　hypoglycemia
　　　food allergies or　obesity
　　　　intolerance
　　Use additional code to identify Body Mass Index
　　　(BMI), if known (V85.0-V85.54)
　　AHA: 4Q, '05, 96

✓5ᵗʰ **V65.4 Other counseling, not elsewhere classified**
　　Health:　　　　　Health:
　　　advice　　　　　instruction
　　　education
　　EXCLUDES　counseling (for):
　　　　　　　contraception (V25.40-V25.49)
　　　　　　　genetic (V26.31-V26.39)
　　　　　　　on behalf of third party (V65.11-
　　　　　　　　V65.19)
　　　　　　　procreative management ▶(V26.41-
　　　　　　　　V26.49)◀

**V65.40 Counseling NOS**

**V65.41 Exercise counseling**

**V65.42 Counseling on substance use and abuse**

**V65.43 Counseling on injury prevention**

**V65.44 Human immunodeficiency virus [HIV] counseling**

**V65.45 Counseling on other sexually transmitted diseases**

**V65.46 Encounter for insulin pump training**

**V65.49 Other specified counseling**
　　AHA: 2Q, '00, 8

**V65.5 Person with feared complaint in whom no diagnosis was made**
　　Feared condition not demonstrated
　　Problem was normal state
　　"Worried well"

**V65.8 Other reasons for seeking consultation**
　　EXCLUDES　specified symptoms
　　AHA: 3Q, '92, 4

**V65.9 Unspecified reason for consultation**

✓4ᵗʰ **V66 Convalescence and palliative care**

² **V66.0 Following surgery**

² **V66.1 Following radiotherapy**

² **V66.2 Following chemotherapy**

² **V66.3 Following psychotherapy and other treatment for mental disorder**

² **V66.4 Following treatment of fracture**

**V66.5 Following other treatment**

² **V66.6 Following combined treatment**

**V66.7 Encounter for palliative care**
　　End of life care　　　Terminal care
　　Hospice care
　　Code first underlying disease
　　AHA: 2Q, '05, 9; 4Q, '03, 107; 1Q, '98, 11; 4Q, '96, 47, 48

**V66.9 Unspecified convalescence**
　　AHA: 4Q, '99, 8

✓4ᵗʰ **V67 Follow-up examination**
　　INCLUDES　surveillance only following completed
　　　　　　　treatment
　　EXCLUDES　surveillance of contraception (V25.40-V25.49)
　　AHA: 2Q, '03, 5

✓5ᵗʰ **V67.0 Following surgery**
　　AHA: 4Q, '00, 56; 4Q, '98, 69; 4Q, '97, 50; 2Q, '95, 8;1Q, '95, 4;
　　　3Q, '92, 11

⁶ **V67.00 Following surgery, unspecified**

⁶ **V67.01 Follow-up vaginal pap smear**　　♀
　　Vaginal pap-smear, status-post
　　　hysterectomy for malignant condition
　　Use additional code to identify:
　　　acquired absence of uterus (V45.77)
　　　personal history of malignant neoplasm
　　　　(V10.40-V10.44)
　　EXCLUDES　vaginal pap smear status-post
　　　　　　　hysterectomy for non-
　　　　　　　malignant condition
　　　　　　　(V76.47)

⁶ **V67.09 Following other surgery**
　　EXCLUDES　sperm count following steril-
　　　　　　　ization reversal (V26.22)
　　　　　　　sperm count for fertility testing
　　　　　　　(V26.21)
　　AHA: 3Q, '03, 16; 3Q, '02, 15

² **V67.1 Following radiotherapy**

² **V67.2 Following chemotherapy**
　　Cancer chemotherapy follow-up

² **V67.3 Following psychotherapy and other treatment for mental disorder**

⁶ **V67.4 Following treatment of healed fracture**
　　EXCLUDES　current (healing) fracture aftercare
　　　　　　　(V54.0-V54.9)
　　AHA: 1Q, '90, 7

✓5ᵗʰ **V67.5 Following other treatment**

² **V67.51 Following completed treatment with high-risk medications, not elsewhere classified**
　　EXCLUDES　long-term (current) drug use
　　　　　　　(V58.61-V58.69)
　　AHA: 1Q, '99, 5, 6;4Q, '95, 61 ; 1Q, '90, 18

² **V67.59 Other**

² **V67.6 Following combined treatment**

**V67.9 Unspecified follow-up examination**

✓4ᵗʰ **V68 Encounters for administrative purposes**

✓5ᵗʰ **V68.0 Issue of medical certificates**
　　EXCLUDES　encounter for general medical
　　　　　　　examination (V70.0-V70.9)

● **V68.01 Disability examination**
　　Use additional code(s) to identify specific
　　　examination(s), screening and testing
　　　performed (V72.0-V82.9)

● **V68.09 Other issue of medical certificates**

**V68.1 Issue of repeat prescriptions**
　　Issue of repeat prescription for:
　　　appliance　　　　　medications
　　　glasses
　　EXCLUDES　repeat prescription for contraceptives
　　　　　　　(V25.41-V25.49)

**V68.2 Request for expert evidence**

✓5ᵗʰ **V68.8 Other specified administrative purpose**

**V68.81 Referral of patient without examination or treatment**

**V68.89 Other**

**V68.9 Unspecified administrative purpose**

✓4ᵗʰ **V69 Problems related to lifestyle**
　　AHA: 4Q, '94, 48

**V69.0 Lack of physical exercise**

---

² These V codes may be used as principal diagnosis on Medicare patients.
⁶ These V codes are acceptable as principal diagnosis and group to DRGs 465-466.

---

N Newborn Age: 0　　P Pediatric Age: 0-17　　M Maternity Age: 12-55　　A Adult Age: 15-124　　CC CC Condition　　MCC Major CC Condition　　HIV HIV Related Dx

356 — Volume 1 • October 2007

© 2007 Ingenix

**V69.1 Inappropriate diet and eating habits**
> EXCLUDES: anorexia nervosa (307.1)
> bulimia (783.6)
> malnutrition and other nutritional deficiencies (260-269.9)
> other and unspecified eating disorders (307.50-307.59)

**V69.2 High-risk sexual behavior**

**V69.3 Gambling and betting**
> EXCLUDES: pathological gambling (312.31)

**V69.4 Lack of adequate sleep**
Sleep deprivation
> EXCLUDES: insomnia (780.52)

**V69.5 Behavioral insomnia of childhood** P
AHA: 4Q, '05, 99

DEF: Behaviors on the part of the child or caregivers that cause negative compliance with a child's sleep schedule; results in lack of adequate sleep.

**V69.8 Other problems related to lifestyle**
Self-damaging behavior

**V69.9 Problem related to lifestyle, unspecified**

## PERSONS WITHOUT REPORTED DIAGNOSIS ENCOUNTERED DURING EXAMINATION AND INVESTIGATION OF INDIVIDUALS AND POPULATIONS (V70-V82)

Note: Nonspecific abnormal findings disclosed at the time of these examinations are classifiable to categories 790-796.

√4th **V70 General medical examination**
Use additional code(s) to identify any special screening examination(s) performed (V73.0-V82.9)

**V70.0 Routine general medical examination at a health care facility**
Health checkup
> EXCLUDES: health checkup of infant or child (V20.2)
> pre-procedural general physical examination (V72.83)

2 **V70.1 General psychiatric examination, requested by the authority**

**V70.2 General psychiatric examination, other and unspecified**

**V70.3 Other medical examination for administrative purposes**
General medical examination for:
admission to old age home
adoption
camp
driving license
immigration and naturalization
insurance certification
marriage
prison
school admission
sports competition
> EXCLUDES: attendance for issue of medical certificates (V68.0)
> pre-employment screening (V70.5)

AHA: 1Q, '90, 6

2 **V70.4 Examination for medicolegal reasons**
Blood-alcohol tests      Paternity testing
Blood-drug tests
> EXCLUDES: examination and observation following:
> accidents (V71.3, V71.4)
> assault (V71.6)
> rape (V71.5)

2 **V70.5 Health examination of defined subpopulations**
Armed forces personnel      Prisoners
Inhabitants of institutions      Prostitutes
Occupational health      Refugees
      examinations      School children
Pre-employment screening      Students
Preschool children

**V70.6 Health examination in population surveys**
> EXCLUDES: special screening (V73.0-V82.9)

2 **V70.7 Examination of participant in clinical trial**
Examination of participant or control in clinical research
AHA: 2Q, '06, 5-6; 4Q, '01, 55

**V70.8 Other specified general medical examinations**
Examination of potential donor of organ or tissue

**V70.9 Unspecified general medical examination**

√4th **V71 Observation and evaluation for suspected conditions not found**
> INCLUDES: This category is to be used when persons without a diagnosis are suspected of having an abnormal condition, without signs or symptoms, which requires study, but after examination and observation, is found not to exist. This category is also for use for administrative and legal observation status.

AHA: 4Q, '94, 47; 2Q, '90, 5; M-A, '87, 1

√5th **V71.0 Observation for suspected mental condition**
2 **V71.01 Adult antisocial behavior** A
Dyssocial behavior or gang activity in adult without manifest psychiatric disorder

2 **V71.02 Childhood or adolescent antisocial behavior**
Dyssocial behavior or gang activity in child or adolescent without manifest psychiatric disorder

2 **V71.09 Other suspected mental condition**

2 **V71.1 Observation for suspected malignant neoplasm**

2 **V71.2 Observation for suspected tuberculosis**

2 **V71.3 Observation following accident at work**

2 **V71.4 Observation following other accident**
Examination of individual involved in motor vehicle traffic accident
AHA: 1Q, '06, 9

2 **V71.5 Observation following alleged rape or seduction**
Examination of victim or culprit

2 **V71.6 Observation following other inflicted injury**
Examination of victim or culprit

2 **V71.7 Observation for suspected cardiovascular disease**
AHA: 1Q, '04, 6; 3Q, '90, 10; S-O, '87, 10

√5th **V71.8 Observation and evaluation for other specified suspected conditions**
AHA: 4Q, '00, 54 ; 1Q, '90, 19

2 **V71.81 Abuse and neglect**
> EXCLUDES: adult abuse and neglect (995.80-995.85)
> child abuse and neglect (995.50-995.59)

AHA: 4Q, '00, 55

2 **V71.82 Observation and evaluation for suspected exposure to anthrax**
AHA: 4Q, '02, 70, 85

2 **V71.83 Observation and evaluation for suspected exposure to other biological agent**
AHA: 4Q, '03, 47

2 **V71.89 Other specified suspected conditions**
AHA: 2Q, '03, 15

**V71.9 Observation for unspecified suspected condition**
AHA: 1Q, '02, 6

√4th **V72 Special investigations and examinations**
> INCLUDES: routine examination of specific system
> EXCLUDES: general medical examination (V70.0-V70.4)
> general screening examination of defined population groups (V70.5, V70.6, V70.7)
> routine examination of infant or child (V20.2)

Use additional code(s) to identify any special screening examination(s) performed (V73.0-V82.9)

2 **V72.0 Examination of eyes and vision**
AHA: 1Q, '04, 15

2 These V codes may be used as principal diagnosis on Medicare patients.

V Codes

V69.1–V72.0

**V Codes**

**V72.1–V76.19**

√5ᵗʰ **V72.1 Examination of ears and hearing**
AHA: 1Q, '04, 15

**V72.11 Encounter for hearing examination following failed hearing screening**
AHA: 4Q, '06, 118

● **V72.12 Encounter for hearing conservation and treatment**

**V72.19 Other examination of ears and hearing**

**V72.2 Dental examination**

√5ᵗʰ **V72.3 Gynecological examination**
EXCLUDES cervical Papanicolaou smear without general gynecological examination (V76.2)
routine examination in contraceptive management (V25.40-V25.49)

² **V72.31 Routine gynecological examination** ♀
General gynecological examination with or without Papanicolaou cervical smear
Pelvic examination (annual) (periodic)
▶Use additional code to identify:
human papillomavirus (HPV) screening (V73.81)
routine vaginal Papanicolaou smear (V76.47)◀
AHA: 2Q, '06, 2-3; 4Q, '05, 9

² **V72.32 Encounter for Papanicolaou cervical smear to confirm findings of recent normal smear following initial abnormal smear** ♀
AHA: 2Q, '06, 4

√5ᵗʰ **V72.4 Pregnancy examination or test**
AHA: 4Q, '05, 98

² **V72.40 Pregnancy examination or test, pregnancy unconfirmed** ♀
Possible pregnancy, not (yet) confirmed

² **V72.41 Pregnancy examination or test, negative result** ♀

² **V72.42 Pregnancy examination or test, positive result** ♀ M

**V72.5 Radiological examination, not elsewhere classified**
Routine chest x-ray
EXCLUDES examination for suspected tuberculosis (V71.2)
AHA: 1Q, '90, 19

**V72.6 Laboratory examination**
EXCLUDES that for suspected disorder (V71.0-V71.9)
AHA: 2Q, '06, 4; 1Q, '90, 22

**V72.7 Diagnostic skin and sensitization tests**
Allergy tests   Skin tests for hypersensitivity
EXCLUDES diagnostic skin tests for bacterial diseases (V74.0-V74.9)

√5ᵗʰ **V72.8 Other specified examinations**
² **V72.81 Pre-operative cardiovascular examination**
Pre-procedural cardiovascular examination

² **V72.82 Pre-operative respiratory examination**
Pre-procedural respiratory examination
AHA: 3Q, '96, 14

² **V72.83 Other specified pre-operative examination**
Other pre-procedural examination
Pre-procedural general physical examination
EXCLUDES routine general medical examination (V70.0)
AHA: 3Q, '96, 14

**V72.84 Pre-operative examination, unspecified**
Pre-procedural examination, unspecified

**V72.85 Other specified examination**
AHA: 4Q, '05, 96; 1Q, '04, 12

**V72.86 Encounter for blood typing**

**V72.9 Unspecified examination**
AHA: 4Q, '06, 117

√4ᵗʰ **V73 Special screening examination for viral and chlamydial diseases**
AHA: 1Q, '04, 11

**V73.0 Poliomyelitis**
**V73.1 Smallpox**
**V73.2 Measles**
**V73.3 Rubella**
**V73.4 Yellow fever**
**V73.5 Other arthropod-borne viral diseases**
Dengue fever   Viral encephalitis:
Hemorrhagic fever   mosquito-borne   tick-borne

**V73.6 Trachoma**
√5ᵗʰ **V73.8 Other specified viral and chlamydial diseases**
● **V73.81 Human papillomavirus [HPV]**
**V73.88 Other specified chlamydial diseases**
**V73.89 Other specified viral diseases**

√5ᵗʰ **V73.9 Unspecified viral and chlamydial disease**
**V73.98 Unspecified chlamydial disease**
**V73.99 Unspecified viral disease**

√4ᵗʰ **V74 Special screening examination for bacterial and spirochetal diseases**
INCLUDES diagnostic skin tests for these diseases
AHA: 1Q, '04, 11

**V74.0 Cholera**
**V74.1 Pulmonary tuberculosis**
**V74.2 Leprosy [Hansen's disease]**
**V74.3 Diphtheria**
**V74.4 Bacterial conjunctivitis**
**V74.5 Venereal disease**
▶Screening for bacterial and spirochetal sexually transmitted diseases
Screening for sexually transmitted diseases NOS◀
EXCLUDES ▶special screening for nonbacterial sexually transmitted diseases (V73.81-V73.89, V75.4, V75.8)◀

**V74.6 Yaws**
**V74.8 Other specified bacterial and spirochetal diseases**
Brucellosis   Tetanus
Leptospirosis   Whooping cough
Plague

**V74.9 Unspecified bacterial and spirochetal disease**
√4ᵗʰ **V75 Special screening examination for other infectious diseases**
AHA: 1Q, '04, 11

**V75.0 Rickettsial diseases**
**V75.1 Malaria**
**V75.2 Leishmaniasis**
**V75.3 Trypanosomiasis**
Chagas' disease   Sleeping sickness
**V75.4 Mycotic infections**
**V75.5 Schistosomiasis**
**V75.6 Filariasis**
**V75.7 Intestinal helminthiasis**
**V75.8 Other specified parasitic infections**
**V75.9 Unspecified infectious disease**
√4ᵗʰ **V76 Special screening for malignant neoplasms**
AHA: 1Q, '04, 11

**V76.0 Respiratory organs**
√5ᵗʰ **V76.1 Breast**
AHA: 4Q, '98, 67

**V76.10 Breast screening, unspecified**
**V76.11 Screening mammogram for high-risk patient** ♀
AHA: 2Q, '03, 4

**V76.12 Other screening mammogram**
AHA: 2Q, '06, 10; 2Q, '03, 3-4

**V76.19 Other screening breast examination**

² These V codes may be used as principal diagnosis on Medicare patients.

N Newborn Age: 0   P Pediatric Age: 0-17   M Maternity Age: 12-55   A Adult Age: 15-124   CC CC Condition   MCC Major CC Condition   HIV HIV Related Dx

| | |
|---|---|
| **V76.2** **Cervix** ♀ | **V78.3** **Other hemoglobinopathies** |
| Routine cervical Papanicolaou smear | **V78.8** **Other disorders of blood and blood-forming organs** |
| EXCLUDES ►*special screening for human papillomavirus (V73.81)*◄ | **V78.9** **Unspecified disorder of blood and blood-forming organs** |

**V76.2** **Cervix** ♀

Routine cervical Papanicolaou smear

EXCLUDES ► *special screening for human papillomavirus (V73.81)*◄

*that as part of a general gynecological examination (V72.31)*

**V76.3** **Bladder**

✓5th **V76.4** **Other sites**

**V76.41** **Rectum**

**V76.42** **Oral cavity**

**V76.43** **Skin**

**V76.44** **Prostate** ♂

**V76.45** **Testis** ♂

**V76.46** **Ovary** ♀

AHA: 4Q, '00, 52

**V76.47** **Vagina** ♀

Vaginal pap smear status-post hysterectomy for non-malignant condition

Use additional code to identify acquired absence of uterus (V45.77)

EXCLUDES *vaginal pap smear status-post hysterectomy for malignant condition (V67.01)*

AHA: 4Q, '00, 52

**V76.49** **Other sites**

AHA: 1Q, '99, 4

✓5th **V76.5** **Intestine**

AHA: 4Q, '00, 52

**V76.50** **Intestine, unspecified**

**V76.51** **Colon**

EXCLUDES *rectum (V76.41)*

AHA: 4Q, '01, 56

**V76.52** **Small intestine**

✓5th **V76.8** **Other neoplasm**

AHA: 4Q, '00, 52

**V76.81** **Nervous system**

**V76.89** **Other neoplasm**

**V76.9** **Unspecified**

✓4th **V77** **Special screening for endocrine, nutritional, metabolic, and immunity disorders**

AHA: 1Q, '04, 11

**V77.0** **Thyroid disorders**

**V77.1** **Diabetes mellitus**

**V77.2** **Malnutrition**

**V77.3** **Phenylketonuria [PKU]**

**V77.4** **Galactosemia**

**V77.5** **Gout**

**V77.6** **Cystic fibrosis**

Screening for mucoviscidosis

**V77.7** **Other inborn errors of metabolism**

**V77.8** **Obesity**

✓5th **V77.9** **Other and unspecified endocrine, nutritional, metabolic, and immunity disorders**

AHA: 4Q, '00, 53

**V77.91** **Screening for lipoid disorders**

Screening for cholesterol level

Screening for hypercholesterolemia

Screening for hyperlipidemia

**V77.99** **Other and unspecified endocrine, nutritional, metabolic, and immunity disorders**

✓4th **V78** **Special screening for disorders of blood and blood-forming organs**

AHA: 1Q, '04, 11

**V78.0** **Iron deficiency anemia**

**V78.1** **Other and unspecified deficiency anemia**

**V78.2** **Sickle cell disease or trait**

**V78.3** **Other hemoglobinopathies**

**V78.8** **Other disorders of blood and blood-forming organs**

**V78.9** **Unspecified disorder of blood and blood-forming organs**

✓4th **V79** **Special screening for mental disorders and developmental handicaps**

AHA: 1Q, '04, 11

**V79.0** **Depression**

**V79.1** **Alcoholism**

**V79.2** **Mental retardation**

**V79.3** **Developmental handicaps in early childhood**

**V79.8** **Other specified mental disorders and developmental handicaps**

**V79.9** **Unspecified mental disorder and developmental handicap**

✓4th **V80** **Special screening for neurological, eye, and ear diseases**

AHA: 1Q, '04, 11

**V80.0** **Neurological conditions**

**V80.1** **Glaucoma**

**V80.2** **Other eye conditions**

Screening for:          Screening for:

cataract                    senile macular lesions

congenital anomaly of eye

EXCLUDES *general vision examination (V72.0)*

**V80.3** **Ear diseases**

EXCLUDES *general hearing examination ►(V72.11-V72.19)*◄

✓4th **V81** **Special screening for cardiovascular, respiratory, and genitourinary diseases**

AHA: 1Q, '04, 11

**V81.0** **Ischemic heart disease**

**V81.1** **Hypertension**

**V81.2** **Other and unspecified cardiovascular conditions**

**V81.3** **Chronic bronchitis and emphysema**

**V81.4** **Other and unspecified respiratory conditions**

EXCLUDES *screening for: lung neoplasm (V76.0) pulmonary tuberculosis (V74.1)*

**V81.5** **Nephropathy**

Screening for asymptomatic bacteriuria

**V81.6** **Other and unspecified genitourinary conditions**

✓4th **V82** **Special screening for other conditions**

AHA: 1Q, '04, 11

**V82.0** **Skin conditions**

**V82.1** **Rheumatoid arthritis**

**V82.2** **Other rheumatic disorders**

**V82.3** **Congenital dislocation of hip**

**V82.4** **Maternal postnatal screening for chromosomal anomalies** ♀

EXCLUDES *antenatal screening by amniocentesis (V28.0)*

**V82.5** **Chemical poisoning and other contamination**

Screening for:

heavy metal poisoning

ingestion of radioactive substance

poisoning from contaminated water supply

radiation exposure

**V82.6** **Multiphasic screening**

✓5th **V82.7** **Genetic screening**

EXCLUDES *genetic testing for procreative management ►(V26.31-V26.39)*◄

**V82.71** **Screening for genetic disease carrier status**

AHA: 4Q, '06, 118

**V82.79** **Other genetic screening**

AHA: 4Q, '06, 118

---

✓4th / ✓5th Additional Digit Required          Unacceptable PDx          Manifestation Code          ►◄ Revised Text          ● New Code          ▲ Revised Code Title

**V Codes**

**V82.8–V86.1**

✓5ᵗʰ **V82.8** **Other specified conditions**
AHA: 4Q, '00, 53

**V82.81 Osteoporosis**
Use additional code to identify:
hormone replacement therapy
(postmenopausal) status (V07.4)
postmenopausal (age-related) (natural)
status (V49.81)

AHA: 4Q, '00, 54

**V82.89 Other specified conditions**

**V82.9 Unspecified condition**

## GENETICS (V83-V84)

✓4ᵗʰ **V83 Genetic carrier status**
AHA: 4Q, '02, 79; 4Q, '01, 54

✓5ᵗʰ **V83.0 Hemophilia A carrier**
**V83.01 Asymptomatic hemophilia A carrier**
**V83.02 Symptomatic hemophilia A carrier**

✓5ᵗʰ **V83.8 Other genetic carrier status**
**V83.81 Cystic fibrosis gene carrier**
**V83.89 Other genetic carrier status**

✓4ᵗʰ **V84 Genetic susceptibility to disease**
INCLUDES   confirmed abnormal gene
Use additional code, if applicable, for any associated family
history of the disease (V16-V19)

AHA: 4Q, '04, 106

✓5ᵗʰ **V84.0 Genetic susceptibility to malignant neoplasm**
Code first, if applicable, any current malignant
neoplasms (140.0-195.8, 200.0-208.9, 230.0-
234.9)
Use additional code, if applicable, for any personal
history of malignant neoplasm (V10.0-V10.9)

**V84.01 Genetic susceptibility to malignant neoplasm of breast**
AHA: 4Q, '04, 107

**V84.02 Genetic susceptibility to malignant neoplasm of ovary**   ♀

**V84.03 Genetic susceptibility to malignant neoplasm of prostate**   ♂

**V84.04 Genetic susceptibility to malignant neoplasm of endometrium**   ♀

**V84.09 Genetic susceptibility to other malignant neoplasm**

✓5ᵗʰ **V84.8 Genetic susceptibility to other disease**
• **V84.81 Genetic susceptibility to multiple endocrine neoplasia [MEN]**
• **V84.89 Genetic susceptibility to other disease**

## BODY MASS INDEX (V85)

✓4ᵗʰ **V85 Body Mass Index [BMI]**
Kilograms per meters squared
Note: BMI adult codes are for use for persons over 20 years
old

AHA: 4Q, '05, 97

**V85.0 Body Mass Index less than 19, adult**   CC A
CC Excl: 278.00-278.01, V77.8, V85.0-V85.54

**V85.1 Body Mass Index between 19-24, adult**   A

✓5ᵗʰ **V85.2 Body Mass Index between 25-29, adult**
**V85.21 Body Mass Index 25.0-25.9, adult**   A
**V85.22 Body Mass Index 26.0-26.9, adult**   A
**V85.23 Body Mass Index 27.0-27.9, adult**   A
**V85.24 Body Mass Index 28.0-28.9, adult**   A
**V85.25 Body Mass Index 29.0-29.9, adult**   A

✓5ᵗʰ **V85.3 Body Mass Index between 30-39, adult**
**V85.30 Body Mass Index 30.0-30.9, adult**   A
**V85.31 Body Mass Index 31.0-31.9, adult**   A
**V85.32 Body Mass Index 32.0-32.9, adult**   A
**V85.33 Body Mass Index 33.0-33.9, adult**   A
**V85.34 Body Mass Index 34.0-34.9, adult**   A
**V85.35 Body Mass Index 35.0-35.9, adult**   A
**V85.36 Body Mass Index 36.0-36.9, adult**   A
**V85.37 Body Mass Index 37.0-37.9, adult**   A
**V85.38 Body Mass Index 38.0-38.9, adult**   A
**V85.39 Body Mass Index 39.0-39.9, adult**   A

**V85.4 Body Mass Index 40 and over, adult**   CC A
CC Excl: 278.00-278.01, 278.1, V85.0-V85.39, V85.51-V85.54

✓5ᵗʰ **V85.5 Body Mass Index, pediatric**
Note: BMI pediatric codes are for use for persons age
2-20 years old. These percentiles are based on
the growth charts published by the Centers for
Disease Control and Prevention (CDC)

AHA: 4Q, '06, 118

**V85.51 Body Mass Index, pediatric, less than 5th percentile for age**   P

**V85.52 Body Mass Index, pediatric, 5th percentile to less than 85th percentile for age**   P

**V85.53 Body Mass Index, pediatric, 85th percentile to less than 95th percentile for age**   P

**V85.54 Body Mass Index, pediatric, greater than or equal to 95th percentile for age**   P

## ESTROGEN RECEPTOR STATUS (V86)

✓4ᵗʰ **V86 Estrogen receptor status**
Code first malignant neoplasm of breast (174.0-174.9, 175.0-
175.9)

AHA: 4Q, '06, 118

**V86.0 Estrogen receptor positive status [ER+]**
**V86.1 Estrogen receptor negative status [ER-]**

---

N Newborn Age: 0    P Pediatric Age: 0-17    M Maternity Age: 12-55    A Adult Age: 15-124    CC CC Condition    MCC Major CC Condition    HIV HIV Related Dx

# SUPPLEMENTARY CLASSIFICATION OF EXTERNAL CAUSES OF INJURY AND POISONING (E800-E999)

This section is provided to permit the classification of environmental events, circumstances, and conditions as the cause of injury, poisoning, and other adverse effects. Where a code from this section is applicable, it is intended that it shall be used in addition to a code from one of the main chapters of ICD-9-CM, indicating the nature of the condition. Certain other conditions which may be stated to be due to external causes are classified in Chapters 1 to 16 of ICD-9-CM. For these, the "E" code classification should be used as an additional code for more detailed analysis.

Machinery accidents [other than those connected with transport] are classifiable to category E919, in which the fourth-digit allows a broad classification of the type of machinery involved. If a more detailed classification of type of machinery is required, it is suggested that the "Classification of Industrial Accidents according to Agency," prepared by the International Labor Office, be used in addition. This is reproduced in Appendix D for optional use.

Categories for "late effects" of accidents and other external causes are to be found at E929, E959, E969, E977, E989, and E999.

## DEFINITIONS AND EXAMPLES RELATED TO TRANSPORT ACCIDENTS

(a) A **transport accident** (E800-E848) is any accident involving a device designed primarily for, or being used at the time primarily for, conveying persons or goods from one place to another.

> **INCLUDES**   accidents involving:
> aircraft and spacecraft (E840-E845)
> watercraft (E830-E838)
> motor vehicle (E810-E825)
> railway (E800-E807)
> other road vehicles (E826-E829)

In classifying accidents which involve more than one kind of transport, the above order of precedence of transport accidents should be used.

Accidents involving agricultural and construction machines, such as tractors, cranes, and bulldozers, are regarded as transport accidents only when these vehicles are under their own power on a highway [otherwise the vehicles are regarded as machinery]. Vehicles which can travel on land or water, such as hovercraft and other amphibious vehicles, are regarded as watercraft when on the water, as motor vehicles when on the highway, and as off-road motor vehicles when on land, but off the highway.

> **EXCLUDES**   *accidents:*
> *in sports which involve the use of transport but where the transport vehicle itself was not involved in the accident*
> *involving vehicles which are part of industrial equipment used entirely on industrial premises*
> *occurring during transportation but unrelated to the hazards associated with the means of transportation [e.g., injuries received in a fight on board ship; transport vehicle involved in a cataclysm such as an earthquake]*
> *to persons engaged in the maintenance or repair of transport equipment or vehicle not in motion, unlesss injured by another vehicle in motion*

(b) A **railway accident** is a transport accident involving a railway train or other railway vehicle operated on rails, whether in motion or not.

> **EXCLUDES**   *accidents:*
> *in repair shops*
> *in roundhouse or on turntable*
> *on railway premises but not involving a train or other railway vehicle*

(c) A **railway train** or **railway vehicle** is any device with or without cars coupled to it, desiged for traffic on a railway.

> **INCLUDES**   interurban:
> electric car ⎫ (operated chiefly on its
> streetcar   ⎬   own right-of-way,
>              ⎭   not open to other
>                  traffic)
>
> railway train, any power [diesel] [electric] [steam]
> funicular
> monorail or two-rail
> subterranean or elevated
> other vehicle designed to run on a railway track
>
> **EXCLUDES**   *interurban electric cars [streetcars] specified to be operating on a right-of-way that forms part of the public street or highway [definition (n)]*

(d) A **railway** or **railroad** is a right-of-way designed for traffic on rails, which is used by carriages or wagons transporting passengers or freight, and by other rolling stock, and which is not open to other public vehicular traffic.

(e) A **motor vehicle accident** is a transport accident involving a motor vehicle. It is defined as a motor vehicle traffic accident or as a motor vehicle nontraffic accident according to whether the accident occurs on a public highway or elsewhere.

> **EXCLUDES**   *injury or damage due to cataclysm*
> *injury or damage while a motor vehicle, not under its own power, is being loaded on, or unloaded from, another conveyance*

(f) A **motor vehicle traffic accident** is any motor vehicle accident occurring on a public highway [i.e., originating, terminating, or involving a vehicle partially on the highway]. A motor vehicle accident is assumed to have occurred on the highway unless another place is specified, except in the case of accidents involving only off-road motor vehicles which are classified as nontraffic accidents unless the contrary is stated.

(g) A **motor vehicle nontraffic accident** is any motor vehicle accident which occurs entirely in any place other than a public highway.

(h) A **public highway [trafficway]** or **street** is the entire width between property lines [or other boundary lines] of every way or place, of which any part is open to the use of the public for purposes of vehicular traffic as a matter of right or custom. A **roadway** is that part of the public highway designed, improved, and ordinarily used, for vehicular travel.

> **INCLUDES**   approaches (public) to:
> docks
> public building
> station
>
> **EXCLUDES**   *driveway (private)*
> *parking lot*
> *ramp*
> *roads in:*
> *airfield*
> *farm*
> *industrial premises*
> *mine*
> *private grounds*
> *quarry*

---

   ▨▨▨ Fourth-digit Required      ▶◀ Revised Text      ● New Code      ▲ Revised Code Title

(i) A **motor vehicle** is any mechanically or electrically powered device, not operated on rails, upon which any person or property may be transported or drawn upon a highway. Any object such as a trailer, coaster, sled, or wagon being towed by a motor vehicle is considerd a part of the motor vehicle.

INCLUDES automobile [any type]
bus
construction machinery, farm and industrial machinery, steam roller, tractor, army tank, highway grader, or similar vehicle on wheels or treads, while in transport under own power
fire engine (motorized)
motorcycle
motorized bicycle [moped] or scooter
trolley bus not operating on rails
truck
van

EXCLUDES *devices used solely to move persons or materials within the confines of a building and its premises, such as:*
*building elevator*
*coal car in mine*
*electric baggage or mail truck used solely within a railroad station*
*electric truck used solely within an industrial plant*
*moving overhead crane*

(j) A **motorcycle** is a two-wheeled motor vehicle having one or two riding saddles and sometimes having a third wheel for the support of a sidecar. The sidecar is considered part of the motorcycle.

INCLUDES motorized:
bicycle [moped]
scooter
tricycle

(k) An **off-road motor vehicle** is a motor vehicle of special design, to enable it to negotiate rough or soft terrain or snow. Examples of special design are high construction, special wheels and tires, driven by treads, or support on a cushion of air.

INCLUDES all terrain vehicle [ATV]
army tank
hovercraft, on land or swamp
snowmobile

(l) A **driver** of a motor vehicle is the occupant of the motor vehicle operating it or intending to operate it. A **motorcyclist** is the driver of a motorcycle. Other authorized occupants of a motor vehicle are **passengers**.

(m) An **other road vehicle** is any device, except a motor vehicle, in, on, or by which any person or property may be transported on a highway.

INCLUDES animal carrying a person or goods
animal-drawn vehicles
animal harnessed to conveyance
bicycle [pedal cycle]
streetcar
tricycle (pedal)

EXCLUDES *pedestrian conveyance [definition (q)]*

(n) A **streetcar** is a device designed and used primarily for transporting persons within a municipality, running on rails, usually subject to normal traffic control signals, and operated principally on a right-of-way that forms part of the traffic way. A trailer being towed by a streetcar is considered a part of the streetcar.

INCLUDES interurban or intraurban electric or streetcar, when specified to be operating on a street or public highway
tram (car)
trolley (car)

(o) A **pedal cycle** is any road transport vehicle operated solely by pedals.

INCLUDES bicycle
pedal cycle
tricycle

EXCLUDES *motorized bicycle [definition (i)]*

(p) A **pedal cyclist** is any person riding on a pedal cycle or in a sidecar attached to such a vehicle.

(q) A **pedestrian conveyance** is any human powered device by which a pedestrian may move other than by walking or by which a walking person may move another pedestrian.

INCLUDES baby carriage
coaster wagon
ice skates
perambulator
pushcart
pushchair
roller skates
scooter
skateboard
skis
sled
wheelchair

(r) A **pedestrian** is any person involved in an accident who was not at the time of the accident riding in or on a motor vehicle, railroad train, streetcar, animal-drawn or other vehicle, or on a bicycle or animal.

INCLUDES person:
changing tire of vehicle
in or operating a pedestrian conveyance
making adjustment to motor of vehicle
on foot

(s) A **watercraft** is any device for transporting passengers or goods on the water.

(t) A **small boat** is any watercraft propelled by paddle, oars, or small motor, with a passenger capacity of less than ten.

INCLUDES boat NOS
canoe
coble
dinghy
punt
raft
rowboat
rowing shell
scull
skiff
small motorboat

EXCLUDES *barge*
*lifeboat (used after abandoning ship)*
*raft (anchored) being used as a diving platform*
*yacht*

(u) An **aircraft** is any device for transporting passengers or goods in the air.

INCLUDES airplane [any type]
balloon
bomber
dirigible
glider (hang)
military aircraft
parachute

(v) A **commercial transport aircraft** is any device for collective passenger or freight transportation by air, whether run on commercial lines for profit or by government authorities, with the exception of military craft.

---

4ᵗʰ Fourth-digit Required ▶◀ Revised Text ● New Code ▲ Revised Code Title

**E Codes**

**E800–E811**

## RAILWAY ACCIDENTS (E800-E807)

Note: For definitions of railway accident and related terms see definitions (a) to (d).

**EXCLUDES** *accidents involving railway train and:*
*aircraft (E840.0-E845.9)*
*motor vehicle (E810.0-E825.9)*
*watercraft (E830.0-E838.9)*

The following fourth-digit subdivisions are for use with categories E800-E807 to identify the injured person:

**.0 Railway employee**
Any person who by virtue of his employment in connection with a railway, whether by the railway company or not, is at increased risk of involvement in a railway accident, such as:
catering staff of train
driver
guard
porter
postal staff on train
railway fireman
shunter
sleeping car attendant

**.1 Passenger on railway**
Any authorized person traveling on a train, except a railway employee.

**EXCLUDES** *intending passenger waiting at station (.8)*
*unauthorized rider on railway vehicle (.8)*

**.2 Pedestrian**
See definition (r)

**.3 Pedal cyclist**
See definition (p)

**.8 Other specified person**
Intending passenger or bystander waiting at station
Unauthorized rider on railway vehicle

**.9 Unspecified person**

✓4ᵗʰ **E800 Railway accident involving collision with rolling stock**
**INCLUDES** collision between railway trains or railway vehicles, any kind
collision NOS on railway
derailment with antecedent collision with rolling stock or NOS

✓4ᵗʰ **E801 Railway accident involving collision with other object**
**INCLUDES** collision of railway train with:
buffers
fallen tree on railway
gates
platform
rock on railway
streetcar
other nonmotor vehicle
other object

**EXCLUDES** *collision with:*
*aircraft (E840.0-E842.9)*
*motor vehicle (E810.0-E810.9, E820.0-E822.9)*

✓4ᵗʰ **E802 Railway accident involving derailment without antecedent collision**

✓4ᵗʰ **E803 Railway accident involving explosion, fire, or burning**
**EXCLUDES** *explosion or fire, with antecedent derailment (E802.0-E802.9)*
*explosion or fire, with mention of antecedent collision (E800.0-E801.9)*

✓4ᵗʰ **E804 Fall in, on, or from railway train**
**INCLUDES** fall while alighting from or boarding railway train
**EXCLUDES** *fall related to collision, derailment, or explosion of railway train (E800.0-E803.9)*

✓4ᵗʰ **E805 Hit by rolling stock**
**INCLUDES** crushed
injured
killed            } by railway train or part
knocked down
run over

**EXCLUDES** *pedestrian hit by object set in motion by railway train (E806.0-E806.9)*

✓4ᵗʰ **E806 Other specified railway accident**
**INCLUDES** hit by object falling in railway train
injured by door or window on railway train
nonmotor road vehicle or pedestrian hit by object set in motion by railway train
railway train hit by falling:
earth NOS
rock
tree
other object

**EXCLUDES** *railway accident due to cataclysm (E908-E909)*

✓4ᵗʰ **E807 Railway accident of unspecified nature**
**INCLUDES** found dead   } on railway right-of-way NOS
injured

railway accident NOS

## MOTOR VEHICLE TRAFFIC ACCIDENTS (E810-E819)

Note: For definitions of motor vehicle traffic accident, and related terms, see definitions (e) to (k).

**EXCLUDES** *accidents involving motor vehicle and aircraft (E840.0-E845.9)*

The following fourth-digit subdivisions are for use with categories E810-E819 to identify the injured person:

**.0 Driver of motor vehicle other than motorcycle**
See definition (1)

**.1 Passenger in motor vehicle other than motorcycle**
See definition (1)

**.2 Motorcyclist**
See definition (1)

**.3 Passenger on motorcycle**
See definition (1)

**.4 Occupant of streetcar**

**.5 Rider of animal; occupant of animal-drawn vehicle**

**.6 Pedal cyclist**
See definition (p)

**.7 Pedestrian**
See definition (r)

**.8 Other specified person**
Occupant of vehicle other than above
Person in railway train involved in accident
Unauthorized rider of motor vehicle

**.9 Unspecified person**

✓4ᵗʰ **E810 Motor vehicle traffic accident involving collision with train**
**EXCLUDES** *motor vehicle collision with object set in motion by railway train (E815.0-E815.9)*
*railway train hit by object set in motion by motor vehicle (E818.0-E818.9)*

✓4ᵗʰ **E811 Motor vehicle traffic accident involving re-entrant collision with another motor vehicle**
**INCLUDES** collision between motor vehicle which accidentally leaves the roadway then re-enters the same roadway, or the opposite roadway on a divided highway, and another motor vehicle
**EXCLUDES** *collision on the same roadway when none of the motor vehicles involved have left and re-entered the highway (E812.0-E812.9)*

---

✓4ᵗʰ Fourth-digit Required    ▶◀ Revised Text    ● New Code    ▲ Revised Code Title

§ ☑4ᵗʰ **E812 Other motor vehicle traffic accident involving collision with motor vehicle**

INCLUDES   collision with another motor vehicle parked, stopped, stalled, disabled, or abandoned on the highway
motor vehicle collision NOS

EXCLUDES   *collision with object set in motion by another motor vehicle (E815.0-E815.9)*
*re-entrant collision with another motor vehicle (E811.0-E811.9)*

§ ☑4ᵗʰ **E813 Motor vehicle traffic accident involving collision with other vehicle**

INCLUDES   collision between motor vehicle, any kind, and:
other road (nonmotor transport) vehicle, such as:
animal carrying a person
animal-drawn vehicle
pedal cycle
streetcar

EXCLUDES   *collision with:*
*object set in motion by nonmotor road vehicle (E815.0-E815.9)*
*pedestrian (E814.0-E814.9)*
*nonmotor road vehicle hit by object set in motion by motor vehicle (E818.0-E818.9)*

§ ☑4ᵗʰ **E814 Motor vehicle traffic accident involving collision with pedestrian**

INCLUDES   collision between motor vehicle, any kind, and pedestrian
pedestrian dragged, hit, or run over by motor vehicle, any kind

EXCLUDES   *pedestrian hit by object set in motion by motor vehicle (E818.0-E818.9)*

§ ☑4ᵗʰ **E815 Other motor vehicle traffic accident involving collision on the highway**

INCLUDES   collision (due to loss of control) (on highway) between motor vehicle, any kind, and:
abutment (bridge) (overpass)
animal (herded) (unattended)
fallen stone, traffic sign, tree, utility pole
guard rail or boundary fence
interhighway divider
landslide (not moving)
object set in motion by railway train or road vehicle (motor) (nonmotor)
object thrown in front of motor vehicle
other object, fixed, movable, or moving
safety island
temporary traffic sign or marker
wall of cut made for road

EXCLUDES   *collision with:*
*any object off the highway (resulting from loss of control) (E816.0-E816.9)*
*any object which normally would have been off the highway and is not stated to have been on it (E816.0-E816.9)*
*motor vehicle parked, stopped, stalled, disabled, or abandoned on highway (E812.0-E812.9)*
*moving landslide (E909)*
*motor vehicle hit by object:*
*set in motion by railway train or road vehicle (motor) (nonmotor) (E818.0-E818.9)*
*thrown into or on vehicle (E818.0-E818.9)*

§ ☑4ᵗʰ **E816 Motor vehicle traffic accident due to loss of control, without collision on the highway**

INCLUDES   motor vehicle:
failing to make curve ⎤ and:
going out of control ⎟ coliding with
(due to): ⎟ object off
blowout ⎟ the high-
burst tire ⎬ way
driver falling ⎟ overturning
asleep ⎟ stopping
driver inattention ⎟ abruptly
excessive speed ⎟ off the
failure of mech- ⎦ highway
anical part

EXCLUDES   *collision on highway following loss of control (E810.0-E815.9)*
*loss of control of motor vehicle following collision on the highway (E810.0-E815.9)*

§ ☑4ᵗʰ **E817 Noncollision motor vehicle traffic accident while boarding or alighting**

INCLUDES   fall down stairs of motor bus ⎤
fall from car in street ⎟
injured by moving part of ⎬ while boarding
the vehicle ⎟ or alighting
trapped by door of motor ⎦
bus

§ ☑4ᵗʰ **E818 Other noncollision motor vehicle traffic accident**

INCLUDES   accidental poisoning from exhaust gas generated by ⎤
breakage of any part of ⎟
explosion of any part of ⎟
fall, jump, or being ⎟
accidentally pushed ⎟
from ⎟
fire starting in ⎬ motor vehicle
hit by object thrown into or ⎟ while
on ⎟ in
injured by being thrown ⎟ motion
against some part of, or ⎟
object in ⎟
injury from moving part of ⎦
object falling in or on
object thrown on

collision of railway train or road vehicle except motor vehicle, with object set in motion by motor vehicle
motor vehicle hit by object set in motion by railway train or road vehicle (motor) (nonmotor)
pedestrian, railway train, or road vehicle (motor) (nonmotor) hit by object set in motion by motor vehicle

EXCLUDES   *collision between motor vehicle and:*
*object set in motion by railway train or road vehicle (motor) (nonmotor) (E815.0-E815.9)*
*object thrown towards the motor vehicle (E815.0-E815.9)*
*person overcome by carbon monoxide generated by stationary motor vehicle off the roadway with motor running (E868.2)*

§ ☑4ᵗʰ **E819 Motor vehicle traffic accident of unspecified nature**

INCLUDES   motor vehicle traffic accident NOS
traffic accident NOS

---

§ Requires fourth-digit. See beginning of section E810-E819 for codes and definitions.

☑4ᵗʰ Fourth-digit Required    ▶◀ Revised Text    ● New Code    ▲ Revised Code Title

## MOTOR VEHICLE NONTRAFFIC ACCIDENTS (E820-E825)

Note: For definitions of motor vehicle nontraffic accident and related terms see definition (a) to (k).

INCLUDES    accidents involving motor vehicles being used in recreational or sporting activities off the highway

collision and noncollision motor vehicle accidents occurring entirely off the highway

EXCLUDES    *accidents involving motor vehicle and:*
*aircraft (E840.0-E845.9)*
*watercraft (E830.0-E838.9)*
*accidents, not on the public highway, involving agricultural and construction machinery but not involving another motor vehicle (E919.0, E919.2, E919.7)*

The following fourth-digit subdivisions are for use with categories E820-E825 to identify the injured person:

**.0 Driver of motor vehicle other than motorcycle**
See definition (l)

**.1 Passenger in motor vehicle other than motorcycle**
See definition (l)

**.2 Motorcyclist**
See definition (l)

**.3 Passenger on motorcycle**
See definition (l)

**.4 Occupant of streetcar**

**.5 Rider of animal; occupant of animal-drawn vehicle**

**.6 Pedal cyclist**
See definition (p)

**.7 Pedestrian**
See definition (r)

**.8 Other specified person**
Occupant of vehicle other than above
Person on railway train involved in accident
Unauthorized rider of motor vehicle

**.9 Unspecified person**

√4ᵗʰ **E820 Nontraffic accident involving motor-driven snow vehicle**

INCLUDES    breakage of part of
fall from
hit by     } motor-driven snow vehicle (not on public highway)
overturning of
run over or dragged by

collision of motor-driven snow vehicle with:
animal (being ridden) (-drawn vehicle)
another off-road motor vehicle
other motor vehicle, not on public highway
railway train
other object, fixed or movable
injury caused by rough landing of motor-driven snow vehicle (after leaving ground on rough terrain)

EXCLUDES    *accident on the public highway involving motor driven snow vehicle (E810.0-E819.9)*

√4ᵗʰ **E821 Nontraffic accident involving other off-road motor vehicle**

INCLUDES    breakage of part of
fall from
hit by
overturning of    } off-road motor vehicle, except snow vehicle (not on public highway)
run over or dragged by
thrown against some
part of or object in

collision with:
animal (being ridden) (-drawn vehicle)
another off-road motor vehicle, except snow vehicle
other motor vehicle, not on public highway
other object, fixed or movable

EXCLUDES    *accident on public highway involving off-road motor vehicle (E810.0-E819.9)*
*collision between motor driven snow vehicle and other off-road motor vehicle (E820.0-E820.9)*
*hovercraft accident on water (E830.0-E838.9)*

√4ᵗʰ **E822 Other motor vehicle nontraffic accident involving collision with moving object**

INCLUDES    collision, not on public highway, between motor vehicle, except off-road motor vehicle and:
animal
nonmotor vehicle
other motor vehicle, except off-road motor vehicle
pedestrian
railway train
other moving object

EXCLUDES    *collision with:*
*motor-driven snow vehicle (E820.0-E820.9)*
*other off-road motor vehicle (E821.0-E821.9)*

√4ᵗʰ **E823 Other motor vehicle nontraffic accident involving collision with stationary object**

INCLUDES    collision, not on public highway, between motor vehicle, except off-road motor vehicle, and any object, fixed or movable, but not in motion

√4ᵗʰ **E824 Other motor vehicle nontraffic accident while boarding and alighting**

INCLUDES    fall
injury from moving part of motor vehicle    } while boarding or alighting from motor vehicle, except off-road motor vehicle, not on public highway
trapped by door of motor vehicle

**E Codes**

**E825–E829**

§ ✓4ᵀᴴ **E825 Other motor vehicle nontraffic accident of other and unspecified nature**

INCLUDES

accidental poisoning from carbon monoxide generated by
breakage of any part of
explosion of any part of
fall, jump, or being accidentally pushed from }
fire starting in
hit by object thrown into, towards, or on
injured by being thrown against some part of, or object in
injury from moving part of
object falling in or on } motor vehicle while in motion, not on public highway

motor vehicle nontraffic accident NOS

EXCLUDES

*fall from or in stationary motor vehicle (E884.9, E885.9)*

*overcome by carbon monoxide or exhaust gas generated by stationary motor vehicle off the roadway with motor running (E868.2)*

*struck by falling object from or in stationary motor vehicle (E916)*

## OTHER ROAD VEHICLE ACCIDENTS (E826-E829)

Note: Other road vehicle accidents are transport accidents involving road vehicles other than motor vehicles. For definitions of other road vehicle and related terms see definitions (m) to (o).

INCLUDES

accidents involving other road vehicles being used in recreational or sporting activities

EXCLUDES

*collision of other road vehicle [any] with:*
  *aircraft (E840.0-E845.9)*
  *motor vehicle (E813.0-E813.9, E820.0-E822.9)*
  *railway train (E801.0-E801.9)*

The following fourth-digit subdivisions are for use with categories E826-E829 to identify the injured person.

    **.0 Pedestrian**
      See definition (r)
    **.1 Pedal cyclist**
      See definition (p)
    **.2 Rider of animal**
    **.3 Occupant of animal-drawn vehicle**
    **.4 Occupant of streetcar**
    **.8 Other specified person**
    **.9 Unspecified person**

✓4ᵀᴴ **E826 Pedal cycle accident**

[0-9]   INCLUDES

breakage of any part of pedal cycle
collision between pedal cycle and:
  animal (being ridden) (herded) (unattended)
  another pedal cycle
  any pedestrian
  nonmotor road vehicle
  other object, fixed, movable, or moving, not set in motion by motor vehicle, railway train, or aircraft
entanglement in wheel of pedal cycle
fall from pedal cycle
hit by object falling or thrown on the pedal cycle
pedal cycle accident NOS
pedal cycle overturned

✓4ᵀᴴ **E827 Animal-drawn vehicle accident**

[0,2-4,8,9]   INCLUDES

breakage of any part of vehicle
collision between animal-drawn vehicle and:
  animal (being ridden) (herded) (unattended)
  nonmotor road vehicle, except pedal cycle
  pedestrian, pedestrian conveyance, or pedestrian vehicle
  other object, fixed, movable, or moving, not set in motion by motor vehicle, railway train, or aircraft

fall from
knocked down by
overturning of } animal-drawn vehicle
run over by
thrown from

EXCLUDES

*collision of animal-drawn vehicle with pedal cycle (E826.0-E826.9)*

✓4ᵀᴴ **E828 Accident involving animal being ridden**

[0,2,4,8,9]   INCLUDES

collision between animal being ridden and:
  another animal
  nonmotor road vehicle, except pedal cycle, and animal-drawn vehicle
  pedestrian, pedestrian conveyance, or pedestrian vehicle
  other object, fixed, movable, or moving, not set in motion by motor vehicle, railway train, or aircraft

fall from
knocked down by
thrown from } animal being ridden
trampled by

ridden animal stumbled and fell

EXCLUDES

*collision of animal being ridden with:*
  *animal-drawn vehicle (E827.0-E827.9)*
  *pedal cycle (E826.0-E826.9)*

✓4ᵀᴴ **E829 Other road vehicle accidents**

[0,4,8,9]   INCLUDES

accident while
  boarding or
  alighting from
blow from object in
breakage of any part of
caught in door of-
derailment of
fall in, on, or from
fire in } streetcar nonmotor road vehicle not classifiable to E826-E828

collision between streetcar or nonmotor road vehicle, except as in E826-E828, and:
  animal (not being ridden)
  another nonmotor road vehicle not classifiable to E826-E828
  pedestrian
  other object, fixed, movable, or moving, not set in motion by motor vehicle, railway train, or aircraft
nonmotor road vehicle accident NOS
streetcar accident NOS

EXCLUDES

*collision with:*
  *animal being ridden (E828.0-E828.9)*
  *animal-drawn vehicle (E827.0-E827.9)*
  *pedal cycle (E826.0-E826.9)*

---

§ Requires fourth-digit. Valid digits are in [brackets] under each code. See beginning of section E820-E825 for codes and definitions.

## WATER TRANSPORT ACCIDENTS (E830-E838)

Note: For definitions of water transport accident and related terms see definitions (a), (s), and (t).

> INCLUDES   watercraft accidents in the course of recreational activities

> EXCLUDES   *accidents involving both aircraft, including objects set in motion by aircraft, and watercraft (E840.0-E845.9)*

The following fourth-digit subdivisions are for use with categories E830-E838 to identify the injured person:

**.0 Occupant of small boat, unpowered**

**.1 Occupant of small boat, powered**
See definition (t)

> EXCLUDES   water skier (.4)

**.2 Occupant of other watercraft — crew**
Persons:
    engaged in operation of watercraft
    providing passenger services [cabin attendants, ship's physician, catering personnel]
    working on ship during voyage in other capacity [musician in band, operators of shops and beauty parlors]

**.3 Occupant of other watercraft — other than crew**
Passenger
Occupant of lifeboat, other than crew, after abandoning ship

**.4 Water skier**

**.5 Swimmer**

**.6 Dockers, stevedores**
Longshoreman employed on the dock in loading and unloading ships

**.8 Other specified person**
Immigration and custom officials on board ship
Person:
    accompanying passenger or member of crew visiting boat
Pilot (guiding ship into port)

**.9 Unspecified person**

### ✓4ᵗʰ E830 Accident to watercraft causing submersion

> INCLUDES   submersion and drowning due to:
> boat overturning
> boat submerging
> falling or jumping from burning ship
> falling or jumping from crushed watercraft
> ship sinking
> other accident to watercraft

### ✓4ᵗʰ E831 Accident to watercraft causing other injury

> INCLUDES   any injury, except submersion and drowning, as a result of an accident to watercraft
> burned while ship on fire
> crushed between ships in collision
> crushed by lifeboat after abandoning ship
> fall due to collision or other accident to watercraft
> hit by falling object due to accident to watercraft
> injured in watercraft accident involving collision
> struck by boat or part thereof after fall or jump from damaged boat

> EXCLUDES   *burns from localized fire or explosion on board ship (E837.0-E837.9)*

### ✓4ᵗʰ E832 Other accidental submersion or drowning in water transport accident

> INCLUDES   submersion or drowning as a result of an accident other than accident to the watercraft, such as:
> fall:
>     from gangplank
>     from ship
>     overboard
> thrown overboard by motion of ship
> washed overboard

> EXCLUDES   *submersion or drowning of swimmer or diver who voluntarily jumps from boat not involved in an accident (E910.0-E910.9)*

### ✓4ᵗʰ E833 Fall on stairs or ladders in water transport

> EXCLUDES   *fall due to accident to watercraft (E831.0-E831.9)*

### ✓4ᵗʰ E834 Other fall from one level to another in water transport

> EXCLUDES   *fall due to accident to watercraft (E831.0-E831.9)*

### ✓4ᵗʰ E835 Other and unspecified fall in water transport

> EXCLUDES   *fall due to accident to watercraft (E831.0-E831.9)*

### ✓4ᵗʰ E836 Machinery accident in water transport

> INCLUDES   injuries in water transport caused by:
> deck
> engine room
> galley     } machinery
> laundry
> loading

### ✓4ᵗʰ E837 Explosion, fire, or burning in watercraft

> INCLUDES   explosion of boiler on steamship
> localized fire on ship

> EXCLUDES   *burning ship (due to collision or explosion) resulting in:*
> *submersion or drowning (E830.0-E830.9)*
> *other injury (E831.0-E831.9)*

### ✓4ᵗʰ E838 Other and unspecified water transport accident

> INCLUDES   accidental poisoning by gases or fumes on ship
> atomic power plant malfunction in watercraft
> crushed between ship and stationary object [wharf]
> crushed between ships without accident to watercraft
> crushed by falling object on ship or while loading or unloading
> hit by boat while water skiing
> struck by boat or part thereof (after fall from boat)
> watercraft accident NOS

## AIR AND SPACE TRANSPORT ACCIDENTS (E840-E845)

Note: For definition of aircraft and related terms see definitions (u) and (v).

The following fourth-digit subdivisions are for use with categories E840-E845 to identify the injured person. Valid fourth digits are in [brackets] under codes E842-E845.

**.0 Occupant of spacecraft**

**.1 Occupant of military aircraft, any**
Crew in military aircraft [air force] [army] [national guard] [navy]
Passenger (civilian) (military) in military aircraft [air force] [army] [national guard] [navy]
Troops in military aircraft [air force] [army] [national guard] [navy]

EXCLUDES *occupants of aircraft operated under jurisdiction of police departments (.5)*
*parachutist (.7)*

**.2 Crew of commercial aircraft (powered) in surface to surface transport**

**.3 Other occupant of commercial aircraft (powered) in surface to surface transport**
Flight personnel:
not part of crew
on familiarization flight
Passenger on aircraft (powered) NOS

**.4 Occupant of commercial aircraft (powered) in surface to air transport**
Occupant [crew] [passenger] of aircraft (powered) engaged in activities, such as:
aerial spraying (crops) (fire retardants)
air drops of emergency supplies
air drops of parachutists, except from military craft
crop dusting
lowering of construction material [bridge or telephone pole]
sky writing

**.5 Occupant of other powered aircraft**
Occupant [crew][passenger] of aircraft [powered] engaged in activities, such as:
aerobatic flying
aircraft racing
rescue operation
storm surveillance
traffic surveillance
Occupant of private plane NOS

**.6 Occupant of unpowered aircraft, except parachutist**
Occupant of aircraft classifiable to E842

**.7 Parachutist (military) (other)**
Person making voluntary descent
EXCLUDES *person making descent after accident to aircraft (.1-.6)*

**.8 Ground crew, airline employee**
Persons employed at airfields (civil) (military) or launching pads, not occupants of aircraft

**.9 Other person**

✓4ᵗʰ **E840 Accident to powered aircraft at takeoff or landing**

INCLUDES
collision of aircraft with any object, fixed, movable, or moving ┐
crash                    │ while taking
explosion on aircraft    │ off or
fire on aircraft         │ landing
forced landing ┘

✓4ᵗʰ **E841 Accident to powered aircraft, other and unspecified**

INCLUDES
aircraft accident NOS
aircraft crash or wreck NOS
any accident to powered aircraft while in transit or when not specified whether in transit, taking off, or landing
collision of aircraft with another aircraft, bird, or any object, while in transit
explosion on aircraft while in transit
fire on aircraft while in transit

✓4ᵗʰ **E842 Accident to unpowered aircraft**
[6-9]   INCLUDES
any accident, except collision with powered aircraft, to:
balloon
glider
hang glider
kite carrying a person
hit by object falling from unpowered aircraft

✓4ᵗʰ **E843 Fall in, on, or from aircraft**
[0-9]   INCLUDES
accident in boarding or alighting from aircraft, any kind
fall in, on, or from aircraft [any kind], while in transit, taking off, or landing, except when as a result of an accident to aircraft

✓4ᵗʰ **E844 Other specified air transport accidents**
[0-9]   INCLUDES
hit by:
aircraft
object falling from aircraft ┐
injury by or from:              │
machinery on aircraft          │ without
rotating propeller             │ accident
voluntary parachute descent    │ to aircraft
poisoning by carbon monoxide from aircraft while in transit │
sucked into jet ┘
any accident involving other transport vehicle (motor) (nonmotor) due to being hit by object set in motion by aircraft (powered)

EXCLUDES *air sickness (E903)*
*effects of:*
*high altitude (E902.0-E902.1)*
*pressure change (E902.0-E902.1)*
*injury in parachute descent due to accident to aircraft (E840.0-E842-9)*

✓4ᵗʰ **E845 Accident involving spacecraft**
[0,8,9]   INCLUDES   launching pad accident
EXCLUDES *effects of weightlessness in spacecraft (E928.0)*

---

✓4ᵗʰ Fourth-digit Required        ▶◀ Revised Text        ● New Code        ▲ Revised Code Title

## VEHICLE ACCIDENTS NOT ELSEWHERE CLASSIFIABLE (E846-E848)

**E846 Accidents involving powered vehicles used solely within the buildings and premises of industrial or commercial establishment**

Accident to, on, or involving:
> battery powered airport passenger vehicle
> battery powered trucks (baggage) (mail)
> coal car in mine
> logging car
> self propelled truck, industrial
> station baggage truck (powered)
> tram, truck, or tub (powered) in mine or quarry

Collision with:
> pedestrian
> other vehicle or object within premises

Explosion of    ⎫
Fall from       ⎬ powered vehicle, industrial
Overturning of   ⎪     or commercial
Struck by      ⎭

> **EXCLUDES**    accidental poisoning by exhaust gas from vehicle not elsewhere classifiable (E868.2)
>               injury by crane, lift (fork), or elevator (E919.2)

**E847 Accidents involving cable cars not running on rails**

Accident to, on, or involving:
> cable car, not on rails
> ski chair-lift
> ski-lift with gondola
> téléférique

Breakage of cable
Caught or dragged by    ⎫
Fall or jump from        ⎬ cable car, not on rails
Object thrown from or in  ⎭

**E848 Accidents involving other vehicles, not elsewhere classifiable**

Accident to, on, or involving:
> ice yacht
> land yacht
> nonmotor, nonroad vehicle NOS

**✓4ᵗʰ E849 Place of occurrence**

> The following category is for use to denote the place where the injury or poisoning occurred.

**E849.0 Home**

| | |
|---|---|
| Apartment | Private: |
| Boarding house | garage |
| Farm house | garden |
| Home premises | home |
| House (residential) | walk |
| Noninstitutional | Swimming pool in private |
|    place of residence |    house or garden |
| Private: | Yard of home |
|    driveway | |

> **EXCLUDES**    home under construction but not yet occupied (E849.3)
>               institutional place of residence (E849.7)

**E849.1 Farm**

Farm:
> buildings
> land under cultivation

> **EXCLUDES**    farm house and home premises of farm (E849.0)

**E849.2 Mine and quarry**

| | |
|---|---|
| Gravel pit | Tunnel under |
| Sand pit |    construction |

**E849.3 Industrial place and premises**

| | |
|---|---|
| Building under | Industrial yard |
|    construction | Loading platform (factory) |
| Dockyard |    (store) |
| Dry dock | Plant, industrial |
| Factory | Railway yard |
|    building | Shop (place of work) |
|    premises | Warehouse |
| Garage (place of work) | Workhouse |

**E849.4 Place for recreation and sport**

| | |
|---|---|
| Amusement park | Public park |
| Baseball field | Racecourse |
| Basketball court | Resort NOS |
| Beach resort | Riding school |
| Cricket ground | Rifle range |
| Fives court | Seashore resort |
| Football field | Skating rink |
| Golf course | Sports palace |
| Gymnasium | Stadium |
| Hockey field | Swimming pool, public |
| Holiday camp | Tennis court |
| Ice palace | Vacation resort |
| Lake resort | |
| Mountain resort | |
| Playground, including school playground | |

> **EXCLUDES**    that in private house or garden (E849.0)

**E849.5 Street and highway**

**E849.6 Public building**

> Building (including adjacent grounds) used by the general public or by a particular group of the public, such as:

| | |
|---|---|
| airport | music hall |
| bank | nightclub |
| café | office |
| casino | office building |
| church | opera house |
| cinema | post office |
| clubhouse | public hall |
| courthouse | radio broadcasting station |
| dance hall | restaurant |
| garage building (for | school (state) (public) |
|    car storage) |    (private) |
| hotel | shop, commercial |
| market (grocery or | station (bus) (railway) |
|    other | store |
|    commodity) | theater |
| movie house | |

> **EXCLUDES**    home garage (E849.0)
>               industrial building or workplace (E849.3)

**E849.7 Residential institution**

| | |
|---|---|
| Children's home | Old people's home |
| Dormitory | Orphanage |
| Hospital | Prison |
| Jail | Reform school |

**E849.8 Other specified places**

| | |
|---|---|
| Beach NOS | Pond or pool (natural) |
| Canal | Prairie |
| Caravan site NOS | Public place NOS |
| Derelict house | Railway line |
| Desert | Reservoir |
| Dock | River |
| Forest | Sea |
| Harbor | Seashore NOS |
| Hill | Stream |
| Lake NOS | Swamp |
| Mountain | Trailer court |
| Parking lot | Woods |
| Parking place | |

**E849.9 Unspecified place**

## ACCIDENTAL POISONING BY DRUGS, MEDICINAL SUBSTANCES, AND BIOLOGICALS (E850-E858)

**INCLUDES**    accidental overdose of drug, wrong drug given or taken in error, and drug taken inadvertently

accidents in the use of drugs and biologicals in medical and surgical procedures

**EXCLUDES**    *administration with suicidal or homicidal intent or intent to harm, or in circumstances classifiable to E980-E989 (E950.0-E950.5, E962.0, E980.0-E980.5)*

*correct drug properly administered in therapeutic or prophylactic dosage, as the cause of adverse effect (E930.0-E949.9)*

See Alphabetic Index for more complete list of specific drugs to be classified under the fourth-digit subdivisions. The American Hospital Formulary numbers can be used to classify new drugs listed by the American Hospital Formulary Service (AHFS). See Appendix C.

**✓4ᵗʰ E850 Accidental poisoning by analgesics, antipyretics, and antirheumatics**

**E850.0 Heroin**
Diacetylmorphine

**E850.1 Methadone**

**E850.2 Other opiates and related narcotics**
Codeine [methylmorphine]    Morphine
Meperidine [pethidine]    Opium (alkaloids)

**E850.3 Salicylates**
Acetylsalicylic acid [aspirin]
Amino derivatives of salicylic acid
Salicylic acid salts

**E850.4 Aromatic analgesics, not elsewhere classified**
Acetanilid
Paracetamol [acetaminophen]
Phenacetin [acetophenetidin]

**E850.5 Pyrazole derivatives**
Aminophenazone [amidopyrine]
Phenylbutazone

**E850.6 Antirheumatics [antiphlogistics]**
Gold salts    Indomethacin
     **EXCLUDES**    *salicylates (E850.3)*
               *steroids (E858.0)*

**E850.7 Other non-narcotic analgesics**
Pyrabital

**E850.8 Other specified analgesics and antipyretics**
Pentazocine

**E850.9 Unspecified analgesic or antipyretic**

**E851 Accidental poisoning by barbiturates**
Amobarbital [amylobarbitone]    Pentobarbital [pentobarbitone]
Barbital [barbitone]    Phenobarbital [phenobarbitone]
Butabarbital [butabarbitone]    Secobarbital [quinalbarbitone]
     **EXCLUDES**    *thiobarbiturates (E855.1)*

**✓4ᵗʰ E852 Accidental poisoning by other sedatives and hypnotics**

**E852.0 Chloral hydrate group**

**E852.1 Paraldehyde**

**E852.2 Bromine compounds**
Bromides    Carbromal (derivatives)

**E852.3 Methaqualone compounds**

**E852.4 Glutethimide group**

**E852.5 Mixed sedatives, not elsewhere classified**

**E852.8 Other specified sedatives and hypnotics**

**E852.9 Unspecified sedative or hypnotic**
Sleeping:
   drug ⎫
   pill  ⎬ NOS
   tablet ⎭

**✓4ᵗʰ E853 Accidental poisoning by tranquilizers**

**E853.0 Phenothiazine-based tranquilizers**
Chlorpromazine    Prochlorperazine
Fluphenazine    Promazine

**E853.1 Butyrophenone-based tranquilizers**
Haloperidol    Trifluperidol
Spiperone

**E853.2 Benzodiazepine-based tranquilizers**
Chlordiazepoxide    Lorazepam
Diazepam    Medazepam
Flurazepam    Nitrazepam

**E853.8 Other specified tranquilizers**
Hydroxyzine    Meprobamate

**E853.9 Unspecified tranquilizer**

**✓4ᵗʰ E854 Accidental poisoning by other psychotropic agents**

**E854.0 Antidepressants**
Amitriptyline
Imipramine
Monoamine oxidase [MAO] inhibitors

**E854.1 Psychodysleptics [hallucinogens]**
Cannabis derivatives    Mescaline
Lysergide [LSD]    Psilocin
Marihuana (derivatives)    Psilocybin

**E854.2 Psychostimulants**
Amphetamine    Caffeine
     **EXCLUDES**    *central appetite depressants (E858.8)*

**E854.3 Central nervous system stimulants**
Analeptics    Opiate antagonists

**E854.8 Other psychotropic agents**

**✓4ᵗʰ E855 Accidental poisoning by other drugs acting on central and autonomic nervous system**

**E855.0 Anticonvulsant and anti-Parkinsonism drugs**
Amantadine
Hydantoin derivatives
Levodopa [L-dopa]
Oxazolidine derivatives [paramethadione]
     [trimethadione]
Succinimides

**E855.1 Other central nervous system depressants**
Ether
Gaseous anesthetics
Halogenated hydrocarbon derivatives
Intravenous anesthetics
Thiobarbiturates, such as thiopental sodium

**E855.2 Local anesthetics**
Cocaine    Procaine
Lidocaine [lignocaine]    Tetracaine

**E855.3 Parasympathomimetics [cholinergics]**
Acetylcholine    Pilocarpine
Anticholinesterase:
   organophosphorus
   reversible

**E855.4 Parasympatholytics [anticholinergics and antimuscarinics] and spasmolytics**
Atropine
Homatropine
Hyoscine [scopolamine]
Quaternary ammonium derivatives

**E855.5 Sympathomimetics [adrenergics]**
Epinephrine [adrenalin]
Levarterenol [noradrenalin]

**E855.6 Sympatholytics [antiadrenergics]**
Phenoxybenzamine
Tolazoline hydrochloride

**E855.8 Other specified drugs acting on central and autonomic nervous systems**

**E855.9 Unspecified drug acting on central and autonomic nervous systems**

**E856 Accidental poisoning by antibiotics**

**E857 Accidental poisoning by other anti-infectives**

**✓4ᵗʰ E858 Accidental poisoning by other drugs**

**E858.0 Hormones and synthetic substitutes**

**E858.1 Primarily systemic agents**

**E858.2 Agents primarily affecting blood constituents**

**E858.3 Agents primarily affecting cardiovascular system**

**E858.4 Agents primarily affecting gastrointestinal system**

---

**✓4ᵗʰ** Fourth-digit Required    ▶◀ Revised Text    ● New Code    ▲ Revised Code Title

E858.5   Water, mineral, and uric acid metabolism drugs

E858.6   Agents primarily acting on the smooth and skeletal muscles and respiratory system

E858.7   Agents primarily affecting skin and mucous membrane, ophthalmological, otorhinolaryngological, and dental drugs

E858.8   Other specified drugs
     Central appetite depressants

E858.9   Unspecified drug

## ACCIDENTAL POISONING BY OTHER SOLID AND LIQUID SUBSTANCES, GASES, AND VAPORS (E860-E869)

Note: Categories in this section are intended primarily to indicate the external cause of poisoning states classifiable to 980-989. They may also be used to indicate external causes of localized effects classifiable to 001-799.

✓4ᵗʰ **E860 Accidental poisoning by alcohol, not elsewhere classified**

E860.0   Alcoholic beverages
     Alcohol in preparations intended for consumption

E860.1   Other and unspecified ethyl alcohol and its products

| Denatured alcohol | Grain alcohol NOS |
| Ethanol NOS | Methylated spirit |

E860.2   Methyl alcohol

| Methanol | Wood alcohol |

E860.3   Isopropyl alcohol

| Dimethyl carbinol | Rubbing alcohol subsitute |
| Isopropanol | Secondary propyl alcohol |

E860.4   Fusel oil

| Alcohol: | Alcohol: |
|   amyl |   propyl |
|   butyl | |

E860.8   Other specified alcohols

E860.9   Unspecified alcohol

✓4ᵗʰ **E861 Accidental poisoning by cleansing and polishing agents, disinfectants, paints, and varnishes**

E861.0   Synthetic detergents and shampoos

E861.1   Soap products

E861.2   Polishes

E861.3   Other cleansing and polishing agents
     Scouring powders

E861.4   Disinfectants
     Household and other disinfectants not ordinarily used on the person
     **EXCLUDES**   *carbolic acid or phenol (E864.0)*

E861.5   Lead paints

E861.6   Other paints and varnishes

| Lacquers | Paints, other than lead |
| Oil colors | White washes |

E861.9   Unspecified

✓4ᵗʰ **E862 Accidental poisoning by petroleum products, other solvents and their vapors, not elsewhere classified**

E862.0   Petroleum solvents

| Petroleum: | Petroleum: |
|   ether |   naphtha |
|   benzine | |

E862.1   Petroleum fuels and cleaners
     Antiknock additives to petroleum fuels
     Gas oils
     Gasoline or petrol
     Kerosene
     **EXCLUDES**   *kerosene insecticides (E863.4)*

E862.2   Lubricating oils

E862.3   Petroleum solids
     Paraffin wax

E862.4   Other specified solvents
     Benzene

E862.9   Unspecified solvent

✓4ᵗʰ **E863 Accidental poisoning by agricultural and horticultural chemical and pharmaceutical preparations other than plant foods and fertilizers**

     **EXCLUDES**   *plant foods and fertilizers (E866.5)*

E863.0   Insecticides of organochlorine compounds

| Benzene hexachloride | Dieldrin |
| Chlordane | Endrine |
| DDT | Toxaphene |

E863.1   Insecticides of organophosphorus compounds

| Demeton | Parathion |
| Diazinon | Phenylsulphthion |
| Dichlorvos | Phorate |
| Malathion | Phosdrin |
| Methyl parathion | |

E863.2   Carbamates

| Aldicarb | Propoxur |
| Carbaryl | |

E863.3   Mixtures of insecticides

E863.4   Other and unspecified insecticides
     Kerosene insecticides

E863.5   Herbicides
     2, 4-Dichlorophenoxyacetic acid [2, 4-D]
     2, 4, 5-Trichlorophenoxyacetic acid [2, 4, 5-T]
     Chlorates
     Diquat
     Mixtures of plant foods and fertilizers with herbicides
     Paraquat

E863.6   Fungicides
     Organic mercurials (used in seed dressing)
     Pentachlorophenols

E863.7   Rodenticides

| Fluoroacetates | Warfarin |
| Squill and derivatives | Zinc phosphide |
| Thallium | |

E863.8   Fumigants

| Cyanides | Phosphine |
| Methyl bromide | |

E863.9   Other and unspecified

✓4ᵗʰ **E864 Accidental poisoning by corrosives and caustics, not elsewhere classified**

     **EXCLUDES**   *those as components of disinfectants (E861.4)*

E864.0   Corrosive aromatics
     Carbolic acid or phenol

E864.1   Acids

| Acid: | Acid: |
|   hydrochloric |   sulfuric |
|   nitric | |

E864.2   Caustic alkalis
     Lye

E864.3   Other specified corrosives and caustics

E864.4   Unspecified corrosives and caustics

✓4ᵗʰ **E865 Accidental poisoning from poisonous foodstuffs and poisonous plants**

     **INCLUDES**   any meat, fish, or shellfish
         plants, berries, and fungi eaten as, or in mistake for, food, or by a child

     **EXCLUDES**   *anaphylactic shock due to adverse food reaction (995.60-995.69)*
         *food poisoning (bacterial) (005.0-005.9)*
         *poisoning and toxic reactions to venomous plants (E905.6-E905.7)*

E865.0   Meat

E865.1   Shellfish

E865.2   Other fish

E865.3   Berries and seeds

E865.4   Other specified plants

E865.5   Mushrooms and other fungi

E865.8   Other specified foods

E865.9   Unspecified foodstuff or poisonous plant

---

✓4ᵗʰ Fourth-digit Required     ▶◀ Revised Text     ● New Code     ▲ Revised Code Title

√4ᵗʰ **E866 Accidental poisoning by other and unspecified solid and liquid substances**

> EXCLUDES   these substances as a component of:
> medicines (E850.0-E858.9)
> paints (E861.5-E861.6)
> pesticides (E863.0-E863.9)
> petroleum fuels (E862.1)

E866.0 **Lead and its compounds and fumes**

E866.1 **Mercury and its compounds and fumes**

E866.2 **Antimony and its compounds and fumes**

E866.3 **Arsenic and its compounds and fumes**

E866.4 **Other metals and their compounds and fumes**

> Beryllium (compounds)    Iron (compounds)
> Brass fumes    Manganese (compounds)
> Cadmium (compounds)    Nickel (compounds)
> Copper salts    Thallium (compounds)

E866.5 **Plant foods and fertilizers**

> EXCLUDES   mixtures with herbicides (E863.5)

E866.6 **Glues and adhesives**

E866.7 **Cosmetics**

E866.8 **Other specified solid or liquid substances**

E866.9 **Unspecified solid or liquid substance**

**E867 Accidental poisoning by gas distributed by pipeline**

> Carbon monoxide from incomplete combustion of piped gas
> Coal gas NOS
> Liquefied petroleum gas distributed through pipes (pure or mixed with air)
> Piped gas (natural) (manufactured)

√4ᵗʰ **E868 Accidental poisoning by other utility gas and other carbon monoxide**

E868.0 **Liquefied petroleum gas distributed in mobile containers**

> Butane
> Liquefied hydrocarbon gas NOS  } or carbon monoxide from incomplete conbustion of these gases
> Propane

E868.1 **Other and unspecified utility gas**

> Acetylene
> Gas NOS used for lighting, heating, or cooking  } or carbon monoxide from incomplete conbustion of these gases
> Water gas

E868.2 **Motor vehicle exhaust gas**

> Exhaust gas from:
> farm tractor, not in transit
> gas engine
> motor pump
> motor vehicle, not in transit
> any type of combustion engine not in watercraft

> EXCLUDES   poisoning by carbon monoxide from:
> aircraft while in transit (E844.0-E844.9)
> motor vehicle while in transit (E818.0-E818.9)
> watercraft whether or not in transit (E838.0-E838.9)

E868.3 **Carbon monoxide from incomplete combustion of other domestic fuels**

> Carbon monoxide from incomplete combustion of:
> coal
> coke
> kerosene  } in domestic stove or fireplace
> wood

> EXCLUDES   carbon monoxide from smoke and fumes due to conflagration (E890.0-E893.9)

E868.8 **Carbon monoxide from other sources**

> Carbon monoxide from:
> blast furnace gas
> incomplete combustion of fuels in industrial use
> kiln vapor

E868.9 **Unspecified carbon monoxide**

√4ᵗʰ **E869 Accidental poisoning by other gases and vapors**

> EXCLUDES   effects of gases used as anesthetics (E855.1, E938.2)
> fumes from heavy metals (E866.0-E866.4)
> smoke and fumes due to conflagration or explosion (E890.0-E899)

E869.0 **Nitrogen oxides**

E869.1 **Sulfur dioxide**

E869.2 **Freon**

E869.3 **Lacrimogenic gas [tear gas]**

> Bromobenzyl cyanide    Ethyliodoacetate
> Chloroacetophenone

E869.4 **Second-hand tobacco smoke**

E869.8 **Other specified gases and vapors**

> Chlorine          Hydrocyanic acid gas

E869.9 **Unspecified gases and vapors**

## MISADVENTURES TO PATIENTS DURING SURGICAL AND MEDICAL CARE (E870-E876)

> EXCLUDES   accidental overdose of drug and wrong drug given in error (E850.0-E858.9)
> surgical and medical procedures as the cause of abnormal reaction by the patient, without mention of misadventure at the time of procedure (E878.0-E879.9)

√4ᵗʰ **E870 Accidental cut, puncture, perforation, or hemorrhage during medical care**

E870.0 **Surgical operation**

E870.1 **Infusion or transfusion**

E870.2 **Kidney dialysis or other perfusion**

E870.3 **Injection or vaccination**

E870.4 **Endoscopic examination**

E870.5 **Aspiration of fluid or tissue, puncture, and catheterization**

> Abdominal paracentesis    Lumbar puncture
> Aspirating needle biopsy    Thoracentesis
> Blood sampling

> EXCLUDES   heart catheterization (E870.6)

E870.6 **Heart catheterization**

E870.7 **Administration of enema**

E870.8 **Other specified medical care**

E870.9 **Unspecified medical care**

√4ᵗʰ **E871 Foreign object left in body during procedure**

E871.0 **Surgical operation**

E871.1 **Infusion or transfusion**

E871.2 **Kidney dialysis or other perfusion**

E871.3 **Injection or vaccination**

E871.4 **Endoscopic examination**

E871.5 **Aspiration of fluid or tissue, puncture, and catheterization**

> Abdominal paracentesis   Lumbar puncture
> Aspiration needle biopsy   Thoracentesis
> Blood sampling

> EXCLUDES   heart catheterization (E871.6)

E871.6 **Heart catheterization**

E871.7 **Removal of catheter or packing**

E871.8 **Other specified procedures**

E871.9 **Unspecified procedure**

√4ᵗʰ **E872 Failure of sterile precautions during procedure**

E872.0 **Surgical operation**

E872.1 **Infusion or transfusion**

E872.2 **Kidney dialysis and other perfusion**

E872.3 **Injection or vaccination**

E872.4 **Endoscopic examination**

E872.5 **Aspiration of fluid or tissue, puncture, and catheterization**

> Abdominal paracentesis    Lumbar puncture
> Aspiration needle biopsy    Thoracentesis
> Blood sampling

> EXCLUDES   heart catheterization (E872.6)

---

√4ᵗʰ Fourth-digit Required     ▶◀ Revised Text     ● New Code     ▲ Revised Code Title

E872.6 **Heart catheterization**

E872.8 **Other specified procedures**

E872.9 **Unspecified procedure**

√4th **E873 Failure in dosage**

> **EXCLUDES** *accidental overdose of drug, medicinal or biological substance (E850.0-E858.9)*

E873.0 **Excessive amount of blood or other fluid during transfusion or infusion**

E873.1 **Incorrect dilution of fluid during infusion**

E873.2 **Overdose of radiation in therapy**

E873.3 **Inadvertent exposure of patient to radiation during medical care**

E873.4 **Failure in dosage in electroshock or insulin-shock therapy**

E873.5 **Inappropriate [too hot or too cold] temperature in local application and packing**

E873.6 **Nonadministration of necessary drug or medicinal substance**

E873.8 **Other specified failure in dosage**

E873.9 **Unspecified failure in dosage**

√4th **E874 Mechanical failure of instrument or apparatus during procedure**

E874.0 **Surgical operation**

E874.1 **Infusion and transfusion**
    Air in system

E874.2 **Kidney dialysis and other perfusion**

E874.3 **Endoscopic examination**

E874.4 **Aspiration of fluid or tissue, puncture, and catheterization**
    Abdominal paracentesis    Lumbar puncture
    Aspiration needle biopsy    Thoracentesis
    Blood sampling
> **EXCLUDES** *heart catheterization (E874.5)*

E874.5 **Heart catheterization**

E874.8 **Other specified procedures**

E874.9 **Unspecified procedure**

√4th **E875 Contaminated or infected blood, other fluid, drug, or biological substance**

> **INCLUDES** presence of:
>     bacterial pyrogens
>     endotoxin-producing bacteria
>     serum hepatitis-producing agent

E875.0 **Contaminated substance transfused or infused**

E875.1 **Contaminated substance injected or used for vaccination**

E875.2 **Contaminated drug or biological substance administered by other means**

E875.8 **Other**

E875.9 **Unspecified**

√4th **E876 Other and unspecified misadventures during medical care**

E876.0 **Mismatched blood in transfusion**

E876.1 **Wrong fluid in infusion**

E876.2 **Failure in suture and ligature during surgical operation**

E876.3 **Endotracheal tube wrongly placed during anesthetic procedure**

E876.4 **Failure to introduce or to remove other tube or instrument**
> **EXCLUDES** *foreign object left in body during procedure (E871.0-E871.9)*

E876.5 **Performance of inappropriate operation**

E876.8 **Other specified misadventures during medical care**
    Performance of inappropriate treatment NEC

E876.9 **Unspecified misadventure during medical care**

## SURGICAL AND MEDICAL PROCEDURES AS THE CAUSE OF ABNORMAL REACTION OF PATIENT OR LATER COMPLICATION, WITHOUT MENTION OF MISADVENTURE AT THE TIME OF PROCEDURE (E878-E879)

> **INCLUDES** procedures as the cause of abnormal reaction, such as:
>     displacement or malfunction of prosthetic device
>     hepatorenal failure, postoperative
>     malfunction of external stoma
>     postoperative intestinal obstruction
>     rejection of transplanted organ

> **EXCLUDES** *anesthetic management properly carried out as the cause of adverse effect (E937.0-E938.9)*
> *infusion and transfusion, without mention of misadventure in the technique of procedure (E930.0-E949.9)*

√4th **E878 Surgical operation and other surgical procedures as the cause of abnormal reaction of patient, or of later complication, without mention of misadventure at the time of operation**

E878.0 **Surgical operation with transplant of whole organ**
    Transplantation of:    Transplantation of:
      heart          liver
      kidney

E878.1 **Surgical operation with implant of artificial internal device**
    Cardiac pacemaker    Heart valve prosthesis
    Electrodes implanted in    Internal orthopedic
      brain          device

E878.2 **Surgical operation with anastomosis, bypass, or graft, with natural or artificial tissues used as implant**
    Anastomosis:    Graft of blood vessel,
      arteriovenous      tendon, or skin
      gastrojejunal
> **EXCLUDES** *external stoma (E878.3)*

E878.3 **Surgical operation with formation of external stoma**
    Colostomy    Gastrostomy
    Cystostomy    Ureterostomy
    Duodenostomy

E878.4 **Other restorative surgery**

E878.5 **Amputation of limb(s)**

E878.6 **Removal of other organ (partial) (total)**

E878.8 **Other specified surgical operations and procedures**

E878.9 **Unspecified surgical operations and procedures**

√4th **E879 Other procedures, without mention of misadventure at the time of procedure, as the cause of abnormal reaction of patient, or of later complication**

E879.0 **Cardiac catheterization**

E879.1 **Kidney dialysis**

E879.2 **Radiological procedure and radiotherapy**
> **EXCLUDES** *radio-opaque dyes for diagnostic x-ray procedures (E947.8)*

E879.3 **Shock therapy**
    Electroshock therapy
    Insulin-shock therapy

E879.4 **Aspiration of fluid**
    Lumbar puncture
    Thoracentesis

E879.5 **Insertion of gastric or duodenal sound**

E879.6 **Urinary catheterization**

E879.7 **Blood sampling**

E879.8 **Other specified procedures**
    Blood transfusion

E879.9 **Unspecified procedure**

---

**E Codes**

**E880–E890.9**

## ACCIDENTAL FALLS (E880–E888)

> **EXCLUDES**    *falls (in or from):*
> *burning building (E890.8, E891.8)*
> *into fire (E890.0-E899)*
> *into water (with submersion or drowning)*
>      *(E910.0-E910.9)*
> *machinery (in operation) (E919.0-E919.9)*
> *on edged, pointed, or sharp object (E920.0-*
>      *E920.9)*
> *transport vehicle (E800.0-E845.9)*
> *vehicle not elsewhere classifiable (E846-E848)*

✓4th **E880 Fall on or from stairs or steps**

   **E880.0 Escalator**

   **E880.1 Fall on or from sidewalk curb**

> **EXCLUDES**    *fall from moving sidewalk (E885.9)*

   **E880.9 Other stairs or steps**

✓4th **E881 Fall on or from ladders or scaffolding**

   **E881.0 Fall from ladder**

   **E881.1 Fall from scaffolding**

**E882 Fall from or out of building or other structure**

Fall from:          Fall from:
   balcony           turret
   bridge            viaduct
   building          wall
   flagpole          window
   tower            Fall through roof

> **EXCLUDES**    *collapse of a building or structure (E916)*
> *fall or jump from burning building (E890.8,*
>      *E891.8)*

✓4th **E883 Fall into hole or other opening in surface**

> **INCLUDES**    fall into:       fall into:
>      cavity         shaft
>      dock          swimming pool
>      hole          tank
>      pit           well
>      quarry

> **EXCLUDES**    *fall into water NOS (E910.9)*
> *that resulting in drowning or submersion*
>      *without mention of injury (E910.0-E910.9)*

   **E883.0 Accident from diving or jumping into water [swimming pool]**

Strike or hit:
   against bottom when jumping or diving into water
   wall or board of swimming pool
   water surface

> **EXCLUDES**    *diving with insufficient air supply*
>      *(E913.2)*
> *effects of air pressure from diving*
>      *(E902.2)*

   **E883.1 Accidental fall into well**

   **E883.2 Accidental fall into storm drain or manhole**

   **E883.9 Fall into other hole or other opening in surface**

✓4th **E884 Other fall from one level to another**

   **E884.0 Fall from playground equipment**

> **EXCLUDES**    *recreational machinery (E919.8)*

   **E884.1 Fall from cliff**

   **E884.2 Fall from chair**

   **E884.3 Fall from wheelchair**

   **E884.4 Fall from bed**

   **E884.5 Fall from other furniture**

   **E884.6 Fall from commode**

     Toilet

   **E884.9 Other fall from one level to another**

Fall from:       Fall from:
   embankment      stationary vehicle
   haystack         tree

✓4th **E885 Fall on same level from slipping, tripping, or stumbling**

   **E885.0 Fall from (nonmotorized) scooter**

   **E885.1 Fall from roller skates**

     In-line skates

   **E885.2 Fall from skateboard**

   **E885.3 Fall from skis**

   **E885.4 Fall from snowboard**

   **E885.9 Fall from other slipping, tripping, or stumbling**

     Fall on moving sidewalk

✓4th **E886 Fall on same level from collision, pushing, or shoving, by or with other person**

> **EXCLUDES**    *crushed or pushed by a crowd or human*
>      *stampede (E917.1, E917.6)*

   **E886.0 In sports**

     Tackles in sports

> **EXCLUDES**    *kicked, stepped on, struck by object, in*
>      *sports (E917.0, E917.5)*

   **E886.9 Other and unspecified**

     Fall from collision of pedestrian (conveyance) with
     another pedestrian (conveyance)

**E887 Fracture, cause unspecified**

✓4th **E888 Other and unspecified fall**

   Accidental fall NOS        Fall on same level NOS

   **E888.0 Fall resulting in striking against sharp object**

     Use additional external cause code to identify object
     (E920)

   **E888.1 Fall resulting in striking against other object**

   **E888.8 Other fall**

   **E888.9 Unspecified fall**

     Fall NOS

## ACCIDENTS CAUSED BY FIRE AND FLAMES (E890–E899)

> **INCLUDES**    asphyxia or poisoning due to conflagration or
>      ignition
> burning by fire
> secondary fires resulting from explosion

> **EXCLUDES**    *arson (E968.0)*
> *fire in or on:*
>      *machinery (in operation) (E919.0-E919.9)*
>      *transport vehicle other than stationary*
>        *vehicle (E800.0-E845.9)*
>      *vehicle not elsewhere classifiable (E846-*
>        *E848)*

✓4th **E890 Conflagration in private dwelling**

> **INCLUDES**    conflagration in:      conflagration in:
>      apartment         lodging house
>      boarding house    mobile home
>      camping place      private garage
>      caravan          rooming house
>      farmhouse        tenement
>      house
> conflagration originating from sources
>      classifiable to E893-E898 in the above
>      buildings

   **E890.0 Explosion caused by conflagration**

   **E890.1 Fumes from combustion of polyvinylchloride [PVC] and similar material in conflagration**

   **E890.2 Other smoke and fumes from conflagration**

     Carbon monoxide
     Fumes NOS     } from conflagration in
     Smoke NOS       private building

   **E890.3 Burning caused by conflagration**

   **E890.8 Other accident resulting from conflagration**

     Collapse of
     Fall from            } burning private
     Hit by object falling from    building
     Jump from

   **E890.9 Unspecified accident resulting from conflagration in private dwelling**

---

✓4th Fourth-digit Required     ►◄ Revised Text     ● New Code     ▲ Revised Code Title

✓4ᵗʰ **E891 Conflagration in other and unspecified building or structure**

Conflagration in:
- barn
- church
- convalescent and other residential home
- dormitory of educational institution
- factory
- farm outbuildings
- hospital
- hotel
- school
- store
- theater

Conflagration originating from sources classifiable to E893-E898, in the above buildings

**E891.0 Explosion caused by conflagration**

**E891.1 Fumes from combustion of polyvinylchloride [PVC] and similar material in conflagration**

**E891.2 Other smoke and fumes from conflagration**

Carbon monoxide } from conflagration in
Fumes NOS }   building or
Smoke NOS }   structure

**E891.3 Burning caused by conflagration**

**E891.8 Other accident resulting from conflagration**

Collapse of }
Fall from }  burning building or
Hit by object falling from } structure
Jump from }

**E891.9 Unspecified accident resulting from conflagration of other and unspecified building or structure**

**E892 Conflagration not in building or structure**

Fire (uncontrolled) (in) (of):
- forest
- grass
- hay
- lumber
- mine

Fire (uncontrolled) (in) (of):
- prairie
- transport vehicle [any], except while in transit
- tunnel

✓4ᵗʰ **E893 Accident caused by ignition of clothing**

EXCLUDES  ignition of clothing:
  from highly inflammable material (E894)
  with conflagration (E890.0-E892)

**E893.0 From controlled fire in private dwelling**

Ignition of clothing from:
normal fire (charcoal) (coal)
  (electric) (gas) (wood) in: } in private
brazier }   dwelling
fireplace }   (as listed
furnace }   in E890)
stove }

**E893.1 From controlled fire in other building or structure**

Ignition of clothing from:
normal fire (charcoal)
  (coal) (electric)
  (gas) (wood) in: } in other building or
brazier }   structure (as
fireplace }   listed in E81)
furnace }
stove }

**E893.2 From controlled fire not in building or structure**

Ignition of clothing from:
- bonfire (controlled)
- brazier fire (controlled), not in building or structure
- trash fire (controlled)

EXCLUDES  conflagration not in building (E892)
  trash fire out of control (E892)

**E893.8 From other specified sources**

Ignition of clothing from:
- blowlamp
- blowtorch
- burning bedspread
- candle
- cigar

Ignition of clothing from:
- cigarette
- lighter
- matches
- pipe
- welding torch

**E893.9 Unspecified source**

Ignition of clothing (from controlled fire NOS) (in building NOS) NOS

**E894 Ignition of highly inflammable material**

Ignition of:
- benzine
- gasoline
- fat
- kerosene
- paraffin
- petrol
} (with ignition of clothing)

EXCLUDES  ignition of highly inflammable material with:
  conflagration (E890.0-E892)
  explosion (E923.0-E923.9)

**E895 Accident caused by controlled fire in private dwelling**

Burning by (flame of) normal fire
  (charcoal) (coal) (electric)
  (gas) (wood) in:
- brazier
- fireplace
- furnace
- stove
} in private dwelling (as listed in E890)

EXCLUDES  burning by hot objects not producing fire or flames (E924.0-E924.9)
  ignition of clothing from these sources (E893.0)
  poisoning by carbon monoxide from incomplete combustion of fuel (E867-E868.9)
  that with conflagration (E890.0-E890.9)

**E896 Accident caused by controlled fire in other and unspecified building or structure**

Burning by (flame of) normal fire (charcoal) (coal) (electric)
  (gas) (wood) in:
- brazier
- fireplace
- furnace
- stove
} in other building or structure (as listed in E891)

EXCLUDES  burning by hot objects not producing fire or flames (E924.0-E924.9)
  ignition of clothing from these sources (E893.1)
  poisoning by carbon monoxide from incomplete combustion of fuel (E867-E868.9)
  that with conflagration (E891.0-E891.9)

**E897 Accident caused by controlled fire not in building or structure**

Burns from flame of:
- bonfire
- brazier fire, not in building or structure
- trash fire
} controlled

EXCLUDES  ignition of clothing from these sources (E893.2)
  trash fire out of control (E892)
  that with conflagration (E892)

✓4ᵗʰ **E898 Accident caused by other specified fire and flames**

EXCLUDES  conflagration (E890.0-E892)
  that with ignition of:
  clothing (E893.0-E893.9)
  highly inflammable material (E894)

**E898.0 Burning bedclothes**

Bed set on fire NOS

**E898.1 Other**

Burning by:
- blowlamp
- blowtorch
- candle
- cigar
- cigarette
- fire in room NOS

Burning by:
- lamp
- lighter
- matches
- pipe
- welding torch

**E899 Accident caused by unspecified fire**

Burning NOS

## ACCIDENTS DUE TO NATURAL AND ENVIRONMENTAL FACTORS (E900-E909)

✓4ᵗʰ **E900 Excessive heat**

**E900.0 Due to weather conditions**

Excessive heat as the external cause of:
- ictus solaris
- siriasis
- sunstroke

**E900.1  Of man-made origin**

Heat (in):                        Heat (in):
  boiler room                       generated in transport
  drying room                         vehicle
  factory                           kitchen
  furnace room

**E900.9  Of unspecified origin**

√4ᵗʰ **E901  Excessive cold**

**E901.0  Due to weather conditions**

Excessive cold as the cause of:
  chilblains NOS
  immersion foot

**E901.1  Of man-made origin**

Contact with or inhalation of:
  dry ice
  liquid air
  liquid hydrogen
  liquid nitrogen
Prolonged exposure in:
  deep freeze unit
  refrigerator

**E901.8  Other specified origin**

**E901.9  Of unspecified origin**

√4ᵗʰ **E902  High and low air pressure and changes in air pressure**

**E902.0  Residence or prolonged visit at high altitude**

Residence or prolonged visit at high altitude as the
  cause of:
  Acosta syndrome
  Alpine sickness
  altitude sickness
  Andes disease
  anoxia, hypoxia
  barotitis, barodontalgia, barosinusitis, otitic
    barotrauma
  hypobarism, hypobaropathy
  mountain sickness
  range disease

**E902.1  In aircraft**

Sudden change in air pressure in aircraft during
  ascent or descent as the cause of:
  aeroneurosis
  aviators' disease

**E902.2  Due to diving**

High air pressure from                 as the cause of:
  rapid descent in water                 caisson disease
Reduction in atmospheric                 divers' disease
  pressure while                         divers' palsy or
  surfacing from deep                      paralysis
  water diving

**E902.8  Due to other specified causes**

Reduction in atmospheric pressure whilesurfacing
  from underground

**E902.9  Unspecified cause**

**E903  Travel and motion**

√4ᵗʰ **E904  Hunger, thirst, exposure, and neglect**

EXCLUDES   any condition resulting from homicidal intent
             (E968.0-E968.9)
           hunger, thirst, and exposure resulting from
             accidents connected with transport
             (E800.0-E848)

**E904.0  Abandonment or neglect of infants and helpless
persons**

Exposure to weather      resulting from
  conditions               abandonment
Hunger or thirst           or neglect

Desertion of newborn
Inattention at or after birth
Lack of care (helpless person) (infant)
EXCLUDES   criminal [purposeful] neglect (E968.4)

**E904.1  Lack of food**

Lack of food as the cause of:
  inanition
  insufficient nourishment
  starvation
EXCLUDES   hunger resulting from abandonment or
             neglect (E904.0)

**E904.2  Lack of water**

Lack of water as the cause of:
  dehydration            inanition
EXCLUDES   dehydration due to acute fluid loss
             (276.51)

**E904.3  Exposure (to weather conditions), not elsewhere
classifiable**

Exposure NOS             Struck by hailstones
Humidity
EXCLUDES   struck by lightning (E907)

**E904.9  Privation, unqualified**

Destitution

√4ᵗʰ **E905  Venomous animals and plants as the cause of poisoning and
toxic reactions**

INCLUDES   chemical released by animal
           insects
           release of venom through fangs, hairs, spines,
             tentacles, and other venom apparatus
EXCLUDES   eating of poisonous animals or plants (E865.0-
             E865.9)

**E905.0  Venomous snakes and lizards**

Cobra                    Mamba
Copperhead snake         Rattlesnake
Coral snake              Sea snake
Fer de lance             Snake (venomous)
Gila monster             Viper
Krait                    Water moccasin
EXCLUDES   bites of snakes and lizards known to
             be nonvenomous (E906.2)

**E905.1  Venomous spiders**

Black widow spider       Tarantula (venomous)
Brown spider

**E905.2  Scorpion**

**E905.3  Hornets, wasps, and bees**

Yellow jacket

**E905.4  Centipede and venomous millipede (tropical)**

**E905.5  Other venomous arthropods**

Sting of:                Sting of:
  ant                      caterpillar

**E905.6  Venomous marine animals and plants**

Puncture by sea          Sting of:
  urchin spine             sea anemone
Sting of:                  sea cucumber
  coral                    other marine animal
  jelly fish                 or plant
  nematocysts
EXCLUDES   bites and other injuries caused by
             nonvenomous marine animal
             (E906.2-E906.8)
           bite of sea snake (venomous) (E905.0)

**E905.7  Poisoning and toxic reactions caused by other
plants**

Injection of poisons or toxins into or through skin by
  plant thorns, spines, or other mechanisms
EXCLUDES   puncture wound NOS by plant thorns
             or spines (E920.8)

**E905.8  Other specified**

**E905.9  Unspecified**

Sting NOS                Venomous bite NOS

√4ᵗʰ **E906  Other injury caused by animals**

EXCLUDES   poisoning and toxic reactions caused by
             venomous animals and insects (E905.0-
             E905.9)
           road vehicle accident involving animals (E827.0-
             E828.9)
           tripping or falling over an animal (E885.9)

E906.0 **Dog bite**

E906.1 **Rat bite**

E906.2 **Bite of nonvenomous snakes and lizards**

E906.3 **Bite of other animal except arthropod**

    Cats        Rodents, except rats

    Moray eel    Shark

E906.4 **Bite of nonvenomous arthropod**

    Insect bite NOS

E906.5 **Bite by unspecified animal**

    Animal bite NOS

E906.8 **Other specified injury caused by animal**

    Butted by animal

    Fallen on by horse or other animal, not being ridden

    Gored by animal

    Implantation of quills of porcupine

    Pecked by bird

    Run over by animal, not being ridden

    Stepped on by animal, not being ridden

        **EXCLUDES** *injury by animal being ridden (E828.0-E828.9)*

E906.9 **Unspecified injury caused by animal**

E907 **Lightning**

    **EXCLUDES** *injury from:*
        *fall of tree or other object caused by lightning (E916)*
        *fire caused by lightning (E890.0-E892)*

✓4ᵗʰ E908 **Cataclysmic storms, and floods resulting from storms**

    **EXCLUDES** *collapse of dam or man-made structure causing flood (E909.3)*

E908.0 **Hurricane**

    Storm surge

    "Tidal wave" caused by storm action

    Typhoon

E908.1 **Tornado**

    Cyclone

    Twisters

E908.2 **Floods**

    Torrential rainfall

    Flash flood

        **EXCLUDES** *collapse of dam or man-made structure causing flood (E909.3)*

E908.3 **Blizzard (snow) (ice)**

E908.4 **Dust storm**

E908.8 **Other cataclysmic storms**

    Cloudburst

E908.9 **Unspecified cataclysmic storms, and floods resulting from storms**

    Storm NOS

✓4ᵗʰ E909 **Cataclysmic earth surface movements and eruptions**

E909.0 **Earthquakes**

E909.1 **Volcanic eruptions**

    Burns from lava

    Ash inhalation

E909.2 **Avalanche, landslide, or mudslide**

E909.3 **Collapse of dam or man-made structure**

E909.4 **Tidalwave caused by earthquake**

    Tidalwave NOS

    Tsunami

        **EXCLUDES** *tidalwave caused by tropical storm (E908.0)*

E909.8 **Other cataclysmic earth surface movements and eruptions**

E909.9 **Unspecified cataclysmic earth surface movements and eruptions**

## ACCIDENTS CAUSED BY SUBMERSION, SUFFOCATION, AND FOREIGN BODIES (E910-E915)

✓4ᵗʰ E910 **Accidental drowning and submersion**

    **INCLUDES**    immersion
                swimmers' cramp

    **EXCLUDES**   *diving accident (NOS) (resulting in injury except drowning) (E883.0)*
        *diving with insufficient air supply (E913.2)*
        *drowning and submersion due to:*
            *cataclysm (E908-E909)*
            *machinery accident (E919.0-E919.9)*
            *transport accident (E800.0-E845.9)*
        *effect of high and low air pressure (E902.2)*
        *injury from striking against objects while in running water (E917.2)*

E910.0 **While water-skiing**

    Fall from water skis with submersion or drowning

        **EXCLUDES** *accident to water-skier involving a watercraft and resulting in submersion or other injury (E830.4, E831.4)*

E910.1 **While engaged in other sport or recreational activity with diving equipment**

    Scuba diving NOS    Underwater spear

    Skin diving NOS      fishing NOS

E910.2 **While engaged in other sport or recreational activity without diving equipment**

    Fishing or hunting, except from boat or with diving equipment

    Ice skating

    Playing in water

    Surfboarding

    Swimming NOS

    Voluntarily jumping from boat, not involved in accident, for swim NOS

    Wading in water

        **EXCLUDES** *jumping into water to rescue another person (E910.3)*

E910.3 **While swimming or diving for purposes other than recreation or sport**

    Marine salvage

    Pearl diving

    Placement of fishing nets

    Rescue (attempt) of another person    } (with diving equipment)

    Underwater construction or repairs

E910.4 **In bathtub**

E910.8 **Other accidental drowning or submersion**

    Drowning in:    Drowning in:

      quenching tank    swimming pool

E910.9 **Unspecified accidental drowning or submersion**

    Accidental fall into water NOS

    Drowning NOS

E911 **Inhalation and ingestion of food causing obstruction of respiratory tract or suffocation**

    Aspiration and inhalation of food [any] (into respiratory tract) NOS

    Asphyxia by

    Choked on    } food [including bone, seed in food, regurgitated food]

    Suffocation by

    Compression of trachea

    Interruption of respiration    } by food lodged in esophagus

    Obstruction of respiration

    Obstruction of pharynx by food (bolus)

        **EXCLUDES** *injury, except asphyxia and obstruction of respiratory passage, caused by food (E915)*
        *obstruction of esophagus by food without mention of asphyxia or obstruction of respiratory passage (E915)*

**E912 Inhalation and ingestion of other object causing obstruction of respiratory tract or suffocation**

Aspiration and inhalation of foreign body except food (into respiratory tract) NOS
Foreign object [bean] [marble] in nose
Obstruction of pharynx by foreign body
Compression
Interruption of respiration } by foreign body in esophagus
Obstruction of respiration

EXCLUDES　injury, except asphyxia and obstruction of respiratory passage, caused by foreign body (E915)
obstruction of esophagus by foreign body without mention of asphyxia or obstruction in respiratory passage (E915)

√4ᵗʰ **E913 Accidental mechanical suffocation**

EXCLUDES　mechanical suffocation from or by:
accidental inhalation or ingestion of:
food (E911)
foreign object (E912)
cataclysm (E908-E909)
explosion (E921.0-E921.9, E923.0-E923.9)
machinery accident (E919.0-E919.9)

**E913.0 In bed or cradle**
EXCLUDES　suffocation by plastic bag (E913.1)

**E913.1 By plastic bag**

**E913.2 Due to lack of air (in closed place)**
Accidentally closed up in refrigerator or other airtight enclosed space
Diving with insufficient air supply
EXCLUDES　suffocation by plastic bag (E913.1)

**E913.3 By falling earth or other substance**
Cave-in NOS
EXCLUDES　cave-in caused by cataclysmic earth surface movements and eruptions (E909)
struck by cave-in without asphyxiation or suffocation (E916)

**E913.8 Other specified means**
Accidental hanging, except in bed or cradle

**E913.9 Unspecified means**
Asphyxia, mechanical NOS　Suffocation NOS
Strangulation NOS

**E914 Foreign body accidentally entering eye and adnexa**
EXCLUDES　corrosive liquid (E924.1)

**E915 Foreign body accidentally entering other orifice**
EXCLUDES　aspiration and inhalation of foreign body, any, (into respiratory tract) NOS (E911-E912)

## OTHER ACCIDENTS (E916-E928)

**E916 Struck accidentally by falling object**
Collapse of building, except on fire
Falling:
rock
snowslide NOS
stone
tree
Object falling from:
machine, not in operation
stationary vehicle

Code first:
collapse of building on fire (E890.0-E891.9)
falling object in:
cataclysm (E908-E909)
machinery accidents (E919.0-E919.9)
transport accidents (E800.0-E845.9)
vehicle accidents not elsewhere classifiable (E846-E848)
object set in motion by:
explosion (E921.0-E921.9, E923.0-E923.9)
firearm (E922.0-E922.9)
projected object (E917.0-E917.9)

√4ᵗʰ **E917 Striking against or struck accidentally by objects or persons**

INCLUDES　bumping into or against
colliding with
kicking against
stepping on
struck by
} object (moving) (projected) (stationary)
pedestrian conveyance
person

EXCLUDES　fall from:
collision with another person, except when caused by a crowd (E886.0-E886.9)
stumbling over object (E885.9)
fall resulting in striking against object (E888.0, E888.1)
injury caused by:
assault (E960.0-E960.1, E967.0-E967.9)
cutting or piercing instrument (E920.0-E920.9)
explosion (E921.0-E921.9, E923.0-E923.9)
firearm (E922.0-E922.9)
machinery (E919.0-E919.9)
transport vehicle (E800.0-E845.9)
vehicle not elsewhere classifiable (E846-E848)

**E917.0 In sports without subsequent fall**
Kicked or stepped on during game (football) (rugby)
Struck by hit or thrown ball
Struck by hockey stick or puck

**E917.1 Caused by a crowd, by collective fear or panic without subsequent fall**
Crushed
Pushed } by crowd or human stampede
Stepped on

**E917.2 In running water without subsequent fall**
EXCLUDES　drowning or submersion (E910.0-E910.9)
that in sports (E917.0, E917.5)

**E917.3 Furniture without subsequent fall**
EXCLUDES　fall from furniture (E884.2, E884.4-E884.5)

**E917.4 Other stationary object without subsequent fall**
Bath tub
Fence
Lamp-post

**E917.5 Object in sports with subsequent fall**
Knocked down while boxing

**E917.6 Caused by a crowd, by collective fear or panic with subsequent fall**

**E917.7 Furniture with subsequent fall**
EXCLUDES　fall from furniture (E884.2, E884.4-E884.5)

**E917.8 Other stationary object with subsequent fall**
Bath tub
Fence
Lamp-post

**E917.9 Other striking against with or without subsequent fall**

**E918 Caught accidentally in or between objects**
Caught, crushed, jammed, or pinched in or between moving or stationary objects, such as:
escalator
folding object
hand tools, appliances, or implements
sliding door and door frame
under packing crate
washing machine wringer
EXCLUDES　injury caused by:
cutting or piercing instrument (E920.0-E920.9)
machinery (E919.0-E919.9)
transport vehicle (E800.0-E845.9)
vehicle not elsewhere classifiable (E846-E848)
struck accidentally by:
falling object (E916)
object (moving) (projected) (E917.0-E917.9)

√4ᵗʰ Fourth-digit Required　►◄ Revised Text　● New Code　▲ Revised Code Title

☑4ᵗʰ **E919 Accidents caused by machinery**

| INCLUDES | burned by | |
|---|---|---|
| | caught in (moving parts of) | |
| | collapse of | |
| | crushed by | |
| | cut or pierced by | |
| | drowning or submersion | |
| |    caused by | |
| | explosion of, on, in | machinery |
| | fall from or into moving | (accident) |
| |    part of | |
| | fire starting in or on | |
| | mechanical suffocation | |
| |    caused by | |
| | object falling from, on, in | |
| |    motion by | |
| | overturning of | |
| | pinned under | |
| | run over by | |
| | struck by | |
| | thrown from | |

caught between machinery and other object
machinery accident NOS

EXCLUDES     *accidents involving machinery, not in operation*
                   *(E884.9, E916-E918)*
             *injury caused by:*
                   *electric current in connection with machinery*
                      *(E925.0-E925.9)*
                   *escalator (E880.0, E918)*
                   *explosion of pressure vessel in connection*
                      *with machinery (E921.0-E921.9)*
                   *moving sidewalk (E885.9)*
                   *powered hand tools, appliances, and*
                      *implements (E916-E918, E920.0-*
                      *E921.9, E923.0-E926.9)*
                   *transport vehicle accidents involving*
                      *machinery (E800.0-E848)*
                   *poisoning by carbon monoxide generated by*
                      *machine (E868.8)*

### E919.0 Agricultural machines

| | |
|---|---|
| Animal-powered | Farm tractor |
|    agricultural machine | Harvester |
| Combine | Hay mower or rake |
| Derrick, hay | Reaper |
| Farm machinery NOS | Thresher |

EXCLUDES     *that in transport under own power on*
                   *the highway (E810.0-E819.9)*
             *that being towed by another vehicle on*
                   *the highway (E810.0-E819.9,*
                   *E827.0-E827.9, E829.0-E829.9)*
             *that involved in accident classifiable to*
                   *E820-E829 (E820.0-E829.9)*

### E919.1 Mining and earth-drilling machinery

| | |
|---|---|
| Bore or drill (land) (seabed) | Shaft lift |
| Shaft hoist | Under-cutter |

EXCLUDES     *coal car, tram, truck, and tub in mine*
                   *(E846)*

### E919.2 Lifting machines and appliances

| | |
|---|---|
| Chain hoist | |
| Crane | |
| Derrick | except in |
| Elevator (building) (grain) | agricultural |
| Forklift truck | or mining |
| Lift | operations |
| Pulley block | |
| Winch | |

EXCLUDES     *that being towed by another vehicle on*
                   *the highway (E810.0-E819.9,*
                   *E827.0-E827.9, E829.0-829.9)*
             *that in transport under own power on*
                   *the highway (E810.0-E819.9)*
             *that involved in accident classifiable to*
                   *E820-E829 (E820.0-E829.9)*

### E919.3 Metalworking machines

| | |
|---|---|
| Abrasive wheel | Metal: |
| Forging machine |    drilling machine |
| Lathe |    milling machine |
| Mechanical shears |    power press |
| |    rolling-mill |
| |    sawing machine |

### E919.4 Woodworking and forming machines

| | |
|---|---|
| Band saw | Overhead plane |
| Bench saw | Powered saw |
| Circular saw | Radial saw |
| Molding machine | Sander |

EXCLUDES     *hand saw (E920.1)*

### E919.5 Prime movers, except electrical motors

Gas turbine
Internal combustion engine
Steam engine
Water driven turbine

EXCLUDES     *that being towed by other vehicle on*
                   *the highway (E810.0-E819.9,*
                   *E827.0-E827.9, E829.0-E829.9)*
             *that in transport under own power on*
                   *the highway (E810.0-E819.9)*

### E919.6 Transmission machinery

| Transmission: | Transmission: |
|---|---|
|    belt |    pinion |
|    cable |    pulley |
|    chain |    shaft |
|    gear | |

### E919.7 Earth moving, scraping, and other excavating machines

| | |
|---|---|
| Bulldozer | Steam shovel |
| Road scraper | |

EXCLUDES     *that being towed by other vehicle on*
                   *the highway (E810.0-E819.9,*
                   *E827.0-E827.9, E829.0-E829.9)*
             *that in transport under own power on*
                   *the highway (E810.0-E819.9)*

### E919.8 Other specified machinery

Machines for manufacture of:
   clothing
   foodstuffs and beverages
   paper
Printing machine
Recreational machinery
Spinning, weaving, and textile machines

### E919.9 Unspecified machinery

☑4ᵗʰ **E920 Accidents caused by cutting and piercing instruments or objects**

| INCLUDES | | object: |
|---|---|---|
| | accidental injury (by) | edged |
| | | pointed |
| | | sharp |

### E920.0 Powered lawn mower

### E920.1 Other powered hand tools

Any powered hand tool [compressed air] [electric]
   [explosive cartridge] [hydraulic power], such as:
   drill
   hand saw
   hedge clipper
   rivet gun
   snow blower
   staple gun

EXCLUDES     *band saw (E919.4)*
             *bench saw (E919.4)*

### E920.2 Powered household appliances and implements

| | |
|---|---|
| Blender | Electric: |
| Electric: |    fan |
|    beater or mixer |    knife |
|    can opener |    sewing machine |
| | Garbage disposal appliance |

### E920.3 Knives, swords, and daggers

**E920.4 Other hand tools and implements**

| | |
|---|---|
| Axe | Paper cutter |
| Can opener NOS | Pitchfork |
| Chisel | Rake |
| Fork | Scissors |
| Hand saw | Screwdriver |
| Hoe | Sewing machine, not powered |
| Ice pick | Shovel |
| Needle (sewing) | |

**E920.5 Hypodermic needle**

Contaminated needle
Needle stick

**E920.8 Other specified cutting and piercing instruments or objects**

| | |
|---|---|
| Arrow | Nail |
| Broken glass | Plant thorn |
| Dart | Splinter |
| Edge of stiff paper | Tin can lid |
| Lathe turnings | |

> **EXCLUDES**   *animal spines or quills (E906.8)*
> *flying glass due to explosion (E921.0-E923.9)*

**E920.9 Unspecified cutting and piercing instrument or object**

**✓4ᵗʰ E921 Accident caused by explosion of pressure vessel**

> **INCLUDES**   accidental explosion of pressure vessels, whether or not part of machinery
>
> **EXCLUDES**   *explosion of pressure vessel on transport vehicle (E800.0-E845.9)*

**E921.0 Boilers**

**E921.1 Gas cylinders**

Air tank
Pressure gas tank

**E921.8 Other specified pressure vessels**

| | |
|---|---|
| Aerosol can | Pressure cooker |
| Automobile tire | |

**E921.9 Unspecified pressure vessel**

**✓4ᵗʰ E922 Accident caused by firearm, and air gun missile**

**E922.0 Handgun**

| | |
|---|---|
| Pistol | Revolver |

> **EXCLUDES**   *Verey pistol (E922.8)*

**E922.1 Shotgun (automatic)**

**E922.2 Hunting rifle**

**E922.3 Military firearms**

| | |
|---|---|
| Army rifle | Machine gun |

**E922.4 Air gun**

BB gun
Pellet gun

**E922.5 Paintball gun**

**E922.8 Other specified firearm missile**

Verey pistol [flare]

**E922.9 Unspecified firearm missile**

Gunshot wound NOS
Shot NOS

**✓4ᵗʰ E923 Accident caused by explosive material**

> **INCLUDES**   flash burns and other injuries resulting from explosion of explosive material
> ignition of highly explosive material with explosion
>
> **EXCLUDES**   *explosion:*
> *in or on machinery (E919.0-E919.9)*
> *on any transport vehicle, except stationary motor vehicle (E800.0-E848)*
> *with conflagration (E890.0, E891.0,E892)*
> *secondary fires resulting from explosion (E890.0-E899)*

**E923.0 Fireworks**

**E923.1 Blasting materials**

Blasting cap
Detonator
Dynamite
Explosive [any] used in blasting operations

**E923.2 Explosive gases**

| | |
|---|---|
| Acetylene | Fire damp |
| Butane | Gasoline fumes |
| Coal gas | Methane |
| Explosion in mine NOS | Propane |

**E923.8 Other explosive materials**

| | |
|---|---|
| Bomb | Torpedo |
| Explosive missile | Explosion in munitions: |
| Grenade | dump |
| Mine | factory |
| Shell | |

**E923.9 Unspecified explosive material**

Explosion NOS

**✓4ᵗʰ E924 Accident caused by hot substance or object, caustic or corrosive material, and steam**

> **EXCLUDES**   *burning NOS (E899)*
> *chemical burn resulting from swallowing a corrosive substance (E860.0-E864.4)*
> *fire caused by these substances and objects (E890.0-E894)*
> *radiation burns (E926.0-E926.9)*
> *therapeutic misadventures (E870.0-E876.9)*

**E924.0 Hot liquids and vapors, including steam**

Burning or scalding by:
  boiling water
  hot or boiling liquids not primarily caustic or corrosive
  liquid metal
  steam
  other hot vapor

> **EXCLUDES**   *hot (boiling) tap water (E924.2)*

**E924.1 Caustic and corrosive substances**

| Burning by: | Burning by: |
|---|---|
| acid [any kind] | corrosive substance |
| ammonia | lye |
| caustic oven cleaner | vitriol |
| or other substance | |

**E924.2 Hot (boiling) tap water**

**E924.8 Other**

Burning by:
  heat from electric heating appliance
  hot object NOS
  light bulb
  steam pipe

**E924.9 Unspecified**

**✓4ᵗʰ E925 Accident caused by electric current**

> **INCLUDES**   electric current from exposed wire, faulty appliance, high voltage cable, live rail, or open electric socket as the cause of:
>   burn
>   cardiac fibrillation
>   convulsion
>   electric shock
>   electrocution
>   puncture wound
>   respiratory paralysis
>
> **EXCLUDES**   *burn by heat from electrical appliance (E924.8)*
> *lightning (E907)*

**E925.0 Domestic wiring and appliances**

**E925.1 Electric power generating plants, distribution stations, transmission lines**

Broken power line

**E925.2 Industrial wiring, appliances, and electrical machinery**

| | |
|---|---|
| Conductors | Electrical equipment and machinery |
| Control apparatus | Transformers |

**E925.8 Other electric current**

Wiring and appliances in or on:
  farm [not farmhouse]
  outdoors
  public building
  residential institutions
  schools

---

✓4ᵗʰ Fourth-digit Required     ►◄ Revised Text     ● New Code     ▲ Revised Code Title

### E925.9  Unspecified electric current
Burns or other injury from electric current NOS
Electric shock NOS
Electrocution NOS

### ✓4ᵗʰ E926  Exposure to radiation
EXCLUDES *abnormal reaction to or complication of*
*treatment without mention of*
*misadventure (E879.2)*
*atomic power plant malfunction in water*
*transport (E838.0-E838.9)*
*misadventure to patient in surgical and medical*
*procedures (E873.2-E873.3)*
*use of radiation in war operations (E996-*
*E997.9)*

### E926.0  Radiofrequency radiation
Overexposure to:     from:
microwave          high-powered radio and
  radiation          television
radar radiation      transmitters
radiofrequency     industrial
radiofrequency       radiofrequency
  radiation           induction heaters
  [any]              radar installations

### E926.1  Infrared heaters and lamps
Exposure to infrared radiation from heaters and
lamps as the cause of:
blistering
burning
charring
inflammatory change
EXCLUDES *physical contact with heater or lamp*
*(E924.8)*

### E926.2  Visible and ultraviolet light sources
Arc lamps            Oxygas welding torch
Black light sources   Sun rays
Electrical welding arc  Tanning bed
EXCLUDES *excessive heat from these sources*
*(E900.1-E900.9)*

### E926.3  X-rays and other electromagnetic ionizing radiation
Gamma rays          X-rays (hard) (soft)

### E926.4  Lasers
### E926.5  Radioactive isotopes
Radiobiologicals     Radiopharmaceuticals

### E926.8  Other specified radiation
Artificially accelerated beams of ionized particles
generated by:
betatrons
synchrotrons

### E926.9  Unspecified radiation
Radiation NOS

### E927  Overexertion and strenuous movements
Excessive physical exercise   Strenuous movements in:
Overexertion (from):            recreational activities
lifting                        other activities
pulling
pushing

### ✓4ᵗʰ E928  Other and unspecified environmental and accidental causes
### E928.0  Prolonged stay in weightless environment
Weightlessness in spacecraft (simulator)

### E928.1  Exposure to noise
Noise (pollution)     Supersonic waves
Sound waves

### E928.2  Vibration
### E928.3  Human bite
### E928.4  External constriction caused by hair
### E928.5  External constriction caused by other object
### E928.6  Environmental exposure to harmful algae and toxins
Algae bloom NOS      Florida red tide
Blue-green algae bloom  Harmful algae bloom
Brown tide           Pfisteria piscicida
Cyanobacteria bloom   Red tide

### E928.8  Other

### E928.9  Unspecified accident
Accident NOS
Blow NOS          } stated as accidentally
Casualty (not due to war)   inflicted
Decapitation

Knocked down
Killed            } stated as accidentally
Injury [any part of body,    inflicted, but
  or unspecified]          not otherwise
Mangled                 specified
Wound
EXCLUDES *fracture, cause unspecified (E887)*
*injuries undetermined whether*
*accidentally or purposely inflicted*
*(E980.0-E989)*

## LATE EFFECTS OF ACCIDENTAL INJURY (E929)
Note: This category is to be used to indicate accidental injury
as the cause of death or disability from late effects,
which are themselves classifiable elsewhere. The "late
effects" include conditions reported as such, or as
sequelae which may occur at any time after the
attempted suicide or self-inflicted injury.

### ✓4ᵗʰ E929  Late effects of accidental injury
EXCLUDES *late effects of:*
*surgical and medical procedures (E870.0-*
*E879.9)*
*therapeutic use of drugs and medicines*
*(E930.0-E949.9)*

### E929.0  Late effects of motor vehicle accident
Late effects of accidents classifiable to E810-E825

### E929.1  Late effects of other transport accident
Late effects of accidents classifiable to E800-E807,
E826-E838, E840-E848

### E929.2  Late effects of accidental poisoning
Late effects of accidents classifiable to E850-E858,
E860-E869

### E929.3  Late effects of accidental fall
Late effects of accidents classifiable to E880-E888

### E929.4  Late effects of accident caused by fire
Late effects of accidents classifiable to E890-E899

### E929.5  Late effects of accident due to natural and environmental factors
Late effects of accidents classifiable to E900-E909

### E929.8  Late effects of other accidents
Late effects of accidents classifiable to E910-E928.8

### E929.9  Late effects of unspecified accident
Late effects of accidents classifiable to E928.9

## DRUGS, MEDICINAL AND BIOLOGICAL SUBSTANCES CAUSING ADVERSE EFFECTS IN THERAPEUTIC USE (E930-E949)
INCLUDES correct drug properly administered in
therapeutic or prophylactic dosage, as
the cause of any adverse effect including
allergic or hypersensitivity reactions
EXCLUDES *accidental overdose of drug and wrong drug*
*given or taken in error (E850.0-E858.9)*
*accidents in the technique of administration of*
*drug or biological substance, such as*
*accidental puncture during injection, or*
*contamination of drug (E870.0-E876.9)*
*administration with suicidal or homicidal intent*
*or intent to harm, or in circumstances*
*classifiable to E980-E989 (E950.0-E950.5,*
*E962.0, E980.0-E980.5)*
See Alphabetic Index for more complete list of specific
drugs to be classified under the fourth-digit subdivisions.
The American Hospital Formulary numbers can be used to
classify new drugs listed by the American Hospital
Formulary Service (AHFS). See Appendix C.

### ✓4ᵗʰ E930  Antibiotics
EXCLUDES *that used as eye, ear, nose, and throat [ENT],*
*and local anti-infectives (E946.0-E946.9)*

---

✓4ᵗʰ  Fourth-digit Required    ▶◀ Revised Text    ● New Code    ▲ Revised Code Title

**E Codes**

**E930.0–E934.3**

**E930.0 Penicillins**
Natural
Synthetic
Semisynthetic, such as:
ampicillin

Semisynthetic, such as:
cloxacillin
nafcillin
oxacillin

**E930.1 Antifungal antibiotics**
Amphotericin B
Griseofulvin

Hachimycin [trichomycin]
Nystatin

**E930.2 Chloramphenicol group**
Chloramphenicol
Thiamphenicol

**E930.3 Erythromycin and other macrolides**
Oleandomycin
Spiramycin

**E930.4 Tetracycline group**
Doxycycline
Minocycline

Oxytetracycline

**E930.5 Cephalosporin group**
Cephalexin
Cephaloglycin

Cephaloridine
Cephalothin

**E930.6 Antimycobacterial antibiotics**
Cycloserine
Kanamycin

Rifampin
Streptomycin

**E930.7 Antineoplastic antibiotics**
Actinomycins, such as:
Bleomycin
Cactinomycin
Dactinomycin

Actinomycins, such as:
Daunorubicin
Mitomycin

> **EXCLUDES** *other antineoplastic drugs (E933.1)*

**E930.8 Other specified antibiotics**

**E930.9 Unspecified antibiotic**

✓4ᵗʰ **E931 Other anti-infectives**
> **EXCLUDES** *ENT, and local anti-infectives (E946.0-E946.9)*

**E931.0 Sulfonamides**
Sulfadiazine
Sulfafurazole

Sulfamethoxazole

**E931.1 Arsenical anti-infectives**

**E931.2 Heavy metal anti-infectives**
Compounds of:
antimony
bismuth

Compounds of:
lead
mercury

> **EXCLUDES** *mercurial diuretics (E944.0)*

**E931.3 Quinoline and hydroxyquinoline derivatives**
Chiniofon
Diiodohydroxyquin
> **EXCLUDES** *antimalarial drugs (E931.4)*

**E931.4 Antimalarials and drugs acting on other blood protozoa**
Chloroquine phosphate
Cycloguanil
Primaquine

Proguanil [chloroguanide]
Pyrimethamine
Quinine (sulphate)

**E931.5 Other antiprotozoal drugs**
Emetine

**E931.6 Anthelmintics**
Hexylresorcinol
Male fern oleoresin

Piperazine
Thiabendazole

**E931.7 Antiviral drugs**
Methisazone
> **EXCLUDES** *amantadine (E936.4)*
> *cytarabine (E933.1)*
> *idoxuridine (E946.5)*

**E931.8 Other antimycobacterial drugs**
Ethambutol
Ethionamide
Isoniazid

Para-aminosalicylic
acid derivatives
Sulfones

**E931.9 Other and unspecified anti-infectives**
Flucytosine
Nitrofuranderivatives

✓4ᵗʰ **E932 Hormones and synthetic substitutes**
**E932.0 Adrenal cortical steroids**
Cortisone derivatives
Desoxycorticosterone derivatives

Fluorinated corticosteroid

**E932.1 Androgens and anabolic congeners**
Nandrolone phenpropionate
Oxymetholone
Testosterone and preparations

**E932.2 Ovarian hormones and synthetic substitutes**
Contraceptives, oral
Estrogens
Estrogens and progestogens combined
Progestogens

**E932.3 Insulins and antidiabetic agents**
Acetohexamide
Biguanide derivatives, oral
Chlorpropamide
Glucagon
Insulin

Phenformin
Sulfonylurea
derivatives,
oral
Tolbutamide

> **EXCLUDES** *adverse effect of insulin administered for shock therapy (E879.3)*

**E932.4 Anterior pituitary hormones**
Corticotropin
Gonadotropin
Somatotropin [growth hormone]

**E932.5 Posterior pituitary hormones**
Vasopressin
> **EXCLUDES** *oxytocic agents (E945.0)*

**E932.6 Parathyroid and parathyroid derivatives**

**E932.7 Thyroid and thyroid derivatives**
Dextrothyroxine
Levothyroxine sodium

Liothyronine
Thyroglobulin

**E932.8 Antithyroid agents**
Iodides
Thiouracil

Thiourea

**E932.9 Other and unspecified hormones and synthetic substitutes**

✓4ᵗʰ **E933 Primarily systemic agents**
**E933.0 Antiallergic and antiemetic drugs**
Antihistamines
Chlorpheniramine
Diphenhydramine

Diphenylpyraline
Thonzylamine
Tripelennamine

> **EXCLUDES** *phenothiazine-based tranquilizers (E939.1)*

**E933.1 Antineoplastic and immunosuppressive drugs**
Azathioprine
Busulfan
Chlorambucil
Cyclophosphamide
Cytarabine
Fluorouracil
Mechlorethamine hydrochloride
Mercaptopurine
Triethylenethiophosphoramide [thio-TEPA]
> **EXCLUDES** *antineoplastic antibiotics (E930.7)*

**E933.2 Acidifying agents**

**E933.3 Alkalizing agents**

**E933.4 Enzymes, not elsewhere classified**
Penicillinase

**E933.5 Vitamins, not elsewhere classified**
Vitamin A
Vitamin D
> **EXCLUDES** *nicotinic acid (E942.2)*
> *vitamin K (E934.3)*

● **E933.6 Oral bisphosphonates**

● **E933.7 Intravenous bisphosphonates**

**E933.8 Other systemic agents, not elsewhere classified**
Heavy metal antagonists

**E933.9 Unspecified systemic agent**

✓4ᵗʰ **E934 Agents primarily affecting blood constituents**
**E934.0 Iron and its compounds**
Ferric salts
Ferrous sulphate and other ferrous salts

**E934.1 Liver preparations and other antianemic agents**
Folic acid

**E934.2 Anticoagulants**
Coumarin
Heparin
Phenindione

Prothrombin synthesis
inhibitor
Warfarin sodium

**E934.3 Vitamin K [phytonadione]**

---

✓4ᵗʰ Fourth-digit Required    ▶◀ Revised Text    ● New Code    ▲ Revised Code Title

**E Codes**

**E934.4 Fibrinolysis-affecting drugs**
  Aminocaproic acid       Streptokinase
  Streptodornase          Urokinase

**E934.5 Anticoagulant antagonists and other coagulants**
  Hexadimethrine bromide
  Protamine sulfate

**E934.6 Gamma globulin**

**E934.7 Natural blood and blood products**
  Blood plasma            Packed red cells
  Human fibrinogen        Whole blood

**E934.8 Other agents affecting blood constituents**
  Macromolecular blood substitutes

**E934.9 Unspecified agent affecting blood constituents**

☑4ᵗʰ **E935 Analgesics, antipyretics, and antirheumatics**

**E935.0 Heroin**
  Diacetylmorphine

**E935.1 Methadone**

**E935.2 Other opiates and related narcotics**
  Codeine [methylmorphine]    Morphine
  Meperidine [pethidine]      Opium (alkaloids)

**E935.3 Salicylates**
  Acetylsalicylic acid [aspirin]
  Amino derivatives of salicylic acid
  Salicylic acid salts

**E935.4 Aromatic analgesics, not elsewhere classified**
  Acetanilid
  Paracetamol [acetaminophen]
  Phenacetin [acetophenetidin]

**E935.5 Pyrazole derivatives**
  Aminophenazone [aminopyrine]
  Phenylbutazone

**E935.6 Antirheumatics [antiphlogistics]**
  Gold salts              Indomethacin
  **EXCLUDES**  *salicylates (E935.3)*
                *steroids (E932.0)*

**E935.7 Other non-narcotic analgesics**
  Pyrabital

**E935.8 Other specified analgesics and antipyretics**
  Pentazocine

**E935.9 Unspecified analgesic and antipyretic**

☑4ᵗʰ **E936 Anticonvulsants and anti-Parkinsonism drugs**

**E936.0 Oxazolidine derivatives**
  Paramethadione
  Trimethadione

**E936.1 Hydantoin derivatives**
  Phenytoin

**E936.2 Succinimides**
  Ethosuximide            Phensuximide

**E936.3 Other and unspecified anticonvulsants**
  Beclamide               Primidone

**E936.4 Anti-Parkinsonism drugs**
  Amantadine
  Ethopropazine [profenamine]
  Levodopa [L-dopa]

☑4ᵗʰ **E937 Sedatives and hypnotics**

**E937.0 Barbiturates**
  Amobarbital [amylobarbitone]
  Barbital [barbitone]
  Butabarbital [butabarbitone]
  Pentobarbital [pentobarbitone]
  Phenobarbital [phenobarbitone]
  Secobarbital [quinalbarbitone]
  **EXCLUDES**  *thiobarbiturates (E938.3)*

**E937.1 Chloral hydrate group**

**E937.2 Paraldehyde**

**E937.3 Bromine compounds**
  Bromide                 Carbromal (derivatives)

**E937.4 Methaqualone compounds**

**E937.5 Glutethimide group**

**E937.6 Mixed sedatives, not elsewhere classified**

**E937.8 Other sedatives and hypnotics**

**E937.9 Unspecified**
  Sleeping:
    drug   ⎤
    pill   ⎬ NOS
    tablet ⎦

☑4ᵗʰ **E938 Other central nervous system depressants and anesthetics**

**E938.0 Central nervous system muscle-tone depressants**
  Chlorphenesin (carbamate)
  Mephenesin
  Methocarbamol

**E938.1 Halothane**

**E938.2 Other gaseous anesthetics**
  Ether
  Halogenated hydrocarbon derivatives, except halothane
  Nitrous oxide

**E938.3 Intravenous anesthetics**
  Ketamine
  Methohexital [methohexitone]
  Thiobarbiturates, such as thiopental sodium

**E938.4 Other and unspecified general anesthetics**

**E938.5 Surface and infiltration anesthetics**
  Cocaine                 Procaine
  Lidocaine [lignocaine]  Tetracaine

**E938.6 Peripheral nerve- and plexus-blocking anesthetics**

**E938.7 Spinal anesthetics**

**E938.9 Other and unspecified local anesthetics**

☑4ᵗʰ **E939 Psychotropic agents**

**E939.0 Antidepressants**
  Amitriptyline
  Imipramine
  Monoamine oxidase [MAO] inhibitors

**E939.1 Phenothiazine-based tranquilizers**
  Chlorpromazine          Prochlorperazine
  Fluphenazine            Promazine
  Phenothiazine

**E939.2 Butyrophenone-based tranquilizers**
  Haloperidol             Trifluperidol
  Spiperone

**E939.3 Other antipsychotics, neuroleptics, and major tranquilizers**

**E939.4 Benzodiazepine-based tranquilizers**
  Chlordiazepoxide        Lorazepam
  Diazepam                Medazepam
  Flurazepam              Nitrazepam

**E939.5 Other tranquilizers**
  Hydroxyzine             Meprobamate

**E939.6 Psychodysleptics [hallucinogens]**
  Cannabis (derivatives)  Mescaline
  Lysergide [LSD]         Psilocin
  Marihuana (derivatives) Psilocybin

**E939.7 Psychostimulants**
  Amphetamine             Caffeine
  **EXCLUDES**  *central appetite depressants (E947.0)*

**E939.8 Other psychotropic agents**

**E939.9 Unspecified psychotropic agent**

☑4ᵗʰ **E940 Central nervous system stimulants**

**E940.0 Analeptics**
  Lobeline                Nikethamide

**E940.1 Opiate antagonists**
  Levallorphan            Naloxone
  Nalorphine

**E940.8 Other specified central nervous system stimulants**

**E940.9 Unspecified central nervous system stimulant**

☑4ᵗʰ **E941 Drugs primarily affecting the autonomic nervous system**

**E941.0 Parasympathomimetics [cholinergics]**
  Acetylcholine
  Anticholinesterase:
    organophosphorus
    reversible
  Pilocarpine

---

☑4ᵗʰ Fourth-digit Required   ►◄ Revised Text   ● New Code   ▲ Revised Code Title

**E Codes**

**E941.1–E948.0**

**E941.1 Parasympatholytics [anticholinergics and antimuscarinics] and spasmolytics**
Atropine    Hyoscine [scopolamine]
Homatropine    Quaternary ammonium derivatives
EXCLUDES   papaverine (E942.5)

**E941.2 Sympathomimetics [adrenergics]**
Epinephrine [adrenalin]   Levarterenol [noradrenalin]

**E941.3 Sympatholytics [antiadrenergics]**
Phenoxybenzamine
Tolazolinehydrochloride

**E941.9 Unspecified drug primarily affecting the autonomic nervous system**

**√4ᵗʰ E942 Agents primarily affecting the cardiovascular system**

**E942.0 Cardiac rhythm regulators**
Practolol    Propranolol
Procainamide    Quinidine

**E942.1 Cardiotonic glycosides and drugs of similar action**
Digitalis glycosides   Strophanthins
Digoxin

**E942.2 Antilipemic and antiarteriosclerotic drugs**
Cholestyramine   Nicotinic acid derivatives
Clofibrate   Sitosterols
EXCLUDES   dextrothyroxine (E932.7)

**E942.3 Ganglion-blocking agents**
Pentamethonium bromide

**E942.4 Coronary vasodilators**
Dipyridamole   Nitrites
Nitrates [nitroglycerin] Prenylamine

**E942.5 Other vasodilators**
Cyclandelate   Hydralazine
Diazoxide   Papaverine

**E942.6 Other antihypertensive agents**
Clonidine   Rauwolfia alkaloids
Guanethidine   Reserpine

**E942.7 Antivaricose drugs, including sclerosing agents**
Monoethanolamine   Zinc salts

**E942.8 Capillary-active drugs**
Adrenochrome derivatives
Bioflavonoids
Metaraminol

**E942.9 Other and unspecified agents primarily affecting the cardiovascular system**

**√4ᵗʰ E943 Agents primarily affecting gastrointestinal system**

**E943.0 Antacids and antigastric secretion drugs**
Aluminum hydroxide
Magnesium trisilicate

**E943.1 Irritant cathartics**
Bisacodyl   Phenolphthalein
Castor oil

**E943.2 Emollient cathartics**
Sodium dioctyl sulfosuccinate

**E943.3 Other cathartics, including intestinal atonia drugs**
Magnesium sulfate

**E943.4 Digestants**
Pancreatin   Pepsin
Papain

**E943.5 Antidiarrheal drugs**
Bismuth subcarbonate Pectin or Kaolin
EXCLUDES   anti-infectives (E930.0-E931.9)

**E943.6 Emetics**

**E943.8 Other specified agents primarily affecting the gastrointestinal system**

**E943.9 Unspecified agent primarily affecting the gastrointestinal system**

**√4ᵗʰ E944 Water, mineral, and uric acid metabolism drugs**

**E944.0 Mercurial diuretics**
Chlormerodrin   Mercurophylline
Mercaptomerin   Mersalyl

**E944.1 Purine derivative diuretics**
Theobromine   Theophylline
EXCLUDES   aminophylline [theophylline ethylenediamine] (E945.7)

**E944.2 Carbonic acid anhydrase inhibitors**
Acetazolamide

**E944.3 Saluretics**
Benzothiadiazides   Chlorothiazide group

**E944.4 Other diuretics**
Ethacrynic acid   Furosemide

**E944.5 Electrolytic, caloric, and water-balance agents**

**E944.6 Other mineral salts, not elsewhere classified**

**E944.7 Uric acid metabolism drugs**
Cinchophen and congeners   Phenoquin
Colchicine   Probenecid

**√4ᵗʰ E945 Agents primarily acting on the smooth and skeletal muscles and respiratory system**

**E945.0 Oxytocic agents**
Ergot alkaloids
Prostaglandins

**E945.1 Smooth muscle relaxants**
Adiphenine
Metaproterenol [orciprenaline]
EXCLUDES   papaverine (E942.5)

**E945.2 Skeletal muscle relaxants**
Alcuronium chloride
Suxamethonium chloride

**E945.3 Other and unspecified drugs acting on muscles**

**E945.4 Antitussives**
Dextromethorphan   Pipazethate hydrochloride

**E945.5 Expectorants**
Acetylcysteine   Ipecacuanha
Cocillana   Terpin hydrate
Guaifenesin [glyceryl guaiacolate]

**E945.6 Anti-common cold drugs**

**E945.7 Antiasthmatics**
Aminophylline [theophylline ethylenediamine]

**E945.8 Other and unspecified respiratory drugs**

**√4ᵗʰ E946 Agents primarily affecting skin and mucous membrane, ophthalmological, otorhinolaryngological, and dental drugs**

**E946.0 Local anti-infectives and anti-inflammatory drugs**

**E946.1 Antipruritics**

**E946.2 Local astringents and local detergents**

**E946.3 Emollients, demulcents, and protectants**

**E946.4 Keratolytics, kerstoplastics, other hair treatment drugs and preparations**

**E946.5 Eye anti-infectives and other eye drugs**
Idoxuridine

**E946.6 Anti-infectives and other drugs and preparations for ear, nose, and throat**

**E946.7 Dental drugs topically applied**

**E946.8 Other agents primarily affecting skin and mucous membrane**
Spermicides

**E946.9 Unspecified agent primarily affecting skin and mucous membrane**

**√4ᵗʰ E947 Other and unspecified drugs and medicinal substances**

**E947.0 Dietetics**

**E947.1 Lipotropic drugs**

**E947.2 Antidotes and chelating agents, not elsewhere classified**

**E947.3 Alcohol deterrents**

**E947.4 Pharmaceutical excipients**

**E947.8 Other drugs and medicinal substances**
Contrast media used for diagnostic x-ray procedures
Diagnostic agents and kits

**E947.9 Unspecified drug or medicinal substance**

**√4ᵗʰ E948 Bacterial vaccines**

**E948.0 BCG vaccine**

√4ᵗʰ Fourth-digit Required    ►◄ Revised Text    ● New Code    ▲ Revised Code Title

E948.1 Typhoid and paratyphoid

E948.2 Cholera

E948.3 Plague

E948.4 Tetanus

E948.5 Diphtheria

E948.6 Pertussis vaccine, including combinations with a pertussis component

E948.8 Other and unspecified bacterial vaccines

E948.9 Mixed bacterial vaccines, except combinations with a pertussis component

☑4ᵗʰ **E949 Other vaccines and biological substances**
> EXCLUDES   *gamma globulin (E934.6)*

E949.0 Smallpox vaccine

E949.1 Rabies vaccine

E949.2 Typhus vaccine

E949.3 Yellow fever vaccine

E949.4 Measles vaccine

E949.5 Poliomyelitis vaccine

E949.6 Other and unspecified viral and rickettsial vaccines
> Mumps vaccine

E949.7 Mixed viral-rickettsial and bacterial vaccines, except combinations with a pertussis component
> EXCLUDES   *combinations with a pertussis component (E948.6)*

E949.9 Other and unspecified vaccines and biological substances

## SUICIDE AND SELF-INFLICTED INJURY (E950-E959)

> INCLUDES   injuries in suicide and attempted suicide
> self-inflicted injuries specified as intentional

☑4ᵗʰ **E950 Suicide and self-inflicted poisoning by solid or liquid substances**

E950.0 Analgesics, antipyretics, and antirheumatics

E950.1 Barbiturates

E950.2 Other sedatives and hypnotics

E950.3 Tranquilizers and other psychotropic agents

E950.4 Other specified drugs and medicinal substances

E950.5 Unspecified drug or medicinal substance

E950.6 Agricultural and horticultural chemical and pharmaceutical preparations other than plant foods and fertilizers

E950.7 Corrosive and caustic substances
> Suicide and self-inflicted poisoning by substances classifiable to E864

E950.8 Arsenic and its compounds

E950.9 Other and unspecified solid and liquid substances

☑4ᵗʰ **E951 Suicide and self-inflicted poisoning by gases in domestic use**

E951.0 Gas distributed by pipeline

E951.1 Liquefied petroleum gas distributed in mobile containers

E951.8 Other utility gas

☑4ᵗʰ **E952 Suicide and self-inflicted poisoning by other gases and vapors**

E952.0 Motor vehicle exhaust gas

E952.1 Other carbon monoxide

E952.8 Other specified gases and vapors

E952.9 Unspecified gases and vapors

☑4ᵗʰ **E953 Suicide and self-inflicted injury by hanging, strangulation, and suffocation**

E953.0 Hanging

E953.1 Suffocation by plastic bag

E953.8 Other specified means

E953.9 Unspecified means

**E954 Suicide and self-inflicted injury by submersion [drowning]**

☑4ᵗʰ **E955 Suicide and self-inflicted injury by firearms, air guns and explosives**

E955.0 Handgun

E955.1 Shotgun

E955.2 Hunting rifle

E955.3 Military firearms

E955.4 Other and unspecified firearm
> Gunshot NOS      Shot NOS

E955.5 Explosives

E955.6 Air gun
> BB gun      Pellet gun

E955.7 Paintball gun

E955.9 Unspecified

**E956 Suicide and self-inflicted injury by cutting and piercing instrument**

☑4ᵗʰ **E957 Suicide and self-inflicted injuries by jumping from high place**

E957.0 Residential premises

E957.1 Other man-made structures

E957.2 Natural sites

E957.9 Unspecified

☑4ᵗʰ **E958 Suicide and self-inflicted injury by other and unspecified means**

E958.0 Jumping or lying before moving object

E958.1 Burns, fire

E958.2 Scald

E958.3 Extremes of cold

E958.4 Electrocution

E958.5 Crashing of motor vehicle

E958.6 Crashing of aircraft

E958.7 Caustic substances, except poisoning
> EXCLUDES   *poisoning by caustic substance (E950.7)*

E958.8 Other specified means

E958.9 Unspecified means

**E959 Late effects of self-inflicted injury**
> Note: This category is to be used to indicate circumstances classifiable to E950-E958 as the cause of death or disability from late effects, which are themselves classifiable elsewhere. The "late effects" include conditions reported as such, or as sequelae which may occur at any time after the attempted suicide or self-inflicted injury.

## HOMICIDE AND INJURY PURPOSELY INFLICTED BY OTHER PERSONS (E960-E969)

> INCLUDES   injuries inflicted by another person with intent to injure or kill, by any means
> EXCLUDES   *injuries due to:*
> *legal intervention (E970-E978)*
> *operations of war (E990-E999)*
> *terrorism (E979)*

☑4ᵗʰ **E960 Fight, brawl, rape**

E960.0 Unarmed fight or brawl
> Beatings NOS
> Brawl or fight with hands, fists, feet
> Injured or killed in fight NOS
> EXCLUDES   *homicidal:*
> *injury by weapons (E965.0-E966, E969)*
> *strangulation (E963)*
> *submersion (E964)*

E960.1 Rape

**E961 Assault by corrosive or caustic substance, except poisoning**
> Injury or death purposely caused by corrosive or caustic substance, such as:
> acid [any]
> corrosive substance
> vitriol
> EXCLUDES   *burns from hot liquid (E968.3)*
> *chemical burns from swallowing a corrosive substance (E962.0-E962.9)*

---

☑4ᵚ Fourth-digit Required     ▶◀ Revised Text     ● New Code     ▲ Revised Code Title

**E Codes**

**E962–E978**

✓4ᵗʰ **E962 Assault by poisoning**

**E962.0 Drugs and medicinal substances**
Homicidal poisoning by any drug or medicinal substance

**E962.1 Other solid and liquid substances**

**E962.2 Other gases and vapors**

**E962.9 Unspecified poisoning**

**E963 Assault by hanging and strangulation**
Homicidal (attempt):   Homicidal (attempt):
  garrotting or ligature   strangulation
  hanging   suffocation

**E964 Assault by submersion [drowning]**

✓4ᵗʰ **E965 Assault by firearms and explosives**

**E965.0 Handgun**
Pistol     Revolver

**E965.1 Shotgun**

**E965.2 Hunting rifle**

**E965.3 Military firearms**

**E965.4 Other and unspecified firearm**

**E965.5 Antipersonnel bomb**

**E965.6 Gasoline bomb**

**E965.7 Letter bomb**

**E965.8 Other specified explosive**
Bomb NOS (placed in):  Dynamite
  car
  house

**E965.9 Unspecified explosive**

**E966 Assault by cutting and piercing instrument**
Assassination (attempt), homicide (attempt) by any instrument classifiable under E920
Homicidal:
  cut
  puncture  ⎫ any part of body
  stab
  Stabbed

✓4ᵗʰ **E967 Perpetrator of child and adult abuse**
Note: Selection of the correct perpetrator code is based on the relationship between the perpetrator and the victim

**E967.0 By father, stepfather, or boyfriend**
Male partner of child's parent or guardian

**E967.1 By other specified person**

**E967.2 By mother, stepmother, or girlfriend**
Female partner of child's parent or guardian

**E967.3 By spouse or partner**
Abuse of spouse or partner by ex-spouse or ex-partner

**E967.4 By child**

**E967.5 By sibling**

**E967.6 By grandparent**

**E967.7 By other relative**

**E967.8 By non-related caregiver**

**E967.9 By unspecified person**

✓4ᵗʰ **E968 Assault by other and unspecified means**

**E968.0 Fire**
Arson
Homicidal burns NOS
**EXCLUDES** *burns from hot liquid (E968.3)*

**E968.1 Pushing from a high place**

**E968.2 Striking by blunt or thrown object**

**E968.3 Hot liquid**
Homicidal burns by scalding

**E968.4 Criminal neglect**
Abandonment of child, infant, or other helpless person with intent to injure or kill

**E968.5 Transport vehicle**
Being struck by other vehicle or run down with intent to injure
Pushed in front of, thrown from, or dragged by moving vehicle with intent to injure

**E968.6 Air gun**
BB gun
Pellet gun

**E968.7 Human bite**

**E968.8 Other specified means**

**E968.9 Unspecified means**
Assassination (attempt) NOS
Homicidal (attempt):
  injury NOS
  wound NOS
Manslaughter (nonaccidental)
Murder (attempt) NOS
Violence, non-accidental

**E969 Late effects of injury purposely inflicted by other person**
Note: This category is to be used to indicate circumstances classifiable to E960-E968 as the cause of death or disability from late effects, which are themselves classifiable elsewhere. The "late effects" include conditions reported as such, or as sequelae which may occur at any time after injury purposely inflicted by another person.

## LEGAL INTERVENTION (E970-E978)

**INCLUDES** injuries inflicted by the police or other law-enforcing agents, including military on duty, in the course of arresting or attempting to arrest lawbreakers, suppressing disturbances, maintaining order, and other legal action
legal execution

**EXCLUDES** *injuries caused by civil insurrections (E990.0-E999)*

**E970 Injury due to legal intervention by firearms**
Gunshot wound    Injury by:
Injury by:     rifle pellet or
  machine gun     rubber bullet
  revolver     shot NOS

**E971 Injury due to legal intervention by explosives**
Injury by:    Injury by:
  dynamite    grenade
  explosive shell    mortar bomb

**E972 Injury due to legal intervention by gas**
Asphyxiation by gas    Poisoning by gas
Injury by tear gas

**E973 Injury due to legal intervention by blunt object**
Hit, struck by:    Hit, struck by:
  baton (nightstick)    stave
  blunt object

**E974 Injury due to legal intervention by cutting and piercing instrument**
Cut    Injured by bayonet
Incised wound    Stab wound

**E975 Injury due to legal intervention by other specified means**
Blow    Manhandling

**E976 Injury due to legal intervention by unspecified means**

**E977 Late effects of injuries due to legal intervention**
Note: This category is to be used to indicate circumstances classifiable to E970-E976 as the cause of death or disability from late effects, which are themselves classifiable elsewhere. The "late effects" include conditions reported as such, or as sequelae, which may occur at any time after the injury due to legal intervention.

**E978 Legal execution**
All executions performed at the behest of the judiciary or ruling authority [whether permanent or temporary] as:
asphyxiation by gas
beheading, decapitation (by guillotine)
capital punishment
electrocution
hanging
poisoning
shooting
other specified means

**✓4ᵗʰ** Fourth-digit Required   ▶◀ Revised Text   ● New Code   ▲ Revised Code Title

## TERRORISM (E979)

✓4ᵗʰ **E979 Terrorism**

Injuries resulting from the unlawful use of force or violence against persons or property to intimidate or coerce a Government, the civilian population, or any segment thereof, in furtherance of political or social objective

**E979.0 Terrorism involving explosion of marine weapons**

Depth-charge
Marine mine
Mine NOS, at sea or in harbour
Sea-based artillery shell
Torpedo
Underwater blast

**E979.1 Terrorism involving destruction of aircraft**

Aircraft used as a weapon
Aircraft:
  burned
  exploded
  shot down
Crushed by falling aircraft

**E979.2 Terrorism involving other explosions and fragments**

Antipersonnel bomb (fragments)
Blast NOS
Explosion (of):
  artillery shell
  breech-block
  cannon block
  mortar bomb
  munitions being used in terrorism
  NOS
Fragments from:
  artillery shell
  bomb
  grenade
  guided missile
  land-mine
  rocket
  shell
  shrapnel
Mine NOS

**E979.3 Terrorism involving fires, conflagration and hot substances**

Burning building or structure:
  collapse of
  fall from
  hit by falling object in
  jump from
Conflagration NOS
Fire (causing):
  Asphyxia
  Burns
  NOS
  Other injury
Melting of fittings and furniture in burning
Petrol bomb
Smouldering building or structure

**E979.4 Terrorism involving firearms**

Bullet:
  carbine
  machine gun
  pistol
  rifle
  rubber (rifle)
Pellets (shotgun)

**E979.5 Terrorism involving nuclear weapons**

Blast effects
Exposure to ionizing radiation from nuclear weapon
Fireball effects
Heat from nuclear weapon
Other direct and secondary effects of nuclear weapons

**E979.6 Terrorism involving biological weapons**

Anthrax
Cholera
Smallpox

**E979.7 Terrorism involving chemical weapons**

Gases, fumes, chemicals
Hydrogen cyanide
Phosgene
Sarin

**E979.8 Terrorism involving other means**

Drowning and submersion
Lasers
Piercing or stabbing instruments
Terrorism NOS

**E979.9 Terrorism, secondary effects**

Note: This code is for use to identify conditions occurring subsequent to a terrorist attack not those that are due to the initial terrorist act

**EXCLUDES** *late effect of terrorist attack (E999.1)*

## INJURY UNDETERMINED WHETHER ACCIDENTALLY OR PURPOSELY INFLICTED (E980-E989)

Note: Categories E980-E989 are for use when it is unspecified or it cannot be determined whether the injuries are accidental (unintentional), suicide (attempted), or assault.

✓4ᵗʰ **E980 Poisoning by solid or liquid substances, undetermined whether accidentally or purposely inflicted**

**E980.0 Analgesics, antipyretics, and antirheumatics**

**E980.1 Barbiturates**

**E980.2 Other sedatives and hypnotics**

**E980.3 Tranquilizers and other psychotropic agents**

**E980.4 Other specified drugs and medicinal substances**

**E980.5 Unspecified drug or medicinal substance**

**E980.6 Corrosive and caustic substances**

Poisoning, undetermined whether accidental or purposeful, by substances classifiable to E864

**E980.7 Agricultural and horticultural chemical and pharmaceutical preparations other than plant foods and fertilizers**

**E980.8 Arsenic and its compounds**

**E980.9 Other and unspecified solid and liquid substances**

✓4ᵗʰ **E981 Poisoning by gases in domestic use, undetermined whether accidentally or purposely inflicted**

**E981.0 Gas distributed by pipeline**

**E981.1 Liquefied petroleum gas distributed in mobile containers**

**E981.8 Other utility gas**

✓4ᵗʰ **E982 Poisoning by other gases, undetermined whether accidentally or purposely inflicted**

**E982.0 Motor vehicle exhaust gas**

**E982.1 Other carbon monoxide**

**E982.8 Other specified gases and vapors**

**E982.9 Unspecified gases and vapors**

✓4ᵗʰ **E983 Hanging, strangulation, or suffocation, undetermined whether accidentally or purposely inflicted**

**E983.0 Hanging**

**E983.1 Suffocation by plastic bag**

**E983.8 Other specified means**

**E983.9 Unspecified means**

**E984 Submersion [drowning], undetermined whether accidentally or purposely inflicted**

✓4ᵗʰ **E985 Injury by firearms, air guns and explosives, undetermined whether accidentally or purposely inflicted**

**E985.0 Handgun**

**E985.1 Shotgun**

**E985.2 Hunting rifle**

**E985.3 Military firearms**

**E985.4 Other and unspecified firearm**

**E985.5 Explosives**

**E985.6 Air gun**

BB gun                    Pellet gun

**E985.7 Paintball gun**

---

✓4ᵗʰ Fourth-digit Required   ▶◀ Revised Text   ● New Code   ▲ Revised Code Title

**E Codes**

**E986 Injury by cutting and piercing instruments, undetermined whether accidentally or purposely inflicted**

✓4th **E987 Falling from high place, undetermined whether accidentally or purposely inflicted**

    **E987.0 Residential premises**

    **E987.1 Other man-made structures**

    **E987.2 Natural sites**

    **E987.9 Unspecified site**

✓4th **E988 Injury by other and unspecified means, undetermined whether accidentally or purposely inflicted**

    **E988.0 Jumping or lying before moving object**

    **E988.1 Burns, fire**

    **E988.2 Scald**

    **E988.3 Extremes of cold**

    **E988.4 Electrocution**

    **E988.5 Crashing of motor vehicle**

    **E988.6 Crashing of aircraft**

    **E988.7 Caustic substances, except poisoning**

    **E988.8 Other specified means**

    **E988.9 Unspecified means**

**E989 Late effects of injury, undetermined whether accidentally or purposely inflicted**

    Note: This category is to be used to indicate circumstances classifiable to E980-E988 as the cause of death or disability from late effects, which are themselves classifiable elsewhere. The "late effects" include conditions reported as such, or as sequelae, which may occur at any time after injury, undetermined whether accidentally or purposely inflicted.

### INJURY RESULTING FROM OPERATIONS OF WAR (E990-E999)

    INCLUDES    injuries to military personnel and civilians caused by war and civil insurrections and occurring during the time of war and insurrection

    EXCLUDES    *accidents during training of military personnel manufacture of war material and transport, unless attributable to enemy action*

✓4th **E990 Injury due to war operations by fires and conflagrations**

    INCLUDES    asphyxia, burns, or other injury originating from fire caused by a fire-producing device or indirectly by any conventional weapon

    **E990.0 From gasoline bomb**

    **E990.9 From other and unspecified source**

✓4th **E991 Injury due to war operations by bullets and fragments**

    **E991.0 Rubber bullets (rifle)**

    **E991.1 Pellets (rifle)**

    **E991.2 Other bullets**

        Bullet [any, except rubber bullets and pellets]
          carbine
          machine gun
          pistol
          rifle
          shotgun

    **E991.3 Antipersonnel bomb (fragments)**

    **E991.9 Other and unspecified fragments**

        Fragments from:      Fragments from:
          artillery shell      land mine
          bombs, except      rockets
            anti-personnel   shell
          grenade      Shrapnel
          guided missile

**E992 Injury due to war operations by explosion of marine weapons**

    Depth charge      Sea-based artillery shell
    Marine mines      Torpedo
    Mine NOS, at sea or in harbor   Underwater blast

**E993 Injury due to war operations by other explosion**

    Accidental explosion of      Explosion of:
      munitions being used        artillery shell
      in war        breech block
    Accidental explosion of own      cannon block
      weapons        mortar bomb
    Air blast NOS      Injury by weapon burst
    Blast NOS
    Explosion NOS

**E994 Injury due to war operations by destruction of aircraft**

    Airplane:      Airplane:
      burned        shot down
      exploded      Crushed by falling
                    airplane

**E995 Injury due to war operations by other and unspecified forms of conventional warfare**

    Battle wounds
    Bayonet injury
    Drowned in war operations

**E996 Injury due to war operations by nuclear weapons**

    Blast effects
    Exposure to ionizing radiation from nuclear weapons
    Fireball effects
    Heat
    Other direct and secondary effects of nuclear weapons

✓4th **E997 Injury due to war operations by other forms of unconventional warfare**

    **E997.0 Lasers**

    **E997.1 Biological warfare**

    **E997.2 Gases, fumes, and chemicals**

    **E997.8 Other specified forms of unconventional warfare**

    **E997.9 Unspecified form of unconventional warfare**

**E998 Injury due to war operations but occurring after cessation of hostilities**

    Injuries due to operations of war but occurring after cessation of hostilities by any means classifiable under E990-E997

    Injuries by explosion of bombs or mines placed in the course of operations of war, if the explosion occurred after cessation of hostilities

✓4th **E999 Late effect of injury due to war operations and terrorism**

    Note: This category is to be used to indicate circumstances classifiable to E979, E990-E998 as the cause of death or disability from late effects, which are themselves classifiable elsewhere. The "late effects" include conditions reported as such, or as sequelae, which may occur at any time after the injury, resulting from operations of war or terrorism

    **E999.0 Late effect of injury due to war operations**

    **E999.1 Late effect of injury due to terrorism**

```
sea anemone sting e905.6
passenger hurt when snowmobile hit tree e820.1
killed by handgun, possible homicide e985.0, e922.0
bicyclist injured by train e806.3
bicyclist collided with wall e826.1
slashed wrists in suicide attempt e956
loss of hearing from rock music e928.1
injured during earthquake e909.0
diving accident, hit bottom of pool e883.0
hurt at campsite, motor home steps collapsed e880.9
thrown from horse & buggy in collision with car e813.59
injured when hot air balloon crashed e842.6
4y/o drank gasoline from pop bottle e862.1
Injured by fireworks e923.0
Overcome by agent orange in Vietnam e997.2
Failure of aortic valve prosthesis, 4days post-op e878.1
Severe reaction, used prescribed dose of eye meds e858.
Burned while tending fireplace at cottage e895
Dehydration, water to home turned off e904.2
Human bites, left arm; 3y/omale e968.7
Drowned when washed overboard during storm e832.9
Infection, contaminated during heart cath. E872.6
Hand slashed by circular saw e919.4
Accidental ether poisoning at fraternity party e862.0
Skin frozen, contact with dry ice e901.1
```

✓4th Fourth-digit Required      ►◄ Revised Text

# Official ICD-9-CM Government Appendixes

## MORPHOLOGY OF NEOPLASMS

The World Health Organization has published an adaptation of the International Classification of Diseases for oncology (ICD-O). It contains a coded nomenclature for the morphology of neoplasms, which is reproduced here for those who wish to use it in conjunction with Chapter 2 of the International Classification of Diseases, 9th Revision, Clinical Modification.

The morphology code numbers consist of five digits; the first four identify the histological type of the neoplasm and the fifth indicates its behavior. The one-digit behavior code is as follows:

- /0 Benign
- /1 Uncertain whether benign or malignant Borderline malignancy
- /2 Carcinoma in situ
  Intraepithelial
  Noninfiltrating
  Noninvasive
- /3 Malignant, primary site
- /6 Malignant, metastatic site
  Secondary site
- /9 Malignant, uncertain whether primary or metastatic site

In the nomenclature below, the morphology code numbers include the behavior code appropriate to the histological type of neoplasm, but this behavior code should be changed if other reported information makes this necessary. For example, "chordoma (M9370/3)" is assumed to be malignant; the term "benign chordoma" should be coded M9370/0. Similarly, "superficial spreading adenocarcinoma (M8143/3)" described as "noninvasive" should be coded M8143/2 and "melanoma (M8720/3)" described as "secondary" should be coded M8720/6.

The following table shows the correspondence between the morphology code and the different sections of Chapter 2:

| Morphology Code Histology/Behavior | | ICD-9-CM Chapter 2 |
|---|---|---|
| Any | 0 | 210-229 Benign neoplasms |
| M8000-M8004 | 1 | 239 Neoplasms of unspecified nature |
| M8010+ | 1 | 235-238 Neoplasms of uncertain behavior |
| Any | 2 | 230-234 Carcinoma in situ |
| Any | 3 | 140-195 200-208 Malignant neoplasms, stated or presumed to be primary |
| Any | 6 | 196-198 Malignant neoplasms, stated or presumed to be secondary |

The ICD-O behavior digit /9 is inapplicable in an ICD context, since all malignant neoplasms are presumed to be primary (/3) or secondary (/6) according to other information on the medical record.

Only the first-listed term of the full ICD-O morphology nomenclature appears against each code number in the list below. The ICD-9-CM Alphabetical Index (Volume 2), however, includes all the ICD-O synonyms as well as a number of other morphological names still likely to be encountered on medical records but omitted from ICD-O as outdated or otherwise undesirable.

A coding difficulty sometimes arises where a morphological diagnosis contains two qualifying adjectives that have different code numbers. An example is "transitional cell epidermoid carcinoma." "Transitional cell carcinoma NOS" is M8120/3 and "epidermoid carcinoma NOS" is M8070/3. In such circumstances, the higher number (M8120/3 in this example) should be used, as it is usually more specific.

## CODED NOMENCLATURE FOR MORPHOLOGY OF NEOPLASMS

| M800 | Neoplasms NOS |
|---|---|
| M8000/0 | Neoplasm, benign |
| M8000/1 | Neoplasm, uncertain whether benign or malignant |
| M8000/3 | Neoplasm, malignant |
| M8000/6 | Neoplasm, metastatic |
| M8000/9 | Neoplasm, malignant, uncertain whether primary or metastatic |
| M8001/0 | Tumor cells, benign |
| M8001/1 | Tumor cells, uncertain whether benign or malignant |
| M8001/3 | Tumor cells, malignant |
| M8002/3 | Malignant tumor, small cell type |
| M8003/3 | Malignant tumor, giant cell type |
| M8004/3 | Malignant tumor, fusiform cell type |
| **M801-M804** | **Epithelial neoplasms NOS** |
| M8010/0 | Epithelial tumor, benign |
| M8010/2 | Carcinoma in situ NOS |
| M8010/3 | Carcinoma NOS |
| M8010/6 | Carcinoma, metastatic NOS |
| M8010/9 | Carcinomatosis |
| M8011/0 | Epithelioma, benign |
| M8011/3 | Epithelioma, malignant |
| M8012/3 | Large cell carcinoma NOS |
| M8020/3 | Carcinoma, undifferentiated type NOS |
| M8021/3 | Carcinoma, anaplastic type NOS |
| M8022/3 | Pleomorphic carcinoma |
| M8030/3 | Giant cell and spindle cell carcinoma |
| M8031/3 | Giant cell carcinoma |
| M8032/3 | Spindle cell carcinoma |
| M8033/3 | Pseudosarcomatous carcinoma |
| M8034/3 | Polygonal cell carcinoma |
| M8035/3 | Spheroidal cell carcinoma |
| M8040/1 | Tumorlet |
| M8041/3 | Small cell carcinoma NOS |
| M8042/3 | Oat cell carcinoma |
| M8043/3 | Small cell carcinoma, fusiform cell type |
| **M805-M808** | **Papillary and squamous cell neoplasms** |
| M8050/0 | Papilloma NOS (except Papilloma of urinary bladder M8120/1) |
| M8050/2 | Papillary carcinoma in situ |
| M8050/3 | Papillary carcinoma NOS |
| M8051/0 | Verrucous papilloma |
| M8051/3 | Verrucous carcinoma NOS |
| M8052/0 | Squamous cell papilloma |
| M8052/3 | Papillary squamous cell carcinoma |
| M8053/0 | Inverted papilloma |
| M8060/0 | Papillomatosis NOS |
| M8070/2 | Squamous cell carcinoma in situ NOS |
| M8070/3 | Squamous cell carcinoma NOS |
| M8070/6 | Squamous cell carcinoma, metastatic NOS |
| M8071/3 | Squamous cell carcinoma, keratinizing type NOS |
| M8072/3 | Squamous cell carcinoma, large cell, nonkeratinizing type |
| M8073/3 | Squamous cell carcinoma, small cell, nonkeratinizing type |
| M8074/3 | Squamous cell carcinoma, spindle cell type |
| M8075/3 | Adenoid squamous cell carcinoma |
| M8076/2 | Squamous cell carcinoma in situ with questionable stromal invasion |
| M8076/3 | Squamous cell carcinoma, microinvasive |
| M8080/2 | Queyrat's erythroplasia |
| M8081/2 | Bowen's disease |
| M8082/3 | Lymphoepithelial carcinoma |
| **M809-M811** | **Basal cell neoplasms** |
| M8090/1 | Basal cell tumor |
| M8090/3 | Basal cell carcinoma NOS |
| M8091/3 | Multicentric basal cell carcinoma |
| M8092/3 | Basal cell carcinoma, morphea type |
| M8093/3 | Basal cell carcinoma, fibroepithelial type |
| M8094/3 | Basosquamous carcinoma |
| M8095/3 | Metatypical carcinoma |
| M8096/0 | Intraepidermal epithelioma of Jadassohn |
| M8100/0 | Trichoepithelioma |
| M8101/0 | Trichofolliculoma |
| M8102/0 | Tricholemmoma |
| M8110/0 | Pilomatrixoma |
| **M812-M813** | **Transitional cell papillomas and carcinomas** |
| M8120/0 | Transitional cell papilloma NOS |
| M8120/1 | Urothelial papilloma |
| M8120/2 | Transitional cell carcinoma in situ |
| M8120/3 | Transitional cell carcinoma NOS |
| M8121/0 | Schneiderian papilloma |
| M8121/1 | Transitional cell papilloma, inverted type |
| M8121/3 | Schneiderian carcinoma |
| M8122/3 | Transitional cell carcinoma, spindle cell type |
| M8123/3 | Basaloid carcinoma |
| M8124/3 | Cloacogenic carcinoma |
| M8130/3 | Papillary transitional cell carcinoma |
| **M814-M838** | **Adenomas and adenocarcinomas** |
| M8140/0 | Adenoma NOS |
| M8140/1 | Bronchial adenoma NOS |
| M8140/2 | Adenocarcinoma in situ |
| M8140/3 | Adenocarcinoma NOS |
| M8140/6 | Adenocarcinoma, metastatic NOS |
| M8141/3 | Scirrhous adenocarcinoma |
| M8142/3 | Linitis plastica |
| M8143/3 | Superficial spreading adenocarcinoma |
| M8144/3 | Adenocarcinoma, intestinal type |
| M8145/3 | Carcinoma, diffuse type |
| M8146/0 | Monomorphic adenoma |
| M8147/0 | Basal cell adenoma |
| M8150/0 | Islet cell adenoma |
| M8150/3 | Islet cell carcinoma |
| M8151/0 | Insulinoma NOS |
| M8151/3 | Insulinoma, malignant |
| M8152/0 | Glucagonoma NOS |
| M8152/3 | Glucagonoma, malignant |
| M8153/1 | Gastrinoma NOS |

**Appendix A: Morphology of Neoplasms**

| | |
|---|---|
| M8153/3 | Gastrinoma, malignant |
| M8154/3 | Mixed islet cell and exocrine adenocarcinoma |
| M8160/0 | Bile duct adenoma |
| M8160/3 | Cholangiocarcinoma |
| M8161/0 | Bile duct cystadenoma |
| M8161/3 | Bile duct cystadenocarcinoma |
| M8170/0 | Liver cell adenoma |
| M8170/3 | Hepatocellular carcinoma NOS |
| M8180/0 | Hepatocholangioma, benign |
| M8180/3 | Combined hepatocellular carcinoma and cholangiocarcinoma |
| M8190/0 | Trabecular adenoma |
| M8190/3 | Trabecular adenocarcinoma |
| M8191/0 | Embryonal adenoma |
| M8200/0 | Eccrine dermal cylindroma |
| M8200/3 | Adenoid cystic carcinoma |
| M8201/3 | Cribriform carcinoma |
| M8210/0 | Adenomatous polyp NOS |
| M8210/3 | Adenocarcinoma in adenomatous polyp |
| M8211/0 | Tubular adenoma NOS |
| M8211/3 | Tubular adenocarcinoma |
| M8220/0 | Adenomatous polyposis coli |
| M8220/3 | Adenocarcinoma in adenomatous polyposis coli |
| M8221/0 | Multiple adenomatous polyps |
| M8230/0 | Solid carcinoma NOS |
| M8231/3 | Carcinoma simplex |
| M8240/1 | Carcinoid tumor NOS |
| M8240/3 | Carcinoid tumor, malignant |
| M8241/1 | Carcinoid tumor, argentaffin NOS |
| M8241/3 | Carcinoid tumor, argentaffin, malignant |
| M8242/1 | Carcinoid tumor, nonargentaffin NOS |
| M8242/3 | Carcinoid tumor, nonargentaffin, malignant |
| M8243/3 | Mucocarcinoid tumor, malignant |
| M8244/3 | Composite carcinoid |
| M8250/1 | Pulmonary adenomatosis |
| M8250/3 | Bronchiolo-alveolar adenocarcinoma |
| M8251/0 | Alveolar adenoma |
| M8251/3 | Alveolar adenocarcinoma |
| M8260/0 | Papillary adenoma NOS |
| M8260/3 | Papillary adenocarcinoma NOS |
| M8261/1 | Villous adenoma NOS |
| M8261/3 | Adenocarcinoma in villous adenoma |
| M8262/3 | Villous adenocarcinoma |
| M8263/0 | Tubulovillous adenoma |
| M8270/0 | Chromophobe adenoma |
| M8270/3 | Chromophobe carcinoma |
| M8280/0 | Acidophil adenoma |
| M8280/3 | Acidophil carcinoma |
| M8281/0 | Mixed acidophil-basophil adenoma |
| M8281/3 | Mixed acidophil-basophil carcinoma |
| M8290/0 | Oxyphilic adenoma |
| M8290/3 | Oxyphilic adenocarcinoma |
| M8300/0 | Basophil adenoma |
| M8300/3 | Basophil carcinoma |
| M8310/0 | Clear cell adenoma |
| M8310/3 | Clear cell adenocarcinoma NOS |
| M8311/1 | Hypernephroid tumor |
| M8312/3 | Renal cell carcinoma |
| M8313/0 | Clear cell adenofibroma |
| M8320/3 | Granular cell carcinoma |
| M8321/0 | Chief cell adenoma |
| M8322/0 | Water-clear cell adenoma |
| M8322/3 | Water-clear cell adenocarcinoma |
| M8323/0 | Mixed cell adenoma |
| M8323/3 | Mixed cell adenocarcinoma |
| M8324/0 | Lipoadenoma |
| M8330/0 | Follicular adenoma |
| M8330/3 | Follicular adenocarcinoma NOS |
| M8331/3 | Follicular adenocarcinoma, well differentiated type |

| | |
|---|---|
| M8332/3 | Follicular adenocarcinoma, trabecular type |
| M8333/0 | Microfollicular adenoma |
| M8334/0 | Macrofollicular adenoma |
| M8340/3 | Papillary and follicular adenocarcinoma |
| M8350/3 | Nonencapsulated sclerosing carcinoma |
| M8360/1 | Multiple endocrine adenomas |
| M8361/1 | Juxtaglomerular tumor |
| M8370/0 | Adrenal cortical adenoma NOS |
| M8370/3 | Adrenal cortical carcinoma |
| M8371/0 | Adrenal cortical adenoma, compact cell type |
| M8372/0 | Adrenal cortical adenoma, heavily pigmented variant |
| M8373/0 | Adrenal cortical adenoma, clear cell type |
| M8374/0 | Adrenal cortical adenoma, glomerulosa cell type |
| M8375/0 | Adrenal cortical adenoma, mixed cell type |
| M8380/0 | Endometrioid adenoma NOS |
| M8380/1 | Endometrioid adenoma, borderline malignancy |
| M8380/3 | Endometrioid carcinoma |
| M8381/0 | Endometrioid adenofibroma NOS |
| M8381/1 | Endometrioid adenofibroma, borderline malignancy |
| M8381/3 | Endometrioid adenofibroma, malignant |

**M839-M842 Adnexal and skin appendage neoplasms**

| | |
|---|---|
| M8390/0 | Skin appendage adenoma |
| M8390/3 | Skin appendage carcinoma |
| M8400/0 | Sweat gland adenoma |
| M8400/1 | Sweat gland tumor NOS |
| M8400/3 | Sweat gland adenocarcinoma |
| M8401/0 | Apocrine adenoma |
| M8401/3 | Apocrine adenocarcinoma |
| M8402/0 | Eccrine acrospiroma |
| M8403/0 | Eccrine spiradenoma |
| M8404/0 | Hidrocystoma |
| M8405/0 | Papillary hydradenoma |
| M8406/0 | Papillary syringadenoma |
| M8407/0 | Syringoma NOS |
| M8410/0 | Sebaceous adenoma |
| M8410/3 | Sebaceous adenocarcinoma |
| M8420/0 | Ceruminous adenoma |
| M8420/3 | Ceruminous adenocarcinoma |

**M843 Mucoepidermoid neoplasms**

| | |
|---|---|
| M8430/1 | Mucoepidermoid tumor |
| M8430/3 | Mucoepidermoid carcinoma |

**M844-M849 Cystic, mucinous, and serous neoplasms**

| | |
|---|---|
| M8440/0 | Cystadenoma NOS |
| M8440/3 | Cystadenocarcinoma NOS |
| M8441/0 | Serous cystadenoma NOS |
| M8441/1 | Serous cystadenoma, borderline malignancy |
| M8441/3 | Serous cystadenocarcinoma NOS |
| M8450/0 | Papillary cystadenoma NOS |
| M8450/1 | Papillary cystadenoma, borderline malignancy |
| M8450/3 | Papillary cystadenocarcinoma NOS |
| M8460/0 | Papillary serous cystadenoma NOS |
| M8460/1 | Papillary serous cystadenoma, borderline malignancy |
| M8460/3 | Papillary serous cystadenocarcinoma |
| M8461/0 | Serous surface papilloma NOS |
| M8461/1 | Serous surface papilloma, borderline malignancy |
| M8461/3 | Serous surface papillary carcinoma |
| M8470/0 | Mucinous cystadenoma NOS |
| M8470/1 | Mucinous cystadenoma, borderline malignancy |

| | |
|---|---|
| M8470/3 | Mucinous cystadenocarcinoma NOS |
| M8471/0 | Papillary mucinous cystadenoma NOS |
| M8471/1 | Papillary mucinous cystadenoma, borderline malignancy |
| M8471/3 | Papillary mucinous cystadenocarcinoma |
| M8480/0 | Mucinous adenoma |
| M8480/3 | Mucinous adenocarcinoma |
| M8480/6 | Pseudomyxoma peritonei |
| M8481/3 | Mucin-producing adenocarcinoma |
| M8490/3 | Signet ring cell carcinoma |
| M8490/6 | Metastatic signet ring cell carcinoma |

**M850-M854 Ductal, lobular, and medullary neoplasms**

| | |
|---|---|
| M8500/2 | Intraductal carcinoma, noninfiltrating NOS |
| M8500/3 | Infiltrating duct carcinoma |
| M8501/2 | Comedocarcinoma, noninfiltrating |
| M8501/3 | Comedocarcinoma NOS |
| M8502/3 | Juvenile carcinoma of the breast |
| M8503/0 | Intraductal papilloma |
| M8503/2 | Noninfiltrating intraductal papillary adenocarcinoma |
| M8504/0 | Intracystic papillary adenoma |
| M8504/2 | Noninfiltrating intracystic carcinoma |
| M8505/0 | Intraductal papillomatosis NOS |
| M8506/0 | Subareolar duct papillomatosis |
| M8510/3 | Medullary carcinoma NOS |
| M8511/3 | Medullary carcinoma with amyloid stroma |
| M8512/3 | Medullary carcinoma with lymphoid stroma |
| M8520/2 | Lobular carcinoma in situ |
| M8520/3 | Lobular carcinoma NOS |
| M8521/3 | Infiltrating ductular carcinoma |
| M8530/3 | Inflammatory carcinoma |
| M8540/3 | Paget's disease, mammary |
| M8541/3 | Paget's disease and infiltrating duct carcinoma of breast |
| M8542/3 | Paget's disease, extramammary (except Paget's disease of bone) |

**M855 Acinar cell neoplasms**

| | |
|---|---|
| M8550/0 | Acinar cell adenoma |
| M8550/1 | Acinar cell tumor |
| M8550/3 | Acinar cell carcinoma |

**M856-M858 Complex epithelial neoplasms**

| | |
|---|---|
| M8560/3 | Adenosquamous carcinoma |
| M8561/0 | Adenolymphoma |
| M8570/3 | Adenocarcinoma with squamous metaplasia |
| M8571/3 | Adenocarcinoma with cartilaginous and osseous metaplasia |
| M8572/3 | Adenocarcinoma with spindle cell metaplasia |
| M8573/3 | Adenocarcinoma with apocrine metaplasia |
| M8580/0 | Thymoma, benign |
| M8580/3 | Thymoma, malignant |

**M859-M867 Specialized gonadal neoplasms**

| | |
|---|---|
| M8590/1 | Sex cord-stromal tumor |
| M8600/0 | Thecoma NOS |
| M8600/3 | Theca cell carcinoma |
| M8610/0 | Luteoma NOS |
| M8620/1 | Granulosa cell tumor NOS |
| M8620/3 | Granulosa cell tumor, malignant |
| M8621/1 | Granulosa cell-theca cell tumor |
| M8630/0 | Androblastoma, benign |
| M8630/1 | Androblastoma NOS |
| M8630/3 | Androblastoma, malignant |
| M8631/0 | Sertoli-Leydig cell tumor |
| M8632/1 | Gynandroblastoma |
| M8640/0 | Tubular androblastoma NOS |
| M8640/3 | Sertoli cell carcinoma |
| M8641/0 | Tubular androblastoma with lipid storage |

| | |
|---|---|
| M8650/0 | Leydig cell tumor, benign |
| M8650/1 | Leydig cell tumor NOS |
| M8650/3 | Leydig cell tumor, malignant |
| M8660/0 | Hilar cell tumor |
| M8670/0 | Lipid cell tumor of ovary |
| M8671/0 | Adrenal rest tumor |

**M868-M871 Paragangliomas and glomus tumors**

| | |
|---|---|
| M8680/1 | Paraganglioma NOS |
| M8680/3 | Paraganglioma, malignant |
| M8681/1 | Sympathetic paraganglioma |
| M8682/1 | Parasympathetic paraganglioma |
| M8690/1 | Glomus jugulare tumor |
| M8691/1 | Aortic body tumor |
| M8692/1 | Carotid body tumor |
| M8693/1 | Extra-adrenal paraganglioma NOS |
| M8693/3 | Extra-adrenal paraganglioma, malignant |
| M8700/0 | Pheochromocytoma NOS |
| M8700/3 | Pheochromocytoma, malignant |
| M8710/3 | Glomangiosarcoma |
| M8711/0 | Glomus tumor |
| M8712/0 | Glomangioma |

**M872-M879 Nevi and melanomas**

| | |
|---|---|
| M8720/0 | Pigmented nevus NOS |
| M8720/3 | Malignant melanoma NOS |
| M8721/3 | Nodular melanoma |
| M8722/0 | Balloon cell nevus |
| M8722/3 | Balloon cell melanoma |
| M8723/0 | Halo nevus |
| M8724/0 | Fibrous papule of the nose |
| M8725/0 | Neuronevus |
| M8726/0 | Magnocellular nevus |
| M8730/0 | Nonpigmented nevus |
| M8730/3 | Amelanotic melanoma |
| M8740/0 | Junctional nevus |
| M8740/3 | Malignant melanoma in junctional nevus |
| M8741/2 | Precancerous melanosis NOS |
| M8741/3 | Malignant melanoma in precancerous melanosis |
| M8742/2 | Hutchinson's melanotic freckle |
| M8742/3 | Malignant melanoma in Hutchinson's melanotic freckle |
| M8743/3 | Superficial spreading melanoma |
| M8750/0 | Intradermal nevus |
| M8760/0 | Compound nevus |
| M8761/1 | Giant pigmented nevus |
| M8761/3 | Malignant melanoma in giant pigmented nevus |
| M8770/0 | Epithelioid and spindle cell nevus |
| M8771/3 | Epithelioid cell melanoma |
| M8772/3 | Spindle cell melanoma NOS |
| M8773/3 | Spindle cell melanoma, type A |
| M8774/3 | Spindle cell melanoma, type B |
| M8775/3 | Mixed epithelioid and spindle cell melanoma |
| M8780/0 | Blue nevus NOS |
| M8780/3 | Blue nevus, malignant |
| M8790/0 | Cellular blue nevus |

**M880 Soft tissue tumors and sarcomas NOS**

| | |
|---|---|
| M8800/0 | Soft tissue tumor, benign |
| M8800/3 | Sarcoma NOS |
| M8800/9 | Sarcomatosis NOS |
| M8801/3 | Spindle cell sarcoma |
| M8802/3 | Giant cell sarcoma (except of bone M9250/3) |
| M8803/3 | Small cell sarcoma |
| M8804/3 | Epithelioid cell sarcoma |

**M881-M883 Fibromatous neoplasms**

| | |
|---|---|
| M8810/0 | Fibroma NOS |
| M8810/3 | Fibrosarcoma NOS |
| M8811/0 | Fibromyxoma |
| M8811/3 | Fibromyxosarcoma |
| M8812/0 | Periosteal fibroma |
| M8812/3 | Periosteal fibrosarcoma |

| | |
|---|---|
| M8813/0 | Fascial fibroma |
| M8813/3 | Fascial fibrosarcoma |
| M8814/3 | Infantile fibrosarcoma |
| M8820/0 | Elastofibroma |
| M8821/1 | Aggressive fibromatosis |
| M8822/1 | Abdominal fibromatosis |
| M8823/1 | Desmoplastic fibroma |
| M8830/0 | Fibrous histiocytoma NOS |
| M8830/1 | Atypical fibrous histiocytoma |
| M8830/3 | Fibrous histiocytoma, malignant |
| M8831/0 | Fibroxanthoma NOS |
| M8831/1 | Atypical fibroxanthoma |
| M8831/3 | Fibroxanthoma, malignant |
| M8832/0 | Dermatofibroma NOS |
| M8832/1 | Dermatofibroma protuberans |
| M8832/3 | Dermatofibrosarcoma NOS |

**M884 Myxomatous neoplasms**

| | |
|---|---|
| M8840/0 | Myxoma NOS |
| M8840/3 | Myxosarcoma |

**M885-M888 Lipomatous neoplasms**

| | |
|---|---|
| M8850/0 | Lipoma NOS |
| M8850/3 | Liposarcoma NOS |
| M8851/0 | Fibrolipoma |
| M8851/3 | Liposarcoma, well differentiated type |
| M8852/0 | Fibromyxolipoma |
| M8852/3 | Myxoid liposarcoma |
| M8853/3 | Round cell liposarcoma |
| M8854/3 | Pleomorphic liposarcoma |
| M8855/3 | Mixed type liposarcoma |
| M8856/0 | Intramuscular lipoma |
| M8857/0 | Spindle cell lipoma |
| M8860/0 | Angiomyolipoma |
| M8860/3 | Angiomyoliposarcoma |
| M8861/0 | Angiolipoma NOS |
| M8861/1 | Angiolipoma, infiltrating |
| M8870/0 | Myelolipoma |
| M8880/0 | Hibernoma |
| M8881/0 | Lipoblastomatosis |

**M889-M892 Myomatous neoplasms**

| | |
|---|---|
| M8890/0 | Leiomyoma NOS |
| M8890/1 | Intravascular leiomyomatosis |
| M8890/3 | Leiomyosarcoma NOS |
| M8891/1 | Epithelioid leiomyoma |
| M8891/3 | Epithelioid leiomyosarcoma |
| M8892/1 | Cellular leiomyoma |
| M8893/0 | Bizarre leiomyoma |
| M8894/0 | Angiomyoma |
| M8894/3 | Angiomyosarcoma |
| M8895/0 | Myoma |
| M8895/3 | Myosarcoma |
| M8900/0 | Rhabdomyoma NOS |
| M8900/3 | Rhabdomyosarcoma NOS |
| M8901/3 | Pleomorphic rhabdomyosarcoma |
| M8902/3 | Mixed type rhabdomyosarcoma |
| M8903/0 | Fetal rhabdomyoma |
| M8904/0 | Adult rhabdomyoma |
| M8910/3 | Embryonal rhabdomyosarcoma |
| M8920/3 | Alveolar rhabdomyosarcoma |

**M893-M899 Complex mixed and stromal neoplasms**

| | |
|---|---|
| M8930/3 | Endometrial stromal sarcoma |
| M8931/1 | Endolymphatic stromal myosis |
| M8932/0 | Adenomyoma |
| M8940/0 | Pleomorphic adenoma |
| M8940/3 | Mixed tumor, malignant NOS |
| M8950/3 | Mullerian mixed tumor |
| M8951/3 | Mesodermal mixed tumor |
| M8960/1 | Mesoblastic nephroma |
| M8960/3 | Nephroblastoma NOS |
| M8961/3 | Epithelial nephroblastoma |
| M8962/3 | Mesenchymal nephroblastoma |
| M8970/3 | Hepatoblastoma |
| M8980/3 | Carcinosarcoma NOS |
| M8981/3 | Carcinosarcoma, embryonal type |
| M8982/0 | Myoepithelioma |
| M8990/0 | Mesenchymoma, benign |

| | |
|---|---|
| M8990/1 | Mesenchymoma NOS |
| M8990/3 | Mesenchymoma, malignant |
| M8991/3 | Embryonal sarcoma |

**M900-M903 Fibroepithelial neoplasms**

| | |
|---|---|
| M9000/0 | Brenner tumor NOS |
| M9000/1 | Brenner tumor, borderline malignancy |
| M9000/3 | Brenner tumor, malignant |
| M9010/0 | Fibroadenoma NOS |
| M9011/0 | Intracanalicular fibroadenoma NOS |
| M9012/0 | Pericanalicular fibroadenoma |
| M9013/0 | Adenofibroma NOS |
| M9014/0 | Serous adenofibroma |
| M9015/0 | Mucinous adenofibroma |
| M9020/0 | Cellular intracanalicular fibroadenoma |
| M9020/1 | Cystosarcoma phyllodes NOS |
| M9020/3 | Cystosarcoma phyllodes, malignant |
| M9030/0 | Juvenile fibroadenoma |

**M904 Synovial neoplasms**

| | |
|---|---|
| M9040/0 | Synovioma, benign |
| M9040/3 | Synovial sarcoma NOS |
| M9041/3 | Synovial sarcoma, spindle cell type |
| M9042/3 | Synovial sarcoma, epithelioid cell type |
| M9043/3 | Synovial sarcoma, biphasic type |
| M9044/3 | Clear cell sarcoma of tendons and aponeuroses |

**M905 Mesothelial neoplasms**

| | |
|---|---|
| M9050/0 | Mesothelioma, benign |
| M9050/3 | Mesothelioma, malignant |
| M9051/0 | Fibrous mesothelioma, benign |
| M9051/3 | Fibrous mesothelioma, malignant |
| M9052/0 | Epithelioid mesothelioma, benign |
| M9052/3 | Epithelioid mesothelioma, malignant |
| M9053/0 | Mesothelioma, biphasic type, benign |
| M9053/3 | Mesothelioma, biphasic type, malignant |
| M9054/0 | Adenomatoid tumor NOS |

**M906-M909 Germ cell neoplasms**

| | |
|---|---|
| M9060/3 | Dysgerminoma |
| M9061/3 | Seminoma NOS |
| M9062/3 | Seminoma, anaplastic type |
| M9063/3 | Spermatocytic seminoma |
| M9064/3 | Germinoma |
| M9070/3 | Embryonal carcinoma NOS |
| M9071/3 | Endodermal sinus tumor |
| M9072/3 | Polyembryoma |
| M9073/1 | Gonadoblastoma |
| M9080/0 | Teratoma, benign |
| M9080/1 | Teratoma NOS |
| M9080/3 | Teratoma, malignant NOS |
| M9081/3 | Teratocarcinoma |
| M9082/3 | Malignant teratoma, undifferentiated type |
| M9083/3 | Malignant teratoma, intermediate type |
| M9084/0 | Dermoid cyst |
| M9084/3 | Dermoid cyst with malignant transformation |
| M9090/0 | Struma ovarii NOS |
| M9090/3 | Struma ovarii, malignant |
| M9091/1 | Strumal carcinoid |

**M910 Trophoblastic neoplasms**

| | |
|---|---|
| M9100/0 | Hydatidiform mole NOS |
| M9100/1 | Invasive hydatidiform mole |
| M9100/3 | Choriocarcinoma |
| M9101/3 | Choriocarcinoma combined with teratoma |
| M9102/3 | Malignant teratoma, trophoblastic |

**M911 Mesonephromas**

| | |
|---|---|
| M9110/0 | Mesonephroma, benign |
| M9110/1 | Mesonephric tumor |
| M9110/3 | Mesonephroma, malignant |
| M9111/1 | Endosalpingioma |

**Appendix A: Morphology of Neoplasms**

**M912-M916  Blood vessel tumors**
M9120/0  Hemangioma NOS
M9120/3  Hemangiosarcoma
M9121/0  Cavernous hemangioma
M9122/0  Venous hemangioma
M9123/0  Racemose hemangioma
M9124/3  Kupffer cell sarcoma
M9130/0  Hemangioendothelioma, benign
M9130/1  Hemangioendothelioma NOS
M9130/3  Hemangioendothelioma, malignant
M9131/0  Capillary hemangioma
M9132/0  Intramuscular hemangioma
M9140/3  Kaposi's sarcoma
M9141/0  Angiokeratoma
M9142/0  Verrucous keratotic hemangioma
M9150/0  Hemangiopericytoma, benign
M9150/1  Hemangiopericytoma NOS
M9150/3  Hemangiopericytoma, malignant
M9160/0  Angiofibroma NOS
M9161/1  Hemangioblastoma
**M917  Lymphatic vessel tumors**
M9170/0  Lymphangioma NOS
M9170/3  Lymphangiosarcoma
M9171/0  Capillary lymphangioma
M9172/0  Cavernous lymphangioma
M9173/0  Cystic lymphangioma
M9174/0  Lymphangiomyoma
M9174/1  Lymphangiomyomatosis
M9175/0  Hemolymphangioma
**M918-M920  Osteomas and osteosarcomas**
M9180/0  Osteoma NOS
M9180/3  Osteosarcoma NOS
M9181/3  Chondroblastic osteosarcoma
M9182/3  Fibroblastic osteosarcoma
M9183/3  Telangiectatic osteosarcoma
M9184/3  Osteosarcoma in Paget's disease of bone
M9190/3  Juxtacortical osteosarcoma
M9191/0  Osteoid osteoma NOS
M9200/0  Osteoblastoma
**M921-M924  Chondromatous neoplasms**
M9210/0  Osteochondroma
M9210/1  Osteochondromatosis NOS
M9220/0  Chondroma NOS
M9220/1  Chondromatosis NOS
M9220/3  Chondrosarcoma NOS
M9221/0  Juxtacortical chondroma
M9221/3  Juxtacortical chondrosarcoma
M9230/0  Chondroblastoma NOS
M9230/3  Chondroblastoma, malignant
M9240/3  Mesenchymal chondrosarcoma
M9241/0  Chondromyxoid fibroma
**M925  Giant cell tumors**
M9250/1  Giant cell tumor of bone NOS
M9250/3  Giant cell tumor of bone, malignant
M9251/1  Giant cell tumor of soft parts NOS
M9251/3  Malignant giant cell tumor of soft parts
**M926  Miscellaneous bone tumors**
M9260/3  Ewing's sarcoma
M9261/3  Adamantinoma of long bones
M9262/0  Ossifying fibroma
**M927-M934  Odontogenic tumors**
M9270/0  Odontogenic tumor, benign
M9270/1  Odontogenic tumor NOS
M9270/3  Odontogenic tumor, malignant
M9271/0  Dentinoma
M9272/0  Cementoma NOS
M9273/0  Cementoblastoma, benign
M9274/0  Cementifying fibroma
M9275/0  Gigantiform cementoma
M9280/0  Odontoma NOS
M9281/0  Compound odontoma
M9282/0  Complex odontoma
M9290/0  Ameloblastic fibro-odontoma
M9290/3  Ameloblastic odontosarcoma
M9300/0  Adenomatoid odontogenic tumor

M9301/0  Calcifying odontogenic cyst
M9310/0  Ameloblastoma NOS
M9310/3  Ameloblastoma, malignant
M9311/0  Odontoameloblastoma
M9312/0  Squamous odontogenic tumor
M9320/0  Odontogenic myxoma
M9321/0  Odontogenic fibroma NOS
M9330/0  Ameloblastic fibroma
M9330/3  Ameloblastic fibrosarcoma
M9340/0  Calcifying epithelial odontogenic tumor
**M935-M937  Miscellaneous tumors**
M9350/1  Craniopharyngioma
M9360/1  Pinealoma
M9361/1  Pineocytoma
M9362/3  Pineoblastoma
M9363/0  Melanotic neuroectodermal tumor
M9370/0  Chordoma
**M938-M948  Gliomas**
M9380/3  Glioma, malignant
M9381/3  Gliomatosis cerebri
M9382/3  Mixed glioma
M9383/1  Subependymal glioma
M9384/1  Subependymal giant cell astrocytoma
M9390/0  Choroid plexus papilloma NOS
M9390/3  Choroid plexus papilloma, malignant
M9391/3  Ependymoma NOS
M9392/3  Ependymoma, anaplastic type
M9393/1  Papillary ependymoma
M9394/1  Myxopapillary ependymoma
M9400/3  Astrocytoma NOS
M9401/3  Astrocytoma, anaplastic type
M9410/3  Protoplasmic astrocytoma
M9411/3  Gemistocytic astrocytoma
M9420/3  Fibrillary astrocytoma
M9421/3  Pilocytic astrocytoma
M9422/3  Spongioblastoma NOS
M9423/3  Spongioblastoma polare
M9430/3  Astroblastoma
M9440/3  Glioblastoma NOS
M9441/3  Giant cell glioblastoma
M9442/3  Glioblastoma with sarcomatous component
M9443/3  Primitive polar spongioblastoma
M9450/3  Oligodendroglioma NOS
M9451/3  Oligodendroglioma, anaplastic type
M9460/3  Oligodendroblastoma
M9470/3  Medulloblastoma NOS
M9471/3  Desmoplastic medulloblastoma
M9472/3  Medullomyoblastoma
M9480/3  Cerebellar sarcoma NOS
M9481/3  Monstrocellular sarcoma
**M949-M952  Neuroepitheliomatous neoplasms**
M9490/0  Ganglioneuroma
M9490/3  Ganglioneuroblastoma
M9491/0  Ganglioneuromatosis
M9500/3  Neuroblastoma NOS
M9501/3  Medulloepithelioma NOS
M9502/3  Teratoid medulloepithelioma
M9503/3  Neuroepithelioma NOS
M9504/3  Spongioneuroblastoma
M9505/1  Ganglioglioma
M9506/0  Neurocytoma
M9507/0  Pacinian tumor
M9510/3  Retinoblastoma NOS
M9511/3  Retinoblastoma, differentiated type
M9512/3  Retinoblastoma, undifferentiated type
M9520/3  Olfactory neurogenic tumor
M9521/3  Esthesioneurocytoma
M9522/3  Esthesioneuroblastoma
M9523/3  Esthesioneuroepithelioma
**M953  Meningiomas**
M9530/0  Meningioma NOS
M9530/1  Meningiomatosis NOS

M9530/3  Meningioma, malignant
M9531/0  Meningotheliomatous meningioma
M9532/0  Fibrous meningioma
M9533/0  Psammomatous meningioma
M9534/0  Angiomatous meningioma
M9535/0  Hemangioblastic meningioma
M9536/0  Hemangiopericytic meningioma
M9537/0  Transitional meningioma
M9538/1  Papillary meningioma
M9539/3  Meningeal sarcomatosis
**M954-M957  Nerve sheath tumor**
M9540/0  Neurofibroma NOS
M9540/1  Neurofibromatosis NOS
M9540/3  Neurofibrosarcoma
M9541/0  Melanotic neurofibroma
M9550/0  Plexiform neurofibroma
M9560/0  Neurilemmoma NOS
M9560/1  Neurinomatosis
M9560/3  Neurilemmoma, malignant
M9570/0  Neuroma NOS
**M958  Granular cell tumors and alveolar soft part sarcoma**
M9580/0  Granular cell tumor NOS
M9580/3  Granular cell tumor, malignant
M9581/3  Alveolar soft part sarcoma
**M959-M963  Lymphomas, NOS or diffuse**
M9590/0  Lymphomatous tumor, benign
M9590/3  Malignant lymphoma NOS
M9591/3  Malignant lymphoma, non Hodgkin's type
M9600/3  Malignant lymphoma, undifferentiated cell type NOS
M9601/3  Malignant lymphoma, stem cell type
M9602/3  Malignant lymphoma, convoluted cell type NOS
M9610/3  Lymphosarcoma NOS
M9611/3  Malignant lymphoma, lymphoplasmacytoid type
M9612/3  Malignant lymphoma, immunoblastic type
M9613/3  Malignant lymphoma, mixed lymphocytic-histiocytic NOS
M9614/3  Malignant lymphoma, centroblastic-centrocytic, diffuse
M9615/3  Malignant lymphoma, follicular center cell NOS
M9620/3  Malignant lymphoma, lymphocytic, well differentiated NOS
M9621/3  Malignant lymphoma, lymphocytic, intermediate differentiation NOS
M9622/3  Malignant lymphoma, centrocytic
M9623/3  Malignant lymphoma, follicular center cell, cleaved NOS
M9630/3  Malignant lymphoma, lymphocytic, poorly differentiated NOS
M9631/3  Prolymphocytic lymphosarcoma
M9632/3  Malignant lymphoma, centroblastic type NOS
M9633/3  Malignant lymphoma, follicular center cell, noncleaved NOS
**M964  Reticulosarcomas**
M9640/3  Reticulosarcoma NOS
M9641/3  Reticulosarcoma, pleomorphic cell type
M9642/3  Reticulosarcoma, nodular
**M965-M966  Hodgkin's disease**
M9650/3  Hodgkin's disease NOS
M9651/3  Hodgkin's disease, lymphocytic predominance
M9652/3  Hodgkin's disease, mixed cellularity
M9653/3  Hodgkin's disease, lymphocytic depletion NOS
M9654/3  Hodgkin's disease, lymphocytic depletion, diffuse fibrosis
M9655/3  Hodgkin's disease, lymphocytic depletion, reticular type

| | |
|---|---|
| M9656/3 | Hodgkin's disease, nodular sclerosis NOS |
| M9657/3 | Hodgkin's disease, nodular sclerosis, cellular phase |
| M9660/3 | Hodgkin's paragranuloma |
| M9661/3 | Hodgkin's granuloma |
| M9662/3 | Hodgkin's sarcoma |

**M969  Lymphomas, nodular or follicular**

| | |
|---|---|
| M9690/3 | Malignant lymphoma, nodular NOS |
| M9691/3 | Malignant lymphoma, mixed lymphocytic-histiocytic, nodular |
| M9692/3 | Malignant lymphoma, centroblastic-centrocytic, follicular |
| M9693/3 | Malignant lymphoma, lymphocytic, well differentiated, nodular |
| M9694/3 | Malignant lymphoma, lymphocytic, intermediate differentiation, nodular |
| M9695/3 | Malignant lymphoma, follicular center cell, cleaved, follicular |
| M9696/3 | Malignant lymphoma, lymphocytic, poorly differentiated, nodular |
| M9697/3 | Malignant lymphoma, centroblastic type, follicular |
| M9698/3 | Malignant lymphoma, follicular center cell, noncleaved, follicular |

**M970  Mycosis fungoides**

| | |
|---|---|
| M9700/3 | Mycosis fungoides |
| M9701/3 | Sezary's disease |

**M971-M972  Miscellaneous reticuloendothelial neoplasms**

| | |
|---|---|
| M9710/3 | Microglioma |
| M9720/3 | Malignant histiocytosis |
| M9721/3 | Histiocytic medullary reticulosis |
| M9722/3 | Letterer-Siwe's disease |

**M973  Plasma cell tumors**

| | |
|---|---|
| M9730/3 | Plasma cell myeloma |
| M9731/0 | Plasma cell tumor, benign |
| M9731/1 | Plasmacytoma NOS |
| M9731/3 | Plasma cell tumor, malignant |

**M974  Mast cell tumors**

| | |
|---|---|
| M9740/1 | Mastocytoma NOS |
| M9740/3 | Mast cell sarcoma |
| M9741/3 | Malignant mastocytosis |

**M975  Burkitt's tumor**

| | |
|---|---|
| M9750/3 | Burkitt's tumor |

**M980-M994  Leukemias**

**M980  Leukemias NOS**

| | |
|---|---|
| M9800/3 | Leukemia NOS |
| M9801/3 | Acute leukemia NOS |
| M9802/3 | Subacute leukemia NOS |
| M9803/3 | Chronic leukemia NOS |
| M9804/3 | Aleukemic leukemia NOS |

**M981  Compound leukemias**

| | |
|---|---|
| M9810/3 | Compound leukemia |

**M982  Lymphoid leukemias**

| | |
|---|---|
| M9820/3 | Lymphoid leukemia NOS |
| M9821/3 | Acute lymphoid leukemia |
| M9822/3 | Subacute lymphoid leukemia |
| M9823/3 | Chronic lymphoid leukemia |
| M9824/3 | Aleukemic lymphoid leukemia |
| M9825/3 | Prolymphocytic leukemia |

**M983  Plasma cell leukemias**

| | |
|---|---|
| M9830/3 | Plasma cell leukemia |

**M984  Erythroleukemias**

| | |
|---|---|
| M9840/3 | Erythroleukemia |
| M9841/3 | Acute erythremia |
| M9842/3 | Chronic erythremia |

**M985  Lymphosarcoma cell leukemias**

| | |
|---|---|
| M9850/3 | Lymphosarcoma cell leukemia |

**M986  Myeloid leukemias**

| | |
|---|---|
| M9860/3 | Myeloid leukemia NOS |
| M9861/3 | Acute myeloid leukemia |
| M9862/3 | Subacute myeloid leukemia |
| M9863/3 | Chronic myeloid leukemia |
| M9864/3 | Aleukemic myeloid leukemia |
| M9865/3 | Neutrophilic leukemia |
| M9866/3 | Acute promyelocytic leukemia |

**M987  Basophilic leukemias**

| | |
|---|---|
| M9870/3 | Basophilic leukemia |

**M988  Eosinophilic leukemias**

| | |
|---|---|
| M9880/3 | Eosinophilic leukemia |

**M989  Monocytic leukemias**

| | |
|---|---|
| M9890/3 | Monocytic leukemia NOS |
| M9891/3 | Acute monocytic leukemia |
| M9892/3 | Subacute monocytic leukemia |
| M9893/3 | Chronic monocytic leukemia |
| M9894/3 | Aleukemic monocytic leukemia |

**M990-M994  Miscellaneous leukemias**

| | |
|---|---|
| M9900/3 | Mast cell leukemia |
| M9910/3 | Megakaryocytic leukemia |
| M9920/3 | Megakaryocytic myelosis |
| M9930/3 | Myeloid sarcoma |
| M9940/3 | Hairy cell leukemia |

**M995-M997  Miscellaneous myeloproliferative and lymphoproliferative disorders**

| | |
|---|---|
| M9950/1 | Polycythemia vera |
| M9951/1 | Acute panmyelosis |
| M9960/1 | Chronic myeloproliferative disease |
| M9961/1 | Myelosclerosis with myeloid metaplasia |
| M9962/1 | Idiopathic thrombocythemia |
| M9970/1 | Chronic lymphoproliferative disease |

Appendix B: Glossary of Mental Disorders

# Appendix B
# was officially deleted
# October 1, 2004

## CLASSIFICATION OF DRUGS BY AMERICAN HOSPITAL FORMULARY SERVICE LIST NUMBER AND THEIR ICD-9-CM EQUIVALENTS

The coding of adverse effects of drugs is keyed to the continually revised Hospital Formulary of the American Hospital Formulary Service (AHFS) published under the direction of the American Society of Hospital Pharmacists.

The following section gives the ICD-9-CM diagnosis code for each AHFS list.

| AHFS* List | ICD-9-CM Diagnosis Code |
|---|---|
| 4:00 ANTIHISTAMINE DRUGS | 963.0 |
| 8:00 ANTI-INFECTIVE AGENTS | |
| 8:04 Amebacides | 961.5 |
| hydroxyquinoline derivatives | 961.3 |
| arsenical anti-infectives | 961.1 |
| 8:08 Anthelmintics | 961.6 |
| quinoline derivatives | 961.3 |
| 8:12.04 Antifungal Antibiotics | 960.1 |
| nonantibiotics | 961.9 |
| 8:12.06 Cephalosporins | 960.5 |
| 8:12.08 Chloramphenicol | 960.2 |
| 8:12.12 The Erythromycins | 960.3 |
| 8:12.16 The Penicillins | 960.0 |
| 8:12.20 The Streptomycins | 960.6 |
| 8:12.24 The Tetracyclines | 960.4 |
| 8:12.28 Other Antibiotics | 960.8 |
| antimycobacterial antibiotics | 960.6 |
| macrolides | 960.3 |
| 8:16 Antituberculars | 961.8 |
| antibiotics | 960.6 |
| 8:18 Antivirals | 961.7 |
| 8:20 Plasmodicides (antimalarials) | 961.4 |
| 8:24 Sulfonamides | 961.0 |
| 8:26 The Sulfones | 961.8 |
| 8:28 Treponemicides | 961.2 |
| 8:32 Trichomonacides | 961.5 |
| hydroxyquinoline derivatives | 961.3 |
| nitrofuran derivatives | 961.9 |
| 8:36 Urinary Germicides | 961.9 |
| quinoline derivatives | 961.3 |
| 8:40 Other Anti-Infectives | 961.9 |
| 10:00 ANTINEOPLASTIC AGENTS | 963.1 |
| antibiotics | 960.7 |
| progestogens | 962.2 |
| 12:00 AUTONOMIC DRUGS | |
| 12:04 Parasympathomimetic (Cholinergic) Agents | 971.0 |
| 12:08 Parasympatholytic (Cholinergic Blocking) Agents | 971.1 |
| 12:12 Sympathomimetic (Adrenergic) Agents | 971.2 |
| 12:16 Sympatholytic (Adrenergic Blocking) Agents | 971.3 |
| 12:20 Skeletal Muscle Relaxants | 975.2 |
| central nervous system muscle-tone depressants | 968.0 |
| 16:00 BLOOD DERIVATIVES | 964.7 |
| 20:00 BLOOD FORMATION AND COAGULATION | |
| 20:04 Antianemia Drugs | 964.1 |
| 20:04.04 Iron Preparations | 964.0 |
| 20:04.08 Liver and Stomach Preparations | 964.1 |
| 20:12.04 Anticoagulants | 964.2 |
| 20:12.08 Antiheparin Agents | 964.5 |
| 20:12.12 Coagulants | 964.5 |
| 20:12.16 Hemostatics | 964.5 |
| capillary-active drugs | 972.8 |
| fibrinolysis-affecting agents | 964.4 |
| natural products | 964.7 |
| 24:00 CARDIOVASCULAR DRUGS | |
| 24:04 Cardiac Drugs | 972.9 |
| cardiotonic agents | 972.1 |
| rhythm regulators | 972.0 |
| 24:06 Antilipemic Agents | 972.2 |
| thyroid derivatives | 962.7 |
| 24:08 Hypotensive Agents | 972.6 |
| adrenergic blocking agents | 971.3 |
| ganglion-blocking agents | 972.3 |
| vasodilators | 972.5 |
| 24:12 Vasodilating Agents | 972.5 |
| coronary | 972.4 |
| nicotinic acid derivatives | 972.2 |

| AHFS* List | ICD-9-CM Diagnosis Code |
|---|---|
| 24:16 Sclerosing Agents | 972.7 |
| 28:00 CENTRAL NERVOUS SYSTEM DRUGS | |
| 28:04 General Anesthetics | 968.4 |
| gaseous anesthetics | 968.2 |
| halothane | 968.1 |
| intravenous anesthetics | 968.3 |
| 28:08 Analgesics and Antipyretics | 965.9 |
| antirheumatics | 965.61-965.69 |
| aromatic analgesics | 965.4 |
| non-narcotics NEC | 965.7 |
| opium alkaloids | 965.00 |
| heroin | 965.01 |
| methadone | 965.02 |
| specified type NEC | 965.09 |
| pyrazole derivatives | 965.5 |
| salicylates | 965.1 |
| specified type NEC | 965.8 |
| 28:10 Narcotic Antagonists | 970.1 |
| 28:12 Anticonvulsants | 966.3 |
| barbiturates | 967.0 |
| benzodiazepine-based tranquilizers | 969.4 |
| bromides | 967.3 |
| hydantoin derivatives | 966.1 |
| oxazolidine derivative | 966.0 |
| succinimides | 966.2 |
| 28:16.04 Antidepressants | 969.0 |
| 28:16.08 Tranquilizers | 969.5 |
| benzodiazepine-based | 969.4 |
| butyrophenone-based | 969.2 |
| major NEC | 969.3 |
| phenothiazine-based | 969.1 |
| 28:16.12 Other Psychotherapeutic Agents | 969.8 |
| 28:20 Respiratory and Cerebral Stimulants | 970.9 |
| analeptics | 970.0 |
| anorexigenic agents | 977.0 |
| psychostimulants | 969.7 |
| specified type NEC | 970.8 |
| 28:24 Sedatives and Hypnotics | 967.9 |
| barbiturates | 967.0 |
| benzodiazepine-based tranquilizers | 969.4 |
| chloral hydrate group | 967.1 |
| glutethamide group | 967.5 |
| intravenous anesthetics | 968.3 |
| methaqualone | 967.4 |
| paraldehyde | 967.2 |
| phenothiazine-based tranquilizers | 969.1 |
| specified type NEC | 967.8 |
| thiobarbiturates | 968.3 |
| tranquilizer NEC | 969.5 |
| 36:00 DIAGNOSTIC AGENTS | 977.8 |
| 40:00 ELECTROLYTE, CALORIC, AND WATER BALANCE AGENTS NEC | 974.5 |
| 40:04 Acidifying Agents | 963.2 |
| 40:08 Alkalinizing Agents | 963.3 |
| 40:10 Ammonia Detoxicants | 974.5 |
| 40:12 Replacement Solutions NEC | 974.5 |
| plasma volume expanders | 964.8 |
| 40:16 Sodium-Removing Resins | 974.5 |
| 40:18 Potassium-Removing Resins | 974.5 |
| 40:20 Caloric Agents | 974.5 |
| 40:24 Salt and Sugar Substitutes | 974.5 |
| 40:28 Diuretics NEC | 974.4 |
| carbonic acid anhydrase inhibitors | 974.2 |
| mercurials | 974.0 |
| purine derivatives | 974.1 |
| saluretics | 974.3 |
| 40:36 Irrigating Solutions | 974.5 |
| 40:40 Uricosuric Agents | 974.7 |
| 44:00 ENZYMES NEC | 963.4 |
| fibrinolysis-affecting agents | 964.4 |
| gastric agents | 973.4 |

**Appendix C: Classification of Drugs by AHFS List**

| AHFS* List | ICD-9-CM Diagnosis Code |
|---|---|
| 48:00 EXPECTORANTS AND COUGH PREPARATIONS | |
|     antihistamine agents | 963.0 |
|     antitussives | 975.4 |
|     codeine derivatives | 965.09 |
|     expectorants | 975.5 |
|     narcotic agents NEC | 965.09 |
| 52:00 EYE, EAR, NOSE, AND THROAT PREPARATIONS | |
| 52:04 Anti-Infectives | |
|     ENT | 976.6 |
|     ophthalmic | 976.5 |
| 52:04.04 Antibiotics | |
|     ENT | 976.6 |
|     ophthalmic | 976.5 |
| 52:04.06 Antivirals | |
|     ENT | 976.6 |
|     ophthalmic | 976.5 |
| 52:04.08 Sulfonamides | |
|     ENT | 976.6 |
|     ophthalmic | 976.5 |
| 52:04.12 Miscellaneous Anti-Infectives | |
|     ENT | 976.6 |
|     ophthalmic | 976.5 |
| 52:08 Anti-Inflammatory Agents | |
|     ENT | 976.6 |
|     ophthalmic | 976.5 |
| 52:10 Carbonic Anhydrase Inhibitors | 974.2 |
| 52:12 Contact Lens Solutions | 976.5 |
| 52:16 Local Anesthetics | 968.5 |
| 52:20 Miotics | 971.0 |
| 52:24 Mydriatics | |
|     adrenergics | 971.2 |
|     anticholinergics | 971.1 |
|     antimuscarinics | 971.1 |
|     parasympatholytics | 971.1 |
|     spasmolytics | 971.1 |
|     sympathomimetics | 971.2 |
| 52:28 Mouth Washes and Gargles | 976.6 |
| 52:32 Vasoconstrictors | 971.2 |
| 52:36 Unclassified Agents | |
|     ENT | 976.6 |
|     ophthalmic | 976.5 |
| 56:00 GASTROINTESTINAL DRUGS | |
| 56:04 Antacids and Absorbents | 973.0 |
| 56:08 Anti-Diarrhea Agents | 973.5 |
| 56:10 Antiflatulents | 973.8 |
| 56:12 Cathartics NEC | 973.3 |
|     emollients | 973.2 |
|     irritants | 973.1 |
| 56:16 Digestants | 973.4 |
| 56:20 Emetics and Antiemetics | |
|     antiemetics | 963.0 |
|     emetics | 973.6 |
| 56:24 Lipotropic Agents | 977.1 |
| 60:00 GOLD COMPOUNDS | 965.69 |
| 64:00 HEAVY METAL ANTAGONISTS | 963.8 |
| 68:00 HORMONES AND SYNTHETIC SUBSTITUTES | |
| 68:04 Adrenals | 962.0 |
| 68:08 Androgens | 962.1 |
| 68:12 Contraceptives | 962.2 |
| 68:16 Estrogens | 962.2 |
| 68:18 Gonadotropins | 962.4 |
| 68:20 Insulins and Antidiabetic Agents | 962.3 |
| 68:20.08 Insulins | 962.3 |
| 68:24 Parathyroid | 962.6 |
| 68:28 Pituitary | |
|     anterior | 962.4 |
|     posterior | 962.5 |
| 68:32 Progestogens | 962.2 |
| 68:34 Other Corpus Luteum Hormones | 962.2 |
| 68:36 Thyroid and Antithyroid | |
|     antithyroid | 962.8 |
|     thyroid | 962.7 |

| AHFS* List | ICD-9-CM Diagnosis Code |
|---|---|
| 72:00 LOCAL ANESTHETICS NEC | 968.9 |
|     topical (surface) agents | 968.5 |
|     infiltrating agents (intradermal) | |
|       (subcutaneous) (submucosal) | 968.5 |
|     nerve blocking agents (peripheral) | |
|       (plexus) (regional) | 968.6 |
|     spinal | 968.7 |
| 76:00 OXYTOCICS | 975.0 |
| 78:00 RADIOACTIVE AGENTS | 990 |
| 80:00 SERUMS, TOXOIDS, AND VACCINES | |
| 80:04 Serums | 979.9 |
|     immune globulin (gamma) (human) | 964.6 |
| 80:08 Toxoids NEC | 978.8 |
|     diphtheria | 978.5 |
|       and tetanus | 978.9 |
|         with pertussis component | 978.6 |
|     tetanus | 978.4 |
|       and diphtheria | 978.9 |
|         with pertussis component | 978.6 |
| 80:12 Vaccines NEC | 979.9 |
|     bacterial NEC | 978.8 |
|       with | |
|         other bacterial component | 978.9 |
|         pertussis component | 978.6 |
|         viral and rickettsial component | 979.7 |
|     rickettsial NEC | 979.6 |
|       with | |
|         bacterial component | 979.7 |
|         pertussis component | 978.6 |
|         viral component | 979.7 |
|     viral NEC | 979.6 |
|       with | |
|         bacterial component | 979.7 |
|         pertussis component | 978.6 |
|         rickettsial component | 979.7 |
| 84:00 SKIN AND MUCOUS MEMBRANE PREPARATIONS | |
| 84:04 Anti-Infectives | 976.0 |
| 84:04.04 Antibiotics | 976.0 |
| 84:04.08 Fungicides | 976.0 |
| 84:04.12 Scabicides and Pediculicides | 976.0 |
| 84:04.16 Miscellaneous Local Anti-Infectives | 976.0 |
| 84:06 Anti-Inflammatory Agents | 976.0 |
| 84:08 Antipruritics and Local Anesthetics | |
|     antipruritics | 976.1 |
|     local anesthetics | 968.5 |
| 84:12 Astringents | 976.2 |
| 84:16 Cell Stimulants and Proliferants | 976.8 |
| 84:20 Detergents | 976.2 |
| 84:24 Emollients, Demulcents, and Protectants | 976.3 |
| 84:28 Keratolytic Agents | 976.4 |
| 84:32 Keratoplastic Agents | 976.4 |
| 84:36 Miscellaneous Agents | 976.8 |
| 86:00 SPASMOLYTIC AGENTS | 975.1 |
|     antiasthmatics | 975.7 |
|     papaverine | 972.5 |
|     theophyllin | 974.1 |
| 88:00 VITAMINS | |
| 88:04 Vitamin A | 963.5 |
| 88:08 Vitamin B Complex | 963.5 |
|     hematopoietic vitamin | 964.1 |
|     nicotinic acid derivatives | 972.2 |
| 88:12 Vitamin C | 963.5 |
| 88:16 Vitamin D | 963.5 |
| 88:20 Vitamin E | 963.5 |
| 88:24 Vitamin K Activity | 964.3 |
| 88:28 Multivitamin Preparations | 963.5 |
| 92:00 UNCLASSIFIED THERAPEUTIC AGENTS | 977.8 |

\* American Hospital Formulary Service

## CLASSIFICATION OF INDUSTRIAL ACCIDENTS ACCORDING TO AGENCY

Annex B to the Resolution concerning Statistics of Employment Injuries adopted by the Tenth International Conference of Labor Statisticians on 12 October 1962

### 1 MACHINES

**11    Prime-Movers, except Electrical Motors**
111    *Steam engines*
112    *Internal combustion engines*
119    *Others*
**12    Transmission Machinery**
121    *Transmission shafts*
122    *Transmission belts, cables, pulleys, pinions, chains, gears*
129    *Others*
**13    Metalworking Machines**
131    *Power presses*
132    *Lathes*
133    *Milling machines*
134    *Abrasive wheels*
135    *Mechanical shears*
136    *Forging machines*
137    *Rolling-mills*
139    *Others*
**14    Wood and Assimilated Machines**
141    *Circular saws*
142    *Other saws*
143    *Molding machines*
144    *Overhand planes*
149    *Others*
**15    Agricultural Machines**
151    *Reapers (including combine reapers)*
152    *Threshers*
159    *Others*
**16    Mining Machinery**
161    *Under-cutters*
169    *Others*
**19    Other Machines Not Elsewhere Classified**
191    *Earth-moving machines, excavating and scraping machines, except means of transport*
192    *Spinning, weaving and other textile machines*
193    *Machines for the manufacture of foodstuffs and beverages*
194    *Machines for the manufacture of paper*
195    *Printing machines*
199    *Others*

### 2 MEANS OF TRANSPORT AND LIFTING EQUIPMENT

**21    Lifting Machines and Appliances**
211    *Cranes*
212    *Lifts and elevators*
213    *Winches*
214    *Pulley blocks*
219    *Others*
**22    Means of Rail Transport**
221    *Inter-urban railways*
222    *Rail transport in mines, tunnels, quarries, industrial establishments, docks, etc.*
229    *Others*
**23    Other Wheeled Means of Transport, Excluding Rail Transport**
231    *Tractors*
232    *Lorries*
233    *Trucks*
234    *Motor vehicles, not elsewhere classified*
235    *Animal-drawn vehicles*
236    *Hand-drawn vehicles*
239    *Others*
**24    Means of Air Transport**
**25    Means of Water Transport**
251    *Motorized means of water transport*
252    *Non-motorized means of water transport*
**26    Other Means of Transport**
261    *Cable-cars*
262    *Mechanical conveyors, except cable-cars*
269    *Others*

### 3 OTHER EQUIPMENT

**31    Pressure Vessels**
311    *Boilers*
312    *Pressurized containers*
313    *Pressurized piping and accessories*
314    *Gas cylinders*
315    *Caissons, diving equipment*
319    *Others*
**32    Furnaces, Ovens, Kilns**
321    *Blast furnaces*
322    *Refining furnaces*
323    *Other furnaces*
324    *Kilns*
325    *Ovens*
**33    Refrigerating Plants**
**34    Electrical Installations, Including Electric Motors, but Excluding Electric Hand Tools**
341    *Rotating machines*
342    *Conductors*
343    *Transformers*
344    *Control apparatus*
349    *Others*
**35    Electric Hand Tools**
**36    Tools, Implements, and Appliances, Except Electric Hand Tools**
361    *Power-driven hand tools, except electric hand tools*
362    *Hand tools, not power-driven*
369    *Others*
**37    Ladders, Mobile Ramps**
**38    Scaffolding**
**39    Other Equipment, Not Elsewhere Classified**

### 4 MATERIALS, SUBSTANCES AND RADIATIONS

**41    Explosives**
**42    Dusts, Gases, Liquids and Chemicals, Excluding Explosives**
421    *Dusts*
422    *Gases, vapors, fumes*
423    *Liquids, not elsewhere classified*
424    *Chemicals, not elsewhere classified*
**43    Flying Fragments**
**44    Radiations**
441    *Ionizing radiations*
449    *Others*
**49    Other Materials and Substances Not Elsewhere Classified**

### 5 WORKING ENVIRONMENT

**51    Outdoor**
511    *Weather*
512    *Traffic and working surfaces*
513    *Water*
519    *Others*
**52    Indoor**
521    *Floors*
522    *Confined quarters*
523    *Stairs*
524    *Other traffic and working surfaces*
525    *Floor openings and wall openings*
526    *Environmental factors (lighting, ventilation, temperature, noise, etc.)*
529    *Others*
**53    Underground**
531    *Roofs and faces of mine roads and tunnels, etc.*
532    *Floors of mine roads and tunnels, etc.*
533    *Working-faces of mines, tunnels, etc.*
534    *Mine shafts*
535    *Fire*
536    *Water*
539    *Others*

### 6 OTHER AGENCIES, NOT ELSEWHERE CLASSIFIED

**61    Animals**
611    *Live animals*
612    *Animal products*
**69    Other Agencies, Not Elsewhere Classified**

### 7 AGENCIES NOT CLASSIFIED FOR LACK OF SUFFICIENT DATA

## LIST OF THREE-DIGIT CATEGORIES

### 1. INFECTIOUS AND PARASITIC DISEASES

**Intestinal infectious diseases (001-009)**
001   Cholera
002   Typhoid and paratyphoid fevers
003   Other salmonella infections
004   Shigellosis
005   Other food poisoning (bacterial)
006   Amebiasis
007   Other protozoal intestinal diseases
008   Intestinal infections due to other organisms
009   Ill-defined intestinal infections

**Tuberculosis (010-018)**
010   Primary tuberculous infection
011   Pulmonary tuberculosis
012   Other respiratory tuberculosis
013   Tuberculosis of meninges and central nervous system
014   Tuberculosis of intestines, peritoneum, and mesenteric glands
015   Tuberculosis of bones and joints
016   Tuberculosis of genitourinary system
017   Tuberculosis of other organs
018   Miliary tuberculosis

**Zoonotic bacterial diseases (020-027)**
020   Plague
021   Tularemia
022   Anthrax
023   Brucellosis
024   Glanders
025   Melioidosis
026   Rat-bite fever
027   Other zoonotic bacterial diseases

**Other bacterial diseases (030-042)**
030   Leprosy
031   Diseases due to other mycobacteria
032   Diphtheria
033   Whooping cough
034   Streptococcal sore throat and scarlatina
035   Erysipelas
036   Meningococcal infection
037   Tetanus
038   Septicemia
039   Actinomycotic infections
040   Other bacterial diseases
041   Bacterial infection in conditions classified elsewhere and of unspecified site

**Human immunodeficiency virus (042)**
042   Human immunodeficiency virus [HIV] disease

**Poliomyelitis and other non-arthropod-borne viral diseases of central nervous system (045-049)**
045   Acute poliomyelitis
046   Slow virus infection of central nervous system
047   Meningitis due to enterovirus
048   Other enterovirus diseases of central nervous system
049   Other non-arthropod-borne viral diseases of central nervous system

**Viral diseases accompanied by exanthem (050-058)**
050   Smallpox
051   Cowpox and paravaccinia
052   Chickenpox
053   Herpes zoster
054   Herpes simplex
055   Measles
056   Rubella
057   Other viral exanthemata
058   Other human herpesvirus

**Arthropod-borne viral diseases (060-066)**
060   Yellow fever
061   Dengue
062   Mosquito-borne viral encephalitis
063   Tick-borne viral encephalitis
064   Viral encephalitis transmitted by other and unspecified arthropods
065   Arthropod-borne hemorrhagic fever
066   Other arthropod-borne viral diseases

**Other diseases due to viruses and Chlamydiae (070-079)**
070   Viral hepatitis
071   Rabies
072   Mumps
073   Ornithosis
074   Specific diseases due to Coxsackievirus
075   Infectious mononucleosis
076   Trachoma
077   Other diseases of conjunctiva due to viruses and Chlamydiae
078   Other diseases due to viruses and Chlamydiae
079   Viral infection in conditions classified elsewhere and of unspecified site

**Rickettsioses and other arthropod-borne diseases (080-088)**
080   Louse-borne [epidemic] typhus
081   Other typhus
082   Tick-borne rickettsioses
083   Other rickettsioses
084   Malaria
085   Leishmaniasis
086   Trypanosomiasis
087   Relapsing fever
088   Other arthropod-borne diseases

**Syphilis and other venereal diseases (090-099)**
090   Congenital syphilis
091   Early syphilis, symptomatic
092   Early syphilis, latent
093   Cardiovascular syphilis
094   Neurosyphilis
095   Other forms of late syphilis, with symptoms
096   Late syphilis, latent
097   Other and unspecified syphilis
098   Gonococcal infections
099   Other venereal diseases

**Other spirochetal diseases (100-104)**
100   Leptospirosis
101   Vincent's angina
102   Yaws
103   Pinta
104   Other spirochetal infection

**Mycoses (110-118)**
110   Dermatophytosis
111   Dermatomycosis, other and unspecified
112   Candidiasis
114   Coccidioidomycosis
115   Histoplasmosis
116   Blastomycotic infection
117   Other mycoses
118   Opportunistic mycoses

**Helminthiases (120-129)**
120   Schistosomiasis [bilharziasis]
121   Other trematode infections
122   Echinococcosis
123   Other cestode infection
124   Trichinosis
125   Filarial infection and dracontiasis
126   Ancylostomiasis and necatoriasis
127   Other intestinal helminthiases
128   Other and unspecified helminthiases
129   Intestinal parasitism, unspecified

**Other infectious and parasitic diseases (130-136)**
130   Toxoplasmosis
131   Trichomoniasis
132   Pediculosis and phthirus infestation
133   Acariasis
134   Other infestation
135   Sarcoidosis
136   Other and unspecified infectious and parasitic diseases

**Late effects of infectious and parasitic diseases (137-139)**
137   Late effects of tuberculosis
138   Late effects of acute poliomyelitis
139   Late effects of other infectious and parasitic diseases

### 2. NEOPLASMS

**Malignant neoplasm of lip, oral cavity, and pharynx (140-149)**
140   Malignant neoplasm of lip
141   Malignant neoplasm of tongue
142   Malignant neoplasm of major salivary glands
143   Malignant neoplasm of gum
144   Malignant neoplasm of floor of mouth
145   Malignant neoplasm of other and unspecified parts of mouth
146   Malignant neoplasm of oropharynx
147   Malignant neoplasm of nasopharynx
148   Malignant neoplasm of hypopharynx
149   Malignant neoplasm of other and ill-defined sites within the lip, oral cavity, and pharynx

**Malignant neoplasm of digestive organs and peritoneum (150-159)**
150   Malignant neoplasm of esophagus
151   Malignant neoplasm of stomach
152   Malignant neoplasm of small intestine, including duodenum
153   Malignant neoplasm of colon
154   Malignant neoplasm of rectum, rectosigmoid junction, and anus
155   Malignant neoplasm of liver and intrahepatic bile ducts
156   Malignant neoplasm of gallbladder and extrahepatic bile ducts
157   Malignant neoplasm of pancreas
158   Malignant neoplasm of retroperitoneum and peritoneum
159   Malignant neoplasm of other and ill-defined sites within the digestive organs and peritoneum

**Malignant neoplasm of respiratory and intrathoracic organs (160-165)**
160   Malignant neoplasm of nasal cavities, middle ear, and accessory sinuses
161   Malignant neoplasm of larynx
162   Malignant neoplasm of trachea, bronchus, and lung
163   Malignant neoplasm of pleura
164   Malignant neoplasm of thymus, heart, and mediastinum
165   Malignant neoplasm of other and ill-defined sites within the respiratory system and intrathoracic organs

**Malignant neoplasm of bone, connective tissue, skin, and breast (170-176)**
170   Malignant neoplasm of bone and articular cartilage
171   Malignant neoplasm of connective and other soft tissue
172   Malignant melanoma of skin
173   Other malignant neoplasm of skin
174   Malignant neoplasm of female breast
175   Malignant neoplasm of male breast
176   Kaposi's sarcoma

**Malignant neoplasm of genitourinary organs (179-189)**
179   Malignant neoplasm of uterus, part unspecified
180   Malignant neoplasm of cervix uteri
181   Malignant neoplasm of placenta
182   Malignant neoplasm of body of uterus
183   Malignant neoplasm of ovary and other uterine adnexa
184   Malignant neoplasm of other and unspecified female genital organs
185   Malignant neoplasm of prostate

186  Malignant neoplasm of testis
187  Malignant neoplasm of penis and other male genital organs
188  Malignant neoplasm of bladder
189  Malignant neoplasm of kidney and other unspecified urinary organs

**Malignant neoplasm of other and unspecified sites (190-199)**
190  Malignant neoplasm of eye
191  Malignant neoplasm of brain
192  Malignant neoplasm of other and unspecified parts of nervous system
193  Malignant neoplasm of thyroid gland
194  Malignant neoplasm of other endocrine glands and related structures
195  Malignant neoplasm of other and ill-defined sites
196  Secondary and unspecified malignant neoplasm of lymph nodes
197  Secondary malignant neoplasm of respiratory and digestive systems
198  Secondary malignant neoplasm of other specified sites
199  Malignant neoplasm without specification of site

**Malignant neoplasm of lymphatic and hematopoietic tissue (200-208)**
200  Lymphosarcoma and reticulosarcoma and other specified malignant tumors of lymphatic tissue
201  Hodgkin's disease
202  Other malignant neoplasm of lymphoid and histiocytic tissue
203  Multiple myeloma and immunoproliferative neoplasms
204  Lymphoid leukemia
205  Myeloid leukemia
206  Monocytic leukemia
207  Other specified leukemia
208  Leukemia of unspecified cell type

**Benign neoplasms (210-229)**
210  Benign neoplasm of lip, oral cavity, and pharynx
211  Benign neoplasm of other parts of digestive system
212  Benign neoplasm of respiratory and intrathoracic organs
213  Benign neoplasm of bone and articular cartilage
214  Lipoma
215  Other benign neoplasm of connective and other soft tissue
216  Benign neoplasm of skin
217  Benign neoplasm of breast
218  Uterine leiomyoma
219  Other benign neoplasm of uterus
220  Benign neoplasm of ovary
221  Benign neoplasm of other female genital organs
222  Benign neoplasm of male genital organs
223  Benign neoplasm of kidney and other urinary organs
224  Benign neoplasm of eye
225  Benign neoplasm of brain and other parts of nervous system
226  Benign neoplasm of thyroid gland
227  Benign neoplasm of other endocrine glands and related structures
228  Hemangioma and lymphangioma, any site
229  Benign neoplasm of other and unspecified sites

**Carcinoma in situ (230-234)**
230  Carcinoma in situ of digestive organs
231  Carcinoma in situ of respiratory system
232  Carcinoma in situ of skin
233  Carcinoma in situ of breast and genitourinary system
234  Carcinoma in situ of other and unspecified sites

**Neoplasms of uncertain behavior (235-238)**
235  Neoplasm of uncertain behavior of digestive and respiratory systems
236  Neoplasm of uncertain behavior of genitourinary organs
237  Neoplasm of uncertain behavior of endocrine glands and nervous system
238  Neoplasm of uncertain behavior of other and unspecified sites and tissues

**Neoplasms of unspecified nature (239)**
239  Neoplasm of unspecified nature

### 3. ENDOCRINE, NUTRITIONAL AND METABOLIC DISEASES, AND IMMUNITY DISORDERS

**Disorders of thyroid gland (240-246)**
240  Simple and unspecified goiter
241  Nontoxic nodular goiter
242  Thyrotoxicosis with or without goiter
243  Congenital hypothyroidism
244  Acquired hypothyroidism
245  Thyroiditis
246  Other disorders of thyroid

**Diseases of other endocrine glands (250-259)**
250  Diabetes mellitus
251  Other disorders of pancreatic internal secretion
252  Disorders of parathyroid gland
253  Disorders of the pituitary gland and its hypothalamic control
254  Diseases of thymus gland
255  Disorders of adrenal glands
256  Ovarian dysfunction
257  Testicular dysfunction
258  Polyglandular dysfunction and related disorders
259  Other endocrine disorders

**Nutritional deficiencies (260-269)**
260  Kwashiorkor
261  Nutritional marasmus
262  Other severe protein-calorie malnutrition
263  Other and unspecified protein-calorie malnutrition
264  Vitamin A deficiency
265  Thiamine and niacin deficiency states
266  Deficiency of B-complex components
267  Ascorbic acid deficiency
268  Vitamin D deficiency
269  Other nutritional deficiencies

**Other metabolic disorders and immunity disorders (270-279)**
270  Disorders of amino-acid transport and metabolism
271  Disorders of carbohydrate transport and metabolism
272  Disorders of lipoid metabolism
273  Disorders of plasma protein metabolism
274  Gout
275  Disorders of mineral metabolism
276  Disorders of fluid, electrolyte, and acid-base balance
277  Other and unspecified disorders of metabolism
278  Overweight, obesity and other hyperalimentation
279  Disorders involving the immune mechanism

### 4. DISEASES OF BLOOD AND BLOOD-FORMING ORGANS (280-289)
280  Iron deficiency anemias
281  Other deficiency anemias
282  Hereditary hemolytic anemias
283  Acquired hemolytic anemias
284  Aplastic anemia
285  Other and unspecified anemias
286  Coagulation defects
287  Purpura and other hemorrhagic conditions
288  Diseases of white blood cells

289  Other diseases of blood and blood-forming organs

### 5. MENTAL DISORDERS

**Organic psychotic conditions (290-294)**
290  Senile and presenile organic psychotic conditions
291  Alcoholic psychoses
292  Drug psychoses
293  Transient organic psychotic conditions
294  Other organic psychotic conditions (chronic)

**Other psychoses (295-299)**
295  Schizophrenic psychoses
296  Affective psychoses
297  Paranoid states
298  Other nonorganic psychoses
299  Psychoses with origin specific to childhood

**Neurotic disorders, personality disorders, and other nonpsychotic mental disorders (300-316)**
300  Neurotic disorders
301  Personality disorders
302  Sexual and gender identity disorders
303  Alcohol dependence syndrome
304  Drug dependence
305  Nondependent abuse of drugs
306  Physiological malfunction arising from mental factors
307  Special symptoms or syndromes, not elsewhere classified
308  Acute reaction to stress
309  Adjustment reaction
310  Specific nonpsychotic mental disorders following organic brain damage
311  Depressive disorder, not elsewhere classified
312  Disturbance of conduct, not elsewhere classified
313  Disturbance of emotions specific to childhood and adolescence
314  Hyperkinetic syndrome of childhood
315  Specific delays in development
316  Psychic factors associated with diseases classified elsewhere

**Mental retardation (317-319)**
317  Mild mental retardation
318  Other specified mental retardation
319  Unspecified mental retardation

### 6. DISEASES OF THE NERVOUS SYSTEM AND SENSE ORGANS

**Inflammatory diseases of the central nervous system (320-326)**
320  Bacterial meningitis
321  Meningitis due to other organisms
322  Meningitis of unspecified cause
323  Encephalitis, myelitis, and encephalomyelitis
324  Intracranial and intraspinal abscess
325  Phlebitis and thrombophlebitis of intracranial venous sinuses
326  Late effects of intracranial abscess or pyogenic infection

**Organic Sleep Disorders (327)**
327  Organic sleep disorders

**Hereditary and degenerative diseases of the central nervous system (330-337)**
330  Cerebral degenerations usually manifest in childhood
331  Other cerebral degenerations
332  Parkinson's disease
333  Other extrapyramidal diseases and abnormal movement disorders
334  Spinocerebellar disease
335  Anterior horn cell disease
336  Other diseases of spinal cord
337  Disorders of the autonomic nervous system

**Pain (338)**
338 Pain, not elsewhere classified

**Other disorders of the central nervous system (340-349)**
340 Multiple sclerosis
341 Other demyelinating diseases of central nervous system
342 Hemiplegia and hemiparesis
343 Infantile cerebral palsy
344 Other paralytic syndromes
345 Epilepsy and recurrent seizures
346 Migraine
347 Cataplexy and narcolepsy
348 Other conditions of brain
349 Other and unspecified disorders of the nervous system

**Disorders of the peripheral nervous system (350-359)**
350 Trigeminal nerve disorders
351 Facial nerve disorders
352 Disorders of other cranial nerves
353 Nerve root and plexus disorders
354 Mononeuritis of upper limb and mononeuritis multiplex
355 Mononeuritis of lower limb
356 Hereditary and idiopathic peripheral neuropathy
357 Inflammatory and toxic neuropathy
358 Myoneural disorders
359 Muscular dystrophies and other myopathies

**Disorders of the eye and adnexa (360-379)**
360 Disorders of the globe
361 Retinal detachments and defects
362 Other retinal disorders
363 Chorioretinal inflammations and scars and other disorders of choroid
364 Disorders of iris and ciliary body
365 Glaucoma
366 Cataract
367 Disorders of refraction and accommodation
368 Visual disturbances
369 Blindness and low vision
370 Keratitis
371 Corneal opacity and other disorders of cornea
372 Disorders of conjunctiva
373 Inflammation of eyelids
374 Other disorders of eyelids
375 Disorders of lacrimal system
376 Disorders of the orbit
377 Disorders of optic nerve and visual pathways
378 Strabismus and other disorders of binocular eye movements
379 Other disorders of eye

**Diseases of the ear and mastoid process (380-389)**
380 Disorders of external ear
381 Nonsuppurative otitis media and Eustachian tube disorders
382 Suppurative and unspecified otitis media
383 Mastoiditis and related conditions
384 Other disorders of tympanic membrane
385 Other disorders of middle ear and mastoid
386 Vertiginous syndromes and other disorders of vestibular system
387 Otosclerosis
388 Other disorders of ear
389 Hearing loss

### 7. DISEASES OF THE CIRCULATORY SYSTEM

**Acute rheumatic fever (390-392)**
390 Rheumatic fever without mention of heart involvement
391 Rheumatic fever with heart involvement
392 Rheumatic chorea

**Chronic rheumatic heart disease (393-398)**
393 Chronic rheumatic pericarditis
394 Diseases of mitral valve
395 Diseases of aortic valve
396 Diseases of mitral and aortic valves
397 Diseases of other endocardial structures
398 Other rheumatic heart disease

**Hypertensive disease (401-405)**
401 Essential hypertension
402 Hypertensive heart disease
403 Hypertensive kidney disease
404 Hypertensive heart and kidney disease
405 Secondary hypertension

**Ischemic heart disease (410-414)**
410 Acute myocardial infarction
411 Other acute and subacute form of ischemic heart disease
412 Old myocardial infarction
413 Angina pectoris
414 Other forms of chronic ischemic heart disease

**Diseases of pulmonary circulation (415-417)**
415 Acute pulmonary heart disease
416 Chronic pulmonary heart disease
417 Other diseases of pulmonary circulation

**Other forms of heart disease (420-429)**
420 Acute pericarditis
421 Acute and subacute endocarditis
422 Acute myocarditis
423 Other diseases of pericardium
424 Other diseases of endocardium
425 Cardiomyopathy
426 Conduction disorders
427 Cardiac dysrhythmias
428 Heart failure
429 Ill-defined descriptions and complications of heart disease

**Cerebrovascular disease (430-438)**
430 Subarachnoid hemorrhage
431 Intracerebral hemorrhage
432 Other and unspecified intracranial hemorrhage
433 Occlusion and stenosis of precerebral arteries
434 Occlusion of cerebral arteries
435 Transient cerebral ischemia
436 Acute but ill-defined cerebrovascular disease
437 Other and ill-defined cerebrovascular disease
438 Late effects of cerebrovascular disease

**Diseases of arteries, arterioles, and capillaries (440-449)**
440 Atherosclerosis
441 Aortic aneurysm and dissection
442 Other aneurysm
443 Other peripheral vascular disease
444 Arterial embolism and thrombosis
445 Atheroembolism
446 Polyarteritis nodosa and allied conditions
447 Other disorders of arteries and arterioles
448 Diseases of capillaries
449 Septic arterial embolism

**Diseases of veins and lymphatics, and other diseases of circulatory system (451-459)**
451 Phlebitis and thrombophlebitis
452 Portal vein thrombosis
453 Other venous embolism and thrombosis
454 Varicose veins of lower extremities
455 Hemorrhoids
456 Varicose veins of other sites
457 Noninfective disorders of lymphatic channels
458 Hypotension
459 Other disorders of circulatory system

### 8. DISEASES OF THE RESPIRATORY SYSTEM

**Acute respiratory infections (460-466)**
460 Acute nasopharyngitis [common cold]
461 Acute sinusitis
462 Acute pharyngitis
463 Acute tonsillitis
464 Acute laryngitis and tracheitis
465 Acute upper respiratory infections of multiple or unspecified sites
466 Acute bronchitis and bronchiolitis

**Other diseases of upper respiratory tract (470-478)**
470 Deviated nasal septum
471 Nasal polyps
472 Chronic pharyngitis and nasopharyngitis
473 Chronic sinusitis
474 Chronic disease of tonsils and adenoids
475 Peritonsillar abscess
476 Chronic laryngitis and laryngotracheitis
477 Allergic rhinitis
478 Other diseases of upper respiratory tract

**Pneumonia and influenza (480-488)**
480 Viral pneumonia
481 Pneumococcal pneumonia [Streptococcus pneumoniae pneumonia]
482 Other bacterial pneumonia
483 Pneumonia due to other specified organism
484 Pneumonia in infectious diseases classified elsewhere
485 Bronchopneumonia, organism unspecified
486 Pneumonia, organism unspecified
487 Influenza
488 Influenza due to identified avian influenza virus

**Chronic obstructive pulmonary disease and allied conditions (490-496)**
490 Bronchitis, not specified as acute or chronic
491 Chronic bronchitis
492 Emphysema
493 Asthma
494 Bronchiectasis
495 Extrinsic allergic alveolitis
496 Chronic airways obstruction, not elsewhere classified

**Pneumoconioses and other lung diseases due to external agents (500-508)**
500 Coal workers' pneumoconiosis
501 Asbestosis
502 Pneumoconiosis due to other silica or silicates
503 Pneumoconiosis due to other inorganic dust
504 Pneumopathy due to inhalation of other dust
505 Pneumoconiosis, unspecified
506 Respiratory conditions due to chemical fumes and vapors
507 Pneumonitis due to solids and liquids
508 Respiratory conditions due to other and unspecified external agents

**Other diseases of respiratory system (510-519)**
510 Empyema
511 Pleurisy
512 Pneumothorax
513 Abscess of lung and mediastinum
514 Pulmonary congestion and hypostasis
515 Postinflammatory pulmonary fibrosis
516 Other alveolar and parietoalveolar pneumopathy
517 Lung involvement in conditions classified elsewhere
518 Other diseases of lung
519 Other diseases of respiratory system

### 9. DISEASES OF THE DIGESTIVE SYSTEM

**Diseases of oral cavity, salivary glands, and jaws (520-529)**
520 Disorders of tooth development and eruption
521 Diseases of hard tissues of teeth
522 Diseases of pulp and periapical tissues
523 Gingival and periodontal diseases
524 Dentofacial anomalies, including malocclusion

**Appendix E: List of Three-Digit Categories**

525 Other diseases and conditions of the teeth and supporting structures
526 Diseases of the jaws
527 Diseases of the salivary glands
528 Diseases of the oral soft tissues, excluding lesions specific for gingiva and tongue
529 Diseases and other conditions of the tongue

### Diseases of esophagus, stomach, and duodenum (530-538)
530 Diseases of esophagus
531 Gastric ulcer
532 Duodenal ulcer
533 Peptic ulcer, site unspecified
534 Gastrojejunal ulcer
535 Gastritis and duodenitis
536 Disorders of function of stomach
537 Other disorders of stomach and duodenum
538 Gastrointestinal mucositis (ulcerative)

### Appendicitis (540-543)
540 Acute appendicitis
541 Appendicitis, unqualified
542 Other appendicitis
543 Other diseases of appendix

### Hernia of abdominal cavity (550-553)
550 Inguinal hernia
551 Other hernia of abdominal cavity, with gangrene
552 Other hernia of abdominal cavity, with obstruction, but without mention of gangrene
553 Other hernia of abdominal cavity without mention of obstruction or gangrene

### Noninfective enteritis and colitis (555-558)
555 Regional enteritis
556 Ulcerative colitis
557 Vascular insufficiency of intestine
558 Other noninfective gastroenteritis and colitis

### Other diseases of intestines and peritoneum (560-569)
560 Intestinal obstruction without mention of hernia
562 Diverticula of intestine
564 Functional digestive disorders, not elsewhere classified
565 Anal fissure and fistula
566 Abscess of anal and rectal regions
567 Peritonitis and retroperitoneal infections
568 Other disorders of peritoneum
569 Other disorders of intestine

### Other diseases of digestive system (570-579)
570 Acute and subacute necrosis of liver
571 Chronic liver disease and cirrhosis
572 Liver abscess and sequelae of chronic liver disease
573 Other disorders of liver
574 Cholelithiasis
575 Other disorders of gallbladder
576 Other disorders of biliary tract
577 Diseases of pancreas
578 Gastrointestinal hemorrhage
579 Intestinal malabsorption

## 10. DISEASES OF THE GENITOURINARY SYSTEM

### Nephritis, nephrotic syndrome, and nephrosis (580-589)
580 Acute glomerulonephritis
581 Nephrotic syndrome
582 Chronic glomerulonephritis
583 Nephritis and nephropathy, not specified as acute or chronic
584 Acute renal failure
585 Chronic kidney disease (CKD)
586 Renal failure, unspecified
587 Renal sclerosis, unspecified
588 Disorders resulting from impaired renal function
589 Small kidney of unknown cause

### Other diseases of urinary system (590-599)
590 Infections of kidney
591 Hydronephrosis
592 Calculus of kidney and ureter
593 Other disorders of kidney and ureter
594 Calculus of lower urinary tract
595 Cystitis
596 Other disorders of bladder
597 Urethritis, not sexually transmitted, and urethral syndrome
598 Urethral stricture
599 Other disorders of urethra and urinary tract

### Diseases of male genital organs (600-608)
600 Hyperplasia of prostate
601 Inflammatory diseases of prostate
602 Other disorders of prostate
603 Hydrocele
604 Orchitis and epididymitis
605 Redundant prepuce and phimosis
606 Infertility, male
607 Disorders of penis
608 Other disorders of male genital organs

### Disorders of breast (610-611)
610 Benign mammary dysplasias
611 Other disorders of breast

### Inflammatory disease of female pelvic organs (614-616)
614 Inflammatory disease of ovary, fallopian tube, pelvic cellular tissue, and peritoneum
615 Inflammatory diseases of uterus, except cervix
616 Inflammatory disease of cervix, vagina, and vulva

### Other disorders of female genital tract (617-629)
617 Endometriosis
618 Genital prolapse
619 Fistula involving female genital tract
620 Noninflammatory disorders of ovary, fallopian tube, and broad ligament
621 Disorders of uterus, not elsewhere classified
622 Noninflammatory disorders of cervix
623 Noninflammatory disorders of vagina
624 Noninflammatory disorders of vulva and perineum
625 Pain and other symptoms associated with female genital organs
626 Disorders of menstruation and other abnormal bleeding from female genital tract
627 Menopausal and postmenopausal disorders
628 Infertility, female
629 Other disorders of female genital organs

## 11. COMPLICATIONS OF PREGNANCY, CHILDBIRTH AND THE PUERPERIUM

### Ectopic and molar pregnancy and other pregnancy with abortive outcome (630-639)
630 Hydatidiform mole
631 Other abnormal product of conception
632 Missed abortion
633 Ectopic pregnancy
634 Spontaneous abortion
635 Legally induced abortion
636 Illegally induced abortion
637 Unspecified abortion
638 Failed attempted abortion
639 Complications following abortion and ectopic and molar pregnancies

### Complications mainly related to pregnancy (640-649)
640 Hemorrhage in early pregnancy
641 Antepartum hemorrhage, abruptio placentae, and placenta previa
642 Hypertension complicating pregnancy, childbirth, and the puerperium
643 Excessive vomiting in pregnancy
644 Early or threatened labor
645 Prolonged pregnancy

646 Other complications of pregnancy, not elsewhere classified
647 Infective and parasitic conditions in the mother classifiable elsewhere but complicating pregnancy, childbirth, and the puerperium
648 Other current conditions in the mother classifiable elsewhere but complicating pregnancy, childbirth, and the puerperium
649 Other conditions or status of the mother complicating pregnancy, childbirth, or puerperium

### Normal delivery, and other indications for care in pregnancy, labor, and delivery (650-659)
650 Normal delivery
651 Multiple gestation
652 Malposition and malpresentation of fetus
653 Disproportion
654 Abnormality of organs and soft tissues of pelvis
655 Known or suspected fetal abnormality affecting management of mother
656 Other fetal and placental problems affecting management of mother
657 Polyhydramnios
658 Other problems associated with amniotic cavity and membranes
659 Other indications for care or intervention related to labor and delivery and not elsewhere classified

### Complications occurring mainly in the course of labor and delivery (660-669)
660 Obstructed labor
661 Abnormality of forces of labor
662 Long labor
663 Umbilical cord complications
664 Trauma to perineum and vulva during delivery
665 Other obstetrical trauma
666 Postpartum hemorrhage
667 Retained placenta or membranes, without hemorrhage
668 Complications of the administration of anesthetic or other sedation in labor and delivery
669 Other complications of labor and delivery, not elsewhere classified

### Complications of the puerperium (670-677)
670 Major puerperal infection
671 Venous complications in pregnancy and the puerperium
672 Pyrexia of unknown origin during the puerperium
673 Obstetrical pulmonary embolism
674 Other and unspecified complications of the puerperium, not elsewhere classified
675 Infections of the breast and nipple associated with childbirth
676 Other disorders of the breast associated with childbirth, and disorders of lactation
677 Late effect of complication of pregnancy, childbirth, and the puerperium

## 12. DISEASES OF THE SKIN AND SUBCUTANEOUS TISSUE

### Infections of skin and subcutaneous tissue (680-686)
680 Carbuncle and furuncle
681 Cellulitis and abscess of finger and toe
682 Other cellulitis and abscess
683 Acute lymphadenitis
684 Impetigo
685 Pilonidal cyst
686 Other local infections of skin and subcutaneous tissue

## Other inflammatory conditions of skin and subcutaneous tissue (690-698)

690  Erythematosquamous dermatosis
691  Atopic dermatitis and related conditions
692  Contact dermatitis and other eczema
693  Dermatitis due to substances taken internally
694  Bullous dermatoses
695  Erythematous conditions
696  Psoriasis and similar disorders
697  Lichen
698  Pruritus and related conditions

## Other diseases of skin and subcutaneous tissue (700-709)

700  Corns and callosities
701  Other hypertrophic and atrophic conditions of skin
702  Other dermatoses
703  Diseases of nail
704  Diseases of hair and hair follicles
705  Disorders of sweat glands
706  Diseases of sebaceous glands
707  Chronic ulcer of skin
708  Urticaria
709  Other disorders of skin and subcutaneous tissue

## 13. DISEASES OF THE MUSCULOSKELETAL SYSTEM AND CONNECTIVE TISSUE

### Arthropathies and related disorders (710-719)

710  Diffuse diseases of connective tissue
711  Arthropathy associated with infections
712  Crystal arthropathies
713  Arthropathy associated with other disorders classified elsewhere
714  Rheumatoid arthritis and other inflammatory polyarthropathies
715  Osteoarthrosis and allied disorders
716  Other and unspecified arthropathies
717  Internal derangement of knee
718  Other derangement of joint
719  Other and unspecified disorder of joint

### Dorsopathies (720-724)

720  Ankylosing spondylitis and other inflammatory spondylopathies
721  Spondylosis and allied disorders
722  Intervertebral disc disorders
723  Other disorders of cervical region
724  Other and unspecified disorders of back

### Rheumatism, excluding the back (725-729)

725  Polymyalgia rheumatica
726  Peripheral enthesopathies and allied syndromes
727  Other disorders of synovium, tendon, and bursa
728  Disorders of muscle, ligament, and fascia
729  Other disorders of soft tissues

### Osteopathies, chondropathies, and acquired musculoskeletal deformities (730-739)

730  Osteomyelitis, periostitis, and other infections involving bone
731  Osteitis deformans and osteopathies associated with other disorders classified elsewhere
732  Osteochondropathies
733  Other disorders of bone and cartilage
734  Flat foot
735  Acquired deformities of toe
736  Other acquired deformities of limbs
737  Curvature of spine
738  Other acquired deformity
739  Nonallopathic lesions, not elsewhere classified

## 14. CONGENITAL ANOMALIES

740  Anencephalus and similar anomalies
741  Spina bifida
742  Other congenital anomalies of nervous system
743  Congenital anomalies of eye
744  Congenital anomalies of ear, face, and neck
745  Bulbus cordis anomalies and anomalies of cardiac septal closure
746  Other congenital anomalies of heart
747  Other congenital anomalies of circulatory system
748  Congenital anomalies of respiratory system
749  Cleft palate and cleft lip
750  Other congenital anomalies of upper alimentary tract
751  Other congenital anomalies of digestive system
752  Congenital anomalies of genital organs
753  Congenital anomalies of urinary system
754  Certain congenital musculoskeletal deformities
755  Other congenital anomalies of limbs
756  Other congenital musculoskeletal anomalies
757  Congenital anomalies of the integument
758  Chromosomal anomalies
759  Other and unspecified congenital anomalies

## 15. CERTAIN CONDITIONS ORIGINATING IN THE PERINATAL PERIOD

### Maternal causes of perinatal morbidity and mortality (760-763)

760  Fetus or newborn affected by maternal conditions which may be unrelated to present pregnancy
761  Fetus or newborn affected by maternal complications of pregnancy
762  Fetus or newborn affected by complications of placenta, cord, and membranes
763  Fetus or newborn affected by other complications of labor and delivery

### Other conditions originating in the perinatal period (764-779)

764  Slow fetal growth and fetal malnutrition
765  Disorders relating to short gestation and unspecified low birthweight
766  Disorders relating to long gestation and high birthweight
767  Birth trauma
768  Intrauterine hypoxia and birth asphyxia
769  Respiratory distress syndrome
770  Other respiratory conditions of fetus and newborn
771  Infections specific to the perinatal period
772  Fetal and neonatal hemorrhage
773  Hemolytic disease of fetus or newborn, due to isoimmunization
774  Other perinatal jaundice
775  Endocrine and metabolic disturbances specific to the fetus and newborn
776  Hematological disorders of fetus and newborn
777  Perinatal disorders of digestive system
778  Conditions involving the integument and temperature regulation of fetus and newborn
779  Other and ill-defined conditions originating in the perinatal period

## 16. SYMPTOMS, SIGNS, AND ILL-DEFINED CONDITIONS

### Symptoms (780-789)

780  General symptoms
781  Symptoms involving nervous and musculoskeletal systems
782  Symptoms involving skin and other integumentary tissue
783  Symptoms concerning nutrition, metabolism, and development
784  Symptoms involving head and neck
785  Symptoms involving cardiovascular system
786  Symptoms involving respiratory system and other chest symptoms
787  Symptoms involving digestive system
788  Symptoms involving urinary system
789  Other symptoms involving abdomen and pelvis

### Nonspecific abnormal findings (790-796)

790  Nonspecific findings on examination of blood
791  Nonspecific findings on examination of urine
792  Nonspecific abnormal findings in other body substances
793  Nonspecific abnormal findings on radiological and other examination of body structure
794  Nonspecific abnormal results of function studies
795  Nonspecific abnormal histological and immunological findings
796  Other nonspecific abnormal findings

### Ill-defined and unknown causes of morbidity and mortality (797-799)

797  Senility without mention of psychosis
798  Sudden death, cause unknown
799  Other ill-defined and unknown causes of morbidity and mortality

## 17. INJURY AND POISONING

### Fracture of skull (800-804)

800  Fracture of vault of skull
801  Fracture of base of skull
802  Fracture of face bones
803  Other and unqualified skull fractures
804  Multiple fractures involving skull or face with other bones

### Fracture of spine and trunk (805-809)

805  Fracture of vertebral column without mention of spinal cord lesion
806  Fracture of vertebral column with spinal cord lesion
807  Fracture of rib(s), sternum, larynx, and trachea
808  Fracture of pelvis
809  Ill-defined fractures of bones of trunk

### Fracture of upper limb (810-819)

810  Fracture of clavicle
811  Fracture of scapula
812  Fracture of humerus
813  Fracture of radius and ulna
814  Fracture of carpal bone(s)
815  Fracture of metacarpal bone(s)
816  Fracture of one or more phalanges of hand
817  Multiple fractures of hand bones
818  Ill-defined fractures of upper limb
819  Multiple fractures involving both upper limbs, and upper limb with rib(s) and sternum

### Fracture of lower limb (820-829)

820  Fracture of neck of femur
821  Fracture of other and unspecified parts of femur
822  Fracture of patella
823  Fracture of tibia and fibula
824  Fracture of ankle
825  Fracture of one or more tarsal and metatarsal bones
826  Fracture of one or more phalanges of foot
827  Other, multiple, and ill-defined fractures of lower limb
828  Multiple fractures involving both lower limbs, lower with upper limb, and lower limb(s) with rib(s) and sternum
829  Fracture of unspecified bones

### Dislocation (830-839)

830  Dislocation of jaw
831  Dislocation of shoulder
832  Dislocation of elbow
833  Dislocation of wrist
834  Dislocation of finger
835  Dislocation of hip
836  Dislocation of knee
837  Dislocation of ankle

838 Dislocation of foot
839 Other, multiple, and ill-defined dislocations

### Sprains and strains of joints and adjacent muscles (840-848)

840 Sprains and strains of shoulder and upper arm
841 Sprains and strains of elbow and forearm
842 Sprains and strains of wrist and hand
843 Sprains and strains of hip and thigh
844 Sprains and strains of knee and leg
845 Sprains and strains of ankle and foot
846 Sprains and strains of sacroiliac region
847 Sprains and strains of other and unspecified parts of back
848 Other and ill-defined sprains and strains

### Intracranial injury, excluding those with skull fracture (850-854)

850 Concussion
851 Cerebral laceration and contusion
852 Subarachnoid, subdural, and extradural hemorrhage, following injury
853 Other and unspecified intracranial hemorrhage following injury
854 Intracranial injury of other and unspecified nature

### Internal injury of chest, abdomen, and pelvis (860-869)

860 Traumatic pneumothorax and hemothorax
861 Injury to heart and lung
862 Injury to other and unspecified intrathoracic organs
863 Injury to gastrointestinal tract
864 Injury to liver
865 Injury to spleen
866 Injury to kidney
867 Injury to pelvic organs
868 Injury to other intra-abdominal organs
869 Internal injury to unspecified or ill-defined organs

### Open wound of head, neck, and trunk (870-879)

870 Open wound of ocular adnexa
871 Open wound of eyeball
872 Open wound of ear
873 Other open wound of head
874 Open wound of neck
875 Open wound of chest (wall)
876 Open wound of back
877 Open wound of buttock
878 Open wound of genital organs (external), including traumatic amputation
879 Open wound of other and unspecified sites, except limbs

### Open wound of upper limb (880-887)

880 Open wound of shoulder and upper arm
881 Open wound of elbow, forearm, and wrist
882 Open wound of hand except finger(s) alone
883 Open wound of finger(s)
884 Multiple and unspecified open wound of upper limb
885 Traumatic amputation of thumb (complete) (partial)
886 Traumatic amputation of other finger(s) (complete) (partial)
887 Traumatic amputation of arm and hand (complete) (partial)

### Open wound of lower limb (890-897)

890 Open wound of hip and thigh
891 Open wound of knee, leg [except thigh], and ankle
892 Open wound of foot except toe(s) alone
893 Open wound of toe(s)
894 Multiple and unspecified open wound of lower limb
895 Traumatic amputation of toe(s) (complete) (partial)
896 Traumatic amputation of foot (complete) (partial)

897 Traumatic amputation of leg(s) (complete) (partial)

### Injury to blood vessels (900-904)

900 Injury to blood vessels of head and neck
901 Injury to blood vessels of thorax
902 Injury to blood vessels of abdomen and pelvis
903 Injury to blood vessels of upper extremity
904 Injury to blood vessels of lower extremity and unspecified sites

### Late effects of injuries, poisonings, toxic effects, and other external causes (905-909)

905 Late effects of musculoskeletal and connective tissue injuries
906 Late effects of injuries to skin and subcutaneous tissues
907 Late effects of injuries to the nervous system
908 Late effects of other and unspecified injuries
909 Late effects of other and unspecified external causes

### Superficial injury (910-919)

910 Superficial injury of face, neck, and scalp except eye
911 Superficial injury of trunk
912 Superficial injury of shoulder and upper arm
913 Superficial injury of elbow, forearm, and wrist
914 Superficial injury of hand(s) except finger(s) alone
915 Superficial injury of finger(s)
916 Superficial injury of hip, thigh, leg, and ankle
917 Superficial injury of foot and toe(s)
918 Superficial injury of eye and adnexa
919 Superficial injury of other, multiple, and unspecified sites

### Contusion with intact skin surface (920-924)

920 Contusion of face, scalp, and neck except eye(s)
921 Contusion of eye and adnexa
922 Contusion of trunk
923 Contusion of upper limb
924 Contusion of lower limb and of other and unspecified sites

### Crushing injury (925-929)

925 Crushing injury of face, scalp, and neck
926 Crushing injury of trunk
927 Crushing injury of upper limb
928 Crushing injury of lower limb
929 Crushing injury of multiple and unspecified sites

### Effects of foreign body entering through orifice (930-939)

930 Foreign body on external eye
931 Foreign body in ear
932 Foreign body in nose
933 Foreign body in pharynx and larynx
934 Foreign body in trachea, bronchus, and lung
935 Foreign body in mouth, esophagus, and stomach
936 Foreign body in intestine and colon
937 Foreign body in anus and rectum
938 Foreign body in digestive system, unspecified
939 Foreign body in genitourinary tract

### Burns (940-949)

940 Burn confined to eye and adnexa
941 Burn of face, head, and neck
942 Burn of trunk
943 Burn of upper limb, except wrist and hand
944 Burn of wrist(s) and hand(s)
945 Burn of lower limb(s)
946 Burns of multiple specified sites
947 Burn of internal organs
948 Burns classified according to extent of body surface involved
949 Burn, unspecified

### Injury to nerves and spinal cord (950-957)

950 Injury to optic nerve and pathways
951 Injury to other cranial nerve(s)
952 Spinal cord injury without evidence of spinal bone injury
953 Injury to nerve roots and spinal plexus
954 Injury to other nerve(s) of trunk excluding shoulder and pelvic girdles
955 Injury to peripheral nerve(s) of shoulder girdle and upper limb
956 Injury to peripheral nerve(s) of pelvic girdle and lower limb
957 Injury to other and unspecified nerves

### Certain traumatic complications and unspecified injuries (958-959)

958 Certain early complications of trauma
959 Injury, other and unspecified

### Poisoning by drugs, medicinals and biological substances (960-979)

960 Poisoning by antibiotics
961 Poisoning by other anti-infectives
962 Poisoning by hormones and synthetic substitutes
963 Poisoning by primarily systemic agents
964 Poisoning by agents primarily affecting blood constituents
965 Poisoning by analgesics, antipyretics, and antirheumatics
966 Poisoning by anticonvulsants and anti-Parkinsonism drugs
967 Poisoning by sedatives and hypnotics
968 Poisoning by other central nervous system depressants and anesthetics
969 Poisoning by psychotropic agents
970 Poisoning by central nervous system stimulants
971 Poisoning by drugs primarily affecting the autonomic nervous system
972 Poisoning by agents primarily affecting the cardiovascular system
973 Poisoning by agents primarily affecting the gastrointestinal system
974 Poisoning by water, mineral, and uric acid metabolism drugs
975 Poisoning by agents primarily acting on the smooth and skeletal muscles and respiratory system
976 Poisoning by agents primarily affecting skin and mucous membrane, ophthalmological, otorhinolaryngological, and dental drugs
977 Poisoning by other and unspecified drugs and medicinals
978 Poisoning by bacterial vaccines
979 Poisoning by other vaccines and biological substances

### Toxic effects of substances chiefly nonmedicinal as to source (980-989)

980 Toxic effect of alcohol
981 Toxic effect of petroleum products
982 Toxic effect of solvents other than petroleum-based
983 Toxic effect of corrosive aromatics, acids, and caustic alkalis
984 Toxic effect of lead and its compounds (including fumes)
985 Toxic effect of other metals
986 Toxic effect of carbon monoxide
987 Toxic effect of other gases, fumes, or vapors
988 Toxic effect of noxious substances eaten as food
989 Toxic effect of other substances, chiefly nonmedicinal as to source

### Other and unspecified effects of external causes (990-995)

990 Effects of radiation, unspecified
991 Effects of reduced temperature
992 Effects of heat and light
993 Effects of air pressure
994 Effects of other external causes

995 Certain adverse effects, not elsewhere classified

## Complications of surgical and medical care, not elsewhere classified (996-999)

996 Complications peculiar to certain specified procedures
997 Complications affecting specified body systems, not elsewhere classified
998 Other complications of procedures, not elsewhere classified
999 Complications of medical care, not elsewhere classified

## SUPPLEMENTARY CLASSIFICATION OF FACTORS INFLUENCING HEALTH STATUS AND CONTACT WITH HEALTH SERVICES

### Persons with potential health hazards related to communicable diseases (V01-V09)

V01 Contact with or exposure to communicable diseases
V02 Carrier or suspected carrier of infectious diseases
V03 Need for prophylactic vaccination and inoculation against bacterial diseases
V04 Need for prophylactic vaccination and inoculation against certain viral diseases
V05 Need for other prophylactic vaccination and inoculation against single diseases
V06 Need for prophylactic vaccination and inoculation against combinations of diseases
V07 Need for isolation and other prophylactic measures
V08 Asymptomatic human immunodeficiency virus [HIV] infection status
V09 Infection with drug-resistant microorganisms

### Persons with potential health hazards related to personal and family history (V10-V19)

V10 Personal history of malignant neoplasm
V11 Personal history of mental disorder
V12 Personal history of certain other diseases
V13 Personal history of other diseases
V14 Personal history of allergy to medicinal agents
V15 Other personal history presenting hazards to health
V16 Family history of malignant neoplasm
V17 Family history of certain chronic disabling diseases
V18 Family history of certain other specific conditions
V19 Family history of other conditions

### Persons encountering health services in circumstances related to reproduction and development (V20-V29)

V20 Health supervision of infant or child
V21 Constitutional states in development
V22 Normal pregnancy
V23 Supervision of high-risk pregnancy
V24 Postpartum care and examination
V25 Encounter for contraceptive management
V26 Procreative management
V27 Outcome of delivery
V28 Antenatal screening
V29 Observation and evaluation of newborns and infants for suspected condition not found

### Liveborn infants according to type of birth (V30-V39)

V30 Single liveborn
V31 Twin, mate liveborn
V32 Twin, mate stillborn
V33 Twin, unspecified
V34 Other multiple, mates all liveborn
V35 Other multiple, mates all stillborn
V36 Other multiple, mates live- and stillborn
V37 Other multiple, unspecified
V39 Unspecified

### Persons with a condition influencing their health status (V40-V49)

V40 Mental and behavioral problems
V41 Problems with special senses and other special functions
V42 Organ or tissue replaced by transplant
V43 Organ or tissue replaced by other means
V44 Artificial opening status
V45 Other postprocedural states
V46 Other dependence on machines
V47 Other problems with internal organs
V48 Problems with head, neck, and trunk
V49 Other conditions influencing health status

### Persons encountering health services for specific procedures and aftercare (V50-V59)

V50 Elective surgery for purposes other than remedying health states
V51 Aftercare involving the use of plastic surgery
V52 Fitting and adjustment of prosthetic device
V53 Fitting and adjustment of other device
V54 Other orthopedic aftercare
V55 Attention to artificial openings
V56 Encounter for dialysis and dialysis catheter care
V57 Care involving use of rehabilitation procedures
V58 Encounter for other and unspecified procedures and aftercare
V59 Donors

### Persons encountering health services in other circumstances (V60-V69)

V60 Housing, household, and economic circumstances
V61 Other family circumstances
V62 Other psychosocial circumstances
V63 Unavailability of other medical facilities for care
V64 Persons encountering health services for specific procedures, not carried out
V65 Other persons seeking consultation
V66 Convalescence and palliative care
V67 Follow-up examination
V68 Encounters for administrative purposes
V69 Problems related to lifestyle

### Persons without reported diagnosis encountered during examination and investigation of individuals and populations (V70-V82)

V70 General medical examination
V71 Observation and evaluation for suspected conditions not found
V72 Special investigations and examinations
V73 Special screening examination for viral and chlamydial diseases
V74 Special screening examination for bacterial and spirochetal diseases
V75 Special screening examination for other infectious diseases
V76 Special screening for malignant neoplasms
V77 Special screening for endocrine, nutritional, metabolic, and immunity disorders
V78 Special screening for disorders of blood and blood-forming organs
V79 Special screening for mental disorders and developmental handicaps
V80 Special screening for neurological, eye, and ear diseases
V81 Special screening for cardiovascular, respiratory, and genitourinary diseases
V82 Special screening for other conditions

### Genetics (V83-V84)

V83 Genetic carrier status
V84 Genetic susceptibility to disease

### Body mass index (V85)

V85 Body Mass Index

### Estrogen receptor status (V86)

V86 Estrogen receptor status

## SUPPLEMENTARY CLASSIFICATION OF EXTERNAL CAUSES OF INJURY AND POISONING

### Railway accidents (E800-E807)

E800 Railway accident involving collision with rolling stock
E801 Railway accident involving collision with other object
E802 Railway accident involving derailment without antecedent collision
E803 Railway accident involving explosion, fire, or burning
E804 Fall in, on, or from railway train
E805 Hit by rolling stock
E806 Other specified railway accident
E807 Railway accident of unspecified nature

### Motor vehicle traffic accidents (E810-E819)

E810 Motor vehicle traffic accident involving collision with train
E811 Motor vehicle traffic accident involving re-entrant collision with another motor vehicle
E812 Other motor vehicle traffic accident involving collision with another motor vehicle
E813 Motor vehicle traffic accident involving collision with other vehicle
E814 Motor vehicle traffic accident involving collision with pedestrian
E815 Other motor vehicle traffic accident involving collision on the highway
E816 Motor vehicle traffic accident due to loss of control, without collision on the highway
E817 Noncollision motor vehicle traffic accident while boarding or alighting
E818 Other noncollision motor vehicle traffic accident
E819 Motor vehicle traffic accident of unspecified nature

### Motor vehicle nontraffic accidents (E820-E825)

E820 Nontraffic accident involving motor-driven snow vehicle
E821 Nontraffic accident involving other off-road motor vehicle
E822 Other motor vehicle nontraffic accident involving collision with moving object
E823 Other motor vehicle nontraffic accident involving collision with stationary object
E824 Other motor vehicle nontraffic accident while boarding and alighting
E825 Other motor vehicle nontraffic accident of other and unspecified nature

### Other road vehicle accidents (E826-E829)

E826 Pedal cycle accident
E827 Animal-drawn vehicle accident
E828 Accident involving animal being ridden
E829 Other road vehicle accidents

### Water transport accidents (E830-E838)

E830 Accident to watercraft causing submersion
E831 Accident to watercraft causing other injury
E832 Other accidental submersion or drowning in water transport accident
E833 Fall on stairs or ladders in water transport
E834 Other fall from one level to another in water transport
E835 Other and unspecified fall in water transport
E836 Machinery accident in water transport
E837 Explosion, fire, or burning in watercraft
E838 Other and unspecified water transport accident

### Air and space transport accidents (E840-E845)

E840 Accident to powered aircraft at takeoff or landing
E841 Accident to powered aircraft, other and unspecified
E842 Accident to unpowered aircraft
E843 Fall in, on, or from aircraft
E844 Other specified air transport accidents
E845 Accident involving spacecraft

### Vehicle accidents, not elsewhere classifiable (E846-E849)

E846 Accidents involving powered vehicles used solely within the buildings and premises of an industrial or commercial establishment
E847 Accidents involving cable cars not running on rails
E848 Accidents involving other vehicles, not elsewhere classifiable
E849 Place of occurrence

### Accidental poisoning by drugs, medicinal substances, and biologicals (E850-E858)

E850 Accidental poisoning by analgesics, antipyretics, and antirheumatics
E851 Accidental poisoning by barbiturates
E852 Accidental poisoning by other sedatives and hypnotics
E853 Accidental poisoning by tranquilizers
E854 Accidental poisoning by other psychotropic agents
E855 Accidental poisoning by other drugs acting on central and autonomic nervous systems
E856 Accidental poisoning by antibiotics
E857 Accidental poisoning by anti-infectives
E858 Accidental poisoning by other drugs

### Accidental poisoning by other solid and liquid substances, gases, and vapors (E860-E869)

E860 Accidental poisoning by alcohol, not elsewhere classified
E861 Accidental poisoning by cleansing and polishing agents, disinfectants, paints, and varnishes
E862 Accidental poisoning by petroleum products, other solvents and their vapors, not elsewhere classified
E863 Accidental poisoning by agricultural and horticultural chemical and pharmaceutical preparations other than plant foods and fertilizers
E864 Accidental poisoning by corrosives and caustics, not elsewhere classified
E865 Accidental poisoning from poisonous foodstuffs and poisonous plants
E866 Accidental poisoning by other and unspecified solid and liquid substances
E867 Accidental poisoning by gas distributed by pipeline
E868 Accidental poisoning by other utility gas and other carbon monoxide
E869 Accidental poisoning by other gases and vapors

### Misadventures to patients during surgical and medical care (E870-E876)

E870 Accidental cut, puncture, perforation, or hemorrhage during medical care
E871 Foreign object left in body during procedure
E872 Failure of sterile precautions during procedure
E873 Failure in dosage
E874 Mechanical failure of instrument or apparatus during procedure
E875 Contaminated or infected blood, other fluid, drug, or biological substance
E876 Other and unspecified misadventures during medical care

### Surgical and medical procedures as the cause of abnormal reaction of patient or later complication, without mention of misadventure at the time of procedure (E878-E879)

E878 Surgical operation and other surgical procedures as the cause of abnormal reaction of patient, or of later complication, without mention of misadventure at the time of operation
E879 Other procedures, without mention of misadventure at the time of procedure, as the cause of abnormal reaction of patient, or of later complication

### Accidental falls (E880-E888)

E880 Fall on or from stairs or steps
E881 Fall on or from ladders or scaffolding
E882 Fall from or out of building or other structure
E883 Fall into hole or other opening in surface
E884 Other fall from one level to another
E885 Fall on same level from slipping, tripping, or stumbling
E886 Fall on same level from collision, pushing or shoving, by or with other person
E887 Fracture, cause unspecified
E888 Other and unspecified fall

### Accidents caused by fire and flames (E890-E899)

E890 Conflagration in private dwelling
E891 Conflagration in other and unspecified building or structure
E892 Conflagration not in building or structure
E893 Accident caused by ignition of clothing
E894 Ignition of highly inflammable material
E895 Accident caused by controlled fire in private dwelling
E896 Accident caused by controlled fire in other and unspecified building or structure
E897 Accident caused by controlled fire not in building or structure
E898 Accident caused by other specified fire and flames
E899 Accident caused by unspecified fire

### Accidents due to natural and environmental factors (E900-E909)

E900 Excessive heat
E901 Excessive cold
E902 High and low air pressure and changes in air pressure
E903 Travel and motion
E904 Hunger, thirst, exposure, and neglect
E905 Venomous animals and plants as the cause of poisoning and toxic reactions
E906 Other injury caused by animals
E907 Lightning
E908 Cataclysmic storms, and floods resulting from storms
E909 Cataclysmic earth surface movements and eruptions

### Accidents caused by submersion, suffocation, and foreign bodies (E910-E915)

E910 Accidental drowning and submersion
E911 Inhalation and ingestion of food causing obstruction of respiratory tract or suffocation
E912 Inhalation and ingestion of other object causing obstruction of respiratory tract or suffocation
E913 Accidental mechanical suffocation
E914 Foreign body accidentally entering eye and adnexa
E915 Foreign body accidentally entering other orifice

### Other accidents (E916-E928)

E916 Struck accidentally by falling object
E917 Striking against or struck accidentally by objects or persons
E918 Caught accidentally in or between objects
E919 Accidents caused by machinery
E920 Accidents caused by cutting and piercing instruments or objects
E921 Accident caused by explosion of pressure vessel
E922 Accident caused by firearm missile
E923 Accident caused by explosive material
E924 Accident caused by hot substance or object, caustic or corrosive material, and steam
E925 Accident caused by electric current
E926 Exposure to radiation
E927 Overexertion and strenuous movements
E928 Other and unspecified environmental and accidental causes

### Late effects of accidental injury (E929)

E929 Late effects of accidental injury

### Drugs, medicinal and biological substances causing adverse effects in therapeutic use (E930-E949)

E930 Antibiotics
E931 Other anti-infectives
E932 Hormones and synthetic substitutes
E933 Primarily systemic agents
E934 Agents primarily affecting blood constituents
E935 Analgesics, antipyretics, and antirheumatics
E936 Anticonvulsants and anti-Parkinsonism drugs
E937 Sedatives and hypnotics
E938 Other central nervous system depressants and anesthetics
E939 Psychotropic agents
E940 Central nervous system stimulants
E941 Drugs primarily affecting the autonomic nervous system
E942 Agents primarily affecting the cardiovascular system
E943 Agents primarily affecting gastrointestinal system
E944 Water, mineral, and uric acid metabolism drugs
E945 Agents primarily acting on the smooth and skeletal muscles and respiratory system
E946 Agents primarily affecting skin and mucous membrane, ophthalmological, otorhinolaryngological, and dental drugs
E947 Other and unspecified drugs and medicinal substances
E948 Bacterial vaccines
E949 Other vaccines and biological substances

### Suicide and self-inflicted injury (E950-E959)

E950 Suicide and self-inflicted poisoning by solid or liquid substances
E951 Suicide and self-inflicted poisoning by gases in domestic use
E952 Suicide and self-inflicted poisoning by other gases and vapors
E953 Suicide and self-inflicted injury by hanging, strangulation, and suffocation
E954 Suicide and self-inflicted injury by submersion [drowning]
E955 Suicide and self-inflicted injury by firearms and explosives
E956 Suicide and self-inflicted injury by cutting and piercing instruments
E957 Suicide and self-inflicted injuries by jumping from high place
E958 Suicide and self-inflicted injury by other and unspecified means
E959 Late effects of self-inflicted injury

### Homicide and injury purposely inflicted by other persons (E960-E969)

E960 Fight, brawl, and rape
E961 Assault by corrosive or caustic substance, except poisoning
E962 Assault by poisoning
E963 Assault by hanging and strangulation
E964 Assault by submersion [drowning]
E965 Assault by firearms and explosives
E966 Assault by cutting and piercing instrument
E967 Child and adult battering and other maltreatment
E968 Assault by other and unspecified means
E969 Late effects of injury purposely inflicted by other person

### Legal intervention (E970-E978)

E970 Injury due to legal intervention by firearms
E971 Injury due to legal intervention by explosives
E972 Injury due to legal intervention by gas
E973 Injury due to legal intervention by blunt object

E974 Injury due to legal intervention by cutting and piercing instruments

E975 Injury due to legal intervention by other specified means

E976 Injury due to legal intervention by unspecified means

E977 Late effects of injuries due to legal intervention

E978 Legal execution

## Terrorism (E979)

E979 Terrorism

## Injury undetermined whether accidentally or purposely inflicted (E980-E989)

E980 Poisoning by solid or liquid substances, undetermined whether accidentally or purposely inflicted

E981 Poisoning by gases in domestic use, undetermined whether accidentally or purposely inflicted

E982 Poisoning by other gases, undetermined whether accidentally or purposely inflicted

E983 Hanging, strangulation, or suffocation, undetermined whether accidentally or purposely inflicted

E984 Submersion [drowning], undetermined whether accidentally or purposely inflicted

E985 Injury by firearms and explosives, undetermined whether accidentally or purposely inflicted

E986 Injury by cutting and piercing instruments, undetermined whether accidentally or purposely inflicted

E987 Falling from high place, undetermined whether accidentally or purposely inflicted

E988 Injury by other and unspecified means, undetermined whether accidentally or purposely inflicted

E989 Late effects of injury, undetermined whether accidentally or purposely inflicted

## Injury resulting from operations of war (E990-E999)

E990 Injury due to war operations by fires and conflagrations

E991 Injury due to war operations by bullets and fragments

E992 Injury due to war operations by explosion of marine weapons

E993 Injury due to war operations by other explosion

E994 Injury due to war operations by destruction of aircraft

E995 Injury due to war operations by other and unspecified forms of conventional warfare

E996 Injury due to war operations by nuclear weapons

E997 Injury due to war operations by other forms of unconventional warfare

E998 Injury due to war operations but occurring after cessation of hostilities

E999 Late effects of injury due to war operations

☑ Additional Digit Required — Refer to the Tabular List for Digit Selection
*2007 Ingenix*
▶◀ Revised Text   ● New Line   ▲ Revised Code
Subterms under main terms may continue to next column or page
**October 2007 · Volume 3 — 1**

**Aneurysmectomy** — *continued*
abdominal
artery 38.66
vein 38.67
aorta (arch) (ascending) (descending) 38.64
atrial, auricular 37.32
head and neck NEC 38.62
heart 37.32
intracranial NEC 38.61
lower limb
artery 38.68
vein 38.69
sinus of Valsalva 35.39
thoracic NEC 38.65
upper limb (artery) (vein) 38.63
ventricle (myocardium) 37.32
**Aneurysmoplasty** — *see* Aneurysmorrhaphy
**Aneurysmorrhaphy** NEC 39.52
by or with
anastomosis — *see* Aneurysmectomy, with anastomosis, by site
clipping 39.51
coagulation 39.52
electrocoagulation 39.52
endovascular graft
abdominal aorta 39.71
lower extremity artery(s) 39.79
thoracic aorta 39.73
upper extremity artery(s) 39.79
excision or resection (*see also* Aneurysmectomy, by site) with
anastomosis — *see* Aneurysmectomy, with anastomosis, by site
graft replacement — *see* Aneurysmectomy, with graft replacement, by site
filipuncture 39.52
graft replacement — *see* Aneurysmectomy, with graft replacement, by site
methyl methacrylate 39.52
suture 39.52
wiring 39.52
wrapping 39.52
Matas' 39.52
**Aneurysmotomy** — *see* Aneurysmectomy
**Angiectomy**
with
anastomosis 38.30
abdominal
artery 38.36
vein 38.37
aorta (arch) (ascending) (descending) 38.34
head and neck NEC 38.32
intracranial NEC 38.31
lower limb
artery 38.38
vein 38.39
thoracic vessel NEC 38.35
upper limb (artery) (vein) 38.33
graft replacement (interposition) 38.40
abdominal
aorta 38.44
artery 38.46
vein 38.47
aorta (arch) (ascending) (descending thoracic)
abdominal 38.44
thoracic 38.45
thoracoabdominal 38.45 [38.44]
head and neck NEC 38.42
intracranial NEC 38.41
lower limb
artery 38.48
vein 38.49
thoracic vessel NEC 38.45

**Angiectomy** — *continued*
with — *continued*
graft replacement — *continued*
upper limb (artery) (vein) 38.43
**Angiocardiography** (selective) 88.50
carbon dioxide (negative contrast) 88.58
combined right and left heart 88.54
intra-operative fluorescence vascular ● 88.59 ●
left heart (aortic valve) (atrium) (ventricle) (ventricular outflow tract) 88.53
combined with right heart 88.54
right heart (atrium) (pulmonary valve) (ventricle) (ventricular outflow tract) 88.52
combined with left heart 88.54
SPY 88.59 ●
vena cava (inferior) (superior) 88.51
**Angiography** (arterial) — *see also* Arteriography 88.40
by radioisotope — *see* Scan, radioisotope, by site
by ultrasound — *see* Ultrasonography, by site
basilar 88.41
brachial 88.49
carotid (internal) 88.41
celiac 88.47
cerebral (posterior circulation) 88.41
coronary NEC 88.57
intra-operative fluorescence vas- ● cular 88.59 ●
eye (fluorescein) 95.12
femoral 88.48
heart 88.50
intra-abdominal NEC 88.47
intracranial 88.41
intrathoracic vessels NEC 88.44
lower extremity NEC 88.48
neck 88.41
placenta 88.46
pulmonary 88.43
renal 88.45
specified artery NEC 88.49
transfemoral 88.48
upper extremity NEC 88.49
veins — *see* Phlebography
vertebral 88.41
**Angioplasty** (laser) — *see also* Repair, blood vessel
balloon (percutaneous transluminal) NEC 39.50
coronary artery 00.66
multiple vessels
coronary 36.09
open chest approach 36.03
percutaneous transluminal (balloon) 00.66

*Note — Also use 00.40, 00.41, 00.42, or 00.43 to show the total number of vessels treated. Use code 00.44 once to show procedure on a bifurcated vessel. In addition, use 00.45, 00.46, 00.47, or 00.48 to show the number of vascular stents inserted.*

percutaneous transluminal (balloon)
basilar 00.61
carotid 00.61
cerebral (intracranial) 00.62
cerebrovascular
cerebral (intracranial) 00.62
precerebral (extracranial) 00.61
carotid 00.61
coronary (balloon) 00.66
femoropopliteal 39.50
iliac 39.50
lower extremity NOS 39.50
mesenteric 39.50
peripheral NEC 39.50
precerebral (extracranial) 00.61
carotid 00.61
renal 39.50
subclavian 39.50
upper extremity NOS 39.50

**Angioplasty** — *see also* Repair, blood vessel — *continued*
percutaneous transluminal — *continued*
vertebral 00.61
specified site 39.50
cerebrovascular
cerebral (intracranial) 00.62
precerebral (extracranial) 00.61
peripheral 39.50
**Angiorrhaphy** 39.30
artery 39.31
vein 39.32
**Angioscopy, percutaneous** 38.22
eye (fluorescein) 95.12
**Angiotomy** 38.00
abdominal
artery 38.06
vein 38.07
aorta (arch) (ascending) (descending) 38.04
head and neck NEC 38.02
intracranial NEC 38.01
lower limb
artery 38.08
vein 38.09
thoracic NEC 38.05
upper limb (artery) (vein) 38.03
**Angiotripsy** 39.98
**Ankylosis, production of** — *see* Arthrodesis
**Annuloplasty** (heart) (posteromedial) 35.33
**Anoplasty** 49.79
with hemorrhoidectomy 49.46
**Anoscopy** 49.21
**Antibiogram** — *see* Examination, microscopic
**Antiembolic filter, vena cava** 38.7
**Antiphobic treatment** 94.39
**Antrectomy**
mastoid 20.49
maxillary 22.39
radical 22.31
pyloric 43.6
**Antrostomy** — *see* Antrotomy
**Antrotomy** (exploratory) (nasal sinus) 22.2
Caldwell-Luc (maxillary sinus) 22.39
with removal of membrane lining 22.31
intranasal 22.2
with external approach (Caldwell-Luc) 22.39
radical 22.31
maxillary (simple) 22.2
with Caldwell-Luc approach 22.39
with removal of membrane lining 22.31
external (Caldwell-Luc approach) 22.39
with removal of membrane lining 22.31
radical (with removal of membrane lining) 22.31
**Antrum window operation** — *see* Antrotomy, maxillary
**Aorticopulmonary window operation** 39.59
**Aortogram, aortography** (abdominal) (retrograde) (selective) (translumbar) 88.42
**Aortoplasty** (aortic valve) (gusset type) 35.11
**Aortotomy** 38.04
**Apexcardiogram** (with ECG lead) 89.57
**Apheresis, therapeutic** — *see* category 99.7 ☑
**Apicectomy**
lung 32.39 ▲
thoracoscopic 32.30 ●
petrous pyramid 20.59
tooth (root) 23.73
with root canal therapy 23.72
**Apicoectomy** 23.73
with root canal therapy 23.72

**Apicolysis** (lung) 33.39
**Apicostomy, alveolar** 24.0
**Aponeurectomy** 83.42
hand 82.33
**Aponeurorrhaphy** — *see also* Suture, tendon 83.64
hand (*see also* Suture, tendon, hand) 82.45
**Aponeurotomy** 83.13
hand 82.11
**Appendectomy** (with drainage) 47.09
incidental 47.19
laparoscopic 47.11
laparoscopic 47.01
**Appendicectomy** (with drainage) 47.09
incidental 47.19
laparoscopic 47.11
laparoscopic 47.01
**Appendicocecostomy** 47.91
**Appendicoenterostomy** 47.91
**Appendicolysis** 54.59
with appendectomy 47.09
laparoscopic 47.01
other 47.09
laparoscopic 54.51
**Appendicostomy** 47.91
closure 47.92
**Appendicotomy** 47.2
**Application**
adhesion barrier substance 99.77
anti-shock trousers 93.58
arch bars (orthodontic) 24.7
for immobilization (fracture) 93.55
barrier substance, adhesion 99.77
Barton's tongs (skull) (with synchronous skeletal traction) 02.94
bone growth stimulator (surface) (transcutaneous) 99.86
bone morphogenetic protein (Infuse™) (OP-1™) (recombinant) (rhBMP) 84.52
Bryant's traction 93.44
with reduction of fracture or dislocation — *see* Reduction, fracture *and* Reduction, dislocation
Buck's traction 93.46
caliper tongs (skull) (with synchronous skeletal traction) 02.94
cast (fiberglass) (plaster) (plastic) NEC 93.53
with reduction of fracture or dislocation — *see* Reduction, fracture *and* Reduction, dislocation
spica 93.51
cervical collar 93.52
with reduction of fracture or dislocation — *see* Reduction, fracture *and* Reduction, dislocation
clamp, cerebral aneurysm (Crutchfield) (Silverstone) 39.51
croupette, croup tent 93.94
crown (artificial) 23.41
Crutchfield tongs (skull) (with synchronous skeletal traction) 02.94
Dunlop's traction 93.44
with reduction of fracture or dislocation — *see* Reduction, fracture *and* Reduction, dislocation
elastic stockings 93.59
electronic gaiter 93.59
external fixator device (bone) 78.10
carpal, metacarpal 78.14
clavicle 78.11
computer assisted (dependent) 84.73
femur 78.15
fibula 78.17
humerus 78.12
hybrid device or system 84.73
Ilizarov type 84.72

☑ Additional Digit Required — Refer to the Tabular List for Digit Selection
*2007 Ingenix*
▶◀ Revised Text ● New Line ▲ Revised Code
ᵂ Subterms under main terms may continue to next column or page
October 2007 · Volume 3 — 3

**Application** — continued
external fixator device — continued
monoplanar system or device 84.71
patella 78.16
pelvic 78.19
phalanges (foot) (hand) 78.19
radius 78.13
ring device or system 84.72
scapula 78.11
Sheffield type 84.72
specified site NEC 78.19
tarsal, metatarsal 78.18
thorax (ribs) (sternum) 78.11
tibia 78.17
ulna 78.13
vertebrae 78.19
forceps, with delivery — see Delivery, forceps
graft — see Graft
gravity (G-) suit 93.59
intermittent pressure device 93.59
Jewett extension brace 93.59
Jobst pumping unit (reduction of edema) 93.59
Lyman Smith traction 93.44
with reduction of fracture or dislocation — see Reduction, fracture and Reduction, dislocation
MAST (military anti-shock trousers) 93.58
Minerva jacket 93.52
minifixator device (bone) — see category 78.1 ☑
neck support (molded) 93.52
obturator (orthodontic) 24.7
orthodontic appliance (obturator) (wiring) 24.7
pelvic sling 93.44
with reduction of fracture or dislocation — see Reduction, fracture and Reduction, dislocation
peridontal splint (orthodontic) 24.7
plaster jacket 93.51
Minerva 93.52
pressure
dressing (bandage) (Gibney) (Robert Jones') (Shanz) 93.56
trousers (anti-shock) (MAST) 93.58
prosthesis for missing ear 18.71
Russell's traction 93.44
with reduction of fracture or dislocation — see Reduction, fracture and Reduction, dislocation
splint, for immobilization (plaster) (pneumatic) (tray) 93.54
with fracture reduction — see Reduction, fracture
stereotactic head frame 93.59
strapping (non-traction) 93.59
substance, adhesion barrier 99.77
Thomas collar 93.52
with reduction of fracture or dislocation — see Reduction, fracture and Reduction, dislocation
traction
with reduction of fracture or dislocation — see Reduction, fracture and Reduction, dislocation
adhesive tape (skin) 93.46
boot 93.46
Bryant's 93.44
Buck's 93.46
Cotrel's 93.42
Dunlop's 93.44
gallows 93.46
Lyman Smith 93.44
Russell's 93.44
skeletal NEC 93.44
intermittent 93.43
skin, limbs NEC 93.46
spinal NEC 93.42

**Application** — continued
traction — continued
spinal — continued
with skull device (halo) (caliper) (Crutchfield) (Gardner-Wells) (Vinke) (tongs) 93.41
with synchronous insertion 02.94
Thomas' splint 93.45
Unna's paste boot 93.53
vasopneumatic device 93.58
Velpeau dressing 93.59
Vinke tongs (skull) (with synchronous skeletal traction) 02.94
wound dressing NEC 93.57
**Aquapheresis** 99.78
**Arc lamp** — see Photocoagulation
**Arrest**
bone growth (epiphyseal) 78.20
by stapling — see Stapling, epiphyseal plate
femur 78.25
fibula 78.27
humerus 78.22
radius 78.23
tibia 78.27
ulna 78.23
cardiac, induced (anoxic) (circulatory) 39.63
circulatory, induced (anoxic) 39.63
hemorrhage — see Control, hemorrhage
**Arslan operation** (fenestration of inner ear) 20.61
**Arteriectomy** 38.60
with
anastomosis 38.30
abdominal 38.36
aorta (arch) (ascending) (descending thoracic) 38.34
head and neck NEC 38.32
intracranial NEC 38.31
lower limb 38.38
thoracic NEC 38.35
upper limb 38.33
graft replacement (interposition) 38.40
abdominal
aorta 38.44
aorta (arch) (ascending) (descending thoracic)
abdominal 38.44
thoracic 38.45
thoracoabdominal 38.45 [38.44]
head and neck NEC 38.42
intracranial NEC 38.41
lower limb 38.48
thoracic NEC 38.45
upper limb 38.43
abdominal 38.66
aorta (arch) (ascending) (descending) 38.64
head and neck NEC 38.62
intracranial NEC 38.61
lower limb 38.68
thoracic NEC 38.65
upper limb 38.63
**Arteriography** (contrast) (fluoroscopic) (retrograde) 88.40
by
radioisotope — see Scan, radioisotope
ultrasound (Doppler) — see Ultrasonography, by site
aorta (arch) (ascending) (descending) 88.42
basilar 88.41
brachial 88.49
carotid (internal) 88.41
cerebral (posterior circulation) 88.41
coronary (direct) (selective) NEC 88.57
double catheter technique (Judkins) (Ricketts and Abrams) 88.56

**Arteriography** — continued
coronary — continued
intra-operative fluorescence vas- ●
cular 88.59 ●
single catheter technique (Sones) 88.55
Doppler (ultrasonic) — see Ultrasonography, by site
femoral 88.48
head and neck 88.41
intra-abdominal NEC 88.47
intrathoracic NEC 88.44
lower extremity 88.48
placenta 88.46
pulmonary 88.43
radioisotope — see Scan, radioisotope
renal 88.45
specified site NEC 88.49
SPY 88.59 ●
superior mesenteric artery 88.47
transfemoral 88.48
ultrasound — see Ultrasonography, by site
upper extremity 88.49
**Arterioplasty** — see Repair, artery
**Arteriorrhaphy** 39.31
**Arteriotomy** 38.00
abdominal 38.06
aorta (arch) (ascending) (descending) 38.04
head and neck NEC 38.02
intracranial NEC 38.01
lower limb 38.08
thoracic NEC 38.05
upper limb 38.03
**Arteriovenostomy** 39.29
for renal dialysis 39.27
**Arthrectomy** 80.90
ankle 80.97
elbow 80.92
foot and toe 80.98
hand and finger 80.94
hip 80.95
intervertebral disc — see category 80.5 ☑
knee 80.96
semilunar cartilage 80.6
shoulder 80.91
specified site NEC 80.99
spine NEC 80.99
wrist 80.93
**Arthrocentesis** 81.91
for arthrography — see Arthrogram
**Arthrodesis** (compression) (extra-articular) (intra-articular) (with bone graft) (with fixation device) 81.20
ankle 81.11
carporadial 81.25
cricoarytenoid 31.69
elbow 81.24
finger 81.28
foot NEC 81.17
hip 81.21
interphalangeal
finger 81.28
toe NEC 77.58
claw toe repair 77.57
hammer toe repair 77.56
ischiofemoral 81.21
knee 81.22
lumbosacral, lumbar NEC 81.08
ALIF (anterior lumbar interbody fusion) 81.06
anterior (interbody), anterolateral technique 81.06
lateral transverse process technique 81.07
PLIF (posterior lumbar interbody fusion) 81.08
posterior (interbody), posterolateral technique 81.08
TLIF (transforaminal lumbar interbody fusion) 81.08
McKeever (metatarsophalangeal) 81.16
metacarpocarpal 81.26
metacarpophalangeal 81.27

**Arthrodesis** — continued
metatarsophalangeal 81.16
midtarsal 81.14
plantar 81.11
sacroiliac 81.08
shoulder 81.23
specified joint NEC 81.29
spinal (see also Fusion, spinal) 81.00
subtalar 81.13
tarsometatarsal 81.15
tibiotalar 81.11
toe NEC 77.58
claw toe repair 77.57
hammer toe repair 77.56
triple 81.12
wrist 81.26
**Arthroendoscopy** — see Arthroscopy
**Arthroereisis, subtalar joint** 81.18
**Arthrogram, arthrography** 88.32
temporomandibular 87.13
**Arthrolysis** 93.26
**Arthroplasty** (with fixation device) (with traction) 81.96
ankle 81.49
carpals 81.75
with prosthetic implant 81.74
carpocarpal, carpometacarpal 81.75
with prosthetic implant 81.74
Carroll and Taber (proximal interphalangeal joint) 81.72
cup (partial hip) 81.52
Curtis (interphalangeal joint) 81.72
elbow 81.85
with prosthetic replacement (total) 81.84
femoral head NEC 81.40
with prosthetic implant 81.52
finger(s) 81.72
with prosthetic implant 81.71
foot (metatarsal) with joint replacement 81.57
Fowler (metacarpophalangeal joint) 81.72
hand (metacarpophalangeal) (interphalangeal) 81.72
with prosthetic implant 81.71
hip (with bone graft) 81.40
cup (partial hip) 81.52
femoral head NEC 81.40
with prosthetic implant 81.52
with total replacement 81.51
partial replacement 81.52
total replacement 81.51
interphalangeal joint 81.72
with prosthetic implant 81.71
Kessler (carpometacarpal joint) 81.74
knee (see also Repair, knee) 81.47
prosthetic replacement (bicompartmental) (hemijoint) (partial) (total) (tricompartmental) (unicompartmental) 81.54
revision 81.55
metacarpophalangeal joint 81.72
with prosthetic implant 81.71
shoulder 81.83
for recurrent dislocation 81.82
prosthetic replacement (partial) 81.81
total 81.80
temporomandibular 76.5
toe NEC 77.58
for hallux valgus repair 77.59
with prosthetic replacement 81.57
wrist 81.75
with prosthetic implant 81.74
total replacement 81.73
**Arthroscopy** 80.20
ankle 80.27
elbow 80.22
finger 80.24
foot 80.28
hand 80.24
hip 80.25
knee 80.26
shoulder 80.21
specified site NEC 80.29

☑ Additional Digit Required — Refer to the Tabular List for Digit Selection

[REF] Subterms under main terms may continue to next column or page

4 — Volume 3 · October 2007
▶◀ Revised Text
● New Line
▲ Revised Code
2007 Ingenix

☑ Additional Digit Required — Refer to the Tabular List for Digit Selection
2007 Ingenix
▶◀ Revised Text   ● New Line   ▲ Revised Code
Subterms under main terms may continue to next column or page
October 2007 · Volume 3 — 5

**Biopsy**
- abdominal wall 54.22
- adenoid 28.11
- adrenal gland NEC 07.11
  - closed 07.11
  - open 07.12
  - percutaneous (aspiration) (needle) 07.11
- alveolus 24.12
- anus 49.23
- appendix 45.26
- artery (any site) 38.21
- aspiration — *see* Biopsy, by site
- bile ducts 51.14
  - closed (endoscopic) 51.14
  - open 51.13
  - percutaneous (needle) 51.12
- bladder 57.33
  - closed 57.33
  - open 57.34
  - transurethral 57.33
- blood vessel (any site) 38.21
- bone 77.40
  - carpal, metacarpal 77.44
  - clavicle 77.41
  - facial 76.11
  - femur 77.45
  - fibula 77.47
  - humerus 77.42
  - marrow 41.31
  - patella 77.46
  - pelvic 77.49
  - phalanges (foot) (hand) 77.49
  - radius 77.43
  - scapula 77.41
  - specified site NEC 77.49
  - tarsal, metatarsal 77.48
  - thorax (ribs) (sternum) 77.41
  - tibia 77.47
  - ulna 77.43
  - vertebrae 77.49
- bowel — *see* Biopsy, intestine
- brain NEC 01.13
  - closed 01.13
  - open 01.14
  - percutaneous (needle) 01.13
- breast 85.11
  - blind 85.11
  - closed 85.11
  - open 85.12
  - percutaneous (needle) (Vimm-Silverman) 85.11
- bronchus NEC 33.24
  - brush 33.24
  - closed (endoscopic) 33.24
  - open 33.25
  - washings 33.24
- bursa 83.21
- cardioesophageal (junction) 44.14
  - closed (endoscopic) 44.14
  - open 44.15
- cecum 45.25
  - brush 45.25
  - closed (endoscopic) 45.25
  - open 45.26
- cerebral meninges NEC 01.11
  - closed 01.11
  - open 01.12
  - percutaneous (needle) 01.11
- cervix (punch) 67.12
  - conization (sharp) 67.2
- chest wall 34.23
- clitoris 71.11
- colon 45.25
  - brush 45.25
  - closed (endoscopic) 45.25
  - open 45.26
- conjunctiva 10.21
- cornea 11.22
- cul-de-sac 70.23
- diaphragm 34.27
- duodenum 45.14
  - brush 45.14
  - closed (endoscopic) 45.14
  - open 45.15
- ear (external) 18.12

**Biopsy** — *continued*
- ear — *continued*
  - middle or inner 20.32
- endocervix 67.11
- endometrium NEC 68.16
  - by
    - aspiration curettage 69.59
    - dilation and curettage 69.09
  - closed (endoscopic) 68.16
  - open 68.13
- epididymis 63.01
- esophagus 42.24
  - closed (endoscopic) 42.24
  - open 42.25
- extraocular muscle or tendon 15.01
- eye 16.23
  - muscle (oblique) (rectus) 15.01
- eyelid 08.11
- fallopian tube 66.11
- fascia 83.21
- fetus 75.33
- gallbladder 51.12
  - closed (endoscopic) 51.14
  - open 51.13
  - percutaneous (needle) 51.12
- ganglion (cranial) (peripheral) NEC 04.11
  - closed 04.11
  - open 04.12
  - percutaneous (needle) 04.11
  - sympathetic nerve 05.11
- gum 24.11
- heart 37.25
- hypophysis (*see also* Biopsy, pituitary gland) 07.15
- ileum 45.14
  - brush 45.14
  - closed (endoscopic) 45.14
  - open 45.15
- intestine NEC 45.27
  - large 45.25
    - brush 45.25
    - closed (endoscopic) 45.25
    - open 45.26
  - small 45.14
    - brush 45.14
    - closed (endoscopic) 45.14
    - open 45.15
- intra-abdominal mass 54.24
  - closed 54.24
  - percutaneous (needle) 54.24
- iris 12.22
- jejunum 45.14
  - brush 45.14
  - closed (endoscopic) 45.14
  - open 45.15
- joint structure (aspiration) 80.30
  - ankle 80.37
  - elbow 80.32
  - foot and toe 80.38
  - hand and finger 80.34
  - hip 80.35
  - knee 80.36
  - shoulder 80.31
  - specified site NEC 80.39
  - spine 80.39
  - wrist 80.33
- kidney 55.23
  - closed 55.23
  - open 55.24
  - percutaneous (aspiration) (needle) 55.23
- labia 71.11
- lacrimal
  - gland 09.11
  - sac 09.12
- larynx 31.43
  - brush 31.43
  - closed (endoscopic) 31.43
  - open 31.45
- lip 27.23
- liver 50.11
  - closed 50.11
  - laparoscopic 50.14  ▲
  - open 50.12

**Biopsy** — *continued*
- liver — *continued*
  - percutaneous (aspiration) (needle) 50.11
  - transjugular 50.13  ●
  - transvenous 50.13  ●
- lung NEC 33.27
  - brush 33.24
  - closed (percutaneous) (needle) 33.26
    - brush 33.24
    - endoscopic 33.27
      - brush 33.24
  - endoscopic 33.27
    - brush 33.24
  - open 33.28
  - thoracoscopic 33.20  ●
  - transbronchial 33.27
  - transthoracic 33.26  ●
- lymphatic structure (channel) (node) (vessel) 40.11
- mediastinum NEC 34.25
  - closed 34.25
  - open 34.26
  - percutaneous (needle) 34.25
- meninges (cerebral) NEC 01.11
  - closed 01.11
  - open 01.12
  - percutaneous (needle) 01.11
  - spinal 03.32
- mesentery 54.23
- mouth NEC 27.24
- muscle 83.21
  - extraocular 15.01
  - ocular 15.01
- nasopharynx 29.12
- nerve (cranial) (peripheral) NEC 04.11
  - closed 04.11
  - open 04.12
  - percutaneous (needle) 04.11
  - sympathetic 05.11
- nose, nasal 21.22
  - sinus 22.11
    - closed (endoscopic) (needle) 22.11
    - open 22.12
- ocular muscle or tendon 15.01
- omentum
  - closed 54.24
  - open 54.23
  - percutaneous (needle) 54.24
- orbit 16.23
  - by aspiration 16.22
- ovary 65.12
  - by aspiration 65.11
  - laparoscopic 65.13
- palate (bony) 27.21
  - soft 27.22
- pancreas 52.11
  - closed (endoscopic) 52.11
  - open 52.12
  - percutaneous (aspiration) (needle) 52.11
- pancreatic duct 52.14
  - closed (endoscopic) 52.14
- parathyroid gland 06.13
- penis 64.11
- perianal tissue 49.22
- pericardium 37.24
- periprostatic 60.15
- perirectal tissue 48.26
- perirenal tissue 59.21
- peritoneal implant
  - closed 54.24
  - open 54.23
  - percutaneous (needle) 54.24
- peritoneum
  - closed 54.24
  - open 54.23
  - percutaneous (needle) 54.24
- periurethral tissue 58.24
- perivesical tissue 59.21
- pharynx, pharyngeal 29.12
- pineal gland 07.17
- pituitary gland 07.15
  - transfrontal approach 07.13

**Biopsy** — *continued*
- pituitary gland — *continued*
  - transsphenoidal approach 07.14
- pleura, pleural 34.24
  - thoracoscopic 34.20  ●
- prostate NEC 60.11
  - closed (transurethral) 60.11
  - open 60.12
  - percutaneous (needle) 60.11
  - transrectal 60.11
- rectum 48.24
  - brush 48.24
  - closed (endoscopic) 48.24
  - open 48.25
- retroperitoneal tissue 54.24
- salivary gland or duct 26.11
  - closed (needle) 26.11
  - open 26.12
- scrotum 61.11
- seminal vesicle NEC 60.13
  - closed 60.13
  - open 60.14
  - percutaneous (needle) 60.13
- sigmoid colon 45.25
  - brush 45.25
  - closed (endoscopic) 45.25
  - open 45.26
- sinus, nasal 22.11
  - closed (endoscopic) (needle) 22.11
  - open 22.12
- skin (punch) 86.11
- skull 01.15
- soft palate 27.22
- soft tissue NEC 83.21
- spermatic cord 63.01
- sphincter of Oddi 51.14
  - closed (endoscopic) 51.14
  - open 51.13
- spinal cord (meninges) 03.32
- spleen 41.32
  - closed 41.32
  - open 41.33
  - percutaneous (aspiration) (needle) 41.32
- stomach 44.14
  - brush 44.14
  - closed (endoscopic) 44.14
  - open 44.15
- subcutaneous tissue (punch) 86.11
- supraglottic mass 29.12
- sympathetic nerve 05.11
- tendon 83.21
  - extraocular 15.01
  - ocular 15.01
- testis NEC 62.11
  - closed 62.11
  - open 62.12
  - percutaneous (needle) 62.11
- thymus 07.16
- thyroid gland NEC 06.11
  - closed 06.11
  - open 06.12
  - percutaneous (aspiration) (needle) 06.11
- tongue 25.01
  - closed (needle) 25.01
  - open 25.02
- tonsil 28.11
- trachea 31.44
  - brush 31.44
  - closed (endoscopic) 31.44
  - open 31.45
- tunica vaginalis 61.11
- umbilicus 54.22
- ureter 56.33
  - closed (percutaneous) 56.32
    - endoscopic 56.33
  - open 56.34
  - transurethral 56.33
- urethra 58.23
- uterus, uterine (endometrial) 68.16
  - by
    - aspiration curettage 69.59
    - dilation and curettage 69.09
  - closed (endoscopic) 68.16
  - ligaments 68.15

**Biopsy** — *continued*
   uterus, uterine — *continued*
     ligaments — *continued*
      closed (endoscopic) 68.15
      open 68.14
     open 68.13
   uvula 27.22
   vagina 70.24
   vas deferens 63.01
   vein (any site) 38.21
   vulva 71.11
**BiPAP** 93.90 ●
**Bischoff operation** (spinal myelotomy) 03.29
**Bischoff operation** (ureteroneocystostomy) 56.74
**Bisection** — *see also* Excision
   hysterectomy 68.39
     laparoscopic 68.31
   ovary 65.29
     laparoscopic 65.25
   stapes foot plate 19.19
     with incus replacement 19.11
**Blalock-Hanlon operation** (creation of atrial septal defect) 35.42
**Blalock operation** (systemic-pulmonary anastomosis) 39.0
**Blalock-Taussig operation** (subclavian-pulmonary anastomosis) 39.0
**Blascovic operation** (resection and advancement of levator palpebrae superioris) 08.33
**Blepharectomy** 08.20
**Blepharoplasty** — *see also* Reconstruction, eyelid 08.70
   extensive 08.44
**Blepharorrhaphy** 08.52
   division or severing 08.02
**Blepharotomy** 08.09
**Blind rehabilitation therapy** NEC 93.78
**Block**
   caudal — *see* Injection, spinal
   celiac ganglion or plexus 05.31
   dissection
     breast
      bilateral 85.46
      unilateral 85.45
     bronchus 32.6
     larynx 30.3
     lymph nodes 40.50
     neck 40.40
     vulva 71.5
   epidural, spinal — *see* Injection, spinal
   gasserian ganglion 04.81
   intercostal nerves 04.81
   intrathecal — *see* Injection, spinal
   nerve (cranial) (peripheral) NEC 04.81
   paravertebral stellate ganglion 05.31
   peripheral nerve 04.81
   spinal nerve root (intrathecal) — *see* Injection, spinal
   stellate (ganglion) 05.31
   subarachnoid, spinal — *see* Injection, spinal
   sympathetic nerve 05.31
   trigeminal nerve 04.81
**Blood**
   flow study, Doppler-type (ultrasound) — *see* Ultrasonography
   patch, spine (epidural) 03.95
   transfusion
     antihemophilic factor 99.06
     autologous
      collected prior to surgery 99.02
      intraoperative 99.00
      perioperative 99.00
      postoperative 99.00
      previously collected 99.02
      salvage 99.00
     blood expander 99.08
     blood surrogate 99.09
     coagulation factors 99.06
     exchange 99.01
     granulocytes 99.09
     hemodilution 99.03

**Blood** — *continued*
   transfusion — *continued*
     other substance 99.09
     packed cells 99.04
     plasma 99.07
     platelets 99.05
     serum, other 99.07
     thrombocytes 99.05
**Blount operation**
   femoral shortening (with blade plate) 78.25
   by epiphyseal stapling 78.25
**Boari operation** (bladder flap) 56.74
**Bobb operation** (cholelithotomy) 51.04
**Bone**
   age studies 88.33
   mineral density study 88.98
**Bonney operation** (abdominal hysterectomy) 68.49
   laparoscopic 68.41
**Borthen operation** (iridotasis) 12.63
**Bost operation**
   plantar dissection 80.48
   radiocarpal fusion 81.26
**Bosworth operation**
   arthroplasty for acromioclavicular separation 81.83
   fusion of posterior lumbar and lumbosacral spine 81.08
     for pseudarthrosis 81.38
   resection of radial head ligaments (for tennis elbow) 80.92
   shelf procedure, hip 81.40
**Bottle repair of hydrocele, tunicavaginalis** 61.2
**Boyd operation** (hip disarticulation) 84.18
**Brachytherapy**
   intravascular 92.27
**Brauer operation** (cardiolysis) 37.10
**Breech extraction** — *see* Extraction, breech
**Bricker operation** (ileoureterostomy) 56.51
**Brisement** (forcé) 93.26
**Bristow operation** (repair of shoulder dislocation) 81.82
**Brockman operation** (soft tissue release for clubfoot) 83.84
**Brock operation** (pulmonary valvotomy) 35.03
**Bronchogram, bronchography** 87.32
   endotracheal 87.31
   transcricoid 87.32
**Bronchoplasty** 33.48
**Bronchorrhaphy** 33.41
**Bronchoscopy** NEC 33.23
   with biopsy 33.24
     lung 33.27
     brush 33.24
   fiberoptic 33.22
     with biopsy 33.24
     lung 33.27
     brush 33.24
   through tracheostomy 33.21
     with biopsy 33.24
     lung 33.27
     brush 33.24
**Bronchospirometry** 89.38
**Bronchostomy** 33.0
   closure 33.42
**Bronchotomy** 33.0
**Browne (-Denis) operation** (hypospadias repair) 58.45
**Brunschwig operation** (temporary gastrostomy) 43.19
**Buckling, scleral** 14.49
   with
     air tamponade 14.49
     implant (silicone) (vitreous) 14.41
     resection of sclera 14.49
     vitrectomy 14.49
     vitreous implant (silicone) 14.41
**Bunionectomy** (radical) 77.59
   with
     arthrodesis 77.52

**Bunionectomy** — *continued*
   with — *continued*
     osteotomy of first metatarsal 77.51
     resection of joint with prosthetic implant 77.59
     soft tissue correction NEC 77.53
**Bunnell operation** (tendon transfer) 82.56
**Burch procedure** (retropubic urethral suspension for urinary stress incontinence) 59.5
**Burgess operation** (amputation of ankle) 84.14
**Burn dressing** 93.57
**Burr holes** 01.24
**Bursectomy** 83.5
   hand 82.31
**Bursocentesis** 83.94
   hand 82.92
**Bursotomy** 83.03
   hand 82.03
**Burying of fimbriae in uterine wall** 66.97
**Bypass**
   abdominal-coronary artery 36.17
   aortocoronary (catheter stent) (with prosthesis) (with saphenous vein graft) (with vein graft) 36.10
     one coronary vessel 36.11
     two coronary vessels 36.12
     three coronary vessels 36.13
     four coronary vessels 36.14
   arterial (graft) (mandril grown graft) (vein graft) NEC 39.29
     carotid-cerebral 39.28
     carotid-vertebral 39.28
     extracranial-intracranial [EC-IC] 39.28
     intra-abdominal NEC 39.26
     intrathoracic NEC 39.23
     peripheral NEC 39.29
   cardiopulmonary 39.61
     open 39.61
     percutaneous (closed) 39.66
   carotid-cerebral 39.28
   carotid-vertebral 39.28
   coronary (*see also* Bypass, aortocoronary) 36.10
   extracranial-intracranial [EC-IC] 39.28
   gastric 44.39
     high 44.31
     laparoscopic 44.38
     Printen and Mason 44.31
   gastroduodenostomy (Jaboulay's) 44.39
     laparoscopic 44.38
   gastroenterostomy 44.39
     laparoscopic 44.38
   gastroepiploic-coronary artery 36.17
   gastrogastrostomy 44.39
     laparoscopic 44.38
   graft, pressurized treatment 00.16
   heart-lung (complete) (partial) 39.61
     open 39.61
     percutaneous (closed) 39.66
   high gastric 44.31
   ileo-jejunal 45.91
   internal mammary-coronary artery (single) 36.15
     double vessel 36.16
   jejunal-ileum 45.91
   pulmonary 39.61
     open 39.61
     percutaneous (closed) 39.66
   shunt
     intestine
      large-to-large 45.94
      small-to-large 45.93
      small-to-small 45.91
     stomach 44.39
      high gastric 44.31
      laparoscopic 44.38
   terminal ileum 45.93
   vascular (arterial) (graft) (mandril grown graft) (vein graft) NEC 39.29

**Bypass** — *continued*
   vascular — *continued*
     aorta-carotid-brachial 39.22
     aorta-iliac-femoral 39.25
     aorta-renal 39.24
     aorta-subclavian-carotid 39.22
     aortic-superior mesenteric 39.26
     aortocarotid 39.22
     aortoceliac 39.26
     aortocoronary (*see also* Bypass, aortocoronary) 36.10
     aortofemoral 39.25
     aortofemoral-popliteal 39.25
     aortoiliac 39.25
      to popliteal 39.25
     aortoiliofemoral 39.25
     aortomesenteric 39.26
     aortopopliteal 39.25
     aortorenal 39.24
     aortosubclavian 39.22
     axillary-brachial 39.29
     axillary-femoral (superficial) 39.29
     axillofemoral (superficial) 39.29
     carotid-cerebral 39.28
     carotid to subclavian artery 39.22
     carotid-vertebral 39.28
     common hepatic-common iliac-renal 39.26
     coronary (*see also* Bypass, aortocoronary) 36.10
     extracranial-intracranial [EC-IC] 39.28
     femoral-femoral 39.29
     femoroperoneal 39.29
     femoropopliteal (reversed saphenous vein) (saphenous) 39.29
     femorotibial (anterior) (posterior) 39.29
     iliofemoral 39.25
     ilioiliac 39.26
     internal mammary-coronary artery (single) 36.15
      double vessel 36.16
     intra-abdominal (arterial) NEC 39.26
     venous NEC 39.1
     intrathoracic NEC 39.23
     peripheral artery NEC 39.29
     popliteal-tibial 39.29
     renal artery 39.24
     splenorenal (venous) 39.1
      arterial 39.26
     subclavian-axillary 39.29
     subclavian-carotid 39.22
     subclavian-subclavian 39.22
     Y graft to renal arteries 39.24

## C

**Caldwell-Luc operation** (maxillary sinusotomy) 22.39
   with removal of membrane lining 22.31
**Caldwell operation** (sulcus extension) 24.91
**Calibration, urethra** 89.29
**Calicectomy** (renal) 55.4
**Callander operation** (knee disarticulation) 84.16
**Caloric test, vestibular function** 95.44
**Calycectomy** (renal) 55.4
**Calyco-ileoneocystostomy** 55.86
**Calycotomy** (renal) 55.11
**Campbell operation**
   bone block, ankle 81.11
   fasciotomy (iliac crest) 83.14
   reconstruction of anterior cruciate ligament 81.45
**Campimetry** 95.05
**Canaliculodacryocystorhinostomy** 09.81
**Canaliculoplasty** 09.73
**Canaliculorhinostomy** 09.81
**Canaloplasty, external auditory meatus** 18.6
**Cannulation** — *see also* Insertion, catheter

**Cannulation** — *see also* Insertion, catheter — *continued*
  ampulla of Vater 51.99
  antrum 22.01
  arteriovenous 39.93
  artery 38.91
  caval-mesenteric vein 39.1
  cisterna chyli 40.61
  Eustachian tube 20.8
  lacrimal apparatus 09.42
  lymphatic duct, left (thoracic) 40.61
  nasal sinus (by puncture) 22.01
    through natural ostium 22.02
  pancreatic duct 52.92
    by retrograde endoscopy (ERP) 52.93
  renoportal 39.1
  sinus (nasal) (by puncture) 22.01
    through natural ostium 22.02
  splenorenal (venous) 39.1
    arterial 39.26
  thoracic duct (cervical approach) (thoracic approach) 40.61
**Cannulization** — *see* Cannulation
**Canthocystostomy** 09.82
**Canthoplasty** 08.59
**Canthorrhaphy** 08.52
  division or severing 08.02
**Canthotomy** 08.51
**Capsulectomy**
  joint (*see also* Arthrectomy) 80.90
  kidney 55.91
  lens 13.65
    with extraction of lens 13.51
  ovary 65.29
    laparoscopic 65.25
**Capsulo-iridectomy** 13.65
**Capsuloplasty** — *see* Arthroplasty
**Capsulorrhaphy** 81.96
  with arthroplasty — *see* Arthroplasty
  ankle 81.94
  foot 81.94
  lower extremity NEC 81.95
  upper extremity 81.93
**Capsulotomy**
  joint (*see also* Division, joint capsule) 80.40
    for claw toe repair 77.57
  lens 13.64
    with
      discission of lens 13.2
      removal of foreign body 13.02
        by magnet extraction 13.01
**Cardiac**
  mapping 37.27
  massage (external) (closed chest) 99.63
    open chest 37.91
  retraining 93.36
**Cardiac support device** (CSD) 37.41
**Cardiectomy** (stomach) 43.5
**Cardiocentesis** 37.0
**Cardiography** — *see also* Angiocardiography 88.50
**Cardiolysis** 37.10
**Cardiomyopexy** 36.39
**Cardiomyotomy** 42.7
**Cardio-omentopexy** 36.39
**Cardiopericardiopexy** 36.39
**Cardioplasty** (stomach and esophagus) 44.65
  stomach alone 44.66
    laparoscopic 44.67
**Cardioplegia** 39.63
**Cardiopneumopexy** 36.39
**Cardiorrhaphy** 37.49
**Cardioschisis** 37.12
**Cardiosplenopexy** 36.39
**Cardiotomy** (exploratory) 37.11
**Cardiovalvulotomy** — *see* Valvulotomy, heart
**Cardioversion** (external) 99.62
  atrial 99.61
**Carotid pulse tracing with ECG lead** 89.56
**Carpectomy** (partial) 77.84

**Carpectomy** — *continued*
  total 77.94
**Carroll and Taber arthroplasty** (proximal interphalangeal joint) 81.72
**Casting** (for immobilization) NEC 93.53
  with fracture-reduction — *see* Reduction, fracture
**Castration**
  female (oophorectomy, bilateral) 65.51
    laparoscopic 65.53
  male 62.41
**C.A.T.** (computerized axial tomography) — *see also* Scan, C.A.T. 88.38
**Catheterization** — *see also* Insertion, catheter
  arteriovenous 39.93
  artery 38.91
  bladder, indwelling 57.94
    percutaneous (cystostomy) 57.17
    suprapubic NEC 57.18
  bronchus 96.05
    with lavage 96.56
  cardiac (right) 37.21
    combined left and right 37.23
    left 37.22
      combined with right heart 37.23
    right 37.21
      combined with left heart 37.23
  central venous NEC 38.93
    peripherally inserted central catheter (PICC) 38.93
  chest 34.04
    revision (with lysis of adhesions) 34.04
      thoracoscopic 34.06   ●
    thoracoscopic 34.06   ●
  Eustachian tube 20.8
  heart (right) 37.21
    combined left and right 37.23
    left 37.22
      combined with right heart 37.23
    right 37.21
      combined with left heart 37.23
  hepatic vein 38.93
  inferior vena cava 38.93
  intercostal space (with water seal), for drainage 34.04
    revision (with lysis of adhesions) 34.04
      thoracoscopic 34.06   ●
    thoracoscopic 34.06   ●
  lacrimonasal duct 09.44
  laryngeal 96.05
  nasolacrimal duct 09.44
  pancreatic cyst 52.01
  renal vein 38.93
  Swan-Ganz (pulmonary) 89.64
  transtracheal for oxygenation 31.99
  umbilical vein 38.92
  ureter (to kidney) 59.8
    for retrograde pyelogram 87.74
  urethra, indwelling 57.94
  vein NEC 38.93
    for renal dialysis 38.95
**Cattell operation** (herniorrhaphy) 53.51
**Cauterization** — *see also* Destruction, lesion, by site
  anus NEC 49.39
    endoscopic 49.31
  Bartholin's gland 71.24
  broad ligament 69.19
  bronchus 32.09
    endoscopic 32.01
  canaliculi 09.73
  cervix 67.32
  chalazion 08.25
  choroid plexus 02.14
  conjunctiva 10.33
    lesion 10.32
  cornea (fistula) (ulcer) 11.42
  ear, external 18.29
  endometrial implant — *see* Excision, lesion, by site
  entropion 08.41
  esophagus 42.39
    endoscopic 42.33

**Cauterization** — *see also* Destruction, lesion, by site — *continued*
  eyelid 08.25
    for entropion or ectropion 08.41
  fallopian tube 66.61
    by endoscopy (hysteroscopy) (laparoscopy) 66.29
  hemorrhoids 49.43
  iris 12.41
  lacrimal
    gland 09.21
    punctum 09.72
      for eversion 09.71
    sac 09.6
  larynx 30.09
  liver 50.29
  lung 32.29
    endoscopic 32.28
  meibomian gland 08.25
  nose, for epistaxis (with packing) 21.03
  ovary 65.29
    laparoscopic 65.25
  palate (bony) 27.31
  pannus (superficial) 11.42
  pharynx 29.39
  punctum, lacrimal 09.72
    for eversion 09.71
  rectum 48.32
    radical 48.31
  round ligament 69.19
  sclera 12.84
    with iridectomy 12.62
  skin 86.3
  subcutaneous tissue 86.3
  tonsillar fossa 28.7
  urethra 58.39
    endoscopic 58.31
  uterosacral ligament 69.19
  uterotubal ostia 66.61
  uterus 68.29
  vagina 70.33
  vocal cords 30.09
  vulva 71.3
**Cavernoscopy** 34.21
**Cavernostomy** 33.1
**Cavernotomy, kidney** 55.39
**Cavography** (inferior vena cava) 88.51
**Cecectomy** (with resection of terminal ileum) 45.72
**Cecil operation** (urethral reconstruction) 58.46
**Cecocoloplicopexy** 46.63
**Cecocolostomy** 45.94
**Cecofixation** 46.64
**Ceco-ileostomy** 45.93
**Cecopexy** 46.64
**Cecoplication** 46.62
**Cecorrhaphy** 46.75
**Cecosigmoidostomy** 45.94
**Cecostomy** (tube) — *see also* Colostomy 46.10
**Cecotomy** 45.03
**Celiocentesis** 54.91
**Celioscopy** 54.21
**Celiotomy, exploratory** 54.11
**Cell block and Papanicolaou smear** — *see* Examination, microscopic
**Cephalogram** 87.17
  dental 87.12
  orthodontic 87.12
**Cephalometry, cephalometrics** 87.17
  echo 88.78
  orthodontic 87.12
  ultrasound (sonar) 88.78
  x-ray 87.81
**Cephalotomy, fetus** 73.8
**Cerclage**
  anus 49.72
  cervix 67.59
    transabdominal 67.51
    transvaginal 67.59
  isthmus uteri (cervix) 67.59
  retinal reattachment (*see also* Buckling, scleral) 14.49

**Cerclage** — *continued*
  sclera (*see also* Buckling, scleral) 14.49
**Cervicectomy** (with synchronous colporrhaphy) 67.4
**Cervicoplasty** 67.69
**Cesarean section** 74.99
  classical 74.0
  corporeal 74.0
  extraperitoneal 74.2
  fundal 74.0
  laparotrachelotomy 74.1
  Latzko 74.2
  low cervical 74.1
  lower uterine segment 74.1
  peritoneal exclusion 74.4
  specified type NEC 74.4
  supravesical 74.2
  transperitoneal 74.4
    classical 74.0
    low cervical 74.1
  upper uterine segment 74.0
  vaginal 74.4
  Waters 74.2
**Chandler operation** (hip fusion) 81.21
**Change** — *see also* Replacement
  cast NEC 97.13
    lower limb 97.12
    upper limb 97.11
  cystostomy catheter or tube 59.94
  gastrostomy tube 97.02
  length
    bone — *see either* category 78.2 ☑ Shortening, bone *or* category 78.3 ☑ Lengthening, bone
    muscle 83.85
      hand 82.55
    tendon 83.85
      hand 82.55
  nephrostomy catheter or tube 55.93
  pyelostomy catheter or tube 55.94
  tracheostomy tube 97.23
  ureterostomy catheter or tube 59.93
  urethral catheter, indwelling 57.95
**Character analysis, psychologic** 94.03
**Charles operation** (correction of lymphedema) 40.9
**Charnley operation** (compression arthrodesis)
  ankle 81.11
  hip 81.21
  knee 81.22
**Cheatle-Henry operation** — *see* Repair, hernia, femoral
**Check**
  automatic implantable cardioverter/defibrillatory (AICD) (interrogation only) 89.49
  CRT-D (cardiac resynchronization defibrillator) (interrogation only) 89.49
  CRT-P (cardiac resynchronization pacemaker) (interrogation only) 89.45
  pacemaker, artificial (cardiac) (function) (interrogation only) (rate) 89.45
    amperage threshold 89.48
    artifact wave form 89.46
    electrode impedance 89.47
    voltage threshold 89.48
  vision NEC 95.09
**Cheiloplasty** 27.59
**Cheilorrhaphy** 27.51
**Cheilostomatoplasty** 27.59
**Cheilotomy** 27.0
**Chemical peel, skin** 86.24
**Chemocauterization** — *see also* Destruction, lesion, by site
  corneal epithelium 11.41
  palate 27.31
**Chemodectomy** 39.8
**Chemoembolization** 99.25
**Chemolysis**
  nerve (peripheral) 04.2
  spinal canal structure 03.8

☑ Additional Digit Required — Refer to the Tabular List for Digit Selection
**2007 Ingenix**
▶◀ Revised Text
● New Line
▲ Revised Code
⬟ Subterms under main terms may continue to next column or page
**Volume 3 — 9**

Chemoneurolysis — Closure

☑ Additional Digit Required — Refer to the Tabular List for Digit Selection

*2007 Ingenix*

▶◀ Revised Text

● New Line

▲ Revised Code

▽ Subterms under main terms may continue to next column or page

October 2007 · Volume 3 — 11

☑ Additional Digit Required — Refer to the Tabular List for Digit Selection

2007 Ingenix

►◄ Revised Text

● New Line    ▲ Revised Code

▽ Subterms under main terms may continue to next column or page

October 2007 · Volume 3 — 13

Decompression — Destruction

**Destruction** — continued
  lesion — continued
    spleen — continued
      by marsupialization 41.41
    stomach NEC 43.49
      by excision 43.42
        endoscopic 43.41
      endoscopic 43.41
    subcutaneous tissue NEC 86.3
    testis 62.2
    tongue 25.1
    urethra (excisional) 58.39
      endoscopic 58.31
    uterus 68.29
  nerve (cranial) (peripheral) (by cryoanalgesia) by radiofrequency) 04.2
  sympathetic, by injection of neurolytic agent 05.32
  neuroma
    acoustic 04.01
      by craniotomy 04.01
      by stereotactic radiosurgery 92.30
        cobalt 60 92.32
        linear accelerator (LINAC) 92.31
        multi-source 92.32
        particle beam 92.33
        particulate 92.33
        radiosurgery NEC 92.39
        single source photon 92.31
    cranial 04.07
    Morton's 04.07
    peripheral
      Morton's 04.07
  prostate (prostatic tissue)
    by
      cryotherapy 60.62
      microwave 60.96
      radiofrequency 60.97
      transurethral microwave thermotherapy (TUMT) 60.96
      transurethral needle ablation (TUNA) 60.97
      TULIP (transurethral (ultrasound) guided laser induced prostatectomy) 60.21
      TUMT (transurethral microwave thermotherapy) 60.96
      TUNA (transurethral needle ablation) 60.97
  semicircular canals, by injection 20.72
  vestibule, by injection 20.72
**Detachment, uterosacral ligaments** 69.3
**Determination**
  mental status (clinical) (medicolegal) (psychiatric) NEC 94.11
  psychologic NEC 94.09
  vital capacity (pulmonary) 89.37
**Detorsion**
  intestine (twisted) (volvulus) 46.80
    large 46.82
      endoscopic (balloon) 46.85
    small 46.81
  kidney 55.84
  ovary 65.95
  spermatic cord 63.52
    with orchiopexy 62.5
  testis 63.52
    with orchiopexy 62.5
  volvulus 46.80
    endoscopic (balloon) 46.85
**Detoxification therapy** 94.25
  alcohol 94.62
    with rehabilitation 94.63
    combined alcohol and drug 94.68
      with rehabilitation 94.69
  drug 94.65
    with rehabilitation 94.66
    combined alcohol and drug 94.68
      with rehabilitation 94.69
**Devascularization, stomach** 44.99
**Device**
  CorCap™ 37.41

**Device** — continued
  external fixator — see Fixator, external
**Dewebbing**
  esophagus 42.01
  syndactyly (fingers) (toes) 86.85
**Dextrorotation** — see Reduction, torsion
**Dialysis**
  hemodiafiltration, hemofiltration (extracorporeal) 39.95
  kidney (extracorporeal) 39.95
  liver 50.92
  peritoneal 54.98
  renal (extracorporeal) 39.95
**Diaphanoscopy**
  nasal sinuses 89.35
  skull (newborn) 89.16
**Diaphysectomy** — see category 77.8 ☑
**Diathermy** 93.34
  choroid — see Diathermy, retina
  nasal turbinates 21.61
  retina
    for
      destruction of lesion 14.21
      reattachment 14.51
      repair of tear 14.31
  surgical — see Destruction, lesion, by site
  turbinates (nasal) 21.61
**Dickson-Diveley operation** (tendon transfer and arthrodesis to correct claw toe) 77.57
**Dickson operation** (fascial transplant) 83.82
**Dieffenbach operation** (hip disarticulation) 84.18
**Dilation**
  achalasia 42.92
  ampulla of Vater 51.81
    endoscopic 51.84
  anus, anal (sphincter) 96.23
  biliary duct
    endoscopic 51.84
    pancreatic duct 52.99
      endoscopic 52.98
    percutaneous (endoscopy) 51.98
    sphincter
      of Oddi 51.81
        endoscopic 51.84
      pancreatic 51.82
        endoscopic 51.85
  bladder 96.25
    neck 57.92
  bronchus 33.91
  cervix (canal) 67.0
    obstetrical 73.1
    to assist delivery 73.1
  choanae (nasopharynx) 29.91
  colon (endoscopic) (balloon) 46.85
  colostomy stoma 96.24
  duodenum (endoscopic) (balloon) 46.85
  endoscopic — see Dilation, by site
  enterostomy stoma 96.24
  esophagus (by bougie) (by sound) 42.92
  fallopian tube 66.96
  foreskin (newborn) 99.95
  frontonasal duct 96.21
  gastrojejunostomy site, endoscopic 44.22
  heart valve — see Valvulotomy, heart
  ileostomy stoma 96.24
  ileum (endoscopic) (balloon) 46.85
  intestinal stoma (artificial) 96.24
  intestine (endoscopic) (balloon) 46.85
  jejunum (endoscopic) (balloon) 46.85
  lacrimal
    duct 09.42
    punctum 09.41
  larynx 31.98
  lymphatic structure(s) (peripheral) 40.9
  nares 21.99
  nasolacrimal duct (retrograde) 09.43

**Dilation** — continued
  nasolacrimal duct — continued
    with insertion of tube or stent 09.44
  nasopharynx 29.91
  pancreatic duct 52.99
    endoscopic 52.98
  pharynx 29.91
  prostatic urethra (transurethral) (balloon) 60.95
  punctum, lacrimal papilla 09.41
  pylorus
    by incision 44.21
    endoscopic 44.22
  rectum 96.22
  salivary duct 26.91
  sphenoid ostia 22.52
  sphincter
    anal 96.23
    cardiac 42.92
    of Oddi 51.81
      endoscopic 51.84
    pancreatic 51.82
      endoscopic 51.85
    pylorus, endoscopic 44.22
      by incision 44.21
  Stenson's duct 26.91
  trachea 31.99
  ureter 59.8
    meatus 56.91
  ureterovesical orifice 59.8
  urethra 58.6
    prostatic (transurethral) (balloon) 60.95
  urethrovesical junction 58.6
  vagina (instrumental) (manual) NEC 96.16
  vesical neck 57.92
  Wharton's duct 26.91
  Wirsung's duct 52.99
    endoscopic 52.98
**Dilation and curettage, uterus** (diagnostic) 69.09
  after
    abortion 69.02
    delivery 69.02
  to terminate pregnancy 69.01
**Diminution, ciliary body** 12.74
**Disarticulation** 84.91
  ankle 84.13
  elbow 84.06
  finger, except thumb 84.01
    thumb 84.02
  hip 84.18
  knee 84.16
  shoulder 84.08
  thumb 84.02
  toe 84.11
  wrist 84.04
**Discectomy** — see Diskectomy
**Discission**
  capsular membrane 13.64
  cataract (Wheeler knife) (Ziegler knife) 13.2
    congenital 13.69
    secondary membrane 13.64
  iris 12.12
  lens (capsule) (Wheeler knife) (Ziegler knife) (with capsulotomy) 13.2
  orbitomaxillary, radical 16.51
  pupillary 13.2
  secondary membrane (after cataract) 13.64
  vitreous strands (posterior approach) 14.74
    anterior approach 14.73
**Discogram, diskogram** 87.21
**Discolysis** (by injection) 80.52
**Diskectomy (discectomy), intervertebral** 80.51
  with corpectomy 80.99
  herniated (nucleus pulposus) 80.51
  percutaneous 80.59
**Dispensing** (with fitting)
  contact lens 95.32
  low vision aids NEC 95.33

**Dispensing** — continued
  spectacles 95.31
**Disruption**
  blood brain barrier via infusion [BBBD] 00.19
**Dissection** — see also Excision
  aneurysm 38.60
  artery-vein-nerve bundle 39.91
  branchial cleft fistula or sinus 29.52
  bronchus 32.1
  femoral hernia 53.29
  groin, radical 40.54
  larynx block (en bloc) 30.3
  mediastinum with pneumonectomy 32.59
    thoracoscopic 32.50
  neck, radical 40.40
    with laryngectomy 30.4
    bilateral 40.42
    unilateral 40.41
  orbital fibrous bands 16.92
  pterygium (with reposition) 11.31
  radical neck — see Dissection, neck, radical
  retroperitoneal NEC 59.00
  thoracic structures (block) (en bloc) (radical) (brachial plexus, bronchus, lobe of lung, ribs, and sympathetic nerves) 32.6
  vascular bundle 39.91
**Distention, bladder** (therapeutic) (intermittent) 96.25
**Diversion**
  biliopancreatic (BPD) 43.7 [45.51] [45.91]
    with duodenal switch 43.89 [45.51] [45.91]
  urinary
    cutaneous 56.61
    ileal conduit 56.51
    internal NEC 56.71
    uretero-ileostomy 56.51
    ureter to
      intestine 56.71
      skin 56.61
**Diversional therapy** 93.81
**Diverticulectomy**
  bladder (suprapubic) 57.59
    transurethral approach 57.49
  duodenum 45.31
    endoscopic 45.30
  esophagomyotomy 42.7
  esophagus 42.31
    endoscopic 42.33
  hypopharyngeal (by cricopharyngeal myotomy) 29.32
  intestine
    large 45.41
      endoscopic 45.43
    small 45.33
  kidney 55.39
  Meckel's 45.33
  pharyngeal (by cricopharyngeal myotomy) 29.32
  pharyngoesophageal (by cricopharyngeal myotomy) 29.32
  stomach 43.42
    endoscopic 43.41
  urethra 58.39
    endoscopic 58.31
**Division**
  Achilles tendon 83.11
  adductor tendon (hip) 83.12
  adhesions — see Lysis, adhesions
  angle of mandible (open) 76.62
    closed 76.61
  anterior synechiae 12.32
  aponeurosis 83.13
  arcuate ligament (spine) — omit code
  arteriovenous fistula (with ligation) 39.53
  artery (with ligation) 38.80
    abdominal 38.86
    aorta (arch) (ascending) (descending) 38.84
    head and neck NEC 38.82

☑ Additional Digit Required — Refer to the Tabular List for Digit Selection

*2007 Ingenix*

▶◀ Revised Text

● New Line

▲ Revised Code

⬛ Subterms under main terms may continue to next column or page

October 2007 · Volume 3 — 17

**Esophagoileostomy** (intrathoracic) NEC 42.54
  with interposition of small bowel 42.53
  antesternal or antethoracic NEC 42.64
    with interposition of small bowel 42.63
**Esophagojejunostomy** (intrathoracic) NEC 42.54
  with
    complete gastrectomy 43.99
    interposition of small bowel 42.53
  antesternal or antethoracic NEC 42.64
    with interposition of small bowel 42.63
**Esophagomyotomy** 42.7
**Esophagoplasty** NEC 42.89
**Esophagorrhaphy** 42.82
**Esophagoscopy** NEC 42.23
  by incision (operative) 42.21
  with closed biopsy 42.24
  through stoma (artificial) 42.22
  transabdominal (operative) 42.21
**Esophagostomy** 42.10
  cervical 42.11
  thoracic 42.19
**Esophagotomy** NEC 42.09
**Estes operation** (ovary) 65.72
  laparoscopic 65.75
**Estlander operation** (thoracoplasty) 33.34
**ESWL** (extracorporeal shockwave lithotripsy) NEC 98.59
  bile duct 98.52
  bladder 98.51
  gallbladder 98.52
  kidney 98.51
  Kock pouch (urinary diversion) 98.51
  renal pelvis 98.51
  specified site NEC 98.59
  ureter 98.51
**Ethmoidectomy** 22.63
**Ethmoidotomy** 22.51
**Evacuation**
  abscess — *see* Drainage, by site
  anterior chamber (eye) (aqueous) (hyphema) 12.91
  cyst (*see also* Excision, lesion, by site)
    breast 85.91
    kidney 55.01
    liver 50.29
  hematoma (*see also* Incision, hematoma)
    obstetrical 75.92
      incisional 75.91
  hemorrhoids (thrombosed) 49.47
  pelvic blood clot (by incision) 54.19
    by
      culdocentesis 70.0
      culdoscopy 70.22
  retained placenta
    with curettage 69.02
    manual 75.4
  streptothrix from lacrimal duct 09.42
**Evaluation** (of)
  audiological 95.43
  cardiac rhythm device (CRT-D) (CRT-P) (AICD) (pacemaker) — *see* Interrogation
  criminal responsibility, psychiatric 94.11
  functional (physical therapy) 93.01
  hearing NEC 95.49
  orthotic (for brace fitting) 93.02
  prosthetic (for artificial limb fitting) 93.03
  psychiatric NEC 94.19
    commitment 94.13
  psychologic NEC 94.08
  testimentary capacity, psychiatric 94.11
**Evans operation** (release of clubfoot) 83.84
**Evisceration**
  eyeball 16.39

**Evisceration** — *continued*
  eyeball — *continued*
    with implant (into scleral shell) 16.31
  ocular contents 16.39
    with implant (into scleral shell) 16.31
  orbit (*see also* Exenteration, orbit) 16.59
  pelvic (anterior) (posterior) (partial) (total) (female) 68.8
    male 57.71
**Evulsion**
  nail (bed) (fold) 86.23
  skin 86.3
  subcutaneous tissue 86.3
**Examination** (for)
  breast
    manual 89.36
    radiographic NEC 87.37
    thermographic 88.85
    ultrasonic 88.73
  cervical rib (by x-ray) 87.43
  colostomy stoma (digital) 89.33
  dental (oral mucosa) (peridontal) 89.31
    radiographic NEC 87.12
  enterostomy stoma (digital) 89.33
  eye 95.09
    color vision 95.06
    comprehensive 95.02
    dark adaptation 95.07
    limited (with prescription of spectacles) 95.01
    under anesthesia 95.04
  fetus, intrauterine 75.35
  general physical 89.7
  glaucoma 95.03
  gynecological 89.26
  hearing 95.47
  microscopic (specimen) (of) 91.9 ☑

*Note — Use the following fourth-digit subclassification with categories 90–91 to identify type of examination:*

| | |
|---|---|
| 1 | *bacterial smear* |
| 2 | *culture* |
| 3 | *culture and sensitivity* |
| 4 | *parasitology* |
| 5 | *toxicology* |
| 6 | *cell block and Papanicolaou smear* |
| 9 | *other microscopic examination* |

    adenoid 90.3 ☑
    adrenal gland 90.1 ☑
    amnion 91.4 ☑
    anus 90.9 ☑
    appendix 90.9 ☑
    bile ducts 91.0 ☑
    bladder 91.3 ☑
    blood 90.5 ☑
    bone 91.5 ☑
      marrow 90.6 ☑
    brain 90.0 ☑
    breast 91.6 ☑
    bronchus 90.4 ☑
    bursa 91.5 ☑
    cartilage 91.5 ☑
    cervix 91.4 ☑
    chest wall 90.4 ☑
    chorion 91.4 ☑
    colon 90.9 ☑
    cul-de-sac 91.1 ☑
    dental 90.8 ☑
    diaphragm 90.4 ☑
    duodenum 90.8 ☑
    ear 90.3 ☑
    endocrine gland NEC 90.1 ☑
    esophagus 90.8 ☑
    eye 90.2 ☑
    fallopian tube 91.4 ☑
    fascia 91.5 ☑
    female genital tract 91.4 ☑

**Examination** — *continued*
  microscopic — *continued*
    fetus 91.4 ☑
    gallbladder 91.0 ☑
    hair 91.6 ☑
    ileum 90.9 ☑
    jejunum 90.9 ☑
    joint fluid 91.5 ☑
    kidney 91.2 ☑
    large intestine 90.9 ☑
    larynx 90.3 ☑
    ligament 91.5 ☑
    liver 91.0 ☑
    lung 90.4 ☑
    lymph (node) 90.7 ☑
    meninges 90.0 ☑
    mesentery 91.1 ☑
    mouth 90.8 ☑
    muscle 91.5 ☑
    musculoskeletal system 91.5 ☑
    nails 91.6 ☑
    nerve 90.0 ☑
    nervous system 90.0 ☑
    nose 90.3 ☑
    omentum 91.1 ☑
    operative wound 91.7 ☑
    ovary 91.4 ☑
    pancreas 91.0 ☑
    parathyroid gland 90.1 ☑
    penis 91.3 ☑
    perirenal tissue 91.2 ☑
    peritoneum (fluid) 91.1 ☑
    periureteral tissue 91.2 ☑
    perivesical (tissue) 91.3 ☑
    pharynx 90.3 ☑
    pineal gland 90.1 ☑
    pituitary gland 90.1 ☑
    placenta 91.4 ☑
    pleura (fluid) 90.4 ☑
    prostate 91.3 ☑
    rectum 90.9 ☑
    retroperitoneum 91.1 ☑
    semen 91.3 ☑
    seminal vesicle 91.3 ☑
    sigmoid 90.9 ☑
    skin 91.6 ☑
    small intestine 90.9 ☑
    specified site NEC 91.8 ☑
    spinal fluid 90.0 ☑
    spleen 90.6 ☑
    sputum 90.4 ☑
    stomach 90.8 ☑
    stool 90.9 ☑
    synovial membrane 91.5 ☑
    tendon 91.5 ☑
    thorax NEC 90.4 ☑
    throat 90.3 ☑
    thymus 90.1 ☑
    thyroid gland 90.1 ☑
    tonsil 90.3 ☑
    trachea 90.4 ☑
    ureter 91.2 ☑
    urethra 91.3 ☑
    urine 91.3 ☑
    uterus 91.4 ☑
    vagina 91.4 ☑
    vas deferens 91.3 ☑
    vomitus 90.8 ☑
    vulva 91.4 ☑
  neurologic 89.13
  neuro-ophthalmology 95.03
  ophthalmoscopic 16.21
  panorex, mandible 87.12
  pelvic (manual) 89.26
    instrumental (by pelvimeter) 88.25
    pelvimetric 88.25
  physical, general 89.7
  postmortem 89.8
  rectum (digital) 89.34
    endoscopic 48.23
      through stoma (artificial) 48.22
      transabdominal 48.21
  retinal disease 95.03
  specified type (manual) NEC 89.39

**Examination** — *continued*
  thyroid field, postoperative 06.02
  uterus (digital) 68.11
    endoscopic 68.12
  vagina 89.26
    endoscopic 70.21
  visual field 95.05
**Exchange transfusion** 99.01
  intrauterine 75.2
**Excision**
  aberrant tissue — *see* Excision, lesion, by site of tissue origin
  abscess — *see* Excision, lesion, by site
  accessory tissue (*see also* Excision, lesion, by site of tissue origin)
    lung 32.29
      endoscopic 32.28
      thoracoscopic 32.20 ●
    spleen 41.93
  adenoids (tag) 28.6
    with tonsillectomy 28.3
  adenoma — *see* Excision, lesion, by site
  adrenal gland (*see also* Adrenalectomy) 07.22
  ampulla of Vater (with reimplantation of common duct) 51.62
  anal papilla 49.39
    endoscopic 49.31
  aneurysm (arteriovenous) (*see also* Aneurysmectomy) 38.60
    coronary artery 36.91
    heart 37.32
    myocardium 37.32
    sinus of Valsalva 35.39
    ventricle (heart) 37.32
  anus (complete) (partial) 49.6
  aortic subvalvular ring 35.35
  apocrine gland 86.3
  aponeurosis 83.42
    hand 82.33
  appendiceal stump 47.09
    laparoscopic 47.01
  appendices epiploicae 54.4
  appendix (*see also* Appendectomy) 47.01, 47.09
    epididymis 63.3
    testis 62.2
  arcuate ligament (spine) — omit code
  arteriovenous fistula (*see also* Aneurysmectomy) 38.60
  artery (*see also* Arteriectomy) 38.60
  Baker's cyst, knee 83.39
  Bartholin's gland 71.24
  basal ganglion 01.59
  bile duct 51.69
    endoscopic 51.64
  bladder (*see also* Cystectomy)
  bleb (emphysematous), lung 32.29
    endoscopic 32.28
    thoracoscopic 32.20 ●
  blood vessel (*see also* Angiectomy) 38.60
  bone (ends) (partial), except facial — *see* category 77.8 ☑
    for graft (autograft) (homograft) — *see* category 77.7 ☑
    facial NEC 76.39
      total 76.45
        with reconstruction 76.44
    fragments (chips) (*see also* Incision, bone) 77.10
    joint (*see also* Arthrotomy) 80.10
    necrotic (*see also* Sequestrectomy, bone) 77.00
    heterotopic, from
      muscle 83.32
        hand 82.22
      skin 86.3
      tendon 83.31
        hand 82.21
    mandible 76.31
      with arthrodesis — *see* Arthrodesis
      total 76.42

Excision — *continued*
  bone, except facial — *see* category —
    *continued*
    mandible — *continued*
      total — *continued*
        with reconstruction 76.41
    spur — *see* Excision, lesion, bone
    total, except facial — *see* category
      77.9 ☑
      facial NEC 76.45
        with reconstruction 76.44
      mandible 76.42
        with reconstruction 76.41
  brain 01.59
    hemisphere 01.52
    lobe 01.53
  branchial cleft cyst or vestige 29.2
  breast (*see also* Mastectomy) 85.41
    aberrant tissue 85.24
    accessory 85.24
    ectopic 85.24
    nipple 85.25
      accessory 85.24
    segmental 85.23
    supernumerary 85.24
    wedge 85.21
  broad ligament 69.19
  bronchogenic cyst 32.09
    endoscopic 32.01
  bronchus (wide sleeve) NEC 32.1
  buccal mucosa 27.49
  bulbourethral gland 58.92
  bulbous tuberosities (mandible)
    (maxilla) (fibrous) (osseous)
    24.31
  bunion (*see also* Bunionectomy) 77.59
  bunionette (with osteotomy) 77.54
  bursa 83.5
    hand 82.31
  canal of Nuck 69.19
  cardioma 37.33
  carotid body (lesion) (partial) (total)
    39.8
  cartilage (*see also* Chondrectomy)
    80.90
    intervertebral — *see* category
      80.5 ☑
    knee (semilunar) 80.6
    larynx 30.29
    nasal (submucous) 21.5
  caruncle, urethra 58.39
    endoscopic 58.31
  cataract (*see also* Extraction, cataract)
    13.19
    secondary membrane (after
      cataract) 13.65
  cervical
    rib 77.91
    stump 67.4
  cervix (stump) NEC 67.4
    cold (knife) 67.2
    conization 67.2
    cryoconization 67.33
    electroconizaton 67.32
  chalazion (multiple) (single) 08.21
  cholesteatoma — *see* Excision, lesion,
    by site
  choroid plexus 02.14
  cicatrix (skin) 86.3
  cilia base 08.20
  ciliary body, prolapsed 12.98
  clavicle (head) (partial) 77.81
    total (complete) 77.91
  clitoris 71.4
  coarctation of aorta (end-to-end
    anastomosis) 38.64
    with
      graft replacement (interposition)
        abdominal 38.44
        thoracic 38.45
        thoracoabdominal
          38.45 *[38.44]*
  common
    duct 51.63

Excision — *continued*
  common — *continued*
    wall between posterior and coro-
      nary sinus (with roofing of
      resultant defect with patch
      graft) 35.82
  condyle — *see* category 77.8 ☑
    mandible 76.5
  conjunctival ring 10.31
  cornea 11.49
    epithelium (with chemocauteriza-
      tion) 11.41
    for smear or culture 11.21
  costal cartilage 80.99
  cul-de-sac (Douglas') 70.92
    with graft or prosthesis 70.93 ●
  cusp, heart valve 35.10
    aortic 35.11
    mitral 35.12
    tricuspid 35.14
  cyst (*see also* Excision, lesion, by site)
    apical (tooth) 23.73
      with root canal therapy 23.72
    Baker's (popliteal) 83.39
    breast 85.21
    broad ligament 69.19
    bronchogenic 32.09
      endoscopic 32.01
    cervix 67.39
    dental 24.4
    dentigerous 24.4
    epididymis 63.2
    fallopian tube 66.61
    Gartner's duct 70.33
    hand 82.29
    labia 71.3
    lung 32.29
      endoscopic 32.28
      thoracoscopic 32.20 ●
    mesonephric duct 69.19
    Morgagni
      female 66.61
      male 62.2
    Müllerian duct 60.73
    nasolabial 27.49
    nasopalatine 27.31
      by wide excision 27.32
    ovary 65.29
      laparoscopic 65.25
    parovarian 69.19
    pericardium 37.31
    periodontal (apical) (lateral) 24.4
    popliteal (Baker's), knee 83.39
    radicular 24.4
    spleen 41.42
    synovial (membrane) 83.39
    thyroglossal (with resection of hy-
      oid bone) 06.7
    urachal (bladder) 57.51
      abdominal wall 54.3
    vagina (Gartner's duct) 70.33
  cystic
    duct remnant 51.61
    hygroma 40.29
  dentinoma 24.4
  diaphragm 34.81
  disc, intervertebral (NOS) 80.50
    herniated (nucleus pulposus) 80.51
    other specified (diskectomy) 80.51
  diverticulum
    ampulla of Vater 51.62
    anus 49.39
      endoscopic 49.31
    bladder 57.59
      transurethral 57.49
    duodenum 45.31
      endoscopic 45.30
    esophagus (local) 42.31
      endoscopic 42.33
    hypopharyngeal (by cricophary-
      geal myotomy) 29.32
    intestine
      large 45.41
        endoscopic 45.43
      small NEC 45.33
    Meckel's 45.33

Excision — *continued*
  diverticulum — *continued*
    pharyngeal (by cricopharyngeal
      myotomy) 29.32
    pharyngoesophageal (by cricopha-
      ryngeal myotomy) 29.32
    stomach 43.42
      endoscopic 43.41
    urethra 58.39
      endoscopic 58.31
    ventricle, heart 37.33
  duct
    Müllerian 69.19
    paramesonephric 69.19
    thyroglossal (with resection of hy-
      oid bone) 06.7
  ear, external (complete) NEC 18.39
    partial 18.29
    radical 18.31
  ectopic
    abdominal fetus 74.3
    tissue (*see also* Excision, lesion, by
      site of tissue origin)
      bone, from muscle 83.32
      breast 85.24
      lung 32.29
        endoscopic 32.28
        thoracoscopic 32.20 ●
      spleen 41.93
  empyema pocket, lung 34.09
  epididymis 63.4
  epiglottis 30.21
  epithelial downgrowth, anterior
    chamber (eye) 12.93
  epulis (gingiva) 24.31
  esophagus (*see also* Esophagectomy)
    42.40
  exostosis (*see also* Excision, lesion,
    bone) 77.60
    auditory canal, external 18.29
    facial bone 76.2
    first metatarsal (hallux valgus re-
      pair) — *see* Bunionectomy
  eye 16.49
    with implant (into Tenon's capsule)
      16.42
      with attachment of muscles
        16.41
  eyelid 08.20
    redundant skin 08.86
  falciform ligament 54.4
  fallopian tube — *see* Salpingectomy
  fascia 83.44
    for graft 83.43
    hand 82.34
    hand 82.35
      for graft 82.34
  fat pad NEC 86.3
    knee (infrapatellar) (prepatellar)
      86.3
    scalene 40.21
  fibroadenoma, breast 85.21
  fissure, anus 49.39
    endoscopic 49.31
  fistula (*see also* Fistulectomy)
    anal 49.12
    arteriovenous (*see also* Aneurys-
      mectomy) 38.60
    ileorectal 46.74
    lacrimal
      gland 09.21
      sac 09.6
    rectal 48.73
    vesicovaginal 57.84
  frenulum, frenum
    labial (lip) 27.41
    lingual (tongue) 25.92
  ganglion (hand) (tendon sheath) (wrist)
    82.21
    gasserian 04.05
    site other than hand or nerve 83.31
    sympathetic nerve 05.29
    trigeminal nerve 04.05
  gastrocolic ligament 54.4
  gingiva 24.31
  glomus jugulare tumor 20.51

Excision — *continued*
  goiter — *see* Thyroidectomy
  gum 24.31
  hallux valgus (*see also* Bunionectomy)
    with prosthetic implant 77.59
  hamartoma, mammary 85.21
  heart assist system — *see* Removal
  hematocele, tunica vaginalis 61.92
  hematoma — *see* Drainage, by site
  hemorrhoids (external) (internal) (tag)
    49.46
  heterotopic bone, from
    muscle 83.32
      hand 82.22
    skin 86.3
    tendon 83.31
      hand 82.21
  hydatid cyst, liver 50.29
  hydatid of Morgagni
    female 66.61
    male 62.2
  hydrocele
    canal of Nuck (female) 69.19
    male 63.1
    round ligament 69.19
    spermatic cord 63.1
    tunica vaginalis 61.2
  hygroma, cystic 40.29
  hymen (tag) 70.31
  hymeno-urethral fusion 70.31
  intervertebral disc — *see* Excision,
    disc, intervertebral (NOS) 80.50
  intestine (*see also* Resection, intestine)
    45.8
    for interposition 45.50
      large 45.52
      small 45.51
    large (total) 45.8
      for interposition 45.52
      local 45.41
        endoscopic 45.43
      segmental 45.79
        multiple 45.71
    small (total) 45.63
      for interposition 45.51
      local 45.33
      partial 45.62
      segmental 45.62
        multiple 45.61
  intraductal papilloma 85.21
  iris prolapse 12.13
  joint (*see also* Arthrectomy) 80.90
  keloid (scar), skin 86.3
  labia — *see* Vulvectomy
  lacrimal
    gland 09.20
      partial 09.22
      total 09.23
    passage 09.6
    sac 09.6
  lesion (local)
    abdominal wall 54.3
    accessory sinus — *see* Excision,
      lesion, nasal sinus
    adenoids 28.92
    adrenal gland(s) 07.21
    alveolus 24.4
    ampulla of Vater 51.62
    anterior chamber (eye) NEC 12.40
    anus 49.39
      endoscopic 49.31
    apocrine gland 86.3
    artery 38.60
      abdominal 38.66
      aorta (arch) (ascending) (de-
        scending thoracic) 38.64
        with end-to-end anastomosis
          38.45
          abdominal 38.44
          thoracic 38.45
          thoracoabdominal
            38.45 *[38.44]*
        with graft interposition graft
          replacement 38.45
          abdominal 38.44
          thoracic 38.45

☑ Additional Digit Required — Refer to the Tabular List for Digit Selection

▽ Subterms under main terms may continue to next column or page

**2007 Ingenix**

▶◀ Revised Text     ● New Line     ▲ Revised Code

**October 2007 · Volume 3 — 19**

Excision — Excision

**Excision** — *continued*
lesion — *continued*
artery — *continued*
aorta — *continued*
with graft interposition graft replacement — *continued*
thoracoabdominal 38.45 *[38.44]*
head and neck NEC 38.62
intracranial NEC 38.61
lower limb 38.68
thoracic NEC 38.65
upper limb 38.63
atrium 37.33
auditory canal or meatus, external 18.29
radical 18.31
auricle, ear 18.29
radical 18.31
biliary ducts 51.69
endoscopic 51.64
bladder (transurethral) 57.49
open 57.59
suprapubic 57.59
blood vessel 38.60
abdominal
artery 38.66
vein 38.67
aorta (arch) (ascending) (descending) 38.64
head and neck NEC 38.62
intracranial NEC 38.61
lower limb
artery 38.68
vein 38.69
thoracic NEC 38.65
upper limb (artery) (vein) 38.63
bone 77.60
carpal, metacarpal 77.64
clavicle 77.61
facial 76.2
femur 77.65
fibula 77.67
humerus 77.62
jaw 76.2
dental 24.4
patella 77.66
pelvic 77.69
phalanges (foot) (hand) 77.69
radius 77.63
scapula 77.61
skull 01.6
specified site NEC 77.69
tarsal, metatarsal 77.68
thorax (ribs) (sternum) 77.61
tibia 77.67
ulna 77.63
vertebrae 77.69
brain (transtemporal approach) NEC 01.59
by stereotactic radiosurgery 92.30
cobalt 60 92.32
linear accelerator (LINAC) 92.31
multi-source 92.32
particle beam 92.33
particulate 92.33
radiosurgery NEC 92.39
single source photon 92.31
breast (segmental) (wedge) 85.21
broad ligament 69.19
bronchus NEC 32.09
endoscopic 32.01
cerebral (cortex) NEC 01.59
meninges 01.51
cervix (myoma) 67.39
chest wall 34.4
choroid plexus 02.14
ciliary body 12.44
colon 45.41
endoscopic NEC 45.43
polypectomy 45.42
conjunctiva 10.31
cornea 11.49

**Excision** — *continued*
lesion — *continued*
cranium 01.6
cul-de-sac (Douglas') 70.32
dental (jaw) 24.4
diaphragm 34.81
duodenum (local) 45.31
endoscopic 45.30
ear, external 18.29
radical 18.31
endometrium 68.29
epicardium 37.31
epididymis 63.3
epiglottis 30.09
esophagus NEC 42.32
endoscopic 42.33
eyebrow (skin) 08.20
eye, eyeball 16.93
anterior segment NEC 12.40
eyelid 08.20
by
halving procedure 08.24
wedge resection 08.24
major
full-thickness 08.24
partial-thickness 08.23
minor 08.22
fallopian tube 66.61
fascia 83.39
hand 82.29
groin region (abdominal wall) (inguinal) 54.3
skin 86.3
subcutaneous tissue 86.3
gum 24.31
heart 37.33
hepatic duct 51.69
inguinal canal 54.3
intestine
large 45.41
endoscopic NEC 45.43
polypectomy 45.42
small NEC 45.33
intracranial NEC 01.59
intranasal 21.31
intraspinal 03.4
iris 12.42
jaw 76.2
dental 24.4
joint 80.80
ankle 80.87
elbow 80.82
foot and toe 80.88
hand and finger 80.84
hip 80.85
knee 80.86
shoulder 80.81
specified site NEC 80.89
spine 80.89
wrist 80.83
kidney 55.39
with partial nephrectomy 55.4
labia 71.3
lacrimal
gland (frontal approach) 09.21
passage 09.6
sac 09.6
larynx 30.09
ligament (joint) (*see also* Excision, lesion, joint) 80.80
broad 69.19
round 69.19
uterosacral 69.19
lip 27.43
by wide excision 27.42
liver 50.29
lung NEC 32.29
by lung volume reduction surgery 32.22
by wide excision 32.39 ▲
thoracoscopic 32.30 ●
endoscopic 32.28
thoracoscopic 32.20 ●
lymph structure(s) (channel) (vessel) NEC 40.29

**Excision** — *continued*
lesion — *continued*
lymph structure(s) — *continued*
node — *see* Excision, lymph, node
mammary duct 85.21
mastoid (bone) 20.49
mediastinum 34.3
meninges (cerebral) 01.51
spinal 03.4
mesentery 54.4
middle ear 20.51
mouth NEC 27.49
muscle 83.32
hand 82.22
ocular 15.13
myocardium 37.33
nail 86.23
nasal sinus 22.60
antrum 22.62
with Caldwell-Luc approach 22.61
specified approach NEC 22.62
ethmoid 22.63
frontal 22.42
maxillary 22.62
with Caldwell-Luc approach 22.61
specified approach NEC 22.62
sphenoid 22.64
nasopharynx 29.3 ☑
nerve (cranial) (peripheral) 04.07
sympathetic 05.29
nonodontogenic 24.31
nose 21.30
intranasal 21.31
polyp 21.31
skin 21.32
specified site NEC 21.32
odontogenic 24.4
omentum 54.4
orbit 16.92
ovary 65.29
by wedge resection 65.22
laparoscopic 65.24
that by laparoscope 65.25
palate (bony) 27.31
by wide excision 27.32
soft 27.49
pancreas (local) 52.22
endoscopic 52.21
parathyroid 06.89
parotid gland or duct NEC 26.29
pelvic wall 54.3
pelvirectal tissue 48.82
penis 64.2
pericardium 37.31
perineum (female) 71.3
male 86.3
periprostatic tissue 60.82
perirectal tissue 48.82
perirenal tissue 59.91
peritoneum 54.4
perivesical tissue 59.91
pharynx 29.39
diverticulum 29.32
pineal gland 07.53
pinna 18.29
radical 18.31
pituitary (gland) (*see also* Hypophysectomy, partial) 07.63
by stereotactic radiosurgery 92.30
cobalt 60 92.32
linear accelerator (LINAC) 92.31
multi-source 92.32
particle beam 92.33
particulate 92.33
radiosurgery NEC 92.39
single source photon 92.31
pleura 34.59
pouch of Douglas 70.32
preauricular (ear) 18.21

**Excision** — *continued*
lesion — *continued*
presacral 54.4
prostate (transurethral) 60.61
pulmonary (fibrosis) 32.29
endoscopic 32.28
thoracoscopic 32.20 ●
rectovaginal septum 48.82
rectum 48.35
polyp (endoscopic) 48.36
retroperitoneum 54.4
salivary gland or duct NEC 26.29
en bloc 26.32
sclera 12.84
scrotum 61.3
sinus (nasal) — *see* Excision, lesion, nasal sinus
Skene's gland 71.3
skin 86.3
breast 85.21
nose 21.32
radical (wide) (involving underlying or adjacent structure) (with flap closure) 86.4
scrotum 61.3
skull 01.6
soft tissue NEC 83.39
hand 82.29
spermatic cord 63.3
sphincter of Oddi 51.62
endoscopic 51.64
spinal cord (meninges) 03.4
spleen (cyst) 41.42
stomach NEC 43.42
endoscopic 43.41
polyp 43.41
polyp (endoscopic) 43.41
subcutaneous tissue 86.3
breast 85.21
subgingival 24.31
sweat gland 86.3
tendon 83.39
hand 82.29
ocular 15.13
sheath 83.31
hand 82.21
testis 62.2
thorax 34.4
thymus
partial (open) (other) 07.81 ●
thoracoscopic 07.83 ●
total (open) (other) 07.82 ●
thoracoscopic 07.84 ●
thyroid 06.31
substernal or transsternal route 06.51
tongue 25.1
tonsil 28.92
trachea 31.5
tunica vaginalis 61.92
ureter 56.41
urethra 58.39
endoscopic 58.31
uterine ligament 69.19
uterosacral ligament 69.19
uterus 68.29
vagina 70.33
vein 38.60
abdominal 38.67
head and neck NEC 38.62
intracranial NEC 38.61
lower limb 38.69
thoracic NEC 38.65
upper limb 38.63
ventricle (heart) 37.33
vocal cords 30.09
vulva 71.3
ligament (*see also* Arthrectomy) 80.90
broad 69.19
round 69.19
uterine 69.19
uterosacral 69.19
ligamentum flavum (spine) — omit code
lingual tonsil 28.5
lip 27.43

---

☑ Additional Digit Required — Refer to the Tabular List for Digit Selection

▽ Subterms under main terms may continue to next column or page

☑ Additional Digit Required — Refer to the Tabular List for Digit Selection

📖 Subterms under main terms may continue to next column or page

☑ Additional Digit Required — Refer to the Tabular List for Digit Selection
Subterms under main terms may continue to next column or page

*2007 Ingenix*
▶◀ Revised Text     ● New Line     ▲ Revised Code
**Volume 3 — 23**

**Fitting** — continued
  prosthesis, prosthetic device
    above knee 84.45
    arm 84.43
      lower (and hand) 84.42
      upper (and shoulder) 84.41
    below knee 84.46
    hand (and lower arm) 84.42
    leg 84.47
      above knee 84.45
      below knee 84.46
    limb NEC 84.40
    ocular 95.34
    penis (external) 64.94
    shoulder (and upper arm) 84.41
  spectacles 95.31
**Five-in-one repair, knee** 81.42
**Fixation**
  bone
    external, without reduction 93.59
      with fracture reduction — see
        Reduction, fracture
      cast immobilization NEC 93.53
      external fixator — see Fixator,
        external
      splint 93.54
      traction (skeletal) NEC 93.44
        intermittent 93.43
    internal (without fracture reduc-
      tion) 78.50
      with fracture reduction — see
        Reduction, fracture
      carpal, metacarpal 78.54
      clavicle 78.51
      femur 78.55
      fibula 78.57
      humerus 78.52
      patella 78.56
      pelvic 78.59
      phalanges (foot) (hand) 78.59
      radius 78.53
      scapula 78.51
      specified site NEC 78.59
      tarsal, metatarsal 78.58
      thorax (ribs) (sternum) 78.51
      tibia 78.57
      ulna 78.53
      vertebrae 78.59
  breast (pendulous) 85.6
  cardinal ligaments 69.22
  cervical collar 93.52
  duodenum 46.62
    to abdominal wall 46.61
  external (without manipulation for re-
    duction) 93.59
      with fracture reduction — see Re-
        duction, fracture
      cast immobilization NEC 93.53
      pressure dressing 93.56
      splint 93.54
      strapping (non-traction) 93.59
      traction (skeletal) NEC 93.44
        intermittent 93.43
  hip 81.40
  ileum 46.62
    to abdominal wall 46.61
  internal
    with fracture reduction — see Re-
      duction, fracture
    without fracture reduction — see
      Fixation, bone, internal
  intestine 46.60
    large 46.64
      to abdominal wall 46.63
    small 46.62
      to abdominal wall 46.61
    to abdominal wall 46.60
  iris (bombé) 12.11
  jejunum 46.62
    to abdominal wall 46.61
  joint — see Arthroplasty
  kidney 55.7
  ligament
    cardinal 69.22
    palpebrae 08.36
  omentum 54.74

**Fixation** — continued
  parametrial 69.22
  plaster jacket 93.51
    other cast 93.53
  rectum (sling) 48.76
  spine, with fusion (see also Fusion,
    spinal) 81.00
  spleen 41.95
  splint 93.54
  tendon 83.88
    hand 82.85
  testis in scrotum 62.5
  tongue 25.59
  urethrovaginal (to Cooper's ligament)
    70.77
    with graft or prosthesis 70.78  ●
  uterus (abdominal) (vaginal) (ventrofix-
    ation) 69.22
  vagina 70.77
    with graft or prosthesis 70.78  ●
**Fixator, external**
  computer assisted (dependent) 84.73
  hybrid device or system 84.73
  Ilizarov type 84.72
  monoplanar system 84.71
  ring device or system 84.72
  Sheffield type 84.72
**Flooding** (psychologic desensitization)
  94.33
**Flowmetry, Doppler** (ultrasonic) — see
  also Ultrasonography
  aortic arch 88.73
  head and neck 88.71
  heart 88.72
  thorax NEC 88.73
**Fluoroscopy** — see Radiography
**Fog therapy** (respiratory) 93.94
**Folding, eye muscle** 15.22
  multiple (two or more muscles) 15.4
**Foley operation** (pyeloplasty) 55.87
**Fontan operation** (creation of conduit
  between right atrium and pulmonary artery) 35.94
**Foraminotomy** 03.09
**Forced extension, limb** 93.25
**Forceps delivery** — see Delivery, forceps
**Formation**
  adhesions
    pericardium 36.39
    pleura 34.6
  anus, artificial (see also Colostomy)
    46.13
    duodenostomy 46.39
    ileostomy (see also Ileostomy)
      46.23
    jejunostomy 46.39
      percutaneous (endoscopic) (PEJ)
        46.32
  arteriovenous fistula (for kidney dialy-
    sis) (peripheral) (shunt) 39.27
    external cannula 39.93
  bone flap, cranial 02.03
  cardiac device (defibrillator) (pacemak-
    er) pocket
    with initial insertion of cardiac de-
      vice — omit code
    new site (skin) (subcutaneous)
      37.79
  colostomy (see also Colostomy) 46.13
  conduit
    ileal (urinary) 56.51
    left ventricle and aorta 35.93
    right atrium and pulmonary artery
      35.94
    right ventricle and pulmonary (dis-
      tal) artery 35.92
    in repair of
      pulmonary artery atresia
        35.92
      transposition of great vessels
        35.92
      truncus arteriosus 35.83
  endorectal ileal pouch (J-pouch) (H-
    pouch) (S-pouch) (with anasto-
    mosis to anus) 45.95

**Formation** — continued
  fistula
    arteriovenous (for kidney dialysis)
      (peripheral shunt) 39.27
      external cannula 39.93
    bladder to skin NEC 57.18
      with bladder flap 57.21
      percutaneous 57.17
    cutaneoperitoneal 54.93
    gastric 43.19
      percutaneous (endoscopic)
        (transabdominal) 43.11
    mucous (see also Colostomy) 46.13
    rectovaginal 48.99
    tracheoesophageal 31.95
    tubulovalvular (Beck-Jianu)
      (Frank's) (Janeway) (Spi-
      vack's) (Ssabanejew-Frank)
      43.19
    urethrovaginal 58.0
  ileal
    bladder
      closed 57.87 [45.51]
      open 56.51
    conduit 56.51
  interatrial fistula 35.42
  mucous fistula (see also Colostomy)
    46.13
  pericardial
    baffle, interatrial 35.91
    window 37.12
  pleural window (for drainage) 34.09
  pocket
    cardiac device (defibrillator) (pace-
      maker)
      with initial insertion of cardiac
        device — omit code
      new site (skin) (subcutaneous)
        37.79
    loop recorder 37.79
    thalamic stimulator pulse genera-
      tor
      with initial insertion of battery
        package — omit code
      new site (skin) (subcutaneous)
        86.09
  pupil 12.39
    by iridectomy 12.14
  rectovaginal fistula 48.99
  reversed gastric tube (intrathoracic)
    (retrosternal) 42.58
    antesternal or antethoracic 42.68
  septal defect, interatrial 35.42
  shunt
    abdominovenous 54.94
    arteriovenous 39.93
    peritoneojugular 54.94
    peritoneo-vascular 54.94
    pleuroperitoneal 34.05
    transjugular intrahepatic portosys-
      temic [TIPS] 39.1
  subcutaneous tunnel
    esophageal 42.86
      with anastomosis — see Anasto-
        mosis, esophagus, an-
        testernal
    pulse generator lead wire 86.99
      with initial procedure — omit
        code
    thalamic stimulator pulse genera-
      tor pocket
      with initial insertion of battery
        package — omit code
      new site (skin) (subcutaneous)
        86.09
  syndactyly (finger) (toe) 86.89
  tracheoesophageal 31.95
  tubulovalvular fistula (Beck-Jianu)
    (Frank's) (Janeway) (Spivack's)
    (Ssabanejew-Frank) 43.19
  uretero-ileostomy, cutaneous 56.51
  ureterostomy, cutaneous 56.61
    ileal 56.51
  urethrovaginal fistula 58.0
  window
    pericardial 37.12

**Formation** — continued
  window — continued
    pleural (for drainage) 34.09
      thoracoscopic 34.06  ●
**Fothergill (-Donald) operation** (uterine
  suspension) 69.22
**Fowler operation**
  arthroplasty of metacarpophalangeal
    joint 81.72
  release (mallet finger repair) 82.84
  tenodesis (hand) 82.85
  thoracoplasty 33.34
**Fox operation** (entropion repair with
  wedge resection) 08.43
**Fracture, surgical** — see also Osteoclasis 78.70
  turbinates (nasal) 21.62
**Fragmentation**
  lithotriptor — see Lithotripsy
  mechanical
    cataract (with aspiration) 13.43
      posterior route 13.42
      secondary membrane 13.66
    secondary membrane (after
      cataract) 13.66
  ultrasonic
    cataract (with aspiration) 13.41
    stones, urinary (Kock pouch) 59.95
    urinary stones 59.95
      percutaneous nephrostomy
        55.04
**Franco operation** (suprapubic cystotomy) 57.18
**Frank operation** 43.19
**Frazier (-Spiller) operation** (subtemporal
  trigeminal rhizotomy) 04.02
**Fredet-Ramstedt operation** (pyloromyotomy) (with wedge resection) 43.3
**Freeing**
  adhesions — see Lysis, adhesions
  anterior synechiae (with injection of
    air or liquid) 12.32
  artery-vein-nerve bundle 39.91
  extraocular muscle, entrapped 15.7
  goniosynechiae (with injection of air
    or liquid) 12.31
  intestinal segment for interposition
    45.50
    large 45.52
    small 45.51
  posterior synechiae 12.33
  synechiae (posterior) 12.33
    anterior (with injection of air or
      liquid) 12.32
  vascular bundle 39.91
  vessel 39.91
**Freezing**
  gastric 96.32
  prostate 60.62
**Frenckner operation** (intrapetrosal
  drainage) 20.22
**Frenectomy**
  labial 27.41
  lingual 25.92
  lip 27.41
  maxillary 27.41
  tongue 25.92
**Frenotomy**
  labial 27.91
  lingual 25.91
**Frenulumectomy** — see Frenectomy
**Frickman operation** (abdominal proctopexy) 48.75
**Frommel operation** (shortening of
  uterosacral ligaments) 69.22
**Fulguration** — see also Electrocoagulation and Destruction, lesion, by site
  adenoid fossa 28.7
  anus 49.39
    endoscopic 49.31
  bladder (transurethral) 57.49
    suprapubic 57.59
  choroid 14.21
  duodenum 45.32
    endoscopic 45.30
  esophagus 42.39

---

☑ Additional Digit Required — Refer to the Tabular List for Digit Selection

▶◀ Revised Text     ● New Line     ▲ Revised Code

▽ Subterms under main terms may continue to next column or page

☑ Additional Digit Required — Refer to the Tabular List for Digit Selection　　　　　　　　　　Subterms under main terms may continue to next column or page

26 — Volume 3 · October 2007　　　▶◀ Revised Text　　　● New Line　　　▲ Revised Code　　　*2007 Ingenix*

**Hemodilution** 99.03
**Hemofiltration** (extracorporeal) 39.95
**Hemorrhage control** — see Control, hemorrhage
**Hemorrhoidectomy** 49.46
  by
    cautery, cauterization 49.43
    crushing 49.45
    cryotherapy, cryosurgery 49.44
    excision 49.46
    injection 49.42
    ligation 49.45
**Hemostasis** — see Control, hemorrhage
**Henley operation** (jejunal transposition) 43.81
**Hepatectomy** (complete) (total) 50.4
  partial or subtotal 50.22
**Hepatic assistance, extracorporeal** 50.92
**Hepaticocholangiojejunostomy** 51.37
**Hepaticocystoduodenostomy** 51.37
**Hepaticodochotomy** 51.59
**Hepaticoduodenostomy** 51.37
**Hepaticojejunostomy** 51.37
**Hepaticolithectomy** 51.49
  endoscopic 51.88
**Hepaticolithotomy** 51.49
  endoscopic 51.88
**Hepaticostomy** 51.59
**Hepaticotomy** 51.59
**Hepatocholangiocystoduodenostomy** 51.37
**Hepatocholedochostomy** 51.43
  endoscopic 51.87
**Hepatoduodenostomy** 50.69
**Hepatogastrostomy** 50.69
**Hepatojejunostomy** 50.69
**Hepatolithotomy**
  hepatic duct 51.49
  liver 50.0
**Hepatopexy** 50.69
**Hepatorrhaphy** 50.61
**Hepatostomy** (external) (internal) 50.69
**Hepatotomy** (with packing) 50.0
**Hernioplasty** — see Repair, hernia
**Herniorrhaphy** — see Repair, hernia
**Herniotomy** — see Repair, hernia
**Heterograft** — see Graft
**Heterotransplant, heterotransplantation** — see Transplant
**Hey-Groves operation** (reconstruction of anterior cruciate ligament) 81.45
**Heyman-Herndon** (-Strong) **operation** (correction of metatarsus varus) 80.48
**Heymen operation** (soft tissue release for clubfoot) 83.84
**Hey operation** (amputation of foot) 84.12
**Hibbs operation** (lumbar spinal fusion) — see Fusion, lumbar
**Higgins operation** — see Repair, hernia, femoral
**High forceps delivery** 72.39
  with episiotomy 72.31
**Hill-Allison operation** (hiatal hernia repair, transpleural approach) 53.80
**Hinging, mitral valve** 35.12
**His bundle recording** 37.29
**Hitchcock operation** (anchoring tendon of biceps) 83.88
**Hofmeister operation** (gastrectomy) 43.7
**Hoke operation**
  midtarsal fusion 81.14
  triple arthrodesis 81.12
**Holth operation**
  iridencleisis 12.63
  sclerectomy 12.65
**Homan operation** (correction of lymphedema) 40.9
**Homograft** — see Graft
**Homotransplant, homotransplantation** — see Transplant
**Hosiery, elastic** 93.59
**Hutch operation** (ureteroneocystostomy) 56.74

**Hybinette-Eden operation** (glenoid bone block) 78.01
**Hydrocelectomy**
  canal of Nuck (female) 69.19
    male 63.1
  round ligament 69.19
  spermatic cord 63.1
  tunica vaginalis 61.2
**Hydrotherapy** 93.33
  assisted exercise in pool 93.31
  whirlpool 93.32
**Hymenectomy** 70.31
**Hymenoplasty** 70.76
**Hymenorrhaphy** 70.76
**Hymenotomy** 70.11
**Hyperalimentation** (parenteral) 99.15
**Hyperbaric oxygenation** 93.95
  wound 93.59
**Hyperextension, joint** 93.25
**Hyperthermia** NEC 93.35
  for cancer treatment (interstitial) (local) (radiofrequency) (regional) (ultrasound) (whole-body) 99.85
**Hypnodrama, psychiatric** 94.32
**Hypnosis** (psychotherapeutic) 94.32
  for anesthesia — omit code
**Hypnotherapy** 94.32
**Hypophysectomy** (complete) (total) 07.69
  partial or subtotal 07.63
    transfrontal approach 07.61
    transsphenoidal approach 07.62
  specified approach NEC 07.68
  transfrontal approach (complete) (total) 07.64
    partial 07.61
  transsphenoidal approach (complete) (total) 07.65
    partial 07.62
**Hypothermia** (central) (local) 99.81
  gastric (cooling) 96.31
    freezing 96.32
  systemic (in open heart surgery) 39.62
**Hypotympanotomy** 20.23
**Hysterectomy** 68.9
  abdominal 68.49
    laparoscopic (total) [TLH] 68.41
    partial or subtotal (supracervical) (supravaginal) 68.39
    radical (modified) (Wertheim's) 68.69
      laparoscopic (total) [TLRH] 68.61
    supracervical 68.39
      classic infrafascial SEMM hysterectomy (CISH) 68.31
      laparoscopically assisted (LASH) 68.31
  vaginal (complete) (partial) (subtotal) (total) 68.59
    laparoscopically assisted (LAVH) 68.51
    radical (Schauta) 68.79
      laparoscopic [LRVH] 68.71
**Hysterocolpectomy** (radical) (vaginal) 68.79
  abdominal 68.69
    laparoscopic 68.61
  laparoscopic 68.71
**Hysterogram** NEC 87.85
  percutaneous 87.84
**Hysterolysis** 54.59
  laparoscopic 54.51
**Hysteromyomectomy** 68.29
**Hysteropexy** 69.22
**Hysteroplasty** 69.49
**Hysterorrhaphy** 69.41
**Hysterosalpingography gas** (contrast) 87.82
  opaque dye (contrast) 87.83
**Hysterosalpingostomy** 66.74
**Hysteroscopy** 68.12
  with
    ablation
      endometrial 68.23
    biopsy 68.16

**Hysterotomy** (with removal of foreign body) (with removal of hydatidiform mole) 68.0
  for intrauterine transfusion 75.2
  obstetrical 74.99
    for termination of pregnancy 74.91
**Hysterotrachelectomy** 67.4
**Hysterotracheloplasty** 69.49
**Hysterotrachelorrhaphy** 69.41
**Hysterotrachelotomy** 69.95

## I

**ICCE** (intracapsular cataract extraction) 13.19
**Ileal**
  bladder
    closed 57.87 *[45.51]*
      open (ileoureterostomy) 56.51
    conduit (ileoureterostomy) 56.51
**Ileocecostomy** 45.93
**Ileocolectomy** 45.73
**Ileocolostomy** 45.93
**Ileocolotomy** 45.00
**Ileocystoplasty** (isolated segment anastomosis) (open loop) 57.87 *[45.51]*
**Ileoduodenotomy** 45.01
**Ileoectomy** (partial) 45.62
  with cecectomy 45.72
**Ileoentectropy** 46.99
**Ileoesophagostomy** 42.54
**Ileoileostomy** 45.91
  proximal to distal segment 45.62
**Ileoloopogram** 87.78
**Ileopancreatostomy** 52.96
**Ileopexy** 46.61
**Ileoproctostomy** 45.93
**Ileorectostomy** 45.93
**Ileorrhaphy** 46.73
**Ileoscopy** 45.13
  through stoma (artificial) 45.12
  transabdominal (operative) 45.11
**Ileosigmoidostomy** 45.93
**Ileostomy** 46.20
  continent (permanent) 46.22
    for urinary diversion 56.51
  delayed opening 46.24
  Hendon (temporary) 46.21
  loop 46.01
  Paul (temporary) 46.21
  permanent 46.23
    continent 46.22
  repair 46.41
  revision 46.41
  tangential (temporary) 46.21
  temporary 46.21
  transplantation to new site 46.23
  tube (temporary) 46.21
  ureteral
    external 56.51
    internal 56.71
**Ileotomy** 45.02
**Ileotransversostomy** 45.93
**Ileoureterostomy** (Bricker's) (ileal bladder) 56.51
**Imaging** (diagnostic)
  diagnostic, not elsewhere classified 88.90
  endovascular ultrasound — see Imaging, intravascular ultrasound
  intraoperative
    iMRI — see Imaging, magnetic resonance
    intravascular — see Imaging, intravascular ultrasound
  intravascular ultrasound (IVUS) 00.29
    aorta 00.22
    aortic arch 00.22
    carotid vessel 00.21
    cerebral vessel, extracranial 00.21
    coronary vessel 00.24
    intrathoracic vessel 00.22
    other specified vessel 00.28
    peripheral vessel 00.23
    renal vessel 00.25
    vena cava (inferior) (superior) 00.22

**Imaging** — continued
  magnetic resonance (nuclear) (proton) NEC 88.97
    abdomen 88.97
    bladder (urinary) 88.95
    bone marrow blood supply 88.94
    brain (brain stem) 88.91
      intraoperative (iMRI) 88.96
      real-time 88.96
    chest (hilar) (mediastinal) 88.92
    computer assisted surgery (CAS) with MR/MRA 00.32
    extremity (upper) (lower) 88.94
    eye orbit 88.97
    face 88.97
    head NEC 88.97
    musculoskeletal 88.94
    myocardium 88.92
    neck 88.97
    orbit of eye 88.97
    prostate 88.95
    specified site NEC 88.97
    spinal canal (cord) (spine) 88.93
**Immobilization** (by)
  with fracture-reduction — see Reduction, fracture
  bandage 93.59
  bone 93.53
  cast NEC 93.53
    with reduction of fracture or dislocation — see Reduction, fracture, and Reduction, dislocation
  device NEC 93.59
  pressure dressing 93.56
  splint (plaster) (tray) 93.54
    with reduction of fracture or dislocation — see Reduction, fracture, and Reduction, dislocation
  stereotactic head frame 93.59
  strapping (non-traction) 93.59
**Immunization** — see also Vaccination
  allergy 99.12
  autoimmune disease 99.13
  BCG 99.33
  brucellosis 99.55
  cholera 99.31
  diphtheria 99.36
  DPT 99.39
  epidemic parotitis 99.46
  German measles 99.47
  Hemophilus influenzae 99.52
  influenza 99.52
  measles 99.45
  meningococcus 99.55
  mumps 99.46
  pertussis 99.37
  plague 99.34
  poliomyelitis 99.41
  rabies 99.44
  rubella 99.47
  salmonella 99.55
  smallpox 99.55
  staphylococcus 99.55
  TAB 99.32
  tetanus 99.38
  triple vaccine 99.48
  tuberculosis 99.33
  tularemia 99.35
  typhoid-paratyphoid 99.32
  typhus 99.55
  viral NEC 99.55
  whooping cough 99.37
  yellow fever 99.43
**Immunoadsorption**
  extracorporeal (ECI) 99.76
**Immunotherapy, antineoplastic** 99.28
  C-Parvum 99.28
  Interferon 99.28
  interleukin-2 (low-dose) 99.28
    high-dose 00.15
  Levamisole 99.28
  Proleukin (low-dose) 99.28
    high-dose 00.15
  Thymosin 99.28

**Implant, implantation**
abdominal artery to coronary artery 36.17
artery
aortic branches to heart muscle 36.2
mammary to ventricular wall (Vineberg) 36.2
baffle, atrial or interatrial 35.91
biliary fistulous tract into stomach or intestine 51.39
bipolar endoprosthesis (femoral head) 81.52
bladder sphincter, artificial (inflatable) 58.93
blood vessels to myocardium 36.2
bone growth stimulator (invasive) (percutaneous) (semi-invasive) — see category 78.9 ☑
bone morphogenetic protein (Infuse™) (OP-1™) (recombinant) (rhBMP) 84.52
bone void filler 84.55
that with kyphoplasty 81.66
that with vertebroplasty 81.65
breast (for augmentation) (bilateral) 85.54
unilateral 85.53
cardiac resynchronization device
defibrillator (biventricular) (BiV ICD) (BiV pacemaker with defibrillator) (BiV pacing with defibrillator) (CRT-D) (device and one or more leads) (total system) 00.51
left ventricular coronary venous lead only 00.52
pulse generator only 00.54
pacemaker (BiV) (biventricular) (CRT-P) (device and one or more leads) (total system) 00.50
left ventricular coronary venous lead only 00.52
pulse generator only 00.53
cardiac support device (CSD) 37.41
cardiomyostimulation system 37.67
cardioverter/defibrillator (automatic) 37.94
leads only (patch electrodes) (sensing) (pacing) 37.95
pulse generator only 37.96
total system 37.94
chest wall (mesh) (silastic) 34.79
chin (polyethylene) (silastic) 76.68
cochlear (electrode) 20.96
prosthetic device (electrode and receiver) 20.96
channel (single) 20.97
multiple 20.98
electrode only 20.99
internal coil only 20.99
CorCap™ 37.41
cornea 11.73
CRT-D (biventricular defibrillator) (BiV ICD) (BiV pacepaker with defibrillator) (BiV pacing with defibrillator) (cardiac resynchronization defibrillator) (device and one or more leads) 00.51
left ventricular coronary venous lead only 00.52
pulse generator only 00.54
CRT-P (biventricular pacemaker) (BiV pacemaker) (cardiac resynchronization pacemaker) (device and one or more leads) 00.50
left ventricular coronary venous lead only 00.52
pulse generator only 00.53
custodis eye 14.41
dental (endosseous) (prosthetic) 23.6
device
adjustable gastric band and port 44.95
bronchial device NOS 33.79

**Implant, implantation** — *continued*
device — *continued*
bronchial substance NOS 33.79
bronchial valve 33.71
cardiac support device (CSD) 37.41
CorCap™ 37.41
epicardial support device 37.41
Lap-Band™ 44.95
left atrial appendage 37.90
left atrial filter 37.90
left atrial occluder 37.90
prosthetic cardiac support device 37.41
subcutaneous for intracardiac hemodynamic monitoring 00.57
vascular access 86.07
ventricular support device 37.41
diaphragmatic pacemaker 34.85
Dynesys® 84.82 ▲
electrode(s)
brain 02.93
depth 02.93
foramen ovale 02.93
sphenoidal 02.96
cardiac (initial) (transvenous) 37.70
atrium (initial) 37.73
replacement 37.76
atrium and ventricle (initial) 37.72
replacement 37.76
epicardium (sternotomy or thoracotomy approach) 37.74
left ventricular coronary venous system 00.52
temporary transvenous pacemaker system 37.78
during and immediately following cardiac surgery 39.64
ventricle (initial) 37.71
replacement 37.76
carotid sinus 39.8 ●
depth 02.93
foramen ovale 02.96
gastric 04.92
heart (see also Implant, electrode(s), cardiac) 37.70
intracranial 02.93
osteogenic (invasive) for bone growth stimulation — see category 78.9 ☑
peripheral nerve 04.92
sacral nerve 04.92
sphenoidal 02.96
spine 03.93
electroencephalographic receiver
brain 02.93
intracranial 02.93
electronic stimulator
anus (subcutaneous) 49.92
bladder 57.96
bone growth (invasive) (percutaneous) (semi-invasive) 78.9 ☑
brain — see Implant, neurostimulator, brain
carotid sinus 39.8
cochlear 20.96
channel (single) 20.97
multiple 20.98
gastric 04.92
intracranial — see Implant, neurostimulator, intracranial
peripheral nerve — see Implant, neurostimulator, peripheral nerve
phrenic nerve 34.85
skeletal muscle 83.92
spine — see Implant, neurostimulator, spine
ureter 56.92
electrostimulator — see Implant, electronic stimulator, by site
endoprosthesis
bile duct 51.87

**Implant, implantation** — *continued*
endoprosthesis — *continued*
femoral head (bipolar) 81.52
pancreatic duct 52.93
endosseous (dental) 23.6
epidural pegs 02.93
epikeratoprosthesis 11.73
estradiol (pellet) 99.23
eye (Iowa type) 16.61
integrated 16.41
facial bone, synthetic (alloplastic) 76.92
fallopian tube (Mulligan hood) (silastic tube) (stent) 66.93
into uterus 66.74
gastroepiploic artery to coronary artery 36.17
half-heart 37.62
hearing device, electromagnetic 20.95
heart
artificial 37.52
total replacement system 37.52
assist system NEC 37.62
external 37.65
extrinsic 37.68
implantable 37.66
non-implantable 37.62
percutaneous external 37.68
pVAD 37.68
auxiliary ventricle 37.62
cardiac support device (CSD) 37.41
circulatory assist system — see Implant, heart, assist system
CorCap™ 37.41
epicardial support device 37.41
pacemaker (see also Implant, pacemaker, cardiac) 37.80
prosthetic cardiac support device 37.41
total replacement system 37.52
valve(s)
prosthesis or synthetic device (partial) (synthetic) (total) 35.20
aortic 35.22
mitral 35.24
pulmonary 35.26
tricuspid 35.28
tissue graft 35.20
aortic 35.21
mitral 35.23
pulmonary 35.25
tricuspid 35.27
ventricular support device 37.41
inert material
breast (for augmentation) (bilateral) 85.54
unilateral 85.53
larynx 31.0
nose 21.85
orbit (eye socket) 16.69
reinsertion 16.62
scleral shell (cup) (with evisceration of eyeball) 16.31
reinsertion 16.62
Tenon's capsule (with enucleation of eyeball) 16.42
with attachment of muscles 16.41
reinsertion 16.62
urethra 59.79
vocal cord(s) 31.0
infusion pump 86.06
interbody spinal fusion device 84.51
intracardiac hemodynamic monitor, subcutaneous 00.57
joint (prosthesis) (silastic) (Swanson type) NEC 81.96
ankle (total) 81.56
revision 81.59
carpocarpal, carpometacarpal 81.74
elbow (total) 81.84
revision 81.97
extremity (bioelectric) (cineplastic) (kineplastic) 84.40

**Implant, implantation** — *continued*
joint — *continued*
extremity — *continued*
lower 84.48
revision 81.59
upper 84.44
revision 81.97
femoral (bipolar endoprosthesis) 81.52
revision NOS 81.53
acetabular and femoral components (total) 00.70
acetabular component only 00.71
acetabular liner and/or femoral head only 00.73
femoral component only 00.72
femoral head only and/or acetabular liner 00.73
total (acetabular and femoral components) 00.70
finger 81.71
hand (metacarpophalangeal) (interphalangeal) 81.71
revision 81.97
hip (partial) 81.52
revision NOS 81.53
acetabular and femoral components (total) 00.70
acetabular component only 00.71
acetabular liner and/or femoral head only 00.73
femoral component only 00.72
femoral head only and/or acetabular liner 00.73
partial
acetabular component only 00.71
acetabular liner and/or femoral head only 00.73
femoral component only 00.72
femoral head only and/or acetabular liner 00.73
total (acetabular and femoral components) 00.70
total 81.51
revision (acetabular and femoral components) 00.70
interphalangeal 81.71
revision 81.97
knee (partial) (total) 81.54
revision NOS 81.55
femoral component 00.82
partial
femoral component 00.82
patellar component 00.83
tibial component 00.81
tibial insert 00.84
patellar component 00.83
tibial component 00.81
tibial insert 00.84
total (all components) 00.80
metacarpophalangeal 81.71
revision 81.97
shoulder (partial) 81.81
revision 81.97
total replacement 81.80
toe 81.57
for hallux valgus repair 77.59
revision 81.59
wrist (partial) 81.74
revision 81.97
total replacement 81.73
kidney, mechanical 55.97
Lap-Band™ 44.95
larynx 31.0

☑ Additional Digit Required — Refer to the Tabular List for Digit Selection                   ᵀᴸ Subterms under main terms may continue to next column or page

28 — Volume 3 · October 2007              ▶◀ Revised Text      ● New Line      ▲ Revised Code          *2007 Ingenix*

**Incision** — *continued*
  abscess (*see also* Incision, by site) —
      *continued*
    subcutaneous tissue 86.04
    subdiaphragmatic 54.19
    subhepatic 54.19
    subphrenic 54.19
    vas deferens 63.6
  adrenal gland 07.41
  alveolus, alveolar bone 24.0
  antecubital fossa 86.09
  anus NEC 49.93
    fistula 49.11
    septum 49.91
  appendix 47.2
  artery 38.00
    abdominal 38.06
      aorta (arch) (ascending) (de-
        scending) 38.04
    head and neck NEC 38.02
    intracranial NEC 38.01
    lower limb 38.08
    thoracic NEC 38.05
    upper limb 38.03
  atrium (heart) 37.11
  auditory canal or meatus, external
      18.02
  auricle 18.09
  axilla 86.09
  Bartholin's gland or cyst 71.22
  bile duct (with T or Y tube insertion)
      NEC 51.59
    for
      exploration 51.59
      relief of obstruction 51.49
    common (exploratory) 51.51
      for
        relief of obstruction NEC
          51.42
        removal of calculus 51.41
  bladder 57.19
    neck (transurethral) 57.91
    percutaneous suprapubic (closed)
      57.17
    suprapubic NEC 57.18
  blood vessel (*see also* Angiotomy)
      38.00
  bone 77.10
    alveolus, alveolar 24.0
    carpals, metacarpals 77.14
    clavicle 77.11
    facial 76.09
    femur 77.15
    fibula 77.17
    humerus 77.12
    patella 77.16
    pelvic 77.19
    phalanges (foot) (hand) 77.19
    radius 77.13
    scapula 77.11
    skull 01.24
    specified site NEC 77.19
    tarsals, metatarsals 77.18
    thorax (ribs) (sternum) 77.11
    tibia 77.17
    ulna 77.13
    vertebrae 77.19
  brain 01.39
    cortical adhesions 02.91
  breast (skin) 85.0
    with removal of tissue expander
      85.96
  bronchus 33.0
  buccal space 27.0
  bulbourethral gland 58.91
  bursa 83.03
    hand 82.03
    pharynx 29.0
  carotid body 39.8
  cerebral (meninges) 01.39
    epidural or extradural space 01.24
    subarachnoid or subdural space
      01.31
  cerebrum 01.39
  cervix 69.95

**Incision** — *continued*
  cervix — *continued*
    to
      assist delivery 73.93
      replace inverted uterus 75.93
  chalazion 08.09
    with removal of capsule 08.21
  cheek 86.09
  chest wall (for extrapleural drainage)
      (for removal of foreign body)
      34.01
    as operative approach — *omit code*
  common bile duct (for exploration)
      51.51
    for
      relief of obstruction 51.42
      removal of calculus 51.41
  common wall between posterior left
      atrium and coronary sinus (with
      roofing of resultant defect with
      patch graft) 35.82
  conjunctiva 10.1
  cornea 11.1
    radial (refractive) 11.75
  cranial sinus 01.21
  craniobuccal pouch 07.72
  cul-de-sac 70.12
  cyst
    dentigerous 24.0
    radicular (apical) (periapical) 24.0
  Dührssen's (cervix, to assist delivery)
      73.93
  duodenum 45.01
  ear
    external 18.09
    inner 20.79
    middle 20.23
  endocardium 37.11
  endolymphatic sac 20.79
  epididymis 63.92
  epidural space, cerebral 01.24
  epigastric region 54.0
    intra-abdominal 54.19
  esophagus, esophageal NEC 42.09
    web 42.01
  exploratory — *see* Exploration
  extradural space (cerebral) 01.24
  extrapleural 34.01
  eyebrow 08.09
  eyelid 08.09
    margin (trichiasis) 08.01
  face 86.09
  fallopian tube 66.01
  fascia 83.09
    with division 83.14
      hand 82.12
    hand 82.09
      with division 82.12
  fascial compartments, head and neck
      27.0
  fistula, anal 49.11
  flank 54.0
  furuncle — *see* Incision, by site
  gallbladder 51.04
  gingiva 24.0
  gluteal 86.09
  groin region (abdominal wall) (in-
      guinal) 54.0
    skin 86.09
    subcutaneous tissue 86.09
  gum 24.0
  hair follicles 86.09
  heart 37.10
    valve — *see* Valvulotomy
  hematoma (*see also* Incision, by site)
    axilla 86.04
    broad ligament 69.98
    ear 18.09
    episiotomy site 75.91
    fossa (superficial) NEC 86.04
    groin region (abdominal wall) (in-
      guinal) 54.0
      skin 86.04
      subcutaneous tissue 86.04
    laparotomy site 54.12
    mediastinum 34.1

**Incision** — *continued*
  hematoma (*see also* Incision, by site)
      — *continued*
    perineum (female) 71.09
      male 86.04
    popliteal space 86.04
    scrotum 61.0
    skin 86.04
    space of Retzius 59.19
    subcutaneous tissue 86.04
    vagina (cuff) 70.14
      episiotomy site 75.91
      obstetrical NEC 75.92
  hepatic ducts 51.59
  hordeolum 08.09
  hygroma (*see also* Incision, by site)
    cystic 40.0
  hymen 70.11
  hypochondrium 54.0
    intra-abdominal 54.19
  hypophysis 07.72
  iliac fossa 54.0
  infratemporal fossa 27.0
  ingrown nail 86.09
  intestine 45.00
    large 45.03
    small 45.02
  intracerebral 01.39
  intracranial (epidural space) (extradu-
      ral space) 01.24
    subarachnoid or subdural space
      01.31
  intraperitoneal 54.19
  ischiorectal tissue 49.02
    abscess 49.01
  joint structures (*see also* Arthrotomy)
      80.10
  kidney 55.01
    pelvis 55.11
  labia 71.09
  lacrimal
    canaliculus 09.52
    gland 09.0
    passage NEC 09.59
    punctum 09.51
    sac 09.53
  larynx NEC 31.3
  ligamentum flavum (spine) — *omit
      code*
  liver 50.0
  lung 33.1
  lymphangioma 40.0
  lymphatic structure (channel) (node)
      (vessel) 40.0
  mastoid 20.21
  mediastinum 34.1
  meibomian gland 08.09
  meninges (cerebral) 01.31
    spinal 03.09
  midpalmar space 82.04
  mouth NEC 27.92
    floor 27.0
  muscle 83.02
    with division 83.19
      hand 82.19
    hand 82.02
      with division 82.19
  myocardium 37.11
  nailbed or nailfold 86.09
  nasolacrimal duct (stricture) 09.59
  neck 86.09
  nerve (cranial) (peripheral) NEC 04.04
    root (spinal) 03.1
  nose 21.1
  omentum 54.19
  orbit (*see also* Orbitotomy) 16.09
  ovary 65.09
    laparoscopic 65.01
  palate 27.1
  palmar space (middle) 82.04
  pancreas 52.09
  pancreatic sphincter 51.82
    endoscopic 51.85
  parapharyngeal (oral) (transcervical)
      28.0
  paronychia 86.09

**Incision** — *continued*
  parotid
    gland or duct 26.0
    space 27.0
  pelvirectal tissue 48.81
  penis 64.92
  perianal (skin) (tissue) 49.02
    abscess 49.01
  perigastric 54.19
  perineum (female) 71.09
    male 86.09
  peripheral vessels
    lower limb
      artery 38.08
      vein 38.09
    upper limb (artery) (vein) 38.03
  periprostatic tissue 60.81
  perirectal tissue 48.81
  perirenal tissue 59.09
  perisplenic 54.19
  peritoneum 54.95
    by laparotomy 54.19
    pelvic (female) 70.12
      male 54.19
  periureteral tissue 59.09
  periurethral tissue 58.91
  perivesical tissue 59.19
  petrous pyramid (air cells) (apex)
      (mastoid) 20.22
  pharynx, pharyngeal (bursa) 29.0
    space, lateral 27.0
  pilonidal sinus (cyst) 86.03
  pineal gland 07.52
  pituitary (gland) 07.72
  pleura NEC 34.09
  popliteal space 86.09
  postzygomatic space 27.0
  pouch of Douglas 70.12
  prostate (perineal approach)
      (transurethral approach) 60.0
  pterygopalatine fossa 27.0
  pulp canal (tooth) 24.0
  Rathke's pouch 07.72
  rectovaginal septum 48.81
  rectum 48.0
    stricture 48.91
  renal pelvis 55.11
  retroperitoneum 54.0
  retropharyngeal (oral) (transcervical)
      28.0
  salivary gland or duct 26.0
  sclera 12.89
  scrotum 61.0
  sebaceous cyst 86.04
  seminal vesicle 60.72
  sinus — *see* Sinusotomy
  Skene's duct or gland 71.09
  skin 86.09
    with drainage 86.04
    breast 85.0
    cardiac pacemaker pocket, new site
      37.79
    ear 18.09
    nose 21.1
    subcutaneous tunnel for pulse
      generator lead wire 86.99
      with initial procedure — *omit
        code*
    thalamic stimulator pulse genera-
      tor pocket, new site 86.09
      with initial insertion of battery
        package — *omit code*
    tunnel, subcutaneous for pulse
      generator lead wire 86.99
      with initial procedure — *omit
        code*
  skull (bone) 01.24
  soft tissue NEC 83.09
    with division 83.19
      hand 82.19
    hand 82.09
      with division 82.19
  space of Retzius 59.19
  spermatic cord 63.93
  sphincter of Oddi 51.82
    endoscopic 51.85

☑ Additional Digit Required — Refer to the Tabular List for Digit Selection                    ▽ Subterms under main terms may continue to next column or page

30 — Volume 3                    ▶◀ Revised Text              ● New Line          ▲ Revised Code                              *2007 Ingenix*

Incision — Injection

☑ Additional Digit Required — Refer to the Tabular List for Digit Selection           ▽ Subterms under main terms may continue to next column or page

*2007 Ingenix*          ▶◀ Revised Text        ● New Line      ▲ Revised Code          **October 2007 · Volume 3 — 31**

**Index**

**Injection — Insertion**

**Injection** — *continued*
  sclerosing agent — *continued*
    pleura — *continued*
      treatment of malignancy — *continued*
        with tetracycline 34.92 [99.21]
    varicose vein 39.92
    vein NEC 39.92
  semicircular canals, for destruction 20.72
  silicone — *see* Implant, inert material
  skin (sclerosing agent) (filling material) 86.02
  soft tissue 83.98
    hand 82.96
  spinal (canal) NEC 03.92
    alcohol 03.8
    anesthetic agent for analgesia 03.91
      for operative anesthesia — *omit code*
    contrast material (for myelogram) 87.21
    destructive agent NEC 03.8
    neurolytic agent NEC 03.8
    phenol 03.8
    proteolytic enzyme (chymopapain) (chymodiactin) 80.52
    saline (hypothermic) 03.92
    steroid 03.92
  spinal nerve root (intrathecal) — *see* Injection, spinal
  steroid NEC 99.23
  subarachnoid, spinal — *see* Injection, spinal
  subconjunctival 10.91
  tendon 83.97
    hand 82.95
  testis 62.92
  therapeutic agent NEC 99.29
  thoracic cavity 34.92
  thrombolytic agent (enzyme) (streptokinase) 99.10
    with percutaneous transluminal angioplasty

*Note: Also use 00.40, 00.41, 00.42, or 00.43 to show the total number of vessels treated.*

      coronary 00.66
      non-coronary vessel(s) 39.50
        specified site NEC 39.50
      direct intracoronary artery 36.04
  trachea 31.94
  tranquilizer 99.26
  tunica vaginalis (with aspiration) 61.91
  tympanum 20.94
  urethra (inert material)
    for repair of urinary stress incontinence
      collagen implant 59.72
      endoscopic injection of implant 59.72
      fat implant 59.72
      polytef implant 59.72
  vaccine
    tumor 99.28
  varices, esophagus (endoscopic) (sclerosing agent) 42.33
  varicose vein (sclerosing agent) 39.92
    esophagus (endoscopic) 42.33
  vestibule, for destruction 20.72
  vitreous substitute (silicone) 14.75
    for reattachment of retina 14.59
  vocal cords 31.0
**Inlay, tooth** 23.3
**Inoculation**
  antitoxins — *see* Administration, antitoxins
  toxoids — *see* Administration, toxoids
  vaccine — *see* Administration, vaccine
**Insemination, artificial** 69.92
**Insertion**
  airway
    esophageal obturator 96.03

**Insertion** — *continued*
  airway — *continued*
    nasopharynx 96.01
    oropharynx 96.02
  Allen-Brown cannula 39.93
  arch bars (orthodontic) 24.7
    for immobilization (fracture) 93.55
  atrial septal umbrella 35.52
  Austin-Moore prosthesis 81.52
  baffle, heart (atrial) (interatrial) (intraatrial) 35.91
  bag, cervix (nonobstetrical) 67.0
    after delivery or abortion 75.8
    to assist delivery or induce labor 73.1
  Baker's (tube) (for stenting) 46.85
  balloon
    gastric 44.93
    heart (pulsation-type) (Kantrowitz) 37.61
    intestine (for decompression) (for dilation) 46.85
  band (adjustable)
    gastric, laparoscopic 44.95
    Lap-Band™ 44.95
  Barton's tongs (skull) (with synchronous skeletal traction) 02.94
  bipolar endoprosthesis (femoral head) 81.52
  Blakemore-Sengstaken tube 96.06
  bone growth stimulator (invasive) (percutaneous) (semi-invasive) — *see* category 78.9 ☑
  bone morphogenetic protein (Infuse™) (OP-1™) (recombinant) (rhBMP) 84.52
  bone void filler 84.55
    that with kyphoplasty 81.66
    that with vertebroplasty 81.65
  bougie, cervix, nonobstetrical 67.0
    to assist delivery or induce labor 73.1
  breast implant (for augmentation) (bilateral) 85.54
    unilateral 85.53
  bridge (dental) (fixed) 23.42
    removable 23.43
  bubble (balloon), stomach 44.93
  caliper tongs (skull) (with synchronous skeletal traction) 02.94
  cannula
    for extracorporeal membrane oxygenation (ECMO) — *omit code*
    Allen-Brown 39.93
    nasal sinus (by puncture) 22.01
      through natural ostium 22.02
    pancreatic duct 52.92
      endoscopic 52.93
    vessel to vessel 39.93
  cardiac resynchronization device
    defibrillator (biventricular defibrillator) (BiV ICD) (BiV pacemaker with defibrillator) (BiV pacing with defibrillator) (CRT-D) (total system) (device and one or more leads) 00.51
      left ventricular coronary venous lead only 00.52
      pulse generator only 00.54
    pacemaker (biventricular pacemaker) (BiV pacemaker) (CRT-P) (total system) (device and one or more leads) 00.50
      left ventricular coronary venous lead only 00.52
      pulse generator only 00.53
  cardiac support device (CSD) (CorCap™) 37.41

**Insertion** — *continued*
  carotid artery stent(s) (stemt graft) 00.63

*Note: Also use 00.40, 00.41, 00.42, or 00.43 to show the total number of vessels treated. Use code 00.44 once to show procedure on a bifurcated vessel. In addition, use 00.45, 00.46, 00.47, or 00.48 to show the number of vascular stents inserted.*

  catheter
    abdomen of fetus, for intrauterine transfusion 75.2
    anterior chamber (eye), for permanent drainage (glaucoma) 12.79
    artery 38.91
    bile duct(s) 51.59
      common 51.51
        endoscopic 51.87
      endoscopic 51.87
    bladder, indwelling 57.94
      suprapubic 57.18
        percutaneous (closed) 57.17
    bronchus 96.05
      with lavage 96.56
    central venous NEC 38.93
      for
        hemodialysis 38.95
        pressure monitoring 89.62
      peripherally inserted central catheter (PICC) 38.93
    chest 34.04
      revision (with lysis of adhesions) 34.04
        thoracoscopic 34.06 ●
      thoracoscopic 34.06 ●
    cranial cavity 01.26
      placement via burr hole(s) 01.28
    esophagus (nonoperative) 96.06
      permanent tube 42.81
    intercostal (with water seal), for drainage 34.04
      revision (with lysis of adhesions) 34.04
        thoracoscopic 34.06 ●
      thoracoscopic 34.06 ●
    intracerebral 01.26
      placement via burr hole(s) 01.28
    spinal canal space (epidural) (subarachnoid) (subdural) for infusion of therapeutic or palliative substances 03.90
    Swan-Ganz (pulmonary) 89.64
    transtracheal for oxygenation 31.99
    vein NEC 38.93
      for renal dialysis 38.95
  chest tube 34.04
    thoracoscopic 34.06 ●
  choledochohepatic tube (for decompression) 51.43
    endoscopic 51.87
  cochlear prosthetic device — *see* Implant, cochlear prosthetic device
  contraceptive device (intrauterine) 69.7
  CorCap™ 37.41
  cordis cannula 54.98
  coronary (artery)

*Note: Also use 00.40, 00.41, 00.42, or 00.43 to show the total number of vessels treated. Use code 00.44 once to show procedure on a bifurcated vessel. In addition, use 00.45, 00.46, 00.47, or 00.48 to show the number of vascular stents inserted.*

    stent, drug-eluting 36.07
    stent, non-drug-eluting 36.06
  Crosby-Cooney button 54.98
  CRT-D (biventricular defibrillator) (BiV ICD) (BiV pacemaker with defibrillator) (BiV pacing with defibrillator) (cardiac resynchronization defibrillator) (device and one or more leads) 00.51

**Insertion** — *continued*
  CRT-D — *continued*
    left ventricular coronary venous lead only 00.52
    pulse generator only 00.54
  CRT-P (biventricular pacemaker) (BiV pacemaker) (cardiac resynchronization pacemaker) (device and one or more leads) 00.50
    left ventricular coronary venous lead only 00.52
    pulse generator only 00.53
  Crutchfield tongs (skull) (with synchronous skeletal traction) 02.94
  Davidson button 54.98
  denture (total) 99.97
  device
    adjustable gastric band and port 44.95
    bronchial device NOS 33.79
    bronchial substance NOS 33.79
    bronchial valve 33.71
    cardiac resynchronization — *see* Insertion, cardiac resynchronization device
    cardiac support device (CSD) 37.41
    CorCap™ 37.41
    epicardial support device 37.41
    Lap-Band™ 44.95
    left atrial appendage 37.90
    left atrial filter 37.90
    left atrial occluder 37.90
    prosthetic cardiac support device 37.41
    vascular access 86.07
    ventricular support device 37.41
  diaphragm, vagina 96.17
  drainage tube
    kidney 55.02
      pelvis 55.12
    renal pelvis 55.12
  Dynesys® 84.82 ▲
  elbow prosthesis (total) 81.84
    revision 81.97
  electrode(s)
    bone growth stimulator (invasive) (percutaneous) (semi-invasive) — *see* category 78.9 ☑
    brain 02.93
      depth 02.93
      foramen ovale 02.93
      sphenoidal 02.96
    depth 02.93
    foramen ovale 02.93
    gastric 04.92
    heart (initial) (transvenous) 37.70
      atrium (initial) 37.73
        replacement 37.76
      atrium and ventricle (initial) 37.72
        replacement 37.76
      epicardium (sternotomy or thoracotomy approach) 37.74
      left ventricular coronary venous system 00.52
      temporary transvenous pacemaker system 37.78
        during and immediately following cardiac surgery 39.64
      ventricle (initial) 37.71
        replacement 37.76
    intracranial 02.93
    osteogenic (for bone growth stimulation) — *see* category 78.9 ☑
    peripheral nerve 04.92
    sacral nerve 04.92
    sphenoidal 02.96
    spine 03.93
  electroencephalographic receiver — *see* Implant, electroencephalographic receiver, by site
  electronic stimulator — *see* Implant, electronic stimulator, by site

☑ Additional Digit Required — Refer to the Tabular List for Digit Selection

ᵂ Subterms under main terms may continue to next column or page

**2007 Ingenix**

▶◀ Revised Text

● New Line

▲ Revised Code

**October 2007 · Volume 3 — 33**

**Insertion** — continued
 prosthesis, prosthetic device — continued
  hip (partial) 81.52
   revision NOS 81.53
    acetabular and femoral com-
     ponents (total) 00.70
    acetabular component only
     00.71
    acetabular liner and/or
     femoral head only
     00.73
    femoral component only
     00.72
    femoral head only and/or
     acetabular liner 00.73
    partial
     acetabular component
      only 00.71
     acetabular liner and/or
      femoral head only
      00.73
     femoral component only
      00.72
     femoral head only and/or
      acetabular liner
      00.73
    total (acetabular and femoral
     components) 00.70
   total 81.51
    revision
     acetabular and femoral
      components (total)
      00.70
     total (acetabular and
      femoral compo-
      nents) 00.70
  joint — see Arthroplasty
  knee (partial) (total) 81.54
   revision NOS 81.55
    femoral component 00.82
    partial
     femoral component 00.82
     patellar component 00.83
     tibial component 00.81
     tibial insert 00.84
    patellar component 00.83
    tibial component 00.81
    tibial insert 00.84
    total (all components) 00.80
  leg (bioelectric) (cineplastic) (kineplastic) 84.48
  lens 13.91
  ocular (secondary) 16.61
   with orbital exenteration 16.42
  outflow tract (gusset type) (heart)
   in
     pulmonary valvuloplasty
      35.26
     total repair of tetralogy of
      Fallot 35.81
  penis (internal) (noninflatable)
   64.95
   with
    construction 64.43
    reconstruction 64.44
   inflatable (internal) 64.97
   Rosen (for urinary incontinence)
    59.79
  shoulder
   partial 81.81
   revision 81.97
   total 81.80
  spine
   artificial disc, NOS 84.60
    cervical 84.62
     nucleus 84.61
     partial 84.61
     total 84.62
    lumbar, lumbosacral 84.65
     nucleus 84.64
     partial 84.64
     total 84.65
    thoracic (partial) (total) 84.63
   other device 84.59

**Insertion** — continued
 prosthesis, prosthetic device — continued
  testicular (bilateral) (unilateral)
   62.7
  toe 81.57
   hallux valgus repair 77.59
  vagina                                    ●
   synthetic 70.95
  pseudophakos (see also Insertion,
   lens) 13.70
  pump, infusion 86.06
  radioactive isotope 92.27
  radium 92.27
  radon seeds 92.27
  Reuter bobbin (with intubation) 20.01
  Rickham reservoir 02.2
  Rosen prosthesis (for urinary incontinence) 59.79
  Scribner shunt 39.93
  Sengstaken-Blakemore tube 96.06
  sensor (lead)
   intra-arterial, for continuous blood
    gas monitoring 89.60
   intracardiac hemodynamic monitor-
    ing 00.56
  sieve, vena cava 38.7
  skeletal muscle stimulator 83.92
  skull
   plate 02.05
   stereotactic frame 93.59
   tongs (Barton) (caliper) (Garder
    Wells) (Vinke) (with syn-
    chronous skeletal traction)
    02.94
  spacer (cement) (joint) ▶(methylmethacrylate)◀ 84.56
   spine 84.51
  sphenoidal electrodes 02.96
  spine
   bone void filler
    that with kyphoplasty 81.66
    that with vertebroplasty 81.65
   cage (BAK) 84.51
   facet replacement device(s) 84.84 ●
   interbody spinal fusion device
    84.51
   interspinous process decompres-
    sion device 84.80             ▲
   non-fusion stabilization device ▶—
    see category 84.8◀
   pedicle-based dynamic stabiliza- ●
    tion device(s) 84.82          ●
   posterior motion preservation      ●
    device(s) — see category        ●
    84.8                            ●
   spacer 84.51
  Spitz-Holter valve 02.2
  Steinmann pin 93.44
   with reduction of fracture or dislo-
    cation — see Reduction,
    fracture and Reduction, dis-
    location
 stent(s) (stent graft)
  artery (bare) (bonded) (drug-coated)
   (non-drug-eluting)

Note — Also use 00.40, 00.41, 00.42,
or 00.43 to show the total number of
vessels treated. Use code 00.44 once to
show procedure on a bifurcated vessel.
In addition, use 00.45, 00.46, 00.47, or
00.48 to show the number of vascular
stents inserted.

   basilar 00.64
   carotid 00.63
   cerebrovascular
    cerebral (intracranial) 00.65
    precerebral (extracranial)
     00.64
    carotid 00.63
   coronary (bare) (bonded) (drug-
    coated) (non-drug-eluting)
    36.06
    drug-eluting 36.07
   extracranial 00.64
   carotid 00.63

**Insertion** — continued
 stent(s) — continued
  artery — continued
   intracranial 00.65
   non-coronary vessel
    basilar 00.64
    carotid 00.63
    extracranial 00.64
    intracranial 00.65
    peripheral 39.90
     bare, drug-coated 39.90
     drug-eluting 00.55
    vertebral 00.64
  bile duct 51.43
   endoscopic 51.87
   percutaneous transhepatic
    51.98
  coronary (artery) (bare) (bonded)
   (drug-coated) (non-drug-
   eluting) 36.06

Note — Also use 00.40, 00.41, 00.42,
or 00.43 to show the total number of
vessels treated. Use code 00.44 once to
show procedure on a bifurcated vessel.
In addition, use 00.45, 00.46, 00.47, or
00.48 to show the number of vascular
stents inserted.

   drug-eluting 36.07
  esophagus (endoscopic) (fluoroscopic) 42.81
  mesenteric 39.90
   bare, drug-coated 39.90
   drug-eluting 00.55
  non-coronary vessel

Note — Also use 00.40, 00.41, 00.42,
or 00.43 to show the total number of
vessels treated. Use code 00.44 once to
show procedure on a bifurcated vessel.
In addition, use 00.45, 00.46, 00.47, or
00.48 to show the number of vascular
stents inserted.

   with angioplasty or atherectomy
    39.50
   with bypass — omit code
   basilar 00.64
   carotid 00.63
   extracranial 00.64
   intracranial 00.65
   mesenteric 39.90
    bare, drug-coated 39.90
    drug-eluting 00.55
   peripheral 39.90
    bare, drug-coated 39.90
    drug-eluting 00.55
   renal 39.90
    bare, drug-coated 39.90
    drug-eluting 00.55
   vertebral 00.64
  pancreatic duct 52.92
   endoscopic 52.93
  peripheral vessel 39.90

Note — Also use 00.40, 00.41, 00.42,
or 00.43 to show the total number of
vessels treated. Use code 00.44 once to
show procedure on a bifurcated vessel.
In addition, use 00.45, 00.46, 00.47, or
00.48 to show the number of vascular
stents inserted.

   bare, drug-coated 39.90
   drug-eluting 00.55
  precerebral 00.64

Note — Also use 00.40, 00.41, 00.42,
or 00.43 to show the total number of
vessels treated. Use code 00.44 once to
show procedure on a bifurcated vessel.
In addition, use 00.45, 00.46, 00.47, or
00.48 to show the number of vascular
stents inserted.

   renal 39.90
    bare, drug-coated 39.90
    drug-eluting 00.55

**Insertion** — continued
 stent(s) — continued
  subclavian 39.90

Note — Also use 00.40, 00.41, 00.42,
or 00.43 to show the total number of
vessels treated. Use code 00.44 once to
show procedure on a bifurcated vessel.
In addition, use 00.45, 00.46, 00.47, or
00.48 to show the number of vascular
stents inserted.

   bare, drug-coated 39.90
   drug-eluting 00.55
   tracheobronchial 96.05
   vertebral 00.64

Note — Also use 00.40, 00.41, 00.42,
or 00.43 to show the total number of
vessels treated. Use code 00.44 once to
show procedure on a bifurcated vessel.
In addition, use 00.45, 00.46, 00.47, or
00.48 to show the number of vascular
stents inserted.

  stimoceiver — see Implant, neurostimulator, by site
  stimulator for bone growth — see
   category 78.9 ☑
  subdural
   grids 02.93
   strips 02.93
  suppository
   prostaglandin (for abortion) 96.49
   vagina 96.49
  Swan-Ganz catheter (pulmonary)
   89.64
  tampon
   esophagus 96.06
   uterus 69.91
   vagina 96.14
    after delivery or abortion 75.8
  Tandem™ heart 37.68
  telescope (IMT) (miniature) 13.91
  testicular prosthesis (bilateral) (unilateral) 62.7
  tissue expander (skin) NEC 86.93
   breast 85.95
  tissue mandril (peripheral vessel)
   (Dacron) (Spark's type) 39.99
   with
    blood vessel repair 39.56
    vascular bypass or shunt — see
     Bypass, vascular
  tongs, skull (with synchronous skeletal traction) 02.94
  totally implanted device for bone
   growth (invasive) — see category
   78.9 ☑
  tube (see also Catheterization and Intubation)
   bile duct 51.43
    endoscopic 51.87
   chest 34.04
    revision (with lysis of adhesions)
     34.04
     thoracoscopic 34.06          ●
     thoracoscopic 34.06          ●
   endotracheal 96.04
   esophagus (nonoperative) (Sen-
    gstaken) 96.06
    permanent (silicone) (Souttar)
     42.81
   feeding
    esophageal 42.81
    gastric 96.6
    nasogastric 96.6
   gastric
    by gastrostomy — see category
     43.1 ☑
    for
     decompression, intestinal
      96.07
     feeding 96.6
   intercostal catheter (with water  ●
    seal), for drainage 34.04       ●
    revision (with lysis of adhe-    ●
     sions) 34.04                    ●
     thoracoscopic 34.06            ●

*Index*

*Insertion — Insertion*

## K

**Kader operation** (temporary gastrostomy) 43.19
**Kasai portoenterostomy** 51.37
**Kaufman operation** (for urinary stress incontinence) 59.79
**Kazanjiian operation** (buccal vestibular sulcus extension) 24.91
**Kehr operation** (hepatopexy) 50.69
**Keller operation** (bunionectomy) 77.59
**Kelly (-Kennedy) operation** (urethrovesical plication) 59.3
**Kelly-Stoeckel operation** (urethrovesical plication) 59.3
**Kelotomy** 53.9
**Keratectomy** (complete) (partial) (superficial) 11.49
   for pterygium 11.39
      with corneal graft 11.32
**Keratocentesis** (for hyphema) 12.91
**Keratomileusis** 11.71
**Keratophakia** 11.72
**Keratoplasty** (tectonic) (with autograft) (with homograft) 11.60
   lamellar (nonpenetrating) (with homograft) 11.62
      with autograft 11.61
   penetrating (full-thickness) (with homograft) 11.64
      with autograft 11.63
   perforating — see Keratoplasty, penetrating
   refractive 11.71
   specified type NEC 11.69
**Keratoprosthesis** 11.73
**Keratotomy** (delimiting) (posterior) 11.1
   radial (refractive) 11.75
**Kerr operation** (low cervical cesarean section) 74.1
**Kessler operation** (arthroplasty, carpometacarpal joint) 81.74
**Kidner operation** (excision of accessory navicular bone) (with tendon transfer) 77.98
**Killian operation** (frontal sinusotomy) 22.41
**Kineplasty** — see Cineplasty
**King-Steelquist operation** (hind-quarter amputation) 84.19
**Kirk operation** (amputation through thigh) 84.17
**Kockogram** (ileal conduitogram) 87.78
**Kockoscopy** 45.12
**Kock pouch**
   bowel anastomosis — omit code
   continent ileostomy 46.22
   cutaneous uretero-ileostomy 56.51
   ESWL (extracorporeal shockwave lithotripsy) 98.51
   removal, calculus 57.19
   revision, cutaneous uretero-ileostomy 56.52
   urinary diversion procedure 56.51
**Kondoleon operation** (correction of lymphedema) 40.9
**Krause operation** (sympathetic denervation) 05.29
**Kroener operation** (partial salpingectomy) 66.69
**Kroenlein operation** (lateral orbitotomy) 16.01
**Krönig operation** (low cervical cesarean section) 74.1
**Krukenberg operation** (reconstruction of below-elbow amputation) 82.89
**Kuhnt-Szymanowski operation** (ectropion repair with lid reconstruction) 08.44
**Kyphoplasty** 81.66

## L

**Labbe operation** (gastrotomy) 43.0
**Labiectomy** (bilateral) 71.62
   unilateral 71.61
**Labyrinthectomy** (transtympanic) 20.79

**Labyrinthotomy** (transtympanic) 20.79
**Ladd operation** (mobilization of intestine) 54.95
**Lagrange operation** (iridosclerectomy) 12.65
**Lambrinudi operation** (triple arthrodesis) 81.12
**Laminectomy** (decompression) (for exploration) 03.09
   as operative approach — omit code
   with
      excision of herniated intervertebral disc (nucleus pulposus) 80.51
      excision of other intraspinal lesion (tumor) 03.4
   reopening of site 03.02
**Laminography** — see Radiography
**Laminoplasty, expansile** 03.09
**Laminotomy** (decompression) (for exploration) 03.09
   as operative approach — omit code
   reopening of site 03.02
**Langenbeck operation** (cleft palate repair) 27.62
**Laparoamnioscopy** 75.31
**Laparorrhaphy** 54.63
**Laparoscopy** 54.21
   with
      biopsy (intra-abdominal) 54.24
         uterine ligaments 68.15
         uterus 68.16
      destruction of fallopian tubes — see Destruction, fallopian tube
**Laparotomy** NEC 54.19
   as operative approach — omit code
   exploratory (pelvic) 54.11
   reopening of recent operative site (for control of hemorrhage) (for exploration) (for incision of hematoma) 54.12
**Laparotrachelotomy** 74.1
**Lapidus operation** (bunionectomy with metatarsal osteotomy) 77.51
**Larry operation** (shoulder disarticulation) 84.08
**Laryngectomy**
   with radical neck dissection (with synchronous thyroidectomy) (with synchronous tracheostomy) 30.4
   complete (with partial laryngectomy) (with synchronous tracheostomy) 30.3
      with radical neck dissection (with synchronous thyroidectomy) (with synchronous tracheostomy) 30.4
   frontolateral partial (extended) 30.29
   glottosupraglottic partial 30.29
   lateral partial 30.29
   partial (frontolateral) (glottosupraglottic) (lateral) (submucous) (supraglottic) (vertical) 30.29
   radical (with synchronous thyroidectomy) (with synchronous tracheostomy) 30.4
   submucous (partial) 30.29
   supraglottic partial 30.29
   total (with partial pharyngectomy) (with synchronous tracheostomy) 30.3
      with radical neck dissection (with synchronous thyroidectomy) (with synchronous tracheostomy) 30.4
   vertical partial 30.29
   wide field 30.3
**Laryngocentesis** 31.3
**Laryngoesophagectomy** 30.4
**Laryngofissure** 30.29
**Laryngogram** 87.09
   contrast 87.07
**Laryngopharyngectomy** (with synchronous tracheostomy) 30.3

**Laryngopharyngectomy** — continued
   radical (with synchronous thyroidectomy) 30.4
**Laryngopharyngoesophagectomy** (with synchronous tracheostomy) 30.3
   with radical neck dissection (with synchronous thyroidectomy) 30.4
**Laryngoplasty** 31.69
**Laryngorrhaphy** 31.61
**Laryngoscopy** (suspension) (through artificial stoma) 31.42
**Laryngostomy** (permanent) 31.29
   revision 31.63
   temporary (emergency) 31.1
**Laryngotomy** 31.3
**Laryngotracheobronchoscopy** 33.23
   with biopsy 33.24
**Laryngotracheoscopy** 31.42
**Laryngotracheostomy** (permanent) 31.29
   temporary (emergency) 31.1
**Laryngotracheotomy** (temporary) 31.1
   permanent 31.29
**Laser** — see also Coagulation, Destruction, and Photocoagulation by site
   angioplasty, percutaneous transluminal 39.59
   coronary — see Angioplasty, coronary
**Lash operation**
   internal cervical os repair 67.59
   laparoscopic supracervical hysterectomy 68.31
**LASIK** (laser-assisted in situ keratomileusis) 11.71
**Latzko operation**
   cesarean section 74.2
   colpocleisis 70.8
**Lavage**
   antral 22.00
   bronchus NEC 96.56
      diagnostic (endoscopic) bronchoalveolar lavage (BAL) 33.24
   endotracheal 96.56
   gastric 96.33
   lung (total) (whole) 33.99
      diagnostic (endoscopic) bronchoalveolar lavage (BAL) 33.24
   nasal sinus(es) 22.00
      by puncture 22.01
      through natural ostium 22.02
   peritoneal (diagnostic) 54.25
   trachea NEC 96.56
**Leadbetter operation** (urethral reconstruction) 58.46
**Leadbetter-Politano operation** (ureteroneocystostomy) 56.74
**LEEP** (loop electrosurgical excision procedure) of cervix 67.32
**Le Fort operation** (colpocleisis) 70.8
**LeMesurier operation** (cleft lip repair) 27.54
**Lengthening**
   bone (with bone graft) 78.30
      for reconstruction of thumb 82.69
      femur 78.35
      specified site NEC (see also category 78.3 ☑)
      tibia 78.37
      ulna 78.33
   extraocular muscle NEC 15.21
      multiple (two or more muscles) 15.4
   fascia 83.89
      hand 82.89
   hamstring NEC 83.85
   heel cord 83.85
   leg
      femur 78.35
      tibia 78.37
   levator palpebrae muscle 08.38
   muscle 83.85
      extraocular 15.21

**Lengthening** — continued
   muscle — continued
      extraocular — continued
         multiple (two or more muscles) 15.4
      hand 82.55
   palate 27.62
      secondary or subsequent 27.63
   tendon 83.85
      for claw toe repair 77.57
      hand 82.55
**Leriche operation** (periarterial sympathectomy) 05.25
**Leucotomy, leukotomy** 01.32
**Leukopheresis, therapeutic** 99.72
**Lid suture operation** (blepharoptosis) 08.31
**Ligation**
   adrenal vessel (artery) (vein) 07.43
   aneurysm 39.52
   appendages, dermal 86.26
   arteriovenous fistula 39.53
      coronary artery 36.99
   artery 38.80
      for control of epistaxis — see Control, epistaxis
      abdominal 38.86
      adrenal 07.43
      aorta (arch) (ascending) (descending) 38.84
      coronary (anomalous) 36.99
      ethmoidal 21.04
      external carotid 21.06
      head and neck NEC 38.82
      intracranial NEC 38.81
      lower limb 38.88
      maxillary (transantral) 21.05
      middle meningeal 02.13
      thoracic NEC 38.85
      thyroid 06.92
      upper limb 38.83
   atrium, heart 37.99
   auricle, heart 37.99
   bleeding vessel — see Control, hemorrhage
   blood vessel 38.80
      abdominal
         artery 38.86
         vein 38.87
      adrenal 07.43
      aorta (arch) (ascending) (descending) 38.84
      esophagus 42.91
         endoscopic 42.33
      head and neck NEC 38.82
      intracranial NEC 38.81
      lower limb
         artery 38.88
         vein 38.89
      meningeal (artery) (longitudinal sinus) 02.13
      thoracic NEC 38.85
      thyroid 06.92
      upper limb (artery) (vein) 38.83
   bronchus 33.92
   cisterna chyli 40.64
   coronary
      artery (anomalous) 36.99
      sinus 36.39
   dermal appendage 86.26
   ductus arteriosus, patent 38.85
   esophageal vessel 42.91
      endoscopic 42.33
   ethmoidal artery 21.04
   external carotid artery 21.06
   fallopian tube (bilateral) (remaining) (solitary) 66.39
      by endoscopy (culdoscopy) (hysteroscopy) (laparoscopy) (peritoneoscopy) 66.29
      with
         crushing 66.31
            by endoscopy (laparoscopy) 66.21
         division 66.32

☑ Additional Digit Required — Refer to the Tabular List for Digit Selection

▶◀ Revised Text    ● New Line    ▲ Revised Code

Subterms under main terms may continue to next column or page

☑ Additional Digit Required — Refer to the Tabular List for Digit Selection
▼ Subterms under main terms may continue to next column or page
*2007 Ingenix*
▶◀ Revised Text
● New Line
▲ Revised Code
October 2007 · Volume 3 — 37

**Lysis** — *continued*
   adhesions — *continued*
      vulva 71.01
      goniosynechiae (with injection of air or liquid) 12.31
      synechiae (posterior) 12.33
         anterior (with injection of air or liquid) 12.32

# M

**Madlener operation** (tubal ligation) 66.31
**Magnet extraction**
   foreign body
      anterior chamber, eye 12.01
      choroid 14.01
      ciliary body 12.01
      conjunctiva 98.22
      cornea 11.0
      eye, eyeball NEC 98.21
         anterior segment 12.01
         posterior segment 14.01
      intraocular (anterior segment) 12.01
      iris 12.01
      lens 13.01
      orbit 98.21
      retina 14.01
      sclera 12.01
      vitreous 14.01
**Magnetic resonance imaging** (nuclear) — *see* Imaging, magnetic resonance
**Magnuson (-Stack) operation** (arthroplasty for recurrent shoulder dislocation) 81.82
**Malleostapediopexy** 19.19
   with incus replacement 19.11
**Malström's vacuum extraction** 72.79
   with episiotomy 72.71
**Mammaplasty** — *see* Mammoplasty
**Mammectomy** — *see also* Mastectomy
   subcutaneous (unilateral) 85.34
      with synchronous implant 85.35
      bilateral 85.36
**Mammilliplasty** 85.87
**Mammography** NEC 87.37
**Mammoplasty** 85.89
   with
      full-thickness graft 85.83
      muscle flap 85.85
      pedicle graft 85.84
      split-thickness graft 85.82
   amputative (reduction) (bilateral) 85.32
      unilateral 85.31
   augmentation 85.50
      with
         breast implant (bilateral) 85.54
            unilateral 85.53
         injection into breast (bilateral) 85.52
            unilateral 85.51
   reduction (bilateral) 85.32
      unilateral 85.31
   revision 85.89
   size reduction (gynecomastia) (bilateral) 85.32
      unilateral 85.31
**Mammotomy** 85.0
**Manchester (-Donald) (-Fothergill) operation** (uterine suspension) 69.22
**Mandibulectomy** (partial) 76.31
   total 76.42
      with reconstruction 76.41
**Maneuver** (method)
   Bracht 72.52
   Credé 73.59
   De Lee (key-in-lock) 72.4
   Kristeller 72.54
   Loveset's (extraction of arms in breech birth) 72.52
   Mauriceau (-Smellie-Veit) 72.52
   Pinard (total breech extraction) 72.54
   Prague 72.52
   Ritgen 73.59
   Scanzoni (rotation) 72.4

**Maneuver** — *continued*
   Van Hoorn 72.52
   Wigand-Martin 72.52
**Manipulation**
   with reduction of fracture or dislocation — *see* Reduction, fracture *and* Reduction, dislocation
   enterostomy stoma (with dilation) 96.24
   intestine (intra-abdominal) 46.80
      large 46.82
      small 46.81
   joint
      adhesions 93.26
         temporomandibular 76.95
      dislocation — *see* Reduction, dislocation
   lacrimal passage (tract) NEC 09.49
   muscle structures 93.27
   musculoskeletal (physical therapy) NEC 93.29
   nasal septum, displaced 21.88
   osteopathic NEC 93.67
      for general mobilization (general articulation) 93.61
      high-velocity, low-amplitude forces (thrusting) 93.62
      indirect forces 93.65
      isotonic, isometric forces 93.64
      low-velocity, high-amplitude forces (springing) 93.63
      to move tissue fluids 93.66
   rectum 96.22
   salivary duct 26.91
   stomach, intraoperative 44.92
   temporomandibular joint NEC 76.95
   ureteral calculus by catheter
      with removal 56.0
      without removal 59.8
   uterus NEC 69.98
      gravid 75.99
      inverted
         manual replacement (following delivery) 75.94
         surgical — *see* Repair, inverted uterus
**Manometry**
   esophageal 89.32
   spinal fluid 89.15
   urinary 89.21
**Manual arts therapy** 93.81
**Mapping**
   cardiac (electrophysiologic) 37.27
      doppler (flow) 88.72
   electrocardiogram only 89.52
**Marckwald operation** (cervical os repair) 67.59
**Marshall-Marchetti (-Krantz) operation** (retropubic urethral suspension) 59.5
**Marsupialization** — *see also* Destruction, lesion, by site
   cyst
      Bartholin's 71.23
      brain 01.59
      cervical (nabothian) 67.31
      dental 24.4
      dentigerous 24.4
      kidney 55.31
      larynx 30.01
      liver 50.21
      ovary 65.21
         laparoscopic 65.23
      pancreas 52.3
      pilonidal (open excision) (with partial closure) 86.21
      salivary gland 26.21
      spinal (intraspinal) (meninges) 03.4
      spleen, splenic 41.41
   lesion
      brain 01.59
      cerebral 01.59
      liver 50.21
   pilonidal cyst or sinus (open excision) (with partial closure) 86.21
   pseudocyst, pancreas 52.3

**Marsupialization** — *see also* Destruction, lesion, by site — *continued*
   ranula, salivary gland 26.21
**Massage**
   cardiac (external) (manual) (closed) 99.63
      open 37.91
   prostatic 99.94
   rectal (for levator spasm) 99.93
**MAST** (military anti-shock trousers) 93.58
**Mastectomy** (complete) (prophylactic) (simple) (unilateral) 85.41
   with
      excision of regional lymph nodes 85.43
         bilateral 85.44
      preservation of skin and nipple 85.34
         with synchronous implant 85.33
         bilateral 85.36
            with synchronous implant 85.35
   bilateral 85.42
   extended
      radical (Urban) (unilateral) 85.47
         bilateral 85.48
      simple (with regional lymphadenectomy) (unilateral) 85.43
         bilateral 85.44
   modified radical (unilateral) 85.43
      bilateral 85.44
   partial 85.23
   radical (Halsted) (Meyer) (unilateral) 85.45
      bilateral 85.46
      extended (Urban) (unilateral) 85.47
         bilateral 85.48
      modified (unilateral) 85.43
         bilateral 85.44
   subcutaneous 85.34
      with synchronous implant 85.33
      bilateral 85.36
         with synchronous implant 85.35
   subtotal 85.23
**Masters' stress test** (two-step) 89.42
**Mastoidectomy** (cortical) (conservative) 20.49
   complete (simple) 20.41
   modified radical 20.49
   radical 20.42
      modified 20.49
   simple (complete) 20.41
**Mastoidotomy** 20.21
**Mastoidotympanectomy** 20.42
**Mastopexy** 85.6
**Mastoplasty** — *see* Mammoplasty
**Mastorrhaphy** 85.81
**Mastotomy** 85.0
**Matas operation** (aneurysmorrhaphy) 39.52
**Mayo operation**
   bunionectomy 77.59
   herniorrhaphy 53.49
   vaginal hysterectomy 68.59
      laparoscopically assisted (LAVH) 68.51
**Mazet operation** (knee disarticulation) 84.16
**McBride operation** (bunionectomy with soft tissue correction) 77.53
**McBurney operation** — *see* Repair, hernia, inguinal
**McCall operation** (enterocele repair) 70.92
**McCauley operation** (release of clubfoot) 83.84
**McDonald operation** (encirclement suture, cervix) 67.59
**McIndoe operation** (vaginal construction) 70.61
   with graft or prosthesis 70.63 ●
**McKeever operation** (fusion of first metatarsophalangeal joint for hallux valgus repair) 77.52

**McKissock operation** (breast reduction) 85.33
**McReynolds operation** (transposition of pterygium) 11.31
**McVay operation**
   femoral hernia — *see* Repair, hernia, femoral
   inguinal hernia — *see* Repair, hernia, inguinal
**Measurement**
   airway resistance 89.38
   anatomic NEC 89.39
   arterial blood gases 89.65
   basal metabolic rate (BMR) 89.39
   blood gases
      arterial 89.65
         continuous intra-arterial 89.60
      venous 89.66
   body 93.07
   cardiac output (by)
      Fick method 89.67
      indicator dilution technique 89.68
      oxygen consumption technique 89.67
      thermodilution indicator 89.68
   cardiovascular NEC 89.59
   central venous pressure 89.62
   coronary blood flow 89.69
   gastric function NEC 89.39
   girth 93.07
   intelligence 94.01
   intracranial pressure 01.10          ▲
   intraocular tension or pressure 89.11
      as part of extended ophthalmologic work-up 95.03
   intrauterine pressure 89.62
   limb length 93.06
   lung volume 89.37
   mixed venous blood gases 89.66
   physiologic NEC 89.39
   portovenous pressure 89.62
   range of motion 93.05
   renal clearance 89.29
   respiratory NEC 89.38
   skin fold thickness 93.07
   skull circumference 93.07
   sphincter of Oddi pressure 51.15
   systemic arterial
      blood gases 89.65
         continuous intra-arterial 89.60
      pressure 89.61
   urine (bioassay) (chemistry) 89.29
   vascular 89.59
   venous blood gases 89.66
   vital capacity (pulmonary) 89.37
**Meatoplasty**
   ear 18.6
   urethra 58.47
**Meatotomy**
   ureter 56.1
   urethra 58.1
      internal 58.5
**Mechanical ventilation** — *see* Ventilation
**Mediastinectomy** 34.3
**Mediastinoscopy** (transpleural) 34.22
**Mediastinotomy** 34.1
   with pneumonectomy 32.59          ▲
      thoracoscopic 32.50          ●
**Meloplasty, facial** 86.82
**Meningeorrhaphy** (cerebral) 02.12
   spinal NEC 03.59
   for
      meningocele 03.51
      myelomeningocele 03.52
**Meniscectomy** (knee) NEC 80.6
   acromioclavicular 80.91
   sternoclavicular 80.91
   temporomandibular (joint) 76.5
   wrist 80.93
**Menstrual extraction or regulation** 69.6
**Mentoplasty** (augmentation) (with graft) (with implant) 76.68
   reduction 76.67
**Mesenterectomy** 54.4
**Mesenteriopexy** 54.75

**Operation** — *continued*
Delorme — *continued*
repair of prolapsed rectum 48.76
thoracoplasty 33.34
Denker (radical maxillary antrotomy) 22.31
Dennis-Varco (herniorrhaphy) — *see* Repair, hernia, femoral
Denonvillier (limited rhinoplasty) 21.86
dental NEC 24.99
orthodontic NEC 24.8
Derlacki (tympanoplasty) 19.4
diaphragm NEC 34.89
Dickson (fascial transplant) 83.82
Dickson-Diveley (tendon transfer and arthrodesis to correct claw toe) 77.57
Dieffenbach (hip disarticulation) 84.18
digestive tract NEC 46.99
Doléris (shortening of round ligaments) 69.22
D'Ombrain (excision of pterygium with corneal graft) 11.32
Dorrance (push-back operation for cleft palate) 27.62
Dotter (transluminal angioplasty) 39.59
Douglas (suture of tongue to lip for micrognathia) 25.59
Doyle (paracervical uterine denervation) 69.3
Duhamel (abdominoperineal pull-through) 48.65
Dührssen (vaginofixation of uterus) 69.22
Dunn (triple arthrodesis) 81.12
duodenum NEC 46.99
Dupuytren
fasciectomy 82.35
fasciotomy 82.12
with excision 82.35
shoulder disarticulation 84.08
Durham (-Caldwell) (transfer of biceps femoris tendon) 83.75
DuToit and Roux (staple capsulorrhaphy of shoulder) 81.82
DuVries (tenoplasty) 83.88
Dwyer
fasciotomy 83.14
soft tissue release NEC 83.84
wedge osteotomy, calcaneus 77.28
Eagleton (extrapetrosal drainage) 20.22
ear (external) NEC 18.9
middle or inner NEC 20.99
Eden-Hybinette (glenoid bone block) 78.01
Effler (heart) 36.2
Eggers
tendon release (patellar retinacula) 83.13
tendon transfer (biceps femoris tendon) (hamstring tendon) 83.75
Elliot (scleral trephination with iridectomy) 12.61
Ellis Jones (repair of peroneal tendon) 83.88
Ellison (reinforcement of collateral ligament) 81.44
Elmslie-Cholmeley (tarsal wedge osteotomy) 77.28
Eloesser
thoracoplasty 33.34
thoracostomy 34.09
Emmet (cervix) 67.61
endorectal pull-through 48.41
epididymis NEC 63.99
esophagus NEC 42.99
Estes (ovary) 65.72
laparoscopic 65.75
Estlander (thoracoplasty) 33.34
Evans (release of clubfoot) 83.84
extraocular muscle NEC 15.9

**Operation** — *continued*
extraocular muscle — *continued*
multiple (two or more muscles) 15.4
with temporary detachment from globe 15.3
revision 15.6
single 15.29
with temporary detachment from globe 15.19
eyeball NEC 16.99
eyelid(s) NEC 08.99
face NEC 27.99
facial bone or joint NEC 76.99
fallopian tube NEC 66.99
Farabeuf (ischiopubiotomy) 77.39
Fasanella-Servatt (blepharoptosis repair) 08.35
fascia NEC 83.99
hand 82.99
female (genital organs) NEC 71.9
hysterectomy NEC 68.9
fenestration (aorta) 39.54
Ferguson (hernia repair) 53.00
Fick (perforation of footplate) 19.0
filtering (for glaucoma) 12.79
with iridectomy 12.65
Finney (pyloroplasty) 44.29
fistulizing, sclera NEC 12.69
Foley (pyeloplasty) 55.87
Fontan (creation of conduit between right atrium and pulmonary artery) 35.94
Fothergill (-Donald) (uterine suspension) 69.22
Fowler
arthroplasty of metacarpophalangeal joint 81.72
release (mallet finger repair) 82.84
tenodesis (hand) 82.85
thoracoplasty 33.34
Fox (entropion repair with wedge resection) 08.43
Franco (suprapubic cystotomy) 57.18
Frank (permanent gastrostomy) 43.19
Frazier (-Spiller) (subtemporal trigeminal rhizotomy) 04.02
Fredet-Ramstedt (pyloromyotomy) (with wedge resection) 43.3
Frenckner (intrapetrosal drainage) 20.22
Frickman (abdominal proctopexy) 48.75
Frommel (shortening of uterosacral ligaments) 69.22
Gabriel (abdominoperineal resection of rectum) 48.5
gallbladder NEC 51.99
ganglia NEC 04.99
sympathetic 05.89
Gant (wedge osteotomy of trochanter) 77.25
Garceau (tibial tendon transfer) 83.75
Gardner (spinal meningocele repair) 03.51
gastric NEC 44.99
Gelman (release of clubfoot) 83.84
genital organ NEC
female 71.9
male 64.99
Ghormley (hip fusion) 81.21
Gifford
destruction of lacrimal sac 09.6
keratotomy (delimiting) 11.1
Gill
arthrodesis of shoulder 81.23
laminectomy 03.09
Gilliam (uterine suspension) 69.22
Gill-Stein (carporadial arthrodesis) 81.25
Girdlestone
laminectomy with spinal fusion 81.00
muscle transfer for claw toe 77.57

**Operation** — *continued*
Girdlestone — *continued*
resection of femoral head and neck (without insertion of joint prosthesis) 77.85
with replacement prosthesis — *see* Implant, joint, hip
resection of hip prosthesis 80.05
with replacement prosthesis — *see* Implant, joint, hip
Girdlestone-Taylor (muscle transfer for claw toe repair) 77.57
glaucoma NEC 12.79
Glenn (anastomosis of superior vena cava to right pulmonary artery) 39.21
globus pallidus NEC 01.42
Goebel-Frangenheim-Stoeckel (urethrovesical suspension) 59.4
Goldner (clubfoot release) 80.48
Goldthwait
ankle stabilization 81.11
patella stabilization 81.44
tendon transfer for patella dislocation 81.44
Goodall-Power (vagina) 70.4
Gordon-Taylor (hindquarter amputation) 84.19
Graber-Duvernay (drilling femoral head) 77.15
Green (scapulopexy) 78.41
Grice (subtalar arthrodesis) 81.13
Gritti-Stokes (knee disarticulation) 84.16
Gross (herniorrhaphy) 53.49
gum NEC 24.39
Guyon (amputation of ankle) 84.13
Hagner (epididymotomy) 63.92
Halsted — *see* Repair, hernia, inguinal
Hampton (anastomosis small intestine to rectal stump) 45.92
hanging hip (muscle release) 83.19
harelip 27.54
Harrison-Richardson (vaginal suspension) 70.77
with graft or prosthesis 70.78   ●
Hartmann — *see* Colectomy, by site
Hauser
achillotenotomy 83.11
bunionectomy with adductor tendon transfer 77.53
stabilization of patella 81.44
Heaney (vaginal hysterectomy) 68.59
laparoscopically assisted (LAVH) 68.51
heart NEC 37.99
valve NEC 35.99
adjacent structure NEC 35.39
Hegar (perineorrhaphy) 71.79
Heine (cyclodialysis) 12.55
Heineke-Mikulicz (pyloroplasty) — *see* category 44.2 ☑
Heller (esophagomyotomy) 42.7
Hellström (transplantation of aberrant renal vessel) 39.55
hemorrhoids NEC 49.49
Henley (jejunal transposition) 43.81
hepatic NEC 50.99
hernia — *see* Repair, hernia
Hey (amputation of foot) 84.12
Hey-Groves (reconstruction of anterior cruciate ligament) 81.45
Heyman (soft tissue release for clubfoot) 83.84
Heyman-Herndon (-Strong) (correction of metatarsus varus) 80.48
Hibbs (lumbar spinal fusion) — *see* Fusion, lumbar
Higgins — *see* Repair, hernia, femoral
Hill-Allison (hiatal hernia repair, transpleural approach) 53.80
Hitchcock (anchoring tendon of biceps) 83.88
Hofmeister (gastrectomy) 43.7
Hoke
midtarsal fusion 81.14

**Operation** — *continued*
Hoke — *continued*
triple arthrodesis 81.12
Holth
iridencleisis 12.63
sclerectomy 12.65
Homan (correction of lymphedema) 40.9
Hutch (ureteroneocystostomy) 56.74
Hybinette-eden (glenoid bone block) 78.01
hymen NEC 70.91
hypopharynx NEC 29.99
hypophysis NEC 07.79
ileal loop 56.51
ileum NEC 46.99
intestine NEC 46.99
iris NEC 12.97
inclusion 12.63
Irving (tubal ligation) 66.32
Irwin (*see also* Osteotomy) 77.30
Jaboulay (gastroduodenostomy) 44.39
laparoscopic 44.38
Janeway (permanent gastrostomy) 43.19
Jatene (arterial switch) 35.84
jejunum NEC 46.99
Johanson (urethral reconstruction) 58.46
joint (capsule) (ligament) (structure) NEC 81.99
facial NEC 76.99
Jones
claw toe (transfer of extensor hallucis longus tendon) 77.57
modified (with arthrodesis) 77.57
dacryocystorhinostomy 09.81
hammer toe (interphalangeal fusion) 77.56
modified (tendon transfer with arthrodesis) 77.57
repair of peroneal tendon 83.88
Joplin (exostectomy with tendon transfer) 77.53
Kader (temporary gastrostomy) 43.19
Kaufman (for urinary stress incontinence) 59.79
Kazanjiian (buccal vestibular sulcus extension) 24.91
Kehr (hepatopexy) 50.69
Keller (bunionectomy) 77.59
Kelly (-Kennedy) (urethrovesical plication) 59.3
Kelly-Stoeckel (urethrovesical plication) 59.3
Kerr (cesarean section) 74.1
Kessler (arthroplasty, carpometacarpal joint) 81.74
Kidner (excision of accessory navicular bone) (with tendon transfer) 77.98
kidney NEC 55.99
Killian (frontal sinusotomy) 22.41
King-Steelquist (hindquarter amputation) 84.19
Kirk (amputation through thigh) 84.17
Kock pouch
bowel anastomosis — *omit code*
continent ileostomy 46.22
cutaneous uretero-ileostomy 56.51
ESWL (electrocorporeal shockwave lithotripsy) 98.51
removal, calculus 57.19
revision, cutaneous uretero-ileostomy 56.52
urinary diversion procedure 56.51
Kondoleon (correction of lymphedema) 40.9
Krause (sympathetic denervation) 05.29
Kroener (partial salpingectomy) 66.69
Kroenlein (lateral orbitotomy) 16.01
Krönig (low cervical cesarean section) 74.1

**Operation** — *continued*

Krukenberg (reconstruction of below-elbow amputation) 82.89

Kuhnt-Szymanowski (ectropion repair with lid reconstruction) 08.44

Labbe (gastrotomy) 43.0

labia NEC 71.8

lacrimal

gland 09.3

system NEC 09.99

Ladd (mobilization of intestine) 54.95

Lagrange (iridosclerectomy) 12.65

Lambrinudi (triple arthrodesis) 81.12

Langenbeck (cleft palate repair) 27.62

Lapidus (bunionectomy with metatarsal osteotomy) 77.51

Larry (shoulder disarticulation) 84.08

larynx NEC 31.98

Lash

internal cervical os repair 67.59

laparoscopic supracervical hysterectomy 68.31

Latzko

cesarean section, extraperitoneal 74.2

colpocleisis 70.8

Leadbetter (urethral reconstruction) 58.46

Leadbetter-Politano (ureteroneocystostomy) 56.74

Le Fort (colpocleisis) 70.8

LeMesurier (cleft lip repair) 27.54

lens NEC 13.90

Leriche (periarterial sympathectomy) 05.25

levator muscle sling

eyelid ptosis repair 08.33

urethrovesical suspension 59.71

urinary stress incontinence 59.71

lid suture (blepharoptosis) 08.31

ligament NEC 81.99

broad NEC 69.98

round NEC 69.98

uterine NEC 69.98

Lindholm (repair of ruptured tendon) 83.88

Linton (varicose vein) 38.59

lip NEC 27.99

Lisfranc

foot amputation 84.12

shoulder disarticulation 84.08

Littlewood (forequarter amputation) 84.09

liver NEC 50.99

Lloyd-Davies (abdominoperineal resection) 48.5

Longmire (bile duct anastomosis) 51.39

Lord

dilation of anal canal for hemorrhoids 49.49

hemorrhoidectomy 49.49

orchidopexy 62.5

Lucas and Murray (knee arthrodesis with plate) 81.22

lung NEC 33.99

lung volume reduction 32.22

biologic lung volume reduction (BLVR) — *see* category 33.7 ☑

lymphatic structure(s) NEC 40.9

duct, left (thoracic) NEC 40.69

Madlener (tubal ligation) 66.31

Magnuson (-Stack) (arthroplasty for recurrent shoulder dislocation) 81.82

male genital organs NEC 64.99

Manchester (-Donald) (-Fothergill) (uterine suspension) 69.22

mandible NEC 76.99

orthognathic 76.64

Marckwald operation (cervical os repair) 67.59

Marshall-Marchetti (-Krantz) (retropubic urethral suspension) 59.5

Matas (aneurysmorrhaphy) 39.52

**Operation** — *continued*

Mayo

bunionectomy 77.59

herniorrhaphy 53.49

vaginal hysterectomy 68.59

laparoscopically assisted (LAVH) 68.51

maze procedure (ablation or destruction of heart tissue)

by incision (open) 37.33

by peripherally inserted catheter 37.34

endovascular approach 37.34

trans-thoracic approach 37.33

Mazet (knee disarticulation) 84.16

McBride (bunionectomy with soft tissue correction) 77.53

McBurney — *see* Repair, hernia, inguinal

McCall (enterocele repair) 70.92

with graft or prosthesis 70.93 ●

McCauley (release of clubfoot) 83.84

McDonald (encirclement suture, cervix) 67.59

McIndoe (vaginal construction) 70.61

with graft or prosthesis 70.63 ●

McKeever (fusion of first metatarsophalangeal joint for hallux valgus repair) 77.52

McKissock (breast reduction) 85.33

McReynolds (transposition of pterygium) 11.31

McVay

femoral hernia — *see* Repair, hernia, femoral

inguinal hernia — *see* Repair, hernia, inguinal

meninges (spinal) NEC 03.99

cerebral NEC 02.99

mesentery NEC 54.99

Mikulicz (exteriorization of intestine) (first stage) 46.03

second stage 46.04

Miles (complete proctectomy) 48.5

Millard (cheiloplasty) 27.54

Miller

midtarsal arthrodesis 81.14

urethrovesical suspension 59.4

Millin-Read (urethrovesical suspension) 59.4

Mitchell (hallux valgus repair) 77.51

Mohs (chemosurgical excision of skin) 86.24

Moore (arthroplasty) 81.52

Moschowitz

enterocele repair 70.92

with graft or prosthesis 70.93 ●

herniorrhaphy — *see* Repair, hernia, femoral

sigmoidopexy 46.63

mouth NEC 27.99

Muller (banding of pulmonary artery) 38.85

Mumford (partial claviculectomy) 77.81

muscle NEC 83.99

extraocular — *see* Operation, extraocular

hand NEC 82.99

papillary heart NEC 35.31

musculoskeletal system NEC 84.99

Mustard (interatrial transposition of venous return) 35.91

nail (finger) (toe) NEC 86.99

nasal sinus NEC 22.9

nasopharynx NEC 29.99

nerve (cranial) (peripheral) NEC 04.99

adrenal NEC 07.49

sympathetic NEC 05.89

nervous system NEC 05.9

Nicola (tenodesis for recurrent dislocation of shoulder) 81.82

nipple NEC 85.99

Nissen (fundoplication of stomach) 44.66

laparoscopic 44.67

**Operation** — *continued*

Noble (plication of small intestine) 46.62

node (lymph) NEC 40.9

Norman Miller (vaginopexy) 70.77

with graft or prosthesis 70.78 ●

Norton (extraperitoneal cesarean operation) 74.2

nose, nasal NEC 21.99

sinus NEC 22.9

Ober (-Yount) (gluteal-iliotibial fasciotomy) 83.14

obstetric NEC 75.99

ocular NEC 16.99

muscle — *see* Operation, extraocular muscle

O'Donoghue (triad knee repair) 81.43

Olshausen (uterine suspension) 69.22

omentum NEC 54.99

ophthalmologic NEC 16.99

oral cavity NEC 27.99

orbicularis muscle sling 08.36

orbit NEC 16.98

oropharynx NEC 29.99

orthodontic NEC 24.8

orthognathic NEC 76.69

Oscar Miller (midtarsal arthrodesis) 81.14

Osmond-Clark (soft tissue release with peroneus brevis tendon transfer) 83.75

ovary NEC 65.99

Oxford (for urinary incontinence) 59.4

palate NEC 27.99

palpebral ligament sling 08.36

Panas (linear proctotomy) 48.0

Pancoast (division of trigeminal nerve at foramen ovale) 04.02

pancreas NEC 52.99

pantaloon (revision of gastric anastomosis) 44.5

papillary muscle (heart) NEC 35.31

Paquin (ureteroneocystostomy) 56.74

parathyroid gland(s) NEC 06.99

parotid gland or duct NEC 26.99

Partsch (marsupialization of dental cyst) 24.4

Pattee (auditory canal) 18.6

Peet (splanchnic resection) 05.29

Pemberton

osteotomy of ilium 77.39

rectum (mobilization and fixation for prolapse repair) 48.76

penis NEC 64.98

Pereyra (paraurethral suspension) 59.6

pericardium NEC 37.99

perineum (female) NEC 71.8

male NEC 86.99

perirectal tissue NEC 48.99

perirenal tissue NEC 59.92

peritoneum NEC 54.99

periurethral tissue NEC 58.99

perivesical tissue NEC 59.92

pharyngeal flap (cleft palate repair) 27.62

secondary or subsequent 27.63

pharynx, pharyngeal (pouch) NEC 29.99

pineal gland NEC 07.59

Pinsker (obliteration of nasoseptal telangiectasia) 21.07

Piper (forceps) 72.6

Pirogoff (ankle amputation through malleoli of tibia and fibula) 84.14

pituitary gland NEC 07.79

plastic — *see* Repair, by site

pleural cavity NEC 34.99

Politano-Leadbetter (ureteroneocystostomy) 56.74

pollicization (with nerves and blood supply) 82.61

Polya (gastrectomy) 43.7

Pomeroy (ligation and division of fallopian tubes) 66.32

**Operation** — *continued*

Poncet

lengthening of Achilles tendon 83.85

urethrostomy, perineal 58.0

Porro (cesarean section) 74.99

posterior chamber (eye) NEC 14.9

Potts-Smith (descending aorta-left pulmonary artery anastomosis) 39.0

Printen and Mason (high gastric bypass) 44.31

prostate NEC (*see also* Prostatectomy) 60.69

specified type 60.99

pterygium 11.39

with corneal graft 11.32

Puestow (pancreaticojejunostomy) 52.96

pull-through NEC 48.49

pulmonary NEC 33.99

push-back (cleft palate repair) 27.62

Putti-Platt (capsulorrhaphy of shoulder for recurrent dislocation) 81.82

pyloric exclusion 44.39

laparoscopic 44.38

pyriform sinus NEC 29.99

"rabbit ear" (anterior urethropexy) (Tudor) 59.79

Ramadier (intrapetrosal drainage) 20.22

Ramstedt (pyloromyotomy) (with wedge resection) 43.3

Rankin

exteriorization of intestine 46.03

proctectomy (complete) 48.5

Rashkind (balloon septostomy) 35.41

Rastelli (creation of conduit between right ventricle and pulmonary artery) 35.92

in repair of

pulmonary artery atresia 35.92

transposition of great vessels 35.92

truncus arteriosus 35.83

Raz-Pereyra procedure (bladder neck suspension) 59.79

rectal NEC 48.99

rectocele NEC 70.52

re-entry (aorta) 39.54

renal NEC 55.99

respiratory (tract) NEC 33.99

retina NEC 14.9

Ripstein (repair of rectal prolapse) 48.75

Rodney Smith (radical subtotal pancreatectomy) 52.53

Roux-en-Y

bile duct 51.36

cholecystojejunostomy 51.32

esophagus (intrathoracic) 42.54

gastroenterostomy 44.39

laparoscopic 44.38

gastrojejunostomy 44.39

laparoscopic 44.38

pancreaticojejunostomy 52.96

Roux-Goldthwait (repair of patellar dislocation) 81.44

Roux-Herzen-Judine (jejunal loop interposition) 42.63

Ruiz-Mora (proximal phalangectomy for hammer toe) 77.99

Russe (bone graft of scaphoid) 78.04

Saemisch (corneal section) 11.1

salivary gland or duct NEC 26.99

Salter (innominate osteotomy) 77.39

Sauer-Bacon (abdominoperineal resection) 48.5

Schanz (femoral osteotomy) 77.35

Schauta (-Amreich) (radical vaginal hysterectomy) 68.79

laparoscopic 68.71

Schede (thoracoplasty) 33.34

Scheie

cautery of sclera 12.62

---

Operation — Orbitotomy

✔ Additional Digit Required — Refer to the Tabular List for Digit Selection

44 — Volume 3    ▶◀ Revised Text    ● New Line    ▲ Revised Code    Subterms under main terms may continue to next column or page    *2007 Ingenix*

**Passage of sounds, urethra** 58.6
**Patch**
blood, spinal (epidural) 03.95
graft — *see* Graft
spinal, blood (epidural) 03.95
subdural, brain 02.12
**Patellapexy** 78.46
**Patellaplasty** NEC 78.46
**Patellectomy** 77.96
partial 77.86
**Pattee operation** (auditory canal) 18.6
**Pectenotomy** — *see also* Sphincterotomy, anal 49.59
**Pedicle flap** — *see* Graft, skin, pedicle
**Peet operation** (splanchnic resection) 05.29
**PEG** (percutaneous endoscopic gastrostomy) 43.11
**PEJ** (percutaneous endoscopic jejunostomy) 46.32
**Pelvectomy, kidney** (partial) 55.4
**Pelvimetry** 88.25
gynecological 89.26
**Peliolithotomy** 55.11
**Pelvioplasty, kidney** 55.87
**Pelviostomy** 55.12
closure 55.82
**Pelviotomy** 77.39
to assist delivery 73.94
**Pelvi-ureteroplasty** 55.87
**Pemberton operation**
osteotomy of ilium 77.39
rectum (mobilization and fixation for prolapse repair) 48.76
**Penectomy** 64.3
**Pereyra operation** (paraurethral suspension) 59.6
**Perforation**
stapes footplate 19.0
**Perfusion** NEC 39.97
for
chemotherapy NEC 99.25
hormone therapy NEC 99.24
carotid artery 39.97
coronary artery 39.97
head 39.97
hyperthermic (lymphatic), localized region or site 93.35
intestine (large) (local) 46.96
small 46.95
kidney, local 55.95
limb (lower) (upper) 39.97
liver, localized 50.93
neck 39.97
subarachnoid (spinal cord) (refrigerated saline) 03.92
total body 39.96
**Pericardiectomy** 37.31
**Pericardiocentesis** 37.0
**Pericardiolysis** 37.12
**Pericardioplasty** 37.49
**Pericardiorrhaphy** 37.49
**Pericardiostomy** (tube) 37.12
**Pericardiotomy** 37.12
**Peridectomy** 10.31
**Perilimbal suction** 89.11
**Perimetry** 95.05
**Perineoplasty** 71.79
**Perineorrhaphy** 71.71
obstetrical laceration (current) 75.69
**Perineotomy** (nonobstetrical) 71.09
to assist delivery — *see* Episiotomy
**Periosteotomy** — *see also* Incision, bone 77.10
facial bone 76.09
**Perirectofistulectomy** 48.93
**Peritectomy** 10.31
**Peritomy** 10.1
**Peritoneocentesis** 54.91
**Peritoneoscopy** 54.21
**Peritoneotomy** 54.19
**Peritoneumectomy** 54.4
**Phacoemulsification** (ultrasonic) (with aspiration) 13.41
**Phacofragmentation** (mechanical) (with aspiration) 13.43

**Phacofragmentation** — *continued*
posterior route 13.42
ultrasonic 13.41
**Phalangectomy** (partial) 77.89
claw toe 77.57
cockup toe 77.58
hammer toe 77.56
overlapping toe 77.58
total 77.99
**Phalangization** (fifth metacarpal) 82.81
**Pharyngeal flap operation** (cleft palate repair) 27.62
secondary or subsequent 27.63
**Pharyngectomy** (partial) 29.33
with laryngectomy 30.3
**Pharyngogram** 87.09
contrast 87.06
**Pharyngolaryngectomy** 30.3
**Pharyngoplasty** (with silastic implant) 29.4
for cleft palate 27.62
secondary or subsequent 27.63
**Pharyngorrhaphy** 29.51
for cleft palate 27.62
**Pharyngoscopy** 29.11
**Pharyngotomy** 29.0
**Phenopeel** (skin) 86.24
**Phlebectomy** 38.60
with
anastomosis 38.30
abdominal 38.37
head and neck NEC 38.32
intracranial NEC 38.31
lower limb 38.39
thoracic NEC 38.35
upper limb 38.33
graft replacement 38.4 ☑
abdominal 38.47
head and neck NEC 38.42
intracranial NEC 38.41
lower limb 38.49
thoracic NEC 38.45
upper limb 38.43
abdominal 38.67
head and neck NEC 38.62
intracranial NEC 38.61
lower limb 38.69
thoracic NEC 38.65
upper limb 38.63
varicose 38.50
abdominal 38.57
head and neck NEC 38.52
intracranial NEC 38.51
lower limb 38.59
thoracic NEC 38.55
upper limb 38.53
**Phlebogoniostomy** 12.52
**Phlebography** (contrast) (retrograde) 88.60
by radioisotope — *see* Scan, radioisotope, by site
adrenal 88.65
femoral 88.66
head 88.61
hepatic 88.64
impedance 88.68
intra-abdominal NEC 88.65
intrathoracic NEC 88.63
lower extremity NEC 88.66
neck 88.61
portal system 88.64
pulmonary 88.62
specified site NEC 88.67
vena cava (inferior) (superior) 88.51
**Phleborrhaphy** 39.32
**Phlebotomy** 38.99
**Phonocardiogram, with ECG lead** 89.55
**Photochemotherapy** NEC 99.83
extracorporeal 99.88
**Photocoagulation**
ciliary body 12.73
eye, eyeball 16.99
iris 12.41
macular hole — *see* Photocoagulation, retina
orbital lesion 16.92

**Photocoagulation** — *continued*
retina
for
destruction of lesion 14.25
reattachment 14.55
repair of tear or defect 14.35
laser (beam)
for
destruction of lesion 14.24
reattachment 14.54
repair of tear or defect 14.34
xenon arc
for
destruction of lesion 14.23
reattachment 14.53
repair of tear or defect 14.33
**Photography** 89.39
fundus 95.11
**Photopheresis, therapeutic** 99.88
**Phototherapy** NEC 99.83
newborn 99.83
ultraviolet 99.82
**Phrenemphraxis** 04.03
for collapse of lung 33.31
**Phrenicectomy** 04.03
for collapse of lung 33.31
**Phrenicoexeresis** 04.03
for collapse of lung 33.31
**Phrenicotomy** 04.03
for collapse of lung 33.31
**Phrenicotripsy** 04.03
for collapse of lung 33.31
**Phrenoplasty** 34.84
**Physical medicine** — *see* Therapy, physical
**Physical therapy** — *see* Therapy, physical
**Physiotherapy, chest** 93.99
**PICC** (peripherally inserted central catheter) 38.93
**Piercing ear, external** (pinna) 18.01
**Pigmenting, skin** 86.02
**Pilojection** (aneurysm) (Gallagher) 39.52
**Pinealectomy** (complete) (total) 07.54
partial 07.53
**Pinealotomy** (with drainage) 07.52
**Pinning**
bone — *see* Fixation, bone, internal
ear 18.5
**Pinsker operation** (obliteration of nasoseptal telangiectasia) 21.07
**Piper operation** (forceps) 72.6
**Pirogoff operation** (ankle amputation through malleoli of tibia and fibula) 84.14
**Pituitectomy** (complete) (total) — *see also* Hypophysectomy 07.69
**Placentogram, placentography** 88.46
with radioisotope (RISA) 92.17
**Planing, skin** 86.25
**Plantation, tooth** (bud) (germ) 23.5
prosthetic 23.6
**Plasma exchange** 99.07
**Plasmapheresis, therapeutic** 99.71
**Plastic repair** — *see* Repair, by site
**Plasty** — *see also* Repair, by site
bladder neck (V-Y) 57.85
skin (without graft) 86.89
subcutaneous tissue 86.89
**Platelet inhibitor** (GP IIb/IIIa inhibitor only), infusion 99.20
**Plateletpheresis, therapeutic** 99.74
**Play**
psychotherapy 94.36
therapy 93.81
**Pleating**
eye muscle 15.22
multiple (two or more muscles) 15.4
sclera, for buckling (*see also* Buckling, scleral) 14.49
**Plethysmogram** (carotid) 89.58
air-filled (pneumatic) 89.58
capacitance 89.58
cerebral 89.58
differential 89.58

**Plethysmogram** — *continued*
oculoplethysmogram 89.58
penile 89.58
photoelectric 89.58
regional 89.58
respiratory function measurement (body) 89.38
segmental 89.58
strain-gauge 89.58
thoracic impedance 89.38
venous occlusion 89.58
water-filled 89.58
**Plethysmography**
CaverMap™ 89.58
penile 89.58
**Pleurectomy** NEC 34.59
**Pleurocentesis** 34.91
**Pleurodesis** 34.6
chemical 34.92
with cancer chemotherapy substance 34.92 [99.25]
tetracycline 34.92 [99.21]
**Pleurolysis** (for collapse of lung) 33.39
**Pleuropexy** 34.99
**Pleurosclerosis** 34.6
chemical 34.92
with cancer chemotherapy substance 34.92 [99.25]
tetracycline 34.92 [99.21]
**Pleurotomy** 34.09
**Plexectomy**
choroid 02.14
hypogastric 05.24
**Plication**
aneurysm
heart 37.32
annulus, heart valve 35.33
bleb (emphysematous), lung 32.21
broad ligament 69.22
diaphragm (for hernia repair) (thoracic approach) (thoracoabdominal approach) 53.81
eye muscle (oblique) (rectus) 15.22
multiple (two or more muscles) 15.4
fascia 83.89
hand 82.89
inferior vena cava 38.7
intestine (jejunum) (Noble) 46.62
Kelly (-Stoeckel) (urethrovesical junction) 59.3
levator, for blepharoptosis 08.34
ligament (*see also* Arthroplasty) 81.96
broad 69.22
round 69.22
uterosacral 69.22
mesentery 54.75
round ligament 69.22
sphincter, urinary bladder 57.85
stomach 44.69
laparoscopic 44.68
superior vena cava 38.7
tendon 83.85
hand 82.55
tricuspid valve (with repositioning) 35.14
ureter 56.89
urethra 58.49
urethrovesical junction 59.3
vein (peripheral) 39.59
vena cava (inferior) (superior) 38.7
ventricle (heart)
aneurysm 37.32
**Plicotomy, tympanum** 20.23
**Plombage, lung** 33.39
**Pneumocentesis** 33.93
**Pneumocisternogram** 87.02
**Pneumoencephalogram** 87.01
**Pneumogram, pneumography**
extraperitoneal 88.15
mediastinal 87.33
orbit 87.14
pelvic 88.13
peritoneum NEC 88.13
presacral 88.15
retroperitoneum 88.15

Passage of sounds, urethra — Pneumogram, pneumography

☑ Additional Digit Required — Refer to the Tabular List for Digit Selection
**2007 Ingenix**
▶◀ Revised Text ● New Line ▲ Revised Code
Subterms under main terms may continue to next column or page
**Volume 3 — 45**

Pneumogynecography — Prostatovesiculectomy

**Pneumogynecography** 87.82
**Pneumomediastinography** 87.33
**Pneumonectomy** (extended) (radical)
(standard) (total) (with mediastinal
dissection) 32.59 ▲
partial
complete excision, one lobe
32.49 ▲
resection (wedge), one lobe
32.39 ▲
thoracoscopic 32.50 ●
**Pneumonolysis** (for collapse of lung)
33.39
**Pneumonotomy** (with exploration) 33.1
**Pneumoperitoneum** (surgically-induced)
54.96
for collapse of lung 33.33
pelvic 88.12
**Pneumothorax** (artificial) (surgical) 33.32
intrapleural 33.32
**Pneumoventriculogram** 87.02
**Politano-Leadbetter operation**
(ureteroneocystostomy) 56.74
**Politerization, Eustachian tube** 20.8
**Pollicization** (with carry over of nerves
and blood supply) 82.61
**Polya operation** (gastrectomy) 43.7
**Polypectomy** — see also Excision, lesion, by site
esophageal 42.32
endoscopic 42.33
gastric (endoscopic) 43.41
large intestine (colon) 45.42
nasal 21.31
rectum (endoscopic) 48.36
**Polysomnogram** 89.17
**Pomeroy operation** (ligation and division
of fallopian tubes) 66.32
**Poncet operation**
lengthening of Achilles tendon 83.85
urethrostomy, perineal 58.0
**Porro operation** (cesarean section) 74.99
**Portoenterostomy** (Kasai) 51.37
**Positrocephalogram** 92.11
**Positron emission tomography** (PET)
— see Scan, radioisotope
**Postmortem examination** 89.8
**Potts-Smith operation** (descending
aorta-left pulmonary artery anastomosis) 39.0
**Poudrage**
intrapericardial 36.39
pleural 34.6
**PPN** (peripheral parenteral nutrition)
99.15
**Preparation** (cutting), pedicle (flap) graft
86.71
**Preputiotomy** 64.91
**Prescription for glasses** 95.31
**Pressure support**
ventilation [PSV] — see category
96.7 ☑
**Pressurized**
graft treatment 00.16
**Printen and Mason operation** (high
gastric bypass) 44.31
**Probing**
canaliculus, lacrimal (with irrigation)
09.42
lacrimal
canaliculi 09.42
punctum (with irrigation) 09.41
nasolacrimal duct (with irrigation)
09.43
with insertion of tube or stent
09.44
salivary duct (for dilation of duct) (for
removal of calculus) 26.91
with incision 26.0
**Procedure** — see also specific procedure
diagnostic NEC
abdomen (region) 54.29
adenoid 28.19
adrenal gland 07.19
alveolus 24.19
amnion 75.35

**Procedure** — see also specific procedure
— continued
diagnostic — continued
anterior chamber, eye 12.29
anus 49.29
appendix 45.28
biliary tract 51.19
bladder 57.39
blood vessel (any site) 38.29
bone 78.80
carpal, metacarpal 78.84
clavicle 78.81
facial 76.19
femur 78.85
fibula 78.87
humerus 78.82
marrow 41.38
patella 78.86
pelvic 78.89
phalanges (foot) (hand) 78.89
radius 78.83
scapula 78.81
specified site NEC 78.89
tarsal, metatarsal 78.88
thorax (ribs) (sternum) 78.81
tibia 78.87
ulna 78.83
vertebrae 78.89
brain 01.18
breast 85.19
bronchus 33.29
buccal 27.24
bursa 83.29
canthus 08.19
cecum 45.28
cerebral meninges 01.18
cervix 67.19
chest wall 34.28
choroid 14.19
ciliary body 12.29
clitoris 71.19
colon 45.28
conjunctiva 10.29
cornea 11.29
cul-de-sac 70.29
dental 24.19
diaphragm 34.28
duodenum 45.19
ear
external 18.19
inner and middle 20.39
epididymis 63.09
esophagus 42.29
Eustachian tube 20.39
extraocular muscle or tendon
15.09
eye 16.29
anterior chamber 12.29
posterior chamber 14.19
eyeball 16.29
eyelid 08.19
fallopian tube 66.19
fascia (any site) 83.29
fetus 75.35
gallbladder 51.19
ganglion (cranial) (peripheral) 04.19
sympathetic 05.19
gastric 44.19
globus pallidus 01.18
gum 24.19
heart 37.29
hepatic 50.19
hypophysis 07.19
ileum 45.19
intestine 45.29
large 45.28
small 45.19
iris 12.29
jejunum 45.19
joint (capsule) (ligament) (structure)
NEC 81.98
facial 76.19
kidney 55.29
labia 71.19
lacrimal (system) 09.19
large intestine 45.28

**Procedure** — see also specific procedure
— continued
diagnostic — continued
larynx 31.48
ligament 81.98
uterine 68.19
liver 50.19
lung 33.29
lymphatic structure (channel)
(gland) (node) (vessel) 40.19
mediastinum 34.29
meninges (cerebral) 01.18
spinal 03.39
mouth 27.29
muscle 83.29
extraocular (oblique) (rectus)
15.09
papillary (heart) 37.29
nail 86.19
nasopharynx 29.19
nerve (cranial) (peripheral) NEC
04.19
sympathetic 05.19
nipple 85.19
nose, nasal 21.29
sinus 22.19
ocular 16.29
muscle 15.09
omentum 54.29
ophthalmologic 16.29
oral (cavity) 27.29
orbit 16.29
orthodontic 24.19
ovary 65.19
laparoscopic 65.14
palate 27.29
pancreas 52.19
papillary muscle (heart) 37.29
parathyroid gland 06.19
penis 64.19
perianal tissue 49.29
pericardium 37.29
periprostatic tissue 60.18
perirectal tissue 48.29
perirenal tissue 59.29
peritoneum 54.29
periurethral tissue 58.29
perivesical tissue 59.29
pharynx 29.19
pineal gland 07.19
pituitary gland 07.19
pleura 34.28
posterior chamber, eye 14.19
prostate 60.18
pulmonary 33.29
rectosigmoid 48.29
rectum 48.29
renal 55.29
respiratory 33.29
retina 14.19
retroperitoneum 59.29
salivary gland or duct 26.19
sclera 12.29
scrotum 61.19
seminal vesicle 60.19
sigmoid 45.28
sinus, nasal 22.19
skin 86.19
skull 01.19
soft tissue 83.29
spermatic cord 63.09
sphincter of Oddi 51.19
spine, spinal (canal) (cord)
(meninges) (structure) 03.39
spleen 41.39
stomach 44.19
subcutaneous tissue 86.19
sympathetic nerve 05.19
tarsus 09.19
tendon NEC 83.29
extraocular 15.09
testicle 62.19
thalamus 01.18
thoracic duct 40.19
thorax 34.28
thymus 07.19

**Procedure** — see also specific procedure
— continued
diagnostic — continued
thyroid gland 06.19
tongue 25.09
tonsils 28.19
tooth 24.19
trachea 31.49
tunica vaginalis 61.19
ureter 56.39
urethra 58.29
uterus and supporting structures
68.19
uvula 27.29
vagina 70.29
vas deferens 63.09
vesical 57.39
vessel (blood) (any site) 38.29
vitreous 14.19
vulva 71.19
fistulizing, sclera NEC 12.69
miscellaneous (nonoperative) NEC
99.99
respiratory (nonoperative) NEC 93.99
surgical — see Operation
**Proctectasis** 96.22
**Proctectomy** (partial) — see also Resection, rectum 48.69
abdominoperineal 48.5
complete (Miles) (Rankin) 48.5
pull-through 48.49
**Proctoclysis** 96.37
**Proctolysis** 48.99
**Proctopexy** (Delorme) 48.76
abdominal (Ripstein) 48.75
**Proctoplasty** 48.79
**Proctorrhaphy** 48.71
**Proctoscopy** 48.23
with biopsy 48.24
through stoma (artificial) 48.22
transabdominal approach 48.21
**Proctosigmoidectomy** — see also Resection, rectum 48.69
**Proctosigmoidopexy** 48.76
**Proctosigmoidoscopy** (rigid) 48.23
with biopsy 48.24
flexible 45.24
through stoma (artificial) 48.22
transabdominal approach 48.21
**Proctostomy** 48.1
**Proctotomy** (decompression) (linear) 48.0
**Production** — see also Formation and
Creation
atrial septal defect 35.42
subcutaneous tunnel for esophageal
anastomosis 42.86
with anastomosis — see Anastomosis, esophagus, antesternal
**Prognathic recession** 76.64
**Prophylaxis, dental** (scaling) (polishing)
96.54
**Prostatectomy** (complete) (partial) NEC
60.69
loop 60.29
perineal 60.62
radical (any approach) 60.5
retropubic (punch) (transcapsular)
60.4
suprapubic (punch) (transvesical) 60.3
transcapsular NEC 60.69
retropubic 60.4
transperineal 60.62
transurethral 60.29
ablation (contact) (noncontact) by
laser 60.21
electrovaporization 60.29
enucleative 60.29
resection of prostate (TURP) 60.29
ultrasound guided laser induced
(TULIP) 60.21
transvesical punch (suprapubic) 60.3
**Prostatocystotomy** 60.0
**Prostatolithotomy** 60.0
**Prostatotomy** (perineal) 60.0
**Prostatovesiculectomy** 60.5

Index

Removal — Removal

**Removal** — *see also* Excision — *continued*
blood clot (*see also* Incision, by site) — *continued*
  bladder — *continued*
    without incision 57.0
  kidney (without incision) 56.0
    by incision 55.01
  ureter
    by incision 56.2
bone fragment (chip) (*see also* Incision, bone) 77.10
  joint (*see also* Arthrotomy) 80.10
  necrotic (*see also* Sequestrectomy, bone) 77.00
    joint (*see also* Arthrotomy) 80.10
  skull 01.25
    with debridement compound fracture 02.02
bone growth stimulator — *see* category 78.6 ☑
bony spicules, spinal canal 03.53
brace 97.88
breast implant 85.94
  tissue expander 85.96
bronchial device or substance
  endoscopic 33.78
calcareous deposit
  bursa 83.03
    hand 82.03
  tendon, intratendinous 83.39
    hand 82.29
calcification, heart valve leaflets — *see* Valvuloplasty, heart
calculus
  bile duct (by incision) 51.49
    endoscopic 51.88
    laparoscopic 51.88
    percutaneous 51.98
  bladder (by incision) 57.19
    without incision 57.0
  common duct (by incision) 51.41
    endoscopic 51.88
    laparoscopic 51.88
    percutaneous 51.96
  gallbladder 51.04
    endoscopic 51.88
    laparoscopic 51.88
  kidney (by incision) 55.01
    without incision (transurethral) 56.0
    percutaneous 55.03
      with fragmentation (ultrasound) 55.04
    renal pelvis (by incision) 55.11
      percutaneous nephrostomy 55.03
        with fragmentation 55.04
      transurethral 56.0
lacrimal
  canaliculi 09.42
    by incision 09.52
  gland 09.3
    by incision 09.0
  passage(s) 09.49
    by incision 09.59
  punctum 09.41
    by incision 09.51
  sac 09.49
    by incision 09.53
pancreatic duct (by incision) 52.09
  endoscopic 52.94
perirenal tissue 59.09
pharynx 29.39
prostate 60.0
salivary gland (by incision) 26.0
  by probe 26.91
ureter (by incision) 56.2
  without incision 56.0
urethra (by incision) 58.0
  without incision 58.6
caliper tongs (skull) 02.95

**Removal** — *see also* Excision — *continued*
cannula
  for extracorporeal membrane oxygenation (ECMO) — omit code
cardiac pacemaker (device) (initial) (permanent) (cardiac resynchronization device, CRT-P) 37.89
  with replacement
    cardiac resynchronization pacemaker (CRT-P)
      device only 00.53
      total system 00.50
    dual-chamber 37.87
    single-chamber device 37.85
    rate responsive 37.86
cardioverter/defibrillator pulse generator without replacement (cardiac resynchronization defibrillator device (CRT-D) 37.79
cast 97.88
  with reapplication 97.13
    lower limb 97.12
    upper limb 97.11
catheter (indwelling) (*see also* Removal, tube)
  bladder 97.64
  cranial cavity 01.27
  middle ear (tympanum) 20.1
  ureter 97.62
  urinary 97.64
  ventricular (cerebral) 02.43
    with synchronous replacement 02.42
cerclage material, cervix 69.96
cerumen, ear 96.52
corneal epithelium 11.41
  for smear or culture 11.21
coronary artery obstruction (thrombus) 36.09
  direct intracoronary artery infusion 36.04
  open chest approach 36.03
  percutaneous transluminal (balloon) 00.66

> *Note* — Also use 00.40, 00.41, 00.42, or 00.43 to show the total number of vessels treated. Use code 00.44 once to show procedure on a bifurcated vessel. In addition, use 00.45, 00.46, 00.47, or 00.48 to show the number of vascular stents inserted.

Crutchfield tongs (skull) 02.95
  with synchronous replacement 02.94
cyst (*see also* Excision, lesion, by site)
  dental 24.4
  lung 32.29
    endoscopic 32.28
    thoracoscopic 32.20 ●
cystic duct remnant 51.61
decidua (by)
  aspiration curettage 69.52
  curettage (D and C) 69.02
  manual 75.4
dental wiring (immobilization device) 97.33
  orthodontic 24.8
device (therapeutic) NEC 97.89
  for musculoskeletal immobilization NEC 97.88
  abdomen NEC 97.86
  bronchus 33.78
    valve 33.78
  digestive system NEC 97.59
  drainage — *see* Removal, tube
  external fixation device 97.88
    mandibular NEC 97.36
    minifixator (bone) — *see* category 78.6 ☑
  genital tract NEC 97.79
  head and neck NEC 97.39
  intrauterine contraceptive 97.71
  spine 80.09
  thorax NEC 97.49

**Removal** — *see also* Excision — *continued*
device — *continued*
  trunk NEC 97.87
  urinary system NEC 97.69
diaphragm, vagina 97.73
drainage device — *see* Removal, tube
dye, spinal canal 03.31
ectopic fetus (from) 66.02
  abdominal cavity 74.3
  extraperitoneal (intraligamentous) 74.3
  fallopian tube (by salpingostomy) 66.02
    by salpingotomy 66.01
    with salpingectomy 66.62
  intraligamentous 74.3
  ovarian 74.3
  peritoneal (following uterine or tubal rupture) 74.3
  site NEC 74.3
  tubal (by salpingostomy) 66.02
    by salpingotomy 66.01
    with salpingectomy 66.62
electrodes
  bone growth stimulator — *see* category 78.6 ☑
  brain 01.22
    depth 01.22
      with synchronous replacement 02.93
    foramen ovale 01.22
      with synchronous replacement 02.93
    sphenoidal — *omit code*
      with synchronous replacement 02.96
  cardiac pacemaker (atrial) (transvenous) (ventricular) 37.77
    with replacement 37.76
  carotid sinus 04.93 ●
    with synchronous replacement ● 04.92 ●
  depth 01.22
    with synchronous replacement 02.93
  epicardial (myocardial) 37.77
    with replacement (by)
      atrial and/or ventricular lead(s) (electrode) 37.76
      epicardial lead 37.74
  epidural pegs 01.22
    with synchronous replacement 02.93
  foramen ovale 01.22
    with synchronous replacement 02.93
  gastric 04.93
    with synchronous replacement 04.92
  intracranial 01.22
    with synchronous replacement 02.93
  peripheral nerve 04.93
    with synchronous replacement 04.92
  sacral nerve 04.93
  sphenoidal — *omit code*
    with synchronous replacement 02.96
  spinal 03.94
    with synchronous replacement 03.93
  temporary transvenous pacemaker system — *omit code*
electroencephalographic receiver (brain) (intracranial) 01.22
  with synchronous replacement 02.93
electronic
  stimulator — *see* Removal, neurostimulator, by site
    bladder 57.98
    bone 78.6 ☑

**Removal** — *see also* Excision — *continued*
electronic — *continued*
  stimulator — *see* Removal, neurostimulator, by site — *continued*
    skeletal muscle 83.93
      with synchronous replacement 83.92
    ureter 56.94
electrostimulator — *see* Removal, electronic, stimulator, by site
embolus 38.00
  with endarterectomy — *see* Endarterectomy
  abdominal
    artery 38.06
    vein 38.07
  aorta (arch) (ascending) (descending) 38.04
  arteriovenous shunt or cannula 39.49
  bovine graft 39.49
  head and neck vessel
    endovascular approach 39.74
    open approach, intracranial vessels 38.01
    open approach, other vessels of head and neck 38.02
  intracranial vessel
    endovascular approach 39.74
    open approach, intracranial vessels 38.01
    open approach, other vessels of head and neck 38.02
  lower limb
    artery 38.08
    vein 38.09
  pulmonary (artery) (vein) 38.05
  thoracic vessel NEC 38.05
  upper limb (artery) (vein) 38.03
embryo — *see* Removal, ectopic fetus
encircling tube, eye (episcleral) 14.6
epithelial downgrowth, anterior chamber 12.93
external fixation device 97.88
  mandibular NEC 97.36
  minifixator (bone) — *see* category 78.6 ☑
extrauterine embryo — *see* Removal, ectopic fetus
eyeball 16.49
  with implant 16.42
    with attachment of muscles 16.41
fallopian tube — *see* Salpingectomy
feces (impacted) (by flushing) (manual) 96.38
fetus, ectopic — *see* Removal, ectopic fetus
fingers, supernumerary 86.26
fixation device
  external 97.88
    mandibular NEC 97.36
    minifixator (bone) — *see* category 78.6 ☑
  internal 78.60
    carpal, metacarpal 78.64
    clavicle 78.61
    facial (bone) 76.97
    femur 78.65
    fibula 78.67
    humerus 78.62
    patella 78.66
    pelvic 78.69
    phalanges (foot) (hand) 78.69
    radius 78.63
    scapula 78.61
    specified site NEC 78.69
    tarsal, metatarsal 78.68
    thorax (ribs) (sternum) 78.61
    tibia 78.67
    ulna 78.63
    vertebrae 78.69
foreign body NEC (*see also* Incision, by site) 98.20

**Removal** — *see also* Excision — *continued*
foreign body (*see also* Incision, by site) — *continued*
abdominal (cavity) 54.92
  wall 54.0
adenoid 98.13
  by incision 28.91
alveolus, alveolar bone 98.22
  by incision 24.0
antecubital fossa 98.27
  by incision 86.05
anterior chamber 12.00
  by incision 12.02
    with use of magnet 12.01
anus (intraluminal) 98.05
  by incision 49.93
artifical stoma (intraluminal) 98.18
auditory canal, external 18.02
axilla 98.27
  by incision 86.05
bladder (without incision) 57.0
  by incision 57.19
bone, except fixation device (*see also* Incision, bone) 77.10
  alveolus, alveolar 98.22
    by incision 24.0
brain 01.39
  without incision into brain 01.24
breast 85.0
bronchus (intraluminal) 98.15
  by incision 33.0
bursa 83.03
  hand 82.03
canthus 98.22
  by incision 08.51
cerebral meninges 01.31
cervix (intraluminal) NEC 98.16
  penetrating 69.97
choroid (by incision) 14.00
  with use of magnet 14.01
  without use of magnet 14.02
ciliary body (by incision) 12.00
  with use of magnet 12.01
  without use of magnet 12.02
conjunctiva (by magnet) 98.22
  by incision 10.0
cornea 98.21
  by
    incision 11.1
    magnet 11.0
duodenum 98.03
  by incision 45.01
ear (intraluminal) 98.11
  with incision 18.09
epididymis 63.92
esophagus (intraluminal) 98.02
  by incision 42.09
extrapleural (by incision) 34.01
eye, eyeball (by magnet) 98.21
  anterior segment (by incision) 12.00
    with use of magnet 12.01
    without use of magnet 12.02
  posterior segment (by incision) 14.00
    with use of magnet 14.01
    without use of magnet 14.02
  superficial 98.21
eyelid 98.22
  by incision 08.09
fallopian tube
  by salpingostomy 66.02
  by salpingotomy 66.01
fascia 83.09
  hand 82.09
foot 98.28
gall bladder 51.04
groin region (abdominal wall) (inguinal) 54.0
gum 98.22
  by incision 24.0
hand 98.26
head and neck NEC 98.22
heart 37.11

**Removal** — *see also* Excision — *continued*
foreign body (*see also* Incision, by site) — *continued*
internal fixation device — *see* Removal, fixation device, internal
intestine
  by incision 45.00
  large (intraluminal) 98.04
    by incision 45.03
  small (intraluminal) 98.03
    by incision 45.02
intraocular (by incision) 12.00
  with use of magnet 12.01
  without use of magnet 12.02
iris (by incision) 12.00
  with use of magnet 12.01
  without use of magnet 12.02
joint structures (*see also* Arthrotomy) 80.10
kidney (transurethral) (by endoscopy) 56.0
  by incision 55.01
  pelvis (transurethral) 56.0
    by incision 55.11
labia 98.23
  by incision 71.09
lacrimal
  canaliculi 09.42
    by incision 09.52
  gland 09.3
    by incision 09.0
  passage(s) 09.49
    by incision 09.59
  punctum 09.41
    by incision 09.51
  sac 09.49
    by incision 09.53
large intestine (intraluminal) 98.04
  by incision 45.03
larynx (intraluminal) 98.14
  by incision 31.3
lens 13.00
  by incision 13.02
    with use of magnet 13.01
liver 50.0
lower limb, except foot 98.29
  foot 98.28
lung 33.1
mediastinum 34.1
meninges (cerebral) 01.31
  spinal 03.01
mouth (intraluminal) 98.01
  by incision 27.92
muscle 83.02
  hand 82.02
nasal sinus 22.50
  antrum 22.2
    with Caldwell-Luc approach 22.39
  ethmoid 22.51
  frontal 22.41
  maxillary 22.2
    with Caldwell-Luc approach 22.39
  sphenoid 22.52
nerve (cranial) (peripheral) NEC 04.04
  root 03.01
nose (intraluminal) 98.12
  by incision 21.1
oral cavity (intraluminal) 98.01
  by incision 27.92
orbit (by magnet) 98.21
  by incision 16.1
palate (penetrating) 98.22
  by incision 27.1
pancreas 52.09
penis 98.24
  by incision 64.92
pericardium 37.12
perineum (female) 98.23
  by incision 71.09
  male 98.25
    by incision 86.05

**Removal** — *see also* Excision — *continued*
foreign body (*see also* Incision, by site) — *continued*
perirenal tissue 59.09
peritoneal cavity 54.92
perivesical tissue 59.19
pharynx (intraluminal) 98.13
  by pharyngotomy 29.0
pleura (by incision) 34.09
popliteal space 98.29
  by incision 86.05
rectum (intraluminal) 98.05
  by incision 48.0
renal pelvis (transurethral) 56.0
  by incision 56.1
retina (by incision) 14.00
  with use of magnet 14.01
  without use of magnet 14.02
retroperitoneum 54.92
sclera (by incision) 12.00
  with use of magnet 12.01
  without use of magnet 12.02
scrotum 98.24
  by incision 61.0
sinus (nasal) 22.50
  antrum 22.2
    with Caldwell-Luc approach 22.39
  ethmoid 22.51
  frontal 22.41
  maxillary 22.2
    with Caldwell-Luc approach 22.39
  sphenoid 22.52
skin NEC 98.20
  by incision 86.05
skull 01.24
  with incision into brain 01.39
small intestine (intraluminal) 98.03
  by incision 45.02
soft tissue NEC 83.09
  hand 82.09
spermatic cord 63.93
spinal (canal) (cord) (meninges) 03.01
stomach (intraluminal) 98.03
  by incision 43.0
  bubble (balloon) 44.94
subconjunctival (by magnet) 98.22
  by incision 10.0
subcutaneous tissue NEC 98.20
  by incision 86.05
supraclavicular fossa 98.27
  by incision 86.05
tendon (sheath) 83.01
  hand 82.01
testis 62.0
thorax (by incision) 34.09
thyroid (field) (gland) (by incision) 06.09
tonsil 98.13
  by incision 28.91
trachea (intraluminal) 98.15
  by incision 31.3
trunk NEC 98.25
tunica vaginalis 98.24
upper limb, except hand 98.27
  hand 98.26
ureter (transurethral) 56.0
  by incision 56.2
urethra (intraluminal) 98.19
  by incision 58.0
uterus (intraluminal) 98.16
vagina (intraluminal) 98.17
  by incision 70.14
vas deferens 63.6
vitreous (by incision) 14.00
  with use of magnet 14.01
  without use of magnet 14.02
vulva 98.23
  by incision 71.09
gallstones
  bile duct (by incision) NEC 51.49
    endoscopic 51.88
  common duct (by incision) 51.41

**Removal** — *see also* Excision — *continued*
gallstones — *continued*
  common duct — *continued*
    endoscopic 51.88
    percutaneous 51.96
  duodenum 45.01
  gallbladder 51.04
    endoscopic 51.88
    laparoscopic 51.88
  hepatic ducts 51.49
    endoscopic 51.88
  intestine 45.00
    large 45.03
    small NEC 45.02
  liver 50.0
Gardner Wells tongs (skull) 02.95
  with synchronous replacement 02.94
gastric band (adjustable), laparoscopic 44.97
gastric bubble (balloon) 44.94
granulation tissue (*see also* Excision, lesion, by site)
  with repair — *see* Repair, by site
  cranial 01.6
  skull 01.6
halo traction device (skull) 02.95
  with synchronous replacement 02.94
heart assist system
  with replacement 37.63
  intra-aortic balloon pump (IABP) 97.44
  nonoperative 97.44
  open removal 37.64
  percutaneous external device 97.44
hematoma — *see* Drainage, by site
Hoffman minifixator device (bone) — *see* category 78.6 ☑
hydatidiform mole 68.0
impacted
  feces (rectum) (by flushing) (manual) 96.38
  tooth 23.19
    from nasal sinus (maxillary) 22.61
implant
  breast 85.94
  cochlear prosthetic device 20.99
  cornea 11.92
  lens (prosthetic) 13.8
  middle ear NEC 20.99
  ocular 16.71
    posterior segment 14.6
  orbit 16.72
  retina 14.6
  tympanum 20.1
implantable hemodynamic sensor (lead) and monitor device 37.79
internal fixation device — *see* Removal, fixation device, internal
intra-aortic balloon pump (IABP) 97.44
intrauterine contraceptive device (IUD) 97.71
joint (structure) NOS 80.90
  ankle 80.97
  elbow 80.92
  foot and toe 80.98
  hand and finger 80.94
  hip 80.95
  knee 80.96
  other specified sites 80.99
  shoulder 80.91
  spine 80.99
  toe 80.98
  wrist 80.93
Kantrowitz heart pump 37.64
  nonoperative 97.44
keel (tantalum plate), larynx 31.98
kidney (*see also* Nephrectomy)
  mechanical 55.98
  transplanted or rejected 55.53
laminaria (tent), uterus 97.79

☑ Additional Digit Required — Refer to the Tabular List for Digit Selection
**2007 Ingenix**
▶◀ Revised Text    ● New Line    ▲ Revised Code
Subterms under main terms may continue to next column or page
**Volume 3 — 51**

**Removal** — see also Excision — continued
tube — continued
mediastinum 97.42
nephrostomy 97.61
pancreas 97.56
peritoneum 97.82
pleural cavity 97.41
pyelostomy 97.61
retroperitoneum 97.81
small intestine 97.52
thoracotomy 97.41
tracheostomy 97.37
tympanostomy 20.1
tympanum 20.1
ureterostomy 97.62
ureteral splint (stent) 97.62
urethral sphincter, artificial 58.99
with replacement 58.93
urinary sphincter, artificial 58.99
with replacement 58.93
utricle 20.79
valve
vas deferens 63.85
ventricular (cerebral) 02.43
vascular graft or prosthesis 39.49
ventricular shunt or reservoir 02.43
with synchronous replacement 02.42
Vinke tongs (skull) 02.95
with synchronous replacement 02.94
vitreous (with replacement) 14.72
anterior approach (partial) 14.71
open sky technique 14.71
Wagner-Brooker minifixator device (bone) — see category 78.6 ☑
wiring, dental (immobilization device) 97.33
orthodontic 24.8
**Renipuncture** (percutaneous) 55.92
**Renogram** 92.03
**Renotransplantation** NEC 55.69

Note — To report donor source:
cadaver 00.93
live non-related donor 00.92
live related donor 00.91
live unrelated donor 00.92

**Reopening** — see also Incision, by site
blepharorrhaphy 08.02
canthorrhaphy 08.02
cilia base 08.71
craniotomy or craniectomy site 01.23
fallopian tube (divided) 66.79
iris in anterior chambers 12.97
laminectomy or laminotomy site 03.02
laparotomy site 54.12
osteotomy site (see also Incision, bone) 77.10
facial bone 76.09
tarsorrhaphy 08.02
thoracotomy site (for control of hemorrhage) (for examination) (for exploration) 34.03
thyroid field wound (for control of hemorrhage) (for examination) (for exploration) (for removal of hematoma) 06.02
**Repacking** — see Replacement, pack, by site
**Repair**
abdominal wall 54.72
adrenal gland 07.44
alveolus, alveolar (process) (ridge) (with graft) (with implant) 24.5
anal sphincter 49.79
artificial sphincter
implantation 49.75
revision 49.75
laceration (by suture) 49.71
obstetric (current) 75.62
old 49.79
aneurysm (false) (true) 39.52
by or with
clipping 39.51
coagulation 39.52

**Repair** — continued
aneurysm — continued
by or with — continued
coil (endovascular approach) 39.79
head and neck 39.72
electrocoagulation 39.52
with
anastomosis — see Aneurysmectomy, with anastomosis, by site
graft replacement — see Aneurysmectomy, with graft replacement, by site
excision or resection of vessel (see also Aneurysmectomy, by site)
endovascular graft 39.79
abdominal aorta 39.71
head and neck 39.72
lower extremity artery(s) 39.79
thoracic aorta 39.73
upper extremity artery(s) 39.79
filipuncture 39.52
graft replacement — see Aneurysmectomy, with graft replacement, by site
ligation 39.52
liquid tissue adhesive (glue) 39.79
endovascular approach 39.79
head and neck 39.72
methyl methacrylate 39.52
endovascular approach 39.79
head and neck 39.72
occlusion 39.52
endovascular approach 39.79
head and neck 39.72
suture 39.52
trapping 39.52
wiring 39.52
wrapping (gauze) (methyl methacrylate) (plastic) 39.52
coronary artery 36.91
heart 37.32
sinus of Valsalva 35.39
thoracic aorta (dissecting), by fenestration 39.54
anomalous pulmonary venous connection (total)
one-stage 35.82
partial — see specific procedure
total 35.82
anus 49.79
laceration (by suture) 49.71
obstetric (current) 75.62
old 49.79
aorta 39.31
aorticopulmonary window 39.59
arteriovenous fistula 39.53
by or with
clipping 39.53
coagulation 39.53
coil (endovascular approach) 39.79
head and neck vessels 39.72
division 39.53
excision or resection (see also Aneurysmectomy, by site)
with
anastomosis — see Aneurysmectomy, with anastomosis, by site
graft replacement — see Aneurysmectomy, with graft replacement, by site

**Repair** — continued
arteriovenous fistula — continued
by or with — continued
ligation 39.53
coronary artery 36.99
occlusion 39.53
endovascular approach 39.79
head and neck 39.72
suture 39.53
artery NEC 39.59
by
endovascular approach
abdominal aorta 39.71
head and neck (embolization or occlusion) 39.72
other repair (of aneurysm) 39.79
percutaneous repair of intracranial vessel(s) (for stent insertion) 00.62

Note — Also use 00.40, 00.41, 00.42, or 00.43 to show the total number of vessels treated. Use code 00.44 once to show procedure on a bifurcated vessel. In addition, use 00.45, 00.46, 00.47, or 00.48 to show the number of vascular stents inserted.

percutaneous repair of precerebral (extracranial) vessel(s) (for stent insertion) 00.61

Note — Also use 00.40, 00.41, 00.42, or 00.43 to show the total number of vessels treated. Use code 00.44 once to show procedure on a bifurcated vessel. In addition, use 00.45, 00.46, 00.47, or 00.48 to show the number of vascular stents inserted.

thoracic aorta 39.73
non-coronary percutaneous transluminal angioplasty or atherectomy

Note — Also use 00.40, 00.41, 00.42, or 00.43 to show the total number of vessels treated. Use code 00.44 once to show procedure on a bifurcated vessel. In addition, use 00.45, 00.46, 00.47, or 00.48 to show the number of vascular stents inserted.

basilar 00.61
carotid 00.61
femoropopliteal 39.50
iliac 39.50
lower extremity NOS 39.50
mesenteric 39.50
renal 39.50
upper extremity NOS 39.50
vertebral 00.61
with
patch graft 39.58
with excision or resection of vessel — see Arteriectomy, with graft replacement, by site
synthetic (Dacron) (Teflon) 39.57
tissue (vein) (autogenous) (homograft) 39.56
suture 39.31
coronary NEC 36.99
by angioplasty — see Angioplasty, coronary
by atherectomy — see Angioplasty, coronary
artificial opening — see Repair, stoma
atrial septal defect 35.71
with
prosthesis (open heart technique) 35.51
closed heart technique 35.52
tissue graft 35.61

**Repair** — continued
atrial septal defect — continued
combined with repair of valvular and ventricular septal defects — see Repair, endocardial cushion defect
in total repair of total anomalous pulmonary venous connection 35.82
atrioventricular canal defect (any type) 35.73
with
prosthesis 35.54
tissue graft 35.63
bifid digit (finger) 82.89
bile duct NEC 51.79
laceration (by suture) NEC 51.79
common bile duct 51.71
bladder NEC 57.89
for stress incontinence — see Repair, stress incontinence
exstrophy 57.86
laceration (by suture) 57.81
obstetric (current) 75.61
old 57.89
neck 57.85
blepharophimosis 08.59
blepharoptosis 08.36
by
frontalis muscle technique (with)
fascial sling 08.32
suture 08.31
levator muscle technique 08.34
with resection or advancement 08.33
orbicularis oculi muscle sling 08.36
tarsal technique 08.35
blood vessel NEC 39.59
with
patch graft 39.58
with excision or resection — see Angiectomy, with graft replacement
synthetic (Dacron) (Teflon) 39.57
tissue (vein) (autogenous) (homograft) 39.56
resection — see Angiectomy
suture 39.30
coronary artery NEC 36.99
by angioplasty — see Angioplasty, coronary
by atherectomy — see Angioplasty, coronary
peripheral vessel NEC 39.59
by angioplasty 39.50

Note — Also use 00.40, 00.41, 00.42, or 00.43 to show the total number of vessels treated. Use code 00.44 once to show procedure on a bifurcated vessel. In addition, use 00.45, 00.46, 00.47, or 00.48 to show the number of vascular stents inserted.

by atherectomy 39.50

Note — Also use 00.40, 00.41, 00.42, or 00.43 to show the total number of vessels treated. Use code 00.44 once to show procedure on a bifurcated vessel. In addition, use 00.45, 00.46, 00.47, or 00.48 to show the number of vascular stents inserted.

by endovascular approach 39.79
bone NEC (see also Osteoplasty) — see category 78.4 ☑
by synostosis technique — see Arthrodesis
for malunion, nonunion, or delayed union of fracture — see Repair, fracture, malunion or nonunion
accessory sinus 22.79
cranium NEC 02.06
with
flap (bone) 02.03

Index — Removal — Repair

☑ Additional Digit Required — Refer to the Tabular List for Digit Selection
2007 Ingenix
▶◀ Revised Text    ● New Line    ▲ Revised Code
Subterms under main terms may continue to next column or page
Volume 3 — 53

**Repair** — *continued*
  bone (*see also* Osteoplasty — *see* category) — *continued*
    cranium — *continued*
      with — *continued*
        graft (bone) 02.04
      nasal 21.89
      skull NEC 02.06
        with
          flap (bone) 02.03
          graft (bone) 02.04
  bottle, hydrocele of tunica vaginalis 61.2
  brain (trauma) NEC 02.92
  breast (plastic) (*see also* Mammoplasty) 85.89
  broad ligament 69.29
  bronchus NEC 33.48
    laceration (by suture) 33.41
  bunionette (with osteotomy) 77.54
  canaliculus, lacrimal 09.73
  canthus (lateral) 08.59
  cardiac pacemaker NEC 37.89
    electrode(s) (lead) NEC 37.75
  cardioverter/defibrillator (automatic)
    pocket (skin) (subcutaneous) 37.99
  cerebral meninges 02.12
  cervix 67.69
    internal os 67.59
      transabdominal 67.51
      transvaginal 67.59
    laceration (by suture) 67.61
      obstetric (current) 75.51
      old 67.69
  chest wall (mesh) (silastic) NEC 34.79
  chordae tendineae 35.32
  choroid NEC 14.9
    with retinal repair — *see* Repair, retina
  cisterna chyli 40.69
  claw toe 77.57
  cleft
    hand 82.82
    laryngotracheal 31.69
    lip 27.54
    palate 27.62
      secondary or subsequent 27.63
  coarctation of aorta — *see* Excision, coarctation of aorta
  cochlear prosthetic device 20.99
    external components only 95.49
  cockup toe 77.58
  colostomy 46.43
  conjunctiva NEC 10.49
    with scleral repair 12.81
    laceration 10.6
      with repair of sclera 12.81
    late effect of trachoma 10.49
  cornea NEC 11.59
    with
      conjunctival flap 11.53
      transplant — *see* Keratoplasty
    postoperative dehiscence 11.52
  coronary artery NEC 36.99
    by angioplasty — *see* Angioplasty, coronary
    by atherectomy — *see* Angioplasty, coronary
  cranium NEC 02.06
    with
      flap (bone) 02.03
      graft (bone) 02.04
  cusp, valve — *see* Repair, heart, valve
  cystocele 70.51
    with graft or prosthesis 70.54 ●
    and rectocele 70.50
      with graft or prosthesis 70.53 ●
  dental arch 24.8
  diaphragm NEC 34.84
  diastasis recti 83.65
  diastematomyelia 03.59
  ear (external) 18.79
    auditory canal or meatus 18.6
    auricle NEC 18.79
    cartilage NEC 18.79

**Repair** — *continued*
  ear — *continued*
    laceration (by suture) 18.4
    lop ear 18.79
    middle NEC 19.9
    prominent or protruding 18.5
  ectropion 08.49
    by or with
      lid reconstruction 08.44
      suture (technique) 08.42
      thermocauterization 08.41
      wedge resection 08.43
  encephalocele (cerebral) 02.12
  endocardial cushion defect 35.73
    with
      prosthesis (grafted to septa) 35.54
      tissue graft 35.63
  enterocele (female) 70.92
    with graft or prosthesis 70.93 ●
    male 53.9
  enterostomy 46.40
  entropion 08.49
    by or with
      lid reconstruction 08.44
      suture (technique) 08.42
      thermocauterization 08.41
      wedge resection 08.43
  epicanthus (fold) 08.59
  epididymis (and spermatic cord) NEC 63.59
    with vas deferens 63.89
  epiglottis 31.69
  episiotomy
    routine following delivery — *see* Episiotomy
    secondary 75.69
  epispadias 58.45
  esophagus, esophageal NEC 42.89
    fistula NEC 42.84
    stricture 42.85
  exstrophy of bladder 57.86
  eyebrow 08.89
    linear 08.81
  eye, eyeball 16.89
    multiple structures 16.82
    rupture 16.82
    socket 16.64
      with graft 16.63
  eyelid 08.89
    full-thickness 08.85
      involving lid margin 08.84
    laceration 08.81
      full-thickness 08.85
        involving lid margin 08.84
      partial-thickness 08.83
        involving lid margin 08.82
    linear 08.81
    partial-thickness 08.83
      involving lid margin 08.82
    retraction 08.38
  fallopian tube (with prosthesis) 66.79
    by
      anastomosis 66.73
      reanastomosis 66.79
      reimplantation into
        ovary 66.72
        uterus 66.74
      suture 66.71
  false aneurysm — *see* Repair, aneurysm
  fascia 83.89
    by or with
      arthroplasty — *see* Arthroplasty
      graft (fascial) (muscle) 83.82
        hand 82.72
        tendon 83.81
          hand 82.79
      suture (direct) 83.65
        hand 82.46
  hand 82.89
    by
      graft NEC 82.79
        fascial 82.72
        muscle 82.72
      suture (direct) 82.46

**Repair** — *continued*
  fascia — *continued*
    joint — *see* Arthroplasty
    filtering bleb (corneal) (scleral) (by excision) 12.82
    by
      corneal graft (*see also* Keratoplasty) 11.60
      scleroplasty 12.82
      suture 11.51
        with conjunctival flap 11.53
  fistula (*see also* Closure, fistula)
    anovaginal 70.73
    arteriovenous 39.53
      clipping 39.53
      coagulation 39.53
        endovascular approach 39.79
        head and neck 39.72
      division 39.53
      excision or resection (*see also* Aneurysmectomy, by site)
        with
          anastomosis — *see* Aneurysmectomy, with anasto-mosis, by site
          graft replacement — *see* Aneurysmectomy, with graft replacement, by site
      ligation 39.53
        coronary artery 36.99
      occlusion 39.53
        endovascular approach 39.79
        head and neck 39.72
      suture 39.53
    cervicovesical 57.84
    cervix 67.62
    choledochoduodenal 51.72
    colovaginal 70.72
    enterovaginal 70.74
    enterovesical 57.83
    esophagocutaneous 42.84
    ileovesical 57.83
    intestinovaginal 70.74
    intestinovesical 57.83
    oroantral 22.71
    perirectal 48.93
    pleuropericardial 37.49
    rectovaginal 70.73
    rectovesical 57.83
    rectovesicovaginal 57.83
    scrotum 61.42
    sigmoidovaginal 70.74
    sinus
      nasal 22.71
      of Valsalva 35.39
    splenocolic 41.95
    urethroperineovesical 57.84
    urethrovesical 57.84
    urethrovesicovaginal 57.84
    uterovesical 57.84
    vagina NEC 70.75
    vaginocutaneous 70.75
    vaginoenteric NEC 70.74
    vaginoileal 70.74
    vaginoperineal 70.75
    vaginovesical 57.84
    vesicocervicovaginal 57.84
    vesicocolic 57.83
    vesicocutaneous 57.84
    vesicoenteric 57.83
    vesicointestinal 57.83
    vesicometrorectal 57.83
    vesicoperineal 57.84
    vesicorectal 57.83
    vesicosigmoidal 57.83
    vesicosigmoidovaginal 57.83
    vesicourethral 57.84
    vesicourethrorectal 57.83
    vesicouterine 57.84
    vesicovaginal 57.84
    vulva 71.72
    vulvorectal 48.73

**Repair** — *continued*
  foramen ovale (patent) 35.71
    with
      prosthesis (open heart technique) 35.51
        closed heart technique 35.52
      tissue graft 35.61
  fracture (*see also* Reduction, fracture)
    larynx 31.64
    malunion or nonunion (delayed) NEC — *see* category 78.4 ☑
      with
        graft — *see* Graft, bone
        insertion (of)
          bone growth stimulator (invasive) — *see* category 78.9 ☑
          internal fixation device 78.5 ☑
        manipulation for realignment — *see* Reduction, fracture, by site, closed
        osteotomy
          with
            correction of alignment — *see* category 77.3 ☑
              with internal fixation device — *see* categories 77.3 ☑ [78.5] ☑
              with intramedullary rod — *see* categories 77.3 ☑ [78.5] ☑
        replacement arthroplasty — *see* Arthroplasty
        sequestrectomy — *see* category 77.0 ☑
        Sofield type procedure — *see* categories 77.3 ☑ [78.5] ☑
        synostosis technique — *see* Arthrodesis
    vertebra 03.53
  funnel chest (with implant) 34.74
  gallbladder 51.91
  gastroschisis 54.71
  great vessels NEC 39.59
    laceration (by suture) 39.30
      artery 39.31
      vein 39.32
  hallux valgus NEC 77.59
    resection of joint with prosthetic implant 77.59
  hammer toe 77.56
  hand 82.89
    with graft or implant 82.79
      fascia 82.72
      muscle 82.72
      tendon 82.79
  heart 37.49
    assist system 37.63
    septum 35.70
      with
        prosthesis 35.50
        tissue graft 35.60
      atrial 35.71
        with
          prosthesis (open heart technique) 35.51
            closed heart technique 35.52
          tissue graft 35.61
      combined with repair of valvular and ventricular septal defects — *see* Repair, endocardial cushion defect
      in total repair of
        tetralogy of Fallot 35.81
        total anomalous pulmonary venous connection 35.82
        truncus arteriosus 35.83

**Repair** — *continued*
 heart — *continued*
  septum — *continued*
   combined with repair of valvular defect — *see* Repair, endocardial cushion defect
   ventricular 35.72
    with
     prosthesis (open heart technique) 35.53
      closed heart technique 35.55
     tissue graft 35.62
    combined with repair of valvular and atrial septal defects — *see* Repair, endocardial cushion defect
    in total repair of
     tetralogy of Fallot 35.81
     total anomalous pulmonary venous connection 35.82
     truncus arteriosus 35.83
  total replacement system 37.52
   implantable battery 37.54
   implantable controller 37.54
   thoracic unit 37.53
   transcutaneous energy transfer (TET) device 37.54
  valve (cusps) (open heart technique) 35.10
   with prosthesis or tissue graft 35.20
   aortic (without replacement) 35.11
    with
     prosthesis 35.22
     tissue graft 35.21
    combined with repair of atrial and ventricular septal defects — *see* Repair, endocardial cushion defect
   mitral (without replacement) 35.12
    with
     prosthesis 35.24
     tissue graft 35.23
   pulmonary (without replacement) 35.13
    with
     prosthesis 35.26
      in total repair of tetralogy of Fallot 35.81
     tissue graft 35.25
   tricuspid (without replacement) 35.14
    with
     prosthesis 35.28
     tissue graft 35.27
 hepatic duct 51.79
 hernia NEC 53.9
  anterior abdominal wall NEC 53.59
   with prosthesis or graft 53.69
  colostomy 46.42
  crural 53.29
  cul-de-sac (Douglas') 70.92
  diaphragmatic
   abdominal approach 53.7
   thoracic, thoracoabdominal approach 53.80
  epigastric 53.59
   with prosthesis or graft 53.69
  esophageal hiatus
   abdominal approach 53.7
   thoracic, thoracoabdominal approach 53.80
  fascia 83.89
   hand 82.89
  femoral (unilateral) 53.29
   with prosthesis or graft 53.21
   bilateral 53.39
    with prosthesis or graft 53.31
  Ferguson 53.00
  Halsted 53.00

**Repair** — *continued*
 hernia — *continued*
  Hill-Allison (hiatal hernia repair, transpleural approach) 53.80
  hypogastric 53.59
   with prosthesis or graft 53.69
  incisional 53.51
   with prosthesis or graft 53.61
  inguinal (unilateral) 53.00
   with prosthesis or graft 53.05
   bilateral 53.10
    with prosthesis or graft 53.17
    direct 53.11
     with prosthesis or graft 53.14
    direct and indirect 53.13
     with prosthesis or graft 53.16
    indirect 53.12
     with prosthesis or graft 53.15
   direct (unilateral) 53.01
    with prosthesis or graft 53.03
    and indirect (unilateral) 53.01
     with prosthesis or graft 53.03
    bilateral 53.13
     with prosthesis or graft 53.16
    bilateral 53.11
     with prosthesis or graft 53.14
   indirect (unilateral) 53.02
    with prosthesis or graft 53.04
    and direct (unilateral) 53.01
     with prosthesis or graft 53.03
    bilateral 53.13
     with prosthesis or graft 53.16
    bilateral 53.12
     with prosthesis or graft 53.15
  internal 53.9
  ischiatic 53.9
  ischiorectal 53.9
  lumbar 53.9
  manual 96.27
  obturator 53.9
  omental 53.9
  paraesophageal 53.7
  parahiatal 53.7
  paraileostomy 46.41
  parasternal 53.82
  paraumbilical 53.49
   with ▶graft or◀ prosthesis 53.41
  pericolostomy 46.42
  perineal (enterocele) 53.9
  preperitoneal 53.29
  pudendal 53.9
  retroperitoneal 53.9
  sciatic 53.9
  scrotal — *see* Repair, hernia, inguinal
  spigelian 53.59
   with prosthesis or graft 53.69
  umbilical 53.49
   with ▶graft or◀ prosthesis 53.41
  uveal 12.39
  ventral 53.59
   incisional 53.51
    with prosthesis or graft 53.61
 hydrocele
  round ligament 69.19
  spermatic cord 63.1
  tunica vaginalis 61.2
 hymen 70.76
 hypospadias 58.45
 ileostomy 46.41
 ingrown toenail 86.23
 intestine, intestinal NEC 46.79
  fistula — *see* Closure, fistula, intestine

**Repair** — *continued*
 intestine, intestinal — *continued*
  laceration
   large intestine 46.75
   small intestine NEC 46.73
   stoma — *see* Repair, stoma
  inverted uterus NEC 69.29
   manual
    nonobstetric 69.94
    obstetric 75.94
   obstetrical
    manual 75.94
    surgical 75.93
   vaginal approach 69.23
  iris (rupture) NEC 12.39
  jejunostomy 46.41
  joint (capsule) (cartilage) NEC (*see also* Arthroplasty) 81.96
  kidney NEC 55.89
  knee (joint) NEC 81.47
   collateral ligaments 81.46
   cruciate ligaments 81.45
   five-in-one 81.42
   triad 81.43
  labia — *see* Repair, vulva
  laceration — *see* Suture, by site
  lacrimal system NEC 09.99
   canaliculus 09.73
   punctum 09.72
    for eversion 09.71
  laryngostomy 31.62
  laryngotracheal cleft 31.69
  larynx 31.69
   fracture 31.64
   laceration 31.61
  leads (cardiac) NEC 37.75
  ligament (*see also* Arthroplasty) 81.96
   broad 69.29
   collateral, knee NEC 81.46
   cruciate, knee NEC 81.45
   round 69.29
   uterine 69.29
  lip NEC 27.59
   cleft 27.54
   laceration (by suture) 27.51
  liver NEC 50.69
   laceration 50.61
  lop ear 18.79
  lung NEC 33.49
  lymphatic (channel) (peripheral) NEC 40.9
   duct, left (thoracic) NEC 40.69
  macrodactyly 82.83
  mallet finger 82.84
  mandibular ridge 76.64
  mastoid (antrum) (cavity) 19.9
  meninges (cerebral) NEC 02.12
   spinal NEC 03.59
    meningocele 03.51
    myelomeningocele 03.52
  meningocele (spinal) 03.51
   cranial 02.12
  mesentery 54.75
  mouth NEC 27.59
   laceration NEC 27.52
  muscle NEC 83.87
   by
    graft or implant (fascia) (muscle) 83.82
     hand 82.72
    tendon 83.81
     hand 82.79
    suture (direct) 83.65
     hand 82.46
    transfer or transplantation (muscle) 83.77
     hand 82.58
   hand 82.89
    by
     graft or implant NEC 82.79
      fascia 82.72
     suture (direct) 82.46
     transfer or transplantation (muscle) 82.58
  musculotendinous cuff, shoulder 83.63

**Repair** — *continued*
 myelomeningocele 03.52
 nasal
  septum (perforation) NEC 21.88
  sinus NEC 22.79
  fistula 22.71
 nasolabial flaps (plastic) 21.86
 nasopharyngeal atresia 29.4
 nerve (cranial) (peripheral) NEC 04.79
  old injury 04.76
  revision 04.75
  sympathetic 05.81
 nipple NEC 85.87
 nose (external) (internal) (plastic) NEC (*see also* Rhinoplasty) 21.89
  laceration (by suture) 21.81
 notched lip 27.59
 omentum 54.74
 omphalocele 53.49
  with ▶graft or◀ prosthesis 53.41
 orbit 16.89
  wound 16.81
 ostium
  primum defect 35.73
   with
    prosthesis 35.54
    tissue graft 35.63
  secundum defect 35.71
   with
    prosthesis (open heart technique) 35.51
     closed heart technique 35.52
    tissue graft 35.61
 ovary 65.79
  with tube 65.73
   laparoscopic 65.76
 overlapping toe 77.58
 pacemaker
  cardiac
   device (permanent) 37.89
   electrode(s) (leads) NEC 37.75
   pocket (skin) (subcutaneous) 37.79
 palate NEC 27.69
  cleft 27.62
   secondary or subsequent 27.63
  laceration (by suture) 27.61
 pancreas NEC 52.95
  Wirsung's duct 52.99
 papillary muscle (heart) 35.31
 patent ductus arteriosus 38.85
 pectus deformity (chest) (carinatum) (excavatum) 34.74
 pelvic floor NEC 70.79
  obstetric laceration (current) 75.69
  old 70.79
 penis NEC 64.49
  for epispadias or hypospadias 58.45
  inflatable prosthesis 64.99
  laceration 64.41
 pericardium 37.49
 perineum (female) 71.79
  laceration (by suture) 71.71
   obstetric (current) 75.69
    old 71.79
  male NEC 86.89
   laceration (by suture) 86.59
 peritoneum NEC 54.73
  by suture 54.64
 pharynx NEC 29.59
  laceration (by suture) 29.51
  plastic 29.4
 pleura NEC 34.93
 postcataract wound dehiscence 11.52
  with conjunctival flap 11.53
 pouch of Douglas 70.52
 primum ostium defect 35.73
  with
   prosthesis 35.54
   tissue graft 35.63
 prostate 60.93
 ptosis, eyelid — *see* Repair, blepharoptosis
 punctum, lacrimal NEC 09.72

☑ Additional Digit Required — Refer to the Tabular List for Digit Selection
▶◀ Revised Text ● New Line ▲ Revised Code
Subterms under main terms may continue to next column or page
*2007 Ingenix* October 2007 · Volume 3 — 55

☑ Additional Digit Required — Refer to the Tabular List for Digit Selection
56 — Volume 3 · October 2007
▶◀ Revised Text   ● New Line   ▲ Revised Code
Subterms under main terms may continue to next column or page
*2007 Ingenix*

**Replacement — Reposition**

☑ Additional Digit Required — Refer to the Tabular List for Digit Selection

*2007 Ingenix*

▶◀ Revised Text      ● New Line      ▲ Revised Code

Subterms under main terms may continue to next column or page

**October 2007 · Volume 3 — 59**

Resection — Revision

Index

Revision — Scan, scanning

☑ Additional Digit Required — Refer to the Tabular List for Digit Selection
▶◀ Revised Text ● New Line ▲ Revised Code
▽ Subterms under main terms may continue to next column or page

**Scan, scanning** — *continued*
  radioisotope — *continued*
    intestine 92.04
    iodine-131 92.01
    kidney 92.03
    liver 92.02
    lung 92.15
    lymphatic system 92.16
    myocardial infarction 92.05
    pancreatic 92.04
    parathyroid 92.13
    pituitary 92.11
    placenta 92.17
    protein-bound iodine 92.01
    pulmonary 92.15
    radio-iodine uptake 92.01
    renal 92.03
    specified site NEC 92.19
    spleen 92.05
    thyroid 92.01
    total body 92.18
    uterus 92.19
  renal 92.03
  thermal — *see* Thermography
**Scapulectomy** (partial) 77.81
  total 77.91
**Scapulopexy** 78.41
**Scarification**
  conjunctiva 10.33
  nasal veins (with packing) 21.03
  pericardium 36.39
  pleura 34.6
    chemical 34.92
      with cancer chemotherapy substance 34.92 [99.25]
      tetracycline 34.92 [99.21]
**Schanz operation** (femoral osteotomy) 77.35
**Schauta (-Amreich) operation** (radical vaginal hysterectomy) 68.79
  laparoscopic 68.71
**Schede operation** (thoracoplasty) 33.34
**Scheie operation**
  cautery of sclera 12.62
  sclerostomy 12.62
**Schlatter operation** (total gastrectomy) 43.99
**Schroeder operation** (endocervical excision) 67.39
**Schuchardt operation** (nonobstetrical episiotomy) 71.09
**Schwartze operation** (simple mastoidectomy) 20.41
**Scintiphotography** — *see* Scan, radioisotope
**Scintiscan** — *see* Scan, radioisotope
**Sclerectomy** (punch) (scissors) 12.65
  for retinal reattachment 14.49
  Holth's 12.65
  trephine 12.61
    with implant 14.41
**Scleroplasty** 12.89
**Sclerosis** — *see* Sclerotherapy
**Sclerostomy** (Scheie's) 12.62
**Sclerotherapy**
  esophageal varices (endoscopic) 42.33
  hemorrhoids 49.42
  pleura 34.92
    treatment of malignancy (cytotoxic agent) 34.92 [99.25]
      with tetracycline 34.92 [99.21]
  varicose vein 39.92
  vein NEC 39.92
**Sclerotomy** (exploratory) 12.89
  anterior 12.89
    with
      iridectomy 12.65
      removal of vitreous 14.71
  posterior 12.89
    with
      iridectomy 12.65
      removal of vitreous 14.72
**Scott operation**
  intestinal bypass for obesity 45.93
  jejunocolostomy (bypass) 45.93

**Scraping**
  corneal epithelium 11.41
    for smear or culture 11.21
  trachoma follicles 10.33
**Scrotectomy** (partial) 61.3
**Scrotoplasty** 61.49
**Scrotorrhaphy** 61.41
**Scrotomy** 61.0
**Scrub, posterior nasal** (adhesions) 21.91
**Sculpturing, heart valve** — *see* Valvuloplasty, heart
**Section** — *see also* Division and Incision
  cesarean — *see* Cesarean section
  ganglion, sympathetic 05.0
  hypophyseal stalk (*see also* Hypophysectomy, partial) 07.63
  ligamentum flavum (spine) — *omit code*
  nerve (cranial) (peripheral) NEC 04.03
    acoustic 04.01
    spinal root (posterior) 03.1
    sympathetic 05.0
    trigeminal tract 04.02
  Saemisch (corneal) 11.1
  spinal ligament 80.49
    arcuate — *omit code*
    flavum — *omit code*
  tooth (impacted) 23.19
**Sedden-Brooks operation** (transfer of pectoralis major tendon) 83.75
**Semb operation** (apicolysis of lung) 33.39
**Senning operation** (correction of transposition of great vessels) 35.91
**Separation**
  twins (attached) (conjoined) (Siamese) 84.93
    asymmetrical (unequal) 84.93
    symmetrical (equal) 84.92
**Septectomy**
  atrial (closed) 35.41
    open 35.42
    transvenous method (balloon) 35.41
  submucous (nasal) 21.5
**Septoplasty** NEC 21.88
  with submucous resection of septum 21.5
**Septorhinoplasty** 21.84
**Septostomy** (atrial) (balloon) 35.41
**Septotomy, nasal** 21.1
**Sequestrectomy**
  bone 77.00
    carpals, metacarpals 77.04
    clavicle 77.01
    facial 76.01
    femur 77.05
    fibula 77.07
    humerus 77.02
    nose 21.32
    patella 77.06
    pelvic 77.09
    phalanges (foot) (hand) 77.09
    radius 77.03
    scapula 77.01
    skull 01.25
    specified site NEC 77.09
    tarsals, metatarsals 77.08
    thorax (ribs) (sternum) 77.01
    tibia 77.07
    ulna 77.03
    vertebrae 77.09
  nose 21.32
  skull 01.25
**Sesamoidectomy** 77.98
**Setback, ear** 18.5
**Severing of blepharorrhaphy** 08.02
**Sever operation** (division of soft tissue of arm) 83.19
**Sewell operation** (heart) 36.2
**Sharrard operation** (iliopsoas muscle transfer) 83.77
**Shaving**
  bone (*see also* Excision, lesion, bone) 77.60
  cornea (epithelium) 11.41

**Shaving** — *continued*
  cornea — *continued*
    for smear or culture 11.21
    patella 77.66
**Shelf operation** (hip arthroplasty) 81.40
**Shirodkar operation** (encirclement suture, cervix) 67.59
**Shock therapy**
  chemical 94.24
  electroconvulsive 94.27
  electrotonic 94.27
  insulin 94.24
  subconvulsive 94.26
**Shortening**
  bone (fusion) 78.20
    femur 78.25
    specified site NEC — *see category* 78.2 ☑
    tibia 78.27
    ulna 78.23
  endopelvic fascia 69.22
  extraocular muscle NEC 15.22
    multiple (two of more muscles) 15.4
  eyelid margin 08.71
  eye muscle NEC 15.22
    multiple (two or more muscles) (with lengthening) 15.4
  finger (macrodactyly repair) 82.83
  heel cord 83.85
  levator palpebrae muscle 08.33
  ligament (*see also* Arthroplasty)
    round 69.22
    uterosacral 69.22
  muscle 83.85
    extraocular 15.22
      multiple (two or more muscles) 15.4
    hand 82.55
  sclera (for repair of retinal detachment) 14.59
    by scleral buckling (*see also* Buckling, scleral) 14.49
  tendon 83.85
    hand 82.55
  ureter (with reimplantation) 56.41
**Shunt** — *see also* Anastomosis and Bypass, vascular
  abdominovenous 54.94
  aorta-coronary sinus 36.39
  aorta (descending)-pulmonary (artery) 39.0
  aortocarotid 39.22
  aortoceliac 39.26
  aortofemoral 39.25
  aortoiliac 39.25
  aortoiliofemoral 39.25
  aortomesenteric 39.26
  aorto-myocardial (graft) 36.2
  aortorenal 39.24
  aortosubclavian 39.22
  apicoaortic 35.93
  arteriovenous NEC 39.29
    for renal dialysis (by)
      anastomosis 39.27
      external cannula 39.93
  ascending aorta to pulmonary artery (Waterston) 39.0
  axillary-femoral 39.29
  carotid-carotid 39.22
  carotid-subclavian 39.22
  caval-mesenteric 39.1
  corpora cavernosa-corpus spongiosum 64.98
  corpora-saphenous 64.98
  descending aorta to pulmonary artery (Potts-Smith) 39.0
  endolymphatic (-subarachnoid) 20.71
  endolymph-perilymph 20.71
  extracranial-intracranial (EC-IC) 39.28
  femoroperoneal 39.29
  femoropopliteal 39.29
  iliofemoral 39.25
  ilioiliac 39.25
  intestinal
    large-to-large 45.94
    small-to-large 45.93

**Shunt** — *see also* Anastomosis and Bypass, vascular — *continued*
  intestinal — *continued*
    small-to-small 45.91
  left subclavian to descending aorta (Blalock-Park) 39.0
  left-to-right (systemic-pulmonary artery) 39.0
  left ventricle (heart) (apex) and aorta 35.93
  lienorenal 39.1
  lumbar-subarachnoid (with valve) NEC 03.79
  mesocaval 39.1
  peritoneal-jugular 54.94
  peritoneo-vascular 54.94
  peritoneovenous 54.94
  pleuroperitoneal 34.05
  pleurothecal (with valve) 03.79
  portacaval (double) 39.1
  portal-systemic 39.1
  portal vein to vena cava 39.1
  pulmonary-innominate 39.0
  pulmonary vein to atrium 35.82
  renoportal 39.1
  right atrium and pulmonary artery 35.94
  right ventricle and pulmonary artery (distal) 35.92
    in repair of
      pulmonary artery atresia 35.92
      transposition of great vessels 35.92
      truncus arteriosus 35.83
  salpingothecal (with valve) 03.79
  semicircular-subarachnoid 20.71
  spinal (thecal) (with valve) NEC 03.79
    subarachnoid-peritoneal 03.71
    subarachnoid-ureteral 03.72
  splenorenal (venous) 39.1
    arterial 39.26
  subarachnoid-peritoneal (with valve) 03.71
  subarachnoid-ureteral (with valve) 03.72
  subclavian-pulmonary 39.0
  subdural-peritoneal (with valve) 02.34
  superior mesenteric-caval 39.1
  systemic-pulmonary artery 39.0
  transjugular intrahepatic portosystemic [TIPS] 39.1
  vena cava to pulmonary artery (Green) 39.21
  ventricular (cerebral) (with valve) 02.2
    to
      abdominal cavity or organ 02.34
      bone marrow 02.39
      cervical subarachnoid space 02.2
      circulatory system 02.32
      cisterna magna 02.2
      extracranial site NEC 02.39
      gallbladder 02.34
      head or neck structure 02.31
      intracerebral site NEC 02.2
      lumbar site 02.39
      mastoid 02.31
      nasopharynx 02.31
      thoracic cavity 02.33
      ureter 02.35
      urinary system 02.35
      venous system 02.32
  ventriculoatrial (with valve) 02.32
  ventriculocaval (with valve) 02.32
  ventriculocisternal (with valve) 02.2
  ventriculolumbar (with valve) 02.39
  ventriculomastoid (with valve) 02.31
  ventriculonasopharyngeal 02.31
  ventriculopleural (with valve) 02.33
**Sialoadenectomy** (parotid) (sublingual) (submaxillary) 26.30
  complete 26.32
  partial 26.31
  radical 26.32
**Sialoadenolithotomy** 26.0
**Sialoadenotomy** 26.0

☑ Additional Digit Required — Refer to the Tabular List for Digit Selection
*2007 Ingenix*
▶◀ Revised Text    ● New Line    ▲ Revised Code
▽ Subterms under main terms may continue to next column or page
**Volume 3 — 61**

☑ Additional Digit Required — Refer to the Tabular List for Digit Selection

▽ Subterms under main terms may continue to next column or page

**2007 Ingenix**

▶◀ Revised Text    ● New Line    ▲ Revised Code

**October 2007 · Volume 3 — 63**

**Study — Syme operation**

**Index**

**Syme operation — Therapy**

**Syme operation** — *continued*
  urethrotomy, external 58.0
**Sympathectomy** NEC 05.29
  cervical 05.22
  cervicothoracic 05.22
  lumbar 05.23
  periarterial 05.25
  presacral 05.24
  renal 05.29
  thoracolumbar 05.23
  tympanum 20.91
**Sympatheticotripsy** 05.0
**Symphysiotomy** 77.39
  assisting delivery (obstetrical) 73.94
  kidney (horseshoe) 55.85
**Symphysis, pleural** 34.6
**Synchondrotomy** — *see also* Division, cartilage 80.40
**Syndactylization** 86.89
**Syndesmotomy** — *see also* Division, ligament 80.40
**Synechiotomy**
  endometrium 68.21
  iris (posterior) 12.33
    anterior 12.32
**Synovectomy** (joint) (complete) (partial) 80.70
  ankle 80.77
  elbow 80.72
  foot and toe 80.78
  hand and finger 80.74
  hip 80.75
  knee 80.76
  shoulder 80.71
  specified site NEC 80.79
  spine 80.79
  tendon sheath 83.42
    hand 82.33
  wrist 80.73
**Syringing**
  lacrimal duct or sac 09.43
  nasolacrimal duct 09.43
    with
      dilation 09.43
      insertion of tube or stent 09.44

**T**

**Taarnhoj operation** (trigeminal nerve root decompression) 04.41
**Tack operation** (sacculotomy) 20.79
**Take-down**
  anastomosis
    arterial 39.49
    blood vessel 39.49
    gastric, gastrointestinal 44.5
    intestine 46.93
    stomach 44.5
    vascular 39.49
    ventricular 02.43
  arterial bypass 39.49
  arteriovenous shunt 39.43
    with creation of new shunt 39.42
  cecostomy 46.52
  colostomy 46.52
  duodenostomy 46.51
  enterostomy 46.50
  esophagostomy 42.83
  gastroduodenostomy 44.5
  gastrojejunostomy 44.5
  ileostomy 46.51
  intestinal stoma 46.50
    large 46.52
    small 46.51
  jejunoileal bypass 46.93
  jejunostomy 46.51
  laryngostomy 31.62
  sigmoidostomy 46.52
  stoma
    bile duct 51.79
    bladder 57.82
    bronchus 33.42
    common duct 51.72
    esophagus 42.83
    gall bladder 51.92
    hepatic duct 51.79
    intestine 46.50

**Take-down** — *continued*
  stoma — *continued*
    intestine — *continued*
      large 46.52
      small 46.51
    kidney 55.82
    larynx 31.62
    rectum 48.72
    stomach 44.62
    thorax 34.72
    trachea 31.72
    ureter 56.83
    urethra 58.42
  systemic-pulmonary artery anastomosis 39.49
    in total repair of tetralogy of Fallot 35.81
  tracheostomy 31.72
  vascular anastomosis or bypass 39.49
  ventricular shunt (cerebral) 02.43
**Talectomy** 77.98
**Talma-Morison operation** (omentopexy) 54.74
**Tamponade**
  esophageal 96.06
  intrauterine (nonobstetric) 69.91
    after delivery or abortion 75.8
    antepartum 73.1
  vagina 96.14
    after delivery or abortion 75.8
    antepartum 73.1
**Tanner operation** (devascularization of stomach) 44.99
**Tap**
  abdomen 54.91
  chest 34.91
  cisternal 01.01
  cranial 01.09
  joint 81.91
  lumbar (diagnostic) (removal of dye) 03.31
  perilymphatic 20.79
  spinal (diagnostic) 03.31
  subdural (through fontanel) 01.09
  thorax 34.91
**Tarsectomy** 08.20
  de Grandmont 08.35
**Tarsoplasty** — *see also* Reconstruction, eyelid 08.70
**Tarsorrhaphy** (lateral) 08.52
  division or severing 08.02
**Tattooing**
  cornea 11.91
  skin 86.02
**Tautening, eyelid for entropion** 08.42
**Telemetry** (cardiac) 89.54
**Teleradiotherapy**
  beta particles 92.25
    intra-operative 92.41
  Betatron 92.24
  cobalt-60 92.23
  electrons 92.25
    intra-operative 92.41
  iodine-125 92.23
  linear accelerator 92.24
  neutrons 92.26
  particulate radiation NEC 92.26
  photons 92.24
  protons 92.26
  radioactive cesium 92.23
  radioisotopes NEC 92.23
**Temperament assessment** 94.02
**Temperature gradient study** — *see also* Thermography 88.89
**Tendinoplasty** — *see* Repair, tendon
**Tendinosuture** (immediate) (primary) — *see also* Suture, tendon 83.64
  hand (*see also* Suture, tendon, hand) 82.45
**Tendolysis** 83.91
  hand 82.91
**Tendoplasty** — *see* Repair, tendon
**Tenectomy** 83.39
  eye 15.13
    levator palpebrae 08.33

**Tenectomy** — *continued*
  eye — *continued*
    multiple (two or more tendons) 15.3
  hand 82.29
  levator palpebrae 08.33
  tendon sheath 83.31
    hand 82.21
**Tenodesis** (tendon fixation to skeletal attachment) 83.88
  Fowler 82.85
  hand 82.85
**Tenolysis** 83.91
  hand 82.91
**Tenomyoplasty** — *see also* Repair, tendon 83.88
  hand (*see also* Repair, tendon, hand) 82.86
**Tenomyotomy** — *see* Tenonectomy
**Tenonectomy** 83.42
  for graft 83.41
    hand 82.32
  hand 82.33
    for graft 82.32
**Tenontomyoplasty** — *see* Repair, tendon
**Tenontoplasty** — *see* Repair, tendon
**Tenoplasty** — *see also* Repair, tendon 83.88
  hand (*see also* Repair, tendon, hand) 82.86
**Tenorrhaphy** — *see also* Suture, tendon 83.64
  hand (*see also* Suture, tendon, hand) 82.45
  to skeletal attachment 83.88
    hand 82.85
**Tenosuspension** 83.88
  hand 82.86
**Tenosuture** — *see also* Suture, tendon 83.64
  hand (*see also* Suture, tendon, hand) 82.45
  to skeletal attachment 83.88
    hand 82.85
**Tenosynovectomy** 83.42
  hand 82.33
**Tenotomy** 83.13
  Achilles tendon 83.11
  adductor (hip) (subcutaneous) 83.12
  eye 15.12
    levator palpebrae 08.38
    multiple (two or more tendons) 15.4
  hand 82.11
  levator palpebrae 08.38
  pectoralis minor tendon (decompression thoracic outlet) 83.13
  stapedius 19.0
  tensor tympani 19.0
**Tenovaginotomy** — *see* Tenotomy
**Tensing, orbicularis oculi** 08.59
**Termination of pregnancy**
  by
    aspiration curettage 69.51
    dilation and curettage 69.01
    hysterectomy — *see* Hysterectomy
    hysterotomy 74.91
    intra-amniotic injection (saline) 75.0
**Test, testing** (for)
  14 C-Urea breath 89.39
  auditory function NEC 95.46
  Bender Visual-Motor Gestalt 94.02
  Benton Visual Retention 94.02
  cardiac (vascular)
    function NEC 89.59
    stress 89.44
      bicycle ergometer 89.43
      Masters' two-step 89.42
      treadmill 89.41
  Denver developmental (screening) 94.02
  fetus, fetal
    nonstress (fetal activity acceleration determinations) 75.34

**Test, testing** — *continued*
  fetus, fetal — *continued*
    oxytocin challenge (contraction stress) 75.35
    sensitivity (to oxytocin) — *omit code*
  function
    cardiac NEC 89.59
    hearing NEC 95.46
    muscle (by)
      electromyography 93.08
      manual 93.04
    neurologic NEC 89.15
    vestibular 95.46
      clinical 95.44
  glaucoma NEC 95.26
  hearing 95.47
    clinical NEC 95.42
  intelligence 94.01
  internal jugular-subclavian venous reflux 89.62
  intracarotid amobarbital (Wada) 89.10
  Masters' two-step stress (cardiac) 89.42
  muscle function (by)
    electromyography 93.08
    manual 93.04
  neurologic function NEC 89.15
  neurophysiologic monitoring   ●
    intra-operative 00.94   ●
  nocturnal penile tumescence 89.29
  provocative, for glaucoma 95.26
  psychologic NEC 94.08
  psychometric 94.01
  radio-cobalt $B_{12}$ Schilling 92.04
  range of motion 93.05
  rotation (Bárány chair) (hearing) 95.45
  sleep disorder function — *see* categories 89.17-89.18
  Stanford-Binet 94.01
  Thallium stress (transesophageal pacing) 89.44
  tuning fork (hearing) 95.42
  Urea breath, (14 C) 89.39
  vestibular function NEC 95.46
    thermal 95.44
  Wada (hemispheric function) 89.10
  whispered speech (hearing) 95.42
**TEVAP** (transurethral electrovaporization of prostate) 60.29
**Thalamectomy** 01.41
**Thalamotomy** 01.41
  by stereotactic radiosurgery 92.32
    cobalt 60 92.32
    linear accelerator (LINAC) 92.31
    multi-source 92.32
    particle beam 92.33
    particulate 92.33
    radiosurgery NEC 92.39
    single source photon 92.31
**Thal operation** (repair of esophageal stricture) 42.85
**Theleplasty** 85.87
**Therapy**
  Antabuse 94.25
  art 93.89
  aversion 94.33
  behavior 94.33
  Bennett respirator — *see* category 96.7 ☑
  blind rehabilitation NEC 93.78
  Byrd respirator — *see* category 96.7 ☑
  carbon dioxide 94.25
  cobalt-60 92.23
  conditioning, psychiatric 94.33
  continuous positive airway pressure (CPAP) 93.90
  croupette, croup tent 93.94
  daily living activities 93.83
    for the blind 93.78
  dance 93.89
  desensitization 94.33
  detoxification 94.25
  diversional 93.81
  domestic tasks 93.83
    for the blind 93.78

Therapy — Tracheotomy

☑ Additional Digit Required — Refer to the Tabular List for Digit Selection    ⬝ Subterms under main terms may continue to next column or page

*2007 Ingenix*    ▶◀ Revised Text    ● New Line    ▲ Revised Code    October 2007 · Volume 3 — 65

☑ Additional Digit Required — Refer to the Tabular List for Digit Selection    ▽ Subterms under main terms may continue to next column or page

**Transplant, transplantation** — *continued*
  ureter to — *continued*
    ileum — *continued*
      internal diversion only 56.71
      intestine 56.71
      skin 56.61
    vein (peripheral) 39.59
      renal, aberrant 39.55
    vitreous 14.72
      anterior approach 14.71
**Transposition**
  extraocular muscles 15.5
  eyelash flaps 08.63
    eye muscle (oblique) (rectus) 15.5
  finger (replacing absent thumb) (same hand) 82.61
    to
      finger, except thumb 82.81
      opposite hand (with amputation) 82.69 [84.01]
  interatrial venous return 35.91
  jejunal (Henley) 43.81
  joint capsule (*see also* Arthroplasty) 81.96
  muscle NEC 83.79
    extraocular 15.5
    hand 82.59
  nerve (cranial) (peripheral) (radial anterior) (ulnar) 04.6
  nipple 85.86
  pterygium 11.31
  tendon NEC 83.76
    hand 82.57
  vocal cords 31.69
**Transureteroureterostomy** 56.75
**Transversostomy** — *see also* Colostomy 46.10
**Trapping, aneurysm** (cerebral) 39.52
**Trauner operation** (lingual sulcus extension) 24.91
**Trephination, trephining**
  accessory sinus — *see* Sinusotomy
  corneoscleral 12.89
  cranium 01.24
  nasal sinus — *see* Sinusotomy
  sclera (with iridectomy) 12.61
**Trial** (failed) forceps 73.3
**Trigonectomy** 57.6
**Trimming, amputation stump** 84.3
**Triple arthrodesis** 81.12
**Trochanterplasty** 81.40
**Tsuge operation** (macrodactyly repair) 82.83
**Tuck, tucking** — *see also* Plication
  eye muscle 15.22
    multiple (two or more muscles) 15.4
    levator palpebrae, for blepharoptosis 08.34
**Tudor "rabbit ear" operation** (anterior urethropexy) 59.79
**Tuffier operation**
  apicolysis of lung 33.39
  vaginal hysterectomy 68.59
    laparoscopically assisted (LAVH) 68.51
**TULIP** (transurethral ultrasound guided laser induced prostatectomy) 60.21
**TUMT (transurethral microwave thermotherapy) of prostate** 60.96
**TUNA** (transurethral needle ablation) of prostate 60.97
**Tunnel, subcutaneous** (antethoracic) 42.86
  with esophageal anastomosis 42.68
  esophageal 42.86
    with anastomosis — *see* Anastomosis, esophagus, antesternal
  pulse generator lead wire 86.99
    with initial procedure — *omit code*
**Turbinectomy** (complete) (partial) NEC 21.69
  by
    cryosurgery 21.61
    diathermy 21.61

**Turbinectomy** — *continued*
  with sinusectomy — *see* Sinusectomy
**Turco operation** (release of joint capsules in clubfoot) 80.48
**TURP** (transurethral resection of prostate) 60.29
**Tylectomy** (breast) (partial) 85.21
**Tympanectomy** 20.59
  with tympanoplasty — *see* Tympanoplasty
**Tympanogram** 95.41
**Tympanomastoidectomy** 20.42
**Tympanoplasty** (type I) (with graft) 19.4
  with
    air pocket over round window 19.54
    fenestra in semicircular canal 19.55
    graft against
      incus or malleus 19.52
      mobile and intact stapes 19.53
    incudostapediopexy 19.52
  epitympanic, type I 19.4
  revision 19.6
  type
    II (graft against incus or malleus) 19.52
    III (graft against mobile and intact stapes) 19.53
    IV (air pocket over round window) 19.54
    V (fenestra in semicircular canal) 19.55
**Tympanosympathectomy** 20.91
**Tympanotomy** 20.09
  with intubation 20.01

**U**

**Uchida operation** (tubal ligation with or without fimbriectomy) 66.32
**UFR** (uroflowmetry) 89.24
**Ultrafiltration** 99.78
  hemodiafiltration 39.95
  hemodialysis (kidney) 39.95
  removal, plasma water 99.78
  therapeutic plasmapheresis 99.71
**Ultrasonography**
  abdomen 88.76
  aortic arch 88.73
  biliary tract 88.74
  breast 88.73
  deep vein thrombosis 88.77
  digestive system 88.74
  eye 95.13
  head and neck 88.71
  heart 88.72
  intestine 88.74
  intravascular — *see* Ultrasound, intravascular (IVUS)
  lung 88.73
  midline shift, brain 88.71
  multiple sites 88.79
  peripheral vascular system 88.77
  retroperitoneum 88.76
  therapeutic — *see* Ultrasound
  thorax NEC 88.73
  total body 88.79
  urinary system 88.75
  uterus 88.79
    gravid 88.78
**Ultrasound**
  diagnostic — *see* Ultrasonography
  fragmentation (of)
    cataract (with aspiration) 13.41
    urinary calculus, stones (Kock pouch) 59.95
  heart (intravascular) 88.72
    intracardiac (heart chambers) (ICE) 37.28
    intravascular (coronary vessels) (IVUS) 00.24
    non-invasive 88.72
  inner ear 20.79
  intravascular (IVUS) 00.29
    aorta 00.22
    aortic arch 00.22

**Ultrasound** — *continued*
  intravascular — *continued*
    cerebral vessel, extracranial 00.21
    coronary vessel 00.24
    intrathoracic vessel 00.22
    other specified vessel 00.28
    peripheral vessel 00.23
    renal vessel 00.25
    vena cava (inferior) (superior) 00.22
  therapeutic
    head 00.01
    heart 00.02
    neck 00.01
    other therapeutic ultrasound 00.09
    peripheral vascular vessels 00.03
    vessels of head and neck 00.01
  therapy 93.35
**Umbilectomy** 54.3
**Unbridling**
  blood vessel, peripheral 39.91
  celiac artery axis 39.91
**Uncovering** — *see* Incision, by site
**Undercutting**
  hair follicle 86.09
  perianal tissue 49.02
**Unroofing** — *see also* Incision, by site
  external
    auditory canal 18.02
    ear NEC 18.09
  kidney cyst 55.39
**UPP** (urethral pressure profile) 89.25
**Upper GI series** (x-ray) 87.62
**UPPP** (uvulopalatopharyngoplasty) 27.69 [29.4]
**Uranoplasty** (for cleft palate repair) 27.62
**Uranorrhaphy** (for cleft palate repair) 27.62
**Uranostaphylorrhaphy** 27.62
**Urban operation** (mastectomy) (unilateral) 85.47
  bilateral 85.48
**Ureterectomy** 56.40
  with nephrectomy 55.51
  partial 56.41
  total 56.42
**Ureterocecostomy** 56.71
**Ureterocelectomy** 56.41
**Ureterocolostomy** 56.71
**Ureterocystostomy** 56.74
**Ureteroenterostomy** 56.71
**Ureteroileostomy** (internal diversion) 56.71
  external diversion 56.51
**Ureterolithotomy** 56.2
**Ureterolysis** 59.02
  with freeing or repositioning of ureter 59.02
  laparoscopic 59.03
**Ureteroneocystostomy** 56.74
**Ureteropexy** 56.85
**Ureteroplasty** 56.89
**Ureteroplication** 56.89
**Ureteroproctostomy** 56.71
**Ureteropyelography** (intravenous) (diuretic infusion) 87.73
  percutaneous 87.75
  retrograde 87.74
**Ureteropyeloplasty** 55.87
**Ureteropyelostomy** 55.86
**Ureterorrhaphy** 56.82
**Ureteroscopy** 56.31
  with biopsy 56.33
**Ureterosigmoidostomy** 56.71
**Ureterostomy** (cutaneous) (external) (tube) 56.61
  closure 56.83
  ileal 56.51
**Ureterotomy** 56.2
**Ureteroureterostomy** (crossed) 56.75
  lumbar 56.41
  resection with end-to-end anastomosis 56.41
  spatulated 56.41
**Urethral catheterization, indwelling** 57.94
**Urethral pressure profile** (UPP) 89.25

**Urethrectomy** (complete) (partial) (radical) 58.39
  with
    complete cystectomy 57.79
    pelvic exenteration 68.8
    radical cystectomy 57.71
**Urethrocystography** (retrograde) (voiding) 87.76
**Urethrocystopexy** (by) 59.79
  levator muscle sling 59.71
  retropubic suspension 59.5
  suprapubic suspension 59.4
**Urethrolithotomy** 58.0
**Urethrolysis** 58.5
**Urethropexy** 58.49
  anterior 59.79
**Urethroplasty** 58.49
  augmentation 59.79
  collagen implant 59.72
  fat implant 59.72
  injection (endoscopic) of implant into urethra 59.72
  polytef implant 59.72
**Urethrorrhaphy** 58.41
**Urethroscopy** 58.22
  for control of hemorrhage of prostate 60.94
  perineal 58.21
**Urethrostomy** (perineal) 58.0
**Urethrotomy** (external) 58.0
  internal (endoscopic) 58.5
**Uroflowmetry** (UFR) 89.24
**Urography** (antegrade) (excretory) (intravenous) 87.73
  retrograde 87.74
**Uteropexy** (abdominal approach) (vaginal approach) 69.22
**UVP** (uvulopalatopharyngoplasty) 27.69 [29.4]
**Uvulectomy** 27.72
**Uvulopalatopharyngoplasty** (UPPP) 27.69 [29.4]
**Uvulotomy** 27.71

**V**

**Vaccination** (prophylactic) (against) 99.59
  anthrax 99.55
  brucellosis 99.55
  cholera 99.31
  common cold 99.51
  disease NEC 99.55
    arthropod-borne viral NEC 99.54
    encephalitis, arthropod-borne viral 99.53
  German measles 99.47
  hydrophobia 99.44
  infectious parotitis 99.46
  influenza 99.52
  measles 99.45
  mumps 99.46
  paratyphoid fever 99.32
  pertussis 99.37
  plague 99.34
  poliomyelitis 99.41
  rabies 99.44
  Rocky Mountain spotted fever 99.55
  rubella 99.47
  rubeola 99.45
  smallpox 99.42
  Staphylococcus 99.55
  Streptococcus 99.55
  tuberculosis 99.33
  tularemia 99.35
  tumor 99.28
  typhoid 99.32
  typhus 99.55
  undulant fever 99.55
  yellow fever 99.43
**Vacuum extraction, fetal head** 72.79
  with episiotomy 72.71
**VAD** (vascular access device) — *see* Implant, heart assist system
**Vagectomy** (subdiaphragmatic) — *see also* Vagotomy 44.00
**Vaginal douche** 96.44

☑ Additional Digit Required — Refer to the Tabular List for Digit Selection
▽ Subterms under main terms may continue to next column or page
68 — Volume 3 · October 2007     ▶◀ Revised Text     ● New Line     ▲ Revised Code     *2007 Ingenix*

## 00. PROCEDURES AND INTERVENTIONS, NOT ELSEWHERE CLASSIFIED (00)

✓3ʳᵈ **00**    **Procedures and interventions, not elsewhere classified**

✓4ᵗʰ    **00.0**    **Therapeutic ultrasound**

> **EXCLUDES**   *diagnostic ultrasound (non-invasive) (88.71-88.79)*
> *intracardiac echocardiography [ICE] (heart chamber(s)) (37.28)*
> *intravascular imaging (adjunctive) (00.21-00.29)*

**AHA:** 4Q, '02, 90

**DEF:** Interventional treatment modality using lower frequency and higher intensity levels of ultrasound energy than used in diagnostic ultrasound modality for the purpose of limiting intimal hyperpalsia, or restenosis, associated with atherosclerotic vascular disease.

**00.01**    **Therapeutic ultrasound of vessels of head and neck**
Anti-restenotic ultrasound
Intravascular non-ablative ultrasound
> **EXCLUDES**   *diagnostic ultrasound of:*
> *eye (95.13)*
> *head and neck (88.71)*
> *that of inner ear (20.79)*
> *ultrasonic:*
> *angioplasty of non-coronary vessel (39.50)*
> *embolectomy (38.01, 38.02)*
> *endarterectomy (38.11, 38.12)*
> *thrombectomy (38.01, 38.02)*

**00.02**    **Therapeutic ultrasound of heart**
Anti-restenotic ultrasound
Intravascular non-ablative ultrasound
> **EXCLUDES**   *diagnostic ultrasound of heart (88.72)*
> *ultrasonic ablation of heart lesion (37.34)*
> *ultrasonic angioplasty of coronary vessels (00.66, 36.09)*

**00.03**    **Therapeutic ultrasound of peripheral vascular vessels**
Anti-restenotic ultrasound
Intravascular non-ablative ultrasound
> **EXCLUDES**   *diagnostic ultrasound of peripheral vascular system (88.77)*
> *ultrasonic angioplasty of: non-coronary vessel (39.50)*

**00.09**    **Other therapeutic ultrasound**
> **EXCLUDES**   *ultrasonic:*
> *fragmentation of urinary stones (59.95)*
> *percutaneous nephrostomy with fragmentation (55.04)*
> *physical therapy (93.35)*
> *transurethral guided laser induced prostatectomy (TULIP) (60.21)*

✓4ᵗʰ    **00.1**    **Pharmaceuticals**

**00.10**    **Implantation of chemotherapeutic agent**
Brain wafer chemotherapy
Interstitial/intracavitary
> **EXCLUDES**   *injection or infusion of cancer chemotherapeutic substance (99.25)*

**AHA:** 4Q, '02, 93

**DEF:** Brain wafer chemotherapy: Placement of wafers containing antineoplastic agent against the wall of the resection cavity subsequent to the surgeon completing a tumor excision to deliver chemotherapy directly to the tumor site; used to treat glioblastoma multiforme (GBM).

**00.11**    **Infusion of drotrecogin alfa (activated)**
Infusion of recombinant protein
**AHA:** 4Q, '02, 93

**00.12**    **Administration of inhaled nitric oxide**
Nitric oxide therapy
**AHA:** 4Q, '02, 94

**00.13**    **Injection or infusion of nesiritide**
*Human B-type natriuretic peptide (hBNP)*
**AHA:** 4Q, '02, 94

**00.14**    **Injection or infusion of oxazolidinone class of antibiotics**
Linezolid injection
**AHA:** 4Q, '02, 95

**00.15**    **High-dose infusion interleukin-2 [IL-2]**
Infusion (IV bolus, CIV) interleukin
Injection of aldesleukin
> **EXCLUDES**   *low-dose infusion interleukin-2 (99.28)*

**AHA:** 4Q, '03, 92

**DEF:** A high-dose anti-neoplastic therapy using a biological response modifier (BRM); the body naturally produces substances called interleukins, which are multi-function cytokines in the generation of an immune response.

**00.16**    **Pressurized treatment of venous bypass graft [conduit] with pharmaceutical substance**
Ex-vivo treatment of vessel
Hyperbaric pressurized graft [conduit]
**DEF:** Ex-vivo process of delivering small nucleic acid molecules that block protein transcription factors essential for the expression of genes controlling cell proliferation into graft tissue under nondistending pressure; reduces intimal hyperplasia and vein graft failure.

**00.17**    **Infusion of vasopressor agent**

**00.18**    **Infusion of immunosuppressive antibody therapy**
Monoclonal antibody therapy
Polyclonal antibody therapy
> **INCLUDES**   ▶during induction phase of solid organ transplantation◀

**AHA:** 4Q, '05, 101

**00.19**    **Disruption of blood brain barrier via infusion [BBBD]**
Infusion of substance to disrupt blood brain barrier
Code also chemotherapy (99.25)
> **EXCLUDES**   *other perfusion (39.97)*

✓4ᵗʰ    **00.2**    **Intravascular imaging of blood vessels**
Note: Real-time imaging of lumen of blood vessel(s) using sound waves
Endovascular ultrasonography
Intravascular [ultrasound] imaging of blood vessels
Intravascular ultrasound (IVUS)
Code also any synchronous diagnostic or therapeutic procedures
> **EXCLUDES**   *adjunct vascular system procedures, number of vessels treated (00.40-00.43)*
> *diagnostic procedures on blood vessels (38.21-38.29)*
> *diagnostic ultrasound of peripheral vascular system (88.77)*
> *magnetic resonance imaging (MRI) (88.91-88.97)*
> *therapeutic ultrasound (00.01-00.09)*

**00.21**    **Intravascular imaging of extracranial cerebral vessels**
Common carotid vessels and branches
Intravascular ultrasound (IVUS), extracranial cerebral vessels
> **EXCLUDES**   *diagnostic ultrasound (non-invasive) of head and neck (88.71)*

**00.22**    **Intravascular imaging of intrathoracic vessels**
Aorta and aortic arch
Intravascular ultrasound (IVUS), intrathoracic vessels
Vena cava (superior) (inferior)
> **EXCLUDES**   *diagnostic ultrasound (non-invasive) of other sites of thorax (88.73)*

---

✓3ʳᵈ / ✓4ᵗʰ Additional Digit Required      Valid OR Procedure      Non-OR Procedure      Adjunct Code

Procedures and Interventions, NEC

00–00.22

**Procedures and Interventions, NEC**

**00.23–00.50**

**00.23   Intravascular imaging of peripheral vessels**
Imaging of:
    vessels of arm(s)
    vessels of leg(s)
Intravascular ultrasound (IVUS), peripheral
    vessels
> **EXCLUDES**   *diagnostic ultrasound (non-invasive) of peripheral vascular system (88.77)*

**00.24   Intravascular imaging of coronary vessels**
Intravascular ultrasound (IVUS), coronary
    vessels
> **EXCLUDES**   *diagnostic ultrasound (non-invasive) of heart (88.72)*
> *intracardiac echocardiography [ICE] (ultrasound of heart chamber(s)) (37.28)*

**AHA:** 3Q, '06, 8

**00.25   Intravascular imaging of renal vessels**
Intravascular ultrasound (IVUS), renal vessels
Renal artery
> **EXCLUDES**   *diagnostic ultrasound (non-invasive) of urinary system (88.75)*

**00.28   Intravascular imaging, other specified vessel(s)**
**00.29   Intravascular imaging, unspecified vessel(s)**

✓4th **00.3   Computer assisted surgery [CAS]**
CT-free navigation
Image guided navigation (IGN)
Image guided surgery (IGS)
Imageless navigation
Code also diagnostic or therapeutic procedure
> **EXCLUDES**   *stereotactic frame application only (93.59)*

**00.31   Computer assisted surgery with CT/CTA**
**AHA:** 4Q, '04, 113

**00.32   Computer assisted surgery with MR/MRA**
**AHA:** 4Q, '04, 113

**00.33   Computer assisted surgery with fluoroscopy**

**00.34   Imageless computer assisted surgery**
**00.35   Computer assisted surgery with multiple datasets**

**00.39   Other computer assisted surgery**
    Computer assisted surgery NOS

✓4th **00.4   Adjunct vascular system procedures**
Note: These codes can apply to both coronary and peripheral vessels. These codes are to be used in conjunction with other therapeutic procedure codes to provide additional information on the number of vessels upon which a procedure was performed and/or the number of stents inserted. As appropriate, code both the number of vessels operated on (00.40-00.43), and the number of stents inserted (00.45-00.48).
Code also any:
    angioplasty or atherectomy (00.61-00.62, 00.66, 39.50)
    endarterectomy (38.10-38.18)
    insertion of vascular stent(s) (00.55, 00.63-00.65, 36.06-36.07, 39.90)
    other removal of coronary artery obstruction (36.09)
**AHA:** 4Q, '05, 101

**00.40   Procedure on single vessel**
Number of vessels, unspecified
> **EXCLUDES**   *(aorto)coronary bypass (36.10-36.19)*
> *intravascular imaging of blood vessels (00.21-00.29)*

**AHA:** ▶1Q, '07, 17;◀ 3Q, '06, 8; 4Q, '05, 71, 106

**00.41   Procedure on two vessels**
> **EXCLUDES**   *(aorto)coronary bypass (36.10-36.19)*
> *intravascular imaging of blood vessels (00.21-00.29)*

**AHA:** 4Q, '06, 119; 4Q, '05, 105

**Stenting Techniques on Vessel Bifurcation**

**00.42   Procedure on three vessels**
> **EXCLUDES**   *(aorto)coronary bypass (36.10-36.19)*
> *intravascular imaging of blood vessels (00.21-00.29)*

**00.43   Procedure on four or more vessels**
> **EXCLUDES**   *(aorto)coronary bypass (36.10-36.19)*
> *intravascular imaging of blood vessels (00.21-00.29)*

**00.44   Procedure on vessel bifurcation**
Note: This code is to be used to identify the presence of a vessel bifurcation; it does not describe a specific bifurcation stent. Use this code only once per operative episode, irrespective of the number of bifurcations in vessels.
**AHA:** 4Q, '06, 119

**00.45   Insertion of one vascular stent**
Number of stents, unspecified
**AHA:** 4Q, '05, 71

**00.46   Insertion of two vascular stents**
**AHA:** 4Q, '05, 105-106

**00.47   Insertion of three vascular stents**
**AHA:** 4Q, '06, 119

**00.48   Insertion of four or more vascular stents**

✓4th **00.5   Other cardiovascular procedures**
**AHA:** 4Q, '02, 95

**00.50   Implantation of cardiac resynchronization pacemaker without mention of defibrillation, total system [CRT-P]**
Note: Device testing during procedure—*omit code*
Biventricular pacemaker
Biventricular pacing without internal cardiac defibrillator
BiV pacemaker
Implantation of cardiac resynchronization (biventricular) pulse generator pacing device, formation of pocket, transvenous leads including placement of lead into left ventricular coronary venous system, and intraoperative procedures for evaluation of lead signals
That with CRT-P generator and one or more leads
> **EXCLUDES**   *implantation of cardiac resynchronization defibrillator, total system [CRT-D] (00.51)*
> *insertion or replacement of any type pacemaker device (37.80-37.87)*
> *replacement of cardiac resynchronization: defibrillator, pulse generator only [CRT-D] (00.54) pacemaker, pulse generator only [CRT-P] (00.53)*

**AHA:** 3Q, '05, 3-9; 4Q, '02, 100
**DEF:** Cardiac resynchronization pacemaker: CRT-P, or biventricular pacing, adds a third lead to traditional pacemaker designs that connects to the left ventricle. The device provides electrical stimulation and coordinates ventricular contractions to improve cardiac output.

---

BI Bilateral Procedure    NC Non-covered Procedure    LC Limited Coverage Procedure    ▶◀ Revised Text    ● New Code    ▲ Revised Code Title

70 — Volume 3 • October 2007          © 2007 Ingenix

**00.51** **Implantation of cardiac resynchronization defibrillator, total system [CRT-D]**

Note: Device testing during procedure—*omit code*

BiV defibrillator

Biventricular defibrillator

Biventricular pacing with internal cardiac defibrillator

BiV ICD

BiV pacemaker with defibrillator

BiV pacing with defibrillator

Implantation of cardiac resynchronization (biventricular) pulse generator with defibrillator [AICD], formation of pocket, transvenous leads, including placement of lead into left ventricular coronary venous system, intraoperative procedures for evaluation of lead signals, and obtaining defibrillator threshold measurements

That with CRT-D generator and one or more leads

> **EXCLUDES**   *implantation of cardiac resynchronization pacemaker, total system [CRT-P] (00.50)*
>
> *implantation or replacement of automatic cardioverter/ defibrillator, total system [AICD] (37.94)*
>
> *replacement of cardiac resynchronization defibrillator, pulse generator only [CRT-D] (00.54)*

**AHA:** ▶1Q, '07, 16, 17;◀ 3Q, '05, 3-9; 4Q, '02, 99, 100

**00.52** **Implantation or replacement of transvenous lead [electrode] into left ventricular coronary venous system**

> **EXCLUDES**   *implantation of cardiac resynchronization:*
>
> *defibrillator, total system [CRT-D] (00.51)*
>
> *pacemaker, total system [CRT-P] (00.50)*
>
> *initial insertion of transvenous lead [electrode] (37.70-37.72)*
>
> *replacement of transvenous atrial and/or ventricular lead(s) [electrodes] (37.76)*

**00.53** **Implantation or replacement of cardiac resynchronization pacemaker, pulse generator only [CRT-P]**

Note: Device testing during procedure—*omit code*

Implantation of CRT-P device with removal of any existing CRT-P or other pacemaker device

> **EXCLUDES**   *implantation of cardiac resynchronization pacemaker, total system [CRT-P] (00.50)*
>
> *implantation or replacement of cardiac resynchronization defibrillator, pulse generator only [CRT-D] (00.54)*
>
> *insertion or replacement of any type pacemaker device (37.80-37.87)*

**AHA:** 3Q, '05, 3-9

**00.54** **Implantation or replacement of cardiac resynchronization defibrillator, pulse generator device only [CRT-D]**

Note: Device testing during procedure—*omit code*

Implantation of CRT-D device with removal of any existing CRT-D, CRT-P, pacemaker, or defibrillator device

> **EXCLUDES**   *implantation of automatic cardioverter/defibrillator pulse generator only (37.96)*
>
> *implantation of cardiac resynchronization defibrillator, total system [CRT-D] (00.51)*
>
> *implantation or replacement of cardiac resynchron- ization pacemaker, pulse generator only [CRT-P] (00.53)*

**AHA:** 3Q, '05, 3-9; 4Q, '02, 100

**00.55** **Insertion of drug-eluting peripheral vessel stent(s)**

Endograft(s)

Endovascular graft(s)

Stent graft(s)

Code also any:

angioplasty or atherectomy of other non-coronary vessel(s) (39.50)

number of vascular stents inserted (00.45-00.48)

number of vessels treated (00.40-00.43)

procedure on vessel bifurcation (00.44)

> **EXCLUDES**   *drug-coated peripheral stents, e.g., heparin coated (39.90)*
>
> *insertion of cerebrovascular stent(s) (00.63-00.65)*
>
> *insertion of drug-eluting coronary artery stent (36.07)*
>
> *insertion of non-drug-eluting stent(s):*
>
> *coronary artery (36.06)*
>
> *peripheral vessel (39.90)*
>
> *that for aneurysm repair (39.71-39.79)*

**AHA:** 4Q, '02, 101

**00.56** **Insertion or replacement of implantable pressure sensor (lead) for intracardiac hemodynamic monitoring**

Code also any associated implantation or replacement of monitor (00.57)

> **EXCLUDES**   *circulatory monitoring (blood gas, arterial or venous pressure, cardiac output and coronary blood flow) (89.60-89.69)*

**AHA:** 4Q, '06, 119

**DEF:** Insertion of an implantable device consisting of a data storage system, a single lead with a pressure sensor tip and a wireless antenna that continuously collects data on heart rate, pressures, physical activity and temperature.

**00.57** **Implantation or replacement of subcutaneous device for intracardiac hemodynamic monitoring**

Implantation of monitoring device with formation of subcutaneous pocket and connection to intracardiac pressure sensor (lead)

Code also any associated insertion or replacement of implanted pressure sensor (lead) (00.56)

**AHA:** 4Q, '06, 119

✓4ᵗʰ **00.6**    **Procedures on blood vessels**

**00.61**    **Percutaneous angioplasty or atherectomy of precerebral (extracranial) vessel(s)**

Basilar
Carotid
Vertebral

Code also any:
  injection or infusion of thrombolytic agent (99.10)
  number of vascular stents inserted (00.45-00.48)
  number of vessels treated (00.40-00.43)
  percutaneous insertion of carotid artery stent(s) (00.63)
  percutaneous insertion of other precerebral artery stent(s) (00.64)
  procedure on vessel bifurcation (00.44)

**EXCLUDES**    *angioplasty or atherectomy of other non-coronary vessel(s) (39.50)*
*removal of cerebrovascular obstruction of vessel(s) by open approach (38.01-38.02, 38.11-38.12, 38.31-38.32, 38.41-38.42)*

7 **00.62**    **Percutaneous angioplasty or atherectomy intracranial vessel(s)**    **NC**

Code also any:
  injection or infusion of thrombolytic agent (99.10)
  number of vascular stents inserted (00.45-00.48)
  number of vessels treated (00.40-00.43)
  percutaneous insertion of intracranial stent(s) (00.65)
  procedure on vessel bifurcation (00.44)

**EXCLUDES**    *angioplasty or atherectomy of other non-coronary vessel(s) (39.50)*
*removal of cerebrovascular obstruction of vessel(s) by open approach (38.01-38.02, 38.11-38.12, 38.31-38.32, 38.41-38.42)*

**00.63**    **Percutaneous insertion of carotid artery stent(s)**

Includes the use of any embolic protection device, distal protection device, filter device, or stent delivery system
Non-drug-eluting stent

Code also any:
  number of vascular stents inserted (00.45-00.48)
  number of vessels treated (00.40-00.43)
  percutaneous angioplasty or atherectomy of precerebral vessel(s) (00.61)
  procedure on vessel bifurcation (00.44)

**EXCLUDES**    *angioplasty or atherectomy of other non-coronary vessel(s) (39.50)*
*insertion of drug-eluting peripheral vessel stent(s) (00.55)*

**00.64**    **Percutaneous insertion of other precerebral (extracranial) artery stent(s)**

Includes the use of any embolic protection device, distal protection device, filter device, or stent delivery system
Basilar stent
Vertebral stent

Code also any:
  number of vascular stents inserted (00.45-00.48)
  number of vessels treated (00.40-00.43)
  percutaneous angioplasty or atherectomy of precerebral vessel(s) (00.61)
  procedure on vessel bifurcation (00.44)

**EXCLUDES**    *angioplasty or atherectomy of other non-coronary vessel(s) (39.50)*
*insertion of drug-eluting peripheral vessel stent(s) (00.55)*

**00.65**    **Percutaneous insertion of intracranial vascular stent(s)**

Includes the use of any embolic protection device, distal protection device, filter device, or stent delivery system

Code also any:
  number of vascular stents inserted (00.45-00.48)
  number of vessels treated (00.40-00.43)
  percutaneous angioplasty or atherectomy of intracranial vessel(s) (00.62)
  procedure on vessel bifurcation (00.44)

**EXCLUDES**    *angioplasty or atherectomy of other non-coronary vessel(s) (39.50)*
*insertion of drug-eluting peripheral vessel stent(s) (00.55)*

**00.66**    **Percutaneous transluminal coronary angioplasty [PTCA] or coronary atherectomy**

Balloon angioplasty of coronary artery
Coronary atherectomy
Percutaneous coronary angioplasty NOS
PTCA NOS

Code also any:
  injection or infusion of thrombolytic agent (99.10)
  insertion of coronary artery stent(s) (36.06-36.07)
  intracoronary artery thrombolytic infusion (36.04)
  number of vascular stents inserted (00.45-00.48)
  number of vessels treated (00.40-00.43)
  procedure on vessel bifurcation (00.44)

**AHA:** ▶1Q, '07, 17;◀ 3Q, '06, 8; 4Q, '05, 71, 101; **The following references pertain to deleted PTCA codes (36.01, 36.02, 36.05):** 1Q, '04, 10; 3Q, '03, 9; 4Q, '02, 114; 3Q, '02, 19; 1Q, '01, 9; 2Q, '01, 24; 1Q, '00, 11; 1Q, '99, 17; 4Q, '98, 74, 85; 1Q, '97, 3; 1Q, '94, 3; 3Q, '91, 24

**DEF:** Balloon angioplasty: Insertion of catheter with inflation of balloon to flatten plaque and widen vessels.

✓4ᵗʰ **00.7**    **Other hip procedures**
**AHA:** 4Q, '05, 106

**PTCA (Balloon Angioplasty)**

7  Noncovered except when reported with code 00.65.

---

**BI** Bilateral Procedure    **NC** Non-covered Procedure    **LC** Limited Coverage Procedure    ▶◀ Revised Text    ● New Code    ▲ Revised Code Title

**72 — Volume 3 • October 2007**                                                    © *2007 Ingenix*

**00.70**   **Revision of hip replacement, both acetabular and femoral components** [BI]

Total hip revision
Code also any:
    removal of (cement) (joint) spacer (84.57)
    type of bearing surface, if known (00.74-00.77)

EXCLUDES   *revision of hip replacement, acetabular component only (00.71)*
*revision of hip replacement, femoral component only (00.72)*
*revision of hip replacement, not otherwise specified (81.53)*
*revision with replacement of acetabular liner and/or femoral head only (00.73)*

**AHA:** 4Q, '05, 113

**00.71**   **Revision of hip replacement, acetabular component**

Partial, acetabular component only
That with:
    exchange of acetabular cup and liner
    exchange of femoral head
Code also any type of bearing surface, if known (00.74-00.77)

EXCLUDES   *revision of hip replacement, both acetabular and femoral components (00.70)*
*revision of hip replacement, femoral component (00.72)*
*revision of hip replacement, not otherwise specified (81.53)*
*revision with replacement of acetabular liner and/or femoral head only (00.73)*

**AHA:** 4Q, '05, 112

**00.72**   **Revision of hip replacement, femoral component**

Partial, femoral component only
That with:
    exchange of acetabular liner
    exchange of femoral stem and head
Code also any type of bearing surface, if known (00.74-00.77)

EXCLUDES   *revision of hip replacement, acetabular component (00.71)*
*revision of hip replacement, both acetabular and femoral components (00.70)*
*revision of hip replacement, not otherwise specified (81.53)*
*revision with replacement of acetabular liner and/or femoral head only (00.73)*

**00.73**   **Revision of hip replacement, acetabular liner and/or femoral head only**

Code also any type of bearing surface, if known (00.74-00.77)

▲   **00.74**   **Hip bearing surface, metal-on-polyethylene**

▲   **00.75**   **Hip bearing surface, metal-on-metal**

**AHA:** 4Q, '06, 121

▲   **00.76**   **Hip bearing surface, ceramic-on-ceramic**

**AHA:** 4Q, '05, 112

▲   **00.77**   **Hip bearing surface, ceramic-on-polyethylene**

**AHA:** 4Q, '06, 120

✓4ᵗʰ   **00.8**   **Other knee and hip procedures**

Note: Report up to two components using 00.81-00.83 to describe revision of knee replacements. If all three components are revised, report 00.80.

**AHA:** 4Q, '05, 1133

**00.80**   **Revision of knee replacement, total (all components)** [BI]

Replacement of femoral, tibial, and patellar components (all components)
Code also any removal of (cement) (joint) spacer (84.57)

EXCLUDES   *revision of only one or two components (tibial, femoral or patellar component) (00.81-00.84)*

**00.81**   **Revision of knee replacement, tibial component**

Replacement of tibial baseplate and tibial insert (liner)

EXCLUDES   *revision of knee replacement, total (all components) (00.80)*

**AHA:** 4Q, '05, 117

**00.82**   **Revision of knee replacement, femoral component**

That with replacement of tibial insert (liner)

EXCLUDES   *revision of knee replacement, total (all components) (00.80)*

**AHA:** 3Q, '06, 9; 4Q, '05, 117

**00.83**   **Revision of knee replacement, patellar component**

EXCLUDES   *revision of knee replacement, total (all components) (00.80)*

**00.84**   **Revision of total knee replacement, tibial insert (liner)**

Replacement of tibial insert (liner)

EXCLUDES   *that with replacement of tibial component (tibial baseplate and liner) (00.81)*

**00.85**   **Resurfacing hip, total, acetabulum and femoral head**

Hip resurfacing arthroplasty, total

**AHA:** 4Q, '06, 121

**00.86**   **Resurfacing hip, partial, femoral head**

Hip resurfacing arthroplasty, NOS
Hip resurfacing arthroplasty, partial, femoral head

EXCLUDES   *that with resurfacing of acetabulum (00.85)*

**AHA:** 4Q, '06, 121

**00.87**   **Resurfacing hip, partial, acetabulum**

Hip resurfacing arthroplasty, partial, acetabulum

EXCLUDES   *that with resurfacing of femoral head (00.85)*

**AHA:** 4Q, '06, 121

✓4ᵗʰ   **00.9**   **Other procedures and interventions**

**00.91**   **Transplant from live related donor**

Code also organ transplant procedure

**00.92**   **Transplant from live non-related donor**

Code also organ transplant procedure

**AHA:** 4Q, '04, 117

**00.93**   **Transplant from cadaver**

Code also organ transplant procedur

**00.94**   **Intra-operative neurophysiologic monitoring**

Intra-operative neurophysiologic testing
IOM
Nerve monitoring
Neuromonitoring

INCLUDES   Cranial nerve, peripheral nerve and spinal cord testing performed intra-operatively

EXCLUDES   *brain temperature monitoring (01.17)*
*intracranial oxygen monitoring (01.16)*
*intracranial pressure monitoring (01.10)*
*plethysmogram (89.58)*

---

✓3ᵗʰ
✓4ᵗʰ Additional Digit Required      Valid OR Procedure      Non-OR Procedure      Adjunct Code

**Operations on the Nervous System**

**01–01.25**

## 1. OPERATIONS ON THE NERVOUS SYSTEM (01-05)

√3rd **01  Incision and excision of skull, brain, and cerebral meninges**

√4th **01.0  Cranial puncture**

**01.01  Cisternal puncture**
Cisternal aspiration
Cisternal tap

EXCLUDES  *pneumocisternogram (87.02)*

DEF: Needle insertion through subarachnoid space to withdraw cerebrospinal fluid.

**01.02  Ventriculopuncture through previously implanted catheter**
Puncture of ventricular shunt tubing

DEF: Piercing of artificial, fluid-diverting tubing in the brain for withdrawal of cerebrospinal fluid.

**01.09  Other cranial puncture**
Aspiration of:
subarachnoid space
subdural space
Cranial aspiration NOS
Puncture of anterior fontanel
Subdural tap (through fontanel)

√4th **01.1  Diagnostic procedures on skull, brain, and cerebral meninges**

● **01.10  Intracranial pressure monitoring**
INCLUDES  insertion of catheter or probe for monitoring

**01.11  Closed [percutaneous] [needle] biopsy of cerebral meninges**
Burr hole approach

DEF: Needle excision of tissue sample through skin into cerebral membranes; no other procedure performed.

**01.12  Open biopsy of cerebral meninges**

DEF: Open surgical excision of tissue sample from cerebral membrane.

**01.13  Closed [percutaneous] [needle] biopsy of brain**
Burr hole approach
Stereotactic method
AHA: M-A, '87, 9

DEF: Removal by needle of brain tissue sample through skin.

**01.14  Open biopsy of brain**

DEF: Open surgical excision of brain tissue sample.

**01.15  Biopsy of skull**

● **01.16  Intracranial oxygen monitoring**
Partial pressure of brain oxygen (PbtO$_2$)
INCLUDES  insertion of catheter or probe for monitoring

● **01.17  Brain temperature monitoring**
INCLUDES  insertion of catheter or probe for monitoring

**01.18  Other diagnostic procedures on brain and cerebral meninges**
EXCLUDES  ► *brain temperature monitoring (01.17)*◄
*cerebral:*
*arteriography (88.41)*
*thermography (88.81)*
*contrast radiogram of brain (87.01-87.02)*
*echoencephalogram (88.71)*
*electroencephalogram (89.14)*
►*intracranial oxygen monitoring (01.16)*
*intracranial pressure monitoring (01.10)*◄
*microscopic examination of specimen from nervous system and of spinal fluid (90.01-90.09)*
*neurologic examination (89.13)*
*phlebography of head and neck (88.61)*
*pneumoencephalogram (87.01)*
*radioisotope scan:*
*cerebral (92.11)*
*head NEC (92.12)*
*tomography of head:*
*C.A.T. scan (87.03)*
*other (87.04)*

AHA: 3Q, '98, 12

**01.19  Other diagnostic procedures on skull**
EXCLUDES  *transillumination of skull (89.16)*
*x-ray of skull (87.17)*

√4th **01.2  Craniotomy and craniectomy**
EXCLUDES  *decompression of skull fracture (02.02)*
*exploration of orbit (16.01-16.09)*
*that as operative approach — omit code*
AHA: 1Q, '91, 1
DEF: Craniotomy: Incision into skull.
DEF: Craniectomy: Excision of part of skull.

**01.21  Incision and drainage of cranial sinus**
DEF: Incision for drainage, including drainage of air cavities in skull bones.

**01.22  Removal of intracranial neurostimulator lead(s)**
Code also any removal of neurostimulator pulse generator (86.05)
EXCLUDES  *removal with synchronous replacement (02.93)*

**01.23  Reopening of craniotomy site**
DEF: Reopening of skull incision.

**01.24  Other craniotomy**
Cranial:
decompression
exploration
trephination
Craniotomy NOS
Craniotomy with removal of:
epidural abscess
extradural hematoma
foreign body of skull
EXCLUDES  *removal of foreign body with incision into brain (01.39)*
AHA: 2Q, '91, 14

**01.25  Other craniectomy**
Debridement of skull NOS
Sequestrectomy of skull
EXCLUDES  *debridement of compound fracture of skull (02.02)*
*strip craniectomy (02.01)*
AHA: 1Q, '06, 6

BI Bilateral Procedure  NC Non-covered Procedure  LC Limited Coverage Procedure  ►◄ Revised Text  ● New Code  ▲ Revised Code Title

74 — Volume 3 • October 2007

© 2007 Ingenix

**01.26  Insertion of catheter(s) into cranial cavity or tissue**
Code also any concomitant procedure (e.g. resection (01.59))
> EXCLUDES  placement of intracerebral catheter(s) via burr hole(s) (01.28)

AHA: 4Q, '05, 117-118

**01.27  Removal of catheter(s) from cranial cavity or tissue**
AHA: 4Q, '05, 117-118

**01.28  Placement of intracerebral catheter(s) via burr hole(s)**
Convection enhanced delivery
Stereotactic placement of intracerebral catheter(s)
Code also infusion of medication
> EXCLUDES  insertion of catheter(s) into cranial cavity or tissue(s) (01.26)

AHA: ▶4Q, '06, 122◀

DEF: ▶The strategic neurosurgical placement of catheters via burr holes into targeted brain tissue, through which therapeutic agents such as antineoplastics are microinfused.◀

**✓4th  01.3  Incision of brain and cerebral meninges**
**01.31  Incision of cerebral meninges**
Drainage of:
  intracranial hygroma
  subarachnoid abscess (cerebral)
  subdural empyema

**01.32  Lobotomy and tractotomy**
Division of:      Percutaneous
  brain tissue    (radiofrequency)
  cerebral tracts  cingulotomy
DEF: Lobotomy: Incision of nerve fibers of brain lobe, usually frontal.
DEF: Tractotomy: Severing of a nerve fiber group to relieve pain.

**01.39  Other incision of brain**
Amygdalohippocampotomy
Drainage of intracerebral hematoma
Incision of brain NOS
> EXCLUDES  division of cortical adhesions (02.91)

**✓4th  01.4  Operations on thalamus and globus pallidus**
**01.41  Operations on thalamus**
Chemothalamectomy  Thalamotomy
> EXCLUDES  that by stereotactic radiosurgery (92.30-92.39)

**01.42  Operations on globus pallidus**
Pallidoansectomy  Pallidotomy
> EXCLUDES  that by stereotactic radiosurgery (92.30-92.39)

**✓4th  01.5  Other excision or destruction of brain and meninges**
AHA: 4Q, '93, 33

**01.51  Excision of lesion or tissue of cerebral meninges**
Decortication       ⎤
Resection           ⎬ of (cerebral) meninges
Stripping of subdural ⎟
  membrane          ⎦
> EXCLUDES  biopsy of cerebral meninges (01.11-01.12)

**01.52  Hemispherectomy**
DEF: Removal of one half of the brain. Most often performed for malignant brain tumors or intractable epilepsy.

**01.53  Lobectomy of brain**
DEF: Excision of a brain lobe.

**01.59  Other excision or destruction of lesion or tissue of brain**
Curettage of brain
Debridement of brain
Marsupialization of brain cyst
Transtemporal (mastoid) excision of brain tumor
> EXCLUDES  biopsy of brain (01.13-01.14)
> that by stereotactic radiosurgery (92.30-92.39)

AHA:  4Q, '05, 118; 3Q, '99, 7; 1Q, '99, 9; 3Q, '98, 12; 1Q, '98, 6

**01.6  Excision of lesion of skull**
Removal of granulation tissue of cranium
> EXCLUDES  biopsy of skull (01.15)
> sequestrectomy (01.25)

**✓3rd  02  Other operations on skull, brain, and cerebral meninges**
**✓4th  02.0  Cranioplasty**
> EXCLUDES  that with synchronous repair of encephalocele (02.12)

**02.01  Opening of cranial suture**
Linear craniectomy
Strip craniectomy

DEF: Opening of the lines of junction between the bones of the skull for removal of strips of skull bone.

**02.02  Elevation of skull fracture fragments**
Debridement of compound fracture of skull
Decompression of skull fracture
Reduction of skull fracture
Code also any synchronous debridement of brain (01.59)
> EXCLUDES  debridement of skull NOS (01.25)
> removal of granulation tissue of cranium (01.6)

**02.03  Formation of cranial bone flap**
Repair of skull with flap

**02.04  Bone graft to skull**
Pericranial graft (autogenous) (heterogenous)

**02.05  Insertion of skull plate**
Replacement of skull plate

**02.06  Other cranial osteoplasty**
Repair of skull NOS
Revision of bone flap of skull
AHA: 1Q, '06, 6; 1Q, '05, 11; 3Q, '98, 9
DEF: Plastic surgery repair of skull bones.

**02.07  Removal of skull plate**
> EXCLUDES  removal with synchronous replacement (02.05)

**✓4th  02.1  Repair of cerebral meninges**
> EXCLUDES  marsupialization of cerebral lesion (01.59)

**02.11  Simple suture of dura mater of brain**
**02.12  Other repair of cerebral meninges**
Closure of fistula of cerebrospinal fluid
Dural graft
Repair of encephalocele including synchronous cranioplasty
Repair of meninges NOS
Subdural patch

**02.13  Ligation of meningeal vessel**
Ligation of:
  longitudinal sinus
  middle meningeal artery

**02.14  Choroid plexectomy**
Cauterization of choroid plexus
DEF: Excision or destruction of the ependymal cells that form the membrane lining in the third, fourth, and lateral ventricles of the brain and secrete cerebrospinal fluid.

**Operations on the Nervous System**

**02.2–03.02**

**02.2**    **Ventriculostomy**

Anastomosis of ventricle to:
cervical subarachnoid space
cisterna magna
Insertion of Holter valve
Ventriculocisternal intubation

DEF: Surgical creation of an opening of ventricle; often performed to drain cerebrospinal fluid in treating hydrocephalus.

√4ᵗʰ **02.3**    **Extracranial ventricular shunt**

INCLUDES    that with insertion of valve

DEF: Placement of shunt or creation of artificial passage leading from skull cavities to site outside skull to relieve excess cerebrospinal fluid created in the chorioid plexuses of the third and fourth ventricles of the brain.

**02.31**   **Ventricular shunt to structure in head and neck**
Ventricle to nasopharynx shunt
Ventriculomastoid anastomosis

**02.32**   **Ventricular shunt to circulatory system**
Ventriculoatrial anastomosis
Ventriculocaval shunt

**02.33**   **Ventricular shunt to thoracic cavity**
Ventriculopleural anastomosis

**02.34**   **Ventricular shunt to abdominal cavity and organs**
Ventriculocholecystostomy
Ventriculoperitoneostomy

**02.35**   **Ventricular shunt to urinary system**
Ventricle to ureter shunt

**02.39**   **Other operations to establish drainage of ventricle**
Ventricle to bone marrow shunt
Ventricular shunt to extracranial site NEC

√4ᵗʰ **02.4**    **Revision, removal, and irrigation of ventricular shunt**

EXCLUDES    revision of distal catheter of ventricular shunt (54.95)

**02.41**   **Irrigation and exploration of ventricular shunt**
Exploration of ventriculoperitoneal shunt at ventricular site
Re-programming of ventriculoperitoneal shunt

**02.42**   **Replacement of ventricular shunt**
Reinsertion of Holter valve
Replacement of ventricular catheter
Revision of ventriculoperitoneal shunt at ventricular site
AHA: N-D, '86, 8

**02.43**   **Removal of ventricular shunt**
AHA: N-D, '86, 8

√4ᵗʰ **02.9**    **Other operations on skull, brain, and cerebral meninges**

EXCLUDES    operations on:
pineal gland (07.17, 07.51-07.59)
pituitary gland [hypophysis] (07.13-07.15, 07.61-07.79)

**02.91**   **Lysis of cortical adhesions**
DEF: Breaking up of fibrous structures in brain outer layer.

**02.92**   **Repair of brain**

**02.93**   **Implantation or replacement of intracranial neurostimulator lead(s)**

Implantation, insertion, placement, or replacement of intracranial:
brain pacemaker [neuropacemaker]
depth electrodes
epidural pegs
electroencephalographic receiver
foramen ovale electrodes
intracranial electrostimulator
subdural grids
subdural strips
Code also any insertion of neurostimulator pulse generator (86.94-86.98)
AHA: 4Q, '97, 57; 4Q, '92, 28

**02.94**   **Insertion or replacement of skull tongs or halo traction device**
AHA: 3Q, '01, 8; 3Q, '96, 14

DEF: Halo traction device: Metal or plastic band encircles the head or neck secured to the skull with four pins and attached to a metal chest plate by rods; provides support and stability for the head and neck.

DEF: Skull tongs: Device inserted into each side of the skull used to apply parallel traction to the long axis of the cervical spine.

**02.95**   **Removal of skull tongs or halo traction device**

**02.96**   **Insertion of sphenoidal electrodes**
AHA: 4Q, '92, 28

**02.99**   **Other**

EXCLUDES    chemical shock therapy (94.24)
electroshock therapy:
subconvulsive (94.26)
other (94.27)

√3ʳᵈ **03**   **Operations on spinal cord and spinal canal structures**
Code also any application or administration of an adhesion barrier substance (99.77)

√4ᵗʰ **03.0**    **Exploration and decompression of spinal canal structures**

**03.01**   **Removal of foreign body from spinal canal**

**03.02**   **Reopening of laminectomy site**

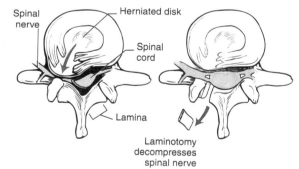

**Laminotomy with Decompression**

Spinal nerve — Herniated disk — Spinal cord — Lamina

Laminotomy decompresses spinal nerve

BI Bilateral Procedure     NC Non-covered Procedure     LC Limited Coverage Procedure     ▶◀ Revised Text     ● New Code     ▲ Revised Code Title

76 — Volume 3                                                                © 2007 Ingenix

**03.09 Other exploration and decompression of spinal canal**

Decompression:
  laminectomy    laminotomy
Expansile laminoplasty
Exploration of spinal nerve root
Foraminotomy
▶Code also any synchronous insertion, replacement and revision of posterior spinal motion preservation device(s), if performed (84.80-84.85)◀

> **EXCLUDES**   *drainage of spinal fluid by anastomosis (03.71-03.79)*
> *laminectomy with excision of intervertebral disc (80.51)*
> *spinal tap (03.31)*
> *that as operative approach — omit code*

**AHA:** ▶1Q, '07, 10;◀ 3Q, '04, 6; 4Q, '02, 109; 2Q, '02, 15; 4Q, '99, 14; 2Q, '97, 6; 2Q, '95, 9; 2Q, '95, 10; 2Q, '90, 22; S-Q, '86, 12

**DEF:** Decompression of spinal canal: Excision of bone pieces, hematoma or other lesion to relieve spinal cord pressure.
**DEF:** Expansile laminoplasty: Lamina is incised at the level of the pedicle to relieve pressure; no tissue is excised.
**DEF:** Foraminotomy: Removal of root opening between vertebrae to relieve nerve root pressure.

**03.1 Division of intraspinal nerve root**

Rhizotomy

**DEF:** Rhizotomy: Surgical severing of spinal nerve roots within spinal canal for pain relief.

**✓4ᵗʰ 03.2 Chordotomy**

**DEF:** Chordotomy: Surgical cutting of lateral spinothalamic tract of spinal cord to relieve pain.

**03.21 Percutaneous chordotomy**

Stereotactic chordotomy

**DEF:** Percutaneous chordotomy: Insertion of hollow needle through skin to interrupt spinal nerve root.

**DEF:** Stereotactic chordotomy: Use of three-dimensional imaging to locate spinal nerve root for surgical interruption.

**03.29 Other chordotomy**

Chordotomy NOS
Tractotomy (one-stage) (two-stage) of spinal cord
Transection of spinal cord tracts

**DEF:** Tractotomy (one stage) (two stages) of the spinal cord: Surgical incision or severing of a nerve tract of spinal cord.

**DEF:** Transection of spinal cord tracts: Use of transverse incision to divide spinal nerve root.

**✓4ᵗʰ 03.3 Diagnostic procedures on spinal cord and spinal canal structures**

**03.31 Spinal tap**

Lumbar puncture for removal of dye

> **EXCLUDES**   *lumbar puncture for injection of dye [myelogram] (87.21)*

**AHA:** 2Q, '90, 22

**DEF:** Puncture into lumbar subarachnoid space to tap cerebrospinal fluid.

**03.32 Biopsy of spinal cord or spinal meninges**

**03.39 Other diagnostic procedures on spinal cord and spinal canal structures**

> **EXCLUDES**   *microscopic examination of specimen from nervous system or of spinal fluid (90.01-90.09)*
> *x-ray of spine (87.21-87.29)*

**03.4 Excision or destruction of lesion of spinal cord or spinal meninges**

Curettage
Debridement        } of spinal cord or
Marsupialization of cyst   } spinal meninges
Resection

> **EXCLUDES**   *biopsy of spinal cord or meninges (03.32)*

**AHA:** 3Q, '95, 5

**✓4ᵗʰ 03.5 Plastic operations on spinal cord structures**

**03.51 Repair of spinal meningocele**

Repair of meningocele NOS

**DEF:** Restoration of hernial protrusion of spinal meninges through defect in vertebral column.

**03.52 Repair of spinal myelomeningocele**

**DEF:** Restoration of hernial protrusion of spinal cord and meninges through defect in vertebral column.

**03.53 Repair of vertebral fracture**

Elevation of spinal bone fragments
Reduction of fracture of vertebrae
Removal of bony spicules from spinal canal

> **EXCLUDES**   *kyphoplasty (81.66)*
> *vertebroplasty (81.65)*

**AHA:** ▶1Q, '07, 20;◀ 4Q, '04, 126; 2Q, '02, 14; 4Q, '99, 11, 12, 13; 3Q, '96, 14

**03.59 Other repair and plastic operations on spinal cord structures**

Repair of:
  diastematomyelia
  spina bifida NOS
  spinal cord NOS
  spinal meninges NOS
  vertebral arch defect

**03.6 Lysis of adhesions of spinal cord and nerve roots**
**AHA:** 2Q, '98, 18

**✓4ᵗʰ 03.7 Shunt of spinal theca**

> **INCLUDES**   that with valve

**DEF:** Surgical passage created from spinal cord dura mater to another channel.

**03.71 Spinal subarachnoid-peritoneal shunt**
**03.72 Spinal subarachnoid-ureteral shunt**
**03.79 Other shunt of spinal theca**

Lumbar-subarachnoid shunt NOS
Pleurothecal anastomosis
Salpingothecal anastomosis
**AHA:** 1Q, '97, 7

**03.8 Injection of destructive agent into spinal canal**

**Lumbar Spinal Puncture**

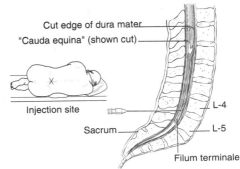

Cut edge of dura mater
"Cauda equina" (shown cut)
Injection site
L-4
Sacrum
L-5
Filum terminale

**Operations on the Nervous System**

**03.9–04.5**

√4th **03.9    Other operations on spinal cord and spinal canal structures**

**03.90    Insertion of catheter into spinal canal for infusion of therapeutic or palliative substances**

Insertion of catheter into epidural, subarachnoid, or subdural space of spine with intermittent or continuous infusion of drug (with creation of any reservoir)

Code also any implantation of infusion pump (86.06)

**03.91    Injection of anesthetic into spinal canal for analgesia**

EXCLUDES    *that for operative anesthesia — omit code*

**AHA:** 3Q, '00, 15; 1Q, '99, 8; 2Q, '98, 18

**03.92    Injection of other agent into spinal canal**

Intrathecal injection of steroid

Subarachnoid perfusion of refrigerated saline

EXCLUDES    *injection of:*
     *contrast material for myelogram (87.21)*
     *destructive agent into spinal canal (03.8)*

**AHA:** 2Q, '03, 6; 3Q, '00, 15; 2Q, '98, 18

**03.93    Implantation or replacement of spinal neurostimulator lead(s)**

Code also any insertion of neurostimulator pulse generator (86.94-86.98)

**AHA:** 1Q, '00, 19

**03.94    Removal of spinal neurostimulator lead(s)**

Code also any removal of neurostimulator pulse generator (86.05)

**03.95    Spinal blood patch**

DEF: Injection of blood into epidural space to patch hole in outer spinal membrane when blood clots.

**03.96    Percutaneous denervation of facet**

**03.97    Revision of spinal thecal shunt**

**AHA:** 2Q, '99, 4

**03.98    Removal of spinal thecal shunt**

**03.99    Other**

√3rd **04    Operations on cranial and peripheral nerves**

√4th **04.0    Incision, division, and excision of cranial and peripheral nerves**

EXCLUDES    *opticociliary neurectomy (12.79)*
     *sympathetic ganglionectomy (05.21-05.29)*

**04.01    Excision of acoustic neuroma**

That by craniotomy

EXCLUDES    *that by stereotactic radiosurgery (92.3)*

**AHA:** 2Q, '98, 20; 2Q, '95, 8; 4Q, '92, 26

**04.02    Division of trigeminal nerve**

Retrogasserian neurotomy

DEF: Transection of sensory root fibers of trigeminal nerve for relief of trigeminal neuralgia.

**04.03    Division or crushing of other cranial and peripheral nerves**

EXCLUDES    *that of:*
     *glossopharyngeal nerve (29.92)*
     *laryngeal nerve (31.91)*
     *nerves to adrenal glands (07.42)*
     *phrenic nerve for collapse of lung (33.31)*
     *vagus nerve (44.00-44.03)*

**AHA:** 2Q, '98, 20

---

**04.04    Other incision of cranial and peripheral nerves**

**04.05    Gasserian ganglionectomy**

**04.06    Other cranial or peripheral ganglionectomy**

EXCLUDES    *sympathetic ganglionectomy (05.21-05.29)*

**04.07    Other excision or avulsion of cranial and peripheral nerves**

Curettage
Debridement  } *of peripheral nerve*
Resection

Excision of peripheral neuroma [Morton's]

EXCLUDES    *biopsy of cranial or peripheral nerve (04.11-04.12)*

**AHA:** 2Q, '95, 8; 4Q, '92, 26

√4th **04.1    Diagnostic procedures on peripheral nervous system**

**04.11    Closed [percutaneous] [needle] biopsy of cranial or peripheral nerve or ganglion**

**04.12    Open biopsy of cranial or peripheral nerve or ganglion**

**04.19    Other diagnostic procedures on cranial and peripheral nerves and ganglia**

EXCLUDES    *microscopic examination of specimen from nervous system (90.01-90.09)*
     *neurologic examination (89.13)*

**04.2    Destruction of cranial and peripheral nerves**

Destruction of cranial or peripheral nerves by:
   cryoanalgesia
   injection of neurolytic agent
   radiofrequency
   Radiofrequency ablation

**AHA:** 3Q, '02, 10, 11; 4Q, '95, 74

DEF: Radiofrequency ablation: High frequency radio waves are applied to injure the nerve resulting in interruption of the pain signal.

**04.3    Suture of cranial and peripheral nerves**

√4th **04.4    Lysis of adhesions and decompression of cranial and peripheral nerves**

**04.41    Decompression of trigeminal nerve root**

**04.42    Other cranial nerve decompression**

**AHA:** 3Q, '02, 13

**04.43    Release of carpal tunnel**

**04.44    Release of tarsal tunnel**

**04.49    Other peripheral nerve or ganglion decompression or lysis of adhesions**

Peripheral nerve neurolysis NOS

**04.5    Cranial or peripheral nerve graft**

**Release of Carpal Tunnel**

Median nerve

(Deep) transverse carpal ligament being cut

---

 Bilateral Procedure      Non-covered Procedure     **LC** Limited Coverage Procedure     ►◄ Revised Text     ● New Code     ▲ Revised Code Title

78 — Volume 3         © 2007 Ingenix

**04.6**    **Transposition of cranial and peripheral nerves**
Nerve transplantation
DEF: Relocation of cranial or peripheral nerves without detaching or severing them.

√4ᵗʰ **04.7**    **Other cranial or peripheral neuroplasty**

**04.71**    **Hypoglossal-facial anastomosis**
DEF: Surgical connection of hypoglossal nerve to facial nerve.

**04.72**    **Accessory-facial anastomosis**
DEF: Surgical connection of accessory nerve to facial nerve.

**04.73**    **Accessory-hypoglossal anastomosis**
DEF: Surgical connection of accessory nerve to hypoglossal nerve.

**04.74**    **Other anastomosis of cranial or peripheral nerve**

**04.75**    **Revision of previous repair of cranial and peripheral nerves**

**04.76**    **Repair of old traumatic injury of cranial and peripheral nerves**

**04.79**    **Other neuroplasty**
AHA: 1Q, '06, 11

√4ᵗʰ **04.8**    **Injection into peripheral nerve**
**EXCLUDES**   *destruction of nerve (by injection of neurolytic agent) (04.2)*

**04.80**    **Peripheral nerve injection, not otherwise specified**

**04.81**    **Injection of anesthetic into peripheral nerve for analgesia**
**EXCLUDES**   *that for operative anesthesia — omit code*
AHA: 1Q, '00, 7

**04.89**    **Injection of other agent, except neurolytic**
**EXCLUDES**   *injection of neurolytic agent (04.2)*

√4ᵗʰ **04.9**    **Other operations on cranial and peripheral nerves**

**04.91**    **Neurectasis**
DEF: Surgical stretching of peripheral or cranial nerve.

**04.92**    **Implantation or replacement of peripheral neurostimulator lead(s)**
Code also any insertion of neurostimulator pulse generator (86.94-86.98)
AHA: ▶2Q, '07, 8;◄ 2Q, '06, 5; 2Q, '04, 7; 3Q, '01, 16; 2Q, '00, 22; 3Q, '96, 12
DEF: Placement of or removal and replacement of neurostimulator lead(s) during the same episode.

**04.93**    **Removal of peripheral neurostimulator lead(s)**
Code also any removal of neurostimulator pulse generator (86.05)
AHA: 3Q, '01, 16

**04.99**    **Other**

√3ʳᵈ **05**    **Operations on sympathetic nerves or ganglia**
**EXCLUDES**   *paracervical uterine denervation (69.3)*

**05.0**    **Division of sympathetic nerve or ganglion**
**EXCLUDES**   *that of nerves to adrenal glands (07.42)*

√4ᵗʰ **05.1**    **Diagnostic procedures on sympathetic nerves or ganglia**

**05.11**    **Biopsy of sympathetic nerve or ganglion**

**05.19**    **Other diagnostic procedures on sympathetic nerves or ganglia**

√4ᵗʰ **05.2**    **Sympathectomy**
DEF: Sympathectomy: Division of nerve pathway at a specific site of a sympathetic nerve.

**05.21**    **Sphenopalatine ganglionectomy**

**05.22**    **Cervical sympathectomy**

**05.23**    **Lumbar sympathectomy**
DEF: Excision, resection of lumber chain nerve group to relieve causalgia, Raynaud's disease, or lower extremity thromboangiitis.

**05.24**    **Presacral sympathectomy**
DEF: Excision or resection of hypogastric nerve network.

**05.25**    **Periarterial sympathectomy**
DEF: Removal of arterial sheath containing sympathetic nerve fibers.

**05.29**    **Other sympathectomy and ganglionectomy**
Excision or avulsion of sympathetic nerve NOS
Sympathetic ganglionectomy NOS
**EXCLUDES**   *biopsy of sympathetic nerve or ganglion (05.11)*
*opticociliary neurectomy (12.79)*
*periarterial sympathectomy (05.25)*
*tympanosympathectomy (20.91)*

√4ᵗʰ **05.3**    **Injection into sympathetic nerve or ganglion**
**EXCLUDES**   *injection of ciliary sympathetic ganglion (12.79)*

**05.31**    **Injection of anesthetic into sympathetic nerve for analgesia**

**05.32**    **Injection of neurolytic agent into sympathetic nerve**

**05.39**    **Other injection into sympathetic nerve or ganglion**

√4ᵗʰ **05.8**    **Other operations on sympathetic nerves or ganglia**

**05.81**    **Repair of sympathetic nerve or ganglion**

**05.89**    **Other**

**05.9**    **Other operations on nervous system**

**Operations on the Endocrine System**

**06–06.99**

## 2. OPERATIONS ON THE ENDOCRINE SYSTEM (06-07)

✓3rd **06**    **Operations on thyroid and parathyroid glands**

**INCLUDES**    incidental resection of hyoid bone

✓4th **06.0**    **Incision of thyroid field**

     **EXCLUDES**    *division of isthmus (06.91)*

   **06.01**    **Aspiration of thyroid field**

      Percutaneous or needle drainage of thyroid field

      **EXCLUDES**    *aspiration biopsy of thyroid (06.11)*

           *drainage by incision (06.09)*

           *postoperative aspiration of field (06.02)*

   **06.02**    **Reopening of wound of thyroid field**

      Reopening of wound of thyroid field for:

      control of (postoperative) hemorrhage

      examination

      exploration

      removal of hematoma

   **06.09**    **Other incision of thyroid field**

      Drainage of hematoma

      Drainage of thyroglossal tract

      Exploration:

        neck             } by incision

        thyroid (field)

      Removal of foreign body

      Thyroidotomy NOS

      **EXCLUDES**    *postoperative exploration (06.02)*

           *removal of hematoma by aspiration (06.01)*

✓4th **06.1**    **Diagnostic procedures on thyroid and parathyroid glands**

   **06.11**    **Closed [percutaneous] [needle] biopsy of thyroid gland**

      Aspiration biopsy of thyroid

      DEF: Insertion of needle-type device for removal of thyroid tissue sample.

   **06.12**    **Open biopsy of thyroid gland**

   **06.13**    **Biopsy of parathyroid gland**

   **06.19**    **Other diagnostic procedures on thyroid and parathyroid glands**

      **EXCLUDES**    *radioisotope scan of:*

           *parathyroid (92.13)*

           *thyroid (92.01)*

           *soft tissue x-ray of thyroid field (87.09)*

**Thyroidectomy**

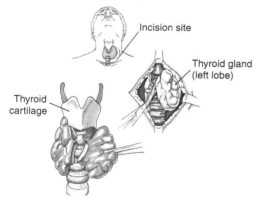

Incision site

Thyroid gland (left lobe)

Thyroid cartilage

 

**06.2**    **Unilateral thyroid lobectomy**

      Complete removal of one lobe of thyroid (with removal of isthmus or portion of other lobe)

      Hemithyroidectomy

      **EXCLUDES**    *partial substernal thyroidectomy (06.51)*

   DEF: Excision of thyroid lobe.

✓4th **06.3**    **Other partial thyroidectomy**

   **06.31**    **Excision of lesion of thyroid**

      **EXCLUDES**    *biopsy of thyroid (06.11-06.12)*

      DEF: Removal of growth on thyroid.

   **06.39**    **Other**

      Isthmectomy      Partial thyroidectomy NOS

      **EXCLUDES**    *partial substernal thyroidectomy (06.51)*

**06.4**    **Complete thyroidectomy**

      **EXCLUDES**    *complete substernal thyroidectomy (06.52)*

           *that with laryngectomy (30.3-30.4)*

✓4th **06.5**    **Substernal thyroidectomy**

   DEF: Removal of thyroid tissue below breastbone.

   **06.50**    **Substernal thyroidectomy, not otherwise specified**

   **06.51**    **Partial substernal thyroidectomy**

   **06.52**    **Complete substernal thyroidectomy**

**06.6**    **Excision of lingual thyroid**

      Excision of thyroid by:

      submental route

      transoral route

   DEF: Excision of thyroid tissue at base of tongue.

**06.7**    **Excision of thyroglossal duct or tract**

✓4th **06.8**    **Parathyroidectomy**

   DEF: Removal of parathyroid glands.

   **06.81**    **Complete parathyroidectomy**

   **06.89**    **Other parathyroidectomy**

      Parathyroidectomy NOS

      Partial parathyroidectomy

      **EXCLUDES**    *biopsy of parathyroid (06.13)*

✓4th **06.9**    **Other operations on thyroid (region) and parathyroid**

   **06.91**    **Division of thyroid isthmus**

      Transection of thyroid isthmus

      DEF: Cutting or division of tissue at narrowest point of thyroid.

   **06.92**    **Ligation of thyroid vessels**

   **06.93**    **Suture of thyroid gland**

   **06.94**    **Thyroid tissue reimplantation**

      Autotransplantation of thyroid tissue

      DEF: Placement of thyroid tissue graft into functional site.

      DEF: Autotransplantation of thyroid tissue: Tissue graft from patient thyroid tissue to another site on thyroid.

   **06.95**    **Parathyroid tissue reimplantation**

      Autotransplantation of parathyroid tissue

      DEF: Placement of parathyroid tissue graft into functional site.

      DEF: Autotransplantation of parathyroid tissue: Use of patient parathyroid tissue for graft.

   **06.98**    **Other operations on thyroid glands**

   **06.99**    **Other operations on parathyroid glands**

---

**BI** Bilateral Procedure     **NC** Non-covered Procedure     **LC** Limited Coverage Procedure     ►◄ Revised Text     ● New Code     ▲ Revised Code Title

✓3ʳᵈ   **07**   **Operations on other endocrine glands**

     **INCLUDES**   operations on:
         adrenal glands    pituitary gland
         pineal gland     thymus

     **EXCLUDES**   operations on:
         *aortic and carotid bodies (39.8)*
         *ovaries (65.0-65.99)*
         *pancreas (52.01-52.99)*
         *testes (62.0-62.99)*

✓4ᵗʰ   **07.0**   **Exploration of adrenal field**

     **EXCLUDES**   *incision of adrenal (gland) (07.41)*

     **07.00**   **Exploration of adrenal field, not otherwise specified**

     **07.01**   **Unilateral exploration of adrenal field**

         DEF: Investigation of one adrenal gland for diagnostic reasons.

     **07.02**   **Bilateral exploration of adrenal field**

         DEF: Investigation of both adrenal glands for diagnostic reasons.

✓4ᵗʰ   **07.1**   **Diagnostic procedures on adrenal glands, pituitary gland, pineal gland, and thymus**

     **07.11**   **Closed [percutaneous] [needle] biopsy of adrenal gland**

     **07.12**   **Open biopsy of adrenal gland**

     **07.13**   **Biopsy of pituitary gland, transfrontal approach**

         DEF: Excision of pituitary gland tissue for exam through frontal bone.

     **07.14**   **Biopsy of pituitary gland, transsphenoidal approach**

         DEF: Excision of pituitary gland tissue for exam through sphenoid bone.

     **07.15**   **Biopsy of pituitary gland, unspecified approach**

     **07.16**   **Biopsy of thymus**

     **07.17**   **Biopsy of pineal gland**

     **07.19**   **Other diagnostic procedures on adrenal glands, pituitary gland, pineal gland, and thymus**

         **EXCLUDES**   *microscopic examination of specimen from endocrine gland (90.11-90.19)*
                *radioisotope scan of pituitary gland (92.11)*

✓4ᵗʰ   **07.2**   **Partial adrenalectomy**

     **07.21**   **Excision of lesion of adrenal gland**

         **EXCLUDES**   *biopsy of adrenal gland (07.11-07.12)*

     **07.22**   **Unilateral adrenalectomy**
         Adrenalectomy NOS

         **EXCLUDES**   *excision of remaining adrenal gland (07.3)*

         DEF: Excision of one adrenal gland.

     **07.29**   **Other partial adrenalectomy**
         Partial adrenalectomy NOS

         **AHA:** 2Q, '05, 4

     **07.3**   **Bilateral adrenalectomy**
         Excision of remaining adrenal gland

         **EXCLUDES**   *bilateral partial adrenalectomy (07.29)*

✓4ᵗʰ   **07.4**   **Other operations on adrenal glands, nerves, and vessels**

     **07.41**   **Incision of adrenal gland**
         Adrenalotomy (with drainage)

     **07.42**   **Division of nerves to adrenal glands**

     **07.43**   **Ligation of adrenal vessels**

     **07.44**   **Repair of adrenal gland**

     **07.45**   **Reimplantation of adrenal tissue**
         Autotransplantation of adrenal tissue

         DEF: Autotransplantation of adrenal tissue: Use of tissue graft from the patient's own body.

     **07.49**   **Other**

✓4ᵗʰ   **07.5**   **Operations on pineal gland**

     **07.51**   **Exploration of pineal field**

         **EXCLUDES**   *that with incision of pineal gland (07.52)*

     **07.52**   **Incision of pineal gland**

     **07.53**   **Partial excision of pineal gland**

         **EXCLUDES**   *biopsy of pineal gland (07.17)*

     **07.54**   **Total excision of pineal gland**
         Pinealectomy (complete) (total)

     **07.59**   **Other operations on pineal gland**

✓4ᵗʰ   **07.6**   **Hypophysectomy**

     DEF: Excision, destruction of pituitary gland.

     **07.61**   **Partial excision of pituitary gland, transfrontal approach**

         Cryohypophysectomy, partial
         Division of hypophyseal stalk
         Excision of lesion of pituitary [hypophysis]     }   transfrontal approach
         Hypophysectomy, subtotal
         Infundibulectomy, hypophyseal

         **EXCLUDES**   *biopsy of pituitary gland, transfrontal approach (07.13)*

         DEF: Removal of pituitary gland, partial, through frontal bone.

     **07.62**   **Partial excision of pituitary gland, transsphenoidal approach**

         **EXCLUDES**   *biopsy of pituitary gland, transsphenoidal approach (07.14)*

         DEF: Removal of pituitary gland, partial, through sphenoid bone.

     **07.63**   **Partial excision of pituitary gland, unspecified approach**

         **EXCLUDES**   *biopsy of pituitary gland NOS (07.15)*

     **07.64**   **Total excision of pituitary gland, transfrontal approach**

         Ablation of pituitary by implantation (strontiumyttrium)     }   transfrontal approach
         Cryohypophysectomy, complete

         DEF: Removal of pituitary gland, total, through frontal bone.

     **07.65**   **Total excision of pituitary gland, transsphenoidal approach**

         DEF: Removal of pituitary gland, total, through sphenoid bone.

     **07.68**   **Total excision of pituitary gland, other specified approach**

         DEF: Destroy or remove pituitary gland by a specified approach, other than those listed.

---

**Operations on the Endocrine System**

**07.69–07.99**

**07.69** **Total excision of pituitary gland, unspecified approach**
Hypophysectomy NOS
Pituitectomy NOS

✓4ᵗʰ **07.7** **Other operations on hypophysis**

**07.71** **Exploration of pituitary fossa**
**EXCLUDES** *exploration with incision of pituitary gland (07.72)*

DEF: Exploration of region of pituitary gland.

**07.72** **Incision of pituitary gland**
Aspiration of:          Aspiration of:
craniobuccal pouch          pituitary gland
craniopharyngioma          Rathke's pouch
hypophysis

**07.79** **Other**
Insertion of pack into sella turcica

✓4ᵗʰ **07.8** **Thymectomy**

**07.80** **Thymectomy, not otherwise specified**

▲ **07.81** **Other partial excision of thymus**
▶Open partial excision of thymus◀
**EXCLUDES** *biopsy of thymus (07.16)*
▶*thoracoscopic partial excision of thymus (07.83)*◀

▲ **07.82** **Other total excision of thymus**
▶Open total excision of thymus◀
**EXCLUDES** ▶*thoracoscopic total excision of thymus (07.84)*◀

● **07.83** **Thoracoscopic partial excision of thymus**
**EXCLUDES** *other partial excision of thymus (07.81)*

● **07.84** **Thoracoscopic total excision of thymus**
**EXCLUDES** *other total excision of thymus (07.82)*

✓4ᵗʰ **07.9** **Other operations on thymus**

**07.91** **Exploration of thymus field**
**EXCLUDES** *exploration with incision of thymus (07.92)*

▲ **07.92** **Other incision of thymus**
▶Open incision of thymus◀
**EXCLUDES** ▶*thoracoscopic incision of thymus (07.95)*◀

**07.93** **Repair of thymus**

**07.94** **Transplantation of thymus**

DEF: Placement of thymus tissue grafts into functional area of gland.

● **07.95** **Thoracoscopic incision of thymus**
**EXCLUDES** *other incision of thymus (07.92)*

● **07.98** **Other and unspecified thoracoscopic operations on thymus**

▲ **07.99** **Other and unspecified operations on thymus**
▶Transcervical thymectomy◀
**EXCLUDES** ▶*other thoracoscopic operations on thymus (07.98)*◀

---

**BI** Bilateral Procedure     **NC** Non-covered Procedure     **LC** Limited Coverage Procedure     ▶◀ Revised Text     ● New Code     ▲ Revised Code Title

82 — Volume 3 • October 2007     © 2007 Ingenix

## 3. OPERATIONS ON THE EYE (08-16)

✓3rd **08**   **Operations on eyelids**
    INCLUDES   operations on the eyebrow

✓4th **08.0**   **Incision of eyelid**

**08.01**   **Incision of lid margin**
    DEF: Cutting into eyelid edge.

**08.02**   **Severing of blepharorrhaphy**
    DEF: Freeing of eyelids previously sutured shut.

**08.09**   **Other incision of eyelid**

✓4th **08.1**   **Diagnostic procedures on eyelid**

**08.11**   **Biopsy of eyelid**

**08.19**   **Other diagnostic procedures on eyelid**

✓4th **08.2**   **Excision or destruction of lesion or tissue of eyelid**
    Code also any synchronous reconstruction (08.61-08.74)
    EXCLUDES   *biopsy of eyelid (08.11)*

**08.20**   **Removal of lesion of eyelid, not otherwise specified**
    Removal of meibomian gland NOS

**08.21**   **Excision of chalazion**

**08.22**   **Excision of other minor lesion of eyelid**
    Excision of:    Excision of:
    verruca         wart

**08.23**   **Excision of major lesion of eyelid, partial-thickness**
    Excision involving one-fourth or more of lid margin, partial-thickness
    DEF: Excision of lesion not in all eyelid layers.

**08.24**   **Excision of major lesion of eyelid, full-thickness**
    Excision involving one-fourth or more of lid margin, full-thickness
    Wedge resection of eyelid
    DEF: Excision of growth in all eyelid layers, full thickness.

**08.25**   **Destruction of lesion of eyelid**

✓4th **08.3**   **Repair of blepharoptosis and lid retraction**

**08.31**   **Repair of blepharoptosis by frontalis muscle technique with suture**
    DEF: Correction of drooping upper eyelid with suture of frontalis muscle.

**08.32**   **Repair of blepharoptosis by frontalis muscle technique with fascial sling**
    DEF: Correction of drooping upper eyelid with fascial tissue sling of frontalis muscle.

**08.33**   **Repair of blepharoptosis by resection or advancement of levator muscle or aponeurosis**
    DEF: Correction of drooping upper eyelid with levator muscle, extended, cut, or by expanded tendon.

**08.34**   **Repair of blepharoptosis by other levator muscle techniques**

**08.35**   **Repair of blepharoptosis by tarsal technique**
    DEF: Correction of drooping upper eyelid with tarsal muscle.

**08.36**   **Repair of blepharoptosis by other techniques**
    Correction of eyelid ptosis NOS
    Orbicularis oculi muscle sling for correction of blepharoptosis

**08.37**   **Reduction of overcorrection of ptosis**
    DEF: Correction, release of previous plastic repair of drooping eyelid.

**08.38**   **Correction of lid retraction**
    DEF: Fixing of withdrawn eyelid into normal position.

✓4th **08.4**   **Repair of entropion or ectropion**

**08.41**   **Repair of entropion or ectropion by thermocauterization**
    DEF: Restoration of eyelid margin to normal position with heat cautery.

**08.42**   **Repair of entropion or ectropion by suture technique**
    DEF: Restoration of eyelid margin to normal position by suture.

**08.43**   **Repair of entropion or ectropion with wedge resection**
    DEF: Restoration of eyelid margin to normal position by removing tissue.

**08.44**   **Repair of entropion or ectropion with lid reconstruction**
    DEF: Reconstruction of eyelid margin.

**08.49**   **Other repair of entropion or ectropion**

✓4th **08.5**   **Other adjustment of lid position**

**08.51**   **Canthotomy**
    DEF: Incision into outer canthus of eye.

**08.52**   **Blepharorrhaphy**
    Canthorrhaphy    Tarsorrhaphy
    DEF: Suture together of eyelids, partial or repair; done to shorten palpebral fissure or protect cornea.

**08.59**   **Other**
    Canthoplasty NOS
    Repair of epicanthal fold

✓4th **08.6**   **Reconstruction of eyelid with flaps or grafts**
    EXCLUDES   *that associated with repair of entropion and ectropion (08.44)*

**08.61**   **Reconstruction of eyelid with skin flap or graft**
    DEF: Rebuild of eyelid by graft or flap method.

**08.62**   **Reconstruction of eyelid with mucous membrane flap or graft**
    DEF: Rebuild of eyelid with mucous membrane by graft or flap method.

**08.63**   **Reconstruction of eyelid with hair follicle graft**
    DEF: Rebuild of eyelid with hair follicle graft.

**08.64**   **Reconstruction of eyelid with tarsoconjunctival flap**
    Transfer of tarsoconjunctival flap from opposing lid
    DEF: Recreation of eyelid with tarsoconjunctival tissue.

**08.69**   **Other reconstruction of eyelid with flaps or grafts**

✓4th **08.7**   **Other reconstruction of eyelid**
    EXCLUDES   *that associated with repair of entropion and ectropion (08.44)*

**08.70**   **Reconstruction of eyelid, not otherwise specified**
    AHA: 2Q, '96, 11

**08.71**   **Reconstruction of eyelid involving lid margin, partial-thickness**
    DEF: Repair of eyelid margin not using all lid layers.

**08.72**   **Other reconstruction of eyelid, partial-thickness**
    DEF: Reshape of eyelid not using all lid layers.

08.73 **Reconstruction of eyelid involving lid margin, full-thickness**
DEF: Repair of eyelid and margin using all tissue layers.

08.74 **Other reconstruction of eyelid, full-thickness**
DEF: Other repair of eyelid using all tissue layers.

√4th 08.8 **Other repair of eyelid**

08.81 **Linear repair of laceration of eyelid or eyebrow**

08.82 **Repair of laceration involving lid margin, partial-thickness**
DEF: Repair of laceration not involving all layers of eyelid margin.

08.83 **Other repair of laceration of eyelid, partial thickness**
DEF: Repair of eyelid tear not involving all eyelid layers.

08.84 **Repair of laceration involving lid margin, full-thickness**
DEF: Repair of eyelid margin tear involving all margin layers.

08.85 **Other repair of laceration of eyelid, full-thickness**
DEF: Repair of eyelid tear involving all layers.

08.86 **Lower eyelid rhytidectomy**
DEF: Removal of wrinkles from lower eyelid.

08.87 **Upper eyelid rhytidectomy**
AHA: 2Q, '96, 11
DEF: Removal of wrinkles from upper eyelid.

08.89 **Other eyelid repair**
AHA: 1Q, '00, 22

√4th 08.9 **Other operations on eyelids**

08.91 **Electrosurgical epilation of eyelid**
DEF: Electrical removal of eyelid hair roots.

08.92 **Cryosurgical epilation of eyelid**
DEF: Removal of eyelid hair roots by freezing.

08.93 **Other epilation of eyelid**

08.99 **Other**

√3rd 09 **Operations on lacrimal system**

09.0 **Incision of lacrimal gland**
Incision of lacrimal cyst (with drainage)

√4th 09.1 **Diagnostic procedures on lacrimal system**

09.11 **Biopsy of lacrimal gland**

09.12 **Biopsy of lacrimal sac**

09.19 **Other diagnostic procedures on lacrimal system**
EXCLUDES contrast dacryocystogram (87.05)
soft tissue x-ray of nasolacrimal duct (87.09)

√4th 09.2 **Excision of lesion or tissue of lacrimal gland**

09.20 **Excision of lacrimal gland, not otherwise specified**

09.21 **Excision of lesion of lacrimal gland**
EXCLUDES biopsy of lacrimal gland (09.11)

09.22 **Other partial dacryoadenectomy**
EXCLUDES biopsy of lacrimal gland (09.11)
DEF: Excision, partial, of tear gland.

09.23 **Total dacryoadenectomy**
DEF: Excision, total, of tear gland.

09.3 **Other operations on lacrimal gland**

√4th 09.4 **Manipulation of lacrimal passage**
INCLUDES removal of calculus
that with dilation
EXCLUDES contrast dacryocystogram (87.05)

09.41 **Probing of lacrimal punctum**
DEF: Exploration of tear duct entrance with flexible rod.

09.42 **Probing of lacrimal canaliculi**
DEF: Exploration of tear duct with flexible rod.

09.43 **Probing of nasolacrimal duct**
EXCLUDES that with insertion of tube or stent (09.44)
DEF: Exploration of passage between tear sac and nose with flexible rod.

09.44 **Intubation of nasolacrimal duct**
Insertion of stent into nasolacrimal duct
AHA: 2Q, '94, 11

09.49 **Other manipulation of lacrimal passage**

√4th 09.5 **Incision of lacrimal sac and passages**

09.51 **Incision of lacrimal punctum**

09.52 **Incision of lacrimal canaliculi**

09.53 **Incision of lacrimal sac**
DEF: Cutting into lacrimal pouch of tear gland.

09.59 **Other incision of lacrimal passages**
Incision (and drainage) of nasolacrimal duct NOS

09.6 **Excision of lacrimal sac and passage**
EXCLUDES biopsy of lacrimal sac (09.12)
DEF: Removal of pouch and passage of tear gland.

√4th 09.7 **Repair of canaliculus and punctum**
EXCLUDES repair of eyelid (08.81-08.89)

09.71 **Correction of everted punctum**
DEF: Repair of an outwardly turned tear duct entrance.

09.72 **Other repair of punctum**

09.73 **Repair of canaliculus**

√4th 09.8 **Fistulization of lacrimal tract to nasal cavity**

09.81 **Dacryocystorhinostomy [DCR]**
DEF: Creation of entrance between tear gland and nasal passage for tear flow.

09.82 **Conjunctivocystorhinostomy**
Conjunctivodacryocystorhinostomy [CDCR]
EXCLUDES that with insertion of tube or stent (09.83)
DEF: Creation of tear drainage path from lacrimal sac to nasal cavity through conjunctiva.

09.83 **Conjunctivorhinostomy with insertion of tube or stent**
DEF: Creation of passage between eye sac membrane and nasal cavity with tube or stent.

√4th 09.9 **Other operations on lacrimal system**

09.91 **Obliteration of lacrimal punctum**
DEF: Destruction, total of tear gland opening in eyelid.

09.99 **Other**
AHA: 2Q, '94, 11

√3rd 10 **Operations on conjunctiva**

10.0 **Removal of embedded foreign body from conjunctiva by incision**
EXCLUDES removal of:
embedded foreign body without incision (98.22)
superficial foreign body (98.21)

10.1 **Other incision of conjunctiva**

BI Bilateral Procedure    NC Non-covered Procedure    LC Limited Coverage Procedure    ▶◀ Revised Text    ● New Code    ▲ Revised Code Title

84 — Volume 3

© 2007 Ingenix

**✓4ᵗʰ 10.2   Diagnostic procedures on conjunctiva**

**10.21   Biopsy of conjunctiva**

**10.29   Other diagnostic procedures on conjunctiva**

**✓4ᵗʰ 10.3   Excision or destruction of lesion or tissue of conjunctiva**

**10.31   Excision of lesion or tissue of conjunctiva**
Excision of ring of conjunctiva around cornea
> **EXCLUDES**   biopsy of conjunctiva (10.21)

AHA: 4Q, '00, 41; 3Q, '96, 7

DEF: Removal of growth or tissue from eye membrane.

**10.32   Destruction of lesion of conjunctiva**
> **EXCLUDES**   excision of lesion (10.31)
> thermocauterization for entropion (08.41)

DEF: Destruction of eye membrane growth; not done by excision.

**10.33   Other destructive procedures on conjunctiva**
Removal of trachoma follicles

**✓4ᵗʰ 10.4   Conjunctivoplasty**
DEF: Correction of conjunctiva by plastic surgery.

**10.41   Repair of symblepharon with free graft**
AHA: 3Q, '96, 7

**10.42   Reconstruction of conjunctival cul-de-sac with free graft**
> **EXCLUDES**   revision of enucleation socket with graft (16.63)

DEF: Rebuilding of eye membrane fold with graft of unattached tissue.

**10.43   Other reconstruction of conjunctival cul-de-sac**
> **EXCLUDES**   revision of enucleation socket (16.64)

**10.44   Other free graft to conjunctiva**

**10.49   Other conjunctivoplasty**
> **EXCLUDES**   repair of cornea with conjunctival flap (11.53)

**10.5   Lysis of adhesions of conjunctiva and eyelid**
Division of symblepharon (with insertion of conformer)

**10.6   Repair of laceration of conjunctiva**
> **EXCLUDES**   that with repair of sclera (12.81)

**✓4ᵗʰ 10.9   Other operations on conjunctiva**

**10.91   Subconjunctival injection**
AHA: 3Q, '96, 7

**10.99   Other**

**✓3ʳᵈ 11   Operations on cornea**

**11.0   Magnetic removal of embedded foreign body from cornea**
> **EXCLUDES**   that with incision (11.1)

**11.1   Incision of cornea**
Incision of cornea for removal of foreign body

**✓4ᵗʰ 11.2   Diagnostic procedures on cornea**

**11.21   Scraping of cornea for smear or culture**

**11.22   Biopsy of cornea**

**11.29   Other diagnostic procedures on cornea**

**✓4ᵗʰ 11.3   Excision of pterygium**

**11.31   Transposition of pterygium**
DEF: Cutting into membranous structure extending from eye membrane to cornea and suturing it in a downward position.

**11.32   Excision of pterygium with corneal graft**
DEF: Surgical removal and repair of membranous structure extending from eye membrane to cornea using corneal tissue transplant.

**11.39   Other excision of pterygium**

**✓4ᵗʰ 11.4   Excision or destruction of tissue or other lesion of cornea**

**11.41   Mechanical removal of corneal epithelium**
That by chemocauterization
> **EXCLUDES**   that for smear or culture (11.21)

AHA: 3Q, '02, 20

DEF: Removal of outer layer of cornea by mechanical means.

**11.42   Thermocauterization of corneal lesion**
DEF: Destruction of corneal lesion by electrical cautery.

**11.43   Cryotherapy of corneal lesion**
DEF: Destruction of corneal lesion with cold therapy.

**11.49   Other removal or destruction of corneal lesion**
Excision of cornea NOS
> **EXCLUDES**   biopsy of cornea (11.22)

**✓4ᵗʰ 11.5   Repair of cornea**

**11.51   Suture of corneal laceration**
AHA: 3Q, '96, 7

**11.52   Repair of postoperative wound dehiscence of cornea**
DEF: Repair of ruptured postoperative corneal wound.

**11.53   Repair of corneal laceration or wound with conjunctival flap**
DEF: Correction corneal wound or tear with conjunctival tissue.

**11.59   Other repair of cornea**

**✓4ᵗʰ 11.6   Corneal transplant**
> **EXCLUDES**   excision of pterygium with corneal graft (11.32)

**11.60   Corneal transplant, not otherwise specified**
Note: To report donor sources — see codes 00.91-00.93
Keratoplasty NOS

**11.61   Lamellar keratoplasty with autograft**
DEF: Restoration of sight using patient's own corneal tissue, partial thickness.

**11.62   Other lamellar keratoplasty**
AHA: S-O, '85, 6

DEF: Restoration of sight using donor corneal tissue, partial thickness.

**11.63   Penetrating keratoplasty with autograft**
Perforating keratoplasty with autograft

**11.64   Other penetrating keratoplasty**
Perforating keratoplasty (with homograft)

**11.69   Other corneal transplant**

**✓4ᵗʰ 11.7   Other reconstructive and refractive surgery on cornea**

**11.71   Keratomileusis**   NC
DEF: Restoration of corneal shape by removing portion of cornea, freezing, reshaping curve and reattaching it.

**11.72   Keratophakia**   NC
DEF: Correction of eye lens loss by dissecting the central zone of the cornea and replacing it with a thickened graft of the cornea.

**11.73   Keratoprosthesis**
DEF: Placement of corneal artificial implant.

**11.74   Thermokeratoplasty**
DEF: Reshaping and reforming cornea by heat application.

**Operations on the Eye**

**10.2–11.74**

---

**Operations on the Eye**

**11.75–12.64**

**11.75  Radial keratotomy** `NC`

DEF: Incisions around cornea radius to correct nearsightedness.

**11.76  Epikeratophakia** `NC`

DEF: Repair lens loss by cornea graft sutured to central corneal zone.

**11.79  Other**

✓4ᵗʰ **11.9  Other operations on cornea**

**11.91  Tattooing of cornea**

**11.92  Removal of artificial implant from cornea**

**11.99  Other**

AHA: 3Q, '02, 20

✓3ʳᵈ **12  Operations on iris, ciliary body, sclera, and anterior chamber**

EXCLUDES   operations on cornea (11.0-11.99)

✓4ᵗʰ **12.0  Removal of intraocular foreign body from anterior segment of eye**

**12.00  Removal of intraocular foreign body from anterior segment of eye, not otherwise specified**

**12.01  Removal of intraocular foreign body from anterior segment of eye with use of magnet**

**12.02  Removal of intraocular foreign body from anterior segment of eye without use of magnet**

✓4ᵗʰ **12.1  Iridotomy and simple iridectomy**

EXCLUDES   iridectomy associated with:
cataract extraction (13.11-13.69)
removal of lesion (12.41-12.42)
scleral fistulization (12.61-12.69)

**12.11  Iridotomy with transfixion**

**12.12  Other iridotomy**

Corectomy
Discission of iris
Iridotomy NOS

DEF: Corectomy: Incision into iris (also called iridectomy).

**12.13  Excision of prolapsed iris**

DEF: Removal of downwardly placed portion of iris.

**12.14  Other iridectomy**

Iridectomy (basal) (peripheral) (total)

DEF: Removal, partial or total of iris.

✓4ᵗʰ **12.2  Diagnostic procedures on iris, ciliary body, sclera, and anterior chamber**

**12.21  Diagnostic aspiration of anterior chamber of eye**

DEF: Suction withdrawal of fluid from anterior eye chamber for diagnostic reasons.

**12.22  Biopsy of iris**

**12.29  Other diagnostic procedures on iris, ciliary body, sclera, and anterior chamber**

✓4ᵗʰ **12.3  Iridoplasty and coreoplasty**

DEF: Correction or abnormal iris or pupil by plastic surgery.

**12.31  Lysis of goniosynechiae**

Lysis of goniosynechiae by injection of air or liquid

DEF: Freeing of fibrous structures between cornea and iris by injecting air or liquid.

**12.32  Lysis of other anterior synechiae**

Lysis of anterior synechiae:
NOS
by injection of air or liquid

**12.33  Lysis of posterior synechiae**

Lysis of iris adhesions NOS

**12.34  Lysis of corneovitreal adhesions**

DEF: Release of adhesions of cornea and vitreous body.

**12.35  Coreoplasty**

Needling of pupillary membrane

DEF: Correction of an iris defect.

**12.39  Other iridoplasty**

✓4ᵗʰ **12.4  Excision or destruction of lesion of iris and ciliary body**

**12.40  Removal of lesion of anterior segment of eye, not otherwise specified**

**12.41  Destruction of lesion of iris, nonexcisional**

Destruction of lesion of iris by:
cauterization
cryotherapy
photocoagulation

**12.42  Excision of lesion of iris**

EXCLUDES   biopsy of iris (12.22)

**12.43  Destruction of lesion of ciliary body, nonexcisional**

**12.44  Excision of lesion of ciliary body**

✓4ᵗʰ **12.5  Facilitation of intraocular circulation**

**12.51  Goniopuncture without goniotomy**

DEF: Stab incision into anterior chamber of eye to relieve optic pressure.

**12.52  Goniotomy without goniopuncture**

DEF: Incision into Schlemm's canal to drain aqueous and relieve pressure.

**12.53  Goniotomy with goniopuncture**

**12.54  Trabeculotomy ab externo**

DEF: Incision into supporting connective tissue strands of eye capsule, via exterior approach.

**12.55  Cyclodialysis**

DEF: Creation of passage between anterior chamber and suprachoroidal space.

**12.59  Other facilitation of intraocular circulation**

✓4ᵗʰ **12.6  Scleral fistulization**

EXCLUDES   exploratory sclerotomy (12.89)

**12.61  Trephination of sclera with iridectomy**

DEF: Cut around sclerocornea to remove part of the iris.

**12.62  Thermocauterization of sclera with iridectomy**

DEF: Destruction of outer eyeball layer with partial excision of iris using heat.

**12.63  Iridencleisis and iridotasis**

DEF: Creation of permanent drain in iris by transposing or stretching iris tissue.

**12.64  Trabeculectomy ab externo**

DEF: Excision of supporting connective tissue strands of eye capsule, via exterior approach.

**Trabeculectomy Ab Externo**

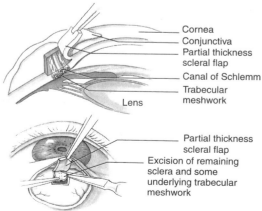

Cornea
Conjunctiva
Partial thickness scleral flap
Canal of Schlemm
Trabecular meshwork
Lens

Partial thickness scleral flap
Excision of remaining sclera and some underlying trabecular meshwork

`BI` Bilateral Procedure    `NC` Non-covered Procedure    `LC` Limited Coverage Procedure    ▶◀ Revised Text    ● New Code    ▲ Revised Code Title

86 — Volume 3

© 2007 Ingenix

**12.65 Other scleral fistulization with iridectomy**
Holth's sclerectomy
DEF: Creation of outer eyeball layer passage with partial excision of iris.

**12.66 Postoperative revision of scleral fistulization procedure**
Revision of filtering bleb
EXCLUDES   *repair of fistula (12.82)*
AHA: 2Q, '01, 16

**12.69 Other fistulizing procedure**

√4ᵗʰ **12.7 Other procedures for relief of elevated intraocular pressure**

**12.71 Cyclodiathermy**
DEF: Destruction of ciliary body tissue with heat.

**12.72 Cyclocryotherapy**
DEF: Destruction of ciliary body tissue by freezing.

**12.73 Cyclophotocoagulation**
DEF: Destruction of ciliary body tissue by high energy light source.

**12.74 Diminution of ciliary body, not otherwise specified**

**12.79 Other glaucoma procedures**
AHA: 2Q, '98, 16

√4ᵗʰ **12.8 Operations on sclera**
EXCLUDES   *those associated with:*
*retinal reattachment (14.41-14.59)*
*scleral fistulization (12.61-12.69)*

**12.81 Suture of laceration of sclera**
Suture of sclera with synchronous repair of conjunctiva

**12.82 Repair of scleral fistula**
EXCLUDES   *postoperative revision of scleral fistulization procedure (12.66)*

**12.83 Revision of operative wound of anterior segment, not elsewhere classified**
EXCLUDES   *postoperative revision of scleral fistulization procedure (12.66)*

**12.84 Excision or destruction of lesion of sclera**

**12.85 Repair of scleral staphyloma with graft**
DEF: Repair of protruding outer eyeball layer with a graft.

**12.86 Other repair of scleral staphyloma**

**12.87 Scleral reinforcement with graft**
DEF: Restoration of outer eyeball shape with tissue graft.

**12.88 Other scleral reinforcement**

**12.89 Other operations on sclera**
Exploratory sclerotomy

√4ᵗʰ **12.9 Other operations on iris, ciliary body, and anterior chamber**

**12.91 Therapeutic evacuation of anterior chamber**
Paracentesis of anterior chamber
EXCLUDES   *diagnostic aspiration (12.21)*

**12.92 Injection into anterior chamber**
Injection of:
air       } into anterior
liquid      } chamber
medication
AHA: J-A, '84, 1

**12.93 Removal or destruction of epithelial downgrowth from anterior chamber**
EXCLUDES   *that with iridectomy (12.41-12.42)*
DEF: Excision or destruction of epithelial overgrowth in anterior eye chamber.

**12.97 Other operations on iris**
**12.98 Other operations on ciliary body**
**12.99 Other operations on anterior chamber**

√3ʳᵈ **13 Operations on lens**

√4ᵗʰ **13.0 Removal of foreign body from lens**
EXCLUDES   *removal of pseudophakos (13.8)*

**13.00 Removal of foreign body from lens, not otherwise specified**

**13.01 Removal of foreign body from lens with use of magnet**

**13.02 Removal of foreign body from lens without use of magnet**

√4ᵗʰ **13.1 Intracapsular extraction of lens**
Code also any synchronous insertion of pseudophakos (13.71)
AHA: S-O, '85, 6

**13.11 Intracapsular extraction of lens by temporal inferior route**
DEF: Extraction of lens and capsule via anterior approach through outer side of eyeball.

**13.19 Other intracapsular extraction of lens**
Cataract extraction NOS
Cryoextraction of lens
Erysiphake extraction of cataract
Extraction of lens NOS

**13.2 Extracapsular extraction of lens by linear extraction technique**
AHA: S-O, '85, 6
DEF: Excision of lens without the posterior capsule at junction between the cornea and outer eyeball layer by means of a linear incision.

**13.3 Extracapsular extraction of lens by simple aspiration (and irrigation) technique**
Irrigation of traumatic cataract
AHA: S-O, '85, 6
DEF: Removal of lens without the posterior capsule by suctioning and flushing out the area.

√4ᵗʰ **13.4 Extracapsular extraction of lens by fragmentation and aspiration technique**
AHA: S-O, '85, 6
DEF: Removal of lens after division into smaller pieces with posterior capsule left intact.

**13.41 Phacoemulsification and aspiration of cataract**
AHA: 3Q, '96, 4; 1Q, '94, 16

**13.42 Mechanical phacofragmentation and aspiration of cataract by posterior route**
Code also any synchronous vitrectomy (14.74)

**Extraction of Lens**
**(with insertion of intraocular lens prosthesis)**

Iris

Lens cataract removed

Iris

Lens

Intraocular lens insertion

**Operations on the Eye**

**13.43–14.49**

### Laser Surgery (YAG)

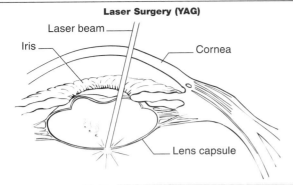

Laser beam
Laser beam
Iris
Cornea
Lens capsule

**13.43** **Mechanical phacofragmentation and other aspiration of cataract**

√4th **13.5** **Other extracapsular extraction of lens**
Code also any synchronous insertion of pseudophakos (13.71)
AHA: S-O, '85, 6

**13.51** **Extracapsular extraction of lens by temporal inferior route**
DEF: Removal of lens through outer eyeball with posterior capsule left intact.

**13.59** **Other extracapsular extraction of lens**

√4th **13.6** **Other cataract extraction**
Code also any synchronous insertion of pseudophakos (13.71)
AHA: S-O, '85, 6

**13.64** **Discission of secondary membrane [after cataract]**
DEF: Breaking up of fibrotic lens capsule developed after previous lens extraction.

**13.65** **Excision of secondary membrane [after cataract]**
Capsulectomy
DEF: Capsulectomy: Excision of lens capsule membrane after previous lens extraction.

**13.66** **Mechanical fragmentation of secondary membrane [after cataract]**
DEF: Breaking up and removal of fibrotic lens capsule developed after previous lens extraction.

**13.69** **Other cataract extraction**

√4th **13.7** **Insertion of prosthetic lens [pseudophakos]**
EXCLUDES *implantation of intraocular telescope prosthesis (13.91)*
AHA: J-A, '84, 1
DEF: Insertion of ocular implant, following lens extraction.

**13.70** **Insertion of pseudophakos, not otherwise specified**

**13.71** **Insertion of intraocular lens prosthesis at time of cataract extraction, one-stage**
Code also synchronous extraction of cataract (13.11-13.69)
AHA: 3Q, '96, 4

**13.72** **Secondary insertion of intraocular lens prosthesis**

**13.8** **Removal of implanted lens**
Removal of pseudophakos

√4th **13.9** **Other operations on lens**
AHA: 1Q, '00, 9

**13.90** **Operation on lens, not elsewhere classified**
AHA: ▶4Q, '06, 123◀

**13.91** **Implantation of intraocular telescope prosthesis**
Implantable miniature telescope
INCLUDES removal of lens, any method
EXCLUDES *secondary insertion of ocular implant (16.61)*
AHA: ▶4Q, '06, 123◀

√3rd **14** **Operations on retina, choroid, vitreous, and posterior chamber**

√4th **14.0** **Removal of foreign body from posterior segment of eye**
EXCLUDES *removal of surgically implanted material (14.6)*

**14.00** **Removal of foreign body from posterior segment of eye, not otherwise specified**

**14.01** **Removal of foreign body from posterior segment of eye with use of magnet**

**14.02** **Removal of foreign body from posterior segment of eye without use of magnet**

√4th **14.1** **Diagnostic procedures on retina, choroid, vitreous, and posterior chamber**

**14.11** **Diagnostic aspiration of vitreous**

**14.19** **Other diagnostic procedures on retina, choroid, vitreous, and posterior chamber**

√4th **14.2** **Destruction of lesion of retina and choroid**
INCLUDES destruction of chorioretinopathy or isolated chorioretinal lesion
EXCLUDES *that for repair of retina (14.31-14.59)*
DEF: Destruction of damaged retina and choroid tissue.

**14.21** **Destruction of chorioretinal lesion by diathermy**

**14.22** **Destruction of chorioretinal lesion by cryotherapy**

**14.23** **Destruction of chorioretinal lesion by xenon arc photocoagulation**

**14.24** **Destruction of chorioretinal lesion by laser photocoagulation**

**14.25** **Destruction of chorioretinal lesion by photocoagulation of unspecified type**

**14.26** **Destruction of chorioretinal lesion by radiation therapy**

**14.27** **Destruction of chorioretinal lesion by implantation of radiation source**

**14.29** **Other destruction of chorioretinal lesion**
Destruction of lesion of retina and choroid NOS

√4th **14.3** **Repair of retinal tear**
INCLUDES repair of retinal defect
EXCLUDES *repair of retinal detachment (14.41-14.59)*

**14.31** **Repair of retinal tear by diathermy**

**14.32** **Repair of retinal tear by cryotherapy**

**14.33** **Repair of retinal tear by xenon arc photocoagulation**

**14.34** **Repair of retinal tear by laser photocoagulation**
AHA: 1Q, '94, 17

**14.35** **Repair of retinal tear by photocoagulation of unspecified type**

**14.39** **Other repair of retinal tear**

√4th **14.4** **Repair of retinal detachment with scleral buckling and implant**
DEF: Placement of material around eye to indent sclera and close a hole or tear or to reduce vitreous traction.

**14.41** **Scleral buckling with implant**
AHA: 3Q, '96, 6

**14.49** **Other scleral buckling**
Scleral buckling with:
air tamponade
resection of sclera
vitrectomy
AHA: 1Q, '94, 16

---

BI Bilateral Procedure    NC Non-covered Procedure    LC Limited Coverage Procedure    ▶◀ Revised Text    ● New Code    ▲ Revised Code Title

✓4ᵗʰ **14.5  Other repair of retinal detachment**
>  INCLUDES  *that with drainage*

**14.51  Repair of retinal detachment with diathermy**

**14.52  Repair of retinal detachment with cryotherapy**

**14.53  Repair of retinal detachment with xenon arc photocoagulation**

**14.54  Repair of retinal detachment with laser photocoagulation**
AHA: N-D, '87, 10

**14.55  Repair of retinal detachment with photocoagulation of unspecified type**

**14.59  Other**

**14.6  Removal of surgically implanted material from posterior segment of eye**

✓4ᵗʰ **14.7  Operations on vitreous**

**14.71  Removal of vitreous, anterior approach**
>  Open sky technique
>  Removal of vitreous, anterior approach (with replacement)

DEF: Removal of all or part of the eyeball fluid via the anterior segment of the eyeball.

**14.72  Other removal of vitreous**
>  Aspiration of vitreous by posterior sclerotomy

**14.73  Mechanical vitrectomy by anterior approach**
AHA: 3Q, '96, 4, 5

DEF: Removal of abnormal tissue in eyeball fluid to control fibrotic overgrowth in severe intraocular injury.

**14.74  Other mechanical vitrectomy**
>  Posterior approach
AHA: 3Q, '96, 4, 5

**14.75  Injection of vitreous substitute**
>  EXCLUDES  *that associated with removal (14.71-14.72)*
AHA: 1Q, '98, 6; 3Q, '96, 4, 5; 1Q, '94, 17

**14.79  Other operations on vitreous**
AHA: 3Q, '99, 12; 1Q, '99, 11; 1Q, '98, 6

**14.9  Other operations on retina, choroid, and posterior chamber**
AHA: 3Q, '96, 5

✓3ʳᵈ **15  Operations on extraocular muscles**

✓4ᵗʰ **15.0  Diagnostic procedures on extraocular muscles or tendons**

**15.01  Biopsy of extraocular muscle or tendon**

**15.09  Other diagnostic procedures on extraocular muscles and tendons**

✓4ᵗʰ **15.1  Operations on one extraocular muscle involving temporary detachment from globe**

**15.11  Recession of one extraocular muscle**
AHA: 3Q, '96, 3

DEF: Detachment of exterior eye muscle with posterior reattachment to correct strabismus.

**15.12  Advancement of one extraocular muscle**
DEF: Detachment of exterior eye muscle with forward reattachment to correct strabismus.

**15.13  Resection of one extraocular muscle**

**15.19  Other operations on one extraocular muscle involving temporary detachment from globe**
>  EXCLUDES  *transposition of muscle (15.5)*

✓4ᵗʰ **15.2  Other operations on one extraocular muscle**

**15.21  Lengthening procedure on one extraocular muscle**
DEF: Extension of exterior eye muscle length.

**Lengthening Procedure on One Extraocular Muscle**

Proposed second cut

Lengthened muscle

Extraocular muscle

**Shortening Procedure on One Extraocular Muscle**

To be resected

Muscle advanced and reattached

Iris

**15.22  Shortening procedure on one extraocular muscle**
DEF: Shortening of exterior eye muscle.

**15.29  Other**

**15.3  Operations on two or more extraocular muscles involving temporary detachment from globe, one or both eyes**
AHA: 3Q, '96, 3

**15.4  Other operations on two or more extraocular muscles, one or both eyes**

**15.5  Transposition of extraocular muscles**
>  EXCLUDES  *that for correction of ptosis (08.31-08.36)*

DEF: Relocation of exterior eye muscle to a more functional site.

**15.6  Revision of extraocular muscle surgery**
DEF: Repair of previous exterior eye muscle surgery.

**15.7  Repair of injury of extraocular muscle**
>  Freeing of entrapped extraocular muscle
>  Lysis of adhesions of extraocular muscle
>  Repair of laceration of extraocular muscle, tendon, or Tenon's capsule

**15.9  Other operations on extraocular muscles and tendons**

✓3ʳᵈ **16  Operations on orbit and eyeball**
>  EXCLUDES  *reduction of fracture of orbit (76.78-76.79)*

✓4ᵗʰ **16.0  Orbitotomy**

**16.01  Orbitotomy with bone flap**
>  Orbitotomy with lateral approach
DEF: Incision into orbital bone with insertion of small bone piece.

**16.02  Orbitotomy with insertion of orbital implant**
>  EXCLUDES  *that with bone flap (16.01)*

**16.09  Other orbitotomy**

**Operations on the Eye**

**16.1–16.99**

**16.1 Removal of penetrating foreign body from eye, not otherwise specified**

> EXCLUDES   removal of nonpenetrating foreign body (98.21)

DEF: Removal of foreign body from an unspecified site in eye.

**✓4th 16.2 Diagnostic procedures on orbit and eyeball**

**16.21 Ophthalmoscopy**

**16.22 Diagnostic aspiration of orbit**

**16.23 Biopsy of eyeball and orbit**

**16.29 Other diagnostic procedures on orbit and eyeball**

> EXCLUDES   examination of form and structure of eye (95.11-95.16)
> general and subjective eye examination (95.01-95.09)
> microscopic examination of specimen from eye (90.21-90.29)
> objective functional tests of eye (95.21-95.26)
> ocular thermography (88.82)
> tonometry (89.11)
> x-ray of orbit (87.14, 87.16)

**✓4th 16.3 Evisceration of eyeball**

DEF: Removal of eyeball, leaving sclera and occasionally cornea.

**16.31 Removal of ocular contents with synchronous implant into scleral shell**

DEF: Removal of eyeball leaving outer eyeball layer with ocular implant into shell.

**16.39 Other evisceration of eyeball**

**✓4th 16.4 Enucleation of eyeball**

DEF: Removal of entire eyeball after severing eye muscles and optic nerves.

**16.41 Enucleation of eyeball with synchronous implant into Tenon's capsule with attachment of muscles**

Integrated implant of eyeball

DEF: Removal of eyeball with insertion of ocular implant and muscle attachment.

**16.42 Enucleation of eyeball with other synchronous implant**

**16.49 Other enucleation of eyeball**

Removal of eyeball NOS

**✓4th 16.5 Exenteration of orbital contents**

**16.51 Exenteration of orbit with removal of adjacent structures**

Radical orbitomaxillectomy

DEF: Removal of contents of bony cavity of eye as well as related tissues and structures.

DEF: Radical orbitomaxillectomy: Removal of contents of bony cavity of eye, related tissues and structures, and a portion of maxillary bone.

**16.52 Exenteration of orbit with therapeutic removal of orbital bone**

**16.59 Other exenteration of orbit**

Evisceration of orbit NOS
Exenteration of orbit with temporalis muscle transplant

**✓4th 16.6 Secondary procedures after removal of eyeball**

> EXCLUDES   that with synchronous:
> enucleation of eyeball (16.41-16.42)
> evisceration of eyeball (16.31)

**16.61 Secondary insertion of ocular implant**

DEF: Insertion of ocular implant after previous eye removal.

**16.62 Revision and reinsertion of ocular implant**

DEF: Reimplant or correction of ocular implant.

**16.63 Revision of enucleation socket with graft**

DEF: Implant of tissue to correct socket after eye removal.

**16.64 Other revision of enucleation socket**

**16.65 Secondary graft to exenteration cavity**

DEF: Implant of tissue in place of eye after removal.

**16.66 Other revision of exenteration cavity**

**16.69 Other secondary procedures after removal of eyeball**

**✓4th 16.7 Removal of ocular or orbital implant**

**16.71 Removal of ocular implant**

**16.72 Removal of orbital implant**

**✓4th 16.8 Repair of injury of eyeball and orbit**

**16.81 Repair of wound of orbit**

> EXCLUDES   reduction of orbital fracture (76.78-76.79)
> repair of extraocular muscles (15.7)

**16.82 Repair of rupture of eyeball**

Repair of multiple structures of eye

> EXCLUDES   repair of laceration of:
> cornea (11.51-11.59)
> sclera (12.81)

**16.89 Other repair of injury of eyeball or orbit**

**✓4th 16.9 Other operations on orbit and eyeball**

> EXCLUDES   irrigation of eye (96.51)
> prescription and fitting of low vision aids (95.31-95.33)
> removal of:
> eye prosthesis NEC (97.31)
> nonpenetrating foreign body from eye without incision (98.21)

**16.91 Retrobulbar injection of therapeutic agent**

> EXCLUDES   injection of radiographic contrast material (87.14)
> opticociliary injection (12.79)

**16.92 Excision of lesion of orbit**

> EXCLUDES   biopsy of orbit (16.23)

**16.93 Excision of lesion of eye, unspecified structure**

> EXCLUDES   biopsy of eye NOS (16.23)

**16.98 Other operations on orbit**

**16.99 Other operations on eyeball**

---

BI Bilateral Procedure     NC Non-covered Procedure     LC Limited Coverage Procedure     ▶◀ Revised Text     ● New Code     ▲ Revised Code Title

90 — Volume 3

© 2007 Ingenix

### 4. OPERATIONS ON THE EAR (18-20)

√3rd **18 Operations on external ear**

INCLUDES operations on:
external auditory canal
skin and cartilage of:
auricle
meatus

√4th **18.0 Incision of external ear**

EXCLUDES *removal of intraluminal foreign body (98.11)*

**18.01 Piercing of ear lobe**
Piercing of pinna

**18.02 Incision of external auditory canal**

**18.09 Other incision of external ear**

√4th **18.1 Diagnostic procedures on external ear**

**18.11 Otoscopy**

DEF: Exam of the ear with instrument designed for visualization.

**18.12 Biopsy of external ear**

**18.19 Other diagnostic procedures on external ear**

EXCLUDES *microscopic examination of specimen from ear (90.31-90.39)*

√4th **18.2 Excision or destruction of lesion of external ear**

**18.21 Excision of preauricular sinus**
Radical excision of preauricular sinus or cyst

EXCLUDES *excision of preauricular remnant [appendage] (18.29)*

DEF: Excision of preauricular sinus or cyst with adjacent tissues.

**18.29 Excision or destruction of other lesion of external ear**
Cauterization
Coagulation
Cryosurgery } of external ear
Curettage
Electrocoagulation
Enucleation

Excision of:
exostosis of external auditory canal
preauricular remnant [appendage]
Partial excision of ear

EXCLUDES *biopsy of external ear (18.12)*
*radical excision of lesion (18.31)*
*removal of cerumen (96.52)*

√4th **18.3 Other excision of external ear**

EXCLUDES *biopsy of external ear (18.12)*

**18.31 Radical excision of lesion of external ear**

EXCLUDES *radical excision of preauricular sinus (18.21)*

DEF: Removal of damaged, diseased ear and adjacent tissue.

**18.39 Other**
Amputation of external ear

EXCLUDES *excision of lesion (18.21-18.29, 18.31)*

**18.4 Suture of laceration of external ear**

**18.5 Surgical correction of prominent ear**
Ear:
pinning
setback

DEF: Reformation of protruding outer ear.

**18.6 Reconstruction of external auditory canal**
Canaloplasty of external auditory meatus
Construction [reconstruction] of external meatus of ear:
osseous portion
skin-lined portion (with skin graft)

DEF: Repair of outer ear canal.

√4th **18.7 Other plastic repair of external ear**

**18.71 Construction of auricle of ear**
Prosthetic appliance for absent ear
Reconstruction:
auricle
ear

DEF: Reformation or repair of external ear flap.

**18.72 Reattachment of amputated ear**

**18.79 Other plastic repair of external ear**
Otoplasty NOS          Repair of lop ear
Postauricular skin graft

AHA: 3Q, '03, 12

DEF: Postauricular skin graft: Graft repair behind ear.

DEF: Repair of lop ear: Reconstruction of ear that is at right angle to head.

**18.9 Other operations on external ear**

EXCLUDES *irrigation of ear (96.52)*
*packing of external auditory canal (96.11)*
*removal of:*
*cerumen (96.52)*
*foreign body (without incision) (98.11)*

√3rd **19 Reconstructive operations on middle ear**

**19.0 Stapes mobilization**
Division, otosclerotic:
material
process
Remobilization of stapes
Stapediolysis
Transcrural stapes mobilization

EXCLUDES *that with synchronous stapedectomy (19.11-19.19)*

DEF: Repair of innermost bone of middle ear to enable movement and response to sound.

√4th **19.1 Stapedectomy**

EXCLUDES *revision of previous stapedectomy (19.21-19.29)*
*stapes mobilization only (19.0)*

DEF: Removal of innermost bone of middle ear.

**19.11 Stapedectomy with incus replacement**
Stapedectomy with incus:
homograft
prosthesis

DEF: Removal of innermost bone of middle ear with autograft or prosthesis replacement.

**19.19 Other stapedectomy**

**Stapedectomy with Incus Replacement**

Incus
Malleus
Tympanic membrane
Stapes with footplate in oval window
Cochlea
Handle of malleus
Wire piston
Tissue seal on oval window
■ Area excised

Operations on the Ear

18–19.19

**Operations on the Ear**

**19.2–20.72**

✓4th **19.2 Revision of stapedectomy**

**19.21 Revision of stapedectomy with incus replacement**

**19.29 Other revision of stapedectomy**

**19.3 Other operations on ossicular chain**

Incudectomy NOS
Ossiculectomy NOS
Reconstruction of ossicles, second stage

DEF: Incudectomy: Excision of middle bone of middle ear, not otherwise specified.

DEF: Ossiculectomy: Excision of middle ear bones, not otherwise specified.

DEF: Reconstruction of ossicles, second stage: Repair of middle ear bones following previous surgery.

**19.4 Myringoplasty**

Epitympanic, type I Myringoplasty by:
Myringoplasty by:    graft
   cauterization    Tympanoplasty (type I)

DEF: Epitympanic, type I: Repair over or upon eardrum.

DEF: Myringoplasty by cauterization: Plastic repair of tympanic membrane of eardrum by heat.

DEF: Graft: Plastic repair using implanted tissue.

DEF: Tympanoplasty (type I): Reconstruction of eardrum to restore hearing.

✓4th **19.5 Other tympanoplasty**

**19.52 Type II tympanoplasty**

Closure of perforation with graft against incus or malleus

**19.53 Type III tympanoplasty**

Graft placed in contact with mobile and intact stapes

**AHA:** M-A, '85, 15

**19.54 Type IV tympanoplasty**

Mobile footplate left exposed with air pocket between round window and graft

**19.55 Type V tympanoplasty**

Fenestra in horizontal semicircular canal covered by graft

**19.6 Revision of tympanoplasty**

DEF: Repair or correction of previous plastic surgery on eardrum.

**19.9 Other repair of middle ear**

Closure of mastoid fistula
Mastoid myoplasty
Obliteration of tympanomastoid cavity

DEF: Closure of mastoid fistula: Closing of abnormal channel in mastoid.

DEF: Mastoid myoplasty: Restoration or repair of mastoid muscle.

DEF: Obliteration of tympanomastoid cavity: Removal, total, of functional elements of middle ear.

✓3rd **20 Other operations on middle and inner ear**

✓4th **20.0 Myringotomy**

DEF: Myringotomy: Puncture of tympanic membrane or eardrum, also called tympanocentesis

**20.01 Myringotomy with insertion of tube**

Myringostomy

**20.09 Other myringotomy**

Aspiration of middle ear NOS

**20.1 Removal of tympanostomy tube**

✓4th **20.2 Incision of mastoid and middle ear**

**20.21 Incision of mastoid**

**20.22 Incision of petrous pyramid air cells**

**20.23 Incision of middle ear**

Atticotomy
Division of tympanum
Lysis of adhesions of middle ear

   **EXCLUDES**    *division of otosclerotic process (19.0)*
*stapediolysis (19.0)*
*that with stapedectomy (19.11-19.19)*

✓4th **20.3 Diagnostic procedures on middle and inner ear**

**20.31 Electrocochleography**

DEF: Measure of electric potential of eighth cranial nerve by electrode applied sound.

**20.32 Biopsy of middle and inner ear**

**20.39 Other diagnostic procedures on middle and inner ear**

   **EXCLUDES**    *auditory and vestibular function tests (89.13, 95.41-95.49)*
*microscopic examination of specimen from ear (90.31-90.39)*

✓4th **20.4 Mastoidectomy**

Code also any:
   skin graft (18.79)
   tympanoplasty (19.4-19.55)

   **EXCLUDES**    *that with implantation of cochlear prosthetic device (20.96-20.98)*

DEF: Mastoidectomy: Excision of bony protrusion behind ear.

**20.41 Simple mastoidectomy**

**20.42 Radical mastoidectomy**

**20.49 Other mastoidectomy**

Atticoantrostomy
Mastoidectomy:
   NOS
   modified radical

DEF: Atticoantrotomy: Opening of cavity of mastoid bone and middle ear.

✓4th **20.5 Other excision of middle ear**

   **EXCLUDES**    *that with synchronous mastoidectomy (20.41-20.49)*

**20.51 Excision of lesion of middle ear**

   **EXCLUDES**    *biopsy of middle ear (20.32)*

**20.59 Other**

Apicectomy of petrous pyramid
Tympanectomy

✓4th **20.6 Fenestration of inner ear**

**20.61 Fenestration of inner ear (initial)**

Fenestration of:
   labyrinth    }   with graft (skin)
   semicircular canals    (vein)
   vestibule

   **EXCLUDES**    *that with tympanoplasty, type V (19.55)*

DEF: Creation of inner ear opening.

**20.62 Revision of fenestration of inner ear**

✓4th **20.7 Incision, excision, and destruction of inner ear**

**20.71 Endolymphatic shunt**

DEF: Insertion of tube to drain fluid in inner ear cavities.

**20.72 Injection into inner ear**

Destruction by injection (alcohol):
   inner ear
   semicircular canals
   vestibule

---

BI Bilateral Procedure    NC Non-covered Procedure    LC Limited Coverage Procedure    ►◄ Revised Text    ● New Code    ▲ Revised Code Title

92 — Volume 3

© 2007 Ingenix

**20.79**   **Other incision, excision, and destruction of inner ear**

Decompression of labyrinth
Drainage of inner ear
Fistulization:
   endolymphatic sac
   labyrinth
Incision of endolymphatic sac
Labyrinthectomy (transtympanic)
Opening of bony labyrinth
Perilymphatic tap

   **EXCLUDES**   *biopsy of inner ear (20.32)*

**DEF:** Decompression of labyrinth: Controlled relief of pressure in cavities of inner ear.

**DEF:** Drainage of inner ear: Removal of fluid from inner ear.

**DEF:** Fistulization of endolymphatic sac: Creation of passage to fluid sac in inner ear cavities.

**DEF:** Fistulization of labyrinth: Creation of passage to inner ear cavities.

**DEF:** Incision of endolymphatic sac: Cutting into fluid sac in inner ear cavities.

**DEF:** Labyrinthectomy (transtympanic): Excision of cavities across eardrum.

**DEF:** Opening of bony labyrinth: Cutting into inner ear bony cavities.

**DEF:** Perilymphatic tap: Puncture or incision into fluid sac of inner ear cavities.

**20.8**   **Operations on Eustachian tube**

Catheterization
Inflation
Injection (Teflon paste)
Insufflation (boric acid-
   salicylic acid)
Intubation
Politzerization
        } of Eustachian tube

**DEF:** Catheterization: Passing catheter into passage between pharynx and middle ear.

**DEF:** Inflation: Blowing air, gas or liquid into passage between pharynx and middle ear to inflate.

**DEF:** Injection (Teflon paste): Forcing fluid (Teflon paste) into passage between pharynx and middle ear.

**DEF:** Insufflation (boric acid-salicylic acid): Blowing gas or liquid into passage between pharynx and middle ear.

**DEF:** Intubation: Placing tube into passage between pharynx and middle ear.

**DEF:** Politzerization: Inflating passage between pharynx and middle ear with Politzer bag.

√4ᵗʰ **20.9**   **Other operations on inner and middle ear**

**20.91**   **Tympanosympathectomy**

**DEF:** Excision or chemical suppression of impulses of middle ear nerves.

**20.92**   **Revision of mastoidectomy**

**AHA:** 2Q, '98, 20

**DEF:** Correction of previous removal of mastoid cells from temporal or mastoid bone.

**20.93**   **Repair of oval and round windows**

Closure of fistula:     Closure of fistula:
   oval window          round window
   perilymph

**DEF:** Restoration of middle ear openings.

**20.94**   **Injection of tympanum**

**20.95**   **Implantation of electromagnetic hearing device**

Bone conduction hearing device

   **EXCLUDES**   *cochlear prosthetic device (20.96-20.98)*

**AHA:** 4Q, '89, 5

**20.96**   **Implantation or replacement of cochlear prosthetic device, not otherwise specified**

Implantation of receiver (within skull) and insertion of electrode(s) in the cochlea

   **INCLUDES**   mastoidectomy
   **EXCLUDES**   *electromagnetic hearing device (20.95)*

**AHA:** 4Q, '89, 5

**20.97**   **Implantation or replacement of cochlear prosthetic device, single channel**

Implantation of receiver (within skull) and insertion of electrode in the cochlea

   **INCLUDES**   mastoidectomy
   **EXCLUDES**   *electromagnetic hearing device (20.95)*

**AHA:** 4Q, '89, 5

**20.98**   **Implantation or replacement of cochlear prosthetic device, multiple channel**

Implantation of receiver (within skull) and insertion of electrodes in the cochlea

   **INCLUDES**   mastoidectomy
   **EXCLUDES**   *electromagnetic hearing device (20.95)*

**AHA:** 4Q, '89, 5

**20.99**   **Other operations on middle and inner ear**

▶Attachment of percutaneous abutment (screw) for prosthetic device◀
Repair or removal of cochlear prosthetic device (receiver) (electrode)

   **EXCLUDES**   *adjustment (external components) of cochlear prosthetic device (95.49)*
               *fitting of hearing aid (95.48)*

**AHA:** 4Q, '89, 7

**Operations on the Nose, Mouth, and Pharynx**

## 5. OPERATIONS ON THE NOSE, MOUTH, AND PHARYNX (21-29)

√3ʳᵈ **21 Operations on nose**

INCLUDES   operations on:
     bone ⎫
     skin ⎬ of nose
        ⎭

AHA: 1Q, '94, 5

√4ᵗʰ **21.0 Control of epistaxis**

  **21.00 Control of epistaxis, not otherwise specified**

  **21.01 Control of epistaxis by anterior nasal packing**

  **21.02 Control of epistaxis by posterior (and anterior) packing**

  **21.03 Control of epistaxis by cauterization (and packing)**

  **21.04 Control of epistaxis by ligation of ethmoidal arteries**

  **21.05 Control of epistaxis by (transantral) ligation of the maxillary artery**

  **21.06 Control of epistaxis by ligation of the external carotid artery**

  **21.07 Control of epistaxis by excision of nasal mucosa and skin grafting of septum and lateral nasal wall**

  **21.09 Control of epistaxis by other means**

**21.1 Incision of nose**

  Chondrotomy      Nasal septotomy
  Incision of skin of nose

DEF: Chondrotomy: Incision or division of nasal cartilage.

DEF: Nasal septotomy: Incision into bone dividing nose into two chambers.

√4ᵗʰ **21.2 Diagnostic procedures on nose**

  **21.21 Rhinoscopy**

    DEF: Visualization of nasal passage with nasal speculum.

  **21.22 Biopsy of nose**

  **21.29 Other diagnostic procedures on nose**

    EXCLUDES   microscopic examination of specimen from nose (90.31-90.39)
        nasal:
          function study (89.12)
          x-ray (87.16)
          rhinomanometry (89.12)

√4ᵗʰ **21.3 Local excision or destruction of lesion of nose**

  EXCLUDES   biopsy of nose (21.22)
         nasal fistulectomy (21.82)

  **21.30 Excision or destruction of lesion of nose, not otherwise specified**

  **21.31 Local excision or destruction of intranasal lesion**

    Nasal polypectomy

  **21.32 Local excision or destruction of other lesion of nose**

    AHA: 2Q, '89, 16

**21.4 Resection of nose**

  Amputation of nose

**21.5 Submucous resection of nasal septum**

DEF: Resection, partial, of nasal septum with mucosa reimplanted after excision.

√4ᵗʰ **21.6 Turbinectomy**

DEF: Removal, partial, or total of turbinate bones; inferior turbinate is most often excised.

  **21.61 Turbinectomy by diathermy or cryosurgery**

    DEF: Destruction of turbinate bone by heat or freezing.

**Excision of Turbinate**

- Middle turbinate
- Superior turbinate
- Inferior turbinate

  **21.62 Fracture of the turbinates**

    DEF: Surgical breaking of turbinate bones.

  **21.69 Other turbinectomy**

    EXCLUDES   turbinectomy associated with sinusectomy (22.31-22.39, 22.42, 22.60-22.64)

√4ᵗʰ **21.7 Reduction of nasal fracture**

  **21.71 Closed reduction of nasal fracture**

  **21.72 Open reduction of nasal fracture**

√4ᵗʰ **21.8 Repair and plastic operations on the nose**

  **21.81 Suture of laceration of nose**

  **21.82 Closure of nasal fistula**

    Nasolabial ⎫
    Nasopharyngeal ⎬ fistulectomy
    Oronasal ⎭

    DEF: Sealing off crack or hole between nose and lip, nose and pharynx, or nose and mouth.

  **21.83 Total nasal reconstruction**

    Reconstruction of nose with:
      arm flap
      forehead flap

    DEF: Reformation, plastic, of nasal structure with tissue flap from arm or forehead.

  **21.84 Revision rhinoplasty**

    Rhinoseptoplasty
    Twisted nose rhinoplasty

    DEF: Rhinoseptoplasty: Repair of nose and the bone dividing the nose into two chambers.

    DEF: Twisted nose rhinoplasty: Repair of nose alignment following reconstructive surgery.

  **21.85 Augmentation rhinoplasty**

    Augmentation rhinoplasty with:
      graft
      synthetic implant

    DEF: Implant of tissue or synthetic graft to enlarge nose.

  **21.86 Limited rhinoplasty**

    Plastic repair of nasolabial flaps
    Tip rhinoplasty

    DEF: Plastic repair of nasolabial flaps: Reconstruction of nasal area above lips.

    DEF: Tip rhinoplasty: Reconstruction or restoration of nasal tip.

  **21.87 Other rhinoplasty**

    Rhinoplasty NOS

---

BI Bilateral Procedure      NC Non-covered Procedure      LC Limited Coverage Procedure      ►◄ Revised Text      ● New Code      ▲ Revised Code Title

**21.88** **Other septoplasty**
Crushing of nasal septum
Repair of septal perforation
> EXCLUDES septoplasty associated with
> submucous resection of
> septum (21.5)

DEF: Crushing of nasal septum: Division and reconstruction of defects in bone dividing nasal chambers.

DEF: Repair of septal perforation: Repair of hole in bone dividing nasal chambers with adjacent tissue.

**21.89** **Other repair and plastic operations on nose**
Reattachment of amputated nose

✓4ᵗʰ **21.9** **Other operations on nose**

**21.91** **Lysis of adhesions of nose**
Posterior nasal scrub

DEF: Posterior nasal scrub: Clearing out of abnormal adhesions in posterior nasal area.

**21.99** **Other**
> EXCLUDES dilation of frontonasal duct
> (96.21)
> irrigation of nasal passages
> (96.53)
> removal of:
> intraluminal foreign body
> without incision
> (98.12)
> nasal packing (97.32)
> replacement of nasal packing
> (97.21)

✓3ʳᵈ **22** **Operations on nasal sinuses**

✓4ᵗʰ **22.0** **Aspiration and lavage of nasal sinus**

**22.00** **Aspiration and lavage of nasal sinus, not otherwise specified**

**22.01** **Puncture of nasal sinus for aspiration or lavage**

**22.02** **Aspiration or lavage of nasal sinus through natural ostium**

DEF: Withdrawal of fluid and washing of nasal cavity through natural opening.

✓4ᵗʰ **22.1** **Diagnostic procedures on nasal sinus**

**22.11** **Closed [endoscopic] [needle] biopsy of nasal sinus**

**22.12** **Open biopsy of nasal sinus**

**22.19** **Other diagnostic procedures on nasal sinuses**
Endoscopy without biopsy
> EXCLUDES transillumination of sinus
> (89.35)
> x-ray of sinus (87.15-87.16)

**22.2** **Intranasal antrotomy**
> EXCLUDES antrotomy with external approach
> (22.31-22.39)

DEF: Incision of intranasal sinus.

✓4ᵗʰ **22.3** **External maxillary antrotomy**

**22.31** **Radical maxillary antrotomy**
Removal of lining membrane of maxillary sinus using Caldwell-Luc approach

DEF: Caldwell-Luc approach: Removal of membrane lining the maxillary cavity through incision above canine teeth.

**22.39** **Other external maxillary antrotomy**
Exploration of maxillary antrum with Caldwell-Luc approach

✓4ᵗʰ **22.4** **Frontal sinusotomy and sinusectomy**

**22.41** **Frontal sinusotomy**

**22.42** **Frontal sinusectomy**
Excision of lesion of frontal sinus
Obliteration of frontal sinus (with fat)
> EXCLUDES biopsy of nasal sinus (22.11-
> 22.12)

✓4ᵗʰ **22.5** **Other nasal sinusotomy**

**22.50** **Sinusotomy, not otherwise specified**

**22.51** **Ethmoidotomy**

**22.52** **Sphenoidotomy**

**22.53** **Incision of multiple nasal sinuses**

✓4ᵗʰ **22.6** **Other nasal sinusectomy**
> INCLUDES that with incidental turbinectomy
> EXCLUDES biopsy of nasal sinus (22.11-22.12)

**22.60** **Sinusectomy, not otherwise specified**

**22.61** **Excision of lesion of maxillary sinus with Caldwell-Luc approach**

**22.62** **Excision of lesion of maxillary sinus with other approach**

**22.63** **Ethmoidectomy**

DEF: Removal of ethmoid cells and bone, partial or total includes excising mucosal lining, partial or total.

**22.64** **Sphenoidectomy**

DEF: Removal of wedge shaped sphenoid bone at base of brain.

✓4ᵗʰ **22.7** **Repair of nasal sinus**

**22.71** **Closure of nasal sinus fistula**
Repair of oro-antral fistula

**22.79** **Other repair of nasal sinus**
Reconstruction of frontonasal duct
Repair of bone of accessory sinus

**22.9** **Other operations on nasal sinuses**
Exteriorization of maxillary sinus
Fistulization of sinus
> EXCLUDES dilation of frontonasal duct (96.21)

DEF: Exteriorization of maxillary sinus: Creation of external maxillary cavity opening.

DEF: Fistulization of sinus: Creation of fistula canal in nasal cavity.

✓3ʳᵈ **23** **Removal and restoration of teeth**

✓4ᵗʰ **23.0** **Forceps extraction of tooth**

**23.01** **Extraction of deciduous tooth**

**23.09** **Extraction of other tooth**
Extraction of tooth NOS

✓4ᵗʰ **23.1** **Surgical removal of tooth**

**23.11** **Removal of residual root**

**23.19** **Other surgical extraction of tooth**
Odontectomy NOS
Removal of impacted tooth
Tooth extraction with elevation of mucoperiosteal flap

**23.2** **Restoration of tooth by filling**

**23.3** **Restoration of tooth by inlay**

DEF: Restoration of tooth by cementing in a molded filling.

✓4ᵗʰ **23.4** **Other dental restoration**

**23.41** **Application of crown**

**23.42** **Insertion of fixed bridge**

**23.43** **Insertion of removable bridge**

**23.49** **Other**

**23.5** **Implantation of tooth**

DEF: Insertion of a sound tooth to replace extracted tooth.

**23.6** **Prosthetic dental implant**
Endosseous dental implant

DEF: Implant of artificial denture within bone covering tooth socket.

✓4ᵗʰ **23.7** **Apicoectomy and root canal therapy**

**23.70** **Root canal, not otherwise specified**

**23.71** **Root canal therapy with irrigation**

---

✓3ʳᵈ Additional Digit Required | Valid OR Procedure | Non-OR Procedure | Adjunct Code
✓4ᵗʰ

**Operations on the Nose, Mouth, and Pharynx**

**23.72–26.0**

**23.72 Root canal therapy with apicoectomy**

DEF: Removal of tooth root to treat damaged root canal tissue.

**23.73 Apicoectomy**

√3rd **24 Other operations on teeth, gums, and alveoli**

**24.0 Incision of gum or alveolar bone**

Apical alveolotomy

√4th **24.1 Diagnostic procedures on teeth, gums, and alveoli**

**24.11 Biopsy of gum**

**24.12 Biopsy of alveolus**

**24.19 Other diagnostic procedures on teeth, gums, and alveoli**

> EXCLUDES dental:
> examination (89.31)
> x-ray:
> full-mouth (87.11)
> other (87.12)
> microscopic examination of dental specimen (90.81-90.89)

**24.2 Gingivoplasty**

Gingivoplasty with bone or soft tissue graft

DEF: Repair of gum tissue.

√4th **24.3 Other operations on gum**

**24.31 Excision of lesion or tissue of gum**

> EXCLUDES biopsy of gum (24.11)
> excision of odontogenic lesion (24.4)

**24.32 Suture of laceration of gum**

**24.39 Other**

**24.4 Excision of dental lesion of jaw**

Excision of odontogenic lesion

**24.5 Alveoloplasty**

Alveolectomy (interradicular) (intraseptal) (radical) (simple) (with graft or implant)

> EXCLUDES biopsy of alveolus (24.12)
> en bloc resection of alveolar process and palate (27.32)

DEF: Repair or correction of bony tooth socket.

**24.6 Exposure of tooth**

**24.7 Application of orthodontic appliance**

Application, insertion, or fitting of:
arch bars                orthodontic wiring
orthodontic obturator    periodontal splint

> EXCLUDES nonorthodontic dental wiring (93.55)

**24.8 Other orthodontic operation**

Closure of diastema       Removal of arch bars
(alveolar) (dental)       Repair of dental arch
Occlusal adjustment

> EXCLUDES removal of nonorthodontic wiring (97.33)

√4th **24.9 Other dental operations**

**24.91 Extension or deepening of buccolabial or lingual sulcus**

**24.99 Other**

> EXCLUDES dental:
> debridement (96.54)
> examination (89.31)
> prophylaxis (96.54)
> scaling and polishing (96.54)
> wiring (93.55)
> fitting of dental appliance [denture] (99.97)
> microscopic examination of dental specimen (90.81-90.89)
> removal of dental:
> packing (97.34)
> prosthesis (97.35)
> wiring (97.33)
> replacement of dental packing (97.22)

√3rd **25 Operations on tongue**

√4th **25.0 Diagnostic procedures on tongue**

**25.01 Closed [needle] biopsy of tongue**

**25.02 Open biopsy of tongue**

Wedge biopsy

**25.09 Other diagnostic procedures on tongue**

**25.1 Excision or destruction of lesion or tissue of tongue**

> EXCLUDES biopsy of tongue (25.01-25.02)
> frenumectomy:
> labial (27.41)
> lingual (25.92)

AHA: 2Q, '02, 5

**25.2 Partial glossectomy**

**25.3 Complete glossectomy**

Glossectomy NOS
Code also any neck dissection (40.40-40.42)

**25.4 Radical glossectomy**

Code also any:
neck dissection (40.40-40.42)
tracheostomy (31.1-31.29)

√4th **25.5 Repair of tongue and glossoplasty**

**25.51 Suture of laceration of tongue**

**25.59 Other repair and plastic operations on tongue**

Fascial sling of tongue
Fusion of tongue (to lip)
Graft of mucosa or skin to tongue

> EXCLUDES lysis of adhesions of tongue (25.93)

AHA: 1Q, '97, 5

√4th **25.9 Other operations on tongue**

**25.91 Lingual frenotomy**

> EXCLUDES labial frenotomy (27.91)

DEF: Extension of groove between cheek and lips or cheek and tongue.

**25.92 Lingual frenectomy**

> EXCLUDES labial frenectomy (27.41)

DEF: Frenectomy: Removal of vertical membrane attaching tongue to floor of mouth.

**25.93 Lysis of adhesions of tongue**

**25.94 Other glossotomy**

**25.99 Other**

√3rd **26 Operations on salivary glands and ducts**

> INCLUDES operations on:
> lesser salivary ⎫
> parotid        ⎬ gland and duct
> sublingual     ⎪
> submaxillary   ⎭

Code also any neck dissection (40.40-40.42)

**26.0 Incision of salivary gland or duct**

BI Bilateral Procedure    NC Non-covered Procedure    LC Limited Coverage Procedure    ▶◀ Revised Text    ● New Code    ▲ Revised Code Title

96 — Volume 3                                                                                    © 2007 Ingenix

☑4ᵗʰ **26.1** **Diagnostic procedures on salivary glands and ducts**

     **26.11** **Closed [needle] biopsy of salivary gland or duct**

     **26.12** **Open biopsy of salivary gland or duct**

     **26.19** **Other diagnostic procedures on salivary glands and ducts**

         **EXCLUDES**   *x-ray of salivary gland (87.09)*

☑4ᵗʰ **26.2** **Excision of lesion of salivary gland**

     **26.21** **Marsupialization of salivary gland cyst**

         DEF: Creation of pouch of salivary gland cyst to drain and promote healing.

     **26.29** **Other excision of salivary gland lesion**

         **EXCLUDES**   *biopsy of salivary gland (26.11-26.12)*

                 *salivary fistulectomy (26.42)*

☑4ᵗʰ **26.3** **Sialoadenectomy**

     DEF: Removal of salivary gland.

     **26.30** **Sialoadenectomy, not otherwise specified**

     **26.31** **Partial sialoadenectomy**

     **26.32** **Complete sialoadenectomy**

         En bloc excision of salivary gland lesion

         Radical sialoadenectomy

☑4ᵗʰ **26.4** **Repair of salivary gland or duct**

     **26.41** **Suture of laceration of salivary gland**

     **26.42** **Closure of salivary fistula**

         DEF: Closing of abnormal opening in salivary gland.

     **26.49** **Other repair and plastic operations on salivary gland or duct**

         Fistulization of salivary gland

         Plastic repair of salivary gland or duct NOS

         Transplantation of salivary duct opening

☑4ᵗʰ **26.9** **Other operations on salivary gland or duct**

     **26.91** **Probing of salivary duct**

     **26.99** **Other**

☑3ʳᵈ **27** **Other operations on mouth and face**

     **INCLUDES**   operations on:

         lips

         palate

         soft tissue of face and mouth, except tongue and gingiva

     **EXCLUDES**   *operations on:*

         *gingiva (24.0-24.99)*

         *tongue (25.01-25.99)*

     **27.0** **Drainage of face and floor of mouth**

         Drainage of:        Drainage of:

         facial region (abscess)      Ludwig's angina

         fascial compartment of face

         **EXCLUDES**   *drainage of thyroglossal tract (06.09)*

     **27.1** **Incision of palate**

☑4ᵗʰ **27.2** **Diagnostic procedures on oral cavity**

     **27.21** **Biopsy of bony palate**

     **27.22** **Biopsy of uvula and soft palate**

     **27.23** **Biopsy of lip**

     **27.24** **Biopsy of mouth, unspecified structure**

     **27.29** **Other diagnostic procedures on oral cavity**

         **EXCLUDES**   *soft tissue x-ray (87.09)*

☑4ᵗʰ **27.3** **Excision of lesion or tissue of bony palate**

     **27.31** **Local excision or destruction of lesion or tissue of bony palate**

         Local excision or destruction of palate by:

         cautery          cryotherapy

         chemotherapy

         **EXCLUDES**   *biopsy of bony palate (27.21)*

     **27.32** **Wide excision or destruction of lesion or tissue of bony palate**

         En bloc resection of alveolar process and palate

☑4ᵗʰ **27.4** **Excision of other parts of mouth**

     **27.41** **Labial frenectomy**

         **EXCLUDES**   *division of labial frenum (27.91)*

         DEF: Removal of mucous membrane fold of lip.

     **27.42** **Wide excision of lesion of lip**

     **27.43** **Other excision of lesion or tissue of lip**

     **27.49** **Other excision of mouth**

         **EXCLUDES**   *biopsy of mouth NOS (27.24)*

         *excision of lesion of:*

           *palate (27.31-27.32)*

           *tongue (25.1)*

           *uvula (27.72)*

         *fistulectomy of mouth (27.53)*

         *frenectomy of:*

           *lip (27.41)*

           *tongue (25.92)*

     AHA: 2Q, '05, 8

☑4ᵗʰ **27.5** **Plastic repair of mouth**

     **EXCLUDES**   *palatoplasty (27.61-27.69)*

     **27.51** **Suture of laceration of lip**

     **27.52** **Suture of laceration of other part of mouth**

     **27.53** **Closure of fistula of mouth**

         **EXCLUDES**   *fistulectomy:*

           *nasolabial (21.82)*

           *oro-antral (22.71)*

           *oronasal (21.82)*

     **27.54** **Repair of cleft lip**

     **27.55** **Full-thickness skin graft to lip and mouth**

     **27.56** **Other skin graft to lip and mouth**

     **27.57** **Attachment of pedicle or flap graft to lip and mouth**

         AHA: 1Q, '96, 14

         DEF: Repair of lip or mouth with tissue pedicle or flap still connected to original vascular base.

     **27.59** **Other plastic repair of mouth**

☑4ᵗʰ **27.6** **Palatoplasty**

     **27.61** **Suture of laceration of palate**

     **27.62** **Correction of cleft palate**

         Correction of cleft palate by push-back operation

         **EXCLUDES**   *revision of cleft palate repair (27.63)*

     **27.63** **Revision of cleft palate repair**

         Secondary:

         attachment of pharyngeal flap

         lengthening of palate

         AHA: 1Q, '96, 14

     **27.64** **Insertion of palatal implant**

         DEF: Nonabsorbable polyester implants into the soft palate at the back of the roof of the mouth; one implant placed at the soft palate midline and two are positioned on either side; to support and stiffen the palate reducing vibration (snoring).

     **27.69** **Other plastic repair of palate**

         Code also any insertion of palatal implant (27.64)

         **EXCLUDES**   *fistulectomy of mouth (27.53)*

         AHA: 3Q, '99, 22; 1Q, '97, 14; 3Q, '92, 18

☑4ᵗʰ **27.7** **Operations on uvula**

     **27.71** **Incision of uvula**

     **27.72** **Excision of uvula**

         **EXCLUDES**   *biopsy of uvula (27.22)*

     **27.73** **Repair of uvula**

         **EXCLUDES**   *that with synchronous cleft palate repair (27.62)*

           *uranostaphylorrhaphy (27.62)*

---

☑3ʳᵈ ☑4ᵗʰ Additional Digit Required      Valid OR Procedure      Non-OR Procedure      Adjunct Code

**Operations on the Nose, Mouth, and Pharynx**

**27.79–29.99**

**27.79 Other operations on uvula**
AHA: 3Q, '92, 18

✓4th **27.9 Other operations on mouth and face**

**27.91 Labial frenotomy**
Division of labial frenum
EXCLUDES   lingual frenotomy (25.91)

DEF: Division of labial frenum: Cutting and separating mucous membrane fold of lip.

**27.92 Incision of mouth, unspecified structure**
EXCLUDES   incision of:
gum (24.0)
palate (27.1)
salivary gland or duct (26.0)
tongue (25.94)
uvula (27.71)

**27.99 Other operations on oral cavity**
Graft of buccal sulcus
EXCLUDES   removal of:
intraluminal foreign body (98.01)
penetrating foreign body from mouth without incision (98.22)

DEF: Graft of buccal sulcus: Implant of tissue into groove of interior cheek lining.

✓3rd **28 Operations on tonsils and adenoids**

**28.0 Incision and drainage of tonsil and peritonsillar structures**
Drainage (oral) (transcervical) of:
parapharyngeal
peritonsillar    } abscess
retropharyngeal
tonsillar

✓4th **28.1 Diagnostic procedures on tonsils and adenoids**
**28.11 Biopsy of tonsils and adenoids**
**28.19 Other diagnostic procedures on tonsils and adenoids**
EXCLUDES   soft tissue x-ray (87.09)

**28.2 Tonsillectomy without adenoidectomy**
AHA: 1Q, '97, 5; 2Q, '90, 23

**28.3 Tonsillectomy with adenoidectomy**
AHA: 2Q, '05, 16

**28.4 Excision of tonsil tag**
**28.5 Excision of lingual tonsil**
**28.6 Adenoidectomy without tonsillectomy**
Excision of adenoid tag

**28.7 Control of hemorrhage after tonsillectomy and adenoidectomy**
AHA: 2Q, '05, 16

✓4th **28.9 Other operations on tonsils and adenoids**
**28.91 Removal of foreign body from tonsil and adenoid by incision**
EXCLUDES   that without incision (98.13)
**28.92 Excision of lesion of tonsil and adenoid**
EXCLUDES   biopsy of tonsil and adenoid (28.11)
**28.99 Other**

✓3rd **29 Operations on pharynx**
INCLUDES   operations on:    operations on:
hypopharynx    pharyngeal pouch
nasopharynx    pyriform sinus
oropharynx

**29.0 Pharyngotomy**
Drainage of pharyngeal bursa
EXCLUDES   incision and drainage of retropharyngeal abscess (28.0)
removal of foreign body (without incision) (98.13)

✓4th **29.1 Diagnostic procedures on pharynx**
**29.11 Pharyngoscopy**
**29.12 Pharyngeal biopsy**
Biopsy of supraglottic mass
**29.19 Other diagnostic procedures on pharynx**
EXCLUDES   x-ray of nasopharynx:
contrast (87.06)
other (87.09)

**29.2 Excision of branchial cleft cyst or vestige**
EXCLUDES   branchial cleft fistulectomy (29.52)

✓4th **29.3 Excision or destruction of lesion or tissue of pharynx**
AHA: 2Q, '89, 18

**29.31 Cricopharyngeal myotomy**
EXCLUDES   that with pharyngeal diverticulectomy (29.32)
DEF: Removal of outward pouching of throat.

**29.32 Pharyngeal diverticulectomy**
**29.33 Pharyngectomy (partial)**
EXCLUDES   laryngopharyngectomy (30.3)
**29.39 Other excision or destruction of lesion or tissue of pharynx**

**29.4 Plastic operation on pharynx**
Correction of nasopharyngeal atresia
EXCLUDES   pharyngoplasty associated with cleft palate repair (27.62-27.63)
AHA: 3Q, '99, 22; 1Q, '97, 5; 3Q, '92, 18

DEF: Correction of nasopharyngeal atresia: Construction of normal opening for throat stricture behind nose.

✓4th **29.5 Other repair of pharynx**
**29.51 Suture of laceration of pharynx**
**29.52 Closure of branchial cleft fistula**
DEF: Sealing off an abnormal opening of the branchial fissure in throat.

**29.53 Closure of other fistula of pharynx**
Pharyngoesophageal fistulectomy
**29.54 Lysis of pharyngeal adhesions**
**29.59 Other**
AHA: 2Q, '89, 18

✓4th **29.9 Other operations on pharynx**
**29.91 Dilation of pharynx**
Dilation of nasopharynx
**29.92 Division of glossopharyngeal nerve**
**29.99 Other**
EXCLUDES   insertion of radium into pharynx and nasopharynx (92.27)
removal of intraluminal foreign body (98.13)

**BI** Bilateral Procedure     **NC** Non-covered Procedure     **LC** Limited Coverage Procedure     ▶◀ Revised Text     ● New Code     ▲ Revised Code Title

98 — Volume 3          © 2007 Ingenix

# 6. OPERATIONS ON THE RESPIRATORY SYSTEM (30-34)

√3ʳᵈ **30 Excision of larynx**

√4ᵗʰ **30.0 Excision or destruction of lesion or tissue of larynx**

**30.01 Marsupialization of laryngeal cyst**

DEF: Incision of cyst of larynx with the edges sutured open to create pouch.

**30.09 Other excision or destruction of lesion or tissue of larynx**

Stripping of vocal cords

EXCLUDES
biopsy of larynx (31.43)
laryngeal fistulectomy (31.62)
laryngotracheal fistulectomy (31.62)

**30.1 Hemilaryngectomy**

DEF: Excision of one side (half) of larynx.

√4ᵗʰ **30.2 Other partial laryngectomy**

**30.21 Epiglottidectomy**

**30.22 Vocal cordectomy**

Excision of vocal cords

**30.29 Other partial laryngectomy**

Excision of laryngeal cartilage

**30.3 Complete laryngectomy**

Block dissection of larynx (with thyroidectomy) (with synchronous tracheostomy)
Laryngopharyngectomy

EXCLUDES
that with radical neck dissection (30.4)

**30.4 Radical laryngectomy**

Complete [total] laryngectomy with radical neck dissection (with thyroidectomy) (with synchronous tracheostomy)

√3ʳᵈ **31 Other operations on larynx and trachea**

**31.0 Injection of larynx**

Injection of inert material into larynx or vocal cords

**31.1 Temporary tracheostomy**

Tracheotomy for assistance in breathing

AHA: 1Q, '97, 6

√4ᵗʰ **31.2 Permanent tracheostomy**

**31.21 Mediastinal tracheostomy**

DEF: Placement of artificial breathing tube in windpipe through mediastinum, for long-term use.

**31.29 Other permanent tracheostomy**

EXCLUDES
that with laryngectomy (30.3-30.4)

AHA: 2Q, '05, 8; 2Q, '02, 6

**31.3 Other incision of larynx or trachea**

EXCLUDES
that for assistance in breathing (31.1-31.29)

√4ᵗʰ **31.4 Diagnostic procedures on larynx and trachea**

**31.41 Tracheoscopy through artificial stoma**

EXCLUDES
that with biopsy (31.43-31.44)

DEF: Exam by scope of trachea through an artificial opening.

**Temporary Tracheostomy**

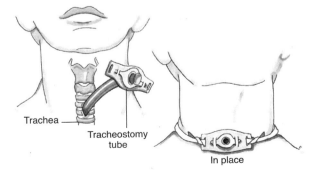

Trachea
Tracheostomy tube
In place

**Closed Endoscopic Biopsy of Larynx**

Laryngoscope
Trachea
Palate

Growth on vocal cord

**31.42 Laryngoscopy and other tracheoscopy**

EXCLUDES
that with biopsy (31.43-31.44)

**31.43 Closed [endoscopic] biopsy of larynx**

**31.44 Closed [endoscopic] biopsy of trachea**

**31.45 Open biopsy of larynx or trachea**

**31.48 Other diagnostic procedures on larynx**

EXCLUDES
contrast laryngogram (87.07)
microscopic examination of specimen from larynx (90.31-90.39)
soft tissue x-ray of larynx NEC (87.09)

**31.49 Other diagnostic procedures on trachea**

EXCLUDES
microscopic examination of specimen from trachea (90.41-90.49)
x-ray of trachea (87.49)

**31.5 Local excision or destruction of lesion or tissue of trachea**

EXCLUDES
biopsy of trachea (31.44-31.45)
laryngotracheal fistulectomy (31.62)
tracheoesophageal fistulectomy (31.73)

√4ᵗʰ **31.6 Repair of larynx**

**31.61 Suture of laceration of larynx**

**31.62 Closure of fistula of larynx**

Laryngotracheal fistulectomy
Take-down of laryngostomy

DEF: Laryngotracheal fistulectomy: Excision and closing of passage between voice box and trachea.

DEF: Take-down of laryngostomy: Removal of laryngostomy tube and restoration of voice box.

**31.63 Revision of laryngostomy**

**31.64 Repair of laryngeal fracture**

DEF: Alignment and positioning of harder structures of larynx such as hyoid bone; following fracture.

**31.69 Other repair of larynx**

Arytenoidopexy
Cordopexy
Graft of larynx
Transposition of vocal cords

EXCLUDES
construction of artificial larynx (31.75)

DEF: Arytenoidopexy: Fixation of pitcher-shaped cartilage in voice box.

DEF: Graft of larynx: Implant of graft tissue into voice box.

DEF: Transposition of the vocal cords: Placement of vocal cords into more functional positions.

√4ᵗʰ **31.7 Repair and plastic operations on trachea**

**31.71 Suture of laceration of trachea**

**31.72 Closure of external fistula of trachea**

Closure of tracheotomy

---

√3ʳᵈ Additional Digit Required
√4ᵗʰ
Valid OR Procedure
Non-OR Procedure
Adjunct Code

© 2007 Ingenix
Volume 3 — 99

**Operations on the Respiratory System**

**31.73–32.30**

**31.73**   **Closure of other fistula of trachea**
Tracheoesophageal fistulectomy
> EXCLUDES   *laryngotracheal fistulectomy (31.62)*

DEF: Tracheoesophageal fistulectomy: Excision and closure of abnormal opening between windpipe and esophagus.

**31.74**   **Revision of tracheostomy**

**31.75**   **Reconstruction of trachea and construction of artificial larynx**
Tracheoplasty with artificial larynx

**31.79**   **Other repair and plastic operations on trachea**

✓4ᵗʰ **31.9**   **Other operations on larynx and trachea**

**31.91**   **Division of laryngeal nerve**

**31.92**   **Lysis of adhesions of trachea or larynx**

**31.93**   **Replacement of laryngeal or tracheal stent**
DEF: Removal and substitution of tubed molding into larynx or trachea.

**31.94**   **Injection of locally-acting therapeutic substance into trachea**

**31.95**   **Tracheoesophageal fistulization**
DEF: Creation of passage between trachea and esophagus.

**31.98**   **Other operations on larynx**
Dilation
Division of congenital web  } of larynx
Removal of keel or stent
> EXCLUDES   *removal of intraluminal foreign body from larynx without incision (98.14)*

DEF: Dilation: Increasing larynx size by stretching.
DEF: Division of congenital web: Cutting and separating congenital membranes around larynx.
DEF: Removal of keel or stent: Removal of prosthetic device from larynx.

**31.99**   **Other operations on trachea**
> EXCLUDES   *removal of:*
> *intraluminal foreign body from trachea without incision (98.15)*
> *tracheostomy tube (97.37)*
> *replacement of tracheostomy tube (97.23)*
> *tracheostomy toilette (96.55)*

AHA: 1Q, '97, 14

✓3ʳᵈ **32**   **Excision of lung and bronchus**
> INCLUDES   rib resection
> sternotomy
> sternum-splitting incision  } as operative approach
> thoracotomy

Code also any synchronous bronchoplasty (33.48)
DEF: Rib resection: Cutting of ribs to access operative field.
DEF: Sternotomy: Cut through breastbone as an operative approach.
DEF: Sternum-splitting incision: Breaking through breastbone to access operative field.

✓4ᵗʰ **32.0**   **Local excision or destruction of lesion or tissue of bronchus**
> EXCLUDES   *biopsy of bronchus (33.24-33.25)*
> *bronchial fistulectomy (33.42)*

AHA: 4Q, '88, 11

**32.01**   **Endoscopic excision or destruction of lesion or tissue of bronchus**

**32.09**   **Other local excision or destruction of lesion or tissue of bronchus**
> EXCLUDES   *that by endoscopic approach (32.01)*

**32.1**   **Other excision of bronchus**
Resection (wide sleeve) of bronchus
> EXCLUDES   *radical dissection [excision] of bronchus (32.6)*

DEF: Resection (wide sleeve) of bronchus: Excision and partial, lengthwise removal of a lung branch.

---

**Lung Volume Reduction**

Chest wall

Diaphragm (dome-shaped)

Normal lungs

Flattened diaphragm

Lungs with emphysema

Original lung area

Staples

Diaphragm resumes a more domed shape

Lungs after surgery

✓4ᵗʰ **32.2**   **Local excision or destruction of lesion or tissue of lung**

**32.20**   **Thoracoscopic excision of lesion or tissue of lung**
Thoracoscopic wedge resection

**32.21**   **Plication of emphysematous bleb**
DEF: Stitching of a swollen vesicle into folds or tuck.

**32.22**   **Lung volume reduction surgery**   LC
AHA: 1Q, '97, 6; 3Q, '96, 20; 4Q, '95, 64
DEF: Excision of portion of lung(s) to reduce respiratory effort in moderate to severe emphysema.

**32.23**   **Open ablation of lung lesion or tissue**
AHA: 4Q, '06, 124

**32.24**   **Percutaneous ablation of lung lesion or tissue**
AHA: 4Q, '06, 124

**32.25**   **Thoracoscopic ablation of lung lesion or tissue**
> EXCLUDES   ▶*thoracoscopic excision of lesion or tissue of lung (32.20)*◀

AHA: 4Q, '06, 124

**32.26**   **Other and unspecified ablation of lung lesion or tissue**
AHA: 4Q, '06, 124

**32.28**   **Endoscopic excision or destruction of lesion or tissue of lung**
> EXCLUDES   *ablation of lung lesion or tissue:*
> *open (32.23)*
> *other (32.26)*
> *percutaneous (32.24)*
> *thoracoscopic (32.25)*
> *biopsy of lung (33.26-33.27)*

**32.29**   **Other local excision or destruction of lesion or tissue of lung**
Resection of lung:     Resection of lung:
NOS              wedge
> EXCLUDES   *ablation of lung lesion or tissue:*
> *open (32.23)*
> *other (32.26)*
> *percutaneous (32.24)*
> *thoracoscopic (32.25)*
> *biopsy of lung (33.26-33.27)*
> *that by endoscopic approach (32.28)*
> ▶*thoracoscopic excision of lesion or tissue of lung (32.20)*◀
> *wide excision of lesion of lung (32.3)*

AHA: 3Q, '99, 3

✓4ᵗʰ **32.3**   **Segmental resection of lung**
Partial lobectomy

**32.30**   **Thoracoscopic segmental resection of lung**

---

BI Bilateral Procedure     NC Non-covered Procedure     LC Limited Coverage Procedure     ▶◀ Revised Text     ● New Code     ▲ Revised Code Title

100 — Volume 3 • October 2007

© 2007 Ingenix

**32.39**    **Other and unspecified segmental resection of lung**
> EXCLUDES    *thoracoscopic segmental resection of lung (32.30)*

✓4ᵗʰ **32.4**    **Lobectomy of lung**
Lobectomy with segmental resection of adjacent lobes of lung
> EXCLUDES    *that with radical dissection [excision] of thoracic structures (32.6)*

**32.41**    **Thoracoscopic lobectomy of lung**

**32.49**    **Other lobectomy of lung**
> EXCLUDES    *thoracoscopic lobectomy of lung (32.41)*

✓4ᵗʰ **32.5**    **Pneumonectomy**
Excision of lung NOS
Pneumonectomy (with mediastinal dissection)
AHA: 1Q, '99, 6

**32.50**    **Thoracoscopic pneumonectomy**

**32.59**    **Other and unspecified pneumonectomy**
> EXCLUDES    *thoracoscopic pneumonectomy (32.50)*

**32.6**    **Radical dissection of thoracic structures**
Block [en bloc] dissection of bronchus, lobe of lung, brachial plexus, intercostal structure, ribs (transverse process), and sympathetic nerves

**32.9**    **Other excision of lung**
> EXCLUDES    *biopsy of lung and bronchus (33.24-33.27)*
> *pulmonary decortication (34.51)*

✓3ʳᵈ **33**    **Other operations on lung and bronchus**
> INCLUDES    rib resection
> sternotomy     } as operative
> sternum-splitting incision   approach
> thoracotomy

**33.0**    **Incision of bronchus**

**33.1**    **Incision of lung**
> EXCLUDES    *puncture of lung (33.93)*

✓4ᵗʰ **33.2**    **Diagnostic procedures on lung and bronchus**

**33.20**    **Thoracoscopic lung biopsy**
> EXCLUDES    *closed endoscopic biopsy of lung (33.27)*
> *closed [percutaneous] [needle] biopsy of lung (33.26)*
> *open biopsy of lung (33.28)*

**33.21**    **Bronchoscopy through artificial stoma**
> EXCLUDES    *that with biopsy (33.24, 33.27)*

DEF: Visual exam of lung and its branches via tube through artificial opening.

**33.22**    **Fiber-optic bronchoscopy**
> EXCLUDES    *that with biopsy (33.24, 33.27)*

AHA: 1Q, '04, 4

DEF: Exam of lung and bronchus via flexible optical instrument for visualization.

**33.23**    **Other bronchoscopy**
> EXCLUDES    *that for:*
> *aspiration (96.05)*
> *biopsy (33.24, 33.27)*

AHA: 3Q, '02, 18; 1Q, '99, 6

**Bronchoscopy with Bite Biopsy**

**33.24**    **Closed [endoscopic] biopsy of bronchus**
Bronchoscopy (fiberoptic) (rigid) with:
brush biopsy of "lung"
brushing or washing for specimen collection
excision (bite) biopsy
Diagnostic bronchoalveolar lavage (BAL)
> EXCLUDES    *closed biopsy of lung, other than brush biopsy of "lung" (33.26, 33.27)*
> *whole lung lavage (33.99)*

AHA: 2Q, '06, 20; 3Q, '04, 9; 3Q, '02, 16; 4Q, '92, 27; 3Q, '91, 15

DEF: Bronchoalveolar lavage (BAL): Saline is introduced into the subsegment of a lobe and retrieved using gentle suction; also called 'liquid biopsy'.

DEF: Brush biopsy: Obtaining cell or tissue samples via bristled instrument without incision.

**33.25**    **Open biopsy of bronchus**
> EXCLUDES    *open biopsy of lung (33.28)*

**33.26**    **Closed [percutaneous] [needle] biopsy of lung**
▶Fine needle aspiration (FNA) of lung
Transthoracic needle biopsy of lung (TTNB)◀
> EXCLUDES    *endoscopic biopsy of lung (33.27)*
> ▶*thoracoscopic lung biopsy (33.20)*◀

AHA: 3Q, '92, 12

**33.27**    **Closed endoscopic biopsy of lung**
Fiber-optic (flexible) bronchoscopy with fluoroscopic guidance with biopsy
Transbronchial lung biopsy
> EXCLUDES    *brush biopsy of "lung" (33.24)*
> *percutaneous biopsy of lung (33.26)*
> ▶*thoracoscopic lung biopsy (33.20)*◀

AHA: 3Q, '04, 9; 3Q, '02, 16; 4Q, '92, 27; 3Q, '91, 15; S-O, '86, 11

**33.28**    **Open biopsy of lung**
AHA: 3Q, '99, 3; 3Q, '92, 12

**33.29**    **Other diagnostic procedures on lung and bronchus**
> EXCLUDES    *contrast bronchogram:*
> *endotracheal (87.31)*
> *other (87.32)*
> *lung scan (92.15)*
> *magnetic resonance imaging (88.92)*
> *microscopic examination of specimen from bronchus or lung (90.41-90.49)*
> *routine chest x-ray (87.44)*
> *ultrasonography of lung (88.73)*
> *vital capacity determination (89.37)*
> *x-ray of bronchus or lung NOS (87.49)*

✓4ᵗʰ **33.3**    **Surgical collapse of lung**

**33.31**    **Destruction of phrenic nerve for collapse of lung**
DEF: Therapeutic deadening or destruction of diaphragmatic nerve to collapse the lung.

**33.32**    **Artificial pneumothorax for collapse of lung**
Thoracotomy for collapse of lung
DEF: Forcing air or gas into diaphragmatic space to achieve therapeutic collapse of lung.
DEF: Thoracotomy for collapse of lung: Incision into chest for therapeutic collapse of lung.

**33.33**    **Pneumoperitoneum for collapse of lung**
DEF: Forcing air or gas into abdominal serous membrane to achieve therapeutic collapse of lung.

**Operations on the Respiratory System**

**33.34–34.23**

**33.34   Thoracoplasty**
DEF: Removal of ribs for therapeutic collapse of lungs.

**33.39   Other surgical collapse of lung**
Collapse of lung NOS

✓4th **33.4   Repair and plastic operation on lung and bronchus**

**33.41   Suture of laceration of bronchus**

**33.42   Closure of bronchial fistula**
Closure of bronchostomy
Fistulectomy:
bronchocutaneous
bronchoesophageal
bronchovisceral

EXCLUDES   *closure of fistula:*
*bronchomediastinal (34.73)*
*bronchopleural (34.73)*
*bronchopleuromediastinal*
*(34.73)*

DEF: Closure of bronchostomy: Removal of bronchostomy tube and repair of surgical wound.
DEF: Fistulectomy: Closure of abnormal passage.
Bronchocutaneous: Between skin and lung branch.
Bronchoesophagus: Between esophagus and lung branch.
Bronchovisceral: Between an internal organ and lung branch.

**33.43   Closure of laceration of lung**

**33.48   Other repair and plastic operations on bronchus**

**33.49   Other repair and plastic operations on lung**
EXCLUDES   *closure of pleural fistula (34.73)*

✓4th **33.5   Lung transplant**
Note: To report donor source — *see* codes 00.91-00.93
Code also cardiopulmonary bypass [extracorporeal circulation] [heart-lung machine] [39.61]
EXCLUDES   *combined heart-lung transplantation (33.6)*
AHA: 4Q, '95, 75

**33.50   Lung transplantation, not otherwise specified**   LC

**33.51   Unilateral lung transplantation**   LC

**33.52   Bilateral lung transplantation**   LC
Double-lung transplantation
En bloc transplantation
DEF: Sequential excision and implant of both lungs.

**33.6   Combined heart-lung transplantation**   LC
Note: To report donor source — *see* codes 00.91-00.93
Code also cardiopulmonary bypass [extracorporeal circulation] [heart-lung machine] (39.61)

✓4th **33.7   Endoscopic insertion, replacement, and removal of therapeutic device or substances in bronchus or lung**
Biologic lung volume reduction (BLVR)
EXCLUDES   *insertion of tracheobronchial stent (96.05)*

**33.71   Endoscopic insertion or replacement of bronchial valve(s)**
Endobronchial airflow redirection valve
Intrabronchial airflow redirection valve
AHA: 4Q, '06, 126

**33.78   Endoscopic removal of bronchial device(s) or substances**
AHA: 4Q, '06, 126

**33.79   Endoscopic insertion of other bronchial device or substances**
Biologic lung volume reduction NOS (BLVR)
AHA: 4Q, '06, 126

✓4th **33.9   Other operations on lung and bronchus**

**33.91   Bronchial dilation**
AHA: 1Q, '97, 14

**33.92   Ligation of bronchus**
DEF: Tying off of a lung branch.

**33.93   Puncture of lung**
EXCLUDES   *needle biopsy (33.26)*
DEF: Piercing of lung with surgical instrument.

**33.98   Other operations on bronchus**
EXCLUDES   *bronchial lavage (96.56)*
*removal of intraluminal foreign body from bronchus without incision (98.15)*

**33.99   Other operations on lung**
Whole lung lavage
EXCLUDES   *other continuous mechanical ventilation (96.70-96.72)*
*respiratory therapy (93.90-93.99)*
AHA: 3Q, '02, 17

✓3rd **34   Operations on chest wall, pleura, mediastinum, and diaphragm**
EXCLUDES   *operations on breast (85.0-85.99)*

✓4th **34.0   Incision of chest wall and pleura**
EXCLUDES   *that as operative approach — omit code*

**34.01   Incision of chest wall**
Extrapleural drainage
EXCLUDES   *incision of pleura (34.09)*
AHA: 3Q, '00, 12; 1Q, '92, 13
DEF: Extrapleural drainage: Incision to drain fluid from external pleura.

**34.02   Exploratory thoracotomy**

**34.03   Reopening of recent thoracotomy site**

**34.04   Insertion of intercostal catheter for drainage**
Chest tube
Closed chest drainage
Revision of intercostal catheter (chest tube) (with lysis of adhesions)
EXCLUDES   ▶ *thoracoscopic drainage of pleural cavity (34.06)* ◀
AHA: 2Q, '03, 7; 1Q, '99, 10; 2Q, '99, 12; 1Q, '95, 5; 1Q, '92, 12
DEF: Insertion of catheter between ribs for drainage.

**34.05   Creation of pleuroperitoneal shunt**
AHA: 4Q, '94, 50

● **34.06   Thoracoscopic drainage of pleural cavity**
Evacuation of empyema

**34.09   Other incision of pleura**
Creation of pleural window for drainage
Intercostal stab
Open chest drainage
EXCLUDES   *thoracoscopy (34.21)*
*thoracotomy for collapse of lung (33.32)*
AHA: ▶ 1Q, '07, 14; ◀ 3Q, '02, 22; 1Q, '94, 7; 4Q, '94, 50
DEF: Creation of pleural window: Creation of circumscribed drainage hole in serous membrane of chest.
DEF: Intercostal stab: Creation of penetrating stab wound between ribs.
DEF: Open chest drainage: Insertion of tube through ribs and serous membrane of chest for drainage.

**34.1   Incision of mediastinum**
EXCLUDES   *mediastinoscopy (34.22)*
*mediastinotomy associated with pneumonectomy (32.5)*

✓4th **34.2   Diagnostic procedures on chest wall, pleura, mediastinum, and diaphragm**

● **34.20   Thoracoscopic pleural biopsy**

**34.21   Transpleural thoracoscopy**
AHA: 3Q, '02, 27
DEF: Exam of chest through serous membrane using scope.

**34.22   Mediastinoscopy**
Code also any lymph node biopsy (40.11)
DEF: Exam of lung cavity and heart using scope.

**34.23   Biopsy of chest wall**

---

BI Bilateral Procedure     NC Non-covered Procedure     LC Limited Coverage Procedure     ▶◀ Revised Text     ● New Code     ▲ Revised Code Title

© *2007 Ingenix*

▲    **34.24**   **Other pleural biopsy**
     *EXCLUDES* ▶ *thoracoscopic pleural biopsy (34.20)*◀
     **AHA:** 3Q, '02, 22, 27; 1Q, '92, 14

**34.25**   **Closed [percutaneous] [needle] biopsy of mediastinum**

**34.26**   **Open biopsy of mediastinum**

**34.27**   **Biopsy of diaphragm**

**34.28**   **Other diagnostic procedures on chest wall, pleura, and diaphragm**
     *EXCLUDES*   *angiocardiography (88.50-88.58)*
     *aortography (88.42)*
     *arteriography of:*
       *intrathoracic vessels NEC (88.44)*
       *pulmonary arteries (88.43)*
     *microscopic examination of specimen from chest wall, pleura, and diaphragm (90.41-90.49)*
     *phlebography of:*
       *intrathoracic vessels NEC (88.63)*
       *pulmonary veins (88.62)*
     *radiological examinations of thorax:*
       *C.A.T. scan (87.41)*
       *diaphragmatic x-ray (87.49)*
       *intrathoracic lymphangiogram (87.34)*
       *routine chest x-ray (87.44)*
       *sinogram of chest wall (87.38)*
       *soft tissue x-ray of chest wall NEC (87.39)*
       *tomogram of thorax NEC (87.42)*
       *ultrasonography of thorax (88.73)*

**34.29**   **Other diagnostic procedures on mediastinum**
     *EXCLUDES*   *mediastinal:*
       *pneumogram (87.33)*
       *x-ray NEC (87.49)*

**34.3**   **Excision or destruction of lesion or tissue of mediastinum**
     *EXCLUDES*   *biopsy of mediastinum (34.25-34.26)*
     *mediastinal fistulectomy (34.73)*

**34.4**   **Excision or destruction of lesion of chest wall**
     Excision of lesion of chest wall NOS (with excision of ribs)
     *EXCLUDES*   *biopsy of chest wall (34.23)*
     *costectomy not incidental to thoracic procedure (77.91)*
     *excision of lesion of:*
       *breast (85.20-85.25)*
       *cartilage (80.89)*
       *skin (86.2-86.3)*
     *fistulectomy (34.73)*

✓4ᵗʰ **34.5**   **Pleurectomy**

**34.51**   **Decortication of lung**
     *EXCLUDES* ▶ *thoracoscopic decortication of lung (34.52)*◀
     **DEF:** Removal of thickened serous membrane for lung expansion.

**34.52**   **Thoracoscopic decortication of lung**

**34.59**   **Other excision of pleura**
     Excision of pleural lesion
     *EXCLUDES*   *biopsy of pleura (34.24)*
     *pleural fistulectomy (34.73)*

**34.6**   **Scarification of pleura**
     Pleurosclerosis
     *EXCLUDES*   *injection of sclerosing agent (34.92)*
     **AHA:** 1Q, '92, 12
     **DEF:** Destruction of fluid-secreting serous membrane cells of chest.

✓4ᵗʰ **34.7**   **Repair of chest wall**

**34.71**   **Suture of laceration of chest wall**
     *EXCLUDES*   *suture of skin and subcutaneous tissue alone (86.59)*

**34.72**   **Closure of thoracostomy**

**34.73**   **Closure of other fistula of thorax**
     Closure of:
       bronchopleural ⎫
       bronchopleurocutaneous ⎬ fistula
       bronchopleuromediastinal ⎭

**34.74**   **Repair of pectus deformity**
     Repair of:
       pectus carinatum ⎫
       pectus excavatum ⎬ (with implant)
     **AHA:** 2Q, '04, 6
     **DEF:** Pectus carinatum repair: Restoration of prominent chest bone defect with implant.
     **DEF:** Pectus excavatum: Restoration of depressed chest bone defect with implant.

**34.79**   **Other repair of chest wall**
     Repair of chest wall NOS
     **AHA:** 2Q, '04, 6; J-F, '87, 13

✓4ᵗʰ **34.8**   **Operations on diaphragm**

**34.81**   **Excision of lesion or tissue of diaphragm**
     *EXCLUDES*   *biopsy of diaphragm (34.27)*

**34.82**   **Suture of laceration of diaphragm**

**34.83**   **Closure of fistula of diaphragm**
     Thoracicoabdominal ⎫
     Thoracicogastric ⎬ fistulectomy
     Thoracicointestinal ⎭
     **DEF:** Fistulectomy: Closure of abnormal passage.

**34.84**   **Other repair of diaphragm**
     *EXCLUDES*   *repair of diaphragmatic hernia (53.7-53.82)*

**34.85**   **Implantation of diaphragmatic pacemaker**

**34.89**   **Other operations on diaphragm**

✓4ᵗʰ **34.9**   **Other operations on thorax**

**34.91**   **Thoracentesis**
     **AHA:** S-O, '85, 6
     **DEF:** Puncture of pleural cavity for fluid aspiration, also called pleurocentesis.

**34.92**   **Injection into thoracic cavity**
     Chemical pleurodesis
     Injection of cytotoxic agent or tetracycline
     Instillation into thoracic cavity
     Requires additional code for any cancer chemotherapeutic substance (99.25)
     *EXCLUDES*   *that for collapse of lung (33.32)*
     **AHA:** ▶1Q, '07, 14;◀ 1Q, '92, 12; 2Q, '89, 17
     **DEF:** Chemical pleurodesis: Tetracycline hydrochloride injections to create adhesions between parietal and visceral pleura for treatment of pleural effusion.

**34.93**   **Repair of pleura**

**34.99**   **Other**
     *EXCLUDES*   *removal of:*
       *mediastinal drain (97.42)*
       *sutures (97.43)*
       *thoracotomy tube (97.41)*
     **AHA:** 1Q, '00, 17; 1Q, '88, 9
     **DEF:** Pleural tent: Extrapleural mobilization of parietal pleura that allows draping of membrane over visceral pleura to eliminate intrapleural dead space and seal visceral pleura.

*Operations on the Respiratory System*

*34.24–34.99*

✓3ʳᵈ / ✓4ᵗʰ Additional Digit Required     Valid OR Procedure     Non-OR Procedure     Adjunct Code

*Operations on the Cardiovascular System*

**35–35.42**

## 7. OPERATIONS ON THE CARDIOVASCULAR SYSTEM (35-39)

√3rd   **35**   **Operations on valves and septa of heart**

INCLUDES   sternotomy (median) (transverse) thoractotomy } as operative approach

Code also cardiopulmonary bypass [extracorporeal circulation] [heart-lung machine] (39.61)

√4th   **35.0**   **Closed heart valvotomy**

EXCLUDES   *percutaneous (balloon) valvuloplasty (35.96)*

DEF: Incision into valve to restore function.

**35.00**   **Closed heart valvotomy, unspecified valve**

**35.01**   **Closed heart valvotomy, aortic valve**

**35.02**   **Closed heart valvotomy, mitral valve**

**35.03**   **Closed heart valvotomy, pulmonary valve**

**35.04**   **Closed heart valvotomy, tricuspid valve**

√4th   **35.1**   **Open heart valvuloplasty without replacement**

INCLUDES   open heart valvotomy

Code also cardiopulmonary bypass, if performed [extracorporeal circulation] [heart-lung machine] (39.61)

EXCLUDES   *that associated with repair of: endocardial cushion defect (35.54,35.63,35.73) percutaneous (balloon) valvuloplasty (35.96) valvular defect associated with atrial and ventricular septal defects (35.54, 35.63, 35.73)*

DEF: Incision into heart for plastic repair of valve without replacing valve.

**35.10**   **Open heart valvuloplasty without replacement, unspecified valve**

**35.11**   **Open heart valvuloplasty of aortic valve without replacement**

**35.12**   **Open heart valvuloplasty of mitral valve without replacement**

AHA: 1Q, '97, 13

**35.13**   **Open heart valvuloplasty of pulmonary valve without replacement**

**35.14**   **Open heart valvuloplasty of tricuspid valve without replacement**

√4th   **35.2**   **Replacement of heart valve**

INCLUDES   excision of heart valve with replacement

Code also cardiopulmonary bypass [extracorporeal circulation] [heart-lung machine] (39.61)

EXCLUDES   *that associated with repair of: endocardial cushion defect (35.54,35.63, 35.73) valvular defect associated with atrial and ventricular septal defects (35.54, 35.63, 35.73)*

DEF: Removal and replacement of valve with tissue from patient, animal, other human, or prosthetic (synthetic) valve.

**35.20**   **Replacement of unspecified heart valve**
Repair of unspecified heart valve with tissue graft or prosthetic implant

**35.21**   **Replacement of aortic valve with tissue graft**
Repair of aortic valve with tissue graft (autograft) (heterograft) (homograft)

AHA: 2Q, '97, 8

**35.22**   **Other replacement of aortic valve**
Repair of aortic valve with replacement:
NOS
prosthetic (partial) (synthetic) (total)

AHA: 1Q, '96, 11

**35.23**   **Replacement of mitral valve with tissue graft**
Repair of mitral valve with tissue graft (autograft) (heterograft) (homograft)

**35.24**   **Other replacement of mitral valve**
Repair of mitral valve with replacement:
NOS
prosthetic (partial) (synthetic) (total)

AHA: 4Q, '97, 55

**35.25**   **Replacement of pulmonary valve with tissue graft**
Repair of pulmonary valve with tissue graft (autograft) (heterograft) (homograft)

AHA: ▶1Q, '07, 14;◀ 1Q, '04, 16; 2Q, '97, 8

**35.26**   **Other replacement of pulmonary valve**
Repair of pulmonary valve with replacement:
NOS
prosthetic (partial) (synthetic) (total)

**35.27**   **Replacement of tricuspid valve with tissue graft**
Repair of tricuspid valve with tissue graft (autograft) (heterograft) (homograft)

**35.28**   **Other replacement of tricuspid valve**
Repair of tricuspid valve with replacement:
NOS
prosthetic (partial) (synthetic) (total)

√4th   **35.3**   **Operations on structures adjacent to heart valves**
Code also cardiopulmonary bypass [extracorporeal circulation] [heart-lung machine] (39.61)

**35.31**   **Operations on papillary muscle**

Division Reattachment Repair } of papillary muscle

**35.32**   **Operations on chordae tendineae**

Division Repair } chordae tendineae

**35.33**   **Annuloplasty**
Plication of annulus

AHA: 1Q, '97, 13; 1Q, '88, 10

DEF: Plication of annulus: Tuck stitched in valvular ring for tightening.

**35.34**   **Infundibulectomy**
Right ventricular infundibulectomy

DEF: Infundibulectomy: Excision of funnel-shaped heart passage.

DEF: Right ventricular infundibulectomy: Excision of funnel-shaped passage in right upper heart chamber.

**35.35**   **Operations on trabeculae carneae cordis**

Division Excision } of trabeculae carneae cordis

Excision of aortic subvalvular ring

**35.39**   **Operations on other structures adjacent to valves of heart**
Repair of sinus of Valsalva (aneurysm)

√4th   **35.4**   **Production of septal defect in heart**

**35.41**   **Enlargement of existing atrial septal defect**
Rashkind procedure
Septostomy (atrial) (balloon)

DEF: Enlargement of partition wall defect in lower heart chamber to improve function.

DEF: Rashkind procedure: Enlargement of partition wall defect between the two lower heart chambers by balloon catheter.

**35.42**   **Creation of septal defect in heart**
Blalock-Hanlon operation

DEF: Blalock-Hanlon operation: Removal of partition wall defect in lower heart chamber.

---

BI Bilateral Procedure    NC Non-covered Procedure    LC Limited Coverage Procedure    ▶◀ Revised Text    ● New Code    ▲ Revised Code Title

104 — Volume 3 • October 2007        © 2007 Ingenix

✓4ᵗʰ **35.5 Repair of atrial and ventricular septa with prosthesis**

INCLUDES repair of septa with synthetic implant or patch

Code also cardiopulmonary bypass [extracorporeal circulation] [heart-lung machine] (39.61)

**35.50 Repair of unspecified septal defect of heart with prosthesis**

EXCLUDES *that associated with repair of:*
*endocardial cushion defect (35.54)*
*septal defect associated with valvular defect (35.54)*

**35.51 Repair of atrial septal defect with prosthesis, open technique**

Atrioseptoplasty
Correction of atrial septal defect
Repair:
   foramen ovale (patent)
   ostium secundum defect
} with prosthesis

EXCLUDES *that associated with repair of:*
*atrial septal defect associated with valvular and ventricular septal defects (35.54)*
*endocardial cushion defect (35.54)*

DEF: Repair of opening or weakening in septum separating the atria; prosthesis implanted through heart incision.

**35.52 Repair of atrial septal defect with prosthesis, closed technique**

Insertion of atrial septal umbrella [King-Mills]
**AHA:** 2Q, '05, 17; 3Q, '98, 11

DEF: Correction of partition wall defect in lower heart chamber with artificial material; without incision into heart.

DEF: Insertion of atrial septal umbrella (King-Mills): Correction of partition wall defect in lower heart chamber with atrial septal umbrella.

**35.53 Repair of ventricular septal defect with prosthesis, open technique**

Correction of ventri-cular septal defect
Repair of supracristal defect
} with prosthesis

EXCLUDES *that associated with repair of:*
*endocardial cushion defect (35.54)*
*ventricular defect assoc-iated with valvular and atrial septal defects (35.54)*

**AHA:** ▶1Q, '07, 14◀

**35.54 Repair of endocardial cushion defect with prosthesis**

Repair:
   atrioventricular canal
   ostium primum defect
   valvular defect assoc-iated with atrial and ventricular septal defects
} with prosthesis (grafted to septa)

EXCLUDES *repair of isolated:*
*atrial septal defect (35.51-35.52)*
*valvular defect (35.20, 35.22, 35.24, 35.26, 35.28)*
*ventricular septal defect (35.53)*

**35.55 Repair of ventricular septal defect with prosthesis, closed technique**

✓4ᵗʰ **35.6 Repair of atrial and ventricular septa with tissue graft**

Code also cardiopulmonary bypass [extracorporeal circulation] [heart-lung machine] (39.61)

**35.60 Repair of unspecified septal defect of heart with tissue graft**

EXCLUDES *that associated with repair of:*
*endocardial cushion defect (35.63)*
*septal defect associated with valvular defect (35.63)*

**35.61 Repair of atrial septal defect with tissue graft**

Atrioseptoplasty
Correction of atrial septal defect
Repair:
   foramen ovale (patent)
   ostium secundum defect
} with tissue graft

EXCLUDES *that associated with repair of:*
*atrial septal defect associated with valvular and ventricular septal defects (35.63)*
*endocardial cushion defect (35.63)*

**35.62 Repair of ventricular septal defect with tissue graft**

Correction of ventricular septal defect
Repair of supracristal defect
} with tissue graft

EXCLUDES *that associated with repair of:*
*endocardial cushion defect (35.63)*
*ventricular defect associated with valvular and atrial septal defects (35.63)*

**35.63 Repair of endocardial cushion defect with tissue graft**

Repair of:
   atrioventricular canal
   ostium primum defect
   valvular defect associated with atrial and ventricular septal defects
} with tissue graft

EXCLUDES *repair of isolated:*
*atrial septal defect (35.61)*
*valvular defect (35.20-35.21, 35.23, 35.25, 35.27)*
*ventricular septal defect (35.62)*

✓4ᵗʰ **35.7 Other and unspecified repair of atrial and ventricular septa**

Code also cardiopulmonary bypass [extracorporeal circulation] [heart-lung machine] (39.61)

**35.70 Other and unspecified repair of unspecified septal defect of heart**

Repair of septal defect NOS

EXCLUDES *that associated with repair of:*
*endocardial cushion defect (35.73)*
*septal defect associated with valvular defect (35.73)*

Operations on the Cardiovascular System

35.5–35.70

**Operations on the Cardiovascular System**

**35.71–35.95**

**35.71**   **Other and unspecified repair of atrial septal defect**

Repair NOS:
    atrial septum
    foramen ovale (patent)
    ostium secundum defect

    **EXCLUDES**    *that associated with repair of:*
        *atrial septal defect assoc-*
        *iated with valvular*
        *and ventricular septal*
        *defects (35.73)*
        *endocardial cushion defect*
        *(35.73)*

**35.72**   **Other and unspecified repair of ventricular septal defect**

Repair NOS:
    supracristal defect
    ventricular septum

    **EXCLUDES**    *that associated with repair of:*
        *endocardial cushion defect*
        *(35.73)*
        *ventricular septal defect*
        *associated with valvular*
        *and atrial septal defects*
        *(35.73)*

**35.73**   **Other and unspecified repair of endocardial cushion defect**

Repair NOS:
    atrioventricular canal
    ostium primum defect
    valvular defect associated with atrial and ventricular septal defects

    **EXCLUDES**    *repair of isolated:*
        *atrial septal defect (35.71)*
        *valvular defect (35.20,*
            *35.22, 35.24, 35.26,*
            *35.28)*
        *ventricular septal defect*
        *(35.72)*

✓4ᵗʰ **35.8**   **Total repair of certain congenital cardiac anomalies**

Note: For partial repair of defect [e.g. repair of atrial septal defect in tetralogy of Fallot] — code to specific procedure

**35.81**   **Total repair of tetralogy of Fallot**

One-stage total correction of tetralogy of Fallot with or without:
    commissurotomy of pulmonary valve
    infundibulectomy
    outflow tract prosthesis
    patch graft of outflow tract
    prosthetic tube for pulmonary artery
    repair of ventricular septal defect (with prosthesis)
    take-down of previous systemic-pulmonary artery anastomosis

**35.82**   **Total repair of total anomalous pulmonary venous connection**

One-stage total correction of total anomalous pulmonary venous connection with or without:
    anastomosis between (horizontal) common pulmonary trunk and posterior wall of left atrium (side-to-side)
    enlargement of foramen ovale
    incision [excision] of common wall between posterior left atrium and coronary sinus and roofing of resultant defect with patch graft (synthetic)
    ligation of venous connection (descending anomalous vein) (to left innominate vein) (to superior vena cava)
    repair of atrial septal defect (with prosthesis)

**35.83**   **Total repair of truncus arteriosus**

One-stage total correction of truncus arteriosus with or without:
    construction (with aortic homograft) (with prosthesis) of a pulmonary artery placed from right ventricle to arteries supplying the lung
    ligation of connections between aorta and pulmonary artery
    repair of ventricular septal defect (with prosthesis)

**35.84**   **Total correction of transposition of great vessels, not elsewhere classified**

Arterial switch operation [Jatene]
Total correction of transposition of great arteries at the arterial level by switching the great arteries, including the left or both coronary arteries, implanted in the wall of the pulmonary artery

    **EXCLUDES**    *baffle operation [Mustard]*
        *[Senning] (35.91)*
        *creation of shunt between*
        *right ventricle and*
        *pulmonary artery*
        *[Rastelli] (35.92)*

✓4ᵗʰ **35.9**   **Other operations on valves and septa of heart**

Code also cardiopulmonary bypass, if performed [extracorporeal circulation] [heart-lung machine] (39.61)

**35.91**   **Interatrial transposition of venous return**

Baffle:        Baffle:
   atrial         interatrial
Mustard's operation
Resection of atrial septum and insertion of patch to direct systemic venous return to tricuspid valve and pulmonary venous return to mitral valve

**DEF:** Atrial baffle: Correction of venous flow of abnormal or deviated lower heart chamber.
**DEF:** Interatrial baffle: Correction of venous flow between abnormal lower heart chambers.
**DEF:** Mustard's operation: Creates intra-atrial baffle using pericardial tissue to correct transposition of the great vessels.

**35.92**   **Creation of conduit between right ventricle and pulmonary artery**

Creation of shunt between right ventricle and (distal) pulmonary artery

    **EXCLUDES**    *that associated with total*
        *repair of truncus*
        *arteriosus (35.83)*

**AHA:** ▶1Q, '07, 14◀

**35.93**   **Creation of conduit between left ventricle and aorta**

Creation of apicoaortic shunt
Shunt between apex of left ventricle and aorta

**35.94**   **Creation of conduit between atrium and pulmonary artery**

Fontan procedure

**35.95**   **Revision of corrective procedure on heart**

Replacement of prosthetic heart valve poppet
Resuture of prosthesis of:
   septum       valve

    **EXCLUDES**    *complete revision — code to*
        *specific procedure*
        *replacement of prosthesis or*
        *graft of:*
            *septum (35.50-35.63)*
            *valve (35.20-35.28)*

**DEF:** Replacement of prosthetic heart valve poppet: Removal and replacement of valve-supporting prosthesis.
**DEF:** Resuture of prosthesis of septum: Restitching of prosthesis in partition wall.
**DEF:** Resuture of prosthesis of valve: Restitching of prosthetic valve.

**BI** Bilateral Procedure     **NC** Non-covered Procedure     **LC** Limited Coverage Procedure     ▶◀ Revised Text     ● New Code     ▲ Revised Code Title

**106 — Volume 3 • October 2007**

© 2007 Ingenix

**35.96**    **Percutaneous valvuloplasty**
Percutaneous balloon valvuloplasty
AHA: 3Q, '04, 10; M-J, '86, 6; N-D, '85, 10

DEF: Repair of valve with catheter.
DEF: Percutaneous balloon valvuloplasty: Repair of valve with inflatable catheter.

**35.98**    **Other operations on septa of heart**
AHA: ▶1Q, '07, 11◀

**35.99**    **Other operations on valves of heart**

√3rd   **36**   **Operations on vessels of heart**

> INCLUDES   sternotomy (median)
> (transverse)     } as operative
> thoracotomy         approach

Code also any:
injection or infusion of platelet inhibitor (99.20)
injection or infusion of thrombolytic agent (99.10)
Code also cardiopulmonary bypass, if performed
[extracorporeal circulation] [heart-lung machine] (39.61)

√4th   **36.0**   **Removal of coronary artery obstruction and insertion of stent(s)**
AHA: 4Q, '95, 66; 2Q, '94, 13; 1Q, '94, 3; 2Q, '90, 23; N-D, '86, 8

**36.03**    **Open chest coronary artery angioplasty**
Coronary (artery):
   endarterectomy (with patch graft)
   thromboendarterectomy (with patch graft)
Open surgery for direct relief of coronary
   artery obstruction
Code also any:
   insertion of drug-eluting coronary stent(s)
     (36.07)
   insertion of non-drug-eluting coronary
     stent(s) (36.06)
   number of vascular stents inserted
     (00.45-00.48)
   number of vessels treated (00.40-00.43)
   procedure on vessel bifurcation (00.44)

> EXCLUDES   *that with coronary artery by-pass graft (36.10-36.19)*

AHA: 2Q, '01, 24; 3Q, '93, 7

DEF: Endarterectomy (with patch graft): Excision of thickened material within coronary artery; repair with patch graft.
DEF: Thromboendarterectomy (with patch graft): Excision of blood clot and thickened material within coronary artery; repair with patch graft.
DEF: Open surgery for direct relief of coronary artery obstruction: Removal of coronary artery obstruction through opening in chest.

**36.04**    **Intracoronary artery thrombolytic infusion**
That by direct coronary artery injection,
   infusion, or catheterization
   enzyme infusion
   platelet inhibitor

> EXCLUDES   *infusion of platelet inhibitor (99.20)*
> *infusion of thrombolytic agent (99.10)*
> *that associated with any procedure in 36.03*

AHA: 4Q, '05, 102; 4Q, '02, 114; 3Q, '02, 20; 2Q, '01, 24; 4Q, '98, 85; 1Q, '97, 3; 4Q, '95, 67

DEF: Infusion of clot breaking solution into intracoronary artery.

**Coronary Bypass**

Right coronary artery
Left coronary artery
Circumflex branch
Descending branch

**Transmyocardial Revascularization**

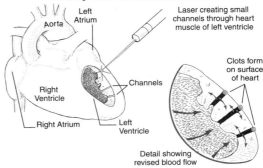

Aorta
Left Atrium
Laser creating small channels through heart muscle of left ventricle
Right Ventricle
Channels
Clots form on surface of heart
Right Atrium
Left Ventricle
Detail showing revised blood flow

**36.06**    **Insertion of non-drug-eluting coronary artery stent(s)**
Bare stent(s)       Endovascular graft(s)
Bonded stent(s)      Stent graft(s)
Drug-coated stent(s),
   e.g., heparin coated
Endograft(s)
Code also any:
   number of vascular stents inserted
     (00.45-00.48)
   number of vessels treated (00.40-00.43)
   open chest coronary artery angioplasty
     (36.03)
   percutaneous transluminal coronary
     angioplasty [PTCA] or coronary
     atherectomy (00.66)
   procedure on vessel bifurcation (00.44)

> EXCLUDES   *insertion of drug-eluting coronary artery stent(s) (36.07)*

AHA: 4Q, '05, 71; 2Q, '04, 3; 4Q, '02, 101; 1Q, '01, 9; 2Q, '01, 24; 1Q, '00, 11; 1Q, '99, 17

DEF: Percutaneous implant via catheter of metal stent, to enlarge, maintain lumen size of coronary artery.

**36.07**    **Insertion of drug-eluting coronary artery stent(s)**
Endograft(s)       Stent graft(s)
Endovascular graft(s)
Code also any:
   number of vascular stents inserted
     (00.45-00.48)
   number of vessels treated (00.40-00.43)
   open chest coronary artery angioplasty
     (36.03)
   percutaneous transluminal coronary
     angioplasty [PTCA] or coronary
     atherectomy (00.66)
   procedure on vessel bifurcation (00.44)

> EXCLUDES   *drug-coated stents, e.g., heparin coated (36.06)*
> *insertion of non-drug-eluting coronary artery stent(s) (36.06)*

AHA: 4Q, '05, 105-106; 4Q, '02, 101

DEF: Drug-eluting stent technology developed to prevent the accumulation of scar tissue that can narrow reopened coronary arteries. A special polymer is used to coat the drug onto the stent, which slowly releases into the coronary artery wall tissue.

**36.09**    **Other removal of coronary artery obstruction**
Coronary angioplasty NOS
Code also any:
   number of vascular stents inserted
     (00.45-00.48)
   number of vessels treated (00.40-00.43)
   procedure on vessel bifurcation (00.44)

> EXCLUDES   *that by open angioplasty (36.03)*
> *that by percutaneous transluminal coronary angioplasty [PTCA] or coronary atherectomy (00.66)*

**Operations on the Cardiovascular System**

**36.1–37.20**

✓4ᵗʰ **36.1    Bypass anastomosis for heart revascularization**
Note: Do not assign codes from series 00.40-00.43 with codes from series 36.10-36.19
Code also:
  cardiopulmonary bypass [extracorporeal circulation] [heart-lung machine] (39.61)
  pressurized treatment of venous bypass graft [conduit] with pharmaceutical substance, if performed (00.16)
**AHA:** 2Q, '96, 7; 3Q, '95, 7; 3Q, '93, 8; 1Q, '91, 7; 2Q, '90, 24; 4Q, '89, 3
**DEF:** Insertion of tube to bypass blocked coronary artery, correct coronary blood flow.

**36.10    Aortocoronary bypass for heart revascularization, not otherwise specified**
Direct revascularization:

| cardiac | |
|---|---|
| coronary | with catheter stent, |
| heart muscle | prosthesis, or |
| myocardial | vein graft |

Heart revascularization NOS
**AHA:** 2Q, '96, 7

**36.11    (Aorto)coronary bypass of one coronary artery**
**AHA:** 3Q, '02, 4, 9; 4Q, '89, 3

**36.12    (Aorto)coronary bypass of two coronary arteries**
**AHA:** 3Q, '02, 8; 4Q, '99, 15; 2Q, '96, 7; 3Q, '97, 14; 4Q, '89, 3

**36.13    (Aorto)coronary bypass of three coronary arteries**
**AHA:** 3Q, '02, 6, 7, 9; 2Q, '96, 7; 4Q, '89, 3

**36.14    (Aorto)coronary bypass of four or more coronary arteries**
**AHA:** 3Q, '02, 5; 2Q, '96, 7; 4Q, '89, 3

**36.15    Single internal mammary-coronary artery bypass**
Anastomosis (single):
  mammary artery to coronary artery
  thoracic artery to coronary artery
**AHA:** 3Q, '02, 4-9; 4Q, '99, 15; 3Q, '97, 14; 2Q, '96, 7

**36.16    Double internal mammary-coronary artery bypass**
Anastomosis, double:
  mammary artery to coronary artery
  thoracic artery to coronary artery
**AHA:** 3Q, '02, 6, 8, 9; 2Q, '96, 7

**36.17    Abdominal-coronary artery bypass**
Anastomosis:
  gastroepiploic artery to coronary artery
**AHA:** 3Q, '97, 14; 4Q, '96, 64

**36.19    Other bypass anastomosis for heart revascularization**
**AHA:** 2Q, '96, 7

**36.2    Heart revascularization by arterial implant**
Implantation of:
  aortic branches [ascending aortic branches] into heart muscle
  blood vessels into myocardium
  internal mammary artery [internal thoracic artery] into:
    heart muscle
    myocardium
    ventricle
    ventricular wall
Indirect heart revascularization NOS

✓4ᵗʰ **36.3    Other heart revascularization**
**36.31    Open chest transmyocardial revascularization**
**DEF:** Transmyocardial revascularization (TMR): Laser creation of channels through myocardium allows oxygenated blood flow from sinusoids to myocardial tissue.

**36.32    Other transmyocardial revascularization**
**AHA:** 4Q, '98, 74

**36.33    Endoscopic transmyocardial revascularization**
Robot-assisted transmyocardial revascularization
Thoracoscopic transmyocardial revascularization
**AHA:** 4Q, '06, 127

**36.34    Percutaneous transmyocardial revascularization**
Endovascular transmyocardial revascularization
**AHA:** 4Q, '06, 127

**36.39    Other heart revascularization**
Abrasion of epicardium
Cardio-omentopexy
Intrapericardial poudrage

| Myocardial graft: | Myocardial graft: |
|---|---|
| mediastinal fat | pectoral muscles |
| omentum | |

**DEF:** Cardio-omentopexy: Suture of omentum segment to heart after drawing segment through incision in diaphragm to improve blood supply.
**DEF:** Intrapericardial poudrage: Application of powder to heart lining to promote fusion.

✓4ᵗʰ **36.9    Other operations on vessels of heart**
Code also cardiopulmonary bypass [extracorporeal circulation] [heart-lung machine] (39.61)

**36.91    Repair of aneurysm of coronary vessel**
**36.99    Other operations on vessels of heart**

| Exploration | |
|---|---|
| Incision | of coronary |
| Ligation | artery |

Repair of arteriovenous fistula
**AHA:** 3Q, '03, 18; 1Q, '94, 3

✓3ʳᵈ **37    Other operations on heart and pericardium**
Code also any injection or infusion of platelet inhibitor (99.20)

**37.0    Pericardiocentesis**
**AHA:** ▶1Q, '07, 11◀
**DEF:** Puncture of the heart lining to withdraw fluid.

✓4ᵗʰ **37.1    Cardiotomy and pericardiotomy**
Code also cardiopulmonary bypass [extracorporeal circulation] [heart-lung machine] (39.61)

**37.10    Incision of heart, not otherwise specified**
Cardiolysis NOS

**37.11    Cardiotomy**

| Incision of: | Incision of: |
|---|---|
| atrium | myocardium |
| endocardium | ventricle |

**37.12    Pericardiotomy**

| Pericardial window | Pericardiolysis |
|---|---|
| operation | Pericardiotomy |

**DEF:** Pericardial window operation: Incision into heart lining for drainage.
**DEF:** Pericardiolysis: Destruction of heart tissue lining.

✓4ᵗʰ **37.2    Diagnostic procedures on heart and pericardium**

**37.20    Non-invasive programmed electrical stimulation [NIPS]**
**EXCLUDES**    catheter based invasive electro-physiologic testing (37.26)
  device interrogation only without arrhythmia induction (bedside check) (89.45-89.49)
  that as part of intraoperative testing—omit code
**AHA:** 4Q, '06, 128
**DEF:** Non-invasive testing of a previously implanted cardioverter-defibrillator to ensure proper lead placement and system function.

---

**BI** Bilateral Procedure     **NC** Non-covered Procedure     **LC** Limited Coverage Procedure     ▶◀ Revised Text     ● New Code     ▲ Revised Code Title

**Intracardiac Echocardiography**

Superior vena cava
Aorta
Inferior vena cava
Right atrium
Left atrium
Left ventricle
Right ventricle
Inferior vena cava
Femoral vein access
Miniaturized ultrasound transducer

### 37.21 Right heart cardiac catheterization
Cardiac catheterization NOS

EXCLUDES    *that with catheterization of left heart (37.23)*

AHA: 3Q, '04, 10; 3Q, '03, 9; 2Q, '90, 23; M-J, '87, 11

### 37.22 Left heart cardiac catheterization

EXCLUDES    *that with catheterization of right heart (37.23)*

AHA: 4Q, '05, 71; 3Q, '05, 14; 3Q, '04, 10; 2Q, '04, 3; 1Q, '00, 21; 2Q, '90, 23; 4Q, '88, 4; M-J, '87, 11

### 37.23 Combined right and left heart cardiac catheterization

AHA: ▶1Q, '07, 11;◀ 2Q, '05, 17; 3Q, '04, 10; 2Q, '01, 8; 1Q, '00, 20; 3Q, '98, 11; 2Q, '90, 23; M-J, '87, 11

### 37.24 Biopsy of pericardium

### 37.25 Biopsy of heart

AHA: 3Q, '03, 16; 3Q, '94, 8

### 37.26 Catheter based invasive electrophysiologic testing
Electrophysiologic studies [EPS]
Code also any concomitant procedure

EXCLUDES    *device interrogation only without arrhythmia induction (bedside check) (89.45-89.49)*
*His bundle recording (37.29)*
*non-invasive programmed electrical stimulation (NIPS) (37.20)*
*that as part of intraoperative testing—omit code*

AHA: 3Q, '03, 23; 2Q, '03, 19; 1Q, '02, 8, 9; 1Q, '99, 3; 2Q, '97, 10; 3Q, '90, 11

DEF: Diagnostic mapping and measurement of intracardiac electrical activity; requires inserting three to six catheters into heart blood vessels and positioning catheters under fluoroscopic guidance to determine site of the tachycardia or abnormal impulse pathway; may also be used to terminate arrhythmias.

### 37.27 Cardiac mapping
Code also any concomitant procedure

EXCLUDES    *electrocardiogram (89.52)*
*His bundle recording (37.29)*

### 37.28 Intracardiac echocardiography
Echocardiography of heart chambers
ICE
Code also any synchronous Doppler flow mapping (88.72)

EXCLUDES    *intravascular imaging of coronary vessels (intravascular ultrasound) (IVUS) (00.24)*

AHA: 4Q, '01, 62

DEF: Creation of a two-dimensional graphic of heart using endoscopic echocardiographic equipment.

### 37.29 Other diagnostic procedures on heart and pericardium

EXCLUDES    *angiocardiography (88.50-88.58)*
*cardiac function tests (89.41-89.69)*
*cardiovascular radioisotopic scan and function study (92.05)*
*coronary arteriography (88.55-88.57)*
*diagnostic pericardiocentesis (37.0)*
*diagnostic ultrasound of heart (88.72)*
*x-ray of heart (87.49)*

AHA: S-O, '87, 3

### ✓4th 37.3 Pericardiectomy and excision of lesion of heart
Code also cardiopulmonary bypass [extracorporeal circulation] [heart-lung machine] (39.61)

### 37.31 Pericardiectomy
Excision of:
adhesions of pericardium
constricting scar of:
epicardium
pericardium

DEF: Excision of a portion of heart lining.

### 37.32 Excision of aneurysm of heart
Repair of aneurysm of heart

### 37.33 Excision or destruction of other lesion or tissue of heart, open approach
Ablation of heart tissue (cryoablation) (electrocurrent) (laser) (microwave) (radiofrequency) (resection), open chest approach
Cox-maze procedure
Maze procedure
Modified maze procedure, trans-thoracic approach

EXCLUDES    *ablation, excision or destruction of lesion or tissue of heart, endovascular approach (37.34)*

AHA: 3Q, '06, 13; 4Q, '03, 93-94; 2Q, '94, 12

### 37.34 Excision or destruction of other lesion or tissue of heart, other approach
Ablation of heart tissue (cryoablation) (electrocurrent) (laser) (microwave) (radiofrequency) (resection), via peripherally inserted catheter
Modified maze procedure, endovascular approach

AHA: 4Q, '03, 93-95; 1Q, '00, 20

DEF: Destruction of heart tissue or lesion by freezing, electric current or resection.

### 37.35 Partial ventriculectomy    NC
Ventricular reduction surgery
Ventricular remodeling
Code also any synchronous:
mitral valve repair (35.02, 35.12)
mitral valve replacement (35.23-35.24)

AHA: 4Q, '97, 54, 55

DEF: Removal of elliptical slice of ventricle between anterior and posterior papillary muscle; also called Batiste operation.

**Ventricular Reduction Surgery**

Superior vena cava
Aorta
Pulmonary artery
Left atrium
Left ventricle
Shape of heart after reduction
Anterior interventricular branch of left coronary artery
Right atrium
Right coronary artery
Right ventricle
New apex
Apex
Posterior interventricular branch of right coronary artery

**Enlarged Heart**

**Removal of Section of Outer Wall of Left Ventricle**
Superior vena cava
Aorta
Circumflex branch

---

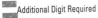 Additional Digit Required      Valid OR Procedure      Non-OR Procedure      Adjunct Code

Operations on the Cardiovascular System    37.21–37.35

*Operations on the Cardiovascular System*

*37.4–37.67*

√4th **37.4**   **Repair of heart and pericardium**
AHA: 2Q, '90, 24

**37.41**   **Implantation of prosthetic cardiac support device around the heart**
Cardiac support device (CSD)
Epicardial support device
Fabric (textile) (mesh) device
Ventricular support device on surface of heart
Code also any:
     cardiopulmonary bypass [extracorporeal circulation] [heart-lung machine] if performed (39.61)
     mitral valve repair (35.02, 35.12)
     mitral valve replacement (35.23-35.24)
     transesophageal echocardiography (88.72)
     **EXCLUDES**   *circulatory assist systems (37.61-37.68)*

AHA: 4Q, '05, 119-120

DEF: Cardiac support device: any device implanted around the ventricles of the heart for cardiac support

DEF: Fabric (textile) (mesh) device: textile mesh net sutured around the heart for support.

**37.49**   **Other repair of heart and pericardium**

√4th **37.5**   **Heart replacement procedures**
AHA: 4Q, '03, 96

**37.51**   **Heart transplantation**   `LC`
     **EXCLUDES**   *combined heart-lung transplantation (33.6)*

AHA: 2Q, '05, 14

**37.52**   **Implantation of total replacement heart system**   `NC`
Artificial heart
Implantation of fully implantable total replacement heart system, including ventriculectomy
     **EXCLUDES**   *implantation of heart assist system [VAD] (37.62, 37.65, 37.66)*

**37.53**   **Replacement or repair of thoracic unit of total replacement heart system**   `NC`
     **EXCLUDES**   *replacement and repair of heart assist system [VAD] (37.63)*

**37.54**   **Replacement or repair of other implantable component of total replacement heart system**   `NC`
Implantable battery
Implantable controller
Transcutaneous energy transfer [TET] device
     **EXCLUDES**   *replacement and repair of heart assist system [VAD] (37.63)*
         *replacement or repair of thoracic unit of total replacement heart system (37.53)*

√4th **37.6**   **Implantation of heart and circulatory assist system**
     **EXCLUDES**   *implantation of prosthetic cardiac support system (37.41)*

AHA: 4Q, '95, 68

DEF: Implant of device for assisting heart in circulating blood.

**37.61**   **Implant of pulsation balloon**
AHA: 3Q, '05, 14

**37.62**   **Insertion of non-implantable heart assist system**
Insertion of heart assist system, NOS
Insertion of heart pump
     **EXCLUDES**   *implantation of total replacement heart system (37.52)*
         *insertion of percutaneous external heart assist device (37.68)*

AHA: 4Q, '03, 116; 2Q, '90, 25

**37.63**   **Repair of heart assist system**
Replacement of parts of an existing ventricular assist device (VAD)
     **EXCLUDES**   *replacement or repair of other implantable component of total replacement heart system [artificial heart] (37.54)*
         *replacement or repair of thoracic unit of total replacement heart system [artificial heart] (37.53)*

**37.64**   **Removal of heart assist system**
     **EXCLUDES**   *explantation [removal] of percutaneous external heart assist device (97.44)*
         *that with replacement of implant (37.63)*
         *nonoperative removal of heart assist system (97.44)*

**37.65**   **Implant of external heart assist system**
Note: Device (outside the body but connected to heart) with external circulation and pump
     **INCLUDES**   open chest (sternotomy) procedure for cannulae attachments
     **EXCLUDES**   *implantation of total replacement heart system (37.52)*
         *implant of pulsation balloon (37.61)*
         *insertion of percutaneous external heart assist device (37.68)*

DEF: Insertion of short-term circulatory support device with pump outside body.

**37.66**   **Insertion of implantable heart assist system**   `LC`
Note:   Device directly connected to the heart and implanted in the upper left quadrant of peritoneal cavity. This device can be used for either destination therapy (DT) or bridge-to-transplant (BTT).
Axial flow heart assist system
Diagonal pump heart assist system
Left ventricular assist device (LVAD)
Pulsatile heart assist system
Right ventricular assist device (RVAD)
Rotary pump heart assist system
Transportable, implantable heart assist system
Ventricular assist device (VAD) not otherwise specified
     **EXCLUDES**   *implantation of total replacement heart system [artificial heart] (37.52)*
         *implant of pulsation balloon (37.61)*
         *insertion of percutaneous external heart assist device (37.68)*

AHA: 4Q, '03, 116; 1Q, '98, 8

DEF: Insertion of long-term circulatory support device with pump in body.

**37.67**   **Implantation of cardiomyostimulation system**
Note: Two-step open procedure consisting of tranfer of one end of the latissimus dorsi muscle; wrapping it around the heart; rib resection; implantation of epicardial cardiac pacing leads into the right ventricle; tunneling and pocket creation for the cardiomyostimulator.
AHA: 4Q, '98, 75; 1Q, '98, 8

`BI` Bilateral Procedure     `NC` Non-covered Procedure     `LC` Limited Coverage Procedure     ◄► Revised Text     ● New Code     ▲ Revised Code Title

110 — Volume 3

© 2007 Ingenix

**37.68   Insertion of percutaneous external heart assist device**
Circulatory assist device
Extrinsic heart assist device
pVAD
Percutaneous heart assist device
| INCLUDES | percutaneous [femoral] insertion of cannulae attachments

✓4th **37.7   Insertion, revision, replacement, and removal of leads; insertion of temporary pacemaker system; or revision of cardiac device pocket**
Code also any insertion and replacement of pacemaker device (37.80-37.87)
| EXCLUDES | implantation or replacement of transvenous lead [electrode] into left ventricular cardiac venous system (00.52)

**AHA:** 1Q, '94, 16; 3Q, '92, 3; M-J, '87, 1

1 **37.70   Initial insertion of lead [electrode], not otherwise specified**
| EXCLUDES | insertion of temporary transvenous pacemaker system (37.78)
replacement of atrial and/or ventricular lead(s) (37.76)

1 **37.71   Initial insertion of transvenous lead [electrode] into ventricle**
| EXCLUDES | insertion of temporary transvenous pacemaker system (37.78)
replacement of atrial and/or ventricular lead(s) (37.76)

2 **37.72   Initial insertion of transvenous leads [electrodes] into atrium and ventricle**
| EXCLUDES | insertion of temporary transvenous pacemaker system (37.78)
replacement of atrial and/or ventricular lead(s) (37.76)

**AHA:** 2Q, '97, 4

1 **37.73   Initial insertion of transvenous lead [electrode] into atrium**
| EXCLUDES | insertion of temporary transvenous pacemaker system (37.78)
replacement of atrial and/or ventricular lead(s) (37.76)

4 **37.74   Insertion or replacement of epicardial lead [electrode] into epicardium**
Insertion or replacement of epicardial lead by:
sternotomy        thoracotomy
| EXCLUDES | replacement of atrial and/or ventricular lead(s) (37.76)

**AHA:** ▶1Q, '07, 20;◀ 3Q, '05, 3-9

**37.75   Revision of lead [electrode]**
Repair of electrode [removal with re-insertion]
Repositioning of lead(s) (AICD) (cardiac device) (CRT-D) (CRT-P) (defibrillator) (pacemaker) (pacing) (sensing) [electrode]
Revision of lead NOS
| EXCLUDES | repositioning of temporary transvenous pacemaker system — omit code

**AHA:** 3Q, '05, 8; 2Q, '99, 11

3 **37.76   Replacement of transvenous atrial and/or ventricular lead(s) [electrode]**
Removal or abandonment of existing transvenous or epicardial lead(s) with transvenous lead(s) replacement
| EXCLUDES | replacement of epicardial lead [electrode] (37.74)

**AHA:** 3Q, '05, 3-9

**37.77   Removal of lead(s) [electrode] without replacement**
Removal:
epicardial lead (transthoracic approach)
transvenous lead(s)
| EXCLUDES | removal of temporary transvenous pacemaker system — omit code
that with replacement of:
atrial and/or ventricular lead(s) [electrode] (37.76)
epicardial lead [electrode] (37.74)

**37.78   Insertion of temporary transvenous pacemaker system**
| EXCLUDES | intraoperative cardiac pacemaker (39.64)

**AHA:** 3Q, '05, 7; 3Q, '93, 12; 1Q, '89, 2

**37.79   Revision or relocation of cardiac device pocket**
Debridement and reforming pocket (skin and subcutaneous tissue)
Insertion of loop recorder
Relocation of pocket [creation of new pocket] pacemaker or CRT-P
Removal of cardiac device/pulse generator without replacement
Removal of the implantable hemodynamic pressure sensor [lead] and monitor device
Removal without replacement of cardiac resynchronization defibrillator device
Repositioning of implantable hemodynamic pressure sensor [lead] and monitor device
Repositioning of pulse generator
Revision of cardioverter/defibrillator (automatic) pocket
Revision of pocket for intracardiac hemodynamic monitoring
Revision or relocation of CRT-D pocket
Revision or relocation of pacemaker, defibrillator, or other implanted cardiac device pocket
| EXCLUDES | removal of loop recorder (86.05)

**AHA:** 3Q, '05, 3-9

✓4th **37.8   Insertion, replacement, removal, and revision of pacemaker device**
Note: Device testing during procedure—omit code
Code also any lead insertion, lead replacement, lead removal and/or lead revision (37.70-37.77)
| EXCLUDES | implantation of cardiac resynchronization pacemaker, total system [CRT-P] (00.50)
implantation or replacement of cardiac resynchronization pacemaker pulse generator only [CRT-P] (00.53)

**AHA:** M-J, '87, 1

**37.80   Insertion of permanent pacemaker, initial or replacement, type of device not specified**

5 **37.81   Initial insertion of single-chamber device, not specified as rate responsive**
| EXCLUDES | replacement of existing pacemaker device (37.85-37.87)

5 **37.82   Initial insertion of single-chamber device, rate responsive**
Rate responsive to physiologic stimuli other than atrial rate
| EXCLUDES | replacement of existing pacemaker device (37.85-37.87)

1 Valid OR procedure code if accompanied by one of the following codes: 37.80, 37.81, 37.82, 37.85, 37.86, 37.87
2 Valid OR procedure code if accompanied by one of the following codes: 37.80, 37.83
3 Valid OR procedure code if accompanied by one of the following codes: 37.80, 37.85, 37.86, 37.87
4 Valid OR procedure code if accompanied by one of the following codes: 37.80, 37.81, 37.82, 37.83, 37.85, 37.86, 37.87
5 Valid OR procedure code if accompanied by one of the following codes: 37.72, 37.76

✓3rd
✓4th Additional Digit Required | Valid OR Procedure | Non-OR Procedure | Adjunct Code

**Operations on the Cardiovascular System**

**37.83–37.98**

### Insertion of Pacemaker

⁶ **37.83　Initial insertion of dual-chamber device**
Atrial ventricular sequential device

**EXCLUDES**　*replacement of existing pacemaker device (37.85-37.87)*

**AHA:** 2Q, '97, 4

**37.85　Replacement of any type pacemaker device with single-chamber device, not specified as rate responsive**

**37.86　Replacement of any type pacemaker device with single-chamber device, rate responsive**
Rate responsive to physiologic stimuli other than atrial rate

**37.87　Replacement of any type pacemaker device with dual-chamber device**
Atrial ventricular sequential device

**37.89　Revision or removal of pacemaker device**
Removal without replacement of cardiac re-synchronization pacemaker device [CRT-P]
Repair of pacemaker device

**EXCLUDES**　*removal of temporary transvenous pacemaker system — omit code*
*replacement of existing pacemaker device (37.85-37.87)*
*replacement of existing pacemaker device with CRT-P pacemaker device (00.53)*

**AHA:** N-D, '86, 1

✓4ᵗʰ **37.9　Other operations on heart and pericardium**
**AHA:** 3Q, '90, 11

**37.90　Insertion of left atrial appendage device**
Left atrial filter　　Transseptal catheter
Left atrial occluder　　technique
**AHA:** 4Q, '04, 121

**DEF:** Implantation of a filtering device within the left atrial appendage (LAA) to block emboli from exiting the LAA causing stroke or systemic thromboembolism.

**37.91　Open chest cardiac massage**

**EXCLUDES**　*closed chest cardiac massage (99.63)*

**AHA:** 4Q, '88, 12
**DEF:** Massage of heart through opening in chest wall to reinstate or maintain circulation.

### Left Atrial Appendage Device Insertion

### Automatic Implantable Cardioverter/Defibrillator

**37.92　Injection of therapeutic substance into heart**
**37.93　Injection of therapeutic substance into pericardium**
**37.94　Implantation or replacement of automatic cardioverter/defibrillator, total system [AICD]**
Note: Device testing during procedure—omit code
Implantation of defibrillator with leads (epicardial patches), formation of pocket (abdominal fascia) (subcutaneous), any transvenous leads, intraoperative procedures for evaluation of lead signals, and obtaining defibrillator threshold measurements
Techniques:
　lateral thoracotomy
　medial sternotomy
　subxiphoid procedure
Code also extracorporeal circulation, if performed (39.61)
Code also any concomitant procedure [e.g., coronary bypass] (36.01-36.19)

**EXCLUDES**　*implantation of cardiac resynchronization defibrillator, total system [CRT-D] (00.51)*

**AHA:** 2Q, '03, 19; 3Q, '01, 5-7; 3Q, '99, 12; 1Q, '99, 3; 3Q, '90, 11; S-O, '87, 5

**DEF:** Direct insertion, of defibrillator/cardioverter system to deliver shock and restore heart rhythm.

**37.95　Implantation of automatic cardioverter/defibrillator lead(s) only**
**AHA:** 3Q, '90, 11

**37.96　Implantation of automatic cardioverter/defibrillator pulse generator only**
Note: Device testing during procedure—omit code

**EXCLUDES**　*implantation or replacement of cardiac resynchronization defibrillator, pulse generator device only [CRT-D] (00.54)*

**AHA:** 3Q, '90, 11

**37.97　Replacement of automatic cardioverter/defibrillator lead(s) only**

**EXCLUDES**　*replacement of epicardial lead [electrode] into epicardium (37.74)*
*replacement of transvenous lead [electrode] into left ventricular coronary venous system (00.52)*

**AHA:** 3Q, '05, 3-9; 3Q, '90, 11

**37.98　Replacement of automatic cardioverter defibrillator pulse generator only**
Note: Device testing during procedure—omit code

**EXCLUDES**　*replacement of cardiac resynchronization defibrillator, pulse generator device only [CRT-D] (00.54)*

**AHA:** 1Q, '99, 3; 3Q, '90, 11

⁶　Valid OR procedure code if accompanied by one of the following codes: 37.70, 37.71, 37.73, 37.76

**BI** Bilateral Procedure　　**NC** Non-covered Procedure　　**LC** Limited Coverage Procedure　　▶◀ Revised Text　　● New Code　　▲ Revised Code Title

**112 — Volume 3**

© 2007 Ingenix

**37.99   Other**

> EXCLUDES *cardiac retraining (93.36)*
> *conversion of cardiac rhythm (99.60-99.69)*
> *implantation of prosthetic cardiac support device (37.41)*
> *insertion of left atrial appendage device (37.90)*
> *maze procedure (Cox-maze), open (37.33)*
> *maze procedure, endovascular approach (37.34)*
> *repositioning of pulse generator (37.79)*
> *revision of lead(s) (37.75)*
> *revision or relocation of pacemaker, defibrillator or other implanted cardiac device pocket (37.79)*

**AHA:** 3Q, '05, 5; 2Q, '05, 14; 1Q, '97, 12; 1Q, '94, 19; 3Q, '90, 11; 1Q, '89, 11

√3rd **38   Incision, excision, and occlusion of vessels**

Code also any application or administration of an adhesion barrier substance (99.77)
Code also cardiopulmonary bypass [extracorporeal circulation] [heart-lung machine] (39.61)

> EXCLUDES *that of coronary vessels (00.66, 36.03, 36.04, 36.09, 36.10-36.99)*

The following fourth-digit subclassification is for use with appropriate categories in section 38.0, 38.1, 38.3, 38.5, 38.6, and 38.8 according to site. Valid fourth-digits are in [brackets] under each code.

**0   unspecified**
**1   intracranial vessels**
> Cerebral (anterior) (middle)
> Circle of Willis
> Posterior communicating artery

**2   other vessels of head and neck**
> Carotid artery (common) (external) (internal)
> Jugular vein (external) (internal)

**3   upper limb vessels**
> Axillary          Radial
> Brachial          Ulnar

**4   aorta**
**5   other thoracic vessels**
> Innominate        Subclavian
> Pulmonary (artery) (vein)    Vena cava, superior

**6   abdominal arteries**
> Celiac            Mesenteric
> Gastric           Renal
> Hepatic           Splenic
> Iliac             Umbilical
> EXCLUDES *abdominal aorta (4)*

**7   abdominal veins**
> Iliac             Splenic
> Portal            Vena cava (inferior)
> Renal

**8   lower limb arteries**
> Femoral (common) (superficial)    Popliteal
>                   Tibial

**9   lower limb veins**
> Femoral           Saphenous
> Popliteal         Tibial

**Endarterectomy of Aortic Bifurcation**

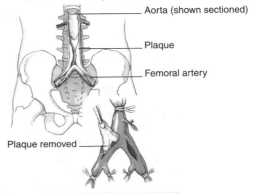

Aorta (shown sectioned)
Plaque
Femoral artery
Plaque removed

§ √4th **38.0   Incision of vessel**
[0-9]
> Embolectomy          Thrombectomy
> EXCLUDES *endovascular removal of obstruction from head and neck vessel(s) (39.74)*
> *puncture or catheterization of any:*
> *artery (38.91, 38.98)*
> *vein (38.92-38.95, 38.99)*

**AHA:** 2Q, '98, 23; **For code 38.08 and 38.09:** 1Q, '03, 17

§ √4th **38.1   Endarterectomy**
[0-6,8]
> Endarterectomy with:
> embolectomy
> patch graft
> temporary bypass during procedure
> thrombectomy
> Code also any:
> number of vascular stents inserted (00.45-00.48)
> number of vessels treated (00.40-00.43)
> procedure on vessel bifurcation (00.44)

**AHA:** 1Q, '00, 16; 2Q, '99, 5; 2Q, '95, 16; **For code 38.12:** 3Q, '06, 20; 1Q, '02, 10

**DEF:** Excision of tunica intima of artery to relieve arterial walls thickened by plaque or chronic inflammation.

√4th **38.2   Diagnostic procedures on blood vessels**
> EXCLUDES *adjunct vascular system procedures (00.40-00.43)*

**38.21   Biopsy of blood vessel**

**38.22   Percutaneous angioscopy**
> EXCLUDES *angioscopy of eye (95.12)*
> **DEF:** Exam, with fiberoptic catheter inserted through peripheral artery to visualize inner lining of blood vessels.

**38.29   Other diagnostic procedures on blood vessels**
> EXCLUDES *blood vessel thermography (88.86)*
> *circulatory monitoring (89.61-89.69)*
> *contrast:*
> *angiocardiography (88.50-88.58)*
> *arteriography (88.40-88.49)*
> *phlebography (88.60-88.67)*
> *impedance phlebography (88.68)*
> *peripheral vascular ultrasonography (88.77)*
> *plethysmogram (89.58)*

**AHA:** 3Q, '00, 16; 1Q, '99, 7

§ √4th **38.3   Resection of vessel with anastomosis**
[0-9]
> Angiectomy
> Excision of:
> aneurysm (arteriovenous) ⎫ with anastomosis
> blood vessel (lesion) ⎭

**DEF:** Reconstruction and reconnection of vessel after partial excision.

§   Requires fourth-digit. Valid digits are in [brackets] under each code. See category 38 for definitions.

√3rd
√4th Additional Digit Required            Valid OR Procedure            Non-OR Procedure            Adjunct Code

**Operations on the Cardiovascular System**

**38.4–38.98**

§§ ☑4th **38.4** **Resection of vessel with replacement**
[0-9]     Angiectomy
          Excision of:
              aneurysm (arteriovenous) or  } with replacement
              blood vessel (lesion)
          Partial resection with replacement
          **EXCLUDES** *endovascular repair of aneurysm (39.71-39.79)*

Requires the use of one of the following fourth-digit subclassifications to identify site:

**0** **unspecified site**
**1** **intracranial vessels**
          Cerebral (anterior) (middle)
          Circle of Willis
          Posterior communicating artery
**2** **other vessels of head and neck**
          Carotid artery (common) (external) (internal)
          Jugular vein (external) (internal)
**3** **upper limb vessels**
          Axillary          Radial
          Brachial          Ulnar
**4** **aorta, abdominal**
          Code also any thoracic vessel involvement
              (thoracoabdominal procedure) (38.45)
**5** **thoracic vessel**
          Aorta (thoracic)
          Innominate        Subclavian
          Pulmonary (artery) (vein)   Vena cava, superior
          Code also any abdominal aorta involvement
              (thoracoabdominal procedure) (38.44)
**6** **abdominal arteries**
          Celiac            Mesenteric
          Gastric           Renal
          Hepatic           Splenic
          Iliac             Umbilical
          **EXCLUDES** *abdominal aorta (4)*
**7** **abdominal veins**
          Iliac             Splenic
          Portal            Vena cava (inferior)
          Renal
**8** **lower limb arteries**
          Femoral (common) (superficial)
          Tibial
**9** **lower limb veins**
          Femoral           Saphenous
          Popliteal         Tibial

AHA: 2Q, '99, 5, 6; **For code 38.44:** 3Q, '06, 15
DEF: Excision of aneurysm (arteriovenous): Excision and replacement of segment of stretched or bulging blood vessel.
DEF: Excision of blood vessel (lesion): Excision and replacement of segment of vessel containing lesion.

§ ☑4th **38.5** **Ligation and stripping of varicose veins**
[0-3,5,7,9] **EXCLUDES** *ligation of varices:*
                *esophageal (42.91)*
                *gastric (44.91)*
AHA: **For code 38.59:** 2Q, '97, 7
DEF: Ligation of varicose veins: Typing off vein with thread or wire to eliminate blood flow; stripping involves excising length of vein.

§ ☑4th **38.6** **Other excision of vessels**
[0-9]     Excision of blood vessel (lesion) NOS
          **EXCLUDES** *excision of vessel for aortocoronary bypass (36.10-36.14)*
                *excision with:*
                    *anastomosis (38.30-38.39)*
                    *graft replacement (38.40-38.49)*
                    *implant (38.40-38.49)*
AHA: 3Q, '90, 17

**38.7** **Interruption of the vena cava**
          Insertion of implant or sieve in vena cava
          Ligation of vena cava (inferior) (superior)
          Plication of vena cava
AHA: ►2Q, '07, 4;◄ 2Q, '94, 9; S-O, '85, 5
DEF: Interruption of the blood flow through the venous heart vessels to prevent clots from reaching the chambers of the heart by means of implanting a sieve or implant, separating off a portion or by narrowing the venous blood vessels.

**Methods of Vessel Anastomoses**

End-to-end          Side-to-side

Oblique cut         Fish mouth

Funnelization       End-to-side

§ ☑4th **38.8** **Other surgical occlusion of vessels**
[0-9]     Clamping
          Division      } of blood vessel
          Ligation
          Occlusion
          **EXCLUDES** *adrenal vessels (07.43)*
                *esophageal varices (42.91)*
                *gastric or duodenal vessel for ulcer (44.40-44.49)*
                *gastric varices (44.91)*
                *meningeal vessel (02.13)*
                *percutaneous transcatheter infusion embolization (99.29)*
                *spermatic vein for varicocele (63.1)*
                *surgical occlusion of vena cava (38.7)*
                *that for chemoembolization (99.25)*
                *that for control of (postoperative) hemorrhage:*
                    *anus (49.95)*
                    *bladder (57.93)*
                    *following vascular procedure (39.41)*
                    *nose (21.00-21.09)*
                    *prostate (60.94)*
                    *tonsil (28.7)*
                    *thyroid vessel (06.92)*
AHA: 2Q, '90, 23; M-A, '87, 9; **For code 38.85:** 1Q, '03, 15; **For code 38.86:** 1Q, '05, 14; N-D, '87, 4

☑4th **38.9** **Puncture of vessel**
          **EXCLUDES** *that for circulatory monitoring (89.60-89.69)*

**38.91** **Arterial catheterization**
AHA: 1Q, '05, 14; 1Q, '97, 3; 1Q, '95, 3; 2Q, '91, 15; 2Q, '90, 23

**38.92** **Umbilical vein catheterization**

**38.93** **Venous catheterization, not elsewhere classified**
          **EXCLUDES** *that for cardiac catheterization (37.21-37.23)*
                *that for renal dialysis (38.95)*
AHA: 3Q, '00, 9; 2Q, '98, 24; 1Q, '96, 3; 2Q, '96, 15; 3Q, '91, 13; 4Q, '90, 14; 2Q, '90, 24; 3Q, '88, 13

**38.94** **Venous cutdown**
DEF: Incision of vein to place needle or catheter.

**38.95** **Venous catheterization for renal dialysis**
          **EXCLUDES** *insertion of totally implantable vascular access device [VAD] (86.07)*
AHA: 3Q, '98, 13; 2Q, '94, 11

**38.98** **Other puncture of artery**
          **EXCLUDES** *that for:*
                *arteriography (88.40-88.49)*
                *coronary arteriography (88.55-88.57)*

§ Requires fourth-digit. Valid digits are in [brackets] under each code. See category 38 for definitions.
§§ Requires fourth-digit. Valid digits are in [brackets] under each code. See subcategory 38.4 for definitions.

**BI** Bilateral Procedure     **NC** Non-covered Procedure     **LC** Limited Coverage Procedure     ►◄ Revised Text     ● New Code     ▲ Revised Code Title

114 — Volume 3 • October 2007

© 2007 Ingenix

**Operations on the Cardiovascular System**

**38.99–39.43**

Typical Venous Cutdown

Vein mobilized, opened by oblique cut, catheter inserted

Distal vein tied

Saphenous vein (typical site) accessed by transverse incision

**38.99 Other puncture of vein**
Phlebotomy
EXCLUDES   that for:
angiography (88.60-88.68)
extracorporeal circulation (39.61, 50.92)
injection or infusion of:
sclerosing solution (39.92)
therapeutic or prophylactic substance (99.11-99.29)
perfusion (39.96, 39.97)
phlebography (88.60-88.68)
transfusion (99.01-99.09)

AHA: 4Q, '94, 50; 1Q, '88, 11

✓3rd **39 Other operations on vessels**
EXCLUDES   those on coronary vessels (36.0-36.99)

**39.0 Systemic to pulmonary artery shunt**
Descending aorta-pulmonary artery
Left to right
Subclavian-pulmonary
} anastomosis (graft)

Code also cardiopulmonary bypass [extracorporeal circulation] [heart-lung machine] (39.61)
DEF: Descending aorta-pulmonary artery anastomosis (graft): Connection of descending main heart artery to pulmonary artery.
DEF: Left to right anastomosis (graft): Connection of systemic arterial blood vessel to venous pulmonary system.
DEF: Subclavian-pulmonary anastomosis (graft): Connection of subclavian artery to pulmonary artery

**39.1 Intra-abdominal venous shunt**
Anastomosis:
mesocaval
portacaval
portal vein to inferior vena cava
splenic and renal veins
transjugular intrahepatic portosystemic shunt [TIPS]
EXCLUDES   peritoneovenous shunt (54.94)
AHA: 2Q, '02, 4; 4Q, '94, 50; 4Q, '93, 31; 2Q, '93, 8
DEF: Connection of two venous blood vessels within abdominal cavity.

✓4th **39.2 Other shunt or vascular bypass**
Code also pressurized treatment of venous bypass graft [conduit] with pharmaceutical substance, if performed (00.16)
DEF: Creation of supplemental blood flow to area with inadequate blood supply due to disease or injury of vessels.

**39.21 Caval-pulmonary artery anastomosis**
Code also cardiopulmonary bypass (39.61)

**39.22 Aorta-subclavian-carotid bypass**
Bypass (arterial):
aorta to carotid and brachial
aorta to subclavian and carotid
carotid to subclavian

**39.23 Other intrathoracic vascular shunt or bypass**
Intrathoracic (arterial) bypass graft NOS
EXCLUDES   coronary artery bypass (36.10-36.19)

**39.24 Aorta-renal bypass**

**39.25 Aorta-iliac-femoral bypass**
Bypass:                 Bypass:
aortofemoral         aortopopliteal
aortoiliac             iliofemoral [iliac-femoral]
aortoiliac to popliteal
AHA: 1Q, '03, 16; 4Q, '90, 27; 1Q, '88, 10

**39.26 Other intra-abdominal vascular shunt or bypass**
Bypass:
aortoceliac
aortic-superior mesenteric
common hepatic-common iliac-renal
Intra-abdominal arterial bypass graft NOS
EXCLUDES   peritoneovenous shunt (54.94)

**39.27 Arteriovenostomy for renal dialysis**
Anastomosis for renal dialysis
Formation of (peripheral) arteriovenous fistula for renal [kidney] dialysis
Code also any renal dialysis (39.95)
AHA: ▶1Q, '07, 18;◄ 1Q, '06, 10

**39.28 Extracranial-intracranial (EC-IC) vascular bypass**   NC
AHA: 2Q, '92, 7; 4Q, '91, 22

**39.29 Other (peripheral) vascular shunt or bypass**
Bypass (graft):
axillary-brachial
axillary-femoral [axillofemora] (superficial)
brachial
femoral-femoral
femoroperoneal
femoropopliteal (arteries)
femorotibial (anterior) (posterior)
popliteal
vascular NOS
EXCLUDES   peritoneovenous shunt (54.94)
AHA: 1Q, '03, 17; 2Q, '02, 8; 1Q, '02, 13; S-O, '85, 13

✓4th **39.3 Suture of vessel**
Repair of laceration of blood vessel
EXCLUDES   any other vascular puncture closure device — omit code
suture of aneurysm (39.52)
that for control of hemorrhage (postoperative):
anus (49.95)
bladder (57.93)
following vascular procedure (39.41)
nose (21.00-21.09)
prostate (60.94)
tonsil (28.7)

**39.30 Suture of unspecified blood vessel**

**39.31 Suture of artery**
AHA: 3Q, '06, 9

**39.32 Suture of vein**

✓4th **39.4 Revision of vascular procedure**

**39.41 Control of hemorrhage following vascular surgery**
EXCLUDES   that for control of hemorrhage (postoperative):
anus (49.95)
bladder (57.93)
nose (21.00-21.09)
prostate (60.94)
tonsil (28.7)

**39.42 Revision of arteriovenous shunt for renal dialysis**
Conversion of renal dialysis:
end-to-end anastomosis to end-to-side
end-to-side anastomosis to end-to-end
vessel-to-vessel cannula to arteriovenous shunt
Removal of old arteriovenous shunt and creation of new shunt
EXCLUDES   replacement of vessel-to-vessel cannula (39.94)
AHA: 2Q, '94, 15; 4Q, '93, 33

**39.43 Removal of arteriovenous shunt for renal dialysis**
EXCLUDES   that with replacement [revision] of shunt (39.42)

**Operations on the Cardiovascular System**

**39.49–39.62**

**39.49　Other revision of vascular procedure**
　　Declotting (graft)
　　Revision of:
　　　anastomosis of blood vessel
　　　vascular procedure (previous)
　　**AHA:** 2Q, '98, 17; 1Q, '97, 3; 2Q, '94, 15
　　**DEF:** Declotting (graft): Removal of clot from graft.

✓4ᵗʰ **39.5　Other repair of vessels**

**39.50　Angioplasty or atherectomy of other non-coronary vessel(s)**
　　Percutaneous transluminal angioplasty (PTA) of non-coronary vessels:
　　　lower extremity vessels
　　　mesenteric artery
　　　renal artery
　　　upper extremity vessels
　　Code also any:
　　　injection or infusion of thrombolytic agent (99.10)
　　　insertion of non-coronary stent(s) or stent grafts(s) (39.90)
　　　number of vascular stents inserted (00.45-00.48)
　　　number of vessels treated (00.40-00.43)
　　　procedure on vessel bifurcation (00.44)
　　　**EXCLUDES**　　*percutaneous angioplasty or atherectomy of precerebral or cerebral vessel(s) (00.61-00.62)*
　　**AHA:** ▶4Q, '06, 119;◀ 3Q, '03, 10; 1Q, '02, 13; 2Q, '01, 23; 2Q, '00, 10; 1Q, '00, 12; 2Q, '98, 17; 1Q, '97, 3; 4Q, '96, 63; 4Q, '95, 66

**39.51　Clipping of aneurysm**
　　**EXCLUDES**　　*clipping of arteriovenous fistula (39.53)*

**39.52　Other repair of aneurysm**
　　Repair of aneurysm by:
　　　coagulation　　　wiring
　　　electrocoagulation　　wrapping
　　　filipuncture
　　　methyl methacrylate
　　　suture
　　　**EXCLUDES**　　*endovascular repair of aneurysm (39.71-39.79)*
　　　　　　　*re-entry operation (aorta) (39.54)*
　　　　　　　*that with:*
　　　　　　　　*graft replacement (38.40-38.49)*
　　　　　　　　*resection (38.30-38.49, 38.60-38.69)*
　　**AHA:** ▶3Q, '06, 15-16;◀ 3Q, '02, 25, 26; 1Q, '99, 15, 16, 17; 1Q, '88, 10
　　**DEF:** Application of device in abnormally stretched blood vessel to prevent movement of material collected in vessel.
　　**DEF:** Repair of aneurysm by: Coagulation: Clotting or solidifying. Electrocoagulation: Electrically produced clotting. Filipuncture: Insertion of wire or thread. Methyl methacrylate: Injection or insertion of plastic material. Suture: Stitching. Wiring: Insertion of wire. Wrapping: Compression.

**39.53　Repair of arteriovenous fistula**
　　Embolization of carotid cavernous fistula
　　Repair of arteriovenous fistula by:
　　　clipping
　　　coagulation
　　　ligation and division
　　　**EXCLUDES**　　*repair of:*
　　　　　　　*arteriovenous shunt for renal dialysis (39.42)*
　　　　　　　*head and neck vessels, endovascular approach (39.72)*
　　　　　　*that with:*
　　　　　　　*graft replacement (38.40-38.49)*
　　　　　　　*resection (38.30-38.49, 38.60-38.69)*
　　**AHA:** 1Q, '00, 8
　　**DEF:** Correction of arteriovenous fistula by application of clamps, causing coagulation or by tying off and dividing the connection.

**39.54　Re-entry operation (aorta)**
　　Fenestration of dissecting aneurysm of thoracic aorta
　　Code also cardiopulmonary bypass [extracorporeal circulation] [heart-lung machine] (39.61)
　　**DEF:** Re-entry operation: Creation of passage between stretched wall of the vessel and major arterial channel to heart.
　　**DEF:** Fenestration of dissecting aneurysm of thoracic aorta: Creation of passage between stretched arterial heart vessel and functional part of vessel.

**39.55　Reimplantation of aberrant renal vessel**
　　**DEF:** Reimplant of renal vessel into normal position.

**39.56　Repair of blood vessel with tissue patch graft**
　　**EXCLUDES**　　*that with resection (38.40-38.49)*
　　**AHA:** 1Q, '04, 16

**39.57　Repair of blood vessel with synthetic patch graft**
　　**EXCLUDES**　　*that with resection (38.40-38.49)*

**39.58　Repair of blood vessel with unspecified type of patch graft**
　　**EXCLUDES**　　*that with resection (38.40-38.49)*

**39.59　Other repair of vessel**
　　Aorticopulmonary window operation
　　Arterioplasty NOS
　　Construction of venous valves (peripheral)
　　Plication of vein (peripheral)
　　Reimplantation of artery
　　Code also cardiopulmonary bypass [extracorporeal circulation] [heart-lung machine] (39.61)
　　**EXCLUDES**　　*interruption of the vena cava (38.7)*
　　　　　　　*reimplantation of renal artery (39.55)*
　　　　　　*that with:*
　　　　　　　*graft (39.56-39.58)*
　　　　　　　*resection (38.30-38.49, 38.60-38.69)*
　　**AHA:** 4Q, '93, 31; 2Q, '89, 17; N-D, '86, 8; S-O, '85, 5; M-A, '85, 15
　　**DEF:** Aorticopulmonary window operation: Repair of abnormal opening between major heart arterial vessel above valves and pulmonary artery.
　　**DEF:** Construction of venous valves (peripheral): Reconstruction of valves within peripheral veins.
　　**DEF:** Plication of vein (peripheral): Shortening of peripheral vein.
　　**DEF:** Reimplantation of artery: Reinsertion of artery into its normal position.

✓4ᵗʰ **39.6　Extracorporeal circulation and procedures auxiliary to heart surgery**
　　**AHA:** 1Q, '95, 5

**39.61　Extracorporeal circulation auxiliary to open heart surgery**
　　Artificial heart and lung
　　Cardiopulmonary bypass
　　Pump oxygenator
　　　**EXCLUDES**　　*extracorporeal hepatic assistance (50.92)*
　　　　　　　*extracorporeal membrane oxygenation [ECMO] (39.65)*
　　　　　　　*hemodialysis (39.95)*
　　　　　　　*percutaneous cardiopulmonary bypass (39.66)*
　　**AHA:** 1Q, '04, 16; 3Q, '02, 5; 4Q, '97, 55; 3Q, '97, 14; 2Q, '97, 8; 2Q, '90, 24

**39.62　Hypothermia (systemic) incidental to open heart surgery**

---

**BI** Bilateral Procedure　　**NC** Non-covered Procedure　　**LC** Limited Coverage Procedure　　◀▶ Revised Text　　● New Code　　▲ Revised Code Title

116 — Volume 3 • February 2007

© 2007 Ingenix

**39.63**   **Cardioplegia**

Arrest:       Arrest:

anoxic       circulatory

DEF: Purposely inducing electromechanical cardiac arrest.

**39.64**   **Intraoperative cardiac pacemaker**

Temporary pacemaker used during and immediately following cardiac surgery

AHA: 1Q, '89, 2; M-J, '87, 3

**39.65**   **Extracorporeal membrane oxygenation [ECMO]**

EXCLUDES   *extracorporeal circulation auxiliary to open heart surgery (39.61)*
*percutaneous cardiopulmonary bypass (39.66)*

AHA: 2Q, '90, 23; 2Q, '89, 17; 4Q, '88, 5

DEF: Creation of closed-chest, heart-lung bypass or Bard cardiopulmonary assist system with tube insertion.

**39.66**   **Percutaneous cardiopulmonary bypass**

Closed chest

EXCLUDES   *extracorporeal circulation auxiliary to open heart surgery (39.61)*
*extracorporeal hepatic assistance (50.92)*
*extracorporeal membrane oxygenation [ECMO] (39.65)*
*hemodialysis (39.95)*

AHA: 3Q, '96, 11

DEF: Use of mechanical pump system to oxygenate and pump blood throughout the body via catheter in the femoral artery and vein.

**√4ᵗʰ**   **39.7**   **Endovascular repair of vessel**

Endoluminal repair

EXCLUDES   *angioplasty or atherectomy of other non-coronary vessel(s) (39.50)*
*insertion of non-drug-eluting peripheral vessel stent(s) (39.90)*
*other repair of aneurysm (39.52)*
*percutaneous insertion of carotid artery stent(s) (00.63)*
*percutaneous insertion of intracranial stent(s) (00.65)*
*percutaneous insertion of other precerebral artery stent(s) (00.64)*
*resection of abdominal aorta with replacement (38.44)*
*resection of lower limb arteries with replacement (38.48)*
*resection of thoracic aorta with replacement (38.45)*
*resection of upper limb vessels with replacement (38.43)*

**39.71**   **Endovascular implantation of graft in abdominal aorta**

Endovascular repair of abdominal aortic aneurysm with graft

Stent graft(s)

AHA: 1Q, '02, 13; 4Q, '00, 63, 64

DEF: Replacement of a section of abdominal aorta with mesh graft; via catheters inserted through femoral arteries.

**Endovascular Repair of Abdominal Aortic Aneurysm**

Renal arteries

Stent

Abdominal aortic aneurysm

Common iliac arteries

**39.72**   **Endovascular repair or occlusion of head and neck vessels**

Coil embolization or occlusion

Endograft(s)

Endovascular graft(s)

Liquid tissue adhesive (glue) embolization or occlusion

Other implant or substance for repair, embolization or occlusion

That for repair of aneurysm, arteriovenous malformation [AVM] or fistula

EXCLUDES   *mechanical thrombectomy of pre-cerebral and cerebral vessels (39.74)*

AHA: 4Q, '02, 103

DEF: Coil embolization or occlusion: Utilizing x-ray guidance a neuro-microcatheter is guided from entry in the femoral artery in the groin to the site of the aneurysm of the head and neck vessels for delivery of micro-coils that stop blood flow to the arteriovenous malfomation (AVM).

**39.73**   **Endovascular implantation of graft in thoracic aorta**

Endograft(s)

Endovascular graft(s)

Endovascular repair of defect of thoracic aorta with graft(s) or device(s)

Stent graft(s) or device(s)

That for repair of aneurysm, dissection, or injury

EXCLUDES   *fenestration of dissecting aneurysm of thoracic aorta (39.54)*

AHA: 4Q, '05, 120

DEF: Intravascular transcatheter deployment of an expanding stent-graft for repair of thoracic aortic aneurysm, performed without opening the chest.

**39.74**   **Endovascular removal of obstruction from head and neck vessel(s)**

Endovascular embolectomy

Endovascular thrombectomy of pre-cerebral and cerebral vessels

Mechanical embolectomy or thrombectomy

Code also:

any injection or infusion of thrombolytic agent (99.10)

number of vessels treated (00.40-00.43)

procedure on vessel bifurcation (00.44)

EXCLUDES   *endarterectomy of intracranial vessels and other vessels of head and neck (38.11-38.12)*
*occlusive endovascular repair of head or neck vessels (39.72)*
*open embolectomy or thrombectomy (38.01-38.02)*

AHA: ▶4Q, '06, 129◀

**External Arteriovenous Shunt**

Cephalic vein

Radial artery

---

**39.79 Other endovascular repair (of aneurysm) of other vessels**

Coil embolization or occlusion
Endograft(s)
Endovascular graft(s)
Liquid tissue adhesive (glue) embolization or occlusion
Other implant or substance for repair, embolization or occlusion

> **EXCLUDES** endovascular implantation of graft in thoracic aorta (39.73)
> endovascular repair or occlusion of head and neck vessels (39.72)
> insertion of drug-eluting peripheral vessel stent(s) (00.55)
> insertion of non-drug-eluting peripheral vessel stent(s) (for other than aneurysm repair) (39.90)
> non-endovascular repair of arteriovenous fistula (39.53)
> other surgical occlusion of vessels–see category 38.8
> percutaneous transcatheter infusion (99.29)
> transcatheter embolization for gastric or duodenal bleeding (44.44)

**AHA:** 2Q, '06, 22, 23; 4Q, '02, 103; 3Q, '01, 17,18; 4Q, '00, 64

▲ **39.8 Operations on carotid body, carotid sinus and other vascular bodies**

Chemodectomy
Denervation of:
    aortic body
    carotid body
►Electronic stimulator◄
Glomectomy, carotid
►Implantation or replacement of carotid sinus baroreflex activation device◄

> **EXCLUDES** excision of glomus jugulare (20.51)
> ►replacement of carotid sinus lead(s) only (04.92)◄

**AHA:** ►2Q, '07, 8◄

**DEF: Chemodectomy:** Removal of a chemoreceptor vascular body.
**DEF: Denervation of aortic body:** Destruction of nerves attending the major heart blood vessels.
**DEF: Denervation of carotid body:** Destruction of nerves of carotid artery.
**DEF: Glomectomy, carotid:** Removal of the carotid artery framework.

✓4ᵗʰ **39.9 Other operations on vessels**

**39.90 Insertion of non-drug-eluting peripheral vessel stent(s)**

Bare stent(s)
Bonded stent(s)
Drug-coated stent(s), i.e., heparin coated
Endograft(s)
Endovascular graft(s)
Endovascular recanalization techniques
Stent graft(s)
Code also any:
    non-coronary angioplasty or atherectomy (39.50)
    number of vascular stents inserted (00.45-00.48)
    number of vessels treated (00.40-00.43)
    procedure on vessel bifurcation (00.44)

> **EXCLUDES** insertion of drug-eluting, peripheral vessel stent(s) (00.55)
> percutaneous insertion of carotid artery stent(s) (00.63)
> percutaneous insertion of intracranial stent(s) (00.65)
> percutaneous insertion of other precerebral artery stent(s) (00.64)
> that for aneurysm repair (39.71-39.79)

**AHA:** 4Q, '06, 119; 4Q, '02, 101; 1Q, '00, 12; 4Q, '96, 63

**39.91 Freeing of vessel**

Dissection and freeing of adherent tissue:
    artery-vein-nerve bundle
    vascular bundle

**AHA:** 3Q, '02, 12

**39.92 Injection of sclerosing agent into vein**

> **EXCLUDES** injection:
> esophageal varices (42.33)
> hemorrhoids (49.42)

**AHA:** 2Q, '92, 17

**39.93 Insertion of vessel-to-vessel cannula**

Formation of:
    arteriovenous:
        fistula ⎫ by external
        shunt ⎬ cannula

Code also any renal dialysis (39.95)

**AHA:** 3Q, '88, 13; S-O, '85, 5 & 12

**39.94 Replacement of vessel-to-vessel cannula**

Revision of vessel-to-vessel cannula

**39.95 Hemodialysis**

Artificial kidney         Hemodiafiltration
Hemofiltration            Renal dialysis

> **EXCLUDES** peritoneal dialysis (54.98)

**AHA:** 1Q, '04, 22; 4Q, '03, 111; 2Q, '01, 2-14; 4Q, '00, 40; 2Q, '98, 20; S-O, '86, 11

**DEF:** Filtration process to treat acute and chronic renal failure by eliminating toxic end products of nitrogen metabolism from blood.

**39.96 Total body perfusion**

Code also substance perfused (99.21-99.29)

**39.97 Other perfusion**

Perfusion NOS            Perfusion, local
Perfusion, local              [regional] of:
    [regional] of:        lower limb
    carotid artery        neck
    coronary artery       upper limb
    head

Code also substance perfused (99.21-99.29)

> **EXCLUDES** perfusion of:
> kidney (55.95)
> large intestine (46.96)
> liver (50.93)
> small intestine (46.95)

**AHA:** 3Q, '96, 11

**39.98 Control of hemorrhage, not otherwise specified**

Angiotripsy
Control of postoperative hemorrhage NOS
Venotripsy

> **EXCLUDES** control of hemorrhage (postoperative):
> anus (49.95)
> bladder (57.93)
> following vascular procedure (39.41)
> nose (21.00-21.09)
> prostate (60.94)
> tonsil (28.7)
> that by:
> ligation (38.80-38.89)
> suture (39.30-39.32)

**DEF: Angiotripsy:** Clamping of tissue to stop arterial blood flow.

**DEF: Venotripsy:** Clamping of tissue to stop venous blood flow.

**39.99 Other operations on vessels**

> **EXCLUDES** injection or infusion of therapeutic or prophylactic substance (99.11-99.29)
> transfusion of blood and blood components (99.01-99.09)

**AHA:** 1Q, '89, 11

---

**BI** Bilateral Procedure   **NC** Non-covered Procedure   **LC** Limited Coverage Procedure   ►◄ Revised Text   ● New Code   ▲ Revised Code Title

# 8. OPERATIONS ON THE HEMIC AND LYMPHATIC SYSTEMS
## (40-41)

√3rd **40**   **Operations on lymphatic system**

   **40.0**    **Incision of lymphatic structures**

√4th **40.1**    **Diagnostic procedures on lymphatic structures**

    **40.11**   **Biopsy of lymphatic structure**

    **40.19**   **Other diagnostic procedures on lymphatic structures**

      EXCLUDES   *lymphangiogram:*
        *abdominal (88.04)*
        *cervical (87.08)*
        *intrathoracic (87.34)*
        *lower limb (88.36)*
        *upper limb (88.34)*
       *microscopic examination of*
        *specimen (90.71-90.79)*
       *radioisotope scan (92.16)*
       *thermography (88.89)*

√4th **40.2**    **Simple excision of lymphatic structure**

      EXCLUDES   *biopsy of lymphatic structure (40.11)*

   DEF: Removal of lymphatic structure only.

    **40.21**   **Excision of deep cervical lymph node**

      AHA: 4Q, '99, 16

    **40.22**   **Excision of internal mammary lymph node**

    **40.23**   **Excision of axillary lymph node**

      AHA: 2Q, '02, 7

    **40.24**   **Excision of inguinal lymph node**

    **40.29**   **Simple excision of other lymphatic structure**

      Excision of:
       cystic hygroma
       lymphangioma
      Simple lymphadenectomy

      AHA: 1Q, '99, 6

      DEF: Lymphangioma: Removal of benign congenital lymphatic malformation.

      DEF: Simple lymphadenectomy: Removal of lymph node.

   **40.3**    **Regional lymph node excision**

      Extended regional lymph node excision
      Regional lymph node excision with excision of lymphatic drainage area including skin, subcutaneous tissue, and fat

   AHA: 2Q, '92, 7

   DEF: Extended regional lymph node excision: Removal of lymph node group, including area around nodes.

√4th **40.4**    **Radical excision of cervical lymph nodes**

      Resection of cervical lymph nodes down to muscle and deep fascia

      EXCLUDES   *that associated with radical laryngectomy (30.4)*

    **40.40**   **Radical neck dissection, not otherwise specified**

    **40.41**   **Radical neck dissection, unilateral**

      AHA: 2Q, '05, 8; 2Q, '99, 6

      DEF: Dissection, total, of cervical lymph nodes on one side of neck.

    **40.42**   **Radical neck dissection, bilateral**

      DEF: Dissection, total, of cervical lymph nodes on both sides of neck.

√4th **40.5**    **Radical excision of other lymph nodes**

      EXCLUDES   *that associated with radical mastectomy (85.45-85.48)*

    **40.50**   **Radical excision of lymph nodes, not otherwise specified**

      Radical (lymph) node dissection NOS

    **40.51**   **Radical excision of axillary lymph nodes**

    **40.52**   **Radical excision of periaortic lymph nodes**

    **40.53**   **Radical excision of iliac lymph nodes**

    **40.54**   **Radical groin dissection**

    **40.59**   **Radical excision of other lymph nodes**

      EXCLUDES   *radical neck dissection (40.40-40.42)*

√4th **40.6**    **Operations on thoracic duct**

    **40.61**   **Cannulation of thoracic duct**

      DEF: Placement of cannula in main lymphatic duct of chest.

    **40.62**   **Fistulization of thoracic duct**

      DEF: Creation of passage in main lymphatic duct of chest.

    **40.63**   **Closure of fistula of thoracic duct**

      DEF: Closure of fistula in main lymphatic duct of chest.

    **40.64**   **Ligation of thoracic duct**

      DEF: Tying off main lymphatic duct of chest.

    **40.69**   **Other operations on thoracic duct**

   **40.9**    **Other operations on lymphatic structures**

      Anastomosis
      Dilation
      Ligation
      Obliteration   }   of peripheral lymphatics
      Reconstruction
      Repair
      Transplantation

      Correction of lymphedema of limb, NOS

      EXCLUDES   *reduction of elephantiasis of scrotum (61.3)*

√3rd **41**   **Operations on bone marrow and spleen**

√4th **41.0**    **Bone marrow or hematopoietic stem cell transplant**

      Note: To report donor source — see codes 00.91-00.93

      EXCLUDES   *aspiration of bone marrow from donor (41.91)*

   AHA: 4Q, '00, 64; 1Q, '91, 3; 4Q, '91, 26

    **41.00**   **Bone marrow transplant, not otherwise specified**

 8    **41.01**   **Autologous bone marrow transplant without purging**   NC

      EXCLUDES   *that with purging (41.09)*

      DEF: Transplant of patient's own bone marrow.

 9    **41.02**   **Allogeneic bone marrow transplant with purging**   NC

      Allograft of bone marrow with in vitro removal (purging) of T-cells

      DEF: Transplant of bone marrow from donor to patient after donor marrow purged of undesirable cells.

 9    **41.03**   **Allogeneic bone marrow transplant without purging**   NC

      Allograft of bone marrow NOS

 8    **41.04**   **Autologous hematopoietic stem cell transplant without purging**   NC

      EXCLUDES   *that with purging (41.07)*

      AHA: 4Q, '94, 52

 9    **41.05**   **Allogeneic hematopoietic stem cell transplant without purging**   NC

      EXCLUDES   *that with purging (41.08)*

      AHA: 4Q, '97, 55

---

8   Non-covered procedure only when the following diagnoses are present as either principal or secondary diagnosis: 204.00, 205.00, 205.10, 205.11, 206.00, 207.00, 208.00

9   Non-covered procedure only when the following diagnoses are present as either principal or secondary diagnosis: 203.00, 203.01

---

√3rd/√4th Additional Digit Required     Valid OR Procedure     Non-OR Procedure     Adjunct Code

*Operations on the Hemic and Lymphatic Systems*

**41.06–41.99**

**Partial Splenectomy**

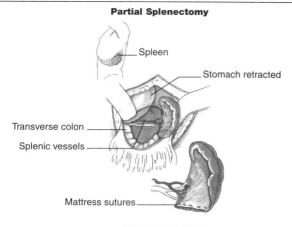

Spleen

Stomach retracted

Transverse colon

Splenic vessels

Mattress sutures

**Total Splenectomy**

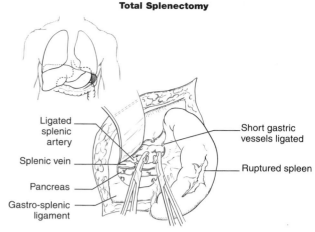

Ligated splenic artery

Splenic vein

Pancreas

Gastro-splenic ligament

Short gastric vessels ligated

Ruptured spleen

**41.06    Cord blood stem cell transplant**
AHA: 4Q, '97, 56

8  **41.07    Autologous hematopoietic stem cell transplant with purging**    [NC]
Cell depletion
AHA: ▶2Q, '06, 20-22◀

9  **41.08    Allogeneic hematopoietic stem cell transplant with purging**    [NC]
Cell depletion

9  **41.09    Autologous bone marrow transplant with purging**    [NC]
With extracorporeal purging of malignant cells from marrow
Cell depletion

**41.1    Puncture of spleen**
EXCLUDES    *aspiration biopsy of spleen (41.32)*

**41.2    Splenotomy**

✓4th  **41.3    Diagnostic procedures on bone marrow and spleen**

**41.31    Biopsy of bone marrow**

**41.32    Closed [aspiration] [percutaneous] biopsy of spleen**
Needle biopsy of spleen

**41.33    Open biopsy of spleen**

**41.38    Other diagnostic procedures on bone marrow**
EXCLUDES    *microscopic examination of specimen from bone marrow (90.61-90.69)*
*radioisotope scan (92.05)*

**41.39    Other diagnostic procedures on spleen**
EXCLUDES    *microscopic examination of specimen from spleen (90.61-90.69)*
*radioisotope scan (92.05)*

✓4th  **41.4    Excision or destruction of lesion or tissue of spleen**
Code also any application or administration of an adhesion barrier substance (99.77)
EXCLUDES    *excision of accessory spleen (41.93)*

**41.41    Marsupialization of splenic cyst**
DEF: Incision of cyst of spleen with edges sutured open to create pouch.

**41.42    Excision of lesion or tissue of spleen**
EXCLUDES    *biopsy of spleen (41.32-41.33)*

**41.43    Partial splenectomy**
DEF: Removal of spleen, partial.

**41.5    Total splenectomy**
Splenectomy NOS
Code also any application or administration of an adhesion barrier substance (99.77)

✓4th  **41.9    Other operations on spleen and bone marrow**
Code also any application or administration of an adhesion barrier substance (99.77)

**41.91    Aspiration of bone marrow from donor for transplant**
EXCLUDES    *biopsy of bone marrow (41.31)*
AHA: 1Q, '91, 3

**41.92    Injection into bone marrow**
EXCLUDES    *bone marrow transplant (41.00-41.03)*
AHA: 3Q, '96, 17

**41.93    Excision of accessory spleen**
**41.94    Transplantation of spleen**
**41.95    Repair and plastic operations on spleen**
**41.98    Other operations on bone marrow**
**41.99    Other operations on spleen**

8  Non-covered procedure only when the following diagnoses are present as either principal or secondary diagnosis: 204.00, 205.00, 205.10, 205.11, 206.00, 207.00, 208.00
9  Non-covered procedure only when the following diagnoses are present as either principal or secondary diagnosis: 203.00, 203.01

[BI] Bilateral Procedure        [NC] Non-covered Procedure        [LC] Limited Coverage Procedure        ▶◀ Revised Text        ● New Code        ▲ Revised Code Title

# 9. OPERATIONS ON THE DIGESTIVE SYSTEM (42-54)

√3rd **42**　**Operations on esophagus**

√4th **42.0**　**Esophagotomy**

**42.01**　**Incision of esophageal web**

　DEF: Cutting into congenital esophageal membrane.

**42.09**　**Other incision of esophagus**

　Esophagotomy NOS

　**EXCLUDES**　*esophagomyotomy (42.7)*
　　　　　　*esophagostomy (42.10-42.19)*

√4th **42.1**　**Esophagostomy**

**42.10**　**Esophagostomy, not otherwise specified**

**42.11**　**Cervical esophagostomy**

　DEF: Creation of opening into upper region of esophagus.

**42.12**　**Exteriorization of esophageal pouch**

　DEF: Transfer of section of esophageal pouch to exterior of the body.

**42.19**　**Other external fistulization of esophagus**

　Thoracic esophagostomy

　Code also any resection (42.40-42.42)

√4th **42.2**　**Diagnostic procedures on esophagus**

**42.21**　**Operative esophagoscopy by incision**

　DEF: Esophageal examination with an endoscope through incision.

**42.22**　**Esophagoscopy through artificial stoma**

　**EXCLUDES**　*that with biopsy (42.24)*

**42.23**　**Other esophagoscopy**

　**EXCLUDES**　*that with biopsy (42.24)*

　AHA: 1Q, '00, 20; 3Q, '98, 11

**42.24**　**Closed [endoscopic] biopsy of esophagus**

　Brushing or washing for specimen collection

　Esophagoscopy with biopsy

　Suction biopsy of the esophagus

　**EXCLUDES**　*esophagogastroduodenoscopy [EGD] with closed biopsy (45.16)*

　DEF: Scope passed through mouth and throat to obtain biopsy specimen, usually by brushing and swabbing.

**42.25**　**Open biopsy of esophagus**

**42.29**　**Other diagnostic procedures on esophagus**

　**EXCLUDES**　*barium swallow (87.61)*
　　　　　　*esophageal manometry (89.32)*
　　　　　　*microscopic examination of specimen from esophagus (90.81-90.89)*

　AHA: 3Q, '96, 12

√4th **42.3**　**Local excision or destruction of lesion or tissue of esophagus**

**42.31**　**Local excision of esophageal diverticulum**

**42.32**　**Local excision of other lesion or tissue of esophagus**

　**EXCLUDES**　*biopsy of esophagus (42.24-42.25)*
　　　　　　*esophageal fistulectomy (42.84)*

**42.33**　**Endoscopic excision or destruction of lesion or tissue of esophagus**

　Ablation of esophageal neoplasm

　Control of esophageal bleeding

　Esophageal polypectomy ⎤

　Esophageal varices ⎟ by endoscopic approach

　Injection of esophageal varices ⎦

　**EXCLUDES**　*biopsy of esophagus (42.24-42.25)*
　　　　　　*fistulectomy (42.84)*
　　　　　　*open ligation of esophageal varices (42.91)*

**42.39**　**Other destruction of lesion or tissue of esophagus**

　**EXCLUDES**　*that by endoscopic approach (42.33)*

√4th **42.4**　**Excision of esophagus**

　**EXCLUDES**　*esophagogastrectomy NOS (43.99)*

**42.40**　**Esophagectomy, not otherwise specified**

**42.41**　**Partial esophagectomy**

　Code also any synchronous:

　　anastomosis other than end-to-end (42.51-42.69)

　　esophagostomy (42.10-42.19)

　　gastrostomy (43.11-43.19)

　DEF: Surgical removal of any part of esophagus.

**42.42**　**Total esophagectomy**

　Code also any synchronous:

　　gastrostomy (43.11-43.19)

　　interposition or anastomosis other than end-to-end (42.51-42.69)

　**EXCLUDES**　*esophagogastrectomy (43.99)*

　AHA: 4Q, '88, 11

　DEF: Surgical removal of entire esophagus.

√4th **42.5**　**Intrathoracic anastomosis of esophagus**

　Code also any synchronous:

　　esophagectomy (42.40-42.42)

　　gastrostomy (43.1)

　DEF: Connection of esophagus to conduit within chest.

**42.51**　**Intrathoracic esophagoesophagostomy**

　DEF: Connection of both ends of esophagus within chest cavity.

**42.52**　**Intrathoracic esophagogastrostomy**

　DEF: Connection of esophagus to stomach within chest; follows esophagogastrectomy.

**42.53**　**Intrathoracic esophageal anastomosis with interposition of small bowel**

**42.54**　**Other intrathoracic esophagoenterostomy**

　Anastomosis of esophagus to intestinal segment NOS

**42.55**　**Intrathoracic esophageal anastomosis with interposition of colon**

**42.56**　**Other intrathoracic esophagocolostomy**

　Esophagocolostomy NOS

**42.58**　**Intrathoracic esophageal anastomosis with other interposition**

　Construction of artificial esophagus

　Retrosternal formation of reversed gastric tube

　DEF: Construction of artificial esophagus: Creation of artificial esophagus.

　DEF: Retrosternal anastomosis of reversed gastric tube: Formation of gastric tube behind breastbone.

**Operations on the Digestive System**

**42.59–43.5**

**42.59** **Other intrathoracic anastomosis of esophagus**
AHA: 4Q, '88, 11

✓4ᵗʰ **42.6** **Antesternal anastomosis of esophagus**
Code also any synchronous:
esophagectomy (42.40-42.42)
gastrostomy (43.1)

**42.61** **Antesternal esophagoesophagostomy**
**42.62** **Antesternal esophagogastrostomy**
**42.63** **Antesternal esophageal anastomosis with interposition of small bowel**
**42.64** **Other antesternal esophagoenterostomy**
Antethoracic:
esophagoenterostomy
esophagoileostomy
esophagojejunostomy
**42.65** **Antesternal esophageal anastomosis with interposition of colon**
DEF: Connection of esophagus with colon segment.
**42.66** **Other antesternal esophagocolostomy**
Antethoracic esophagocolostomy
**42.68** **Other antesternal esophageal anastomosis with interposition**
**42.69** **Other antesternal anastomosis of esophagus**

**42.7** **Esophagomyotomy**
DEF: Division of esophageal muscle, usually distal.

✓4ᵗʰ **42.8** **Other repair of esophagus**
**42.81** **Insertion of permanent tube into esophagus**
AHA: 1Q, '97, 15
**42.82** **Suture of laceration of esophagus**
**42.83** **Closure of esophagostomy**
**42.84** **Repair of esophageal fistula, not elsewhere classified**
EXCLUDES repair of fistula:
bronchoesophageal (33.42)
esophagopleurocutaneous (34.73)
pharyngoesophageal (29.53)
tracheoesophageal (31.73)
**42.85** **Repair of esophageal stricture**
**42.86** **Production of subcutaneous tunnel without esophageal anastomosis**
DEF: Surgical formation of esophageal passage, without cutting, and reconnection.
**42.87** **Other graft of esophagus**
EXCLUDES antesternal esophageal anastomosis with interposition of:
colon (42.65)
small bowel (42.63)
antesternal esophageal anastomosis with other interposition (42.68)
intrathoracic esophageal anastomosis with interposition of:
colon (42.55)
small bowel (42.53)
intrathoracic esophageal anastomosis with other interposition (42.58)
**42.89** **Other repair of esophagus**

✓4ᵗʰ **42.9** **Other operations on esophagus**
**42.91** **Ligation of esophageal varices**
EXCLUDES that by endoscopic approach (42.33)
DEF: Destruction of dilated veins by suture strangulation.

**42.92** **Dilation of esophagus**
Dilation of cardiac sphincter
EXCLUDES intubation of esophagus (96.03, 96.06-96.08)
DEF: Passing of balloon or hydrostatic dilators through esophagus to enlarge esophagus and relieve obstruction.

**42.99** **Other**
EXCLUDES insertion of Sengstaken tube (96.06)
intubation of esophagus (96.03, 96.06-96.08)
removal of intraluminal foreign body from esophagus without incision (98.02)
tamponade of esophagus (96.06)

✓3ʳᵈ **43** **Incision and excision of stomach**
Code also any application or administration of an adhesion barrier substance (99.77)

**43.0** **Gastrotomy**
EXCLUDES gastrostomy (43.11-43.19)
that for control of hemorrhage (44.49)
AHA: 3Q, '89, 14

✓4ᵗʰ **43.1** **Gastrostomy**
AHA: S-O, '85, 5
**43.11** **Percutaneous [endoscopic] gastrostomy [PEG]**
Percutaneous transabdominal gastrostomy
DEF: Endoscopic positioning of tube through abdominal wall into stomach.
**43.19** **Other gastrostomy**
EXCLUDES percutaneous [endoscopic] gastrostomy [PEG] (43.11)
AHA: 1Q, '92, 14; 3Q, '89, 14

**43.3** **Pyloromyotomy**
DEF: Cutting into longitudinal and circular muscular membrane between stomach and small intestine.

✓4ᵗʰ **43.4** **Local excision or destruction of lesion or tissue of stomach**
**43.41** **Endoscopic excision or destruction of lesion or tissue of stomach**
Gastric polypectomy by endoscopic approach
Gastric varices by endoscopic approach
EXCLUDES biopsy of stomach (44.14-44.15)
control of hemorrhage (44.43)
open ligation of gastric varices (44.91)
AHA: 3Q, '96, 10
**43.42** **Local excision of other lesion or tissue of stomach**
EXCLUDES biopsy of stomach (44.14-44.15)
gastric fistulectomy (44.62-44.63)
partial gastrectomy (43.5-43.89)
**43.49** **Other destruction of lesion or tissue of stomach**
EXCLUDES that by endoscopic approach (43.41)
AHA: N-D, '87, 5; S-O, '85, 6

**43.5** **Partial gastrectomy with anastomosis to esophagus**
Proximal gastrectomy

**BI** Bilateral Procedure    **NC** Non-covered Procedure    **LC** Limited Coverage Procedure    ▶◀ Revised Text    ● New Code    ▲ Revised Code Title

**122 — Volume 3**

© 2007 Ingenix

**Biliopancreatic Diversion Without Duodenal Switch**

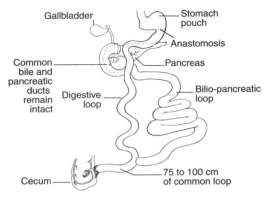

**43.6**    **Partial gastrectomy with anastomosis to duodenum**
Billroth I operation    Gastropylorectomy
Distal gastrectomy

**43.7**    **Partial gastrectomy with anastomosis to jejunum**
Billroth II operation
**AHA:** 3Q, '03, 7

✓4ᵗʰ **43.8**    **Other partial gastrectomy**
   **43.81**   **Partial gastrectomy with jejunal transposition**
     Henley jejunal transposition operation
     Code also any synchronous intestinal resection (45.51)
   **43.89**   **Other**
     Partial gastrectomy with bypass gastrogastrostomy
     Sleeve resection of stomach
   **AHA:** 3Q, '03, 6-8

✓4ᵗʰ **43.9**    **Total gastrectomy**
   **43.91**   **Total gastrectomy with intestinal interposition**
   **43.99**   **Other total gastrectomy**
     Complete gastroduodenectomy
     Esophagoduodenostomy with complete gastrectomy
     Esophagogastrectomy NOS
     Esophagojejunostomy with complete gastrectomy
     Radical gastrectomy

✓3ʳᵈ **44**   **Other operations on stomach**
   Code also any application or administration of an adhesion barrier substance (99.77)

✓4ᵗʰ **44.0**    **Vagotomy**
   **44.00**   **Vagotomy, not otherwise specified**
     Division of vagus nerve NOS
     **DEF:** Cutting of vagus nerve to reduce acid production.
   **44.01**   **Truncal vagotomy**
     **DEF:** Surgical removal of vagus nerve segment near stomach branches.

**Biliopancreatic Diversion with Duodenal Switch**

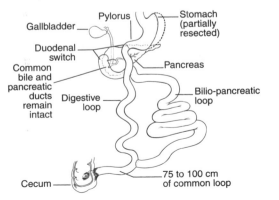

**Partial Gastrectomy with Anastomosis to Duodenum**

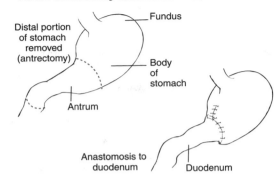

   **44.02**   **Highly selective vagotomy**
     Parietal cell vagotomy
     Selective proximal vagotomy
     **DEF:** Cutting select gastric branches of vagus nerve to reduce acid production and preserve other nerve functions.
   **44.03**   **Other selective vagotomy**

✓4ᵗʰ **44.1**    **Diagnostic procedures on stomach**
   **44.11**   **Transabdominal gastroscopy**
     Intraoperative gastroscopy
     **EXCLUDES**   *that with biopsy (44.14)*
   **44.12**   **Gastroscopy through artificial stoma**
     **EXCLUDES**   *that with biopsy (44.14)*
   **44.13**   **Other gastroscopy**
     **EXCLUDES**   *that with biopsy (44.14)*
   **AHA:** 1Q, '88, 15; N-D, '87, 5
   **44.14**   **Closed [endoscopic] biopsy of stomach**
     Brushing or washing for specimen collection
     **EXCLUDES**   *esophagogastroduodenoscopy [EGD] with closed biopsy (45.16)*
   **AHA:** 1Q, '88, 15; N-D, '87, 5
   **44.15**   **Open biopsy of stomach**
   **44.19**   **Other diagnostic procedures on stomach**
     **EXCLUDES**   *gastric lavage (96.33)*
      *microscopic examination of specimen from stomach (90.81-90.89)*
      *upper GI series (87.62)*

✓4ᵗʰ **44.2**    **Pyloroplasty**
   **44.21**   **Dilation of pylorus by incision**
     **DEF:** Cutting and suturing pylorus to relieve obstruction.
   **44.22**   **Endoscopic dilation of pylorus**
     Dilation with balloon endoscope
     Endoscopic dilation of gastrojejunostomy site
   **AHA:** 2Q, '01, 17

**Types of Vagotomy Procedures**

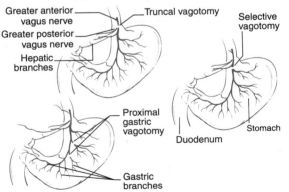

**Operations on the Digestive System**

**44.29–44.69**

**44.29**   **Other pyloroplasty**
Pyloroplasty NOS
Revision of pylorus
**AHA:** 3Q, '99, 3

✓4th **44.3**   **Gastroenterostomy without gastrectomy**

**44.31**   **High gastric bypass**
Printen and Mason gastric bypass
**AHA:** M-J, '85, 17

DEF: Connection of middle part of small intestine to upper stomach to divert food passage from upper intestine.

**44.32**   **Percutaneous [endoscopic] gastrojejunostomy**
Endoscopic conversion of gastrostomy to jejunostomy

DEF: Percutaneous placement of a thin feeding tube through a gastrostomy tube and then pulling the tube into the proximal end of the jejunum.

**44.38**   **Laparoscopic gastroenterostomy**
Bypass:
gastroduodenostomy
gastroenterostomy
gastrogastrostomy
Laparoscopic gastrojejunostomy without gastrectomy NEC
**EXCLUDES**   *gastroenterostomy, open approach (44.39)*

**44.39**   **Other gastroenterostomy**
Bypass:
gastroduodenostomy
gastroenterostomy
gastrogastrostomy
Gastrojejunostomy without gastrectomy NOS
**AHA:** 3Q, '03, 6; 1Q, '01, 16, 17

✓4th **44.4**   **Control of hemorrhage and suture of ulcer of stomach or duodenum**

**44.40**   **Suture of peptic ulcer, not otherwise specified**

**44.41**   **Suture of gastric ulcer site**
**EXCLUDES**   *ligation of gastric varices (44.91)*

**44.42**   **Suture of duodenal ulcer site**
**AHA:** J-F, '87, 11

**44.43**   **Endoscopic control of gastric or duodenal bleeding**
**AHA:** 2Q, '04, 12; 2Q, '92, 17; N-D, '87, 4

**44.44**   **Transcatheter embolization for gastric or duodenal bleeding**
**EXCLUDES**   *surgical occlusion of abdominal vessels (38.86-38.87)*
**AHA:** 1Q, '88, 15; N-D, '87, 4

DEF: Therapeutic blocking of stomach or upper small intestine blood vessel to stop hemorrhaging; accomplished by introducing various substances using a catheter.

**44.49**   **Other control of hemorrhage of stomach or duodenum**
That with gastrotomy

**44.5**   **Revision of gastric anastomosis**
Closure of:
gastric anastomosis
gastroduodenostomy
gastrojejunostomy
Pantaloon operation

✓4th **44.6**   **Other repair of stomach**

**44.61**   **Suture of laceration of stomach**
**EXCLUDES**   *that of ulcer site (44.41)*

**44.62**   **Closure of gastrostomy**

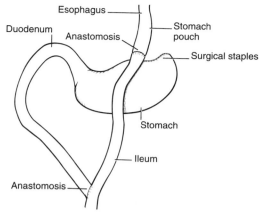

**Roux-en-Y Operation (Gastrojejunostomy without gastrectomy)**

Esophagus — 
Duodenum — 
Anastomosis — 
Stomach pouch — 
Surgical staples — 
Stomach — 
Ileum — 
Anastomosis — 

**44.63**   **Closure of other gastric fistula**
Closure of:
gastrocolic fistula
gastrojejunocolic fistula

**44.64**   **Gastropexy**
**AHA:** M-J, '85, 17

DEF: Suturing of stomach into position.

**44.65**   **Esophagogastroplasty**
Belsey operation
Esophagus and stomach cardioplasty
**AHA:** M-J, '85, 17

**44.66**   **Other procedures for creation of esophagogastric sphincteric competence**
Fundoplication
Gastric cardioplasty
Nissen's fundoplication
Restoration of cardio-esophageal angle
**EXCLUDES**   *that by laparoscopy (44.67)*
**AHA:** 2Q, '03, 12; 2Q, '01, 3, 5, 6; 3Q, '98, 10; M-J, '85, 17

**44.67**   **Laparoscopic procedures for creation of esophagogastric sphincteric competence**
Fundoplication
Gastric cardioplasty
Nissen's fundoplication
Restoration of cardio-esophageal angle

**44.68**   **Laparoscopic gastroplasty**
Banding
Silastic vertical banding
Vertical banded gastroplasty (VBG)
Code also any synchronous laparoscopic gastroenterostomy (44.38)
**EXCLUDES**   *insertion, laparoscopic adjustable gastric band (restrictive procedure) (44.95)*
*other repair of stomach, open approach (44.61-44.65, 44.69)*

**44.69**   **Other**
Inversion of gastric diverticulum
Repair of stomach NOS
**AHA:** 3Q, '03, 8; 2Q, '01, 3; 3Q, '99, 3; M-J, '85, 17; N-D, '84, 13

DEF: Inversion of gastric diverticulum: Turning stomach inward to repair outpouch of wall.

---

**BI** Bilateral Procedure     **NC** Non-covered Procedure     **LC** Limited Coverage Procedure     ▶◀ Revised Text     ● New Code     ▲ Revised Code Title

**✓4ᵗʰ 44.9    Other operations on stomach**

**44.91   Ligation of gastric varices**

> **EXCLUDES**   *that by endoscopic approach (43.41)*

> DEF: Destruction of dilated veins by suture or strangulation.

**44.92   Intraoperative manipulation of stomach**
> Reduction of gastric volvulus

**44.93   Insertion of gastric bubble (balloon)**   NC
**44.94   Removal of gastric bubble (balloon)**
**44.95   Laparoscopic gastric restrictive procedure**
> Adjustable gastric band and port insertion

> **EXCLUDES**   *laparoscopic gastroplasty (44.68)*
>            *other repair of stomach (44.69)*

**44.96   Laparoscopic revision of gastric restrictive procedure**
> Revision or replacement of:
>    adjustable gastric band
>    subcutaneous gastric port device

**44.97   Laparoscopic removal of gastric restrictive device(s)**
> Removal of either or both:
>    adjustable gastric band
>    subcutaneous port device

> **EXCLUDES**   *nonoperative removal of gastric restrictive device(s) (97.86)*
>            *open removal of gastric restrictive device(s) (44.99)*

**44.98   (Laparoscopic) adjustment of size of adjustable gastric restrictive device**
> Infusion of saline for device tightening
> Withdrawal of saline for device loosening
> Code also any:
>    abdominal ultrasound (88.76)
>    abdominal wall fluoroscopy (88.09)
>    barium swallow (87.61)

**44.99   Other**

> **EXCLUDES**   *change of gastrostomy tube (97.02)*
>            *dilation of cardiac sphincter (42.92)*
>            *gastric:*
>              *cooling (96.31)*
>              *freezing (96.32)*
>              *gavage (96.35)*
>              *hypothermia (96.31)*
>              *lavage (96.33)*
>            *insertion of nasogastric tube (96.07)*
>            *irrigation of gastrostomy (96.36)*
>            *irrigation of nasogastric tube (96.34)*
>            *removal of:*
>              *gastrostomy tube (97.51)*
>              *intraluminal foreign body from stomach without incision (98.03)*
>            *replacement of:*
>              *gastrostomy tube (97.02)*
>              *(naso-)gastric tube (97.01)*

> AHA: 3Q, '04, 5

**✓3ʳᵈ 45   Incision, excision, and anastomosis of intestine**
> Code also any application or administration of an adhesion barrier substance (99.77)

**✓4ᵗʰ 45.0    Enterotomy**

> **EXCLUDES**   *duodenocholedochotomy (51.41-51.42, 51.51)*
>            *that for destruction of lesion (45.30-45.34)*
>            *that of exteriorized intestine (46.14, 46.24, 46.31)*

**45.00   Incision of intestine not otherwise specified**
**45.01   Incision of duodenum**
**45.02   Other incision of small intestine**
**45.03   Incision of large intestine**

> **EXCLUDES**   *proctotomy (48.0)*

**✓4ᵗʰ 45.1   Diagnostic procedures on small intestine**
> Code also any laparotomy (54.11-54.19)

**45.11   Transabdominal endoscopy of small intestine**
> Intraoperative endoscopy of small intestine

> **EXCLUDES**   *that with biopsy (45.14)*

> DEF: Endoscopic exam of small intestine through abdominal wall.

> DEF: Intraoperative endoscope of small intestine: Endoscopic exam of small intestine during surgery.

**45.12   Endoscopy of small intestine through artificial stoma**

> **EXCLUDES**   *that with biopsy (45.14)*

> AHA: M-J, '85, 17

**45.13   Other endoscopy of small intestine**
> Esophagogastroduodenoscopy [EGD]

> **EXCLUDES**   *that with biopsy (45.14, 45.16)*

> AHA: 3Q, '04, 5; N-D, '87, 5

**45.14   Closed [endoscopic] biopsy of small intestine**
> Brushing or washing for specimen collection

> **EXCLUDES**   *esophagogastroduodenoscopy [EGD] with closed biopsy (45.16)*

**45.15   Open biopsy of small intestine**

> AHA: 2Q, '05, 12

**45.16   Esophagogastroduodenoscopy [EGD] with closed biopsy**
> Biopsy of one or more sites involving esophagus, stomach, and/or duodenum

> AHA: 3Q, '05, 17; 2Q, '01, 9

**45.19   Other diagnostic procedures on small intestine**

> **EXCLUDES**   *microscopic examination of specimen from small intestine (90.91-90.99)*
>            *radioisotope scan (92.04)*
>            *ultrasonography (88.74)*
>            *x-ray (87.61-87.69)*

**✓4ᵗʰ 45.2   Diagnostic procedures on large intestine**
> Code also any laparotomy (54.11-54.19)

**45.21   Transabdominal endoscopy of large intestine**
> Intraoperative endoscopy of large intestine

> **EXCLUDES**   *that with biopsy (45.25)*

> DEF: Endoscopic exam of large intestine through abdominal wall.

> DEF: Intraoperative endoscopy of large intestine: Endoscopic exam of large intestine during surgery.

**Esophagogastroduodenoscopy**

Esophagus
Duodenum
Stomach

**Operations on the Digestive System**

**45.22–45.52**

**45.22 Endoscopy of large intestine through artificial stoma**

EXCLUDES that with biopsy (45.25)

DEF: Endoscopic exam of large intestine lining from rectum to cecum via colostomy stoma.

**45.23 Colonoscopy**

Flexible fiberoptic colonoscopy

EXCLUDES endoscopy of large intestine through artificial stoma (45.22)
flexible sigmoidoscopy (45.24)
rigid proctosigmoidoscopy (48.23)
transabdominal endoscopy of large intestine (45.21)

AHA: 3Q, '05, 17; S-O, '85, 5

DEF: Endoscopic exam of descending colon, splenic flexure, transverse colon, hepatic flexure and cecum.

**45.24 Flexible sigmoidoscopy**

Endoscopy of descending colon

EXCLUDES rigid proctosigmoidoscopy (48.23)

DEF: Endoscopic exam of anus, rectum and sigmoid colon.

**45.25 Closed [endoscopic] biopsy of large intestine**

Biopsy, closed, of unspecified intestinal site
Brushing or washing for specimen collection
Colonoscopy with biopsy

EXCLUDES proctosigmoidoscopy with biopsy (48.24)

AHA: 1Q, '03, 10

**45.26 Open biopsy of large intestine**
**45.27 Intestinal biopsy, site unspecified**
**45.28 Other diagnostic procedures on large intestine**
**45.29 Other diagnostic procedures on intestine, site unspecified**

EXCLUDES microscopic examination of specimen (90.91-90.99)
scan and radioisotope function study (92.04)
ultrasonography (88.74)
x-ray (87.61-87.69)

√4ᵗʰ **45.3 Local excision or destruction of lesion or tissue of small intestine**

**45.30 Endoscopic excision or destruction of lesion of duodenum**

EXCLUDES biopsy of duodenum (45.14-45.15)
control of hemorrhage (44.43)
fistulectomy (46.72)

**45.31 Other local excision of lesion of duodenum**

EXCLUDES biopsy of duodenum (45.14-45.15)
fistulectomy (46.72)
multiple segmental resection (45.61)
that by endoscopic approach (45.30)

**45.32 Other destruction of lesion of duodenum**

EXCLUDES that by endoscopic approach (45.30)

AHA: N-D, '87, 5; S-O, '85, 6

**45.33 Local excision of lesion or tissue of small intestine, except duodenum**

Excision of redundant mucosa of ileostomy

EXCLUDES biopsy of small intestine (45.14-45.15)
fistulectomy (46.74)
multiple segmental resection (45.61)

**45.34 Other destruction of lesion of small intestine, except duodenum**

√4ᵗʰ **45.4 Local excision or destruction of lesion or tissue of large intestine**

AHA: N-D, '87, 11

**45.41 Excision of lesion or tissue of large intestine**

Excision of redundant mucosa of colostomy

EXCLUDES biopsy of large intestine (45.25-45.27)
endoscopic polypectomy of large intestine (45.42)
fistulectomy (46.76)
multiple segmental resection (45.71)
that by endoscopic approach (45.42-45.43)

**45.42 Endoscopic polypectomy of large intestine**

EXCLUDES that by open approach (45.41)

AHA: 2Q, '05, 16; 2Q, '90, 25

DEF: Endoscopic removal of polyp from large intestine.

**45.43 Endoscopic destruction of other lesion or tissue of large intestine**

Endoscopic ablation of tumor of large intestine
Endoscopic control of colonic bleeding

EXCLUDES endoscopic polypectomy of large intestine (45.42)

AHA: 4Q, '02, 61

**45.49 Other destruction of lesion of large intestine**

EXCLUDES that by endoscopic approach (45.43)

√4ᵗʰ **45.5 Isolation of intestinal segment**

Code also any synchronous:
anastomosis other than end-to-end (45.90-45.94)
enterostomy (46.10-46.39)

**45.50 Isolation of intestinal segment, not otherwise specified**

Isolation of intestinal pedicle flap
Reversal of intestinal segment

DEF: Isolation of small intestinal pedicle flap: Separation of intestinal pedicle flap.

DEF: Reversal of intestinal segment: Separation of intestinal segment.

**45.51 Isolation of segment of small intestine**

Isolation of ileal loop
Resection of small intestine for interposition

AHA: 2Q, '05, 12; 3Q, '03, 6-8; 2Q, '03, 11; 3Q, '00, 7

**45.52 Isolation of segment of large intestine**

Resection of colon for interposition

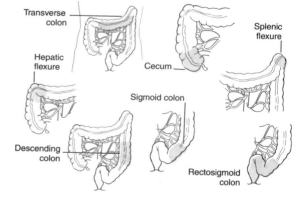

**Colectomy**

Transverse colon
Splenic flexure
Hepatic flexure
Cecum
Sigmoid colon
Descending colon
Rectosigmoid colon

BI Bilateral Procedure    NC Non-covered Procedure    LC Limited Coverage Procedure    ►◄ Revised Text    ● New Code    ▲ Revised Code Title

© 2007 Ingenix

**Operations on the Digestive System**

**45.6–46.24**

√4ᵗʰ **45.6**   **Other excision of small intestine**
Code also any synchronous:
anastomosis other than end-to-end (45.90-45.93, 45.95)
colostomy (46.10-46.13)
enterostomy (46.10-46.39)

> EXCLUDES   cecectomy (45.72)
> enterocolectomy (45.79)
> gastroduodenectomy (43.6-43.99)
> ileocolectomy (45.73)
> pancreatoduodenectomy (52.51-52.7)

**45.61**   **Multiple segmental resection of small intestine**
Segmental resection for multiple traumatic lesions of small intestine

**45.62**   **Other partial resection of small intestine**
Duodenectomy   Jejunectomy
Ileectomy

> EXCLUDES   duodenectomy with synchronous pancreatectomy (52.51-52.7)
> resection of cecum and terminal ileum (45.72)

AHA: 1Q, '04, 10; 1Q, '03, 18

**45.63**   **Total removal of small intestine**

√4ᵗʰ **45.7**   **Partial excision of large intestine**
Code also any synchronous:
anastomosis other than end-to-end (45.92-45.94)
enterostomy (46.10-46.39)

AHA: 4Q, '92, 27

**45.71**   **Multiple segmental resection of large intestine**
Segmental resection for multiple traumatic lesions of large intestine

**45.72**   **Cecectomy**
Resection of cecum and terminal ileum

**45.73**   **Right hemicolectomy**
Ileocolectomy
Right radical colectomy

AHA: 3Q, '99, 10

**45.74**   **Resection of transverse colon**

**45.75**   **Left hemicolectomy**

> EXCLUDES   proctosigmoidectomy (48.41-48.69)
> second stage Mikulicz operation (46.04)

DEF: Excision of left descending large intestine.

**45.76**   **Sigmoidectomy**
AHA: 1Q, '96, 9; 3Q, '89, 15

**45.79**   **Other partial excision of large intestine**
Enterocolectomy NEC
AHA: 1Q, '03, 18; 3Q, '97, 9; 2Q, '91, 16

**45.8**   **Total intra-abdominal colectomy**
Excision of cecum, colon, and sigmoid

> EXCLUDES   coloproctectomy (48.41-48.69)

**Intestinal Anastomosis**

Area to be excised

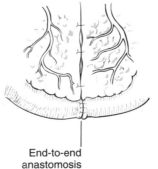

End-to-end anastomosis

√4ᵗʰ **45.9**   **Intestinal anastomosis**
Code also any synchronous resection (45.31-45.8, 48.41-48.69)

> EXCLUDES   end-to-end anastomosis — omit code

**45.90**   **Intestinal anastomosis, not otherwise specified**

**45.91**   **Small-to-small intestinal anastomosis**
AHA: 3Q, '03, 6-8; M-J, '85, 17

**45.92**   **Anastomosis of small intestine to rectal stump**
Hampton procedure

**45.93**   **Other small-to-large intestinal anastomosis**
AHA: 1Q, '03, 18; N-D, '86, 11

**45.94**   **Large-to-large intestinal anastomosis**

> EXCLUDES   rectorectostomy (48.74)

AHA: 3Q, '89, 15

**45.95**   **Anastomosis to anus**
Formation of endorectal ileal pouch (J-pouch) (H-pouch) (S-pouch) with anastomosis of small intestine to anus
AHA: 2Q, '05, 13

√3ʳᵈ **46**   **Other operations on intestine**
Code also any application or administration of an adhesion barrier substance (99.77)

√4ᵗʰ **46.0**   **Exteriorization of intestine**

> INCLUDES   loop enterostomy
> multiple stage resection of intestine

DEF: Bringing intestinal segment to body surface.

**46.01**   **Exteriorization of small intestine**
Loop ileostomy

**46.02**   **Resection of exteriorized segment of small intestine**

**46.03**   **Exteriorization of large intestine**
Exteriorization of intestine NOS
First stage Mikulicz exteriorization of intestine
Loop colostomy

**46.04**   **Resection of exteriorized segment of large intestine**
Resection of exteriorized segment of intestine NOS
Second stage Mikulicz operation

√4ᵗʰ **46.1**   **Colostomy**
Code also any synchronous resection (45.49, 45.71-45.79, 45.8)

> EXCLUDES   loop colostomy (46.03)
> that with abdominoperineal resection of rectum (48.5)
> that with synchronous anterior rectal resection (48.62)

DEF: Creation of opening from large intestine through abdominal wall to body surface.

**46.10**   **Colostomy, not otherwise specified**

**46.11**   **Temporary colostomy**

**46.13**   **Permanent colostomy**

**46.14**   **Delayed opening of colostomy**

√4ᵗʰ **46.2**   **Ileostomy**
Code also any synchronous resection (45.34, 45.61-45.63)

> EXCLUDES   loop ileostomy (46.01)

DEF: Creation of artificial anus by bringing ileum through abdominal wall to body surface.

**46.20**   **Ileostomy, not otherwise specified**

**46.21**   **Temporary ileostomy**

**46.22**   **Continent ileostomy**
AHA: M-J, '85, 17

DEF: Creation of opening from third part of small intestine through abdominal wall, with pouch outside abdomen.

**46.23**   **Other permanent ileostomy**

**46.24**   **Delayed opening of ileostomy**

---

√3ʳᵈ √4ᵗʰ Additional Digit Required      Valid OR Procedure      Non-OR Procedure      Adjunct Code

**Operations on the Digestive System**

**46.3–46.97**

☑4ᵗʰ **46.3 Other enterostomy**
Code also any synchronous resection (45.61-45.8)

**46.31 Delayed opening of other enterostomy**

**46.32 Percutaneous (endoscopic) jejunostomy [PEJ]**

DEF: Endoscopic placement of tube in midsection of small intestine through abdominal wall.

**46.39 Other**
Duodenostomy    Feeding enterostomy

AHA: 3Q, '89, 15

☑4ᵗʰ **46.4 Revision of intestinal stoma**
DEF: Revision of opening surgically created from intestine through abdominal wall, to skin surface.

**46.40 Revision of intestinal stoma, not otherwise specified**
Plastic enlargement of intestinal stoma
Reconstruction of stoma of intestine
Release of scar tissue of intestinal stoma
**EXCLUDES** excision of redundant mucosa (45.41)

**46.41 Revision of stoma of small intestine**
**EXCLUDES** excision of redundant mucosa (45.33)

AHA: 2Q, '05, 11

**46.42 Repair of pericolostomy hernia**

**46.43 Other revision of stoma of large intestine**
**EXCLUDES** excision of redundant mucosa (45.41)

AHA: 2Q, '02, 9

☑4ᵗʰ **46.5 Closure of intestinal stoma**
Code also any synchronous resection (45.34, 45.49, 45.61-45.8)

**46.50 Closure of intestinal stoma, not otherwise specified**

**46.51 Closure of stoma of small intestine**

**46.52 Closure of stoma of large intestine**
Closure or take-down of cecostomy
Closure or take-down of colostomy
Closure or take-down of sigmoidostomy
AHA: 2Q, '05, 4; 3Q, '97, 9; 2Q, '91, 16; N-D, '87, 8

☑4ᵗʰ **46.6 Fixation of intestine**

**46.60 Fixation of intestine not otherwise specified**
Fixation of intestine to abdominal wall

**46.61 Fixation of small intestine to abdominal wall**
Ileopexy

**46.62 Other fixation of small intestine**
Noble plication of small intestine
Plication of jejunum

DEF: Noble plication of small intestine: Fixing small intestine into place with tuck in small intestine.
DEF: Plication of jejunum: Fixing small intestine into place with tuck in midsection.

**46.63 Fixation of large intestine to abdominal wall**
Cecocoloplicopexy
Sigmoidopexy    (Moschowitz)

**46.64 Other fixation of large intestine**
Cecofixation    Colofixation

☑4ᵗʰ **46.7 Other repair of intestine**
**EXCLUDES** closure of:
    ulcer of duodenum (44.42)
    vesicoenteric fistula (57.83)

**46.71 Suture of laceration of duodenum**

**46.72 Closure of fistula of duodenum**

**46.73 Suture of laceration of small intestine, except duodenum**

**46.74 Closure of fistula of small intestine, except duodenum**
**EXCLUDES** closure of:
    artificial stoma (46.51)
    vaginal fistula (70.74)
    repair of gastrojejunocolic fistula (44.63)

**46.75 Suture of laceration of large intestine**

**46.76 Closure of fistula of large intestine**
**EXCLUDES** closure of:
    gastrocolic fistula (44.63)
    rectal fistula (48.73)
    sigmoidovesical fistula (57.83)
    stoma (46.52)
    vaginal fistula (70.72-70.73)
    vesicocolic fistula (57.83)
    vesicosigmoidovaginal fistula (57.83)

AHA: 3Q, '99, 8

**46.79 Other repair of intestine**
Duodenoplasty
AHA: 3Q, '02, 11

☑4ᵗʰ **46.8 Dilation and manipulation of intestine**
AHA: 1Q, '03, 14

**46.80 Intra-abdominal manipulation of intestine, not otherwise specified**
Correction of intestinal malrotation
Reduction of:
    intestinal torsion
    intestinal volvulus
    intussusception
**EXCLUDES** reduction of intussusception with:
    fluoroscopy (96.29)
    ionizing radiation enema (96.29)
    ultrasonography guidance (96.29)

AHA: 4Q, '98, 82

DEF: Correction of intestinal malrotation: Repair of abnormal rotation.
DEF: Reduction of:
    Intestinal torsion: Repair of twisted segment.
    Intestinal volvulus: Repair of a knotted segment.
    Intussusception: Repair of prolapsed segment.

**46.81 Intra-abdominal manipulation of small intestine**

**46.82 Intra-abdominal manipulation of large intestine**

**46.85 Dilation of intestine**
Dilation (balloon) of duodenum
Dilation (balloon) of jejunum
Endoscopic dilation (balloon) of large intestine
That through rectum or colostomy
AHA: 3Q, '89, 15

☑4ᵗʰ **46.9 Other operations on intestines**

**46.91 Myotomy of sigmoid colon**

**46.92 Myotomy of other parts of colon**

**46.93 Revision of anastomosis of small intestine**

**46.94 Revision of anastomosis of large intestine**

**46.95 Local perfusion of small intestine**
Code also substance perfused (99.21-99.29)

**46.96 Local perfusion of large intestine**
Code also substance perfused (99.21-99.29)

**46.97 Transplant of intestine**    **LC**
Note: To report donor source — see codes 00.91-00.93
AHA: 4Q, '00, 66

BI Bilateral Procedure      NC Non-covered Procedure      LC Limited Coverage Procedure      ▶◀ Revised Text      ● New Code      ▲ Revised Code Title

128 — Volume 3 • October 2007

© 2007 Ingenix

**46.99　Other**
Ileoentectropy
　EXCLUDES　*diagnostic procedures on intestine (45.11-45.29)*
　　　　*dilation of enterostomy stoma (96.24)*
　　　　*intestinal intubation (96.08)*
　　　　*removal of:*
　　　　　*intraluminal foreign body from large intestine without incision (98.04)*
　　　　　*intraluminal foreign body from small intestine without incision (98.03)*
　　　　　*tube from large intestine (97.53)*
　　　　　*tube from small intestine (97.52)*
　　　　*replacement of:*
　　　　　*large intestine tube or enterostomy device (97.04)*
　　　　　*small intestine tube or enterostomy device (97.03)*
　　**AHA:** 3Q, '99, 11; 1Q, '89, 11

**✓3rd 47　Operations on appendix**
　INCLUDES　appendiceal stump
　Code also any application or administration of an adhesion barrier substance (99.77)

**✓4th 47.0　Appendectomy**
　EXCLUDES　*incidental appendectomy, so described (47.11, 47.19)*
　**AHA:** 4Q, '96, 64; 3Q, '92, 12

　**47.01　Laparoscopic appendectomy**
　　**AHA:** 1Q, '01, 15; 4Q, '96, 64

　**47.09　Other appendectomy**
　　**AHA:** 4Q, '97, 52

**✓4th 47.1　Incidental appendectomy**
　**DEF:** Removal of appendix during abdominal surgery as prophylactic measure, without significant appendiceal pathology.

　**47.11　Laparoscopic incidental appendectomy**
　**47.19　Other incidental appendectomy**
　　**AHA:** 4Q, '96, 65

　**47.2　Drainage of appendiceal abscess**
　　EXCLUDES　*that with appendectomy (47.0)*

**✓4th 47.9　Other operations on appendix**
　**47.91　Appendicostomy**
　**47.92　Closure of appendiceal fistula**
　**47.99　Other**
　　Anastomosis of appendix
　　EXCLUDES　*diagnostic procedures on appendix (45.21-45.29)*
　　**AHA:** 3Q, '01, 16

**✓3rd 48　Operations on rectum, rectosigmoid, and perirectal tissue**
　Code also any application or administration of an adhesion barrier substance (99.77)

　**48.0　Proctotomy**
　　Decompression of imperforate anus
　　Panas' operation [linear proctotomy]
　　EXCLUDES　*incision of perirectal tissue (48.81)*
　　**AHA:** 3Q, '99, 8
　　**DEF:** Incision into rectal portion of large intestine.
　　**DEF:** Decompression of imperforate anus: opening a closed anus by means of an incision.
　　**DEF:** Panas' operation (linear proctotomy): Linear incision into rectal portion of large intestine

　**48.1　Proctostomy**

**✓4th 48.2　Diagnostic procedures on rectum, rectosigmoid, and perirectal tissue**
　**48.21　Transabdominal proctosigmoidoscopy**
　　Intraoperative proctosigmoidoscopy
　　EXCLUDES　*that with biopsy (48.24)*

　**48.22　Proctosigmoidoscopy through artificial stoma**
　　EXCLUDES　*that with biopsy (48.24)*

　**48.23　Rigid proctosigmoidoscopy**
　　EXCLUDES　*flexible sigmoidoscopy (45.24)*
　　**AHA:** 1Q, '01, 8
　　**DEF:** Endoscopic exam of anus, rectum and lower sigmoid colon.

　**48.24　Closed [endoscopic] biopsy of rectum**
　　Brushing or washing for specimen collection
　　Proctosigmoidoscopy with biopsy
　　**AHA:** 1Q, '03, 14

　**48.25　Open biopsy of rectum**
　**48.26　Biopsy of perirectal tissue**
　**48.29　Other diagnostic procedures on rectum, rectosigmoid, and perirectal tissue**
　　EXCLUDES　*digital examination of rectum (89.34)*
　　　　*lower GI series (87.64)*
　　　　*microscopic examination of specimen from rectum (90.91-90.99)*

**✓4th 48.3　Local excision or destruction of lesion or tissue of rectum**
　**48.31　Radical electrocoagulation of rectal lesion or tissue**
　　**DEF:** Destruction of lesion or tissue of large intestine, rectal part.

　**48.32　Other electrocoagulation of rectal lesion or tissue**
　　**AHA:** 2Q, '98, 18

　**48.33　Destruction of rectal lesion or tissue by laser**
　**48.34　Destruction of rectal lesion or tissue by cryosurgery**
　**48.35　Local excision of rectal lesion or tissue**
　　EXCLUDES　*biopsy of rectum (48.24-48.25)*
　　　　*[endoscopic] polypectomy of rectum (48.36)*
　　　　*excision of perirectal tissue (48.82)*
　　　　*hemorrhoidectomy (49.46)*
　　　　*rectal fistulectomy (48.73)*

　**48.36　[Endoscopic] polypectomy of rectum**
　　**AHA:** 4Q, '95, 65

**✓4th 48.4　Pull-through resection of rectum**
　Code also any synchronous anastomosis other than end-to-end (45.90, 45.92-45.95)
　**48.41　Soave submucosal resection of rectum**
　　Endorectal pull-through operation
　　**DEF:** Soave submucosal resection: Resection of submucosal rectal part of large intestine by pull-through technique.
　　**DEF:** Endorectal pull-through operation: Resection of interior large intestine by pull-through technique.

　**48.49　Other pull-through resection of rectum**
　　Abdominoperineal pull-through
　　Altemeier operation
　　Swenson proctectomy
　　EXCLUDES　*Duhamel abdominoperineal pull-through (48.65)*
　　**AHA:** 3Q, '01, 8; 2Q, '99, 13
　　**DEF:** Abdominoperineal pull-through: Resection of large intestine, latter part, by pull-through of abdomen, scrotum or vulva and anus.
　　**DEF:** Swenson proctatectomy: Excision of large intestine, rectal by pull-through and preserving muscles that close the anus.

---

✓3rd
✓4th　Additional Digit Required　　　Valid OR Procedure　　　Non-OR Procedure　　　Adjunct Code

**Operations on the Digestive System**

**48.5–49.23**

**48.5** **Abdominoperineal resection of rectum**
Combined abdominoendorectal resection
Complete proctectomy
Code also any synchronous anastomosis other than end-to-end (45.90, 45.92-45.95)

INCLUDES    with synchronous colostomy

EXCLUDES    *Duhamel abdominoperineal pull-through (48.65)*
*that as part of pelvic exenteration (68.8)*

AHA: 2Q, '97, 5

DEF: Rectal excision through cavities formed by abdomen, anus, vulva or scrotum.

✓4ᵗʰ **48.6** **Other resection of rectum**
Code also any synchronous anastomosis other than end-to-end (45.90, 45.92-45.95)

**48.61** **Transsacral rectosigmoidectomy**
DEF: Excision through sacral bone area of sigmoid and last parts of large intestine.

**48.62** **Anterior resection of rectum with synchronous colostomy**
DEF: Resection of front terminal end of large intestine and creation of colostomy.

**48.63** **Other anterior resection of rectum**
EXCLUDES    *that with synchronous colostomy (48.62)*

AHA: 1Q, '96, 9

**48.64** **Posterior resection of rectum**
**48.65** **Duhamel resection of rectum**
Duhamel abdominoperineal pull-through

**48.69** **Other**
Partial proctectomy
Rectal resection NOS

AHA: 2Q, '05, 13; J-F, '87, 11; N-D, '86, 11

✓4ᵗʰ **48.7** **Repair of rectum**
EXCLUDES    *repair of:*
*current obstetric laceration (75.62)*
*vaginal rectocele (70.50, 70.52)*

**48.71** **Suture of laceration of rectum**
**48.72** **Closure of proctostomy**
**48.73** **Closure of other rectal fistula**
EXCLUDES    *fistulectomy:*
*perirectal (48.93)*
*rectourethral (58.43)*
*rectovaginal (70.73)*
*rectovesical (57.83)*
*rectovesicovaginal (57.83)*

**48.74** **Rectorectostomy**
Rectal anastomosis NOS
▶Stapled transanal rectal resection (STARR)◀
DEF: Rectal anastomosis: Connection of two cut portions of large intestine, rectal end.

**48.75** **Abdominal proctopexy**
Frickman procedure
Ripstein repair of rectal prolapse
DEF: Fixation of rectum to adjacent abdominal structures.

**48.76** **Other proctopexy**
Delorme repair of prolapsed rectum
Proctosigmoidopexy
Puborectalis sling operation
EXCLUDES    *manual reduction of rectal prolapse (96.26)*

DEF: Delorme repair of prolapsed rectum: Fixation of collapsed large intestine, rectal part.

DEF: Proctosigmoidopexy: Suturing of twisted large intestine, rectal part.

DEF: Puborectalis sling operation: Fixation of large intestine, rectal part by forming puborectalis muscle into sling.

**48.79** **Other repair of rectum**
Repair of old obstetric laceration of rectum
EXCLUDES    *anastomosis to:*
*large intestine (45.94)*
*small intestine (45.92-45.93)*
*repair of:*
*current obstetrical laceration (75.62)*
*vaginal rectocele (70.50, 70.52)*

✓4ᵗʰ **48.8** **Incision or excision of perirectal tissue or lesion**
INCLUDES    pelvirectal tissue
rectovaginal septum

**48.81** **Incision of perirectal tissue**
Incision of rectovaginal septum

**48.82** **Excision of perirectal tissue**
EXCLUDES    *perirectal biopsy (48.26)*
*perirectofistulectomy (48.93)*
*rectal fistulectomy (48.73)*

✓4ᵗʰ **48.9** **Other operations on rectum and perirectal tissue**
**48.91** **Incision of rectal stricture**
**48.92** **Anorectal myectomy**
DEF: Excision of anorectal muscle.

**48.93** **Repair of perirectal fistula**
EXCLUDES    *that opening into rectum (48.73)*

AHA: ▶1Q, '07, 13◀

DEF: Closure of abdominal passage in tissue around large intestine, rectal part.

**48.99** **Other**
EXCLUDES    *digital examination of rectum (89.34)*
*dilation of rectum (96.22)*
*insertion of rectal tube (96.09)*
*irrigation of rectum (96.38-96.39)*
*manual reduction of rectal prolapse (96.26)*
*proctoclysis (96.37)*
*rectal massage (99.93)*
*rectal packing (96.19)*
*removal of:*
*impacted feces (96.38)*
*intraluminal foreign body from rectum without incision (98.05)*
*rectal packing (97.59)*
*transanal enema (96.39)*

✓3ʳᵈ **49** **Operations on anus**
Code also any application or administration of an adhesion barrier substance (99.77)

✓4ᵗʰ **49.0** **Incision or excision of perianal tissue**
**49.01** **Incision of perianal abscess**
AHA: 2Q, '05, 10

**49.02** **Other incision of perianal tissue**
Undercutting of perianal tissue
EXCLUDES    *anal fistulotomy (49.11)*

**49.03** **Excision of perianal skin tags**
**49.04** **Other excision of perianal tissue**
EXCLUDES    *anal fistulectomy (49.12)*
*biopsy of perianal tissue (49.22)*

AHA: 1Q, '01, 8

✓4ᵗʰ **49.1** **Incision or excision of anal fistula**
EXCLUDES    *closure of anal fistula (49.73)*

**49.11** **Anal fistulotomy**
**49.12** **Anal fistulectomy**

✓4ᵗʰ **49.2** **Diagnostic procedures on anus and perianal tissue**
**49.21** **Anoscopy**
**49.22** **Biopsy of perianal tissue**
**49.23** **Biopsy of anus**

BI  Bilateral Procedure    NC  Non-covered Procedure    LC  Limited Coverage Procedure    ▶◀ Revised Text    ● New Code    ▲ Revised Code Title

**49.29** **Other diagnostic procedures on anus and perianal tissue**

> EXCLUDES *microscopic examination of specimen from anus (90.91-90.99)*

✓4ᵗʰ **49.3** **Local excision or destruction of other lesion or tissue of anus**

Anal cryptotomy
Cauterization of lesion of anus

> EXCLUDES *biopsy of anus (49.23)*
> *control of (postoperative) hemorrhage of anus (49.95)*
> *hemorrhoidectomy (49.46)*

**49.31** **Endoscopic excision or destruction of lesion or tissue of anus**

**49.39** **Other local excision or destruction of lesion or tissue of anus**

> EXCLUDES *that by endoscopic approach (49.31)*

AHA: 1Q, '01, 8

✓4ᵗʰ **49.4** **Procedures on hemorrhoids**

**49.41** **Reduction of hemorrhoids**
DEF: Manual manipulation to reduce hemorrhoids.

**49.42** **Injection of hemorrhoids**

**49.43** **Cauterization of hemorrhoids**
Clamp and cautery of hemorrhoids

**49.44** **Destruction of hemorrhoids by cryotherapy**

**49.45** **Ligation of hemorrhoids**

**49.46** **Excision of hemorrhoids**
Hemorrhoidectomy NOS
AHA: ▶1Q, '07, 13◀

**49.47** **Evacuation of thrombosed hemorrhoids**
DEF: Removal of clotted material from hemorrhoid.

**49.49** **Other procedures on hemorrhoids**
Lord procedure

✓4ᵗʰ **49.5** **Division of anal sphincter**

**49.51** **Left lateral anal sphincterotomy**

**49.52** **Posterior anal sphincterotomy**

**49.59** **Other anal sphincterotomy**
Division of sphincter NOS

**49.6** **Excision of anus**

✓4ᵗʰ **49.7** **Repair of anus**

> EXCLUDES *repair of current obstetric laceration (75.62)*

**49.71** **Suture of laceration of anus**

**49.72** **Anal cerclage**
DEF: Encircling anus with ring or sutures.

**49.73** **Closure of anal fistula**

> EXCLUDES *excision of anal fistula (49.12)*

**49.74** **Gracilis muscle transplant for anal incontinence**
DEF: Moving pubic attachment of gracilis muscle to restore anal control.

**49.75** **Implantation or revision of artificial anal sphincter**
Removal with subsequent replacement
Replacement during same or subsequent operative episode
AHA: 4Q, '02, 105

**49.76** **Removal of artificial anal sphincter**
Explantation or removal without replacement

> EXCLUDES *revision with implantation during same operative episode (49.75)*

AHA: 4Q, '02, 105

**49.79** **Other repair of anal sphincter**
Repair of old obstetric laceration of anus

> EXCLUDES *anoplasty with synchronous hemorrhoidectomy (49.46)*
> *repair of current obstetric laceration (75.62)*

AHA: 2Q, '98, 16; 1Q, '97, 9

✓4ᵗʰ **49.9** **Other operations on anus**

> EXCLUDES *dilation of anus (sphincter) (96.23)*

**49.91** **Incision of anal septum**

**49.92** **Insertion of subcutaneous electrical anal stimulator**

**49.93** **Other incision of anus**
Removal of:
　foreign body from anus with incision
　seton from anus

> EXCLUDES *anal fistulotomy (49.11)*
> *removal of intraluminal foreign body without incision (98.05)*

**49.94** **Reduction of anal prolapse**

> EXCLUDES *manual reduction of rectal prolapse (96.26)*

DEF: Manipulation of displaced anal tissue to normal position.

**49.95** **Control of (postoperative) hemorrhage of anus**

**49.99** **Other**

✓3ʳᵈ **50** **Operations on liver**
Code also any application or administration of an adhesion barrier substance (99.77)

**50.0** **Hepatotomy**
Incision of abscess of liver
Removal of gallstones from liver
Stromeyer-Little operation

✓4ᵗʰ **50.1** **Diagnostic procedures on liver**

**50.11** **Closed (percutaneous) (needle) biopsy of liver**
Diagnostic aspiration of liver
AHA: 3Q, '05, 24; 4Q, '88, 12

**50.12** **Open biopsy of liver**
Wedge biopsy
AHA: 3Q, '05, 24; 2Q, '05, 13

**50.13** **Transjugular liver biopsy**
Transvenous liver biopsy

> EXCLUDES *closed (percutaneous) [needle] biopsy of liver (50.11)*
> *laparoscopic liver biopsy (50.14)*

**50.14** **Laparoscopic liver biopsy**

> EXCLUDES *closed (percutaneous) [needle] biopsy of liver (50.11)*
> *open biopsy of liver (50.12)*
> *transjugular liver biopsy (50.13)*

**Dynamic Graciloplasty**

Rectum
Generator
Electrodes
Gracilis muscle
(transpositional)
Neosphincter
Anal opening

**Closed Liver Biopsy**

8
9
Inserted along
midaxillary line 10
11
(12 behind)

### Liver Biopsy (Open, Wedge)

Right lobe

Left lobe

Liver

Caudate lobe

Gallbladder

**Typical wedge biopsy sites**

**50.19   Other diagnostic procedures on liver**
> **EXCLUDES** ► laparoscopic liver biopsy
> (50.14)◄
> liver scan and radioisotope
> function study (92.02)
> microscopic examination of
> specimen from liver
> (91.01-91.09)
> ►transjugular liver biopsy
> (50.13)◄

√4ᵗʰ **50.2   Local excision or destruction of liver tissue or lesion**

**50.21   Marsupialization of lesion of liver**
DEF: Exteriorizing lesion by incision and suturing cut edges to skin to create opening.

**50.22   Partial hepatectomy**
Wedge resection of liver
> **EXCLUDES** biopsy of liver (50.11-50.12)
> hepatic lobectomy (50.3)

**50.23   Open ablation of liver lesion or tissue**
AHA: 4Q, '06, 124

**50.24   Percutaneous ablation of liver lesion or tissue**
AHA: 4Q, '06, 124

**50.25   Laparoscopic ablation of liver lesion or tissue**
AHA: 4Q, '06, 124

**50.26   Other and unspecified ablation of liver lesion or tissue**
AHA: 4Q, '06, 124

**50.29   Other destruction of lesion of liver**
Cauterization
Enucleation } of hepatic lesion
Evacuation
> **EXCLUDES** ablation of liver lesion or
> tissue:
> laparoscopic (50.25)
> open (50.23)
> other (50.26)
> percutaneous (50.24)
> percutaneous aspiration of
> lesion (50.91)

AHA: 2Q, '03, 9

**50.3   Lobectomy of liver**
Total hepatic lobectomy with partial excision of other lobe

**50.4   Total hepatectomy**

√4ᵗʰ **50.5   Liver transplant**
Note: To report donor source — see codes 00.91-00.93

**50.51   Auxiliary liver transplant**    NC
Auxiliary hepatic transplantation leaving patient's own liver in situ

**50.59   Other transplant of liver**    LC

√4ᵗʰ **50.6   Repair of liver**

**50.61   Closure of laceration of liver**

**50.69   Other repair of liver**
Hepatopexy

√4ᵗʰ **50.9   Other operations on liver**
> **EXCLUDES** lysis of adhesions (54.5)

**50.91   Percutaneous aspiration of liver**
> **EXCLUDES** percutaneous biopsy (50.11)
DEF: Incision into liver through body wall to withdraw fluid.

**50.92   Extracorporeal hepatic assistance**
Liver dialysis
AHA: 2Q, '01, 21
DEF: Devices used outside body to assist liver function.

**50.93   Localized perfusion of liver**

**50.94   Other injection of therapeutic substance into liver**

**50.99   Other**

√3ʳᵈ **51   Operations on gallbladder and biliary tract**
> **INCLUDES** operations on:
> ampulla of Vater
> common bile duct
> cystic duct
> hepatic duct
> intrahepatic bile duct
> sphincter of Oddi
Code also any application or administration of an adhesion barrier substance (99.77)

√4ᵗʰ **51.0   Cholecystotomy and cholecystostomy**

**51.01   Percutaneous aspiration of gallbladder**
Percutaneous cholecystotomy for drainage
That by: needle or catheter
> **EXCLUDES** needle biopsy (51.12)

**51.02   Trocar cholecystostomy**
AHA: 3Q, '89, 18
DEF: Creating opening in gallbladder with catheter.

**51.03   Other cholecystostomy**

**51.04   Other cholecystostomy**
Cholelithotomy NOS

√4ᵗʰ **51.1   Diagnostic procedures on biliary tract**
> **EXCLUDES** that for endoscopic procedures classifi-
> able to 51.64, 51.84-51.88, 52.14,
> 52.21, 52.93 -52.94, 52.97-52.98

AHA: 2Q, '97, 7

**51.10   Endoscopic retrograde cholangiopancreatography [ERCP]**
> **EXCLUDES** endoscopic retrograde:
> cholangiography [ERC]
> (51.11)
> pancreatography [ERP]
> (52.13)

AHA: 4Q, '03, 118; 3Q, '03, 17; 1Q, '01, 8; 2Q, '99, 13
DEF: Endoscopic and radioscopic exam of pancreatic and common bile ducts with contrast material injected in opposite direction of normal flow through catheter.

**51.11   Endoscopic retrograde cholangiography [ERC]**
Laparoscopic exploration of common bile duct
> **EXCLUDES** endoscopic retrograde:
> cholangiopancreatography
> [ERCP] (51.10)
> pancreatography [ERP]
> (52.13)

AHA: 1Q, '96, 12; 3Q, '89, 18; 4Q, '88, 7
DEF: Endoscopic and radioscopic exam of common bile ducts with contrast material injected in opposite direction of normal flow through catheter.

**51.12   Percutaneous biopsy of gallbladder or bile ducts**
Needle biopsy of gallbladder

**51.13   Open biopsy of gallbladder or bile ducts**

**51.14   Other closed [endoscopic] biopsy of biliary duct or sphincter of Oddi**
Brushing or washing for specimen collection
Closed biopsy of biliary duct or sphincter of Oddi by procedures classifiable to 51.10-51.11, 52.13
DEF: Endoscopic biopsy of muscle tissue around pancreatic and common bile ducts.

---

BI Bilateral Procedure    NC Non-covered Procedure    LC Limited Coverage Procedure    ►◄ Revised Text    ● New Code    ▲ Revised Code Title

**51.15** **Pressure measurement of sphincter of Oddi**
Pressure measurement of sphincter by procedures classifiable to 51.10-51.11, 52.13
DEF: Pressure measurement tests of muscle tissue surrounding pancreatic and common bile ducts.

**51.19** **Other diagnostic procedures on biliary tract**
EXCLUDES     biliary tract x-ray (87.51-87.59)
microscopic examination of specimen from biliary tract (91.01-91.09)

✓4th **51.2** **Cholecystectomy**
AHA: 1Q, '93, 17; 4Q, '91, 26; 3Q, '89, 18

**51.21** **Other partial cholecystectomy**
Revision of prior cholecystectomy
EXCLUDES     that by laparoscope (51.24)
AHA: 4Q, '96, 69

**51.22** **Cholecystectomy**
EXCLUDES     laparoscopic cholecystectomy (51.23)
AHA: 4Q, '97, 52; 2Q, '91, 16

**51.23** **Laparoscopic cholecystectomy**
That by laser
AHA: 3Q, '98, 10; 4Q, '97, 52; 1Q, '96, 12; 2Q, '95, 11; 4Q, '91, 26
DEF: Endoscopic removal of gallbladder.

**51.24** **Laparoscopic partial cholecystectomy**
AHA: 4Q, '96, 69

✓4th **51.3** **Anastomosis of gallbladder or bile duct**
EXCLUDES     resection with end-to-end anastomosis (51.61-51.69)

**51.31** **Anastomosis of gallbladder to hepatic ducts**
**51.32** **Anastomosis of gallbladder to intestine**
**51.33** **Anastomosis of gallbladder to pancreas**
**51.34** **Anastomosis of gallbladder to stomach**
**51.35** **Other gallbladder anastomosis**
Gallbladder anastomosis NOS

**51.36** **Choledochoenterostomy**
DEF: Connection of common bile duct to intestine.

**51.37** **Anastomosis of hepatic duct to gastrointestinal tract**
Kasai portoenterostomy
AHA: 2Q, '02, 12
DEF: Kaisi portoenterostomy: A duct to drain bile from the liver is formed by anastomosing the porta hepatis to a loop of bowel.

**51.39** **Other bile duct anastomosis**
Anastomosis of bile duct NOS
Anastomosis of unspecified bile duct to:
    intestine      pancreas
    liver         stomach

✓4th **51.4** **Incision of bile duct for relief of obstruction**
**51.41** **Common duct exploration for removal of calculus**
EXCLUDES     percutaneous extraction (51.96)
AHA: 1Q, '96, 12; 3Q, '89, 18; 4Q, '88, 7

**Laparoscopic Cholecystectomy by Laser**

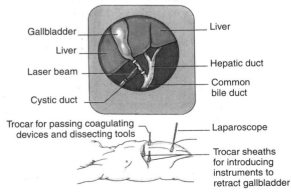

Gallbladder — Liver
Liver —
Laser beam — Hepatic duct
Cystic duct — Common bile duct
Trocar for passing coagulating devices and dissecting tools — Laparoscope
Trocar sheaths for introducing instruments to retract gallbladder

**51.42** **Common duct exploration for relief of other obstruction**
AHA: 3Q, '89, 18

**51.43** **Insertion of choledochohepatic tube for decompression**
Hepatocholedochostomy
AHA: 3Q, '89, 18; 4Q, '88, 7

**51.49** **Incision of other bile ducts for relief of obstruction**
AHA: 3Q, '89, 18

✓4th **51.5** **Other incision of bile duct**
EXCLUDES     that for relief of obstruction (51.41-51.49)

**51.51** **Exploration of common duct**
Incision of common bile duct
AHA: 2Q, '97, 16; 1Q, '96, 12

**51.59** **Incision of other bile duct**
AHA: 2Q, '97, 16; 3Q, '89, 18

✓4th **51.6** **Local excision or destruction of lesion or tissue of biliary ducts and sphincter of Oddi**
Code also anastomosis other than end-to-end (51.31, 51.36-51.39)
EXCLUDES     biopsy of bile duct (51.12-51.13)

**51.61** **Excision of cystic duct remnant**
AHA: 3Q, '89, 18

**51.62** **Excision of ampulla of Vater (with reimplantation of common duct)**

**51.63** **Other excision of common duct**
Choledochectomy
EXCLUDES     fistulectomy (51.72)

**51.64** **Endoscopic excision or destruction of lesion of biliary ducts or sphincter of Oddi**
Excision or destruction of lesion of biliary duct by procedures classifiable to 51.10-51.11, 52.13

**51.69** **Excision of other bile duct**
Excision of lesion of bile duct NOS
EXCLUDES     fistulectomy (51.79)

✓4th **51.7** **Repair of bile ducts**
**51.71** **Simple suture of common bile duct**
**51.72** **Choledochoplasty**
Repair of fistula of common bile duct

**51.79** **Repair of other bile ducts**
Closure of artificial opening of bile duct NOS
Suture of bile duct NOS
EXCLUDES     operative removal of prosthetic device (51.95)

✓4th **51.8** **Other operations on biliary ducts and sphincter of Oddi**
**51.81** **Dilation of sphincter of Oddi**
Dilation of ampulla of Vater
EXCLUDES     that by endoscopic approach (51.84)
DEF: Dilation of muscle around common bile and pancreatic ducts; to mitigate constriction obstructing bile flow.

**51.82** **Pancreatic sphincterotomy**
Incision of pancreatic sphincter
Transduodenal ampullary sphincterotomy
EXCLUDES     that by endoscopic approach (51.85)
DEF: Pancreatic sphincterotomy: Division of muscle around common bile and pancreatic ducts.
DEF: Transduodenal ampullary sphincterotomy: Incision into muscle around common bile and pancreatic ducts; closing approach through first section of small intestine.

**51.83** **Pancreatic sphincteroplasty**
**51.84** **Endoscopic dilation of ampulla and biliary duct**
Dilation of ampulla and biliary duct by procedures classifiable to 51.10-51.11, 52.13

✓3rd **Additional Digit Required**
✓4th
    Valid OR Procedure        Non-OR Procedure        Adjunct Code

**51.85 Endoscopic sphincterotomy and papillotomy**

Sphincterotomy and papillotomy by procedures classifiable to 51.10-51.11, 52.13

**AHA:** 4Q, '03, 118; 3Q, '03, 17; 2Q, '97, 7

**DEF:** Incision of muscle around common bile and pancreatic ducts and closing the duodenal papilla.

**51.86 Endoscopic insertion of nasobiliary drainage tube**

Insertion of nasobiliary tube by procedures classifiable to 51.10-51.11, 52.13

**51.87 Endoscopic insertion of stent (tube) into bile duct**

Endoprosthesis of bile duct

Insertion of stent into bile duct by procedures classifiable to 51.10-51.11, 52.13

**EXCLUDES** *nasobiliary drainage tube (51.86)*
*replacement of stent (tube) (97.05)*

**AHA:** 3Q, '03, 17

**51.88 Endoscopic removal of stone(s) from biliary tract**

Laparoscopic removal of stone(s) from biliary tract

Removal of biliary tract stone(s) by procedures classifiable to 51.10-51.11, 52.13

**EXCLUDES** *percutaneous extraction of common duct stones (51.96)*

**AHA:** 2Q, '00, 11; 2Q, '97, 7

**51.89 Other operations on sphincter of Oddi**

✓4ᵗʰ **51.9 Other operations on biliary tract**

**51.91 Repair of laceration of gallbladder**

**51.92 Closure of cholecystostomy**

**51.93 Closure of other biliary fistula**

Cholecystogastroenteric fistulectomy

**51.94 Revision of anastomosis of biliary tract**

**51.95 Removal of prosthetic device from bile duct**

**EXCLUDES** *nonoperative removal (97.55)*

**51.96 Percutaneous extraction of common duct stones**

**AHA:** 4Q, '88, 7

**51.98 Other percutaneous procedures on biliary tract**

Percutaneous biliary endoscopy via existing T-tube or other tract for:
dilation of biliary duct stricture
removal of stone(s) except common duct stone
exploration (postoperative)

Percutaneous transhepatic biliary drainage

**EXCLUDES** *percutaneous aspiration of gallbladder (51.01)*
*percutaneous biopsy and/or collection of specimen by brushing or washing (51.12)*
*percutaneous removal of common duct stone(s) (51.96)*

**AHA:** 1Q, '97, 14; 3Q, '89, 18; N-D, '87, 1

**51.99 Other**

Insertion or replacement of biliary tract prosthesis

**EXCLUDES** *biopsy of gallbladder (51.12-51.13)*
*irrigation of cholecystostomy and other biliary tube (96.41)*
*lysis of peritoneal adhesions (54.5)*
*nonoperative removal of: cholecystostomy tube (97.54)*
*tube from biliary tract or liver (97.55)*

✓3ʳᵈ **52 Operations on pancreas**

**INCLUDES** operations on pancreatic duct

Code also any application or administration of an adhesion barrier substance (99.77)

✓4ᵗʰ **52.0 Pancreatotomy**

**52.01 Drainage of pancreatic cyst by catheter**

**52.09 Other pancreatotomy**

Pancreatolithotomy

**EXCLUDES** *drainage by anastomosis (52.4, 52.96)*
*incision of pancreatic sphincter (51.82)*
*marsupialization of cyst (52.3)*

**DEF:** Pancreatolithotomy: Incision into pancreas to remove stones.

✓4ᵗʰ **52.1 Diagnostic procedures on pancreas**

**52.11 Closed [aspiration] [needle] [percutaneous] biopsy of pancreas**

**52.12 Open biopsy of pancreas**

**52.13 Endoscopic retrograde pancreatography [ERP]**

**EXCLUDES** *endoscopic retrograde: cholangiography [ERC] (51.11)*
*cholangiopancreatography [ERCP] (51.10)*
*that for procedures classifiable to 51.14-51.15, 51.64, 51.84-51.88, 52.14, 52.21, 52.92-52.94, 52.97-52.98*

**52.14 Closed [endoscopic] biopsy of pancreatic duct**

Closed biopsy of pancreatic duct by procedures classifiable to 51.10-51.11, 52.13

**52.19 Other diagnostic procedures on pancreas**

**EXCLUDES** *contrast pancreatogram (87.66)*
*endoscopic retrograde pancreatography [ERP] (52.13)*
*microscopic examination of specimen from pancreas (91.01-91.09)*

✓4ᵗʰ **52.2 Local excision or destruction of pancreas and pancreatic duct**

**EXCLUDES** *biopsy of pancreas (52.11-52.12, 52.14)*
*pancreatic fistulectomy (52.95)*

**52.21 Endoscopic excision or destruction of lesion or tissue of pancreatic duct**

Excision or destruction of lesion or tissue of pancreatic duct by procedures classifiable to 51.10-51.11, 52.13

**52.22 Other excision or destruction of lesion or tissue of pancreas or pancreatic duct**

**52.3 Marsupialization of pancreatic cyst**

**EXCLUDES** *drainage of cyst by catheter (52.01)*

**DEF:** Incision into pancreas and suturing edges to form pocket; promotes drainage and healing.

**52.4 Internal drainage of pancreatic cyst**

Pancreaticocystoduodenostomy
Pancreaticocystogastrostomy
Pancreaticocystojejunostomy

**DEF:** Withdrawing fluid from pancreatic cyst by draining it through a created passage to another organ.

**DEF:** Pancreaticocystoduodenostomy: Creation of passage from pancreatic cyst to first portion of small intestine.

**DEF:** Pancreaticocystogastrostomy: Creation of passage from pancreatic cyst to stomach.

**DEF:** Pancreaticocystojejunostomy: Creation of passage from pancreatic cyst to midsection of small intestine.

✓4ᵗʰ **52.5** **Partial pancreatectomy**
>  EXCLUDES  *pancreatic fistulectomy (52.95)*

**52.51** **Proximal pancreatectomy**
> Excision of head of pancreas (with part of body)
> Proximal pancreatectomy with synchronous duodenectomy

**52.52** **Distal pancreatectomy**
> Excision of tail of pancreas (with part of body)

**52.53** **Radical subtotal pancreatectomy**

**52.59** **Other partial pancreatectomy**

**52.6** **Total pancreatectomy**
> Pancreatectomy with synchronous duodenectomy

AHA: 4Q, '96, 71

**52.7** **Radical pancreaticoduodenectomy**
> One-stage pancreaticoduodenal resection with choledochojejunal anastomosis, pancreaticojejunal anastomosis, and gastrojejunostomy
> Two-stage pancreaticoduodenal resection (first stage) (second stage)
> Radical resection of the pancreas
> Whipple procedure
>  EXCLUDES  *radical subtotal pancreatectomy (52.53)*

AHA: 1Q, '01, 13

DEF: Whipple procedure: pancreaticoduodenectomy involving the removal of the head of the pancreas and part of the small intestines; pancreaticojejunostomy, choledochojejunal anastomosis, and gastrojejunostomy included in the procedure.

✓4ᵗʰ **52.8** **Transplant of pancreas**
> Note: To report donor source—*see* codes 00.91-00.93

¹⁰ **52.80** **Pancreatic transplant, not otherwise specified** NC LC

**52.81** **Reimplantation of pancreatic tissue**

¹⁰ **52.82** **Homotransplant of pancreas** NC LC

**52.83** **Heterotransplant of pancreas** NC

**52.84** **Autotransplantation of cells of islets of Langerhans**
> Homotransplantation of islet cells of pancreas

AHA: 4Q, '96, 70, 71

DEF: Transplantation of Islet cells from pancreas to another location of same patient.

**52.85** **Allotransplantation of cells of islets of Langerhans**
> Heterotransplantation of islet cells of pancreas

AHA: 4Q, '96, 70, 71

DEF: Transplantation of Islet cells from one individual to another.

**52.86** **Transplantation of cells of islets of Langerhans, not otherwise specified**

AHA: 4Q, '96, 70

✓4ᵗʰ **52.9** **Other operations on pancreas**
> DEF: Placement of tube into pancreatic duct, without an endoscope.

**52.92** **Cannulation of pancreatic duct**
>  EXCLUDES  *that by endoscopic approach (52.93)*

**52.93** **Endoscopic insertion of stent (tube) into pancreatic duct**
> Insertion of cannula or stent into pancreatic duct by procedures classifiable to 51.10-51.11, 52.13
>  EXCLUDES  *endoscopic insertion of nasopancreatic drainage tube (52.97)*
> *replacement of stent (tube) (97.05)*

AHA: 2Q, '97, 7

**52.94** **Endoscopic removal of stone(s) from pancreatic duct**
> Removal of stone(s) from pancreatic duct by procedures classifiable to 51.10-51.11, 52.13

**52.95** **Other repair of pancreas**
> Fistulectomy ⎫
> Simple suture ⎬ of pancreas

**52.96** **Anastomosis of pancreas**
> Anastomosis of pancreas (duct) to:
> intestine        stomach
> jejunum
>  EXCLUDES  *anastomosis to:*
> *bile duct (51.39)*
> *gallbladder (51.33)*

**52.97** **Endoscopic insertion of nasopancreatic drainage tube**
> Insertion of nasopancreatic drainage tube by procedures classifiable to 51.10-51.11, 52.13
>  EXCLUDES  *drainage of pancreatic cyst by catheter (52.01)*
> *replacement of stent (tube) (97.05)*

**52.98** **Endoscopic dilation of pancreatic duct**
> Dilation of Wirsung's duct by procedures classifiable to 51.10-51.11, 52.13

**52.99** **Other**
> Dilation of pancreatic ⎫
> [Wirsung's] duct    ⎬ by open
> Repair of pancreatic ⎪ approach
> [Wirsung's] duct    ⎭
>  EXCLUDES  *irrigation of pancreatic tube (96.42)*
> *removal of pancreatic tube (97.56)*

✓3ʳᵈ **53** **Repair of hernia**
>  INCLUDES  hernioplasty        herniotomy
> herniorrhaphy
> Code also any application or administration of an adhesion barrier substance (99.77)
>  EXCLUDES  *manual reduction of hernia (96.27)*

AHA: 3Q, '94, 8

DEF: Repair of hernia: Restoration of abnormally protruding organ or tissue.
DEF: Herniorrhaphy: Repair of hernia.
DEF: Herniotomy: Division of constricted, strangulated, irreducible hernia.

✓4ᵗʰ **53.0** **Unilateral repair of inguinal hernia**
**53.00** **Unilateral repair of inguinal hernia, not otherwise specified**
> Inguinal herniorrhaphy NOS

AHA: 3Q, '03, 10

**53.01** **Repair of direct inguinal hernia**

AHA: 4Q, '96, 66

**Indirect Repair of Hernia**

Incision
Internal ring
Internal ring
Internal ring
Herniating peritoneal sac
Sac twisted and sewn shut
External ring

¹⁰ Noncovered procedure unless reported with code 55.69 and a diagnosis code from 250.x0 or 250.x2 with 403.x1, 404.x2, 404.x3, 585.x, V42.0 or V42.89; or reported with a diagnosis code 250.x1 or 250.x3.

✓3ʳᵈ
✓4ᵗʰ  Additional Digit Required | Valid OR Procedure | Non-OR Procedure | Adjunct Code

**Operations on the Digestive System**

**53.02–54.19**

53.02   **Repair of indirect inguinal hernia**

53.03   **Repair of direct inguinal hernia with graft or prosthesis**

53.04   **Repair of indirect inguinal hernia with graft or prosthesis**

53.05   **Repair of inguinal hernia with graft or prosthesis, not otherwise specified**

√4ᵗʰ **53.1**   **Bilateral repair of inguinal hernia**

53.10   **Bilateral repair of inguinal hernia, not otherwise specified**

53.11   **Bilateral repair of direct inguinal hernia**

53.12   **Bilateral repair of indirect inguinal hernia**

53.13   **Bilateral repair of inguinal hernia, one direct and one indirect**

53.14   **Bilateral repair of direct inguinal hernia with graft or prosthesis**

53.15   **Bilateral repair of indirect inguinal hernia with graft or prosthesis**

53.16   **Bilateral repair of inguinal hernia, one direct and one indirect, with graft or prosthesis**

53.17   **Bilateral inguinal hernia repair with graft or prosthesis, not otherwise specified**

√4ᵗʰ **53.2**   **Unilateral repair of femoral hernia**

53.21   **Unilateral repair of femoral hernia with graft or prosthesis**

53.29   **Other unilateral femoral herniorrhaphy**

√4ᵗʰ **53.3**   **Bilateral repair of femoral hernia**

53.31   **Bilateral repair of femoral hernia with graft or prosthesis**

53.39   **Other bilateral femoral herniorrhaphy**

√4ᵗʰ **53.4**   **Repair of umbilical hernia**

**EXCLUDES**   *repair of gastroschisis (54.71)*

▲

53.41   **Repair of umbilical hernia with graft or prosthesis**

53.49   **Other umbilical herniorrhaphy**

√4ᵗʰ **53.5**   **Repair of other hernia of anterior abdominal wall (without graft or prosthesis)**

53.51   **Incisional hernia repair**

AHA: 3Q, '03, 6

53.59   **Repair of other hernia of anterior abdominal wall**

Repair of hernia:
epigastric    spigelian
hypogastric    ventral

AHA: 2Q, '06, 10; 3Q, '03, 6; 3Q, '96, 15

√4ᵗʰ **53.6**   **Repair of other hernia of anterior abdominal wall with graft or prosthesis**

▲

53.61   **Incisional hernia repair with graft or prosthesis**

AHA: 3Q, '03, 11

▲

53.69   **Repair of other hernia of anterior abdominal wall with graft or prosthesis**

**53.7**   **Repair of diaphragmatic hernia, abdominal approach**

√4ᵗʰ **53.8**   **Repair of diaphragmatic hernia, thoracic approach**

DEF: Repair of diaphragmatic hernia though abdomen and thorax.

53.80   **Repair of diaphragmatic hernia with thoracic approach, not otherwise specified**

Thoracoabdominal repair of diaphragmatic hernia

53.81   **Plication of the diaphragm**

DEF: Tuck repair of diaphragmatic hernia.

53.82   **Repair of parasternal hernia**

DEF: Repair of hernia protruding into breastbone area.

**53.9**   **Other hernia repair**

Repair of hernia:     Repair of hernia:
ischiatic     omental
ischiorectal     retroperitoneal
lumbar     sciatic
obturator

**EXCLUDES**   *relief of strangulated hernia with exteriorization of intestine (46.01, 46.03)*
*repair of pericolostomy hernia (46.42)*
*repair of vaginal enterocele (70.92)*

√3ʳᵈ **54**   **Other operations on abdominal region**

**INCLUDES**   operations on:    operations on:
epigastric region    mesentery
flank    omentum
groin region    ▶pelvic cavity◀
hypochondrium    peritoneum
inguinal region    retroperitoneal
loin region    tissue space

Code also any application or administration of an adhesion barrier substance (99.77)

**EXCLUDES**   *hernia repair (53.00-53.9)*
*obliteration of cul-de-sac (70.92)*
*retroperitoneal tissue dissection (59.00-59.09)*
*skin and subcutaneous tissue of abdominal wall (86.01-86.99)*

**54.0**   **Incision of abdominal wall**

Drainage of:
abdominal wall
extraperitoneal abscess
retroperitoneal abscess

**EXCLUDES**   *incision of peritoneum (54.95)*
*laparotomy (54.11-54.19)*

AHA: 2Q, '06, 23; 4Q, '05, 77; 1Q, '97, 11; N-D, '87, 12

√4ᵗʰ **54.1**   **Laparotomy**

AHA: 1Q, '92, 13

DEF: Incision into abdomen.

54.11   **Exploratory laparotomy**

**EXCLUDES**   *exploration incidental to intra-abdominal surgery — omit code*

AHA: 3Q, '89, 14; 4Q, '88, 12

DEF: Exam of peritoneal cavity through incision into abdomen.

54.12   **Reopening of recent laparotomy site**

Reopening of recent laparotomy site for:
control of hemorrhage
exploration
incision of hematoma

54.19   **Other laparotomy**

Drainage of intraperitoneal abscess or hematoma

**EXCLUDES**   *culdocentesis (70.0)*
*drainage of appendiceal abscess (47.2)*
*exploration incidental to intra-abdominal surgery — omit code*
*Ladd operation (54.95)*
*percutaneous drainage of abdomen (54.91)*
*removal of foreign body (54.92)*

AHA: 3Q, '03, 17

---

**BI** Bilateral Procedure    **NC** Non-covered Procedure    **LC** Limited Coverage Procedure    ▶◀ Revised Text    ● New Code    ▲ Revised Code Title

√4ᵗʰ **54.2** **Diagnostic procedures of abdominal region**
**54.21** **Laparoscopy**
Peritoneoscopy
**EXCLUDES** *laparoscopic cholecystectomy (51.23)*
*that incidental to destruction of fallopian tubes (66.21-66.29)*

DEF: Endoscopic exam of peritoneal cavity through abdominal incision.

**54.22** **Biopsy of abdominal wall or umbilicus**
**54.23** **Biopsy of peritoneum**
Biopsy of:
mesentery
omentum
peritoneal implant
**EXCLUDES** *closed biopsy of:*
*omentum (54.24)*
*peritoneum (54.24)*

**54.24** **Closed [percutaneous] [needle] biopsy of intra-abdominal mass**
Closed biopsy of:
omentum
peritoneal implant
peritoneum
**EXCLUDES** *that of:*
*fallopian tube (66.11)*
*ovary (65.11)*
*uterine ligaments (68.15)*
*uterus (68.16)*

AHA: 4Q, '97, 57

**54.25** **Peritoneal lavage**
Diagnostic peritoneal lavage
**EXCLUDES** *peritoneal dialysis (54.98)*

AHA: 2Q, '98, 19; 4Q, '93, 28

DEF: Irrigation of peritoneal cavity with siphoning of liquid contents for analysis.

**54.29** **Other diagnostic procedures on abdominal region**
**EXCLUDES** *abdominal lymphangiogram (88.04)*
*abdominal x-ray NEC (88.19)*
*angiocardiography of venae cavae (88.51)*
*C.A.T. scan of abdomen (88.01)*
*contrast x-ray of abdominal cavity (88.11-88.15)*
*intra-abdominal arteriography NEC (88.47)*
*microscopic examination of peritoneal and retroperitoneal specimen (91.11-91.19)*
*phlebography of:*
*intra-abdominal vessels NEC (88.65)*
*portal venous system (88.64)*
*sinogram of abdominal wall (88.03)*
*soft tissue x-ray of abdominal wall NEC (88.09)*
*tomography of abdomen NEC (88.02)*
*ultrasonography of abdomen and retroperitoneum (88.76)*

**54.3** **Excision or destruction of lesion or tissue of abdominal wall or umbilicus**
Debridement of abdominal wall
Omphalectomy
**EXCLUDES** *biopsy of abdominal wall or umbilicus (54.22)*
*size reduction operation (86.83)*
*that of skin of abdominal wall (86.22, 86.26, 86.3)*

AHA: 1Q, '89, 11

**54.4** **Excision or destruction of peritoneal tissue**
Excision of:
appendices epiploicae
falciform ligament
gastrocolic ligament
lesion of:
mesentery
omentum
peritoneum
presacral lesion NOS
retroperitoneal lesion NOS
**EXCLUDES** *biopsy of peritoneum (54.23)*
*endometrectomy of cul-de-sac (70.32)*

√4ᵗʰ **54.5** **Lysis of peritoneal adhesions**
Freeing of adhesions of:
biliary tract
intestines
liver
pelvic peritoneum
peritoneum
spleen
uterus
**EXCLUDES** *lysis of adhesions of:*
*bladder (59.11)*
*fallopian tube and ovary (65.81, 65.89)*
*kidney (59.02)*
*ureter (59.02-59.03)*

AHA: 3Q, '94, 8; 4Q, '90, 18

**54.51** **Laparoscopic lysis of peritoneal adhesions**
AHA: ▶4Q, '06, 134;◀ 3Q, '03, 6-7; 4Q, '96, 65

**54.59** **Other lysis of peritoneal adhesions**
AHA: ▶3Q, '06, 15;◀ 3Q, '03, 11; 1Q, '03, 14; 4Q, '96, 66

√4ᵗʰ **54.6** **Suture of abdominal wall and peritoneum**
**54.61** **Reclosure of postoperative disruption of abdominal wall**
**54.62** **Delayed closure of granulating abdominal wound**
Tertiary subcutaneous wound closure

DEF: Closure of outer layers of abdominal wound; follows procedure to close initial layers of wound.

**54.63** **Other suture of abdominal wall**
Suture of laceration of abdominal wall
**EXCLUDES** *closure of operative wound — omit code*

**54.64** **Suture of peritoneum**
Secondary suture of peritoneum
**EXCLUDES** *closure of operative wound — omit code*

√4ᵗʰ **54.7** **Other repair of abdominal wall and peritoneum**
**54.71** **Repair of gastroschisis**
AHA: 2Q, '02, 9

DEF: Repair of congenital fistula of abdominal wall.

**54.72** **Other repair of abdominal wall**
**54.73** **Other repair of peritoneum**
Suture of gastrocolic ligament

**54.74**   **Other repair of omentum**
Epiplorrhaphy
Graft of omentum
Omentopexy
Reduction of torsion of omentum

> **EXCLUDES**   cardio-omentopexy (36.39)

**AHA:** J-F, '87, 11

DEF: Epiplorrhaphy: Suture of abdominal serous membrane.

DEF: Graft of omentum: Implantation of tissue into abdominal serous membrane.

DEF: Omentopexy: Anchoring of abdominal serous membrane.

DEF: Reduction of torsion of omentum: Reduction of twisted abdominal serous membrane.

**54.75**   **Other repair of mesentery**
Mesenteric plication
Mesenteropexy

DEF: Creation of folds in mesentery for shortening.

DEF: Mesenteriopexy: Fixation of torn, incised mesentery.

**✓4ᵗʰ 54.9**   **Other operations of abdominal region**

> **EXCLUDES**   removal of ectopic pregnancy (74.3)

**54.91**   **Percutaneous abdominal drainage**
Paracentesis

> **EXCLUDES**   creation of cutaneoperitoneal fistula (54.93)

**AHA:** 3Q, '99, 9; 2Q, '99, 14; 3Q, '98, 12; 1Q, '92, 14; 2Q, '90, 25

DEF: Puncture for removal of fluid.

**54.92**   **Removal of foreign body from peritoneal cavity**

**AHA:** 1Q, '89, 11

**54.93**   **Creation of cutaneoperitoneal fistula**

**AHA:** 2Q, '95, 10; N-D, '84, 6

DEF: Creation of opening between skin and peritoneal cavity.

**54.94**   **Creation of peritoneovascular shunt**
Peritoneovenous shunt

**AHA:** 1Q, '94, 7; 1Q, '88, 9; S-O, '85, 6

DEF: Peritoneal vascular shunt: Construction of shunt to connect peritoneal cavity with vascular system.

DEF: Peritoneovenous shunt: Construction of shunt to connect peritoneal cavity with vein.

**54.95**   **Incision of peritoneum**
Exploration of ventriculoperitoneal shunt at peritoneal site
Ladd operation
Revision of distal catheter of ventricular shunt
Revision of ventriculoperitoneal shunt at peritoneal site

> **EXCLUDES**   that incidental to laparotomy (54.11-54.19)

**AHA:** 4Q, '95, 65

DEF: Ladd operation: Peritoneal attachment of incompletely rotated cecum, obstructing duodenum.

**54.96**   **Injection of air into peritoneal cavity**
Pneumoperitoneum

> **EXCLUDES**   that for:
> collapse of lung (33.33)
> radiography (88.12-88.13, 88.15)

**54.97**   **Injection of locally-acting therapeutic substance into peritoneal cavity**

> **EXCLUDES**   peritoneal dialysis (54.98)

**54.98**   **Peritoneal dialysis**

> **EXCLUDES**   peritoneal lavage (diagnostic) (54.25)

**AHA:** 4Q, '93, 28; N-D, '84, 6

DEF: Separation of blood elements by diffusion through membrane.

**54.99**   **Other**

> **EXCLUDES**   removal of:
> abdominal wall sutures (97.83)
> peritoneal drainage device (97.82)
> retroperitoneal drainage device (97.81)

**AHA:** 1Q, '99, 4

**BI** Bilateral Procedure    **NC** Non-covered Procedure    **LC** Limited Coverage Procedure    ▶◀ Revised Text    ● New Code    ▲ Revised Code Title

138 — Volume 3

© 2007 Ingenix

## 10. OPERATIONS ON THE URINARY SYSTEM (55-59)

### ✓3rd 55 Operations on kidney

INCLUDES operations on renal pelvis

Code also any application or administration of an adhesion barrier substance (99.77)

EXCLUDES perirenal tissue (59.00-59.09, 59.21-59.29, 59.91-59.92)

#### ✓4th 55.0 Nephrotomy and nephrostomy

EXCLUDES drainage by:
anastomosis (55.86)
aspiration (55.92)

**55.01 Nephrotomy**
Evacuation of renal cyst
Exploration of kidney
Nephrolithotomy

DEF: Nephrotomy: Incision into kidney.

DEF: Evacuation of renal cyst: Draining contents of cyst.

DEF: Exploration of kidney: Exploration through incision.

DEF: Nephrolithotomy: Removal of kidney stone through incision.

**55.02 Nephrostomy**
AHA: 2Q, '97, 4

**55.03 Percutaneous nephrostomy without fragmentation**
Nephrostolithotomy, percutaneous (nephroscopic)
Percutaneous removal of kidney stone(s) by:
forceps extraction (nephroscopic)
basket extraction
Pyelostolithotomy, percutaneous (nephroscopic)
With placement of catheter down ureter

EXCLUDES percutaneous removal by fragmentation (55.04)
repeat nephroscopic removal during current episode (55.92)

AHA: 2Q, '96, 5

DEF: Insertion of tube through abdominal wall without breaking up stones.

DEF: Nephrostolithotomy: Insertion of tube through the abdominal wall to remove stones.

DEF: Basket extraction: Removal, percutaneous of stone with grasping forceps.

DEF: Pyelostolithotomy: Removal, percutaneous of stones from funnel-shaped portion of kidney.

**55.04 Percutaneous nephrostomy with fragmentation**
Percutaneous nephrostomy with disruption of kidney stone by ultrasonic energy and extraction (suction) through endoscope
With placement of catheter down ureter
With fluoroscopic guidance

EXCLUDES repeat fragmentation during current episode (59.95)

AHA: 1Q, '89, 1; S-O, '86, 11

DEF: Insertion of tube through abdominal wall into kidney to break up stones.

#### ✓4th 55.1 Pyelotomy and pyelostomy

EXCLUDES drainage by anastomosis (55.86)
percutaneous pyelostolithotomy (55.03)
removal of calculus without incision (56.0)

**55.11 Pyelotomy**
Exploration of renal pelvis
Pyelolithotomy

**55.12 Pyelostomy**
Insertion of drainage tube into renal pelvis

#### ✓4th 55.2 Diagnostic procedures on kidney

**55.21 Nephroscopy**
DEF: Endoscopic exam of renal pelvis; retrograde through ureter, percutaneous or open exposure.

**55.22 Pyeloscopy**
DEF: Fluoroscopic exam of kidney pelvis, calyces and ureters; follows IV or retrograde injection of contrast.

**55.23 Closed [percutaneous] [needle] biopsy of kidney**
Endoscopic biopsy via existing nephrostomy, nephrotomy, pyelostomy, or pyelotomy

**55.24 Open biopsy of kidney**

**55.29 Other diagnostic procedures on kidney**

EXCLUDES microscopic examination of specimen from kidney (91.21-91.29)
pyelogram:
intravenous (87.73)
percutaneous (87.75)
retrograde (87.74)
radioisotope scan (92.03)
renal arteriography (88.45)
tomography:
C.A.T scan (87.71)
other (87.72)

#### ✓4th 55.3 Local excision or destruction of lesion or tissue of kidney

**55.31 Marsupialization of kidney lesion**
DEF: Exteriorization of lesion by incising anterior wall and suturing cut edges to create open pouch.

**55.32 Open ablation of renal lesion or tissue**
AHA: ▶4Q, '06, 124◀

**55.33 Percutaneous ablation of renal lesion or tissue**
AHA: ▶4Q, '06, 124◀

**55.34 Laparoscopic ablation of renal lesion or tissue**
AHA: ▶4Q, '06, 124◀

**55.35 Other and unspecified ablation of renal lesion or tissue**
AHA: ▶4Q, '06, 124◀

**55.39 Other local destruction or excision of renal lesion or tissue**
Obliteration of calyceal diverticulum

EXCLUDES ablation of renal lesion or tissue:
laparoscopic (55.34)
open (55.32)
other (55.35)
percutaneous (55.33)
biopsy of kidney (55.23-55.24)
partial nephrectomy (55.4)
percutaneous aspiration of kidney (55.92)
wedge resection of kidney (55.4)

### 55.4 Partial nephrectomy
Calycectomy
Wedge resection of kidney
Code also any synchronous resection of ureter (56.40-56.42)

DEF: Surgical removal of a part of the kidney.

DEF: Calycectomy: Removal of indentations in kidney.

---

**Operations on the Urinary System**

**55.5–56.2**

✓4ᵗʰ **55.5** **Complete nephrectomy**

Code also any synchronous excision of:
adrenal gland (07.21-07.3)
bladder segment (57.6)
lymph nodes (40.3, 40.52-40.59)

**55.51** **Nephroureterectomy**

Nephroureterectomy with bladder cuff
Total nephrectomy (unilateral)

**EXCLUDES** *removal of transplanted
kidney (55.53)*

AHA: 2Q, '05, 4

DEF: Complete removal of the kidney and all or portion of
the ureter.

DEF: Nephroureterectomy with bladder cuff: Removal of
kidney, ureter, and portion of bladder attached to ureter.

DEF: Total nephrectomy (unilateral): Complete excision of
one kidney.

**55.52** **Nephrectomy of remaining kidney**

Removal of solitary kidney

**EXCLUDES** *removal of transplanted
kidney (55.53)*

**55.53** **Removal of transplanted or rejected kidney**

**55.54** **Bilateral nephrectomy**

**EXCLUDES** *complete nephrectomy NOS
(55.51)*

DEF: Removal of both kidneys same operative session.

✓4ᵗʰ **55.6** **Transplant of kidney**

Note: To report donor source — see codes 00.91-
00.93

**55.61** **Renal autotransplantation**

**55.69** **Other kidney transplantation**    LC

AHA: 4Q, '04, 117; 4Q, '96, 71

**55.7** **Nephropexy**

Fixation or suspension of movable [floating] kidney

✓4ᵗʰ **55.8** **Other repair of kidney**

**55.81** **Suture of laceration of kidney**

**55.82** **Closure of nephrostomy and pyelostomy**

DEF: Removal of tube from kidney and closure of site of
tube insertion.

**55.83** **Closure of other fistula of kidney**

**55.84** **Reduction of torsion of renal pedicle**

DEF: Restoration of twisted renal pedicle into normal
position.

**55.85** **Symphysiotomy for horseshoe kidney**

DEF: Division of congenitally malformed kidney into two
parts.

**55.86** **Anastomosis of kidney**

Nephropyeloureterostomy
Pyeloureterovesical anastomosis
Ureterocalyceal anastomosis

**EXCLUDES** *nephrocystanastomosis NOS
(56.73)*

DEF: Nephropyeloureterostomy: Creation of passage
between kidney and ureter.

DEF: Pyeloureterovesical anastomosis: Creation of
passage between kidney and bladder.

DEF: Ureterocalyceal anastomosis: Creation of passage
between ureter and kidney indentations.

**55.87** **Correction of ureteropelvic junction**

**55.89** **Other**

✓4ᵗʰ **55.9** **Other operations on kidney**

**EXCLUDES** *lysis of perirenal adhesions (59.02)*

**55.91** **Decapsulation of kidney**

Capsulectomy ⎫
Decortication ⎬ of kidney
       ⎭

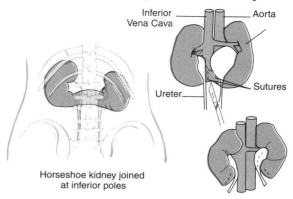

**Symphysiostomy for Horseshoe Kidney**

Inferior Vena Cava — Aorta

Ureter — Sutures

Horseshoe kidney joined
at inferior poles

**55.92** **Percutaneous aspiration of kidney (pelvis)**

Aspiration of renal cyst    Renipuncture

**EXCLUDES** *percutaneous biopsy of kidney
(55.23)*

AHA: N-D, '84, 20

DEF: Insertion of needle into kidney to withdraw fluid.

**55.93** **Replacement of nephrostomy tube**

**55.94** **Replacement of pyelostomy tube**

**55.95** **Local perfusion of kidney**

DEF: Fluid passage through kidney.

**55.96** **Other injection of therapeutic substance
into kidney**

Injection into renal cyst

**55.97** **Implantation or replacement of mechanical
kidney**

**55.98** **Removal of mechanical kidney**

**55.99** **Other**

**EXCLUDES** *removal of pyelostomy or
nephrostomy tube
(97.61)*

✓3ʳᵈ **56** **Operations on ureter**

Code also any application or administration of an adhesion
barrier substance (99.77)

**56.0** **Transurethral removal of obstruction from ureter
and renal pelvis**

Removal of:
blood clot    ⎫
calculus     ⎬ from ureter or renal pelvis
foreign body ⎭     without incision

**EXCLUDES** *manipulation without removal of
obstruction (59.8)
that by incision (55.11,56.2)
transurethral insertion of ureteral stent
for passage of calculus (59.8)*

AHA: 1Q, '89, 1; S-O, '86, 12

DEF: Removal of obstruction by tube inserted through urethra to
ureter.

**56.1** **Ureteral meatotomy**

DEF: Incision into ureteral meatus to enlarge passage.

**56.2** **Ureterotomy**

Incision of ureter for:   Incision of ureter for:
drainage            removal of calculus
exploration

**EXCLUDES** *cutting of ureterovesical orifice (56.1)
removal of calculus without incision
(56.0)
transurethral insertion of ureteral stent
for passage of calculus (59.8)
urinary diversion (56.51-56.79)*

AHA: S-O, '86, 10

---

✓4th **56.3** **Diagnostic procedures on ureter**

**56.31** **Ureteroscopy**

**56.32** **Closed percutaneous biopsy of ureter**
EXCLUDES *endoscopic biopsy of ureter (56.33)*

**56.33** **Closed endoscopic biopsy of ureter**
Cystourethroscopy with ureteral biopsy
Transurethral biopsy of ureter
Ureteral endoscopy with biopsy through ureterotomy
Ureteroscopy with biopsy
EXCLUDES *percutaneous biopsy of ureter (56.32)*

**56.34** **Open biopsy of ureter**

**56.35** **Endoscopy (cystoscopy) (looposcopy) of ileal conduit**
DEF: Endoscopic exam of created opening between ureters and one end of small intestine; other end used to form artificial opening.

**56.39** **Other diagnostic procedures on ureter**
EXCLUDES *microscopic examination of specimen from ureter (91.21-91.29)*

✓4th **56.4** **Ureterectomy**
Code also anastomosis other than end-to-end (56.51-56.79)
EXCLUDES *fistulectomy (56.84)*
*nephroureterectomy (55.51-55.54)*

**56.40** **Ureterectomy, not otherwise specified**

**56.41** **Partial ureterotomy**
Excision of lesion of ureter
Shortening of ureter with reimplantation
EXCLUDES *biopsy of ureter (56.32-56.34)*

**56.42** **Total ureterectomy**

✓4th **56.5** **Cutaneous uretero-ileostomy**

**56.51** **Formation of cutaneous uretero-ileostomy**
Construction of ileal conduit
External ureteral ileostomy
Formation of open ileal bladder
Ileal loop operation
Ileoureterostomy (Bricker's) (ileal bladder)
Transplantation of ureter into ileum with external diversion
EXCLUDES *closed ileal bladder (57.87)*
*replacement of ureteral defect by ileal segment (56.89)*

DEF: Creation of urinary passage by connecting the terminal end of small intestine to ureter then connected to opening through abdominal wall.

DEF: Construction of ileal conduit: Formation of conduit from terminal end of small intestine.

**56.52** **Revision of cutaneous uretero-ileostomy**
AHA: 3Q, '96, 15; 4Q, '88, 7

✓4th **56.6** **Other external urinary diversion**

**56.61** **Formation of other cutaneous ureterostomy**
Anastomosis of ureter to skin
Ureterostomy NOS

**56.62** **Revision of other cutaneous ureterostomy**
Revision of ureterostomy stoma
EXCLUDES *nonoperative removal of ureterostomy tube (97.62)*

✓4th **56.7** **Other anastomosis or bypass of ureter**
EXCLUDES *ureteropyelostomy (55.86)*

**56.71** **Urinary diversion to intestine**
Anastomosis of ureter to intestine
Internal urinary diversion NOS
Code also any synchronous colostomy (46.10-46.13)
EXCLUDES *external ureteral ileostomy (56.51)*

**56.72** **Revision of ureterointestinal anastomosis**
EXCLUDES *revision of external ureteral ileostomy (56.52)*

**56.73** **Nephrocystanastomosis, not otherwise specified**
DEF: Connection of kidney to bladder.

**56.74** **Ureteroneocystostomy**
Replacement of ureter with bladder flap
Ureterovesical anastomosis
DEF: Transfer of ureter to another site in bladder.
DEF: Ureterovesical anastomosis: Implantation of ureter into bladder.

**56.75** **Transureteroureterostomy**
EXCLUDES *ureteroureterostomy associated with partial resection (56.41)*
DEF: Separating one ureter and joining the ends to the opposite ureter.

**56.79** **Other**

✓4th **56.8** **Repair of ureter**

**56.81** **Lysis of intraluminal adhesions of ureter**
EXCLUDES *lysis of periureteral adhesions (59.01-59.02)*
*ureterolysis (59.02-59.03)*
DEF: Destruction of adhesions within urethral cavity.

**56.82** **Suture of laceration of ureter**

**56.83** **Closure of ureterostomy**

**56.84** **Closure of other fistula of ureter**

**56.85** **Ureteropexy**

**56.86** **Removal of ligature from ureter**

**56.89** **Other repair of ureter**
Graft of ureter
Replacement of ureter with ileal segment implanted into bladder
Ureteroplication
DEF: Graft of ureter: Tissue from another site for graft replacement or repair of ureter.
DEF: Replacement of ureter with ileal segment implanted into bladder and ureter replacement with terminal end of small intestine.
DEF: Ureteroplication: Creation of tucks in ureter.

✓4th **56.9** **Other operations on ureter**

**56.91** **Dilation of ureteral meatus**

**56.92** **Implantation of electronic ureteral stimulator**

**56.93** **Replacement of electronic ureteral stimulator**

**56.94** **Removal of electronic ureteral stimulator**
EXCLUDES *that with synchronous replacement (56.93)*

**56.95** **Ligation of ureter**

**56.99** **Other**
EXCLUDES *removal of ureterostomy tube and ureteral catheter (97.62)*
*ureteral catheterization (59.8)*

✓3rd **57** **Operations on urinary bladder**
Code also any application or administration of an adhesion barrier substance (99.77)
EXCLUDES *perivesical tissue (59.11-59.29, 59.91-59.92)*
*ureterovesical orifice (56.0-56.99)*

**57.0** **Transurethral clearance of bladder**
Drainage of bladder without incision
Removal of:
blood clot
calculus } from bladder without incision
foreign body
EXCLUDES *that by incision (57.19)*
AHA: S-O, '86, 11
DEF: Insertion of device through urethra to cleanse bladder.

✓3rd
✓4th Additional Digit Required
Valid OR Procedure
Non-OR Procedure
Adjunct Code
© 2007 Ingenix
October 2007 • Volume 3 — 141

Operations on the Urinary System

56.3–57.0

**Operations on the Urinary System**

**57.1–57.6**

✓4ᵗʰ **57.1**   **Cystotomy and cystostomy**

> EXCLUDES   *cystotomy and cystostomy as operative approach — omit code*

DEF: Cystotomy: Incision of bladder.

DEF: Cystostomy: Creation of opening into bladder.

**57.11**   **Percutaneous aspiration of bladder**

**57.12**   **Lysis of intraluminal adhesions with incision into bladder**

> EXCLUDES   *transurethral lysis of intraluminal adhesions (57.41)*

DEF: Incision into bladder to destroy lesions.

**57.17**   **Percutaneous cystostomy**

Closed cystostomy
Percutaneous suprapubic cystostomy

> EXCLUDES   *removal of cystostomy tube (97.63)*
> *replacement of cystostomy tube (59.94)*

DEF: Incision through body wall into bladder to insert tube.

DEF: Percutaneous (closed) suprapubic cystostomy: Incision above pubic arch, through body wall, into the bladder to insert tube.

**57.18**   **Other suprapubic cystostomy**

> EXCLUDES   *percutaneous cystostomy (57.17)*
> *removal of cystostomy tube (97.63)*
> *replacement of cystostomy tube (59.94)*

**57.19**   **Other cystotomy**

Cystolithotomy

> EXCLUDES   *percutaneous cystostomy (57.17)*
> *suprapubic cystostomy (57.18)*

AHA: 4Q, '95, 73; S-O, '86, 11

✓4ᵗʰ **57.2**   **Vesicostomy**

> EXCLUDES   *percutaneous cystostomy (57.17)*
> *suprapubic cystostomy (57.18)*

**57.21**   **Vesicostomy**

Creation of permanent opening from bladder to skin using a bladder flap

DEF: Creation of permanent opening from the bladder to the skin.

**57.22**   **Revision or closure of vesicostomy**

> EXCLUDES   *closure of cystostomy (57.82)*

✓4ᵗʰ **57.3**   **Diagnostic procedures on bladder**

**57.31**   **Cystoscopy through artificial stoma**

**57.32**   **Other cystoscopy**

Transurethral cystoscopy

> EXCLUDES   *cystourethroscopy with ureteral biopsy (56.33)*
> *retrograde pyelogram (87.74)*
> *that for control of hemorrhage (postoperative):*
> *bladder (57.93)*
> *prostate (60.94)*

AHA: 1Q, '01, 14

**57.33**   **Closed [transurethral] biopsy of bladder**

**57.34**   **Open biopsy of bladder**

AHA: 2Q, '05, 12

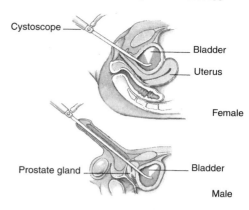

**Transurethral Cystourethroscopy**

Cystoscope — Bladder / Uterus / Female

Prostate gland — Bladder / Male

**57.39**   **Other diagnostic procedures on bladder**

> EXCLUDES   *cystogram NEC (87.77)*
> *microscopic examination of specimen from bladder (91.31-91.39)*
> *retrograde cystourethrogram (87.76)*
> *therapeutic distention of bladder (96.25)*

✓4ᵗʰ **57.4**   **Transurethral excision or destruction of bladder tissue**

DEF: Destruction of bladder tissue with instrument inserted into urethra.

**57.41**   **Transurethral lysis of intraluminal adhesions**

**57.49**   **Other transurethral excision or destruction of lesion or tissue of bladder**

Endoscopic resection of bladder lesion

> EXCLUDES   *transurethral biopsy of bladder (57.33)*
> *transurethral fistulectomy (57.83-57.84)*

✓4ᵗʰ **57.5**   **Other excision or destruction of bladder tissue**

> EXCLUDES   *that with transurethral approach (57.41-57.49)*

**57.51**   **Excision of urachus**

Excision of urachal sinus of bladder

> EXCLUDES   *excision of urachal cyst of abdominal wall (54.3)*

**57.59**   **Open excision or destruction of other lesion or tissue of bladder**

Endometrectomy of bladder
Suprapubic excision of bladder lesion

> EXCLUDES   *biopsy of bladder (57.33-57.34)*
> *fistulectomy of bladder (57.83-57.84)*

DEF: Endometrectomy of bladder: Removal of inner lining.

DEF: Suprapubic excision of bladder lesion: Removal of lesion by excision above suprapubic bone arch.

**57.6**   **Partial cystectomy**

Excision of bladder dome
Trigonectomy
Wedge resection of bladder

BI Bilateral Procedure     NC Non-covered Procedure     LC Limited Coverage Procedure     ▶◀ Revised Text     ● New Code     ▲ Revised Code Title

**142 — Volume 3**

© 2007 Ingenix

√4ᵗʰ **57.7**    **Total cystectomy**

     INCLUDES    total cystectomy with urethrectomy

     **57.71**    **Radical cystectomy**

         Pelvic exenteration in male

         Removal of bladder, prostate, seminal vesicles and fat

         Removal of bladder, urethra, and fat in a female

         Code also any:

            lymph node dissection (40.3, 40.5)

            urinary diversion (56.51-56.79)

         EXCLUDES   that as part of pelvic exenteration in female (68.8)

         DEF: Radical cystectomy: Removal of bladder and surrounding tissue.

         DEF: Pelvic exenteration in male: Excision of bladder, prostate, seminal vessels and fat.

     **57.79**    **Other total cystectomy**

√4ᵗʰ **57.8**   **Other repair of urinary bladder**

         EXCLUDES   repair of:

            current obstetric laceration (75.61)

            cystocele (70.50-70.51)

            that for stress incontinence (59.3-59.79)

     **57.81**    **Suture of laceration of bladder**

     **57.82**    **Closure of cystostomy**

     **57.83**    **Repair of fistula involving bladder and intestine**

         Rectovesicovaginal      ⎫

         Vesicosigmoidovaginal  ⎬ fistulectomy

     **57.84**    **Repair of other fistula of bladder**

         Cervicovesical          ⎫

         Urethroperineovesical  ⎬

         Uterovesical            ⎬ fistulectomy

         Vaginovesical          ⎭

         EXCLUDES   vesicoureterovaginal fistulectomy (56.84)

     **57.85**    **Cystourethroplasty and plastic repair of bladder neck**

         Plication of sphincter of urinary bladder

         V-Y plasty of bladder neck

         DEF: Cystourethroplasty: Reconstruction of narrowed portion of bladder.

         DEF: Plication of sphincter or urinary bladder: Creation of tuck in bladder sphincter.

         DEF: V-Y plasty of bladder neck: Surgical reconstruction of the narrowed portion of bladder by V-Y technique.

     **57.86**    **Repair of bladder exstrophy**

         DEF: Surgical correction of a congenital bladder wall defect.

     **57.87**    **Reconstruction of urinary bladder**

         Anastomosis of bladder with isolated segment of ileum

         Augmentation of bladder

         Replacement of bladder with ileum or sigmoid [closed ileal bladder]

         Code also resection of intestine (45.50-45.52)

         AHA: 2Q, '05, 12; 2Q, '03, 11; 3Q, '00, 7

         DEF: Anastomosis of bladder with isolated segment of ileum: Creation of connection between bladder and separated terminal end of small intestine.

     **57.88**    **Other anastomosis of bladder**

         Anastomosis of bladder to intestine NOS

         Cystocolic anastomosis

         EXCLUDES   formation of closed ileal bladder (57.87)

     **57.89**    **Other repair of bladder**

         Bladder suspension, not elsewhere classified

         Cystopexy NOS

         Repair of old obstetric laceration of bladder

         EXCLUDES   repair of current obstetric laceration (75.61)

√4ᵗʰ **57.9**   **Other operations on bladder**

     **57.91**    **Sphincterotomy of bladder**

         Division of bladder neck

         AHA: 2Q, '90, 26

     **57.92**    **Dilation of bladder neck**

     **57.93**    **Control of (postoperative) hemorrhage of bladder**

     **57.94**    **Insertion of indwelling urinary catheter**

     **57.95**    **Replacement of indwelling urinary catheter**

     **57.96**    **Implantation of electronic bladder stimulator**   NC

     **57.97**    **Replacement of electronic bladder stimulator**   NC

     **57.98**    **Removal of electronic bladder stimulator**

         EXCLUDES   that with synchronous replacement (57.97)

     **57.99**    **Other**

         EXCLUDES   irrigation of:

            cystostomy (96.47)

            other indwelling urinary catheter (96.48)

         lysis of external adhesions (59.11)

         removal of:

            cystostomy tube (97.63)

            other urinary drainage device (97.64)

         therapeutic distention of bladder (96.25)

√3ʳᵈ **58**   **Operations on urethra**

     INCLUDES   operations on:

         bulbourethral gland [Cowper's gland]

         periurethral tissue

   Code also any application or administration of an adhesion barrier substance (99.77)

     **58.0**    **Urethrotomy**

         Excision of urethral septum

         Formation of urethrovaginal fistula

         Perineal urethrostomy

         Removal of calculus from urethra by incision

         EXCLUDES   drainage of bulbourethral gland or periurethral tissue (58.91)

            internal urethral meatotomy (58.5)

            removal of urethral calculus without incision (58.6)

     **58.1**    **Urethral meatotomy**

         EXCLUDES   internal urethral meatotomy (58.5)

         DEF: Incision of urethra to enlarge passage.

√4ᵗʰ **58.2**   **Diagnostic procedures on urethra**

     **58.21**    **Perineal urethroscopy**

     **58.22**    **Other urethroscopy**

     **58.23**    **Biopsy of urethra**

     **58.24**    **Biopsy of periurethral tissue**

         DEF: Removal for biopsy of tissue around urethra.

     **58.29**    **Other diagnostic procedures on urethra and periurethral tissue**

         EXCLUDES   microscopic examination of specimen from urethra (91.31-91.39)

            retrograde cystourethrogram (87.76)

            urethral pressure profile (89.25)

            urethral sphincter electromyogram (89.23)

**Operations on the Urinary System**

**57.7–58.29**

**Operations on the Urinary System**

**58.3–59.3**

√4ᵗʰ **58.3** **Excision or destruction of lesion or tissue of urethra**

EXCLUDES    biopsy of urethra (58.23)
excision of bulbourethral gland (58.92)
fistulectomy (58.43)
urethrectomy as part of:
complete cystectomy (57.79)
pelvic evisceration (68.8)
radical cystectomy (57.71)

**58.31** **Endoscopic excision or destruction of lesion or tissue of urethra**
Fulguration of urethral lesion

**58.39** **Other local excision or destruction of lesion or tissue of urethra**
Excision of:
congenital valve ⎫
lesion            ⎬ of urethra
stricture         ⎭

Urethrectomy
EXCLUDES    that by endoscopic appoach (58.31)

√4ᵗʰ **58.4** **Repair of urethra**
EXCLUDES    repair of current obstetric laceration (75.61)

**58.41** **Suture of laceration of urethra**

**58.42** **Closure of urethrostomy**

**58.43** **Closure of other fistula of urethra**
EXCLUDES    repair of urethroperineovesical fistula (57.84)

**58.44** **Reanastomosis of urethra**
Anastomosis of urethra
DEF: Repair of severed urethra.

**58.45** **Repair of hypospadias or epispadias**
AHA: 3Q, '97, 6; 4Q, '96, 35
DEF: Repair of abnormal urethral opening.

**58.46** **Other reconstruction of urethra**
Urethral construction

**58.47** **Urethral meatoplasty**
DEF: Reconstruction of urethral opening.

**58.49** **Other repair of urethra**
Benenenti rotation of bulbous urethra
Repair of old obstetric laceration of urethra
Urethral plication
EXCLUDES    repair of:
current obstetric laceration (75.61)
urethrocele (70.50-70.51)

**58.5** **Release of urethral stricture**
Cutting of urethral sphincter
Internal urethral meatotomy
Urethrolysis
AHA: 1Q, '97, 13

**58.6** **Dilation of urethra**
Dilation of urethrovesical junction
Passage of sounds through urethra
Removal of calculus from urethra without incision
EXCLUDES    urethral calibration (89.29)
AHA: 1Q, '01, 14; 1Q, '97, 13

√4ᵗʰ **58.9** **Other operations on urethra and periurethral tissue**

**58.91** **Incision of periurethral tissue**
Drainage of bulbourethral gland
DEF: Incision of tissue around urethra.

**58.92** **Excision of periurethral tissue**
EXCLUDES    biopsy of periurethral tissue (58.24)
lysis of periurethral adhesions (59.11-59.12)

**58.93** **Implantation of artificial urinary sphincter [AUS]**
Placement of inflatable:
urethral sphincter
bladder sphincter
Removal with replacement of sphincter device [AUS]
With pump and/or reservoir

**58.99** **Other**
Repair of inflatable sphincter pump and/or reservoir
Surgical correction of hydraulic pressure of inflatable sphincter device
Removal of inflatable urinary sphincter without replacement
EXCLUDES    removal of:
intraluminal foreign body from urethra without incision (98.19)
urethral stent (97.65)

√3ʳᵈ **59** **Other operations on urinary tract**
Code also any application or administration of an adhesion barrier substance (99.77)

√4ᵗʰ **59.0** **Dissection of retroperitoneal tissue**

**59.00** **Retroperitoneal dissection, not otherwise specified**

**59.02** **Other lysis of perirenal or periureteral adhesions**
EXCLUDES    that by laparoscope (59.03)

**59.03** **Laparoscopic lysis of perirenal or periureteral adhesions**
AHA: ▶4Q, '06, 134◀

**59.09** **Other incision of perirenal or periureteral tissue**
Exploration of perinephric area
Incision of perirenal abscess
DEF: Exploration of the perinephric area: Exam of tissue around the kidney by incision.
DEF: Incision of perirenal abscess: Incising abscess in tissue around kidney.

√4ᵗʰ **59.1** **Incision of perivesical tissue**
DEF: Incising tissue around bladder.

**59.11** **Other lysis of perivesical adhesions**

**59.12** **Laparoscopic lysis of perivesical adhesions**

**59.19** **Other incision of perivesical tissue**
Exploration of perivesical tissue
Incision of hematoma of space of Retzius
Retropubic exploration

√4ᵗʰ **59.2** **Diagnostic procedures on perirenal and perivesical tissue**

**59.21** **Biopsy of perirenal or perivesical tissue**

**59.29** **Other diagnostic procedures on perirenal tissue, perivesical tissue, and retroperitoneum**
EXCLUDES    microscopic examination of specimen from:
perirenal tissue (91.21-91.29)
perivesical tissue (91.31-91.39)
retroperitoneum NEC (91.11-91.19)
retroperitoneal x-ray (88.14-88.16)

**59.3** **Plication of urethrovesical junction**
Kelly-Kennedy operation on urethra
Kelly-Stoeckel urethral plication
DEF: Suturing a tuck in tissues around urethra at junction with bladder; changes angle of junction and provides support.

---

BI Bilateral Procedure        NC Non-covered Procedure        LC Limited Coverage Procedure        ▶◀ Revised Text        ● New Code        ▲ Revised Code Title

**59.4**    **Suprapubic sling operation**
     Goebel-Frangenheim-Stoeckel urethrovesical
       suspension
     Millin-Read urethrovesical suspension
     Oxford operation for urinary incontinence
     Urethrocystopexy by suprapubic suspension

DEF: Suspension of urethra from suprapubic periosteum to restore
support to bladder and urethra.

**59.5**    **Retropubic urethral suspension**
     Burch procedure
     Marshall-Marchetti-Krantz operation
     Suture of periurethral tissue to symphysis pubis
     Urethral suspension NOS

AHA: 1Q, '97, 11

DEF: Suspension of urethra from pubic bone with suture placed
from symphysis pubis to paraurethral tissues; elevates
urethrovesical angle, restores urinary continence.

**59.6**    **Paraurethral suspension**
     Pereyra paraurethral suspension
     Periurethral suspension

DEF: Suspension of bladder neck from fibrous membranes of
anterior abdominal wall; upward traction applied; changes angle of
urethra, improves urinary control.

√4ᵗʰ **59.7**    **Other repair of urinary stress incontinence**

    **59.71**    **Levator muscle operation for urethrovesical suspension**
       Cystourethropexy with levator muscle sling
       Gracilis muscle transplant for
         urethrovesical suspension
       Pubococcygeal sling

    **59.72**    **Injection of implant into urethra and/or bladder neck**
       Collagen implant
       Endoscopic injection of implant
       Fat implant
       Polytef implant

AHA: 4Q, '95, 72, 73

DEF: Injection of collagen into submucosal tissues to
increase tissue bulk and improve urinary control.

    **59.79**    **Other**
       Anterior urethropexy
       Repair of stress incontinence NOS
       Tudor "rabbit ear" urethropexy

AHA: 2Q, '01, 20; 1Q, '00, 14, 15, 19

DEF: Pubovaginal sling for treatment of stress
incontinence: A strip of fascia is harvested and the
vaginal epithelium is mobilized and then sutured to the
midline at the urethral level to the rectus muscle to
create a sling supporting the bladder.

DEF: Vaginal wall sling with bone anchors for treatment
of stress incontinence: A sling for the bladder is formed
by a suture attachment of vaginal wall to the abdominal
wall. In addition, a suture is run from the vagina to a
bone anchor placed in the pubic bone.

DEF: Transvaginal endoscopic bladder neck suspension
for treatment of stress incontinence: Endoscopic surgical
suturing of the vaginal epithelium and the pubocervical
fascia at the bladder neck level on both sides of the
urethra. Two supporting sutures are run from the vagina
to an anchor placed in the pubic bone on each side.

**59.8**    **Ureteral catheterization**
     Drainage of kidney by catheter
     Insertion of ureteral stent
     Ureterovesical orifice dilation
     Code also any ureterotomy (56.2)

     **EXCLUDES**   *that for:*
       *transurethral removal of calculus or*
       *clot from ureter and renal*
       *pelvis (56.0)*
       *retrograde pyelogram (87.74)*

AHA: 2Q, '05, 12; 2Q, '03, 11; 3Q, '00, 7; 1Q, '89, 1; S-O, '86, 10

√4ᵗʰ **59.9**    **Other operations on urinary system**
     **EXCLUDES**   *nonoperative removal of therapeutic*
       *device (97.61-97.69)*

    **59.91**    **Excision of perirenal or perivesical tissue**
       **EXCLUDES**   *biopsy of perirenal or*
         *perivesical tissue (59.21)*

    **59.92**    **Other operations on perirenal or perivesical tissue**

    **59.93**    **Replacement of ureterostomy tube**
       Change of ureterostomy tube
       Reinsertion of ureterostomy tube
       **EXCLUDES**   *nonoperative removal of*
         *ureterostomy tube*
         *(97.62)*

    **59.94**    **Replacement of cystostomy tube**
       **EXCLUDES**   *nonoperative removal of*
         *cystostomy tube (97.63)*

    **59.95**    **Ultrasonic fragmentation of urinary stones**
       Shattered urinary stones
       **EXCLUDES**   *percutaneous nephrostomy*
         *with fragmentation*
         *(55.04)*
         *shockwave disintegration*
         *(98.51)*

AHA: 1Q, '89, 1; S-O, '86, 11

    **59.99**    **Other**
       **EXCLUDES**   *instillation of medication into*
         *urinary tract (96.49)*
         *irrigation of urinary tract*
         *(96.45-96.48)*

**Operations on the Male Genital Organs**

**60–60.79**

## 11. OPERATIONS ON THE MALE GENITAL ORGANS (60-64)

**✓3rd 60   Operations on prostate and seminal vesicles**

Code also any application or administration of an adhesion barrier substance (99.77)

INCLUDES   operations on periprostatic tissue

EXCLUDES   *that associated with radical cystectomy (57.71)*

**60.0   Incision of prostate** ♂

Drainage of prostatic abscess

Prostatolithotomy

EXCLUDES   *drainage of periprostatic tissue only (60.81)*

**✓4th 60.1   Diagnostic procedures on prostate and seminal vesicles**

**60.11   Closed [percutaneous] [needle] biopsy of prostate** ♂

Approach:
     transrectal      Punch biopsy
     transurethral

DEF: Excision of prostate tissue by closed technique for biopsy.

**60.12   Open biopsy of prostate** ♂

**60.13   Closed [percutaneous] biopsy of seminal vesicles** ♂

Needle biopsy of seminal vesicles

**60.14   Open biopsy of seminal vesicles** ♂

**60.15   Biopsy of periprostatic tissue** ♂

**60.18   Other diagnostic procedures on prostate and periprostatic tissue** ♂

EXCLUDES   *microscopic examination of specimen from prostate (91.31-91.39)*
      *x-ray of prostate (87.92)*

**60.19   Other diagnostic procedures on seminal vesicles** ♂

EXCLUDES   *microscopic examination of specimen from seminal vesicles (91.31-91.39)*
      *x-ray:*
        *contrast seminal vesiculogram (87.91)*
        *other (87.92)*

**✓4th 60.2   Transurethral prostatectomy**

EXCLUDES   *local excision of lesion of prostate (60.61)*

AHA: 2Q, '94, 9; 3Q, '92, 13

**60.21   Transurethral (ultrasound) guided laser induced prostatectomy (TULIP)** ♂

Ablation (contact) (noncontact) by laser

AHA: 4Q, '95, 7

**60.29   Other transurethral prostatectomy** ♂

Excision of median bar by transurethral approach

Transurethral electrovaporization of prostate (TEVAP)

Transurethral enucleative procedure

Transurethral prostatectomy NOS

Transurethral resection of prostate (TURP)

DEF: Excision of median bar by transurethral approach: Removal of fibrous structure of prostate.

DEF: Transurethral enucleative procedure: Transurethral prostatectomy.

AHA: 3Q, '97, 3

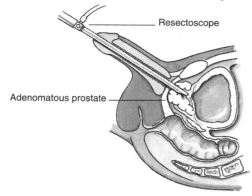

**Transurethral Prostatectomy**

Resectoscope

Adenomatous prostate

**60.3   Suprapubic prostatectomy** ♂

Transvesical prostatectomy

EXCLUDES   *local excision of lesion of prostate (60.61)*
      *radical prostatectomy (60.5)*

DEF: Resection of prostate through incision in abdomen above pubic arch.

**60.4   Retropubic prostatectomy** ♂

EXCLUDES   *local excision of lesion of prostate (60.61)*
      *radical prostatectomy (60.5)*

DEF: Removal of the prostate using an abdominal approach with direct cutting into prostatic capsule.

**60.5   Radical prostatectomy** ♂

Prostatovesiculectomy

Radical prostatectomy by any approach

EXCLUDES   *cystoprostatectomy (57.71)*

AHA: 3Q, '93, 12

DEF: Removal of prostate, epididymis and vas ampullae.

DEF: Prostatovesiculectomy: Removal of prostate and epididymis.

**✓4th 60.6   Other prostatectomy**

**60.61   Local excision of lesion of prostate** ♂

Excision of prostatic lesion by any approach

EXCLUDES   *biopsy of prostate (60.11-60.12)*

**60.62   Perineal prostatectomy** ♂

Cryoablation of prostate

Cryoprostatectomy

Cryosurgery of prostate

Radical cryosurcial ablation of prostate (RCSA)

EXCLUDES   *local excision of lesion of prostate (60.61)*

AHA: 4Q, '95, 71

DEF: Excision of prostate tissue through incision between scrotum and anus.

**60.69   Other** ♂

**✓4th 60.7   Operations on seminal vesicles**

**60.71   Percutaneous aspiration of seminal vesicle** ♂

EXCLUDES   *needle biopsy of seminal vesicle (60.13)*

**60.72   Incision of seminal vesicle** ♂

**60.73   Excision of seminal vesicle** ♂

Excision of Müllerian duct cyst

Spermatocystectomy

EXCLUDES   *biopsy of seminal vesicle (60.13-60.14)*
      *prostatovesiculectomy (60.5)*

**60.79   Other operations on seminal vesicles** ♂

BI Bilateral Procedure      NC Non-covered Procedure      LC Limited Coverage Procedure      ►◄ Revised Text      ● New Code      ▲ Revised Code Title

146 — Volume 3

© 2007 Ingenix

✓4th **60.8**  **Incision or excision of periprostatic tissue**

**60.81**  **Incision of periprostatic tissue**  ♂
Drainage of periprostatic abscess

**60.82**  **Excision of periprostatic tissue**  ♂
Excision of lesion of periprostatic tissue
**EXCLUDES**  *biopsy of periprostatic tissue (60.15)*

✓4th **60.9**  **Other operations on prostate**

**60.91**  **Percutaneous aspiration of prostate**  ♂
**EXCLUDES**  *needle biopsy of prostate (60.11)*

**60.92**  **Injection into prostate**  ♂

**60.93**  **Repair of prostate**  ♂

**60.94**  **Control of (postoperative) hemorrhage of prostate**  ♂
Coagulation of prostatic bed
Cystoscopy for control of prostatic hemorrhage

**60.95**  **Transurethral balloon dilation of the prostatic urethra**  ♂
**AHA:** 4Q, '91, 23

DEF: Insertion and inflation of balloon to stretch prostate passage.

**60.96**  **Transurethral destruction of prostate tissue by microwave thermotherapy**  ♂
Transurethral microwave thermotherapy (TUMT) of prostate
**EXCLUDES**  *Prostatectomy:*
*other (60.61-60.69)*
*radical (60.5)*
*retropubic (60.4)*
*suprapubic (60.3)*
*transurethral (60.21-60.29)*

**AHA:** 4Q, '00, 67

**60.97**  **Other transurethral destruction of prostate tissue by other thermotherapy**  ♂
Radiofrequency thermotherapy
Transurethral needle ablation (TUNA) of prostate
**EXCLUDES**  *Prostatectomy:*
*other (60.61-60.69)*
*radical (60.5)*
*retropubic (60.4)*
*suprapubic (60.3)*
*transurethral (60.21-60.29)*

**AHA:** 4Q, '00, 67

**60.99**  **Other**  ♂
**EXCLUDES**  *prostatic massage (99.94)*
**AHA:** 3Q, '90, 12

✓3rd **61**  **Operations on scrotum and tunica vaginalis**

**61.0**  **Incision and drainage of scrotum and tunica vaginalis**  ♂
**EXCLUDES**  *percutaneous aspiration of hydrocele (61.91)*

✓4th **61.1**  **Diagnostic procedures on scrotum and tunica vaginalis**

**61.11**  **Biopsy of scrotum or tunica vaginalis**  ♂

**61.19**  **Other diagnostic procedures on scrotum and tunica vaginalis**  ♂

**61.2**  **Excision of hydrocele (of tunica vaginalis)**  ♂
Bottle repair of hydrocele of tunica vaginalis
**EXCLUDES**  *percutaneous aspiration of hydrocele (61.91)*

DEF: Removal of fluid collected in serous membrane of testes.

**Hydrocelectomy**

Scrotal skin incised
Sac opened
Fluid-filled sac mobilized
Excess tissue trimmed
Testis
Remaining sacular tissue folded back and sewn to itself to preclude recurrence ("bottle" procedure)

**61.3**  **Excision or destruction of lesion or tissue of scrotum**  ♂
Fulguration of lesion
Reduction of elephantiasis } of scrotum
Partial scrotectomy
**EXCLUDES**  *biopsy of scrotum (61.11)*
*scrotal fistulectomy (61.42)*

✓4th **61.4**  **Repair of scrotum and tunica vaginalis**

**61.41**  **Suture of laceration of scrotum and tunica vaginalis**  ♂

**61.42**  **Repair of scrotal fistula**  ♂

**61.49**  **Other repair of scrotum and tunica vaginalis**  ♂
Reconstruction with rotational or pedicle flaps

✓4th **61.9**  **Other operations on scrotum and tunica vaginalis**

**61.91**  **Percutaneous aspiration of tunica vaginalis**  ♂
Aspiration of hydrocele of tunica vaginalis

**61.92**  **Excision of lesion of tunica vaginalis other than hydrocele**  ♂
Excision of hematocele of tunica vaginalis
DEF: Removal of blood collected in tunica vaginalis.

**61.99**  **Other**  ♂
**EXCLUDES**  *removal of foreign body from scrotum without incision (98.24)*

✓3rd **62**  **Operations on testes**

**62.0**  **Incision of testis**  ♂

✓4th **62.1**  **Diagnostic procedures on testes**

**62.11**  **Closed [percutaneous] [needle] biopsy of testis**  ♂

**62.12**  **Open biopsy of testis**  ♂

**62.19**  **Other diagnostic procedures on testes**  ♂

**62.2**  **Excision or destruction of testicular lesion**  ♂
Excision of appendix testis
Excision of cyst of Morgagni in the male
Excision of hydatid of Morgagni in the male
**EXCLUDES**  *biopsy of testis (62.11-62.12)*

**62.3**  **Unilateral orchiectomy**  ♂
Orchidectomy (with epididymectomy) NOS

✓4th **62.4**  **Bilateral orchiectomy**
Male castration
Radical bilateral orchiectomy (with epididymectomy)
Code also any synchronous lymph node dissection (40.3, 40.5)

DEF: Removal of both testes.

DEF: Radical bilateral orchiectomy (with epididymectomy): Excision of both testes and structures that store sperm.

**62.41**  **Removal of both testes at same operative episode**  ♂
Bilateral orchidectomy NOS

**62.42**  **Removal of remaining testis**  ♂
Removal of solitary testis

**Operations on the Male Genital Organs**

**62.5–63.89**

▶Orchiopexy with Detorsion of Testes◀

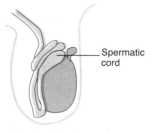

Torsion of testis

Spermatic cord

Testes after correction showing bilateral fixation

Varicocelectomy

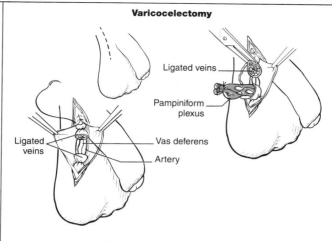

Ligated veins

Pampiniform plexus

Ligated veins

Vas deferens

Artery

**62.5**    **Orchiopexy**    ♂
Mobilization and replacement of testis in scrotum
Orchiopexy with detorsion of testis
Torek (-Bevan) operation (orchidopexy) (first stage) (second stage)
Transplantation to and fixation of testis in scrotum
DEF: Fixation of testis in scrotum.

DEF: Orchiopexy with detorsion of testis: Fixation and placement of testis in scrotum after correcting angle.

DEF: Torek operation (first stage) (second stage): Transfer of congenitally undescended testis from inguinal canal to scrotum.

DEF: Transplantation to and fixation of testis in scrotum: Transfer of displaced testis to scrotum.

✓4ᵗʰ **62.6**    **Repair of testes**
     **EXCLUDES**   *reduction of torsion (63.52)*
   **62.61**    **Suture of laceration of testis**    ♂
   **62.69**    **Other repair of testis**    ♂
       Testicular graft

**62.7**    **Insertion of testicular prosthesis**    ♂

✓4ᵗʰ **62.9**    **Other operations on testes**
   **62.91**    **Aspiration of testis**    ♂
       **EXCLUDES**   *percutaneous biopsy of testis (62.11)*
   **62.92**    **Injection of therapeutic substance into testis**    ♂
   **62.99**    **Other**    ♂

✓3ʳᵈ **63**    **Operations on spermatic cord, epididymis, and vas deferens**

✓4ᵗʰ **63.0**    **Diagnostic procedures on spermatic cord, epididymis, and vas deferens**
   **63.01**    **Biopsy of spermatic cord, epididymis, or vas deferens**    ♂
   **63.09**    **Other diagnostic procedures on spermatic cord, epididymis, and vas deferens**    ♂
       **EXCLUDES**   *contrast epididymogram (87.93)*
            *contrast vasogram (87.94)*
            *other x-ray of epididymis and vas deferens (87.95)*

**63.1**    **Excision of varicocele and hydrocele of spermatic cord**    ♂
High ligation of spermatic vein
Hydrocelectomy of canal of Nuck
DEF: Removal of a swollen vein and collected fluid from spermatic cord.

DEF: High ligation of spermatic vein: Tying off of spermatic vein.

DEF: Hydrocelectomy of canal of Nuck: Removal of fluid collected from serous membrane of inguinal canal.

**63.2**    **Excision of cyst of epididymis**    ♂
Spermatocelectomy

**63.3**    **Excision of other lesion or tissue of spermatic cord and epididymis**    ♂
Excision of appendix epididymis
     **EXCLUDES**   *biopsy of spermatic cord or epididymis (63.01)*

**63.4**    **Epididymectomy**    ♂
     **EXCLUDES**   *that synchronous with orchiectomy (62.3-62.42)*

✓4ᵗʰ **63.5**    **Repair of spermatic cord and epididymis**
   **63.51**    **Suture of laceration of spermatic cord and epididymis**    ♂
   **63.52**    **Reduction of torsion of testis or spermatic cord**    ♂
       **EXCLUDES**   *that associated with orchiopexy (62.5)*
       DEF: Correction of twisted testicle or spermatic cord.
   **63.53**    **Transplantation of spermatic cord**    ♂
   **63.59**    **Other repair of spermatic cord and epididymis**    ♂

**63.6**    **Vasotomy**    ♂
Vasostomy
DEF: Vasotomy: Incision of ducts carrying sperm from testicles.

DEF: Vasostomy: Creation of an opening into duct.

✓4ᵗʰ **63.7**    **Vasectomy and ligation of vas deferens**
   **63.70**    **Male sterilization procedure, not otherwise specified**    NC ♂
   **63.71**    **Ligation of vas deferens**    NC ♂
       Crushing of vas deferens
       Division of vas deferens
   **63.72**    **Ligation of spermatic cord**    NC ♂
   **63.73**    **Vasectomy**    NC ♂
       AHA: 2Q, '98, 13

✓4ᵗʰ **63.8**    **Repair of vas deferens and epididymis**
   **63.81**    **Suture of laceration of vas deferens and epididymis**    ♂
   **63.82**    **Reconstruction of surgically divided vas deferens**    ♂
   **63.83**    **Epididymovasostomy**    ♂
       DEF: Creation of new connection between vas deferens and epididymis.
   **63.84**    **Removal of ligature from vas deferens**    ♂
   **63.85**    **Removal of valve from vas deferens**    ♂
   **63.89**    **Other repair of vas deferens and epididymis**    ♂

✓4ᵗʰ **63.9 Other operations on spermatic cord, epididymis, and vas deferens**

**63.91 Aspiration of spermatocele** ♂
DEF: Puncture of cystic distention of epididymis.

**63.92 Epididymotomy** ♂
DEF: Incision of epididymis.

**63.93 Incision of spermatic cord** ♂
DEF: Incision into sperm storage structure.

**63.94 Lysis of adhesions of spermatic cord** ♂

**63.95 Insertion of valve in vas deferens** ♂

**63.99 Other** ♂

✓3ʳᵈ **64 Operations on penis**

INCLUDES operations on:
corpora cavernosa
glans penis
prepuce

**64.0 Circumcision** ♂
DEF: Removal of penis foreskin.

✓4ᵗʰ **64.1 Diagnostic procedures on the penis**

**64.11 Biopsy of penis** ♂

**64.19 Other diagnostic procedures on penis** ♂

**64.2 Local excision or destruction of lesion of penis** ♂
EXCLUDES biopsy of penis (64.11)

**64.3 Amputation of penis** ♂

✓4ᵗʰ **64.4 Repair and plastic operation on penis**

**64.41 Suture of laceration of penis** ♂

**64.42 Release of chordee** ♂
AHA: 4Q, '96, 34
DEF: Correction of downward displacement of penis.

**64.43 Construction of penis** ♂

**64.44 Reconstruction of penis** ♂

**64.45 Replantation of penis** ♂
Reattachment of amputated penis

**64.49 Other repair of penis** ♂
EXCLUDES repair of epispadias and hypospadias (58.45)

**64.5 Operations for sex transformation, not elsewhere classified** NC ♂

✓4ᵗʰ **64.9 Other operations on male genital organs**

**64.91 Dorsal or lateral slit of prepuce** ♂

**64.92 Incision of penis** ♂

**64.93 Division of penile adhesions** ♂

**64.94 Fitting of external prosthesis of penis** ♂
Penile prosthesis NOS

**64.95 Insertion or replacement of non-inflatable penile prosthesis** ♂
Insertion of semi-rigid rod prosthesis into shaft of penis
EXCLUDES external penile prosthesis (64.94)
inflatable penile prosthesis (64.97)
plastic repair, penis (64.43-64.49)
that associated with:
construction (64.43)
reconstruction (64.44)

**64.96 Removal of internal prosthesis of penis** ♂
Removal without replacement of non-inflatable or inflatable penile prosthesis

**64.97 Insertion or replacement of inflatable penile prosthesis** ♂
Insertion of cylinders into shaft of penis and placement of pump and reservoir
EXCLUDES external penile prosthesis (64.94)
non-inflatable penile prosthesis (64.95)
plastic repair, penis (64.43-64.49)

**64.98 Other operations on penis** ♂
Corpora cavernosa-corpus spongiosum shunt
Corpora-saphenous shunt
Irrigation of corpus cavernosum
EXCLUDES removal of foreign body:
intraluminal (98.19)
without incision (98.24)
stretching of foreskin (99.95)

AHA: 3Q, '92, 9

DEF: Corpora cavernosa-corpus spongiosum shunt: Insertion of shunt between erectile tissues of penis.

DEF: Corpora-saphenous shunt: Insertion of shunt between erectile tissue and vein of penis.

DEF: Irrigation of corpus cavernosum: Washing of erectile tissue forming dorsum and side of penis.

**64.99 Other** ♂
EXCLUDES collection of sperm for artificial insemination (99.96)

✓3ʳᵈ
✓4ᵗʰ Additional Digit Required

Valid OR Procedure

Non-OR Procedure

Adjunct Code

© 2007 Ingenix

**Volume 3 — 149**

**Operations on the Female Genital Organs**

**65—65.99**

## 12. OPERATIONS ON THE FEMALE GENITAL ORGANS (65-71)

√3rd **65**   **Operations on ovary**

     Code also any application or administration of an adhesion barrier substance (99.77)

√4th **65.0**   **Oophorotomy**

     Salpingo-oophorotomy

     DEF: Incision into ovary.

     DEF: Salpingo-oophorotomy: Incision into ovary and the fallopian tube.

     **65.01**   **Laparoscopic oophorotomy**   ♀

     **65.09**   **Other oophorotomy**   ♀

√4th **65.1**   **Diagnostic procedures on ovaries**

     **65.11**   **Aspiration biopsy of ovary**   ♀

     **65.12**   **Other biopsy of ovary**   ♀

     **65.13**   **Laparoscopic biopsy of ovary**   ♀

         AHA: 4Q, '96, 67

     **65.14**   **Other laparoscopic diagnostic procedures on ovaries**   ♀

     **65.19**   **Other diagnostic procedures on ovaries**   ♀

         EXCLUDES   microscopic examination of specimen from ovary (91.41-91.49)

√4th **65.2**   **Local excision or destruction of ovarian lesion or tissue**

     **65.21**   **Marsupialization of ovarian cyst**   ♀

         EXCLUDES   that by laparoscope (65.23)

         DEF: Exteriorized cyst to outside by incising anterior wall and suturing cut edges to create open pouch.

     **65.22**   **Wedge resection of ovary**   ♀

         EXCLUDES   that by laparoscope (65.24)

     **65.23**   **Laparoscopic marsupialization of ovarian cyst**   ♀

     **65.24**   **Laparoscopic wedge resection of ovary**   ♀

     **65.25**   **Other laparoscopic local excision or destruction of ovary**   ♀

     **65.29**   **Other local excision or destruction of ovary**   ♀

         Bisection
         Cauterization } of ovary
         Partial excision

         EXCLUDES   biopsy of ovary (65.11-65.13)
         that by laparoscope (65.25)

√4th **65.3**   **Unilateral oophorectomy**

     **65.31**   **Laparoscopic unilateral oophorectomy**   ♀

     **65.39**   **Other unilateral oophorectomy**   ♀

         EXCLUDES   that by laparoscope (65.31)

         AHA: 4Q, '96, 66

√4th **65.4**   **Unilateral salpingo-oophorectomy**

     **65.41**   **Laparoscopic unilateral salpingo-oophorectomy**   ♀

         AHA: 4Q, '96, 67

     **65.49**   **Other unilateral salpingo-oophorectomy**   ♀

     **Oophorectomy**

Fallopian tube

Fimbria

Ovary

Ovarian cyst

√4th **65.5**   **Bilateral oophorectomy**

     **65.51**   **Other removal of both ovaries at same operative episode**   ♀

         Female castration

         EXCLUDES   that by laparoscope (65.53)

     **65.52**   **Other removal of remaining ovary**   ♀

         Removal of solitary ovary

         EXCLUDES   that by laparoscope (65.54)

     **65.53**   **Laparoscopic removal of both ovaries at same operative eisode**   ♀

     **65.54**   **Laparoscopic removal of remaining ovary**   ♀

√4th **65.6**   **Bilateral salpingo-oophorectomy**

     **65.61**   **Other removal of both ovaries and tubes at same operative episode**   ♀

         EXCLUDES   that by laparoscope (65.53)

         AHA: 4Q, '96, 65

     **65.62**   **Other removal of remaining ovary and tube**   ♀

         Removal of solitary ovary and tube

         EXCLUDES   that by laparoscope (65.54)

     **65.63**   **Laparoscopic removal of both ovaries and tubes at the same operative episode**   ♀

         AHA: ▶4Q, '06, 133, 134;◀ 4Q, '96, 68

     **65.64**   **Laparoscopic removal of remaining ovary and tube**   ♀

√4th **65.7**   **Repair of ovary**

     EXCLUDES   salpingo-oophorostomy (66.72)

     **65.71**   **Other simple suture of ovary**   ♀

         EXCLUDES   that by laparoscope (65.74)

     **65.72**   **Other reimplantation of ovary**   ♀

         EXCLUDES   that by laparoscope (65.75)

         DEF: Grafting and repositioning of ovary at same site.

     **65.73**   **Other salpingo-oophoroplasty**   ♀

         EXCLUDES   that by laparoscope (65.76)

     **65.74**   **Laparoscopic simple suture of ovary**   ♀

     **65.75**   **Laparoscopic reimplantation of ovary**   ♀

     **65.76**   **Laparoscopic salpingo-oophoroplasty**   ♀

     **65.79**   **Other repair of ovary**   ♀

         Oophoropexy

√4th **65.8**   **Lysis of adhesions of ovary and fallopian tube**

     **65.81**   **Laparoscopic lysis of adhesions of ovary and fallopian tube**   ♀

         AHA: 4Q, '96, 67

     **65.89**   **Other lysis of adhesions of ovary and fallopian tube**   ♀

         EXCLUDES   that by laparoscope (65.81)

√4th **65.9**   **Other operations on ovary**

     **65.91**   **Aspiration of ovary**   ♀

         EXCLUDES   aspiration biopsy of ovary (65.11)

     **65.92**   **Transplantation of ovary**   ♀

         EXCLUDES   reimplantation of ovary (65.72, 65.75)

     **65.93**   **Manual rupture of ovarian cyst**   ♀

         DEF: Breaking up an ovarian cyst using manual technique or blunt instruments.

     **65.94**   **Ovarian denervation**   ♀

         DEF: Destruction of nerve tracts to ovary.

     **65.95**   **Release of torsion of ovary**   ♀

     **65.99**   **Other**   ♀

         Ovarian drilling

         AHA: N-D, '86, 9

---

**BI** Bilateral Procedure    **NC** Non-covered Procedure    **LC** Limited Coverage Procedure    ▶◀ Revised Text    ● New Code    ▲ Revised Code Title

**Endoscopic Ligation of Fallopian Tubes**

Uterus
Ovary
Ligated fallopian tube
Monitor view
Laparoscopic procedure

√3ʳᵈ **66　Operations on fallopian tubes**
Code also any application or administration of an adhesion barrier substance (99.77)

√4ᵗʰ **66.0　Salpingotomy and salpingostomy**
　　**66.01　Salpingotomy**　　♀
　　**66.02　Salpingostomy**　　♀

√4ᵗʰ **66.1　Diagnostic procedures on fallopian tubes**
　　**66.11　Biopsy of fallopian tube**　　♀
　　**66.19　Other diagnostic procedures on fallopian tubes**　　♀
　　　　EXCLUDES　*microscopic examination of specimen from fallopian tubes (91.41-91.49)*
　　　　　　*radiography of fallopian tubes (87.82-87.83, 87.85)*
　　　　　　*Rubin's test (66.8)*

√4ᵗʰ **66.2　Bilateral endoscopic destruction or occlusion of fallopian tubes**
　　　　INCLUDES　bilateral endoscopic destruction or occlusion of fallopian tubes by:
　　　　　　culdoscopy　　　laparoscopy
　　　　　　endoscopy　　　peritoneoscopy
　　　　　　hysteroscopy
　　　　　　endoscopic destruction of solitary fallopian tube

DEF: Endoscopic blockage or destruction of both fallopian tubes.

DEF: Bilateral endoscopic destruction or occlusion of fallopian tubes by:

　Culdoscopy: Endoscopic insertion through posterior structure of vagina.

　Hysteroscopy: Endoscopic insertion through uterus.

　Laparoscopy: Endoscopic insertion through abdomen.

　Peritoneoscopy: Endoscopic insertion through abdominal serous membrane cavity.

　Endoscopic destruction of solitary fallopian tube: Endoscopic destruction of one fallopian tube.

　　**66.21　Bilateral endoscopic ligation and crushing of fallopian tubes**　　NC♀
　　**66.22　Bilateral endoscopic ligation and division of fallopian tubes**　　NC♀
　　**66.29　Other bilateral endoscopic destruction or occlusion of fallopian tubes**　　NC♀

√4ᵗʰ **66.3　Other bilateral destruction or occlusion of fallopian tubes**
　　　　INCLUDES　destruction of solitary fallopian tube
　　　　EXCLUDES　*endoscopic destruction or occlusion of fallopian tubes (66.21-66.29)*
　　**66.31　Other bilateral ligation and crushing of fallopian tubes**　　NC♀
　　**66.32　Other bilateral ligation and division of fallopian tubes**　　NC♀
　　　　Pomeroy operation

　　**66.39　Other bilateral destruction or occlusion of fallopian tubes**　　NC♀
　　　　Female sterilization operation NOS
**66.4　Total unilateral salpingectomy**　　♀

√4ᵗʰ **66.5　Total bilateral salpingectomy**
　　　　EXCLUDES　*bilateral partial salpingectomy for sterilization (66.39)*
　　　　　　*that with oophorectomy (65.61-65.64)*
　　**66.51　Removal of both fallopian tubes at same operative episode**　　♀
　　**66.52　Removal of remaining fallopian tube**　　♀
　　　　Removal of solitary fallopian tube

√4ᵗʰ **66.6　Other salpingectomy**
　　　　INCLUDES　salpingectomy by:
　　　　　　cauterization
　　　　　　coagulation
　　　　　　electrocoagulation
　　　　　　excision
　　　　EXCLUDES　*fistulectomy (66.73)*
　　**66.61　Excision or destruction of lesion of fallopian tube**　　♀
　　　　EXCLUDES　*biopsy of fallopian tube (66.11)*
　　**66.62　Salpingectomy with removal of tubal pregnancy**　　♀
　　　　Code also any synchronous oophorectomy (65.31, 65.39)
　　　　AHA: 3Q, '95, 15; S-O, '85, 14

　　**66.63　Bilateral partial salpingectomy, not otherwise specified**　　♀
　　**66.69　Other partial salpingectomy**　　♀

√4ᵗʰ **66.7　Repair of fallopian tube**
　　**66.71　Simple suture of fallopian tube**　　♀
　　**66.72　Salpingo-oophorostomy**　　♀
　　**66.73　Salpingo-salpingostomy**　　♀
　　**66.74　Salpingo-uterostomy**　　♀
　　**66.79　Other repair of fallopian tube**　　♀
　　　　Graft of fallopian tube
　　　　Reopening of divided fallopian tube
　　　　Salpingoplasty
　　　　AHA: 2Q, '95, 10

　　　　DEF: Graft of fallopian: Repair of fallopian tube with implanted graft.

　　　　DEF: Reopening of divided fallopian tube: Reconnection of severed fallopian tube to restore patency.

　　　　DEF: Salpingoplasty: Plastic reconstruction of fallopian tube defect.

**66.8　Insufflation of fallopian tube**　　♀
　　Insufflation of fallopian tube with:
　　　air
　　　dye
　　　gas
　　　saline
　　　Rubin's test
　　　　EXCLUDES　*insufflation of therapeutic agent (66.95)*
　　　　　　*that for hysterosalpingography (87.82-87.83)*

　　DEF: Forceful blowing of gas or liquid into fallopian tubes.

　　DEF: Rubin's test: Introduction of carbon dioxide gas into fallopian tubes.

√4ᵗʰ **66.9　Other operations on fallopian tubes**
　　**66.91　Aspiration of fallopian tube**　　♀
　　**66.92　Unilateral destruction or occlusion of fallopian tube**　　♀
　　　　EXCLUDES　*that of solitary tube (66.21-66.39)*
　　**66.93　Implantation or replacement of prosthesis of fallopian tube**　　♀
　　**66.94　Removal of prosthesis of fallopian tube**　　♀

√3ʳᵈ
√4ᵗʰ Additional Digit Required　　　　Valid OR Procedure　　　　Non-OR Procedure　　　　Adjunct Code

**Operations on the Female Genital Organs**

**66–66.94**

**66.95 Insufflation of therapeutic agent into fallopian tubes** ♀

**66.96 Dilation of fallopian tube** ♀

**66.97 Burying of fimbriae in uterine wall** ♀

DEF: Implantation of fallopian tube, fringed edges into uterine wall.

**66.99 Other** ♀

EXCLUDES    lysis of adhesions of ovary and tube (65.81, 65.89)

AHA: 2Q, '94, 11

√3rd **67    Operations on cervix**

Code also any application or administration of an adhesion barrier substance (99.77)

**67.0 Dilation of cervical canal** ♀

EXCLUDES    dilation and curettage (69.01-69.09)
that for induction of labor (73.1)

√4th **67.1 Diagnostic procedures on cervix**

**67.11 Endocervical biopsy** ♀

EXCLUDES    conization of cervix (67.2)

**67.12 Other cervical biopsy** ♀

Punch biopsy of cervix NOS

EXCLUDES    conization of cervix (67.2)

**67.19 Other diagnostic procedures on cervix** ♀

EXCLUDES    microscopic examination of specimen from cervix (91.41-91.49)

**67.2 Conization of cervix** ♀

EXCLUDES    that by:
cryosurgery (67.33)
electrosurgery (67.32)

DEF: Removal of cone-shaped section from distal cervix; cervical function preserved.

√4th **67.3 Other excision or destruction of lesion or tissue of cervix**

**67.31 Marsupialization of cervical cyst** ♀

DEF: Incision and then suturing open of a cyst in the neck of the uterus.

**67.32 Destruction of lesion of cervix by cauterization** ♀

Electroconization of cervix
LEEP (loop electrosurgical excision procedure)
LLETZ (large loop excision of the transformation zone)

AHA: 1Q, '98, 3

DEF: Destruction of lesion of uterine neck by applying intense heat.

DEF: Electroconization of cervix: Electrocautery excision of multilayer cone-shaped section from uterine neck.

**67.33 Destruction of lesion of cervix by cryosurgery** ♀

Cryoconization of cervix

DEF: Destruction of lesion of uterine neck by freezing.

DEF: Cryoconization of cervix: Excision by freezing of multilayer cone-shaped section of abnormal tissue in uterine neck.

**67.39 Other excision or destruction of lesion or tissue of cervix** ♀

EXCLUDES    biopsy of cervix (67.11-67.12)
cervical fistulectomy (67.62)
conization of cervix (67.2)

**67.4 Amputation of cervix** ♀

Cervicectomy with synchronous colporrhaphy

DEF: Excision of lower uterine neck.
DEF: Cervicectomy with synchronous colporrhaphy: Excision of lower uterine neck with suture of vaginal stump.

√4th **67.5 Repair of internal cervical os**

AHA: 4Q, '01, 63; 3Q, '00, 11

DEF: Repair of cervical opening defect.

**67.51 Transabdominal cerclage of cervix** ♀

Cerclage of Cervix

Suture material is inserted around cervix and tightened

Uterus

Cervix and cervical canal

Cervix and cervical canal

**67.59 Other repair of internal cervical os** ♀

Cerclage of isthmus uteri
McDonald operation
Shirodkar operation
Transvaginal cerclage

EXCLUDES    laparoscopically assisted supracervical hysterectomy [LASH] (68.31)
transabdominal cerclage of cervix (67.51)

DEF: Cerclage of isthmus uteri: Placement of encircling suture between neck and body of uterus.

DEF: Shirodkar operation: Placement of purse-string suture in internal cervical opening.

√4th **67.6 Other repair of cervix**

EXCLUDES    repair of current obstetric laceration (75.51)

**67.61 Suture of laceration of cervix** ♀

**67.62 Repair of fistula of cervix** ♀

Cervicosigmoidal fistulectomy

EXCLUDES    fistulectomy:
cervicovesical (57.84)
ureterocervical (56.84)
vesicocervicovaginal (57.84)

DEF: Closure of fistula in lower uterus.

DEF: Cervicosigmoidal fistulectomy: Excision of abnormal passage between uterine neck and torsion of large intestine.

**67.69 Other repair of cervix** ♀

Repair of old obstetric laceration of cervix

√3rd **68    Other incision and excision of uterus**

Code also any application or administration of an adhesion barrier substance (99.77)

**68.0 Hysterotomy** ♀

Hysterotomy with removal of hydatidiform mole

EXCLUDES    hysterotomy for termination of pregnancy (74.91)

DEF: Incision into the uterus.

√4th **68.1 Diagnostic procedures on uterus and supporting structures**

**68.11 Digital examination of uterus** ♀

EXCLUDES    pelvic examination, so described (89.26)
postpartal manual exploration of uterine cavity (75.7)

**68.12 Hysteroscopy** ♀

EXCLUDES    that with biopsy (68.16)

**68.13 Open biopsy of uterus** ♀

EXCLUDES    closed biopsy of uterus (68.16)

**68.14 Open biopsy of uterine ligaments** ♀

EXCLUDES    closed biopsy of uterine ligaments (68.15)

**68.15 Closed biopsy of uterine ligaments** ♀

Endoscopic (laparoscopy) biopsy of uterine adnexa, except ovary and fallopian tube

BI Bilateral Procedure    NC Non-covered Procedure    LC Limited Coverage Procedure    ►◄ Revised Text    ● New Code    ▲ Revised Code Title

**68.16  Closed biopsy of uterus**  ♀
Endoscopic (laparoscopy) (hysteroscopy) biopsy of uterus
> EXCLUDES   *open biopsy of uterus (68.13)*

**68.19  Other diagnostic procedures on uterus and supporting structures**  ♀
> EXCLUDES   *diagnostic:*
> *aspiration curettage (69.59)*
> *dilation and curettage (69.09)*
> *microscopic examination of specimen from uterus (91.41-91.49)*
> *pelvic examination (89.26)*
> *radioisotope scan of:*
> *placenta (92.17)*
> *uterus (92.19)*
> *ultrasonography of uterus (88.78-88.79)*
> *x-ray of uterus (87.81-87.89)*

✓4ᵗʰ **68.2  Excision or destruction of lesion or tissue of uterus**

**68.21  Division of endometrial synechiae**  ♀
Lysis of intraluminal uterine adhesions
DEF: Separation of uterine adhesions.
DEF: Lysis of intraluminal uterine adhesion: Surgical destruction of adhesive, fibrous structures inside uterine cavity.

**68.22  Incision or excision of congenital septum of uterus**  ♀

**68.23  Endometrial ablation**  ♀
Dilation and curettage
Hysteroscopic endometrial ablation
AHA: 4Q, '96, 68
DEF: Removal or destruction of uterine lining; usually by electrocautery or loop electrosurgical excision procedure (LEEP).

**68.29  Other excision or destruction of lesion of uterus**  ♀
Uterine myomectomy
> EXCLUDES   *biopsy of uterus (68.13)*
> *uterine fistulectomy (69.42)*
AHA: ▶3Q, '06, 18;◀ 1Q, '96, 14

✓4ᵗʰ **68.3  Subtotal abdominal hysterectomy**

**68.31  Laparoscopic supracervical hysterectomy [LSH]**  ♀
Classic infrafascial SEMM hysterectomy [CISH]
Laparoscopically assisted supracervical hysterectomy [LASH]
AHA: 4Q, '03, 98-99
DEF: A hysterectomy that spares the cervix and maintains the integrity of the pelvic floor; SEMM version of the supracervical hysterectomy, also called the classic infrafascial SEMM hysterectomy [CISH], the cardinal ligaments, or lateral cervical ligaments that merge with the pelvic diaphragm remain intact.

**68.39  Other and unspecified subtotal abdominal hysterectomy**  ♀
Supracervical hysterectomy
> EXCLUDES   *classic infrafascial SEMM hysterectomy [CISH] (68.31)*
> *laparoscopic supracervical hysterectomy [LSH] (68.31)*
AHA: 4Q, '03, 98

✓4ᵗʰ **68.4  Total abdominal hysterectomy**
Code also any synchronous removal of tubes and ovaries (65.31-65.64)
> EXCLUDES   *laparoscopic total abdominal hysterectomy (68.41)*
> *radical abdominal hysterectomy, any approach (68.61-68.69)*
AHA: 4Q, '96, 65
DEF: Complete excision of uterus and uterine neck through abdominal approach.

**Vaginal Hysterectomy**

Total hysterectomy (uterus only removed)

Total hysterectomy with bilateral salpingectomy (uterus and tubes removed)

Total hysterectomy with bilateral salpingo-oophorectomy (uterus, tubes, and ovaries removed)

**68.41  Laparoscopic total abdominal hysterectomy**  ♀
Total laparoscopic hysterectomy [TLH]
AHA: ▶4Q, '06, 130, 133◀

**68.49  Other and unspecified total abdominal hysterectomy**  ♀
Hysterectomy:
extended
AHA: ▶4Q, '06, 130◀

✓4ᵗʰ **68.5  Vaginal hysterectomy**
Code also any synchronous:
removal of tubes and ovaries (65.31-65.64)
repair of cystocele or rectocele (70.50-70.52)
repair of pelvic floor (70.79)
DEF: Complete excision of the uterus by a vaginal approach.

**68.51  Laparoscopically assisted vaginal hysterectomy (LAVH)**  ♀
AHA: 4Q, '96, 68

**68.59  Other and unspecified vaginal hysterectomy**  ♀
> EXCLUDES   *laparoscopically assisted vaginal hysterectomy (68.51)*
> *radical vaginal hysterectomy (68.71-68.79)*

✓4ᵗʰ **68.6  Radical abdominal hysterectomy**
Code also any synchronous:
lymph gland dissection (40.3, 40.5)
removal of tubes and ovaries (65.31-65.64)
> EXCLUDES   *pelvic evisceration (68.8)*
DEF: Excision of uterus, loose connective tissue and smooth muscle around uterus and vagina via abdominal approach.

**68.61  Laparoscopic radical abdominal hysterectomy**  ♀
Laparoscopic modified radical hysterectomy
Total laparoscopic radical hysterectomy [TLRH]
AHA: ▶4Q, '06, 130, 134◀

**68.69  Other and unspecified radical abdominal hysterectomy**  ♀
Modified radical hysterectomy
Wertheim's operation
> EXCLUDES   *laparoscopic total abdominal hysterectomy (68.41)*
> *laparoscopic radical abdominal hysterectomy (68.61)*
AHA: ▶4Q, '06, 130◀

✓4ᵗʰ **68.7  Radical vaginal hysterectomy**
Code also any synchronous:
lymph gland dissection (40.3, 40.5)
removal of tubes and ovaries (65.31-65.64)
> EXCLUDES   *abdominal hysterectomy, any approach (68.31-68.39, 68.41-68.49, 68.61-68.69, 68.9)*
DEF: Excision of uterus, loose connective tissue and smooth muscle around uterus and vagina via vaginal approach.

**68.71  Laparoscopic radical vaginal hysterectomy [LRVH]**  ♀
AHA: ▶4Q, '06, 130◀

---

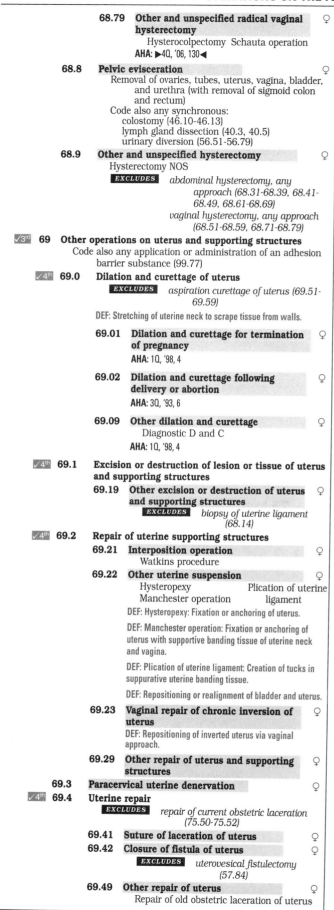

**68.79 Other and unspecified radical vaginal hysterectomy** ♀
  Hysterocolpectomy  Schauta operation
  **AHA:** ▶4Q, '06, 130◀

**68.8 Pelvic evisceration** ♀
  Removal of ovaries, tubes, uterus, vagina, bladder, and urethra (with removal of sigmoid colon and rectum)
  Code also any synchronous:
    colostomy (46.10-46.13)
    lymph gland dissection (40.3, 40.5)
    urinary diversion (56.51-56.79)

**68.9 Other and unspecified hysterectomy** ♀
  Hysterectomy NOS
  **EXCLUDES** *abdominal hysterectomy, any approach (68.31-68.39, 68.41-68.49, 68.61-68.69)*
    *vaginal hysterectomy, any approach (68.51-68.59, 68.71-68.79)*

√3rd **69 Other operations on uterus and supporting structures**
  Code also any application or administration of an adhesion barrier substance (99.77)

√4th **69.0 Dilation and curettage of uterus**
  **EXCLUDES** *aspiration curettage of uterus (69.51-69.59)*
  **DEF:** Stretching of uterine neck to scrape tissue from walls.

  **69.01 Dilation and curettage for termination of pregnancy** ♀
    **AHA:** 1Q, '98, 4

  **69.02 Dilation and curettage following delivery or abortion** ♀
    **AHA:** 3Q, '93, 6

  **69.09 Other dilation and curettage** ♀
    Diagnostic D and C
    **AHA:** 1Q, '98, 4

√4th **69.1 Excision or destruction of lesion or tissue of uterus and supporting structures**

  **69.19 Other excision or destruction of uterus and supporting structures** ♀
    **EXCLUDES** *biopsy of uterine ligament (68.14)*

√4th **69.2 Repair of uterine supporting structures**

  **69.21 Interposition operation** ♀
    Watkins procedure

  **69.22 Other uterine suspension** ♀
    Hysteropexy          Plication of uterine
    Manchester operation     ligament
    **DEF:** Hysteropexy: Fixation or anchoring of uterus.
    **DEF:** Manchester operation: Fixation or anchoring of uterus with supportive banding tissue of uterine neck and vagina.
    **DEF:** Plication of uterine ligament: Creation of tucks in suppurative uterine banding tissue.
    **DEF:** Repositioning or realignment of bladder and uterus.

  **69.23 Vaginal repair of chronic inversion of uterus** ♀
    **DEF:** Repositioning of inverted uterus via vaginal approach.

  **69.29 Other repair of uterus and supporting structures** ♀

**69.3 Paracervical uterine denervation** ♀

√4th **69.4 Uterine repair**
  **EXCLUDES** *repair of current obstetric laceration (75.50-75.52)*

  **69.41 Suture of laceration of uterus** ♀
  **69.42 Closure of fistula of uterus** ♀
    **EXCLUDES** *uterovesical fistulectomy (57.84)*

  **69.49 Other repair of uterus** ♀
    Repair of old obstetric laceration of uterus

**Dilation and Curettage**

Fallopian tube — Cervix (being dilated)
Ovary — Curetting endometrium
— Cervix
— Vagina

√4th **69.5 Aspiration curettage of uterus**
  **EXCLUDES** *menstrual extraction (69.6)*

  **69.51 Aspiration curettage of uterus for termination of pregnancy** ♀
    Therapeutic abortion NOS

  **69.52 Aspiration curettage following delivery or abortion** ♀

  **69.59 Other aspiration curettage of uterus** ♀
    **AHA:** 1Q, '98, 7

**69.6 Menstrual extraction or regulation** ♀
  **DEF:** Induction of menstruation by low pressure suction.

**69.7 Insertion of intrauterine contraceptive device** ♀

√4th **69.9 Other operations on uterus, cervix, and supporting structures** ♀
  **EXCLUDES** *obstetric dilation or incision of cervix (73.1, 73.93)*

  **69.91 Insertion of therapeutic device into uterus** ♀
    **EXCLUDES** *insertion of:*
      *intrauterine contraceptive device (69.7)*
      *laminaria (69.93)*
      *obstetric insertion of bag, bougie, or pack (73.1)*

  **69.92 Artificial insemination** ♀

  **69.93 Insertion of laminaria** ♀
    **DEF:** Placement of laminaria, a sea kelp, in cervical os to induce labor; applied for six to 12 hours.

  **69.94 Manual replacement of inverted uterus** ♀
    **EXCLUDES** *that in immediate postpartal period (75.94)*

  **69.95 Incision of cervix** ♀
    **EXCLUDES** *that to assist delivery (73.93)*

  **69.96 Removal of cerclage material from cervix**
    **DEF:** Removal of ring inserted to restore uterine neck competency.

  **69.97 Removal of other penetrating foreign body from cervix** ♀
    **EXCLUDES** *removal of intraluminal foreign body from cervix (98.16)*

  **69.98 Other operations on supporting structures of uterus** ♀
    **EXCLUDES** *biopsy of uterine ligament (68.14)*

  **69.99 Other operations on cervix and uterus** ♀
    **EXCLUDES** *removal of:*
      *foreign body (98.16)*
      *intrauterine contraceptive device (97.71)*
      *obstetric bag, bougie, or pack (97.72)*
      *packing (97.72)*

**BI** Bilateral Procedure   **NC** Non-covered Procedure   **LC** Limited Coverage Procedure   ▶◀ Revised Text   ● New Code   ▲ Revised Code Title

**154** — Volume 3 • February 2007

© 2007 Ingenix

**Operations on the Female Genital Organs**

**70–70.8**

√3ʳᵈ **70 Operations on vagina and cul-de-sac**
Code also any application or administration of an adhesion barrier substance (99.77)

**70.0 Culdocentesis** ♀
AHA: 2Q, '90, 26
DEF: Insertion of needle into upper vaginal vault encircling cervix to withdraw fluid.

√4ᵗʰ **70.1 Incision of vagina and cul-de-sac**

**70.11 Hymenotomy** ♀

**70.12 Culdotomy** ♀
DEF: Incision into pocket between terminal end of large intestine and posterior uterus.

**70.13 Lysis of intraluminal adhesions of vagina** ♀

**70.14 Other vaginotomy** ♀
Division of vaginal septum
Drainage of hematoma of vaginal cuff
DEF: Division of vaginal septum: Incision into partition of vaginal walls.
DEF: Drainage of hematoma of vaginal cuff: Incision into vaginal tissue to drain collected blood.

√4ᵗʰ **70.2 Diagnostic procedures on vagina and cul-de-sac**

**70.21 Vaginoscopy** ♀

**70.22 Culdoscopy** ♀
DEF: Endoscopic exam of pelvic viscera through incision in posterior vaginal wall.

**70.23 Biopsy of cul-de-sac** ♀

**70.24 Vaginal biopsy** ♀

**70.29 Other diagnostic procedures on vagina and cul-de-sac** ♀

√4ᵗʰ **70.3 Local excision or destruction of vagina and cul-de-sac**

**70.31 Hymenectomy** ♀

**70.32 Excision or destruction of lesion of cul-de-sac** ♀
Endometrectomy of cul-de-sac
EXCLUDES   biopsy of cul-de-sac (70.23)

**70.33 Excision or destruction of lesion of vagina** ♀
EXCLUDES   biopsy of vagina (70.24)
vaginal fistulectomy (70.72-70.75)

**70.4 Obliteration and total excision of vagina** ♀
Vaginectomy
EXCLUDES   obliteration of vaginal vault (70.8)
DEF: Vaginectomy: Removal of vagina.

√4ᵗʰ **70.5 Repair of cystocele and rectocele**

**70.50 Repair of cystocele and rectocele** ♀
DEF: Repair of anterior and posterior vaginal wall bulges.

**70.51 Repair of cystocele** ♀
Anterior colporrhaphy (with urethrocele repair)
AHA: N-D, '84, 20

**70.52 Repair of rectocele** ♀
Posterior colporrhaphy
EXCLUDES ► STARR procedure (48.74)◄
AHA: 1Q, '06, 12

**70.53 Repair of cystocele and rectocele with graft or prosthesis** ♀
Use additional code for biological substance (70.94) or synthetic substance (70.95), if known

**70.54 Repair of cystocele with graft or prosthesis** ♀
Anterior colporrhaphy (with urethrocele repair)
Use additional code for biological substance (70.94) or synthetic substance (70.95), if known

**70.55 Repair of rectocele with graft or prosthesis** ♀
Posterior colporrhaphy
Use additional code for biological substance (70.94) or synthetic substance (70.95), if known

√4ᵗʰ **70.6 Vaginal construction and reconstruction**

**70.61 Vaginal construction** ♀
AHA: 3Q, '06, 18

**70.62 Vaginal reconstruction** ♀
AHA: N-D, '84, 20

**70.63 Vaginal construction with graft or prosthesis** ♀
Use additional code for biological substance (70.94) or synthetic substance (70.95), if known
EXCLUDES   vaginal construction (70.61)

**70.64 Vaginal reconstruction with graft or prosthesis** ♀
Use additional code for biological substance (70.94) or synthetic substance (70.95), if known
EXCLUDES   vaginal reconstruction (70.62)

√4ᵗʰ **70.7 Other repair of vagina**
EXCLUDES   lysis of intraluminal adhesions (70.13)
repair of current obstetric laceration (75.69)
that associated with cervical amputation (67.4)

**70.71 Suture of laceration of vagina** ♀
AHA: N-D, '84, 20

**70.72 Repair of colovaginal fistula** ♀
DEF: Correction of abnormal opening between midsection of large intestine and vagina.

**70.73 Repair of rectovaginal fistula** ♀
DEF: Correction of abnormal opening between last section of large intestine and vagina.

**70.74 Repair of other vaginoenteric fistula** ♀
DEF: Correction of abnormal opening between vagina and intestine; other than mid or last sections.

**70.75 Repair of other fistula of vagina** ♀
EXCLUDES   repair of fistula:
rectovesicovaginal (57.83)
ureterovaginal (56.84)
urethrovaginal (58.43)
uterovaginal (69.42)
vesicocervicovaginal (57.84)
vesicosigmoidovaginal (57.83)
vesicoureterovaginal (56.84)
vesicovaginal (57.84)

**70.76 Hymenorrhaphy** ♀
DEF: Closure of vagina with suture of hymenal ring or hymenal remnant flaps.

**70.77 Vaginal suspension and fixation** ♀
DEF: Repair of vaginal protrusion, sinking or laxity by suturing vagina into position.

**70.78 Vaginal suspension and fixation with graft or prosthesis** ♀
Use additional code for biological substance (70.94) or synthetic substance (70.95), if known

**70.79 Other repair of vagina** ♀
Colpoperineoplasty
Repair of old obstetric laceration of vagina

**70.8 Obliteration of vaginal vault** ♀
LeFort operation
DEF: LeFort operation: Uniting or sewing together vaginal walls.

√3ʳᵈ
√4ᵗʰ Additional Digit Required      Valid OR Procedure      Non-OR Procedure      Adjunct Code

**Operations on the Female Genital Organs**

**70.9–71.9**

√4ᵗʰ **70.9 Other operations on vagina and cul-de-sac**

    **70.91 Other operations on vagina** ♀

        **EXCLUDES** *insertion of:*
            *diaphragm (96.17)*
            *mold (96.15)*
            *pack (96.14)*
            *pessary (96.18)*
            *suppository (96.49)*
        *removal of:*
            *diaphragm (97.73)*
            *foreign body (98.17)*
            *pack (97.75)*
            *pessary (97.74)*
        *replacement of:*
            *diaphragm (97.24)*
            *pack (97.26)*
            *pessary (97.25)*
        *vaginal dilation (96.16)*
        *vaginal douche (96.44)*

    **70.92 Other operations on cul-de-sac** ♀
        Obliteration of cul-de-sac
        Repair of vaginal enterocele
        **AHA:** 4Q, '94, 54
        **DEF:** Repair of vaginal enterocele: Elimination of herniated cavity within pouch between last part of large intestine and posterior uterus.

•     **70.93 Other operations on cul-de-sac with graft or prosthesis** ♀
        Repair of vaginal enterocele with graft or prosthesis
        Use additional code for biological substance (70.94) or synthetic substance (70.95), if known

•     **70.94 Insertion of biological graft** ♀
        Allogenic material or substance
        Allograft
        Autograft
        Autologous material or substance
        Heterograft
        Xenogenic material or substance
        Code first these procedures when done with graft or prosthesis:
          Other operations on cul-de-sac (70.93)
          Repair of cystocele (70.54)
          Repair of cystocele and rectocele (70.53)
          Repair of rectocele (70.55)
          Vaginal construction (70.63)
          Vaginal reconstruction (70.64)
          Vaginal suspension and fixation (70.78)

•     **70.95 Insertion of synthetic graft or prosthesis** ♀
        Artificial tissue
        Code first these procedures when done with graft or prosthesis:
          Other operations on cul-de-sac (70.93)
          Repair of cystocele (70.54)
          Repair of cystocele and rectocele (70.53)
          Repair of rectocele (70.55)
          Vaginal construction (70.63)
          Vaginal reconstruction (70.64)
          Vaginal suspension and fixation (70.78)

√3ʳᵈ **71 Operations on vulva and perineum**
    Code also any application or administration of an adhesion barrier substance (99.77)

√4ᵗʰ **71.0 Incision of vulva and perineum**
    **71.01 Lysis of vulvar adhesions** ♀
    **71.09 Other incision of vulva and perineum** ♀
        Enlargement of introitus NOS
        **EXCLUDES** *removal of foreign body without incision (98.23)*

√4ᵗʰ **71.1 Diagnostic procedures on vulva**
    **71.11 Biopsy of vulva** ♀
    **71.19 Other diagnostic procedures on vulva** ♀

√4ᵗʰ **71.2 Operations on Bartholin's gland**
    **71.21 Percutaneous aspiration of Bartholin's gland (cyst)** ♀

---

**Marsupialization**

Portion of cyst and overlying skin to be excised

Cyst "unroofed"

Cyst walls sutured to skin

    **71.22 Incision of Bartholin's gland (cyst)** ♀
    **71.23 Marsupialization of Bartholin's gland (cyst)** ♀
        **DEF:** Incision and suturing opening of a cyst in Bartholin's gland.

    **71.24 Excision or other destruction of Bartholin's gland (cyst)** ♀
    **71.29 Other operations on Bartholin's gland** ♀

**71.3 Other local excision or destruction of vulva and perineum** ♀
    Division of Skene's gland
    **EXCLUDES** *biopsy of vulva (71.11)*
            *vulvar fistulectomy (71.72)*

**71.4 Operations on clitoris** ♀
    Amputation of clitoris     Female circumcision
    Clitoridotomy
    **DEF:** Amputation of clitoris: Removal of clitoris.
    **DEF:** Clitoridotomy: Incision into clitoris.
    **DEF:** Female circumcision: Incision of skin fold over clitoris.

**71.5 Radical vulvectomy** ♀
    Code also any synchronous lymph gland dissection (40.3, 40.5)
    **DEF:** Removal of over 80 percent of deep tissue from vulva, including tissue of abdomen, groin, labia minora, labia majora, clitoris, mons veneris, and terminal portions of urethra, vagina and other vulvar organs.

√4ᵗʰ **71.6 Other vulvectomy**
    **71.61 Unilateral vulvectomy** ♀
        **AHA:** 2Q, '06, 19
    **71.62 Bilateral vulvectomy** ♀
        Vulvectomy NOS

√4ᵗʰ **71.7 Repair of vulva and perineum**
    **EXCLUDES** *repair of current obstetric laceration (75.69)*
    **71.71 Suture of laceration of vulva or perineum** ♀
    **71.72 Repair of fistula of vulva or perineum** ♀
        **EXCLUDES** *repair of fistula:*
            *urethroperineal (58.43)*
            *urethroperineovesical (57.84)*
            *vaginoperineal (70.75)*
    **71.79 Other repair of vulva and perineum** ♀
        Repair of old obstetric laceration of vulva or perineum
        **AHA:** 1Q, '97, 9

**71.8 Other operations on vulva** ♀
    **EXCLUDES** *removal of:*
        *foreign body without incision (98.23)*
        *packing (97.75)*
        *replacement of packing (97.26)*

**71.9 Other operations on female genital organs** ♀
    **AHA:** 4Q, '04, 90; 1Q, '03, 13

---

**BI** Bilateral Procedure     **NC** Non-covered Procedure     **LC** Limited Coverage Procedure     �▶◀ Revised Text     ● New Code     ▲ Revised Code Title

## 13. OBSTETRICAL PROCEDURES (72-75)

√3rd **72** **Forceps, vacuum, and breech delivery**

**72.0** **Low forceps operation** ♀
Outlet forceps operation

**72.1** **Low forceps operation with episiotomy** ♀
Outlet forceps operation with episiotomy

√4th **72.2** **Mid forceps operation**

**72.21** **Mid forceps operation with episiotomy** ♀

**72.29** **Other mid forceps operation** ♀

√4th **72.3** **High forceps operation**

**72.31** **High forceps operation with episiotomy** ♀

**72.39** **Other high forceps operation** ♀

**72.4** **Forceps rotation of fetal head** ♀
DeLee maneuver
Key-in-lock rotation
Kielland rotation
Scanzoni's maneuver
Code also any associated forceps extraction (72.0-72.39)

√4th **72.5** **Breech extraction**

**72.51** **Partial breech extraction with forceps to aftercoming head** ♀

**72.52** **Other partial breech extraction** ♀

**72.53** **Total breech extraction with forceps to aftercoming head** ♀

**72.54** **Other total breech extraction** ♀

**72.6** **Forceps application to aftercoming head** ♀
Piper forceps operation
   **EXCLUDES**    *partial breech extraction with forceps to aftercoming head (72.51)*
      *total breech extraction with forceps to aftercoming head (72.53)*

√4th **72.7** **Vacuum extraction**
   **INCLUDES**    Malström's extraction

**72.71** **Vacuum extraction with episiotomy** ♀

**72.79** **Other vacuum extraction** ♀
**AHA:** ▶2Q, '06, 5◀

**72.8** **Other specified instrumental delivery** ♀

**72.9** **Unspecified instrumental delivery** ♀

√3rd **73** **Other procedures inducing or assisting delivery**

√4th **73.0** **Artificial rupture of membranes**

**73.01** **Induction of labor by artificial rupture of membranes** ♀
Surgical induction NOS
   **EXCLUDES**    *artificial rupture of membranes after onset of labor (73.09)*

**AHA:** 3Q, '00, 5

**73.09** **Other artificial rupture of membranes** ♀
Artificial rupture of membranes at time of delivery

### Breech Extraction

Breech presentation

Delivery of legs

Baby rotated for delivery of arms

Umbilicus

**73.1** **Other surgical induction of labor** ♀
Induction by cervical dilation
   **EXCLUDES**    *injection for abortion (75.0)*
      *insertion of suppository for abortion (96.49)*

√4th **73.2** **Internal and combined version and extraction**

**73.21** **Internal and combined version without extraction** ♀
Version NOS

**73.22** **Internal and combined version with extraction** ♀

**73.3** **Failed forceps** ♀
Application of forceps without delivery
Trial forceps

**73.4** **Medical induction of labor** ♀
   **EXCLUDES**    *medication to augment active labor — omit code*

√4th **73.5** **Manually assisted delivery** ♀

**73.51** **Manual rotation of fetal head** ♀

**73.59** **Other manually assisted delivery** ♀
Assisted spontaneous delivery
Credé maneuver
**AHA:** 4Q, '98, 76

**73.6** **Episiotomy** ♀
Episioproctotomy
Episiotomy with subsequent episiorrhaphy
   **EXCLUDES**    *that with:*
      *high forceps (72.31)*
      *low forceps (72.1)*
      *mid forceps (72.21)*
      *outlet forceps (72.1)*
      *vacuum extraction (72.71)*

**AHA:** 1Q, '92, 10

**73.8** **Operations on fetus to facilitate delivery** ♀
Clavicotomy on fetus
Destruction of fetus
Needling of hydrocephalic head

√4th **73.9** **Other operations assisting delivery**

**73.91** **External version** ♀

**73.92** **Replacement of prolapsed umbilical cord** ♀

**73.93** **Incision of cervix to assist delivery** ♀
Dührssen's incisions

**73.94** **Pubiotomy to assist delivery** ♀
Obstetrical symphysiotomy

**73.99** **Other** ♀
   **EXCLUDES**    *dilation of cervix, obstetrical, to induce labor (73.1)*
      *insertion of bag or bougie to induce labor (73.1)*
      *removal of cerclage material (69.96)*

√3rd **74** **Cesarean section and removal of fetus**
Code also any synchronous:
hysterectomy (68.3-68.4, 68.6, 68.8)
myomectomy (68.29)
sterilization (66.31-66.39, 66.63)
**AHA:** ▶2Q, '06, 5◀

**74.0** **Classical cesarean section** ♀
Transperitoneal classical cesarean section

**74.1** **Low cervical cesarean section** ♀
Lower uterine segment cesarean section
**AHA:** 1Q, '01, 11

**74.2** **Extraperitoneal cesarean section** ♀
Supravesical cesarean section

**Obstetrical Procedures**

74.3–75.99

**74.3**   **Removal of extratubal ectopic pregnancy** ♀
Removal of:
     ectopic abdominal pregnancy
     fetus from peritoneal or extraperitoneal cavity
         following uterine or tubal rupture
     EXCLUDES   *that by salpingostomy (66.02)*
                *that by salpingotomy (66.01)*
                *that with synchronous salpingectomy (66.62)*

AHA: 4Q, '92, 25; 2Q, '90, 25; 2Q, '90, 27; 1Q, '89, 11

**74.4**   **Cesarean section of other specified type** ♀
Peritoneal exclusion cesareansection
Transperitoneal cesarean section NOS
Vaginal cesarean section

√4th **74.9**   **Cesarean section of unspecified type**

    **74.91**   **Hysterotomy to terminate pregnancy** ♀
         Therapeutic abortion by hysterotomy

    **74.99**   **Other cesarean section of unspecified type** ♀
         Cesarean section NOS
         Obstetrical abdominouterotomy
         Obstetrical hysterotomy

√3rd **75**   **Other obstetric operations**

**75.0**   **Intra-amniotic injection for abortion** ♀
Injection of:
    prostaglandin   ⎫  for induction of
    saline              ⎬  abortion

Termination of pregnancy by intrauterine injection
     EXCLUDES   *insertion of prostaglandin suppository for abortion (96.49)*

**75.1**   **Diagnostic amniocentesis** ♀

**75.2**   **Intrauterine transfusion** ♀
Exchange transfusion in utero
Insertion of catheter into abdomen of fetus for transfusion
Code also any hysterotomy approach (68.0)

√4th **75.3**   **Other intrauterine operations on fetus and amnion**
Code also any hysterotomy approach (68.0)

    **75.31**   **Amnioscopy** ♀
         Fetoscopy
         Laparoamnioscopy
         AHA: 3Q, '06, 16-17

    **75.32**   **Fetal EKG (scalp)** ♀
    **75.33**   **Fetal blood sampling and biopsy** ♀
    **75.34**   **Other fetal monitoring** ♀
         Antepartum fetal nonstress test
         Fetal monitoring, not otherwise specified
         EXCLUDES   *fetal pulse oximetry (75.38)*

    **75.35**   **Other diagnostic procedures on fetus and amnion** ♀
         Intrauterine pressure determination
         EXCLUDES   *amniocentesis (75.1)*
                 *diagnostic procedures on gravid uterus and placenta (87.81, 88.46, 88.78, 92.17)*

         AHA: 3Q, '06, 16-17

    **75.36**   **Correction of fetal defect** ♀
    **75.37**   **Amnioinfusion**
         Code also injection of antibiotic (99.21)
         AHA: 4Q, '98, 76

    **75.38**   **Fetal pulse oximetry**
         Transcervical fetal oxygen saturation monitoring
         Transcervical fetal SpO$_2$ monitoring
         DEF: Single-use sensor inserted through the birth canal and positioned to rest against the fetal cheek, forehead, or temple; infrared beam of light aimed at the fetal skin is reflected back through the sensor for analysis.
         AHA: 4Q, '01, 64

**Amniocentesis**

Aspiration of amniotic fluid

**75.4**   **Manual removal of retained placenta** ♀
     EXCLUDES   *aspiration curettage (69.52)*
                *dilation and curettage (69.02)*

AHA: 3Q, '06, 11

√4th **75.5**   **Repair of current obstetric laceration of uterus**

    **75.50**   **Repair of current obstetric laceration of uterus, not otherwise specified**

    **75.51**   **Repair of current obstetric laceration of cervix** ♀

    **75.52**   **Repair of current obstetric laceration of corpus uteri** ♀

√4th **75.6**   **Repair of other current obstetric laceration**
AHA: 1Q, '92, 11

    **75.61**   **Repair of current obstetric laceration of bladder and urethra** ♀

    **75.62**   **Repair of current obstetric laceration of rectum and sphincter ani** ♀

    **75.69**   **Repair of other current obstetric laceration** ♀
         Episioperineorrhaphy
         Repair of:
            pelvic floor
            perineum
            vagina
            vulva
         Secondary repair of episiotomy
         EXCLUDES   *repair of routine episiotomy (73.6)*

**75.7**   **Manual exploration of uterine cavity, postpartum** ♀

**75.8**   **Obstetric tamponade of uterus or vagina** ♀
     EXCLUDES   *antepartum tamponade (73.1)*

√4th **75.9**   **Other obstetric operations**

    **75.91**   **Evacuation of obstetrical incisional hematoma of perineum** ♀
         Evacuation of hematoma of:
            episiotomy
            perineorrhaphy

    **75.92**   **Evacuation of other hematoma of vulva or vagina** ♀

    **75.93**   **Surgical correction of inverted uterus** ♀
         Spintelli operation
         EXCLUDES   *vaginal repair of chronic inversion of uterus (69.23)*

    **75.94**   **Manual replacement of inverted uterus** ♀
    **75.99**   **Other** ♀
         AHA: 3Q, '06, 16-17

---

BI Bilateral Procedure     NC Non-covered Procedure     LC Limited Coverage Procedure     ►◄ Revised Text     ● New Code     ▲ Revised Code Title

## 14. OPERATIONS ON THE MUSCULOSKELETAL SYSTEM
### (76-84)

**✓3rd 76   Operations on facial bones and joints**
> **EXCLUDES**   accessory sinuses (22.00-22.9)
> nasal bones (21.00-21.99)
> skull (01.01-02.99)

**✓4th 76.0   Incision of facial bone without division**
**76.01   Sequestrectomy of facial bone**
Removal of necrotic bone chip from facial bone

**76.09   Other incision of facial bone**
Reopening of osteotomy site of facial bone
> **EXCLUDES**   osteotomy associated with
> orthognathic surgery
> (76.61-76.69)
> removal of internal fixation
> device (76.97)

**✓4th 76.1   Diagnostic procedures on facial bones and joints**
**76.11   Biopsy of facial bone**
**76.19   Other diagnostic procedures on facial bones and joints**
> **EXCLUDES**   contrast arthrogram of
> temporomandibular joint
> (87.13)
> other x-ray (87.11-87.12,
> 87.14-87.16)

AHA: N-D, '87, 12

**76.2   Local excision or destruction of lesion of facial bone**
> **EXCLUDES**   biopsy of facial bone (76.11)
> excision of odontogenic lesion (24.4)

**✓4th 76.3   Partial ostectomy of facial bone**
**76.31   Partial mandibulectomy**
Hemimandibulectomy
> **EXCLUDES**   that associated with
> temporomandibular
> arthroplasty (76.5)

AHA: 2Q, '05, 8

DEF: Excision, partial of lower jawbone.

DEF: Hemimandibulectomy: Excision of one-half of lower jawbone.

**76.39   Partial ostectomy of other facial bone**
Hemimaxillectomy (with bonegraft or prosthesis)

AHA: J-F, '87, 14

DEF: Excision, partial of facial bone; other than lower jawbone.

DEF: Hemimaxillectomy (with bone graft or prosthesis): Excision of one side of upper jawbone and restoration with bone graft or prosthesis.

**✓4th 76.4   Excision and reconstruction of facial bones**
**76.41   Total mandibulectomy with synchronous reconstruction**
**76.42   Other total mandibulectomy**
**76.43   Other reconstruction of mandible**
> **EXCLUDES**   genioplasty (76.67-76.68)
> that with synchronous total
> mandibulectomy (76.41)

AHA: 2Q, '03, 13

**76.44   Total ostectomy of other facial bone with synchronous reconstruction**
AHA: 3Q, '93, 6

DEF: Excision, facial bone, total with reconstruction during same operative session.

**76.45   Other total ostectomy of other facial bone**
**76.46   Other reconstruction of other facial bone**
> **EXCLUDES**   that with synchronous total
> ostectomy (76.44)

**76.5   Temporomandibular arthroplasty**
AHA: 4Q, '99, 20

**✓4th 76.6   Other facial bone repair and orthognathic surgery**
Code also any synchronous:
bone graft (76.91)
synthetic implant (76.92)
> **EXCLUDES**   reconstruction of facial bones (76.41-
> 76.46)

**76.61   Closed osteoplasty [osteotomy] of mandibular ramus**
Gigli saw osteotomy

DEF: Reshaping and restoration of lower jawbone projection; closed surgical field.

DEF: Gigli saw osteotomy: Plastic repair using a flexible wire with saw teeth.

**76.62   Open osteoplasty [osteotomy] of mandibular ramus**
**76.63   Osteoplasty [osteotomy] of body of mandible**
**76.64   Other orthognathic surgery on mandible**
Mandibular osteoplasty NOS
Segmental or subapical osteotomy

AHA: 2Q, '04, 9, 10

**76.65   Segmental osteoplasty [osteotomy] of maxilla**
Maxillary osteoplasty NOS
**76.66   Total osteoplasty [osteotomy] of maxilla**
**76.67   Reduction genioplasty**
Reduction mentoplasty

DEF: Reduction of protruding chin or lower jawbone.

**76.68   Augmentation genioplasty**
Mentoplasty:
NOS
with graft or implant

DEF: Extension of the lower jawbone to a functional position by means of plastic surgery.

**76.69   Other facial bone repair**
Osteoplasty of facial bone NOS

**✓4th 76.7   Reduction of facial fracture**
> **INCLUDES**   internal fixation
Code also any synchronous:
bone graft (76.91)
synthetic implant (76.92)
> **EXCLUDES**   that of nasal bones (21.71-21.72)

**76.70   Reduction of facial fracture, not otherwise specified**
**76.71   Closed reduction of malar and zygomatic fracture**
**76.72   Open reduction of malar and zygomatic fracture**
**76.73   Closed reduction of maxillary fracture**
**76.74   Open reduction of maxillary fracture**
**76.75   Closed reduction of mandibular fracture**
**76.76   Open reduction of mandibular fracture**
**76.77   Open reduction of alveolar fracture**
Reduction of alveolar fracture with stabilization of teeth

**76.78   Other closed reduction of facial fracture**
Closed reduction of orbital fracture
> **EXCLUDES**   nasal bone (21.71)

**76.79   Other open reduction of facial fracture**
Open reduction of orbit rim or wall
> **EXCLUDES**   nasal bone (21.72)

**✓4th 76.9   Other operations on facial bones and joints**
**76.91   Bone graft to facial bone**
Autogenous
Bone bank          } graft to facial bone
Heterogenous

**76.92   Insertion of synthetic implant in facial bone**
Alloplastic implant to facial bone

**Operations on the Musculoskeletal System**

**76.93–77.7**

**76.93**   **Closed reduction of temporomandibular dislocation**

**76.94**   **Open reduction of temporomandibular dislocation**

**76.95**   **Other manipulation of temporomandibular joint**

**76.96**   **Injection of therapeutic substance into temporomandibular joint**

**76.97**   **Removal of internal fixation device from facial bone**

> EXCLUDES   *removal of:*
> *dental wiring (97.33)*
> *external mandibular*
> *fixation device NEC*
> *(97.36)*

**76.99**   **Other**

**√3rd 77**   **Incision, excision, and division of other bones**

> EXCLUDES   *laminectomy for decompression (03.09)*
> *operations on:*
> *accessory sinuses (22.00-22.9)*
> *ear ossicles (19.0-19.55)*
> *facial bones (76.01-76.99)*
> *joint structures (80.00-81.99)*
> *mastoid (19.9-20.99)*
> *nasal bones (21.00-21.99)*
> *skull (01.01-02.99)*

The following fourth-digit subclassification is for use with appropriate categories in section 77 to identify the site. Valid fourth-digit categories are in [brackets] under each code.

   **0**   **unspecified site**
   **1**   **scapula, clavicle, and thorax [ribs and sternum]**
   **2**   **humerus**
   **3**   **radius and ulna**
   **4**   **carpals and metacarpals**
   **5**   **femur**
   **6**   **patella**
   **7**   **tibia and fibula**
   **8**   **tarsals and metatarsals**
   **9**   **other**
       Pelvic bones
       Phalanges (of foot) (of hand)
       Vertebrae

§   √4th **77.0**   **Sequestrectomy**
    [0-9]   DEF: Excision and removal of dead bone.

§   √4th **77.1**   **Other incision of bone without division**
    [0-9]      Reopening of osteotomy site
> EXCLUDES   *aspiration of bone marrow, (41.31, 41.91)*
> *removal of internal fixation device (78.60-78.69)*

      **AHA:** For code **77.17:** 1Q, '02, 3

      DEF: Incision into bone without division of site.

§   √4th **77.2**   **Wedge osteotomy**
    [0-9]   EXCLUDES   *that for hallux valgus (77.51)*
      DEF: Removal of wedge-shaped piece of bone.

§   √4th **77.3**   **Other division of bone**
    [0-9]      Osteoarthrotomy
> EXCLUDES   *clavicotomy of fetus (73.8)*
> *laminotomy or incision of vertebra (03.01-03.09)*
> *pubiotomy to assist delivery (73.94)*
> *sternotomy incidental to thoracic operation — omit code*

§   √4th **77.4**   **Biopsy of bone**
    [0-9]   **AHA:** 2Q, '98, 12; **For code 77.49:** 3Q, '06, 13

**Repair of Hammer Toe**

Corn

Hemiphalengectomy

Hammertoe

Callus

After

**√4th 77.5**   **Excision and repair of bunion and other toe deformities**

**77.51**   **Bunionectomy with soft tissue correction and osteotomy of the first metatarsal**
      DEF: Incision and removal of big toe bony prominence and reconstruction with soft tissue.

**77.52**   **Bunionectomy with soft tissue correction and arthrodesis**
      DEF: Removal of big toe bony prominence and reconstruction with soft tissue and joint fixation.

**77.53**   **Other bunionectomy with soft tissue correction**

**77.54**   **Excision or correction of bunionette**
      That with osteotomy
      DEF: Resection of fifth metatarsal head via exposure of joint; includes imbrication of capsule.

**77.56**   **Repair of hammer toe**
      Filleting
      Fusion          } of hammer toe
      Phalangectomy (partial)

      DEF: Repair of clawlike toe defect by joint fusion, or partial removal of toe via traction technique.

**77.57**   **Repair of claw toe**
      Capsulotomy
      Fusion
      Phalangectomy (partial)    } of claw toe
      Tendon lengthening

      DEF: Repair of clawlike toe defect by joint fusion, partial removal of toe, joint capsule incision or lengthening of fibrous muscle attachment.

**77.58**   **Other excision, fusion, and repair of toes**
      Cockup toe repair
      Overlapping toe repair
      That with use of prosthetic materials

**77.59**   **Other bunionectomy**
      Resection of hallux valgus joint with insertion of prosthesis
      DEF: Resection of hallux valgus joint with insertion of prosthesis: Cutting away part of big toe with prosthesis insertion to correct bony prominence.

§   √4th **77.6**   **Local excision of lesion or tissue of bone**
    [0-9]   EXCLUDES   *biopsy of bone (77.40-77.49)*
> *debridement of compound fracture (79.60-79.69)*

      **AHA:** For code **77.61:** 3Q, '01, 9; **For code 77.65:** 4Q, '04, 128; S-O, '85, 4; **For code 77.67:** 1Q, '02, 3; 1Q, '99, 8; **For code 77.69:** 2Q, '00, 18

§   √4th **77.7**   **Excision of bone for graft**
    [0-9]   **AHA:** ▶2Q, '07, 5;◀ 4Q, '99, 11, 13; **For code 77.71:** 3Q, '03, 19; **For code 77.79:** 2Q, '03, 13; 4Q, '02, 107, 109-110; 2Q, '02, 16; 2Q, '00 12, 13; 4Q, '99, 11, 13

---

§   Requires fourth-digit. Valid digits are in [brackets] under each code. See category 77 for definitions.

**BI** Bilateral Procedure     **NC** Non-covered Procedure     **LC** Limited Coverage Procedure     ▶◀ Revised Text     ● New Code     ▲ Revised Code Title

§ ✓4th **77.8** **Other partial ostectomy**
[0-9]    Condylectomy
    EXCLUDES   *amputation (84.00-84.19, 84.91)*
     *arthrectomy (80.90-80.99)*
     *excision of bone ends associated with:*
      *arthrodesis (81.00-81.29)*
      *arthroplasty (81.51-81.59, 81.71-*
       *81.81, 81.84)*
     *excision of cartilage (80.5-80.6, 80.80-*
      *80.99)*
     *excision of head of femur with syn-*
      *chronous replacement (00.70-*
      *00.73, 81.51-81.53)*
     *hemilaminectomy (03.01-03.09)*
     *laminectomy (03.01-03.09)*
     *ostectomy for hallux valgus (77.51-*
      *77.59)*
     *partial amputation:*
      *finger (84.01)*
      *thumb (84.02)*
      *toe (84.11)*
     *resection of ribs incidental to thoracic*
      *operation — omit code*
     *that incidental to other operation —*
      *omit code*

     **AHA:** For code **77.89:** 2Q, '02, 8

§ ✓4th **77.9** **Total ostectomy**
[0-9]    EXCLUDES   *amputation of limb (84.00-84.19, 84.91)*
     *that incidental to other operation —*
      *omit code*

✓3rd **78** **Other operations on bones, except facial bones**
   EXCLUDES   *operations on:*
     *accessory sinuses (22.00-22.9)*
     *facial bones (76.01-76.99)*
     *joint structures (80.00-81.99)*
     *nasal bones (21.00-21.99)*
     *skull (01.01-02.99)*

The following fourth-digit subclassification is for use with categories in section 78 to identify the site. Valid fourth-digit categories are in [brackets] under each code.

   **0**  **unspecified site**
   **1**  **scapula, clavicle, and thorax [ribs and sternum]**
   **2**  **humerus**
   **3**  **radius and ulna**
   **4**  **carpals and metacarpals**
   **5**  **femur**
   **6**  **patella**
   **7**  **tibia and fibula**
   **8**  **tarsals and metatarsals**
   **9**  **other**
     Pelvic bones          Vertebrae
     Phalanges (of foot) (of hand)

✓4th **78.0** **Bone graft**
[0-9]    Bone:
     bank graft
     graft (autogenous) (heterogenous)
   That with debridement of bone graft site (removal of sclerosed, fibrous, or necrotic bone or tissue)
   Transplantation of bone
   Code also any excision of bone for graft (77.70-77.79)
     EXCLUDES   *that for bone lengthening (78.30-78.39)*
     **AHA:** 2Q, '02, 11; 2Q, '98, 12; 3Q, '94, 10; 1Q, '91, 3

✓4th **78.1** **Application of external fixator device**
[0-9]    Fixator with insertion of pins/wires/screws into bone
   Code also any type of fixator device, if known (84.71-84.73)
     EXCLUDES   *other immobilization, pressure, and attention to wound (93.51-93.59)*
     **AHA:** 2Q, '94, 4; For code **78.12:** 4Q, '05, 129

✓4th **78.2** **Limb shortening procedures**
[0,2-5,7-9] Epiphyseal stapling
     Open epiphysiodesis
     Percutaneous epiphysiodesis
     Resection/osteotomy

✓4th **78.3** **Limb lengthening procedures**
[0,2-5,7-9] Bone graft with or without internal fixation devices or osteotomy
     Distraction technique with or without corticotomy/osteotomy
     Code also any application of an external fixation device (78.10-78.19)

✓4th **78.4** **Other repair or plastic operations on bone**
[0-9]    Other operation on bone NEC
   Repair of malunion or nonunion fracture NEC
     EXCLUDES   *application of external fixation device (78.10-78.19)*
      *limb lengthening procedures (78.30-78.39)*
      *limb shortening procedures (78.20-78.29)*
      *osteotomy (77.3)*
      *reconstruction of thumb (82.61-82.69)*
      *repair of pectus deformity (34.74)*
      *repair with bone graft (78.00-78.09)*
   **AHA:** 3Q, '91, 20; 4Q, '88, 11; For code **78.41:** 2Q, '02, 16; For code **78.47:** 3Q, '91, 20; For code **78.49:** 3Q, '04, 9; 2Q, '03, 22; 3Q, '02, 12; 2Q, '02, 14, 15; 4Q, '99, 22; 1Q, '97, 5

✓4th **78.5** **Internal fixation of bone without fracture reduction**
[0-9]    Internal fixation of bone (prophylactic)
   Reinsertion of internal fixation device
   Revision of displaced or broken fixation device
     EXCLUDES   *arthroplasty and arthrodesis (81.00-81.85)*
      *bone graft (78.00-78.09)*
      *limb shortening procedures (78.20-78.29)*
      *that for fracture reduction (79.10-79.19, 79.30-79.59)*
   **AHA:** 2Q, '99, 11; 2Q, '94, 4; For code **78.59:** 3Q, '04, 6; 2Q, '03, 15; 4Q, '99, 13

✓4th **78.6** **Removal of implanted devices from bone**
[0-9]    External fixator device (invasive)
   Internal fixation device
   Removal of bone growth stimulator (invasive)
   Removal of internal limb lengthening device
   ▶Removal of pedicle screw(s) used in spinal fusion◀
     EXCLUDES   *removal of cast, splint, and traction device (Kirschner wire) (Steinmann pin) (97.88)*
      ▶*removal of posterior spinal motion preservation (facet replacement, pedicle-based dynamic stabilization, interspinous process) device(s) (80.09)*◀
      *removal of skull tongs or halo traction device (02.95)*
   **AHA:** 1Q, '00, 15; For code **78.67** 2Q, '03, 14; For code **78.69:** 4Q, '02, 110; 2Q, '00, 18

✓4th **78.7** **Osteoclasis**
[0-9]    DEF: Surgical breaking or rebreaking of bone.

✓4th **78.8** **Diagnostic procedures on bone, not elsewhere classified**
[0-9]    EXCLUDES   *biopsy of bone (77.40-77.49)*
     *magnetic resonance imaging (88.94)*
     *microscopic examination of specimen from bone (91.51-91.59)*
     *radioisotope scan (92.14)*
     *skeletal x-ray (87.21-87.29, 87.43, 88.21-88.33)*
     *thermography (88.83)*

§   Requires fourth-digit. Valid digits are in [brackets] under each code. See category 77 for definitions.

✓3rd ✓4th Additional Digit Required      Valid OR Procedure      Non-OR Procedure      Adjunct Code

§ ✓4th **78.9 Insertion of bone growth stimulator**
[0-9]     Insertion of:
          bone stimulator (electrical) to aid bone healing
          osteogenic electrodes for bone growth stimulation
          totally implanted device (invasive)
          **EXCLUDES** *non-invasive (transcutaneous) (surface)*
                      *stimulator (99.86)*

✓3rd **79 Reduction of fracture and dislocation**
     **INCLUDES** application of cast or splint
               reduction with insertion of traction device
                   (Kirschner wire) (Steinmann pin)
     Code also any:
         application of external fixator device (78.10-78.19)
         type of fixator device, if known (84.71-84.73)
     **EXCLUDES** *external fixation alone for immobilization of*
                 *fracture (93.51-93.56, 93.59)*
                 *internal fixation without reduction of fracture*
                 *(78.50-78.59)*
                 *operations on:*
                     *facial bones (76.70-76.79)*
                     *nasal bones (21.71-21.72)*
                     *orbit (76.78-76.79)*
                     *skull (02.02)*
                     *vertebrae (03.53)*
                 *removal of cast or splint (97.88)*
                 *replacement of cast or splint (97.11-97.14)*
                 *traction alone for reduction of fracture (93.41-*
                 *93.46)*

The following fourth-digit subclassification is for use with appropriate
categories in section 79 to identify the site. Valid fourth-digit
categories are in [brackets] under each code.
    0  **unspecified site**
    1  **humerus**
    2  **radius and ulna**
           Arm NOS
    3  **carpals and metacarpals**
           Hand NOS
    4  **phalanges of hand**
    5  **femur**
    6  **tibia and fibula**
           Leg NOS
    7  **tarsals and metatarsals**
           Foot NOS
    8  **phalanges of foot**
    9  **other specified bone**

✓4th **79.0 Closed reduction of fracture without internal**
[0-9]     **fixation**
          **EXCLUDES** *that for separation of epiphysis*
                      *(79.40-79.49)*
     **AHA:** 2Q, '94, 3; 3Q, '89, 17; 4Q, '88, 11;
          **For code 79.01:** 4Q, '05, 129; **For code 79.05:** 3Q, '89, 16

     DEF: Manipulative realignment of fracture; without incision or
     internal fixation.

✓4th **79.1 Closed reduction of fracture with internal**
[0-9]     **fixation**
          **EXCLUDES** *that for separation of epiphysis*
                      *(79.40-79.49)*
     **AHA:** 2Q, '94, 4; 4Q, '93, 35; 1Q, '93, 27

     DEF: Manipulative realignment of fracture; with internal fixation but
     without incision.

✓4th **79.2 Open reduction of fracture without internal**
[0-9]     **fixation**
          **EXCLUDES** *that for separation of epiphysis*
                      *(79.50-79.59)*
     **AHA:** 2Q, '94, 3

✓4th **79.3 Open reduction of fracture with internal**
[0-9]     **fixation**
          **EXCLUDES** *that for separation of epiphysis*
                      *(79.50-79.59)*
     **AHA:** 2Q, '98, 12; 3Q, '94, 10; 2Q, '94, 3; 4Q, '93, 35
          **For code 79.32:** ▶1Q, '07, 7;◀ **For code 79.35:** ▶1Q, '07, 4◀
     DEF: Realignment of fracture with incision and internal fixation.

✓4th **79.4 Closed reduction of separated epiphysis**
[0-2,5,6,9] Reduction with or without internal fixation
     DEF: Manipulative reduction of expanded joint end of long bone to
     normal position without incision.

✓4th **79.5 Open reduction of separated epiphysis**
[0-2,5,6,9] Reduction with or without internal fixation
     DEF: Reduction of expanded joint end of long bone with incision.

✓4th **79.6 Debridement of open fracture site**
[0-9]     Debridement of compound fracture
     **AHA:** 3Q, '95, 12; 3Q, '89, 16
     DEF: Removal of damaged tissue at fracture site.

✓4th **79.7 Closed reduction of dislocation**
          **INCLUDES** closed reduction (with external
                      traction device)
          **EXCLUDES** *closed reduction of dislocation of*
                      *temporomandibular joint (76.93)*
     DEF: Manipulative reduction of displaced joint without incision;
     with or without external traction.

     **79.70 Closed reduction of dislocation of**
            **unspecified site**
     **79.71 Closed reduction of dislocation of shoulder**
     **79.72 Closed reduction of dislocation of elbow**
     **79.73 Closed reduction of dislocation of wrist**
     **79.74 Closed reduction of dislocation of hand and**
            **finger**
     **79.75 Closed reduction of dislocation of hip**
     **79.76 Closed reduction of dislocation of knee**
            **AHA:** N-D, '86, 7
     **79.77 Closed reduction of dislocation of ankle**
     **79.78 Closed reduction of dislocation of foot and toe**
     **79.79 Closed reduction of dislocation of other**
            **specified sites**

✓4th **79.8 Open reduction of dislocation**
          **INCLUDES** open reduction (with internal and
                      external fixation devices)
          **EXCLUDES** *open reduction of dislocation of*
                      *temporomandibular joint (76.94)*
     DEF: Reduction of displaced joint via incision; with or without
     internal and external fixation.

     **79.80 Open reduction of dislocation of**
            **unspecified site**
     **79.81 Open reduction of dislocation of shoulder**
     **79.82 Open reduction of dislocation of elbow**
     **79.83 Open reduction of dislocation of wrist**
     **79.84 Open reduction of dislocation of hand and**
            **finger**
     **79.85 Open reduction of dislocation of hip**
     **79.86 Open reduction of dislocation of knee**
     **79.87 Open reduction of dislocation of ankle**
     **79.88 Open reduction of dislocation of foot and toe**
     **79.89 Open reduction of dislocation of other**
            **specified sites**

✓4th **79.9 Unspecified operation on bone injury**
[0-9]

§  Requires fourth-digit. Valid digits are in [brackets] under each code. See category 78 for definitions.

**BI** Bilateral Procedure    **NC** Non-covered Procedure    **LC** Limited Coverage Procedure    ▶◀ Revised Text    ● New Code    ▲ Revised Code Title

√3rd **80 Incision and excision of joint structures**

INCLUDES   operations on:
     capsule of joint
     cartilage
     condyle
     ligament
     meniscus
     synovial membrane

EXCLUDES   *cartilage of:*
     *ear (18.01-18.9)*
     *nose (21.00-21.99)*
     *temporomandibular joint (76.01-76.99)*

The following fourth-digit subclassification is for use with appropriate categories in section 80 to identify the site:

   **0 unspecified site**
   **1 shoulder**
   **2 elbow**
   **3 wrist**
   **4 hand and finger**
   **5 hip**
   **6 knee**
   **7 ankle**
   **8 foot and toe**
   **9 other specified sites**
      Spine

√4th **80.0 Arthrotomy for removal of prosthesis**

INCLUDES   ►removal of posterior spinal motion preservation (dynamic stabilization, facet replacement, interspinous process) device(s)◄

Code also any:
   insertion of (cement) (joint)
     ►(methylmethacrylate)◄ spacer (84.56)
   removal of (cement) (joint)
     ►(methylmethacrylate)◄ spacer (84.57)

EXCLUDES   ► *removal of pedicle screws used in spinal fusion (78.69)*◄

AHA: For code 80.06: 2Q, '97, 10

DEF: Incision into joint to remove prosthesis.

√4th **80.1 Other arthrotomy**
   Arthrostomy

EXCLUDES   *that for:*
     *arthrography (88.32)*
     *arthroscopy (80.20-80.29)*
     *injection of drug (81.92)*
     *operative approach — omit code*

AHA: For code 80.15: 3Q, '06, 22-23; For code 80.16: 3Q, '06, 23

DEF: Incision into joint; other than to remove prosthesis.
DEF: Arthrostomy: Creation of opening into joint.

√4th **80.2 Arthroscopy**
AHA: 3Q, '93, 5; 1Q, '93, 23

√4th **80.3 Biopsy of joint structure**
   Aspiration biopsy
AHA: For code 80.39: 3Q, '05, 13-14

√4th **80.4 Division of joint capsule, ligament, or cartilage**
   Goldner clubfoot release
   Heyman-Herndon(-Strong) correction of metatarsus varus
   Release of:
     adherent or constrictive joint capsule
     joint
     ligament

EXCLUDES   *symphysiotomy to assist delivery (73.94)*
     *that for:*
      *carpal tunnel syndrome (04.43)*
      *tarsal tunnel syndrome (04.44)*

AHA: For code 80.49: 2Q, '02, 16

DEF: Incision and separation of joint tissues, including capsule, fibrous bone attachment or cartilage.

√4th **80.5 Excision or destruction of intervertebral disc**

**80.50 Excision or destruction of intervertebral disc, unspecified**
     Unspecified as to excision or destruction

**80.51 Excision of intervertebral disc**
   Code also any concurrent spinal fusion (81.00-81.08)
   Diskectomy
   Level:
     cervical
     thoracic
     lumbar (lumbosacral)
   Removal of herniated nucleus pulposus
   That by laminotomy or hemilaminectomy
   That with decompression of spinal nerve root at same level
   Requires additional code for any concomitant decompression of spinal nerve root at different level from excision site

EXCLUDES   *intervertebral chemonucleolysis (80.52)*
     *laminectomy for exploration of intraspinal canal (03.09)*
     *laminotomy for decompression of spinal nerve root only (03.09)*
     *that for insertion of (non-fusion) spinal disc replacement device (84.60-84.69)*
     *that with corpectomy, (vertebral) (80.99)*

AHA: ►1Q, '07, 9;◄ 1Q, '06, 12; 4Q, '04, 133; 3Q, '03, 12; 1Q, '96, 7; 2Q, '95, 9; 2Q, '90, 27; S-O, '86, 12

DEF: Diskectomy: Removal of intervertebral disc.
DEF: Removal of a herniated nucleus pulposus: Removal of displaced intervertebral disc, central part.

**80.52 Intervertebral chemonucleolysis**
   With aspiration of disc fragments
   With diskography
   Injection of proteolytic enzyme into intervertebral space (chymopapain)

EXCLUDES   *injection of anesthestic substance (03.91)*
     *injection of other substances (03.92)*

DEF: Destruction of intervertebral disc via injection of enzyme.

**80.59 Other destruction of intervertebral disc**
   Destruction NEC
   That by laser
AHA: 3Q, '02, 10

**80.6 Excision of semilunar cartilage of knee**
   Excision of meniscus of knee
AHA: 2Q, '03, 18; 3Q, '00, 4; 2Q, '96, 3; 1Q, '93, 23

√4th **80.7 Synovectomy**
   Complete or partial resection of synovial membrane

EXCLUDES   *excision of Baker's cyst (83.39)*

DEF: Excision of inner membrane of joint capsule.

**Types of Grafts for Anterior Arthrodesis**

Anteroposterior

Anteroposterior

Anteroposterior

Lateral

Lateral

Lateral

§ ✓4ᵗʰ **80.8**   **Other local excision or destruction of lesion of joint**

§ ✓4ᵗʰ **80.9**   **Other excision of joint**

> **EXCLUDES**   *cheilectomy of joint (77.80-77.89)*
> *excision of bone ends (77.80-77.89)*

**AHA: For code 80.99** ▶1Q, '07, 20◀

✓3ʳᵈ **81**   **Repair and plastic operations on joint structures**

✓4ᵗʰ **81.0**   **Spinal fusion**

> **INCLUDES**   arthrodesis of spine with:
>      bone graft
>      internal fixation

Code also any:
     insertion of interbody spinal fusion device (84.51)
     insertion of recombinant bone morphogenetic
       protein (84.52)
     ▶synchronous excision of (locally) harvested bone
       for graft (77.70-77.79)◀

Code also the total number of vertebrae fused
     (81.62-81.64)

> **EXCLUDES**   *corrections of pseudarthrosis of spine*
> *(81.30-81.39)*
> *refusion of spine (81.30-81.39)*

**AHA: 4Q, '03, 99**

**DEF:** Spinal fusion: Immobilization of spinal column.

**DEF:** Anterior interbody fusion: Arthrodesis by excising disc and cartilage end plates with bone graft insertion between two vertebrae.

**DEF:** Lateral fusion: Arthrodesis by decorticating and bone grafting lateral surface of zygapophysial joint, pars interarticularis and transverse process.

**DEF:** Posterior fusion: Arthrodesis by decorticating and bone grafting of neural arches between right and left zygapophysial joints.

**DEF:** Posterolateral fusion: Arthrodesis by decorticating and bone grafting zygapophysial joint, pars interarticularis and transverse processes

**81.00**   **Spinal fusion, not otherwise specified**

**81.01**   **Atlas-axis spinal fusion**

> Craniocervical fusion ⎫ by anterior trans-
> C1-C2 fusion       ⎬ oral or poster-
> Occiput C2 fusion ⎭ ior technique

**81.02**   **Other cervical fusion, anterior technique**
Arthrodesis of C2 level or below:
     anterior (interbody) technique
     anterolateral technique

**AHA: 4Q, '03, 101; 1Q, '01, 6; 1Q, '96, 7**

**81.03**   **Other cervical fusion, posterior technique**
Arthrodesis of C2 level or below:
     posterior (interbody) technique
     posterolateral technique

**81.04**   **Dorsal and dorsolumbar fusion, anterior technique**
Arthrodesis of thoracic or thoracolumbar
     region:
     anterior (interbody) technique
     anterolateral technique

**AHA: 3Q, '03, 19**

**81.05**   **Dorsal and dorsolumbar fusion, posterior technique**
Arthrodesis of thoracic or thoracolumbar
     region:
     posterior (interbody) technique
     posterolateral technique

**AHA: 2Q, '02, 16; 4Q, '99, 11**

**81.06**   **Lumbar and lumbosacral fusion, anterior technique**
Anterior lumbar interbody fusion (ALIF)
Arthrodesis of lumbar or lumbosacral
     region:
     anterior (interbody) technique
     anterolateral technique

**AHA:** ▶1Q, '07, 20;◀ 4Q, '05, 122; 4Q, '02, 107; 4Q, '99, 11

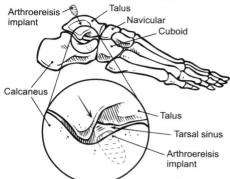

**Subtalar Joint Arthroereisis**

Arthroereisis implant — Talus
Navicular
Cuboid
Calcaneus
Talus
Tarsal sinus
Arthroereisis implant

**81.07**   **Lumbar and lumbosacral fusion, lateral transverse process technique**

**AHA: 4Q, '02, 108**

**81.08**   **Lumbar and lumbosacral fusion, posterior technique**
Arthrodesis of lumbar or lumbosacral region:
     posterior (interbody) technique
     posterolateral technique
Posterior lumbar interbody fusion (PLIF)
Transforaminal lumbar interbody fusion
     (TLIF)

**AHA:** 1Q, '06, 12, 13; 4Q, '05, 122-123; 4Q, '02, 107, 109;
     2Q, '00, 12, 13; 4Q, '99, 13; 2Q, '95, 9

✓4ᵗʰ **81.1**   **Arthrodesis and arthroereisis of foot and ankle**

> **INCLUDES**   arthrodesis of foot and ankle with:
>      bone graft
>      external fixation device

**DEF:** Fixation of foot or ankle joints.

**81.11**   **Ankle fusion**
Tibiotalar fusion

**81.12**   **Triple arthrodesis**
Talus to calcaneus and calcaneus to cuboid
     and navicular

**81.13**   **Subtalar fusion**

> **EXCLUDES**   *arthroereisis (81.18)*

**81.14**   **Midtarsal fusion**

**81.15**   **Tarsometatarsal fusion**

**81.16**   **Metatarsophalangeal fusion**

**81.17**   **Other fusion of foot**

**81.18**   **Subtalar joint arthroereisis**

**AHA: 4Q, '05, 124**

**DEF:** Insertion of an endoprostheses to limit excessive valgus motion of the subtalar joint; nonfusion procedure to prevent pronation.

✓4ᵗʰ **81.2**   **Arthrodesis of other joint**

> **INCLUDES**   arthrodesis with:
>      bone graft
>      external fixation device
>      excision of bone ends and
>        compression

**81.20**   **Arthrodesis of unspecified joint**

**81.21**   **Arthrodesis of hip**

**81.22**   **Arthrodesis of knee**

**81.23**   **Arthrodesis of shoulder**

**81.24**   **Arthrodesis of elbow**

**81.25**   **Carporadial fusion**

**81.26**   **Metacarpocarpal fusion**

**81.27**   **Metacarpophalangeal fusion**

**81.28**   **Interphalangeal fusion**

**81.29**   **Arthrodesis of other specified joints**

---

§   Requires fourth-digit. Valid digits are in [brackets] under each code. See category 80 for definitions.

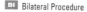 Bilateral Procedure     NC Non-covered Procedure     LC Limited Coverage Procedure     ▶◀ Revised Text     ● New Code     ▲ Revised Code Title

164 — Volume 3 • October 2007                    © 2007 Ingenix

√4ᵗʰ **81.3**    **Refusion of spine**

> **INCLUDES**   arthrodesis of spine with:
> > bone graft
> > internal fixation
> > correction of pseudarthrosis of spine
>
> Code also any:
> > insertion of interbody spinal fusion device (84.51)
> > insertion of recombinant bone morphogenetic
> > > protein (84.52)
> > ▶synchronous excision of (locally) harvested bone
> > > for graft (77.70-77.79)◄
> Code also the total number of vertebrae fused
> > (81.62-81.64)

**AHA:** 4Q, '03, 99; 4Q, '01, 64

**81.30**    **Refusion of spine, nototherwise specified**

**81.31**    **Refusion of atlas-axis spine**

> Craniocervical
> > fusion
>
> C1-C2 fusion    }   by anterior transoral
> > or posterior
> Occiput C2 fusion      technique

**81.32**    **Refusion of other cervical spine, anterior technique**
> Arthrodesis of C2 level or below:
> > anterior (interbody) technique
> > anterolateral technique

**81.33**    **Refusion of other cervical spine, posterior technique**
> Arthrodesis of C2 level or below:
> > posterior (interbody) technique
> > posterolateral technique

**81.34**    **Refusion of dorsal and dorsolumbar spine, anterior technique**
> Arthrodesis of thoracic or thoracolumbar
> > region:
> > anterior (interbody) technique
> > anterolateral technique

**81.35**    **Refusion of dorsal and dorsolumbar spine, posterior technique**
> Arthrodesis of thoracic or thoracolumbar
> > region:
> > posterior (interbody) technique
> > posterolateral technique

**81.36**    **Refusion of lumbar and lumbosacral spine, anterior technique**
> Anterior lumbar interbody fusion (ALIF)
> Arthrodesis of lumbar or lumbosacral
> > region:
> > anterior (interbody) technique
> > anterolateral technique

**AHA:** 4Q, '05, 122-123

**81.37**    **Refusion of lumbar and lumbosacral spine, lateral transverse process technique**

**81.38**    **Refusion of lumbar and lumbosacral spine, posterior technique**
> Arthrodesis of lumbar or lumbosacral
> > region:
> > posterior (interbody) technique
> > posterolateral technique
> Posterior lumbar interbody fusion (PLIF)
> Transforaminal lumbar interbody fusion
> > (TLIF)

**AHA:** 4Q, '05, 122-123; 4Q, '02, 110

**81.39**    **Refusion of spine, not elsewhere classified**

√4ᵗʰ **81.4**    **Other repair of joint of lower extremity**

> **INCLUDES**   arthroplasty of lower extremity with:
> > external traction or fixation
> > graft of bone (chips) or cartilage
> > internal fixation device

**AHA:** S-O, '85, 4

**81.40**    **Repair of hip, not elsewhere classified**

**81.42**    **Five-in-one repair of knee**
> Medial meniscectomy, medial collateral
> > ligament repair, vastus medialis
> > advancement, semitendinosus
> > advancement, and pes anserinus
> > transfer

**81.43**    **Triad knee repair**
> Medial meniscectomy with repair of the
> > anterior cruciate ligament and the
> > medial collateral ligament
> O'Donoghue procedure

**81.44**    **Patellar stabilization**
> Roux-Goldthwait operation for recurrent
> > dislocation of patella
>
> **DEF:** Roux-Goldthwait operation: Stabilization of patella
> via lateral ligament transposed at insertion beneath
> undisturbed medial insertion; excision of capsule ellipse
> and medial patella retinaculum; capsule reefed for
> lateral patella hold.

**81.45**    **Other repair of the cruciate ligaments**
> **AHA:** M-A, '87, 12

**81.46**    **Other repair of the collateral ligaments**

**81.47**    **Other repair of knee**
> **AHA:** 2Q, '06, 13; 2Q, '03, 18; 1Q, '00, 12, 13; 1Q, '96, 3; 3Q, '93, 5

**81.49**    **Other repair of ankle**
> **AHA:** 2Q, '01, 15; 3Q, '00, 4

√4ᵗʰ **81.5**    **Joint replacement of lower extremity**

> **INCLUDES**   arthroplasty of lower extremity with:
> > external traction or fixation
> > graft of bone (chips) or cartilage
> > internal fixation device or prosthesis

**AHA:** S-O, '85, 4

**81.51**    **Total hip replacement**     **BI**
> Replacement of both femoral head and
> > acetabulum by prosthesis
> Total reconstruction of hip
> Code also any type of bearing surface, if
> > known (00.74-00.77)
>
> **AHA:** 4Q, '04, 113; 2Q, '91, 18
>
> **DEF:** Repair of both surfaces of hip joint with prosthesis.

**Partial Hip Replacement**

Acetabulum
remains intact

Prosthesis

**Total Hip Replacement**

Damaged femur head ("ball")
in degenerated socket (acetabulum)

Cuplike acetabular
component of
prosthesis fixed
into hip bone

Prosthesis anchored
into shaft of long bone

Damaged femur head
replaced with prosthesis

---

**Operations on the Musculoskeletal System**

**81.3–81.51**

**Operations on the Musculoskeletal System**

**81.52–81.81**

### Total Knee Replacement

### Vertebroplasty

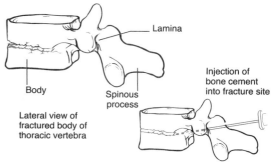

Lateral view of fractured body of thoracic vertebra

### Kyphoplasty

The cavity is filled with bone cement

---

**81.52**   **Partial hip replacement**    `BI`
Bipolar endoprosthesis
Code also any type of bearing surface, if known (00.74-00.77)
**AHA:** 2Q, '91, 18
**DEF:** Repair of single surface of hip joint with prosthesis.

**81.53**   **Revision of hip replacement, not otherwise specified**
Revision of hip replacement, not specified as to component(s) replaced, (acetabular, femoral or both)
Code also any:
   removal of (cement) (joint) spacer (84.57)
   type of bearing surface, if known (00.74-00.77)
> `EXCLUDES`   revision of hip replacement, components specified (00.70-00.73)

**AHA:** 4Q, '05, 125; 3Q, '97, 12

**81.54**   **Total knee replacement**    `BI`
Bicompartmental
Tricompartmental
Unicompartmental (hemijoint)
**DEF:** Repair of a knee joint with prosthetic implant in one, two, or three compartments.

**81.55**   **Revision of knee replacement, not otherwise specified**
Code also any removal of (cement) (joint) spacer (84.57)
> `EXCLUDES`   arthrodesis of knee (81.22)
> revision of knee replacement, components specified (00.80-00.84)

**AHA:** 4Q, '05, 113; 2Q, '97, 10

**81.56**   **Total ankle replacement**    `BI`
**81.57**   **Replacement of joint of foot and toe**
**81.59**   **Revision of joint replacement of lower extremity, not elsewhere classified**

`√4ᵗʰ` **81.6**   **Other procedures on spine**
**Note: Number of vertebrae**
The vertebral spine consists of 25 vertebrae in the following order and number:
   Cervical: C1 (atlas), C2 (axis), C3, C4, C5, C6, C7
   Thoracic or Dorsal: T1, T2, T3, T4, T5, T6, T7, T8, T9, T10, T11, T12
   Lumbar and Sacral: L1, L2, L3, L4, L5, S1
Coders should report only one code from the series 81.62-81.64 to show the total number of vertebrae fused on the patient.
Code also the level and approach of the fusion or refusion (81.00-81.08, 81.30-81.39)
**AHA:** 4Q, '03, 99
**DEF:** A combined posterior and anterior fusion performed by a surgeon through one incision: lateral transverse, posterior, or anterior.

**81.62**   **Fusion or refusion of 2-3 vertebrae**
**AHA:** 1Q, '06, 12, 13; 4Q, '05, 123; 4Q, '03, 99

**81.63**   **Fusion or refusion of 4-8 vertebrae**
**AHA:** ▶1Q, '07, 20;◀ 1Q, '03, 99-101

**81.64**   **Fusion or refusion of 9 or more vertebrae**
**AHA:** 4Q, '03, 99

---

**81.65**   **Vertebroplasty**
Injection of bone void filler (cement) (poly-methylmethacrylate) (PMMA) into the diseased or fractured vertebral body
> `EXCLUDES`   kyphoplasty (81.66)

**81.66**   **Kyphoplasty**
Insertion of inflatable balloon, bone tamp, or other device to create a cavity for partial restoration of height of diseased or fractured vertebral body prior to injection of bone void filler (cement) (polymethylmethacrylate) (PMMA)
> `EXCLUDES`   vertebroplasty (81.65)

**AHA:** ▶1Q, '07, 5, 7;◀ 3Q, '06, 13; 4Q, '04, 126

`√4ᵗʰ` **81.7**   **Arthroplasty and repair of hand, fingers, and wrist**
> `INCLUDES`   arthroplasty of hand and finger with:
>    external traction or fixation
>    graft of bone (chips) or cartilage
>    internal fixation device or prosthesis

> `EXCLUDES`   operations on muscle, tendon, and fascia of hand (82.01-82.99)

**DEF:** Plastic surgery of hand, fingers and wrist joints.

**81.71**   **Arthroplasty of metacarpophalangeal and interphalangeal joint with implant**
**81.72**   **Arthroplasty of metacarpophalangeal and interphalangeal joint without implant**
**AHA:** 1Q, '93, 28

**81.73**   **Total wrist replacement**
**81.74**   **Arthroplasty of carpocarpal or carpometacarpal joint with implant**
**81.75**   **Arthroplasty of carpocarpal or carpometacarpal joint without implant**
**AHA:** 3Q, '93, 8

**81.79**   **Other repair of hand, fingers, and wrist**

`√4ᵗʰ` **81.8**   **Arthroplasty and repair of shoulder and elbow**
> `INCLUDES`   arthroplasty of upper limb NEC with:
>    external traction or fixation
>    graft of bone (chips) or cartilage
>    internal fixation device or prosthesis

**81.80**   **Total shoulder replacement**
**81.81**   **Partial shoulder replacement**

---

`BI` Bilateral Procedure    `NC` Non-covered Procedure    `LC` Limited Coverage Procedure    ▶◀ Revised Text    ● New Code    ▲ Revised Code Title

**81.82 Repair of recurrent dislocation of shoulder**
AHA: 3Q, '95, 15

**81.83 Other repair of shoulder**
Revision of arthroplasty of shoulder
AHA: 1Q, '02, 9; 4Q, '01, 51; 2Q, '00, 14; 3Q, '93, 5

**81.84 Total elbow replacement**

**81.85 Other repair of elbow**

√4th **81.9 Other operations on joint structures**

**81.91 Arthrocentesis**
Joint aspiration
**EXCLUDES** that for:
arthrography (88.32)
biopsy of joint structure
(80.30-80.39)
injection of drug (81.92)
DEF: Insertion of needle to withdraw fluid from joint.

**81.92 Injection of therapeutic substance into joint or ligament**
AHA: 2Q, '00, 14; 3Q, '89, 16

**81.93 Suture of capsule or ligament of upper extremity**
**EXCLUDES** that associated with arthroplasty (81.71-81.75, 81.80-81.81, 81.84)

**81.94 Suture of capsule or ligament of ankle and foot**
**EXCLUDES** that associated with arthroplasty (81.56-81.59)

**81.95 Suture of capsule or ligament of other lower extremity**
**EXCLUDES** that associated with arthroplasty (81.51-81.55, 81.59)

**81.96 Other repair of joint**

**81.97 Revision of joint replacement of upper extremity**
Partial      Total
Removal of cement spacer
AHA: 1Q, '04, 12

**81.98 Other diagnostic procedures on joint structures**
**EXCLUDES** arthroscopy (80.20-80.29)
biopsy of joint structure
(80.30-80.39)
microscopic examination of
specimen from joint
(91.51-91.59)
thermography (88.83)
x-ray (87.21-87.29, 88.21-88.33)

**81.99 Other**
AHA: 4Q, '05, 124

√3rd **82 Operations on muscle, tendon, and fascia of hand**
**INCLUDES** operations on:
aponeurosis
synovial membrane (tendon sheath)
tendon sheath

√4th **82.0 Incision of muscle, tendon, fascia, and bursa of hand**

**82.01 Exploration of tendon sheath of hand**
Incision of   } tendon sheath
Removal of rice bodies in } of hand
**EXCLUDES** division of tendon (82.11)
DEF: Incision into and exploring the hand's muscle and its accompanying supportive, connective tissue, bands, and sacs.

**82.02 Myotomy of hand**
**EXCLUDES** myotomy for division (82.19)
DEF: Incision into hand muscle.

**82.03 Bursotomy of hand**

**82.04 Incision and drainage of palmar or thenar space**

**Arthrocentesis**

**82.09 Other incision of soft tissue of hand**
**EXCLUDES** incision of skin and
subcutaneous tissue
alone (86.01-86.09)
AHA: N-D, '87, 10

√4th **82.1 Division of muscle, tendon, and fascia of hand**

**82.11 Tenotomy of hand**
Division of tendon of hand

**82.12 Fasciotomy of hand**
Division of fascia of hand

**82.19 Other division of soft tissue of hand**
Division of muscle of hand

√4th **82.2 Excision of lesion of muscle, tendon, and fascia of hand**

**82.21 Excision or lesion of tendon sheath of hand**
Ganglionectomy of tendon sheath (wrist)

**82.22 Excision of lesion of muscle of hand**

**82.29 Excision of other lesion of soft tissue of hand**
**EXCLUDES** excision of lesion of skin and
subcutaneous tissue
(86.21-86.3)

√4th **82.3 Other excision of soft tissue of hand**
Code also any skin graft (86.61-86.62, 86.73)
**EXCLUDES** excision of skin and subcutaneous
tissue (86.21-86.3)

**82.31 Bursectomy of hand**

**82.32 Excision of tendon of hand for graft**
DEF: Resection and excision of fibrous tissue connecting bone to hand muscle for grafting.

**82.33 Other tenonectomy of hand**
Tenosynovectomy of hand
**EXCLUDES** excision of lesion of:
tendon (82.29)
sheath (82.21)
DEF: Removal of fibrous bands connecting muscle to bone of hand.
DEF: Tenosynovectomy of hand: Excision of fibrous band connecting muscle and bone of hand and removal of coverings.

**82.34 Excision of muscle or fascia of hand for graft**

**82.35 Other fasciectomy of hand**
Release of Dupuytren's contracture
**EXCLUDES** excision of lesion of fascia
(82.29)
DEF: Excision of fibrous connective tissue; other than for grafting or removing lesion.
DEF: Release of Dupuytren's contracture: Excision of fibrous connective tissue to correct flexion of fingers.

**82.36 Other myectomy of hand**
**EXCLUDES** excision of lesion of muscle
(82.22)

**82.39 Other excision of soft tissue of hand**
**EXCLUDES** excision of skin (86.21-86.3)
excision of soft tissue lesion
(82.29)

√4th **82.4 Suture of muscle, tendon, and fascia of hand**

**82.41 Suture of tendon sheath of hand**

**Operations on the Musculoskeletal System**

**82.42–83.12**

**82.42 Delayed suture of flexor tendon of hand**
DEF: Suture of fibrous band between flexor muscle and bone; following initial repair.

**82.43 Delayed suture of other tendon of hand**

**82.44 Other suture of flexor tendon of hand**
EXCLUDES   *delayed suture of flexor tendon of hand (82.42)*

**82.45 Other suture of other tendon of hand**
EXCLUDES   *delayed suture of other tendon of hand (82.43)*

**82.46 Suture of muscle or fascia of hand**

√4th **82.5 Transplantation of muscle and tendon of hand**
AHA: 1Q, '93, 28

**82.51 Advancement of tendon of hand**
DEF: Detachment of fibrous connective muscle band and bone with reattachment at advanced point of hand.

**82.52 Recession of tendon of hand**
DEF: Detachment of fibrous band of muscle and bone with reattachment at drawn-back point of hand.

**82.53 Reattachment of tendon of hand**

**82.54 Reattachment of muscle of hand**

**82.55 Other change in hand muscle or tendon length**

**82.56 Other hand tendon transfer or transplantation**
EXCLUDES   *pollicization of thumb (82.61)*
*transfer of finger, except thumb (82.81)*
AHA: 2Q, '99, 10; 4Q, '98, 40

**82.57 Other hand tendon transposition**
AHA: 1Q, '93, 28; 3Q, '93, 8

**82.58 Other hand muscle transfer or transplantation**

**82.59 Other hand muscle transposition**

√4th **82.6 Reconstruction of thumb**
INCLUDES   digital transfer to act as thumb
Code also any amputation for digital transfer (84.01, 84.11)

**82.61 Pollicization operation carrying over nerves and blood supply**
DEF: Creation or reconstruction of a thumb with another digit, commonly the index finger.

**82.69 Other reconstruction of thumb**
"Cocked-hat" procedure [skin flap and bone]
Grafts:
bone
skin (pedicle) } to thumb

√4th **82.7 Plastic operation on hand with graft or implant**

**82.71 Tendon pulley reconstruction**
Reconstruction for opponensplasty
DEF: Reconstruction of fibrous band between muscle and bone of hand.

**82.72 Plastic operation on hand with graft of muscle or fascia**

**82.79 Plastic operation on hand with other graft or implant**
Tendon graft to hand
AHA: J-F, '87, 6

√4th **82.8 Other plastic operations on hand**

**82.81 Transfer of finger, except thumb**
EXCLUDES   *pollicization of thumb (82.61)*
AHA: 2Q, '05, 7

**82.82 Repair of cleft hand**
DEF: Correction of fissure defect of hand.

**82.83 Repair of macrodactyly**
DEF: Reduction in size of abnormally large fingers.

**82.84 Repair of mallet finger**
DEF: Repair of flexed little finger.

**82.85 Other tenodesis of hand**
Tendon fixation of hand NOS
DEF: Fixation of fibrous connective band between muscle and bone of hand.

**82.86 Other tenoplasty of hand**
Myotenoplasty of hand
DEF: Myotenoplasty of hand: Plastic repair of muscle and fibrous band connecting muscle to bone.

**82.89 Other plastic operations on hand**
Plication of fascia
Repair of fascial hernia
EXCLUDES   *that with graft or implant (82.71-82.79)*

√4th **82.9 Other operations on muscle, tendon, and fascia of hand**
EXCLUDES   *diagnostic procedures on soft tissue of hand (83.21-83.29)*

**82.91 Lysis of adhesions of hand**
Freeing of adhesions of fascia, muscle, and tendon of hand
EXCLUDES   *decompression of carpal tunnel (04.43)*
*that by stretching or manipulation only (93.26)*

**82.92 Aspiration of bursa of hand**

**82.93 Aspiration of other soft tissue of hand**
EXCLUDES   *skin and subcutaneous tissue (86.01)*

**82.94 Injection of therapeutic substance into bursa of hand**

**82.95 Injection of therapeutic substance into tendon of hand**

**82.96 Other injection of locally-acting therapeutic substance into soft tissue of hand**
EXCLUDES   *subcutaneous or intramuscular injection (99.11-99.29)*

**82.99 Other operations on muscle, tendon, and fascia of hand**

√3rd **83 Operations on muscle, tendon, fascia, and bursa, except hand**
INCLUDES   operations on:
aponeurosis
synovial membrane of bursa and tendon sheaths
tendon sheaths
EXCLUDES   *diaphragm (34.81-34.89)*
*hand (82.01-82.99)*
*muscles of eye (15.01-15.9)*

√4th **83.0 Incision of muscle, tendon, fascia, and bursa**

**83.01 Exploration of tendon sheath**
Incision of tendon sheath
Removal of rice bodies from tendon sheath
DEF: Incision of external covering of fibrous cord for exam.
DEF: Removal of rice bodies from tendon sheath: Incision and removal of small bodies resembling grains of rice.

**83.02 Myotomy**
EXCLUDES   *cricopharyngeal myotomy (29.31)*
AHA: 2Q, '89, 18

**83.03 Bursotomy**
Removal of calcareous deposit of bursa
EXCLUDES   *aspiration of bursa (percutaneous) (83.94)*

**83.09 Other incision of soft tissue**
Incision of fascia
EXCLUDES   *incision of skin and subcutaneous tissue alone (86.01-86.09)*

√4th **83.1 Division of muscle, tendon, and fascia**

**83.11 Achillotenotomy**

**83.12 Adductor tenotomy of hip**
DEF: Incision into fibrous attachment between adductor muscle and hip bone.

---

**BI** Bilateral Procedure    **NC** Non-covered Procedure    **LC** Limited Coverage Procedure    ►◄ Revised Text    ● New Code    ▲ Revised Code Title

168 — Volume 3

© 2007 Ingenix

**83.13 Other tenotomy**

Aponeurotomy     Tendon transection
Division of tendon     Tenotomy for thoracic
Tendon release         outlet decom-
                        pression

DEF: Aponeurotomy: Incision and separation of fibrous cords attaching a muscle to bone to aid movement.

DEF: Division of tendon: Separation of fibrous band connecting muscle to bone.

DEF: Tendon release: Surgical detachment of fibrous band from muscle and/or bone.

DEF: Tendon transection: Incision across width of fibrous bands between muscle and bone.

DEF: Tenotomy for thoracic outlet decompression: Incision of fibrous muscle with separation from bone to relieve compressed thoracic outlet.

**83.14 Fasciotomy**

Division of fascia
Division of iliotibial band
Fascia stripping
Release of Volkmann's contracture by
    fasciotomy

AHA: ▶4Q, '06, 102;◀ 3Q, '98, 8

DEF: Division of fascia: Incision to separate fibrous connective tissue.

DEF: Division of iliotibial band: Incision to separate fibrous band connecting tibial bone to muscle in flank.

DEF: Fascia stripping: Incision and lengthwise separation of fibrous connective tissue.

DEF: Release of Volkmann's contracture by fasciotomy: Divisional incision of connective tissue to correct defect in flexion of finger(s).

**83.19 Other division of soft tissue**

Division of muscle
Muscle release
Myotomy for thoracic outlet decompression
Myotomy with division
Scalenotomy
Transection of muscle

✓4ᵗʰ **83.2 Diagnostic procedures on muscle, tendon, fascia, and bursa, including that of hand**

**83.21 Biopsy of soft tissue**

EXCLUDES   biopsy of chest wall (34.23)
              biopsy of skin and subcutan-
                 eous tissue (86.11)

**83.29 Other diagnostic procedures on muscle, tendon, fascia, and bursa, including that of hand**

EXCLUDES   microscopic examination of
              specimen (91.51-91.-59)
              soft tissue x-ray (87.09, 87.38-
              87.39, 88.09, 88.35,
              88.37)
              thermography of muscle (88.84)

✓4ᵗʰ **83.3 Excision of lesion of muscle, tendon, fascia, and bursa**

EXCLUDES   biopsy of soft tissue (83.21)

**83.31 Excision of lesion of tendon sheath**

Excision of ganglion of tendon sheath,
    except of hand

**83.32 Excision of lesion of muscle**

Excision of:
    heterotopic bone
    muscle scar for release of Volkmann's
       contracture
    myositis ossificans

DEF: Heterotopic bone: Bone lesion in muscle.

DEF: Muscle scar for release of Volkmann's contracture: Scarred muscle tissue interfering with finger flexion.

DEF: Myositis ossificans: Bony deposits in muscle.

**83.39 Excision of lesion of other soft tissue**

Excision of Baker's cyst
EXCLUDES   bursectomy (83.5)
              excision of lesion of skin and
               subcutaneous tissue
               (86.3)
              synovectomy (80.70-80.79)
AHA: 2Q, '05, 3; 2Q, '97, 6

✓4ᵗʰ **83.4 Other excision of muscle, tendon, and fascia**

**83.41 Excision of tendon for graft**

**83.42 Other tenonectomy**

Excision of:       Tenosynovectomy
   aponeurosis
   tendon sheath

**83.43 Excision of muscle or fascia for graft**

**83.44 Other fasciectomy**

DEF: Excision of fascia; other than for graft.

**83.45 Other myectomy**

Debridement of muscle NOS
Scalenectomy
AHA: 1Q, '99, 8

DEF: Scalenectomy: Removal of thoracic scaleni muscle tissue.

**83.49 Other excision of soft tissue**

**83.5 Bursectomy**

AHA: ▶2Q, '06, 15;◀ 2Q, '99, 11

✓4ᵗʰ **83.6 Suture of muscle, tendon, and fascia**

**83.61 Suture of tendon sheath**

**83.62 Delayed suture of tendon**

**83.63 Rotator cuff repair**

AHA: 1Q, '06, 6; 2Q, '93, 8

DEF: Repair of musculomembranous structure around shoulder joint capsule.

**83.64 Other suture of tendon**

Achillorrhaphy     Aponeurorrhaphy
EXCLUDES   delayed suture of tendon
              (83.62)

DEF: Achillorrhaphy: Suture of fibrous band connecting Achilles tendon to heel bone.

DEF: Aponeurorrhaphy: Suture of fibrous cords connecting muscle to bone.

**83.65 Other suture of muscle or fascia**

Repair of diastasis recti

✓4ᵗʰ **83.7 Reconstruction of muscle and tendon**

EXCLUDES   reconstruction of muscle and tendon
              associated with arthroplasty

**83.71 Advancement of tendon**

DEF: Detaching fibrous cord between muscle and bone with reattachment at advanced point.

**83.72 Recession of tendon**

DEF: Detaching fibrous cord between muscle and bone with reattachment at drawn-back point.

**83.73 Reattachment of tendon**

**83.74 Reattachment of muscle**

**83.75 Tendon transfer or transplantation**

**83.76 Other tendon transposition**

**83.77 Muscle transfer or transplantation**

Release of Volkmann's contracture by
    muscle transplantation

**83.79 Other muscle transposition**

✓4ᵗʰ **83.8 Other plastic operations on muscle, tendon, and fascia**

EXCLUDES   plastic operations on muscle, tendon,
              and fascia associated with
              arthroplasty

**83.81 Tendon graft**

**83.82 Graft of muscle or fascia**

AHA: 3Q, '01, 9

**83.83 Tendon pulley reconstruction**

DEF: Reconstruction of fibrous cord between muscle and bone; at any site other than hand.

**Operations on the Musculoskeletal System**

**83.84–84.10**

**83.84**   **Release of clubfoot, not elsewhere classified**
Evans operation on clubfoot

**83.85**   **Other change in muscle or tendon length**
Hamstring lengthening
Heel cord shortening
Plastic achillotenotomy
Tendon plication

DEF: Plastic achillotenotomy: Increase in heel cord length.

DEF: Tendon plication: Surgical tuck of tendon.

**83.86**   **Quadricepsplasty**

DEF: Correction of quadriceps femoris muscle.

**83.87**   **Other plastic operations on muscle**
Musculoplasty     Myoplasty

AHA: 1Q, '97, 9

**83.88**   **Other plastic operations on tendon**
Myotenoplasty     Tenodesis
Tendon fixation     Tenoplasty

**83.89**   **Other plastic operations on fascia**
Fascia lengthening
Fascioplasty
Plication of fascia

✓4th   **83.9**   **Other operations on muscle, tendon, fascia, and bursa**

EXCLUDES   nonoperative:
manipulation (93.25-93.29)
stretching (93.27-93.29)

**83.91**   **Lysis of adhesions of muscle, tendon, fascia, and bursa**

EXCLUDES   that for tarsal tunnel
syndrome (04.44)

DEF: Separation of created fibrous structures from muscle, connective tissues, bands and sacs.

**83.92**   **Insertion or replacement of skeletal muscle stimulator**
Implantation, insertion, placement, or replacement of skeletal muscle:
electrodes
stimulator

AHA: 2Q, '99, 10

**83.93**   **Removal of skeletal muscle stimulator**

**83.94**   **Aspiration of bursa**

**83.95**   **Aspiration of other soft tissue**

EXCLUDES   that of skin and subcutaneous
tissue (86.01)

**83.96**   **Injection of therapeutic substance into bursa**

**83.97**   **Injection of therapeutic substance into tendon**

**83.98**   **Injection of locally-acting therapeutic substance into other soft tissue**

EXCLUDES   subcutaneous or
intramuscular injection
(99.11-99.29)

AHA: 2Q, '06, 11

**83.99**   **Other operations on muscle, tendon, fascia, and bursa**
Suture of bursa

✓3rd   **84**   **Other procedures on musculoskeletal system**

✓4th   **84.0**   **Amputation of upper limb**

EXCLUDES   revision of amputation stump (84.3)

**84.00**   **Upper limb amputation, not otherwise specified**

Closed flap amputation
Kineplastic amputation
Open or guillotine
amputation     } of upper limb NOS
Revision of current
traumatic
amputation

DEF: Closed flap amputation: Sewing a created skin flap over stump end of upper limb.

DEF: Kineplastic amputation: Amputation and preparation of stump of upper limb to permit movement.

DEF: Open or guillotine amputation: Straight incision across upper limb; used when primary closure is contraindicated.

DEF: Revision of current traumatic amputation: Reconstruction of traumatic amputation of upper limb to enable closure.

**84.01**   **Amputation and disarticulation of finger**

EXCLUDES   ligation of supernumerary
finger (86.26)

**84.02**   **Amputation and disarticulation of thumb**

**84.03**   **Amputation through hand**
Amputation through carpals

**84.04**   **Disarticulation of wrist**

**84.05**   **Amputation through forearm**
Forearm amputation

**84.06**   **Disarticulation of elbow**

DEF: Amputation of forearm through elbow joint.

**84.07**   **Amputation through humerus**
Upper arm amputation

**84.08**   **Disarticulation of shoulder**

DEF: Amputation of arm through shoulder joint.

**84.09**   **Interthoracoscapular amputation**
Forequarter amputation

DEF: Removal of upper arm, shoulder bone and collarbone.

✓4th   **84.1**   **Amputation of lower limb**

EXCLUDES   revision of amputation stump (84.3)

**84.10**   **Lower limb amputation, not otherwise specified**

Closed flap amputation
Kineplastic amputation
Open or guillotine
amputation     } of lower limb NOS
Revision of current
traumatic
amputation

DEF: Closed flap amputation: Sewing a created skin flap over stump of lower limb.

DEF: Kineplastic amputation: Amputation and preparation of stump of lower limb to permit movement.

DEF: Open or guillotine amputation: Straight incision across lower limb; used when primary closure is contraindicated.

DEF: Revision of current traumatic amputation: Reconstruction of traumatic amputation of lower limb to enable closure.

BI   Bilateral Procedure     NC   Non-covered Procedure     LC   Limited Coverage Procedure     ►◄ Revised Text     ● New Code     ▲ Revised Code Title

170 — Volume 3 • October 2007

© 2007 Ingenix

**84.11**   **Amputation of toe**

Amputation through metatarsophalangeal joint

Disarticulation of toe

Metatarsal head amputation

Ray amputation of foot (disarticulation of the metatarsal head of the toe extending across the forefoot, just proximal to the metatarsophalangeal crease)

> **EXCLUDES**   ligation of supernumerary toe (86.26)

AHA: 2Q, '05, 7; 4Q, '99, 19

**84.12**   **Amputation through foot**

Amputation of forefoot

Amputation through middle of foot

Chopart's amputation

Midtarsal amputation

Transmetatarsal amputation (amputation of the forefoot, including the toes)

> **EXCLUDES**   Ray amputation of foot (84.11)

AHA: 4Q, '99, 19

DEF: Amputation of forefoot: Removal of foot in front of joint between toes and body of foot.

DEF: Chopart's amputation: Removal of foot with retention of heel, ankle and other associated ankle bones.

DEF: Midtarsal amputation: Amputation of foot through tarsals.

DEF: Transmetatarsal amputation: Amputation of foot through metatarsals.

**84.13**   **Disarticulation of ankle**

DEF: Removal of foot through ankle bone.

**84.14**   **Amputation of ankle through malleoli of tibia and fibula**

**84.15**   **Other amputation below knee**

Amputation of leg through tibia and fibula NOS

**84.16**   **Disarticulation of knee**

Batch, Spitler, and McFaddin amputation

Mazet amputation

S.P. Roger's amputation

DEF: Removal of lower leg through knee joint.

**84.17**   **Amputation above knee**

Amputation of leg through femur

Amputation of thigh

Conversion of below-knee amputation into above-knee amputation

Supracondylar above-knee amputation

AHA: 1Q, '05, 16; 1Q, '05, 16; 3Q, '03, 14

**84.18**   **Disarticulation of hip**

DEF: Removal of leg through hip joint.

**84.19**   **Abdominopelvic amputation**

Hemipelvectomy

Hindquarter amputation

DEF: Removal of leg and portion of pelvic bone.

DEF: Hemipelvectomy: Removal of leg and lateral pelvis.

✓4ᵗʰ **84.2**   **Reattachment of extremity**

AHA: 1Q, '95, 8

**84.21**   **Thumb reattachment**

**84.22**   **Finger reattachment**

**84.23**   **Forearm, wrist, or hand reattachment**

**84.24**   **Upper arm reattachment**

Reattachment of arm NOS

**84.25**   **Toe reattachment**

**84.26**   **Foot reattachment**

**84.27**   **Lower leg or ankle reattachment**

Reattachment of leg NOS

**84.28**   **Thigh reattachment**

**84.29**   **Other reattachment**

**84.3**   **Revision of amputation stump**

Reamputation ⎫

Secondary closure ⎬ of stump

Trimming ⎭

> **EXCLUDES**   revision of current traumatic amputation [revision by further amputation of current injury] (84.00-84.19, 84.91)

AHA: 4Q, '99, 15; 2Q, '98, 15; 4Q, '88, 12

✓4ᵗʰ **84.4**   **Implantation or fitting of prosthetic limb device**

**84.40**   **Implantation or fitting of prosthetic limb device, not otherwise specified**

**84.41**   **Fitting of prosthesis of upper arm and shoulder**

**84.42**   **Fitting of prosthesis of lower arm and hand**

**84.43**   **Fitting of prosthesis of arm, not otherwise specified**

**84.44**   **Implantation of prosthetic device of arm**

**84.45**   **Fitting of prosthesis above knee**

**84.46**   **Fitting of prosthesis below knee**

**84.47**   **Fitting of prosthesis of leg, not otherwise specified**

**84.48**   **Implantation of prosthetic device of leg**

✓4ᵗʰ **84.5**   **Implantation of other musculoskeletal devices and substances**

> **EXCLUDES**   insertion of (non-fusion) spinal disc replacement device (84.60-84.69)

**84.51**   **Insertion of interbody spinal fusion device**

Insertion of:

cages (carbn, ceramic, metal, plastic or titanium)

interbody fusion cage

synthetic cages or spacers

threaded bone dowels

Code also refusion of spine (81.30-81.39)

Code also spinal fusion (81.00-81.08)

AHA:▶1Q, '07, 20;◀ 4Q, '05, 123; 1Q, '04, 21; 4Q, '02, 108-110

**84.52**   **Insertion of recombinant bone morphogenetic protein**

rhBMP

That via collagen sponge, coral, ceramic and other carriers

Code also primary procedure performed:

fracture repair (79.00-79.99)

spinal fusion (81.00-81.08)

spinal refusion (81.30-81.39)

AHA: 4Q, '02, 110

DEF: Surgical implantation of bone morphogenetic proteins (BMP) and recombinant BMP (rhBMP) to induce new bone growth formation; clinical applications include delayed unions and nonunions, fractures, and spinal fusions.

**Spinal Fusion with Metal Cage**

Metal cages support spine until fusion occurs

Anterior view

Lateral view

Spinal fusion with metal cages

Detail

**Operations on the Musculoskeletal System**

**84.53–84.72**

**84.53 Implantation of internal limb lengthening device with kinetic distraction**
Code also limb lengthening procedure (78.30-78.39)

**84.54 Implantation of other internal limb lengthening device**
Implantation of internal limb lengthening device, not otherwise specified (NOS)
Code also limb lengthening procedure (78.30-78.39)

**84.55 Insertion of bone void filler**
Insertion of:
acrylic cement (PMMA)
bone void cement
calcium based bone void filler
polymethylmethacrylate (PMMA)
EXCLUDES   *that with kyphoplasty (81.66)*
*that with vertebroplasty (81.65)*

**AHA:** 4Q, '04, 128

**84.56 Insertion of (cement) spacer**
Insertion of joint ▶(methylmethacrylate)◀ spacer

**AHA:** 4Q, '05, 124

DEF: Implantation of an interspinous process decompressive (IPD) device between the spinous processes to limit extension; nonfusion, posterior approach procedure.

**84.57 Removal of (cement) spacer**
Removal of joint ▶(methylmethacrylate)◀ spacer

**AHA:** 4Q, '05, 113, 124-125

**84.59 Insertion of other spinal devices**
EXCLUDES ▶ *initial insertion of pedicle screws with spinal fusion — omit code*
*insertion of facet replacement device(s) (84.84)*
*insertion of interspinous process device(s) (84.80)*
*insertion of pedicle-based dynamic stabilization device(s) (84.82)◀*

**AHA:** ▶1Q, '07, 9, 10◀

☑4th **84.6 Replacement of spinal disc**
INCLUDES   non-fusion arthroplasty of the spine with insertion of artificial disc prosthesis

**84.60 Insertion of spinal disc prosthesis, not otherwise specified**
Replacement of spinal disc, NOS
INCLUDES   diskectomy (discectomy)

**84.61 Insertion of partial spinal disc prosthesis, cervical**
Nuclear replacement device, cervical
Partial artificial disc prosthesis (flexible), cervical
Replacement of nuclear disc (nucleus pulposus), cervical
INCLUDES   diskectomy (discectomy)

**84.62 Insertion of total spinal disc prosthesis, cervical**
Replacement of cervical spinal disc, NOS
Replacement of total spinal disc, cervical
Total artificial disc prosthesis (flexible), cervical
INCLUDES   diskectomy (discectomy)

**84.63 Insertion of spinal disc prosthesis, thoracic**
Artificial disc prosthesis (flexible), thoracic
Replacement of thoracic spinal disc, partial or total
INCLUDES   diskectomy (discectomy)

**84.64 Insertion of partial spinal disc prosthesis, lumbosacral**
Nuclear replacement device, lumbar
Partial artificial disc prosthesis (flexible), lumbar
Replacement of nuclear disc (nucleus pulposus), lumbar
INCLUDES   diskectomy (discectomy)

[11] **84.65 Insertion of total spinal disc prosthesis, lumbosacral**   NC
Replacement of lumbar spinal disc, NOS
Replacement of total spinal disc, lumbar
Total artificial disc prosthesis (flexible), lumbar
INCLUDES   diskectomy (discectomy)

**AHA:** 4Q, '04, 133

**84.66 Revision or replacement of artificial spinal disc prosthesis, cervical**
Removal of (partial) (total) spinal disc prosthesis with synchronous insertion of new (partial) (total) spinal disc prosthesis, cervical
Repair of previously inserted spinal disc prosthesis, cervical

**84.67 Revision or replacement of artificial spinal disc prosthesis, thoracic**
Removal of (partial) (total) spinal disc prosthesis with synchronous insertion of new (partial) (total) spinal disc prosthesis, thoracic
Repair of previously inserted spinal disc prosthesis, thoracic

**84.68 Revision or replacement of artificial spinal disc prosthesis, lumbosacral**
Removal of (partial) (total) spinal disc prosthesis with synchronous insertion of new (partial) (total) spinal disc prosthesis, lumbosacral
Repair of previously inserted spinal disc prosthesis, lumbosacral

**84.69 Revision or replacement of artificial spinal disc prosthesis, not otherwise specified**
Removal of (partial) (total) spinal disc prosthesis with synchronous insertion of new (partial) (total) spinal disc prosthesis
Repair of previously inserted spinal disc prosthesis

☑4th **84.7 Adjunct codes for external fixator devices**
Code also any primary procedure performed:
application of external fixator device (78.10, 78.12-78.13, 78.15, 78.17-78.19)
reduction of fracture and dislocation (79.00-79.89)

**AHA:** 4Q, '05, 127-129

**84.71 Application of external fixator device, monoplanar system**
EXCLUDES   *other hybrid device or system (84.73)*
*ring device or system (84.72)*

**AHA:** 4Q, '05, 129

DEF: Instrumentation that provides percutaneous neutralization, compression, and /or distraction of bone in a single plane by applying force within that plane.

**84.72 Application of external fixator device, ring system**
Ilizarov type
Sheffield type
EXCLUDES   *monoplanar device or system (84.71)*
*other hybrid device or system (84.73)*

DEF: Instrumentation that provides percutaneous neutralization, compression, and/or distraction of bone through 360 degrees of force application.

[11] Noncovered except when patient is 60 years or less.

BI   Bilateral Procedure     NC   Non-covered Procedure     LC   Limited Coverage Procedure     ▶◀ Revised Text     ● New Code     ▲ Revised Code Title

© 2007 Ingenix

**External Fixator Devices**

Monoplanar     Ring system     Hybrid

**84.73**   **Application of hybrid external fixator device**

Computer (assisted) (dependent) external fixator device

Hybrid system using both ring and monoplanar devices

> **EXCLUDES**   *monoplanar device or system, when used alone (84.71)*
> *ring device or system, when used alone (84.72)*

DEF: Instrumentation that provides percutaneous neutralization, compression, and /or distraction of bone by applying multiple external forces using monoplanar and ring device combinations.

✓4ᵗʰ **84.8**   **Insertion, replacement and revision of posterior spinal motion preservation device(s)**

Dynamic spinal stabilization device(s)

> **INCLUDES**   any synchronous facetectomy (partial, total) performed at the same level

Code also any synchronous surgical decompression (foraminotomy, laminectomy, laminotomy), if performed (03.09)

> **EXCLUDES**   *fusion of spine (81.00-81.08, 81.30-81.39)*
> *insertion of artificial disc prosthesis (84.60-84.69)*
> *insertion of interbody spinal fusion device (84.51)*

**84.80**   **Insertion or replacement of interspinous process device(s)**

Interspinous process decompression device(s)

Interspinous process distraction device(s)

> **EXCLUDES**   *insertion or replacement of facet replacement device (84.84)*
> *insertion or replacement of pedicle-based dynamic stabilization device (84.82)*

**84.81**   **Revision of interspinous process device(s)**

Repair of previously inserted interspinous process device(s)

> **EXCLUDES**   *revision of facet replacement device(s) (84.85)*
> *revision of pedicle-based dynamic stabilization device (84.83)*

**84.82**   **Insertion or replacement of pedicle-based dynamic stabilization device(s)**

> **EXCLUDES**   *initial insertion of pedicle screws with spinal fusion — omit code*
> *insertion or replacement of facet replacement device(s) (84.84)*
> *insertion or replacement of interspinous process device(s) (84.80)*
> *replacement of pedicle screws used in spinal fusion (78.59)*

**84.83**   **Revision of pedicle-based dynamic stabilization device(s)**

Repair of previously inserted pedicle-based dynamic stabilization device(s)

> **EXCLUDES**   *removal of pedicle screws used in spinal fusion (78.69)*
> *replacement of pedicle screws used in spinal fusion (78.59)*
> *revision of facet replacement device(s) (84.85)*
> *revision of interspinous process device(s) (84.81)*

**84.84**   **Insertion or replacement of facet replacement device(s)**

Facet arthroplasty

> **EXCLUDES**   *initial insertion of pedicle screws with spinal fusion — omit code*
> *insertion or replacement of interspinous process device(s) (84.80)*
> *insertion or replacement of pedicle-based dynamic stabilization device(s) (84.82)*
> *replacement of pedicle screws used in spinal fusion (78.59)*

**84.85**   **Revision of facet replacement device(s)**

Repair of previously inserted facet replacement device(s)

> **EXCLUDES**   *removal of pedicle screws used in spinal fusion (78.69)*
> *replacement of pedicle screws used in spinal fusion (78.59)*
> *revision of interspinous process device(s) (84.81)*
> *revision of pedicle-based dynamic stabilization device(s) (84.83)*

✓4ᵗʰ **84.9**   **Other operations on musculoskeletal system**

> **EXCLUDES**   *nonoperative manipulation (93.25-93.29)*

**84.91**   **Amputation, not otherwise specified**

**84.92**   **Separation of equal conjoined twins**

**84.93**   **Separation of unequal conjoined twins**

Separation of conjoined twins NOS

**84.99**   **Other**

**Operations on the Musculoskeletal System**     **84.73–84.99**

**Operations on the Integumentary System**

**85–85.45**

## 15. OPERATIONS ON THE INTEGUMENTARY SYSTEM (85-86)

**√3rd 85**   **Operations on the breast**

    **INCLUDES**   operations on the skin and subcutaneous
tissue of:

      breast                 }   female or
      previous mastectomy site }   male

      revision of previous mastectomy site

**85.0**   **Mastotomy**

      Incision of breast (skin)
      Mammotomy

      **EXCLUDES**   *aspiration of breast (85.91)*
                        *removal of implant (85.94)*

      **AHA:** 1Q, '04, 3; 2Q, '90, 27

**√4th 85.1**   **Diagnostic procedures on breast**

**85.11**   **Closed [percutaneous] [needle] biopsy of breast**

      **AHA:** 2Q, '00, 10; 3Q, '89, 17

      DEF: Mammatome biopsy: Excision of breast tissue using
a needle inserted through a small incision; followed by a
full cut circle of tissue surrounding the core biopsy to
obtain; multiple contiguous directional sampling for
definitive diagnosis and staging of cancer.

**85.12**   **Open biopsy of breast**

      **AHA:** 3Q, '89, 17; M-A, '86, 11

      DEF: Excision of breast tissue for examination.

**85.19**   **Other diagnostic procedures on breast**

      **EXCLUDES**   *mammary ductogram (87.35)*
                    *mammography NEC (87.37)*
                    *manual examination (89.36)*
                    *microscopic examination of*
                       *specimen (91.61-91.69)*
                    *thermography (88.85)*
                    *ultrasonography (88.73)*
                    *xerography (87.36)*

**√4th 85.2**   **Excision or destruction of breast tissue**

      **EXCLUDES**   *mastectomy (85.41-85.48)*
                    *reduction mammoplasty (85.31-85.32)*

**85.20**   **Excision or destruction of breast tissue, not otherwise specified**

**85.21**   **Local excision of lesion of breast**

      Lumpectomy
      Removal of area of fibrosis from breast

      **EXCLUDES**   *biopsy of breast (85.11-85.12)*

      **AHA:** 2Q, '90, 27; 3Q, '89, 17; M-A, '86, 11

**85.22**   **Resection of quadrant of breast**

**85.23**   **Subtotal mastectomy**

      **EXCLUDES**   *quadrant resection (85.22)*

      **AHA:** 2Q, '92, 7

      DEF: Excision of a large portion of breast tissue.

**85.24**   **Excision of ectopic breast tissue**

      Excision of accessory nipple

      DEF: Excision of breast tissue outside normal breast
region.

**85.25**   **Excision of nipple**

      **EXCLUDES**   *excision of accessory nipple (85.24)*

**√4th 85.3**   **Reduction mammoplasty and subcutaneous mammectomy**

      **AHA:** 4Q, '95, 79, 80

**85.31**   **Unilateral reduction mammoplasty**

      Unilateral:
         amputative mammoplasty
         size reduction mammoplasty

**85.32**   **Bilateral reduction mammoplasty**

      Amputative mammoplasty
      Biesenberger operation
      Reduction mammoplasty (for gynecomastia)

**85.33**   **Unilateral subcutaneous mammectomy with synchronous implant**

      **EXCLUDES**   *that without synchronous implant (85.34)*

      DEF: Removal of mammary tissue, leaving skin and nipple
intact with implant of prosthesis.

**85.34**   **Other unilateral subcutaneous mammectomy**

      Removal of breast tissue with preservation
of skin and nipple
      Subcutaneous mammectomy NOS

      DEF: Excision of mammary tissue, leaving skin and nipple
intact.

**85.35**   **Bilateral subcutaneous mammectomy with synchronous implant**

      **EXCLUDES**   *that without synchronous implant (85.36)*

      DEF: Excision of mammary tissue, both breasts, leaving
skin and nipples intact; with prosthesis.

**85.36**   **Other bilateral subcutaneous mammectomy**

**√4th 85.4**   **Mastectomy**

**85.41**   **Unilateral simple mastectomy**

      Mastectomy:      Mastectomy:
         NOS                complete

      DEF: Removal of one breast.

**85.42**   **Bilateral simple mastectomy**

      Bilateral complete mastectomy

      DEF: Removal of both breasts.

**85.43**   **Unilateral extended simple mastectomy**

      Extended simple mastectomy NOS
      Modified radical mastectomy
      Simple mastectomy with excision of regional
lymph nodes

      **AHA:** 2Q, '92, 7; 3Q, '91, 24; 2Q, '91, 21

      DEF: Removal of one breast and lymph nodes under arm.

**85.44**   **Bilateral extended simple mastectomy**

      **AHA:** 2Q, '92, 7; 3Q, '91, 24; 2Q, '91, 21

**85.45**   **Unilateral radical mastectomy**

      Excision of breast, pectoral muscles, and
regional lymph nodes [axillary,
clavicular, supraclavicular]
      Radical mastectomy NOS

      **AHA:** 2Q, '91, 21

      DEF: Removal of one breast and regional lymph nodes,
pectoral muscle and adjacent tissue.

      **Mastectomy**

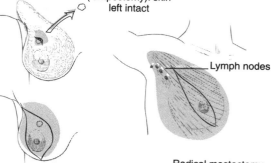

Partial mastectomy
(lumpectomy): skin
left intact

Lymph nodes

Simple mastectomy           Radical mastectomy

**BI** Bilateral Procedure      **NC** Non-covered Procedure      **LC** Limited Coverage Procedure      ▶◀ Revised Text      ● New Code      ▲ Revised Code Title

174 — Volume 3

© 2007 Ingenix

**85.46** **Bilateral radical mastectomy**
AHA: 2Q, '91, 21

**85.47** **Unilateral extended radical mastectomy**
Excision of breast, muscles, and lymph nodes [axillary, clavicular, supraclavicular, internal mammary, and mediastinal]
Extended radical mastectomy NOS

DEF: Removal of one breast, regional and middle chest lymph nodes, chest muscle and adjacent tissue.

**85.48** **Bilateral extended radical mastectomy**
DEF: Removal of both breasts, regional and middle chest lymph nodes, chest muscle and adjacent tissue.

✓4th **85.5** **Augmentation mammoplasty**
EXCLUDES   *that associated with subcutaneous mammectomy (85.33, 85.35)*

AHA: 3Q, '97, 12; 4Q, '95, 76, 80

DEF: Plastic surgery to increase breast size.

**85.50** **Augmentation mammoplasty, not otherwise specified**

**85.51** **Unilateral injection into breast for augmentation**

**85.52** **Bilateral injection into breast for augmentation**
Injection into breast for augmentation NOS

**85.53** **Unilateral breast implant**
AHA: 2Q, '00 18; 2Q, '98, 14

**85.54** **Bilateral breast implant**
Breast implant NOS

**85.6** **Mastopexy**
DEF: Anchoring of pendulous breast.

**85.7** **Total reconstruction of breast**
AHA: 4Q, '95, 77; 1Q, '93, 27

✓4th **85.8** **Other repair and plastic operations on breast**
EXCLUDES   *that for:*
*augmentation (85.50-85.54)*
*reconstruction (85.7)*
*reduction (85.31-85.32)*

AHA: 4Q, '95, 77

**85.81** **Suture of laceration of breast**
**85.82** **Split-thickness graft to breast**
**85.83** **Full-thickness graft to breast**
AHA: 4Q, '95, 77

**85.84** **Pedicle graft to breast**
AHA: 4Q, '95, 77

DEF: Implantation of transferred muscle tissue still connected to vascular source.

**85.85** **Muscle flap graft to breast**
AHA: 4Q, '95, 77

DEF: Relocation of nipple.

**85.86** **Transposition of nipple**
AHA: 4Q, '95, 78

**85.87** **Other repair or reconstruction of nipple**
AHA: 4Q, '95, 78

**85.89** **Other mammoplasty**

✓4th **85.9** **Other operations on the breast**
**85.91** **Aspiration of breast**
EXCLUDES   *percutaneous biopsy of breast (85.11)*

**85.92** **Injection of therapeutic agent into breast**
EXCLUDES   *that for augmentation of breast (85.51-85.52)*

**85.93** **Revision of implant of breast**
AHA: 2Q, '98, 14; 4Q, '95, 76

**85.94** **Removal of implant of breast**
AHA: 2Q, '98, 14; 3Q, '92, 4

**85.95** **Insertion of breast tissue expander**
Insertion (soft tissue) of tissue expander (one or more) under muscle or platysma to develop skin flaps for donor use

**85.96** **Removal of breast tissue expander(s)**
AHA: 2Q, '00, 18; 4Q, '95, 77

**85.99** **Other**

✓3rd **86** **Operations on skin and subcutaneous tissue**
INCLUDES   operations on:    operations on:
   hair follicles    subcutaneous fat pads
   male perineum    sudoriferous glands
   nails    superficial fossae
   sebaceous glands

EXCLUDES   *those on skin of:*
*anus (49.01-49.99)*
*breast (mastectomy site) (85.0-85.99)*
*ear (18.01-18.9)*
*eyebrow (08.01-08.99)*
*eyelid (08.01-08.99)*
*female perineum (71.01-71.9)*
*lips (27.0-27.99)*
*nose (21.00-21.99)*
*penis (64.0-64.99)*
*scrotum (61.0-61.99)*
*vulva (71.01-71.9)*

✓4th **86.0** **Incision of skin and subcutaneous tissue**
**86.01** **Aspiration of skin and subcutaneous tissue**
Aspiration of:
   abscess  } of nail, skin, or
   hematoma  } subcutaneous
   seroma  } tissue

AHA: 3Q, '89, 16

**86.02** **Injection or tattooing of skin lesion or defect**
   Insertion  } of filling material
   Injection  }

   Pigmenting of skin

DEF: Pigmenting of skin: Adding color to skin.

**86.03** **Incision of pilonidal sinus or cyst**
EXCLUDES   *marsupialization (86.21)*

**86.04** **Other incision with drainage of skin and subcutaneous tissue**
EXCLUDES   *drainage of:*
*fascial compartments of face and mouth (27.0)*
*palmar or thenar space (82.04)*
*pilonidal sinus or cyst (86.03)*

AHA: 4Q, '04, 76

**86.05** **Incision with removal of foreign body or device from skin and subcutaneous tissue**
▶Removal of carotid sinus baroreflex activation device◀
Removal of loop recorder
Removal of neurostimulator pulse generator (single array, dual array)
Removal of tissue expander(s) from skin or soft tissue other than breast tissue
EXCLUDES   *removal of foreign body without incision (98.20-98.29)*

AHA: 2Q, '96, 15; N-D, '87, 10; N-D, '86, 9

**86.06** **Insertion of totally implantable infusion pump**

Code also any associated catheterization

**EXCLUDES** *insertion of totally implantable vascular access device (86.07)*

**AHA:** 2Q, '99, 4; 4Q, '90, 14

**86.07** **Insertion of totally implantable vascular access device [VAD]**

Totally implanted port

**EXCLUDES** *insertion of totally implantable infusion pump (86.06)*

**AHA:** 1Q, '01, 13; 1Q, '96, 3; 2Q, '94, 11; 3Q, '91, 13; 4Q, '90, 15

**DEF:** Placement of vascular access infusion catheter system under skin to allow for frequent manual infusions into blood vessel.

**86.09** **Other incision of skin and subcutaneous tissue**

Creation of thalamic stimulator pulse generator pocket, new site
Escharotomy
Exploration:
sinus tract, skin
superficial fossa
Relocation of subcutaneous device pocket NEC
Reopening subcutaneous pocket for device revision without replacement
Undercutting of hair follicle

**EXCLUDES** *that of:*
*cardiac pacemaker pocket, new site (37.79)*
*creation of loop recorder pocket, new site and insertion/relocation of device (37.79)*
*creation of pocket for implantable, patient-activated cardiac event recorder and insertion/relocation of device (37.79)*
*fascial compartments of face and mouth (27.0)*
*removal of catheter from cranial cavity (01.27)*

**AHA:** 1Q, '05, 17; 2Q, '04, 7, 8; 4Q, '00, 68; 4Q, '99, 21; 4Q, '97, 57; 3Q, '89, 17; N-D, '86, 1; N-D, '84, 6

✓4ᵗʰ **86.1** **Diagnostic procedures on skin and subcutaneous tissue**

**86.11** **Biopsy of skin and subcutaneous tissue**

**86.19** **Other diagnostic procedures on skin and subcutaneous tissue**

**EXCLUDES** *microscopic examination of specimen from skin and subcutaneous tissue (91.61-91.79)*

✓4ᵗʰ **86.2** **Excision or destruction of lesion or tissue of skin and subcutaneous tissue**

**86.21** **Excision of pilonidal cyst or sinus**

Marsupialization of cyst

**EXCLUDES** *incision of pilonidal cyst or sinus (86.03)*

**DEF:** Marsupialization of cyst: Incision of cyst and suturing edges to skin to open site.

**86.22** **Excisional debridement of wound, infection, or burn**

Removal by excision of:
devitalized tissue
necrosis
slough

**EXCLUDES** *debridement of:*
*abdominal wall (wound) (54.3)*
*bone (77.60-77.69)*
*muscle (83.45)*
*of hand (82.36)*
*nail (bed) (fold) (86.27)*
*nonexcisional debridement of wound, infection, or burn (86.28)*
*open fracture site (79.60-79.69)*
*pedicle or flap graft (86.75)*

**AHA:** 3Q, '06, 19; 2Q, '06, 11; 1Q, '05, 14; 4Q, '04, 138; 3Q, '02, 23; 2Q, '00, 9; 1Q, '99, 8; 2Q, '92, 17; 3Q, '91, 18; 3Q, '89, 16; 4Q, '88, 5; N-D, '86, 1

**86.23** **Removal of nail, nailbed, or nail fold**

**86.24** **Chemosurgery of skin**

Chemical peel of skin

**DEF:** Chemicals applied to destroy skin tissue.

**DEF:** Chemical peel of skin: Chemicals used to peel skin layers.

**86.25** **Dermabrasion**

That with laser

**EXCLUDES** *dermabrasion of wound to remove embedded debris (86.28)*

**DEF:** Removal of wrinkled or scarred skin; with fine sandpaper, wire, brushes or laser.

**86.26** **Ligation of dermal appendage**

**EXCLUDES** *excision of preauricular appendage (18.29)*

**DEF:** Tying off extra skin.

**86.27** **Debridement of nail, nail bed, or nail fold**

Removal of:
necrosis
slough

**EXCLUDES** *removal of nail, nail bed, or nail fold (86.23)*

**86.28** **Nonexcisional debridement of wound, infection, or burn**

Debridement NOS
Maggot therapy
Removal of devitalized tissue, necrosis, and slough by such methods as:
brushing
irrigation (under pressure)
scrubbing
washing
Water scalpel (jet)

**AHA:** ▶1Q, '07, 10, 11;◀1Q, '05, 14; 2Q, '04, 5, 6; 4Q, '03, 110; 2Q, '03, 15; 3Q, '02, 23; 2Q, '01, 18; 3Q, '91, 18; 4Q, '88, 5

**DEF:** Removal of damaged skin; by methods other than excision.

**86.3** **Other local excision or destruction of lesion or tissue of skin and subcutaneous tissue**

Destruction of skin by:       Destruction of skin by:
cauterization                 fulguration
cryosurgery                   laser beam
That with Z-plasty

**EXCLUDES** *adipectomy (86.83)*
*biopsy of skin (86.11)*
*wide or radical excision of skin (86.4)*
*Z-plasty without excision (86.84)*

**AHA:** 1Q, '96, 15; 2Q, '90, 27; 1Q, '89, 12; 3Q, '89, 18; 4Q, '88, 7

**BI** Bilateral Procedure    **NC** Non-covered Procedure    **LC** Limited Coverage Procedure    ►◄ Revised Text    ● New Code    ▲ Revised Code Title

176 — Volume 3 • October 2007

© *2007 Ingenix*

**86.4** **Radical excision of skin lesion**
Wide excision of skin lesion involving underlying or adjacent structure
Code also any lymph node dissection (40.3-40.5)

✓4ᵗʰ **86.5** **Suture or other closure of skin and subcutaneous tissue**

**86.51** **Replantation of scalp**

**86.59** **Closure of skin and subcutaneous tissue of other sites**
Adhesives (surgical) (tissue)
Staples
Sutures
**EXCLUDES** *application of adhesive strips (butterfly) — omit code*

AHA: 4Q, '99, 23

✓4ᵗʰ **86.6** **Free skin graft**
**INCLUDES** excision of skin for autogenous graft
**EXCLUDES** *construction or reconstruction of:*
*penis (64.43-64.44)*
*trachea (31.75)*
*vagina ▶(70.61-70.64)◀*
DEF: Transplantation of skin to another site.

**86.60** **Free skin graft, not otherwise specified**

**86.61** **Full-thickness skin graft to hand**
**EXCLUDES** *heterograft (86.65)*
*homograft (86.66)*

**86.62** **Other skin graft to hand**
**EXCLUDES** *heterograft (86.65)*
*homograft (86.66)*

**86.63** **Full-thickness skin graft to other sites**
**EXCLUDES** *heterograft (86.65)*
*homograft (86.66)*

**86.64** **Hair transplant**
**EXCLUDES** *hair follicle transplant to eyebrow or eyelash (08.63)*

**86.65** **Heterograft to skin**
Pigskin graft     Porcine graft
**EXCLUDES** *application of dressing only (93.57)*

AHA: 3Q,'02, 23

DEF: Implantation of nonhuman tissue.

**86.66** **Homograft to skin**
Graft to skin of:
amnionic membrane
skin    } from donor

DEF: Implantation of tissue from human donor.

**86.67** **Dermal regenerative graft**
Artificial skin, NOS
Creation of "neodermis"
Decellularized allodermis
Integumentary matrix implants
Prosthetic implant of dermal layer of skin
Regenerate dermal layer of skin
**EXCLUDES** *heterograft to skin (86.65)*
*homograft to skin (86.66)*

AHA: 3Q, '06, 19; 4Q, '98, 76, 79

DEF: Replacement of dermis and epidermal layer of skin by cultured or regenerated autologous tissue; used to treat full-thickness or deep partial-thickness burns; also called cultured epidermal autograft (CEA).

**86.69** **Other skin graft to other sites**
**EXCLUDES** *heterograft (86.65)*
*homograft (86.66)*

AHA: 4Q, '99, 15

✓4ᵗʰ **86.7** **Pedicle grafts or flaps**
**EXCLUDES** *construction or reconstruction of:*
*penis (64.43-64.44)*
*trachea (31.75)*
*vagina ▶(70.61-70.64)◀*
DEF: Full thickness skin and subcutaneous tissue partially attached to the body by a narrow strip of tissue so that it retains its blood supply. The unattached portion is sutured to the defect.

**86.70** **Pedicle or flap graft, not otherwise specified**

**86.71** **Cutting and preparation of pedicle grafts or flaps**
Elevation of pedicle from its bed
Flap design and raising
Partial cutting of pedicle or tube
Pedicle delay
**EXCLUDES** *pollicization or digital transfer (82.61,82.81)*
*revision of pedicle (86.75)*

AHA: 4Q, '01, 66

DEF: Elevation of pedicle from its bed: Separation of tissue implanted from its bed.

DEF: Flap design and raising: Planing and elevation of tissue to be implanted.

DEF: Pedicle delay: Elevation and preparation of tissue still attached to vascular bed; delayed implant.

**86.72** **Advancement of pedicle graft**
AHA: 3Q, '99, 9, 10

**86.73** **Attachment of pedicle or flap graft to hand**
**EXCLUDES** *pollicization or digital transfer (82.61, 82.81)*

**86.74** **Attachment of pedicle or flap graft to other sites**
Attachment by:     Attachment by:
advanced flap     rotating flap
double pedicled flap     sliding flap
pedicle graft     tube graft
AHA: 3Q, '99, 9; 1Q, '96, 15
DEF: Attachment by:
Advanced flap: Sliding tissue implant into new position.
Double pedicle flap: Implant connected to two vascular beds.
Pedicle graft: Implant connected to vascular bed.
Rotating flap: Implant rotated along curved incision.
Sliding flap: Sliding implant to site.
Tube graft: Double tissue implant to form tube with base connected to original site.

**86.75** **Revision of pedicle or flap graft**
Debridement
Defatting    } of pedicle or flap graft

DEF: Connection of implant still attached to its vascular tissue.

✓4ᵗʰ **86.8** **Other repair and reconstruction of skin and subcutaneous tissue**
DEF: Revision and tightening of excess, wrinkled facial skin.

**86.81** **Repair for facial weakness**

**86.82** **Facial rhytidectomy**
Face lift
**EXCLUDES** *rhytidectomy of eyelid (08.86-08.87)*

Operations on the Integumentary System

86.4–86.82

**Operations on the Integumentary System**

**86.83–86.99**

**86.83  Size reduction plastic operation**
Liposuction
Reduction of adipose tissue of:
   abdominal wall (pendulous)
   arms (batwing)
   buttock
   thighs (trochanteric lipomatosis)
   **EXCLUDES**    breast (85.31-85.32)

AHA: 2Q, '06, 10

DEF: Excision and plastic repair of excess skin and
underlying tissue.

**86.84  Relaxation of scar or web contracture of skin**
Z-plasty of skin
   **EXCLUDES**    Z-plasty with excision of lesion (86.3)

**86.85  Correction of syndactyly**
DEF: Plastic repair of webbed fingers or toes.

**86.86  Onychoplasty**
DEF: Plastic repair of nail or nail bed.

**86.89  Other repair and reconstruction of skin and subcutaneous tissue**
   **EXCLUDES**    mentoplasty (76.67-76.68)
AHA: 4Q, '02, 107; 1Q, '00, 26; 2Q, '98, 20; 2Q, '93, 11;
       2Q, '92, 17

✓4ᵗʰ **86.9  Other operations on skin and subcutaneous tissue**

**86.91  Excision of skin for graft**
Excision of skin with closure of donor site
   **EXCLUDES**    that with graft at same operative episode (86.60-86.69)

**86.92  Electrolysis and other epilation of skin**
   **EXCLUDES**    epilation of eyelid (08.91-08.93)

**86.93  Insertion of tissue expander**
Insertion (subcutaneous) (soft tissue) of
   expander (one or more) in scalp
   (subgaleal space), face, neck, trunk
   except breast, and upper and lower
   extremities for development of skin
   flaps for donor use
   **EXCLUDES**    flap graft preparation (86.71)
                    tissue expander, breast (85.95)

**86.94  Insertion or replacement of single array neurostimulator pulse generator, not specified as rechargeable**
Pulse generator (single array, single
   channel) for intracranial, spinal, and
   peripheral neurostimulator
Code also any associated lead implantation
   (02.93, 03.93, 04.92)
   **EXCLUDES**    insertion or replacement of single array recharge-able neurostimulator pulse generator (86.97)

AHA: 4Q, '04, 135

**86.95  Insertion or replacement of dual array neurostimulator pulse generator, not specified as rechargeable**
Pulse generator (dual array, dual channel)
   for intracranial, spinal, and peripheral
   neurostimulator
Code also any associated lead implantation
   (02.93, 03.93, 04.92)
   **EXCLUDES**    insertion or replacement of dual array rechargeable neurostimulator pulse generator (86.98)

**86.96  Insertion or replacement of other neurostimulator pulse generator**
Code also any associated lead implantation
   (02.93, 03.93, 04.92)
   **EXCLUDES**    insertion of dual array neuro-stimulator pulse gener-ator (86.95, 86.98)
                    insertion of single array neuro-stimulator pulse gener-ator (86.94, 86.97)

AHA: ▶2Q, '07, 8;◀ 2Q, '06, 5-6

**86.97  Insertion or replacement of single array rechargeable neurostimulator pulse generator**
Rechargeable pulse generator (single array,
   single channel) for intracranial, spinal,
   and peripheral neurostimulator
Code also any associated lead implantation
   (02.93, 03.93, 04.92)

AHA: 4Q, '05, 130

**86.98  Insertion or replacement of dual array rechargeable neurostimulator pulse generator**
Rechargeable pulse generator (dual array,
   dual channel) for intracranial, spinal,
   and peripheral neurostimulator
Code also any associated lead implantation
   (02.93, 03.93, 04.92)

AHA: 4Q, '05, 130

**86.99  Other**
   **EXCLUDES**    removal of sutures from:
                    abdomen (97.83)
                    head and neck (97.38)
                    thorax (97.43)
                    trunk NEC (97.84)
                    wound catheter:
                    irrigation (96.58)
                    replacement (97.15)

AHA: 4Q, '97, 57; N-D, '86, 1

---

BI Bilateral Procedure        NC Non-covered Procedure        LC Limited Coverage Procedure        ▶◀ Revised Text        ● New Code        ▲ Revised Code Title

## 16. MISCELLANEOUS DIAGNOSTIC AND THERAPEUTIC PROCEDURES (87-99)

√3rd **87 Diagnostic radiology**

√4th **87.0 Soft tissue x-ray of face, head, and neck**

> EXCLUDES *angiography (88.40-88.68)*

**87.01 Pneumoencephalogram**
DEF: Radiographic exam of cerebral ventricles and subarachnoid spaces; with injection of air or gas for contrast.

**87.02 Other contrast radiogram of brain and skull**
Pneumocisternogram
Pneumoventriculogram
Posterior fossa myelogram
DEF: Pneumocisternogram: radiographic exam of subarachnoid spaces after injection of gas or contrast.

DEF: Pneumoventriculography: radiographic exam of cerebral ventricles after injection of gas or contrast.

DEF: Posterior fossa myelogram: radiographic exam of posterior channel of spinal cord after injection of gas or contrast.

**87.03 Computerized axial tomography of head**
C.A.T. scan of head
**AHA:** 3Q, '05, 12; 3Q, '99, 7

**87.04 Other tomography of head**

**87.05 Contrast dacryocystogram**
DEF: Radiographic exam of tear sac after injection of contrast.

**87.06 Contrast radiogram of nasopharynx**

**87.07 Contrast laryngogram**

**87.08 Cervical lymphangiogram**
DEF: Radiographic exam of lymph vessels of neck; with or without contrast.

**87.09 Other soft tissue x-ray of face, head, and neck**
Noncontrast x-ray of:    Noncontrast x-ray of:
  adenoid                          salivary gland
  larynx                             thyroid region
  nasolacrimal duct            uvula
  nasopharynx
> EXCLUDES *x-ray study of eye (95.14)*

√4th **87.1 Other x-ray of face, head, and neck**
> EXCLUDES *angiography (88.40-88.68)*

**87.11 Full-mouth x-ray of teeth**

**87.12 Other dental x-ray**
Orthodontic cephalogram or cephalometrics
Panorex examination of mandible
Root canal x-ray

**87.13 Temporomandibular contrast arthrogram**

**87.14 Contrast radiogram of orbit**

**87.15 Contrast radiogram of sinus**

**87.16 Other x-ray of facial bones**
X-ray of:           X-ray of:
  frontal area        orbit
  mandible            supraorbital area
  maxilla              symphysis menti
  nasal sinuses     zygomaticomaxillary
  nose                   complex

**87.17 Other x-ray of skull**
Lateral projection
Sagittal projection    } of skull
Tangential projection

DEF: Lateral projection: Side to side view of head.

DEF: Sagittal projection: View of body in plane running midline from front to back.

DEF: Tangential projection: Views from adjacent skull surfaces.

√4th **87.2 X-ray of spine**

**87.21 Contrast myelogram**
DEF: Radiographic exam of space between middle and outer spinal cord coverings after injection of contrast.

**87.22 Other x-ray of cervical spine**

**87.23 Other x-ray of thoracic spine**

**87.24 Other x-ray of lumbosacral spine**
Sacrococcygeal x-ray

**87.29 Other x-ray of spine**
Spinal x-ray NOS

√4th **87.3 Soft tissue x-ray of thorax**
> EXCLUDES *angiocardiography (88.50-88.58)*
> *angiography (88.40-88.68)*

**87.31 Endotracheal bronchogram**
DEF: Radiographic exam of lung, main branch, with contrast introduced through windpipe.

**87.32 Other contrast bronchogram**
Transcricoid bronchogram
DEF: Transcricoid bronchogram: Radiographic exam of lung, main branch, with contrast introduced through cartilage of neck.

**87.33 Mediastinal pneumogram**
DEF: Radiographic exam of cavity containing heart, esophagus and adjacent structures.

**87.34 Intrathoracic lymphangiogram**
DEF: Radiographic exam of lymphatic vessels within chest; with or without contrast.

**87.35 Contrast radiogram of mammary ducts**
DEF: Radiographic exam of mammary ducts; with contrast.

**87.36 Xerography of breast**
DEF: Radiographic exam of breast via selenium-coated plates.

**87.37 Other mammography**
**AHA:** 3Q, '89, 17; 2Q, '90, 28; N-D, '87, 1

**87.38 Sinogram of chest wall**
Fistulogram of chest wall
DEF: Fistulogram of chest wall: Radiographic exam of abnormal opening in chest.

**87.39 Other soft tissue x-ray of chest wall**

√4th **87.4 Other x-ray of thorax**
> EXCLUDES *angiocardiography (88.50-88.58)*
> *angiography (88.40-88.68)*

**87.41 Computerized axial tomography of thorax**
C.A.T. scan
Crystal linea scan of x-ray
  beam
Electronic subtraction          } of thorax
Photoelectric response
Tomography with use of
  computer, x-rays, and
  camera

**87.42 Other tomography of thorax**
Cardiac tomogram
DEF: Radiographic exam of chest plane.

**87.43 X-ray of ribs, sternum, and clavicle**
Examination for:
  cervical rib
  fracture

**87.44 Routine chest x-ray, so described**
X-ray of chest NOS

**87.49 Other chest x-ray**
X-ray of:              X-ray of:
  bronchus NOS      lung NOS
  diaphragm NOS    mediastinum NOS
  heart NOS            trachea NOS

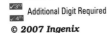

Diagnostic and Therapeutic Procedures

87–87.49

√4th **87.5**   **Biliary tract x-ray**

    **87.51**   **Percutaneous hepatic cholangiogram**
AHA: 2Q, '90, 28; N-D, '87, 1

      DEF: Radiographic exam of bile tract of gallbladder; with needle injection of contrast into bile duct of liver.

    **87.52**   **Intravenous cholangiogram**
      DEF: Radiographic exam of bile ducts; with intravenous contrast injection.

    **87.53**   **Intraoperative cholangiogram**
AHA: 1Q, '96, 12; 2Q, '90, 28; 3Q, '89, 18; 4Q, '88, 7

      DEF: Radiographic exam of bile ducts; with contrast; following gallbladder removal.

    **87.54**   **Other cholangiogram**

    **87.59**   **Other biliary tract x-ray**
      Cholecystogram

√4th **87.6**   **Other x-ray of digestive system**

    **87.61**   **Barium swallow**

    **87.62**   **Upper GI series**

    **87.63**   **Small bowel series**

    **87.64**   **Lower GI series**

    **87.65**   **Other x-ray of intestine**

    **87.66**   **Contrast pancreatogram**

    **87.69**   **Other digestive tract x-ray**

√4th **87.7**   **X-ray of urinary system**
      **EXCLUDES**   angiography of renal vessels (88.45, 88.65)

    **87.71**   **Computerized axial tomography of kidney**
      C.A.T. scan of kidney

    **87.72**   **Other nephrotomogram**
      DEF: Radiographic exam of kidney plane.

    **87.73**   **Intravenous pyelogram**
      Diuretic infusion pyelogram
      DEF: Radiographic exam of lower kidney, with intravenous contrast injection.

      DEF: Diuretic infusion pyelogram: Radiographic exam of lower kidney with diuretic contrast.

    **87.74**   **Retrograde pyelogram**

    **87.75**   **Percutaneous pyelogram**

    **87.76**   **Retrograde cystourethrogram**
      DEF: Radiographic exam of bladder and urethra with contrast injected through catheter into bladder.

    **87.77**   **Other cystogram**

    **87.78**   **Ileal conduitogram**
AHA: M-J, '87, 11

      DEF: Radiographic exam of passage created between ureter and artificial opening into abdomen.

    **87.79**   **Other x-ray of the urinary system**
      KUB x-ray

**Ureteropyelography**

Renal pelvis; Fat and abdominal wall; Ureter; Kidney; Minor calyces; Major calyces; Renal pelvis; Percutaneous injection; Cutaway schematic; Ureter; Bladder

√4th **87.8**   **X-ray of female genital organs**

    **87.81**   **X-ray of gravid uterus** ♀
      Intrauterine cephalometry by x-ray

    **87.82**   **Gas contrast hysterosalpingogram** ♀
      DEF: Radiographic exam of uterus and fallopian tubes; with gas contrast.

    **87.83**   **Opaque dye contrast hysterosal-pingogram** ♀

    **87.84**   **Percutaneous hysterogram** ♀
      DEF: Radiographic exam of uterus with contrast injected through body wall.

    **87.85**   **Other x-ray of fallopian tubes and uterus** ♀

    **87.89**   **Other x-ray of female genital organs** ♀

√4th **87.9**   **X-ray of male genital organs**

    **87.91**   **Contrast seminal vesiculogram** ♂

    **87.92**   **Other x-ray of prostate and seminal vesicles** ♂

    **87.93**   **Contrast epididymogram** ♂

    **87.94**   **Contrast vasogram** ♂

    **87.95**   **Other x-ray of epididymis and vas deferens** ♂

    **87.99**   **Other x-ray of male genital organs** ♂

√3rd **88**   **Other diagnostic radiology and related techniques**

√4th **88.0**   **Soft tissue x-ray of abdomen**
      **EXCLUDES**   angiography (88.40-88.68)

    **88.01**   **Computerized axial tomography of abdomen**
      C.A.T. scan of abdomen
      **EXCLUDES**   C.A.T. scan of kidney (87.71)
      AHA: 2Q, '98, 13

    **88.02**   **Other abdomen tomography**
      **EXCLUDES**   nephrotomogram (87.72)

    **88.03**   **Sinogram of abdominal wall**
      Fistulogram of abdominal wall
      DEF: Radiographic exam of abnormal abdominal passage.

    **88.04**   **Abdominal lymphangiogram**
      DEF: Radiographic exam of abdominal lymphatic vessels; with contrast.

    **88.09**   **Other soft tissue x-ray of abdominal wall**

√4th **88.1**   **Other x-ray of abdomen**

    **88.11**   **Pelvic opaque dye contrast radiography**

    **88.12**   **Pelvic gas contrast radiography**
      Pelvic pneumoperitoneum

    **88.13**   **Other peritoneal pneumogram**

    **88.14**   **Retroperitoneal fistulogram**

    **88.15**   **Retroperitoneal pneumogram**

    **88.16**   **Other retroperitoneal x-ray**

    **88.19**   **Other x-ray of abdomen**
      Flat plate of abdomen
      AHA: 3Q, '99, 9

√4th **88.2**   **Skeletal x-ray of extremities and pelvis**
      **EXCLUDES**   contrast radiogram of joint (88.32)

    **88.21**   **Skeletal x-ray of shoulder and upper arm**

    **88.22**   **Skeletal x-ray of elbow and forearm**

    **88.23**   **Skeletal x-ray of wrist and hand**

    **88.24**   **Skeletal x-ray of upper limb, not otherwise specified**

    **88.25**   **Pelvimetry**
      DEF: Imaging of pelvic bones to measure pelvic capacity.

    **88.26**   **Other skeletal x-ray of pelvis and hip**

    **88.27**   **Skeletal x-ray of thigh, knee, and lower leg**

    **88.28**   **Skeletal x-ray of ankle and foot**

    **88.29**   **Skeletal x-ray of lower limb, not otherwise specified**

---

**BI** Bilateral Procedure    **NC** Non-covered Procedure    **LC** Limited Coverage Procedure    ►◄ Revised Text    ● New Code    ▲ Revised Code Title

√4ᵗʰ **88.3**    **Other x-ray**

**88.31**   **Skeletal series**
X-ray of whole skeleton

**88.32**   **Contrast arthrogram**
EXCLUDES   *that of temporomandibular joint (87.13)*

**88.33**   **Other skeletal x-ray**
EXCLUDES   *skeletal x-ray of: extremities and pelvis (88.21-88.29) face, head, and neck (87.11-87.17) spine (87.21-87.29) thorax (87.43)*

**88.34**   **Lymphangiogram of upper limb**

**88.35**   **Other soft tissue x-ray of upper limb**

**88.36**   **Lymphangiogram of lower limb**

**88.37**   **Other soft tissue x-ray of lower limb**
EXCLUDES   *femoral angiography (88.48, 88.66)*

**88.38**   **Other computerized axial tomography**
C.A.T. scan NOS
EXCLUDES   *C.A.T. scan of: abdomen (88.01) head (87.03) kidney (87.71) thorax (87.41)*
**AHA:** 3Q, '05, 13-14

**88.39**   **X-ray, other and unspecified**

√4ᵗʰ **88.4**    **Arteriography using contrast material**
Note: The fourth-digit subclassification identifies the site to be viewed, not the site of injection.
INCLUDES   angiography of arteries
arterial puncture for injection of contrast material
radiography of arteries (by fluoroscopy)
retrograde arteriography
EXCLUDES   *arteriography using: radioisotopes or radionuclides (92.01-92.19) ultrasound (88.71-88.79) fluorescein angiography of eye (95.12)*
**AHA:** N-D, '85, 14

DEF: Electromagnetic wave photography of arteries; with contrast.

**88.40**   **Arteriography using contrast material, unspecified site**

**88.41**   **Arteriography of cerebral arteries**
Angiography of:
basilar artery
carotid (internal)
posterior cerebral circulation
vertebral artery
**AHA:** 1Q, '00, 16; 1Q, '99, 7; 1Q, '97, 3

**88.42**   **Aortography**
Arteriography of aorta and aortic arch
**AHA:** 1Q, '99, 17

**88.43**   **Arteriography of pulmonary arteries**

**88.44**   **Arteriography of other intrathoracic vessels**
EXCLUDES   *angiocardiography (88.50-88.58) arteriography of coronary arteries (88.55-88.57)*

**88.45**   **Arteriography of renal arteries**

**88.46**   **Arteriography of placenta**    ♀
Placentogram using contrast material

**88.47**   **Arteriography of other intra-abdominal arteries**
**AHA:** 1Q, '00, 18; N-D, '87, 4

**88.48**   **Arteriography of femoral and other lower extremity arteries**
**AHA:** 2Q, '06, 23; 3Q, '03, 10; 1Q, '03, 17; 2Q, '96, 6; 2Q, '89, 17

**88.49**   **Arteriography of other specified sites**

√4ᵗʰ **88.5**    **Angiocardiography using contrast material**
INCLUDES   arterial puncture and insertion of arterial catheter for injection of contrast material
cineangiocardiography
selective angiocardiography
Code also synchronous cardiac catheterization (37.21-37.23)
EXCLUDES   *angiography of pulmonary vessels (88.43, 88.62)*
**AHA:** 3Q, '92, 10; M-J, '87, 11

DEF: Electromagnetic wave photography of heart and great vessels; with contrast.

**88.50**   **Angiocardiography, not otherwise specified**

**88.51**   **Angiocardiography of venae cavae**
Inferior vena cavography
Phlebography of vena cava (inferior) (superior)

**88.52**   **Angiocardiography of right heart structures**
Angiocardiography of:
pulmonary valve
right atrium
right ventricle (outflow tract)
EXCLUDES   ▶*intra-operative fluorescence vascular angiography (88.59)*◀
*that combined with left heart angiocardiography (88.54)*
**AHA:** ▶1Q, '07, 16◀

**88.53**   **Angiocardiography of left heart structures**
Angiocardiography of:
aortic valve
left atrium
left ventricle (outflow tract)
EXCLUDES   ▶*intra-operative fluorescence vascular angiography (88.59)*◀
*that combined with right heart angiocardiography (88.54)*
**AHA:**▶1Q, '07, 11, 17;◀4Q, '05, 71; 3Q, '05, 14; 1Q, '00, 20; 4Q, '88, 4

**88.54**   **Combined right and left heart angiocardiography**
EXCLUDES   ▶*intra-operative fluorescence vascular angiography (88.59)*◀

**88.55**   **Coronary arteriography using a single catheter**
Coronary arteriography by Sones technique
Direct selective coronary arteriography using a single catheter
EXCLUDES   ▶*intra-operative fluorescence vascular angiography (88.59)*◀
**AHA:** 2Q, '06, 25-26; 3Q, '02, 20

**88.56**   **Coronary arteriography using two catheters**
Coronary arteriography by:
Judkins technique
Ricketts and Abrams technique
Direct selective coronary arteriography using two catheters
EXCLUDES   ▶*intra-operative fluorescence vascular angiography (88.59)*◀
**AHA:** 3Q, '06, 8; 1Q, '00, 20; 4Q, '88, 4

√3ʳᵈ √4ᵗʰ Additional Digit Required     Valid OR Procedure     Non-OR Procedure     Adjunct Code

**Diagnostic and Therapeutic Procedures**

**88.57–88.93**

**88.57 Other and unspecified coronary arteriography**
Coronary arteriography NOS
EXCLUDES ▶ intra-operative fluorescence vascular angiography (88.59)◀
AHA:▶1Q, '07, 15;◀ 2Q, '06, 25; 4Q, '05, 71; 3Q, '05, 14; 2Q, '05, 17; 1Q, '00, 21

**88.58 Negative-contrast cardiac roentgenography**
Cardiac roentgenography with injection of carbon dioxide

● **88.59 Intra-operative fluorescence vascular angiography**
Intraoperative laser arteriogram (SPY)
SPY arteriogram
SPY arteriography

✓4ᵗʰ **88.6 Phlebography**
Note: The fourth-digit subclassification (88.60-88.67) identifies the site to be viewed, not the site of injection.
INCLUDES angiography of veins
radiography of veins (by fluoroscopy)
retrograde phlebography
venipuncture for injection of contrast material
venography using contrast material
EXCLUDES angiography using:
radioisotopes or radionuclides (92.01-92.19)
ultrasound (88.71-88.79)
fluorescein angiography of eye (95.12)
DEF: Electromagnetic wave photography of veins; with contrast.

**88.60 Phlebography using contrast material, unspecified site**

**88.61 Phlebography of veins of head and neck using contrast material**

**88.62 Phlebography of pulmonary veins using contrast material**

**88.63 Phlebography of other intrathoracic veins using contrast material**

**88.64 Phlebography of the portal venous system using contrast material**
Splenoportogram (by splenic arteriography)

**88.65 Phlebography of other intra-abdominal veins using contrast material**

**88.66 Phlebography of femoral and other lower extremity veins using contrast material**
AHA: 2Q, '06, 23

**88.67 Phlebography of other specified sites using contrast material**

**88.68 Impedance phlebography**

✓4ᵗʰ **88.7 Diagnostic ultrasound**
INCLUDES echography
non-invasive ultrasound
ultrasonic angiography
ultrasonography
EXCLUDES intravascular imaging (adjunctive) (IVUS) (00.21-00.29)
therapeutic ultrasound (00.01-00.09)
DEF: Graphic recording of anatomical structures via high frequency, sound-wave imaging and computer graphics.

**88.71 Diagnostic ultrasound of head and neck**
Determination of midline shift of brain
Echoencephalography
EXCLUDES eye (95.13)
AHA: 1Q, '02, 10; 1Q, '92, 11

**88.72 Diagnostic ultrasound of heart**
Echocardiography
Transesophageal echocardiography
EXCLUDES echocardiography of heart chambers (37.28)
intracardiac echocardiography (ICE) (37.28)
intravascular (IVUS) imaging of coronary vessels (00.24)
AHA:▶1Q, '07, 11;◀ 3Q, '05, 14; 2Q, '05, 17; 4Q, '04, 121; 1Q, '04, 16; 1Q, '00, 20, 21; 1Q, '99, 6; 3Q, '98, 11

**88.73 Diagnostic ultrasound of other sites of thorax**
Aortic arch ⎫
Breast ⎬ ultrasonography
Lung ⎭

**88.74 Diagnostic ultrasound of digestive system**

**88.75 Diagnostic ultrasound of urinary system**

**88.76 Diagnostic ultrasound of abdomen and retroperitoneum**
AHA: 2Q, '99, 14

**88.77 Diagnostic ultrasound of peripheral vascular system**
Deep vein thrombosis ultrasonic scanning
EXCLUDES adjunct vascular system procedures (00.40-00.43)
AHA: 4Q, '99, 17; 1Q, '99, 12; 1Q, '92, 11

**88.78 Diagnostic ultrasound of gravid uterus** ♀
Intrauterine cephalometry:
echo
ultrasonic
Placental localization by ultrasound

**88.79 Other diagnostic ultrasound**
Ultrasonography of:
multiple sites
nongravid uterus
total body

✓4ᵗʰ **88.8 Thermography**
DEF: Infrared photography to determine various body temperatures.

**88.81 Cerebral thermography**

**88.82 Ocular thermography**

**88.83 Bone thermography**
Osteoarticular thermography

**88.84 Muscle thermography**

**88.85 Breast thermography**

**88.86 Blood vessel thermography**
Deep vein thermography

**88.89 Thermographay of other sites**
Lymph gland thermography
Thermography NOS

✓4ᵗʰ **88.9 Other diagnostic imaging**

**88.90 Diagnostic imaging, not elsewhere classified**
AHA: 2Q, '06, 25-26

**88.91 Magnetic resonance imaging of brain and brain stem**
EXCLUDES intraoperative magnetic resonance imaging (88.96)
real-time magnetic resonance imaging (88.96)

**88.92 Magnetic resonance imaging of chest and myocardium**
For evaluation of hilar and mediastinal lymphadenopathy

**88.93 Magnetic resonance imaging of spinal canal**
Spinal cord levels:
cervical
thoracic
lumbar (lumbosacral)
Spinal cord
Spine

---

BI Bilateral Procedure    NC Non-covered Procedure    LC Limited Coverage Procedure    ▶◀ Revised Text    ● New Code    ▲ Revised Code Title

**88.94** **Magnetic resonance imaging of musculoskeletal**
Bone marrow blood supply
Extremities (upper) (lower)

**88.95** **Magnetic resonance imaging of pelvis, prostate, and bladder**

**88.96** **Other intraoperative magnetic resonance imaging**
iMRI
Real-time magnetic resonance imaging
AHA: 4Q, '02, 111

**88.97** **Magnetic resonance imaging of other and unspecified sites**
Abdomen      Face
Eye orbit      Neck

**88.98** **Bone mineral density studies**
Dual photon absorptiometry
Quantitative computed tomography (CT) studies
Radiographic densitometry
Single photon absorptiometry
DEF: Dual photon absorptiometry: Measurement of bone mineral density by comparing dissipation of emission from two separate photoelectric energy peaks.
DEF: Quantitative computed tomography (CT) studies: Computer assisted analysis of x-ray absorption through bone to determine density.
DEF: Radiographic densimetry: Measurement of bone mineral density by degree of bone radiopacity.
DEF: Single photon absorptiometry: Measurement of bone mineral density by degree of dissipation of emission from one photoelectric energy peaks emitted by gadolinium 153.

✓3rd **89** **Interview, evaluation, consultation, and examination**

✓4th **89.0** **Diagnostic interview, consultation, and evaluation**
EXCLUDES   psychiatric diagnostic interview (94.11-94.19)

**89.01** **Interview and evaluation, described as brief**
Abbreviated history and evaluation

**89.02** **Interview and evaluation, described as limited**
Interval history and evaluation

**89.03** **Interview and evaluation, described as comprehensive**
History and evaluation of new problem

**89.04** **Other interview and evaluation**

**89.05** **Diagnostic interview and evaluation, not otherwise specified**

**89.06** **Consultation, described as limited**
Consultation on a single organ system

**89.07** **Consultation, described as comprehensive**

**89.08** **Other consultation**

**89.09** **Consulation, not otherwise specified**

✓4th **89.1** **Anatomic and physiologic measurements and manual examinations — nervous system and sense organs**
EXCLUDES   ear examination (95.41-95.49)
eye examination (95.01-95.26)
the listed procedures when done as part of a general physical examination (89.7)

**89.10** **Intracarotid amobarbital test**
Wada test
DEF: Amobarbital injections into internal carotid artery to induce hemiparalysis to determine the hemisphere that controls speech and language.

**89.11** **Tonometry**
DEF: Pressure measurements inside eye.

**89.12** **Nasal function study**
Rhinomanometry
DEF: Rhinomanometry: Measure of degree of nasal cavity obstruction.

**89.13** **Neurologic examination**

**89.14** **Electroencephalogram**
EXCLUDES   that with polysomnogram (89.17)
AHA: 3Q, '05, 12
DEF: Recording of electrical currents in brain via electrodes to detect epilepsy, lesions and other encephalopathies.

**89.15** **Other nonoperative neurologic function tests**
AHA: 3Q, '95, 5; 2Q, '91, 14; J-F, '87, 16; N-D, '84, 6

**89.16** **Transillumination of newborn skull**
DEF: Light passed through newborn skull for diagnostic purposes.

**89.17** **Polysomnogram**
Sleep recording
DEF: Graphic studies of sleep patterns.

**89.18** **Other sleep disorder function tests**
Multiple sleep latency test [MSLT]

**89.19** **Video and radio-telemetered electroencephalographic monitoring**
Radiographic
Video   } EEG Monitoring
AHA: 1Q, '92, 17; 2Q, '90, 27

✓4th **89.2** **Anatomic and physiologic measurements and manual examinations — genitourinary system**
EXCLUDES   the listed procedures when done as part of a general physical examination (89.7)
AHA: 1Q, '90, 27

**89.21** **Urinary manometry**
Manometry through:
indwelling ureteral catheter
nephrostomy
pyelostomy
ureterostomy
DEF: Measurement of urinary pressure.
DEF: Manometry through:
Indwelling urinary catheter: Semipermanent urinary catheter.
Nephrostomy: Opening into pelvis of kidney.
Pyelostomy: Opening in lower kidney.
Ureterostomy: Opening into ureter.

**89.22** **Cystometrogram**
DEF: Pressure recordings at various stages of bladder filling.

**89.23** **Urethral sphincter electromyogram**

**89.24** **Uroflowmetry [UFR]**
DEF: Continuous recording of urine flow.

**89.25** **Urethral pressure profile [UPP]**

**89.26** **Gynecological examination**     ♀
Pelvic examination

**89.29** **Other nonoperative genitourinary system measurements**
Bioassay of urine    Urine chemistry
Renal clearance
AHA: N-D, '84, 6

✓4th **89.3** **Other anatomic and physiologic measurements and manual examinations**
EXCLUDES   the listed procedures when done as part of a general physical examination (89.7)

**89.31** **Dental examination**
Oral mucosal survey
Periodontal survey

**89.32** **Esophageal manometry**
AHA: 3Q, '96, 13
DEF: Measurement of esophageal fluid and gas pressures.

**89.33  Digital examination of enterostomy stoma**
Digital examination of colostomy stoma

**89.34  Digital examination of rectum**

**89.35  Transillumination of nasal sinuses**

**89.36  Manual examination of breast**

**89.37  Vital capacity determination**
DEF: Measurement of expelled gas volume after full inhalation.

**89.38  Other nonoperative respiratory measurements**
Plethysmography for measurement of respiratory function
Thoracic impedance plethysmography
AHA: S-O, '87, 6
DEF: Plethysmography for measurement of respiratory function: Registering changes in respiratory function as noted in blood circulation.

**89.39  Other nonoperative measurements and examinations**
[14] C-Urea breath test
Basal metabolic rate [BMR]
Gastric:
    analysis
    function NEC
> EXCLUDES  *body measurement (93.07)*
> *cardiac tests (89.41-89.69)*
> *fundus photography (95.11)*
> *limb length measurement (93.06)*

AHA:  2Q, '01, 9; 3Q, '00, 9; 3Q, '96, 12; 1Q, '94, 18; N-D, '84, 6

**✓4ᵗʰ  89.4  Cardiac stress tests, pacemaker and defibrillator checks**

**89.41  Cardiovascular stress test using treadmill**
AHA: 1Q, '88, 11

**89.42  Masters' two-step stress test**
AHA: 1Q, '88, 11

**89.43  Cardiovascular stress test using bicycle ergometer**
AHA: 1Q, '88, 11
DEF: Electrocardiogram during exercise on bicycle with device capable of measuring muscular, metabolic and respiratory effects of exercise.

**89.44  Other cardiovascular stress test**
Thallium stress test with or without transesophageal pacing

**89.45  Artificial pacemaker rate check**
Artificial pacemaker function check NOS
Bedside device check of pacemaker or cardiac resynchronization pacemaker [CRT-P]
Interrogation only without arrhythmia induction
> EXCLUDES  *catheter based invasive electrophysiologic testing (37.26)*
> *non-invasive programmed electrical stimulation [NIPS] (arrhythmia induction) (37.20)*

AHA: 1Q, '02, 3

**89.46  Artificial pacemaker artifact wave form check**

**89.47  Artificial pacemaker electrode impedance check**

**89.48  Artificial pacemaker voltage or amperage threshold check**

**89.49  Automatic implantable cardioverter/ defibrillator (AICD) check**
Bedside check of an AICD or cardiac resynchronization defibrillator [CRT-D]
Checking pacing thresholds of device
Interrogation only without arrhythmia induction
> EXCLUDES  *catheter based invasive electrophysiologic testing (37.26)*
> *non-invasive programmed electrical stimulation [NIPS] (arrhythmia induction) (37.20)*

AHA: 4Q, '04, 136

**✓4ᵗʰ  89.5  Other nonoperative cardiac and vascular diagnostic procedures**
> EXCLUDES  *fetal EKG (75.32)*

**89.50  Ambulatory cardiac monitoring**
Analog devices [Holter-type]
AHA: 4Q, '99, 21; 4Q, '91, 23

**89.51  Rhythm electrocardiogram**
Rhythm EKG (with one to three leads)

**89.52  Electrocardiogram**
ECG NOS       EKG (with 12 or more leads)
AHA: 1Q, '88, 11; S-O, '87, 6

**89.53  Vectorcardiogram (with ECG)**

**89.54  Electrographic monitoring**
Telemetry
> EXCLUDES  *ambulatory cardiac monitoring (89.50)*
> *electrographic monitoring during surgery — omit code*

AHA: 4Q, '91, 23; 1Q, '88, 11
DEF: Evaluation of heart electrical activity by continuous screen monitoring.
DEF: Telemetry: Evaluation of heart electrical activity; with radio signals at distance from patient.

**89.55  Phonocardiogram with ECG lead**

**89.56  Carotid pulse tracing with ECG lead**
> EXCLUDES  *oculoplethysmography (89.58)*

**89.57  Apexcardiogram (with ECG lead)**
AHA: J-F, '87, 16

**89.58  Plethysmogram**
Penile plethysmography with nerve stimulation
> EXCLUDES  *plethysmography (for):*
> *measurement of respiratory function (89.38)*
> *thoracic impedance (89.38)*

AHA: S-O, '87, 7
DEF: Determination and recording of blood pressure variations present or passing through an organ.

**89.59  Other nonoperative cardiac and vascular measurements**
AHA: 3Q, '05, 21; 3Q, '03, 23; 2Q, '92, 12

**✓4ᵗʰ  89.6  Circulatory monitoring**
> EXCLUDES  *electrocardiographic monitoring during surgery — omit code*
> *implantation or replacement of subcutaneous device for intracardiac hemodynamic monitoring (00.57)*
> *insertion or replacement of implantable pressure sensor (lead) for intracardiac hemodynamic monitoring (00.56)*

AHA: M-J, '87, 11

**89.60  Continuous intra-arterial blood gas monitoring**
Insertion of blood gas monitoring system and continuous monitoring of blood gases through an intra-arterial sensor
AHA: 4Q, '02, 111

---

BI Bilateral Procedure    NC Non-covered Procedure    LC Limited Coverage Procedure    ▶◀ Revised Text    ● New Code    ▲ Revised Code Title

**Central Venous Pressure Monitoring**

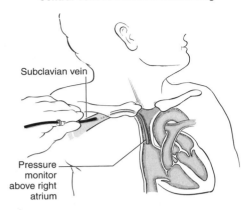

Subclavian vein

Pressure monitor above right atrium

**89.61**   **Systemic arterial pressure monitoring**

**89.62**   **Central venous pressure monitoring**

**89.63**   **Pulmonary artery pressure monitoring**

> **EXCLUDES**   *pulmonary artery wedge monitoring (89.64)*

**89.64**   **Pulmonary artery wedge monitoring**
> Pulmonary capillary wedge [PCW] monitoring
> Swan-Ganz catheterization
>
> DEF: Monitoring pulmonary artery pressure via catheter inserted through right lower and upper heart chambers into pulmonary artery and advancing the balloon-tip to wedge it in the distal pulmonary artery branch.

**89.65**   **Measurement of systemic arterial blood gases**

> **EXCLUDES**   *continuous intra-arterial blood gas monitoring (89.60)*

**89.66**   **Measurement of mixed venous blood gases**

**89.67**   **Monitoring of cardiac output by oxygen consumption technique**
> Fick method
>
> DEF: Fick method: Indirect measure of cardiac output through blood volume flow over pulmonary capillaries; determines oxygen absorption by measurement of arterial oxygen content versus venous oxygen content.

**89.68**   **Monitoring of cardiac output by other technique**
> Cardiac output monitor by thermodilution indicator
>
> DEF: Cardiac output monitor by thermodilution indicator: Injection of ice cold dextrose solution into right lower heart chamber; temperature sensitive catheter monitors disappearance from beat to beat to measure expelled blood volume.

**89.69**   **Monitoring of coronary blood flow**
> Coronary blood flow monitoring by coincidence counting technique

**89.7**   **General physical examination**

**89.8**   **Autopsy**

√3rd **90**   **Microscopic examination - I**

The following fourth-digit subclassification is for use with categories in section 90 to identify type of examination:

1   bacterial smear
2   culture
3   culture and sensitivity
4   parasitology
5   toxicology
6   cell block and Papanicolaou smear
9   other microscopic examination

√4th **90.0**   **Microscopic examination of specimen from nervous system and of spinal fluid**

√4th **90.1**   **Microscopic examination of specimen from endocrine gland, not elsewhere classified**

√4th **90.2**   **Microscopic examination of specimen from eye**

√4th **90.3**   **Microscopic examination of specimen from ear, nose, throat, and larynx**

√4th **90.4**   **Microscopic examination of specimen from trachea, bronchus, pleura, lung, and other thoracic specimen, and of sputum**

√4th **90.5**   **Microscopic examination of blood**

√4th **90.6**   **Microscopic examination of specimen from spleen and of bone marrow**

√4th **90.7**   **Microscopic examination of specimen from lymph node and of lymph**

√4th **90.8**   **Microscopic examination of specimen from upper gastrointestinal tract and of vomitus**

√4th **90.9**   **Microscopic examination of specimen from lower gastrointestinal tract and of stool**

√3rd **91**   **Microscopic examination - II**

The following fourth-digit subclassification is for use with categories in section 91 to identify type of examination:

1   bacterial smear
2   culture
3   culture and sensitivity
4   parasitology
5   toxicology
6   cell block and Papanicolaou smear
9   other microscopic examination

√4th **91.0**   **Microscopic examination of specimen from liver, biliary tract, and pancreas**

√4th **91.1**   **Microscopic examination of peritoneal and retroperitoneal specimen**

√4th **91.2**   **Microscopic examination of specimen from kidney, ureter, perirenal and periureteral tissue**

√4th **91.3**   **Microscopic examination of specimen from bladder, urethra, prostate, seminal vesicle, perivesical tissue, and of urine and semen**

√4th **91.4**   **Microscopic examination of specimen from female genital tract**     ♀
> Amnionic sac     Fetus

√4th **91.5**   **Microscopic examination of specimen from musculoskeletal system and of joint fluid**
> Microscopic examination of:
> bone          ligament
> bursa         muscle
> cartilage     synovial membrane
> fascia        tendon

√4th **91.6**   **Microscopic examination of specimen from skin and other integument**
> Microscopic examination of:
> hair
> nails
> skin
>
> **EXCLUDES**   *mucous membrane — code to organ site that of operative wound (91.71-91.79)*

√4th **91.7**   **Microscopic examination of specimen from operative wound**

√4th **91.8**   **Microscopic examination of specimen from other site**

√4th **91.9**   **Microscopic examination of specimen from unspecified site**

√3rd **92**   **Nuclear medicine**

√4th **92.0**   **Radioisotope scan and function study**

    **92.01**   **Thyroid scan and radioisotope function studies**
> Iodine-131 uptake     Radio-iodine uptake
> Protein-bound iodine

    **92.02**   **Liver scan and radioisotope function study**

    **92.03**   **Renal scan and radioisotope function study**
> Renal clearance study

    **92.04**   **Gastrointestinal scan and radioisotope function study**
> Radio-cobalt $B_{12}$ Schilling test
> Radio-iodinated triolein study

**Diagnostic and Therapeutic Procedures**

**92.05–93.14**

**92.05** **Cardiovascular and hematopoietic scan and radioisotope function study**

Bone marrow
Cardiac output
Circulation time    } scan or function study
Radionuclide cardiac ventriculogram
Spleen

AHA: 2Q, '92, 7; 1Q, '88, 11

**92.09** **Other radioisotope function studies**

✓4ᵗʰ **92.1** **Other radioisotope scan**

**92.11** **Cerebral scan**
Pituitary

**92.12** **Scan of other sites of head**
EXCLUDES    *eye (95.16)*

**92.13** **Parathyroid scan**

**92.14** **Bone scan**

**92.15** **Pulmonary scan**

**92.16** **Scan of lymphatic system**

**92.17** **Placental scan**      ♀

**92.18** **Total body scan**

**92.19** **Scan of other sites**

✓4ᵗʰ **92.2** **Therapeutic radiology and nuclear medicine**
EXCLUDES    *that for:*
*ablation of pituitary gland (07.64-07.69)*
*destruction of chorioretinal lesion (14.26-14.27)*

AHA: 3Q, '92, 5
DEF: Radiation and nuclear isotope treatment of diseased tissue.

**92.20** **Infusion of liquid brachytherapy radioisotope**
I-125 radioisotope
Intracavitary brachytherapy
INCLUDES    removal of radioisotope

AHA: 4Q, '05, 117-118

**92.21** **Superficial radiation**
Contact radiation [up to 150 KVP]

**92.22** **Orthovoltage radiation**
Deep radiation [200-300 KVP]

**92.23** **Radioisotopic teleradiotherapy**
Teleradiotherapy using:
cobalt-60
iodine-125
radioactive cesium

**92.24** **Teleradiotherapy using photons**
Megavoltage NOS    Use of:
Supervoltage NOS    Betatron
linear accelerator

**92.25** **Teleradiotherapy using electrons**
Beta particles
EXCLUDES  ▶ *intra-operative electron radiation therapy (92.41)*◀

**92.26** **Teleradiotherapy of other particulate radiation**
Neutrons    Protons NOS

**92.27** **Implantation or insertion of radioactive elements**
Intravascular brachytherapy
Code also incision of site
EXCLUDES    *infusion of liquid brachytherapy radioisotope (92.20)*

AHA: 1Q, '04, 3-4; 1Q, '00, 11, 12; 3Q, '94, 11; 1Q, '88, 4

**92.28** **Injection or instillation of radioisotopes**
Injection or infusion of radioimmunoconjugate
Intracavitary injection or instillation
Intravenous injection or instillation
Iodine-131 [I-131] tositumomab
Radioimmunotherapy
Ytrium-90 [Y-90] ibritumomab tiuxetan
EXCLUDES    *infusion of liquid brachytherapy radioisotope (92.20)*

**92.29** **Other radiotherapeutic procedure**
AHA: 3Q, '06, 14-15

✓4ᵗʰ **92.3** **Stereotactic radiosurgery**
Code also stereotactic head frame application (93.59)
EXCLUDES    *stereotactic biopsy*

AHA: 4Q, '98, 79; 4Q, '95, 70
DEF: Ablation of deep intracranial lesions; single procedure; placement of head frame for 3-D analysis of lesion, followed by radiation treatment from helmet attached to frame.

**92.30** **Stereotactic radiosurgery, not otherwise specified**

**92.31** **Single source photon radiosurgery**
High energy x-rays
Linear accelerator (LINAC)

**92.32** **Multi-source photon radiosurgery**
Cobalt 60 radiation
Gamma irradiation
AHA: 4Q, '04, 113

**92.33** **Particulate radiosurgery**
Particle beam radiation (cyclotron)
Proton accelerator

**92.39** **Stereotactic radiosurgery, not elsewhere classified**

● ✓4ᵗʰ **92.4** **Intra-operative radiation procedures**

● **92.41** **Intra-operative electron radiation therapy**
IOERT
That using a mobile linear accelerator

✓3ʳᵈ **93** **Physical therapy, respiratory therapy, rehabilitation, and related procedures**

✓4ᵗʰ **93.0** **Diagnostic physical therapy**
AHA: N-D, '86, 7

**93.01** **Functional evaluation**

**93.02** **Orthotic evaluation**

**93.03** **Prosthetic evaluation**

**93.04** **Manual testing of muscle function**
AHA: J-F, '87, 16

**93.05** **Range of motion testing**
AHA: J-F, '87, 16

**93.06** **Measurement of limb length**

**93.07** **Body measurement**
Girth measurement
Measurement of skull circumference

**93.08** **Electromyography**
EXCLUDES    *eye EMG (95.25)*
*that with polysomnogram (89.17)*
*urethral sphincter EMG (89.23)*

AHA: J-F, '87, 16
DEF: Graphic recording of electrical activity of muscle.

**93.09** **Other diagnostic physical therapy procedure**

✓4ᵗʰ **93.1** **Physical therapy exercises**
AHA: J-F, '87, 16; N-D, '86, 7

**93.11** **Assisting exercise**
EXCLUDES    *assisted exercise in pool (93.31)*

**93.12** **Other active musculoskeletal exercise**

**93.13** **Resistive exercise**

**93.14** **Training in joint movements**

---

BI Bilateral Procedure    NC Non-covered Procedure    LC Limited Coverage Procedure    ▶◀ Revised Text    ● New Code    ▲ Revised Code Title

**93.15 Mobilization of spine**

**93.16 Mobilization of other joints**
> EXCLUDES   manipulation of temporo-mandibular joint (76.95)

**93.17 Other passive musculoskeletal exercise**

**93.18 Breathing exercise**

**93.19 Exercise, not elsewhere classified**

✓4th **93.2 Other physical therapy musculoskeletal manipulation**
AHA: N-D, '86, 7

**93.21 Manual and mechanical traction**
> EXCLUDES   skeletal traction (93.43-93.44)
> skin traction (93.45-93.46)
> spinal traction (93.41-93.42)

**93.22 Ambulation and gait training**

**93.23 Fitting of orthotic device**

**93.24 Training in use of prosthetic or orthotic device**
> Training in crutch walking

**93.25 Forced extension of limb**

**93.26 Manual rupture of joint adhesions**
DEF: Therapeutic application of force to rupture adhesions restricting movement.

**93.27 Stretching of muscle or tendon**

**93.28 Stretching of fascia**

**93.29 Other forcible correction of deformity**
AHA: N-D, '85, 11

✓4th **93.3 Other physical therapy therapeutic procedures**

**93.31 Assisted exercise in pool**

**93.32 Whirlpool treatment**

**93.33 Other hydrotherapy**

**93.34 Diathermy**

**93.35 Other heat therapy**
> Acupuncture with smouldering moxa
> Hot packs
> Hyperthermia NEC
> Infrared irradiation
> Moxibustion
> Paraffin bath
> EXCLUDES   hyperthermia for treatment of cancer (99.85)

DEF: Moxibustion: Igniting moxa, a Chinese plant, for counterirritation of skin.
DEF: Paraffin bath: Hot wax treatment.

**93.36 Cardiac retraining**
DEF: Cardiac rehabilitation regimen following myocardial infarction or coronary bypass graft procedure.

**93.37 Prenatal training**
> Training for natural childbirth

**93.38 Combined physical therapy without mention of the components**

**93.39 Other physical therapy**
AHA: 2Q, '05, 6; 4Q, '03, 105 -106, 108-110; 3Q, '97, 12; 3Q, '91, 15

✓4th **93.4 Skeletal traction and other traction**

**93.41 Spinal traction using skull device**
> Traction using:    Traction using:
> caliper tongs    halo device
> Crutchfield tongs    Vinke tongs
> EXCLUDES   insertion of tongs or halo traction device (02.94)

AHA: 3Q, '01, 8; 3Q, '96, 14; 2Q, '94, 3
DEF: Applying device to head to exert pulling force on spine.

**93.42 Other spinal traction**
> Cotrel's traction
> EXCLUDES   cervical collar (93.52)

DEF: Pulling force exerted on spine without skull device.

**93.43 Intermittent skeletal traction**

**93.44 Other skeletal traction**
> Bryant's ⎫
> Dunlop's ⎬ traction
> Lyman Smith ⎪
> Russell's ⎭

**93.45 Thomas' splint traction**
DEF: Thomas splint: Placement of ring around thigh, attached to rods running length of leg for therapeutic purposes.

**93.46 Other skin traction of limbs**
> Adhesive tape traction    Buck's traction
> Boot traction    Gallows traction

✓4th **93.5 Other immobilization, pressure, and attention to wound**
> EXCLUDES   external fixator device (84.71-84.73)
> wound cleansing (96.58-96.59)

**93.51 Application of plaster jacket**
> EXCLUDES   Minerva jacket (93.52)

**93.52 Application of neck support**
> Application of:    Application of:
> cervical collar    molded neck support
> Minerva jacket

**93.53 Application of other cast**

**93.54 Application of splint**
> Plaster splint    Tray splint
> EXCLUDES   periodontal splint (24.7)

**93.55 Dental wiring**
> EXCLUDES   that for orthodontia (24.7)

**93.56 Application of pressure dressing**
> Application of:
> Gibney bandage
> Robert Jones' bandage
> Shanz dressing

**93.57 Application of other wound dressing**
> Porcine wound dressing
AHA: 3Q, '02, 23

**93.58 Application of pressure trousers**
> Application of:
> anti-shock trousers
> MAST trousers
> vasopneumatic device
AHA: 3Q, '96, 13

**93.59 Other immobilization, pressure, and attention to wound**
> Elastic stockings
> Electronic gaiter
> Intermittent pressure device
> Oxygenation of wound (hyperbaric)
> Stereotactic head frame application
> Strapping (non-traction)
> Velpeau dressing
AHA: 3Q, '99, 7; 1Q, '99, 12, 13; 1Q, '91, 11; 1Q, '89, 12

✓4th **93.6 Osteopathic manipulative treatment**

**93.61 Osteopathic manipulative treatment for general mobilization**
> General articulatory treatment

**93.62 Osteopathic manipulative treatment using high-velocity, low-amplitude forces**
> Thrusting forces

**93.63 Osteopathic manipulative treatment using low-velocity, high-amplitude forces**
> Springing forces

**93.64 Osteopathic manipulative treatment using isotonic, isometric forces**

**93.65 Osteopathic manipulative treatment using indirect forces**

**93.66 Osteopathic manipulative treatment to move tissue fluids**
> Lymphatic pump

**93.67 Other specified osteopathic manipulative treatment**

---

✓3rd
✓4th Additional Digit Required      Valid OR Procedure      Non-OR Procedure      Adjunct Code

**Diagnostic and Therapeutic Procedures**

**93.7–94.33**

√4th **93.7 Speech and reading rehabilitation and rehabilitation of the blind**

**93.71 Dyslexia training**

**93.72 Dysphasia training**
DEF: Speech training to coordinate and arrange words in proper sequence.

**93.73 Esophageal speech training**
DEF: Speech training after voice box removal; sound is produced by vibration of air column in esophagus against the cricopharangeal sphincter.

**93.74 Speech defect training**

**93.75 Other speech training and therapy**
AHA: 4Q, '03, 105, 109; 4Q, '97, 36; 3Q, '97, 12

**93.76 Training in use of lead dog for the blind**

**93.77 Training in braille or Moon**

**93.78 Other rehabilitation for the blind**

√4th **93.8 Other rehabilitation therapy**

**93.81 Recreational therapy**
Diversional therapy    Play therapy
EXCLUDES   play psychotherapy (94.36)

**93.82 Educational therapy**
Education of bed-bound children
Special schooling for the handicapped

**93.83 Occupational therapy**
Daily living activities therapy
EXCLUDES   training in activities of daily living for the blind (93.78)
AHA: 2Q, '05, 6; 4Q, '03, 105-106, 108, 110; 3Q, '97, 12

**93.84 Music therapy**

**93.85 Vocational rehabilitation**
Sheltered employment
Vocational:
     assessment
     retraining
     training

**93.89 Rehabilitation, not elsewhere classified**
AHA: 2Q, '05, 6

√4th **93.9 Respiratory therapy**
EXCLUDES   insertion of airway (96.01-96.05)
other continuous mechanical ventilation (96.70-96.72)

**93.90 Continuous positive airway pressure [CPAP]**
Bi-level airway pressure
Non-invasive positive pressure (NIPPV)
AHA: 3Q, '04, 3; 1Q, '02, 12, 13; 3Q, '98, 14; 4Q, '91, 21

DEF: Noninvasive ventilation support system that augments the ability to breathe spontaneously without the insertion of an endotracheal tube or tracheostomy.

**93.91 Intermittent positive pressure breathing [IPPB]**
AHA: 4Q, '91, 21

**93.93 Nonmechanical methods of resuscitation**
Artificial respiration
Manual resuscitation
Mouth-to-mouth resuscitition
AHA: 2Q, '03, 17

**93.94 Respiratory medication administered by nebulizer**
Mist therapy

**93.95 Hyperbaric oxygenation**
EXCLUDES   oxygenation of wound (93.59)

**93.96 Other oxygen enrichment**
Catalytic oxygen therapy
Cytoreductive effect
Oxygenators
Oxygen therapy
EXCLUDES   oxygenation of wound (93.59)

**93.97 Decompression chamber**

**93.98 Other control of atmospheric pressure and composition**
Antigen-free air conditioning
Helium therapy
EXCLUDES   inhaled nitric oxide therapy (INO) (00.12)
AHA: 1Q, '02, 14

**93.99 Other respiratory procedures**
Continuous negative pressure ventilation [CNP]
Postural drainage
AHA: 4Q, '03, 108; 3Q, '99, 11; 4Q, '91, 22

√3rd **94 Procedures related to the psyche**

√4th **94.0 Psychologic evaluation and testing**

**94.01 Administration of intelligence test**
Administration of:
     Stanford-Binet
     Wechsler Adult Intelligence Scale
     Wechsler Intelligence Scale for Children

**94.02 Administration of psychologic test**
Administration of:
     Bender Visual-Motor Gestalt Test
     Benton Visual Retention Test
     Minnesota Multiphasic Personality Inventory
     Wechsler Memory Scale

**94.03 Character analysis**

**94.08 Other psychologic evaluation and testing**

**94.09 Psychologic mental status determination, not otherwise specified**

√4th **94.1 Psychiatric interviews, consultations, and evaluations**

**94.11 Psychiatric mental status determination**
Clinical psychiatric mental status determination
Evaluation for criminal responsibility
Evaluation for testimentary capacity
Medicolegal mental status determination
Mental status determination NOS

**94.12 Routine psychiatric visit, not otherwise specified**

**94.13 Psychiatric commitment evaluation**
Pre-commitment interview

**94.19 Other psychiatric interview and evaluation**
Follow-up psychiatric interview NOS

√4th **94.2 Psychiatric somatotherapy**

DEF: Biological treatment of mental disorders.

**94.21 Narcoanalysis**
Narcosynthesis

**94.22 Lithium therapy**

**94.23 Neuroleptic therapy**

**94.24 Chemical shock therapy**

**94.25 Other psychiatric drug therapy**
AHA: S-O, '86, 4

**94.26 Subconvulsive electroshock therapy**

**94.27 Other electroshock therapy**
Electroconvulsive therapy (ECT)
EST

**94.29 Other psychiatric somatotherapy**

√4th **94.3 Individual psychotherapy**

**94.31 Psychoanalysis**

**94.32 Hypnotherapy**
Hypnodrome    Hypnosis

**94.33 Behavior therapy**
Aversion therapy
Behavior modification
Desensitization therapy
Extinction therapy
Relaxation training
Token economy

---

BI Bilateral Procedure     NC Non-covered Procedure     LC Limited Coverage Procedure     ▶◀ Revised Text     ● New Code     ▲ Revised Code Title

**94.34** Individual therapy for psychosexual dysfunction

> EXCLUDES   that performed in group setting (94.41)

**94.35** Crisis intervention
**94.36** Play psychotherapy
**94.37** Exploratory verbal psychotherapy
**94.38** Supportive verbal psychotherapy
**94.39** Other individual psychotherapy
> Biofeedback

✓4th **94.4** Other psychotherapy and counseling
**94.41** Group therapy for psychosexual dysfunction
**94.42** Family therapy
**94.43** Psychodrama
**94.44** Other group therapy
**94.45** Drug addiction counseling
**94.46** Alcoholism counseling
**94.49** Other counseling

✓4th **94.5** Referral for psychologic rehabilitation
**94.51** Referral for psychotherapy
**94.52** Referral for psychiatric aftercare
> That in:
> halfway house
> outpatient (clinic) facility

**94.53** Referral for alcoholism rehabilitation
**94.54** Referral for drug addiction rehabilitation
**94.55** Referral for vocational rehabilitation
**94.59** Referral for other psychologic rehabilitation

✓4th **94.6** Alcohol and drug rehabilitation and detoxification
> AHA: 2Q, '91, 12

**94.61** Alcohol rehabilitation
> DEF: Program designed to restore social and physical functioning, free of the dependence of alcohol.

**94.62** Alcohol detoxification
> DEF: Treatment of physical symptoms during withdrawal from alcohol dependence.

**94.63** Alcohol rehabilitation and detoxification
**94.64** Drug rehabilitation
> DEF: Program designed to restore social and physical functioning, free of the dependence of drugs.

**94.65** Drug detoxification
> DEF: Treatment of physical symptoms during withdrawal from drug dependence.

**94.66** Drug rehabilitation and detoxification
**94.67** Combined alcohol and drug rehabilitation
**94.68** Combined alcohol and drug detoxification
**94.69** Combined alcohol and drug rehabilitation and detoxification

✓3rd **95** Ophthalmologic and otologic diagnosis and treatment

✓4th **95.0** General and subjective eye examination
**95.01** Limited eye examination
> Eye examination with prescription of spectacles

**95.02** Comprehensive eye examination
> Eye examination covering all aspects of the visual system

**95.03** Extended ophthalmologic work-up
> Examination (for):
> glaucoma
> neuro-ophthalmology
> retinal disease

**95.04** Eye examination under anesthesia
> Code also type of examination

**95.05** Visual field study
**95.06** Color vision study
**95.07** Dark adaptation study
> DEF: Exam of eye's adaption to dark.

**95.09** Eye examination, not otherwise specified
> Vision check NOS

✓4th **95.1** Examinations of form and structure of eye
**95.11** Fundus photography
**95.12** Fluorescein angiography or angioscopy of eye
**95.13** Ultrasound study of eye
**95.14** X-ray study of eye
**95.15** Ocular motility study
**95.16** $P_{32}$ and other tracer studies of eye

✓4th **95.2** Objective functional tests of eye

> EXCLUDES   that with polysomnogram (89.17)

**95.21** Electroretinogram [ERG]
**95.22** Electro-oculogram [EOG]
**95.23** Visual evoked potential [VEP]
> DEF: Measuring and recording evoked visual responses of body and senses.

**95.24** Electronystagmogram [ENG]
> DEF: Monitoring of brain waves to record induced and spontaneous eye movements.

**95.25** Electromyogram of eye [EMG]
**95.26** Tonography, provocative tests, and other glaucoma testing

✓4th **95.3** Special vision services
**95.31** Fitting and dispensing of spectacles
**95.32** Prescription, fitting, and dispensing of contact lens
**95.33** Dispensing of other low vision aids
**95.34** Ocular prosthetics
**95.35** Orthoptic training
**95.36** Ophthalmologic counselling and instruction
> Counselling in:
> adaptation to visual loss
> use of low vision aids

✓4th **95.4** Nonoperative procedures related to hearing
**95.41** Audiometry
> Békésy 5-tone audiometry
> Impedance audiometry
> Stapedial reflex response
> Subjective audiometry
> Tympanogram

**95.42** Clinical test of hearing
> Tuning fork test     Whispered speech test

**95.43** Audiological evaluation
> Audiological evaluation by:
> Bárány noise machine
> blindfold test
> delayed feedback
> masking
> Weber lateralization

**95.44** Clinical vestibular function tests
> Thermal test of vestibular function

**95.45** Rotation tests
> Bárány chair
> DEF: Irrigation of ear canal with warm or cold water to evaluate vestibular function.

**95.46** Other auditory and vestibular function tests
**95.47** Hearing examination, not otherwise specified
**95.48** Fitting of hearing aid

> EXCLUDES   implantation of electromagnetic hearing device (20.95)

> AHA: 4Q, '89, 5

**95.49** Other nonoperative procedures related to hearing
> Adjustment (external components) of cochlear prosthetic device

✓3rd **96** Nonoperative intubation and irrigation
✓4th **96.0** Nonoperative intubation of gastrointestinal and respiratory tracts
**96.01** Insertion of nasopharyngeal airway
**96.02** Insertion of oropharyngeal airway

✓3rd
✓4th  Additional Digit Required        Valid OR Procedure        Non-OR Procedure        Adjunct Code

**Diagnostic and Therapeutic Procedures**

**96.03–96.6**

**Endotracheal Intubation**

Laryngoscope

Larynx

Trachea

Balloon inflated above carina

**96.03**    **Insertion of esophageal obturator airway**

**96.04**    **Insertion of endotracheal tube**
AHA:▶1Q, '07, 11;◄ 2Q, '06, 8; 4Q, '05, 88; 3Q, '05, 10; 2Q, '05, 19

**96.05**    **Other intubation of respiratory tract**
> EXCLUDES   endoscopic insertion or replacement of bronchial device or substance (33.71, 33.79)

AHA: 1Q, '97, 14

**96.06**    **Insertion of Sengstaken tube**
Esophageal tamponade
DEF: Insertion of Sengstaken tube: Nonsurgical emergency measure to stop esophageal bleeding using compression exerted by inflated balloons; additional tube ports to aspirate blood and clots.

**96.07**    **Insertion of other (naso-) gastric tube**
Intubation for decompression
> EXCLUDES   that for enteral infusion of nutritional substance (96.6)

**96.08**    **Insertion of (naso-) intestinal tube**
Miller-Abbott tube (for decompression)

**96.09**    **Insertion of rectal tube**
Replacement of rectal tube

✓4ᵗʰ **96.1**    **Other nonoperative insertion**
> EXCLUDES   nasolacrimal intubation (09.44)

**96.11**    **Packing of external auditory canal**
**96.14**    **Vaginal packing**    ♀
**96.15**    **Insertion of vaginal mold**    ♀
**96.16**    **Other vaginal dilation**    ♀
**96.17**    **Insertion of vaginal diaphragm**    ♀
**96.18**    **Insertion of other vaginal pessary**    ♀
**96.19**    **Rectal packing**

✓4ᵗʰ **96.2**    **Nonoperative dilation and manipulation**
**96.21**    **Dilation of frontonasal duct**
**96.22**    **Dilation of rectum**
**96.23**    **Dilation of anal sphincter**
**96.24**    **Dilation and manipulation of enterostomy stoma**
**96.25**    **Therapeutic distention of bladder**
Intermittent distention of bladder
**96.26**    **Manual reduction of rectal prolapse**
**96.27**    **Manual reduction of hernia**
**96.28**    **Manual reduction of enterostomy prolapse**
AHA: N-D, '87, 11
**96.29**    **Reduction of intussusception of alimentary tract**
With:
   fluoroscopy
   ionizing radiation enema
   ultrasonography guidance
Hydrostatic reduction
Pneumatic reduction
> EXCLUDES   intra-abdominal manipulation of intestine, not otherwise specified (46.80)

AHA: 4Q, '98, 82

✓4ᵗʰ **96.3**    **Nonoperative alimentary tract irrigation, cleaning, and local instillation**
**96.31**    **Gastric cooling**
Gastric hypothermia
DEF: Reduction of internal stomach temperature.
**96.32**    **Gastric freezing**
**96.33**    **Gastric lavage**
**96.34**    **Other irrigation of (naso-)gastric tube**
**96.35**    **Gastric gavage**
DEF: Food forced into stomach.
**96.36**    **Irrigation of gastrostomy or enterostomy**
**96.37**    **Proctoclysis**
DEF: Slow introduction of large amounts of fluids into lower large intestine.7
**96.38**    **Removal of impacted feces**
Removal of impaction:
   by flushing manually
**96.39**    **Other transanal enema**
Rectal irrigation
> EXCLUDES   reduction of intussusception of alimentary tract by ionizing radiation enema (96.29)

✓4ᵗʰ **96.4**    **Nonoperative irrigation, cleaning, and local instillation of other digestive and genitourinary organs**
**96.41**    **Irrigation of cholecystostomy and other biliary tube**
**96.42**    **Irrigation of pancreatic tube**
**96.43**    **Digestive tract instillation, except gastric gavage**
**96.44**    **Vaginal douche**    ♀
**96.45**    **Irrigation of nephrostomy and pyelostomy**
**96.46**    **Irrigation of ureterostomy and ureteral catheter**
**96.47**    **Irrigation of cystostomy**
**96.48**    **Irrigation of other indwelling urinary catheter**
**96.49**    **Other genitourinary instillation**
Insertion of prostaglandin suppository
AHA: 1Q, '01, 5

✓4ᵗʰ **96.5**    **Other nonoperative irrigation and cleaning**
**96.51**    **Irrigation of eye**
Irrigation of cornea
> EXCLUDES   irrigation with removal of foreign body (98.21)

**96.52**    **Irrigation of ear**
Irrigation with removal of cerumen
**96.53**    **Irrigation of nasal passages**
**96.54**    **Dental scaling, polishing, and debridement**
Dental prophylaxis    Plaque removal
**96.55**    **Tracheostomy toilette**
**96.56**    **Other lavage of bronchus and trachea**
> EXCLUDES   diagnostic bronchoalveolar lavage (BAL) (33.24)   whole lung lavage (33.99)

AHA: 3Q, '02, 18
**96.57**    **Irrigation of vascular catheter**
AHA: 3Q, '93, 5
**96.58**    **Irrigation of wound catheter**
**96.59**    **Other irrigation of wound**
Wound cleaning NOS
> EXCLUDES   debridement (86.22, 86.27-86.28)

AHA: S-O, '85, 7

**96.6**    **Enteral infusion of concentrated-nutritional substances**

**BI** Bilateral Procedure    **NC** Non-covered Procedure    **LC** Limited Coverage Procedure    ▶◀ Revised Text    ● New Code    ▲ Revised Code Title

190 — Volume 3 • October 2007

© 2007 Ingenix

√4ᵗʰ **96.7**   **Other continuous mechanical ventilation**

     INCLUDES   Endotracheal respiratory assistance
           Intermittent mandatory ventilation
            [IMV]
           Positive end expiratory pressure
            [PEEP]
           Pressure support ventilation [PSV]
           That by tracheostomy
           Weaning of an intubated (endotracheal
            tube) patient

     EXCLUDES ▶ *bi-level positive airway pressure*
            *[BiPAP] (93.90)*◀
           *continuous negative pressure*
            *ventilation [CNP] (iron lung)*
            *(cuirass) (93.99)*
           *continuous positive airway pressure*
            *[CPAP] (93.90)*
           *intermittent positive pressure breathing*
            *[IPPB] (93.91)*
           *non-invasive positive pressure (NIPPV)*
            *(93.90)*
           *that by face mask (93.90-93.99)*
           *that by nasal cannula (93.90-93.99)*
           *that by nasal catheter (93.90-93.99)*

     Code also any associated:
        endotracheal tube insertion (96.04)
        tracheostomy (31.1-31.29)

**Note:**   **Endotracheal intubation**

To calculate the number of hours (duration) of continuous mechanical ventilation during a hospitalization, begin the count from the start of the (endotracheal) intubation. The duration ends with (endotracheal) extubation.

If a patient is intubated prior to admission, begin counting the duration from the time of the admission. If a patient is transferred (discharged) while intubated, the duration would end at the time of transfer (discharge).

For patients who begin on (endotracheal) intubation and subsequently have a tracheostomy performed for mechanical ventilation, the duration begins with the (endotracheal) intubation and ends when the mechanical ventilation is turned off (after the weaning period).

     **Tracheostomy**

To calculate the number of hours of continuous mechanical ventilation during a hospitalization, begin counting the duration when mechanical ventilation is started. The duration ends when the mechanical ventilator is turned off (after the weaning period).

If a patient has received a tracheostomy prior to admission and is on mechanical ventilation at the time of admission, begin counting the duration from the time of admission. If a patient is transferred (discharged) while still on mechanical ventilation via tracheostomy, the duration would end at the time of the transfer (discharge).

     **AHA:** 3Q, '04, 3; 2Q, '92, 13; 4Q, '91, 16; 4Q, '91, 18; 4Q, '91, 21

     **96.70**   **Continuous mechanical ventilation of unspecified duration**
           Mechanical ventilation NOS

     **96.71**   **Continuous mechanical ventilation for less than 96 consecutive hours**
           **AHA:** 2Q, '06, 8; 3Q, '05, 10; 3Q, '04, 11; 2Q, '02, 19; 1Q, '02, 12; 1Q, '01, 6

     **96.72**   **Continuous mechanical ventilation for 96 consecutive hours or more**
           **AHA:** 2Q, '05, 19; 1Q, '04, 23

√3ʳᵈ **97**   **Replacement and removal of therapeutic appliances**

√4ᵗʰ **97.0**   **Nonoperative replacement of gastrointestinal appliance**

     **97.01**   **Replacement of (naso-)gastric or esophagostomy tube**

     **97.02**   **Replacement of gastrostomy tube**
           **AHA:** 1Q, '97, 11

     **97.03**   **Replacement of tube or enterostomy device of small intestine**
           **AHA:** 1Q, '03, 10

     **97.04**   **Replacement of tube or enterostomy device of large intestine**

     **97.05**   **Replacement of stent (tube) in biliary or pancreatic duct**
           **AHA:** 2Q, '99, 13

√4ᵗʰ **97.1**   **Nonoperative replacement of musculoskeletal and integumentary system appliance**

     **97.11**   **Replacement of cast on upper limb**

     **97.12**   **Replacement of cast on lower limb**

     **97.13**   **Replacement of other cast**

     **97.14**   **Replacement of other device for musculoskeletal immobilization**

     **97.15**   **Replacement of wound catheter**

     **97.16**   **Replacement of wound packing or drain**
         EXCLUDES   *repacking of:*
            *dental wound (97.22)*
            *vulvar wound (97.26)*

√4ᵗʰ **97.2**   **Other nonoperative replacement**

     **97.21**   **Replacement of nasal packing**

     **97.22**   **Replacement of dental packing**

     **97.23**   **Replacement of tracheostomy tube**
           **AHA:** N-D, '87, 11

     **97.24**   **Replacement and refitting of vagina diaphragm**   ♀

     **97.25**   **Replacement of other vaginal pessary**   ♀

     **97.26**   **Replacement of vaginal or vulvar packing or drain**   ♀

     **97.29**   **Other nonoperative replacements**
           **AHA:** 3Q, '99, 9; 3Q, '98, 12

√4ᵗʰ **97.3**   **Nonoperative removal of therapeutic device from head and neck**

     **97.31**   **Removal of eye prosthesis**
         EXCLUDES   *removal of ocular implant*
            *(16.71)*
           *removal of orbital implant*
            *(16.72)*

     **97.32**   **Removal of nasal packing**

     **97.33**   **Removal of dental wiring**

     **97.34**   **Removal of dental packing**

     **97.35**   **Removal of dental prosthesis**

     **97.36**   **Removal of other external mandibular fixation device**

     **97.37**   **Removal of tracheostomy tube**

     **97.38**   **Removal of sutures from head and neck**

     **97.39**   **Removal of other therapeutic device from head and neck**
         EXCLUDES   *removal of skull tongs (02.94)*

√4ᵗʰ **97.4**   **Nonoperative removal of therapeutic device from thorax**

     **97.41**   **Removal of thoracotomy tube or pleural cavity drain**
           **AHA:** 1Q, '99, 10

     **97.42**   **Removal of mediastinal drain**

       **Intraaortic Balloon Pump**

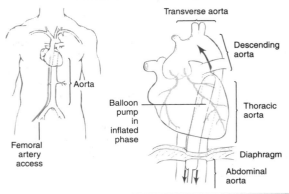

Transverse aorta

Descending aorta

Aorta

Balloon pump in inflated phase

Thoracic aorta

Femoral artery access

Diaphragm

Abdominal aorta

---

√3ᵗʰ √4ᵗʰ   Additional Digit Required      Valid OR Procedure      Non-OR Procedure      Adjunct Code

**Diagnostic and Therapeutic Procedures**

**97.43–98.24**

**97.43** Removal of sutures from thorax

**97.44** Nonoperative removal of heart assist system

Explantation [removal] of circulatory assist device

Explantation [removal] of percutaneous external heart assist device

Removal of extrinsic heart assist device

Removal of pVAD

Removal of percutaneous heart assist device

**AHA: 4Q, '01, 65**

**DEF:** Non-invasive removal of ventricular assist systems, or intraaortic balloon pump, which is a balloon catheter placed into the descending thoracic aorta and timed to inflate and deflate with the patient's own heart rhythm to aid in blood circulation.

**97.49** Removal of other device from thorax

> EXCLUDES ► endoscopic removal of bronchial device(s) or substances (33.78)◄

**AHA: N-D, '86, 9**

✓4ᵗʰ **97.5** Nonoperative removal of therapeutic device from digestive system

**97.51** Removal of gastrostomy tube

**97.52** Removal of tube from small intestine

**97.53** Removal of tube from large intestine or appendix

**97.54** Removal of cholecystostomy tube

**97.55** Removal of T-tube, other bile duct tube, or liver tube

Removal of bile duct stent

**AHA: 1Q, '01, 8**

**97.56** Removal of pancreatic tube or drain

**97.59** Removal of other device from digestive system

Removal of rectal packing

✓4ᵗʰ **97.6** Nonoperative removal of therapeutic device from urinary system

**97.61** Removal of pyelostomy and nephrostomy tube

**DEF:** Nonsurgical removal of tubes from lower part of kidney.

**97.62** Removal of ureterostomy tube and ureteral catheter

**97.63** Removal of cystostomy tube

**97.64** Removal of other urinary drainage device

Removal of indwelling urinary catheter

**97.65** Removal of urethral stent

**97.69** Removal of other device from urinary system

✓4ᵗʰ **97.7** Nonoperative removal of therapeutic device from genital system

**97.71** Removal of intrauterine contraceptive device ♀

**97.72** Removal of intrauterine pack ♀

**97.73** Removal of vaginal diaphragm ♀

**97.74** Removal of other vaginal pessary ♀

**97.75** Removal of vaginal or vulvar packing ♀

**97.79** Removal of other device from genital tract

Removal of sutures

✓4ᵗʰ **97.8** Other nonoperative removal of therapeutic device

**97.81** Removal of retroperitoneal drainage device

**97.82** Removal of peritoneal drainage device

**AHA: 2Q, '90, 28; S-O, '86, 12**

**97.83** Removal of abdominal wall sutures

**97.84** Removal of sutures from trunk, not elsewhere classified

**97.85** Removal of packing from trunk, not elsewhere classified

**97.86** Removal of other device from abdomen

**97.87** Removal of other device from trunk

**97.88** Removal of external immobilization device

Removal of:     Removal of:
brace          splint
cast

**97.89** Removal of other therapeutic device

✓3ʳᵈ **98** Nonoperative removal of foreign body or calculus

✓4ᵗʰ **98.0** Removal of intraluminal foreign body from digestive system without incision

> EXCLUDES removal of therapeutic device (97.51-97.59)

DEF: Retrieval of foreign body from digestive system lining without incision.

**98.01** Removal of intraluminal foreign body from mouth without incision

**98.02** Removal of intraluminal foreign body from esophagus without incision

**98.03** Removal of intraluminal foreign body from stomach and small intestine without incision

**98.04** Removal of intraluminal foreign body from large intestine without incision

**98.05** Removal of intraluminal foreign body from rectum and anus without incision

✓4ᵗʰ **98.1** Removal of intraluminal foreign body from other sites without incision

> EXCLUDES removal of therapeutic device (97.31-97.49, 97.61-97.89)

**98.11** Removal of intraluminal foreign body from ear without incision

**98.12** Removal of intraluminal foreign body from nose without incision

**98.13** Removal of intraluminal foreign body from pharynx without incision

**98.14** Removal of intraluminal foreign body from larynx without incision

**98.15** Removal of intraluminal foreign body from trachea and bronchus without incision

> EXCLUDES ► endoscopic removal of bronchial device(s) or substances (33.78)◄

**98.16** Removal of intraluminal foreign body from uterus without incision ♀

> EXCLUDES removal of intrauterine contraceptive device (97.71)

**98.17** Removal of intraluminal foreign body from vagina without incision ♀

**98.18** Removal of intraluminal foreign body from artificial stoma without incision

**98.19** Removal of intraluminal foreign body from urethra without incision

✓4ᵗʰ **98.2** Removal of other foreign body without incision

> EXCLUDES removal of intraluminal foreign body (98.01-98.19)

**98.20** Removal of foreign body, not otherwise specified

**98.21** Removal of superficial foreign body from eye without incision

**98.22** Removal of other foreign body without incision from head and neck

Removal of embedded foreign body from eyelid or conjunctiva without incision

**98.23** Removal of foreign body from vulva without incision ♀

**98.24** Removal of foreign body from scrotum or penis without incision ♂

---

BI Bilateral Procedure     NC Non-covered Procedure     LC Limited Coverage Procedure     ►◄ Revised Text     ● New Code     ▲ Revised Code Title

**Extracorporeal Shock Wave Lithotripsy**

Radiographic monitors

Shock wave exit area

Water cushion

Shock wave entry area

Kidney

Lithotripsy unit

**98.25**   **Removal of other foreign body without incision from trunk except scrotum, penis, or vulva**

**98.26**   **Removal of foreign body from hand without incision**
> AHA: N-D, '87, 10

**98.27**   **Removal of foreign body without incision from upper limb, except hand**

**98.28**   **Removal of foreign body from foot without incision**

**98.29**   **Removal of foreign body without incision from lower limb, except foot**

√4th **98.5**   **Extracorporeal shockwave lithotripsy [ESWL]**
> Lithotriptor tank procedure
> Disintegration of stones by extracorporeal induced shockwaves
> That with insertion of stent
> DEF: Breaking of stones with high voltage condenser device synchronized with patient R waves.

**98.51**   **Extracorporeal shockwave lithotripsy [ESWL] of the kidney, ureter and/or bladder**
> AHA: 4Q, '95, 73; 1Q, '89, 2

**98.52**   **Extracorporeal shockwave lithotripsy [ESWL] of the gallbladder and/or bile duct** `NC`

**98.59**   **Extracorporeal shockwave lithotripsy of other sites** `NC`

√3rd **99**   **Other nonoperative procedures**

√4th **99.0**   **Transfusion of blood and blood components**
> Use additional code for that done via catheter or cutdown (38.92-38.94)

**99.00**   **Perioperative autologous transfusion of whole blood or blood components**
> Intraoperative blood collection
> Postoperative blood collection
> Salvage
> AHA: 4Q, '95, 69
> DEF: Salvaging patient blood with reinfusion during perioperative period.

**99.01**   **Exchange transfusion**
> Transfusion:    Transfusion:
>    exsanguination    replacement
> AHA: 2Q, '89, 15
> DEF: Repetitive withdrawal of blood, replaced by donor blood.

**99.02**   **Transfusion of previously collected autologous blood**
> Blood component
> AHA: 4Q, '95, 69; 1Q, '90, 10; J-A, '85, 16
> DEF: Transfusion with patient's own previously withdrawn and stored blood.

**99.03**   **Other transfusion of whole blood**
> Transfusion:    Transfusion:
>    blood NOS    NOS
>    hemodilution

**99.04**   **Transfusion of packed cells**

**99.05**   **Transfusion of platelets**
> Transfusion of thrombocytes

**99.06**   **Transfusion of coagulation factors**
> Transfusion of antihemophilic factor

**99.07**   **Transfusion of other serum**
> Transfusion of plasma
> EXCLUDES   injection [transfusion] of:
>      antivenin (99.16)
>      gamma globulin (99.14)

**99.08**   **Transfusion of blood expander**
> Transfusion of Dextran

**99.09**   **Transfusion of other substance**
> Transfusion of:
>    blood surrogate
>    granulocytes
> EXCLUDES   transplantation [transfusion] of: bone marrow (41.0)

√4th **99.1**   **Injection or infusion of therapeutic or prophylactic substance**
> INCLUDES   injection or infusion given:
>    hypodermically
>    intramuscularly } acting locally or systemically
>    intravenously

**99.10**   **Injection or infusion of thrombolytic agent**
> Alteplase
> Anistreplase
> Reteplase
> Streptokinase
> Tenecteplase
> Tissue plasminogen activator (TPA)
> Urokinase
> EXCLUDES   aspirin — omit code
>      GP IIb/IIIa platelet inhibitors (99.20)
>      heparin (99.19)
>      warfarin — omit code
> AHA: 2Q, '06, 22; 4Q, '05, 101-103; 2Q, '01, 7-9, 23; 4Q, '98, 83

**99.11**   **Injection of Rh immune globulin**
> Injection of:
>    Anti-D (Rhesus) globulin
>    RhoGAM

**99.12**   **Immunization for allergy**
> Desensitization

**99.13**   **Immunization for autoimmune disease**

**99.14**   **Injection or infusion of gamma globulin**
> Injection of immune sera

**99.15**   **Parenteral infusion of concentrated nutritional substances**
> Hyperalimentation
> Total parenteral nutrition [TPN]
> Peripheral parenteral nutrition [PPN]
> AHA: 4Q, '03, 104
> DEF: Administration of greater than necessary amount of nutrients via other than the alimentary canal (e.g., infusion).

**99.16**   **Injection of antidote**
> Injection of:    Injection of:
>    antivenin    heavy metal antagonist

**99.17**   **Injection of insulin**

**99.18**   **Injection or infusion of electrolytes**

**99.19**   **Injection of anticoagulant**
> EXCLUDES   infusion of drotrecogin alfa (activated) (00.11)

▲

---

√4ᵗʰ **99.2    Injection or infusion of other therapeutic or prophylactic substance**

INCLUDES    injection or infusion given:

    hypodermically
    intramuscularly  } acting locally or systemically
    intravenously

Use additional code for:

| injection (into): | injection (into): |
|---|---|
| breast (85.92) | kidney (55.96) |
| bursa (82.94, 83.96) | liver (50.94) |
| intraperitoneal | orbit (16.91) |
| (cavity) (54.97) | other sites — see |
| intrathecal (03.92) | Alphabetic Index |
| joint (76.96, 81.92) | |
| perfusion: | perfusion: |
| NOS (39.97) | liver (50.93) |
| intestine (46.95, 46.96) | total body (39.96) |
| kidney (55.95) | |

**99.20    Injection or infusion of platelet inhibitor**

Glycoprotein IIb/IIIa inhibitor
GP IIb-IIIa inhibitor
GP IIb/IIIa inhibitor

EXCLUDES    infusion of heparin (99.19)
injection or infusion of thrombolytic agent (99.10)

AHA: 3Q, '06, 8; 2Q, '04, 3; 4Q, '02, 114; 4Q, '98, 85

**99.21    Injection of antibiotic**

EXCLUDES    injection or infusion of oxazolidinone class of antibiotics (00.14)

AHA: 4Q, '98, 76; 2Q, '90, 24; M-A, '87, 9

**99.22    Injection of other anti-infective**

EXCLUDES    injection or infusion of oxazolidinone class of antibiotics (00.14)

**99.23    Injection of steroid**

Injection of cortisone
Subdermal implantation of progesterone

AHA: 3Q, '00, 15; 1Q, '99, 8; 3Q, '96, 7; 3Q, '92, 9; S-O, '85, 7

**99.24    Injection of other hormone**

AHA: 1Q, '06, 9

**99.25    Injection or infusion of cancer chemotherapeutic substance**

Chemoembolization
Injection or infusion of antineoplastic agent
►Use additional code for disruption of blood brain barrier, if performed [BBBD] (00.19)◄

EXCLUDES    immunotherapy, antineoplastic (00.15, 99.28)
implantation of chemotherapeutic agent (00.10)
injection of radioisotope (92.28)
injection or infusion of biological response modifier [BRM] as an antineoplastic agent (99.28)

AHA: 2Q, '03, 6, 16; 4Q, '02, 93; 1Q, '99, 4; 1Q, '98, 6; 3Q, '96, 11; 4Q, '95, 67; 2Q, '92, 7; 1Q, '92, 12; 1Q, '88, 8; N-D, '86, 11

**99.26    Injection of tranquilizer**

**99.27    Iontophoresis**

DEF: Iontophoresis: Introduction of soluble salts into tissues via electric current.

**99.28    Injection or infusion of biological response modifier [BRM] as an antineoplastic agent**

Immunotherapy, antineoplastic
Infusion of cintredekin besudotox
Interleukin therapy
Low-dose interleukin-2 [IL-2] therapy
Tumor vaccine

EXCLUDES    high-dose infusion interleukin-2 [IL-2] (00.15)

AHA: 4Q, '06, 123; 4Q, '03, 92; 2Q, '99, 8; 2Q, '98, 10; 4Q, '94, 51

**99.29    Injection or infusion of other therapeutic or prophylactic substance**

EXCLUDES    administration of neuroprotective agent (99.75)
immunization (99.31-99.59)
►infusion of blood brain barrier disruption substance (00.19)◄
injection of sclerosing agent into:
esophageal varices (42.33)
hemorrhoids (49.42)
veins (39.92)
injection or infusion of:
human B-type natriuretic peptide (hBNP) (00.13)
nesiritide (00.13)
platelet inhibitor (99.20)
thrombolytic agent (99.10)

AHA:►1Q, '07, 11;◄ 2Q, '03, 10; 3Q, '02, 19, 24; 1Q, '01, 15; 2Q, '00, 14; 1Q, '00, 8, 18, 23; 4Q, '99, 17; 3Q, '99, 21; 4Q, '98, 83; 2Q, '98, 17, 18, 23, 24; 1Q, '98, 6; 2Q, '97, 11; 1Q, '97, 3; 4Q, '95, 67; 2Q, '95, 12; 4Q, '90, 14; 2Q, '90, 23; 2Q, '89, 17; 1Q, '88, 9; N-D, '87, 4; S-O, '87, 11

√4ᵗʰ **99.3    Prophylactic vaccination and inoculation against certain bacterial diseases**

DEF: Administration of a killed bacteria suspension to produce immunity.

**99.31    Vaccination against cholera**

**99.32    Vaccination against typhoid and paratyphoid fever**

Administration of TAB vaccine

**99.33    Vaccination against tuberculosis**

Administration of BCG vaccine

**99.34    Vaccination against plague**

**99.35    Vaccination against tularemia**

**99.36    Administration of diphtheria toxoid**

EXCLUDES    administration of:
diphtheria antitoxin (99.58)
diphtheria-tetanus-pertussis, combined (99.39)

**99.37    Vaccination against pertussis**

EXCLUDES    administration of diphtheria-tetanus-pertussis, combined (99.39)

**99.38    Administration of tetanus toxoid**

EXCLUDES    administration of:
diphtheria-tetanus-pertussis, combined (99.39)
tetanus antitoxin (99.56)

**99.39    Administration of diphtheria-tetanus-pertussis, combined**

BI Bilateral Procedure    NC Non-covered Procedure    LC Limited Coverage Procedure    ►◄ Revised Text    ● New Code    ▲ Revised Code Title

194 — Volume 3 • October 2007

© 2007 Ingenix

✓4ᵗʰ **99.4** **Prophylactic vaccination and inoculation against certain viral diseases**

DEF: Administration of a killed virus suspension to produce immunity.

**99.41** **Administration of poliomyelitis vaccine**

**99.42** **Vaccination against smallpox**

**99.43** **Vaccination against yellow fever**

**99.44** **Vaccination against rabies**

**99.45** **Vaccination against measles**

　　EXCLUDES　*administration of measles-mumps-rubella vaccine (99.48)*

**99.46** **Vaccination against mumps**

　　EXCLUDES　*administration of measles-mumps-rubella vaccine (99.48)*

**99.47** **Vaccination against rubella**

　　EXCLUDES　*administration of measles-mumps-rubella vaccine (99.48)*

**99.48** **Administration of measles-mumps-rubella vaccine**

✓4ᵗʰ **99.5** **Other vaccination and inoculation**

**99.51** **Prophylactic vaccination against the common cold**

**99.52** **Prophylactic vaccination against influenza**

**99.53** **Prophylactic vaccination against arthropod-borne viral encephalitis**

**99.54** **Prophylactic vaccination against other arthropod-borne viral diseases**

**99.55** **Prophylactic administration of vaccine against other diseases**

Vaccination against:　　Vaccination against:
　anthrax　　　　　　　Staphylococcus
　brucellosis　　　　　Streptococcus
　Rocky Mountain　　typhus
　　spotted fever

AHA: 2Q, '00, 9; 1Q, '94, 10

**99.56** **Administration of tetanus antitoxin**

**99.57** **Administration of botulism antitoxin**

**99.58** **Administration of other antitoxins**

Administration of:
　diphtheria antitoxin
　gas gangrene antitoxin
　scarlet fever antitoxin

**99.59** **Other vaccination and inoculation**

Vaccination NOS

　　EXCLUDES　*injection of:*
　　　*gamma globulin (99.14)*
　　　*Rh immune globulin (99.11)*
　　*immunization for:*
　　　*allergy (99.12)*
　　　*autoimmune disease (99.13)*

✓4ᵗʰ **99.6** **Conversion of cardiac rhythm**

　　EXCLUDES　*open chest cardiac:*
　　　*electric stimulation (37.91)*
　　　*massage (37.91)*

DEF: Correction of cardiac rhythm.

**99.60** **Cardiopulmonary resuscitation, not otherwise specified**

AHA: 1Q, '94, 16

**99.61** **Atrial cardioversion**

DEF: Application of electric shock to upper heart chamber to restore normal heart rhythm.

**99.62** **Other electric countershock of heart**

Cardioversion:
　NOS
　external
Conversion to sinus rhythm
Defibrillation
External electrode stimulation

AHA: ▶1Q, '07, 17◀

**99.63** **Closed chest cardiac massage**

Cardiac massage NOS
Manual external cardiac massage

DEF: Application of alternating manual pressure over breastbone to restore normal heart rhythm.

**99.64** **Carotid sinus stimulation**

**99.69** **Other conversion of cardiac rhythm**

AHA: 4Q, '88, 11

✓4ᵗʰ **99.7** **Therapeutic apheresis or other injection, administration, or infusion of other therapeutic or prophylactic substance**

**99.71** **Therapeutic plasmapheresis**

　　EXCLUDES　*extracorporeal immuno-adsorption [ECI] (99.76)*

**99.72** **Therapeutic leukopheresis**

Therapeutic leukocytapheresis

**99.73** **Therapeutic erythrocytapheresis**

Therapeutic erythropheresis

AHA: 1Q, '94, 20

**99.74** **Therapeutic plateletpheresis**

**99.75** **Administration of neuroprotective agent**

AHA: 4Q, '00, 68

DEF: Direct application of neuroprotective agent (e.g., nimodipine) to miinimize ischemic injury by inhibiting toxic neurotransmitters, blocking free ions, removing free radicals, and causing vasodilation.

**99.76** **Extracorporeal immunoadsorption**

Removal of antibodies from plasma with protein A columns

AHA: 4Q, '02, 112

**99.77** **Application or administration of adhesion barrier substance**

AHA: 4Q, '02, 113

**99.78** **Aquapheresis**

Plasma water removal
Ultrafiltration [for water removal]

　　EXCLUDES　*hemodiafiltration (39.95)*
　　　*hemodialysis (39.95)*
　　　*therapeutic plasmapheresis (99.71)*

**99.79** **Other**

Apheresis (harvest) of stem cells

AHA: 1Q, '06, 12, 13; 1Q, '05, 16; 4Q, '97, 55

✓4ᵗʰ **99.8** **Miscellaneous physical procedures**

**99.81** **Hypothermia (central) (local)**

　　EXCLUDES　*gastric cooling (96.31)*
　　　*gastric freezing (96.32)*
　　　*that incidental to open heart surgery (39.62)*

**99.82** **Ultraviolet light therapy**

Actinotherapy

**99.83** **Other phototherapy**

Phototherapy of the newborn

　　EXCLUDES　*extracorporeal photochemo-therapy (99.88)*
　　　*photocoagulation of retinal lesion (14.23-14.25, 14.33-14.35, 14.53-14.55)*

AHA: 2Q, '89, 15

DEF: Treating disease with light rays of various concentrations.

Diagnostic and Therapeutic Procedures

99.4–99.83

**Diagnostic and Therapeutic Procedures**

**99.84–99.99**

**99.84**   **Isolation**
  Isolation after contact with infectious disease
  Protection of individual from his surroundings
  Protection of surroundings from individual

**99.85**   **Hyperthermia for treatment of cancer**
  Hyperthermia (adjunct therapy) induced by microwave, ultrasound, low energy radio frequency, probes (interstitial), or other means in the treatment of cancer
  Code also any concurrent chemotherapy or radiation therapy
  **AHA:** 3Q, '96, 11; 3Q, '89, 17

**99.86**   **Non-invasive placement of bone growth stimulator**
  Transcutaneous (surface) placement of pads or patches for stimulation to aid bone healing
  **EXCLUDES**   *insertion of invasive or semi-invasive bone growth stimulators (device) (percutaneous electrodes) (78.90-78.99)*

**99.88**   **Therapeutic photopheresis**
  Extracorporeal photochemotherapy
  Extracorporeal photopheresis
  **EXCLUDES**   *other phototherapy (99.83)*
  *ultraviolet light therapy (99.82)*
  **AHA:** 2Q, '99, 7
  DEF: Extracorporeal photochemotherapy: Treating disease with drugs that react to ultraviolet radiation or sunlight.

✓4ᵗʰ   **99.9**   **Other miscellaneous procedures**

**99.91**   **Acupuncture for anesthesia**

**99.92**   **Other acupuncture**
  **EXCLUDES**   *that with smouldering moxa (93.35)*

**99.93**   **Rectal massage (for levator spasm)**

**99.94**   **Prostatic massage**   ♂

**99.95**   **Stretching of foreskin**   ♂

**99.96**   **Collection of sperm for artificial insemination**   ♂

**99.97**   **Fitting of denture**

**99.98**   **Extraction of milk from lactating breast**   ♀

**99.99**   **Other**
  Leech therapy

# DRG Mapping Table

The table below contains a map with the Medicare Severity (MS) DRGs (version 25) mapped back to their corresponding CMS DRGs, version 24. Please note that there are three alternative DRG cluster groupings in MS-DRGs: 1) three subgroups: with MCC, with CC, w/o CC/MCC; 2) two subgroups: with MCC, w/o MCC; or 3) two subgroups: with CC/MCC, w/o CC/MCC. There are several instances in which diagnosis codes were mapped to more than one MS-DRG cluster, which are denoted with footnotes. There are also several procedure codes that are always grouped to the highest weighted MS-DRG in the cluster, regardless of severity level; these are also designated with footnotes. This information was derived from the CMS Crosswalk from CMS-DRG to MS-DRG mapping file that can be found at http://www.cms.hhs.gov/AcuteInpatientPPS/FFD.

| MDC | Med/Surg | CMS-DRG | MS-DRG | MS-DRG Title |
|---|---|---|---|---|
| PRE | S | 103 | 001, 002 | Heart transplant or implant of heart assist system w MCC, w/o MCC |
| PRE | S | 541 | 003 | ECMO or trach w MV 96+ hrs or PDX exc face, mouth & neck w maj O.R. |
| PRE | S | 542 | 004 | Trach w MV 96+ hrs or PDX exc face, mouth & neck w/o maj O.R. |
| PRE | S | 480 | [1]005, 006 | Liver transplant w or w/o MCC or intestinal transplant |
| PRE | S | 495 | 007 | Lung transplant |
| PRE | S | 512 | 008 | Simultaneous pancreas/kidney transplant |
| PRE | S | 481 | 009 | Bone marrow transplant |
| PRE | S | 513 | 010 | Pancreas transplant |
| PRE | S | 482 | 011, 012, 013 | Tracheostomy for face, mouth & neck diagnoses w MCC, w CC, w/o CC/MCC |
| 01 | S | 528 | 020, 021, 022 | Intracranial vascular procedures w PDX hemorrhage w MCC, w CC, w/o CC/MCC |
| 01 | S | 543 | [2]023, 024 | Craniotomy w major device implant or acute complex CNS PDX w MCC or with chemo implant, w/o MCC |
| 01 | S | 001, 002, [3]003 | 025, 026, 027 | Craniotomy & endovascular intracranial procedures w MCC, w CC, w/o CC/MCC |
| 01 | S | 531, 532 | 028, [4]029, 030 | Spinal procedures w MCC, w CC or with spinal neurostimulators, w/o CC/MCC |
| 01 | S | 529, 530 | 031, 032, 033 | Ventricular shunt procedures w MCC, w CC, w/o CC/MCC |
| 01 | S | 577 | 034, 035, 036 | Carotid artery stent procedure w MCC, w CC, w/o CC/MCC |
| 01 | S | 533, 534 | 037, 038, 039 | Extracranial procedures w MCC, w CC, w/o CC/MCC |
| 01 | S | 006, 007, 008 | 040, [5]041, 042 | Periph & cranial nerve & other nerv syst proc w MCC, w CC or with peripheral neurostimulators, w/o CC/MCC |
| 01 | M | 009 | 052, 053 | Spinal disorders & injuries w CC/MCC, w/o CC/MCC |
| 01 | M | 010, 011 | 054, 055 | Nervous system neoplasms w MCC, w/o MCC |
| 01 | M | 012 | 056, 057 | Degenerative nervous system disorders w MCC, w/o MCC |
| 01 | M | 013 | 058, 059, 060 | Multiple sclerosis & cerebellar ataxia w MCC, w CC, w/o CC/MCC |
| 01 | M | 559 | 061, 062, 063 | Acute ischemic stroke w use of thrombolytic agent w MCC, w CC, w/o CC/MCC |
| 01 | M | 014 | 064, 065, 066 | Intracranial hemorrhage or cerebral infarction w MCC, w CC, w/o CC/MCC |
| 01 | M | 015 | 067, 068 | Nonspecific cva & precerebral occlusion w/o infarct w MCC, w/o MCC |
| 01 | M | 524 | 069 | Transient ischemia |
| 01 | M | 016, 017 | 070, 071, 072 | Nonspecific cerebrovascular disorders w MCC, w CC, w/o CC/MCC |
| 01 | M | 018, 019 | 073, 074 | Cranial & peripheral nerve disorders w MCC, w/o MCC |
| 01 | M | 021 | 075, 076 | Viral meningitis w CC/MCC, w/o CC/MCC |
| 01 | M | 022 | 077, 078, 079 | Hypertensive encephalopathy w MCC, w CC, w/o CC/MCC |
| 01 | M | 023 | 080, 081 | Nontraumatic stupor & coma w MCC, w/o MCC |
| 01 | M | 027 | 082, 083, 084 | Traumatic stupor & coma, coma >1 hr w MCC, w CC, w/o CC/MCC |
| 01 | M | 028, 029, 030 | 085, 086, 087 | Traumatic stupor & coma, coma <1 hr w MCC, w CC, w/o CC/MCC |
| 01 | M | 031, 032, 033 | 088, 089, 090 | Concussion w MCC, w CC, w/o CC/MCC |
| 01 | M | 034, 035 | 091, 092, 093 | Other disorders of nervous system w MCC, w CC, w/o CC/MCC |
| 01 | M | 560 | 094, 095, 096 | Bacterial & tuberculous infections of nervous system w MCC, w CC, w/o CC/MCC |
| 01 | M | 561 | 097, 098, 099 | Non-bacterial infect of nervous sys exc viral meningitis w MCC, w CC, w/o CC/MCC |
| 01 | M | [6]026, 562, 563 | 100, 101 | Seizures w MCC, w/o MCC |
| 01 | M | 564 | 102, 103 | Headaches w MCC, w/o MCC |
| 02 | S | 037 | 113, 114 | Orbital procedures w CC/MCC, w/o CC/MCC |
| 02 | S | 040, 041 | 115 | Extraocular procedures except orbit |
| 02 | S | 036, 038, 039, 042 | 116, 117 | Intraocular procedures w CC/MCC, w/o CC/MCC |
| 02 | M | 044 | 121, 122 | Acute major eye infections w CC/MCC, w/o CC/MCC |
| 02 | M | 045 | 123 | Neurological eye disorders |
| 02 | M | 043, 046, 047, 048 | 124, 125 | Other disorders of the eye w MCC, w/o MCC |
| 03 | S | 049 | [7]129, 130 | Major head & neck procedures w CC/MCC, w/o CC/MCC or with major device |
| 03 | S | 056-063 | 131, 132 | Cranial/facial procedures w CC/MCC, w/o CC/MCC |
| 03 | S | 052, 055 | 133, 134 | Other ear, nose, mouth & throat O.R. procedures w CC/MCC, w/o CC/MCC |
| 03 | S | 053, 054 | 135,136 | Sinus & mastoid procedures w CC/MCC, w/o CC/MCC |
| 03 | S | 168, 169 | 137, 138 | Mouth procedures w CC/MCC, w/o CC/MCC |
| 03 | S | 050, 051 | 139 | Salivary gland procedures |
| 03 | M | 064 | 146, 147, 148 | Ear, nose, mouth & throat malignancy w MCC, w CC, w/o CC/MCC |

[1] Procedure 46.87 [Transplant of intestine] is always grouped to MS-DRG 005 regardless of severity level

[2] Cases with code 00.10 (chemo implant) will always group to DRG 023, regardless of severity level

[3] CMS-DRG 003 procedures are split between MS-DRGs 025, 026, 027, 031, 032, 033

[4] Cases with code 86.94, 86.95, 86.97, 86.98, when in combination with 03.93 for spinal neurostimulators, are always assigned to DRG 029, regardless of severity level

[5] Cases with code 86.94, 86.95, 86.97, 86.98, when in combination with 04.92 for peripheral neurostimulators, are always assigned to DRG 041, regardless of severity level

[6] CMS-DRG 026 PDX are split between MS-DRGs 100, 101, 102, 103

[7] Procedures 20.96, 20.97, 20.98 (cochlear implants) are always assigned to MS-DRG 129 regardless of severity level

| MDC | Med/Surg | CMS-DRG | MS-DRG | MS-DRG Title |
|-----|----------|---------|--------|--------------|
| 03 | M | 065 | 149 | Dysequilibrium |
| 03 | M | 066 | 150, 151 | Epistaxis w MCC, w/o MCC |
| 03 | M | 067-071 | 152, 153 | Otitis media & URI w MCC, w/o MCC |
| 03 | M | 072, 073, 074 | 154, 155, 156 | Nasal trauma & deformity w MCC, w CC, w/o CC/MCC |
| 03 | M | 185, 186, 187 | 157, 158, 159 | Dental & oral diseases w MCC, w CC, w/o CC/MCC |
| 04 | S | 075 | 163, 164, 165 | Major chest procedures w MCC, w CC, w/o CC/MCC |
| 04 | S | 076, 077 | 166, 167, 168 | Other resp system O.R. procedures w MCC, w CC, w/o CC/MCC |
| 04 | M | 078 | 175, 176 | Pulmonary embolism w MCC, w/o MCC |
| 04 | M | 079, 080, 081 | 177, 178, 179 | Respiratory infections & inflammations w MCC, w CC, w/o CC/MCC |
| 04 | M | 082 | 180, 181, 182 | Respiratory neoplasms w MCC, w CC, w/o CC/MCC |
| 04 | M | 083, 084 | 183, 184, 185 | Major chest trauma w MCC, w CC, w/o CC/MCC |
| 04 | M | 085, 086 | 186, 187, 188 | Pleural effusion w MCC, w CC, w/o CC/MCC |
| 04 | M | 087 | 189 | Pulmonary edema & respiratory failure |
| 04 | M | 088 | 190, 191, 192 | Chronic obstructive pulmonary disease w MCC, w CC, w/o CC/MCC |
| 04 | M | 089, 090, 091 | 193, 194, 195 | Simple pneumonia & pleurisy w MCC, w CC, w/o CC/MCC |
| 04 | M | 092, 093 | 196, 197, 198 | Interstitial lung disease w MCC, w CC, w/o CC/MCC |
| 04 | M | 094, 095 | 199, 200, 201 | Pneumothorax w MCC, w CC, w/o CC/MCC |
| 04 | M | 096, 097, 098 | 202, 203 | Bronchitis & asthma w CC/MCC, w/o CC/MCC |
| 04 | M | 099, 100 | 204 | Respiratory signs & symptoms |
| 04 | M | 101, 102 | 205, 206 | Other respiratory system diagnoses w MCC, w/o MCC |
| 04 | M | 565 | 207 | Respiratory system diagnosis w ventilator support 96+ hours |
| 04 | M | 566 | 208 | Respiratory system diagnosis w ventilator support <96 hours |
| 05 | S | 525 | 215 | Other heart assist system implant |
| 05 | S | 104 | 216, 217, 218 | Cardiac valve & oth maj cardiothoracic proc w card cath w MCC, w CC, w/o CC/MCC |
| 05 | S | 105 | 219, 220, 221 | Cardiac valve & oth maj cardiothoracic proc w/o card cath w MCC, w CC, w/o CC/MCC |
| 05 | S | 535 | 222, 223 | Cardiac defib implant w cardiac cath w AMI/HF/shock w MCC, w/o MCC |
| 05 | S | 536 | 224, 225 | Cardiac defib implant w cardiac cath w/o AMI/HF/shock w MCC, w/o MCC |
| 05 | S | 515 | 226, 227 | Cardiac defibrillator implant w/o cardiac cath w MCC, w/o MCC |
| 05 | S | 108 | 228, 229, 230 | Other cardiothoracic procedures w MCC, w CC, w/o CC/MCC |
| 05 | S | 106 | 231, 232 | Coronary bypass w PTCA w MCC, w/o MCC |
| 05 | S | 547, 548 | 233, 234 | Coronary bypass w cardiac cath w MCC, w/o MCC |
| 05 | S | 549, 550 | 235, 236 | Coronary bypass w/o cardiac cath w MCC, w/o MCC |
| 05 | S | 110, 111 | [8]237, 238 | Major cardiovascular procedures w MCC or with thoracic aortic aneurysm repair, w/o MCC |
| 05 | S | 113 | 239, 240, 241 | Amputation for circ sys disorders exc upper limb & toe w MCC, w CC, w/o CC/MCC |
| 05 | S | 551, 552 | 242, 243, 244, 245 | Permanent cardiac pacemaker implant w MCC, w CC, w/o CC/MCC or AICD lead, genrtr proc |
| 05 | S | 557, 558 | [9]246, 247 | Percutaneous cardiovascular proc w drug-eluting stent w MCC or 4+ vessels/stents, w/o MCC |
| 05 | S | 555, 556 | [10]248, 249 | Percutaneous cardiovasc proc w non-drug-eluting stent w MCC or 4+ vessels/stents, w/o MCC |
| 05 | S | 518 | 250, 251 | Perc cardiovasc proc w/o coronary artery stent or AMI w MCC, w/o MCC |
| 05 | S | 479, 553, 554 | 252, 253, 254 | Other vascular procedures w MCC, w CC, w/o CC/MCC |
| 05 | S | 114 | 255, 256, 257 | Upper limb & toe amputation for circ system disorders w MCC, w CC, w/o CC/MCC |
| 05 | S | 118 | 258, 259 | Cardiac pacemaker device replacement w MCC, w/o MCC |
| 05 | S | 117 | 260, 261, 262 | Cardiac pacemaker revision except device replacement w MCC, w CC, w/o CC/MCC |
| 05 | S | 119 | 263 | Vein ligation & stripping |
| 05 | S | 120 | 264 | Other circulatory system O.R. procedures |
| 05 | M | 121, 122 | 280, 281, 282 | Acute myocardial infarction, discharged alive w MCC, w CC, w/o CC/MCC |
| 05 | M | 123 | 283, 284, 285 | Acute myocardial infarction, expired w MCC, w CC, w/o CC/MCC |
| 05 | M | 124, 125 | 286, 287 | Circulatory disorders except AMI, w card cath w MCC, w/o MCC |
| 05 | M | 126 | 288, 289, 290 | Acute & subacute endocarditis w MCC, w CC, w/o CC/MCC |
| 05 | M | 127 | 291, 292, 293 | Heart failure & shock w MCC, w CC, w/o CC/MCC |
| 05 | M | 128 | 294, 295 | Deep vein thrombophlebitis w CC/MCC, w/o CC/MCC |
| 05 | M | 129 | 296, 297, 298 | Cardiac arrest, unexplained w MCC, w CC, w/o CC/MCC |
| 05 | M | 130, 131 | 299, 300, 301 | Peripheral vascular disorders w MCC, w CC, w/o CC/MCC |
| 05 | M | 132, 133 | 302, 303 | Atherosclerosis w MCC, w/o MCC |

[8] Cases with code 39.73 (endovascular implant of graft in thoracic aorta) are always assigned to DRG 237, regardless of severity level

[9] Cases with codes 00.66, 36.07 and 00.43 or 00.48 (PTCA or stenting on 4 or more vessels) are always assigned to DRG 246, regardless of severity level

[10] Cases with codes 00.66, 36.06 and 00.43 or 00.48 (PTCA or stenting on 4 or more vessels) are always assigned to DRG 248, regardless of severity level

| MDC | Med/Surg | CMS-DRG | MS-DRG | MS-DRG Title |
|-----|----------|---------|--------|--------------|
| 05 | M | 134 | 304, 305 | Hypertension w MCC, w/o MCC |
| 05 | M | 135, 136, 137 | 306, 307 | Cardiac congenital & valvular disorders w MCC, w/o MCC |
| 05 | M | 138, 139 | 308, 309, 310 | Cardiac arrhythmia & conduction disorders w MCC, w CC, w/o CC/MCC |
| 05 | M | 140 | 311 | Angina pectoris |
| 05 | M | 141, 142 | 312 | Syncope & collapse |
| 05 | M | 143 | 313 | Chest pain |
| 05 | M | 144, 145 | 314, 315, 316 | Other circulatory system diagnoses w MCC, w CC, w/o CC/MCC |
| 06 | S | 155, 156, 567, 568 | 326, 327, 328 | Stomach, esophageal & duodenal proc w MCC, w CC, w/o CC/MCC |
| 06 | S | 149, 569, 570 | 329, 330, 331 | Major small & large bowel procedures w MCC, w CC, w/o CC/MCC |
| 06 | S | 146, 147 | 332, 333, 334 | Rectal resection w MCC, w CC, w/o CC/MCC |
| 06 | S | 150, 151 | 335, 336, 337 | Peritoneal adhesiolysis w MCC, w CC, w/o CC/MCC |
| 06 | S | 164, 165 | 338, 339, 340 | Appendectomy w complicated principal diag w MCC, w CC, w/o CC/MCC |
| 06 | S | 166, 167 | 341, 342, 343 | Appendectomy w/o complicated principal diag w MCC, w CC, w/o CC/MCC |
| 06 | S | 152, 153 | 344, 345, 346 | Minor small & large bowel procedures w MCC, w CC, w/o CC/MCC |
| 06 | S | 157, 158 | 347, 348, 349 | Anal & stomal procedures w MCC, w CC, w/o CC/MCC |
| 06 | S | 161, 162, [11]163 | 350, 351, 352 | Inguinal & femoral hernia procedures w MCC, w CC, w/o CC/MCC |
| 06 | S | 159, 160 | 353, 354, 355 | Hernia procedures except inguinal & femoral w MCC, w CC, w/o CC/MCC |
| 06 | S | 170, 171 | 356, 357, 358 | Other digestive system O.R. procedures w MCC, w CC, w/o CC/MCC |
| 06 | M | 571 | 368, 369, 370 | Major esophageal disorders w MCC, w CC, w/o CC/MCC |
| 06 | M | 572 | 371, 372, 373 | Major gastrointestinal disorders & peritoneal infections w MCC, w CC, w/o CC/MCC |
| 06 | M | 172, 173 | 374, 375, 376 | Digestive malignancy w MCC, w CC, w/o CC/MCC |
| 06 | M | 174, 175 | 377, 378, 379 | G.I. hemorrhage w MCC, w CC, w/o CC/MCC |
| 06 | M | 176 | 380, 381, 382 | Complicated peptic ulcer w MCC, w CC, w/o CC/MCC |
| 06 | M | 177, 178 | 383, 384 | Uncomplicated peptic ulcer w MCC, w/o MCC |
| 06 | M | 179 | 385, 386, 387 | Inflammatory bowel disease w MCC, w CC, w/o CC/MCC |
| 06 | M | 180, 181 | 388, 389, 390 | G.I. obstruction w MCC, w CC, w/o CC/MCC |
| 06 | M | 182, 183, 184 | 391, 392 | Esophagitis, gastroent & misc digest disorders w MCC, w/o MCC |
| 06 | M | 188, 189, 190 | 393, 394, 395 | Other digestive system diagnoses w MCC, w CC, w/o CC/MCC |
| 07 | S | 191, 192 | 405, 406, 407 | Pancreas, liver & shunt procedures w MCC, w CC, w/o CC/MCC |
| 07 | S | 193, 194 | 408, 409, 410 | Biliary tract proc except only cholecyst w or w/o c.d.e. w MCC, w CC, w/o CC/MCC |
| 07 | S | 195, 196 | 411, 412, 413 | Cholecystectomy w c.d.e. w MCC, w CC, w/o CC/MCC |
| 07 | S | 197, 198 | 414, 415, 416 | Cholecystectomy except by laparoscope w/o c.d.e. w MCC, w CC, w/o CC/MCC |
| 07 | S | 493, 494 | 417, 418, 419 | Laparoscopic cholecystectomy w/o c.d.e. w MCC, w CC, w/o CC/MCC |
| 07 | S | 199, 200 | 420, 421, 422 | Hepatobiliary diagnostic procedures w MCC, w CC, w/o CC/MCC |
| 07 | S | 201 | 423, 424, 425 | Other hepatobiliary or pancreas O.R. procedures w MCC, w CC, w/o CC/MCC |
| 07 | M | 202 | 432, 433, 434 | Cirrhosis & alcoholic hepatitis w MCC, w CC, w/o CC/MCC |
| 07 | M | 203 | 435, 436, 437 | Malignancy of hepatobiliary system or pancreas w MCC, w CC, w/o CC/MCC |
| 07 | M | 204 | 438, 439, 440 | Disorders of pancreas except malignancy w MCC, w CC, w/o CC/MCC |
| 07 | M | 205, 206 | 441, 442, 443 | Disorders of liver except malig,cirr,alc hepa w MCC, w CC, w/o CC/MCC |
| 07 | M | 207, 208 | 444, 445, 446 | Disorders of the biliary tract w MCC, w CC, w/o CC/MCC |
| 08 | S | 496 | 453, 454, 455 | Combined anterior/posterior spinal fusion w MCC, w CC, w/o CC/MCC |
| 08 | S | 546 | 456, 457, 458 | Spinal fusion exc cerv w spinal curvature/infection, malig or 9+ fusions w MCC, w CC, w/o CC/MCC |
| 08 | S | 497, 498 | 459, 460 | Spinal fusion except cervical w MCC, w/o MCC |
| 08 | S | 471 | 461, 462 | Bilateral or multiple major joint procs of lower extremity w MCC, w/o MCC |
| 08 | S | 217 | 463, 464, 465 | Wnd debrid & skn grft exc hand, for musculo-conn tiss dis w MCC, w CC, w/o CC/MCC |
| 08 | S | 545 | 466, 467, 468 | Revision of hip or knee replacement w MCC, w CC, w/o CC/MCC |
| 08 | S | 544 | 469, 470 | Major joint replacement or reattachment of lower extremity w MCC, w/o MCC |
| 08 | S | 519, 520 | 471, 472, 473 | Cervical spinal fusion w MCC, w CC, w/o CC/MCC |
| 08 | S | 213 | 474, 475, 476 | Amputation for musculoskeletal sys & conn tissue dis w MCC, w CC, w/o CC/MCC |
| 08 | S | 216 | 477, 478, 479 | Biopsies of musculoskeletal system & connective tissue w MCC, w CC, w/o CC/MCC |
| 08 | S | 210, 211, 212 | 480, 481, 482 | Hip & femur procedures except major joint w MCC, w CC, w/o CC/MCC |
| 08 | S | 491 | 483, 484 | Major joint & limb reattachment proc of upper extremity w CC/MCC, w/o CC/MCC |
| 08 | S | 501, 502 | 485, 486, 487 | Knee procedures w pdx of infection w MCC, w CC, w/o CC/MCC |
| 08 | S | 503 | 488, 489 | Knee procedures w/o pdx of infection w CC/MCC, w/o CC/MCC |

[11] CMS DRG 163 procedures are split between MS-DRGs 350, 351, 352, 353, 354, 355

| MDC | Med/Surg | CMS-DRG | MS-DRG | MS-DRG Title |
|---|---|---|---|---|
| 08 | S | 499, 500 | [12]490, 491 | Back & neck procedures except spinal fusion w CC/MCC, w/o CC/MCC or with disc devices/ neurostimulators |
| 08 | S | 218, 219, 220 | 492, 493, 494 | Lower extrem & humer proc except hip,foot,femur w MCC, w CC, w/o CC/MCC |
| 08 | S | 537, 538 | 495, 496, 497 | Local excision & removal int fix devices exc hip & femur w MCC, w CC, w/o CC/MCC |
| 08 | S | 230 | 498, 499 | Local excision & removal int fix devices of hip & femur w CC/MCC, w/o CC/MCC |
| 08 | S | 226, 227 | 500, 501, 502 | Soft tissue procedures w MCC, w CC, w/o CC/MCC |
| 08 | S | 225 | 503, 504, 505 | Foot procedures w MCC, w CC, w/o CC/MCC |
| 08 | S | 228 | 506 | Major thumb or joint procedures |
| 08 | S | 223 | 507, 508 | Major shoulder or elbow joint procedures w CC/MCC, w/o CC/MCC |
| 08 | S | 232 | 509 | Arthroscopy |
| 08 | S | 224 | 510, 511, 512 | Shoulder,elbow or forearm proc,exc major joint proc w MCC, w CC, w/o CC/MCC |
| 08 | S | 229 | 513, 514 | Hand or wrist proc, except major thumb or joint proc w CC/MCC, w/o CC/MCC |
| 08 | S | 233, 234 | 515, 516, 517 | Other musculoskelet sys & conn tiss O.R. proc w MCC, w CC, w/o CC/MCC |
| 08 | M | 235 | 533, 534 | Fractures of femur w MCC, w/o MCC |
| 08 | M | 236 | 535, 536 | Fractures of hip & pelvis w MCC, w/o MCC |
| 08 | M | 237 | 537,538 | Sprains, strains, & dislocations of hip, pelvis & thigh w CC/MCC, w/o CC/MCC |
| 08 | M | 238 | 539, 540,541 | Osteomyelitis w MCC, w CC, w/o CC/MCC |
| 08 | M | 239 | 542,543,544 | Pathological fractures & musculoskelet & conn tiss malig w MCC, w CC, w/o CC/MCC |
| 08 | M | 240, 241 | 545, 546, 547 | Connective tissue disorders w MCC, w CC, w/o CC/MCC |
| 08 | M | 242 | 548, 549, 550 | Septic arthritis w MCC, w CC, w/o CC/MCC |
| 08 | M | 243 | 551,552 | Medical back problems w MCC, w/o MCC |
| 08 | M | 244, 245, 246 | 553,554 | Bone diseases & arthropathies w MCC, w/o MCC |
| 08 | M | 247 | 555,556 | Signs & symptoms of musculoskeletal system & conn tissue w MCC, w/o MCC |
| 08 | M | 248 | 557, 558 | Tendonitis, myositis & bursitis w MCC, w/o MCC |
| 08 | M | 249 | 559, 560, 561 | Aftercare, musculoskeletal system & connective tissue w MCC, w CC, w/o CC/MCC |
| 08 | M | 250-255 | 562, 563 | Fx, sprn, strn & disl except femur, hip, pelvis & thigh w MCC, w/o MCC |
| 08 | M | 256 | 564, 565, 566 | Other musculoskeletal sys & connective tissue diagnoses w MCC, w CC, w/o CC/MCC |
| 09 | S | 263,264 | 573,574,575 | Skin graft &/or debrid for skn ulcer or cellulitis w MCC, w CC, w/o CC/MCC |
| 09 | S | 265,266 | 576,577,578 | Skin graft &/or debrid exc for skin ulcer or cellulitis w MCC, w CC, w/o CC/MCC |
| 09 | S | 267-270 | 579,580,581 | Other skin, subcut tiss & breast proc w MCC, w CC, w/o CC/MCC |
| 09 | S | 257,258 | 582,583 | Mastectomy for malignancy w CC/MCC, w/o CC/MCC |
| 09 | S | 259-262 | 584,585 | Breast biopsy, local excision & other breast procedures w CC/MCC, w/o CC/MCC |
| 09 | M | 271 | 592, 593, 594 | Skin ulcers w MCC, w CC, w/o CC/MCC |
| 09 | M | 272, 273 | 595,596 | Major skin disorders w MCC, w/o MCC |
| 09 | M | 274, 275 | 597, 598, 599 | Malignant breast disorders w MCC, w CC, w/o CC/MCC |
| 09 | M | 276 | 600, 601 | Non-malignant breast disorders w CC/MCC, w/o CC/MCC |
| 09 | M | 277,278,279 | 602, 603 | Cellulitis w MCC, w/o MCC |
| 09 | M | 280,281,282 | 604,605 | Trauma to the skin, subcut tiss & breast w MCC, w/o MCC |
| 09 | M | 283,284 | 606,607 | Minor skin disorders w MCC, w/o MCC |
| 10 | S | 286 | 614, 615 | Adrenal & pituitary procedures w CC/MCC, w/o CC/MCC |
| 10 | S | 285 | 616,617, 618 | Amputat of lower limb for endocrine,nutrit,& metabol dis w MCC, w CC, w/o CC/MCC |
| 10 | S | 288 | 619,620,621 | O.R. procedures for obesity w MCC, w CC, w/o CC/MCC |
| 10 | S | 287 | 622,623,624 | Skin grafts & wound debrid for endoc, nutrit & metab dis w MCC, w CC, w/o CC/MCC |
| 10 | S | 289,290,291 | 625,626,627 | Thyroid, parathyroid & thyroglossal procedures w MCC, w CC, w/o CC/MCC |
| 10 | S | 292, 293 | 628,629,630 | Other endocrine, nutrit & metab O.R. proc w MCC, w CC, w/o CC/MCC |
| 10 | M | 294,295 | 637,638,639 | Diabetes w MCC, w CC, w/o CC/MCC |
| 10 | M | 296,297,298 | 640,641 | Nutritional & misc metabolic disorders w MCC, w/o MCC |
| 10 | M | 299 | 642 | Inborn errors of metabolism |
| 10 | M | 300,301 | 643,644,645 | Endocrine disorders w MCC, w CC, w/o CC/MCC |
| 11 | S | 302 | 652 | Kidney transplant |
| 11 | S | 573 | 653,654,655 | Major bladder procedures w MCC, w CC, w/o CC/MCC |
| 11 | S | 303 | 656,657,658 | Kidney & ureter procedures for neoplasm w MCC, w CC, w/o CC/MCC |
| 11 | S | 304,305 | 659,660,661 | Kidney & ureter procedures for non-neoplasm w MCC, w CC, w/o CC/MCC |
| 11 | S | 308, 309 | 662,663,664 | Minor bladder procedures w MCC, w CC, w/o CC/MCC |
| 11 | S | 306,307 | 665,666, 667 | Prostatectomy w MCC, w CC, w/o CC/MCC |

[12] Procedures 84.58, 84.59, 84.65 are always assigned to MS-DRG 490 regardless of severity level; Combination 03.93 with (86.94 or 86.95 or 86.97 or 86.98) is always assigned to MS-DRG 490 regardless of severity level

| MDC | Med/Surg | CMS-DRG | MS-DRG | MS-DRG Title |
|---|---|---|---|---|
| 11 | S | 310,311 | 668,669,670 | Transurethral procedures w MCC, w CC, w/o CC/MCC |
| 11 | S | 312,313,314 | 671,672 | Urethral procedures w CC/MCC, w/o CC/MCC |
| 11 | S | 315 | 673,674,675 | Other kidney & urinary tract procedures w MCC, w CC, w/o CC/MCC |
| 11 | M | 316 | 682,683,684 | Renal failure w MCC, w CC, w/o CC/MCC |
| 11 | M | 317 | 685 | Admit for renal dialysis |
| 11 | M | 318, 319 | 686,687,688 | Kidney & urinary tract neoplasms w MCC, w CC, w/o CC/MCC |
| 11 | M | 320,321,322 | 689,690 | Kidney & urinary tract infections w MCC, w/o MCC |
| 11 | M | 323 | 691,692 | Urinary stones w esw lithotripsy w CC/MCC, w/o CC/MCC |
| 11 | M | 324 | 693,694 | Urinary stones w/o esw lithotripsy w MCC, w/o MCC |
| 11 | M | 325,326,327 | 695,696 | Kidney & urinary tract signs & symptoms w MCC, w/o MCC |
| 11 | M | 328,329,330 | 697 | Urethral stricture |
| 11 | M | 331,332,333 | 698,699,700 | Other kidney & urinary tract diagnoses w MCC, w CC, w/o CC/MCC |
| 12 | S | 334,335 | 707,708 | Major male pelvic procedures w CC/MCC, w/o CC/MCC |
| 12 | S | 341 | 709,710 | Penis procedures w CC/MCC, w/o CC/MCC |
| 12 | S | 338,339,340 | 711,712 | Testes procedures w CC/MCC, w/o CC/MCC |
| 12 | S | 336,337 | 713, 714 | Transurethral prostatectomy w CC/MCC, w/o CC/MCC |
| 12 | S | 344 | 715,716 | Other male reproductive system O.R. proc for malignancy w CC/MCC, w/o CC/MCC |
| 12 | S | 345 | 717,718 | Other male reproductive system O.R. proc exc malignancy w CC/MCC, w/o CC/MCC |
|  |  | 342,[13]343 |  | Deleted |
| 12 | M | 346,347 | 722,723,724 | Malignancy, male reproductive system w MCC, w CC, w/o CC/MCC |
| 12 | M | 348,349 | 725,726 | Benign prostatic hypertrophy w MCC, w/o MCC |
| 12 | M | 350 | 727,728 | Inflammation of the male reproductive system w MCC, w/o MCC |
| 12 | M | 351,352 | 729,730 | Other male reproductive system diagnoses w CC/MCC, w/o CC/MCC |
| 13 | S | 353 | 734,735 | Pelvic evisceration, rad hysterectomy & rad vulvectomy w CC/MCC, w/o CC/MCC |
| 13 | S | 357 | 736,737,738 | Uterine & adnexa proc for ovarian or adnexal malignancy w MCC, w CC, w/o CC/MCC |
| 13 | S | 354,355 | 739,740,741 | Uterine,adnexa proc for non-ovarian/adnexal malig w MCC, w CC, w/o CC/MCC |
| 13 | S | 358,359 | 742,743 | Uterine & adnexa proc for non-malignancy w CC/MCC, w/oCC/MCC |
| 13 | S | 361-364 | 744, 745 | D&C, conization, laparoscopy & tubal interruption w CC/MCC, w/o CC/MCC |
| 13 | S | 360 | 746,747 | Vagina, cervix & vulva procedures w CC/MCC, w/o CC/MCC |
| 13 | S | 356 | 748 | Female reproductive system reconstructive procedures |
| 13 | S | 365 | 749,750 | Other female reproductive system O.R. procedures w CC/MCC, w/o CC/MCC |
| 13 | M | 366,367 | 754,755,756 | Malignancy, female reproductive system w MCC, w CC, w/o CC/MCC |
| 13 | M | 368 | 757,758,759 | Infections, female reproductive system w MCC, w CC, w/o CC/MCC |
| 13 | M | 369 | 760,761 | Menstrual & other female reproductive system disorders w CC/MCC, w/o CC/MCC |
| 14 | S | 370, 371 | 765,766 | Cesarean section w CC/MCC, w/o CC/MCC |
| 14 | S | 374 | 767 | Vaginal delivery w sterilization &/or D&C |
| 14 | S | 375 | 768 | Vaginal delivery w O.R. proc except steril &/or D&C |
| 14 | S | 377 | 769 | Postpartum & post abortion diagnoses w O.R. procedure |
| 14 | S | 381 | 770 | Abortion w D&C, aspiration curettage or hysterotomy |
| 14 | M | 372 | 774 | Vaginal delivery w complicating diagnoses |
| 14 | M | 373 | 775 | Vaginal delivery w/o complicating diagnoses |
| 14 | M | 376 | 776 | Postpartum & post abortion diagnoses w/o O.R. procedure |
| 14 | M | 378 | 777 | Ectopic pregnancy |
| 14 | M | 379 | 778 | Threatened abortion |
| 14 | M | 380 | 779 | Abortion w/o D&C |
| 14 | M | 382 | 780 | False labor |
| 14 | M | 383 | 781 | Other antepartum diagnoses w medical complications |
| 14 | M | 384 | 782 | Other antepartum diagnoses w/o medical complications |
| 15 | M | 385 | 789 | Neonates, died or transferred to another acute care facility |
| 15 | M | 386 | 790 | Extreme immaturity or respiratory distress syndrome, neonate |
| 15 | M | 387 | 791 | Prematurity w major problems |
| 15 | M | 388 | 792 | Prematurity w/o major problems |
| 15 | M | 389 | 793 | Full term neonate w major problems |
| 15 | M | 390 | 794 | Neonate w other significant problems |
| 15 | M | 391 | 795 | Normal newborn |

[13] OR procedure 64.0 (Circumcision) changed to non-OR and DRGs 342 & 343 deleted

| MDC | Med/Surg | CMS-DRG | MS-DRG | MS-DRG Title |
|---|---|---|---|---|
| 16 | S | 392, 393 | 799, 800,801 | Splenectomy w MCC, w CC, w/o CC/MCC |
| 16 | S | 394 | 802, 803,804 | Other O.R. proc of the blood & blood forming organs w MCC, w CC, w/o CC/MCC |
| 16 | M | 574 | 808, 809, 810 | Major hematol/immun diag exc sickle cell crisis & coagul w MCC, w CC, w/o CC/MCC |
| 16 | M | 395, 396 | 811, 812 | Red blood cell disorders w MCC, w/o MCC |
| 16 | M | 397 | 813 | Coagulation disorders |
| 16 | M | 398, 399 | 814, 815,816 | Reticuloendothelial & immunity disorders w MCC, w CC, w/o CC/MCC |
| 17 | S | 539, 540 | 820, 821,822 | Lymphoma & leukemia w major O.R. procedure w MCC, w CC, w/o CC/MCC |
| 17 | S | 401, 402 | 823, 824, 825 | Lymphoma & non-acute leukemia w other O.R. proc w MCC, w CC, w/o CC/MCC |
| 17 | S | 406, 407 | 826, 827,828 | Myeloprolif disord or poorly diff neopl w maj O.R. proc w MCC, w CC, w/o CC/MCC |
| 17 | S | 408 | 829, 830 | Myeloprolif disord or poorly diff neopl w other O.R. proc w CC/MCC, w/o CC/MCC |
| 17 | M | 405, 473 | 834, 835,836 | Acute leukemia w/o major O.R. procedure w MCC, w CC, w/o CC/MCC |
| 17 | M | [14]492 | 837, 838,839 | Chemo w acute leukemia as sdx or w  high dose chemo agent w MCC, w CC, w/o CC/MCC (no high dose chemo) |
| 17 | M | 403, 404 | 840, 841, 842 | Lymphoma & non-acute leukemia w MCC, w CC, w/o CC/MCC |
| 17 | M | 411-414 | 843,844,845 | Other myeloprolif dis or poorly diff neopl diag w MCC, w CC, w/o CC/MCC |
| 17 | M | 410 | 846, 847,848 | Chemotherapy w/o acute leukemia as secondary diagnosis w MCC, w CC, w/o CC/MCC |
| 17 | M | 409 | 849 | Radiotherapy |
| 18 | S | 578 | 853,854,855 | Infectious & parasitic diseases w O.R. procedure w MCC, w CC, w/o CC/MCC |
| 18 | S | 579 | 856,857,858 | Postoperative or post-traumatic infections w O.R. proc w MCC, w CC, w/o CC/MCC |
| 18 | M | 418 | 862,863 | Postoperative & post-traumatic infections w MCC, w/o MCC |
| 18 | M | 419,420 | 864 | Fever of unknown origin |
| 18 | M | 421, [15]422 | 865, 866 | Viral illness w MCC, w/o MCC |
| 18 | M | 423 | 867,868,869 | Other infectious & parasitic diseases diagnoses w MCC, w CC, w/o CC/MCC |
| 18 | M | 417, 575 | 870 | Septicemia w MV 96+ hours |
| 18 | M | 576 | 871, 872 | Septicemia w/o MV 96+ hours w MCC, w/o MCC |
| 19 | S | 424 | 876 | O.R. procedure w principal diagnoses of mental illness |
| 19 | M | 425 | 880 | Acute adjustment reaction & psychosocial dysfunction |
| 19 | M | 426 | 881 | Depressive neuroses |
| 19 | M | 427 | 882 | Neuroses except depressive |
| 19 | M | 428 | 883 | Disorders of personality & impulse control |
| 19 | M | 429 | 884 | Organic disturbances & mental retardation |
| 19 | M | 430 | 885 | Psychoses |
| 19 | M | 431 | 886 | Behavioral & developmental disorders |
| 19 | M | 432 | 887 | Other mental disorder diagnoses |
| 20 | M | 433 | 894 | Alcohol/drug abuse or dependence, left ama |
| 20 | M | 521,522 | 895 | Alcohol/drug abuse or dependence w rehabilitation therapy |
| 20 | M | 523 | 896, 897 | Alcohol/drug abuse or dependence w/o rehabilitation therapy w MCC, w/o MCC |
| 21 | S | 440 | 901, 902, 903 | Wound debridements for injuries w MCC, w CC, w/o CC/MCC |
| 21 | S | 439 | 904, 905 | Skin grafts for injuries w CC/MCC, w/o CC/MCC |
| 21 | S | 441 | 906 | Hand procedures for injuries |
| 21 | S | 442, 443 | 907, 908, 909 | Other O.R. procedures for injuries w MCC, w CC, w/o CC/MCC |
| 21 | M | 444, 445, 446 | 913, 914 | Traumatic injury w MCC, w/o MCC |
| 21 | M | 447, 448 | 915, 916 | Allergic reactions w MCC, w/o MCC |
| 21 | M | 449, 450, 451 | 917, 918 | Poisoning & toxic effects of drugs w MCC, w/o MCC |
| 21 | M | 452,453 | 919, 920, 921 | Complications of treatment w MCC, w CC, w/o CC/MCC |
| 21 | M | 454, 455 | 922, 923 | Other injury, poisoning & toxic effect diag w MCC, w/o MCC |
| 22 | S | 504 | 927 | Extensive burns or full thickness burns w MV 96+ hrs w skin graft |
| 22 | S | 506, 507 | 928, 929 | Full thickness burn w skin graft or inhal inj w CC/MCC, w/o CC/MCC |
| 22 | M | 505 | 933 | Extensive burns or full thickness burns w MV 96+ hrs w/o skin graft |
| 22 | M | 508, 509 | 934 | Full thickness burn w/o skin grft or inhal inj |
| 22 | M | 510, 511 | 935 | Non-extensive burns |
| 23 | S | 461 | 939, 940, 941 | O.R. proc w diagnoses of other contact w health services w MCC, w CC, w/o CC/MCC |
| 23 | M | 462 | 945, 946 | Rehabilitation w CC/MCC, w/o CC/MCC |
| 23 | M | 463, 464 | 947, 948 | Signs & symptoms w MCC, w/o MCC |
| 23 | M | 465, 466 | 949, 950 | Aftercare w CC/MCC, w/o CC/MCC |

[14] Cases with code 00.15 (High-dose infusion IL-2) are always assigned to either DRG 837 & 838

[15] CMS-DRG 422 PDX split between MS-DRGs 864,865, 866

| MDC | Med/Surg | CMS-DRG | MS-DRG | MS-DRG Title |
|-----|----------|---------|--------|--------------|
| 23 | M | 467 | 951 | Other factors influencing health status |
| 24 | S | 484 | 955 | Craniotomy for multiple significant trauma |
| 24 | S | 485 | 956 | Limb reattachment, hip & femur proc for multiple significant trauma |
| 24 | S | 486 | 957, 958, 959 | Other O.R. procedures for multiple significant trauma w MCC, w CC, w/o CC/MCC |
| 24 | M | 487 | 963, 964, 965 | Other multiple significant trauma w MCC, w CC, w/o CC/MCC |
| 25 | S | 488 | 969, 970 | HIV w extensive O.R. procedure w MCC, w/o MCC |
| 25 | M | 489 | 974, 975, 976 | HIV w major related condition w MCC, w CC, w/o CC/MCC |
| 25 | M | 490 | 977 | HIV w or w/o other related condition |
|  | S | 468 | 981, 982, 983 | Extensive O.R. procedure unrelated to principal diagnosis w MCC, w CC, w/o CC/MCC |
|  | S | 476 | 984, 985, 986 | Prostatic O.R. procedure unrelated to principal diagnosis w MCC, w CC, w/o CC/MCC |
|  | S | 477 | 987, 988, 989 | Non-extensive O.R. proc unrelated to principal diagnosis w MCC, w CC, w/o CC/MCC |
|  | * | 469 | 998 | Principal diagnosis invalid as discharge diagnosis |
|  | * | 470 | 999 | Ungroupable |

# Diagnosis Code/MDC/DRG List

The following list provides the MDC and **Medical** DRG(s) to which the diagnosis code is assigned when listed as the principal diagnosis with the exception of principal diagnosis in combination with secondary diagnosis causing assignment to MDC 24 or the secondary diagnosis causing assignment to MDC 25. The resources used to compile this list are the Medicare Program; Changes to the Hospital Inpatient Prospective Payment System: Final Rule *Federal Register*, August 22, 2007) and the CMS Crosswalk from CMS-DRG to MS-DRG mapping file that can be found at http://www.cms.hhs.gov/AcuteInpatientPPS/FFD.

| DX ...MDC ..DRG | DX ...MDC ..DRG | DX ...MDC ..DRG | DX ...MDC ..DRG | DX ...MDC ..DRG |
|---|---|---|---|---|
| **Infectious and Parastic Diseases** | 008.49 ..06 .371-373 | 011.33 ..04 ..177-179 | 012.30 ..03 ..154-156 | 013.84 ..01 ..094-096 |
| 001.0 ...06 .371-373 | 008.5 ...06 .371-373 | 011.34 ..04 ..177-179 | 012.31 ..03 ..154-156 | 013.85 ..01 ..094-096 |
| 001.1 ...06 .371-373 | 008.61 ..06 .391-392 | 011.35 ..04 ..177-179 | 012.32 ..03 ..154-156 | 013.86 ..01 ..094-096 |
| 001.9 ...06 .371-373 | 008.62 ..06 .391-392 | 011.36 ..04 ..177-179 | 012.33 ..03 ..154-156 | 013.90 ..01 ..094-096 |
| 002.0 ...18 .867-869 | 008.63 ..06 .391-392 | 011.40 ..04 ..177-179 | 012.34 ..03 ..154-156 | 013.91 ..01 ..094-096 |
| 002.1 ...18 .867-869 | 008.64 ..06 .391-392 | 011.41 ..04 ..177-179 | 012.35 ..03 ..154-156 | 013.92 ..01 ..094-096 |
| 002.2 ...18 .867-869 | 008.65 ..06 .391-392 | 011.42 ..04 ..177-179 | 012.36 ..03 ..154-156 | 013.93 ..01 ..094-096 |
| 002.3 ...18 .867-869 | 008.66 ..06 .391-392 | 011.43 ..04 ..177-179 | 012.80 ..04 ..177-179 | 013.94 ..01 ..094-096 |
| 002.9 ...18 .867-869 | 008.67 ..06 .391-392 | 011.44 ..04 ..177-179 | 012.81 ..04 ..177-179 | 013.95 ..01 ..094-096 |
| 003.0 ...06 .371-373 | 008.69 ..06 .391-392 | 011.45 ..04 ..177-179 | 012.82 ..04 ..177-179 | 013.96 ..01 ..094-096 |
| 003.1 ...18 .870-872 | 008.8 ...06 .391-392 | 011.46 ..04 ..177-179 | 012.83 ..04 ..177-179 | 014.00 ..06 .371-373 |
| 003.20 ..18 .867-869 | 009.0 ...06 .391-392 | 011.50 ..04 ..177-179 | 012.84 ..04 ..177-179 | 014.01 ..06 .371-373 |
| 003.21 ..01 ..094-096 | 009.1 ...06 .391-392 | 011.51 ..04 ..177-179 | 012.85 ..04 ..177-179 | 014.02 ..06 .371-373 |
| 003.22 ..04 ..177-179 | 009.2 ...06 .391-392 | 011.52 ..04 ..177-179 | 012.86 ..04 ..177-179 | 014.03 ..06 .371-373 |
| 003.23 ..08 .548-550 | 009.3 ...06 .391-392 | 011.53 ..04 ..177-179 | 013.00 ..01 ..094-096 | 014.04 ..06 .371-373 |
| 003.24 ..08 .539-541 | 010.00 ..04 ..177-179 | 011.54 ..04 ..177-179 | 013.01 ..01 ..094-096 | 014.05 ..06 .371-373 |
| 003.29 ..18 .867-869 | 010.01 ..04 ..177-179 | 011.55 ..04 ..177-179 | 013.02 ..01 ..094-096 | 014.06 ..06 .371-373 |
| 003.8 ...18 .867-869 | 010.02 ..04 ..177-179 | 011.56 ..04 ..177-179 | 013.03 ..01 ..094-096 | 014.80 ..06 .371-373 |
| 003.9 ...18 .867-869 | 010.03 ..04 ..177-179 | 011.60 ..04 ..177-179 | 013.04 ..01 ..094-096 | 014.81 ..06 .371-373 |
| 004.0 ...06 .371-373 | 010.04 ..04 ..177-179 | 011.61 ..04 ..177-179 | 013.05 ..01 ..094-096 | 014.82 ..06 .371-373 |
| 004.1 ...06 .371-373 | 010.05 ..04 ..177-179 | 011.62 ..04 ..177-179 | 013.06 ..01 ..094-096 | 014.83 ..06 .371-373 |
| 004.2 ...06 .371-373 | 010.06 ..04 ..177-179 | 011.63 ..04 ..177-179 | 013.10 ..01 ..094-096 | 014.84 ..06 .371-373 |
| 004.3 ...06 .371-373 | 010.10 ..04 ..177-179 | 011.64 ..04 ..177-179 | 013.11 ..01 ..094-096 | 014.85 ..06 .371-373 |
| 004.8 ...06 .371-373 | 010.11 ..04 ..177-179 | 011.65 ..04 ..177-179 | 013.12 ..01 ..094-096 | 014.86 ..06 .371-373 |
| 004.9 ...06 .371-373 | 010.12 ..04 ..177-179 | 011.66 ..04 ..177-179 | 013.13 ..01 ..094-096 | 015.00 ..08 .539-541 |
| 005.0 ...06 .371-373 | 010.13 ..04 ..177-179 | 011.70 ..04 ..177-179 | 013.14 ..01 ..094-096 | 015.01 ..08 .539-541 |
| 005.1 ...18 .867-869 | 010.14 ..04 ..177-179 | 011.71 ..04 ..177-179 | 013.15 ..01 ..094-096 | 015.02 ..08 .539-541 |
| 005.2 ...06 .371-373 | 010.15 ..04 ..177-179 | 011.72 ..04 ..177-179 | 013.16 ..01 ..094-096 | 015.03 ..08 .539-541 |
| 005.3 ...06 .371-373 | 010.16 ..04 ..177-179 | 011.73 ..04 ..177-179 | 013.20 ..01 ..094-096 | 015.04 ..08 .539-541 |
| 005.4 ...06 .371-373 | 010.80 ..04 ..177-179 | 011.74 ..04 ..177-179 | 013.21 ..01 ..094-096 | 015.05 ..08 .539-541 |
| 005.81 ..06 .371-373 | 010.81 ..04 ..177-179 | 011.75 ..04 ..177-179 | 013.22 ..01 ..094-096 | 015.06 ..08 .539-541 |
| 005.89 ..06 .371-373 | 010.82 ..04 ..177-179 | 011.76 ..04 ..177-179 | 013.23 ..01 ..094-096 | 015.10 ..08 .548-550 |
| 005.9 ...06 .391-392 | 010.83 ..04 ..177-179 | 011.80 ..04 ..177-179 | 013.24 ..01 ..094-096 | 015.11 ..08 .548-550 |
| 006.0 ...06 .371-373 | 010.84 ..04 ..177-179 | 011.81 ..04 ..177-179 | 013.25 ..01 ..094-096 | 015.12 ..08 .548-550 |
| 006.1 ...06 .371-373 | 010.85 ..04 ..177-179 | 011.82 ..04 ..177-179 | 013.26 ..01 ..094-096 | 015.13 ..08 .548-550 |
| 006.2 ...06 .371-373 | 010.86 ..04 ..177-179 | 011.83 ..04 ..177-179 | 013.30 ..01 ..094-096 | 015.14 ..08 .548-550 |
| 006.3 ...07 .441-443 | 010.90 ..04 ..177-179 | 011.84 ..04 ..177-179 | 013.31 ..01 ..094-096 | 015.15 ..08 .548-550 |
| 006.4 ...04 ..177-179 | 010.91 ..04 ..177-179 | 011.85 ..04 ..177-179 | 013.32 ..01 ..094-096 | 015.16 ..08 .548-550 |
| 006.5 ...01 ..097-099 | 010.92 ..04 ..177-179 | 011.86 ..04 ..177-179 | 013.33 ..01 ..094-096 | 015.20 ..08 .548-550 |
| 006.6 ...09 .606-607 | 010.93 ..04 ..177-179 | 011.90 ..04 ..177-179 | 013.34 ..01 ..094-096 | 015.21 ..08 .548-550 |
| 006.8 ...18 .867-869 | 010.94 ..04 ..177-179 | 011.91 ..04 ..177-179 | 013.35 ..01 ..094-096 | 015.22 ..08 .548-550 |
| 006.9 ...18 .867-869 | 010.95 ..04 ..177-179 | 011.92 ..04 ..177-179 | 013.36 ..01 ..094-096 | 015.23 ..08 .548-550 |
| 007.0 ...06 .371-373 | 010.96 ..04 ..177-179 | 011.93 ..04 ..177-179 | 013.40 ..01 ..094-096 | 015.24 ..08 .548-550 |
| 007.1 ...06 .371-373 | 011.00 ..04 ..177-179 | 011.94 ..04 ..177-179 | 013.41 ..01 ..094-096 | 015.25 ..08 .548-550 |
| 007.2 ...06 .371-373 | 011.01 ..04 ..177-179 | 011.95 ..04 ..177-179 | 013.42 ..01 ..094-096 | 015.26 ..08 .548-550 |
| 007.3 ...06 .371-373 | 011.02 ..04 ..177-179 | 011.96 ..04 ..177-179 | 013.43 ..01 ..094-096 | 015.50 ..08 .539-541 |
| 007.4 ...06 .371-373 | 011.03 ..04 ..177-179 | 012.00 ..04 ..177-179 | 013.44 ..01 ..094-096 | 015.51 ..08 .539-541 |
| 007.5 ...06 .371-373 | 011.04 ..04 ..177-179 | 012.01 ..04 ..177-179 | 013.45 ..01 ..094-096 | 015.52 ..08 .539-541 |
| 007.8 ...06 .371-373 | 011.05 ..04 ..177-179 | 012.02 ..04 ..177-179 | 013.46 ..01 ..094-096 | 015.53 ..08 .539-541 |
| 007.9 ...06 .371-373 | 011.06 ..04 ..177-179 | 012.03 ..04 ..177-179 | 013.50 ..01 ..094-096 | 015.54 ..08 .539-541 |
| 008.00 ..06 .371-373 | 011.10 ..04 ..177-179 | 012.04 ..04 ..177-179 | 013.51 ..01 ..094-096 | 015.55 ..08 .539-541 |
| 008.01 ..06 .371-373 | 011.11 ..04 ..177-179 | 012.05 ..04 ..177-179 | 013.52 ..01 ..094-096 | 015.56 ..08 .539-541 |
| 008.02 ..06 .371-373 | 011.12 ..04 ..177-179 | 012.06 ..04 ..177-179 | 013.53 ..01 ..094-096 | 015.60 ..03 ..154-156 |
| 008.03 ..06 .371-373 | 011.13 ..04 ..177-179 | 012.10 ..04 ..177-179 | 013.54 ..01 ..094-096 | 015.61 ..03 ..154-156 |
| 008.04 ..06 .371-373 | 011.14 ..04 ..177-179 | 012.11 ..04 ..177-179 | 013.55 ..01 ..094-096 | 015.62 ..03 ..154-156 |
| 008.09 ..06 .371-373 | 011.15 ..04 ..177-179 | 012.12 ..04 ..177-179 | 013.56 ..01 ..094-096 | 015.63 ..03 ..154-156 |
| 008.1 ...06 .371-373 | 011.16 ..04 ..177-179 | 012.13 ..04 ..177-179 | 013.60 ..01 ..094-096 | 015.64 ..03 ..154-156 |
| 008.2 ...06 .371-373 | 011.20 ..04 ..177-179 | 012.14 ..04 ..177-179 | 013.61 ..01 ..094-096 | 015.65 ..03 ..154-156 |
| 008.3 ...06 .371-373 | 011.21 ..04 ..177-179 | 012.15 ..04 ..177-179 | 013.62 ..01 ..094-096 | 015.66 ..03 ..154-156 |
| 008.41 ..06 .371-373 | 011.22 ..04 ..177-179 | 012.16 ..04 ..177-179 | 013.63 ..01 ..094-096 | 015.70 ..08 .539-541 |
| 008.42 ..06 .371-373 | 011.23 ..04 ..177-179 | 012.20 ..04 ..177-179 | 013.64 ..01 ..094-096 | 015.71 ..08 .539-541 |
| 008.43 ..06 .371-373 | 011.24 ..04 ..177-179 | 012.21 ..04 ..177-179 | 013.65 ..01 ..094-096 | 015.72 ..08 .539-541 |
| 008.44 ..06 .371-373 | 011.25 ..04 ..177-179 | 012.22 ..04 ..177-179 | 013.66 ..01 ..094-096 | 015.73 ..08 .539-541 |
| 008.45 ..06 .371-373 | 011.26 ..04 ..177-179 | 012.23 ..04 ..177-179 | 013.80 ..01 ..094-096 | 015.74 ..08 .539-541 |
| 008.46 ..06 .371-373 | 011.30 ..04 ..177-179 | 012.24 ..04 ..177-179 | 013.81 ..01 ..094-096 | 015.75 ..08 .539-541 |
| 008.47 ..06 .371-373 | 011.31 ..04 ..177-179 | 012.25 ..04 ..177-179 | 013.82 ..01 ..094-096 | 015.76 ..08 .539-541 |
|  | 011.32 ..04 ..177-179 | 012.26 ..04 ..177-179 | 013.83 ..01 ..094-096 | 015.80 ..08 .548-550 |

| DX ...MDC ..DRG | DX ...MDC ..DRG | DX ...MDC ..DRG | DX ...MDC ..DRG | DX ...MDC ..DRG |
|---|---|---|---|---|
| 015.81 ..08 ..548-550 | 017.01 ..09 ..606-607 | 018.81 ..18 ..867-869 | 035 .....09 ..602-603 | 045.21 ..18 ..864-866 |
| 015.82 ..08 ..548-550 | 017.02 ..09 ..606-607 | 018.82 ..18 ..867-869 | 036.0 ..01 ..094-096 | 045.22 ..18 ..864-866 |
| 015.83 ..08 ..548-550 | 017.03 ..09 ..606-607 | 018.83 ..18 ..867-869 | 036.1 ..01 ..094-096 | 045.23 ..18 ..864-866 |
| 015.84 ..08 ..548-550 | 017.04 ..09 ..606-607 | 018.84 ..18 ..867-869 | 036.2 ..18 ..870-872 | 045.90 ..01 ..097-099 |
| 015.85 ..08 ..548-550 | 017.05 ..09 ..606-607 | 018.85 ..18 ..867-869 | 036.3 ..18 ..870-872 | 045.91 ..01 ..097-099 |
| 015.86 ..08 ..548-550 | 017.06 ..09 ..606-607 | 018.86 ..18 ..867-869 | 036.40 ..05 ..314-316 | 045.92 ..01 ..097-099 |
| 015.90 ..08 ..548-550 | 017.10 ..09 ..595-596 | 018.90 ..18 ..867-869 | 036.41 ..05 ..314-316 | 045.93 ..01 ..097-099 |
| 015.91 ..08 ..548-550 | 017.11 ..09 ..595-596 | 018.91 ..18 ..867-869 | 036.42 ..05 ..288-290 | 046.0 ..01 ..056-057 |
| 015.92 ..08 ..548-550 | 017.12 ..09 ..595-596 | 018.92 ..18 ..867-869 | 036.43 ..05 ..314-316 | 046.1 ..01 ..056-057 |
| 015.93 ..08 ..548-550 | 017.13 ..09 ..595-596 | 018.93 ..18 ..867-869 | 036.81 ..02 ..123 | 046.2 ..01 ..056-057 |
| 015.94 ..08 ..548-550 | 017.14 ..09 ..595-596 | 018.94 ..18 ..867-869 | 036.82 ..08 ..548-550 | 046.3 ..01 ..056-057 |
| 015.95 ..08 ..548-550 | 017.15 ..09 ..595-596 | 018.95 ..18 ..867-869 | 036.89 ..18 ..870-872 | 046.8 ..01 ..056-057 |
| 015.96 ..08 ..548-550 | 017.16 ..09 ..595-596 | 018.96 ..18 ..867-869 | 036.9 ..18 ..870-872 | 046.9 ..01 ..056-057 |
| 016.00 ..11 ..689-690 | 017.20 ..16 ..814-816 | 020.0 ...18 ..867-869 | 037 .....18 ..867-869 | 047.0 ..01 ..075-076 |
| 016.01 ..11 ..689-690 | 017.21 ..16 ..814-816 | 020.1 ...18 ..867-869 | 038.0 ...18 ..870-872 | 047.1 ..01 ..075-076 |
| 016.02 ..11 ..689-690 | 017.22 ..16 ..814-816 | 020.2 ..18 ..870-872 | 038.10 ..18 ..870-872 | 047.8 ..01 ..075-076 |
| 016.03 ..11 ..689-690 | 017.23 ..16 ..814-816 | 020.3 ..04 ..177-179 | 038.11 ..18 ..870-872 | 047.9 ..01 ..075-076 |
| 016.04 ..11 ..689-690 | 017.24 ..16 ..814-816 | 020.4 ..04 ..177-179 | 038.19 ..18 ..870-872 | 048 .....01 ..075-076 |
| 016.05 ..11 ..689-690 | 017.25 ..16 ..814-816 | 020.5 ..04 ..177-179 | 038.2 ..18 ..870-872 | 049.0 ..01 ..075-076 |
| 016.06 ..11 ..689-690 | 017.26 ..16 ..814-816 | 020.8 ..18 ..867-869 | 038.3 ..18 ..870-872 | 049.1 ..01 ..075-076 |
| 016.10 ..11 ..689-690 | 017.30 ..02 ..124-125 | 020.9 ..18 ..867-869 | 038.40 ..18 ..870-872 | 049.8 ..01 ..097-099 |
| 016.11 ..11 ..689-690 | 017.31 ..02 ..124-125 | 021.0 ..18 ..867-869 | 038.41 ..18 ..870-872 | 049.9 ..01 ..097-099 |
| 016.12 ..11 ..689-690 | 017.32 ..02 ..124-125 | 021.1 ..06 ..371-373 | 038.42 ..18 ..870-872 | 050.0 ...18 ..864-866 |
| 016.13 ..11 ..689-690 | 017.33 ..02 ..124-125 | 021.2 ..04 ..177-179 | 038.43 ..18 ..870-872 | 050.1 ...18 ..864-866 |
| 016.14 ..11 ..689-690 | 017.34 ..02 ..124-125 | 021.3 ..18 ..867-869 | 038.44 ..18 ..870-872 | 050.2 ...18 ..864-866 |
| 016.15 ..11 ..689-690 | 017.35 ..02 ..124-125 | 021.8 ..18 ..867-869 | 038.49 ..18 ..870-872 | 050.9 ...18 ..864-866 |
| 016.16 ..11 ..689-690 | 017.36 ..02 ..124-125 | 021.9 ..18 ..867-869 | 038.8 ..18 ..870-872 | 051.0 ...18 ..864-866 |
| 016.20 ..11 ..689-690 | 017.40 ..03 ..154-156 | 022.0 ..09 ..606-607 | 038.9 ..18 ..870-872 | 051.1 ...09 ..606-607 |
| 016.21 ..11 ..689-690 | 017.41 ..03 ..154-156 | 022.1 ..04 ..177-179 | 039.0 ...09 ..606-607 | 051.2 ...09 ..606-607 |
| 016.22 ..11 ..689-690 | 017.42 ..03 ..154-156 | 022.2 ..06 ..371-373 | 039.1 ...04 ..177-179 | 051.9 ...18 ..864-866 |
| 016.23 ..11 ..689-690 | 017.43 ..03 ..154-156 | 022.3 ..18 ..870-872 | 039.2 ...06 ..371-373 | 052.0 ...01 ..097-099 |
| 016.24 ..11 ..689-690 | 017.44 ..03 ..154-156 | 022.8 ..18 ..867-869 | 039.3 ...09 ..606-607 | 052.1 ...04 ..177-179 |
| 016.25 ..11 ..689-690 | 017.45 ..03 ..154-156 | 022.9 ..18 ..867-869 | 039.4 ...09 ..606-607 | 052.2 ...01 ..097-099 |
| 016.26 ..11 ..689-690 | 017.46 ..03 ..154-156 | 023.0 ..18 ..867-869 | 039.8 ...18 ..867-869 | 052.7 ...18 ..864-866 |
| 016.30 ..11 ..689-690 | 017.50 ..10 ..643-645 | 023.1 ..18 ..867-869 | 039.9 ...18 ..867-869 | 052.8 ...18 ..864-866 |
| 016.31 ..11 ..689-690 | 017.51 ..10 ..643-645 | 023.2 ..18 ..867-869 | 040.0 ...18 ..867-869 | 052.9 ...18 ..864-866 |
| 016.32 ..11 ..689-690 | 017.52 ..10 ..643-645 | 023.3 ..18 ..867-869 | 040.1 ...18 ..867-869 | 053.0 ...01 ..075-076 |
| 016.33 ..11 ..689-690 | 017.53 ..10 ..643-645 | 023.8 ..18 ..867-869 | 040.2 ...06 ..393-395 | 053.10 ..01 ..073-074 |
| 016.34 ..11 ..689-690 | 017.54 ..10 ..643-645 | 023.9 ..18 ..867-869 | 040.3 ...18 ..867-869 | 053.11 ..01 ..073-074 |
| 016.35 ..11 ..689-690 | 017.55 ..10 ..643-645 | 024 .....18 ..867-869 | 040.41 ..18 ..867-869 | 053.12 ..01 ..073-074 |
| 016.36 ..11 ..689-690 | 017.56 ..10 ..643-645 | 025 .....18 ..867-869 | 040.42 ..18 ..867-869 | 053.13 ..01 ..073-074 |
| 016.40 ..12 ..727-728 | 017.60 ..10 ..643-645 | 026.0 ..18 ..867-869 | 040.81 ..08 ..557-558 | 053.14 ..01 ..097-099 |
| 016.41 ..12 ..727-728 | 017.61 ..10 ..643-645 | 026.1 ..18 ..867-869 | 040.82 ..18 ..867-869 | 053.19 ..01 ..073-074 |
| 016.42 ..12 ..727-728 | 017.62 ..10 ..643-645 | 026.9 ..18 ..867-869 | 040.89 ..18 ..867-869 | 053.20 ..02 ..124-125 |
| 016.43 ..12 ..727-728 | 017.63 ..10 ..643-645 | 027.0 ..18 ..867-869 | 041.00 ..18 ..867-869 | 053.21 ..02 ..124-125 |
| 016.44 ..12 ..727-728 | 017.64 ..10 ..643-645 | 027.1 ..18 ..867-869 | 041.01 ..18 ..867-869 | 053.22 ..02 ..124-125 |
| 016.45 ..12 ..727-728 | 017.65 ..10 ..643-645 | 027.2 ..18 ..867-869 | 041.02 ..18 ..867-869 | 053.29 ..02 ..124-125 |
| 016.46 ..12 ..727-728 | 017.66 ..10 ..643-645 | 027.8 ..18 ..867-869 | 041.03 ..18 ..867-869 | 053.71 ..03 ..154-156 |
| 016.50 ..12 ..727-728 | 017.70 ..16 ..814-816 | 027.9 ..18 ..867-869 | 041.04 ..18 ..867-869 | 053.79 ..18 ..864-866 |
| 016.51 ..12 ..727-728 | 017.71 ..16 ..814-816 | 030.0 ..18 ..867-869 | 041.05 ..18 ..867-869 | 053.8 ...18 ..864-866 |
| 016.52 ..12 ..727-728 | 017.72 ..16 ..814-816 | 030.1 ..18 ..867-869 | 041.09 ..18 ..867-869 | 053.9 ...09 ..595-596 |
| 016.53 ..12 ..727-728 | 017.73 ..16 ..814-816 | 030.2 ..18 ..867-869 | 041.10 ..18 ..867-869 | 054.0 ...09 ..606-607 |
| 016.54 ..12 ..727-728 | 017.74 ..16 ..814-816 | 030.3 ..18 ..867-869 | 041.11 ..18 ..867-869 | 054.10 ..12 ..727-728 |
| 016.55 ..12 ..727-728 | 017.75 ..16 ..814-816 | 030.8 ..18 ..867-869 | 041.19 ..18 ..867-869 | 054.10 ..13 ..757-759 |
| 016.56 ..12 ..727-728 | 017.76 ..16 ..814-816 | 030.9 ..18 ..867-869 | 041.2 ..18 ..867-869 | 054.11 ..13 ..757-759 |
| 016.60 ..13 ..757-759 | 017.80 ..06 ..368-370 | 031.0 ..04 ..177-179 | 041.3 ..18 ..867-869 | 054.12 ..13 ..757-759 |
| 016.61 ..13 ..757-759 | 017.81 ..06 ..368-370 | 031.1 ..09 ..606-607 | 041.4 ..18 ..867-869 | 054.13 ..12 ..727-728 |
| 016.62 ..13 ..757-759 | 017.82 ..06 ..368-370 | 031.2 ..18 ..867-869 | 041.5 ..18 ..867-869 | 054.19 ..12 ..727-728 |
| 016.63 ..13 ..757-759 | 017.83 ..06 ..368-370 | 031.8 ..18 ..867-869 | 041.6 ..18 ..867-869 | 054.19 ..13 ..757-759 |
| 016.64 ..13 ..757-759 | 017.84 ..06 ..368-370 | 031.9 ..18 ..867-869 | 041.7 ..18 ..867-869 | 054.2 ...03 ..157-159 |
| 016.65 ..13 ..757-759 | 017.85 ..06 ..368-370 | 032.0 ..03 ..154-156 | 041.81 ..18 ..867-869 | 054.3 ...01 ..097-099 |
| 016.66 ..13 ..757-759 | 017.86 ..06 ..368-370 | 032.1 ..03 ..154-156 | 041.82 ..18 ..867-869 | 054.40 ..02 ..124-125 |
| 016.70 ..13 ..757-759 | 017.90 ..18 ..867-869 | 032.2 ..03 ..154-156 | 041.83 ..18 ..867-869 | 054.41 ..02 ..124-125 |
| 016.71 ..13 ..757-759 | 017.91 ..18 ..867-869 | 032.3 ..03 ..154-156 | 041.84 ..18 ..867-869 | 054.42 ..02 ..124-125 |
| 016.72 ..13 ..757-759 | 017.92 ..18 ..867-869 | 032.81 ..02 ..124-125 | 041.85 ..18 ..867-869 | 054.43 ..02 ..124-125 |
| 016.73 ..13 ..757-759 | 017.93 ..18 ..867-869 | 032.82 ..05 ..314-316 | 041.86 ..18 ..867-869 | 054.44 ..02 ..124-125 |
| 016.74 ..13 ..757-759 | 017.94 ..18 ..867-869 | 032.83 ..06 ..371-373 | 041.89 ..18 ..867-869 | 054.49 ..02 ..124-125 |
| 016.75 ..13 ..757-759 | 017.95 ..18 ..867-869 | 032.84 ..11 ..689-690 | 041.9 ...18 ..867-869 | 054.5 ...18 ..870-872 |
| 016.76 ..13 ..757-759 | 017.96 ..18 ..867-869 | 032.85 ..09 ..606-607 | 045.00 ..01 ..097-099 | 054.6 ...09 ..606-607 |
| 016.90 ..11 ..689-690 | 018.00 ..18 ..867-869 | 032.89 ..18 ..867-869 | 045.01 ..01 ..097-099 | 054.71 ..06 ..393-395 |
| 016.91 ..11 ..689-690 | 018.01 ..18 ..867-869 | 032.9 ..18 ..867-869 | 045.02 ..01 ..097-099 | 054.72 ..01 ..075-076 |
| 016.92 ..11 ..689-690 | 018.02 ..18 ..867-869 | 033.0 ..04 ..202-203 | 045.03 ..01 ..097-099 | 054.73 ..03 ..154-156 |
| 016.93 ..11 ..689-690 | 018.03 ..18 ..867-869 | 033.1 ...04 ..202-203 | 045.10 ..01 ..097-099 | 054.74 ..01 ..097-099 |
| 016.94 ..11 ..689-690 | 018.04 ..18 ..867-869 | 033.8 ...04 ..202-203 | 045.11 ..01 ..097-099 | 054.79 ..18 ..864-866 |
| 016.95 ..11 ..689-690 | 018.05 ..18 ..867-869 | 033.9 ...04 ..202-203 | 045.12 ..01 ..097-099 | 054.8 ...18 ..864-866 |
| 016.96 ..11 ..689-690 | 018.06 ..18 ..867-869 | 034.0 ...03 ..152-153 | 045.13 ..01 ..097-099 | 054.9 ...09 ..606-607 |
| 017.00 ..09 ..606-607 | 018.80 ..18 ..867-869 | 034.1 ...18 ..867-869 | 045.20 ..18 ..864-866 | 055.0 ...01 ..097-099 |

| DX | MDC | DRG | DX | MDC | DRG | DX | MDC | DRG | DX | MDC | DRG | DX | MDC | DRG |
|---|---|---|---|---|---|---|---|---|---|---|---|---|---|---|
| 055.1 | 04 | 177-179 | 070.53 | 07 | 441-443 | 082.0 | 18 | 867-869 | 093.0 | 05 | 306-307 | 098.83 | 05 | 314-316 |
| 055.2 | 03 | 152-153 | 070.54 | 07 | 441-443 | 082.1 | 18 | 867-869 | 093.1 | 05 | 306-307 | 098.84 | 05 | 288-290 |
| 055.71 | 02 | 124-125 | 070.59 | 07 | 441-443 | 082.2 | 18 | 867-869 | 093.20 | 05 | 288-290 | 098.85 | 05 | 314-316 |
| 055.79 | 18 | 864-866 | 070.6 | 07 | 441-443 | 082.3 | 18 | 867-869 | 093.21 | 05 | 306-307 | 098.86 | 06 | 371-373 |
| 055.8 | 18 | 864-866 | 070.70 | 07 | 441-443 | 082.40 | 18 | 867-869 | 093.22 | 05 | 306-307 | 098.89 | 18 | 867-869 |
| 055.9 | 18 | 864-866 | 070.71 | 07 | 441-443 | 082.41 | 18 | 867-869 | 093.23 | 05 | 306-307 | 099.0 | 12 | 727-728 |
| 056.00 | 01 | 073-074 | 070.9 | 07 | 441-443 | 082.49 | 18 | 867-869 | 093.24 | 05 | 306-307 | 099.0 | 13 | 757-759 |
| 056.01 | 01 | 097-099 | 071 | 01 | 097-099 | 082.8 | 18 | 867-869 | 093.81 | 05 | 314-316 | 099.1 | 12 | 727-728 |
| 056.09 | 01 | 097-099 | 072.0 | 12 | 727-728 | 082.9 | 18 | 867-869 | 093.82 | 05 | 314-316 | 099.1 | 13 | 757-759 |
| 056.71 | 08 | 553-554 | 072.1 | 01 | 075-076 | 083.0 | 18 | 867-869 | 093.89 | 05 | 314-316 | 099.2 | 12 | 727-728 |
| 056.79 | 18 | 864-866 | 072.2 | 01 | 097-099 | 083.1 | 18 | 867-869 | 093.9 | 05 | 314-316 | 099.2 | 13 | 757-759 |
| 056.8 | 18 | 864-866 | 072.3 | 07 | 438-440 | 083.2 | 18 | 867-869 | 094.0 | 01 | 056-057 | 099.3 | 08 | 545-547 |
| 056.9 | 18 | 864-866 | 072.71 | 07 | 441-443 | 083.8 | 18 | 867-869 | 094.1 | 01 | 056-057 | 099.40 | 12 | 727-728 |
| 057.0 | 18 | 864-866 | 072.72 | 01 | 073-074 | 083.9 | 18 | 867-869 | 094.2 | 01 | 097-099 | 099.40 | 13 | 757-759 |
| 057.8 | 18 | 864-866 | 072.79 | 18 | 864-866 | 084.0 | 18 | 867-869 | 094.3 | 01 | 097-099 | 099.41 | 12 | 727-728 |
| 057.9 | 18 | 864-866 | 072.8 | 18 | 864-866 | 084.1 | 18 | 867-869 | 094.81 | 01 | 097-099 | 099.41 | 13 | 757-759 |
| 058.10 | 18 | 865-866 | 072.9 | 18 | 864-866 | 084.2 | 18 | 867-869 | 094.82 | 01 | 056-057 | 099.49 | 12 | 727-728 |
| 058.11 | 18 | 865-866 | 073.0 | 04 | 177-179 | 084.3 | 18 | 867-869 | 094.83 | 02 | 124-125 | 099.49 | 13 | 757-759 |
| 058.12 | 18 | 865-866 | 073.7 | 18 | 864-866 | 084.4 | 18 | 867-869 | 094.84 | 02 | 124-125 | 099.50 | 12 | 727-728 |
| 058.21 | 01 | 097-099 | 073.8 | 18 | 864-866 | 084.5 | 18 | 867-869 | 094.85 | 01 | 056-057 | 099.50 | 13 | 757-759 |
| 058.29 | 01 | 097-099 | 073.9 | 18 | 864-866 | 084.6 | 18 | 867-869 | 094.86 | 03 | 154-156 | 099.51 | 03 | 152-153 |
| 058.81 | 09 | 606-607 | 074.0 | 03 | 152-153 | 084.7 | 18 | 867-869 | 094.87 | 01 | 091-093 | 099.52 | 06 | 393-395 |
| 058.82 | 09 | 606-607 | 074.1 | 04 | 193-195 | 084.8 | 18 | 867-869 | 094.89 | 01 | 056-057 | 099.53 | 12 | 727-728 |
| 058.89 | 09 | 606-607 | 074.20 | 05 | 314-316 | 084.9 | 18 | 867-869 | 094.9 | 01 | 056-057 | 099.53 | 13 | 757-759 |
| 060.0 | 18 | 864-866 | 074.21 | 05 | 314-316 | 085.0 | 18 | 867-869 | 095 | 02 | 124-125 | 099.54 | 11 | 689-690 |
| 060.1 | 18 | 864-866 | 074.22 | 05 | 306-307 | 085.1 | 09 | 606-607 | 095.1 | 04 | 177-179 | 099.55 | 12 | 727-728 |
| 060.9 | 18 | 864-866 | 074.23 | 05 | 314-316 | 085.2 | 09 | 606-607 | 095.2 | 06 | 371-373 | 099.55 | 13 | 757-759 |
| 061 | 18 | 864-866 | 074.3 | 18 | 864-866 | 085.3 | 09 | 606-607 | 095.3 | 07 | 441-443 | 099.56 | 06 | 393-395 |
| 062.0 | 01 | 097-099 | 074.8 | 18 | 864-866 | 085.4 | 09 | 606-607 | 095.4 | 11 | 689-690 | 099.59 | 12 | 727-728 |
| 062.1 | 01 | 097-099 | 075 | 18 | 864-866 | 085.5 | 09 | 606-607 | 095.5 | 08 | 539-541 | 099.59 | 13 | 757-759 |
| 062.2 | 01 | 097-099 | 076.0 | 02 | 124-125 | 085.9 | 18 | 867-869 | 095.6 | 08 | 557-558 | 099.8 | 12 | 727-728 |
| 062.3 | 01 | 097-099 | 076.1 | 02 | 124-125 | 086.0 | 05 | 314-316 | 095.7 | 08 | 557-558 | 099.8 | 13 | 757-759 |
| 062.4 | 01 | 097-099 | 076.9 | 02 | 124-125 | 086.1 | 18 | 867-869 | 095.8 | 18 | 867-869 | 099.9 | 12 | 727-728 |
| 062.5 | 01 | 097-099 | 077.0 | 02 | 124-125 | 086.2 | 18 | 867-869 | 095.9 | 18 | 867-869 | 099.9 | 13 | 757-759 |
| 062.8 | 01 | 097-099 | 077.1 | 02 | 124-125 | 086.3 | 18 | 867-869 | 096 | 18 | 867-869 | 100.0 | 18 | 867-869 |
| 062.9 | 01 | 097-099 | 077.2 | 02 | 124-125 | 086.4 | 18 | 867-869 | 097.0 | 18 | 867-869 | 100.81 | 01 | 097-099 |
| 063.0 | 01 | 097-099 | 077.3 | 02 | 124-125 | 086.5 | 18 | 867-869 | 097.1 | 18 | 867-869 | 100.89 | 01 | 097-099 |
| 063.1 | 01 | 097-099 | 077.4 | 02 | 124-125 | 086.9 | 18 | 867-869 | 097.9 | 18 | 867-869 | 100.9 | 18 | 867-869 |
| 063.2 | 01 | 097-099 | 077.8 | 02 | 124-125 | 087.0 | 18 | 867-869 | 098.0 | 12 | 727-728 | 101 | 03 | 152-153 |
| 063.8 | 01 | 097-099 | 077.98 | 02 | 124-125 | 087.1 | 18 | 867-869 | 098.0 | 13 | 757-759 | 102.0 | 09 | 606-607 |
| 063.9 | 01 | 097-099 | 077.99 | 02 | 124-125 | 087.9 | 18 | 867-869 | 098.10 | 12 | 727-728 | 102.1 | 09 | 606-607 |
| 064 | 01 | 097-099 | 078.0 | 09 | 606-607 | 088.0 | 18 | 867-869 | 098.10 | 13 | 757-759 | 102.2 | 09 | 606-607 |
| 065.0 | 18 | 864-866 | 078.10 | 09 | 606-607 | 088.81 | 18 | 867-869 | 098.11 | 11 | 689-690 | 102.3 | 09 | 606-607 |
| 065.1 | 18 | 864-866 | 078.11 | 09 | 606-607 | 088.82 | 18 | 867-869 | 098.12 | 12 | 727-728 | 102.4 | 09 | 606-607 |
| 065.2 | 18 | 864-866 | 078.19 | 09 | 606-607 | 088.89 | 18 | 867-869 | 098.13 | 12 | 727-728 | 102.5 | 03 | 154-156 |
| 065.3 | 18 | 864-866 | 078.2 | 18 | 864-866 | 088.9 | 18 | 867-869 | 098.14 | 12 | 727-728 | 102.6 | 08 | 548-550 |
| 065.4 | 18 | 864-866 | 078.3 | 16 | 814-816 | 090.0 | 18 | 867-869 | 098.15 | 13 | 757-759 | 102.7 | 18 | 867-869 |
| 065.8 | 18 | 864-866 | 078.4 | 18 | 864-866 | 090.1 | 18 | 867-869 | 098.16 | 13 | 757-759 | 102.8 | 18 | 867-869 |
| 065.9 | 18 | 864-866 | 078.5 | 18 | 864-866 | 090.2 | 18 | 867-869 | 098.17 | 13 | 757-759 | 102.9 | 18 | 867-869 |
| 066.0 | 18 | 864-866 | 078.6 | 11 | 689-690 | 090.3 | 02 | 124-125 | 098.19 | 12 | 727-728 | 103.0 | 09 | 606-607 |
| 066.1 | 18 | 864-866 | 078.7 | 18 | 864-866 | 090.40 | 01 | 097-099 | 098.19 | 13 | 757-759 | 103.1 | 09 | 606-607 |
| 066.2 | 01 | 097-099 | 078.81 | 01 | 091-093 | 090.41 | 01 | 097-099 | 098.2 | 12 | 727-728 | 103.2 | 18 | 867-869 |
| 066.3 | 18 | 864-866 | 078.82 | 06 | 391-392 | 090.42 | 01 | 097-099 | 098.2 | 13 | 757-759 | 103.3 | 09 | 606-607 |
| 066.40 | 18 | 864-866 | 078.88 | 18 | 864-866 | 090.49 | 01 | 097-099 | 098.30 | 11 | 689-690 | 103.9 | 18 | 867-869 |
| 066.41 | 18 | 864-866 | 078.89 | 18 | 864-866 | 090.5 | 18 | 867-869 | 098.31 | 11 | 689-690 | 104.0 | 18 | 867-869 |
| 066.42 | 18 | 864-866 | 079.0 | 18 | 864-866 | 090.6 | 18 | 867-869 | 098.32 | 12 | 727-728 | 104.8 | 18 | 867-869 |
| 066.49 | 18 | 864-866 | 079.1 | 18 | 864-866 | 090.7 | 18 | 867-869 | 098.33 | 12 | 727-728 | 104.9 | 18 | 867-869 |
| 066.8 | 18 | 864-866 | 079.2 | 18 | 864-866 | 090.9 | 18 | 867-869 | 098.34 | 12 | 727-728 | 110.0 | 09 | 606-607 |
| 066.9 | 18 | 864-866 | 079.3 | 18 | 864-866 | 091.0 | 12 | 727-728 | 098.35 | 13 | 757-759 | 110.1 | 09 | 606-607 |
| 070.0 | 07 | 441-443 | 079.4 | 18 | 864-866 | 091.0 | 13 | 757-759 | 098.36 | 13 | 757-759 | 110.2 | 09 | 606-607 |
| 070.71 | 07 | 441-443 | 079.50 | 18 | 864-866 | 091.1 | 06 | 393-395 | 098.37 | 13 | 757-759 | 110.3 | 09 | 606-607 |
| 070.1 | 07 | 441-443 | 079.51 | 18 | 864-866 | 091.2 | 18 | 867-869 | 098.39 | 12 | 727-728 | 110.4 | 09 | 606-607 |
| 070.20 | 07 | 441-443 | 079.52 | 18 | 864-866 | 091.3 | 09 | 606-607 | 098.39 | 13 | 757-759 | 110.5 | 09 | 606-607 |
| 070.21 | 07 | 441-443 | 079.53 | 18 | 864-866 | 091.4 | 16 | 814-816 | 098.40 | 02 | 124-125 | 110.6 | 09 | 606-607 |
| 070.22 | 07 | 441-443 | 079.59 | 18 | 864-866 | 091.50 | 02 | 124-125 | 098.41 | 02 | 124-125 | 110.8 | 09 | 606-607 |
| 070.23 | 07 | 441-443 | 079.6 | 18 | 864-866 | 091.51 | 02 | 124-125 | 098.42 | 02 | 124-125 | 110.9 | 09 | 606-607 |
| 070.30 | 07 | 441-443 | 079.81 | 18 | 864-866 | 091.52 | 02 | 124-125 | 098.43 | 02 | 124-125 | 111.0 | 09 | 606-607 |
| 070.31 | 07 | 441-443 | 079.83 | 18 | 865-866 | 091.61 | 08 | 539-541 | 098.49 | 02 | 124-125 | 111.1 | 09 | 606-607 |
| 070.32 | 07 | 441-443 | 079.88 | 18 | 864-866 | 091.62 | 07 | 441-443 | 098.50 | 08 | 548-550 | 111.2 | 09 | 606-607 |
| 070.33 | 07 | 441-443 | 079.89 | 18 | 864-866 | 091.69 | 06 | 393-395 | 098.51 | 08 | 548-550 | 111.3 | 09 | 606-607 |
| 070.41 | 07 | 441-443 | 079.98 | 18 | 864-866 | 091.7 | 18 | 867-869 | 098.52 | 08 | 548-550 | 111.8 | 09 | 606-607 |
| 070.42 | 07 | 441-443 | 079.99 | 18 | 864-866 | 091.81 | 01 | 097-099 | 098.53 | 08 | 539-541 | 111.9 | 09 | 606-607 |
| 070.43 | 07 | 441-443 | 080 | 18 | 867-869 | 091.82 | 09 | 606-607 | 098.59 | 08 | 548-550 | 112.0 | 03 | 157-159 |
| 070.44 | 07 | 441-443 | 081.0 | 18 | 867-869 | 091.89 | 18 | 867-869 | 098.6 | 03 | 152-153 | 112.1 | 13 | 757-759 |
| 070.49 | 07 | 441-443 | 081.1 | 18 | 867-869 | 091.9 | 18 | 867-869 | 098.7 | 06 | 393-395 | 112.2 | 12 | 727-728 |
| 070.51 | 07 | 441-443 | 081.2 | 18 | 867-869 | 092.0 | 18 | 867-869 | 098.81 | 02 | 124-125 | 112.2 | 13 | 757-759 |
| 070.52 | 07 | 441-443 | 081.9 | 18 | 867-869 | 092.9 | 18 | 867-869 | 098.82 | 01 | 094-096 | 112.3 | 09 | 606-607 |

| DX . . .MDC . .DRG | DX . . .MDC . .DRG | DX . . .MDC . .DRG | DX . . .MDC . .DRG | DX . . .MDC . .DRG |
|---|---|---|---|---|
| 112.4 . . .04 . .177-179 | 123.1 . . .06 . .371-373 | 136.5 . . .18 . .867-869 | 149.8 . . .03 . .146-148 | 162.2 . . .04 . .180-182 |
| 112.5 . . .18 . .867-869 | 123.2 . . .06 . .391-392 | 136.8 . . .18 . .867-869 | 149.9 . . .03 . .146-148 | 162.3 . . .04 . .180-182 |
| 112.81 . .05 . .288-290 | 123.3 . . .06 . .391-392 | 136.9 . . .18 . .867-869 | 150.0 . . .06 . .374-376 | 162.4 . . .04 . .180-182 |
| 112.82 . .03 . .154-156 | 123.4 . . .06 . .391-392 | 137.0 . . .04 . .196-198 | 150.1 . . .06 . .374-376 | 162.5 . . .04 . .180-182 |
| 112.83 . .01 . .097-099 | 123.5 . . .06 . .371-373 | 137.1 . . .01 . .091-093 | 150.2 . . .06 . .374-376 | 162.8 . . .04 . .180-182 |
| 112.84 . .06 . .368-370 | 123.6 . . .06 . .371-373 | 137.2 . . .11 . .689-690 | 150.3 . . .06 . .374-376 | 162.9 . . .04 . .180-182 |
| 112.85 . .06 . .391-392 | 123.8 . . .06 . .371-373 | 137.3 . . .08 . .564-566 | 150.4 . . .06 . .374-376 | 163.0 . . .04 . .180-182 |
| 112.89 . .18 . .867-869 | 123.9 . . .06 . .371-373 | 137.4 . . .18 . .867-869 | 150.5 . . .06 . .374-376 | 163.1 . . .04 . .180-182 |
| 112.9 . . .18 . .867-869 | 124 . . . . .18 . .867-869 | 138 . . . . .01 . .091-093 | 150.8 . . .06 . .374-376 | 163.8 . . .04 . .180-182 |
| 114.0 . . .04 . .177-179 | 125.0 . . .18 . .867-869 | 139.0 . . .01 . .091-093 | 150.9 . . .06 . .374-376 | 163.9 . . .04 . .180-182 |
| 114.1 . . .09 . .606-607 | 125.1 . . .18 . .867-869 | 139.1 . . .02 . .124-125 | 151.0 . . .06 . .374-376 | 164.0 . . .17 . .843-845 |
| 114.2 . . .01 . .097-099 | 125.2 . . .18 . .867-869 | 139.8 . . .18 . .867-869 | 151.1 . . .06 . .374-376 | 164.1 . . .05 . .314-316 |
| 114.3 . . .18 . .867-869 | 125.3 . . .18 . .867-869 | | 151.2 . . .06 . .374-376 | 164.2 . . .04 . .180-182 |
| 114.4 . . .04 . .177-179 | 125.4 . . .18 . .867-869 | **Neoplasms** | 151.3 . . .06 . .374-376 | 164.3 . . .04 . .180-182 |
| 114.5 . . .04 . .177-179 | 125.5 . . .18 . .867-869 | 140.0 . . .03 . .146-148 | 151.4 . . .06 . .374-376 | 164.8 . . .04 . .180-182 |
| 114.9 . . .18 . .867-869 | 125.6 . . .18 . .867-869 | 140.1 . . .03 . .146-148 | 151.5 . . .06 . .374-376 | 164.9 . . .04 . .180-182 |
| 115.00 . .18 . .867-869 | 125.7 . . .18 . .867-869 | 140.3 . . .03 . .146-148 | 151.6 . . .06 . .374-376 | 165.0 . . .03 . .146-148 |
| 115.01 . .01 . .097-099 | 125.9 . . .18 . .867-869 | 140.4 . . .03 . .146-148 | 151.8 . . .06 . .374-376 | 165.8 . . .04 . .180-182 |
| 115.02 . .02 . .124-125 | 126.0 . . .06 . .371-373 | 140.5 . . .03 . .146-148 | 151.9 . . .06 . .374-376 | 165.9 . . .04 . .180-182 |
| 115.03 . .05 . .314-316 | 126.1 . . .06 . .371-373 | 140.6 . . .03 . .146-148 | 152.0 . . .06 . .374-376 | 170.0 . . .08 . .542-544 |
| 115.04 . .05 . .288-290 | 126.2 . . .06 . .371-373 | 140.8 . . .03 . .146-148 | 152.1 . . .06 . .374-376 | 170.1 . . .08 . .542-544 |
| 115.05 . .04 . .177-179 | 126.3 . . .06 . .371-373 | 140.9 . . .03 . .146-148 | 152.2 . . .06 . .374-376 | 170.2 . . .08 . .542-544 |
| 115.09 . .18 . .867-869 | 126.8 . . .06 . .371-373 | 141.0 . . .03 . .146-148 | 152.3 . . .06 . .374-376 | 170.3 . . .08 . .542-544 |
| 115.10 . .18 . .867-869 | 126.9 . . .06 . .371-373 | 141.1 . . .03 . .146-148 | 152.8 . . .06 . .374-376 | 170.4 . . .08 . .542-544 |
| 115.11 . .01 . .097-099 | 127.0 . . .06 . .391-392 | 141.2 . . .03 . .146-148 | 152.9 . . .06 . .374-376 | 170.5 . . .08 . .542-544 |
| 115.12 . .02 . .124-125 | 127.1 . . .06 . .391-392 | 141.3 . . .03 . .146-148 | 153.0 . . .06 . .374-376 | 170.6 . . .08 . .542-544 |
| 115.13 . .05 . .314-316 | 127.2 . . .06 . .391-392 | 141.4 . . .03 . .146-148 | 153.1 . . .06 . .374-376 | 170.7 . . .08 . .542-544 |
| 115.14 . .05 . .288-290 | 127.3 . . .06 . .391-392 | 141.5 . . .03 . .146-148 | 153.2 . . .06 . .374-376 | 170.8 . . .08 . .542-544 |
| 115.15 . .04 . .177-179 | 127.4 . . .06 . .391-392 | 141.6 . . .03 . .146-148 | 153.3 . . .06 . .374-376 | 170.9 . . .08 . .542-544 |
| 115.19 . .18 . .867-869 | 127.5 . . .06 . .391-392 | 141.8 . . .03 . .146-148 | 153.4 . . .06 . .374-376 | 171.0 . . .08 . .542-544 |
| 115.90 . .18 . .867-869 | 127.6 . . .06 . .391-392 | 141.9 . . .03 . .146-148 | 153.5 . . .06 . .374-376 | 171.2 . . .08 . .542-544 |
| 115.91 . .01 . .097-099 | 127.7 . . .06 . .391-392 | 142.0 . . .03 . .146-148 | 153.6 . . .06 . .374-376 | 171.3 . . .08 . .542-544 |
| 115.92 . .02 . .124-125 | 127.8 . . .18 . .867-869 | 142.1 . . .03 . .146-148 | 153.7 . . .06 . .374-376 | 171.4 . . .08 . .542-544 |
| 115.93 . .05 . .314-316 | 127.9 . . .06 . .391-392 | 142.2 . . .03 . .146-148 | 153.8 . . .06 . .374-376 | 171.5 . . .08 . .542-544 |
| 115.94 . .05 . .288-290 | 128.0 . . .18 . .867-869 | 142.8 . . .03 . .146-148 | 153.9 . . .06 . .374-376 | 171.6 . . .08 . .542-544 |
| 115.95 . .04 . .177-179 | 128.1 . . .18 . .867-869 | 142.9 . . .03 . .146-148 | 154.0 . . .06 . .374-376 | 171.7 . . .08 . .542-544 |
| 115.99 . .18 . .867-869 | 128.8 . . .18 . .867-869 | 143.0 . . .03 . .146-148 | 154.1 . . .06 . .374-376 | 171.8 . . .08 . .542-544 |
| 116.0 . . .18 . .867-869 | 128.9 . . .18 . .867-869 | 143.1 . . .03 . .146-148 | 154.2 . . .06 . .374-376 | 171.9 . . .08 . .542-544 |
| 116.1 . . .18 . .867-869 | 129 . . . . .06 . .391-392 | 143.8 . . .03 . .146-148 | 154.3 . . .06 . .374-376 | 172.0 . . .09 . .595-596 |
| 116.2 . . .18 . .867-869 | 130.0 . . .01 . .097-099 | 143.9 . . .03 . .146-148 | 154.8 . . .06 . .374-376 | 172.1 . . .02 . .124-125 |
| 117.0 . . .18 . .867-869 | 130.1 . . .02 . .124-125 | 144.0 . . .03 . .146-148 | 155.0 . . .07 . .435-437 | 172.2 . . .09 . .595-596 |
| 117.1 . . .18 . .867-869 | 130.2 . . .02 . .124-125 | 144.1 . . .03 . .146-148 | 155.1 . . .07 . .435-437 | 172.3 . . .09 . .595-596 |
| 117.2 . . .18 . .867-869 | 130.3 . . .05 . .314-316 | 144.8 . . .03 . .146-148 | 155.2 . . .07 . .435-437 | 172.4 . . .09 . .595-596 |
| 117.3 . . .18 . .867-869 | 130.4 . . .04 . .177-179 | 144.9 . . .03 . .146-148 | 156.0 . . .07 . .435-437 | 172.5 . . .09 . .595-596 |
| 117.4 . . .18 . .867-869 | 130.5 . . .07 . .441-443 | 145.0 . . .03 . .146-148 | 156.1 . . .07 . .435-437 | 172.6 . . .09 . .595-596 |
| 117.5 . . .18 . .867-869 | 130.7 . . .18 . .867-869 | 145.1 . . .03 . .146-148 | 156.2 . . .07 . .435-437 | 172.7 . . .09 . .595-596 |
| 117.6 . . .18 . .867-869 | 130.8 . . .18 . .867-869 | 145.2 . . .03 . .146-148 | 156.8 . . .07 . .435-437 | 172.8 . . .09 . .595-596 |
| 117.7 . . .18 . .867-869 | 130.9 . . .18 . .867-869 | 145.3 . . .03 . .146-148 | 156.9 . . .07 . .435-437 | 172.9 . . .09 . .595-596 |
| 117.8 . . .18 . .867-869 | 131.00 . .12 . .727-728 | 145.4 . . .03 . .146-148 | 157.0 . . .07 . .435-437 | 173.0 . . .09 . .606-607 |
| 117.9 . . .18 . .867-869 | 131.00 . .13 . .757-759 | 145.5 . . .03 . .146-148 | 157.1 . . .07 . .435-437 | 173.1 . . .02 . .124-125 |
| 118 . . . . .18 . .867-869 | 131.01 . .13 . .757-759 | 145.6 . . .03 . .146-148 | 157.2 . . .07 . .435-437 | 173.2 . . .09 . .606-607 |
| 120.0 . . .11 . .689-690 | 131.02 . .12 . .727-728 | 145.8 . . .03 . .146-148 | 157.3 . . .07 . .435-437 | 173.3 . . .09 . .606-607 |
| 120.1 . . .07 . .441-443 | 131.02 . .13 . .757-759 | 145.9 . . .03 . .146-148 | 157.4 . . .07 . .435-437 | 173.4 . . .09 . .606-607 |
| 120.2 . . .18 . .867-869 | 131.03 . .12 . .727-728 | 146.0 . . .03 . .146-148 | 157.8 . . .07 . .435-437 | 173.5 . . .09 . .606-607 |
| 120.3 . . .09 . .606-607 | 131.09 . .12 . .727-728 | 146.1 . . .03 . .146-148 | 157.9 . . .07 . .435-437 | 173.6 . . .09 . .606-607 |
| 120.8 . . .18 . .867-869 | 131.09 . .13 . .757-759 | 146.2 . . .03 . .146-148 | 158.0 . . .17 . .843-845 | 173.7 . . .09 . .606-607 |
| 120.9 . . .18 . .867-869 | 131.8 . . .18 . .867-869 | 146.3 . . .03 . .146-148 | 158.8 . . .06 . .374-376 | 173.8 . . .09 . .606-607 |
| 121.0 . . .07 . .441-443 | 131.9 . . .18 . .867-869 | 146.4 . . .03 . .146-148 | 158.9 . . .06 . .374-376 | 173.9 . . .09 . .606-607 |
| 121.1 . . .07 . .441-443 | 132.0 . . .09 . .606-607 | 146.5 . . .03 . .146-148 | 159.0 . . .06 . .374-376 | 174.0 . . .09 . .597-599 |
| 121.2 . . .04 . .177-179 | 132.1 . . .09 . .606-607 | 146.6 . . .03 . .146-148 | 159.1 . . .17 . .840-842 | 174.1 . . .09 . .597-599 |
| 121.3 . . .07 . .441-443 | 132.2 . . .09 . .606-607 | 146.7 . . .03 . .146-148 | 159.8 . . .06 . .374-376 | 174.2 . . .09 . .597-599 |
| 121.4 . . .07 . .441-443 | 132.3 . . .09 . .606-607 | 146.8 . . .03 . .146-148 | 159.9 . . .06 . .374-376 | 174.3 . . .09 . .597-599 |
| 121.5 . . .18 . .867-869 | 132.9 . . .09 . .606-607 | 146.9 . . .03 . .146-148 | 160.0 . . .03 . .146-148 | 174.4 . . .09 . .597-599 |
| 121.6 . . .18 . .867-869 | 133.0 . . .09 . .606-607 | 147.0 . . .03 . .146-148 | 160.1 . . .03 . .146-148 | 174.5 . . .09 . .597-599 |
| 121.8 . . .18 . .867-869 | 133.8 . . .09 . .606-607 | 147.1 . . .03 . .146-148 | 160.2 . . .03 . .146-148 | 174.6 . . .09 . .597-599 |
| 121.9 . . .18 . .867-869 | 133.9 . . .09 . .606-607 | 147.2 . . .03 . .146-148 | 160.3 . . .03 . .146-148 | 174.8 . . .09 . .597-599 |
| 122.0 . . .07 . .441-443 | 134.0 . . .09 . .606-607 | 147.3 . . .03 . .146-148 | 160.4 . . .03 . .146-148 | 174.9 . . .09 . .597-599 |
| 122.1 . . .04 . .177-179 | 134.1 . . .09 . .606-607 | 147.8 . . .03 . .146-148 | 160.5 . . .03 . .146-148 | 175.0 . . .09 . .597-599 |
| 122.2 . . .10 . .643-645 | 134.2 . . .09 . .606-607 | 147.9 . . .03 . .146-148 | 160.8 . . .03 . .146-148 | 175.9 . . .09 . .597-599 |
| 122.3 . . .18 . .867-869 | 134.8 . . .09 . .606-607 | 148.0 . . .03 . .146-148 | 160.9 . . .03 . .146-148 | 176.0 . . .09 . .606-607 |
| 122.4 . . .18 . .867-869 | 134.9 . . .09 . .606-607 | 148.1 . . .03 . .146-148 | 161.0 . . .03 . .146-148 | 176.1 . . .09 . .606-607 |
| 122.5 . . .07 . .441-443 | 135 . . . . .04 . .196-198 | 148.2 . . .03 . .146-148 | 161.1 . . .03 . .146-148 | 176.2 . . .03 . .146-148 |
| 122.6 . . .18 . .867-869 | 136.0 . . .18 . .867-869 | 148.3 . . .03 . .146-148 | 161.2 . . .03 . .146-148 | 176.3 . . .06 . .374-376 |
| 122.7 . . .18 . .867-869 | 136.1 . . .08 . .545-547 | 148.8 . . .03 . .146-148 | 161.3 . . .03 . .146-148 | 176.4 . . .04 . .180-182 |
| 122.8 . . .07 . .441-443 | 136.2 . . .18 . .867-869 | 148.9 . . .03 . .146-148 | 161.8 . . .03 . .146-148 | 176.5 . . .17 . .840-842 |
| 122.9 . . .18 . .867-869 | 136.3 . . .04 . .177-179 | 149.0 . . .03 . .146-148 | 161.9 . . .03 . .146-148 | 176.8 . . .09 . .606-607 |
| 123.0 . . .06 . .391-392 | 136.4 . . .18 . .867-869 | 149.1 . . .03 . .146-148 | 162.0 . . .04 . .180-182 | 176.9 . . .09 . .606-607 |

| DX | MDC | DRG | DX | MDC | DRG | DX | MDC | DRG | DX | MDC | DRG | DX | MDC | DRG |
|---|---|---|---|---|---|---|---|---|---|---|---|---|---|---|
| 179 | 13 | 754-756 | 192.9 | 01 | 054-055 | 200.31 | 17 | 840-842 | 201.26 | 17 | 840-842 | 202.32 | 17 | 840-842 |
| 180.0 | 13 | 754-756 | 193 | 10 | 643-645 | 200.32 | 17 | 840-842 | 201.27 | 17 | 840-842 | 202.33 | 17 | 840-842 |
| 180.1 | 13 | 754-756 | 194.0 | 10 | 643-645 | 200.33 | 17 | 840-842 | 201.28 | 17 | 840-842 | 202.34 | 17 | 840-842 |
| 180.8 | 13 | 754-756 | 194.1 | 10 | 643-645 | 200.34 | 17 | 840-842 | 201.40 | 17 | 840-842 | 202.35 | 17 | 840-842 |
| 180.9 | 13 | 754-756 | 194.3 | 10 | 643-645 | 200.35 | 17 | 840-842 | 201.41 | 17 | 840-842 | 202.36 | 17 | 840-842 |
| 181. | 13 | 754-756 | 194.4 | 01 | 054-055 | 200.36 | 17 | 840-842 | 201.42 | 17 | 840-842 | 202.37 | 17 | 840-842 |
| 182.0 | 13 | 754-756 | 194.5 | 01 | 054-055 | 200.37 | 17 | 840-842 | 201.43 | 17 | 840-842 | 202.38 | 17 | 840-842 |
| 182.1 | 13 | 754-756 | 194.6 | 01 | 054-055 | 200.38 | 17 | 840-842 | 201.44 | 17 | 840-842 | 202.40 | 17 | 840-842 |
| 182.8 | 13 | 754-756 | 194.8 | 10 | 643-645 | 200.30 | 17 | 840-842 | 201.45 | 17 | 840-842 | 202.41 | 17 | 840-842 |
| 183.0 | 13 | 754-756 | 194.9 | 10 | 643-645 | 200.41 | 17 | 840-842 | 201.46 | 17 | 840-842 | 202.42 | 17 | 840-842 |
| 183.2 | 13 | 754-756 | 195.0 | 03 | 146-148 | 200.42 | 17 | 840-842 | 201.47 | 17 | 840-842 | 202.43 | 17 | 840-842 |
| 183.3 | 13 | 754-756 | 195.1 | 04 | 180-182 | 200.43 | 17 | 840-842 | 201.48 | 17 | 840-842 | 202.44 | 17 | 840-842 |
| 183.4 | 13 | 754-756 | 195.2 | 06 | 374-376 | 200.44 | 17 | 840-842 | 201.50 | 17 | 840-842 | 202.45 | 17 | 840-842 |
| 183.5 | 13 | 754-756 | 195.3 | 12 | 722-724 | 200.45 | 17 | 840-842 | 201.51 | 17 | 840-842 | 202.46 | 17 | 840-842 |
| 183.8 | 13 | 754-756 | 195.3 | 13 | 754-756 | 200.46 | 17 | 840-842 | 201.52 | 17 | 840-842 | 202.47 | 17 | 840-842 |
| 183.9 | 13 | 754-756 | 195.4 | 17 | 843-845 | 200.47 | 17 | 840-842 | 201.53 | 17 | 840-842 | 202.48 | 17 | 840-842 |
| 184.0 | 13 | 754-756 | 195.5 | 17 | 843-845 | 200.48 | 17 | 840-842 | 201.54 | 17 | 840-842 | 202.50 | 17 | 843-845 |
| 184.1 | 13 | 754-756 | 195.8 | 17 | 843-845 | 200.50 | 17 | 840-842 | 201.55 | 17 | 840-842 | 202.51 | 17 | 843-845 |
| 184.2 | 13 | 754-756 | 196.0 | 17 | 840-842 | 200.51 | 17 | 840-842 | 201.56 | 17 | 840-842 | 202.52 | 17 | 843-845 |
| 184.3 | 13 | 754-756 | 196.1 | 17 | 840-842 | 200.52 | 17 | 840-842 | 201.57 | 17 | 840-842 | 202.53 | 17 | 843-845 |
| 184.4 | 13 | 754-756 | 196.2 | 17 | 840-842 | 200.53 | 17 | 840-842 | 201.58 | 17 | 840-842 | 202.54 | 17 | 843-845 |
| 184.8 | 13 | 754-756 | 196.3 | 17 | 840-842 | 200.54 | 17 | 840-842 | 201.60 | 17 | 840-842 | 202.55 | 17 | 843-845 |
| 184.9 | 13 | 754-756 | 196.5 | 17 | 840-842 | 200.55 | 17 | 840-842 | 201.61 | 17 | 840-842 | 202.56 | 17 | 843-845 |
| 185. | 12 | 722-724 | 196.6 | 17 | 840-842 | 200.56 | 17 | 840-842 | 201.62 | 17 | 840-842 | 202.57 | 17 | 843-845 |
| 186.0 | 12 | 722-724 | 196.8 | 17 | 840-842 | 200.57 | 17 | 840-842 | 201.63 | 17 | 840-842 | 202.58 | 17 | 843-845 |
| 186.9 | 12 | 722-724 | 196.9 | 17 | 840-842 | 200.58 | 17 | 840-842 | 201.64 | 17 | 840-842 | 202.60 | 17 | 840-842 |
| 187.1 | 12 | 722-724 | 197.0 | 04 | 180-182 | 200.60 | 17 | 840-842 | 201.65 | 17 | 840-842 | 202.61 | 17 | 840-842 |
| 187.2 | 12 | 722-724 | 197.1 | 04 | 180-182 | 200.61 | 17 | 840-842 | 201.66 | 17 | 840-842 | 202.62 | 17 | 840-842 |
| 187.3 | 12 | 722-724 | 197.2 | 04 | 180-182 | 200.62 | 17 | 840-842 | 201.67 | 17 | 840-842 | 202.63 | 17 | 840-842 |
| 187.4 | 12 | 722-724 | 197.3 | 04 | 180-182 | 200.63 | 17 | 840-842 | 201.68 | 17 | 840-842 | 202.64 | 17 | 840-842 |
| 187.5 | 12 | 722-724 | 197.4 | 06 | 374-376 | 200.64 | 17 | 840-842 | 201.70 | 17 | 840-842 | 202.65 | 17 | 840-842 |
| 187.6 | 12 | 722-724 | 197.5 | 06 | 374-376 | 200.65 | 17 | 840-842 | 201.71 | 17 | 840-842 | 202.66 | 17 | 840-842 |
| 187.7 | 12 | 722-724 | 197.6 | 06 | 374-376 | 200.66 | 17 | 840-842 | 201.72 | 17 | 840-842 | 202.67 | 17 | 840-842 |
| 187.8 | 12 | 722-724 | 197.7 | 07 | 435-437 | 200.67 | 17 | 840-842 | 201.73 | 17 | 840-842 | 202.68 | 17 | 840-842 |
| 187.9 | 12 | 722-724 | 197.8 | 06 | 374-376 | 200.68 | 17 | 840-842 | 201.74 | 17 | 840-842 | 202.70 | 17 | 840-842 |
| 188.0 | 11 | 686-688 | 198.0 | 11 | 686-688 | 200.70 | 17 | 840-842 | 201.75 | 17 | 840-842 | 202.71 | 17 | 840-842 |
| 188.1 | 11 | 686-688 | 198.1 | 11 | 686-688 | 200.71 | 17 | 840-842 | 201.76 | 17 | 840-842 | 202.72 | 17 | 840-842 |
| 188.2 | 11 | 686-688 | 198.2 | 09 | 597-599 | 200.72 | 17 | 840-842 | 201.77 | 17 | 840-842 | 202.73 | 17 | 840-842 |
| 188.3 | 11 | 686-688 | 198.3 | 01 | 054-055 | 200.73 | 17 | 840-842 | 201.78 | 17 | 840-842 | 202.74 | 17 | 840-842 |
| 188.4 | 11 | 686-688 | 198.4 | 01 | 054-055 | 200.74 | 17 | 840-842 | 201.90 | 17 | 840-842 | 202.75 | 17 | 840-842 |
| 188.5 | 11 | 686-688 | 198.5 | 08 | 542-544 | 200.75 | 17 | 840-842 | 201.91 | 17 | 840-842 | 202.76 | 17 | 840-842 |
| 188.6 | 11 | 686-688 | 198.6 | 13 | 754-756 | 200.76 | 17 | 840-842 | 201.92 | 17 | 840-842 | 202.77 | 17 | 840-842 |
| 188.7 | 11 | 686-688 | 198.7 | 10 | 643-645 | 200.77 | 17 | 840-842 | 201.93 | 17 | 840-842 | 202.78 | 17 | 840-842 |
| 188.8 | 11 | 686-688 | 198.81 | 09 | 597-599 | 200.78 | 17 | 840-842 | 201.94 | 17 | 840-842 | 202.80 | 17 | 840-842 |
| 188.9 | 11 | 686-688 | 198.82 | 12 | 722-724 | 200.80 | 17 | 840-842 | 201.95 | 17 | 840-842 | 202.81 | 17 | 840-842 |
| 189.0 | 11 | 686-688 | 198.82 | 13 | 754-756 | 200.81 | 17 | 840-842 | 201.96 | 17 | 840-842 | 202.82 | 17 | 840-842 |
| 189.1 | 11 | 686-688 | 198.89 | 17 | 843-845 | 200.82 | 17 | 840-842 | 201.97 | 17 | 840-842 | 202.83 | 17 | 840-842 |
| 189.2 | 11 | 686-688 | 199.0 | 17 | 843-845 | 200.83 | 17 | 840-842 | 201.98 | 17 | 840-842 | 202.84 | 17 | 840-842 |
| 189.3 | 11 | 686-688 | 199.1 | 17 | 843-845 | 200.84 | 17 | 840-842 | 202.00 | 17 | 840-842 | 202.85 | 17 | 840-842 |
| 189.4 | 11 | 686-688 | 200.00 | 17 | 840-842 | 200.85 | 17 | 840-842 | 202.01 | 17 | 840-842 | 202.86 | 17 | 840-842 |
| 189.8 | 11 | 686-688 | 200.01 | 17 | 840-842 | 200.86 | 17 | 840-842 | 202.02 | 17 | 840-842 | 202.87 | 17 | 840-842 |
| 189.9 | 11 | 686-688 | 200.02 | 17 | 840-842 | 200.87 | 17 | 840-842 | 202.03 | 17 | 840-842 | 202.88 | 17 | 840-842 |
| 190.0 | 02 | 124-125 | 200.03 | 17 | 840-842 | 200.88 | 17 | 840-842 | 202.04 | 17 | 840-842 | 202.90 | 17 | 840-842 |
| 190.1 | 02 | 124-125 | 200.04 | 17 | 840-842 | 201.00 | 17 | 840-842 | 202.05 | 17 | 840-842 | 202.91 | 17 | 840-842 |
| 190.2 | 02 | 124-125 | 200.05 | 17 | 840-842 | 201.01 | 17 | 840-842 | 202.06 | 17 | 840-842 | 202.92 | 17 | 840-842 |
| 190.3 | 02 | 124-125 | 200.06 | 17 | 840-842 | 201.02 | 17 | 840-842 | 202.07 | 17 | 840-842 | 202.93 | 17 | 840-842 |
| 190.4 | 02 | 124-125 | 200.07 | 17 | 840-842 | 201.03 | 17 | 840-842 | 202.08 | 17 | 840-842 | 202.94 | 17 | 840-842 |
| 190.5 | 02 | 124-125 | 200.08 | 17 | 840-842 | 201.04 | 17 | 840-842 | 202.10 | 17 | 840-842 | 202.95 | 17 | 840-842 |
| 190.6 | 02 | 124-125 | 200.10 | 17 | 840-842 | 201.05 | 17 | 840-842 | 202.11 | 17 | 840-842 | 202.96 | 17 | 840-842 |
| 190.7 | 02 | 124-125 | 200.11 | 17 | 840-842 | 201.06 | 17 | 840-842 | 202.12 | 17 | 840-842 | 202.97 | 17 | 840-842 |
| 190.8 | 02 | 124-125 | 200.12 | 17 | 840-842 | 201.07 | 17 | 840-842 | 202.13 | 17 | 840-842 | 202.98 | 17 | 840-842 |
| 190.9 | 02 | 124-125 | 200.13 | 17 | 840-842 | 201.08 | 17 | 840-842 | 202.14 | 17 | 840-842 | 203.00 | 17 | 840-842 |
| 191.0 | 01 | 054-055 | 200.14 | 17 | 840-842 | 201.10 | 17 | 840-842 | 202.15 | 17 | 840-842 | 203.01 | 17 | 840-842 |
| 191.1 | 01 | 054-055 | 200.15 | 17 | 840-842 | 201.11 | 17 | 840-842 | 202.16 | 17 | 840-842 | 203.10 | 17 | 840-842 |
| 191.2 | 01 | 054-055 | 200.16 | 17 | 840-842 | 201.12 | 17 | 840-842 | 202.17 | 17 | 840-842 | 203.11 | 17 | 840-842 |
| 191.3 | 01 | 054-055 | 200.17 | 17 | 840-842 | 201.13 | 17 | 840-842 | 202.18 | 17 | 840-842 | 203.80 | 17 | 840-842 |
| 191.4 | 01 | 054-055 | 200.18 | 17 | 840-842 | 201.14 | 17 | 840-842 | 202.20 | 17 | 840-842 | 203.81 | 17 | 840-842 |
| 191.5 | 01 | 054-055 | 200.20 | 17 | 840-842 | 201.15 | 17 | 840-842 | 202.21 | 17 | 840-842 | 204.00 | 17 | 834-836 |
| 191.6 | 01 | 054-055 | 200.21 | 17 | 840-842 | 201.16 | 17 | 840-842 | 202.22 | 17 | 840-842 | 204.01 | 17 | 834-836 |
| 191.7 | 01 | 054-055 | 200.22 | 17 | 840-842 | 201.17 | 17 | 840-842 | 202.23 | 17 | 840-842 | 204.10 | 17 | 840-842 |
| 191.8 | 01 | 054-055 | 200.23 | 17 | 840-842 | 201.18 | 17 | 840-842 | 202.24 | 17 | 840-842 | 204.11 | 17 | 840-842 |
| 191.9 | 01 | 054-055 | 200.24 | 17 | 840-842 | 201.20 | 17 | 840-842 | 202.25 | 17 | 840-842 | 204.20 | 17 | 840-842 |
| 192.0 | 01 | 054-055 | 200.25 | 17 | 840-842 | 201.21 | 17 | 840-842 | 202.26 | 17 | 840-842 | 204.21 | 17 | 840-842 |
| 192.1 | 01 | 054-055 | 200.26 | 17 | 840-842 | 201.22 | 17 | 840-842 | 202.27 | 17 | 840-842 | 204.80 | 17 | 840-842 |
| 192.2 | 01 | 054-055 | 200.27 | 17 | 840-842 | 201.23 | 17 | 840-842 | 202.28 | 17 | 840-842 | 204.81 | 17 | 840-842 |
| 192.3 | 01 | 054-055 | 200.28 | 17 | 840-842 | 201.24 | 17 | 840-842 | 202.30 | 17 | 840-842 | 204.90 | 17 | 840-842 |
| 192.8 | 01 | 054-055 | 200.30 | 17 | 840-842 | 201.25 | 17 | 840-842 | 202.31 | 17 | 840-842 | 204.91 | 17 | 840-842 |

| DX | MDC | DRG | DX | MDC | DRG | DX | MDC | DRG | DX | MDC | DRG | DX | MDC | DRG |
|---|---|---|---|---|---|---|---|---|---|---|---|---|---|---|
| 205.00 | 17 | 834-836 | 213.7 | 08 | 564-566 | 227.1 | 10 | 643-645 | 236.99 | 11 | 686-688 | 246.2 | 10 | 643-645 |
| 205.01 | 17 | 834-836 | 213.8 | 08 | 564-566 | 227.3 | 10 | 643-645 | 237.0 | 10 | 643-645 | 246.3 | 10 | 643-645 |
| 205.10 | 17 | 840-842 | 213.9 | 08 | 564-566 | 227.4 | 01 | 054-055 | 237.1 | 01 | 054-055 | 246.8 | 10 | 643-645 |
| 205.11 | 17 | 840-842 | 214.0 | 09 | 606-607 | 227.5 | 01 | 054-055 | 237.2 | 10 | 643-645 | 246.9 | 10 | 643-645 |
| 205.20 | 17 | 840-842 | 214.1 | 09 | 606-607 | 227.6 | 01 | 054-055 | 237.3 | 01 | 054-055 | 250.00 | 10 | 637-639 |
| 205.21 | 17 | 840-842 | 214.2 | 04 | 180-182 | 227.8 | 10 | 643-645 | 237.4 | 10 | 643-645 | 250.01 | 10 | 637-639 |
| 205.30 | 17 | 840-842 | 214.3 | 06 | 393-395 | 227.9 | 10 | 643-645 | 237.5 | 01 | 054-055 | 250.02 | 10 | 637-639 |
| 205.31 | 17 | 840-842 | 214.4 | 12 | 729-730 | 228.00 | 05 | 314-316 | 237.6 | 01 | 054-055 | 250.03 | 10 | 637-639 |
| 205.80 | 17 | 840-842 | 214.8 | 09 | 606-607 | 228.01 | 09 | 606-607 | 237.70 | 01 | 091-093 | 250.10 | 10 | 637-639 |
| 205.81 | 17 | 840-842 | 214.9 | 09 | 606-607 | 228.02 | 01 | 091-093 | 237.71 | 01 | 091-093 | 250.11 | 10 | 637-639 |
| 205.90 | 17 | 840-842 | 215.0 | 08 | 564-566 | 228.03 | 02 | 124-125 | 237.72 | 01 | 091-093 | 250.12 | 10 | 637-639 |
| 205.91 | 17 | 840-842 | 215.2 | 08 | 564-566 | 228.04 | 06 | 391-392 | 237.9 | 01 | 054-055 | 250.13 | 10 | 637-639 |
| 206.00 | 17 | 834-836 | 215.3 | 08 | 564-566 | 228.09 | 05 | 314-316 | 238.0 | 08 | 542-544 | 250.20 | 10 | 637-639 |
| 206.01 | 17 | 834-836 | 215.4 | 08 | 564-566 | 228.1 | 16 | 814-816 | 238.1 | 08 | 564-566 | 250.21 | 10 | 637-639 |
| 206.10 | 17 | 840-842 | 215.5 | 08 | 564-566 | 229.0 | 16 | 814-816 | 238.2 | 09 | 606-607 | 250.22 | 10 | 637-639 |
| 206.11 | 17 | 840-842 | 215.6 | 08 | 564-566 | 229.8 | 17 | 843-845 | 238.3 | 09 | 597-599 | 250.23 | 10 | 637-639 |
| 206.20 | 17 | 840-842 | 215.7 | 08 | 564-566 | 229.9 | 17 | 843-845 | 238.4 | 17 | 840-842 | 250.30 | 10 | 637-639 |
| 206.21 | 17 | 840-842 | 215.8 | 08 | 564-566 | 230.0 | 03 | 146-148 | 238.5 | 17 | 840-842 | 250.31 | 10 | 637-639 |
| 206.80 | 17 | 840-842 | 215.9 | 08 | 564-566 | 230.1 | 06 | 374-376 | 238.6 | 17 | 840-842 | 250.32 | 10 | 637-639 |
| 206.81 | 17 | 840-842 | 216.0 | 09 | 606-607 | 230.2 | 06 | 374-376 | 238.71 | 16 | 814-816 | 250.33 | 10 | 637-639 |
| 206.90 | 17 | 840-842 | 216.1 | 02 | 124-125 | 230.3 | 06 | 374-376 | 238.72 | 16 | 811-812 | 250.40 | 11 | 698-700 |
| 206.91 | 17 | 840-842 | 216.2 | 09 | 606-607 | 230.4 | 06 | 374-376 | 238.73 | 16 | 811-812 | 250.41 | 11 | 698-700 |
| 207.00 | 17 | 834-836 | 216.3 | 09 | 606-607 | 230.5 | 06 | 374-376 | 238.74 | 16 | 811-812 | 250.42 | 11 | 698-700 |
| 207.01 | 17 | 834-836 | 216.4 | 09 | 606-607 | 230.6 | 06 | 374-376 | 238.75 | 16 | 811-812 | 250.43 | 11 | 698-700 |
| 207.10 | 17 | 840-842 | 216.5 | 09 | 606-607 | 230.7 | 06 | 374-376 | 238.76 | 17 | 840-842 | 250.50 | 02 | 124-125 |
| 207.11 | 17 | 840-842 | 216.6 | 09 | 606-607 | 230.8 | 07 | 435-437 | 238.79 | 17 | 840-842 | 250.51 | 02 | 124-125 |
| 207.20 | 17 | 840-842 | 216.7 | 09 | 606-607 | 230.9 | 06 | 374-376 | 238.8 | 17 | 843-845 | 250.52 | 02 | 124-125 |
| 207.21 | 17 | 840-842 | 216.8 | 09 | 606-607 | 231.0 | 03 | 146-148 | 238.9 | 17 | 843-845 | 250.53 | 02 | 124-125 |
| 207.80 | 17 | 840-842 | 216.9 | 09 | 606-607 | 231.1 | 04 | 180-182 | 239.0 | 06 | 374-376 | 250.60 | 01 | 073-074 |
| 207.81 | 17 | 840-842 | 217 | 09 | 606-607 | 231.2 | 04 | 180-182 | 239.1 | 04 | 180-182 | 250.61 | 01 | 073-074 |
| 208.00 | 17 | 834-836 | 218.0 | 13 | 760-761 | 231.8 | 04 | 180-182 | 239.2 | 08 | 564-566 | 250.62 | 01 | 073-074 |
| 208.01 | 17 | 834-836 | 218.1 | 13 | 760-761 | 231.9 | 04 | 180-182 | 239.3 | 09 | 600-601 | 250.63 | 01 | 073-074 |
| 208.10 | 17 | 840-842 | 218.2 | 13 | 760-761 | 232.0 | 09 | 606-607 | 239.4 | 11 | 686-688 | 250.70 | 05 | 299-301 |
| 208.11 | 17 | 840-842 | 218.9 | 13 | 760-761 | 232.1 | 02 | 124-125 | 239.5 | 11 | 686-688 | 250.71 | 05 | 299-301 |
| 208.20 | 17 | 840-842 | 219.0 | 13 | 760-761 | 232.2 | 09 | 606-607 | 239.6 | 01 | 054-055 | 250.72 | 05 | 299-301 |
| 208.21 | 17 | 840-842 | 219.1 | 13 | 760-761 | 232.3 | 09 | 606-607 | 239.7 | 10 | 643-645 | 250.73 | 05 | 299-301 |
| 208.80 | 17 | 840-842 | 219.8 | 13 | 760-761 | 232.4 | 09 | 606-607 | 239.8 | 17 | 843-845 | 250.80 | 10 | 637-639 |
| 208.81 | 17 | 840-842 | 219.9 | 13 | 760-761 | 232.5 | 09 | 606-607 | 239.9 | 17 | 843-845 | 250.81 | 10 | 637-639 |
| 208.90 | 17 | 840-842 | 220 | 13 | 760-761 | 232.6 | 09 | 606-607 |  |  |  | 250.82 | 10 | 637-639 |
| 208.91 | 17 | 840-842 | 221.0 | 13 | 760-761 | 232.7 | 09 | 606-607 | **Endocrine, Nutritional and Metabolic Diseases, and Immunity Diseases** | | | 250.83 | 10 | 637-639 |
| 210.0 | 03 | 157-159 | 221.1 | 13 | 760-761 | 232.8 | 09 | 606-607 | 240.0 | 10 | 643-645 | 250.90 | 10 | 637-639 |
| 210.1 | 03 | 157-159 | 221.2 | 13 | 760-761 | 232.9 | 09 | 606-607 | 240.9 | 10 | 643-645 | 250.91 | 10 | 637-639 |
| 210.2 | 03 | 154-156 | 221.8 | 13 | 760-761 | 233.0 | 09 | 597-599 | 241.0 | 10 | 643-645 | 250.92 | 10 | 637-639 |
| 210.3 | 03 | 157-159 | 221.9 | 13 | 760-761 | 233.1 | 13 | 754-756 | 241.1 | 10 | 643-645 | 250.93 | 10 | 637-639 |
| 210.4 | 03 | 157-159 | 222.0 | 12 | 729-730 | 233.2 | 13 | 754-756 | 241.9 | 10 | 643-645 | 251.0 | 10 | 640-641 |
| 210.5 | 03 | 154-156 | 222.1 | 12 | 729-730 | 233.30 | 13 | 754-756 | 242.00 | 10 | 643-645 | 251.1 | 10 | 643-645 |
| 210.6 | 03 | 154-156 | 222.2 | 12 | 729-730 | 233.31 | 13 | 754-756 | 242.01 | 10 | 643-645 | 251.2 | 10 | 640-641 |
| 210.7 | 03 | 154-156 | 222.3 | 12 | 729-730 | 233.32 | 13 | 754-756 | 242.10 | 10 | 643-645 | 251.3 | 10 | 640-641 |
| 210.8 | 03 | 154-156 | 222.4 | 12 | 729-730 | 233.39 | 13 | 754-756 | 242.11 | 10 | 643-645 | 251.4 | 10 | 643-645 |
| 210.9 | 03 | 154-156 | 222.8 | 12 | 729-730 | 233.4 | 12 | 722-724 | 242.20 | 10 | 643-645 | 251.5 | 06 | 380-382 |
| 211.0 | 06 | 393-395 | 222.9 | 12 | 729-730 | 233.5 | 12 | 722-724 | 242.21 | 10 | 643-645 | 251.8 | 10 | 643-645 |
| 211.1 | 06 | 393-395 | 223.0 | 11 | 686-688 | 233.6 | 12 | 722-724 | 242.30 | 10 | 643-645 | 251.9 | 10 | 643-645 |
| 211.2 | 06 | 393-395 | 223.1 | 11 | 686-688 | 233.7 | 11 | 686-688 | 242.31 | 10 | 643-645 | 252.00 | 10 | 643-645 |
| 211.3 | 06 | 393-395 | 223.2 | 11 | 686-688 | 233.9 | 11 | 686-688 | 242.40 | 10 | 643-645 | 252.01 | 10 | 643-645 |
| 211.4 | 06 | 393-395 | 223.3 | 11 | 686-688 | 234.0 | 02 | 124-125 | 242.41 | 10 | 643-645 | 252.02 | 10 | 643-645 |
| 211.5 | 07 | 441-443 | 223.81 | 11 | 686-688 | 234.8 | 17 | 843-845 | 242.80 | 10 | 643-645 | 252.08 | 10 | 643-645 |
| 211.6 | 07 | 438-440 | 223.89 | 11 | 686-688 | 234.9 | 17 | 843-845 | 242.81 | 10 | 643-645 | 252.1 | 10 | 643-645 |
| 211.7 | 10 | 643-645 | 223.9 | 11 | 686-688 | 235.0 | 03 | 146-148 | 242.90 | 10 | 643-645 | 252.8 | 10 | 643-645 |
| 211.8 | 06 | 393-395 | 224.0 | 02 | 124-125 | 235.1 | 03 | 146-148 | 242.91 | 10 | 643-645 | 252.9 | 10 | 643-645 |
| 211.9 | 06 | 393-395 | 224.1 | 02 | 124-125 | 235.2 | 06 | 374-376 | 243 | 10 | 643-645 | 253.0 | 10 | 643-645 |
| 212.0 | 03 | 154-156 | 224.2 | 02 | 124-125 | 235.3 | 07 | 435-437 | 244.0 | 10 | 643-645 | 253.1 | 10 | 643-645 |
| 212.1 | 03 | 154-156 | 224.3 | 02 | 124-125 | 235.4 | 06 | 374-376 | 244.1 | 10 | 643-645 | 253.2 | 10 | 643-645 |
| 212.2 | 04 | 180-182 | 224.4 | 02 | 124-125 | 235.5 | 06 | 374-376 | 244.2 | 10 | 643-645 | 253.3 | 10 | 643-645 |
| 212.3 | 04 | 180-182 | 224.5 | 02 | 124-125 | 235.6 | 03 | 146-148 | 244.3 | 10 | 643-645 | 253.4 | 10 | 643-645 |
| 212.4 | 04 | 180-182 | 224.6 | 02 | 124-125 | 235.7 | 04 | 180-182 | 244.8 | 10 | 643-645 | 253.5 | 10 | 643-645 |
| 212.5 | 04 | 180-182 | 224.7 | 02 | 124-125 | 235.8 | 04 | 180-182 | 244.9 | 10 | 643-645 | 253.6 | 10 | 643-645 |
| 212.6 | 16 | 814-816 | 224.8 | 02 | 124-125 | 235.9 | 04 | 180-182 | 245.0 | 10 | 643-645 | 253.7 | 10 | 643-645 |
| 212.7 | 05 | 314-316 | 224.9 | 02 | 124-125 | 236.0 | 13 | 754-756 | 245.1 | 10 | 643-645 | 253.8 | 10 | 643-645 |
| 212.8 | 04 | 180-182 | 225.0 | 01 | 054-055 | 236.1 | 13 | 754-756 | 245.2 | 10 | 643-645 | 253.9 | 10 | 643-645 |
| 212.9 | 04 | 180-182 | 225.1 | 01 | 054-055 | 236.2 | 13 | 754-756 | 245.3 | 10 | 643-645 | 254.0 | 16 | 814-816 |
| 213.0 | 08 | 564-566 | 225.2 | 01 | 054-055 | 236.3 | 13 | 754-756 | 245.4 | 10 | 643-645 | 254.1 | 16 | 814-816 |
| 213.1 | 03 | 157-159 | 225.3 | 01 | 054-055 | 236.4 | 12 | 722-724 | 245.8 | 10 | 643-645 | 254.8 | 16 | 814-816 |
| 213.2 | 08 | 564-566 | 225.4 | 01 | 054-055 | 236.5 | 12 | 722-724 | 245.9 | 10 | 643-645 | 254.9 | 16 | 814-816 |
| 213.3 | 04 | 180-182 | 225.8 | 01 | 054-055 | 236.6 | 12 | 722-724 | 246.0 | 10 | 643-645 | 255.0 | 10 | 643-645 |
| 213.4 | 08 | 564-566 | 225.9 | 01 | 054-055 | 236.7 | 11 | 686-688 | 246.1 | 10 | 643-645 | 255.10 | 10 | 643-645 |
| 213.5 | 08 | 564-566 | 226 | 10 | 643-645 | 236.90 | 11 | 686-688 |  |  |  | 255.11 | 10 | 643-645 |
| 213.6 | 08 | 564-566 | 227.0 | 10 | 643-645 | 236.91 | 11 | 686-688 |  |  |  | 255.12 | 10 | 643-645 |

| DX | MDC | DRG |
|---|---|---|
| 255.13 | 10 | 643-645 |
| 255.14 | 10 | 643-645 |
| 255.2 | 10 | 643-645 |
| 255.3 | 10 | 643-645 |
| 255.41 | 10 | 643-645 |
| 255.42 | 10 | 643-645 |
| 255.5 | 10 | 643-645 |
| 255.6 | 10 | 643-645 |
| 255.8 | 10 | 643-645 |
| 255.9 | 10 | 643-645 |
| 256.0 | 13 | 760-761 |
| 256.1 | 13 | 760-761 |
| 256.2 | 13 | 760-761 |
| 256.31 | 13 | 760-761 |
| 256.39 | 13 | 760-761 |
| 256.4 | 13 | 760-761 |
| 256.8 | 13 | 760-761 |
| 256.9 | 13 | 760-761 |
| 257.0 | 10 | 643-645 |
| 257.1 | 10 | 643-645 |
| 257.2 | 10 | 643-645 |
| 257.8 | 10 | 643-645 |
| 257.9 | 10 | 643-645 |
| 258.01 | 10 | 643-645 |
| 258.02 | 10 | 643-645 |
| 258.03 | 10 | 643-645 |
| 258.1 | 10 | 643-645 |
| 258.8 | 10 | 643-645 |
| 258.9 | 10 | 643-645 |
| 259.0 | 10 | 643-645 |
| 259.1 | 10 | 643-645 |
| 259.2 | 10 | 643-645 |
| 259.3 | 10 | 643-645 |
| 259.4 | 10 | 643-645 |
| 259.5 | 10 | 643-645 |
| 259.8 | 10 | 643-645 |
| 259.9 | 10 | 643-645 |
| 260 | 10 | 640-641 |
| 261 | 10 | 640-641 |
| 262 | 10 | 640-641 |
| 263.0 | 10 | 640-641 |
| 263.1 | 10 | 640-641 |
| 263.2 | 10 | 640-641 |
| 263.8 | 10 | 640-641 |
| 263.9 | 10 | 640-641 |
| 264.0 | 02 | 124-125 |
| 264.1 | 02 | 124-125 |
| 264.2 | 02 | 124-125 |
| 264.3 | 02 | 124-125 |
| 264.4 | 02 | 124-125 |
| 264.5 | 02 | 124-125 |
| 264.6 | 02 | 124-125 |
| 264.7 | 02 | 124-125 |
| 264.8 | 10 | 640-641 |
| 264.9 | 10 | 640-641 |
| 265.0 | 10 | 640-641 |
| 265.1 | 10 | 640-641 |
| 265.2 | 10 | 640-641 |
| 266.0 | 10 | 640-641 |
| 266.1 | 10 | 640-641 |
| 266.2 | 10 | 640-641 |
| 266.9 | 10 | 640-641 |
| 267 | 10 | 640-641 |
| 268.0 | 08 | 553-554 |
| 268.1 | 08 | 553-554 |
| 268.2 | 08 | 553-554 |
| 268.9 | 10 | 640-641 |
| 269.0 | 10 | 640-641 |
| 269.1 | 10 | 640-641 |
| 269.2 | 10 | 640-641 |
| 269.3 | 10 | 640-641 |
| 269.8 | 10 | 640-641 |
| 269.9 | 10 | 640-641 |
| 270.0 | 10 | 642 |
| 270.1 | 10 | 642 |
| 270.2 | 10 | 642 |
| 270.3 | 10 | 642 |
| 270.4 | 10 | 642 |
| 270.5 | 10 | 642 |
| 270.6 | 10 | 642 |
| 270.7 | 10 | 642 |
| 270.8 | 10 | 642 |
| 270.9 | 10 | 642 |
| 271.0 | 10 | 642 |
| 271.1 | 10 | 642 |
| 271.2 | 06 | 391-392 |
| 271.3 | 06 | 391-392 |
| 271.4 | 10 | 642 |
| 271.8 | 10 | 642 |
| 271.9 | 10 | 642 |
| 272.0 | 10 | 642 |
| 272.1 | 10 | 642 |
| 272.2 | 10 | 642 |
| 272.3 | 10 | 642 |
| 272.4 | 10 | 642 |
| 272.5 | 10 | 642 |
| 272.6 | 10 | 642 |
| 272.7 | 10 | 642 |
| 272.8 | 10 | 642 |
| 272.9 | 10 | 642 |
| 273.0 | 16 | 814-816 |
| 273.1 | 16 | 814-816 |
| 273.2 | 17 | 840-842 |
| 273.3 | 17 | 840-842 |
| 273.4 | 10 | 642 |
| 273.8 | 17 | 843-845 |
| 273.9 | 17 | 843-845 |
| 274.0 | 08 | 553-554 |
| 274.10 | 11 | 698-700 |
| 274.11 | 11 | 691-694 |
| 274.19 | 11 | 698-700 |
| 274.81 | 08 | 553-554 |
| 274.82 | 08 | 553-554 |
| 274.89 | 08 | 553-554 |
| 274.9 | 08 | 553-554 |
| 275.0 | 10 | 642 |
| 275.1 | 10 | 642 |
| 275.2 | 10 | 640-641 |
| 275.3 | 10 | 642 |
| 275.40 | 10 | 640-641 |
| 275.41 | 10 | 640-641 |
| 275.42 | 10 | 640-641 |
| 275.49 | 10 | 640-641 |
| 275.8 | 10 | 642 |
| 275.9 | 10 | 642 |
| 276.0 | 10 | 640-641 |
| 276.1 | 10 | 640-641 |
| 276.2 | 10 | 640-641 |
| 276.3 | 10 | 640-641 |
| 276.4 | 10 | 640-641 |
| 276.50 | 10 | 640-641 |
| 276.51 | 10 | 640-641 |
| 276.52 | 10 | 640-641 |
| 276.6 | 10 | 640-641 |
| 276.7 | 10 | 640-641 |
| 276.8 | 10 | 640-641 |
| 276.9 | 10 | 640-641 |
| 277.00 | 10 | 640-641 |
| 277.01 | 15 | 791, 793 |
| 277.02 | 04 | 177-179 |
| 277.03 | 06 | 393-395 |
| 277.09 | 10 | 640-641 |
| 277.1 | 10 | 642 |
| 277.2 | 10 | 642 |
| 277.30 | 08 | 545-547 |
| 277.31 | 08 | 545-547 |
| 277.39 | 08 | 545-547 |
| 277.4 | 07 | 441-443 |
| 277.5 | 10 | 642 |
| 277.6 | 10 | 642 |
| 277.7 | 10 | 642 |
| 277.81 | 10 | 642 |
| 277.82 | 10 | 642 |
| 277.83 | 10 | 642 |
| 277.84 | 10 | 642 |
| 277.85 | 10 | 642 |
| 277.86 | 10 | 642 |
| 277.87 | 10 | 642 |
| 277.89 | 10 | 642 |
| 277.9 | 10 | 642 |
| 278.00 | 10 | 640-641 |
| 278.01 | 10 | 640-641 |
| 278.02 | 10 | 640-641 |
| 278.1 | 10 | 640-641 |
| 278.2 | 10 | 640-641 |
| 278.3 | 10 | 640-641 |
| 278.4 | 10 | 640-641 |
| 278.8 | 10 | 640-641 |
| 279.00 | 16 | 814-816 |
| 279.01 | 16 | 814-816 |
| 279.02 | 16 | 814-816 |
| 279.03 | 16 | 814-816 |
| 279.04 | 16 | 814-816 |
| 279.05 | 16 | 814-816 |
| 279.06 | 16 | 814-816 |
| 279.09 | 16 | 814-816 |
| 279.10 | 16 | 814-816 |
| 279.11 | 16 | 808-810 |
| 279.12 | 16 | 808-810 |
| 279.13 | 16 | 808-810 |
| 279.19 | 16 | 808-810 |
| 279.2 | 16 | 808-810 |
| 279.3 | 16 | 814-816 |
| 279.4 | 08 | 545-547 |
| 279.8 | 16 | 814-816 |
| 279.9 | 16 | 814-816 |

**Diseases of the Blood and Blood Forming Organs**

| DX | MDC | DRG |
|---|---|---|
| 280.0 | 16 | 811-812 |
| 280.1 | 16 | 811-812 |
| 280.8 | 16 | 811-812 |
| 280.9 | 16 | 811-812 |
| 281.0 | 16 | 811-812 |
| 281.1 | 16 | 811-812 |
| 281.2 | 16 | 811-812 |
| 281.3 | 16 | 811-812 |
| 281.4 | 16 | 811-812 |
| 281.8 | 16 | 811-812 |
| 281.9 | 16 | 811-812 |
| 282.0 | 16 | 811-812 |
| 282.1 | 16 | 811-812 |
| 282.2 | 16 | 811-812 |
| 282.3 | 16 | 811-812 |
| 282.41 | 16 | 811-812 |
| 282.42 | 16 | 811-812 |
| 282.49 | 16 | 811-812 |
| 282.5 | 16 | 811-812 |
| 282.60 | 16 | 811-812 |
| 282.61 | 16 | 811-812 |
| 282.62 | 16 | 811-812 |
| 282.63 | 16 | 811-812 |
| 282.64 | 16 | 811-812 |
| 282.68 | 16 | 811-812 |
| 282.69 | 16 | 811-812 |
| 282.7 | 16 | 811-812 |
| 282.8 | 16 | 811-812 |
| 282.9 | 16 | 811-812 |
| 283.0 | 16 | 808-810 |
| 283.10 | 16 | 808-810 |
| 283.11 | 16 | 811-812 |
| 283.19 | 16 | 808-810 |
| 283.2 | 16 | 808-810 |
| 283.9 | 16 | 808-810 |
| 284.01 | 16 | 808-810 |
| 284.09 | 16 | 808-810 |
| 284.1 | 16 | 811-812 |
| 284.2 | 17 | 840-842 |
| 284.81 | 16 | 808-810 |
| 284.89 | 16 | 808-810 |
| 284.9 | 16 | 808-810 |
| 285.0 | 16 | 811-812 |
| 285.1 | 16 | 811-812 |
| 285.21 | 16 | 811-812 |
| 285.22 | 16 | 811-812 |
| 285.29 | 16 | 811-812 |
| 285.8 | 16 | 811-812 |
| 285.9 | 16 | 811-812 |
| 286.0 | 16 | 813 |
| 286.1 | 16 | 813 |
| 286.2 | 16 | 813 |
| 286.3 | 16 | 813 |
| 286.4 | 16 | 813 |
| 286.5 | 16 | 813 |
| 286.6 | 16 | 813 |
| 286.7 | 16 | 813 |
| 286.9 | 16 | 813 |
| 287.0 | 16 | 813 |
| 287.1 | 16 | 813 |
| 287.2 | 16 | 813 |
| 287.30 | 16 | 813 |
| 287.31 | 16 | 813 |
| 287.32 | 16 | 813 |
| 287.33 | 16 | 813 |
| 287.39 | 16 | 813 |
| 287.4 | 16 | 813 |
| 287.5 | 16 | 813 |
| 287.8 | 16 | 813 |
| 287.9 | 16 | 813 |
| 288.00 | 16 | 808-810 |
| 288.01 | 16 | 808-810 |
| 288.02 | 16 | 808-810 |
| 288.03 | 16 | 808-810 |
| 288.04 | 16 | 808-810 |
| 288.09 | 16 | 808-810 |
| 288.1 | 16 | 808-810 |
| 288.2 | 16 | 808-810 |
| 288.3 | 16 | 814-816 |
| 288.4 | 16 | 814-816 |
| 288.50 | 16 | 814-816 |
| 288.51 | 16 | 814-816 |
| 288.59 | 16 | 814-816 |
| 288.60 | 16 | 814-816 |
| 288.61 | 16 | 814-816 |
| 288.62 | 16 | 814-816 |
| 288.63 | 16 | 814-816 |
| 288.64 | 16 | 814-816 |
| 288.65 | 16 | 814-816 |
| 288.66 | 16 | 814-816 |
| 288.69 | 16 | 814-816 |
| 288.8 | 16 | 814-816 |
| 288.9 | 16 | 814-816 |
| 289.0 | 16 | 814-816 |
| 289.1 | 16 | 814-816 |
| 289.2 | 06 | 393-395 |
| 289.3 | 16 | 814-816 |
| 289.4 | 16 | 814-816 |
| 289.50 | 16 | 814-816 |
| 289.51 | 16 | 814-816 |
| 289.52 | 16 | 814-816 |
| 289.53 | 16 | 814-816 |
| 289.59 | 16 | 814-816 |
| 289.6 | 16 | 814-816 |
| 289.7 | 16 | 811-812 |
| 289.81 | 16 | 814-816 |
| 289.82 | 16 | 814-816 |
| 289.83 | 17 | 840-842 |
| 289.89 | 16 | 814-816 |
| 289.9 | 16 | 814-816 |

**Mental Disorders**

| DX | MDC | DRG |
|---|---|---|
| 290.0 | 19 | 884 |
| 290.10 | 19 | 884 |
| 290.11 | 19 | 884 |
| 290.12 | 19 | 884 |
| 290.13 | 19 | 884 |
| 290.20 | 19 | 884 |
| 290.21 | 19 | 884 |
| 290.3 | 19 | 884 |
| 290.40 | 19 | 884 |
| 290.41 | 19 | 884 |
| 290.42 | 19 | 884 |
| 290.43 | 19 | 884 |
| 290.8 | 19 | 884 |
| 290.9 | 19 | 884 |
| 291.0 | 20 | 895-897 |
| 291.1 | 20 | 895-897 |
| 291.2 | 20 | 895-897 |
| 291.3 | 20 | 895-897 |
| 291.4 | 20 | 895-897 |
| 291.5 | 20 | 895-897 |
| 291.81 | 20 | 895-897 |
| 291.82 | 20 | 895-897 |
| 291.89 | 20 | 895-897 |
| 291.9 | 20 | 895-897 |
| 292.0 | 20 | 895-897 |
| 292.11 | 20 | 895-897 |
| 292.12 | 20 | 895-897 |
| 292.2 | 20 | 895-897 |
| 292.81 | 20 | 895-897 |
| 292.82 | 20 | 895-897 |
| 292.83 | 20 | 895-897 |
| 292.84 | 20 | 895-897 |
| 292.85 | 20 | 895-897 |
| 292.89 | 20 | 895-897 |
| 292.9 | 20 | 895-897 |
| 293 | 19 | 880 |
| 293.1 | 19 | 880 |
| 293.81 | 19 | 884 |
| 293.82 | 19 | 884 |
| 293.83 | 19 | 884 |
| 293.84 | 19 | 884 |
| 293.89 | 19 | 884 |
| 293.9 | 19 | 880 |
| 294.10 | 19 | 884 |
| 294.11 | 19 | 884 |
| 294.8 | 19 | 884 |
| 294.9 | 19 | 884 |
| 295.00 | 19 | 885 |
| 295.01 | 19 | 885 |
| 295.02 | 19 | 885 |
| 295.03 | 19 | 885 |
| 295.04 | 19 | 885 |
| 295.05 | 19 | 885 |
| 295.10 | 19 | 885 |
| 295.11 | 19 | 885 |
| 295.12 | 19 | 885 |
| 295.13 | 19 | 885 |
| 295.14 | 19 | 885 |
| 295.15 | 19 | 885 |
| 295.20 | 19 | 885 |
| 295.21 | 19 | 885 |
| 295.22 | 19 | 885 |
| 295.23 | 19 | 885 |
| 295.24 | 19 | 885 |
| 295.25 | 19 | 885 |
| 295.30 | 19 | 885 |
| 295.31 | 19 | 885 |
| 295.32 | 19 | 885 |
| 295.33 | 19 | 885 |
| 295.34 | 19 | 885 |
| 295.35 | 19 | 885 |
| 295.40 | 19 | 885 |
| 295.41 | 19 | 885 |
| 295.42 | 19 | 885 |
| 295.43 | 19 | 885 |
| 295.44 | 19 | 885 |
| 295.45 | 19 | 885 |
| 295.50 | 19 | 885 |
| 295.51 | 19 | 885 |
| 295.52 | 19 | 885 |
| 295.53 | 19 | 885 |
| 295.54 | 19 | 885 |
| 295.55 | 19 | 885 |
| 295.60 | 19 | 885 |

| DX ...MDC ..DRG | DX ...MDC ..DRG | DX ...MDC ..DRG | DX ...MDC ..DRG | DX ...MDC ..DRG |
|---|---|---|---|---|
| 295.61 ..19 ..885 | 296.90 ..19 ..885 | 302.52 ..19 ..887 | 305.32 ..20 ..895-897 | 309.21 ..19 ..882 |
| 295.62 ..19 ..885 | 296.99 ..19 ..885 | 302.53 ..19 ..887 | 305.33 ..20 ..895-897 | 309.22 ..19 ..882 |
| 295.63 ..19 ..885 | 297.0 ...19 ..885 | 302.6 ...19 ..887 | 305.40 ..20 ..895-897 | 309.23 ..19 ..882 |
| 295.64 ..19 ..885 | 297.1 ...19 ..885 | 302.70 ..19 ..887 | 305.41 ..20 ..895-897 | 309.24 ..19 ..882 |
| 295.65 ..19 ..885 | 297.2 ...19 ..885 | 302.71 ..19 ..887 | 305.42 ..20 ..895-897 | 309.28 ..19 ..882 |
| 295.70 ..19 ..885 | 297.3 ...19 ..885 | 302.72 ..19 ..887 | 305.43 ..20 ..895-897 | 309.29 ..19 ..882 |
| 295.71 ..19 ..885 | 297.8 ...19 ..885 | 302.73 ..19 ..887 | 305.50 ..20 ..895-897 | 309.3 ...19 ..882 |
| 295.72 ..19 ..885 | 297.9 ...19 ..885 | 302.74 ..19 ..887 | 305.51 ..20 ..895-897 | 309.4 ...19 ..882 |
| 295.73 ..19 ..885 | 298.0 ...19 ..885 | 302.75 ..19 ..887 | 305.52 ..20 ..895-897 | 309.81 ..19 ..882 |
| 295.74 ..19 ..885 | 298.1 ...19 ..885 | 302.76 ..19 ..887 | 305.53 ..20 ..895-897 | 309.82 ..19 ..882 |
| 295.75 ..19 ..885 | 298.2 ...19 ..887 | 302.79 ..19 ..887 | 305.60 ..20 ..895-897 | 309.83 ..19 ..882 |
| 295.80 ..19 ..885 | 298.3 ...19 ..885 | 302.81 ..19 ..887 | 305.61 ..20 ..895-897 | 309.89 ..19 ..882 |
| 295.81 ..19 ..885 | 298.4 ...19 ..885 | 302.82 ..19 ..887 | 305.62 ..20 ..895-897 | 309.9 ...19 ..882 |
| 295.82 ..19 ..885 | 298.8 ...19 ..885 | 302.83 ..19 ..887 | 305.63 ..20 ..895-897 | 310.0 ...19 ..884 |
| 295.83 ..19 ..885 | 298.9 ...19 ..885 | 302.84 ..19 ..887 | 305.70 ..20 ..895-897 | 310.1 ...19 ..884 |
| 295.84 ..19 ..885 | 299.00 ..19 ..884 | 302.85 ..19 ..887 | 305.71 ..20 ..895-897 | 310.2 ...01 ..100-103 |
| 295.85 ..19 ..885 | 299.01 ..19 ..884 | 302.89 ..19 ..887 | 305.72 ..20 ..895-897 | 310.8 ...19 ..884 |
| 295.90 ..19 ..885 | 299.10 ..19 ..884 | 302.9 ...19 ..887 | 305.73 ..20 ..895-897 | 310.9 ...19 ..884 |
| 295.91 ..19 ..885 | 299.11 ..19 ..884 | 303.00 ..20 ..895-897 | 305.80 ..20 ..895-897 | 311 .....19 ..881 |
| 295.92 ..19 ..885 | 299.80 ..19 ..885 | 303.01 ..20 ..895-897 | 305.81 ..20 ..895-897 | 312.00 ..19 ..886 |
| 295.93 ..19 ..885 | 299.81 ..19 ..885 | 303.02 ..20 ..895-897 | 305.82 ..20 ..895-897 | 312.01 ..19 ..886 |
| 295.94 ..19 ..885 | 299.90 ..19 ..885 | 303.03 ..20 ..895-897 | 305.83 ..20 ..895-897 | 312.02 ..19 ..886 |
| 295.95 ..19 ..885 | 299.91 ..19 ..885 | 303.90 ..20 ..895-897 | 305.90 ..20 ..895-897 | 312.03 ..19 ..886 |
| 296.00 ..19 ..885 | 300.00 ..19 ..880 | 303.91 ..20 ..895-897 | 305.91 ..20 ..895-897 | 312.10 ..19 ..886 |
| 296.01 ..19 ..885 | 300.01 ..19 ..880 | 303.92 ..20 ..895-897 | 305.92 ..20 ..895-897 | 312.11 ..19 ..886 |
| 296.02 ..19 ..885 | 300.02 ..19 ..880 | 303.93 ..20 ..895-897 | 305.93 ..20 ..895-897 | 312.12 ..19 ..886 |
| 296.03 ..19 ..885 | 300.09 ..19 ..880 | 304.00 ..20 ..895-897 | 306.0 ...08 ..557-558 | 312.13 ..19 ..886 |
| 296.04 ..19 ..885 | 300.10 ..19 ..880 | 304.01 ..20 ..895-897 | 306.1 ...04 ..205-206 | 312.20 ..19 ..886 |
| 296.05 ..19 ..885 | 300.11 ..19 ..880 | 304.02 ..20 ..895-897 | 306.2 ...05 ..314-316 | 312.21 ..19 ..886 |
| 296.06 ..19 ..885 | 300.12 ..19 ..880 | 304.03 ..20 ..895-897 | 306.3 ...09 ..606-607 | 312.22 ..19 ..886 |
| 296.10 ..19 ..885 | 300.13 ..19 ..880 | 304.10 ..20 ..895-897 | 306.4 ...06 ..391-392 | 312.23 ..19 ..886 |
| 296.11 ..19 ..885 | 300.14 ..19 ..883 | 304.11 ..20 ..895-897 | 306.50 ..11 ..698-700 | 312.30 ..19 ..886 |
| 296.12 ..19 ..885 | 300.15 ..19 ..880 | 304.12 ..20 ..895-897 | 306.51 ..13 ..760-761 | 312.31 ..19 ..883 |
| 296.13 ..19 ..885 | 300.16 ..19 ..880 | 304.13 ..20 ..895-897 | 306.52 ..13 ..760-761 | 312.32 ..19 ..883 |
| 296.14 ..19 ..885 | 300.19 ..19 ..880 | 304.20 ..20 ..895-897 | 306.53 ..11 ..698-700 | 312.33 ..19 ..886 |
| 296.15 ..19 ..885 | 300.20 ..19 ..882 | 304.21 ..20 ..895-897 | 306.59 ..11 ..698-700 | 312.34 ..19 ..883 |
| 296.16 ..19 ..885 | 300.21 ..19 ..882 | 304.22 ..20 ..895-897 | 306.6 ...10 ..643-645 | 312.35 ..19 ..883 |
| 296.20 ..19 ..885 | 300.22 ..19 ..882 | 304.23 ..20 ..895-897 | 306.7 ...19 ..882 | 312.39 ..19 ..883 |
| 296.21 ..19 ..885 | 300.23 ..19 ..882 | 304.30 ..20 ..895-897 | 306.8 ...19 ..887 | 312.4 ...19 ..886 |
| 296.22 ..19 ..885 | 300.29 ..19 ..882 | 304.31 ..20 ..895-897 | 306.9 ...19 ..882 | 312.81 ..19 ..886 |
| 296.23 ..19 ..885 | 300.3 ...19 ..882 | 304.32 ..20 ..895-897 | 307.0 ...19 ..887 | 312.82 ..19 ..886 |
| 296.24 ..19 ..885 | 300.4 ...19 ..881 | 304.33 ..20 ..895-897 | 307.1 ...19 ..883 | 312.89 ..19 ..886 |
| 296.25 ..19 ..885 | 300.5 ...19 ..882 | 304.40 ..20 ..895-897 | 307.20 ..01 ..091-093 | 312.9 ...19 ..886 |
| 296.26 ..19 ..885 | 300.6 ...19 ..882 | 304.41 ..20 ..895-897 | 307.21 ..01 ..091-093 | 313.0 ...19 ..882 |
| 296.30 ..19 ..885 | 300.7 ...19 ..882 | 304.42 ..20 ..895-897 | 307.22 ..01 ..091-093 | 313.1 ...19 ..882 |
| 296.31 ..19 ..885 | 300.81 ..19 ..882 | 304.43 ..20 ..895-897 | 307.23 ..01 ..091-093 | 313.21 ..19 ..886 |
| 296.32 ..19 ..885 | 300.82 ..19 ..882 | 304.50 ..20 ..895-897 | 307.3 ...19 ..887 | 313.22 ..19 ..886 |
| 296.33 ..19 ..885 | 300.89 ..19 ..882 | 304.51 ..20 ..895-897 | 307.40 ..19 ..887 | 313.23 ..19 ..886 |
| 296.34 ..19 ..885 | 300.9 ...19 ..880 | 304.52 ..20 ..895-897 | 307.41 ..19 ..887 | 313.3 ...19 ..886 |
| 296.35 ..19 ..885 | 301.0 ...19 ..883 | 304.53 ..20 ..895-897 | 307.42 ..19 ..887 | 313.81 ..19 ..886 |
| 296.36 ..19 ..885 | 301.10 ..19 ..883 | 304.60 ..20 ..895-897 | 307.43 ..19 ..887 | 313.82 ..19 ..886 |
| 296.40 ..19 ..885 | 301.11 ..19 ..883 | 304.61 ..20 ..895-897 | 307.44 ..19 ..887 | 313.83 ..19 ..886 |
| 296.41 ..19 ..885 | 301.12 ..19 ..881 | 304.62 ..20 ..895-897 | 307.45 ..19 ..887 | 313.89 ..19 ..886 |
| 296.42 ..19 ..885 | 301.13 ..19 ..883 | 304.63 ..20 ..895-897 | 307.46 ..19 ..887 | 313.9 ...19 ..886 |
| 296.43 ..19 ..885 | 301.20 ..19 ..883 | 304.70 ..20 ..895-897 | 307.47 ..19 ..887 | 314.00 ..19 ..886 |
| 296.44 ..19 ..885 | 301.21 ..19 ..883 | 304.71 ..20 ..895-897 | 307.48 ..19 ..887 | 314.01 ..19 ..886 |
| 296.45 ..19 ..885 | 301.22 ..19 ..883 | 304.72 ..20 ..895-897 | 307.49 ..19 ..887 | 314.1 ...19 ..886 |
| 296.46 ..19 ..885 | 301.3 ...19 ..883 | 304.73 ..20 ..895-897 | 307.50 ..19 ..887 | 314.2 ...19 ..886 |
| 296.50 ..19 ..885 | 301.4 ...19 ..883 | 304.80 ..20 ..895-897 | 307.51 ..19 ..887 | 314.8 ...19 ..886 |
| 296.51 ..19 ..885 | 301.50 ..19 ..883 | 304.81 ..20 ..895-897 | 307.52 ..19 ..886 | 314.9 ...19 ..886 |
| 296.52 ..19 ..885 | 301.51 ..19 ..883 | 304.82 ..20 ..895-897 | 307.53 ..19 ..882 | 315.00 ..19 ..886 |
| 296.53 ..19 ..885 | 301.59 ..19 ..883 | 304.83 ..20 ..895-897 | 307.54 ..19 ..882 | 315.01 ..19 ..886 |
| 296.54 ..19 ..885 | 301.6 ...19 ..883 | 304.90 ..20 ..895-897 | 307.59 ..19 ..887 | 315.02 ..19 ..886 |
| 296.55 ..19 ..885 | 301.7 ...19 ..883 | 304.91 ..20 ..895-897 | 307.6 ...19 ..886 | 315.09 ..19 ..886 |
| 296.56 ..19 ..885 | 301.81 ..19 ..883 | 304.92 ..20 ..895-897 | 307.7 ...19 ..886 | 315.1 ...19 ..886 |
| 296.60 ..19 ..885 | 301.82 ..19 ..883 | 304.93 ..20 ..895-897 | 307.80 ..19 ..882 | 315.2 ...19 ..886 |
| 296.61 ..19 ..885 | 301.83 ..19 ..883 | 305.00 ..20 ..895-897 | 307.81 ..01 ..100-103 | 315.31 ..19 ..886 |
| 296.62 ..19 ..885 | 301.84 ..19 ..883 | 305.01 ..20 ..895-897 | 307.89 ..19 ..882 | 315.32 ..19 ..886 |
| 296.63 ..19 ..885 | 301.89 ..19 ..883 | 305.02 ..20 ..895-897 | 307.9 ...19 ..884 | 315.34 ..19 ..886 |
| 296.64 ..19 ..885 | 301.9 ...19 ..883 | 305.03 ..20 ..895-897 | 308.0 ...19 ..880 | 315.39 ..19 ..886 |
| 296.65 ..19 ..885 | 302.0 ...19 ..887 | 305.1 ...23 ..951 | 308.1 ...19 ..880 | 315.4 ...19 ..886 |
| 296.66 ..19 ..885 | 302.1 ...19 ..887 | 305.20 ..20 ..895-897 | 308.2 ...19 ..880 | 315.5 ...19 ..886 |
| 296.7 ...19 ..885 | 302.2 ...19 ..887 | 305.21 ..20 ..895-897 | 308.3 ...19 ..880 | 315.8 ...19 ..886 |
| 296.80 ..19 ..885 | 302.3 ...19 ..887 | 305.22 ..20 ..895-897 | 308.4 ...19 ..880 | 315.9 ...19 ..886 |
| 296.81 ..19 ..885 | 302.4 ...19 ..887 | 305.23 ..20 ..895-897 | 308.9 ...19 ..880 | 316 .....19 ..884 |
| 296.82 ..19 ..885 | 302.50 ..19 ..887 | 305.30 ..20 ..895-897 | 309.0 ...19 ..881 | 317 .....19 ..884 |
| 296.89 ..19 ..885 | 302.51 ..19 ..887 | 305.31 ..20 ..895-897 | 309.1 ...19 ..881 | 318.0 ...19 ..884 |

| DX | MDC | DRG |
|---|---|---|
| 318.1 | 19 | 884 |
| 318.2 | 19 | 884 |
| 319 | 19 | 884 |

### Diseases of the Nervous System and Sense Organs

| DX | MDC | DRG |
|---|---|---|
| 320.0 | 01 | 094-096 |
| 320.1 | 01 | 094-096 |
| 320.2 | 01 | 094-096 |
| 320.3 | 01 | 094-096 |
| 320.7 | 01 | 094-096 |
| 320.81 | 01 | 094-096 |
| 320.82 | 01 | 094-096 |
| 320.89 | 01 | 094-096 |
| 320.9 | 01 | 094-096 |
| 321.0 | 01 | 097-099 |
| 321.1 | 01 | 097-099 |
| 321.2 | 01 | 097-099 |
| 321.3 | 01 | 097-099 |
| 321.4 | 01 | 097-099 |
| 321.8 | 01 | 097-099 |
| 322.0 | 01 | 097-099 |
| 322.1 | 01 | 097-099 |
| 322.2 | 01 | 097-099 |
| 322.9 | 01 | 097-099 |
| 323.01 | 01 | 097-099 |
| 323.02 | 01 | 097-099 |
| 323.1 | 01 | 097-099 |
| 323.2 | 01 | 097-099 |
| 323.41 | 01 | 097-099 |
| 323.42 | 01 | 097-099 |
| 323.51 | 01 | 097-099 |
| 323.52 | 01 | 097-099 |
| 323.61 | 01 | 097-099 |
| 323.62 | 01 | 097-099 |
| 323.63 | 01 | 097-099 |
| 323.71 | 01 | 091-093 |
| 323.72 | 01 | 091-093 |
| 323.81 | 01 | 097-099 |
| 323.82 | 01 | 097-099 |
| 323.9 | 01 | 097-099 |
| 324.0 | 01 | 094-096 |
| 324.1 | 01 | 094-096 |
| 324.9 | 01 | 094-096 |
| 325 | 01 | 091-093 |
| 326 | 01 | 091-093 |
| 327.00 | 19 | 887 |
| 327.01 | 19 | 887 |
| 327.02 | 19 | 887 |
| 327.09 | 19 | 887 |
| 327.10 | 19 | 887 |
| 327.11 | 19 | 887 |
| 327.12 | 19 | 887 |
| 327.13 | 19 | 887 |
| 327.14 | 19 | 887 |
| 327.15 | 19 | 887 |
| 327.19 | 19 | 887 |
| 327.20 | 03 | 154-156 |
| 327.21 | 01 | 091-093 |
| 327.22 | 04 | 204 |
| 327.23 | 03 | 154-156 |
| 327.24 | 03 | 154-156 |
| 327.25 | 01 | 091-093 |
| 327.26 | 03 | 154-156 |
| 327.27 | 01 | 091-093 |
| 327.29 | 03 | 154-156 |
| 327.30 | 01 | 091-093 |
| 327.31 | 01 | 091-093 |
| 327.32 | 01 | 091-093 |
| 327.33 | 01 | 091-093 |
| 327.34 | 01 | 091-093 |
| 327.35 | 01 | 091-093 |
| 327.36 | 01 | 091-093 |
| 327.37 | 01 | 091-093 |
| 327.39 | 01 | 091-093 |
| 327.40 | 03 | 154-156 |
| 327.41 | 01 | 091-093 |
| 327.42 | 03 | 154-156 |
| 327.43 | 01 | 091-093 |
| 327.44 | 03 | 154-156 |
| 327.49 | 03 | 154-156 |
| 327.51 | 01 | 091-093 |
| 327.52 | 01 | 091-093 |
| 327.53 | 03 | 154-156 |
| 327.59 | 03 | 154-156 |
| 327.8 | 03 | 154-156 |
| 330.0 | 01 | 056-057 |
| 330.1 | 01 | 056-057 |
| 330.2 | 01 | 056-057 |
| 330.3 | 01 | 056-057 |
| 330.8 | 01 | 056-057 |
| 330.9 | 01 | 056-057 |
| 331.0 | 01 | 056-057 |
| 331.11 | 01 | 056-057 |
| 331.19 | 01 | 056-057 |
| 331.2 | 01 | 056-057 |
| 331.3 | 01 | 056-057 |
| 331.4 | 01 | 056-057 |
| 331.5 | 01 | 056-057 |
| 331.7 | 01 | 056-057 |
| 331.81 | 01 | 091-093 |
| 331.82 | 01 | 056-057 |
| 331.83 | 01 | 056-057 |
| 331.89 | 01 | 056-057 |
| 331.9 | 01 | 056-057 |
| 332.0 | 01 | 056-057 |
| 332.1 | 01 | 056-057 |
| 333.0 | 01 | 056-057 |
| 333.1 | 01 | 091-093 |
| 333.2 | 01 | 091-093 |
| 333.3 | 01 | 091-093 |
| 333.4 | 01 | 056-057 |
| 333.5 | 01 | 056-057 |
| 333.6 | 01 | 056-057 |
| 333.71 | 01 | 056-057 |
| 333.72 | 01 | 091-093 |
| 333.79 | 01 | 091-093 |
| 333.81 | 02 | 124-125 |
| 333.82 | 01 | 091-093 |
| 333.83 | 01 | 091-093 |
| 333.84 | 01 | 091-093 |
| 333.85 | 01 | 091-093 |
| 333.89 | 01 | 091-093 |
| 333.90 | 01 | 056-057 |
| 333.91 | 01 | 091-093 |
| 333.92 | 01 | 091-093 |
| 333.93 | 01 | 091-093 |
| 333.94 | 01 | 056-057 |
| 333.99 | 01 | 056-057 |
| 334.0 | 01 | 058-060 |
| 334.1 | 01 | 058-060 |
| 334.2 | 01 | 058-060 |
| 334.3 | 01 | 058-060 |
| 334.4 | 01 | 058-060 |
| 334.8 | 01 | 058-060 |
| 334.9 | 01 | 058-060 |
| 335.0 | 01 | 056-057 |
| 335.10 | 01 | 056-057 |
| 335.11 | 01 | 056-057 |
| 335.19 | 01 | 056-057 |
| 335.20 | 01 | 056-057 |
| 335.21 | 01 | 056-057 |
| 335.22 | 01 | 056-057 |
| 335.23 | 01 | 056-057 |
| 335.24 | 01 | 056-057 |
| 335.29 | 01 | 056-057 |
| 335.8 | 01 | 056-057 |
| 335.9 | 01 | 056-057 |
| 336.0 | 01 | 056-057 |
| 336.1 | 01 | 091-093 |
| 336.2 | 01 | 091-093 |
| 336.3 | 01 | 091-093 |
| 336.8 | 01 | 091-093 |
| 336.9 | 01 | 091-093 |
| 337.0 | 01 | 073-074 |
| 337.1 | 01 | 073-074 |
| 337.20 | 01 | 073-074 |
| 337.21 | 01 | 073-074 |
| 337.22 | 01 | 073-074 |
| 337.29 | 01 | 073-074 |
| 337.3 | 01 | 073-074 |
| 337.9 | 01 | 073-074 |
| 338.0 | 01 | 091-093 |
| 338.11 | 23 | 947-948 |
| 338.12 | 23 | 947-948 |
| 338.18 | 23 | 947-948 |
| 338.19 | 23 | 947-948 |
| 338.21 | 01 | 091-093 |
| 338.22 | 01 | 091-093 |
| 338.28 | 01 | 091-093 |
| 338.29 | 01 | 091-093 |
| 338.3 | 23 | 947-948 |
| 338.4 | 01 | 091-093 |
| 340 | 01 | 058-060 |
| 341.0 | 01 | 058-060 |
| 341.1 | 01 | 058-060 |
| 341.20 | 01 | 097-099 |
| 341.21 | 01 | 097-099 |
| 341.22 | 01 | 097-099 |
| 341.8 | 01 | 058-060 |
| 341.9 | 01 | 058-060 |
| 342.00 | 01 | 056-057 |
| 342.01 | 01 | 056-057 |
| 342.02 | 01 | 056-057 |
| 342.10 | 01 | 056-057 |
| 342.11 | 01 | 056-057 |
| 342.12 | 01 | 056-057 |
| 342.80 | 01 | 056-057 |
| 342.81 | 01 | 056-057 |
| 342.82 | 01 | 056-057 |
| 342.90 | 01 | 056-057 |
| 342.91 | 01 | 056-057 |
| 342.92 | 01 | 056-057 |
| 343.0 | 01 | 052-053 |
| 343.1 | 01 | 052-053 |
| 343.2 | 01 | 052-053 |
| 343.3 | 01 | 091-093 |
| 343.4 | 01 | 052-053 |
| 343.8 | 01 | 091-093 |
| 343.9 | 01 | 091-093 |
| 344.00 | 01 | 052-053 |
| 344.01 | 01 | 052-053 |
| 344.02 | 01 | 052-053 |
| 344.03 | 01 | 052-053 |
| 344.04 | 01 | 052-053 |
| 344.09 | 01 | 052-053 |
| 344.1 | 01 | 052-053 |
| 344.2 | 01 | 052-053 |
| 344.30 | 01 | 091-093 |
| 344.31 | 01 | 091-093 |
| 344.32 | 01 | 091-093 |
| 344.40 | 01 | 091-093 |
| 344.41 | 01 | 091-093 |
| 344.42 | 01 | 091-093 |
| 344.5 | 01 | 091-093 |
| 344.60 | 01 | 073-074 |
| 344.61 | 11 | 698-700 |
| 344.81 | 01 | 091-093 |
| 344.89 | 01 | 091-093 |
| 344.9 | 01 | 091-093 |
| 345.00 | 01 | 100-103 |
| 345.01 | 01 | 100-103 |
| 345.10 | 01 | 100-103 |
| 345.11 | 01 | 100-103 |
| 345.2 | 01 | 100-103 |
| 345.3 | 01 | 100-103 |
| 345.40 | 01 | 100-103 |
| 345.41 | 01 | 100-103 |
| 345.50 | 01 | 100-103 |
| 345.51 | 01 | 100-103 |
| 345.60 | 01 | 100-103 |
| 345.61 | 01 | 100-103 |
| 345.70 | 01 | 100-103 |
| 345.71 | 01 | 100-103 |
| 345.80 | 01 | 100-103 |
| 345.81 | 01 | 100-103 |
| 345.90 | 01 | 100-103 |
| 345.91 | 01 | 100-103 |
| 346.00 | 01 | 100-103 |
| 346.01 | 01 | 100-103 |
| 346.10 | 01 | 100-103 |
| 346.11 | 01 | 100-103 |
| 346.20 | 01 | 100-103 |
| 346.21 | 01 | 100-103 |
| 346.80 | 01 | 100-103 |
| 346.81 | 01 | 100-103 |
| 346.90 | 01 | 100-103 |
| 346.91 | 01 | 100-103 |
| 347.00 | 01 | 091-093 |
| 347.01 | 01 | 091-093 |
| 347.10 | 01 | 091-093 |
| 347.11 | 01 | 091-093 |
| 348.0 | 01 | 091-093 |
| 348.1 | 01 | 091-093 |
| 348.2 | 01 | 100-103 |
| 348.30 | 01 | 070-072 |
| 348.31 | 01 | 070-072 |
| 348.39 | 01 | 070-072 |
| 348.4 | 01 | 080-081 |
| 348.5 | 01 | 080-081 |
| 348.8 | 01 | 070-072 |
| 348.9 | 01 | 070-072 |
| 349.0 | 01 | 100-103 |
| 349.1 | 01 | 091-093 |
| 349.2 | 01 | 091-093 |
| 349.81 | 01 | 091-093 |
| 349.82 | 01 | 091-093 |
| 349.89 | 01 | 070-072 |
| 349.9 | 01 | 070-072 |
| 350.1 | 01 | 073-074 |
| 350.2 | 01 | 073-074 |
| 350.8 | 01 | 073-074 |
| 350.9 | 01 | 073-074 |
| 351.0 | 01 | 073-074 |
| 351.1 | 01 | 073-074 |
| 351.8 | 01 | 073-074 |
| 351.9 | 01 | 073-074 |
| 352.0 | 01 | 073-074 |
| 352.1 | 01 | 073-074 |
| 352.2 | 01 | 073-074 |
| 352.3 | 01 | 073-074 |
| 352.4 | 01 | 073-074 |
| 352.5 | 01 | 073-074 |
| 352.6 | 01 | 073-074 |
| 352.9 | 01 | 073-074 |
| 353.0 | 01 | 073-074 |
| 353.1 | 01 | 073-074 |
| 353.2 | 01 | 073-074 |
| 353.3 | 01 | 073-074 |
| 353.4 | 01 | 073-074 |
| 353.5 | 01 | 073-074 |
| 353.6 | 01 | 073-074 |
| 353.8 | 01 | 073-074 |
| 353.9 | 01 | 073-074 |
| 354.0 | 01 | 073-074 |
| 354.1 | 01 | 073-074 |
| 354.2 | 01 | 073-074 |
| 354.3 | 01 | 073-074 |
| 354.4 | 01 | 073-074 |
| 354.5 | 01 | 073-074 |
| 354.8 | 01 | 073-074 |
| 354.9 | 01 | 073-074 |
| 355.0 | 01 | 073-074 |
| 355.1 | 01 | 073-074 |
| 355.2 | 01 | 073-074 |
| 355.3 | 01 | 073-074 |
| 355.4 | 01 | 073-074 |
| 355.5 | 01 | 073-074 |
| 355.6 | 01 | 073-074 |
| 355.71 | 01 | 073-074 |
| 355.79 | 01 | 073-074 |
| 355.8 | 01 | 073-074 |
| 355.9 | 01 | 073-074 |
| 356.0 | 01 | 073-074 |
| 356.1 | 01 | 073-074 |
| 356.2 | 01 | 073-074 |
| 356.3 | 01 | 091-093 |
| 356.4 | 01 | 073-074 |
| 356.8 | 01 | 073-074 |
| 356.9 | 01 | 073-074 |
| 357.0 | 01 | 094-096 |
| 357.1 | 01 | 073-074 |
| 357.2 | 01 | 073-074 |
| 357.3 | 01 | 073-074 |
| 357.4 | 01 | 073-074 |
| 357.5 | 01 | 073-074 |
| 357.6 | 01 | 073-074 |
| 357.7 | 01 | 073-074 |
| 357.81 | 01 | 073-074 |
| 357.82 | 01 | 073-074 |
| 357.89 | 01 | 073-074 |
| 357.9 | 01 | 073-074 |
| 358.00 | 01 | 056-057 |
| 358.01 | 01 | 056-057 |
| 358.1 | 01 | 056-057 |
| 358.2 | 01 | 073-074 |
| 358.8 | 01 | 073-074 |
| 358.9 | 01 | 073-074 |
| 359.0 | 01 | 091-093 |
| 359.1 | 01 | 091-093 |
| 359.21 | 01 | 091-093 |
| 359.22 | 01 | 091-093 |
| 359.23 | 01 | 091-093 |
| 359.24 | 01 | 091-093 |
| 359.29 | 01 | 091-093 |
| 359.3 | 01 | 091-093 |
| 359.4 | 01 | 091-093 |
| 359.5 | 01 | 091-093 |
| 359.6 | 01 | 091-093 |
| 359.81 | 01 | 091-093 |
| 359.89 | 01 | 091-093 |
| 359.9 | 01 | 091-093 |
| 360.00 | 02 | 121-122 |
| 360.01 | 02 | 121-122 |
| 360.02 | 02 | 121-122 |
| 360.03 | 02 | 124-125 |
| 360.04 | 02 | 121-122 |
| 360.11 | 02 | 124-125 |
| 360.12 | 02 | 124-125 |
| 360.13 | 02 | 121-122 |
| 360.14 | 02 | 124-125 |
| 360.19 | 02 | 121-122 |
| 360.20 | 02 | 124-125 |
| 360.21 | 02 | 124-125 |
| 360.23 | 02 | 124-125 |
| 360.24 | 02 | 124-125 |
| 360.29 | 02 | 124-125 |
| 360.30 | 02 | 124-125 |
| 360.31 | 02 | 124-125 |
| 360.32 | 02 | 124-125 |
| 360.33 | 02 | 124-125 |
| 360.34 | 02 | 124-125 |
| 360.40 | 02 | 124-125 |
| 360.41 | 02 | 124-125 |
| 360.42 | 02 | 124-125 |
| 360.43 | 02 | 124-125 |
| 360.44 | 02 | 124-125 |
| 360.50 | 02 | 124-125 |
| 360.51 | 02 | 124-125 |
| 360.52 | 02 | 124-125 |
| 360.53 | 02 | 124-125 |
| 360.54 | 02 | 124-125 |
| 360.55 | 02 | 124-125 |
| 360.59 | 02 | 124-125 |
| 360.60 | 02 | 124-125 |

| DX ...MDC ..DRG | DX ...MDC ..DRG | DX ...MDC ..DRG | DX ...MDC ..DRG | DX ...MDC ..DRG |
|---|---|---|---|---|
| 360.61 ..02 ..124-125 | 362.71 ..02 ..124-125 | 364.56 ..02 ..124-125 | 366.32 ..02 ..124-125 | 369.11 ..02 ..124-125 |
| 360.62 ..02 ..124-125 | 362.72 ..02 ..124-125 | 364.57 ..02 ..124-125 | 366.33 ..02 ..124-125 | 369.12 ..02 ..124-125 |
| 360.63 ..02 ..124-125 | 362.73 ..02 ..124-125 | 364.59 ..02 ..124-125 | 366.34 ..02 ..124-125 | 369.13 ..02 ..124-125 |
| 360.64 ..02 ..124-125 | 362.74 ..02 ..124-125 | 364.60 ..02 ..124-125 | 366.41 ..02 ..124-125 | 369.14 ..02 ..124-125 |
| 360.65 ..02 ..124-125 | 362.75 ..02 ..124-125 | 364.61 ..02 ..124-125 | 366.42 ..02 ..124-125 | 369.15 ..02 ..124-125 |
| 360.69 ..02 ..124-125 | 362.76 ..02 ..124-125 | 364.62 ..02 ..124-125 | 366.43 ..02 ..124-125 | 369.16 ..02 ..124-125 |
| 360.81 ..02 ..124-125 | 362.77 ..02 ..124-125 | 364.63 ..02 ..124-125 | 366.44 ..02 ..124-125 | 369.17 ..02 ..124-125 |
| 360.89 ..02 ..124-125 | 362.81 ..02 ..124-125 | 364.64 ..02 ..124-125 | 366.45 ..02 ..124-125 | 369.18 ..02 ..124-125 |
| 360.9 ...02 ..124-125 | 362.82 ..02 ..124-125 | 364.70 ..02 ..124-125 | 366.46 ..02 ..124-125 | 369.20 ..02 ..124-125 |
| 361.00 ..02 ..124-125 | 362.83 ..02 ..124-125 | 364.71 ..02 ..124-125 | 366.50 ..02 ..124-125 | 369.21 ..02 ..124-125 |
| 361.01 ..02 ..124-125 | 362.84 ..02 ..124-125 | 364.72 ..02 ..124-125 | 366.51 ..02 ..124-125 | 369.22 ..02 ..124-125 |
| 361.02 ..02 ..124-125 | 362.85 ..02 ..124-125 | 364.73 ..02 ..124-125 | 366.52 ..02 ..124-125 | 369.23 ..02 ..124-125 |
| 361.03 ..02 ..124-125 | 362.89 ..02 ..124-125 | 364.74 ..02 ..124-125 | 366.53 ..02 ..124-125 | 369.24 ..02 ..124-125 |
| 361.04 ..02 ..124-125 | 362.9 ...02 ..124-125 | 364.75 ..02 ..124-125 | 366.8 ..02 ..124-125 | 369.25 ..02 ..124-125 |
| 361.05 ..02 ..124-125 | 363.00 ..02 ..124-125 | 364.76 ..02 ..124-125 | 366.9 ...02 ..124-125 | 369.3 ...02 ..124-125 |
| 361.06 ..02 ..124-125 | 363.01 ..02 ..124-125 | 364.77 ..02 ..124-125 | 367.0 ...02 ..124-125 | 369.4 ...02 ..124-125 |
| 361.07 ..02 ..124-125 | 363.03 ..02 ..124-125 | 364.81 ..02 ..124-125 | 367.1 ...02 ..124-125 | 369.60 ..02 ..124-125 |
| 361.10 ..02 ..124-125 | 363.04 ..02 ..124-125 | 364.89 ..02 ..124-125 | 367.20 ..02 ..124-125 | 369.61 ..02 ..124-125 |
| 361.11 ..02 ..124-125 | 363.05 ..02 ..124-125 | 364.9 ...02 ..124-125 | 367.21 ..02 ..124-125 | 369.62 ..02 ..124-125 |
| 361.12 ..02 ..124-125 | 363.06 ..02 ..124-125 | 365.00 ..02 ..124-125 | 367.22 ..02 ..124-125 | 369.63 ..02 ..124-125 |
| 361.13 ..02 ..124-125 | 363.07 ..02 ..124-125 | 365.01 ..02 ..124-125 | 367.31 ..02 ..124-125 | 369.64 ..02 ..124-125 |
| 361.14 ..02 ..124-125 | 363.08 ..02 ..124-125 | 365.02 ..02 ..124-125 | 367.32 ..02 ..124-125 | 369.65 ..02 ..124-125 |
| 361.19 ..02 ..124-125 | 363.10 ..02 ..124-125 | 365.03 ..02 ..124-125 | 367.4 ...02 ..124-125 | 369.66 ..02 ..124-125 |
| 361.2 ...02 ..124-125 | 363.11 ..02 ..124-125 | 365.04 ..02 ..124-125 | 367.51 ..02 ..124-125 | 369.67 ..02 ..124-125 |
| 361.30 ..02 ..124-125 | 363.12 ..02 ..124-125 | 365.10 ..02 ..124-125 | 367.52 ..02 ..123 | 369.68 ..02 ..124-125 |
| 361.31 ..02 ..124-125 | 363.13 ..02 ..124-125 | 365.11 ..02 ..124-125 | 367.53 ..02 ..124-125 | 369.69 ..02 ..124-125 |
| 361.32 ..02 ..124-125 | 363.14 ..02 ..124-125 | 365.12 ..02 ..123 | 367.81 ..02 ..124-125 | 369.70 ..02 ..124-125 |
| 361.33 ..02 ..124-125 | 363.15 ..02 ..124-125 | 365.13 ..02 ..124-125 | 367.89 ..02 ..124-125 | 369.71 ..02 ..124-125 |
| 361.81 ..02 ..124-125 | 363.20 ..02 ..124-125 | 365.14 ..02 ..124-125 | 367.9 ...02 ..124-125 | 369.72 ..02 ..124-125 |
| 361.89 ..02 ..124-125 | 363.21 ..02 ..124-125 | 365.15 ..02 ..124-125 | 368.00 ..02 ..124-125 | 369.73 ..02 ..124-125 |
| 361.9 ...02 ..124-125 | 363.22 ..02 ..124-125 | 365.20 ..02 ..124-125 | 368.01 ..02 ..124-125 | 369.74 ..02 ..124-125 |
| 362.01 ..02 ..124-125 | 363.30 ..02 ..124-125 | 365.21 ..02 ..124-125 | 368.02 ..02 ..124-125 | 369.75 ..02 ..124-125 |
| 362.02 ..02 ..124-125 | 363.31 ..02 ..124-125 | 365.22 ..02 ..124-125 | 368.03 ..02 ..124-125 | 369.76 ..02 ..124-125 |
| 362.03 ..02 ..124-125 | 363.32 ..02 ..124-125 | 365.23 ..02 ..124-125 | 368.10 ..02 ..124-125 | 369.8 ...02 ..124-125 |
| 362.04 ..02 ..124-125 | 363.33 ..02 ..124-125 | 365.24 ..02 ..124-125 | 368.11 ..02 ..123 | 369.9 ...02 ..124-125 |
| 362.05 ..02 ..124-125 | 363.34 ..02 ..124-125 | 365.31 ..02 ..124-125 | 368.12 ..02 ..123 | 370.00 ..02 ..121-122 |
| 362.06 ..02 ..124-125 | 363.35 ..02 ..124-125 | 365.32 ..02 ..124-125 | 368.13 ..02 ..124-125 | 370.01 ..02 ..124-125 |
| 362.07 ..02 ..124-125 | 363.40 ..02 ..124-125 | 365.41 ..02 ..124-125 | 368.14 ..02 ..124-125 | 370.02 ..02 ..124-125 |
| 362.10 ..02 ..124-125 | 363.41 ..02 ..124-125 | 365.42 ..02 ..124-125 | 368.15 ..02 ..124-125 | 370.03 ..02 ..121-122 |
| 362.11 ..02 ..124-125 | 363.42 ..02 ..124-125 | 365.43 ..02 ..124-125 | 368.16 ..02 ..124-125 | 370.04 ..02 ..121-122 |
| 362.12 ..02 ..124-125 | 363.43 ..02 ..124-125 | 365.44 ..02 ..124-125 | 368.2 ..02 ..123 | 370.05 ..02 ..121-122 |
| 362.13 ..02 ..124-125 | 363.50 ..02 ..124-125 | 365.51 ..02 ..124-125 | 368.30 ..02 ..124-125 | 370.06 ..02 ..121-122 |
| 362.14 ..02 ..124-125 | 363.51 ..02 ..124-125 | 365.52 ..02 ..124-125 | 368.31 ..02 ..124-125 | 370.07 ..02 ..124-125 |
| 362.15 ..02 ..124-125 | 363.52 ..02 ..124-125 | 365.59 ..02 ..124-125 | 368.32 ..02 ..124-125 | 370.20 ..02 ..124-125 |
| 362.16 ..02 ..124-125 | 363.53 ..02 ..124-125 | 365.60 ..02 ..124-125 | 368.33 ..02 ..124-125 | 370.21 ..02 ..124-125 |
| 362.17 ..02 ..124-125 | 363.54 ..02 ..124-125 | 365.61 ..02 ..124-125 | 368.34 ..02 ..124-125 | 370.22 ..02 ..124-125 |
| 362.18 ..02 ..124-125 | 363.55 ..02 ..124-125 | 365.62 ..02 ..124-125 | 368.40 ..02 ..123 | 370.23 ..02 ..124-125 |
| 362.21 ..02 ..124-125 | 363.56 ..02 ..124-125 | 365.63 ..02 ..124-125 | 368.41 ..02 ..123 | 370.24 ..02 ..124-125 |
| 362.29 ..02 ..124-125 | 363.57 ..02 ..124-125 | 365.64 ..02 ..124-125 | 368.42 ..02 ..124-125 | 370.31 ..02 ..124-125 |
| 362.30 ..02 ..123 | 363.61 ..02 ..124-125 | 365.65 ..02 ..124-125 | 368.43 ..02 ..123 | 370.32 ..02 ..124-125 |
| 362.31 ..02 ..123 | 363.62 ..02 ..124-125 | 365.81 ..02 ..124-125 | 368.44 ..02 ..123 | 370.33 ..02 ..124-125 |
| 362.32 ..02 ..123 | 363.63 ..02 ..124-125 | 365.82 ..02 ..124-125 | 368.45 ..02 ..123 | 370.34 ..02 ..124-125 |
| 362.33 ..02 ..123 | 363.70 ..02 ..124-125 | 365.83 ..02 ..124-125 | 368.46 ..02 ..123 | 370.35 ..02 ..124-125 |
| 362.34 ..02 ..123 | 363.71 ..02 ..124-125 | 365.89 ..02 ..124-125 | 368.47 ..02 ..123 | 370.40 ..02 ..124-125 |
| 362.35 ..02 ..123 | 363.72 ..02 ..124-125 | 365.9 ...02 ..124-125 | 368.51 ..02 ..124-125 | 370.44 ..02 ..124-125 |
| 362.36 ..02 ..123 | 363.8 ...02 ..124-125 | 366.00 ..02 ..124-125 | 368.52 ..02 ..124-125 | 370.49 ..02 ..124-125 |
| 362.37 ..02 ..123 | 363.9 ...02 ..124-125 | 366.01 ..02 ..124-125 | 368.53 ..02 ..124-125 | 370.50 ..02 ..124-125 |
| 362.40 ..02 ..124-125 | 364.00 ..02 ..124-125 | 366.02 ..02 ..124-125 | 368.54 ..02 ..124-125 | 370.52 ..02 ..124-125 |
| 362.41 ..02 ..124-125 | 364.01 ..02 ..124-125 | 366.03 ..02 ..124-125 | 368.55 ..02 ..123 | 370.54 ..02 ..124-125 |
| 362.42 ..02 ..124-125 | 364.02 ..02 ..124-125 | 366.04 ..02 ..124-125 | 368.59 ..02 ..124-125 | 370.55 ..02 ..121-122 |
| 362.43 ..02 ..124-125 | 364.03 ..02 ..124-125 | 366.09 ..02 ..124-125 | 368.60 ..02 ..124-125 | 370.59 ..02 ..124-125 |
| 362.50 ..02 ..124-125 | 364.04 ..02 ..124-125 | 366.10 ..02 ..124-125 | 368.61 ..02 ..124-125 | 370.60 ..02 ..124-125 |
| 362.51 ..02 ..124-125 | 364.05 ..02 ..124-125 | 366.11 ..02 ..124-125 | 368.62 ..02 ..124-125 | 370.61 ..02 ..124-125 |
| 362.52 ..02 ..124-125 | 364.10 ..02 ..124-125 | 366.12 ..02 ..124-125 | 368.63 ..02 ..124-125 | 370.62 ..02 ..124-125 |
| 362.53 ..02 ..124-125 | 364.11 ..02 ..124-125 | 366.13 ..02 ..124-125 | 368.69 ..02 ..124-125 | 370.63 ..02 ..124-125 |
| 362.54 ..02 ..124-125 | 364.21 ..02 ..124-125 | 366.14 ..02 ..124-125 | 368.8 ..02 ..124-125 | 370.64 ..02 ..124-125 |
| 362.55 ..02 ..124-125 | 364.22 ..02 ..124-125 | 366.15 ..02 ..124-125 | 368.9 ...02 ..124-125 | 370.8 ...02 ..124-125 |
| 362.56 ..02 ..124-125 | 364.23 ..02 ..124-125 | 366.16 ..02 ..124-125 | 369.00 ..02 ..124-125 | 370.9 ...02 ..124-125 |
| 362.57 ..02 ..124-125 | 364.24 ..02 ..124-125 | 366.17 ..02 ..124-125 | 369.01 ..02 ..124-125 | 371.00 ..02 ..124-125 |
| 362.60 ..02 ..124-125 | 364.3 ...02 ..124-125 | 366.18 ..02 ..124-125 | 369.02 ..02 ..124-125 | 371.01 ..02 ..124-125 |
| 362.61 ..02 ..124-125 | 364.41 ..02 ..124-125 | 366.19 ..02 ..124-125 | 369.03 ..02 ..124-125 | 371.02 ..02 ..124-125 |
| 362.62 ..02 ..124-125 | 364.42 ..02 ..124-125 | 366.20 ..02 ..124-125 | 369.04 ..02 ..124-125 | 371.03 ..02 ..124-125 |
| 362.63 ..02 ..124-125 | 364.51 ..02 ..124-125 | 366.21 ..02 ..124-125 | 369.05 ..02 ..124-125 | 371.04 ..02 ..124-125 |
| 362.64 ..02 ..124-125 | 364.52 ..02 ..124-125 | 366.22 ..02 ..124-125 | 369.06 ..02 ..124-125 | 371.05 ..02 ..124-125 |
| 362.65 ..02 ..124-125 | 364.53 ..02 ..124-125 | 366.23 ..02 ..124-125 | 369.07 ..02 ..124-125 | 371.10 ..02 ..124-125 |
| 362.66 ..02 ..124-125 | 364.54 ..02 ..124-125 | 366.30 ..02 ..124-125 | 369.08 ..02 ..124-125 | 371.11 ..02 ..124-125 |
| 362.70 ..02 ..124-125 | 364.55 ..02 ..124-125 | 366.31 ..02 ..124-125 | 369.10 ..02 ..124-125 | 371.12 ..02 ..124-125 |

| DX | MDC | DRG | DX | MDC | DRG | DX | MDC | DRG | DX | MDC | DRG | DX | MDC | DRG |
|---|---|---|---|---|---|---|---|---|---|---|---|---|---|---|
| 371.13 | 02 | 124-125 | 372.64 | 02 | 124-125 | 375.21 | 02 | 124-125 | 377.41 | 02 | 123 | 379.04 | 02 | 124-125 |
| 371.14 | 02 | 124-125 | 372.71 | 02 | 124-125 | 375.22 | 02 | 124-125 | 377.42 | 02 | 123 | 379.05 | 02 | 124-125 |
| 371.15 | 02 | 124-125 | 372.72 | 02 | 124-125 | 375.30 | 02 | 124-125 | 377.43 | 02 | 123 | 379.06 | 02 | 124-125 |
| 371.16 | 02 | 124-125 | 372.73 | 02 | 124-125 | 375.31 | 02 | 121-122 | 377.49 | 02 | 123 | 379.07 | 02 | 124-125 |
| 371.20 | 02 | 124-125 | 372.74 | 02 | 124-125 | 375.32 | 02 | 121-122 | 377.51 | 01 | 091-093 | 379.09 | 02 | 124-125 |
| 371.21 | 02 | 124-125 | 372.75 | 02 | 124-125 | 375.33 | 02 | 124-125 | 377.52 | 01 | 091-093 | 379.11 | 02 | 124-125 |
| 371.22 | 02 | 124-125 | 372.81 | 02 | 124-125 | 375.41 | 02 | 124-125 | 377.53 | 01 | 091-093 | 379.12 | 02 | 124-125 |
| 371.23 | 02 | 124-125 | 327.89 | 02 | 124-125 | 375.42 | 02 | 124-125 | 377.54 | 01 | 091-093 | 379.13 | 02 | 124-125 |
| 371.24 | 02 | 124-125 | 372.9 | 02 | 124-125 | 375.43 | 02 | 124-125 | 377.61 | 01 | 091-093 | 379.14 | 02 | 124-125 |
| 371.30 | 02 | 124-125 | 373.00 | 02 | 124-125 | 375.51 | 02 | 124-125 | 377.62 | 01 | 091-093 | 379.15 | 02 | 124-125 |
| 371.31 | 02 | 124-125 | 373.01 | 02 | 124-125 | 375.52 | 02 | 124-125 | 377.63 | 01 | 091-093 | 379.16 | 02 | 124-125 |
| 371.32 | 02 | 124-125 | 373.02 | 02 | 124-125 | 375.53 | 02 | 124-125 | 377.71 | 01 | 091-093 | 379.19 | 02 | 124-125 |
| 371.33 | 02 | 124-125 | 373.11 | 02 | 124-125 | 375.54 | 02 | 124-125 | 377.72 | 01 | 091-093 | 379.21 | 02 | 124-125 |
| 371.40 | 02 | 124-125 | 373.12 | 02 | 124-125 | 375.55 | 02 | 124-125 | 377.73 | 01 | 091-093 | 379.22 | 02 | 124-125 |
| 371.41 | 02 | 124-125 | 373.13 | 02 | 124-125 | 375.56 | 02 | 124-125 | 377.75 | 01 | 091-093 | 379.23 | 02 | 124-125 |
| 371.42 | 02 | 124-125 | 373.2 | 02 | 124-125 | 375.57 | 02 | 124-125 | 377.9 | 01 | 091-093 | 379.24 | 02 | 124-125 |
| 371.43 | 02 | 124-125 | 373.31 | 02 | 124-125 | 375.61 | 02 | 124-125 | 378.00 | 02 | 124-125 | 379.25 | 02 | 124-125 |
| 371.44 | 02 | 124-125 | 373.32 | 02 | 124-125 | 375.69 | 02 | 124-125 | 378.01 | 02 | 124-125 | 379.26 | 02 | 124-125 |
| 371.45 | 02 | 124-125 | 373.33 | 02 | 124-125 | 375.81 | 02 | 124-125 | 378.02 | 02 | 124-125 | 379.29 | 02 | 124-125 |
| 371.46 | 02 | 124-125 | 373.34 | 02 | 124-125 | 375.89 | 02 | 124-125 | 378.03 | 02 | 124-125 | 379.31 | 02 | 124-125 |
| 371.48 | 02 | 124-125 | 373.4 | 02 | 124-125 | 375.9 | 02 | 124-125 | 378.04 | 02 | 124-125 | 379.32 | 02 | 124-125 |
| 371.49 | 02 | 124-125 | 373.5 | 02 | 124-125 | 376.00 | 02 | 124-125 | 378.05 | 02 | 124-125 | 379.33 | 02 | 124-125 |
| 371.50 | 02 | 124-125 | 373.6 | 02 | 124-125 | 376.01 | 02 | 121-122 | 378.06 | 02 | 124-125 | 379.34 | 02 | 124-125 |
| 371.51 | 02 | 124-125 | 373.8 | 02 | 124-125 | 376.02 | 02 | 121-122 | 378.07 | 02 | 124-125 | 379.39 | 02 | 124-125 |
| 371.52 | 02 | 124-125 | 373.9 | 02 | 124-125 | 376.03 | 02 | 121-122 | 378.08 | 02 | 124-125 | 379.40 | 02 | 123 |
| 371.53 | 02 | 124-125 | 374.00 | 02 | 124-125 | 376.04 | 02 | 121-122 | 378.10 | 02 | 124-125 | 379.41 | 02 | 123 |
| 371.54 | 02 | 124-125 | 374.01 | 02 | 124-125 | 376.10 | 02 | 124-125 | 378.11 | 02 | 124-125 | 379.42 | 02 | 123 |
| 371.55 | 02 | 124-125 | 374.02 | 02 | 124-125 | 376.11 | 02 | 124-125 | 378.12 | 02 | 124-125 | 379.43 | 02 | 123 |
| 371.56 | 02 | 124-125 | 374.03 | 02 | 124-125 | 376.12 | 02 | 124-125 | 378.13 | 02 | 124-125 | 379.45 | 01 | 056-057 |
| 371.57 | 02 | 124-125 | 374.04 | 02 | 124-125 | 376.13 | 02 | 124-125 | 378.14 | 02 | 124-125 | 379.46 | 02 | 123 |
| 371.58 | 02 | 124-125 | 374.05 | 02 | 124-125 | 376.21 | 02 | 124-125 | 378.15 | 02 | 124-125 | 379.49 | 02 | 123 |
| 371.60 | 02 | 124-125 | 374.10 | 02 | 124-125 | 376.22 | 02 | 124-125 | 378.16 | 02 | 124-125 | 379.50 | 02 | 123 |
| 371.61 | 02 | 124-125 | 374.11 | 02 | 124-125 | 376.30 | 02 | 124-125 | 378.17 | 02 | 124-125 | 379.51 | 02 | 124-125 |
| 371.62 | 02 | 124-125 | 374.12 | 02 | 124-125 | 376.31 | 02 | 124-125 | 378.18 | 02 | 124-125 | 379.52 | 02 | 123 |
| 371.70 | 02 | 124-125 | 374.13 | 02 | 124-125 | 376.32 | 02 | 124-125 | 378.20 | 02 | 124-125 | 379.53 | 02 | 124-125 |
| 371.71 | 02 | 124-125 | 374.14 | 02 | 124-125 | 376.33 | 02 | 124-125 | 378.21 | 02 | 124-125 | 379.54 | 02 | 123 |
| 371.72 | 02 | 124-125 | 374.20 | 02 | 124-125 | 376.34 | 02 | 123 | 378.22 | 02 | 124-125 | 379.55 | 02 | 123 |
| 371.73 | 02 | 124-125 | 374.21 | 02 | 124-125 | 376.35 | 02 | 123 | 378.23 | 02 | 124-125 | 379.56 | 02 | 124-125 |
| 371.81 | 02 | 124-125 | 374.22 | 02 | 124-125 | 376.36 | 02 | 123 | 378.24 | 02 | 124-125 | 379.57 | 02 | 123 |
| 371.82 | 02 | 124-125 | 374.23 | 02 | 124-125 | 376.40 | 02 | 124-125 | 378.30 | 02 | 124-125 | 379.58 | 02 | 123 |
| 371.89 | 02 | 124-125 | 374.30 | 02 | 123 | 376.41 | 02 | 124-125 | 378.31 | 02 | 124-125 | 379.59 | 02 | 124-125 |
| 371.9 | 02 | 124-125 | 374.31 | 02 | 123 | 376.42 | 02 | 124-125 | 378.32 | 02 | 124-125 | 379.60 | 02 | 124-125 |
| 372.00 | 02 | 124-125 | 374.32 | 02 | 123 | 376.43 | 02 | 124-125 | 378.33 | 02 | 124-125 | 379.61 | 02 | 124-125 |
| 372.01 | 02 | 124-125 | 374.33 | 02 | 124-125 | 376.44 | 02 | 124-125 | 378.34 | 02 | 124-125 | 379.62 | 02 | 124-125 |
| 372.02 | 02 | 124-125 | 374.34 | 02 | 124-125 | 376.45 | 02 | 124-125 | 378.35 | 02 | 124-125 | 379.63 | 02 | 124-125 |
| 372.03 | 02 | 124-125 | 374.41 | 02 | 124-125 | 376.46 | 02 | 124-125 | 378.40 | 02 | 124-125 | 379.8 | 02 | 124-125 |
| 372.04 | 02 | 124-125 | 374.43 | 02 | 124-125 | 376.47 | 02 | 124-125 | 378.41 | 02 | 124-125 | 379.90 | 02 | 124-125 |
| 372.05 | 02 | 124-125 | 374.44 | 02 | 124-125 | 376.50 | 02 | 124-125 | 378.42 | 02 | 124-125 | 379.91 | 02 | 124-125 |
| 372.10 | 02 | 124-125 | 374.45 | 02 | 123 | 376.51 | 02 | 124-125 | 378.43 | 02 | 124-125 | 379.92 | 02 | 124-125 |
| 372.11 | 02 | 124-125 | 374.46 | 02 | 124-125 | 376.52 | 02 | 124-125 | 378.44 | 02 | 124-125 | 379.93 | 02 | 124-125 |
| 372.12 | 02 | 124-125 | 374.50 | 02 | 124-125 | 376.6 | 02 | 124-125 | 378.45 | 02 | 124-125 | 379.99 | 02 | 124-125 |
| 372.13 | 02 | 124-125 | 374.51 | 09 | 606-607 | 376.81 | 02 | 124-125 | 378.50 | 02 | 123 | 380.00 | 03 | 152-153 |
| 372.14 | 02 | 124-125 | 374.52 | 02 | 124-125 | 376.82 | 02 | 123 | 378.51 | 02 | 123 | 380.01 | 08 | 564-566 |
| 372.15 | 02 | 124-125 | 374.53 | 02 | 124-125 | 376.89 | 02 | 124-125 | 378.52 | 02 | 123 | 380.02 | 08 | 564-566 |
| 372.20 | 02 | 124-125 | 374.54 | 02 | 124-125 | 376.9 | 02 | 124-125 | 378.53 | 02 | 123 | 380.03 | 08 | 564-566 |
| 372.21 | 02 | 124-125 | 374.55 | 02 | 124-125 | 377.00 | 01 | 091-093 | 378.54 | 02 | 123 | 380.10 | 03 | 154-156 |
| 372.22 | 02 | 124-125 | 374.56 | 02 | 124-125 | 377.01 | 01 | 091-093 | 378.55 | 02 | 123 | 380.11 | 03 | 154-156 |
| 372.30 | 02 | 124-125 | 374.81 | 02 | 124-125 | 377.02 | 02 | 124-125 | 378.56 | 02 | 123 | 380.12 | 03 | 154-156 |
| 372.31 | 02 | 124-125 | 374.82 | 02 | 124-125 | 377.03 | 02 | 124-125 | 378.60 | 02 | 124-125 | 380.13 | 03 | 154-156 |
| 372.33 | 02 | 124-125 | 374.83 | 02 | 124-125 | 377.04 | 01 | 091-093 | 378.61 | 02 | 124-125 | 380.14 | 03 | 154-156 |
| 372.39 | 02 | 124-125 | 374.84 | 02 | 124-125 | 377.10 | 02 | 123 | 378.62 | 02 | 124-125 | 380.15 | 03 | 154-156 |
| 372.40 | 02 | 124-125 | 374.85 | 02 | 124-125 | 377.11 | 02 | 123 | 378.63 | 02 | 124-125 | 380.16 | 03 | 154-156 |
| 372.41 | 02 | 124-125 | 374.86 | 02 | 124-125 | 377.12 | 02 | 123 | 378.71 | 02 | 124-125 | 380.21 | 03 | 154-156 |
| 372.42 | 02 | 124-125 | 374.87 | 02 | 124-125 | 377.13 | 02 | 124-125 | 378.72 | 02 | 123 | 380.22 | 03 | 154-156 |
| 372.43 | 02 | 124-125 | 374.89 | 02 | 124-125 | 377.14 | 02 | 124-125 | 378.73 | 02 | 123 | 380.23 | 03 | 154-156 |
| 372.44 | 02 | 124-125 | 374.9 | 02 | 124-125 | 377.15 | 02 | 123 | 378.81 | 02 | 124-125 | 380.30 | 03 | 154-156 |
| 372.45 | 02 | 124-125 | 375.00 | 02 | 124-125 | 377.16 | 02 | 123 | 378.82 | 02 | 124-125 | 380.31 | 03 | 154-156 |
| 372.50 | 02 | 124-125 | 375.01 | 02 | 121-122 | 377.21 | 02 | 123 | 378.83 | 02 | 124-125 | 380.32 | 03 | 154-156 |
| 372.51 | 02 | 124-125 | 375.02 | 02 | 124-125 | 377.22 | 02 | 124-125 | 378.84 | 02 | 124-125 | 380.39 | 03 | 154-156 |
| 372.52 | 02 | 124-125 | 375.03 | 02 | 124-125 | 377.23 | 02 | 124-125 | 378.85 | 02 | 124-125 | 380.4 | 03 | 154-156 |
| 372.53 | 02 | 124-125 | 375.11 | 02 | 124-125 | 377.24 | 02 | 123 | 378.86 | 01 | 091-093 | 380.50 | 03 | 154-156 |
| 372.54 | 02 | 124-125 | 375.12 | 02 | 124-125 | 377.30 | 02 | 123 | 378.87 | 02 | 123 | 380.51 | 03 | 154-156 |
| 372.55 | 02 | 124-125 | 375.13 | 02 | 124-125 | 377.31 | 02 | 123 | 378.9 | 02 | 124-125 | 380.52 | 03 | 154-156 |
| 372.56 | 02 | 124-125 | 375.14 | 02 | 124-125 | 377.32 | 02 | 123 | 379.00 | 02 | 124-125 | 380.53 | 03 | 154-156 |
| 372.61 | 02 | 124-125 | 375.15 | 02 | 124-125 | 377.33 | 02 | 123 | 379.01 | 02 | 124-125 | 380.81 | 03 | 154-156 |
| 372.62 | 02 | 124-125 | 375.16 | 02 | 124-125 | 377.34 | 02 | 123 | 379.02 | 02 | 124-125 | 380.89 | 03 | 154-156 |
| 372.63 | 02 | 124-125 | 375.20 | 02 | 124-125 | 377.39 | 02 | 123 | 379.03 | 02 | 124-125 | 380.9 | 03 | 154-156 |

| DX . . .MDC . .DRG | DX . . .MDC . .DRG | DX . . .MDC . .DRG | DX . . .MDC . .DRG | DX . . .MDC . .DRG |
|---|---|---|---|---|
| 381.00 . .03 . .152-153 | 385.35 . .03 . .154-156 | 389.13 . .03 . .154-156 | 404.91 . .05 . .280-281, 286, 291-293 | 420.90 . .05 . .286, 314-316 |
| 381.01 . .03 . .152-153 | 385.82 . .03 . .154-156 | 389.14 . .03 . .154-156 | 404.92 . .11 . .682-684 | 420.91 . .05 . .286, 314-316 |
| 381.02 . .03 . .152-153 | 385.83 . .03 . .154-156 | 389.15 . .03 . .154-156 | 404.93 . .05 . .280-281, 286, 291-293 | 420.99 . .05 . .286, 314-316 |
| 381.03 . .03 . .152-153 | 385.89 . .03 . .154-156 | 389.16 . .03 . .154-156 | | 421.0 . . .05 . .286, 288-290 |
| 381.04 . .03 . .152-153 | 385.9 . . .03 . .154-156 | 389.17 . .03 . .154-156 | 405.01 . .05 . .304-305 | 421.1 . . .05 . .286, 288-290 |
| 381.05 . .03 . .152-153 | 386.00 . .03 . .149 | 389.18 . .03 . .154-156 | 405.09 . .05 . .304-305 | 421.9 . . .05 . .286, 288-290 |
| 381.06 . .03 . .152-153 | 386.01 . .03 . .149 | 389.20 . .03 . .154-156 | 405.11 . .05 . .304-305 | 422. . . .05 . .286, 314-316 |
| 381.10 . .03 . .152-153 | 386.02 . .03 . .149 | 389.21 . .03 . .154-156 | 405.19 . .05 . .304-305 | 422.90 . .05 . .286, 314-316 |
| 381.19 . .03 . .152-153 | 386.03 . .03 . .149 | 389.22 . .03 . .154-156 | 405.91 . .05 . .304-305 | 422.91 . .05 . .286, 314-316 |
| 381.20 . .03 . .152-153 | 386.04 . .03 . .149 | 389.7 . . .03 . .154-156 | 405.99 . .05 . .304-305 | 422.92 . .05 . .286, 314-316 |
| 381.29 . .03 . .152-153 | 386.10 . .03 . .149 | 389.8 . . .03 . .154-156 | 410.00 . .05 . .314-316 | 422.93 . .05 . .286, 314-316 |
| 381.3 . . .03 . .152-153 | 386.11 . .03 . .149 | 389.9 . . .03 . .154-156 | 410.01 . .05 . .280-285 | 422.99 . .05 . .286, 314-316 |
| 381.4 . . .03 . .152-153 | 386.12 . .03 . .149 | | 410.02 . .05 . .314-316 | 423.0 . . .05 . .286, 314-316 |
| 381.50 . .03 . .152-153 | 386.19 . .03 . .149 | **Diseases of the Circulartory** | 410.10 . .05 . .314-316 | 423.1 . . .05 . .314-316 |
| 381.51 . .03 . .152-153 | 386.2 . . .03 . .149 | **System** | 410.11 . .05 . .280-285 | 423.2 . . .05 . .314-316 |
| 381.52 . .03 . .152-153 | 386.30 . .03 . .149 | 390 . . . . .08 . .545-547 | 410.12 . .05 . .314-316 | 423.3 . . .05 . .314-316 |
| 381.60 . .03 . .154-156 | 386.31 . .03 . .149 | 391.0 . . .05 . .314-316 | 410.20 . .05 . .314-316 | 423.8 . . .05 . .314-316 |
| 381.61 . .03 . .154-156 | 386.32 . .03 . .149 | 391.1 . . .05 . .306-307 | 410.21 . .05 . .280-285 | 423.9 . . .05 . .314-316 |
| 381.62 . .03 . .154-156 | 386.33 . .03 . .149 | 391.2 . . .05 . .314-316 | 410.22 . .05 . .314-316 | 424.0 . . .05 . .306-307 |
| 381.63 . .03 . .154-156 | 386.34 . .03 . .149 | 391.8 . . .05 . .314-316 | 410.30 . .05 . .314-316 | 424.1 . . .05 . .306-307 |
| 381.7 . . .03 . .154-156 | 386.35 . .03 . .149 | 391.9 . . .05 . .314-316 | 410.31 . .05 . .280-285 | 424.2 . . .05 . .306-307 |
| 381.81 . .03 . .154-156 | 386.40 . .03 . .154-156 | 392.0 . . .05 . .314-316 | 410.32 . .05 . .314-316 | 424.3 . . .05 . .306-307 |
| 381.89 . .03 . .154-156 | 386.41 . .03 . .154-156 | 392.9 . . .05 . .314-316 | 410.40 . .05 . .314-316 | 424.90 . .05 . .286, 306-307 |
| 381.9 . . .03 . .154-156 | 386.42 . .03 . .154-156 | 393 . . .05 . .314-316 | 410.41 . .05 . .280-285 | 424.91 . .05 . .286, 306-307 |
| 382.00 . .03 . .152-153 | 386.43 . .03 . .154-156 | 394.0 . . .05 . .306-307 | 410.42 . .05 . .314-316 | 424.99 . .05 . .306-307 |
| 382.01 . .03 . .152-153 | 386.48 . .03 . .154-156 | 394.1 . . .05 . .306-307 | 410.50 . .05 . .314-316 | 425.0 . . .05 . .314-316 |
| 382.02 . .03 . .152-153 | 386.50 . .03 . .149 | 394.2 . . .05 . .306-307 | 410.51 . .05 . .280-285 | 425.1 . . .05 . .314-316 |
| 382.1 . . .03 . .152-153 | 386.51 . .03 . .149 | 394.9 . . .05 . .306-307 | 410.52 . .05 . .314-316 | 425.2 . . .05 . .286, 314-316 |
| 382.2 . . .03 . .152-153 | 386.52 . .03 . .149 | 395.0 . . .05 . .306-307 | 410.60 . .05 . .314-316 | 425.3 . . .05 . .286, 314-316 |
| 382.3 . . .03 . .152-153 | 386.53 . .03 . .149 | 395.1 . . .05 . .306-307 | 410.61 . .05 . .280-285 | 425.4 . . .05 . .286, 314-316 |
| 382.4 . . .03 . .152-153 | 386.54 . .03 . .149 | 395.2 . . .05 . .306-307 | 410.62 . .05 . .314-316 | 425.5 . . .05 . .286, 314-316 |
| 382.9 . . .03 . .152-153 | 386.55 . .03 . .149 | 395.9 . . .05 . .306-307 | 410.70 . .05 . .314-316 | 425.7 . . .05 . .286, 314-316 |
| 383.00 . .03 . .152-153 | 386.56 . .03 . .149 | 396.0 . . .05 . .306-307 | 410.71 . .05 . .280-285 | 425.8 . . .05 . .286, 314-316 |
| 383.01 . .03 . .152-153 | 386.58 . .03 . .149 | 396.1 . . .05 . .306-307 | 410.72 . .05 . .314-316 | 425.9 . . .05 . .286, 314-316 |
| 383.02 . .03 . .152-153 | 386.8 . . .03 . .149 | 396.2 . . .05 . .306-307 | 410.80 . .05 . .314-316 | 426.0 . . .05 . .280-281, 308-310 |
| 383.1 . . .03 . .152-153 | 386.9 . . .03 . .149 | 396.3 . . .05 . .306-307 | 410.81 . .05 . .280-285 | 426.10 . .05 . .280-281, 308-310 |
| 383.20 . .03 . .152-153 | 387.0 . . .03 . .154-156 | 396.8 . . .05 . .306-307 | 410.82 . .05 . .314-316 | 426.11 . .05 . .308-310 |
| 383.21 . .03 . .152-153 | 387.1 . . .03 . .154-156 | 396.9 . . .05 . .306-307 | 410.90 . .05 . .314-316 | 426.12 . .05 . .280-281, 308-310 |
| 383.22 . .03 . .152-153 | 387.2 . . .03 . .154-156 | 397.0 . . .05 . .306-307 | 410.91 . .05 . .280-285 | 426.13 . .05 . .280-281, 308-310 |
| 383.30 . .03 . .154-156 | 387.8 . . .03 . .154-156 | 397.1 . . .05 . .306-307 | 410.92 . .05 . .314-316 | 426.2 . . .05 . .308-310 |
| 383.31 . .03 . .154-156 | 387.9 . . .03 . .154-156 | 397.9 . . .05 . .306-307 | 411.0 . . .05 . .280-281, 314-316 | 426.3 . . .05 . .280-281, 308-310 |
| 383.32 . .03 . .154-156 | 388.00 . .03 . .154-156 | 398.0 . . .05 . .314-316 | 411.1 . . .05 . .286, 311 | 426.4 . . .05 . .308-310 |
| 383.33 . .03 . .154-156 | 388.01 . .03 . .154-156 | 398.90 . .05 . .314-316 | 411.81 . .05 . .286, 311 | 426.50 . .05 . .308-310 |
| 383.81 . .03 . .154-156 | 388.02 . .03 . .154-156 | 398.91 . .05 . .280-281, 286,291-293 | 411.89 . .05 . .286, 311 | 426.51 . .05 . .280-281, 308-310 |
| 383.89 . .03 . .154-156 | 388.10 . .03 . .154-156 | | 412. . . .05 . .302-303 | 426.52 . .05 . .280-281, 308-310 |
| 383.9 . . .03 . .152-153 | 388.11 . .03 . .154-156 | 398.99 . .05 . .314-316 | 413.0 . . .05 . .311 | 426.53 . .05 . .280-281, 308-310 |
| 384.00 . .03 . .152-153 | 388.12 . .03 . .154-156 | 401.0 . . .05 . .304-305 | 413.1 . . .05 . .311 | 426.54 . .05 . .280-281, 308-310 |
| 384.01 . .03 . .152-153 | 388.2 . . .03 . .154-156 | 401.1 . . .05 . .304-305 | 413.9 . . .05 . .311 | 426.6 . . .05 . .308-310 |
| 384.09 . .03 . .152-153 | 388.30 . .03 . .154-156 | 401.9 . . .05 . .304-305 | 414.00 . .05 . .302-303 | 426.7 . . .05 . .308-310 |
| 384.1 . . .03 . .152-153 | 388.31 . .03 . .154-156 | 402.00 . .05 . .304-305 | 414.01 . .05 . .302-303 | 426.81 . .05 . .308-310 |
| 384.20 . .03 . .154-156 | 388.32 . .03 . .154-156 | 402.01 . .05 . .280-281, 286, 291-293 | 414.02 . .05 . .302-303 | 426.82 . .05 . .308-310 |
| 384.21 . .03 . .154-156 | 388.40 . .03 . .154-156 | | 414.03 . .05 . .302-303 | 426.89 . .05 . .308-310 |
| 384.22 . .03 . .154-156 | 388.41 . .03 . .154-156 | 402.10 . .05 . .304-305 | 414.04 . .05 . .302-303 | 426.9 . . .05 . .308-310 |
| 384.23 . .03 . .154-156 | 388.42 . .03 . .154-156 | 402.11 . .05 . .280-281, 286, 291-293 | 414.05 . .05 . .302-303 | 427.0 . . .05 . .280-281, 308-310 |
| 384.24 . .03 . .154-156 | 388.43 . .03 . .154-156 | | 414.06 . .05 . .302-303 | 427.1 . . .05 . .280-281, 286, 308-310 |
| 384.25 . .03 . .154-156 | 388.44 . .03 . .154-156 | 402.90 . .05 . .304-305 | 414.07 . .05 . .302-303 | |
| 384.81 . .03 . .154-156 | 388.45 . .19 . .886 | 402.91 . .05 . .280-281, 286, 291-293 | 414.10 . .05 . .280-281, 314-316 | 427.2 . . .05 . .280-281, 308-310 |
| 384.82 . .03 . .154-156 | 388.5 . . .03 . .154-156 | | 414.11 . .05 . .280-281, 314-316 | 427.31 . .05 . .280-281, 308-310 |
| 384.9 . . .03 . .154-156 | 388.60 . .03 . .154-156 | 403.00 . .11 . .698-700 | 414.12 . .05 . .280-281, 314-316 | 427.32 . .05 . .280-281, 308-310 |
| 385.00 . .03 . .154-156 | 388.61 . .01 . .091-093 | 403.01 . .11 . .682-684 | 414.19 . .05 . .280-281, 314-316 | 427.41 . .05 . .280-281, 308-310 |
| 385.01 . .03 . .154-156 | 388.69 . .03 . .154-156 | 403.10 . .11 . .698-700 | 414.2 . . .05 . .302-303 | 427.42 . .05 . .280-281, 308-310 |
| 385.02 . .03 . .154-156 | 388.70 . .03 . .154-156 | 403.11 . .11 . .682-684 | 414.8 . . .05 . .302-303 | 427.5 . . .05 . .280-281, 286, 296-298 |
| 385.03 . .03 . .154-156 | 388.71 . .03 . .154-156 | 403.90 . .11 . .698-700 | 414.9 . . .05 . .302-303 | |
| 385.09 . .03 . .154-156 | 388.72 . .03 . .154-156 | 403.91 . .11 . .682-684 | 415.0 . . .05 . .280-281, 314-316 | 427.60 . .05 . .308-310 |
| 385.10 . .03 . .154-156 | 388.8 . . .03 . .154-156 | 404.00 . .05 . .304-305 | 415.11 . .04 . .175-176 | 427.61 . .05 . .308-310 |
| 385.11 . .03 . .154-156 | 388.9 . . .03 . .154-156 | 404.01 . .05 . .280-281, 286, 291-293 | 415.12 . .04 . .175-176 | 427.69 . .05 . .308-310 |
| 385.12 . .03 . .154-156 | 389.00 . .03 . .154-156 | | 415.19 . .04 . .175-176 | 427.81 . .05 . .308-310 |
| 385.13 . .03 . .154-156 | 389.01 . .03 . .154-156 | 404.02 . .11 . .682-684 | 416.0 . . .05 . .280-281, 314-316 | 427.89 . .05 . .308-310 |
| 385.19 . .03 . .154-156 | 389.02 . .03 . .154-156 | 404.03 . .05 . .280-281, 286, 291-293 | 416.1 . . .05 . .314-316 | 427.9 . . .05 . .308-310 |
| 385.21 . .03 . .154-156 | 389.03 . .03 . .154-156 | | 416.8 . . .05 . .314-316 | 428.0 . . .05 . .280-281, 286, 291-293 |
| 385.22 . .03 . .154-156 | 389.04 . .03 . .154-156 | 404.10 . .05 . .304-305 | 416.9 . . .05 . .314-316 | |
| 385.23 . .03 . .154-156 | 389.05 . .03 . .154-156 | 404.11 . .05 . .280-281, 286, 291-293 | 417.0 . . .05 . .314-316 | 428.1 . . .05 . .280-281, 286, 291-293 |
| 385.24 . .03 . .154-156 | 389.06 . .03 . .154-156 | | 417.1 . . .05 . .314-316 | |
| 385.30 . .03 . .154-156 | 389.08 . .03 . .154-156 | 404.12 . .11 . .682-684 | 417.8 . . .05 . .314-316 | 428.9 . . .05 . .280-281, 286, 291-293 |
| 385.31 . .03 . .154-156 | 389.10 . .03 . .154-156 | 404.13 . .05 . .280-281, 286, 291-293 | 417.9 . . .05 . .314-316 | |
| 385.32 . .03 . .154-156 | 389.11 . .03 . .154-156 | | 420.0 . . .05 . .286, 314-316 | 428.20 . .05 . .280-281, 286, 291-293 |
| 385.33 . .03 . .154-156 | 389.12 . .03 . .154-156 | 404.90 . .05 . .304-305 | | |

| DX | MDC | DRG |
|---|---|---|
| 428.21 | .05 | .280-281, 286, 291-293 |
| 428.22 | .05 | .280-281, 286, 291-293 |
| 428.23 | .05 | .280-281, 286, 291-293 |
| 428.30 | .05 | .280-281, 286, 291-293 |
| 428.31 | .05 | .280-281, 286, 291-293 |
| 428.32 | .05 | .280-281, 286, 291-293 |
| 428.33 | .05 | .280-281, 286, 291-293 |
| 428.40 | .05 | .280-281, 286, 291-293 |
| 428.41 | .05 | .280-281, 286, 291-293 |
| 428.42 | .05 | .280-281, 286, 291-293 |
| 428.43 | .05 | .280-281, 286, 291-293 |
| 428.9 | .05 | .280-281, 286, 291-293 |
| 429.0 | .05 | .314-316 |
| 429.1 | .05 | .314-316 |
| 429.2 | .05 | .302-303 |
| 429.3 | .05 | .302-303 |
| 429.4 | .05 | .286, 314-316 |
| 429.5 | .05 | .280-281, 286, 306-307 |
| 429.6 | .05 | .280-281, 286, 306-307 |
| 429.71 | .05 | .286, 314-316 |
| 429.79 | .05 | .286, 314-316 |
| 429.81 | .05 | .280-281, 286, 306-307 |
| 429.82 | .05 | .286, 314-316 |
| 429.83 | .05 | .314-316 |
| 429.89 | .05 | .302-303 |
| 429.9 | .05 | .302-303 |
| 430 | .01 | .064-066 |
| 431 | .01 | .064-066 |
| 432.0 | .01 | .064-066 |
| 432.1 | .01 | .064-066 |
| 432.9 | .01 | .064-066 |
| 433.00 | .01 | .067-068 |
| 433.01 | .01 | .061-066 |
| 433.10 | .01 | .067-068 |
| 433.11 | .01 | .061-066 |
| 433.20 | .01 | .067-068 |
| 433.21 | .01 | .061-066 |
| 433.30 | .01 | .067-068 |
| 433.31 | .01 | .061-066 |
| 433.80 | .01 | .067-068 |
| 433.81 | .01 | .061-066 |
| 433.90 | .01 | .067-068 |
| 433.91 | .01 | .061-066 |
| 434.00 | .01 | .067-068 |
| 434.01 | .01 | .061-066 |
| 434.10 | .01 | .067-068 |
| 434.11 | .01 | .061-066 |
| 434.90 | .01 | .067-068 |
| 434.91 | .01 | .061-066 |
| 435.0 | .01 | .069 |
| 435.1 | .01 | .069 |
| 435.2 | .01 | .069 |
| 435.8 | .01 | .069 |
| 435.9 | .01 | .069 |
| 436 | .01 | .067-068 |
| 437.0 | .01 | .070-072 |
| 437.1 | .01 | .069 |
| 437.2 | .01 | .077-079 |
| 437.3 | .01 | .091-093 |
| 437.4 | .01 | .100-103 |
| 437.5 | .01 | .091-093 |
| 437.6 | .01 | .091-093 |
| 437.7 | .01 | .070-072 |
| 437.8 | .01 | .070-072 |
| 437.9 | .01 | .070-072 |
| 438.0 | .01 | .056-057 |
| 438.10 | .01 | .056-057 |
| 438.11 | .01 | .056-057 |
| 438.12 | .01 | .056-057 |
| 438.19 | .01 | .056-057 |
| 438.20 | .01 | .056-057 |
| 438.21 | .01 | .056-057 |
| 438.22 | .01 | .056-057 |
| 438.30 | .01 | .056-057 |
| 438.31 | .01 | .056-057 |
| 438.32 | .01 | .056-057 |
| 438.40 | .01 | .056-057 |
| 438.41 | .01 | .056-057 |
| 438.42 | .01 | .056-057 |
| 438.50 | .01 | .056-057 |
| 438.51 | .01 | .056-057 |
| 438.52 | .01 | .056-057 |
| 438.53 | .01 | .056-057 |
| 438.6 | .01 | .056-057 |
| 438.7 | .01 | .056-057 |
| 438.81 | .01 | .056-057 |
| 438.82 | .01 | .056-057 |
| 438.83 | .01 | .056-057 |
| 438.84 | .01 | .056-057 |
| 438.85 | .01 | .056-057 |
| 438.89 | .01 | .056-057 |
| 438.9 | .01 | .056-057 |
| 440.0 | .05 | .299-301 |
| 440.1 | .11 | .698-700 |
| 440.20 | .05 | .299-301 |
| 440.21 | .05 | .299-301 |
| 440.22 | .05 | .299-301 |
| 440.23 | .05 | .299-301 |
| 440.24 | .05 | .299-301 |
| 440.29 | .05 | .299-301 |
| 440.30 | .05 | .299-301 |
| 440.31 | .05 | .299-301 |
| 440.32 | .05 | .299-301 |
| 440.4 | .05 | .299-301 |
| 440.8 | .05 | .299-301 |
| 440.9 | .05 | .299-301 |
| 441.00 | .05 | .280-281, 299-301 |
| 441.01 | .05 | .280-281, 299-301 |
| 441.02 | .05 | .280-281, 299-301 |
| 441.03 | .05 | .280-281, 299-301 |
| 441.1 | .05 | .299-301 |
| 441.2 | .05 | .299-301 |
| 441.3 | .05 | .299-301 |
| 441.4 | .05 | .299-301 |
| 441.5 | .05 | .299-301 |
| 441.6 | .05 | .299-301 |
| 441.7 | .05 | .299-301 |
| 441.9 | .05 | .299-301 |
| 442.0 | .05 | .299-301 |
| 442.1 | .11 | .698-700 |
| 442.2 | .05 | .299-301 |
| 442.3 | .05 | .299-301 |
| 442.81 | .05 | .299-301 |
| 442.82 | .05 | .299-301 |
| 442.83 | .05 | .299-301 |
| 442.84 | .05 | .299-301 |
| 442.89 | .05 | .299-301 |
| 442.9 | .05 | .299-301 |
| 443.0 | .08 | .545-547 |
| 443.1 | .05 | .299-301 |
| 443.21 | .05 | .299-301 |
| 443.22 | .05 | .299-301 |
| 443.23 | .11 | .698-700 |
| 443.24 | .05 | .299-301 |
| 443.29 | .05 | .299-301 |
| 443.81 | .05 | .299-301 |
| 443.82 | .05 | .299-301 |
| 443.89 | .05 | .299-301 |
| 443.9 | .05 | .299-301 |
| 444.0 | .05 | .299-301 |
| 444.1 | .05 | .299-301 |
| 444.21 | .05 | .299-301 |
| 444.22 | .05 | .299-301 |
| 444.81 | .05 | .299-301 |
| 444.89 | .05 | .299-301 |
| 444.9 | .05 | .299-301 |
| 445.01 | .05 | .299-301 |
| 445.02 | .05 | .299-301 |
| 445.81 | .11 | .698-700 |
| 445.89 | .05 | .299-301 |
| 446.0 | .08 | .545-547 |
| 446.1 | .08 | .545-547 |
| 446.20 | .08 | .545-547 |
| 446.21 | .08 | .545-547 |
| 446.29 | .08 | .545-547 |
| 446.3 | .08 | .542-544 |
| 446.4 | .08 | .542-543 |
| 446.5 | .08 | .545-547 |
| 446.6 | .08 | .545-547 |
| 446.7 | .08 | .545-547 |
| 447.0 | .05 | .299-301 |
| 447.1 | .05 | .299-301 |
| 447.2 | .05 | .299-301 |
| 447.3 | .11 | .698-700 |
| 447.4 | .06 | .391-392 |
| 447.5 | .05 | .299-301 |
| 447.6 | .08 | .545-547 |
| 447.8 | .05 | .299-301 |
| 447.9 | .05 | .299-301 |
| 448.0 | .05 | .299-301 |
| 448.1 | .09 | .606-607 |
| 448.9 | .05 | .299-301 |
| 449 | .05 | .299-301 |
| 451.0 | .05 | .299-301 |
| 451.11 | .05 | .294-295 |
| 451.19 | .05 | .294-295 |
| 451.2 | .05 | .294-295 |
| 451.81 | .05 | .294-295 |
| 451.82 | .05 | .299-301 |
| 451.83 | .05 | .299-301 |
| 451.84 | .05 | .299-301 |
| 451.89 | .05 | .299-301 |
| 451.9 | .05 | .299-301 |
| 452 | .07 | .441-443 |
| 453.0 | .07 | .441-443 |
| 453.1 | .05 | .299-301 |
| 453.2 | .05 | .294-295 |
| 453.3 | .11 | .698-700 |
| 453.40 | .05 | .299-301 |
| 453.41 | .05 | .299-301 |
| 453.42 | .05 | .299-301 |
| 453.8 | .05 | .299-301 |
| 453.9 | .05 | .299-301 |
| 454.0 | .05 | .299-301 |
| 454.1 | .05 | .299-301 |
| 454.2 | .05 | .299-301 |
| 454.8 | .05 | .299-301 |
| 454.9 | .05 | .299-301 |
| 455.0 | .06 | .393-395 |
| 455.1 | .06 | .393-395 |
| 455.2 | .06 | .393-395 |
| 455.3 | .06 | .393-395 |
| 455.4 | .06 | .393-395 |
| 455.5 | .06 | .393-395 |
| 455.6 | .06 | .393-395 |
| 455.7 | .06 | .393-395 |
| 455.8 | .06 | .393-395 |
| 455.9 | .06 | .393-395 |
| 456.0 | .06 | .368-370 |
| 456.1 | .06 | .368-370 |
| 456.20 | .06 | .368-370 |
| 456.21 | .06 | .393-395 |
| 456.3 | .05 | .299-301 |
| 456.4 | .12 | .729-730 |
| 456.5 | .12 | .729-730 |
| 456.5 | .13 | .760-761 |
| 456.6 | .13 | .760-761 |
| 456.8 | .05 | .299-301 |
| 457.0 | .09 | .600-601 |
| 457.1 | .09 | .606-607 |
| 457.2 | .09 | .602-603 |
| 457.8 | .16 | .814-816 |
| 457.9 | .16 | .814-816 |
| 458.0 | .05 | .312 |
| 458.1 | .05 | .314-316 |
| 458.21 | .05 | .312 |
| 458.29 | .05 | .312 |
| 458.8 | .05 | .280-281, 314-316 |
| 458.9 | .05 | .280-281, 314-316 |
| 459.0 | .05 | .314-316 |
| 459.1 | .05 | .299-301 |
| 459.2 | .05 | .299-301 |
| 459.10 | .05 | .299-301 |
| 459.11 | .05 | .299-301 |
| 459.12 | .05 | .299-301 |
| 459.13 | .05 | .299-301 |
| 459.19 | .05 | .299-301 |
| 459.30 | .05 | .299-301 |
| 459.31 | .05 | .299-301 |
| 459.32 | .05 | .299-301 |
| 459.33 | .05 | .299-301 |
| 459.39 | .05 | .299-301 |
| 459.81 | .05 | .299-301 |
| 459.89 | .05 | .302-303 |
| 459.9 | .05 | .302-303 |

**Diseases of the Respiratory System**

| DX | MDC | DRG |
|---|---|---|
| 460 | .03 | .152-153 |
| 461.0 | .03 | .152-153 |
| 461.1 | .03 | .152-153 |
| 461.2 | .03 | .152-153 |
| 461.3 | .03 | .152-153 |
| 461.8 | .03 | .152-153 |
| 461.9 | .03 | .152-153 |
| 462 | .03 | .152-153 |
| 463 | .03 | .152-153 |
| 464.00 | .03 | .152-153 |
| 464.01 | .03 | .152-153 |
| 464.10 | .04 | .202-203 |
| 464.11 | .04 | .202-203 |
| 464.20 | .03 | .152-153 |
| 464.21 | .03 | .152-153 |
| 464.30 | .03 | .152-153 |
| 464.31 | .03 | .152-153 |
| 464.4 | .03 | .152-153 |
| 464.50 | .03 | .152-153 |
| 464.51 | .03 | .152-153 |
| 465.0 | .03 | .152-153 |
| 465.8 | .03 | .152-153 |
| 465.9 | .03 | .152-153 |
| 466.0 | .04 | .202-203 |
| 466.11 | .04 | .202-203 |
| 466.19 | .04 | .202-203 |
| 470 | .03 | .154-156 |
| 471.0 | .03 | .154-156 |
| 471.1 | .03 | .154-156 |
| 471.8 | .03 | .154-156 |
| 471.9 | .03 | .154-156 |
| 472.0 | .03 | .152-153 |
| 472.1 | .03 | .152-153 |
| 472.2 | .03 | .152-153 |
| 473.0 | .03 | .152-153 |
| 473.1 | .03 | .152-153 |
| 473.2 | .03 | .152-153 |
| 473.3 | .03 | .152-153 |
| 473.8 | .03 | .152-153 |
| 473.9 | .03 | .152-153 |
| 474.00 | .03 | .152-153 |
| 474.01 | .03 | .152-153 |
| 474.02 | .03 | .152-153 |
| 474.10 | .03 | .154-156 |
| 474.11 | .03 | .154-156 |
| 474.12 | .03 | .154-156 |
| 474.2 | .03 | .154-156 |
| 474.8 | .03 | .154-156 |
| 474.9 | .03 | .154-156 |
| 475 | .03 | .152-153 |
| 476.0 | .03 | .152-153 |
| 476.1 | .03 | .152-153 |
| 477.0 | .03 | .152-153 |
| 477.1 | .03 | .152-153 |
| 477.2 | .03 | .152-153 |
| 477.8 | .03 | .152-153 |
| 477.9 | .03 | .152-153 |
| 478.0 | .03 | .154-156 |
| 478.11 | .03 | .154-156 |
| 478.19 | .03 | .154-156 |
| 478.20 | .03 | .154-156 |
| 478.21 | .03 | .152-153 |
| 478.22 | .03 | .152-153 |
| 478.24 | .03 | .152-153 |
| 478.25 | .03 | .154-156 |
| 478.26 | .03 | .154-156 |
| 478.29 | .03 | .154-156 |
| 478.30 | .03 | .154-156 |
| 478.31 | .03 | .154-156 |
| 478.32 | .03 | .154-156 |
| 478.33 | .03 | .154-156 |
| 478.34 | .03 | .154-156 |
| 478.4 | .03 | .154-156 |
| 478.5 | .03 | .154-156 |
| 478.6 | .03 | .154-156 |
| 478.70 | .03 | .154-156 |
| 478.71 | .03 | .152-153 |
| 478.74 | .03 | .154-156 |
| 478.75 | .03 | .154-156 |
| 478.79 | .03 | .154-156 |
| 478.8 | .03 | .152-153 |
| 478.9 | .03 | .152-153 |
| 480.0 | .04 | .193-195 |
| 480.1 | .04 | .193-195 |
| 480.2 | .04 | .193-195 |
| 480.8 | .04 | .193-195 |
| 480.9 | .04 | .193-195 |
| 481 | .04 | .193-195 |
| 482.0 | .04 | .177-179 |
| 482.1 | .04 | .177-179 |
| 482.2 | .04 | .193-195 |
| 482.30 | .04 | .193-195 |
| 482.31 | .04 | .193-195 |
| 482.32 | .04 | .193-195 |
| 482.39 | .04 | .193-195 |
| 482.40 | .04 | .177-179 |
| 482.40 | .05 | .280-281 |
| 482.40 | .15 | .791, 793 |
| 482.41 | .04 | .177-179 |
| 482.41 | .05 | .280-281 |
| 482.41 | .15 | .791, 793 |
| 482.49 | .04 | .177-179 |
| 482.49 | .05 | .280-281 |
| 482.49 | .15 | .791, 793 |
| 482.81 | .04 | .177-179 |
| 482.81 | .15 | .791, 793 |
| 482.82 | .04 | .177-179 |
| 482.82 | .15 | .791, 793 |
| 482.83 | .04 | .177-179 |
| 482.83 | .15 | .791, 793 |
| 482.84 | .04 | .177-179 |
| 482.89 | .04 | .177-179 |
| 482.89 | .15 | .791, 793 |
| 482.9 | .04 | .193-195 |
| 483.0 | .04 | .193-195 |
| 483.1 | .04 | .193-195 |
| 483.1 | .15 | .791, 793 |
| 483.8 | .04 | .193-195 |
| 484.1 | .04 | .177-179 |
| 484.3 | .04 | .177-179 |
| 484.5 | .04 | .177-179 |
| 484.6 | .04 | .177-179 |

| DX ...MDC ..DRG | DX ...MDC ..DRG | DX ...MDC ..DRG | DX ...MDC ..DRG | DX ...MDC ..DRG |
|---|---|---|---|---|
| 484.7 ...04 ..177-179 | 516.0 ...04 ..196-198 | 521.49 ..03 ..157-159 | 524.56 ..03 ..157-159 | 527.4 ...03 ..154-156 |
| 484.8 ...04 ..177-179 | 516.1 ...04 ..196-198 | 521.5 ..03 ..157-159 | 524.57 ..03 ..157-159 | 527.5 ...03 ..154-156 |
| 485 .....04 ..193-195 | 516.2 ...04 ..196-198 | 521.6 ..03 ..157-159 | 524.59 ..03 ..157-159 | 527.6 ...03 ..154-156 |
| 486 .....04 ..193-195 | 516.3 ...04 ..196-198 | 521.7 ..03 ..157-159 | 524.60 ..03 ..157-159 | 527.7 ...03 ..154-156 |
| 487.0 ...04 ..193-195 | 516.8 ...04 ..196-198 | 521.81 ..03 .157-159 | 524.61 ..03 ..157-159 | 527.8 ...03 ..154-156 |
| 487.1 ...03 ..152-153 | 516.9 ...04 ..196-198 | 521.89 ..03 .157-159 | 524.62 ..03 ..157-159 | 527.9 ...03 ..154-156 |
| 487.8 ...18 ..864-866 | 517.1 ...04 ..196-198 | 521.9 ..03 ..157-159 | 524.63 ..03 ..157-159 | 528.00 ..03 ..157-159 |
| 488 .....03 ..152-153 | 517.2 ...04 ..196-198 | 522.0 ..03 ..157-159 | 524.64 ..03 ..157-159 | 528.01 ..03 ..157-159 |
| 490 .....04 ..202-203 | 517.3 ...04 ..196-198 | 522.1 ..03 ..157-159 | 524.69 ..03 ..157-159 | 528.02 ..03 ..157-159 |
| 491.0 ...04 ..202-203 | 517.8 ...04 ..196-198 | 522.2 ..03 ..157-159 | 524.70 ..03 ..157-159 | 528.09 ..03 ..157-159 |
| 491.1 ...04 ..190-192 | 518.0 ...04 ..205-206 | 522.3 ..03 ..157-159 | 524.71 ..03 ..157-159 | 528.1 ...03 ..157-159 |
| 491.20 ..04 ..190-192 | 518.1 ...04 ..199-201 | 522.4 ..03 ..157-159 | 524.72 ..03 ..157-159 | 528.2 ...03 ..157-159 |
| 491.21 ..04 ..190-192 | 518.2 ...04 ..205-206 | 522.5 ..03 ..157-159 | 524.73 ..03 ..157-159 | 528.3 ...03 ..157-159 |
| 491.22 ..04 ..190-192 | 518.3 ...04 ..196-198 | 522.6 ..03 ..157-159 | 524.74 ..03 ..157-159 | 528.4 ...03 ..157-159 |
| 491.8 ...04 ..190-192 | 518.4 ...04 ..189 | 522.7 ..03 ..157-159 | 524.75 ..03 ..157-159 | 528.5 ...03 ..157-159 |
| 491.9 ...04 ..190-192 | 518.5 ...04 ..189 | 522.8 ..03 ..157-159 | 524.76 ..03 ..157-159 | 528.6 ...03 ..157-159 |
| 492.0 ...04 ..190-192 | 518.6 ...04 ..196-198 | 522.9 ..03 ..157-159 | 524.79 ..03 ..157-159 | 528.71 ..03 ..157-159 |
| 492.8 ...04 ..190-192 | 518.7 ...04 ..205-206 | 523.00 ..03 ..157-159 | 524.81 ..03 ..157-159 | 528.72 ..03 ..157-159 |
| 493.00 ..04 ..202-203 | 518.81 ..04 ..189 | 523.01 ..03 ..157-159 | 524.82 ..03 ..157-159 | 528.79 ..03 ..157-159 |
| 493.01 ..04 ..202-203 | 518.82 ..04 ..204 | 523.10 ..03 ..157-159 | 524.89 ..03 ..157-159 | 528.8 ...03 ..157-159 |
| 493.02 ..04 ..202-203 | 518.83 ..04 ..189 | 523.11 ..03 ..157-159 | 524.9 ...03 ..157-159 | 528.9 ...03 ..157-159 |
| 493.10 ..04 ..202-203 | 518.84 ..04 ..189 | 523.20 ..03 ..157-159 | 525.0 ...03 ..157-159 | 529.0 ...03 ..157-159 |
| 493.11 ..04 ..202-203 | 518.89 ..04 ..205-206 | 523.21 ..03 ..157-159 | 525.10 ..03 ..157-159 | 529.1 ...03 ..157-159 |
| 493.12 ..04 ..202-203 | 519.00 ..04 ..205-206 | 523.22 ..03 ..157-159 | 525.11 ..03 ..157-159 | 529.2 ...03 ..157-159 |
| 493.20 ..04 ..190-192 | 519.0 ...04 ..205-206 | 523.23 ..03 ..157-159 | 525.12 ..03 ..157-159 | 529.3 ...03 ..157-159 |
| 493.21 ..04 ..190-192 | 519.02 ..04 ..205-206 | 523.24 ..03 ..157-159 | 525.13 ..03 ..157-159 | 529.4 ...03 ..157-159 |
| 493.22 ..04 ..190-192 | 519.09 ..04 ..205-206 | 523.25 ..03 ..157-159 | 525.19 ..03 ..157-159 | 529.5 ...03 ..157-159 |
| 493.81 ..04 ..202-203 | 519.11 ..04 ..202-203 | 523.30 ..03 ..157-159 | 525.20 ..03 ..157-159 | 529.6 ...03 ..157-159 |
| 493.82 ..04 ..202-203 | 519.19 ..04 ..202-203 | 523.31 ..03 ..157-159 | 525.21 ..03 ..157-159 | 529.8 ...03 ..157-159 |
| 493.90 ..04 ..202-203 | 519.2 ...04 ..177-179 | 523.32 ..03 ..157-159 | 525.22 ..03 ..157-159 | 529.9 ...03 ..157-159 |
| 493.91 ..04 ..202-203 | 519.3 ...04 ..205-206 | 523.33 ..03 ..157-159 | 525.23 ..03 ..157-159 | 530 .....06 ..391-392 |
| 493.92 ..04 ..202-203 | 519.4 ...04 ..205-206 | 523.40 ..03 ..157-159 | 525.24 ..03 ..157-159 | 530.10 ..06 ..391-392 |
| 494.0 ...04 ..190-192 | 519.8 ...04 ..205-206 | 523.41 ..03 ..157-159 | 525.25 ..03 ..157-159 | 530.11 ..06 ..391-392 |
| 494.1 ...04 ..190-192 | 519.9 ...04 ..205-206 | 523.42 ..03 ..157-159 | 525.26 ..03 ..157-159 | 530.12 ..06 ..391-392 |
| 495.0 ...04 ..196-198 | | 523.5 ..03 ..157-159 | 525.3 ...03 ..157-159 | 530.19 ..06 ..391-392 |
| 495.1 ...04 ..196-198 | **Diseases of the Digestive** | 523.6 ..03 ..157-159 | 525.40 ..03 ..157-159 | 530.20 ..06 ..380-382 |
| 495.2 ...04 ..196-198 | **Sysem** | 523.8 ..03 ..157-159 | 525.41 ..03 ..157-159 | 530.21 ..06 ..380-382 |
| 495.3 ...04 ..196-198 | 520.0 ...03 ..157-159 | 523.9 ..03 ..157-159 | 525.42 ..03 ..157-159 | 530.3 ...06 ..391-392 |
| 495.4 ...04 ..196-198 | 520.1 ...03 ..157-159 | 524.00 ..03 ..157-159 | 525.43 ..03 ..157-159 | 530.4 ...06 ..368-370 |
| 495.5 ...04 ..196-198 | 520.2 ...03 ..157-159 | 524.01 ..03 ..157-159 | 525.44 ..03 ..157-159 | 530.5 ...06 ..391-392 |
| 495.6 ...04 ..196-198 | 520.3 ...03 ..157-159 | 524.02 ..03 ..157-159 | 525.50 ..03 ..157-159 | 530.6 ...06 ..391-392 |
| 495.7 ...04 ..196-198 | 520.4 ...03 ..157-159 | 524.03 ..03 ..157-159 | 525.51 ..03 ..157-159 | 530.7 ...06 ..368-370 |
| 495.8 ...04 ..196-198 | 520.5 ...03 ..157-159 | 524.04 ..03 ..157-159 | 525.52 ..03 ..157-159 | 530.81 ..06 ..391-392 |
| 495.9 ...04 ..196-198 | 520.6 ...03 ..157-159 | 524.05 ..03 ..157-159 | 525.53 ..03 ..157-159 | 530.82 ..06 ..368-370 |
| 496 .....04 ..190-192 | 520.7 ...03 ..157-159 | 524.06 ..03 ..157-159 | 525.54 ..03 ..157-159 | 530.83 ..06 ..391-392 |
| 500 .....04 ..196-198 | 520.8 ...03 ..157-159 | 524.07 ..03 ..157-159 | 525.60 ..03 ..157-159 | 530.84 ..06 ..368-370 |
| 501 .....04 ..196-198 | 520.9 ...03 ..157-159 | 524.09 ..03 ..157-159 | 525.61 ..03 ..157-159 | 530.85 ..06 ..380-382 |
| 502 .....04 ..196-198 | 521.00 ..03 ..157-159 | 524.10 ..03 ..157-159 | 525.62 ..03 ..157-159 | 530.86 ..06 ..393-395 |
| 503 .....04 ..196-198 | 521.01 ..03 ..157-159 | 524.11 ..03 ..157-159 | 525.63 ..03 ..157-159 | 530.87 ..06 ..393-395 |
| 504 .....04 ..196-198 | 521.02 ..03 ..157-159 | 524.12 ..03 ..157-159 | 525.64 ..03 ..157-159 | 530.89 ..06 ..391-392 |
| 505 .....04 ..196-198 | 521.03 ..03 ..157-159 | 524.19 ..03 ..157-159 | 525.65 ..03 ..157-159 | 530.9 ...06 ..391-392 |
| 506.0 ...04 ..205-206 | 521.04 ..03 ..157-159 | 524.20 ..03 ..157-159 | 525.66 ..03 ..157-159 | 531.00 ..06 ..377-379 |
| 506.1 ...04 ..189 | 521.06 ..03 ..157-159 | 524.21 ..03 ..157-159 | 525.67 ..03 ..157-159 | 531.01 ..06 ..377-379 |
| 506.2 ...04 ..205-206 | 521.07 ..03 ..157-159 | 524.22 ..03 ..157-159 | 525.69 ..03 ..157-159 | 531.10 ..06 ..380-382 |
| 506.3 ...04 ..205-206 | 521.08 ..03 ..157-159 | 524.23 ..03 ..157-159 | 525.71 ..03 ..157-159 | 531.11 ..06 ..380-382 |
| 506.4 ...04 ..190-192 | 521.09 ..03 ..157-159 | 524.24 ..03 ..157-159 | 525.72 ..03 ..157-159 | 531.20 ..06 ..377-379 |
| 506.9 ...04 ..190-192 | 521.10 ..03 ..157-159 | 524.25 ..03 ..157-159 | 525.73 ..03 ..157-159 | 531.21 ..06 ..377-379 |
| 507.0 ...04 ..177-179 | 521.11 ..03 ..157-159 | 524.26 ..03 ..157-159 | 525.79 ..03 ..157-159 | 531.30 ..06 ..383-384 |
| 507.1 ...04 ..177-179 | 521.12 ..03 ..157-159 | 524.27 ..03 ..157-159 | 525.8 ...03 ..157-159 | 531.31 ..06 ..380-382 |
| 507.8 ...04 ..177-179 | 521.13 ..03 ..157-159 | 524.28 ..03 ..157-159 | 525.9 ...03 ..157-159 | 531.40 ..06 ..377-379 |
| 508.0 ...04 ..205-206 | 521.14 ..03 ..157-159 | 524.29 ..03. ..157-159 | 526.0 ...03 ..157-159 | 531.41 ..06 ..377-379 |
| 508.1 ...04 ..196-198 | 521.15 ..03 ..157-159 | 524.30 ..03 ..157-159 | 526.1 ...03 ..157-159 | 531.50 ..06 ..380-382 |
| 508.8 ...04 ..205-206 | 521.20 ..03 ..157-159 | 524.31 ..03 ..157-159 | 526.2 ...03 ..157-159 | 531.51 ..06 ..380-382 |
| 508.9 ...04 ..205-206 | 521.21 ..03 ..157-159 | 524.32 ..03 ..157-159 | 526.3 ...03 ..157-159 | 531.60 ..06 ..377-379 |
| 510.0 ...04 ..177-179 | 521.22 ..03 ..157-159 | 524.33 ..03 ..157-159 | 526.4 ...03 ..157-159 | 531.61 ..06 ..377-379 |
| 510.9 ...04 ..177-179 | 521.23 ..03 ..157-159 | 524.34 ..03 ..157-159 | 526.5 ...03 ..157-159 | 531.70 ..06 ..383-384 |
| 511.0 ...04 ..193-195 | 521.24 ..03 ..157-159 | 524.35 ..03 ..157-159 | 526.61 ..03 ..157-159 | 531.71 ..06 ..380-382 |
| 511.1 ...04 ..177-179 | 521.25 ..03 ..157-159 | 524.36 ..03 ..157-159 | 526.62 ..03 ..157-159 | 531.90 ..06 ..383-384 |
| 511.8 ...04 ..186-188 | 521.30 ..03 ..157-159 | 524.37 ..03 ..157-159 | 526.63 ..03 ..157-159 | 531.91 ..06 ..380-382 |
| 511.9 ...04 ..186-188 | 521.31 ..03 ..157-159 | 524.39 ..03 ..157-159 | 526.69 ..03 ..157-159 | 532.00 ..06 ..377-379 |
| 512.0 ...04 ..199-201 | 521.32 ..03 ..157-159 | 524.4 ...03 ..157-159 | 526.81 ..03 ..157-159 | 532.01 ..06 ..377-379 |
| 512.1 ...04 ..199-201 | 521.33 ..03 ..157-159 | 524.50 ..03 ..157-159 | 526.89 ..03 ..157-159 | 532.10 ..06 ..380-382 |
| 512.8 ...04 ..199-201 | 521.34 ..03 ..157-159 | 524.51 ..03 ..157-159 | 526.9 ...03 ..157-159 | 532.11 ..06 ..380-382 |
| 513.0 ...04 ..177-179 | 521.35 ..03 ..157-159 | 524.52 ..03 ..157-159 | 527.0 ...03 ..154-156 | 532.20 ..06 ..377-379 |
| 513.1 ...04 ..177-179 | 521.40 ..03 ..157-159 | 524.53 ..03 ..157-159 | 527.1 ...03 ..154-156 | 532.21 ..06 ..377-379 |
| 514 .....04 ..189 | 521.41 ..03 ..157-159 | 524.54 ..03 ..157-159 | 527.2 ...03 ..154-156 | 532.30 ..06 ..383-384 |
| 515 .....04 ..196-198 | 521.42 ..03 ..157-159 | 524.55 ..03 ..157-159 | 527.3 ...03 ..154-156 | 532.31 ..06 ..380-382 |

| DX | MDC | DRG |
|---|---|---|
| 532.40 | .06 | .377-379 |
| 532.41 | .06 | .377-379 |
| 532.50 | .06 | .380-382 |
| 532.51 | .06 | .380-382 |
| 532.60 | .06 | .377-379 |
| 532.61 | .06 | .377-379 |
| 532.70 | .06 | .383-384 |
| 532.71 | .06 | .380-382 |
| 532.90 | .06 | .383-384 |
| 532.91 | .06 | .380-382 |
| 533.00 | .06 | .377-379 |
| 533.01 | .06 | .377-379 |
| 533.10 | .06 | .380-382 |
| 533.11 | .06 | .380-382 |
| 533.20 | .06 | .377-379 |
| 533.21 | .06 | .377-379 |
| 533.30 | .06 | .383-384 |
| 533.31 | .06 | .380-382 |
| 533.40 | .06 | .377-379 |
| 533.41 | .06 | .377-379 |
| 533.50 | .06 | .380-382 |
| 533.51 | .06 | .380-382 |
| 533.60 | .06 | .377-379 |
| 533.61 | .06 | .377-379 |
| 533.70 | .06 | .383-384 |
| 533.71 | .06 | .380-382 |
| 533.90 | .06 | .383-384 |
| 533.91 | .06 | .380-382 |
| 534.00 | .06 | .377-379 |
| 534.01 | .06 | .377-379 |
| 534.10 | .06 | .380-382 |
| 534.11 | .06 | .380-382 |
| 534.20 | .06 | .377-379 |
| 534.21 | .06 | .377-379 |
| 534.30 | .06 | .380-382 |
| 534.31 | .06 | .380-382 |
| 534.40 | .06 | .377-379 |
| 534.41 | .06 | .377-379 |
| 534.50 | .06 | .380-382 |
| 534.51 | .06 | .380-382 |
| 534.60 | .06 | .377-379 |
| 534.61 | .06 | .377-379 |
| 534.70 | .06 | .380-382 |
| 534.71 | .06 | .380-382 |
| 534.90 | .06 | .380-382 |
| 534.91 | .06 | .380-382 |
| 535.00 | .06 | .391-392 |
| 535.01 | .06 | .377-379 |
| 535.10 | .06 | .391-392 |
| 535.11 | .06 | .377-379 |
| 535.20 | .06 | .391-392 |
| 535.21 | .06 | .377-379 |
| 535.30 | .06 | .391-392 |
| 535.31 | .06 | .377-379 |
| 535.40 | .06 | .391-392 |
| 535.41 | .06 | .377-379 |
| 535.50 | .06 | .391-392 |
| 535.51 | .06 | .377-379 |
| 535.60 | .06 | .391-392 |
| 535.61 | .06 | .377-379 |
| 536.0 | .06 | .391-392 |
| 536.1 | .06 | .391-392 |
| 536.2 | .06 | .391-392 |
| 536.3 | .06 | .391-392 |
| 536.40 | .06 | .393-395 |
| 536.41 | .06 | .393-395 |
| 536.42 | .06 | .393-395 |
| 536.49 | .06 | .393-395 |
| 536.8 | .06 | .391-392 |
| 536.9 | .06 | .391-392 |
| 537.0 | .06 | .380-382 |
| 537.1 | .06 | .391-392 |
| 537.2 | .06 | .391-392 |
| 537.3 | .06 | .380-382 |
| 537.4 | .06 | .391-392 |
| 537.5 | .06 | .391-392 |
| 537.6 | .06 | .391-392 |

| DX | MDC | DRG |
|---|---|---|
| 537.81 | .06 | .391-392 |
| 537.82 | .06 | .391-392 |
| 537.83 | .06 | .377-379 |
| 537.84 | .06 | .377-379 |
| 537.89 | .06 | .391-392 |
| 537.9 | .06 | .391-392 |
| 538 | .06 | .391-392 |
| 540.0 | .06 | .371-373 |
| 540.1 | .06 | .371-373 |
| 540.9 | .06 | .393-395 |
| 541 | .06 | .393-395 |
| 542 | .06 | .393-395 |
| 543.0 | .06 | .393-395 |
| 543.9 | .06 | .393-395 |
| 550.00 | .06 | .393-395 |
| 550.01 | .06 | .393-395 |
| 550.02 | .06 | .393-395 |
| 550.03 | .06 | .393-395 |
| 550.10 | .06 | .393-395 |
| 550.11 | .06 | .393-395 |
| 550.12 | .06 | .393-395 |
| 550.13 | .06 | .393-395 |
| 550.90 | .06 | .393-395 |
| 550.91 | .06 | .393-395 |
| 550.92 | .06 | .393-395 |
| 550.93 | .06 | .393-395 |
| 551.00 | .06 | .393-395 |
| 551.01 | .06 | .393-395 |
| 551.02 | .06 | .393-395 |
| 551.03 | .06 | .393-395 |
| 551.1 | .06 | .393-395 |
| 551.20 | .06 | .393-395 |
| 551.21 | .06 | .393-395 |
| 551.29 | .06 | .393-395 |
| 551.3 | .06 | .393-395 |
| 551.8 | .06 | .393-395 |
| 551.9 | .06 | .393-395 |
| 552.00 | .06 | .393-395 |
| 552.01 | .06 | .393-395 |
| 552.02 | .06 | .393-395 |
| 552.03 | .06 | .393-395 |
| 552.1 | .06 | .393-395 |
| 552.20 | .06 | .393-395 |
| 552.21 | .06 | .393-395 |
| 552.29 | .06 | .393-395 |
| 552.3 | .06 | .391-392 |
| 552.8 | .06 | .393-395 |
| 552.9 | .06 | .393-395 |
| 553.00 | .06 | .393-395 |
| 553.01 | .06 | .393-395 |
| 553.02 | .06 | .393-395 |
| 553.03 | .06 | .393-395 |
| 553.1 | .06 | .393-395 |
| 553.20 | .06 | .393-395 |
| 553.21 | .06 | .393-395 |
| 553.29 | .06 | .393-395 |
| 553.3 | .06 | .391-392 |
| 553.8 | .06 | .393-395 |
| 553.9 | .06 | .393-395 |
| 555.0 | .06 | .385-387 |
| 555.1 | .06 | .385-387 |
| 555.2 | .06 | .385-387 |
| 555.9 | .06 | .385-387 |
| 556.0 | .06 | .385-387 |
| 556.1 | .06 | .385-387 |
| 556.2 | .06 | .385-387 |
| 556.3 | .06 | .385-387 |
| 556.4 | .06 | .385-387 |
| 556.5 | .06 | .385-387 |
| 556.6 | .06 | .385-387 |
| 556.8 | .06 | .385-387 |
| 556.9 | .06 | .385-387 |
| 557.0 | .06 | .393-395 |
| 557.1 | .06 | .393-395 |
| 557.9 | .06 | .393-395 |
| 558.1 | .06 | .393-395 |
| 558.2 | .06 | .393-395 |

| DX | MDC | DRG |
|---|---|---|
| 558.3 | .06 | .391-392 |
| 558.9 | .06 | .391-392 |
| 560.0 | .06 | .388-390 |
| 560.1 | .06 | .388-390 |
| 560.2 | .06 | .388-390 |
| 560.30 | .06 | .388-390 |
| 560.31 | .06 | .388-390 |
| 560.39 | .06 | .388-390 |
| 560.81 | .06 | .388-390 |
| 560.89 | .06 | .388-390 |
| 560.9 | .06 | .388-390 |
| 562.00 | .06 | .391-392 |
| 562.01 | .06 | .391-392 |
| 562.02 | .06 | .377-379 |
| 562.03 | .06 | .377-379 |
| 562.10 | .06 | .391-392 |
| 562.11 | .06 | .391-392 |
| 562.12 | .06 | .377-379 |
| 562.13 | .06 | .377-379 |
| 564.00 | .06 | .391-392 |
| 564.01 | .06 | .391-392 |
| 564.02 | .06 | .391-392 |
| 564.09 | .06 | .391-392 |
| 564.1 | .06 | .391-392 |
| 564.2 | .06 | .391-392 |
| 564.3 | .06 | .391-392 |
| 564.4 | .06 | .391-392 |
| 564.5 | .06 | .391-392 |
| 564.6 | .06 | .391-392 |
| 564.7 | .06 | .393-395 |
| 564.81 | .06 | .391-392 |
| 564.89 | .06 | .391-392 |
| 564.9 | .06 | .391-392 |
| 565.0 | .06 | .393-395 |
| 565.1 | .06 | .393-395 |
| 566 | .06 | .393-395 |
| 567.0 | .06 | .371-373 |
| 567.1 | .06 | .371-373 |
| 567.21 | .06 | .371-373 |
| 567.22 | .06 | .371-373 |
| 567.23 | .06 | .371-373 |
| 567.29 | .06 | .371-373 |
| 567.31 | .06 | .371-373 |
| 567.38 | .06 | .371-373 |
| 567.39 | .06 | .371-373 |
| 567.81 | .06 | .393-395 |
| 567.82 | .06 | .393-395 |
| 567.89 | .06 | .393-395 |
| 567.9 | .06 | .393-395 |
| 568.0 | .06 | .393-395 |
| 568.81 | .06 | .393-395 |
| 568.82 | .06 | .393-395 |
| 568.89 | .06 | .371-373 |
| 568.9 | .06 | .371-373 |
| 569.0 | .06 | .393-395 |
| 569.1 | .06 | .393-395 |
| 569.2 | .06 | .393-395 |
| 569.3 | .06 | .377-379 |
| 569.41 | .06 | .393-395 |
| 569.42 | .06 | .393-395 |
| 569.43 | .06 | .393-395 |
| 569.49 | .06 | .393-395 |
| 569.5 | .06 | .371-373 |
| 569.60 | .06 | .393-395 |
| 569.61 | .06 | .393-395 |
| 569.62 | .06 | .393-395 |
| 569.69 | .06 | .393-395 |
| 569.81 | .06 | .393-395 |
| 569.82 | .06 | .393-395 |
| 569.83 | .06 | .393-395 |
| 569.84 | .06 | .393-395 |
| 569.85 | .06 | .377-379 |
| 569.86 | .06 | .393-395 |
| 569.89 | .06 | .393-395 |
| 569.9 | .06 | .393-395 |
| 570 | .07 | .441-443 |
| 571.0 | .07 | .441-443 |

| DX | MDC | DRG |
|---|---|---|
| 571.1 | .07 | .432-434 |
| 571.2 | .07 | .432-434 |
| 571.3 | .07 | .432-434 |
| 571.40 | .07 | .441-443 |
| 571.41 | .07 | .441-443 |
| 571.49 | .07 | .441-443 |
| 571.5 | .07 | .432-434 |
| 571.6 | .07 | .432-434 |
| 571.8 | .07 | .441-443 |
| 571.9 | .07 | .441-443 |
| 572.0 | .07 | .441-443 |
| 572.1 | .07 | .441-443 |
| 572.2 | .07 | .441-443 |
| 572.3 | .07 | .441-443 |
| 572.4 | .07 | .441-443 |
| 572.8 | .07 | .441-443 |
| 573.0 | .07 | .441-443 |
| 573.1 | .07 | .441-443 |
| 573.2 | .07 | .441-443 |
| 573.3 | .07 | .441-443 |
| 573.4 | .07 | .441-443 |
| 573.8 | .07 | .441-443 |
| 573.9 | .07 | .441-443 |
| 574.00 | .07 | .444-446 |
| 574.01 | .07 | .444-446 |
| 574.10 | .07 | .444-446 |
| 574.11 | .07 | .444-446 |
| 574.20 | .07 | .444-446 |
| 574.21 | .07 | .444-446 |
| 574.30 | .07 | .444-446 |
| 574.31 | .07 | .444-446 |
| 574.40 | .07 | .444-446 |
| 574.41 | .07 | .444-446 |
| 574.50 | .07 | .444-446 |
| 574.51 | .07 | .444-446 |
| 574.60 | .07 | .444-446 |
| 574.61 | .07 | .444-446 |
| 574.70 | .07 | .444-446 |
| 574.71 | .07 | .444-446 |
| 574.80 | .07 | .444-446 |
| 574.81 | .07 | .444-446 |
| 574.90 | .07 | .444-446 |
| 574.91 | .07 | .444-446 |
| 575.0 | .07 | .444-446 |
| 575.10 | .07 | .444-446 |
| 575.11 | .07 | .444-446 |
| 575.12 | .07 | .444-446 |
| 575.2 | .07 | .444-446 |
| 575.3 | .07 | .444-446 |
| 575.4 | .07 | .444-446 |
| 575.5 | .07 | .444-446 |
| 575.6 | .07 | .444-446 |
| 575.8 | .07 | .444-446 |
| 575.9 | .07 | .444-446 |
| 576.0 | .07 | .444-446 |
| 576.1 | .07 | .444-446 |
| 576.2 | .07 | .444-446 |
| 576.3 | .07 | .444-446 |
| 576.4 | .07 | .444-446 |
| 576.5 | .07 | .444-446 |
| 576.8 | .07 | .444-446 |
| 576.9 | .07 | .444-446 |
| 577.0 | .07 | .438-440 |
| 577.1 | .07 | .438-440 |
| 577.2 | .07 | .438-440 |
| 577.8 | .07 | .438-440 |
| 577.9 | .07 | .438-440 |
| 578.0 | .06 | .377-379 |
| 578.1 | .06 | .377-379 |
| 578.9 | .06 | .377-379 |
| 579.0 | .06 | .391-392 |
| 579.1 | .06 | .391-392 |
| 579.2 | .06 | .391-392 |
| 579.3 | .06 | .391-392 |
| 579.4 | .06 | .391-392 |
| 579.8 | .06 | .391-392 |
| 579.9 | .06 | .391-392 |

| DX | MDC | DRG |
|---|---|---|
| **Diseases of the Genitourinary System** | | |
| 580.0 | .11 | .698-700 |
| 580.4 | .11 | .698-700 |
| 580.81 | .11 | .698-700 |
| 580.89 | .11 | .698-700 |
| 580.9 | .11 | .698-700 |
| 581.0 | .11 | .698-700 |
| 581.1 | .11 | .698-700 |
| 581.2 | .11 | .698-700 |
| 581.3 | .11 | .698-700 |
| 581.81 | .11 | .698-700 |
| 581.89 | .11 | .698-700 |
| 581.9 | .11 | .698-700 |
| 582.0 | .11 | .698-700 |
| 582.1 | .11 | .698-700 |
| 582.2 | .11 | .698-700 |
| 582.4 | .11 | .698-700 |
| 582.81 | .11 | .698-700 |
| 582.89 | .11 | .698-700 |
| 582.9 | .11 | .698-700 |
| 583.0 | .11 | .698-700 |
| 583.1 | .11 | .698-700 |
| 583.2 | .11 | .698-700 |
| 583.4 | .11 | .698-700 |
| 583.6 | .11 | .698-700 |
| 583.7 | .11 | .698-700 |
| 583.81 | .11 | .698-700 |
| 583.89 | .11 | .698-700 |
| 583.9 | .11 | .698-700 |
| 584.5 | .11 | .682-684 |
| 584.6 | .11 | .682-684 |
| 584.7 | .11 | .682-684 |
| 584.8 | .11 | .682-684 |
| 584.9 | .11 | .682-684 |
| 585.1 | .11 | .682-684 |
| 585.2 | .11 | .682-684 |
| 585.3 | .11 | .682-684 |
| 585.4 | .11 | .682-684 |
| 585.5 | .11 | .682-684 |
| 585.6 | .11 | .682-684 |
| 585.9 | .11 | .682-684 |
| 586 | .11 | .682-684 |
| 587 | .11 | .698-700 |
| 588.0 | .11 | .698-700 |
| 588.1 | .11 | .698-700 |
| 588.81 | .11 | .698-700 |
| 588.89 | .11 | .698-700 |
| 588.9 | .11 | .698-700 |
| 589.0 | .11 | .698-700 |
| 589.1 | .11 | .698-700 |
| 589.9 | .11 | .698-700 |
| 590.00 | .11 | .689-690 |
| 590.01 | .11 | .689-690 |
| 590.10 | .11 | .689-690 |
| 590.11 | .11 | .689-690 |
| 590.2 | .11 | .689-690 |
| 590.3 | .11 | .689-690 |
| 590.80 | .11 | .689-690 |
| 590.81 | .11 | .689-690 |
| 590.9 | .11 | .689-690 |
| 591 | .11 | .691-694 |
| 592.0 | .11 | .691-694 |
| 592.1 | .11 | .691-694 |
| 592.9 | .11 | .691-694 |
| 593.0 | .11 | .698-700 |
| 593.1 | .11 | .698-700 |
| 593.2 | .11 | .698-700 |
| 593.3 | .11 | .698-700 |
| 593.4 | .11 | .691-694 |
| 593.5 | .11 | .691-694 |
| 593.6 | .11 | .698-700 |
| 593.70 | .11 | .698-700 |
| 593.71 | .11 | .698-700 |
| 593.72 | .11 | .698-700 |
| 593.73 | .11 | .698-700 |
| 593.81 | .11 | .698-700 |

| DX . . .MDC . .DRG | DX . . .MDC . .DRG | DX . . .MDC . .DRG | DX . . .MDC . .DRG | DX . . .MDC . .DRG |
|---|---|---|---|---|
| 593.82 ..11 ..698-700 | 602.3 ...12 ..729-730 | 616.0 ...13 ..757-759 | 622.7 ...13 ..760-761 | 633.11 ..14 ..777 |
| 593.89 ..11 ..698-700 | 602.8 ...12 ..729-730 | 616.10 ..13 ..757-759 | 622.8 ...13 ..760-761 | 633.20 ..14 ..777 |
| 593.9 ...11 ..698-700 | 602.9 ...12 ..729-730 | 616.11 ..13 ..757-759 | 622.9 ...13 ..760-761 | 633.21 ..14 ..777 |
| 594.0 ...11 ..698-700 | 603.0 ...12 ..729-730 | 616.2 ...13 ..760-761 | 623.0 ...13 ..760-761 | 633.80 ..14 ..777 |
| 594.1 ...11 ..691-694 | 603.1 ...12 ..727-728 | 616.3 ...13 ..757-759 | 623.1 ...13 ..760-761 | 633.81 ..14 ..777 |
| 594.2 ...11 ..691-694 | 603.8 ...12 ..729-730 | 616.4 ...13 ..757-759 | 623.2 ...13 ..760-761 | 633.90 ..14 ..777 |
| 594.8 ...11 ..691-694 | 603.9 ...12 ..729-730 | 616.50 ..13 ..760-761 | 623.3 ...13 ..760-761 | 633.91 ..14 ..777 |
| 594.9 ...11 ..691-694 | 604.0 ...12 ..727-728 | 616.51 ..13 ..760-761 | 623.4 ...13 ..760-761 | 633.0 ...14 ..777 |
| 595.0 ...11 ..689-690 | 604.90 ..12 ..727-728 | 616.81 ..13 ..757-759 | 623.5 ...13 ..760-761 | 633.1 ...14 ..777 |
| 595.1 ...11 ..689-690 | 604.91 ..12 ..727-728 | 616.89 ..13 ..757-759 | 623.6 ...13 ..760-761 | 633.2 ...14 ..777 |
| 595.2 ...11 ..689-690 | 604.99 ..12 ..727-728 | 616.9 ...13 ..757-759 | 623.7 ...13 ..760-761 | 633.8 ...14 ..777 |
| 595.3 ...11 ..689-690 | 605 .....12 ..727-728 | 617.0 ...13 ..760-761 | 623.8 ...13 ..760-761 | 633.9 ...14 ..777 |
| 595.4 ...11 ..689-690 | 606.0 ...12 ..729-730 | 617.1 ...13 ..760-761 | 623.9 ...13 ..760-761 | 634.00 ..14 ..779 |
| 595.81 ..11 ..689-690 | 606.1 ...12 ..729-730 | 617.2 ...13 ..760-761 | 624.01 ..13 ..760-761 | 634.01 ..14 ..779 |
| 595.82 ..11 ..698-700 | 606.8 ...12 ..729-730 | 617.3 ...13 ..760-761 | 624.02 ..13 ..760-761 | 634.02 ..14 ..779 |
| 595.89 ..11 ..689-690 | 606.9 ...12 ..729-730 | 617.4 ...13 ..760-761 | 624.09 ..13 ..760-761 | 634.10 ..14 ..779 |
| 595.9 ...11 ..689-690 | 607.0 ...12 ..729-730 | 617.5 ...06 ..391-392 | 624.1 ...13 ..760-761 | 634.11 ..14 ..779 |
| 596.0 ...11 ..698-700 | 607.1 ...12 ..727-728 | 617.6 ...09 ..606-607 | 624.2 ...13 ..760-761 | 634.12 ..14 ..779 |
| 596.1 ...11 ..698-700 | 607.2 ...12 ..727-728 | 617.8 ...13 ..760-761 | 624.3 ...13 ..760-761 | 634.20 ..14 ..779 |
| 596.2 ...11 ..698-700 | 607.3 ...12 ..729-730 | 617.9 ...13 ..760-761 | 624.4 ...13 ..760-761 | 634.21 ..14 ..779 |
| 596.3 ...11 ..698-700 | 607.81 ..12 ..727-728 | 618.00 ..13 ..760-761 | 624.5 ...13 ..760-761 | 634.22 ..14 ..779 |
| 596.4 ...11 ..698-700 | 607.82 ..12 ..729-730 | 618.01 ..13 ..760-761 | 624.6 ...13 ..760-761 | 634.30 ..14 ..779 |
| 596.51 ..11 ..698-700 | 607.83 ..12 ..729-730 | 618.02 ..13 ..760-761 | 624.8 ...13 ..760-761 | 634.31 ..14 ..779 |
| 596.52 ..11 ..698-700 | 607.84 ..12 ..729-730 | 618.03 ..13 ..760-761 | 624.9 ...13 ..760-761 | 634.32 ..14 ..779 |
| 596.53 ..11 ..698-700 | 607.85 ..12 ..729-730 | 618.04 ..13 ..760-761 | 625.0 ...13 ..760-761 | 634.40 ..14 ..779 |
| 596.54 ..11 ..698-700 | 607.89 ..12 ..729-730 | 618.05 ..13 ..760-761 | 625.1 ...13 ..760-761 | 634.41 ..14 ..779 |
| 596.55 ..11 ..698-700 | 607.9 ...12 ..729-730 | 618.09 ..13 ..760-761 | 625.2 ...13 ..760-761 | 634.42 ..14 ..779 |
| 596.59 ..11 ..698-700 | 608.0 ...12 ..727-728 | 618.1 ...13 ..760-761 | 625.3 ...13 ..760-761 | 634.50 ..14 ..779 |
| 596.6 ...11 ..698-700 | 608.1 ...12 ..729-730 | 618.2 ...13 ..760-761 | 625.4 ...13 ..760-761 | 634.51 ..14 ..779 |
| 596.7 ...11 ..698-700 | 608.20 ..12 ..729-730 | 618.3 ...13 ..760-761 | 625.5 ...13 ..760-761 | 634.52 ..14 ..779 |
| 596.8 ...11 ..698-700 | 608.21 ..12 ..729-730 | 618.4 ...13 ..760-761 | 625.6 ...13 ..760-761 | 634.60 ..14 ..779 |
| 596.9 ...11 ..698-700 | 608.22 ..12 ..729-730 | 618.5 ...13 ..760-761 | 625.8 ...13 ..760-761 | 634.61 ..14 ..779 |
| 597.0 ...11 ..689-690 | 608.23 ..12 ..729-730 | 618.6 ...13 ..760-761 | 625.9 ...13 ..760-761 | 634.62 ..14 ..779 |
| 597.80 ..11 ..689-690 | 608.24 ..12 ..729-730 | 618.7 ...13 ..760-761 | 626.0 ...13 ..760-761 | 634.70 ..14 ..779 |
| 597.81 ..11 ..689-690 | 608.3 ...12 ..729-730 | 618.81 ..13 ..760-761 | 626.1 ...13 ..760-761 | 634.71 ..14 ..779 |
| 597.89 ..11 ..689-690 | 608.4 ...12 ..727-728 | 618.82 ..13 ..760-761 | 626.2 ...13 ..760-761 | 634.72 ..14 ..779 |
| 598.00 ..11 ..697 | 608.81 ..12 ..729-730 | 618.83 ..13 ..760-761 | 626.3 ...13 ..760-761 | 634.80 ..14 ..779 |
| 598.01 ..11 ..697 | 608.82 ..12 ..729-730 | 618.84 ..13 ..760-761 | 626.4 ...13 ..760-761 | 634.81 ..14 ..779 |
| 598.1 ...11 ..697 | 608.83 ..12 ..729-730 | 618.89 ..13 ..760-761 | 626.5 ...13 ..760-761 | 634.82 ..14 ..779 |
| 598.2 ...11 ..697 | 608.84 ..12 ..729-730 | 618.9 ...13 ..760-761 | 626.6 ...13 ..760-761 | 634.90 ..14 ..779 |
| 598.8 ...11 ..697 | 608.85 ..12 ..729-730 | 619.0 ...13 ..760-761 | 626.7 ...13 ..760-761 | 634.91 ..14 ..779 |
| 598.9 ...11 ..697 | 608.86 ..12 ..729-730 | 619.1 ...06 ..393-395 | 626.8 ...13 ..760-761 | 634.92 ..14 ..779 |
| 599.0 ...11 ..689-690 | 608.87 ..12 ..729-730 | 619.2 ...13 ..760-761 | 626.9 ...13 ..760-761 | 635.00 ..14 ..779 |
| 599.1 ...11 ..698-700 | 608.89 ..12 ..729-730 | 619.8 ...13 ..760-761 | 627.0 ...13 ..760-761 | 635.01 ..14 ..779 |
| 599.2 ...11 ..698-700 | 608.9 ...12 ..729-730 | 619.9 ...13 ..760-761 | 627.1 ...13 ..760-761 | 635.02 ..14 ..779 |
| 599.3 ...11 ..698-700 | 610.0 ...09 ..600-601 | 620.0 ...13 ..760-761 | 627.2 ...13 ..760-761 | 635.10 ..14 ..779 |
| 599.4 ...11 ..698-700 | 610.1 ...09 ..600-601 | 620.1 ...13 ..760-761 | 627.3 ...13 ..760-761 | 635.11 ..14 ..779 |
| 599.5 ...11 ..698-700 | 610.2 ...09 ..600-601 | 620.2 ...13 ..760-761 | 627.4 ...13 ..760-761 | 635.12 ..14 ..779 |
| 599.60 ..11 ..698-700 | 610.3 ...09 ..600-601 | 620.3 ...13 ..760-761 | 627.8 ...13 ..760-761 | 635.20 ..14 ..779 |
| 599.69 ..11 ..698-700 | 610.4 ...09 ..600-601 | 620.4 ...13 ..760-761 | 627.9 ...13 ..760-761 | 635.21 ..14 ..779 |
| 599.7 ...11 ..695-696 | 610.8 ...09 ..600-601 | 620.5 ...13 ..760-761 | 628.0 ...13 ..760-761 | 635.22 ..14 ..779 |
| 599.81 ..11 ..698-700 | 610.9 ...09 ..600-601 | 620.6 ...13 ..760-761 | 628.1 ...13 ..760-761 | 635.30 ..14 ..779 |
| 599.82 ..11 ..698-700 | 611.0 ...09 ..600-601 | 620.7 ...13 ..760-761 | 628.2 ...13 ..760-761 | 635.31 ..14 ..779 |
| 599.83 ..11 ..698-700 | 611.1 ...09 ..600-601 | 620.8 ...13 ..760-761 | 628.3 ...13 ..760-761 | 635.32 ..14 ..779 |
| 599.84 ..11 ..698-700 | 611.2 ...09 ..600-601 | 620.9 ...13 ..760-761 | 628.4 ...13 ..760-761 | 635.40 ..14 ..779 |
| 599.89 ..11 ..698-700 | 611.3 ...09 ..600-601 | 621.0 ...13 ..760-761 | 628.8 ...13 ..760-761 | 635.41 ..14 ..779 |
| 599.9 ...11 ..698-700 | 611.4 ...09 ..600-601 | 621.1 ...13 ..760-761 | 628.9 ...13 ..760-761 | 635.42 ..14 ..779 |
| 600.00 ..12 ..725-726 | 611.5 ...09 ..600-601 | 621.2 ...13 ..760-761 | 629.0 ...13 ..760-761 | 635.50 ..14 ..779 |
| 600.01 ..12 ..725-726 | 611.6 ...09 ..600-601 | 621.30 ..13 ..760-761 | 629.1 ...13 ..760-761 | 635.51 ..14 ..779 |
| 600.10 ..12 ..725-726 | 611.71 ..09 ..600-601 | 621.31 ..13 ..760-761 | 629.20 ..13 ..760-761 | 635.52 ..14 ..779 |
| 600.11 ..12 ..725-726 | 611.72 ..09 ..600-601 | 621.32 ..13 ..760-761 | 629.21 ..13 ..760-761 | 635.60 ..14 ..779 |
| 600.20 ..12 ..725-726 | 611.79 ..09 ..600-601 | 621.33 ..13 ..760-761 | 629.22 ..13 ..760-761 | 635.61 ..14 ..779 |
| 600.21 ..12 ..725-726 | 611.8 ...09 ..600-601 | 621.4 ...13 ..760-761 | 629.23 ..13 ..760-761 | 635.62 ..14 ..779 |
| 600.30 ..12 ..725-726 | 611.9 ...09 ..600-601 | 621.5 ...13 ..760-761 | 629.29 ..13 ..760-761 | 635.70 ..14 ..779 |
| 600.31 ..12 ..725-726 | 614.0 ...13 ..757-759 | 621.6 ...13 ..760-761 | 629.81 ..13 ..757-759 | 635.71 ..14 ..779 |
| 600.90 ..12 ..725-726 | 614.1 ...13 ..757-759 | 621.7 ...13 ..760-761 | 629.89 ..13 ..757-759 | 635.72 ..14 ..779 |
| 600.91 ..12 ..725-726 | 614.2 ...13 ..757-759 | 621.8 ...13 ..760-761 | 629.9 ...13 ..760-761 | 635.80 ..14 ..779 |
| 601.0 ...12 ..727-728 | 614.3 ...13 ..757-759 | 621.9 ...13 ..760-761 | | 635.81 ..14 ..779 |
| 601.1 ...12 ..727-728 | 614.4 ...13 ..757-759 | 622.0 ...13 ..760-761 | **Complications of** | 635.82 ..14 ..779 |
| 601.2 ...12 ..727-728 | 614.5 ...13 ..757-759 | 622.10 ..13 ..760-761 | **Pregnancy, Childbirth and** | 635.90 ..14 ..779 |
| 601.3 ...12 ..727-728 | 614.6 ...13 ..760-761 | 622.11 ..13 ..760-761 | **the Puerperium** | 635.91 ..14 ..779 |
| 601.4 ...12 ..727-728 | 614.7 ...13 ..757-759 | 622.12 ..13 ..760-761 | 630 .....14 ..781-782 | 635.92 ..14 ..779 |
| 601.8 ...12 ..727-728 | 614.8 ...13 ..757-759 | 622.2 ...13 ..760-761 | 631 .....14 ..781-782 | 636.00 ..14 ..779 |
| 601.9 ...12 ..727-728 | 614.9 ...13 ..757-759 | 622.3 ...13 ..760-761 | 632 .....14 ..779 | 636.01 ..14 ..779 |
| 602.0 ...12 ..729-730 | 615.0 ...13 ..757-759 | 622.4 ...13 ..760-761 | 633.00 ..14 ..777 | 636.02 ..14 ..779 |
| 602.1 ...12 ..729-730 | 615.1 ...13 ..757-759 | 622.5 ...13 ..760-761 | 633.01 ..14 ..777 | 636.10 ..14 ..779 |
| 602.2 ...12 ..729-730 | 615.9 ...13 ..757-759 | 622.6 ...13 ..760-761 | 633.10 ..14 ..777 | 636.11 ..14 ..779 |

| DX | MDC | DRG | DX | MDC | DRG | DX | MDC | DRG | DX | MDC | DRG | DX | MDC | DRG |
|---|---|---|---|---|---|---|---|---|---|---|---|---|---|---|
| 636.12 | 14 | 779 | 640.80 | 14 | 778 | 643.23 | 14 | 781 | 647.31 | 14 | 774 | 648.93 | 14 | 781 |
| 636.20 | 14 | 779 | 640.81 | 14 | 774-775 | 643.80 | 14 | 998 | 647.32 | 14 | 774 | 648.94 | 14 | 776 |
| 636.21 | 14 | 779 | 640.83 | 14 | 778 | 643.81 | 14 | 774-775 | 647.33 | 14 | 781 | 649.00 | 14 | 998 |
| 636.22 | 14 | 779 | 640.90 | 14 | 778 | 643.83 | 14 | 781 | 647.34 | 14 | 776 | 649.01 | 14 | 774-775 |
| 636.30 | 14 | 779 | 640.91 | 14 | 774-775 | 643.90 | 14 | 998 | 647.40 | 14 | 998 | 649.02 | 14 | 774-775 |
| 636.31 | 14 | 779 | 640.93 | 14 | 778 | 643.91 | 14 | 774-775 | 647.41 | 14 | 774 | 649.03 | 14 | 781-782 |
| 636.32 | 14 | 779 | 641.00 | 14 | 998 | 643.93 | 14 | 781 | 647.42 | 14 | 774 | 649.04 | 14 | 776 |
| 636.40 | 14 | 779 | 641.01 | 14 | 774 | 644.00 | 14 | 778 | 647.43 | 14 | 781 | 649.10 | 14 | 998 |
| 636.41 | 14 | 779 | 641.03 | 14 | 781-782 | 644.03 | 14 | 778 | 647.44 | 14 | 776 | 649.11 | 14 | 774-775 |
| 636.42 | 14 | 779 | 641.10 | 14 | 998 | 644.10 | 14 | 780 | 647.50 | 14 | 998 | 649.12 | 14 | 774-775 |
| 636.50 | 14 | 779 | 641.11 | 14 | 774 | 644.13 | 14 | 780 | 647.51 | 14 | 774 | 649.13 | 14 | 781-782 |
| 636.51 | 14 | 779 | 641.13 | 14 | 781-782 | 644.20 | 14 | 781-782 | 647.52 | 14 | 774 | 649.14 | 14 | 776 |
| 636.52 | 14 | 779 | 641.20 | 14 | 998 | 644.21 | 14 | 774-775 | 647.53 | 14 | 781 | 649.20 | 14 | 998 |
| 636.60 | 14 | 779 | 641.21 | 14 | 774 | 645.10 | 14 | 998 | 647.54 | 14 | 776 | 649.21 | 14 | 774-775 |
| 636.61 | 14 | 779 | 641.23 | 14 | 781-782 | 645.11 | 14 | 774-775 | 647.60 | 14 | 998 | 649.22 | 14 | 774-775 |
| 636.62 | 14 | 779 | 641.30 | 14 | 998 | 645.13 | 14 | 781-782 | 647.61 | 14 | 774 | 649.23 | 14 | 781-782 |
| 636.70 | 14 | 779 | 641.31 | 14 | 774 | 645.20 | 14 | 998 | 647.62 | 14 | 774 | 649.24 | 14 | 776 |
| 636.71 | 14 | 779 | 641.33 | 14 | 781 | 645.21 | 14 | 774-775 | 647.63 | 14 | 781 | 649.30 | 14 | 998 |
| 636.72 | 14 | 779 | 641.80 | 14 | 998 | 645.23 | 14 | 781-782 | 647.64 | 14 | 776 | 649.31 | 14 | 774-775 |
| 636.80 | 14 | 779 | 641.81 | 14 | 774 | 646.00 | 14 | 774-775 | 647.80 | 14 | 998 | 649.32 | 14 | 774-775 |
| 636.81 | 14 | 779 | 641.83 | 14 | 781-782 | 646.01 | 14 | 774-775 | 647.81 | 14 | 774 | 649.33 | 14 | 781-782 |
| 636.82 | 14 | 779 | 641.90 | 14 | 998 | 646.03 | 14 | 781-782 | 647.82 | 14 | 774 | 649.34 | 14 | 776 |
| 636.90 | 14 | 779 | 641.91 | 14 | 774 | 646.10 | 14 | 998 | 647.83 | 14 | 781 | 649.40 | 14 | 998 |
| 636.91 | 14 | 779 | 641.93 | 14 | 781-782 | 646.11 | 14 | 774-775 | 647.84 | 14 | 776 | 649.41 | 14 | 774-775 |
| 636.92 | 14 | 779 | 642.00 | 14 | 998 | 646.12 | 14 | 774-775 | 647.90 | 14 | 998 | 649.42 | 14 | 774-775 |
| 637.00 | 14 | 779 | 642.01 | 14 | 774 | 646.13 | 14 | 781 | 647.91 | 14 | 774 | 649.43 | 14 | 781-782 |
| 637.01 | 14 | 779 | 642.02 | 14 | 774 | 646.14 | 14 | 776 | 647.92 | 14 | 774 | 649.44 | 14 | 776 |
| 637.02 | 14 | 779 | 642.03 | 14 | 781 | 646.20 | 14 | 998 | 647.93 | 14 | 781 | 649.50 | 14 | 998 |
| 637.10 | 14 | 779 | 642.04 | 14 | 776 | 646.21 | 14 | 774-775 | 647.94 | 14 | 776 | 649.51 | 14 | 774-775 |
| 637.11 | 14 | 779 | 642.10 | 14 | 998 | 646.22 | 14 | 774-775 | 648.00 | 14 | 998 | 649.53 | 14 | 781-782 |
| 637.12 | 14 | 779 | 642.11 | 14 | 774 | 646.23 | 14 | 781 | 648.01 | 14 | 774 | 649.60 | 14 | 998 |
| 637.20 | 14 | 779 | 642.12 | 14 | 774 | 646.24 | 14 | 776 | 648.02 | 14 | 774 | 649.61 | 14 | 774-775 |
| 637.21 | 14 | 779 | 642.13 | 14 | 781 | 646.30 | 14 | 998 | 648.03 | 14 | 781 | 649.62 | 14 | 774-775 |
| 637.22 | 14 | 779 | 642.14 | 14 | 776 | 646.31 | 14 | 774-775 | 648.04 | 14 | 776 | 649.63 | 14 | 781-782 |
| 637.30 | 14 | 779 | 642.20 | 14 | 998 | 646.33 | 14 | 781-782 | 648.10 | 14 | 998 | 649.64 | 14 | 776 |
| 637.31 | 14 | 779 | 642.21 | 14 | 774 | 646.40 | 14 | 998 | 648.11 | 14 | 774-775 | 650 | 14 | 774-775 |
| 637.32 | 14 | 779 | 642.22 | 14 | 774 | 646.41 | 14 | 774-775 | 648.12 | 14 | 774-775 | 651.00 | 14 | 998 |
| 637.40 | 14 | 779 | 642.23 | 14 | 781 | 646.42 | 14 | 774-775 | 648.13 | 14 | 781 | 651.01 | 14 | 774-775 |
| 637.41 | 14 | 779 | 642.24 | 14 | 776 | 646.43 | 14 | 781 | 648.14 | 14 | 776 | 651.03 | 14 | 781-782 |
| 637.42 | 14 | 779 | 642.30 | 14 | 998 | 646.44 | 14 | 776 | 648.20 | 14 | 998 | 651.10 | 14 | 998 |
| 637.50 | 14 | 779 | 642.31 | 14 | 774-775 | 646.50 | 14 | 998 | 648.21 | 14 | 774-775 | 651.11 | 14 | 774-775 |
| 637.51 | 14 | 779 | 642.32 | 14 | 774-775 | 646.51 | 14 | 774-775 | 648.22 | 14 | 774-775 | 651.13 | 14 | 781-782 |
| 637.52 | 14 | 779 | 642.33 | 14 | 781-782 | 646.52 | 14 | 774-775 | 648.23 | 14 | 781 | 651.20 | 14 | 998 |
| 637.60 | 14 | 779 | 642.34 | 14 | 776 | 646.53 | 14 | 781-782 | 648.24 | 14 | 776 | 651.21 | 14 | 774-775 |
| 637.61 | 14 | 779 | 642.40 | 14 | 998 | 646.54 | 14 | 776 | 648.30 | 14 | 998 | 651.23 | 14 | 781-782 |
| 637.62 | 14 | 779 | 642.41 | 14 | 774 | 646.60 | 14 | 998 | 648.31 | 14 | 774-775 | 651.30 | 14 | 998 |
| 637.70 | 14 | 779 | 642.42 | 14 | 774 | 646.61 | 14 | 774-775 | 648.32 | 14 | 774-775 | 651.31 | 14 | 774-775 |
| 637.71 | 14 | 779 | 642.43 | 14 | 781 | 646.62 | 14 | 774-775 | 648.33 | 14 | 781 | 651.33 | 14 | 781-782 |
| 637.72 | 14 | 779 | 642.44 | 14 | 776 | 646.63 | 14 | 781 | 648.34 | 14 | 776 | 651.40 | 14 | 998 |
| 637.80 | 14 | 779 | 642.50 | 14 | 998 | 646.64 | 14 | 776 | 648.40 | 14 | 998 | 651.41 | 14 | 774-775 |
| 637.81 | 14 | 779 | 642.51 | 14 | 774 | 646.70 | 14 | 998 | 648.41 | 14 | 774-775 | 651.43 | 14 | 781-782 |
| 637.82 | 14 | 779 | 642.52 | 14 | 774 | 646.71 | 14 | 774-775 | 648.42 | 14 | 774-775 | 651.50 | 14 | 998 |
| 637.90 | 14 | 779 | 642.53 | 14 | 781 | 646.73 | 14 | 781 | 648.43 | 14 | 781 | 651.51 | 14 | 774-775 |
| 637.91 | 14 | 779 | 642.54 | 14 | 776 | 646.80 | 14 | 998 | 648.44 | 14 | 776 | 651.53 | 14 | 781-782 |
| 637.92 | 14 | 779 | 642.60 | 14 | 998 | 646.81 | 14 | 774-775 | 648.50 | 14 | 998 | 651.60 | 14 | 998 |
| 638.0 | 14 | 779 | 642.61 | 14 | 774 | 646.82 | 14 | 774-775 | 648.51 | 14 | 774 | 651.61 | 14 | 774-775 |
| 638.1 | 14 | 779 | 642.62 | 14 | 774 | 646.83 | 14 | 781 | 648.52 | 14 | 774 | 651.63 | 14 | 781-782 |
| 638.2 | 14 | 779 | 642.63 | 14 | 781 | 646.84 | 14 | 776 | 648.53 | 14 | 781 | 651.70 | 14 | 998 |
| 638.3 | 14 | 779 | 642.64 | 14 | 776 | 646.90 | 14 | 998 | 648.54 | 14 | 776 | 651.71 | 14 | 774-775 |
| 638.4 | 14 | 779 | 642.70 | 14 | 998 | 646.91 | 14 | 774-775 | 648.60 | 14 | 998 | 651.73 | 14 | 781-782 |
| 638.5 | 14 | 779 | 642.71 | 14 | 774 | 646.93 | 14 | 781-782 | 648.61 | 14 | 774 | 651.80 | 14 | 998 |
| 638.6 | 14 | 779 | 642.72 | 14 | 774 | 647.00 | 14 | 998 | 648.62 | 14 | 774 | 651.81 | 14 | 774-775 |
| 638.7 | 14 | 779 | 642.73 | 14 | 781 | 647.01 | 14 | 774 | 648.63 | 14 | 781 | 651.83 | 14 | 781-782 |
| 638.8 | 14 | 779 | 642.74 | 14 | 776 | 647.02 | 14 | 774 | 648.64 | 14 | 776 | 651.90 | 14 | 998 |
| 638.9 | 14 | 779 | 642.90 | 14 | 998 | 647.03 | 14 | 781 | 648.70 | 14 | 998 | 651.91 | 14 | 774-775 |
| 639.0 | 14 | 776 | 642.91 | 14 | 774 | 647.04 | 14 | 776 | 648.71 | 14 | 774-775 | 651.93 | 14 | 781-782 |
| 639.1 | 14 | 776 | 642.92 | 14 | 774 | 647.10 | 14 | 998 | 648.72 | 14 | 774-775 | 652.00 | 14 | 998 |
| 639.2 | 14 | 776 | 642.93 | 14 | 781 | 647.11 | 14 | 774 | 648.73 | 14 | 781 | 652.01 | 14 | 774-775 |
| 639.3 | 14 | 776 | 642.94 | 14 | 776 | 647.12 | 14 | 774 | 648.74 | 14 | 776 | 652.03 | 14 | 781-782 |
| 639.4 | 14 | 776 | 643.00 | 14 | 998 | 647.13 | 14 | 781 | 648.80 | 14 | 998 | 652.10 | 14 | 998 |
| 639.5 | 14 | 776 | 643.01 | 14 | 774-775 | 647.14 | 14 | 776 | 648.81 | 14 | 774-775 | 652.11 | 14 | 774-775 |
| 639.6 | 14 | 776 | 643.03 | 14 | 781 | 647.20 | 14 | 998 | 648.82 | 14 | 774-775 | 652.13 | 14 | 781-782 |
| 639.8 | 14 | 776 | 643.10 | 14 | 998 | 647.21 | 14 | 774 | 648.83 | 14 | 781 | 652.20 | 14 | 998 |
| 639.9 | 14 | 776 | 643.11 | 14 | 774 | 647.22 | 14 | 774 | 648.84 | 14 | 776 | 652.21 | 14 | 774-775 |
| 640.00 | 14 | 778 | 643.13 | 14 | 781 | 647.23 | 14 | 781 | 648.90 | 14 | 998 | 652.23 | 14 | 781-782 |
| 640.01 | 14 | 774-775 | 643.20 | 14 | 998 | 647.24 | 14 | 776 | 648.91 | 14 | 774-775 | 652.30 | 14 | 998 |
| 640.03 | 14 | 778 | 643.21 | 14 | 774-775 | 647.30 | 14 | 998 | 648.92 | 14 | 774-775 | 652.31 | 14 | 774-775 |

| DX ...MDC ..DRG | DX ...MDC ..DRG | DX ...MDC ..DRG | DX ...MDC ..DRG | DX ...MDC ..DRG |
|---|---|---|---|---|
| 652.33 ..14 ..781-782 | 654.60 ..14 ..998 | 656.90 ..14 ..998 | 660.63 ..14 ..781-782 | 664.31 ..14 ..774-775 |
| 652.40 ..14 ..998 | 654.61 ..14 ..774-775 | 656.91 ..14 ..774-775 | 660.70 ..14 ..774-775 | 664.34 ..14 ..776 |
| 652.41 ..14 ..774-775 | 654.62 ..14 ..774-775 | 656.93 ..14 ..781-782 | 660.71 ..14 ..774-775 | 664.40 ..14 ..774-775 |
| 652.43 ..14 ..781-782 | 654.63 ..14 ..781-782 | 657.00 ..14 ..998 | 660.73 ..14 ..781-782 | 664.41 ..14 ..774-775 |
| 652.50 ..14 ..998 | 654.64 ..14 ..776 | 657.01 ..14 ..774-775 | 660.80 ..14 ..774-775 | 664.44 ..14 ..776 |
| 652.51 ..14 ..774-775 | 654.70 ..14 ..998 | 657.03 ..14 ..781-782 | 660.81 ..14 ..774-775 | 664.50 ..14 ..774-775 |
| 652.53 ..14 ..781-782 | 654.71 ..14 ..774-775 | 658.00 ..14 ..998 | 660.83 ..14 ..781-782 | 664.51 ..14 ..774-775 |
| 652.60 ..14 ..998 | 654.72 ..14 ..774-775 | 658.01 ..14 ..774-775 | 660.90 ..14 ..774-775 | 664.54 ..14 ..776 |
| 652.61 ..14 ..774-775 | 654.73 ..14 ..781-782 | 658.03 ..14 ..781-782 | 660.91 ..14 ..774-775 | 664.60 ..14 ..774-775 |
| 652.63 ..14 ..781-782 | 654.74 ..14 ..776 | 658.10 ..14 ..774-775 | 660.93 ..14 ..781-782 | 664.61 ..14 ..774-775 |
| 652.70 ..14 ..998 | 654.80 ..14 ..998 | 658.11 ..14 ..774-775 | 661.00 ..14 ..774-775 | 664.64 ..14 ..776 |
| 652.71 ..14 ..774-775 | 654.81 ..14 ..774-775 | 658.13 ..14 ..781-782 | 661.01 ..14 ..774-775 | 664.80 ..14 ..774-775 |
| 652.73 ..14 ..781-782 | 654.82 ..14 ..774-775 | 658.20 ..14 ..774-775 | 661.03 ..14 ..781-782 | 664.81 ..14 ..774-775 |
| 652.80 ..14 ..998 | 654.83 ..14 ..781-782 | 658.21 ..14 ..774-775 | 661.10 ..14 ..774-775 | 664.84 ..14 ..776 |
| 652.81 ..14 ..774-775 | 654.84 ..14 ..776 | 658.23 ..14 ..781-782 | 661.11 ..14 ..774-775 | 664.90 ..14 ..774-775 |
| 652.83 ..14 ..781-782 | 654.90 ..14 ..998 | 658.30 ..14 ..774-775 | 661.13 ..14 ..781-782 | 664.91 ..14 ..774-775 |
| 652.90 ..14 ..998 | 654.91 ..14 ..774-775 | 658.31 ..14 ..774-775 | 661.20 ..14 ..774-775 | 664.94 ..14 ..776 |
| 652.91 ..14 ..774-775 | 654.92 ..14 ..774-775 | 658.33 ..14 ..781-782 | 661.21 ..14 ..774-775 | 665.00 ..14 ..774-775 |
| 652.93 ..14 ..781-782 | 654.93 ..14 ..781-782 | 658.40 ..14 ..774-775 | 661.23 ..14 ..781-782 | 665.01 ..14 ..774-775 |
| 653.00 ..14 ..998 | 654.94 ..14 ..776 | 658.41 ..14 ..774-775 | 661.30 ..14 ..774-775 | 665.03 ..14 ..781-782 |
| 653.01 ..14 ..774-775 | 655.00 ..14 ..998 | 658.43 ..14 ..781-782 | 661.31 ..14 ..774-775 | 665.10 ..14 ..774-775 |
| 653.03 ..14 ..781-782 | 655.01 ..14 ..774-775 | 658.80 ..14 ..998 | 661.33 ..14 ..781-782 | 665.11 ..14 ..774-775 |
| 653.10 ..14 ..998 | 655.03 ..14 ..781-782 | 658.81 ..14 ..774-775 | 661.40 ..14 ..774-775 | 665.20 ..14 ..774-775 |
| 653.11 ..14 ..774-775 | 655.10 ..14 ..998 | 658.83 ..14 ..781-782 | 661.41 ..14 ..774-775 | 665.22 ..14 ..774-775 |
| 653.13 ..14 ..781-782 | 655.11 ..14 ..774-775 | 658.90 ..14 ..998 | 661.43 ..14 ..781-782 | 665.24 ..14 ..776 |
| 653.20 ..14 ..998 | 655.13 ..14 ..781-782 | 658.91 ..14 ..774-775 | 661.90 ..14 ..774-775 | 665.30 ..14 ..774-775 |
| 653.21 ..14 ..774-775 | 655.20 ..14 ..998 | 658.93 ..14 ..781-782 | 661.91 ..14 ..774-775 | 665.31 ..14 ..774-775 |
| 653.23 ..14 ..781-782 | 655.21 ..14 ..774-775 | 659.00 ..14 ..774-775 | 661.93 ..14 ..781-782 | 665.34 ..14 ..776 |
| 653.30 ..14 ..998 | 655.23 ..14 ..781-782 | 659.01 ..14 ..774-775 | 662.00 ..14 ..774-775 | 665.40 ..14 ..774-775 |
| 653.31 ..14 ..774-775 | 655.30 ..14 ..998 | 659.03 ..14 ..781-782 | 662.01 ..14 ..774-775 | 665.41 ..14 ..774-775 |
| 653.33 ..14 ..781-782 | 655.31 ..14 ..774-775 | 659.10 ..14 ..774-775 | 662.03 ..14 ..781-782 | 665.44 ..14 ..776 |
| 653.40 ..14 ..998 | 655.33 ..14 ..781-782 | 659.11 ..14 ..774-775 | 662.10 ..14 ..774-775 | 665.50 ..14 ..774-775 |
| 653.41 ..14 ..774-775 | 655.40 ..14 ..998 | 659.13 ..14 ..781-782 | 662.11 ..14 ..774-775 | 665.51 ..14 ..774-775 |
| 653.43 ..14 ..781-782 | 655.41 ..14 ..774-775 | 659.20 ..14 ..774-775 | 662.13 ..14 ..781-782 | 665.54 ..14 ..776 |
| 653.50 ..14 ..998 | 655.43 ..14 ..781-782 | 659.21 ..14 ..774-775 | 662.20 ..14 ..774-775 | 665.60 ..14 ..774-775 |
| 653.51 ..14 ..774-775 | 655.50 ..14 ..998 | 659.23 ..14 ..781-782 | 662.21 ..14 ..774-775 | 665.61 ..14 ..774-775 |
| 653.53 ..14 ..781-782 | 655.51 ..14 ..774-775 | 659.30 ..14 ..774-775 | 662.23 ..14 ..781-782 | 665.64 ..14 ..776 |
| 653.60 ..14 ..998 | 655.53 ..14 ..781-782 | 659.31 ..14 ..774-775 | 662.30 ..14 ..774-775 | 665.70 ..14 ..774-775 |
| 653.61 ..14 ..774-775 | 655.60 ..14 ..998 | 659.33 ..14 ..781-782 | 662.31 ..14 ..774-775 | 665.71 ..14 ..774-775 |
| 653.63 ..14 ..781-782 | 655.61 ..14 ..774-775 | 659.40 ..14 ..998 | 662.33 ..14 ..781-782 | 665.72 ..14 ..774-775 |
| 653.70 ..14 ..998 | 655.63 ..14 ..781-782 | 659.41 ..14 ..774-775 | 663.00 ..14 ..774-775 | 665.74 ..14 ..776 |
| 653.71 ..14 ..774-775 | 655.70 ..14 ..998 | 659.43 ..14 ..781-782 | 663.01 ..14 ..774-775 | 665.80 ..14 ..774-775 |
| 653.73 ..14 ..781-782 | 655.71 ..14 ..774-775 | 659.50 ..14 ..774-775 | 663.03 ..14 ..781-782 | 665.81 ..14 ..774-775 |
| 653.80 ..14 ..998 | 655.73 ..14 ..781-782 | 659.51 ..14 ..774-775 | 663.10 ..14 ..774-775 | 665.82 ..14 ..774-775 |
| 653.81 ..14 ..774-775 | 655.80 ..14 ..998 | 659.53 ..14 ..781-782 | 663.11 ..14 ..774-775 | 665.83 ..14 ..781-782 |
| 653.83 ..14 ..781-782 | 655.81 ..14 ..774-775 | 659.60 ..14 ..774-775 | 663.13 ..14 ..781-782 | 665.84 ..14 ..776 |
| 653.90 ..14 ..998 | 655.83 ..14 ..781-782 | 659.61 ..14 ..774-775 | 663.20 ..14 ..774-775 | 665.90 ..14 ..774-775 |
| 653.91 ..14 ..774-775 | 655.90 ..14 ..998 | 659.63 ..14 ..781-782 | 663.21 ..14 ..774-775 | 665.91 ..14 ..774-775 |
| 653.93 ..14 ..781-782 | 655.91 ..14 ..774-775 | 659.70 ..14 ..774-775 | 663.23 ..14 ..781-782 | 665.92 ..14 ..774-775 |
| 654.00 ..14 ..998 | 655.93 ..14 ..781-782 | 659.71 ..14 ..774-775 | 663.30 ..14 ..774-775 | 665.93 ..14 ..781-782 |
| 654.01 ..14 ..774-775 | 656.00 ..14 ..998 | 659.73 ..14 ..781-782 | 663.31 ..14 ..774-775 | 665.94 ..14 ..776 |
| 654.02 ..14 ..774-775 | 656.01 ..14 ..774-775 | 659.80 ..14 ..774-775 | 663.33 ..14 ..781-782 | 666.00 ..14 ..998 |
| 654.03 ..14 ..781-782 | 656.03 ..14 ..781-782 | 659.81 ..14 ..774-775 | 663.40 ..14 ..774-775 | 666.02 ..14 ..774 |
| 654.04 ..14 ..776 | 656.10 ..14 ..998 | 659.83 ..14 ..781-782 | 663.41 ..14 ..774-775 | 666.04 ..14 ..776 |
| 654.10 ..14 ..998 | 656.11 ..14 ..774-775 | 659.90 ..14 ..774-775 | 663.43 ..14 ..781-782 | 666.10 ..14 ..998 |
| 654.11 ..14 ..774-775 | 656.13 ..14 ..781-782 | 659.91 ..14 ..774-775 | 663.50 ..14 ..774-775 | 666.12 ..14 ..774 |
| 654.12 ..14 ..774-775 | 656.20 ..14 ..998 | 659.93 ..14 ..781-782 | 663.51 ..14 ..774-775 | 666.14 ..14 ..776 |
| 654.13 ..14 ..781-782 | 656.21 ..14 ..774-775 | 660.00 ..14 ..774-775 | 663.53 ..14 ..781-782 | 666.20 ..14 ..998 |
| 654.14 ..14 ..776 | 656.23 ..14 ..781-782 | 660.01 ..14 ..774-775 | 663.60 ..14 ..774-775 | 666.22 ..14 ..774 |
| 654.20 ..14 ..998 | 656.30 ..14 ..774-775 | 660.03 ..14 ..781-782 | 663.61 ..14 ..774-775 | 666.24 ..14 ..776 |
| 654.21 ..14 ..774-775 | 656.31 ..14 ..774-775 | 660.10 ..14 ..774-775 | 663.63 ..14 ..781-782 | 666.30 ..14 ..998 |
| 654.23 ..14 ..781-782 | 656.33 ..14 ..781-782 | 660.11 ..14 ..774-775 | 663.80 ..14 ..774-775 | 666.32 ..14 ..774 |
| 654.30 ..14 ..998 | 656.40 ..14 ..774-775 | 660.13 ..14 ..781-782 | 663.81 ..14 ..774-775 | 666.34 ..14 ..776 |
| 654.31 ..14 ..774-775 | 656.41 ..14 ..774-775 | 660.20 ..14 ..774-775 | 663.83 ..14 ..781-782 | 667.00 ..14 ..998 |
| 654.32 ..14 ..774-775 | 656.43 ..14 ..781-782 | 660.21 ..14 ..774-775 | 663.90 ..14 ..774-775 | 667.02 ..14 ..774 |
| 654.33 ..14 ..781-782 | 656.50 ..14 ..998 | 660.23 ..14 ..781-782 | 663.91 ..14 ..774-775 | 667.04 ..14 ..776 |
| 654.34 ..14 ..776 | 656.51 ..14 ..774-775 | 660.30 ..14 ..774-775 | 663.93 ..14 ..781-782 | 667.10 ..14 ..998 |
| 654.40 ..14 ..998 | 656.53 ..14 ..781-782 | 660.31 ..14 ..774-775 | 664.00 ..14 ..774-775 | 667.12 ..14 ..774 |
| 654.41 ..14 ..774-775 | 656.60 ..14 ..998 | 660.33 ..14 ..781-782 | 664.01 ..14 ..774-775 | 667.14 ..14 ..776 |
| 654.42 ..14 ..774-775 | 656.61 ..14 ..774-775 | 660.40 ..14 ..774-775 | 664.04 ..14 ..776 | 668.00 ..14 ..774-775 |
| 654.43 ..14 ..781-782 | 656.63 ..14 ..781-782 | 660.41 ..14 ..774-775 | 664.10 ..14 ..774-775 | 668.01 ..14 ..774 |
| 654.44 ..14 ..776 | 656.70 ..14 ..998 | 660.43 ..14 ..781-782 | 664.11 ..14 ..774-775 | 668.02 ..14 ..774 |
| 654.50 ..14 ..998 | 656.71 ..14 ..774-775 | 660.50 ..14 ..774-775 | 664.14 ..14 ..776 | 668.03 ..14 ..781-782 |
| 654.51 ..14 ..774-775 | 656.73 ..14 ..781-782 | 660.51 ..14 ..774-775 | 664.20 ..14 ..774-775 | 668.04 ..14 ..776 |
| 654.52 ..14 ..774-775 | 656.80 ..14 ..998 | 660.53 ..14 ..781-782 | 664.21 ..14 ..774-775 | 668.10 ..14 ..774-775 |
| 654.53 ..14 ..781-782 | 656.81 ..14 ..774-775 | 660.60 ..14 ..774-775 | 664.24 ..14 ..776 | 668.11 ..14 ..774 |
| 654.54 ..14 ..776 | 656.83 ..14 ..781-782 | 660.61 ..14 ..774-775 | 664.30 ..14 ..774-775 | 668.12 ..14 ..774 |

| DX . . .MDC . .DRG | DX . . .MDC . .DRG | DX . . .MDC . .DRG | DX . . .MDC . .DRG | DX . . .MDC . .DRG |
|---|---|---|---|---|
| 668.13 . .14 . .781-782 | 671.42 . .14 . .774 | 675.04 . .14 . .776 | 680.7 . . .09 . .602-603 | 695.81 . .09 . .595-596 |
| 668.14 . .14 . .776 | 671.44 . .14 . .776 | 675.10 . .14 . .998 | 680.8 . . .09 . .602-603 | 695.89 . .09 . .606-607 |
| 668.20 . .14 . .774-775 | 671.50 . .14 . .998 | 675.11 . .14 . .774 | 680.9 . . .09 . .602-603 | 695.9 . . .09 . .606-607 |
| 668.21 . .14 . .774 | 671.51 . .14 . .774 | 675.12 . .14 . .774 | 681.00 . .09 . .602-603 | 696.0 . . .08 . .545-547 |
| 668.22 . .14 . .774 | 671.52 . .14 . .774 | 675.13 . .14 . .781-782 | 681.01 . .09 . .602-603 | 696.1 . . .09 . .595-596 |
| 668.23 . .14 . .781-782 | 671.53 . .14 . .781-782 | 675.14 . .14 . .776 | 681.02 . .09 . .602-603 | 696.2 . . .09 . .595-596 |
| 668.24 . .14 . .776 | 671.54 . .14 . .776 | 675.20 . .14 . .998 | 681.10 . .09 . .602-603 | 696.3 . . .09 . .606-607 |
| 668.80 . .14 . .774-775 | 671.80 . .14 . .998 | 675.21 . .14 . .774 | 681.11 . .09 . .602-603 | 696.4 . . .09 . .606-607 |
| 668.81 . .14 . .774 | 671.81 . .14 . .774-775 | 675.22 . .14 . .774 | 681.9 . . .09 . .602-603 | 696.5 . . .09 . .606-607 |
| 668.82 . .14 . .774 | 671.82 . .14 . .774-775 | 675.23 . .14 . .781-782 | 682.0 . . .09 . .602-603 | 696.8 . . .09 . .606-607 |
| 668.83 . .14 . .781-782 | 671.83 . .14 . .781-782 | 675.24 . .14 . .776 | 682.1 . . .09 . .602-603 | 697.0 . . .09 . .606-607 |
| 668.84 . .14 . .776 | 671.84 . .14 . .776 | 675.80 . .14 . .998 | 682.2 . . .09 . .602-603 | 697.1 . . .09 . .606-607 |
| 668.90 . .14 . .774-775 | 671.90 . .14 . .998 | 675.81 . .14 . .774-775 | 682.3 . . .09 . .602-603 | 697.8 . . .09 . .606-607 |
| 668.91 . .14 . .774 | 671.91 . .14 . .774-775 | 675.82 . .14 . .774-775 | 682.4 . . .09 . .602-603 | 697.9 . . .09 . .606-607 |
| 668.92 . .14 . .774 | 671.92 . .14 . .774-775 | 675.83 . .14 . .781-782 | 682.5 . . .09 . .602-603 | 698.0 . . .09 . .606-607 |
| 668.93 . .14 . .781-782 | 671.93 . .14 . .781-782 | 675.84 . .14 . .776 | 682.6 . . .09 . .602-603 | 698.1 . . .12 . .729-730 |
| 668.94 . .14 . .776 | 671.94 . .14 . .776 | 675.90 . .14 . .998 | 682.7 . . .09 . .602-603 | 698.1 . . .13 . .757-759 |
| 669.00 . .14 . .774-775 | 672.00 . .14 . .998 | 675.91 . .14 . .774-775 | 682.8 . . .09 . .602-603 | 698.2 . . .09 . .606-607 |
| 669.01 . .14 . .774-775 | 672.02 . .14 . .774 | 675.92 . .14 . .774-775 | 682.9 . . .09 . .602-603 | 698.3 . . .09 . .606-607 |
| 669.02 . .14 . .774-775 | 672.04 . .14 . .776 | 675.93 . .14 . .781-782 | 683 . . . . .16 . .814-816 | 698.4 . . .09 . .606-607 |
| 669.03 . .14 . .781-782 | 673.00 . .14 . .998 | 675.94 . .14 . .776 | 684 . . . . .09 . .602-603 | 698.8 . . .09 . .606-607 |
| 669.04 . .14 . .776 | 673.01 . .14 . .774 | 676.00 . .14 . .998 | 685.0 . . .09 . .602-603 | 698.9 . . .09 . .606-607 |
| 669.10 . .14 . .774-775 | 673.02 . .14 . .774 | 676.01 . .14 . .774-775 | 685.1 . . .09 . .602-603 | 700 . . . . .09 . .606-607 |
| 669.11 . .14 . .774 | 673.03 . .14 . .781-782 | 676.02 . .14 . .774-775 | 686.00 . .09 . .602-603 | 701.0 . . .09 . .606-607 |
| 669.12 . .14 . .774 | 673.04 . .14 . .776 | 676.03 . .14 . .781-782 | 686.01 . .09 . .602-603 | 701.1 . . .09 . .606-607 |
| 669.13 . .14 . .781-782 | 673.10 . .14 . .998 | 676.04 . .14 . .776 | 686.09 . .09 . .602-603 | 701.2 . . .09 . .606-607 |
| 669.14 . .14 . .776 | 673.11 . .14 . .774 | 676.10 . .14 . .998 | 686.1 . . .09 . .602-603 | 701.3 . . .09 . .606-607 |
| 669.20 . .14 . .774-775 | 673.12 . .14 . .774 | 676.11 . .14 . .774-775 | 686.8 . . .09 . .602-603 | 701.4 . . .09 . .606-607 |
| 669.21 . .14 . .774-775 | 673.13 . .14 . .781-782 | 676.12 . .14 . .774-775 | 686.9 . . .09 . .602-603 | 701.5 . . .09 . .606-607 |
| 669.22 . .14 . .774-775 | 673.14 . .14 . .776 | 676.13 . .14 . .781-782 | 690.10 . .09 . .606-607 | 701.8 . . .09 . .606-607 |
| 669.23 . .14 . .781-782 | 673.20 . .14 . .998 | 676.14 . .14 . .776 | 690.11 . .09 . .606-607 | 701.9 . . .09 . .606-607 |
| 669.24 . .14 . .776 | 673.21 . .14 . .774 | 676.20 . .14 . .998 | 690.12 . .09 . .606-607 | 702.0 . . .09 . .606-607 |
| 669.30 . .14 . .774-775 | 673.22 . .14 . .774 | 676.21 . .14 . .774-775 | 690.18 . .09 . .606-607 | 702.11 . .09 . .606-607 |
| 669.32 . .14 . .774 | 673.23 . .14 . .781-782 | 676.22 . .14 . .774-775 | 690.8 . . .09 . .606-607 | 702.19 . .09 . .606-607 |
| 669.34 . .14 . .776 | 673.24 . .14 . .776 | 676.23 . .14 . .781-782 | 691.0 . . .09 . .606-607 | 702.8 . . .09 . .606-607 |
| 669.40 . .14 . .774-775 | 673.30 . .14 . .998 | 676.24 . .14 . .776 | 691.8 . . .09 . .606-607 | 703.0 . . .09 . .606-607 |
| 669.41 . .14 . .774 | 673.31 . .14 . .774 | 676.30 . .14 . .998 | 692.0 . . .09 . .606-607 | 703.8 . . .09 . .606-607 |
| 669.42 . .14 . .774 | 673.32 . .14 . .774 | 676.31 . .14 . .774-775 | 692.1 . . .09 . .606-607 | 703.9 . . .09 . .606-607 |
| 669.44 . .14 . .776 | 673.33 . .14 . .781-782 | 676.32 . .14 . .774-775 | 692.2 . . .09 . .606-607 | 704.00 . .09 . .606-607 |
| 669.50 . .14 . .774-775 | 673.34 . .14 . .776 | 676.33 . .14 . .781-782 | 692.3 . . .09 . .606-607 | 704.01 . .09 . .606-607 |
| 669.51 . .14 . .774-775 | 673.80 . .14 . .998 | 676.34 . .14 . .776 | 692.4 . . .09 . .606-607 | 704.02 . .09 . .606-607 |
| 669.60 . .14 . .774-775 | 673.81 . .14 . .774 | 676.40 . .14 . .998 | 692.5 . . .09 . .606-607 | 704.09 . .09 . .606-607 |
| 669.61 . .14 . .774-775 | 673.82 . .14 . .774 | 676.41 . .14 . .774-775 | 692.6 . . .09 . .606-607 | 704.1 . . .09 . .606-607 |
| 669.70 . .14 . .774-775 | 673.83 . .14 . .781-782 | 676.42 . .14 . .774-775 | 692.70 . .09 . .606-607 | 704.2 . . .09 . .606-607 |
| 669.71 . .14 . .774-775 | 673.84 . .14 . .776 | 676.43 . .14 . .781-782 | 692.71 . .09 . .606-607 | 704.3 . . .09 . .606-607 |
| 669.80 . .14 . .774-775 | 674.00 . .14 . .998 | 676.44 . .14 . .776 | 692.72 . .09 . .606-607 | 704.8 . . .09 . .606-607 |
| 669.81 . .14 . .774-775 | 674.01 . .14 . .774 | 676.50 . .14 . .998 | 692.73 . .09 . .606-607 | 704.9 . . .09 . .606-607 |
| 669.82 . .14 . .774-775 | 674.02 . .14 . .774 | 676.51 . .14 . .774-775 | 692.74 . .09 . .606-607 | 705.0 . . .09 . .606-607 |
| 669.83 . .14 . .781-782 | 674.03 . .14 . .781-782 | 676.52 . .14 . .774-775 | 692.75 . .09 . .606-607 | 705.1 . . .09 . .606-607 |
| 669.84 . .14 . .776 | 674.04 . .14 . .776 | 676.53 . .14 . .781-782 | 692.76 . .09 . .606-607 | 705.21 . .09 . .606-607 |
| 669.90 . .14 . .774-775 | 674.10 . .14 . .998 | 676.54 . .14 . .776 | 692.77 . .09 . .606-607 | 705.22 . .09 . .606-607 |
| 669.91 . .14 . .774-775 | 674.12 . .14 . .774 | 676.60 . .14 . .998 | 692.79 . .09 . .606-607 | 705.81 . .09 . .606-607 |
| 669.92 . .14 . .774-775 | 674.14 . .14 . .776 | 676.61 . .14 . .774-775 | 692.81 . .09 . .606-607 | 705.82 . .09 . .606-607 |
| 669.93 . .14 . .781-782 | 674.20 . .14 . .998 | 676.62 . .14 . .774-775 | 692.82 . .09 . .606-607 | 705.83 . .09 . .606-607 |
| 669.94 . .14 . .776 | 674.22 . .14 . .774 | 676.63 . .14 . .781-782 | 692.83 . .09 . .606-607 | 705.89 . .09 . .606-607 |
| 670.00 . .14 . .998 | 674.24 . .14 . .776 | 676.64 . .14 . .776 | 692.84 . .09 . .606-607 | 705.9 . . .09 . .606-607 |
| 670.02 . .14 . .774 | 674.30 . .14 . .998 | 676.80 . .14 . .998 | 692.89 . .09 . .606-607 | 706.0 . . .09 . .606-607 |
| 670.04 . .14 . .776 | 674.32 . .14 . .774 | 676.81 . .14 . .774-775 | 692.9 . . .09 . .606-607 | 706.1 . . .09 . .606-607 |
| 671.00 . .14 . .998 | 674.34 . .14 . .776 | 676.82 . .14 . .774-775 | 693.0 . . .09 . .606-607 | 706.2 . . .09 . .606-607 |
| 671.01 . .14 . .774-775 | 674.40 . .14 . .998 | 676.83 . .14 . .781-782 | 693.1 . . .09 . .606-607 | 706.3 . . .09 . .606-607 |
| 671.02 . .14 . .774-775 | 674.42 . .14 . .774-775 | 676.84 . .14 . .776 | 693.8 . . .09 . .606-607 | 706.8 . . .09 . .606-607 |
| 671.03 . .14 . .781-782 | 674.44 . .14 . .776 | 676.90 . .14 . .998 | 693.9 . . .09 . .606-607 | 706.9 . . .09 . .606-607 |
| 671.04 . .14 . .776 | 674.50 . .14 . .998 | 676.91 . .14 . .774-775 | 694.0 . . .09 . .606-607 | 707.00 . .09 . .592-594 |
| 671.10 . .14 . .998 | 674.51 . .14 . .774 | 676.92 . .14 . .774-775 | 694.1 . . .09 . .606-607 | 707.01 . .09 . .592-594 |
| 671.11 . .14 . .774-775 | 674.52 . .14 . .774 | 676.93 . .14 . .781-782 | 694.2 . . .09 . .606-607 | 707.02 . .09 . .592-594 |
| 671.12 . .14 . .774-775 | 674.53 . .14 . .781-782 | 676.94 . .14 . .776 | 694.3 . . .09 . .606-607 | 707.03 . .09 . .592-594 |
| 671.13 . .14 . .781-782 | 674.54 . .14 . .776 | 677 . . . . .14 . .998 | 694.4 . . .09 . .595-596 | 707.04 . .09 . .592-594 |
| 671.14 . .14 . .776 | 674.80 . .14 . .998 |  | 694.5 . . .09 . .595-596 | 707.05 . .09 . .592-594 |
| 671.20 . .14 . .998 | 674.82 . .14 . .774 | **Diseases of the Skin and** | 694.60 . .09 . .595-596 | 707.06 . .09 . .592-594 |
| 671.21 . .14 . .774-775 | 674.84 . .14 . .776 | **Subcantaneous Tissue** | 694.61 . .02 . .124-125 | 707.07 . .09 . .592-594 |
| 671.22 . .14 . .774-775 | 674.90 . .14 . .998 | 680.0 . . .09 . .602-603 | 694.8 . . .09 . .595-596 | 707.09 . .09 . .592-594 |
| 671.23 . .14 . .781-782 | 674.92 . .14 . .774-775 | 680.1 . . .09 . .602-603 | 694.9 . . .09 . .595-596 | 707.10 . .09 . .592-594 |
| 671.24 . .14 . .776 | 674.94 . .14 . .776 | 680.2 . . .09 . .602-603 | 695.0 . . .09 . .595-596 | 707.11 . .09 . .592-594 |
| 671.30 . .14 . .998 | 675.00 . .14 . .998 | 680.3 . . .09 . .602-603 | 695.1 . . .09 . .595-596 | 707.12 . .09 . .592-594 |
| 671.31 . .14 . .774 | 675.01 . .14 . .774 | 680.4 . . .09 . .602-603 | 695.2 . . .09 . .595-596 | 707.13 . .09 . .592-594 |
| 671.33 . .14 . .781-782 | 675.02 . .14 . .774 | 680.5 . . .09 . .602-603 | 695.3 . . .09 . .606-607 | 707.14 . .09 . .592-594 |
| 671.40 . .14 . .998 | 675.03 . .14 . .781-782 | 680.6 . . .09 . .602-603 | 695.4 . . .09 . .595-596 | 707.15 . .09 . .592-594 |

| DX | MDC | DRG |
|---|---|---|
| 707.19 | 09 | 592-594 |
| 707.8 | 09 | 592-594 |
| 707.9 | 09 | 592-594 |
| 708.0 | 09 | 606-607 |
| 708.1 | 09 | 606-607 |
| 708.2 | 09 | 606-607 |
| 708.3 | 09 | 606-607 |
| 708.4 | 09 | 606-607 |
| 708.5 | 09 | 606-607 |
| 708.8 | 09 | 606-607 |
| 708.9 | 09 | 606-607 |
| 709.00 | 09 | 606-607 |
| 709.01 | 09 | 606-607 |
| 709.09 | 09 | 606-607 |
| 709.1 | 09 | 606-607 |
| 709.2 | 09 | 606-607 |
| 709.3 | 09 | 606-607 |
| 709.4 | 09 | 606-607 |
| 709.8 | 09 | 606-607 |
| 709.9 | 09 | 606-607 |

**Diseases of the Musculoskeletal System and Connective Tissue**

| DX | MDC | DRG |
|---|---|---|
| 710.0 | 08 | 545-547 |
| 710.1 | 08 | 545-547 |
| 710.2 | 08 | 545-547 |
| 710.3 | 08 | 545-547 |
| 710.4 | 08 | 545-547 |
| 710.5 | 08 | 545-547 |
| 710.8 | 08 | 545-547 |
| 710.9 | 08 | 545-547 |
| 711.00 | 08 | 548-550 |
| 711.01 | 08 | 548-550 |
| 711.02 | 08 | 548-550 |
| 711.03 | 08 | 548-550 |
| 711.04 | 08 | 548-550 |
| 711.05 | 08 | 548-550 |
| 711.06 | 08 | 548-550 |
| 711.07 | 08 | 548-550 |
| 711.08 | 08 | 548-550 |
| 711.09 | 08 | 548-550 |
| 711.10 | 08 | 545-547 |
| 711.11 | 08 | 545-547 |
| 711.12 | 08 | 545-547 |
| 711.13 | 08 | 545-547 |
| 711.14 | 08 | 545-547 |
| 711.15 | 08 | 545-547 |
| 711.16 | 08 | 545-547 |
| 711.17 | 08 | 545-547 |
| 711.18 | 08 | 545-547 |
| 711.19 | 08 | 545-547 |
| 711.20 | 08 | 545-547 |
| 711.21 | 08 | 545-547 |
| 711.22 | 08 | 545-547 |
| 711.23 | 08 | 545-547 |
| 711.24 | 08 | 545-547 |
| 711.25 | 08 | 545-547 |
| 711.26 | 08 | 545-547 |
| 711.27 | 08 | 545-547 |
| 711.28 | 08 | 545-547 |
| 711.29 | 08 | 545-547 |
| 711.30 | 08 | 553-554 |
| 711.31 | 08 | 553-554 |
| 711.32 | 08 | 553-554 |
| 711.33 | 08 | 553-554 |
| 711.34 | 08 | 553-554 |
| 711.35 | 08 | 553-554 |
| 711.36 | 08 | 553-554 |
| 711.37 | 08 | 553-554 |
| 711.38 | 08 | 553-554 |
| 711.39 | 08 | 553-554 |
| 711.40 | 08 | 548-550 |
| 711.41 | 08 | 548-550 |
| 711.42 | 08 | 548-550 |
| 711.43 | 08 | 548-550 |
| 711.44 | 08 | 548-550 |
| 711.45 | 08 | 548-550 |
| 711.46 | 08 | 548-550 |
| 711.47 | 08 | 548-550 |
| 711.48 | 08 | 548-550 |
| 711.49 | 08 | 548-550 |
| 711.50 | 08 | 553-554 |
| 711.51 | 08 | 553-554 |
| 711.52 | 08 | 553-554 |
| 711.53 | 08 | 553-554 |
| 711.54 | 08 | 553-554 |
| 711.55 | 08 | 553-554 |
| 711.56 | 08 | 553-554 |
| 711.57 | 08 | 553-554 |
| 711.58 | 08 | 553-554 |
| 711.59 | 08 | 553-554 |
| 711.60 | 08 | 548-550 |
| 711.61 | 08 | 548-550 |
| 711.62 | 08 | 548-550 |
| 711.63 | 08 | 548-550 |
| 711.64 | 08 | 548-550 |
| 711.65 | 08 | 548-550 |
| 711.66 | 08 | 548-550 |
| 711.67 | 08 | 548-550 |
| 711.68 | 08 | 548-550 |
| 711.69 | 08 | 548-550 |
| 711.70 | 08 | 548-550 |
| 711.71 | 08 | 548-550 |
| 711.72 | 08 | 548-550 |
| 711.73 | 08 | 548-550 |
| 711.74 | 08 | 548-550 |
| 711.75 | 08 | 548-550 |
| 711.76 | 08 | 548-550 |
| 711.77 | 08 | 548-550 |
| 711.78 | 08 | 548-550 |
| 711.79 | 08 | 548-550 |
| 711.80 | 08 | 548-550 |
| 711.81 | 08 | 548-550 |
| 711.82 | 08 | 548-550 |
| 711.83 | 08 | 548-550 |
| 711.84 | 08 | 548-550 |
| 711.85 | 08 | 548-550 |
| 711.86 | 08 | 548-550 |
| 711.87 | 08 | 548-550 |
| 711.88 | 08 | 548-550 |
| 711.89 | 08 | 548-550 |
| 711.90 | 08 | 548-550 |
| 711.91 | 08 | 548-550 |
| 711.92 | 08 | 548-550 |
| 711.93 | 08 | 548-550 |
| 711.94 | 08 | 548-550 |
| 711.95 | 08 | 548-550 |
| 711.96 | 08 | 548-550 |
| 711.97 | 08 | 548-550 |
| 711.98 | 08 | 548-550 |
| 711.99 | 08 | 548-550 |
| 712.10 | 08 | 553-554 |
| 712.11 | 08 | 553-554 |
| 712.12 | 08 | 553-554 |
| 712.13 | 08 | 553-554 |
| 712.14 | 08 | 553-554 |
| 712.15 | 08 | 553-554 |
| 712.16 | 08 | 553-554 |
| 712.17 | 08 | 553-554 |
| 712.18 | 08 | 553-554 |
| 712.19 | 08 | 553-554 |
| 712.20 | 08 | 553-554 |
| 712.21 | 08 | 553-554 |
| 712.22 | 08 | 553-554 |
| 712.23 | 08 | 553-554 |
| 712.24 | 08 | 553-554 |
| 712.25 | 08 | 553-554 |
| 712.26 | 08 | 553-554 |
| 712.27 | 08 | 553-554 |
| 712.28 | 08 | 553-554 |
| 712.29 | 08 | 553-554 |
| 712.30 | 08 | 553-554 |
| 712.31 | 08 | 553-554 |
| 712.32 | 08 | 553-554 |
| 712.33 | 08 | 553-554 |
| 712.34 | 08 | 553-554 |
| 712.35 | 08 | 553-554 |
| 712.36 | 08 | 553-554 |
| 712.37 | 08 | 553-554 |
| 712.38 | 08 | 553-554 |
| 712.39 | 08 | 553-554 |
| 712.80 | 08 | 553-554 |
| 712.81 | 08 | 553-554 |
| 712.82 | 08 | 553-554 |
| 712.83 | 08 | 553-554 |
| 712.84 | 08 | 553-554 |
| 712.85 | 08 | 553-554 |
| 712.86 | 08 | 553-554 |
| 712.87 | 08 | 553-554 |
| 712.88 | 08 | 553-554 |
| 712.89 | 08 | 553-554 |
| 712.90 | 08 | 553-554 |
| 712.91 | 08 | 553-554 |
| 712.92 | 08 | 553-554 |
| 712.93 | 08 | 553-554 |
| 712.94 | 08 | 553-554 |
| 712.95 | 08 | 553-554 |
| 712.96 | 08 | 553-554 |
| 712.97 | 08 | 553-554 |
| 712.98 | 08 | 553-554 |
| 712.99 | 08 | 553-554 |
| 713.0 | 08 | 553-554 |
| 713.1 | 08 | 553-554 |
| 713.2 | 08 | 553-554 |
| 713.3 | 08 | 553-554 |
| 713.4 | 08 | 553-554 |
| 713.5 | 08 | 553-554 |
| 713.6 | 08 | 553-554 |
| 713.7 | 08 | 553-554 |
| 713.8 | 08 | 553-554 |
| 714.0 | 08 | 545-547 |
| 714.1 | 08 | 545-547 |
| 714.2 | 08 | 545-547 |
| 714.30 | 08 | 545-547 |
| 714.31 | 08 | 545-547 |
| 714.32 | 08 | 545-547 |
| 714.33 | 08 | 545-547 |
| 714.4 | 08 | 553-554 |
| 714.81 | 04 | 196-198 |
| 714.89 | 08 | 545-547 |
| 714.9 | 08 | 553-554 |
| 715.00 | 08 | 553-554 |
| 715.04 | 08 | 553-554 |
| 715.09 | 08 | 553-554 |
| 715.10 | 08 | 553-554 |
| 715.11 | 08 | 553-554 |
| 715.12 | 08 | 553-554 |
| 715.13 | 08 | 553-554 |
| 715.14 | 08 | 553-554 |
| 715.15 | 08 | 553-554 |
| 715.16 | 08 | 553-554 |
| 715.17 | 08 | 553-554 |
| 715.18 | 08 | 553-554 |
| 715.20 | 08 | 553-554 |
| 715.21 | 08 | 553-554 |
| 715.22 | 08 | 553-554 |
| 715.23 | 08 | 553-554 |
| 715.24 | 08 | 553-554 |
| 715.25 | 08 | 553-554 |
| 715.26 | 08 | 553-554 |
| 715.27 | 08 | 553-554 |
| 715.28 | 08 | 553-554 |
| 715.30 | 08 | 553-554 |
| 715.31 | 08 | 553-554 |
| 715.32 | 08 | 553-554 |
| 715.33 | 08 | 553-554 |
| 715.34 | 08 | 553-554 |
| 715.35 | 08 | 553-554 |
| 715.36 | 08 | 553-554 |
| 715.37 | 08 | 553-554 |
| 715.38 | 08 | 553-554 |
| 715.80 | 08 | 553-554 |
| 715.89 | 08 | 553-554 |
| 715.90 | 08 | 553-554 |
| 715.91 | 08 | 553-554 |
| 715.92 | 08 | 553-554 |
| 715.93 | 08 | 553-554 |
| 715.94 | 08 | 553-554 |
| 715.95 | 08 | 553-554 |
| 715.96 | 08 | 553-554 |
| 715.97 | 08 | 553-554 |
| 715.98 | 08 | 553-554 |
| 716.00 | 08 | 553-554 |
| 716.01 | 08 | 553-554 |
| 716.02 | 08 | 553-554 |
| 716.03 | 08 | 553-554 |
| 716.04 | 08 | 553-554 |
| 716.05 | 08 | 553-554 |
| 716.06 | 08 | 553-554 |
| 716.07 | 08 | 553-554 |
| 716.08 | 08 | 553-554 |
| 716.09 | 08 | 553-554 |
| 716.10 | 08 | 553-554 |
| 716.11 | 08 | 553-554 |
| 716.12 | 08 | 553-554 |
| 716.13 | 08 | 553-554 |
| 716.14 | 08 | 553-554 |
| 716.15 | 08 | 553-554 |
| 716.16 | 08 | 553-554 |
| 716.17 | 08 | 553-554 |
| 716.18 | 08 | 553-554 |
| 716.19 | 08 | 553-554 |
| 716.20 | 08 | 553-554 |
| 716.21 | 08 | 553-554 |
| 716.22 | 08 | 553-554 |
| 716.23 | 08 | 553-554 |
| 716.24 | 08 | 553-554 |
| 716.25 | 08 | 553-554 |
| 716.26 | 08 | 553-554 |
| 716.27 | 08 | 553-554 |
| 716.28 | 08 | 553-554 |
| 716.29 | 08 | 553-554 |
| 716.30 | 08 | 553-554 |
| 716.31 | 08 | 553-554 |
| 716.32 | 08 | 553-554 |
| 716.33 | 08 | 553-554 |
| 716.34 | 08 | 553-554 |
| 716.35 | 08 | 553-554 |
| 716.36 | 08 | 553-554 |
| 716.37 | 08 | 553-554 |
| 716.38 | 08 | 553-554 |
| 716.39 | 08 | 553-554 |
| 716.40 | 08 | 553-554 |
| 716.41 | 08 | 553-554 |
| 716.42 | 08 | 553-554 |
| 716.43 | 08 | 553-554 |
| 716.44 | 08 | 553-554 |
| 716.45 | 08 | 553-554 |
| 716.46 | 08 | 553-554 |
| 716.47 | 08 | 553-554 |
| 716.48 | 08 | 553-554 |
| 716.49 | 08 | 553-554 |
| 716.50 | 08 | 553-554 |
| 716.51 | 08 | 553-554 |
| 716.52 | 08 | 553-554 |
| 716.53 | 08 | 553-554 |
| 716.54 | 08 | 553-554 |
| 716.55 | 08 | 553-554 |
| 716.56 | 08 | 553-554 |
| 716.57 | 08 | 553-554 |
| 716.58 | 08 | 553-554 |
| 716.59 | 08 | 553-554 |
| 716.60 | 08 | 553-554 |
| 716.61 | 08 | 553-554 |
| 716.62 | 08 | 553-554 |
| 716.63 | 08 | 553-554 |
| 716.64 | 08 | 553-554 |
| 716.65 | 08 | 553-554 |
| 716.66 | 08 | 553-554 |
| 716.67 | 08 | 553-554 |
| 716.68 | 08 | 553-554 |
| 716.80 | 08 | 553-554 |
| 716.81 | 08 | 553-554 |
| 716.82 | 08 | 553-554 |
| 716.83 | 08 | 553-554 |
| 716.84 | 08 | 553-554 |
| 716.85 | 08 | 553-554 |
| 716.86 | 08 | 553-554 |
| 716.87 | 08 | 553-554 |
| 716.88 | 08 | 553-554 |
| 716.89 | 08 | 553-554 |
| 716.90 | 08 | 553-554 |
| 716.91 | 08 | 553-554 |
| 716.92 | 08 | 553-554 |
| 716.93 | 08 | 553-554 |
| 716.94 | 08 | 553-554 |
| 716.95 | 08 | 553-554 |
| 716.96 | 08 | 553-554 |
| 716.97 | 08 | 553-554 |
| 716.98 | 08 | 553-554 |
| 716.99 | 08 | 553-554 |
| 717.0 | 08 | 562-563 |
| 717.1 | 08 | 562-563 |
| 717.2 | 08 | 562-563 |
| 717.3 | 08 | 562-563 |
| 717.40 | 08 | 562-563 |
| 717.41 | 08 | 562-563 |
| 717.42 | 08 | 562-563 |
| 717.43 | 08 | 562-563 |
| 717.49 | 08 | 562-563 |
| 717.5 | 08 | 562-563 |
| 717.6 | 08 | 564-566 |
| 717.7 | 08 | 562-563 |
| 717.81 | 08 | 562-563 |
| 717.82 | 08 | 562-563 |
| 717.83 | 08 | 562-563 |
| 717.84 | 08 | 562-563 |
| 717.85 | 08 | 562-563 |
| 717.89 | 08 | 562-563 |
| 717.9 | 08 | 562-563 |
| 718.00 | 08 | 564-566 |
| 718.01 | 08 | 562-563 |
| 718.02 | 08 | 562-563 |
| 718.03 | 08 | 562-563 |
| 718.04 | 08 | 562-563 |
| 718.05 | 08 | 564-566 |
| 718.07 | 08 | 562-563 |
| 718.08 | 08 | 564-566 |
| 718.09 | 08 | 564-566 |
| 718.10 | 08 | 564-566 |
| 718.11 | 08 | 564-566 |
| 718.12 | 08 | 564-566 |
| 718.13 | 08 | 564-566 |
| 718.14 | 08 | 564-566 |
| 718.15 | 08 | 564-566 |
| 718.17 | 08 | 564-566 |
| 718.18 | 08 | 564-566 |
| 718.19 | 08 | 564-566 |
| 718.20 | 08 | 562-563 |
| 718.21 | 08 | 562-563 |
| 718.22 | 08 | 562-563 |
| 718.23 | 08 | 562-563 |
| 718.24 | 08 | 562-563 |
| 718.25 | 08 | 564-566 |
| 718.26 | 08 | 562-563 |
| 718.27 | 08 | 562-563 |
| 718.28 | 08 | 564-566 |
| 718.29 | 08 | 564-566 |
| 718.30 | 08 | 564-566 |
| 718.31 | 08 | 562-563 |
| 718.32 | 08 | 562-563 |
| 718.33 | 08 | 562-563 |
| 718.34 | 08 | 562-563 |
| 718.35 | 08 | 564-566 |

| DX ...MDC ..DRG | DX ...MDC ..DRG | DX ...MDC ..DRG | DX ...MDC ..DRG | DX ...MDC ..DRG |
|---|---|---|---|---|
| 718.36 ..08 .562-563 | 719.22 ..08 .553-554 | 721.2 ..08 .551-552 | 726.64 ..08 .557-558 | 729.72 ..08 .557-558 |
| 718.37 ..08 .562-563 | 719.23 ..08 .553-554 | 721.3 ..08 .551-552 | 726.65 ..08 .557-558 | 729.73 ..08 .557-558 |
| 718.38 ..08 .564-566 | 719.24 ..08 .553-554 | 721.41 ..08 .551-552 | 726.69 ..08 .557-558 | 729.79 ..08 .557-558 |
| 718.39 ..08 .564-566 | 719.25 ..08 .553-554 | 721.42 ..08 .551-552 | 726.70 ..08 .557-558 | 729.81 ..08 .555-556 |
| 718.40 ..08 .564-566 | 719.26 ..08 .553-554 | 721.5 ..08 .551-552 | 726.71 ..08 .557-558 | 729.82 ..08 .555-556 |
| 718.41 ..08 .564-566 | 719.27 ..08 .553-554 | 721.6 ..08 .551-552 | 726.72 ..08 .557-558 | 729.89 ..08 .555-556 |
| 718.42 ..08 .564-566 | 719.28 ..08 .553-554 | 721.7 ..08 .551-552 | 726.73 ..08 .564-566 | 729.9 ...08 .555-556 |
| 718.43 ..08 .564-566 | 719.29 ..08 .553-554 | 721.8 ..08 .551-552 | 726.79 ..08 .557-558 | 730.00 ..08 .539-541 |
| 718.44 ..08 .564-566 | 719.30 ..08 .553-554 | 721.90 ..08 .551-552 | 726.8 ..08 .557-558 | 730.01 ..08 .539-541 |
| 718.45 ..08 .564-566 | 719.31 ..08 .553-554 | 721.91 ..08 .551-552 | 726.90 ..08 .557-558 | 730.02 ..08 .539-541 |
| 718.46 ..08 .564-566 | 719.32 ..08 .553-554 | 722.0 ..08 .551-552 | 726.91 ..08 .557-558 | 730.03 ..08 .539-541 |
| 718.47 ..08 .564-566 | 719.33 ..08 .553-554 | 722.10 ..08 .551-552 | 727.00 ..08 .557-558 | 730.04 ..08 .539-541 |
| 718.48 ..08 .564-566 | 719.34 ..08 .553-554 | 722.11 ..08 .551-552 | 727.01 ..08 .557-558 | 730.05 ..08 .539-541 |
| 718.49 ..08 .564-566 | 719.35 ..08 .553-554 | 722.2 ..08 .551-552 | 727.02 ..08 .557-558 | 730.06 ..08 .539-541 |
| 718.50 ..08 .553-554 | 719.36 ..08 .553-554 | 722.30 ..08 .551-552 | 727.03 ..08 .557-558 | 730.07 ..08 .539-541 |
| 718.51 ..08 .553-554 | 719.37 ..08 .553-554 | 722.31 ..08 .551-552 | 727.04 ..08 .557-558 | 730.08 ..08 .539-541 |
| 718.52 ..08 .553-554 | 719.38 ..08 .553-554 | 722.32 ..08 .551-552 | 727.05 ..08 .557-558 | 730.09 ..08 .539-541 |
| 718.53 ..08 .553-554 | 719.39 ..08 .553-554 | 722.39 ..08 .551-552 | 727.06 ..08 .557-558 | 730.10 ..08 .539-541 |
| 718.54 ..08 .553-554 | 719.40 ..08 .555-556 | 722.4 ...08 .551-552 | 727.09 ..08 .557-558 | 730.11 ..08 .539-541 |
| 718.55 ..08 .553-554 | 719.41 ..08 .555-556 | 722.51 ..08 .551-552 | 727.1 ...08 .564-566 | 730.12 ..08 .539-541 |
| 718.56 ..08 .553-554 | 719.42 ..08 .555-556 | 722.52 ..08 .551-552 | 727.2 ..08 .557-558 | 730.13 ..08 .539-541 |
| 718.57 ..08 .553-554 | 719.43 ..08 .555-556 | 722.6 ...08 .551-552 | 727.3 ..08 .557-558 | 730.14 ..08 .539-541 |
| 718.58 ..08 .553-554 | 719.44 ..08 .555-556 | 722.70 ..08 .551-552 | 727.40 ..08 .557-558 | 730.15 ..08 .539-541 |
| 718.59 ..08 .553-554 | 719.45 ..08 .555-556 | 722.71 ..08 .551-552 | 727.41 ..08 .557-558 | 730.16 ..08 .539-541 |
| 718.60 ..08 .564-566 | 719.46 ..08 .555-556 | 722.72 ..08 .551-552 | 727.42 ..08 .557-558 | 730.17 ..08 .539-541 |
| 718.65 ..08 .564-566 | 719.47 ..08 .555-556 | 722.73 ..08 .551-552 | 727.43 ..08 .557-558 | 730.18 ..08 .539-541 |
| 718.70 ...08 .564-566 | 719.48 ..08 .555-556 | 722.80 ..08 .551-552 | 727.49 ..08 .557-558 | 730.19 ..08 .539-541 |
| 718.71 ..08 .564-566 | 719.49 ..08 .555-556 | 722.81 ..08 .551-552 | 727.50 ..08 .557-558 | 730.20 ..08 .539-541 |
| 718.72 ..08 .564-566 | 719.50 ..08 .555-556 | 722.82 ..08 .551-552 | 727.51 ..08 .557-558 | 730.21 ..08 .539-541 |
| 718.73 ..08 .564-566 | 719.51 ..08 .555-556 | 722.83 ..08 .551-552 | 727.59 ..08 .557-558 | 730.22 ..08 .539-541 |
| 718.74 ..08 .564-566 | 719.52 ..08 .555-556 | 722.90 ..08 .551-552 | 727.60 ..08 .557-558 | 730.23 ..08 .539-541 |
| 718.75 ..08 .564-566 | 719.53 ..08 .555-556 | 722.91 ..08 .551-552 | 727.61 ..08 .557-558 | 730.24 ..08 .539-541 |
| 718.76 ..08 .564-566 | 719.54 ..08 .555-556 | 722.92 ..08 .551-552 | 727.62 ..08 .557-558 | 730.25 ..08 .539-541 |
| 718.77 ..08 .564-566 | 719.55 ..08 .555-556 | 722.93 ..08 .551-552 | 727.63 ..08 .557-558 | 730.26 ..08 .539-541 |
| 718.78 ..08 .564-566 | 719.56 ..08 .555-556 | 723.0 ...08 .551-552 | 727.64 ..08 .557-558 | 730.27 ..08 .539-541 |
| 718.79 ..08 .564-566 | 719.57 ..08 .555-556 | 723.1 ...08 .551-552 | 727.65 ..08 .557-558 | 730.28 ..08 .539-541 |
| 718.80 ..08 .564-566 | 719.58 ..08 .555-556 | 723.2 ...01 .073-074 | 727.66 ..08 .557-558 | 730.29 ..08 .539-541 |
| 718.81 ..08 .564-566 | 719.59 ..08 .555-556 | 723.3 ...01 .073-074 | 727.67 ..08 .557-558 | 730.30 ..08 .553-554 |
| 718.82 ..08 .564-566 | 719.60 ..08 .555-556 | 723.4 ...01 .073-074 | 727.68 ..08 .557-558 | 730.31 ..08 .553-554 |
| 718.83 ..08 .564-566 | 719.61 ..08 .555-556 | 723.5 ...08 .551-552 | 727.69 ..08 .557-558 | 730.32 ..08 .553-554 |
| 718.84 ..08 .564-566 | 719.62 ..08 .555-556 | 723.6 ...09 .606-607 | 727.81 ..08 .557-558 | 730.33 ..08 .553-554 |
| 718.85 ..08 .564-566 | 719.63 ..08 .555-556 | 723.7 ...08 .551-552 | 727.82 ..08 .557-558 | 730.34 ..08 .553-554 |
| 718.86 ..08 .564-566 | 719.64 ..08 .555-556 | 723.8 ...08 .551-552 | 727.83 ..08 .557-558 | 730.35 ..08 .553-554 |
| 718.87 ..08 .564-566 | 719.65 ..08 .555-556 | 723.9 ...08 .551-552 | 727.89 ..08 .557-558 | 730.36 ..08 .553-554 |
| 718.88 ..08 .564-566 | 719.66 ..08 .555-556 | 724.00 ..08 .551-552 | 727.9 ...08 .557-558 | 730.37 ..08 .564-566 |
| 718.89 ..08 .564-566 | 719.67 ..08 .555-556 | 724.01 ..08 .551-552 | 728.0 ..08 .557-558 | 730.38 ..08 .564-566 |
| 718.90 ..08 .564-566 | 719.68 ..08 .555-556 | 724.02 ..08 .551-552 | 728.10 ..08 .557-558 | 730.39 ..08 .564-566 |
| 718.91 ..08 .564-566 | 719.69 ..08 .555-556 | 724.09 ..08 .551-552 | 728.11 ..08 .557-558 | 730.70 ..08 .564-566 |
| 718.92 ..08 .564-566 | 719.7 ...08 .555-556 | 724.1 ...08 .551-552 | 728.12 ..08 .557-558 | 730.71 ..08 .564-566 |
| 718.93 ..08 .564-566 | 719.80 ..08 .555-556 | 724.2 ..08 .551-552 | 728.13 ..08 .557-558 | 730.72 ..08 .564-566 |
| 718.94 ..08 .564-566 | 719.81 ..08 .555-556 | 724.3 ...08 .551-552 | 728.19 ..08 .557-558 | 730.73 ..08 .564-566 |
| 718.95 ..08 .564-566 | 719.82 ..08 .555-556 | 724.4 ...08 .551-552 | 728.2 ..08 .557-558 | 730.74 ..08 .564-566 |
| 718.97 ..08 .564-566 | 719.83 ..08 .555-556 | 724.5 ...08 .551-552 | 728.3 ..08 .557-558 | 730.75 ..08 .564-566 |
| 718.98 ..08 .564-566 | 719.84 ..08 .555-556 | 724.6 ...08 .551-552 | 728.4 ..08 .557-558 | 730.76 ..08 .564-566 |
| 718.99 ..08 .564-566 | 719.85 ..08 .555-556 | 724.70 ..08 .551-552 | 728.5 ..08 .557-558 | 730.77 ..08 .564-566 |
| 719.00 ..08 .564-566 | 719.86 ..08 .555-556 | 724.71 ..08 .551-552 | 728.6 ..08 .557-558 | 730.78 ..08 .564-566 |
| 719.01 ..08 .564-566 | 719.87 ..08 .555-556 | 724.79 ..08 .551-552 | 728.71 ..08 .557-558 | 730.79 ..08 .564-566 |
| 719.02 ..08 .564-566 | 719.88 ..08 .555-556 | 724.8 ...08 .551-552 | 728.79 ..08 .557-558 | 730.80 ..08 .539-541 |
| 719.03 ..08 .564-566 | 719.89 ..08 .555-556 | 724.9 ...08 .551-552 | 728.81 ..08 .557-558 | 730.81 ..08 .539-541 |
| 719.04 ..08 .564-566 | 719.90 ..08 .555-556 | 725. ....08 .545-547 | 728.82 ..08 .557-558 | 730.82 ..08 .539-541 |
| 719.05 ..08 .564-566 | 719.91 ..08 .555-556 | 726.0 ..08 .557-558 | 728.83 ..08 .557-558 | 730.83 ..08 .539-541 |
| 719.06 ..08 .564-566 | 719.92 ..08 .555-556 | 726.10 ..08 .557-558 | 728.84 ..08 .557-558 | 730.84 ..08 .539-541 |
| 719.07 ..08 .564-566 | 719.93 ..08 .555-556 | 726.11 ..08 .557-558 | 728.85 ..08 .555-556 | 730.85 ..08 .539-541 |
| 719.08 ..08 .564-566 | 719.94 ..08 .555-556 | 726.12 ..08 .557-558 | 728.87 ..08 .555-556 | 730.86 ..08 .539-541 |
| 719.09 ..08 .564-566 | 719.95 ..08 .555-556 | 726.19 ..08 .557-558 | 728.88 ..08 .557-558 | 730.87 ..08 .539-541 |
| 719.10 ..08 .553-554 | 719.96 ..08 .555-556 | 726.2 ...08 .557-558 | 728.89 ..08 .557-558 | 730.88 ..08 .539-541 |
| 719.11 ..08 .553-554 | 719.97 ..08 .555-556 | 726.30 ..08 .557-558 | 728.9 ..08 .557-558 | 730.89 ..08 .539-541 |
| 719.12 ..08 .553-554 | 719.98 ..08 .555-556 | 726.31 ..08 .557-558 | 729.0 ..08 .555-556 | 730.90 ..08 .539-541 |
| 719.13 ..08 .553-554 | 719.99 ..08 .555-556 | 726.32 ..08 .557-558 | 729.1 ...08 .555-556 | 730.91 ..08 .539-541 |
| 719.14 ..08 .553-554 | 720.0 ..08 .545-547 | 726.33 ..08 .557-558 | 729.2 ...01 .073-074 | 730.92 ..08 .539-541 |
| 719.15 ..08 .553-554 | 720.1 ..08 .551-552 | 726.39 ..08 .557-558 | 729.30 ..09 .606-607 | 730.93 ..08 .539-541 |
| 719.16 ..08 .553-554 | 720.2 ..08 .551-552 | 726.4 ...08 .557-558 | 729.31 ..09 .606-607 | 730.94 ..08 .539-541 |
| 719.17 ..08 .553-554 | 720.81 ..08 .551-552 | 726.5 ...08 .557-558 | 729.39 ..09 .606-607 | 730.95 ..08 .539-541 |
| 719.18 ..08 .553-554 | 720.89 ..08 .551-552 | 726.60 ..08 .557-558 | 729.4 ...08 .557-558 | 730.96 ..08 .539-541 |
| 719.19 ..08 .553-554 | 720.9 ..08 .551-552 | 726.61 ..08 .557-558 | 729.5 ...08 .555-556 | 730.97 ..08 .539-541 |
| 719.20 ..08 .553-554 | 721.0 ..08 .551-552 | 726.62 ..08 .557-558 | 729.6 ...08 .564-566 | 730.98 ..08 .539-541 |
| 719.21 ..08 .553-554 | 721.1 ..08 .551-552 | 726.63 ..08 .557-558 | 729.71 ..08 .557-558 | 730.99 ..08 .539-541 |

| DX ...MDC ..DRG | DX ...MDC ..DRG | DX ...MDC ..DRG | DX ...MDC ..DRG | DX ...MDC ..DRG |
|---|---|---|---|---|
| 731.0 ...08 ..553-554 | 736.32 ..08 ..564-566 | 742.3 ...01 ..091-093 | 744.89 ..03 ..154-156 | 749.11 ..03 ..157-159 |
| 731.1 ...08 ..553-554 | 736.39 ..08 ..564-566 | 742.4 ...01 ..091-093 | 744.9 ...09 ..606-607 | 749.12 ..03 ..157-159 |
| 731.2 ..08 ..553-554 | 736.41 ..08 ..564-566 | 742.51 ..01 ..091-093 | 745.0 ...05 ..306-307 | 749.13 ..03 ..157-159 |
| 731.3 ..08 ..553-554 | 736.42 ..08 ..564-566 | 742.53 ..01 ..091-093 | 745.10 ..05 ..306-307 | 749.14 ..03 ..157-159 |
| 731.8 ..08 ..553-554 | 736.5 ..08 ..564-566 | 742.59 ..01 ..091-093 | 745.11 ..05 ..306-307 | 749.20 ..03 ..157-159 |
| 732.0 ..08 ..553-554 | 736.6 ..08 ..564-566 | 742.8 ...01 ..091-093 | 745.12 ..05 ..306-307 | 749.21 ..03 ..157-159 |
| 732.1 ..08 ..553-554 | 736.70 ..08 ..564-566 | 742.9 ...01 ..091-093 | 745.19 ..05 ..306-307 | 749.22 ..03 ..157-159 |
| 732.2 ..08 ..553-554 | 736.71 ..08 ..564-566 | 743.00 ..02 ..124-125 | 745.2 ...05 ..306-307 | 749.23 ..03 ..157-159 |
| 732.3 ..08 ..553-554 | 736.72 ..08 ..564-566 | 743.03 ..02 ..124-125 | 745.3 ...05 ..306-307 | 749.24 ..03 ..157-159 |
| 732.4 ..08 ..553-554 | 736.73 ..08 ..564-566 | 743.06 ..02 ..124-125 | 745.4 ...05 ..306-307 | 749.25 ..03 ..157-159 |
| 732.5 ..08 ..553-554 | 736.74 ..01 ..073-074 | 743.10 ..02 ..124-125 | 745.5 ...05 ..306-307 | 750.0 ...03 ..157-159 |
| 732.6 ..08 ..553-554 | 736.75 ..08 ..564-566 | 743.11 ..02 ..124-125 | 745.60 ..05 ..306-307 | 750.10 ..03 ..157-159 |
| 732.7 ..08 ..553-554 | 736.76 ..08 ..564-566 | 743.12 ..02 ..124-125 | 745.61 ..05 ..306-307 | 750.11 ..03 ..157-159 |
| 732.8 ..08 ..553-554 | 736.79 ..08 ..564-566 | 743.20 ..02 ..124-125 | 745.69 ..05 ..306-307 | 750.12 ..03 ..157-159 |
| 732.9 ..08 ..553-554 | 736.81 ..08 ..564-566 | 743.21 ..02 ..124-125 | 745.7 ...05 ..306-307 | 750.13 ..03 ..157-159 |
| 733.00 ..08 ..553-554 | 736.89 ..08 ..564-566 | 743.22 ..02 ..124-125 | 745.8 ...05 ..306-307 | 750.15 ..03 ..157-159 |
| 733.01 ..08 ..553-554 | 736.9 ...08 ..564-566 | 743.30 ..02 ..124-125 | 745.9 ...05 ..306-307 | 750.16 ..03 ..157-159 |
| 733.02 ..08 ..553-554 | 737.0 ...08 ..551-552 | 743.31 ..02 ..124-125 | 746.00 ..05 ..306-307 | 750.19 ..03 ..157-159 |
| 733.03 ..08 ..553-554 | 737.10 ..08 ..551-552 | 743.32 ..02 ..124-125 | 746.01 ..05 ..306-307 | 750.21 ..03 ..154-156 |
| 733.09 ......553-554 | 737.11 ..08 ..551-552 | 743.33 ..02 ..124-125 | 746.02 ..05 ..306-307 | 750.22 ..03 ..154-156 |
| 733.10 ..08 ..542-544 | 737.12 ..08 ..551-552 | 743.34 ..02 ..124-125 | 746.09 ..05 ..306-307 | 750.23 ..03 ..154-156 |
| 733.11 ..08 ..542-544 | 737.19 ..08 ..551-552 | 743.35 ..02 ..124-125 | 746.1 ...05 ..306-307 | 750.24 ..03 ..157-159 |
| 733.12 ..08 ..542-544 | 737.20 ..08 ..551-552 | 743.36 ..02 ..124-125 | 746.2 ...05 ..306-307 | 750.25 ..03 ..157-159 |
| 733.13 ..08 ..542-544 | 737.21 ..08 ..551-552 | 743.37 ..02 ..124-125 | 746.3 ...05 ..306-307 | 750.26 ..03 ..157-159 |
| 733.14 ..08 ..542-544 | 737.22 ..08 ..551-552 | 743.39 ..02 ..124-125 | 746.4 ...05 ..306-307 | 750.27 ..03 ..154-156 |
| 733.15 ..08 ..542-544 | 737.29 ..08 ..551-552 | 743.41 ..02 ..124-125 | 746.5 ...05 ..306-307 | 750.29 ..03 ..154-156 |
| 733.16 ..08 ..542-544 | 737.30 ..08 ..551-552 | 743.42 ..02 ..124-125 | 746.6 ...05 ..306-307 | 750.3 ...06 ..368-370 |
| 733.19 ..08 ..542-544 | 737.31 ..08 ..551-552 | 743.43 ..02 ..124-125 | 746.7 ...05 ..306-307 | 750.4 ...06 ..368-370 |
| 733.20 ..08 ..553-554 | 737.32 ..08 ..551-552 | 743.44 ..02 ..124-125 | 746.81 ..05 ..306-307 | 750.5 ...06 ..393-395 |
| 733.21 ..08 ..553-554 | 737.33 ..08 ..551-552 | 743.45 ..02 ..124-125 | 746.82 ..05 ..306-307 | 750.6 ...06 ..393-395 |
| 733.22 ..08 ..553-554 | 737.34 ..08 ..551-552 | 743.46 ..02 ..124-125 | 746.83 ..05 ..306-307 | 750.7 ...06 ..393-395 |
| 733.29 ..08 ..553-554 | 737.39 ..08 ..551-552 | 743.47 ..02 ..124-125 | 746.84 ..05 ..306-307 | 750.8 ...06 ..393-395 |
| 733.3 ..08 ..564-566 | 737.40 ..08 ..551-552 | 743.48 ..02 ..124-125 | 746.85 ..05 ..306-307 | 750.9 ...06 ..393-395 |
| 733.40 ..08 ..553-554 | 737.41 ..08 ..551-552 | 743.49 ..02 ..124-125 | 746.86 ..05 ..308-310 | 751.0 ...06 ..380-382 |
| 733.41 ..08 ..553-554 | 737.42 ..08 ..551-552 | 743.51 ..02 ..124-125 | 746.87 ..05 ..306-307 | 751.1 ...06 ..393-395 |
| 733.42 ..08 ..553-554 | 737.43 ..08 ..551-552 | 743.52 ..02 ..124-125 | 746.89 ..05 ..306-307 | 751.2 ...06 ..393-395 |
| 733.43 ..08 ..553-554 | 737.8 ..08 ..551-552 | 743.53 ..02 ..124-125 | 746.9 ...05 ..306-307 | 751.3 ...06 ..393-395 |
| 733.44 ..08 ..553-554 | 737.9 ..08 ..551-552 | 743.54 ..02 ..124-125 | 747.0 ...05 ..306-307 | 751.4 ...06 ..393-395 |
| 733.45 ..08 ..553-554 | 738.0 ...03 ..154-156 | 743.55 ..02 ..124-125 | 747.10 ..05 ..306-307 | 751.5 ...06 ..393-395 |
| 733.49 ..08 ..553-554 | 738.10 ..08 ..564-566 | 743.56 ..02 ..124-125 | 747.11 ..05 ..306-307 | 751.60 ..07 ..444-446 |
| 733.5 ...08 ..553-554 | 738.11 ..08 ..564-566 | 743.57 ..02 ..124-125 | 747.20 ..05 ..306-307 | 751.61 ..07 ..444-446 |
| 733.6 ...04 ..205-206 | 738.12 ..08 ..564-566 | 743.58 ..02 ..124-125 | 747.21 ..05 ..306-307 | 751.62 ..07 ..441-443 |
| 733.7 ..08 ..564-566 | 738.19 ..08 ..564-566 | 743.59 ..02 ..124-125 | 747.22 ..05 ..306-307 | 751.69 ..07 ..441-443 |
| 733.81 ..08 ..564-566 | 738.2 ...08 ..564-566 | 743.61 ..02 ..124-125 | 747.29 ..05 ..306-307 | 751.7 ...07 ..438-440 |
| 733.82 ..08 ..564-566 | 738.3 ...08 ..564-566 | 743.62 ..02 ..124-125 | 747.3 ...05 ..306-307 | 751.8 ...06 ..393-395 |
| 733.90 ..08 ..564-566 | 738.4 ...08 ..551-552 | 743.63 ..02 ..124-125 | 747.40 ..05 ..306-307 | 751.9 ...06 ..393-395 |
| 733.91 ..08 ..564-566 | 738.5 ...08 ..551-552 | 743.64 ..02 ..124-125 | 747.41 ..05 ..306-307 | 752.0 ...13 ..760-761 |
| 733.92 ..08 ..553-554 | 738.6 ...08 ..564-566 | 743.65 ..02 ..124-125 | 747.42 ..05 ..306-307 | 752.10 ..13 ..760-761 |
| 733.93 ..08 ..542-544 | 738.7 ...03 ..154-156 | 743.66 ..02 ..124-125 | 747.49 ..05 ..306-307 | 752.11 ..13 ..760-761 |
| 733.94 ..08 ..542-544 | 738.8 ...08 ..564-566 | 743.69 ..02 ..124-125 | 747.5 ...05 ..299-301 | 752.19 ..13 ..760-761 |
| 733.95 ..08 ..542-544 | 738.9 ...08 ..564-566 | 743.8 ...02 ..124-125 | 747.60 ..05 ..299-301 | 752.2 ...13 ..760-761 |
| 733.99 ..08 ..564-566 | 739.0 ...08 ..555-556 | 743.9 ...02 ..124-125 | 747.61 ..05 ..299-301 | 752.3 ...13 ..760-761 |
| 734 ....08 ..564-566 | 739.1 ...08 ..551-552 | 744.00 ..03 ..154-156 | 747.62 ..05 ..299-301 | 752.40 ..13 ..760-761 |
| 735.0 ..08 ..564-566 | 739.2 ...08 ..551-552 | 744.01 ..03 ..154-156 | 747.63 ..05 ..299-301 | 752.41 ..13 ..760-761 |
| 735.1 ..08 ..564-566 | 739.3 ...08 ..551-552 | 744.02 ..03 ..154-156 | 747.64 ..05 ..299-301 | 752.42 ..13 ..760-761 |
| 735.2 ..08 ..564-566 | 739 ....08 ..551-552 | 744.03 ..03 ..154-156 | 747.69 ..05 ..299-301 | 752.49 ..13 ..760-761 |
| 735.3 ..08 ..564-566 | 739.5 ...08 ..555-556 | 744.04 ..03 ..154-156 | 747.81 ..01 ..091-093 | 752.51 ..12 ..729-730 |
| 735.4 ..08 ..564-566 | 739.6 ...08 ..555-556 | 744.05 ..03 ..154-156 | 747.83 ..15 ..791-793 | 752.52 ..12 ..729-730 |
| 735.5 ..08 ..564-566 | 739.7 ...08 ..555-556 | 744.09 ..03 ..154-156 | 747.89 ..05 ..299-301 | 752.61 ..12 ..729-730 |
| 735.8 ..08 ..564-566 | 739.8 ...08 ..555-556 | 744.1 ...03 ..154-156 | 747.9 ...05 ..299-301 | 752.62 ..12 ..729-730 |
| 735.9 ..08 ..564-566 | 739.9 ...08 ..555-556 | 744.21 ..03 ..154-156 | 748.0 ...03 ..154-156 | 752.63 ..12 ..729-730 |
| 736.00 ..08 ..564-566 | | 744.22 ..03 ..154-156 | 748.1 ...03 ..154-156 | 752.64 ..12 ..729-730 |
| 736.01 ..08 ..564-566 | **Congenital Anomalies** | 744.23 ..03 ..154-156 | 748.2 ...03 ..154-156 | 752.65 ..12 ..729-730 |
| 736.02 ..08 ..564-566 | 740.0 ...01 ..091-093 | 744.24 ..03 ..154-156 | 748.3 ...03 ..154-156 | 752.69 ..12 ..729-730 |
| 736.03 ..08 ..564-566 | 740.1 ...01 ..091-093 | 744.29 ..03 ..154-156 | 748.4 ...04 ..205-206 | 752.7 ...12 ..729-730 |
| 736.04 ..08 ..564-566 | 740.2 ...01 ..091-093 | 744.3 ...03 ..154-156 | 748.5 ...04 ..205-206 | 752.7 ...13 ..760-761 |
| 736.05 ..01 ..073-074 | 741.00 ..01 ..091-093 | 744.41 ..03 ..154-156 | 748.60 ..04 ..205-206 | 752.81 ..12 ..729-730 |
| 736.06 ..01 ..073-074 | 741.01 ..01 ..091-093 | 744.42 ..03 ..154-156 | 748.61 ..04 ..190-192 | 752.89 ..12 ..729-730 |
| 736.07 ..01 ..073-074 | 741.02 ..01 ..091-093 | 744.43 ..03 ..154-156 | 748.69 ..04 ..205-206 | 752.8 ...13 ..760-761 |
| 736.09 ..08 ..564-566 | 741.03 ..01 ..091-093 | 744.46 ..03 ..154-156 | 748.8 ...04 ..205-206 | 752.9 ...12 ..729-730 |
| 736.1 ..08 ..564-566 | 741.90 ..01 ..091-093 | 744.47 ..03 ..154-156 | 748.9 ...04 ..205-206 | 752.9 ...13 ..760-761 |
| 736.20 ..08 ..564-566 | 741.91 ..01 ..091-093 | 744.49 ..03 ..154-156 | 749.00 ..03 ..157-159 | 753.0 ...11 ..698-700 |
| 736.21 ..08 ..564-566 | 741.92 ..01 ..091-093 | 744.5 ...09 ..606-607 | 749.01 ..03 ..157-159 | 753.10 ..11 ..698-700 |
| 736.22 ..08 ..564-566 | 741.93 ..01 ..091-093 | 744.81 ..03 ..157-159 | 749.02 ..03 ..157-159 | 753.11 ..11 ..698-700 |
| 736.29 ..08 ..564-566 | 742.0 ...01 ..091-093 | 744.82 ..03 ..157-159 | 749.03 ..03 ..157-159 | 753.12 ..11 ..698-700 |
| 736.30 ..08 ..564-566 | 742.1 ...01 ..091-093 | 744.83 ..03 ..157-159 | 749.04 ..03 ..157-159 | 753.13 ..11 ..698-700 |
| 736.31 ..08 ..564-566 | 742.2 ...01 ..091-093 | 744.84 ..03 ..157-159 | 749.10 ..03 ..157-159 | 753.14 ..11 ..698-700 |

| DX | MDC | DRG |
|---|---|---|
| 753.15 | 11 | 698-700 |
| 753.16 | 11 | 698-700 |
| 753.17 | 11 | 698-700 |
| 753.19 | 11 | 698-700 |
| 753.20 | 11 | 698-700 |
| 753.21 | 11 | 698-700 |
| 753.22 | 11 | 698-700 |
| 753.23 | 11 | 698-700 |
| 753.29 | 11 | 698-700 |
| 753.3 | 11 | 698-700 |
| 753.4 | 11 | 698-700 |
| 753.5 | 11 | 698-700 |
| 753.6 | 11 | 698-700 |
| 753.7 | 11 | 698-700 |
| 753.8 | 11 | 698-700 |
| 753.9 | 11 | 698-700 |
| 754.0 | 08 | 564-566 |
| 754.1 | 08 | 564-566 |
| 754.2 | 08 | 564-566 |
| 754.30 | 08 | 564-566 |
| 754.31 | 08 | 564-566 |
| 754.32 | 08 | 564-566 |
| 754.33 | 08 | 564-566 |
| 754.35 | 08 | 564-566 |
| 754.40 | 08 | 564-566 |
| 754.41 | 08 | 562-563 |
| 754.42 | 08 | 564-566 |
| 754.43 | 08 | 564-566 |
| 754.44 | 08 | 564-566 |
| 754.50 | 08 | 564-566 |
| 754.51 | 08 | 564-566 |
| 754.52 | 08 | 564-566 |
| 754.53 | 08 | 564-566 |
| 754.59 | 08 | 564-566 |
| 754.60 | 08 | 564-566 |
| 754.61 | 08 | 564-566 |
| 754.62 | 08 | 564-566 |
| 754.69 | 08 | 564-566 |
| 754.70 | 08 | 564-566 |
| 754.71 | 08 | 564-566 |
| 754.79 | 08 | 564-566 |
| 754.81 | 04 | 205-206 |
| 754.82 | 04 | 205-206 |
| 754.89 | 08 | 564-566 |
| 755.00 | 08 | 564-566 |
| 755.01 | 08 | 564-566 |
| 755.02 | 08 | 564-566 |
| 755.10 | 08 | 564-566 |
| 755.11 | 08 | 564-566 |
| 755.12 | 08 | 564-566 |
| 755.13 | 08 | 564-566 |
| 755.14 | 08 | 564-566 |
| 755.20 | 08 | 564-566 |
| 755.21 | 08 | 564-566 |
| 755.22 | 08 | 564-566 |
| 755.23 | 08 | 564-566 |
| 755.24 | 08 | 564-566 |
| 755.25 | 08 | 564-566 |
| 755.26 | 08 | 564-566 |
| 755.27 | 08 | 564-566 |
| 755.28 | 08 | 564-566 |
| 755.29 | 08 | 564-566 |
| 755.30 | 08 | 564-566 |
| 755.31 | 08 | 564-566 |
| 755.32 | 08 | 564-566 |
| 755.33 | 08 | 564-566 |
| 755.34 | 08 | 564-566 |
| 755.35 | 08 | 564-566 |
| 755.36 | 08 | 564-566 |
| 755.37 | 08 | 564-566 |
| 755.38 | 08 | 564-566 |
| 755.39 | 08 | 564-566 |
| 755.4 | 08 | 564-566 |
| 755.50 | 08 | 564-566 |
| 755.51 | 08 | 564-566 |
| 755.52 | 08 | 564-566 |
| 755.53 | 08 | 564-566 |

| DX | MDC | DRG |
|---|---|---|
| 755.54 | 08 | 564-566 |
| 755.55 | 08 | 564-566 |
| 755.56 | 08 | 564-566 |
| 755.57 | 08 | 564-566 |
| 755.58 | 08 | 564-566 |
| 755.59 | 08 | 564-566 |
| 755.60 | 08 | 564-566 |
| 755.61 | 08 | 564-566 |
| 755.62 | 08 | 564-566 |
| 755.63 | 08 | 564-566 |
| 755.64 | 08 | 564-566 |
| 755.65 | 08 | 564-566 |
| 755.66 | 08 | 564-566 |
| 755.67 | 08 | 564-566 |
| 755.69 | 08 | 564-566 |
| 755.8 | 08 | 564-566 |
| 755.9 | 08 | 564-566 |
| 756.0 | 08 | 564-566 |
| 756.10 | 08 | 551-552 |
| 756.11 | 08 | 551-552 |
| 756.12 | 08 | 551-552 |
| 756.13 | 08 | 551-552 |
| 756.14 | 08 | 551-552 |
| 756.15 | 08 | 551-552 |
| 756.16 | 08 | 564-566 |
| 756.17 | 01 | 091-093 |
| 756.19 | 08 | 551-552 |
| 756.2 | 08 | 564-566 |
| 756.3 | 04 | 205-206 |
| 756.4 | 08 | 564-566 |
| 756.50 | 08 | 564-566 |
| 756.51 | 08 | 564-566 |
| 756.52 | 08 | 564-566 |
| 756.53 | 08 | 564-566 |
| 756.54 | 08 | 564-566 |
| 756.55 | 08 | 564-566 |
| 756.56 | 08 | 564-566 |
| 756.59 | 08 | 564-566 |
| 756.6 | 04 | 205-206 |
| 756.70 | 06 | 393-395 |
| 756.71 | 06 | 393-395 |
| 756.79 | 06 | 393-395 |
| 756.81 | 08 | 564-566 |
| 756.82 | 08 | 564-566 |
| 756.83 | 08 | 564-566 |
| 756.89 | 08 | 564-566 |
| 756.9 | 08 | 564-566 |
| 757.0 | 09 | 606-607 |
| 757.1 | 09 | 606-607 |
| 757.2 | 09 | 606-607 |
| 757.31 | 09 | 606-607 |
| 757.32 | 09 | 606-607 |
| 757.33 | 09 | 606-607 |
| 757.39 | 09 | 606-607 |
| 757.4 | 09 | 606-607 |
| 757.5 | 09 | 606-607 |
| 757.6 | 09 | 600-601 |
| 757.8 | 09 | 606-607 |
| 757.9 | 09 | 606-607 |
| 758.0 | 19 | 884 |
| 758.1 | 19 | 884 |
| 758.2 | 19 | 884 |
| 758.31 | 19 | 884 |
| 758.32 | 19 | 884 |
| 758.33 | 19 | 884 |
| 758.39 | 19 | 884 |
| 758.4 | 23 | 951 |
| 758.5 | 23 | 951 |
| 758.6 | 12 | 729-730 |
| 758.6 | 13 | 760-761 |
| 758.7 | 12 | 729-730 |
| 758.8 | 12 | 729-730 |
| 758.81 | 12 | 729-730 |
| 758.81 | 13 | 760-761 |
| 758.89 | 12 | 729-730 |
| 758.89 | 13 | 760-761 |
| 758.9 | 23 | 951 |

| DX | MDC | DRG |
|---|---|---|
| 759.0 | 16 | 814-816 |
| 759.1 | 10 | 643-645 |
| 759.2 | 10 | 643-645 |
| 759.3 | 06 | 393-395 |
| 759.4 | 06 | 393-395 |
| 759.5 | 01 | 091-093 |
| 759.6 | 17 | 843-845 |
| 759.7 | 08 | 564-566 |
| 759.81 | 08 | 564-566 |
| 759.82 | 05 | 306-307 |
| 759.83 | 19 | 884 |
| 759.89 | 08 | 564-566 |
| 759.9 | 23 | 951 |

**Certain Conditions Originating in the Perinatal Period**

| DX | MDC | DRG |
|---|---|---|
| 760.0 | 15 | 794 |
| 760.1 | 15 | 794 |
| 760.2 | 15 | 794 |
| 760.3 | 15 | 794 |
| 760.4 | 15 | 794 |
| 760.5 | 15 | 794 |
| 760.6 | 15 | 794 |
| 760.70 | 15 | 794 |
| 760.71 | 15 | 794 |
| 760.72 | 15 | 794 |
| 760.73 | 15 | 794 |
| 760.74 | 15 | 794 |
| 760.75 | 15 | 794 |
| 760.77 | 15 | 794 |
| 760.78 | 15 | 794 |
| 760.79 | 15 | 794 |
| 760.8 | 15 | 794 |
| 760.9 | 15 | 794 |
| 761.0 | 15 | 794 |
| 761.1 | 15 | 794 |
| 761.2 | 15 | 794 |
| 761.3 | 15 | 794 |
| 761.4 | 15 | 794 |
| 761.5 | 15 | 794 |
| 761.6 | 15 | 794 |
| 761.7 | 15 | 794 |
| 761.8 | 15 | 794 |
| 761.9 | 15 | 794 |
| 762.0 | 15 | 794 |
| 762.1 | 15 | 794 |
| 762.2 | 15 | 794 |
| 762.3 | 15 | 794 |
| 762.4 | 15 | 795 |
| 762.5 | 15 | 795 |
| 762.6 | 15 | 795 |
| 762.7 | 15 | 794 |
| 762.8 | 15 | 794 |
| 762.9 | 15 | 794 |
| 763.0 | 15 | 795 |
| 763.1 | 15 | 795 |
| 763.2 | 15 | 795 |
| 763.3 | 15 | 795 |
| 763.4 | 15 | 791, 793 |
| 763.5 | 15 | 794 |
| 763.6 | 15 | 795 |
| 763.7 | 15 | 794 |
| 763.81 | 15 | 794 |
| 763.82 | 15 | 794 |
| 763.83 | 15 | 794 |
| 763.84 | 15 | 794 |
| 763.89 | 15 | 794 |
| 763.9 | 15 | 795 |
| 764.00 | 15 | 794 |
| 764.01 | 15 | 794 |
| 764.02 | 15 | 794 |
| 764.03 | 15 | 794 |
| 764.04 | 15 | 794 |
| 764.05 | 15 | 794 |
| 764.06 | 15 | 794 |
| 764.07 | 15 | 794 |

| DX | MDC | DRG |
|---|---|---|
| 764.08 | 15 | 794 |
| 764.09 | 15 | 795 |
| 764.10 | 15 | 794 |
| 764.11 | 15 | 791, 793 |
| 764.12 | 15 | 791, 793 |
| 764.13 | 15 | 791, 793 |
| 764.14 | 15 | 791, 793 |
| 764.15 | 15 | 791, 793 |
| 764.16 | 15 | 791, 793 |
| 764.17 | 15 | 791, 793 |
| 764.18 | 15 | 791, 793 |
| 764.19 | 15 | 794 |
| 764.20 | 15 | 794 |
| 764.21 | 15 | 791, 793 |
| 764.22 | 15 | 791, 793 |
| 764.23 | 15 | 791, 793 |
| 764.24 | 15 | 791, 793 |
| 764.25 | 15 | 791, 793 |
| 764.26 | 15 | 791, 793 |
| 764.27 | 15 | 791, 793 |
| 764.28 | 15 | 791, 793 |
| 764.29 | 15 | 794 |
| 764.90 | 15 | 794 |
| 764.91 | 15 | 794 |
| 764.92 | 15 | 794 |
| 764.93 | 15 | 794 |
| 764.93 | 15 | 794 |
| 764.94 | 15 | 794 |
| 764.95 | 15 | 794 |
| 764.96 | 15 | 794 |
| 764.97 | 15 | 794 |
| 764.98 | 15 | 795 |
| 764.99 | 15 | 795 |
| 765.00 | 15 | 791-792 |
| 765.01 | 15 | 790 |
| 765.02 | 15 | 790 |
| 765.03 | 15 | 790 |
| 765.04 | 15 | 790 |
| 765.05 | 15 | 790 |
| 765.06 | 15 | 791-792 |
| 765.07 | 15 | 791-792 |
| 765.08 | 15 | 791-792 |
| 765.09 | 15 | 999 |
| 765.10 | 15 | 791-792 |
| 765.11 | 15 | 791-792 |
| 765.12 | 15 | 791-792 |
| 765.13 | 15 | 791-792 |
| 765.14 | 15 | 791-792 |
| 765.15 | 15 | 791-792 |
| 765.16 | 15 | 791-792 |
| 765.17 | 15 | 791-792 |
| 765.18 | 15 | 791-792 |
| 765.19 | 15 | 791-792 |
| 765.20 | 15 | 795 |
| 765.21 | 15 | 790 |
| 765.22 | 15 | 790 |
| 765.23 | 15 | 790 |
| 765.24 | 15 | 791-792 |
| 765.25 | 15 | 791-792 |
| 765.26 | 15 | 791-792 |
| 765.27 | 15 | 791-792 |
| 765.28 | 15 | 791-792 |
| 765.29 | 15 | 795 |
| 766.0 | 15 | 795 |
| 766.1 | 15 | 795 |
| 766.21 | 15 | 795 |
| 766.22 | 15 | 795 |
| 767.0 | 15 | 791, 793 |
| 767.11 | 15 | 793 |
| 767.19 | 15 | 795 |
| 767.2 | 15 | 794 |
| 767.3 | 15 | 794 |
| 767.4 | 15 | 791, 793 |
| 767.5 | 15 | 794 |
| 767.6 | 15 | 794 |
| 767.7 | 15 | 791, 793 |
| 767.8 | 15 | 794 |

| DX | MDC | DRG |
|---|---|---|
| 767.9 | 15 | 794 |
| 768.0 | 15 | 794 |
| 768.1 | 15 | 794 |
| 768.2 | 15 | 794 |
| 768.3 | 15 | 794 |
| 768.4 | 15 | 794 |
| 768.5 | 15 | 791, 793 |
| 768.6 | 15 | 795 |
| 768.7 | 15 | 794 |
| 768.9 | 15 | 794 |
| 769 | 15 | 793 |
| 770.0 | 15 | 791, 793 |
| 770.10 | 15 | 791, 793 |
| 770.11 | 15 | 791, 793 |
| 770.12 | 15 | 791, 793 |
| 770.13 | 15 | 791, 793 |
| 770.14 | 15 | 791, 793 |
| 770.15 | 15 | 791, 793 |
| 770.16 | 15 | 791, 793 |
| 770.17 | 15 | 791, 793 |
| 770.18 | 15 | 791, 793 |
| 770.2 | 15 | 791, 793 |
| 770.3 | 15 | 791, 793 |
| 770.4 | 15 | 791, 793 |
| 770.5 | 15 | 794 |
| 770.6 | 15 | 794 |
| 770.7 | 04 | 196-198 |
| 770.8 | 15 | 791, 793 |
| 770.81 | 15 | 794 |
| 770.82 | 15 | 794 |
| 770.83 | 15 | 794 |
| 770.84 | 15 | 791, 793 |
| 770.85 | 15 | 791, 793 |
| 770.86 | 15 | 791, 793 |
| 770.87 | 15 | 794 |
| 770.88 | 15 | 794 |
| 770.89 | 15 | 794 |
| 770.9 | 15 | 794 |
| 771.0 | 15 | 791, 793 |
| 771.1 | 15 | 791, 793 |
| 771.2 | 15 | 791, 793 |
| 771.3 | 15 | 794 |
| 771.4 | 15 | 791, 793 |
| 771.5 | 15 | 791, 793 |
| 771.6 | 15 | 794 |
| 771.7 | 15 | 794 |
| 771.8 | 15 | 791, 793 |
| 771.81 | 15 | 791, 793 |
| 771.82 | 15 | 791, 793 |
| 771.83 | 15 | 791, 793 |
| 771.89 | 15 | 791, 793 |
| 772.0 | 15 | 791, 793 |
| 772.10 | 15 | 791, 793 |
| 772.11 | 15 | 791, 793 |
| 772.12 | 15 | 791, 793 |
| 772.13 | 15 | 791, 793 |
| 772.14 | 15 | 791, 793 |
| 772.2 | 15 | 791, 793 |
| 772.3 | 15 | 794 |
| 772.4 | 15 | 791, 793 |
| 772.5 | 15 | 791, 793 |
| 772.6 | 15 | 794 |
| 772.8 | 15 | 794 |
| 772.9 | 15 | 794 |
| 773.0 | 15 | 794 |
| 773.1 | 15 | 794 |
| 773.2 | 15 | 791, 793 |
| 773.3 | 15 | 791, 793 |
| 773.4 | 15 | 791, 793 |
| 773.5 | 15 | 791, 793 |
| 774.0 | 15 | 791, 793 |
| 774.1 | 15 | 791, 793 |
| 774.2 | 15 | 791, 793 |
| 774.30 | 15 | 791, 793 |
| 774.31 | 15 | 791, 793 |
| 774.39 | 15 | 791, 793 |
| 774.4 | 15 | 791, 793 |

| DX ...MDC ..DRG | DX ...MDC ..DRG | DX ...MDC ..DRG | DX ...MDC ..DRG | DX ...MDC ..DRG |
|---|---|---|---|---|
| 774.5 ...15 ..791, 793 | 780.56 ..19 ..887 | 785.59 ..18 ..870-872 | 789.1 ...07 ..441-443 | 793.91 ..23 ..947-948 |
| 774.6 ...15 ..795 | 780.57 ..03 ..154-156 | 785.6 ...16 ..814-816 | 789.2 ...16 ..814-816 | 793.99 ..23 ..947-948 |
| 774.7 ...15 ..791, 793 | 780.58 ..19 ..887 | 785.9 ...05 ..314-316 | 789.30 ..06 ..391-392 | 794.00 ..01 ..091-093 |
| 775.0 ...15 ..794 | 780.59 ..19 ..887 | 786.00 ..04 ..204 | 789.31 ..06 ..391-392 | 794.01 ..01 ..091-093 |
| 775.1 ...15 ..791, 793 | 780.6 ...18 .. | 786.01 ..04 ..204 | 789.32 ..06 ..391-392 | 794.02 ..01 ..091-093 |
| 775.2 ...15 ..791, 793 | 780.71 ..23 ..947-948 | 786.02 ..04 ..204 | 789.33 ..06 ..391-392 | 794.09 ..01 ..091-093 |
| 775.3 ...15 ..791, 793 | 780.79 ..23 ..947-948 | 786.03 ..04 ..204 | 789.34 ..06 ..391-392 | 794.10 ..01 ..091-093 |
| 775.4 ...15 ..791, 793 | 780.8 ...09 ..606-607 | 786.04 ..04 ..204 | 789.35 ..06 ..391-392 | 794.11 ..02 ..124-125 |
| 775.5 ...15 ..791, 793 | 780.91 ..23 ..947-948 | 786.05 ..04 ..204 | 789.36 ..06 ..391-392 | 794.12 ..02 ..124-125 |
| 775.6 ...15 ..791, 793 | 780.92 ..23 ..947-948 | 786.06 ..04 ..204 | 789.37 ..06 ..391-392 | 794.13 ..02 ..124-125 |
| 775.7 ...15 ..791, 793 | 780.93 ..23 ..947-948 | 786.07 ..04 ..204 | 789.39 ..06 ..391-392 | 794.14 ..02 ..124-125 |
| 775.81 .15 ..794 | 780.94 ..23 ..947-948 | 786.09 ..04 ..204 | 789.40 ..06 ..393-395 | 794.15 ..03 ..154-156 |
| 775.89 .15 ..794 | 780.95 ..23 ..947-948 | 786.1 ...04 ..204 | 789.41 ..06 ..393-395 | 794.16 ..03 ..154-156 |
| 775.9 ...15 ..794 | 780.96 ..23 ..947-948 | 786.2 ...04 ..204 | 789.42 ..06 ..393-395 | 794.17 ..08 ..564-566 |
| 776.0 ...15 ..791, 793 | 780.97 ..23 ..947-948 | 786.3 ...04 ..204 | 789.43 ..06 ..393-395 | 794.19 ..01 ..091-093 |
| 776.1 ...15 ..791, 793 | 780.99 ..23 ..947-948 | 786.4 ...04 ..204 | 789.44 ..06 ..393-395 | 794.2 ...04 ..205-206 |
| 776.2 ...15 ..791, 793 | 781.0 ...01 ..091-093 | 786.50 ..05 ..313 | 789.45 ..06 ..393-395 | 794.30 ..05 ..314-316 |
| 776.3 ...15 ..791, 793 | 781.1 ...01 ..091-093 | 786.51 ..05 ..313 | 789.46 ..06 ..393-395 | 794.31 ..05 ..314-316 |
| 776.4 ...15 ..794 | 781.2 ...01 ..091-093 | 786.52 ..04 ..204 | 789.47 ..06 ..393-395 | 794.39 ..05 ..314-316 |
| 776.5 ...15 ..794 | 781.3 ...01 ..091-093 | 786.59 ..05 ..313 | 789.49 ..06 ..393-395 | 794.4 ...11 ..695-696 |
| 776.6 ...15 ..791, 793 | 781.4 ...01 ..091-093 | 786.6 ...04 ..204 | 789.51 ..23 ..947-948 | 794.5 ...10 ..643-645 |
| 776.7 ...15 ..794 | 781.5 ...04 ..205-206 | 786.7 ...04 ..204 | 789.59 ..23 ..947-948 | 794.6 ...10 ..643-645 |
| 776.8 ...15 ..794 | 781.6 ...01 ..091-093 | 786.8 ...04 ..204 | 789.60 ..06 ..391-392 | 794.7 ...10 ..643-645 |
| 776.9 ...15 ..794 | 781.7 ...10 ..640-641 | 786.9 ...04 ..204 | 789.61 ..06 ..391-392 | 794.8 ...07 ..441-443 |
| 777.1 ...15 ..791, 793 | 781.91 ..01 ..091-093 | 787.01 ..06 ..391-392 | 789.62 ..06 ..391-392 | 794.9 ...11 ..695-696 |
| 777.2 ...15 ..791, 793 | 781.92 ..01 ..091-093 | 787.02 ..06 ..391-392 | 789.63 ..06 ..391-392 | 795.00 ..13 ..760-761 |
| 777.3 ...15 ..794 | 781.93 ..08 ..551-552 | 787.03 ..06 ..391-392 | 789.64 ..06 ..391-392 | 795.01 ..13 ..760-761 |
| 777.4 ...15 ..794 | 781.94 ..01 ..091-093 | 787.1 ...06 ..391-392 | 789.65 ..06 ..391-392 | 795.02 ..13 ..760-761 |
| 777.5 ...15 ..791, 793 | 781.99 ..01 ..091-093 | 787.20 ..06 ..391-392 | 789.66 ..06 ..391-392 | 795.03 ..13 ..760-761 |
| 777.6 ...15 ..791, 793 | 782.0 ...01 ..091-093 | 787.21 ..06 ..391-392 | 789.67 ..06 ..391-392 | 795.04 ..13 ..760-761 |
| 777.8 ...15 ..794 | 782.1 ...09 ..606-607 | 787.22 ..06 ..391-392 | 789.69 ..06 ..391-392 | 795.05 ..13 ..760-761 |
| 777.9 ...15 ..794 | 782.2 ...09 ..606-607 | 787.23 ..06 ..391-392 | 789.9 ...06 ..391-392 | 795.06 ..13 ..760-761 |
| 778.0 ...15 ..791, 793 | 782.3 ...23 ..947-948 | 787.24 ..06 ..391-392 | 790.01 ..16 ..811-812 | 795.08 ..13 ..760-761 |
| 778.1 ...15 ..794 | 782.4 ...07 ..441-443 | 787.29 ..06 ..391-392 | 790.09 ..16 ..811-812 | 795.09 ..13 ..760-761 |
| 778.2 ...15 ..794 | 782.5 ...23 ..947-948 | 787.3 ...06 ..391-392 | 790.1 ...23 ..947-948 | 795.1 ...04 ..180-182 |
| 778.3 ...15 ..794 | 782.61 ..23 ..947-948 | 787.4 ...06 ..391-392 | 790.21 ..10 ..640-641 | 795.2 ...23 ..951 |
| 778.4 ...15 ..794 | 782.62 ..23 ..947-948 | 787.5 ...06 ..391-392 | 790.22 ..10 ..640-641 | 795.31 ..18 ..867-869 |
| 778.5 ...15 ..794 | 782.7 ...16 ..813 | 787.6 ...06 ..391-392 | 790.29 ..10 ..640-641 | 795.39 ..18 ..867-869 |
| 778.6 ...15 ..794 | 782.8 ...09 ..606-607 | 787.7 ...06 ..391-392 | 790.3 ...20 ..895-897 | 795.4 ...23 ..947-948 |
| 778.7 ...15 ..794 | 782.9 ...09 ..606-607 | 787.9 ...06 ..391-392 | 790.4 ...23 ..947-948 | 795.5 ...04 ..177-179 |
| 778.8 ...15 ..794 | 783.0 ...10 ..640-641 | 788.0 ...11 ..691-694 | 790.5 ...23 ..947-948 | 795.6 ...08 ..545-547 |
| 778.9 ...15 ..794 | 783.1 ...10 ..640-641 | 788.1 ...11 ..695-696 | 790.6 ...23 ..947-948 | 795.71 ..16 ..814-816 |
| 779.0 ...15 ..791, 793 | 783.21 ..10 ..640-641 | 788.20 ..11 ..695-696 | 790.7 ...18 ..870-872 | 795.79 ..16 ..814-816 |
| 779.1 ...15 ..791, 793 | 783.22 ..10 ..640-641 | 788.21 ..11 ..695-696 | 790.8 ...18 ..864-866 | 795.81 ..23 ..947-948 |
| 779.2 ...15 ..791, 793 | 783.40 ..10 ..640-641 | 788.29 ..11 ..695-696 | 790.91 ..23 ..947-948 | 795.82 ..23 ..947-948 |
| 779.3 ...15 ..795 | 783.41 ..10 ..640-641 | 788.30 ..11 ..695-696 | 790.92 ..23 ..947-948 | 795.89 ..23 ..947-948 |
| 779.4 ...15 ..791, 793 | 783.42 ..10 ..640-641 | 788.31 ..11 ..695-696 | 790.93 ..23 ..947-948 | 796.0 ...21 ..922-923 |
| 779.5 ...15 ..791, 793 | 783.43 ..10 ..640-641 | 788.32 ..11 ..695-696 | 790.94 ..23 ..947-948 | 796.1 ...01 ..091-093 |
| 779.6 ...15 ..794 | 783.5 ...10 ..640-641 | 788.33 ..11 ..695-696 | 790.95 ..23 ..947-948 | 796.2 ...05 ..314-316 |
| 779.7 ...01 ..091-093 | 783.6 ...10 ..640-641 | 788.34 ..11 ..695-696 | 790.99 ..23 ..947-948 | 796.3 ...05 ..314-316 |
| 779.8 ...15 ..794 | 783.7 ...10 ..640-641 | 788.35 ..11 ..695-696 | 791.0 ...11 ..695-696 | 796.4 ...23 ..947-948 |
| 779.81 .15 ..794 | 783.9 ...10 ..640-641 | 788.36 ..11 ..695-696 | 791.1 ...11 ..695-696 | 796.5 ...14 ..781-782 |
| 779.82 .15 ..794 | 784.0 ...01 ..100-103 | 788.37 ..11 ..695-696 | 791.2 ...11 ..695-696 | 796.6 ...23 ..947-948 |
| 779.83 .15 ..795 | 784.1 ...03 ..154-156 | 788.38 ..11 ..695-696 | 791.3 ...23 ..947-948 | 796.9 ...23 ..947-948 |
| 779.84 .15 ..794 | 784.2 ...09 ..606-607 | 788.39 ..11 ..695-696 | 791.4 ...07 ..441-443 | 797 .....19 ..884 |
| 779.85 .15 ..791, 793 | 784.3 ...01 ..091-093 | 788.41 ..11 ..695-696 | 791.5 ...10 ..637-639 | 798.0 ...01 ..091-093 |
| 779.89 .15 ..794 | 784.40 ..03 ..154-156 | 788.42 ..11 ..695-696 | 791.6 ...10 ..640-641 | 798.1 ...05 ..296-298 |
| 779.9 ...15 ..794 | 784.41 ..03 ..154-156 | 788.43 ..11 ..695-696 | 791.7 ...11 ..695-696 | 798.2 ...05 ..296-298 |
| | 784.49 ..03 ..154-156 | 788.5 ...11 ..682-684 | 791.9 ...11 ..695-696 | 798.9 ...23 ..951 |
| **Symptoms, Signs and Ill-defined Conditions** | 784.5 ...01 ..091-093 | 788.61 ..11 ..695-696 | 792.0 ...01 ..091-093 | 799.01 ..4 ...205-206 |
| 780.01 ..01 ..080-081 | 784.60 ..19 ..887 | 788.62 ..11 ..695-696 | 792.1 ...06 ..391-392 | 799.02 ..4 ...205-206 |
| 780.02 ..19 ..884 | 784.61 ..19 ..886 | 788.63 ..11 ..695-696 | 792.2 ...12 ..729-730 | 799.1 ...04 ..205-206 |
| 780.03 ..01 ..080-081 | 784.69 ..19 ..886 | 788.64 ..11 .695-696 | 792.3 ...14 ..781-782 | 799.2 ...19 ..880 |
| 780.09 ..01 ..080-081 | 784.7 ...03 ..151 | 788.65 ..11 ..695-696 | 792.4 ...03 ..154-156 | 799.3 ...23 ..947-948 |
| 780.1 ...19 ..880 | 784.8 ...03 ..154-156 | 788.69 ..11 ..695-696 | 792.5 ...23 ..947-948 | 799.4 ...23 ..947-948 |
| 780.2 ...05 ..312 | 784.91 ..03 ..154-156 | 788.7 ...11 ..695-696 | 792.9 ...23 ..947-948 | 799.81 ..23 ..951 |
| 780.31 ..01 ..100-103 | 784.99 ..03 ..154-156 | 788.8 ...11 ..695-696 | 793.0 ...01 ..091-093 | 799.89 ..23 ..951 |
| 780.32 ..01 ..100-103 | 785.0 ...05 ..308-310 | 788.9 ...11 ..695-696 | 793.1 ...04 ..204 | 799.9 ...23 ..951 |
| 780.39 ..01 ..100-103 | 785.1 ...05 ..308-310 | 789.00 ..06 ..391-392 | 793.2 ...05 ..302-303 | |
| 780.4 ...03 ..149 | 785.2 ...05 ..306-307 | 789.01 ..06 ..391-392 | 793.3 ...07 ..444-446 | **Injury and Poisoning** |
| 780.50 ..19 ..887 | 785.3 ...05 ..314-316 | 789.02 ..06 ..391-392 | 793.4 ...06 ..391-392 | 800.00 ..01 ..082-087 |
| 780.51 ..03 ..154-156 | 785.4 ...05 ..299-301 | 789.03 ..06 ..391-392 | 793.5 ...11 ..695-696 | 800.01 ..01 ..082-087 |
| 780.52 ..19 ..887 | 785.50 ..05 ..280-281, 286, 291-293 | 789.04 ..06 ..391-392 | 793.6 ...06 ..391-392 | 800.02 ..01 ..082-087 |
| 780.53 ..03 ..154-156 | | 789.05 ..06 ..391-392 | 793.7 ...08 ..564-566 | 800.03 ..01 ..082-084 |
| 780.54 ..19 ..887 | 785.51 ..05 ..280-281, 286, 291-293 | 789.06 ..06 ..391-392 | 793.80 ..09 ..600-601 | 800.04 ..01 ..082-084 |
| 780.55 ..19 ..887 | | 789.07 ..06 ..391-392 | 793.81 ..09 ..600-601 | 800.05 ..01 ..082-084 |
| | 785.52 ..18 ..870-872 | 789.09 ..06 ..391-392 | 793.89 ..09 ..600-601 | 800.06 ..01 ..082-084 |

| DX | MDC | DRG | DX | MDC | DRG | DX | MDC | DRG | DX | MDC | DRG | DX | MDC | DRG |
|---|---|---|---|---|---|---|---|---|---|---|---|---|---|---|
| 800.09 | 01 | 082-087 | 801.04 | 01 | 082-084 | 802.1 | 03 | 154-156 | 803.62 | 01 | 082-087 | 804.59 | 01 | 082-087 |
| 800.10 | 01 | 082-087 | 801.05 | 01 | 082-084 | 802.20 | 03 | 157-159 | 803.63 | 01 | 082-084 | 804.60 | 01 | 082-087 |
| 800.11 | 01 | 082-087 | 801.06 | 01 | 082-084 | 802.21 | 03 | 157-159 | 803.64 | 01 | 082-084 | 804.61 | 01 | 082-087 |
| 800.12 | 01 | 082-087 | 801.09 | 01 | 082-087 | 802.22 | 03 | 157-159 | 803.65 | 01 | 082-084 | 804.62 | 01 | 082-087 |
| 800.13 | 01 | 082-084 | 801.10 | 01 | 082-087 | 802.23 | 03 | 157-159 | 803.66 | 01 | 082-084 | 804.63 | 01 | 082-084 |
| 800.14 | 01 | 082-084 | 801.11 | 01 | 082-087 | 802.24 | 03 | 157-159 | 803.69 | 01 | 082-087 | 804.64 | 01 | 082-084 |
| 800.15 | 01 | 082-084 | 801.12 | 01 | 082-087 | 802.25 | 03 | 157-159 | 803.70 | 01 | 082-087 | 804.65 | 01 | 082-084 |
| 800.16 | 01 | 082-087 | 801.13 | 01 | 082-084 | 802.26 | 03 | 157-159 | 803.71 | 01 | 082-087 | 804.66 | 01 | 082-084 |
| 800.19 | 01 | 082-087 | 801.14 | 01 | 082-084 | 802.27 | 03 | 157-159 | 803.72 | 01 | 082-087 | 804.69 | 01 | 082-087 |
| 800.20 | 01 | 082-087 | 801.15 | 01 | 082-084 | 802.28 | 03 | 157-159 | 803.73 | 01 | 082-084 | 804.70 | 01 | 082-087 |
| 800.21 | 01 | 082-087 | 801.16 | 01 | 082-084 | 802.29 | 03 | 157-159 | 803.74 | 01 | 082-084 | 804.71 | 01 | 082-087 |
| 800.22 | 01 | 082-087 | 801.19 | 01 | 082-087 | 802.30 | 03 | 157-159 | 803.75 | 01 | 082-084 | 804.72 | 01 | 082-087 |
| 800.23 | 01 | 082-084 | 801.20 | 01 | 082-087 | 802.31 | 03 | 157-159 | 803.76 | 01 | 082-084 | 804.73 | 01 | 082-084 |
| 800.24 | 01 | 082-084 | 801.21 | 01 | 082-087 | 802.32 | 03 | 157-159 | 803.79 | 01 | 082-087 | 804.74 | 01 | 082-084 |
| 800.25 | 01 | 082-084 | 801.22 | 01 | 082-087 | 802.33 | 03 | 157-159 | 803.80 | 01 | 082-087 | 804.75 | 01 | 082-084 |
| 800.26 | 01 | 082-084 | 801.23 | 01 | 082-084 | 802.34 | 03 | 157-159 | 803.81 | 01 | 082-087 | 804.76 | 01 | 082-084 |
| 800.29 | 01 | 082-087 | 801.24 | 01 | 082-084 | 802.35 | 03 | 157-159 | 803.82 | 01 | 082-087 | 804.79 | 01 | 082-087 |
| 800.30 | 01 | 082-087 | 801.25 | 01 | 082-084 | 802.36 | 03 | 157-159 | 803.83 | 01 | 082-084 | 804.80 | 01 | 082-087 |
| 800.31 | 01 | 082-087 | 801.26 | 01 | 082-084 | 802.37 | 03 | 157-159 | 803.84 | 01 | 082-084 | 804.81 | 01 | 082-087 |
| 800.32 | 01 | 082-087 | 801.29 | 01 | 082-087 | 802.38 | 03 | 157-159 | 803.85 | 01 | 082-084 | 804.82 | 01 | 082-087 |
| 800.33 | 01 | 082-084 | 801.30 | 01 | 082-087 | 802.39 | 03 | 157-159 | 803.86 | 01 | 082-084 | 804.83 | 01 | 082-084 |
| 800.34 | 01 | 082-084 | 801.31 | 01 | 082-087 | 802.4 | 03 | 157-159 | 803.89 | 01 | 082-087 | 804.84 | 01 | 082-084 |
| 800.35 | 01 | 082-084 | 801.32 | 01 | 082-087 | 802.5 | 03 | 157-159 | 803.90 | 01 | 082-087 | 804.85 | 01 | 082-084 |
| 800.36 | 01 | 082-084 | 801.33 | 01 | 082-084 | 802.6 | 02 | 124-125 | 803.91 | 01 | 082-087 | 804.86 | 01 | 082-084 |
| 800.39 | 01 | 082-087 | 801.34 | 01 | 082-084 | 802.7 | 02 | 124-125 | 803.92 | 01 | 082-087 | 804.89 | 01 | 082-087 |
| 800.40 | 01 | 082-087 | 801.35 | 01 | 082-084 | 802.8 | 08 | 564-566 | 803.93 | 01 | 082-084 | 804.90 | 01 | 082-087 |
| 800.41 | 01 | 082-087 | 801.36 | 01 | 082-084 | 802.9 | 08 | 564-566 | 803.94 | 01 | 082-084 | 804.91 | 01 | 082-087 |
| 800.42 | 01 | 082-087 | 801.39 | 01 | 082-087 | 803.00 | 01 | 082-087 | 803.95 | 01 | 082-084 | 804.92 | 01 | 082-087 |
| 800.43 | 01 | 082-084 | 801.40 | 01 | 082-087 | 803.01 | 01 | 082-087 | 803.96 | 01 | 082-084 | 804.93 | 01 | 082-084 |
| 800.44 | 01 | 082-084 | 801.41 | 01 | 082-087 | 803.02 | 01 | 082-087 | 803.99 | 01 | 082-087 | 804.94 | 01 | 082-084 |
| 800.45 | 01 | 082-084 | 801.42 | 01 | 082-087 | 803.03 | 01 | 082-084 | 804.00 | 01 | 082-087 | 804.95 | 01 | 082-084 |
| 800.46 | 01 | 082-084 | 801.43 | 01 | 082-084 | 803.04 | 01 | 082-084 | 804.01 | 01 | 082-087 | 804.96 | 01 | 082-084 |
| 800.49 | 01 | 082-087 | 801.44 | 01 | 082-084 | 803.05 | 01 | 082-084 | 804.02 | 01 | 082-087 | 804.99 | 01 | 082-087 |
| 800.50 | 01 | 082-087 | 801.45 | 01 | 082-084 | 803.06 | 01 | 082-084 | 804.03 | 01 | 082-084 | 805.00 | 08 | 551-552 |
| 800.51 | 01 | 082-087 | 801.46 | 01 | 082-084 | 803.09 | 01 | 082-087 | 804.04 | 01 | 082-084 | 805.01 | 08 | 551-552 |
| 800.52 | 01 | 082-087 | 801.49 | 01 | 082-087 | 803.10 | 01 | 082-087 | 804.05 | 01 | 082-084 | 805.02 | 08 | 551-552 |
| 800.53 | 01 | 082-084 | 801.50 | 01 | 082-087 | 803.11 | 01 | 082-087 | 804.06 | 01 | 082-084 | 805.03 | 08 | 551-552 |
| 800.54 | 01 | 082-084 | 801.51 | 01 | 082-087 | 803.12 | 01 | 082-087 | 804.09 | 01 | 082-087 | 805.04 | 08 | 551-552 |
| 800.55 | 01 | 082-084 | 801.52 | 01 | 082-087 | 803.13 | 01 | 082-084 | 804.10 | 01 | 082-087 | 805.05 | 08 | 551-552 |
| 800.56 | 01 | 082-084 | 801.53 | 01 | 082-084 | 803.14 | 01 | 082-084 | 804.11 | 01 | 082-087 | 805.06 | 08 | 551-552 |
| 800.59 | 01 | 082-087 | 801.54 | 01 | 082-084 | 803.15 | 01 | 082-084 | 804.12 | 01 | 082-087 | 805.07 | 08 | 551-552 |
| 800.60 | 01 | 082-087 | 801.55 | 01 | 082-084 | 803.16 | 01 | 082-084 | 804.13 | 01 | 082-084 | 805.08 | 08 | 551-552 |
| 800.61 | 01 | 082-087 | 801.56 | 01 | 082-084 | 803.19 | 01 | 082-087 | 804.14 | 01 | 082-084 | 805.10 | 08 | 551-552 |
| 800.62 | 01 | 082-087 | 801.59 | 01 | 082-087 | 803.20 | 01 | 082-087 | 804.15 | 01 | 082-084 | 805.11 | 08 | 551-552 |
| 800.63 | 01 | 082-084 | 801.60 | 01 | 082-087 | 803.21 | 01 | 082-087 | 804.16 | 01 | 082-084 | 805.12 | 08 | 551-552 |
| 800.64 | 01 | 082-084 | 801.61 | 01 | 082-087 | 803.22 | 01 | 082-087 | 804.19 | 01 | 082-087 | 805.13 | 08 | 551-552 |
| 800.65 | 01 | 082-084 | 801.62 | 01 | 082-087 | 803.23 | 01 | 082-084 | 804.20 | 01 | 082-087 | 805.14 | 08 | 551-552 |
| 800.66 | 01 | 082-084 | 801.63 | 01 | 082-084 | 803.24 | 01 | 082-084 | 804.21 | 01 | 082-087 | 805.15 | 08 | 551-552 |
| 800.69 | 01 | 082-087 | 801.64 | 01 | 082-084 | 803.25 | 01 | 082-084 | 804.22 | 01 | 082-087 | 805.16 | 08 | 551-552 |
| 800.70 | 01 | 082-087 | 801.65 | 01 | 082-084 | 803.26 | 01 | 082-084 | 804.23 | 01 | 082-084 | 805.17 | 08 | 551-552 |
| 800.71 | 01 | 082-087 | 801.66 | 01 | 082-084 | 803.29 | 01 | 082-087 | 804.24 | 01 | 082-087 | 805.18 | 08 | 551-552 |
| 800.72 | 01 | 082-087 | 801.69 | 01 | 082-087 | 803.30 | 01 | 082-087 | 804.25 | 01 | 082-084 | 805.2 | 08 | 551-552 |
| 800.73 | 01 | 082-084 | 801.70 | 01 | 082-087 | 803.31 | 01 | 082-087 | 804.26 | 01 | 082-084 | 805.3 | 08 | 551-552 |
| 800.74 | 01 | 082-084 | 801.71 | 01 | 082-087 | 803.32 | 01 | 082-087 | 804.29 | 01 | 082-087 | 805.4 | 08 | 551-552 |
| 800.75 | 01 | 082-084 | 801.72 | 01 | 082-087 | 803.33 | 01 | 082-084 | 804.30 | 01 | 082-087 | 805.5 | 08 | 551-552 |
| 800.76 | 01 | 082-084 | 801.73 | 01 | 082-084 | 803.34 | 01 | 082-084 | 804.31 | 01 | 082-087 | 805.6 | 08 | 551-552 |
| 800.79 | 01 | 082-087 | 801.74 | 01 | 082-084 | 803.35 | 01 | 082-084 | 804.32 | 01 | 082-087 | 805.7 | 08 | 551-552 |
| 800.80 | 01 | 082-087 | 801.75 | 01 | 082-084 | 803.36 | 01 | 082-084 | 804.33 | 01 | 082-084 | 805.8 | 08 | 551-552 |
| 800.81 | 01 | 082-087 | 801.76 | 01 | 082-084 | 803.39 | 01 | 082-087 | 804.34 | 01 | 082-084 | 805.9 | 08 | 551-552 |
| 800.82 | 01 | 082-087 | 801.79 | 01 | 082-087 | 803.40 | 01 | 082-087 | 804.35 | 01 | 082-084 | 806.00 | 01 | 052-053 |
| 800.83 | 01 | 082-084 | 801.80 | 01 | 082-087 | 803.41 | 01 | 082-087 | 804.36 | 01 | 082-084 | 806.01 | 01 | 052-053 |
| 800.84 | 01 | 082-084 | 801.81 | 01 | 082-087 | 803.42 | 01 | 082-087 | 804.39 | 01 | 082-087 | 806.02 | 01 | 052-053 |
| 800.85 | 01 | 082-084 | 801.82 | 01 | 082-087 | 803.43 | 01 | 082-084 | 804.40 | 01 | 082-087 | 806.03 | 01 | 052-053 |
| 800.86 | 01 | 082-084 | 801.83 | 01 | 082-084 | 803.44 | 01 | 082-084 | 804.41 | 01 | 082-087 | 806.04 | 01 | 052-053 |
| 800.89 | 01 | 082-087 | 801.84 | 01 | 082-084 | 803.45 | 01 | 082-084 | 804.42 | 01 | 082-087 | 806.05 | 01 | 052-053 |
| 800.90 | 01 | 082-087 | 801.85 | 01 | 082-084 | 803.46 | 01 | 082-084 | 804.43 | 01 | 082-084 | 806.06 | 01 | 052-053 |
| 800.91 | 01 | 082-087 | 801.86 | 01 | 082-084 | 803.49 | 01 | 082-087 | 804.44 | 01 | 082-084 | 806.07 | 01 | 052-053 |
| 800.92 | 01 | 082-087 | 801.89 | 01 | 082-087 | 803.50 | 01 | 082-087 | 804.45 | 01 | 082-087 | 806.08 | 01 | 052-053 |
| 800.93 | 01 | 082-084 | 801.90 | 01 | 082-087 | 803.51 | 01 | 082-087 | 804.46 | 01 | 082-084 | 806.09 | 01 | 052-053 |
| 800.94 | 01 | 082-084 | 801.91 | 01 | 082-087 | 803.52 | 01 | 082-087 | 804.49 | 01 | 082-087 | 806.10 | 01 | 052-053 |
| 800.95 | 01 | 082-084 | 801.92 | 01 | 082-087 | 803.53 | 01 | 082-084 | 804.50 | 01 | 082-087 | 806.11 | 01 | 052-053 |
| 800.96 | 01 | 082-084 | 801.93 | 01 | 082-084 | 803.54 | 01 | 082-084 | 804.51 | 01 | 082-087 | 806.12 | 01 | 052-053 |
| 800.99 | 01 | 082-087 | 801.94 | 01 | 082-084 | 803.55 | 01 | 082-084 | 804.52 | 01 | 082-087 | 806.13 | 01 | 052-053 |
| 801.00 | 01 | 082-087 | 801.95 | 01 | 082-084 | 803.56 | 01 | 082-084 | 804.53 | 01 | 082-084 | 806.14 | 01 | 052-053 |
| 801.01 | 01 | 082-087 | 801.96 | 01 | 082-084 | 803.59 | 01 | 082-087 | 804.54 | 01 | 082-084 | 806.15 | 01 | 052-053 |
| 801.02 | 01 | 082-087 | 801.99 | 01 | 082-087 | 803.60 | 01 | 082-087 | 804.55 | 01 | 082-084 | 806.16 | 01 | 052-053 |
| 801.03 | 01 | 082-084 | 802.0 | 03 | 154-156 | 803.61 | 01 | 082-087 | 804.56 | 01 | 082-084 | 806.17 | 01 | 052-053 |

| DX ...MDC ..DRG | DX ...MDC ..DRG | DX ...MDC ..DRG | DX ...MDC ..DRG | DX ...MDC ..DRG |
|---|---|---|---|---|
| 806.18 ..01 ..052-053 | 810.02 ..08 ..562-563 | 813.53 ..08 ..562-563 | 821.11 ..08 ..533-534 | 831.11 ..08 ..562-563 |
| 806.19 ..01 ..052-053 | 810.03 ..08 ..562-563 | 813.54 ..08 ..562-563 | 821.20 ..08 ..533-534 | 831.12 ..08 ..562-563 |
| 806.20 ..01 ..052-053 | 810.10 ..08 ..562-563 | 813.80 ..08 ..562-563 | 821.21 ..08 ..533-534 | 831.13 ..08 ..562-563 |
| 806.21 ..01 ..052-053 | 810.11 ..08 ..562-563 | 813.81 ..08 ..562-563 | 821.22 ..08 ..533-534 | 831.14 ..08 ..562-563 |
| 806.22 ..01 ..052-053 | 810.12 ..08 ..562-563 | 813.82 ..08 ..562-563 | 821.23 ..08 ..533-534 | 831.19 ..08 ..562-563 |
| 806.23 ..01 ..052-053 | 810.13 ..08 ..562-563 | 813.83 ..08 ..562-563 | 821.29 ..08 ..533-534 | 832.00 ..08 ..562-563 |
| 806.24 ..01 ..052-053 | 811.00 ..08 ..562-563 | 813.90 ..08 ..562-563 | 821.30 ..08 ..533-534 | 832.01 ..08 ..562-563 |
| 806.25 ..01 ..052-053 | 811.01 ..08 ..562-563 | 813.91 ..08 ..562-563 | 821.31 ..08 ..533-534 | 832.02 ..08 ..562-563 |
| 806.26 ..01 ..052-053 | 811.02 ..08 ..562-563 | 813.92 ..08 ..562-563 | 821.32 ..08 ..533-534 | 832.03 ..08 ..562-563 |
| 806.27 ..01 ..052-053 | 811.03 ..08 ..562-563 | 813.93 ..08 ..562-563 | 821.33 ..08 ..533-534 | 832.04 ..08 ..562-563 |
| 806.28 ..01 ..052-053 | 811.09 ..08 ..564-566 | 814.00 ..08 ..562-563 | 821.39 ..08 ..533-534 | 832.09 ..08 ..562-563 |
| 806.29 ..01 ..052-053 | 811.10 ..08 ..562-563 | 814.01 ..08 ..562-563 | 822.0 ..08 ..562-563 | 832.10 ..08 ..562-563 |
| 806.30 ..01 ..052-053 | 811.11 ..08 ..562-563 | 814.02 ..08 ..562-563 | 822.1 ..08 ..562-563 | 832.11 ..08 ..562-563 |
| 806.31 ..01 ..052-053 | 811.12 ..08 ..562-563 | 814.03 ..08 ..562-563 | 823.00 ..08 ..562-563 | 832.12 ..08 ..562-563 |
| 806.32 ..01 ..052-053 | 811.13 ..08 ..562-563 | 814.04 ..08 ..562-563 | 823.01 ..08 ..562-563 | 832.13 ..08 ..562-563 |
| 806.33 ..01 ..052-053 | 811.19 ..08 ..564-566 | 814.05 ..08 ..562-563 | 823.02 ..08 ..562-563 | 832.14 ..08 ..562-563 |
| 806.34 ..01 ..052-053 | 812.00 ..08 ..562-563 | 814.06 ..08 ..562-563 | 823.10 ..08 ..562-563 | 832.19 ..08 ..562-563 |
| 806.35 ..01 ..052-053 | 812.01 ..08 ..562-563 | 814.07 ..08 ..562-563 | 823.11 ..08 ..562-563 | 833.00 ..08 ..562-563 |
| 806.36 ..01 ..052-053 | 812.02 ..08 ..562-563 | 814.08 ..08 ..562-563 | 823.12 ..08 ..562-563 | 833.01 ..08 ..562-563 |
| 806.37 ..01 ..052-053 | 812.03 ..08 ..562-563 | 814.09 ..08 ..562-563 | 823.20 ..08 ..562-563 | 833.02 ..08 ..562-563 |
| 806.38 ..01 ..052-053 | 812.09 ..08 ..562-563 | 814.10 ..08 ..562-563 | 823.21 ..08 ..562-563 | 833.03 ..08 ..562-563 |
| 806.39 ..01 ..052-053 | 812.10 ..08 ..562-563 | 814.11 ..08 ..562-563 | 823.22 ..08 ..562-563 | 833.04 ..08 ..562-563 |
| 806.4 ...01 ..052-053 | 812.11 ..08 ..562-563 | 814.12 ..08 ..562-563 | 823.30 ..08 ..562-563 | 833.05 ..08 ..562-563 |
| 806.5 ...01 ..052-053 | 812.12 ..08 ..562-563 | 814.13 ..08 ..562-563 | 823.31 ..08 ..562-563 | 833.09 ..08 ..562-563 |
| 806.60 ..01 ..052-053 | 812.13 ..08 ..562-563 | 814.14 ..08 ..562-563 | 823.32 ..08 ..562-563 | 833.10 ..08 ..562-563 |
| 806.61 ..01 ..052-053 | 812.19 ..08 ..562-563 | 814.15 ..08 ..562-563 | 823.40 ..08 ..562-563 | 833.11 ..08 ..562-563 |
| 806.62 ..01 ..052-053 | 812.20 ..08 ..562-563 | 814.16 ..08 ..562-563 | 823.41 ..08 ..562-563 | 833.12 ..08 ..562-563 |
| 806.69 ..01 ..052-053 | 812.21 ..08 ..562-563 | 814.17 ..08 ..562-563 | 823.42 ..08 ..562-563 | 833.13 ..08 ..562-563 |
| 806.70 ..01 ..052-053 | 812.30 ..08 ..562-563 | 814.18 ..08 ..562-563 | 823.80 ..08 ..562-563 | 833.14 ..08 ..562-563 |
| 806.71 ..01 ..052-053 | 812.31 ..08 ..562-563 | 814.19 ..08 ..562-563 | 823.81 ..08 ..562-563 | 833.15 ..08 ..562-563 |
| 806.72 ..01 ..052-053 | 812.40 ..08 ..562-563 | 815.00 ..08 ..562-563 | 823.82 ..08 ..562-563 | 833.19 ..08 ..562-563 |
| 806.79 ..01 ..052-053 | 812.41 ..08 ..562-563 | 815.01 ..08 ..562-563 | 823.90 ..08 ..562-563 | 834.00 ..08 ..562-563 |
| 806.8 ...01 ..052-053 | 812.42 ..08 ..562-563 | 815.02 ..08 ..562-563 | 823.91 ..08 ..562-563 | 834.01 ..08 ..562-563 |
| 806.9 ...01 ..052-053 | 812.43 ..08 ..562-563 | 815.03 ..08 ..562-563 | 823.92 ..08 ..562-563 | 834.02 ..08 ..562-563 |
| 807.00 ..04 ..205-206 | 812.44 ..08 ..562-563 | 815.04 ..08 ..562-563 | 824.0 ..08 ..562-563 | 834.10 ..08 ..562-563 |
| 807.01 ..04 ..205-206 | 812.49 ..08 ..562-563 | 815.09 ..08 ..562-563 | 824.1 ..08 ..562-563 | 834.11 ..08 ..562-563 |
| 807.02 ..04 ..205-206 | 812.50 ..08 ..562-563 | 815.10 ..08 ..562-563 | 824.2 ..08 ..562-563 | 834.12 ..08 ..562-563 |
| 807.03 ..04 ..183-185 | 812.51 ..08 ..562-563 | 815.11 ..08 ..562-563 | 824.3 ..08 ..562-563 | 835.00 ..08 ..537-538 |
| 807.04 ..04 ..183-185 | 812.52 ..08 ..562-563 | 815.12 ..08 ..562-563 | 824.4 ..08 ..562-563 | 835.01 ..08 ..537-538 |
| 807.05 ..04 ..183-185 | 812.53 ..08 ..562-563 | 815.13 ..08 ..562-563 | 824.5 ..08 ..562-563 | 835.02 ..08 ..537-538 |
| 807.06 ..04 ..183-185 | 812.54 ..08 ..562-563 | 815.14 ..08 ..562-563 | 824.6 ..08 ..562-563 | 835.03 ..08 ..537-538 |
| 807.07 ..04 ..183-185 | 812.59 ..08 ..562-563 | 815.19 ..08 ..562-563 | 824.7 ..08 ..562-563 | 835.10 ..08 ..537-538 |
| 807.08 ..04 ..183-185 | 813.00 ..08 ..562-563 | 816.00 ..08 ..562-563 | 824.8 ..08 ..562-563 | 835.11 ..08 ..537-538 |
| 807.09 ..04 ..183-185 | 813.01 ..08 ..562-563 | 816.01 ..08 ..562-563 | 824.9 ..08 ..562-563 | 835.12 ..08 ..537-538 |
| 807.10 ..04 ..183-185 | 813.02 ..08 ..562-563 | 816.02 ..08 ..562-563 | 825.0 ..08 ..562-563 | 835.13 ..08 ..537-538 |
| 807.11 ..04 ..183-185 | 813.03 ..08 ..562-563 | 816.03 ..08 ..562-563 | 825.1 ..08 ..562-563 | 836.0 ...08 ..562-563 |
| 807.12 ..04 ..183-185 | 813.04 ..08 ..562-563 | 816.10 ..08 ..562-563 | 825.20 ..08 ..562-563 | 836.1 ...08 ..562-563 |
| 807.13 ..04 ..183-185 | 813.05 ..08 ..562-563 | 816.11 ..08 ..562-563 | 825.21 ..08 ..562-563 | 836.2 ...08 ..562-563 |
| 807.14 ..04 ..183-185 | 813.06 ..08 ..562-563 | 816.12 ..08 ..562-563 | 825.22 ..08 ..562-563 | 836.3 ...08 ..562-563 |
| 807.15 ..04 ..183-185 | 813.07 ..08 ..562-563 | 816.13 ..08 ..562-563 | 825.23 ..08 ..562-563 | 836.4 ...08 ..562-563 |
| 807.16 ..04 ..183-185 | 813.08 ..08 ..562-563 | 817.0 ...08 ..562-563 | 825.24 ..08 ..562-563 | 836.50 ..08 ..562-563 |
| 807.17 ..04 ..183-185 | 813.10 ..08 ..562-563 | 817.1 ...08 ..562-563 | 825.25 ..08 ..562-563 | 836.51 ..08 ..562-563 |
| 807.18 ..04 ..183-185 | 813.11 ..08 ..562-563 | 818.0 ...08 ..562-563 | 825.29 ..08 ..562-563 | 836.52 ..08 ..562-563 |
| 807.19 ..04 ..183-185 | 813.12 ..08 ..562-563 | 818.1 ...08 ..562-563 | 825.30 ..08 ..562-563 | 836.53 ..08 ..562-563 |
| 807.2 ...04 ..183-185 | 813.13 ..08 ..562-563 | 819.0 ...21 ..913-914 | 825.31 ..08 ..562-563 | 836.54 ..08 ..562-563 |
| 807.3 ...04 ..183-185 | 813.14 ..08 ..562-563 | 819.1 ...21 ..913-914 | 825.32 ..08 ..562-563 | 836.59 ..08 ..562-563 |
| 807.4 ...04 ..183-185 | 813.15 ..08 ..562-563 | 820.00 ..08 ..535-536 | 825.33 ..08 ..562-563 | 836.60 ..08 ..562-563 |
| 807.5 ...03 ..154-156 | 813.16 ..08 ..562-563 | 820.01 ..08 ..535-536 | 825.34 ..08 ..562-563 | 836.61 ..08 ..562-563 |
| 807.6 ...03 ..154-156 | 813.17 ..08 ..562-563 | 820.02 ..08 ..535-536 | 825.35 ..08 ..562-563 | 836.62 ..08 ..562-563 |
| 808.0 ...08 ..535-536 | 813.18 ..08 ..562-563 | 820.03 ..08 ..535-536 | 825.39 ..08 ..562-563 | 836.63 ..08 ..562-563 |
| 808.1 ...08 ..535-536 | 813.20 ..08 ..562-563 | 820.09 ..08 ..535-536 | 826.0 ..08 ..562-563 | 836.64 ..08 ..562-563 |
| 808.2 ...08 ..535-536 | 813.21 ..08 ..562-563 | 820.10 ..08 ..535-536 | 826.1 ..08 ..562-563 | 836.69 ..08 ..562-563 |
| 808.3 ...08 ..535-536 | 813.22 ..08 ..562-563 | 820.11 ..08 ..535-536 | 827.0 ..08 ..562-563 | 837.0 ...08 ..562-563 |
| 808.41 ..08 ..535-536 | 813.23 ..08 ..562-563 | 820.12 ..08 ..535-536 | 827.1 ..08 ..562-563 | 837.1 ...08 ..562-563 |
| 808.42 ..08 ..535-536 | 813.30 ..08 ..562-563 | 820.13 ..08 ..535-536 | 828.0 ..21 ..913-914 | 838.00 ..08 ..562-563 |
| 808.43 ..08 ..535-536 | 813.31 ..08 ..562-563 | 820.19 ..08 ..535-536 | 828.1 ..21 ..913-914 | 838.01 ..08 ..562-563 |
| 808.49 ..08 ..535-536 | 813.32 ..08 ..562-563 | 820.20 ..08 ..535-536 | 829.0 ..08 ..562-563 | 838.02 ..08 ..562-563 |
| 808.51 ..08 ..535-536 | 813.33 ..08 ..562-563 | 820.21 ..08 ..535-536 | 829.1 ..08 ..562-563 | 838.03 ..08 ..562-563 |
| 808.52 ..08 ..535-536 | 813.40 ..08 ..562-563 | 820.22 ..08 ..535-536 | 830.0 ...03 ..157-159 | 838.04 ..08 ..562-563 |
| 808.53 ..08 ..535-536 | 813.41 ..08 ..562-563 | 820.30 ..08 ..535-536 | 830.1 ...03 ..157-159 | 838.05 ..08 ..562-563 |
| 808.59 ..08 ..535-536 | 813.42 ..08 ..562-563 | 820.31 ..08 ..535-536 | 831.00 ..08 ..562-563 | 838.06 ..08 ..562-563 |
| 808.8 ...08 ..535-536 | 813.43 ..08 ..562-563 | 820.32 ..08 ..535-536 | 831.01 ..08 ..562-563 | 838.09 ..08 ..562-563 |
| 808.9 ...08 ..535-536 | 813.44 ..08 ..562-563 | 820.8 ...08 ..535-536 | 831.02 ..08 ..562-563 | 838.10 ..08 ..562-563 |
| 809.0 ...08 ..564-566 | 813.45 ..08 ..562-563 | 820.9 ...08 ..535-536 | 831.03 ..08 ..562-563 | 838.11 ..08 ..562-563 |
| 809.1 ...08 ..564-566 | 813.50 ..08 ..562-563 | 821.00 ..08 ..533-534 | 831.04 ..08 ..562-563 | 838.12 ..08 ..562-563 |
| 810.00 ..08 ..562-563 | 813.51 ..08 ..562-563 | 821.01 ..08 ..533-534 | 831.09 ..08 ..562-563 | 838.13 ..08 ..562-563 |
| 810.01 ..08 ..562-563 | 813.52 ..08 ..562-563 | 821.10 ..08 ..533-534 | 831.10 ..08 ..562-563 | 838.14 ..08 ..562-563 |

| DX | MDC | DRG |
|---|---|---|
| 838.15 | 08 | 562-563 |
| 838.16 | 08 | 562-563 |
| 838.19 | 08 | 562-563 |
| 839.00 | 08 | 551-552 |
| 839.01 | 08 | 551-552 |
| 839.02 | 08 | 551-552 |
| 839.03 | 08 | 551-552 |
| 839.04 | 08 | 551-552 |
| 839.05 | 08 | 551-552 |
| 839.06 | 08 | 551-552 |
| 839.07 | 08 | 551-552 |
| 839.08 | 08 | 551-552 |
| 839.10 | 08 | 551-552 |
| 839.11 | 08 | 551-552 |
| 839.12 | 08 | 551-552 |
| 839.13 | 08 | 551-552 |
| 839.14 | 08 | 551-552 |
| 839.15 | 08 | 551-552 |
| 839.16 | 08 | 551-552 |
| 839.17 | 08 | 551-552 |
| 839.18 | 08 | 551-552 |
| 839.20 | 08 | 551-552 |
| 839.21 | 08 | 551-552 |
| 839.30 | 08 | 551-552 |
| 839.31 | 08 | 551-552 |
| 839.40 | 08 | 551-552 |
| 839.41 | 08 | 551-552 |
| 839.42 | 08 | 551-552 |
| 839.49 | 08 | 551-552 |
| 839.50 | 08 | 551-552 |
| 839.51 | 08 | 551-552 |
| 839.52 | 08 | 551-552 |
| 839.59 | 08 | 551-552 |
| 839.61 | 04 | 183-185 |
| 839.69 | 08 | 562-563 |
| 839.71 | 04 | 183-185 |
| 839.79 | 08 | 562-563 |
| 839.8 | 08 | 562-563 |
| 839.9 | 08 | 562-563 |
| 840.0 | 08 | 562-563 |
| 840.1 | 08 | 562-563 |
| 840.2 | 08 | 562-563 |
| 840.3 | 08 | 562-563 |
| 840.4 | 08 | 562-563 |
| 840.5 | 08 | 562-563 |
| 840.6 | 08 | 562-563 |
| 840.7 | 08 | 562-563 |
| 840.8 | 08 | 562-563 |
| 840.9 | 08 | 562-563 |
| 841.0 | 08 | 562-563 |
| 841.1 | 08 | 562-563 |
| 841.2 | 08 | 562-563 |
| 841.3 | 08 | 562-563 |
| 841.8 | 08 | 562-563 |
| 841.9 | 08 | 562-563 |
| 842.00 | 08 | 562-563 |
| 842.01 | 08 | 562-563 |
| 842.02 | 08 | 562-563 |
| 842.09 | 08 | 562-563 |
| 842.10 | 08 | 562-563 |
| 842.11 | 08 | 562-563 |
| 842.12 | 08 | 562-563 |
| 842.13 | 08 | 562-563 |
| 842.19 | 08 | 562-563 |
| 843.0 | 08 | 537-538 |
| 843.1 | 08 | 537-538 |
| 843.8 | 08 | 537-538 |
| 843.9 | 08 | 537-538 |
| 844.0 | 08 | 562-563 |
| 844.1 | 08 | 562-563 |
| 844.2 | 08 | 562-563 |
| 844.3 | 08 | 562-563 |
| 844.8 | 08 | 562-563 |
| 844.9 | 08 | 562-563 |
| 845.00 | 08 | 562-563 |
| 845.01 | 08 | 562-563 |
| 845.02 | 08 | 562-563 |
| 845.03 | 08 | 562-563 |
| 845.09 | 08 | 562-563 |
| 845.10 | 08 | 562-563 |
| 845.11 | 08 | 562-563 |
| 845.12 | 08 | 562-563 |
| 845.13 | 08 | 562-563 |
| 845.19 | 08 | 562-563 |
| 846.0 | 08 | 551-552 |
| 846.1 | 08 | 551-552 |
| 846.2 | 08 | 551-552 |
| 846.3 | 08 | 551-552 |
| 846.8 | 08 | 551-552 |
| 846.9 | 08 | 551-552 |
| 847.0 | 08 | 551-552 |
| 847.1 | 08 | 551-552 |
| 847.2 | 08 | 551-552 |
| 847.3 | 08 | 551-552 |
| 847.4 | 08 | 551-552 |
| 847.9 | 08 | 551-552 |
| 848.0 | 08 | 564-566 |
| 848.1 | 03 | 157-159 |
| 848.2 | 08 | 564-566 |
| 848.3 | 04 | 205-206 |
| 848.40 | 04 | 205-206 |
| 848.41 | 04 | 205-206 |
| 848.42 | 04 | 205-206 |
| 848.49 | 04 | 205-206 |
| 848.5 | 08 | 537-538 |
| 848.8 | 08 | 562-563 |
| 848.9 | 08 | 562-563 |
| 850.0 | 01 | 088-090 |
| 850.11 | 01 | 088-090 |
| 850.12 | 01 | 088-090 |
| 850.2 | 01 | 088-090 |
| 850.3 | 01 | 088-090 |
| 850.4 | 01 | 088-090 |
| 850.5 | 01 | 088-090 |
| 850.9 | 01 | 088-090 |
| 851.00 | 01 | 082-087 |
| 851.01 | 01 | 082-087 |
| 851.02 | 01 | 082-087 |
| 851.03 | 01 | 082-084 |
| 851.05 | 01 | 082-084 |
| 851.06 | 01 | 082-084 |
| 851.09 | 01 | 082-087 |
| 851.10 | 01 | 082-087 |
| 851.11 | 01 | 082-087 |
| 851.12 | 01 | 082-087 |
| 851.13 | 01 | 082-084 |
| 851.14 | 01 | 082-084 |
| 851.15 | 01 | 082-084 |
| 851.16 | 01 | 082-084 |
| 851.19 | 01 | 082-087 |
| 851.20 | 01 | 082-087 |
| 851.21 | 01 | 082-087 |
| 851.22 | 01 | 082-087 |
| 851.23 | 01 | 082-084 |
| 851.24 | 01 | 082-084 |
| 851.25 | 01 | 082-084 |
| 851.26 | 01 | 082-084 |
| 851.29 | 01 | 082-087 |
| 851.30 | 01 | 082-087 |
| 851.31 | 01 | 082-087 |
| 851.32 | 01 | 082-087 |
| 851.33 | 01 | 082-084 |
| 851.34 | 01 | 082-084 |
| 851.35 | 01 | 082-084 |
| 851.36 | 01 | 082-084 |
| 851.39 | 01 | 082-087 |
| 851.40 | 01 | 082-087 |
| 851.41 | 01 | 082-087 |
| 851.42 | 01 | 082-087 |
| 851.43 | 01 | 082-084 |
| 851.44 | 01 | 082-084 |
| 851.45 | 01 | 082-084 |
| 851.46 | 01 | 082-084 |
| 851.49 | 01 | 082-087 |
| 851.50 | 01 | 082-087 |
| 851.51 | 01 | 082-087 |
| 851.52 | 01 | 082-087 |
| 851.53 | 01 | 082-084 |
| 851.54 | 01 | 082-084 |
| 851.55 | 01 | 082-084 |
| 851.56 | 01 | 082-084 |
| 851.59 | 01 | 082-087 |
| 851.60 | 01 | 082-087 |
| 851.61 | 01 | 082-087 |
| 851.62 | 01 | 082-087 |
| 851.63 | 01 | 082-084 |
| 851.64 | 01 | 082-084 |
| 851.65 | 01 | 082-084 |
| 851.66 | 01 | 082-084 |
| 851.69 | 01 | 082-087 |
| 851.70 | 01 | 082-087 |
| 851.71 | 01 | 082-087 |
| 851.72 | 01 | 082-087 |
| 851.73 | 01 | 082-084 |
| 851.74 | 01 | 082-084 |
| 851.75 | 01 | 082-084 |
| 851.76 | 01 | 082-084 |
| 851.79 | 01 | 082-087 |
| 851.80 | 01 | 082-087 |
| 851.81 | 01 | 082-087 |
| 851.82 | 01 | 082-087 |
| 851.83 | 01 | 082-084 |
| 851.84 | 01 | 082-084 |
| 851.85 | 01 | 082-084 |
| 851.86 | 01 | 082-084 |
| 851.89 | 01 | 082-087 |
| 851.90 | 01 | 082-087 |
| 851.91 | 01 | 082-087 |
| 851.92 | 01 | 082-087 |
| 851.93 | 01 | 082-084 |
| 851.94 | 01 | 082-084 |
| 851.95 | 01 | 082-084 |
| 851.96 | 01 | 082-084 |
| 851.99 | 01 | 082-087 |
| 852.00 | 01 | 082-087 |
| 852.01 | 01 | 082-087 |
| 852.02 | 01 | 082-087 |
| 852.03 | 01 | 082-084 |
| 852.04 | 01 | 082-084 |
| 852.05 | 01 | 082-084 |
| 852.06 | 01 | 082-084 |
| 852.09 | 01 | 082-087 |
| 852.10 | 01 | 082-087 |
| 852.11 | 01 | 082-087 |
| 852.12 | 01 | 082-087 |
| 852.13 | 01 | 082-084 |
| 852.14 | 01 | 082-084 |
| 852.15 | 01 | 082-084 |
| 852.16 | 01 | 082-084 |
| 852.19 | 01 | 082-087 |
| 852.20 | 01 | 082-087 |
| 852.21 | 01 | 082-087 |
| 852.22 | 01 | 082-087 |
| 852.23 | 01 | 082-084 |
| 852.24 | 01 | 082-084 |
| 852.25 | 01 | 082-084 |
| 852.26 | 01 | 082-084 |
| 852.29 | 01 | 082-087 |
| 852.30 | 01 | 082-087 |
| 852.31 | 01 | 082-087 |
| 852.32 | 01 | 082-087 |
| 852.33 | 01 | 082-084 |
| 852.34 | 01 | 082-084 |
| 852.35 | 01 | 082-084 |
| 852.36 | 01 | 082-084 |
| 852.39 | 01 | 082-087 |
| 852.40 | 01 | 082-087 |
| 852.41 | 01 | 082-087 |
| 852.42 | 01 | 082-087 |
| 852.43 | 01 | 082-084 |
| 852.44 | 01 | 082-084 |
| 852.45 | 01 | 082-084 |
| 852.46 | 01 | 082-084 |
| 852.49 | 01 | 082-087 |
| 852.50 | 01 | 082-087 |
| 852.51 | 01 | 082-087 |
| 852.52 | 01 | 082-087 |
| 852.53 | 01 | 082-084 |
| 852.54 | 01 | 082-084 |
| 852.55 | 01 | 082-084 |
| 852.56 | 01 | 082-084 |
| 852.59 | 01 | 082-087 |
| 853.00 | 01 | 082-087 |
| 853.01 | 01 | 082-087 |
| 853.02 | 01 | 082-087 |
| 853.03 | 01 | 082-084 |
| 853.04 | 01 | 082-084 |
| 853.05 | 01 | 082-084 |
| 853.06 | 01 | 082-084 |
| 853.09 | 01 | 082-087 |
| 853.10 | 01 | 082-087 |
| 853.11 | 01 | 082-087 |
| 853.12 | 01 | 082-087 |
| 853.13 | 01 | 082-084 |
| 853.14 | 01 | 082-084 |
| 853.15 | 01 | 082-084 |
| 853.16 | 01 | 082-084 |
| 853.19 | 01 | 082-087 |
| 854.00 | 01 | 082-087 |
| 854.01 | 01 | 082-087 |
| 854.02 | 01 | 082-087 |
| 854.03 | 01 | 082-084 |
| 854.04 | 01 | 082-084 |
| 854.05 | 01 | 082-084 |
| 854.06 | 01 | 082-084 |
| 854.09 | 01 | 082-087 |
| 854.10 | 01 | 082-087 |
| 854.11 | 01 | 082-087 |
| 854.12 | 01 | 082-087 |
| 854.13 | 01 | 082-084 |
| 854.14 | 01 | 082-084 |
| 854.15 | 01 | 082-084 |
| 854.16 | 01 | 082-084 |
| 854.19 | 01 | 082-087 |
| 860.0 | 04 | 199-201 |
| 860.1 | 04 | 199-201 |
| 860.2 | 04 | 199-201 |
| 860.3 | 04 | 199-201 |
| 860.4 | 04 | 199-201 |
| 860.5 | 04 | 199-201 |
| 861.00 | 05 | 314-316 |
| 861.01 | 05 | 314-316 |
| 861.02 | 05 | 314-316 |
| 861.03 | 05 | 314-316 |
| 861.10 | 05 | 314-316 |
| 861.11 | 05 | 314-316 |
| 861.12 | 05 | 314-316 |
| 861.13 | 05 | 314-316 |
| 861.20 | 04 | 205-206 |
| 861.21 | 04 | 205-206 |
| 861.22 | 04 | 183-185 |
| 861.30 | 04 | 205-206 |
| 861.31 | 04 | 205-206 |
| 861.32 | 04 | 183-185 |
| 862.0 | 04 | 183-185 |
| 862.1 | 04 | 183-185 |
| 862.21 | 04 | 183-185 |
| 862.22 | 06 | 368-370 |
| 862.29 | 04 | 205-206 |
| 862.31 | 04 | 183-185 |
| 862.32 | 06 | 393-395 |
| 862.39 | 04 | 205-206 |
| 862.8 | 21 | 913-914 |
| 862.9 | 21 | 913-914 |
| 863.0 | 06 | 393-395 |
| 863.1 | 06 | 393-395 |
| 863.20 | 06 | 393-395 |
| 863.21 | 06 | 393-395 |
| 863.29 | 06 | 393-395 |
| 863.30 | 06 | 393-395 |
| 863.31 | 06 | 393-395 |
| 863.39 | 06 | 393-395 |
| 863.40 | 06 | 393-395 |
| 863.41 | 06 | 393-395 |
| 863.42 | 06 | 393-395 |
| 863.43 | 06 | 393-395 |
| 863.44 | 06 | 393-395 |
| 863.45 | 06 | 393-395 |
| 863.46 | 06 | 393-395 |
| 863.49 | 06 | 393-395 |
| 863.50 | 06 | 393-395 |
| 863.51 | 06 | 393-395 |
| 863.52 | 06 | 393-395 |
| 863.53 | 06 | 393-395 |
| 863.54 | 06 | 393-395 |
| 863.55 | 06 | 393-395 |
| 863.56 | 06 | 393-395 |
| 863.59 | 06 | 393-395 |
| 863.80 | 06 | 393-395 |
| 863.81 | 07 | 438-440 |
| 863.82 | 07 | 438-440 |
| 863.83 | 07 | 438-440 |
| 863.84 | 07 | 438-440 |
| 863.85 | 06 | 393-395 |
| 863.89 | 06 | 393-395 |
| 863.90 | 06 | 393-395 |
| 863.91 | 07 | 438-440 |
| 863.92 | 07 | 438-440 |
| 863.93 | 07 | 438-440 |
| 863.94 | 07 | 438-440 |
| 863.95 | 06 | 393-395 |
| 863.99 | 06 | 393-395 |
| 864.00 | 07 | 441-443 |
| 864.01 | 07 | 441-443 |
| 864.02 | 07 | 441-443 |
| 864.03 | 07 | 441-443 |
| 864.04 | 07 | 441-443 |
| 864.05 | 07 | 441-443 |
| 864.09 | 07 | 441-443 |
| 864.10 | 07 | 441-443 |
| 864.11 | 07 | 441-443 |
| 864.12 | 07 | 441-443 |
| 864.13 | 07 | 441-443 |
| 864.14 | 07 | 441-443 |
| 864.15 | 07 | 441-443 |
| 864.19 | 07 | 441-443 |
| 865.00 | 16 | 814-816 |
| 865.01 | 16 | 814-816 |
| 865.02 | 16 | 814-816 |
| 865.03 | 16 | 814-816 |
| 865.04 | 16 | 814-816 |
| 865.09 | 16 | 814-816 |
| 865.10 | 16 | 814-816 |
| 865.11 | 16 | 814-816 |
| 865.12 | 16 | 814-816 |
| 865.13 | 16 | 814-816 |
| 865.14 | 16 | 814-816 |
| 865.19 | 16 | 814-816 |
| 866.00 | 11 | 698-700 |
| 866.01 | 11 | 698-700 |
| 866.02 | 11 | 698-700 |
| 866.03 | 11 | 698-700 |
| 866.10 | 11 | 698-700 |
| 866.11 | 11 | 698-700 |
| 866.12 | 11 | 698-700 |
| 866.13 | 11 | 698-700 |
| 867.0 | 11 | 698-700 |
| 867.1 | 11 | 698-700 |
| 867.2 | 11 | 698-700 |
| 867.3 | 11 | 698-700 |
| 867.4 | 13 | 760-761 |
| 867.5 | 13 | 760-761 |
| 867.6 | 12 | 729-730 |
| 867.6 | 13 | 760-761 |

| DX | MDC | DRG | DX | MDC | DRG | DX | MDC | DRG | DX | MDC | DRG | DX | MDC | DRG |
|---|---|---|---|---|---|---|---|---|---|---|---|---|---|---|
| 867.7 | 12 | 729-730 | 873.59 | 09 | 604-605 | 881.12 | 21 | 913-914 | 902.11 | 21 | 913-914 | 906.8 | 09 | 604-605 |
| 867.7 | 13 | 760-761 | 873.60 | 03 | 157-159 | 881.20 | 08 | 564-566 | 902.19 | 21 | 913-914 | 906.9 | 09 | 604-605 |
| 867.8 | 12 | 729-730 | 873.61 | 03 | 157-159 | 881.21 | 08 | 564-566 | 902.20 | 21 | 913-914 | 907.0 | 01 | 091-093 |
| 867.8 | 13 | 760-761 | 873.62 | 03 | 157-159 | 881.22 | 08 | 564-566 | 902.21 | 21 | 913-914 | 907.1 | 01 | 091-093 |
| 867.9 | 12 | 729-730 | 873.63 | 03 | 157-159 | 882.0 | 09 | 604-605 | 902.22 | 21 | 913-914 | 907.2 | 01 | 052-053 |
| 867.9 | 13 | 760-761 | 873.64 | 03 | 157-159 | 882.1 | 21 | 913-914 | 902.23 | 21 | 913-914 | 907.3 | 01 | 091-093 |
| 868.00 | 06 | 393-395 | 873.65 | 03 | 157-159 | 882.2 | 08 | 564-566 | 902.24 | 21 | 913-914 | 907.4 | 01 | 091-093 |
| 868.01 | 10 | 643-645 | 873.69 | 03 | 157-159 | 883.0 | 09 | 604-605 | 902.25 | 21 | 913-914 | 907.5 | 01 | 091-093 |
| 868.02 | 07 | 444-446 | 873.70 | 03 | 157-159 | 883.1 | 21 | 913-914 | 902.26 | 21 | 913-914 | 907.9 | 01 | 091-093 |
| 868.03 | 06 | 393-395 | 873.71 | 03 | 157-159 | 883.2 | 08 | 564-566 | 902.27 | 21 | 913-914 | 908.0 | 04 | 205-206 |
| 868.04 | 11 | 698-700 | 873.72 | 03 | 157-159 | 884.0 | 09 | 604-605 | 902.29 | 21 | 913-914 | 908.1 | 06 | 393-395 |
| 868.09 | 21 | 913-914 | 873.73 | 03 | 157-159 | 884.1 | 21 | 913-914 | 902.31 | 21 | 913-914 | 908.2 | 12 | 729-730 |
| 868.10 | 06 | 393-395 | 873.74 | 03 | 157-159 | 884.2 | 08 | 564-566 | 902.32 | 21 | 913-914 | 908.2 | 13 | 760-761 |
| 868.11 | 10 | 643-645 | 873.75 | 03 | 157-159 | 885.0 | 21 | 913-914 | 902.33 | 21 | 913-914 | 908.3 | 05 | 299-301 |
| 868.12 | 07 | 444-446 | 873.79 | 03 | 157-159 | 885.1 | 21 | 913-914 | 902.34 | 21 | 913-914 | 908.4 | 05 | 299-301 |
| 868.13 | 06 | 393-395 | 873.8 | 09 | 604-605 | 886.0 | 21 | 913-914 | 902.39 | 21 | 913-914 | 908.5 | 21 | 913-914 |
| 868.14 | 11 | 698-700 | 873.9 | 09 | 604-605 | 886.1 | 21 | 913-914 | 902.40 | 21 | 913-914 | 908.6 | 21 | 913-914 |
| 868.19 | 21 | 913-914 | 874.00 | 03 | 154-156 | 887.0 | 21 | 913-914 | 902.41 | 21 | 913-914 | 908.9 | 21 | 913-914 |
| 869.0 | 21 | 913-914 | 874.01 | 03 | 154-156 | 887.1 | 21 | 913-914 | 902.42 | 21 | 913-914 | 909.0 | 21 | 922-923 |
| 869.1 | 21 | 913-914 | 874.02 | 04 | 183-185 | 887.2 | 21 | 913-914 | 902.49 | 21 | 913-914 | 909.1 | 21 | 922-923 |
| 870.0 | 02 | 124-125 | 874.10 | 03 | 154-156 | 887.3 | 21 | 913-914 | 902.50 | 21 | 913-914 | 909.2 | 21 | 922-923 |
| 870.1 | 02 | 124-125 | 874.11 | 03 | 154-156 | 887.4 | 21 | 913-914 | 902.51 | 21 | 913-914 | 909.3 | 21 | 922-923 |
| 870.2 | 02 | 124-125 | 874.12 | 04 | 183-185 | 887.5 | 21 | 913-914 | 902.52 | 21 | 913-914 | 909.4 | 21 | 922-923 |
| 870.3 | 02 | 124-125 | 874.2 | 10 | 643-645 | 887.6 | 21 | 913-914 | 902.53 | 21 | 913-914 | 909.9 | 21 | 922-923 |
| 870.4 | 02 | 124-125 | 874.3 | 10 | 643-645 | 887.7 | 21 | 913-914 | 902.54 | 21 | 913-914 | 910.0 | 09 | 604-605 |
| 870.8 | 02 | 124-125 | 874.4 | 03 | 154-156 | 890.0 | 09 | 604-605 | 902.55 | 21 | 913-914 | 910.1 | 09 | 602-603 |
| 870.9 | 02 | 124-125 | 874.5 | 03 | 154-156 | 890.1 | 21 | 913-914 | 902.56 | 21 | 913-914 | 910.2 | 09 | 606-607 |
| 871.0 | 02 | 124-125 | 874.8 | 09 | 604-605 | 890.2 | 08 | 564-566 | 902.59 | 21 | 913-914 | 910.3 | 09 | 606-607 |
| 871.1 | 02 | 124-125 | 874.9 | 09 | 604-605 | 891.0 | 09 | 604-605 | 902.81 | 21 | 913-914 | 910.4 | 09 | 606-607 |
| 871.2 | 02 | 124-125 | 875.0 | 09 | 604-605 | 891.1 | 21 | 913-914 | 902.82 | 21 | 913-914 | 910.5 | 09 | 602-603 |
| 871.3 | 02 | 124-125 | 875.1 | 21 | 913-914 | 891.2 | 08 | 564-566 | 902.87 | 21 | 913-914 | 910.6 | 09 | 604-605 |
| 871.4 | 02 | 124-125 | 876.0 | 09 | 604-605 | 892.0 | 09 | 604-605 | 902.89 | 21 | 913-914 | 910.7 | 09 | 602-603 |
| 871.5 | 02 | 124-125 | 876.1 | 09 | 604-605 | 892.1 | 21 | 913-914 | 902.9 | 21 | 913-914 | 910.8 | 09 | 604-605 |
| 871.6 | 02 | 124-125 | 877.0 | 09 | 604-605 | 892.2 | 08 | 564-566 | 903.00 | 21 | 913-914 | 910.9 | 09 | 602-603 |
| 871.7 | 02 | 124-125 | 877.1 | 09 | 604-605 | 893.0 | 09 | 604-605 | 903.01 | 21 | 913-914 | 911.0 | 09 | 604-605 |
| 871.9 | 02 | 124-125 | 878.0 | 12 | 729-730 | 893.1 | 21 | 913-914 | 903.02 | 21 | 913-914 | 911.1 | 09 | 602-603 |
| 872.00 | 03 | 154-156 | 878.1 | 12 | 729-730 | 893.2 | 08 | 564-566 | 903.1 | 21 | 913-914 | 911.2 | 09 | 606-607 |
| 872.01 | 03 | 154-156 | 878.2 | 12 | 729-730 | 894.0 | 09 | 604-605 | 903.2 | 21 | 913-914 | 911.3 | 09 | 602-603 |
| 872.02 | 03 | 154-156 | 878.3 | 12 | 729-730 | 894.1 | 21 | 913-914 | 903.3 | 21 | 913-914 | 911.4 | 09 | 606-607 |
| 872.10 | 03 | 154-156 | 878.4 | 13 | 760-761 | 894.2 | 08 | 564-566 | 903.4 | 21 | 913-914 | 911.5 | 09 | 602-603 |
| 872.11 | 03 | 154-156 | 878.5 | 13 | 760-761 | 895.0 | 21 | 913-914 | 903.5 | 21 | 913-914 | 911.6 | 09 | 604-605 |
| 872.12 | 03 | 154-156 | 878.6 | 13 | 760-761 | 895.1 | 21 | 913-914 | 903.8 | 21 | 913-914 | 911.7 | 09 | 602-603 |
| 872.61 | 03 | 154-156 | 878.7 | 13 | 760-761 | 896.0 | 21 | 913-914 | 903.9 | 21 | 913-914 | 911.8 | 09 | 604-605 |
| 872.62 | 03 | 154-156 | 878.8 | 12 | 729-730 | 896.1 | 21 | 913-914 | 904.0 | 21 | 913-914 | 911.9 | 09 | 602-603 |
| 872.63 | 03 | 154-156 | 878.8 | 13 | 760-761 | 896.2 | 21 | 913-914 | 904.1 | 21 | 913-914 | 912.0 | 09 | 604-605 |
| 872.64 | 03 | 154-156 | 878.9 | 12 | 729-730 | 896.3 | 21 | 913-914 | 904.2 | 21 | 913-914 | 912.1 | 09 | 602-603 |
| 872.69 | 03 | 154-156 | 878.9 | 13 | 760-761 | 897.0 | 21 | 913-914 | 904.3 | 21 | 913-914 | 912.2 | 09 | 604-605 |
| 872.71 | 03 | 154-156 | 879.0 | 09 | 604-605 | 897.1 | 21 | 913-914 | 904.40 | 21 | 913-914 | 912.3 | 09 | 602-603 |
| 872.72 | 03 | 154-156 | 879.1 | 09 | 604-605 | 897.2 | 21 | 913-914 | 904.41 | 21 | 913-914 | 912.4 | 09 | 606-607 |
| 872.73 | 03 | 154-156 | 879.2 | 09 | 604-605 | 897.3 | 21 | 913-914 | 904.42 | 21 | 913-914 | 912.5 | 09 | 602-603 |
| 872.74 | 03 | 154-156 | 879.3 | 21 | 913-914 | 897.4 | 21 | 913-914 | 904.50 | 21 | 913-914 | 912.6 | 09 | 604-605 |
| 872.79 | 03 | 154-156 | 879.4 | 09 | 604-605 | 897.5 | 21 | 913-914 | 904.51 | 21 | 913-914 | 912.7 | 09 | 602-603 |
| 872.8 | 03 | 154-156 | 879.5 | 21 | 913-914 | 897.6 | 21 | 913-914 | 904.52 | 21 | 913-914 | 912.8 | 09 | 604-605 |
| 872.9 | 03 | 154-156 | 879.6 | 09 | 604-605 | 897.7 | 21 | 913-914 | 904.53 | 21 | 913-914 | 912.9 | 09 | 602-603 |
| 873.0 | 09 | 604-605 | 879.7 | 21 | 913-914 | 900.00 | 21 | 913-914 | 904.54 | 21 | 913-914 | 913.0 | 09 | 604-605 |
| 873.1 | 09 | 604-605 | 879.8 | 09 | 604-605 | 900.01 | 21 | 913-914 | 904.6 | 21 | 913-914 | 913.1 | 09 | 602-603 |
| 873.20 | 03 | 154-156 | 879.9 | 21 | 913-914 | 900.02 | 21 | 913-914 | 904.7 | 21 | 913-914 | 913.2 | 09 | 606-607 |
| 873.21 | 03 | 154-156 | 880.00 | 09 | 604-605 | 900.03 | 21 | 913-914 | 904.8 | 21 | 913-914 | 913.3 | 09 | 602-603 |
| 873.22 | 03 | 154-156 | 880.01 | 09 | 604-605 | 900.1 | 21 | 913-914 | 904.9 | 21 | 913-914 | 913.4 | 09 | 606-607 |
| 873.23 | 03 | 154-156 | 880.02 | 09 | 604-605 | 900.81 | 21 | 913-914 | 905.0 | 01 | 091-093 | 913.5 | 09 | 602-603 |
| 873.29 | 03 | 154-156 | 880.03 | 09 | 604-605 | 900.82 | 21 | 913-914 | 905.1 | 08 | 551-552 | 913.6 | 09 | 604-605 |
| 873.30 | 03 | 154-156 | 880.09 | 09 | 604-605 | 900.89 | 21 | 913-914 | 905.2 | 08 | 559-561 | 913.7 | 09 | 602-603 |
| 873.31 | 03 | 154-156 | 880.10 | 21 | 913-914 | 900.9 | 21 | 913-914 | 905.3 | 08 | 559-561 | 913.8 | 09 | 604-605 |
| 873.32 | 03 | 154-156 | 880.11 | 21 | 913-914 | 901.0 | 21 | 913-914 | 905.4 | 08 | 559-561 | 913.9 | 09 | 602-603 |
| 873.33 | 03 | 154-156 | 880.12 | 21 | 913-914 | 901.1 | 21 | 913-914 | 905.5 | 08 | 559-561 | 914.0 | 09 | 604-605 |
| 873.39 | 03 | 154-156 | 880.13 | 21 | 913-914 | 901.2 | 21 | 913-914 | 905.6 | 08 | 562-563 | 914.1 | 09 | 602-603 |
| 873.40 | 09 | 604-605 | 880.19 | 21 | 913-914 | 901.3 | 21 | 913-914 | 905.7 | 08 | 562-563 | 914.2 | 09 | 606-607 |
| 873.41 | 09 | 604-605 | 880.20 | 08 | 564-566 | 901.40 | 21 | 913-914 | 905.8 | 08 | 559-561 | 914.3 | 09 | 602-603 |
| 873.42 | 09 | 604-605 | 880.21 | 08 | 564-566 | 901.41 | 21 | 913-914 | 905.9 | 08 | 559-561 | 914.4 | 09 | 606-607 |
| 873.43 | 03 | 157-159 | 880.22 | 08 | 564-566 | 901.42 | 21 | 913-914 | 906.0 | 09 | 604-605 | 914.5 | 09 | 602-603 |
| 873.44 | 03 | 157-159 | 880.23 | 08 | 564-566 | 901.81 | 21 | 913-914 | 906.1 | 09 | 604-605 | 914.6 | 09 | 604-605 |
| 873.49 | 09 | 604-605 | 880.29 | 08 | 564-566 | 901.82 | 21 | 913-914 | 906.2 | 09 | 604-605 | 914.7 | 09 | 602-603 |
| 873.50 | 09 | 604-605 | 881.00 | 09 | 604-605 | 901.83 | 21 | 913-914 | 906.3 | 09 | 604-605 | 914.8 | 09 | 604-605 |
| 873.51 | 09 | 604-605 | 881.01 | 09 | 604-605 | 901.89 | 21 | 913-914 | 906.4 | 09 | 604-605 | 914.9 | 09 | 602-603 |
| 873.52 | 09 | 604-605 | 881.02 | 09 | 604-605 | 901.9 | 21 | 913-914 | 906.5 | 09 | 604-605 | 915.0 | 09 | 604-605 |
| 873.53 | 03 | 157-159 | 881.10 | 21 | 913-914 | 902.0 | 21 | 913-914 | 906.6 | 09 | 604-605 | 915.1 | 09 | 602-603 |
| 873.54 | 03 | 157-159 | 881.11 | 21 | 913-914 | 902.10 | 21 | 913-914 | 906.7 | 09 | 604-605 | 915.2 | 09 | 606-607 |

| DX | MDC | DRG | DX | MDC | DRG | DX | MDC | DRG | DX | MDC | DRG | DX | MDC | DRG |
|---|---|---|---|---|---|---|---|---|---|---|---|---|---|---|
| 915.3 | 09 | 602-603 | 924.5 | 09 | 604-605 | 941.11 | 22 | 935 | 942.40 | 22 | 934 | 944.16 | 22 | 935 |
| 915.4 | 09 | 606-607 | 924.8 | 09 | 604-605 | 941.12 | 02 | 124-125 | 942.41 | 22 | 934 | 944.17 | 22 | 935 |
| 915.5 | 09 | 602-603 | 924.9 | 09 | 604-605 | 941.13 | 22 | 935 | 942.42 | 22 | 934 | 944.18 | 22 | 935 |
| 915.6 | 09 | 604-605 | 925.1 | 21 | 913-914 | 941.14 | 22 | 935 | 942.43 | 22 | 934 | 944.20 | 22 | 935 |
| 915.7 | 09 | 602-603 | 925.2 | 21 | 913-914 | 941.15 | 22 | 935 | 942.44 | 22 | 934 | 944.21 | 22 | 935 |
| 915.8 | 09 | 604-605 | 926.0 | 12 | 729-730 | 941.16 | 22 | 935 | 942.45 | 22 | 934 | 944.22 | 22 | 935 |
| 915.9 | 09 | 602-603 | 926.0 | 13 | 760-761 | 941.17 | 22 | 935 | 942.49 | 22 | 934 | 944.23 | 22 | 935 |
| 916.0 | 09 | 604-605 | 926.11 | 21 | 913-914 | 941.18 | 22 | 935 | 942.50 | 22 | 934 | 944.24 | 22 | 935 |
| 916.1 | 09 | 602-603 | 926.12 | 21 | 913-914 | 941.19 | 22 | 935 | 942.51 | 22 | 934 | 944.25 | 22 | 935 |
| 916.2 | 09 | 606-607 | 926.19 | 21 | 913-914 | 941.20 | 22 | 935 | 942.52 | 22 | 934 | 944.26 | 22 | 935 |
| 916.3 | 09 | 602-603 | 926.8 | 21 | 913-914 | 941.21 | 22 | 935 | 942.53 | 22 | 934 | 944.27 | 22 | 935 |
| 916.4 | 09 | 606-607 | 926.9 | 21 | 913-914 | 941.22 | 02 | 124-125 | 942.54 | 22 | 934 | 944.28 | 22 | 935 |
| 916.5 | 09 | 602-603 | 927.00 | 21 | 913-914 | 941.23 | 22 | 935 | 942.55 | 22 | 934 | 944.30 | 22 | 934 |
| 916.6 | 09 | 604-605 | 927.01 | 21 | 913-914 | 941.24 | 22 | 935 | 942.59 | 22 | 934 | 944.31 | 22 | 934 |
| 916.7 | 09 | 602-603 | 927.02 | 21 | 913-914 | 941.25 | 22 | 935 | 943.00 | 22 | 935 | 944.32 | 22 | 934 |
| 916.8 | 09 | 604-605 | 927.03 | 21 | 913-914 | 941.26 | 22 | 935 | 943.01 | 22 | 935 | 944.33 | 22 | 934 |
| 916.9 | 09 | 602-603 | 927.09 | 21 | 913-914 | 941.27 | 22 | 935 | 943.02 | 22 | 935 | 944.34 | 22 | 934 |
| 917.0 | 09 | 604-605 | 927.10 | 21 | 913-914 | 941.28 | 22 | 935 | 943.03 | 22 | 935 | 944.35 | 22 | 934 |
| 917.1 | 09 | 602-603 | 927.11 | 21 | 913-914 | 941.29 | 22 | 935 | 943.04 | 22 | 935 | 944.36 | 22 | 934 |
| 917.2 | 09 | 606-607 | 927.20 | 21 | 913-914 | 941.30 | 22 | 934 | 943.05 | 22 | 935 | 944.37 | 22 | 934 |
| 917.3 | 09 | 602-603 | 927.21 | 21 | 913-914 | 941.31 | 22 | 934 | 943.06 | 22 | 935 | 944.38 | 22 | 934 |
| 917.4 | 09 | 606-607 | 927.3 | 21 | 913-914 | 941.32 | 02 | 124-125 | 943.09 | 22 | 935 | 944.40 | 22 | 934 |
| 917.5 | 09 | 602-603 | 927.8 | 21 | 913-914 | 941.33 | 22 | 934 | 943.10 | 22 | 935 | 944.41 | 22 | 934 |
| 917.6 | 09 | 604-605 | 927.9 | 21 | 913-914 | 941.34 | 22 | 934 | 943.11 | 22 | 935 | 944.42 | 22 | 934 |
| 917.7 | 09 | 602-603 | 928.00 | 21 | 913-914 | 941.35 | 22 | 934 | 943.12 | 22 | 935 | 944.43 | 22 | 934 |
| 917.8 | 09 | 604-605 | 928.01 | 21 | 913-914 | 941.36 | 22 | 934 | 943.13 | 22 | 935 | 944.44 | 22 | 934 |
| 917.9 | 09 | 602-603 | 928.10 | 21 | 913-914 | 941.37 | 22 | 934 | 943.14 | 22 | 935 | 944.45 | 22 | 934 |
| 918.0 | 02 | 124-125 | 928.11 | 21 | 913-914 | 941.38 | 22 | 934 | 943.15 | 22 | 935 | 944.46 | 22 | 934 |
| 918.1 | 02 | 124-125 | 928.20 | 21 | 913-914 | 941.39 | 22 | 934 | 943.16 | 22 | 935 | 944.47 | 22 | 934 |
| 918.2 | 02 | 124-125 | 928.21 | 21 | 913-914 | 941.40 | 22 | 934 | 943.19 | 22 | 935 | 944.48 | 22 | 934 |
| 918.9 | 02 | 124-125 | 928.3 | 21 | 913-914 | 941.41 | 22 | 934 | 943.20 | 22 | 935 | 944.50 | 22 | 934 |
| 919.0 | 09 | 604-605 | 928.8 | 21 | 913-914 | 941.42 | 02 | 124-125 | 943.21 | 22 | 935 | 944.51 | 22 | 934 |
| 919.1 | 09 | 602-603 | 928.9 | 21 | 913-914 | 941.43 | 22 | 934 | 943.22 | 22 | 935 | 944.52 | 22 | 934 |
| 919.2 | 09 | 606-607 | 929.0 | 21 | 913-914 | 941.44 | 22 | 934 | 943.23 | 22 | 935 | 944.53 | 22 | 934 |
| 919.3 | 09 | 602-603 | 929.9 | 21 | 913-914 | 941.45 | 22 | 934 | 943.24 | 22 | 935 | 944.54 | 22 | 934 |
| 919.4 | 09 | 606-607 | 930.0 | 02 | 124-125 | 941.46 | 22 | 934 | 943.25 | 22 | 935 | 944.55 | 22 | 934 |
| 919.5 | 09 | 602-603 | 930.1 | 02 | 124-125 | 941.47 | 22 | 934 | 943.26 | 22 | 935 | 944.56 | 22 | 934 |
| 919.6 | 09 | 604-605 | 930.2 | 02 | 124-125 | 941.48 | 22 | 934 | 943.29 | 22 | 935 | 944.57 | 22 | 934 |
| 919.7 | 09 | 602-603 | 930.8 | 02 | 124-125 | 941.49 | 22 | 934 | 943.30 | 22 | 934 | 944.58 | 22 | 934 |
| 919.8 | 09 | 604-605 | 930.9 | 02 | 124-125 | 941.50 | 22 | 934 | 943.31 | 22 | 934 | 945.00 | 22 | 935 |
| 919.9 | 09 | 602-603 | 931 | 03 | 154-156 | 941.51 | 22 | 934 | 943.32 | 22 | 934 | 945.01 | 22 | 935 |
| 920. | 09 | 604-605 | 932 | 03 | 154-156 | 941.52 | 02 | 124-125 | 943.33 | 22 | 934 | 945.02 | 22 | 935 |
| 921.0 | 02 | 124-125 | 933.0 | 03 | 154-156 | 941.53 | 22 | 934 | 943.34 | 22 | 934 | 945.03 | 22 | 935 |
| 921.1 | 02 | 124-125 | 933.1 | 03 | 154-156 | 941.54 | 22 | 934 | 943.35 | 22 | 934 | 945.04 | 22 | 935 |
| 921.2 | 02 | 124-125 | 934.0 | 04 | 205-206 | 941.55 | 22 | 934 | 943.36 | 22 | 934 | 945.05 | 22 | 935 |
| 921.3 | 02 | 124-125 | 934.1 | 04 | 205-206 | 941.56 | 22 | 934 | 943.39 | 22 | 934 | 945.06 | 22 | 935 |
| 921.9 | 02 | 124-125 | 934.8 | 04 | 205-206 | 941.57 | 22 | 934 | 943.40 | 22 | 934 | 945.09 | 22 | 935 |
| 922.0 | 09 | 604-605 | 934.9 | 04 | 205-206 | 941.58 | 22 | 934 | 943.41 | 22 | 934 | 945.10 | 22 | 935 |
| 922.1 | 09 | 604-605 | 935.0 | 03 | 157-159 | 941.59 | 22 | 934 | 943.42 | 22 | 934 | 945.11 | 22 | 935 |
| 922.2 | 09 | 604-605 | 935.1 | 06 | 393-395 | 942.00 | 22 | 935 | 943.43 | 22 | 934 | 945.12 | 22 | 935 |
| 922.31 | 09 | 604-605 | 935.2 | 06 | 393-395 | 942.01 | 22 | 935 | 943.44 | 22 | 934 | 945.13 | 22 | 935 |
| 922.32 | 09 | 604-605 | 936 | 06 | 393-395 | 942.02 | 22 | 935 | 943.45 | 22 | 934 | 945.14 | 22 | 935 |
| 922.33 | 09 | 604-605 | 937 | 06 | 393-395 | 942.03 | 22 | 935 | 943.46 | 22 | 934 | 945.15 | 22 | 935 |
| 922.4 | 12 | 729-730 | 938 | 06 | 393-395 | 942.04 | 22 | 935 | 943.49 | 22 | 934 | 945.16 | 22 | 935 |
| 922.4 | 13 | 760-761 | 939.0 | 11 | 698-700 | 942.05 | 22 | 935 | 943.50 | 22 | 934 | 945.19 | 22 | 935 |
| 922.8 | 09 | 604-605 | 939.1 | 13 | 760-761 | 942.09 | 22 | 935 | 943.51 | 22 | 934 | 945.20 | 22 | 935 |
| 922.9 | 09 | 604-605 | 939.2 | 13 | 760-761 | 942.10 | 22 | 935 | 943.52 | 22 | 934 | 945.21 | 22 | 935 |
| 923.00 | 09 | 604-605 | 939.3 | 12 | 729-730 | 942.11 | 22 | 935 | 943.53 | 22 | 934 | 945.22 | 22 | 935 |
| 923.01 | 09 | 604-605 | 939.9 | 11 | 698-700 | 942.12 | 22 | 935 | 943.54 | 22 | 934 | 945.23 | 22 | 935 |
| 923.02 | 09 | 604-605 | 940.0 | 02 | 124-125 | 942.13 | 22 | 935 | 943.55 | 22 | 934 | 945.24 | 22 | 935 |
| 923.03 | 09 | 604-605 | 940.1 | 02 | 124-125 | 942.14 | 22 | 935 | 943.56 | 22 | 934 | 945.25 | 22 | 935 |
| 923.09 | 09 | 604-605 | 940.2 | 02 | 124-125 | 942.15 | 22 | 935 | 943.59 | 22 | 934 | 945.26 | 22 | 935 |
| 923.10 | 09 | 604-605 | 940.3 | 02 | 124-125 | 942.19 | 22 | 935 | 944.00 | 22 | 935 | 945.29 | 22 | 935 |
| 923.11 | 09 | 604-605 | 940.4 | 02 | 124-125 | 942.20 | 22 | 935 | 944.01 | 22 | 935 | 945.30 | 22 | 934 |
| 923.20 | 09 | 604-605 | 940.5 | 02 | 124-125 | 942.21 | 22 | 935 | 944.02 | 22 | 935 | 945.31 | 22 | 934 |
| 923.21 | 09 | 604-605 | 940.9 | 02 | 124-125 | 942.22 | 22 | 935 | 944.03 | 22 | 935 | 945.32 | 22 | 934 |
| 923.3 | 09 | 604-605 | 941.00 | 22 | 935 | 942.23 | 22 | 935 | 944.04 | 22 | 935 | 945.33 | 22 | 934 |
| 923.8 | 09 | 604-605 | 941.01 | 22 | 935 | 942.24 | 22 | 935 | 944.05 | 22 | 935 | 945.34 | 22 | 934 |
| 923.9 | 09 | 604-605 | 941.02 | 02 | 124-125 | 942.25 | 22 | 935 | 944.06 | 22 | 935 | 945.35 | 22 | 934 |
| 924.00 | 09 | 604-605 | 941.03 | 22 | 935 | 942.29 | 22 | 935 | 944.07 | 22 | 935 | 945.36 | 22 | 934 |
| 924.01 | 09 | 604-605 | 941.04 | 22 | 935 | 942.30 | 22 | 934 | 944.08 | 22 | 935 | 945.39 | 22 | 934 |
| 924.10 | 09 | 604-605 | 941.05 | 22 | 935 | 942.31 | 22 | 934 | 944.10 | 22 | 935 | 945.40 | 22 | 934 |
| 924.11 | 09 | 604-605 | 941.06 | 22 | 935 | 942.32 | 22 | 934 | 944.11 | 22 | 935 | 945.41 | 22 | 934 |
| 924.20 | 09 | 604-605 | 941.07 | 22 | 935 | 942.33 | 22 | 934 | 944.12 | 22 | 935 | 945.42 | 22 | 934 |
| 924.21 | 09 | 604-605 | 941.08 | 22 | 935 | 942.34 | 22 | 934 | 944.13 | 22 | 935 | 945.43 | 22 | 934 |
| 924.3 | 09 | 604-605 | 941.09 | 22 | 935 | 942.35 | 22 | 934 | 944.14 | 22 | 935 | 945.44 | 22 | 934 |
| 924.4 | 09 | 604-605 | 941.10 | 22 | 935 | 942.39 | 22 | 934 | 944.15 | 22 | 935 | 945.45 | 22 | 934 |

| DX | MDC | DRG | DX | MDC | DRG | DX | MDC | DRG | DX | MDC | DRG | DX | MDC | DRG |
|---|---|---|---|---|---|---|---|---|---|---|---|---|---|---|
| 945.46 | 22 | 934 | 948.99 | 22 | 933 | 957.0 | 01 | 073-074 | 964.6 | 21 | 917-918 | 974.0 | 21 | 917-918 |
| 945.49 | 22 | 934 | 949.0 | 22 | 935 | 957.1 | 01 | 073-074 | 964.7 | 21 | 917-918 | 974.1 | 21 | 917-918 |
| 945.50 | 22 | 934 | 949.1 | 22 | 935 | 957.8 | 01 | 073-074 | 964.8 | 21 | 917-918 | 974.2 | 21 | 917-918 |
| 945.51 | 22 | 934 | 949.2 | 22 | 935 | 957.9 | 01 | 073-074 | 964.9 | 21 | 917-918 | 974.3 | 21 | 917-918 |
| 945.52 | 22 | 934 | 949.3 | 22 | 934 | 958.0 | 04 | 175-176 | 965.00 | 21 | 917-918 | 974.4 | 21 | 917-918 |
| 945.53 | 22 | 934 | 949.4 | 22 | 934 | 958.1 | 04 | 175-176 | 965.01 | 21 | 917-918 | 974.5 | 21 | 917-918 |
| 945.54 | 22 | 934 | 949.5 | 22 | 934 | 958.2 | 21 | 922-923 | 965.02 | 21 | 917-918 | 974.6 | 21 | 917-918 |
| 945.55 | 22 | 934 | 950.0 | 02 | 124-125 | 958.3 | 18 | 862-863 | 965.09 | 21 | 917-918 | 974.7 | 21 | 917-918 |
| 945.56 | 22 | 934 | 950.1 | 01 | 091-093 | 958.4 | 21 | 922-923 | 965.1 | 21 | 917-918 | 975.0 | 21 | 917-918 |
| 945.59 | 22 | 934 | 950.2 | 01 | 091-093 | 958.5 | 11 | 682-684 | 965.4 | 21 | 917-918 | 975.1 | 21 | 917-918 |
| 946.0 | 22 | 935 | 950.3 | 01 | 091-093 | 958.6 | 08 | 564-566 | 965.5 | 21 | 917-918 | 975.2 | 21 | 917-918 |
| 946.1 | 22 | 935 | 950.9 | 01 | 091-093 | 958.7 | 04 | 199-201 | 965.61 | 21 | 917-918 | 975.3 | 21 | 917-918 |
| 946.2 | 22 | 935 | 951.0 | 01 | 073-074 | 958.8 | 21 | 922-923 | 965.69 | 21 | 917-918 | 975.4 | 21 | 917-918 |
| 946.3 | 22 | 934 | 951.1 | 01 | 073-074 | 958.90 | 21 | 922-923 | 965.7 | 21 | 917-918 | 975.5 | 21 | 917-918 |
| 946.4 | 22 | 934 | 951.2 | 01 | 073-074 | 958.91 | 21 | 922-923 | 965.8 | 21 | 917-918 | 975.6 | 21 | 917-918 |
| 946.5 | 22 | 934 | 951.3 | 01 | 073-074 | 958.92 | 21 | 922-923 | 965.9 | 21 | 917-918 | 975.7 | 21 | 917-918 |
| 947.0 | 03 | 154-156 | 951.4 | 01 | 073-074 | 958.93 | 21 | 922-923 | 966.0 | 21 | 917-918 | 975.8 | 21 | 917-918 |
| 947.1 | 04 | 205-206 | 951.5 | 03 | 154-156 | 958.99 | 21 | 922-923 | 966.1 | 21 | 917-918 | 976.0 | 21 | 917-918 |
| 947.2 | 06 | 368-370 | 951.6 | 01 | 073-074 | 959.01 | 21 | 913-914 | 966.2 | 21 | 917-918 | 976.1 | 21 | 917-918 |
| 947.3 | 06 | 393-395 | 951.7 | 01 | 073-074 | 959.09 | 21 | 913-914 | 966.3 | 21 | 917-918 | 976.2 | 21 | 917-918 |
| 947.4 | 13 | 760-761 | 951.8 | 01 | 073-074 | 959.11 | 21 | 913-914 | 966.4 | 21 | 917-918 | 976.3 | 21 | 917-918 |
| 947.8 | 22 | 935 | 951.9 | 01 | 073-074 | 959.12 | 21 | 913-914 | 967.0 | 21 | 917-918 | 976.4 | 21 | 917-918 |
| 947.9 | 22 | 935 | 952.00 | 01 | 052-053 | 959.13 | 21 | 913-914 | 967.1 | 21 | 917-918 | 976.5 | 02 | 124-125 |
| 948.00 | 22 | 935 | 952.01 | 01 | 052-053 | 959.14 | 21 | 913-914 | 967.2 | 21 | 917-918 | 976.6 | 21 | 917-918 |
| 948.10 | 22 | 935 | 952.02 | 01 | 052-053 | 959.19 | 21 | 913-914 | 967.3 | 21 | 917-918 | 976.7 | 21 | 917-918 |
| 948.11 | 22 | 934 | 952.03 | 01 | 052-053 | 959.2 | 21 | 913-914 | 967.4 | 21 | 917-918 | 976.8 | 21 | 917-918 |
| 948.20 | 22 | 935 | 952.04 | 01 | 052-053 | 959.3 | 21 | 913-914 | 967.5 | 21 | 917-918 | 976.9 | 21 | 917-918 |
| 948.21 | 22 | 933 | 952.05 | 01 | 052-053 | 959.4 | 21 | 913-914 | 967.6 | 21 | 917-918 | 977.0 | 21 | 917-918 |
| 948.22 | 22 | 933 | 952.06 | 01 | 052-053 | 959.5 | 21 | 913-914 | 967.8 | 21 | 917-918 | 977.1 | 21 | 917-918 |
| 948.30 | 22 | 935 | 952.07 | 01 | 052-053 | 959.6 | 21 | 913-914 | 967.9 | 21 | 917-918 | 977.2 | 21 | 917-918 |
| 948.31 | 22 | 933 | 952.08 | 01 | 052-053 | 959.7 | 21 | 913-914 | 968.0 | 21 | 917-918 | 977.3 | 21 | 917-918 |
| 948.32 | 22 | 933 | 952.09 | 01 | 052-053 | 959.8 | 21 | 913-914 | 968.1 | 21 | 917-918 | 977.4 | 21 | 917-918 |
| 948.33 | 22 | 933 | 952.10 | 01 | 052-053 | 959.9 | 21 | 913-914 | 968.2 | 21 | 917-918 | 977.8 | 21 | 917-918 |
| 948.40 | 22 | 935 | 952.11 | 01 | 052-053 | 960.0 | 21 | 917-918 | 968.3 | 21 | 917-918 | 977.9 | 21 | 917-918 |
| 948.41 | 22 | 933 | 952.12 | 01 | 052-053 | 960.1 | 21 | 917-918 | 968.4 | 21 | 917-918 | 978.0 | 21 | 917-918 |
| 948.42 | 22 | 933 | 952.13 | 01 | 052-053 | 960.2 | 21 | 917-918 | 968.5 | 21 | 917-918 | 978.1 | 21 | 917-918 |
| 948.43 | 22 | 933 | 952.14 | 01 | 052-053 | 960.3 | 21 | 917-918 | 968.6 | 21 | 917-918 | 978.2 | 21 | 917-918 |
| 948.44 | 22 | 933 | 952.15 | 01 | 052-053 | 960.4 | 21 | 917-918 | 968.7 | 21 | 917-918 | 978.3 | 21 | 917-918 |
| 948.50 | 22 | 935 | 952.16 | 01 | 052-053 | 960.5 | 21 | 917-918 | 968.9 | 21 | 917-918 | 978.4 | 21 | 917-918 |
| 948.51 | 22 | 933 | 952.17 | 01 | 052-053 | 960.6 | 21 | 917-918 | 969.0 | 21 | 917-918 | 978.5 | 21 | 917-918 |
| 948.52 | 22 | 933 | 952.18 | 01 | 052-053 | 960.7 | 21 | 917-918 | 969.1 | 21 | 917-918 | 978.6 | 21 | 917-918 |
| 948.53 | 22 | 933 | 952.19 | 01 | 052-053 | 960.8 | 21 | 917-918 | 969.2 | 21 | 917-918 | 978.8 | 21 | 917-918 |
| 948.54 | 22 | 933 | 952.2 | 01 | 052-053 | 960.9 | 21 | 917-918 | 969.3 | 21 | 917-918 | 978.9 | 21 | 917-918 |
| 948.55 | 22 | 933 | 952.3 | 01 | 052-053 | 961.0 | 21 | 917-918 | 969.4 | 21 | 917-918 | 979.0 | 21 | 917-918 |
| 948.60 | 22 | 935 | 952.4 | 01 | 052-053 | 961.1 | 21 | 917-918 | 969.5 | 21 | 917-918 | 979.1 | 21 | 917-918 |
| 948.61 | 22 | 933 | 952.8 | 01 | 052-053 | 961.2 | 21 | 917-918 | 969.6 | 21 | 917-918 | 979.2 | 21 | 917-918 |
| 948.62 | 22 | 933 | 952.9 | 01 | 052-053 | 961.3 | 21 | 917-918 | 969.7 | 21 | 917-918 | 979.3 | 21 | 917-918 |
| 948.63 | 22 | 933 | 953.0 | 01 | 073-074 | 961.4 | 21 | 917-918 | 969.8 | 21 | 917-918 | 979.4 | 21 | 917-918 |
| 948.64 | 22 | 933 | 953.1 | 01 | 073-074 | 961.5 | 21 | 917-918 | 969.9 | 21 | 917-918 | 979.5 | 21 | 917-918 |
| 948.65 | 22 | 933 | 953.2 | 01 | 073-074 | 961.6 | 21 | 917-918 | 970.0 | 21 | 917-918 | 979.6 | 21 | 917-918 |
| 948.66 | 22 | 933 | 953.3 | 01 | 073-074 | 961.7 | 21 | 917-918 | 970.1 | 21 | 917-918 | 979.7 | 21 | 917-918 |
| 948.70 | 22 | 935 | 953.4 | 01 | 073-074 | 961.8 | 21 | 917-918 | 970.8 | 21 | 917-918 | 979.9 | 21 | 917-918 |
| 948.71 | 22 | 933 | 953.5 | 01 | 073-074 | 961.9 | 21 | 917-918 | 970.9 | 21 | 917-918 | 980.0 | 21 | 917-918 |
| 948.72 | 22 | 933 | 953.8 | 01 | 073-074 | 962.0 | 21 | 917-918 | 971.0 | 21 | 917-918 | 980.1 | 21 | 917-918 |
| 948.73 | 22 | 933 | 953.9 | 01 | 073-074 | 962.1 | 21 | 917-918 | 971.1 | 21 | 917-918 | 980.2 | 21 | 917-918 |
| 948.74 | 22 | 933 | 954.0 | 01 | 073-074 | 962.2 | 21 | 917-918 | 971.2 | 21 | 917-918 | 980.3 | 21 | 917-918 |
| 948.75 | 22 | 933 | 954.1 | 01 | 073-074 | 962.3 | 21 | 917-918 | 971.3 | 21 | 917-918 | 980.8 | 21 | 917-918 |
| 948.76 | 22 | 933 | 954.8 | 01 | 073-074 | 962.4 | 21 | 917-918 | 971.9 | 21 | 917-918 | 980.9 | 21 | 917-918 |
| 948.77 | 22 | 933 | 954.9 | 01 | 073-074 | 962.5 | 21 | 917-918 | 972.0 | 21 | 917-918 | 981 | 21 | 917-918 |
| 948.80 | 22 | 935 | 955.0 | 01 | 073-074 | 962.6 | 21 | 917-918 | 972.1 | 21 | 917-918 | 982.0 | 21 | 917-918 |
| 948.81 | 22 | 933 | 955.1 | 01 | 073-074 | 962.7 | 21 | 917-918 | 972.2 | 21 | 917-918 | 982.1 | 21 | 917-918 |
| 948.82 | 22 | 933 | 955.2 | 01 | 073-074 | 962.8 | 21 | 917-918 | 972.3 | 21 | 917-918 | 982.2 | 21 | 917-918 |
| 948.83 | 22 | 933 | 955.3 | 01 | 073-074 | 962.9 | 21 | 917-918 | 972.4 | 21 | 917-918 | 982.3 | 21 | 917-918 |
| 948.84 | 22 | 933 | 955.4 | 01 | 073-074 | 963.0 | 21 | 917-918 | 972.5 | 21 | 917-918 | 982.4 | 21 | 917-918 |
| 948.85 | 22 | 933 | 955.5 | 01 | 073-074 | 963.1 | 21 | 917-918 | 972.6 | 21 | 917-918 | 982.8 | 21 | 917-918 |
| 948.86 | 22 | 933 | 955.6 | 01 | 073-074 | 963.2 | 21 | 917-918 | 972.7 | 21 | 917-918 | 983.0 | 21 | 917-918 |
| 948.87 | 22 | 933 | 955.7 | 01 | 073-074 | 963.3 | 21 | 917-918 | 972.8 | 21 | 917-918 | 983.1 | 21 | 917-918 |
| 948.88 | 22 | 933 | 955.8 | 01 | 073-074 | 963.4 | 21 | 917-918 | 972.9 | 21 | 917-918 | 983.2 | 21 | 917-918 |
| 948.90 | 22 | 935 | 955.9 | 01 | 073-074 | 963.5 | 21 | 917-918 | 973.0 | 21 | 917-918 | 983.9 | 21 | 917-918 |
| 948.91 | 22 | 933 | 956.0 | 01 | 073-074 | 963.8 | 21 | 917-918 | 973.1 | 21 | 917-918 | 984.0 | 21 | 917-918 |
| 948.92 | 22 | 933 | 956.1 | 01 | 073-074 | 963.9 | 21 | 917-918 | 973.2 | 21 | 917-918 | 984.1 | 21 | 917-918 |
| 948.93 | 22 | 933 | 956.2 | 01 | 073-074 | 964.0 | 21 | 917-918 | 973.3 | 21 | 917-918 | 984.8 | 21 | 917-918 |
| 948.94 | 22 | 933 | 956.3 | 01 | 073-074 | 964.1 | 21 | 917-918 | 973.4 | 21 | 917-918 | 984.9 | 21 | 917-918 |
| 948.95 | 22 | 933 | 956.4 | 01 | 073-074 | 964.2 | 21 | 917-918 | 973.5 | 21 | 917-918 | 985.0 | 21 | 917-918 |
| 948.96 | 22 | 933 | 956.5 | 01 | 073-074 | 964.3 | 21 | 917-918 | 973.6 | 21 | 917-918 | 985.1 | 21 | 917-918 |
| 948.97 | 22 | 933 | 956.8 | 01 | 073-074 | 964.4 | 21 | 917-918 | 973.8 | 21 | 917-918 | 985.2 | 21 | 917-918 |
| 948.98 | 22 | 933 | 956.9 | 01 | 073-074 | 964.5 | 21 | 917-918 | 973.9 | 21 | 917-918 | 985.3 | 21 | 917-918 |

| DX . . .MDC . .DRG | DX . . .MDC . .DRG | DX . . .MDC . .DRG | DX . . .MDC . .DRG | DX . . .MDC . .DRG |
|---|---|---|---|---|
| 985.4 . . .21 . .917-918 | 995.23 . .21 . .917-918 | 996.72 . .05 . .280-281, 314-315 | V01.0 . . .23 . .951 | V09.1 . . .18 . .867-869 |
| 985.5 . . .21 . .917-918 | 995.27 . .21 . .917-918 | 996.73 . .05 . .314-316 | V01.1 . . .23 . .951 | V09.2 . . .18 . .867-869 |
| 985.6 . . .21 . .917-918 | 995.29 . .21 . .917-918 | 996.74 . .05 . .314-316 | V01.2 . . .23 . .951 | V09.3 . . .18 . .867-869 |
| 985.8 . . .21 . .917-918 | 995.3 . .21 . .915-916 | 996.75 . .01 . .091-093 | V01.3 . . .23 . .951 | V09.4 . . .18 . .867-869 |
| 985.9 . . .21 . .917-918 | 995.4 . .21 . .922-923 | 996.76 . .11 . .698-700 | V01.4 . . .23 . .951 | V09.50 . .18 . .867-869 |
| 986 . . . . .21 . .917-918 | 995.50 . .21 . .922-923 | 996.77 . .08 . .559-561 | V01.5 . . .23 . .951 | V09.51 . .18 . .867-869 |
| 987.0 . . .21 . .917-918 | 995.51 . .21 . .922-923 | 996.78 . .08 . .559-561 | V01.6 . . .23 . .951 | V09.6 . . .18 . .867-869 |
| 987.1 . . .21 . .917-918 | 995.52 . .21 . .922-923 | 996.79 . .21 . .919-921 | V01.71 . .23 . .951 | V09.70 . .18 . .867-869 |
| 987.2 . . .21 . .917-918 | 995.53 . .21 . .922-923 | 996.80 . .21 . .919-921 | V01.79 . .23 . .951 | V09.71 . .18 . .867-869 |
| 987.3 . . .21 . .917-918 | 995.54 . .21 . .922-923 | 996.81 . .11 . .698-700 | V01.81 . .15 . .795 | V09.80 . .18 . .867-869 |
| 987.4 . . .21 . .917-918 | 995.55 . .21 . .922-923 | 996.82 . .07 . .441-443 | V01.81 . .23 . .951 | V09.81 . .18 . .867-869 |
| 987.5 . . .21 . .917-918 | 995.59 . .21 . .922-923 | 996.83 . .05 . .314-316 | V01.83 . .23 . .951 | V09.90 . .18 . .867-869 |
| 987.6 . . .21 . .917-918 | 995.60 . .21 . .915-916 | 996.84 . .04 . .205-206 | V01.84 . .23 . .951 | V09.91 . .18 . .867-869 |
| 987.7 . . .21 . .917-918 | 995.61 . .21 . .915-916 | 996.85 . .16 . .808-810 | V01.89 . .23 . .951 | V10.00 . .17 . .843-845 |
| 987.8 . . .21 . .917-918 | 995.62 . .21 . .915-916 | 996.86 . .07 . .438-440 | V01.9 . . .23 . .951 | V10.01 . .17 . .843-845 |
| 987.9 . . .21 . .917-918 | 995.63 . .21 . .915-916 | 996.87 . .21 . .919-921 | V02.0 . . .23 . .951 | V10.02 . .17 . .843-845 |
| 988.0 . . .21 . .917-918 | 995.64 . .21 . .915-916 | 996.89 . .21 . .919-921 | V02.1 . . .23 . .951 | V10.03 . .17 . .843-845 |
| 988.1 . . .21 . .917-918 | 995.65 . .21 . .915-916 | 996.90 . .08 . .559-561 | V02.2 . . .23 . .951 | V10.04 . .17 . .843-845 |
| 988.2 . . .21 . .917-918 | 995.66 . .21 . .915-916 | 996.91 . .08 . .559-561 | V02.3 . . .23 . .951 | V10.05 . .17 . .843-845 |
| 988.8 . . .21 . .917-918 | 995.67 . .21 . .915-916 | 996.92 . .08 . .559-561 | V02.4 . . .23 . .951 | V10.06 . .17 . .843-845 |
| 988.9 . . .21 . .917-918 | 995.68 . .21 . .915-916 | 996.93 . .08 . .559-561 | V02.51 . .23 . .951 | V10.07 . .17 . .843-845 |
| 989.0 . . .21 . .917-918 | 995.69 . .21 . .915-916 | 996.94 . .08 . .559-561 | V02.52 . .23 . .951 | V10.09 . .17 . .843-845 |
| 989.1 . . .21 . .917-918 | 995.7 . .21 . .922-923 | 996.95 . .08 . .559-561 | V02.59 . .23 . .951 | V10.11 . .17 . .843-845 |
| 989.2 . . .21 . .917-918 | 995.80 . .21 . .922-923 | 996.96 . .08 . .559-561 | V02.60 . .07 . .441-443 | V10.12 . .17 . .843-845 |
| 989.3 . . .21 . .917-918 | 995.81 . .21 . .922-923 | 996.99 . .08 . .559-561 | V02.61 . .07 . .441-443 | V10.20 . .17 . .843-845 |
| 989.4 . . .21 . .917-918 | 995.82 . .21 . .922-923 | 997.00 . .01 . .091-093 | V02.62 . .07 . .441-443 | V10.21 . .17 . .843-845 |
| 989.5 . . .21 . .917-918 | 995.83 . .21 . .922-923 | 997.01 . .01 . .091-093 | V02.69 . .07 . .441-443 | V10.22 . .17 . .843-845 |
| 989.6 . . .21 . .917-918 | 995.84 . .21 . .922-923 | 997.02 . .01 . .091-093 | V02.7 . . .23 . .951 | V10.29 . .17 . .843-845 |
| 989.7 . . .21 . .917-918 | 995.85 . .21 . .922-923 | 997.09 . .01 . .091-093 | V02.8 . . .23 . .951 | V10.3 . . .17 . .843-845 |
| 989.81 . .21 . .917-918 | 995.86 . .21 . .922-923 | 997.1 . . .05 . .314-316 | V02.9 . . .23 . .951 | V10.40 . .17 . .843-845 |
| 989.82 . .21 . .917-918 | 995.89 . .21 . .922-923 | 997.2 . . .05 . .299-301 | V03.0 . . .23 . .951 | V10.41 . .17 . .843-845 |
| 989.83 . .21 . .917-918 | 995.90 . .18 . .870-872 | 997.3 . . .04 . .205-206 | V03.1 . . .23 . .951 | V10.42 . .17 . .843-845 |
| 989.84 . .21 . .917-918 | 995.91 . .18 . .870-872 | 997.4 . . .06 . .393-395 | V03.2 . . .23 . .951 | V10.43 . .17 . .843-845 |
| 989.89 . .21 . .917-918 | 995.92 . .18 . .870-872 | 997.5 . . .11 . .698-700 | V03.3 . . .23 . .951 | V10.44 . .17 . .843-845 |
| 989.9 . . .21 . .917-918 | 995.93 . .18 . .870-872 | 997.60 . .08 . .564-566 | V03.4 . . .23 . .951 | V10.45 . .17 . .843-845 |
| 990 . . . . .21 . .922-923 | 995.94 . .18 . .870-872 | 997.61 . .08 . .564-566 | V03.5 . . .23 . .951 | V10.46 . .17 . .843-845 |
| 991.0 . . .21 . .922-923 | 996.00 . .05 . .314-316 | 997.62 . .08 . .564-566 | V03.6 . . .23 . .951 | V10.47 . .17 . .843-845 |
| 991.1 . . .21 . .922-923 | 996.01 . .05 . .308-310 | 997.69 . .08 . .564-566 | V03.7 . . .23 . .951 | V10.48 . .17 . .843-845 |
| 991.2 . . .21 . .922-923 | 996.02 . .05 . .306-307 | 997.71 . .06 . .393-395 | V03.81 . .23 . .951 | V10.49 . .17 . .843-845 |
| 991.3 . . .21 . .922-923 | 996.03 . .05 . .314-316 | 997.72 . .11 . .698-700 | V03.82 . .23 . .951 | V10.50 . .17 . .843-845 |
| 991.4 . . .21 . .922-923 | 996.04 . .05 . .308-310 | 997.79 . .05 . .299-301 | V03.89 . .23 . .951 | V10.51 . .17 . .843-845 |
| 991.5 . . .21 . .922-923 | 996.09 . .05 . .314-316 | 997.91 . .21 . .919-921 | V03.9 . . .23 . .951 | V10.52 . .17 . .843-845 |
| 991.6 . . .21 . .922-923 | 996.1 . . .05 . .314-316 | 997.99 . .21 . .919-921 | V04.0 . . .23 . .951 | V10.53 . .17 . .843-845 |
| 991.8 . . .21 . .922-923 | 996.2 . . .01 . .091-093 | 998.0 . . .21 . .919-921 | V04.1 . . .23 . .951 | V10.59 . .17 . .843-845 |
| 991.9 . . .21 . .922-923 | 996.30 . .11 . .698-700 | 998.11 . .21 . .919-921 | V04.2 . . .23 . .951 | V10.60 . .17 . .843-845 |
| 992.0 . . .21 . .922-923 | 996.31 . .11 . .698-700 | 998.12 . .21 . .919-921 | V04.3 . . .23 . .951 | V10.61 . .17 . .843-845 |
| 992.1 . . .21 . .922-923 | 996.32 . .13 . .760-761 | 998.13 . .21 . .919-921 | V04.4 . . .23 . .951 | V10.62 . .17 . .843-845 |
| 992.2 . . .21 . .922-923 | 996.39 . .11 . .698-700 | 998.2 . . .21 . .919-921 | V04.5 . . .23 . .951 | V10.63 . .17 . .843-845 |
| 992.3 . . .21 . .922-923 | 996.40 . .08 . .559-561 | 998.31 . .21 . .919-921 | V04.6 . . .23 . .951 | V10.69 . .17 . .843-845 |
| 992.4 . . .21 . .922-923 | 996.41 . .08 . .559-561 | 998.32 . .21 . .919-921 | V04.7 . . .23 . .951 | V10.71 . .17 . .843-845 |
| 992.5 . . .21 . .922-923 | 996.42 . .08 . .559-561 | 998.4 . . .21 . .919-921 | V04.81 . .23 . .951 | V10.72 . .17 . .843-845 |
| 992.6 . . .21 . .922-923 | 996.43 . .08 . .559-561 | 998.51 . .18 . .862-863 | V04.82 . .23 . .951 | V10.79 . .17 . .843-845 |
| 992.7 . . .21 . .922-923 | 996.44 . .08 . .559-561 | 998.59 . .18 . .862-863 | V04.89 . .23 . .951 | V10.81 . .17 . .843-845 |
| 992.8 . . .21 . .922-923 | 996.45 . .08 . .559-561 | 998.6 . . .21 . .919-921 | V05.0 . . .23 . .951 | V10.82 . .17 . .843-845 |
| 992.9 . . .21 . .922-923 | 996.46 . .08 . .559-561 | 998.7 . . .21 . .919-921 | V05.1 . . .23 . .951 | V10.83 . .17 . .843-845 |
| 993.0 . . .03 . .152-153 | 996.47 . .08 . .559-561 | 998.81 . .21 . .919-921 | V05.2 . . .23 . .951 | V10.84 . .17 . .843-845 |
| 993.1 . . .03 . .152-153 | 996.49 . .08 . .559-561 | 998.82 . .02 . .124-125 | V05.3 . . .23 . .951 | V10.85 . .17 . .843-845 |
| 993.2 . . .21 . .922-923 | 996.51 . .02 . .124-125 | 998.83 . .21 . .919-921 | V05.4 . . .23 . .951 | V10.86 . .17 . .843-845 |
| 993.3 . . .21 . .922-923 | 996.52 . .21 . .919-921 | 998.89 . .21 . .919-921 | V05.8 . . .23 . .951 | V10.87 . .17 . .843-845 |
| 993.4 . . .21 . .922-923 | 996.53 . .02 . .124-125 | 998.9 . . .21 . .919-921 | V05.9 . . .23 . .951 | V10.88 . .17 . .843-845 |
| 993.8 . . .21 . .922-923 | 996.54 . .09 . .600-601 | 999.0 . . .18 . .864-866 | V06.0 . . .23 . .951 | V10.89 . .17 . .843-845 |
| 993.9 . . .21 . .922-923 | 996.55 . .21 . .919-921 | 999.1 . . .04 . .175-176 | V06.1 . . .23 . .951 | V10.9 . . .17 . .843-845 |
| 994.0 . . .21 . .922-923 | 996.56 . .21 . .919-921 | 999.2 . . .05 . .314-316 | V06.2 . . .23 . .951 | V11.0 . . .23 . .951 |
| 994.1 . . .21 . .922-923 | 996.57 . .21 . .919-921 | 999.31 . .05 . .314-316 | V06.3 . . .23 . .951 | V11.1 . . .23 . .951 |
| 994.2 . . .21 . .922-923 | 996.59 . .21 . .919-921 | 999.39 . .18 . .867-869 | V06.4 . . .23 . .951 | V11.2 . . .23 . .951 |
| 994.3 . . .21 . .922-923 | 996.60 . .21 . .919-921 | 999.4 . . .21 . .915-916 | V06.5 . . .23 . .951 | V11.3 . . .23 . .951 |
| 994.4 . . .21 . .922-923 | 996.61 . .05 . .314-316 | 999.5 . . .21 . .915-916 | V06.6 . . .23 . .951 | V11.8 . . .23 . .951 |
| 994.5 . . .21 . .922-923 | 996.62 . .05 . .280-281, 314-316 | 999.6 . . .16 . .811-812 | V06.8 . . .23 . .951 | V11.9 . . .23 . .951 |
| 994.6 . . .03 . .149 | 996.63 . .01 . .091-093 | 999.7 . . .16 . .811-812 | V06.9 . . .23 . .951 | V12.00 . .23 . .951 |
| 994.7 . . .21 . .922-923 | 996.64 . .11 . .698-700 | 999.8 . . .16 . .811-812 | V07.0 . . .23 . .951 | V12.01 . .23 . .951 |
| 994.8 . . .21 . .922-923 | 996.65 . .11 . .698-700 | 999.9 . . .21 . .919-920 | V07.1 . . .23 . .951 | V12.02 . .23 . .951 |
| 994.9 . . .21 . .922-923 | 996.66 . .08 . .559-561 | | V07.2 . . .23 . .951 | V12.03 . .23 . .951 |
| 995.0 . . .21 . .915-916 | 996.67 . .08 . .559-561 | **Supplementary Classification of Factors Influencing Health Status and Contact with Health Services** | V07.31 . .23 . .951 | V12.09 . .23 . .951 |
| 995.1 . . .21 . .915-916 | 996.68 . .21 . .919-921 | | V07.39 . .23 . .951 | V12.1 . . .23 . .951 |
| 995.20 . .21 . .917-918 | 996.69 . .21 . .919-921 | | V07.4 . . .23 . .951 | V12.2 . . .23 . .951 |
| 995.21 . .21 . .917-918 | 996.70 . .21 . .919-921 | | V07.8 . . .23 . .951 | V12.3 . . .23 . .951 |
| 995.22 . .21 . .917-918 | 996.71 . .05 . .314-316 | | V09.0 . . .18 . .867-869 | V12.40 . .23 . .951 |

| DX | MDC | DRG |
|---|---|---|
| V12.41 | 23 | 951 |
| V12.42 | 23 | 951 |
| V12.49 | 23 | 951 |
| V12.50 | 23 | 951 |
| V12.51 | 23 | 951 |
| V12.52 | 23 | 951 |
| V12.53 | 23 | 951 |
| V12.54 | 23 | 951 |
| V12.59 | 23 | 951 |
| V12.60 | 23 | 951 |
| V12.61 | 23 | 951 |
| V12.69 | 23 | 951 |
| V12.70 | 23 | 951 |
| V12.71 | 23 | 951 |
| V12.72 | 23 | 951 |
| V12.79 | 23 | 951 |
| V13.00 | 23 | 951 |
| V13.01 | 23 | 951 |
| V13.02 | 23 | 951 |
| V13.03 | 23 | 951 |
| V13.09 | 23 | 951 |
| V13.1 | 23 | 951 |
| V13.21 | 23 | 951 |
| V13.22 | 17 | 843-845 |
| V13.29 | 23 | 951 |
| V13.3 | 23 | 951 |
| V13.4 | 23 | 951 |
| V13.5 | 23 | 951 |
| V13.61 | 23 | 951 |
| V13.69 | 23 | 951 |
| V13.7 | 23 | 951 |
| V13.8 | 23 | 951 |
| V13.9 | 23 | 951 |
| V14.0 | 23 | 951 |
| V14.1 | 23 | 951 |
| V14.2 | 23 | 951 |
| V14.3 | 23 | 951 |
| V14.4 | 23 | 951 |
| V14.5 | 23 | 951 |
| V14.6 | 23 | 951 |
| V14.7 | 23 | 951 |
| V14.8 | 23 | 951 |
| V14.9 | 23 | 951 |
| V15.01 | 23 | 951 |
| V15.02 | 23 | 951 |
| V15.03 | 23 | 951 |
| V15.04 | 23 | 951 |
| V15.05 | 23 | 951 |
| V15.06 | 23 | 951 |
| V15.07 | 23 | 951 |
| V15.08 | 23 | 951 |
| V15.09 | 23 | 951 |
| V15.1 | 23 | 951 |
| V15.2 | 23 | 951 |
| V15.3 | 23 | 951 |
| V15.41 | 23 | 951 |
| V15.42 | 23 | 951 |
| V15.49 | 23 | 951 |
| V15.5 | 23 | 951 |
| V15.6 | 23 | 951 |
| V15.7 | 23 | 951 |
| V15.81 | 23 | 951 |
| V15.82 | 23 | 951 |
| V15.84 | 23 | 951 |
| V15.85 | 23 | 951 |
| V15.86 | 23 | 951 |
| V15.87 | 23 | 951 |
| V15.88 | 23 | 951 |
| V15.89 | 23 | 951 |
| V15.9 | 23 | 951 |
| V16.0 | 23 | 951 |
| V16.1 | 23 | 951 |
| V16.2 | 23 | 951 |
| V16.3 | 23 | 951 |
| V16.40 | 23 | 951 |
| V16.41 | 23 | 951 |
| V16.42 | 23 | 951 |
| V16.43 | 23 | 951 |
| V16.49 | 23 | 951 |
| V16.51 | 23 | 951 |
| V16.52 | 23 | 951 |
| V16.59 | 23 | 951 |
| V16.6 | 23 | 951 |
| V16.7 | 23 | 951 |
| V16.8 | 23 | 951 |
| V16.9 | 23 | 951 |
| V17.0 | 23 | 951 |
| V17.1 | 23 | 951 |
| V17.2 | 23 | 951 |
| V17.3 | 23 | 951 |
| V17.41 | 23 | 951 |
| V17.49 | 23 | 951 |
| V17.5 | 23 | 951 |
| V17.6 | 23 | 951 |
| V17.7 | 23 | 951 |
| V17.81 | 23 | 951 |
| V17.89 | 23 | 951 |
| V18.0 | 23 | 951 |
| V18.11 | 23 | 951 |
| V18.19 | 23 | 951 |
| V18.2 | 23 | 951 |
| V18.3 | 23 | 951 |
| V18.4 | 23 | 951 |
| V18.51 | 23 | 951 |
| V18.59 | 23 | 951 |
| V18.61 | 23 | 951 |
| V18.69 | 23 | 951 |
| V18.7 | 23 | 951 |
| V18.8 | 23 | 951 |
| V18.9 | 23 | 951 |
| V19.0 | 23 | 951 |
| V19.1 | 23 | 951 |
| V19.2 | 23 | 951 |
| V19.3 | 23 | 951 |
| V19.4 | 23 | 951 |
| V19.5 | 23 | 951 |
| V19.6 | 23 | 951 |
| V19.7 | 23 | 951 |
| V19.8 | 23 | 951 |
| V20.0 | 23 | 951 |
| V20.1 | 23 | 951 |
| V20.2 | 23 | 951 |
| V21.0 | 23 | 951 |
| V21.1 | 23 | 951 |
| V21.2 | 23 | 951 |
| V21.30 | 23 | 951 |
| V21.31 | 23 | 951 |
| V21.32 | 23 | 951 |
| V21.33 | 23 | 951 |
| V21.34 | 23 | 951 |
| V21.35 | 23 | 951 |
| V21.8 | 23 | 951 |
| V21.9 | 23 | 951 |
| V22.0 | 23 | 951 |
| V22.1 | 23 | 951 |
| V22.2 | 23 | 951 |
| V23.0 | 14 | 998 |
| V23.1 | 14 | 998 |
| V23.2 | 14 | 998 |
| V23.3 | 14 | 998 |
| V23.41 | 14 | 998 |
| V23.49 | 14 | 998 |
| V23.5 | 14 | 998 |
| V23.7 | 14 | 998 |
| V23.81 | 14 | 998 |
| V23.82 | 14 | 998 |
| V23.83 | 14 | 998 |
| V23.84 | 14 | 998 |
| V23.89 | 14 | 998 |
| V23.9 | 14 | 998 |
| V24.0 | 14 | 776 |
| V24.1 | 23 | 951 |
| V24.2 | 23 | 951 |
| V25.01 | 23 | 951 |
| V25.02 | 23 | 951 |
| V25.03 | 23 | 951 |
| V25.04 | 23 | 951 |
| V25.09 | 23 | 951 |
| V25.1 | 23 | 951 |
| V25.2 | 12 | 729 |
| V25.2 | 13 | 760-761 |
| V25.3 | 13 | 760-761 |
| V25.40 | 23 | 951 |
| V25.41 | 23 | 951 |
| V25.42 | 23 | 951 |
| V25.43 | 23 | 951 |
| V25.49 | 23 | 951 |
| V25.5 | 23 | 951 |
| V25.8 | 23 | 951 |
| V25.9 | 23 | 951 |
| V26.0 | 12 | 729-730 |
| V26.0 | 13 | 760-761 |
| V26.1 | 23 | 951 |
| V26.21 | 23 | 951 |
| V26.22 | 23 | 951 |
| V26.29 | 23 | 951 |
| V26.31 | 23 | 951 |
| V26.32 | 23 | 951 |
| V26.33 | 23 | 951 |
| V26.34 | 23 | 951 |
| V26.35 | 23 | 951 |
| V26.39 | 23 | 951 |
| V26.41 | 23 | 951 |
| V26.49 | 23 | 951 |
| V26.51 | 23 | 951 |
| V26.52 | 23 | 951 |
| V26.81 | 23 | 951 |
| V26.89 | 23 | 951 |
| V26.9 | 23 | 951 |
| V27.0 | 23 | 951 |
| V27.1 | 23 | 951 |
| V27.2 | 23 | 951 |
| V27.3 | 23 | 951 |
| V27.4 | 23 | 951 |
| V27.5 | 23 | 951 |
| V27.6 | 23 | 951 |
| V27.7 | 23 | 951 |
| V27.9 | 23 | 951 |
| V28.0 | 14 | 781-782 |
| V28.1 | 14 | 781-782 |
| V28.2 | 14 | 781-782 |
| V28.3 | 23 | 951 |
| V28.4 | 23 | 951 |
| V28.5 | 23 | 951 |
| V28.6 | 23 | 951 |
| V28.8 | 23 | 951 |
| V28.9 | 23 | 951 |
| V29.0 | 23 | 951 |
| V29.1 | 23 | 951 |
| V29.2 | 23 | 951 |
| V29.3 | 23 | 951 |
| V29.8 | 23 | 951 |
| V29.9 | 23 | 951 |
| V30.00 | 15 | 795 |
| V30.01 | 15 | 795 |
| V30.1 | 15 | 795 |
| V30.2 | 15 | 998 |
| V31.00 | 15 | 795 |
| V31.01 | 15 | 795 |
| V31.1 | 15 | 795 |
| V31.2 | 15 | 998 |
| V32.00 | 15 | 795 |
| V32.01 | 15 | 795 |
| V32.1 | 15 | 795 |
| V32.2 | 15 | 998 |
| V33.00 | 15 | 795 |
| V33.01 | 15 | 795 |
| V33.1 | 15 | 795 |
| V33.2 | 15 | 998 |
| V34.00 | 15 | 795 |
| V34.01 | 15 | 795 |
| V34.1 | 15 | 795 |
| V34.2 | 15 | 998 |
| V35.00 | 15 | 795 |
| V35.01 | 15 | 795 |
| V35.1 | 15 | 795 |
| V35.2 | 15 | 998 |
| V36.00 | 15 | 795 |
| V36.01 | 15 | 795 |
| V36.1 | 15 | 795 |
| V36.2 | 15 | 998 |
| V37.00 | 15 | 795 |
| V37.01 | 15 | 795 |
| V37.1 | 15 | 795 |
| V37.2 | 15 | 998 |
| V39.00 | 15 | 795 |
| V39.01 | 15 | 795 |
| V39.1 | 15 | 795 |
| V39.2 | 15 | 998 |
| V40.0 | 23 | 951 |
| V40.1 | 23 | 951 |
| V40.2 | 23 | 951 |
| V40.3 | 23 | 951 |
| V40.9 | 23 | 951 |
| V41.0 | 23 | 951 |
| V41.1 | 23 | 951 |
| V41.2 | 23 | 951 |
| V41.3 | 23 | 951 |
| V41.4 | 23 | 951 |
| V41.5 | 23 | 951 |
| V41.6 | 23 | 951 |
| V41.7 | 23 | 951 |
| V41.8 | 23 | 951 |
| V41.9 | 23 | 951 |
| V42.0 | 11 | 698-700 |
| V42.1 | 05 | 314-316 |
| V42.2 | 05 | 314-316 |
| V42.3 | 09 | 606-607 |
| V42.4 | 08 | 564-566 |
| V42.5 | 02 | 124-125 |
| V42.6 | 04 | 205-206 |
| V42.7 | 07 | 441-443 |
| V42.81 | 16 | 814-816 |
| V42.82 | 16 | 814-816 |
| V42.83 | 07 | 951 |
| V42.84 | 07 | 951 |
| V42.89 | 23 | 951 |
| V42.9 | 23 | 951 |
| V43.0 | 02 | 124-125 |
| V43.1 | 02 | 124-125 |
| V43.21 | 05 | 314-316 |
| V43.22 | 05 | 314-316 |
| V43.3 | 05 | 314-316 |
| V43.4 | 05 | 314-316 |
| V43.5 | 11 | 698-700 |
| V43.60 | 08 | 564-566 |
| V43.61 | 08 | 564-566 |
| V43.62 | 08 | 564-566 |
| V43.63 | 08 | 564-566 |
| V43.64 | 08 | 564-566 |
| V43.65 | 08 | 564-566 |
| V43.66 | 08 | 564-566 |
| V43.69 | 08 | 564-566 |
| V43.7 | 08 | 564-566 |
| V43.81 | 23 | 951 |
| V43.82 | 23 | 951 |
| V43.83 | 23 | 951 |
| V43.89 | 23 | 951 |
| V44.0 | 23 | 951 |
| V44.1 | 23 | 951 |
| V44.2 | 23 | 951 |
| V44.3 | 23 | 951 |
| V44.4 | 23 | 951 |
| V44.50 | 23 | 951 |
| V44.51 | 23 | 951 |
| V44.52 | 23 | 951 |
| V44.59 | 23 | 951 |
| V44.6 | 23 | 951 |
| V44.7 | 23 | 951 |
| V44.8 | 23 | 951 |
| V44.9 | 23 | 951 |
| V45.00 | 23 | 951 |
| V45.01 | 23 | 951 |
| V45.02 | 23 | 951 |
| V45.09 | 23 | 951 |
| V45.1 | 23 | 951 |
| V45.2 | 23 | 951 |
| V45.3 | 23 | 951 |
| V45.4 | 23 | 951 |
| V45.51 | 23 | 951 |
| V45.52 | 23 | 951 |
| V45.59 | 23 | 951 |
| V45.61 | 23 | 951 |
| V45.69 | 23 | 951 |
| V45.71 | 23 | 951 |
| V45.72 | 23 | 951 |
| V45.73 | 23 | 951 |
| V45.74 | 11 | 698-700 |
| V45.75 | 23 | 951 |
| V45.76 | 04 | 205-206 |
| V45.77 | 12 | 729-730 |
| V45.77 | 13 | 760-761 |
| V45.78 | 02 | 124-125 |
| V45.79 | 23 | 951 |
| V45.81 | 23 | 951 |
| V45.82 | 23 | 951 |
| V45.83 | 23 | 951 |
| V45.84 | 23 | 951 |
| V45.85 | 23 | 951 |
| V45.86 | 23 | 951 |
| V45.89 | 23 | 951 |
| V46.0 | 23 | 951 |
| V46.11 | 23 | 951 |
| V46.12 | 23 | 951 |
| V46.13 | 23 | 951 |
| V46.14 | 23 | 951 |
| V46.2 | 23 | 951 |
| V46.8 | 23 | 951 |
| V46.9 | 23 | 951 |
| V47.0 | 23 | 951 |
| V47.1 | 23 | 951 |
| V47.2 | 23 | 951 |
| V47.3 | 23 | 951 |
| V47.4 | 23 | 951 |
| V47.5 | 23 | 951 |
| V47.9 | 23 | 951 |
| V48.0 | 23 | 951 |
| V48.1 | 23 | 951 |
| V48.2 | 23 | 951 |
| V48.3 | 23 | 951 |
| V48.4 | 23 | 951 |
| V48.5 | 23 | 951 |
| V48.6 | 23 | 951 |
| V48.7 | 23 | 951 |
| V48.8 | 23 | 951 |
| V48.9 | 23 | 951 |
| V49.0 | 23 | 951 |
| V49.1 | 23 | 951 |
| V49.2 | 23 | 951 |
| V49.3 | 23 | 951 |
| V49.4 | 23 | 951 |
| V49.5 | 23 | 951 |
| V49.60 | 23 | 951 |
| V49.61 | 23 | 951 |
| V49.62 | 23 | 951 |
| V49.63 | 23 | 951 |
| V49.64 | 23 | 951 |
| V49.65 | 23 | 951 |
| V49.66 | 23 | 951 |
| V49.67 | 23 | 951 |
| V49.70 | 23 | 951 |
| V49.71 | 23 | 951 |
| V49.72 | 23 | 951 |
| V49.73 | 23 | 951 |
| V49.74 | 23 | 951 |

| DX | MDC | DRG | DX | MDC | DRG | DX | MDC | DRG | DX | MDC | DRG | DX | MDC | DRG |
|---|---|---|---|---|---|---|---|---|---|---|---|---|---|---|
| V49.75 | 23 | 951 | V55.9 | 23 | 951 | V61.10 | 23 | 951 | V67.09 | 23 | 949-950 | V73.81 | 23 | 951 |
| V49.76 | 23 | 951 | V56.0 | 11 | 685 | V61.11 | 23 | 951 | V67.1 | 17 | 849 | V73.88 | 23 | 951 |
| V49.77 | 23 | 951 | V56.1 | 11 | 685 | V61.12 | 23 | 951 | V67.2 | 17 | 837-839, 846-848 | V73.89 | 23 | 951 |
| V49.81 | 23 | 951 | V56.2 | 11 | 685 | V61.20 | 23 | 951 | V67.3 | 23 | 951 | V73.98 | 23 | 951 |
| V49.82 | 23 | 951 | V56.31 | 11 | 685 | V61.21 | 23 | 951 | V67.4 | 23 | 949-950 | V73.99 | 23 | 951 |
| V49.83 | 23 | 951 | V56.32 | 11 | 685 | V61.22 | 23 | 951 | V67.51 | 23 | 951 | V74.0 | 23 | 951 |
| V49.84 | 23 | 951 | V56.8 | 11 | 685 | V61.29 | 23 | 951 | V67.59 | 23 | 951 | V74.1 | 23 | 951 |
| V49.85 | 23 | 951 | V57.0 | 23 | 951 | V61.3 | 23 | 951 | V67.6 | 23 | 951 | V74.2 | 23 | 951 |
| V49.89 | 23 | 951 | V57.1 | 23 | 945-946 | V61.41 | 23 | 951 | V67.9 | 23 | 951 | V74.3 | 23 | 951 |
| V49.9 | 23 | 951 | V57.21 | 23 | 945-946 | V61.49 | 23 | 951 | V68.01 | 23 | 951 | V74.4 | 23 | 951 |
| V50.0 | 09 | 606-607 | V57.22 | 23 | 945-946 | V61.5 | 13 | 760-761 | V68.09 | 23 | 951 | V74.5 | 23 | 951 |
| V50.1 | 09 | 606-607 | V57.3 | 23 | 945-946 | V61.6 | 14 | 781-782 | V68.1 | 23 | 951 | V74.6 | 23 | 951 |
| V50.2 | 12 | 727-728 | V57.4 | 23 | 951 | V61.7 | 14 | 779 | V68.2 | 23 | 951 | V74.8 | 23 | 951 |
| V50.3 | 23 | 951 | V57.81 | 23 | 951 | V61.8 | 23 | 951 | V68.81 | 23 | 951 | V74.9 | 23 | 951 |
| V50.41 | 9 | 600-601 | V57.89 | 23 | 945-946 | V61.9 | 23 | 951 | V68.89 | 23 | 951 | V75.0 | 23 | 951 |
| V50.42 | 13 | 760-761 | V57.9 | 23 | 945-946 | V62.0 | 23 | 951 | V68.9 | 23 | 951 | V75.1 | 23 | 951 |
| V50.49 | 23 | 951 | V58.0 | 17 | 849 | V62.1 | 23 | 951 | V69.0 | 23 | 951 | V75.2 | 23 | 951 |
| V50.8 | 23 | 951 | V58.11 | 17 | 837-839, 846-848 | V62.2 | 23 | 951 | V69.1 | 23 | 951 | V75.3 | 23 | 951 |
| V50.9 | 23 | 951 | V58.12 | 17 | 837-839, 846-848 | V62.3 | 23 | 951 | V69.2 | 23 | 951 | V75.4 | 23 | 951 |
| V51 | 09 | 606-607 | V58.2 | 23 | 951 | V62.4 | 23 | 951 | V69.3 | 23 | 951 | V75.5 | 23 | 951 |
| V52.0 | 08 | 559-561 | V58.30 | 23 | 951 | V62.5 | 23 | 951 | V69.4 | 23 | 951 | V75.6 | 23 | 951 |
| V52.1 | 08 | 559-561 | V58.31 | 23 | 951 | V62.6 | 23 | 951 | V69.5 | 23 | 951 | V75.7 | 23 | 951 |
| V52.2 | 23 | 951 | V58.32 | 23 | 951 | V62.81 | 23 | 951 | V69.8 | 23 | 951 | V75.8 | 23 | 951 |
| V52.3 | 23 | 951 | V58.41 | 23 | 949-950 | V62.82 | 23 | 951 | V69.9 | 23 | 951 | V75.9 | 23 | 951 |
| V52.4 | 23 | 951 | V58.42 | 23 | 949-950 | V62.83 | 23 | 951 | V70.0 | 23 | 951 | V76.0 | 23 | 951 |
| V52.8 | 23 | 945-946 | V58.43 | 23 | 949-950 | V62.84 | 19 | 880 | V70.1 | 23 | 951 | V76.10 | 23 | 951 |
| V52.9 | 23 | 945-946 | V58.44 | 23 | 949-950 | V62.89 | 23 | 951 | V70.2 | 23 | 951 | V76.11 | 23 | 951 |
| V53.01 | 01 | 091-093 | V58.49 | 23 | 949-950 | V62.9 | 23 | 951 | V70.3 | 23 | 951 | V76.12 | 23 | 951 |
| V53.02 | 01 | 091-093 | V58.5 | 23 | 949-950 | V63.0 | 23 | 951 | V70.4 | 23 | 951 | V76.19 | 23 | 951 |
| V53.09 | 01 | 091-093 | V58.61 | 23 | 949-950 | V63.1 | 23 | 951 | V70.5 | 23 | 951 | V76.2 | 23 | 951 |
| V53.1 | 23 | 951 | V58.62 | 23 | 949-950 | V63.2 | 23 | 951 | V70.6 | 23 | 951 | V76.3 | 23 | 951 |
| V53.2 | 23 | 951 | V58.63 | 23 | 949-950 | V63.8 | 23 | 951 | V70.7 | 23 | 951 | V76.41 | 23 | 951 |
| V53.31 | 05 | 314-316 | V58.64 | 23 | 949-950 | V63.9 | 23 | 951 | V70.8 | 23 | 951 | V76.42 | 23 | 951 |
| V53.32 | 05 | 314-316 | V58.65 | 23 | 949-950 | V64.00 | 23 | 951 | V70.9 | 23 | 951 | V76.43 | 23 | 951 |
| V53.39 | 05 | 314-316 | V58.66 | 23 | 949-950 | V64.01 | 23 | 951 | V71.01 | 19 | 880 | V76.44 | 23 | 951 |
| V53.4 | 23 | 951 | V58.67 | 23 | 949-950 | V64.02 | 23 | 951 | V71.02 | 19 | 880 | V76.45 | 23 | 951 |
| V53.5 | 06 | 393-395 | V58.69 | 23 | 949-950 | V64.03 | 23 | 951 | V71.09 | 19 | 887 | V76.46 | 23 | 951 |
| V53.6 | 11 | 698-700 | V58.71 | 23 | 949-950 | V64.04 | 23 | 951 | V71.1 | 17 | 843-845 | V76.47 | 23 | 951 |
| V53.7 | 08 | 559-561 | V58.72 | 23 | 949-950 | V64.05 | 23 | 951 | V71.2 | 04 | 177-179 | V76.49 | 23 | 951 |
| V53.8 | 23 | 951 | V58.73 | 23 | 949-950 | V64.06 | 23 | 951 | V71.3 | 21 | 922-923 | V76.50 | 23 | 951 |
| V53.90 | 23 | 951 | V58.74 | 23 | 949-950 | V64.07 | 23 | 951 | V71.4 | 21 | 922-923 | V76.51 | 23 | 951 |
| V53.91 | 23 | 951 | V58.75 | 23 | 949-950 | V64.08 | 23 | 951 | V71.5 | 23 | 951 | V76.52 | 23 | 951 |
| V53.99 | 23 | 951 | V58.76 | 23 | 949-950 | V64.09 | 23 | 951 | V71.6 | 21 | 922-923 | V76.81 | 23 | 951 |
| V54.01 | 08 | 559-561 | V58.77 | 23 | 949-950 | V64.1 | 23 | 951 | V71.7 | 05 | 313 | V76.89 | 23 | 951 |
| V54.02 | 08 | 559-561 | V58.78 | 23 | 949-950 | V64.2 | 23 | 951 | V71.81 | 23 | 951 | V76.9 | 23 | 951 |
| V54.09 | 08 | 559-561 | V58.81 | 23 | 949-950 | V64.3 | 23 | 951 | V71.82 | 23 | 951 | V77.0 | 23 | 951 |
| V54.10 | 08 | 559-561 | V58.83 | 23 | 949-950 | V64.41 | 23 | 951 | V71.83 | 23 | 951 | V77.1 | 23 | 951 |
| V54.11 | 08 | 559-561 | V58.82 | 23 | 949-950 | V64.42 | 23 | 951 | V71.89 | 23 | 951 | V77.2 | 23 | 951 |
| V54.12 | 08 | 559-561 | V58.89 | 23 | 949-950 | V64.43 | 23 | 951 | V71.9 | 23 | 951 | V77.3 | 23 | 951 |
| V54.13 | 08 | 559-561 | V58.9 | 23 | 949-950 | V65.0 | 23 | 951 | V72.0 | 23 | 951 | V77.4 | 23 | 951 |
| V54.14 | 08 | 559-561 | V59.01 | 23 | 951 | V65.11 | 23 | 951 | V72.11 | 23 | 951 | V77.5 | 23 | 951 |
| V54.15 | 08 | 559-561 | V59.02 | 23 | 951 | V65.19 | 23 | 951 | V72.12 | 23 | 951 | V77.6 | 23 | 951 |
| V54.16 | 08 | 559-561 | V59.09 | 23 | 951 | V65.2 | 23 | 951 | V72.19 | 23 | 951 | V77.7 | 23 | 951 |
| V54.17 | 08 | 559-561 | V59.1 | 09 | 606-607 | V65.3 | 23 | 951 | V72.2 | 23 | 951 | V77.8 | 23 | 951 |
| V54.19 | 08 | 559-561 | V59.2 | 08 | 564-566 | V65.40 | 23 | 951 | V72.31 | 23 | 951 | V77.91 | 23 | 951 |
| V54.20 | 08 | 559-561 | V59.3 | 23 | 951 | V65.41 | 23 | 951 | V72.32 | 23 | 951 | V77.99 | 23 | 951 |
| V54.21 | 08 | 559-561 | V59.4 | 11 | 698-700 | V65.42 | 23 | 951 | V72.40 | 23 | 951 | V78.0 | 23 | 951 |
| V54.22 | 08 | 559-561 | V59.5 | 23 | 951 | V65.43 | 23 | 951 | V72.41 | 23 | 951 | V78.1 | 23 | 951 |
| V54.23 | 08 | 559-561 | V59.6 | 23 | 951 | V65.44 | 23 | 951 | V72.42 | 23 | 951 | V78.2 | 23 | 951 |
| V54.24 | 08 | 559-561 | V59.70 | 23 | 951 | V65.45 | 23 | 951 | V72.5 | 23 | 951 | V78.3 | 23 | 951 |
| V54.25 | 08 | 559-561 | V59.71 | 23 | 951 | V65.46 | 23 | 951 | V72.6 | 23 | 951 | V78.8 | 23 | 951 |
| V54.26 | 08 | 559-561 | V59.72 | 23 | 951 | V65.49 | 23 | 951 | V72.7 | 23 | 951 | V78.9 | 23 | 951 |
| V54.27 | 08 | 559-561 | V59.73 | 23 | 951 | V65.5 | 23 | 951 | V72.81 | 23 | 951 | V79.0 | 23 | 951 |
| V54.29 | 08 | 559-561 | V59.74 | 23 | 951 | V65.8 | 23 | 951 | V72.82 | 23 | 951 | V79.1 | 23 | 951 |
| V54.81 | 08 | 559-561 | V59.8 | 23 | 951 | V65.9 | 23 | 951 | V72.83 | 23 | 951 | V79.2 | 23 | 951 |
| V54.89 | 08 | 559-561 | V59.9 | 23 | 951 | V66.0 | 23 | 951 | V72.84 | 23 | 951 | V79.3 | 23 | 951 |
| V54.9 | 08 | 559-561 | V60.0 | 23 | 951 | V66.1 | 23 | 951 | V72.85 | 23 | 951 | V79.8 | 23 | 951 |
| V55.0 | 04 | 205-206 | V60.1 | 23 | 951 | V66.2 | 23 | 951 | V72.86 | 23 | 951 | V79.9 | 23 | 951 |
| V55.1 | 06 | 393-395 | V60.2 | 23 | 951 | V66.3 | 23 | 951 | V72.9 | 23 | 951 | V80.0 | 23 | 951 |
| V55.2 | 06 | 393-395 | V60.3 | 23 | 951 | V66.4 | 23 | 951 | V73.0 | 23 | 951 | V80.1 | 23 | 951 |
| V55.3 | 06 | 393-395 | V60.4 | 23 | 951 | V66.5 | 23 | 951 | V73.1 | 23 | 951 | V80.2 | 23 | 951 |
| V55.4 | 06 | 393-395 | V60.5 | 23 | 951 | V66.6 | 23 | 951 | V73.2 | 23 | 951 | V80.3 | 23 | 951 |
| V55.5 | 11 | 698-700 | V60.6 | 23 | 951 | V66.7 | 23 | 951 | V73.3 | 23 | 951 | V81.0 | 23 | 951 |
| V55.6 | 11 | 698-700 | V60.8 | 23 | 951 | V66.9 | 23 | 951 | V73.4 | 23 | 951 | V81.1 | 23 | 951 |
| V55.7 | 13 | 760-761 | V60.9 | 23 | 951 | V67.00 | 23 | 949-950 | V73.5 | 23 | 951 | V81.2 | 23 | 951 |
| V55.8 | 23 | 951 | V61.0 | 23 | 951 | V67.01 | 23 | 949-950 | V73.6 | 23 | 951 | V81.3 | 23 | 951 |

| DX | MDC | DRG |
|---|---|---|
| V81.4 | 23 | 951 |
| V81.5 | 23 | 951 |
| V81.6 | 23 | 951 |
| V82.0 | 23 | 951 |
| V82.1 | 23 | 951 |
| V82.2 | 23 | 951 |
| V82.3 | 23 | 951 |
| V82.4 | 23 | 951 |
| V82.5 | 23 | 951 |
| V82.6 | 23 | 951 |
| V82.71 | 23 | 951 |

| DX | MDC | DRG |
|---|---|---|
| V82.79 | 23 | 951 |
| V82.81 | 23 | 951 |
| V82.89 | 23 | 951 |
| V82.9 | 23 | 951 |
| V83.01 | 23 | 951 |
| V83.02 | 23 | 951 |
| V83.81 | 23 | 951 |
| V83.89 | 23 | 951 |
| V84.01 | 23 | 951 |
| V84.02 | 23 | 951 |
| V84.03 | 23 | 951 |

| DX | MDC | DRG |
|---|---|---|
| V84.04 | 23 | 951 |
| V84.09 | 23 | 951 |
| V84.81 | 23 | 951 |
| V84.89 | 23 | 951 |
| V85.0 | 23 | 951 |
| V85.1 | 23 | 951 |
| V85.21 | 23 | 951 |
| V85.22 | 23 | 951 |
| V85.23 | 23 | 951 |
| V85.24 | 23 | 951 |
| V85.25 | 23 | 951 |

| DX | MDC | DRG |
|---|---|---|
| V85.30 | 23 | 951 |
| V85.31 | 23 | 951 |
| V85.32 | 23 | 951 |
| V85.33 | 23 | 951 |
| V85.34 | 23 | 951 |
| V85.35 | 23 | 951 |
| V85.36 | 23 | 951 |
| V85.37 | 23 | 951 |
| V85.38 | 23 | 951 |
| V85.39 | 23 | 951 |
| V85.4 | 10 | 640-641 |

| DX | MDC | DRG |
|---|---|---|
| V85.51 | 23 | 951 |
| V85.52 | 23 | 951 |
| V85.53 | 23 | 951 |
| V85.54 | 23 | 951 |
| V86.0 | 23 | 951 |
| V86.1 | 23 | 951 |

# Major Complication & Comorbidity (MCC) Code List

The following is the standards list of conditions considered to be major complications and comorbidities that when present as a secondary diagnosis may affect DRG assignment under the Medicare Severity DRG (MS-DRG) system version 25.0. An asterisk (*) indicates that a code range is represented.

| | | | | | | | |
|---|---|---|---|---|---|---|---|
| 003.1 | 094.2 | *323.6 | 452 | 534.31 | 634.61 | 671.44 | 767.0 |
| 003.21 | 094.81 | *323.7 | 453.0 | *534.4 | 634.62 | 673.01 | 768.5 |
| 003.22 | 094.87 | *323.8 | 453.2 | *534.5 | 635.30 | 673.02 | 768.7 |
| 006.3 | 098.82 | 323.9 | 456.0 | *534.6 | 635.31 | 673.03 | 769 |
| 006.4 | 098.83 | *324 | 456.20 | 534.71 | 635.32 | 673.04 | 770.0 |
| 006.5 | 098.84 | 325 | 464.01 | 534.91 | *635.5 | 673.11 | 770.12 |
| *011.6 | 100.81 | 331.81 | 464.11 | 535.01 | *635.6 | 673.12 | 770.14 |
| *013.0 | 112.4 | 333.92 | 464.21 | 535.11 | *636.3 | 673.13 | 770.16 |
| *013.1 | 112.5 | 336.1 | 464.31 | 535.21 | *636.5 | 673.14 | 770.18 |
| *013.2 | 112.81 | 343.2 | 464.51 | 535.31 | *636.6 | 673.21 | 770.2 |
| *013.3 | 112.83 | *344.0 | *480 | 535.41 | *637.3 | 673.22 | 770.3 |
| *013.4 | 114.2 | 344.81 | 481 | 535.51 | *637.5 | 673.23 | 770.7 |
| *013.5 | 115.01 | 345.2 | *482 | 535.61 | *637.6 | 673.24 | 770.84 |
| *013.6 | 115.03 | 345.3 | *483 | 537.83 | 638.3 | 673.31 | 770.86 |
| *013.8 | 115.04 | 345.71 | *484 | 537.84 | 638.5 | 673.32 | 770.87 |
| *013.9 | 115.05 | *348.3 | 485 | 540.0 | 638.6 | 673.33 | 771.1 |
| *014.0 | 115.11 | 348.4 | 486 | 540.1 | 639.3 | 673.34 | 771.2 |
| *018.0 | 115.13 | 348.5 | 487.0 | *550.0 | 639.5 | 673.81 | 771.3 |
| *018.8 | 115.14 | 349.82 | 506.1 | *551.0 | 639.6 | 673.82 | 771.81 |
| *018.9 | 115.15 | 358.01 | *507 | 551.1 | 641.11 | 673.83 | 772.13 |
| *020 | 115.91 | 410.01 | *510 | *551.2 | 641.13 | 673.84 | 772.14 |
| 022.1 | 115.93 | 410.11 | 511.1 | 551.3 | 641.21 | 674.01 | 772.2 |
| 022.3 | 115.94 | 410.21 | 511.8 | 551.8 | 641.31 | 674.50 | 772.4 |
| *036 | 115.95 | 410.31 | 512.0 | 551.9 | 641.33 | 674.51 | 773.3 |
| 037 | 117.7 | 410.41 | 513.0 | 557.0 | 642.11 | 674.52 | 773.4 |
| 038.0 | 130.0 | 410.51 | 513.1 | 560.2 | 642.12 | 674.53 | 774.4 |
| *038.1 | 130.3 | 410.61 | 518.4 | 562.02 | 642.42 | 674.54 | 774.7 |
| 038.2 | 130.4 | 410.71 | 518.5 | 562.03 | 642.51 | 707.02 | 775.7 |
| 038.3 | 130.8 | 410.81 | 518.81 | 562.12 | 642.52 | 707.03 | 776.1 |
| *038.4 | 136.2 | 410.91 | 518.84 | 562.13 | 642.53 | 707.04 | 776.2 |
| 038.8 | 136.3 | 414.12 | 519.2 | 567.0 | 642.54 | 707.05 | 776.7 |
| 038.9 | 242.01 | *415 | 530.21 | 567.1 | 642.61 | 707.06 | 777.5 |
| 040.0 | 242.11 | 421.0 | 530.4 | *567.2 | 642.62 | 707.07 | 777.6 |
| 040.82 | 242.21 | 421.1 | 530.7 | *567.3 | 642.63 | 728.86 | 778.0 |
| 042 | 242.31 | 421.9 | 530.82 | 567.81 | 642.64 | 740.0 | 779.0 |
| *045.0 | 242.41 | 422.0 | 530.84 | 567.89 | 642.71 | 740.1 | 779.2 |
| *045.1 | 242.81 | *422.9 | *531.0 | 567.9 | 642.72 | 740.2 | 779.7 |
| 052.0 | 242.91 | *427.4 | *531.1 | 568.81 | 642.73 | 742.2 | 779.85 |
| 052.1 | *250.1 | 427.5 | *531.2 | 569.83 | 642.74 | 745.0 | 780.01 |
| 052.2 | *250.2 | 428.21 | 531.21 | 569.85 | 644.03 | 745.10 | 785.51 |
| 053.0 | *250.3 | 428.23 | 531.31 | 569.86 | 644.21 | 745.11 | 785.52 |
| 053.14 | 260 | 428.31 | *531.4 | 570 | 648.01 | 745.19 | 785.59 |
| 054.3 | 261 | 428.33 | *531.5 | 572.0 | 648.02 | 745.2 | 799.1 |
| 054.5 | 262 | 428.41 | *531.6 | 572.1 | 654.51 | 745.3 | 800.03 |
| 054.72 | 277.01 | 428.43 | 531.71 | 572.2 | 654.52 | 745.7 | 800.04 |
| 054.74 | 277.02 | 429.5 | 531.91 | 572.4 | 654.53 | 746.01 | 800.05 |
| 055.0 | 282.42 | 429.6 | *532.0 | 573.4 | 654.54 | 746.1 | *800.1 |
| 055.1 | 282.62 | 430 | *532.1 | 574.81 | 658.41 | 746.2 | *800.2 |
| 056.01 | 282.64 | 431 | *532.2 | 575.4 | 658.43 | 746.7 | *800.3 |
| 058.21 | 282.69 | 432.0 | 532.31 | 576.2 | 659.31 | 746.81 | 800.43 |
| 058.29 | 283.11 | 432.1 | *532.4 | 576.3 | 659.33 | 746.82 | 800.44 |
| *062 | *284.8 | 433.01 | *532.5 | 577.0 | 665.01 | 746.84 | 800.45 |
| *063 | 286.0 | 433.11 | *532.6 | 580.0 | 665.03 | 746.86 | *800.5 |
| 064 | 286.1 | 433.21 | 532.71 | 580.4 | 665.11 | 747.11 | *800.6 |
| *066.4 | 286.6 | 433.31 | 532.91 | 580.81 | 669.11 | 747.3 | *800.7 |
| 070.0 | *320 | 433.81 | *533.0 | 580.89 | 669.12 | 747.81 | *800.8 |
| *070.2 | *320.8 | 433.91 | *533.1 | 580.9 | 669.13 | 747.83 | *800.9 |
| *070.4 | 320.9 | 434.01 | *533.2 | 583.4 | 669.14 | 748.5 | 801.03 |
| 070.6 | *321 | 434.11 | 533.31 | 583.6 | 669.21 | 750.3 | 801.04 |
| 070.71 | 322.0 | 434.91 | 533.71 | *584 | 669.22 | 751.61 | 801.05 |
| 072.1 | 322.1 | *441.0 | *533.4 | 585.6 | 669.32 | 755.55 | *801.1 |
| 072.2 | 322.9 | 441.1 | *533.5 | 590.11 | 669.34 | 756.6 | *801.2 |
| 073.0 | *323.0 | 441.3 | *533.6 | 590.2 | 670.02 | 756.70 | *801.3 |
| 084.0 | 323.1 | 441.5 | 533.71 | 596.6 | 670.04 | 756.71 | 801.43 |
| 090.41 | 323.2 | 441.6 | 533.91 | 614.5 | 671.31 | 756.79 | 801.44 |
| 090.42 | *323.4 | *443.2 | *534.0 | *634.3 | 671.33 | 758.32 | 801.45 |
| 091.81 | *323.5 | 446.6 | *534.1 | *634.5 | 671.42 | 759.4 | *801.5 |

| | | | | | | | |
|---|---|---|---|---|---|---|---|
| *801.6 | *804.6 | 808.9 | *851.2 | 862.22 | 896.3 | 948.33 | 948.88 |
| *801.7 | *804.7 | 809.1 | *851.3 | *862.3 | 897.6 | 948.41 | 948.91 |
| *801.8 | *804.8 | *812.1 | 851.45 | 862.9 | 897.7 | 948.42 | 948.92 |
| *801.9 | 804.93 | *812.3 | *851.5 | 863.1 | 901.0 | 948.43 | 948.93 |
| 803.03 | 804.94 | *812.5 | *851.6 | *863.3 | 901.1 | 948.44 | 948.94 |
| 803.04 | 804.95 | *813.1 | *851.7 | *863.5 | 901.2 | 948.51 | 948.95 |
| 803.05 | *805.1 | *813.3 | *851.8 | *863.9 | 901.3 | 948.52 | 948.96 |
| *803.1 | 805.3 | *813.5 | *851.9 | 864.03 | *901.4 | 948.53 | 948.97 |
| *803.2 | 805.5 | *813.9 | *852.0 | 864.04 | 901.83 | 948.54 | 948.98 |
| *803.3 | 805.7 | *820 | *852.1 | *864.1 | 902.0 | 948.55 | 948.99 |
| 803.43 | 805.9 | *821.0 | *852.2 | 865.03 | *902.1 | 948.61 | *952.0 |
| 803.44 | *806.0 | *821.1 | *852.3 | 865.04 | *902.2 | 948.62 | *952.1 |
| 803.45 | *806.1 | *821.3 | *852.4 | *865.1 | *902.3 | 948.63 | 952.2 |
| *803.5 | *806.2 | *823.1 | *852.5 | 866.03 | *902.4 | 948.64 | 952.3 |
| *803.6 | *806.3 | *823.3 | *853.0 | 866.10 | 902.50 | 948.65 | 952.4 |
| *803.7 | 806.4 | *823.9 | *853.1 | 866.11 | 902.51 | 948.66 | 952.8 |
| *803.8 | 806.5 | 828.0 | 854.05 | 866.12 | 902.52 | 948.71 | 958.0 |
| *803.9 | *806.6 | 828.1 | *854.1 | 866.13 | 902.53 | 948.72 | 958.1 |
| 804.03 | *806.7 | 835.10 | 860.1 | 867.1 | 902.54 | 948.73 | 958.4 |
| 804.04 | 806.8 | 835.11 | 860.2 | 867.3 | 902.59 | 948.74 | 958.5 |
| 804.05 | 806.9 | 835.12 | 860.3 | 867.5 | 902.87 | 948.75 | 995.91 |
| *804.1 | *807.1 | 835.13 | 860.4 | 867.7 | *903.0 | 948.76 | 995.92 |
| *804.2 | 807.3 | *839.1 | 860.5 | 867.9 | 904.0 | 948.77 | 995.94 |
| *804.3 | 807.4 | *839.3 | 861.02 | *868.1 | 904.1 | 948.81 | 999.1 |
| 804.43 | 807.5 | 839.50 | 861.03 | 869.1 | 904.2 | 948.82 | |
| 804.44 | 807.6 | 839.59 | *861.1 | *874.0 | *904.4 | 948.83 | |
| 804.45 | 808.0 | 839.71 | 861.22 | *874.1 | 948.21 | 948.84 | |
| 804.53 | 808.1 | 850.4 | *861.3 | 887.6 | 948.22 | 948.85 | |
| 804.54 | 808.3 | 851.05 | 862.1 | 887.7 | 948.31 | 948.86 | |
| 804.55 | *808.5 | *851.1 | 862.21 | 896.2 | 948.32 | 948.87 | |

# Complication & Comorbidity (CC) Code List

The following is the standards list of conditions considered to be complications and comorbidities that when present as a secondary diagnosis may affect DRG assignment under the Medicare Severity DRG (MS-DRG) system version 25.0. An astersisk (*) indicates that a code range is represented.

| | | | | | | | | |
|---|---|---|---|---|---|---|---|---|
| *001 | *016.6 | *055.7 | 091.7 | 117.9 | *201.7 | 271.0 | 292.82 | |
| *002 | *016.7 | 056.00 | 091.82 | 118 | *201.9 | 271.1 | 293.0 | |
| 003.0 | *016.9 | 056.09 | 091.89 | *120 | *202.0 | 271.8 | 293.1 | |
| 003.23 | *017.0 | *056.7 | 091.9 | 121.0 | *202.1 | 274.11 | 293.81 | |
| 003.24 | *017.2 | 057.0 | 093.0 | 121.1 | *202.2 | 276.0 | 293.82 | |
| 003.29 | *017.3 | *060 | 093.1 | 121.2 | *202.3 | 276.1 | 293.9 | |
| 003.8 | *017.4 | 061 | 093.20 | 121.3 | *202.4 | 276.2 | 294.11 | |
| 003.9 | *017.5 | *065 | 093.21 | 121.4 | *202.5 | 276.3 | 295.00 | |
| 004.0 | *017.6 | 066.0 | 093.22 | 121.5 | *202.6 | 276.4 | 295.01 | |
| 005.0 | *017.7 | 066.1 | 093.23 | 121.6 | *202.7 | 277.00 | 295.02 | |
| 005.1 | *017.8 | 066.2 | 093.24 | 121.8 | *202.8 | 277.03 | 295.03 | |
| 005.2 | *017.9 | 066.3 | *093.8 | *122 | *202.9 | 277.09 | 295.04 | |
| 005.3 | *021 | 066.8 | 093.9 | 123.0 | *203.0 | 277.1 | 295.10 | |
| 005.4 | 022.0 | 066.9 | 094.0 | 123.1 | *203.1 | 277.2 | 295.11 | |
| 005.81 | 022.2 | 070.1 | 094.1 | 123.2 | *203.8 | *277.3 | 295.12 | |
| 005.89 | 022.8 | 070.30 | 094.3 | 123.3 | *204.0 | 277.5 | 295.13 | |
| 006.0 | 022.9 | 070.31 | 094.82 | 123.4 | *204.1 | 277.85 | 295.14 | |
| 006.1 | 023.8 | 070.32 | 094.83 | 123.5 | *204.2 | 277.86 | 295.20 | |
| 006.2 | 023.9 | 070.33 | 094.84 | 123.6 | *204.8 | 277.87 | 295.21 | |
| 006.8 | 024 | 070.51 | 094.85 | 123.8 | *204.9 | 277.89 | 295.22 | |
| 007.1 | 025 | 070.52 | 094.86 | 124 | *205.0 | *279.0 | 295.23 | |
| 007.2 | *026 | 070.53 | 094.89 | *125 | *205.1 | *279.1 | 295.24 | |
| 007.4 | 027.0 | 070.59 | 094.9 | *126 | *205.2 | 279.2 | 295.30 | |
| 007.5 | 027.2 | 070.9 | 095.0 | *127 | *205.3 | 279.3 | 295.31 | |
| 007.8 | 027.8 | 071 | 095.1 | 130.1 | *205.8 | 282.8 | 295.32 | |
| 007.9 | 027.9 | 072.0 | 095.2 | 130.2 | *205.9 | 282.9 | 295.33 | |
| *008.0 | *030 | 072.3 | 095.3 | 130.5 | *206.0 | 283.0 | 295.34 | |
| 008.1 | *031 | *072.7 | 095.4 | 130.7 | *206.1 | 283.10 | 295.40 | |
| 008.2 | *032 | 072.8 | 095.5 | 130.9 | *206.2 | 283.19 | 295.41 | |
| 008.3 | *033 | 073.7 | 095.6 | 136.4 | *206.8 | 283.9 | 295.42 | |
| *008.4 | 034.1 | 073.8 | 095.7 | 136.5 | *206.9 | *284.0 | 295.43 | |
| 008.5 | *036.8 | 073.9 | 095.8 | *150 | *207.0 | 284.1 | 295.44 | |
| *008.6 | 036.9 | *074.2 | 095.9 | *151 | *207.1 | 284.2 | 295.53 | |
| 009.0 | *039 | 078.3 | 098.0 | *152 | *207.2 | 284.9 | 295.54 | |
| 009.1 | 040.2 | 078.5 | *098.1 | *153 | *207.8 | 285.1 | 295.60 | |
| 009.2 | 040.3 | 078.6 | *098.4 | *154 | *208.0 | 286.2 | 295.61 | |
| 009.3 | 040.41 | 078.7 | *098.5 | *155 | *208.1 | 286.3 | 295.62 | |
| *010.0 | 040.42 | 079.51 | 098.81 | *156 | *208.2 | 286.4 | 295.63 | |
| *010.1 | 040.81 | 079.52 | 098.85 | *157 | *208.8 | 286.5 | 295.64 | |
| *010.8 | 046.0 | 079.53 | 098.86 | *158 | *208.9 | 286.7 | 295.71 | |
| *010.9 | 046.1 | *079.8 | 098.89 | *162 | 238.5 | 286.9 | 295.72 | |
| *011.0 | 046.2 | 080 | 099.56 | *163 | 238.6 | 287.0 | 295.73 | |
| *011.1 | 046.3 | *081 | 100.0 | *164 | 238.73 | 287.31 | 295.74 | |
| *011.2 | 046.8 | *082 | 100.89 | *170 | 238.74 | 287.32 | 295.80 | |
| *011.3 | 046.9 | *083 | 100.9 | *171 | 238.76 | 287.33 | 295.81 | |
| *011.4 | *047 | 084.1 | 101 | *176 | 238.79 | 288.4 | 295.82 | |
| *011.5 | 048 | 084.2 | 112.0 | 183.0 | 245.0 | 289.7 | 295.83 | |
| *011.7 | *049 | 084.3 | 112.2 | *189 | 246.3 | 289.81 | 295.84 | |
| *011.8 | *050 | 084.4 | 112.82 | *191 | 251.0 | 289.82 | 295.91 | |
| *011.9 | 052.7 | 084.5 | 112.84 | *192 | 251.3 | 289.83 | 295.92 | |
| *012.0 | 052.8 | 084.6 | 112.85 | *194 | 253.1 | 290.11 | 295.93 | |
| *012.1 | 052.9 | 084.7 | 112.89 | *196 | 253.2 | 290.12 | 295.94 | |
| *012.2 | 053.10 | 084.8 | 114.0 | *197 | 253.5 | 290.13 | 296.00 | |
| *012.3 | 053.11 | 084.9 | 114.1 | *198 | 253.6 | 290.20 | 296.01 | |
| *012.8 | 053.12 | *085 | 114.3 | 199.0 | 254.1 | 290.21 | 296.02 | |
| *014.8 | 053.13 | *086 | 114.4 | *200.0 | 255.0 | 290.3 | 296.03 | |
| *015.0 | 053.19 | *087 | 114.5 | *200.1 | 255.3 | 290.41 | 296.04 | |
| *015.1 | *053.2 | 088.0 | 114.9 | *200.2 | 255.41 | 290.42 | 296.10 | |
| *015.2 | 053.71 | 088.81 | 115.02 | *200.3 | 255.42 | 290.43 | 296.11 | |
| *015.5 | 053.79 | 088.82 | 115.09 | *200.4 | 255.5 | 290.8 | 296.12 | |
| *015.6 | 053.8 | 090.0 | 115.12 | *200.5 | 255.6 | 290.9 | 296.13 | |
| *015.7 | 054.2 | 090.2 | 115.19 | *200.6 | 259.2 | 291.0 | 296.14 | |
| *015.8 | 054.40 | 090.3 | 115.92 | *200.7 | 263.2 | 291.2 | 296.20 | |
| *015.9 | 054.41 | 090.40 | 116.0 | *200.8 | 263.8 | 291.3 | 296.21 | |
| *016.0 | 054.42 | 090.49 | 116.1 | *201.0 | 263.9 | 291.81 | 296.22 | |
| *016.1 | 054.43 | 090.5 | 117.3 | *201.1 | 265.0 | 291.89 | 296.23 | |
| *016.2 | 054.44 | 091.3 | 117.4 | *201.2 | 265.1 | 291.9 | 296.24 | |
| *016.3 | 054.49 | 091.4 | 117.5 | *201.4 | 266.0 | 292.0 | 296.30 | |
| *016.4 | 054.71 | *091.5 | 117.6 | *201.5 | 268.0 | *292.1 | 296.31 | |
| *016.5 | 054.79 | *091.6 | 117.8 | *201.6 | *270 | 292.81 | 296.32 | |

| | | | | | | | |
|---|---|---|---|---|---|---|---|
| 296.33 | 345.11 | 398.91 | 446.7 | 536.1 | 579.2 | 635.71 | 646.63 |
| 296.34 | 345.40 | 401.0 | 447.2 | 536.41 | 579.3 | 635.72 | 646.64 |
| 296.40 | 345.41 | *402.0 | 447.4 | 536.42 | 579.4 | 635.80 | 646.71 |
| 296.41 | 345.50 | *403.0 | 447.5 | 537.0 | 579.8 | 635.81 | 646.73 |
| 296.42 | 345.51 | 403.11 | 449 | 537.3 | 579.9 | 635.82 | 647.01 |
| 296.43 | 345.60 | 403.91 | 451.11 | 537.4 | 581.0 | 636.00 | 647.02 |
| 296.44 | 345.61 | *404.0 | 451.19 | 538 | 581.1 | 636.01 | 647.03 |
| 296.50 | 345.70 | 404.11 | 451.81 | 540.9 | 581.2 | 636.02 | 647.04 |
| 296.51 | 345.80 | 404.12 | 451.83 | 550.10 | 581.3 | 636.20 | 647.11 |
| 296.52 | 345.81 | 404.13 | 451.89 | 550.11 | 581.81 | 636.21 | 647.12 |
| 296.53 | 345.91 | 404.91 | 453.1 | 550.12 | 581.89 | 636.22 | 647.13 |
| 296.54 | 348.1 | 404.92 | 453.3 | 550.13 | 581.9 | 636.40 | 647.14 |
| 296.60 | 349.1 | 404.93 | *453.4 | *552.0 | *582 | 636.41 | 647.21 |
| 296.61 | 349.81 | *405.0 | 453.8 | 552.1 | 583.0 | 636.42 | 647.22 |
| 296.62 | 356.3 | *411 | 453.9 | *552.2 | 583.1 | 636.70 | 647.23 |
| 296.63 | 357.0 | 413.0 | 454.2 | 552.3 | 583.2 | 636.71 | 647.24 |
| 296.64 | 357.81 | 413.1 | 456.1 | 552.8 | 583.7 | 636.72 | 647.31 |
| 296.89 | 357.82 | 414.02 | 456.21 | 552.9 | 585.4 | 636.80 | 647.32 |
| 296.99 | 358.1 | 414.03 | 459.11 | *555 | 585.5 | 636.81 | 647.33 |
| 298.0 | 359.0 | 414.04 | 459.13 | *556 | 588.1 | 636.82 | 647.34 |
| 298.1 | 359.1 | 414.06 | 459.2 | 557.1 | 588.81 | 637.00 | 647.41 |
| 298.3 | 359.4 | 414.07 | 459.31 | 557.9 | 590.01 | 637.01 | 647.42 |
| 298.4 | 359.6 | 414.10 | 459.33 | 558.1 | 590.10 | 637.02 | 647.43 |
| *299 | 359.81 | 414.19 | 464.30 | 558.2 | 590.3 | 637.20 | 647.44 |
| 301.51 | 360.00 | 416.0 | *466.1 | 560.0 | *590.8 | 637.21 | 647.51 |
| 304.01 | 360.01 | 416.1 | 475 | 560.1 | 591 | 637.22 | 647.52 |
| 304.11 | 360.02 | 417.0 | 478.21 | *560.3 | 592.1 | 637.40 | 647.53 |
| 304.21 | 360.04 | 417.1 | 478.22 | *560.8 | 593.4 | 637.41 | 647.54 |
| 304.41 | 360.11 | 420.0 | 478.24 | 560.9 | 593.5 | 637.42 | 647.61 |
| 304.51 | 360.12 | 420.90 | 478.34 | 562.01 | 593.81 | 637.70 | 647.62 |
| 304.61 | 360.13 | 420.91 | 478.71 | 562.11 | 593.82 | 637.71 | 647.63 |
| 304.71 | 360.19 | 420.99 | 491.21 | 564.7 | 595.0 | 637.72 | 647.64 |
| 304.81 | 361.2 | *423 | 491.22 | 564.81 | 595.82 | 637.80 | 647.81 |
| 304.91 | *361.8 | *424.9 | 493.01 | 566 | 596.1 | 637.81 | 647.82 |
| 307.1 | 361.9 | *425 | 493.02 | 567.82 | 596.2 | 637.82 | 647.83 |
| 307.51 | 362.30 | 426.0 | 493.11 | 568.82 | 596.7 | 638.0 | 647.84 |
| 318.1 | 362.31 | 426.12 | 493.12 | 569.3 | 597.0 | 638.1 | 647.91 |
| 318.2 | 362.32 | 426.53 | 493.21 | 569.41 | 599.0 | 638.2 | 647.92 |
| 322.2 | 362.33 | 426.54 | 493.22 | 569.5 | 599.1 | 638.4 | 647.93 |
| 330.0 | 362.34 | 426.89 | 493.91 | 569.61 | 601.0 | 638.7 | 647.94 |
| 330.1 | 362.35 | 427.0 | 493.92 | 569.62 | 601.2 | 638.8 | 648.00 |
| 330.2 | 362.40 | 427.1 | 494.1 | 569.69 | 603.1 | 639.0 | 648.03 |
| 330.3 | 362.42 | 427.32 | 495.7 | 569.81 | 604.0 | 639.1 | 648.04 |
| 330.8 | 362.43 | 428.1 | 495.8 | 569.82 | 607.3 | 639.2 | 648.31 |
| 330.9 | 362.84 | 428.20 | 495.9 | 572.3 | 607.82 | 639.4 | 648.32 |
| 331.3 | *363.1 | 428.22 | 506.0 | 573.1 | *608.2 | 639.8 | 648.33 |
| 331.4 | 363.20 | 428.30 | 508.0 | 573.2 | 614.0 | 639.9 | 648.34 |
| 331.5 | 363.63 | 428.32 | 508.1 | 574.00 | 614.3 | 640.01 | 648.51 |
| 332.1 | *363.7 | 428.40 | 511.9 | 574.01 | 614.7 | 640.03 | 648.52 |
| 333.0 | 364.00 | 428.42 | 512.1 | 574.10 | 615.0 | 640.93 | 648.53 |
| 333.4 | 364.01 | *429.7 | 512.8 | 574.11 | 616.3 | 641.01 | 648.54 |
| 333.71 | 364.02 | 429.81 | 514 | 574.21 | 616.4 | 641.03 | 648.61 |
| 333.72 | 364.03 | 429.82 | *516 | 574.30 | 616.81 | 641.23 | 648.62 |
| 333.79 | 364.22 | 429.83 | 517.1 | 574.31 | *619 | 642.01 | 648.63 |
| 333.90 | 364.3 | 432.9 | 517.2 | 574.40 | 620.5 | 642.02 | 648.64 |
| 333.91 | 365.22 | *435 | 517.3 | 574.41 | *633 | 642.03 | 648.71 |
| *334 | 368.11 | 436 | 518.0 | 574.51 | *634.0 | 642.13 | 648.72 |
| *335 | 368.12 | 437.1 | 518.3 | 574.60 | *634.2 | 642.14 | 648.73 |
| 336.0 | 376.01 | 437.2 | 518.6 | 574.61 | *634.4 | 642.31 | 648.74 |
| 336.2 | 376.02 | 437.4 | 518.7 | 574.70 | 634.60 | 642.32 | 649.30 |
| 336.3 | 376.03 | 437.5 | 518.82 | 574.71 | 634.70 | 642.41 | 649.31 |
| 336.8 | 377.00 | 437.6 | 518.83 | 574.80 | 634.71 | 642.43 | 649.32 |
| 336.9 | 377.01 | *438.2 | *519.0 | 574.91 | 634.72 | 642.44 | 649.33 |
| 337.0 | *377.3 | 440.24 | 522.0 | 575.0 | 634.80 | 642.91 | 649.34 |
| 337.1 | *377.5 | 444.0 | 522.4 | 575.12 | 634.81 | 642.92 | 649.41 |
| *337.2 | *377.6 | 444.1 | 527.3 | 575.2 | 634.82 | 642.93 | 649.42 |
| *341 | 377.71 | *444.2 | 527.4 | 575.3 | 635.00 | 642.94 | 649.43 |
| *342 | 377.72 | *444.8 | 528.3 | 575.5 | 635.01 | 644.13 | 649.44 |
| 343.0 | 377.73 | 444.9 | 530.12 | 576.1 | 635.02 | 644.20 | 651.01 |
| 343.1 | 380.14 | *445.0 | 530.20 | 576.4 | 635.20 | 646.21 | 651.11 |
| 343.4 | *383.0 | *445.8 | 530.86 | 577.1 | 635.21 | 646.22 | 651.13 |
| 344.1 | 388.61 | 446.0 | 530.87 | 577.2 | 635.22 | 646.23 | 651.21 |
| 344.2 | *391 | 446.1 | 531.30 | 578.0 | 635.40 | 646.24 | 651.23 |
| 344.60 | *392 | *446.2 | 532.30 | 578.1 | 635.41 | 646.31 | 651.41 |
| 344.61 | 393 | 446.3 | 533.30 | 578.9 | 635.42 | 646.61 | 651.43 |
| 345.01 | 398.0 | 446.4 | 534.30 | 579.1 | 635.70 | 646.62 | 651.51 |

| | | | | | | | |
|---|---|---|---|---|---|---|---|
| 651.53 | *711.4 | 758.1 | 801.02 | 823.00 | 867.8 | 925.2 | 996.30 |
| 651.81 | *711.5 | 758.2 | 801.06 | 823.02 | *868.0 | 928.00 | 996.39 |
| 651.83 | *711.6 | 758.31 | 801.09 | 823.20 | 869.0 | 928.01 | *996.4 |
| 656.13 | *711.7 | 758.33 | 801.40 | 823.22 | 870.2 | 934.0 | *996.5 |
| 656.31 | *711.8 | 758.39 | 801.41 | 823.40 | 870.3 | 934.1 | *996.6 |
| 656.41 | *711.9 | 759.0 | 801.42 | 823.42 | 870.4 | 934.8 | 996.71 |
| 656.43 | 714.31 | 759.3 | 801.46 | 823.80 | 870.8 | 940.5 | 996.72 |
| 656.51 | *719.1 | 759.5 | 801.49 | 823.82 | 870.9 | *941.3 | 996.73 |
| 657.01 | 721.1 | 759.6 | 802.1 | 824.1 | 871.0 | *941.4 | 996.74 |
| 658.01 | *721.4 | 759.7 | *802.2 | 824.3 | 871.1 | *941.5 | 996.75 |
| 658.03 | 721.7 | 759.81 | *802.3 | 824.5 | 871.2 | *942.3 | 996.76 |
| 658.81 | 721.91 | 759.82 | 802.4 | 824.7 | 871.3 | *942.4 | 996.77 |
| 659.21 | 722.71 | 759.89 | 802.5 | 824.9 | 871.5 | *942.5 | 996.78 |
| 660.03 | 722.72 | 767.11 | 802.6 | 825.1 | 871.6 | *943.3 | 996.79 |
| 662.11 | 722.73 | 770.4 | 802.7 | *825.3 | 871.9 | *943.4 | *996.8 |
| 664.21 | 728.0 | 770.5 | 802.8 | 827.1 | 872.12 | *943.5 | *996.9 |
| 664.31 | 728.88 | 770.81 | 802.9 | 830.1 | *872.6 | *944.3 | *997.0 |
| 664.61 | 729.71 | 770.82 | 803.00 | *831.1 | *872.7 | *944.4 | 997.1 |
| 664.64 | 729.72 | 770.83 | 803.01 | *832.1 | 873.23 | *944.5 | 997.2 |
| 665.22 | 729.73 | 771.0 | 803.02 | *833.1 | 873.33 | *945.3 | 997.3 |
| 665.31 | 729.79 | 771.4 | 803.06 | 835.00 | 874.2 | *945.4 | 997.4 |
| 665.41 | *730.0 | 771.5 | 803.09 | 835.01 | 874.3 | *945.5 | 997.62 |
| 665.51 | *730.1 | 771.82 | 803.40 | 835.02 | 874.4 | 946.3 | *997.7 |
| 665.61 | *730.2 | 771.83 | 803.41 | 835.03 | 874.5 | 946.4 | 997.99 |
| 665.71 | *730.8 | 771.89 | 803.42 | 836.4 | 875.0 | 946.5 | 998.0 |
| 665.72 | *730.9 | 772.10 | 803.46 | *836.6 | 875.1 | 947.1 | *998.1 |
| 666.02 | *733.1 | 772.11 | 803.49 | 837.1 | *880.2 | 947.2 | 998.2 |
| 666.04 | *733.4 | 772.12 | 804.00 | *839.0 | *881.2 | 947.3 | *998.3 |
| 666.12 | *733.8 | 772.5 | 804.01 | 839.51 | 882.2 | 947.4 | 998.4 |
| 666.14 | *741.0 | 775.1 | 804.02 | 839.52 | 883.2 | 948.10 | *998.5 |
| 666.22 | 742.0 | 775.2 | 804.06 | 839.61 | 884.2 | 948.11 | 998.6 |
| 666.24 | 742.4 | 775.3 | 804.09 | 839.79 | 887.0 | 948.20 | 998.7 |
| 666.32 | 745.12 | 775.4 | 804.40 | 839.9 | 887.1 | 948.30 | 998.83 |
| 669.24 | 745.4 | 775.81 | 804.41 | 850.11 | 887.2 | 948.40 | 999.0 |
| 671.20 | 745.5 | 775.89 | 804.42 | 850.12 | 887.3 | 948.50 | 999.2 |
| 671.21 | *745.6 | 776.0 | 804.46 | 850.2 | 887.4 | 948.60 | 999.3 |
| 671.22 | 746.00 | 776.3 | 804.49 | 850.3 | 887.5 | 948.70 | 999.4 |
| 671.23 | 746.02 | 776.5 | 804.50 | 850.5 | 890.2 | 948.80 | 999.5 |
| 671.24 | 746.09 | 776.6 | 804.51 | 851.02 | 891.2 | 948.90 | 999.6 |
| 671.30 | 746.3 | 777.4 | 804.52 | 851.03 | 892.2 | 949.3 | 999.7 |
| 671.40 | 746.4 | 778.1 | 804.56 | 851.04 | 893.2 | 949.4 | 999.8 |
| *671.5 | 746.5 | 778.5 | 804.59 | 851.06 | 894.2 | 949.5 | V42.0 |
| *671.8 | 746.6 | 779.4 | 804.90 | 851.42 | 896.0 | *950 | V42.1 |
| 671.90 | 746.83 | 779.5 | 804.91 | 851.43 | 896.1 | *951 | V42.6 |
| 671.91 | 746.85 | 780.03 | 804.92 | 851.44 | 897.0 | 958.2 | V42.7 |
| 671.92 | 746.87 | 780.1 | 804.96 | 851.46 | 897.1 | 958.3 | V42.81 |
| 672.02 | 747.0 | 780.31 | 804.99 | 854.02 | 897.2 | 958.7 | V42.82 |
| 672.04 | 747.10 | 780.32 | *805.0 | 854.03 | 897.3 | *958.9 | V42.83 |
| 673.30 | *747.2 | 781.4 | 805.2 | 854.04 | 897.4 | 991.0 | V42.84 |
| 674.02 | *747.4 | 781.6 | 805.4 | 854.06 | 897.5 | 991.1 | *V43.2 |
| 674.03 | 747.82 | 781.7 | 805.6 | 860.0 | *900.0 | 991.2 | *V46.1 |
| 674.04 | 747.89 | 781.8 | 805.8 | 861.00 | 900.1 | 991.3 | V55.1 |
| 675.11 | 747.9 | 782.4 | *807.0 | 861.01 | *900.8 | 991.4 | V62.84 |
| 675.12 | 748.3 | 784.3 | 807.2 | 861.20 | 900.9 | 992.0 | V85.0 |
| *682 | 748.4 | 785.4 | 808.2 | 861.21 | 901.81 | 993.3 | V85.4 |
| 685.0 | 748.61 | 785.50 | *808.4 | 862.0 | 901.82 | 994.1 | |
| 686.01 | 750.4 | 786.04 | 808.8 | 862.29 | 901.89 | 994.7 | |
| 694.4 | 751.1 | 786.3 | 809.0 | 862.8 | 901.9 | 995.0 | |
| 694.5 | 751.2 | 788.8 | *810.1 | 863.0 | 902.55 | 995.4 | |
| 695.0 | 751.3 | *789.5 | *811.1 | *863.2 | 902.56 | 995.50 | |
| 695.1 | 751.4 | 790.01 | *812.0 | *863.4 | 902.81 | 995.51 | |
| 707.00 | 751.5 | 790.7 | *812.2 | *863.8 | 902.82 | 995.52 | |
| 707.01 | 751.60 | 791.1 | *812.4 | 864.00 | 902.89 | 995.53 | |
| 707.09 | 751.62 | 791.3 | *813.2 | 864.01 | 902.9 | 995.54 | |
| 707.10 | 751.69 | 799.01 | *813.4 | 864.02 | 903.1 | 995.55 | |
| 707.11 | 751.7 | 799.4 | 813.80 | 864.05 | 903.2 | 995.59 | |
| 707.12 | 753.0 | 800.00 | 813.82 | 864.09 | 903.3 | *995.6 | |
| 707.13 | *753.1 | 800.01 | 813.83 | 865.00 | 903.4 | 995.80 | |
| 707.14 | *753.2 | 800.02 | *814.1 | 865.01 | 903.5 | 995.81 | |
| 707.19 | 753.5 | 800.06 | *815.1 | 865.02 | 903.8 | 995.83 | |
| 710.3 | 753.6 | 800.09 | *816.1 | 865.09 | 903.9 | 995.84 | |
| 710.4 | 754.2 | 800.40 | 817.1 | 866.00 | 904.3 | 995.85 | |
| 710.5 | 754.89 | 800.41 | 818.1 | 866.01 | *904.5 | 995.86 | |
| 710.8 | 756.13 | 800.42 | 819.0 | 866.02 | 904.6 | 995.90 | |
| *711.0 | 756.3 | 800.46 | 819.1 | 867.0 | 904.7 | 995.93 | |
| *711.1 | 756.51 | 800.49 | *821.2 | 867.2 | 904.8 | *996.0 | |
| *711.2 | 756.52 | 801.00 | 822.0 | 867.4 | 904.9 | 996.1 | |
| *711.3 | 756.83 | 801.01 | 822.1 | 867.6 | 925.1 | 996.2 | |

# Pharmacological Listings

## Pharmacology Considerations

Medications are listed by classification and brand name for each of the chapters of ICD-9-CM. The list includes many of the common medications and should not be considered exhaustive. The pharmacology considerations that follow are presented as guidance only for the recognition of the link between implication of disease process and treatment.

## Infectious and Parasitic Diseases (001-139)

### AIDS Related Complex (ARC) Therapeutic Agents

| | |
|---|---|
| Agenerase | Crixivan |
| Epivir | Fortovase |
| Hivid | Intron A |
| Invirase | Norvir |
| Pentam | Rescriptor |
| Retrovir | Rimactane |
| Roferon-A | Sustiva |
| Videx | Viracept |
| Vitravene | Zerit |
| Ziagen | Zovirax |

### Antibiotics

| | |
|---|---|
| Achromycin-V | Amikin |
| Amoxicillin | Amoxil |
| Ampicillin | Ancef |
| Augmentin | Azactam |
| Bactrim | Bicillin |
| Biocef | Ceclor |
| Cefizox• | Cefobid |
| Cefotan | Ceftin |
| Chloromycetin | Cipro |
| Claforan | Cleocin |
| Duricef | E-Mycin |
| ERYC | Ery-Tab |
| Erythromycin | Factive |
| Floxin | Fortaz |
| Garamycin | Levaquin |
| Macrobid | Maxipime |
| Mefoxin | Minocin |
| Nebcin | Neo-fradin |
| PCE Dispertab | Penicillin G |
| Penicillin V | Pfizerpen |
| Pipracil | Primaxin |
| Proloprim | Septra |
| Spectrobid | Suprax |
| Synersid | Tazicef |
| Tazidime | Terramycin |
| Tetracycline HCl | Ticar |
| Timentin | Totacillin |
| Trimox | Trimpex |
| Unasyn | Unipen |
| Vancocin | Vibramycin |
| Vibra-Tabs | Wycillin |
| Zefazone | Zinacef |
| Zithromax | Zosyn |
| Zymar | |

### Antiparasitics

| | |
|---|---|
| Antiminth | Aralen |
| Daraprim | Flagyl |
| G-well | Helidac |
| MepronnebuPent | Pentam 300 |
| Penticarinat | Pin-X |
| Protostat | Vermox |

### Corticosteroids

| | |
|---|---|
| Aristocort | Celestone |
| Cortastat | Cortef |
| Cortenema | Cortone Acetate |
| Dalalone | Decadron |
| Deltasone | Depo-Medrol |
| Florinef acetate | Hydeltrasol |
| Hydrocortisone | Hydrocortone |
| Medralone | Medrol |
| Orasone | Predalone |
| Prednisone | Prelone |
| Protocort | Solu-Cortef |

### Fungal Medications

| | |
|---|---|
| Abelcet | AmBisome |
| Amphocin | Amphotec |
| Ancobon | Diflucan |
| Fulvicin P/G | Fungilin |
| Fungizone | Fungoid |
| Grifulvin | Grisactin |
| Gris-PEG | Lamisil |
| Lotrimin | Lotrisone |
| Monistat | Mycelex-G |
| Mycolog | Mycostatin |
| Nilstst | Nizoral |
| Spectazole | Sporanox |

### Tuberculosis Preparations

| | |
|---|---|
| Capastat | INH Tablets |
| Lamprene | Laniazid |
| Myambutol | Mycobutin |
| Priftin | Pyrazinamide |
| Rifadin | Rifamate |
| Rimactane | Seromycin |
| Sodium P.A.S. | Streptomycin |
| Trecator-SC | |

### Viral Agents

| | |
|---|---|
| Abreva | Agenerase |
| Combivir | Crixivan |
| Cytovene | Emtriva |
| Epivir | Famvir |
| Flumadine | Fortovase |
| Foscavir | Fuzeon |
| Herplex | Hepsera |
| Hivid | Invirase |
| Lexiva | Norvir |
| Relenza | Rescriptor |
| Retrovir | Reyataz |
| Sustiva | Symmetrel |
| Tamiflu | Valtrex |
| Videx | Viracept |
| Viramune | Virazole |
| Vistide | Vitravene |
| Zerit | Ziagen |
| Zovirax | |

## Neoplasms (140-239)

### Adjunct

| | |
|---|---|
| Anzemet | Arrestin |
| Compazine | Epogen |
| Ergamisol | Kytril |
| Leukine | Martinol |
| Metastron | Neumega |
| Neupogen | Procrit |
| Prokine | Quadramet |
| Reglan | Relcomide |
| Salagen | Sandostatin |
| Zinecard | Zofran |

### Androgen Inhibitor

| | |
|---|---|
| Casodex | Eulexin |
| Lupron | Nilandron |
| Zoladex | |

### Antibiotic Derivatives

| | |
|---|---|
| Adriamycin | Blenoxane |
| Cerubidine | Cosmegen |
| Doxorubicin | Idamycin |
| Mutamycin | Mithracin |
| Nipent | Novantrone |
| Pacis | Rubex |
| TheraCys | |

### Antiestrogen

| | |
|---|---|
| Femara | Nolvadex |

### Antimetabolites

| | |
|---|---|
| Adrucil | Cytarabine |
| Cytosar-U | Droxia |
| Efudex | Folex |
| Fludara | Fluoroplex |
| Fluorouracil | FUDR |
| Intron A | Leustatin |
| Methotrexate | Purinethol |
| Roferon-A | Thioguanine |
| Xeloda | |

### Cytotoxic Agents

| | |
|---|---|
| Adriamycin | BiCNU |
| CeeNU | Cerubidine |
| Cytosar-U | Doxorubicin |
| Gemzar | Hexalen |
| Hydrea | Intron A |
| Matulane | Mutamycin |
| Myleran | Novantrone |
| Paraplatin | Platinol |
| Zanosar | |

### Hormones

| | |
|---|---|
| Arimidex | Aromasin |
| Depo-Provera | Eligard |
| Emcyt | Estinyl |
| Estradurin | Fareston |
| Lupron | Megace |
| Stilphostrol | Teslac |
| Zoladex | |

### Nitrogen Mustard Derivatives

| | |
|---|---|
| Alkeran | Cytoxan |
| Leukeran | Mustargen |
| Neosar | Thiotepa |

### Steroids and Combinations

Celestone Soluspan

### Other

| | |
|---|---|
| Camptosar | DTIC-Dome |
| Elspar | Etopophos |
| Iressa | Navelbine |
| Oncaspar | Oncovin |
| Phosphocol P32 | Photofrin |
| Proleukin | Rituxan |
| Semzar | Taxol |
| Taxotere | TICE |
| Velban | Velcade |
| VePesid | Vesanoid |
| Vumon | |

## Endocrine, Nutritional and Metabolic Diseases and Immunity Disorders (240-279)

### Acidifier and Alkalinizers

| | |
|---|---|
| Ammonium chloride | Citrocarbonate |
| Sodium bicarbonate | Sodium lactate |
| Tham | |

### Antigout Agents

| | |
|---|---|
| Anturane | Benemid |
| Colchicine | Probalan |
| Zyloprim | |

### Antilipemics

| | |
|---|---|
| atorvastatin calcium | fluvastatin sodium |
| Lescol | Lipitor |
| lovastatin | Mevacor |
| Pravachol | pravastatin sodium |
| simvastatin | Tricor |
| Vytorin | Zetia |
| Zocor | |

### Antioxidants
| | |
|---|---|
| Aquasol E | Calcium-D |
| Calcium Health Packs | Carotene-E |
| Carotene Health Packs | Glutathione |
| Performance Packs | Pure-E |

### Appetite Suppressants
| | |
|---|---|
| Adipex-P | Adipost |
| Biphetamine | Bontril |
| Desoxyn | Didrex |
| Fastin | Ionamin |
| Mazanor | Meridia |
| Phentride | Plegine |
| Pondimin | Prelu-2 |
| Sanorex | Tenuate |

### Diabetic Agents and Glucagon
| | |
|---|---|
| Actos | Amaryl |
| Avandia | DiaBeta |
| Diabinese | Glucagon |
| Glucophage | Glucotrol |
| Glynase | Glyset |
| Humulin R | Iletin II |
| Lantus | Lispro (Humalog) |
| Micronase | Novolin |
| NovoLog | Prandin |
| Precose | Rezulin |
| Riomet | Ultralente |
| Velosulin | |

### Electrolytes and Replacement Solutions
| | |
|---|---|
| Calcium acetate | Calcium carbonate |
| Calcium chloride | Calcium citrate |
| Calcium gluconate | Calcium lactate |
| Calcium phosphate, dibasic | Calcium phosphate, tribasic |
| Dextran | Gendex |
| Hespan | Magnesium chloride |
| Magnesium sulfate | Phoslo |
| Potassium acetate | |

Potassium bicarbonate (K+ Care ET, Klor-Con/EF, K-Vescent)

Potassium chloride (Kaochlor, Kaon-Cl, Kato Powder, Kay Ciel, K-Lease, K-Lor, Klor-10%, Klor-Con, Klorvess, Klotrix, K-Lyte/Cl, K-Tab, Micro-K Extencaps, SK-Potassium Chloride, Slow-K, Ten-K)

Potassium gluconate (Glu-K, Kaon, Kayliker, K-G Elixir)

| | |
|---|---|
| Slow-mag | Ringer's Injection |

### Hormones
| | |
|---|---|
| Anadrol-50 | Android |
| A.P.L. | Combipatch |
| Delatestryl | Depo-Provers |
| Estrace | Estraderm |
| Estratab | Estrovis |
| Factrel | Halotestin |
| Micronor | Norplant |
| Ogen | Ortho-Est |
| Ortho-Novum | Orvette |
| Pregnyl | premarin |
| Proscar | Provera |
| Testoderm | Testred |

### Parathyroid-like Agents
| | |
|---|---|
| Aredia | Calcimar |
| Calderol | Cibacalcin |
| Didronel | E-Vista |
| Fosamax | Miacalcin |
| Osteocalcin | Rocaltrol |
| Salmonine | |

### Pituitary Hormones
| | |
|---|---|
| ACTH | Acthar |
| Cortrosyn | Diapid |
| Genotropin | Humatrope |
| Pegvisomant | Pitressin |
| Protropin | Somavert |
| Stimate | |

### Thyroid Antagonists
| | |
|---|---|
| Pima | Tapazole |

### Thyroid Hormones
| | |
|---|---|
| Cytomel | Euthroid |
| Levothroid | Levoxine |
| Levoxyl | Triostat |
| Synthroid | |

### Vitamins
Vitamin A

Vitamin B complex (including cyanocobalamin, hydroxocobalamin, folic acid, leucovorin calcium, niacin, niacinamide, pyridoxine hydrochloride, riboflavin, thiamine hydrochloride)

Vitamin C

Vitamin D (cholecalciferol, ergocalciferol)

Vitamin E

Vitamin K analogs (menadione/menadiol sodium diphosphate, phytonadione, sodium fluoride)

Trace elements (chromium, copper, iodine, manganese, selenium, zinc)

## Blood and Blood-Forming Organs (280-289)
### Anticoagulants
| | |
|---|---|
| abciximab | Aggrastat |
| cilostazol | clopidrogrel bisulfate |
| eptifibatide | Integrilin |
| Plavix | Pletal |
| RepPro | Ticlid |
| ticlopidine hydrochloride | tirofiban hydrochloride |

### Coagulants
AlphaNine Coagulation Factor
Profilate OSD Antihemophilic Factor
Trasylol

### Hematinics
**Ferrous fumarate:**
| | |
|---|---|
| Femiron | Feostat |
| Hemocyte | Ircon |
| Nephro-Fer | Novofumar |
| Vitron-C | |

**Ferrous gluconate:**
| | |
|---|---|
| Fergon | Feratab |
| Fer-Gen-Sol | |

**Ferrous sulfate:**
| | |
|---|---|
| ED-IN-SOL | Fe50 |
| Feosol | Fer-In-Sol |
| Fer-Iron | Slow Fe |

**Iron dextran:**
| | |
|---|---|
| DexFerrum | INFeD |

### Others
Konyne-HT Factor IX Complex    Nu-Iron
Monoclate-P Factor VIII:C, Antihemophilic Factor

## Mental Disorders (290-319)
### Central Nervous System Stimulants
| | |
|---|---|
| Adderall XR | Atomoxetine HCI |
| Concerta | Cylert |
| Desoxyn | Dexedrine |
| Dopram | Methylin |
| Provigil | Ritalin |
| Strattera | Vivarin |

### Cerebral Metabolic Enhancer
| | |
|---|---|
| Ergostat | Hydergine |
| Migranal | |

### Alzheimer's Dementia Agents
| | |
|---|---|
| Aricept | Cognex |
| Exelon | Namenda |
| Reminyl | |

### Anti-anxiety
| | |
|---|---|
| Atarax | Ativan |
| BuSpar | Libritabs |
| Librium | Miltown |
| Serax | Tranxene |
| Valium | Versed |
| Xanax | |

### Anti-depressants
| | |
|---|---|
| Anafranil | Asendin |
| Aventyl | Celexa |
| Desyrel | Effexor |
| Elavil | Lexapro |
| Nardil | Norpramin |
| Pamelor | Parnate |
| Paxil | Prozac |

| | |
|---|---|
| Remeron | Serzone |
| Sinequan | Surmontil |
| Tofranillbutrin | Trialodine |
| Wellbutrin | Zoloft |

### Anti-psychotics
| | |
|---|---|
| Clozaril | Etrafon |
| Haldol | Loxitane |
| Mellaril | Navane |
| Orap | Prolixin |
| Risperdal | Serentil |
| Seroquel | Serpasil |
| Stelazine | Thorazine |
| Triavil | Trilafon |
| Zyprexa | |

### Sedatives
| | |
|---|---|
| Ambien | Dalmane |
| Diprivan | Mebaral |
| Nembutal | Precedex |
| ProSom | Restoril |
| Seconal Sodium | Sonata |
| Tuinal | Unisom |

### Other Psychotrophics
| | |
|---|---|
| Antabuse | Cibalith-S |
| Eskalith | Lithane |
| Lithium Carbonate | Lithobid |
| Luvox | Meridia |
| Methadone | Zomig |
| Zyban | |

## Nervous System and Sense Organs (320-389)
### Antibiotics Central Nervous System Agents:
| | |
|---|---|
| Amikin | Ancef |
| Cefizox | Fortaz |
| Garamycin | Kefurox |
| Nebcin | Rocephin |
| Tazidime | |

### Anticonvulsants
| | |
|---|---|
| Celontin | Cerebyx |
| Depakene | Depakote |
| Dilantin | Felbatol |
| Keppra | Klonopin |
| Lamictal | Mebaral |
| Mesantoin | Milontin |
| Mysoline | Neurontin |
| Peganone | Phenobarbital |
| Phenytoin | Phenurone |
| Tegretol | Tranxene |
| Tridione | Zarontin |

### Dopamine Receptor Agonist
| | |
|---|---|
| Eldepryl | Mirapex |
| Parlodel | Permax |
| Requip | Sinemet |
| Stalevo | Symmetrel |
| Tasmar | |

### Miscellaneous Ophthalmics
| | |
|---|---|
| Alphagan | Betoptic |
| Emadine | Iopidine |
| Lacrisert | Lumigan |
| Opticrom | OptiPranolol |
| OPTIVAR | Propine |
| Timoptic | Trusopt |
| Zaditor | |

### Migraine Agents
| | |
|---|---|
| Amerge | Cafergot |
| Depakote | Ergostat |
| Imitrex | Inderal |
| Isocom | Maxalt |
| Midrin | Migranal |
| Relpax | Sansert |
| Wigraine | Zomig |

### Miotics
| | |
|---|---|
| Carboptic | Miochol-E |
| Miostat | Pilocar |
| Pilostat | Phospholine Iodide |

### Mydriatics
| | |
|---|---|
| AK-Dilate | AK-Nefrin |
| AK-Pentolate | Atropisol |

Cyclogyl
Epinal
Homatropine
Isopto Atropine
Isopto Homatropine
Minims
Mydriacyl

Epifrin
Eppy/N
Glaucon
Isopto Frin
Isopto Hyoscine
Mydfrin

## Ophthalmic Antiinfectives

AK-Tracin
Chloromycetin
Garamycin
Polymyxin B Sulfate
Sodium Sulamyd
Tobrex
Vira-A

Bleph-10 Liqifilm
Ciloxan
Ilotycin
Oculflox
Tobradex
Vigamox
Zymar

## Ophthalmic Antiinflammatory Agents

Acular
Flarex
Maxidex
Voltarin

Decadron Phosphate
Fluor-Op
Ocufen

## Otics

Augmentin
Cerumex
Coly-Mycin S
Cotrim
Murine Ear
PediOtic

Auro-Dri
Chloromycetin Otic
Cortisporin
LazerSporin-C
OticTridesilon
Septra

## Parasympathomimetics

Duvoid
Mestinon
Tensilon

Evoxac
Prostigmin
Urecholine

## Parkinsonism Agents

Akineton
Benztropine
Comtan
Larodopa
Parlodel
Requip
Symmetrel

Artane
Cogentin
Dopar
Mirapex
Permax
Sinemet

## Skeletal Muscle Relaxants

Dantrium
Lioresal
Zaraflex

Flexeril
Vanadom

## Vertigo Agents

Antivert

Vergon

# Circulatory System (390-459)

## Alpha Adrenoceptor Agonists

Aldomet
Combipres

Catapres
Wytensin

## Alpha Receptor Blocking Agents

Cardura
Minipress
Trandate

Hytrin
Regitine

## Anginal Preparations

Calan
Cardizem
Inderal
Isordil
Nitro-Dur
Nitrogard
Procardia
Transderm-Nitro

Cardia XT
Dilitrate-SR
Isoptin
Nitro-Bid
Nitrodisc
Nitrostat IV
Sorbitrate

## Angiotensin Converting Enzyme Inhibitors

Accupril
Avapro
Capozide
Lotensin
Monopril
Univasc
Zestril

Altace
Capoten
Cozaar
Mavik
Prinivil
Vasotec

## Antihypertensives

Aldactazide
Aldomet
Atacard
Avapro
Calan

Aldactone
Apresoline
Atenolol
Benicar HCT
Capoten

---

Cardizem
Catapres
Cozaar
HydroDIURIL
Hytrin
Inderal
Levatol
Minipress
Procardia
Temex
Teveten
Wytensin

Cardura
Corlopam
Diuril
Hyperstat
Hyzaar
Isoptin
Lopressor
Monopril
Renese
Tenormin
Vasotec
Zestric

## Arrhythmia Medications

Betapace
Cardioquin
Inderal
Mexitil
Procan
Quinaglute
Tonocard

Calan
Cordarone
Isoptin
Norpace
Pronestyl
Rythmol

## Beta Blocking Agents

Blocadren
Coreg
Corzide
Kerlone
Lopressor
Sectral
Tenormin
Trandate
Zebeta

Cartrol
Corgard
Inderal
Levatol
Normodyne
Tenoretic
Toprol XL
Visken

## Calcium Channel Blockers

Adalat
Cardene
DynaCirc
Norvasc
Posicor
Sular
Verelan
Lanoxin (Digoxin)

Calan
Cardizem
Isoptin
Plendil
Procardia
Vascor
Cardiac Glycosides

## Diuretics

Aldactazide
Bumex
Demadex
Dyazide
Esidrix
Furosemide
Rauzide
Zaroxolyn

Aldoril
Combipres
Diuril
Edecrin
Esimil
Lasix
Renese

## Thrombolytic Enzymes

Abbokinase
Kabikinase
Streptase

Activase
Retavase

## Vasodilators, Cerebral

Pavabid

## Vasodilators, Coronary

Cardilate
Nitro-Bid
Nitrolingual Spray
Pavabid
Sorbitrate

Isordil
Nitro-Dur
Nitrostat IV
Peritrate
Transderm-Nitro

## Vasodilators, Peripheral

Apresoline
Esimil
Loniten

Dibenzyline
Hyperstat IV
Pavabid

# Respiratory System (460-519)

## Allergy Relief Products

Antihist-1
Brexin
Clarinex
Naldecon
Trimeton

Benadryl
Bromphen
Dristan
Tavist

## Antibiotics

Achromycin
Amoxicillin
Ampicillin
Augmentin
Bactrim

Amikin
Amoxil
Ancef
Azactam
Biaxin

---

Bicillin
Cefizox
Cefotan
Cipro
Duricef
E-Mycin
ERYC
Factive
Fortaz
Geocillin
Iotycin
Keftab
Levaquin
Mefoxin
Mezlin
Nebcin
PCE Dispertab
Penicillin V
Primaxin
Rocephin
Spectrobid
Tazicef
Tetracycline HCl
Timentin
Wycillin
Zefazone
Zithromax

Ceclor
Cefobid
Ceftin
Claforan
Dynabec
Ery-Tab
Erythromycin
Floxin
Garamycin
Ilosone
Keflex
Kefurox
Mandol
Meropen
Minocin
Netromycin
Penicillin G
Pipracil
Raxar
Septra
Suprax
Tazidime
Ticar
Trovan
Zagam
Zinacef

## Antihistamines

Actifed
Allerest
Benadryl
Chlor-Trimeton
Coricidin
Four-Way
Tavist
Zyrtec

Allegra
Atarax
Bromphen
Claritin
Deconamine
Periactin
Triaminic

## Asthma Preparations

Accolate
Alupent
Beclovent
Bronkaid
Crolom
Flovent
Maxair
Primatene
Serevent
TheoDur
Tornalate
Ventolin

AeroBid
Aminophylline
Brethine
Choledyl SA
Dilor
Intal
Metaprel
Proventil
Singulair
Tilade
Vanceril
Zyflo

## Bronchial Dilators

Accolate
Alupent
Asbron G
Brethaire Inhaler
Bronkephrine
Combivent
Isuprel
Marax
Medihaler-Iso
Primatene
Quadrinal
Serevent
Slo-bid
Theolair
Ventolin
Xopenex

Advair Diskus
Aminophylline
Atrovent
Bricanyl
Bronkometer
Choledyl
Lufyllin
Maxair
Prez-D
Proventil
Quibron
Singulair
Tedral
Tornalate
Xolair
Zyflo

## Cold, Cough Preparations and Mucolytics

Calcidrine
Comtrex
Dimetane
Guaifed
Hycomine
Novahistine
Ornade
Quibron
Rondec
Rynatan
Sine-Aid
Tuss-Ornade
Tussionex

Cheracol
Dimetapp
Entex
Humibid
Naldecon
Nucofed
Quelidrine
Robitussin
Ru-Tuss
Rynatuss
Triaminic
Tussi-Organdin

### Corticosteroids

| | |
|---|---|
| Aristocort | Celestone |
| Cortone Acetate | Deltasone |
| Depo-Medrol | Hydeltrasol |
| Hydrocortone | Prednisone |
| Solu-Cortef | Solu-Medrol |

### Nasal Preparations

| | |
|---|---|
| Adrenalin Chloride | Afrin |
| Beconase | Decadron Phosphate |
| Dopram Injectable | Flonase |
| Nasacort | Nasalide |
| Nasarel | Otrivin |
| Privine | Respiratory Stimulants |
| Rhinocort | Turbinaire |
| Vancenase | |

### Respiratory Therapy Agents

| | |
|---|---|
| Alupent | Arm-a-Med Isoetharine |
| Survanta | |

## Digestive System (520-579)

### Anorectal Products

| | |
|---|---|
| Analpram-HC | Proctofoam-HC |
| Rowasa | |

### Antacids

| | |
|---|---|
| Alka-Seltzer | Amphojel |
| Basaljel | Di-Gel |
| Gaviscon | Maalox |
| Mylanta | Polycitra |
| Riopan | Tums |

### Antibiotics and Antibacterials

| | |
|---|---|
| Amikin | Ancef |
| Azactam | Cefizox |
| Cefobid | Cefotan |
| Claforan | Fortaz |
| Furoxone | Kefzol |
| Mandol | Mefoxin |
| Nebcin | Netromycin |
| Pipracil | Primaxin |
| Tazicef | Tazidime |
| Ticar | Unasyn |
| Vancocin | Zefazone |

### Antispasmodics and Anticholinergics

| | |
|---|---|
| Bentyl | Darabid |
| Donnatal | Levsin |
| Librax | Prilosec |
| Pro-Banthine | Quarzan |
| Reglan | Robinul |

### Antiulcer

| | |
|---|---|
| cimetidine | esomeprazole magnesium |
| famotidine | iansoprazole |
| Nexium | omeprazole |
| Pepcid AC | Prevacid |
| Prilosec | ranitidine hydrochloride |
| Tagamet | Zantac |

### Corticosteroids

| | |
|---|---|
| Alinia | Aristocort |
| Cortenema | Decadron |
| Deltasone | Depo-Medrol |
| Hydeltrasol | Hydrocortone |
| Prednisone | Solu-Cortef |
| Solu-Medrol | |

### Diarrhea Medications

| | |
|---|---|
| Alinia | Arco-Lase Plus |
| Charcoal Plus | Donnagel |
| Furoxone | Kaopectate |
| Kapectolin | Imodium |
| Lomotil | Mitrolan |
| Motofen | Pepto-Bismol |

### Digestants

| | |
|---|---|
| Cotazym | Donnazyme |
| Entozyme | Ku-Zyme |
| Lactaid | Pancrease |
| Pancreatin | Ultrase |
| Viokase | |

### Flatulence Relief

| | |
|---|---|
| Flatulex | Gas-X |
| Kutrase | Mylicon |
| Phazyme | |

### Gallstone Dissolution Agent

Actigall Capsules

### Gastric Acid Secretion Inhibitor

| | |
|---|---|
| Axid | Cytotec |
| Prevacid | Zantac |

### Gastrointestinal Antigranulomatous Disease

| | |
|---|---|
| Azulfidine Tablets, EN-tabs | Dipentum Capsules |
| Mesasal | Pentasa |
| Remicade | Rowasa |

### Nausea and Vertigo Medications

| | |
|---|---|
| Aloxi | Anzeme |
| Anfernet | Antivert |
| Aprepitant | Bonine |
| Bucladin-S Softab | Compazine |
| Dramamine | Emend |
| Kytril | Marinol |
| Reglan | Tigan |
| Torecan | Vergon |
| Zofran | |

### Parasympatholytics

| | |
|---|---|
| Bellergal-S | Bentyl |
| Cantil | Levsin |
| Robinul | |

## Genitourinary System (580-629)

### Alpha-adrenergic blockers

| | |
|---|---|
| Flomax | Tamsulosin HCL |

### Antibiotics

| | |
|---|---|
| Achromycin | Ancef |
| Augmentin | Azactam |
| Azo Gantanol | Azo Gantrisin |
| Bactrim | Ceclor |
| Cefizox | Cefobid |
| Cefotan | Ceftin |
| Ceptaz | Cipro |
| Claforan | Duricef |
| E-Mycin | Ery-tab |
| Floxin | Fortaz |
| Garamycin | Keftab |
| Kefurox | Mefoxin |
| Mezlin | Monuril |
| Nebcin | Netromycin |
| Noroxin | PCE Dispertab |
| Penetrex | Primaxin |
| Rocephin | Septra |
| Sumycin | Suprax |
| Tazidime | Timentin |
| Unasyn | Zinacef |

### Gonadotropin Inhibitors

| | |
|---|---|
| Antagon | Danocrine Capsules |
| Synarel Nasal Solution | |

### Hormones

**Androgen and estrogen combinations:**

| | |
|---|---|
| Estratest | |
| Premarin with Methyltestosterone | |
| Premphase | Prempro |

**Estrogens:**

| | |
|---|---|
| Climara | Estrace |
| Estraderm | Estrofem |
| Femring | Levolet |
| Menest | Ogen |
| Premarin | Seasonale |

**Gonadotropin:**

| | |
|---|---|
| Lutrepulse | Pregnyl |
| Profasi | Synarel |

**Menotropins:**

| | |
|---|---|
| Humegon | Pergonal |
| Repronex | |

**Progesterone:**

| | |
|---|---|
| Cycrin | Provera |

**Progestogen:**

| | |
|---|---|
| Aygestin | Micronor |

### Urinary Tract Agents

**Analgesics:**

| | |
|---|---|
| Pyridium | Rimso-50 |

**Antibacterials:**

| | |
|---|---|
| Bactrim | Cipro |
| Furadantin | Gantanol |
| Gantrisin | Macrobid |
| Macrodantin | NegGram |
| Neosporin | Noroxin |
| Proloprim | Septra |
| Thiosulfil | Trimpex |
| Uroqid Acid No. 2 | |

**Antispasmodics:**

| | |
|---|---|
| Cystospaz | Levsin |
| Oxytrol | Urised |
| Urispas | UroXatral |

### Vaginal Preparations

**Antifungal agents:**

| | |
|---|---|
| Betadine Douche | Femstat |
| Gyne-Lotrimin | Monistat |
| Mycelex | Terazol |
| Vagistat | Yeast-X |

**Capsules, tablets:**

| | |
|---|---|
| Mycelex-G | Sultrin |

**Creams:**

| | |
|---|---|
| Amino-Cerv | Estrace |
| Mycostatin | Nystex |
| Premarin | Trysul |

**Inserts, suppositories:**

| | |
|---|---|
| Terazol | Vagisec Plus |

**Jellies, ointments:**

Aci-Jel

## Pregnancy, Childbirth, Puerperium (630-677)

### Antibiotics

| | |
|---|---|
| Amikin | Ancef |
| Azactam | Ceclor |
| Cefizox | Cefobid |
| Cefotan | Claforan |
| E-Mycin | Fortaz |
| Garamycin | Keftab |
| Kefzol | Mefoxin |
| Nebcin | PCE Dispertab |
| Primaxin | Rocephin |
| Tazidime | Ticar |
| Timentin | Trobicin |
| Unasyn | Zefazone |
| Zolicef | Zyvox |

### Antihypertensives

| | |
|---|---|
| Adalat | Aldactazide |
| Aldactone | Aldomet |
| Apresoline | Calan |
| Cardizem | Catapres |
| Deponit | Diuril |
| Esidrix | Hydralazine |
| HydroDIURIL | Hygroton |
| Hyperstat | Hytrin |
| Inderal | Isoptin |
| Levatol | Lopressor |
| Midamor | Minipress |
| Minoxidil | Nitrostat |
| Procardia | Renese |
| Tenormin | Tridil |
| Vasotec | Wytensin |

### Diuretics

| | |
|---|---|
| Aldactazide | AldactoneAldoril |
| Bumex | Demadex Diuril |
| Dyazide | |
| Dyrenium | Edecrin |
| Esidrix | Esimil |
| HydroDIURIL | Lasix |
| Lozol | Maxzide |
| Rauzide | Renese |
| Zaroxolyn | |

## Galactokinetic Agents
Syntocinon Nasal Spray

## Nausea Medication
| | |
|---|---|
| Antivert | Arrestin |
| Bonine | Compazine |
| Emetrol | Norzine |
| Tigan | Torecan |

## Oxytocics
| | |
|---|---|
| Hemabate | Cervidil |
| Methergine | Oxytocin |
| Pitocin | Syntocinon |

## Uterine Relaxants
Yutopar

---

# Skin and Subcutaneous Tissue (680-709)

## Abradants
Ureacin

## Acne Preparations
| | |
|---|---|
| Accutane Tablets | Azelex |
| Benzac | Benzamycin |
| Cleocin | Clinda-Derm |
| Desquam | Emgel |
| Erycette | Novacet |
| Persa-Gel | Retin-A |
| Staticin | Sulfacet-R Acne |
| Theramycin Z | Xerac |

## Antibacterials, Antifungals and Combinations
| | |
|---|---|
| Benzamycin | Fungi-Nail |
| Loprox | Lotrisone |
| Neosporin | Nizoral |
| Sporanox | |

## Antibiotics
| | |
|---|---|
| Amikin | Ancef |
| Azactam | Bactroban |
| Ceclor | Cefizox |
| Cefobid | Cefotan |
| Ceftin | Cipro |
| Cubicin | Duricef |
| ERYC | Erythromycin |
| Floxin | Furacin |
| Garamycin | Ilosone |
| Ilotycin | Keflex |
| Keftab | Kefzol |
| Mandol | Mefoxin |
| Mezlin | Netromycin |
| Pipracil | Primaxin |
| Rocephin | Silvadene |
| Spectrobid | Tazidime |
| Ticar | Timentin |
| Ultracef | Zefazone |
| Zinacef | |

## Antiinflammatory Agents
| | |
|---|---|
| Aclovate | Aristocort |
| Cortisporin | Cutivate |
| Cyclocort | Decadron |
| Diprolene | Elocon |
| Halog | Kenalog |
| Lidex | Lotrisone |
| Mantadil | NeoDecadron |
| Nutracort | Synacort |
| Synalar | Temovate |
| Topicort | Tridesilon |
| Ultravate | Westcort |

## Corticosteroids
| | |
|---|---|
| Amcort | Celestone |
| Cortef | Deltasone |
| Depo-Medrol | Hydeltrasol |
| Solu-Cortef | Solu-Medrol |

## Depigmenting Agents
| | |
|---|---|
| Benoquin Cream | Eldopaque |
| Eldoquin | |

## Dermatologicals

### Dermatitis Herpetiformis:
Dapsone USP

### Dermatitis Relief:
| | |
|---|---|
| Decaspray | Elidel |
| Florone | Hytone |

| | |
|---|---|
| Locoid | Mytrex |
| Psorcon | |

### Epidermal and Cellular Growth:
Lazer Cream

## Fungicides:
| | |
|---|---|
| Amphotec | Abelcet |
| BAZA Cream | Clioquinol |
| Exelderm | Fungoid Creme |
| Grisactin | Halotex |
| Lamisil | Loprox |
| Lotrimin | Lotrisone |
| Mycelex | Mycolog-11 |
| Mycostatin | Spectazole |

## Keratolytics:
| | |
|---|---|
| Adrucil | Fluoroplex |
| Keralyt Gel | Occlusal-HP |

## Pruritis Medications:
| | |
|---|---|
| Alphatrex | Betatrex |
| Dermoplast | Eldecort |
| Eurax | Florone |
| Hytone | Hyzine-50 |
| Locoid | Mytrex |
| Periactin | Pramosone |
| Psorcon | Vistaril |

## Psoriasis Agents:
| | |
|---|---|
| Amevive | Anthra-Derm |
| Cormax | Denorex |
| DHS Tar | Dovonex |
| Drithocreme | Dritho-Scalp |
| Enbrel | Hunira |
| Pentrax | Raptiva |
| Tazorac | Temovate |
| Zetar | |

## Steroids and Combinations:
| | |
|---|---|
| Neo-Synalar | Psorcon |
| Synalar | Synemol |
| Vanoxide-HC | Vytone |

## Wart Removers:
| | |
|---|---|
| Compound W | Condylox |
| LazerFormalyde | Occlusal |
| Podocon-25 | Sal-Acid Plasters |
| Sal-Plant Gel | Trans-Plantar |
| Trans-Ver-Sal | Verr-Canth |
| Verrex | Verrusol |
| Viranol Gel | |

---

# Musculoskeletal System and Connective Tissue (710-739)

## Analgesics
| | |
|---|---|
| Advil | Anacin |
| Anaprox | Anexsia |
| Ansaid | Ascriptin |
| Bufferin | Butazolidin |
| Clinoril | Darvocet |
| Darvon | Datril |
| Disalcid | Dolobid |
| Easprin | Ecotrin |
| Empirin/Codeine | Equagesic |
| Esgic | Exedrin |
| Feldene | Flexeril |
| Hydrocodone | Indocin |
| Lortab/Lorcet | Meclomen |
| Medipren | Mono-Gesic |
| Motrin | Nalfon |
| Naprosyn | Norflex |
| Norgesic | Orudis |
| Parafon Forte | Ponstel |
| Percocet | Percodan |
| Phenaphen/Codeine | Rufen |
| Salflex | Sarapin |
| Synalgos-DC | Talacen |
| Talwin | Tolectin |
| Trilisate | Tylenol |
| Tylenol/Codeine | Tylox |
| Vicodin | Wygesic |

## Antibiotics (Osteomyelitis Treatments)
| | |
|---|---|
| Amikin | Ancef |
| Cefizox | Cefotan |
| Cipro | Clindamycin |
| Floxin | Fortaz |
| Garamycin | Keflex |
| Keftab | Kefurox |
| Kefzol | Mandol |
| Mefoxin | Monocid |
| Pipracil | Rocephin |
| Timentin | Vancocin |
| Zinacef | |

## Antiinflammatory Agents, Steroids and Combinations
| | |
|---|---|
| Aristocort | Bextra |
| Celebrex | Cortone |
| Decadron | Deltasone |
| Depo-Medrol | Hydeltra-T.B.A. |
| Hydeltrasol | Hydrocortone |
| Kenalog | Lodine |
| Lexiva | Medrol |
| Relafen | Remicade |
| Voltren | |

## Antirheumatic, Disease Modifying Agent
| | |
|---|---|
| Enbrel | Etanercept |

## Calcium Preparations
| | |
|---|---|
| Calcium-D | Calphosan |
| Caltrate | Citracal |
| Dical-D | Neo-Calglucon |
| Nephro-Calci | Os-Cal |
| Phos-Ex | Posture |

## Muscle Relaxants
| | |
|---|---|
| Actonel | Flexeril |
| Forteo | Paraflex |
| Parafon Forte | Robaxin |
| Robaxisal | Skelaxin |
| Soma | Valium |
| Valrelease | |

## Osteoporosis Preparations
| | |
|---|---|
| Aredia | Boniva |
| Calcimar | Didronel |
| Evista | Fosamax |
| Gerimed | Lexiva |
| Miacalcin | |

---

# Congenital Anomalies (740-759)
A pharmacological reference list cannot be presented for this chapter because most conditions listed are treatable only by surgical methods and are not affected by medications.

# Conditions in the Perinatal Period (760-779)

## Antibiotics
| | |
|---|---|
| Amoxcillin | Biaxin |
| Bicillin | Cloxacillin |
| Dicloxacillin | E-Mycin |
| Fortaz | Garamycin |
| Kefzol | Mandol |
| Mezlin | Nebcin |
| Rocephin | Spectrobid |
| Tazicef | Tazidime |
| Ticar | Vibramycin |
| Zithromax | |

## Bronchodilators
| | |
|---|---|
| Aerolate Jr. | Asbron G |
| Bronkephrine | Choledyl |
| Dilor | Proventil |
| Quadrinal | Somophyllin |
| Theolair | Ventolin |

## Corticosteroids
| | |
|---|---|
| Aristocort | Celeston |
| Cortone Acetate | Decadron |
| Deltasone | Depo-Medrol |
| Hydeltrasol | Prednisone |
| Solu-Cortef | Solu-Medrol |

## Electrolytes
| | |
|---|---|
| Infalyte | Oralyte |
| Pedialyte | Rehydralyte |

### Galactokinetics (Milk Flow Stimulants)
Syntocinon Nasal Spray

### Galactorrhea (Lactation) Inhibitors
Parlodel

### Neonatal Respiratory Distress Syndrome Agents
Exosurf          Survanta

### Ophthalmic Ointments, Antibiotics
Ilotycin

### Rh Hemolytic Disease-Related Agents
Gamulin Rh
HypRho-D Full Dose (for baby)
HypRho-D Mini-Dose (for mother)
Win Rho-SD          Gamulin Rh
HypRho-D Full Dose (for baby)
HypRho-D Mini-Dose (for mother)          Win Rho-SD

### Uterine Contractants
Oxytocin

### Vitamins
AquaMEPHYTON

## Symptoms, Signs and Ill-Defined Conditions (780-799)

### Analgesics

**Acetaminophens and combinations:**

| | |
|---|---|
| Acetaminophen | Anacin—Aspirin-Free |
| Anexsia | Bufferin |
| Datril | Excedrin |
| Feverall | Isocom |
| Midrin | Tylenol |

**Aspirins:**

| | |
|---|---|
| Easprin | Ecotrin |
| Forprin | |

**Aspirin combinations:**

| | |
|---|---|
| Anacin | Ascriptin A/D |
| Bufferin | Equagesic |
| Norgesic | |

**Narcotics, synthetics and combinations:**

| | |
|---|---|
| Alfenta | Anexsia |
| Astramorph/PF | Azdone |
| B&O Supprettes | Dalgan |
| Damason-P | Darvocet-N |
| Darvon | Demerol |
| Dilaudid | Dolophine |
| Duramorph | Esgic |
| Fioricet | Fiorinal |
| Hydrocet | Infumorph |
| Levo-Dromoran | Lortab |
| Lurline | Mepergan |
| Methadone-HCl | MS-Contin |
| MSIR | Nubain |
| Numorphan | Oralet |
| Oramorph | Percocet |
| Percodan | Phenaphen/Codeine |
| Phrenilin | Roxanol |
| Roxicodone | Sedapap |
| Stadol | Sublimaze |
| Sufenta | Synalgos-DC |
| Talacen | Talwin-NX |
| Tylox | Vicodin |

**Nonsteroidal antiinflammatory drugs (NSAIDs):**

| | |
|---|---|
| Advil | Anaprox |
| Daypro | Duract |
| Feldene | Indocin |
| Lodine | Meclomen |
| Medipren | Motrin |
| Nalfon | Naprosyn |
| Nuprin | Orudis |
| Ponstel | Rufen |
| Tolectin | Toradol |
| Voltaren | |

**Other:**

| | |
|---|---|
| Alka-Seltzer | Dolobid |
| Empirin/Codeine | Mono-Gesic |
| Norflex | Parafon Forte |

### Antacids

| | |
|---|---|
| Salflex | Sarapin |
| Trilisate | |
| Alka-Seltzer | Amphojel |
| Basaljel | Maalox |
| Mylanta | Riopan |

### Anticonvulsives

| | |
|---|---|
| Depakane | Depakote |
| Dilantin | Jabatril |
| Lamictal | Nurontin |
| Phenobarbital | Tegretol |
| Topamax | |

### Antiflatulents and Antigas Medications

| | |
|---|---|
| Flatulex | Kutrase |
| Mylicon | |

### Antipyretics

| | |
|---|---|
| Acetaminophen | Ascriptin A/D |
| Feverall | PediaProfen |
| Rufen | Trilisate |
| Tylenol | |

### Antispasmodics and Anticholinergics

| | |
|---|---|
| Arco-Lase | Bentyl |
| Cantil | Darabid |
| Donnatal | Kinesed |
| Kutrase | Levsin |
| Levsinex | Librax |
| Prilosec | Pro-Banthine |
| Quarzan | Robinul |
| Valpin-50 | |

### Appetite Suppressants

**Amphetamines:**

| | |
|---|---|
| Biphetamine | Desoxyn |
| Dexedrine | Didrex |

**Nonamphetamines:**

| | |
|---|---|
| Adipex-P | Bontril |
| Fastin | Ionamin |
| Plegine | Pondimin |
| Prelu-2 | Redux |
| Sanorex | Tenuate |

### Digestives

| | |
|---|---|
| Cotazym | Donnazyme |
| Ku-Zyme | Pancrease |
| Pancreatin | Viokase |

### Diuretics

| | |
|---|---|
| Aldactazide | Aldactone |
| Bumex | Capozide |
| Corzide | Demadex |
| Diamox | Diulo |
| Diuril | Dyazide |
| Dyrenium | Edecrin |
| Enduron | Enduronyl |
| Esidrex | Exna |
| HydroDIURIL | Hydromox |
| Lasix | Lozol |
| Maxzide | Midamor |
| Moduretic | Naturetin |
| Oretic | Prinzide |
| Rauzide | Renese |
| Saluron | Thalitone |
| Vaseretic | Zestoretic |

### Nausea and Vertigo Agents

| | |
|---|---|
| Aloxi | Antivert |
| Bonine | Compazine |
| Emend | Emetrol |
| Kytril | Norzine |
| Phenergan | Tigan |
| Torecan | Zofran |

### Sleep Aids

| | |
|---|---|
| Ambien | Chloral hydrate |
| Dalmane | Doriden |
| Halcion | Lunesta |
| Restoril | Valmid |

### Hypnotics:

| | |
|---|---|
| Butisol | Mebaral |
| Phenobarbital | |

### Sedatives (barbiturates):

| | |
|---|---|
| Benadryl | BufferinAF |
| Excedrin PM | Magonate |
| Mepergan | Phenergan |
| Tylenol PM | Unisom |
| Versed | |

### Sedatives (nonbarbiturates):

| | |
|---|---|
| Eldertonic | Niferex |
| Nu-Iron | |

### Tonics
Inderal

### Tremor Preparations

| | |
|---|---|
| Eldertonic | Niferex |
| Nu-Iron | Inderal |

## Injury and Poisoning (800-999)

### Agents Used in Poisonings

| | |
|---|---|
| Amyl nitrate | Antilirium |
| Antizole | BAL |
| Benadryl | Desferal |
| Digibind | Ipecac Syrup |
| Narcan (Naloxone) | Penicillamine |
| Pralidoxime | Protopam Chloride |
| Revex | Romazicon |
| Sodium nitrite | |

### Analgesics

**Acetaminophens and combinations:**

| | |
|---|---|
| Acetaminophen | Anexsia |
| Aspirin-Free Anacin | Excedrin |
| Feverall | Isocom |
| Midrin | Tylenol |
| Tylenol with codeine | |

**Aspirins:**

| | |
|---|---|
| Aspirin | Easprin |
| Ecotrin | |

**Aspirin combinations:**

| | |
|---|---|
| Anacin | Ascriptin A/D |
| Bufferin | Equagesic |
| Norgesic | |

**Narcotics, synthetics and combinations:**

| | |
|---|---|
| Alfenta | Anexsia |
| Astromorph PF | Azdone |
| B&O Supprettes | Dalgan |
| Damason-P | Darvocet-N |
| Darvon | Demerol |
| Dilaudid | Dolophine |
| Duramorph | Esgic |
| Fioricet | Fiorinal |
| Hydrocet | Infumorph |
| Levo-Dromoran | Lortab/Lorcet |
| Lurline | Mepergan |
| Methadone HCl | MS Contin |
| MSIR | Nubain |
| Numorphan | Oramorph |
| Percocet | Percodan |
| Phrenilin | Roxanol |
| Roxicodone | Sedapap |
| Stadol | Sublimaze |
| Sufenta | Synalgos-DC |
| Talacen | Talwin |
| Tegretol | Tylox |
| Vicodin | Wygesic |
| Zydone | |

**Nonsteroidal antiinflammatory drugs (NSAIDs):**

| | |
|---|---|
| Advil | Anaprox |
| Ansaid | Cataflam |
| Clinoril | Daypro |
| Feldene | Ibuprofen |
| Lodine | Meclamen |
| Medipren | Motrin |
| Nalfon | Naprosyn |
| Nuprin | Orudis |
| Ponstel | Relafen |
| Rufen | Tolectin |
| Toradol | Voltaren |

## Antibiotics

| | |
|---|---|
| Achromycin | Amikin |
| Amoxicillin | Amoxil |
| Ancef | Augmentin |
| Azactam | Ceclor |
| Cefizox | Cefobid |
| Cefotan | Cipro |
| Claforan | Floxin |
| Garamycin | Keflex |
| Keftab | Kefurox |
| Kefzol | Mefoxin |
| Mezlin | Nebcin |
| Netromycin | Pipracil |
| Tazidime | Timentin |
| Zefazone | Zinacef |

## Anticoagulants

| | |
|---|---|
| Calciparine | Coumadin |
| Dicumarol | Fragmin |
| Heparin Sodium | Lovenox |
| Organan | Panwarfin |

## Antihistamines

| | |
|---|---|
| Allegra | Atarax/Vistaril |
| Benadryl | Chlor-Trimeton |
| Claritin | Dimetap |
| Extendryl | Hismanal |
| Optimine | Seldane |
| Tacaryl | Temaril |
| Zyrtec | |

## Antivertigo Medications

| | |
|---|---|
| Antivert | Bonine |
| Bucladin-S | Meclizine |
| Vontrol | |

## Burn Agents

| | |
|---|---|
| Americaine | Aquaphor |
| Butesin Picrate | Chloresium |
| Collagenase Santyl | Dermoplast |
| Eucerin | Nupercainal |
| Panafil | Prophyllin |
| Silvadine | Sween Cream |
| Tronothane | |

## Corticoster\

Aristocort
Decadron
Depo-Medrol
Hydrocortone
Solu-Cortef

## Detoxifying Ager\

Mesnex Injection

## Skin Wound Prepa\

Betadine
DuoDERM

## Wound Dressings

| | |
|---|---|
| Aquaphor | |
| Critic-Aid | |
| DuoDERM | ( |
| Lazer | Pa |
| SSD | |

# Valid Three-digit ICD-9-CM Codes

Three-digit ICD-9-CM codes are used to identify a condition or disease only when a fourth or fifth digit is not available. The following are the only ICD-9-CM codes that are valid without further specificity.

024  Glanders

025  Melioidosis

035  Erysipelas

037  Tetanus

042  Human immunodeficiency virus (HIV) disease

048  Other enterovirus diseases of central nervous system

061  Dengue

064  Viral encephalitis transmitted by other and unspecified arthropods

071  Rabies

075  Infectious mononucleosis

080  Louse-borne [epidemic] typhus

096  Late syphilis, latent

101  Vincent's angina

118  Opportunistic mycoses

124  Trichinosis

129  Intestinal parasitism, unspecified

135  Sarcoidosis

138  Late effects of acute poliomyelitis

179  Malignant neoplasm of uterus, part unspecified

181  Malignant neoplasm of placenta

185  Malignant neoplasm of prostate

193  Malignant neoplasm of thyroid gland

217  Benign neoplasm of breast

220  Benign neoplasm of ovary

226  Benign neoplasm of thyroid glands

243  Congenital hypothyroidism

260  Kwashiorkor

261  Nutritional marasmus

262  Other severe, protein-calorie malnutrition

267  Ascorbic acid deficiency

311  Depressive disorder, not elsewhere classified

316  Psychic factors associated with diseases classified elsewhere

317  Mild mental retardation

319  Unspecified mental retardation

325  Phlebitis and thrombophlebitis of intracranial venous sinuses

326  Late effects of intracranial abscess or pyogenic infection

340  Multiple sclerosis

390  Rheumatic fever without mention of heart involvement

393  Chronic rheumatic pericarditis

412  Old myocardial infarction

430  Subarachnoid hemorrhage

431  Intracerebral hemorrhage

436  Acute, but ill-defined, cerebrovascular disease

452  Portal vein thrombosis

460  Acute nasopharyngitis [common cold]

462  Acute pharyngitis

463  Acute tonsillitis

470  Deviated nasal septum

475  Peritonsillar abscess

481  Pneumococcal pneumonia [streptococcus pneumoniae pneumonia]

485  Bronchopneumonia, organism unspecified

486  Pneumonia, organism unspecified

490  Bronchitis, not specified as acute or chronic

496  Chronic airway obstruction, not elsewhere classified

500  Coal workers' pneumoconiosis

501  Asbestosis

502  Pneumoconiosis due to other silica or silicates

503  Pneumoconiosis due to other inorganic dust

504  Pneumoconopathy due to inhalation of other dust

505  Pneumoconiosis, unspecified

514  Pulmonary congestion and hypostasis

515  Postinflammatory pulmonary fibrosis

538  Gastrointestinal mucostitis (ulcerative)

541  Appendicitis, unqualified

542  Other appendicitis

566  Abscess of anal and rectal regions

570  Acute and subacute necrosis of liver

586  Renal failure, unspecified

587  Renal sclerosis, unspecified

591  Hydronephrosis

605  Redundant prepuce and phimosis

630  Hydatidiform mole

631  Other abnormal product of conception

632  Missed abortion

650  Normal delivery

677  Late effect of complication of pregnancy, childbirth, and the puerperium

683  Acute lymphadenitis

684  Impetigo

700  Corns and callosities

725  Polymyalgia rheumatica

734  Flat foot

769  Respiratory distress syndrome

797  Senility without mention of psychosis

920  Contusion of face, scalp, and neck except eye(s)

931  Foreign body in ear

932  Foreign body in nose

936  Foreign body in intestine and colon

937  Foreign body in anus and rectum

938  Foreign body in digestive system, unspecified

981  Toxic effect of petroleum products

986  Toxic effect of carbon monoxide

990  Effects of radiation, unspecified

V08  Asymptomatic HIV infection status

V51  Aftercare involving the use of plastic surgery

# Present on Admission (POA) Tutorial

## Background

The Deficit Reduction Act of 2005 (DRA), section 5001(C), requires that CMS implement Present on Admission (POA) indicators for all diagnoses and external causes of injury on Medicare claims for inpatient acute care discharges beginning October 1, 2007. Critical access hospitals, Maryland waiver hospitals, long term care hospitals, cancer hospitals, and children's inpatient facilities are exempt from this requirement.

## Claim Submission Requirements

Beginning in October 1, 2007, all inpatient acute care hospital discharges must be reported using POA indicators on all diagnoses and external causes of injury codes in order to group cases to the appropriate DRG. An exception is made for claims submitted via direct data entry (DDE). DDE claims will not be ready to accept the POA indicators until January 1, 2008.

Hospital that fail to submit claims for discharges beginning January 1, 2008 with POA indicators will receive remittance advice remarks only. After April 1, 2008, claims will be returned for completion with POA indicators.

CMS is also required to identify at least two conditions will be designated such that when the POA indicator reflects that they developed during the admission, they will not be recognized as complication/comorbidity (CC) conditions under the DRG inpatient prospective payment system (IPPS). These conditions will have met the following criteria:

- high cost and/or high volume
- represent conditions that could have been avoided using evidence-based practice guidelines
- when present with other secondary diagnoses on the claim result in higher DRG payment weight

Effective October 1, 2008 (FY2009), hospitals will not receive additional payment for claims with codes that represent one of the selected conditions when not indicated as present on admission, meaning it developed during the acute care inpatient stay. The regulation effectively deactivates the CC or MCC status of the code, but hospital staff should be aware that other conditions on the case may carry valid CC or MCC status. Refer to page 45 of this tutorial, which provides a list of the eight conditions that CMS has designated as "Hospital Acquired Conditions" and will be included in the policy for FY2009.

## General Guidelines

The POA indicator guidelines are not intended to replace the official ICD-9-CM reporting guidelines. Nor will the POA guidelines supersede the Uniform Hospital Discharge Data Set (UHDDS) definition of principal diagnosis. A principal diagnosis remains defined as the condition established after study to be chiefly responsible for occasioning the admission of the patient to the hospital. The definition of "Other Diagnoses' also remains the same. Coders must report all conditions that coexist at the time of admission, develop subsequently, or that affect the treatment received and/or the length of stay. This has significant impact on the practice of assigning the POA indicators.

Because the POA indicator selection should accurately reflect the patient's conditions upon admission, review of POA guidelines and official coding guidelines is required. Consistent, complete documentation in the medical record is of the utmost importance. Lack of complete documentation may impact DRG case grouping and reimbursement. It is incumbent upon the provider to resolve any documentation issues.

The following is a summary of the basic POA Indicator Guidelines:

- The POA indictor requirement applies only to acute care hospital inpatient admissions or other facilities, as required by regulation for public health reporting.

- A POA condition is defined not only as one that is clearly present at the time of admission, but also those that were clearly present, but not diagnosed until after the time of admission.
- Present on admission is defined as present at the time the order for an inpatient admission is made, regardless of whether the patient's episode of care originated in the emergency department, ambulatory surgery area, or other outpatient area. Conditions that develop during an outpatient encounter are considered present on admission.
- The POA guidelines are not intended to replace any of the other *ICD-9-CM Official Guidelines for Coding and Reporting.*
- Guidelines are not intended to determine whether or not a condition should be coded, but rather how to apply the POA indicator.

The following options should be used to indicate whether a condition was POA:

Y Yes

N No

U Unknown

W Clinically undetermined

U Unreported/not used – (Exempt from POA reporting) – CMS has developed a standard "exempt' list of conditions and external causes. For these codes the POA indicator field is left blank. *See Appendix I of the ICD-9-CM Official Guidelines for Coding and Reporting for the complete list of exempt codes.*

When using the options listed above, the following definitions should be used:

Y present at the time of inpatient admission

N not present at the time of inpatient admission

U documentation is insufficient to determine if condition is present on admission

W Provider is unable to clinically determine whether condition was present on admission or not

Most ICD-9-CM diagnosis codes and E codes require POA indicator assignment. However, there are some diagnoses that are considered exempt from the POA reporting. To view exempt codes, refer to the *ICD-9-CM Official Guidelines for Coding and Reporting.* The list reflects those conditions that either do not represent a current disease or are always considered POA.

## Specific Guidelines

Before instituting a policy and procedure for assigning POA indicators, review and educational activities should be conducted, with ongoing feedback to the coders. Complete and accurate medical record documentation is a critical aspect of the review and training that must take place. The *ICD-9-CM Official Guidelines for Coding and Reporting* indicate that to achieve accurate and complete documentation, code assignment, and reporting of diagnoses and procedures, documentation must be a collaborative effort between healthcare provider and the coder. To assist the coder in determining which documentation in the medical record may be used for code selection, an Official Guidelines for Source Documentation Table is provided at the end of this section.

Assignment of POA indicators may be confusing for several types of cases, particularly if the documentation is not clear. The following are examples of POA guidelines and case scenarios illustrating various coding situations:

**Note:** As always, query the physician for a definitive diagnosis when documentation is inconsistent. The tips are presented as a guide to what information a coder might review in the process of verifying a diagnosis before assigning a POA indicator. The HIM department should work closely with the medical staff to develop a list of criteria for all conditions that are frequently queried.

- **Combination codes:** Assign "N" if any part of the combination code was not present at the time of admission.

Example: Obstructive chronic bronchitis with acute exacerbation

Tips: The POA indicator "N" would be assigned if the exacerbation did not happen until after the admission (code 491.21).

Definition of acute exacerbation: the presence of one or more of the following findings are indications of acute exacerbation: increase in sputum purulence, increase in sputum volume, tightening of chest, fluid retention and worsening of dyspnea or shortness of breath and/or wheezing.

Indicators of an acute exacerbation of COPD might be the documentation of either of the following treatments:

- Bronchodilator: Nebulised beta2-agonist or ipratropium bromide. If no response, IV aminophylline or nebulised beta2-agonist and ipratropium bromide in combination
- Oxygen: Given in ambulance or on arrival, 24-28% by mask or 2 ltr/min by nasal prongs.

Source Documents: Laboratory report, physician orders, nursing notes

- **Impending Conditions:** If a threatened or impending condition is present prior to or at the time of admission, report "Y" for the POA indicator.

Example: An impending acute myocardial infarction (code 411.1)

Tips: Impending acute myocardial infarction is also documented as unstable angina. This condition is a type of acute chest pain that occurs when the heart does not get enough oxygen. Patients with atherosclerosis, which is the most common cause of unstable angina, may accelerate to unstable angina. Unstable angina is acute worsening of chest pain.

The chest pain that:
- Occurs without cause
- Lasts longer than 15 to 20 minutes
- Does not go away with nitroglycerine
- May occur along with a drop in blood pressure or significant shortness of breath

Tests to diagnose angina include:
- Blood tests to check the levels of creatine phosphokinase (CPK), myoglobin, and troponin I and T
- Coronary angiography
- ECG ( transient ST- or T-wave changes that develop during a symptomatic episode at rest and resolve when the patient becomes asymptomatic strongly suggest unstable angina)
- Echocardiography

Drug treatment associated with Impending myocardial infarction:
- Aspirin: 324 mg
- Heparin: 80 units/kg IV bolus with constant IV infusion at 18 units/kg/hr titrated to maintain a PTT between 46 and 70 seconds
- Nitrates: Sublingual (1-3 tablets); IV (5-100 micro-g/min)
- Beta Blockers: Oral dose appropriate for specific drug: IV metoprolol (1-5 m slow IV every 5 minutes to 15 mg total); IV propranolol 0.5 to 1.0 mg; IV atenolol 5 mg every minute to 10 mg total
- Narcotics: Morphine sulfate 2 to 5 mg IV

Source Documents: Laboratory reports, physician orders, EKG

- **Two or more Contrasting Conditions:** If the symptoms related to the two conditions were present at the time of admission, the POA indicators for both are "Y."

Example: Diverticulitis versus chronic appendicitis (codes 562.11, 542)

Tip: A patient may present with acute abdominal pain but may improve clinically and be discharged or transferred before a definitive determination of the final diagnosis can be made.

Tests to diagnose diverticulitis include:
- Abdominal palpation, which may indicate left lower quadrant mass

- CT scan may reveal thickening of the inflamed area or bowel spasm if irritable bowel syndrome accompanies diverticular disease
- Lab studies may indicate elevated white blood count

Diverticular disease may be diagnosed via barium enema or sigmoidoscopy or colonoscopy services, but these studies are typically not performed if the acute inflamed diverticulitis phase of the disease is present, since these procedures may cause bowel rupture or require strenuous bowel prep.

Tests to diagnose appendicitis include:
- Abdominal palpation, which may indicate right lower quadrant pain, which typically worsens when the patient is asked to cough or upon gentle percussion
- Lab studies may indicate a moderately elevated white blood count, with increased numbers of immature cells
- Enema studies with a contrast agent may be helpful; appendicitis is present if the appendix does not fill with contrast agent

In this example, the POA indicator for codes representing both the diverticulitis and the chronic appendicitis should be "Y," since it was thought that the presenting symptom was caused by one of these conditions.

Source Documents: Radiology reports, laboratory results, physician documentation of abdominal examination findings

- **Symptom Followed by Comparative or Contrasting Conditions:** If a symptom followed by comparative or contrasting conditions is present prior to or at the time of admission, all indicators are reported as "Y."

Example: Chills due to either pneumonia or urinary tract infection. (codes 780.99, 486, 599.0).

Tips: A patient may present with chills but may improve clinically and be discharged or transferred before a definitive determination of the final diagnosis can be made.

A patient presenting with chills is typically worked-up for an infectious disease process. Chest X-rays or other radiological studies may be performed to rule out the presence of pneumonia, but coders should be aware that in some cases, the first chest X-ray may not show any consolidation indicative of pneumonia. After the patient is admitted and hydrated, the follow-up chest X-ray may show signs of pneumonia, but this disease process may have been present at the time of admission. The determination must be made by the physician, who may have documented clinical signs of pneumonia in the initial physical examination.

The search for the underlying cause of an infectious disease process is also typically aided by laboratory studies, which may include sputum or urine cultures. The coder should not assign any diagnosis code based on laboratory findings only, but these findings are clues that help focus the clinical picture for each patient. Coders must also be aware that some cultures may contain contaminated material that does not represent an infectious process. This is particularly problematic with *Staphylococcus aureus* , which is a bacteria very commonly found on skin surfaces. Culture and sensitivity studies help determine which antibiotics would be most effective in treating the particular infection. Again, the coder may not assign any diagnosis code based on treatment options, but they can provide clues to the type of infectious process that may be present. For example, if a patient presents with fever and chills, is found to have consolidation on chest X-ray and is treated with Sporanox, an antifungal agent, this is indicative of a fungal pneumonia and the physician documentation should specify such.

Source Documents: Physical examination, radiology reports, laboratory findings, including urine, sputum or blood cultures, sputum gram stain, biopsy results

In this example, codes for all the presenting diagnoses would be represented with a "Y" POA indicator.

- **External Cause of Injury Codes:** If an injury or poisoning occurred prior to or at the time of admission, both the code for the injury/poisoning and the corresponding E code are reported with POA indicator "Y."

Example: Intertrochanteric fracture of the hip due to fall down stairs (codes 820.21, E880.9).

Tips: Typically most trauma cases are very straight-forward and it is very clear which injuries were present at the time of admission. However, in cases of multiple trauma, one or several injuries may not be diagnosed initially, but may have been present at the time of admission. For example, if a patient suffers a closed head injury and internal abdominal injuries, a comparatively minor fractured extremity may not be diagnosed or treated initially, during the life-saving treatment phase. But if the injury was sustained in the original injury, the POA indicator should remain "Y."

Coders should be extremely careful in assigning the appropriate POA indicator if a patient suffers an injury while an inpatient. For example, if a patient falls from the hospital bed and fractures a hip, the codes representing that injury (along with the appropriate E code) should be designated "N" in the corresponding POA indicator assignment.

Source Documents: Emergency Department reports, radiology reports, History and Physical report, consultation reports (particularly orthopedic), physician orders

The following guidelines may be helpful when assigning POA indicators for obstetrical patients.

Coders should also keep in mind that several of the obstetrical related codes (such as code 650, Normal delivery) are found on the POA exemption list and do not require POA indicator assignment.

- **Antepartum Conditions:** If an antepartum condition is present prior to or at the time of the current admission, report "Y" for the POA indicator.

Example: Pregnancy with fetal distress, antepartum (code 656.33).

Tip: Most obstetrical departments in acute care facilities use pre-printed forms specifically designed for pregnant patients. These forms should include designations for labor-related conditions that were present at the time the patient was admitted. Other forms are used to detail a patient's course as she progresses from labor through delivery. Although nursing staff document most of the information on these forms, the physician should also document any complication of labor, along with treatment provided.

Source Documents: Obstetrical Intake Record, History & Physical, Labor Record

- **Pre-existing Chronic Conditions:** If a pregnant patient has a chronic condition that was present prior to or at the time of admission, the POA indicator is "Y."

Example: Pregnancy with pre-existing hypertension, delivered (code 642.01).

Tip: The POA guideline related to pre-existing chronic conditions for pregnant patients follows that for other patients. Any pre-existing chronic condition should be coded with POA indicator "Y," denoting that the condition was present before or at the time the patient was admitted. Coders should keep in mind that there may be a specific pregnancy related code for the condition.

Source Documents: Obstetrical Intake Record, History & Physical, Labor Record

- **Acute Conditions:** If a pregnant patient has an acute condition that develops during delivery and it was not present prior to or at the time of admission, the POA indicator is "N."

Example: Second degree perineal laceration, delivered (code 664.11);

Tip: Many of the conditions that are a result of the delivery process itself are, by their very definition, not present on admission. At admission, the pregnant patient has not progressed to the point of delivery or sustained a condition such as a perineal laceration. All conditions that develop as a result of the delivery process itself should be considered not present on admission and designated with POA indicator "N."

Source Documents: Obstetrical Intake Record, History & Physical, Labor Record, Delivery Record, Discharge Summary

- **Co-existing Conditions:** If a patient has a condition that is diagnosed on the current admission but the documentation does not indicate whether it was present at the time of admission, the provider should be queried. If no answer can be determined, the POA indicator is "U."

Example: Pregnant patient delivers and is also found to have a breast nipple abscess (code 675.01).

Tip: In only very limited circumstances should a POA indicator of "U" be assigned, and only if the physician cannot be reached for clarification. Conditions that are pregnancy related should be clearly documented concerning whether they were present at the time of admission. It is typically conditions related to other body systems that may not contain specific enough detail to determine whether they were present at the time of admission. Most acute care facilities have physician query processes in place to address these issues, but in some limited cases, a POA indicator of "U" must be assigned.

Source Documents: Obstetrical Intake Record, History & Physical, Labor Record, Delivery Record, Discharge Summary

The following guidelines may be helpful when assigning POA indicators for V codes:

- **Birth or Outcome of Delivery:** If a V code represents a birth or outcome of delivery (mother's record) for the current admission, the POA indicator is "Y."

Example: Normal single liveborn infant, born in hospital, delivered vaginally; single liveborn infant (outcome of delivery) (code V30.00 or V27.0).

Tip: The two V codes that represent either a birth or an outcome of delivery for the mother's medical record should always be considered "Y" for POA assignment. These are routine cases with expected outcomes.

Source Documents: Labor Record, Delivery Record, Discharge Summary

- **Reason for Encounter:** If a V code indicates the reason that the patient was admitted for the encounter, the POA indicator is "Y."

Example: A patient is admitted for radiation therapy (code V58.0).

Tip: A V code representing a reason for a patient encounter would always be considered "Y" POA indicator since it was obviously a planned admission and the circumstances were known at the time of admission.

Source Documents: History & Physical, physician orders

- **Status or History:** When a V code represents a status or history at the time of the current admission, the POA indicator is Y.

Example: Personal history of breast carcinoma or tracheostomy status (code V10.3 or V44.0).

Tip: V codes representing either history or patient status should always be considered "Y" POA indicator since the condition has already happened and was known at the time of admission.

Source Documents: History & Physical, physician orders

One of the most significant challenges to correct POA indicator assignment may be ensuring complete, consistent and appropriate physician documentation at the time of initial coding. While some cases, particularly those for surgical patients admitted for a specific procedure, are very straight-forward and it is clear which conditions were present at the time of admission, many other cases are much more vague. Coders should keep in mind that a patient may present to the hospital with ambiguous signs or symptoms of a disease that could take several days to accurately diagnose. If the presenting signs or symptoms were related to the subsequently diagnosed condition, the POA indicator should be "Y," but only the provider may make this connection and it must be clearly documented in the medical record. The POA Reporting Guidelines include: "Issues related to inconsistent, missing, conflicting or unclear documentation must still be resolved by the provider." This may involve physician queries either during or following the patient encounter; medical record documentation from any provider involved in the care and treatment of the patient may be used to support the determination of whether a condition was present on admission or not. To assist the coder in determining which documentation in the medical record may be used for code selection, the following Official Guidelines for Source Documentation Table was developed. The table includes AHA's Coding Clinic for ICD-9-CM official guidelines related to medical record documentation.

## Selected Hospital Acquired Conditions for FY2009

In the IPPS Final Rule for FY2008, released on August 22, 2007, CMS designated the following eight conditions to be subject to the 'Hospital Acquired Conditions' provision affecting reimbursement, effective October 1, 2008 (FY2009):

- Serious Preventable Event – Object Left in Surgery
- Serious Preventable Event – Air Embolism
- Serious Preventable Event – Blood Incompatibility
- Catheter-Associated Urinary Tract Infections
- Pressure Ulcers (Decubitus Ulcers)
- Vascular Catheter-Associated Infection
- Surgical Site Infection – Mediastinitis After Coronary Artery Bypass Graft (CABG) Surgery
- Hospital-Acquired Injuries – Fractures, Dislocations, Intracranial Injury, Crushing Injury, Burn, and Other Unspecified Effects of External Causes

CMS also indicated that they will be working to address issues surrounding the possible inclusion of the following conditions to be included in the FY2009 list of potential additional conditions:

- Ventilator Associated Pneumonia (VAP)
- *Staphylococcus Aureus* Septicemia
- Deep Vein Thrombosis (DVT)/ Pulmonary Embolism (PE)

# Source Documentation Official Guidelines Table

| Issues | Guideline | POA Impact | Coding Clinic Source |
|---|---|---|---|
| Internal Coding Guidelines | A facility's internal guidelines may not conflict with the *Official ICD-9-CM Guidelines for Coding & Reporting* and may not be used in place of actual physician documentation in the medical record used to substantiate code assignment. | A physician must be queried concerning the presence of a diagnosis if there are abnormal lab values or other documentation indicating the possibility of a condition either present on admission or developing later. | 2Q, '04, 13-14; 3Q, '00, 6; 1Q, '00, 24 |
| Information from MD other than attending physician | Code assignment may be based on information documented by another physician as long as it doesn't conflict with that from the attending physician. | Medical record documentation provided by any physician other than the attending physician should be carefully reviewed to ensure that all conditions present and treated are coded appropriately. | 1Q, '04, 18-19 |
| Mid-level provider documentation | Codes may be assigned based on documentation by nurse practitioners or physician assistants who provide diagnoses and provide care, if they are considered legally accountable for establishing a diagnosis within the regulations governing the provider and the facility. | Coders should be aware of the admitting and attending regulations for their facility and always review nurse practitioner and physician assistant medical record entries carefully for documentation of codable diagnoses. | 4Q, '04, 138 |
| Coding diagnoses from pathology reports (inpatient visits) | When a pathology report reflects a completely different diagnosis than the physician documented (e.g. CA breast vs breast mass), the coder must query the physician for additional clarifying information to resolve the conflict. If the pathology report adds greater detail to a diagnosis made by the attending physician, it may be used for coding purposes. | Coders should ensure that any postoperative diagnosis that is found on a pathology report is also documented elsewhere in the record by the physician. It should also be determined whether the condition in question was actually present on admission, even if the postoperative condition differs from the preoperative condition. | 1Q, '04, 20-21 |
| Coding diagnoses from autopsy reports (inpatient visits) | The information provided on an autopsy report may be used for coding purposes if it clarifies, or provides greater detail or specificity to the diagnoses provided by the attending physician. The autopsy report is completed by a pathologist, who is a physician. | If an autopsy report is available at the time of coding, the coder must ensure that any diagnoses contained in it are substantiated by the attending physician documentation. Any conflicts should be clarified by the attending physician. | 1Q, '01, 5 |
| Anesthesia record diagnosis documentation | An anesthesiologist is a physician and diagnostic information may be coded from the anesthesiology report unless it conflicts with information provided by the attending physician, in which case the attending should be queried. | Anesthesia reports should be regularly reviewed as part of the coding process. This evaluation can also be helpful in determining the onset of various diagnoses, pertinent in the assignment of the POA indicator. | 2Q, '00, 15 |

## Source Documentation Official Guidelines Table (*continued*)

| Issues | Guideline | POA Impact | Coding Clinic Source |
|---|---|---|---|
| Diagnoses found in the body of the medical record | Documentation of codable diagnoses is not limited to the final diagnostic statement, discharge summary, H&P or other specific report. If a physician has documented the diagnosis and it does not conflict with diagnostic information listed elsewhere, it may be coded. | Coders should not limit their review to only those medical record reports that most often contain diagnostic information. Codable diagnoses may be found in any area of the record that contains documentation by a physician or other licensed caregiver. | 2Q, '00, 17-18 |
| Adding specificity from radiology reports | When a physician has documented a general diagnosis and a radiology report adds specificity to that diagnosis, without any conflicting information concerning the original diagnosis, the specific information may be used in code selection. | Coders should review all diagnostic or therapeutic reports that carry diagnoses by a physician. If the diagnosis does not conflict with that provided by the attending physician, it may be used to aid in code specificity. | 1Q, '99, 5 |
| Diagnoses based on physician orders | When a physician orders a prescribed medication for a patient without supporting documentation of a related diagnosis, he or she must be queried concerning the presence of a corresponding diagnosis. | Coders may not assign diagnosis codes based on documentation of physician orders for medications. The query process should include information related to asking the physician to document each condition treated and whether it was a long-standing, chronic or new condition. | 3Q, '05, 18-20 |
| Pneumonia coding | While laboratory results can aid in the diagnosis of pneumonia, it is the physician documentation of physical findings, along with supporting information, that substantiates the diagnosis for coding purposes. Coders may not assign a pneumonia code based on laboratory or radiology findings alone, or on treatment by antibiotics or antifungal medications. | Coders must review laboratory, radiology and treatment related documentation and may query the physician based on information contained in these reports. The physician must also document whether the patient had signs or symptoms of the disease process at the time of admission in order to assign the most appropriate POA indicator. | 2Q, '98, 3-6 |
| Abnormal lab values | The physician must substantiate that an abnormal lab value represents an actual condition before it may be coded. If the findings are outside the normal range and there is an indication that the physician has ordered further work-up or treatment, the physician should be queried. | No secondary diagnoses should be assigned based on lab values alone. The coder may review the lab and the dates on which the lab studies were performed in order to formulate a physician query to identify whether the patient has a particular condition and whether it was present on admission. | *Official Coding Guidelines* 11/15/06: Section III.B; 2Q, '90, 16 |